D0707558

INCLUDES NETTER'S ANATOMY ART

BUCK'S

2020

ICD-10-CM

FOR PHYSICIANS

Jackie L. Koesterman, CPC
Coding and Reimbursement Specialist
JDK Medical Coding EDU, LLC
Grand Forks, North Dakota

SEVIER

Elsevier
3251 Riverport Lane
St. Louis, Missouri 63043

BUCK'S 2020 ICD-10-CM FOR PHYSICIANS ISBN: 978-0-323-69439-1

Notice

Practitioners and researchers must always rely on their own experience and knowledge in evaluating and using any information, methods, compounds or experiments described herein. Because of rapid advances in the medical sciences, in particular, independent verification of diagnoses and drug dosages should be made. To the fullest extent of the law, no responsibility is assumed by Elsevier, authors, editors or contributors for any injury and/or damage to persons or property as a matter of products liability, negligence or otherwise, or from any use or operation of any methods, products, instructions, or ideas contained in the material herein.

Previous editions copyrighted 2019, 2018, 2017, 2016, 2015, 2014, 2013, 2010

International Standard Book Number: 978-0-323-69439-1

Content Strategist: Brandi Graham
Senior Content Development Manager: Luke E. Held
Senior Content Development Specialist: Joshua S. Rapplean
Publishing Services Manager: Julie Eddy
Senior Project Manager: Tracey Schriefer
Senior Book Designer: Maggie Reid

Printed in Canada

Last digit is the print number: 9 8 7 6 5 4 3 2

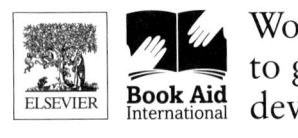

DEDICATION

To all the brave medical coders who transitioned the nation into a new coding system.
Decades of waiting finally concluded with the implementation of I-10,
and you have been the pioneers leading the way.

With greatest appreciations for your efforts!

Carol J. Buck, MS

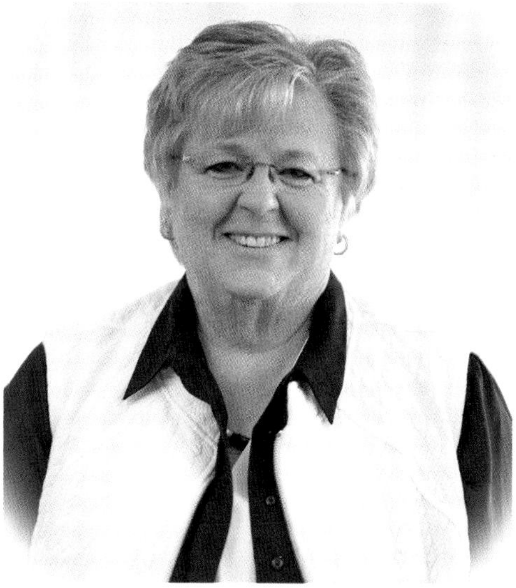

CONTENTS

ICD-10-CM

Guide to Using the 2020 ICD-10-CM for Physicians vi
Symbols and Conventions viii
Guide to the 2020 ICD-10-CM Updates xiii

Part I Introduction 1

ICD-10-CM Official Guidelines for Coding and Reporting 2020 1
Anatomy Illustrations 51

Part II Alphabetic Index 83

Index to Diseases and Injuries 84
Table of Neoplasms 467
Table of Drugs and Chemicals 495
External Cause of Injuries Index 591

Part III Tabular List of Diseases and Injuries 635

Chapter 1 Certain Infectious and Parasitic Diseases (A00-B99) 636
Chapter 2 Neoplasms (C00-D49) 665
Chapter 3 Diseases of the Blood and Blood-Forming Organs and Certain Disorders Involving the Immune Mechanism (D50-D89) 712
Chapter 4 Endocrine, Nutritional and Metabolic Diseases (E00-E89) 723
Chapter 5 Mental, Behavioral and Neurodevelopmental Disorders (F01-F99) 749
Chapter 6 Diseases of the Nervous System (G00-G99) 778
Chapter 7 Diseases of the Eye and Adnexa (H00-H59) 800
Chapter 8 Diseases of the Ear and Mastoid Process (H60-H95) 845
Chapter 9 Diseases of the Circulatory System (I00-I99) 858
Chapter 10 Diseases of the Respiratory System (J00-J99) 907
Chapter 11 Diseases of the Digestive System (K00-K95) 924
Chapter 12 Diseases of the Skin and Subcutaneous Tissue (L00-L99) 951
Chapter 13 Diseases of the Musculoskeletal System and Connective Tissue (M00-M99) 976
Chapter 14 Diseases of the Genitourinary System (N00-N99) 1,077
Chapter 15 Pregnancy, Childbirth, and the Puerperium (O00-O9A) 1,098
Chapter 16 Certain Conditions Originating in the Perinatal Period (P00-P96) 1,142
Chapter 17 Congenital Malformations, Deformations, and Chromosomal Abnormalities (Q00-Q99) 1,156
Chapter 18 Symptoms, Signs, and Abnormal Clinical and Laboratory Findings, Not Elsewhere Classified (R00-R99) 1,177
Chapter 19 Injury, Poisoning and Certain Other Consequences of External Causes (S00-T88) 1,200
Chapter 20 External Causes of Morbidity (V00-Y99) 1,444
Chapter 21 Factors Influencing Health Status and Contact with Health Services (Z00-Z99) 1,530

GUIDE TO USING THE 2020 ICD-10-CM FOR PHYSICIANS

Medical coding has long been a part of the health care profession. Through the years medical coding systems have become more complex and extensive. Today, medical coding is an intricate and immense process that is present in every health care setting. The increased use of electronic submissions for health care services only increases the need for coders who understand the coding process.

2020 ICD-10-CM for Physicians, Professional Edition was developed to help meet the needs of coding professionals at all levels by offering a comprehensive coding text at a reasonable price.

All material strictly adheres to the latest government versions available at the time of printing. Updates from the *Definitions of Medicare Code Edits* (MCE) will be posted to the companion website (www. codingupdates.com) when available.

Illustrations and Items

The ICD-10-CM Tabular List contains illustrations, pictures, and items to assist you in understanding difficult terminology, diseases/conditions, or coding in a specific category. Items are always printed in [redacted] ink so that the added material is not mistaken for official notations or instructions. [redacted] ink is used for other annotations in the text. Your ideas on what other descriptions or illustrations should be in future editions of this text are always appreciated.

Instructional Notations

Includes Notes

Includes

The word "Includes" appears immediately under certain categories to further define, or give examples of, the content of the category.

Excludes Notes

The ICD-10-CM has two types of excludes notes. Each note has a different definition for use, but they are both similar in that they indicate that codes excluded from each other are independent of each other.

Excludes1

A type 1 Excludes note is a pure excludes. It means "NOT CODED HERE!" An Excludes1 note indicates that the code excluded should never be used at the same time as the code above the Excludes1 note. An Excludes1 is for use when two conditions cannot occur together, such as a congenital form versus an acquired form of the same condition.

Excludes2

A type 2 Excludes note represents "NOT INCLUDED HERE." An Excludes2 note indicates that the condition excluded is not part of the condition it is excluded from, but a patient may have both conditions at the same time. When an Excludes2 note appears under a code, it is acceptable to use both the code and the excluded code together.

Code First/Use Additional Code notes (etiology/manifestation paired codes)

Certain conditions have both an underlying etiology and multiple body system manifestations due to the underlying etiology. For such conditions the ICD-10-CM has a coding convention that requires the underlying condition be sequenced first, followed by the manifestation. Wherever such a combination exists, there is a "use additional code" note at the etiology code, and a "code first" note at the manifestation code. These instructional notes indicate the proper sequencing order of the codes, etiology followed by manifestation.

In most cases the manifestation codes will have in the code title, "in diseases classified elsewhere." Codes with this title are a component of the etiology/manifestation convention. The code title indicates that it is a manifestation code. "In diseases classified elsewhere" codes are never permitted to be used as first-listed or principal diagnosis codes. They must be used in conjunction with an underlying condition code, and they must be listed following the underlying condition.

Use additional

The words indicate an instructional note that another code may be needed.

Code first

The words indicate an instructional note that directs the coder to sequence the underlying condition before the manifestation.

Code also

A "code also" note instructs that two codes may be required to fully describe a condition, but the sequencing of the two codes is discretionary, depending on the severity of the conditions and the reason for the encounter.

7th characters and placeholder X

For codes less than 6 characters that require a 7th character, a placeholder X should be assigned for all characters less than 6. The 7th character must always be the 7th character of a code.

Annotated

Throughout the manual, revisions, additions, and deleted codes or words are indicated by the following symbols:

Revised: Revisions within the line or code from the previous edition are indicated by the arrow.

▶ **New:** Additions to the previous edition are indicated by the triangle.

~~deleted~~ **Deleted:** Deletions from the previous edition are struck through.

ICD-10-CM Tabular List Symbols

● **Use Additional Character(s):** The red stop sign cautions that the code requires additional character(s) to ensure the greatest specificity.

X For codes less than 6 characters that require a 7th character, a placeholder X should be assigned for all characters less than 6. The 7th character must always be the 7th character of a code.

OGCR The ***Official Guidelines for Coding and Reporting*** symbol includes the placement of a portion of a guideline as that guideline pertains to the code by which it is located. The complete OGCR are located in Part I.

The **Hierarchical condition category (HCC)** was initiated in 2004 for the reimbursement for patients with Medicare Advantage plans (Medicare Part C). HCC is based on a list of chronic or severity of illness diagnosis codes that CMS uses to determine reimbursements to Medicare Advantage plans. The HCC risk adjustment factor data is calculated for an entire year for encounters of the patient's care.

Manifestation Code: Describes the manifestation of an underlying disease, not the disease itself, and therefore should not be assigned as a principal diagnosis, according to the *Definitions of Medicare Code Edits* (MCE).

Age conflict: The *Definitions of Medicare Code Edits* (MCE) detects inconsistencies between a patient's age and diagnosis. For example, a 5-year-old patient with benign prostatic hypertrophy or a 78-year-old pregnant female.

The diagnosis is clinically and virtually impossible in a patient of the stated age. Therefore, either the diagnosis or the age is presumed to be incorrect. There are four age categories for diagnoses in the *Definitions of Medicare Code Edits* (MCE):

N
- Newborn. Age of 0 years; a subset of diagnoses intended only for newborns and neonates (e.g., fetal distress, perinatal jaundice).

P
- Pediatric. Age range is 0-17 years inclusive (e.g., Reye's syndrome, routine child health exam).

M
- Maternity. Age range is 12-55 years inclusive (e.g., diabetes in pregnancy, antepartum pulmonary complication).

A
- Adult. Age range is 15-124 years inclusive (e.g., senile delirium, mature cataract).

♀♂ **Sex conflict:** *Definitions of Medicare Code Edits* (MCE) detects inconsistencies between a patient's sex and any diagnosis or procedure on the patient's record. For example, a male patient with cervical cancer (diagnosis) or a female patient with a prostatectomy (procedure). In both instances, the indicated diagnosis or the procedure conflicts with the stated sex of the patient. Therefore, either the patient's diagnosis, procedure, or sex is presumed to be incorrect.

Key words

Highlight identifies key words within similar code descriptions in a particular category.

Coding Clinic Identifies the year, quarter, and page number that presents information about an ICD-10-CM code in the American Hospital Association's *Coding Clinic®* for ICD-10-CM.

Visit codingupdates.com for the full list of 2019 Present on Admission codes.

SYMBOLS AND CONVENTIONS

ICD-10-CM Tabular

Use Additional Character(s): The red stop sign cautions you that the code requires additional character(s) to ensure greatest specificity.

Volume 1, Tabular List

● K22 Other diseases of esophagus
Excludes2 esophageal varices (I85.-)

Placeholder X: The red X reminds you that for codes less than 6 characters that require a 7th character, a placeholder X should be assigned to all characters less than 6.

X● V00.01 Pedestrian on foot injured in collision with roller-skater

A02.20 Localized salmonella infection, unspecified

Unspecified: These codes are for use when the information in the medical record is insufficient to assign a more specific code. For those categories for which an unspecified code is not provided, the "other specified" code may represent both other and unspecified.

Unacceptable Principal Diagnosis: These codes have a blue dot before them and are not permitted as a first-listed or principal diagnosis. They must be assigned in conjunction with an underlying condition code, and they must be listed following the underlying condition.

● B95.0 Streptococcus, group A, as the cause of diseases classified elsewhere

A48.3 Toxic shock syndrome
Use additional code to identify the organism (B95, B96)

Use additional code: Located at the etiology code and directs you to assign a manifestation code.

Code first indicates the etiology code is to be first-listed before the manifestation code.

B39 Histoplasmosis
Code first associated AIDS (B20)

Notes define terms or give coding instructions.

E34.0 Carcinoid syndrome
Note: May be used as an additional code to identify functional activity associated with a carcinoid tumor.

Codes or index entries are for purposes of illustration only and may not be current.

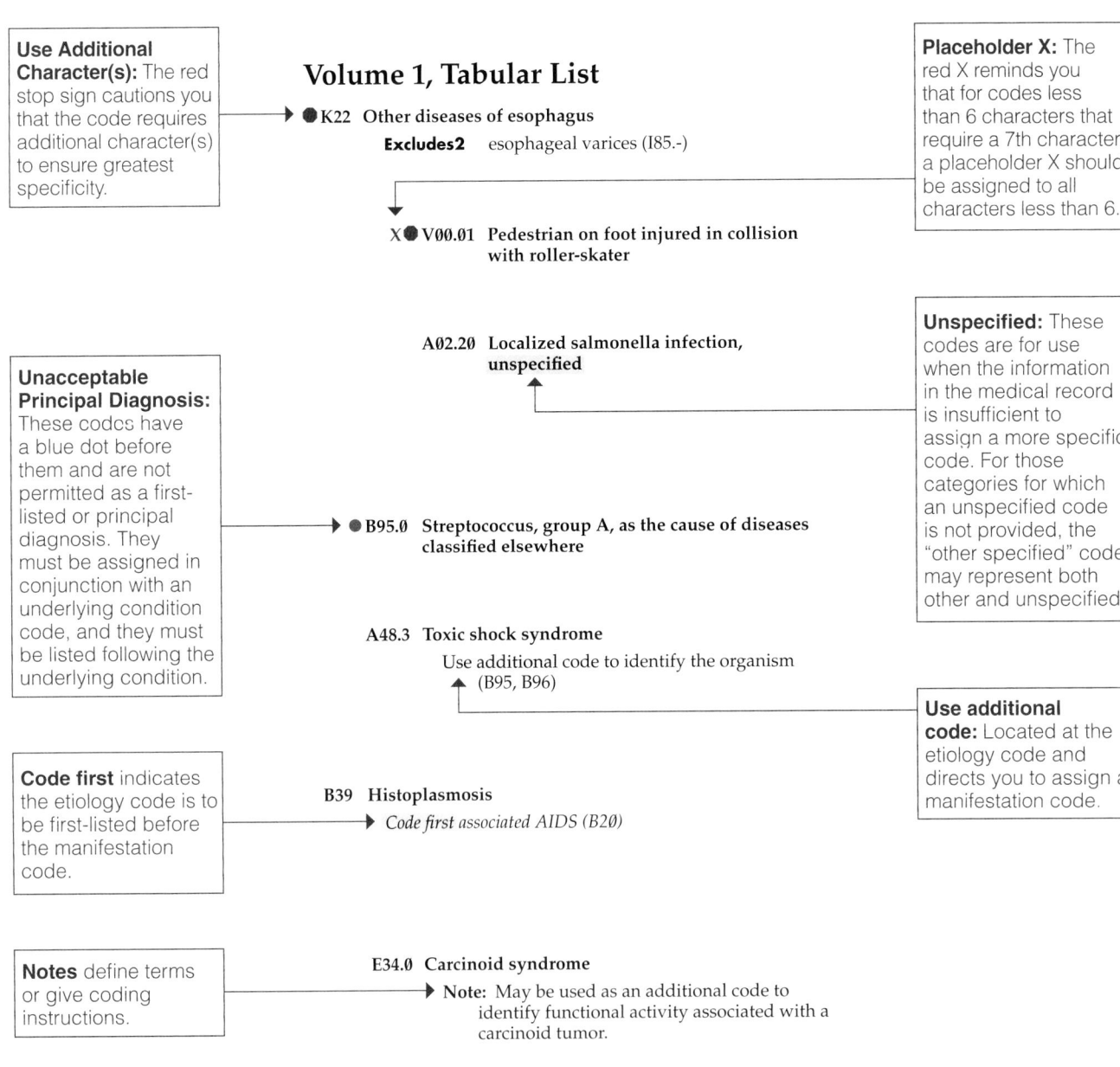

OGCR Section I.C.6.B.5.

Neoplasm Related Pain Code G89.3 is assigned to pain documented as being related, associated or due to cancer, primary or secondary malignancy, or tumor. This code is assigned regardless of whether the pain is acute or chronic.

OGCR: The *Official Guidelines for Coding and Reporting* are placed near the codes to which they refer and are highlighted.

I70.2 Atherosclerosis of native arteries of the extremities
Mönckeberg's (medial) sclerosis
Use additional code, if applicable, to identify chronic total occlusion of artery of extremity (I70.92)

code, if applicable, directs the coder to other conditions that may be appropriate to report.

The word "and" should be interpreted to mean either "and" or "or" when it appears in a statement.

I74 Arterial embolism and thrombosis
Includes embolic infarction
embolic occlusion
thrombotic infarction
thrombotic occlusion

Bold typeface is used on all codes and titles.

I83.001 Varicose veins of unspecified lower extremity with ulcer of thigh

"with" should be interpreted to mean "associated with" or "due to."

K73.2 Chronic active hepatitis, not elsewhere classified

"not elsewhere classified" or **NEC** identifies a code that is assigned only when the information at hand specifies a condition for which no more specific code is available.

"not otherwise specified" or **NOS** is equivalent to unspecified.

W13.9 Fall from, out of or through building, not otherwise specified

Codes or index entries are for purposes of illustration only and may not be current.

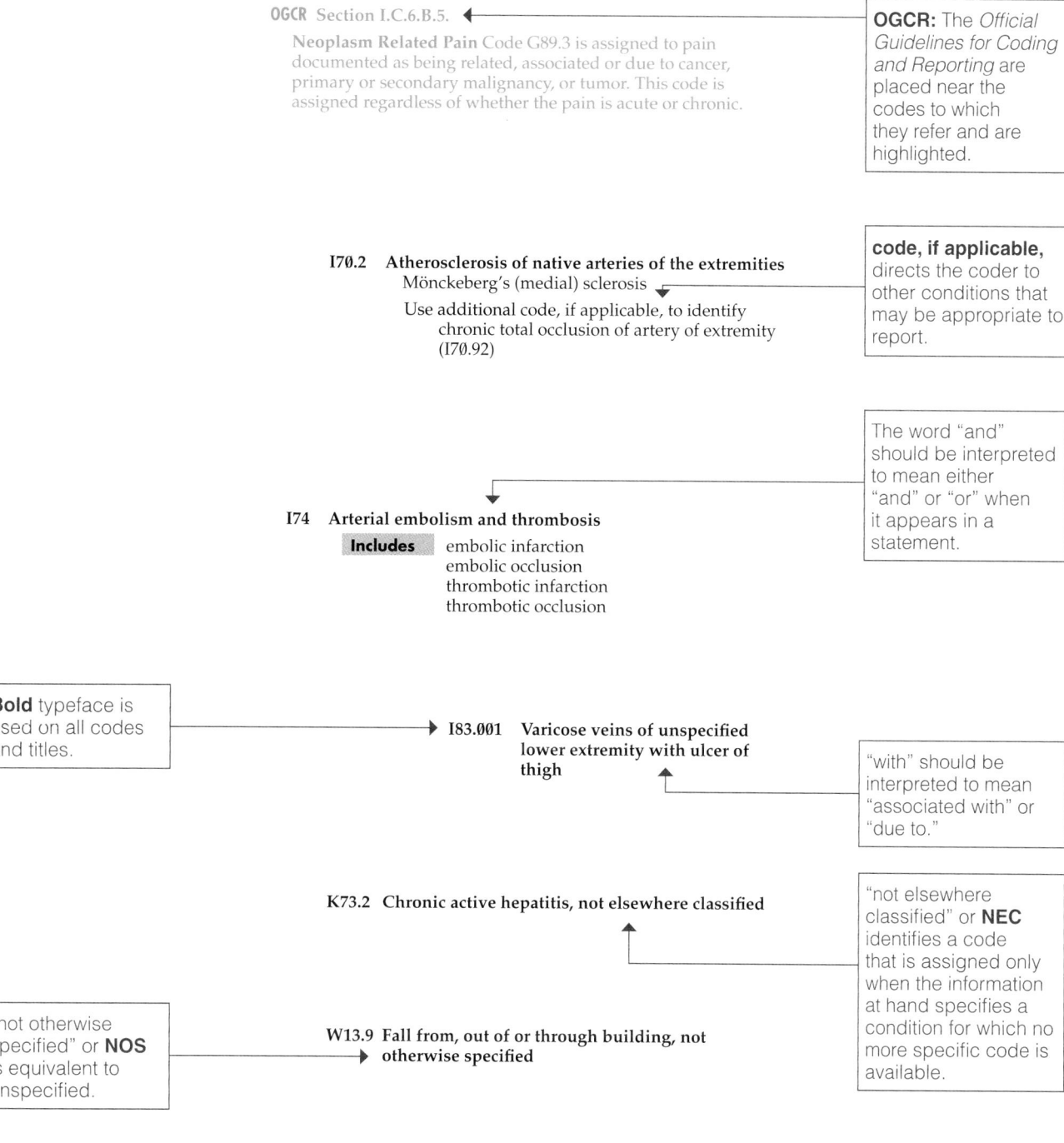

Excludes1 means "NOT CODED HERE!" An Excludes1 note indicates that the code excluded should never be assigned at the same time as the code above the Excludes1 note.

M19 Other and unspecified osteoarthritis
Excludes1 polyarthritis (M15.-)
Excludes2 arthrosis of spine (M47.-)
hallux rigidus (M2Ø.2)
osteoarthritis of spine (M47.-)

Excludes2 represents "NOT INCLUDED HERE." An Excludes2 note indicates that the condition excluded is not part of the condition represented by the code, but a patient may have both conditions at the same time and it is acceptable to use both the code and the excluded code together, when appropriate.

Includes: This note appears immediately under a three-character code title to further define, or give examples of, the content.

AØ6 Amebiasis
Includes infection due to Entamoeba histolytica

E26.Ø1 Conn's syndrome
Code also adrenal adenoma (D35.Ø)

Code also instructs that two codes may be required to fully describe a condition, but this note does not provide sequencing direction.

Codes titled "other" or "other specified" are for use when the information in the medical record provides detail for which a specific code does not exist.

E25.8 Other adrenogenital disorders

OØØ.2 Ovarian pregnancy M

Maternity DX (Diagnosis) for ages 12-55 according to the *Definitions of Medicare Code Edits* (MCE).

PØ2.2Ø Newborn (suspected to be) affected by unspecified morphological and functional abnormalities of placenta N

Newborn, Age Ø, according to the *Definitions of Medicare Code Edits* (MCE).

L21.Ø Seborrhea capitis P
Cradle cap

Pediatric Age, Ø-17, according to the *Definitions of Medicare Code Edits* (MCE).

G3Ø.1 Alzheimer's disease with late onset A

Adult Age, 15-124, according to the *Definitions of Medicare Code Edits* (MCE).

B37.3 Candidiasis of vulva and vagina ♀

Females Only according to the *Definitions of Medicare Code Edits* (MCE).

C6Ø.1 Malignant neoplasm of glans penis ♂

Males Only according to the *Definitions of Medicare Code Edits* (MCE).

Codes or index entries are for purposes of illustration only and may not be current.

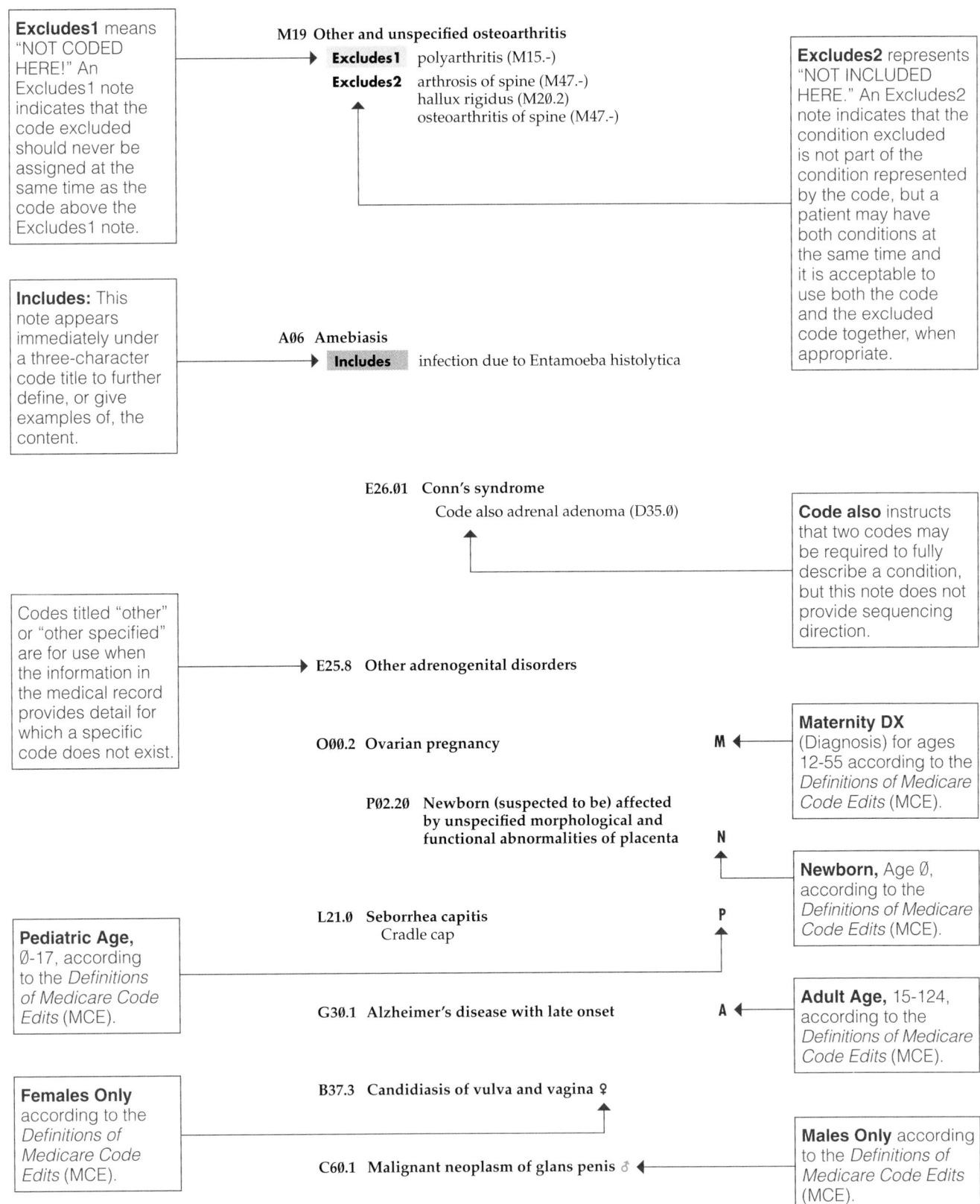

Manifestation according to the *Definitions of Medicare Code Edits* (MCE).

◗ *H22 Disorders of iris and ciliary body in diseases classified elsewhere*

Code first underlying disease, such as:
gout (M1A-, M1Ø.-)

Key Term Highlight identifies key words within similar code descriptions in a particular category.

F1Ø.21 Alcohol dependence, in remission

Coding Clinic identifies the year, quarter, and page number that presents information about an ICD-10-PCS code in the American Hospital Association's *Coding Clinic®*.

B96.5 Pseudomonas (aeruginosa) (mallei) (pseudomallei) as the cause of diseases classified elsewhere
Coding Clinic: 2Ø15, Q1, P18

Codes or index entries are for purposes of illustration only and may not be current.

Alphabetic Index

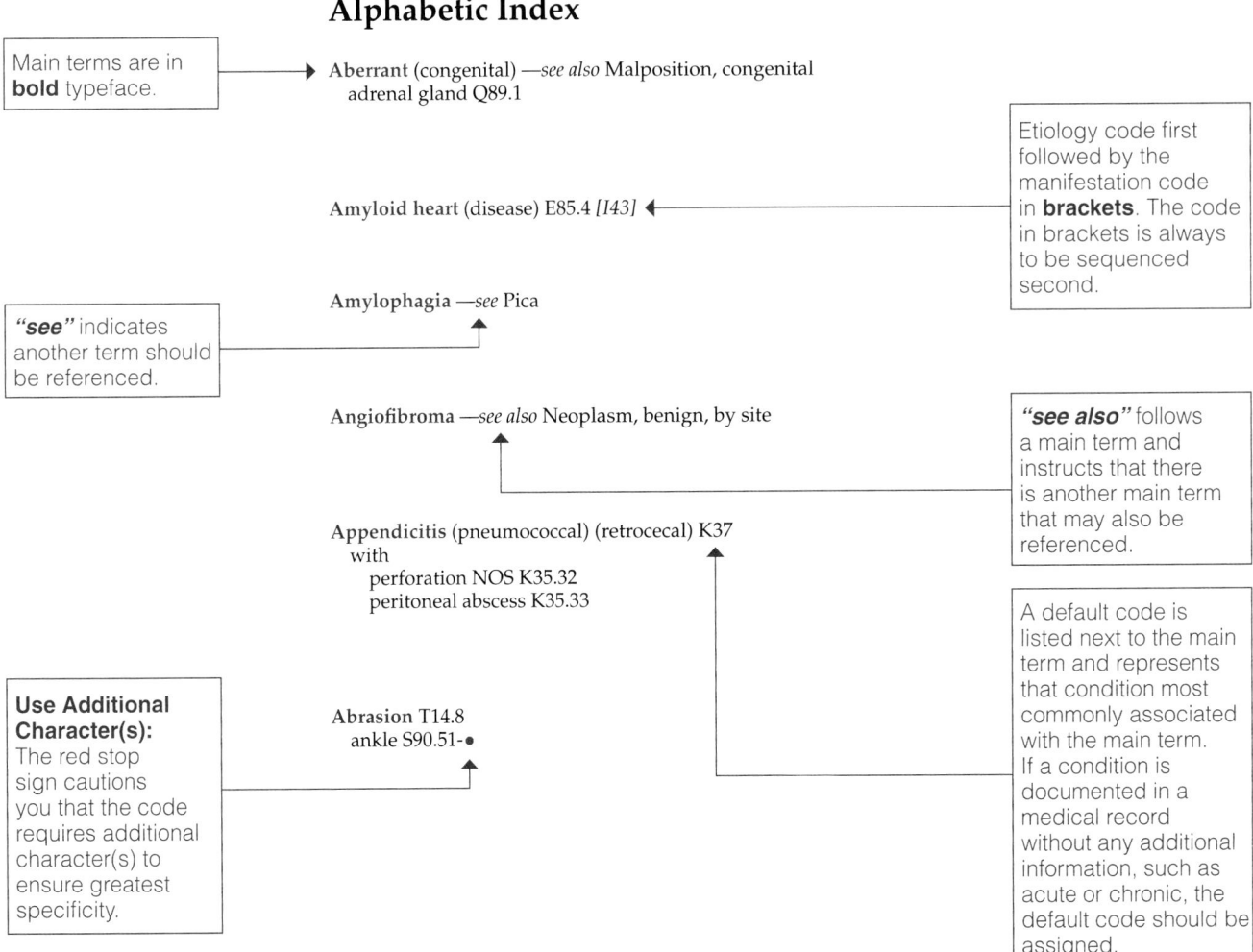

Main terms are in **bold** typeface.

Aberrant (congenital) —*see also* Malposition, congenital
adrenal gland Q89.1

Amyloid heart (disease) E85.4 *[I43]*

Etiology code first followed by the manifestation code in **brackets**. The code in brackets is always to be sequenced second.

Amylophagia —*see* Pica

"see" indicates another term should be referenced.

Angiofibroma —*see also* Neoplasm, benign, by site

"see also" follows a main term and instructs that there is another main term that may also be referenced.

Appendicitis (pneumococcal) (retrocecal) K37
with
perforation NOS K35.32
peritoneal abscess K35.33

A default code is listed next to the main term and represents that condition most commonly associated with the main term. If a condition is documented in a medical record without any additional information, such as acute or chronic, the default code should be assigned.

Abrasion T14.8
ankle S90.51-●

Use Additional Character(s): The red stop sign cautions you that the code requires additional character(s) to ensure greatest specificity.

Codes or index entries are for purposes of illustration only and may not be current.

GUIDE TO THE 2020 ICD-10-CM UPDATES

No Change **CHAPTER 1**

No Change **CERTAIN INFECTIOUS AND PARASITIC DISEASES (A00-B99)**

No Change **TUBERCULOSIS (A15-A19)**

No Change **A18 Tuberculosis of other organs**
No Change **A18.4 Tuberculosis of skin and subcutaneous tissue**
No Change **Excludes2**
Delete lupus NOS (M32.9)
Revise from systemic (M32.-)
Revise to systemic lupus erythematosus (M32.-)

No Change **BACTERIAL AND VIRAL INFECTIOUS AGENTS (B95-B97)**

No Change **B96 Other bacterial agents as the cause of diseases classified elsewhere**
No Change **B96.2 Escherichia coli [E. coli] as the cause of diseases classified elsewhere**
Revise from **B96.21 Shiga toxin-producing Escherichia coli [E. coli] (STEC) O157 as the cause of diseases classified elsewhere**
Revise to **B96.21 Shiga toxin-producing Escherichia coli [E. coli] [STEC] O157 as the cause of diseases classified elsewhere**
Revise from **B96.22 Other specified Shiga toxin-producing Escherichia coli [E. coli] (STEC) as the cause of diseases classified elsewhere**
Revise to **B96.22 Other specified Shiga toxin-producing Escherichia coli [E. coli] [STEC] as the cause of diseases classified elsewhere**
Revise from **B96.23 Unspecified Shiga toxin-producing Escherichia coli [E. coli] (STEC) as the cause of diseases classified elsewhere**
Revise to **B96.23 Unspecified Shiga toxin-producing Escherichia coli [E. coli] [STEC] as the cause of diseases classified elsewhere**

No Change **B97 Viral agents as the cause of diseases classified elsewhere**
No Change **B97.4 Respiratory syncytial virus as the cause of diseases classified elsewhere**
Add RSV as the cause of diseases classified elsewhere
Add *Code first related disorders, such as:*
Add otitis media (H65.-)
Add upper respiratory infection (J06.9)
Add **Excludes2** acute bronchiolitis due to respiratory syncytial virus (RSV) (J21.0)
Add acute bronchitis due to respiratory syncytial virus (RSV) (J20.5)
Add respiratory syncytial virus (RSV) pneumonia (J12.1)

No Change **CHAPTER 2**

No Change **NEOPLASMS (C00-D49)**

No Change **MALIGNANT NEOPLASMS OF LYMPHOID, HEMATOPOIETIC AND RELATED TISSUE (C81-C96)**

No Change **C91 Lymphoid leukemia**
No Change **C91.0 Acute lymphoblastic leukemia [ALL]**
No Change Note:
Revise from Code C91.0 should only be used for T-cell and B-cell precursor leukemia
Revise to Codes in subcategory C91.0 should only be used for T-cell and B-cell precusor leukemia

No Change **IN SITU NEOPLASMS (D00-D09)**

No Change **D04 Carcinoma in situ of skin**
No Change **D04.0 Carcinoma in situ of skin of lip**
Delete **Excludes1** carcinoma in situ of vermilion border of lip (D00.01)
Add **Excludes2** carcinoma in situ of vermilion border of lip (D00.01)

No Change **BENIGN NEOPLASMS, EXCEPT BENIGN NEUROENDOCRINE TUMORS (D10-D36)**

No Change **D12 Benign neoplasm of colon, rectum, anus and anal canal**
Add **Excludes1** polyp of colon NOS (K63.5)
No Change **D12.6 Benign neoplasm of colon, unspecified**
Delete **Excludes1** polyp of colon NOS (K63.5)

No Change **D21 Other benign neoplasms of connective and other soft tissue**
No Change **D21.6 Benign neoplasm of connective and other soft tissue of trunk, unspecified**
Revise from Benign neoplasm of back NOS
Revise to Benign neoplasm of connective and other soft tissue back NOS

No Change **D23 Other benign neoplasms of skin**
Delete **Excludes1** melanocytic nevi (D22.-)
Add **Excludes2** melanocytic nevi (D22.-)

No Change **D36 Benign neoplasm of other and unspecified sites**
No Change **D36.7 Benign neoplasm of other specified sites**
Add Benign neoplasm of back NOS

No Change **CHAPTER 3**

No Change **DISEASES OF THE BLOOD AND BLOOD-FORMING ORGANS AND CERTAIN DISORDERS INVOLVING THE IMMUNE MECHANISM (D50-D89)**

No Change **HEMOLYTIC ANEMIAS (D55-D59)**

No Change **D55 Anemia due to enzyme disorders**
No Change **D55.0 Anemia due to glucose-6-phosphate dehydrogenase [G6PD] deficiency**
Add **Excludes1** glucose-6-phosphate dehydrogenase (G6PD) deficiency without anemia (D75.A)

No Change **OTHER DISORDERS OF BLOOD AND BLOOD-FORMING ORGANS (D7Ø-D77)**

No Change D75 **Other and unspecified diseases of blood and blood-forming organs**

Add D75.A **Glucose-6-phosphate dehydrogenase (G6PD) deficiency without anemia**

Add **Excludes1** glucose-6-phosphate dehydrogenase (G6PD) deficiency with anemia (D55.Ø)

No Change **CERTAIN DISORDERS INVOLVING THE IMMUNE MECHANISM (D8Ø-D89)**

No Change D81 **Combined immunodeficiencies**

No Change D81.3 **Adenosine deaminase [ADA] deficiency**

Add D81.3Ø **Adenosine deaminase deficiency, unspecified**

Add ADA deficiency NOS

Add D81.31 **Severe combined immunodeficiency due to adenosine deaminase deficiency**

Add ADA deficiency with SCID

Add Adenosine deaminase [ADA] deficiency with severe combined immunodeficiency

Add D81.32 **Adenosine deaminase 2 deficiency**

Add ADA2 deficiency

Add Adenosine deaminase deficiency type 2

Add *Code also, if applicable, any associated manifestations, such as:*

Add polyarteritis nodosa (M3Ø.Ø)

Add stroke (I63.-)

Add D81.39 **Other adenosine deaminase deficiency**

Add Adenosine deaminase [ADA] deficiency type 1, NOS

Add Adenosine deaminase [ADA] deficiency type 1, without SCID

Add Adenosine deaminase [ADA] deficiency type 1, without severe combined immunodeficiency

Add Partial ADA deficiency (type 1)

Add Partial adenosine deaminase deficiency (type 1)

No Change CHAPTER 4

No Change ENDOCRINE, NUTRITIONAL AND METABOLIC DISEASES (EØØ-E89)

No Change **DISORDERS OF OTHER ENDOCRINE GLANDS (E2Ø-E35)**

No Change E23 **Hypofunction and other disorders of the pituitary gland**

No Change E23.3 **Hypothalamic dysfunction, not elsewhere classified**

No Change **Excludes1**

Revise from Prader-Willi syndrome (Q87.1)

Revise to Prader-Willi syndrome (Q87.11)

Revise from Russell-Silver syndrome (Q87.1)

Revise to Russell-Silver syndrome (Q87.19)

No Change E34 **Other endocrine disorders**

No Change E34.3 **Short stature due to endocrine disorder**

No Change **Excludes1**

Revise from Russell-Silver syndrome (Q87.1)

Revise to Russell-Silver syndrome (Q87.19)

No Change **OVERWEIGHT, OBESITY AND OTHER HYPERALIMENTATION (E65-E68)**

No Change E66 **Overweight and obesity**

No Change **Excludes1**

Revise from Prader-Willi syndrome (Q87.1)

Revise to Prader-Willi syndrome (Q87.11)

No Change **METABOLIC DISORDERS (E7Ø-E88)**

No Change **Excludes1**

Revise from Ehlers-Danlos syndrome (Q79.6)

Revise to Ehlers-Danlos syndrome (Q79.6-)

No Change E79 **Disorders of purine and pyrimidine metabolism**

No Change **Excludes1**

Revise from Ataxia-telangiectasia (Q87.1)

Revise to Ataxia-telangiectasia (Q87.19)

Revise from Cockayne's syndrome (Q87.1)

Revise to Cockayne's syndrome (Q87.19)

No Change E88 **Other and unspecified metabolic disorders**

No Change E88.Ø **Disorders of plasma-protein metabolism, not elsewhere classified**

No Change E88.Ø2 **Plasminogen deficiency**

Delete Use additional ligneous conjunctivitis (H1Ø.51)

No Change CHAPTER 6

No Change DISEASES OF THE NERVOUS SYSTEM (GØØ-G99)

No Change **SYSTEMIC ATROPHIES PRIMARILY AFFECTING THE CENTRAL NERVOUS SYSTEM (G1Ø-G14)**

No Change G11 **Hereditary ataxia**

No Change G11.3 **Cerebellar ataxia with defective DNA repair**

No Change **Excludes2**

Revise from Cockayne's syndrome (Q87.1)

Revise to Cockayne's syndrome (Q87.19)

No Change **OTHER DEGENERATIVE DISEASES OF THE NERVOUS SYSTEM (G3Ø-G32)**

No Change G31 **Other degenerative diseases of nervous system, not elsewhere classified**

No Change Use additional

Revise from code to identify:

Revise to For codes G31.Ø-G31.83, G31.85-G31.9, use additional code to identify:

No Change **EPISODIC AND PAROXYSMAL DISORDERS (G4Ø-G47)**

No Change G43 **Migraine**

No Change G43.A **Cyclical vomiting**

Add **Excludes1** cyclical vomiting syndrome unrelated to migraine (R11.15)

Revise from G43.AØ **Cyclical vomiting, not intractable**

Revise to G43.AØ **Cyclical vomiting, in migraine, not intractable**

Revise from G43.A1 **Cyclical vomiting, intractable**

Revise to G43.A1 **Cyclical vomiting, in migraine, intractable**

No Change **POLYNEUROPATHIES AND OTHER DISORDERS OF THE PERIPHERAL NERVOUS SYSTEM (G6Ø-G65)**

No Change G63 **Polyneuropathy in diseases classified elsewhere**

No Change **Excludes1**

Revise from rheumatoid arthritis (MØ5.33)

Revise to rheumatoid arthritis (MØ5.5-)

No Change CHAPTER 7

No Change DISEASES OF THE EYE AND ADNEXA (HØØ-H59)

No Change **DISORDERS OF OPTIC NERVE AND VISUAL PATHWAYS (H46-H47)**

No Change H47 **Other disorders of optic [2nd] nerve and visual pathways**

No Change H47.6 **Disorders of visual cortex**

No Change **Excludes1**

Revise from injury to visual cortex SØ4.Ø4

Revise to injury to visual cortex SØ4.Ø4-

No Change **CHAPTER 8**

No Change **DISEASES OF THE EAR AND MASTOID PROCESS (H60-H95)**

No Change **DISEASES OF MIDDLE EAR AND MASTOID (H65-H75)**

No Change **H65** **Nonsuppurative otitis media**
No Change Use additional
Revise from code to identify:
Revise to code, if available, to identify:
Add infectious agent (B95-B97)

No Change **DISEASES OF INNER EAR (H80-H83)**

No Change **H81** **Disorders of vestibular function**
No Change **H81.4** **Vertigo of central origin**
Delete **H81.41** **Vertigo of central origin, right ear**
Delete **H81.42** **Vertigo of central origin, left ear**
Delete **H81.43** **Vertigo of central origin, bilateral**
Delete **H81.49** **Vertigo of central origin, unspecified ear**

No Change **CHAPTER 9**

No Change **DISEASES OF THE CIRCULATORY SYSTEM (I00-I99)**

No Change **ISCHEMIC HEART DISEASES (I20-I25)**

No Change **I21** **Acute myocardial infarction**
No Change **I21.A** **Other type of myocardial infarction**
No Change **I21.A1** **Myocardial infarction type 2**
Delete Code also the underlying cause, if known and applicable, such as:
Delete anemia (D50.0-D64.9)
Delete chronic obstructive pulmonary disease (J44.-)
Delete heart failure (I50.-)
Delete paroxysmal tachycardia (I47.0-I47.9)
Delete renal failure (N17.0-N19)
Delete shock (R57.0-R57.9)
Add *Code first the underlying cause, such as:*
Add anemia (D50.0-D64.9)
Add chronic obstructive pulmonary disease (J44.-)
Add paroxysmal tachycardia (I47.0-I47.9)
Add shock (R57.0-R57.9)
No Change **I21.A9** **Other myocardial infarction type**
No Change Code also
Revise from (acute) stent stenosis (T82.857-)
Revise to (acute) stent stenosis (T82.855-)

No Change **I25** **Chronic ischemic heart disease**
No Change **I25.8** **Other forms of chronic ischemic heart disease**
No Change **I25.81** **Atherosclerosis of other coronary vessels without angina pectoris**
Delete **Excludes1** atherosclerotic heart disease of native coronary artery without angina pectoris (I25.10)
Add **Excludes2** atherosclerotic heart disease of native coronary artery without angina pectoris (I25.10)

No Change **PULMONARY HEART DISEASE AND DISEASES OF PULMONARY CIRCULATION (I26-I28)**

No Change **I26** **Pulmonary embolism**
No Change **I26.9** **Pulmonary embolism without acute cor pulmonale**
Add **I26.93** **Single subsegmental pulmonary embolism without acute cor pulmonale**
Add Subsegmental pulmonary embolism NOS
Add **I26.94** **Multiple subsegmental pulmonary emboli without acute cor pulmonale**

No Change **OTHER FORMS OF HEART DISEASE (I30-I52)**

No Change **I48** **Atrial fibrillation and flutter**
No Change **I48.1** **Persistent atrial fibrillation**
Add **Excludes1** Permanent atrial fibrillation (I48.21)
Add **I48.11** **Longstanding persistent atrial fibrillation**
Add **I48.19** **Other persistent atrial fibrillation**
Add Chronic persistent atrial fibrillation
Add Persistent atrial fibrillation, NOS
No Change **I48.2** **Chronic atrial fibrillation**
Delete Permanent atrial fibrillation
Add **I48.20** **Chronic atrial fibrillation, unspecified**
Add **Excludes1** Chronic persistent atrial fibrillation (I48.19)
Add **I48.21** **Permanent atrial fibrillation**

No Change **I50** **Heart failure**
No Change **I50.9** **Heart failure, unspecified**
No Change **Excludes2**
Revise from fluid overload (E87.70)
Revise to fluid overload unrelated to congestive heart failure (E87.70)

No Change **DISEASES OF ARTERIES, ARTERIOLES AND CAPILLARIES (I70-I79)**

No Change **I70** **Atherosclerosis**
No Change **I70.2** **Atherosclerosis of native arteries of the extremities**
No Change **I70.23** **Atherosclerosis of native arteries of right leg with ulceration**
Revise from **I70.238** **Atherosclerosis of native arteries of right leg with ulceration of other part of lower right leg**
Revise to **I70.238** **Atherosclerosis of native arteries of right leg with ulceration of other part of lower leg**
No Change **I70.24** **Atherosclerosis of native arteries of left leg with ulceration**
Revise from **I70.248** **Atherosclerosis of native arteries of left leg with ulceration of other part of lower left leg**
Revise to **I70.248** **Atherosclerosis of native arteries of left leg with ulceration of other part of lower leg**

No Change **DISEASES OF VEINS, LYMPHATIC VESSELS AND LYMPH NODES, NOT ELSEWHERE CLASSIFIED (I80-I89)**

No Change **I80** **Phlebitis and thrombophlebitis**
No Change **I80.1** **Phlebitis and thrombophlebitis of femoral vein**
Add Phlebitis and thrombophlebitis of common femoral vein
Add Phlebitis and thrombophlebitis of deep femoral vein

No Change **I80.2 Phlebitis and thrombophlebitis of other and unspecified deep vessels of lower extremities**

No Change **I80.21 Phlebitis and thrombophlebitis of iliac vein**

Add Phlebitis and thrombophlebitis of common iliac vein

Add Phlebitis and thrombophlebitis of external iliac vein

Add Phlebitis and thrombophlebitis of internal iliac vein

No Change **I80.23 Phlebitis and thrombophlebitis of tibial vein**

Add Phlebitis and thrombophlebitis of anterior tibial vein

Add Phlebitis and thrombophlebitis of posterior tibial vein

Add **I80.24 Phlebitis and thrombophlebitis of peroneal vein**

Add **I80.241 Phlebitis and thrombophlebitis of right peroneal vein**

Add **I80.242 Phlebitis and thrombophlebitis of left peroneal vein**

Add **I80.243 Phlebitis and thrombophlebitis of peroneal vein, bilateral**

Add **I80.249 Phlebitis and thrombophlebitis of unspecified peroneal vein**

Add **I80.25 Phlebitis and thrombophlebitis of calf muscular vein**

Add Phlebitis and thrombophlebitis of calf muscular vein, NOS

Add Phlebitis and thrombophlebitis of gastrocnemial vein

Add Phlebitis and thrombophlebitis of soleal vein

Add **I80.251 Phlebitis and thrombophlebitis of right calf muscular vein**

Add **I80.252 Phlebitis and thrombophlebitis of left calf muscular vein**

Add **I80.253 Phlebitis and thrombophlebitis of calf muscular vein, bilateral**

Add **I80.259 Phlebitis and thrombophlebitis of unspecified calf muscular vein**

No Change **I82 Other venous embolism and thrombosis**

No Change **I82.4 Acute embolism and thrombosis of deep veins of lower extremity**

No Change **I82.41 Acute embolism and thrombosis of femoral vein**

Add Acute embolism and thrombosis of common femoral vein

Add Acute embolism and thrombosis of deep femoral vein

No Change **I82.42 Acute embolism and thrombosis of iliac vein**

Add Acute embolism and thrombosis of common iliac vein

Add Acute embolism and thrombosis of external iliac vein

Add Acute embolism and thrombosis of internal iliac vein

No Change **I82.44 Acute embolism and thrombosis of tibial vein**

Add Acute embolism and thrombosis of anterior tibial vein

Add Acute embolism and thrombosis of posterior tibial vein

Add **I82.45 Acute embolism and thrombosis of peroneal vein**

Add **I82.451 Acute embolism and thrombosis of right peroneal vein**

Add **I82.452 Acute embolism and thrombosis of left peroneal vein**

Add **I82.453 Acute embolism and thrombosis of peroneal vein, bilateral**

Add **I82.459 Acute embolism and thrombosis of unspecified peroneal vein**

Add **I82.46 Acute embolism and thrombosis of calf muscular vein**

Add Acute embolism and thrombosis of calf muscular vein, NOS

Add Acute embolism and thrombosis of gastrocnemial vein

Add Acute embolism and thrombosis of soleal vein

Add **I82.461 Acute embolism and thrombosis of right calf muscular vein**

Add **I82.462 Acute embolism and thrombosis of left calf muscular vein**

Add **I82.463 Acute embolism and thrombosis of calf muscular vein, bilateral**

Add **I82.469 Acute embolism and thrombosis of unspecified calf muscular vein**

No Change **I82.5 Chronic embolism and thrombosis of deep veins of lower extremity**

No Change **I82.51 Chronic embolism and thrombosis of femoral vein**

Add Chronic embolism and thrombosis of common femoral vein

Add Chronic embolism and thrombosis of deep femoral vein

No Change **I82.52 Chronic embolism and thrombosis of iliac vein**

Add Chronic embolism and thrombosis of common iliac vein

Add Chronic embolism and thrombosis of external iliac vein

Add Chronic embolism and thrombosis of internal iliac vein

No Change **I82.54 Chronic embolism and thrombosis of tibial vein**

Add Chronic embolism and thrombosis of anterior tibial vein

Add Chronic embolism and thrombosis of posterior tibial vein

Add **I82.55 Chronic embolism and thrombosis of peroneal vein**

Add **I82.551 Chronic embolism and thrombosis of right peroneal vein**

Add **I82.552 Chronic embolism and thrombosis of left peroneal vein**

Add **I82.553 Chronic embolism and thrombosis of peroneal vein, bilateral**

Add **I82.559 Chronic embolism and thrombosis of unspecified peroneal vein**

Add I82.56 **Chronic embolism and thrombosis of calf muscular vein**
Add Chronic embolism and thrombosis of calf muscular vein NOS
Add Chronic embolism and thrombosis of gastrocnemial vein
Add Chronic embolism and thrombosis of soleal vein
Add I82.561 **Chronic embolism and thrombosis of right calf muscular vein**
Add I82.562 **Chronic embolism and thrombosis of left calf muscular vein**
Add I82.563 **Chronic embolism and thrombosis of calf muscular vein, bilateral**
Add I82.569 **Chronic embolism and thrombosis of unspecified calf muscular vein**

No Change **CHAPTER 10**

No Change **DISEASES OF THE RESPIRATORY SYSTEM (J00-J99)**

No Change **ACUTE UPPER RESPIRATORY INFECTIONS (J00-J06)**

No Change J06 **Acute upper respiratory infections of multiple and unspecified sites**
No Change J06.9 **Acute upper respiratory infection, unspecified**
Add Use additional code (B95-B97) to identify infectious agent, if known, such as:
Add respiratory syncytial virus (RSV) (B97.4)

No Change **INFLUENZA AND PNEUMONIA (J09-J18)**

No Change J12 **Viral pneumonia, not elsewhere classified**
No Change J12.1 **Respiratory syncytial virus pneumonia**
Add RSV pneumonia

No Change **OTHER ACUTE LOWER RESPIRATORY INFECTIONS (J20-J22)**

No Change J20 **Acute bronchitis**
No Change J20.5 **Acute bronchitis due to respiratory syncytial virus**
Add Acute bronchitis due to RSV

No Change J21 **Acute bronchiolitis**
No Change J21.0 **Acute bronchiolitis due to respiratory syncytial virus**
Add Acute bronchitis due to RSV

No Change **CHRONIC LOWER RESPIRATORY DISEASES (J40-J47)**

No Change J44 **Other chronic obstructive pulmonary disease**
Revise from J44.0 **J44.0 Chronic obstructive pulmonary disease with acute lower respiratory infection**
Revise to J44.0 **Chronic obstructive pulmonary disease with (acute) lower respiratory infection**

No Change **CHAPTER 11**

No Change **DISEASES OF THE DIGESTIVE SYSTEM (K00-K95)**

No Change **OTHER DISEASES OF INTESTINES (K55-K64)**

No Change K59 **Other functional intestinal disorders**
No Change K59.0 **Constipation**
Delete Use additional code for adverse effect, if applicable, to identify drug (T36-T50 with fifth or sixth character 5)

No Change K63 **Other diseases of intestine**
No Change K63.5 **Polyp of colon**
No Change **Excludes1**
Revise from adenomatous polyp of colon (D12.6)
Revise to adenomatous polyp of colon (D12.-)

No Change **DISEASES OF LIVER (K70-K77)**

No Change K74 **Fibrosis and cirrhosis of liver**
No Change K74.3 **Primary biliary cirrhosis**
No Change **Excludes2**
Revise from primary schlerosing cholangitis (K83.01)
Revise to primary sclerosing cholangitis (K83.01)

No Change **CHAPTER 12**

No Change **DISEASES OF THE SKIN AND SUBCUTANEOUS TISSUE (L00-L99)**

No Change **URTICARIA AND ERYTHEMA (L49-L54)**

No Change L49 **Exfoliation due to erythematous conditions according to extent of body surface involved**
No Change *Code first*
Revise from (Staphylococcal) scalded skin syndrom (L00)
Revise to (Staphylococcal) scalded skin syndrome (L00)

No Change L50 **Urticaria**
No Change **Excludes1**
Revise from urticaria pigmentosa (Q82.2)
Revise to urticaria pigmentosa (D47.01)

No Change **OTHER DISORDERS OF THE SKIN AND SUBCUTANEOUS TISSUE (L80-L99)**

No Change L89 **Pressure ulcer**
No Change L89.0 **Pressure ulcer of elbow**
No Change L89.00 **Pressure ulcer of unspecified elbow**
Add L89.006 **Pressure-induced deep tissue damage of unspecified elbow**
No Change L89.01 **Pressure ulcer of right elbow**
Add L89.016 **Pressure-induced deep tissue damage of right elbow**
No Change L89.02 **Pressure ulcer of left elbow**
Add L89.026 **Pressure-induced deep tissue damage of left elbow**
No Change L89.1 **Pressure ulcer of back**
No Change L89.10 **Pressure ulcer of unspecified part of back**
Add L89.106 **Pressure-induced deep tissue damage of unspecified part of back**
No Change L89.11 **Pressure ulcer of right upper back**
Add L89.116 **Pressure-induced deep tissue damage of right upper back**
No Change L89.12 **Pressure ulcer of left upper back**
Add L89.126 **Pressure-induced deep tissue damage of left upper back**
No Change L89.13 **Pressure ulcer of right lower back**
Add L89.136 **Pressure-induced deep tissue damage of right lower back**
No Change L89.14 **Pressure ulcer of left lower back**
Add L89.146 **Pressure-induced deep tissue damage of left lower back**
No Change L89.15 **Pressure ulcer of sacral region**
Add L89.156 **Pressure-induced deep tissue damage of sacral region**

No Change L89.2 Pressure ulcer of hip

No Change L89.2Ø Pressure ulcer of unspecified hip

Add L89.2Ø6 Pressure-induced deep tissue damage of unspecified hip

No Change L89.21 Pressure ulcer of right hip

Add L89.216 Pressure-induced deep tissue damage of right hip

No Change L89.22 Pressure ulcer of left hip

Add L89.226 Pressure-induced deep tissue damage of left hip

No Change L89.3 Pressure ulcer of buttock

No Change L89.3Ø Pressure ulcer of unspecified buttock

Add L89.3Ø6 Pressure-induced deep tissue damage of unspecified buttock

No Change L89.31 Pressure ulcer of right buttock

Add L89.316 Pressure-induced deep tissue damage of right buttock

No Change L89.32 Pressure ulcer of left buttock

Add L89.326 Pressure-induced deep tissue damage of left buttock

No Change L89.4 Pressure ulcer of contiguous site of back, buttock and hip

Add L89.46 Pressure-induced deep tissue damage of contiguous site of back, buttock and hip

No Change L89.5 Pressure ulcer of ankle

No Change L89.5Ø Pressure ulcer of unspecified ankle

Add L89.5Ø6 Pressure-induced deep tissue damage of unspecified ankle

No Change L89.51 Pressure ulcer of right ankle

Add L89.516 Pressure-induced deep tissue damage of right ankle

No Change L89.52 Pressure ulcer of left ankle

Add L89.526 Pressure-induced deep tissue damage of left ankle

No Change L89.6 Pressure ulcer of heel

No Change L89.6Ø Pressure ulcer of unspecified heel

Add L89.6Ø6 Pressure-induced deep tissue damage of unspecified heel

No Change L89.61 Pressure ulcer of right heel

Add L89.616 Pressure-induced deep tissue damage of right heel

No Change L89.62 Pressure ulcer of left heel

Add L89.626 Pressure-induced deep tissue damage of left heel

No Change L89.8 Pressure ulcer of other site

No Change L89.81 Pressure ulcer of head

Add L89.816 Pressure-induced deep tissue damage of head

No Change L89.89 Pressure ulcer of other site

Add L89.896 Pressure-induced deep tissue damage of other site

No Change L89.9 Pressure ulcer of unspecified site

Add L89.96 Pressure-induced deep tissue damage of unspecified site

No Change CHAPTER 13

No Change DISEASES OF THE MUSCULOSKELETAL SYSTEM AND CONNECTIVE TISSUE (MØØ-M99)

No Change **OTHER JOINT DISORDERS (M2Ø-M25)**

No Change M21 Other acquired deformities of limbs

No Change M21.Ø Valgus deformity, not elsewhere classified

No Change **Excludes1**

Revise from talipes calcaneovalgus (Q66.4)

Revise to talipes calcaneovalgus (Q66.4-)

No Change M21.1 Varus deformity, not elsewhere classified

No Change **Excludes1**

Revise from metatarsus varus (Q66.22)

Revise to metatarsus varus (Q66.22-)

No Change M24 Other specific joint derangements

No Change M24.2 Disorder of ligament

No Change **Excludes2**

Revise from internal derangement of knee (M23.5-M23.89)

Revise to internal derangement of knee (M23.5-M23.8X9)

No Change **SYSTEMIC CONNECTIVE TISSUE DISORDERS (M3Ø-M36)**

No Change M34 Systemic sclerosis [scleroderma]

No Change **Excludes1**

Revise from neonatal scleroderma (P83.8)

Revise to neonatal scleroderma (P83.88)

No Change M35 Other systemic involvement of connective tissue

No Change M35.7 Hypermobility syndrome

No Change **Excludes1**

Revise from Ehlers-Danlos syndrome (Q79.6)

Revise to Ehlers-Danlos syndrome (Q79.6-)

No Change **SPONDYLOPATHIES (M45-M49)**

No Change M47 Spondylosis

No Change M47.1 Other spondylosis with myelopathy

No Change **Excludes1**

Revise from vertebral subluxation (M43.3-M43.59)

Revise to vertebral subluxation (M43.3-M43.5X9)

No Change **OTHER DORSOPATHIES (M5Ø-M54)**

No Change M5Ø Cervical disc disorders

No Change M5Ø.1 Cervical disc disorder with radiculopathy

No Change M5Ø.12 Cervical disc disorder with radiculopathy, mid-cervical region

Revise from M5Ø.12Ø Mid-cervical disc disorder, unspecified

Revise to M5Ø.12Ø Mid-cervical disc disorder, unspecified level

No Change **DISORDERS OF SYNOVIUM AND TENDON (M65-M67)**

No Change M66 Spontaneous rupture of synovium and tendon

No Change M66.8 Spontaneous rupture of other tendons

Revise from M66.88 Spontaneous rupture of other tendons, other

Revise to M66.88 Spontaneous rupture of other tendons, other sites

No Change M67 Other disorders of synovium and tendon

No Change M67.8 Other specified disorders of synovium and tendon

No Change M67.83 Other specified disorders of synovium and tendon, wrist

Revise from M67.839 Other specified disorders of synovium and tendon, unspecified forearm

Revise to M67.839 Other specified disorders of synovium and tendon, unspecified wrist

No Change **OTHER SOFT TISSUE DISORDERS (M70-M79)**

No Change M77 Other enthesopathies
Revise from M77.5 Other enthesopathy of foot
Revise to M77.5 Other enthesopathy of foot and ankle
Revise from M77.50 Other enthesopathy of unspecified foot
Revise to M77.50 Other enthesopathy of unspecified foot and ankle
Revise from M77.51 Other enthesopathy of right foot
Revise to M77.51 Other enthesopathy of right foot and ankle
Revise from M77.52 Other enthesopathy of left foot
Revise to M77.52 Other enthesopathy of left foot and ankle

No Change CHAPTER 14

No Change DISEASES OF THE GENITOURINARY SYSTEM (N00-N99)

No Change **OTHER DISEASES OF THE URINARY SYSTEM (N30-N39)**

No Change N35 Urethral stricture
No Change N35.8 Other urethral stricture
No Change N35.81 Other urethral stricture, male
Revise from N35.814 Other anterior urethral stricture, male, anterior
Revise to N35.814 Other anterior urethral stricture, male

No Change N39 Other disorders of urinary system
No Change N39.0 Urinary tract infection, site not specified
Add **Excludes1** pyuria (R82.81)

No Change **DISORDERS OF BREAST (N60-N65)**

No Change N63 Unspecified lump in breast
No Change N63.1 Unspecified lump in the right breast
Add N63.15 Unspecified lump in the right breast, overlapping quadrants
No Change N63.2 Unspecified lump in the left breast
Add N63.25 Unspecified lump in the left breast, overlapping quadrants

No Change **NONINFLAMMATORY DISORDERS OF FEMALE GENITAL TRACT (N80-N98)**

No Change N92 Excessive, frequent and irregular menstruation
No Change N92.4 Excessive bleeding in the premenopausal period
Add Perimenopausal bleeding
Add Perimenopausal menorrhagia or metrorrhagia

No Change **INTRAOPERATIVE AND POSTPROCEDURAL COMPLICATIONS AND DISORDERS OF GENITOURINARY SYSTEM, NOT ELSEWHERE CLASSIFIED (N99)**

No Change N99 Intraoperative and postprocedural complications and disorders of genitourinary system, not elsewhere classified
No Change N99.8 Other intraoperative and postprocedural complications and disorders of genitourinary system
Add N99.85 Post endometrial ablation syndrome

No Change CHAPTER 15

No Change PREGNANCY, CHILDBIRTH, AND THE PUERPERIUM (O00-O9A)

No Change **MATERNAL CARE RELATED TO THE FETUS AND AMNIOTIC CAVITY AND POSSIBLE DELIVERY PROBLEMS (O30-O48)**

No Change O36 Maternal care for other fetal problems
No Change O36.8 Maternal care for other specified fetal problems
No Change O36.83 Maternal care for abnormalities of the fetal heart rate or rhythm
Add Maternal care for depressed fetal heart rate tones
Add Maternal care for fetal bradycardia
Add Maternal care for fetal heart rate abnormal variability
Add Maternal care for fetal heart rate decelerations
Add Maternal care for fetal heart rate irregularity
Add Maternal care for fetal tachycardia
Add Maternal care for non-reassuring fetal heart rate or rhythm

No Change **COMPLICATIONS PREDOMINANTLY RELATED TO THE PUERPERIUM (O85-O92)**

No Change O86 Other puerperal infections
No Change O86.0 Infection of obstetric surgical wound
No Change O86.02 Infection of obstetric surgical wound, deep incisional site
Revise from Sub-fascial abscess following a procedure
Revise to Sub-fascial abscess following an obstetrical procedure

No Change **OTHER OBSTETRIC CONDITIONS, NOT ELSEWHERE CLASSIFIED (O94-O9A)**

No Change O99 Other maternal diseases classifiable elsewhere but complicating pregnancy, childbirth and the puerperium
No Change O99.3 Mental disorders and diseases of the nervous system complicating pregnancy, childbirth and the puerperium
No Change O99.34 Other mental disorders complicating pregnancy, childbirth, and the puerperium
Revise from Conditions in F01-F09 and F20-F99
Revise to Conditions in F01-F09, F20-F99 and F54-F99
No Change O99.8 Other specified diseases and conditions complicating pregnancy, childbirth and the puerperium
No Change **Excludes2**
Revise from infection of genitourinary tract following delivery (O86.1-O86.3)
Revise to infection of genitourinary tract following delivery (O86.1-O86.4)

No Change CHAPTER 16

No Change CERTAIN CONDITIONS ORIGINATING IN THE PERINATAL PERIOD (P00-P96)

No Change **NEWBORN AFFECTED BY MATERNAL FACTORS AND BY COMPLICATIONS OF PREGNANCY, LABOR, AND DELIVERY (P00–P04)**

No Change P04 Newborn affected by noxious substances transmitted via placenta or breast milk
No Change P04.4 Newborn affected by maternal use of drugs of addiction
No Change P04.41 Newborn affected by maternal use of cocaine
Delete "Crack baby"

No Change **RESPIRATORY AND CARDIOVASCULAR DISORDERS SPECIFIC TO THE PERINATAL PERIOD (P19-P29)**

No Change P22 Respiratory distress of newborn
Excludes1 respiratory arrest of newborn (P28.81)
Delete respiratory failure of newborn NOS (P28.5)

No Change P22.Ø Respiratory distress syndrome of newborn
Add **Excludes2** respiratory arrest of newborn (P28.81)
Add respiratory failure of newborn NOS (P28.5)

No Change P22.8 Other respiratory distress of newborn
Add **Excludes1** respiratory arrest of newborn (P28.81)
Add respiratory failure of newborn NOS (P28.5)

No Change P22.9 Respiratory distress of newborn, unspecified
Add **Excludes1** respiratory arrest of newborn (P28.81)
Add respiratory failure of newborn NOS (P28.5)

No Change **TRANSITORY ENDOCRINE AND METABOLIC DISORDERS SPECIFIC TO NEWBORN (P7Ø-P74)**

No Change P74 Other transitory neonatal electrolyte and metabolic disturbances
No Change P74.4 Other transitory electrolyte disturbances of newborn
No Change P74.42 Disturbances of chlorine balance of newborn
No Change P74.421 Hyperchloremia of newborn
No Change **Excludes2**
Revise from late metabolic acidosis of the newborn (P77.Ø)
Revise to late metabolic acidosis of the newborn (P74.Ø)

No Change **CHAPTER 17**

No Change **CONGENITAL MALFORMATIONS, DEFORMATIONS, AND CHROMOSOMAL ABNORMALITIES (QØØ-Q99)**

No Change **CONGENITAL MALFORMATIONS OF THE NERVOUS SYSTEM (QØØ–QØ7)**

No Change QØ2 Microcephaly
Delete Use additional code, if applicable, to identify congenital Zika virus disease
Add *Code first, if applicable, congenital Zika virus disease*

No Change **CONGENITAL MALFORMATIONS AND DEFORMATIONS OF THE MUSCULOSKELETAL SYSTEM (Q65-Q79)**

No Change Q66 Congenital deformities of feet
No Change Q66.Ø Congenital talipes equinovarus
Add Q66.ØØ Congenital talipes equinovarus, unspecified foot
Add Q66.Ø1 Congenital talipes equinovarus, right foot
Add Q66.Ø2 Congenital talipes equinovarus, left foot
No Change Q66.1 Congenital talipes calcaneovarus
Add Q66.1Ø Congenital talipes calcaneovarus, unspecified foot
Add Q66.11 Congenital talipes calcaneovarus, right foot
Add Q66.12 Congenital talipes calcaneovarus, left foot
No Change Q66.2 Congenital metatarsus (primus) varus
No Change Q66.21 Congenital metatarsus primus varus
Add Q66.211 Congenital metatarsus primus varus, right foot
Add Q66.212 Congenital metatarsus primus varus, left foot
Add Q66.219 Congenital metatarsus primus varus, unspecified foot
No Change Q66.22 Congenital metatarsus adductus
Add Q66.221 Congenital metatarsus adductus, right foot
Add Q66.222 Congenital metatarsus adductus, left foot
Add Q66.229 Congenital metatarsus adductus, unspecified foot
No Change Q66.3 Other congenital varus deformities of feet
Add Q66.3Ø Other congenital varus deformities of feet, unspecified foot
Add Q66.31 Other congenital varus deformities of feet, right foot
Add Q66.32 Other congenital varus deformities of feet, left foot
No Change Q66.4 Congenital talipes calcaneovalgus
Add Q66.4Ø Congenital talipes calcaneovalgus, unspecified foot
Add Q66.41 Congenital talipes calcaneovalgus, right foot
Add Q66.42 Congenital talipes calcaneovalgus, left foot
No Change Q66.7 Congenital pes cavus
Add Q66.7Ø Congenital pes cavus, unspecified foot
Add Q66.71 Congenital pes cavus, right foot
Add Q66.72 Congenital pes cavus, left foot
No Change Q66.9 Congenital deformity of feet, unspecified
Add Q66.9Ø Congenital deformity of feet, unspecified, unspecified foot
Add Q66.91 Congenital deformity of feet, unspecified, right foot
Add Q66.92 Congenital deformity of feet, unspecified, left foot

No Change Q79 Congenital malformations of musculoskeletal system, not elsewhere classified
Revise from Q79.6 Ehlers-Danlos syndrome
Revise to Q79.6 Ehlers-Danlos syndromes
Add Q79.6Ø Ehlers-Danlos syndrome, unspecified
Add Q79.61 Classical Ehlers-Danlos syndrome
Add Classical EDS (cEDS)
Add Q79.62 Hypermobile Ehlers-Danlos syndrome
Add Hypermobile EDS (hEDS)
Add Q79.63 Vascular Ehlers-Danlos syndrome
Add Vascular EDS (vEDS)
Add Q79.69 Other Ehlers-Danlos syndromes

No Change **OTHER CONGENITAL MALFORMATIONS (Q8Ø-Q89)**

No Change Q81 Epidermolysis bullosa
No Change Q81.Ø Epidermolysis bullosa simplex
No Change **Excludes1**
Revise from Cockayne's syndrome (Q87.1)
Revise to Cockayne's syndrome (Q87.19)

No Change Q82 **Other congenital malformations of skin**
No Change Q82.8 **Other specified congenital malformations of skin**
No Change **Excludes1**
Revise from Ehlers-Danlos syndrome (Q79.6)
Revise to Ehlers-Danlos syndrome (Q79.6-)

No Change Q87 **Other specified congenital malformation syndromes affecting multiple systems**
No Change Q87.1 **Congenital malformation syndromes predominantly associated with short stature**
Delete Aarskog syndrome
Delete Cockayne syndrome
Delete De Lange syndrome
Delete Dubowitz syndrome
Delete Noonan syndrome
Delete Prader-Willi syndrome
Delete Robinow-Silverman-Smith syndrome
Delete Russell-Silver syndrome
Delete Seckel syndrome
Add Q87.11 **Prader-Willi syndrome**
Add Q87.19 **Other congenital malformation syndromes predominantly associated with shortstature**
Add Aarskog syndrome
Add Cockayne syndrome
Add De Lange syndrome
Add Dubowitz syndrome
Add Noonan syndrome
Add Robinow-Silverman-Smith syndrome
Add Russell-Silver syndrome
Add Seckel syndrome

No Change **CHROMOSOMAL ABNORMALITIES, NOT ELSEWHERE CLASSIFIED (Q90-Q99)**

No Change Q96 **Turner's syndrome**
No Change **Excludes1**
Revise from Noonan syndrome (Q87.1)
Revise to Noonan syndrome (Q87.19)

No Change CHAPTER 18

No Change SYMPTOMS, SIGNS, AND ABNORMAL CLINICAL AND LABORATORY FINDINGS, NOT ELSEWHERE CLASSIFIED (R00-R99)

No Change **SYMPTOMS AND SIGNS INVOLVING THE CIRCULATORY AND RESPIRATORY SYSTEMS (R10-R19)**

No Change R11 **Nausea and vomiting**
No Change R11.1 **Vomiting**
Add R11.15 **Cyclical vomiting syndrome unrelated to migraine**
Add Cyclic vomiting syndrome NOS
Add Persistent vomiting
Add **Excludes1** cyclical vomiting in migraine (G43.A-)
Add **Excludes2** bulimia nervosa (F50.2)
Add diabetes mellitus due to underlying condition (E08.-)

No Change **GENERAL SYMPTOMS AND SIGNS (R50-R69)**

No Change R63 **Symptoms and signs concerning food and fluid intake**
Delete **Excludes1** eating disorders of nonorganic origin (F50.-)
Delete malnutrition (E40-E46)

No Change R65 **Symptoms and signs specifically associated with systemic inflammation and infection**
No Change R65.1 **Systemic inflammatory response syndrome (SIRS) of non-infectious origin**
No Change *Code first*
Revise from heatstroke (T67.0)
Revise to heatstroke (T67.0-)

No Change **ABNORMAL FINDINGS ON EXAMINATION OF BLOOD, WITHOUT DIAGNOSIS (R80-R82)**

No Change R82 **Other and unspecified abnormal findings in urine**
No Change R82.8 **Abnormal findings on cytological and histological examination of urine**
Add R82.81 **Pyuria**
Add Sterile pyuria
Add R82.89 **Other abnormal findings on cytological and histological examination of urine**
No Change R82.9 **Other and unspecified abnormal findings in urine**
No Change R82.99 **Other abnormal findings in urine**
Revise from R82.993 **Hyperuricoscuria**
Revise to R82.993 **Hyperuricosuria**

No Change CHAPTER 19

No Change INJURY, POISONING AND CERTAIN OTHER CONSEQUENCES OF EXTERNAL CAUSES (S00-T88)

No Change **INJURIES TO THE HEAD (S00-S09)**

No Change S02 **Fracture of skull and facial bones**
No Change S02.1 **Fracture of base of skull**
Delete **Excludes1** orbit NOS (S02.8)
Add **Excludes2** lateral orbital wall (S02.84-)
Add medial orbital wall (S02.83-)
Add S02.12 **Fracture of orbital roof**
Add S02.121 **Fracture of orbital roof, right side**
Add S02.122 **Fracture of orbital roof, left side**
Add S02.129 **Fracture of orbital roof, unspecified side**
No Change S02.19 **Other fracture of base of skull**
Delete Fracture of orbital roof
No Change S02.3 **Fracture of orbital floor**
Add Fracture of inferior orbital wall
No Change **Excludes1**
Revise from orbit NOS (S02.8)
Revise to orbit NOS (S02.85)
Add **Excludes2** lateral orbital wall (S02.84-)
Add medial orbital wall (S02.83-)
No Change S02.8 **Fractures of other specified skull and facial bones**
Delete Fracture of orbit NOS
Delete **Excludes1** fracture of orbital floor (S02.3-)
Delete fracture of orbital roof (S02.1-)
Add **Excludes2** fracture of orbital floor (S02.3-)
Add fracture of orbital roof (S02.12-)
Add S02.83 **Fracture of medial orbital wall**
Add **Excludes2** orbital floor (S02.3-)
Add orbital roof (S02.12-)
Add S02.831 **Fracture of medial orbital wall, right side**
Add S02.832 **Fracture of medial orbital wall, left side**
Add S02.839 **Fracture of medial orbital wall, unspecified side**

Add S02.84 Fracture of lateral orbital wall
Add **Excludes2** orbital floor (S02.3-)
Add orbital roof (S02.12-)
Add **S02.841 Fracture of lateral orbital wall, right side**
Add **S02.842 Fracture of lateral orbital wall, left side**
Add **S02.849 Fracture of lateral orbital wall, unspecified side**
Add S02.85 Fracture of orbit, unspecified
Add Fracture of orbit NOS
Add Fracture of orbit wall NOS
Add **Excludes1** lateral orbital wall (S02.84-)
Add medial orbital wall (S02.83-)
Add orbital floor (S02.3-)
Add orbital roof (S02.12-)

No Change **BURNS AND CORROSIONS CONFINED TO EYE AND INTERNAL ORGANS (T26-T28)**

No Change T27 Burn and corrosion of respiratory tract
No Change T27.5 Corrosion involving larynx and trachea with lung
Add *Code first (T51-T65) to identify chemical and intent*

No Change T28 Burn and corrosion of other internal organs
No Change T28.4 Burns of other and unspecified internal organs
Delete *Code first (T51-T65) to identify chemical and intent*

No Change **POISONING BY, ADVERSE EFFECTS OF AND UNDERDOSING OF DRUGS MEDICAMENTS AND BIOLOGICAL SUBSTANCES (T36-T50)**

No Change T40 Poisoning by, adverse effect of and underdosing of narcotics and psychodysleptics [hallucinogens]
No Change T40.9 Poisoning by, adverse effect of and underdosing of other and unspecified psychodysleptics [hallucinogens]
No Change **T40.90 Poisoning by, adverse effect of and underdosing of unspecified psychodysleptics [hallucinogens]**
Revise from **T40.906 Underdosing of unspecified psychodysleptics**
Revise to **T40.906 Underdosing of unspecified psychodysleptics [hallucinogens]**
No Change **T40.99 Poisoning by, adverse effect of and underdosing of other psychodysleptics [hallucinogens]**
Revise from **T40.996 Underdosing of other psychodysleptics**
Revise to **T40.996 Underdosing of other psychodysleptics [hallucinogens]**

No Change T44 Poisoning by, adverse effect of and underdosing of drugs primarily affecting the autonomic nervous system
No Change T44.1 Poisoning by, adverse effect of and underdosing of other parasympathomimetics [cholinergics]
No Change **T44.1X Poisoning by, adverse effect of and underdosing of other parasympathomimetics [cholinergics]**
Revise from **T44.1X6 Underdosing of other parasympathomimetics**
Revise to **T44.1X6 Underdosing of other parasympathomimetics [cholinergics]**

No Change T50 **Poisoning by, adverse effect of and underdosing of diuretics and other and unspecified drugs, medicaments and biological substances**
No Change T50.9 **Poisoning by, adverse effect of and underdosing of other and unspecified drugs, medicaments and biological substances**
Add **T50.91 Poisoning by, adverse effect of and underdosing of multiple unspecified drugs, medicaments and biological substances**
Add Multiple drug ingestion NOS
Add Code also any specific drugs, medicaments and biological substances
Add **T50.911 Poisoning by multiple unspecified drugs, medicaments and biological substances, accidental (unintentional)**
Add **T50.912 Poisoning by multiple unspecified drugs, medicaments and biological substances, intentional self-harm**
Add **T50.913 Poisoning by multiple unspecified drugs, medicaments and biological substances, assault**
Add **T50.914 Poisoning by multiple unspecified drugs, medicaments and biological substances, undetermined**
Add **T50.915 Adverse effect of multiple unspecified drugs, medicaments and biological substances**
Add **T50.916 Underdosing of multiple unspecified drugs, medicaments and biological substances**

No Change **OTHER AND UNSPECIFIED EFFECTS OF EXTERNAL CAUSES (T66-T78)**

No Change T67 Effects of heat and light
No Change T67.0 Heatstroke and sunstroke
Delete Heat apoplexy
Delete Heat pyrexia
Delete Siriasis
Delete Thermoplegia
Add Use additional rhabdomyolysis (M62.82)
Add **T67.01 Heatstroke and sunstroke**
Add Heat apoplexy
Add Heat pyrexia
Add Siriasis
Add Thermoplegia
Add **T67.02 Exertional heatstroke**
Add **T67.09 Other heatstroke and sunstroke**

No Change **CERTAIN EARLY COMPLICATIONS OF TRAUMA (T79)**

No Change T79 Certain early complications of trauma, not elsewhere classified
No Change T79.A Traumatic compartment syndrome
Delete **Excludes1** traumatic ischemic infarction of muscle (T79.6)
Add **Excludes2** traumatic ischemic infarction of muscle (T79.6)

No Change **CHAPTER 2Ø**

No Change **EXTERNAL CAUSES OF MORBIDITY (VØØ-Y99)**

No Change **CAR OCCUPANT INJURED IN TRANSPORT ACCIDENT (V4Ø-V49)**

No Change V43 Car occupant injured in collision with car, pick-up truck or van

No Change V43.1 Car passenger injured in collision with car, pick-up truck or van in nontraffic accident

Revise from V43.13 Car passenger injured in collision with pick-up in nontraffic accident

Revise to V43.13 Car passenger injured in collision with pick-up truck in nontraffic accident

No Change **OTHER LAND TRANSPORT ACCIDENTS (V8Ø-V89)**

No Change V86 Occupant of special all-terrain or other off-road motor vehicle, injured in transport accident

No Change V86.Ø Driver of special all-terrain or other off-road motor vehicle injured in traffic accident

No Change V86.Ø9 Driver of other off-road special all-terrain or other off-road vehicle injured in traffic accident

Delete Driver of dirt bike injured in traffic accident

No Change V86.1 Passenger of special all-terrain or other off-road motor vehicle injured in traffic accident

No Change V86.19 Passenger of other off-road special all-terrain or other off-road off-road motor vehicle injured in traffic accident

Delete Passenger of dirt bike injured in traffic accident

No Change V86.2 Person on outside of special all-terrain or other off-road motor vehicle injured in traffic accident

No Change V86.29 Person on outside of other special all-terrain or other off-road motor vehicle injured in traffic accident

Delete Person on outside of dirt bike injured in traffic accident

No Change V86.3 Unspecified occupant of special all-terrain or other off-road motor vehicle injured in traffic accident

No Change V86.39 Unspecified occupant of other special all-terrain or other off-road motor vehicle injured in traffic accident

Delete Unspecified occupant of dirt bike injured in traffic accident

No Change V86.4 Person injured while boarding or alighting from special all-terrain or other off-road motor vehicle

No Change V86.49 Person injured while boarding or alighting from other special all-terrain or other off-road motor vehicle

Delete Person injured while boarding or alighting from dirt bike

No Change V86.5 Driver of special all-terrain or other off-road motor vehicle injured in nontraffic accident

No Change V86.59 Driver of other off-road special all-terrain or other off-road motor vehicle injured in nontraffic accident

Delete Driver of dirt bike injured in nontraffic accident

No Change V86.6 Passenger of special all-terrain or other off-road motor vehicle injured in nontraffic accident

No Change V86.69 Passenger of other special all-terrain or other off-road vehicle injured in nontraffic accident

Delete Passenger of dirt bike injured in nontraffic accident

No Change V86.7 Person on outside of special all-terrain or other off-road motor vehicle injured in nontraffic accident

No Change V86.79 Person on outside of other special all-terrain or other off-road motor vehicles injured in nontraffic accident

Delete Person on outside of dirt bike injured in nontraffic accident

No Change **EXPOSURE TO INANIMATE MECHANICAL FORCES (W2Ø-W49)**

No Change W25 Contact with sharp glass

No Change **Excludes1**

Revise from fall on same level due to slipping, tripping and stumbling with subsequent striking against sharp glass (WØ1.1Ø)

Revise to fall on same level due to slipping, tripping and stumbling with subsequent striking against sharp glass (WØ1.11Ø)

No Change **LEGAL INTERVENTION, OPERATIONS OF WAR, MILITARY OPERATIONS, AND TERRORISM (Y35-Y38)**

No Change Y35 Legal intervention

No Change Y35.Ø Legal intervention involving firearm discharge

No Change Y35.ØØ Legal intervention involving unspecified firearm discharge

Add Y35.ØØ9 Legal intervention involving unspecified firearm discharge, unspecified person injured

No Change Y35.Ø1 Legal intervention involving injury by machine gun

Add Y35.Ø19 Legal intervention involving injury by machine gun, unspecified person Injured

No Change Y35.Ø2 Legal intervention involving injury by handgun

Add Y35.Ø29 Legal intervention involving injury by handgun, unspecified person Injured

No Change Y35.Ø3 Legal intervention involving injury by rifle pellet

Add Y35.Ø39 Legal intervention involving injury by rifle pellet, unspecified person Injured

No Change Y35.Ø4 Legal intervention involving injury by rubber bullet

Add Y35.Ø49 Legal intervention involving injury by rubber bullet, unspecified person injured

No Change Y35.Ø9 Legal intervention involving other firearm discharge

Add Y35.Ø99 Legal intervention involving other firearm discharge, unspecified person Injured

No Change Y35.1 Legal intervention involving explosives

No Change Y35.1Ø Legal intervention involving unspecified explosives

Add Y35.1Ø9 Legal intervention involving unspecified explosives, unspecified person injured

No Change Y35.11 Legal intervention involving injury by dynamite

Add Y35.119 Legal intervention involving injury by dynamite, unspecified person injured

No Change Y35.12 Legal intervention involving injury by explosive shell

Add Y35.129 Legal intervention involving other explosives, unspecified person injured

No Change Y35.19 Legal intervention involving other explosives

Add Y35.199 Legal intervention involving other explosives, unspecified person injured

No Change Y35.2 Legal intervention involving gas
No Change Y35.20 Legal intervention involving unspecified gas
Add Y35.209 Legal intervention involving unspecified gas, unspecified person injured
No Change Y35.21 Legal intervention involving injury by tear gas
Add Y35.219 Legal intervention involving injury by tear gas, unspecified person Injured
No Change Y35.29 Legal intervention involving other gas
Add Y35.299 Legal intervention involving other gas, unspecified person injured
No Change Y35.3 Legal intervention involving blunt objects
No Change Y35.30 Legal intervention involving unspecified blunt objects
Add Y35.309 Legal intervention involving unspecified blunt objects, unspecified person injured
No Change Y35.31 Legal intervention involving baton
Add Y35.319 Legal intervention involving baton, unspecified person injured
No Change Y35.39 Legal intervention involving other blunt objects
Add Y35.399 Legal intervention involving other blunt objects, unspecified person injured
No Change Y35.4 Legal intervention involving sharp objects
No Change Y35.40 Legal intervention involving unspecified sharp objects
Add Y35.409 Legal intervention involving unspecified sharp objects, unspecified person injured
No Change Y35.41 Legal intervention involving bayonet
Add Y35.419 Legal intervention involving bayonet, unspecified person injured
No Change Y35.49 Legal intervention involving other sharp objects
Add Y35.499 Legal intervention involving other sharp objects, unspecified person Injured
No Change Y35.8 Legal intervention involving other specified means
No Change Y35.81 Legal intervention involving manhandling
Add Y35.819 Legal intervention involving manhandling, unspecified person injured
Add Y35.83 Legal intervention involving a conducted energy device
Add Electroshock device (taser)
Add Stun gun
Add Y35.831 Legal intervention involving a conducted energy device, law enforcement official injured
Add Y35.832 Legal intervention involving a conducted energy device, bystander injured
Add Y35.833 Legal intervention involving a conducted energy device, suspect injured
Add Y35.839 Legal intervention involving a conducted energy device, unspecified person injured
No Change Y35.9 Legal intervention, means unspecified
Add Y35.99 Legal intervention, means unspecified, unspecified person injured

No Change CHAPTER 21

No Change
FACTORS INFLUENCING HEALTH STATUS AND CONTACT WITH HEALTH SERVICES (Z00-Z99)

No Change
PERSONS ENCOUNTERING HEALTH SERVICES FOR EXAMINATIONS (Z00-Z13)

No Change Z01 Encounter for other special examination without complaint, suspected or reported diagnosis
No Change Z01.0 Encounter for examination of eyes and vision
Add Z01.02 Encounter for examination of eyes and vision following failed vision screening
Add **Excludes1** examination for examination of eyes and vision with abnormal findings (Z01.01)
Add examination for examination of eyes and vision without abnormal findings (Z01.00)
Add Z01.020 Encounter for examination of eyes and vision following failed vision screening without abnormal findings
Add Z01.021 Encounter for examination of eyes and vision following failed vision screening with abnormal findings
Add Use additional code to identify abnormal findings

No Change Z11 Encounter for screening for infectious and parasitic diseases
No Change Z11.1 Encounter for screening for respiratory tuberculosis
Add Encounter for screening for active tuberculosis disease
Add Z11.7 Encounter for testing for latent tuberculosis infection

No Change
PERSONS WITH POTENTIAL HEALTH HAZARDS RELATED TO COMMUNICABLE DISEASES (Z20-Z29)

No Change Z22 Carrier of infectious disease
Add Z22.7 Latent tuberculosis
Add Latent tuberculosis infection (LTBI)
Add **Excludes1** nonspecific reaction to cell mediated immunity measurement of gamma interferon antigen response without active tuberculosis (R76.12)
Add nonspecific reaction to tuberculin skin test without active tuberculosis (R76.11)

No Change
ENCOUNTERS FOR OTHER SPECIFIC HEALTH CARE (Z40-Z53)

No Change Z45 Encounter for adjustment and management of implanted device
No Change Z45.0 Encounter for adjustment and management of cardiac device
No Change Z45.01 Encounter for adjustment and management of cardiac pacemaker

No Change Z45.Ø18 **Encounter for adjustment and management of other part of cardiac pacemaker**

Add **Excludes1** presence of other part of cardiac pacemaker (Z95.Ø)

No Change **Excludes2**

Revise from presence of prosthetic and other devices (Z95.1-Z97)

Revise to presence of prosthetic and other devices (Z95.1-Z95.5, Z95.811-Z97)

No Change Z45.4 **Encounter for adjustment and management of implanted nervous system device**

Revise from Z45.42 **Encounter for adjustment and management of neuropacemaker (brain) (peripheral nerve) (spinal cord)**

Revise to Z45.42 **Encounter for adjustment and management of neurostimulator**

Add Encounter for adjustment and management of brain neurostimulator

Add Encounter for adjustment and management of gastric neurostimulator

Add Encounter for adjustment and management of peripheral nerve neurostimulator

Add Encounter for adjustment and management of sacral nerve neurostimulator

Add Encounter for adjustment and management of spinal cord neurostimulator

Add Encounter for adjustment and management of vagus nerve neurostimulator

No Change Z45.8 **Encounter for adjustment and management of other implanted devices**

No Change Z45.81 **Encounter for adjustment or removal of breast implant**

Revise from Encounter removal of tissue expander without synchronous insertion of permanent implant

Revise to Encounter removal of tissue expander with or without synchronous insertion of permanent implant

No Change **BODY MASS INDEX [BMI] (Z68)**

No Change Z68 **Body mass index [BMI]**

No Change **Note:**

Revise from BMI adult codes are for use for persons 21 years of age or older.

Revise to BMI adult codes are for use for persons 2Ø years of age or older.

Revise from BMI pediatric codes are for use for persons 2-2Ø years of age. These percentiles are based on the growth charts published by the Centers for Disease Control and Prevention (CDC)

Revise to BMI pediatric codes are for use for persons 2-19 years of age.

Add These percentiles are based on the growth charts published by the Centers for Disease Control and Prevention (CDC)

No Change Z68.4 **Body mass index (BMI) 4Ø or greater, adult**

Revise from Z68.43 **Body mass index (BMI) 5Ø-59.9, adult**

Revise to Z68.43 **Body mass index (BMI) 5Ø.Ø-59.9, adult**

No Change **PERSONS ENCOUNTERING HEALTH SERVICES IN OTHER CIRCUMSTANCES (Z69-Z76)**

No Change Z69 **Encounter for mental health services for victim and perpetrator of abuse**

No Change Z69.8 **Encounter for mental health services for victim or perpetrator of other abuse**

No Change Z69.81 **Encounter for mental health services for victim of other abuse**

Delete Encounter for mental health services for perpetrator of non-spousal adult abuse

No Change Z69.82 **Encounter for mental health services for perpetrator of other abuse**

Delete Encounter for mental health services for perpetrator of non-spousal adult abuse

No Change Z71 **Persons encountering health services for other counseling and medical advice, not elsewhere classified**

No Change Z71.8 **Other specified counseling**

Add Z71.84 **Encounter for health counseling related to travel**

Add Encounter for health risk and safety counseling for (international) travel

Add Code also, if applicable, encounter for immunization (Z23)

Add **Excludes2** encounter for administrative examination (ZØ2.-)

Add encounter for other special examination without complaint, suspected or reported diagnosis (ZØ1.-)

No Change **PERSONS WITH POTENTIAL HEALTH HAZARDS RELATED TO FAMILY AND PERSONAL HISTORY AND CERTAIN CONDITIONS INFLUENCING HEALTH STATUS (Z77-Z99)**

No Change Z86 **Personal history of certain other diseases**

No Change Z86.Ø **Personal history of in-situ and benign neoplasms and neoplasms of uncertain behavior**

No Change Z86.ØØ **Personal history of in-situ neoplasm**

No Change Z86.ØØØ **Personal history of in-situ neoplasm of breast**

Add Conditions classifiable to DØ5

No Change Z86.ØØ1 **Personal history of in-situ neoplasm of cervix uteri**

Add Conditions classifiable to DØ6

Add Z86.ØØ2 **Personal history of in-situ neoplasm of other and unspecified genital organs**

Add Conditions classifiable to DØ7

Add Personal history of high-grade prostatic intraepithelial neoplasia III [HGPIN III]

Add Personal history of vaginal intraepithelial neoplasia III [VAIN III]

Add Personal history of vulvar intraepithelial neoplasia III [VIN III]

Z86.ØØ3 **Personal history of in-situ neoplasm of oral cavity, esophagus and stomach**

Add Conditions classifiable to DØØ

Add **Z86.004 Personal history of in-situ neoplasm of other and unspecified digestive organs**
Add Conditions classifiable to D01
Add Personal history of anal intraepithelial neoplasia (AIN III)
Add **Z86.005 Personal history of in-situ neoplasm of middle ear and respiratory system**
Add Conditions classifiable to D02
Add **Z86.006 Personal history of melanoma in-situ**
Add Conditions classifiable to D03
Add **Excludes2** sites other than skin - code to personal history of in-situ neoplasm of the site
Add **Z86.007 Personal history of in-situ neoplasm of skin**
Add Conditions classifiable to D04
Add Personal history of carcinoma in situ of skin
No Change **Z86.008 Personal history of in-situ neoplasm of other site**
Delete Personal history of vaginal intraepithelial neoplasia III [VAIN III]
Delete Personal history of vulvar intraepithelial neoplasia III [VIN III]
Add Conditions classifiable to D09

No Change **Z86.1 Personal history of infectious and parasitic diseases**
Add **Z86.15 Personal history of latent tuberculosis infection**

No Change **Z90 Acquired absence of organs, not elsewhere classified**
No Change **Z90.4 Acquired absence of other specified parts of digestive tract**
No Change **Z90.41 Acquired absence of pancreas**
No Change Use additional
Delete insulin use (Z79.4)
Delete diabetes mellitus, postpancreatectomy (E13.-)
Add diabetes mellitus, postpancreatectomy (E13.-)
Add insulin use (Z79.4)

No Change **Z96 Presence of other functional implants**
No Change **Z96.8 Presence of other specified functional implants**
Add **Z96.82 Presence of neurostimulator**
Add Presence of brain neurostimulator
Add Presence of gastric neurostimulator
Add Presence of peripheral nerve neurostimulator
Add Presence of sacral nerve neurostimulator
Add Presence of spinal cord neurostimulator
Add Presence of vagus nerve neurostimulator

No Change **Z97 Presence of other devices**
Delete **Excludes1** fitting and adjustment of prosthetic and other devices (Z44-Z46)
Add **Excludes2** fitting and adjustment of prosthetic and other devices (Z44-Z46)

PART I

Introduction

ICD-10-CM Official Guidelines for Coding and Reporting 2020
Narrative changes appear in **bold** text
Items <u>underlined</u> have been moved within the guidelines since the 2019 version
Italics are used to indicate revisions to heading changes

The Centers for Medicare and Medicaid Services (CMS) and the National Center for Health Statistics (NCHS), two departments within the U.S. Federal Government's Department of Health and Human Services (DHHS), provide the following guidelines for coding and reporting using the International Classification of Diseases, 10th Revision, Clinical Modification (ICD-10-CM). These guidelines should be used as a companion document to the official version of the ICD-10-CM as published on the NCHS website. The ICD-10-CM is a morbidity classification published by the United States for classifying diagnoses and reason for visits in all health care settings. The ICD-10-CM is based on the ICD-10, the statistical classification of disease published by the World Health Organization (WHO).

These guidelines have been approved by the four organizations that make up the Cooperating Parties for the ICD-10-CM: the American Hospital Association (AHA), the American Health Information Management Association (AHIMA), CMS, and NCHS.

These guidelines are a set of rules that have been developed to accompany and complement the official conventions and instructions provided within the ICD-10-CM itself. The instructions and conventions of the classification take precedence over guidelines. These guidelines are based on the coding and sequencing instructions in the Tabular List and Alphabetic Index of ICD-10-CM, but provide additional instruction. Adherence to these guidelines when assigning ICD-10-CM diagnosis codes is required under the Health Insurance Portability and Accountability Act (HIPAA). The diagnosis codes (Tabular List and Alphabetic Index)

have been adopted under HIPAA for all health care settings. A joint effort between the health care provider and the coder is essential to achieve complete and accurate documentation, code assignment, and reporting of diagnoses and procedures. These guidelines have been developed to assist both the health care provider and the coder in identifying those diagnoses that are to be reported. The importance of consistent, complete documentation in the medical record cannot be overemphasized. Without such documentation accurate coding cannot be achieved. The entire record should be reviewed to determine the specific reason for the encounter and the conditions treated.

The term "encounter" is used for all settings, including hospital admissions. In the context of these guidelines, the term "provider" is used throughout the guidelines to mean physician or any qualified health care practitioner who is legally accountable for establishing the patient's diagnosis. Only this set of guidelines, approved by the Cooperating Parties, is official.

The guidelines are organized into sections. Section I includes the structure and conventions of the classification and general guidelines that apply to the entire classification, and chapter-specific guidelines that correspond to the chapters as they are arranged in the classification. Section II includes guidelines for selection of principal diagnosis for non-outpatient settings. Section III includes guidelines for reporting additional diagnoses in non-outpatient settings. Section IV is for outpatient coding and reporting. It is necessary to review all sections of the guidelines to fully understand all of the rules and instructions needed to code properly.

ICD-10-CM Official Guidelines for Coding and Reporting

Section I. Conventions, General Coding Guidelines and Chapter Specific Guidelines

A. Conventions for the ICD-10-CM
1. The Alphabetic Index and Tabular List
2. Format and Structure:
3. Use of codes for reporting purposes
4. Placeholder character
5. 7th Characters
6. Abbreviations
   a. Alphabetic Index abbreviations
   b. Tabular List abbreviations
7. Punctuation
8. Use of "and"
9. Other and Unspecified codes
   a. "Other" codes
   b. "Unspecified" codes
10. Includes Notes
11. Inclusion terms
12. Excludes Notes
    a. Excludes1
    b. Excludes2
13. Etiology/manifestation convention ("code first", "use additional code" and "in diseases classified elsewhere" notes)
14. "And"
15. "With"
16. "See" and "See Also"
17. "Code also note"
18. Default codes
19. Code assignment and Clinical Criteria

B. General Coding Guidelines
1. Locating a code in the ICD-10-CM
2. Level of Detail in Coding
3. Code or codes from A00.0 through T88.9, Z00-Z99.8
4. Signs and symptoms
5. Conditions that are an integral part of a disease process
6. Conditions that are not an integral part of a disease process
7. Multiple coding for a single condition
8. Acute and Chronic Conditions
9. Combination Code
10. Sequela (Late Effects)
11. Impending or Threatened Condition
12. Reporting Same Diagnosis Code More than Once
13. Laterality
14. Documentation *by Clinicians Other than the Patient's Provider*
15. Syndromes
16. Documentation of Complications of Care
17. Borderline Diagnosis
18. Use of Sign/Symptom/Unspecified Codes
19. Coding for Healthcare Encounters in Hurricane Aftermath
    a. Use of External Cause of Morbidity Codes
    b. Sequencing of External Causes of Morbidity Codes
    c. Other External Causes of Morbidity Code Issues
    d. Use of Z codes

C. Chapter-Specific Coding Guidelines
1. Chapter 1: Certain Infectious and Parasitic Diseases (A00-B99)
   a. Human Immunodeficiency Virus (HIV) Infections
   b. Infectious agents as the cause of diseases classified to other chapters
   c. Infections resistant to antibiotics
   d. Sepsis, Severe Sepsis, and Septic Shock
   e. Methicillin Resistant *Staphylococcus aureus* (MRSA) Conditions
   f. Zika virus infection
2. Chapter 2: Neoplasms (C00-D49)
   a. Treatment directed at the malignancy
   b. Treatment of secondary site
   c. Coding and sequencing of complications
   d. Primary malignancy previously excised
   e. Admissions/Encounters involving chemotherapy, immunotherapy and radiation therapy
   f. Admission/encounter to determine extent of malignancy
   g. Symptoms, signs, and abnormal findings listed in Chapter 18 associated with neoplasms
   h. Admission/encounter for pain control/management
   i. Malignancy in two or more noncontiguous sites
   j. Disseminated malignant neoplasm, unspecified
   k. Malignant neoplasm without specification of site
   l. Sequencing of neoplasm codes
   m. Current malignancy versus personal history of malignancy
   n. Leukemia, Multiple Myeloma, and Malignant Plasma Cell Neoplasms in remission versus personal history
   o. Aftercare following surgery for neoplasm
   p. Follow-up care for completed treatment of a malignancy
   q. Prophylactic organ removal for prevention of malignancy
   r. Malignant neoplasm associated with transplanted organ
3. Chapter 3: Disease of the Blood and Blood-Forming Organs and Certain Disorders Involving the Immune Mechanism (D50-D89)
4. Chapter 4: Endocrine, Nutritional, and Metabolic Diseases (E00-E89)
   a. Diabetes mellitus
5. Chapter 5: Mental, Behavioral, and Neurodevelopmental disorders (F01 – F99)
   a. Pain disorders related to psychological factors
   b. Mental and behavioral disorders due to psychoactive substance use
   c. Factitious Disorder
6. Chapter 6: Diseases of the Nervous System (G00-G99)
   a. Dominant/nondominant side
   b. Pain - Category G89
7. Chapter 7: Diseases of the Eye and Adnexa (H00-H59)
   a. Glaucoma
   b. Blindness
8. Chapter 8: Diseases of the Ear and Mastoid Process (H60-H95)

9. Chapter 9: Diseases of the Circulatory System (I00-I99)
   a. Hypertension
   b. Atherosclerotic Coronary Artery Disease and Angina
   c. Intraoperative and Postprocedural Cerebrovascular Accident
   d. Sequelae of Cerebrovascular Disease
   e. Acute myocardial infarction (AMI)
10. Chapter 10: Diseases of the Respiratory System (J00-J99)
   a. Chronic Obstructive Pulmonary Disease [COPD] and Asthma
   b. Acute Respiratory Failure
   c. Influenza due to certain identified influenza viruses
   d. Ventilator associated Pneumonia
11. Chapter 11: Diseases of the Digestive System (K00-K95)
12. Chapter 12: Diseases of the Skin and Subcutaneous Tissue (L00-L99)
   a. Pressure ulcer stage codes
   b. Non-Pressure Chronic Ulcers
13. Chapter 13: Diseases of the Musculoskeletal System and Connective Tissue (M00-M99)
   a. Site and laterality
   b. Acute traumatic versus chronic or recurrent musculoskeletal conditions
   c. Coding of Pathologic Fractures
   d. Osteoporosis
14. Chapter 14: Diseases of Genitourinary System (N00-N99)
   a. Chronic kidney disease
15. Chapter 15: Pregnancy, Childbirth, and the Puerperium (O00-O9A)
   a. General Rules for Obstetric Cases
   b. Selection of OB Principal or First-listed Diagnosis
   c. Pre-existing conditions versus conditions due to the pregnancy
   d. Pre-existing hypertension in pregnancy
   e. Fetal Conditions Affecting the Management of the Mother
   f. HIV Infection in Pregnancy, Childbirth and the Puerperium
   g. Diabetes mellitus in pregnancy
   h. Long term use of insulin and oral hypoglycemics
   i. Gestational (pregnancy induced) diabetes
   j. Sepsis and septic shock complicating abortion, pregnancy, childbirth and the puerperium
   k. Puerperal sepsis
   l. Alcohol, tobacco *and drug* use during pregnancy, childbirth and the puerperium
   m. Poisoning, toxic effects, adverse effects and underdosing in a pregnant patient
   n. Normal Delivery, Code O80
   o. The Peripartum and Postpartum Periods
   p. Code O94, Sequelae of complication of pregnancy, childbirth, and the puerperium
   q. Termination of Pregnancy and Spontaneous abortions
   r. Abuse in a pregnant patient

16. Chapter 16: Certain Conditions Originating in the Perinatal Period (P00-P96)
   a. General Perinatal Rules
   b. Observation and Evaluation of Newborns for Suspected Conditions not Found
   c. Coding Additional Perinatal Diagnoses
   d. Prematurity and Fetal Growth Retardation
   e. Low birth weight and immaturity status
   f. Bacterial Sepsis of Newborn
   g. Stillbirth
17. Chapter 17: Congenital Malformations, Deformations, and Chromosomal Abnormalities (Q00-Q99)
18. Chapter 18: Symptoms, Signs, and Abnormal Clinical and Laboratory Findings, Not Elsewhere Classified (R00-R99)
   a. Use of symptom codes
   b. Use of a symptom code with a definitive diagnosis code
   c. Combination codes that include symptoms
   d. Repeated falls
   e. Coma scale
   f. Functional quadriplegia
   g. SIRS due to Non-Infectious Process
   h. Death NOS
   i. NIHSS Stroke Scale
19. Chapter 19: Injury, Poisoning, and Certain Other Consequences of External Causes (S00-T88)
   a. Application of 7th Characters in Chapter 19
   b. Coding of Injuries
   c. Coding of Traumatic Fractures
   d. Coding of Burns and Corrosions
   e. Adverse Effects, Poisoning, Underdosing and Toxic Effects
   f. Adult and child abuse, neglect and other maltreatment
   g. Complications of care
20. Chapter 20: External Causes of Morbidity (V00-Y99)
   a. General External Cause Coding Guidelines
   b. Place of Occurrence Guideline
   c. Activity Code
   d. Place of Occurrence, Activity, and Status Codes Used with other External Cause Code
   e. If the Reporting Format Limits the Number of External Cause Codes
   f. Multiple External Cause Coding Guidelines
   g. Child and Adult Abuse Guideline
   h. Unknown or Undetermined Intent Guideline
   i. Sequelae (Late Effects) of External Cause Guidelines
   j. Terrorism Guidelines
   k. External cause status
21. Chapter 21: Factors Influencing Health Status and Contact with Health Services (Z00-Z99)
   a. Use of Z codes in any healthcare setting
   b. Z Codes indicate a reason for an encounter
   c. Categories of Z Codes

Section II. Selection of Principal Diagnosis

A. Codes for symptoms, signs, and ill-defined conditions
B. Two or more interrelated conditions, each potentially meeting the definition for principal diagnosis
C. Two or more diagnoses that equally meet the definition for principal diagnosis
D. Two or more comparative or contrasting conditions
E. A symptom(s) followed by contrasting/comparative diagnoses
F. Original treatment plan not carried out
G. Complications of surgery and other medical care
H. Uncertain Diagnosis
I. Admission from Observation Unit
   1. Admission Following Medical Observation
   2. Admission Following Post-Operative Observation
J. Admission from Outpatient Surgery
K. Admissions/Encounters for Rehabilitation

Section III. Reporting Additional Diagnoses

A. Previous conditions
B. Abnormal findings
C. Uncertain Diagnosis

Section IV. Diagnostic Coding and Reporting Guidelines for Outpatient Services

A. Selection of first-listed condition
   1. Outpatient Surgery
   2. Observation Stay
B. Codes from A00.0 through T88.9, Z00-Z99
C. Accurate reporting of ICD-10-CM diagnosis codes
D. Codes that describe symptoms and signs
E. Encounters for circumstances other than a disease or injury
F. Level of Detail in Coding
   1. ICD-10-CM codes with 3, 4, 5, 6, or 7 characters
   2. Use of full number of characters required for a code
G. ICD-10-CM code for the diagnosis, condition, problem, or other reason for encounter/visit
H. Uncertain diagnosis
I. Chronic diseases
J. Code all documented conditions that coexist
K. Patients receiving diagnostic services only
L. Patients receiving therapeutic services only
M. Patients receiving preoperative evaluations only
N. Ambulatory surgery
O. Routine outpatient prenatal visits
P. Encounters for general medical examinations with abnormal findings
Q. Encounters for routine health screenings

Appendix I: Present on Admission Reporting Guidelines

Section I. Conventions, General Coding Guidelines, and Chapter Specific Guidelines

The conventions, general guidelines, and chapter-specific guidelines are applicable to all health care settings unless otherwise indicated. The conventions and instructions of the classification take precedence over guidelines.

A. Conventions for the ICD-10-CM

The conventions for the ICD-10-CM are the general rules for use of the classification independent of the guidelines. These conventions are incorporated within the Alphabetic Index and Tabular List of the ICD-10-CM as instructional notes.

1. The Alphabetic Index and Tabular List

The ICD-10-CM is divided into the Alphabetic Index, an alphabetical list of terms and their corresponding code, and the Tabular List, a structured list of codes divided into chapters based on body system or condition. The Alphabetic Index consists of the following parts: the Index of Diseases and Injury, the Index of External Causes of Injury, the Table of Neoplasms, and the Table of Drugs and Chemicals.

See Section I.C2. General guidelines

See Section I.C.19. Adverse effects, poisoning, underdosing and toxic effects

2. Format and Structure:

The ICD-10-CM Tabular List contains categories, subcategories and codes. Characters for categories, subcategories and codes may be either a letter or a number. All categories are 3 characters. A 3-character category that has no further subdivision is equivalent to a code. Subcategories are either 4 or 5 characters. Codes may be 3, 4, 5, 6 or 7 characters. That is, each level of subdivision after a category is a subcategory. The final level of subdivision is a code. Codes that have applicable 7th characters are still referred to as codes, not subcategories. A code that has an applicable 7th character is considered invalid without the 7th character.

The ICD-10-CM uses an indented format for ease in reference

3. Use of codes for reporting purposes

For reporting purposes only codes are permissible, not categories or subcategories, and any applicable 7th character is required.

4. Placeholder character

The ICD-10-CM utilizes a placeholder character "X". The "X" is used as a placeholder at certain codes to allow for future expansion. An example of this is at the poisoning, adverse effect and underdosing codes, categories T36-T50. Where a placeholder exists, the X must be used in order for the code to be considered a valid code.

5. 7th Characters

Certain ICD-10-CM categories have applicable 7th characters. The applicable 7th character is required for all codes within the category, or as the notes in the Tabular List instruct. The 7th character must always be the 7th character in the data field. If a code that requires a 7th character is not 6 characters, a placeholder X must be used to fill in the empty characters.

6. Abbreviations

a. Alphabetic Index abbreviations

NEC "Not elsewhere classifiable"

This abbreviation in the Alphabetic Index represents "other specified". When a specific code is not available for a condition the Alphabetic Index directs the coder to the "other specified" code in the Tabular List.

NOS "Not otherwise specified"
This abbreviation is the equivalent of unspecified.

b. Tabular List abbreviations

NEC "Not elsewhere classifiable"
This abbreviation in the Tabular List represents "other specified". When a specific code is not available for a condition, the Tabular List includes an NEC entry under a code to identify the code as the "other specified" code.

NOS "Not otherwise specified"
This abbreviation is the equivalent of unspecified.

7. Punctuation

[ ] Brackets are used in the Tabular List to enclose synonyms, alternative wording or explanatory phrases. Brackets are used in the Alphabetic Index to identify manifestation codes.

( ) Parentheses are used in both the Alphabetic Index and Tabular List to enclose supplementary words that may be present or absent in the statement of a disease or procedure without affecting the code number to which it is assigned. The terms within the parentheses are referred to as nonessential modifiers. The nonessential modifiers in the Alphabetic Index to Diseases apply to subterms following a main term except when a nonessential modifier and a subentry are mutually exclusive, the subentry takes precedence. For example, in the ICD-10-CM Alphabetic Index under the main term Enteritis, "acute" is a nonessential modifier and "chronic" is a subentry. In this case, the nonessential modifier "acute" does not apply to the subentry "chronic".

: Colons are used in the Tabular List after an incomplete term which needs one or more of the modifiers following the colon to make it assignable to a given category.

8. Use of "and".
See Section I.A.14. Use of the term "And"

9. Other and Unspecified codes

a. "Other" codes
Codes titled "other" or "other specified" are for use when the information in the medical record provides detail for which a specific code does not exist. Alphabetic Index entries with NEC in the line designate "other" codes in the Tabular List. These Alphabetic Index entries represent specific disease entities for which no specific code exists so the term is included within an "other" code.

b. "Unspecified" codes
Codes titled "unspecified" are for use when the information in the medical record is insufficient to assign a more specific code. For those categories for which an unspecified code is not provided, the "other specified" code may represent both other and unspecified.
See Section I.B.18 Use of signs/symptoms/unspecified codes

10. Includes Notes
This note appears immediately under a 3-character code title to further define, or give examples of, the content of the category.

11. Inclusion terms
List of terms is included under some codes. These terms are the conditions for which that code is to be used. The terms may be synonyms of the code title, or, in the case of "other specified" codes, the terms are a list of the various conditions assigned to that code. The inclusion terms are not necessarily exhaustive. Additional terms found only in the Alphabetic Index may also be assigned to a code.

12. Excludes Notes
The ICD-10-CM has two types of excludes notes. Each type of note has a different definition for use but they are all similar in that they indicate that codes excluded from each other are independent of each other.

a. Excludes1
A type 1 Excludes note is a pure excludes note. It means "NOT CODED HERE!" An Excludes1 note indicates that the code excluded should never be used at the same time as the code above the Excludes1 note. An Excludes1 is used when two conditions cannot occur together, such as a congenital form versus an acquired form of the same condition.

An exception to the Excludes1 definition is the circumstance when the two conditions are unrelated to each other. If it is not clear whether the two conditions involving an Excludes1 note are related or not, query the provider. For example, code F45.8, Other somatoform disorders, has an Excludes1 note for "sleep related teeth grinding (G47.63)" because "teeth grinding" is an inclusion term under F45.8. Only one of these two codes should be assigned for teeth grinding. However, psychogenic dysmenorrhea is also an inclusion term under F45.8, and a patient could have both this condition and sleep-related teeth grinding. In this case, the two conditions are clearly unrelated to each other, and so it would be appropriate to report F45.8 and G47.63 together.

b. Excludes2
A Type 2 Excludes note represents "Not included here." An excludes2 note indicates that the condition excluded is not part of the condition represented by the code, but a patient may have both conditions at the same time. When an Excludes2 note appears under a code, it is acceptable to use both the code and the excluded code together, when appropriate.

13. **Etiology/manifestation convention ("code first", "use additional code" and "in diseases classified elsewhere" notes)**
Certain conditions have both an underlying etiology and multiple body system manifestations due to the underlying etiology. For such conditions, the ICD-10-CM has a coding convention that requires the underlying condition be sequenced first, if applicable, followed by the manifestation. Wherever such a combination exists, there is a "use additional code" note at the etiology code, and a "code first" note at the manifestation code. These instructional notes indicate the proper sequencing order of the codes, etiology followed by manifestation.
In most cases the manifestation codes will have in the code title, "in diseases classified elsewhere." Codes with this title are a component of the etiology/manifestation convention. The code title indicates that it is a manifestation code. "In diseases classified elsewhere" codes are never permitted to be used as first-listed or principal diagnosis codes. They must be used in conjunction with an underlying condition code and they must be listed following the underlying condition. See category FØ2, Dementia in other diseases classified elsewhere, for an example of this convention.
There are manifestation codes that do not have "in diseases classified elsewhere" in the title. For such codes, there is a "use additional code" note at the etiology code and a "code first" note at the manifestation code and the rules for sequencing apply.
In addition to the notes in the Tabular List, these conditions also have a specific Alphabetic Index entry structure. In the Alphabetic Index both conditions are listed together with the etiology code first followed by the manifestation codes in brackets. The code in brackets is always to be sequenced second.
An example of the etiology/manifestation convention is dementia in Parkinson's disease. In the Alphabetic Index, code G2Ø is listed first, followed by code FØ2.8Ø or FØ2.81 in brackets. Code G2Ø represents the underlying etiology, Parkinson's disease, and must be sequenced first, whereas code FØ2.8Ø and FØ2.81 represent the manifestation of dementia in diseases classified elsewhere, with or without behavioral disturbance.
"Code first" and "Use additional code" notes are also used as sequencing rules in the classification for certain codes that are not part of an etiology/manifestation combination.
See Section I.B.7. Multiple coding for a single condition.

14. **"And"**
The word "and" should be interpreted to mean either "and" or "or" when it appears in a title.
For example, cases of "tuberculosis of bones", "tuberculosis of joints" and "tuberculosis of bones and joints" are classified to subcategory A18.Ø, Tuberculosis of bones and joints.

15. **"With"**
The word "with" or "in" should be interpreted to mean "associated with" or "due to" when it appears in a code title, the Alphabetic Index, (either under a main term or subterm) or an instructional note in the Tabular List. The classification presumes a causal relationship between the two conditions linked by these terms in the Alphabetic Index or Tabular List. These conditions should be coded as related even in the absence of provider documentation explicitly linking them, unless the documentation clearly states the conditions are unrelated or when another guideline exists that specifically requires a documented linkage between two conditions (e.g., sepsis guideline for "acute organ dysfunction that is not clearly associated with the sepsis").
For conditions not specifically linked by these relational terms in the classification or when a guideline requires that a linkage between two conditions be explicitly documented provider documentation must link the conditions in order to code them as related.
The word "with" in the Alphabetic Index is sequenced immediately following the main term **or subterm**, not in alphabetical order.

16. **"See" and "See Also"**
The "see" instruction following a main term in the Alphabetic Index indicates that another term should be referenced. It is necessary to go to the main term referenced with the "see" note to locate the correct code.
A "see also" instruction following a main term in the Alphabetic Index instructs that there is another main term that may also be referenced that may provide additional Alphabetic Index entries that may be useful. It is not necessary to follow the "see also" note when the original main term provides the necessary code.

17. **"Code also" note**
A "code also" note instructs that two codes may be required to fully describe a condition, but this note does not provide sequencing direction. The sequencing depends on the circumstances of the encounter.

18. **Default codes**
A code listed next to a main term in the ICD-10-CM Alphabetic Index is referred to as a default code. The default code represents that condition that is most commonly associated with the main term, or is the unspecified code for the condition. If a condition is documented in a medical record (for example, appendicitis) without any additional information, such as acute or chronic, the default code should be assigned.

19. **Code assignment and Clinical Criteria**
The assignment of a diagnosis code is based on the provider's diagnostic statement that the condition exists. The provider's statement that the patient has a particular condition is sufficient. Code assignment is not based on clinical criteria used by the provider to establish the diagnosis.

B. General Coding Guidelines

1. Locating a code in the ICD-10-CM

To select a code in the classification that corresponds to a diagnosis or reason for visit documented in a medical record, first locate the term in the Alphabetic Index, and then verify the code in the Tabular List. Read and be guided by instructional notations that appear in both the Alphabetic Index and the Tabular List.

It is essential to use both the Alphabetic Index and Tabular List when locating and assigning a code. The Alphabetic Index does not always provide the full code. Selection of the full code, including laterality and any applicable 7th character can only be done in the Tabular List. A dash (-) at the end of an Alphabetic Index entry indicates that additional characters are required. Even if a dash is not included at the Alphabetic Index entry, it is necessary to refer to the Tabular List to verify that no 7th character is required.

2. Level of Detail in Coding

Diagnosis codes are to be used and reported at their highest number of characters available.

ICD-10-CM diagnosis codes are composed of codes with 3, 4, 5, 6, or 7 characters. Codes with three characters are included in ICD-10-CM as the heading of a category of codes that may be further subdivided by the use of 4th and/or 5th characters and/or 6th characters, which provide greater detail.

A 3-character code is to be used only if it is not further subdivided. A code is invalid if it has not been coded to the full number of characters required for that code, including the 7th character, if applicable.

3. Code or codes from A00.0 through T88.9, Z00-Z99.8

The appropriate code or codes from A00.0 through T88.9, Z00-Z99.8 must be used to identify diagnoses, symptoms, conditions, problems, complaints or other reason(s) for the encounter/visit.

4. Signs and symptoms

Codes that describe symptoms and signs, as opposed to diagnoses, are acceptable for reporting purposes when a related definitive diagnosis has not been established (confirmed) by the provider. Chapter 18 of ICD-10-CM, Symptoms, Signs, and Abnormal Clinical and Laboratory Findings, Not Elsewhere Classified (codes R00.0 - R99) contains many, but not all codes for symptoms.

See Section I.B.18 Use of signs/symptoms/ unspecified codes

5. Conditions that are an integral part of a disease process

Signs and symptoms that are associated routinely with a disease process should not be assigned as additional codes, unless otherwise instructed by the classification.

6. Conditions that are not an integral part of a disease process

Additional signs and symptoms that may not be associated routinely with a disease process should be coded when present.

7. Multiple coding for a single condition

In addition to the etiology/manifestation convention that requires two codes to fully describe a single condition that affects multiple body systems, there are other single conditions that also require more than one code. "Use additional code" notes are found in the Tabular List at codes that are not part of an etiology/manifestation pair where a secondary code is useful to fully describe a condition. The sequencing rule is the same as the etiology/manifestation pair, "use additional code" indicates that a secondary code should be added, if known.

For example, for bacterial infections that are not included in Chapter 1, a secondary code from category B95, Streptococcus, Staphylococcus, and Enterococcus, as the cause of diseases classified elsewhere, or B96, Other bacterial agents as the cause of diseases classified elsewhere, may be required to identify the bacterial organism causing the infection. A "use additional code" note will normally be found at the infectious disease code, indicating a need for the organism code to be added as a secondary code.

"Code first" notes are also under certain codes that are not specifically manifestation codes but may be due to an underlying cause. When there is a "code first" note and an underlying condition is present, the underlying condition should be sequenced first, if known.

"Code, if applicable, any causal condition first," notes indicate that this code may be assigned as a principal diagnosis when the causal condition is unknown or not applicable. If a causal condition is known, then the code for that condition should be sequenced as the principal or first-listed diagnosis.

Multiple codes may be needed for sequela, complication codes and obstetric codes to more fully describe a condition. See the specific guidelines for these conditions for further instruction.

8. Acute and Chronic Conditions

If the same condition is described as both acute (subacute) and chronic, and separate subentries exist in the Alphabetic Index at the same indentation level, code both and sequence the acute (subacute) code first.

9. Combination Code

A combination code is a single code used to classify:
Two diagnoses, or
A diagnosis with an associated secondary process (manifestation)
A diagnosis with an associated complication
Combination codes are identified by referring to subterm entries in the Alphabetic Index and by reading the inclusion and exclusion notes in the Tabular List.

GUIDELINES (ICD-10-CM)

Assign only the combination code when that code fully identifies the diagnostic conditions involved or when the Alphabetic Index so directs. Multiple coding should not be used when the classification provides a combination code that clearly identifies all of the elements documented in the diagnosis. When the combination code lacks necessary specificity in describing the manifestation or complication, an additional code should be used as a secondary code.

10. **Sequela (Late Effects)**
A sequela is the residual effect (condition produced) after the acute phase of an illness or injury has terminated. There is no time limit on when a sequela code can be used. The residual may be apparent early, such as in cerebral infarction, or it may occur months or years later, such as that due to a previous injury. Examples of sequela include: scar formation resulting from a burn, deviated septum due to a nasal fracture, and infertility due to tubal occlusion from old tuberculosis. Coding of sequela generally requires two codes sequenced in the following order: the condition or nature of the sequela is sequenced first. The sequela code is sequenced second.

An exception to the above guidelines are those instances where the code for the sequela is followed by a manifestation code identified in the Tabular List and title, or the sequela code has been expanded (at the 4th, 5th, or 6th character levels) to include the manifestation(s). The code for the acute phase of an illness or injury that led to the sequela is never used with a code for the late effect.
See Section I.C.9. Sequelae of cerebrovascular disease
See Section I.C.15. Sequelae of complication of pregnancy, childbirth and the puerperium
See Section I.C.19. Application of 7th characters for Chapter 19

11. **Impending or Threatened Condition**
Code any condition described at the time of discharge as "impending" or "threatened" as follows:
If it did occur, code as confirmed diagnosis.
If it did not occur, reference the Alphabetic Index to determine if the condition has a subentry term for "impending" or "threatened" and also reference main term entries for "Impending" and for "Threatened."
If the subterms are listed, assign the given code.
If the subterms are not listed, code the existing underlying condition(s) and not the condition described as impending or threatened.

12. **Reporting Same Diagnosis Code More Than Once**
Each unique ICD-10-CM diagnosis code may be reported only once for an encounter. This applies to bilateral conditions when there are no distinct codes identifying laterality or two different conditions classified to the same ICD-10-CM diagnosis code.

13. **Laterality**
Some ICD-10-CM codes indicate laterality, specifying whether the condition occurs on the left, right or is bilateral. If no bilateral code is provided and the condition is bilateral, assign separate codes for both the left and right side. If the side is not identified in the medical record, assign the code for the unspecified side.

When a patient has a bilateral condition and each side is treated during separate encounters, assign the "bilateral" code (as the condition still exists on both sides), including for the encounter to treat the first side. For the second encounter for treatment after one side has previously been treated and the condition no longer exists on that side, assign the appropriate unilateral code for the side where the condition still exists (e.g., cataract surgery performed on each eye in separate encounters). The bilateral code would not be assigned for the subsequent encounter, as the patient no longer has the condition in the previously-treated site. If the treatment on the first side did not completely resolve the condition, then the bilateral code would still be appropriate.

14. **Documentation by Clinicians Other than the Patient's Provider**
Code assignment is based on the documentation by patient's provider (i.e., physician or other qualified healthcare practitioner legally accountable for establishing the patient's diagnosis). There are a few exceptions, such as codes for the Body Mass Index (BMI), depth of non-pressure chronic ulcers, pressure ulcer stage, coma scale, and NIH stroke scale (NIHSS) codes, code assignment may be based on medical record documentation from clinicians who are not the patient's provider (i.e., physician or other qualified healthcare practitioner legally accountable for establishing the patient's diagnosis), since this information is typically documented by other clinicians involved in the care of the patient (e.g., a dietitian often documents the BMI, a nurse often documents the pressure ulcer stages, and an emergency medical technician often documents the coma scale). However, the associated diagnosis (such as overweight, obesity, acute stroke, or pressure ulcer) must be documented by the patient's provider. If there is conflicting medical record documentation, either from the same clinician or different clinicians, the patient's attending provider should be queried for clarification.

For social determinants of health, such as information found in categories Z55-Z65, Persons with potential health hazards related to socioeconomic and psychosocial circumstances, code assignment may be based on medical record documentation from clinicians involved in the care of the patient who are not the patient's provider since this information represents social information, rather than medical diagnoses.

The BMI, coma scale, and NIHSS codes and categories Z55-Z65 should only be reported as secondary diagnoses.

15. Syndromes
Follow the Alphabetic Index guidance when coding syndromes. In the absence of Alphabetic Index guidance, assign codes for the documented manifestations of the syndrome. Additional codes for manifestations that are not an integral part of the disease process may also be assigned when the condition does not have a unique code.

16. Documentation of Complications of Care
Code assignment is based on the provider's documentation of the relationship between the condition and the care or procedure, unless otherwise instructed by the classification. The guideline extends to any complications of care, regardless of the chapter the code is located in. It is important to note that not all conditions that occur during or following medical care or surgery are classified as complications. There must be a cause-and-effect relationship between the care provided and the condition, and an indication in the documentation that it is a complication. Query the provider for clarification, if the complication is not clearly documented.

17. Borderline Diagnosis
If the provider documents a "borderline" diagnosis at the time of discharge, the diagnosis is coded as confirmed, unless the classification provides a specific entry (e.g., borderline diabetes). If a borderline condition has a specific index entry in ICD-10-CM, it should be coded as such. Since borderline conditions are not uncertain diagnoses, no distinction is made between the care setting (inpatient versus outpatient). Whenever the documentation is unclear regarding a borderline condition, coders are encouraged to query for clarification.

18. Use of Sign/Symptom/Unspecified Codes
Sign/symptom and "unspecified" codes have acceptable, even necessary, uses. While specific diagnosis codes should be reported when they are supported by the available medical record documentation and clinical knowledge of the patient's health condition, there are instances when signs/symptoms or unspecified codes are the best choices for accurately reflecting the healthcare encounter. Each healthcare encounter should be coded to the level of certainty known for that encounter.

If a definitive diagnosis has not been established by the end of the encounter, it is appropriate to report codes for sign(s) and/or symptom(s) in lieu of a definitive diagnosis. When sufficient clinical information isn't known or available about a particular health condition to assign a more specific code, it is acceptable to report the appropriate "unspecified" code (e.g., a diagnosis of pneumonia has been determined, but not the specific type). Unspecified codes should be reported when they are the codes that most accurately reflect what is known about the patient's condition at the time of that particular encounter. It would be inappropriate to select a specific code that is not supported by the medical record documentation or conduct medically unnecessary diagnostic testing in order to determine a more specific code.

19. Coding for Healthcare Encounters in Hurricane Aftermath

a. Use of External Cause of Morbidity Codes
An external cause of morbidity code should be assigned to identify the cause of the injury(ies) incurred as a result of the hurricane. The use of external cause of morbidity codes is supplemental to the application of ICD-10-CM codes. External cause of morbidity codes are never to be recorded as a principal diagnosis (first-listed in non-inpatient settings). The appropriate injury code should be sequenced before any external cause codes. The external cause of morbidity codes capture how the injury or health condition happened (cause), the intent (unintentional or accidental; or intentional, such as suicide or assault), the place where the event occurred, the activity of the patient at the time of the event, and the person's status (e.g., civilian, military). They should not be assigned for encounters to treat hurricane victims' medical conditions when no injury, adverse effect or poisoning is involved. External cause of morbidity codes should be assigned for each encounter for care and treatment of the injury. External cause of morbidity codes may be assigned in all health care settings. For the purpose of capturing complete and accurate ICD-10-CM data in the aftermath of the hurricane, a healthcare setting should be considered as any location where medical care is provided by licensed healthcare professionals.

b. Sequencing of External Causes of Morbidity Codes
Codes for cataclysmic events, such as a hurricane, take priority over all other external cause codes except child and adult abuse and terrorism and should be sequenced before other external cause of injury codes. Assign as many external cause of morbidity codes as necessary to fully explain each cause. For example, if an injury occurs as a result of a building collapse during the hurricane, external cause codes for both the hurricane and the building collapse should be assigned, with the external causes code for hurricane being sequenced as the first external cause code. For injuries incurred as a direct result of the hurricane, assign the appropriate code(s) for the injuries, followed by the code X37.Ø-, Hurricane (with the appropriate 7th character), and any other applicable external cause of injury codes. Code X37.Ø- also should be assigned when an injury is incurred as a result of flooding caused by a levee breaking related to the hurricane. Code X38.-, Flood (with the appropriate 7th character), should be assigned when an injury is from flooding

GUIDELINES (ICD-10-CM)

resulting directly from the storm. Code X36.Ø.-, Collapse of dam or man-made structure, should not be assigned when the cause of the collapse is due to the hurricane. Use of code X36.Ø- is limited to collapses of man-made structures due to earth surface movements, not due to storm surges directly from a hurricane.

c. Other External Causes of Morbidity Code Issues

For injuries that are not a direct result of the hurricane, such as an evacuee that has incurred an injury as a result of a motor vehicle accident, assign the appropriate external cause of morbidity code(s) to describe the cause of the injury, but do not assign code X37.Ø-, Hurricane. If it is not clear whether the injury was a direct result of the hurricane, assume the injury is due to the hurricane and assign code X37.Ø-, Hurricane, as well as any other applicable external cause of morbidity codes. In addition to code X37.Ø-, Hurricane, other possible applicable external cause of morbidity codes include:

W54.Ø-	Bitten by dog
X3Ø-	Exposure to excessive natural heat
X31-	Exposure to excessive natural cold
X38-	Flood

d. Use of Z codes

Z codes (other reasons for healthcare encounters) may be assigned as appropriate to further explain the reasons for presenting for healthcare services, including transfers between healthcare facilities. The ICD-10-CM Official Guidelines for Coding and Reporting identify which codes maybe assigned as principal or first-listed diagnosis only, secondary diagnosis only, or principal/first-listed or secondary (depending on the circumstances). Possible applicable Z codes include:

Z59.Ø	Homelessness
Z59.1	Inadequate housing
Z59.5	Extreme poverty
Z75.1	Person awaiting admission to adequate facility elsewhere
Z75.3	Unavailability and inaccessibility of health-care facilities
Z75.4	Unavailability and inaccessibility of other helping agencies
Z76.2	Encounter for health supervision and care of other healthy infant and child
Z99.12	Encounter for respirator [ventilator] dependence during power failure

The external cause of morbidity codes and the Z codes listed above are not an all-inclusive list. Other codes may be applicable to the encounter based upon the documentation. Assign as many codes as necessary to fully explain each healthcare encounter. Since patient history information may be very limited, use any available documentation to assign the appropriate external cause of morbidity and Z codes.

C. Chapter-Specific Coding Guidelines

In addition to general coding guidelines, there are guidelines for specific diagnoses and/or conditions in the classification. Unless otherwise indicated, these guidelines apply to all health care settings. Please refer to Section II for guidelines on the selection of principal diagnosis.

1. Chapter 1: Certain Infectious and Parasitic Diseases (AØØ-B99)

a. Human Immunodeficiency Virus (HIV) Infections

1) Code only confirmed cases

Code only confirmed cases of HIV infection/illness. This is an exception to the hospital inpatient guideline Section II, H.

In this context, "confirmation" does not require documentation of positive serology or culture for HIV; the provider's diagnostic statement that the patient is HIV positive, or has an HIV-related illness is sufficient.

2) Selection and sequencing of HIV codes

(a) Patient admitted for HIV-related condition

If a patient is admitted for an HIV-related condition, the principal diagnosis should be B2Ø, Human immunodeficiency virus [HIV] disease followed by additional diagnosis codes for all reported HIV-related conditions.

(b) Patient with HIV disease admitted for unrelated condition

If a patient with HIV disease is admitted for an unrelated condition (such as a traumatic injury), the code for the unrelated condition (e.g., the nature of injury code) should be the principal diagnosis. Other diagnoses would be B2Ø followed by additional diagnosis codes for all reported HIV-related conditions.

(c) Whether the patient is newly diagnosed

Whether the patient is newly diagnosed or has had previous admissions/encounters for HIV conditions is irrelevant to the sequencing decision.

(d) Asymptomatic human immunodeficiency virus

Z21, Asymptomatic human immunodeficiency virus [HIV] infection status, is to be applied when the patient without any documentation of symptoms is listed as being "HIV positive," "known HIV," "HIV test positive," or similar terminology. Do not use this code if the term "AIDS" is used or if the patient is treated for any HIV-related illness or is described as having any condition(s) resulting from his/her HIV positive status; use B2Ø in these cases.

(e) Patients with inconclusive HIV serology

Patients with inconclusive HIV serology, but no definitive diagnosis or manifestations of the illness, may be assigned code R75, Inconclusive laboratory evidence of human immunodeficiency virus [HIV].

(f) **Previously diagnosed HIV-related illness**

Patients with any known prior diagnosis of an HIV-related illness should be coded to B2Ø. Once a patient has developed an HIV-related illness, the patient should always be assigned code B2Ø on every subsequent admission/encounter. Patients previously diagnosed with any HIV illness (B2Ø) should never be assigned to R75 or Z21, Asymptomatic human immunodeficiency virus [HIV] infection status.

(g) **HIV Infection in Pregnancy, Childbirth and the Puerperium**

During pregnancy, childbirth or the puerperium, a patient admitted (or presenting for a health care encounter) because of an HIV-related illness should receive a principal diagnosis code of O98.7-, Human immunodeficiency [HIV] disease complicating pregnancy, childbirth and the puerperium, followed by B2Ø and the code(s) for the HIV-related illness(es). Codes from Chapter 15 always take sequencing priority.

Patients with asymptomatic HIV infection status admitted (or presenting for a health care encounter) during pregnancy, childbirth, or the puerperium should receive codes of O98.7- and Z21.

(h) **Encounters for testing for HIV**

If a patient is being seen to determine his/her HIV status, use code Z11.4, Encounter for screening for human immunodeficiency virus [HIV]. Use additional codes for any associated high-risk behavior.

If a patient with signs or symptoms is being seen for HIV testing, code the signs and symptoms. An additional counseling code Z71.7, Human immunodeficiency virus [HIV] counseling, may be used if counseling is provided during the encounter for the test.

When a patient returns to be informed of his/her HIV test results and the test result is negative, use code Z71.7, Human immunodeficiency virus [HIV] counseling.

If the results are positive, see previous guidelines and assign codes as appropriate.

b. **Infectious agents as the cause of diseases classified to other chapters**

Certain infections are classified in chapters other than Chapter 1 and no organism is identified as part of the infection code. In these instances, it is necessary to use an additional code from Chapter 1 to identify the organism. A code from category B95, Streptococcus, Staphylococcus, and Enterococcus as the cause of diseases classified to other chapters, B96, Other bacterial agents as the cause of diseases classified to other chapters, or B97, Viral agents as the cause of diseases classified to other chapters, is to be used as an additional code to identify the organism. An instructional note will be found at the infection code advising that an additional organism code is required.

c. **Infections resistant to antibiotics**

Many bacterial infections are resistant to current antibiotics. It is necessary to identify all infections documented as antibiotic resistant. Assign a code from category Z16, Resistance to antimicrobial drugs, following the infection code only if the infection code does not identify drug resistance.

d. **Sepsis, Severe Sepsis, and Septic Shock**

1) **Coding of Sepsis and Severe Sepsis**

(a) **Sepsis**

For a diagnosis of sepsis, assign the appropriate code for the underlying systemic infection. If the type of infection or causal organism is not further specified, assign code A41.9, Sepsis, unspecified organism.

A code from subcategory R65.2, Severe sepsis, should not be assigned unless severe sepsis or an associated acute organ dysfunction is documented.

(i) Negative or inconclusive blood cultures and sepsis
Negative or inconclusive blood cultures do not preclude a diagnosis of sepsis in patients with clinical evidence of the condition, however, the provider should be queried.

(ii) Urosepsis
The term urosepsis is a nonspecific term. It is not to be considered synonymous with sepsis. It has no default code in the Alphabetic Index. Should a provider use this term, he/she must be queried for clarification.

(iii) Sepsis with organ dysfunction
If a patient has sepsis and associated acute organ dysfunction or multiple organ dysfunction (MOD), follow the instructions for coding severe sepsis.

(iv) Acute organ dysfunction that is not clearly associated with the sepsis
If a patient has sepsis and an acute organ dysfunction, but the medical record documentation indicates that the acute organ dysfunction is related to a medical condition other than the sepsis, do not assign a code from subcategory R65.2, Severe sepsis. An acute organ dysfunction must be associated with the sepsis in order to assign the severe sepsis code. If the documentation is not clear as to whether an acute organ dysfunction is related to the sepsis or another medical condition, query the provider.

(b) **Severe sepsis**

The coding of severe sepsis requires a minimum of 2 codes: first a code for the underlying systemic infection, followed by a code from subcategory

R65.2, Severe sepsis. If the causal organism is not documented, assign code A41.9, Sepsis, unspecified organism, for the infection. Additional code(s) for the associated acute organ dysfunction are also required.

Due to the complex nature of severe sepsis, some cases may require querying the provider prior to assignment of the codes.

2) Septic shock

(a) Septic shock generally refers to circulatory failure associated with severe sepsis, and therefore, it represents a type of acute organ dysfunction.

For all cases of septic shock, the code for the systemic infection should be sequenced first, followed by code R65.21, Severe sepsis with septic shock or code T81.12, Postprocedural septic shock. Any additional codes for the other acute organ dysfunctions should also be assigned. As noted in the sequencing instructions in the Tabular List, the code for septic shock cannot be assigned as a principal diagnosis.

3) Sequencing of severe sepsis

If severe sepsis is present on admission, and meets the definition of principal diagnosis, the underlying systemic infection should be assigned as principal diagnosis followed by the appropriate code from subcategory R65.2 as required by the sequencing rules in the Tabular List. A code from subcategory R65.2 can never be assigned as a principal diagnosis.

When severe sepsis develops during an encounter (it was not present on admission) the underlying systemic infection and the appropriate code from subcategory R65.2 should be assigned as secondary diagnoses.

Severe sepsis may be present on admission but the diagnosis may not be confirmed until sometime after admission. If the documentation is not clear whether severe sepsis was present on admission, the provider should be queried.

4) Sepsis *or* severe sepsis with a localized infection

If the reason for admission is sepsis or severe sepsis and a localized infection, such as pneumonia or cellulitis, a code(s) for the underlying systemic infection should be assigned first and the code for the localized infection should be assigned as a secondary diagnosis. If the patient has severe sepsis, a code from subcategory R65.2 should also be assigned as a secondary diagnosis. If the patient is admitted with a localized infection, such as pneumonia, and sepsis/severe sepsis doesn't develop until after admission, the localized infection should be assigned first, followed by the appropriate sepsis/severe sepsis codes.

5) Sepsis due to a postprocedural infection

(a) Documentation of causal relationship

As with all postprocedural complications, code assignment is based on the provider's documentation of the relationship between the infection and the procedure.

(b) Sepsis due to a postprocedural infection

For infections following a procedure, a code from T81.4Ø, to T81.43. Infection following a procedure, or a code from O86.ØØ to O86.Ø3, Infection of obstetric surgical wound, that identifies the site of the infection should be coded first, if known. Assign an additional code for sepsis following a procedure (T81.44) or sepsis following an obstetrical procedure (O86.Ø4). Use an additional code to identify the infectious agent. If the patient has severe sepsis the appropriate code from subcategory R65.2 should also be assigned with the additional code(s) for any acute organ dysfunction.

For infections following infusion, transfusion, therapeutic injection, or immunization, a code from subcategory T8Ø.2, Infections following infusion, transfusion, and therapeutic injection, or code T88.Ø-, Infection following immunization, should be coded first, followed by the code for the specific infection. If the patient has severe sepsis, the appropriate code from subcategory R65.2 should also be assigned, with the additional codes(s) for any acute organ dysfunction.

(c) Postprocedural infection and postprocedural septic shock

If a postprocedural infection has resulted in postprocedural septic shock, assign the codes indicated above for sepsis due to a postprocedural infection, followed by code T81.12-, Postprocedural septic shock. Do not assign code R65.21, Severe sepsis with septic shock. Additional code(s) should be assigned for any acute organ dysfunction.

6) Sepsis and severe sepsis associated with a noninfectious process (condition)

In some cases a noninfectious process (condition), such as trauma, may lead to an infection which can result in sepsis or severe sepsis. If sepsis or severe sepsis is documented as associated with a noninfectious condition, such as a burn or serious injury, and this condition meets the definition for principal diagnosis, the code for the noninfectious condition should be sequenced first, followed by the code for the resulting infection. If severe sepsis is present, a code from subcategory R65.2 should also be assigned with any associated organ dysfunction(s) codes. It is not necessary to assign a code from subcategory R65.1, Systemic inflammatory response syndrome (SIRS) of non-infectious origin, for these cases.

If the infection meets the definition of principal diagnosis it should be sequenced before the non-infectious condition. When both the associated non-infectious condition and the infection meet the definition of principal diagnosis either may be assigned as principal diagnosis.

Only one code from category R65, Symptoms and signs specifically associated with systemic inflammation and infection, should be assigned. Therefore, when a non-infectious condition leads to an infection resulting in severe sepsis, assign the appropriate code from subcategory R65.2, Severe sepsis. Do not additionally assign a code from subcategory R65.1, Systemic inflammatory response syndrome (SIRS) of non-infectious origin.

See Section I.C.18. SIRS due to non-infectious process

7) Sepsis and septic shock complicating abortion, pregnancy, childbirth, and the puerperium

See Section I.C.15. Sepsis and septic shock complicating abortion, pregnancy, childbirth and the puerperium

8) Newborn sepsis

See Section I.C.16. f. Bacterial sepsis of Newborn

e. Methicillin Resistant Staphylococcus aureus (MRSA) Conditions

1) Selection and sequencing of MRSA codes

(a) Combination codes for MRSA infection

When a patient is diagnosed with an infection that is due to methicillin resistant *Staphylococcus aureus* (MRSA), and that infection has a combination code that includes the causal organism (e.g., sepsis, pneumonia) assign the appropriate combination code for the condition (e.g., code A41.02, Sepsis due to Methicillin resistant Staphylococcus aureus or code J15.212, Pneumonia due to Methicillin resistant Staphylococcus aureus). Do not assign code B95.62, Methicillin resistant Staphylococcus aureus infection as the cause of diseases classified elsewhere, as an additional code because the combination code includes the type of infection and the MRSA organism. Do not assign a code from subcategory Z16.11, Resistance to penicillins, as an additional diagnosis.

See Section C.1. for instructions on coding and sequencing of sepsis and severe sepsis.

(b) Other codes for MRSA infection

When there is documentation of a current infection (e.g., wound infection, stitch abscess, urinary tract infection) due to MRSA, and that infection does not have a combination code that includes the causal organism, assign the appropriate code to identify the condition along with code B95.62, Methicillin resistant Staphylococcus aureus infection as the cause of diseases classified elsewhere for the MRSA infection. Do not assign a code from subcategory Z16.11, Resistance to penicillins.

(c) Methicillin susceptible Staphylococcus aureus (MSSA) and MRSA colonization

The condition or state of being colonized or carrying MSSA or MRSA is called colonization or carriage, while an individual person is described as being colonized or being a carrier. Colonization means that MSSA or MSRA is present on or in the body without necessarily causing illness. A positive MRSA colonization test might be documented by the provider as "MRSA screen positive" or "MRSA nasal swab positive".

Assign code Z22.322, Carrier or suspected carrier of Methicillin resistant Staphylococcus

aureus, for patients documented as having MRSA colonization. Assign code Z22.321, Carrier or suspected carrier of Methicillin susceptible Staphylococcus aureus, for patients documented as having MSSA colonization. Colonization is not necessarily indicative of a disease process or as the cause of a specific condition the patient may have unless documented as such by the provider.

(d) MRSA colonization and infection

If a patient is documented as having both MRSA colonization and infection during a hospital admission, code Z22.322, Carrier or suspected carrier of Methicillin resistant Staphylococcus aureus, and a code for the MRSA infection may both be assigned.

f. Zika virus infections

1) Code only confirmed cases

Code only a confirmed diagnosis of Zika virus (A92.5, Zika virus disease) as documented by the provider. This is an exception to the hospital inpatient guideline Section II, H.

In this context, "confirmation" does not require documentation of the type of test performed; the **provider's** diagnostic statement that the condition is confirmed is sufficient. This code should be assigned regardless of the stated mode of transmission.

If the provider documents "suspected", "possible" or "probable" Zika, do not assign code A92.5. Assign a code(s) explaining the reason for encounter (such as fever, rash, or joint pain) or Z20.821, Contact with and (suspected) exposure to Zika virus.

2. Chapter 2: Neoplasms (C00-D49)
General guidelines

Chapter 2 of the ICD-10-CM contains the codes for most benign and all malignant neoplasms. Certain benign neoplasms, such as prostatic adenomas, may be found in the specific body system chapters. To properly code a neoplasm it is necessary to determine from the record if the neoplasm is benign, in-situ, malignant, or of uncertain histologic behavior. If malignant, any secondary (metastatic) sites should also be determined.

Primary malignant neoplasms overlapping site boundaries

A primary malignant neoplasm that overlaps two or more contiguous (next to each other) sites should be classified to the subcategory/code .8 ("overlapping lesion"), unless the combination is specifically indexed elsewhere. For multiple neoplasms of the same site that are not contiguous such as tumors in different quadrants of the same breast, codes for each site should be assigned.

Malignant neoplasm of ectopic tissue

Malignant neoplasms of ectopic tissue are to be coded to the site of origin mentioned (e.g., ectopic pancreatic malignant neoplasms involving the stomach are coded to malignant neoplasm of pancreas, unspecified) (C25.9).

The neoplasm table in the Alphabetic Index should be referenced first. However, if the histological term is documented, that term should be referenced first, rather than going immediately to the Neoplasm Table, in order to determine which column in the Neoplasm Table is appropriate. For example, if the documentation indicates "adenoma," refer to the term in the Alphabetic Index to review the entries under this term and the instructional note to "see also neoplasm, by site, benign." The table provides the proper code based on the type of neoplasm and the site. It is important to select the proper column in the table that corresponds to the type of neoplasm. The Tabular List should then be referenced to verify that the correct code has been selected from the table and that a more specific site code does not exist.

See Section I.C.21. Factors influencing health status and contact with health services, Status, for information regarding Z15.Ø, codes for genetic susceptibility to cancer.

a. Treatment directed at the malignancy

If the treatment is directed at the malignancy, designate the malignancy as the principal diagnosis.

The only exception to this guideline is if a patient admission/encounter is solely for the administration of chemotherapy, immunotherapy or external beam radiation therapy, assign the appropriate Z51.— code as the first-listed or principal diagnosis, and the diagnosis or problem for which the service is being performed as a secondary diagnosis.

b. Treatment of secondary site

When a patient is admitted because of a primary neoplasm with metastasis and treatment is directed toward the secondary site only, the secondary neoplasm is designated as the principal diagnosis even though the primary malignancy is still present.

c. Coding and sequencing of complications

Coding and sequencing of complications associated with the malignancies or with the therapy thereof are subject to the following guidelines:

1) Anemia associated with malignancy

When admission/encounter is for management of an anemia associated with the malignancy, and the treatment is only for anemia, the appropriate code for the malignancy is sequenced as the principal or first-listed diagnosis followed by the appropriate code for the anemia (such as code D63.Ø, Anemia in neoplastic disease).

2) Anemia associated with chemotherapy, immunotherapy and radiation therapy

When the admission/encounter is for management of an anemia associated with an adverse effect of the administration of chemotherapy or immunotherapy and the only treatment is for the anemia, the anemia code is sequenced first followed by the appropriate codes for the

neoplasm and the adverse effect (T45.1X5, Adverse effect of antineoplastic and immunosuppressive drugs).

When the admission/encounter is for management of an anemia associated with an adverse effect of radiotherapy, the anemia code should be sequenced first, followed by the appropriate neoplasm code and code Y84.2, Radiological procedure and radiotherapy as the cause of abnormal reaction of the patient, or of later complication, without mention of misadventure at the time of the procedure.

3) Management of dehydration due to the malignancy

When the admission/encounter is for management of dehydration due to the malignancy and only the dehydration is being treated (intravenous rehydration), the dehydration is sequenced first, followed by the code(s) for the malignancy.

4) Treatment of a complication resulting from a surgical procedure

When the admission/encounter is for treatment of a complication resulting from a surgical procedure, designate the complication as the principal or first-listed diagnosis if treatment is directed at resolving the complication.

d. Primary malignancy previously excised

When a primary malignancy has been previously excised or eradicated from its site and there is no further treatment directed to that site and there is no evidence of any existing primary malignancy, at that site a code from category Z85, Personal history of malignant neoplasm, should be used to indicate the former site of the malignancy. Any mention of extension, invasion, or metastasis to another site is coded as a secondary malignant neoplasm to that site. The secondary site may be the principal or first-listed **diagnosis** with the Z85 code used as a secondary code.

e. Admissions/Encounters involving chemotherapy, immunotherapy and radiation therapy

1) Episode of care involves surgical removal of neoplasm

When an episode of care involves the surgical removal of a neoplasm, primary or secondary site, followed by adjunct chemotherapy or radiation treatment during the same episode of care, the code for the neoplasm should be assigned as principal or first-listed diagnosis.

2) Patient admission/encounter solely for administration of chemotherapy, immunotherapy and radiation therapy

If a patient admission/encounter is solely for the administration of chemotherapy, immunotherapy or external beam radiation therapy assign code Z51.Ø, Encounter for antineoplastic radiation therapy, or Z51.11, Encounter for antineoplastic chemotherapy, or Z51.12, Encounter for antineoplastic immunotherapy as the first-listed or principal diagnosis. If a patient receives more than one of these therapies during the same admission more than one of these codes may be assigned, in any sequence.

The malignancy for which the therapy is being administered should be assigned as a secondary diagnosis.

If a patient admission/encounter is for the insertion or implantation of radioactive elements (e.g., brachytherapy) the appropriate code for the malignancy is sequenced as the principal or first-listed diagnosis. Code Z51.0 should not be assigned.

3) Patient admitted for radiation therapy, chemotherapy or immunotherapy and develops complications

When a patient is admitted for the purpose of external beam radiotherapy, immunotherapy or chemotherapy and develops complications such as uncontrolled nausea and vomiting or dehydration, the principal or first-listed diagnosis is Z51.0, Encounter for antineoplastic radiation therapy, or Z51.11, Encounter for antineoplastic chemotherapy, or Z51.12, Encounter for antineoplastic immunotherapy followed by any codes for the complications.

When a patient is admitted for the purpose of insertion or implantation of radioactive elements (e.g., brachytherapy) and develops complications such as uncontrolled nausea and vomiting or dehydration, the principal or first-listed diagnosis is the appropriate code for the malignancy followed by any codes for the complications.

f. Admission/encounter to determine extent of malignancy

When the reason for admission/encounter is to determine the extent of the malignancy, or for a procedure such as paracentesis or thoracentesis, the primary malignancy or appropriate metastatic site is designated as the principal or first-listed diagnosis, even though chemotherapy or radiotherapy is administered.

g. Symptoms, signs, and abnormal findings listed in Chapter 18 associated with neoplasms

Symptoms, signs, and ill-defined conditions listed in Chapter 18 characteristic of, or associated with, an existing primary or secondary site malignancy cannot be used to replace the malignancy as principal or first-listed diagnosis, regardless of the number of admissions or encounters for treatment and care of the neoplasm.

See Section I.C.21. Factors influencing health status and contact with health services, Encounter for prophylactic organ removal.

h. Admission/encounter for pain control/management

See Section I.C.6. for information on coding admission/encounter for pain control/management.

i. Malignancy in two or more noncontiguous sites

A patient may have more than one malignant tumor in the same organ. These tumors may represent different primaries or metastatic disease, depending on the site. Should the documentation be unclear, the provider should be queried as to the status of each tumor so that the correct codes can be assigned.

j. Disseminated malignant neoplasm, unspecified

Code C80.0, Disseminated malignant neoplasm, unspecified, is for use only in those cases where the patient has advanced metastatic disease and no known primary or secondary sites are specified. It should not be used in place of assigning codes for the primary site and all known secondary sites.

k. Malignant neoplasm without specification of site

Code C80.1, Malignant (primary) neoplasm, unspecified, equates to Cancer, unspecified. This code should only be used when no determination can be made as to the primary site of a malignancy. This code should rarely be used in the inpatient setting.

l. Sequencing of neoplasm codes

1) Encounter for treatment of primary malignancy

If the reason for the encounter is for treatment of a primary malignancy, assign the malignancy as the principal/first-listed diagnosis. The primary site is to be sequenced first, followed by any metastatic sites.

2) Encounter for treatment of secondary malignancy

When an encounter is for a primary malignancy with metastasis and treatment is directed toward the metastatic (secondary) site(s) only, the metastatic site(s) is designated as the principal/first-listed diagnosis. The primary malignancy is coded as an additional code.

3) Malignant neoplasm in a pregnant patient

When a pregnant woman has a malignant neoplasm, a code from subcategory O9A.1-, Malignant neoplasm complicating pregnancy, childbirth, and the puerperium, should be sequenced first, followed by the appropriate code from Chapter 2 to indicate the type of neoplasm.

4) Encounter for complication associated with a neoplasm

When an encounter is for management of a complication associated with a neoplasm, such as dehydration, and the treatment is only for the complication, the complication is coded first, followed by the appropriate code(s) for the neoplasm.

The exception to this guideline is anemia. When the admission/encounter is for management of an anemia associated with the malignancy, and the treatment is only for anemia, the appropriate code for the malignancy is sequenced as the principal or first-listed diagnosis followed by code D63.0, Anemia in neoplastic disease.

5) Complication from surgical procedure for treatment of a neoplasm

When an encounter is for treatment of a complication resulting from a surgical procedure performed for the treatment of the neoplasm, designate the complication as the principal/first-listed diagnosis. See **the** guideline regarding the coding of a current malignancy versus personal history to determine if the code for the neoplasm should also be assigned.

6) Pathologic fracture due to a neoplasm

When an encounter is for a pathological fracture due to a neoplasm, and the focus of treatment is the fracture, a code from subcategory M84.5, Pathological fracture in neoplastic disease, should be sequenced first, followed by the code for the neoplasm.

If the focus of treatment is the neoplasm with an associated pathological fracture, the neoplasm code should be sequenced first, followed by a code from M84.5 for the pathological fracture.

m. Current malignancy versus personal history of malignancy

When a primary malignancy has been excised but further treatment, such as an additional surgery for the malignancy, radiation therapy or chemotherapy is directed to that site, the primary malignancy code should be used until treatment is completed.

When a primary malignancy has been previously excised or eradicated from its site, there is no further treatment (of the malignancy) directed to that site, and there is no evidence of any existing primary malignancy at that site, a code from category Z85, Personal history of malignant neoplasm, should be used to indicate the former site of the malignancy.

Subcategories Z85.Ø – Z85.7 should only be assigned for the former site of a primary malignancy, not the site of a secondary malignancy. Codes from subcategory Z85.8-, may be assigned for the former site(s) of either a primary or secondary malignancy included in this subcategory.

See Section I.C.21. Factors influencing health status and contact with health services, History (of)

n. Leukemia, Multiple Myeloma, and Malignant Plasma Cell Neoplasms in remission versus personal history

The categories for leukemia, and category C9Ø, Multiple myeloma and malignant plasma cell neoplasms, have codes indicating whether or not the leukemia has achieved remission. There are also codes Z85.6, Personal history of leukemia, and Z85.79, Personal history of other malignant neoplasms of lymphoid, hematopoietic and related tissues. If the documentation is unclear, as to whether the leukemia has achieved remission, the provider should be queried.

See Section I.C.21. Factors influencing health status and contact with health services, History (of)

o. Aftercare following surgery for neoplasm

See Section I.C.21. Factors influencing health status and contact with health services, Aftercare

p. Follow-up care for completed treatment of a malignancy

See Section I.C.21. Factors influencing health status and contact with health services, Follow-up

q. Prophylactic organ removal for prevention of malignancy

See Section I.C. 21, Factors influencing health status and contact with health services, Prophylactic organ removal

r. Malignant neoplasm associated with transplanted organ

A malignant neoplasm of a transplanted organ should be coded as a transplant complication. Assign first the appropriate code from category T86.-, Complications of transplanted organs and tissue, followed by code C8Ø.2, Malignant neoplasm associated with transplanted organ. Use an additional code for the specific malignancy.

3. Chapter 3: Disease of the blood and blood-forming organs and certain disorders involving the immune mechanism (D5Ø-D89)

Reserved for future guideline expansion

4. Chapter 4: Endocrine, Nutritional, and Metabolic Diseases (EØØ-E89)

a. Diabetes mellitus

The diabetes mellitus codes are combination codes that include the type of diabetes mellitus, the body system affected, and the complications affecting that body system. As many codes within a particular category as are necessary to describe all of the complications of the disease may be used. They should be sequenced based on the reason for a particular encounter. Assign as many codes from categories EØ8 – E13 as needed to identify all of the associated conditions that the patient has.

1) Type of diabetes

The age of a patient is not the sole determining factor, though most type 1 diabetics develop the condition before reaching puberty. For this reason type 1 diabetes mellitus is also referred to as juvenile diabetes.

2) Type of diabetes mellitus not documented

If the type of diabetes mellitus is not documented in the medical record the default is E11.-, Type 2 diabetes mellitus.

3) Diabetes mellitus and the use of insulin oral hypoglycemics

If the documentation in a medical record does not indicate the type of diabetes but does indicate that the patient uses insulin, code E11, Type 2 diabetes mellitus, should be assigned. An additional code should be assigned from category Z79 to identify the long-term (current) use of insulin or oral hypoglycemic drugs. If the patient is treated with both oral medications and insulin, only the code for long-term (current) use of insulin should be assigned. Code Z79.4 should not be assigned if insulin is given temporarily to bring a type 2 patient's blood sugar under control during an encounter.

4) Diabetes mellitus in pregnancy and gestational diabetes

See Section I.C.15. Diabetes mellitus in pregnancy.

See Section I.C.15. Gestational (pregnancy induced) diabetes

5) **Complications due to insulin pump malfunction**

(a) **Underdose of insulin due to insulin pump failure**

An underdose of insulin due to an insulin pump failure should be assigned to a code from subcategory T85.6, Mechanical complication of other specified internal and external prosthetic devices, implants and grafts, that specifies the type of pump malfunction, as the principal or first-listed code, followed by code T38.3X6-, Underdosing of insulin and oral hypoglycemic [antidiabetic] drugs. Additional codes for the type of diabetes mellitus and any associated complications due to the underdosing should also be assigned.

(b) **Overdose of insulin due to insulin pump failure**

The principal or first-listed code for an encounter due to an insulin pump malfunction resulting in an overdose of insulin, should also be T85.6-, Mechanical complication of other specified internal and external prosthetic devices, implants and grafts, followed by code T38.3X1-, Poisoning by insulin and oral hypoglycemic [antidiabetic] drugs, accidental (unintentional).

6) **Secondary diabetes mellitus**

Codes under categories EØ8, Diabetes mellitus due to underlying condition, EØ9, Drug or chemical induced diabetes mellitus and E13, Other specified diabetes mellitus, identify complications/manifestations associated with secondary diabetes mellitus. Secondary diabetes is always caused by another condition or event (e.g., cystic fibrosis, malignant neoplasm of pancreas, pancreatectomy, adverse effect of drug, or poisoning).

(a) **Secondary diabetes mellitus and the use of insulin or hypoglycemic drugs**

For patients with secondary diabetes mellitus who routinely use insulin or oral hypoglycemic drugs, an additional code from category Z79 should be assigned to identify the long-term (current) use of insulin or oral hypoglycemic drugs. If the patient is treated with both oral medications and insulin, only the code for long-term (current) use of insulin should be assigned. Code Z79.4 should not be assigned if insulin is given temporarily to bring a type 2 patient's blood sugar under control during an encounter.

(b) **Assigning and sequencing secondary diabetes codes and its causes**

The sequencing of the secondary diabetes codes in relationship to codes for the cause of the diabetes is based on the Tabular List instructions for categories EØ8, EØ9 and E13.

(i) **Secondary diabetes mellitus due to pancreatectomy** For postpancreatectomy diabetes mellitus (lack of insulin due to the surgical removal of all or part of the pancreas), assign code E89.1, Postprocedural hypoinsulinemia. Assign a code from category E13 and a code from subcategory Z9Ø.41-, Acquired absence of pancreas, as additional codes.

(ii) **Secondary diabetes due to drugs** Secondary diabetes may be caused by an adverse effect of correctly administered medications, poisoning or sequela of poisoning.

See Section I.C.19.e for coding of adverse effects and poisoning, and Section I.C.2Ø for external cause code reporting.

5. **Chapter 5: Mental, Behavioral and Neurodevelopmental disorders (FØ1 – F99)**

a. **Pain disorders related to psychological factors**

Assign code F45.41, for pain that is exclusively related to psychological disorders. As indicated by the Excludes1 note under category G89, a code from category G89 should not be assigned with code F45.41

Code F45.42, Pain disorders with related psychological factors, should be used with a code from category G89, Pain, not elsewhere classified, if there is documentation of a psychological component for a patient with acute or chronic pain.

See Section I.C.6. Pain

b. **Mental and behavioral disorders due to psychoactive substance use**

1) **In Remission**

Selection of codes for "in remission" for categories F1Ø-F19, Mental and behavioral disorders due to psychoactive substance use (categories F1Ø-F19 with -11, -.21) requires the provider's clinical judgment. The appropriate codes for "in remission" are assigned only on the basis of provider documentation (as defined in the Official Guidelines for Coding and Reporting), unless otherwise instructed by the classification.

Mild substance use disorders in early or sustained remission are classified to the appropriate codes for substance abuse in remission, and moderate or severe substance use disorders in early or sustained remission are classified to the appropriate codes for substance dependence in remission.

2) **Psychoactive Substance Use, Abuse and Dependence**

When the provider documentation refers to use, abuse and dependence of the same substance (e.g., alcohol, opioid, cannabis, etc.), only one code should be assigned to identify the pattern of use based on the following hierarchy:

- If both use and abuse are documented, assign only the code for abuse
- If both abuse and dependence are documented, assign only the code for dependence
- If use, abuse and dependence are all documented, assign only the code for dependence
- If both use and dependence are documented, assign only the code for dependence.

GUIDELINES (ICD-10-CM)

3) Psychoactive Substance Use, Unspecified

As with all other unspecified diagnoses, the codes for unspecified psychoactive substance use disorders (F10.9-, F11.9-, F12.9-, F13.9-, F14.9-, F15.9-, F16.9-, F18.9-, F19.9-) should only be assigned based on provider documentation and when they meet the definition of a reportable diagnosis (see Section III, Reporting Additional Diagnoses). These codes are to be used only when the psychoactive substance use is associated with a physical, mental or behavioral disorder, and such a relationship is documented by the provider.

c. Factitious Disorder

Factitious disorder imposed on self or Munchausen's syndrome is a disorder in which a person falsely reports or causes his or her own physical or psychological signs or symptoms. For patients with documented factitious disorder on self or Munchausen's syndrome, assign the appropriate code from subcategory F68.1-, Factitious disorder imposed on self.

Munchausen's syndrome by proxy (MSBP) is a disorder in which a caregiver (perpetrator) falsely reports or causes an illness or injury in another person (victim) under his or her care, such as a child, an elderly adult, or a person who has a disability. The condition is also referred to as "factitious disorder imposed on another" or "factitious disorder by proxy." The perpetrator, not the victim, receives this diagnosis. Assign code F68.A, Factitious disorder imposed on another, to the perpetrator's record. For the victim of a patient suffering from MSBP, assign the appropriate code from categories T74, Adult and child abuse, neglect and other maltreatment, confirmed, or T76, Adult and child abuse, neglect and other maltreatment, suspected.

See Section I.C.19.f. Adult and child abuse, neglect and other maltreatment

6. Chapter 6: Diseases of the Nervous System (G00-G99)

a. Dominant/nondominant side

Codes from category G81, Hemiplegia and hemiparesis, and subcategories, G83.1, Monoplegia of lower limb, G83.2, Monoplegia of upper limb, and G83.3, Monoplegia, unspecified, identify whether the dominant or nondominant side is affected. Should the affected side be documented, but not specified as dominant or nondominant, and the classification system does not indicate a default, code selection is as follows:

- For ambidextrous patients, the default should be dominant.
- If the left side is affected, the default is non-dominant.
- If the right side is affected, the default is dominant.

b. Pain - Category G89

1) General coding information

Codes in category G89, Pain, not elsewhere classified, may be used in conjunction with codes from other categories and chapters to provide more detail about acute or chronic pain and neoplasm-related pain, unless otherwise indicated below.

If the pain is not specified as acute or chronic, post-thoracotomy, postprocedural, or neoplasm-related, do not assign codes from category G89.

A code from category G89 should not be assigned if the underlying (definitive) diagnosis is known, unless the reason for the encounter is pain control/management and not management of the underlying condition.

When an admission or encounter is for a procedure aimed at treating the underlying condition (e.g., spinal fusion, kyphoplasty), a code for the underlying condition (e.g., vertebral fracture, spinal stenosis) should be assigned as the principal diagnosis. No code from category G89 should be assigned.

(a) Category G89 Codes as Principal or First-Listed Diagnosis

Category G89 codes are acceptable as principal diagnosis or the first-listed code:

- When pain control or pain management is the reason for the admission/encounter (e.g., a patient with displaced intervertebral disc, nerve impingement and severe back pain presents for injection of steroid into the spinal canal). The underlying cause of the pain should be reported as an additional diagnosis, if known.
- When a patient is admitted for the insertion of a neurostimulator for pain control, assign the appropriate pain code as the principal or first-listed diagnosis. When an admission or encounter is for a procedure aimed at treating the underlying condition and a neurostimulator is inserted for pain control during the same admission/encounter, a code for the underlying condition should be assigned as the principal diagnosis and the appropriate pain code should be assigned as a secondary diagnosis.

(b) Use of Category G89 Codes in Conjunction with Site-Specific Pain Codes

(i) Assigning Category G89 and Site-Specific Pain Codes

Codes from category G89 may be used in conjunction with codes that identify the site of pain (including codes from Chapter 18) if the category G89 code provides additional information. For example, if the code describes the site of the pain, but does not fully describe whether the pain is acute or chronic, then both codes should be assigned.

(ii) Sequencing of Category G89 Codes with Site-Specific Pain Codes

The sequencing of category G89 codes with site-specific pain codes (including Chapter 18 codes), is dependent on the circumstances of the encounter/admission as follows:

- If the encounter is for pain control or pain management, assign the code from category G89 followed by the code identifying the specific site of pain (e.g., encounter for pain management for acute neck pain from trauma is assigned code G89.11, Acute pain due to trauma, followed by code M54.2, Cervicalgia, to identify the site of pain).
- If the encounter is for any other reason except pain control or pain management, and a related definitive diagnosis has not been established (confirmed) by the provider, assign the code for the specific site of pain first, followed by the appropriate code from category G89.

2) Pain due to devices, implants and grafts
See Section I.C.19. Pain due to medical devices

3) Postoperative Pain
The provider's documentation should be used to guide the coding of postoperative pain, as well as *Section III. Reporting Additional Diagnoses* and *Section IV. Diagnostic Coding and Reporting in the Outpatient Setting.*

The default for post-thoracotomy and other postoperative pain not specified as acute or chronic is the code for the acute form.

Routine or expected postoperative pain immediately after surgery should not be coded.

(a) Postoperative pain not associated with specific postoperative complication
Postoperative pain not associated with a specific postoperative complication is assigned to the appropriate postoperative pain code in category G89.

(b) Postoperative pain associated with specific postoperative complication
Postoperative pain associated with a specific postoperative complication (such as painful wire sutures) is assigned to the appropriate code(s) found in Chapter 19, Injury, poisoning, and certain other consequences of external causes. If appropriate, use additional code(s) from category G89 to identify acute or chronic pain (G89.18 or G89.28).

4) Chronic pain
Chronic pain is classified to subcategory G89.2. There is no time frame defining when pain becomes chronic pain. The provider's documentation should be used to guide use of these codes.

5) Neoplasm Related Pain
Code G89.3 is assigned to pain documented as being related, associated or due to cancer, primary or secondary malignancy, or tumor. This code is assigned regardless of whether the pain is acute or chronic.

This code may be assigned as the principal or first-listed code when the stated reason for the admission/encounter is documented as pain control/pain management. The underlying neoplasm should be reported as an additional diagnosis.

When the reason for the admission/encounter is management of the neoplasm and the pain associated with the neoplasm is also documented, code G89.3 may be assigned as an additional diagnosis. It is not necessary to assign an additional code for the site of the pain.

See Section I.C.2 for instructions on the sequencing of neoplasms for all other stated reasons for the admission/encounter (except for pain control/pain management).

6) Chronic pain syndrome
Central pain syndrome (G89.Ø) and chronic pain syndrome (G89.4) are different than the term "chronic pain," and therefore codes should only be used when the provider has specifically documented this condition.

See Section I.C.5. Pain disorders related to psychological factors

7. Chapter 7: Diseases of the Eye and Adnexa (H00-H59)

a. Glaucoma

1) Assigning Glaucoma Codes
Assign as many codes from category H4Ø, Glaucoma, as needed to identify the type of glaucoma, the affected eye, and the glaucoma stage.

2) Bilateral glaucoma with same type and stage
When a patient has bilateral glaucoma and both eyes are documented as being the same type and stage, and there is a code for bilateral glaucoma, report only the code for the type of glaucoma, bilateral, with the seventh character for the stage.

When a patient has bilateral glaucoma and both eyes are documented as being the same type and stage, and the classification does not provide a code for bilateral glaucoma (i.e., subcategories H4Ø.1Ø, H4Ø.11 and H4Ø.2Ø) report only one code for the type of glaucoma with the appropriate seventh character for the stage.

3) Bilateral glaucoma stage with different types or stages
When a patient has bilateral glaucoma and each eye is documented as having a different type or stage, and the classification distinguishes laterality, assign the appropriate code for each eye rather than the code for bilateral glaucoma.

When a patient has bilateral glaucoma and each eye is documented as having a different type, and the classification does not distinguish laterality (i.e., subcategories H4Ø.1Ø, H4Ø.11 and H4Ø.2Ø), assign one code for each type of glaucoma with the appropriate 7th character for the stage.

When a patient has bilateral glaucoma and each eye is documented as having the same type, but different stage, and the classification does not distinguish laterality (i.e., subcategories H4Ø.1Ø, H4Ø.11 and H4Ø.2Ø), assign a code for the type of glaucoma for each eye with the 7th character for the specific glaucoma stage documented for each eye.

4) Patient admitted with glaucoma and stage evolves during the admission

If a patient is admitted with glaucoma and the stage progresses during the admission, assign the code for highest stage documented.

5) Indeterminate stage glaucoma

Assignment of the 7th character "4" for "indeterminate stage" should be based on the clinical documentation. The 7th character "4" is used for glaucomas whose stage cannot be clinically determined. This 7th character should not be confused with the 7th character "Ø", unspecified, which should be assigned when there is no documentation regarding the stage of the glaucoma.

b. Blindness

If "blindness" or "low vision" of both eyes is documented but the visual impairment category is not documented, assign code H54.3, Unqualified visual loss, both eyes. If "blindness" or "low vision" in one eye is documented but the visual impairment category is not documented, assign a code from H54.6-, Unqualified visual loss, one eye. If "blindness" or "visual loss" is documented without any information about whether one or both eyes are affected, assign code H54.7, Unspecified visual loss.

8. Chapter 8: Diseases of the Ear and Mastoid Process (H6Ø-H95)

Reserved for future guideline expansion

9. Chapter 9: Diseases of the Circulatory System (IØØ-I99)

a. Hypertension

The classification presumes a causal relationship between hypertension and heart involvement and between hypertension and kidney involvement, as the two conditions are linked by the term "with" in the Alphabetic Index. These conditions should be coded as related even in the absence of provider documentation explicitly linking them, unless the documentation clearly states the conditions are unrelated.

For hypertension and conditions not specifically linked by relational terms such as "with," "associated with" or "due to" in the classification, provider documentation must link the conditions in order to code them as related.

1) Hypertension with Heart Disease

Hypertension with heart conditions classified to I5Ø.- or I51.4-I51.7, I51.89, I51.9, are assigned to, a code from category I11, Hypertensive heart disease. Use additional code(s) from category I5Ø, Heart failure, to identify the type(s) of heart failure in those patients with heart failure.

The same heart conditions (I5Ø.-, I51.4-I51.7, I51.89, I51.9) with hypertension are coded separately if the provider has documented they are unrelated to the hypertension. Sequence according to the circumstances of the admission/encounter.

2) Hypertensive Chronic Kidney Disease

Assign codes from category I12, Hypertensive chronic kidney disease, when both hypertension and a condition classifiable to category N18, Chronic kidney disease (CKD), are present. CKD should not be coded as hypertensive if the provider indicates the CKD is not related to the hypertension.

The appropriate code from category N18 should be used as a secondary code with a code from category I12 to identify the stage of chronic kidney disease.

See Section I.C.14. Chronic kidney disease.

If a patient has hypertensive chronic kidney disease and acute renal failure, an additional code for the acute renal failure is required.

3) Hypertensive Heart and Chronic Kidney Disease

Assign codes from combination category I13, Hypertensive heart and chronic kidney disease, when there is hypertension with both heart and kidney involvement. If heart failure is present, assign an additional code from category I5Ø to identify the type of heart failure.

The appropriate code from category N18, Chronic kidney disease, should be used as a secondary code with a code from category I13 to identify the stage of chronic kidney disease.

See Section I.C.14. Chronic kidney disease.

The codes in category I13, Hypertensive heart and chronic kidney disease, are combination codes that include hypertension, heart disease and chronic kidney disease. The Includes note at I13 specifies that the conditions included at I11 and I12 are included together in I13. If a patient has hypertension, heart disease and chronic kidney disease then a code from I13 should be used, not individual codes for hypertension, heart disease and chronic kidney disease, or codes from I11 or I12.

For patients with both acute renal failure and chronic kidney disease an additional code for acute renal failure is required.

4) Hypertensive Cerebrovascular Disease

For hypertensive cerebrovascular disease, first assign the appropriate code from categories I6Ø-I69, followed by the appropriate hypertension code.

5) Hypertensive Retinopathy

Subcategory H35.Ø, Background retinopathy and retinal vascular changes, should be used with a code from category I1Ø – I15, Hypertensive disease to include the systemic hypertension. The sequencing is based on the reason for the encounter.

6) Hypertension, Secondary

Secondary hypertension is due to an underlying condition. Two codes are required: one to identify the underlying etiology and one from category I15 to identify the hypertension. Sequencing of codes is determined by the reason for admission/encounter.

7) Hypertension, Transient

Assign code RØ3.Ø, Elevated blood pressure reading without diagnosis of hypertension, unless patient has an established diagnosis of hypertension. Assign code O13.-, Gestational [pregnancy-induced] hypertension without significant proteinuria, or O14.-, Pre-eclampsia, for transient hypertension of pregnancy.

8) Hypertension, Controlled
This diagnostic statement usually refers to an existing state of hypertension under control by therapy. Assign the appropriate code from categories I10-I15, Hypertensive diseases.

9) Hypertension, Uncontrolled
Uncontrolled hypertension may refer to untreated hypertension or hypertension not responding to current therapeutic regimen. In either case, assign the appropriate code from categories I10-I15, Hypertensive diseases.

10) Hypertensive Crisis
Assign a code from category I16, Hypertensive crisis, for documented hypertensive urgency, hypertensive emergency or unspecified hypertensive crisis. Code also any identified hypertensive disease (I10-I15). The sequencing is based on the reason for the encounter.

11) Pulmonary Hypertension
Pulmonary hypertension is classified to category I27, Other pulmonary heart diseases. For secondary pulmonary hypertension (I27.1, I27.2-), code also any associated conditions or adverse effects of drugs or toxins. The sequencing is based on the reason for the encounter, except for adverse effects of drugs.
See Section I.C.19.e

b. Atherosclerotic Coronary Artery Disease and Angina
ICD-10-CM has combination codes for atherosclerotic heart disease with angina pectoris. The subcategories for these codes are I25.11, Atherosclerotic heart disease of native coronary artery with angina pectoris and I25.7, Atherosclerosis of coronary artery bypass graft(s) and coronary artery of transplanted heart with angina pectoris.

When using one of these combination codes it is not necessary to use an additional code for angina pectoris. A causal relationship can be assumed in a patient with both atherosclerosis and angina pectoris, unless the documentation indicates the angina is due to something other than the atherosclerosis.

If a patient with coronary artery disease is admitted due to an acute myocardial infarction (AMI), the AMI should be sequenced before the coronary artery disease.
See Section I.C.9. Acute myocardial infarction (AMI)

c. Intraoperative and Postprocedural Cerebrovascular Accident
Medical record documentation should clearly specify the cause-and-effect relationship between the medical intervention and the cerebrovascular accident in order to assign a code for intraoperative or postprocedural cerebrovascular accident.

Proper code assignment depends on whether it was an infarction or hemorrhage and whether it occurred intraoperatively or postoperatively. If it was a cerebral hemorrhage, code assignment depends on the type of procedure performed.

d. Sequelae of Cerebrovascular Disease
1) Category I69, Sequelae of Cerebrovascular disease
Category I69 is used to indicate conditions classifiable to categories I60-I67 as the causes of sequela (neurologic deficits), themselves classified elsewhere. These "late effects" include neurologic deficits that persist after initial onset of conditions classifiable to categories I60-I67. The neurologic deficits caused by cerebrovascular disease may be present from the onset or may arise at any time after the onset of the condition classifiable to categories I60-I67.

Codes from category I69, Sequelae of cerebrovascular disease, that specify hemiplegia, hemiparesis and monoplegia identify whether the dominant or nondominant side is affected. Should the affected side be documented, but not specified as dominant or nondominant, and the classification system does not indicate a default, code selection is as follows:
- For ambidextrous patients, the default should be dominant.
- If the left side is affected, the default is non-dominant.
- If the right side is affected, the default is dominant.

2) Codes from category I69 with codes from I60-I67
Codes from category I69 may be assigned on a health care record with codes from I60-I67, if the patient has a current cerebrovascular disease and deficits from an old cerebrovascular disease.

3) Codes from category I69 and Personal history of transient ischemic attack (TIA) and cerebral infarction (Z86.73)
Codes from category I69 should not be assigned if the patient does not have neurologic deficits.
See Section I.C.21. 4. History (of) for use of personal history codes

e. Acute myocardial infarction (AMI)
1) Type 1 ST elevation myocardial infarction (STEMI) and non ST elevation myocardial infarction (NSTEMI)
The ICD-10-CM codes for type 1 acute myocardial infarction (AMI) identify the site, such as anterolateral wall or true posterior wall. Subcategories I21.0-I21.2 and code I21.3 are used for type 1 ST elevation myocardial infarction (STEMI). Code I21.4, Non-ST elevation (NSTEMI) myocardial infarction, is used for type 1 non ST elevation myocardial infarction (NSTEMI) and nontransmural MIs.

If a type 1 NSTEMI evolves to STEMI, assign the STEMI code. If a type 1 STEMI converts to NSTEMI due to thrombolytic therapy, it is still coded as STEMI.

For encounters occurring while the myocardial infarction is equal to, or less than, 4 weeks old, including transfers to another acute setting or a postacute setting, and the myocardial infarction meets the definition for "other diagnoses" (see Section III, Reporting Additional Diagnoses), codes from category I21 may continue to be reported. For encounters after the 4 week time frame and the patient is still receiving care related to the myocardial infarction, the appropriate aftercare code should be assigned, rather than a code from category I21. For old or healed myocardial infarctions not requiring further care, code I25.2, Old myocardial infarction, may be assigned.

2) Acute myocardial infarction, unspecified

Code I21.9, Acute myocardial infarction, unspecified, is the default for unspecified acute myocardial infarction or unspecified type. If only type 1 STEMI or transmural MI without the site is documented, assign code I21.3, ST elevation (STEMI) myocardial infarction of unspecified site.

3) AMI documented as nontransmural or subendocardial but site provided

If an AMI is documented as nontransmural or subendocardial, but the site is provided, it is still coded as a subendocardial AMI.

See Section I.C.21.3 for information on coding status post administration of tPA in a different facility within the last 24 hours.

4) Subsequent acute myocardial infarction

A code from category I22, Subsequent ST elevation (STEMI) and non ST elevation (NSTEMI) myocardial infarction, is to be used when a patient who has suffered a type 1 or unspecified AMI has a new AMI within the 4 week time frame of the initial AMI. A code from category I22 must be used in conjunction with a code from category I21. The sequencing of the I22 and I21 codes depends on the circumstances of the encounter.

Do not assign code I22 for subsequent myocardial infarctions other than type 1 or unspecified. For subsequent type 2 AMI assign only code I21.A1. For subsequent type 4 or type 5 AMI, assign only code I21.A9.

If a subsequent myocardial infarction of one type occurs within 4 weeks of a myocardial infarction of a different type, assign the appropriate codes from category I21 to identify each type. Do not assign a code from I22. Codes from category I22 should only be assigned if both the initial and subsequent myocardial infarctions are type 1 or unspecified.

5) Other Types of Myocardial Infarction

The ICD-10-CM provides codes for different types of myocardial infarction. Type 1 myocardial infarctions are assigned to codes I21.Ø-I21.4.

Type 2 myocardial infarction (myocardial infarction due to demand ischemia or secondary to ischemic **imbalance**) is assigned to code I21.A1, Myocardial infarction type 2 with the underlying cause **coded first**. Do not assign code I24.8, Other forms of acute ischemic heart disease**,** for the demand ischemia. **If a** type 2 AMI is described as NSTEMI or STEMI, only assign code I21.A1. Codes I21.Ø1-I21.4 should only be assigned for type 1 AMIs.

Acute myocardial infarctions type 3, 4a, 4b, 4c, and 5 are assigned to code I21.A9, Other myocardial infarction type.

The "Code also" and "Code first" notes should be followed related to complications, and for coding of postprocedural myocardial infarctions during or following cardiac surgery.

1Ø. Chapter 1Ø: Diseases of the Respiratory System (JØØ-J99)

a. Chronic Obstructive Pulmonary Disease [COPD] and Asthma

1) Acute exacerbation of chronic obstructive bronchitis and asthma

The codes in categories J44 and J45 distinguish between uncomplicated cases and those in acute exacerbation. An acute exacerbation is a worsening or a decompensation of a chronic condition. An acute exacerbation is not equivalent to an infection superimposed on a chronic condition, though an exacerbation may be triggered by an infection.

b. Acute Respiratory Failure

1) Acute respiratory failure as principal diagnosis

A code from subcategory J96.Ø, Acute respiratory failure, or subcategory J96.2, Acute and chronic respiratory failure, may be assigned as a principal diagnosis when it is the condition established after study to be chiefly responsible for occasioning the admission to the hospital, and the selection is supported by the Alphabetic Index and Tabular List. However, chapter-specific coding guidelines (such as obstetrics, poisoning, HIV, newborn) that provide sequencing direction take precedence.

2) Acute respiratory failure as secondary diagnosis

Respiratory failure may be listed as a secondary diagnosis if it occurs after admission, or if it is present on admission, but does not meet the definition of principal diagnosis.

3) Sequencing of acute respiratory failure and another acute condition

When a patient is admitted with respiratory failure and another acute condition (e.g., myocardial infarction, cerebrovascular accident, aspiration pneumonia), the principal diagnosis will not be the same in every situation. This applies whether the other acute condition is a respiratory or nonrespiratory condition. Selection of the principal diagnosis will be dependent on the circumstances of admission. If both the respiratory failure and the other acute condition are equally responsible for occasioning the admission to the hospital, and there are no chapter-specific sequencing rules, the guideline regarding two or more diagnoses that equally meet the definition for principal diagnosis *(Section II, C.)* may be applied in these situations.

If the documentation is not clear as to whether acute respiratory failure and another condition are equally responsible for occasioning the admission, query the provider for clarification.

c. Influenza due to certain identified influenza viruses

Code only confirmed cases of influenza due to certain identified influenza viruses (category J09), and due to other identified influenza virus (category J10). This is an exception to the hospital inpatient guideline Section II, H. (Uncertain Diagnosis).

In this context, "confirmation" does not require documentation of positive laboratory testing specific for avian or other novel influenza A or other identified influenza virus. However, coding should be based on the provider's diagnostic statement that the patient has avian influenza, or other novel influenza A, for category J09, or has another particular identified strain of influenza, such as H1N1 or H3N2, but not identified as novel or variant, for category J10.

If the provider records "suspected" or "possible" or "probable" avian influenza, or novel influenza, or other identified influenza, then the appropriate influenza code from category J11, Influenza due to unidentified influenza virus, should be assigned. A code from category J09, Influenza due to certain identified influenza viruses, should not be assigned nor should a code from category J10, Influenza due to other identified influenza virus.

d. Ventilator associated Pneumonia

1) Documentation of Ventilator associated Pneumonia

As with all procedural or postprocedural complications, code assignment is based on the provider's documentation of the relationship between the condition and the procedure.

Code J95.851, Ventilator associated pneumonia, should be assigned only when the provider has documented ventilator associated pneumonia (VAP). An additional code to identify the organism (e.g., Pseudomonas aeruginosa, code B96.5) should also be assigned. Do not assign an additional code from categories J12-J18 to identify the type of pneumonia.

Code J95.851 should not be assigned for cases where the patient has pneumonia and is on a mechanical ventilator and the provider has not specifically stated that the pneumonia is ventilator-associated pneumonia. If the documentation is unclear as to whether the patient has a pneumonia that is a complication attributable to the mechanical ventilator, query the provider.

2) Ventilator associated Pneumonia Develops after Admission

A patient may be admitted with one type of pneumonia (e.g., code J13, Pneumonia due to Streptococcus pneumonia) and subsequently develop VAP. In this instance, the principal diagnosis would be the appropriate code from categories J12-J18 for the pneumonia diagnosed at the time of admission. Code J95.851, Ventilator associated pneumonia, would be assigned as an additional diagnosis when the provider has also documented the presence of ventilator associated pneumonia.

11. Chapter 11: Diseases of the Digestive System (K00-K95)

Reserved for future guideline expansion

12. Chapter 12: Diseases of the Skin and Subcutaneous Tissue (L00-L99)

a. Pressure ulcer stage codes

1) Pressure ulcer stages

Codes **in** category L89, Pressure ulcer, identify the site **and stage** of the pressure ulcer.

The ICD-10-CM classifies pressure ulcer stages based on severity, which is designated by stages 1-4, **deep tissue pressure injury,** unspecified stage, and unstageable.

Assign as many codes from category L89 as needed to identify all the pressure ulcers the patient has, if applicable.

See Section I.B.14 for pressure ulcer stage documentation by clinicians other than patient's provider

2) Unstageable pressure ulcers

Assignment of the code for unstageable pressure ulcer (L89.--0) should be based on the clinical documentation. These codes are used for pressure ulcers whose stage cannot be clinically determined (e.g., the ulcer is covered by eschar or has been treated with a skin or muscle graft). This code should not be confused with the codes for unspecified stage (L89.--9). When there is no documentation regarding the stage of the pressure ulcer, assign the appropriate code for unspecified stage (**L89.9**).

3) Documented pressure ulcer stage

Assignment of the pressure ulcer stage code should be guided by clinical documentation of the stage or documentation of the terms found in the Alphabetic Index. For clinical terms describing the stage that are not found in the Alphabetic Index, and there is no documentation of the stage, the provider should be queried.

4) Patients admitted with pressure ulcers documented as healed

No code is assigned if the documentation states that the pressure ulcer is completely healed **at the time of admission**.

5) *Pressure ulcers documented as healing*

Pressure ulcers described as healing should be assigned the appropriate pressure ulcer stage code based on the documentation in the medical record. If the documentation does not provide information about the stage of the healing pressure ulcer, assign the appropriate code for unspecified stage.

If the documentation is unclear as to whether the patient has a current (new) pressure ulcer or if the patient is being treated for a healing pressure ulcer, query the provider.

For ulcers that were present on admission but healed at the time of discharge, assign the code for the site and stage of the pressure ulcer at the time of admission.

> #### 6) Patient admitted with pressure ulcer evolving into another stage during the admission

If a patient is admitted to an inpatient hospital with a pressure ulcer at one stage and it progresses to a higher stage, two separate codes should be assigned: one code for the site and stage of the ulcer on admission and a second code for the same ulcer site and the highest stage reported during the stay.

> #### 7) *Pressure-induced deep tissue damage*
> **For pressure-induced deep tissue damage or deep tissue pressure injury, assign only the appropriate code for pressure-induced deep tissue damage (L89.--6).**

b. Non-Pressure Chronic Ulcers

> #### 1) Patients admitted with non-pressure ulcers documented as healed

No code is assigned if the documentation states that the non-pressure ulcer is completely healed **at the time of admission**.

> #### 2) Non-pressure ulcers documented as healing

Non-pressure ulcers described as healing should be assigned the appropriate non-pressure ulcer code based on the documentation in the medical record. If the documentation does not provide information about the severity of the healing non-pressure ulcer, assign the appropriate code for unspecified severity.

If the documentation is unclear as to whether the patient has a current (new) non-pressure ulcer or if the patient is being treated for a healing non-pressure ulcer, query the provider.

For ulcers that were present on admission but healed at the time of discharge, assign the code for the site and severity of the non-pressure ulcer at the time of admission.

> #### 3) Patient admitted with non-pressure ulcer that progresses to another severity level during the admission

If a patient is admitted to an inpatient hospital with a non-pressure ulcer at one severity level and it progresses to a higher severity level, two separate codes should be assigned: one code for the site and severity level of the ulcer on admission and a second code for the same ulcer site and the highest severity level reported during the stay.

See Section I.B.14 for pressure ulcer stage documentation by clinicians other than patient's provider

13. Chapter 13: Diseases of the Musculoskeletal System and Connective Tissue (M00-M99)

a. Site and laterality

Most of the codes within Chapter 13 have site and laterality designations. The site represents the bone, joint or the muscle involved. For some conditions where more than one bone, joint or muscle is usually involved, such as osteoarthritis, there is a "multiple sites" code available. For categories where no multiple site code is provided and more than one bone, joint or muscle is involved, multiple codes should be used to indicate the different sites involved.

> #### 1) Bone versus joint
For certain conditions, the bone may be affected at the upper or lower end (e.g., avascular necrosis of bone, M87, Osteoporosis, M80, M81). Though the portion of the bone affected may be at the joint, the site designation will be the bone, not the joint.

b. Acute traumatic versus chronic or recurrent musculoskeletal conditions

Many musculoskeletal conditions are a result of previous injury or trauma to a site, or are recurrent conditions. Bone, joint or muscle conditions that are the result of a healed injury are usually found in Chapter 13. Recurrent bone, joint or muscle conditions are also usually found in Chapter 13. Any current, acute injury should be coded to the appropriate injury code from Chapter 19. Chronic or recurrent conditions should generally be coded with a code from Chapter 13. If it is difficult to determine from the documentation in the record which code is best to describe a condition, query the provider.

c. Coding of Pathologic Fractures

Seventh character A is for use as long as the patient is receiving active treatment for the fracture. While the patient may be seen by a new or different provider over the course of treatment for a pathological fracture, assignment of the 7th character is based on whether the patient is undergoing active treatment and not whether the provider is seeing the patient for the first time.

Seventh character, D is to be used for encounters after the patient has completed active treatment for the fracture and is receiving routine care for the fracture during the healing or recovery phase. The other 7th characters, listed under each subcategory in the Tabular List, are to be used for subsequent encounters for treatment of problems associated with the healing, such as malunions, nonunions, and sequelae.

Care for complications of surgical treatment for fracture repairs during the healing or recovery phase should be coded with the appropriate complication codes.

See Section I.C.19. Coding of traumatic fractures

d. Osteoporosis

Osteoporosis is a systemic condition, meaning that all bones of the musculoskeletal system are affected. Therefore, site is not a component of the codes under category M81, Osteoporosis without current pathological fracture. The site codes under category M80, Osteoporosis with current pathological fracture, identify the site of the fracture, not the osteoporosis.

1) Osteoporosis without pathological fracture

Category M81, Osteoporosis without current pathological fracture, is for use for patients with osteoporosis who do not currently have a pathologic fracture due to the osteoporosis, even if they have had a fracture in the past. For patients with a history of osteoporosis fractures, status code Z87.31Ø, Personal history of (healed) osteoporosis fracture, should follow the code from M81.

2) Osteoporosis with current pathological fracture

Category M8Ø, Osteoporosis with current pathological fracture, is for patients who have a current pathologic fracture at the time of an encounter. The codes under M8Ø identify the site of the fracture. A code from category M8Ø, not a traumatic fracture code, should be used for any patient with known osteoporosis who suffers a fracture, even if the patient had a minor fall or trauma, if that fall or trauma would not usually break a normal, healthy bone.

14. Chapter 14: Diseases of Genitourinary System (NØØ-N99)

a. Chronic kidney disease

1) Stages of chronic kidney disease (CKD)

The ICD-10-CM classifies CKD based on severity. The severity of CKD is designated by stages 1-5. Stage 2, code N18.2, equates to mild CKD; stage 3, code N18.3, equates to moderate CKD; and stage 4, code N18.4, equates to severe CKD. Code N18.6, End stage renal disease (ESRD), is assigned when the provider has documented end-stage-renal disease (ESRD).

If both a stage of CKD and ESRD are documented, assign code N18.6 only.

2) Chronic kidney disease and kidney transplant status

Patients who have undergone kidney transplant may still have some form of chronic kidney disease (CKD) because the kidney transplant may not fully restore kidney function. Therefore, the presence of CKD alone does not constitute a transplant complication. Assign the appropriate N18 code for the patient's stage of CKD and code Z94.Ø, Kidney transplant status. If a transplant complication such as failure or rejection or other transplant complication is documented, see Section I.C.19.g for information on coding complications of a kidney transplant. If the documentation is unclear as to whether the patient has a complication of the transplant, query the provider.

3) Chronic kidney disease with other conditions

Patients with CKD may also suffer from other serious conditions, most commonly diabetes mellitus and hypertension. The sequencing of the CKD code in relationship to codes for other contributing conditions is based on the conventions in the Tabular List.

See I.C.9. Hypertensive chronic kidney disease.

See I.C.19. Chronic kidney disease and kidney transplant complications.

15. Chapter 15: Pregnancy, Childbirth, and the Puerperium (OØØ-O9A)

a. General Rules for Obstetric Cases

1) Codes from Chapter 15 and sequencing priority

Obstetric cases require codes from Chapter 15, codes in the range OØØ-O9A, Pregnancy, Childbirth, and the Puerperium. Chapter 15 codes have sequencing priority over codes from other chapters. Additional codes from other chapters may be used in conjunction with Chapter 15 codes to further specify conditions. Should the provider document that the pregnancy is incidental to the encounter, then code Z33.1, Pregnant state, incidental, should be used in place of any Chapter 15 codes. It is the provider's responsibility to state that the condition being treated is not affecting the pregnancy.

2) Chapter 15 codes used only on the maternal record

Chapter 15 codes are to be used only on the maternal record, never on the record of the newborn.

3) Final character for trimester

The majority of codes in Chapter 15 have a final character indicating the trimester of pregnancy. The time frames for the trimesters are indicated at the beginning of the chapter. If trimester is not a component of a code it is because the condition always occurs in a specific trimester, or the concept of trimester of pregnancy is not applicable. Certain codes have characters for only certain trimesters because the condition does not occur in all trimesters, but it may occur in more than just one.

Assignment of the final character for trimester should be based on the provider's documentation of the trimester (or number of weeks) for the current admission/encounter. This applies to the assignment of trimester for pre-existing conditions as well as those that develop during or are due to the pregnancy. The provider's documentation of the number of weeks may be used to assign the appropriate code identifying the trimester.

Whenever delivery occurs during the current admission, and there is an "in childbirth" option for the obstetric complication being coded, the "in childbirth" code should be assigned.

4) Selection of trimester for inpatient admissions that encompass more than one trimester

In instances when a patient is admitted to a hospital for complications of pregnancy during one trimester and remains in the hospital into a subsequent trimester, the trimester character for the antepartum complication code should be assigned on the basis of the trimester when the complication developed, not the trimester of the discharge. If the condition developed prior to the current admission/encounter or represents a pre-existing condition, the trimester character for the trimester at the time of the admission/encounter should be assigned.

5) Unspecified trimester

Each category that includes codes for trimester has a code for "unspecified trimester." The "unspecified trimester" code should rarely be used, such as when the documentation in the record is insufficient to determine the trimester and it is not possible to obtain clarification.

6) 7th character for Fetus Identification

Where applicable, a 7th character is to be assigned for certain categories (O31, O32, O33.3 - O33.6, O35, O36, O4Ø, O41, O6Ø.1, O6Ø.2, O64, and O69) to identify the fetus for which the complication code applies.

Assign 7th character "Ø":

- For single gestations
- When the documentation in the record is insufficient to determine the fetus affected and it is not possible to obtain clarification.
- When it is not possible to clinically determine which fetus is affected.

b. Selection of OB Principal or First-listed Diagnosis

1) Routine outpatient prenatal visits

For routine outpatient prenatal visits when no complications are present, a code from category Z34, Encounter for supervision of normal pregnancy, should be used as the first-listed diagnosis. These codes should not be used in conjunction with Chapter 15 codes.

2) Supervision of High-Risk Pregnancy

Codes from category OØ9, Supervision of high-risk pregnancy, are intended for use only during the prenatal period. For complications during the labor or delivery episode as a result of a high-risk pregnancy, assign the applicable complication codes from Chapter 15. If there are no complications during the labor or delivery episode, assign code O8Ø, Encounter for full-term uncomplicated delivery.

For routine prenatal outpatient visits for patients with high-risk pregnancies, a code from category OØ9, Supervision of high-risk pregnancy, should be used as the first-listed diagnosis. Secondary Chapter 15 codes may be used in conjunction with these codes if appropriate.

3) Episodes when no delivery occurs

In episodes when no delivery occurs, the principal diagnosis should correspond to the principal complication of the pregnancy which necessitated the encounter. Should more than one complication exist, all of which are treated or monitored, any of the complication codes may be sequenced first.

4) When a delivery occurs

When an obstetric patient is admitted and delivers during that admission, the condition that prompted the admission should be sequenced as the principal diagnosis. If multiple conditions prompted the admission, sequence the one most related to the delivery as the principal diagnosis. A code for any complication of the delivery should be assigned as an additional diagnosis. In cases of cesarean delivery, if the patient was admitted with a condition that resulted in the performance of a cesarean procedure, that condition should be selected as the principal diagnosis. If the reason for the admission was unrelated to the condition resulting in the cesarean delivery, the condition related to the reason for the admission should be selected as the principal diagnosis.

5) Outcome of delivery

A code from category Z37, Outcome of delivery, should be included on every maternal record when a delivery has occurred. These codes are not to be used on subsequent records or on the newborn record.

c. Pre-existing conditions versus conditions due to the pregnancy

Certain categories in Chapter 15 distinguish between conditions of the mother that existed prior to pregnancy (pre-existing) and those that are a direct result of pregnancy. When assigning codes from Chapter 15, it is important to assess if a condition was pre-existing prior to pregnancy or developed during or due to the pregnancy in order to assign the correct code.

Categories that do not distinguish between pre-existing and pregnancy-related conditions may be used for either. It is acceptable to use codes specifically for the puerperium with codes complicating pregnancy and childbirth if a condition arises postpartum during the delivery encounter.

d. Pre-existing hypertension in pregnancy

Category O1Ø, Pre-existing hypertension complicating pregnancy, childbirth and the puerperium, includes codes for hypertensive heart and hypertensive chronic kidney disease. When assigning one of the O1Ø codes that includes hypertensive heart disease or hypertensive chronic kidney disease, it is necessary to add a secondary code from the appropriate hypertension category to specify the type of heart failure or chronic kidney disease.

See Section I.C.9. Hypertension.

e. Fetal Conditions Affecting the Management of the Mother

1) Codes from categories O35 and O36

Codes from categories O35, Maternal care for known or suspected fetal abnormality and damage, and O36, Maternal care for other fetal problems, are assigned only when the fetal condition is actually responsible for modifying the management of the mother, i.e., by requiring diagnostic studies, additional observation, special care, or termination of pregnancy. The fact that the fetal condition exists does not justify assigning a code from this series to the mother's record.

2) In utero surgery

In cases when surgery is performed on the fetus, a diagnosis code from category O35, Maternal care for known or suspected fetal abnormality and damage, should be assigned identifying the fetal condition. Assign the appropriate procedure code for the procedure performed.

No code from Chapter 16, the perinatal codes, should be used on the mother's record to identify fetal conditions. Surgery performed in utero on a fetus is still to be coded as an obstetric encounter.

f. HIV Infection in Pregnancy, Childbirth and the Puerperium

During pregnancy, childbirth or the puerperium, a patient admitted because of an HIV-related illness should receive a principal diagnosis from subcategory O98.7-, Human immunodeficiency [HIV] disease complicating pregnancy, childbirth and the puerperium, followed by the code(s) for the HIV-related illness(es).

Patients with asymptomatic HIV infection status admitted during pregnancy, childbirth, or the puerperium should receive codes of O98.7- and Z21, Asymptomatic human immunodeficiency virus [HIV] infection status.

g. Diabetes mellitus in pregnancy

Diabetes mellitus is a significant complicating factor in pregnancy. Pregnant women who are diabetic should be assigned a code from category O24, Diabetes mellitus in pregnancy, childbirth, and the puerperium, first, followed by the appropriate diabetes code(s) (E08-E13) from Chapter 4.

h. Long-term use of insulin and oral hypoglycemics

See Section I.C.4.a.3 for information on the long term use of insulin and oral hypoglycemic.

i. Gestational (pregnancy induced) diabetes

Gestational (pregnancy induced) diabetes can occur during the second and third trimester of pregnancy in women who were not diabetic prior to pregnancy. Gestational diabetes can cause complications in the pregnancy similar to those of pre-existing diabetes mellitus. It also puts the woman at greater risk of developing diabetes after the pregnancy. Codes for gestational diabetes are in subcategory O24.4, Gestational diabetes mellitus. No other code from category O24, Diabetes mellitus in pregnancy, childbirth, and the puerperium, should be used with a code from O24.4.

The codes under subcategory O24.4 include diet controlled, insulin controlled, and controlled by oral hypoglycemic drugs. If a patient with gestational diabetes is treated with both diet and insulin, only the code for insulin-controlled is required. If a patient with gestational diabetes is treated with both diet and oral hypoglycemic medications, only the code for "controlled by oral hypoglycemic drugs" is required. Code Z79.4, Long-term (current) use of insulin or code Z79.84, Long-term (current) use of oral hypoglycemic drugs, should not be assigned with codes from subcategory O24.4.

An abnormal glucose tolerance in pregnancy is assigned a code from subcategory O99.81, Abnormal glucose complicating pregnancy, childbirth, and the puerperium.

j. Sepsis and septic shock complicating abortion, pregnancy, childbirth and the puerperium

When assigning a Chapter 15 code for sepsis complicating abortion, pregnancy, childbirth, and the puerperium, a code for the specific type of infection should be assigned as an additional diagnosis. If severe sepsis is present, a code from subcategory R65.2, Severe sepsis, and code(s) for associated organ dysfunction(s) should also be assigned as additional diagnoses.

k. Puerperal sepsis

Code O85, Puerperal sepsis, should be assigned with a secondary code to identify the causal organism (e.g., for a bacterial infection, assign a code from category B95-B96, Bacterial infections in conditions classified elsewhere). A code from category A40, Streptococcal sepsis, or A41, Other sepsis, should not be used for puerperal sepsis. If applicable, use additional codes to identify severe sepsis (R65.2-) and any associated acute organ dysfunction.

l. Alcohol, tobacco and drug use during pregnancy, childbirth and the puerperium

1) Alcohol use during pregnancy, childbirth and the puerperium

Codes under subcategory O99.31, Alcohol use complicating pregnancy, childbirth, and the puerperium, should be assigned for any pregnancy case when a mother uses alcohol during the pregnancy or postpartum. A secondary code from category F10, Alcohol related disorders, should also be assigned to identify manifestations of the alcohol use.

2) Tobacco use during pregnancy, childbirth and the puerperium

Codes under subcategory O99.33, Smoking (tobacco) complicating pregnancy, childbirth, and the puerperium, should be assigned for any pregnancy case when a mother uses any type of tobacco product during the pregnancy or postpartum. A secondary code from category F17, Nicotine dependence, should also be assigned to identify the type of nicotine dependence.

3) Drug use during pregnancy, childbirth and the puerperium

Codes under subcategory O99.32, Drug use complicating pregnancy, childbirth, and the puerperium, should be assigned for any pregnancy case when a mother uses drugs during the pregnancy or postpartum. This can involve illegal drugs, or inappropriate use or abuse of prescription drugs. Secondary code(s) from categories F11-F16 and **F18-F19** should also be assigned to identify manifestations of the drug use.

m. Poisoning, toxic effects, adverse effects and underdosing in a pregnant patient

A code from subcategory O9A.2, Injury, poisoning and certain other consequences of external causes complicating pregnancy, childbirth, and the puerperium, should be sequenced first, followed by the appropriate injury, poisoning, toxic effect, adverse effect or underdosing code, and then the additional code(s) that specifies the condition caused by the poisoning, toxic effect, adverse effect or underdosing.

See Section I.C.19. Adverse effects, poisoning, underdosing and toxic effects.

n. Normal Delivery, Code O8Ø

1) Encounter for full term uncomplicated delivery

Code O8Ø should be assigned when a woman is admitted for a full-term normal delivery and delivers a single, healthy infant without any complications antepartum, during the delivery, or postpartum during the delivery episode. Code O8Ø is always a principal diagnosis. It is not to be used if any other code from Chapter 15 is needed to describe a current complication of the antenatal, delivery, or **postnatal** period. Additional codes from other chapters may be used with code O8Ø if they are not related to or are in any way complicating the pregnancy.

2) Uncomplicated delivery with resolved antepartum complication

Code O8Ø may be used if the patient had a complication at some point during the pregnancy, but the complication is not present at the time of the admission for delivery.

3) Outcome of delivery for O8Ø

Z37.Ø, Single live birth, is the only outcome of delivery code appropriate for use with O8Ø.

o. The Peripartum and Postpartum Periods

1) Peripartum and Postpartum periods

The postpartum period begins immediately after delivery and continues for 6 weeks following delivery. The peripartum period is defined as the last month of pregnancy to 5 months postpartum.

2) Peripartum and postpartum complication

A postpartum complication is any complication occurring within the 6-week period.

3) Pregnancy-related complications after 6-week period

Chapter 15 codes may also be used to describe pregnancy-related complications after the peripartum or postpartum period if the provider documents that a condition is pregnancy related.

4) Admission for routine postpartum care following delivery outside hospital

When the mother delivers outside the hospital prior to admission and is admitted for routine postpartum care and no complications are noted, code Z39.Ø, Encounter for care and examination of mother immediately after delivery, should be assigned as the principal diagnosis.

5) Pregnancy associated cardiomyopathy

Pregnancy associated cardiomyopathy, code O9Ø.3, is unique in that it may be diagnosed in the third trimester of pregnancy but may continue to progress months after delivery. For this reason, it is referred to as peripartum cardiomyopathy. Code O9Ø.3 is only for use when the cardiomyopathy develops as a result of pregnancy in a woman who did not have pre-existing heart disease.

p. Code O94, Sequelae of complication of pregnancy, childbirth, and the puerperium

1) Code O94

Code O94, Sequelae of complication of pregnancy, childbirth, and the puerperium, is for use in those cases when an initial complication of a pregnancy develops a sequelae requiring care or treatment at a future date.

2) After the initial postpartum period

This code may be used at any time after the initial postpartum period.

3) Sequencing of Code O94

This code, like all sequela codes, is to be sequenced following the code describing the sequelae of the complication.

q. Termination of Pregnancy and Spontaneous abortions

1) Abortion with Liveborn Fetus

When an attempted termination of pregnancy results in a liveborn fetus assign code Z33.2, Encounter for elective termination of pregnancy and a code from category Z37, Outcome of Delivery.

2) Retained Products of Conception following an abortion

Subsequent encounters for retained products of conception following a spontaneous abortion or elective termination of pregnancy, without complications are assigned OØ3.4, Incomplete spontaneous, abortion without complication or codes OØ7.4, Failed attempted termination of pregnancy without complication. This advice is appropriate even when the patient was discharged previously with a discharge diagnosis of complete abortion. If the patient has a specific complication associated with the spontaneous abortion or elective termination of pregnancy in addition to retained products of conception, assign the appropriate complication **code (e.g., OØ3.-, OØ4.-, OØ7.-)** instead of code OØ3.4 or OØ7.4

3) Complications leading to abortion

Codes from Chapter 15 may be used as additional codes to identify any documented complications of the pregnancy in conjunction with codes in categories in OØ4, OØ7 and OØ8.

r. Abuse in a pregnant patient

For suspected or confirmed cases of abuse of a pregnant patient, a code(s) from subcategories O9A.3, Physical abuse complicating pregnancy, childbirth, and the puerperium, O9A.4, Sexual abuse complicating pregnancy, childbirth, and the puerperium, and O9A.5, Psychological abuse complicating pregnancy, childbirth, and the puerperium, should be sequenced first, followed by the appropriate codes (if applicable) to identify any associated current injury due to physical abuse, sexual abuse, and the perpetrator of abuse.

See Section I.C.19. Adult and child abuse, neglect and other maltreatment.

16. **Chapter 16: Certain Conditions Originating in the Perinatal Period (PØØ-P96)**

For coding and reporting purposes the perinatal period is defined as before birth through the 28th day following birth. The following guidelines are provided for reporting purposes

a. **General Perinatal Rules**

1) **Use of Chapter 16 Codes**

Codes in this chapter are for use on the maternal record. Codes from Chapter 15, the obstetric chapter, are never permitted on the newborn record. Chapter 16 codes may be used throughout the life of the patient if the condition is still present.

2) **Principal Diagnosis for Birth Record**

When coding the birth episode in a newborn record, assign a code from category Z38, Liveborn infants according to place of birth and type of delivery, as the principal diagnosis. A code from category Z38 is assigned only once, to a newborn at the time of birth. If a newborn is transferred to another institution, a code from category Z38 should not be used at the receiving hospital.

A code from category Z38 is used only on the newborn record, not on the mother's record.

3) **Use of Codes from other Chapters with Codes from Chapter 16**

Codes from other chapters may be used with codes from Chapter 16 if the codes from the other chapters provide more specific detail. Codes for signs and symptoms may be assigned when a definitive diagnosis has not been established. If the reason for the encounter is a perinatal condition, the code from Chapter 16 should be sequenced first.

4) **Use of Chapter 16 Codes after the Perinatal Period**

Should a condition originate in the perinatal period, and continue throughout the life of the patient, the perinatal code should continue to be used regardless of the patient's age.

5) **Birth process or community acquired conditions**

If a newborn has a condition that may be either due to the birth process or community acquired and the documentation does not indicate which it is, the default is due to the birth process and the code from Chapter 16 should be used. If the condition is community-acquired, a code from Chapter 16 should not be assigned.

6) **Code all clinically significant conditions**

All clinically significant conditions noted on routine newborn examination should be coded. A condition is clinically significant if it requires:

- clinical evaluation; or
- therapeutic treatment; or
- diagnostic procedures; or
- extended length of hospital stay; or
- increased nursing care and/or monitoring; or
- has implications for future health care needs

Note: The perinatal guidelines listed above are the same as the general coding guidelines for "additional diagnoses", except for the final point regarding implications for future health care needs. Codes should be assigned for conditions that have been specified by the provider as having implications for future health care needs.

b. **Observation and Evaluation of Newborns for Suspected Conditions not Found**

1) **Use of ZØ5 codes**

Assign a code from category ZØ5, Observation and evaluation of newborns and infants for suspected conditions ruled out, to identify those instances when a healthy newborn is evaluated for a suspected condition that is determined after study not to be present. Do not use a code from category ZØ5 when the patient has identified signs or symptoms of a suspected problem; in such cases code the sign or symptom.

2) **ZØ5 on other than the birth record**

A code from category ZØ5 may also be assigned as a principal or first-listed code for readmissions or encounters when the code from category Z38 code no longer applies. Codes from category ZØ5 are for use only for healthy newborns and infants for which no condition after study is found to be present.

3) **ZØ5 on a birth record**

A code from category ZØ5 is to be used as a secondary code after the code from category Z38, Liveborn infants according to place of birth and type of delivery.

c. **Coding Additional Perinatal Diagnoses**

1) **Assigning codes for conditions that require treatment**

Assign codes for conditions that require treatment or further investigation, prolong the length of stay, or require resource utilization.

2) **Codes for conditions specified as having implications for future health care needs**

Assign codes for conditions that have been specified by the provider as having implications for future health care needs.

Note: This guideline should not be used for adult patients.

d. **Prematurity and Fetal Growth Retardation**

Providers utilize different criteria in determining prematurity. A code for prematurity should not be assigned unless it is documented. Assignment of codes in categories PØ5, Disorders of newborn related to slow fetal growth and fetal malnutrition, and P07, Disorders of newborn related to short gestation and low birth weight, not elsewhere classified, should be based on the recorded birth weight and estimated gestational age.

When both birth weight and gestational age are available, two codes from category P07 should be assigned, with the code for birth weight sequenced before the code for gestational age.

e. Low birth weight and immaturity status

Codes from category P07, Disorders of newborn related to short gestation and low birth weight, not elsewhere classified, are for use for a child or adult who was premature or had a low birth weight as a newborn and this is affecting the patient's current health status.

See Section I.C.21. Factors influencing health status and contact with health services, Status.

f. Bacterial Sepsis of Newborn

Category P36, Bacterial sepsis of newborn, includes congenital sepsis. If a perinate is documented as having sepsis without documentation of congenital or community acquired, the default is congenital and a code from category P36 should be assigned. If the P36 code includes the causal organism, an additional code from category B95, Streptococcus, Staphylococcus, and Enterococcus as the cause of diseases classified elsewhere, or B96, Other bacterial agents as the cause of diseases classified elsewhere, should not be assigned. If the P36 code does not include the causal organism, assign an additional code from category B96. If applicable, use additional codes to identify severe sepsis (R65.2-) and any associated acute organ dysfunction.

g. Stillbirth

Code P95, Stillbirth, is only for use in institutions that maintain separate records for stillbirths. No other code should be used with P95. Code P95 should not be used on the mother's record.

17. Chapter 17: Congenital Malformations, Deformations, and Chromosomal Abnormalities (Q00-Q99)

Assign an appropriate code(s) from categories Q00-Q99, Congenital malformations, deformations, and chromosomal abnormalities when a malformation/deformation or chromosomal abnormality is documented. A malformation/deformation/or chromosomal abnormality may be the principal/first-listed diagnosis on a record or a secondary diagnosis.

When a malformation/deformation/or chromosomal abnormality does not have a unique code assignment, assign additional code(s) for any manifestations that may be present.

When the code assignment specifically identifies the malformation/deformation/or chromosomal abnormality, manifestations that are an inherent component of the anomaly should not be coded separately. Additional codes should be assigned for manifestations that are not an inherent component.

Codes from Chapter 17 may be used throughout the life of the patient. If a congenital malformation or deformity has been corrected, a personal history code should be used to identify the history of the malformation or deformity. Although present at birth, **a** malformation/deformation/or chromosomal abnormality may not be identified until later in life. Whenever the condition is diagnosed by the **provider**, it is appropriate to assign a code from codes Q00-Q99.

For the birth admission, the appropriate code from category Z38, Liveborn infants, according to place of birth and type of delivery, should be sequenced as the principal diagnosis, followed by any congenital anomaly codes, Q00-Q99.

18. Chapter 18: Symptoms, Signs, and Abnormal Clinical and Laboratory Findings, Not Elsewhere Classified (R00-R99)

Chapter 18 includes symptoms, signs, abnormal results of clinical or other investigative procedures, and ill-defined conditions regarding which no diagnosis classifiable elsewhere is recorded. Signs and symptoms that point to a specific diagnosis have been assigned to a category in other chapters of the classification.

a. Use of symptom codes

Codes that describe symptoms and signs are acceptable for reporting purposes when a related definitive diagnosis has not been established (confirmed) by the provider.

b. Use of a symptom code with a definitive diagnosis code

Codes for signs and symptoms may be reported in addition to a related definitive diagnosis when the sign or symptom is not routinely associated with that diagnosis, such as the various signs and symptoms associated with complex syndromes. The definitive diagnosis code should be sequenced before the symptom code.

Signs or symptoms that are associated routinely with a disease process should not be assigned as additional codes, unless otherwise instructed by the classification.

c. Combination codes that include symptoms

ICD-10-CM contains a number of combination codes that identify both the definitive diagnosis and common symptoms of that diagnosis. When using one of these combination codes, an additional code should not be assigned for the symptom.

d. Repeated falls

Code R29.6, Repeated falls, is for use for encounters when a patient has recently fallen and the reason for the fall is being investigated.

Code Z91.81, History of falling, is for use when a patient has fallen in the past and is at risk for future falls. When appropriate, both codes R29.6 and Z91.81 may be assigned together.

e. Coma scale

The coma scale codes (R40.2-) can be used in conjunction with traumatic brain injury codes, acute cerebrovascular disease or sequelae of cerebrovascular disease codes. These codes are primarily for use by trauma registries, but they may be used in any setting where this information is collected. The coma scale may also be used to assess the status of the central nervous system for other non-trauma conditions, such as monitoring patients in the intensive care unit regardless of medical condition. The coma scale codes should be sequenced after the diagnosis code(s).

These codes, one from each subcategory, are needed to complete the scale. The 7th character indicates when the scale was recorded. The 7th character should match for all three codes.

At a minimum, report the initial score documented on presentation at your facility. This may be a score from the emergency medicine technician (EMT) or in the emergency department. If desired, a facility may choose to capture multiple coma scale scores.

Assign code R40.24, Glasgow coma scale, total score, when only the total score is documented in the medical record and not the individual score(s).

Do not report codes for individual or total Glasgow coma scale scores for a patient with a medically induced coma or a sedated patient.

See Section I.B.14 for coma scale documentation by clinicians other than patient's provider

f. Functional quadriplegia
GUIDELINE HAS BEEN DELETED EFFECTIVE OCTOBER 1, 2017

g. SIRS due to Non-Infectious Process
The systemic inflammatory response syndrome (SIRS) can develop as a result of certain non-infectious disease processes, such as trauma, malignant neoplasm, or pancreatitis. When SIRS is documented with a noninfectious condition, and no subsequent infection is documented, the code for the underlying condition, such as an injury, should be assigned, followed by code R65.10, Systemic inflammatory response syndrome (SIRS) of non-infectious origin without acute organ dysfunction, or code R65.11, Systemic inflammatory response syndrome (SIRS) of non-infectious origin with acute organ dysfunction. If an associated acute organ dysfunction is documented, the appropriate code(s) for the specific type of organ dysfunction(s) should be assigned in addition to code R65.11. If acute organ dysfunction is documented, but it cannot be determined if the acute organ dysfunction is associated with SIRS or due to another condition (e.g., directly due to the trauma), the provider should be queried.

h. Death NOS
Code R99, Ill-defined and unknown cause of mortality, is only for use in the very limited circumstance when a patient who has already died is brought into an emergency department or other healthcare facility and is pronounced dead upon arrival. It does not represent the discharge disposition of death.

i. NIHSS Stroke Scale
The NIH stroke scale (NIHSS) codes (R29.7- -) can be used in conjunction with acute stroke codes (I63) to identify the patient's neurological status and the severity of the stroke. The stroke scale codes should be sequenced after the acute stroke diagnosis code(s).

At a minimum, report the initial score documented. If desired, a facility may choose to capture multiple stroke scale scores.

See Section I.B.14 for NIHSS stroke scale documentation by clinicians other than patient's provider

19. Chapter 19: Injury, Poisoning, and Certain Other Consequences of External Causes (S00-T88)

a. Application of 7th Characters in Chapter 19
Most categories in Chapter 19 have a 7th character requirement for each applicable code. Most categories in this chapter have three 7th character values (with the exception of fractures): A, initial encounter, D, subsequent encounter and S, sequela. Categories for traumatic fractures have additional 7th character values. While the patient may be seen by a new or different provider over the course of treatment for an injury, assignment of the 7th character is based on whether the patient is undergoing active treatment and not whether the provider is seeing the patient for the first time.

For complication codes, active treatment refers to treatment for the condition described by the code, even though it may be related to an earlier precipitating problem. For example, code T84.50XA, Infection and inflammatory reaction due to unspecified internal joint prosthesis, initial encounter, is used when active treatment is provided for the infection, even though the condition relates to the prosthetic device, implant or graft that was placed at a previous encounter.

7th character "A", initial encounter is used for each encounter where the patient is receiving active treatment for the condition.

7th character "D" subsequent encounter is used for encounters after the patient has completed active treatment of the condition and is receiving routine care for the condition during the healing or recovery phase.

The aftercare Z codes should not be used for aftercare for conditions such as injuries or poisonings, where 7th characters are provided to identify subsequent care. For example, for aftercare of an injury, assign the acute injury code with the 7th character "D" (subsequent encounter).

7th character "S", sequela, is for use for complications or conditions that arise as a direct result of a condition, such as scar formation after a burn. The scars are sequelae of the burn. When using 7th character "S", it is necessary to use both the injury code that precipitated the sequela and the code for the sequela itself. The "S" is added only to the injury code, not the sequela code. The 7th character "S" identifies the injury responsible for the sequela. The specific type of sequela (e.g., scar) is sequenced first, followed by the injury code.

See Section I.B.10. Sequelae, (Late Effects)

b. Coding of Injuries

When coding injuries, assign separate codes for each injury unless a combination code is provided, in which case the combination code is assigned. Codes from category T07, Unspecified multiple injuries should not be assigned in the inpatient setting unless information for a more specific code is not available. Traumatic injury codes (S00-T14.9) are not to be used for normal, healing surgical wounds or to identify complications of surgical wounds.

The code for the most serious injury, as determined by the provider and the focus of treatment, is sequenced first.

1) Superficial injuries

Superficial injuries such as abrasions or contusions are not coded when associated with more severe injuries of the same site.

2) Primary injury with damage to nerves/ blood vessels

When a primary injury results in minor damage to peripheral nerves or blood vessels, the primary injury is sequenced first with additional code(s) for injuries to nerves and spinal cord (such as category S04), and/or injury to blood vessels (such as category S15). When the primary injury is to the blood vessels or nerves, that injury should be sequenced first.

3) *Iatrogenic injuries*

Injury codes from Chapter 19 should not be assigned for injuries that occur during, or as a result of, a medical intervention. Assign the appropriate complication code(s).

c. Coding of Traumatic Fractures

The principles of multiple coding of injuries should be followed in coding fractures. Fractures of specified sites are coded individually by site in accordance with both the provisions within categories S02, S12, S22, S32, S42, S49, S52, S59, S62, S72, S79, S82, S89, S92 and the level of detail furnished by medical record content.

A fracture not indicated as open or closed should be coded to closed. A fracture not indicated whether displaced or not displaced should be coded to displaced.

More specific guidelines are as follows:

1) Initial vs. subsequent encounter for fractures

Traumatic fractures are coded using the appropriate 7th character for initial encounter (A, B, C) for each encounter where the patient is receiving active treatment for the fracture. The appropriate 7th character for initial encounter should also be assigned for a patient who delayed seeking treatment for the fracture or nonunion.

Fractures are coded using the appropriate 7th character for subsequent care for encounters after the patient has completed active treatment of the fracture and is receiving routine care for the fracture during the healing or recovery phase.

Care for complications of surgical treatment for fracture repairs during the healing or recovery phase should be coded with the appropriate complication codes.

Care of complications of fractures, such as malunion and nonunion, should be reported with the appropriate 7th character for subsequent care with nonunion (K, M, N,) or subsequent care with malunion (P, Q, R).

Malunion/nonunion: The appropriate 7th character for initial encounter should also be assigned for a patient who delayed seeking treatment for the fracture or nonunion.

The open fracture designations in the assignment of the 7th character for fractures of the forearm, femur and lower leg, including ankle are based on the Gustilo open fracture classification. When the Gustilo classification type is not specified for an open fracture, the 7th character for open fracture type I or II should be assigned (B, E, H, M, Q).

A code from category M80, not a traumatic fracture code, should be used for any patient with known osteoporosis who suffers a fracture, even if the patient had a minor fall or trauma, if that fall or trauma would not usually break a normal, healthy bone.

See Section I.C.13. Osteoporosis.

The aftercare Z codes should not be used for aftercare for traumatic fractures. For aftercare of a traumatic fracture, assign the acute fracture code with the appropriate 7th character.

2) Multiple fractures sequencing

Multiple fractures are sequenced in accordance with the severity of the fracture.

3) *Physeal fractures*

For physeal fractures, assign only the code identifying the type of physeal fracture. Do not assign a separate code to identify the specific bone that is fractured.

d. Coding of Burns and Corrosions

The ICD-10-CM makes a distinction between burns and corrosions. The burn codes are for thermal burns, except sunburns, that come from a heat source, such as a fire or hot appliance. The burn codes are also for burns resulting from electricity and radiation. Corrosions are burns due to chemicals. The guidelines are the same for burns and corrosions.

Current burns (T20-T25) are classified by depth, extent and by agent (X code). Burns are classified by depth as first degree (erythema), second degree (blistering), and third degree (full-thickness involvement). Burns of the eye and internal organs (T26-T28) are classified by site, but not by degree.

1) Sequencing of burn and related condition codes

Sequence first the code that reflects the highest degree of burn when more than one burn is present.

- a. When the reason for the admission or encounter is for treatment of external multiple burns, sequence first the code that reflects the burn of the highest degree.
- b. When a patient has both internal and external burns, the circumstances of admission govern the selection of the principal diagnosis or first-listed diagnosis.

c. When a patient is admitted for burn injuries and other related conditions such as smoke inhalation and/or respiratory failure, the circumstances of admission govern the selection of the principal or first-listed diagnosis.

2) Burns of the same anatomic site

Classify burns of the same anatomic site and on the same side but of different degrees to the subcategory identifying the highest degree recorded in the diagnosis (e.g., for second and third degree burns of right thigh, assign only code T24.311-).

3) Non-healing burns

Non-healing burns are coded as acute burns.

Necrosis of burned skin should be coded as a non-healed burn.

4) Infected burn

For any documented infected burn site, use an additional code for the infection.

5) Assign separate codes for each burn site

When coding burns, assign separate codes for each burn site. Category T3Ø, Burn and corrosion, body region unspecified is extremely vague and should rarely be used.

Codes for burns of "multiple sites" should only be assigned when the medical record documentation does not specify the individual sites.

6) Burns and corrosions classified according to extent of body surface involved

Assign codes from category T31, Burns classified according to extent of body surface involved, or T32, Corrosions classified according to extent of body surface involved, when the site of the burn is not specified or when there is a need for additional data. It is advisable to use category T31 as additional coding when needed to provide data for evaluating burn mortality, such as that needed by burn units. It is also advisable to use category T31 as an additional code for reporting purposes when there is mention of a third-degree burn involving 2Ø percent or more of the body surface.

Categories T31 and T32 are based on the classic "rule of nines" in estimating body surface involved: head and neck are assigned nine percent, each arm nine percent, each leg 18 percent, the anterior trunk 18 percent, posterior trunk 18 percent, and genitalia 1 percent. Providers may change these percentage assignments where necessary to accommodate infants and children who have proportionately larger heads than adults, and patients who have large buttocks, thighs, or abdomen that involve burns.

7) Encounters for treatment of sequela of burns

Encounters for the treatment of the late effects of burns or corrosions (i.e., scars or joint contractures) should be coded with a burn or corrosion code with the 7th character "S" for sequela.

8) Sequelae with a late effect code and current burn

When appropriate, both a code for a current burn or corrosion with 7th character "A" or "D" and a burn or corrosion code with 7th character "S" may be assigned on the same record (when both a current burn and sequelae of an old burn exist). Burns and corrosions do not heal at the same rate and a current healing wound may still exist with sequela of a healed burn or corrosion.

See Section I.B.1Ø. Sequela, (Late Effects)

9) Use of an external cause code with burns and corrosions

An external cause code should be used with burns and corrosions to identify the source and intent of the burn, as well as the place where it occurred.

e. Adverse Effects, Poisoning, Underdosing and Toxic Effects

Codes in categories T36-T65 are combination codes that include the substance that was taken as well as the intent. No additional external cause code is required for poisonings, toxic effects, adverse effects and underdosing codes.

1) Do not code directly from the Table of Drugs

Do not code directly from the Table of Drugs and Chemicals. Always refer back to the Tabular List.

2) Use as many codes as necessary to describe

Use as many codes as necessary to describe completely all drugs, medicinal or biological substances.

3) If the same code would describe the causative agent

If the same code would describe the causative agent for more than one adverse reaction, poisoning, toxic effect or underdosing, assign the code only once.

4) If two or more drugs, medicinal or biological substances

If two or more drugs, medicinal or biological substances are **taken**, code each individually unless a combination code is listed in the Table of Drugs and Chemicals.

If multiple unspecified drugs, medicinal or biological substances were taken, assign the appropriate code from subcategory T5Ø.91, Poisoning by, adverse effect of and underdosing of multiple unspecified drugs, medicaments and biological substances.

5) The occurrence of drug toxicity is classified in ICD-1Ø-CM as follows:

(a) Adverse Effect

When coding an adverse effect of a drug that has been correctly prescribed and properly administered, assign the appropriate code for the nature of the adverse effect followed by the appropriate code for the adverse effect of the drug (T36-T5Ø). The code for the drug should have a 5th or 6th character "5" (for example T36.ØX5-) Examples of the nature of an adverse effect are tachycardia, delirium, gastrointestinal hemorrhaging, vomiting, hypokalemia, hepatitis, renal failure, or respiratory failure.

(b) Poisoning

When coding a poisoning or reaction to the improper use of a medication (e.g., overdose, wrong substance given or taken in error, wrong route of administration), first assign the appropriate code from categories T36-T5Ø. The poisoning codes have an associated intent as their 5th or 6th character (accidental, intentional self-harm, assault and undetermined). If the intent of the poisoning is unknown or unspecified, code the intent as accidental intent. The undetermined intent is only for use if the documentation in the record specifies that the intent cannot be determined. Use additional code(s) for all manifestations of poisonings.

If there is also a diagnosis of abuse or dependence of the substance, the abuse or dependence is assigned as an additional code.

Examples of poisoning include:

(i) Error was made in drug prescription Errors made in drug prescription or in the administration of the drug by provider, nurse, patient, or other person.

(ii) Overdose of a drug intentionally taken If an overdose of a drug was intentionally taken or administered and resulted in drug toxicity, it would be coded as a poisoning.

(iii) Nonprescribed drug taken with correctly prescribed and properly administered drug.
If a nonprescribed drug or medicinal agent was taken in combination with a correctly prescribed and properly administered drug, any drug toxicity or other reaction resulting from the interaction of the two drugs would be classified as a poisoning.

(iv) Interaction of drug(s) and alcohol. When a reaction results from the interaction of a drug(s) and alcohol, this would be classified as poisoning.

See Section I.C.4. if poisoning is the result of insulin pump malfunctions.

(c) Underdosing

Underdosing refers to taking less of a medication than is prescribed by a provider or a manufacturer's instruction. Discontinuing the use of a prescribed medication on the patient's own initiative (not directed by the patient's provider) is also classified as an underdosing. For underdosing, assign the code from categories T36-T5Ø (5th or 6th character "6").

Codes for underdosing should never be assigned as principal or first-listed codes. If a patient has a relapse or exacerbation of the medical condition for which the drug is prescribed because of the reduction in dose, then the medical condition itself should be coded.

Noncompliance (Z91.12-, Z91.13- and Z91.14-) or complication of care (Y63.6-Y63.9) codes are to be used with an underdosing code to indicate intent, if known.

(d) Toxic Effects

When a harmful substance is ingested or comes in contact with a person, this is classified as a toxic effect. The toxic effect codes are in categories T51-T65.

Toxic effect codes have an associated intent: accidental, intentional self-harm, assault and undetermined.

f. Adult and child abuse, neglect and other maltreatment

Sequence first the appropriate code from categories T74 (Adult and child abuse, neglect and other maltreatment, confirmed) or T76 (Adult and child abuse, neglect and other maltreatment, suspected) for abuse, neglect and other maltreatment, followed by any accompanying mental health or injury code(s).

If the documentation in the medical record states abuse or neglect it is coded as confirmed (T74.-). It is coded as suspected if it is documented as suspected (T76.-).

For cases of confirmed abuse or neglect an external cause code from the assault section (X92-YØ9) should be added to identify the cause of any physical injuries. A perpetrator code (YØ7) should be added when the perpetrator of the abuse is known. For suspected cases of abuse or neglect, do not report external cause or perpetrator code.

If a suspected case of abuse, neglect or mistreatment is ruled out during an encounter code ZØ4.71, Encounter for examination and observation following alleged physical adult abuse, ruled out, or code ZØ4.72, Encounter for examination and observation following alleged child physical abuse, ruled out, should be used, not a code from T76.

If a suspected case of alleged rape or sexual abuse is ruled out during an encounter code ZØ4.41, Encounter for examination and observation following alleged adult rape or code ZØ4.42, Encounter for examination and observation following alleged child rape, should be used, not a code from T76.

If a suspected case of forced sexual exploitation or forced labor exploitation is ruled out during an encounter, code ZØ4.81, Encounter for examination and observation of victim following forced sexual exploitation, or code ZØ4.82, Encounter for examination and observation of victim following forced labor exploitation, should be used, not a code from T76.

See Section I.C.15. Abuse in a pregnant patient.

g. Complications of care

1) General guidelines for complications of care

(a) Documentation of complications of care

See Section I.B.16. for information on documentation of complications of care.

2) Pain due to medical devices

Pain associated with devices, implants or grafts left in a surgical site (for example painful hip prosthesis) is assigned to the appropriate code(s) found in Chapter 19, Injury, poisoning, and certain other consequences of external causes. Specific codes for pain due to medical devices are found in the T code section of the ICD-10-CM. Use additional code(s) from category G89 to identify acute or chronic pain due to presence of the device, implant or graft (G89.18 or G89.28).

3) Transplant complications

(a) Transplant complications other than kidney

Codes under category T86, Complications of transplanted organs and tissues, are for use for both complications and rejection of transplanted organs. A transplant complication code is only assigned if the complication affects the function of the transplanted organ. Two codes are required to fully describe a transplant complication: the appropriate code from category T86 and a secondary code that identifies the complication.

Pre-existing conditions or conditions that develop after the transplant are not coded as complications unless they affect the function of the transplanted organs.

See Section I.C.21. for transplant organ removal status
See Section I.C.2. for malignant neoplasm associated with transplanted organ.

(b) Kidney transplant complications

Patients who have undergone kidney transplant may still have some form of chronic kidney disease (CKD) because the kidney transplant may not fully restore kidney function. Code T86.1- should be assigned for documented complications of a kidney transplant, such as transplant failure or rejection or other transplant complication. Code T86.1- should not be assigned for post kidney transplant patients who have chronic kidney (CKD) unless a transplant complication such as transplant failure or rejection is documented. If the documentation is unclear as to whether the patient has a complication of the transplant, query the provider.

Conditions that affect the function of the transplanted kidney, other than CKD, should be assigned a code from subcategory T86.1, Complications of transplanted organ, Kidney, and a secondary code that identifies the complication.

For patients with CKD following a kidney transplant, but who do not have a complication such as failure or rejection, *see Section I.C.14. Chronic kidney disease and kidney transplant status.*

4) Complication codes that include the external cause

As with certain other T codes, some of the complications of care codes have the external cause included in the code. The code includes the nature of the complication as well as the type of procedure that caused the complication. No external cause code indicating the type of procedure is necessary for these codes.

5) Complications of care codes within the body system chapters

Intraoperative and postprocedural complication codes are found within the body system chapters with codes specific to the organs and structures of that body system. These codes should be sequenced first, followed by a code(s) for the specific complication, if applicable.

Complication codes from the body system chapters should be assigned for intraoperative and postprocedural complications (e.g., the appropriate complication code from Chapter 9 would be assigned for a vascular intraoperative or postprocedural complication) unless the complication is specifically indexed to a T code in Chapter 19.

20. Chapter 20: External Causes of Morbidity (V00-Y99)

The external causes of morbidity codes should never be sequenced as the first-listed or principal diagnosis.

External cause codes are intended to provide data for injury research and evaluation of injury prevention strategies. These codes capture how the injury or health condition happened (cause), the intent (unintentional or accidental; or intentional, such as suicide or assault), the place where the event occurred the activity of the patient at the time of the event, and the person's status (e.g., civilian, military).

There is no national requirement for mandatory ICD-10-CM external cause code reporting. Unless a provider is subject to a state-based external cause code reporting mandate or these codes are required by a particular payer, reporting of ICD-10-CM codes in Chapter 20, External Causes of Morbidity, is not required. In the absence of a mandatory reporting requirement, providers are encouraged to voluntarily report external cause codes, as they provide valuable data for injury research and evaluation of injury prevention strategies.

a. General External Cause Coding Guidelines

1) Used with any code in the range of A00.0-T88.9, Z00-Z99

An external cause code may be used with any code in the range of A00.0-T88.9, Z00-Z99, classification that represents a health condition due to an external cause. Though they are most applicable to injuries, they are also valid for use with such things as infections or diseases due to an external source, and other health conditions, such as a heart attack that occurs during strenuous physical activity.

2) External cause code used for length of treatment

Assign the external cause code, with the appropriate 7th character (initial encounter, subsequent encounter or sequela) for each encounter for which the injury or condition is being treated.

Most categories in Chapter 20 have a 7th character requirement for each applicable code. Most categories in this chapter have three 7th character values: A, initial encounter, D, subsequent encounter and S, sequela. While the patient may be seen by a new or different provider over the course of treatment for an injury or condition, assignment of the 7th character for external cause should match the 7th character of the code assigned for the associated injury or condition for the encounter.

3) Use the full range of external cause codes
Use the full range of external cause codes to completely describe the cause, the intent, the place of occurrence and if applicable, the activity of the patient at the time of the event, and the patient's status, for all injuries, and other health conditions due to an external cause.

4) Assign as many external cause codes as necessary
Assign as many external cause codes as necessary to fully explain each cause. If only one external code can be recorded, assign the code most related to the principal diagnosis.

5) The selection of the appropriate external cause code
The selection of the appropriate external cause code is guided by the Alphabetic Index of External Causes and by Inclusion and Exclusion notes in the Tabular List.

6) External cause code can never be a principal diagnosis
An external cause code can never be a principal (first-listed) diagnosis.

7) Combination external cause codes
Certain of the external cause codes are combination codes that identify sequential events that result in an injury, such as a fall which results in striking against an object. The injury may be due to either event or both. The combination external cause code used should correspond to the sequence of events regardless of which caused the most serious injury.

8) No external cause code needed in certain circumstances
No external cause code from Chapter 2Ø is needed if the external cause and intent are included in a code from another chapter (e.g., T36.ØX1- Poisoning by penicillins, accidental (unintentional)).

b. Place of Occurrence Guideline
Codes from category Y92, Place of occurrence of the external cause, are secondary codes for use after other external cause codes to identify the location of the patient at the time of injury or other condition.

Generally, a place of occurrence code is assigned only once, at the initial encounter for treatment. However, in the rare instance that a new injury occurs during hospitalization, an additional place of occurrence code may be assigned. No 7th characters are used for Y92. Only one code from Y92 should be recorded on a medical record.

Do not use place of occurrence code Y92.9 if the place is not stated or is not applicable.

c. Activity Code
Assign a code from category Y93, Activity code, to describe the activity of the patient at the time the injury or other health condition occurred.

An activity code is used only once, at the initial encounter for treatment. Only one code from Y93 should be recorded on a medical record.

The activity codes are not applicable to poisonings, adverse effects, misadventures or sequela.

Do not assign Y93.9, Unspecified activity, if the activity is not stated.

A code from category Y93 is appropriate for use with external cause and intent codes if identifying the activity provides additional information about the event.

d. Place of Occurrence, Activity, and Status Codes Used with other External Cause Code
When applicable, place of occurrence, activity, and external cause status codes are sequenced after the main external cause code(s). Regardless of the number of external cause codes assigned, there should be only one place of occurrence code, one activity code, and one external cause status code assigned to an encounter.

e. If the Reporting Format Limits the Number of External Cause Codes
If the reporting format limits the number of external cause codes that can be used in reporting clinical data, report the code for the cause/intent most related to the principal diagnosis. If the format permits capture of additional external cause codes, the cause/intent, including medical misadventures, of the additional events should be reported rather than the codes for place, activity, or external status.

f. Multiple External Cause Coding Guidelines
More than one external cause code is required to fully describe the external cause of an illness or injury. The assignment of external cause codes should be sequenced in the following priority:

If two or more events cause separate injuries, an external cause code should be assigned for each cause. The first-listed external cause code will be selected in the following order:

External codes for child and adult abuse take priority over all other external cause codes.

See Section I.C.19., Child and Adult abuse guidelines.

External codes for terrorism events take priority over all other external cause codes except child and adult abuse.

External cause codes for cataclysmic events take priority over all other external cause codes except child and adult abuse and terrorism.

External cause codes for transport accidents take priority over all other external cause codes except cataclysmic events, child and adult abuse and terrorism.

Activity and external cause status codes are assigned following all causal (intent) external cause codes.

The first-listed external cause code should correspond to the cause of the most serious diagnosis due to an assault, accident, or self-harm, following the order of hierarchy listed above.

g. Child and Adult Abuse Guideline
Adult and child abuse, neglect and maltreatment are classified as assault. Any of the assault codes may be used to indicate the external cause of any injury resulting from the confirmed abuse.

For confirmed cases of abuse, neglect and maltreatment, when the perpetrator is known, a code from YØ7, Perpetrator of maltreatment and neglect, should accompany any other assault codes.

See Section I.C.19. Adult and child abuse, neglect and other maltreatment

h. Unknown or Undetermined Intent Guideline

If the intent (accident, self-harm, assault) of the cause of an injury or other condition is unknown or unspecified, code the intent as accidental intent. All transport accident categories assume accidental intent.

1) Use of undetermined intent

External cause codes for events of undetermined intent are only for use if the documentation in the record specifies that the intent cannot be determined.

i. Sequelae (Late Effects) of External Cause Guidelines

1) Sequelae external cause codes

Sequela are reported using the external cause code with the 7th character "S" for sequela. These codes should be used with any report of a late effect or sequela resulting from a previous injury.

See Section I.B.10. Sequela (Late Effects)

2) Sequela external cause code with a related current injury

A sequela external cause code should never be used with a related current nature of injury code.

3) Use of sequela external cause codes for subsequent visits

Use a late effect external cause code for subsequent visits when a late effect of the initial injury is being treated. Do not use a late effect external cause code for subsequent visits for follow-up care (e.g., to assess healing, to receive rehabilitative therapy) of the injury when no late effect of the injury has been documented.

j. Terrorism Guidelines

1) Cause of injury identified by the Federal Government (FBI) as terrorism

When the cause of an injury is identified by the Federal Government (FBI) as terrorism, the first-listed external cause code should be a code from category Y38, Terrorism. The definition of terrorism employed by the FBI is found at the inclusion note at the beginning of category Y38. Use additional code for place of occurrence (Y92.-). More than one Y38 code may be assigned if the injury is the result of more than one mechanism of terrorism.

2) Cause of an injury is suspected to be the result of terrorism

When the cause of an injury is suspected to be the result of terrorism a code from category Y38 should not be assigned. Suspected cases should be classified as assault.

3) Code Y38.9, Terrorism, secondary effects

Assign code Y38.9, Terrorism, secondary effects, for conditions occurring subsequent to the terrorist event. This code should not be assigned for conditions that are due to the initial terrorist act.

It is acceptable to assign code Y38.9 with another code from Y38 if there is an injury due to the initial terrorist event and an injury that is a subsequent result of the terrorist event.

k. External Cause Status

A code from category Y99, External cause status, should be assigned whenever any other external cause code is assigned for an encounter, including an Activity code, except for the events noted below. Assign a code from category Y99, External cause status, to indicate the work status of the person at the time the event occurred. The status code indicates whether the event occurred during military activity, whether a non-military person was at work, whether an individual including a student or volunteer was involved in a non-work activity at the time of the causal event.

A code from Y99, External cause status, should be assigned, when applicable, with other external cause codes, such as transport accidents and falls. The external cause status codes are not applicable to poisonings, adverse effects, misadventures or late effects.

Do not assign a code from category Y99 if no other external cause codes (cause, activity) are applicable for the encounter.

An external cause status code is used only once, at the initial encounter for treatment. Only one code from Y99 should be recorded on a medical record.

Do not assign code Y99.9, Unspecified external cause status, if the status is not stated.

21. Chapter 21: Factors Influencing Health Status and Contact with Health Services (Z00-Z99)

Note: The chapter-specific guidelines provide additional information about the use of Z codes for specified encounters.

a. Use of Z Codes in Any Healthcare Setting

Z codes are for use in any healthcare setting. Z codes may be used as either a first-listed (principal diagnosis code in the inpatient setting) or secondary code, depending on the circumstances of the encounter. Certain Z codes may only be used as first-listed or principal diagnosis.

b. Z Codes Indicate a Reason for an Encounter

Z codes are not procedure codes. A corresponding procedure code must accompany a Z code to describe any procedure performed.

c. Categories of Z Codes

1) Contact/Exposure

Category Z20 indicates contact with, and suspected exposure to, communicable diseases. These codes are for patients who do not show any sign or symptom of a disease but are suspected to have been exposed to it by close personal contact with an infected individual or are in an area where a disease is epidemic.

Category Z77, Other contact with and (suspected) exposures hazardous to health, indicates contact with and suspected exposures hazardous to health.

Contact/exposure codes may be used as a first-listed code to explain an encounter for testing, or, more commonly, as a secondary code to identify a potential risk.

GUIDELINES (ICD-10-CM)

2) Inoculations and vaccinations

Code Z23 is for encounters for inoculations and vaccinations. It indicates that a patient is being seen to receive a prophylactic inoculation against a disease. Procedure codes are required to identify the actual administration of the injection and the type(s) of immunizations given. Code Z23 may be used as a secondary code if the inoculation is given as a routine part of preventive health care, such as a well-baby visit.

3) Status

Status codes indicate that a patient is either a carrier of a disease or has the sequelae or residual of a past disease or condition. This includes such things as the presence of prosthetic or mechanical devices resulting from past treatment. A status code is informative, because the status may affect the course of treatment and its outcome. A status code is distinct from a history code. The history code indicates that the patient no longer has the condition.

A status code should not be used with a diagnosis code from one of the body system chapters, if the diagnosis code includes the information provided by the status code. For example, code Z94.1, Heart transplant status, should not be used with a code from subcategory T86.2, Complications of heart transplant. The status code does not provide additional information. The complication code indicates that the patient is a heart transplant patient.

For encounters for weaning from a mechanical ventilator, assign a code from subcategory J96.1, Chronic respiratory failure, followed by code Z99.11, Dependence on respirator [ventilator] status.

The status Z codes/categories are:

Z14 Genetic carrier

Genetic carrier status indicates that a person carries a gene, associated with a particular disease, which may be passed to offspring who may develop that disease. The person does not have the disease and is not at risk of developing the disease.

Z15 Genetic susceptibility to disease Genetic susceptibility indicates that a person has a gene that increases the risk of that person developing the disease.

Codes from category Z15 should not be used as principal or first-listed codes. If the patient has the condition to which he/she is susceptible, and that condition is the reason for the encounter, the code for the current condition should be sequenced first. If the patient is being seen for follow-up after completed treatment for this condition, and the condition no longer exists, a follow-up code should be sequenced first, followed by the appropriate personal history and genetic susceptibility codes. If the purpose of the encounter is genetic counseling associated with procreative management, code Z31.5, Encounter for genetic counseling, should be assigned as the first-listed code, followed by a code from category Z15. Additional codes should be assigned for any applicable family or personal history.

Z16 Resistance to antimicrobial drugs

This code indicates that a patient has a condition that is resistant to antimicrobial drug treatment. Sequence the infection code first.

Z17 Estrogen receptor status

Z18 Retained foreign body fragments

Z19 Hormone sensitivity malignancy status

Z21 Asymptomatic HIV infection status This code indicates that a patient has tested positive for HIV but has manifested no signs or symptoms of the disease.

Z22 Carrier of infectious disease Carrier status indicates that a person harbors the specific organisms of a disease without manifest symptoms and is capable of transmitting the infection.

Z28.3 Underimmunization status

Z33.1 Pregnant state, incidental This code is a secondary code only for use when the pregnancy is in no way complicating the reason for visit. Otherwise, a code from the obstetric chapter is required.

Z66 Do not resuscitate

This code may be used when it is documented by the provider that a patient is on do not resuscitate status at any time during the stay.

Z67 Blood type

Z68 Body mass index (BMI)

BMI codes should only be assigned when **there is an** associated reportable diagnosis (**such as obesity**). Do not assign BMI codes during pregnancy.

See Section I.B.14 for BMI documentation by clinicians other than the patient's provider.

Z74.01 Bed confinement status

Z76.82 Awaiting organ transplant status

Z78 Other specified health status

Code Z78.1, Physical restraint status, may be used when it is documented by the provider that a patient has been put in restraints during the current encounter. Please note that this code should not be reported when it is documented by the provider that a patient is temporarily restrained during a procedure.

Z79 Long-term (current) drug therapy

Codes from this category indicate a patient's continuous use of a prescribed drug (including such things as aspirin therapy) for the long-term treatment of a condition or for prophylactic use. It is not for use for patients who have addictions to drugs. This subcategory is not for use of medications for detoxification or maintenance programs to prevent withdrawal symptoms in patients with drug dependence (e.g., methadone maintenance for opiate dependence). Assign the appropriate code for the drug dependence instead.

Assign a code from Z79 if the patient is receiving a medication for an extended period as a prophylactic measure (such as for the prevention of deep vein thrombosis) or as treatment of a chronic condition (such as arthritis) or a disease requiring a lengthy course of treatment (such as cancer). Do not assign a code from category Z79 for medication being administered for a brief period of time to treat an acute illness or injury (such as a course of antibiotics to treat acute bronchitis).

- Z88 Allergy status to drugs, medicaments and biological substances Except: Z88.9, Allergy status to unspecified drugs, medicaments and biological substances status
- Z89 Acquired absence of limb
- Z9Ø Acquired absence of organs, not elsewhere classified
- Z91.Ø- Allergy status, other than to drugs and biological substances
- Z92.82 Status post administration of tPA (rtPA) in a different facility within the last 24 hours prior to admission to a current facility Assign code Z92.82, Status post administration of tPA (rtPA) in a different facility within the last 24 hours prior to admission to current facility, as a secondary diagnosis when a patient is received by transfer into a facility and documentation indicates they were administered tissue plasminogen activator (tPA) within the last 24 hours prior to admission to the current facility. This guideline applies even if the patient is still receiving the tPA at the time they are received into the current facility. The appropriate code for the condition for which the tPA was administered (such as cerebrovascular disease or myocardial infarction) should be assigned first. Code Z92.82 is only applicable to the receiving facility record and not to the transferring facility record.
- Z93 Artificial opening status
- Z94 Transplanted organ and tissue status
- Z95 Presence of cardiac and vascular implants and grafts
- Z96 Presence of other functional implants
- Z97 Presence of other devices
- Z98 Other postprocedural states

Assign code Z98.85, Transplanted organ removal status, to indicate that a transplanted organ has been previously removed. This code should not be assigned for the encounter in which the transplanted organ is removed. The complication necessitating removal of the transplant organ should be assigned for that encounter.

See Section I.C.19. for information on the coding of organ transplant complications.

- Z99 Dependence on enabling machines and devices, not elsewhere classified

Note: Categories Z89-Z9Ø and Z93-Z99 are for use only if there are no complications or malfunctions of the organ or tissue replaced, the amputation site or the equipment on which the patient is dependent.

4) History (of)

There are two types of history Z codes, personal and family. Personal history codes explain a patient's past medical condition that no longer exists and is not receiving any treatment, but that has the potential for recurrence, and therefore may require continued monitoring.

Family history codes are for use when a patient has a family member(s) who has had a particular disease that causes the patient to be at higher risk of also contracting the disease.

Personal history codes may be used in conjunction with follow-up codes and family history codes may be used in conjunction with screening codes to explain the need for a test or procedure. History codes are also acceptable on any medical record regardless of the reason for visit. A history of an illness, even if no longer present, is important information that may alter the type of treatment ordered.

The history Z code categories are:

- Z8Ø Family history of primary malignant neoplasm
- Z81 Family history of mental and behavioral disorders
- Z82 Family history of certain disabilities and chronic diseases (leading to disablement)
- Z83 Family history of other specific disorders
- Z84 Family history of other conditions
- Z85 Personal history of malignant neoplasm
- Z86 Personal history of certain other diseases
- Z87 Personal history of other diseases and conditions
- Z91.4- Personal history of psychological trauma, not elsewhere classified
- Z91.5 Personal history of self-harm
- Z91.81 History of falling
- Z91.82 Personal history of military deployment
- Z92 Personal history of medical treatment Except: Z92.Ø, Personal history of contraception Except: Z92.82, Status post administration of tPA (rtPA) in a different facility within the last 24 hours prior to admission to a current facility

5) Screening

Screening is the testing for disease or disease precursors in seemingly well individuals so that early detection and treatment can be provided for those who test positive for the disease (e.g., screening mammogram).

The testing of a person to rule out or confirm a suspected diagnosis because the patient has some sign or symptom is a diagnostic examination, not a screening. In these cases, the sign or symptom is used to explain the reason for the test.

A screening code may be a first-listed code if the reason for the visit is specifically the screening exam. It may also be used as an additional code if the screening is done during an office visit for other health problems. A screening code is not necessary if the screening is inherent to a routine examination, such as a pap smear done during a routine pelvic examination.

Should a condition be discovered during the screening then the code for the condition may be assigned as an additional diagnosis.

The Z code indicates that a screening exam is planned. A procedure code is required to confirm that the screening was performed.

The screening Z codes/categories:

Z11	Encounter for screening for infectious and parasitic diseases
Z12	Encounter for screening for malignant neoplasms
Z13	Encounter for screening for other diseases and disorders Except: Z13.9, Encounter for screening, unspecified
Z36	Encounter for antenatal screening for mother

6) Observation

There are three observation Z code categories. They are for use in very limited circumstances when a person is being observed for a suspected condition that is ruled out. The observation codes are not for use if an injury or illness or any signs or symptoms related to the suspected condition are present. In such cases the diagnosis/symptom code is used with the corresponding external cause code.

The observation codes are to be used as principal diagnosis only. The only exception to this is when the principal diagnosis is required to be a code from category Z38, Liveborn infants according to place of birth and type of delivery. Then a code from category Z05, Encounter for observation and evaluation of newborn for suspected diseases and conditions ruled out, is sequenced after the Z38 code. Additional codes may be used in addition to the observation code, but only if they are unrelated to the suspected condition being observed.

Codes from subcategory Z03.7 Encounter for suspected maternal and fetal conditions ruled out, may either be used as a first-listed or as an additional code assignment depending on the case. They are for use in very limited circumstances on a maternal record when an encounter is for a suspected maternal or fetal condition that is ruled out during that encounter (for example, a maternal or fetal condition may be suspected due to an abnormal test result). These codes should not be used when the condition is confirmed. In those cases, the confirmed condition should be coded. In addition, these codes are not for use if an illness or any signs or symptoms related to the suspected condition or problem are present. In such cases the diagnosis/symptom code is used.

Additional codes may be used in addition to the code from subcategory Z03.7, but only if they are unrelated to the suspected condition being evaluated.

Codes from subcategory Z03.7 may not be used for encounters for antenatal screening of mother. *See Section I.C.21. Screening.*

For encounters for suspected fetal condition that are inconclusive following testing and evaluation, assign the appropriate code from category O35, O36, O40 or O41.

The observation Z code categories:

Z03	Encounter for medical observation for suspected diseases and conditions ruled out
Z04	Encounter for examination and observation for other reasons Except: Z04.9, Encounter for examination and observation for unspecified reason
Z05	Encounter for observation and evaluation of newborn for suspected diseases and conditions ruled out

7) Aftercare

Aftercare visit codes cover situations when the initial treatment of a disease has been performed and the patient requires continued care during the healing or recovery phase, or for the long-term consequences of the disease. The aftercare Z code should not be used if treatment is directed at a current, acute disease. The diagnosis code is to be used in these cases.

Exceptions to this rule are codes Z51.0, Encounter for antineoplastic radiation therapy, and codes from subcategory Z51.1, Encounter for antineoplastic chemotherapy and immunotherapy. These codes are to be first-listed, followed by the diagnosis code when a patient's encounter is solely to receive radiation therapy, chemotherapy, or immunotherapy for the treatment of a neoplasm. If the reason for the encounter is more than one type of antineoplastic therapy, code Z51.0 and a code from subcategory Z51.1 may be assigned together, in which case one of these codes would be reported as a secondary diagnosis.

The aftercare Z codes should also not be used for aftercare for injuries. For aftercare of an injury, assign the acute injury code with the appropriate 7th character (for subsequent encounter).

The aftercare codes are generally first-listed to explain the specific reason for the encounter. An aftercare code may be used as an additional code when some type of aftercare is provided in addition to the reason for admission and no diagnosis code is applicable. An example of this would be the closure of a colostomy during an encounter for treatment of another condition.

Aftercare codes should be used in conjunction with other aftercare codes or diagnosis codes to provide better detail on the specifics of an aftercare encounter visit, unless otherwise directed by the classification. The sequencing of multiple aftercare codes depends on the circumstances of the encounter.

Certain aftercare Z code categories need a secondary diagnosis code to describe the resolving condition or sequelae. For others, the condition is included in the code title.

Additional Z code aftercare category terms include fitting and adjustment, and attention to artificial openings.

Status Z codes may be used with aftercare Z codes to indicate the nature of the aftercare. For example code Z95.1, Presence of aortocoronary bypass graft, may be used with code Z48.812, Encounter for surgical aftercare following surgery on the circulatory system, to indicate the surgery for which the aftercare is being performed. A status code should not be used when the aftercare code indicates the type of status, such as using Z43.Ø, Encounter for attention to tracheostomy, with Z93.Ø, Tracheostomy status.

The aftercare Z category/codes:

- Z42 Encounter for plastic and reconstructive surgery following medical procedure or healed injury
- Z43 Encounter for attention to artificial openings
- Z44 Encounter for fitting and adjustment of external prosthetic device
- Z45 Encounter for adjustment and management of implanted device
- Z46 Encounter for fitting and adjustment of other devices
- Z47 Orthopedic aftercare
- Z48 Encounter for other postprocedural aftercare
- Z49 Encounter for care involving renal dialysis
- Z51 Encounter for other aftercare and medical care

8) Follow-up

The follow-up codes are used to explain continuing surveillance following completed treatment of a disease, condition, or injury. They imply that the condition has been fully treated and no longer exists. They should not be confused with aftercare codes, or injury codes with a 7th character for subsequent encounter, that explain ongoing care of a healing condition or its sequelae. Follow-up codes may be used in conjunction with history codes to provide the full picture of the healed condition and its treatment. The follow-up code is sequenced first, followed by the history code.

A follow-up code may be used to explain multiple visits. Should a condition be found to have recurred on the follow-up visit, then the diagnosis code for the condition should be assigned in place of the follow-up code.

The follow-up Z code categories:

- ZØ8 Encounter for follow-up examination after completed treatment for malignant neoplasm
- ZØ9 Encounter for follow-up examination after completed treatment for conditions other than malignant neoplasm
- Z39 Encounter for maternal postpartum care and examination

9) Donor

Codes in category Z52, Donors of organs and tissues, are used for living individuals who are donating blood or other body tissue. These codes are only for individuals donating for others, not for self-donations. They are not used to identify cadaveric donations.

1Ø) Counseling

Counseling Z codes are used when a patient or family member receives assistance in the aftermath of an illness or injury, or when support is required in coping with family or social problems.

The counseling Z codes/categories:

- Z3Ø.Ø- Encounter for general counseling and advice on contraception
- Z31.5 Encounter for procreative genetic counseling
- Z31.6- Encounter for general counseling and advice on procreation
- Z32.2 Encounter for childbirth instruction
- Z32.3 Encounter for childcare instruction
- Z69 Encounter for mental health services for victim and perpetrator of abuse
- Z7Ø Counseling related to sexual attitude, behavior and orientation
- Z71 Persons encountering health services for other counseling and medical advice, not elsewhere classified
  Note: **Code Z71.84, Encounter for health counseling related to travel, is to be used for health risk and safety counseling for future travel purposes.**
- Z76.81 Expectant mother prebirth pediatrician visit

11) Encounters for Obstetrical and Reproductive Services

See Section I.C.15. Pregnancy, childbirth, and the puerperium, for further instruction on the use of these codes.

Z codes for pregnancy are for use in those circumstances when none of the problems or complications included in the codes from the Obstetrics chapter exist (a routine prenatal visit or postpartum care). Codes in category Z34, Encounter for supervision of normal pregnancy, are always first listed and are not to be used with any other code from the OB chapter.

Codes in category Z3A, Weeks of gestation, may be assigned to provide additional information about the pregnancy. Category Z3A codes should not be assigned for pregnancies with abortive outcomes (categories OØØ-OØ8), elective termination of pregnancy (code Z33.2), nor for postpartum conditions, as category Z3A is not applicable to these conditions. The date of the admission should be used to determine weeks of gestation for inpatient admissions that encompass more than one gestational week.

The outcome of delivery, category Z37, should be included on all maternal delivery records. It is always a secondary code. Codes in category Z37 should not be used on the newborn record.

Z codes for family planning (contraceptive) or procreative management and counseling should be included on an obstetric record either during the pregnancy or the postpartum stage, if applicable.

Z codes/categories for obstetrical and reproductive services:

Z3Ø	Encounter for contraceptive management
Z31	Encounter for procreative management
Z32.2	Encounter for childbirth instruction
Z32.3	Encounter for childcare instruction
Z33	Pregnant state
Z34	Encounter for supervision of normal pregnancy
Z36	Encounter for antenatal screening of mother
Z3A	Weeks of gestation
Z37	Outcome of delivery
Z39	Encounter for maternal postpartum care and examination
Z76.81	Expectant mother prebirth pediatrician visit

12) Newborns and Infants

See Section I.C.16. Newborn (Perinatal) guidelines, for further instruction on the use of these codes.

Newborn Z codes/categories:

Z76.1	Encounter for health supervision and care of foundling
ZØØ.1-	Encounter for routine child health examination
Z38	Liveborn infants according to place of birth and type of delivery

13) Routine and Administrative Examinations

The Z codes allow for the description of encounters for routine examinations, such as, a general check-up, or, examinations for administrative purposes, such as, a pre-employment physical. The codes are not to be used if the examination is for diagnosis of a suspected condition or for treatment purposes. In such cases the diagnosis code is used. During a routine exam, should a diagnosis or condition be discovered, it should be coded as an additional code. Pre-existing and chronic conditions and history codes may also be included as additional codes as long as the examination is for administrative purposes and not focused on any particular condition.

Some of the codes for routine health examinations distinguish between "with" and "without" abnormal findings. Code assignment depends on the information that is known at the time the encounter is being coded. For example, if no abnormal findings were found during the examination, but the encounter is being coded before test results are back, it is acceptable to assign the code for "without abnormal findings." When assigning a code for "with abnormal findings," additional code(s) should be assigned to identify the specific abnormal finding(s).

Pre-operative examination and pre-procedural laboratory examination Z codes are for use only in those situations when a patient is being cleared for a procedure or surgery and no treatment is given.

The Z codes/categories for routine and administrative examinations:

ZØØ	Encounter for general examination without complaint, suspected or reported diagnosis
ZØ1	Encounter for other special examination without complaint, suspected or reported diagnosis
ZØ2	Encounter for administrative examination Except: ZØ2.9, Encounter for administrative examinations, unspecified
Z32.Ø-	Encounter for pregnancy test

14) Miscellaneous Z Codes

The miscellaneous Z codes capture a number of other health care encounters that do not fall into one of the other categories. Certain of these codes identify the reason for the encounter; others are for use as additional codes that provide useful information on circumstances that may affect a patient's care and treatment.

Prophylactic Organ Removal

For encounters specifically for prophylactic removal of an organ (such as prophylactic removal of breasts due to a genetic susceptibility to cancer or a family history of cancer), the principal or first-listed code should be a code from category Z4Ø, Encounter for prophylactic surgery, followed by the appropriate codes to identify the associated risk factor (such as genetic susceptibility or family history).

If the patient has a malignancy of one site and is having prophylactic removal at another site to prevent either a new primary malignancy or metastatic disease, a code for the malignancy should also be assigned in addition to a code from subcategory Z4Ø.Ø, Encounter for prophylactic surgery for risk factors related to malignant neoplasms. A Z4Ø.Ø code should not be assigned if the patient is having organ removal for treatment of a malignancy, such as the removal of the testes for the treatment of prostate cancer.

Miscellaneous Z codes/categories:

Z28	Immunization not carried out Except: Z28.3, Underimmunization status
Z29	Encounter for other prophylactic measures
Z4Ø	Encounter for prophylactic surgery
Z41	Encounter for procedures for purposes other than remedying health state Except: Z41.9, Encounter for procedure for purposes other than remedying health state, unspecified

Z53 Persons encountering health services for specific procedures and treatment, not carried out
Z55 Problems related to education and literacy
Z56 Problems related to employment and unemployment
Z57 Occupational exposure to risk factors
Z58 Problems related to physical environment
Z59 Problems related to housing and economic circumstances
Z60 Problems related to social environment
Z62 Problems related to upbringing
Z63 Other problems related to primary support group, including family circumstances
Z64 Problems related to certain psychosocial circumstances
Z65 Problems related to other psychosocial circumstances
Z72 Problems related to lifestyle
Note: These codes should be assigned only when the documentation specifies that the patient has an associated problem
Z73 Problems related to life management difficulty
Z74 Problems related to care provider dependency Except: Z74.01, Bed confinement status
Z75 Problems related to medical facilities and other health care
Z76.0 Encounter for issue of repeat prescription
Z76.3 Healthy person accompanying sick person
Z76.4 Other boarder to healthcare facility
Z76.5 Malingerer [conscious simulation]
Z91.1- Patient's noncompliance with medical treatment and regimen
Z91.83 Wandering in diseases classified elsewhere
Z91.84- Oral health risk factors
Z91.89 Other specified personal risk factors, not elsewhere classified

See Section I.B.14 for Z55-Z65 Persons with potential health hazards related to socioeconomic and psychosocial circumstances, documentation by clinicians other than the patient's provider

15) Nonspecific Z Codes

Certain Z codes are so non-specific, or potentially redundant with other codes in the classification, that there can be little justification for their use in the inpatient setting. Their use in the outpatient setting should be limited to those instances when there is no further documentation to permit more precise coding. Otherwise, any sign or symptom or any other reason for visit that is captured in another code should be used.

Nonspecific Z codes/categories:
Z02.9 Encounter for administrative examinations, unspecified
Z04.9 Encounter for examination and observation for unspecified reason
Z13.9 Encounter for screening, unspecified
Z41.9 Encounter for procedure for purposes other than remedying health state, unspecified
Z52.9 Donor of unspecified organ or tissue
Z86.59 Personal history of other mental and behavioral disorders
Z88.9 Allergy status to unspecified drugs, medicaments and biological substances status
Z92.0 Personal history of contraception

16) Z Codes That May Only be Principal/First-Listed Diagnosis

The following Z codes/categories may only be reported as the principal/first-listed diagnosis, except when there are multiple encounters on the same day and the medical records for the encounters are combined:
Z00 Encounter for general examination without complaint, suspected or reported diagnosis
Except: Z00.6
Z01 Encounter for other special examination without complaint, suspected or reported diagnosis
Z02 Encounter for administrative examination
Z03 Encounter for medical observation for suspected diseases and conditions ruled out
Z04 Encounter for examination and observation for other reasons
Z33.2 Encounter for elective termination of pregnancy
Z31.81 Encounter for male factor infertility in female patient
Z31.83 Encounter for assisted reproductive fertility procedure cycle
Z31.84 Encounter for fertility preservation procedure
Z34 Encounter for supervision of normal pregnancy
Z39 Encounter for maternal postpartum care and examination
Z38 Liveborn infants according to place of birth and type of delivery
Z40 Encounter for prophylactic surgery
Z42 Encounter for plastic and reconstructive surgery following medical procedure or healed injury
Z51.0 Encounter for antineoplastic radiation therapy
Z51.1- Encounter for antineoplastic chemotherapy and immunotherapy
Z52 Donors of organs and tissues Except: Z52.9, Donor of unspecified organ or tissue
Z76.1 Encounter for health supervision and care of foundling
Z76.2 Encounter for health supervision and care of other healthy infant and child
Z99.12 Encounter for respirator [ventilator] dependence during power failure

Section II. Selection of Principal Diagnosis

The circumstances of inpatient admission always govern the selection of principal diagnosis. The principal diagnosis is defined in the Uniform Hospital Discharge Data Set (UHDDS) as "that condition established after study to be chiefly responsible for occasioning the admission of the patient to the hospital for care."

The UHDDS definitions are used by hospitals to report inpatient data elements in a standardized manner. These data elements and their definitions can be found in the July 31, 1985, Federal Register (Vol. 50, No, 147), pp. 31038-40.

Since that time the application of the UHDDS definitions has been expanded to include all nonoutpatient settings (acute care, short term, long-term care and psychiatric hospitals; home health agencies; rehab facilities; nursing homes, etc). The UHDDS definitions also apply to hospice services (all levels of care).

In determining principal diagnosis, coding conventions in the ICD-10-CM, the Tabular List and Alphabetic Index take precedence over these official coding guidelines.
(See Section I.A., Conventions for the ICD-10-CM)

The importance of consistent, complete documentation in the medical record cannot be overemphasized. Without such documentation the application of all coding guidelines is a difficult, if not impossible, task.

A. **Codes for symptoms, signs, and ill-defined conditions**
   Codes for symptoms, signs, and ill-defined conditions from Chapter 18 are not to be used as principal diagnosis when a related definitive diagnosis has been established.

B. **Two or more interrelated conditions, each potentially meeting the definition for principal diagnosis.**
   When there are two or more interrelated conditions (such as diseases in the same ICD-10-CM chapter or manifestations characteristically associated with a certain disease) potentially meeting the definition of principal diagnosis, either condition may be sequenced first, unless the circumstances of the admission, the therapy provided, the Tabular List, or the Alphabetic Index indicate otherwise.

C. **Two or more diagnoses that equally meet the definition for principal diagnosis**
   In the unusual instance when two or more diagnoses equally meet the criteria for principal diagnosis as determined by the circumstances of admission, diagnostic workup and/or therapy provided, and the Alphabetic Index, Tabular List, or another coding guidelines does not provide sequencing direction, any one of the diagnoses may be sequenced first.

D. **Two or more comparative or contrasting conditions.**
   In those rare instances when two or more contrasting or comparative diagnoses are documented as "either/or" (or similar terminology), they are coded as if the diagnoses were confirmed and the diagnoses are sequenced according to the circumstances of the admission. If no further determination can be made as to which diagnosis should be principal, either diagnosis may be sequenced first.

E. **A symptom(s) followed by contrasting/ comparative diagnoses**
   GUIDELINE HAS BEEN DELETED EFFECTIVE OCTOBER 1, 2014

F. **Original treatment plan not carried out**
   Sequence as the principal diagnosis the condition, which after study occasioned the admission to the hospital, even though treatment may not have been carried out due to unforeseen circumstances.

G. **Complications of surgery and other medical care**
   When the admission is for treatment of a complication resulting from surgery or other medical care, the complication code is sequenced as the principal diagnosis. If the complication is classified to the T80-T88 series and the code lacks the necessary specificity in describing the complication, an additional code for the specific complication should be assigned.

H. **Uncertain Diagnosis**
   If the diagnosis documented at the time of discharge is qualified as "probable," "suspected," "likely," "questionable," "possible," or "still to be ruled out," **"compatible with," "consistent with,"** or other similar terms indicating uncertainty, code the condition as if it existed or was established. The bases for these guidelines are the diagnostic workup, arrangements for further workup or observation, and initial therapeutic approach that correspond most closely with the established diagnosis.
   Note: This guideline is applicable only to inpatient admissions to short-term, acute, long-term care and psychiatric hospitals.

I. **Admission from Observation Unit**
   1. **Admission Following Medical Observation**
   When a patient is admitted to an observation unit for a medical condition, which either worsens or does not improve, and is subsequently admitted as an inpatient of the same hospital for this same medical condition, the principal diagnosis would be the medical condition which led to the hospital admission.
   2. **Admission Following Post-Operative Observation**
   When a patient is admitted to an observation unit to monitor a condition (or complication) that develops following outpatient surgery, and then is subsequently admitted as an inpatient of the same hospital, hospitals should apply the Uniform Hospital Discharge Data Set (UHDDS) definition of principal diagnosis as "that condition established after study to be chiefly responsible for occasioning the admission of the patient to the hospital for care."

J. **Admission from Outpatient Surgery**
   When a patient receives surgery in the hospital's outpatient surgery department and is subsequently admitted for continuing inpatient care at the

same hospital, the following guidelines should be followed in selecting the principal diagnosis for the inpatient admission:
- If the reason for the inpatient admission is a complication, assign the complication as the principal diagnosis.
- If no complication, or other condition, is documented as the reason for the inpatient admission, assign the reason for the outpatient surgery as the principal diagnosis.
- If the reason for the inpatient admission is another condition unrelated to the surgery, assign the unrelated condition as the principal diagnosis.

K. Admissions/Encounters for Rehabilitation

When the purpose for the admission/encounter is rehabilitation, sequence first the code for the condition for which the service is being performed. For example, for an admission/encounter for rehabilitation for right-sided dominant hemiplegia following a cerebrovascular infarction, report code I69.351, Hemiplegia and hemiparesis following cerebral infarction affecting right dominant side, as the first-listed or principal diagnosis.

If the condition for which the rehabilitation service is no longer present, report the appropriate aftercare code as the first-listed or principal diagnosis, unless the rehabilitation service is being provided following an injury. For rehabilitation services following active treatment of an injury, assign the injury code with the appropriate seventh character for subsequent encounter as the first-listed or principal diagnosis. For example, if a patient with severe degenerative osteoarthritis of the hip, underwent hip replacement and the current encounter/admission is for rehabilitation, report code Z47.1, Aftercare following joint replacement surgery, as the first-listed or principal diagnosis. If the patient requires rehabilitation post hip replacement for right intertrochanteric femur fracture, report code S72.141D, Displaced intertrochanteric fracture of right femur, subsequent encounter for closed fracture with routine healing, as the first-listed or principal diagnosis.

See Section I.C.21.c.7, Factors influencing health states and contact with health services, Aftercare.

See Section I.C.19.a for additional information about the use of 7th characters for injury codes.

Section III. Reporting Additional Diagnoses

GENERAL RULES FOR OTHER (ADDITIONAL) DIAGNOSES

For reporting purposes the definition for "other diagnoses" is interpreted as additional conditions that affect patient care in terms of requiring:

    clinical evaluation; or

    therapeutic treatment; or

    diagnostic procedures; or

    extended length of hospital stay; or

    increased nursing care and/or monitoring.

The UHDDS item #11-b defines Other Diagnoses as "all conditions that coexist at the time of admission, that develop subsequently, or that affect the treatment received and/or the length of stay. Diagnoses that relate to an earlier episode which have no bearing on the current hospital stay are to be excluded." UHDDS definitions apply to inpatients in acute care, short-term, long term care and psychiatric hospital setting. The UHDDS definitions are used by acute care short-term hospitals to report inpatient data elements in a standardized manner. These data elements and their definitions can be found in the July 31, 1985, Federal Register (Vol. 50, No, 147), pp. 31038-40.

Since that time the application of the UHDDS definitions has been expanded to include all nonoutpatient settings (acute care, short term, long term care and psychiatric hospitals; home health agencies; rehab facilities; nursing homes, etc.). The UHDDS definitions also apply to hospice services (all levels of care).

The following guidelines are to be applied in designating "other diagnoses" when neither the Alphabetic Index nor the Tabular List in ICD-10-CM provide direction. The listing of the diagnoses in the patient record is the responsibility of the attending provider.

A. Previous conditions

If the provider has included a diagnosis in the final diagnostic statement, such as the discharge summary or the face sheet, it should ordinarily be coded. Some providers include in the diagnostic statement resolved conditions or diagnoses and status-post procedures from previous admission that have no bearing on the current stay. Such conditions are not to be reported and are coded only if required by hospital policy.

However, history codes (categories Z80-Z87) may be used as secondary codes if the historical condition or family history has an impact on current care or influences treatment.

B. Abnormal findings

Abnormal findings (laboratory, x-ray, pathologic, and other diagnostic results) are not coded and reported unless the provider indicates their clinical significance. If the findings are outside the normal range and the attending provider has ordered other tests to evaluate the condition or prescribed treatment, it is appropriate to ask the provider whether the abnormal finding should be added.

Please note: This differs from the coding practices in the outpatient setting for coding encounters for diagnostic tests that have been interpreted by a provider.

C. Uncertain Diagnosis

If the diagnosis documented at the time of discharge is qualified as "probable," "suspected," "likely," "questionable," "possible," or "still to be ruled out," **"compatible with," "consistent with,"** or other similar terms indicating uncertainty, code the condition as if it existed or was established. The bases for these guidelines are the diagnostic workup, arrangements for further workup or observation, and initial therapeutic approach that correspond most closely with the established diagnosis.

Note: This guideline is applicable only to inpatient admissions to short-term, acute, long-term care and psychiatric hospitals.

Section IV. Diagnostic Coding and Reporting Guidelines for Outpatient Services

These coding guidelines for outpatient diagnoses have been approved for use by hospitals/ providers in coding and reporting hospital-based outpatient services and provider-based office visits. Guidelines in Section I, Conventions, general coding guidelines and chapter-specific guidelines, should also be applied for outpatient services and office visits.

Information about the use of certain abbreviations, punctuation, symbols, and other conventions used in the ICD-10-CM Tabular List (code numbers and titles), can be found in Section IA of these guidelines, under "Conventions Used in the Tabular List." Section I.B. contains general guidelines that apply to the entire classification. Section I.C. contains chapter-specific guidelines that correspond to the chapters as they are arranged in the classification. Information about the correct sequence to use in finding a code is also described in Section I.

The terms encounter and visit are often used interchangeably in describing outpatient service contacts and, therefore, appear together in these guidelines without distinguishing one from the other.

Though the conventions and general guidelines apply to all settings, coding guidelines for outpatient and provider reporting of diagnoses will vary in a number of instances from those for inpatient diagnoses, recognizing that:

The Uniform Hospital Discharge Data Set (UHDDS) definition of principal diagnosis does not apply to hospital-based outpatient services and provider-based office visits.

Coding guidelines for inconclusive diagnoses (probable, suspected, rule out, etc.) were developed for inpatient reporting and do not apply to outpatients.

A. Selection of first-listed condition

In the outpatient setting, the term first-listed diagnosis is used in lieu of principal diagnosis.

In determining the first-listed diagnosis the coding conventions of ICD-10-CM, as well as the general and disease specific guidelines take precedence over the outpatient guidelines.

Diagnoses often are not established at the time of the initial encounter/visit. It may take two or more visits before the diagnosis is confirmed.

The most critical rule involves beginning the search for the correct code assignment through the Alphabetic Index. Never begin searching initially in the Tabular List as this will lead to coding errors.

1. Outpatient Surgery

When a patient presents for outpatient surgery (same day surgery), code the reason for the surgery as the first-listed diagnosis (reason for the encounter), even if the surgery is not performed due to a contraindication.

2. Observation Stay

When a patient is admitted for observation for a medical condition, assign a code for the medical condition as the first-listed diagnosis.

When a patient presents for outpatient surgery and develops complications requiring admission to observation, code the reason for the surgery as the first reported diagnosis (reason for the encounter), followed by codes for the complications as secondary diagnoses.

B. Codes from A00.0 through T88.9, Z00-Z99

The appropriate code(s) from A00.0 through T88.9, Z00-Z99 must be used to identify diagnoses, symptoms, conditions, problems, complaints, or other reason(s) for the encounter/visit.

C. Accurate reporting of ICD-10-CM diagnosis codes

For accurate reporting of ICD-10-CM diagnosis codes, the documentation should describe the patient's condition, using terminology which includes specific diagnoses as well as symptoms, problems, or reasons for the encounter. There are ICD-10-CM codes to describe all of these.

D. Codes that describe symptoms and signs

Codes that describe symptoms and signs, as opposed to diagnoses, are acceptable for reporting purposes when a diagnosis has not been established (confirmed) by the provider. Chapter 18 of ICD-10-CM, Symptoms, Signs, and Abnormal Clinical and Laboratory Findings Not Elsewhere Classified (codes R00-R99) contains many, but not all codes for symptoms.

E. Encounters for circumstances other than a disease or injury

ICD-10-CM provides codes to deal with encounters for circumstances other than a disease or injury. The Factors Influencing Health Status and Contact with Health Services codes (Z00-Z99) are provided to deal with occasions when circumstances other than a disease or injury are recorded as diagnosis or problems.

See Section I.C.21., Factors influencing health status and contact with health services.

F. Level of Detail in Coding

1. ICD-10-CM codes with 3, 4, 5, 6 or 7 characters

ICD-10-CM is composed of codes with 3, 4, 5, 6 or 7 characters. Codes with three characters are included in ICD-10-CM as the heading of a category of codes that may be further subdivided by the use of 4th, 5th, 6th or 7th characters to provide greater specificity.

2. Use of full number of characters required for a code

A 3-character code is to be used only if it is not further subdivided. A code is invalid if it has not been coded to the full number of characters required for that code, including the 7th character, if applicable.

G. ICD-10-CM code for the diagnosis, condition, problem, or other reason for encounter/visit

List first the ICD-10-CM code for the diagnosis, condition, problem, or other reason for encounter/visit shown in the medical record to be chiefly responsible for the services provided. List additional codes that describe any coexisting conditions. In some cases the first-listed diagnosis may be a symptom when a diagnosis has not been established (confirmed) by the **provider**.

H. Uncertain diagnosis
Do not code diagnoses documented as "probable," "suspected," "questionable," "ruled out," **"compatible with," "consistent with,"** or "working diagnosis" or other similar terms indicating uncertainty. Rather, code the condition(s) to the highest degree of certainty for that encounter/visit, such as symptoms, signs, abnormal test results, or other reason for the visit.

Please note: This differs from the coding practices used by short-term, acute care, long-term care and psychiatric hospitals.

I. Chronic diseases
Chronic diseases treated on an ongoing basis may be coded and reported as many times as the patient receives treatment and care for the condition(s)

J. Code all documented conditions that coexist
Code all documented conditions that coexist at the time of the encounter/visit, and require or affect patient care treatment or management. Do not code conditions that were previously treated and no longer exist. However, history codes (categories Z8Ø-Z87) may be used as secondary codes if the historical condition or family history has an impact on current care or influences treatment.

K. Patients receiving diagnostic services only
For patients receiving diagnostic services only during an encounter/visit, sequence first the diagnosis, condition, problem, or other reason for encounter/visit shown in the medical record to be chiefly responsible for the outpatient services provided during the encounter/visit. Codes for other diagnoses (e.g., chronic conditions) may be sequenced as additional diagnoses.

For encounters for routine laboratory/radiology testing in the absence of any signs, symptoms, or associated diagnosis, assign ZØ1.89, Encounter for other specified special examinations. If routine testing is performed during the same encounter as a test to evaluate a sign, symptom, or diagnosis, it is appropriate to assign both the Z code and the code describing the reason for the non-routine test.

For outpatient encounters for diagnostic tests that have been interpreted by a physician, and the final report is available at the time of coding, code any confirmed or definitive diagnosis(es) documented in the interpretation. Do not code related signs and symptoms as additional diagnoses.

Please note: This differs from the coding practice in the hospital inpatient setting regarding abnormal findings on test results.

L. Patients receiving therapeutic services only
For patients receiving therapeutic services only during an encounter/visit, sequence first the diagnosis, condition, problem, or other reason for encounter/visit shown in the medical record to be chiefly responsible for the outpatient services provided during the encounter/visit. Codes for other diagnoses (e.g., chronic conditions) may be sequenced as additional diagnoses.

The only exception to this rule is that when the primary reason for the admission/encounter is chemotherapy or radiation therapy, the appropriate Z code for the service is listed first, and the diagnosis or problem for which the service is being performed listed second.

M. Patients receiving preoperative evaluations only
For patients receiving preoperative evaluations only, sequence first a code from subcategory ZØ1.81, Encounter for pre-procedural examinations, to describe the pre-op consultations. Assign a code for the condition to describe the reason for the surgery as an additional diagnosis. Code also any findings related to the pre-op evaluation.

N. Ambulatory surgery
For ambulatory surgery, code the diagnosis for which the surgery was performed. If the postoperative diagnosis is known to be different from the preoperative diagnosis at the time the diagnosis is confirmed, select the postoperative diagnosis for coding, since it is the most definitive.

O. Routine outpatient prenatal visits
See Section I.C.15., Routine outpatient prenatal visits.

P. Encounters for general medical examinations with abnormal findings
The subcategories for encounters for general medical examinations, ZØØ.Ø- and encounter for routine child health examination, ZØØ.12-, provide codes for with and without abnormal findings. Should a general medical examination result in an abnormal finding, the code for general medical examination with abnormal finding should be assigned as the first-listed diagnosis. An examination with abnormal findings refers to a condition/diagnosis that is newly identified or a change in severity of a chronic condition (such as uncontrolled hypertension, or an acute exacerbation of chronic obstructive pulmonary disease) during a routine physical examination. A secondary code for the abnormal finding should also be coded.

Q. Encounters for routine health screenings
See Section I.C.21., Factors influencing health status and contact with health services, Screening

Appendix I
Present on Admission Reporting Guidelines

Introduction

These guidelines are to be used as a supplement to the *ICD-10-CM Official Guidelines for Coding and Reporting* to facilitate the assignment of the Present on Admission (POA) indicator for each diagnosis and external cause of injury code reported on claim forms (UB-04 and 837 Institutional).

These guidelines are not intended to replace any guidelines in the main body of the *ICD-10-CM Official Guidelines for Coding and Reporting*. The POA guidelines are not intended to provide guidance on when a condition should be coded, but rather, how to apply the POA indicator to the final set of diagnosis codes that have been assigned in accordance with Sections I, II, and III of the official coding guidelines. Subsequent to the assignment of the ICD-10-CM codes, the POA indicator should then be assigned to those conditions that have been coded.

As stated in the Introduction to the ICD-10-CM Official Guidelines for Coding and Reporting, a joint effort between the healthcare provider and the coder is essential to achieve complete and accurate documentation, code assignment, and reporting of diagnoses and procedures. The importance of consistent, complete documentation in the medical record cannot be overemphasized. Medical record documentation from any provider involved in the care and treatment of the patient may be used to support the determination of whether a condition was present on admission or not. In the context of the official coding guidelines, the term "provider" means a physician or any qualified healthcare practitioner who is legally accountable for establishing the patient's diagnosis.

These guidelines are not a substitute for the provider's clinical judgment as to the determination of whether a condition was/was not present on admission. The provider should be queried regarding issues related to the linking of signs/symptoms, timing of test results, and the timing of findings.

Please see the CDC website for the detailed list of ICD-10-CM codes that do not require the use of a POA indicator (https://www.cdc.gov/nchs/icd/icd10cm.htm) (https://www.cms.gov/Medicare/Coding/ICD10/2018-ICD-10-CM-and-GEMs.html). The codes and categories on this exempt list are for circumstances regarding the healthcare encounter or factors influencing health status that do not represent a current disease or injury or that describe conditions that are always present on admission.

General Reporting Requirements

All claims involving inpatient admissions to general acute care hospitals or other facilities that are subject to a law or regulation mandating collection of present on admission information.

Present on admission is defined as present at the time the order for inpatient admission occurs—conditions that develop during an outpatient encounter, including emergency department, observation, or outpatient surgery, are considered as present on admission.

POA indicator is assigned to principal and secondary diagnoses (as defined in Section II of the Official Guidelines for Coding and Reporting) and the external cause of injury codes.

Issues related to inconsistent, missing, conflicting or unclear documentation must still be resolved by the provider.

If a condition would not be coded and reported based on UHDDS definitions and current official coding guidelines, then the POA indicator would not be reported.

Reporting Options

Y - Yes

N - No

U - Unknown

W - Clinically undetermined

Unreported/Not used - (Exempt from POA reporting)

Reporting Definitions

Y = present at the time of inpatient admission

N = not present at the time of inpatient admission

U = documentation is insufficient to determine if condition is present on admission

W = provider is unable to clinically determine whether condition was present on admission or not

Timeframe for POA Identification and Documentation

There is no required timeframe as to when a provider (per the definition of "provider" used in these guidelines) must identify or document a condition to be present on admission. In some clinical situations, it may not be possible for a provider to make a definitive diagnosis (or a condition may not be recognized or reported by the patient) for a period of time after admission. In some cases it may be several days before the provider arrives at a definitive diagnosis. This does not mean that the condition was not present on admission. Determination of whether the condition was present on admission or not will be based on the applicable POA guideline as identified in this document, or on the provider's best clinical judgment.

If at the time of code assignment the documentation is unclear as to whether a condition was present on admission or not, it is appropriate to query the provider for clarification.

Assigning the POA Indicator

Condition is on the "Exempt from Reporting" list

Leave the "present on admission" field blank if the condition is on the list of ICD-10-CM codes for which this field is not applicable. This is the only circumstance in which the field may be left blank.

POA Explicitly Documented

Assign "Y" for any condition the provider explicitly documents as being present on admission.

Assign "N" for any condition the provider explicitly documents as not present at the time of admission.

Conditions diagnosed prior to inpatient admission

Assign "Y" for conditions that were diagnosed prior to admission (example: hypertension, diabetes mellitus, asthma)

Conditions diagnosed during the admission but clearly present before admission

Assign "Y" for conditions diagnosed during the admission that were clearly present but not diagnosed until after admission occurred.

Diagnoses subsequently confirmed after admission are considered present on admission if at the time of admission they are documented as suspected, possible, rule out, differential diagnosis, or constitute an underlying cause of a symptom that is present at the time of admission.

Condition develops during outpatient encounter prior to inpatient admission

Assign "Y" for any condition that develops during an outpatient encounter prior to a written order for inpatient admission.

Documentation does not indicate whether condition was present on admission

Assign "U" when the medical record documentation is unclear as to whether the condition was present on admission. "U" should not be routinely assigned and used only in very limited circumstances. Coders are encouraged to query the providers when the documentation is unclear.

Documentation states that it cannot be determined whether the condition was or was not present on admission

Assign "W" when the medical record documentation indicates that it cannot be clinically determined whether or not the condition was present on admission.

Chronic condition with acute exacerbation during the admission

If a single code identifies both the chronic condition and the acute exacerbation, see POA guidelines pertaining to codes that contain multiple clinical concepts.

If a single code only identifies the chronic condition and not the acute exacerbation (e.g., acute exacerbation of chronic leukemia), assign "Y."

Conditions documented as possible, probable, suspected, or rule out at the time of discharge

If the final diagnosis contains a possible, probable, suspected, or rule out diagnosis, and this diagnosis was based on signs, symptoms or clinical findings suspected at the time of inpatient admission, assign "Y."

If the final diagnosis contains a possible, probable, suspected, or rule out diagnosis, and this diagnosis was based on signs, symptoms or clinical findings that were not present on admission, assign "N".

Conditions documented as impending or threatened at the time of discharge

If the final diagnosis contains an impending or threatened diagnosis, and this diagnosis is based on symptoms or clinical findings that were present on admission, assign "Y".

If the final diagnosis contains an impending or threatened diagnosis, and this diagnosis is based on symptoms or clinical findings that were not present on admission, assign "N".

Acute and Chronic Conditions

Assign "Y" for acute conditions that are present at time of admission and "N" for acute conditions that are not present at time of admission.

Assign "Y" for chronic conditions, even though the condition may not be diagnosed until after admission.

If a single code identifies both an acute and chronic condition, see the POA guidelines for codes that contain multiple clinical concepts.

Codes That Contain Multiple Clinical Concepts

Assign "N" if at least one of the clinical concepts included in the code was not present on admission (e.g., COPD with acute exacerbation and the exacerbation was not present on admission; gastric ulcer that does not start bleeding until after admission; asthma patient develops status asthmaticus after admission).

Assign "Y" if all of the clinical concepts included in the code were present on admission (e.g., duodenal ulcer that perforates prior to admission).

For infection codes that include the causal organism, assign "Y" if the infection (or signs of the infection) were present on admission, even though the culture results may not be known until after admission (e.g., patient is admitted with pneumonia and the provider documents Pseudomonas as the causal organism a few days later).

Same Diagnosis Code for Two or More Conditions

When the same ICD-10-CM diagnosis code applies to two or more conditions during the same encounter (e.g., two separate conditions classified to the same ICD-10-CM diagnosis code):

Assign "Y" if all conditions represented by the single ICD-10-CM code were present on admission (e.g., bilateral unspecified age-related cataracts).

Assign "N" if any of the conditions represented by the single ICD-10-CM code was not present on admission (e.g., traumatic secondary and recurrent hemorrhage and seroma is assigned to a single code T79.2, but only one of the conditions was present on admission).

Obstetrical conditions

Whether or not the patient delivers during the current hospitalization does not affect assignment of the POA indicator. The determining factor for POA assignment is whether the pregnancy complication or obstetrical condition described by the code was present at the time of admission or not.

If the pregnancy complication or obstetrical condition was present on admission (e.g., patient admitted in preterm labor), assign "Y".

If the pregnancy complication or obstetrical condition was not present on admission (e.g., 2nd degree laceration during delivery, postpartum hemorrhage that occurred during current hospitalization, fetal distress develops after admission), assign "N".

If the obstetrical code includes more than one diagnosis and any of the diagnoses identified by the code were not present on admission assign "N".

(e.g., Category O11, Pre-existing hypertension with pre-eclampsia)

Perinatal conditions

Newborns are not considered to be admitted until after birth. Therefore, any condition present at birth or that developed in utero is considered present at admission and should be assigned "Y". This includes conditions that occur during delivery (e.g., injury during delivery, meconium aspiration, exposure to streptococcus B in the vaginal canal).

Congenital conditions and anomalies

Assign "Y" for congenital conditions and anomalies except for categories QØØ-Q99, Congenital anomalies, which are on the exempt list. Congenital conditions are always considered present on admission.

External cause of injury codes

Assign "Y" for any external cause code representing an external cause of morbidity that occurred prior to inpatient admission (e.g., patient fell out of bed at home, patient fell out of bed in emergency room prior to admission).

Assign "N" for any external cause code representing an external cause of morbidity that occurred during inpatient hospitalization (e.g., patient fell out of hospital bed during hospital stay, patient experienced an adverse reaction to a medication administered after inpatient admission).

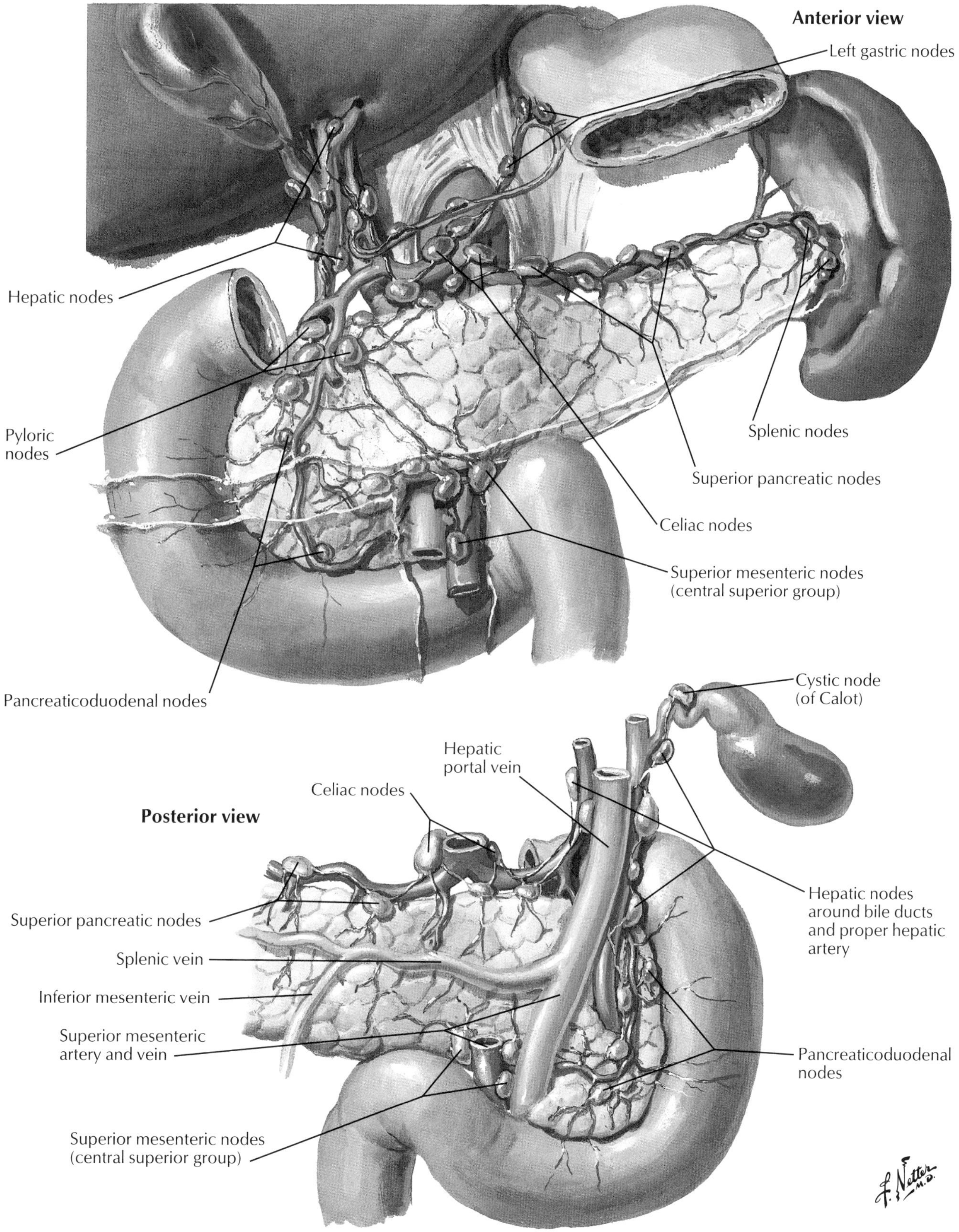

Plate 1 Lymph Vessels and Nodes of Pancreas. (Netter: Atlas of Human Anatomy, 4 ed, 2006, Saunders. Plate 315)

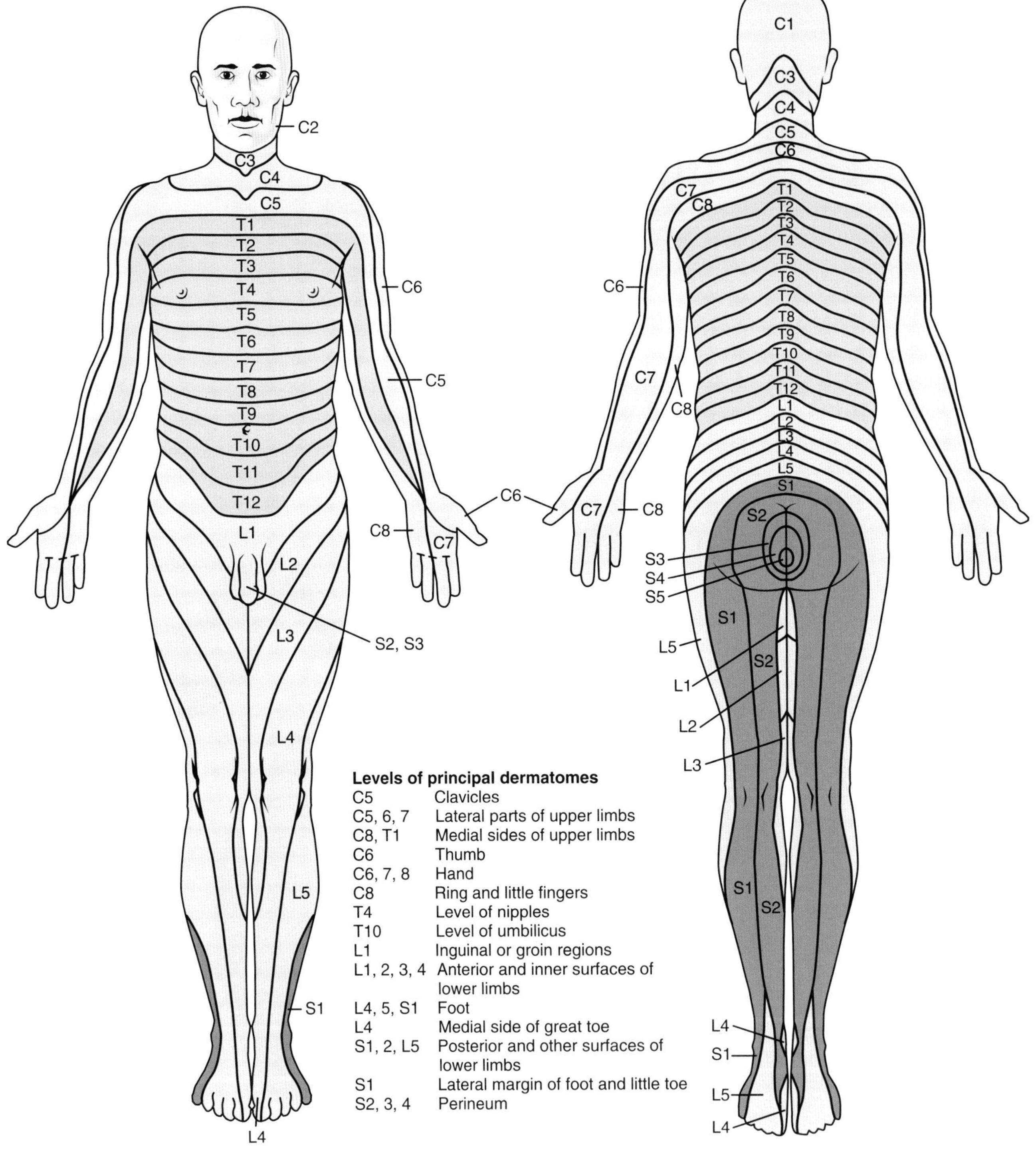

Levels of principal dermatomes

C5	Clavicles
C5, 6, 7	Lateral parts of upper limbs
C8, T1	Medial sides of upper limbs
C6	Thumb
C6, 7, 8	Hand
C8	Ring and little fingers
T4	Level of nipples
T10	Level of umbilicus
L1	Inguinal or groin regions
L1, 2, 3, 4	Anterior and inner surfaces of lower limbs
L4, 5, S1	Foot
L4	Medial side of great toe
S1, 2, L5	Posterior and other surfaces of lower limbs
S1	Lateral margin of foot and little toe
S2, 3, 4	Perineum

Plate 2 Schematic demarcation of Dermatomes. (Miller MD, Hart JA, MacKnight JM: Essential Orthopaedics, ed 2, Philadelphia, 2020, Elsevier.)

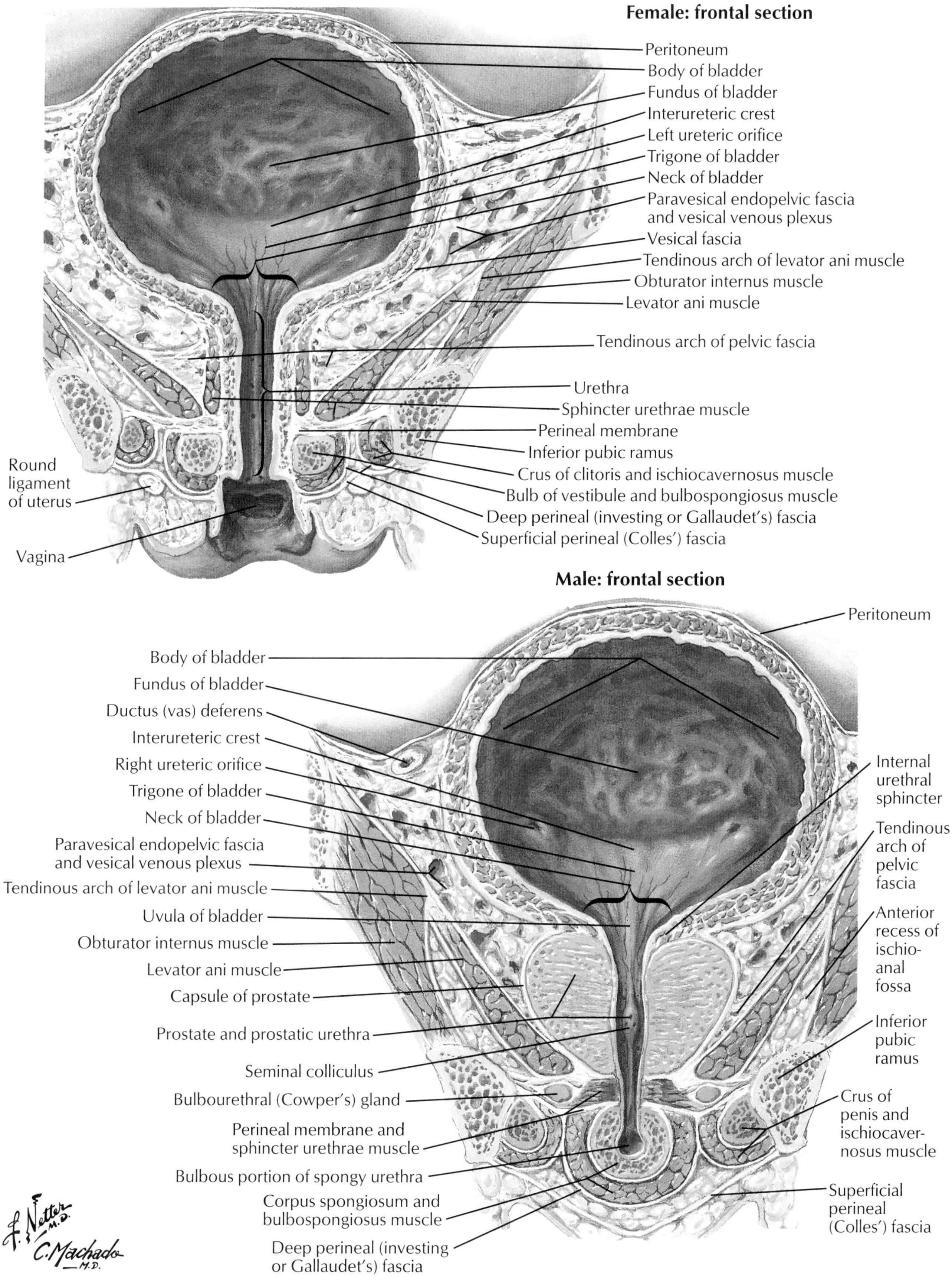
Female: frontal section
Peritoneum
Body of bladder
Fundus of bladder
Interureteric crest
Left ureteric orifice
Trigone of bladder
Neck of bladder
Paravesical endopelvic fascia and vesical venous plexus
Vesical fascia
Tendinous arch of levator ani muscle
Obturator internus muscle
Levator ani muscle
Tendinous arch of pelvic fascia
Urethra
Sphincter urethrae muscle
Perineal membrane
Inferior pubic ramus
Crus of clitoris and ischiocavernosus muscle
Bulb of vestibule and bulbospongiosus muscle
Deep perineal (investing or Gallaudet's) fascia
Superficial perineal (Colles') fascia
Round ligament of uterus
Vagina
Male: frontal section
Peritoneum
Body of bladder
Fundus of bladder
Ductus (vas) deferens
Interureteric crest
Right ureteric orifice
Trigone of bladder
Neck of bladder
Paravesical endopelvic fascia and vesical venous plexus
Tendinous arch of levator ani muscle
Uvula of bladder
Obturator internus muscle
Levator ani muscle
Capsule of prostate
Prostate and prostatic urethra
Seminal colliculus
Bulbourethral (Cowper's) gland
Perineal membrane and sphincter urethrae muscle
Bulbous portion of spongy urethra
Corpus spongiosum and bulbospongiosus muscle
Deep perineal (investing or Gallaudet's) fascia
Internal urethral sphincter
Tendinous arch of pelvic fascia
Anterior recess of ischio-anal fossa
Inferior pubic ramus
Crus of penis and ischiocavernosus muscle
Superficial perineal (Colles') fascia
F. Netter M.D.
C. Machado M.D.

Plate 3 Urinary Bladder: Female and Male. (Netter: Atlas of Human Anatomy, 4 ed, 2006, Saunders. Plate 366.)

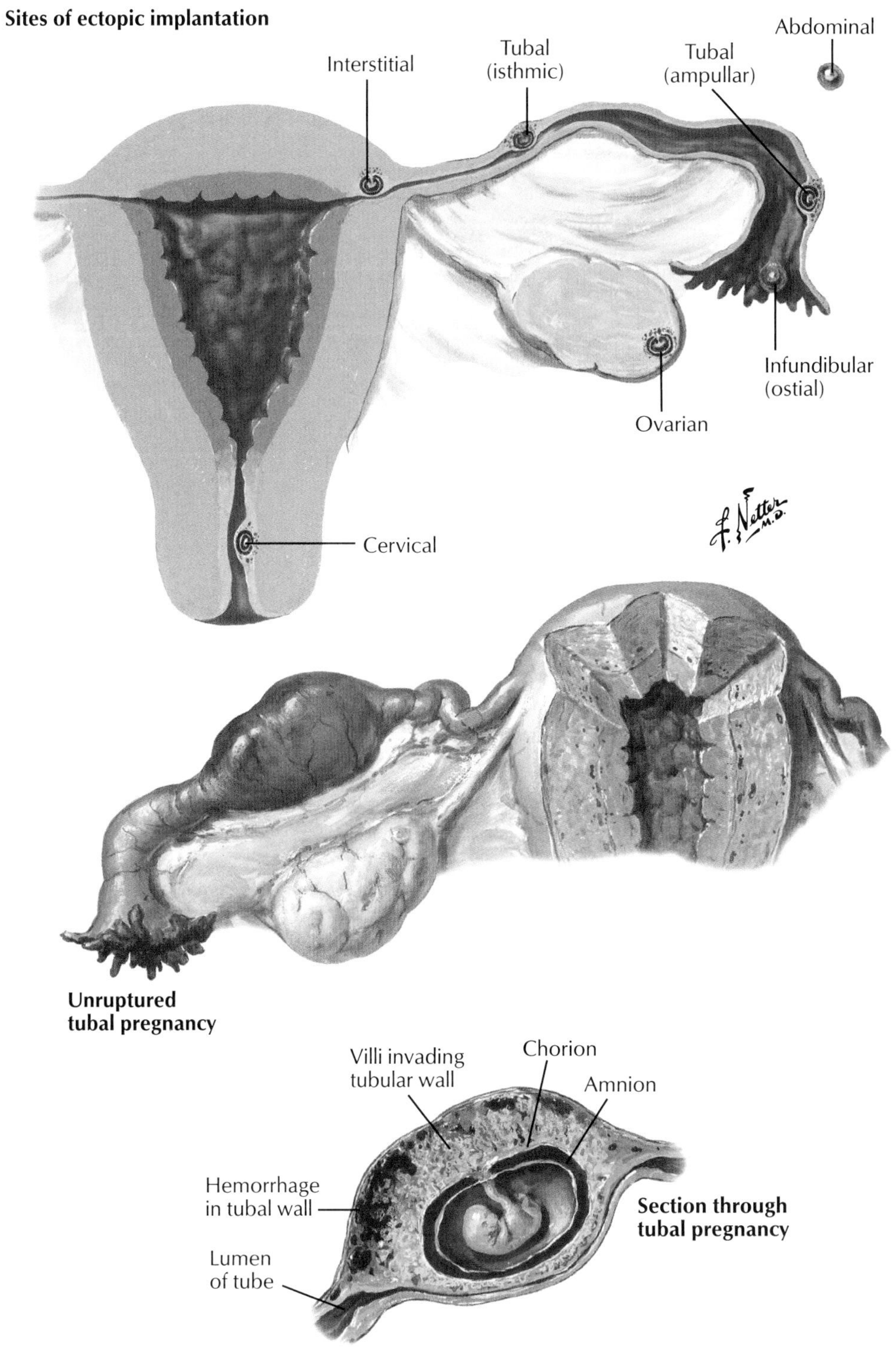

Plate 4 Ectopic Pregnancy. (Netter: Atlas of Human Anatomy, 4 ed, 2006, Saunders. Plate 375)

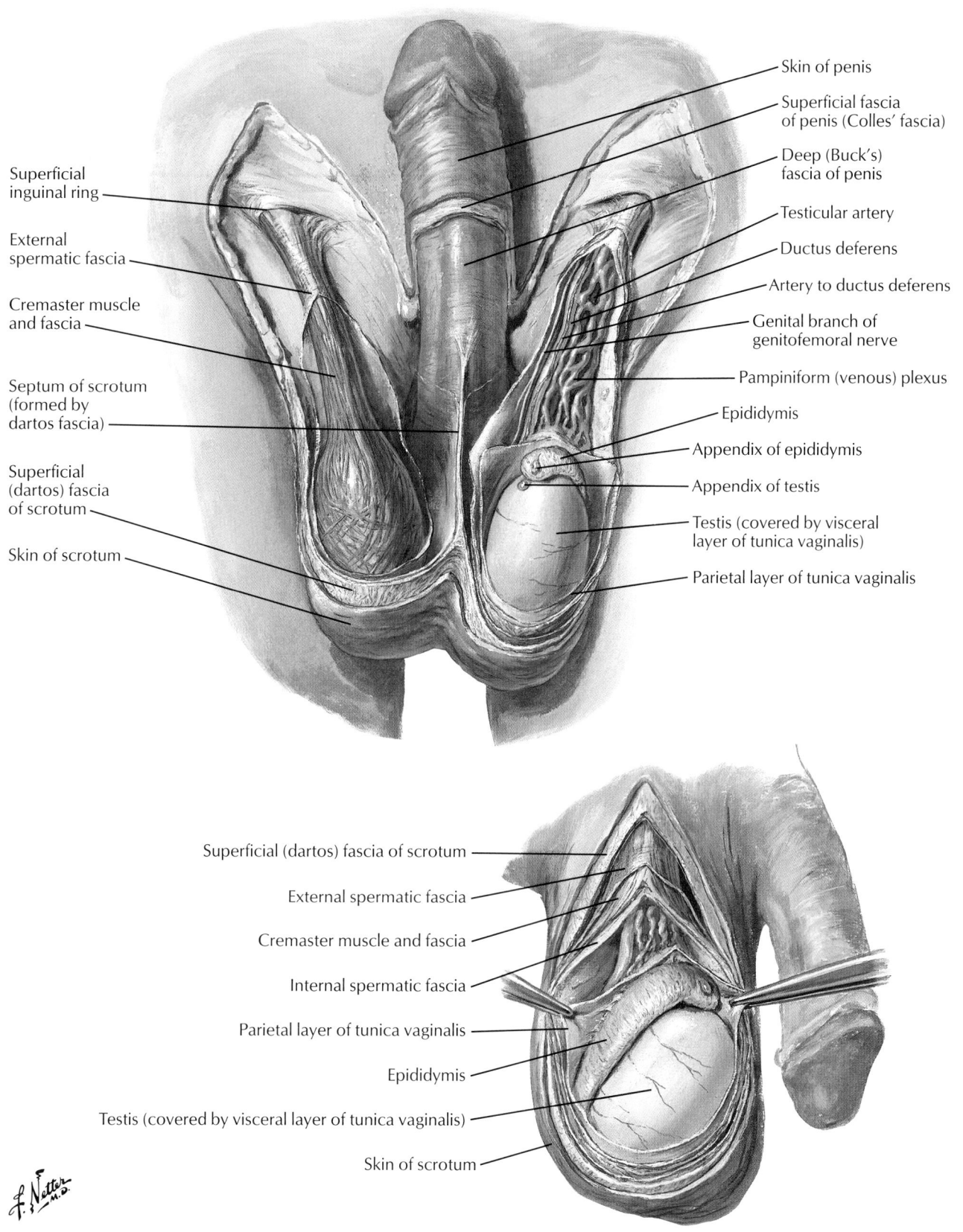

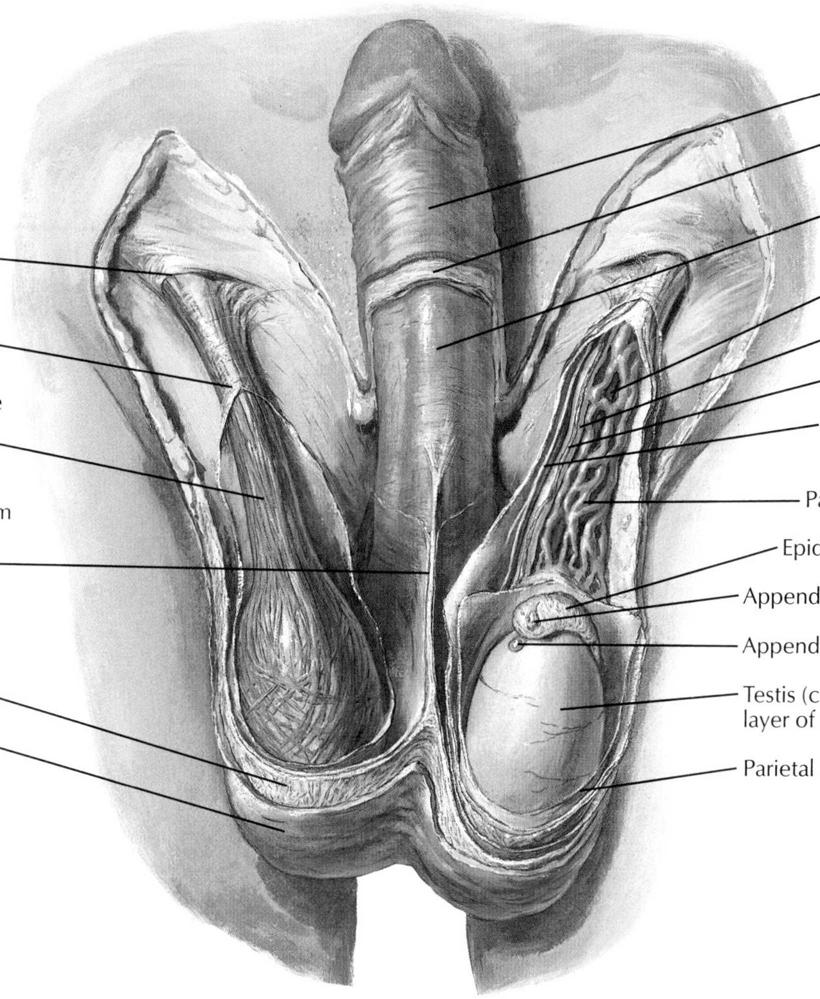
Skin of penis
Superficial fascia of penis (Colles' fascia)
Deep (Buck's) fascia of penis
Testicular artery
Ductus deferens
Artery to ductus deferens
Genital branch of genitofemoral nerve
Pampiniform (venous) plexus
Epididymis
Appendix of epididymis
Appendix of testis
Testis (covered by visceral layer of tunica vaginalis)
Parietal layer of tunica vaginalis
Superficial inguinal ring
External spermatic fascia
Cremaster muscle and fascia
Septum of scrotum (formed by dartos fascia)
Superficial (dartos) fascia of scrotum
Skin of scrotum

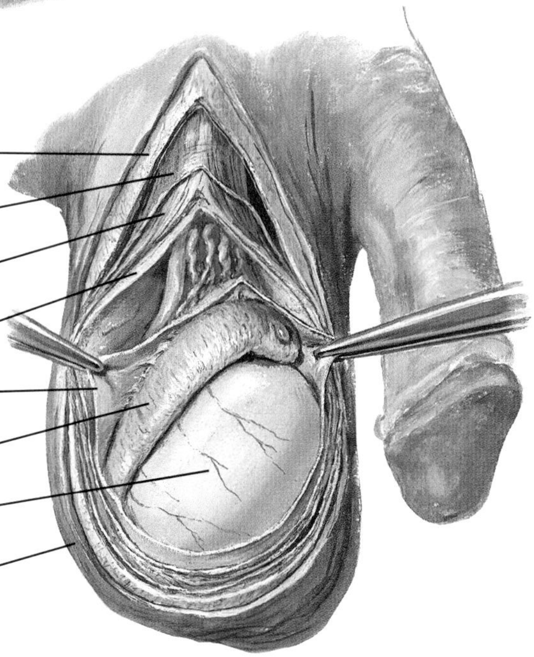
Superficial (dartos) fascia of scrotum
External spermatic fascia
Cremaster muscle and fascia
Internal spermatic fascia
Parietal layer of tunica vaginalis
Epididymis
Testis (covered by visceral layer of tunica vaginalis)
Skin of scrotum
F. Netter M.D.

Plate 5 Scrotum and Contents. (Netter: Atlas of Human Anatomy, 4 ed, 2006, Saunders. Plate 387)

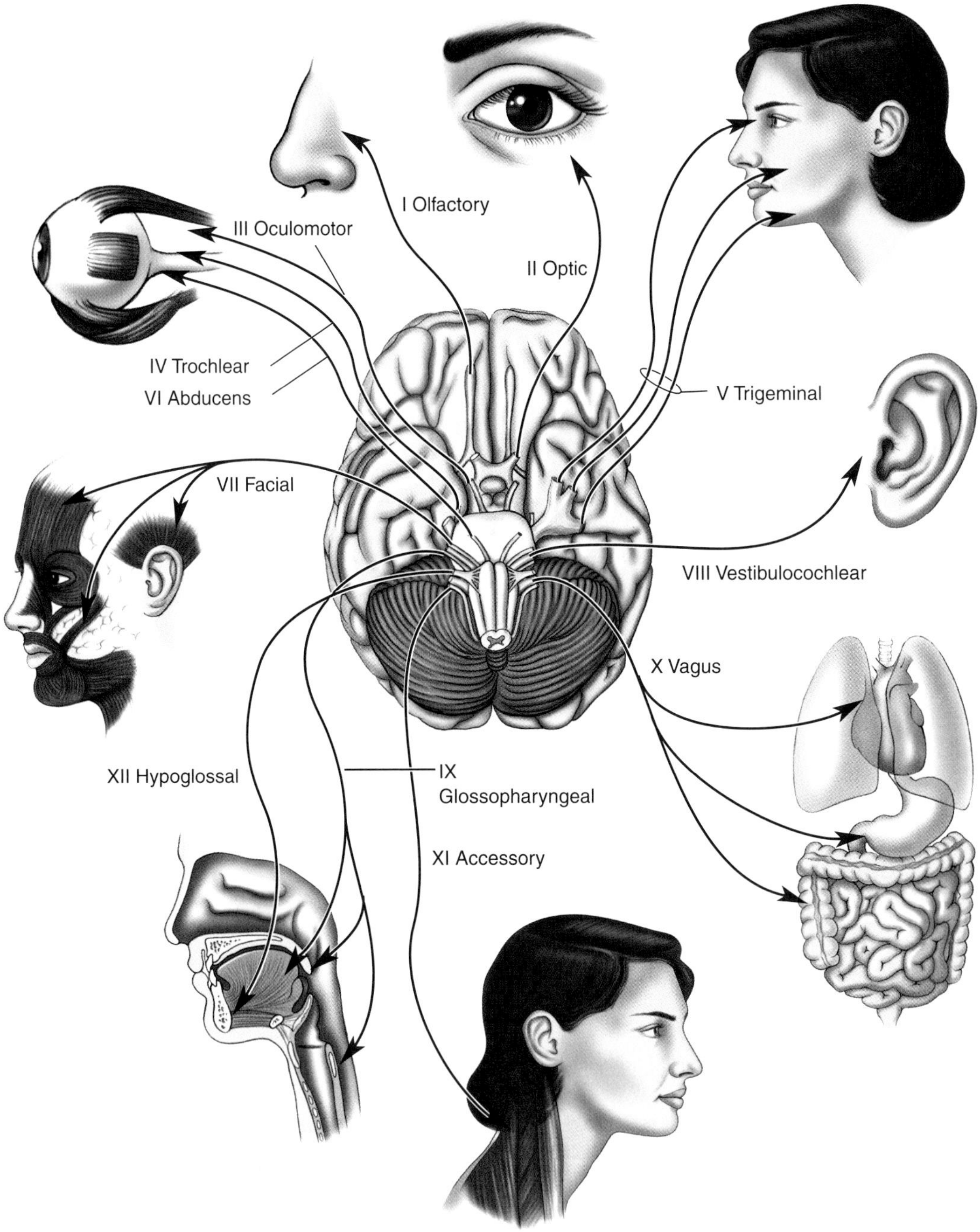

Plate 6 Cranial Nerves (12 pairs) are known by their numbers (Roman numerals) and names. (Herlihy BL: The Human Body in Health and Illness, ed 6, St. Louis, 2018, Elsevier.)

Superior view

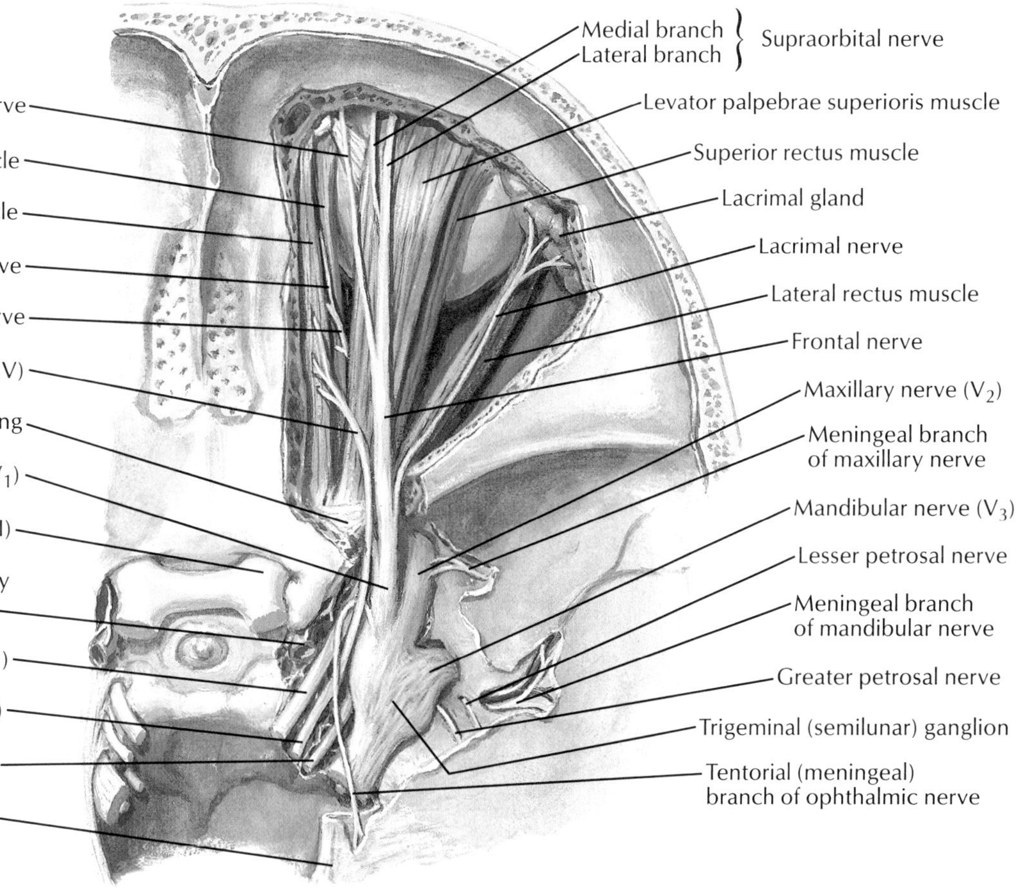

Superior view:
levator palpebrae superioris, superior rectus, and superior oblique muscles partially cut away

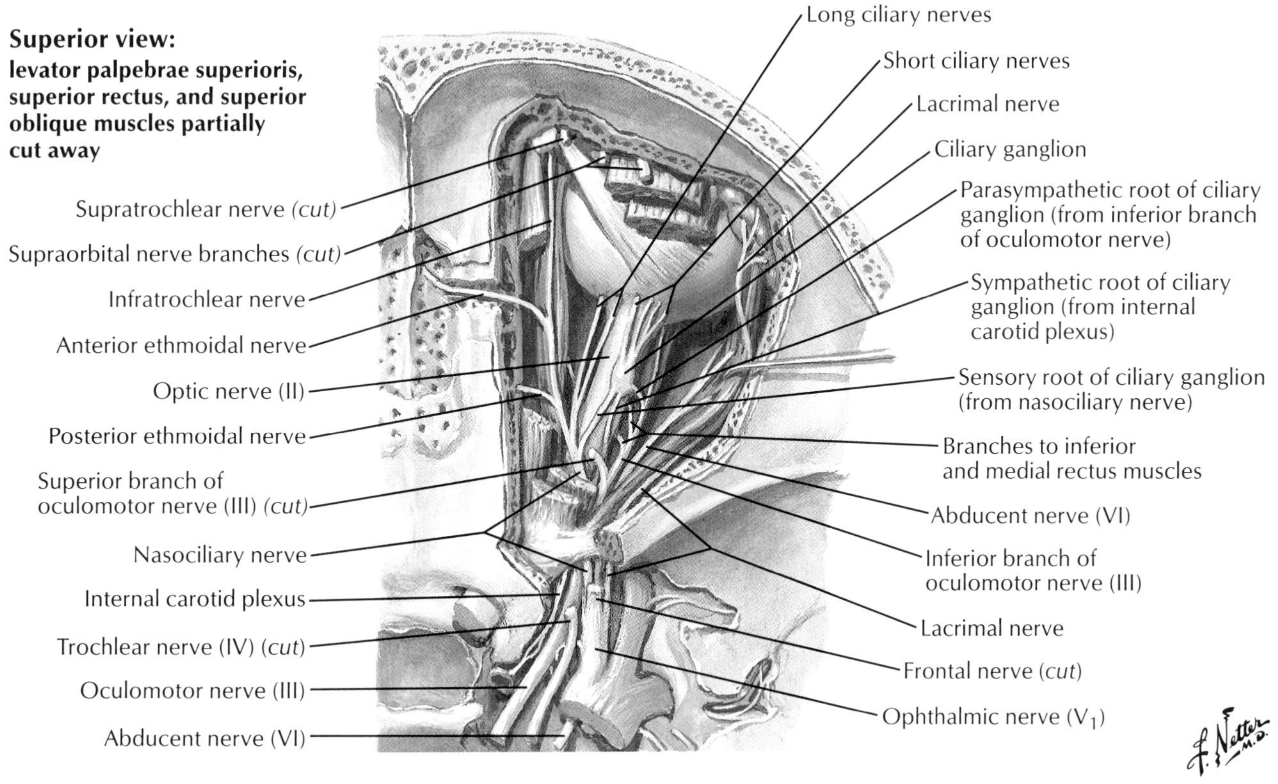

Plate 7 Nerves of Orbit. (Netter: Atlas of Human Anatomy, 4 ed, 2006, Saunders. Plate 86)

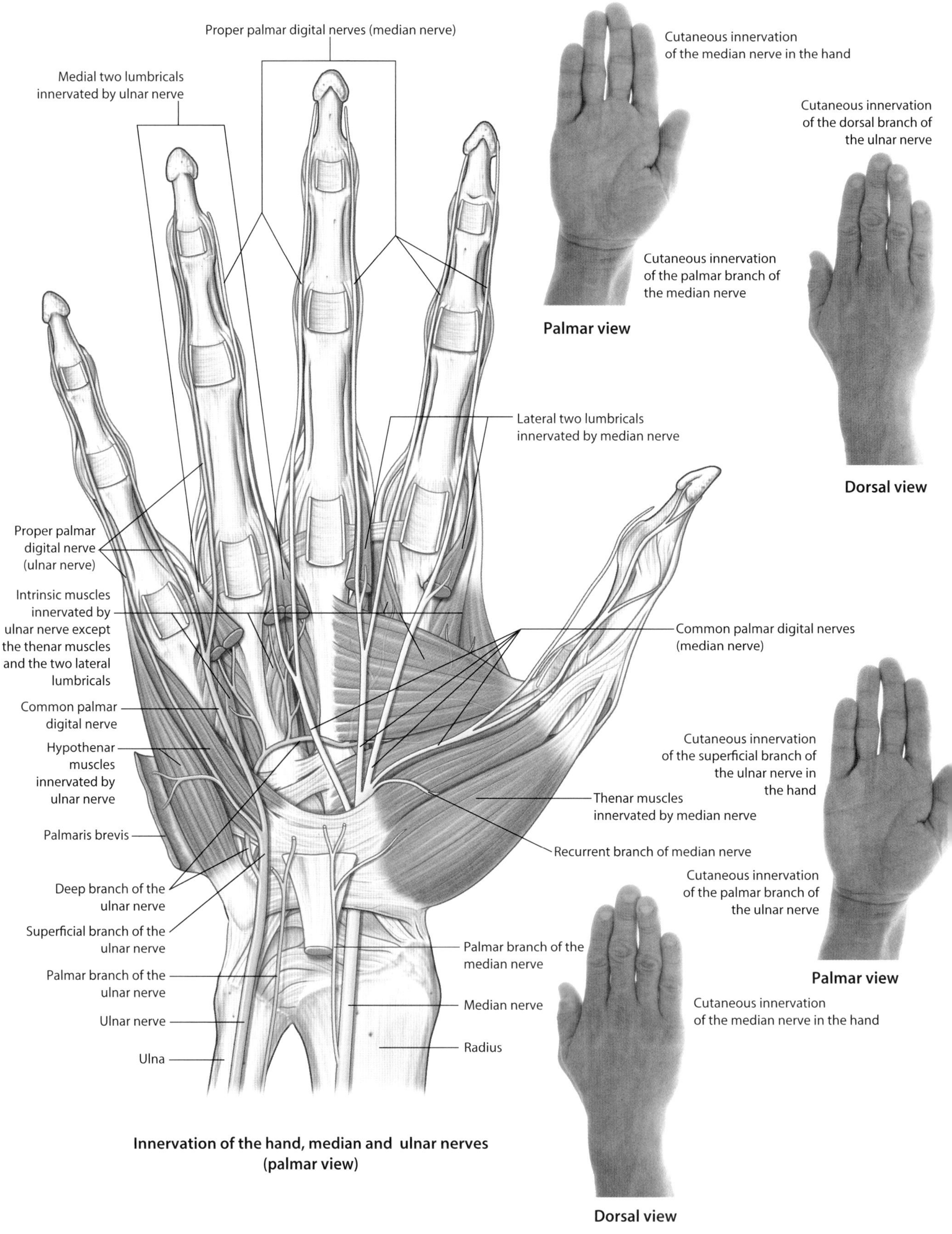

Plate 8 Innervation of the Hand: Median and Ulnar Nerves (From Drake RL, Vogl AW, Mitchell AWM, Tibbitts RM, Richardson PE: Gray's Atlas of Anatomy, ed 2, Philadelphia, 2015, Churchill Livingstone.)

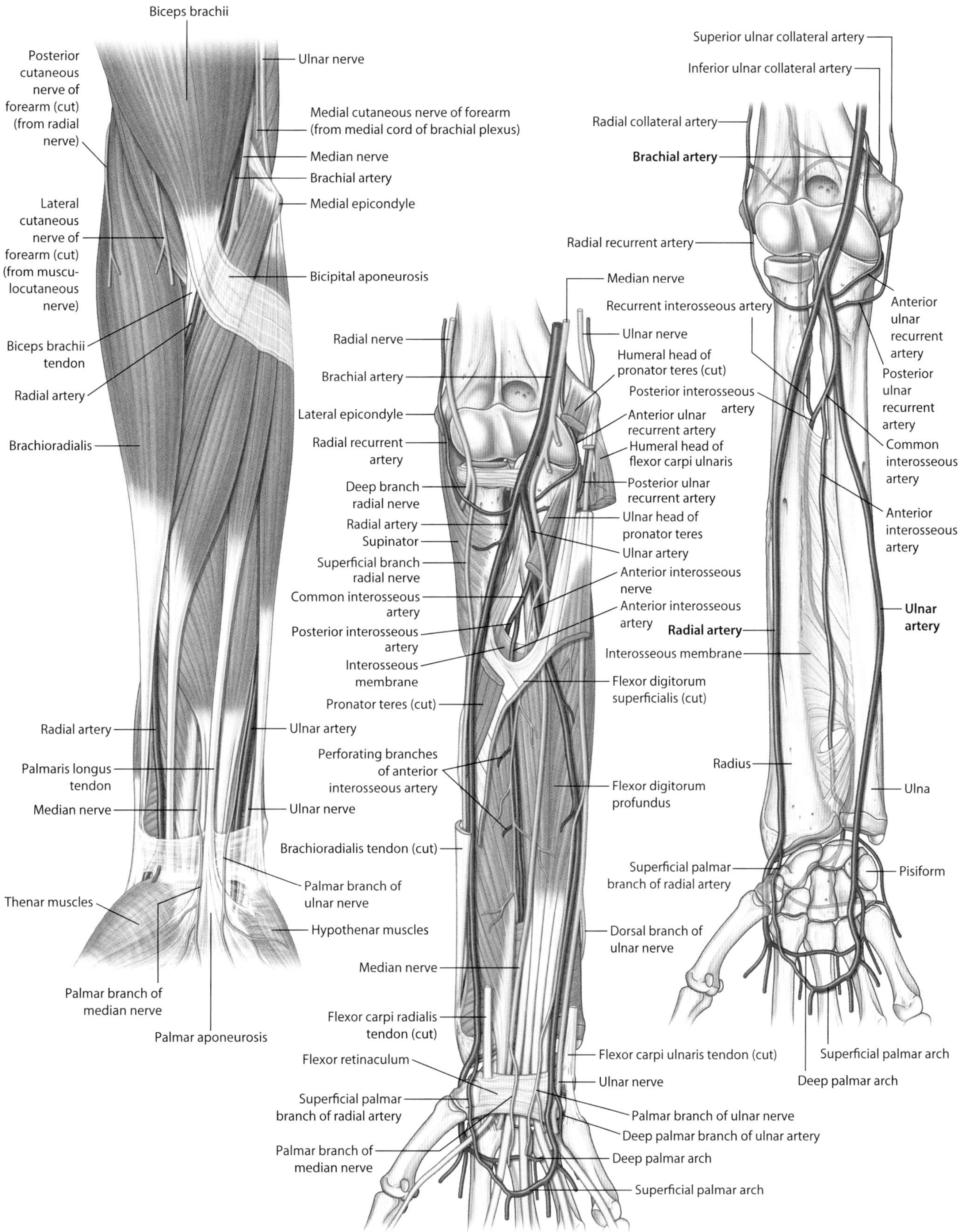

Arteries and nerves of forearm (anterior view)

Plate 9 Arteries and Nerves of the Forearm (Anterior View) (From Drake RL, Vogl AW, Mitchell AWM, Tibbitts RM, Richardson PE: Gray's Atlas of Anatomy, ed 2, Philadelphia, 2015, Churchill Livingstone.)

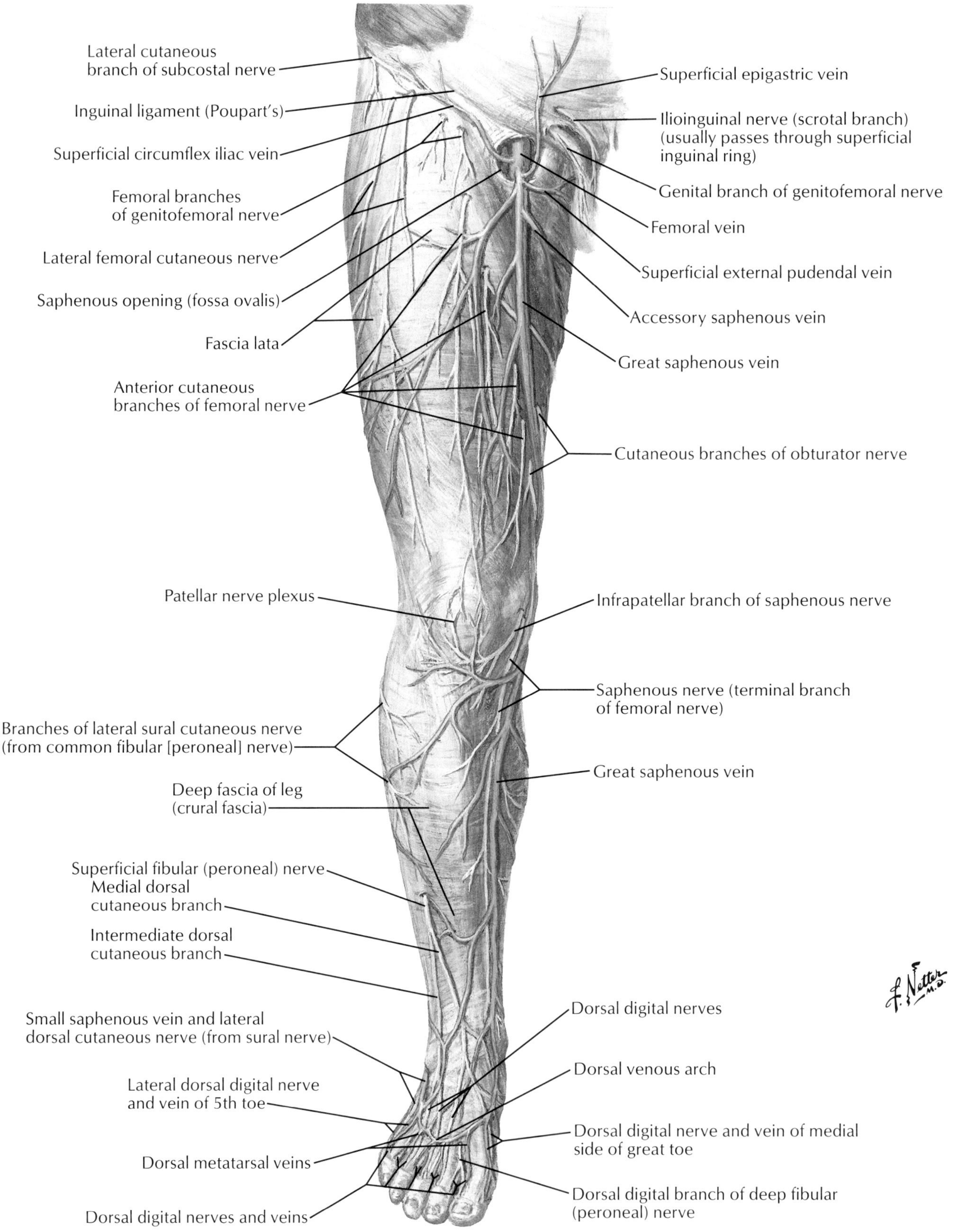
Lateral cutaneous branch of subcostal nerve
Inguinal ligament (Poupart's)
Superficial circumflex iliac vein
Femoral branches of genitofemoral nerve
Lateral femoral cutaneous nerve
Saphenous opening (fossa ovalis)
Fascia lata
Anterior cutaneous branches of femoral nerve
Superficial epigastric vein
Ilioinguinal nerve (scrotal branch) (usually passes through superficial inguinal ring)
Genital branch of genitofemoral nerve
Femoral vein
Superficial external pudendal vein
Accessory saphenous vein
Great saphenous vein
Cutaneous branches of obturator nerve
Patellar nerve plexus
Infrapatellar branch of saphenous nerve
Saphenous nerve (terminal branch of femoral nerve)
Branches of lateral sural cutaneous nerve (from common fibular [peroneal] nerve)
Great saphenous vein
Deep fascia of leg (crural fascia)
Superficial fibular (peroneal) nerve
Medial dorsal cutaneous branch
Intermediate dorsal cutaneous branch
Small saphenous vein and lateral dorsal cutaneous nerve (from sural nerve)
Lateral dorsal digital nerve and vein of 5th toe
Dorsal metatarsal veins
Dorsal digital nerves and veins
Dorsal digital nerves
Dorsal venous arch
Dorsal digital nerve and vein of medial side of great toe
Dorsal digital branch of deep fibular (peroneal) nerve
F. Netter M.D.

Plate 10 Superficial Nerves and Veins of Lower Limb: Anterior View. (Netter: Atlas of Human Anatomy, 4 ed, 2006, Saunders. Plate 544)

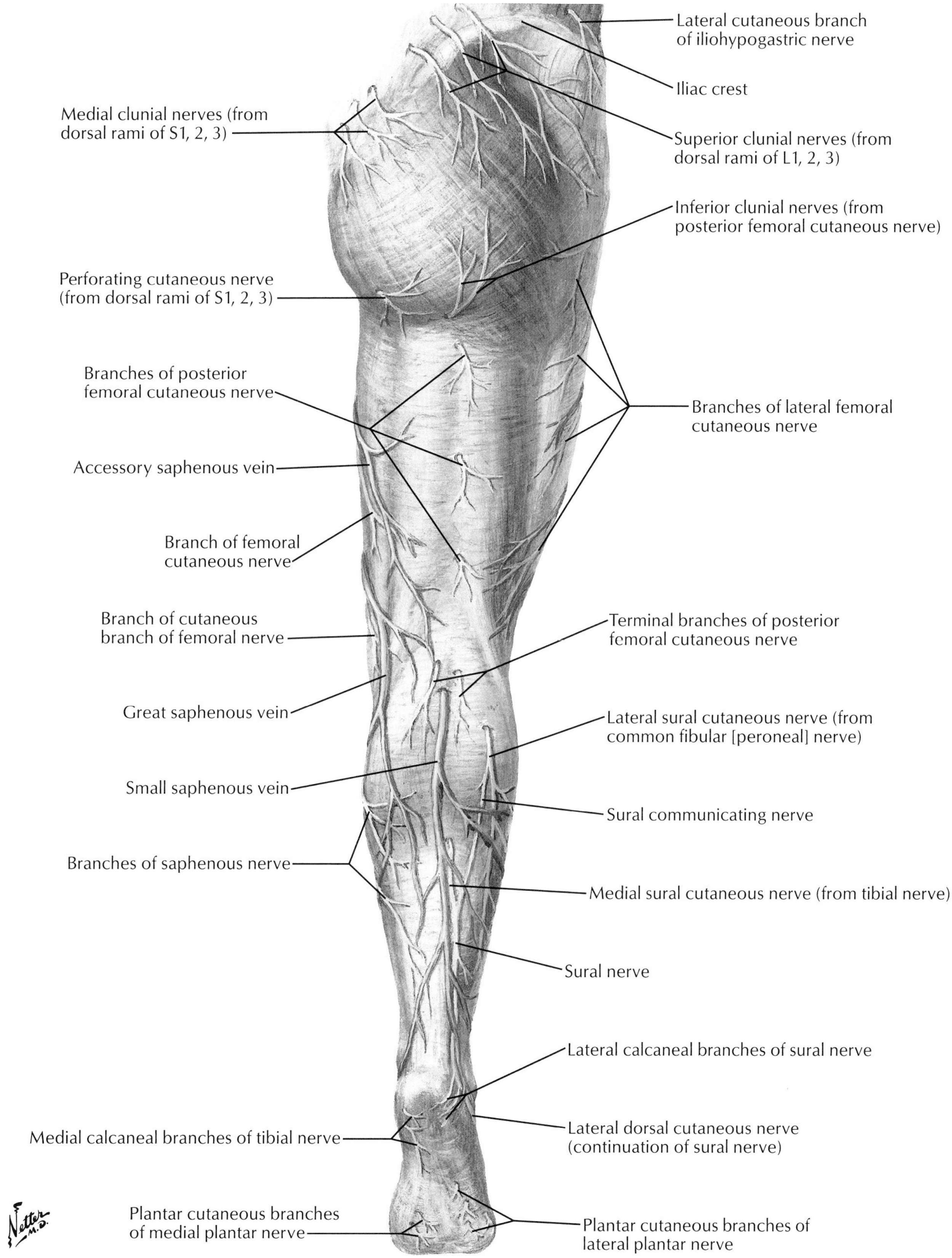

Plate 11 Superficial Nerves and Veins of Lower Limb: Posterior View. (Netter: Atlas of Human Anatomy, 4 ed, 2006, Saunders. Plate 545)

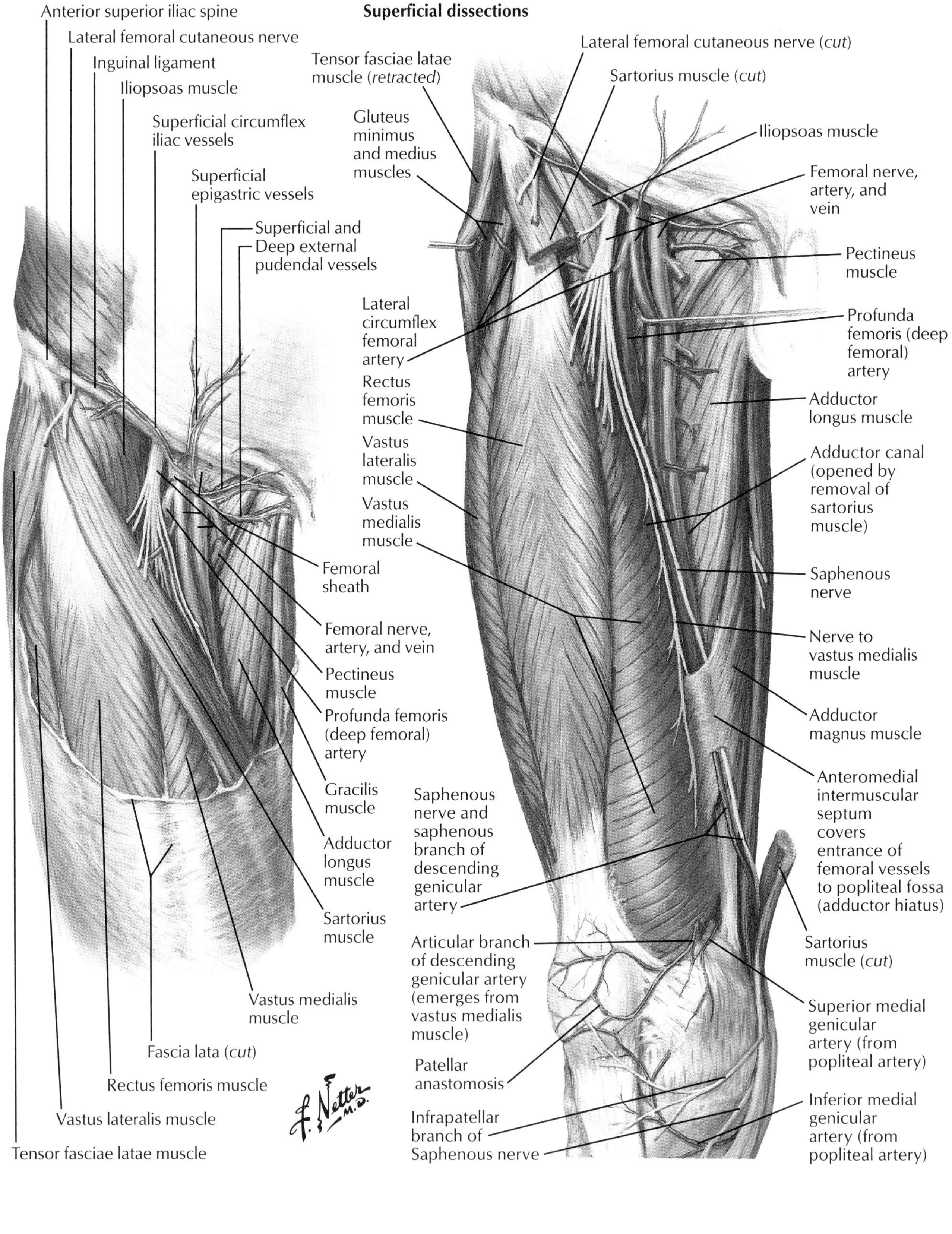
Superficial dissections
Anterior superior iliac spine
Lateral femoral cutaneous nerve
Inguinal ligament
Iliopsoas muscle
Superficial circumflex iliac vessels
Superficial epigastric vessels
Superficial and Deep external pudendal vessels
Femoral sheath
Femoral nerve, artery, and vein
Pectineus muscle
Profunda femoris (deep femoral) artery
Gracilis muscle
Adductor longus muscle
Sartorius muscle
Vastus medialis muscle
Fascia lata (cut)
Rectus femoris muscle
Vastus lateralis muscle
Tensor fasciae latae muscle
Tensor fasciae latae muscle (retracted)
Gluteus minimus and medius muscles
Lateral circumflex femoral artery
Rectus femoris muscle
Vastus lateralis muscle
Vastus medialis muscle
Saphenous nerve and saphenous branch of descending genicular artery
Articular branch of descending genicular artery (emerges from vastus medialis muscle)
Patellar anastomosis
Infrapatellar branch of Saphenous nerve
Lateral femoral cutaneous nerve (cut)
Sartorius muscle (cut)
Iliopsoas muscle
Femoral nerve, artery, and vein
Pectineus muscle
Profunda femoris (deep femoral) artery
Adductor longus muscle
Adductor canal (opened by removal of sartorius muscle)
Saphenous nerve
Nerve to vastus medialis muscle
Adductor magnus muscle
Anteromedial intermuscular septum covers entrance of femoral vessels to popliteal fossa (adductor hiatus)
Sartorius muscle (cut)
Superior medial genicular artery (from popliteal artery)
Inferior medial genicular artery (from popliteal artery)

Plate 12 Arteries and Nerves of Thigh: Anterior Views. (Netter: Atlas of Human Anatomy, 4 ed, 2006, Saunders. Plate 500)

Deep dissection

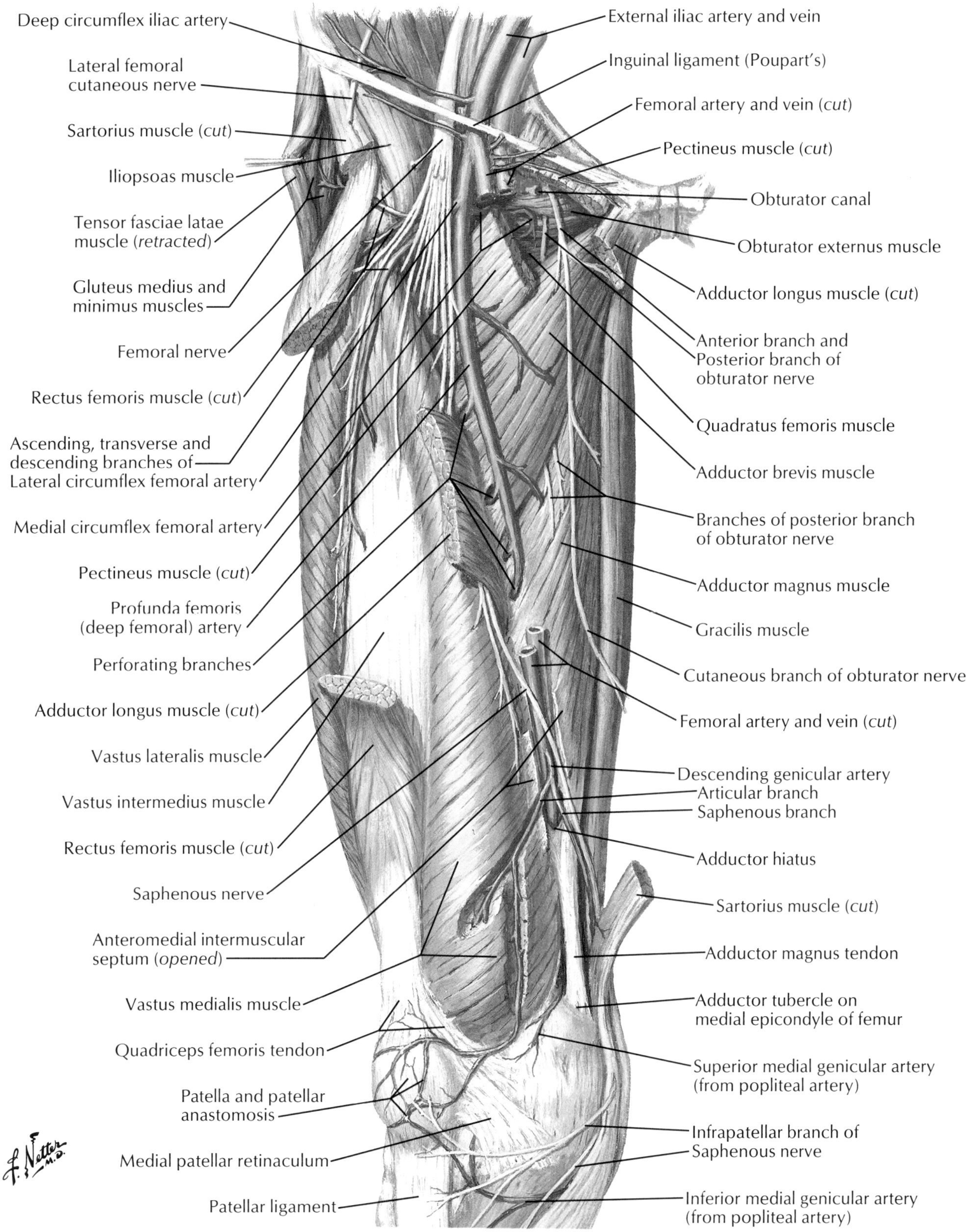
Deep circumflex iliac artery
Lateral femoral cutaneous nerve
Sartorius muscle (cut)
Iliopsoas muscle
Tensor fasciae latae muscle (retracted)
Gluteus medius and minimus muscles
Femoral nerve
Rectus femoris muscle (cut)
Ascending, transverse and descending branches of Lateral circumflex femoral artery
Medial circumflex femoral artery
Pectineus muscle (cut)
Profunda femoris (deep femoral) artery
Perforating branches
Adductor longus muscle (cut)
Vastus lateralis muscle
Vastus intermedius muscle
Rectus femoris muscle (cut)
Saphenous nerve
Anteromedial intermuscular septum (opened)
Vastus medialis muscle
Quadriceps femoris tendon
Patella and patellar anastomosis
Medial patellar retinaculum
Patellar ligament
External iliac artery and vein
Inguinal ligament (Poupart's)
Femoral artery and vein (cut)
Pectineus muscle (cut)
Obturator canal
Obturator externus muscle
Adductor longus muscle (cut)
Anterior branch and Posterior branch of obturator nerve
Quadratus femoris muscle
Adductor brevis muscle
Branches of posterior branch of obturator nerve
Adductor magnus muscle
Gracilis muscle
Cutaneous branch of obturator nerve
Femoral artery and vein (cut)
Descending genicular artery
Articular branch
Saphenous branch
Adductor hiatus
Sartorius muscle (cut)
Adductor magnus tendon
Adductor tubercle on medial epicondyle of femur
Superior medial genicular artery (from popliteal artery)
Infrapatellar branch of Saphenous nerve
Inferior medial genicular artery (from popliteal artery)
F. Netter M.D.

Plate 13 Arteries and Nerves of Thigh: Posterior View. (Netter: Atlas of Human Anatomy, 4 ed, 2006, Saunders. Plate 501)

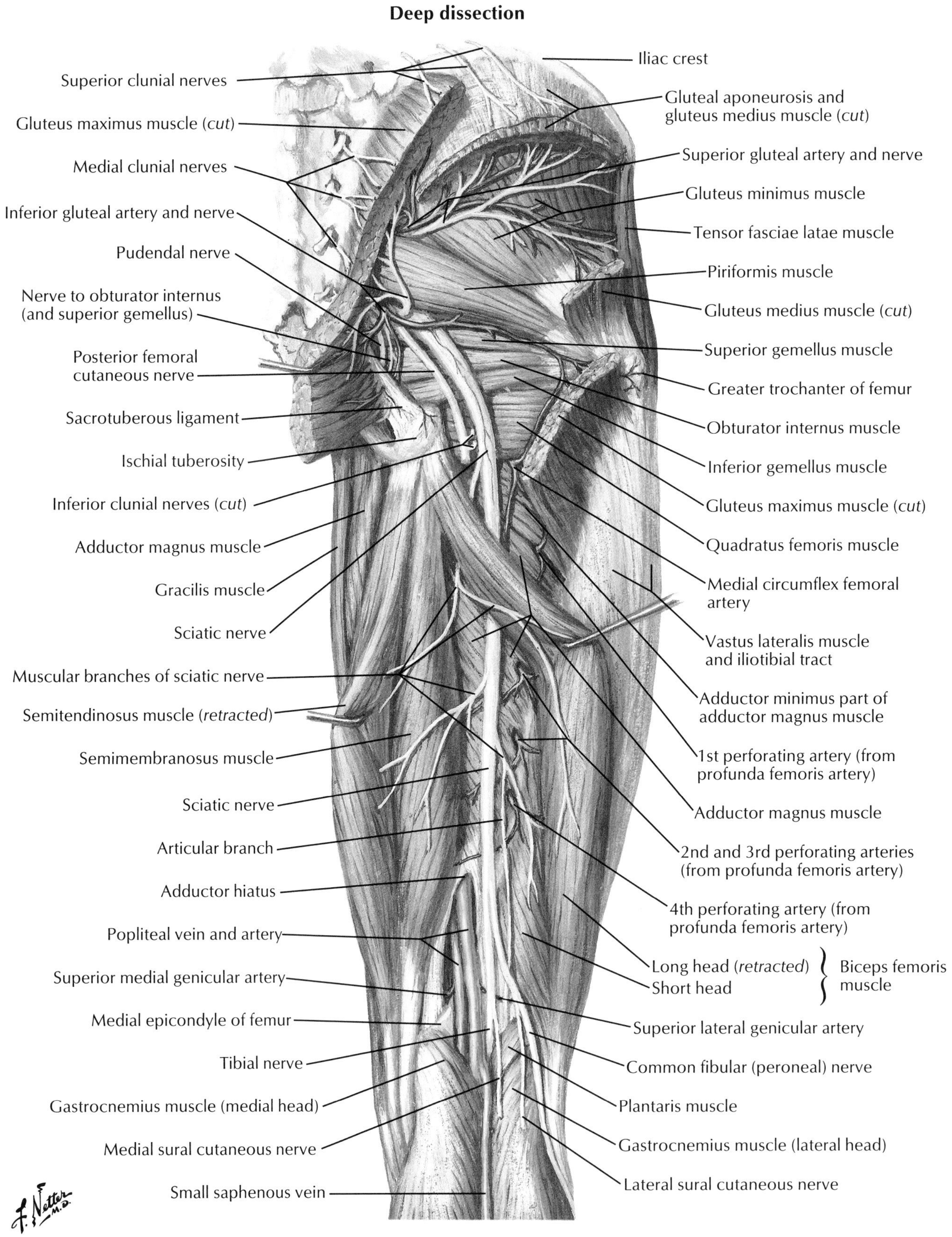
Deep dissection
Superior clunial nerves
Gluteus maximus muscle (*cut*)
Medial clunial nerves
Inferior gluteal artery and nerve
Pudendal nerve
Nerve to obturator internus (and superior gemellus)
Posterior femoral cutaneous nerve
Sacrotuberous ligament
Ischial tuberosity
Inferior clunial nerves (*cut*)
Adductor magnus muscle
Gracilis muscle
Sciatic nerve
Muscular branches of sciatic nerve
Semitendinosus muscle (*retracted*)
Semimembranosus muscle
Sciatic nerve
Articular branch
Adductor hiatus
Popliteal vein and artery
Superior medial genicular artery
Medial epicondyle of femur
Tibial nerve
Gastrocnemius muscle (medial head)
Medial sural cutaneous nerve
Small saphenous vein
Iliac crest
Gluteal aponeurosis and gluteus medius muscle (*cut*)
Superior gluteal artery and nerve
Gluteus minimus muscle
Tensor fasciae latae muscle
Piriformis muscle
Gluteus medius muscle (*cut*)
Superior gemellus muscle
Greater trochanter of femur
Obturator internus muscle
Inferior gemellus muscle
Gluteus maximus muscle (*cut*)
Quadratus femoris muscle
Medial circumflex femoral artery
Vastus lateralis muscle and iliotibial tract
Adductor minimus part of adductor magnus muscle
1st perforating artery (from profunda femoris artery)
Adductor magnus muscle
2nd and 3rd perforating arteries (from profunda femoris artery)
4th perforating artery (from profunda femoris artery)
Long head (*retracted*)
Short head
Biceps femoris muscle
Superior lateral genicular artery
Common fibular (peroneal) nerve
Plantaris muscle
Gastrocnemius muscle (lateral head)
Lateral sural cutaneous nerve
F. Netter M.D.

Plate 14 Arteries and Nerves of Thigh: Posterior View. (Netter: Atlas of Human Anatomy, 4 ed, 2006, Saunders. Plate 502)

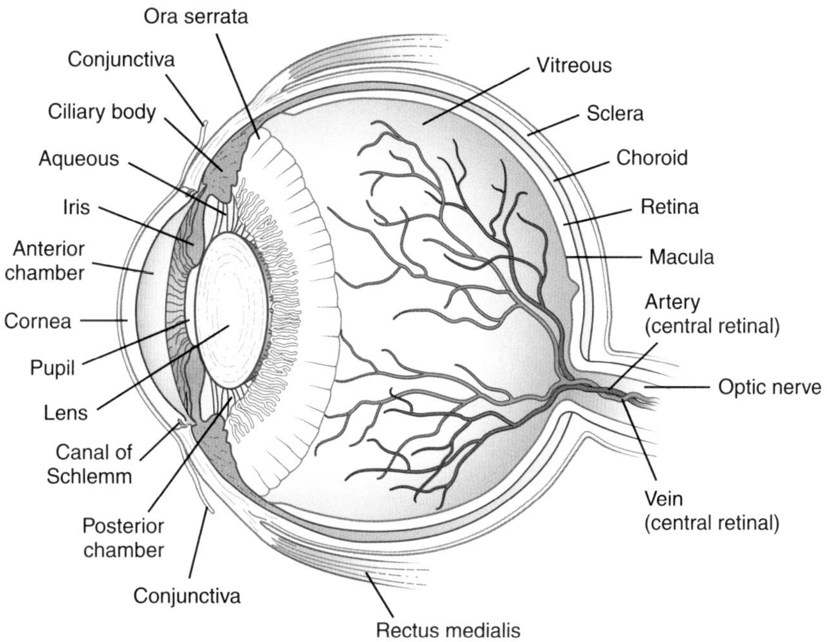

Plate 15 Anatomy of the eye. (Dehn RW, Asprey DP: Essential Clinical Procedures, ed 3, Philadelphia, 2013, Saunders.)

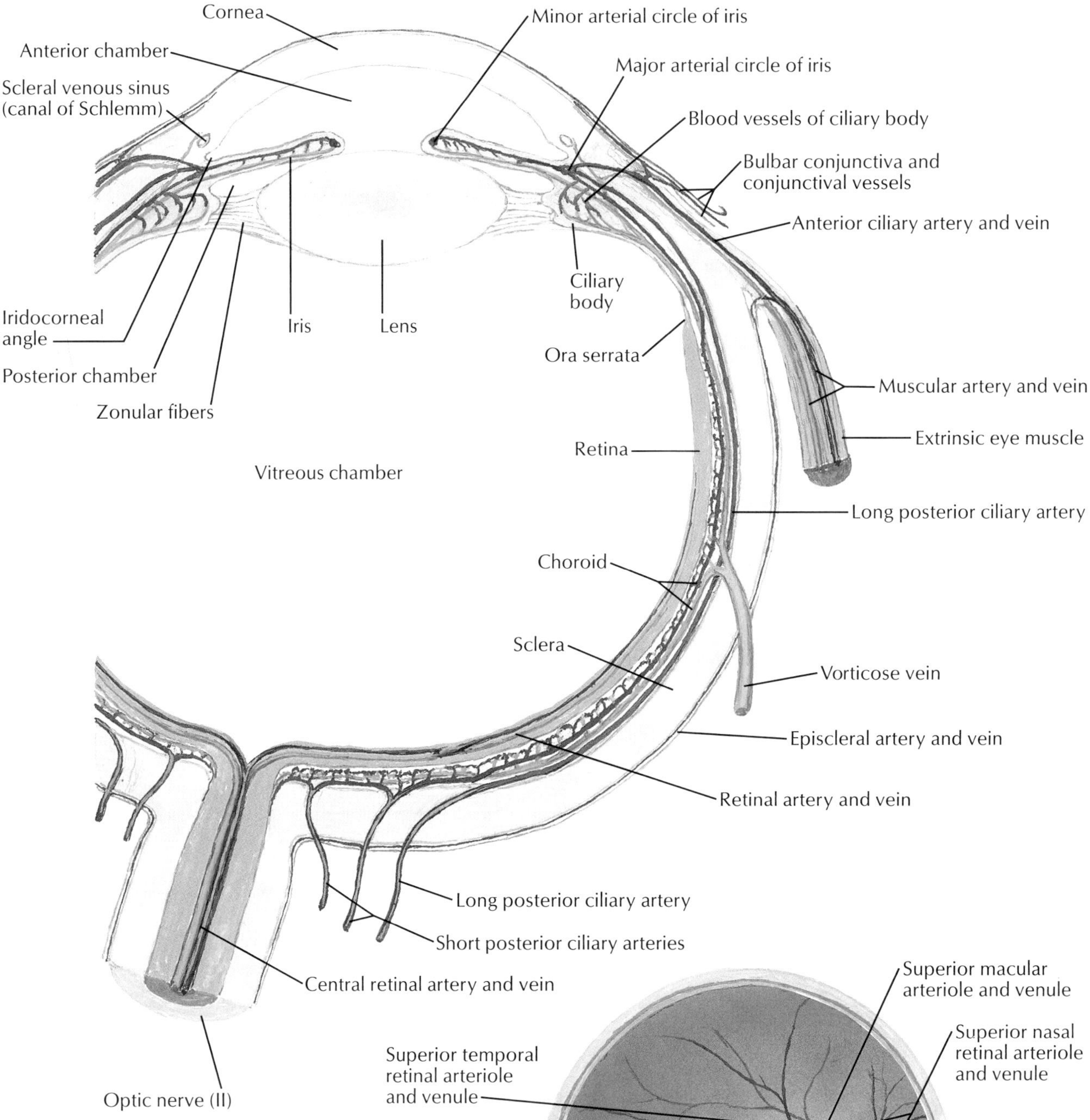

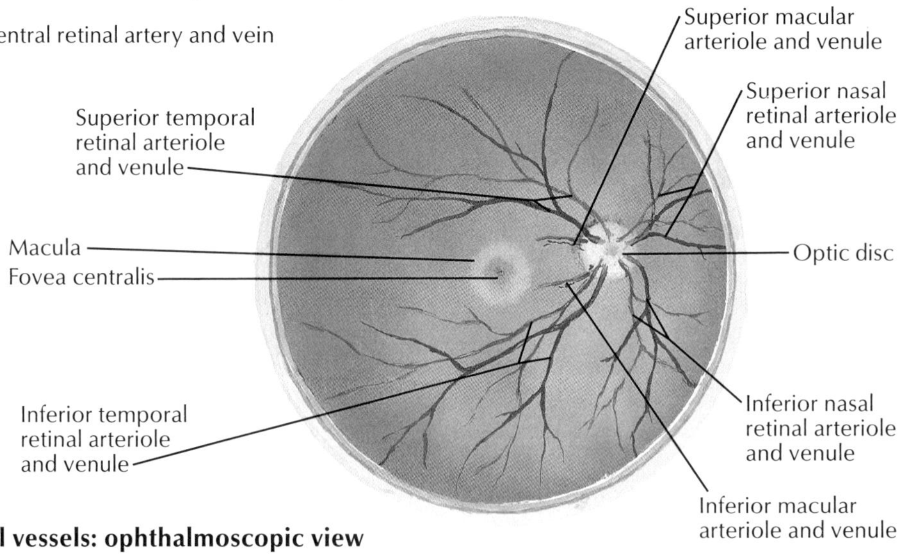

Right retinal vessels: ophthalmoscopic view

Plate 16 Intrinsic Arteries and Veins of Eye. (Netter: Atlas of Human Anatomy, 4 ed, 2006, Saunders. Plate 90)

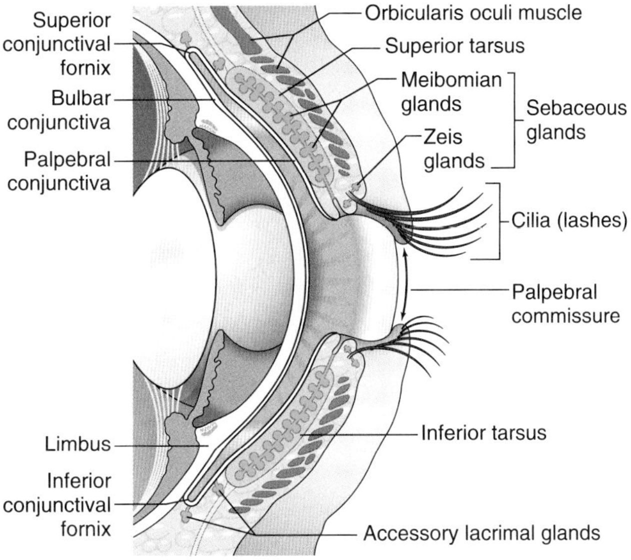

Plate 17 Anatomy of the conjunctiva and eyelids. (Kumar V, Abbas AK, Aster JC: Robbins and Cotran Pathologic Basis of Disease, ed 9, Philadelphia, 2015, Saunders.)

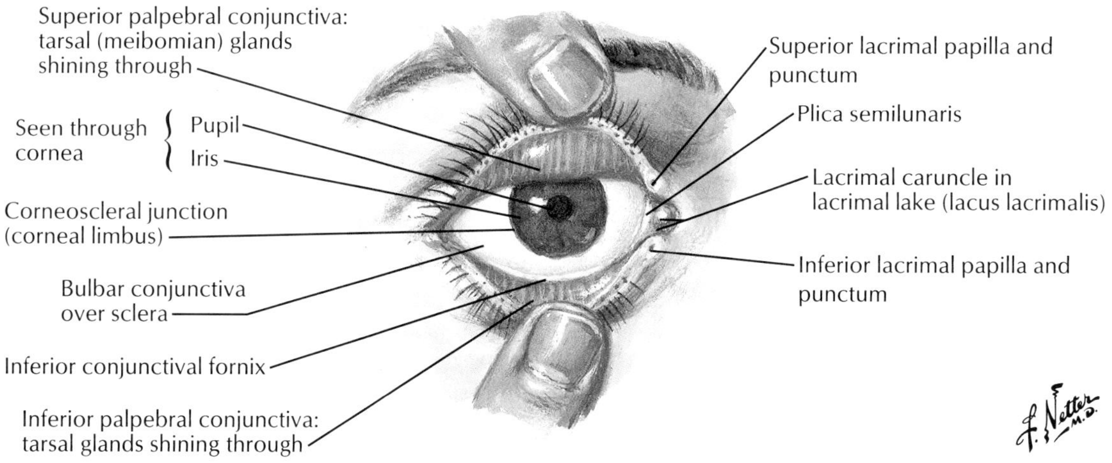

Plate 18 Eyelid. (Netter: Atlas of Human Anatomy, 4 ed, 2006, Saunders. Plate 81, Upper)

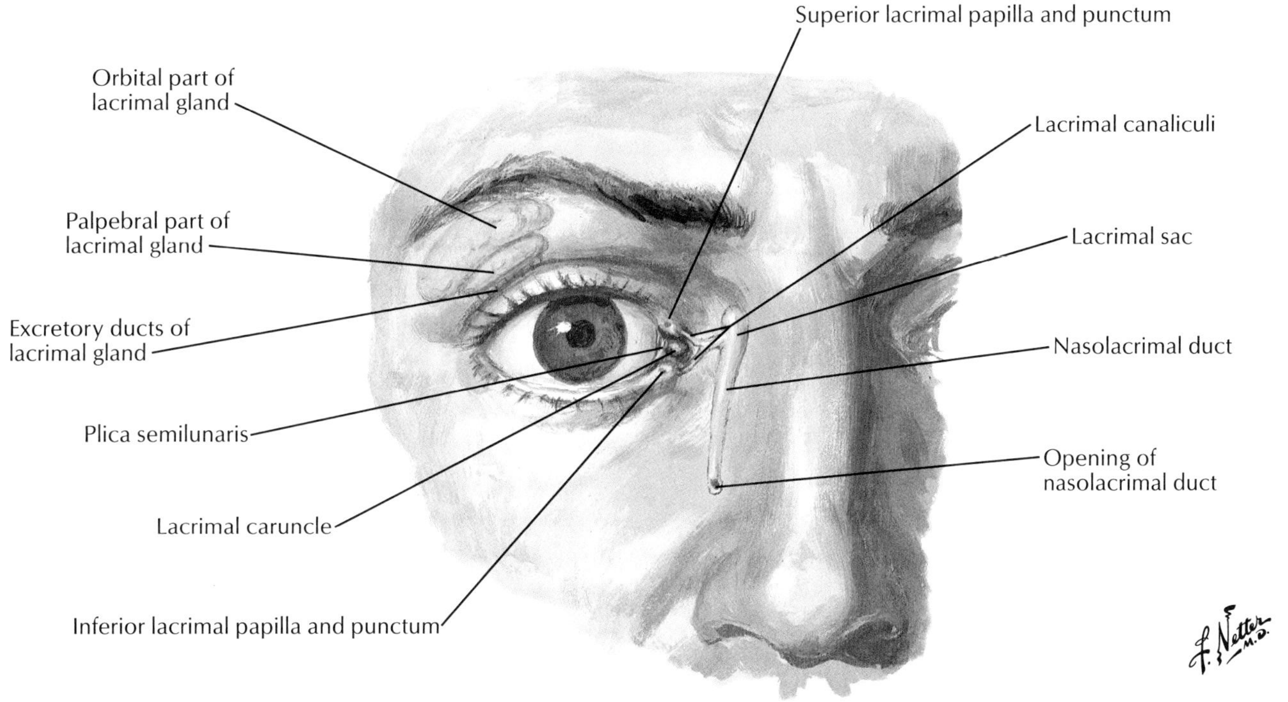

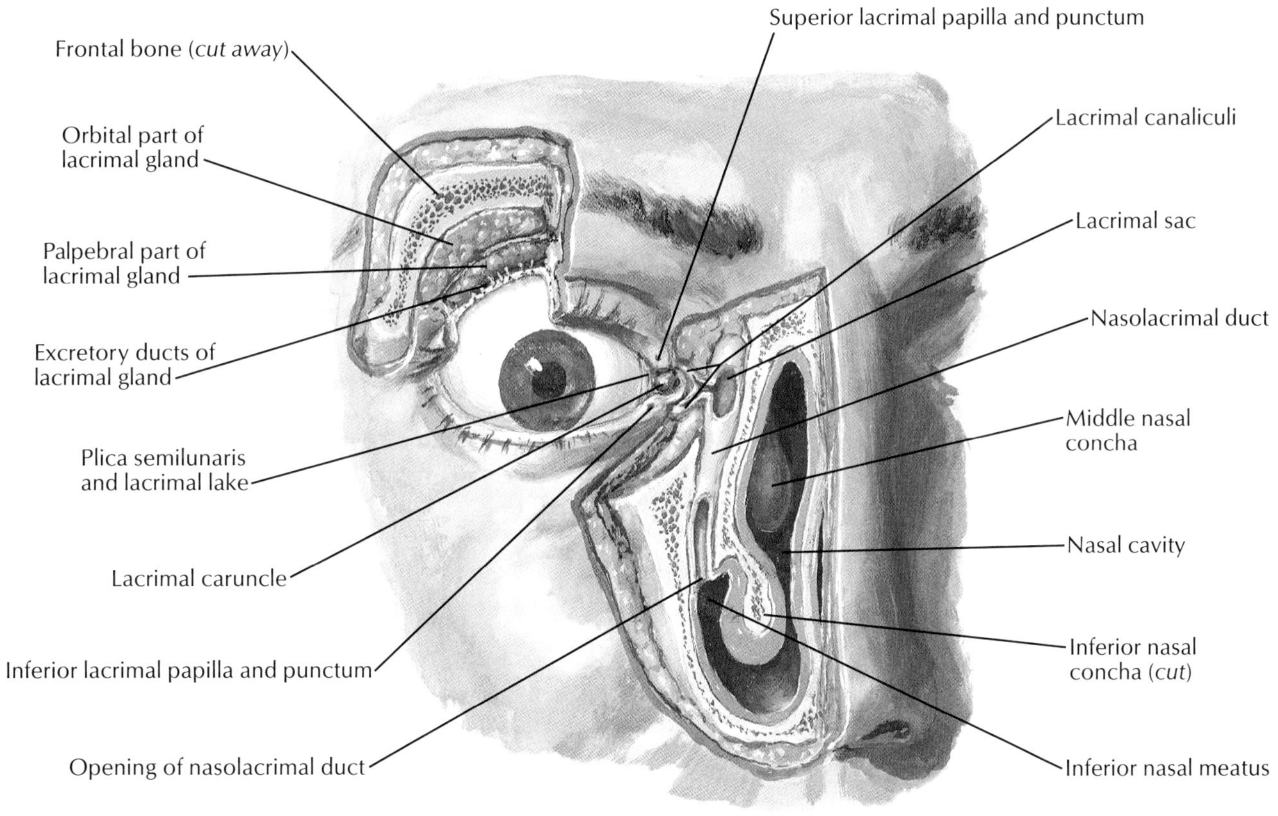

Plate 19 Lacrimal Apparatus. (Netter: Atlas of Human Anatomy, 4 ed, 2006, Saunders. Plate 82)

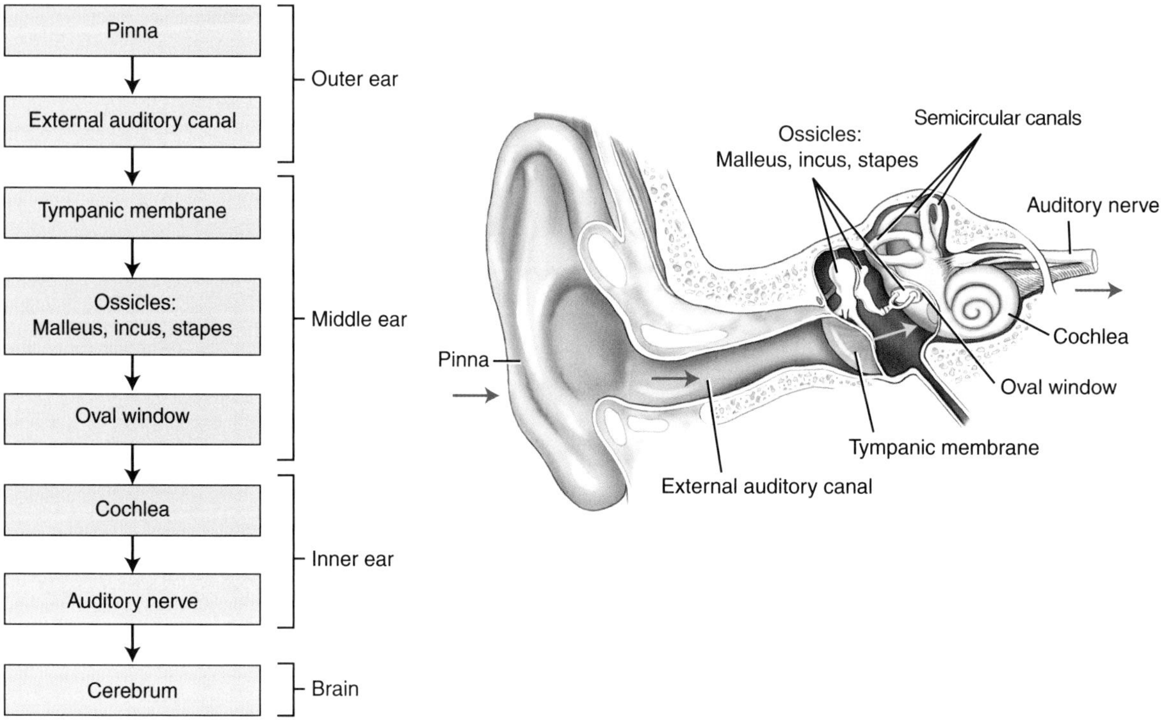

Plate 20 Pathway of Sound. (LaFleur Brooks D, LaFleur Brooks M: Basic Medical Language, ed 4, St. Louis, 2013, Mosby.)

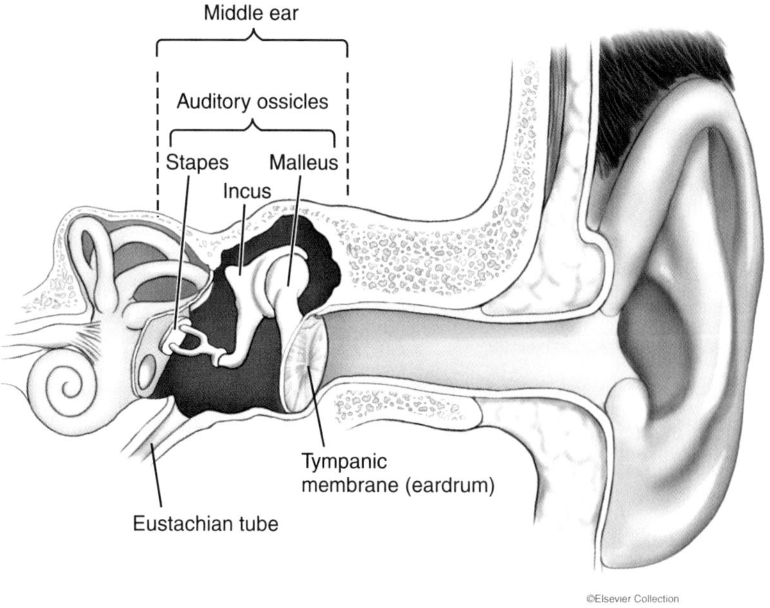

Plate 21 Middle ear structures. (©Elsevier Collection.)

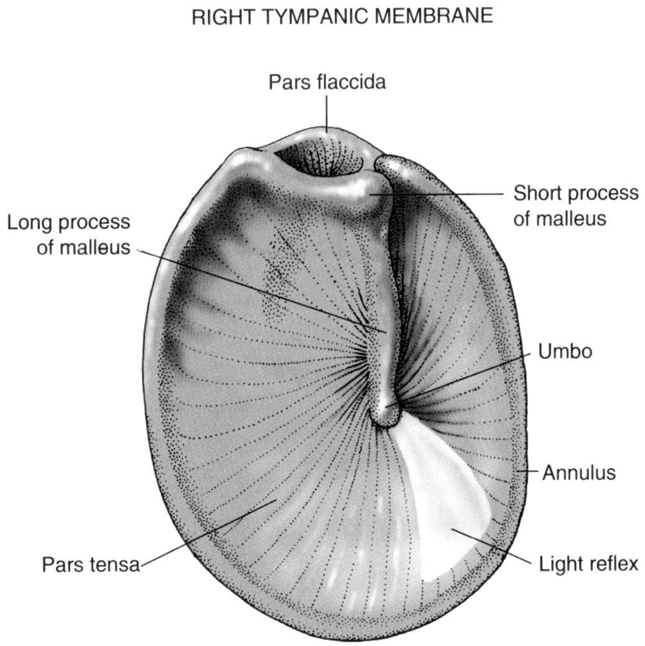

Plate 22 Structural landmarks of tympanic membrane. (Ignatavicius DD, Workman ML: Medical-Surgical Nursing: Patient-Centered Collaborative Care, ed 7, St. Louis, 2013, Saunders.)

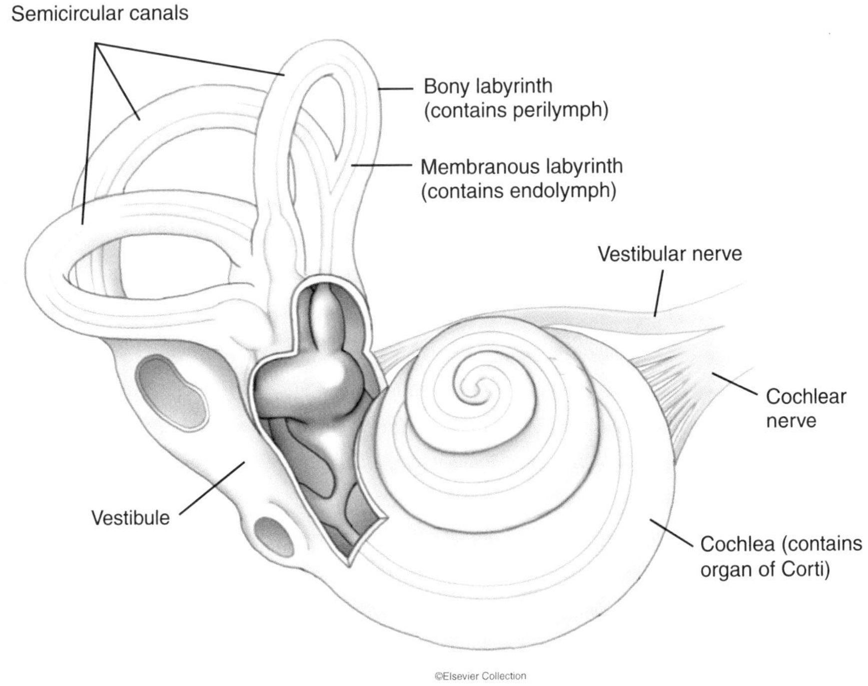

Plate 23 Inner ear structures. (©Elsevier Collection.)

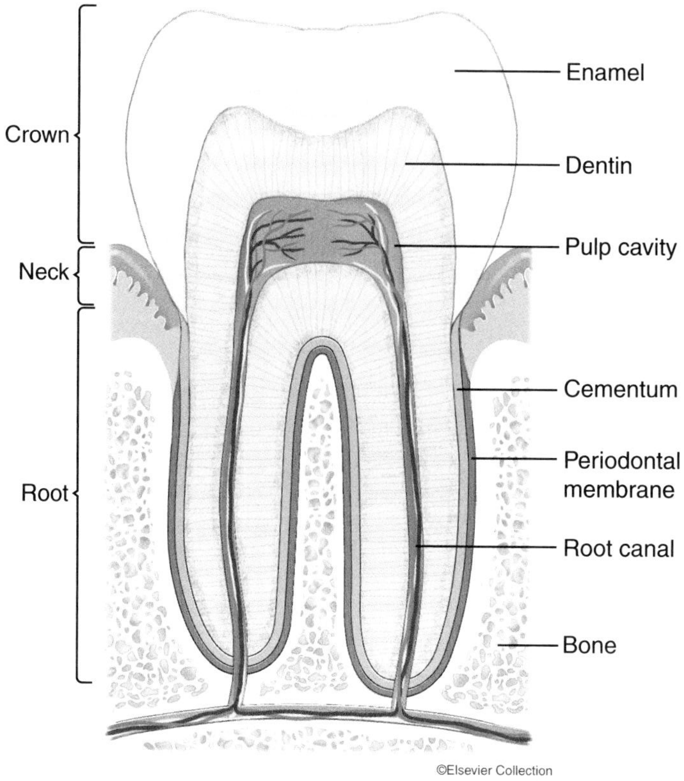

Plate 24 The Tooth. (©Elsevier Collection).

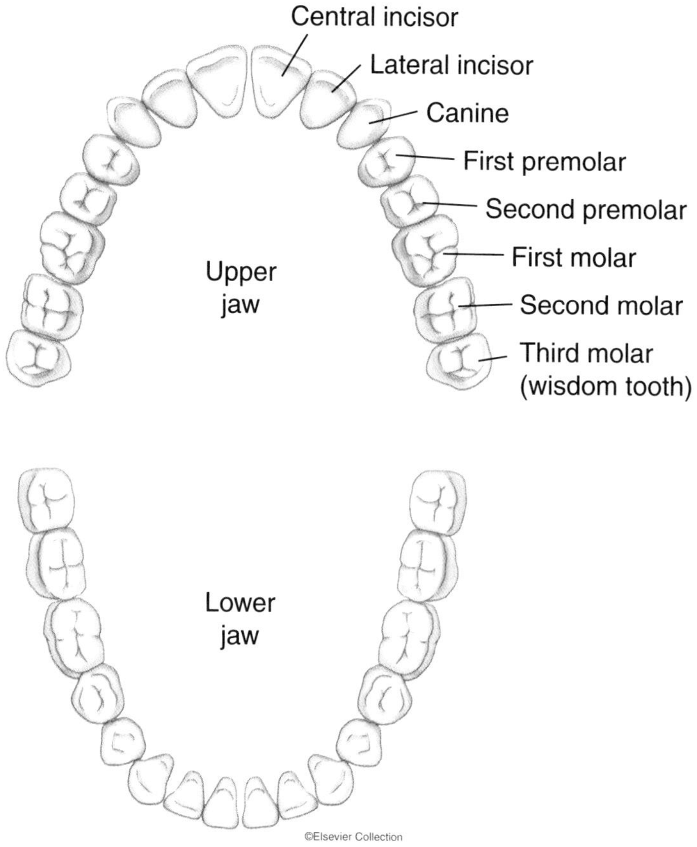

Plate 25 Adult Teeth. (©Elsevier Collection).

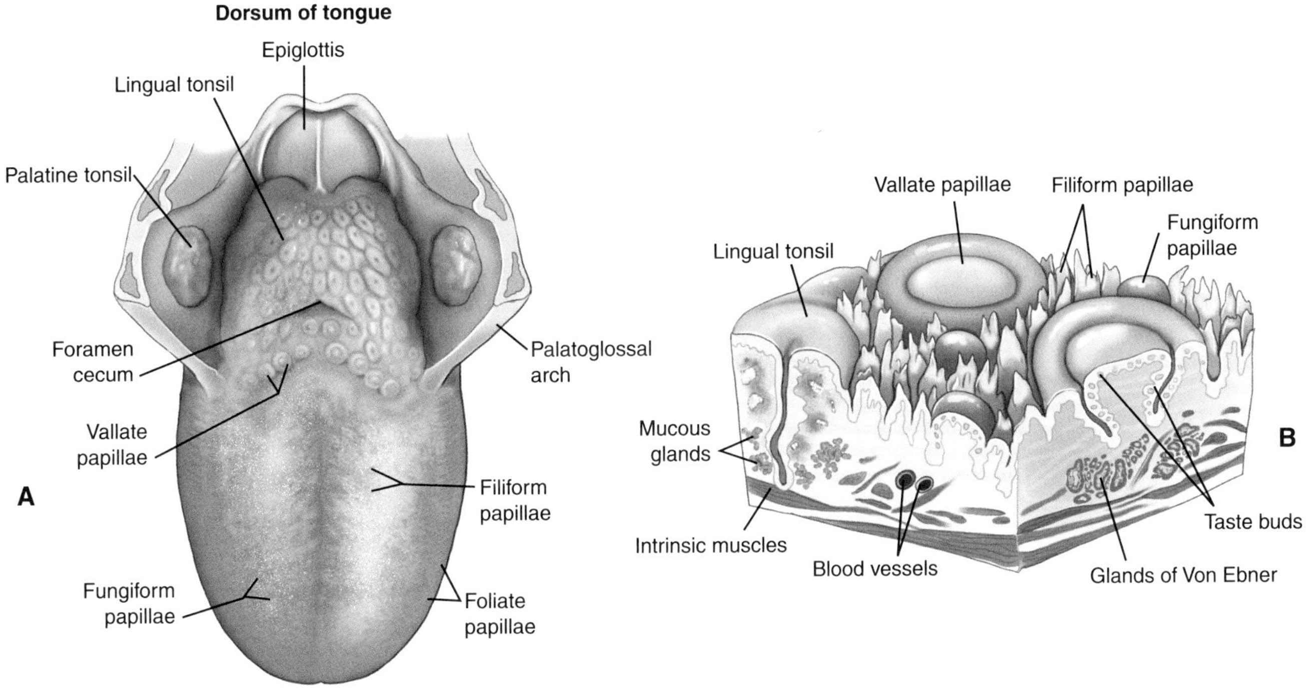

Plate 26 A, Dorsal view of tongue showing the roughened large lingual tonsils on the posterior of the tongue and the foliate papillae on the side. B, Section of dorsal of the tongue showing a cutaway through lingual papillae and showing von Ebner's glands at the base of the vallate papilla. (Brand RW, Isselhard DE: Anatomy of Orofacial Structures: A Comprehensive Approach, ed 8, St. Louis, 2019, Elsevier.)

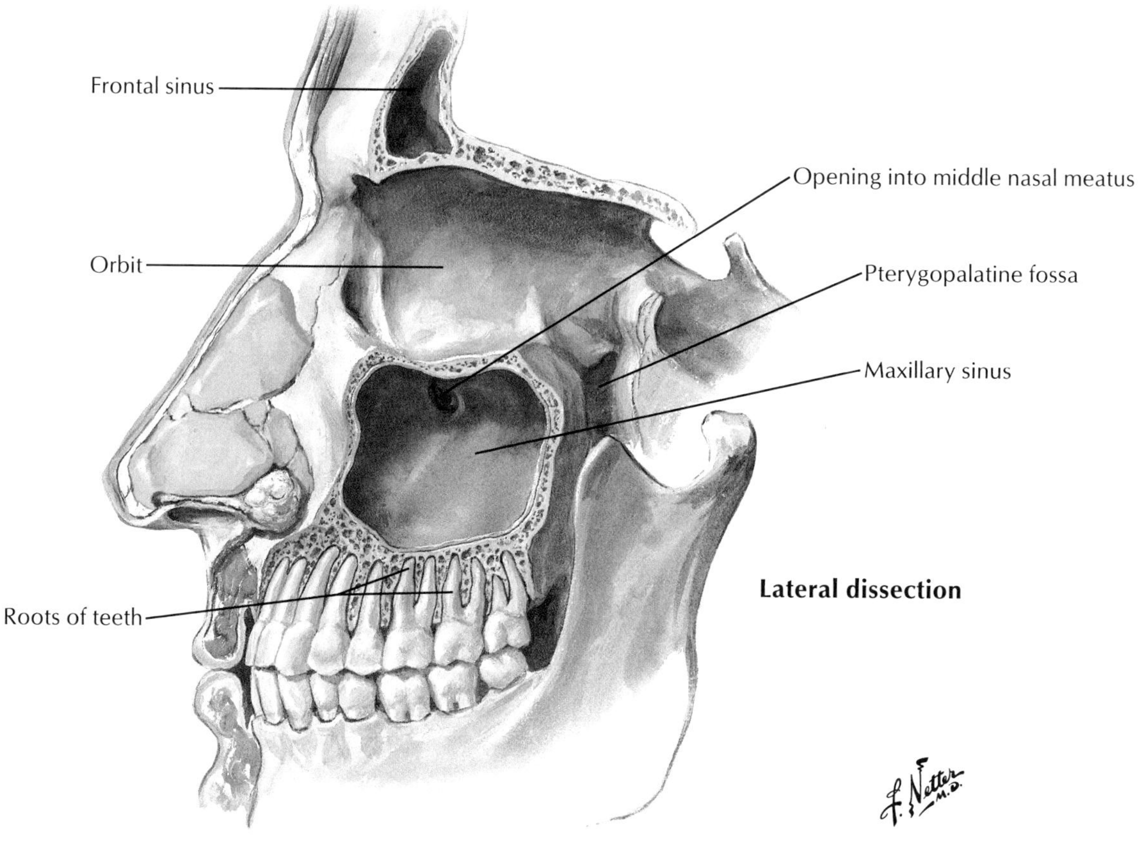

Plate 27 Paranasal Sinuses. (Netter: Atlas of Human Anatomy, 4 ed, 2006, Saunders. Plate 49)

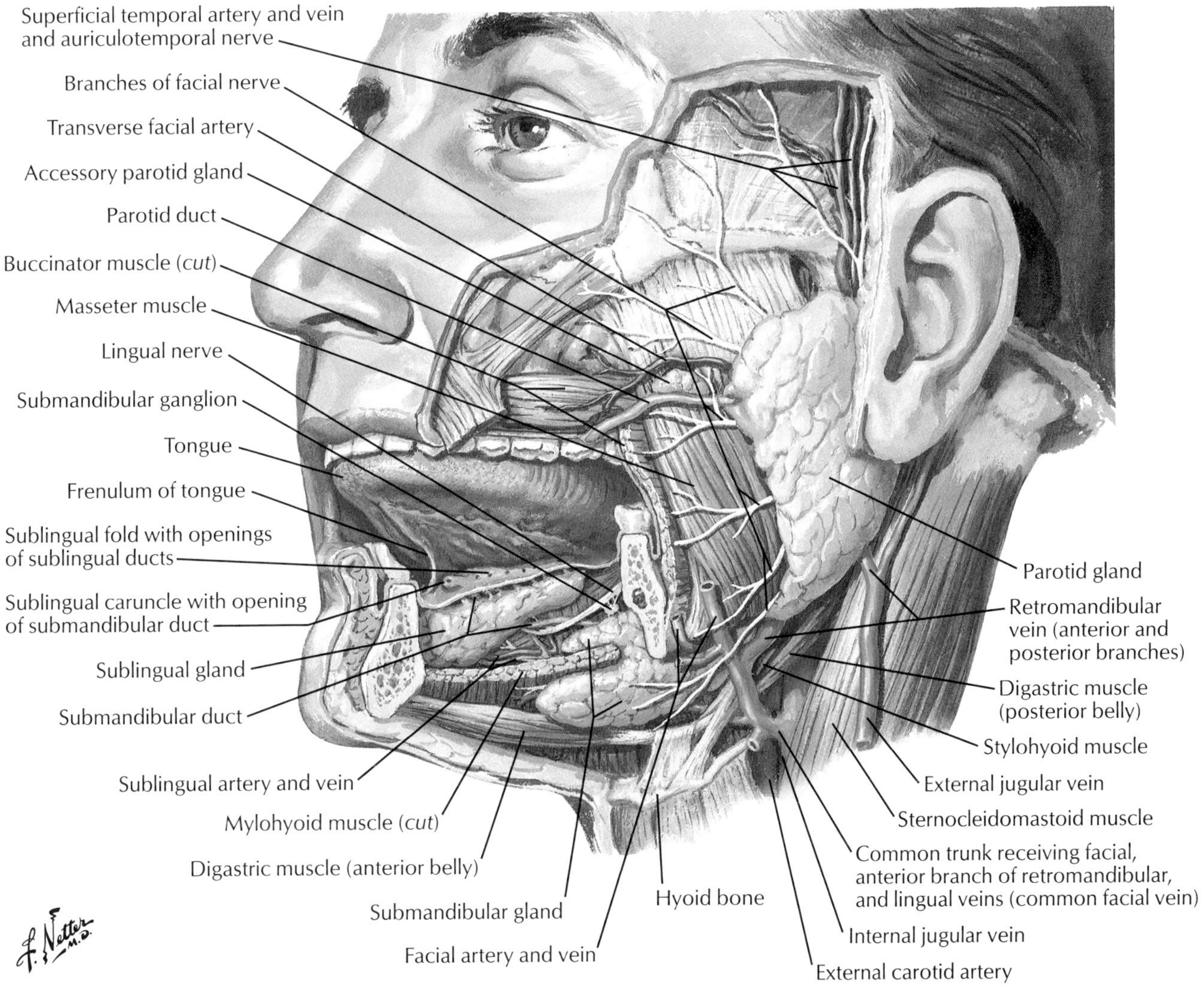

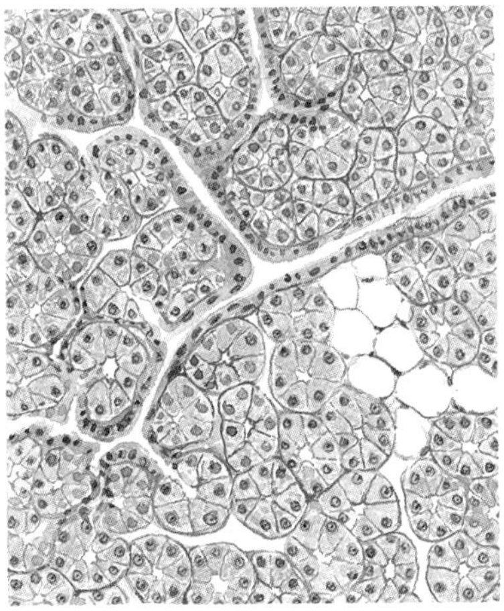
Parotid gland: totally serous

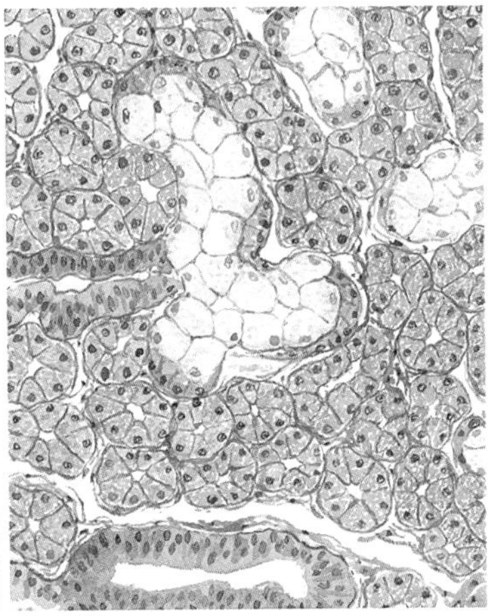
Submandibular gland: mostly serous, partially mucous

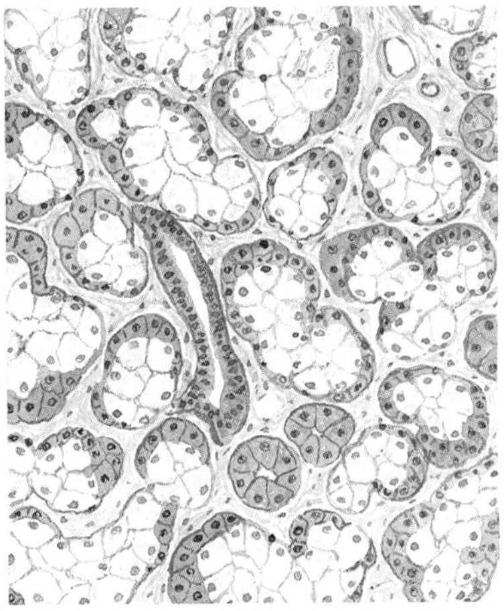
Sublingual gland: almost completely mucous

Plate 28 Salivary Glands. (Netter: Atlas of Human Anatomy, 4 ed, 2006, Saunders. Plate 61)

Coronary Arteries: Arteriographic Views

Right coronary artery: left anterior oblique view

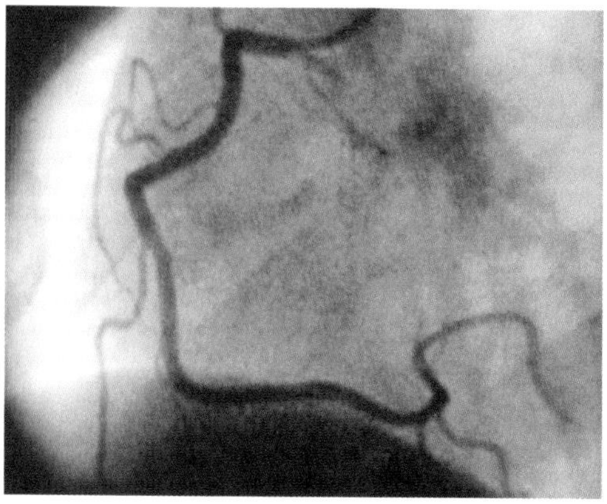

Arteriogram

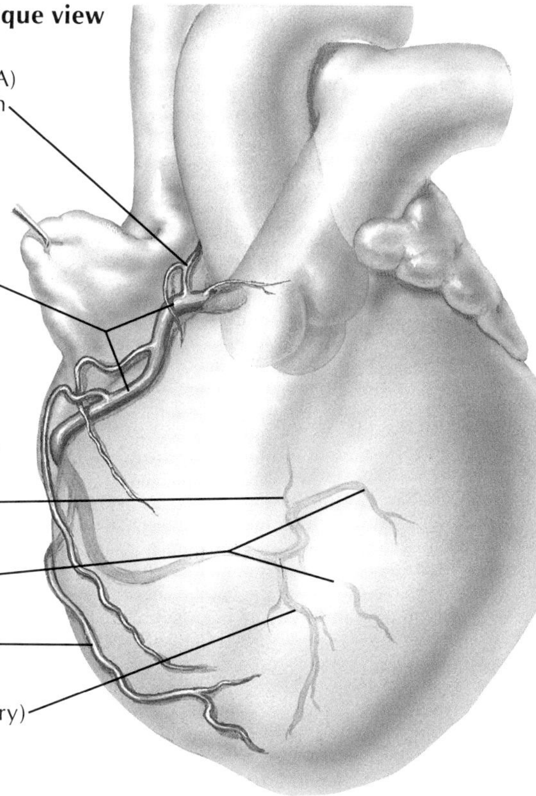

Right coronary artery: right anterior oblique view

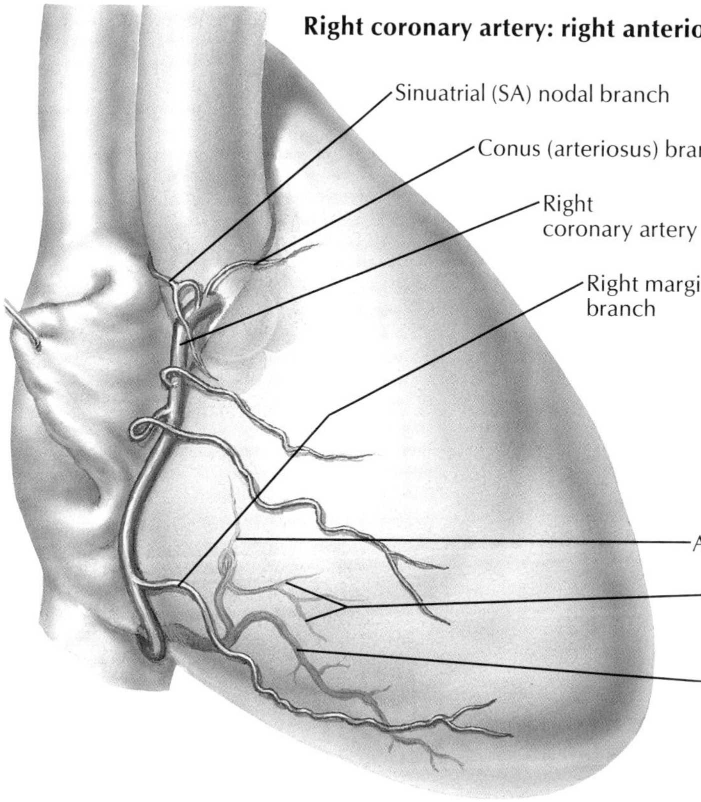

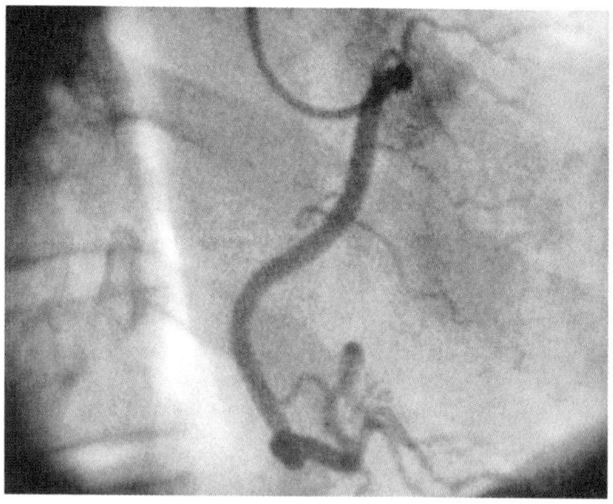

Arteriogram

F. Netter M.D.
© ICON LEARNING SYSTEMS

Plate 29 Coronary Arteries: Arteriographic Views. (Netter: Atlas of Human Anatomy, 4 ed, 2006, Saunders. Plate 218)

Left coronary artery: left anterior oblique view

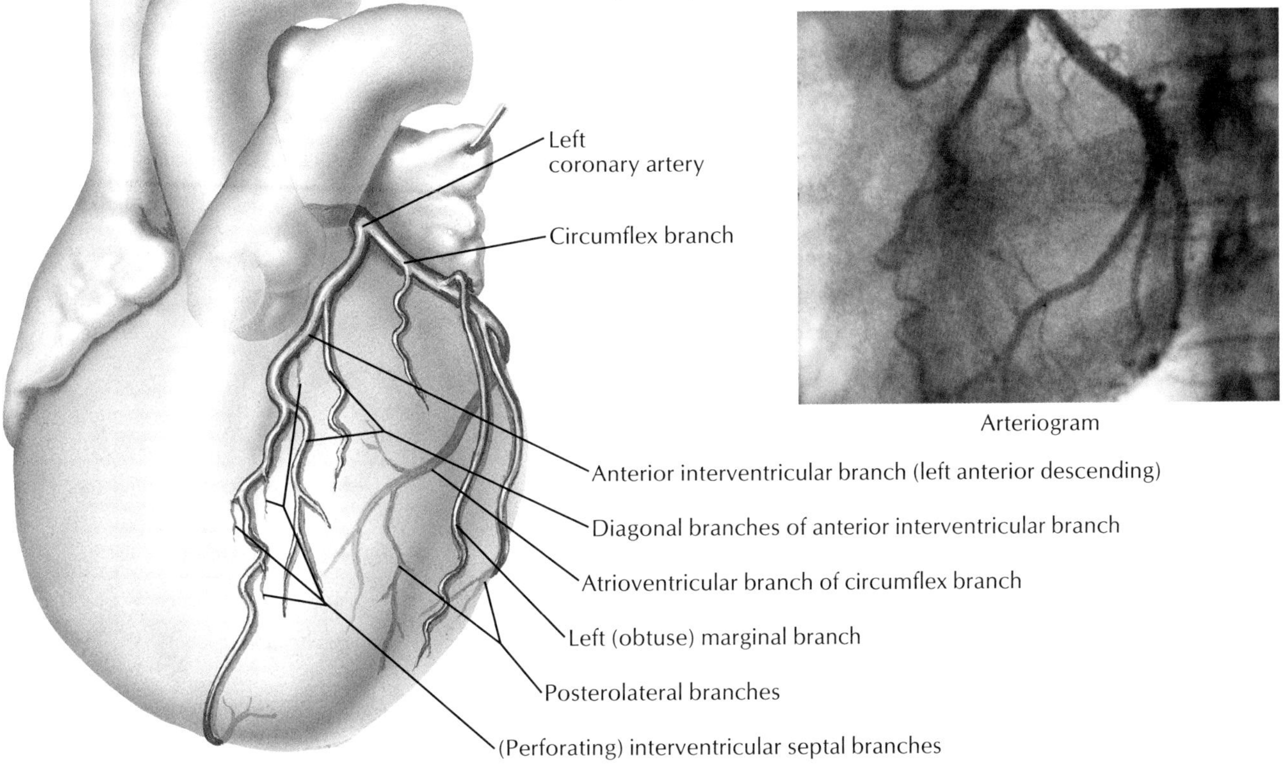

Left coronary artery: right anterior oblique view

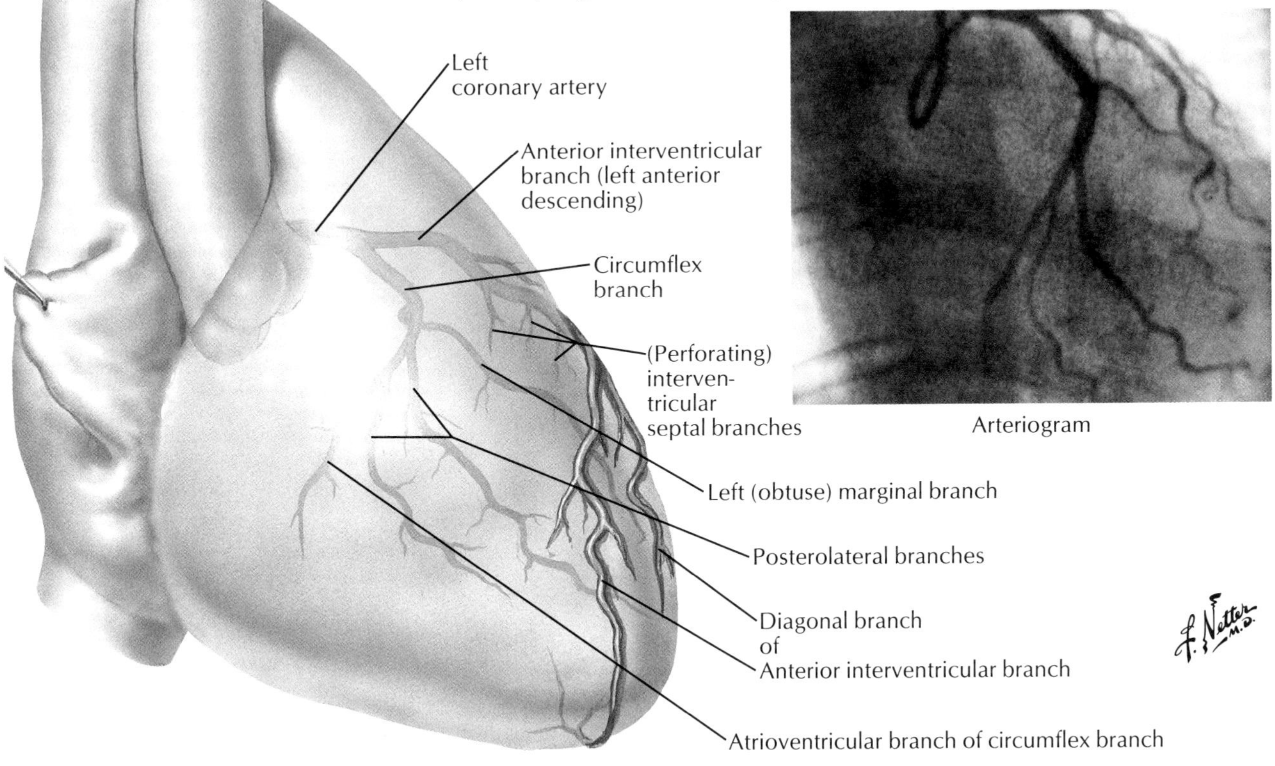

Plate 30 Coronary Arteries: Arteriographic Views. (Netter: Atlas of Human Anatomy, 4 ed, 2006, Saunders. Plate 219)

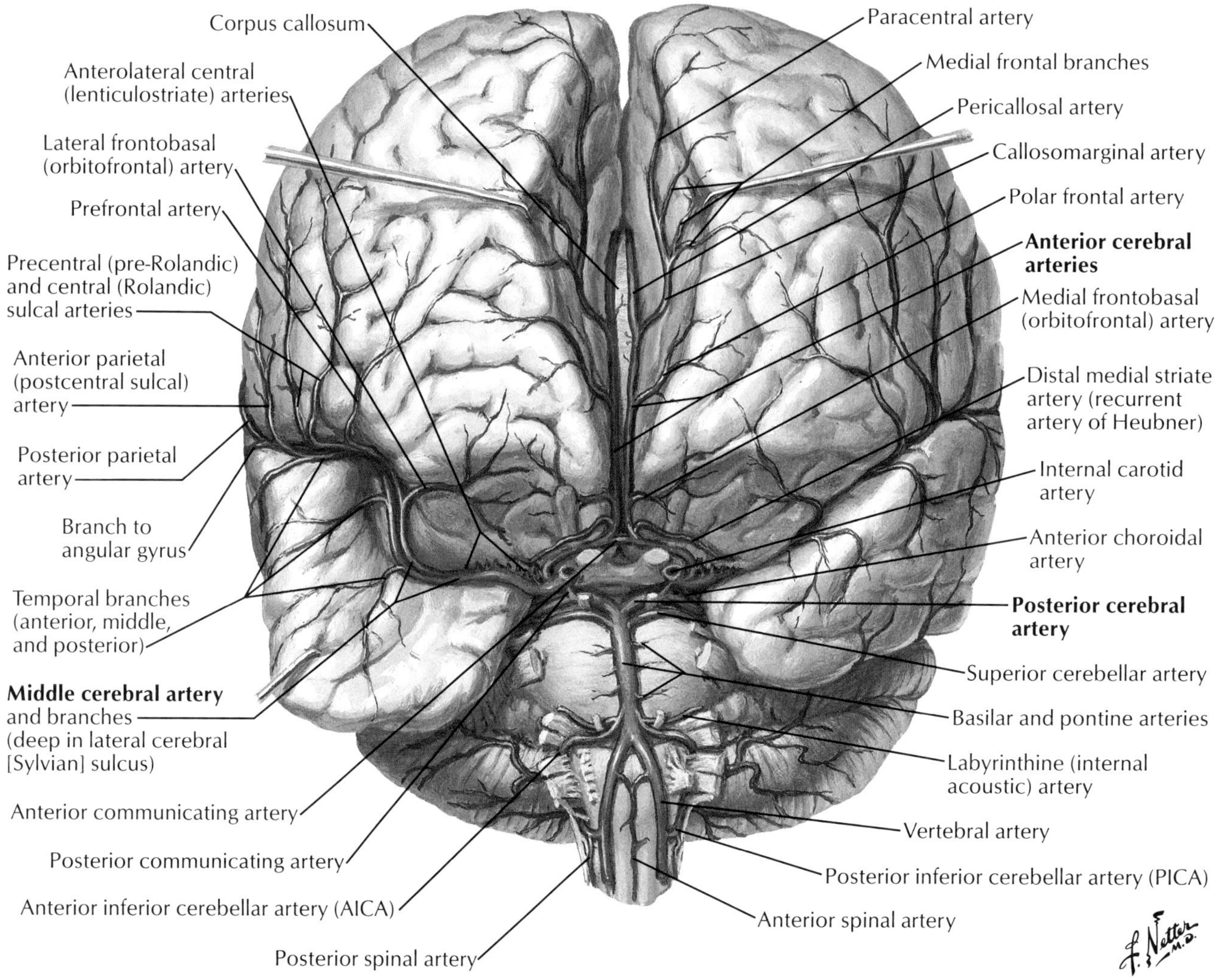
Corpus callosum
Anterolateral central (lenticulostriate) arteries
Lateral frontobasal (orbitofrontal) artery
Prefrontal artery
Precentral (pre-Rolandic) and central (Rolandic) sulcal arteries
Anterior parietal (postcentral sulcal) artery
Posterior parietal artery
Branch to angular gyrus
Temporal branches (anterior, middle, and posterior)
Middle cerebral artery and branches (deep in lateral cerebral [Sylvian] sulcus)
Anterior communicating artery
Posterior communicating artery
Anterior inferior cerebellar artery (AICA)
Posterior spinal artery
Paracentral artery
Medial frontal branches
Pericallosal artery
Callosomarginal artery
Polar frontal artery
Anterior cerebral arteries
Medial frontobasal (orbitofrontal) artery
Distal medial striate artery (recurrent artery of Heubner)
Internal carotid artery
Anterior choroidal artery
Posterior cerebral artery
Superior cerebellar artery
Basilar and pontine arteries
Labyrinthine (internal acoustic) artery
Vertebral artery
Posterior inferior cerebellar artery (PICA)
Anterior spinal artery
F. Netter M.D.

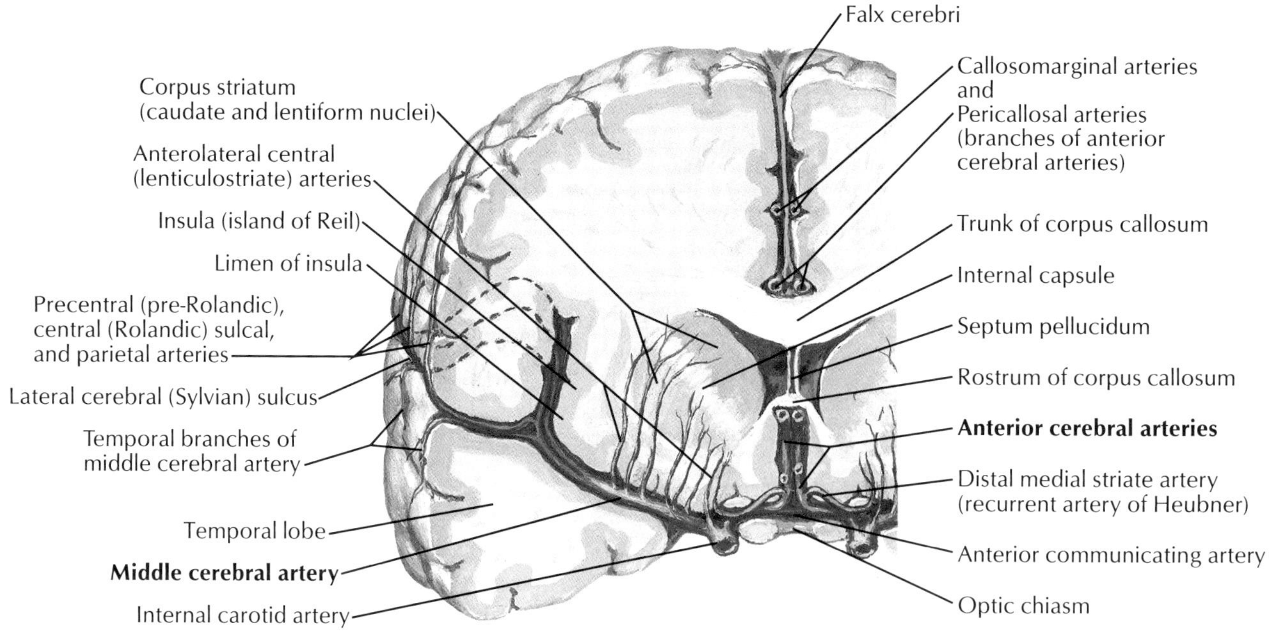
Falx cerebri
Corpus striatum (caudate and lentiform nuclei)
Anterolateral central (lenticulostriate) arteries
Insula (island of Reil)
Limen of insula
Precentral (pre-Rolandic), central (Rolandic) sulcal, and parietal arteries
Lateral cerebral (Sylvian) sulcus
Temporal branches of middle cerebral artery
Temporal lobe
Middle cerebral artery
Internal carotid artery
Callosomarginal arteries and Pericallosal arteries (branches of anterior cerebral arteries)
Trunk of corpus callosum
Internal capsule
Septum pellucidum
Rostrum of corpus callosum
Anterior cerebral arteries
Distal medial striate artery (recurrent artery of Heubner)
Anterior communicating artery
Optic chiasm

Plate 31 Arteries of Brain: Frontal View and Section. (Netter: Atlas of Human Anatomy, 4 ed, 2006, Saunders. Plate 141)

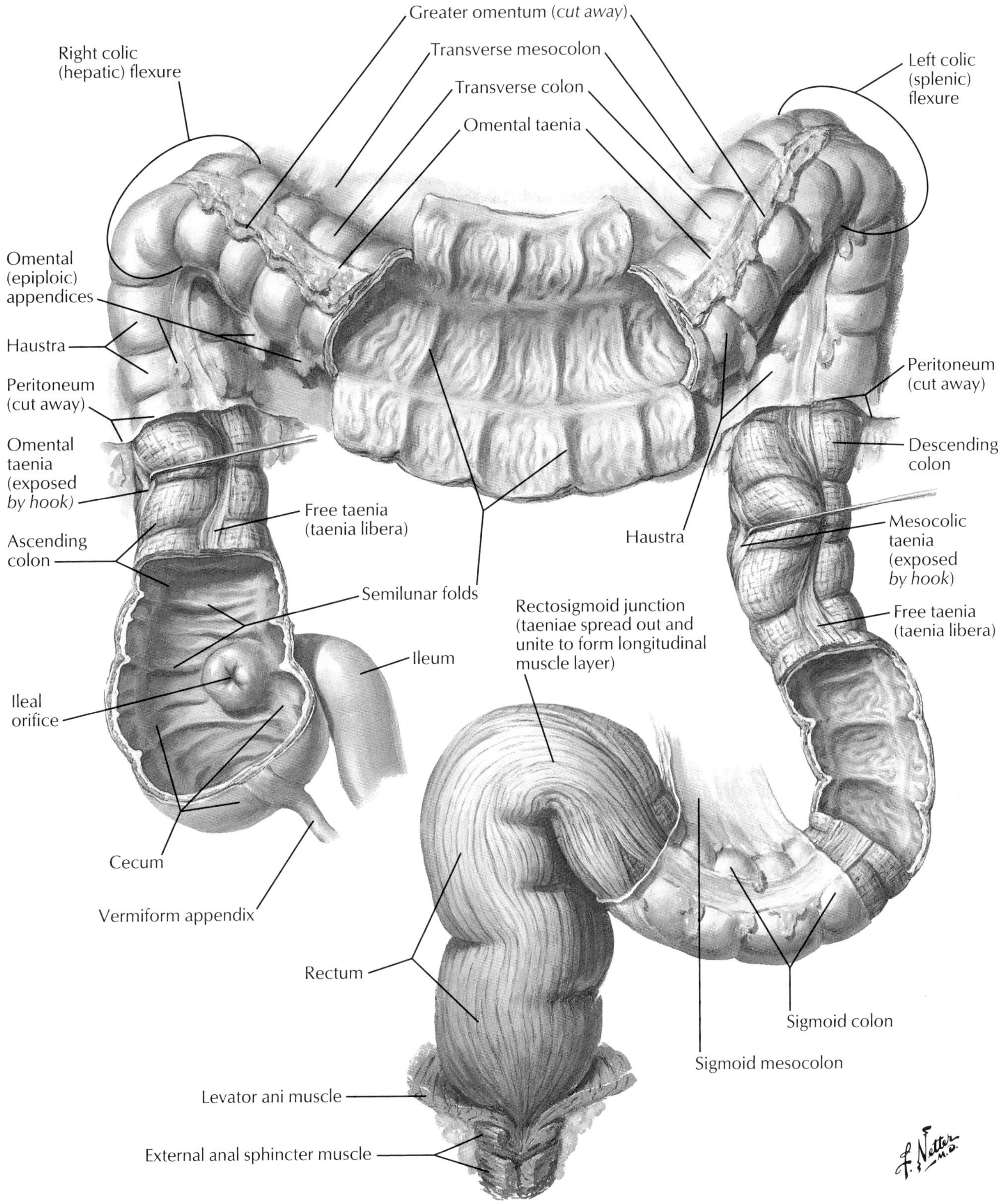

Plate 32 Mucosa and Musculature of Large Intestine. (Netter: Atlas of Human Anatomy, 4 ed, 2006, Saunders. Plate 284)

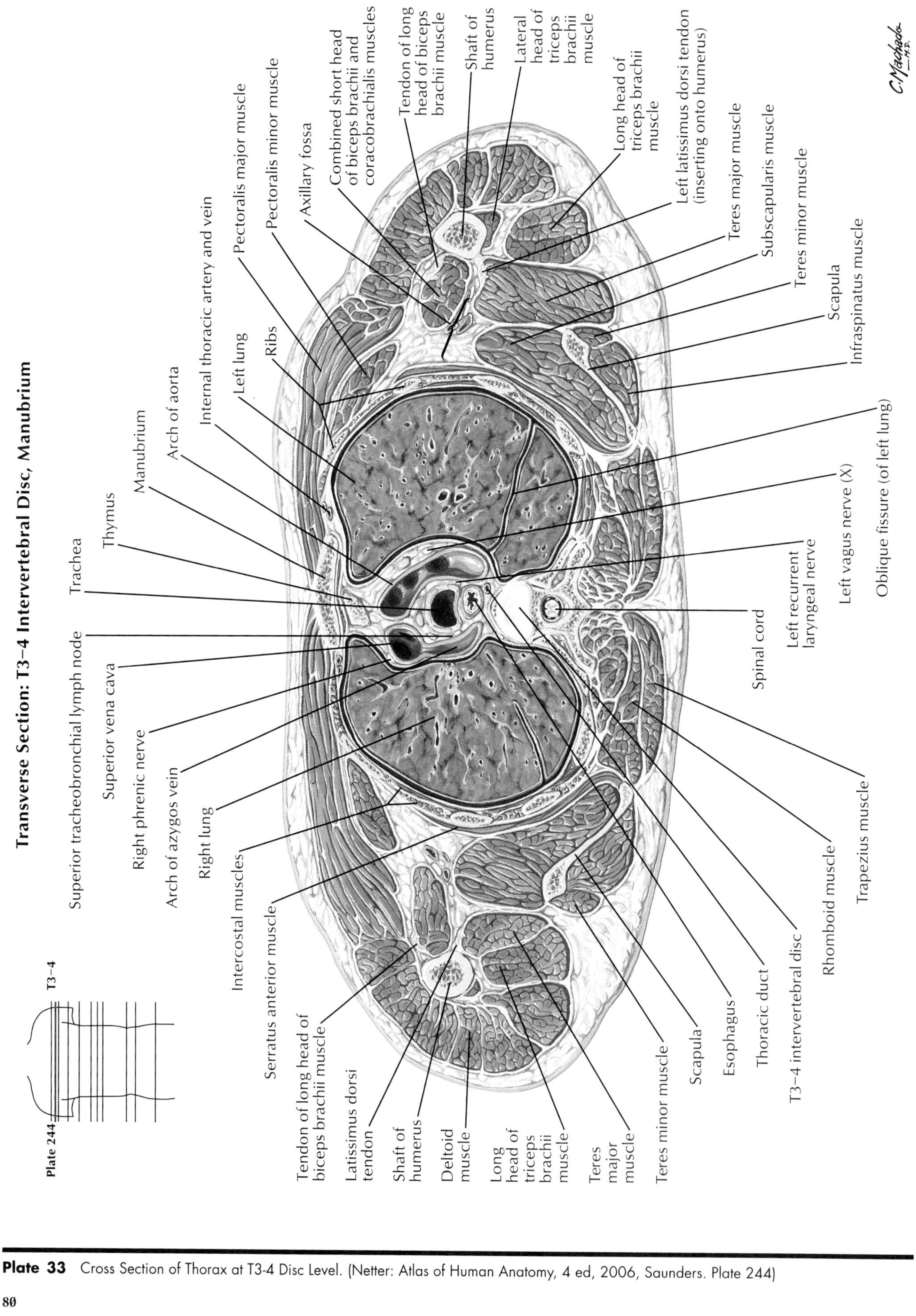
Transverse Section: T3–4 Intervertebral Disc, Manubrium
Plate 244
T3–4
Superior tracheobronchial lymph node
Superior vena cava
Right phrenic nerve
Arch of azygos vein
Right lung
Intercostal muscles
Serratus anterior muscle
Tendon of long head of biceps brachii muscle
Latissimus dorsi tendon
Shaft of humerus
Deltoid muscle
Long head of triceps brachii muscle
Teres major muscle
Teres minor muscle
Trachea
Thymus
Manubrium
Arch of aorta
Internal thoracic artery and vein
Left lung
Ribs
Pectoralis major muscle
Pectoralis minor muscle
Axillary fossa
Combined short head of biceps brachii and coracobrachialis muscles
Tendon of long head of biceps brachii muscle
Shaft of humerus
Lateral head of triceps brachii muscle
Long head of triceps brachii muscle
Left latissimus dorsi tendon (inserting onto humerus)
Teres major muscle
Subscapularis muscle
Teres minor muscle
Scapula
Infraspinatus muscle
Oblique fissure (of left lung)
Left vagus nerve (X)
Left recurrent laryngeal nerve
Spinal cord
Trapezius muscle
Rhomboid muscle
T3–4 intervertebral disc
Thoracic duct
Esophagus
Scapula
C.Machado M.D.

Plate 33 Cross Section of Thorax at T3-4 Disc Level. (Netter: Atlas of Human Anatomy, 4 ed, 2006, Saunders. Plate 244)

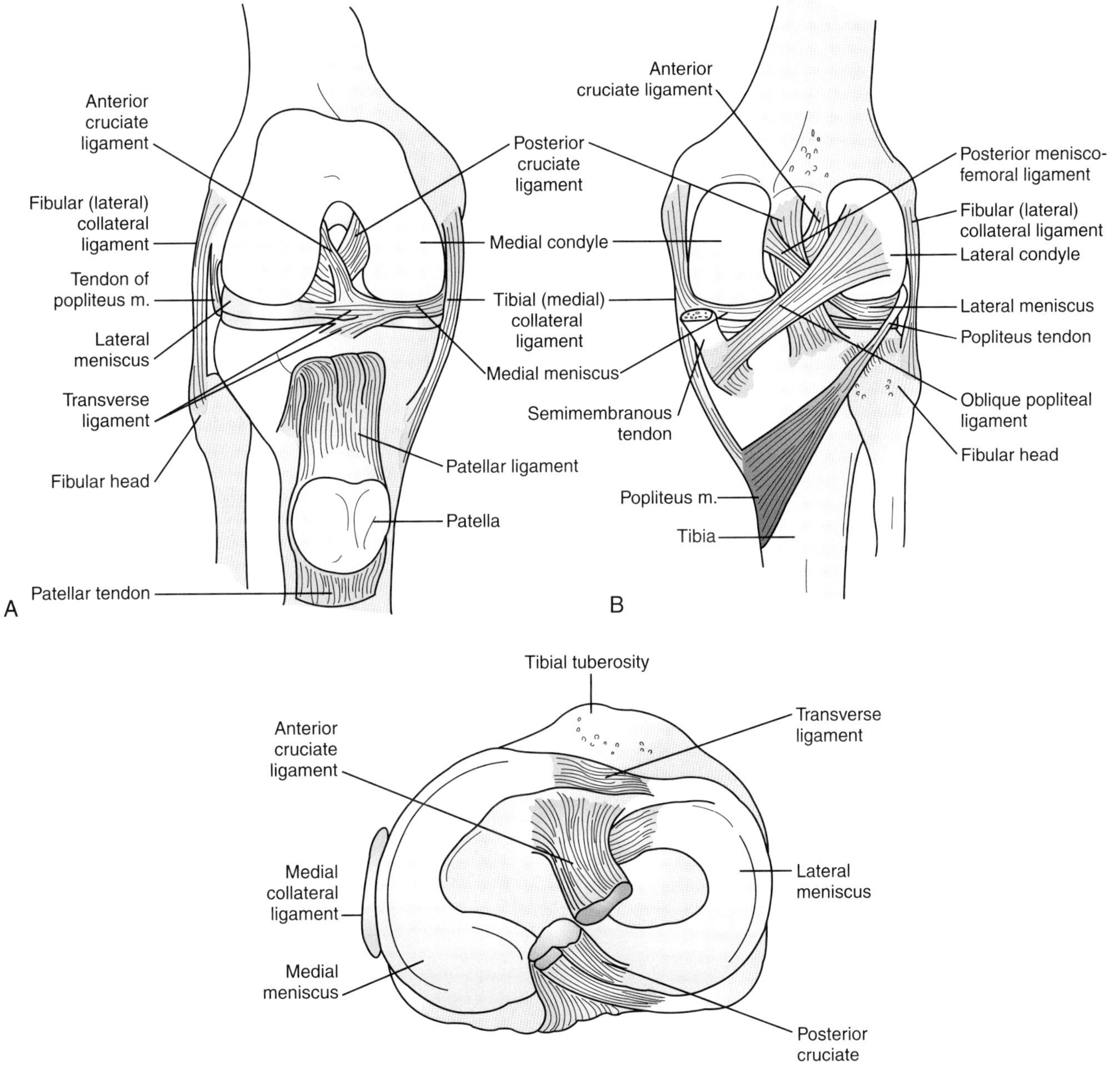

Plate 34 Knee joint opened; anterior, posterior, and proximal views. A, Anterior view of the knee joint, opened by folding the patella and patellar ligament inferiorly. On the lateral side is the fibular collateral ligament, separated by the popliteal tendon from the lateral meniscus. On the medial side, the tibial collateral ligament is attached to the medial meniscus. The anterior and posterior cruciate ligaments are seen between the femoral condyles. B, Posterior view of the opened knee joint with a more complete view of the posterior cruciate ligament. C, The femur is removed, showing the proximal (articular) end of the right tibia. On the medial side is the gently curved medial meniscus; on the lateral side is the more tightly curved lateral meniscus. The anterior end of the medial meniscus is anchored to the surface of the tibia by the transverse ligament. The cut ends of the anterior and posterior cruciate ligaments are shown, as well as the meniscofemoral ligament. (Fritz S: Mosby's Essential Sciences for Therapeutic Massage: Anatomy, Physiology, Biomechanics, and Pathology, ed 5, St. Louis, 2017, Elsevier.)

Paramedian (sagittal) dissection

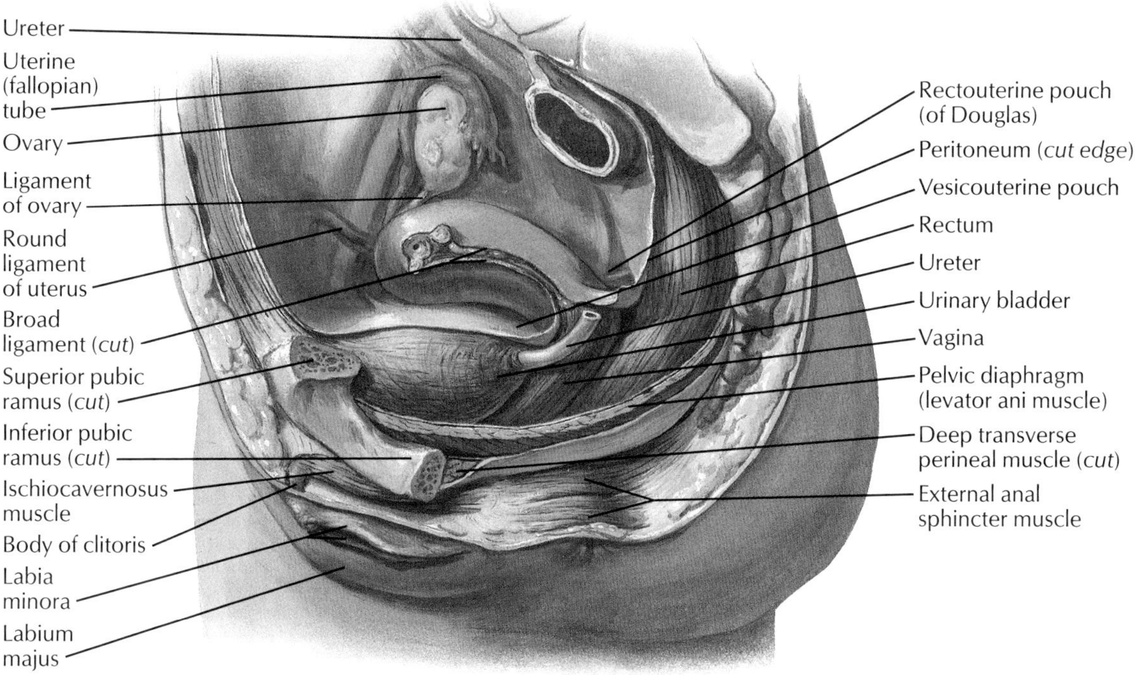

Median (sagittal) section

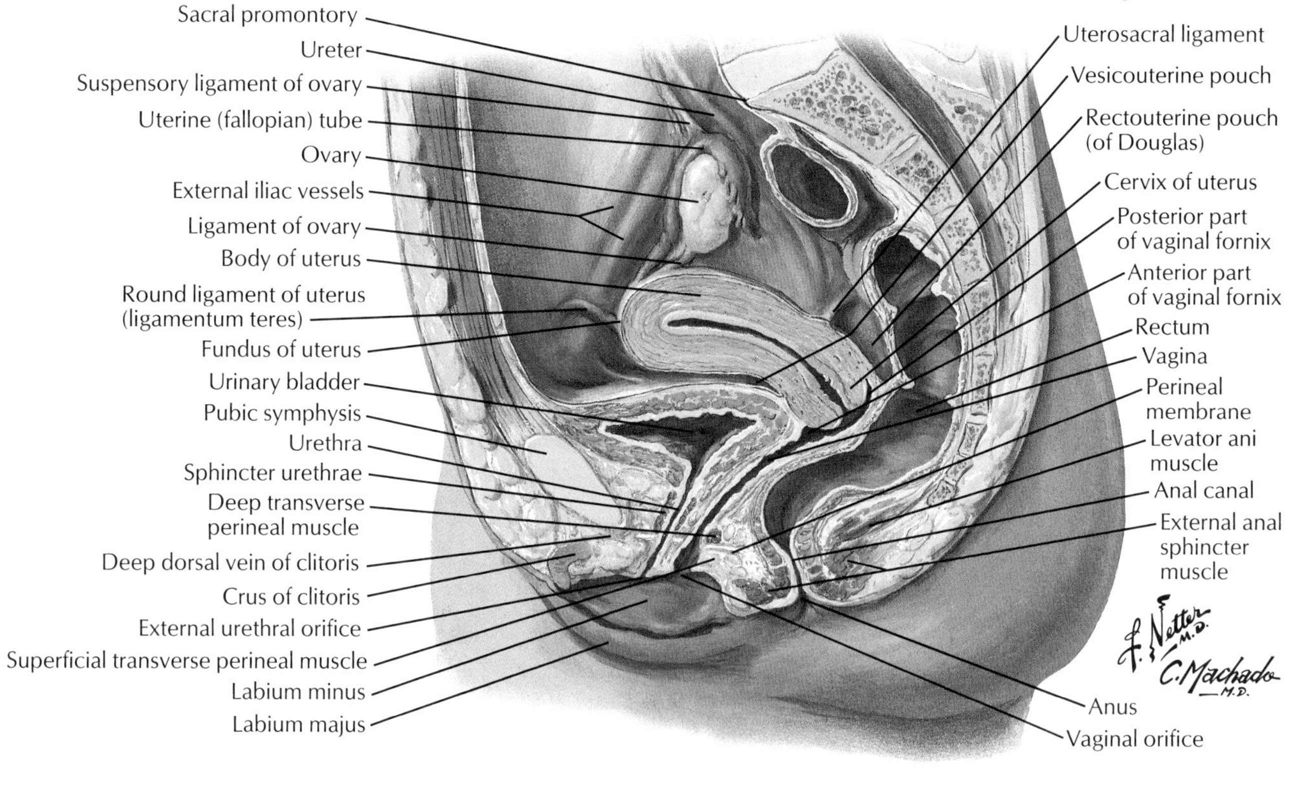

Plate 35 Pelvic Viscera and Perineum: Female. (Netter: Atlas of Human Anatomy, 4 ed, 2006, Saunders. Plate 360)

PART II

Alphabetic Index

A

- Aarskog's syndrome Q87.19
- Abandonment *—see* Maltreatment
- Abasia (-astasia) (hysterical) F44.4
- Abderhalden-Kaufmann-Lignac syndrome (cystinosis) E72.Ø4
- Abdomen, abdominal *—see also* condition
  - acute R1Ø.Ø
  - angina K55.1
  - muscle deficiency syndrome Q79.4
- Abdominalgia *—see* Pain, abdominal
- Abduction contracture, hip or other joint *—see* Contraction, joint
- Aberrant (congenital) *—see also* Malposition, congenital
  - adrenal gland Q89.1
  - artery (peripheral) Q27.8
    - basilar NEC Q28.1
    - cerebral Q28.3
    - coronary Q24.5
    - digestive system Q27.8
    - eye Q15.8
    - lower limb Q27.8
    - precerebral Q28.1
    - pulmonary Q25.79
    - renal Q27.2
    - retina Q14.1
    - specified site NEC Q27.8
    - subclavian Q27.8
    - upper limb Q27.8
    - vertebral Q28.1
  - breast Q83.8
  - endocrine gland NEC Q89.2
  - hepatic duct Q44.5
  - pancreas Q45.3
  - parathyroid gland Q89.2
  - pituitary gland Q89.2
  - sebaceous glands, mucous membrane, mouth, congenital Q38.6
  - spleen Q89.Ø9
  - subclavian artery Q27.8
  - thymus (gland) Q89.2
  - thyroid gland Q89.2
  - vein (peripheral) NEC Q27.8
    - cerebral Q28.3
    - digestive system Q27.8
    - lower limb Q27.8
    - precerebral Q28.1
    - specified site NEC Q27.8
    - upper limb Q27.8
- Aberration
  - distantial *—see* Disturbance, visual
  - mental F99
- Abetalipoproteinemia E78.6
- Abiotrophy R68.89
- Ablatio, ablation
  - retinae *—see* Detachment, retina
- Ablepharia, ablepharon Q1Ø.3
- Abnormal, abnormality, abnormalities *—see also* Anomaly
  - acid-base balance (mixed) E87.4
  - albumin R77.Ø
  - alphafetoprotein R77.2
  - alveolar ridge KØ8.9
  - anatomical relationship Q89.9
  - apertures, congenital, diaphragm Q79.1
  - auditory perception H93.29-●
    - diplacusis *—see* Diplacusis
    - hyperacusis *—see* Hyperacusis
    - recruitment *—see* Recruitment, auditory
    - threshold shift *—see* Shift, auditory threshold
  - autosomes Q99.9
    - fragile site Q95.5
  - basal metabolic rate R94.8
  - biosynthesis, testicular androgen E29.1
  - bleeding time R79.1

Abnormal, abnormality, abnormalities *—(Continued)*

  - blood level (of)
    - cobalt R79.Ø
    - copper R79.Ø
    - iron R79.Ø
    - lithium R78.89
    - magnesium R79.Ø
    - mineral NEC R79.Ø
    - zinc R79.Ø
  - blood pressure
    - elevated RØ3.Ø
    - low reading (nonspecific) RØ3.1
  - blood sugar R73.Ø9
  - blood-gas level R79.81
  - bowel sounds R19.15
    - absent R19.11
    - hyperactive R19.12
  - brain scan R94.Ø2
  - breathing RØ6.9
  - caloric test R94.138
  - cerebrospinal fluid R83.9
    - cytology R83.6
    - drug level R83.2
    - enzyme level R83.Ø
    - hormones R83.1
    - immunology R83.4
    - microbiology R83.5
    - nonmedicinal level R83.3
    - specified type NEC R83.8
  - chemistry, blood R79.9
    - C-reactive protein R79.82
    - drugs *—see* Findings, abnormal, in blood
    - gas level R79.81
    - minerals R79.Ø
    - pancytopenia D61.818
    - PTT R79.1
    - specified NEC R79.89
    - toxins *—see* Findings, abnormal, in blood
  - chest sounds (friction) (rales) RØ9.89
  - chromosome, chromosomal Q99.9
    - with more than three X chromosomes, female Q97.1
    - analysis result R89.8
      - bronchial washings R84.8
      - cerebrospinal fluid R83.8
      - cervix uteri NEC R87.89
      - nasal secretions R84.8
      - nipple discharge R89.8
      - peritoneal fluid R85.89
      - pleural fluid R84.8
      - prostatic secretions R86.8
      - saliva R85.89
      - seminal fluid R86.8
      - sputum R84.8
      - synovial fluid R89.8
      - throat scrapings R84.8
      - vagina R87.89
      - vulva R87.89
      - wound secretions R89.8
    - dicentric replacement Q93.2
    - ring replacement Q93.2
    - sex Q99.8
      - female phenotype Q97.9
        - specified NEC Q97.8
      - male phenotype Q98.9
        - specified NEC Q98.8
      - structural male Q98.6
    - specified NEC Q99.8
  - clinical findings NEC R68.89
  - coagulation D68.9
    - newborn, transient P61.6
    - profile R79.1
    - time R79.1
  - communication *—see* Fistula
  - conjunctiva, vascular H11.41-●
  - coronary artery Q24.5
  - cortisol-binding globulin E27.8
  - course, eustachian tube Q17.8

Abnormal, abnormality, abnormalities *—(Continued)*

  - creatinine clearance R94.4
  - cytology
    - anus R85.619
      - atypical squamous cells cannot exclude high grade squamous intraepithelial lesion (ASC-H) R85.611
      - atypical squamous cells of undetermined significance (ASC-US) R85.61Ø
      - cytologic evidence of malignancy R85.614
      - high grade squamous intraepithelial lesion (HGSIL) R85.613
      - human papillomavirus (HPV) DNA test
        - high risk positive R85.81
        - low risk postive R85.82
      - inadequate smear R85.615
      - low grade squamous intraepithelial lesion (LGSIL) R85.612
      - satisfactory anal smear but lacking transformation zone R85.616
      - specified NEC R85.618
      - unsatisfactory smear R85.615
    - female genital organs *—see* Abnormal, Papanicolaou (smear)
  - dark adaptation curve H53.61
  - dentofacial NEC *—see* Anomaly, dentofacial
  - development, developmental Q89.9
    - central nervous system QØ7.9
  - diagnostic imaging
    - abdomen, abdominal region NEC R93.5
    - biliary tract R93.2
    - bladder R93.41
    - breast R92.8
    - central nervous system NEC R9Ø.89
    - cerebrovascular NEC R9Ø.89
    - coronary circulation R93.1
    - digestive tract NEC R93.3
    - gastrointestinal (tract) R93.3
    - genitourinary organs R93.89
    - head R93.Ø
    - heart R93.1
    - intrathoracic organ NEC R93.89
    - kidney R93.42-●
    - limbs R93.6
    - liver R93.2
    - lung (field) R91.8
    - musculoskeletal system NEC R93.7
    - renal pelvis R93.41
    - retroperitoneum R93.5
    - site specified NEC R93.89
    - skin and subcutaneous tissue R93.89
    - skull R93.Ø9
    - testis R93.81-●
    - urinary organs specified NEC R93.49
    - ureter R93.41
  - direction, teeth, fully erupted M26.3Ø
  - ear ossicles, acquired NEC H74.39-●
    - ankylosis *—see* Ankylosis, ear ossicles
    - discontinuity *—see* Discontinuity, ossicles, ear
    - partial loss *—see* Loss, ossicles, ear (partial)
  - Ebstein Q22.5
  - echocardiogram R93.1
  - echoencephalogram R9Ø.81
  - echogram *—see* Abnormal, diagnostic imaging
  - electrocardiogram [ECG] [EKG] R94.31
  - electroencephalogram [EEG] R94.Ø1
  - electrolyte *—see* Imbalance, electrolyte
  - electromyogram [EMG] R94.131
  - electro-oculogram [EOG] R94.11Ø
  - electrophysiological intracardiac studies R94.39
  - electroretinogram [ERG] R94.111
  - erythrocytes
    - congenital, with perinatal jaundice D58.9
  - feces (color) (contents) (mucus) R19.5

A

Abnormal, abnormality, abnormalities — *(Continued)*
finding —*see* Findings, abnormal, without diagnosis
fluid
amniotic —*see* Abnormal, specimen, specified
cerebrospinal —*see* Abnormal, cerebrospinal fluid
peritoneal —*see* Abnormal, specimen, digestive organs
pleural —*see* Abnormal, specimen, respiratory organs
synovial —*see* Abnormal, specimen, specified
thorax (bronchial washings) (pleural fluid) —*see* Abnormal, specimen, respiratory organs
vaginal —*see* Abnormal, specimen, female genital organs
form
teeth KØØ.2
uterus —*see* Anomaly, uterus
function studies
auditory R94.12Ø
bladder R94.8
brain R94.Ø9
cardiovascular R94.3Ø
ear R94.128
endocrine NEC R94.7
eye NEC R94.118
kidney R94.4
liver R94.5
nervous system
central NEC R94.Ø9
peripheral NEC R94.138
pancreas R94.8
placenta R94.8
pulmonary R94.2
special senses NEC R94.128
spleen R94.8
thyroid R94.6
vestibular R94.121
gait —*see* Gait
hysterical F44.4
gastrin secretion E16.4
globulin R77.1
cortisol-binding E27.8
thyroid-binding EØ7.89
glomerular, minor —*see also* NØØ-NØ7 with fourth character .Ø NØ5.Ø
glucagon secretion E16.3
glucose tolerance (test) (non-fasting) R73.Ø9
gravitational (G) forces or states (effect of) T75.81
hair (color) (shaft) L67.9
specified NEC L67.8
hard tissue formation in pulp (dental) KØ4.3
head movement R25.Ø
heart
rate RØØ.9
specified NEC RØØ.8
shadow R93.1
sounds NEC RØ1.2
hemoglobin (disease) —*see also* Disease, hemoglobin D58.2
trait —*see* Trait, hemoglobin, abnormal
histology NEC R89.7
immunological findings R89.4
in serum R76.9
specified NEC R76.8
increase in appetite R63.2
involuntary movement —*see* Abnormal, movement, involuntary
jaw closure M26.51
karyotype R89.8
kidney function test R94.4
knee jerk R29.2
leukocyte (cell) (differential) NEC D72.9

Abnormal, abnormality, abnormalities — *(Continued)*
liver function test R94.5
loss of
height R29.89Ø
weight R63.4
mammogram NEC R92.8
calcification (calculus) R92.1
microcalcification R92.Ø
Mantoux test R76.11
movement (disorder) —*see also* Disorder, movement
head R25.Ø
involuntary R25.9
fasciculation R25.3
of head R25.Ø
spasm R25.2
specified type NEC R25.8
tremor R25.1
myoglobin (Aberdeen) (Annapolis) R89.7
neonatal screening PØ9
oculomotor study R94.113
palmar creases Q82.8
Papanicolaou (smear)
anus R85.619
atypical squamous cells cannot exclude high grade squamous intraepithelial lesion (ASC-H) R85.611
atypical squamous cells of undetermined significance (ASC-US) R85.61Ø
cytologic evidence of malignancy R85.614
high grade squamous intraepithelial lesion (HGSIL) R85.613
human papillomavirus (HPV) DNA test
high risk positive R85.81
low risk postive R85.82
inadequate smear R85.615
low grade squamous intraepithelial lesion (LGSIL) R85.612
satisfactory anal smear but lacking transformation zone R85.616
specified NEC R85.618
unsatisfactory smear R85.615
bronchial washings R84.6
cerebrospinal fluid R83.6
cervix R87.619
atypical squamous cells cannot exclude high grade squamous intraepithelial lesion (ASC-H) R87.611
atypical squamous cells of undetermined significance (ASC-US) R87.61Ø
cytologic evidence of malignancy R87.614
high grade squamous intraepithelial lesion (HGSIL) R87.613
inadequate smear R87.615
low grade squamous intraepithelial lesion (LGSIL) R87.612
non-atypical endometrial cells R87.618
satisfactory cervical smear but lacking transformation zone R87.616
specified NEC R87.618
thin preparaton R87.619
unsatisfactory smear R87.615
nasal secretions R84.6
nipple discharge R89.6
peritoneal fluid R85.69
pleural fluid R84.6
prostatic secretions R86.6
saliva R85.69
seminal fluid R86.6
sites NEC R89.6
sputum R84.6
synovial fluid R89.6
throat scrapings R84.6

Abnormal, abnormality, abnormalities — *(Continued)*
Papanicolaou (smear) *(Continued)*
vagina R87.629
atypical squamous cells cannot exclude high grade squamous intraepithelial lesion (ASC-H) R87.621
atypical squamous cells of undetermined significance (ASC-US) R87.62Ø
cytologic evidence of malignancy R87.624
high grade squamous intraepithelial lesion (HGSIL) R87.623
inadequate smear R87.625
low grade squamous intraepithelial lesion (LGSIL) R87.622
specified NEC R87.628
thin preparation R87.629
unsatisfactory smear R87.625
vulva R87.69
wound secretions R89.6
partial thromboplastin time (PTT) R79.1
pelvis (bony) —*see* Deformity, pelvis
percussion, chest (tympany) RØ9.89
periods (grossly) —*see* Menstruation
phonocardiogram R94.39
plantar reflex R29.2
plasma
protein R77.9
specified NEC R77.8
viscosity R7Ø.1
pleural (folds) Q34.Ø
posture R29.3
product of conception OØ2.9
specified type NEC OØ2.89
prothrombin time (PT) R79.1
pulmonary
artery, congenital Q25.79
function, newborn P28.89
test results R94.2
pulsations in neck RØØ.2
pupillary H21.56- •
function (reaction) (reflex) —*see* Anomaly, pupil, function
radiological examination —*see* Abnormal, diagnostic imaging
red blood cell(s) (morphology) (volume) R71.8
reflex —*see* Reflex
renal function test R94.4
response to nerve stimulation R94.13Ø
retinal correspondence H53.31
retinal function study R94.111
rhythm, heart —*see also* Arrhythmia
saliva —*see* Abnormal, specimen, digestive organs
scan
kidney R94.4
liver R93.2
thyroid R94.6
secretion
gastrin E16.4
glucagon E16.3
semen, seminal fluid —*see* Abnormal, specimen, male genital organs
serum level (of)
acid phosphatase R74.8
alkaline phosphatase R74.8
amylase R74.8
enzymes R74.9
specified NEC R74.8
lipase R74.8
triacylglycerol lipase R74.8
shape
gravid uterus —*see* Anomaly, uterus
sinus venosus Q21.1
size, tooth, teeth KØØ.2
spacing, tooth, teeth, fully erupted M26.3Ø

A

Abnormal, abnormality, abnormalities — *(Continued)*
specimen
digestive organs (peritoneal fluid) (saliva) R85.9
cytology R85.69
drug level R85.2
enzyme level R85.Ø
histology R85.7
hormones R85.1
immunology R85.4
microbiology R85.5
nonmedicinal level R85.3
specified type NEC R85.89
female genital organs (secretions) (smears) R87.9
cytology R87.69
cervix R87.619
human papillomavirus (HPV) DNA test
high risk positive R87.81Ø
low risk positive R87.82Ø
inadequate (unsatisfactory) smear R87.615
non-atypical endometrial cells R87.618
specified NEC R87.618
vagina R87.629
human papillomavirus (HPV) DNA test
high risk positive R87.811
low risk positive R87.821
inadequate (unsatisfactory) smear R87.625
vulva R87.69
drug level R87.2
enzyme level R87.Ø
histological R87.7
hormones R87.1
immunology R87.4
microbiology R87.5
nonmedicinal level R87.3
specified type NEC R87.89
male genital organs (prostatic secretions) (semen) R86.9
cytology R86.6
drug level R86.2
enzyme level R86.Ø
histological R86.7
hormones R86.1
immunology R86.4
microbiology R86.5
nonmedicinal level R86.3
specified type NEC R86.8
nipple discharge —*see* Abnormal, specimen, specified
respiratory organs (bronchial washings) (nasal secretions) (pleural fluid) (sputum) R84.9
cytology R84.6
drug level R84.2
enzyme level R84.Ø
histology R84.7
hormones R84.1
immunology R84.4
microbiology R84.5
nonmedicinal level R84.3
specified type NEC R84.8
specified organ, system and tissue NOS R89.9
cytology R89.6
drug level R89.2
enzyme level R89.Ø
histology R89.7
hormones R89.1
immunology R89.4
microbiology R89.5
nonmedicinal level R89.3
specified type NEC R89.8
synovial fluid —*see* Abnormal, specimen, specified

Abnormal, abnormality, abnormalities — *(Continued)*
specimen *(Continued)*
thorax (bronchial washings) (pleural fluids) —*see* Abnormal, specimen, respiratory organs
vagina (secretion) (smear) R87.629
vulva (secretion) (smear) R87.69
wound secretion —*see* Abnormal, specimen, specified
spermatozoa —*see* Abnormal, specimen, male genital organs
sputum (amount) (color) (odor) RØ9.3
stool (color) (contents) (mucus) R19.5
bloody K92.1
guaiac positive R19.5
synchondrosis Q78.8
thermography —*see also* Abnormal, diagnostic imaging R93.89
thyroid-binding globulin EØ7.89
tooth, teeth (form) (size) KØØ.2
toxicology (findings) R78.9
transport protein E88.Ø9
tumor marker NEC R97.8
ultrasound results —*see* Abnormal, diagnostic imaging
umbilical cord complicating delivery O69.9
urination NEC R39.198
urine (constituents) R82.9Ø
bile R82.2
➡ cytological examination R82.89
drugs R82.5
fat R82.Ø
glucose R81
heavy metals R82.6
hemoglobin R82.3
➡ histological examination R82.89
ketones R82.4
microbiological examination (culture) R82.79
myoglobin R82.1
positive culture R82.79
protein —*see* Proteinuria
specified substance NEC R82.998
chromoabnormality NEC R82.91
substances nonmedical R82.6
uterine hemorrhage —*see* Hemorrhage, uterus
vectorcardiogram R94.39
visually evoked potential (VEP) R94.112
white blood cells D72.9
specified NEC D72.89
X-ray examination —*see* Abnormal, diagnostic imaging
Abnormity (any organ or part) —*see* Anomaly
Abocclusion M26.29
hemolytic disease (newborn) P55.1
incompatibility reaction ABO —*see* Complication(s), transfusion, incompatibility reaction, ABO
Abolition, language R48.8
Aborter, habitual or recurrent —*see* Loss (of), pregnancy, recurrent
Abortion (complete) (spontaneous) OØ3.9
with
retained products of conception —*see* Abortion, incomplete
attempted (elective) (failed) OØ7.4
complicated by OØ7.3Ø
afibrinogenemia OØ7.1
cardiac arrest OØ7.36
chemical damage of pelvic organ(s) OØ7.34
circulatory collapse OØ7.31
cystitis OØ7.38
defibrination syndrome OØ7.1
electrolyte imbalance OØ7.33
embolism (air) (amniotic fluid) (blood clot) (fat) (pulmonary) (septic) (soap) OØ7.2
endometritis OØ7.Ø

Abortion *(Continued)*
attempted *(Continued)*
complicated by *(Continued)*
genital tract and pelvic infection OØ7.Ø
hemolysis OØ7.1
hemorrhage (delayed) (excessive) OØ7.1
infection
genital tract or pelvic OØ7.Ø
urinary tract tract OØ7.38
intravascular coagulation OØ7.1
laceration of pelvic organ(s) OØ7.34
metabolic disorder OØ7.33
oliguria OØ7.32
oophoritis OØ7.Ø
parametritis OØ7.Ø
pelvic peritonitis OØ7.Ø
perforation of pelvic organ(s) OØ7.34
renal failure or shutdown OØ7.32
salpingitis or salpingo-oophoritis OØ7.Ø
sepsis OØ7.37
shock OØ7.31
specified condition NEC OØ7.39
tubular necrosis (renal) OØ7.32
uremia OØ7.32
urinary tract infection OØ7.38
venous complication NEC OØ7.35
embolism (air) (amniotic fluid) (blood clot) (fat) (pulmonary) (septic) (soap) OØ7.2
complicated (by) (following) OØ3.8Ø
afibrinogenemia OØ3.6
cardiac arrest OØ3.86
chemical damage of pelvic organ(s) OØ3.84
circulatory collapse OØ3.81
cystitis OØ3.88
defibrination syndrome OØ3.6
electrolyte imbalance OØ3.83
embolism (air) (amniotic fluid) (blood clot) (fat) (pulmonary) (septic) (soap) OØ3.7
endometritis OØ3.5
genital tract and pelvic infection OØ3.5
hemolysis OØ3.6
hemorrhage (delayed) (excessive) OØ3.6
infection
genital tract or pelvic OØ3.5
urinary tract OØ3.88
intravascular coagulation OØ3.6
laceration of pelvic organ(s) OØ3.84
metabolic disorder OØ3.83
oliguria OØ3.82
oophoritis OØ3.5
parametritis OØ3.5
pelvic peritonitis OØ3.5
perforation of pelvic organ(s) OØ3.84
renal failure or shutdown OØ3.82
salpingitis or salpingo-oophoritis OØ3.5
sepsis OØ3.87
shock OØ3.81
specified condition NEC OØ3.89
tubular necrosis (renal) OØ3.82
uremia OØ3.82
urinary tract infection OØ3.88
venous complication NEC OØ3.85
embolism (air) (amniotic fluid) (blood clot) (fat) (pulmonary) (septic) (soap) OØ3.7
failed —*see* Abortion, attempted
habitual or recurrent N96
with current abortion —*see* categories OØ3-OØ4
without current pregnancy N96
care in current pregnancy O26.2- •
incomplete (spontaneous) OØ3.4
complicated (by) (following) OØ3.3Ø
afibrinogenemia OØ3.1
cardiac arrest OØ3.36
chemical damage of pelvic organ(s) OØ3.34
circulatory collapse OØ3.31
cystitis OØ3.38

Abortion *(Continued)*
incomplete *(Continued)*
complicated *(Continued)*
defibrination syndrome O03.1
electrolyte imbalance O03.33
embolism (air) (amniotic fluid) (blood clot) (fat) (pulmonary) (septic) (soap) O03.2
endometritis O03.0
genital tract and pelvic infection O03.0
hemolysis O03.1
hemorrhage (delayed) (excessive) O03.1
infection
genital tract or pelvic O03.0
urinary tract O03.38
intravascular coagulation O03.1
laceration of pelvic organ(s) O03.34
metabolic disorder O03.33
oliguria O03.32
oophoritis O03.0
parametritis O03.0
pelvic peritonitis O03.0
perforation of pelvic organ(s) O03.34
renal failure or shutdown O03.32
salpingitis or salpingo-oophoritis O03.0
sepsis O03.37
shock O03.31
specified condition NEC O03.39
tubular necrosis (renal) O03.32
uremia O03.32
urinary infection O03.38
venous complication NEC O03.35
embolism (air) (amniotic fluid) (blood clot) (fat) (pulmonary) (septic) (soap) O03.2
induced (encounter for) Z33.2
complicated by O04.80
afibrinogenemia O04.6
cardiac arrest O04.86
chemical damage of pelvic organ(s) O04.84
circulatory collapse O04.81
cystitis O04.88
defibrination syndrome O04.6
electrolyte imbalance O04.83
embolism (air) (amniotic fluid) (blood clot) (fat) (pulmonary) (septic) (soap) O04.7
endometritis O04.5
genital tract and pelvic infection O04.5
hemolysis O04.6
hemorrhage (delayed) (excessive) O04.6
infection
genital tract or pelvic O04.5
urinary tract O04.88
intravascular coagulation O04.6
laceration of pelvic organ(s) O04.84
metabolic disorder O04.83
oliguria O04.82
oophoritis O04.5
parametritis O04.5
pelvic peritonitis O04.5
perforation of pelvic organ(s) O04.84
renal failure or shutdown O04.82
salpingitis or salpingo-oophoritis O04.5
sepsis O04.87
shock O04.81
specified condition NEC O04.89
tubular necrosis (renal) O04.82
uremia O04.82
urinary tract infection O04.88
venous complication NEC O04.85
embolism (air) (amniotic fluid) (blood clot) (fat) (pulmonary) (septic) (soap) O04.7
missed O02.1
spontaneous *—see* Abortion (complete) (spontaneous)
threatened O20.0
threatened (spontaneous) O20.0

Abortion *(Continued)*
tubal O00.10-●
with intrauterine pregnancy O00.11-
Abortus fever A23.1
Aboulomania F60.7
Abrami's disease D59.8
Abramov-Fiedler myocarditis (acute isolated myocarditis) I40.1
Abrasion T14.8
abdomen, abdominal (wall) S30.811
alveolar process S00.512
ankle S90.51-●
antecubital space *—see* Abrasion, elbow
anus S30.817
arm (upper) S40.81-●
auditory canal *—see* Abrasion, ear
auricle *—see* Abrasion, ear
axilla *—see* Abrasion, arm
back, lower S30.810
breast S20.11-●
brow S00.81
buttock S30.810
calf *—see* Abrasion, leg
canthus *—see* Abrasion, eyelid
cheek S00.81
internal S00.512
chest wall *—see* Abrasion, thorax
chin S00.81
clitoris S30.814
cornea S05.0-●
costal region *—see* Abrasion, thorax
dental K03.1
digit(s)
foot *—see* Abrasion, toe
hand *—see* Abrasion, finger
ear S00.41-●
elbow S50.31-●
epididymis S30.813
epigastric region S30.811
epiglottis S10.11
esophagus (thoracic) S27.818
cervical S10.11
eyebrow *—see* Abrasion, eyelid
eyelid S00.21-●
face S00.81
finger(s) S60.41-●
index S60.41-●
little S60.41-●
middle S60.41-●
ring S60.41-●
flank S30.811
foot (except toe(s) alone) S90.81-●
toe *—see* Abrasion, toe
forearm S50.81-●
elbow only *—see* Abrasion, elbow
forehead S00.81
genital organs, external
female S30.816
male S30.815
groin S30.811
gum S00.512
hand S60.51-●
head S00.91
ear *—see* Abrasion, ear
eyelid *—see* Abrasion, eyelid
lip S00.511
nose S00.31
oral cavity S00.512
scalp S00.01
specified site NEC S00.81
heel *—see* Abrasion, foot
hip S70.21-●
inguinal region S30.811
interscapular region S20.419
jaw S00.81
knee S80.21-●
labium (majus) (minus) S30.814
larynx S10.11
leg (lower) S80.81-●
knee *—see* Abrasion, knee
upper *—see* Abrasion, thigh

Abrasion *(Continued)*
lip S00.511
lower back S30.810
lumbar region S30.810
malar region S00.81
mammary *—see* Abrasion, breast
mastoid region S00.81
mouth S00.512
nail
finger *—see* Abrasion, finger
toe *—see* Abrasion, toe
nape S10.81
nasal S00.31
neck S10.91
specified site NEC S10.81
throat S10.11
nose S00.31
occipital region S00.01
oral cavity S00.512
orbital region *—see* Abrasion, eyelid
palate S00.512
palm *—see* Abrasion, hand
parietal region S00.01
pelvis S30.810
penis S30.812
perineum
female S30.814
male S30.810
periocular area *—see* Abrasion, eyelid
phalanges
finger *—see* Abrasion, finger
toe *—see* Abrasion, toe
pharynx S10.11
pinna *—see* Abrasion, ear
popliteal space *—see* Abrasion, knee
prepuce S30.812
pubic region S30.810
pudendum
female S30.816
male S30.815
sacral region S30.810
scalp S00.01
scapular region *—see* Abrasion, shoulder
scrotum S30.813
shin *—see* Abrasion, leg
shoulder S40.21-●
skin NEC T14.8
sternal region S20.319
submaxillary region S00.81
submental region S00.81
subungual
finger(s) *—see* Abrasion, finger
toe(s) *—see* Abrasion, toe
supraclavicular fossa S10.81
supraorbital S00.81
temple S00.81
temporal region S00.81
testis S30.813
thigh S70.31-●
thorax, thoracic (wall) S20.91
back S20.41-●
front S20.31-●
throat S10.11
thumb S60.31-●
toe(s) (lesser) S90.416
great S90.41-●
tongue S00.512
tooth, teeth (dentifrice) (habitual) (hard tissues) (occupational) (ritual) (traditional) K03.1
trachea S10.11
tunica vaginalis S30.813
tympanum, tympanic membrane *—see* Abrasion, ear
uvula S00.512
vagina S30.814
vocal cords S10.11
vulva S30.814
wrist S60.81-●
Abrism *—see* Poisoning, food, noxious, plant

- **Abruptio placentae** O45.9-•
  - with
    - afibrinogenemia O45.Ø1-•
    - coagulation defect O45.ØØ-•
      - specified NEC O45.Ø9-•
    - disseminated intravascular coagulation O45.Ø2-•
    - hypofibrinogenemia O45.Ø1-•
  - specified NEC O45.8-•
- **Abruption, placenta** —*see* Abruptio placentae
- **Abscess** (connective tissue) (embolic) (fistulous) (infective) (metastatic) (multiple) (pernicious) (pyogenic) (septic) LØ2.91
  - with
    - diverticular disease (intestine) K57.8Ø
      - with bleeding K57.81
      - large intestine K57.2Ø
        - with
          - bleeding K57.21
          - small intestine K57.4Ø
            - with bleeding K57.41
      - small intestine K57.ØØ
        - with
          - bleeding K57.Ø1
          - large intestine K57.4Ø
            - with bleeding K57.41
    - lymphangitis - code by site under Abscess
  - abdomen, abdominal
    - cavity K65.1
    - wall LØ2.211
  - abdominopelvic K65.1
  - accessory sinus —*see* Sinusitis
  - adrenal (capsule) (gland) E27.8
  - alveolar KØ4.7
    - with sinus KØ4.6
  - amebic AØ6.4
    - brain (and liver or lung abscess) AØ6.6
    - genitourinary tract AØ6.82
    - liver (without mention of brain or lung abscess) AØ6.4
    - lung (and liver) (without mention of brain abscess) AØ6.5
    - specified site NEC AØ6.89
    - spleen AØ6.89
  - anerobic A48.Ø
  - ankle —*see* Abscess, lower limb
  - anorectal K61.2
  - antecubital space —*see* Abscess, upper limb
  - antrum (chronic) (Highmore) —*see* Sinusitis, maxillary
  - anus K61.Ø
  - apical (tooth) KØ4.7
    - with sinus (alveolar) KØ4.6
  - appendix K35.33
  - areola (acute) (chronic) (nonpuerperal) N61.1
    - puerperal, postpartum or gestational —*see* Infection, nipple
  - arm (any part) —*see* Abscess, upper limb
  - artery (wall) I77.89
  - atheromatous I77.2
  - auricle, ear —*see* Abscess, ear, external
  - axilla (region) LØ2.41-•
    - lymph gland or node LØ4.2
  - back (any part, except buttock) LØ2.212
  - Bartholin's gland N75.1
    - with
      - abortion —*see* Abortion, by type complicated by, sepsis
      - ectopic or molar pregnancy OØ8.Ø
    - following ectopic or molar pregnancy OØ8.Ø
  - Bezold's —*see* Mastoiditis, acute
  - bilharziasis B65.1
  - bladder (wall) —*see* Cystitis, specified type NEC
  - bone (subperiosteal) —*see also* Osteomyelitis, specified type NEC
    - accessory sinus (chronic) —*see* Sinusitis
    - chronic or old —*see* Osteomyelitis, chronic
    - jaw (lower) (upper) M27.2

Abscess *(Continued)*
  - bone *(Continued)*
    - mastoid —*see* Mastoiditis, acute, subperiosteal
    - petrous —*see* Petrositis
    - spinal (tuberculous) A18.Ø1
      - nontuberculous —*see* Osteomyelitis, vertebra
  - bowel K63.Ø
  - brain (any part) (cystic) (otogenic) GØ6.Ø
    - amebic (with abscess of any other site) AØ6.6
    - gonococcal A54.82
    - pheomycotic (chromomycotic) B43.1
    - tuberculous A17.81
  - breast (acute) (chronic) (nonpuerperal) N61.1
    - newborn P39.Ø
    - puerperal, postpartum, gestational —*see* Mastitis, obstetric, purulent
  - broad ligament N73.2
    - acute N73.Ø
    - chronic N73.1
  - Brodie's (localized) (chronic) M86.8X-•
  - bronchi J98.Ø9
  - buccal cavity K12.2
  - bulbourethral gland N34.Ø
  - bursa M71.ØØ
    - ankle M71.Ø7-•
    - elbow M71.Ø2-•
    - foot M71.Ø7-•
    - hand M71.Ø4-•
    - hip M71.Ø5-•
    - knee M71.Ø6-•
    - multiple sites M71.Ø9
    - pharyngeal J39.1
    - shoulder M71.Ø1-•
    - specified site NEC M71.Ø8
    - wrist M71.Ø3-•
  - buttock LØ2.31
  - canthus —*see* Blepharoconjunctivitis
  - cartilage —*see* Disorder, cartilage, specified type NEC
  - cecum K35.33
  - cerebellum, cerebellar GØ6.Ø
    - sequelae GØ9
  - cerebral (embolic) GØ6.Ø
    - sequelae GØ9
  - cervical (meaning neck) LØ2.11
    - lymph gland or node LØ4.Ø
  - cervix (stump) (uteri) —*see* Cervicitis
  - cheek (external) LØ2.Ø1
    - inner K12.2
  - chest J86.9
    - with fistula J86.Ø
    - wall LØ2.213
  - chin LØ2.Ø1
  - choroid —*see* Inflammation, chorioretinal
  - circumtonsillar J36
  - cold (lung) (tuberculous) —*see also* Tuberculosis, abscess, lung
    - articular —*see* Tuberculosis, joint
  - colon (wall) K63.Ø
  - colostomy K94.Ø2
  - conjunctiva —*see* Conjunctivitis, acute
  - cornea H16.31-•
  - corpus
    - cavernosum N48.21
    - luteum —*see* Oophoritis
  - Cowper's gland N34.Ø
  - cranium GØ6.Ø
  - cul-de-sac (Douglas') (posterior) —*see* Peritonitis, pelvic, female
  - cutaneous —*see* Abscess, by site
  - dental KØ4.7
    - with sinus (alveolar) KØ4.6
  - dentoalveolar KØ4.7
    - with sinus KØ4.6
  - diaphragm, diaphragmatic K65.1
  - Douglas' cul-de-sac or pouch —*see* Peritonitis, pelvic, female
  - Dubois A5Ø.59

Abscess *(Continued)*
  - ear (middle) —*see also* Otitis, media, suppurative
    - acute —*see* Otitis, media, suppurative, acute
    - external H6Ø.Ø-•
  - entamebic —*see* Abscess, amebic
  - enterostomy K94.12
  - epididymis N45.4
  - epidural GØ6.2
    - brain GØ6.Ø
    - spinal cord GØ6.1
  - epiglottis J38.7
  - epiploon, epiploic K65.1
  - erysipelatous —*see* Erysipelas
  - esophagus K2Ø.8
  - ethmoid (bone) (chronic) (sinus) J32.2
  - external auditory canal —*see* Abscess, ear, external
  - extradural GØ6.2
    - brain GØ6.Ø
      - sequelae GØ9
    - spinal cord GØ6.1
  - extraperitoneal K68.19
  - eye —*see* Endophthalmitis, purulent
  - eyelid HØØ.Ø3-•
  - face (any part, except ear, eye and nose) LØ2.Ø1
  - fallopian tube —*see* Salpingitis
  - fascia M72.8
  - fauces J39.1
  - fecal K63.Ø
  - femoral (region) —*see* Abscess, lower limb
  - filaria, filarial —*see* Infestation, filarial
  - finger (any) —*see also* Abscess, hand
    - nail —*see* Cellulitis, finger
  - foot LØ2.61-•
  - forehead LØ2.Ø1
  - frontal sinus (chronic) J32.1
  - gallbladder K81.Ø
  - genital organ or tract
    - female (external) N76.4
    - male N49.9
      - multiple sites N49.8
      - specified NEC N49.8
  - gestational mammary O91.11-•
  - gestational subareolar O91.11-•
  - gingival —*see* Periodontitis, localized
  - gland, glandular (lymph) (acute) —*see* Lymphadenitis, acute
  - gluteal (region) LØ2.31
  - gonorrheal —*see* Gonococcus
  - groin LØ2.214
  - gum —*see* Periodontitis, localized
  - hand LØ2.51-•
  - head NEC LØ2.811
    - face (any part, except ear, eye and nose) LØ2.Ø1
  - heart —*see* Carditis
  - heel —*see* Abscess, foot
  - helminthic —*see* Infestation, helminth
  - hepatic (cholangitic) (hematogenic) (lymphogenic) (pylephlebitic) K75.Ø
    - amebic AØ6.4
  - hip (region) —*see* Abscess, lower limb
  - horseshoe K61.31
  - ileocecal K35.33
  - ileostomy (bud) K94.12
  - iliac (region) LØ2.214
    - fossa K35.33
  - infraclavicular (fossa) —*see* Abscess, upper limb
  - inguinal (region) LØ2.214
    - lymph gland or node LØ4.1
  - intersphincteric K61.4
  - intestine, intestinal NEC K63.Ø
    - rectal K61.1
  - intra-abdominal —*see also* Abscess, peritoneum K65.1
    - following procedure T81.43
      - obstetrical O86.Ø3
    - postprocedural T81.49
      - retroperitoneal K68.11

Abscess *(Continued)*
intracranial GØ6.Ø
intramammary *—see* Abscess, breast
intramuscular, following procedure T81.44
obstetrical O86.Ø2
intraorbital *—see* Abscess, orbit
intraperitoneal K65.1
intrasphincteric (anus) K61.4
intraspinal GØ6.1
intratonsillar J36
ischiorectal (fossa) (specified NEC) K61.39
jaw (bone) (lower) (upper) M27.2
joint *—see* Arthritis, pyogenic or pyemic
spine (tuberculous) A18.Ø1
nontuberculous *—see* Spondylopathy, infective
kidney N15.1
with calculus N2Ø.Ø
with hydronephrosis N13.6
puerperal (postpartum) O86.21
knee *—see also* Abscess, lower limb
joint MØØ.9
labium (majus) (minus) N76.4
lacrimal
caruncle *—see* Inflammation, lacrimal, passages, acute
gland *—see* Dacryoadenitis
passages (duct) (sac) *—see* Inflammation, lacrimal, passages, acute
lacunar N34.Ø
larynx J38.7
lateral (alveolar) KØ4.7
with sinus KØ4.6
leg (any part) *—see* Abscess, lower limb
lens H27.8
lingual K14.Ø
tonsil J36
lip K13.Ø
Littre's gland N34.Ø
liver (cholangitic) (hematogenic) (lymphogenic) (pylephlebitic) (pyogenic) K75.Ø
amebic (due to Entamoeba histolytica) (dysenteric) (tropical) AØ6.4
with
brain abscess (and liver or lung abscess) AØ6.6
lung abscess AØ6.5
loin (region) LØ2.211
lower limb LØ2.41- •
lumbar (tuberculous) A18.Ø1
nontuberculous LØ2.212
lung (miliary) (putrid) J85.2
with pneumonia J85.1
due to specified organism (*see* Pneumonia, in (due to))
amebic (with liver abscess) AØ6.5
with
brain abscess AØ6.6
pneumonia AØ6.5
lymph, lymphatic, gland or node (acute) *—see also* Lymphadenitis, acute
mesentery I88.Ø
malar M27.2
mammary gland *—see* Abscess, breast
marginal, anus K61.Ø
mastoid *—see* Mastoiditis, acute
maxilla, maxillary M27.2
molar (tooth) KØ4.7
with sinus KØ4.6
premolar KØ4.7
sinus (chronic) J32.Ø
mediastinum J85.3
meibomian gland *—see* Hordeolum
meninges GØ6.2
mesentery, mesenteric K65.1
mesosalpinx *—see* Salpingitis
mons pubis LØ2.215
mouth (floor) K12.2
muscle *—see* Myositis, infective
myocardium I4Ø.Ø
nabothian (follicle) *—see* Cervicitis
nasal J32.9
nasopharyngeal J39.1

Abscess *(Continued)*
navel LØ2.216
newborn P38.9
with mild hemorrhage P38.1
without hemorrhage P38.9
neck (region) LØ2.11
lymph gland or node LØ4.Ø
nephritic *—see* Abscess, kidney
nipple N61.1
associated with
lactation *—see* Pregnancy, complicated by
pregnancy *—see* Pregnancy, complicated by
nose (external) (fossa) (septum) J34.Ø
sinus (chronic) *—see* Sinusitis
omentum K65.1
operative wound T81.49
orbit, orbital *—see* Cellulitis, orbit
otogenic GØ6.Ø
ovary, ovarian (corpus luteum) *—see* Oophoritis
oviduct *—see* Oophoritis
palate (soft) K12.2
hard M27.2
palmar (space) *—see* Abscess, hand
pancreas (duct) *—see* Pancreatitis, acute
parafrenal N48.21
parametric, parametrium N73.2
acute N73.Ø
chronic N73.1
paranephric N15.1
parapancreatic *—see* Pancreatitis, acute
parapharyngeal J39.Ø
pararectal K61.1
parasinus *—see* Sinusitis
parauterine (*see also* Disease, pelvis, inflammatory) N73.2
paravaginal *—see* Vaginitis
parietal region (scalp) LØ2.811
parodontal *—see* Periodontitis, aggressive, localized
parotid (duct) (gland) K11.3
region K12.2
pectoral (region) LØ2.213
pelvis, pelvic
female *—see* Disease, pelvis, inflammatory
male, peritoneal K65.1
penis N48.21
gonococcal (accessory gland) (periurethral) A54.1
perianal K61.Ø
periapical KØ4.7
with sinus (alveolar) KØ4.6
periappendicular K35.33
pericardial I3Ø.1
pericecal K35.33
pericemental *—see* Periodontitis, aggressive, localized
pericholecystic *—see* Cholecystitis, acute
pericoronal *—see* Periodontitis, aggressive, localized
peridental *—see* Periodontitis, aggressive, localized
perimetric *—see also* Disease, pelvis, inflammatory N73.2
perinephric, perinephritic *—see* Abscess, kidney
perineum, perineal (superficial) LØ2.215
urethra N34.Ø
periodontal (parietal) *—see* Periodontitis, aggressive, localized
apical KØ4.7
periosteum, periosteal *—see also* Osteomyelitis, specified type NEC
with osteomyelitis *—see also* Osteomyelitis, specified type NEC
acute *—see* Osteomyelitis, acute
chronic *—see* Osteomyelitis, chronic
peripharyngeal J39.Ø
peripleuritic J86.9
with fistula J86.Ø
periprostatic N41.2

Abscess *(Continued)*
perirectal K61.1
perirenal (tissue) *—see* Abscess, kidney
perisinuous (nose) *—see* Sinusitis
peritoneum, peritoneal (perforated) (ruptured) K65.1
with appendicitis (*see also* Appendicitis) K35.33
pelvic
female *—see* Peritonitis, pelvic, female
male K65.1
postoperative T81.49
puerperal, postpartum, childbirth O85
tuberculous A18.31
peritonsillar J36
perityphlic K35.33
periureteral N28.89
periurethral N34.Ø
gonococcal (accessory gland) (periurethral) A54.1
periuterine *—see also* Disease, pelvis, inflammatory N73.2
perivesical *—see* Cystitis, specified type NEC
petrous bone *—see* Petrositis
phagedenic NOS LØ2.91
chancroid A57
pharynx, pharyngeal (lateral) J39.1
pilonidal LØ5.Ø1
pituitary (gland) E23.6
pleura J86.9
with fistula J86.Ø
popliteal *—see* Abscess, lower limb
postcecal K35.33
postlaryngeal J38.7
postnasal J34.Ø
postoperative (any site) (*see also* Infection, postoperative wound) T81.49
retroperitoneal K68.11
postpharyngeal J39.Ø
posttonsillar J36
post-typhoid AØ1.Ø9
pouch of Douglas *—see* Peritonitis, pelvic, female
premammary *—see* Abscess, breast
prepatellar *—see* Abscess, lower limb
prostate N41.2
gonococcal (acute) (chronic) A54.22
psoas muscle K68.12
puerperal - code by site under Puerperal, abscess
pulmonary *—see* Abscess, lung
pulp, pulpal (dental) KØ4.Ø1
irreversible KØ4.Ø2
reversible KØ4.Ø1
rectovaginal septum K63.Ø
rectovesical *—see* Cystitis, specified type NEC
rectum K61.1
renal *—see* Abscess, kidney
retina *—see* Inflammation, chorioretinal
retrobulbar *—see* Abscess, orbit
retrocecal K65.1
retrolaryngeal J38.7
retromammary *—see* Abscess, breast
retroperitoneal NEC K68.19
postprocedural K68.11
retropharyngeal J39.Ø
retrouterine *—see* Peritonitis, pelvic, female
retrovesical *—see* Cystitis, specified type NEC
root, tooth KØ4.7
with sinus (alveolar) KØ4.6
round ligament *—see also* Disease, pelvis, inflammatory N73.2
rupture (spontaneous) NOS LØ2.91
sacrum (tuberculous) A18.Ø1
nontuberculous M46.28
salivary (duct) (gland) K11.3
scalp (any part) LØ2.811
scapular *—see* Osteomyelitis, specified type NEC
sclera *—see* Scleritis
scrofulous (tuberculous) A18.2
scrotum N49.2

Abscess *(Continued)*
- seminal vesicle N49.Ø
- septal, dental KØ4.7
  - with sinus (alveolar) KØ4.6
- serous *—see* Periostitis
- shoulder (region) *—see* Abscess, upper limb
- sigmoid K63.Ø
- sinus (accessory) (chronic) (nasal) *—see also* Sinusitis
  - intracranial venous (any) GØ6.Ø
- Skene's duct or gland N34.Ø
- skin *—see* Abscess, by site
- specified site NEC LØ2.818
- spermatic cord N49.1
- sphenoidal (sinus) (chronic) J32.3
- spinal cord (any part) (staphylococcal) GØ6.1
  - tuberculous A17.81
- spine (column) (tuberculous) A18.Ø1
  - epidural GØ6.1
  - nontuberculous *—see* Osteomyelitis, vertebra
- spleen D73.3
  - amebic AØ6.89
- stitch T81.41
  - following an obstetrical procedure O86.Ø1
- subarachnoid GØ6.2
  - brain GØ6.Ø
  - spinal cord GØ6.1
- subareolar *—see* Abscess, breast
- subcecal K35.33
- subcutaneous *—see also* Abscess, by site
  - following procedure T81.41
    - obstetrical O86.Ø1
  - pheomycotic (chromomycotic) B43.2
- subdiaphragmatic K65.1
- subdural GØ6.2
  - brain GØ6.Ø
    - sequelae GØ9
  - spinal cord GØ6.1
- sub-fascial, following an obstetrical procedure O86.Ø2
- subgaleal LØ2.811
- subhepatic K65.1
- sublingual K12.2
  - gland K11.3
- submammary *—see* Abscess, breast
- submandibular (region) (space) (triangle) K12.2
  - gland K11.3
- submaxillary (region) LØ2.Ø1
  - gland K11.3
- submental LØ2.Ø1
  - gland K11.3
- subperiosteal *—see* Osteomyelitis, specified type NEC
- subphrenic K65.1
  - following an obstetrical procedure O86.Ø3
  - postoperative T81.43
- suburethral N34.Ø
- sudoriparous L75.8
- supraclavicular (fossa) *—see* Abscess, upper limb
- supralevator K61.5
- suprapelvic, acute N73.Ø
- suprarenal (capsule) (gland) E27.8
- sweat gland L74.8
- tear duct *—see* Inflammation, lacrimal, passages, acute
- temple LØ2.Ø1
- temporal region LØ2.Ø1
- temporosphenoidal GØ6.Ø
- tendon (sheath) M65.ØØ
  - ankle M65.Ø7- •
  - foot M65.Ø7- •
  - forearm M65.Ø3- •
  - hand M65.Ø4- •
  - lower leg M65.Ø6- •
  - pelvic region M65.Ø5- •
  - shoulder region M65.Ø1- •
  - specified site NEC M65.Ø8
  - thigh M65.Ø5- •
  - upper arm M65.Ø2- •
- testis N45.4
- thigh *—see* Abscess, lower limb

Abscess *(Continued)*
- thorax J86.9
  - with fistula J86.Ø
- throat J39.1
- thumb *—see also* Abscess, hand
  - nail *—see* Cellulitis, finger
- thymus (gland) E32.1
- thyroid (gland) EØ6.Ø
- toe (any) *—see also* Abscess, foot
  - nail *—see* Cellulitis, toe
- tongue (staphylococcal) K14.Ø
- tonsil(s) (lingual) J36
- tonsillopharyngeal J36
- tooth, teeth (root) KØ4.7
  - with sinus (alveolar) KØ4.6
  - supporting structures NEC *—see* Periodontitis, aggressive, localized
- trachea J39.8
- trunk LØ2.219
  - abdominal wall LØ2.211
  - back LØ2.212
  - chest wall LØ2.213
  - groin LØ2.214
  - perineum LØ2.215
  - umbilicus LØ2.216
- tubal *—see* Salpingitis
- tuberculous *—see* Tuberculosis, abscess
- tubo-ovarian *—see* Salpingo-oophoritis
- tunica vaginalis N49.1
- umbilicus LØ2.216
- upper
  - limb LØ2.41- •
  - respiratory J39.8
- urethral (gland) N34.Ø
- urinary N34.Ø
- uterus, uterine (wall) *—see also* Endometritis
  - ligament *—see also* Disease, pelvis, inflammatory N73.2
  - neck *—see* Cervicitis
- uvula K12.2
- vagina (wall) *—see* Vaginitis
- vaginorectal *—see* Vaginitis
- vas deferens N49.1
- vermiform appendix K35.33
- vertebra (column) (tuberculous) A18.Ø1
  - nontuberculous *—see* Osteomyelitis, vertebra
- vesical *—see* Cystitis, specified type NEC
- vesico-uterine pouch *—see* Peritonitis, pelvic, female
- vitreous (humor) *—see* Endophthalmitis, purulent
- vocal cord J38.3
- von Bezold's *—see* Mastoiditis, acute
- vulva N76.4
- vulvovaginal gland N75.1
- web space *—see* Abscess, hand
- wound T81.49
- wrist *—see* Abscess, upper limb

Absence (of) (organ or part) (complete or partial)
- adrenal (gland) (congenital) Q89.1
  - acquired E89.6
- albumin in blood E88.Ø9
- alimentary tract (congenital) Q45.8
  - upper Q4Ø.8
- alveolar process (acquired) *—see* Anomaly, alveolar
- ankle (acquired) Z89.44- •
- anus (congenital) Q42.3
  - with fistula Q42.2
- aorta (congenital) Q25.41
- appendix, congenital Q42.8
- arm (acquired) Z89.2Ø- •
  - above elbow Z89.22- •
    - congenital (with hand present) *—see* Agenesis, arm, with hand present
      - and hand *—see* Agenesis, forearm, and hand
  - below elbow Z89.21- •
    - congenital (with hand present) *—see* Agenesis, arm, with hand present
      - and hand *—see* Agenesis, forearm, and hand

Absence *(Continued)*
- arm *(Continued)*
  - congenital *—see* Defect, reduction, upper limb
  - shoulder (following explantation of shoulder joint prosthesis) (joint) (with or without presence of antibiotic-impregnated cement spacer) Z89.23- •
    - congenital (with hand present) *—see* Agenesis, arm, with hand present
- artery (congenital) (peripheral) Q27.8
  - brain Q28.3
  - coronary Q24.5
  - pulmonary Q25.79
  - specified NEC Q27.8
  - umbilical Q27.Ø
- atrial septum (congenital) Q21.1
- auditory canal (congenital) (external) Q16.1
- auricle (ear), congenital Q16.Ø
- bile, biliary duct, congenital Q44.5
- bladder (acquired) Z9Ø.6
  - congenital Q64.5
- bowel sounds R19.11
- brain QØØ.Ø
  - part of QØ4.3
- breast(s) (and nipple(s)) (acquired) Z9Ø.1- •
  - congenital Q83.8
- broad ligament Q5Ø.6
- bronchus (congenital) Q32.4
- canaliculus lacrimalis, congenital Q1Ø.4
- cerebellum (vermis) QØ4.3
- cervix (acquired) (with uterus) Z9Ø.71Ø
  - with remaining uterus Z9Ø.712
  - congenital Q51.5
- chin, congenital Q18.8
- cilia (congenital) Q1Ø.3
  - acquired *—see* Madarosis
- clitoris (congenital) Q52.6
- coccyx, congenital Q76.49
- cold sense R2Ø.8
- congenital
  - lumen *—see* Atresia
  - organ or site NEC *—see* Agenesis
  - septum *—see* Imperfect, closure
- corpus callosum QØ4.Ø
- cricoid cartilage, congenital Q31.8
- diaphragm (with hernia), congenital Q79.1
- digestive organ(s) or tract, congenital Q45.8
  - acquired NEC Z9Ø.49
  - upper Q4Ø.8
- ductus arteriosus Q28.8
- duodenum (acquired) Z9Ø.49
  - congenital Q41.Ø
- ear, congenital Q16.9
  - acquired H93.8- •
  - auricle Q16.Ø
  - external Q16.Ø
  - inner Q16.5
  - lobe, lobule Q17.8
  - middle, except ossicles Q16.4
    - ossicles Q16.3
  - ossicles Q16.3
- ejaculatory duct (congenital) Q55.4
- endocrine gland (congenital) NEC Q89.2
  - acquired E89.89
- epididymis (congenital) Q55.4
  - acquired Z9Ø.79
- epiglottis, congenital Q31.8
- esophagus (congenital) Q39.8
  - acquired (partial) Z9Ø.49
- eustachian tube (congenital) Q16.2
- extremity (acquired) Z89.9
  - congenital Q73.Ø
  - knee (following explantation of knee joint prosthesis) (joint) (with or without presence of antibiotic-impregnated cement spacer) Z89.52- •
  - lower (above knee) Z89.619
    - below knee Z89.51- •
  - upper *—see* Absence, arm
- eye (acquired) Z9Ø.Ø1
  - congenital Q11.1
  - muscle (congenital) Q1Ø.3

A

Absence *(Continued)*
eyeball (acquired) Z90.01
eyelid (fold) (congenital) Q10.3
acquired Z90.01
face, specified part NEC Q18.8
fallopian tube(s) (acquired) Z90.79
congenital Q50.6
family member (causing problem in home) NEC —*see also* Disruption, family Z63.32
femur, congenital —*see* Defect, reduction, lower limb, longitudinal, femur
fibrinogen (congenital) D68.2
acquired D65
finger(s) (acquired) Z89.02-●
congenital —*see* Agenesis, hand
foot (acquired) Z89.43-●
congenital —*see* Agenesis, foot
forearm (acquired) —*see* Absence, arm, below elbow
gallbladder (acquired) Z90.49
congenital Q44.0
gamma globulin in blood D80.1
hereditary D80.0
genital organs
acquired (female) (male) Z90.79
female, congenital Q52.8
external Q52.71
internal NEC Q52.8
male, congenital Q55.8
genitourinary organs, congenital NEC
female Q52.8
male Q55.8
globe (acquired) Z90.01
congenital Q11.1
glottis, congenital Q31.8
hand and wrist (acquired) Z89.11-●
congenital —*see* Agenesis, hand
head, part (acquired) NEC Z90.09
heat sense R20.8
hip (following explantation of hip joint prosthesis) (joint) (with or without presence of antibiotic-impregnated cement spacer) Z89.62-●
hymen (congenital) Q52.4
ileum (acquired) Z90.49
congenital Q41.2
immunoglobulin, isolated NEC D80.3
IgA D80.2
IgG D80.3
IgM D80.4
incus (acquired) —*see* Loss, ossicles, ear
congenital Q16.3
inner ear, congenital Q16.5
intestine (acquired) (small) Z90.49
congenital Q41.9
specified NEC Q41.8
large Z90.49
congenital Q42.9
specified NEC Q42.8
iris, congenital Q13.1
jejunum (acquired) Z90.49
congenital Q41.1
joint
acquired
hip (following explantation of hip joint prosthesis) (with or without presence of antibiotic-impregnated cement spacer) Z89.62-●
knee (following explantation of knee joint prosthesis) (with or without presence of antibiotic-impregnated cement spacer) Z89.52-●
shoulder (following explantation of shoulder joint prosthesis) (with or without presence of antibiotic-impregnated cement spacer) Z89.23-●
congenital NEC Q74.8
kidney(s) (acquired) Z90.5
congenital Q60.2
bilateral Q60.1
unilateral Q60.0

Absence *(Continued)*
knee (following explantation of knee joint prosthesis) (joint) (with or without presence of antibiotic-impregnated cement spacer) Z89.52-●
labyrinth, membranous Q16.5
larynx (congenital) Q31.8
acquired Z90.02
leg (acquired) (above knee) Z89.61-●
below knee (acquired) Z89.51-●
congenital —*see* Defect, reduction, lower limb
lens (acquired) —*see also* Aphakia
congenital Q12.3
post cataract extraction Z98.4-●
limb (acquired) —*see* Absence, extremity
lip Q38.6
liver (congenital) Q44.7
lung (fissure) (lobe) (bilateral) (unilateral) (congenital) Q33.3
acquired (any part) Z90.2
menstruation —*see* Amenorrhea
muscle (congenital) (pectoral) Q79.8
ocular Q10.3
neck, part Q18.8
neutrophil —*see* Agranulocytosis
nipple(s) (with breast(s)) (acquired) Z90.1-●
congenital Q83.2
nose (congenital) Q30.1
acquired Z90.09
organ
of Corti, congenital Q16.5
or site, congenital NEC Q89.8
acquired NEC Z90.89
osseous meatus (ear) Q16.4
ovary (acquired)
bilateral Z90.722
congenital
bilateral Q50.02
unilateral Q50.01
unilateral Z90.721
oviduct (acquired)
bilateral Z90.722
congenital Q50.6
unilateral Z90.721
pancreas (congenital) Q45.0
acquired Z90.410
complete Z90.410
partial Z90.411
total Z90.410
parathyroid gland (acquired) E89.2
congenital Q89.2
patella, congenital Q74.1
penis (congenital) Q55.5
acquired Z90.79
pericardium (congenital) Q24.8
pituitary gland (congenital) Q89.2
acquired E89.3
prostate (acquired) Z90.79
congenital Q55.4
pulmonary valve Q22.0
punctum lacrimale (congenital) Q10.4
radius, congenital —*see* Defect, reduction, upper limb, longitudinal, radius
rectum (congenital) Q42.1
with fistula Q42.0
acquired Z90.49
respiratory organ NOS Q34.9
rib (acquired) Z90.89
congenital Q76.6
sacrum, congenital Q76.49
salivary gland(s), congenital Q38.4
scrotum, congenital Q55.29
seminal vesicles (congenital) Q55.4
acquired Z90.79
septum
atrial (congenital) Q21.1
between aorta and pulmonary artery Q21.4
ventricular (congenital) Q20.4
sex chromosome
female phenotype Q97.8
male phenotype Q98.8

Absence *(Continued)*
skull bone (congenital) Q75.8
with
anencephaly Q00.0
encephalocele —*see* Encephalocele
hydrocephalus Q03.9
with spina bifida —*see* Spina bifida, by site, with hydrocephalus
microcephaly Q02
spermatic cord, congenital Q55.4
spine, congenital Q76.49
spleen (congenital) Q89.01
acquired Z90.81
sternum, congenital Q76.7
stomach (acquired) (partial) Z90.3
congenital Q40.2
superior vena cava, congenital Q26.8
teeth, tooth (congenital) K00.0
acquired (complete) K08.109
class I K08.101
class II K08.102
class III K08.103
class IV K08.104
due to
caries K08.139
class I K08.131
class II K08.132
class III K08.133
class IV K08.134
periodontal disease K08.129
class I K08.121
class II K08.122
class III K08.123
class IV K08.124
specified NEC K08.199
class I K08.191
class II K08.192
class III K08.193
class IV K08.194
trauma K08.119
class I K08.111
class II K08.112
class III K08.113
class IV K08.114
partial K08.409
class I K08.401
class II K08.402
class III K08.403
class IV K08.404
due to
caries K08.439
class I K08.431
class II K08.432
class III K08.433
class IV K08.434
periodontal disease K08.429
class I K08.421
class II K08.422
class III K08.423
class IV K08.424
specified NEC K08.499
class I K08.491
class II K08.492
class III K08.493
class IV K08.494
trauma K08.419
class I K08.411
class II K08.412
class III K08.413
class IV K08.414
tendon (congenital) Q79.8
testis (congenital) Q55.0
acquired Z90.79
thumb (acquired) Z89.01-●
congenital —*see* Agenesis, hand
thymus gland Q89.2
thyroid (gland) (acquired) E89.0
cartilage, congenital Q31.8
congenital E03.1
toe(s) (acquired) Z89.42-●
with foot —*see* Absence, foot and ankle
congenital —*see* Agenesis, foot
great Z89.41-●

Absence *(Continued)*
tongue, congenital Q38.3
trachea (cartilage), congenital Q32.1
transverse aortic arch, congenital Q25.49
tricuspid valve Q22.4
umbilical artery, congenital Q27.Ø
upper arm and forearm with hand present, congenital —*see* Agenesis, arm, with hand present
ureter (congenital) Q62.4
acquired Z9Ø.6
urethra, congenital Q64.5
uterus (acquired) Z9Ø.71Ø
with cervix Z9Ø.71Ø
with remaining cervical stump Z9Ø.711
congenital Q51.Ø
uvula, congenital Q38.5
vagina, congenital Q52.Ø
vas deferens (congenital) Q55.4
acquired Z9Ø.79
vein (peripheral) congenital NEC Q27.8
cerebral Q28.3
digestive system Q27.8
great Q26.8
lower limb Q27.8
portal Q26.5
precerebral Q28.1
specified site NEC Q27.8
upper limb Q27.8
vena cava (inferior) (superior), congenital Q26.8
ventricular septum Q2Ø.4
vertebra, congenital Q76.49
vulva, congenital Q52.71
wrist (acquired) Z89.12- •
Absorbent system disease I87.8
Absorption
carbohydrate, disturbance K9Ø.49
chemical —*see* Table of Drugs and Chemicals
through placenta (newborn) PØ4.9
environmental substance PØ4.6
nutritional substance PØ4.5
obstetric anesthetic or analgesic drug PØ4.Ø
drug NEC —*see* Table of Drugs and Chemicals
addictive
through placenta (newborn) (*see also* Newborn, affected by, maternal, use of) PØ4.4Ø
cocaine PØ4.41
hallucinogens PØ4.42
specified drug NEC PØ4.49
medicinal
through placenta (newborn) PØ4.19
through placenta (newborn) PØ4.19
obstetric anesthetic or analgesic drug PØ4.Ø
fat, disturbance K9Ø.49
pancreatic K9Ø.3
noxious substance —*see* Table of Drugs and Chemicals
protein, disturbance K9Ø.49
starch, disturbance K9Ø.49
toxic substance —*see* Table of Drugs and Chemicals
uremic —*see* Uremia
Abstinence symptoms, syndrome
alcohol F1Ø.239
with delirium F1Ø.231
cocaine F14.23
neonatal P96.1
nicotine —*see* Dependence, drug, nicotine, with, withdrawal
opioid F11.93
with dependence F11.23
psychoactive NEC F19.939
with
delirium F19.931
dependence F19.239
with
delirium F19.231
perceptual disturbance F19.232
uncomplicated F19.23Ø
perceptual disturbance F19.932
uncomplicated F19.93Ø

Abstinence symptoms, syndrome *(Continued)*
sedative F13.939
with
delirium F13.931
dependence F13.239
with
delirium F13.231
perceptual disturbance F13.232
uncomplicated F13.23Ø
perceptual disturbance F13.932
uncomplicated F13.93Ø
stimulant NEC F15.93
with dependence F15.23
Abulia R68.89
Abulomania F6Ø.7
Abuse
adult —*see* Maltreatment, adult
as reason for
couple seeking advice (including offender) Z63.Ø
alcohol (non-dependent) F1Ø.1Ø
with
anxiety disorder F1Ø.18Ø
intoxication F1Ø.129
with delirium F1Ø.121
uncomplicated F1Ø.12Ø
mood disorder F1Ø.14
other specified disorder F1Ø.188
psychosis F1Ø.159
delusions F1Ø.15Ø
hallucinations F1Ø.151
sexual dysfunction F1Ø.181
sleep disorder F1Ø.182
unspecified disorder F1Ø.19
counseling and surveillance Z71.41
in remission (early) (sustained) F1Ø.11
➡ amphetamine (or related substance) —*see also* Abuse, drug, stimulant NEC
▶ stimulant NEC F15.1Ø
▶ with
▶ anxiety disorder F15.18Ø
▶ intoxication F15.129
▶ with
▶ delirium F15.121
▶ perceptual disturbance F15.122
analgesics (non-prescribed) (over the counter) F55.8
antacids F55.Ø
antidepressants —*see* Abuse, drug, psychoactive NEC
anxiolytic —*see* Abuse, drug, sedative
barbiturates —*see* Abuse, drug, sedative
caffeine —*see* Abuse, drug, stimulant NEC
cannabis, cannabinoids —*see* Abuse, drug, cannabis
child —*see* Maltreatment, child
cocaine —*see* Abuse, drug, cocaine
drug NEC (non-dependent) F19.1Ø
with sleep disorder F19.182
amphetamine type —*see* Abuse, drug, stimulant NEC
analgesics (non-prescribed) (over the counter) F55.8
antacids F55.Ø
antidepressants —*see* Abuse, drug, psychoactive NEC
anxiolytics —*see* Abuse, drug, sedative
barbiturates —*see* Abuse, drug, sedative
caffeine —*see* Abuse, drug, stimulant NEC
cannabis F12.1Ø
with
anxiety disorder F12.18Ø
intoxication F12.129
with
delirium F12.121
perceptual disturbance F12.122
uncomplicated F12.12Ø
other specified disorder F12.188
psychosis F12.159
delusions F12.15Ø
hallucinations F12.151
unspecified disorder F12.19
in remission (early) (sustained) F12.11

Abuse *(Continued)*
drug NEC *(Continued)*
cocaine F14.1Ø
with
anxiety disorder F14.18Ø
intoxication F14.129
with
delirium F14.121
perceptual disturbance F14.122
uncomplicated F14.12Ø
mood disorder F14.14
other specified disorder F14.188
psychosis F14.159
delusions F14.15Ø
hallucinations F14.151
sexual dysfunction F14.181
sleep disorder F14.182
unspecified disorder F14.19
in remission (early) (sustained) F14.11
counseling and surveillance Z71.51
hallucinogen F16.1Ø
with
anxiety disorder F16.18Ø
flashbacks F16.183
intoxication F16.129
with
delirium F16.121
perceptual disturbance F16.122
uncomplicated F16.12Ø
mood disorder F16.14
other specified disorder F16.188
perception disorder, persisting F16.183
psychosis F16.159
delusions F16.15Ø
hallucinations F16.151
unspecified disorder F16.19
in remission (early) (sustained) F16.11
hashish —*see* Abuse, drug, cannabis
herbal or folk remedies F55.1
hormones F55.3
hypnotics —*see* Abuse, drug, sedative
inhalant F18.1Ø
with
anxiety disorder F18.18Ø
dementia, persisting F18.17
intoxication F18.129
with delirium F18.121
uncomplicated F18.12Ø
mood disorder F18.14
other specified disorder F18.188
psychosis F18.159
delusions F18.15Ø
hallucinations F18.151
unspecified disorder F18.19
in remission (early) (sustained) F18.11
in remission (early) (sustained) F19.11
laxatives F55.2
LSD —*see* Abuse, drug, hallucinogen
marihuana —*see* Abuse, drug, cannabis
morphine type (opioids) —*see* Abuse, drug, opioid
opioid F11.1Ø
with
intoxication F11.129
with
delirium F11.121
perceptual disturbance F11.122
uncomplicated F11.12Ø
mood disorder F11.14
other specified disorder F11.188
psychosis F11.159
delusions F11.15Ø
hallucinations F11.151
sexual dysfunction F11.181
sleep disorder F11.182
unspecified disorder F11.19
in remission (early) (sustained) F11.11
PCP (phencyclidine) (or related substance) —*see* Abuse, drug, hallucinogen

- **Abuse** *(Continued)*
  - drug NEC *(Continued)*
    - psychoactive NEC F19.1Ø
      - with
        - amnestic disorder F19.16
        - anxiety disorder F19.18Ø
        - dementia F19.17
        - intoxication F19.129
          - with
            - delirium F19.121
            - perceptual disturbance F19.122
          - uncomplicated F19.12Ø
        - mood disorder F19.14
        - other specified disorder F19.188
        - psychosis F19.159
          - delusions F19.15Ø
          - hallucinations F19.151
        - sexual dysfunction F19.181
        - sleep disorder F19.182
        - unspecified disorder F19.19
    - sedative, hypnotic or anxiolytic F13.1Ø
      - with
        - anxiety disorder F13.18Ø
        - intoxication F13.129
          - with delirium F13.121
          - uncomplicated F13.12Ø
        - mood disorder F13.14
        - other specified disorder F13.188
        - psychosis F13.159
          - delusions F13.15Ø
          - hallucinations F13.151
        - sexual dysfunction F13.181
        - sleep disorder F13.182
        - unspecified disorder F13.19
      - in remission (early) (sustained) F13.11
    - solvent —*see* Abuse, drug, inhalant
    - steroids F55.3
    - stimulant NEC F15.1Ø
      - with
        - anxiety disorder F15.18Ø
        - intoxication F15.129
          - with
            - delirium F15.121
            - perceptual disturbance F15.122
          - uncomplicated F15.12Ø
        - mood disorder F15.14
        - other specified disorder F15.188
        - psychosis F15.159
          - delusions F15.15Ø
          - hallucinations F15.151
        - sexual dysfunction F15.181
        - sleep disorder F15.182
        - unspecified disorder F15.19
      - in remission (early) (sustained) F15.11
    - tranquilizers —*see* Abuse, drug, sedative
    - vitamins F55.4
  - hallucinogens —*see* Abuse, drug, hallucinogen
  - hashish —*see* Abuse, drug, cannabis
  - herbal or folk remedies F55.1
  - hormones F55.3
  - hypnotic —*see* Abuse, drug, sedative
  - inhalant —*see* Abuse, drug, inhalant
  - laxatives F55.2
  - LSD —*see* Abuse, drug, hallucinogen
  - marihuana —*see* Abuse, drug, cannabis
  - morphine type (opioids) —*see* Abuse, drug, opioid
  - non-psychoactive substance NEC F55.8
    - antacids F55.Ø
    - folk remedies F55.1
    - herbal remedies F55.1
    - hormones F55.3
    - laxatives F55.2
    - steroids F55.3
    - vitamins F55.4
  - opioids —*see* Abuse, drug, opioid
  - PCP (phencyclidine) (or related substance) —*see* Abuse, drug, hallucinogen
  - physical (adult) (child) —*see* Maltreatment
  - psychoactive substance —*see* Abuse, drug, psychoactive NEC
- **Abuse** *(Continued)*
  - psychological (adult) (child) —*see* Maltreatment
  - sedative —*see* Abuse, drug, sedative
  - sexual —*see* Maltreatment
  - solvent —*see* Abuse, drug, inhalant
  - steroids F55.3
  - vitamins F55.4
- **Acalculia** R48.8
  - developmental F81.2
- **Acanthamebiasis** (with) B6Ø.1Ø
  - conjunctiva B6Ø.12
  - keratoconjunctivitis B6Ø.13
  - meningoencephalitis B6Ø.11
  - other specified B6Ø.19
- **Acanthocephaliasis** B83.8
- **Acanthocheilonemiasis** B74.4
- **Acanthocytosis** E78.6
- **Acantholysis** L11.9
- **Acanthosis** (acquired) (nigricans) L83
  - benign Q82.8
  - congenital Q82.8
  - seborrheic L82.1
    - inflamed L82.Ø
  - tongue K14.3
- **Acapnia** E87.3
- **Acarbia** E87.2
- **Acardia, acardius** Q89.8
- **Acardiacus amorphus** Q89.8
- **Acardiotrophia** I51.4
- **Acariasis** B88.Ø
  - scabies B86
- **Acarodermatitis** (urticarioides) B88.Ø
- **Acarophobia** F4Ø.218
- **Acatalasemia, acatalasia** E8Ø.3
- **Acathisia** (drug induced) G25.71
- **Accelerated atrioventricular conduction** I45.6
- **Accentuation of personality traits** (type A) Z73.1
- **Accessory** (congenital)
  - adrenal gland Q89.1
  - anus Q43.4
  - appendix Q43.4
  - atrioventricular conduction I45.6
  - auditory ossicles Q16.3
  - auricle (ear) Q17.Ø
  - biliary duct or passage Q44.5
  - bladder Q64.79
  - blood vessels NEC Q27.9
    - coronary Q24.5
  - bone NEC Q79.8
  - breast tissue, axilla Q83.1
  - carpal bones Q74.Ø
  - cecum Q43.4
  - chromosome(s) NEC (nonsex) Q92.9
    - with complex rearrangements NEC Q92.5
      - seen only at prometaphase Q92.8
    - 13 —*see* Trisomy, 13
    - 18 —*see* Trisomy, 18
    - 21 —*see* Trisomy, 21
    - partial Q92.9
    - sex
      - female phenotype Q97.8
  - coronary artery Q24.5
  - cusp(s), heart valve NEC Q24.8
    - pulmonary Q22.3
  - cystic duct Q44.5
  - digit(s) Q69.9
  - ear (auricle) (lobe) Q17.Ø
  - endocrine gland NEC Q89.2
  - eye muscle Q1Ø.3
  - eyelid Q1Ø.3
  - face bone(s) Q75.8
  - fallopian tube (fimbria) (ostium) Q5Ø.6
  - finger(s) Q69.Ø
  - foreskin N47.8
  - frontonasal process Q75.8
  - gallbladder Q44.1
  - genital organ(s)
    - female Q52.8
      - external Q52.79
      - internal NEC Q52.8
    - male Q55.8
- **Accessory** *(Continued)*
  - genitourinary organs NEC Q89.8
    - female Q52.8
    - male Q55.8
  - hallux Q69.2
  - heart Q24.8
    - valve NEC Q24.8
      - pulmonary Q22.3
  - hepatic ducts Q44.5
  - hymen Q52.4
  - intestine (large) (small) Q43.4
  - kidney Q63.Ø
  - lacrimal canal Q1Ø.6
  - leaflet, heart valve NEC Q24.8
  - ligament, broad Q5Ø.6
  - liver Q44.7
    - duct Q44.5
  - lobule (ear) Q17.Ø
  - lung (lobe) Q33.1
  - muscle Q79.8
  - navicular of carpus Q74.Ø
  - nervous system, part NEC QØ7.8
  - nipple Q83.3
  - nose Q3Ø.8
  - organ or site not listed —*see* Anomaly, by site
  - ovary Q5Ø.31
  - oviduct Q5Ø.6
  - pancreas Q45.3
  - parathyroid gland Q89.2
  - parotid gland (and duct) Q38.4
  - pituitary gland Q89.2
  - preauricular appendage Q17.Ø
  - prepuce N47.8
  - renal arteries (multiple) Q27.2
  - rib Q76.6
    - cervical Q76.5
  - roots (teeth) KØØ.2
  - salivary gland Q38.4
  - sesamoid bones Q74.8
    - foot Q74.2
    - hand Q74.Ø
  - skin tags Q82.8
  - spleen Q89.Ø9
  - sternum Q76.7
  - submaxillary gland Q38.4
  - tarsal bones Q74.2
  - teeth, tooth KØØ.1
  - tendon Q79.8
  - thumb Q69.1
  - thymus gland Q89.2
  - thyroid gland Q89.2
  - toes Q69.2
  - tongue Q38.3
  - tooth, teeth KØØ.1
  - tragus Q17.Ø
  - ureter Q62.5
  - urethra Q64.79
  - urinary organ or tract NEC Q64.8
  - uterus Q51.28
  - vagina Q52.1Ø
  - valve, heart NEC Q24.8
    - pulmonary Q22.3
  - vertebra Q76.49
  - vocal cords Q31.8
  - vulva Q52.79
- **Accident**
  - birth —*see* Birth, injury
  - cardiac —*see* Infarct, myocardium
  - cerebral I63.9
  - cerebrovascular (embolic) (ischemic) (thrombotic) I63.9
    - aborted I63.9
    - hemorrhagic —*see* Hemorrhage, intracranial, intracerebral
    - old (without sequelae) Z86.73
      - with sequelae (of) —*see* Sequelae, infarction, cerebral
  - coronary —*see* Infarct, myocardium
  - craniovascular I63.9
  - vascular, brain I63.9
- **Accidental** —*see* condition

A

Accommodation (disorder) —*see also* condition
  hysterical paralysis of F44.89
  insufficiency of H52.4
  paresis —*see* Paresis, of accommodation
  spasm —*see* Spasm, of accommodation
Accouchement —*see* Delivery
Accreta placenta O43.21-●
Accretio cordis (nonrheumatic) I31.Ø
Accretions, tooth, teeth KØ3.6
Acculturation difficulty Z6Ø.3
Accumulation secretion, prostate N42.89
Acephalia, acephalism, acephalus, acephaly QØØ.Ø
Acephalobrachia monster Q89.8
Acephalochirus monster Q89.8
Acephalogaster Q89.8
Acephalostomus monster Q89.8
Acephalothorax Q89.8
Acerophobia F4Ø.298
Acetonemia R79.89
  in Type 1 diabetes E1Ø.1Ø
    with coma E1Ø.11
Acetonuria R82.4
Achalasia (cardia) (esophagus) K22.Ø
  congenital Q39.5
  pylorus Q4Ø.Ø
  sphincteral NEC K59.8
Ache(s) —*see* Pain
Acheilia Q38.6
Achillobursitis —*see* Tendinitis, Achilles
Achillodynia —*see* Tendinitis, Achilles
Achlorhydria, achlorhydric (neurogenic) K31.83
  anemia D5Ø.8
  diarrhea K31.83
  psychogenic F45.8
  secondary to vagotomy K91.1
Achluophobia F4Ø.228
Acholia K82.8
Acholuric jaundice (familial) (splenomegalic) —*see also* Spherocytosis
  acquired D59.8
Achondrogenesis Q77.Ø
Achondroplasia (osteosclerosis congenita) Q77.4
Achroma, cutis L8Ø
Achromat (ism), achromatopsia (acquired) (congenital) H53.51
Achromia, congenital —*see* Albinism
Achromia parasitica B36.Ø
Achylia gastrica K31.89
  psychogenic F45.8
Acid
  burn —*see* Corrosion
  deficiency
    amide nicotinic E52
    ascorbic E54
    folic E53.8
    nicotinic E52
    pantothenic E53.8
  intoxication E87.2
  peptic disease K3Ø
  phosphatase deficiency E83.39
  stomach K3Ø
    psychogenic F45.8
Acidemia E87.2
  argininosuccinic E72.22
  isovaleric E71.11Ø
  metabolic (newborn) P19.9
    first noted before onset of labor P19.Ø
    first noted during labor P19.1
    noted at birth P19.2
  methylmalonic E71.12Ø
  pipecolic E72.3
  propionic E71.121
Acidity, gastric (high) K3Ø
  psychogenic F45.8
Acidocytopenia —*see* Agranulocytosis
Acidocytosis D72.1
Acidopenia —*see* Agranulocytosis
Acidosis (lactic) (respiratory) E87.2
  in Type 1 diabetes E1Ø.1Ø
    with coma E1Ø.11
  kidney, tubular N25.89
Acidosis *(Continued)*
  lactic E87.2
  metabolic NEC E87.2
    hyperchloremic, of newborn P74.421
    with respiratory acidosis E87.4
    late, of newborn P74.Ø
  mixed metabolic and respiratory, newborn P84
  newborn P84
  renal (hyperchloremic) (tubular) N25.89
  respiratory E87.2
    complicated by
      metabolic
        acidosis E87.4
        alkalosis E87.4
Aciduria
  4-hydroxybutyric E72.81
  argininosuccinic E72.22
  gamma-hydroxybutyric E72.81
  glutaric (type I) E72.3
    type II E71.313
    type III E71.5-●
  orotic (congenital) (hereditary) (pyrimidine deficiency) E79.8
    anemia D53.Ø
Acladiosis (skin) B36.Ø
Aclasis, diaphyseal Q78.6
Acleistocardia Q21.1
Aclusion —*see* Anomaly, dentofacial, malocclusion
Acne L7Ø.9
  artificialis L7Ø.8
  atrophica L7Ø.2
  cachecticorum (Hebra) L7Ø.8
  conglobata L7Ø.1
  cystic L7Ø.Ø
  decalvans L66.2
  excoriée (des jeunes filles) L7Ø.5
  frontalis L7Ø.2
  indurata L7Ø.Ø
  infantile L7Ø.4
  keloid L73.Ø
  lupoid L7Ø.2
  necrotic, necrotica (miliaris) L7Ø.2
  neonatal L7Ø.4
  nodular L7Ø.Ø
  occupational L7Ø.8
  picker's L7Ø.5
  pustular L7Ø.Ø
  rodens L7Ø.2
  rosacea L71.9
  specified NEC L7Ø.8
  tropica L7Ø.3
  varioliformis L7Ø.2
  vulgaris L7Ø.Ø
Acnitis (primary) A18.4
Acosta's disease T7Ø.29
Acoustic —*see* condition
Acousticophobia F4Ø.298
Acquired —*see also* condition
  immunodeficiency syndrome (AIDS) B2Ø
Acrania QØØ.Ø
Acroangiodermatitis I78.9
Acroasphyxia, chronic I73.89
Acrobystitis N47.7
Acrocephalopolysyndactyly Q87.Ø
Acrocephalosyndactyly Q87.Ø
Acrocephaly Q75.Ø
Acrochondrohyperplasia —*see* Syndrome, Marfan's
Acrocyanosis I73.89
  newborn P28.2
    meaning transient blue hands and feet - omit code
Acrodermatitis L3Ø.8
  atrophicans (chronica) L9Ø.4
  continua (Hallopeau) L4Ø.2
  enteropathica (hereditary) E83.2
  Hallopeau's L4Ø.2
  infantile papular L44.4
  perstans L4Ø.2
  pustulosa continua L4Ø.2
  recalcitrant pustular L4Ø.2
Acrodynia —*see* Poisoning, mercury
Acromegaly, acromegalia E22.Ø
Acromelalgia I73.81
Acromicria, acromikria Q79.8
Acronyx L6Ø.Ø
Acropachy, thyroid —*see* Thyrotoxicosis
Acroparesthesia (simple) (vasomotor) I73.89
Acropathy, thyroid —*see* Thyrotoxicosis
Acrophobia F4Ø.241
Acroposthitis N47.7
Acroscleriasis, acroscleroderma, acrosclerosis —*see* Sclerosis, systemic
Acrosphacelus I96
Acrospiroma, eccrine —*see* Neoplasm, skin, benign
Acrostealgia —*see* Osteochondropathy
Acrotrophodynia —*see* Immersion
ACTH ectopic syndrome E24.3
Actinic —*see* condition
Actinobacillosis, actinobacillus A28.8
  mallei A24.Ø
  muris A25.1
Actinomyces israelii (infection) —*see* Actinomycosis
Actinomycetoma (foot) B47.1
Actinomycosis, actinomycotic A42.9
  with pneumonia A42.Ø
  abdominal A42.1
  cervicofacial A42.2
  cutaneous A42.89
  gastrointestinal A42.1
  pulmonary A42.Ø
  sepsis A42.7
  specified site NEC A42.89
Actinoneuritis G62.82
Action, heart
  disorder I49.9
  irregular I49.9
    psychogenic F45.8
Activated protein C resistance D68.51
Activation
  mast cell (disorder) (syndrome) D89.4Ø
    idiopathic D89.42
    monoclonal D89.41
    secondary D89.43
    specified type NEC D89.49
Active —*see* condition
Acute —*see also* condition
  abdomen R1Ø.Ø
  gallbladder —*see* Cholecystitis, acute
Acyanotic heart disease (congenital) Q24.9
Acystia Q64.5
Adair-Dighton syndrome (brittle bones and blue sclera, deafness) Q78.Ø
Adamantinoblastoma —*see* Ameloblastoma
Adamantinoma —*see also* Cyst, calcifying odontogenic
  long bones C4Ø.9Ø
    lower limb C4Ø.2-●
    upper limb C4Ø.Ø-●
  malignant C41.1
    jaw (bone) (lower) C41.1
      upper C41.Ø
  tibial C4Ø.2-●
Adamantoblastoma —*see* Ameloblastoma
Adams-Stokes (-Morgagni) disease or syndrome I45.9
Adaption reaction —*see* Disorder, adjustment
Addiction —*see also* Dependence F19.2Ø
  alcohol, alcoholic (ethyl) (methyl) (wood) (without remission) F1Ø.2Ø
    with remission F1Ø.21
  drug —*see* Dependence, drug
  ethyl alcohol (without remission) F1Ø.2Ø
    with remission F1Ø.21
  heroin —*see* Dependence, drug, opioid
  methyl alcohol (without remission) F1Ø.2Ø
    with remission F1Ø.21
  methylated spirit (without remission) F1Ø.2Ø
    with remission F1Ø.21

A

New Revised ~~deleted~~ Deleted ● Use Additional Character(s)

Addiction *(Continued)*
morphine(-like substances) —*see* Dependence, drug, opioid
nicotine —*see* Dependence, drug, nicotine
opium and opioids —*see* Dependence, drug, opioid
tobacco —*see* Dependence, drug, nicotine
Addisonian crisis E27.2
Addison's
anemia (pernicious) D51.Ø
disease (bronze) or syndrome E27.1
tuberculous A18.7
keloid L94.Ø
Addison-Biermer anemia (pernicious) D51.Ø
Addison-Schilder complex E71.528
Additional —*see also* Accessory
chromosome(s) Q99.8
21 —*see* Trisomy, 21
sex —*see* Abnormal, chromosome, sex
Adduction contracture, hip or other joint —*see* Contraction, joint
Adenitis —*see also* Lymphadenitis
acute, unspecified site LØ4.9
axillary I88.9
acute LØ4.2
chronic or subacute I88.1
Bartholin's gland N75.8
bulbourethral gland —*see* Urethritis
cervical I88.9
acute LØ4.Ø
chronic or subacute I88.1
chancroid (Hemophilus ducreyi) A57
chronic, unspecified site I88.1
Cowper's gland —*see* Urethritis
due to Pasteurella multocida (P. septica) A28.Ø
epidemic, acute B27.Ø9
gangrenous LØ4.9
gonorrheal NEC A54.89
groin I88.9
acute LØ4.1
chronic or subacute I88.1
infectious (acute) (epidemic) B27.Ø9
inguinal I88.9
acute LØ4.1
chronic or subacute I88.1
lymph gland or node, except mesenteric I88.9
acute —*see* Lymphadenitis, acute
chronic or subacute I88.1
mesenteric (acute) (chronic) (nonspecific) (subacute) I88.Ø
parotid gland (suppurative) —*see* Sialoadenitis
salivary gland (any) (suppurative) —*see* Sialoadenitis
scrofulous (tuberculous) A18.2
Skene's duct or gland —*see* Urethritis
strumous, tuberculous A18.2
subacute, unspecified site I88.1
sublingual gland (suppurative) —*see* Sialoadenitis
submandibular gland (suppurative) —*see* Sialoadenitis
submaxillary gland (suppurative) —*see* Sialoadenitis
tuberculous —*see* Tuberculosis, lymph gland
urethral gland —*see* Urethritis
Wharton's duct (suppurative) —*see* Sialoadenitis
Adenoacanthoma —*see* Neoplasm, malignant, by site
Adenoameloblastoma —*see* Cyst, calcifying odontogenic
Adenocarcinoid (tumor) —*see* Neoplasm, malignant, by site
Adenocarcinoma —*see also* Neoplasm, malignant, by site
acidophil
specified site —*see* Neoplasm, malignant, by site
unspecified site C75.1

Adenocarcinoma *(Continued)*
adrenal cortical C74.Ø- ●
alveolar —*see* Neoplasm, lung, malignant
apocrine
breast —*see* Neoplasm, breast, malignant
in situ
breast DØ5.8- ●
specified site NEC —*see* Neoplasm, skin, in situ
unspecified site DØ4.9
specified site NEC —*see* Neoplasm, skin, malignant
unspecified site C44.99
basal cell
specified site —*see* Neoplasm, skin, malignant
unspecified site CØ8.9
basophil
specified site —*see* Neoplasm, malignant, by site
unspecified site C75.1
bile duct type C22.1
liver C22.1
specified site NEC —*see* Neoplasm, malignant, by site
unspecified site C22.1
bronchiolar —*see* Neoplasm, lung, malignant
bronchioloalveolar —*see* Neoplasm, lung, malignant
ceruminous C44.29- ●
cervix, in situ (*see also* Carcinoma, cervix uteri, in situ) DØ6.9
chromophobe
specified site —*see* Neoplasm, malignant, by site
unspecified site C75.1
diffuse type
specified site —*see* Neoplasm, malignant, by site
unspecified site C16.9
duct
infiltrating
with Paget's disease —*see* Neoplasm, breast, malignant
specified site —*see* Neoplasm, malignant, by site
unspecified site (female) C5Ø.91- ●
male C5Ø.92- ●
specified site —*see* Neoplasm, malignant, by site
unspecified site
female C56.9
male C61
eosinophil
specified site —*see* Neoplasm, malignant, by site
unspecified site C75.1
follicular
with papillary C73
moderately differentiated C73
specified site —*see* Neoplasm, malignant, by site
trabecular C73
unspecified site C73
well differentiated C73
Hurthle cell C73
in
adenomatous
polyposis coli C18.9
infiltrating duct
with Paget's disease —*see* Neoplasm, breast, malignant
specified site —*see* Neoplasm, malignant, by site
unspecified site (female) C5Ø.91- ●
male C5Ø.92- ●
inflammatory
specified site —*see* Neoplasm, malignant, by site
unspecified site (female) C5Ø.91- ●
male C5Ø.92- ●

Adenocarcinoma *(Continued)*
intestinal type
specified site —*see* Neoplasm, malignant, by site
unspecified site C16.9
intracystic papillary
intraductal
breast DØ5.1- ●
noninfiltrating
breast DØ5.1- ●
papillary
with invasion
specified site —*see* Neoplasm, malignant, by site
unspecified site (female) C5Ø.91- ●
male C5Ø.92- ●
breast DØ5.1- ●
specified site NEC —*see* Neoplasm, in situ, by site
unspecified site DØ5.1- ●
specified site NEC —*see* Neoplasm, in situ, by site
unspecified site DØ5.1- ●
papillary
with invasion
specified site —*see* Neoplasm, malignant, by site
unspecified site (female) C5Ø.91- ●
male C5Ø.92- ●
breast DØ5.1- ●
specified site —*see* Neoplasm, in situ, by site
unspecified site DØ5.1- ●
specified site NEC —*see* Neoplasm, in situ, by site
unspecified site DØ5.1- ●
islet cell
with exocrine, mixed
specified site —*see* Neoplasm, malignant, by site
unspecified site C25.9
pancreas C25.4
specified site NEC —*see* Neoplasm, malignant, by site
unspecified site C25.4
lobular
in situ
breast DØ5.Ø- ●
specified site NEC —*see* Neoplasm, in situ, by site
unspecified site DØ5.Ø- ●
specified site —*see* Neoplasm, malignant, by site
unspecified site (female) C5Ø.91- ●
male C5Ø.92- ●
mucoid —*see also* Neoplasm, malignant, by site
cell
specified site —*see* Neoplasm, malignant, by site
unspecified site C75.1
nonencapsulated sclerosing C73
papillary
with follicular C73
follicular variant C73
intraductal (noninfiltrating)
with invasion
specified site —*see* Neoplasm, malignant, by site
unspecified site (female) C5Ø.91- ●
male C5Ø.92- ●
breast DØ5.1- ●
specified site NEC —*see* Neoplasm, in situ, by site
unspecified site DØ5.1- ●
serous
specified site —*see* Neoplasm, malignant, by site
unspecified site C56.9
papillocystic
specified site —*see* Neoplasm, malignant, by site
unspecified site C56.9

Adenocarcinoma *(Continued)*
pseudomucinous
specified site —*see* Neoplasm, malignant, by site
unspecified site C56.9
renal cell C64-●
sebaceous —*see* Neoplasm, skin, malignant, by site
serous —*see also* Neoplasm, malignant, by site
papillary
specified site —*see* Neoplasm, malignant, by site
unspecified site C56.9
sweat gland —*see* Neoplasm, skin, malignant
water-clear cell C75.Ø
Adenocarcinoma-in-situ —*see also* Neoplasm, in situ, by site
breast DØ5.9-●
Adenofibroma
clear cell —*see* Neoplasm, benign, by site
endometrioid D27.9
borderline malignancy D39.1Ø
malignant C56-●
mucinous
specified site —*see* Neoplasm, benign, by site
unspecified site D27.9
papillary
specified site —*see* Neoplasm, benign, by site
unspecified site D27.9
prostate —*see* Enlargement, enlarged, prostate
serous
specified site —*see* Neoplasm, benign, by site
unspecified site D27.9
specified site —*see* Neoplasm, benign, by site
unspecified site D27.9
Adenofibrosis
breast —*see* Fibroadenosis, breast
endometrioid N8Ø.Ø
Adenoiditis (chronic) J35.Ø2
with tonsillitis J35.Ø3
acute JØ3.9Ø
recurrent JØ3.91
specified organism NEC JØ3.8Ø
recurrent JØ3.81
staphylococcal JØ3.8Ø
recurrent JØ3.81
streptococcal JØ3.ØØ
recurrent JØ3.Ø1
Adenoids —*see* condition
Adenolipoma —*see* Neoplasm, benign, by site
Adenolipomatosis, Launois-Bensaude E88.89
Adenolymphoma
specified site —*see* Neoplasm, benign, by site
unspecified site D11.9
Adenoma —*see also* Neoplasm, benign, by site
acidophil
specified site —*see* Neoplasm, benign, by site
unspecified site D35.2
acidophil-basophil, mixed
specified site —*see* Neoplasm, benign, by site
unspecified site D35.2
adrenal (cortical) D35.ØØ
clear cell D35.ØØ
compact cell D35.ØØ
glomerulosa cell D35.ØØ
heavily pigmented variant D35.ØØ
mixed cell D35.ØØ
alpha-cell
pancreas D13.7
specified site NEC —*see* Neoplasm, benign, by site
unspecified site D13.7
alveolar D14.3Ø

Adenoma *(Continued)*
apocrine
breast D24-●
specified site NEC —*see* Neoplasm, skin, benign, by site
unspecified site D23.9
basal cell D11.9
basophil
specified site —*see* Neoplasm, benign, by site
unspecified site D35.2
basophil-acidophil, mixed
specified site —*see* Neoplasm, benign, by site
unspecified site D35.2
beta-cell
pancreas D13.7
specified site NEC —*see* Neoplasm, benign, by site
unspecified site D13.7
bile duct D13.4
common D13.5
extrahepatic D13.5
intrahepatic D13.4
specified site NEC —*see* Neoplasm, benign, by site
unspecified site D13.4
black D35.ØØ
bronchial D38.1
cylindroid type —*see* Neoplasm, lung, malignant
ceruminous D23.2-●
chief cell D35.1
chromophobe
specified site —*see* Neoplasm, benign, by site
unspecified site D35.2
colloid
specified site —*see* Neoplasm, benign, by site
unspecified site D34
duct
eccrine, papillary —*see* Neoplasm, skin, benign
endocrine, multiple
single specified site —*see* Neoplasm, uncertain behavior, by site
two or more specified sites D44-●
unspecified site D44.9
endometrioid —*see also* Neoplasm, benign
borderline malignancy —*see* Neoplasm, uncertain behavior, by site
eosinophil
specified site —*see* Neoplasm, malignant, by site
unspecified site D35.2
fetal
specified site —*see* Neoplasm, benign, by site
unspecified site D34
follicular
specified site —*see* Neoplasm, benign, by site
unspecified site D34
hepatocellular D13.4
Hurthle cell D34
islet cell
pancreas D13.7
specified site NEC —*see* Neoplasm, benign, by site
unspecified site D13.7
liver cell D13.4
macrofollicular
specified site —*see* Neoplasm, benign, by site
unspecified site D34
malignant, malignum —*see* Neoplasm, malignant, by site
microcystic
pancreas D13.6
specified site NEC —*see* Neoplasm, benign, by site
unspecified site D13.6

Adenoma *(Continued)*
microfollicular
specified site —*see* Neoplasm, benign, by site
unspecified site D34
mucoid cell
specified site —*see* Neoplasm, benign, by site
unspecified site D35.2
multiple endocrine
single specified site —*see* Neoplasm, uncertain behavior, by site
two or more specified sites D44-●
unspecified site D44.9
nipple D24-●
papillary —*see also* Neoplasm, benign, by site
eccrine —*see* Neoplasm, skin, benign, by site
Pick's tubular
specified site —*see* Neoplasm, benign, by site
unspecified site
female D27.9
male D29.2Ø
pleomorphic
carcinoma in —*see* Neoplasm, salivary gland, malignant
specified site —*see* Neoplasm, malignant, by site
unspecified site CØ8.9
polypoid —*see also* Neoplasm, benign
adenocarcinoma in —*see* Neoplasm, malignant, by site
adenocarcinoma in situ —*see* Neoplasm, in situ, by site
prostate —*see* Neoplasm, benign, prostate
rete cell D29.2Ø
sebaceous —*see* Neoplasm, skin, benign
Sertoli cell
specified site —*see* Neoplasm, benign, by site
unspecified site
female D27.9
male D29.2Ø
skin appendage —*see* Neoplasm, skin, benign
sudoriferous gland —*see* Neoplasm, skin, benign
sweat gland —*see* Neoplasm, skin, benign
testicular
specified site —*see* Neoplasm, benign, by site
unspecified site
female D27.9
male D29.2Ø
tubular —*see also* Neoplasm, benign, by site
adenocarcinoma in —*see* Neoplasm, malignant, by site
adenocarcinoma in situ —*see* Neoplasm, in situ, by site
Pick's
specified site —*see* Neoplasm, benign
unspecified site
female D27.9
male D29.2Ø
tubulovillous —*see also* Neoplasm, benign, by site
adenocarcinoma in —*see* Neoplasm, malignant, by site
adenocarcinoma in situ —*see* Neoplasm, in situ, by site
villous —*see* Neoplasm, uncertain behavior, by site
adenocarcinoma in —*see* Neoplasm, malignant, by site
adenocarcinoma in situ —*see* Neoplasm, in situ, by site
water-clear cell D35.1
Adenomatosis
endocrine (multiple) E31.2Ø
single specified site —*see* Neoplasm, uncertain behavior, by site

Adenomatosis *(Continued)*
erosive of nipple D24-●
pluriendocrine —*see* Adenomatosis, endocrine
pulmonary D38.1
malignant —*see* Neoplasm, lung, malignant
specified site —*see* Neoplasm, benign, by site
unspecified site D12.6
Adenomatous
goiter (nontoxic) E04.9
with hyperthyroidism —*see* Hyperthyroidism, with, goiter, nodular
toxic —*see* Hyperthyroidism, with, goiter, nodular
Adenomyoma —*see also* Neoplasm, benign, by site
prostate —*see* Enlarged, prostate
Adenomyometritis N80.0
Adenomyosis N80.0
Adenopathy (lymph gland) R59.9
generalized R59.1
inguinal R59.0
localized R59.0
mediastinal R59.0
mesentery R59.0
syphilitic (secondary) A51.49
tracheobronchial R59.0
tuberculous A15.4
primary (progressive) A15.7
tuberculous —*see also* Tuberculosis, lymph gland
tracheobronchial A15.4
primary (progressive) A15.7
Adenosalpingitis —*see* Salpingitis
Adenosarcoma —*see* Neoplasm, malignant, by site
Adenosclerosis I88.8
Adenosis (sclerosing) breast —*see* Fibroadenosis, breast
Adenovirus, as cause of disease classified elsewhere B97.0
Adentia (complete) (partial) —*see* Absence, teeth
Adherent —*see also* Adhesions
labia (minora) N90.89
pericardium (nonrheumatic) I31.0
rheumatic I09.2
placenta (with hemorrhage) O72.0
without hemorrhage O73.0
prepuce, newborn N47.0
scar (skin) L90.5
tendon in scar L90.5
Adhesions, adhesive (postinfective) K66.0
with intestinal obstruction K56.50
complete K56.52
incomplete K56.51
partial K56.51
abdominal (wall) —*see* Adhesions, peritoneum
appendix K38.8
bile duct (common) (hepatic) K83.8
bladder (sphincter) N32.89
bowel —*see* Adhesions, peritoneum
cardiac I31.0
rheumatic I09.2
cecum —*see* Adhesions, peritoneum
cervicovaginal N88.1
congenital Q52.8
postpartal O90.89
old N88.1
cervix N88.1
ciliary body NEC —*see* Adhesions, iris
clitoris N90.89
colon —*see* Adhesions, peritoneum
common duct K83.8
congenital —*see also* Anomaly, by site
fingers —*see* Syndactylism, complex, fingers
omental, anomalous Q43.3
peritoneal Q43.3
tongue (to gum or roof of mouth) Q38.3
conjunctiva (acquired) H11.21-●
congenital Q15.8

Adhesions, adhesive *(Continued)*
cystic duct K82.8
diaphragm —*see* Adhesions, peritoneum
due to foreign body —*see* Foreign body
duodenum —*see* Adhesions, peritoneum
ear
middle H74.1-●
epididymis N50.89
epidural —*see* Adhesions, meninges
epiglottis J38.7
eyelid H02.59
female pelvis N73.6
gallbladder K82.8
globe H44.89
heart I31.0
rheumatic I09.2
ileocecal (coil) —*see* Adhesions, peritoneum
ileum —*see* Adhesions, peritoneum
intestine —*see also* Adhesions, peritoneum
with obstruction K56.50
complete K56.52
incomplete K56.51
partial K56.51
intra-abdominal —*see* Adhesions, peritoneum
iris H21.50-●
anterior H21.51-●
goniosynechiae H21.52-●
posterior H21.54-●
to corneal graft T85.898
joint —*see* Ankylosis
knee M23.8X
temporomandibular M26.61-●
labium (majus) (minus), congenital Q52.5
liver —*see* Adhesions, peritoneum
lung J98.4
mediastinum J98.59
meninges (cerebral) (spinal) G96.12
congenital Q07.8
tuberculous (cerebral) (spinal) A17.0
mesenteric —*see* Adhesions, peritoneum
nasal (septum) (to turbinates) J34.89
ocular muscle —*see* Strabismus, mechanical
omentum —*see* Adhesions, peritoneum
ovary N73.6
congenital (to cecum, kidney or omentum) Q50.39
paraovarian N73.6
pelvic (peritoneal)
female N73.6
postprocedural N99.4
male —*see* Adhesions, peritoneum
postpartal (old) N73.6
tuberculous A18.17
penis to scrotum (congenital) Q55.8
periappendiceal —*see also* Adhesions, peritoneum
pericardium (nonrheumatic) I31.0
focal I31.8
rheumatic I09.2
tuberculous A18.84
pericholecystic K82.8
perigastric —*see* Adhesions, peritoneum
periovarian N73.6
periprostatic N42.89
perirectal —*see* Adhesions, peritoneum
perirenal N28.89
peritoneum, peritoneal (postinfective) K66.0
with obstruction (intestinal) K56.50
complete K56.52
incomplete K56.51
partial K56.51
congenital Q43.3
pelvic, female N73.6
postprocedural N99.4
postpartal, pelvic N73.6
postprocedural K66.0
to uterus N73.6
peritubal N73.6
periureteral N28.89
periuterine N73.6
perivesical N32.89

Adhesions, adhesive *(Continued)*
perivesicular (seminal vesicle) N50.89
pleura, pleuritic J94.8
tuberculous NEC A15.6
pleuropericardial J94.8
postoperative (gastrointestinal tract) K66.0
with obstruction —*see also* Obstruction, intestine, postoperative K91.30
due to foreign body accidentally left in wound —*see* Foreign body, accidentally left during a procedure
pelvic peritoneal N99.4
urethra —*see* Stricture, urethra, postprocedural
vagina N99.2
postpartal, old (vulva or perineum) N90.89
preputial, prepuce N47.5
pulmonary J98.4
pylorus —*see* Adhesions, peritoneum
sciatic nerve —*see* Lesion, nerve, sciatic
seminal vesicle N50.89
shoulder (joint) —*see* Capsulitis, adhesive
sigmoid flexure —*see* Adhesions, peritoneum
spermatic cord (acquired) N50.89
congenital Q55.4
spinal canal G96.12
stomach —*see* Adhesions, peritoneum
subscapular —*see* Capsulitis, adhesive
temporomandibular M26.61-●
tendinitis —*see also* Tenosynovitis, specified type NEC
shoulder —*see* Capsulitis, adhesive
testis N44.8
tongue, congenital (to gum or roof of mouth) Q38.3
acquired K14.8
trachea J39.8
tubo-ovarian N73.6
tunica vaginalis N44.8
uterus N73.6
internal N85.6
to abdominal wall N73.6
vagina (chronic) N89.5
postoperative N99.2
vitreomacular H43.82-●
vitreous H43.89
vulva N90.89
Adiaspiromycosis B48.8
Adie (-Holmes) pupil or syndrome —*see* Anomaly, pupil, function, tonic pupil
Adiponecrosis neonatorum P83.88
Adiposis —*see also* Obesity
cerebralis E23.6
dolorosa E88.2
Adiposity —*see also* Obesity
heart —*see* Degeneration, myocardial
localized E65
Adiposogenital dystrophy E23.6
Adjustment
disorder —*see* Disorder, adjustment
implanted device —*see* Encounter (for), adjustment (of)
prosthesis, external —*see* Fitting
reaction —*see* Disorder, adjustment
Administration of tPA (rtPA) in a different facility within the last 24 hours prior to admission to current facility Z92.82
Admission (for) —*see also* Encounter (for)
adjustment (of)
artificial
arm Z44.00-●
complete Z44.01-●
partial Z44.02-●
eye Z44.2
leg Z44.10-●
complete Z44.11-●
partial Z44.12-●
brain neuropacemaker Z46.2
implanted Z45.42
breast
implant Z45.81
prosthesis (external) Z44.3

A

- Admission *(Continued)*
  - adjustment *(Continued)*
    - colostomy belt Z46.89
    - contact lenses Z46.Ø
    - cystostomy device Z46.6
    - dental prosthesis Z46.3
    - device NEC
      - abdominal Z46.89
      - implanted Z45.89
        - cardiac Z45.Ø9
          - ➡defibrillator (with synchronous cardiac pacemaker) Z45.Ø2
          - pacemaker (cardiac resynchronization therapy (CRT-P)) Z45.Ø18
            - pulse generator Z45.Ø1Ø
          - resynchronization therapy defibrillator (CRT-D) Z45.Ø2
        - hearing device Z45.328
          - bone conduction Z45.32Ø
          - cochlear Z45.321
        - infusion pump Z45.1
        - nervous system Z45.49
          - CSF drainage Z45.41
          - hearing device —*see* Admission, adjustment, device, implanted, hearing device
          - neuropacemaker Z45.42
          - visual substitution Z45.31
        - specified NEC Z45.89
        - vascular access Z45.2
        - visual substitution Z45.31
      - nervous system Z46.2
        - implanted —*see* Admission, adjustment, device, implanted, nervous system
      - orthodontic Z46.4
      - prosthetic Z44.9
        - arm —*see* Admission, adjustment, artificial, arm
        - breast Z44.3
        - dental Z46.3
        - eye Z44.2
        - leg —*see* Admission, adjustment, artificial, leg
        - specified type NEC Z44.8
      - substitution
        - auditory Z46.2
          - implanted —*see* Admission, adjustment, device, implanted, hearing device
        - nervous system Z46.2
          - implanted —*see* Admission, adjustment, device, implanted, nervous system
        - visual Z46.2
          - implanted Z45.31
      - urinary Z46.6
    - hearing aid Z46.1
      - implanted —*see* Admission, adjustment, device, implanted, hearing device
    - ileostomy device Z46.89
    - intestinal appliance or device NEC Z46.89
    - neuropacemaker (brain) (peripheral nerve) (spinal cord) Z46.2
      - implanted Z45.42
    - orthodontic device Z46.4
    - orthopedic (brace) (cast) (device) (shoes) Z46.89
    - pacemaker (cardiac resynchronization therapy (CRT-P))
      - cardiac Z45.Ø18
        - pulse generator Z45.Ø1Ø
      - nervous system Z46.2
        - implanted Z45.42
    - portacath (port-a-cath) Z45.2
    - prosthesis Z44.9
      - arm —*see* Admission, adjustment, artificial, arm
      - breast Z44.3
      - dental Z46.3
      - eye Z44.2

- Admission *(Continued)*
  - adjustment *(Continued)*
    - prosthesis *(Continued)*
      - leg —*see* Admission, adjustment, artificial, leg
      - specified NEC Z44.8
    - spectacles Z46.Ø
  - aftercare (*see also* Aftercare) Z51.89
    - postpartum
      - immediately after delivery Z39.Ø
      - routine follow-up Z39.2
    - radiation therapy (antineoplastic) Z51.Ø
  - attention to artificial opening (of) Z43.9
    - artificial vagina Z43.7
    - colostomy Z43.3
    - cystostomy Z43.5
    - enterostomy Z43.4
    - gastrostomy Z43.1
    - ileostomy Z43.2
    - jejunostomy Z43.4
    - nephrostomy Z43.6
    - specified site NEC Z43.8
      - intestinal tract Z43.4
      - urinary tract Z43.6
    - tracheostomy Z43.Ø
    - ureterostomy Z43.6
    - urethrostomy Z43.6
  - breast augmentation or reduction Z41.1
  - breast reconstruction following mastectomy Z42.1
  - change of
    - dressing (nonsurgical) Z48.ØØ
    - neuropacemaker device (brain) (peripheral nerve) (spinal cord) Z46.2
      - implanted Z45.42
    - surgical dressing Z48.Ø1
  - circumcision, ritual or routine (in absence of diagnosis) Z41.2
  - clinical research investigation (control) (normal comparison) (participant) ZØØ.6
  - contraceptive management Z3Ø.9
  - cosmetic surgery NEC Z41.1
  - counseling (*see also* Counseling)
    - dietary Z71.3
    - gestational carrier Z31.7
    - HIV Z71.7
    - human immunodeficiency virus Z71.7
    - nonattending third party Z71.Ø
    - procreative management NEC Z31.69
  - delivery, full-term, uncomplicated O8Ø
    - cesarean, without indication O82
  - desensitization to allergens Z51.6
  - dietary surveillance and counseling Z71.3
  - ear piercing Z41.3
  - examination at health care facility (adult) —*see also* Examination ZØØ.ØØ
    - with abnormal findings ZØØ.Ø1
    - clinical research investigation (control) (normal comparison) (participant) ZØØ.6
    - dental ZØ1.2Ø
      - with abnormal findings ZØ1.21
    - donor (potential) ZØØ.5
    - ear ZØ1.1Ø
      - with abnormal findings NEC ZØ1.118
      - ▶following failed vision screening ZØ1.Ø2Ø
        - ▶with abnormal findings ZØ1.Ø21
    - eye ZØ1.ØØ
      - with abnormal findings ZØ1.Ø1
    - general, specified reason NEC ZØØ.8
    - hearing ZØ1.1Ø
      - with abnormal findings NEC ZØ1.118
      - infant or child (over 28 days old) ZØØ.129
        - with abnormal findings ZØØ.121
    - postpartum checkup Z39.2
    - psychiatric (general) ZØØ.8
      - requested by authority ZØ4.6
    - vision ZØ1.ØØ
      - with abnormal findings ZØ1.Ø1
      - ▶following failed vision screening ZØ1.Ø2Ø
        - ▶with abnormal findings ZØ1.Ø21

- Admission *(Continued)*
  - examination at health care facility *(Continued)*
    - vision *(Continued)*
      - infant or child (over 28 days old) ZØØ.129
        - with abnormal findings ZØØ.121
  - fitting (of)
    - artificial
      - arm —*see* Admission, adjustment, artificial, arm
      - eye Z44.2
      - leg —*see* Admission, adjustment, artificial, leg
    - brain neuropacemaker Z46.2
      - implanted Z45.42
    - breast prosthesis (external) Z44.3
    - colostomy belt Z46.89
    - contact lenses Z46.Ø
    - cystostomy device Z46.6
    - dental prosthesis Z46.3
    - dentures Z46.3
    - device NEC
      - abdominal Z46.89
      - nervous system Z46.2
        - implanted —*see* Admission, adjustment, device, implanted, nervous system
      - orthodontic Z46.4
      - prosthetic Z44.9
        - breast Z44.3
        - dental Z46.3
        - eye Z44.2
      - substitution
        - auditory Z46.2
          - implanted —*see* Admission, adjustment, device, implanted, hearing device
        - nervous system Z46.2
          - implanted —*see* Admission, adjustment, device, implanted, nervous system
        - visual Z46.2
          - implanted Z45.31
    - hearing aid Z46.1
    - ileostomy device Z46.89
    - intestinal appliance or device NEC Z46.89
    - neuropacemaker (brain) (peripheral nerve) (spinal cord) Z46.2
      - implanted Z45.42
    - orthodontic device Z46.4
    - orthopedic device (brace) (cast) (shoes) Z46.89
    - prosthesis Z44.9
      - arm —*see* Admission, adjustment, artificial, arm
      - breast Z44.3
      - dental Z46.3
      - eye Z44.2
      - leg —*see* Admission, adjustment, artificial, leg
      - specified type NEC Z44.8
    - spectacles Z46.Ø
  - follow-up examination ZØ9
  - intrauterine device management Z3Ø.431
    - initial prescription Z3Ø.Ø14
  - mental health evaluation ZØØ.8
    - requested by authority ZØ4.6
  - observation —*see* Observation
  - Papanicolaou smear, cervix Z12.4
    - for suspected malignant neoplasm Z12.4
  - plastic and reconstructive surgery following medical procedure or healed injury NEC Z42.8
  - plastic surgery, cosmetic NEC Z41.1
  - postpartum observation
    - immediately after delivery Z39.Ø
    - routine follow-up Z39.2
  - poststerilization (for restoration) Z31.Ø
    - aftercare Z31.42
  - procreative management Z31.9

A

Admission *(Continued)*
prophylactic (measure) —*see also* Encounter, prophylactic measures
organ removal Z40.00
breast Z40.01
fallopian tube(s) Z40.03
with ovary(s) Z40.02
ovary(s) Z40.02
specified organ NEC Z40.09
testes Z40.09
vaccination Z23
psychiatric examination (general) Z00.8
requested by authority Z04.6
radiation therapy (antineoplastic) Z51.0
reconstructive surgery following medical procedure or healed injury NEC Z42.8
removal of
cystostomy catheter Z43.5
drains Z48.03
dressing (nonsurgical) Z48.00
implantable subdermal contraceptive Z30.46
intrauterine contraceptive device Z30.432
neuropacemaker (brain) (peripheral nerve) (spinal cord) Z46.2
implanted Z45.42
staples Z48.02
surgical dressing Z48.01
sutures Z48.02
ureteral stent Z46.6
respirator [ventilator] use during power failure Z99.12
restoration of organ continuity (poststerilization) Z31.0
aftercare Z31.42
sensitivity test —*see also* Test, skin
allergy NEC Z01.82
Mantoux Z11.1
tuboplasty following previous sterilization Z31.0
aftercare Z31.42
vasoplasty following previous sterilization Z31.0
aftercare Z31.42
vision examination Z01.00
with abnormal findings Z01.01
▶following failed vision screening Z01.020
▶with abnormal findings Z01.021
infant or child (over 28 days old) Z00.129
with abnormal findings Z00.121
waiting period for admission to other facility Z75.1
Adnexitis (suppurative) —*see* Salpingo-oophoritis
Adolescent X-linked adrenoleukodystrophy E71.521
Adrenal (gland) —*see* condition
Adrenalism, tuberculous A18.7
Adrenalitis, adrenitis E27.8
autoimmune E27.1
meningococcal, hemorrhagic A39.1
Adrenarche, premature E27.0
Adrenocortical syndrome —*see* Cushing's, syndrome
Adrenogenital syndrome E25.9
acquired E25.8
congenital E25.0
salt loss E25.0
Adrenogenitalism, congenital E25.0
Adrenoleukodystrophy E71.529
neonatal E71.511
X-linked E71.529
Addison only phenotype E71.528
Addison-Schilder E71.528
adolescent E71.521
adrenomyeloneuropathy E71.522
childhood cerebral E71.520
other specified E71.528
Adrenomyeloneuropathy E71.522
Adventitious bursa —*see* Bursopathy, specified type NEC
Adverse effect —*see* Table of Drugs and Chemicals, categories T36-T50, with 6th character 5
Advice —*see* Counseling
Adynamia (episodica) (hereditary) (periodic) G72.3
Aeration lung imperfect, newborn —*see* Atelectasis
Aerobullosis T70.3
Aerocele —*see* Embolism, air
Aerodermectasia
subcutaneous (traumatic) T79.7
Aerodontalgia T70.29
Aeroembolism T70.3
Aerogenes capsulatus infection A48.0
Aero-otitis media T70.0
Aerophagy, aerophagia (psychogenic) F45.8
Aerophobia F40.228
Aerosinusitis T70.1
Aerotitis T70.0
Affection —*see* Disease
Afibrinogenemia —*see also* Defect, coagulation D68.8
acquired D65
congenital D68.2
following ectopic or molar pregnancy O08.1
in abortion —*see* Abortion, by type, complicated by, afibrinogenemia
puerperal O72.3
African
sleeping sickness B56.9
tick fever A68.1
trypanosomiasis B56.9
gambian B56.0
rhodesian B56.1
Aftercare —*see also* Care Z51.89
following surgery (for) (on)
amputation Z47.81
attention to
drains Z48.03
dressings (nonsurgical) Z48.00
surgical Z48.01
sutures Z48.02
circulatory system Z48.812
delayed (planned) wound closure Z48.1
digestive system Z48.815
explantation of joint prosthesis (staged procedure)
hip Z47.32
knee Z47.33
shoulder Z47.31
genitourinary system Z48.816
joint replacement Z47.1
neoplasm Z48.3
nervous system Z48.811
oral cavity Z48.814
organ transplant
bone marrow Z48.290
heart Z48.21
heart-lung Z48.280
kidney Z48.22
liver Z48.23
lung Z48.24
multiple organs NEC Z48.288
specified NEC Z48.298
orthopedic NEC Z47.89
planned wound closure Z48.1
removal of internal fixation device Z47.2
respiratory system Z48.813
scoliosis Z47.82
sense organs Z48.810
skin and subcutaneous tissue Z48.817
specified body system
circulatory Z48.812
digestive Z48.815
genitourinary Z48.816
nervous Z48.811
oral cavity Z48.814
respiratory Z48.813
sense organs Z48.810
skin and subcutaneous tissue Z48.817
teeth Z48.814
Aftercare *(Continued)*
following surgery *(Continued)*
specified NEC Z48.89
spinal Z47.89
teeth Z48.814
fracture — code to fracture with seventh character D
involving
removal of
drains Z48.03
dressings (nonsurgical) Z48.00
staples Z48.02
surgical dressings Z48.01
sutures Z48.02
neuropacemaker (brain) (peripheral nerve) (spinal cord) Z46.2
implanted Z45.42
orthopedic NEC Z47.89
postprocedural —*see* Aftercare, following surgery
After-cataract —*see* Cataract, secondary
Agalactia (primary) O92.3
elective, secondary or therapeutic O92.5
Agammaglobulinemia (acquired (secondary)) (nonfamilial) D80.1
with
immunoglobulin-bearing B-lymphocytes D80.1
lymphopenia D81.9
autosomal recessive (Swiss type) D80.0
Bruton's X-linked D80.0
common variable (CVAgamma) D80.1
congenital sex-linked D80.0
hereditary D80.0
lymphopenic D81.9
Swiss type (autosomal recessive) D80.0
X-linked (with growth hormone deficiency) (Bruton) D80.0
Aganglionosis (bowel) (colon) Q43.1
Age (old) —*see* Senility
Agenesis
adrenal (gland) Q89.1
alimentary tract (complete) (partial) NEC Q45.8
upper Q40.8
anus, anal (canal) Q42.3
with fistula Q42.2
aorta Q25.41
appendix Q42.8
arm (complete) Q71.0-●
with hand present Q71.1-●
artery (peripheral) Q27.9
brain Q28.3
coronary Q24.5
pulmonary Q25.79
specified NEC Q27.8
umbilical Q27.0
auditory (canal) (external) Q16.1
auricle (ear) Q16.0
bile duct or passage Q44.5
bladder Q64.5
bone Q79.9
brain Q00.0
part of Q04.3
breast (with nipple present) Q83.8
with absent nipple Q83.0
bronchus Q32.4
canaliculus lacrimalis Q10.4
carpus —*see* Agenesis, hand
cartilage Q79.9
cecum Q42.8
cerebellum Q04.3
cervix Q51.5
chin Q18.8
cilia Q10.3
circulatory system, part NOS Q28.9
clavicle Q74.0
clitoris Q52.6
coccyx Q76.49
colon Q42.9
specified NEC Q42.8

A

Agenesis *(Continued)*
  corpus callosum Q04.0
  cricoid cartilage Q31.8
  diaphragm (with hernia) Q79.1
  digestive organ(s) or tract (complete) (partial) NEC Q45.8
    upper Q40.8
  ductus arteriosus Q28.8
  duodenum Q41.0
  ear Q16.9
    auricle Q16.0
    lobe Q17.8
  ejaculatory duct Q55.4
  endocrine (gland) NEC Q89.2
  epiglottis Q31.8
  esophagus Q39.8
  eustachian tube Q16.2
  eye Q11.1
    adnexa Q15.8
  eyelid (fold) Q10.3
  face
    bones NEC Q75.8
    specified part NEC Q18.8
  fallopian tube Q50.6
  femur —*see* Defect, reduction, lower limb, longitudinal, femur
  fibula —*see* Defect, reduction, lower limb, longitudinal, fibula
  finger (complete) (partial) —*see* Agenesis, hand
  foot (and toes) (complete) (partial) Q72.3-●
  forearm (with hand present) —*see* Agenesis, arm, with hand present
    and hand Q71.2-●
  gallbladder Q44.0
  gastric Q40.2
  genitalia, genital (organ(s))
    female Q52.8
      external Q52.71
      internal NEC Q52.8
    male Q55.8
  glottis Q31.8
  hair Q84.0
  hand (and fingers) (complete) (partial) Q71.3-●
  heart Q24.8
    valve NEC Q24.8
      pulmonary Q22.0
  hepatic Q44.7
  humerus —*see* Defect, reduction, upper limb
  hymen Q52.4
  ileum Q41.2
  incus Q16.3
  intestine (small) Q41.9
    large Q42.9
      specified NEC Q42.8
  iris (dilator fibers) Q13.1
  jaw M26.09
  jejunum Q41.1
  kidney(s) (partial) Q60.2
    bilateral Q60.1
    unilateral Q60.0
  labium (majus) (minus) Q52.71
  labyrinth, membranous Q16.5
  lacrimal apparatus Q10.4
  larynx Q31.8
  leg (complete) Q72.0-●
    with foot present Q72.1-●
    lower leg (with foot present) —*see* Agenesis, leg, with foot present
      and foot Q72.2-●
  lens Q12.3
  limb (complete) Q73.0
    lower —*see* Agenesis, leg
    upper —*see* Agenesis, arm
  lip Q38.0
  liver Q44.7
  lung (fissure) (lobe) (bilateral) (unilateral) Q33.3
  mandible, maxilla M26.09
  metacarpus —*see* Agenesis, hand
  metatarsus —*see* Agenesis, foot

Agenesis *(Continued)*
  muscle Q79.8
    eyelid Q10.3
    ocular Q15.8
  musculoskeletal system NEC Q79.8
  nail(s) Q84.3
  neck, part Q18.8
  nerve Q07.8
  nervous system, part NEC Q07.8
  nipple Q83.2
  nose Q30.1
  nuclear Q07.8
  organ
    of Corti Q16.5
    or site not listed —*see* Anomaly, by site
  osseous meatus (ear) Q16.1
  ovary
    bilateral Q50.02
    unilateral Q50.01
  oviduct Q50.6
  pancreas Q45.0
  parathyroid (gland) Q89.2
  parotid gland(s) Q38.4
  patella Q74.1
  pelvic girdle (complete) (partial) Q74.2
  penis Q55.5
  pericardium Q24.8
  pituitary (gland) Q89.2
  prostate Q55.4
  punctum lacrimale Q10.4
  radioulnar —*see* Defect, reduction, upper limb
  radius —*see* Defect, reduction, upper limb, longitudinal, radius
  rectum Q42.1
    with fistula Q42.0
  renal Q60.2
    bilateral Q60.1
    unilateral Q60.0
  respiratory organ NEC Q34.8
  rib Q76.6
  roof of orbit Q75.8
  round ligament Q52.8
  sacrum Q76.49
  salivary gland Q38.4
  scapula Q74.0
  scrotum Q55.29
  seminal vesicles Q55.4
  septum
    atrial Q21.1
    between aorta and pulmonary artery Q21.4
    ventricular Q20.4
  shoulder girdle (complete) (partial) Q74.0
  skull (bone) Q75.8
    with
      anencephaly Q00.0
      encephalocele —*see* Encephalocele
      hydrocephalus Q03.9
        with spina bifida —*see* Spina bifida, by site, with hydrocephalus
      microcephaly Q02
  spermatic cord Q55.4
  spinal cord Q06.0
  spine Q76.49
  spleen Q89.01
  sternum Q76.7
  stomach Q40.2
  submaxillary gland(s) (congenital) Q38.4
  tarsus —*see* Agenesis, foot
  tendon Q79.8
  testicle Q55.0
  thymus (gland) Q89.2
  thyroid (gland) E03.1
    cartilage Q31.8
  tibia —*see* Defect, reduction, lower limb, longitudinal, tibia
  tibiofibular —*see* Defect, reduction, lower limb, specified type NEC
  toe (and foot) (complete) (partial) —*see* Agenesis, foot
  tongue Q38.3
  trachea (cartilage) Q32.1

Agenesis *(Continued)*
  ulna —*see* Defect, reduction, upper limb, longitudinal, ulna
  upper limb —*see* Agenesis, arm
  ureter Q62.4
  urethra Q64.5
  urinary tract NEC Q64.8
  uterus Q51.0
  uvula Q38.5
  vagina Q52.0
  vas deferens Q55.4
  vein(s) (peripheral) Q27.9
    brain Q28.3
    great NEC Q26.8
    portal Q26.5
  vena cava (inferior) (superior) Q26.8
  vermis of cerebellum Q04.3
  vertebra Q76.49
  vulva Q52.71
Ageusia R43.2
Agitated —*see* condition
Agitation R45.1
Aglossia (congenital) Q38.3
Aglossia-adactylia syndrome Q87.0
Aglycogenosis E74.00
Agnosia (body image) (other senses) (tactile) R48.1
  developmental F88
  verbal R48.1
    auditory R48.1
      developmental F80.2
    developmental F80.2
  visual (object) R48.3
Agoraphobia F40.00
  with panic disorder F40.01
  without panic disorder F40.02
Agrammatism R48.8
Agranulocytopenia —*see* Agranulocytosis
Agranulocytosis (chronic) (cyclical) (genetic) (infantile) (periodic) (pernicious) (*see also* Neutropenia) D70.9
  congenital D70.0
  cytoreductive cancer chemotherapy sequela D70.1
  drug-induced D70.2
    due to cytoreductive cancer chemotherapy D70.1
  due to infection D70.3
  secondary D70.4
    drug-induced D70.2
      due to cytoreductive cancer chemotherapy D70.1
Agraphia (absolute) R48.8
  with alexia R48.0
  developmental F81.81
Ague (dumb) —*see* Malaria
Agyria Q04.3
Ahumada-del Castillo syndrome E23.0
Aichomophobia F40.298
AIDS (related complex) B20
Ailment heart —*see* Disease, heart
Ailurophobia F40.218
Ainhum (disease) L94.6
AIN —*see* Neoplasia, intraepithelial, anal
AIPHI (acute idiopathic pulmonary hemorrhage in infants (over 28 days old)) R04.81
Air
  anterior mediastinum J98.2
  compressed, disease T70.3
  conditioner lung or pneumonitis J67.7
  embolism (artery) (cerebral) (any site) T79.0
    with ectopic or molar pregnancy O08.2
    due to implanted device NEC —*see* Complications, by site and type, specified NEC
    following
      abortion —*see* Abortion by type, complicated by, embolism
      ectopic or molar pregnancy O08.2
      infusion, therapeutic injection or transfusion T80.0

- **Air** *(Continued)*
  - embolism *(Continued)*
    - in pregnancy, childbirth or puerperium —*see* Embolism, obstetric
    - traumatic T79.0
  - hunger, psychogenic F45.8
  - rarefied, effects of —*see* Effect, adverse, high altitude
  - sickness T75.3
- **Airplane sickness** T75.3
- **Akathisia** (drug-induced) (treatment- induced) G25.71
  - neuroleptic induced (acute) G25.71
  - tardive G25.71
- **Akinesia** R29.898
- **Akinetic mutism** R41.89
- **Akureyri's disease** G93.3
- **Alactasia, congenital** E73.0
- **Alagille's syndrome** Q44.7
- **Alastrim** B03
- **Albers-Schönberg syndrome** Q78.2
- **Albert's syndrome** —*see* Tendinitis, Achilles
- **Albinism, albino** E70.30
  - with hematologic abnormality E70.339
    - Chédiak-Higashi syndrome E70.330
    - Hermansky-Pudlak syndrome E70.331
    - other specified E70.338
  - I E70.320
  - II E70.321
  - ocular E70.319
    - autosomal recessive E70.311
    - other specified E70.318
    - X-linked E70.310
  - oculocutaneous E70.329
    - other specified E70.328
    - tyrosinase (ty) negative E70.320
    - tyrosinase (ty) positive E70.321
  - other specified E70.39
- **Albinismus** E70.30
- **Albright (-McCune)(-Sternberg) syndrome** Q78.1
- **Albuminous** —*see* condition
- **Albuminuria, albuminuric** (acute) (chronic) (subacute) —*see also* Proteinuria R80.9
  - complicating pregnancy —*see* Proteinuria, gestational
    - with
      - gestational hypertension —*see* Pre-eclampsia
      - pre-existing hypertension —*see* Hypertension, complicating pregnancy, pre-existing, with, pre-eclampsia
  - gestational —*see* Proteinuria, gestational
    - with
      - gestational hypertension —*see* Pre-eclampsia
      - pre-existing hypertension —*see* Hypertension, complicating pregnancy, pre-existing, with, pre-eclampsia
  - orthostatic R80.2
  - postural R80.2
  - pre-eclamptic —*see* Pre-eclampsia
  - scarlatinal A38.8
- **Albuminurophobia** F40.298
- **Alcaptonuria** E70.29
- **Alcohol, alcoholic, alcohol-induced**
  - addiction (without remission) F10.20
    - with remission F10.21
  - amnestic disorder, persisting F10.96
    - with dependence F10.26
  - anxiety disorder F10.980
  - bipolar and related disorder F10.94
  - brain syndrome, chronic F10.97
    - with dependence F10.27
  - cardiopathy I42.6
  - counseling and surveillance Z71.41
    - family member Z71.42
- **Alcohol, alcoholic, alcohol-induced** *(Continued)*
  - delirium (acute) (tremens) (withdrawal) F10.231
    - with intoxication F10.921
      - in
        - abuse F10.121
        - dependence F10.221
  - dementia F10.97
    - with dependence F10.27
  - depressive disorder F10.94
  - deterioration F10.97
    - with dependence F10.27
  - hallucinosis (acute) F10.951
    - in
      - abuse F10.151
      - dependence F10.251
  - insanity F10.959
  - intoxication (acute) (without dependence) F10.129
    - with
      - delirium F10.121
      - dependence F10.229
        - with delirium F10.221
        - uncomplicated F10.220
    - uncomplicated F10.120
  - jealousy F10.988
  - Korsakoff's, Korsakov's, Korsakow's F10.26
  - liver K70.9
    - acute —*see* Disease, liver, alcoholic, hepatitis
  - major neurocognitive disorder, amnestic-confabulatory type F10.96
  - major neurocognitive disorder, nonamnestic-confabulatory type F10.97
  - mania (acute) (chronic) F10.959
  - mild neurocognitive disorder F10.988
  - paranoia, paranoid (type) psychosis F10.950
  - pellagra E52
  - poisoning, accidental (acute) NEC —*see* Table of Drugs and Chemicals, alcohol, poisoning
  - psychosis —*see* Psychosis, alcoholic
  - psychotic disorder F10.959
  - sexual dysfunction F10.981
  - sleep disorder F10.982
  - withdrawal (without convulsions) F10.239
    - with delirium F10.231
- **Alcoholism** (chronic) (without remission) F10.20
  - with
    - psychosis —*see* Psychosis, alcoholic
    - remission F10.21
  - Korsakov's F10.96
    - with dependence F10.26
- **Alder (-Reilly) anomaly or syndrome** (leukocyte granulation) D72.0
- **Aldosteronism** E26.9
  - familial (type I) E26.02
  - glucocorticoid-remediable E26.02
  - primary (due to (bilateral) adrenal hyperplasia) E26.09
  - primary NEC E26.09
  - secondary E26.1
  - specified NEC E26.89
- **Aldosteronoma** D44.10
- **Aldrich(-Wiskott) syndrome** (eczema-thrombocytopenia) D82.0
- **Alektorophobia** F40.218
- **Aleppo boil** B55.1
- **Aleukemic** —*see* condition Aleukia
  - congenital D70.0
  - hemorrhagica D61.9
    - congenital D61.09
  - splenica D73.1
- **Alexia** R48.0
  - developmental F81.0
  - secondary to organic lesion R48.0
- **Algoneurodystrophy** M89.00
  - ankle M89.07- •
  - foot M89.07- •
  - forearm M89.03- •
- **Algoneurodystrophy** *(Continued)*
  - hand M89.04- •
  - lower leg M89.06- •
  - multiple sites M89.0- •
  - shoulder M89.01- •
  - specified site NEC M89.08
  - thigh M89.05- •
  - upper arm M89.02- •
- **Algophobia** F40.298
- **Alienation, mental** —*see* Psychosis
- **Alkalemia** E87.3
- **Alkalosis** E87.3
  - metabolic E87.3
    - with respiratory acidosis E87.4
  - of newborn P74.41
  - respiratory E87.3
- **Alkaptonuria** E70.29
- **Allen-Masters syndrome** N83.8
- **Allergy, allergic** (reaction) (to) T78.40
  - air-borne substance NEC (rhinitis) J30.89
  - alveolitis (extrinsic) J67.9
    - due to
      - Aspergillus clavatus J67.4
      - Cryptostroma corticale J67.6
      - organisms (fungal, thermophilic actinomycete) growing in ventilation (air conditioning) systems J67.7
    - specified type NEC J67.8
  - anaphylactic reaction or shock T78.2
  - angioneurotic edema T78.3
  - animal (dander) (epidermal) (hair) (rhinitis) J30.81
  - bee sting (anaphylactic shock) —*see* Toxicity, venom, arthropod, bee
  - biological —*see* Allergy, drug
  - colitis —*see also* Colitis, allergic K52.29
  - dander (animal) (rhinitis) J30.81
  - dandruff (rhinitis) J30.81
  - dental restorative material (existing) K08.55
  - dermatitis —*see* Dermatitis, contact, allergic
  - diathesis —*see* History, allergy
  - drug, medicament & biological (any) (external) (internal) T78.40
    - correct substance properly administered —*see* Table of Drugs and Chemicals, by drug, adverse effect
    - wrong substance given or taken NEC (by accident) —*see* Table of Drugs and Chemicals, by drug, poisoning
  - due to pollen J30.1
  - dust (house) (stock) (rhinitis) J30.89
    - with asthma —*see* Asthma, allergic extrinsic
  - eczema —*see* Dermatitis, contact, allergic
  - epidermal (animal) (rhinitis) J30.81
  - feathers (rhinitis) J30.89
  - food (any) (ingested) NEC T78.1
    - anaphylactic shock —*see* Shock, anaphylactic, due to food
    - dermatitis —*see* Dermatitis, due to, food
    - dietary counseling and surveillance Z71.3
    - in contact with skin L23.6
    - rhinitis J30.5
    - status (without reaction) Z91.018
      - eggs Z91.012
      - milk products Z91.011
      - peanuts Z91.010
      - seafood Z91.013
      - specified NEC Z91.018
  - gastrointestinal —*see also* specific type of allergic reaction
    - meaning colitis —*see also* Colitis, allergic) K52.29
    - meaning gastroenteritis —*see also* Gastroenteritis, allergic) K52.29
    - meaning other adverse food reaction not elsewhere classified T78.1
  - grain J30.1
  - grass (hay fever) (pollen) J30.1
    - asthma —*see* Asthma, allergic extrinsic
  - hair (animal) (rhinitis) J30.81
  - history (of) —*see* History, allergy

A

Allergy, allergic (Continued)
horse serum —see Allergy, serum
inhalant (rhinitis) J30.89
pollen J30.1
kapok (rhinitis) J30.89
medicine —see Allergy, drug
milk protein —see also Allergy, food Z91.011
anaphylactic reaction T78.07
dermatitis L27.2
enterocolitis syndrome K52.21
enteropathy K52.22
gastroenteritis K52.29
gastroesophageal reflux —see also Reaction, adverse, food) K21.9
with esophagitis K21.0
proctocolitis K52.82]
nasal, seasonal due to pollen J30.1
pneumonia J82
pollen (any) (hay fever) J30.1
asthma —see Asthma, allergic extrinsic
primrose J30.1
primula J30.1
proctocolitis K52.82
purpura D69.0
ragweed (hay fever) (pollen) J30.1
asthma —see Asthma, allergic extrinsic
rose (pollen) J30.1
seasonal NEC J30.2
Senecio jacobae (pollen) J30.1
serum —see also Reaction, serum T80.69
anaphylactic shock T80.59
shock (anaphylactic) T78.2
due to
administration of blood and blood products T80.51
adverse effect of correct medicinal substance properly administered T88.6
immunization T80.52
serum NEC T80.59
vaccination T80.52
specific NEC T78.49
tree (any) (hay fever) (pollen) J30.1
asthma —see Asthma, allergic extrinsic
upper respiratory J30.9
urticaria L50.0
vaccine —see Allergy, serum
wheat —see Allergy, food
Allescheriasis B48.2
Alligator skin disease Q80.9
Allocheiria, allochiria R20.8
Almeida's disease —see Paracoccidioidomycosis
Alopecia (hereditaria) (seborrheica) L65.9
androgenic L64.9
drug-induced L64.0
specified NEC L64.8
areata L63.9
ophiasis L63.2
specified NEC L63.8
totalis L63.0
universalis L63.1
cicatricial L66.9
specified NEC L66.8
circumscripta L63.9
congenital, congenitalis Q84.0
due to cytotoxic drugs NEC L65.8
mucinosa L65.2
postinfective NEC L65.8
postpartum L65.0
premature L64.8
specific (syphilitic) A51.32
specified NEC L65.8
syphilitic (secondary) A51.32
totalis (capitis) L63.0
universalis (entire body) L63.1
X-ray L58.1
Alpers' disease G31.81
Alpine sickness T70.29
Alport syndrome Q87.81
ALTE (apparent life threatening event) in newborn and infant R68.13
Alteration (of), Altered
awareness
transient R40.4
unintended under general anesthesia, during procedure T88.53
mental status R41.82
pattern of family relationships affecting child Z62.898
sensation
following
cerebrovascular disease I69.998
cerebral infarction I69.398
intracerebral hemorrhage I69.198
nontraumatic intracranial hemorrhage NEC I69.298
specified disease NEC I69.898
subarachnoid hemorrhage I69.098
Alternating —see condition
Altitude, high (effects) —see Effect, adverse, high altitude
Aluminosis (of lung) J63.0
Alveolitis
allergic (extrinsic) —see Pneumonitis, hypersensitivity
due to
Aspergillus clavatus J67.4
Cryptostroma corticale J67.6
fibrosing (cryptogenic) (idiopathic) J84.112
jaw M27.3
sicca dolorosa M27.3
Alveolus, alveolar —see condition
Alymphocytosis D72.810
thymic (with immunodeficiency) D82.1
Alymphoplasia, thymic D82.1
Alzheimer's disease or sclerosis —see Disease, Alzheimer's
Amastia (with nipple present) Q83.8
with absent nipple Q83.0
Amathophobia F40.228
Amaurosis (acquired) (congenital) —see also Blindness
fugax G45.3
hysterical F44.6
Leber's congenital H35.50
uremic —see Uremia
Amaurotic idiocy (infantile) (juvenile) (late) E75.4
Amaxophobia F40.248
Ambiguous genitalia Q56.4
Amblyopia (congenital) (ex anopsia) (partial) (suppression) H53.00-●
anisometropic —see Amblyopia, refractive
deprivation H53.01-●
hysterical F44.6
nocturnal —see also Blindness, night
vitamin A deficiency E50.5
refractive H53.02-●
strabismic H53.03-●
suspect H53.04-●
tobacco H53.8
toxic NEC H53.8
uremic —see Uremia
Ameba, amebic (histolytica) —see also Amebiasis
abscess (liver) A06.4
Amebiasis A06.9
with abscess —see Abscess, amebic
acute A06.0
chronic (intestine) A06.1
with abscess —see Abscess, amebic
cutaneous A06.7
cutis A06.7
cystitis A06.81
genitourinary tract NEC A06.82
hepatic —see Abscess, liver, amebic
intestine A06.0
nondysenteric colitis A06.2
skin A06.7
specified site NEC A06.89
Ameboma (of intestine) A06.3
Amelia Q73.0
lower limb —see Agenesis, leg
upper limb —see Agenesis, arm
Ameloblastoma —see also Cyst, calcifying odontogenic
long bones C40.9-●
lower limb C40.2-●
upper limb C40.0-●
malignant C41.1
jaw (bone) (lower) C41.1
upper C41.0
tibial C40.2-●
Amelogenesis imperfecta K00.5
nonhereditaria (segmentalis) K00.4
Amenorrhea N91.2
hyperhormonal E28.8
primary N91.0
secondary N91.1
Amentia —see Disability, intellectual
Meynert's (nonalcoholic) F04
American
leishmaniasis B55.2
mountain tick fever A93.2
Ametropia —see Disorder, refraction
AMH (asymptomatic microscopic hematuria) R31.21
Amianthosis J61
Amimia R48.8
Amino-acid disorder E72.9
anemia D53.0
Aminoacidopathy E72.9
Aminoaciduria E72.9
Amnes (t)ic syndrome (post-traumatic) F04
induced by
alcohol F10.96
with dependence F10.26
psychoactive NEC F19.96
with
abuse F19.16
dependence F19.26
sedative F13.96
with dependence F13.26
Amnesia R41.3
anterograde R41.1
auditory R48.8
dissociative F44.0
with dissociative fugue F44.1
hysterical F44.0
postictal in epilepsy —see Epilepsy
psychogenic F44.0
retrograde R41.2
transient global G45.4
Amnion, amniotic —see condition
Amnionitis —see Pregnancy, complicated by
Amok F68.8
Amoral traits F60.89
Amphetamine (or other stimulant) —induced
anxiety disorder F15.980
bipolar and related disorder F15.94
delirium F15.921
depressive disorder F15.94
obsessive-compulsive and related disorder F15.988
psychotic disorder F15.959
sexual dysfunction F15.981
sleep disorder F15.982
stimulant withdrawal F15.23
Ampulla
lower esophagus K22.8
phrenic K22.8
Amputation —see also Absence, by site, acquired
neuroma (postoperative) (traumatic) —see Complications, amputation stump, neuroma
stump (surgical)
abnormal, painful, or with complication (late) —see Complications, amputation stump
healed or old NOS Z89.9

A

Amputation (Continued)
traumatic (complete) (partial)
arm (upper) (complete) S48.91-●
at
elbow S58.01-●
partial S58.02-●
shoulder joint (complete) S48.01-●
partial S48.02-●
between
elbow and wrist (complete) S58.11-●
partial S58.12-●
shoulder and elbow (complete) S48.11-●
partial S48.12-●
partial S48.92-●
breast (complete) S28.21-●
partial S28.22-●
clitoris (complete) S38.211
partial S38.212
ear (complete) S08.11-●
partial S08.12-●
finger (complete) (metacarpophalangeal) S68.11-●
index S68.11-●
little S68.11-●
middle S68.11-●
partial S68.12-●
index S68.12-●
little S68.12-●
middle S68.12-●
ring S68.12-●
ring S68.11-●
thumb —*see* Amputation, traumatic, thumb
transphalangeal (complete) S68.61-●
index S68.61-●
little S68.61-●
middle S68.61-●
partial S68.62-●
index S68.62-●
little S68.62-●
middle S68.62-●
ring S68.62-●
ring S68.61-●
foot (complete) S98.91-●
at ankle level S98.01-●
partial S98.02-●
midfoot S98.31-●
partial S98.32-●
partial S98.92-●
forearm (complete) S58.91-●
at elbow level (complete) S58.01-●
partial S58.02-●
between elbow and wrist (complete) S58.11-●
partial S58.12-●
partial S58.92-●
genital organ(s) (external)
female (complete) S38.211
partial S38.212
male
penis (complete) S38.221
partial S38.222
scrotum (complete) S38.231
partial S38.232
testes (complete) S38.231
partial S38.232
hand (complete) (wrist level) S68.41-●
finger(s) alone —*see* Amputation, traumatic, finger
partial S68.42-●
thumb alone —*see* Amputation, traumatic, thumb
transmetacarpal (complete) S68.71-●
partial S68.72-●
head
ear —*see* Amputation, traumatic, ear
nose (partial) S08.812
complete S08.811
part S08.89
scalp S08.0

Amputation (Continued)
traumatic (Continued)
hip (and thigh) (complete) S78.91-●
at hip joint (complete) S78.01-●
partial S78.02-●
between hip and knee (complete) S78.11-●
partial S78.12-●
partial S78.92-●
labium (majus) (minus) (complete) S38.21-●
partial S38.21-●
leg (lower) S88.91-●
at knee level S88.01-●
partial S88.02-●
between knee and ankle S88.11-●
partial S88.12-●
partial S88.92-●
nose (partial) S08.812
complete S08.811
penis (complete) S38.221
partial S38.222
scrotum (complete) S38.231
partial S38.232
shoulder —*see* Amputation, traumatic, arm
at shoulder joint —*see* Amputation, traumatic, arm, at shoulder joint
testes (complete) S38.231
partial S38.232
thigh —*see* Amputation, traumatic, hip
thorax, part of S28.1
breast —*see* Amputation, traumatic, breast
thumb (complete) (metacarpophalangeal) S68.01-●
partial S68.02-●
transphalangeal (complete) S68.51-●
partial S68.52-●
toe (lesser) S98.13-●
great S98.11-●
partial S98.12-●
more than one S98.21-●
partial S98.22-●
partial S98.14-●
vulva (complete) S38.211
partial S38.212
Amputee (bilateral) (old) Z89.9
Amsterdam dwarfism Q87.19
Amusia R48.8
developmental F80.89
Amyelencephalus, amyelencephaly Q00.0
Amyelia Q06.0
Amygdalitis —*see* Tonsillitis
Amygdalolith J35.8
Amyloid heart (disease) E85.4 *[I43]*
Amyloidosis (generalized) (primary) E85.9
with lung involvement E85.4 *[J99]*
familial E85.2
genetic E85.2
heart E85.4 *[I43]*
hemodialysis-associated E85.3
light chain (AL) E85.81
liver E85.4 *[K77]*
localized E85.4
neuropathic heredofamilial E85.1
non-neuropathic heredofamilial E85.0
organ limited E85.4
Portuguese E85.1
pulmonary E85.4 *[J99]*
secondary systemic E85.3
senile systemic (SSA) E85.82
skin (lichen) (macular) E85.4 *[L99]*
specified NEC E85.89
subglottic E85.4 *[J99]*
wild-type transthyretin-related (ATTR) E85.82
Amylopectinosis (brancher enzyme deficiency) E74.03
Amylophagia —*see* Pica
Amyoplasia congenita Q79.8
Amyotonia M62.89
congenita G70.2

Amyotrophia, amyotrophy, amyotrophic G71.8
congenita Q79.8
diabetic —*see* Diabetes, amyotrophy
lateral sclerosis G12.21
neuralgic G54.5
spinal progressive G12.25
Anacidity, gastric K31.83
psychogenic F45.8
Anaerosis of newborn P28.89
Analbuminemia E88.09
Analgesia —*see* Anesthesia
Analphalipoproteinemia E78.6
Anaphylactic
purpura D69.0
shock or reaction —*see* Shock, anaphylactic
Anaphylactoid shock or reaction —*see* Shock, anaphylactic
Anaphylactoid syndrome of pregnancy O88.01-●
Anaphylaxis —*see* Shock, anaphylactic
Anaplasia cervix —*see also* Dysplasia, cervix N87.9
Anaplasmosis, human A77.49
Anarthria R47.1
Anasarca R60.1
cardiac —*see* Failure, heart, congestive
lung J18.2
newborn P83.2
nutritional E43
pulmonary J18.2
renal N04.9
Anastomosis
aneurysmal —*see* Aneurysm
arteriovenous ruptured brain I60.8
intestinal K63.89
complicated NEC K91.89
involving urinary tract N99.89
▶ intracerebral I61.8
▶ intraparenchymal I61.8
▶ intraventricular I61.5
retinal and choroidal vessels (congenital) Q14.8
▶ subarachnoid I60.8
Anatomical narrow angle H40.03-●
Ancylostoma, ancylostomiasis (braziliense) (caninum) (ceylanicum) (duodenale) B76.0
Necator americanus B76.1
Andersen's disease (glycogen storage) E74.09
Anderson-Fabry disease E75.21
Andes disease T70.29
Andrews' disease (bacterid) L08.89
Androblastoma
benign
specified site —*see* Neoplasm, benign, by site
unspecified site
female D27.9
male D29.20
malignant
specified site —*see* Neoplasm, malignant, by site
unspecified site
female C56.9
male C62.90
specified site —*see* Neoplasm, uncertain behavior, by site
tubular
with lipid storage
specified site —*see* Neoplasm, benign, by site
unspecified site
female D27.9
male D29.20
specified site —*see* Neoplasm, benign, by site
unspecified site
female D27.9
male D29.20
unspecified site
female D39.10
male D40.10
Androgen insensitivity syndrome —*see* Syndrome, androgen insensitivity E

A

Androgen resistance syndrome —*see also* Syndrome, androgen insensitivity E34.50
Android pelvis Q74.2
with disproportion (fetopelvic) O33.3
causing obstructed labor O65.3
Androphobia F40.290
Anectasis, pulmonary (newborn) —*see* Atelectasis
Anemia (essential) (general) (hemoglobin deficiency) (infantile) (primary) (profound) D64.9
with (due to) (in)
disorder of
anaerobic glycolysis D55.2
pentose phosphate pathway D55.1
koilonychia D50.9
achlorhydric D50.8
achrestic D53.1
Addison (-Biermer) (pernicious) D51.0
agranulocytic —*see* Agranulocytosis
amino-acid-deficiency D53.0
aplastic D61.9
congenital D61.09
drug-induced D61.1
due to
drugs D61.1
external agents NEC D61.2
infection D61.2
radiation D61.2
idiopathic D61.3
red cell (pure) D60.9
chronic D60.0
congenital D61.01
specified type NEC D60.8
transient D60.1
specified type NEC D61.89
toxic D61.2
aregenerative
congenital D61.09
asiderotic D50.9
atypical (primary) D64.9
Baghdad spring D55.0
Balantidium coli A07.0
Biermer's (pernicious) D51.0
blood loss (chronic) D50.0
acute D62
bothriocephalus B70.0 *[D63.8]*
brickmaker's B76.9 *[D63.8]*
cerebral I67.89
childhood D58.9
chlorotic D50.8
chronic
blood loss D50.0
hemolytic D58.9
idiopathic D59.9
simple D53.9
chronica congenita aregenerativa D61.09
combined system disease NEC D51.0 *[G32.0]*
due to dietary vitamin B12 deficiency D51.3 *[G32.0]*
complicating pregnancy, childbirth or puerperium —*see* Pregnancy, complicated by (management affected by), anemia
congenital P61.4
aplastic D61.09
due to isoimmunization NOS P55.9
dyserythropoietic, dyshematopoietic D64.4
following fetal blood loss P61.3
Heinz body D58.2
hereditary hemolytic NOS D58.9
pernicious D51.0
spherocytic D58.0
Cooley's (erythroblastic) D56.1
cytogenic D51.0
deficiency D53.9
2, 3 diphosphoglycurate mutase D55.2
2, 3 PG D55.2
6 phosphogluconate dehydrogenase D55.1
6-PGD D55.1
amino-acid D53.0
combined B12 and folate D53.1
Anemia *(Continued)*
deficiency *(Continued)*
enzyme D55.9
drug-induced (hemolytic) D59.2
glucose-6-phosphate dehydrogenase (G6PD) D55.0
glycolytic D55.2
nucleotide metabolism D55.3
related to hexose monophosphate (HMP) shunt pathway NEC D55.1
specified type NEC D55.8
erythrocytic glutathione D55.1
folate D52.9
dietary D52.0
drug-induced D52.1
folic acid D52.9
dietary D52.0
drug-induced D52.1
G SH D55.1
G6PD D55.0
GGS-R D55.1
glucose-6-phosphate dehydrogenase D55.0
glutathione reductase D55.1
glyceraldehyde phosphate dehydrogenase D55.2
hexokinase D55.2
iron D50.9
secondary to blood loss (chronic) D50.0
nutritional D53.9
with
poor iron absorption D50.8
specified deficiency NEC D53.8
phosphofructo-aldolase D55.2
phosphoglycerate kinase D55.2
PK D55.2
protein D53.0
pyruvate kinase D55.2
transcobalamin II D51.2
triose-phosphate isomerase D55.2
vitamin B12 NOS D51.9
dietary D51.3
due to
intrinsic factor deficiency D51.0
selective vitamin B12 malabsorption with proteinuria D51.1
pernicious D51.0
specified type NEC D51.8
Diamond-Blackfan (congenital hypoplastic) D61.01
dibothriocephalus B70.0 *[D63.8]*
dimorphic D53.1
diphasic D53.1
Diphyllobothrium (Dibothriocephalus) B70.0 *[D63.8]*
due to (in) (with)
antineoplastic chemotherapy D64.81
blood loss (chronic) D50.0
acute D62
chemotherapy, antineoplastic D64.81
chronic disease classified elsewhere NEC D63.8
chronic kidney disease D63.1
deficiency
amino-acid D53.0
copper D53.8
folate (folic acid) D52.9
dietary D52.0
drug-induced D52.1
molybdenum D53.8
protein D53.0
zinc D53.8
dietary vitamin B12 deficiency D51.3
disorder of
glutathione metabolism D55.1
nucleotide metabolism D55.3
drug —*see* Anemia, by type —*see also* Table of Drugs and Chemicals
end stage renal disease D63.1
enzyme disorder D55.9
fetal blood loss P61.3
fish tapeworm (D latum) infestation B70.0 *[D63.8]*
Anemia *(Continued)*
due to *(Continued)*
hemorrhage (chronic) D50.0
acute D62
impaired absorption D50.9
loss of blood (chronic) D50.0
acute D62
myxedema E03.9 *[D63.8]*
Necator americanus B76.1 *[D63.8]*
prematurity P61.2
selective vitamin B12 malabsorption with proteinuria D51.1
transcobalamin II deficiency D51.2
Dyke-Young type (secondary) (symptomatic) D59.1
dyserythropoietic (congenital) D64.4
dyshematopoietic (congenital) D64.4
Egyptian B76.9 *[D63.8]*
elliptocytosis —*see* Elliptocytosis
enzyme-deficiency, drug-induced D59.2
epidemic —*see also* Ancylostomiasis B76.9 *[D63.8]*
erythroblastic
familial D56.1
newborn —*see also* Disease, hemolytic P55.9
of childhood D56.1
erythrocytic glutathione deficiency D55.1
erythropoietin-resistant anemia (EPO resistant anemia) D63.1
Faber's (achlorhydric anemia) D50.9
factitious (self-induced blood letting) D50.0
familial erythroblastic D56.1
Fanconi's (congenital pancytopenia) D61.09
favism D55.0
fish tapeworm (D. latum) infestation B70.0 *[D63.8]*
folate (folic acid) deficiency D52.9
glucose-6-phosphate dehydrogenase (G6PD) deficiency D55.0
glutathione-reductase deficiency D55.1
goat's milk D52.0
granulocytic —*see* Agranulocytosis
Heinz body, congenital D58.2
hemolytic D58.9
acquired D59.9
with hemoglobinuria NEC D59.6
autoimmune NEC D59.1
infectious D59.4
specified type NEC D59.8
toxic D59.4
acute D59.9
due to enzyme deficiency specified type NEC D55.8
Lederer's D59.1
autoimmune D59.1
drug-induced D59.0
chronic D58.9
idiopathic D59.9
cold type (secondary) (symptomatic) D59.1
congenital (spherocytic) —*see* Spherocytosis
due to
cardiac conditions D59.4
drugs (nonautoimmune) D59.2
autoimmune D59.0
enzyme disorder D55.9
drug-induced D59.2
presence of shunt or other internal prosthetic device D59.4
familial D58.9
hereditary D58.9
due to enzyme disorder D55.9
specified type NEC D55.8
specified type NEC D58.8
idiopathic (chronic) D59.9
mechanical D59.4
microangiopathic D59.4
nonautoimmune D59.4
drug-induced D59.2

Anemia *(Continued)*
hemolytic *(Continued)*
nonspherocytic
congenital or hereditary NEC D55.8
glucose-6-phosphate dehydrogenase deficiency D55.0
pyruvate kinase deficiency D55.2
type
I D55.1
II D55.2
type
I D55.1
II D55.2
secondary D59.4
autoimmune D59.1
specified (hereditary) type NEC D58.8
Stransky-Regala type —*see also* Hemoglobinopathy D58.8
symptomatic D59.4
autoimmune D59.1
toxic D59.4
warm type (secondary) (symptomatic) D59.1
hemorrhagic (chronic) D50.0
acute D62
Herrick's D57.1
hexokinase deficiency D55.2
hookworm B76.9 *[D63.8]*
hypochromic (idiopathic) (microcytic) (normoblastic) D50.9
due to blood loss (chronic) D50.0
acute D62
familial sex-linked D64.0
pyridoxine-responsive D64.3
sideroblastic, sex-linked D64.0
hypoplasia, red blood cells D61.9
congenital or familial D61.01
hypoplastic (idiopathic) D61.9
congenital or familial (of childhood) D61.01
hypoproliferative (refractive) D61.9
idiopathic D64.9
aplastic D61.3
hemolytic, chronic D59.9
in (due to) (with)
chronic kidney disease D63.1
end stage renal disease D63.1
failure, kidney (renal) D63.1
neoplastic disease —*see also* Neoplasm D63.0
intertropical —*see also* Ancylostomiasis D63.8
iron deficiency D50.9
secondary to blood loss (chronic) D50.0
acute D62
specified type NEC D50.8
Joseph-Diamond-Blackfan (congenital hypoplastic) D61.01
Lederer's (hemolytic) D59.1
leukoerythroblastic D61.82
macrocytic D53.9
nutritional D52.0
tropical D52.8
malarial (*see also* Malaria) B54 *[D63.8]*
malignant (progressive) D51.0
malnutrition D53.9
marsh (*see also* Malaria) B54 *[D63.8]*
Mediterranean (with other hemoglobinopathy) D56.9
megaloblastic D53.1
combined B12 and folate deficiency D53.1
hereditary D51.1
nutritional D52.0
orotic aciduria D53.0
refractory D53.1
specified type NEC D53.1
megalocytic D53.1
microcytic (hypochromic) D50.9
due to blood loss (chronic) D50.0
acute D62
familial D56.8
microdrepanocytosis D57.40

Anemia *(Continued)*
microelliptopoikilocytic (Rietti-Greppi-Micheli) D56.9
miner's B76.9 *[D63.8]*
myelodysplastic D46.9
myelofibrosis D75.81
myelogenous D64.89
myelopathic D64.89
myelophthisic D61.82
myeloproliferative D47.Z9
newborn P61.4
due to
ABO (antibodies, isoimmunization, maternal/fetal incompatibility) P55.1
Rh (antibodies, isoimmunization, maternal/fetal incompatibility) P55.0
following fetal blood loss P61.3
posthemorrhagic (fetal) P61.3
nonspherocytic hemolytic —*see* Anemia, hemolytic, nonspherocytic
normocytic (infectional) D64.9
due to blood loss (chronic) D50.0
acute D62
myelophthisic D61.82
nutritional (deficiency) D53.9
with
poor iron absorption D50.8
specified deficiency NEC D53.8
megaloblastic D52.0
of prematurity P61.2
orotaciduric (congenital) (hereditary) D53.0
osteosclerotic D64.89
ovalocytosis (hereditary) —*see* Elliptocytosis
paludal —*see also* Malaria B54 *[D63.8]*
pernicious (congenital) (malignant) (progressive) D51.0
pleochromic D64.89
of sprue D52.8
posthemorrhagic (chronic) D50.0
acute D62
newborn P61.3
postoperative (postprocedural)
due to (acute) blood loss D62
chronic blood loss D50.0
specified NEC D64.9
postpartum O90.81
pressure D64.89
progressive D64.9
malignant D51.0
pernicious D51.0
protein-deficiency D53.0
pseudoleukemica infantum D64.89
pure red cell D60.9
congenital D61.01
pyridoxine-responsive D64.3
pyruvate kinase deficiency D55.2
refractory D46.4
with
excess of blasts D46.20
1 (RAEB 1) D46.21
2 (RAEB 2) D46.22
in transformation (RAEB T) —*see* Leukemia, acute myeloblastic
hemochromatosis D46.1
sideroblasts (ring) (RARS) D46.1
without ring sideroblasts, so stated D46.0
without sideroblasts without excess of blasts D46.0
megaloblastic D53.1
sideroblastic D46.1
sideropenic D50.9
Rietti-Greppi-Micheli D56.9
scorbutic D53.2
secondary to
blood loss (chronic) D50.0
acute D62
hemorrhage (chronic) D50.0
acute D62
semiplastic D61.89

Anemia *(Continued)*
sickle-cell —*see* Disease, sickle-cell
sideroblastic D64.3
hereditary D64.0
hypochromic, sex-linked D64.0
pyridoxine-responsive NEC D64.3
refractory D46.1
secondary (due to)
disease D64.1
drugs and toxins D64.2
specified type NEC D64.3
sideropenic (refractory) D50.9
due to blood loss (chronic) D50.0
acute D62
simple chronic D53.9
specified type NEC D64.89
spherocytic (hereditary) —*see* Spherocytosis
splenic D64.89
splenomegalic D64.89
stomatocytosis D58.8
syphilitic (acquired) (late) A52.79 *[D63.8]*
target cell D64.89
thalassemia D56.9
thrombocytopenic —*see* Thrombocytopenia
toxic D61.2
tropical B76.9 *[D63.8]*
macrocytic D52.8
tuberculous A18.89 *[D63.8]*
vegan D51.3
vitamin
B6-responsive D64.3
B12 deficiency (dietary) pernicious D51.0
von Jaksch's D64.89
Witts' (achlorhydric anemia) D50.8
Anemophobia F40.228
Anencephalus, anencephaly Q00.0
Anergasia —*see* Psychosis, organic
Anesthesia, anesthetic R20.0
complication or reaction NEC —*see also* Complications, anesthesia T88.59
due to
correct substance properly administered —*see* Table of Drugs and Chemicals, by drug, adverse effect
overdose or wrong substance given —*see* Table of Drugs and Chemicals, by drug, poisoning
unintended awareness under general anesthesia during procedure T88.53
personal history of Z92.84
cornea H18.81-●
dissociative F44.6
functional (hysterical) F44.6
hyperesthetic, thalamic G89.0
hysterical F44.6
local skin lesion R20.0
sexual (psychogenic) F52.1
shock (due to) T88.2
skin R20.0
testicular N50.9
Anetoderma (maculosum) (of) L90.8
Jadassohn-Pellizzari L90.2
Schweniger-Buzzi L90.1
Aneurin deficiency E51.9
Aneurysm (anastomotic) (artery) (cirsoid) (diffuse) (false) (fusiform) (multiple) (saccular) I72.9
abdominal (aorta) I71.4
ruptured I71.3
syphilitic A52.01
aorta, aortic (nonsyphilitic) I71.9
abdominal I71.4
ruptured I71.3
arch I71.2
ruptured I71.1
arteriosclerotic I71.9
ruptured I71.8
ascending I71.2
ruptured I71.1

Aneurysm *(Continued)*
aorta, aortic (nonsyphilitic) *(Continued)*
congenital Q25.43
descending I71.9
abdominal I71.4
ruptured I71.3
ruptured I71.8
thoracic I71.2
ruptured I71.1
root Q25.43
ruptured I71.8
sinus, congenital Q25.43
syphilitic A52.Ø1
thoracic I71.2
ruptured I71.1
thoracoabdominal I71.6
ruptured I71.5
thorax, thoracic (arch) I71.2
ruptured I71.1
transverse I71.2
ruptured I71.1
valve (heart) —*see also* Endocarditis, aortic I35.8
arteriosclerotic I72.9
cerebral I67.1
ruptured —*see* Hemorrhage, intracranial, subarachnoid
arteriovenous (congenital) —*see also* Malformation, arteriovenous
acquired I77.Ø
brain I67.1
▶ruptured —*see* Aneurysm, arteriorvenous, brain, ruptured
coronary I25.41
pulmonary I28.Ø
brain Q28.2
ruptured I6Ø.8
▶intracerebral I61.8
▶intraparenchymal I61.8
▶intraventricular I61.5
▶subarachnoid I6Ø.8
peripheral —*see* Malformation, arteriovenous, peripheral
precerebral vessels Q28.Ø
specified site NEC —*see also* Malformation, arteriovenous
acquired I77.Ø
basal —*see* Aneurysm, brain
basilar (trunk) I72.5
berry (congenital) (nonruptured) I67.1
ruptured I6Ø.7
brain I67.1
arteriosclerotic I67.1
ruptured —*see* Hemorrhage, intracranial, subarachnoid
arteriovenous (congenital) (nonruptured) Q28.2
acquired I67.1
ruptured —*see* Aneurysm, arteriorvenous, brain, ruptured I6Ø.8
ruptured —*see* Aneurysm, arteriorvenous, brain, ruptured I6Ø.8
berry (congenital) (nonruptured) I67.1
ruptured —*see also* Hemorrhage, intracranial, subarachnoid I6Ø.7
congenital Q28.3
aorta (root) (sinus) Q25.43
ruptured I6Ø.7
meninges I67.1
ruptured I6Ø.8
miliary (congenital) (nonruptured) I67.1
ruptured —*see also* Hemorrhage, intracranial, subarachnoid I6Ø.7
mycotic I33.Ø
ruptured —*see* Hemorrhage, intracranial, subarachnoid
syphilitic (hemorrhage) A52.Ø5
cardiac (false) —*see also* Aneurysm, heart I25.3

Aneurysm *(Continued)*
carotid artery (common) (external) I72.Ø
internal (intracranial) I67.1
extracranial portion I72.Ø
ruptured into brain I6Ø.Ø- •
syphilitic A52.Ø9
intracranial A52.Ø5
cavernous sinus I67.1
arteriovenous (congenital) (nonruptured) Q28.3
ruptured I6Ø.8
celiac I72.8
central nervous system, syphilitic A52.Ø5
cerebral —*see* Aneurysm, brain
chest —*see* Aneurysm, thorax
circle of Willis I67.1
congenital Q28.3
ruptured I6Ø.6
ruptured I6Ø.6
common iliac artery I72.3
congenital (peripheral) Q27.8
aorta (root) (sinus) Q25.43
brain Q28.3
ruptured I6Ø.7
coronary Q24.5
digestive system Q27.8
lower limb Q27.8
pulmonary Q25.79
retina Q14.1
specified site NEC Q27.8
upper limb Q27.8
conjunctiva —*see* Abnormality, conjunctiva, vascular
conus arteriosus —*see* Aneurysm, heart
coronary (arteriosclerotic) (artery) I25.41
arteriovenous, congenital Q24.5
congenital Q24.5
ruptured —*see* Infarct, myocardium
syphilitic A52.Ø6
vein I25.89
cylindroid (aorta) I71.9
ruptured I71.8
syphilitic A52.Ø1
ductus arteriosus Q25.Ø
endocardial, infective (any valve) I33.Ø
femoral (artery) (ruptured) I72.4
gastroduodenal I72.8
gastroepiploic I72.8
heart (wall) (chronic or with a stated duration of over 4 weeks) I25.3
valve —*see* Endocarditis
hepatic I72.8
iliac (common) (artery) (ruptured) I72.3
infective I72.9
endocardial (any valve) I33.Ø
innominate (nonsyphilitic) I72.8
syphilitic A52.Ø9
interauricular septum —*see* Aneurysm, heart
interventricular septum —*see* Aneurysm, heart
intrathoracic (nonsyphilitic) I71.2
ruptured I71.1
syphilitic A52.Ø1
lower limb I72.4
lung (pulmonary artery) I28.1
mediastinal (nonsyphilitic) I72.8
syphilitic A52.Ø9
miliary (congenital) I67.1
ruptured —*see* Hemorrhage, intracerebral, subarachnoid, intracranial
mitral (heart) (valve) I34.8
mural —*see* Aneurysm, heart
mycotic I72.9
endocardial (any valve) I33.Ø
ruptured, brain —*see* Hemorrhage, intracerebral, subarachnoid
myocardium —*see* Aneurysm, heart
neck I72.Ø
pancreaticoduodenal I72.8
patent ductus arteriosus Q25.Ø

Aneurysm *(Continued)*
peripheral NEC I72.8
congenital Q27.8
digestive system Q27.8
lower limb Q27.8
specified site NEC Q27.8
upper limb Q27.8
popliteal (artery) (ruptured) I72.4
precerebral
congenital (nonruptured) Q28.1
specified site, NEC I72.5
pulmonary I28.1
arteriovenous Q25.72
acquired I28.Ø
syphilitic A52.Ø9
valve (heart) —*see* Endocarditis, pulmonary
racemose (peripheral) I72.9
congenital —*see* Aneurysm, congenital
radial I72.1
Rasmussen NEC A15.Ø
renal (artery) I72.2
retina —*see also* Disorder, retina, microaneurysms
congenital Q14.1
diabetic —*see* EØ8-E13 with .3- •
sinus of Valsalva Q25.49
specified NEC I72.8
spinal (cord) I72.8
syphilitic (hemorrhage) A52.Ø9
splenic I72.8
subclavian (artery) (ruptured) I72.8
syphilitic A52.Ø9
superior mesenteric I72.8
syphilitic (aorta) A52.Ø1
central nervous system A52.Ø5
congenital (late) A5Ø.54 *[I79.Ø]*
spine, spinal A52.Ø9
thoracoabdominal (aorta) I71.6
ruptured I71.5
syphilitic A52.Ø1
thorax, thoracic (aorta) (arch) (nonsyphilitic) I71.2
ruptured I71.1
syphilitic A52.Ø1
traumatic (complication) (early), specified site —*see* Injury, blood vessel
tricuspid (heart) (valve) IØ7.8
ulnar I72.1
upper limb (ruptured) I72.1
valve, valvular —*see* Endocarditis
visceral NEC I72.8
venous —*see also* Varix I86.8
congenital Q27.8
digestive system Q27.8
lower limb Q27.8
specified site NEC Q27.8
upper limb Q27.8
ventricle —*see* Aneurysm, heart
vertebral artery I72.6
visceral NEC I72.8
Angelman syndrome Q93.51
Anger R45.4
Angiectasis, angiectopia I99.8
Angiitis I77.6
allergic granulomatous M3Ø.1
hypersensitivity M31.Ø
necrotizing M31.9
specified NEC M31.8
nervous system, granulomatous I67.7
Angina (attack) (cardiac) (chest) (heart) (pectoris) (syndrome) (vasomotor) I2Ø.9
with
atherosclerotic heart disease —*see* Arteriosclerosis, coronary (artery)
documented spasm I2Ø.1
abdominal K55.1
accelerated —*see* Angina, unstable
agranulocytic —*see* Agranulocytosis
angiospastic —*see* Angina, with documented spasm
aphthous BØ8.5

Angina *(Continued)*
- crescendo —*see* Angina, unstable
- croupous J05.0
- cruris I73.9
- de novo effort —*see* Angina, unstable
- diphtheritic, membranous A36.0
- equivalent I20.8
- exudative, chronic J37.0
- following acute myocardial infarction I23.7
- gangrenous diphtheritic A36.0
- intestinal K55.1
- Ludovici K12.2
- Ludwig's K12.2
- malignant diphtheritic A36.0
- membranous J05.0
  - diphtheritic A36.0
  - Vincent's A69.1
- mesenteric K55.1
- monocytic —*see* Mononucleosis, infectious
- of effort —*see* Angina, specified NEC
- phlegmonous J36
  - diphtheritic A36.0
- post-infarctional I23.7
- pre-infarctional —*see* Angina, unstable
- Prinzmetal —*see* Angina, with documented spasm
- progressive —*see* Angina, unstable
- pseudomembranous A69.1
- pultaceous, diphtheritic A36.0
- spasm-induced —*see* Angina, with documented spasm
- specified NEC I20.8
- stable I20.8
- stenocardia —*see* Angina, specified NEC
- stridulous, diphtheritic A36.2
- tonsil J36
- trachealis J05.0
- unstable I20.0
- variant —*see* Angina, with documented spasm
- Vincent's A69.1
- worsening effort —*see* Angina, unstable

Angioblastoma —*see* Neoplasm, connective tissue, uncertain behavior

Angiocholecystitis —*see* Cholecystitis, acute

Angiocholitis —*see also* Cholecystitis, acute K83.09

Angiodysgenesis spinalis G95.19

Angiodysplasia (cecum) (colon) K55.20
- with bleeding K55.21
- duodenum (and stomach) K31.819
  - with bleeding K31.811
- stomach (and duodenum) K31.819
  - with bleeding K31.811

Angioedema (allergic) (any site) (with urticaria) T78.3
- hereditary D84.1

Angioendothelioma —*see* Neoplasm, uncertain behavior, by site
- benign D18.00
  - intra-abdominal D18.03
  - intracranial D18.02
  - skin D18.01
  - specified site NEC D18.09
- bone —*see* Neoplasm, bone, malignant
- Ewing's —*see* Neoplasm, bone, malignant

Angioendotheliomatosis C85.8-●

Angiofibroma —*see also* Neoplasm, benign, by site
- juvenile
  - specified site —*see* Neoplasm, benign, by site
  - unspecified site D10.6

Angiohemophilia (A) (B) D68.0

Angioid streaks (choroid) (macula) (retina) H35.33

Angiokeratoma —*see* Neoplasm, skin, benign
- corporis diffusum E75.21

Angioleiomyoma —*see* Neoplasm, connective tissue, benign

Angiolipoma —*see also* Lipoma
- infiltrating —*see* Lipoma

Angioma —*see also* Hemangioma, by site
- capillary I78.1
- hemorrhagicum hereditaria I78.0
- intra-abdominal D18.03
- intracranial D18.02
- malignant —*see* Neoplasm, connective tissue, malignant
- plexiform D18.00
  - intra-abdominal D18.03
  - intracranial D18.02
  - skin D18.01
  - specified site NEC D18.09
- senile I78.1
- serpiginosum L81.7
- skin D18.01
- specified site NEC D18.09
- spider I78.1
- stellate I78.1
- venous Q28.3

Angiomatosis Q82.8
- bacillary A79.89
- encephalotrigeminal Q85.8
- hemorrhagic familial I78.0
- hereditary familial I78.0
- liver K76.4

Angiomyolipoma —*see* Lipoma

Angiomyoliposarcoma —*see* Neoplasm, connective tissue, malignant

Angiomyoma —*see* Neoplasm, connective tissue, benign

Angiomyosarcoma —*see* Neoplasm, connective tissue, malignant

Angiomyxoma —*see* Neoplasm, connective tissue, uncertain behavior

Angioneurosis F45.8

Angioneurotic edema (allergic) (any site) (with urticaria) T78.3
- hereditary D84.1

Angiopathia, angiopathy I99.9
- cerebral I67.9
  - amyloid E85.4 *[I68.0]*
- diabetic (peripheral) —*see* Diabetes, angiopathy
- peripheral I73.9
  - diabetic —*see* Diabetes, angiopathy
  - specified type NEC I73.89
- retinae syphilitica A52.05
- retinalis (juvenilis)
  - diabetic —*see* Diabetes, retinopathy
  - proliferative —*see* Retinopathy, proliferative

Angiosarcoma —*see also* Neoplasm, connective tissue, malignant
- liver C22.3

Angiosclerosis —*see* Arteriosclerosis

Angiospasm (peripheral) (traumatic) (vessel) I73.9
- brachial plexus G54.0
- cerebral G45.9
- cervical plexus G54.2
- nerve
  - arm —*see* Mononeuropathy, upper limb
    - axillary G54.0
    - median —*see* Lesion, nerve, median
    - ulnar —*see* Lesion, nerve, ulnar
  - axillary G54.0
  - leg —*see* Mononeuropathy, lower limb
  - median —*see* Lesion, nerve, median
  - plantar —*see* Lesion, nerve, plantar
  - ulnar —*see* Lesion, nerve, ulnar

Angiospastic disease or edema I73.9

Angiostrongyliasis
- due to
  - Parastrongylus
    - cantonensis B83.2
    - costaricensis B81.3
- intestinal B81.3

Anguillulosis —*see* Strongyloidiasis

Angulation
- cecum —*see* Obstruction, intestine
- coccyx (acquired) —*see also* subcategory M43.8
  - congenital NEC Q76.49
- femur (acquired) —*see also* Deformity, limb, specified type NEC, thigh
  - congenital Q74.2
- intestine (large) (small) —*see* Obstruction, intestine
- sacrum (acquired) —*see also* subcategory M43.8
  - congenital NEC Q76.49
- sigmoid (flexure) —*see* Obstruction, intestine
- spine —*see* Dorsopathy, deforming, specified NEC
- tibia (acquired) —*see also* Deformity, limb, specified type NEC, lower leg
  - congenital Q74.2
- ureter N13.5
  - with infection N13.6
- wrist (acquired) —*see also* Deformity, limb, specified type NEC, forearm
  - congenital Q74.0

Angulus infectiosus (lips) K13.0

Anhedonia R45.84
- sexual F52.0

Anhidrosis L74.4

Anhydration E86.0

Anhydremia E86.0

Anidrosis L74.4

Aniridia (congenital) Q13.1

Anisakiasis (infection) (infestation) B81.0

Anisakis larvae infestation B81.0

Aniseikonia H52.32

Anisocoria (pupil) H57.02
- congenital Q13.2

Anisocytosis R71.8

Anisometropia (congenital) H52.31

Ankle —*see* condition

Ankyloblepharon (eyelid) (acquired) —*see also* Blepharophimosis
- filiforme (adnatum) (congenital) Q10.3
- total Q10.3

Ankyloglossia Q38.1

Ankylosis (fibrous) (osseous) (joint) M24.60
- ankle M24.67-●
- arthrodesis status Z98.1
- cricoarytenoid (cartilage) (joint) (larynx) J38.7
- dental K03.5
- ear ossicles H74.31-●
- elbow M24.62-●
- foot M24.67-●
- hand M24.64-●
- hip M24.65-●
- incostapedial joint (infectional) —*see* Ankylosis, ear ossicles
- jaw (temporomandibular) M26.61-●
- knee M24.66-●
- lumbosacral (joint) M43.27
- postoperative (status) Z98.1
- produced by surgical fusion, status Z98.1
- sacro-iliac (joint) M43.28
- shoulder M24.61-●
- spine (joint) —*see also* Fusion, spine
  - spondylitic —*see* Spondylitis, ankylosing
- surgical Z98.1
- temporomandibular M26.61-●
- tooth, teeth (hard tissues) K03.5
- wrist M24.63-●

Ankylostoma —*see* Ancylostoma

Ankylostomiasis —*see* Ancylostomiasis

Ankylurethria —*see* Stricture, urethra

Annular —*see also* condition
- detachment, cervix N88.8
- organ or site, congenital NEC —*see* Distortion
- pancreas (congenital) Q45.1

Anodontia (complete) (partial) (vera) K00.0
- acquired K08.10

Anomaly, anomalous (congenital) (unspecified type) Q89.9
- abdominal wall NEC Q79.59
- acoustic nerve Q07.8
- adrenal (gland) Q89.1
- Alder (-Reilly) (leukocyte granulation) D72.0

A

Anomaly, anomalous (Continued)
alimentary tract Q45.9
upper Q40.9
alveolar M26.70
hyperplasia M26.79
mandibular M26.72
maxillary M26.71
hypoplasia M26.79
mandibular M26.74
maxillary M26.73
ridge (process) M26.79
specified NEC M26.79
ankle (joint) Q74.2
anus Q43.9
aorta (arch) NEC Q25.40
coarctation (preductal) (postductal) Q25.1
aortic cusp or valve Q23.9
appendix Q43.8
apple peel syndrome Q41.1
aqueduct of Sylvius Q03.0
with spina bifida —*see* Spina bifida, with hydrocephalus
arm Q74.0
arteriovenous NEC
coronary Q24.5
gastrointestinal Q27.33
acquired —*see* Angiodysplasia
artery (peripheral) Q27.9
basilar NEC Q28.1
cerebral Q28.3
coronary Q24.5
digestive system Q27.8
eye Q15.8
great Q25.9
specified NEC Q25.8
lower limb Q27.8
peripheral Q27.9
specified NEC Q27.8
pulmonary NEC Q25.79
renal Q27.2
retina Q14.1
specified site NEC Q27.8
subclavian Q27.8
origin Q25.48
umbilical Q27.0
upper limb Q27.8
vertebral NEC Q28.1
aryteno-epiglottic folds Q31.8
atrial
bands or folds Q20.8
septa Q21.1
atrioventricular
excitation I45.6
septum Q21.0
auditory canal Q17.8
auricle
ear Q17.8
causing impairment of hearing Q16.9
heart Q20.8
Axenfeld's Q15.0
back Q89.9
band
atrial Q20.8
heart Q24.8
ventricular Q24.8
Bartholin's duct Q38.4
biliary duct or passage Q44.5
bladder Q64.70
absence Q64.5
diverticulum Q64.6
exstrophy Q64.10
cloacal Q64.12
extroversion Q64.19
specified type NEC Q64.19
supravesical fissure Q64.11
neck obstruction Q64.31
specified type NEC Q64.79
bone Q79.9
arm Q74.0
face Q75.9
leg Q74.2

Anomaly, anomalous (Continued)
bone (Continued)
pelvic girdle Q74.2
shoulder girdle Q74.0
skull Q75.9
with
anencephaly Q00.0
encephalocele —*see* Encephalocele
hydrocephalus Q03.9
with spina bifida —*see* Spina bifida, by site, with hydrocephalus
microcephaly Q02
brain (multiple) Q04.9
vessel Q28.3
breast Q83.9
broad ligament Q50.6
bronchus Q32.4
bulbus cordis Q21.9
bursa Q79.9
canal of Nuck Q52.4
canthus Q10.3
capillary Q27.9
cardiac Q24.9
chambers Q20.9
specified NEC Q20.8
septal closure Q21.9
specified NEC Q21.8
valve NEC Q24.8
pulmonary Q22.3
cardiovascular system Q28.8
carpus Q74.0
caruncle, lacrimal Q10.6
cascade stomach Q40.2
cauda equina Q06.3
cecum Q43.9
cerebral Q04.9
vessels Q28.3
cervix Q51.9
Chédiak-Higashi(-Steinbrinck) (congenital gigantism of peroxidase granules) E70.330
cheek Q18.9
chest wall Q67.8
bones Q76.9
chin Q18.9
chordae tendineae Q24.8
choroid Q14.3
plexus Q07.8
chromosomes, chromosomal Q99.9
D (1) —*see* condition, chromosome 13
E (3) —*see* condition, chromosome 18
G —*see* condition, chromosome 21
sex
female phenotype Q97.8
gonadal dysgenesis (pure) Q99.1
Klinefelter's Q98.4
male phenotype Q98.9
Turner's Q96.9
specified NEC Q99.8
cilia Q10.3
circulatory system Q28.9
clavicle Q74.0
clitoris Q52.6
coccyx Q76.49
colon Q43.9
common duct Q44.5
communication
coronary artery Q24.5
left ventricle with right atrium Q21.0
concha (ear) Q17.3
connection
portal vein Q26.5
pulmonary venous Q26.4
partial Q26.3
total Q26.2
renal artery with kidney Q27.2
cornea (shape) Q13.4
coronary artery or vein Q24.5
cranium —*see* Anomaly, skull
cricoid cartilage Q31.8
cystic duct Q44.5

Anomaly, anomalous (Continued)
dental
alveolar —*see* Anomaly, alveolar
arch relationship M26.20
specified NEC M26.29
dentofacial M26.9
alveolar —*see* Anomaly, alveolar
dental arch relationship M26.20
specified NEC M26.29
functional M26.50
specified NEC M26.59
jaw-cranial base relationship M26.10
asymmetry M26.12
maxillary M26.11
specified type NEC M26.19
jaw size M26.00
macrogenia M26.05
mandibular
hyperplasia M26.03
hypoplasia M26.04
maxillary
hyperplasia M26.01
hypoplasia M26.02
microgenia M26.06
specified type NEC M26.09
malocclusion M26.4
dental arch relationship NEC M26.29
jaw-cranial base relationship —*see* Anomaly, dentofacial, jaw-cranial base relationship
jaw size —*see* Anomaly, dentofacial, jaw size
specified type NEC M26.89
temporomandibular joint M26.60- ●
adhesions M26.61- ●
ankylosis M26.61- ●
arthralgia M26.62- ●
articular disc M26.63- ●
specified type NEC M26.69
tooth position, fully erupted M26.30
specified NEC M26.39
dermatoglyphic Q82.8
diaphragm (apertures) NEC Q79.1
digestive organ(s) or tract Q45.9
lower Q43.9
upper Q40.9
distance, interarch (excessive) (inadequate) M26.25
distribution, coronary artery Q24.5
ductus
arteriosus Q25.0
botalli Q25.0
duodenum Q43.9
dura (brain) Q04.9
spinal cord Q06.9
ear (external) Q17.9
causing impairment of hearing Q16.9
inner Q16.5
middle (causing impairment of hearing) Q16.4
ossicles Q16.3
Ebstein's (heart) (tricuspid valve) Q22.5
ectodermal Q82.9
Eisenmenger's (ventricular septal defect) Q21.8
ejaculatory duct Q55.4
elbow Q74.0
endocrine gland NEC Q89.2
epididymis Q55.4
epiglottis Q31.8
esophagus Q39.9
eustachian tube Q17.8
eye Q15.9
anterior segment Q13.9
specified NEC Q13.89
posterior segment Q14.9
specified NEC Q14.8
ptosis (eyelid) Q10.0
specified NEC Q15.8
eyebrow Q18.8
eyelid Q10.3
ptosis Q10.0

A

Anomaly, anomalous *(Continued)*
  face Q18.9
    bone(s) Q75.9
  fallopian tube Q5Ø.6
  fascia Q79.9
  femur NEC Q74.2
  fibula NEC Q74.2
  finger Q74.Ø
  fixation, intestine Q43.3
  flexion (joint) NOS Q74.9
    hip or thigh Q65.89
  foot NEC Q74.2
    varus (congenital) Q66.3- •
  foramen
    Botalli Q21.1
    ovale Q21.1
  forearm Q74.Ø
  forehead Q75.8
  form, teeth KØØ.2
  fovea centralis Q14.1
  frontal bone —*see* Anomaly, skull
  gallbladder (position) (shape) (size) Q44.1
  Gartner's duct Q52.4
  gastrointestinal tract Q45.9
  genitalia, genital organ(s) or system
    female Q52.9
      external Q52.7Ø
      internal NOS Q52.9
    male Q55.9
      hydrocele P83.5
      specified NEC Q55.8
  genitourinary NEC
    female Q52.9
    male Q55.9
  Gerbode Q21.Ø
  glottis Q31.8
  granulation or granulocyte, genetic (constitutional) (leukocyte) D72.Ø
  gum Q38.6
  gyri QØ7.9
  hair Q84.2
  hand Q74.Ø
  hard tissue formation in pulp KØ4.3
  head —*see* Anomaly, skull
  heart Q24.9
    auricle Q2Ø.8
    bands or folds Q24.8
    fibroelastosis cordis I42.4
    obstructive NEC Q22.6
    patent ductus arteriosus (Botalli) Q25.Ø
    septum Q21.9
      auricular Q21.1
      interatrial Q21.1
      interventricular Q21.Ø
        with pulmonary stenosis or atresia, dextraposition of aorta and hypertrophy of right ventricle Q21.3
      specified NEC Q21.8
      ventricular Q21.Ø
        with pulmonary stenosis or atresia, dextraposition of aorta and hypertrophy of right ventricle Q21.3
    tetralogy of Fallot Q21.3
    valve NEC Q24.8
      aortic
        bicuspid valve Q23.1
        insufficiency Q23.1
        stenosis Q23.Ø
          subaortic Q24.4
      mitral
        insufficiency Q23.3
        stenosis Q23.2
      pulmonary Q22.3
        atresia Q22.Ø
        insufficiency Q22.2
        stenosis Q22.1
          infundibular Q24.3
          subvalvular Q24.3

Anomaly, anomalous *(Continued)*
  heart *(Continued)*
    valve NEC *(Continued)*
      tricuspid
        atresia Q22.4
        stenosis Q22.4
    ventricle Q2Ø.8
  heel NEC Q74.2
  Hegglin's D72.Ø
  hemianencephaly QØØ.Ø
  hemicephaly QØØ.Ø
  hemicrania QØØ.Ø
  hepatic duct Q44.5
  hip NEC Q74.2
  hourglass stomach Q4Ø.2
  humerus Q74.Ø
  hydatid of Morgagni
    female Q5Ø.5
    male (epididymal) Q55.4
      testicular Q55.29
  hymen Q52.4
  hypersegmentation of neutrophils, hereditary D72.Ø
  hypophyseal Q89.2
  ileocecal (coil) (valve) Q43.9
  ileum Q43.9
  ilium NEC Q74.2
  integument Q84.9
    specified NEC Q84.8
  interarch distance (excessive) (inadequate) M26.25
  intervertebral cartilage or disc Q76.49
  intestine (large) (small) Q43.9
    with anomalous adhesions, fixation or malrotation Q43.3
  iris Q13.2
  ischium NEC Q74.2
  jaw —*see* Anomaly, dentofacial
    alveolar —*see* Anomaly, alveolar
  jaw-cranial base relationship —*see* Anomaly, dentofacial, jaw-cranial base relationship
  jejunum Q43.8
  joint Q74.9
    specified NEC Q74.8
  Jordan's D72.Ø
  kidney(s) (calyx) (pelvis) Q63.9
    artery Q27.2
    specified NEC Q63.8
  Klippel-Feil (brevicollis) Q76.1
  knee Q74.1
  labium (majus) (minus) Q52.7Ø
  labyrinth, membranous Q16.5
  lacrimal apparatus or duct Q1Ø.6
  larynx, laryngeal (muscle) Q31.9
    web (bed) Q31.Ø
  lens Q12.9
  leukocytes, genetic D72.Ø
    granulation (constitutional) D72.Ø
  lid (fold) Q1Ø.3
  ligament Q79.9
    broad Q5Ø.6
    round Q52.8
  limb Q74.9
    lower NEC Q74.2
      reduction deformity —*see* Defect, reduction, lower limb
    upper Q74.Ø
  lip Q38.Ø
  liver Q44.7
    duct Q44.5
  lower limb NEC Q74.2
  lumbosacral (joint) (region) Q76.49
    kyphosis —*see* Kyphosis, congenital
    lordosis —*see* Lordosis, congenital
  lung (fissure) (lobe) Q33.9
  mandible —*see* Anomaly, dentofacial
  maxilla —*see* Anomaly, dentofacial
  May (-Hegglin) D72.Ø
  meatus urinarius NEC Q64.79
  meningeal bands or folds QØ7.9
    constriction of QØ7.8
    spinal QØ6.9

Anomaly, anomalous *(Continued)*
  meninges QØ7.9
    cerebral QØ4.8
    spinal QØ6.9
  meningocele QØ5.9
  mesentery Q45.9
  metacarpus Q74.Ø
  metatarsus NEC Q74.2
  middle ear Q16.4
    ossicles Q16.3
  mitral (leaflets) (valve) Q23.9
    insufficiency Q23.3
    specified NEC Q23.8
    stenosis Q23.2
  mouth Q38.6
  Müllerian —*see also* Anomaly, by site
    uterus NEC Q51.818
  multiple NEC Q89.7
  muscle Q79.9
    eyelid Q1Ø.3
  musculoskeletal system, except limbs Q79.9
  myocardium Q24.8
  nail Q84.6
  narrowness, eyelid Q1Ø.3
  nasal sinus (wall) Q3Ø.8
  neck (any part) Q18.9
  nerve QØ7.9
    acoustic QØ7.8
    optic QØ7.8
  nervous system (central) QØ7.9
  nipple Q83.9
  nose, nasal (bones) (cartilage) (septum) (sinus) Q3Ø.9
    specified NEC Q3Ø.8
  ocular muscle Q15.8
  omphalomesenteric duct Q43.Ø
  opening, pulmonary veins Q26.4
  optic
    disc Q14.2
    nerve QØ7.8
  opticociliary vessels Q13.2
  orbit (eye) Q1Ø.7
  organ Q89.9
    of Corti Q16.5
  origin
    artery
      innominate Q25.8
      pulmonary Q25.79
      renal Q27.2
      subclavian Q25.48
  osseous meatus (ear) Q16.1
  ovary Q5Ø.39
  oviduct Q5Ø.6
  palate (hard) (soft) NEC Q38.5
  pancreas or pancreatic duct Q45.3
  papillary muscles Q24.8
  parathyroid gland Q89.2
  paraurethral ducts Q64.79
  parotid (gland) Q38.4
  patella Q74.1
  Pelger-Huët (hereditary hyposegmentation) D72.Ø
  pelvic girdle NEC Q74.2
  pelvis (bony) NEC Q74.2
    rachitic E64.3
  penis (glans) Q55.69
  pericardium Q24.8
  peripheral vascular system Q27.9
  Peter's Q13.4
  pharynx Q38.8
  pigmentation L81.9
    congenital Q82.8
  pituitary (gland) Q89.2
  pleural (folds) Q34.Ø
  portal vein Q26.5
    connection Q26.5
  position, tooth, teeth, fully erupted M26.3Ø
    specified NEC M26.39
  precerebral vessel Q28.1
  prepuce Q55.69
  prostate Q55.4

A

- **Anomaly, anomalous** *(Continued)*
  - pulmonary Q33.9
    - artery NEC Q25.79
    - valve Q22.3
      - atresia Q22.0
      - insufficiency Q22.2
      - specified type NEC Q22.3
      - stenosis Q22.1
        - infundibular Q24.3
        - subvalvular Q24.3
    - venous connection Q26.4
      - partial Q26.3
      - total Q26.2
  - pupil Q13.2
    - function H57.00
      - anisocoria H57.02
      - Argyll Robertson pupil H57.01
      - miosis H57.03
      - mydriasis H57.04
      - specified type NEC H57.09
      - tonic pupil H57.05-•
  - pylorus Q40.3
  - radius Q74.0
  - rectum Q43.9
  - reduction (extremity) (limb)
    - femur (longitudinal) —*see* Defect, reduction, lower limb, longitudinal, femur
    - fibula (longitudinal) —*see* Defect, reduction, lower limb, longitudinal, fibula
    - lower limb —*see* Defect, reduction, lower limb
    - radius (longitudinal) —*see* Defect, reduction, upper limb, longitudinal, radius
    - tibia (longitudinal) —*see* Defect, reduction, lower limb, longitudinal, tibia
    - ulna (longitudinal) —*see* Defect, reduction, upper limb, longitudinal, ulna
    - upper limb —*see* Defect, reduction, upper limb
  - refraction —*see* Disorder, refraction
  - renal Q63.9
    - artery Q27.2
    - pelvis Q63.9
      - specified NEC Q63.8
  - respiratory system Q34.9
    - specified NEC Q34.8
  - retina Q14.1
  - rib Q76.6
    - cervical Q76.5
  - Rieger's Q13.81
  - rotation —*see* Malrotation
    - hip or thigh Q65.89
  - round ligament Q52.8
  - sacroiliac (joint) NEC Q74.2
  - sacrum NEC Q76.49
    - kyphosis —*see* Kyphosis, congenital
    - lordosis —*see* Lordosis, congenital
  - saddle nose, syphilitic A50.57
  - salivary duct or gland Q38.4
  - scapula Q74.0
  - scrotum —*see* Malformation, testis and scrotum
  - sebaceous gland Q82.9
  - seminal vesicles Q55.4
  - sense organs NEC Q07.8
  - sex chromosomes NEC —*see also* Anomaly, chromosomes
    - female phenotype Q97.8
    - male phenotype Q98.9
  - shoulder (girdle) (joint) Q74.0
  - sigmoid (flexure) Q43.9
  - simian crease Q82.8
  - sinus of Valsalva Q25.49
  - skeleton generalized Q78.9
  - skin (appendage) Q82.9
  - skull Q75.9
    - with
      - anencephaly Q00.0
      - encephalocele —*see* Encephalocele
- **Anomaly, anomalous** *(Continued)*
  - skull *(Continued)*
    - with *(Continued)*
      - hydrocephalus Q03.9
        - with spina bifida —*see* Spina bifida, by site, with hydrocephalus
      - microcephaly Q02
  - specified organ or site NEC Q89.8
  - spermatic cord Q55.4
  - spine, spinal NEC Q76.49
    - column NEC Q76.49
      - kyphosis —*see* Kyphosis, congenital
      - lordosis —*see* Lordosis, congenital
    - cord Q06.9
    - nerve root Q07.8
  - spleen Q89.09
    - agenesis Q89.01
  - stenonian duct Q38.4
  - sternum NEC Q76.7
  - stomach Q40.3
  - submaxillary gland Q38.4
  - tarsus NEC Q74.2
  - tendon Q79.9
  - testis —*see* Malformation, testis and scrotum
  - thigh NEC Q74.2
  - thorax (wall) Q67.8
    - bony Q76.9
  - throat Q38.8
  - thumb Q74.0
  - thymus gland Q89.2
  - thyroid (gland) Q89.2
    - cartilage Q31.8
  - tibia NEC Q74.2
    - saber A50.56
  - toe Q74.2
  - tongue Q38.3
  - tooth, teeth K00.9
    - eruption K00.6
    - position, fully erupted M26.30
    - spacing, fully erupted M26.30
  - trachea (cartilage) Q32.1
  - tragus Q17.9
  - tricuspid (leaflet) (valve) Q22.9
    - atresia or stenosis Q22.4
    - Ebstein's Q22.5
  - Uhl's (hypoplasia of myocardium, right ventricle) Q24.8
  - ulna Q74.0
  - umbilical artery Q27.0
  - union
    - cricoid cartilage and thyroid cartilage Q31.8
    - thyroid cartilage and hyoid bone Q31.8
    - trachea with larynx Q31.8
  - upper limb Q74.0
  - urachus Q64.4
  - ureter Q62.8
    - obstructive NEC Q62.39
      - cecoureterocele Q62.32
      - orthotopic ureterocele Q62.31
  - urethra Q64.70
    - absence Q64.5
    - double Q64.74
    - fistula to rectum Q64.73
    - obstructive Q64.39
      - stricture Q64.32
    - prolapse Q64.71
    - specified type NEC Q64.79
  - urinary tract Q64.9
  - uterus Q51.9
    - with only one functioning horn Q51.4
  - uvula Q38.5
  - vagina Q52.4
  - valleculae Q31.8
  - valve (heart) NEC Q24.8
    - coronary sinus Q24.5
    - inferior vena cava Q24.8
    - pulmonary Q22.3
    - sinus coronario Q24.5
    - venae cavae inferioris Q24.8
  - vas deferens Q55.4
- **Anomaly, anomalous** *(Continued)*
  - vascular Q27.9
    - brain Q28.3
    - ring Q25.45
  - vein(s) (peripheral) Q27.9
    - brain Q28.3
    - cerebral Q28.3
    - coronary Q24.5
    - developmental Q28.3
    - great Q26.9
      - specified NEC Q26.8
  - vena cava (inferior) (superior) Q26.9
  - venous —*see* Anomaly, vein(s)
  - venous return Q26.8
  - ventricular
    - bands or folds Q24.8
    - septa Q21.0
  - vertebra Q76.49
    - kyphosis —*see* Kyphosis, congenital
    - lordosis —*see* Lordosis, congenital
  - vesicourethral orifice Q64.79
  - vessel(s) Q27.9
    - optic papilla Q14.2
    - precerebral Q28.1
  - vitelline duct Q43.0
  - vitreous body or humor Q14.0
  - vulva Q52.70
  - wrist (joint) Q74.0
- **Anomia** R48.8
- **Anonychia** (congenital) Q84.3
  - acquired L60.8
- **Anophthalmos, anophthalmus** (congenital) (globe) Q11.1
  - acquired Z90.01
- **Anopia, anopsia** H53.46-•
  - quadrant H53.46-•
- **Anorchia, anorchism, anorchidism** Q55.0
- **Anorexia** R63.0
  - hysterical F44.89
  - nervosa F50.00
    - atypical F50.9
    - binge-eating type F50.2
      - with purging F50.02
    - restricting type F50.01
- **Anorgasmy,** psychogenic (female) F52.31
  - male F52.32
- **Anosmia** R43.0
  - hysterical F44.6
  - postinfectional J39.8
- **Anosognosia** R41.89
- **Anosteoplasia** Q78.9
- **Anovulatory cycle** N97.0
- **Anoxemia** R09.02
  - newborn P84
- **Anoxia** (pathological) R09.02
  - altitude T70.29
  - cerebral G93.1
    - complicating
      - anesthesia (general) (local) or other sedation T88.59
        - in labor and delivery O74.3
        - in pregnancy O29.21-•
        - postpartum, puerperal O89.2
      - delivery (cesarean) (instrumental) O75.4
    - during a procedure G97.81
    - newborn P84
    - resulting from a procedure G97.82
  - due to
    - drowning T75.1
    - high altitude T70.29
  - heart —*see* Insufficiency, coronary
  - intrauterine P84
  - myocardial —*see* Insufficiency, coronary
  - newborn P84
  - spinal cord G95.11
  - systemic (by suffocation) (low content in atmosphere) —*see* Asphyxia, traumatic
- **Anteflexion** —*see* Anteversion

Antenatal
care (normal pregnancy) Z34.9Ø
screening (encounter for) of mother *—see also* Encounter, antenatal screening Z36.9
Antepartum *—see* condition
Anterior *—see* condition
Antero-occlusion M26.22Ø
Anteversion
cervix *—see* Anteversion, uterus
femur (neck), congenital Q65.89
uterus, uterine (cervix) (postinfectional) (postpartal, old) N85.4
congenital Q51.818
in pregnancy or childbirth *—see* Pregnancy, complicated by
Anthophobia F4Ø.228
Anthracosilicosis J6Ø
Anthracosis (lung) (occupational) J6Ø
lingua K14.3
Anthrax A22.9
with pneumonia A22.1
cerebral A22.8
colitis A22.2
cutaneous A22.Ø
gastrointestinal A22.2
inhalation A22.1
intestinal A22.2
meningitis A22.8
pulmonary A22.1
respiratory A22.1
sepsis A22.7
specified manifestation NEC A22.8
Anthropoid pelvis Q74.2
with disproportion (fetopelvic) O33.Ø
Anthropophobia F4Ø.1Ø
generalized F4Ø.11
Antibodies, maternal (blood group) *—see* Isoimmunization, affecting management of pregnancy
anti-D *—see* Isoimmunization, affecting management of pregnancy, Rh
newborn P55.Ø
Antibody
anticardiolipin R76.Ø
with
hemorrhagic disorder D68.312
hypercoagulable state D68.61
antiphosphatidylglycerol R76.Ø
with
hemorrhagic disorder D68.312
hypercoagulable state D68.61
antiphosphatidylinositol R76.Ø
with
hemorrhagic disorder D68.312
hypercoagulable state D68.61
antiphosphatidylserine R76.Ø
with
hemorrhagic disorder D68.312
hypercoagulable state D68.61
antiphospholipid R76.Ø
with
hemorrhagic disorder D68.312
hypercoagulable state D68.61
Anticardiolipin syndrome D68.61
Anticoagulant, circulating (intrinsic) *—see also* - Disorder, hemorrhagic D68.318
drug-induced (extrinsic) *—see also* - Disorder, hemorrhagic D68.32
iatrogenic D68.32
Antidiuretic hormone syndrome E22.2
Antimonial cholera *—see* Poisoning, antimony
Antiphospholipid
antibody
with hemorrhagic disorder D68.312
syndrome D68.61
Antisocial personality F6Ø.2
Antithrombinemia *—see* Circulating anticoagulants
Antithromboplastinemia D68.318
Antithromboplastinogenemia D68.318
Antitoxin complication or reaction *—see* Complications, vaccination
Antlophobia F4Ø.228
Antritis J32.Ø
maxilla J32.Ø
acute JØ1.ØØ
recurrent JØ1.Ø1
stomach K29.6Ø
with bleeding K29.61
Antrum, antral *—see* condition
Anuria R34
calculous (impacted) (recurrent) *—see also* Calculus, urinary N2Ø.9
following
abortion *—see* Abortion by type complicated by, renal failure
ectopic or molar pregnancy OØ8.4
newborn P96.Ø
postprocedural N99.Ø
postrenal N13.8
traumatic (following crushing) T79.5
Anus, anal *—see* condition
Anusitis K62.89
Anxiety F41.9
depression F41.8
episodic paroxysmal F41.Ø
generalized F41.1
hysteria F41.8
neurosis F41.1
panic type F41.Ø
reaction F41.1
separation, abnormal (of childhood) F93.Ø
specified NEC F41.8
state F41.1
Aorta, aortic *—see* condition
Aortectasia *—see* Ectasia, aorta
with aneurysm *—see* Aneurysm, aorta
Aortitis (nonsyphilitic) (calcific) I77.6
arteriosclerotic I7Ø.Ø
Doehle-Heller A52.Ø2
luetic A52.Ø2
rheumatic *—see* Endocarditis, acute, rheumatic
specific (syphilitic) A52.Ø2
syphilitic A52.Ø2
congenital A5Ø.54 *[I79.1]*
Apathetic thyroid storm *—see* Thyrotoxicosis
Apathy R45.3
Apeirophobia F4Ø.228
Apepsia K3Ø
psychogenic F45.8
Aperistalsis, esophagus K22.Ø
Apertognathia M26.29
Apert's syndrome Q87.Ø
Aphagia R13.Ø
psychogenic F5Ø.9
Aphakia (acquired) (postoperative) H27.Ø- •
congenital Q12.3
Aphasia (amnestic) (global) (nominal) (semantic) (syntactic) R47.Ø1
acquired, with epilepsy (Landau-Kleffner syndrome) *—see* Epilepsy, specified NEC
auditory (developmental) F8Ø.2
developmental (receptive type) F8Ø.2
expressive type F8Ø.1
Wernicke's F8Ø.2
following
cerebrovascular disease I69.92Ø
cerebral infarction I69.32Ø
intracerebral hemorrhage I69.12Ø
nontraumatic intracranial hemorrhage NEC I69.22Ø
specified disease NEC I69.82Ø
subarachnoid hemorrhage I69.Ø2Ø
primary progressive G31.Ø1 *[FØ2.8Ø]*
with behavioral disturbance G31.Ø1 *[FØ2.81]*
progressive isolated G31.Ø1 *[FØ2.8Ø]*
with behavioral disturbance G31.Ø1 *[FØ2.81]*
Aphasia *(Continued)*
sensory F8Ø.2
syphilis, tertiary A52.19
Wernicke's (developmental) F8Ø.2
Aphonia (organic) R49.1
hysterical F44.4
psychogenic F44.4
Aphthae, aphthous *—see also* condition
Bednar's K12.Ø
cachectic K14.Ø
epizootic BØ8.8
fever BØ8.8
oral (recurrent) K12.Ø
stomatitis (major) (minor) K12.Ø
thrush B37.Ø
ulcer (oral) (recurrent) K12.Ø
genital organ(s) NEC
female N76.6
male N5Ø.89
larynx J38.7
Apical *—see* condition
Apiphobia F4Ø.218
Aplasia *—see also* Agenesis
abdominal muscle syndrome Q79.4
alveolar process (acquired) *—see* Anomaly, alveolar
congenital Q38.6
aorta (congenital) Q25.41
axialis extracorticalis (congenita) E75.29
bone marrow (myeloid) D61.9
congenital D61.Ø1
brain QØØ.Ø
part of QØ4.3
bronchus Q32.4
cementum KØØ.4
cerebellum QØ4.3
cervix (congenital) Q51.5
congenital pure red cell D61.Ø1
corpus callosum QØ4.Ø
cutis congenita Q84.8
erythrocyte congenital D61.Ø1
extracortical axial E75.29
eye Q11.1
fovea centralis (congenital) Q14.1
gallbladder, congenital Q44.Ø
iris Q13.1
labyrinth, membranous Q16.5
limb (congenital) Q73.8
lower *—see* Defect, reduction, lower limb
upper *—see* Agenesis, arm
lung, congenital (bilateral) (unilateral) Q33.3
pancreas Q45.Ø
parathyroid-thymic D82.1
Pelizaeus-Merzbacher E75.29
penis Q55.5
prostate Q55.4
red cell (with thymoma) D6Ø.9
acquired D6Ø.9
due to drugs D6Ø.9
adult D6Ø.9
chronic D6Ø.Ø
congenital D61.Ø1
constitutional D61.Ø1
due to drugs D6Ø.9
hereditary D61.Ø1
of infants D61.Ø1
primary D61.Ø1
pure D61.Ø1
due to drugs D6Ø.9
specified type NEC D6Ø.8
transient D6Ø.1
round ligament Q52.8
skin Q84.8
spermatic cord Q55.4
spleen Q89.Ø1
testicle Q55.Ø
thymic, with immunodeficiency D82.1
thyroid (congenital) (with myxedema) EØ3.1
uterus Q51.Ø
ventral horn cell QØ6.1

A

Apnea, apneic (of) (spells) RØ6.81
newborn NEC P28.4
obstructive P28.4
sleep (central) (obstructive) (primary) P28.3
prematurity P28.4
sleep G47.3Ø
central (primary) G47.31
idiopathic G47.31
in conditions classified elsewhere G47.37
obstructive (adult) (pediatric) G47.33
hypopnea G47.33
primary central G47.31
specified NEC G47.39
Apneumatosis, newborn P28.Ø
Apocrine metaplasia (breast) —*see* Dysplasia, mammary, specified type NEC
Apophysitis (bone) —*see also* Osteochondropathy
calcaneus M92.8
juvenile M92.9
Apoplectiform convulsions (cerebral ischemia) I67.82
Apoplexia, apoplexy, apoplectic
adrenal A39.1
heart (auricle) (ventricle) —*see* Infarct, myocardium
➡ heat T67.Ø1
hemorrhagic (stroke) —*see* Hemorrhage, intracranial
meninges, hemorrhagic —*see* Hemorrhage, intracranial, subarachnoid
uremic N18.9 *[I68.8]*
Appearance
bizarre R46.1
specified NEC R46.89
very low level of personal hygiene R46.Ø
Appendage
epididymal (organ of Morgagni) Q55.4
intestine (epiploic) Q43.8
preauricular Q17.Ø
testicular (organ of Morgagni) Q55.29
Appendicitis (pneumococcal) (retrocecal) K37
with
gangrene K35.891
perforation NOS K35.32
peritoneal abscess K35.33
peritonitis NEC K35.33
generalized (with perforation or rupture) K35.2Ø
with abscess K35.21
localized K35.3Ø
with
gangrene K35.32
perforation K35.32
and abscess K35.33
ruptured NOS (with localized peritonitis) K35.32
acute (catarrhal) (fulminating) (gangrenous) (obstructive) (retrocecal) (suppurative) K35.8Ø
with
gangrene K35.891
peritoneal abscess K35.33
peritonitis NEC K35.33
generalized (with perforation or rupture) K35.2Ø
with abscess K35.21
localized K35.3Ø
with
gangrene K35.32
perforation K35.32
and abscess K35.33
specified NEC K35.89Ø
with gangrene K35.891
amebic AØ6.89
chronic (recurrent) K36
exacerbation —*see* Appendicitis, acute
gangrenous —*see* Appendicitis, acute
healed (obliterative) K36
interval K36
neurogenic K36
Appendicitis *(Continued)*
obstructive K36
recurrent K36
relapsing K36
ruptured NOS (with localized peritonitis) K35.32
subacute (adhesive) K36
subsiding K36
suppurative —*see* Appendicitis, acute
tuberculous A18.32
Appendicopathia oxyurica B8Ø
Appendix, appendicular —*see also* condition
epididymis Q55.4
Morgagni
female Q5Ø.5
male (epididymal) Q55.4
testicular Q55.29
testis Q55.29
Appetite
depraved —*see* Pica
excessive R63.2
lack or loss —*see also* Anorexia R63.Ø
nonorganic origin F5Ø.89
psychogenic F5Ø.89
perverted (hysterical) —*see* Pica
Apple peel syndrome Q41.1
Apprehension state F41.1
Apprehensiveness, abnormal F41.9
Approximal wear KØ3.Ø
Apraxia (classic) (ideational) (ideokinetic) (ideomotor) (motor) (verbal) R48.2
following
cerebrovascular disease I69.99Ø
cerebral infarction I69.39Ø
intracerebral hemorrhage I69.19Ø
nontraumatic intracranial hemorrhage NEC I69.29Ø
specified disease NEC I69.89Ø
subarachnoid hemorrhage I69.Ø9Ø
oculomotor, congenital H51.8
Aptyalism K11.7
Apudoma —*see* Neoplasm, uncertain behavior, by site
Aqueous misdirection H4Ø.83-●
Arabicum elephantiasis —*see* Infestation, filarial
Arachnitis —*see* Meningitis
Arachnodactyly —*see* Syndrome, Marfan's
Arachnoiditis (acute) (adhesive) (basal) (brain) (cerebrospinal) —*see* Meningitis
Arachnophobia F4Ø.21Ø
Arboencephalitis, Australian A83.4
Arborization block (heart) I45.5
ARC (AIDS-related complex) B2Ø
Arch
aortic Q25.49
bovine Q25.49
Arches —*see* condition
Arcuate uterus Q51.81Ø
Arcuatus uterus Q51.81Ø
Arcus (cornea) **senilis** —*see* Degeneration, cornea, senile
Arc-welder's lung J63.4
Areflexia R29.2
Areola —*see* condition
Argentaffinoma —*see also* Neoplasm, uncertain behavior, by site
malignant —*see* Neoplasm, malignant, by site
syndrome E34.Ø
Argininemia E72.21
Arginosuccinic aciduria E72.22
Argyll Robertson phenomenon, pupil or syndrome (syphilitic) A52.19
atypical H57.Ø9
nonsyphilitic H57.Ø9
Argyria, argyriasis
conjunctival H11.13-●
from drug or medicament —*see* Table of Drugs and Chemicals, by substance
Argyrosis, conjunctival H11.13-●
Arhinencephaly QØ4.1
Ariboflavinosis E53.Ø
Arm —*see* condition
Arnold-Chiari disease, obstruction or syndrome (type II) QØ7.ØØ
with
hydrocephalus QØ7.Ø2
with spina bifida QØ7.Ø3
spina bifida QØ7.Ø1
with hydrocephalus QØ7.Ø3
type III —*see* Encephalocele
type IV QØ4.8
Aromatic amino-acid metabolism disorder E7Ø.9
specified NEC E7Ø.8
Arousals, confusional G47.51
Arrest, arrested
cardiac I46.9
complicating
abortion —*see* Abortion, by type, complicated by, cardiac arrest
anesthesia (general) (local) or other sedation —*see* Table of Drugs and Chemicals, by drug
in labor and delivery O74.2
in pregnancy O29.11-●
postpartum, puerperal O89.1
delivery (cesarean) (instrumental) O75.4
due to
cardiac condition I46.2
specified condition NEC I46.8
intraoperative I97.71-●
newborn P29.81
personal history, successfully resuscitated Z86.74
postprocedural I97.12-●
obstetric procedure O75.4
cardiorespiratory —*see* Arrest, cardiac
circulatory —*see* Arrest, cardiac
deep transverse O64.Ø
development or growth
bone —*see* Disorder, bone, development or growth
child R62.5Ø
tracheal rings Q32.1
epiphyseal
complete
femur M89.15-●
humerus M89.12-●
tibia M89.16-●
ulna M89.13-●
forearm M89.13-●
specified NEC M89.13-●
ulna —*see* Arrest, epiphyseal, by type, ulna
lower leg M89.16-●
specified NEC M89.168
tibia —*see* Arrest, epiphyseal, by type, tibia
partial
femur M89.15-●
humerus M89.12-●
tibia M89.16-●
ulna M89.13-●
specified NEC M89.18
granulopoiesis —*see* Agranulocytosis
growth plate —*see* Arrest, epiphyseal
heart —*see* Arrest, cardiac
legal, anxiety concerning Z65.3
physeal —*see* Arrest, epiphyseal
respiratory RØ9.2
newborn P28.81
sinus I45.5
spermatogenesis (complete) —*see* Azoospermia
incomplete —*see* Oligospermia
transverse (deep) O64.Ø
Arrhenoblastoma
benign
specified site —*see* Neoplasm, benign, by site
unspecified site
female D27.9
male D29.2Ø

Arrhenoblastoma *(Continued)*
malignant
specified site —*see* Neoplasm, malignant, by site
unspecified site
female C56.9
male C62.90
specified site —*see* Neoplasm, uncertain behavior, by site
unspecified site
female D39.10
male D40.10
Arrhythmia (auricle)(cardiac) (juvenile)(nodal) (reflex)(sinus)(supraventricular)(transitory) (ventricle) I49.9
block I45.9
extrasystolic I49.49
newborn
bradycardia P29.12
occurring before birth P03.819
before onset of labor P03.810
during labor P03.811
tachycardia P29.11
psychogenic F45.8
specified NEC I49.8
vagal R55
ventricular re-entry I47.0
Arrillaga-Ayerza syndrome (pulmonary sclerosis with pulmonary hypertension) I27.0
Arsenical pigmentation L81.8
from drug or medicament —*see* Table of Drugs and Chemicals
Arsenism —*see* Poisoning, arsenic
Arterial —*see* condition
Arteriofibrosis —*see* Arteriosclerosis
Arteriolar sclerosis —*see* Arteriosclerosis
Arteriolith —*see* Arteriosclerosis
Arteriolitis I77.6
necrotizing, kidney I77.5
renal —*see* Hypertension, kidney
Arteriolosclerosis —*see* Arteriosclerosis
Arterionephrosclerosis —*see* Hypertension, kidney
Arteriopathy I77.9
cerebral autosomal dominant, with subcortical infarcts and leukoencephalopathy (CADASIL) I67.850
Arteriosclerosis, arteriosclerotic (diffuse) (obliterans) (of) (senile) (with calcification) I70.90
aorta I70.0
arteries of extremities —*see* Arteriosclerosis, extremities
brain I67.2
bypass graft
coronary —*see* Arteriosclerosis, coronary, bypass graft
extremities —*see* Arteriosclerosis, extremities, bypass graft
cardiac —*see* Disease, heart, ischemic, atherosclerotic
cardiopathy —*see* Disease, heart, ischemic, atherosclerotic
cardiorenal —*see* Hypertension, cardiorenal
cardiovascular —*see* Disease, heart, ischemic, atherosclerotic
carotid —*see also* Occlusion, artery, carotid I65.2-•
central nervous system I67.2
cerebral I67.2
cerebrovascular I67.2
coronary (artery) I25.10
bypass graft I25.810
with
angina pectoris I25.709
with documented spasm I25.701
specified type NEC I25.708
unstable I25.700
ischemic chest pain I25.709

Arteriosclerosis, arteriosclerotic *(Continued)*
coronary *(Continued)*
bypass graft *(Continued)*
autologous artery I25.810
with
angina pectoris I25.729
with documented spasm I25.721
specified type I25.728
unstable I25.720
ischemic chest pain I25.729
autologous vein I25.810
with
angina pectoris I25.719
with documented spasm I25.711
specified type I25.718
unstable I25.710
ischemic chest pain I25.719
nonautologous biological I25.810
with
angina pectoris I25.739
with documented spasm I25.731
specified type I25.738
unstable I25.730
ischemic chest pain I25.739
specified type NEC I25.810
with
angina pectoris I25.799
with documented spasm I25.791
specified type I25.798
unstable I25.790
ischemic chest pain I25.799
due to
calcified coronary lesion (severely) I25.84
lipid rich plaque I25.83
native vessel
with
angina pectoris I25.119
with documented spasm I25.111
specified type NEC I25.118
unstable I25.110
ischemic chest pain I25.119
transplanted heart I25.811
bypass graft I25.812
with
angina pectoris I25.769
with documented spasm I25.761
specified type I25.768
unstable I25.760
ischemic chest pain I25.769
native coronary artery I25.811
with
angina pectoris I25.759
with documented spasm I25.751
specified type I25.758
unstable I25.750
ischemic chest pain I25.759
extremities (native arteries) I70.209
bypass graft I70.309
autologous vein graft I70.409
leg I70.409
with
gangrene (and intermittent claudication, rest pain and ulcer) I70.469
intermittent claudication I70.419
rest pain (and intermittent claudication) I70.429
bilateral I70.403
with
gangrene (and intermittent claudication, rest pain and ulcer) I70.463
intermittent claudication I70.413
rest pain (and intermittent claudication) I70.423
specified type NEC I70.493

Arteriosclerosis, arteriosclerotic *(Continued)*
extremities *(Continued)*
bypass graft *(Continued)*
autologous vein graft *(Continued)*
leg *(Continued)*
left I70.402
with
gangrene (and intermittent claudication, rest pain and ulcer) I70.462
intermittent claudication I70.412
rest pain (and intermittent claudication) I70.422
ulceration (and intermittent claudication and rest pain) I70.449
ankle I70.443
calf I70.442
foot site NEC I70.445
heel I70.444
lower leg NEC I70.448
midfoot I70.444
thigh I70.441
specified type NEC I70.492
right I70.401
with
gangrene (and intermittent claudication, rest pain and ulcer) I70.461
intermittent claudication I70.411
rest pain (and intermittent claudication) I70.421
ulceration (and intermittent claudication and rest pain) I70.439
ankle I70.433
calf I70.432
foot site NEC I70.435
heel I70.434
lower leg NEC I70.438
midfoot I70.434
thigh I70.431
specified type NEC I70.491
specified type NEC I70.499
specified NEC I70.408
with
gangrene (and intermittent claudication, rest pain and ulcer) I70.468
intermittent claudication I70.418
rest pain (and intermittent claudication) I70.428
ulceration (and intermittent claudication and rest pain) I70.45
specified type NEC I70.498
leg I70.309
with
gangrene (and intermittent claudication, rest pain and ulcer) I70.369
intermittent claudication I70.319
rest pain (and intermittent claudication) I70.329
bilateral I70.303
with
gangrene (and intermittent claudication, rest pain and ulcer) I70.363
intermittent claudication I70.313
rest pain (and intermittent claudication) I70.323
specified type NEC I70.393
left I70.302
with
gangrene (and intermittent claudication, rest pain and ulcer) I70.362
intermittent claudication I70.312

A

Arteriosclerosis, arteriosclerotic *(Continued)*
extremities *(Continued)*
bypass graft *(Continued)*
leg *(Continued)*
left *(Continued)*
with *(Continued)*
rest pain (and intermittent claudication) I70.322
ulceration (and intermittent claudication and rest pain) I70.349
ankle I70.343
calf I70.342
foot site NEC I70.345
heel I70.344
lower leg NEC I70.348
midfoot I70.344
thigh I70.341
specified type NEC I70.392
right I70.301
with
gangrene (and intermittent claudication, rest pain and ulcer) I70.361
intermittent claudication I70.311
rest pain (and intermittent claudication) I70.321
ulceration (and intermittent claudication and rest pain) I70.339
ankle I70.333
calf I70.332
foot site NEC I70.335
heel I70.334
lower leg NEC I70.338
midfoot I70.334
thigh I70.331
specified type NEC I70.391
specified type NEC I70.399
nonautologous biological graft I70.509
leg I70.509
with
gangrene (and intermittent claudication, rest pain and ulcer) I70.569
intermittent claudication I70.519
rest pain (and intermittent claudication) I70.529
bilateral I70.503
with
gangrene (and intermittent claudication, rest pain and ulcer) I70.563
intermittent claudication I70.513
rest pain (and intermittent claudication) I70.523
specified type NEC I70.593
left I70.502
with
gangrene (and intermittent claudication, rest pain and ulcer) I70.562
intermittent claudication I70.512
rest pain (and intermittent claudication) I70.522
ulceration (and intermittent claudication and rest pain) I70.549
ankle I70.543
calf I70.542
foot site NEC I70.545
heel I70.544
lower leg NEC I70.548
midfoot I70.544
thigh I70.541
specified type NEC I70.592

Arteriosclerosis, arteriosclerotic *(Continued)*
extremities *(Continued)*
bypass graft *(Continued)*
nonautologous biological graft *(Continued)*
leg *(Continued)*
right I70.501
with
gangrene (and intermittent claudication, rest pain and ulcer) I70.561
intermittent claudication I70.511
rest pain (and intermittent claudication) I70.521
ulceration (and intermittent claudication and rest pain) I70.539
ankle I70.533
calf I70.532
foot site NEC I70.535
heel I70.534
lower leg NEC I70.538
midfoot I70.534
thigh I70.531
specified type NEC I70.591
specified type NEC I70.599
specified NEC I70.508
with
gangrene (and intermittent claudication, rest pain and ulcer) I70.568
intermittent claudication I70.518
rest pain (and intermittent claudication) I70.528
ulceration (and intermittent claudication and rest pain) I70.55
specified type NEC I70.598
nonbiological graft I70.609
leg I70.609
with
gangrene (and intermittent claudication, rest pain and ulcer) I70.669
intermittent claudication I70.619
rest pain (and intermittent claudication) I70.629
bilateral I70.603
with
gangrene (and intermittent claudication, rest pain and ulcer) I70.663
intermittent claudication I70.613
rest pain (and intermittent claudication) I70.623
specified type NEC I70.693
left I70.602
with
gangrene (and intermittent claudication, rest pain and ulcer) I70.662
intermittent claudication I70.612
rest pain (and intermittent claudication) I70.622
ulceration (and intermittent claudication and rest pain) I70.649
ankle I70.643
calf I70.642
foot site NEC I70.645
heel I70.644
lower leg NEC I70.648
midfoot I70.644
thigh I70.641
specified type NEC I70.692
right I70.601
with
gangrene (and intermittent claudication, rest pain and ulcer) I70.661

Arteriosclerosis, arteriosclerotic *(Continued)*
extremities *(Continued)*
bypass graft *(Continued)*
nonbiological graft *(Continued)*
leg *(Continued)*
right *(Continued)*
with *(Continued)*
intermittent claudication I70.611
rest pain (and intermittent claudication) I70.621
ulceration (and intermittent claudication and rest pain) I70.639
ankle I70.633
calf I70.632
foot site NEC I70.635
heel I70.634
lower leg NEC I70.638
midfoot I70.634
thigh I70.631
specified type NEC I70.691
specified type NEC I70.699
specified NEC I70.608
with
gangrene (and intermittent claudication, rest pain and ulcer) I70.668
intermittent claudication I70.618
rest pain (and intermittent claudication) I70.628
ulceration (and intermittent claudication and rest pain) I70.65
specified type NEC I70.698
specified graft NEC I70.709
leg I70.709
with
gangrene (and intermittent claudication, rest pain and ulcer) I70.769
intermittent claudication I70.719
rest pain (and intermittent claudication) I70.729
bilateral I70.703
with
gangrene (and intermittent claudication, rest pain and ulcer) I70.763
intermittent claudication I70.713
rest pain (and intermittent claudication) I70.723
specified type NEC I70.793
left I70.702
with
gangrene (and intermittent claudication, rest pain and ulcer) I70.762
intermittent claudication I70.712
rest pain (and intermittent claudication) I70.722
ulceration (and intermittent claudication and rest pain) I70.749
ankle I70.743
calf I70.742
foot site NEC I70.745
heel I70.744
lower leg NEC I70.748
midfoot I70.744
thigh I70.741
specified type NEC I70.792
right I70.701
with
gangrene (and intermittent claudication, rest pain and ulcer) I70.761
intermittent claudication I70.711
rest pain (and intermittent claudication) I70.721

A

Arteriosclerosis, arteriosclerotic *(Continued)*
extremities *(Continued)*
bypass graft *(Continued)*
specified graft NEC *(Continued)*
leg *(Continued)*
right *(Continued)*
with *(Continued)*
ulceration (and intermittent claudication and rest pain) I7Ø.739
ankle I7Ø.733
calf I7Ø.732
foot site NEC I7Ø.735
heel I7Ø.734
lower leg NEC I7Ø.738
midfoot I7Ø.734
thigh I7Ø.731
specified type NEC I7Ø.791
specified type NEC I7Ø.799
specified NEC I7Ø.7Ø8
with
gangrene (and intermittent claudication, rest pain and ulcer) I7Ø.768
intermittent claudication I7Ø.718
rest pain (and intermittent claudication) I7Ø.728
ulceration (and intermittent claudication and rest pain) I7Ø.75
specified type NEC I7Ø.798
specified NEC I7Ø.3Ø8
with
gangrene (and intermittent claudication, rest pain and ulcer) I7Ø.368
intermittent claudication I7Ø.318
rest pain (and intermittent claudication) I7Ø.328
ulceration (and intermittent claudication and rest pain) I7Ø.35
specified type NEC I7Ø.398
leg I7Ø.2Ø9
with
gangrene (and intermittent claudication, rest pain and ulcer) I7Ø.269
intermittent claudication I7Ø.219
rest pain (and intermittent claudication) I7Ø.229
bilateral I7Ø.2Ø3
with
gangrene (and intermittent claudication, rest pain and ulcer) I7Ø.263
intermittent claudication I7Ø.213
rest pain (and intermittent claudication) I7Ø.223
specified type NEC I7Ø.293
left I7Ø.2Ø2
with
gangrene (and intermittent claudication, rest pain and ulcer) I7Ø.262
intermittent claudication I7Ø.212
rest pain (and intermittent claudication) I7Ø.222
ulceration (and intermittent claudication and rest pain) I7Ø.249
ankle I7Ø.243
calf I7Ø.242
foot site NEC I7Ø.245
heel I7Ø.244
lower leg NEC I7Ø.248
midfoot I7Ø.244
thigh I7Ø.241
specified type NEC I7Ø.292

Arteriosclerosis, arteriosclerotic *(Continued)*
extremities *(Continued)*
leg *(Continued)*
right I7Ø.2Ø1
with
gangrene (and intermittent claudication, rest pain and ulcer) I7Ø.261
intermittent claudication I7Ø.211
rest pain (and intermittent claudication) I7Ø.221
ulceration (and intermittent claudication and rest pain) I7Ø.239
ankle I7Ø.233
calf I7Ø.232
foot site NEC I7Ø.235
heel I7Ø.234
lower leg NEC I7Ø.238
midfoot I7Ø.234
thigh I7Ø.231
specified type NEC I7Ø.291
specified type NEC I7Ø.299
specified site NEC I7Ø.2Ø8
with
gangrene (and intermittent claudication, rest pain and ulcer) I7Ø.268
intermittent claudication I7Ø.218
rest pain (and intermittent claudication) I7Ø.228
ulceration (and intermittent claudication and rest pain) I7Ø.25
specified type NEC I7Ø.298
generalized I7Ø.91
heart (disease) —*see* Arteriosclerosis, coronary (artery)
kidney —*see* Hypertension, kidney
medial —*see* Arteriosclerosis, extremities
mesenteric (artery) K55.1
Mönckeberg's —*see* Arteriosclerosis, extremities
myocarditis I51.4
peripheral (of extremities) —*see* Arteriosclerosis, extremities
pulmonary (idiopathic) I27.Ø
renal (arterioles) —*see also* Hypertension, kidney
artery I7Ø.1
retina (vascular) I7Ø.8 *[H35.Ø-•]*
specified artery NEC I7Ø.8
spinal (cord) G95.19
vertebral (artery) I67.2
Arteriospasm I73.9
Arteriovenous —*see* condition
Arteritis I77.6
allergic M31.Ø
aorta (nonsyphilitic) I77.6
syphilitic A52.Ø2
aortic arch M31.4
brachiocephalic M31.4
brain I67.7
syphilitic A52.Ø4
cerebral I67.7
in
diseases classified elsewhere I68.2
systemic lupus erythematosus M32.19
listerial A32.89
syphilitic A52.Ø4
tuberculous A18.89
coronary (artery) I25.89
rheumatic IØ1.8
chronic IØ9.89
syphilitic A52.Ø6
cranial (left) (right), giant cell M31.6
deformans —*see* Arteriosclerosis
giant cell NEC M31.6
with polymyalgia rheumatica M31.5
necrosing or necrotizing M31.9
specified NEC M31.8
nodosa M3Ø.Ø
obliterans —*see* Arteriosclerosis
pulmonary I28.8

Arteritis *(Continued)*
rheumatic —*see* Fever, rheumatic
senile —*see* Arteriosclerosis
suppurative I77.2
syphilitic (general) A52.Ø9
brain A52.Ø4
coronary A52.Ø6
spinal A52.Ø9
temporal, giant cell M31.6
young female aortic arch syndrome M31.4
Artery, arterial —*see also* condition
abscess I77.89
single umbilical Q27.Ø
Arthralgia (allergic) —*see also* Pain, joint
in caisson disease T7Ø.3
temporomandibular M26.62
Arthritis, arthritic (acute) (chronic) (nonpyogenic) (subacute) M19.9Ø
allergic —*see* Arthritis, specified form NEC
ankylosing (crippling) (spine) —*see also* Spondylitis, ankylosing
sites other than spine —*see* Arthritis, specified form NEC
atrophic —*see* Osteoarthritis
spine —*see* Spondylitis, ankylosing
back —*see* Spondylopathy, inflammatory
blennorrhagic (gonococcal) A54.42
Charcot's —*see* Arthropathy, neuropathic
diabetic —*see* Diabetes, arthropathy, neuropathic
syringomyelic G95.Ø
chylous (filarial) —*see also* category MØ1 B74.9
climacteric (any site) NEC —*see* Arthritis, specified form NEC
crystal (-induced) —*see* Arthritis, in, crystals
deformans —*see* Osteoarthritis
degenerative —*see* Osteoarthritis
due to or associated with
acromegaly E22.Ø
brucellosis —*see* Brucellosis
caisson disease T7Ø.3
diabetes —*see* Diabetes, arthropathy
dracontiasis —*see also* category MØ1 B72
enteritis NEC
regional —*see* Enteritis, regional
erysipelas —*see also* category MØ1 A46
erythema
epidemic A25.1
nodosum L52
filariasis NOS B74.9
glanders A24.Ø
helminthiasis —*see also* category MØ1 B83.9
hemophilia D66 *[M36.2]*
Henoch-(Schönlein) purpura D69.Ø *[M36.4]*
human parvovirus —*see also* category MØ1 B97.6
infectious disease NEC —*see* category MØ1
leprosy (*see also* category MØ1) —*see also* Leprosy A3Ø.9
Lyme disease A69.23
mycobacteria —*see also* category MØ1 A31.8
parasitic disease NEC —*see also* category MØ1 B89
paratyphoid fever (*see also* category MØ1) —*see also* Fever, paratyphoid AØ1.4
rat bite fever —*see also* category MØ1 A25.1
regional enteritis —*see* Enteritis, regional
respiratory disorder NOS J98.9
serum sickness —*see also* Reaction, serum T8Ø.69
syringomyelia G95.Ø
typhoid fever AØ1.Ø4
epidemic erythema A25.1
febrile —*see* Fever, rheumatic
gonococcal A54.42
gouty (acute) —*see* Gout
in (due to)
acromegaly —*see also* subcategory M14.8-• E22.Ø
amyloidosis —*see also* subcategory M14.8-• E85.4

A

Arthritis, arthritic *(Continued)*
in *(Continued)*
bacterial disease *—see also* subcategory M01 A49.9
Behçet's syndrome M35.2
caisson disease *—see also* subcategory M14.8-● T70.3
coliform bacilli (Escherichia coli) *—see* Arthritis, in, pyogenic organism NEC
crystals M11.9
dicalcium phosphate *—see* Arthritis, in, crystals, specified type NEC
hydroxyapatite M11.0-●
pyrophosphate *—see* Arthritis, in, crystals, specified type NEC
specified type NEC M11.80
ankle M11.87-●
elbow M11.82-●
foot joint M11.87-●
hand joint M11.84-●
hip M11.85-●
knee M11.86-●
multiple sites M11.8-●
shoulder M11.81-●
vertebrae M11.88
wrist M11.83-●
dermatoarthritis, lipoid E78.81
dracontiasis (dracunculiasis) *—see also* category M01 B72
endocrine disorder NEC *—see also* subcategory M14.8-● E34.9
enteritis, infectious NEC *—see also* category M01 A09
specified organism NEC *—see also* category M01 A08.8
erythema
multiforme *—see also* subcategory M14.8-● L51.9
nodosum *—see also* subcategory M14.8-● L52
gout *—see* Gout
helminthiasis NEC *—see also* category M01 B83.9
hemochromatosis *—see also* subcategory M14.8-● E83.118
hemoglobinopathy NEC D58.2 *[M36.3]*
hemophilia NEC D66 *[M36.2]*
Hemophilus influenzae M00.8-● *[B96.3]*
Henoch(-Schönlein) purpura D69.0 *[M36.4]*
hyperparathyroidism NEC *—see also* subcategory M14.8-● E21.3
hypersensitivity reaction NEC T78.49 *[M36.4]*
hypogammaglobulinemia *—see also* subcategory M14.8-● D80.1
hypothyroidism NEC *—see also* subcategory M14.8-● E03.9
infection *—see* Arthritis, pyogenic or pyemic
spine *—see* Spondylopathy, infective
infectious disease NEC *—see* category M01
leprosy *—see also* category M01 A30.9
leukemia NEC C95.9-● *[M36.1]*
lipoid dermatoarthritis E78.81
Lyme disease A69.23
Mediterranean fever, familial *—see also* subcategory M14.8-● M04.1
Meningococcus A39.83
metabolic disorder NEC *—see also* subcategory M14.8-● E88.9
multiple myelomatosis C90.0-● *[M36.1]*
mumps B26.85
mycosis NEC *—see also* category M01 B49
myelomatosis (multiple) C90.0-● *[M36.1]*
neurological disorder NEC G98.0
ochronosis *—see also* subcategory M14.8-● E70.29
O'nyong-nyong *—see also* category M01 A92.1
parasitic disease NEC *—see also* category M01 B89

Arthritis, arthritic *(Continued)*
in *(Continued)*
paratyphoid fever *—see also* category M01 A01.4
Pseudomonas *—see* Arthritis, pyogenic, bacterial NEC
psoriasis L40.50
pyogenic organism NEC *—see* Arthritis, pyogenic, bacterial NEC
Reiter's disease *—see* Reiter's disease
respiratory disorder NEC *—see also* subcategory M14.8-● J98.9
reticulosis, malignant *—see also* subcategory M14.8-● C86.0
rubella B06.82
Salmonella (arizonae) (cholerae-suis) (enteritidis) (typhimurium) A02.23
sarcoidosis D86.86
specified bacteria NEC *—see* Arthritis, pyogenic, bacterial NEC
sporotrichosis B42.82
syringomyelia G95.0
thalassemia NEC D56.9 *[M36.3]*
tuberculosis *—see* Tuberculosis, arthritis
typhoid fever A01.04
urethritis, Reiter's *—see* Reiter's disease
viral disease NEC *—see also* category M01 B34.9
infectious or infective *—see also* Arthritis, pyogenic or pyemic
spine *—see* Spondylopathy, infective
juvenile M08.90
with systemic onset *—see* Still's disease
ankle M08.97-●
elbow M08.92-●
foot joint M08.97-●
hand joint M08.94-●
hip M08.95-●
knee M08.96-●
multiple site M08.99
pauciarticular M08.40
ankle M08.47-●
elbow M08.42-●
foot joint M08.47-●
hand joint M08.44-●
hip M08.45-●
knee M08.46-●
shoulder M08.41-●
vertebrae M08.48
wrist M08.43-●
psoriatic L40.54
rheumatoid *—see* Arthritis, rheumatoid, juvenile
shoulder M08.91-●
specified type NEC M08.80
ankle M08.87-●
elbow M08.82-●
foot joint M08.87-●
hand joint M08.84-●
hip M08.85-●
knee M08.86-●
multiple site M08.89
shoulder M08.81-●
specified joint NEC M08.88
vertebrae M08.88
wrist M08.83-●
vertebra M08.98
wrist M08.93-●
meaning osteoarthritis *—see* Osteoarthritis
meningococcal A39.83
menopausal (any site) NEC *—see* Arthritis, specified form NEC
mutilans (psoriatic) L40.52
mycotic NEC *—see also* category M01 B49
neuropathic (Charcot) *—see* Arthropathy, neuropathic
diabetic *—see* Diabetes, arthropathy, neuropathic
nonsyphilitic NEC G98.0
syringomyelic G95.0
ochronotic *—see also* subcategory M14.8-● E70.29

Arthritis, arthritic *(Continued)*
palindromic (any site) *—see* Rheumatism, palindromic
pneumococcal M00.10
ankle M00.17-●
elbow M00.12-●
foot joint *—see* Arthritis, pneumococcal, ankle
hand joint M00.14-●
hip M00.15-●
knee M00.16-●
multiple site M00.19
shoulder M00.11-●
vertebra M00.18
wrist M00.13-●
postdysenteric *—see* Arthropathy, postdysenteric
postmeningococcal A39.84
postrheumatic, chronic *—see* Arthropathy, postrheumatic, chronic
primary progressive *—see also* Arthritis, specified form NEC
spine *—see* Spondylitis, ankylosing
psoriatic L40.50
purulent (any site except spine) *—see* Arthritis, pyogenic or pyemic
spine *—see* Spondylopathy, infective
pyogenic or pyemic (any site except spine) M00.9
bacterial NEC M00.80
ankle M00.87-●
elbow M00.82-●
foot joint *—see* Arthritis, pyogenic, bacterial NEC, ankle
hand joint M00.84-●
hip M00.85-●
knee M00.86-●
multiple site M00.89
shoulder M00.81-●
vertebra M00.88
wrist M00.83-●
pneumococcal *—see* Arthritis, pneumococcal
spine *—see* Spondylopathy, infective
staphylococcal *—see* Arthritis, staphylococcal
streptococcal *—see* Arthritis, streptococcal NEC
pneumococcal *—see* Arthritis, pneumococcal
reactive *—see* Reiter's disease
rheumatic *—see also* Arthritis, rheumatoid
acute or subacute *—see* Fever, rheumatic
rheumatoid M06.9
with
carditis *—see* Rheumatoid, carditis
endocarditis *—see* Rheumatoid, carditis
heart involvement NEC *—see* Rheumatoid, carditis
lung involvement *—see* Rheumatoid, lung
myocarditis *—see* Rheumatoid, carditis
myopathy *—see* Rheumatoid, myopathy
pericarditis *—see* Rheumatoid, carditis
polyneuropathy *—see* Rheumatoid, polyneuropathy
rheumatoid factor *—see* Arthritis, rheumatoid, seropositive
splenoadenomegaly and leukopenia *— see* Felty's syndrome
vasculitis *—see* Rheumatoid, vasculitis
visceral involvement NEC *—see* Rheumatoid, arthritis, with involvement of organs NEC
juvenile (with or without rheumatoid factor) M08.00
ankle M08.07-●
elbow M08.02-●
foot joint M08.07-●
hand joint M08.04-●
hip M08.05-●
knee M08.06-●

A

Arthritis, arthritic *(Continued)*
rheumatoid *(Continued)*
juvenile *(Continued)*
multiple site MØ8.Ø9
shoulder MØ8.Ø1-•
vertebra MØ8.Ø8
wrist MØ8.Ø3-•
seronegative MØ6.ØØ
ankle MØ6.Ø7-•
elbow MØ6.Ø2-•
foot joint MØ6.Ø7-•
hand joint MØ6.Ø4-•
hip MØ6.Ø5-•
knee MØ6.Ø6-•
multiple sites MØ6.Ø9
shoulder MØ6.Ø1-•
vertebra MØ6.Ø8
wrist MØ6.Ø3-•
seropositive MØ5.9
without organ involvement MØ5.7Ø
ankle MØ5.77-•
elbow MØ5.72-•
foot joint MØ5.77-•
hand joint MØ5.74-•
hip MØ5.75-•
knee MØ5.76-•
multiple sites MØ5.79
shoulder MØ5.71-•
vertebra —*see* Spondylitis, ankylosing
wrist MØ5.73-•
specified NEC MØ5.8Ø
ankle MØ5.87-•
elbow MØ5.82-•
foot joint MØ5.87-•
hand joint MØ5.84-•
hip MØ5.85-•
knee MØ5.86-•
multiple sites MØ5.89
shoulder MØ5.81-•
vertebra —*see* Spondylitis, ankylosing
wrist MØ5.83-•
specified type NEC MØ6.8Ø
ankle MØ6.87-•
elbow MØ6.82-•
foot joint MØ6.87-•
hand joint MØ6.84-•
hip MØ6.85-•
knee MØ6.86-•
multiple site MØ6.89
shoulder MØ6.81-•
vertebra MØ6.88
wrist MØ6.83-•
spine —*see* Spondylitis, ankylosing
rubella BØ6.82
scorbutic —*see also* subcategory M14.8-• E54
senile or senescent —*see* Osteoarthritis
septic (any site except spine) —*see* Arthritis, pyogenic or pyemic
spine —*see* Spondylopathy, infective
serum (nontherapeutic) (therapeutic) —*see* Arthropathy, postimmunization
specified form NEC M13.8Ø
ankle M13.87-•
elbow M13.82-•
foot joint M13.87-•
hand joint M13.84-•
hip M13.85-•
knee M13.86-•
multiple site M13.89
shoulder M13.81-•
specified joint NEC M13.88
wrist M13.83-•
spine —*see also* Spondylopathy, inflammatory
infectious or infective NEC —*see* Spondylopathy, infective
Marie-Strümpell —*see* Spondylitis, ankylosing
pyogenic —*see* Spondylopathy, infective
rheumatoid —*see* Spondylitis, ankylosing
traumatic (old) —*see* Spondylopathy, traumatic
tuberculous A18.Ø1

Arthritis, arthritic *(Continued)*
staphylococcal MØØ.ØØ
ankle MØØ.Ø7-•
elbow MØØ.Ø2-•
foot joint —*see* Arthritis, staphylococcal, ankle
hand joint MØØ.Ø4-•
hip MØØ.Ø5-•
knee MØØ.Ø6-•
multiple site MØØ.Ø9
shoulder MØØ.Ø1-•
vertebra MØØ.Ø8
wrist MØØ.Ø3-•
streptococcal NEC MØØ.2Ø
ankle MØØ.27-•
elbow MØØ.22-•
foot joint —*see* Arthritis, streptococcal, ankle
hand joint MØØ.24-•
hip MØØ.25-•
knee MØØ.26-•
multiple site MØØ.29
shoulder MØØ.21-•
vertebra MØØ.28
wrist MØØ.23-•
suppurative —*see* Arthritis, pyogenic or pyemic
syphilitic (late) A52.16
congenital A5Ø.55 *[M12.8Ø]*
syphilitica deformans (Charcot) A52.16
temporomandibular M26.69
toxic of menopause (any site) —*see* Arthritis, specified form NEC
transient —*see* Arthropathy, specified form NEC
traumatic (chronic) —*see* Arthropathy, traumatic
tuberculous A18.Ø2
spine A18.Ø1
uratic —*see* Gout
urethritica (Reiter's) —*see* Reiter's disease
vertebral —*see* Spondylopathy, inflammatory
villous (any site) —*see* Arthropathy, specified form NEC
Arthrocele —*see* Effusion, joint
Arthrodesis status Z98.1
Arthrodynia —*see also* Pain, joint
Arthrodysplasia Q74.9
Arthrofibrosis, joint —*see* Ankylosis
Arthrogryposis (congenital) Q68.8
multiplex congenita Q74.3
Arthrokatadysis M24.7
Arthropathy (*see also* Arthritis) M12.9
Charcot's —*see* Arthropathy, neuropathic
diabetic —*see* Diabetes, arthropathy, neuropathic
syringomyelic G95.Ø
cricoarytenoid J38.7
crystal(-induced) —*see* Arthritis, in, crystals
diabetic NEC —*see* Diabetes, arthropathy
distal interphalangeal, psoriatic L4Ø.51
enteropathic MØ7.6Ø
ankle MØ7.67-•
elbow MØ7.62-•
foot joint MØ7.67-•
hand joint MØ7.64-•
hip MØ7.65-•
knee MØ7.66-•
multiple site MØ7.69
shoulder MØ7.61-•
vertebra MØ7.68
wrist MØ7.63-•
following intestinal bypass MØ2.ØØ
ankle MØ2.Ø7-•
elbow MØ2.Ø2-•
foot joint MØ2.Ø7-•
hand joint MØ2.Ø4-•
hip MØ2.Ø5-•
knee MØ2.Ø6-•
multiple site MØ2.Ø9
shoulder MØ2.Ø1-•
vertebra MØ2.Ø8
wrist MØ2.Ø3-•

Arthropathy *(Continued)*
gouty —*see also* Gout
in (due to)
Lesch-Nyhan syndrome E79.1 *[M14.8-•]*
sickle-cell disorders D57-• *[M14.8-•]*
hemophilic NEC D66 *[M36.2]*
in (due to)
hyperparathyroidism NEC E21.3 *[M14.8-•]*
metabolic disease NOS E88.9 *[M14.8-•]*
in (due to)
acromegaly E22.Ø *[M14.8-•]*
amyloidosis E85.4 *[M14.8-•]*
blood disorder NOS D75.9 *[M36.3]*
diabetes —*see* Diabetes, arthropathy
endocrine disease NOS E34.9 *[M14.8-•]*
erythema
multiforme L51.9 *[M14.8-•]*
nodosum L52 *[M14.8-•]*
hemochromatosis E83.118 *[M14.8-•]*
hemoglobinopathy NEC D58.2 *[M36.3]*
hemophilia NEC D66 *[M36.2]*
Henoch-Schönlein purpura D69.Ø *[M36.4]*
hyperthyroidism EØ5.9Ø *[M14.8-•]*
hypothyroidism EØ3.9 *[M14.8-•]*
infective endocarditis I33.Ø *[M12.8Ø]*
leukemia NEC C95.9-• *[M36.1]*
malignant histiocytosis C96.A *[M36.1]*
metabolic disease NOS E88.9 *[M14.8-•]*
multiple myeloma C9Ø.Ø-• *[M36.1]*
neoplastic disease NOS (*see also* Neoplasm) D49.9 *[M36.1]*
nutritional deficiency —*see also* subcategory M14.8-• E63.9
psoriasis NOS L4Ø.5Ø
sarcoidosis D86.86
syphilis (late) A52.77
congenital A5Ø.55 *[M12.8Ø]*
thyrotoxicosis —*see also* subcategory M14.8-• EØ5.9Ø
ulcerative colitis K51.9Ø *[MØ7.6Ø]*
viral hepatitis (postinfectious) NEC B19.9 *[M12.8Ø]*
Whipple's disease —*see also* subcategory M14.8-• K9Ø.81
Jaccoud —*see* Arthropathy, postrheumatic, chronic
juvenile —*see* Arthritis, juvenile
psoriatic L4Ø.54
mutilans (psoriatic) L4Ø.52
neuropathic (Charcot) M14.6Ø
ankle M14.67-•
diabetic —*see* Diabetes, arthropathy, neuropathic
elbow M14.62-•
foot joint M14.67-•
hand joint M14.64-•
hip M14.65-•
knee M14.66-•
multiple site M14.69
nonsyphilitic NEC G98.Ø
shoulder M14.61-•
syringomyelic G95.Ø
vertebra M14.68
wrist M14.63-•
osteopulmonary —*see* Osteoarthropathy, hypertrophic, specified NEC
postdysenteric MØ2.1Ø
ankle MØ2.17-•
elbow MØ2.12-•
foot joint MØ2.17-•
hand joint MØ2.14-•
hip MØ2.15-•
knee MØ2.16-•
multiple site MØ2.19
shoulder MØ2.11-•
vertebra MØ2.18
wrist MØ2.13-•
postimmunization MØ2.2Ø
ankle MØ2.27-•
elbow MØ2.22-•

Arthropathy *(Continued)*
postimmunization *(Continued)*
foot joint M02.27-●
hand joint M02.24-●
hip M02.25-●
knee M02.26-●
multiple site M02.29
shoulder M02.21-●
vertebra M02.28
wrist M02.23-●
postinfectious NEC B99 *[M12.80]*
in (due to)
enteritis due to Yersinia enterocolitica A04.6 *[M12.80]*
syphilis A52.77
viral hepatitis NEC B19.9 *[M12.80]*
postrheumatic, chronic (Jaccoud) M12.00
ankle M12.07-●
elbow M12.02-●
foot joint M12.07-●
hand joint M12.04-●
hip M12.05-●
knee M12.06-●
multiple site M12.09
shoulder M12.01-●
specified joint NEC M12.08
vertebrae M12.08
wrist M12.03-●
psoriatic NEC L40.59
interphalangeal, distal L40.51
reactive M02.9
in (due to)
infective endocarditis I33.0 *[M02.9]*
specified type NEC M02.80
ankle M02.87-●
elbow M02.82-●
foot joint M02.87-●
hand joint M02.84-●
hip M02.85-●
knee M02.86-●
multiple site M02.89
shoulder M02.81-●
vertebra M02.88
wrist M02.83-●
specified form NEC M12.80
ankle M12.87-●
elbow M12.82-●
foot joint M12.87-●
hand joint M12.84-●
hip M12.85-●
knee M12.86-●
multiple site M12.89
shoulder M12.81-●
specified joint NEC M12.88
vertebrae M12.88
wrist M12.83-●
syringomyelic G95.0
tabes dorsalis A52.16
tabetic A52.16
transient *—see* Arthropathy, specified form NEC
traumatic M12.50
ankle M12.57-●
elbow M12.52-●
foot joint M12.57-●
hand joint M12.54-●
hip M12.55-●
knee M12.56-●
multiple site M12.59
shoulder M12.51-●
specified joint NEC M12.58
vertebrae M12.58
wrist M12.53-●
Arthropyosis *—see* Arthritis, pyogenic or pyemic
Arthrosis (deformans) (degenerative) (localized) *—see also* Osteoarthritis M19.90
spine *—see* Spondylosis
Arthus' phenomenon or reaction T78.41
due to
drug *—see* Table of Drugs and Chemicals, by drug
Articular *—see* condition
Articulation, reverse (teeth) M26.24
Artificial
insemination complication *—see* Complications, artificial, fertilization
opening status (functioning) (without complication) Z93.9
anus (colostomy) Z93.3
colostomy Z93.3
cystostomy Z93.50
appendico-vesicostomy Z93.52
cutaneous Z93.51
specified NEC Z93.59
enterostomy Z93.4
gastrostomy Z93.1
ileostomy Z93.2
intestinal tract NEC Z93.4
jejunostomy Z93.4
nephrostomy Z93.6
specified site NEC Z93.8
tracheostomy Z93.0
ureterostomy Z93.6
urethrostomy Z93.6
urinary tract NEC Z93.6
vagina Z93.8
vagina status Z93.8
Arytenoid *—see* condition
Asbestosis (occupational) J61
ASC-H (atypical squamous cells cannot exclude high grade squamous intraepithelial lesion on cytologic smear)
anus R85.611
cervix R87.611
vagina R87.621
ASC-US (atypical squamous cells of undetermined significance on cytologic smear)
anus R85.610
cervix R87.610
vagina R87.620
Ascariasis B77.9
with
complications NEC B77.89
intestinal complications B77.0
pneumonia, pneumonitis B77.81
Ascaridosis, ascaridiasis *—see* Ascariasis
Ascaris (infection) (infestation) (lumbricoides) *—see* Ascariasis
Ascending *—see* condition
Aschoff's bodies *—see* Myocarditis, rheumatic
Ascites (abdominal) R18.8
cardiac *—see also* Failure, heart, right I50.810
chylous (nonfilarial) I89.8
filarial *—see* Infestation, filarial
due to
cirrhosis, alcoholic K70.31
hepatitis
alcoholic K70.11
chronic active K71.51
S. japonicum B65.2
heart *—see also* Failure, heart, right I50.810
malignant R18.0
pseudochylous R18.8
syphilitic A52.74
tuberculous A18.31
Aseptic *—see* condition
Asherman's syndrome N85.6
Asialia K11.7
Asiatic cholera *—see* Cholera
Asimultagnosia (simultanagnosia) R48.3
Askin's tumor *—see* Neoplasm, connective tissue, malignant
Asocial personality F60.2
Asomatognosia R41.4
Aspartylglucosaminuria E77.1
Asperger's disease or syndrome F84.5
Aspergilloma *—see* Aspergillosis
Aspergillosis (with pneumonia) B44.9
bronchopulmonary, allergic B44.81
disseminated B44.7
generalized B44.7
Aspergillosis *(Continued)*
pulmonary NEC B44.1
allergic B44.81
invasive B44.0
specified NEC B44.89
tonsillar B44.2
Aspergillus (flavus) (fumigatus) (infection) (terreus) *—see* Aspergillosis
Aspermatogenesis *—see* Azoospermia
Aspermia (testis) *—see* Azoospermia
Asphyxia, asphyxiation (by) R09.01
antenatal P84
birth P84
bunny bag *—see* Asphyxia, due to, mechanical threat to breathing, trapped in bed clothes
crushing S28.0
drowning T75.1
gas, fumes, or vapor *—see* Table of Drugs and Chemicals
inhalation *—see* Inhalation
intrauterine P84
local I73.00
with gangrene I73.01
mucus *—see also* Foreign body, respiratory tract, causing asphyxia
newborn P84
pathological R09.01
postnatal P84
mechanical *—see* Asphyxia, due to, mechanical threat to breathing
prenatal P84
reticularis R23.1
strangulation *—see* Asphyxia, due to, mechanical threat to breathing
submersion T75.1
traumatic T71.9
due to
crushed chest S28.0
foreign body (in) *—see* Foreign body, respiratory tract, causing asphyxia
low oxygen content of ambient air T71.20
due to
being trapped in
low oxygen environment T71.29
in car trunk T71.221
circumstances undetermined T71.224
done with intent to harm by
another person T71.223
self T71.222
in refrigerator T71.231
circumstances undetermined T71.234
done with intent to harm by
another person T71.233
self T71.232
cave-in T71.21
mechanical threat to breathing (accidental) T71.191
circumstances undetermined T71.194
done with intent to harm by
another person T71.193
self T71.192
hanging T71.161
circumstances undetermined T71.164
done with intent to harm by
another person T71.163
self T71.162
plastic bag T71.121
circumstances undetermined T71.124
done with intent to harm by
another person T71.123
self T71.122

Asphyxia, asphyxiation *(Continued)*
traumatic *(Continued)*
due to *(Continued)*
mechanical threat to breathing *(Continued)*
smothering
in furniture T71.151
circumstances undetermined T71.154
done with intent to harm by
another person T71.153
self T71.152
under
another person's body T71.141
circumstances undetermined T71.144
done with intent to harm T71.143
pillow T71.111
circumstances undetermined T71.114
done with intent to harm by
another person T71.113
self T71.112
trapped in bed clothes T71.131
circumstances undetermined T71.134
done with intent to harm by
another person T71.133
self T71.132
vomiting, vomitus —*see* Foreign body, respiratory tract, causing asphyxia
Aspiration
amniotic (clear) fluid (newborn) P24.10
with
pneumonia (pneumonitis) P24.11
respiratory symptoms P24.11
blood
newborn (without respiratory symptoms) P24.20
with
pneumonia (pneumonitis) P24.21
respiratory symptoms P24.21
specified age NEC —*see* Foreign body, respiratory tract
bronchitis J69.0
food or foreign body (with asphyxiation) —*see* Asphyxia, food
liquor (amnii) (newborn) P24.10
with
pneumonia (pneumonitis) P24.11
respiratory symptoms P24.11
meconium (newborn) (without respiratory symptoms) P24.00
with
pneumonitis (pneumonitis) P24.01
respiratory symptoms P24.01
milk (newborn) (without respiratory symptoms) P24.30
with
pneumonia (pneumonitis) P24.31
respiratory symptoms P24.31
specified age NEC —*see* Foreign body, respiratory tract
mucus —*see also* Foreign body, by site, causing asphyxia
newborn P24.10
with
pneumonia (pneumonitis) P24.11
respiratory symptoms P24.11
neonatal P24.9
specific NEC (without respiratory symptoms) P24.80
with
pneumonia (pneumonitis) P24.81
respiratory symptoms P24.81
newborn P24.9
specific NEC (without respiratory symptoms) P24.80
with
pneumonia (pneumonitis) P24.81
respiratory symptoms P24.81

Aspiration *(Continued)*
pneumonia J69.0
pneumonitis J69.0
syndrome of newborn —*see* Aspiration, by substance, with pneumonia
vernix caseosa (newborn) P24.80
with
pneumonia (pneumonitis) P24.81
respiratory symptoms P24.81
vomitus —*see also* Foreign body, respiratory tract
newborn (without respiratory symptoms) P24.30
with
pneumonia (pneumonitis) P24.31
respiratory symptoms P24.31
Asplenia (congenital) Q89.01
postsurgical Z90.81
Assam fever B55.0
Assault, sexual —*see* Maltreatment
Assmann's focus NEC A15.0
Astasia (-abasia) (hysterical) F44.4
Asteatosis cutis L85.3
Astereognosia, astereognosis R48.1
Asterixis R27.8
in liver disease K71.3
Asteroid hyalitis —*see* Deposit, crystalline
Asthenia, asthenic R53.1
cardiac —*see also* Failure, heart I50.9
psychogenic F45.8
cardiovascular —*see also* Failure, heart I50.9
psychogenic F45.8
heart —*see also* Failure, heart I50.9
psychogenic F45.8
hysterical F44.4
myocardial —*see also* Failure, heart I50.9
psychogenic F45.8
nervous F48.8
neurocirculatory F45.8
neurotic F48.8
psychogenic F48.8
psychoneurotic F48.8
psychophysiologic F48.8
reaction (psychophysiologic) F48.8
senile R54
Asthenopia —*see also* Discomfort, visual
hysterical F44.6
psychogenic F44.6
Asthenospermia —*see* Abnormal, specimen, male genital organs
Asthma, asthmatic (bronchial) (catarrh) (spasmodic) J45.909
with
chronic obstructive bronchitis J44.9
with
acute lower respiratory infection J44.0
exacerbation (acute) J44.1
chronic obstructive pulmonary disease J44.9
with
acute lower respiratory infection J44.0
exacerbation (acute) J44.1
exacerbation (acute) J45.901
hay fever —*see* Asthma, allergic extrinsic
rhinitis, allergic —*see* Asthma, allergic extrinsic
status asthmaticus J45.902
allergic extrinsic J45.909
with
exacerbation (acute) J45.901
status asthmaticus J45.902
atopic —*see* Asthma, allergic extrinsic
cardiac —*see* Failure, ventricular, left
cardiobronchial I50.1
childhood J45.909
with
exacerbation (acute) J45.901
status asthmaticus J45.902
chronic obstructive J44.9
with
acute lower respiratory infection J44.0
exacerbation (acute) J44.1

Asthma, asthmatic *(Continued)*
collier's J60
cough variant J45.991
detergent J69.8
due to
detergent J69.8
inhalation of fumes J68.3
eosinophilic J82
extrinsic, allergic —*see* Asthma, allergic extrinsic
grinder's J62.8
hay —*see* Asthma, allergic extrinsic
heart I50.1
idiosyncratic —*see* Asthma, nonallergic
intermittent (mild) J45.20
with
exacerbation (acute) J45.21
status asthmaticus J45.22
intrinsic, nonallergic —*see* Asthma, nonallergic
Kopp's E32.8
late-onset J45.909
with
exacerbation (acute) J45.901
status asthmaticus J45.902
mild intermittent J45.20
with
exacerbation (acute) J45.21
status asthmaticus J45.22
mild persistent J45.30
with
exacerbation (acute) J45.31
status asthmaticus J45.32
Millar's (laryngismus stridulus) J38.5
miner's J60
mixed J45.909
with
exacerbation (acute) J45.901
status asthmaticus J45.902
moderate persistent J45.40
with
exacerbation (acute) J45.41
status asthmaticus J45.42
nervous —*see* Asthma, nonallergic
nonallergic (intrinsic) J45.909
with
exacerbation (acute) J45.901
status asthmaticus J45.902
persistent
mild J45.30
with
exacerbation (acute) J45.31
status asthmaticus J45.32
moderate J45.40
with
exacerbation (acute) J45.41
status asthmaticus J45.42
severe J45.50
with
exacerbation (acute) J45.51
status asthmaticus J45.52
platinum J45.998
pneumoconiotic NEC J64
potter's J62.8
predominantly allergic J45.909
psychogenic F54
pulmonary eosinophilic J82
red cedar J67.8
Rostan's I50.1
sandblaster's J62.8
sequoiosis J67.8
severe persistent J45.50
with
exacerbation (acute) J45.51
status asthmaticus J45.52
specified NEC J45.998
stonemason's J62.8
thymic E32.8
tuberculous —*see* Tuberculosis, pulmonary
Wichmann's (laryngismus stridulus) J38.5
wood J67.8

Astigmatism (compound) (congenital) H52.2Ø-•
  irregular H52.21-•
  regular H52.22-•
Astraphobia F4Ø.22Ø
Astroblastoma
  specified site —*see* Neoplasm, malignant, by site
  unspecified site C71.9
Astrocytoma (cystic)
  anaplastic
    specified site —*see* Neoplasm, malignant, by site
    unspecified site C71.9
  fibrillary
    specified site —*see* Neoplasm, malignant, by site
    unspecified site C71.9
  fibrous
    specified site —*see* Neoplasm, malignant, by site
    unspecified site C71.9
  gemistocytic
    specified site —*see* Neoplasm, malignant, by site
    unspecified site C71.9
  juvenile
    specified site —*see* Neoplasm, malignant, by site
    unspecified site C71.9
  pilocytic
    specified site —*see* Neoplasm, malignant, by site
    unspecified site C71.9
  piloid
    specified site —*see* Neoplasm, malignant, by site
    unspecified site C71.9
  protoplasmic
    specified site —*see* Neoplasm, malignant, by site
    unspecified site C71.9
  specified site NEC —*see* Neoplasm, malignant, by site
  subependymal D43.2
    giant cell
      specified site —*see* Neoplasm, uncertain behavior, by site
      unspecified site D43.2
    specified site —*see* Neoplasm, uncertain behavior, by site
    unspecified site D43.2
  unspecified site C71.9
Astroglioma
  specified site —*see* Neoplasm, malignant, by site
  unspecified site C71.9
Asymbolia R48.8
Asymmetry —*see also* Distortion
  between native and reconstructed breast N65.1
  face Q67.Ø
  jaw (lower) —*see* Anomaly, dentofacial, jaw-cranial base relationship, asymmetry
Asynergia, asynergy R27.8
  ventricular I51.89
Asystole (heart) —*see* Arrest, cardiac
At risk
  for
    dental caries Z91.849
      high Z91.843
      low Z91.841
      moderate Z91.842
    falling Z91.81
Ataxia, ataxy, ataxic R27.Ø
  acute R27.8
  brain (hereditary) G11.9
  cerebellar (hereditary) G11.9
    with defective DNA repair G11.3
    alcoholic G31.2
    early-onset G11.1
Ataxia, ataxy, ataxic *(Continued)*
  cerebellar (hereditary) *(Continued)*
    in
      alcoholism G31.2
      myxedema EØ3.9 *[G13.2]*
      neoplastic disease —*see also* Neoplasm D49.9 *[G32.81]*
      specified disease NEC G32.81
    late-onset (Marie's) G11.2
  cerebral (hereditary) G11.9
  congenital nonprogressive G11.Ø
  family, familial —*see* Ataxia, hereditary
  following
    cerebrovascular disease I69.993
      cerebral infarction I69.393
      intracerebral hemorrhage I69.193
      nontraumatic intracranial hemorrhage NEC I69.293
      specified disease NEC I69.893
      subarachnoid hemorrhage I69.Ø93
  Friedreich's (heredofamilial) (cerebellar) (spinal) G11.1
  gait R26.Ø
    hysterical F44.4
  general R27.8
  gluten M35.9 *[G32.81]*
    with celiac disease K9Ø.Ø *[G32.81]*
  hereditary G11.9
    with neuropathy G6Ø.2
    cerebellar —*see* Ataxia, cerebellar
    spastic G11.4
    specified NEC G11.8
    spinal (Friedreich's) G11.1
  heredofamilial —*see* Ataxia, hereditary
  Hunt's G11.1
  hysterical F44.4
  locomotor (progressive) (syphilitic) (partial) (spastic) A52.11
    diabetic —*see* Diabetes, ataxia
  Marie's (cerebellar) (heredofamilial) (late- onset) G11.2
  nonorganic origin F44.4
  nonprogressive, congenital G11.Ø
  psychogenic F44.4
  Roussy-Lévy G6Ø.Ø
  Sanger-Brown's (hereditary) G11.2
  spastic hereditary G11.4
  spinal
    hereditary (Friedreich's) G11.1
    progressive (syphilitic) A52.11
  spinocerebellar, X-linked recessive G11.1
  telangiectasia (Louis-Bar) G11.3
Ataxia-telangiectasia (Louis-Bar) G11.3
Atelectasis (massive) (partial) (pressure) (pulmonary) J98.11
  newborn P28.1Ø
    due to resorption P28.11
    partial P28.19
    primary P28.Ø
    secondary P28.19
  primary (newborn) P28.Ø
  tuberculous —*see* Tuberculosis, pulmonary
Atelocardia Q24.9
Atelomyelia QØ6.1
Atheroembolism
  of
    extremities
      lower I75.Ø2-•
      upper I75.Ø1-•
    kidney I75.81
    specified NEC I75.89
Atheroma, atheromatous —*see also* Arteriosclerosis I7Ø.9Ø
  aorta, aortic I7Ø.Ø
    valve —*see also* Endocarditis, aortic I35.8
  aorto-iliac I7Ø.Ø
  artery —*see* Arteriosclerosis
  basilar (artery) I67.2
  carotid (artery) (common) (internal) I67.2
  cerebral (arteries) I67.2
Atheroma, atheromatous *(Continued)*
  coronary (artery) I25.1Ø
    with angina pectoris —*see* Arteriosclerosis, coronary (artery)
  degeneration —*see* Arteriosclerosis
  heart, cardiac —*see* Disease, heart, ischemic, atherosclerotic
  mitral (valve) I34.8
  myocardium, myocardial —*see* Disease, heart, ischemic, atherosclerotic
  pulmonary valve (heart) —*see also* Endocarditis, pulmonary I37.8
  tricuspid (heart) (valve) I36.8
  valve, valvular —*see* Endocarditis
  vertebral (artery) I67.2
Atheromatosis —*see* Arteriosclerosis
Atherosclerosis —*see also* Arteriosclerosis
  coronary
    artery I25.1Ø
      with angina pectoris —*see* Arteriosclerosis, coronary (artery),
      due to
        calcified coronary lesion (severely) I25.84
        lipid rich plaque I25.83
  transplanted heart I25.811
    bypass graft I25.812
      with angina pectoris —*see* Arteriosclerosis, coronary (artery)
    native coronary artery I25.811
      with angina pectoris —*see* Arteriosclerosis, coronary (artery)
Athetosis (acquired) R25.8
  bilateral (congenital) G8Ø.3
  congenital (bilateral) (double) G8Ø.3
  double (congenital) G8Ø.3
  unilateral R25.8
Athlete's
  foot B35.3
  heart I51.7
Athrepsia E41
Athyrea (acquired) —*see also* Hypothyroidism
  congenital EØ3.1
Atonia, atony, atonic
  bladder (sphincter) (neurogenic) N31.2
  capillary I78.8
  cecum K59.8
    psychogenic F45.8
  colon —*see* Atony, intestine
  congenital P94.2
  esophagus K22.8
  intestine K59.8
    psychogenic F45.8
  stomach K31.89
    neurotic or psychogenic F45.8
  uterus (during labor) O62.2
    with hemorrhage (postpartum) O72.1
    postpartum (with hemorrhage) O72.1
      without hemorrhage O75.89
Atopy —*see* History, allergy
Atransferrinemia, congenital E88.Ø9
Atresia, atretic
  alimentary organ or tract NEC Q45.8
    upper Q4Ø.8
  ani, anus, anal (canal) Q42.3
    with fistula Q42.2
  aorta (ring) Q25.29
  aortic (orifice) (valve) Q23.Ø
    arch Q25.21
    congenital with hypoplasia of ascending aorta and defective development of left ventricle (with mitral stenosis) Q23.4
    in hypoplastic left heart syndrome Q23.4
  aqueduct of Sylvius QØ3.Ø
    with spina bifida —*see* Spina bifida, with hydrocephalus
  artery NEC Q27.8
    cerebral Q28.3
    coronary Q24.5
    digestive system Q27.8

A

Atresia, atretic *(Continued)*
artery NEC *(Continued)*
eye Q15.8
lower limb Q27.8
pulmonary Q25.5
specified site NEC Q27.8
umbilical Q27.0
upper limb Q27.8
auditory canal (external) Q16.1
bile duct (common) (congenital) (hepatic) Q44.2
acquired —*see* Obstruction, bile duct
bladder (neck) Q64.39
obstruction Q64.31
bronchus Q32.4
cecum Q42.8
cervix (acquired) N88.2
congenital Q51.828
in pregnancy or childbirth —*see* Anomaly, cervix, in pregnancy or childbirth
causing obstructed labor O65.5
choana Q30.0
colon Q42.9
specified NEC Q42.8
common duct Q44.2
cricoid cartilage Q31.8
cystic duct Q44.2
acquired K82.8
with obstruction K82.0
digestive organs NEC Q45.8
duodenum Q41.0
ear canal Q16.1
ejaculatory duct Q55.4
epiglottis Q31.8
esophagus Q39.0
with tracheoesophageal fistula Q39.1
eustachian tube Q17.8
fallopian tube (congenital) Q50.6
acquired N97.1
follicular cyst N83.0-●
foramen of
Luschka Q03.1
with spina bifida —*see* Spina bifida, with hydrocephalus
Magendie Q03.1
with spina bifida —*see* Spina bifida, with hydrocephalus
gallbladder Q44.1
genital organ
external
female Q52.79
male Q55.8
internal
female Q52.8
male Q55.8
glottis Q31.8
gullet Q39.0
with tracheoesophageal fistula Q39.1
heart valve NEC Q24.8
pulmonary Q22.0
tricuspid Q22.4
hymen Q52.3
acquired (postinfective) N89.6
ileum Q41.2
intestine (small) Q41.9
large Q42.9
specified NEC Q42.8
iris, filtration angle Q15.0
jejunum Q41.1
lacrimal apparatus Q10.4
larynx Q31.8
meatus urinarius Q64.33
mitral valve Q23.2
in hypoplastic left heart syndrome Q23.4
nares (anterior) (posterior) Q30.0
nasopharynx Q34.8
nose, nostril Q30.0
acquired J34.89
organ or site NEC Q89.8
osseous meatus (ear) Q16.1
oviduct (congenital) Q50.6
acquired N97.1

Atresia, atretic *(Continued)*
parotid duct Q38.4
acquired K11.8
pulmonary (artery) Q25.5
valve Q22.0
pulmonic Q22.0
pupil Q13.2
rectum Q42.1
with fistula Q42.0
salivary duct Q38.4
acquired K11.8
sublingual duct Q38.4
acquired K11.8
submandibular duct Q38.4
acquired K11.8
submaxillary duct Q38.4
acquired K11.8
thyroid cartilage Q31.8
trachea Q32.1
tricuspid valve Q22.4
ureter Q62.10
pelvic junction Q62.11
vesical orifice Q62.12
ureteropelvic junction Q62.11
ureterovesical orifice Q62.12
urethra (valvular) Q64.39
stricture Q64.32
urinary tract NEC Q64.8
uterus Q51.818
acquired N85.8
vagina (congenital) Q52.4
acquired (postinfectional) (senile) N89.5
vas deferens Q55.3
vascular NEC Q27.8
cerebral Q28.3
digestive system Q27.8
lower limb Q27.8
specified site NEC Q27.8
upper limb Q27.8
vein NEC Q27.8
digestive system Q27.8
great Q26.8
lower limb Q27.8
portal Q26.5
pulmonary Q26.4
partial Q26.3
total Q26.2
specified site NEC Q27.8
upper limb Q27.8
vena cava (inferior) (superior) Q26.8
vesicourethral orifice Q64.31
vulva Q52.79
acquired N90.5
Atrichia, atrichosis —*see* Alopecia
Atrophia —*see also* Atrophy
cutis senilis L90.8
due to radiation L57.8
gyrata of choroid and retina H31.23
senilis R54
dermatological L90.8
due to radiation (nonionizing) (solar) L57.8
unguium L60.3
congenita Q84.6
Atrophie blanche (en plaque) (de Milian) L95.0
Atrophoderma, atrophodermia (of) L90.9
diffusum (idiopathic) L90.4
maculatum L90.8
et striatum L90.8
due to syphilis A52.79
syphilitic A51.39
neuriticum L90.8
Pasini and Pierini L90.3
pigmentosum Q82.1
reticulatum symmetricum faciei L66.4
senile L90.8
due to radiation (nonionizing) (solar) L57.8
vermiculata (cheeks) L66.4
Atrophy, atrophic (of)
adrenal (capsule) (gland) E27.49
primary (autoimmune) E27.1
alveolar process or ridge (edentulous) K08.20

Atrophy, atrophic *(Continued)*
anal sphincter (disuse) N81.84
appendix K38.8
arteriosclerotic —*see* Arteriosclerosis
bile duct (common) (hepatic) K83.8
bladder N32.89
neurogenic N31.8
blanche (en plaque) (of Milian) L95.0
bone (senile) NEC —*see also* Disorder, bone, specified type NEC
due to
tabes dorsalis (neurogenic) A52.11
brain (cortex) (progressive) G31.9
frontotemporal circumscribed G31.01 *[F02.80]*
with behavioral disturbance G31.01 *[F02.81]*
senile NEC G31.1
breast N64.2
obstetric —*see* Disorder, breast, specified type NEC
buccal cavity K13.79
cardiac —*see* Degeneration, myocardial
cartilage (infectional) (joint) —*see* Disorder, cartilage, specified NEC
cerebellar —*see* Atrophy, brain
cerebral —*see* Atrophy, brain
cervix (mucosa) (senile) (uteri) N88.8
menopausal N95.8
Charcot-Marie-Tooth G60.0
choroid (central) (macular) (myopic) (retina) H31.10-●
diffuse secondary H31.12-●
gyrate H31.23
senile H31.11-●
ciliary body —*see* Atrophy, iris
conjunctiva (senile) H11.89
corpus cavernosum N48.89
cortical —*see* Atrophy, brain
cystic duct K82.8
Déjérine-Thomas G23.8
disuse NEC —*see* Atrophy, muscle
Duchenne-Aran G12.21
ear H93.8-●
edentulous alveolar ridge K08.20
endometrium (senile) N85.8
cervix N88.8
enteric K63.89
epididymis N50.89
eyeball —*see* Disorder, globe, degenerated condition, atrophy
eyelid (senile) —*see* Disorder, eyelid, degenerative
facial (skin) L90.9
fallopian tube (senile) N83.32-●
with ovary N83.33-●
fascioscapulohumeral (Landouzy-Déjérine) G71.02
fatty, thymus (gland) E32.8
gallbladder K82.8
gastric K29.40
with bleeding K29.41
gastrointestinal K63.89
glandular I89.8
globe H44.52-●
gum —*see* Recession, gingival
hair L67.8
heart (brown) —*see* Degeneration, myocardial
hemifacial Q67.4
Romberg G51.8
infantile E41
paralysis, acute —*see* Poliomyelitis, paralytic
intestine K63.89
iris (essential) (progressive) H21.26-●
specified NEC H21.29
kidney (senile) (terminal) —*see also* Sclerosis, renal N26.1
congenital or infantile Q60.5
bilateral Q60.4
unilateral Q60.3
hydronephrotic —*see* Hydronephrosis

A

- **Atrophy, atrophic** *(Continued)*
  - lacrimal gland (primary) H04.14-•
    - secondary H04.15-•
  - Landouzy-Déjérine G71.02
  - laryngitis, infective J37.0
  - larynx J38.7
  - Leber's optic (hereditary) H47.22
  - lip K13.0
  - liver (yellow) K72.90
    - with coma K72.91
    - acute, subacute K72.00
      - with coma K72.01
    - chronic K72.10
      - with coma K72.11
  - lung (senile) J98.4
  - macular (dermatological) L90.8
    - syphilitic, skin A51.39
      - striated A52.79
  - mandible (edentulous) K08.20
    - minimal K08.21
    - moderate K08.22
    - severe K08.23
  - maxilla K08.20
    - minimal K08.24
    - moderate K08.25
    - severe K08.26
  - muscle, muscular (diffuse) (general) (idiopathic) (primary) M62.50
    - ankle M62.57-•
    - Duchenne-Aran G12.21
    - foot M62.57-•
    - forearm M62.53-•
    - hand M62.54-•
    - infantile spinal G12.0
    - lower leg M62.56-•
    - multiple sites M62.59
    - myelopathic —*see* Atrophy, muscle, spinal
    - myotonic G71.11
    - neuritic G58.9
    - neuropathic (peroneal) (progressive) G60.0
    - pelvic (disuse) N81.84
    - peroneal G60.0
    - progressive (bulbar) G12.21
      - adult G12.1
      - infantile (spinal) G12.0
      - spinal G12.25
        - adult G12.1
        - infantile G12.0
    - pseudohypertrophic G71.02
    - shoulder region M62.51-•
    - specified site NEC M62.58
    - spinal G12.9
      - adult form G12.1
      - Aran-Duchenne G12.21
      - childhood form, type II G12.1
      - distal G12.1
      - hereditary NEC G12.1
      - infantile, type I (Werdnig-Hoffmann) G12.0
      - juvenile form, type III (Kugelberg-Welander) G12.1
      - progressive G12.25
      - scapuloperoneal form G12.1
      - specified NEC G12.8
    - syphilitic A52.78
    - thigh M62.55-•
    - upper arm M62.52-•
  - myocardium —*see* Degeneration, myocardial
  - myometrium (senile) N85.8
    - cervix N88.8
  - myopathic NEC —*see* Atrophy, muscle
  - myotonia G71.11
  - nail L60.3
  - nasopharynx J31.1
  - nerve —*see also* Disorder, nerve
    - abducens —*see* Strabismus, paralytic, sixth nerve
    - accessory G52.8
    - acoustic or auditory —*see* subcategory H93.3
- **Atrophy, atrophic** *(Continued)*
  - nerve *(Continued)*
    - cranial G52.9
      - eighth (auditory) —*see* subcategory H93.3
      - eleventh (accessory) G52.8
      - fifth (trigeminal) G50.8
      - first (olfactory) G52.0
      - fourth (trochlear) —*see* Strabismus, paralytic, fourth nerve
      - second (optic) H47.20
      - sixth (abducens) —*see* Strabismus, paralytic, sixth nerve
      - tenth (pneumogastric) (vagus) G52.2
      - third (oculomotor) —*see* Strabismus, paralytic, third nerve
      - twelfth (hypoglossal) G52.3
    - hypoglossal G52.3
    - oculomotor —*see* Strabismus, paralytic, third nerve
    - olfactory G52.0
    - optic (papillomacular bundle)
      - syphilitic (late) A52.15
        - congenital A50.44
    - pneumogastric G52.2
    - trigeminal G50.8
    - trochlear —*see* Strabismus, paralytic, fourth nerve
    - vagus (pneumogastric) G52.2
  - neurogenic, bone, tabetic A52.11
  - nutritional E41
  - old age R54
  - olivopontocerebellar G23.8
  - optic (nerve) H47.20
    - glaucomatous H47.23-•
    - hereditary H47.22
    - primary H47.21-•
    - specified type NEC H47.29-•
    - syphilitic (late) A52.15
      - congenital A50.44
  - orbit H05.31-•
  - ovary (senile) N83.31-•
    - with fallopian tube N83.33-•
  - oviduct (senile) —*see* Atrophy, fallopian tube
  - palsy, diffuse (progressive) G12.22
  - pancreas (duct) (senile) K86.89
  - parotid gland K11.0
  - pelvic muscle N81.84
  - penis N48.89
  - pharynx J39.2
  - pluriglandular E31.8
    - autoimmune E31.0
  - polyarthritis M15.9
  - prostate N42.89
  - pseudohypertrophic (muscle) G71.02
  - renal —*see also* Sclerosis, renal N26.1
  - retina, retinal (postinfectional) H35.89
  - rhinitis J31.0
  - salivary gland K11.0
  - scar L90.5
  - sclerosis, lobar (of brain) G31.09 *[F02.80]*
    - with behavioral disturbance G31.09 *[F02.81]*
  - scrotum N50.89
  - seminal vesicle N50.89
  - senile R54
    - due to radiation (nonionizing) (solar) L57.8
  - skin (patches) (spots) L90.9
    - degenerative (senile) L90.8
    - due to radiation (nonionizing) (solar) L57.8
    - senile L90.8
  - spermatic cord N50.89
  - spinal (acute) (cord) G95.89
    - muscular —*see* Atrophy, muscle, spinal
    - paralysis G12.20
      - acute —*see* Poliomyelitis, paralytic
      - meaning progressive muscular atrophy G12.25
  - spine (column) —*see* Spondylopathy, specified NEC
  - spleen (senile) D73.0
- **Atrophy, atrophic** *(Continued)*
  - stomach K29.40
    - with bleeding K29.41
  - striate (skin) L90.6
    - syphilitic A52.79
  - subcutaneous L90.9
  - sublingual gland K11.0
  - submandibular gland K11.0
  - submaxillary gland K11.0
  - Sudeck's —*see* Algoneurodystrophy
  - suprarenal (capsule) (gland) E27.49
    - primary E27.1
  - systemic affecting central nervous system
    - in
      - myxedema E03.9 *[G13.2]*
      - neoplastic disease —*see also* Neoplasm D49.9 *[G13.1]*
      - specified disease NEC G13.8
  - tarso-orbital fascia, congenital Q10.3
  - testis N50.0
  - thenar, partial —*see* Syndrome, carpal tunnel
  - thymus (fatty) E32.8
  - thyroid (gland) (acquired) E03.4
    - with cretinism E03.1
    - congenital (with myxedema) E03.1
  - tongue (senile) K14.8
    - papillae K14.4
  - trachea J39.8
  - tunica vaginalis N50.89
  - turbinate J34.89
  - tympanic membrane (nonflaccid) H73.82-•
    - flaccid H73.81-•
  - upper respiratory tract J39.8
  - uterus, uterine (senile) N85.8
    - cervix N88.8
    - due to radiation (intended effect) N85.8
      - adverse effect or misadventure N99.89
  - vagina (senile) N95.2
  - vas deferens N50.89
  - vascular I99.8
  - vertebra (senile) —*see* Spondylopathy, specified NEC
  - vulva (senile) N90.5
  - Werdnig-Hoffmann G12.0
  - yellow —*see* Failure, hepatic
- **Attack, attacks**
  - with alteration of consciousness (with automatisms) —*see* Epilepsy, localization-related, symptomatic, with complex partial seizures
  - without alteration of consciousness —*see* Epilepsy, localization-related, symptomatic, with simple partial seizures
  - Adams-Stokes I45.9
  - akinetic —*see* Epilepsy, generalized, specified NEC
  - angina —*see* Angina
  - atonic —*see* Epilepsy, generalized, specified NEC
  - benign shuddering G25.83
  - cataleptic —*see* Catalepsy
  - coronary —*see* Infarct, myocardium
  - cyanotic, newborn P28.2
  - drop NEC R55
  - epileptic —*see* Epilepsy
  - heart —*see* infarct, myocardium
  - hysterical F44.9
  - jacksonian —*see* Epilepsy, localization-related, symptomatic, with simple partial seizures
  - myocardium, myocardial —*see* Infarct, myocardium
  - myoclonic —*see* Epilepsy, generalized, specified NEC
  - panic F41.0
  - psychomotor —*see* Epilepsy, localization-related, symptomatic, with complex partial seizures
  - salaam —*see* Epilepsy, spasms
  - schizophreniform, brief F23
  - shuddering, benign G25.83

A

Attack, attacks *(Continued)*
Stokes-Adams I45.9
syncope R55
transient ischemic (TIA) G45.9
specified NEC G45.8
unconsciousness R55
hysterical F44.89
vasomotor R55
vasovagal (paroxysmal) (idiopathic) R55
Attention (to)
artificial
opening (of) Z43.9
digestive tract NEC Z43.4
colon Z43.3
ilium Z43.2
stomach Z43.1
specified NEC Z43.8
trachea Z43.Ø
urinary tract NEC Z43.6
cystostomy Z43.5
nephrostomy Z43.6
ureterostomy Z43.6
urethrostomy Z43.6
vagina Z43.7
colostomy Z43.3
cystostomy Z43.5
deficit disorder or syndrome F98.8
with hyperactivity —*see* Disorder, attention-deficit hyperactivity
gastrostomy Z43.1
ileostomy Z43.2
jejunostomy Z43.4
nephrostomy Z43.6
surgical dressings Z48.Ø1
sutures Z48.Ø2
tracheostomy Z43.Ø
ureterostomy Z43.6
urethrostomy Z43.6
Attrition
gum —*see* Recession, gingival
tooth, teeth (excessive) (hard tissues) KØ3.Ø
Atypical, atypism —*see also* condition
cells (on cytolgocial smear) (endocervical) (endometrial) (glandular)
cervix R87.619
vagina R87.629
cervical N87.9
endometrium N85.9
hyperplasia N85.ØØ
parenting situation Z62.9
Auditory —*see* condition
Aujeszky's disease B33.8
Aurantiasis, cutis E67.1
Auricle, auricular —*see also* condition
cervical Q18.2
Auriculotemporal syndrome G5Ø.8
Austin Flint murmur (aortic insufficiency) I35.1
Australian
Q fever A78
X disease A83.4
Autism, autistic (childhood) (infantile) F84.Ø
atypical F84.9
spectrum disorder F84.Ø
Autodigestion R68.89
Autoerythrocyte sensitization (syndrome) D69.2
Autographism L5Ø.3
Autoimmune
disease (systemic) M35.9
inhibitors to clotting factors D68.311
lymphoproliferative syndrome [ALPS] D89.82
thyroiditis EØ6.3
Autointoxication R68.89
Automatism G93.89
with temporal sclerosis G93.81
epileptic —*see* Epilepsy, localization- related, symptomatic, with complex partial seizures
paroxysmal, idiopathic —*see* Epilepsy, localization-related, symptomatic, with complex partial seizures
Autonomic, autonomous
bladder (neurogenic) N31.2
hysteria seizure F44.5
Autosensitivity, erythrocyte D69.2
Autosensitization, cutaneous L3Ø.2
Autosome —*see* condition by chromosome involved
Autotopagnosia R48.1
Autotoxemia R68.89
Autumn —*see* condition
Avellis' syndrome G46.8
Aversion
oral R63.3
newborn P92.-●
nonorganic origin F98.2
sexual F52.1
Aviator's
disease or sickness —*see* Effect, adverse, high altitude
ear T7Ø.Ø
Avitaminosis (multiple) —*see also* Deficiency, vitamin E56.9
B E53.9
with
beriberi E51.11
pellagra E52
B2 E53.Ø
B6 E53.1
B12 E53.8
D E55.9
with rickets E55.Ø
G E53.Ø
K E56.1
nicotinic acid E52
AVNRT (atrioventricular nodal re-entrant tachycardia) I47.1
AVRT (atrioventricular nodal re-entrant tachycardia) I47.1
Avulsion (traumatic)
blood vessel —*see* Injury, blood vessel
bone —*see* Fracture, by site
cartilage —*see also* Dislocation, by site
symphyseal (inner), complicating delivery O71.6
external site other than limb —*see* Wound, open, by site
eye SØ5.7-●
head (intracranial)
external site NEC SØ8.89
scalp SØ8.Ø
internal organ or site —*see* Injury, by site
joint —*see also* Dislocation, by site
capsule —*see* Sprain, by site
kidney S37.Ø6-●
ligament —*see* Sprain, by site
limb —*see also* Amputation, traumatic, by site
skin and subcutaneous tissue —*see* Wound, open, by site
muscle —*see* Injury, muscle
nerve (root) —*see* Injury, nerve
scalp SØ8.Ø
skin and subcutaneous tissue —*see* Wound, open, by site
spleen S36.Ø32
symphyseal cartilage (inner), complicating delivery O71.6
tendon —*see* Injury, muscle
tooth SØ3.2
Awareness of heart beat RØØ.2
Axenfeld's
anomaly or syndrome Q15.Ø
degeneration (calcareous) Q13.4
Axilla, axillary —*see also* condition
breast Q83.1
Axonotmesis —*see* Injury, nerve
Ayerza's disease or syndrome (pulmonary artery sclerosis with pulmonary hypertension) I27.Ø
Azoospermia (organic) N46.Ø1
due to
drug therapy N46.Ø21
efferent duct obstruction N46.Ø23
infection N46.Ø22
radiation N46.Ø24
specified cause NEC N46.Ø29
systemic disease N46.Ø25
Azotemia R79.89
meaning uremia N19
Aztec ear Q17.3
Azygos
continuation inferior vena cava Q26.8
lobe (lung) Q33.1

B

Baastrup's disease —*see* Kissing spine
Babesiosis B6Ø.Ø
Babington's disease (familial hemorrhagic telangiectasia) I78.Ø
Babinski's syndrome A52.79
Baby
  crying constantly R68.11
  floppy (syndrome) P94.2
Bacillary —*see* condition
Bacilluria R82.71
Bacillus —*see also* Infection, bacillus
  abortus infection A23.1
  anthracis infection A22.9
  coli infection —*see also* Escherichia coli B96.2Ø
  Flexner's AØ3.1
  mallei infection A24.Ø
  Shiga's AØ3.Ø
  suipestifer infection —*see* Infection, salmonella
Back —*see* condition
Backache (postural) M54.9
  sacroiliac M53.3
  specified NEC M54.89
Backflow —*see* Reflux
Backward reading (dyslexia) F81.Ø
Bacteremia R78.81
  with sepsis —*see* Sepsis
Bactericholia —*see* Cholecystitis, acute
Bacterid, bacteride (pustular) L4Ø.3
Bacterium, bacteria, bacterial
  agent NEC, as cause of disease classified elsewhere B96.89
  in blood —*see* Bacteremia
  in urine —*see* Bacteriuria
Bacteriuria, bacteruria R82.71
  asymptomatic R82.71
Bacteroides
  fragilis, as cause of disease classified elsewhere B96.6
Bad
  heart —*see* Disease, heart
  trip
    due to drug abuse —*see* Abuse, drug, hallucinogen
    due to drug dependence —*see* Dependence, drug, hallucinogen
Baelz's disease (cheilitis glandularis apostematosa) K13.Ø
Baerensprung's disease (eczema marginatum) B35.6
Bagasse disease or pneumonitis J67.1
Bagassosis J67.1
Baker's cyst —*see* Cyst, Baker's
Bakwin-Krida syndrome (metaphyseal dysplasia) Q78.5
Balancing side interference M26.56
Balanitis (circinata) (erosiva) (gangrenosa) (phagedenic) (vulgaris) N48.1
  amebic AØ6.82
  candidal B37.42
  due to Haemophilus ducreyi A57
  gonococcal (acute) (chronic) A54.23
  xerotica obliterans N48.Ø
Balanoposthitis N47.6
  gonococcal (acute) (chronic) A54.23
  ulcerative (specific) A63.8
Balanorrhagia —*see* Balanitis
Balantidiasis, balantidiosis AØ7.Ø
Bald tongue K14.4
Baldness —*see also* Alopecia
  male-pattern —*see* Alopecia, androgenic
Balkan grippe A78
Balloon disease —*see* Effect, adverse, high altitude
Balo's disease (concentric sclerosis) G37.5
Bamberger-Marie disease —*see* Osteoarthropathy, hypertrophic, specified type NEC
Bancroft's filariasis B74.Ø
Band(s)
  adhesive —*see* Adhesions, peritoneum
  anomalous or congenital —*see also* Anomaly, by site
    heart (atrial) (ventricular) Q24.8
    intestine Q43.3
    omentum Q43.3
  cervix N88.1
  constricting, congenital Q79.8
  gallbladder (congenital) Q44.1
  intestinal (adhesive) —*see* Adhesions, peritoneum
  obstructive
    intestine K56.5Ø
      complete K56.52
      incomplete K56.51
      partial K56.51
    peritoneum K56.5Ø
      complete K56.52
      incomplete K56.51
      partial K56.51
  periappendiceal, congenital Q43.3
  peritoneal (adhesive) —*see* Adhesions, peritoneum
  uterus N73.6
    internal N85.6
  vagina N89.5
Bandemia D72.825
Bandl's ring (contraction), **complicating delivery** O62.4
Bangkok hemorrhagic fever A91
Bang's disease (brucella abortus) A23.1
Bankruptcy, anxiety concerning Z59.8
Bannister's disease T78.3
  hereditary D84.1
Banti's disease or syndrome (with cirrhosis) (with portal hypertension) K76.6
Bar, median, prostate —*see* Enlargement, enlarged, prostate
Barcoo disease or rot —*see* Ulcer, skin
Barlow's disease E54
Barodontalgia T7Ø.29
Baron Münchausen syndrome —*see* Disorder, factitious
Barosinusitis T7Ø.1
Barotitis T7Ø.Ø
Barotrauma T7Ø.29
  odontalgia T7Ø.29
  otitic T7Ø.Ø
  sinus T7Ø.1
Barraquer (-Simons) **disease or syndrome** (progressive lipodystrophy) E88.1
Barré-Guillain disease or syndrome G61.Ø
Barré-Liéou syndrome (posterior cervical sympathetic) M53.Ø
Barrel chest M95.4
Barrett's
  disease —*see* Barrett's, esophagus
  esophagus K22.7Ø
    with dysplasia K22.719
      high grade K22.711
      low grade K22.71Ø
    without dysplasia K22.7Ø
  syndrome —*see* Barrett's, esophagus
  ulcer K22.1Ø
    with bleeding K22.11
    without bleeding K22.1Ø
Barth syndrome E78.71
Bársony (-Polgár) (-Teschendorf) **syndrome** (corkscrew esophagus) K22.4
Bartholinitis (suppurating) N75.8
  gonococcal (acute) (chronic) (with abscess) A54.1
Bartonellosis A44.9
  cutaneous A44.1
  mucocutaneous A44.1
  specified NEC A44.8
  systemic A44.Ø
Barton's fracture S52.56-•
Bartter's syndrome E26.81
Basal —*see* condition
Basan's (hidrotic) **ectodermal dysplasia** Q82.4
Baseball finger —*see* Dislocation, finger
Basedow's disease (exophthalmic goiter) —*see* Hyperthyroidism, with, goiter
Basic —*see* condition
Basilar —*see* condition
Bason's (hidrotic) **ectodermal dysplasia** Q82.4
Basopenia —*see* Agranulocytosis
Basophilia D72.824
Basophilism (cortico-adrenal) (Cushing's) (pituitary) E24.Ø
Bassen-Kornzweig disease or syndrome E78.6
Bat ear Q17.5
Bateman's
  disease BØ8.1
  purpura (senile) D69.2
Bathing cramp T75.1
Bathophobia F4Ø.248
Batten (-Mayou) **disease** E75.4
  retina E75.4 *[H36]*
Batten-Steinert syndrome G71.11
Battered —*see* Maltreatment
Battey Mycobacterium infection A31.Ø
Battle exhaustion F43.Ø
Battledore placenta O43.19-•
Baumgarten-Cruveilhier cirrhosis, disease or syndrome K74.69
Bauxite fibrosis (of lung) J63.1
Bayle's disease (general paresis) A52.17
Bazin's disease (primary) (tuberculous) A18.4
Beach ear —*see* Swimmer's, ear
Beaded hair (congenital) Q84.1
Béal conjunctivitis or syndrome B3Ø.2
Beard's disease (neurasthenia) F48.8
Beat(s)
  atrial, premature I49.1
  ectopic I49.49
  elbow —*see* Bursitis, elbow
  escaped, heart I49.49
  hand —*see* Bursitis, hand
  knee —*see* Bursitis, knee
  premature I49.4Ø
    atrial I49.1
    auricular I49.1
    supraventricular I49.1
Beau's
  disease or syndrome —*see* Degeneration, myocardial
  lines (transverse furrows on fingernails) L6Ø.4
Bechterev's syndrome —*see* Spondylitis, ankylosing
Beck's syndrome (anterior spinal artery occlusion) I65.8
Becker's
  cardiomyopathy I42.8
  disease
    idiopathic mural endomyocardial disease I42.3
    myotonia congenita, recessive form G71.12
  dystrophy G71.Ø1
  pigmented hairy nevus D22.5
Beckwith-Wiedemann syndrome Q87.3
Bed confinement status Z74.Ø1
Bed sore —*see* Ulcer, pressure, by site
Bedbug bite(s) —*see* Bite(s), by site, superficial, insect
Bedclothes, asphyxiation or suffocation by —*see* Asphyxia, traumatic, due to, mechanical, trapped
Bednar's
  aphthae K12.Ø
  tumor —*see* Neoplasm, malignant, by site
Bedridden Z74.Ø1
Bedsore —*see* Ulcer, pressure, by site
Bedwetting —*see* Enuresis
Bee sting (with allergic or anaphylactic shock) —*see* Toxicity, venom, arthropod, bee
Beer drinker's heart (disease) I42.6
Begbie's disease (exophthalmic goiter) —*see* Hyperthyroidism, with, goiter

Behavior
- antisocial
  - adult Z72.811
  - child or adolescent Z72.810
- disorder, disturbance —*see* Disorder, conduct
- disruptive —*see* Disorder, conduct
- drug seeking Z76.5
- inexplicable R46.2
- marked evasiveness R46.5
- obsessive-compulsive R46.81
- overactivity R46.3
- poor responsiveness R46.4
- self-damaging (life-style) Z72.89
- sleep-incompatible Z72.821
- slowness R46.4
- specified NEC R46.89
- strange (and inexplicable) R46.2
- suspiciousness R46.5
- type A pattern Z73.1
- undue concern or preoccupation with stressful events R46.6
- verbosity and circumstantial detail obscuring reason for contact R46.7

Behcet's disease or syndrome M35.2
Behr's disease —*see* Degeneration, macula
Beigel's disease or morbus (white piedra) B36.2
Bejel A65
Bekhterev's syndrome —*see* Spondylitis, ankylosing
Belching —*see* Eructation
Bell's
- mania F30.8
- palsy, paralysis G51.0
  - infant or newborn P11.3
- spasm G51.3-●

Bence Jones albuminuria or proteinuria NEC R80.3
Bends T70.3
Benedikt's paralysis or syndrome G46.3
Benign (*see also* condition)
- prostatic hyperplasia —*see* Hyperplasia, prostate

Bennett's fracture (displaced) S62.21-●
Benson's disease —*see* Deposit, crystalline
Bent
- back (hysterical) F44.4
- nose M95.0
  - congenital Q67.4

Bereavement (uncomplicated) Z63.4
Bergeron's disease (hysterical chorea) F44.4
Berger's disease —*see* Nephropathy, IgA
Beriberi (dry) E51.11
- heart (disease) E51.12
- polyneuropathy E51.11
- wet E51.12
  - involving circulatory system E51.11

Berlin's disease or edema (traumatic) S05.8X-●
Berlock (berloque) **dermatitis** L56.2
Bernard-Horner syndrome G90.2
Bernard-Soulier disease or thrombopathia D69.1
Bernhardt (-Roth) **disease** —*see* Mononeuropathy, lower limb, meralgia paresthetica
Bernheim's syndrome —*see* Failure, heart, right
Bertielliasis B71.8
Berylliosis (lung) J63.2
Besnier-Boeck (-Schaumann) **disease** —*see* Sarcoidosis
Besnier's
- lupus pernio D86.3
- prurigo L20.0

Bestiality F65.89
Best's disease H35.50
Beta-mercaptolactate-cysteine disulfiduria E72.09
Betalipoproteinemia, broad or floating E78.2
Betting and gambling Z72.6
- pathological (compulsive) F63.0

Bezoar T18.9
- intestine T18.3
- stomach T18.2

Bezold's abscess —*see* Mastoiditis, acute
Bianchi's syndrome R48.8
Bicornate or bicornis uterus Q51.3
- in pregnancy or childbirth O34.00
  - causing obstructed labor O65.5

Bicuspid aortic valve Q23.1
Biedl-Bardet syndrome Q87.89
Bielschowsky (-Jansky) **disease** E75.4
Biermer's (pernicious) **anemia or disease** D51.0
Biett's disease L93.0
Bifid (congenital)
- apex, heart Q24.8
- clitoris Q52.6
- kidney Q63.8
- nose Q30.2
- patella Q74.1
- scrotum Q55.29
- toe NEC Q74.2
- tongue Q38.3
- ureter Q62.8
- uterus Q51.3
- uvula Q35.7

Biforis uterus (suprasimplex) Q51.3
Bifurcation (congenital)
- gallbladder Q44.1
- kidney pelvis Q63.8
- renal pelvis Q63.8
- rib Q76.6
- tongue, congenital Q38.3
- trachea Q32.1
- ureter Q62.8
- urethra Q64.74
- vertebra Q76.49

Big spleen syndrome D73.1
Bigeminal pulse R00.8
Bilateral —*see* condition
Bile
- duct —*see* condition
- pigments in urine R82.2

Bilharziasis —*see also* Schistosomiasis
- chyluria B65.0
- cutaneous B65.3
- galacturia B65.0
- hematochyluria B65.0
- intestinal B65.1
- lipemia B65.9
- lipuria B65.0
- oriental B65.2
- piarhemia B65.9
- pulmonary NOS B65.9 *[J99]*
  - pneumonia B65.9 *[J17]*
- tropical hematuria B65.0
- vesical B65.0

Biliary —*see* condition
Bilirubin metabolism disorder E80.7
- specified NEC E80.6

Bilirubinemia, familial nonhemolytic E80.4
Bilirubinuria R82.2
Biliuria R82.2
Bilocular stomach K31.2
Binswanger's disease I67.3
Biparta, bipartite
- carpal scaphoid Q74.0
- patella Q74.1
- vagina Q52.10

Bird
- face Q75.8
- fancier's disease or lung J67.2

Birt-Hogg-Dube syndrome Q87.89
Birth
- complications in mother —*see* Delivery, complicated
- compression during NOS P15.9
- defect —*see* Anomaly
- immature (less than 37 completed weeks) —*see* Preterm, newborn
  - extremely (less than 28 completed weeks) —*see* Immaturity, extreme

Birth *(Continued)*
- inattention, at or after —*see* Maltreatment, child, neglect
- injury NOS P15.9
  - basal ganglia P11.1
  - brachial plexus NEC P14.3
  - brain (compression) (pressure) P11.2
  - central nervous system NOS P11.9
  - cerebellum P11.1
  - cerebral hemorrhage P10.1
  - external genitalia P15.5
  - eye P15.3
  - face P15.4
  - fracture
    - bone P13.9
      - specified NEC P13.8
    - clavicle P13.4
    - femur P13.2
    - humerus P13.3
    - long bone, except femur P13.3
    - radius and ulna P13.3
    - skull P13.0
    - spine P11.5
    - tibia and fibula P13.3
  - intracranial P11.2
    - laceration or hemorrhage P10.9
      - specified NEC P10.8
  - intraventricular hemorrhage P10.2
  - laceration
    - brain P10.1
    - by scalpel P15.8
    - peripheral nerve P14.9
  - liver P15.0
  - meninges
    - brain P11.1
    - spinal cord P11.5
  - nerve
    - brachial plexus P14.3
    - cranial NEC (except facial) P11.4
    - facial P11.3
    - peripheral P14.9
    - phrenic (paralysis) P14.2
  - paralysis
    - facial nerve P11.3
    - spinal P11.5
  - penis P15.5
  - rupture
    - spinal cord P11.5
  - scalp P12.9
  - scalpel wound P15.8
  - scrotum P15.5
  - skull NEC P13.1
    - fracture P13.0
  - specified type NEC P15.8
  - spinal cord P11.5
  - spine P11.5
  - spleen P15.1
  - sternomastoid (hematoma) P15.2
  - subarachnoid hemorrhage P10.3
  - subcutaneous fat necrosis P15.6
  - subdural hemorrhage P10.0
  - tentorial tear P10.4
  - testes P15.5
  - vulva P15.5
- lack of care, at or after —*see* Maltreatment, child, neglect
- neglect, at or after —*see* Maltreatment, child, neglect
- palsy or paralysis, newborn, NOS (birth injury) P14.9
- premature (infant) —*see* Preterm, newborn
- shock, newborn P96.89
- trauma —*see* Birth, injury
- weight
  - 4000 grams to 4499 grams P08.1
  - 4500 grams or more P08.0
  - low (2499 grams or less) —*see* Low, birthweight
    - extremely (999 grams or less) —*see* Low, birthweight, extreme

Birthmark Q82.5

B

- **Bisalbuminemia** E88.09
- **Biskra's button** B55.1
- **Bite(s)** (animal) (human)
  - abdomen, abdominal
    - wall S31.159
      - with penetration into peritoneal cavity S31.659
      - epigastric region S31.152
        - with penetration into peritoneal cavity S31.652
      - left
        - lower quadrant S31.154
          - with penetration into peritoneal cavity S31.654
        - upper quadrant S31.151
          - with penetration into peritoneal cavity S31.651
      - periumbilic region S31.155
        - with penetration into peritoneal cavity S31.655
      - right
        - lower quadrant S31.153
          - with penetration into peritoneal cavity S31.653
        - upper quadrant S31.150
          - with penetration into peritoneal cavity S31.650
      - superficial NEC S30.871
        - insect S30.861
  - alveolar (process) —*see* Bite, oral cavity
  - amphibian (venomous) —*see* Venom, bite, amphibian
  - animal —*see also* Bite, by site
    - venomous —*see* Venom
  - ankle S91.05- ●
    - superficial NEC S90.57- ●
      - insect S90.56- ●
  - antecubital space —*see* Bite, elbow
  - anus S31.835
    - superficial NEC S30.877
      - insect S30.867
  - arm (upper) S41.15- ●
    - lower —*see* Bite, forearm
    - superficial NEC S40.87- ●
      - insect S40.86- ●
  - arthropod NEC —*see* Venom, bite, arthropod
  - auditory canal (external) (meatus) —*see* Bite, ear
  - auricle, ear —*see* Bite, ear
  - axilla —*see* Bite, arm
  - back —*see also* Bite, thorax, back
    - lower S31.050
      - with penetration into retroperitoneal space S31.051
      - superficial NEC S30.870
        - insect S30.860
  - bedbug —*see* Bite(s), by site, superficial, insect
  - breast S21.05- ●
    - superficial NEC S20.17- ●
      - insect S20.16- ●
  - brow —*see* Bite, head, specified site NEC
  - buttock S31.805
    - left S31.825
    - right S31.815
    - superficial NEC S30.870
      - insect S30.860
  - calf —*see* Bite, leg
  - canaliculus lacrimalis —*see* Bite, eyelid
  - canthus, eye —*see* Bite, eyelid
  - centipede —*see* Toxicity, venom, arthropod, centipede
  - cheek (external) S01.45- ●
    - internal —*see* Bite, oral cavity
    - superficial NEC S00.87
      - insect S00.86
  - chest wall —*see* Bite, thorax
  - chigger B88.0
  - chin —*see* Bite, head, specified site NEC
  - clitoris —*see* Bite, vulva
  - costal region —*see* Bite, thorax

Bite *(Continued)*
  - digit(s)
    - hand —*see* Bite, finger
    - toe —*see* Bite, toe
  - ear (canal) (external) S01.35- ●
    - superficial NEC S00.47- ●
      - insect S00.46- ●
  - elbow S51.05- ●
    - superficial NEC S50.37- ●
      - insect S50.36- ●
  - epididymis —*see* Bite, testis
  - epigastric region —*see* Bite, abdomen
  - epiglottis —*see* Bite, neck, specified site NEC
  - esophagus, cervical S11.25
    - superficial NEC S10.17
      - insect S10.16
  - eyebrow —*see* Bite, eyelid
  - eyelid S01.15- ●
    - superficial NEC S00.27- ●
      - insect S00.26- ●
  - face NEC —*see* Bite, head, specified site NEC
  - finger(s) S61.259
    - with
      - damage to nail S61.359
    - index S61.258
      - with
        - damage to nail S61.358
      - left S61.251
        - with
          - damage to nail S61.351
      - right S61.250
        - with
          - damage to nail S61.350
      - superficial NEC S60.478
        - insect S60.46- ●
    - little S61.25- ●
      - with
        - damage to nail S61.35- ●
      - superficial NEC S60.47- ●
        - insect S60.46- ●
    - middle S61.25- ●
      - with
        - damage to nail S61.35- ●
      - superficial NEC S60.47- ●
        - insect S60.46- ●
    - ring S61.25- ●
      - with
        - damage to nail S61.35- ●
      - superficial NEC S60.47- ●
        - insect S60.46- ●
    - superficial NEC S60.479
      - insect S60.469
    - thumb —*see* Bite, thumb
  - flank —*see* Bite, abdomen, wall
  - flea —*see* Bite, by site, superficial, insect
  - foot (except toe(s) alone) S91.35- ●
    - superficial NEC S90.87- ●
      - insect S90.86- ●
    - toe —*see* Bite, toe
  - forearm S51.85- ●
    - elbow only —*see* Bite, elbow
    - superficial NEC S50.87- ●
      - insect S50.86- ●
  - forehead —*see* Bite, head, specified site NEC
  - genital organs, external
    - female S31.552
      - superficial NEC S30.876
        - insect S30.866
      - vagina and vulva —*see* Bite, vulva
    - male S31.551
      - penis —*see* Bite, penis
      - scrotum —*see* Bite, scrotum
      - superficial NEC S30.875
        - insect S30.865
      - testes —*see* Bite, testis
  - groin —*see* Bite, abdomen, wall
  - gum —*see* Bite, oral cavity

Bite *(Continued)*
  - hand S61.45- ●
    - finger —*see* Bite, finger
    - superficial NEC S60.57- ●
      - insect S60.56- ●
    - thumb —*see* Bite, thumb
  - head S01.95
    - cheek —*see* Bite, cheek
    - ear —*see* Bite, ear
    - eyelid —*see* Bite, eyelid
    - lip —*see* Bite, lip
    - nose —*see* Bite, nose
    - oral cavity —*see* Bite, oral cavity
    - scalp —*see* Bite, scalp
    - specified site NEC S01.85
      - superficial NEC S00.87
        - insect S00.86
    - superficial NEC S00.97
      - insect S00.96
    - temporomandibular area —*see* Bite, cheek
  - heel —*see* Bite, foot
  - hip S71.05- ●
    - superficial NEC S70.27- ●
      - insect S70.26- ●
  - hymen S31.45
  - hypochondrium —*see* Bite, abdomen, wall
  - hypogastric region —*see* Bite, abdomen, wall
  - inguinal region —*see* Bite, abdomen, wall
  - insect —*see* Bite, by site, superficial, insect
  - instep —*see* Bite, foot
  - interscapular region —*see* Bite, thorax, back
  - jaw —*see* Bite, head, specified site NEC
  - knee S81.05- ●
    - superficial NEC S80.27- ●
      - insect S80.26- ●
  - labium (majus) (minus) —*see* Bite, vulva
  - lacrimal duct —*see* Bite, eyelid
  - larynx S11.015
    - superficial NEC S10.17
      - insect S10.16
  - leg (lower) S81.85- ●
    - ankle —*see* Bite, ankle
    - foot —*see* Bite, foot
    - knee —*see* Bite, knee
    - superficial NEC S80.87- ●
      - insect S80.86- ●
    - toe —*see* Bite, toe
    - upper —*see* Bite, thigh
  - lip S01.551
    - superficial NEC S00.571
      - insect S00.561
  - lizard (venomous) —*see* Venom, bite, reptile
  - loin —*see* Bite, abdomen, wall
  - lower back —*see* Bite, back, lower
  - lumbar region —*see* Bite, back, lower
  - malar region —*see* Bite, head, specified site NEC
  - mammary —*see* Bite, breast
  - marine animals (venomous) —*see* Toxicity, venom, marine animal
  - mastoid region —*see* Bite, head, specified site NEC
  - mouth —*see* Bite, oral cavity
  - nail
    - finger —*see* Bite, finger
    - toe —*see* Bite, toe
  - nape —*see* Bite, neck, specified site NEC
  - nasal (septum) (sinus) —*see* Bite, nose
  - nasopharynx —*see* Bite, head, specified site NEC
  - neck S11.95
    - involving
      - cervical esophagus —*see* Bite, esophagus, cervical
      - larynx —*see* Bite, larynx
      - pharynx —*see* Bite, pharynx
      - thyroid gland S11.15
      - trachea —*see* Bite, trachea
    - specified site NEC S11.85
      - superficial NEC S10.87
        - insect S10.86

- **Bite** *(Continued)*
  - neck *(Continued)*
    - superficial NEC S10.97
      - insect S10.96
    - throat S11.85
      - superficial NEC S10.17
        - insect S10.16
  - nose (septum) (sinus) S01.25
    - superficial NEC S00.37
      - insect S00.36
  - occipital region —*see* Bite, scalp
  - oral cavity S01.552
    - superficial NEC S00.572
      - insect S00.562
  - orbital region —*see* Bite, eyelid
  - palate —*see* Bite, oral cavity
  - palm —*see* Bite, hand
  - parietal region —*see* Bite, scalp
  - pelvis S31.050
    - with penetration into retroperitoneal space S31.051
    - superficial NEC S30.870
      - insect S30.860
  - penis S31.25
    - superficial NEC S30.872
      - insect S30.862
  - perineum
    - female —*see* Bite, vulva
    - male —*see* Bite, pelvis
  - periocular area (with or without lacrimal passages) —*see* Bite, eyelid
  - phalanges
    - finger —*see* Bite, finger
    - toe —*see* Bite, toe
  - pharynx S11.25
    - superficial NEC S10.17
      - insect S10.16
  - pinna —*see* Bite, ear
  - poisonous —*see* Venom
  - popliteal space —*see* Bite, knee
  - prepuce —*see* Bite, penis
  - pubic region —*see* Bite, abdomen, wall
  - rectovaginal septum —*see* Bite, vulva
  - red bug B88.0
  - reptile NEC —*see also* Venom, bite, reptile
    - nonvenomous —*see* Bite, by site
    - snake —*see* Venom, bite, snake
  - sacral region —*see* Bite, back, lower
  - sacroiliac region —*see* Bite, back, lower
  - salivary gland —*see* Bite, oral cavity
  - scalp S01.05
    - superficial NEC S00.07
      - insect S00.06
  - scapular region —*see* Bite, shoulder
  - scrotum S31.35
    - superficial NEC S30.873
      - insect S30.863
  - sea-snake (venomous) —*see* Toxicity, venom, snake, sea snake
  - shin —*see* Bite, leg
  - shoulder S41.05-●
    - superficial NEC S40.27-●
      - insect S40.26-●
  - snake —*see also* Venom, bite, snake
    - nonvenomous —*see* Bite, by site
  - spermatic cord —*see* Bite, testis
  - spider (venomous) —*see* Toxicity, venom, spider
    - nonvenomous —*see* Bite, by site, superficial, insect
  - sternal region —*see* Bite, thorax, front
  - submaxillary region —*see* Bite, head, specified site NEC
  - submental region —*see* Bite, head, specified site NEC
  - subungual
    - finger(s) —*see* Bite, finger
    - toe —*see* Bite, toe
  - superficial —*see* Bite, by site, superficial
  - supraclavicular fossa S11.85
- **Bite** *(Continued)*
  - supraorbital —*see* Bite, head, specified site NEC
  - temple, temporal region —*see* Bite, head, specified site NEC
  - temporomandibular area —*see* Bite, cheek
  - testis S31.35
    - superficial NEC S30.873
      - insect S30.863
  - thigh S71.15-●
    - superficial NEC S70.37-●
      - insect S70.36-●
  - thorax, thoracic (wall) S21.95
    - back S21.25-●
      - with penetration into thoracic cavity S21.45-●
    - breast —*see* Bite, breast
    - front S21.15-●
      - with penetration into thoracic cavity S21.35-●
    - superficial NEC S20.97
      - back S20.47-●
      - front S20.37-●
      - insect S20.96
        - back S20.46-●
        - front S20.36-●
  - throat —*see* Bite, neck, throat
  - thumb S61.05-●
    - with
      - damage to nail S61.15-●
    - superficial NEC S60.37-●
      - insect S60.36-●
  - thyroid S11.15
    - superficial NEC S10.87
      - insect S10.86
  - toe(s) S91.15-●
    - with
      - damage to nail S91.25-●
    - great S91.15-●
      - with
        - damage to nail S91.25-●
    - lesser S91.15-●
      - with
        - damage to nail S91.25-●
    - superficial NEC S90.47-●
      - great S90.47-●
      - insect S90.46-●
        - great S90.46-●
  - tongue S01.552
  - trachea S11.025
    - superficial NEC S10.17
      - insect S10.16
  - tunica vaginalis —*see* Bite, testis
  - tympanum, tympanic membrane —*see* Bite, ear
  - umbilical region S31.155
  - uvula —*see* Bite, oral cavity
  - vagina —*see* Bite, vulva
  - venomous —*see* Venom
  - vocal cords S11.035
    - superficial NEC S10.17
      - insect S10.16
  - vulva S31.45
    - superficial NEC S30.874
      - insect S30.864
  - wrist S61.55-●
    - superficial NEC S60.87-●
      - insect S60.86-●
- **Biting, cheek or lip** K13.1
- **Biventricular failure** (heart) I50.82
- **Björck** (-Thorson) **syndrome** (malignant carcinoid) E34.0
- **Black**
  - death A20.9
  - eye S00.1-●
  - hairy tongue K14.3
  - heel (foot) S90.3-●
  - lung (disease) J60
  - palm (hand) S60.22-●
- **Blackfan-Diamond anemia or syndrome** (congenital hypoplastic anemia) D61.01
- **Blackhead** L70.0
- **Blackout** R55
- **Bladder** —*see* condition
- **Blast** (air) (hydraulic) (immersion) (underwater)
  - blindness S05.8X-●
  - injury
    - abdomen or thorax —*see* Injury, by site
    - ear (acoustic nerve trauma) —*see* Injury, nerve, acoustic, specified type NEC
  - syndrome NEC T70.8
- **Blastoma** —*see* Neoplasm, malignant, by site
  - pulmonary —*see* Neoplasm, lung, malignant
- **Blastomycosis, blastomycotic** B40.9
  - Brazilian —*see* Paracoccidioidomycosis
  - cutaneous B40.3
  - disseminated B40.7
  - European —*see* Cryptococcosis
  - generalized B40.7
  - keloidal B48.0
  - North American B40.9
  - primary pulmonary B40.0
  - pulmonary B40.2
    - acute B40.0
    - chronic B40.1
  - skin B40.3
  - South American —*see* Paracoccidioidomycosis
  - specified NEC B40.89
- **Bleb(s)** R23.8
  - emphysematous (lung) (solitary) J43.9
  - endophthalmitis H59.43
  - filtering (vitreous), after glaucoma surgery Z98.83
  - inflammed (infected), postprocedural H59.40
    - stage 1 H59.41
    - stage 2 H59.42
    - stage 3 H59.43
  - lung (ruptured) J43.9
    - congenital —*see* Atelectasis
    - newborn P25.8
  - subpleural (emphysematous) J43.9
- **Blebitis, postprocedural** H59.40
  - stage 1 H59.41
  - stage 2 H59.42
  - stage 3 H59.43
- **Bleeder** (familial) (hereditary) —*see* Hemophilia
- **Bleeding** —*see also* Hemorrhage
  - anal K62.5
  - anovulatory N97.0
  - atonic, following delivery O72.1
  - capillary I78.8
    - puerperal O72.2
  - contact (postcoital) N93.0
  - due to uterine subinvolution N85.3
  - ear —*see* Otorrhagia
  - excessive, associated with menopausal onset N92.4
  - familial —*see* Defect, coagulation
  - following intercourse N93.0
  - gastrointestinal K92.2
  - hemorrhoids —*see* Hemorrhoids
  - intermenstrual (regular) N92.3
    - irregular N92.1
  - intraoperative —*see* Complication, intraoperative, hemorrhage
  - irregular N92.6
  - menopausal N92.4
  - newborn, intraventricular —*see* Newborn, affected by, hemorrhage, intraventricular
  - nipple N64.59
  - nose R04.0
  - ovulation N92.3
  - ▶ perimenopausal N92.4
  - postclimacteric N95.0
  - postcoital N93.0
  - postmenopausal N95.0
  - postoperative —*see* Complication, postprocedural, hemorrhage
  - preclimacteric N92.4
  - pre-pubertal vaginal N93.1
  - puberty (excessive, with onset of menstrual periods) N92.2

Bleeding (Continued)
  rectum, rectal K62.5
    newborn P54.2
  tendencies —see Defect, coagulation
  throat RØ4.1
  tooth socket (post-extraction) K91.84Ø
  umbilical stump P51.9
  uterus, uterine NEC N93.9
    climacteric N92.4
    dysfunctional or functional N93.8
    menopausal N92.4
    preclimacteric or premenopausal N92.4
    unrelated to menstrual cycle N93.9
  vagina, vaginal (abnormal) N93.9
    dysfunctional or functional N93.8
    newborn P54.6
    pre-pubertal N93.1
  vicarious N94.89
Blennorrhagia, blennorrhagic —see Gonorrhea
Blennorrhea (acute) (chronic) —see also Gonorrhea
  inclusion (neonatal) (newborn) P39.1
  lower genitourinary tract (gonococcal) A54.ØØ
  neonatorum (gonococcal ophthalmia) A54.31
Blepharelosis —see Entropion
Blepharitis (angularis) (ciliaris) (eyelid) (marginal) (nonulcerative) HØ1.ØØ9
  herpes zoster BØ2.39
  left HØ1.ØØ6
    lower HØ1.ØØ5
    upper HØ1.ØØ4
    upper and lower HØ1.ØØB
  right HØ1.ØØ3
    lower HØ1.ØØ2
    upper HØ1.ØØ1
    upper and lower HØ1.ØØA
  squamous HØ1.Ø29
    left HØ1.Ø26
      lower HØ1.Ø25
      upper HØ1.Ø24
      upper and lower HØ1.Ø2B
    right HØ1.Ø23
      lower HØ1.Ø22
      upper HØ1.Ø21
      upper and lower HØ1.Ø2A
  ulcerative HØ1.Ø19
    left HØ1.Ø16
      lower HØ1.Ø15
      upper HØ1.Ø14
      upper and lower HØ1.Ø1B
    right HØ1.Ø13
      lower HØ1.Ø12
      upper HØ1.Ø11
      upper and lower HØ1.Ø1B
Blepharochalasis HØ2.3Ø
  congenital Q1Ø.Ø
  left HØ2.36
    lower HØ2.35
    upper HØ2.34
  right HØ2.33
    lower HØ2.32
    upper HØ2.31
Blepharoclonus HØ2.59
Blepharoconjunctivitis H1Ø.5Ø-●
  angular H1Ø.52-●
  contact H1Ø.53-●
  ligneous H1Ø.51-●
Blepharophimosis (eyelid) HØ2.529
  congenital Q1Ø.3
  left HØ2.526
    lower HØ2.525
    upper HØ2.524
  right HØ2.523
    lower HØ2.522
    upper HØ2.521
Blepharoptosis HØ2.4Ø-●
  congenital Q1Ø.Ø
  mechanical HØ2.41-●
  myogenic HØ2.42-●
  neurogenic HØ2.43-●
  paralytic HØ2.43-●
Blepharopyorrhea, gonococcal A54.39
Blepharospasm G24.5
  drug induced G24.Ø1
Blighted ovum OØ2.Ø
Blind —see also Blindness
  bronchus (congenital) Q32.4
  loop syndrome K9Ø.2
    congenital Q43.8
  sac, fallopian tube (congenital) Q5Ø.6
  spot, enlarged —see Defect, visual field, localized, scotoma, blind spot area
  tract or tube, congenital NEC —see Atresia, by site
Blindness (acquired) (congenital) (both eyes) H54.ØX-●
  blast SØ5.8X-●
  color —see Deficiency, color vision
  concussion SØ5.8X-●
  cortical H47.619
    left brain H47.612
    right brain H47.611
  day H53.11
  due to injury (current episode) SØ5.9-●
    sequelae — code to injury with seventh character S
  eclipse (total) —see Retinopathy, solar
  emotional (hysterical) F44.6
  face H53.16
  hysterical F44.6
  legal (both eyes) (USA definition) H54.8
  mind R48.8
  night H53.6Ø
    abnormal dark adaptation curve H53.61
    acquired H53.62
    congenital H53.63
    specified type NEC H53.69
    vitamin A deficiency E5Ø.5
  one eye (other eye normal) H54.4Ø
    left (normal vision on right) H54.42-●
      low vision on right H54.12-●
    low vision, other eye H54.1Ø
    right (normal vision on left) H54.41-●
      low vision on left H54.11-●
  psychic R48.8
  river B73.Ø1
  snow —see Photokeratitis
  sun, solar —see Retinopathy, solar
  transient —see Disturbance, vision, subjective, loss, transient
  traumatic (current episode) SØ5.9-●
  word (developmental) F81.Ø
    acquired R48.Ø
    secondary to organic lesion R48.Ø
Blister (nonthermal)
  abdominal wall S3Ø.821
  alveolar process SØØ.522
  ankle S9Ø.52-●
  antecubital space —see Blister, elbow
  anus S3Ø.827
  arm (upper) S4Ø.82-●
  auditory canal —see Blister, ear
  auricle —see Blister, ear
  axilla —see Blister, arm
  back, lower S3Ø.82Ø
  beetle dermatitis L24.89
  breast S2Ø.12-●
  brow SØØ.82
  calf —see Blister, leg
  canthus —see Blister, eyelid
  cheek SØØ.82
    internal SØØ.522
  chest wall —see Blister, thorax
  chin SØØ.82
  costal region —see Blister, thorax
  digit(s)
    foot —see Blister, toe
    hand —see Blister, finger
  due to burn —see Burn, by site, second degree
  ear SØØ.42-●
  elbow S5Ø.32-●
  epiglottis S1Ø.12
  esophagus, cervical S1Ø.12
  eyebrow —see Blister, eyelid
Blister (Continued)
  eyelid SØØ.22-●
  face SØØ.82
  fever BØØ.1
  finger(s) S6Ø.429
    index S6Ø.42-●
    little S6Ø.42-●
    middle S6Ø.42-●
    ring S6Ø.42-●
  foot (except toe(s) alone) S9Ø.82-●
    toe —see Blister, toe
  forearm S5Ø.82-●
    elbow only —see Blister, elbow
  forehead SØØ.82
  fracture - omit code
  genital organ
    female S3Ø.826
    male S3Ø.825
  gum SØØ.522
  hand S6Ø.52-●
  head SØØ.92
    ear —see Blister, ear
    eyelid —see Blister, eyelid
    lip SØØ.521
    nose SØØ.32
    oral cavity SØØ.522
    scalp SØØ.Ø2
    specified site NEC SØØ.82
  heel —see Blister, foot
  hip S7Ø.22-●
  interscapular region S2Ø.429
  jaw SØØ.82
  knee S8Ø.22-●
  larynx S1Ø.12
  leg (lower) S8Ø.82-●
    knee —see Blister, knee
    upper —see Blister, thigh
  lip SØØ.521
  malar region SØØ.82
  mammary —see Blister, breast
  mastoid region SØØ.82
  mouth SØØ.522
  multiple, skin, nontraumatic R23.8
  nail
    finger —see Blister, finger
    toe —see Blister, toe
  nasal SØØ.32
  neck S1Ø.92
    specified site NEC S1Ø.82
    throat S1Ø.12
  nose SØØ.32
  occipital region SØØ.Ø2
  oral cavity SØØ.522
  orbital region —see Blister, eyelid
  palate SØØ.522
  palm —see Blister, hand
  parietal region SØØ.Ø2
  pelvis S3Ø.82Ø
  penis S3Ø.822
  periocular area —see Blister, eyelid
  phalanges
    finger —see Blister, finger
    toe —see Blister, toe
  pharynx S1Ø.12
  pinna —see Blister, ear
  popliteal space —see Blister, knee
  scalp SØØ.Ø2
  scapular region —see Blister, shoulder
  scrotum S3Ø.823
  shin —see Blister, leg
  shoulder S4Ø.22-●
  sternal region S2Ø.329
  submaxillary region SØØ.82
  submental region SØØ.82
  subungual
    finger(s) —see Blister, finger
    toe(s) —see Blister, toe
  supraclavicular fossa S1Ø.82
  supraorbital SØØ.82
  temple SØØ.82
  temporal region SØØ.82
  testis S3Ø.823

Blister *(Continued)*
thermal *—see* Burn, second degree, by site
thigh S70.32-●
thorax, thoracic (wall) S20.92
back S20.42-●
front S20.32-●
throat S10.12
thumb S60.32-●
toe(s) S90.42-●
great S90.42-●
tongue S00.522
trachea S10.12
tympanum, tympanic membrane *—see* Blister, ear
upper arm *—see* Blister, arm (upper)
uvula S00.522
vagina S30.824
vocal cords S10.12
vulva S30.824
wrist S60.82-●
Bloating R14.0
Bloch-Sulzberger disease or syndrome Q82.3
Block, blocked
alveolocapillary J84.10
arborization (heart) I45.5
arrhythmic I45.9
atrioventricular (incomplete) (partial) I44.30
with atrioventricular dissociation I44.2
complete I44.2
congenital Q24.6
congenital Q24.6
first degree I44.0
second degree (types I and II) I44.1
specified NEC I44.39
third degree I44.2
types I and II I44.1
auriculoventricular *—see* Block, atrioventricular
bifascicular (cardiac) I45.2
bundle-branch (complete) (false) (incomplete) I45.4
bilateral I45.2
left I44.7
with right bundle branch block I45.2
hemiblock I44.60
anterior I44.4
posterior I44.5
incomplete I44.7
with right bundle branch block I45.2
right I45.10
with
left bundle branch block I45.2
left fascicular block I45.2
specified NEC I45.19
Wilson's type I45.19
cardiac I45.9
conduction I45.9
complete I44.2
fascicular (left) I44.60
anterior I44.4
posterior I44.5
right I45.0
specified NEC I44.69
foramen Magendie (acquired) G91.1
congenital Q03.1
with spina bifida *—see* Spina bifida, by site, with hydrocephalus
heart I45.9
bundle branch I45.4
bilateral I45.2
complete (atrioventricular) I44.2
congenital Q24.6
first degree (atrioventricular) I44.0
second degree (atrioventricular) I44.1
specified type NEC I45.5
third degree (atrioventricular) I44.2
hepatic vein I82.0
intraventricular (nonspecific) I45.4
bundle branch
bilateral I45.2
kidney N28.9
postcystoscopic or postprocedural N99.0

Block, blocked *(Continued)*
Mobitz (types I and II) I44.1
myocardial *—see* Block, heart
nodal I45.5
organ or site, congenital NEC *—see* Atresia, by site
portal (vein) I81
second degree (types I and II) I44.1
sinoatrial I45.5
sinoauricular I45.5
third degree I44.2
trifascicular I45.3
tubal N97.1
vein NOS I82.90
Wenckebach (types I and II) I44.1
Blockage *—see* Obstruction
Blocq's disease F44.4
Blood
constituents, abnormal R78.9
disease D75.9
donor *—see* Donor, blood
dyscrasia D75.9
with
abortion *—see* Abortion, by type, complicated by, hemorrhage
ectopic pregnancy O08.1
molar pregnancy O08.1
following ectopic or molar pregnancy O08.1
newborn P61.9
puerperal, postpartum O72.3
flukes NEC *—see* Schistosomiasis
in
feces K92.1
occult R19.5
urine *—see* Hematuria
mole O02.0
occult in feces R19.5
pressure
decreased, due to shock following injury T79.4
examination only Z01.30
fluctuating I99.8
high *—see* Hypertension
borderline R03.0
incidental reading, without diagnosis of hypertension R03.0
low *—see also* Hypotension
incidental reading, without diagnosis of hypotension R03.1
spitting *—see* Hemoptysis
staining cornea *—see* Pigmentation, cornea, stromal
transfusion
reaction or complication *—see* Complications, transfusion
type
A (Rh positive) Z67.10
Rh negative Z67.11
AB (Rh positive) Z67.30
Rh negative Z67.31
B (Rh positive) Z67.20
Rh negative Z67.21
O (Rh positive) Z67.40
Rh negative Z67.41
Rh (positive) Z67.90
negative Z67.91
vessel rupture *—see* Hemorrhage
vomiting *—see* Hematemesis
Blood-forming organs, disease D75.9
Bloodgood's disease *—see* Mastopathy, cystic
Bloom (-Machacek)(-Torre) **syndrome** Q82.8
Blount's disease or osteochondrosis *—see* Osteochondrosis, juvenile, tibia
Blue
baby Q24.9
diaper syndrome E72.09
dome cyst (breast) *—see* Cyst, breast
dot cataract Q12.0
nevus D22.9

Blue *(Continued)*
sclera Q13.5
with fragility of bone and deafness Q78.0
toe syndrome I75.02-●
Blueness *—see* Cyanosis
Blues, postpartal O90.6
baby O90.6
Blurring, visual H53.8
Blushing (abnormal) (excessive) R23.2
BMI *—see* Body, mass index
Boarder, hospital NEC Z76.4
accompanying sick person Z76.3
healthy infant or child Z76.2
foundling Z76.1
Bockhart's impetigo L01.02
Bodechtel-Guttman disease (subacute sclerosing panencephalitis) A81.1
Boder-Sedgwick syndrome (ataxia-telangiectasia) G11.3
Body, bodies
Aschoff's *—see* Myocarditis, rheumatic
asteroid, vitreous *—see* Deposit, crystalline
cytoid (retina) *—see* Occlusion, artery, retina
drusen (degenerative) (macula) (retinal) *—see also* Degeneration, macula, drusen
optic disc *—see* Drusen, optic disc
foreign *—see* Foreign body
loose
joint, except knee *—see* Loose, body, joint
knee M23.4-●
sheath, tendon *—see* Disorder, tendon, specified type NEC
mass index (BMI)
adult
19.9 or less Z68.1
20.0-20.9 Z68.20
21.0-21.9 Z68.21
22.0-22.9 Z68.22
23.0-23.9 Z68.23
24.0-24.9 Z68.24
25.0-25.9 Z68.25
26.0-26.9 Z68.26
27.0-27.9 Z68.27
28.0-28.9 Z68.28
29.0-29.9 Z68.29
30.0-30.9 Z68.30
31.0-31.9 Z68.31
32.0-32.9 Z68.32
33.0-33.9 Z68.33
34.0-34.9 Z68.34
35.0-35.9 Z68.35
36.0-36.9 Z68.36
37.0-37.9 Z68.37
38.0-38.9 Z68.38
39.0-39.9 Z68.39
40.0-44.9 Z68.41
45.0-49.9 Z68.42
50.0-59.9 Z68.43
60.0-69.9 Z68.44
70 and over Z68.45
pediatric
5th percentile to less than 85th percentile for age Z68.52
85th percentile to less than 95th percentile for age Z68.53
greater than or equal to ninety-fifth percentile for age Z68.54
less than fifth percentile for age Z68.51
Mooser's A75.2
rice *—see also* Loose, body, joint
knee M23.4-●
rocking F98.4
Boeck's
disease or sarcoid *—see* Sarcoidosis
lupoid (miliary) D86.3
Boerhaave's syndrome (spontaneous esophageal rupture) K22.3
Boggy
cervix N88.8
uterus N85.8

Boil —*see also* Furuncle, by site
  Aleppo B55.1
  Baghdad B55.1
  Delhi B55.1
  lacrimal
    gland —*see* Dacryoadenitis
    passages (duct) (sac) —*see* Inflammation, lacrimal, passages, acute
  Natal B55.1
  orbit, orbital —*see* Abscess, orbit
  tropical B55.1
Bold hives —*see* Urticaria
Bombé, iris —*see* Membrane, pupillary
Bone —*see* condition
Bonnevie-Ullrich syndrome —*see also* Turner's syndrome Q87.19
Bonnier's syndrome —*see* subcategory H81.8
Bonvale dam fever T73.3
Bony block of joint —*see* Ankylosis
BOOP (bronchiolitis obliterans organized pneumonia) J84.89
Borderline
  diabetes mellitus R73.03
  hypertension R03.0
  osteopenia M85.8-●
  pelvis, with obstruction during labor O65.1
  personality F60.3
Borna disease A83.9
Bornholm disease B33.0
Boston exanthem A88.0
Botalli, ductus (patent) (persistent) Q25.0
Bothriocephalus latus infestation B70.0
Botulism (foodborne intoxication) A05.1
  infant A48.51
  non-foodborne A48.52
  wound A48.52
Bouba —*see* Yaws
Bouchard's nodes (with arthropathy) M15.2
Bouffée délirante F23
Bouillaud's disease or syndrome (rheumatic heart disease) I01.9
Bourneville's disease Q85.1
Boutonniere deformity (finger) —*see* Deformity, finger, boutonniere
Bouveret (-Hoffmann) syndrome (paroxysmal tachycardia) I47.9
Bovine heart —*see* Hypertrophy, cardiac
Bowel —*see* condition
Bowen's
  dermatosis (precancerous) —*see* Neoplasm, skin, in situ
  disease —*see* Neoplasm, skin, in situ
  epithelioma —*see* Neoplasm, skin, in situ
  type
    epidermoid carcinoma-in-situ —*see* Neoplasm, skin, in situ
    intraepidermal squamous cell carcinoma —*see* Neoplasm, skin, in situ
Bowing
  femur —*see also* Deformity, limb, specified type NEC, thigh
    congenital Q68.3
  fibula —*see also* Deformity, limb, specified type NEC, lower leg
    congenital Q68.4
  forearm —*see* Deformity, limb, specified type NEC, forearm
  leg(s), long bones, congenital Q68.5
  radius —*see* Deformity, limb, specified type NEC, forearm
  tibia —*see also* Deformity, limb, specified type NEC, lower leg
    congenital Q68.4
Bowleg(s) (acquired) M21.16-●
  congenital Q68.5
  rachitic E64.3
Boyd's dysentery A03.2
Brachial —*see* condition
Brachycardia R00.1
Brachycephaly Q75.0
Bradley's disease A08.19
Bradyarrhythmia, cardiac I49.8
Bradycardia (sinoatrial) (sinus) (vagal) R00.1
  neonatal P29.12
  reflex G90.09
  tachycardia syndrome I49.5
Bradykinesia R25.8
Bradypnea R06.89
Bradytachycardia I49.5
Brailsford's disease or osteochondrosis —*see* Osteochondrosis, juvenile, radius
Brain —*see also* condition
  death G93.82
  syndrome —*see* Syndrome, brain
Branched-chain amino-acid disorder E71.2
Branchial —*see* condition
  cartilage, congenital Q18.2
Branchiogenic remnant (in neck) Q18.0
Brandt's syndrome (acrodermatitis enteropathica) E83.2
Brash (water) R12
Bravais-Jacksonian epilepsy —*see* Epilepsy, localization-related, symptomatic, with simple partial seizures
Braxton Hicks contractions —*see* False, labor
Brazilian leishmaniasis B55.2
BRBPR K62.5
Break, retina (without detachment) H33.30-●
  with retinal detachment —*see* Detachment, retina
  horseshoe tear H33.31-●
  multiple H33.33-●
  round hole H33.32-●
Breakdown
  device, graft or implant —*see also* Complications, by site and type, mechanical T85.618
    arterial graft NEC —*see* Complication, cardiovascular device, mechanical, vascular
    breast (implant) T85.41
    catheter NEC T85.618
      cystostomy T83.010
      dialysis (renal) T82.41
        intraperitoneal T85.611
      Hopkins T83.018
      ileostomy T83.018
      infusion NEC T82.514
        cranial T85.610
        epidural T85.610
        intrathecal T85.610
        spinal T85.610
        subarachnoid T85.610
        subdural T85.610
      nephrostomy T83.012
      urethral indwelling T83.011
      urinary NEC T83.018
      urostomy T83.018
    electronic (electrode) (pulse generator) (stimulator)
      bone T84.310
      cardiac T82.119
        electrode T82.110
        pulse generator T82.111
        specified type NEC T82.118
      nervous system —*see* Complication, prosthetic device, mechanical, electronic nervous system stimulator
      urinary —*see* Complication, genitourinary, device, urinary, mechanical
    fixation, internal (orthopedic) NEC —*see* Complication, fixation device, mechanical
    gastrointestinal —*see* Complications, prosthetic device, mechanical, gastrointestinal device
    genital NEC T83.418
      intrauterine contraceptive device T83.31
      penile prosthesis (cylinder) (implanted) (pump) (resevoir) T83.410
      testicular prosthesis T83.411
Breakdown *(Continued)*
  device, graft or implant *(Continued)*
    heart NEC —*see* Complication, cardiovascular device, mechanical
    intrathecal infusion pump T85.615
    joint prosthesis —*see* Complications..., joint prosthesis,internal, mechanical, by site
    nervous system, specified device NEC T85.615
    ocular NEC —*see* Complications, prosthetic device, mechanical, ocular device
    orthopedic NEC —*see* Complication, orthopedic, device, mechanical
    specified NEC T85.618
    subcutaneous device pocket
      nervous system prosthetic device, implant, or graft T85.890
      other internal prosthetic device, implant, or graft T85.898
    sutures, permanent T85.612
      used in bone repair —*see* Complications, fixation device, internal (orthopedic), mechanical
    urinary NEC T83.118
      graft T83.21
      sphincter, implanted T83.111
      stent (ileal conduit) (nephroureteral) T83.113
        ureteral indwelling T83.112
    vascular NEC —*see* Complication, cardiovascular device, mechanical
    ventricular intracranial shunt T85.01
  nervous F48.8
  perineum O90.1
  respirator J95.850
    specified NEC J95.859
  ventilator J95.850
    specified NEC J95.859
Breast —*see also* condition
  buds E30.1
    in newborn P96.89
  dense R92.2
  nodule —*see also* Lump, breast N63.0
Breath
  foul R19.6
  holder, child R06.89
  holding spell R06.89
  shortness R06.02
Breathing
  labored —*see* Hyperventilation
  mouth R06.5
    causing malocclusion M26.5
  periodic R06.3
    high altitude G47.32
Breathlessness R06.81
Breda's disease —*see* Yaws
Breech presentation (mother) O32.1
  causing obstructed labor O64.1
  footling O32.8
    causing obstructed labor O64.8
  incomplete O32.8
    causing obstructed labor O64.8
Breisky's disease N90.4
Brennemann's syndrome I88.0
Brenner
  tumor (benign) D27.9
    borderline malignancy D39.1-●
    malignant C56
    proliferating D39.1
Bretonneau's disease or angina A36.0
Breus' mole O02.0
Brevicollis Q76.49
Brickmakers' anemia B76.9 *[D63.8]*
Bridge, myocardial Q24.5
Bright red blood per rectum (BRBPR) K62.5
Bright's disease —*see also* Nephritis
  arteriosclerotic —*see* Hypertension, kidney
Brill (-Zinsser) disease (recrudescent typhus) A75.1
  ~~flea-borne A75.2~~
  ~~louse-borne A75.1~~

B

Brill-Symmers' disease C82.90
Brion-Kayser disease —*see* Fever, parathyroid
Briquet's disorder or syndrome F45.0
Brissaud's
infantilism or dwarfism E23.0
motor-verbal tic F95.2
Brittle
bones disease Q78.0
nails L60.3
congenital Q84.6
Broad —*see also* condition
beta disease E78.2
ligament laceration syndrome N83.8
Broad- or floating-betalipoproteinemia E78.2
Brock's syndrome (atelectasis due to enlarged lymph nodes) J98.19
Brocq-Duhring disease (dermatitis herpetiformis) L13.0
Brodie's abscess or disease M86.8X-●
Broken
arches —*see also* Deformity, limb, flat foot
arm (meaning upper limb) —*see* Fracture, arm
back —*see* Fracture, vertebra
bone —*see* Fracture
implant or internal device —*see* Complications, by site and type, mechanical
leg (meaning lower limb) —*see* Fracture, leg
nose S02.2
tooth, teeth —*see* Fracture, tooth
Bromhidrosis, bromidrosis L75.0
Bromidism, bromism G92
chronic (dependence) F13.20
due to
correct substance properly administered —*see* Table of Drugs and Chemicals, by drug, adverse effect
overdose or wrong substance given or taken —*see* Table of Drugs and Chemicals, by drug, poisoning
Bromidrosiphobia F40.298
Bronchi, bronchial —*see* condition
Bronchiectasis (cylindrical) (diffuse) (fusiform) (localized) (saccular) J47.9
with
acute
bronchitis J47.0
lower respiratory infection J47.0
exacerbation (acute) J47.1
congenital Q33.4
tuberculous NEC —*see* Tuberculosis, pulmonary
Bronchiolectasis —*see* Bronchiectasis
Bronchiolitis (acute) (infective) (subacute) J21.9
with
bronchospasm or obstruction J21.9
influenza, flu or grippe —*see* Influenza, with, respiratory manifestations NEC
chemical (chronic) J68.4
acute J68.0
chronic (fibrosing) (obliterative) J44.9
due to
external agent —*see* Bronchitis, acute, due to
human metapneumovirus J21.1
➧respiratory syncytial virus (RSV) J21.0
specified organism NEC J21.8
fibrosa obliterans J44.9
influenzal —*see* Influenza, with, respiratory manifestations NEC
obliterans J42
with organizing pneumonia (BOOP) J84.89
obliterative (chronic) (subacute) J44.9
due to chemicals, gases, fumes or vapors (inhalation) J68.4
due to fumes or vapors J68.4
respiratory, interstitial lung disease J84.115
Bronchitis (diffuse) (fibrinous) (hypostatic) (infective) (membranous) J40
with
influenza, flu or grippe —*see* Influenza, with, respiratory manifestations NEC
Bronchitis *(Continued)*
with *(Continued)*
obstruction (airway) (lung) J44.9
tracheitis (15 years of age and above) J40
acute or subacute J20.9
chronic J42
under 15 years of age J20.9
acute or subacute (with bronchospasm or obstruction) J20.9
with
bronchiectasis J47.0
chronic obstructive pulmonary disease J44.0
chemical (due to gases, fumes or vapors) J68.0
due to
fumes or vapors J68.0
Haemophilus influenzae J20.1
Mycoplasma pneumoniae J20.0
radiation J70.0
specified organism NEC J20.8
Streptococcus J20.2
virus
coxsackie J20.3
echovirus J20.7
parainfluenzae J20.4
➧respiratory syncytial (RSV) J20.5
rhinovirus J20.6
viral NEC J20.8
allergic (acute) J45.909
with
exacerbation (acute) J45.901
status asthmaticus J45.902
arachidic T17.528
aspiration (due to fumes or vapors) J68.0
asthmatic J45.9
chronic J44.9
with
acute lower respiratory infection J44.0
exacerbation (acute) J44.1
capillary —*see* Pneumonia, broncho
caseous (tuberculous) A15.5
Castellani's A69.8
catarrhal (15 years of age and above) J40
acute —*see* Bronchitis, acute
chronic J41.0
under 15 years of age J20.9
chemical (acute) (subacute) J68.0
chronic J68.4
due to fumes or vapors J68.0
chronic J68.4
chronic J42
with
airways obstruction J44.9
tracheitis (chronic) J42
asthmatic (obstructive) J44.9
catarrhal J41.0
chemical (due to fumes or vapors) J68.4
due to
chemicals, gases, fumes or vapors (inhalation) J68.4
radiation J70.1
tobacco smoking J41.0
emphysematous J44.9
mucopurulent J41.1
non-obstructive J41.0
obliterans J44.9
obstructive J44.9
purulent J41.1
simple J41.0
croupous —*see* Bronchitis, acute
due to gases, fumes or vapors (chemical) J68.0
emphysematous (obstructive) J44.9
exudative —*see* Bronchitis, acute
fetid J41.1
grippal —*see* Influenza, with, respiratory manifestations NEC
in those under 15 years age —*see* Bronchitis, acute
chronic —*see* Bronchitis, chronic
Bronchitis *(Continued)*
influenzal —*see* Influenza, with, respiratory manifestations NEC
mixed simple and mucopurulent J41.8
moulder's J62.8
mucopurulent (chronic) (recurrent) J41.1
acute or subacute J20.9
simple (mixed) J41.8
obliterans (chronic) J44.9
obstructive (chronic) (diffuse) J44.9
pituitous J41.1
pneumococcal, acute or subacute J20.2
pseudomembranous, acute or subacute —*see* Bronchitis, acute
purulent (chronic) (recurrent) J41.1
acute or subacute —*see* Bronchitis, acute
putrid J41.1
senile (chronic) J42
simple and mucopurulent (mixed) J41.8
smokers' J41.0
spirochetal NEC A69.8
subacute —*see* Bronchitis, acute
suppurative (chronic) J41.1
acute or subacute —*see* Bronchitis, acute
tuberculous A15.5
under 15 years of age —*see* Bronchitis, acute
chronic —*see* Bronchitis, chronic
viral NEC, acute or subacute —*see also* Bronchitis, acute J20.8
Bronchoalveolitis J18.0
Bronchoaspergillosis B44.1
Bronchocele meaning goiter E04.0
Broncholithiasis J98.09
tuberculous NEC A15.5
Bronchomalacia J98.09
congenital Q32.2
Bronchomycosis NOS B49 *[J99]*
candidal B37.1
Bronchopleuropneumonia —*see* Pneumonia, broncho
Bronchopneumonia —*see* Pneumonia, broncho
Bronchopneumonitis —*see* Pneumonia, broncho
Bronchopulmonary —*see* condition
Bronchopulmonitis —*see* Pneumonia, broncho
Bronchorrhagia (*see* Hemoptysis)
Bronchorrhea J98.09
acute J20.9
chronic (infective) (purulent) J42
Bronchospasm (acute) J98.01
with
bronchiolitis, acute J21.9
bronchitis, acute (conditions in J20) —*see* Bronchitis, acute
due to external agent —*see* condition, respiratory, acute, due to
exercise induced J45.990
Bronchospirochetosis A69.8
Castellani A69.8
Bronchostenosis J98.09
Bronchus —*see* condition
Brontophobia F40.220
Bronze baby syndrome P83.88
Brooke's tumor —*see* Neoplasm, skin, benign
Brown enamel of teeth (hereditary) K00.5
Brown's sheath syndrome H50.61-●
Brown-Séquard disease, paralysis or syndrome G83.81
Bruce sepsis A23.0
Brucellosis (infection) A23.9
abortus A23.1
canis A23.3
dermatitis A23.9
melitensis A23.0
mixed A23.8
sepsis A23.9
melitensis A23.0
specified NEC A23.8
suis A23.2
➧Bruck-de Lange disease Q87.19
Bruck's disease —*see* Deformity, limb

B

BRUE (brief resolved unexplained event) R68.13
Brugsch's syndrome Q82.8
Bruise (skin surface intact) —*see also* Contusion
with
open wound —*see* Wound, open
internal organ —*see* Injury, by site
newborn P54.5
scalp, due to birth injury, newborn P12.3
umbilical cord O69.5
Bruit (arterial) R09.89
cardiac R01.1
Brush burn —*see* Abrasion, by site
Bruton's X-linked agammaglobulinemia D80.0
Bruxism
psychogenic F45.8
sleep related G47.63
Bubbly lung syndrome P27.0
Bubo I88.8
blennorrhagic (gonococcal) A54.89
chancroidal A57
climatic A55
due to Haemophilus ducreyi A57
gonococcal A54.89
indolent (nonspecific) I88.8
inguinal (nonspecific) I88.8
chancroidal A57
climatic A55
due to H. ducreyi A57
infective I88.8
scrofulous (tuberculous) A18.2
soft chancre A57
suppurating —*see* Lymphadenitis, acute
syphilitic (primary) A51.0
congenital A50.07
tropical A55
virulent (chancroidal) A57
Bubonic plague A20.0
Bubonocele —*see* Hernia, inguinal
Buccal —*see* condition
Buchanan's disease or osteochondrosis M91.0
Buchem's syndrome (hyperostosis corticalis) M85.2
Bucket-handle fracture or tear (semilunar cartilage) —*see* Tear, meniscus
Budd-Chiari syndrome (hepatic vein thrombosis) I82.0
Budgerigar fancier's disease or lung J67.2
Buds
breast E30.1
in newborn P96.89
Buerger's disease (thromboangiitis obliterans) I73.1
Bulbar —*see* condition
Bulbus cordis (left ventricle) (persistent) Q21.8
Bulimia (nervosa) F50.2
atypical F50.9
normal weight F50.9
Bulky
stools R19.5
uterus N85.2
Bulla (e) R23.8
lung (emphysematous) (solitary) J43.9
newborn P25.8
Bullet wound —*see also* Wound, open
fracture - code as Fracture, by site
internal organ —*see* Injury, by site
Bundle
branch block (complete) (false) (incomplete) —*see* Block, bundle-branch
of His —*see* condition
Bunion M21.61-●
tailor's M21.62-●
Bunionette M21.62-●
Buphthalmia, buphthalmos (congenital) Q15.0
Burdwan fever B55.0
Bürger-Grütz disease or syndrome E78.3
Buried
penis (congenital) Q55.64
acquired N48.83
roots K08.3
Burke's syndrome K86.89
Burkitt
cell leukemia C91.0-●
lymphoma (malignant) C83.7-●
small noncleaved, diffuse C83.7-●
spleen C83.77
undifferentiated C83.7-●
tumor C83.7-●
type
acute lymphoblastic leukemia C91.0-●
undifferentiated C83.7-●
Burn (electricity) (flame) (hot gas, liquid or hot object) (radiation) (steam) (thermal) T30.0
abdomen, abdominal (muscle) (wall) T21.02
first degree T21.12
second degree T21.22
third degree T21.32
above elbow T22.039
first degree T22.139
left T22.032
first degree T22.132
second degree T22.232
third degree T22.332
right T22.031
first degree T22.131
second degree T22.231
third degree T22.331
second degree T22.239
third degree T22.339
acid (caustic) (external) (internal) —*see* Corrosion, by site
alimentary tract NEC T28.2
esophagus T28.1
mouth T28.0
pharynx T28.0
alkaline (caustic) (external) (internal) —*see* Corrosion, by site
ankle T25.019
first degree T25.119
left T25.012
first degree T25.112
second degree T25.212
third degree T25.312
multiple with foot —*see* Burn, lower, limb, multiple, ankle and foot
right T25.011
first degree T25.111
second degree T25.211
third degree T25.311
second degree T25.219
third degree T25.319
anus —*see* Burn, buttock
arm (lower) (upper) —*see* Burn, upper, limb
axilla T22.049
first degree T22.149
left T22.042
first degree T22.142
second degree T22.242
third degree T22.342
right T22.041
first degree T22.141
second degree T22.241
third degree T22.341
second degree T22.249
third degree T22.349
back (lower) T21.04
first degree T21.14
second degree T21.24
third degree T21.34
upper T21.03
first degree T21.13
second degree T21.23
third degree T21.33
blisters - code as Burn, second degree, by site
breast(s) —*see* Burn, chest wall
buttock(s) T21.05
first degree T21.15
second degree T21.25
third degree T21.35
Burn *(Continued)*
calf T24.039
first degree T24.139
left T24.032
first degree T24.132
second degree T24.232
third degree T24.332
right T24.031
first degree T24.131
second degree T24.231
third degree T24.331
second degree T24.239
third degree T24.339
canthus (eye) —*see* Burn, eyelid
caustic acid or alkaline —*see* Corrosion, by site
cervix T28.3
cheek T20.06
first degree T20.16
second degree T20.26
third degree T20.36
chemical (acids) (alkalines) (caustics) (external) (internal) —*see* Corrosion, by site
chest wall T21.01
first degree T21.11
second degree T21.21
third degree T21.31
chin T20.03
first degree T20.13
second degree T20.23
third degree T20.33
colon T28.2
conjunctiva (and cornea) —*see* Burn, cornea
cornea (and conjunctiva) T26.1-●
chemical —*see* Corrosion, cornea
corrosion (external) (internal) —*see* Corrosion, by site
deep necrosis of underlying tissue - code as Burn, third degree, by site
dorsum of hand T23.069
first degree T23.169
left T23.062
first degree T23.162
second degree T23.262
third degree T23.362
right T23.061
first degree T23.161
second degree T23.261
third degree T23.361
second degree T23.269
third degree T23.369
due to ingested chemical agent —*see* Corrosion, by site
ear (auricle) (external) (canal) T20.01
first degree T20.11
second degree T20.21
third degree T20.31
elbow T22.029
first degree T22.129
left T22.022
first degree T22.122
second degree T22.222
third degree T22.322
right T22.021
first degree T22.121
second degree T22.221
third degree T22.321
second degree T22.229
third degree T22.329
epidermal loss - code as Burn, second degree, by site
erythema, erythematous - code as Burn, first degree, by site
esophagus T28.1
extent (percentage of body surface)
less than 10 percent T31.0
10-19 percent T31.10
with 0-9 percent third degree burns T31.10
with 10-19 percent third degree burns T31.11

Burn (Continued)
extent (Continued)
20-29 percent T31.20
with 0-9 percent third degree burns T31.20
with 10-19 percent third degree burns T31.21
with 20-29 percent third degree burns T31.22
30-39 percent T31.30
with 0-9 percent third degree burns T31.30
with 10-19 percent third degree burns T31.31
with 20-29 percent third degree burns T31.32
with 30-39 percent third degree burns T31.33
40-49 percent T31.40
with 0-9 percent third degree burns T31.40
with 10-19 percent third degree burns T31.41
with 20-29 percent third degree burns T31.42
with 30-39 percent third degree burns T31.43
with 40-49 percent third degree burns T31.44
50-59 percent T31.50
with 0-9 percent third degree burns T31.50
with 10-19 percent third degree burns T31.51
with 20-29 percent third degree burns T31.52
with 30-39 percent third degree burns T31.53
with 40-49 percent third degree burns T31.54
with 50-59 percent third degree burns T31.55
60-69 percent T31.60
with 0-9 percent third degree burns T31.60
with 10-19 percent third degree burns T31.61
with 20-29 percent third degree burns T31.62
with 30-39 percent third degree burns T31.63
with 40-49 percent third degree burns T31.64
with 50-59 percent third degree burns T31.65
with 60-69 percent third degree burns T31.66
70-79 percent T31.70
with 0-9 percent third degree burns T31.70
with 10-19 percent third degree burns T31.71
with 20-29 percent third degree burns T31.72
with 30-39 percent third degree burns T31.73
with 40-49 percent third degree burns T31.74
with 50-59 percent third degree burns T31.75
with 60-69 percent third degree burns T31.76
with 70-79 percent third degree burns T31.77
80-89 percent T31.80
with 0-9 percent third degree burns T31.80
with 10-19 percent third degree burns T31.81
with 20-29 percent third degree burns T31.82
with 30-39 percent third degree burns T31.83
with 40-49 percent third degree burns T31.84

Burn (Continued)
extent (Continued)
80-89 percent T31.80 (Continued)
with 50-59 percent third degree burns T31.85
with 60-69 percent third degree burns T31.86
with 70-79 percent third degree burns T31.87
with 80-89 percent third degree burns T31.88
90 percent or more T31.90
with 0-9 percent third degree burns T31.90
with 10-19 percent third degree burns T31.91
with 20-29 percent third degree burns T31.92
with 30-39 percent third degree burns T31.93
with 40-49 percent third degree burns T31.94
with 50-59 percent third degree burns T31.95
with 60-69 percent third degree burns T31.96
with 70-79 percent third degree burns T31.97
with 80-89 percent third degree burns T31.98
with 90 percent or more third degree burns T31.99
extremity —*see* Burn, limb
eye(s) and adnexa T26.4-●
with resulting rupture and destruction of eyeball T26.2-●
conjunctival sac —*see* Burn, cornea
cornea —*see* Burn, cornea
lid —*see* Burn, eyelid
periocular area —*see* Burn, eyelid
specified site NEC T26.3-●
eyeball —*see* Burn, eye
eyelid(s) T26.0-●
chemical —*see* Corrosion, eyelid
face —*see* Burn, head
finger T23.029
first degree T23.129
left T23.022
first degree T23.122
second degree T23.222
third degree T23.322
multiple sites (without thumb) T23.039
with thumb T23.049
first degree T23.149
left T23.042
first degree T23.142
second degree T23.242
third degree T23.342
right T23.041
first degree T23.141
second degree T23.241
third degree T23.341
second degree T23.249
third degree T23.349
first degree T23.139
left T23.032
first degree T23.132
second degree T23.232
third degree T23.332
right T23.031
first degree T23.131
second degree T23.231
third degree T23.331
second degree T23.239
third degree T23.339
right T23.021
first degree T23.121
second degree T23.221
third degree T23.321
second degree T23.229
third degree T23.329
flank —*see* Burn, abdominal wall

Burn (Continued)
foot T25.029
first degree T25.129
left T25.022
first degree T25.122
second degree T25.222
third degree T25.322
multiple with ankle —*see* Burn, lower, limb, multiple, ankle and foot
right T25.021
first degree T25.121
second degree T25.221
third degree T25.321
second degree T25.229
third degree T25.329
forearm T22.019
first degree T22.119
left T22.012
first degree T22.112
second degree T22.212
third degree T22.312
right T22.011
first degree T22.111
second degree T22.211
third degree T22.311
second degree T22.219
third degree T22.319
forehead T20.06
first degree T20.16
second degree T20.26
third degree T20.36
fourth degree - code as Burn, third degree, by site
friction —*see* Burn, by site
from swallowing caustic or corrosive substance NEC —*see* Corrosion, by site
full thickness skin loss - code as Burn, third degree, by site
gastrointestinal tract NEC T28.2
from swallowing caustic or corrosive substance T28.7
genital organs
external
female T21.07
first degree T21.17
second degree T21.27
third degree T21.37
male T21.06
first degree T21.16
second degree T21.26
third degree T21.36
internal T28.3
from caustic or corrosive substance T28.8
groin —*see* Burn, abdominal wall
hand(s) T23.009
back —*see* Burn, dorsum of hand
finger —*see* Burn, finger
first degree T23.109
left T23.002
first degree T23.102
second degree T23.202
third degree T23.302
multiple sites with wrist T23.099
first degree T23.199
left T23.092
first degree T23.192
second degree T23.292
third degree T23.392
right T23.091
first degree T23.191
second degree T23.291
third degree T23.391
second degree T23.299
third degree T23.399
palm —*see* Burn, palm
right T23.001
first degree T23.101
second degree T23.201
third degree T23.301

Burn (Continued)
hand (Continued)
second degree T23.2Ø9
third degree T23.3Ø9
thumb —see Burn, thumb
head (and face) (and neck) T2Ø.ØØ
cheek —see Burn, cheek
chin —see Burn, chin
ear —see Burn, ear
eye(s) only —see Burn, eye
first degree T2Ø.1Ø
forehead —see Burn, forehead
lip —see Burn, lip
multiple sites T2Ø.Ø9
first degree T2Ø.19
second degree T2Ø.29
third degree T2Ø.39
neck —see Burn, neck
nose —see Burn, nose
scalp —see Burn, scalp
second degree T2Ø.2Ø
third degree T2Ø.3Ø
hip(s) —see Burn, thigh
inhalation —see Burn, respiratory tract
caustic or corrosive substance (fumes) —see Corrosion, respiratory tract
internal organ(s) T28.4Ø
alimentary tract T28.2
esophagus T28.1
eardrum T28.41
esophagus T28.1
from caustic or corrosive substance (swallowing) NEC —see Corrosion, by site
genitourinary T28.3
mouth T28.Ø
pharynx T28.Ø
respiratory tract —see Burn, respiratory tract
specified organ NEC T28.49
interscapular region —see Burn, back, upper
intestine (large) (small) T28.2
knee T24.Ø29
first degree T24.129
left T24.Ø22
first degree T24.122
second degree T24.222
third degree T24.322
right T24.Ø21
first degree T24.121
second degree T24.221
third degree T24.321
second degree T24.229
third degree T24.329
labium (majus) (minus) —see Burn, genital organs, external, female
lacrimal apparatus, duct, gland or sac —see Burn, eye, specified site NEC
larynx T27.Ø
with lung T27.1
leg(s) (lower) (upper) —see Burn, lower, limb
lightning —see Burn, by site
limb(s)
lower (except ankle or foot alone) —see Burn, lower, limb
upper —see Burn, upper limb
lip(s) T2Ø.Ø2
first degree T2Ø.12
second degree T2Ø.22
third degree T2Ø.32
lower
back —see Burn, back
limb T24.ØØ9
ankle —see Burn, ankle
calf —see Burn, calf
first degree T24.1Ø9
foot —see Burn, foot
hip —see Burn, thigh
knee —see Burn, knee

Burn (Continued)
lower (Continued)
limb (Continued)
left T24.ØØ2
first degree T24.1Ø2
second degree T24.2Ø2
third degree T24.3Ø2
multiple sites, except ankle and foot T24.Ø99
ankle and foot T25.Ø99
first degree T25.199
left T25.Ø92
first degree T25.192
second degree T25.292
third degree T25.392
right T25.Ø91
first degree T25.191
second degree T25.291
third degree T25.391
second degree T25.299
third degree T25.399
first degree T24.199
left T24.Ø92
first degree T24.192
second degree T24.292
third degree T24.392
right T24.Ø91
first degree T24.191
second degree T24.291
third degree T24.391
second degree T24.299
third degree T24.399
right T24.ØØ1
first degree T24.1Ø1
second degree T24.2Ø1
third degree T24.3Ø1
second degree T24.2Ø9
thigh —see Burn, thigh
third degree T24.3Ø9
toe —see Burn, toe
lung (with larynx and trachea) T27.1
mouth T28.Ø
neck T2Ø.Ø7
first degree T2Ø.17
second degree T2Ø.27
third degree T2Ø.37
nose (septum) T2Ø.Ø4
first degree T2Ø.14
second degree T2Ø.24
third degree T2Ø.34
ocular adnexa —see Burn, eye
orbit region —see Burn, eyelid
palm T23.Ø59
first degree T23.159
left T23.Ø52
first degree T23.152
second degree T23.252
third degree T23.352
right T23.Ø51
first degree T23.151
second degree T23.251
third degree T23.351
second degree T23.259
third degree T23.359
partial thickness - code as Burn, degree, by site
pelvis —see Burn, trunk
penis —see Burn, genital organs, external, male
perineum
female —see Burn, genital organs, external, female
male —see Burn, genital organs, external, male
periocular area —see Burn, eyelid
pharynx T28.Ø
rectum T28.2
respiratory tract T27.3
larynx —see Burn, larynx
specified part NEC T27.2
trachea —see Burn, trachea

Burn (Continued)
sac, lacrimal —see Burn, eye, specified site NEC
scalp T2Ø.Ø5
first degree T2Ø.15
second degree T2Ø.25
third degree T2Ø.35
scapular region T22.Ø69
first degree T22.169
left T22.Ø62
first degree T22.162
second degree T22.262
third degree T22.362
right T22.Ø61
first degree T22.161
second degree T22.261
third degree T22.361
second degree T22.269
third degree T22.369
sclera —see Burn, eye, specified site NEC
scrotum —see Burn, genital organs, external, male
shoulder T22.Ø59
first degree T22.159
left T22.Ø52
first degree T22.152
second degree T22.252
third degree T22.352
right T22.Ø51
first degree T22.151
second degree T22.251
third degree T22.351
second degree T22.259
third degree T22.359
stomach T28.2
temple —see Burn, head
testis —see Burn, genital organs, external, male
thigh T24.Ø19
first degree T24.119
left T24.Ø12
first degree T24.112
second degree T24.212
third degree T24.312
right T24.Ø11
first degree T24.111
second degree T24.211
third degree T24.311
second degree T24.219
third degree T24.319
thorax (external) —see Burn, trunk
throat (meaning pharynx) T28.Ø
thumb(s) T23.Ø19
first degree T23.119
left T23.Ø12
first degree T23.112
second degree T23.212
third degree T23.312
multiple sites with fingers T23.Ø49
first degree T23.149
left T23.Ø42
first degree T23.142
second degree T23.242
third degree T23.342
right T23.Ø41
first degree T23.141
second degree T23.241
third degree T23.341
second degree T23.249
third degree T23.349
right T23.Ø11
first degree T23.111
second degree T23.211
third degree T23.311
second degree T23.219
third degree T23.319
toe T25.Ø39
first degree T25.139
left T25.Ø32
first degree T25.132
second degree T25.232
third degree T25.332

Burn *(Continued)*
  toe *(Continued)*
    right T25.Ø31
      first degree T25.131
      second degree T25.231
      third degree T25.331
    second degree T25.239
    third degree T25.339
  tongue T28.Ø
  tonsil(s) T28.Ø
  trachea T27.Ø
    with lung T27.1
  trunk T21.ØØ
    abdominal wall —*see* Burn, abdominal wall
    anus —*see* Burn, buttock
    axilla —*see* Burn, upper limb
    back —*see* Burn, back
    breast —*see* Burn, chest wall
    buttock —*see* Burn, buttock
    chest wall —*see* Burn, chest wall
    first degree T21.1Ø
    flank —*see* Burn, abdominal wall
    genital
      female —*see* Burn, genital organs, external, female
      male —*see* Burn, genital organs, external, male
    groin —*see* Burn, abdominal wall
    interscapular region —*see* Burn, back, upper
    labia —*see* Burn, genital organs, external, female
    lower back —*see* Burn, back
    penis —*see* Burn, genital organs, external, male
    perineum
      female —*see* Burn, genital organs, external, female
      male —*see* Burn, genital organs, external, male
    scapula region —*see* Burn, scapular region
    scrotum —*see* Burn, genital organs, external, male
    second degree T21.2Ø
    specified site NEC T21.Ø9
      first degree T21.19
      second degree T21.29
      third degree T21.39
    testes —*see* Burn, genital organs, external, male
    third degree T21.3Ø
    upper back —*see* Burn, back, upper
    vulva —*see* Burn, genital organs, external, female
  unspecified site with extent of body surface involved specified
    less than 1Ø percent T31.Ø
    1Ø-19 percent (Ø-9 percent third degree) T31.1Ø
      with 1Ø-19 percent third degree T31.11
    2Ø-29 percent (Ø-9 percent third degree) T31.2Ø
      with
        1Ø-19 percent third degree T31.21
        2Ø-29 percent third degree T31.22
    3Ø-39 percent (Ø-9 percent third degree) T31.3Ø
      with
        1Ø-19 percent third degree T31.31
        2Ø-29 percent third degree T31.32
        3Ø-39 percent third degree T31.33
    4Ø-49 percent (Ø-9 percent third degree) T31.4Ø
      with
        1Ø-19 percent third degree T31.41
        2Ø-29 percent third degree T31.42
        3Ø-39 percent third degree T31.43
        4Ø-49 percent third degree T31.44

Burn *(Continued)*
  unspecified site with extent of body surface involved specified *(Continued)*
    5Ø-59 percent (Ø-9 percent third degree) T31.5Ø
      with
        1Ø-19 percent third degree T31.51
        2Ø-29 percent third degree T31.52
        3Ø-39 percent third degree T31.53
        4Ø-49 percent third degree T31.54
        5Ø-59 percent third degree T31.55
    6Ø-69 percent (Ø-9 percent third degree) T31.6Ø
      with
        1Ø-19 percent third degree T31.61
        2Ø-29 percent third degree T31.62
        3Ø-39 percent third degree T31.63
        4Ø-49 percent third degree T31.64
        5Ø-59 percent third degree T31.65
        6Ø-69 percent third degree T31.66
    7Ø-79 percent (Ø-9 percent third degree) T31.7Ø
      with
        1Ø-19 percent third degree T31.71
        2Ø-29 percent third degree T31.72
        3Ø-39 percent third degree T31.73
        4Ø-49 percent third degree T31.74
        5Ø-59 percent third degree T31.75
        6Ø-69 percent third degree T31.76
        7Ø-79 percent third degree T31.77
    8Ø-89 percent (Ø-9 percent third degree) T31.8Ø
      with
        1Ø-19 percent third degree T31.81
        2Ø-29 percent third degree T31.82
        3Ø-39 percent third degree T31.83
        4Ø-49 percent third degree T31.84
        5Ø-59 percent third degree T31.85
        6Ø-69 percent third degree T31.86
        7Ø-79 percent third degree T31.87
        8Ø-89 percent third degree T31.88
    9Ø percent or more (Ø-9 percent third degree) T31.9Ø
      with
        1Ø-19 percent third degree T31.91
        2Ø-29 percent third degree T31.92
        3Ø-39 percent third degree T31.93
        4Ø-49 percent third degree T31.94
        5Ø-59 percent third degree T31.95
        6Ø-69 percent third degree T31.96
        7Ø-79 percent third degree T31.97
        8Ø-89 percent third degree T31.98
        9Ø-99 percent third degree T31.99
  upper limb T22.ØØ
    above elbow —*see* Burn, above elbow
    axilla —*see* Burn, axilla
    elbow —*see* Burn, elbow
    first degree T22.1Ø
    forearm —*see* Burn, forearm
    hand —*see* Burn, hand
    interscapular region —*see* Burn, back, upper
    multiple sites T22.Ø99
      first degree T22.199
      left T22.Ø92
        first degree T22.192
        second degree T22.292
        third degree T22.392
      right T22.Ø91
        first degree T22.191
        second degree T22.291
        third degree T22.391
      second degree T22.299
      third degree T22.399
    scapular region —*see* Burn, scapular region
    second degree T22.2Ø
    shoulder —*see* Burn, shoulder
    third degree T22.3Ø
    wrist —*see* Burn, wrist
  uterus T28.3
  vagina T28.3

Burn *(Continued)*
  vulva —*see* Burn, genital organs, external, female
  wrist T23.Ø79
    first degree T23.179
    left T23.Ø72
      first degree T23.172
      second degree T23.272
      third degree T23.372
    multiple sites with hand T23.Ø99
      first degree T23.199
      left T23.Ø92
        first degree T23.192
        second degree T23.292
        third degree T23.392
      right T23.Ø91
        first degree T23.191
        second degree T23.291
        third degree T23.391
      second degree T23.299
      third degree T23.399
    right T23.Ø71
      first degree T23.171
      second degree T23.271
      third degree T23.371
    second degree T23.279
    third degree T23.379
Burnett's syndrome E83.52
Burning
  feet syndrome E53.9
  sensation R2Ø.8
  tongue K14.6
Burn-out (state) Z73.Ø
Burns' disease or osteochondrosis —*see* Osteochondrosis, juvenile, ulna
Bursa —*see* condition
Bursitis M71.9
  Achilles —*see* Tendinitis, Achilles
  adhesive —*see* Bursitis, specified NEC
  ankle —*see* Enthesopathy, lower limb, ankle, specified type NEC
  calcaneal —*see* Enthesopathy, foot, specified type NEC
  collateral ligament, tibial —*see* Bursitis, tibial collateral
  due to use, overuse, pressure —*see also* Disorder, soft tissue, due to use, specified type NEC
    specified NEC —*see* Disorder, soft tissue, due to use, specified NEC
  Duplay's M75.Ø
  elbow NEC M7Ø.3- •
    olecranon M7Ø.2- •
  finger —*see* Disorder, soft tissue, due to use, specified type NEC, hand
  foot —*see* Enthesopathy, foot, specified type NEC
  gonococcal A54.49
  gouty —*see* Gout
  hand M7Ø.1- •
  hip NEC M7Ø.7- •
    trochanteric M7Ø.6- •
  infective NEC M71.1Ø
    abscess —*see* Abscess, bursa
    ankle M71.17- •
    elbow M71.12- •
    foot M71.17- •
    hand M71.14- •
    hip M71.15- •
    knee M71.16- •
    multiple sites M71.19
    shoulder M71.11- •
    specified site NEC M71.18
    wrist M71.13- •
  ischial —*see* Bursitis, hip
  knee NEC M7Ø.5- •
    prepatellar M7Ø.4- •
  occupational NEC —*see also* Disorder, soft tissue, due to, use
  olecranon —*see* Bursitis, elbow, olecranon
  pharyngeal J39.1

B

Bursitis *(Continued)*
popliteal *—see* Bursitis, knee
prepatellar M70.4-●
radiohumeral M77.8
rheumatoid M06.20
ankle M06.27-●
elbow M06.22-●
foot joint M06.27-●
hand joint M06.24-●
hip M06.25-●
knee M06.26-●
multiple site M06.29
shoulder M06.21-●
vertebra M06.28
wrist M06.23-●
scapulohumeral *—see* Bursitis, shoulder
semimembranous muscle (knee) *—see* Bursitis, knee
shoulder M75.5-●
adhesive *—see* Capsulitis, adhesive
specified NEC M71.50
ankle M71.57-●
due to use, overuse or pressure *—see* Disorder, soft tissue, due to, use
elbow M71.52-●
foot M71.57-●
hand M71.54-●

Bursitis *(Continued)*
specified NEC *(Continued)*
hip M71.55-●
knee M71.56-●
shoulder *—see* Bursitis, shoulder
specified site NEC M71.58
tibial collateral M76.4-●
wrist M71.53-●
subacromial *—see* Bursitis, shoulder
subcoracoid *—see* Bursitis, shoulder
subdeltoid *—see* Bursitis, shoulder
syphilitic A52.78
Thornwaldt, Tornwaldt J39.2
tibial collateral M76.4-●
toe *—see* Enthesopathy, foot, specified type NEC
trochanteric (area) *—see* Bursitis, hip, trochanteric
wrist *—see* Bursitis, hand
Bursopathy M71.9
specified type NEC M71.80
ankle M71.87-●
elbow M71.82-●
foot M71.87-●
hand M71.84-●
hip M71.85-●
knee M71.86-●

Bursopathy *(Continued)*
specified type NEC *(Continued)*
multiple sites M71.89
shoulder M71.81-●
specified site NEC M71.88
wrist M71.83-●
Burst stitches or sutures (complication of surgery) T81.31
external operation wound T81.31
internal operation wound T81.32
Buruli ulcer A31.1
Bury's disease L95.1
Buschke's
disease B45.3
scleredema *—see* Sclerosis, systemic
Busse-Buschke disease B45.3
Buttock *—see* condition
Button
Biskra B55.1
Delhi B55.1
oriental B55.1
Buttonhole deformity (finger) *—see* Deformity, finger, boutonniere
Bwamba fever A92.8
Byssinosis J66.0
Bywaters' syndrome T79.5

▶ New ➠ Revised ~~deleted~~ Deleted ● Use Additional Character(s)

C

Cachexia R64
cancerous R64
cardiac —*see* Disease, heart
dehydration E86.0
due to malnutrition R64
exophthalmic —*see* Hyperthyroidism
heart —*see* Disease, heart
hypophyseal E23.0
hypopituitary E23.0
lead —*see* Poisoning, lead
malignant R64
marsh —*see* Malaria
nervous F48.8
old age R54
paludal —*see* Malaria
pituitary E23.0
renal N28.9
saturnine —*see* Poisoning, lead
senile R54
Simmonds' E23.0
splenica D73.0
strumipriva E03.4
tuberculous NEC —*see* Tuberculosis
CADASIL (cerebral autosomal dominant arteriopathy with subcortical infarcts and leukoencephalopathy) I67.850
Café au lait spots L81.3
Caffeine-induced
anxiety disorder F15.980
sleep disorder F15.982
Caffey's syndrome Q78.8
Caisson disease T70.3
Cake kidney Q63.1
Caked breast (puerperal, postpartum) O92.79
Calabar swelling B74.3
Calcaneal spur —*see* Spur, bone, calcaneal
Calcaneo-apophysitis M92.8
Calcareous —*see* condition
Calcicosis J62.8
Calciferol (vitamin D) deficiency E55.9
with rickets E55.0
Calcification
adrenal (capsule) (gland) E27.49
tuberculous E35 *[B90.8]*
aorta I70.0
artery (annular) —*see* Arteriosclerosis
auricle (ear) —*see* Disorder, pinna, specified type NEC
basal ganglia G23.8
bladder N32.89
due to Schistosoma hematobium B65.0
brain (cortex) —*see* Calcification, cerebral
bronchus J98.09
bursa M71.40
ankle M71.47- •
elbow M71.42- •
foot M71.47- •
hand M71.44- •
hip M71.45- •
knee M71.46- •
multiple sites M71.49
shoulder M75.3- •
specified site NEC M71.48
wrist M71.43- •
cardiac —*see* Degeneration, myocardial
cerebral (cortex) G93.89
artery I67.2
cervix (uteri) N88.8
choroid plexus G93.89
conjunctiva —*see* Concretion, conjunctiva
corpora cavernosa (penis) N48.89
cortex (brain) —*see* Calcification, cerebral
dental pulp (nodular) K04.2
dentinal papilla K00.4
fallopian tube N83.8
falx cerebri G96.19
gallbladder K82.8
general E83.59
heart —*see also* Degeneration, myocardial
valve —*see* Endocarditis
Calcification *(Continued)*
idiopathic infantile arterial (IIAC) Q28.8
intervertebral cartilage or disc (postinfective) —*see* Disorder, disc, specified NEC
intracranial —*see* Calcification, cerebral
joint —*see* Disorder, joint, specified type NEC
kidney N28.89
tuberculous N29 *[B90.1]*
larynx (senile) J38.7
lens —*see* Cataract, specified NEC
lung (active) (postinfectional) J98.4
tuberculous B90.9
lymph gland or node (postinfectional) I89.8
tuberculous —*see also* Tuberculosis, lymph gland B90.8
mammographic R92.1
massive (paraplegic) —*see* Myositis, ossificans, in, quadriplegia
medial —*see* Arteriosclerosis, extremities
meninges (cerebral) (spinal) G96.19
metastatic E83.59
Mönckeberg's —*see* Arteriosclerosis, extremities
muscle M61.9
due to burns —*see* Myositis, ossificans, in, burns
paralytic —*see* Myositis, ossificans, in, quadriplegia
specified type NEC M61.40
ankle M61.47- •
foot M61.47- •
forearm M61.43- •
hand M61.44- •
lower leg M61.46- •
multiple sites M61.49
pelvic region M61.45- •
shoulder region M61.41- •
specified site NEC M61.48
thigh M61.45- •
upper arm M61.42- •
myocardium, myocardial —*see* Degeneration, myocardial
ovary N83.8
pancreas K86.89
penis N48.89
periarticular —*see* Disorder, joint, specified type NEC
pericardium —*see also* Pericarditis I31.1
pineal gland E34.8
pleura J94.8
postinfectional J94.8
tuberculous NEC B90.9
pulpal (dental) (nodular) K04.2
sclera H15.89
spleen D73.89
subcutaneous L94.2
suprarenal (capsule) (gland) E27.49
tendon (sheath) —*see also* Tenosynovitis, specified type NEC
with bursitis, synovitis or tenosynovitis —*see* Tendinitis, calcific
trachea J39.8
ureter N28.89
vitreous —*see* Deposit, crystalline
Calcified —*see* Calcification
Calcinosis (interstitial) (tumoral) (universalis) E83.59
with Raynaud's phenomenon, esophageal dysfunction, sclerodactyly, telangiectasia (CREST syndrome) M34.1
circumscripta (skin) L94.2
cutis L94.2
Calciphylaxis —*see also* Calcification, by site E83.59
Calcium
deposits —*see* Calcification, by site
metabolism disorder E83.50
salts or soaps in vitreous —*see* Deposit, crystalline
Calciuria R82.994
Calculi —*see* Calculus
Calculosis, intrahepatic —*see* Calculus, bile duct
Calculus, calculi, calculous
ampulla of Vater —*see* Calculus, bile duct
anuria (impacted) (recurrent) —*see also* Calculus, urinary N20.9
appendix K38.1
bile duct (common) (hepatic) K80.50
with
calculus of gallbladder —*see* Calculus, gallbladder and bile duct
cholangitis K80.30
with
cholecystitis —*see* Calculus, bile duct, with cholecystitis
obstruction K80.31
acute K80.32
with
chronic cholangitis K80.36
with obstruction K80.37
obstruction K80.33
chronic K80.34
with
acute cholangitis K80.36
with obstruction K80.37
obstruction K80.35
cholecystitis (with cholangitis) K80.40
with obstruction K80.41
acute K80.42
with
chronic cholecystitis K80.46
with obstruction K80.47
obstruction K80.43
chronic K80.44
with
acute cholecystitis K80.46
with obstruction K80.47
obstruction K80.45
obstruction K80.51
biliary —*see also* Calculus, gallbladder
specified NEC K80.80
with obstruction K80.81
bilirubin, multiple —*see* Calculus, gallbladder
bladder (encysted) (impacted) (urinary) (diverticulum) N21.0
bronchus J98.09
calyx (kidney) (renal) —*see* Calculus, kidney
cholesterol (pure) (solitary) —*see* Calculus, gallbladder
common duct (bile) —*see* Calculus, bile duct
conjunctiva —*see* Concretion, conjunctiva
cystic N21.0
duct —*see* Calculus, gallbladder
dental (subgingival) (supragingival) K03.6
diverticulum
bladder N21.0
kidney N20.0
epididymis N50.89
gallbladder K80.20
with
bile duct calculus —*see* Calculus, gallbladder and bile duct
cholecystitis K80.10
with obstruction K80.11
acute K80.00
with
chronic cholecystitis K80.12
with obstruction K80.13
obstruction K80.01
chronic K80.10
with
acute cholecystitis K80.12
with obstruction K80.13
obstruction K80.11
specified NEC K80.18
with obstruction K80.19
obstruction K80.21

C

- Calculus, calculi, calculous *(Continued)*
  - gallbladder and bile duct K8Ø.7Ø
    - with
      - cholecystitis K8Ø.6Ø
        - with obstruction K8Ø.61
        - acute K8Ø.62
          - with
            - chronic cholecystitis K8Ø.66
              - with obstruction K8Ø.67
            - obstruction K8Ø.63
        - chronic K8Ø.64
          - with
            - acute cholecystitis K8Ø.66
              - with obstruction K8Ø.67
            - obstruction K8Ø.65
      - obstruction K8Ø.71
  - hepatic (duct) *—see* Calculus, bile duct
  - hepatobiliary K8Ø.8Ø
    - with obstruction K8Ø.81
  - ileal conduit N21.8
  - intestinal (impaction) (obstruction) K56.49
  - kidney (impacted) (multiple) (pelvis) (recurrent) (staghorn) N2Ø.Ø
    - with calculus, ureter N2Ø.2
    - congenital Q63.8
  - lacrimal passages *—see* Dacryolith
  - liver (impacted) *—see* Calculus, bile duct
  - lung J98.4
  - mammographic R92.1
  - nephritic (impacted) (recurrent) *—see* Calculus, kidney
  - nose J34.89
  - pancreas (duct) K86.89
  - parotid duct or gland K11.5
  - pelvis, encysted *—see* Calculus, kidney
  - prostate N42.Ø
  - pulmonary J98.4
  - pyelitis (impacted) (recurrent) N2Ø.Ø
    - with hydronephrosis N13.6
  - pyelonephritis (impacted) (recurrent) *—see* category N2Ø
    - with hydronephrosis N13.6
  - renal (impacted) (recurrent) *—see* Calculus, kidney
  - salivary (duct) (gland) K11.5
  - seminal vesicle N5Ø.89
  - staghorn *—see* Calculus, kidney
  - Stensen's duct K11.5
  - stomach K31.89
  - sublingual duct or gland K11.5
    - congenital Q38.4
  - submandibular duct, gland or region K11.5
  - submaxillary duct, gland or region K11.5
  - suburethral N21.8
  - tonsil J35.8
  - tooth, teeth (subgingival) (supragingival) KØ3.6
  - tunica vaginalis N5Ø.89
  - ureter (impacted) (recurrent) N2Ø.1
    - with calculus, kidney N2Ø.2
      - with hydronephrosis N13.2
        - with infection N13.6
  - urethra (impacted) N21.1
  - urinary (duct) (impacted) (passage) (tract) N2Ø.9
    - with hydronephrosis N13.2
      - with infection N13.6
    - in (due to)
    - lower N21.9
      - specified NEC N21.8
  - vagina N89.8
  - vesical (impacted) N21.Ø
  - Wharton's duct K11.5
  - xanthine E79.8 *[N22]*
- Calicectasis N28.89
- Caliectasis N28.89
- California
  - disease B38.9
  - encephalitis A83.5
- Caligo cornea *—see* Opacity, cornea, central
- Callositas, callosity (infected) L84
- Callus (infected) L84
  - bone *—see* Osteophyte
    - excessive, following fracture - code as Sequelae of fracture
- CALME (childhood asymmetric labium majus enlargement) N9Ø.61
- Calorie deficiency or malnutrition *—see also* Malnutrition E46
- Calvé-Perthes disease *—see* Legg-Calve-Perthes disease
- Calvé's disease *—see* Osteochondrosis, juvenile, spine
- Calvities *—see* Alopecia, androgenic
- Cameroon fever *—see* Malaria
- Camptocormia (hysterical) F44.4
- Camurati-Engelmann syndrome Q78.3
- Canal *—see also* condition
  - atrioventricular common Q21.2
- Canaliculitis (lacrimal) (acute) (subacute) HØ4.33-•
  - Actinomyces A42.89
  - chronic HØ4.42-•
- Canavan's disease E75.29
- Canceled procedure (surgical) Z53.9
  - because of
    - contraindication Z53.Ø9
      - smoking Z53.Ø1
    - left against medical advice (AMA) Z53.29
    - patient's decision Z53.2Ø
      - for reasons of belief or group pressure Z53.1
      - specified reason NEC Z53.29
    - specified reason NEC Z53.8
- Cancer *—see also* Neoplasm, by site, malignant
  - bile duct type, liver C22.1
  - blood *—see* Leukemia
  - breast *—see also* Neoplasm, breast, malignant C5Ø.91-•
  - hepatocellular C22.Ø
  - lung *—see also* Neoplasm, lung, malignant C34.9Ø-•
  - ovarian *—see also* Neoplasm, ovary, malignant C56.9-•
  - unspecified site (primary) C8Ø.1
- Cancer (o)phobia F45.29
- Cancerous *—see* Neoplasm, malignant, by site
- Cancrum oris A69.Ø
- Candidiasis, candidal B37.9
  - balanitis B37.42
  - bronchitis B37.1
  - cheilitis B37.83
  - congenital P37.5
  - cystitis B37.41
  - disseminated B37.7
  - endocarditis B37.6
  - enteritis B37.82
  - esophagitis B37.81
  - intertrigo B37.2
  - lung B37.1
  - meningitis B37.5
  - mouth B37.Ø
  - nails B37.2
  - neonatal P37.5
  - onychia B37.2
  - oral B37.Ø
  - osteomyelitis B37.89
  - otitis externa B37.84
  - paronychia B37.2
  - perionyxis B37.2
  - pneumonia B37.1
  - proctitis B37.82
  - pulmonary B37.1
  - pyelonephritis B37.49
  - sepsis B37.7
  - skin B37.2
  - specified site NEC B37.89
  - stomatitis B37.Ø
  - systemic B37.7
  - urethritis B37.41
  - urogenital site NEC B37.49
  - vagina B37.3
  - vulva B37.3
  - vulvovaginitis B37.3
- Candidid L3Ø.2
- Candidosis *—see* Candidiasis
- Candiru infection or infestation B88.8
- Canities (premature) L67.1
  - congenital Q84.2
- Canker (mouth) (sore) K12.Ø
  - rash A38.9
- Cannabinosis J66.2
- Cannabis induced
  - anxiety disorder F12.98Ø
  - psychotic disorder F12.959
  - sleep disorder F12.988
- Canton fever A75.9
- Cantrell's syndrome Q87.89
- Capillariasis (intestinal) B81.1
  - hepatic B83.8
- Capillary *—see* condition
- Caplan's syndrome *—see* Rheumatoid, lung
- Capsule *—see* condition
- Capsulitis (joint) *—see also* Enthesopathy
  - adhesive (shoulder) M75.Ø-•
  - hepatic K65.8
  - labyrinthine *—see* Otosclerosis, specified NEC
  - thyroid EØ6.9
- Caput
  - crepitus Q75.8
  - medusae I86.8
  - succedaneum P12.81
- Car sickness T75.3
- Carapata (disease) A68.Ø
- Carate *—see* Pinta
- Carbon lung J6Ø
- Carbuncle LØ2.93
  - abdominal wall LØ2.231
  - anus K61.Ø
  - auditory canal, external *—see* Abscess, ear, external
  - auricle ear *—see* Abscess, ear, external
  - axilla LØ2.43-•
  - back (any part) LØ2.232
  - breast N61.1
  - buttock LØ2.33
  - cheek (external) LØ2.Ø3
  - chest wall LØ2.233
  - chin LØ2.Ø3
  - corpus cavernosum N48.21
  - ear (any part) (external) (middle) *—see* Abscess, ear, external
  - external auditory canal *—see* Abscess, ear, external
  - eyelid *—see* Abscess, eyelid
  - face NEC LØ2.Ø3
  - femoral (region) *—see* Carbuncle, lower limb
  - finger *—see* Carbuncle, hand
  - flank LØ2.231
  - foot LØ2.63-•
  - forehead LØ2.Ø3
  - genital *—see* Abscess, genital
  - gluteal (region) LØ2.33
  - groin LØ2.234
  - hand LØ2.53-•
  - head NEC LØ2.831
  - heel *—see* Carbuncle, foot
  - hip *—see* Carbuncle, lower limb
  - kidney *—see* Abscess, kidney
  - knee *—see* Carbuncle, lower limb
  - labium (majus) (minus) N76.4
  - lacrimal
    - gland *—see* Dacryoadenitis
    - passages (duct) (sac) *—see* Inflammation, lacrimal, passages, acute
  - leg *—see* Carbuncle, lower limb
  - lower limb LØ2.43-•
  - malignant A22.Ø
  - navel LØ2.236
  - neck LØ2.13
  - nose (external) (septum) J34.Ø
  - orbit, orbital *—see* Abscess, orbit
  - palmar (space) *—see* Carbuncle, hand
  - partes posteriores LØ2.33
  - pectoral region LØ2.233
  - penis N48.21

▶ New ➠ Revised ~~deleted~~ Deleted • Use Additional Character(s)

Carbuncle *(Continued)*
- perineum L02.235
- pinna *—see* Abscess, ear, external
- popliteal *—see* Carbuncle, lower limb
- scalp L02.831
- seminal vesicle N49.0
- shoulder *—see* Carbuncle, upper limb
- specified site NEC L02.838
- temple (region) L02.03
- thumb *—see* Carbuncle, hand
- toe *—see* Carbuncle, foot
- trunk L02.239
  - abdominal wall L02.231
  - back L02.232
  - chest wall L02.233
  - groin L02.234
  - perineum L02.235
  - umbilicus L02.236
- umbilicus L02.236
- upper limb L02.43- •
- urethra N34.0
- vulva N76.4

Carbunculus *—see* Carbuncle

Carcinoid (tumor) *—see* Tumor, carcinoid

Carcinoidosis E34.0

Carcinoma (malignant) *—see also* Neoplasm, by site, malignant
- acidophil
  - specified site *—see* Neoplasm, malignant, by site
  - unspecified site C75.1
- acidophil-basophil, mixed
  - specified site *—see* Neoplasm, malignant, by site
  - unspecified site C75.1
- adnexal (skin) *—see* Neoplasm, skin, malignant
- adrenal cortical C74.0- •
- alveolar *—see* Neoplasm, lung, malignant
  - cell *—see* Neoplasm, lung, malignant
- ameloblastic C41.1
  - upper jaw (bone) C41.0
- apocrine
  - breast *—see* Neoplasm, breast, malignant
  - specified site NEC *—see* Neoplasm, skin, malignant
  - unspecified site C44.99
- basal cell (pigmented) (*see also* Neoplasm, skin, malignant) C44.91
  - fibro-epithelial *—see* Neoplasm, skin, malignant
  - morphea *—see* Neoplasm, skin, malignant
  - multicentric *—see* Neoplasm, skin, malignant
- basaloid
- basal-squamous cell, mixed *—see* Neoplasm, skin, malignant
- basophil
  - specified site *—see* Neoplasm, malignant, by site
  - unspecified site C75.1
- basophil-acidophil, mixed
  - specified site *—see* Neoplasm, malignant, by site
  - unspecified site C75.1
- basosquamous *—see* Neoplasm, skin, malignant
- bile duct
  - with hepatocellular, mixed C22.0
  - liver C22.1
  - specified site NEC *—see* Neoplasm, malignant, by site
  - unspecified site C22.1
- branchial or branchiogenic C10.4
- bronchial or bronchogenic *—see* Neoplasm, lung, malignant
- bronchiolar *—see* Neoplasm, lung, malignant
- bronchioloalveolar *—see* Neoplasm, lung, malignant
- C cell
  - specified site *—see* Neoplasm, malignant, by site
  - unspecified site C73
- ceruminous C44.29- •

Carcinoma *(Continued)*
- cervix uteri
  - in situ D06.9
    - endocervix D06.0
    - exocervix D06.1
    - specified site NEC D06.7
- chorionic
  - specified site *—see* Neoplasm, malignant, by site
  - unspecified site
    - female C58
    - male C62.90
- chromophobe
  - specified site *—see* Neoplasm, malignant, by site
  - unspecified site C75.1
- cloacogenic
  - specified site *—see* Neoplasm, malignant, by site
  - unspecified site C21.2
- diffuse type
  - specified site *—see* Neoplasm, malignant, by site
  - unspecified site C16.9
- duct (cell)
  - with Paget's disease *—see* Neoplasm, breast, malignant
  - infiltrating
    - with lobular carcinoma (in situ)
      - specified site *—see* Neoplasm, malignant, by site
      - unspecified site (female) C50.91- •
        - male C50.92- •
    - specified site *—see* Neoplasm, malignant, by site
    - unspecified site (female) C50.91- •
      - male C50.92- •
- ductal
  - with lobular
    - specified site *—see* Neoplasm, malignant, by site
    - unspecified site (female) C50.91- •
      - male C50.92- •
- ductular, infiltrating
  - specified site *—see* Neoplasm, malignant, by site
  - unspecified site (female) C50.91- •
    - male C50.92- •
- embryonal
  - liver C22.7
- endometrioid
  - specified site *—see* Neoplasm, malignant, by site
  - unspecified site
    - female C56.9
    - male C61
- eosinophil
  - specified site *—see* Neoplasm, malignant, by site
  - unspecified site C75.1
- epidermoid *—see also* Neoplasm, skin malignant
  - in situ, Bowen's type *—see* Neoplasm, skin, in situ
- fibroepithelial, basal cell *—see* Neoplasm, skin, malignant
- follicular
  - with papillary (mixed) C73
  - moderately differentiated C73
  - pure follicle C73
  - specified site *—see* Neoplasm, malignant, by site
  - trabecular C73
  - unspecified site C73
  - well differentiated C73
- generalized, with unspecified primary site C80.0
- glycogen-rich *—see* Neoplasm, breast, malignant
- granulosa cell C56- •
- hepatic cell C22.0

Carcinoma *(Continued)*
- hepatocellular C22.0
  - with bile duct, mixed C22.0
  - fibrolamellar C22.0
- hepatocholangiolitic C22.0
- Hurthle cell C73
- in
  - adenomatous
    - polyposis coli C18.9
  - pleomorphic adenoma *—see* Neoplasm, salivary glands, malignant
  - situ *—see* Carcinoma-in-situ
- infiltrating
  - duct
    - with lobular
      - specified site *—see* Neoplasm, malignant, by site
      - unspecified site (female) C50.91- •
        - male C50.92- •
    - with Paget's disease *—see* Neoplasm, breast, malignant
    - specified site *—see* Neoplasm, malignant
    - unspecified site (female) C50.91- •
      - male C50.92- •
  - ductular
    - specified site *—see* Neoplasm, malignant
    - unspecified site (female) C50.91- •
      - male C50.92- •
  - lobular
    - specified site *—see* Neoplasm, malignant
    - unspecified site (female) C50.91- •
      - male C50.92- •
- inflammatory
  - specified site *—see* Neoplasm, malignant
  - unspecified site (female) C50.91- •
    - male C50.92- •
- intestinal type
  - specified site *—see* Neoplasm, malignant, by site
  - unspecified site C16.9
- intracystic
  - noninfiltrating *—see* Neoplasm, in situ, by site
- intraductal (noninfiltrating)
  - with Paget's disease *—see* Neoplasm, breast, malignant
  - breast D05.1- •
  - papillary
    - with invasion
      - specified site *—see* Neoplasm, malignant, by site
      - unspecified site (female) C50.91- •
        - male C50.92- •
    - breast D05.1- •
    - specified site NEC *—see* Neoplasm, in situ, by site
    - unspecified site (female) D05.1- •
  - specified site NEC *—see* Neoplasm, in situ, by site
  - unspecified site (female) D05.1- •
- intraepidermal *—see* Neoplasm, in situ
  - squamous cell, Bowen's type *—see* Neoplasm, skin, in situ
- intraepithelial *—see* Neoplasm, in situ, by site
  - squamous cell *—see* Neoplasm, in situ, by site
- intraosseous C41.1
  - upper jaw (bone) C41.0
- islet cell
  - with exocrine, mixed
    - specified site *—see* Neoplasm, malignant, by site
    - unspecified site C25.9
  - pancreas C25.4
  - specified site NEC *—see* Neoplasm, malignant, by site
  - unspecified site C25.4

Carcinoma *(Continued)*
juvenile, breast —*see* Neoplasm, breast, malignant
large cell
small cell
specified site —*see* Neoplasm, malignant, by site
unspecified site C34.9Ø
Leydig cell (testis)
specified site —*see* Neoplasm, malignant, by site
unspecified site
female C56.9
male C62.9Ø
lipid-rich (female) C5Ø.91-●
male C5Ø.92-●
liver cell C22.Ø
liver NEC C22.7
lobular (infiltrating)
with intraductal
specified site —*see* Neoplasm, malignant, by site
unspecified site (female) C5Ø.91-●
male C5Ø.92-●
noninfiltrating
breast DØ5.Ø-●
specified site NEC —*see* Neoplasm, in situ, by site
unspecified site DØ5.Ø-●
specified site —*see* Neoplasm, malignant, by site
unspecified site (female) C5Ø.91-●
male C5Ø.92-●
medullary
with
amyloid stroma
specified site —*see* Neoplasm, malignant, by site
unspecified site C73
lymphoid stroma
specified site —*see* Neoplasm, malignant, by site
unspecified site (female) C5Ø.91-●
male C5Ø.92-●
Merkel cell C4A.9
anal margin C4A.51
anal skin C4A.51
canthus C4A.1-●
ear and external auricular canal C4A.2-●
external auricular canal C4A.2-●
eyelid, including canthus C4A.1-●
face C4A.3Ø
specified NEC C4A.39
hip C4A.7-●
lip C4A.Ø
lower limb, including hip C4A.7-●
neck C4A.4
nodal presentation C7B.1
nose C4A.31
overlapping sites C4A.8
perianal skin C4A.51
scalp C4A.4
secondary C7B.1
shoulder C4A.6-●
skin of breast C4A.52
trunk NEC C4A.59
upper limb, including shoulder C4A.6-●
visceral metastatic C7B.1
metastatic —*see* Neoplasm, secondary
metatypical —*see* Neoplasm, skin, malignant
morphea, basal cell —*see* Neoplasm, skin, malignant
mucoid
cell
specified site —*see* Neoplasm, malignant, by site
unspecified site C75.1
neuroendocrine —*see also* Tumor, neuroendocrine
high grade, any site C7A.1
poorly differentiated, any site C7A.1

Carcinoma *(Continued)*
nonencapsulated sclerosing C73
noninfiltrating
intracystic —*see* Neoplasm, in situ, by site
intraductal
breast DØ5.1-●
papillary
breast DØ5.1-●
specified site NEC —*see* Neoplasm, in situ, by site
unspecified site DØ5.1-●
specified site —*see* Neoplasm, in situ, by site
unspecified site DØ5.1-●
lobular
breast DØ5.Ø-●
specified site NEC —*see* Neoplasm, in situ, by site
unspecified site (female) DØ5.Ø-●
oat cell
specified site —*see* Neoplasm, malignant, by site
unspecified site C34.9Ø
odontogenic C41.1
upper jaw (bone) C41.Ø
papillary
with follicular (mixed) C73
follicular variant C73
intraductal (noninfiltrating)
with invasion
specified site —*see* Neoplasm, malignant, by site
unspecified site (female) C5Ø.91-●
male C5Ø.92-●
breast DØ5.1-●
specified site NEC —*see* Neoplasm, in situ, by site
unspecified site DØ5.1-●
serous
specified site —*see* Neoplasm, malignant, by site
surface
specified site —*see* Neoplasm, malignant, by site
unspecified site C56.9
unspecified site C56.9
papillocystic
specified site —*see* Neoplasm, malignant, by site
unspecified site C56.9
parafollicular cell
specified site —*see* Neoplasm, malignant, by site
unspecified site C73
pilomatrix —*see* Neoplasm, skin, malignant
pseudomucinous
specified site —*see* Neoplasm, malignant, by site
unspecified site C56.9
renal cell C64-●
Schmincke —*see* Neoplasm, nasopharynx, malignant
Schneiderian
specified site —*see* Neoplasm, malignant, by site
unspecified site C3Ø.Ø
sebaceous —*see* Neoplasm, skin, malignant
secondary —*see also* Neoplasm, secondary, by site
Merkel cell C7B.1
secretory, breast —*see* Neoplasm, breast, malignant
serous
papillary
specified site —*see* Neoplasm, malignant, by site
unspecified site C56.9
surface, papillary
specified site —*see* Neoplasm, malignant, by site
unspecified site C56.9

Carcinoma *(Continued)*
Sertoli cell
specified site —*see* Neoplasm, malignant, by site
unspecified site C62.9Ø
female C56.9
male C62.9Ø
skin appendage —*see* Neoplasm, skin, malignant
small cell
fusiform cell
specified site —*see* Neoplasm, malignant, by site
unspecified site C34.9Ø
intermediate cell
specified site —*see* Neoplasm, malignant, by site
unspecified site C34.9Ø
large cell
specified site —*see* Neoplasm, malignant, by site
unspecified site C34.9Ø
solid
with amyloid stroma
specified site —*see* Neoplasm, malignant, by site
unspecified site C73
microinvasive
specified site —*see* Neoplasm, malignant, by site
unspecified site C53.9
sweat gland —*see* Neoplasm, skin, malignant
theca cell C56.-●
thymic C37
unspecified site (primary) C8Ø.1
water-clear cell C75.Ø
Carcinoma-in-situ —*see also* Neoplasm, in situ, by site
breast NOS DØ5.9-●
specified type NEC DØ5.8-●
epidermoid —*see also* Neoplasm, in situ, by site
with questionable stromal invasion
cervix DØ6.9
specified site NEC —*see* Neoplasm, in situ, by site
unspecified site DØ6.9
Bowen's type —*see* Neoplasm, skin, in situ
intraductal
breast DØ5.1-●
specified site NEC —*see* Neoplasm, in situ, by site
unspecified site DØ5.1-●
lobular
with
infiltrating duct
breast (female) C5Ø.91-●
male C5Ø.92-●
specified site NEC —*see* Neoplasm, malignant
unspecified site (female) C5Ø.91-●
male C5Ø.92-●
intraductal
breast DØ5.8-●
specified site NEC —*see* Neoplasm, in situ, by site
unspecified site (female) DØ5.8-●
breast DØ5.Ø-●
specified site NEC —*see* Neoplasm, in situ, by site
unspecified site DØ5.Ø-●
squamous cell —*see also* Neoplasm, in situ, by site
with questionable stromal invasion
cervix DØ6.9
specified site NEC —*see* Neoplasm, in situ, by site
unspecified site DØ6.9
Carcinomaphobia F45.29

Carcinomatosis C80.0
  peritonei C78.6
  unspecified site (primary) (secondary) C80.0
Carcinosarcoma —*see* Neoplasm, malignant, by site
  embryonal —*see* Neoplasm, malignant, by site
Cardia, cardial —*see* condition
Cardiac —*see also* condition
  death, sudden —*see* Arrest, cardiac
  pacemaker
    in situ Z95.0
    management or adjustment Z45.018
  tamponade I31.4
Cardialgia —*see* Pain, precordial
Cardiectasis —*see* Hypertrophy, cardiac
Cardiochalasia K21.9
Cardiomalacia I51.5
Cardiomegalia glycogenica diffusa E74.02 *[I43]*
Cardiomegaly —*see also* Hypertrophy, cardiac
  congenital Q24.8
  glycogen E74.02 *[I43]*
  idiopathic I51.7
Cardiomyoliposis I51.5
Cardiomyopathy (familial) (idiopathic) I42.9
  alcoholic I42.6
  amyloid E85.4 *[I43]*
    ➡ transthyretin-related (ATTR) familial E85.4 *[I43]*
  arteriosclerotic —*see* Disease, heart, ischemic, atherosclerotic
  beriberi E51.12
  cobalt-beer I42.6
  congenital I42.4
  congestive I42.0
  constrictive NOS I42.5
  dilated I42.0
  due to
    alcohol I42.6
    beriberi E51.12
    cardiac glycogenosis E74.02 *[I43]*
    drugs I42.7
    external agents NEC I42.7
    Friedreich's ataxia G11.1
    myotonia atrophica G71.11 *[I43]*
    progressive muscular dystrophy G71.09 *[I43]*
  glycogen storage E74.02 *[I43]*
  hypertensive —*see* Hypertension, heart
  hypertrophic (nonobstructive) I42.2
    obstructive I42.1
      congenital Q24.8
  in
    Chagas' disease (chronic) B57.2
      acute B57.0
    sarcoidosis D86.85
  ischemic I25.5
  metabolic E88.9 *[I43]*
    thyrotoxic E05.90 *[I43]*
      with thyroid storm E05.91 *[I43]*
  newborn I42.8
    congenital I42.4
  ▶ non-ischemic (*see also* by cause) I42.8
  nutritional E63.9 *[I43]*
    beriberi E51.12
  obscure of Africa I42.8
  peripartum O90.3
  postpartum O90.3
  restrictive NEC I42.5
  rheumatic I09.0
  secondary I42.9
  ▶ specified NEC I42.8
  stress induced I51.81
  takotsubo I51.81
  thyrotoxic E05.90 *[I43]*
    with thyroid storm E05.91 *[I43]*
  toxic NEC I42.7
  transthyretin-related (ATTR) familial amyloid E85.4
  tuberculous A18.84
  viral B33.24
Cardionephritis —*see* Hypertension, cardiorenal
Cardionephropathy —*see* Hypertension, cardiorenal
Cardionephrosis —*see* Hypertension, cardiorenal
Cardiopathia nigra I27.0
Cardiopathy —*see also* Disease, heart I51.9
  idiopathic I42.9
  mucopolysaccharidosis E76.3 *[I52]*
Cardiopericarditis —*see* Pericarditis
Cardiophobia F45.29
Cardiorenal —*see* condition
Cardiorrhexis —*see* Infarct, myocardium
Cardiosclerosis —*see* Disease, heart, ischemic, atherosclerotic
Cardiosis —*see* Disease, heart
Cardiospasm (esophagus) (reflex) (stomach) K22.0
  congenital Q39.5
    with megaesophagus Q39.5
Cardiostenosis —*see* Disease, heart
Cardiosymphysis I31.0
Cardiovascular —*see* condition
Carditis (acute) (bacterial) (chronic) (subacute) I51.89
  meningococcal A39.50
  rheumatic —*see* Disease, heart, rheumatic
  rheumatoid —*see* Rheumatoid, carditis
  viral B33.20
Care (of) (for) (following)
  child (routine) Z76.2
  family member (handicapped) (sick)
    creating problem for family Z63.6
    provided away from home for holiday relief Z75.5
    unavailable, due to
      absence (person rendering care) (sufferer) Z74.2
      inability (any reason) of person rendering care Z74.2
  foundling Z76.1
  holiday relief Z75.5
  improper —*see* Maltreatment
  lack of (at or after birth) (infant) —*see* Maltreatment, child, neglect
  lactating mother Z39.1
  palliative Z51.5
  postpartum
    immediately after delivery Z39.0
    routine follow-up Z39.2
  respite Z75.5
  unavailable, due to
    absence of person rendering care Z74.2
    inability (any reason) of person rendering care Z74.2
  well-baby Z76.2
Caries
  bone NEC A18.03
  dental (dentino enamel junction) (early childhood) (of dentine) (pre-eruptive) (recurrent) (to the pulp) K02.9
    arrested (coronal) (root) K02.3
    chewing surface
      limited to enamel K02.51
      penetrating into dentin K02.52
      penetrating into pulp K02.53
    coronal surface
      chewing surface
        limited to enamel K02.51
        penetrating into dentin K02.52
        penetrating into pulp K02.53
      pit and fissure surface
        limited to enamel K02.51
        penetrating into dentin K02.52
        penetrating into pulp K02.53
      smooth surface
        limited to enamel K02.61
        penetrating into dentin K02.62
        penetrating into pulp K02.63
    pit and fissure surface
      limited to enamel K02.51
      penetrating into dentin K02.52
      penetrating into pulp K02.53
Caries *(Continued)*
  dental *(Continued)*
    primary, cervical origin K02.52
    root K02.7
    smooth surface
      limited to enamel K02.61
      penetrating into dentin K02.62
      penetrating into pulp K02.63
  external meatus —*see* Disorder, ear, external, specified type NEC
  hip (tuberculous) A18.02
  initial (tooth)
    chewing surface K02.51
    pit and fissure surface K02.51
    smooth surface K02.61
  knee (tuberculous) A18.02
  labyrinth —*see* subcategory H83.8
  limb NEC (tuberculous) A18.03
  mastoid process (chronic) —*see* Mastoiditis, chronic
    tuberculous A18.03
  middle ear —*see* subcategory H74.8
  nose (tuberculous) A18.03
  orbit (tuberculous) A18.03
  ossicles, ear —*see* Abnormal, ear ossicles
  petrous bone —*see* Petrositis
  root (dental) (tooth) K02.7
  sacrum (tuberculous) A18.01
  spine, spinal (column) (tuberculous) A18.01
  syphilitic A52.77
    congenital (early) A50.02 *[M90.80]*
  tooth, teeth —*see* Caries, dental
  tuberculous A18.03
  vertebra (column) (tuberculous) A18.01
Carious teeth —*see* Caries, dental
Carneous mole O02.0
Carnitine insufficiency E71.40
Carotenemia (dietary) E67.1
Carotenosis (cutis) (skin) E67.1
Carotid body or sinus syndrome G90.01
Carotidynia G90.01
Carpal tunnel syndrome —*see* Syndrome, carpal tunnel
Carpenter's syndrome Q87.0
Carpopedal spasm —*see* Tetany
Carr-Barr-Plunkett syndrome Q97.1
Carrier (suspected) **of**
  amebiasis Z22.1
  bacterial disease NEC Z22.39
    diphtheria Z22.2
    intestinal infectious NEC Z22.1
      typhoid Z22.0
    meningococcal Z22.31
    sexually transmitted Z22.4
    specified NEC Z22.39
    staphylococcal (Methicillin susceptible) Z22.321
      Methicillin resistant Z22.322
    streptococcal Z22.338
      group B Z22.330
        complicating pregnancy or delivery O99.82- •
    typhoid Z22.0
  cholera Z22.1
  diphtheria Z22.2
  gastrointestinal pathogens NEC Z22.1
  genetic Z14.8
    cystic fibrosis Z14.1
    hemophilia A (asymptomatic) Z14.01
      symptomatic Z14.02
  gestational, pregnant Z33.1
  gonorrhea Z22.4
  HAA (hepatitis Australian-antigen) B18.8
  HB (c)(s)-AG B18.1
  hepatitis (viral) B18.9
    Australia-antigen (HAA) B18.8
    B surface antigen (HBsAg) B18.1
      with acute delta- (super)infection B17.0
    C B18.2
    specified NEC B18.8
  human T-cell lymphotropic virus type-1 (HTLV-1) infection Z22.6

Carrier of *(Continued)*
infectious organism Z22.9
specified NEC Z22.8
meningococci Z22.31
Salmonella typhosa Z22.0
serum hepatitis —*see* Carrier, hepatitis
staphylococci (Methicillin susceptible) Z22.321
Methicillin resistant Z22.322
streptococci Z22.338
group B Z22.330
complicating pregnancy or delivery O99.82-●
syphilis Z22.4
typhoid Z22.0
venereal disease NEC Z22.4
Carrion's disease A44.0
Carter's relapsing fever (Asiatic) A68.1
Cartilage —*see* condition
Caruncle (inflamed)
conjunctiva (acute) —*see* Conjunctivitis, acute
labium (majus) (minus) N90.89
lacrimal —*see* Inflammation, lacrimal, passages
myrtiform N89.8
urethral (benign) N36.2
Cascade stomach K31.2
Caseation lymphatic gland (tuberculous) A18.2
Cassidy (-Scholte) **syndrome** (malignant carcinoid) E34.0
Castellani's disease A69.8
Castration, traumatic, male S38.231
Casts in urine R82.998
Cat
cry syndrome Q93.4
ear Q17.3
eye syndrome Q92.8
Catabolism, senile R54
Catalepsy (hysterical) F44.2
schizophrenic F20.2
Cataplexy (idiopathic) —*see* Narcolepsy
Cataract (cortical) (immature) (incipient) H26.9
with
neovascularization —*see* Cataract, complicated
age-related —*see* Cataract, senile
anterior
and posterior axial embryonal Q12.0
pyramidal Q12.0
associated with
galactosemia E74.21 *[H28]*
myotonic disorders G71.19 *[H28]*
blue Q12.0
central Q12.0
cerulean Q12.0
complicated H26.20
with
neovascularization H26.21-●
ocular disorder H26.22-●
glaucomatous flecks H26.23-●
congenital Q12.0
coraliform Q12.0
coronary Q12.0
crystalline Q12.0
diabetic —*see* Diabetes, cataract
drug-induced H26.3-●
due to
ocular disorder —*see* Cataract, complicated
radiation H26.8
electric H26.8
extraction status Z98.4-●
glass-blower's H26.8
heat ray H26.8
heterochromic —*see* Cataract, complicated
hypermature —*see* Cataract, senile, morgagnian type
in (due to)
chronic iridocyclitis —*see* Cataract, complicated
diabetes —*see* Diabetes, cataract
endocrine disease E34.9 *[H28]*
eye disease —*see* Cataract, complicated

Cataract *(Continued)*
in (due to) *(Continued)*
hypoparathyroidism E20.9 *[H28]*
malnutrition-dehydration E46 *[H28]*
metabolic disease E88.9 *[H28]*
myotonic disorders G71.19 *[H28]*
nutritional disease E63.9 *[H28]*
infantile —*see* Cataract, presenile
irradiational —*see* Cataract, specified NEC
juvenile —*see* Cataract, presenile
malnutrition-dehydration E46 *[H28]*
morgagnian —*see* Cataract, senile, morgagnian type
myotonic G71.19 *[H28]*
myxedema E03.9 *[H28]*
nuclear
embryonal Q12.0
sclerosis —*see* Cataract, senile, nuclear
presenile H26.00-●
combined forms H26.06-●
cortical H26.01-●
lamellar —*see* Cataract, presenile, cortical
nuclear H26.03-●
specified NEC H26.09
subcapsular polar (anterior) H26.04-●
posterior H26.05-●
zonular —*see* Cataract, presenile, cortical
secondary H26.40
Soemmering's ring H26.41-●
specified NEC H26.49-●
to eye disease —*see* Cataract, complicated
senile H25.9
brunescens —*see* Cataract, senile, nuclear
combined forms H25.81-●
coronary —*see* Cataract, senile, incipient
cortical H25.01-●
hypermature —*see* Cataract, senile, morgagnian type
incipient (mature) (total) H25.09-●
cortical —*see* Cataract, senile, cortical
subcapsular —*see* Cataract, senile, subcapsular
morgagnian type (hypermature) H25.2-●
nuclear (sclerosis) H25.1-●
polar subcapsular (anterior) (posterior) —*see* Cataract, senile, incipient
punctate —*see* Cataract, senile, incipient
specified NEC H25.89
subcapsular polar (anterior) H25.03-●
posterior H25.04-●
snowflake —*see* Diabetes, cataract
specified NEC H26.8
toxic —*see* Cataract, drug-induced
traumatic H26.10-●
localized H26.11-●
partially resolved H26.12-●
total H26.13-●
zonular (perinuclear) Q12.0
Cataracta —*see also* Cataract
brunescens —*see* Cataract, senile, nuclear
centralis pulverulenta Q12.0
cerulea Q12.0
complicata —*see* Cataract, complicated
congenita Q12.0
coralliformis Q12.0
coronaria Q12.0
diabetic —*see* Diabetes, cataract
membranacea
accreta —*see* Cataract, secondary
congenita Q12.0
nigra —*see* Cataract, senile, nuclear
sunflower —*see* Cataract, complicated
Catarrh, catarrhal (acute) (febrile) (infectious) (inflammation) (*see also* condition) J00
bronchial —*see* Bronchitis
chest —*see* Bronchitis
chronic J31.0
due to congenital syphilis A50.03
enteric —*see* Enteritis
eustachian H68.009
fauces —*see* Pharyngitis

Catarrh, catarrhal *(Continued)*
gastrointestinal —*see* Enteritis
gingivitis K05.00
nonplaque induced K05.01
plaque induced K05.00
hay —*see* Fever, hay
intestinal —*see* Enteritis
larynx, chronic J37.0
liver B15.9
with hepatic coma B15.0
lung —*see* Bronchitis
middle ear, chronic —*see* Otitis, media, nonsuppurative, chronic, serous
mouth K12.1
nasal (chronic) —*see* Rhinitis
nasobronchial J31.1
nasopharyngeal (chronic) J31.1
acute J00
pulmonary —*see* Bronchitis
spring (eye) (vernal) —*see* Conjunctivitis, acute, atopic
summer (hay) —*see* Fever, hay
throat J31.2
tubotympanal —*see also* Otitis, media, nonsuppurative
chronic —*see* Otitis, media, nonsuppurative, chronic, serous
Catatonia (schizophrenic) F20.2
Catatonic
disorder due to known physiologic condition F06.1
schizophrenia F20.2
stupor R40.1
Cat-scratch —*see also* Abrasion
disease or fever A28.1
Cauda equina —*see* condition
Cauliflower ear M95.1-●
Causalgia (upper limb) G56.4-●
lower limb G57.7-●
Cause
external, general effects T75.89
Caustic burn —*see* Corrosion, by site
Cavare's disease (familial periodic paralysis) G72.3
Cave-in, injury
crushing (severe) —*see* Crush
suffocation —*see* Asphyxia, traumatic, due to low oxygen, due to cave-in
Cavernitis (penis) N48.29
Cavernositis N48.29
Cavernous —*see* condition
Cavitation of lung —*see also* Tuberculosis, pulmonary
nontuberculous J98.4
Cavities, dental —*see* Caries, dental
Cavity
lung —*see* Cavitation of lung
optic papilla Q14.2
pulmonary —*see* Cavitation of lung
Cavovarus foot, congenital Q66.1-●
Cavus foot (congenital) Q66.7-●
acquired —*see* Deformity, limb, foot, specified NEC
Cazenave's disease L10.2
Cecitis K52.9
with perforation, peritonitis, or rupture K65.8
Cecoureterocele Q62.32
Cecum —*see* condition
Celiac
artery compression syndrome I77.4
disease (with steatorrhea) K90.0
infantilism K90.0
Cell(s), cellular —*see also* condition
in urine R82.998
Cellulitis (diffuse) (phlegmonous) (septic) (suppurative) L03.90
abdominal wall L03.311
anaerobic A48.0
ankle —*see* Cellulitis, lower limb
anus K61.0
arm —*see* Cellulitis, upper limb
auricle (ear) —*see* Cellulitis, ear

C

Cellulitis *(Continued)*
axilla LØ3.11-●
back (any part) LØ3.312
breast (acute) (nonpuerperal) (subacute) N61.Ø
nipple N61.Ø
broad ligament
acute N73.Ø
buttock LØ3.317
cervical (meaning neck) LØ3.221
cervix (uteri) —*see* Cervicitis
cheek (external) LØ3.211
internal K12.2
chest wall LØ3.313
chronic LØ3.9Ø
clostridial A48.Ø
corpus cavernosum N48.22
digit
finger —*see* Cellulitis, finger
toe —*see* Cellulitis, toe
Douglas' cul-de-sac or pouch
acute N73.Ø
drainage site (following operation) T81.49
ear (external) H6Ø.1-●
eosinophilic (granulomatous) L98.3
erysipelatous —*see* Erysipelas
external auditory canal —*see* Cellulitis, ear
eyelid —*see* Abscess, eyelid
face NEC LØ3.211
finger (intrathecal) (periosteal) (subcutaneous) (subcuticular) LØ3.Ø1-●
foot —*see* Cellulitis, lower limb
gangrenous —*see* Gangrene
genital organ NEC
female (external) N76.4
male N49.9
multiple sites N49.8
specified NEC N49.8
gluteal (region) LØ3.317
gonococcal A54.89
groin LØ3.314
hand —*see* Cellulitis, upper limb
head NEC LØ3.811
face (any part, except ear, eye and nose) LØ3.211
heel —*see* Cellulitis, lower limb
hip —*see* Cellulitis, lower limb
jaw (region) LØ3.211
knee —*see* Cellulitis, lower limb
labium (majus) (minus) —*see* Vulvitis
lacrimal passages —*see* Inflammation, lacrimal, passages
larynx J38.7
leg —*see* Cellulitis, lower limb
lip K13.Ø
lower limb LØ3.11-●
toe —*see* Cellulitis, toe
mouth (floor) K12.2
multiple sites, so stated LØ3.9Ø
nasopharynx J39.1
navel LØ3.316
newborn P38.9
with mild hemorrhage P38.1
without hemorrhage P38.9
neck (region) LØ3.221
nipple (acute) (nonpuerperal) (subacute) N61.Ø
nose (septum) (external) J34.Ø
orbit, orbital HØ5.Ø1-●
palate (soft) K12.2
pectoral (region) LØ3.313
pelvis, pelvic (chronic)
female —*see also* Disease, pelvis, inflammatory N73.2
acute N73.Ø
following ectopic or molar pregnancy OØ8.Ø
male K65.Ø
penis N48.22
perineal, perineum LØ3.315
periorbital LØ3.213

Cellulitis *(Continued)*
perirectal K61.1
peritonsillar J36
periurethral N34.Ø
periuterine —*see also* Disease, pelvis, inflammatory N73.2
acute N73.Ø
pharynx J39.1
preseptal LØ3.213
rectum K61.1
retroperitoneal K68.9
round ligament
acute N73.Ø
scalp (any part) LØ3.811
scrotum N49.2
seminal vesicle N49.Ø
shoulder —*see* Cellulitis, upper limb
specified site NEC LØ3.818
submandibular (region) (space) (triangle) K12.2
gland K11.3
submaxillary (region) K12.2
gland K11.3
thigh —*see* Cellulitis, lower limb
thumb (intrathecal) (periosteal) (subcutaneous) (subcuticular) —*see* Cellulitis, finger
toe (intrathecal) (periosteal) (subcutaneous) (subcuticular) LØ3.Ø3-●
tonsil J36
trunk LØ3.319
abdominal wall LØ3.311
back (any part) LØ3.312
buttock LØ3.317
chest wall LØ3.313
groin LØ3.314
perineal, perineum LØ3.315
umbilicus LØ3.316
tuberculous (primary) A18.4
umbilicus LØ3.316
upper limb LØ3.11-●
axilla —*see* Cellulitis, axilla
finger —*see* Cellulitis, finger
thumb —*see* Cellulitis, finger
vaccinal T88.Ø
vocal cord J38.3
vulva —*see* Vulvitis
wrist —*see* Cellulitis, upper limb
Cementoblastoma, benign —*see* Cyst, calcifying odontogenic
Cementoma —*see* Cyst, calcifying odontogenic
Cementoperiostitis —*see* Periodontitis
Cementosis KØ3.4
Central auditory processing disorder H93.25
Central pain syndrome G89.Ø
Cephalematocele, cephal (o)**hematocele**
newborn P52.8
birth injury P1Ø.8
traumatic —*see* Hematoma, brain
Cephalematoma, cephalhematoma (calcified)
newborn (birth injury) P12.Ø
traumatic —*see* Hematoma, brain
Cephalgia, cephalalgia —*see also* Headache
histamine G44.ØØ9
intractable G44.ØØ1
not intractable G44.ØØ9
trigeminal autonomic (TAC) NEC G44.Ø99
intractable G44.Ø91
not intractable G44.Ø99
Cephalic —*see* condition
Cephalitis —*see* Encephalitis
Cephalocele —*see* Encephalocele
Cephalomenia N94.89
Cephalopelvic —*see* condition
Cerclage (with cervical incompetence) **in pregnancy** —*see* Incompetence, cervix, in pregnancy
Cerebellitis —*see* Encephalitis
Cerebellum, cerebellar —*see* condition
Cerebral —*see* condition
Cerebritis —*see* Encephalitis

Cerebro-hepato-renal syndrome Q87.89
Cerebromalacia —*see* Softening, brain
sequelae of cerebrovascular disease I69.398
Cerebroside lipidosis E75.22
Cerebrospasticity (congenital) G8Ø.1
Cerebrospinal —*see* condition
Cerebrum —*see* condition
Ceroid-lipofuscinosis, neuronal E75.4
Cerumen (accumulation) (impacted) H61.2-●
Cervical —*see also* condition
auricle Q18.2
dysplasia in pregnancy —*see* Abnormal, cervix, in pregnancy or childbirth
erosion in pregnancy —*see* Abnormal, cervix, in pregnancy or childbirth
fibrosis in pregnancy —*see* Abnormal, cervix, in pregnancy or childbirth
fusion syndrome Q76.1
rib Q76.5
shortening (complicating pregnancy) O26.87-●
Cervicalgia M54.2
Cervicitis (acute) (chronic) (nonvenereal) (senile (atrophic)) (subacute) (with ulceration) N72
with
abortion —*see* Abortion, by type complicated by genital tract and pelvic infection
ectopic pregnancy OØ8.Ø
molar pregnancy OØ8.Ø
chlamydial A56.Ø9
gonococcal A54.Ø3
herpesviral A6Ø.Ø3
puerperal (postpartum) O86.11
syphilitic A52.76
trichomonal A59.Ø9
tuberculous A18.16
Cervicocolpitis (emphysematosa) (*see also* Cervicitis) N72
Cervix —*see* condition
Cesarean delivery, previous, affecting management of pregnancy O34.219
classical (vertical) scar O34.212
low transverse scar O34.211
Céstan (-Chenais) **paralysis or syndrome** G46.3
Céstan-Raymond syndrome I65.8
Cestode infestation B71.9
specified type NEC B71.8
Cestodiasis B71.9
Chabert's disease A22.9
Chacaleh E53.8
Chafing L3Ø.4
Chagas' (-Mazza) **disease** (chronic) B57.2
with
cardiovascular involvement NEC B57.2
digestive system involvement B57.3Ø
megacolon B57.32
megaesophagus B57.31
other specified B57.39
megacolon B57.32
megaesophagus B57.31
myocarditis B57.2
nervous system involvement B57.4Ø
meningitis B57.41
meningoencephalitis B57.42
other specified B57.49
specified organ involvement NEC B57.5
acute (with) B57.1
cardiovascular NEC B57.Ø
myocarditis B57.Ø
Chagres fever B5Ø.9
Chairridden Z74.Ø9
Chalasia (cardiac sphincter) K21.9
Chalazion HØØ.19
left HØØ.16
lower HØØ.15
upper HØØ.14
right HØØ.13
lower HØØ.12
upper HØØ.11

- **Chalcosis** —*see also* Disorder, globe, degenerative, chalcosis
  - cornea —*see* Deposit, cornea
  - crystalline lens —*see* Cataract, complicated
  - retina H35.89
- **Chalicosis** (pulmonum) J62.8
- **Chancre** (any genital site) (hard) (hunterian) (mixed) (primary) (seronegative) (seropositive) (syphilitic) A51.Ø
  - congenital A5Ø.Ø7
  - conjunctiva NEC A51.2
  - Ducrey's A57
  - extragenital A51.2
  - eyelid A51.2
  - lip A51.2
  - nipple A51.2
  - Nisbet's A57
  - of
    - carate A67.Ø
    - pinta A67.Ø
    - yaws A66.Ø
  - palate, soft A51.2
  - phagedenic A57
  - simple A57
  - soft A57
    - bubo A57
    - palate A51.2
  - urethra A51.Ø
  - yaws A66.Ø
- **Chancroid** (anus) (genital) (penis) (perineum) (rectum) (urethra) (vulva) A57
- **Chandler's disease** (osteochondritis dissecans, hip) —*see* Osteochondritis, dissecans, hip
- **Change**(s) (in) (of) —*see also* Removal
  - arteriosclerotic —*see* Arteriosclerosis
  - bone —*see also* Disorder, bone
    - diabetic —*see* Diabetes, bone change
  - bowel habit R19.4
  - cardiorenal (vascular) —*see* Hypertension, cardiorenal
  - cardiovascular —*see* Disease, cardiovascular
  - circulatory I99.9
  - cognitive (mild) (organic) R41.89
  - color, tooth, teeth
    - during formation KØØ.8
    - posteruptive KØ3.7
  - contraceptive device Z3Ø.433
  - corneal membrane H18.3Ø
    - Bowman's membrane fold or rupture H18.31-●
    - Descemet's membrane
      - fold H18.32-●
      - rupture H18.33-●
  - coronary —*see* Disease, heart, ischemic
  - degenerative, spine or vertebra —*see* Spondylosis
  - dental pulp, regressive KØ4.2
  - dressing (nonsurgical) Z48.ØØ
    - surgical Z48.Ø1
  - heart —*see* Disease, heart
  - hip joint —*see* Derangement, joint, hip
  - hyperplastic larynx J38.7
  - hypertrophic
    - nasal sinus J34.89
    - turbinate, nasal J34.3
    - upper respiratory tract J39.8
  - indwelling catheter Z46.6
  - inflammatory —*see also* Inflammation
    - sacroiliac M46.1
  - job, anxiety concerning Z56.1
  - joint —*see* Derangement, joint
  - life —*see* Menopause
  - mental status R41.82
  - minimal (glomerular) —*see also* NØØ-NØ7
    - with fourth character .Ø NØ5.Ø
  - myocardium, myocardial —*see* Degeneration, myocardial - of life —*see* Menopause
  - pacemaker Z45.Ø18
    - pulse generator Z45.Ø1Ø
- **Change** *(Continued)*
  - personality (enduring) F68.8
    - due to (secondary to)
      - general medical condition FØ7.Ø
    - secondary (nonspecific) F6Ø.89
  - regressive, dental pulp KØ4.2
  - renal —*see* Disease, renal
  - retina H35.9
    - myopic —*see also* Myopia, degenerative H44.2-●
  - sacroiliac joint M53.3
  - senile —*see also* condition R54
  - sensory R2Ø.8
  - skin R23.9
    - acute, due to ultraviolet radiation L56.9
      - specified NEC L56.8
    - chronic, due to nonionizing radiation L57.9
      - specified NEC L57.8
    - cyanosis R23.Ø
    - flushing R23.2
    - pallor R23.1
    - petechiae R23.3
    - specified change NEC R23.8
    - swelling —*see* Mass, localized
    - texture R23.4
  - trophic
    - arm —*see* Mononeuropathy, upper limb
    - leg —*see* Mononeuropathy, lower limb
  - vascular I99.9
  - vasomotor I73.9
  - voice R49.9
    - psychogenic F44.4
    - specified NEC R49.8
- **Changing sleep-work schedule, affecting sleep** G47.26
- **Changuinola fever** A93.1
- **Chapping skin** T69.8
- **Charcot-Marie-Tooth disease, paralysis or syndrome** G6Ø.Ø
- **Charcot's**
  - arthropathy —*see* Arthropathy, neuropathic
  - cirrhosis K74.3
  - disease (tabetic arthropathy) A52.16
  - joint (disease) (tabetic) A52.16
    - diabetic —*see* Diabetes, with, arthropathy
    - syringomyelic G95.Ø
  - syndrome (intermittent claudication) I73.9
- **CHARGE association** Q89.8
- **Charley-horse** (quadriceps) M62.831
  - traumatic (quadriceps) S76.11-●
- **Charlouis' disease** —*see* Yaws
- **Cheadle's disease** E54
- **Checking** (of)
  - cardiac pacemaker (battery) (electrode(s)) Z45.Ø18
    - pulse generator Z45.Ø1Ø
  - implantable subdermal contraceptive Z3Ø.46
  - intrauterine contraceptive device Z3Ø.431
  - wound Z48.Ø-●
    - due to injury - code to Injury, by site, using appropriate seventh character for subsequent encounter
- **Check-up** —*see* Examination
- **Chédiak-Higashi** (-Steinbrinck) **syndrome** (congenital gigantism of peroxidase granules) E7Ø.33Ø
- **Cheek** —*see* condition
- **Cheese itch** B88.Ø
- **Cheese-washer's lung** J67.8
- **Cheese-worker's lung** J67.8
- **Cheilitis** (acute) (angular) (catarrhal) (chronic) (exfoliative) (gangrenous) (glandular) (infectional) (suppurative) (ulcerative) (vesicular) K13.Ø
  - actinic (due to sun) L56.8
    - other than from sun L59.8
  - candidal B37.83
- **Cheilodynia** K13.Ø
- **Cheiloschisis** —*see* Cleft, lip
- **Cheilosis** (angular) K13.Ø
  - with pellagra E52
  - due to
    - vitamin B2 (riboflavin) deficiency E53.Ø
- **Cheiromegaly** M79.89
- **Cheiropompholyx** L3Ø.1
- **Cheloid** —*see* Keloid
- **Chemical burn** —*see* Corrosion, by site
- **Chemodectoma** —*see* Paraganglioma, nonchromaffin
- **Chemosis, conjunctiva** —*see* Edema, conjunctiva
- **Chemotherapy** (session) (for)
  - cancer Z51.11
  - neoplasm Z51.11
- **Cherubism** M27.8
- **Chest** —*see* condition
- **Cheyne-Stokes breathing** (respiration) RØ6.3
- **Chiari's**
  - disease or syndrome (hepatic vein thrombosis) I82.Ø
  - malformation
    - type I G93.5
    - type II —*see* Spina bifida
  - net Q24.8
- **Chicago disease** B4Ø.9
- **Chickenpox** —*see* Varicella
- **Chiclero ulcer or sore** B55.1
- **Chigger** (infestation) B88.Ø
- **Chignon** (disease) B36.8
  - newborn (from vacuum extraction) (birth injury) P12.1
- **Chilaiditi's syndrome** (subphrenic displacement, colon) Q43.3
- **Chilblain**(s) (lupus) T69.1
- **Child**
  - custody dispute Z65.3
- **Childbirth** —*see* Delivery
- **Childhood**
  - cerebral X-linked adrenoleukodystrophy E71.52Ø
  - period of rapid growth ZØØ.2
- **Chill**(s) R68.83
  - with fever R5Ø.9
  - without fever R68.83
  - congestive in malarial regions B54
- **Chilomastigiasis** AØ7.8
- **Chimera 46,XX/46,XY** Q99.Ø
- **Chin** —*see* condition
- **Chinese dysentery** AØ3.9
- **Chionophobia** F4Ø.228
- **Chitral fever** A93.1
- **Chlamydia, chlamydial** A74.9
  - cervicitis A56.Ø9
  - conjunctivitis A74.Ø
  - cystitis A56.Ø1
  - endometritis A56.11
  - epididymitis A56.19
  - female
    - pelvic inflammatory disease A56.11
    - pelviperitonitis A56.11
  - orchitis A56.19
  - peritonitis A74.81
  - pharyngitis A56.4
  - proctitis A56.3
  - psittaci (infection) A7Ø
  - salpingitis A56.11
  - sexually-transmitted infection NEC A56.8
  - specified NEC A74.89
  - urethritis A56.Ø1
  - vulvovaginitis A56.Ø2
- **Chlamydiosis** —*see* Chlamydia
- **Chloasma** (skin) (idiopathic) (symptomatic) L81.1
  - eyelid HØ2.719
    - hyperthyroid EØ5.9Ø *[HØ2.719]*
      - with thyroid storm EØ5.91 *[HØ2.719]*
    - left HØ2.716
      - lower HØ2.715
      - upper HØ2.714
    - right HØ2.713
      - lower HØ2.712
      - upper HØ2.711
- **Chloroma** C92.3-●
- **Chlorosis** D5Ø.9
  - Egyptian B76.9 *[D63.8]*
  - miner's B76.9 *[D63.8]*

Chlorotic anemia D5Ø.8
Chocolate cyst (ovary) N8Ø.1
Choked
- disc or disk —*see* Papilledema
- on food, phlegm, or vomitus NOS —*see* Foreign body, by site
- while vomiting NOS —*see* Foreign body, by site

Chokes (resulting from bends) T7Ø.3
Choking sensation RØ9.89
Cholangiectasis K83.8
Cholangiocarcinoma
- with hepatocellular carcinoma, combined C22.Ø
- liver C22.1
- specified site NEC —*see* Neoplasm, malignant, by site
- unspecified site C22.1

Cholangiohepatitis K83.8
- due to fluke infestation B66.1

Cholangiohepatoma C22.Ø
Cholangiolitis (acute) (chronic) (extrahepatic) (gangrenous) (intrahepatic) K83.Ø9
- paratyphoidal —*see* Fever, paratyphoid
- typhoidal AØ1.Ø9

Cholangioma D13.4
- malignant —*see* Cholangiocarcinoma

Cholangitis (ascending) (primary) (recurrent) (sclerosing) (secondary) (stenosing) (suppurative) K83.Ø9
- with calculus, bile duct —*see* Calculus, bile duct, with cholangitis
- chronic nonsuppurative destructive K74.3
- primary K83.Ø9
  - sclerosing K83.Ø1
- sclerosing K83.Ø9

Cholecystectasia K82.8
Cholecystitis K81.9
- with
  - calculus, stones in
    - bile duct (common) (hepatic) —*see* Calculus, bile duct, with cholecystitis
    - cystic duct —*see* Calculus, gallbladder, with cholecystitis
    - gallbladder —*see* Calculus, gallbladder, with cholecystitis
  - choledocholithiasis —*see* Calculus, bile duct, with cholecystitis
  - cholelithiasis —*see* Calculus, gallbladder, with cholecystitis
  - gangrene of gallbladder K82.A1
  - perforation of gallbladder K82.A2
- acute (emphysematous) (gangrenous) (suppurative) K81.Ø
  - with
    - calculus, stones in
      - cystic duct —*see* Calculus, gallbladder, with cholecystitis, acute
      - gallbladder —*see* Calculus, gallbladder, with cholecystitis, acute
    - choledocholithiasis —*see* Calculus, bile duct, with cholecystitis, acute
    - cholelithiasis —*see* Calculus, gallbladder, with cholecystitis, acute
    - chronic cholecystitis K81.2
      - with gallbladder calculus K8Ø.12
        - with obstruction K8Ø.13
- chronic K81.1
  - with acute cholecystitis K81.2
    - with gallbladder calculus K8Ø.12
      - with obstruction K8Ø.13
- emphysematous (acute) —*see* Cholecystitis, acute
- gangrenous —*see* Cholecystitis, acute
- paratyphoidal, current AØ1.4
- suppurative —*see* Cholecystitis, acute
- typhoidal AØ1.Ø9

Cholecystolithiasis —*see* Calculus, gallbladder
Choledochitis (suppurative) K83.Ø9
Choledocholith —*see* Calculus, bile duct
Choledocholithiasis (common duct) (hepatic duct) —*see* Calculus, bile duct
- cystic —*see* Calculus, gallbladder
- typhoidal AØ1.Ø9

Cholelithiasis (cystic duct) (gallbladder) (impacted) (multiple) —*see* Calculus, gallbladder
- bile duct (common) (hepatic) —*see* Calculus, bile duct
- hepatic duct —*see* Calculus, bile duct
- specified NEC K8Ø.8Ø
  - with obstruction K8Ø.81

Cholemia —*see also* Jaundice
- familial (simple) (congenital) E8Ø.4
- Gilbert's E8Ø.4

Choleperitoneum, choleperitonitis K65.3
Cholera (Asiatic) (epidemic) (malignant) AØØ.9
- antimonial —*see* Poisoning, antimony
- classical AØØ.Ø
- due to Vibrio cholerae Ø1 AØØ.9
  - biovar cholerae AØØ.Ø
  - biovar eltor AØØ.1
  - el tor AØØ.1
- el tor AØØ.1

Cholerine —*see* Cholera
Cholestasis NEC K83.1
- with hepatocyte injury K71.Ø
- due to total parenteral nutrition (TPN) K76.89
- pure K71.Ø

Cholesteatoma (ear) (middle) (with reaction) H71.9-●
- attic H71.Ø-●
- external ear (canal) H6Ø.4-●
- mastoid H71.2-●
- postmastoidectomy cavity (recurrent) —*see* Complications, postmastoidectomy, recurrent cholesteatoma
- recurrent (postmastoidectomy) —*see* Complications, postmastoidectomy, recurrent cholesteatoma
- tympanum H71.1-●

Cholesteatosis, diffuse H71.3-●
Cholesteremia E78.ØØ
Cholesterin in vitreous —*see* Deposit, crystalline
Cholesterol
- deposit
  - retina H35.89
  - vitreous —*see* Deposit, crystalline
- elevated (high) E78.ØØ
  - with elevated (high) triglycerides E78.2
  - screening for Z13.22Ø
- imbibition of gallbladder K82.4

Cholesterolemia (essential) (pure) E78.ØØ
- familial E78.Ø1
- hereditary E78.Ø1

Cholesterolosis, cholesterosis (gallbladder) K82.4
- cerebrotendinous E75.5

Cholocolic fistula K82.3
Choluria R82.2
Chondritis M94.8X9
- aurical H61.Ø3-●
- costal (Tietze's) M94.Ø
- external ear H61.Ø3-●
- patella, posttraumatic —*see* Chondromalacia, patella
- pinna H61.Ø3-●
- purulent M94.8X-●
- tuberculous NEC A18.Ø2
  - intervertebral A18.Ø1

Chondroblastoma —*see also* Neoplasm, bone, benign
- malignant —*see* Neoplasm, bone, malignant

Chondrocalcinosis M11.2Ø
- ankle M11.27-●
- elbow M11.22-●
- familial M11.1Ø
  - ankle M11.17-●
  - elbow M11.12-●
  - foot joint M11.17-●
  - hand joint M11.14-●
  - hip M11.15-●
  - knee M11.16-●
  - multiple site M11.19
  - shoulder M11.11-●
  - vertebrae M11.18
  - wrist M11.13-●
- foot joint M11.27-●
- hand joint M11.24-●
- hip M11.25-●
- knee M11.26-●
- multiple site M11.29
- shoulder M11.21-●
- specified type NEC M11.2Ø
  - ankle M11.27-●
  - elbow M11.22-●
  - foot joint M11.27-●
  - hand joint M11.24-●
  - hip M11.25-●
  - knee M11.26-●
  - multiple site M11.29
  - shoulder M11.21-●
  - vertebrae M11.28
  - wrist M11.23-●
- vertebrae M11.28
- wrist M11.23-●

Chondrodermatitis nodularis helicis or anthelicis —*see* Perichondritis, ear
Chondrodysplasia Q78.9
- with hemangioma Q78.4
- calcificans congenita Q77.3
- fetalis Q77.4
- metaphyseal (Jansen's) (McKusick's) (Schmid's) Q78.8
- punctata Q77.3

Chondrodystrophy, chondrodystrophia (familial) (fetalis) (hypoplastic) Q78.9
- calcificans congenita Q77.3
- myotonic (congenital) G71.13
- punctata Q77.3

Chondroectodermal dysplasia Q77.6
Chondrogenesis imperfecta Q77.4
Chondrolysis M94.35-●
Chondroma —*see also* Neoplasm, cartilage, benign
- juxtacortical —*see* Neoplasm, bone, benign
- periosteal —*see* Neoplasm, bone, benign

Chondromalacia (systemic) M94.2Ø
- acromioclavicular joint M94.21-●
- ankle M94.27-●
- elbow M94.22-●
- foot joint M94.27-●
- glenohumeral joint M94.21-●
- hand joint M94.24-●
- hip M94.25-●
- knee M94.26-●
  - patella M22.4-●
- multiple sites M94.29
- patella M22.4-●
- rib M94.28
- sacroiliac joint M94.259
- shoulder M94.21-●
- sternoclavicular joint M94.21-●
- vertebral joint M94.28
- wrist M94.23-●

Chondromatosis —*see also* Neoplasm, cartilage, uncertain behavior
- internal Q78.4

Chondromyxosarcoma —*see* Neoplasm, cartilage, malignant
Chondro-osteodysplasia (Morquio-Brailsford type) E76.219
Chondro-osteodystrophy E76.29
Chondro-osteoma —*see* Neoplasm, bone, benign
Chondropathia tuberosa M94.Ø
Chondrosarcoma —*see* Neoplasm, cartilage, malignant
- juxtacortical —*see* Neoplasm, bone, malignant
- mesenchymal —*see* Neoplasm, connective tissue, malignant
- myxoid —*see* Neoplasm, cartilage, malignant

- **Chordee** (nonvenereal) N48.89
  - congenital Q54.4
  - gonococcal A54.09
- **Chorditis** (fibrinous) (nodosa) (tuberosa) J38.2
- **Chordoma** —*see* Neoplasm, vertebral (column), malignant
- **Chorea** (chronic) (gravis) (posthemiplegic) (senile) (spasmodic) G25.5
  - with
    - heart involvement I02.0
      - active or acute (conditions in I01-•) I02.0
      - rheumatic I02.9
        - with valvular disorder I02.0
    - rheumatic heart disease (chronic) (inactive) (quiescent) — code to rheumatic heart condition involved
  - drug-induced G25.4
  - habit F95.8
  - hereditary G10
  - Huntington's G10
  - hysterical F44.4
  - minor I02.9
    - with heart involvement I02.0
  - progressive G25.5
    - hereditary G10
  - rheumatic (chronic) I02.9
    - with heart involvement I02.0
  - Sydenham's I02.9
    - with heart involvement —*see* Chorea, with rheumatic heart disease
    - nonrheumatic G25.5
- **Choreoathetosis** (paroxysmal) G25.5
- **Chorioadenoma** (destruens) D39.2
- **Chorioamnionitis** O41.12-•
- **Chorioangioma** D26.7
- **Choriocarcinoma** —*see* Neoplasm, malignant, by site
  - combined with
    - embryonal carcinoma —*see* Neoplasm, malignant, by site
    - other germ cell elements —*see* Neoplasm, malignant, by site
    - teratoma —*see* Neoplasm, malignant, by site
  - specified site —*see* Neoplasm, malignant, by site
  - unspecified site
    - female C58
    - male C62.90
- **Chorioencephalitis** (acute) (lymphocytic) (serous) A87.2
- **Chorioepithelioma** —*see* Choriocarcinoma
- **Choriomeningitis** (acute) (lymphocytic) (serous) A87.2
- **Chorionepithelioma** —*see* Choriocarcinoma
- **Chorioretinitis** —*see also* Inflammation, chorioretinal
  - disseminated —*see also* Inflammation, chorioretinal, disseminated
    - in neurosyphilis A52.19
  - Egyptian B76.9 *[D63.8]*
  - focal —*see also* Inflammation, chorioretinal, focal
  - histoplasmic B39.9 *[H32]*
  - in (due to)
    - histoplasmosis B39.9 *[H32]*
    - syphilis (secondary) A51.43
      - late A52.71
    - toxoplasmosis (acquired) B58.01
      - congenital (active) P37.1 *[H32]*
    - tuberculosis A18.53
  - juxtapapillary, juxtapapillaris —*see* Inflammation, chorioretinal, focal, juxtapapillary
  - leprous A30.9 *[H32]*
  - miner's B76.9 *[D63.8]*
  - progressive myopia (degeneration) —*see also* Myopia, degenerative H44.2-•
  - syphilitic (secondary) A51.43
    - congenital (early) A50.01 *[H32]*
      - late A50.32
    - late A52.71
  - tuberculous A18.53
- **Chorioretinopathy, central serous** H35.71-•
- **Choroid** —*see* condition
- **Choroideremia** H31.21
- **Choroiditis** —*see* Chorioretinitis
- **Choroidopathy** —*see* Disorder, choroid
- **Choroidoretinitis** —*see* Chorioretinitis
- **Choroidoretinopathy, central serous** —*see* Chorioretinopathy, central serous
- **Christian-Weber disease** M35.6
- **Christmas disease** D67
- **Chromaffinoma** —*see also* Neoplasm, benign, by site
  - malignant —*see* Neoplasm, malignant, by site
- **Chromatopsia** —*see* Deficiency, color vision
- **Chromhidrosis, chromidrosis** L75.1
- **Chromoblastomycosis** —*see* Chromomycosis
- **Chromoconversion** R82.91
- **Chromomycosis** B43.9
  - brain abscess B43.1
  - cerebral B43.1
  - cutaneous B43.0
  - skin B43.0
  - specified NEC B43.8
  - subcutaneous abscess or cyst B43.2
- **Chromophytosis** B36.0
- **Chromosome** —*see* condition by chromosome involved
  - D (1) —*see* condition, chromosome 13
  - E (3) —*see* condition, chromosome 18
  - G —*see* condition, chromosome 21
- **Chromotrichomycosis** B36.8
- **Chronic** —*see* condition
  - fracture —*see* Fracture, pathological
- **Churg-Strauss syndrome** M30.1
- **Chyle cyst, mesentery** I89.8
- **Chylocele** (nonfilarial) I89.8
  - filarial —*see also* Infestation, filarial B74.9 *[N51]*
  - tunica vaginalis N50.89
    - filarial —*see also* Infestation, filarial B74.9 *[N51]*
- **Chylomicronemia** (fasting) (with hyperprebetalipoproteinemia) E78.3
- **Chylopericardium** I31.3
  - acute I30.9
- **Chylothorax** (nonfilarial) I89.8
  - filarial —*see also* Infestation, filarial B74.9 *[J91.8]*
- **Chylous** —*see* condition
- **Chyluria** (nonfilarial) R82.0
  - due to
    - bilharziasis B65.0
    - Brugia (malayi) B74.1
      - timori B74.2
    - schistosomiasis (bilharziasis) B65.0
    - Wuchereria (bancrofti) B74.0
  - filarial —*see* Infestation, filarial
- **Cicatricial** (deformity) —*see* Cicatrix
- **Cicatrix** (adherent) (contracted) (painful) (vicious) —*see also* Scar L90.5
  - adenoid (and tonsil) J35.8
  - alveolar process M26.79
  - anus K62.89
  - auricle —*see* Disorder, pinna, specified type NEC
  - bile duct (common) (hepatic) K83.8
  - bladder N32.89
  - bone —*see* Disorder, bone, specified type NEC
  - brain G93.89
  - cervix (postoperative) (postpartal) N88.1
  - common duct K83.8
  - cornea H17.9
    - tuberculous A18.59
  - duodenum (bulb), obstructive K31.5
  - esophagus K22.2
  - eyelid —*see* Disorder, eyelid function
  - hypopharynx J39.2
  - lacrimal passages —*see* Obstruction, lacrimal
  - larynx J38.7
  - lung J98.4
  - middle ear —*see* subcategory H74.8
  - mouth K13.79

Cicatrix *(Continued)*
  - muscle M62.89
    - with contracture —*see* Contraction, muscle NEC
  - nasopharynx J39.2
  - palate (soft) K13.79
  - penis N48.89
  - pharynx J39.2
  - prostate N42.89
  - rectum K62.89
  - retina —*see* Scar, chorioretinal
  - semilunar cartilage —*see* Derangement, meniscus
  - seminal vesicle N50.89
  - skin L90.5
    - infected L08.89
    - postinfective L90.5
    - tuberculous B90.8
  - specified site NEC L90.5
  - throat J39.2
  - tongue K14.8
  - tonsil (and adenoid) J35.8
  - trachea J39.8
  - tuberculous NEC B90.9
  - urethra N36.8
  - uterus N85.8
  - vagina N89.8
    - postoperative N99.2
  - vocal cord J38.3
  - wrist, constricting (annular) L90.5
- **CIDP** (chronic inflammatory demyelinating polyneuropathy) G61.81
- **CIN** —*see* Neoplasia, intraepithelial, cervix
- **CINCA** (chronic infantile neurological, cutaneous and articular syndrome) M04.2
- **Cinchonism** —*see* Deafness, ototoxic
  - correct substance properly administered —*see* Table of Drugs and Chemicals, by drug, adverse effect
  - overdose or wrong substance given or taken —*see* Table of Drugs and Chemicals, by drug, poisoning
- **Circle of Willis** —*see* condition
- **Circular** —*see* condition
- **Circulating anticoagulants** —*see also* - Disorder, hemorrhagic D68.318
  - due to drugs —*see also* - Disorder, hemorrhagic D68.32
  - following childbirth O72.3
- **Circulation**
  - collateral, any site I99.8
  - defective (lower extremity) I99.9
    - congenital Q28.9
  - embryonic Q28.9
  - failure (peripheral) R57.9
    - newborn P29.89
  - fetal, persistent P29.38
  - heart, incomplete Q28.9
- **Circulatory system** —*see* condition
- **Circulus senilis** (cornea) —*see* Degeneration, cornea, senile
- **Circumcision** (in absence of medical indication) (ritual) (routine) Z41.2
- **Circumscribed** —*see* condition
- **Circumvallate placenta** O43.11-•
- **Cirrhosis, cirrhotic** (hepatic) (liver) K74.60
  - alcoholic K70.30
    - with ascites K70.31
  - atrophic —*see* Cirrhosis, liver
  - Baumgarten-Cruveilhier K74.69
  - biliary (cholangiolitic) (cholangitic) (hypertrophic) (obstructive) (pericholangiolitic) K74.5
    - due to
      - Clonorchiasis B66.1
      - flukes B66.3
    - primary K74.3
    - secondary K74.4
  - cardiac (of liver) K76.1
  - Charcot's K74.3

Cirrhosis, cirrhotic *(Continued)*
cholangiolitic, cholangitic, cholostatic (primary) K74.3
congestive K76.1
Cruveilhier-Baumgarten K74.69
cryptogenic (liver) K74.69
due to
hepatolenticular degeneration E83.01
Wilson's disease E83.01
xanthomatosis E78.2
fatty K76.0
alcoholic K70.0
Hanot's (hypertrophic) K74.3
hepatic —*see* Cirrhosis, liver
hypertrophic K74.3
Indian childhood K74.69
kidney —*see* Sclerosis, renal
Laennec's K70.30
with ascites K70.31
alcoholic K70.30
with ascites K70.31
nonalcoholic K74.69
liver K74.60
alcoholic K70.30
with ascites K70.31
fatty K70.0
congenital P78.81
syphilitic A52.74
lung (chronic) J84.10
macronodular K74.69
alcoholic K70.30
with ascites K70.31
micronodular K74.69
alcoholic K70.30
with ascites K70.31
mixed type K74.69
monolobular K74.3
nephritis —*see* Sclerosis, renal
nutritional K74.69
alcoholic K70.30
with ascites K70.31
obstructive —*see* Cirrhosis, biliary
ovarian N83.8
pancreas (duct) K86.89
pigmentary E83.110
portal K74.69
alcoholic K70.30
with ascites K70.31
postnecrotic K74.69
alcoholic K70.30
with ascites K70.31
pulmonary J84.10
renal —*see* Sclerosis, renal
spleen D73.2
stasis K76.1
Todd's K74.3
unilobar K74.3
xanthomatous (biliary) K74.5
due to xanthomatosis (familial) (metabolic) (primary) E78.2
Cistern, subarachnoid R93.0
Citrullinemia E72.23
Citrullinuria E72.23
Civatte's disease or poikiloderma L57.3
Clam digger's itch B65.3
Clammy skin R23.1
Clap —*see* Gonorrhea
Clarke-Hadfield syndrome (pancreatic infantilism) K86.89
Clark's paralysis G80.9
Clastothrix L67.8
Claude Bernard-Horner syndrome G90.2
traumatic —*see* Injury, nerve, cervical sympathetic
Claude's disease or syndrome G46.3
Claudicatio venosa intermittens I87.8
Claudication (intermittent) I73.9
cerebral (artery) G45.9
spinal cord (arteriosclerotic) G95.19
syphilitic A52.09
venous (axillary) I87.8
Claustrophobia F40.240
Clavus (infected) L84
Clawfoot (congenital) Q66.89
acquired —*see* Deformity, limb, clawfoot
Clawhand (acquired) —*see also* Deformity, limb, clawhand
congenital Q68.1
Clawtoe (congenital) Q66.89
acquired —*see* Deformity, toe, specified NEC
Clay eating —*see* Pica
Cleansing of artificial opening —*see* Attention to, artificial, opening
Cleft (congenital) —*see also* Imperfect, closure
alveolar process M26.79
branchial (persistent) Q18.2
cyst Q18.0
fistula Q18.0
sinus Q18.0
cricoid cartilage, posterior Q31.8
foot Q72.7
hand Q71.6
lip (unilateral) Q36.9
with cleft palate Q37.9
hard Q37.1
with soft Q37.5
soft Q37.3
with hard Q37.5
bilateral Q36.0
with cleft palate Q37.8
hard Q37.0
with soft Q37.4
soft Q37.2
with hard Q37.4
median Q36.1
nose Q30.2
palate Q35.9
with cleft lip (unilateral) Q37.9
bilateral Q37.8
hard Q35.1
with
cleft lip (unilateral) Q37.1
bilateral Q37.0
soft Q35.5
with cleft lip (unilateral) Q37.5
bilateral Q37.4
medial Q35.5
soft Q35.3
with
cleft lip (unilateral) Q37.3
bilateral Q37.2
hard Q35.5
with cleft lip (unilateral) Q37.5
bilateral Q37.4
penis Q55.69
scrotum Q55.29
thyroid cartilage Q31.8
uvula Q35.7
Cleidocranial dysostosis Q74.0
Cleptomania F63.2
Clicking hip (newborn) R29.4
Climacteric (female) —*see also* Menopause
arthritis (any site) NEC —*see* Arthritis, specified form NEC
depression (single episode) F32.89
recurrent episode F33.8
male (symptoms) (syndrome) NEC N50.89
melancholia (single episode) F32.89
recurrent episode F33.8
paranoid state F22
polyarthritis NEC —*see* Arthritis, specified form NEC
symptoms (female) N95.1
Clinical research investigation (clinical trial) (control subject) (normal comparison) (participant) Z00.6
Clitoris —*see* condition **Cloaca** (persistent) Q43.7
Clonorchiasis, clonorchis infection (liver) B66.1
Clonus R25.8
Closed bite M26.29
Clostridium (C.) perfringens, as cause of disease classified elsewhere B96.7
Closure
congenital, nose Q30.0
cranial sutures, premature Q75.0
defective or imperfect NEC —*see* Imperfect, closure
fistula, delayed —*see* Fistula
foramen ovale, imperfect Q21.1
hymen N89.6
interauricular septum, defective Q21.1
interventricular septum, defective Q21.0
lacrimal duct —*see also* Stenosis, lacrimal, duct
congenital Q10.5
nose (congenital) Q30.0
acquired M95.0
of artificial opening —*see* Attention to, artificial, opening
primary angle, without glaucoma damage H40.06-●
vagina N89.5
valve —*see* Endocarditis
vulva N90.5
Clot (blood) —*see also* Embolism
artery (obstruction) (occlusion) —*see* Embolism
bladder N32.89
brain (intradural or extradural) —*see* Occlusion, artery, cerebral
circulation I74.9
heart —*see also* Infarct, myocardium
not resulting in infarction I51.3
vein —*see* Thrombosis
Clouded state R40.1
epileptic —*see* Epilepsy, specified NEC
paroxysmal —*see* Epilepsy, specified NEC
Cloudy antrum, antra J32.0
Clouston's (hidrotic) ectodermal dysplasia Q82.4
Clubbed nail pachydermoperiostosis M89.40 *[L62]*
Clubbing of finger(s) (nails) R68.3
Clubfinger R68.3
congenital Q68.1
Clubfoot (congenital) Q66.89
acquired —*see* Deformity, limb, clubfoot
➡equinovarus Q66.0-●
paralytic —*see* Deformity, limb, clubfoot
Clubhand (congenital) (radial) Q71.4-●
acquired —*see* Deformity, limb, clubhand
Clubnail R68.3
congenital Q84.6
Clump, kidney Q63.1
Clumsiness, clumsy child syndrome F82
Cluttering F98.81
Clutton's joints A50.51 *[M12.80]*
Coagulation, intravascular (diffuse) (disseminated) —*see also* Defibrination syndrome
complicating abortion —*see* Abortion, by type, complicated by, intravascular coagulation
following ectopic or molar pregnancy O08.1
Coagulopathy —*see also* Defect, coagulation
consumption D65
intravascular D65
newborn P60
Coalition
calcaneo-scaphoid Q66.89
tarsal Q66.89
Coalminer's
elbow —*see* Bursitis, elbow, olecranon
lung or pneumoconiosis J60
Coalworker's lung or pneumoconiosis J60
Coarctation
aorta (preductal) (postductal) Q25.1
pulmonary artery Q25.71
Coated tongue K14.3

Coats' disease (exudative retinopathy) —*see* Retinopathy, exudative
Cocaine-induced
anxiety disorder F14.980
bipolar and related disorder F14.94
depressive disorder F14.94
obsessive-compulsive and related disorder F14.988
psychotic disorder F14.959
sleep disorder F14.982
sexual dysfunction F14.981
Cocainism —*see* Disorder, cocaine use
Coccidioidomycosis B38.9
cutaneous B38.3
disseminated B38.7
generalized B38.7
meninges B38.4
prostate B38.81
pulmonary B38.2
acute B38.0
chronic B38.1
skin B38.3
specified NEC B38.89
Coccidioidosis —*see* Coccidioidomycosis
Coccidiosis (intestinal) A07.3
Coccydynia, coccygodynia M53.3
Coccyx —*see* condition
Cochin-China diarrhea K90.1
Cockayne's syndrome Q87.19
Cocked up toe —*see* Deformity, toe, specified NEC
Cock's peculiar tumor L72.3
Codman's tumor —*see* Neoplasm, bone, benign
Coenurosis B71.8
Coffee-worker's lung J67.8
Cogan's syndrome H16.32-●
oculomotor apraxia H51.8
Coitus, painful (female) N94.10
male N53.12
psychogenic F52.6
Cold J00
with influenza, flu, or grippe —*see* Influenza, with, respiratory manifestations NEC
agglutinin disease or hemoglobinuria (chronic) D59.1
bronchial —*see* Bronchitis
chest —*see* Bronchitis
common (head) J00
effects of T69.9
specified effect NEC T69.8
excessive, effects of T69.9
specified effect NEC T69.8
exhaustion from T69.8
exposure to T69.9
specified effect NEC T69.8
head J00
injury syndrome (newborn) P80.0
on lung —*see* Bronchitis
rose J30.1
sensitivity, auto-immune D59.1
symptoms J00
virus J00
Coldsore B00.1
Colibacillosis A49.8
as the cause of other disease (*see also* Escherichia coli) B96.20
generalized A41.50
Colic (bilious) (infantile) (intestinal) (recurrent) (spasmodic) R10.83
abdomen R10.83
psychogenic F45.8
appendix, appendicular K38.8
bile duct —*see* Calculus, bile duct
biliary —*see* Calculus, bile duct
common duct —*see* Calculus, bile duct
cystic duct —*see* Calculus, gallbladder
Devonshire NEC —*see* Poisoning, lead
gallbladder —*see* Calculus, gallbladder
gallstone —*see* Calculus, gallbladder
gallbladder or cystic duct —*see* Calculus, gallbladder
Colic *(Continued)*
hepatic (duct) —*see* Calculus, bile duct
hysterical F45.8
kidney N23
lead NEC —*see* Poisoning, lead
mucous K58.9
with diarrhea K58.0
psychogenic F54
nephritic N23
painter's NEC —*see* Poisoning, lead
pancreas K86.89
psychogenic F45.8
renal N23
saturnine NEC —*see* Poisoning, lead
ureter N23
urethral N36.8
due to calculus N21.1
uterus NEC N94.89
menstrual —*see* Dysmenorrhea
worm NOS B83.9
Colicystitis —*see* Cystitis
Colitis (acute) (catarrhal) (chronic) (noninfective) (hemorrhagic) (*see also* Enteritis) K52.9
allergic K52.29
with
food protein-induced enterocolitis syndrome K52.21
proctocolitis K52.82
amebic (acute) —*see also* Amebiasis A06.0
nondysenteric A06.2
anthrax A22.2
bacillary —*see* Infection, Shigella
balantidial A07.0
Clostridium difficile
not specified as recurrent A04.72
recurrent A04.71
coccidial A07.3
collagenous K52.831
cystica superficialis K52.89
dietary counseling and surveillance (for) Z71.3
dietetic —*see also* Colitis, allergic K52.29
drug-induced K52.1
due to radiation K52.0
eosinophilic K52.82
food hypersensitivity —*see also* Colitis, allergic K52.29
giardial A07.1
granulomatous —*see* Enteritis, regional, large intestine
infectious —*see* Enteritis, infectious
indeterminate, so stated K52.3
ischemic K55.9
acute (subacute) —*see also* Ischemia, intestine, acute K55.039
chronic K55.1
due to mesenteric artery insufficiency K55.1
fulminant (acute) —*see also* Ischemia, intestine, acute K55.039
left sided K51.50
with
abscess K51.514
complication K51.519
specified NEC K51.518
fistula K51.513
obstruction K51.512
rectal bleeding K51.511
lymphocytic K52.832
membranous
psychogenic F54
microscopic K52.839
specified NEC K52.838
mucous —*see* Syndrome, irritable, bowel
psychogenic F54
noninfective K52.9
specified NEC K52.89
polyposa —*see* Polyp, colon, inflammatory
protozoal A07.9
pseudomembranous
not specified as recurrent A04.72
recurrent A04.71
Colitis *(Continued)*
pseudomucinous —*see* Syndrome, irritable, bowel
regional —*see* Enteritis, regional, large intestine
infectious A09
segmental —*see* Enteritis, regional, large intestine
septic —*see* Enteritis, infectious
spastic K58.9
with diarrhea K58.0
psychogenic F54
staphylococcal A04.8
foodborne A05.0
subacute ischemic —*see also* Ischemia, intestine, acute K55.039
thromboulcerative —*see also* Ischemia, intestine, acute K55.039
toxic NEC K52.1
due to Clostridium difficile
not specified as recurrent A04.72
recurrent A04.71
transmural —*see* Enteritis, regional, large intestine
trichomonal A07.8
tuberculous (ulcerative) A18.32
ulcerative (chronic) K51.90
with
complication K51.919
abscess K51.914
fistula K51.913
obstruction K51.912
rectal bleeding K51.911
specified complication NEC K51.918
enterocolitis —*see* Enterocolitis, ulcerative
ileocolitis —*see* Ileocolitis, ulcerative
mucosal proctocolitis —*see* Proctocolitis, mucosal
proctitis —*see* Proctitis, ulcerative
pseudopolyposis —*see* Polyp, colon, inflammatory
psychogenic F54
rectosigmoiditis —*see* Rectosigmoiditis, ulcerative
specified type NEC K51.80
with
complication K51.819
abscess K51.814
fistula K51.813
obstruction K51.812
rectal bleeding K51.811
specified complication NEC K51.818
Collagenosis, collagen disease (nonvascular) (vascular) M35.9
cardiovascular I42.8
reactive perforating L87.1
specified NEC M35.8
Collapse R55
adrenal E27.2
cardiorespiratory R57.0
cardiovascular R57.0
newborn P29.89
circulatory (peripheral) R57.9
during or after labor and delivery O75.1
following ectopic or molar pregnancy O08.3
newborn P29.89
during or
after labor and delivery O75.1
resulting from a procedure, not elsewhere classified T81.10
external ear canal —*see* Stenosis, external ear canal
general R55
heart —*see* Disease, heart
heat T67.1
hysterical F44.89
labyrinth, membranous (congenital) Q16.5
lung (massive) —*see also* Atelectasis J98.19
pressure due to anesthesia (general) (local) or other sedation T88.2
during labor and delivery O74.1
in pregnancy O29.02-●
postpartum, puerperal O89.09

C

Collapse *(Continued)*
myocardial —*see* Disease, heart
nervous F48.8
neurocirculatory F45.8
nose M95.Ø
postoperative T81.1Ø
pulmonary —*see also* Atelectasis J98.19
newborn —*see* Atelectasis
trachea J39.8
tracheobronchial J98.Ø9
valvular —*see* Endocarditis
vascular (peripheral) R57.9
during or after labor and delivery O75.1
following ectopic or molar pregnancy OØ8.3
newborn P29.89
vertebra M48.5Ø-•
cervical region M48.52-•
cervicothoracic region M48.53-•
in (due to)
metastasis —*see* Collapse, vertebra, in, specified disease NEC
osteoporosis —*see also* Osteoporosis M8Ø.88
cervical region M8Ø.88
cervicothoracic region M8Ø.88
lumbar region M8Ø.88
lumbosacral region M8Ø.88
multiple sites M8Ø.88
occipito-atlanto-axial region M8Ø.88
sacrococcygeal region M8Ø.88
thoracic region M8Ø.88
thoracolumbar region M8Ø.88
specified disease NEC M48.5Ø-•
cervical region M48.52-•
cervicothoracic region M48.53-•
lumbar region M48.56-•
lumbosacral region M48.57-•
occipito-atlanto-axial region M48.51-•
sacrococcygeal region M48.58-•
thoracic region M48.54-•
thoracolumbar region M48.55-•
lumbar region M48.56-•
lumbosacral region M48.57-•
occipito-atlanto-axial region M48.51-•
sacrococcygeal region M48.58-•
thoracic region M48.54-•
thoracolumbar region M48.55-•
Collateral —*see also* condition
circulation (venous) I87.8
dilation, veins I87.8
Colles' fracture S52.53-•
Collet (-Sicard) **syndrome** G52.7
Collier's asthma or lung J6Ø
Collodion baby Q8Ø.2
Colloid nodule (of thyroid) (cystic) EØ4.1
Coloboma (iris) Q13.Ø
eyelid Q1Ø.3
fundus Q14.8
lens Q12.2
optic disc (congenital) Q14.2
acquired H47.31-•
Coloenteritis —*see* Enteritis
Colon —*see* condition
Colonization
MRSA (Methicillin resistant Staphylococcus aureus) Z22.322
MSSA (Methicillin susceptible Staphylococcus aureus) Z22.321
status —*see* Carrier (suspected) of
Coloptosis K63.4
Color blindness —*see* Deficiency, color vision
Colostomy
attention to Z43.3
fitting or adjustment Z46.89
malfunctioning K94.Ø3
status Z93.3
Colpitis (acute) —*see* Vaginitis
Colpocele N81.5
Colpocystitis —*see* Vaginitis
Colpospasm N94.2
Column, spinal, vertebral —*see* condition

Coma R4Ø.2Ø
with
motor response (none) R4Ø.231
abnormal R4Ø.233
abnormal extensor posturing to pain or noxious stimuli (<2 years of age) R4Ø.232
abnormal flexure posturing to pain or noxious stimuli (Ø-5 years of age) R4Ø.233
extension R4Ø.232
extensor posturing to pain or noxious stimuli (2-5 years of age) R4Ø.232
flexion/decorticate posturing (<2 years of age) R4Ø.233
flexion withdrawal R4Ø.234
localizes pain (2-5 years of age) R4Ø.235
normal or spontaneous movement (<2 years of age) R4Ø.236
obeys commands (2-5 years of age) R4Ø.236
score of
1 R4Ø.231
2 R4Ø.232
3 R4Ø.233
4 R4Ø.234
5 R4Ø.235
6 R4Ø.236
withdraws from pain or noxious stimuli (Ø-5 years of age) R4Ø.234
withdraws to touch (<2 years of age) R4Ø.235
opening of eyes (never) R4Ø.211
in response to
pain R4Ø.212
sound R4Ø.213
score of
1 R4Ø.211
2 R4Ø.212
3 R4Ø.213
4 R4Ø.214
spontaneous R4Ø.214
verbal response (none) R4Ø.221
confused conversation R4Ø.224
cooing or babbling or crying appropriately (<2 years of age) R4Ø.225
inappropriate crying or screaming (<2 years of age) R4Ø.223
inappropriate words R4Ø.223
inappropriate words (2-5 years of age) R4Ø.224
incomprehensible sounds (2-5 years of age) R4Ø.222
incomprehensible words R4Ø.222
irritable cries (<2 years of age) R4Ø.224
moans/grunts to pain; restless (<2 years old) R4Ø.222
oriented R4Ø.225
score of
1 R4Ø.221
2 R4Ø.222
3 R4Ø.223
4 R4Ø.224
5 R4Ø.225
screaming (2-5 years of age) R4Ø.223
uses appropriate words (2-5 years of age) R4Ø.225
eclamptic —*see* Eclampsia
epileptic —*see* Epilepsy
Glasgow, scale score —*see* Glasgow coma scale
hepatic —*see* Failure, hepatic, by type, with coma
hyperglycemic (diabetic) —*see* Diabetes, by type, with hyperosmolarity, with coma
hyperosmolar (diabetic) —*see* Diabetes, by type, with hyperosmolarity, with coma
hypoglycemic (diabetic) —*see* Diabetes, by type, with hypoglycemia, with coma
nondiabetic E15

Coma *(Continued)*
in diabetes —*see* Diabetes, coma
insulin-induced —*see* Coma, hypoglycemic
ketoacidotic (diabetic) —*see* Diabetes, by type, with ketoacidosis, with coma
myxedematous EØ3.5
newborn P91.5
persistent vegetative state R4Ø.3
specified NEC, without documented Glasgow coma scale score, or with partial Glasgow coma scale score reported R4Ø.244
Comatose —*see* Coma
Combat fatigue F43.Ø
Combined —*see* condition
Comedo, comedones (giant) L7Ø.Ø
Comedocarcinoma —*see also* Neoplasm, breast, malignant
noninfiltrating
breast DØ5.8-•
specified site —*see* Neoplasm, in situ, by site
unspecified site DØ5.8-•
Comedomastitis —*see* Ectasia, mammary duct
Comminuted fracture - code as Fracture, closed
Common
arterial trunk Q2Ø.Ø
atrioventricular canal Q21.2
atrium Q21.1
cold (head) JØØ
truncus (arteriosus) Q2Ø.Ø
variable immunodeficiency —*see* Immunodeficiency, common variable
ventricle Q2Ø.4
Commotio, commotion (current)
brain —*see* Injury, intracranial, concussion
cerebri —*see* Injury, intracranial, concussion
retinae SØ5.8X-•
spinal cord —*see* Injury, spinal cord, by region
spinalis —*see* Injury, spinal cord, by region
Communication
between
base of aorta and pulmonary artery Q21.4
left ventricle and right atrium Q2Ø.5
pericardial sac and pleural sac Q34.8
pulmonary artery and pulmonary vein, congenital Q25.72
congenital between uterus and digestive or urinary tract Q51.7
Compartment syndrome (deep) (posterior) (traumatic) T79.AØ
abdomen T79.A3
lower extremity (hip, buttock, thigh, leg, foot, toes) T79.A2
nontraumatic
abdomen M79.A3
lower extremity (hip, buttock, thigh, leg, foot, toes) M79.A2-•
specified site NEC M79.A9
upper extremity (shoulder, arm, forearm, wrist, hand, fingers) M79.A1-•
specified site NEC T79.A9
upper extremity (shoulder, arm, forearm, wrist, hand, fingers) T79.A1
Compensation
failure —*see* Disease, heart
neurosis, psychoneurosis —*see* Disorder, factitious
Complaint —*see also* Disease
bowel, functional K59.9
psychogenic F45.8
intestine, functional K59.9
psychogenic F45.8
kidney —*see* Disease, renal
miners' J6Ø
Complete —*see* condition
Complex
Addison-Schilder E71.528
cardiorenal —*see* Hypertension, cardiorenal
Costen's M26.69
disseminated mycobacterium avium-intracellulare (DMAC) A31.2

Complex *(Continued)*
Eisenmenger's (ventricular septal defect) I27.83
hypersexual F52.8
jumped process, spine —*see* Dislocation, vertebra
primary, tuberculous A15.7
Schilder-Addison E71.528
subluxation (vertebral) M99.19
abdomen M99.19
acromioclavicular M99.17
cervical region M99.11
cervicothoracic M99.11
costochondral M99.18
costovertebral M99.18
head region M99.1Ø
hip M99.15
lower extremity M99.16
lumbar region M99.13
lumbosacral M99.13
occipitocervical M99.1Ø
pelvic region M99.15
pubic M99.15
rib cage M99.18
sacral region M99.14
sacrococcygeal M99.14
sacroiliac M99.14
specified NEC M99.19
sternochondral M99.18
sternoclavicular M99.17
thoracic region M99.12
thoracolumbar M99.12
upper extremity M99.17
Taussig-Bing (transposition, aorta and overriding pulmonary artery) Q2Ø.1
Complication(s) (from) (of)
accidental puncture or laceration during a procedure (of) —*see* Complications, intraoperative (intraprocedural), puncture or laceration
amputation stump (surgical) (late) NEC T87.9
dehiscence T87.81
infection or inflammation T87.4Ø
lower limb T87.4-●
upper limb T87.4-●
necrosis T87.5Ø
lower limb T87.5-●
upper limb T87.5-●
neuroma T87.3Ø
lower limb T87.3-●
upper limb T87.3-●
specified type NEC T87.89
anastomosis (and bypass) —*see also* Complications, prosthetic device or implant
intestinal (internal) NEC K91.89
involving urinary tract N99.89
urinary tract (involving intestinal tract) N99.89
vascular —*see* Complications, cardiovascular device or implant
anesthesia, anesthetic —*see also* Anesthesia, complication T88.59
brain, postpartum, puerperal O89.2
cardiac
in
labor and delivery O74.2
pregnancy O29.19-●
postpartum, puerperal O89.1
central nervous system
in
labor and delivery O74.3
pregnancy O29.29-●
postpartum, puerperal O89.2
difficult or failed intubation T88.4
in pregnancy O29.6-●
failed sedation (conscious) (moderate) during procedure T88.52
general, unintended awareness during procedure T88.53
hyperthermia, malignant T88.3
hypothermia T88.51
intubation failure T88.4

Complication *(Continued)*
anesthesia, anesthetic *(Continued)*
malignant hyperthermia T88.3
pulmonary
in
labor and delivery O74.1
pregnancy NEC O29.Ø9-●
postpartum, puerperal O89.Ø9
shock T88.2
spinal and epidural
in
labor and delivery NEC O74.6
headache O74.5
pregnancy NEC O29.5X-●
postpartum, puerperal NEC O89.5
headache O89.4
unintended awareness under general anesthesia during procedure T88.53
anti-reflux device —*see* Complications, esophageal anti-reflux device
aortic (bifurcation) graft —*see* Complications, graft, vascular
aortocoronary (bypass) graft —*see* Complications, coronary artery (bypass) graft
aortofemoral (bypass) graft —*see* Complications, extremity artery (bypass) graft
arteriovenous
fistula, surgically created T82.9
embolism T82.818
fibrosis T82.828
hemorrhage T82.838
infection or inflammation T82.7
mechanical
breakdown T82.51Ø
displacement T82.52Ø
leakage T82.53Ø
malposition T82.52Ø
obstruction T82.59Ø
perforation T82.59Ø
protrusion T82.59Ø
pain T82.848
specified type NEC T82.898
stenosis T82.858
thrombosis T82.868
shunt, surgically created T82.9
embolism T82.818
fibrosis T82.828
hemorrhage T82.838
infection or inflammation T82.7
mechanical
breakdown T82.511
displacement T82.521
leakage T82.531
malposition T82.521
obstruction T82.591
perforation T82.591
protrusion T82.591
pain T82.848
specified type NEC T82.898
stenosis T82.858
thrombosis T82.868
arthroplasty —*see* Complications, joint prosthesis
artificial
fertilization or insemination N98.9
attempted introduction (of)
embryo in embryo transfer N98.3
ovum following in vitro fertilization N98.2
hyperstimulation of ovaries N98.1
infection N98.Ø
specified NEC N98.8
heart T82.9
embolism T82.817
fibrosis T82.827
hemorrhage T82.837
infection or inflammation T82.7
mechanical
breakdown T82.512
displacement T82.522
leakage T82.532

Complication *(Continued)*
artificial *(Continued)*
heart *(Continued)*
mechanical *(Continued)*
malposition T82.522
obstruction T82.592
perforation T82.592
protrusion T82.592
pain T82.847
specified type NEC T82.897
stenosis T82.857
thrombosis T82.867
opening
cecostomy —*see* Complications, colostomy
colostomy —*see* Complications, colostomy
cystostomy —*see* Complications, cystostomy
enterostomy —*see* Complications, enterostomy
gastrostomy —*see* Complications, gastrostomy
ileostomy —*see* Complications, enterostomy
jejunostomy —*see* Complications, enterostomy
nephrostomy —*see* Complications, stoma, urinary tract
tracheostomy —*see* Complications, tracheostomy
ureterostomy —*see* Complications, stoma, urinary tract
urethrostomy —*see* Complications, stoma, urinary tract
balloon implant or device
gastrointestinal T85.9
embolism T85.818
fibrosis T85.828
hemorrhage T85.838
infection and inflammation T85.79
pain T85.848
specified type NEC T85.898
stenosis T85.858
thrombosis T85.868
vascular (counterpulsation) T82.9
embolism T82.818
fibrosis T82.828
hemorrhage T82.838
infection or inflammation T82.7
mechanical
breakdown T82.513
displacement T82.523
leakage T82.533
malposition T82.523
obstruction T82.593
perforation T82.593
protrusion T82.593
pain T82.848
specified type NEC T82.898
stenosis T82.858
thrombosis T82.868
bariatric procedure
gastric band procedure K95.Ø9
infection K95.Ø1
specified procedure NEC K95.89
infection K95.81
bile duct implant (prosthetic) T85.9
embolism T85.818
fibrosis T85.828
hemorrhage T85.838
infection and inflammation T85.79
mechanical
breakdown T85.51Ø
displacement T85.52Ø
malfunction T85.51Ø
malposition T85.52Ø
obstruction T85.59Ø
perforation T85.59Ø
protrusion T85.59Ø
specified NEC T85.59Ø
pain T85.848
specified type NEC T85.898

C

Complication *(Continued)*
bile duct implant *(Continued)*
stenosis T85.858
thrombosis T85.868
bladder device (auxiliary) —*see* Complications, genitourinary, device or implant, urinary system
bleeding (postoperative) —*see* Complication, postoperative, hemorrhage
intraoperative —*see* Complication, intraoperative, hemorrhage
blood vessel graft —*see* Complications, graft, vascular
bone
device NEC T84.9
embolism T84.81
fibrosis T84.82
hemorrhage T84.83
infection or inflammation T84.7
mechanical
breakdown T84.318
displacement T84.328
malposition T84.328
obstruction T84.398
perforation T84.398
protrusion T84.398
pain T84.84
specified type NEC T84.89
stenosis T84.85
thrombosis T84.86
graft —*see* Complications, graft, bone
growth stimulator (electrode) —*see* Complications, electronic stimulator device, bone
marrow transplant —*see* Complications, transplant, bone, marrow
brain neurostimulator (electrode) —*see* Complications, electronic stimulator device, brain
breast implant (prosthetic) T85.9
capsular contracture T85.44
embolism T85.818
fibrosis T85.828
hemorrhage T85.838
infection and inflammation T85.79
mechanical
breakdown T85.41
displacement T85.42
leakage T85.43
malposition T85.42
obstruction T85.49
perforation T85.49
protrusion T85.49
specified NEC T85.49
pain T85.848
specified type NEC T85.898
stenosis T85.858
thrombosis T85.868
bypass —*see also* Complications, prosthetic device or implant
aortocoronary —*see* Complications, coronary artery (bypass) graft
arterial —*see also* Complications, graft, vascular
extremity —*see* Complications, extremity artery (bypass) graft
cardiac —*see also* Disease, heart
device, implant or graft T82.9
embolism T82.817
fibrosis T82.827
hemorrhage T82.837
infection or inflammation T82.7
valve prosthesis T82.6
mechanical
breakdown T82.519
specified device NEC T82.518
displacement T82.529
specified device NEC T82.528
leakage T82.539
specified device NEC T82.538
malposition T82.529
specified device NEC T82.528

Complication *(Continued)*
cardiac *(Continued)*
device, implant or graft *(Continued)*
mechanical *(Continued)*
obstruction T82.599
specified device NEC T82.598
perforation T82.599
specified device NEC T82.598
protrusion T82.599
specified device NEC T82.598
pain T82.847
specified type NEC T82.897
stenosis T82.857
thrombosis T82.867
cardiovascular device, graft or implant T82.9
aortic graft —*see* Complications, graft, vascular
arteriovenous
fistula, artificial —*see* Complication, arteriovenous, fistula, surgically created
shunt —*see* Complication, arteriovenous, shunt, surgically created
artificial heart —*see* Complication, artificial, heart
balloon (counterpulsation) device —*see* Complication, balloon implant, vascular
carotid artery graft —*see* Complications, graft, vascular
coronary bypass graft —*see* Complication, coronary artery (bypass) graft
dialysis catheter (vascular) —*see* Complication, catheter, dialysis
electronic T82.9
electrode T82.9
embolism T82.817
fibrosis T82.827
hemorrhage T82.837
infection T82.7
mechanical
breakdown T82.110
displacement T82.120
leakage T82.190
obstruction T82.190
perforation T82.190
protrusion T82.190
specified type NEC T82.190
pain T82.847
specified NEC T82.897
stenosis T82.857
thrombosis T82.867
embolism T82.817
fibrosis T82.827
hemorrhage T82.837
infection T82.7
mechanical
breakdown T82.119
displacement T82.129
leakage T82.199
obstruction T82.199
perforation T82.199
protrusion T82.199
specified type NEC T82.199
pain T82.847
pulse generator T82.9
embolism T82.817
fibrosis T82.827
hemorrhage T82.837
infection T82.7
mechanical
breakdown T82.111
displacement T82.121
leakage T82.191
obstruction T82.191
perforation T82.191
protrusion T82.191
specified type NEC T82.191
pain T82.847
specified NEC T82.897
stenosis T82.857
thrombosis T82.867

Complication *(Continued)*
cardiovascular device, graft or implant *(Continued)*
electronic *(Continued)*
specified condition NEC T82.897
specified device NEC T82.9
embolism T82.817
fibrosis T82.827
hemorrhage T82.837
infection T82.7
mechanical
breakdown T82.118
displacement T82.128
leakage T82.198
obstruction T82.198
perforation T82.198
protrusion T82.198
specified type NEC T82.198
pain T82.847
specified NEC T82.897
stenosis T82.857
thrombosis T82.867
stenosis T82.857
thrombosis T82.867
extremity artery graft —*see* Complication, extremity artery (bypass) graft
femoral artery graft —*see* Complication, extremity artery (bypass) graft
heart
transplant —*see* Complication, transplant, heart
valve —*see* Complication, prosthetic device, heart valve
graft —*see* Complication, heart, valve, graft
heart-lung transplant —*see* Complication, transplant, heart, with lung
infection or inflammation T82.7
umbrella device —*see* Complication, umbrella device, vascular
vascular graft (or anastomosis) —*see* Complication, graft, vascular
carotid artery (bypass) graft —*see* Complications, graft, vascular
catheter (device) NEC —*see also* Complications, prosthetic device or implant
cranial infusion
infection and inflammation T85.735
mechanical
breakdown T85.610
displacement T85.620
leakage T85.630
malfunction T85.690
malposition T85.620
obstruction T85.690
perforation T85.690
protrusion T85.690
specified NEC T85.690
cystostomy T83.9
embolism T83.81
fibrosis T83.82
hemorrhage T83.83
infection and inflammation T83.510
mechanical
breakdown T83.010
displacement T83.020
leakage T83.030
malposition T83.020
obstruction T83.090
perforation T83.090
protrusion T83.090
specified NEC T83.090
pain T83.84
specified type NEC T83.89
stenosis T83.85
thrombosis T83.86
dialysis (vascular) T82.9
embolism T82.818
fibrosis T82.828
hemorrhage T82.838

Complication *(Continued)*
catheter NEC *(Continued)*
dialysis *(Continued)*
infection and inflammation T82.7
intraperitoneal —*see* Complications, catheter, intraperitoneal
mechanical
breakdown T82.41
displacement T82.42
leakage T82.43
malposition T82.42
obstruction T82.49
perforation T82.49
protrusion T82.49
pain T82.848
specified type NEC T82.898
stenosis T82.858
thrombosis T82.868
epidural infusion T85.9
embolism T85.810
fibrosis T85.820
hemorrhage T85.830
infection and inflammation T85.735
mechanical
breakdown T85.610
displacement T85.620
leakage T85.630
malfunction T85.610
malposition T85.620
obstruction T85.690
perforation T85.690
protrusion T85.690
specified NEC T85.690
pain T85.840
specified type NEC T85.890
stenosis T85.850
thrombosis T85.860
intraperitoneal dialysis T85.9
embolism T85.818
fibrosis T85.828
hemorrhage T85.838
infection and inflammation T85.71
mechanical
breakdown T85.611
displacement T85.621
leakage T85.631
malfunction T85.611
malposition T85.621
obstruction T85.691
perforation T85.691
protrusion T85.691
specified NEC T85.691
pain T85.848
specified type NEC T85.898
stenosis T85.858
thrombosis T85.868
intrathecal infusion
infection and inflammation T85.735
mechanical
breakdown T85.610
displacement T85.620
leakage T85.630
malfunction T85.690
malposition T85.620
obstruction T85.690
perforation T85.690
protrusion T85.690
specified NEC T85.690
intravenous infusion T82.9
embolism T82.818
fibrosis T82.828
hemorrhage T82.838
infection or inflammation T82.7
mechanical
breakdown T82.514
displacement T82.524
leakage T82.534
malposition T82.524
obstruction T82.594
perforation T82.594
protrusion T82.594
pain T82.848

Complication *(Continued)*
catheter NEC *(Continued)*
intravenous infusion *(Continued)*
specified type NEC T82.898
stenosis T82.858
thrombosis T82.868
spinal infusion
infection and inflammation T85.735
mechanical
breakdown T85.610
displacement T85.620
leakage T85.630
malfunction T85.690
malposition T85.620
obstruction T85.690
perforation T85.690
protrusion T85.690
specified NEC T85.690
subarachnoid infusion
infection and inflammation T85.735
mechanical
breakdown T85.610
displacement T85.620
leakage T85.630
malfunction T85.690
malposition T85.620
obstruction T85.690
perforation T85.690
protrusion T85.690
specified NEC T85.690
subdural infusion T85.9
embolism T85.810
fibrosis T85.820
hemorrhage T85.830
infection and inflammation T85.735
mechanical
breakdown T85.610
displacement T85.620
leakage T85.630
malfunction T85.610
malposition T85.620
obstruction T85.690
perforation T85.690
protrusion T85.690
specified NEC T85.690
pain T85.840
specified type NEC T85.890
stenosis T85.850
thrombosis T85.860
urethral T83.9
displacement T83.028
embolism T83.81
fibrosis T83.82
hemorrhage T83.83
indwelling
breakdown T83.011
displacement T83.021
infection and inflammation T83.511
leakage T83.031
specified complication NEC T83.091
infection and inflammation T83.511
leakage T83.038
malposition T83.028
mechanical
breakdown T83.011
obstruction (mechanical) T83.091
pain T83.84
perforation T83.091
protrusion T83.091
specified type NEC T83.091
stenosis T83.85
thrombosis T83.86
urinary NEC
breakdown T83.018
displacement T83.028
infection and inflammation T83.518
leakage T83.038
specified complication NEC T83.098
cecostomy (stoma) —*see* Complications, colostomy

Complication *(Continued)*
cesarean delivery wound NEC O90.89
disruption O90.0
hematoma O90.2
infection (following delivery) O86.00
chemotherapy (antineoplastic) NEC T88.7
chin implant (prosthetic) —*see* Complication, prosthetic device or implant, specified NEC
circulatory system I99.8
intraoperative I97.88
postprocedural I97.89
following cardiac surgery —*see also* Infarct, myocardium, associated with revascularization procedure I97.19- •
postcardiotomy syndrome I97.0
hypertension I97.3
lymphedema after mastectomy I97.2
postcardiotomy syndrome I97.0
specified NEC I97.89
colostomy (stoma) K94.00
hemorrhage K94.01
infection K94.02
malfunction K94.03
mechanical K94.03
specified complication NEC K94.09
contraceptive device, intrauterine —*see* Complications, intrauterine, contraceptive device
cord (umbilical) —*see* Complications, umbilical cord
corneal graft —*see* Complications, graft, cornea
coronary artery (bypass) graft T82.9
atherosclerosis —*see* Arteriosclerosis, coronary (artery)
embolism T82.818
fibrosis T82.828
hemorrhage T82.838
infection and inflammation T82.7
mechanical
breakdown T82.211
displacement T82.212
leakage T82.213
malposition T82.212
obstruction T82.218
perforation T82.218
protrusion T82.218
specified NEC T82.218
pain T82.848
specified type NEC T82.898
stenosis T82.858
thrombosis T82.868
counterpulsation device (balloon), intra-aortic —*see* Complications, balloon implant, vascular
cystostomy (stoma) N99.518
catheter —*see* Complications, catheter, cystostomy
hemorrhage N99.510
infection N99.511
malfunction N99.512
specified type NEC N99.518
delivery —*see also* Complications, obstetric O75.9
procedure (instrumental) (manual) (surgical) O75.4
specified NEC O75.89
dialysis (peritoneal) (renal) —*see also* Complications, infusion
catheter (vascular) —*see* Complication, catheter, dialysis
peritoneal, intraperitoneal —*see* Complications, catheter, intraperitoneal
dorsal column (spinal) neurostimulator —*see* Complications, electronic stimulator device, spinal cord
drug NEC T88.7
ear procedure —*see also* Disorder, ear
intraoperative H95.88- •
hematoma —*see* Complications, intraoperative, hematoma (of), ear

C

▶ New ➡ Revised ~~deleted~~ Deleted • Use Additional Character(s)

Complication *(Continued)*
ear procedure *(Continued)*
intraoperative *(Continued)*
hemorrhage —*see* Complications, intraoperative, hemorrhage (of), ear
laceration —*see* Complications, intraoperative, puncture or laceration..., ear
seroma —*see* Complications, postprocedural, seroma (of), mastoid process
specified NEC H95.88- •
postoperative H95.89- •
external ear canal stenosis H95.81- •
hematoma —*see* Complications, postprocedural, hemorrhage (hematoma) (of), ear
hemorrhage —*see* Complications, postprocedural, hemorrhage (hematoma) (of), ear
postmastoidectomy —*see* Complications, postmastoidectomy
specified NEC H95.89- •
ectopic pregnancy O08.9
damage to pelvic organs O08.6
embolism O08.2
genital infection O08.0
hemorrhage (delayed) (excessive) O08.1
metabolic disorder O08.5
renal failure O08.4
shock O08.3
specified type NEC O08.0
venous complication NEC O08.7
electronic stimulator device
bladder (urinary) —*see* Complications, electronic stimulator device, urinary
bone T84.9
breakdown T84.310
displacement T84.320
embolism T84.81
fibrosis T84.82
hemorrhage T84.83
infection or inflammation T84.7
malfunction T84.310
malposition T84.320
mechanical NEC T84.390
obstruction T84.390
pain T84.84
perforation T84.390
protrusion T84.390
specified type NEC T84.89
stenosis T84.85
thrombosis T84.86
brain T85.9
embolism T85.810
fibrosis T85.820
hemorrhage T85.830
infection and inflammation T85.731
mechanical
breakdown T85.110
displacement T85.120
leakage T85.190
malposition T85.120
obstruction T85.190
perforation T85.190
protrusion T85.190
specified NEC T85.190
pain T85.840
specified type NEC T85.890
stenosis T85.850
thrombosis T85.860
cardiac (defibrillator) (pacemaker) —*see* Complications, cardiovascular device or implant, electronic
generator (brain) (gastric) (peripheral) (sacral) (spinal)
breakdown T85.113
displacement T85.123
leakage T85.193
malposition T85.123
obstruction T85.193

Complication *(Continued)*
electronic stimulator device *(Continued)*
generator *(Continued)*
perforation T85.193
protrusion T85.193
specified type NEC T85.193
muscle T84.9
breakdown T84.418
displacement T84.428
embolism T84.81
fibrosis T84.82
hemorrhage T84.83
infection or inflammation T84.7
mechanical NEC T84.498
pain T84.84
specified type NEC T84.89
stenosis T84.85
thrombosis T84.86
nervous system T85.9
brain —*see* Complications, electronic stimulator device, brain
cranial nerve —*see* Complications, electronic stimulator device, peripheral nerve
embolism T85.810
fibrosis T85.820
gastric nerve —*see* Complications, electronic stimulator device, peripheral nerve
hemorrhage T85.830
infection and inflammation T85.738
mechanical
breakdown T85.118
displacement T85.128
leakage T85.199
malposition T85.128
obstruction T85.199
perforation T85.199
protrusion T85.199
specified NEC T85.199
pain T85.840
peripheral nerve —*see* Complications, electronic stimulator device, peripheral nerve
sacral nerve —*see* Complications, electronic stimulator device, peripheral nerve
specified type NEC T85.890
spinal cord —*see* Complications, electronic stimulator device, spinal cord
stenosis T85.850
thrombosis T85.860
vagal nerve —*see* Complications, electronic stimulator device, peripheral nerve
peripheral nerve T85.9
embolism T85.810
fibrosis T85.820
hemorrhage T85.830
infection and inflammation T85.732
mechanical
breakdown T85.111
displacement T85.121
leakage T85.191
malposition T85.121
obstruction T85.191
perforation T85.191
protrusion T85.191
specified NEC T85.191
pain T85.840
specified type NEC T85.890
stenosis T85.850
thrombosis T85.860
spinal cord T85.9
embolism T85.810
fibrosis T85.820
hemorrhage T85.830
infection and inflammation T85.733
mechanical
breakdown T85.112
displacement T85.122

Complication *(Continued)*
electronic stimulator device *(Continued)*
spinal cord *(Continued)*
mechanical *(Continued)*
leakage T85.192
malposition T85.122
obstruction T85.192
perforation T85.192
protrusion T85.192
specified NEC T85.192
pain T85.840
specified type NEC T85.890
stenosis T85.850
thrombosis T85.860
urinary T83.9
embolism T83.81
fibrosis T83.82
hemorrhage T83.83
infection and inflammation T83.598
mechanical
breakdown T83.110
displacement T83.120
malposition T83.120
perforation T83.190
protrusion T83.190
specified NEC T83.190
pain T83.84
specified type NEC T83.89
stenosis T83.85
thrombosis T83.86
electroshock therapy T88.9
specified NEC T88.8
endocrine E34.9
postprocedural
adrenal hypofunction E89.6
hypoinsulinemia E89.1
hypoparathyroidism E89.2
hypopituitarism E89.3
hypothyroidism E89.0
ovarian failure E89.40
asymptomatic E89.40
symptomatic E89.41
specified NEC E89.89
testicular hypofunction E89.5
endodontic treatment NEC M27.59
enterostomy (stoma) K94.10
hemorrhage K94.11
infection K94.12
malfunction K94.13
mechanical K94.13
specified complication NEC K94.19
episiotomy, disruption O90.1
esophageal anti-reflux device T85.9
embolism T85.818
fibrosis T85.828
hemorrhage T85.838
infection and inflammation T85.79
mechanical
breakdown T85.511
displacement T85.521
malfunction T85.511
malposition T85.521
obstruction T85.591
perforation T85.591
protrusion T85.591
specified NEC T85.591
pain T85.848
specified type NEC T85.898
stenosis T85.858
thrombosis T85.868
esophagostomy K94.30
hemorrhage K94.31
infection K94.32
malfunction K94.33
mechanical K94.33
specified complication NEC K94.39
extracorporeal circulation T80.90
extremity artery (bypass) graft T82.9
arteriosclerosis —*see* Arteriosclerosis, extremities, bypass graft
embolism T82.818
fibrosis T82.828

C

- Complication *(Continued)*
  - extremity artery (bypass) graft *(Continued)*
    - hemorrhage T82.838
    - infection and inflammation T82.7
    - mechanical
      - breakdown T82.318
        - femoral artery T82.312
      - displacement T82.328
        - femoral artery T82.322
      - leakage T82.338
        - femoral artery T82.332
      - malposition T82.328
        - femoral artery T82.322
      - obstruction T82.398
        - femoral artery T82.392
      - perforation T82.398
        - femoral artery T82.392
      - protrusion T82.398
        - femoral artery T82.392
    - pain T82.848
    - specified type NEC T82.898
    - stenosis T82.858
    - thrombosis T82.868
  - eye H57.9
    - corneal graft —*see* Complications, graft, cornea
    - implant (prosthetic) T85.9
      - embolism T85.818
      - fibrosis T85.828
      - hemorrhage T85.838
      - infection and inflammation T85.79
      - mechanical
        - breakdown T85.318
        - displacement T85.328
        - leakage T85.398
        - malposition T85.328
        - obstruction T85.398
        - perforation T85.398
        - protrusion T85.398
        - specified NEC T85.398
      - pain T85.848
      - specified type NEC T85.898
      - stenosis T85.858
      - thrombosis T85.868
    - intraocular lens —*see* Complications, intraocular lens
    - orbital prosthesis —*see* Complications, orbital prosthesis
  - female genital N94.9
    - device, implant or graft NEC —*see* Complications, genitourinary, device or implant, genital tract
  - femoral artery (bypass) graft —*see* Complication, extremity artery (bypass) graft
  - fixation device, internal (orthopedic) T84.9
    - infection and inflammation T84.60
      - arm T84.61-●
        - humerus T84.61-●
        - radius T84.61-●
        - ulna T84.61-●
      - leg T84.629
        - femur T84.62-●
        - fibula T84.62-●
        - tibia T84.62-●
      - specified site NEC T84.69
      - spine T84.63
    - mechanical
      - breakdown
        - limb T84.119
          - carpal T84.210
          - femur T84.11-●
          - fibula T84.11-●
          - humerus T84.11-●
          - metacarpal T84.210
          - metatarsal T84.213
          - phalanx
            - foot T84.213
            - hand T84.210
          - radius T84.11-●
          - tarsal T84.213

- Complication *(Continued)*
  - fixation device, internal *(Continued)*
    - mechanical *(Continued)*
      - breakdown *(Continued)*
        - limb *(Continued)*
          - tibia T84.11-●
          - ulna T84.11-●
        - specified bone NEC T84.218
        - spine T84.216
      - displacement
        - limb T84.129
          - carpal T84.220
          - femur T84.12-●
          - fibula T84.12-●
          - humerus T84.12-●
          - metacarpal T84.220
          - metatarsal T84.223
          - phalanx
            - foot T84.223
            - hand T84.220
          - radius T84.12-●
          - tarsal T84.223
          - tibia T84.12-●
          - ulna T84.12-●
        - specified bone NEC T84.228
        - spine T84.226
      - malposition —*see* Complications, fixation device, internal, mechanical, displacement
      - obstruction —*see* Complications, fixation device, internal, mechanical, specified type NEC
      - perforation —*see* Complications, fixation device, internal, mechanical, specified type NEC
      - protrusion —*see* Complications, fixation device, internal, mechanical, specified type NEC
      - specified type NEC
        - limb T84.199
          - carpal T84.290
          - femur T84.19-●
          - fibula T84.19-●
          - humerus T84.19-●
          - metacarpal T84.290
          - metatarsal T84.293
          - phalanx
            - foot T84.293
            - hand T84.290
          - radius T84.19-●
          - tarsal T84.293
          - tibia T84.19-●
          - ulna T84.19-●
        - specified bone NEC T84.298
        - vertebra T84.296
    - specified type NEC T84.89
      - embolism T84.81
      - fibrosis T84.82
      - hemorrhage T84.83
      - pain T84.84
      - specified complication NEC T84.89
      - stenosis T84.85
      - thrombosis T84.86
  - following
    - acute myocardial infarction NEC I23.8
      - aneurysm (false) (of cardiac wall) (of heart wall) (ruptured) I23.3
      - angina I23.7
      - atrial
        - septal defect I23.1
        - thrombosis I23.6
      - cardiac wall rupture I23.3
      - chordae tendinae rupture I23.4
      - defect
        - septal
          - atrial (heart) I23.1
          - ventricular (heart) I23.2
      - hemopericardium I23.0
      - papillary muscle rupture I23.5
      - rupture
        - cardiac wall I23.3
          - with hemopericardium I23.0

- Complication *(Continued)*
  - following *(Continued)*
    - acute myocardial infarction NEC *(Continued)*
      - rupture *(Continued)*
        - chordae tendineae I23.4
        - papillary muscle I23.5
      - specified NEC I23.8
      - thrombosis
        - atrium I23.6
        - auricular appendage I23.6
        - ventricle (heart) I23.6
      - ventricular
        - septal defect I23.2
        - thrombosis I23.6
    - ectopic or molar pregnancy O08.9
      - cardiac arrest O08.81
      - sepsis O08.82
      - specified type NEC O08.89
      - urinary tract infection O08.83
    - termination of pregnancy —*see* Abortion
  - gastrointestinal K92.9
    - bile duct prosthesis —*see* Complications, bile duct implant
    - esophageal anti-reflux device —*see* Complications, esophageal anti-reflux device
    - postoperative
      - colostomy —*see* Complications, colostomy
      - dumping syndrome K91.1
      - enterostomy —*see* Complications, enterostomy
      - gastrostomy —*see* Complications, gastrostomy
      - malabsorption NEC K91.2
      - obstruction —*see also* Obstruction, intestine, postoperative K91.30
      - postcholecystectomy syndrome K91.5
      - specified NEC K91.89
      - vomiting after GI surgery K91.0
    - prosthetic device or implant
      - bile duct prosthesis —*see* Complications, bile duct implant
      - esophageal anti-reflux device —*see* Complications, esophageal anti-reflux device
      - specified type NEC
        - embolism T85.818
        - fibrosis T85.828
        - hemorrhage T85.838
        - mechanical
          - breakdown T85.518
          - displacement T85.528
          - malfunction T85.518
          - malposition T85.528
          - obstruction T85.598
          - perforation T85.598
          - protrusion T85.598
          - specified NEC T85.598
        - pain T85.848
        - specified complication NEC T85.898
        - stenosis T85.858
        - thrombosis T85.868
  - gastrostomy (stoma) K94.20
    - hemorrhage K94.21
    - infection K94.22
    - malfunction K94.23
    - mechanical K94.23
    - specified complication NEC K94.29
  - genitourinary
    - device or implant T83.9
      - genital tract T83.9
        - infection or inflammation T83.69
        - intrauterine contraceptive device —*see* Complications, intrauterine, contraceptive device
        - mechanical —*see* Complications, by device, mechanical
        - ➡ mesh —*see* Complications, prosthetic device or implant, mesh
        - penile prosthesis —*see* Complications, prosthetic device, penile

Complication (Continued)
genitourinary (Continued)
device or implant (Continued)
genital tract (Continued)
specified type NEC T83.89
embolism T83.81
fibrosis T83.82
hemorrhage T83.83
pain T83.84
specified complication NEC T83.89
stenosis T83.85
thrombosis T83.86
vaginal mesh —see Complications, prosthetic device or implant, mesh
urinary system T83.9
cystostomy catheter —see Complication, catheter, cystostomy
electronic stimulator —see Complications, electronic stimulator device, urinary
indwelling urethral catheter —see Complications, catheter, urethral, indwelling
infection or inflammation T83.598
indwelling urethral catheter T83.511
kidney transplant —see Complication, transplant, kidney
organ graft —see Complication, graft, urinary organ
specified type NEC T83.89
embolism T83.81
fibrosis T83.82
hemorrhage T83.83
mechanical T83.198
breakdown T83.118
displacement T83.128
malfunction T83.118
malposition T83.128
obstruction T83.198
perforation T83.198
protrusion T83.198
specified NEC T83.198
sphincter, implanted T83.191
stent (ileal conduit) (nephroureteral) T83.193
ureteral indwelling T83.192
pain T83.84
specified complication NEC T83.89
stenosis T83.85
thrombosis T83.86
sphincter implant —see Complications, implant, urinary sphincter
postprocedural
pelvic peritoneal adhesions N99.4
renal failure N99.Ø
specified NEC N99.89
stoma —see Complications, stoma, urinary tract
urethral stricture —see Stricture, urethra, postprocedural
vaginal
adhesions N99.2
vault prolapse N99.3
graft (bypass) (patch) —see also Complications, prosthetic device or implant
aorta —see Complications, graft, vascular
arterial —see Complication, graft, vascular
bone T86.839
failure T86.831
infection T86.832
mechanical T84.318
breakdown T84.318
displacement T84.328
protrusion T84.398
specified type NEC T84.398
rejection T86.83Ø
specified type NEC T86.838
carotid artery —see Complications, graft, vascular

Complication (Continued)
graft (Continued)
cornea T86.849
failure T86.841
infection T86.842
mechanical T85.398
breakdown T85.318
displacement T85.328
protrusion T85.398
specified type NEC T85.398
rejection T86.84Ø
retroprosthetic membrane T85.398
specified type NEC T86.848
femoral artery (bypass) —see Complication, extremity artery (bypass) graft
genital organ or tract —see Complications, genitourinary, device or implant, genital tract
muscle T84.9
breakdown T84.41Ø
displacement T84.42Ø
embolism T84.81
fibrosis T84.82
hemorrhage T84.83
infection and inflammation T84.7
mechanical NEC T84.49Ø
pain T84.84
specified type NEC T84.89
stenosis T84.85
thrombosis T84.86
nerve —see Complication, prosthetic device or implant, specified NEC
skin —see Complications, prosthetic device or implant, skin graft
tendon T84.9
breakdown T84.41Ø
displacement T84.42Ø
embolism T84.81
fibrosis T84.82
hemorrhage T84.83
infection and inflammation T84.7
mechanical NEC T84.49Ø
pain T84.84
specified type NEC T84.89
stenosis T84.85
thrombosis T84.86
urinary organ T83.9
embolism T83.81
fibrosis T83.82
hemorrhage T83.83
infection and inflammation T83.598
indwelling urethral catheter T83.511
mechanical
breakdown T83.21
displacement T83.22
erosion T83.24
exposure T83.25
leakage T83.23
malposition T83.22
obstruction T83.29
perforation T83.29
protrusion T83.29
specified NEC T83.29
pain T83.84
specified type NEC T83.89
stenosis T83.85
thrombosis T83.86
vascular T82.9
embolism T82.818
femoral artery —see Complication, extremity artery (bypass) graft
fibrosis T82.828
hemorrhage T82.838
mechanical
breakdown T82.319
aorta (bifurcation) T82.31Ø
carotid artery T82.311
specified vessel NEC T82.318
displacement T82.329
aorta (bifurcation) T82.32Ø
carotid artery T82.321
specified vessel NEC T82.328

Complication (Continued)
graft (Continued)
vascular (Continued)
mechanical (Continued)
leakage T82.339
aorta (bifurcation) T82.33Ø
carotid artery T82.331
specified vessel NEC T82.338
malposition T82.329
aorta (bifurcation) T82.32Ø
carotid artery T82.321
specified vessel NEC T82.328
obstruction T82.399
aorta (bifurcation) T82.39Ø
carotid artery T82.391
specified vessel NEC T82.398
perforation T82.399
aorta (bifurcation) T82.39Ø
carotid artery T82.391
specified vessel NEC T82.398
protrusion T82.399
aorta (bifurcation) T82.39Ø
carotid artery T82.391
specified vessel NEC T82.398
pain T82.848
specified complication NEC T82.898
stenosis T82.858
thrombosis T82.868
heart I51.9
assist device
infection and inflammation T82.7
following acute myocardial infarction —see Complications, following, acute myocardial infarction
postoperative —see Complications, circulatory system
transplant —see Complication, transplant, heart
and lung(s) —see Complications, transplant, heart, with lung
valve
graft (biological) T82.9
embolism T82.817
fibrosis T82.827
hemorrhage T82.837
infection and inflammation T82.7
mechanical T82.228
breakdown T82.221
displacement T82.222
leakage T82.223
malposition T82.222
obstruction T82.228
perforation T82.228
protrusion T82.228
pain T82.847
specified type NEC T82.897
stenosis T82.857
thrombosis T82.867
prosthesis T82.9
embolism T82.817
fibrosis T82.827
hemorrhage T82.837
infection or inflammation T82.6
mechanical T82.Ø9
breakdown T82.Ø1
displacement T82.Ø2
leakage T82.Ø3
malposition T82.Ø2
obstruction T82.Ø9
perforation T82.Ø9
protrusion T82.Ø9
pain T82.847
specified type NEC T82.897
mechanical T82.Ø9
stenosis T82.857
thrombosis T82.867
hematoma
intraoperative —see Complication, intraoperative, hemorrhage
postprocedural —see Complication, postprocedural, hematoma
hemodialysis —see Complications, dialysis

Complication *(Continued)*
hemorrhage
intraoperative —*see* Complication, intraoperative, hemorrhage
postprocedural —*see* Complication, postprocedural, hemorrhage
ileostomy (stoma) —*see* Complications, enterostomy
immunization (procedure) —*see* Complications, vaccination
implant —*see also* Complications, by site and type
urinary sphincter T83.9
embolism T83.81
fibrosis T83.82
hemorrhage T83.83
infection and inflammation T83.591
mechanical
breakdown T83.111
displacement T83.121
leakage T83.191
malposition T83.121
obstruction T83.191
perforation T83.191
protrusion T83.191
specified NEC T83.191
pain T83.84
specified type NEC T83.89
stenosis T83.85
thrombosis T83.86
infusion (procedure) T8Ø.9Ø
air embolism T8Ø.Ø
blood —*see* Complications, transfusion
catheter —*see* Complications, catheter
infection T8Ø.29
pump —*see* Complications, cardiovascular, device or implant
sepsis T8Ø.29
serum reaction —*see also* Reaction, serum T8Ø.69
anaphylactic shock —*see also* Shock, anaphylactic T8Ø.59
specified type NEC T8Ø.89
inhalation therapy NEC T81.81
injection (procedure) T8Ø.9Ø
drug reaction —*see* Reaction, drug
infection T8Ø.29
sepsis T8Ø.29
serum (prophylactic) (therapeutic) —*see* Complications, vaccination
specified type NEC T8Ø.89
vaccine (any) —*see* Complications, vaccination
inoculation (any) —*see* Complications, vaccination
insulin pump
infection and inflammation T85.72
mechanical
breakdown T85.614
displacement T85.624
leakage T85.633
malposition T85.624
obstruction T85.694
perforation T85.694
protrusion T85.694
specified NEC T85.694
intestinal pouch NEC K91.858
intraocular lens (prosthetic) T85.9
embolism T85.818
fibrosis T85.828
hemorrhage T85.838
infection and inflammation T85.79
mechanical
breakdown T85.21
displacement T85.22
malposition T85.22
obstruction T85.29
perforation T85.29
protrusion T85.29
specified NEC T85.29
pain T85.848
specified type NEC T85.898

Complication *(Continued)*
intraocular lens *(Continued)*
stenosis T85.858
thrombosis T85.868
intraoperative (intraprocedural)
cardiac arrest —*see also* Infarct, myocardium, associated with revascularization procedure
during cardiac surgery I97.71Ø
during other surgery I97.711
cardiac functional disturbance NEC —*see also* Infarct, myocardium, associated with revascularization procedure
during cardiac surgery I97.79Ø
during other surgery I97.791
hemorrhage (hematoma) (of)
circulatory system organ or structure
during cardiac bypass I97.411
during cardiac catheterization I97.41Ø
during other circulatory system procedure I97.418
during other procedure I97.42
digestive system organ
during procedure on digestive system K91.61
during procedure on other organ K91.62
ear
during procedure on ear and mastoid process H95.21
during procedure on other organ H95.22
endocrine system organ or structure
during procedure on endocrine system organ or structure E36.Ø1
during procedure on other organ E36.Ø2
eye and adnexa
during ophthalmic procedure H59.11-●
during other procedure H59.12-●
genitourinary organ or structure
during procedure on genitourinary organ or structure N99.61
during procedure on other organ N99.62
mastoid process
during procedure on ear and mastoid process H95.21
during procedure on other organ H95.22
musculoskeletal structure
during musculoskeletal surgery M96.81Ø
during non-orthopedic surgery M96.811
during orthopedic surgery M96.81Ø
nervous system
during a nervous system procedure G97.31
during other procedure G97.32
respiratory system
during other procedure J95.62
during procedure on respiratory system organ or structure J95.61
skin and subcutaneous tissue
during a dermatologic procedure L76.Ø1
during a procedure on other organ L76.Ø2
spleen
during a procedure on other organ D78.Ø2
during a procedure on the spleen D78.Ø1
puncture or laceration (accidental) (unintentional) (of)
brain
during a nervous system procedure G97.48
during other procedure G97.49

Complication *(Continued)*
intraoperative *(Continued)*
puncture or laceration *(Continued)*
circulatory system organ or structure
during circulatory system procedure I97.51
during other procedure I97.52
digestive system
during procedure on digestive system K91.71
during procedure on other organ K91.72
ear
during procedure on ear and mastoid process H95.31
during procedure on other organ H95.32
endocrine system organ or structure
during procedure on endocrine system organ or structure E36.11
during procedure on other organ E36.12
eye and adnexa
during ophthalmic procedure H59.21-●
during other procedure H59.22-●
genitourinary organ or structure
during procedure on genitourinary organ or structure N99.71
during procedure on other organ N99.72
mastoid process
during procedure on ear and mastoid process H95.31
during procedure on other organ H95.32
musculoskeletal structure
during musculoskeletal surgery M96.82Ø
during non-orthopedic surgery M96.821
during orthopedic surgery M96.82Ø
nervous system
during a nervous system procedure G97.48
during other procedure G97.49
respiratory system
during other procedure J95.72
during procedure on respiratory system organ or structure J95.71
skin and subcutaneous tissue
during a dermatologic procedure L76.11
during a procedure on other organ L76.12
spleen
during a procedure on other organ D78.12
during a procedure on the spleen D78.11
specified NEC
circulatory system I97.88
digestive system K91.81
ear H95.88
endocrine system E36.8
eye and adnexa H59.88
genitourinary system N99.81
mastoid process H95.88
musculoskeletal structure M96.89
nervous system G97.81
respiratory system J95.88
skin and subcutaneous tissue L76.81
spleen D78.81
intraperitoneal catheter (dialysis) (infusion) —*see* Complications, catheter, intraperitoneal
intrathecal infusion pump
infection and inflammation T85.738
mechanical
breakdown T85.615
displacement T85.625
leakage T85.635
malfunction T85.695
malposition T85.625
obstruction T85.695

- Complication *(Continued)*
  - intrathecal infusion pump *(Continued)*
    - mechanical *(Continued)*
      - perforation T85.695
      - protrusion T85.695
      - specified NEC T85.695
  - intrauterine
    - contraceptive device
      - embolism T83.81
      - fibrosis T83.82
      - hemorrhage T83.83
      - infection and inflammation T83.69
      - mechanical
        - breakdown T83.31
        - displacement T83.32
        - malposition T83.32
        - obstruction T83.39
        - perforation T83.39
        - protrusion T83.39
        - specified NEC T83.39
      - pain T83.84
      - specified type NEC T83.89
      - stenosis T83.85
      - thrombosis T83.86
    - procedure (fetal), to newborn P96.5
  - jejunostomy (stoma) —*see* Complications, enterostomy
  - joint prosthesis, internal T84.9
    - breakage (fracture) T84.01- ●
    - dislocation T84.02- ●
    - fracture T84.01- ●
    - infection or inflammation T84.50
      - hip T84.5- ●
      - knee T84.5- ●
      - specified joint NEC T84.59
    - instability T84.02- ●
    - malposition —*see* Complications, joint prosthesis, mechanical, displacement
    - mechanical
      - breakage, broken T84.01- ●
      - dislocation T84.02- ●
      - fracture T84.01- ●
      - instability T84.02- ●
      - leakage —*see* Complications, joint prosthesis, mechanical, specified NEC
      - loosening T84.039
        - hip T84.03- ●
        - knee T84.03- ●
        - specified joint NEC T84.038
      - obstruction —*see* Complications, joint prosthesis, mechanical, specified NEC
      - perforation —*see* Complications, joint prosthesis, mechanical, specified NEC
        - osteolysis T84.059
          - hip T84.05- ●
          - knee T84.05- ●
          - other specified joint T84.058
      - ▶ periprosthetic T84.059
      - protrusion —*see* Complications, joint prosthesis, mechanical, specified NEC
      - specified complication NEC T84.099
        - hip T84.09- ●
        - knee T84.09- ●
        - other specified joint T84.098
      - subluxation T84.02- ●
      - wear of articular bearing surface T84.069
        - hip T84.06- ●
        - knee T84.06- ●
        - other specified joint T84.068
    - specified joint NEC T84.89
      - embolism T84.81
      - fibrosis T84.82
      - hemorrhage T84.83
      - pain T84.84
      - specified complication NEC T84.89
      - stenosis T84.85
      - thrombosis T84.86
    - subluxation T84.02- ●

- Complication *(Continued)*
  - kidney transplant —*see* Complications, transplant, kidney
  - labor O75.9
    - specified NEC O75.89
  - liver transplant (immune or nonimmune) —*see* Complications, transplant, liver
  - lumbar puncture G97.1
    - cerebrospinal fluid leak G97.0
    - headache or reaction G97.1
  - lung transplant —*see* Complications, transplant, lung
    - and heart —*see* Complications, transplant, lung, with heart
  - male genital N50.9
    - device, implant or graft —*see* Complications, genitourinary, device or implant, genital tract
    - postprocedural or postoperative —*see* Complications, genitourinary, postprocedural
      - specified NEC N99.89
  - mastoid (process) procedure
    - intraoperative H95.88- ●
      - hematoma —*see* Complications, intraoperative, hemorrhage (hematoma) (of), mastoid process
      - hemorrhage —*see* Complications, intraoperative, hemorrhage (hematoma) (of), mastoid process
      - laceration —*see* Complications, intraoperative, puncture or laceration..., mastoid process
      - specified NEC H95.88- ●
    - postmastoidectomy —*see* Complications, postmastoidectomy
    - postoperative H95.89- ●
      - external ear canal stenosis H95.81- ●
      - hematoma —*see* Complications..., postprocedural, hematoma (of), mastoid process
      - hemorrhage —*see* Complications..., postprocedural, hemorrhage (of), mastoid process
      - postmastoidectomy —*see* Complications, postmastoidectomy
      - seroma —*see* Complications, postprocedural, seroma (of), mastoid process
      - specified NEC H95.89- ●
  - mastoidectomy cavity —*see* Complications, postmastoidectomy
  - mechanical —*see* Complications, by site and type, mechanical
  - medical procedures (*see also* Complication(s), intraoperative) T88.9
  - metabolic E88.9
    - postoperative E89.89
      - specified NEC E89.89
  - molar pregnancy NOS O08.9
    - damage to pelvic organs O08.6
    - embolism O08.2
    - genital infection O08.0
    - hemorrhage (delayed) (excessive) O08.1
    - metabolic disorder O08.5
    - renal failure O08.4
    - shock O08.3
    - specified type NEC O08.0
    - venous complication NEC O08.7
  - musculoskeletal system —*see also* Complication, intraoperative (intraprocedural), by site
    - device, implant or graft NEC —*see* Complications, orthopedic, device or implant
    - internal fixation (nail) (plate) (rod) —*see* Complications, fixation device, internal
    - joint prosthesis —*see* Complications, joint prosthesis

- Complication *(Continued)*
  - musculoskeletal system *(Continued)*
    - postoperative (postprocedural) M96.89
      - with osteoporosis —*see* Osteoporosis
      - fracture following insertion of device —*see* Fracture, following insertion of orthopedic implant, joint prosthesis or bone plate
      - joint instability after prosthesis removal M96.89
      - lordosis M96.4
      - postlaminectomy syndrome NEC M96.1
        - kyphosis M96.2
      - pseudarthrosis M96.0
      - specified complication NEC M96.89
    - post radiation M96.89
      - kyphosis M96.3
      - scoliosis M96.5
      - specified complication NEC M96.89
  - nephrostomy (stoma) —*see* Complications, stoma, urinary tract, external NEC
  - nervous system G98.8
    - central G96.9
    - device, implant or graft —*see also* Complication, prosthetic device or implant, specified NEC
      - electronic stimulator (electrode(s)) —*see* Complications, electronic stimulator device
      - specified NEC
        - infection and inflammation T85.738
        - mechanical T85.695
          - breakdown T85.615
          - displacement T85.625
          - leakage T85.635
          - malfunction T85.695
          - malposition T85.625
          - obstruction T85.695
          - perforation T85.695
          - protrusion T85.695
          - specified NEC T85.695
      - ventricular shunt —*see* Complications, ventricular shunt
    - electronic stimulator (electrode(s)) —*see* Complications, electronic stimulator device
    - postprocedural G97.82
      - intracranial hypotension G97.2
      - specified NEC G97.82
      - spinal fluid leak G97.0
  - newborn, due to intrauterine (fetal) procedure P96.5
  - nonabsorbable (permanent) sutures —*see* Complication, sutures, permanent
  - obstetric O75.9
    - procedure (instrumental) (manual) (surgical) specified NEC O75.4
    - specified NEC O75.89
    - surgical wound NEC O90.89
      - hematoma O90.2
      - infection O86.00
  - ocular lens implant —*see* Complications, intraocular lens
  - ophthalmologic
    - postprocedural bleb —*see* Blebitis
  - orbital prosthesis T85.9
    - embolism T85.818
    - fibrosis T85.828
    - hemorrhage T85.838
    - infection and inflammation T85.79
    - mechanical
      - breakdown T85.31- ●
      - displacement T85.32- ●
      - malposition T85.32- ●
      - obstruction T85.39- ●
      - perforation T85.39- ●
      - protrusion T85.39- ●
      - specified NEC T85.39- ●
    - pain T85.848
    - specified type NEC T85.898
    - stenosis T85.858
    - thrombosis T85.868

Complication *(Continued)*
organ or tissue transplant (partial) (total) —*see* Complications, transplant
orthopedic —*see also* Disorder, soft tissue
device or implant T84.9
bone
device or implant —*see* Complication, bone, device NEC
graft —*see* Complication, graft, bone
breakdown T84.418
displacement T84.428
electronic bone stimulator —*see* Complications, electronic stimulator device, bone
embolism T84.81
fibrosis T84.82
fixation device —*see* Complication, fixation device, internal
hemorrhage T84.83
infection or inflammation T84.7
joint prosthesis —*see* Complication, joint prosthesis, internal
malfunction T84.418
malposition T84.428
mechanical NEC T84.498
muscle graft —*see* Complications, graft, muscle
obstruction T84.498
pain T84.84
perforation T84.498
protrusion T84.498
specified complication NEC T84.89
stenosis T84.85
tendon graft —*see* Complications, graft, tendon
thrombosis T84.86
fracture (following insertion of device) —*see* Fracture, following insertion of orthopedic implant, joint prosthesis or bone plate
postprocedural M96.89
fracture —*see* Fracture, following insertion of orthopedic implant, joint prosthesis or bone plate
postlaminectomy syndrome NEC M96.1
kyphosis M96.3
lordosis M96.4
postradiation
kyphosis M96.2
scoliosis M96.5
pseudarthrosis post-fusion M96.0
specified type NEC M96.89
pacemaker (cardiac) —*see* Complications, cardiovascular device or implant, electronic
pancreas transplant —*see* Complications, transplant, pancreas
penile prosthesis (implant) —*see* Complications, prosthetic device, penile
perfusion NEC T80.90
perineal repair (obstetrical) NEC O90.89
disruption O90.1
hematoma O90.2
infection (following delivery) O86.09
phototherapy T88.9
specified NEC T88.8
postmastoidectomy NEC H95.19-●
cyst, mucosal H95.13-●
granulation H95.12-●
inflammation, chronic H95.11-●
recurrent cholesteatoma H95.0-●
postoperative —*see* Complications, postprocedural
circulatory —*see* Complications, circulatory system
ear —*see* Complications, ear
endocrine —*see* Complications, endocrine
eye —*see* Complications, eye
lumbar puncture G97.1
cerebrospinal fluid leak G97.0

Complication *(Continued)*
postoperative *(Continued)*
nervous system (central) (peripheral) —*see* Complications, nervous system
respiratory system —*see* Complications, respiratory system
postprocedural —*see also* Complications, surgical procedure
cardiac arrest —*see also* Infarct, myocardium, associated with revascularization procedure
following cardiac surgery I97.120
following other surgery I97.121
cardiac functional disturbance NEC —*see also* Infarct, myocardium, associated with revascularization procedure
following cardiac surgery I97.190
following other surgery I97.191
cardiac insufficiency
following cardiac surgery I97.110
following other surgery I97.111
chorioretinal scars following retinal surgery H59.81-●
following cataract surgery
cataract (lens) fragments H59.02-●
cystoid macular edema H59.03-●
specified NEC H59.09-●
vitreous (touch) syndrome H59.01-●
heart failure
following cardiac surgery I97.130
following other surgery I97.131
hematoma (of)
circulatory system organ or structure
following cardiac bypass I97.631
following cardiac catheterization I97.630
following other circulatory system procedure I97.638
following other procedure I97.621
digestive system
following procedure on digestive system K91.870
following procedure on other organ K91.871
ear
following other procedure H95.52
following procedure on ear and mastoid process H95.51
endocrine system
following endocrine system procedure E89.820
following other procedure E89.821
eye and adnexa
following ophthalmic procedure H59.33-●
following other procedure H59.34-●
genitourinary organ or structure
following procedure on genitourinary organ or structure N99.840
following procedure on other organ N99.841
mastoid process
following other procedure H95.52
following procedure on ear and mastoid process H95.51
musculoskeletal structure
following musculoskeletal surgery M96.840
following non-orthopedic surgery M96.841
following orthopedic surgery M96.840
nervous system
following nervous system procedure G97.61
following other procedure G97.62
respiratory system
following other procedure J95.861
following procedure on respiratory system organ or structure J95.860
skin and subcutaneous tissue
following dermatologic procedure L76.31

Complication *(Continued)*
postprocedural *(Continued)*
hematoma *(Continued)*
skin and subcutaneous tissue *(Continued)*
following procedure on other organ L76.32
spleen
following procedure on other organ D78.32
following procedure on the spleen D78.31
hemorrhage (of)
circulatory system organ or structure
following cardiac bypass I97.611
following cardiac catheterization I97.610
following other circulatory system procedure I97.618
following other procedure I97.620
digestive system
following procedure on digestive system K91.840
following procedure on other organ K91.841
ear
following other procedure H95.42
following procedure on ear and mastoid process H95.41
endocrine system
following endocrine system procedure E89.810
following other procedure E89.811
eye and adnexa
following ophthalmic procedure H59.31-●
following other procedure H59.32-●
genitourinary organ or structure
following procedure on genitourinary organ or structure N99.820
following procedure on other organ N99.821
mastoid process
following other procedure H95.42
following procedure on ear and mastoid process H95.41
musculoskeletal structure
following musculoskeletal surgery M96.830
following non-orthopedic surgery M96.831
following orthopedic surgery M96.830
nervous system
following nervous system procedure G97.51
following other procedure G97.52
respiratory system
following other procedure J95.831
following procedure on respiratory system organ or structure J95.830
skin and subcutaneous tissue
following dermatologic procedure L76.21
following a procedure on other organ L76.22
spleen
following procedure on other organ D78.22
following procedure on the spleen D78.21
seroma (of)
circulatory system organ or structure
following cardiac bypass I97.641
following cardiac catheterization I97.640
following other circulatory system procedure I97.648
following other procedure I97.622
digestive system
following procedure on digestive system K91.872
following procedure on other organ K91.873

C

- Complication *(Continued)*
  - postprocedural *(Continued)*
    - seroma *(Continued)*
      - ear
        - following other procedure H95.54
        - following procedure on ear and mastoid process H95.53
      - endocrine system
        - following endocrine system procedure E89.822
        - following other procedure E89.823
      - eye and adnexa
        - following ophthalmic procedure H59.35-●
        - following other procedure H59.36-●
      - genitourinary organ or structure
        - following procedure on genitourinary organ or structure N99.842
        - following procedure on other organ N99.843
      - mastoid process
        - following other procedure H95.54
        - following procedure on ear and mastoid process H95.53
      - musculoskeletal structure
        - following musculoskeletal surgery M96.842
        - following non-orthopedic surgery M96.843
        - following orthopedic surgery M96.842
      - nervous system
        - following nervous system procedure G97.63
        - following other procedure G97.64
      - respiratory system
        - following other procedure J95.863
        - following procedure on respiratory system organ or structure J95.862
      - skin and subcutaneous tissue
        - following dermatologic procedure L76.33
        - following procedure on other organ L76.34
      - spleen
        - following procedure on other organ D78.34
        - following procedure on the spleen D78.33
    - specified NEC
      - circulatory system I97.89
      - digestive K91.89
      - ear H95.89
      - endocrine E89.89
      - eye and adnexa H59.89
      - genitourinary N99.89
      - mastoid process H95.89
      - metabolic E89.89
      - musculoskeletal structure M96.89
      - nervous system G97.82
      - respiratory system J95.89
      - skin and subcutaneous tissue L76.82
      - spleen D78.89
  - pregnancy NEC —*see* Pregnancy, complicated by
  - prosthetic device or implant T85.9
    - bile duct —*see* Complications, bile duct implant
    - breast —*see* Complications, breast implant
    - bulking agent
      - ureteral
        - erosion T83.714
        - exposure T83.724
      - urethral
        - erosion T83.713
        - exposure T83.723
    - cardiac and vascular NEC —*see* Complications, cardiovascular device or implant
    - corneal transplant —*see* Complications, graft, cornea

- Complication *(Continued)*
  - prosthetic device or implant *(Continued)*
    - electronic nervous system stimulator —*see* Complications, electronic stimulator device
    - epidural infusion catheter —*see* Complications, catheter, epidural
    - esophageal anti-reflux device —*see* Complications, esophageal anti-reflux device
    - genital organ or tract —*see* Complications, genitourinary, device or implant, genital tract
      - specified NEC T83.79
    - heart valve —*see* Complications, heart, valve, prosthesis
    - infection or inflammation T85.79
      - intestine transplant T86.892
      - liver transplant T86.43
      - lung transplant T86.812
      - pancreas transplant T86.892
      - skin graft T86.822
    - intraocular lens —*see* Complications, intraocular lens
    - intraperitoneal (dialysis) catheter —*see* Complications, catheter, intraperitoneal
    - joint —*see* Complications, joint prosthesis, internal
    - mechanical NEC T85.698
      - dialysis catheter (vascular) —*see also* Complication, catheter, dialysis, mechanical
        - peritoneal —*see* Complication, catheter, intraperitoneal, mechanical
      - gastrointestinal device T85.598
      - ocular device T85.398
      - subdural (infusion) catheter T85.690
      - suture, permanent T85.692
        - that for bone repair —*see* Complications, fixation device, internal (orthopedic), mechanical
      - ventricular shunt
        - breakdown T85.01
        - displacement T85.02
        - leakage T85.03
        - malposition T85.02
        - obstruction T85.09
        - perforation T85.09
        - protrusion T85.09
        - specified NEC T85.09
    - mesh
      - erosion (to surrounding organ or tissue) T83.718
        - urethral (into pelvic floor muscles) T83.712
        - vaginal (into pelvic floor muscles) T83.711
      - exposure (into surrounding organ or tissue) T83.728
        - urethral (through urethral wall) T83.722
        - vaginal (into vagina) (through vaginal wall) T83.721
    - orbital —*see* Complications, orbital prosthesis
    - penile T83.9
      - embolism T83.81
      - fibrosis T83.82
      - hemorrhage T83.83
      - infection and inflammation T83.61
      - mechanical
        - breakdown T83.410
        - displacement T83.420
        - leakage T83.490
        - malposition T83.420
        - obstruction T83.490
        - perforation T83.490
        - protrusion T83.490
        - specified NEC T83.490
      - pain T83.84

- Complication *(Continued)*
  - prosthetic device or implant *(Continued)*
    - penile *(Continued)*
      - specified type NEC T83.89
      - stenosis T83.85
      - thrombosis T83.86
    - prosthetic materials NEC
      - erosion (to surrounding organ or tissue) T83.718
      - exposure (into surrounding organ or tissue) T83.728
    - skin graft T86.829
      - artificial skin or decellularized allodermis
        - embolism T85.818
        - fibrosis T85.828
        - hemorrhage T85.838
        - infection and inflammation T85.79
        - mechanical
          - breakdown T85.613
          - displacement T85.623
          - malfunction T85.613
          - malposition T85.623
          - obstruction T85.693
          - perforation T85.693
          - protrusion T85.693
          - specified NEC T85.693
        - pain T85.848
        - specified type NEC T85.898
        - stenosis T85.858
        - thrombosis T85.868
      - failure T86.821
      - infection T86.822
      - rejection T86.820
      - specified NEC T86.828
    - sling
      - urethral (female) (male)
        - erosion T83.712
        - exposure T83.722
    - specified NEC T85.9
      - embolism T85.818
      - fibrosis T85.828
      - hemorrhage T85.838
      - infection and inflammation T85.79
      - mechanical
        - breakdown T85.618
        - displacement T85.628
        - leakage T85.638
        - malfunction T85.618
        - malposition T85.628
        - obstruction T85.698
        - perforation T85.698
        - protrusion T85.698
        - specified NEC T85.698
      - pain T85.848
      - specified type NEC T85.898
      - stenosis T85.858
      - thrombosis T85.868
    - subdural infusion catheter —*see* Complications, catheter, subdural
    - sutures —*see* Complications, sutures
    - urinary organ or tract NEC —*see* Complications, genitourinary, device or implant, urinary system
    - vascular —*see* Complications, cardiovascular device or implant
    - ventricular shunt —*see* Complications, ventricular shunt (device)
  - puerperium —*see* Puerperal
  - puncture, spinal G97.1
    - cerebrospinal fluid leak G97.0
    - headache or reaction G97.1
  - pyelogram N99.89
  - radiation
    - kyphosis M96.2
    - scoliosis M96.5
  - reattached
    - extremity (infection) (rejection)
      - lower T87.1X-●
      - upper T87.0X-●
    - specified body part NEC T87.2

Complication (Continued)
reconstructed breast
asymmetry between native and reconstructed breast N65.1
deformity N65.Ø
disproportion between native and reconstructed breast N65.1
excess tissue N65.Ø
misshappen N65.Ø
reimplant NEC —see also Complications, prosthetic device or implant
limb (infection) (rejection) —see Complications, reattached, extremity
organ (partial) (total) —see Complications, transplant
prosthetic device NEC —see Complications, prosthetic device
renal N28.9
allograft —see Complications, transplant, kidney
dialysis —see Complications, dialysis
respirator
mechancial J95.85Ø
specified NEC J95.859
respiratory system J98.9
device, implant or graft —see Complication, prosthetic device or implant, specified NEC
lung transplant —see Complications, prosthetic device or implant, lung transplant
postoperative J95.89
air leak J95.812
Mendelson's syndrome (chemical pneumonitis) J95.4
pneumothorax J95.811
pulmonary insufficiency (acute) (after nonthoracic surgery) J95.2
chronic J95.3
following thoracic surgery J95.1
respiratory failure (acute) J95.821
acute and chronic J95.822
specified NEC J95.89
subglottic stenosis J95.5
tracheostomy complication —see Complications, tracheostomy
therapy T81.89
sedation during labor and delivery O74.9
cardiac O74.2
central nervous system O74.3
pulmonary NEC O74.1
shunt —see also Complications, prosthetic device or implant
arteriovenous —see Complications, arteriovenous, shunt
ventricular (communicating) —see Complications, ventricular shunt
skin
graft T86.829
failure T86.821
infection T86.822
rejection T86.82Ø
specified type NEC T86.828
spinal
anesthesia —see Complications, anesthesia, spinal
catheter (epidural) (subdural) —see Complications, catheter
puncture or tap G97.1
cerebrospinal fluid leak G97.Ø
headache or reaction G97.1
stent
bile duct —see Complications, bile duct prosthesis
ureteral indwelling
breakdown T83.112
displacement T83.122
leakage T83.192
malposition T83.122

Complication (Continued)
stent (Continued)
ureteral indwelling (Continued)
obstruction T83.192
perforation T83.192
protrusion T83.192
specified NEC T83.192
urinary (ileal conduit) (nephroureteral) T83.193
embolism T83.81
fibrosis T83.82
hemorrhage T83.83
infection and inflammation T83.593
mechanical
breakdown T83.113
displacement T83.123
leakage T83.193
malposition T83.123
obstruction T83.193
perforation T83.193
protrusion T83.193
specified NEC T83.193
pain T83.84
specified type NEC T83.89
stenosis T83.85
thrombosis T83.86
vascular
end stent stenosis —see Restenosis, stent
in stent stenosis —see Restenosis, stent
stoma
digestive tract
colostomy —see Complications, colostomy
enterostomy —see Complications, enterostomy
esophagostomy —see Complications, esophagostomy
gastrostomy —see Complications, gastrostomy
urinary tract N99.528
continent N99.538
hemorrhage N99.53Ø
herniation N99.533
infection N99.531
malfunction N99.532
specified type NEC N99.538
stenosis N99.534
cystostomy —see Complications, cystostomy
external NOS N99.528
hemorrhage N99.52Ø
herniation N99.523
incontinent N99.528
hemorrhage N99.52Ø
herniation N99.523
infection N99.521
malfunction N99.522
specified type NEC N99.528
stenosis N99.524
infection N99.521
malfunction N99.522
specified type NEC N99.528
stenosis N99.524
stomach banding —see Complication(s), bariatric procedure
stomach stapling —see Complication(s), bariatric procedure
surgical material, nonabsorbable —see Complication, suture, permanent
surgical procedure (on) T81.9
amputation stump (late) —see Complications, amputation stump
cardiac —see Complications, circulatory system
cholesteatoma, recurrent —see Complications, postmastoidectomy, recurrent cholesteatoma
circulatory (early) —see Complications, circulatory system

Complication (Continued)
surgical procedure (Continued)
digestive system —see Complications, gastrointestinal
dumping syndrome (postgastrectomy) K91.1
ear —see Complications, ear
elephantiasis or lymphedema I97.89
postmastectomy I97.2
emphysema (surgical) T81.82
endocrine —see Complications, endocrine
eye —see Complications, eye
fistula (persistent postoperative) T81.83
foreign body inadvertently left in wound (sponge) (suture) (swab) —see Foreign body, accidentally left during a procedure
gastrointestinal —see Complications, gastrointestinal
genitourinary NEC N99.89
hematoma
intraoperative —see Complication, intraoperative, hemorrhage
postprocedural —see Complication, postprocedural, hematoma
hemorrhage
intraoperative —see Complication, intraoperative, hemorrhage
postprocedural —see Complication, postprocedural, hemorrhage
hepatic failure K91.82
hyperglycemia (postpancreatectomy) E89.1
hypoinsulinemia (postpancreatectomy) E89.1
hypoparathyroidism (postparathyroidectomy) E89.2
hypopituitarism (posthypophysectomy) E89.3
hypothyroidism (post-thyroidectomy) E89.Ø
intestinal obstruction —see also Obstruction, intestine, postoperative K91.3Ø
intracranial hypotension following ventricular shunting (ventriculostomy) G97.2
lymphedema I97.89
postmastectomy I97.2
malabsorption (postsurgical) NEC K91.2
osteoporosis —see Osteoporosis, postsurgical malabsorption
mastoidectomy cavity NEC —see Complications, postmastoidectomy
metabolic E89.89
specified NEC E89.89
musculoskeletal —see Complications, musculoskeletal system
nervous system (central) (peripheral) —see Complications, nervous system
ovarian failure E89.4Ø
asymptomatic E89.4Ø
symptomatic E89.41
peripheral vascular —see Complications, surgical procedure, vascular
postcardiotomy syndrome I97.Ø
postcholecystectomy syndrome K91.5
postcommissurotomy syndrome I97.Ø
postgastrectomy dumping syndrome K91.1
postlaminectomy syndrome NEC M96.1
kyphosis M96.3
postmastectomy lymphedema syndrome I97.2
postmastoidectomy cholesteatoma —see Complications, postmastoidectomy, recurrent cholesteatoma
postvagotomy syndrome K91.1
postvalvulotomy syndrome I97.Ø
pulmonary insufficiency (acute) J95.2
chronic J95.3
following thoracic surgery J95.1

C

Complication (Continued)
surgical procedure (Continued)
reattached body part —see Complications, reattached
respiratory —see Complications, respiratory system
shock (hypovolemic) T81.19
spleen (postoperative) D78.89
intraoperative D78.81
stitch abscess T81.41
subglottic stenosis (postsurgical) J95.5
testicular hypofunction E89.5
transplant —see Complications, organ or tissue transplant
urinary NEC N99.89
vaginal vault prolapse (posthysterectomy) N99.3
vascular (peripheral)
artery T81.719
mesenteric T81.71Ø
renal T81.711
specified NEC T81.718
vein T81.72
wound infection T81.49
suture, permanent (wire) NEC T85.9
with repair of bone —see Complications, fixation device, internal
embolism T85.818
fibrosis T85.828
hemorrhage T85.838
infection and inflammation T85.79
mechanical
breakdown T85.612
displacement T85.622
malfunction T85.612
malposition T85.622
obstruction T85.692
perforation T85.692
protrusion T85.692
specified NEC T85.692
pain T85.848
specified type NEC T85.898
stenosis T85.858
thrombosis T85.868
tracheostomy J95.ØØ
granuloma J95.Ø9
hemorrhage J95.Ø1
infection J95.Ø2
malfunction J95.Ø3
mechanical J95.Ø3
obstruction J95.Ø3
specified type NEC J95.Ø9
tracheo-esophageal fistula J95.Ø4
transfusion (blood) (lymphocytes) (plasma) T8Ø.92
air embolism T8Ø.Ø
circulatory overload E87.71
febrile nonhemolytic transfusion reaction R5Ø.84
hemochromatosis E83.111
hemolysis T8Ø.89
hemolytic reaction (antigen unspecified) T8Ø.919
incompatibility reaction (antigen unspecified) T8Ø.919
ABO T8Ø.3Ø
delayed serologic (DSTR) T8Ø.39
hemolytic transfusion reaction (HTR) (unspecified time after transfusion) T8Ø.319
acute (AHTR) (less than 24 hours after transfusion) T8Ø.31Ø
delayed (DHTR) (24 hours or more after transfusion) T8Ø.311
specified NEC T8Ø.39
acute (antigen unspecified) T8Ø.91Ø
delayed (antigen unspecified) T8Ø.911
delayed serologic (DSTR) T8Ø.89

Complication (Continued)
transfusion (Continued)
incompatibility reaction (Continued)
Non-ABO (minor antigens (Duffy) (K) (Kell) (Kidd) (Lewis) (M) (N) (P) (S)) T8Ø.AØ
delayed serologic (DSTR) T8Ø.A9
hemolytic transfusion reaction (HTR) (unspecified time after transfusion) T8Ø.A19
acute (AHTR) (less than 24 hours after transfusion) T8Ø.A1Ø
delayed (DHTR) (24 hours or more after transfusion) T8Ø.A11
specified NEC T8Ø.A9
Rh (antigens (C) (c) (D) (E) (e)) (factor) T8Ø.4Ø
delayed serologic (DSTR) T8Ø.49
hemolytic transfusion reaction (HTR) (unspecified time after transfusion) T8Ø.419
acute (AHTR) (less than 24 hours after transfusion) T8Ø.41Ø
delayed (DHTR) (24 hours or more after transfusion) T8Ø.411
specified NEC T8Ø.49
infection T8Ø.29
acute T8Ø.22
reaction NEC T8Ø.89
sepsis T8Ø.29
shock T8Ø.89
transplant T86.9Ø
bone T86.839
failure T86.831
infection T86.832
rejection T86.83Ø
specified type NEC T86.838
bone marrow T86.ØØ
failure T86.Ø2
infection T86.Ø3
rejection T86.Ø1
specified type NEC T86.Ø9
cornea T86.849
failure T86.841
infection T86.842
rejection T86.84Ø
specified type NEC T86.848
failure T86.92
heart T86.2Ø
with lung T86.3Ø
cardiac allograft vasculopathy T86.29Ø
failure T86.32
infection T86.33
rejection T86.31
specified type NEC T86.39
failure T86.22
infection T86.23
rejection T86.21
specified type NEC T86.298
infection T86.93
intestine T86.859
failure T86.851
infection T86.852
rejection T86.85Ø
specified type NEC T86.858
kidney T86.1Ø
failure T86.12
infection T86.13
rejection T86.11
specified type NEC T86.19
liver T86.4Ø
failure T86.42
infection T86.43
rejection T86.41
specified type NEC T86.49
lung T86.819
with heart T86.3Ø
failure T86.32
infection T86.33
rejection T86.31
specified type NEC T86.39

Complication (Continued)
transplant (Continued)
lung (Continued)
failure T86.811
infection T86.812
rejection T86.81Ø
specified type NEC T86.818
malignant neoplasm C8Ø.2
pancreas T86.899
failure T86.891
infection T86.892
rejection T86.89Ø
specified type NEC T86.898
peripheral blood stem cells T86.5
post-transplant lymphoproliferative disorder (PTLD) D47.Z1
rejection T86.91
skin T86.829
failure T86.821
infection T86.822
rejection T86.82Ø
specified type NEC T86.828
specified
tissue T86.899
failure T86.891
infection T86.892
rejection T86.89Ø
specified type NEC T86.898
type NEC T86.99
stem cell (from peripheral blood) (from umbilical cord) T86.5
umbilical cord stem cells T86.5
trauma (early) T79.9
specified NEC T79.8
ultrasound therapy NEC T88.9
umbilical cord NEC
complicating delivery O69.9
specified NEC O69.89
umbrella device, vascular T82.9
embolism T82.818
fibrosis T82.828
hemorrhage T82.838
infection or inflammation T82.7
mechanical
breakdown T82.515
displacement T82.525
leakage T82.535
malposition T82.525
obstruction T82.595
perforation T82.595
protrusion T82.595
pain T82.848
specified type NEC T82.898
stenosis T82.858
thrombosis T82.868
urethral catheter —see Complications, catheter, urethral, indwelling
vaccination T88.1
anaphylaxis NEC T8Ø.52
arthropathy —see Arthropathy, postimmunization
cellulitis T88.Ø
encephalitis or encephalomyelitis GØ4.Ø2
infection (general) (local) NEC T88.Ø
meningitis GØ3.8
myelitis GØ4.Ø2
protein sickness T8Ø.62
rash T88.1
reaction (allergic) T88.1
serum T8Ø.62
sepsis T88.Ø
serum intoxication, sickness, rash, or other serum reaction NEC T8Ø.62
anaphylactic shock T8Ø.52
shock (allergic) (anaphylactic) T8Ø.52
vaccinia (generalized) (localized) T88.1
vas deferens device or implant —see Complications, genitourinary, device or implant, genital tract

Complication (Continued)
vascular I99.9
device or implant T82.9
embolism T82.818
fibrosis T82.828
hemorrhage T82.838
infection or inflammation T82.7
mechanical
breakdown T82.519
specified device NEC T82.518
displacement T82.529
specified device NEC T82.528
leakage T82.539
specified device NEC T82.538
malposition T82.529
specified device NEC T82.528
obstruction T82.599
specified device NEC T82.598
perforation T82.599
specified device NEC T82.598
protrusion T82.599
specified device NEC T82.598
pain T82.848
specified type NEC T82.898
stenosis T82.858
thrombosis T82.868
dialysis catheter —*see* Complication, catheter, dialysis
following infusion, therapeutic injection or transfusion T80.1
graft T82.9
embolism T82.818
fibrosis T82.828
hemorrhage T82.838
mechanical
breakdown T82.319
aorta (bifurcation) T82.310
carotid artery T82.311
specified vessel NEC T82.318
displacement T82.329
aorta (bifurcation) T82.320
carotid artery T82.321
specified vessel NEC T82.328
leakage T82.339
aorta (bifurcation) T82.330
carotid artery T82.331
specified vessel NEC T82.338
malposition T82.329
aorta (bifurcation) T82.320
carotid artery T82.321
specified vessel NEC T82.328
obstruction T82.399
aorta (bifurcation) T82.390
carotid artery T82.391
specified vessel NEC T82.398
perforation T82.399
aorta (bifurcation) T82.390
carotid artery T82.391
specified vessel NEC T82.398
protrusion T82.399
aorta (bifurcation) T82.390
carotid artery T82.391
specified vessel NEC T82.398
pain T82.848
specified complication NEC T82.898
stenosis T82.858
thrombosis T82.868
postoperative —*see* Complications, postoperative, circulatory
vena cava device (filter) (sieve) (umbrella) —*see* Complications, umbrella device, vascular
ventilation therapy NEC T81.81
ventilator
mechanical J95.850
specified NEC J95.859
ventricular (communicating) shunt (device) T85.9
embolism T85.810
fibrosis T85.820
hemorrhage T85.830

Complication (Continued)
ventricular shunt (Continued)
infection and inflammation T85.730
mechanical
breakdown T85.01
displacement T85.02
leakage T85.03
malposition T85.02
obstruction T85.09
perforation T85.09
protrusion T85.09
specified NEC T85.09
pain T85.840
specified type NEC T85.890
stenosis T85.850
thrombosis T85.860
wire suture, permanent (implanted) —*see* Complications, suture, permanent
Compressed air disease T70.3
Compression
with injury - code by Nature of injury
artery I77.1
celiac, syndrome I77.4
brachial plexus G54.0
brain (stem) G93.5
due to
contusion (diffuse) —*see* Injury, intracranial, diffuse
focal —*see* Injury, intracranial, focal
injury NEC —*see* Injury, intracranial, diffuse
traumatic —*see* Injury, intracranial, diffuse
bronchus J98.09
cauda equina G83.4
celiac (artery) (axis) I77.4
cerebral —*see* Compression, brain
cervical plexus G54.2
cord
spinal —*see* Compression, spinal
umbilical —*see* Compression, umbilical cord
cranial nerve G52.9
eighth —*see* subcategory H93.3
eleventh G52.8
fifth G50.8
first G52.0
fourth —*see* Strabismus, paralytic, fourth nerve
ninth G52.1
second —*see* Disorder, nerve, optic
seventh G51.8
sixth —*see* Strabismus, paralytic, sixth nerve
tenth G52.2
third —*see* Strabismus, paralytic, third nerve
twelfth G52.3
diver's squeeze T70.3
during birth (newborn) P15.9
esophagus K22.2
eustachian tube —*see* Obstruction, eustachian tube, cartilaginous
facies Q67.1
fracture
nontraumatic NOS —*see* Collapse, vertebra
pathological —*see* Fracture, pathological
traumatic —*see* Fracture, traumatic
heart —*see* Disease, heart
intestine —*see* Obstruction, intestine
laryngeal nerve, recurrent G52.2
with paralysis of vocal cords and larynx J38.00
bilateral J38.02
unilateral J38.01
lumbosacral plexus G54.1
lung J98.4
lymphatic vessel I89.0
medulla —*see* Compression, brain
nerve —*see also* Disorder, nerve G58.9
arm NEC —*see* Mononeuropathy, upper limb

Compression (Continued)
nerve (Continued)
axillary G54.0
cranial —*see* Compression, cranial nerve
leg NEC —*see* Mononeuropathy, lower limb
median (in carpal tunnel) —*see* Syndrome, carpal tunnel
optic —*see* Disorder, nerve, optic
plantar —*see* Lesion, nerve, plantar
posterior tibial (in tarsal tunnel) —*see* Syndrome, tarsal tunnel
root or plexus NOS (in) G54.9
intervertebral disc disorder NEC —*see* Disorder, disc, with, radiculopathy
with myelopathy —*see* Disorder, disc, with, myelopathy
neoplastic disease —*see also* Neoplasm D49.9 *[G55]*
spondylosis —*see* Spondylosis, with radiculopathy
sciatic (acute) —*see* Lesion, nerve, sciatic
sympathetic G90.8
traumatic —*see* Injury, nerve
ulnar —*see* Lesion, nerve, ulnar
upper extremity NEC —*see* Mononeuropathy, upper limb
spinal (cord) G95.20
by displacement of intervertebral disc NEC —*see also* Disorder, disc, with, myelopathy
nerve root NOS G54.9
due to displacement of intervertebral disc NEC —*see* Disorder, disc, with, radiculopathy
with myelopathy —*see* Disorder, disc, with, myelopathy
specified NEC G95.29
spondylogenic (cervical) (lumbar, lumbosacral) (thoracic) —*see* Spondylosis, with myelopathy NEC
anterior —*see* Syndrome, anterior, spinal artery, compression
traumatic —*see* Injury, spinal cord, by region
subcostal nerve (syndrome) —*see* Mononeuropathy, upper limb, specified NEC
sympathetic nerve NEC G90.8
syndrome T79.5
trachea J39.8
ulnar nerve (by scar tissue) —*see* Lesion, nerve, ulnar
umbilical cord
complicating delivery O69.2
cord around neck O69.1
prolapse O69.0
specified NEC O69.2
ureter N13.5
vein I87.1
vena cava (inferior) (superior) I87.1
Compulsion, compulsive
gambling F63.0
neurosis F42.8
personality F60.5
states F42.8
swearing F42.8
in Gilles de la Tourette's syndrome F95.2
tics and spasms F95.9
Concato's disease (pericardial polyserositis) A19.9
nontubercular I31.1
pleural —*see* Pleurisy, with effusion
Concavity chest wall M95.4
Concealed penis Q55.64
Concern (normal) **about sick person in family** Z63.6
Concrescence (teeth) K00.2
Concretio cordis I31.1
rheumatic I09.2

- **Concretion** —*see also* Calculus
  - appendicular K38.1
  - canaliculus —*see* Dacryolith
  - clitoris N90.89
  - conjunctiva H11.12-●
  - eyelid —*see* Disorder, eyelid, specified type NEC
  - lacrimal passages —*see* Dacryolith
  - prepuce (male) N47.8
  - salivary gland (any) K11.5
  - seminal vesicle N50.89
  - tonsil J35.8
- **Concussion** (brain) (cerebral) (current) S06.0X9
  - with
    - loss of consciousness of 30 minutes or less S06.0X1
    - loss of consciousness of unspecified duration S06.0X9
  - blast (air) (hydraulic) (immersion) (underwater)
    - abdomen or thorax —*see* Injury, blast, by site
    - ear with acoustic nerve injury —*see* Injury, nerve, acoustic, specified type NEC
  - cauda equina S34.3
  - conus medullaris S34.02
  - ocular S05.8X-●
  - spinal (cord)
    - cervical S14.0
    - lumbar S34.01
    - sacral S34.02
    - thoracic S24.0
  - syndrome F07.81
  - ▶without loss of consciousness S06.0X0
  - ~~Without loss of consciousness S06.0X0~~
- **Condition** —*see* Disease
- **Conditions arising in the perinatal period** —*see* Newborn, affected by
- **Conduct disorder** —*see* Disorder, conduct
- **Condyloma** A63.0
  - acuminatum A63.0
  - gonorrheal A54.09
  - latum A51.31
  - syphilitic A51.31
    - congenital A50.07
  - venereal, syphilitic A51.31
- **Conflagration** —*see also* Burn
  - asphyxia (by inhalation of gases, fumes or vapors) —*see also* Table of Drugs and Chemicals T59.9-●
- **Conflict** (with) —*see also* Discord
  - family Z73.9
  - marital Z63.0
    - involving divorce or estrangement Z63.5
  - parent-child Z62.820
    - parent-adopted child Z62.821
    - parent-biological child Z62.820
    - parent-foster child Z62.822
  - social role NEC Z73.5
- **Confluent** —*see* condition
- **Confusion, confused** R41.0
  - epileptic F05
  - mental state (psychogenic) F44.89
  - psychogenic F44.89
  - reactive (from emotional stress, psychological trauma) F44.89
- **Confusional arousals** G47.51
- **Congelation** T69.9
- **Congenital** —*see also* condition
  - aortic septum Q25.49
  - intrinsic factor deficiency D51.0
  - malformation —*see* Anomaly
- **Congestion, congestive**
  - bladder N32.89
  - bowel K63.89
  - brain G93.89
  - breast N64.59
  - bronchial J98.09
  - catarrhal J31.0
  - chest R09.89
  - chill, malarial —*see* Malaria

Congestion, congestive *(Continued)*
  - circulatory NEC I99.8
  - duodenum K31.89
  - eye —*see* Hyperemia, conjunctiva
  - facial, due to birth injury P15.4
  - general R68.89
  - glottis J37.0
  - heart —*see* Failure, heart, congestive
  - hepatic K76.1
  - hypostatic (lung) —*see* Edema, lung
  - intestine K63.89
  - kidney N28.89
  - labyrinth —*see* subcategory H83.8
  - larynx J37.0
  - liver K76.1
  - lung R09.89
    - active or acute —*see* Pneumonia
  - malaria, malarial —*see* Malaria
  - nasal R09.81
  - nose R09.81
  - orbit, orbital —*see also* Exophthalmos
    - inflammatory (chronic) —*see* Inflammation, orbit
  - ovary N83.8
  - pancreas K86.89
  - pelvic, female N94.89
  - pleural J94.8
  - prostate (active) N42.1
  - pulmonary —*see* Congestion, lung
  - renal N28.89
  - retina H35.81
  - seminal vesicle N50.1
  - spinal cord G95.19
  - spleen (chronic) D73.2
  - stomach K31.89
  - trachea —*see* Tracheitis
  - urethra N36.8
  - uterus N85.8
    - with subinvolution N85.3
  - venous (passive) I87.8
  - viscera R68.89
- **Congestive** —*see* Congestion
- **Conical**
  - cervix (hypertrophic elongation) N88.4
  - cornea —*see* Keratoconus
  - teeth K00.2
- **Conjoined twins** Q89.4
- **Conjugal maladjustment** Z63.0
  - involving divorce or estrangement Z63.5
- **Conjunctiva** —*see* condition
- **Conjunctivitis** (staphylococcal) (streptococcal) NOS H10.9
  - Acanthamoeba B60.12
  - acute H10.3-●
    - atopic H10.1-●
    - chemical —*see also* Corrosion, cornea H10.21-●
    - mucopurulent H10.02-●
      - follicular H10.01-●
    - pseudomembranous H10.22-●
    - serous except viral H10.23-●
      - viral —*see* Conjunctivitis, viral
    - toxic H10.21-●
  - adenoviral (acute) (follicular) B30.1
  - allergic (acute) —*see* Conjunctivitis, acute, atopic
    - chronic H10.45
      - vernal H10.44
  - anaphylactic —*see* Conjunctivitis, acute, atopic
  - Apollo B30.3
  - atopic (acute) —*see* Conjunctivitis, acute, atopic
  - Béal's B30.2
  - blennorrhagic (gonococcal) (neonatorum) A54.31
  - chemical (acute) —*see also* Corrosion, cornea H10.21-●
  - chlamydial A74.0
    - due to trachoma A71.1
    - neonatal P39.1

Conjunctivitis *(Continued)*
  - chronic (nodosa) (petrificans) (phlyctenular) H10.40-●
    - allergic H10.45
      - vernal H10.44
    - follicular H10.43-●
    - giant papillary H10.41-●
    - simple H10.42-●
    - vernal H10.44
  - coxsackievirus 24 B30.3
  - diphtheritic A36.86
  - due to
    - dust —*see* Conjunctivitis, acute, atopic
    - filariasis B74.9
    - mucocutaneous leishmaniasis B55.2
  - enterovirus type 70 (hemorrhagic) B30.3
  - epidemic (viral) B30.9
    - hemorrhagic B30.3
  - gonococcal (neonatorum) A54.31
  - granular (trachomatous) A71.1
    - sequelae (late effect) B94.0
  - hemorrhagic (acute) (epidemic) B30.3
  - herpes zoster B02.31
  - in (due to)
    - Acanthamoeba B60.12
    - adenovirus (acute) (follicular) B30.1
    - Chlamydia A74.0
    - coxsackievirus 24 B30.3
    - diphtheria A36.86
    - enterovirus type 70 (hemorrhagic) B30.3
    - filariasis B74.9
    - gonococci A54.31
    - herpes (simplex) virus B00.53
      - zoster B02.31
    - infectious disease NEC B99
    - meningococci A39.89
    - mucocutaneous leishmaniasis B55.2
    - rosacea H10.82-●
    - syphilis (late) A52.71
    - zoster B02.31
  - inclusion A74.0
  - infantile P39.1
    - gonococcal A54.31
  - Koch-Weeks' —*see* Conjunctivitis, acute, mucopurulent
  - light —*see* Conjunctivitis, acute, atopic
  - ligneous —*see* Blepharoconjunctivitis, ligneous
  - meningococcal A39.89
  - mucopurulent —*see* Conjunctivitis, acute, mucopurulent
  - neonatal P39.1
    - gonococcal A54.31
  - Newcastle B30.8
  - of Béal B30.2
  - parasitic
    - filariasis B74.9
    - mucocutaneous leishmaniasis B55.2
  - Parinaud's H10.89
  - petrificans H10.89
  - rosacea H10.82-●
  - specified NEC H10.89
  - swimming-pool B30.1
  - trachomatous A71.1
    - acute A71.0
    - sequelae (late effect) B94.0
  - traumatic NEC H10.89
  - tuberculous A18.59
  - tularemic A21.1
  - tularensis A21.1
  - viral B30.9
    - due to
      - adenovirus B30.1
      - enterovirus B30.3
    - specified NEC B30.8
- **Conjunctivochalasis** H11.82-●
- **Connective tissue** —*see* condition
- **Conn's syndrome** E26.01
- **Conradi (-Hunermann) disease** Q77.3
- **Consanguinity** Z84.3
  - counseling Z71.89

C

Conscious simulation (of illness) Z76.5
Consecutive —*see* condition
Consolidation lung (base) —*see* Pneumonia, lobar
Constipation (atonic) (neurogenic) (simple) (spastic) K59.00
- chronic K59.09
  - idiopathic K59.04
- drug-induced K59.03
- functional K59.04
- outlet dysfunction K59.02
- psychogenic F45.8
- slow transit K59.01
- specified NEC K59.09

Constitutional —*see also* condition
- substandard F60.7

Constitutionally substandard F60.7
Constriction —*see also* Stricture
- auditory canal —*see* Stenosis, external ear canal
- bronchial J98.09
- duodenum K31.5
- esophagus K22.2
- external
  - abdomen, abdominal (wall) S30.841
  - alveolar process S00.542
  - ankle S90.54-●
  - antecubital space —*see* Constriction, external, forearm
  - arm (upper) S40.84-●
  - auricle —*see* Constriction, external, ear
  - axilla —*see* Constriction, external, arm
  - back, lower S30.840
  - breast S20.14-●
  - brow S00.84
  - buttock S30.840
  - calf —*see* Constriction, external, leg
  - canthus —*see* Constriction, external, eyelid
  - cheek S00.84
    - internal S00.542
  - chest wall —*see* Constriction, external, thorax
  - chin S00.84
  - clitoris S30.844
  - costal region —*see* Constriction, external, thorax
  - digit(s)
    - foot —*see* Constriction, external, toe
    - hand —*see* Constriction, external, finger
  - ear S00.44-●
  - elbow S50.34-●
  - epididymis S30.843
  - epigastric region S30.841
  - esophagus, cervical S10.14
  - eyebrow —*see* Constriction, external, eyelid
  - eyelid S00.24-●
  - face S00.84
  - finger(s) S60.44-●
    - index S60.44-●
    - little S60.44-●
    - middle S60.44-●
    - ring S60.44-●
  - flank S30.841
  - foot (except toe(s) alone) S90.84-●
    - toe —*see* Constriction, external, toe
  - forearm S50.84-●
    - elbow only —*see* Constriction, external, elbow
  - forehead S00.84
  - genital organs, external
    - female S30.846
    - male S30.845
  - groin S30.841
  - gum S00.542
  - hand S60.54-●
  - head S00.94
    - ear —*see* Constriction, external, ear
    - eyelid —*see* Constriction, external, eyelid
    - lip S00.541
    - nose S00.34
    - oral cavity S00.542

Constriction *(Continued)*
- external *(Continued)*
  - head *(Continued)*
    - scalp S00.04
    - specified site NEC S00.84
  - heel —*see* Constriction, external, foot
  - hip S70.24-●
  - inguinal region S30.841
  - interscapular region S20.449
  - jaw S00.84
  - knee S80.24-●
  - labium (majus) (minus) S30.844
  - larynx S10.14
  - leg (lower) S80.84-●
    - knee —*see* Constriction, external, knee
    - upper —*see* Constriction, external, thigh
  - lip S00.541
  - lower back S30.840
  - lumbar region S30.840
  - malar region S00.84
  - mammary —*see* Constriction, external, breast
  - mastoid region S00.84
  - mouth S00.542
  - nail
    - finger —*see* Constriction, external, finger
    - toe —*see* Constriction, external, toe
  - nasal S00.34
  - neck S10.94
    - specified site NEC S10.84
    - throat S10.14
  - nose S00.34
  - occipital region S00.04
  - oral cavity S00.542
  - orbital region —*see* Constriction, external, eyelid
  - palate S00.542
  - palm —*see* Constriction, external, hand
  - parietal region S00.04
  - pelvis S30.840
  - penis S30.842
  - perineum
    - female S30.844
    - male S30.840
  - periocular area —*see* Constriction, external, eyelid
  - phalanges
    - finger —*see* Constriction, external, finger
    - toe —*see* Constriction, external, toe
  - pharynx S10.14
  - pinna —*see* Constriction, external, ear
  - popliteal space —*see* Constriction, external, knee
  - prepuce S30.842
  - pubic region S30.840
  - pudendum
    - female S30.846
    - male S30.845
  - sacral region S30.840
  - scalp S00.04
  - scapular region —*see* Constriction, external, shoulder
  - scrotum S30.843
  - shin —*see* Constriction, external, leg
  - shoulder S40.24-●
  - sternal region S20.349
  - submaxillary region S00.84
  - submental region S00.84
  - subungual
    - finger(s) —*see* Constriction, external, finger
    - toe(s) —*see* Constriction, external, toe
  - supraclavicular fossa S10.84
  - supraorbital S00.84
  - temple S00.84
  - temporal region S00.84
  - testis S30.843
  - thigh S70.34-●
  - thorax, thoracic (wall) S20.94
    - back S20.44-●
    - front S20.34-●

Constriction *(Continued)*
- external *(Continued)*
  - throat S10.14
  - thumb S60.34-●
  - toe(s) (lesser) S90.44-●
    - great S90.44-●
  - tongue S00.542
  - trachea S10.14
  - tunica vaginalis S30.843
  - uvula S00.542
  - vagina S30.844
  - vulva S30.844
  - wrist S60.84-●
- gallbladder —*see* Obstruction, gallbladder
- intestine —*see* Obstruction, intestine
- larynx J38.6
  - congenital Q31.8
    - specified NEC Q31.8
    - subglottic Q31.1
- organ or site, congenital NEC —*see* Atresia, by site
- prepuce (acquired) (congenital) N47.1
- pylorus (adult hypertrophic) K31.1
  - congenital or infantile Q40.0
  - newborn Q40.0
- ring dystocia (uterus) O62.4
- spastic —*see also* Spasm
  - ureter N13.5
- ureter N13.5
  - with infection N13.6
- urethra —*see* Stricture, urethra
- visual field (peripheral) (functional) —*see* Defect, visual field

Constrictive —*see* condition
Consultation
- without complaint or sickness Z71.9
  - feared complaint unfounded Z71.1
  - specified reason NEC Z71.89
- medical —*see* Counseling, medical
- religious Z71.81
- specified reason NEC Z71.89
- spiritual Z71.81

Consumption —*see* Tuberculosis
Contact (with) —*see also* Exposure (to)
- acariasis Z20.7
- AIDS virus Z20.6
- air pollution Z77.110
- algae and algae toxins Z77.121
- algae bloom Z77.121
- anthrax Z20.810
- aromatic (hazardous) compounds NEC Z77.028
- aromatic amines Z77.020
- aromatic dyes NOS Z77.028
- arsenic Z77.010
- asbestos Z77.090
- bacterial disease NEC Z20.818
- benzene Z77.021
- blue-green algae bloom Z77.121
- body fluids (potentially hazardous) Z77.21
- brown tide Z77.121
- chemicals (chiefly nonmedicinal) (hazardous) NEC Z77.098
- cholera Z20.09
- chromium compounds Z77.018
- communicable disease Z20.9
  - bacterial NEC Z20.818
  - specified NEC Z20.89
  - viral NEC Z20.828
  - Zika virus Z20.821
- cyanobacteria bloom Z77.121
- dyes Z77.098
- Escherichia coli (E. coli) Z20.01
- fiberglass —*see* Table of Drugs and Chemicals, fiberglass
- German measles Z20.4
- gonorrhea Z20.2
- hazardous metals NEC Z77.018
- hazardous substances NEC Z77.29
- hazards in the physical environment NEC Z77.128
- hazards to health NEC Z77.9

Contact *(Continued)*
HIV Z20.6
HTLV-III/LAV Z20.6
human immunodeficiency virus (HIV) Z20.6
infection Z20.9
specified NEC Z20.89
infestation (parasitic) NEC Z20.7
intestinal infectious disease NEC Z20.09
Escherichia coli (E. coli) Z20.01
lead Z77.011
meningococcus Z20.811
mold (toxic) Z77.120
nickel dust Z77.018
noise Z77.122
parasitic disease Z20.7
pediculosis Z20.7
pfiesteria piscicida Z77.121
poliomyelitis Z20.89
pollution
air Z77.110
environmental NEC Z77.118
soil Z77.112
water Z77.111
polycyclic aromatic hydrocarbons Z77.028
rabies Z20.3
radiation, naturally occurring NEC Z77.123
radon Z77.123
red tide (Florida) Z77.121
rubella Z20.4
sexually-transmitted disease Z20.2
smallpox (laboratory) Z20.89
syphilis Z20.2
tuberculosis Z20.1
uranium Z77.012
varicella Z20.820
venereal disease Z20.2
viral disease NEC Z20.828
viral hepatitis Z20.5
water pollution Z77.111
Zika virus Z20.821
Contamination, food —*see* Intoxication, foodborne
Contraception, contraceptive
advice Z30.09
counseling Z30.09
device (intrauterine) (in situ) Z97.5
causing menorrhagia T83.83
checking Z30.431
complications —*see* Complications, intrauterine, contraceptive device
in place Z97.5
initial prescription Z30.014
reinsertion Z30.433
removal Z30.432
replacement Z30.433
emergency (postcoital) Z30.012
initial prescription Z30.019
barrier Z30.018
diaphragm Z30.018
injectable Z30.013
intrauterine device Z30.014
pills Z30.011
postcoital (emergency) Z30.012
specified type NEC Z30.018
subdermal implantable Z30.017
transdermal patch hormonal Z30.016
vaginal ring hormonal Z30.015
maintenance Z30.40
barrier Z30.49
diaphragm Z30.49
examination Z30.8
injectable Z30.42
intrauterine device Z30.431
pills Z30.41
specified type NEC Z30.49
subdermal implantable Z30.46
transdermal patch hormonal Z30.45
vaginal ring hormonal Z30.44
management Z30.9
specified NEC Z30.8
postcoital (emergency) Z30.012
prescription Z30.019
repeat Z30.40
Contraception, contraceptive *(Continued)*
sterilization Z30.2
surveillance (drug) —*see* Contraception, maintenance
Contraction(s), contracture, contracted
Achilles tendon —*see also* Short, tendon, Achilles
congenital Q66.89
amputation stump (surgical) (flexion) (late) next proximal joint T87.89
anus K59.8
bile duct (common) (hepatic) K83.8
bladder N32.89
neck or sphincter N32.0
bowel, cecum, colon or intestine, any part —*see* Obstruction, intestine
Braxton Hicks —*see* False, labor
breast implant, capsular T85.44
bronchial J98.09
burn (old) —*see* Cicatrix
cervix —*see* Stricture, cervix
cicatricial —*see* Cicatrix
conjunctiva, trachomatous, active A71.1
sequelae (late effect) B94.0
Dupuytren's M72.0
eyelid —*see* Disorder, eyelid function
fascia (lata) (postural) M72.8
Dupuytren's M72.0
palmar M72.0
plantar M72.2
finger NEC —*see also* Deformity, finger
congenital Q68.1
joint —*see* Contraction, joint, hand
flaccid —*see* Contraction, paralytic
gallbladder K82.0
heart valve —*see* Endocarditis
hip —*see* Contraction, joint, hip
hourglass
bladder N32.89
congenital Q64.79
gallbladder K82.0
congenital Q44.1
stomach K31.89
congenital Q40.2
psychogenic F45.8
uterus (complicating delivery) O62.4
hysterical F44.4
internal os —*see* Stricture, cervix
joint (abduction) (acquired) (adduction) (flexion) (rotation) M24.50
ankle M24.57- ●
congenital NEC Q68.8
hip Q65.89
elbow M24.52- ●
foot joint M24.57- ●
hand joint M24.54- ●
hip M24.55- ●
congenital Q65.89
hysterical F44.4
knee M24.56- ●
shoulder M24.51- ●
wrist M24.53- ●
kidney (granular) (secondary) N26.9
congenital Q63.8
hydronephritic —*see* Hydronephrosis
Page N26.2
pyelonephritic —*see* Pyelitis, chronic
tuberculous A18.11
ligament —*see also* Disorder, ligament
congenital Q79.8
muscle (postinfective) (postural) NEC M62.40
with contracture of joint —*see* Contraction, joint
ankle M62.47- ●
congenital Q79.8
sternocleidomastoid Q68.0
extraocular —*see* Strabismus
eye (extrinsic) —*see* Strabismus
foot M62.47- ●
forearm M62.43- ●
hand M62.44- ●
Contraction, contracture, contracted *(Continued)*
muscle *(Continued)*
hysterical F44.4
ischemic (Volkmann's) T79.6
lower leg M62.46- ●
multiple sites M62.49
pelvic region M62.45- ●
posttraumatic —*see* Strabismus, paralytic
psychogenic F45.8
conversion reaction F44.4
shoulder region M62.41- ●
specified site NEC M62.48
thigh M62.45- ●
upper arm M62.42- ●
neck —*see* Torticollis
ocular muscle —*see* Strabismus
organ or site, congenital NEC —*see* Atresia, by site
outlet (pelvis) —*see* Contraction, pelvis
palmar fascia M72.0
paralytic
joint —*see* Contraction, joint
muscle —*see also* Contraction, muscle NEC
ocular —*see* Strabismus, paralytic
pelvis (acquired) (general) M95.5
with disproportion (fetopelvic) O33.1
causing obstructed labor O65.1
inlet O33.2
mid-cavity O33.3
outlet O33.3
plantar fascia M72.2
premature
atrium I49.1
auriculoventricular I49.49
heart I49.49
junctional I49.2
supraventricular I49.1
ventricular I49.3
prostate N42.89
pylorus NEC —*see also* Pylorospasm
psychogenic F45.8
rectum, rectal (sphincter) K59.8
ring (Bandl's) (complicating delivery) O62.4
scar —*see* Cicatrix
spine —*see* Dorsopathy, deforming
sternocleidomastoid (muscle), congenital Q68.0
stomach K31.89
hourglass K31.89
congenital Q40.2
psychogenic F45.8
psychogenic F45.8
tendon (sheath) M62.40
with contracture of joint —*see* Contraction, joint
Achilles —*see* Short, tendon, Achilles
ankle M62.47- ●
Achilles —*see* Short, tendon, Achilles
foot M62.47- ●
forearm M62.43- ●
hand M62.44- ●
lower leg M62.46- ●
multiple sites M62.49
neck M62.48
pelvic region M62.45- ●
shoulder region M62.41- ●
specified site NEC M62.48
thigh M62.45- ●
thorax M62.48
trunk M62.48
upper arm M62.42- ●
toe —*see* Deformity, toe, specified NEC
ureterovesical orifice (postinfectional) N13.5
with infection N13.6
urethra —*see also* Stricture, urethra
orifice N32.0
uterus N85.8
abnormal NEC O62.9
clonic (complicating delivery) O62.4
dyscoordinate (complicating delivery) O62.4

Contraction, contracture, contracted *(Continued)*
uterus *(Continued)*
hourglass (complicating delivery) O62.4
hypertonic O62.4
hypotonic NEC O62.2
inadequate
primary O62.Ø
secondary O62.1
incoordinate (complicating delivery) O62.4
poor O62.2
tetanic (complicating delivery) O62.4
vagina (outlet) N89.5
vesical N32.89
neck or urethral orifice N32.Ø
visual field —*see* Defect, visual field, generalized
Volkmann's (ischemic) T79.6
Contusion (skin surface intact) T14.8
abdomen, abdominal (muscle) (wall) S3Ø.1
adnexa, eye NEC SØ5.8X-•
adrenal gland S37.812
alveolar process SØØ.532
ankle S9Ø.Ø-•
antecubital space —*see* Contusion, forearm
anus S3Ø.3
arm (upper) S4Ø.Ø2-•
lower (with elbow) —*see* Contusion, forearm
auditory canal —*see* Contusion, ear
auricle —*see* Contusion, ear
axilla —*see* Contusion, arm, upper
back —*see also* Contusion, thorax, back
lower S3Ø.Ø
bile duct S36.13
bladder S37.22
bone NEC T14.8
brain (diffuse) —*see* Injury, intracranial, diffuse
focal —*see* Injury, intracranial, focal
brainstem SØ6.38-•
breast S2Ø.Ø-•
broad ligament S37.892
brow SØØ.83
buttock S3Ø.Ø
canthus, eye SØØ.1-•
cauda equina S34.3
cerebellar, traumatic SØ6.37-•
cerebral SØ6.33-•
left side SØ6.32-•
right side SØ6.31-•
cheek SØØ.83
internal SØØ.532
chest (wall) —*see* Contusion, thorax
chin SØØ.83
clitoris S3Ø.23
colon —*see* Injury, intestine, large, contusion
common bile duct S36.13
conjunctiva SØ5.1-•
with foreign body (in conjunctival sac) —*see* Foreign body, conjunctival sac
conus medullaris (spine) S34.139
cornea —*see* Contusion, eyeball
with foreign body —*see* Foreign body, cornea
corpus cavernosum S3Ø.21
cortex (brain) (cerebral) —*see* Injury, intracranial, diffuse
focal —*see* Injury, intracranial, focal
costal region —*see* Contusion, thorax
cystic duct S36.13
diaphragm S27.8Ø2
duodenum S36.42Ø
ear SØØ.43-•
elbow S5Ø.Ø-•
with forearm —*see* Contusion, forearm
epididymis S3Ø.22
epigastric region S3Ø.1
epiglottis S1Ø.Ø
esophagus (thoracic) S27.812
cervical S1Ø.Ø
eyeball SØ5.1-•

Contusion *(Continued)*
eyebrow SØØ.1-•
eyelid (and periocular area) SØØ.1-•
face NEC SØØ.83
fallopian tube S37.529
bilateral S37.522
unilateral S37.521
femoral triangle S3Ø.1
finger(s) S6Ø.ØØ
with damage to nail (matrix) S6Ø.1Ø
index S6Ø.Ø2-•
with damage to nail S6Ø.12-•
little S6Ø.Ø5-•
with damage to nail S6Ø.15-•
middle S6Ø.Ø3-•
with damage to nail S6Ø.13-•
ring S6Ø.Ø4-•
with damage to nail S6Ø.14-•
thumb —*see* Contusion, thumb
flank S3Ø.1
foot (except toe(s) alone) S9Ø.3-•
toe —*see* Contusion, toe
forearm S5Ø.1-•
elbow only —*see* Contusion, elbow
forehead SØØ.83
gallbladder S36.122
genital organs, external
female S3Ø.2Ø2
male S3Ø.2Ø1
globe (eye) —*see* Contusion, eyeball
groin S3Ø.1
gum SØØ.532
hand S6Ø.22-•
finger(s) —*see* Contusion, finger
wrist —*see* Contusion, wrist
head SØØ.93
ear —*see* Contusion, ear
eyelid —*see* Contusion, eyelid
lip SØØ.531
nose SØØ.33
oral cavity SØØ.532
scalp SØØ.Ø3
specified part NEC SØØ.83
heart —*see also* Injury, heart S26.91
heel —*see* Contusion, foot
hepatic duct S36.13
hip S7Ø.Ø-•
ileum S36.428
iliac region S3Ø.1
inguinal region S3Ø.1
interscapular region S2Ø.229
intra-abdominal organ S36.92
colon —*see* Injury, intestine, large, contusion
liver S36.112
pancreas —*see* Contusion, pancreas
rectum S36.62
small intestine —*see* Injury, intestine, small, contusion
specified organ NEC S36.892
spleen —*see* Contusion, spleen
stomach S36.32
iris (eye) —*see* Contusion, eyeball
jaw SØØ.83
jejunum S36.428
kidney S37.Ø1-•
major (greater than 2 cm) S37.Ø2-•
minor (less than 2 cm) S37.Ø1-•
knee S8Ø.Ø-•
labium (majus) (minus) S3Ø.23
lacrimal apparatus, gland or sac SØ5.8X-•
larynx S1Ø.Ø
leg (lower) S8Ø.1-•
knee —*see* Contusion, knee
lens —*see* Contusion, eyeball
lip SØØ.531
liver S36.112
lower back S3Ø.Ø
lumbar region S3Ø.Ø
lung S27.329
bilateral S27.322
unilateral S27.321

Contusion *(Continued)*
malar region SØØ.83
mastoid region SØØ.83
membrane, brain —*see* Injury, intracranial, diffuse
focal —*see* Injury, intracranial, focal
mesentery S36.892
mesosalpinx S37.892
mouth SØØ.532
muscle —*see* Contusion, by site
nail
finger —*see* Contusion, finger, with damage to nail
toe —*see* Contusion, toe, with damage to nail
nasal SØØ.33
neck S1Ø.93
specified site NEC S1Ø.83
throat S1Ø.Ø
nerve —*see* Injury, nerve
newborn P54.5
nose SØØ.33
occipital
lobe (brain) —*see* Injury, intracranial, diffuse
focal —*see* Injury, intracranial, focal
region (scalp) SØØ.Ø3
orbit (region) (tissues) SØ5.1-•
ovary S37.429
bilateral S37.422
unilateral S37.421
palate SØØ.532
pancreas S36.229
body S36.221
head S36.22Ø
tail S36.222
parietal
lobe (brain) —*see* Injury, intracranial, diffuse
focal —*see* Injury, intracranial, focal
region (scalp) SØØ.Ø3
pelvic organ S37.92
adrenal gland S37.812
bladder S37.22
fallopian tube —*see* Contusion, fallopian tube
kidney —*see* Contusion, kidney
ovary —*see* Contusion, ovary
prostate S37.822
specified organ NEC S37.892
ureter S37.12
urethra S37.32
uterus S37.62
pelvis S3Ø.Ø
penis S3Ø.21
perineum
female S3Ø.23
male S3Ø.Ø
periocular area SØØ.1-•
peritoneum S36.81
periurethral tissue —*see* Contusion, urethra
pharynx S1Ø.Ø
pinna —*see* Contusion, ear
popliteal space —*see* Contusion, knee
prepuce S3Ø.21
prostate S37.822
pubic region S3Ø.1
pudendum
female S3Ø.2Ø2
male S3Ø.2Ø1
quadriceps femoris —*see* Contusion, thigh
rectum S36.62
retroperitoneum S36.892
round ligament S37.892
sacral region S3Ø.Ø
scalp SØØ.Ø3
due to birth injury P12.3
scapular region —*see* Contusion, shoulder
sclera —*see* Contusion, eyeball

Contusion *(Continued)*
scrotum S30.22
seminal vesicle S37.892
shoulder S40.01-●
skin NEC T14.8
small intestine —*see* Injury, intestine, small, contusion
spermatic cord S30.22
spinal cord —*see* Injury, spinal cord, by region
cauda equina S34.3
conus medullaris S34.139
spleen S36.029
major S36.021
minor S36.020
sternal region S20.219
stomach S36.32
subconjunctival S05.1-●
subcutaneous NEC T14.8
submaxillary region S00.83
submental region S00.83
subperiosteal NEC T14.8
subungual
finger —*see* Contusion, finger, with damage to nail
toe —*see* Contusion, toe, with damage to nail
supraclavicular fossa S10.83
supraorbital S00.83
suprarenal gland S37.812
temple (region) S00.83
temporal
lobe (brain) —*see* Injury, intracranial, diffuse
focal —*see* Injury, intracranial, focal
region S00.83
testis S30.22
thigh S70.1-●
thorax (wall) S20.20
back S20.22-●
front S20.21-●
throat S10.0
thumb S60.01-●
with damage to nail S60.11-●
toe(s) (lesser) S90.12-●
with damage to nail S90.22-●
great S90.11-●
with damage to nail S90.21-●
tongue S00.532
trachea (cervical) S10.0
thoracic S27.52
tunica vaginalis S30.22
tympanum, tympanic membrane —*see* Contusion, ear
ureter S37.12
urethra S37.32
urinary organ NEC S37.892
uterus S37.62
uvula S00.532
vagina S30.23
vas deferens S37.892
vesical S37.22
vocal cord(s) S10.0
vulva S30.23
wrist S60.21-●
Conus (congenital) (any type) Q14.8
cornea —*see* Keratoconus
medullaris syndrome G95.81
Conversion hysteria, neurosis or reaction F44.9
Converter, tuberculosis (test reaction) R76.11
Conviction (legal), **anxiety concerning** Z65.0
with imprisonment Z65.1
Convulsions (idiopathic) —*see also* Seizure(s) R56.9
apoplectiform (cerebral ischemia) I67.82
dissociative F44.5
epileptic —*see* Epilepsy
epileptiform, epileptoid —*see* Seizure, epileptiform

Convulsions *(Continued)*
ether (anesthetic) —*see* Table of Drugs and Chemicals, by drug
febrile R56.00
with status epilepticus G40.901
complex R56.01
with status epilepticus G40.901
simple R56.00
hysterical F44.5
infantile P90
epilepsy —*see* Epilepsy
jacksonian —*see* Epilepsy, localization-related, symptomatic, with simple partial seizures
myoclonic G25.3
newborn P90
obstetrical (nephritic) (uremic) —*see* Eclampsia
paretic A52.17
post traumatic R56.1
psychomotor —*see* Epilepsy, localization-related, symptomatic, with complex partial seizures
recurrent R56.9
reflex R25.8
scarlatinal A38.8
tetanus, tetanic —*see* Tetanus
thymic E32.8
Convulsive —*see also* Convulsions
Cooley's anemia D56.1
Coolie itch B76.9
Cooper's
disease —*see* Mastopathy, cystic
hernia —*see* Hernia, abdomen, specified site NEC
Copra itch B88.0
Coprophagy F50.89
Coprophobia F40.298
Coproporphyria, hereditary E80.29
Cor
biloculare Q20.8
bovis, bovinum —*see* Hypertrophy, cardiac
pulmonale (chronic) I27.81
acute I26.09
triatriatum, triatrium Q24.2
triloculare Q20.8
biatrium Q20.4
biventriculare Q21.1
Corbus' disease (gangrenous balanitis) N48.1
Cord —*see also* condition
around neck
complicating delivery O69.81
with compression O69.1
bladder G95.89
tabetic A52.19
Cordis ectopia Q24.8
Corditis (spermatic) N49.1
Corectopia Q13.2
Cori's disease (glycogen storage) E74.03
Corkhandler's disease or lung J67.3
Corkscrew esophagus K22.4
Corkworker's disease or lung J67.3
Corn (infected) L84
Cornea —*see also* condition
donor Z52.5
plana Q13.4
Cornelia de Lange syndrome Q87.19
Cornu cutaneum L85.8
Cornual gestation or pregnancy O00.80
with intrauterine pregnancy O00.81
Coronary (artery) —*see* condition
Coronavirus, as cause of disease classified elsewhere B97.29
SARS-associated B97.21
Corpora —*see also* condition
amylacea, prostate N42.89
cavernosa —*see* condition
Corpulence —*see* Obesity
Corpus —*see* condition
Corrected transposition Q20.5

Corrosion (injury) (acid) (caustic) (chemical) (lime) (external) (internal) T30.4
abdomen, abdominal (muscle) (wall) T21.42
first degree T21.52
second degree T21.62
third degree T21.72
above elbow T22.439
first degree T22.539
left T22.432
first degree T22.532
second degree T22.632
third degree T22.732
right T22.431
first degree T22.531
second degree T22.631
third degree T22.731
second degree T22.639
third degree T22.739
alimentary tract NEC T28.7
ankle T25.419
first degree T25.519
left T25.412
first degree T25.512
second degree T25.612
third degree T25.712
multiple with foot —*see* Corrosion, lower, limb, multiple, ankle and foot
right T25.411
first degree T25.511
second degree T25.611
third degree T25.711
second degree T25.619
third degree T25.719
anus —*see* Corrosion, buttock
arm(s) (meaning upper limb(s)) —*see* Corrosion, upper limb
axilla T22.449
first degree T22.549
left T22.442
first degree T22.542
second degree T22.642
third degree T22.742
right T22.441
first degree T22.541
second degree T22.641
third degree T22.741
second degree T22.649
third degree T22.749
back (lower) T21.44
first degree T21.54
second degree T21.64
third degree T21.74
upper T21.43
first degree T21.53
second degree T21.63
third degree T21.73
blisters - code as Corrosion, second degree, by site
breast(s) —*see* Corrosion, chest wall
buttock(s) T21.45
first degree T21.55
second degree T21.65
third degree T21.75
calf T24.439
first degree T24.539
left T24.432
first degree T24.532
second degree T24.632
third degree T24.732
right T24.431
first degree T24.531
second degree T24.631
third degree T24.731
second degree T24.639
third degree T24.739
canthus (eye) —*see* Corrosion, eyelid
cervix T28.8
cheek T20.46
first degree T20.56
second degree T20.66
third degree T20.76

Corrosion *(Continued)*
chest wall T21.41
first degree T21.51
second degree T21.61
third degree T21.71
chin T20.43
first degree T20.53
second degree T20.63
third degree T20.73
colon T28.7
conjunctiva (and cornea) —*see* Corrosion, cornea
cornea (and conjunctiva) T26.6-•
deep necrosis of underlying tissue - code as Corrosion, third degree, by site
dorsum of hand T23.469
first degree T23.569
left T23.462
first degree T23.562
second degree T23.662
third degree T23.762
right T23.461
first degree T23.561
second degree T23.661
third degree T23.761
second degree T23.669
third degree T23.769
ear (auricle) (external) (canal) T20.41
drum T28.91
first degree T20.51
second degree T20.61
third degree T20.71
elbow T22.429
first degree T22.529
left T22.422
first degree T22.522
second degree T22.622
third degree T22.722
right T22.421
first degree T22.521
second degree T22.621
third degree T22.721
second degree T22.629
third degree T22.729
entire body —*see* Corrosion, multiple body regions
epidermal loss - code as Corrosion, second degree, by site
epiglottis T27.4
erythema, erythematous - code as Corrosion, first degree, by site
esophagus T28.6
extent (percentage of body surface)
less than 10 percent T32.0
10-19 percent (0-9 percent third degree) T32.10
with 10-19 percent third degree T32.11
20-29 percent (0-9 percent third degree) T32.20
with
10-19 percent third degree T32.21
20-29 percent third degree T32.22
30-39 percent (0-9 percent third degree) T32.30
with
10-19 percent third degree T32.31
20-29 percent third degree T32.32
30-39 percent third degree T32.33
40-49 percent (0-9 percent third degree) T32.40
with
10-19 percent third degree T32.41
20-29 percent third degree T32.42
30-39 percent third degree T32.43
40-49 percent third degree T32.44
50-59 percent (0-9 percent third degree) T32.50
with
10-19 percent third degree T32.51
20-29 percent third degree T32.52

Corrosion *(Continued)*
extent *(Continued)*
50-59 percent *(Continued)*
with *(Continued)*
30-39 percent third degree T32.53
40-49 percent third degree T32.54
50-59 percent third degree T32.55
60-69 percent (0-9 percent third degree) T32.60
with
10-19 percent third degree T32.61
20-29 percent third degree T32.62
30-39 percent third degree T32.63
40-49 percent third degree T32.64
50-59 percent third degree T32.65
60-69 percent third degree T32.66
70-79 percent (0-9 percent third degree) T32.70
with
10-19 percent third degree T32.71
20-29 percent third degree T32.72
30-39 percent third degree T32.73
40-49 percent third degree T32.74
50-59 percent third degree T32.75
60-69 percent third degree T32.76
70-79 percent third degree T32.77
80-89 percent (0-9 percent third degree) T32.80
with
10-19 percent third degree T32.81
20-29 percent third degree T32.82
30-39 percent third degree T32.83
40-49 percent third degree T32.84
50-59 percent third degree T32.85
60-69 percent third degree T32.86
70-79 percent third degree T32.87
80-89 percent third degree T32.88
90 percent or more (0-9 percent third degree) T32.90
with
10-19 percent third degree T32.91
20-29 percent third degree T32.92
30-39 percent third degree T32.93
40-49 percent third degree T32.94
50-59 percent third degree T32.95
60-69 percent third degree T32.96
70-79 percent third degree T32.97
80-89 percent third degree T32.98
90-99 percent third degree T32.99
extremity —*see* Corrosion, limb
eye(s) and adnexa T26.9-•
with resulting rupture and destruction of eyeball T26.7-•
conjunctival sac —*see* Corrosion, cornea
cornea —*see* Corrosion, cornea
lid —*see* Corrosion, eyelid
periocular area —*see* Corrosion eyelid
specified site NEC T26.8-•
eyeball —*see* Corrosion, eye
eyelid(s) T26.5-•
face —*see* Corrosion, head
finger T23.429
first degree T23.529
left T23.422
first degree T23.522
second degree T23.622
third degree T23.722
multiple sites (without thumb) T23.439
with thumb T23.449
first degree T23.549
left T23.442
first degree T23.542
second degree T23.642
third degree T23.742
right T23.441
first degree T23.541
second degree T23.641
third degree T23.741
second degree T23.649
third degree T23.749

Corrosion *(Continued)*
finger *(Continued)*
multiple sites *(Continued)*
first degree T23.539
left T23.432
first degree T23.532
second degree T23.632
third degree T23.732
right T23.431
first degree T23.531
second degree T23.631
third degree T23.731
second degree T23.639
third degree T23.739
right T23.421
first degree T23.521
second degree T23.621
third degree T23.721
second degree T23.629
third degree T23.729
flank —*see* Corrosion, abdomen
foot T25.429
first degree T25.529
left T25.422
first degree T25.522
second degree T25.622
third degree T25.722
multiple with ankle —*see* Corrosion, lower, limb, multiple, ankle and foot
right T25.421
first degree T25.521
second degree T25.621
third degree T25.721
second degree T25.629
third degree T25.729
forearm T22.419
first degree T22.519
left T22.412
first degree T22.512
second degree T22.612
third degree T22.712
right T22.411
first degree T22.511
second degree T22.611
third degree T22.711
second degree T22.619
third degree T22.719
forehead T20.46
first degree T20.56
second degree T20.66
third degree T20.76
fourth degree - code as Corrosion, third degree, by site
full thickness skin loss - code as Corrosion, third degree, by site
gastrointestinal tract NEC T28.7
genital organs
external
female T21.47
first degree T21.57
second degree T21.67
third degree T21.77
male T21.46
first degree T21.56
second degree T21.66
third degree T21.76
internal T28.8
groin —*see* Corrosion, abdominal wall
hand(s) T23.409
back —*see* Corrosion, dorsum of hand
finger —*see* Corrosion, finger
first degree T23.509
left T23.402
first degree T23.502
second degree T23.602
third degree T23.702
multiple sites with wrist T23.499
first degree T23.599
left T23.492
first degree T23.592
second degree T23.692
third degree T23.792

C

▶ New ➠ Revised ~~deleted~~ Deleted • Use Additional Character(s)

Corrosion (Continued)
  hand(s) (Continued)
    multiple sites (Continued)
      right T23.491
        first degree T23.591
        second degree T23.691
        third degree T23.791
      second degree T23.699
      third degree T23.799
    palm —see Corrosion, palm
    right T23.401
      first degree T23.501
      second degree T23.601
      third degree T23.701
    second degree T23.609
    third degree T23.709
    thumb —see Corrosion, thumb
  head (and face) (and neck) T20.40
    cheek —see Corrosion, cheek
    chin —see Corrosion, chin
    ear —see Corrosion, ear
    eye(s) only —see Corrosion, eye
    first degree T20.50
    forehead —see Corrosion, forehead
    lip —see Corrosion, lip
    multiple sites T20.49
      first degree T20.59
      second degree T20.69
      third degree T20.79
    neck —see Corrosion, neck
    nose —see Corrosion, nose
    scalp —see Corrosion, scalp
    second degree T20.60
    third degree T20.70
  hip(s) —see Corrosion, lower, limb
  inhalation —see Corrosion, respiratory tract
  internal organ(s) (see also Corrosion, by site) T28.90
    alimentary tract T28.7
      esophagus T28.6
    esophagus T28.6
    genitourinary T28.8
    mouth T28.5
    pharynx T28.5
    specified organ NEC T28.99
  interscapular region —see Corrosion, back, upper
  intestine (large) (small) T28.7
  knee T24.429
    first degree T24.529
    left T24.422
      first degree T24.522
      second degree T24.622
      third degree T24.722
    right T24.421
      first degree T24.521
      second degree T24.621
      third degree T24.721
    second degree T24.629
    third degree T24.729
  labium (majus) (minus) —see Corrosion, genital organs, external, female
  lacrimal apparatus, duct, gland or sac —see Corrosion, eye, specified site NEC
  larynx T27.4
    with lung T27.5
  leg(s) (meaning lower limb(s)) —see Corrosion, lower limb
  limb(s)
    lower —see Corrosion, lower, limb
    upper —see Corrosion, upper limb
  lip(s) T20.42
    first degree T20.52
    second degree T20.62
    third degree T20.72
  lower
    back —see Corrosion, back
    limb T24.409
      ankle —see Corrosion, ankle
      calf —see Corrosion, calf

Corrosion (Continued)
  lower (Continued)
    limb (Continued)
      first degree T24.509
      foot —see Corrosion, foot
      hip —see Corrosion, thigh
      knee —see Corrosion, knee
      left T24.402
        first degree T24.502
        second degree T24.602
        third degree T24.702
      multiple sites, except ankle and foot T24.499
        ankle and foot T25.499
          first degree T25.599
          left T25.492
            first degree T25.592
            second degree T25.692
            third degree T25.792
          right T25.491
            first degree T25.591
            second degree T25.691
            third degree T25.791
          second degree T25.699
          third degree T25.799
        first degree T24.599
        left T24.492
          first degree T24.592
          second degree T24.692
          third degree T24.792
        right T24.491
          first degree T24.591
          second degree T24.691
          third degree T24.791
        second degree T24.699
        third degree T24.799
      right T24.401
        first degree T24.501
        second degree T24.601
        third degree T24.701
      second degree T24.609
      thigh —see Corrosion, thigh
      third degree T24.709
  lung (with larynx and trachea) T27.5
  mouth T28.5
  neck T20.47
    first degree T20.57
    second degree T20.67
    third degree T20.77
  nose (septum) T20.44
    first degree T20.54
    second degree T20.64
    third degree T20.74
  ocular adnexa —see Corrosion, eye
  orbit region —see Corrosion, eyelid
  palm T23.459
    first degree T23.559
    left T23.452
      first degree T23.552
      second degree T23.652
      third degree T23.752
    right T23.451
      first degree T23.551
      second degree T23.651
      third degree T23.751
    second degree T23.659
    third degree T23.759
  partial thickness - code as Corrosion, unspecified degree, by site
  pelvis —see Corrosion, trunk
  penis —see Corrosion, genital organs, external, male
  perineum
    female —see Corrosion, genital organs, external, female
    male —see Corrosion, genital organs, external, male
  periocular area —see Corrosion, eyelid
  pharynx T28.5
  rectum T28.7

Corrosion (Continued)
  respiratory tract T27.7
    larynx —see Corrosion, larynx
    specified part NEC T27.6
    trachea —see Corrosion, larynx
  sac, lacrimal —see Corrosion, eye, specified site NEC
  scalp T20.45
    first degree T20.55
    second degree T20.65
    third degree T20.75
  scapular region T22.469
    first degree T22.569
    left T22.462
      first degree T22.562
      second degree T22.662
      third degree T22.762
    right T22.461
      first degree T22.561
      second degree T22.661
      third degree T22.761
    second degree T22.669
    third degree T22.769
  sclera —see Corrosion, eye, specified site NEC
  scrotum —see Corrosion, genital organs, external, male
  shoulder T22.459
    first degree T22.559
    left T22.452
      first degree T22.552
      second degree T22.652
      third degree T22.752
    right T22.451
      first degree T22.551
      second degree T22.651
      third degree T22.751
    second degree T22.659
    third degree T22.759
  stomach T28.7
  temple —see Corrosion, head
  testis —see Corrosion, genital organs, external, male
  thigh T24.419
    first degree T24.519
    left T24.412
      first degree T24.512
      second degree T24.612
      third degree T24.712
    right T24.411
      first degree T24.511
      second degree T24.611
      third degree T24.711
    second degree T24.619
    third degree T24.719
  thorax (external) —see Corrosion, trunk
  throat (meaning pharynx) T28.5
  thumb(s) T23.419
    first degree T23.519
    left T23.412
      first degree T23.512
      second degree T23.612
      third degree T23.712
    multiple sites with fingers T23.449
      first degree T23.549
      left T23.442
        first degree T23.542
        second degree T23.642
        third degree T23.742
      right T23.441
        first degree T23.541
        second degree T23.641
        third degree T23.741
      second degree T23.649
      third degree T23.749
    right T23.411
      first degree T23.511
      second degree T23.611
      third degree T23.711
    second degree T23.619
    third degree T23.719

Corrosion *(Continued)*
- toe T25.439
  - first degree T25.539
  - left T25.432
    - first degree T25.532
    - second degree T25.632
    - third degree T25.732
  - right T25.431
    - first degree T25.531
    - second degree T25.631
    - third degree T25.731
  - second degree T25.639
  - third degree T25.739
- tongue T28.5
- tonsil(s) T28.5
- total body —*see* Corrosion, multiple body regions
- trachea T27.4
  - with lung T27.5
- trunk T21.40
  - abdominal wall —*see* Corrosion, abdominal wall
  - anus —*see* Corrosion, buttock
  - axilla —*see* Corrosion, upper limb
  - back —*see* Corrosion, back
  - breast —*see* Corrosion, chest wall
  - buttock —*see* Corrosion, buttock
  - chest wall —*see* Corrosion, chest wall
  - first degree T21.50
  - flank —*see* Corrosion, abdominal wall
  - genital
    - female —*see* Corrosion, genital organs, external, female
    - male —*see* Corrosion, genital organs, external, male
  - groin —*see* Corrosion, abdominal wall
  - interscapular region —*see* Corrosion, back, upper
  - labia —*see* Corrosion, genital organs, external, female
  - lower back —*see* Corrosion, back
  - penis —*see* Corrosion, genital organs, external, male
  - perineum
    - female —*see* Corrosion, genital organs, external, female
    - male —*see* Corrosion, genital organs, external, male
  - scapular region —*see* Corrosion, upper limb
  - scrotum —*see* Corrosion, genital organs, external, male
  - second degree T21.60
  - shoulder —*see* Corrosion, upper limb
  - specified site NEC T21.49
    - first degree T21.59
    - second degree T21.69
    - third degree T21.79
  - testes —*see* Corrosion, genital organs, external, male
  - third degree T21.70
  - upper back —*see* Corrosion, back, upper
  - vagina T28.8
  - vulva —*see* Corrosion, genital organs, external, female
- unspecified site with extent of body surface involved specified
  - less than 10 percent T32.0
  - 10-19 percent (0-9 percent third degree) T32.10
    - with 10-19 percent third degree T32.11
  - 20-29 percent (0-9 percent third degree) T32.20
    - with
      - 10-19 percent third degree T32.21
      - 20-29 percent third degree T32.22
  - 30-39 percent (0-9 percent third degree) T32.30
    - with
      - 10-19 percent third degree T32.31
      - 20-29 percent third degree T32.32
      - 30-39 percent third degree T32.33

Corrosion *(Continued)*
- unspecified site with extent of body surface involved specified *(Continued)*
  - 40-49 percent (0-9 percent third degree) T32.40
    - with
      - 10-19 percent third degree T32.41
      - 20-29 percent third degree T32.42
      - 30-39 percent third degree T32.43
      - 40-49 percent third degree T32.44
  - 50-59 percent (0-9 percent third degree) T32.50
    - with
      - 10-19 percent third degree T32.51
      - 20-29 percent third degree T32.52
      - 30-39 percent third degree T32.53
      - 40-49 percent third degree T32.54
      - 50-59 percent third degree T32.55
  - 60-69 percent (0-9 percent third degree) T32.60
    - with
      - 10-19 percent third degree T32.61
      - 20-29 percent third degree T32.62
      - 30-39 percent third degree T32.63
      - 40-49 percent third degree T32.64
      - 50-59 percent third degree T32.65
      - 60-69 percent third degree T32.66
  - 70-79 percent (0-9 percent third degree) T32.70
    - with
      - 10-19 percent third degree T32.71
      - 20-29 percent third degree T32.72
      - 30-39 percent third degree T32.73
      - 40-49 percent third degree T32.74
      - 50-59 percent third degree T32.75
      - 60-69 percent third degree T32.76
      - 70-79 percent third degree T32.77
  - 80-89 percent (0-9 percent third degree) T32.80
    - with
      - 10-19 percent third degree T32.81
      - 20-29 percent third degree T32.82
      - 30-39 percent third degree T32.83
      - 40-49 percent third degree T32.84
      - 50-59 percent third degree T32.85
      - 60-69 percent third degree T32.86
      - 70-79 percent third degree T32.87
      - 80-89 percent third degree T32.88
  - 90 percent or more (0-9 percent third degree) T32.90
    - with
      - 10-19 percent third degree T32.91
      - 20-29 percent third degree T32.92
      - 30-39 percent third degree T32.93
      - 40-49 percent third degree T32.94
      - 50-59 percent third degree T32.95
      - 60-69 percent third degree T32.96
      - 70-79 percent third degree T32.97
      - 80-89 percent third degree T32.98
      - 90-99 percent third degree T32.99
- upper limb (axilla) (scapular region) T22.40
  - above elbow —*see* Corrosion, above elbow
  - axilla —*see* Corrosion, axilla
  - elbow —*see* Corrosion, elbow
  - first degree T22.50
  - forearm —*see* Corrosion, forearm
  - hand —*see* Corrosion, hand
  - interscapular region —*see* Corrosion, back, upper
  - multiple sites T22.499
    - first degree T22.599
    - left T22.492
      - first degree T22.592
      - second degree T22.692
      - third degree T22.792
    - right T22.491
      - first degree T22.591
      - second degree T22.691
      - third degree T22.791
    - second degree T22.699
    - third degree T22.799

Corrosion *(Continued)*
- upper limb (axilla) (scapular region) *(Continued)*
  - scapular region —*see* Corrosion, scapular region
  - second degree T22.60
  - shoulder —*see* Corrosion, shoulder
  - third degree T22.70
  - wrist —*see* Corrosion, hand
- uterus T28.8
- vagina T28.8
- vulva —*see* Corrosion, genital organs, external, female
- wrist T23.479
  - first degree T23.579
  - left T23.472
    - first degree T23.572
    - second degree T23.672
    - third degree T23.772
  - multiple sites with hand T23.499
    - first degree T23.599
    - left T23.492
      - first degree T23.592
      - second degree T23.692
      - third degree T23.792
    - right T23.491
      - first degree T23.591
      - second degree T23.691
      - third degree T23.791
    - second degree T23.699
    - third degree T23.799
  - right T23.471
    - first degree T23.571
    - second degree T23.671
    - third degree T23.771
  - second degree T23.679
  - third degree T23.779

Corrosive burn —*see* Corrosion

Corsican fever —*see* Malaria

Cortical —*see* condition

Cortico-adrenal —*see* condition

Coryza (acute) J00
- with grippe or influenza —*see* Influenza, with, respiratory manifestations NEC
- syphilitic
  - congenital (chronic) A50.05

Costen's syndrome or complex M26.69

Costiveness —*see* Constipation

Costochondritis M94.0

Cot death R99

Cotard's syndrome F22

Cotia virus B08.8

Cotton wool spots (retinal) H35.81

Cotungo's disease —*see* Sciatica

Cough (affected) (chronic) (epidemic) (nervous) R05
- with hemorrhage —*see* Hemoptysis
- bronchial R05
  - with grippe or influenza —*see* Influenza, with, respiratory manifestations NEC
- functional F45.8
- hysterical F45.8
- laryngeal, spasmodic R05
- psychogenic F45.8
- smokers' J41.0
- tea taster's B49

Counseling (for) Z71.9
- abuse NEC
  - perpetrator Z69.82
  - victim Z69.81
- alcohol abuser Z71.41
  - family Z71.42
- child abuse
  - nonparental
    - perpetrator Z69.021
    - victim Z69.020
  - parental
    - perpetrator Z69.011
    - victim Z69.010

▶ New ➡ Revised ~~deleted~~ Deleted ● Use Additional Character(s)

Counseling *(Continued)*
consanguinity Z71.89
contraceptive Z3Ø.Ø9
dietary Z71.3
drug abuser Z71.51
family member Z71.52
exercise Z71.82
family Z71.89
fertility preservation (prior to cancer therapy) (prior to removal of gonads) Z31.62
for non-attending third party Z71.Ø
related to sexual behavior or orientation Z7Ø.2
genetic
nonprocreative Z71.83
procreative NEC Z31.5
gestational carrier Z31.7
health (advice) (education) (instruction) —*see* Counseling, medical
▶ risk for travel (international) Z71.84
human immunodeficiency virus (HIV) Z71.7
impotence Z7Ø.1
insulin pump use Z46.81
medical (for) Z71.9
boarding school resident Z59.3
consanguinity Z71.89
feared complaint and no disease found Z71.1
human immunodeficiency virus (HIV) Z71.7
institutional resident Z59.3
on behalf of another Z71.Ø
related to sexual behavior or orientation Z7Ø.2
person living alone Z6Ø.2
specified reason NEC Z71.89
natural family planning
procreative Z31.61
to avoid pregnancy Z3Ø.Ø2
perpetrator (of)
abuse NEC Z69.82
child abuse
non-parental Z69.Ø21
parental Z69.Ø11
rape NEC Z69.82
spousal abuse Z69.12
procreative NEC Z31.69
fertility preservation (prior to cancer therapy) (prior to removal of gonads) Z31.62
using natural family planning Z31.61
promiscuity Z7Ø.1
rape victim Z69.81
religious Z71.81
▶ safety for travel (international) Z71.84
sex, sexual (related to) Z7Ø.9
attitude(s) Z7Ø.Ø
behavior or orientation Z7Ø.1
combined concerns Z7Ø.3
non-responsiveness Z7Ø.1
on behalf of third party Z7Ø.2
specified reason NEC Z7Ø.8
specified reason NEC Z71.89
spiritual Z71.81
spousal abuse (perpetrator) Z69.12
victim Z69.11
substance abuse Z71.89
alcohol Z71.41
drug Z71.51
tobacco Z71.6
▶ travel (international) Z71.84
tobacco use Z71.6
use (of)
insulin pump Z46.81
victim (of)
abuse Z69.81
child abuse
by parent Z69.Ø1Ø
non-parental Z69.Ø2Ø
rape NEC Z69.81
Coupled rhythm RØØ.8
Couvelaire syndrome or uterus (complicating delivery) O45.8X-●
Cowperitis —*see* Urethritis
Cowper's gland —*see* condition
Cowpox BØ8.Ø1Ø
due to vaccination T88.1
Coxa
magna M91.4-●
plana M91.2-●
valga (acquired) —*see also* Deformity, limb, specified type NEC, thigh
congenital Q65.81
sequelae (late effect) of rickets E64.3
vara (acquired) —*see also* Deformity, limb, specified type NEC, thigh
congenital Q65.82
sequelae (late effect) of rickets E64.3
Coxalgia, coxalgic (nontuberculous) —*see also* Pain, joint, hip
tuberculous A18.Ø2
Coxitis —*see* Monoarthritis, hip
Coxsackie (virus) (infection) B34.1
as cause of disease classified elsewhere B97.11
carditis B33.2Ø
central nervous system NEC A88.8
endocarditis B33.21
enteritis AØ8.39
meningitis (aseptic) A87.Ø
myocarditis B33.22
pericarditis B33.23
pharyngitis BØ8.5
pleurodynia B33.Ø
specific disease NEC B33.8
Crabs, meaning pubic lice B85.3
Crack baby PØ4.41
Cracked nipple N64.Ø
associated with
lactation O92.13
pregnancy O92.11-●
puerperium O92.12
Cracked tooth KØ3.81
Cradle cap L21.Ø
Craft neurosis F48.8
Cramp(s) R25.2
abdominal —*see* Pain, abdominal
bathing T75.1
colic R1Ø.83
psychogenic F45.8
due to immersion T75.1
fireman T67.2
heat T67.2
immersion T75.1
intestinal —*see* Pain, abdominal
psychogenic F45.8
leg, sleep related G47.62
limb (lower) (upper) NEC R25.2
sleep related G47.62
linotypist's F48.8
organic G25.89
muscle (limb) (general) R25.2
due to immersion T75.1
psychogenic F45.8
occupational (hand) F48.8
organic G25.89
salt-depletion E87.1
sleep related, leg G47.62
stoker's T67.2
swimmer's T75.1
telegrapher's F48.8
organic G25.89
typist's F48.8
organic G25.89
uterus N94.89
menstrual —*see* Dysmenorrhea
writer's F48.8
organic G25.89
Cranial —*see* condition
Craniocleidodysostosis Q74.Ø
Craniofenestria (skull) Q75.8
Craniolacunia (skull) Q75.8
Craniopagus Q89.4
Craniopathy, metabolic M85.2
Craniopharyngeal —*see* condition
Craniopharyngioma D44.4
Craniorachischisis (totalis) QØØ.1
Cranioschisis Q75.8
Craniostenosis Q75.Ø
Craniosynostosis Q75.Ø
Craniotabes (cause unknown) M83.8
neonatal P96.3
rachitic E64.3
syphilitic A5Ø.56
Cranium —*see* condition
Craw-craw —*see* Onchocerciasis
Creaking joint —*see* Derangement, joint, specified type NEC
Creeping
eruption B76.9
palsy or paralysis G12.22
Crenated tongue K14.8
Creotoxism AØ5.9
Crepitus
caput Q75.8
joint —*see* Derangement, joint, specified type NEC
Crescent or conus choroid, congenital Q14.3
CREST syndrome M34.1
Cretin, cretinism (congenital) (endemic) (nongoitrous) (sporadic) EØØ.9
pelvis
with disproportion (fetopelvic) O33.Ø
causing obstructed labor O65.Ø
type
hypothyroid EØØ.1
mixed EØØ.2
myxedematous EØØ.1
neurological EØØ.Ø
Creutzfeldt-Jakob disease or syndrome (with dementia) A81.ØØ
familial A81.Ø9
iatrogenic A81.Ø9
specified NEC A81.Ø9
sporadic A81.Ø9
variant (vCJD) A81.Ø1
Crib death R99
Cribriform hymen Q52.3
Cri-du-chat syndrome Q93.4
Crigler-Najjar disease or syndrome E8Ø.5
Crime, victim of Z65.4
Crimean hemorrhagic fever A98.Ø
Criminalism F6Ø.2
Crisis
abdomen R1Ø.Ø
acute reaction F43.Ø
addisonian E27.2
adrenal (cortical) E27.2
celiac K9Ø.Ø
Dietl's N13.8
emotional —*see also* Disorder, adjustment
acute reaction to stress F43.Ø
specific to childhood and adolescence F93.8
glaucomatocyclitic —*see* Glaucoma, secondary, inflammation
heart —*see* Failure, heart
nitritoid I95.2
correct substance properly administered —*see* Table of Drugs and Chemicals, by drug, adverse effect
overdose or wrong substance given or taken —*see* Table of Drugs and Chemicals, by drug, poisoning
oculogyric H51.8
psychogenic F45.8
Pel's (tabetic) A52.11
psychosexual identity F64.2
renal N28.Ø
sickle-cell D57.ØØ
with
acute chest syndrome D57.Ø1
splenic sequestration D57.Ø2
state (acute reaction) F43.Ø
tabetic A52.11
thyroid —*see* Thyrotoxicosis with thyroid storm
thyrotoxic —*see* Thyrotoxicosis with thyroid storm

Crocq's disease (acrocyanosis) I73.89
Crohn's disease —*see* Enteritis, regional
Crooked septum, nasal J34.2
Cross syndrome E7Ø.328
Crossbite (anterior) (posterior) M26.24
Cross-eye —*see* Strabismus, convergent concomitant
Croup, croupous (catarrhal) (infectious) (inflammatory) (nondiphtheritic) JØ5.Ø
  bronchial J2Ø.9
  diphtheritic A36.2
  false J38.5
  spasmodic J38.5
    diphtheritic A36.2
  stridulous J38.5
    diphtheritic A36.2
Crouzon's disease Q75.1
Crowding, tooth, teeth, fully erupted M26.31
CRST syndrome M34.1
Cruchet's disease A85.8
Cruelty in children —*see also* Disorder, conduct
Crural ulcer —*see* Ulcer, lower limb
Crush, crushed, crushing T14.8
  abdomen S38.1
  ankle S97.Ø- ●
  arm (upper) (and shoulder) S47.- ●
  axilla —*see* Crush, arm
  back, lower S38.1
  buttock S38.1
  cheek SØ7.Ø
  chest S28.Ø
  cranium SØ7.1
  ear SØ7.Ø
  elbow S57.Ø- ●
  extremity
    lower
      ankle —*see* Crush, ankle
      below knee —*see* Crush, leg
      foot —*see* Crush, foot
      hip —*see* Crush, hip
      knee —*see* Crush, knee
      thigh —*see* Crush, thigh
      toe —*see* Crush, toe
    upper
      below elbow S67.9- ●
      elbow —*see* Crush, elbow
      finger —*see* Crush, finger
      forearm —*see* Crush, forearm
      hand —*see* Crush, hand
      thumb —*see* Crush, thumb
      upper arm —*see* Crush, arm
      wrist —*see* Crush, wrist
  face SØ7.Ø
  finger(s) S67.1- ●
    with hand (and wrist) —*see* Crush, hand, specified site NEC
    index S67.19- ●
    little S67.19- ●
    middle S67.19- ●
    ring S67.19- ●
    thumb —*see* Crush, thumb
  foot S97.8- ●
    toe —*see* Crush, toe
  forearm S57.8- ●
  genitalia, external
    female S38.ØØ2
      vagina S38.Ø3
      vulva S38.Ø3
    male S38.ØØ1
      penis S38.Ø1
      scrotum S38.Ø2
      testis S38.Ø2
  hand (except fingers alone) S67.2- ●
    with wrist S67.4- ●
  head SØ7.9
    specified NEC SØ7.8
  heel —*see* Crush, foot
  hip S77.Ø- ●
    with thigh S77.2- ●
  internal organ (abdomen, chest, or pelvis) NEC T14.8
Crush, crushed, crushing *(Continued)*
  knee S87.Ø- ●
  labium (majus) (minus) S38.Ø3
  larynx S17.Ø
  leg (lower) S87.8- ●
    knee —*see* Crush, knee
  lip SØ7.Ø
  lower
    back S38.1
    leg —*see* Crush, leg
  neck S17.9
  nerve —*see* Injury, nerve
  nose SØ7.Ø
  pelvis S38.1
  penis S38.Ø1
  scalp SØ7.8
  scapular region —*see* Crush, arm
  scrotum S38.Ø2
  severe, unspecified site T14.8
  shoulder (and upper arm) —*see* Crush, arm
  skull SØ7.1
  syndrome (complication of trauma) T79.5
  testis S38.Ø2
  thigh S77.1- ●
    with hip S77.2- ●
  throat S17.8
  thumb S67.Ø- ●
    with hand (and wrist) —*see* Crush, hand, specified site NEC
  toe(s) S97.1Ø- ●
    great S97.11- ●
    lesser S97.12- ●
  trachea S17.Ø
  vagina S38.Ø3
  vulva S38.Ø3
  wrist S67.3- ●
    with hand S67.4- ●
Crusta lactea L21.Ø
Crusts R23.4
Crutch paralysis —*see* Injury, brachial plexus
Cruveilhier-Baumgarten cirrhosis, disease or syndrome K74.69
Cruveilhier's atrophy or disease G12.8
Crying (constant) (continuous) (excessive)
  child, adolescent, or adult R45.83
  infant (baby) (newborn) R68.11
Cryofibrinogenemia D89.2
Cryoglobulinemia (essential) (idiopathic) (mixed) (primary) (purpura) (secondary) (vasculitis) D89.1
  with lung involvement D89.1 *[J99]*
Cryptitis (anal) (rectal) K62.89
Cryptococcosis, cryptococcus (infection) (neoformans) B45.9
  bone B45.3
  cerebral B45.1
  cutaneous B45.2
  disseminated B45.7
  generalized B45.7
  meningitis B45.1
  meningocerebralis B45.1
  osseous B45.3
  pulmonary B45.Ø
  skin B45.2
  specified NEC B45.8
Cryptopapillitis (anus) K62.89
Cryptophthalmos Q11.2
  syndrome Q87.Ø
Cryptorchid, cryptorchism, cryptorchidism Q53.9
  bilateral Q53.2Ø
    abdominal Q53.211
    perineal Q53.22
  unilateral Q53.1Ø
    abdominal Q53.111
    perineal Q53.12
Cryptosporidiosis AØ7.2
  hepatobiliary B88.8
  respiratory B88.8
Cryptostromosis J67.6
Crystalluria R82.998
Cubitus
  congenital Q68.8
  valgus (acquired) M21.Ø- ●
    congenital Q68.8
    sequelae (late effect) of rickets E64.3
  varus (acquired) M21.1- ●
    congenital Q68.8
    sequelae (late effect) of rickets E64.3
Cultural deprivation or shock Z6Ø.3
Curling esophagus K22.4
Curling's ulcer —*see* Ulcer, peptic, acute
Curschmann (-Batten) (-Steinert) disease or syndrome G71.11
Curse, Ondine's —*see* Apnea, sleep
Curvature
  organ or site, congenital NEC —*see* Distortion
  penis (lateral) Q55.61
  Pott's (spinal) A18.Ø1
  radius, idiopathic, progressive (congenital) Q74.Ø
  spine (acquired) (angular) (idiopathic) (incorrect) (postural) —*see* Dorsopathy, deforming
    congenital Q67.5
    due to or associated with
      Charcot-Marie-Tooth disease —*see also* subcategory M49.8 G6Ø.Ø
      osteitis
        deformans M88.88
        fibrosa cystica —*see also* subcategory M49.8 E21.Ø
      tuberculosis (Pott's curvature) A18.Ø1
    sequelae (late effect) of rickets E64.3
    tuberculous A18.Ø1
Cushingoid due to steroid therapy E24.2
  correct substance properly administered —*see* Table of Drugs and Chemicals, by drug, adverse effect
  overdose or wrong substance given or taken —*see* Table of Drugs and Chemicals, by drug, poisoning
Cushing's
  syndrome or disease E24.9
    drug-induced E24.2
    iatrogenic E24.2
    pituitary-dependent E24.Ø
    specified NEC E24.8
  ulcer —*see* Ulcer, peptic, acute
Cusp, Carabelli - omit code
Cut (external) —*see also* Laceration
  muscle —*see* Injury, muscle
Cutaneous —*see also* condition
  hemorrhage R23.3
  larva migrans B76.9
Cutis —*see also* condition
  hyperelastica Q82.8
    acquired L57.4
  laxa (hyperelastica) —*see* Dermatolysis
  marmorata R23.8
  osteosis L94.2
  pendula —*see* Dermatolysis
  rhomboidalis nuchae L57.2
  verticis gyrata Q82.8
    acquired L91.8
Cyanosis R23.Ø
  due to
    patent foramen botalli Q21.1
    persistent foramen ovale Q21.1
  enterogenous D74.8
  paroxysmal digital —*see* Raynaud's disease
    with gangrene I73.Ø1
  retina, retinal H35.89
Cyanotic heart disease I24.9
  congenital Q24.9
Cycle
  anovulatory N97.Ø
  menstrual, irregular N92.6
Cyclencephaly QØ4.9
Cyclical vomiting, in migraine (*see also* Vomiting, cyclical) G43.AØ
  psychogenic F5Ø.89

C

New   Revised   ~~deleted~~ Deleted   ● Use Additional Character(s)

Cyclitis —*see also* Iridocyclitis H2Ø.9
  chronic —*see* Iridocyclitis, chronic
  Fuchs' heterochromic H2Ø.81-●
  granulomatous —*see* Iridocyclitis, chronic
  lens-induced —*see* Iridocyclitis, lens-induced
  posterior H3Ø.2-●
Cycloid personality F34.Ø
Cyclophoria H5Ø.54
Cyclopia, cyclops Q87.Ø
Cyclopism Q87.Ø
Cyclosporiasis AØ7.4
Cyclothymia F34.Ø
Cyclothymic personality F34.Ø
Cyclotropia H5Ø.41-●
Cylindroma —*see also* Neoplasm, malignant, by site
  eccrine dermal —*see* Neoplasm, skin, benign
  skin —*see* Neoplasm, skin, benign
Cylindruria R82.998
Cynanche
  diphtheritic A36.2
  tonsillaris J36
Cynophobia F4Ø.218
Cynorexia R63.2
Cyphosis —*see* Kyphosis
Cyprus fever —*see* Brucellosis
Cyst (colloid) (mucous) (simple) (retention)
  adenoid (infected) J35.8
  adrenal gland E27.8
    congenital Q89.1
  air, lung J98.4
  allantoic Q64.4
  alveolar process (jaw bone) M27.4Ø
  amnion, amniotic O41.8X-●
  aneurysmal M27.49
  anterior
    chamber (eye) —*see* Cyst, iris
    nasopalatine KØ9.1
  antrum J34.1
  anus K62.89
  apical (tooth) (periodontal) KØ4.8
  appendix K38.8
  arachnoid, brain (acquired) G93.Ø
    congenital QØ4.6
  arytenoid J38.7
  Baker's M71.2-●
    ruptured M66.Ø
    tuberculous A18.Ø2
  Bartholin's gland N75.Ø
  bile duct (common) (hepatic) K83.5
  bladder (multiple) (trigone) N32.89
  blue dome (breast) —*see* Cyst, breast
  bone (local) NEC M85.6Ø
    aneurysmal M85.5Ø
      ankle M85.57-●
      foot M85.57-●
      forearm M85.53-●
      hand M85.54-●
      jaw M27.49
      lower leg M85.56-●
      multiple site M85.59
      neck M85.58
      rib M85.58
      shoulder M85.51-●
      skull M85.58
      specified site NEC M85.58
      thigh M85.55-●
      toe M85.57-●
      upper arm M85.52-●
      vertebra M85.58
    solitary M85.4Ø
      ankle M85.47-●
      fibula M85.46-●
      foot M85.47-●
      hand M85.44-●
      humerus M85.42-●
      jaw M27.49
      neck M85.48
      pelvis M85.45-●

Cyst *(Continued)*
  bone NEC *(Continued)*
    solitary *(Continued)*
      radius M85.43-●
      rib M85.48
      shoulder M85.41-●
      skull M85.48
      specified site NEC M85.48
      tibia M85.46-●
      toe M85.47-●
      ulna M85.43-●
      vertebra M85.48
    specified type NEC M85.6Ø
      ankle M85.67-●
      foot M85.67-●
      forearm M85.63-●
      hand M85.64-●
      jaw M27.4Ø
        developmental (nonodontogenic) KØ9.1
          odontogenic KØ9.Ø
        latent M27.Ø
      lower leg M85.66-●
      multiple site M85.69
      neck M85.68
      rib M85.68
      shoulder M85.61-●
      skull M85.68
      specified site NEC M85.68
      thigh M85.65-●
      toe M85.67-●
      upper arm M85.62-●
      vertebra M85.68
  brain (acquired) G93.Ø
    congenital QØ4.6
    hydatid B67.99 *[G94]*
    third ventricle (colloid), congenital QØ4.6
  branchial (cleft) Q18.Ø
  branchiogenic Q18.Ø
  breast (benign) (blue dome) (pedunculated) (solitary) N6Ø.Ø-●
    involution —*see* Dysplasia, mammary, specified type NEC
    sebaceous —*see* Dysplasia, mammary, specified type NEC
  broad ligament (benign) N83.8
  bronchogenic (mediastinal) (sequestration) J98.4
    congenital Q33.Ø
  buccal KØ9.8
  bulbourethral gland N36.8
  bursa, bursal NEC M71.3Ø
    with rupture —*see* Rupture, synovium
    ankle M71.37-●
    elbow M71.32-●
    foot M71.37-●
    hand M71.34-●
    hip M71.35-●
    multiple sites M71.39
    pharyngeal J39.2
    popliteal space —*see* Cyst, Baker's
    shoulder M71.31-●
    specified site NEC M71.38
    wrist M71.33-●
  calcifying odontogenic D16.5
    upper jaw (bone) (maxilla) D16.4
  canal of Nuck (female) N94.89
    congenital Q52.4
  canthus —*see* Cyst, conjunctiva
  carcinomatous —*see* Neoplasm, malignant, by site
  cauda equina G95.89
  cavum septi pellucidi —*see* Cyst, brain
  celomic (pericardium) Q24.8
  cerebellopontine (angle) —*see* Cyst, brain
  cerebellum —*see* Cyst, brain
  cerebral —*see* Cyst, brain
  cervical lateral Q18.Ø
  cervix NEC N88.8
    embryonic Q51.6
    nabothian N88.8

Cyst *(Continued)*
  chiasmal optic NEC —*see* Disorder, optic, chiasm
  chocolate (ovary) N8Ø.1
  choledochus, congenital Q44.4
  chorion O41.8X-●
  choroid plexus G93.Ø
    ▶congenital QØ4.6
  ciliary body —*see* Cyst, iris
  clitoris N9Ø.7
  colon K63.89
  common (bile) duct K83.5
  congenital NEC Q89.8
    adrenal gland Q89.1
    epiglottis Q31.8
    esophagus Q39.8
    fallopian tube Q5Ø.4
    kidney Q61.ØØ
      more than one (multiple) Q61.Ø2
        specified as polycystic Q61.3
          adult type Q61.2
          infantile type NEC Q61.19
            collecting duct dilation Q61.11
      solitary Q61.Ø1
    larynx Q31.8
    liver Q44.6
    lung Q33.Ø
    mediastinum Q34.1
    ovary Q5Ø.1
    oviduct Q5Ø.4
    periurethral (tissue) Q64.79
    prepuce Q55.69
    salivary gland (any) Q38.4
    sublingual Q38.6
    submaxillary gland Q38.6
    thymus (gland) Q89.2
    tongue Q38.3
    ureterovesical orifice Q62.8
    vulva Q52.79
  conjunctiva H11.44-●
  cornea H18.89-●
  corpora quadrigemina G93.Ø
  corpus
    albicans N83.29-●
    luteum (hemorrhagic) (ruptured) N83.1-●
  Cowper's gland (benign) (infected) N36.8
  cranial meninges G93.Ø
  craniobuccal pouch E23.6
  craniopharyngeal pouch E23.6
  cystic duct K82.8
  Cysticercus —*see* Cysticercosis
  Dandy-Walker QØ3.1
    with spina bifida —*see* Spina bifida
  dental (root) KØ4.8
    developmental KØ9.Ø
    eruption KØ9.Ø
    primordial KØ9.Ø
  dentigerous (mandible) (maxilla) KØ9.Ø
  dermoid —*see* Neoplasm, benign, by site
    with malignant transformation C56.-●
    implantation
      external area or site (skin) NEC L72.Ø
      iris —*see* Cyst, iris, implantation
      vagina N89.8
      vulva N9Ø.7
    mouth KØ9.8
    oral soft tissue KØ9.8
    sacrococcygeal —*see* Cyst, pilonidal
  developmental KØ9.1
    odontogenic KØ9.Ø
    oral region (nonodontogenic) KØ9.1
    ovary, ovarian Q5Ø.1
  dura (cerebral) G93.Ø
    spinal G96.19
  ear (external) Q18.1
  echinococcal —*see* Echinococcus
  embryonic
    cervix uteri Q51.6
    fallopian tube Q5Ø.4
    vagina Q52.4
  endometrium, endometrial (uterus) N85.8
    ectopic —*see* Endometriosis

C

Cyst *(Continued)*
  enterogenous Q43.8
  epidermal, epidermoid (inclusion) (*see also* Cyst, skin) L72.Ø
    mouth KØ9.8
    oral soft tissue KØ9.8
  epididymis N5Ø.3
  epiglottis J38.7
  epiphysis cerebri E34.8
  epithelial (inclusion) L72.Ø
  epoophoron Q5Ø.5
  eruption KØ9.Ø
  esophagus K22.8
  ethmoid sinus J34.1
  external female genital organs NEC N9Ø.7
  eye NEC H57.89
    congenital Q15.8
  eyelid (sebaceous) HØ2.829
    infected —*see* Hordeolum
    left HØ2.826
      lower HØ2.825
      upper HØ2.824
    right HØ2.823
      lower HØ2.822
      upper HØ2.821
  fallopian tube N83.8
    congenital Q5Ø.4
  fimbrial (twisted) Q5Ø.4
  fissural (oral region) KØ9.1
  follicle (graafian) (hemorrhagic) N83.Ø- •
    nabothian N88.8
  follicular (atretic) (hemorrhagic) (ovarian) N83.Ø- •
    dentigerous KØ9.Ø
    odontogenic KØ9.Ø
    skin L72.9
      specified NEC L72.8
  frontal sinus J34.1
  gallbladder K82.8
  ganglion —*see* Ganglion
  Gartner's duct Q52.4
  gingiva KØ9.Ø
  gland of Moll —*see* Cyst, eyelid
  globulomaxillary KØ9.1
  graafian follicle (hemorrhagic) N83.Ø- •
  granulosal lutein (hemorrhagic) N83.1- •
  hemangiomatous D18.ØØ
    intra-abdominal D18.Ø3
    intracranial D18.Ø2
    skin D18.Ø1
    specified site NEC D18.Ø9
  hemorrhagic M27.49
  hydatid —*see also* Echinococcus B67.9Ø
    brain B67.99 *[G94]*
    liver —*see also* Cyst, liver, hydatid B67.8
    lung NEC B67.99 *[J99]*
    Morgagni
      female Q5Ø.5
      male (epididymal) Q55.4
        testicular Q55.29
    specified site NEC B67.99
  hymen N89.8
    embryonic Q52.4
  hypopharynx J39.2
  hypophysis, hypophyseal (duct) (recurrent) E23.6
    cerebri E23.6
  implantation (dermoid)
    external area or site (skin) NEC L72.Ø
    iris —*see* Cyst, iris, implantation
    vagina N89.8
    vulva N9Ø.7
  incisive canal KØ9.1
  inclusion (epidermal) (epithelial) (epidermoid) (squamous) L72.Ø
    not of skin - code under Cyst, by site
  intestine (large) (small) K63.89
  intracranial —*see* Cyst, brain
  intraligamentous —*see also* Disorder, ligament
    knee —*see* Derangement, knee

Cyst *(Continued)*
  intrasellar E23.6
  iris H21.3Ø9
    exudative H21.31- •
    idiopathic H21.3Ø- •
    implantation H21.32- •
    parasitic H21.33- •
    pars plana (primary) H21.34- •
      exudative H21.35- •
  jaw (bone) M27.4Ø
    aneurysmal M27.49
    developmental (odontogenic) KØ9.Ø
    fissural KØ9.1
    hemorrhagic M27.49
    traumatic M27.49
  joint NEC —*see* Disorder, joint, specified type NEC
  kidney (acquired) N28.1
    calyceal —*see* Hydronephrosis
    congenital Q61.ØØ
    more than one (multiple) Q61.Ø2
      specified as polycystic Q61.3
        adult type (autosomal dominant) Q61.2
        infantile type (autosomal recessive) NEC Q61.19
          collecting duct dilation Q61.11
    pyelogenic —*see* Hydronephrosis
    simple N28.1
    solitary (single) Q61.Ø1
      acquired N28.1
  labium (majus) (minus) N9Ø.7
    sebaceous N9Ø.7
  lacrimal —*see also* Disorder, lacrimal system, specified NEC
    gland HØ4.13- •
    passages or sac —*see* Disorder, lacrimal system, specified NEC
  larynx J38.7
  lateral periodontal KØ9.Ø
  lens H27.8
    congenital Q12.8
  lip (gland) K13.Ø
  liver (idiopathic) (simple) K76.89
    congenital Q44.6
    hydatid B67.8
      granulosus B67.Ø
      multilocularis B67.5
  lung J98.4
    congenital Q33.Ø
    giant bullous J43.9
  lutein N83.1- •
  lymphangiomatous D18.1
  lymphoepithelial, oral soft tissue KØ9.8
  macula —*see* Degeneration, macula, hole
  malignant —*see* Neoplasm, malignant, by site
  mammary gland —*see* Cyst, breast
  mandible M27.4Ø
    dentigerous KØ9.Ø
    radicular KØ4.8
  maxilla M27.4Ø
    dentigerous KØ9.Ø
    radicular KØ4.8
  medial, face and neck Q18.8
  median
    anterior maxillary KØ9.1
    palatal KØ9.1
  mediastinum, congenital Q34.1
  meibomian (gland) —*see* Chalazion
    infected —*see* Hordeolum
  membrane, brain G93.Ø
  meninges (cerebral) G93.Ø
    spinal G96.19
  meniscus, knee —*see* Derangement, knee, meniscus, cystic
  mesentery, mesenteric K66.8
    chyle I89.8
  mesonephric duct
    female Q5Ø.5
    male Q55.4
  milk N64.89

Cyst *(Continued)*
  Morgagni (hydatid)
    female Q5Ø.5
    male (epididymal) Q55.4
      testicular Q55.29
  mouth KØ9.8
  Müllerian duct Q5Ø.4
    appendix testis Q55.29
    cervix Q51.6
    fallopian tube Q5Ø.4
    female Q5Ø.4
    male Q55.29
    prostatic utricle Q55.4
    vagina (embryonal) Q52.4
  multilocular (ovary) D39.1Ø
    benign —*see* Neoplasm, benign, by site
  myometrium N85.8
  nabothian (follicle) (ruptured) N88.8
  nasoalveolar KØ9.1
  nasolabial KØ9.1
  nasopalatine (anterior) (duct) KØ9.1
  nasopharynx J39.2
  neoplastic —*see* Neoplasm, uncertain behavior, by site
    benign —*see* Neoplasm, benign, by site
  nervous system NEC G96.8
  neuroenteric (congenital) QØ6.8
  nipple —*see* Cyst, breast
  nose (turbinates) J34.1
    sinus J34.1
  odontogenic, developmental KØ9.Ø
  omentum (lesser) K66.8
    congenital Q45.8
  ora serrata —*see* Cyst, retina, ora serrata
  oral
    region KØ9.9
      developmental (nonodontogenic) KØ9.1
      specified NEC KØ9.8
    soft tissue KØ9.9
      specified NEC KØ9.8
  orbit HØ5.81- •
  ovary, ovarian (twisted) N83.2Ø- •
    adherent N83.2Ø- •
    chocolate N8Ø.1
    corpus
      albicans N83.29- •
      luteum (hemorrhagic) N83.1- •
    dermoid D27.9
    developmental Q5Ø.1
    due to failure of involution NEC N83.2Ø- •
    endometrial N8Ø.1
    follicular (graafian) (hemorrhagic) N83.Ø- •
    hemorrhagic N83.2Ø- •
    in pregnancy or childbirth O34.8- •
      with obstructed labor O65.5
    multilocular D39.1Ø
    pseudomucinous D27.9
    retention N83.29- •
    serous N83.2Ø- •
    specified NEC N83.29- •
    theca lutein (hemorrhagic) N83.1- •
    tuberculous A18.18
  oviduct N83.8
  palate (median) (fissural) KØ9.1
  palatine papilla (jaw) KØ9.1
  pancreas, pancreatic (hemorrhagic) (true) K86.2
    congenital Q45.2
    false K86.3
  paralabral
    hip M24.85- •
    shoulder S43.43- •
  paramesonephric duct Q5Ø.4
    female Q5Ø.4
    male Q55.29
  paranephric N28.1
  paraphysis, cerebri, congenital QØ4.6
  parasitic B89
  parathyroid (gland) E21.4
  paratubal N83.8
  paraurethral duct N36.8
  paroophoron Q5Ø.5

Cyst *(Continued)*
parotid gland K11.6
parovarian Q5Ø.5
pelvis, female N94.89
in pregnancy or childbirth O34.8- ●
causing obstructed labor O65.5
penis (sebaceous) N48.89
periapical KØ4.8
pericardial (congenital) Q24.8
acquired (secondary) I31.8
pericoronal KØ9.Ø
periodontal KØ4.8
lateral KØ9.Ø
peripelvic (lymphatic) N28.1
peritoneum K66.8
chylous I89.8
periventricular, acquired, newborn P91.1
pharynx (wall) J39.2
pilar L72.11
pilonidal (infected) (rectum) LØ5.91
with abscess LØ5.Ø1
malignant C44.59- ●
pituitary (duct) (gland) E23.6
placenta O43.19- ●
pleura J94.8
popliteal —*see* Cyst, Baker's
porencephalic QØ4.6
acquired G93.Ø
postanal (infected) —*see* Cyst, pilonidal
postmastoidectomy cavity (mucosal) —*see* Complications, postmastoidectomy, cyst
preauricular Q18.1
prepuce N47.4
congenital Q55.69
primordial (jaw) KØ9.Ø
prostate N42.83
pseudomucinous (ovary) D27.9
pupillary, miotic H21.27- ●
radicular (residual) KØ4.8
radiculodental KØ4.8
ranular K11.8
Rathke's pouch E23.6
rectum (epithelium) (mucous) K62.89
renal —*see* Cyst, kidney
residual (radicular) KØ4.8
retention (ovary) N83.29- ●
salivary gland K11.6
retina H33.19- ●
ora serrata H33.11- ●
parasitic H33.12- ●
retroperitoneal K68.9
sacrococcygeal (dermoid) —*see* Cyst, pilonidal
salivary gland or duct (mucous extravasation or retention) K11.6
Sampson's N8Ø.1
sclera H15.89
scrotum L72.9
sebaceous L72.3
sebaceous (duct) (gland) L72.3
breast —*see* Dysplasia, mammary, specified type NEC
eyelid —*see* Cyst, eyelid
genital organ NEC
female N94.89
male N5Ø.89
scrotum L72.3
semilunar cartilage (knee) (multiple) —*see* Derangement, knee, meniscus, cystic
seminal vesicle N5Ø.89
serous (ovary) N83.2Ø- ●
sinus (accessory) (nasal) J34.1
Skene's gland N36.8
skin L72.9
breast —*see* Dysplasia, mammary, specified type NEC
epidermal, epidermoid L72.Ø
epithelial L72.Ø
eyelid —*see* Cyst, eyelid
genital organ NEC
female N9Ø.7
male N5Ø.89

Cyst *(Continued)*
skin *(Continued)*
inclusion L72.Ø
scrotum L72.9
sebaceous L72.3
sweat gland or duct L74.8
solitary
bone —*see* Cyst, bone, solitary
jaw M27.4Ø
kidney N28.1
spermatic cord N5Ø.89
sphenoid sinus J34.1
spinal meninges G96.19
spleen NEC D73.4
congenital Q89.Ø9
hydatid —*see also* Echinococcus B67.99 *[D77]*
Stafne's M27.Ø
subarachnoid intrasellar R93.Ø
subcutaneous, pheomycotic (chromomycotic) B43.2
subdural (cerebral) G93.Ø
spinal cord G96.19
sublingual gland K11.6
submandibular gland K11.6
submaxillary gland K11.6
suburethral N36.8
suprarenal gland E27.8
suprasellar —*see* Cyst, brain
sweat gland or duct L74.8
synovial —*see also* Cyst, bursa
ruptured —*see* Rupture, synovium
tarsal —*see* Chalazion
tendon (sheath) —*see* Disorder, tendon, specified type NEC
testis N44.2
tunica albuginea N44.1
theca lutein (ovary) N83.1- ●
Thornwaldt's J39.2
thymus (gland) E32.8
thyroglossal duct (infected) (persistent) Q89.2
thyroid (gland) EØ4.1
thyrolingual duct (infected) (persistent) Q89.2
tongue K14.8
tonsil J35.8
tooth —*see* Cyst, dental
Tornwaldt's J39.2
trichilemmal (proliferating) L72.12
trichodermal L72.12
tubal (fallopian) N83.8
inflammatory —*see* Salpingitis, chronic
tubo-ovarian N83.8
inflammatory N7Ø.13
tunica
albuginea testis N44.1
vaginalis N5Ø.89
turbinate (nose) J34.1
Tyson's gland N48.89
urachus, congenital Q64.4
ureter N28.89
ureterovesical orifice N28.89
urethra, urethral (gland) N36.8
uterine ligament N83.8
uterus (body) (corpus) (recurrent) N85.8
embryonic Q51.818
cervix Q51.6
vagina, vaginal (implantation) (inclusion) (squamous cell) (wall) N89.8
embryonic Q52.4
vallecula, vallecular (epiglottis) J38.7
vesical (orifice) N32.89
vitreous body H43.89
vulva (implantation) (inclusion) N9Ø.7
congenital Q52.79
sebaceous gland N9Ø.7
vulvovaginal gland N9Ø.7
wolffian
female Q5Ø.5
male Q55.4

Cystadenocarcinoma —*see* Neoplasm, malignant, by site
bile duct C22.1
endometrioid —*see* Neoplasm, malignant, by site
specified site —*see* Neoplasm, malignant, by site
unspecified site
female C56.9
male C61
mucinous
papillary
specified site —*see* Neoplasm, malignant, by site
unspecified site C56.9
specified site —*see* Neoplasm, malignant, by site
unspecified site C56.9
papillary
mucinous
specified site —*see* Neoplasm, malignant, by site
unspecified site C56.9
pseudomucinous
specified site —*see* Neoplasm, malignant, by site
unspecified site C56.9
serous
specified site —*see* Neoplasm, malignant, by site
unspecified site C56.9
specified site —*see* Neoplasm, malignant, by site
unspecified site C56.9
pseudomucinous
papillary
specified site —*see* Neoplasm, malignant, by site
unspecified site C56.9
specified site —*see* Neoplasm, malignant, by site
unspecified site C56.9
serous
papillary
specified site —*see* Neoplasm, malignant, by site
unspecified site C56.9
specified site —*see* Neoplasm, malignant, by site
unspecified site C56.9
Cystadenofibroma
clear cell —*see* Neoplasm, benign, by site
endometrioid D27.9
borderline malignancy D39.1- ●
malignant C56.- ●
mucinous
specified site —*see* Neoplasm, benign, by site
unspecified site D27.9
serous
specified site —*see* Neoplasm, benign, by site
unspecified site D27.9
specified site —*see* Neoplasm, benign, by site
unspecified site D27.9
Cystadenoma —*see also* Neoplasm, benign, by site
bile duct D13.4
endometrioid —*see* Neoplasm, benign, by site
borderline malignancy —*see* Neoplasm, uncertain behavior, by site
malignant —*see* Neoplasm, malignant, by site
mucinous
borderline malignancy
ovary C56.- ●
specified site NEC —*see* Neoplasm, uncertain behavior, by site
unspecified site C56.9
papillary
borderline malignancy
ovary C56.- ●
specified site NEC —*see* Neoplasm, uncertain behavior, by site
unspecified site C56.9

- **Cystadenoma** *(Continued)*
  - mucinous *(Continued)*
    - papillary *(Continued)*
      - specified site —*see* Neoplasm, benign, by site
      - unspecified site D27.9
    - specified site —*see* Neoplasm, benign, by site
    - unspecified site D27.9
  - papillary
    - borderline malignancy
      - ovary C56-●
      - specified site NEC —*see* Neoplasm, uncertain behavior, by site
      - unspecified site C56.9
    - lymphomatosum
      - specified site —*see* Neoplasm, benign, by site
      - unspecified site D11.9
    - mucinous
      - borderline malignancy
        - ovary C56.-●
        - specified site NEC —*see* Neoplasm, uncertain behavior, by site
        - unspecified site C56.9
      - specified site —*see* Neoplasm, benign, by site
      - unspecified site D27.9
    - pseudomucinous
      - borderline malignancy
        - ovary C56.-●
        - specified site NEC —*see* Neoplasm, uncertain behavior, by site
        - unspecified site C56.9
      - specified site —*see* Neoplasm, benign, by site
      - unspecified site D27.9
    - serous
      - borderline malignancy
        - ovary C56.-●
        - specified site NEC —*see* Neoplasm, uncertain behavior, by site
        - unspecified site C56.9
      - specified site —*see* Neoplasm, benign, by site
      - unspecified site D27.9
    - specified site —*see* Neoplasm, benign, by site
    - unspecified site D27.9
  - pseudomucinous
    - borderline malignancy
      - ovary C56.-●
      - specified site NEC —*see* Neoplasm, uncertain behavior, by site
      - unspecified site C56.9
    - papillary
      - borderline malignancy
        - ovary C56.-●
        - specified site NEC —*see* Neoplasm, uncertain behavior, by site
        - unspecified site C56.9
      - specified site —*see* Neoplasm, benign, by site
      - unspecified site D27.9
    - specified site —*see* Neoplasm, benign, by site
    - unspecified site D27.9
  - serous
    - borderline malignancy
      - ovary C56.-●
      - specified site NEC —*see* Neoplasm, uncertain behavior, by site
      - unspecified site C56.9
    - papillary
      - borderline malignancy
        - ovary C56.-●
        - specified site NEC —*see* Neoplasm, uncertain behavior, by site
        - unspecified site C56.9
      - specified site —*see* Neoplasm, benign, by site
      - unspecified site D27.9
    - specified site —*see* Neoplasm, benign, by site
    - unspecified site D27.9
- **Cystathionine synthase deficiency** E72.11
- **Cystathioninemia** E72.19
- **Cystathioninuria** E72.19
- **Cystic** —*see also* condition
  - breast (chronic) —*see* Mastopathy, cystic
  - corpora lutea (hemorrhagic) N83.1-●
  - duct —*see* condition
  - eyeball (congenital) Q11.0
  - fibrosis —*see* Fibrosis, cystic
  - kidney (congenital) Q61.9
    - adult type Q61.2
    - infantile type NEC Q61.19
      - collecting duct dilatation Q61.11
    - medullary Q61.5
  - liver, congenital Q44.6
  - lung disease J98.4
    - congenital Q33.0
  - mastitis, chronic —*see* Mastopathy, cystic
  - medullary, kidney Q61.5
  - meniscus —*see* Derangement, knee, meniscus, cystic
  - ovary N83.20-●
- **Cysticercosis, cysticerciasis** B69.9
  - with
    - epileptiform fits B69.0
    - myositis B69.81
  - brain B69.0
  - central nervous system B69.0
  - cerebral B69.0
  - ocular B69.1
  - specified NEC B69.89
- **Cysticercus cellulose infestation** —*see* Cysticercosis
- **Cystinosis** (malignant) E72.04
- **Cystinuria** E72.01
- **Cystitis** (exudative) (hemorrhagic) (septic) (suppurative) N30.90
  - with
    - fibrosis —*see* Cystitis, chronic, interstitial
    - hematuria N30.91
    - leukoplakia —*see* Cystitis, chronic, interstitial
    - malakoplakia —*see* Cystitis, chronic, interstitial
    - metaplasia —*see* Cystitis, chronic, interstitial
    - prostatitis N41.3
  - acute N30.00
    - with hematuria N30.01
    - of trigone N30.30
      - with hematuria N30.31
  - allergic —*see* Cystitis, specified type NEC
  - amebic A06.81
  - bilharzial B65.9 *[N33]*
  - blennorrhagic (gonococcal) A54.01
  - bullous —*see* Cystitis, specified type NEC
  - calculous N21.0
  - chlamydial A56.01
  - chronic N30.20
    - with hematuria N30.21
    - interstitial N30.10
      - with hematuria N30.11
    - of trigone N30.30
      - with hematuria N30.31
    - specified NEC N30.20
      - with hematuria N30.21
  - cystic (a) —*see* Cystitis, specified type NEC
  - diphtheritic A36.85
  - echinococcal
    - granulosus B67.39
    - multilocularis B67.69
  - emphysematous —*see* Cystitis, specified type NEC
  - encysted —*see* Cystitis, specified type NEC
  - eosinophilic —*see* Cystitis, specified type NEC
  - follicular —*see* Cystitis, of trigone
  - gangrenous —*see* Cystitis, specified type NEC
  - glandularis —*see* Cystitis, specified type NEC
- **Cystitis** *(Continued)*
  - gonococcal A54.01
  - incrusted —*see* Cystitis, specified type NEC
  - interstitial (chronic) —*see* Cystitis, chronic, interstitial
  - irradiation N30.40
    - with hematuria N30.41
  - irritation —*see* Cystitis, specified type NEC
  - malignant —*see* Cystitis, specified type NEC
  - of trigone N30.30
    - with hematuria N30.31
  - panmural —*see* Cystitis, chronic, interstitial
  - polyposa —*see* Cystitis, specified type NEC
  - prostatic N41.3
  - puerperal (postpartum) O86.22
  - radiation —*see* Cystitis, irradiation
  - specified type NEC N30.80
    - with hematuria N30.81
  - subacute —*see* Cystitis, chronic
  - submucous —*see* Cystitis, chronic, interstitial
  - syphilitic (late) A52.76
  - trichomonal A59.03
  - tuberculous A18.12
  - ulcerative —*see* Cystitis, chronic, interstitial
- **Cystocele** (-urethrocele)
  - female N81.10
    - with prolapse of uterus —*see* Prolapse, uterus
    - lateral N81.12
    - midline N81.11
    - paravaginal N81.12
  - in pregnancy or childbirth O34.8-●
    - causing obstructed labor O65.5
  - male N32.89
- **Cystolithiasis** N21.0
- **Cystoma** —*see also* Neoplasm, benign, by site
  - endometrial, ovary N80.1
  - mucinous
    - specified site —*see* Neoplasm, benign, by site
    - unspecified site D27.9
  - serous
    - specified site —*see* Neoplasm, benign, by site
    - unspecified site D27.9
  - simple (ovary) N83.29-●
- **Cystoplegia** N31.2
- **Cystoptosis** N32.89
- **Cystopyelitis** —*see* Pyelonephritis
- **Cystorrhagia** N32.89
- **Cystosarcoma phyllodes** D48.6-●
  - benign D24-●
  - malignant —*see* Neoplasm, breast, malignant
- **Cystostomy**
  - attention to Z43.5
  - complication —*see* Complications, cystostomy
  - status Z93.50
    - appendico-vesicostomy Z93.52
    - cutaneous Z93.51
    - specified NEC Z93.59
- **Cystourethritis** —*see* Urethritis
- **Cystourethrocele** —*see also* Cystocele
  - female N81.10
    - with uterine prolapse —*see* Prolapse, uterus
    - lateral N81.12
    - midline N81.11
    - paravaginal N81.12
  - male N32.89
- **Cytomegalic inclusion disease**
  - congenital P35.1
- **Cytomegalovirus infection** B25.9
- **Cytomycosis** (reticuloendothelial) B39.4
- **Cytopenia** D75.9
  - refractory
    - with multilineage dysplasia D46.A
      - and ring sideroblasts (RCMD RS) D46.B
- **Czerny's disease** (periodic hydrarthrosis of the knee) —*see* Effusion, joint, knee

C

D

- **Daae** (-Finsen) disease (epidemic pleurodynia) B33.Ø
- **Dabney's grip** B33.Ø
- **Da Costa's syndrome** F45.8
- **Dacryoadenitis, dacryadenitis** HØ4.ØØ-●
  - acute HØ4.Ø1-●
  - chronic HØ4.Ø2-●
- **Dacryocystitis** HØ4.3Ø-●
  - acute HØ4.32-●
  - chronic HØ4.41-●
  - neonatal P39.1
  - phlegmonous HØ4.31-●
  - syphilitic A52.71
    - congenital (early) A5Ø.Ø1
  - trachomatous, active A71.1
    - sequelae (late effect) B94.Ø
- **Dacryocystoblenorrhea** —*see* Inflammation, lacrimal, passages, chronic
- **Dacryocystocele** —*see* Disorder, lacrimal system, changes
- **Dacryolith, dacryolithiasis** HØ4.51-●
- **Dacryoma** —*see* Disorder, lacrimal system, changes
- **Dacryopericystitis** —*see* Dacryocystitis
- **Dacryops** HØ4.11-●
- **Dacryostenosis** —*see also* Stenosis, lacrimal
  - congenital Q1Ø.5
- **Dactylitis**
  - bone —*see* Osteomyelitis
  - sickle-cell D57.ØØ
    - Hb C D57.219
    - Hb SS D57.ØØ
    - specified NEC D57.819
  - skin LØ8.9
  - syphilitic A52.77
  - tuberculous A18.Ø3
- **Dactylolysis spontanea** (ainhum) L94.6
- **Dactylosymphysis** Q7Ø.9
  - fingers —*see* Syndactylism, complex, fingers
  - toes —*see* Syndactylism, complex, toes
- **Damage**
  - arteriosclerotic —*see* Arteriosclerosis
  - brain (nontraumatic) G93.9
    - anoxic, hypoxic G93.1
      - resulting from a procedure G97.82
    - child NEC G8Ø.9
    - due to birth injury P11.2
  - cardiorenal (vascular) —*see* Hypertension, cardiorenal
  - cerebral NEC —*see* Damage, brain
  - coccyx, complicating delivery O71.6
  - coronary —*see* Disease, heart, ischemic
  - ▶deep tissue, pressure-induced —*see also* L89 with final character .6
  - eye, birth injury P15.3
  - liver (nontraumatic) K76.9
    - alcoholic K7Ø.9
    - due to drugs —*see* Disease, liver, toxic
    - toxic —*see* Disease, liver, toxic
  - medication T88.7
  - pelvic
    - joint or ligament, during delivery O71.6
    - organ NEC
      - during delivery O71.5
      - following ectopic or molar pregnancy OØ8.6
  - renal —*see* Disease, renal
  - subendocardium, subendocardial —*see* Degeneration, myocardial
  - vascular I99.9
- **Dana-Putnam syndrome** (subacute combined sclerosis with pernicious anemia) —*see* Degeneration, combined
- **Danbolt** (-Cross) **syndrome** (acrodermatitis enteropathica) E83.2
- **Dandruff** L21.Ø
- **Dandy-Walker syndrome** QØ3.1
  - with spina bifida —*see* Spina bifida
- ➡**Danlos' syndrome** (see also Syndrome, Ehler-Danlos) Q79.6Ø
- **Darier** (-White) **disease** (congenital) Q82.8
  - meaning erythema annulare centrifugum L53.1
- **Darier-Roussy sarcoid** D86.3
- **Darling's disease or histoplasmosis** B39.4
- **Darwin's tubercle** Q17.8
- **Dawson's** (inclusion body) **encephalitis** A81.1
- **De Beurmann** (-Gougerot) **disease** B42.1
- **De la Tourette's syndrome** F95.2
- ➡**De Lange's syndrome** Q87.19
- **De Morgan's spots** (senile angiomas) I78.1
- **De Quervain's**
  - disease (tendon sheath) M65.4
  - syndrome E34.51
  - thyroiditis (subacute granulomatous thyroiditis) EØ6.1
- **De Toni-Fanconi** (-Debré) **syndrome** E72.Ø9
  - with cystinosis E72.Ø4
- **Dead**
  - fetus, retained (mother) O36.4
    - early pregnancy OØ2.1
  - labyrinth —*see* subcategory H83.2
  - ovum, retained OØ2.Ø
- **Deaf nonspeaking NEC** H91.3
- **Deafmutism** (acquired) (congenital) NEC H91.3
  - hysterical F44.6
  - syphilitic, congenital —*see also* subcategory H94.8 A5Ø.Ø9
- **Deafness** (acquired) (complete) (hereditary) (partial) H91.9-●
  - with blue sclera and fragility of bone Q78.Ø
  - auditory fatigue —*see* Deafness, specified type NEC
  - aviation T7Ø.Ø
    - nerve injury —*see* Injury, nerve, acoustic, specified type NEC
  - boilermaker's —*see* subcategory H83.3
  - central —*see* Deafness, sensorineural
  - conductive H9Ø.2
    - and sensorineural
      - mixed H9Ø.8
        - bilateral H9Ø.6
    - bilateral H9Ø.Ø
    - unilateral H9Ø.1-●
      - with restricted hearing on the contralateral side H9Ø.A-●
  - congenital H9Ø.5
    - with blue sclera and fragility of bone Q78.Ø
  - due to toxic agents —*see* Deafness, ototoxic
  - emotional (hysterical) F44.6
  - functional (hysterical) F44.6
  - high frequency H91.9-●
  - hysterical F44.6
  - low frequency H91.9-●
  - mental R48.8
  - mixed conductive and sensorineural H9Ø.8
    - bilateral H9Ø.6
    - unilateral H9Ø.7-●
  - nerve —*see* Deafness, sensorineural
  - neural —*see* Deafness, sensorineural
  - noise-induced —*see also* subcategory H83.3
    - nerve injury —*see* Injury, nerve, acoustic, specified type NEC
  - nonspeaking H91.3
  - ototoxic —*see* subcategory H91.Ø
  - perceptive —*see* Deafness, sensorineural
  - psychogenic (hysterical) F44.6
  - sensorineural H9Ø.5
    - and conductive
      - mixed H9Ø.8
        - bilateral H9Ø.6
    - bilateral H9Ø.3
    - unilateral H9Ø.4-●
      - with restricted hearing on the contralateral side H9Ø.A-●
  - sensory —*see* Deafness, sensorineural
  - specified type NEC —*see* subcategory H91.8
  - sudden (idiopathic) H91.2-●
  - syphilitic A52.15
  - transient ischemic H93.Ø1-●

Deafness *(Continued)*

  - traumatic —*see* Injury, nerve, acoustic, specified type NEC
  - word (developmental) H93.25
- **Death** (cause unknown) (of) (unexplained) (unspecified cause) R99
  - brain G93.82
  - cardiac (sudden) (with successful resuscitation) — code to underlying disease
    - family history of Z82.41
    - personal history of Z86.74
  - family member (assumed) Z63.4
- **Debility** (chronic) (general) (nervous) R53.81
  - congenital or neonatal NOS P96.9
  - nervous R53.81
  - old age R54
  - senile R54
- **Débove's disease** (splenomegaly) R16.1
- **Decalcification**
  - bone —*see* Osteoporosis
  - teeth KØ3.89
- **Decapsulation, kidney** N28.89
- **Decay**
  - dental —*see* Caries, dental
  - senile R54
  - tooth, teeth —*see* Caries, dental
- **Deciduitis** (acute)
  - following ectopic or molar pregnancy OØ8.Ø
- **Decline** (general) —*see* Debility
  - cognitive, age-associated R41.81
- **Decompensation**
  - cardiac (acute) (chronic) —*see* Disease, heart
  - cardiovascular —*see* Disease, cardiovascular
  - heart —*see* Disease, heart
  - hepatic —*see* Failure, hepatic
  - myocardial (acute) (chronic) —*see* Disease, heart
  - respiratory J98.8
- **Decompression sickness** T7Ø.3
- **Decrease** (d)
  - absolute neutrophile count —*see* Neutropenia
  - blood
    - platelets —*see* Thrombocytopenia
    - pressure RØ3.1
      - due to shock following
        - injury T79.4
        - operation T81.19
  - estrogen E28.39
    - postablative E89.4Ø
      - asymptomatic E89.4Ø
      - symptomatic E89.41
  - fragility of erythrocytes D58.8
  - function
    - lipase (pancreatic) K9Ø.3
    - ovary in hypopituitarism E23.Ø
    - parenchyma of pancreas K86.89
    - pituitary (gland) (anterior) (lobe) E23.Ø
      - posterior (lobe) E23.Ø
  - functional activity R68.89
  - glucose R73.Ø9
  - hematocrit R71.Ø
  - hemoglobin R71.Ø
  - leukocytes D72.819
    - specified NEC D72.818
  - libido R68.82
  - lymphocytes D72.81Ø
  - platelets D69.6
  - respiration, due to shock following injury T79.4
  - sexual desire R68.82
  - tear secretion NEC —*see* Syndrome, dry eye
  - tolerance
    - fat K9Ø.49
    - glucose R73.Ø9
    - pancreatic K9Ø.3
    - salt and water E87.8
  - vision NEC H54.7
  - white blood cell count D72.819
    - specified NEC D72.818
- **Decubitus** (ulcer) —*see* Ulcer, pressure, by site
  - cervix N86

Deepening acetabulum —*see* Derangement, joint, specified type NEC, hip
Defect, defective Q89.9
 3-beta-hydroxysteroid dehydrogenase E25.Ø
 11-hydroxylase E25.Ø
 21-hydroxylase E25.Ø
 abdominal wall, congenital Q79.59
 antibody immunodeficiency D8Ø.9
 aorticopulmonary septum Q21.4
 atrial septal (ostium secundum type) Q21.1
  following acute myocardial infarction (current complication) I23.1
  ostium primum type Q21.2
 atrioventricular
  canal Q21.2
  septum Q21.2
 auricular septal Q21.1
 bilirubin excretion NEC E8Ø.6
 biosynthesis, androgen (testicular) E29.1
 bulbar septum Q21.Ø
 catalase E8Ø.3
 cell membrane receptor complex (CR3) D71
 circulation I99.9
  congenital Q28.9
  newborn Q28.9
 coagulation (factor) —*see also* Deficiency, factor D68.9
  with
   ectopic pregnancy OØ8.1
   molar pregnancy OØ8.1
  acquired D68.4
  antepartum with hemorrhage —*see* Hemorrhage, antepartum, with coagulation defect
  due to
   liver disease D68.4
   vitamin K deficiency D68.4
  hereditary NEC D68.2
  intrapartum O67.Ø
  newborn, transient P61.6
  postpartum O99.13
   with hemorrhage O72.3
  specified type NEC D68.8
 complement system D84.1
 conduction (heart) I45.9
  bone —*see* Deafness, conductive
 congenital, organ or site not listed —*see* Anomaly, by site
 coronary sinus Q21.1
 cushion, endocardial Q21.2
 degradation, glycoprotein E77.1
 dental bridge, crown, fillings —*see* Defect, dental restoration
 dental restoration KØ8.5Ø
  specified NEC KØ8.59
 dentin (hereditary) KØØ.5
 Descemet's membrane, congenital Q13.89
 developmental —*see also* Anomaly
  cauda equina QØ6.3
 diaphragm
  with elevation, eventration or hernia —*see* Hernia, diaphragm
  congenital Q79.1
   with hernia Q79.Ø
   gross (with hernia) Q79.Ø
 ectodermal, congenital Q82.9
 Eisenmenger's Q21.8
 enzyme
  catalase E8Ø.3
  peroxidase E8Ø.3
 esophagus, congenital Q39.9
 extensor retinaculum M62.89
 fibrin polymerization D68.2
 filling
  bladder R93.41
  kidney R93.42- •
  renal pelvis R93.41
  stomach R93.3
  ureter R93.41
  urinary organs, specified NEC R93.49
 GABA (gamma aminobutyric acid) metabolic E72.81

Defect, defective *(Continued)*
 Gerbode Q21.Ø
 glycoprotein degradation E77.1
 Hageman (factor) D68.2
 hearing —*see* Deafness
 high grade F7Ø
 interatrial septal Q21.1
 interauricular septal Q21.1
 interventricular septal Q21.Ø
  with dextroposition of aorta, pulmonary stenosis and hypertrophy of right ventricle Q21.3
  in tetralogy of Fallot Q21.3
 learning (specific) —*see* Disorder, learning
 lymphocyte function antigen-1 (LFA-1) D84.Ø
 lysosomal enzyme, post-translational modification E77.Ø
 major osseous M89.7Ø
  ankle M89.77- •
  carpus M89.74- •
  clavicle M89.71- •
  femur M89.75- •
  fibula M89.76- •
  fingers M89.74- •
  foot M89.77- •
  forearm M89.73- •
  hand M89.74- •
  humerus M89.72- •
  lower leg M89.76- •
  metacarpus M89.74- •
  metatarsus M89.77- •
  multiple sites M89.79
  pelvic region M89.75- •
  pelvis M89.75- •
  radius M89.73- •
  scapula M89.71- •
  shoulder region M89.71- •
  specified NEC M89.78
  tarsus M89.77- •
  thigh M89.75- •
  tibia M89.76- •
  toes M89.77- •
  ulna M89.73- •
 mental —*see* Disability, intellectual
 modification, lysosomal enzymes, post-translational E77.Ø
 obstructive, congenital
  renal pelvis Q62.39
  ureter Q62.39
   atresia —*see* Atresia, ureter
   cecoureterocele Q62.32
   megaureter Q62.2
   orthotopic ureterocele Q62.31
 osseous, major M89.7Ø
  ankle M89.77- •
  carpus M89.74- •
  clavicle M89.71- •
  femur M89.75- •
  fibula M89.76- •
  fingers M89.74- •
  foot M89.77- •
  forearm M89.73- •
  hand M89.74- •
  humerus M89.72- •
  lower leg M89.76- •
  metacarpus M89.74- •
  metatarsus M89.77- •
  multiple sites M89.9
  pelvic region M89.75- •
  pelvis M89.75- •
  radius M89.73- •
  scapula M89.71- •
  shoulder region M89.71- •
  specified NEC M89.78
  tarsus M89.77- •
  thigh M89.75- •
  tibia M89.76- •
  toes M89.77- •
  ulna M89.73- •
 osteochondral NEC —*see also* Deformity M95.8- •

Defect, defective *(Continued)*
 ostium
  primum Q21.2
  secundum Q21.1
 peroxidase E8Ø.3
 placental blood supply —*see* Insufficiency, placental
 platelets, qualitative D69.1
  constitutional D68.Ø
 postural NEC, spine —*see* Dorsopathy, deforming
 reduction
  limb Q73.8
   lower Q72.9- •
    absence —*see* Agenesis, leg
     foot —*see* Agenesis, foot
    longitudinal
     femur Q72.4- •
     fibula Q72.6- •
     tibia Q72.5- •
    specified type NEC Q72.89- •
    split foot Q72.7- •
   specified type NEC Q73.8
   upper Q71.9- •
    absence —*see* Agenesis, arm
     forearm —*see* Agenesis, forearm
     hand —*see* Agenesis, hand
    lobster-claw hand Q71.6- •
    longitudinal
     radius Q71.4- •
     ulna Q71.5- •
    specified type NEC Q71.89- •
 renal pelvis Q63.8
  obstructive Q62.39
 respiratory system, congenital Q34.9
 restoration, dental KØ8.5Ø
  specified NEC KØ8.59
 retinal nerve bundle fibers H35.89
 septal (heart) NOS Q21.9
  acquired (atrial) (auricular) (ventricular) (old) I51.Ø
  atrial Q21.1
   concurrent with acute myocardial infarction —*see* Infarct, myocardium
   following acute myocardial infarction (current complication) I23.1
  ventricular —*see also* Defect, ventricular septal Q21.Ø
 sinus venosus Q21.1
 speech R47.9
  developmental F8Ø.9
  specified NEC R47.89
 Taussig-Bing (aortic transposition and overriding pulmonary artery) Q2Ø.1
 teeth, wedge KØ3.1
 vascular (local) I99.9
  congenital Q27.9
 ventricular septal Q21.Ø
  concurrent with acute myocardial infarction —*see* Infarct, myocardium
  following acute myocardial infarction (current complication) I23.2
  in tetralogy of Fallot Q21.3
 vision NEC H54.7
 visual field H53.4Ø
  bilateral
   heteronymous H53.47
   homonymous H53.46- •
  generalized contraction H53.48- •
  localized
   arcuate H53.43- •
   scotoma (central area) H53.41- •
    blind spot area H53.42- •
   sector H53.43- •
   specified type NEC H53.45- •
 voice R49.9
  specified NEC R49.8
 wedge, tooth, teeth (abrasion) KØ3.1
Deferentitis N49.1
 gonorrheal (acute) (chronic) A54.23

Defibrination (syndrome) D65
  antepartum —*see* Hemorrhage, antepartum, with coagulation defect, disseminated intravascular coagulation
  following ectopic or molar pregnancy OØ8.1
  intrapartum O67.Ø
  newborn P6Ø
  postpartum O72.3
Deficiency, deficient
  3-beta hydroxysteroid dehydrogenase E25.Ø
  11-hydroxylase E25.Ø
  21-hydroxylase E25.Ø
  5-alpha reductase (with male pseudohermaphroditism) E29.1
  abdominal muscle syndrome Q79.4
  AC globulin (congenital) (hereditary) D68.2
    acquired D68.4
  accelerator globulin (Ac G) (blood) D68.2
  acid phosphatase E83.39
  activating factor (blood) D68.2
  ▶ADA2 (adenosine deaminase 2) D81.32
  ➡adenosine deaminase (ADA) D81.3Ø
    ▶with severe combined immunodeficiency (SCID) D81.31
    ▶partial (type 1) D81.39
    ▶specified NEC D81.39
    ▶type 1 (without SCID) (without severe combined immunodeficiency) D81.39
    ▶type 2 D81.32
  aldolase (hereditary) E74.19
  alpha-1-antitrypsin E88.Ø1
  amino-acids E72.9
  anemia —*see* Anemia
  aneurin E51.9
  antibody with
    hyperimmunoglobulinemia D8Ø.6
    near-normal immunoglobins D8Ø.6
  antidiuretic hormone E23.2
  anti-hemophilic
    factor (A) D66
      B D67
      C D68.1
    globulin (AHG) NEC D66
  antithrombin (antithrombin III) D68.59
  ascorbic acid E54
  attention (disorder) (syndrome) F98.8
    with hyperactivity —*see* Disorder, attention-deficit hyperactivity
  autoprothrombin
    I D68.2
    II D67
    C D68.2
  beta-glucuronidase E76.29
  biotin E53.8
  biotin-dependent carboxylase D81.819
  biotinidase D81.81Ø
  brancher enzyme (amylopectinosis) E74.Ø3
  C1 esterase inhibitor (C1-INH) D84.1
  calciferol E55.9
    with
      adult osteomalacia M83.8
      rickets —*see* Rickets
  calcium (dietary) E58
  calorie, severe E43
    with marasmus E41
      and kwashiorkor E42
  cardiac —*see* Insufficiency, myocardial
  carnitine E71.4Ø
    due to
      hemodialysis E71.43
      inborn errors of metabolism E71.42
      Valproic acid therapy E71.43
    iatrogenic E71.43
    muscle palmityltransferase E71.314
    primary E71.41
    secondary E71.448
  carotene E5Ø.9
  central nervous system G96.8
  ceruloplasmin (Wilson) E83.Ø1
  choline E53.8
  Christmas factor D67
  chromium E61.4

Deficiency, deficient *(Continued)*
  clotting (blood) —*see also* Deficiency, coagulation factor D68.9
  clotting factor NEC (hereditary) —*see also* Deficiency, factor D68.2
  coagulation NOS D68.9
    with
      ectopic pregnancy OØ8.1
      molar pregnancy OØ8.1
    acquired (any) D68.4
    antepartum hemorrhage —*see* Hemorrhage, antepartum, with coagulation defect
    clotting factor NEC —*see also* Deficiency, factor D68.2
    due to
      hyperprothrombinemia D68.4
      liver disease D68.4
      vitamin K deficiency D68.4
    newborn, transient P61.6
    postpartum O72.3
    specified NEC D68.8
  cognitive FØ9
  color vision H53.5Ø
    achromatopsia H53.51
    acquired H53.52
    deuteranomaly H53.53
    protanomaly H53.54
    specified type NEC H53.59
    tritanomaly H53.55
  combined glucocorticoid and mineralocorticoid E27.49
  contact factor D68.2
  copper (nutritional) E61.Ø
  corticoadrenal E27.4Ø
    primary E27.1
  craniofacial axis Q75.Ø
  cyanocobalamin E53.8
  debrancher enzyme (limit dextrinosis) E74.Ø3
  dehydrogenase
    long chain/very long chain acyl CoA E71.31Ø
    medium chain acyl CoA E71.311
    short chain acyl CoA E71.312
  diet E63.9
  dihydropyrimidine dehydrogenase (DPD) E88.89
  disaccharidase E73.9
  edema —*see* Malnutrition, severe
  endocrine E34.9
  energy-supply —*see* Malnutrition
  enzymes, circulating NEC E88.Ø9
  ergosterol E55.9
    with
      adult osteomalacia M83.8
      rickets —*see* Rickets
  essential fatty acid (EFA) E63.Ø
  factor —*see also* Deficiency, coagulation
    Hageman D68.2
    I (congenital) (hereditary) D68.2
    II (congenital) (hereditary) D68.2
    IX (congenital) (functional) (hereditary) (with functional defect) D67
    multiple (congenital) D68.8
      acquired D68.4
    V (congenital) (hereditary) D68.2
    VII (congenital) (hereditary) D68.2
    VIII (congenital) (functional) (hereditary) (with functional defect) D66
      with vascular defect D68.Ø
    X (congenital) (hereditary) D68.2
    XI (congenital) (hereditary) D68.1
    XII (congenital) (hereditary) D68.2
    XIII (congenital) (hereditary) D68.2
  femoral, proximal focal (congenital) —*see* Defect, reduction, lower limb, longitudinal, femur
  fibrin-stabilizing factor (congenital) (hereditary) D68.2
    acquired D68.4
  fibrinase D68.2
  fibrinogen (congenital) (hereditary) D68.2
    acquired D65
  folate E53.8

Deficiency, deficient *(Continued)*
  folic acid E53.8
  foreskin N47.3
  fructokinase E74.11
  fructose 1,6-diphosphatase E74.19
  fructose-1-phosphate aldolase E74.19
  GABA (gamma aminobutyric acid) transaminase E72.81
  GABA-T (gamma aminobutyric acid transaminase) E72.81
  galactokinase E74.29
  galactose-1-phosphate uridyl transferase E74.29
  gammaglobulin in blood D8Ø.1
    hereditary D8Ø.Ø
  glass factor D68.2
  glucocorticoid E27.49
    mineralocorticoid E27.49
  glucose-6-phosphatase E74.Ø1
  ➡glucose-6-phosphate dehydrogenase anemia
    ➡anemia D55.Ø
    ➡without anemia D75.A
  glucuronyl transferase E8Ø.5
  glycogen synthetase E74.Ø9
  gonadotropin (isolated) E23.Ø
  growth hormone (idiopathic) (isolated) E23.Ø
  Hageman factor D68.2
  hemoglobin D64.9
  hepatophosphorylase E74.Ø9
  homogentisate 1,2-dioxygenase E7Ø.29
  hormone
    anterior pituitary (partial) NEC E23.Ø
      growth E23.Ø
    growth (isolated) E23.Ø
    pituitary E23.Ø
    testicular E29.1
  hypoxanthine-(guanine)-phosphoribosyltransferase (HG-PRT) (total HG-PRT) E79.1
  immunity D84.9
    cell-mediated D84.8
      with thrombocytopenia and eczema D82.Ø
    combined D81.9
    humoral D8Ø.9
    IgA (secretory) D8Ø.2
    IgG D8Ø.3
    IgM D8Ø.4
  immuno —*see* Immunodeficiency
  immunoglobulin, selective
    A (IgA) D8Ø.2
    G (IgG) (subclasses) D8Ø.3
    M (IgM) D8Ø.4
  inositol (B complex) E53.8
  intrinsic
    factor (congenital) D51.Ø
    sphincter N36.42
      with urethral hypermobility N36.43
  iodine E61.8
    congenital syndrome —*see* Syndrome, iodine-deficiency, congenital
  iron E61.1
    anemia D5Ø.9
  kalium E87.6
  kappa-light chain D8Ø.8
  labile factor (congenital) (hereditary) D68.2
    acquired D68.4
  lacrimal fluid (acquired) —*see also* Syndrome, dry eye
    congenital Q1Ø.6
  lactase
    congenital E73.Ø
    secondary E73.1
  Laki-Lorand factor D68.2
  lecithin cholesterol acyltransferase E78.6
  lipocaic K86.89
  lipoprotein (familial) (high density) E78.6
  liver phosphorylase E74.Ø9
  lysosomal alpha-1, 4 glucosidase E74.Ø2
  magnesium E61.2
  major histocompatibility complex
    class I D81.6
    class II D81.7

D

Deficiency, deficient *(Continued)*
manganese E61.3
menadione (vitamin K) E56.1
newborn P53
mental (familial) (hereditary) —*see* Disability, intellectual
methylenetetrahydrofolate reductase (MTHFR) E72.12
mevalonate kinase MØ4.1
mineral NEC E61.8
mineralocorticoid E27.49
with glucocorticoid E27.49
molybdenum (nutritional) E61.5
moral F6Ø.2
multiple nutrient elements E61.7
multiple sulfatase (MSD) E75.26
muscle
carnitine (palmityltransferase) E71.314
phosphofructokinase E74.Ø9
myoadenylate deaminase E79.2
myocardial —*see* Insufficiency, myocardial
myophosphorylase E74.Ø4
NADH diaphorase or reductase (congenital) D74.Ø
NADH-methemoglobin reductase (congenital) D74.Ø
natrium E87.1
niacin (amide) (-tryptophan) E52
nicotinamide E52
nicotinic acid E52
number of teeth —*see* Anodontia
nutrient element E61.9
multiple E61.7
specified NEC E61.8
nutrition, nutritional E63.9
sequelae —*see* Sequelae, nutritional deficiency
specified NEC E63.8
of interleukin 1 receptor antagonist [DIRA] MØ4.8
ornithine transcarbamylase E72.4
ovarian E28.39
oxygen —*see* Anoxia
pantothenic acid E53.8
parathyroid (gland) E2Ø.9
perineum (female) N81.89
phenylalanine hydroxylase E7Ø.1
phosphoenolpyruvate carboxykinase E74.4
phosphofructokinase E74.19
phosphomannomutuse E74.8
phosphomannose isomerase E74.8
phosphomannosyl mutase E74.8
phosphorylase kinase, liver E74.Ø9
pituitary hormone (isolated) E23.Ø
plasma thromboplastin
antecedent (PTA) D68.1
component (PTC) D67
plasminogen (type 1) (type 2) E88.Ø2
platelet NEC D69.1
constitutional D68.Ø
polyglandular E31.8
autoimmune E31.Ø
potassium (K) E87.6
prepuce N47.3
proaccelerin (congenital) (hereditary) D68.2
acquired D68.4
proconvertin factor (congenital) (hereditary) D68.2
acquired D68.4
protein —*see also* Malnutrition E46
anemia D53.Ø
C D68.59
S D68.59
prothrombin (congenital) (heredItary) D68.2
acquired D68.4
Prower factor D68.2
pseudocholinesterase E88.Ø9
PTA (plasma thromboplastin antecedent) D68.1
PTC (plasma thromboplastin component) D67
purine nucleoside phosphorylase (PNP) D81.5
pyracin (alpha) (beta) E53.1
pyridoxal E53.1

Deficiency, deficient *(Continued)*
pyridoxamine E53.1
pyridoxine (derivatives) E53.1
pyruvate
carboxylase E74.4
dehydrogenase E74.4
riboflavin (vitamin B2) E53.Ø
salt E87.1
secretion
ovary E28.39
salivary gland (any) K11.7
urine R34
selenium (dietary) E59
serum antitrypsin, familial E88.Ø1
short stature homeobox gene (SHOX)
with
dyschondrosteosis Q78.8
short stature (idiopathic) E34.3
Turner's syndrome Q96.9
sodium (Na) E87.1
SPCA (factor VII) D68.2
sphincter, intrinsic N36.42
with urethral hypermobility N36.43
stable factor (congenital) (hereditary) D68.2
acquired D68.4
Stuart-Prower (factor X) D68.2
succinic semialdehyde dehydrogenase E72.81
sucrase E74.39
sulfatase E75.26
sulfite oxidase E72.19
thiamin, thiaminic (chloride) E51.9
beriberi (dry) E51.11
wet E51.12
thrombokinase D68.2
newborn P53
thyroid (gland) —*see* Hypothyroidism
tocopherol E56.Ø
tooth bud KØØ.Ø
transcobalamine II (anemia) D51.2
vanadium E61.6
vascular I99.9
vasopressin E23.2
vertical ridge KØ6.8
viosterol —*see* Deficiency, calciferol
vitamin (multiple) NOS E56.9
A E5Ø.9
with
Bitot's spot (corneal) E5Ø.1
follicular keratosis E5Ø.8
keratomalacia E5Ø.4
manifestations NEC E5Ø.8
night blindness E5Ø.5
scar of cornea, xerophthalmic E5Ø.6
xeroderma E5Ø.8
xerophthalmia E5Ø.7
xerosis
conjunctival E5Ø.Ø
and Bitot's spot E5Ø.1
cornea E5Ø.2
and ulceration E5Ø.3
sequelae E64.1
B (complex) NOS E53.9
with
beriberi (dry) E51.11
wet E51.12
pellagra E52
B1 NOS E51.9
beriberi (dry) E51.11
with circulatory system manifestations E51.11
wet E51.12
B12 E53.8
B2 (riboflavin) E53.Ø
B6 E53.1
C E54
sequelae E64.2
D E55.9
with
adult osteomalacia M83.8
rickets —*see* Rickets
25-hydroxylase E83.32
E E56.Ø

Deficiency, deficient *(Continued)*
vitamin *(Continued)*
folic acid E53.8
G E53.Ø
group B E53.9
specified NEC E53.8
H (biotin) E53.8
K E56.1
of newborn P53
nicotinic E52
P E56.8
PP (pellagra-preventing) E52
specified NEC E56.8
thiamin E51.9
beriberi —*see* Beriberi
zinc, dietary E6Ø
Deficit —*see also* Deficiency
attention and concentration R41.84Ø
following
cerebral infarction I69.31Ø
cerebrovascular disease I69.91Ø
specified disease NEC I69.81Ø
nontraumatic
intracerebral hemorrhage I69.11Ø
specified intracranial hemorrhage NEC I69.21Ø
subarachnoid hemorrhage I69.Ø1Ø
disorder —*see* Attention, deficit
cognitive
communication R41.841
emotional
following
cerebral infarction I69.315
cerebrovascular disease I69.915
specified disease NEC I69.815
nontraumatic
intracerebral hemorrhage I69.115
specified intracranial hemorrhage NEC I69.215
subarachnoid hemorrhage I69.Ø15
following
cerebral infarction I69.319
cerebrovascular disease I69.919
specified disease NEC I69.819
nontraumatic
intracerebral hemorrhage I69.119
specified intracranial hemorrhage NEC I69.219
subarachnoid hemorrhage I69.Ø19
social
following
cerebral infarction I69.315
cerebrovascular disease I69.915
specified disease NEC I69.815
nontraumatic
intracerebral hemorrhage I69.115
specified intracranial hemorrhage NEC I69.215
subarachnoid hemorrhage I69.Ø15
cognitive NEC R41.89
following
cerebral infarction I69.318
cerebrovascular disease I69.918
specified disease NEC I69.818
nontraumatic
intracerebral hemorrhage I69.118
specified intracranial hemorrhage NEC I69.218
subarachnoid hemorrhage I69.Ø18
concentration R41.84Ø
executive function R41.844
following
cerebral infarction I69.314
cerebrovascular disease I69.914
specified disease NEC I69.814
nontraumatic
intracerebral hemorrhage I69.114
specified intracranial hemorrhage NEC I69.214
subarachnoid hemorrhage I69.Ø14

Deficit (Continued)
frontal lobe R41.844
following
cerebral infarction I69.314
cerebrovascular disease I69.914
specified disease NEC I69.814
nontraumatic
intracerebral hemorrhage I69.114
specified intracranial hemorrhage NEC I69.214
subarachnoid hemorrhage I69.Ø14
memory
following
cerebral infarction I69.311
cerebrovascular disease I69.911
specified disease NEC I69.811
nontraumatic
intracerebral hemorrhage I69.111
specified intracranial hemorrhage NEC I69.211
subarachnoid hemorrhage I69.Ø11
neurologic NEC R29.818
ischemic
reversible (RIND) I63.9
prolonged (PRIND) I63.9
oxygen RØ9.Ø2
prolonged reversible ischemic neurologic (PRIND) I63.9
psychomotor R41.843
following
cerebral infarction I69.313
cerebrovascular disease I69.913
specified disease NEC I69.813
nontraumatic
intracerebral hemorrhage I69.113
specified intracranial hemorrhage NEC I69.213
subarachnoid hemorrhage I69.Ø13
visuospatial R41.842
following
cerebral infarction I69.312
cerebrovascular disease I69.912
specified disease NEC I69.812
nontraumatic
intracerebral hemorrhage I69.112
specified intracranial hemorrhage NEC I69.212
subarachnoid hemorrhage I69.Ø12
Deflection
radius —*see* Deformity, limb, specified type NEC, forearm
septum (acquired) (nasal) (nose) J34.2
spine —*see* Curvature, spine
turbinate (nose) J34.2
Defluvium
capillorum —*see* Alopecia
ciliorum —*see* Madarosis
unguium L6Ø.8
Deformity Q89.9
abdomen, congenital Q89.9
abdominal wall
acquired M95.8
congenital Q79.59
acquired (unspecified site) M95.9
adrenal gland Q89.1
alimentary tract, congenital Q45.9
upper Q4Ø.9
ankle (joint) (acquired) —*see also* Deformity, limb, lower leg
abduction —*see* Contraction, joint, ankle
congenital Q68.8
contraction —*see* Contraction, joint, ankle
specified type NEC —*see* Deformity, limb, foot, specified NEC
anus (acquired) K62.89
congenital Q43.9
aorta (arch) (congenital) Q25.4Ø
acquired I77.89

Deformity (Continued)
aortic
arch, acquired I77.89
cusp or valve (congenital) Q23.8
acquired —*see also* Endocarditis, aortic I35.8
arm (acquired) (upper) —*see also* Deformity, limb, upper arm
congenital Q68.8
forearm —*see* Deformity, limb, forearm
artery (congenital) (peripheral) NOS Q27.9
acquired I77.89
coronary (acquired) I25.9
congenital Q24.5
umbilical Q27.Ø
atrial septal Q21.1
auditory canal (external) (congenital) —*see also* Malformation, ear, external
acquired —*see* Disorder, ear, external, specified type NEC
auricle
ear (congenital) —*see also* Malformation, ear, external
acquired —*see* Disorder, pinna, deformity
back —*see* Dorsopathy, deforming
bile duct (common) (congenital) (hepatic) Q44.5
acquired K83.8
biliary duct or passage (congenital) Q44.5
acquired K83.8
bladder (neck) (trigone) (sphincter) (acquired) N32.89
congenital Q64.79
bone (acquired) NOS M95.9
congenital Q79.9
turbinate M95.Ø
brain (congenital) QØ4.9
acquired G93.89
reduction QØ4.3
breast (acquired) N64.89
congenital Q83.9
reconstructed N65.Ø
bronchus (congenital) Q32.4
acquired NEC J98.Ø9
bursa, congenital Q79.9
canaliculi (lacrimalis) (acquired) —*see also* Disorder, lacrimal system, changes
congenital Q1Ø.6
canthus, acquired —*see* Disorder, eyelid, specified type NEC
capillary (acquired) I78.8
cardiovascular system, congenital Q28.9
caruncle, lacrimal (acquired) —*see also* Disorder, lacrimal system, changes
congenital Q1Ø.6
cascade, stomach K31.2
cecum (congenital) Q43.9
acquired K63.89
cerebral, acquired G93.89
congenital QØ4.9
cervix (uterus) (acquired) NEC N88.8
congenital Q51.9
cheek (acquired) M95.2
congenital Q18.9
chest (acquired) (wall) M95.4
congenital Q67.8
sequelae (late effect) of rickets E64.3
chin (acquired) M95.2
congenital Q18.9
choroid (congenital) Q14.3
acquired H31.8
plexus QØ7.8
acquired G96.19
cicatricial —*see* Cicatrix
cilia, acquired —*see* Disorder, eyelid, specified type NEC
clavicle (acquired) M95.8
congenital Q68.8
clitoris (congenital) Q52.6
acquired N9Ø.89

Deformity (Continued)
clubfoot —*see* Clubfoot
coccyx (acquired) —*see* subcategory M43.8
colon (congenital) Q43.9
acquired K63.89
concha (ear), congenital —*see also* Malformation, ear, external
acquired —*see* Disorder, pinna, deformity
cornea (acquired) H18.7Ø
congenital Q13.4
descemetocele —*see* Descemetocele
ectasia —*see* Ectasia, cornea
specified NEC H18.79- ●
staphyloma —*see* Staphyloma, cornea
coronary artery (acquired) I25.9
congenital Q24.5
cranium (acquired) —*see* Deformity, skull
cricoid cartilage (congenital) Q31.8
acquired J38.7
cystic duct (congenital) Q44.5
acquired K82.8
Dandy-Walker QØ3.1
with spina bifida —*see* Spina bifida
diaphragm (congenital) Q79.1
acquired J98.6
digestive organ NOS Q45.9
ductus arteriosus Q25.Ø
duodenal bulb K31.89
duodenum (congenital) Q43.9
acquired K31.89
dura —*see* Deformity, meninges
ear (acquired) —*see also* Disorder, pinna, deformity
congenital (external) Q17.9
internal Q16.5
middle Q16.4
ossicles Q16.3
ossicles Q16.3
ectodermal (congenital) NEC Q84.9
ejaculatory duct (congenital) Q55.4
acquired N5Ø.89
elbow (joint) (acquired) —*see also* Deformity, limb, upper arm
congenital Q68.8
contraction —*see* Contraction, joint, elbow
endocrine gland NEC Q89.2
epididymis (congenital) Q55.4
acquired N5Ø.89
epiglottis (congenital) Q31.8
acquired J38.7
esophagus (congenital) Q39.9
acquired K22.8
eustachian tube (congenital) NEC Q17.8
eye, congenital Q15.9
eyebrow (congenital) Q18.8
eyelid (acquired) —*see also* Disorder, eyelid, specified type NEC
congenital Q1Ø.3
face (acquired) M95.2
congenital Q18.9
fallopian tube, acquired N83.8
femur (acquired) —*see* Deformity, limb, specified type NEC, thigh
fetal
with fetopelvic disproportion O33.7
causing obstructed labor O66.3
finger (acquired) M2Ø.ØØ- ●
boutonniere M2Ø.Ø2- ●
congenital Q68.1
flexion contracture —*see* Contraction, joint, hand
mallet finger M2Ø.Ø1- ●
specified NEC M2Ø.Ø9- ●
swan-neck M2Ø.Ø3- ●
flexion (joint) (acquired) —*see also* Deformity, limb, flexion M21.2Ø
congenital NOS Q74.9
hip Q65.89
foot (acquired) —*see also* Deformity, limb, lower leg
➡ cavovarus (congenital) Q66.1- ●

Deformity *(Continued)*
  foot *(Continued)*
    congenital NOS Q66.9- •
      specified type NEC Q66.89
    specified type NEC *—see* Deformity, limb, foot, specified NEC
    valgus (congenital) Q66.6
      acquired *—see* Deformity, valgus, ankle
    varus (congenital) NEC Q66.3- •
      acquired *—see* Deformity, varus, ankle
  forearm (acquired) *—see also* Deformity, limb, forearm
    congenital Q68.8
  forehead (acquired) M95.2
    congenital Q75.8
  frontal bone (acquired) M95.2
    congenital Q75.8
  gallbladder (congenital) Q44.1
    acquired K82.8
  gastrointestinal tract (congenital) NOS Q45.9
    acquired K63.89
  genitalia, genital organ(s) or system NEC
    female (congenital) Q52.9
      acquired N94.89
      external Q52.7Ø
    male (congenital) Q55.9
      acquired N5Ø.89
  globe (eye) (congenital) Q15.8
    acquired H44.89
  gum, acquired NEC KØ6.8
  hand (acquired) *—see* Deformity, limb, hand
    congenital Q68.1
  head (acquired) M95.2
    congenital Q75.8
  heart (congenital) Q24.9
    septum Q21.9
      auricular Q21.1
      ventricular Q21.Ø
    valve (congenital) NEC Q24.8
      acquired *—see* Endocarditis
  heel (acquired) *—see* Deformity, foot
  hepatic duct (congenital) Q44.5
    acquired K83.8
  hip (joint) (acquired) *—see also* Deformity, limb, thigh
    congenital Q65.9
    due to (previous) juvenile osteochondrosis *—see* Coxa, plana
    flexion *—see* Contraction, joint, hip
  hourglass *—see* Contraction, hourglass
  humerus (acquired) M21.82- •
    congenital Q74.Ø
  hypophyseal (congenital) Q89.2
  ileocecal (coil) (valve) (acquired) K63.89
    congenital Q43.9
  ileum (congenital) Q43.9
    acquired K63.89
  ilium (acquired) M95.5
    congenital Q74.2
  integument (congenital) Q84.9
  intervertebral cartilage or disc (acquired) *—see* Disorder, disc, specified NEC
  intestine (large) (small) (congenital) NOS Q43.9
    acquired K63.89
  intrinsic minus or plus (hand) *—see* Deformity, limb, specified type NEC, forearm
  iris (acquired) H21.89
    congenital Q13.2
  ischium (acquired) M95.5
    congenital Q74.2
  jaw (acquired) (congenital) M26.9
  joint (acquired) NEC M21.9Ø
    congenital Q68.8
    elbow M21.92- •
    hand M21.94- •
    hip M21.95- •
    knee M21.96- •
    shoulder M21.92- •
    wrist M21.93- •

Deformity *(Continued)*
  kidney(s) (calyx) (pelvis) (congenital) Q63.9
    acquired N28.89
    artery (congenital) Q27.2
      acquired I77.89
  Klippel-Feil (brevicollis) Q76.1
  knee (acquired) NEC *—see also* Deformity, limb, lower leg
    congenital Q68.2
  labium (majus) (minus) (congenital) Q52.79
    acquired N9Ø.89
  lacrimal passages or duct (congenital) NEC Q1Ø.6
    acquired *—see* Disorder, lacrimal system, changes
  larynx (muscle) (congenital) Q31.8
    acquired J38.7
    web (glottic) Q31.Ø
  leg (upper) (acquired) NEC *—see also* Deformity, limb, thigh
    congenital Q68.8
    lower leg *—see* Deformity, limb, lower leg
  lens (acquired) H27.8
    congenital Q12.9
  lid (fold) (acquired) *—see also* Disorder, eyelid, specified type NEC
    congenital Q1Ø.3
  ligament (acquired) *—see* Disorder, ligament
    congenital Q79.9
  limb (acquired) M21.9Ø
    clawfoot M21.53- •
    clawhand M21.51- •
    clubfoot M21.54- •
    clubhand M21.52- •
    congenital, except reduction deformity Q74.9
    flat foot M21.4- •
    flexion M21.2Ø
      ankle M21.27- •
      elbow M21.22- •
      finger M21.24- •
      hip M21.25- •
      knee M21.26- •
      shoulder M21.21- •
      toe M21.27- •
      wrist M21.23- •
    foot
      claw *—see* Deformity, limb, clawfoot
      club *—see* Deformity, limb, clubfoot
      drop M21.37- •
      flat *—see* Deformity, limb, flat foot
      specified NEC M21.6X- •
    forearm M21.93- •
    hand M21.94- •
    lower leg M21.96- •
    specified type NEC M21.8Ø
      forearm M21.83- •
      lower leg M21.86- •
      thigh M21.85- •
      upper arm M21.82- •
    thigh M21.95- •
    unequal length M21.7Ø
      short site is
        femur M21.75- •
        fibula M21.76- •
        humerus M21.72- •
        radius M21.73- •
        tibia M21.76- •
        ulna M21.73- •
    upper arm M21.92- •
    valgus *—see* Deformity, valgus
    varus *—see* Deformity, varus
    wrist drop M21.33- •
  lip (acquired) NEC K13.Ø
    congenital Q38.Ø
  liver (congenital) Q44.7
    acquired K76.89
  lumbosacral (congenital) (joint) (region) Q76.49
    acquired *—see* subcategory M43.8
    kyphosis *—see* Kyphosis, congenital
    lordosis *—see* Lordosis, congenital

Deformity *(Continued)*
  lung (congenital) Q33.9
    acquired J98.4
  lymphatic system, congenital Q89.9
  Madelung's (radius) Q74.Ø
  mandible (acquired) (congenital) M26.9
  maxilla (acquired) (congenital) M26.9
  meninges or membrane (congenital) QØ7.9
    cerebral QØ4.8
      acquired G96.19
    spinal cord (congenital) G96.19
      acquired G96.19
  metacarpus (acquired) *—see* Deformity, limb, forearm
    congenital Q74.Ø
  metatarsus (acquired) *—see* Deformity, foot
    congenital Q66.9- •
  middle ear (congenital) Q16.4
    ossicles Q16.3
  mitral (leaflets) (valve) IØ5.8
    parachute Q23.2
    stenosis, congenital Q23.2
  mouth (acquired) K13.79
    congenital Q38.6
  multiple, congenital NEC Q89.7
  muscle (acquired) M62.89
    congenital Q79.9
      sternocleidomastoid Q68.Ø
  musculoskeletal system (acquired) M95.9
    congenital Q79.9
    specified NEC M95.8
  nail (acquired) L6Ø.8
    congenital Q84.6
  nasal *—see* Deformity, nose
  neck (acquired) M95.3
    congenital Q18.9
      sternocleidomastoid Q68.Ø
  nervous system (congenital) QØ7.9
  nipple (congenital) Q83.9
    acquired N64.89
  nose (acquired) (cartilage) M95.Ø
    bone (turbinate) M95.Ø
    congenital Q3Ø.9
      bent or squashed Q67.4
    saddle M95.Ø
      syphilitic A5Ø.57
    septum (acquired) J34.2
      congenital Q3Ø.8
    sinus (wall) (congenital) Q3Ø.8
      acquired M95.Ø
    syphilitic (congenital) A5Ø.57
      late A52.73
  ocular muscle (congenital) Q1Ø.3
    acquired *—see* Strabismus, mechanical
  opticociliary vessels (congenital) Q13.2
  orbit (eye) (acquired) HØ5.3Ø
    atrophy *—see* Atrophy, orbit
    congenital Q1Ø.7
    due to
      bone disease NEC HØ5.32- •
      trauma or surgery HØ5.33- •
    enlargement *—see* Enlargement, orbit
    exostosis *—see* Exostosis, orbit
  organ of Corti (congenital) Q16.5
  ovary (congenital) Q5Ø.39
    acquired N83.8
  oviduct, acquired N83.8
  palate (congenital) Q38.5
    acquired M27.8
    cleft (congenital) *—see* Cleft, palate
  pancreas (congenital) Q45.3
    acquired K86.89
  parathyroid (gland) Q89.2
  parotid (gland) (congenital) Q38.4
    acquired K11.8
  patella (acquired) *—see* Disorder, patella, specified NEC
  pelvis, pelvic (acquired) (bony) M95.5
    with disproportion (fetopelvic) O33.Ø
      causing obstructed labor O65.Ø

Deformity *(Continued)*
pelvis, pelvic *(Continued)*
congenital Q74.2
rachitic sequelae (late effect) E64.3
penis (glans) (congenital) Q55.69
acquired N48.89
pericardium (congenital) Q24.8
acquired —*see* Pericarditis
pharynx (congenital) Q38.8
acquired J39.2
pinna, acquired —*see also* Disorder, pinna, deformity
congenital Q17.9
pituitary (congenital) Q89.2
posture —*see* Dorsopathy, deforming
prepuce (congenital) Q55.69
acquired N47.8
prostate (congenital) Q55.4
acquired N42.89
pupil (congenital) Q13.2
acquired —*see* Abnormality, pupillary
pylorus (congenital) Q4Ø.3
acquired K31.89
rachitic (acquired), old or healed E64.3
radius (acquired) —*see also* Deformity, limb, forearm
congenital Q68.8
rectum (congenital) Q43.9
acquired K62.89
reduction (extremity) (limb), congenital (*see also* condition and site) Q73.8
brain QØ4.3
lower —*see* Defect, reduction, lower limb
upper —*see* Defect, reduction, upper limb
renal —*see* Deformity, kidney
respiratory system (congenital) Q34.9
rib (acquired) M95.4
congenital Q76.6
cervical Q76.5
rotation (joint) (acquired) —*see* Deformity, limb, specified site NEC
congenital Q74.9
hip —*see* Deformity, limb, specified type NEC, thigh
congenital Q65.89
sacroiliac joint (congenital) Q74.2
acquired —*see* subcategory M43.8
sacrum (acquired) —*see* subcategory M43.8
saddle
back —*see* Lordosis
nose M95.Ø
syphilitic A5Ø.57
salivary gland or duct (congenital) Q38.4
acquired K11.8
scapula (acquired) M95.8
congenital Q68.8
scrotum (congenital) —*see also* Malformation, testis and scrotum
acquired N5Ø.89
seminal vesicles (congenital) Q55.4
acquired N5Ø.89
septum, nasal (acquired) J34.2
shoulder (joint) (acquired) —*see* Deformity, limb, upper arm
congenital Q74.Ø
contraction —*see* Contraction, joint, shoulder
sigmoid (flexure) (congenital) Q43.9
acquired K63.89
skin (congenital) Q82.9
skull (acquired) M95.2
congenital Q75.8
with
anencephaly QØØ.Ø
encephalocele —*see* Encephalocele
hydrocephalus QØ3.9
with spina bifida —*see* Spina bifida, by site, with hydrocephalus
microcephaly QØ2

Deformity *(Continued)*
soft parts, organs or tissues (of pelvis)
in pregnancy or childbirth NEC O34.8-●
causing obstructed labor O65.5
spermatic cord (congenital) Q55.4
acquired N5Ø.89
torsion —*see* Torsion, spermatic cord
spinal —*see* Dorsopathy, deforming
column (acquired) —*see* Dorsopathy, deforming
congenital Q67.5
cord (congenital) QØ6.9
acquired G95.89
nerve root (congenital) QØ7.9
spine (acquired) —*see also* Dorsopathy, deforming
congenital Q67.5
rachitic E64.3
specified NEC —*see* Dorsopathy, deforming, specified NEC
spleen
acquired D73.89
congenital Q89.Ø9
Sprengel's (congenital) Q74.Ø
sternocleidomastoid (muscle), congenital Q68.Ø
sternum (acquired) M95.4
congenital NEC Q76.7
stomach (congenital) Q4Ø.3
acquired K31.89
submandibular gland (congenital) Q38.4
submaxillary gland (congenital) Q38.4
acquired K11.8
talipes —*see* Talipes
testis (congenital) —*see also* Malformation, testis and scrotum
acquired N44.8
torsion —*see* Torsion, testis
thigh (acquired) —*see also* Deformity, limb, thigh
congenital NEC Q68.8
thorax (acquired) (wall) M95.4
congenital Q67.8
sequelae of rickets E64.3
thumb (acquired) —*see also* Deformity, finger
congenital NEC Q68.1
thymus (tissue) (congenital) Q89.2
thyroid (gland) (congenital) Q89.2
cartilage Q31.8
acquired J38.7
tibia (acquired) —*see also* Deformity, limb, specified type NEC, lower leg
congenital NEC Q68.8
saber (syphilitic) A5Ø.56
toe (acquired) M2Ø.6-●
congenital Q66.9-●
hallux rigidus M2Ø.2-●
hallux valgus M2Ø.1-●
hallux varus M2Ø.3-●
hammer toe M2Ø.4-●
specified NEC M2Ø.5X-●
tongue (congenital) Q38.3
acquired K14.8
tooth, teeth KØØ.2
trachea (rings) (congenital) Q32.1
acquired J39.8
transverse aortic arch (congenital) Q25.49
tricuspid (leaflets) (valve) IØ7.8
atresia or stenosis Q22.4
Ebstein's Q22.5
trunk (acquired) M95.8
congenital Q89.9
ulna (acquired) —*see also* Deformity, limb, forearm
congenital NEC Q68.8
urachus, congenital Q64.4
ureter (opening) (congenital) Q62.8
acquired N28.89
urethra (congenital) Q64.79
acquired N36.8

Deformity *(Continued)*
urinary tract (congenital) Q64.9
urachus Q64.4
uterus (congenital) Q51.9
acquired N85.8
uvula (congenital) Q38.5
vagina (acquired) N89.8
congenital Q52.4
valgus NEC M21.ØØ
ankle M21.Ø7-●
elbow M21.Ø2-●
hip M21.Ø5-●
knee M21.Ø6-●
valve, valvular (congenital) (heart) Q24.8
acquired —*see* Endocarditis
varus NEC M21.1Ø
ankle M21.17-●
elbow M21.12-●
hip M21.15
knee M21.16-●
tibia —*see* Osteochondrosis, juvenile, tibia
vas deferens (congenital) Q55.4
acquired N5Ø.89
vein (congenital) Q27.9
great Q26.9
vertebra —*see* Dorsopathy, deforming
vertical talus (congenital) Q66.8Ø
left foot Q66.82
right foot Q66.81
vesicourethral orifice (acquired) N32.89
congenital NEC Q64.79
vessels of optic papilla (congenital) Q14.2
visual field (contraction) —*see* Defect, visual field
vitreous body, acquired H43.89
vulva (congenital) Q52.79
acquired N9Ø.89
wrist (joint) (acquired) —*see also* Deformity, limb, forearm
congenital Q68.8
contraction —*see* Contraction, joint, wrist
Degeneration, degenerative
adrenal (capsule) (fatty) (gland) (hyaline) (infectional) E27.8
amyloid —*see also* Amyloidosis E85.9
anterior cornua, spinal cord G12.29
anterior labral S43.49-●
aorta, aortic I7Ø.Ø
fatty I77.89
aortic valve (heart) —*see* Endocarditis, aortic
arteriovascular —*see* Arteriosclerosis
artery, arterial (atheromatous) (calcareous) —*see also* Arteriosclerosis
cerebral, amyloid E85.4 *[I68.Ø]*
medial —*see* Arteriosclerosis, extremities
articular cartilage NEC —*see* Derangement, joint, articular cartilage, by site
atheromatous —*see* Arteriosclerosis
basal nuclei or ganglia G23.9
specified NEC G23.8
bone NEC —*see* Disorder, bone, specified type NEC
brachial plexus G54.Ø
brain (cortical) (progressive) G31.9
alcoholic G31.2
arteriosclerotic I67.2
childhood G31.9
specified NEC G31.89
cystic G31.89
congenital QØ4.6
in
alcoholism G31.2
beriberi E51.2
cerebrovascular disease I67.9
congenital hydrocephalus QØ3.9
with spina bifida —*see also* Spina bifida
Fabry-Anderson disease E75.21
Gaucher's disease E75.22
Hunter's syndrome E76.1

Degeneration, degenerative *(Continued)*
brain *(Continued)*
in *(Continued)*
lipidosis
cerebral E75.4
generalized E75.6
mucopolysaccharidosis —*see* Mucopolysaccharidosis
myxedema E03.9 *[G32.89]*
neoplastic disease —*see also* Neoplasm D49.6 *[G32.89]*
Niemann-Pick disease E75.249 *[G32.89]*
sphingolipidosis E75.3 *[G32.89]*
vitamin B12 deficiency E53.8 *[G32.89]*
senile NEC G31.1
breast N64.89
Bruch's membrane —*see* Degeneration, choroid
capillaries (fatty) I78.8
amyloid E85.89 *[I79.8]*
cardiac —*see also* Degeneration, myocardial
valve, valvular —*see* Endocarditis
cardiorenal —*see* Hypertension, cardiorenal
cardiovascular —*see also* Disease, cardiovascular
renal —*see* Hypertension, cardiorenal
cerebellar NOS G31.9
alcoholic G31.2
primary (hereditary) (sporadic) G11.9
cerebral —*see* Degeneration, brain
cerebrovascular I67.9
due to hypertension I67.4
cervical plexus G54.2
cervix N88.8
due to radiation (intended effect) N88.8
adverse effect or misadventure N99.89
chamber angle H21.21-●
changes, spine or vertebra —*see* Spondylosis
chorioretinal —*see also* Degeneration, choroid
hereditary H31.20
choroid (colloid) (drusen) H31.10-●
atrophy —*see* Atrophy, choroidal
hereditary —*see* Dystrophy, choroidal, hereditary
ciliary body H21.22-●
cochlear —*see* subcategory H83.8
combined (spinal cord) (subacute) E53.8 *[G32.0]*
with anemia (pernicious) D51.0 *[G32.0]*
due to dietary vitamin B12 deficiency D51.3 *[G32.0]*
in (due to)
vitamin B12 deficiency E53.8 *[G32.0]*
anemia D51.9 *[G32.0]*
conjunctiva H11.10
concretions —*see* Concretion, conjunctiva
deposits —*see* Deposit, conjunctiva
pigmentations —*see* Pigmentation, conjunctiva
pinguecula —*see* Pinguecula
xerosis —*see* Xerosis, conjunctiva
cornea H18.40
calcerous H18.43
band keratopathy H18.42-●
familial, hereditary —*see* Dystrophy, cornea
hyaline (of old scars) H18.49
keratomalacia —*see* Keratomalacia
nodular H18.45-●
peripheral H18.46-●
senile H18.41-●
specified type NEC H18.49
cortical (cerebellar) (parenchymatous) G31.89
alcoholic G31.2
diffuse, due to arteriopathy I67.2
corticobasal G31.85
cutis L98.8
amyloid E85.4 *[L99]*
dental pulp K04.2
disc disease —*see* Degeneration, intervertebral disc NEC

Degeneration, degenerative *(Continued)*
dorsolateral (spinal cord) —*see* Degeneration, combined
extrapyramidal G25.9
eye, macular —*see also* Degeneration, macula
congenital or hereditary —*see* Dystrophy, retina
facet joints —*see* Spondylosis
fatty
liver NEC K76.0
alcoholic K70.0
grey matter (brain) (Alpers') G31.81
heart —*see also* Degeneration, myocardial
amyloid E85.4 *[I43]*
atheromatous —*see* Disease, heart, ischemic, atherosclerotic
ischemic —*see* Disease, heart, ischemic
hepatolenticular (Wilson's) E83.01
hepatorenal K76.7
hyaline (diffuse) (generalized)
localized —*see* Degeneration, by site
infrapatellar fat pad M79.4
intervertebral disc NOS
with
myelopathy —*see* Disorder, disc, with, myelopathy
radiculitis or radiculopathy —*see* Disorder, disc, with, radiculopathy
cervical, cervicothoracic —*see* Disorder, disc, cervical, degeneration
with
myelopathy —*see* Disorder, disc, cervical, with myelopathy
neuritis, radiculitis or radiculopathy —*see* Disorder, disc, cervical, with neuritis
lumbar region M51.36
with
myelopathy M51.06
neuritis, radiculitis, radiculopathy or sciatica M51.16
lumbosacral region M51.37
with
neuritis, radiculitis, radiculopathy or sciatica M51.17
sacrococcygeal region M53.3
thoracic region M51.34
with
myelopathy M51.04
neuritis, radiculitis, radiculopathy M51.14
thoracolumbar region M51.35
with
myelopathy M51.05
neuritis, radiculitis, radiculopathy M51.15
intestine, amyloid E85.4
iris (pigmentary) H21.23-●
ischemic —*see* Ischemia
joint disease —*see* Osteoarthritis
kidney N28.89
amyloid E85.4 *[N29]*
cystic, congenital Q61.9
fatty N28.89
polycystic Q61.3
adult type (autosomal dominant) Q61.2
infantile type (autosomal recessive) NEC Q61.19
collecting duct dilatation Q61.11
Kuhnt-Junius —*see also* Degeneration, macula H35.32-●
lens —*see* Cataract
lenticular (familial) (progressive) (Wilson's) (with cirrhosis of liver) E83.01
liver (diffuse) NEC K76.89
amyloid E85.4 *[K77]*
cystic K76.89
congenital Q44.6
fatty NEC K76.0
alcoholic K70.0

Degeneration, degenerative *(Continued)*
liver *(Continued)*
hypertrophic K76.89
parenchymatous, acute or subacute K72.00
with coma K72.01
pigmentary K76.89
toxic (acute) K71.9
lung J98.4
lymph gland I89.8
hyaline I89.8
macula, macular (acquired) (age-related) (senile) H35.30
angioid streaks H35.33
atrophic age-related H35.31-●
congenital or hereditary —*see* Dystrophy, retina
cystoid H35.35-●
drusen H35.36-●
dry age-related H35.31-●
exudative H35.32-●
hole H35.34-●
nonexudative H35.31-●
puckering H35.37-●
toxic H35.38-●
wet age-related H35.32-●
membranous labyrinth, congenital (causing impairment of hearing) Q16.5
meniscus —*see* Derangement, meniscus
mitral —*see* Insufficiency, mitral
Mönckeberg's —*see* Arteriosclerosis, extremities
motor centers, senile G31.1
multi-system G90.3
mural —*see* Degeneration, myocardial
muscle (fatty) (fibrous) (hyaline) (progressive) M62.89
heart —*see* Degeneration, myocardial
myelin, central nervous system G37.9
myocardial, myocardium (fatty) (hyaline) (senile) I51.5
with rheumatic fever (conditions in I00) I09.0
active, acute or subacute I01.2
with chorea I02.0
inactive or quiescent (with chorea) I09.0
hypertensive —*see* Hypertension, heart
rheumatic —*see* Degeneration, myocardial, with rheumatic fever
syphilitic A52.06
nasal sinus (mucosa) J32.9
frontal J32.1
maxillary J32.0
nerve —*see* Disorder, nerve
nervous system G31.9
alcoholic G31.2
amyloid E85.4 *[G99.8]*
autonomic G90.9
fatty G31.89
specified NEC G31.89
nipple N64.89
olivopontocerebellar (hereditary) (familial) G23.8
osseous labyrinth —*see* subcategory H83.8
ovary N83.8
cystic N83.20-●
microcystic N83.20-●
pallidal pigmentary (progressive) G23.0
pancreas K86.89
tuberculous A18.83
penis N48.89
pigmentary (diffuse) (general)
localized —*see* Degeneration, by site
pallidal (progressive) G23.0
pineal gland E34.8
pituitary (gland) E23.6
popliteal fat pad M79.4
posterolateral (spinal cord) —*see* Degeneration, combined
pulmonary valve (heart) I37.8
pulp (tooth) K04.2

Degeneration, degenerative *(Continued)*
pupillary margin H21.24-●
renal —*see* Degeneration, kidney
retina H35.9
hereditary (cerebroretinal) (congenital) (juvenile) (macula) (peripheral) (pigmentary) —*see* Dystrophy, retina
Kuhnt-Junius —*see also* Degeneration, macula H35.32-●
macula (cystic) (exudative) (hole) (nonexudative) (pseudohole) (senile) (toxic) —*see* Degeneration, macula
peripheral H35.40
lattice H35.41-●
microcystoid H35.42-●
paving stone H35.43-●
secondary
pigmentary H35.45-●
vitreoretinal H35.46-●
senile reticular H35.44-●
pigmentary (primary) —*see also* Dystrophy, retina
secondary —*see* Degeneration, retina, peripheral, secondary
posterior pole —*see* Degeneration, macula
saccule, congenital (causing impairment of hearing) Q16.5
senile R54
brain G31.1
cardiac, heart or myocardium —*see* Degeneration, myocardial
motor centers G31.1
vascular —*see* Arteriosclerosis
sinus (cystic) —*see also* Sinusitis
polypoid J33.1
skin L98.8
amyloid E85.4 *[L99]*
colloid L98.8
spinal (cord) G31.89
amyloid E85.4 *[G32.89]*
combined (subacute) —*see* Degeneration, combined
dorsolateral —*see* Degeneration, combined
familial NEC G31.89
fatty G31.89
funicular —*see* Degeneration, combined
posterolateral —*see* Degeneration, combined
subacute combined —*see* Degeneration, combined
tuberculous A17.81
spleen D73.Ø
amyloid E85.4 *[D77]*
stomach K31.89
striatonigral G23.2
suprarenal (capsule) (gland) E27.8
synovial membrane (pulpy) —*see* Disorder, synovium, specified type NEC
tapetoretinal —*see* Dystrophy, retina
thymus (gland) E32.8
fatty E32.8
thyroid (gland) EØ7.89
tricuspid (heart) (valve) IØ7.9
tuberculous NEC —*see* Tuberculosis
turbinate J34.89
uterus (cystic) N85.8
vascular (senile) —*see* Arteriosclerosis
hypertensive —*see* Hypertension
vitreoretinal, secondary —*see* Degeneration, retina, peripheral, secondary, vitreoretinal
vitreous (body) H43.81-●
Wallerian —*see* Disorder, nerve
Wilson's hepatolenticular E83.Ø1
Deglutition
paralysis R13.Ø
hysterical F44.4
pneumonia J69.Ø
Degos' disease I77.89
Dehiscence (of)
amputation stump T87.81
cesarean wound O9Ø.Ø
Dehiscence *(Continued)*
closure of
cornea T81.31
craniotomy T81.32
fascia (muscular) (superficial) T81.32
internal organ or tissue T81.32
laceration (external) (internal) T81.33
ligament T81.32
mucosa T81.31
muscle or muscle flap T81.32
ribs or rib cage T81.32
skin and subcutaneous tissue (full-thickness) (superficial) T81.31
skull T81.32
sternum (sternotomy) T81.32
tendon T81.32
traumatic laceration (external) (internal) T81.33
episiotomy O9Ø.1
operation wound NEC T81.31
external operation wound (superficial) T81.31
internal operation wound (deep) T81.32
perineal wound (postpartum) O9Ø.1
traumatic injury wound repair T81.33
wound T81.3Ø
traumatic repair T81.33
Dehydration E86.Ø
newborn P74.1
Déjérine-Roussy syndrome G93.89
Déjérine-Sottas disease or neuropathy (hypertrophic) G6Ø.Ø
Déjérine-Thomas atrophy G23.8
Delay, delayed
any plane in pelvis
complicating delivery O66.9
birth or delivery NOS O63.9
closure, ductus arteriosus (Botalli) P29.38
coagulation —*see* Defect, coagulation
conduction (cardiac) (ventricular) I45.9
delivery, second twin, triplet, etc O63.2
development R62.5Ø
global F88
intellectual (specific) F81.9
language F8Ø.9
due to hearing loss F8Ø.4
learning F81.9
pervasive F84.9
physiological R62.5Ø
specified stage NEC R62.Ø
reading F81.Ø
sexual E3Ø.Ø
speech F8Ø.9
due to hearing loss F8Ø.4
spelling F81.81
ejaculation F52.32
gastric emptying K3Ø
menarche E3Ø.Ø
menstruation (cause unknown) N91.Ø
milestone R62.Ø
passage of meconium (newborn) P76.Ø
primary respiration P28.9
puberty (constitutional) E3Ø.Ø
separation of umbilical cord P96.82
sexual maturation, female E3Ø.Ø
sleep phase syndrome G47.21
union, fracture —*see* Fracture, by site
vaccination Z28.9
Deletion(s)
autosome Q93.9
identified by fluorescence in situ hybridization (FISH) Q93.89
identified by in situ hybridization (ISH) Q93.89
chromosome
with complex rearrangements NEC Q93.7
part of NEC Q93.59
seen only at prometaphase Q93.89
Deletion *(Continued)*
chromosome *(Continued)*
short arm
4 Q93.3
5p Q93.4
22q11.2 Q93.81
specified NEC Q93.89
long arm chromosome 18 or 21 Q93.89
with complex rearrangements NEC Q93.7
microdeletions NEC Q93.88
Delhi boil or button B55.1
Delinquency (juvenile) (neurotic) F91.8
group Z72.81Ø
Delinquent immunization status Z28.3
Delirious (acute or subacute) (not alcohol or drug-induced) (with dementia) R41.Ø
alcoholic (acute) (tremens) (withdrawal) F1Ø.921
with intoxication F1Ø.921
in
abuse F1Ø.121
dependence F1Ø.221
due to (secondary to)
alcohol
intoxication F1Ø.921
in
abuse F1Ø.121
dependence F1Ø.221
withdrawal F1Ø.231
amphetamine intoxication F15.921
in
abuse F15.121
dependence F15.221
anxiolytic
intoxication F13.921
in
abuse F13.121
dependence F13.221
withdrawal F13.231
cannabis intoxication (acute) F12.921
in
abuse F12.121
dependence F12.221
cocaine intoxication (acute) F14.921
in
abuse F14.121
dependence F14.221
general medical condition FØ5
hallucinogen intoxication F16.921
in
abuse F16.121
dependence F16.221
hypnotic
intoxication F13.921
in
abuse F13.121
dependence F13.221
withdrawal F13.231
inhalant intoxication (acute) F18.921
in
abuse F18.121
dependence F18.221
multiple etiologies FØ5
opioid intoxication (acute) F11.921
in
abuse F11.121
dependence F11.221
other (or unknown) substance F19.921
phencyclidine intoxication (acute) F16.921
in
abuse F16.121
dependence F16.221
psychoactive substance NEC intoxication (acute) F19.921
in
abuse F19.121
dependence F19.221

Delirious *(Continued)*
  due to *(Continued)*
    sedative
      intoxication F13.921
        in
          abuse F13.121
          dependence F13.221
      withdrawal F13.231
  unknown etiology R41.Ø
  exhaustion F43.Ø
  hysterical F44.89
  postprocedural (postoperative) FØ5
  puerperal FØ5
  thyroid *—see* Thyrotoxicosis with thyroid storm
  traumatic *—see* Injury, intracranial
  tremens (alcohol-induced) F1Ø.231
    sedative-induced F13.231
Delivery (childbirth) (labor)
  arrested active phase O62.1
  cesarean (for)
    without indication O82
    abnormal
      pelvis (bony) (deformity) (major) NEC
        with disproportion (fetopelvic) O33.Ø
        with obstructed labor O65.Ø
      presentation or position O32.9
    abruptio placentae *—see also* Abruptio placentae Ø45.9-●
    acromion presentation O32.2
    atony, uterus O62.2
    breech presentation O32.1
      incomplete O32.8
    brow presentation O32.3
    cephalopelvic disproportion O33.9
    cerclage O34.3-●
    chin presentation O32.3
    cicatrix of cervix O34.4-●
    contracted pelvis (general)
      inlet O33.2
      outlet O33.3
    cord presentation or prolapse O69.Ø
    cystocele O34.8-●
    deformity (acquired) (congenital)
      pelvic organs or tissues NEC O34.8-●
      pelvis (bony) NEC O33.Ø
    disproportion NOS O33.9
    eclampsia *—see* Eclampsia
    face presentation O32.3
    failed
      forceps O66.5
      induction of labor O61.9
        instrumental O61.1
        mechanical O61.1
        medical O61.Ø
        specified NEC O61.8
        surgical O61.1
      trial of labor NOS O66.4Ø
        following previous cesarean delivery O66.41
      vacuum extraction O66.5
      ventouse O66.5
    fetal-maternal hemorrhage O43.Ø1-●
    hemorrhage (intrapartum) O67.9
      with coagulation defect O67.Ø
      specified cause NEC O67.8
    high head at term O32.4
    hydrocephalic fetus O33.6
    incarceration of uterus O34.51-●
    incoordinate uterine action O62.4
    increased size, fetus O33.5
    inertia, uterus O62.2
      primary O62.Ø
      secondary O62.1
    lateroversion, uterus O34.59-●
    mal lie O32.9
    malposition
      fetus O32.9
      pelvic organs or tissues NEC O34.8-●
      uterus NEC O34.59-●

Delivery *(Continued)*
  cesarean *(Continued)*
    malpresentation NOS O32.9
    oblique presentation O32.2
    occurring after 37 completed weeks of gestation but before 39 completed weeks gestation due to (spontaneous) onset of labor O75.82
    oversize fetus O33.5
    pelvic tumor NEC O34.8-●
    placenta previa O44.Ø-●
      complete O44.Ø-●
        with hemorrhage O44.1-●
    placental insufficiency O36.51-●
    planned, occurring after 37 completed weeks of gestation but before 39 completed weeks gestation due to (spontaneous) onset of labor O75.82
    polyp, cervix O34.4-●
      causing obstructed labor O65.5
    poor dilatation, cervix O62.Ø
    pre-eclampsia O14.94
      mild O14.Ø4
      moderate O14.Ø4
      severe O14.14
        with hemolysis, elevated liver enzymes and low platelet count (HELLP) O14.24
    previous
      cesarean delivery O34.219
        classical (vertical) scar O34.212
        low transverse scar O34.211
      surgery (to)
        cervix O34.4-●
        gynecological NEC O34.8-●
        rectum O34.7-●
        uterus O34.29
        vagina O34.6-●
    prolapse
      arm or hand O32.2
      uterus O34.52-●
    prolonged labor NOS O63.9
    rectocele O34.8-●
    retroversion
      uterus O34.53-●
    rigid
      cervix O34.4-●
      pelvic floor O34.8-●
      perineum O34.7-●
      vagina O34.6-●
      vulva O34.7-●
    sacculation, pregnant uterus O34.59-●
    scar(s)
      cervix O34.4-●
      cesarean delivery O34.219
        classical (vertical) O34.212
        low transverse O34.211
      transmural uterine O34.29
      uterus O34.29
    Shirodkar suture in situ O34.3-●
    shoulder presentation O32.2
    stenosis or stricture, cervix O34.4-●
    streptococcus group B (GBS) carrier state O99.824
    transmural uterine scar O34.29
    transverse presentation or lie O32.2
    tumor, pelvic organs or tissues NEC O34.8-●
      cervix O34.4-●
    umbilical cord presentation or prolapse O69.Ø
  completely normal case O8Ø
  complicated O75.9
    by
      abnormal, abnormality (of)
        forces of labor O62.9
          specified type NEC O62.8
        glucose O99.814
        uterine contractions NOS O62.9
      abruptio placentae *—see also* Abruptio placentae O45.9-●

Delivery *(Continued)*
  complicated *(Continued)*
    by *(Continued)*
      abuse
        physical O9A.32
        psychological O9A.52
        sexual O9A.42
      adherent placenta O72.Ø
        without hemorrhage O73.Ø
      alcohol use O99.314
      anemia (pre-existing) O99.Ø2
      anesthetic death O74.8
      annular detachment of cervix O71.3
      atony, uterus O62.2
      attempted vacuum extraction and forceps O66.5
      Bandl's ring O62.4
      bariatric surgery status O99.844
      biliary tract disorder O26.62
      bleeding *—see* Delivery, complicated by, hemorrhage
      blood disorder NEC O99.12
      cervical dystocia (hypotonic) O62.2
        primary O62.Ø
        secondary O62.1
      circulatory system disorder O99.42
      compression of cord (umbilical) NEC O69.2
      condition NEC O99.89
      contraction, contracted ring O62.4
      cord (umbilical)
        around neck
          with compression O69.1
          without compression O69.81
        bruising O69.5
        complication O69.9
          specified NEC O69.89
        compression NEC O69.2
        entanglement O69.2
          without compression O69.82
        hematoma O69.5
        presentation O69.Ø
        prolapse O69.Ø
        short O69.3
        thrombosis (vessels) O69.5
        vascular lesion O69.5
      Couvelaire uterus O45.8X-●
      damage to (injury to) NEC
        perineum O71.82
        periurethral tissue O71.82
        vulva O71.82
      delay following rupture of membranes (spontaneous) *—see* Pregnancy, complicated by, premature rupture of membranes
      depressed fetal heart tones O76
      diabetes O24.92
        gestational O24.429
          diet controlled O24.42Ø
          insulin controlled O24.424
          oral drug controlled (antidiabetic) (hypoglycemic) O24.425
        pre-existing O24.32
          specified NEC O24.82
          type 1 O24.Ø2
          type 2 O24.12
      diastasis recti (abdominis) O71.89
      dilatation
        bladder O66.8
        cervix incomplete, poor or slow O62.Ø
      disease NEC O99.89
      disruptio uteri *—see* Delivery, complicated by, rupture, uterus
      drug use O99.324
      dysfunction, uterus NOS O62.9
        hypertonic O62.4
        hypotonic O62.2
          primary O62.Ø
          secondary O62.1
        incoordinate O62.4
      eclampsia O15.1

- Delivery *(Continued)*
  - complicated *(Continued)*
    - by *(Continued)*
      - embolism (pulmonary) —*see* Embolism, obstetric
      - endocrine, nutritional or metabolic disease NEC O99.284
      - failed
        - attempted vaginal birth after previous cesarean delivery O66.41
        - induction of labor O61.9
          - instrumental O61.1
          - mechanical O61.1
          - medical O61.Ø
          - specified NEC O61.8
          - surgical O61.1
        - trial of labor O66.4Ø
      - female genital mutilation O65.5
      - fetal
        - abnormal acid-base balance O68
        - acidemia O68
        - acidosis O68
        - alkalosis O68
        - death, early OØ2.1
        - deformity O66.3
        - heart rate or rhythm (abnormal) (non-reassuring) O76
        - hypoxia O77.8
        - stress O77.9
          - due to drug administration O77.1
          - electrocardiographic evidence of O77.8
          - specified NEC O77.8
          - ultrasound evidence of O77.8
      - fever during labor O75.2
      - gastric banding status O99.844
      - gastric bypass status O99.844
      - gastrointestinal disease NEC O99.62
      - gestational
        - diabetes O24.429
          - diet controlled O24.42Ø
          - insulin (and diet) controlled O24.424
          - oral drug controlled (antidiabetic) (hypoglycemic) O24.425
        - edema O12.Ø4
          - with proteinuria O12.24
        - proteinuria O12.14
      - gonorrhea O98.22
      - hematoma O71.7
        - ischial spine O71.7
        - pelvic O71.7
        - vagina O71.7
        - vulva or perineum O71.7
      - hemorrhage (uterine) O67.9
        - associated with
          - afibrinogenemia O67.Ø
          - coagulation defect O67.Ø
          - hyperfibrinolysis O67.Ø
          - hypofibrinogenemia O67.Ø
        - due to
          - low implantation of placenta O44.5-●
          - low-lying placenta O44.5-●
          - placenta previa O44.1-●
            - marginal O44.3-●
            - partial O44.3-●
          - premature separation of placenta (normally implanted) (*see also* Abruptio placentae) O45.9-●
          - retained placenta O72.Ø
          - uterine leiomyoma O67.8
        - placenta NEC O67.8
        - postpartum NEC (atonic) (immediate) O72.1
          - with retained or trapped placenta O72.Ø
          - delayed O72.2
          - secondary O72.2
          - third stage O72.Ø

- Delivery *(Continued)*
  - complicated *(Continued)*
    - by *(Continued)*
      - hourglass contraction, uterus O62.4
      - hypertension, hypertensive (pre-existing) —*see* Hypertension, complicated by, childbirth (labor)
      - hypotension O26.5-●
      - incomplete dilatation (cervix) O62.Ø
      - incoordinate uterus contractions O62.4
      - inertia, uterus O62.2
        - during latent phase of labor O62.Ø
        - primary O62.Ø
        - secondary O62.1
      - infection (maternal) O98.92
        - carrier state NEC O99.834
        - gonorrhea O98.22
        - human immunodeficiency virus (HIV) O98.72
        - sexually transmitted NEC O98.32
        - specified NEC O98.82
        - syphilis O98.12
        - tuberculosis O98.Ø2
        - viral hepatitis O98.42
        - viral NEC O98.52
      - injury (to mother) (*see also* Delivery, complicated, by, damage to) O71.9
        - nonobstetric O9A.22
          - caused by abuse —*see* Delivery, complicated by, abuse
      - intrauterine fetal death, early OØ2.1
      - inversion, uterus O71.2
      - laceration (perineal) O7Ø.9
        - anus (sphincter) O7Ø.4
          - with third degree laceration —*see also* Delivery, complicated, by, laceration, perineum, third degree O7Ø.2Ø
            - with mucosa O7Ø.3
          - without third degree laceration O7Ø.4
        - bladder (urinary) O71.5
        - bowel O71.5
        - cervix (uteri) O71.3
        - fourchette O7Ø.Ø
        - hymen O7Ø.Ø
        - labia O7Ø.Ø
        - pelvic
          - floor O7Ø.1
          - organ NEC O71.5
        - perineum, perineal O7Ø.9
          - first degree O7Ø.Ø
          - fourth degree O7Ø.3
          - muscles O7Ø.1
          - second degree O7Ø.1
          - skin O7Ø.Ø
          - slight O7Ø.Ø
          - third degree O7Ø.2Ø
            - with
              - both external anal sphincter (EAS) and internal anal sphincter (IAS) torn (IIIc) O7Ø.23
              - less than 5Ø% of external anal sphincter (EAS) thickness torn (IIIa) O7Ø.21
              - more than 5Ø% external anal sphincter (EAS) thickness torn (IIIb) O7Ø.22
            - IIIa O7Ø.21
            - IIIb O7Ø.22
            - IIIc O7Ø.23
        - peritoneum (pelvic) O71.5
        - rectovaginal (septum) (without perineal laceration) O71.4
          - with perineum —*see also* Delivery, complicated, by, laceration, perineum, third degree O7Ø.2Ø
            - with anal or rectal mucosa O7Ø.3

- Delivery *(Continued)*
  - complicated *(Continued)*
    - by *(Continued)*
      - laceration *(Continued)*
        - specified NEC O71.89
        - sphincter ani —*see* Delivery, complicated, by, laceration, anus (sphincter)
        - urethra O71.5
        - uterus O71.81
          - before labor O71.81
        - vagina, vaginal (deep) (high) (without perineal laceration) O71.4
          - with perineum O7Ø.Ø
          - muscles, with perineum O7Ø.1
        - vulva O7Ø.Ø
      - liver disorder O26.62
      - malignancy O9A.12
      - malnutrition O25.2
      - malposition, malpresentation
        - without obstruction O32.9 —*see also* Delivery, complicated by, obstruction
          - breech O32.1
          - compound O32.6
          - face (brow) (chin) O32.3
          - footling O38.8
          - high head O32.4
          - oblique O32.2
          - specified NEC O32.8
          - transverse O32.2
          - unstable lie O32.Ø
        - placenta O44.Ø-●
          - with hemorrhage O44.1-●
        - uterus or cervix O65.5
      - meconium in amniotic fluid O77.Ø
      - mental disorder NEC O99.344
      - metrorrhexis —*see* Delivery, complicated by, rupture, uterus
      - nervous system disorder O99.354
      - obesity (pre-existing) O99.214
      - obesity surgery status O99.844
      - obstetric trauma O71.9
        - specified NEC O71.89
      - obstructed labor
        - due to
          - breech (complete) (frank) presentation O64.1
            - incomplete O64.8
          - brow presenation O64.3
          - buttock presentation O64.1
          - chin presentation O64.2
          - compound presentation O64.5
          - contracted pelvis O65.1
          - deep transverse arrest O64.Ø
          - deformed pelvis O65.Ø
          - dystocia (fetal) O66.9
            - due to
              - conjoined twins O66.3
              - fetal
                - abnormality NEC O66.3
                - ascites O66.3
                - hydrops O66.3
                - meningomyelocele O66.3
                - sacral teratoma O66.3
                - tumor O66.3
              - hydrocephalic fetus O66.3
            - shoulder O66.Ø
          - face presentation O64.2
          - fetopelvic disproportion O65.4
          - footling presentation O64.8
          - impacted shoulders O66.Ø
          - incomplete rotation of fetal head O64.Ø
          - large fetus O66.2
          - locked twins O66.1
          - malposition O64.9
            - specified NEC O64.8
          - malpresentation O64.9
            - specified NEC O64.8

Delivery (Continued)
complicated (Continued)
by (Continued)
obstructed labor (Continued)
due to (Continued)
multiple fetuses NEC O66.6
pelvic
abnormality (maternal) O65.9
organ O65.5
specified NEC O65.8
contraction
inlet O65.2
mid-cavity O65.3
outlet O65.3
persistent (position)
occipitoiliac O64.0
occipitoposterior O64.0
occipitosacral O64.0
occipitotransverse O64.0
prolapsed arm O64.4
shoulder presentation O64.4
specified NEC O66.8
pathological retraction ring, uterus O62.4
penetration, pregnant uterus by instrument O71.1
perforation —see Delivery, complicated by, laceration
placenta, placental
ablatio —see also Abruptio placentae O45.9-●
abnormality O43.9-●
specified NEC O43.89-●
abruptio —see also Abruptio placentae O45.9-●
accreta O43.21-●
adherent (with hemorrhage) O72.0
without hemorrhage O73.0
detachment (premature) —see also Abruptio placentae O45.9-●
disorder O43.9-●
specified NEC O43.89-●
hemorrhage NEC O67.8
increta O43.22-●
low (implantation) (lying) O44.4-●
with hemorrhage O44.5-●
malformation O43.10-●
malposition O44.0-●
without hemorrhage O44.1-●
percreta O43.23-●
previa (central) (complete) (lateral) (total) O44.0-●
with hemorrhage O44.1-●
marginal O44.2-●
with hemorrhage O44.3-●
partial O44.2-●
with hemorrhage O44.3-●
retained (with hemorrhage) O72.0
without hemorrhage O73.0
separation (premature) O45.9-●
specified NEC O45.8X-●
vicious insertion O44.1-●
precipitate labor O62.3
premature rupture, membranes (see also Pregnancy, complicated by, premature rupture of membranes) O42.90
prolapse
arm or hand O32.2
cord (umbilical) O69.0
foot or leg O32.8
uterus O34.52-●
prolonged labor O63.9
first stage O63.0
second stage O63.1
protozoal disease (maternal) O98.62
respiratory disease NEC O99.52
retained membranes or portions of placenta O72.2
without hemorrhage O73.1
retarded birth O63.9

Delivery (Continued)
complicated (Continued)
by (Continued)
retention of secundines (with hemorrhage) O72.0
without hemorrhage O73.0
partial O72.2
without hemorrhage O73.1
rupture
bladder (urinary) O71.5
cervix O71.3
pelvic organ NEC O71.5
urethra O71.5
uterus (during or after labor) O71.1
before labor O71.0-●
separation, pubic bone (symphysis pubis) O71.6
shock O75.1
shoulder presentation O64.4
skin disorder NEC O99.72
spasm, cervix O62.4
stenosis or stricture, cervix O65.5
streptococcus group B (GBS) carrier state O99.824
subluxation of symphysis (pubis) O26.72
syphilis (maternal) O98.12
tear —see Delivery, complicated by, laceration
tetanic uterus O62.4
trauma (obstetrical) —see also Delivery, complicated, by, damage to O71.9
non-obstetric O9A.22
periurethral O71.82
specified NEC O71.89
tuberculosis (maternal) O98.02
tumor, pelvic organs or tissues NEC O65.5
umbilical cord around neck
with compression O69.1
without compression O69.81
uterine inertia O62.2
during latent phase of labor O62.0
primary O62.0
secondary O62.1
vasa previa O69.4
velamentous insertion of cord O43.12-●
specified complication NEC O75.89
delayed NOS O63.9
following rupture of membranes
artificial O75.5
second twin, triplet, etc. O63.2
forceps, low following failed vacuum extraction O66.5
missed (at or near term) O36.4
normal O80
obstructed —see Delivery, complicated by, obstructed labor
precipitate O62.3
preterm —see also Pregnancy, complicated by, preterm labor O60.10
spontaneous O80
term pregnancy NOS O80
uncomplicated O80
vaginal, following previous cesarean delivery O34.219
classical (vertical) scar O34.212
low transverse scar O34.211
Delusions (paranoid) —see Disorder, delusional
Dementia (degenerative (primary)) (old age) (persisting) F03.90
with
aggressive behavior F03.91
behavioral disturbance F03.91
combative behavior F03.91
Lewy bodies G31.83 [F02.80]
with behavioral disturbance G31.83 [F02.81]
Parkinson's disease G20 [F02.80]
with behavioral disturbance G20 [F02.81]

Dementia (Continued)
with (Continued)
Parkinsonism G31.83 [F02.80]
with behavioral disturbance G31.83 [F02.81]
violent behavior F03.91
alcoholic F10.97
with dependence F10.27
Alzheimer's type —see Disease, Alzheimer's
arteriosclerotic —see Dementia, vascular
atypical, Alzheimer's type —see Disease, Alzheimer's, specified NEC
congenital —see Disability, intellectual
frontal (lobe) G31.09 [F02.80]
with behavioral disturbance G31.09 [F02.81]
frontotemporal G31.09 [F02.80]
with behavioral disturbance G31.09 [F02.81]
specified NEC G31.09 [F02.80]
with behavioral disturbance G31.09 [F02.81]
in (due to)
alcohol F10.97
with dependence F10.27
Alzheimer's disease —see Disease, Alzheimer's
arteriosclerotic brain disease —see Dementia, vascular
cerebral lipidoses E75.-● [F02.80]
with behavioral disturbance E75.-● [F02.81]
Creutzfeldt-Jakob disease —see also Creutzfeldt-Jakob disease or syndrome (with dementia) A81.00
epilepsy G40.-● [F02.80]
with behavioral disturbance G40.-● [F02.81]
hepatolenticular degeneration E83.01 [F02.80]
with behavioral disturbance E83.01 [F02.81]
human immunodeficiency virus (HIV) disease B20 [F02.80]
with behavioral disturbance B20 [F02.81]
Huntington's disease or chorea G10 [F02.80]
with behavioral disturbance G10 [F02.81]
hypercalcemia E83.52 [F02.80]
with behavioral disturbance E83.52 [F02.81]
hypothyroidism, acquired E03.9 [F02.80]
with behavioral disturbance E03.9 [F02.81]
due to iodine deficiency E01.8 [F02.80]
with behavioral disturbance E01.8 [F02.81]
inhalants F18.97
with dependence F18.27
multiple
etiologies F03
sclerosis G35 [F02.80]
with behavioral disturbance G35 [F02.81]
neurosyphilis A52.17 [F02.80]
with behavioral disturbance A52.17 [F02.81]
juvenile A50.49 [F02.80]
with behavioral disturbance A50.49 [F02.81]
niacin deficiency E52 [F02.80]
with behavioral disturbance E52 [F02.81]
paralysis agitans G20 [F02.80]
with behavioral disturbance G20 [F02.81]
Parkinson's disease G20 [F02.80]
pellagra E52 [F02.80]
with behavioral disturbance E52 [F02.81]
Pick's G31.01 [F02.80]
with behavioral disturbance G31.01 [F02.81]
polyarteritis nodosa M30.0 [F02.80]
with behavioral disturbance M30.0 [F02.81]

Dementia *(Continued)*
in *(Continued)*
psychoactive drug F19.97
with dependence F19.27
inhalants F18.97
with dependence F18.27
sedatives, hypnotics or anxiolytics F13.97
with dependence F13.27
sedatives, hypnotics or anxiolytics F13.97
with dependence F13.27
systemic lupus erythematosus M32.-● *[F02.80]*
with behavioral disturbance M32.-● *[F02.81]*
trypanosomiasis
African B56.9 *[F02.80]*
with behavioral disturbance B56.9 *[F02.81]*
unknown etiology F03
vitamin B12 deficiency E53.8 *[F02.80]*
with behavioral disturbance E53.8 *[F02.81]*
volatile solvents F18.97
with dependence F18.27
infantile, infantilis F84.3
Lewy body G31.83 *[F02.80]*
with behavioral disturbance G31.83 *[F02.81]*
multi-infarct *—see* Dementia, vascular
paralytica, paralytic (syphilitic) A52.17 *[F02.80]*
with behavioral disturbance A52.17 *[F02.81]*
juvenilis A50.45
paretic A52.17
praecox *—see* Schizophrenia
presenile F03
Alzheimer's type *—see* Disease, Alzheimer's, early onset
primary degenerative F03
progressive, syphilitic A52.17
senile F03
with acute confusional state F05
Alzheimer's type *—see* Disease, Alzheimer's, late onset
depressed or paranoid type F03
vascular (acute onset) (mixed) (multi-infarct) (subcortical) F01.50
with behavioral disturbance F01.51
Demineralization, bone *—see* Osteoporosis
Demodex folliculorum (infestation) B88.0
Demophobia F40.248
Demoralization R45.3
Demyelination, demyelinization
central nervous system G37.9
specified NEC G37.8
corpus callosum (central) G37.1
disseminated, acute G36.9
specified NEC G36.8
global G35
in optic neuritis G36.0
Dengue (classical) (fever) A90
hemorrhagic A91
sandfly A93.1
Dennie-Marfan syphilitic syndrome A50.45
Dens evaginatus, in dente or invaginatus K00.2
Dense breasts R92.2
Density
increased, bone (disseminated) (generalized) (spotted) *—see* Disorder, bone, density and structure, specified type NEC
lung (nodular) J98.4
Dental *—see also* condition
examination Z01.20
with abnormal findings Z01.21
restoration
aesthetically inadequate or displeasing K08.56
Dental *(Continued)*
restoration *(Continued)*
defective K08.50
specified NEC K08.59
failure of marginal integrity K08.51
failure of periodontal anatomical integrity K08.54
Dentia praecox K00.6
Denticles (pulp) K04.2
Dentigerous cyst K09.0
Dentin
irregular (in pulp) K04.3
opalescent K00.5
secondary (in pulp) K04.3
sensitive K03.89
Dentinogenesis imperfecta K00.5
Dentinoma *—see* Cyst, calcifying odontogenic
Dentition (syndrome) K00.7
delayed K00.6
difficult K00.7
precocious K00.6
premature K00.6
retarded K00.6
Dependence (on) (syndrome) F19.20
with remission F19.21
alcohol (ethyl) (methyl) (without remission) F10.20
with
amnestic disorder, persisting F10.26
anxiety disorder F10.280
dementia, persisting F10.27
intoxication F10.229
with delirium F10.221
uncomplicated F10.220
mood disorder F10.24
psychotic disorder F10.259
with
delusions F10.250
hallucinations F10.251
remission F10.21
sexual dysfunction F10.281
sleep disorder F10.282
specified disorder NEC F10.288
withdrawal F10.239
with
delirium F10.231
perceptual disturbance F10.232
uncomplicated F10.230
counseling and surveillance Z71.41
amobarbital *—see* Dependence, drug, sedative
amphetamine(s) (type) *—see* Dependence, drug, stimulant NEC
amytal (sodium) *—see* Dependence, drug, sedative
analgesic NEC F55.8
anesthetic (agent) (gas) (general) (local) NEC *—see* Dependence, drug, psychoactive NEC
anxiolytic NEC *—see* Dependence, drug, sedative
barbital(s) *—see* Dependence, drug, sedative
barbiturate(s) (compounds) (drugs classifiable to T42) *—see* Dependence, drug, sedative
benzedrine *—see* Dependence, drug, stimulant NEC
bhang *—see* Dependence, drug, cannabis
bromide(s) NEC *—see* Dependence, drug, sedative
caffeine *—see* Dependence, drug, stimulant NEC
cannabis (sativa) (indica) (resin) (derivatives) (type) *—see* Dependence, drug, cannabis
chloral (betaine) (hydrate) *—see* Dependence, drug, sedative
chlordiazepoxide *—see* Dependence, drug, sedative
coca (leaf) (derivatives) *—see* Dependence, drug, cocaine
cocaine *—see* Dependence, drug, cocaine
Dependence *(Continued)*
codeine *—see* Dependence, drug, opioid
combinations of drugs F19.20
dagga *—see* Dependence, drug, cannabis
demerol *—see* Dependence, drug, opioid
dexamphetamine *—see* Dependence, drug, stimulant NEC
dexedrine *—see* Dependence, drug, stimulant NEC
dextromethorphan *—see* Dependence, drug, opioid
dextromoramide *—see* Dependence, drug, opioid
dextro-nor-pseudo-ephedrine *—see* Dependence, drug, stimulant NEC
dextrorphan *—see* Dependence, drug, opioid
diazepam *—see* Dependence, drug, sedative
dilaudid *—see* Dependence, drug, opioid
D-lysergic acid diethylamide *—see* Dependence, drug, hallucinogen
drug NEC F19.20
with sleep disorder F19.282
cannabis F12.20
with
anxiety disorder F12.280
intoxication F12.229
with
delirium F12.221
perceptual disturbance F12.222
uncomplicated F12.220
other specified disorder F12.288
psychosis F12.259
delusions F12.250
hallucinations F12.251
unspecified disorder F12.29
withdrawal F12.23
in remission F12.21
cocaine F14.20
with
anxiety disorder F14.280
intoxication F14.229
with
delirium F14.221
perceptual disturbance F14.222
uncomplicated F14.220
mood disorder F14.24
other specified disorder F14.288
psychosis F14.259
delusions F14.250
hallucinations F14.251
sexual dysfunction F14.281
sleep disorder F14.282
unspecified disorder F14.29
withdrawal F14.23
in remission F14.21
withdrawal symptoms in newborn P96.1
counseling and surveillance Z71.51
hallucinogen F16.20
with
anxiety disorder F16.280
flashbacks F16.283
intoxication F16.229
with delirium F16.221
uncomplicated F16.220
mood disorder F16.24
other specified disorder F16.288
perception disorder, persisting F16.283
psychosis F16.259
delusions F16.250
hallucinations F16.251
unspecified disorder F16.29
in remission F16.21
in remission F19.21
inhalant F18.20
with
anxiety disorder F18.280
dementia, persisting F18.27
intoxication F18.229
with delirium F18.221
uncomplicated F18.220
mood disorder F18.24

Dependence (Continued)
drug NEC (Continued)
inhalant (Continued)
with (Continued)
other specified disorder F18.288
psychosis F18.259
delusions F18.250
hallucinations F18.251
unspecified disorder F18.29
in remission F18.21
nicotine F17.200
with disorder F17.209
in remission F17.201
specified disorder NEC F17.208
withdrawal F17.203
chewing tobacco F17.220
with disorder F17.229
in remission F17.221
specified disorder NEC F17.228
withdrawal F17.223
cigarettes F17.210
with disorder F17.219
in remission F17.211
specified disorder NEC F17.218
withdrawal F17.213
specified product NEC F17.290
with disorder F17.299
remission F17.291
specified disorder NEC F17.298
withdrawal F17.293
opioid F11.20
with
intoxication F11.229
with
delirium F11.221
perceptual disturbance F11.222
uncomplicated F11.220
mood disorder F11.24
other specified disorder F11.288
psychosis F11.259
delusions F11.250
hallucinations F11.251
sexual dysfunction F11.281
sleep disorder F11.282
unspecified disorder F11.29
withdrawal F11.23
in remission F11.21
psychoactive NEC F19.20
with
amnestic disorder F19.26
anxiety disorder F19.280
dementia F19.27
intoxication F19.229
with
delirium F19.221
perceptual disturbance F19.222
uncomplicated F19.220
mood disorder F19.24
other specified disorder F19.288
psychosis F19.259
delusions F19.250
hallucinations F19.251
sexual dysfunction F19.281
sleep disorder F19.282
unspecified disorder F19.29
withdrawal F19.239
with
delirium F19.231
perceptual disturbance F19.232
uncomplicated F19.230
sedative, hypnotic or anxiolytic F13.20
with
amnestic disorder F13.26
anxiety disorder F13.280
dementia, persisting F13.27
intoxication F13.229
with delirium F13.221
uncomplicated F13.220
mood disorder F13.24
other specified disorder F13.288

Dependence (Continued)
drug NEC (Continued)
sedative, hypnotic or anxiolytic (Continued)
with (Continued)
psychosis F13.259
delusions F13.250
hallucinations F13.251
sexual dysfunction F13.281
sleep disorder F13.282
unspecified disorder F13.29
withdrawal F13.239
with
delirium F13.231
perceptual disturbance F13.232
uncomplicated F13.230
in remission F13.21
stimulant NEC F15.20
with
anxiety disorder F15.280
intoxication F15.229
with
delirium F15.221
perceptual disturbance F15.222
uncomplicated F15.220
mood disorder F15.24
other specified disorder F15.288
psychosis F15.259
delusions F15.250
hallucinations F15.251
sexual dysfunction F15.281
sleep disorder F15.282
unspecified disorder F15.29
withdrawal F15.23
in remission F15.21
ethyl
alcohol (without remission) F10.20
with remission F10.21
bromide —*see* Dependence, drug, sedative
carbamate F19.20
chloride F19.20
morphine —*see* Dependence, drug, opioid
ganja —*see* Dependence, drug, cannabis
glue (airplane) (sniffing) —*see* Dependence, drug, inhalant
glutethimide —*see* Dependence, drug, sedative
hallucinogenics —*see* Dependence, drug, hallucinogen
hashish —*see* Dependence, drug, cannabis
hemp —*see* Dependence, drug, cannabis
heroin (salt) (any) —*see* Dependence, drug, opioid
hypnotic NEC —*see* Dependence, drug, sedative
Indian hemp —*see* Dependence, drug, cannabis
inhalants —*see* Dependence, drug, inhalant
khat —*see* Dependence, drug, stimulant NEC
laudanum —*see* Dependence, drug, opioid
LSD (-25) (derivatives) —*see* Dependence, drug, hallucinogen
luminal —*see* Dependence, drug, sedative
lysergic acid —*see* Dependence, drug, hallucinogen
maconha —*see* Dependence, drug, cannabis
marihuana —*see* Dependence, drug, cannabis
meprobamate —*see* Dependence, drug, sedative
mescaline —*see* Dependence, drug, hallucinogen
methadone —*see* Dependence, drug, opioid
methamphetamine(s) —*see* Dependence, drug, stimulant NEC
methaqualone —*see* Dependence, drug, sedative
methyl
alcohol (without remission) F10.20
with remission F10.21
bromide —*see* Dependence, drug, sedative
morphine —*see* Dependence, drug, opioid

Dependence (Continued)
methyl (Continued)
phenidate —*see* Dependence, drug, stimulant NEC
sulfonal —*see* Dependence, drug, sedative
morphine (sulfate) (sulfite) (type) —*see* Dependence, drug, opioid
narcotic (drug) NEC —*see* Dependence, drug, opioid
nembutal —*see* Dependence, drug, sedative
neraval —*see* Dependence, drug, sedative
neravan —*see* Dependence, drug, sedative
neurobarb —*see* Dependence, drug, sedative
nicotine —*see* Dependence, drug, nicotine
nitrous oxide F19.20
nonbarbiturate sedatives and tranquilizers with similar effect —*see* Dependence, drug, sedative
on
artificial heart (fully implantable) (mechanical) Z95.812
aspirator Z99.0
care provider (because of) Z74.9
impaired mobility Z74.09
need for
assistance with personal care Z74.1
continuous supervision Z74.3
no other household member able to render care Z74.2
specified reason NEC Z74.8
machine Z99.89
enabling NEC Z99.89
specified type NEC Z99.89
renal dialysis (hemodialysis) (peritoneal) Z99.2
respirator Z99.11
ventilator Z99.11
wheelchair Z99.3
opiate —*see* Dependence, drug, opioid
opioids —*see* Dependence, drug, opioid
opium (alkaloids) (derivatives) (tincture) —*see* Dependence, drug, opioid
oxygen (long-term) (supplemental) Z99.81
paraldehyde —*see* Dependence, drug, sedative
paregoric —*see* Dependence, drug, opioid
PCP (phencyclidine) (or related substance) —*see* Dependence, drug, hallucinogen
pentobarbital —*see* Dependence, drug, sedative
pentobarbitone (sodium) —*see* Dependence, drug, sedative
pentothal —*see* Dependence, drug, sedative
peyote —*see* Dependence, drug, hallucinogen
phencyclidine (PCP) (or related substance) —*see* Dependence, drug, hallucinogen
phenmetrazine —*see* Dependence, drug, stimulant NEC
phenobarbital —*see* Dependence, drug, sedative
polysubstance F19.20
psilocibin, psilocin, psilocyn, psilocyline —*see* Dependence, drug, hallucinogen
psychostimulant NEC —*see* Dependence, drug, stimulant NEC
secobarbital —*see* Dependence, drug, sedative
seconal —*see* Dependence, drug, sedative
sedative NEC —*see* Dependence, drug, sedative
specified drug NEC —*see* Dependence, drug
stimulant NEC —*see* Dependence, drug, stimulant NEC
substance NEC —*see* Dependence, drug
supplemental oxygen Z99.81
tobacco —*see* Dependence, drug, nicotine
counseling and surveillance Z71.6
tranquilizer NEC —*see* Dependence, drug, sedative
vitamin B6 E53.1
volatile solvents —*see* Dependence, drug, inhalant

D

Dependency
care-provider Z74.9
passive F60.7
reactions (persistent) F60.7
Depersonalization (in neurotic state) (neurotic) (syndrome) F48.1
Depletion
extracellular fluid E86.9
plasma E86.1
potassium E87.6
nephropathy N25.89
salt or sodium E87.1
causing heat exhaustion or prostration T67.4
nephropathy N28.9
volume NOS E86.9
Deployment (current) (military) status Z56.82
in theater or in support of military war, peacekeeping and humanitarian operations Z56.82
personal history of Z91.82
military war, peacekeeping and humanitarian deployment (current or past conflict) Z91.82
returned from Z91.82
Depolarization, premature I49.40
atrial I49.1
junctional I49.2
specified NEC I49.49
ventricular I49.3
Deposit
bone in Boeck's sarcoid D86.89
calcareous, calcium —*see* Calcification
cholesterol
retina H35.89
vitreous (body) (humor) —*see* Deposit, crystalline
conjunctiva H11.11-●
cornea H18.00-●
argentous H18.02-●
due to metabolic disorder H18.03-●
Kayser-Fleischer ring H18.04-●
pigmentation —*see* Pigmentation, cornea
crystalline, vitreous (body) (humor) H43.2-●
hemosiderin in old scars of cornea —*see* Pigmentation, cornea, stromal
metallic in lens —*see* Cataract, specified NEC
skin R23.8
tooth, teeth (betel) (black) (green) (materia alba) (orange) (tobacco) K03.6
urate, kidney —*see* Calculus, kidney
Depraved appetite —*see* Pica
Depressed
HDL cholesterol E78.6
Depression (acute) (mental) F32.9
agitated (single episode) F32.2
anaclitic —*see* Disorder, adjustment
anxiety F41.8
persistent F34.1
arches —*see also* Deformity, limb, flat foot
atypical (single episode) F32.89
recurrent episode F33.8
basal metabolic rate R94.8
bone marrow D75.89
central nervous system R09.2
cerebral R29.818
newborn P91.4
cerebrovascular I67.9
chest wall M95.4
climacteric (single episode) F32.89
recurrent episode F33.8
endogenous (without psychotic symptoms) F33.2
with psychotic symptoms F33.3
functional activity R68.89
hysterical F44.89
involutional (single episode) F32.89
recurrent episode F33.8
major F32.9
with psychotic symptoms F32.3
recurrent —*see* Disorder, depressive, recurrent
Depression *(Continued)*
manic-depressive —*see* Disorder, depressive, recurrent
masked (single episode) F32.89
medullary G93.89
menopausal (single episode) F32.89
recurrent episode F33.8
metatarsus —*see* Depression, arches
monopolar F33.9
nervous F34.1
neurotic F34.1
nose M95.0
postnatal (NOS) F53.0
postpartum (NOS) F53.0
post-psychotic of schizophrenia F32.89
post-schizophrenic F32.89
psychogenic (reactive) (single episode) F32.9
psychoneurotic F34.1
psychotic (single episode) F32.3
recurrent F33.3
reactive (psychogenic) (single episode) F32.9
psychotic (single episode) F32.3
recurrent —*see* Disorder, depressive, recurrent
respiratory center G93.89
seasonal —*see* Disorder, depressive, recurrent
senile F03
severe, single episode F32.2
situational F43.21
skull Q67.4
specified NEC (single episode) F32.89
sternum M95.4
visual field —*see* Defect, visual field
vital (recurrent) (without psychotic symptoms) F33.2
with psychotic symptoms F33.3
single episode F32.2
Deprivation
cultural Z60.3
effects NOS T73.9
specified NEC T73.8
emotional NEC Z65.8
affecting infant or child —*see* Maltreatment, child, psychological
food T73.0
protein —*see* Malnutrition
sleep Z72.820
social Z60.4
affecting infant or child —*see* Maltreatment, child, psychological
specified NEC T73.8
vitamins —*see* Deficiency, vitamin
water T73.1
Derangement
ankle (internal) —*see* Derangement, joint, ankle
cartilage (articular) NEC —*see* Derangement, joint, articular cartilage, by site
recurrent —*see* Dislocation, recurrent
cruciate ligament, anterior, current injury —*see* Sprain, knee, cruciate, anterior
elbow (internal) —*see* Derangement, joint, elbow
hip (joint) (internal) (old) —*see* Derangement, joint, hip
joint (internal) M24.9
ankylosis —*see* Ankylosis
articular cartilage M24.10
ankle M24.17-●
elbow M24.12-●
foot M24.17-●
hand M24.14-●
hip M24.15-●
knee NEC M23.9-●
loose body —*see* Loose, body
shoulder M24.11-●
wrist M24.13-●
contracture —*see* Contraction, joint
current injury —*see also* Dislocation
knee, meniscus or cartilage —*see* Tear, meniscus
Derangement *(Continued)*
joint *(Continued)*
dislocation
pathological —*see* Dislocation, pathological
recurrent —*see* Dislocation, recurrent
knee —*see* Derangement, knee
ligament —*see* Disorder, ligament
loose body —*see* Loose, body
recurrent —*see* Dislocation, recurrent
specified type NEC M24.80
ankle M24.87-●
elbow M24.82-●
foot joint M24.87-●
hand joint M24.84-●
hip M24.85-●
shoulder M24.81-●
wrist M24.83-●
temporomandibular M26.69
knee (recurrent) M23.9-●
ligament disruption, spontaneous M23.60-●
anterior cruciate M23.61-●
capsular M23.67-●
instability, chronic M23.5-●
lateral collateral M23.64-●
medial collateral M23.63-●
posterior cruciate M23.62-●
loose body M23.4-●
meniscus M23.30-●
cystic M23.00-●
lateral M23.002
anterior horn M23.04-●
posterior horn M23.05-●
specified NEC M23.06-●
medial M23.005
anterior horn M23.01-●
posterior horn M23.02-●
specified NEC M23.03-●
degenerate —*see* Derangement, knee, meniscus, specified NEC
detached —*see* Derangement, knee, meniscus, specified NEC
due to old tear or injury M23.20-●
lateral M23.20-●
anterior horn M23.24-●
posterior horn M23.25-●
specified NEC M23.26-●
medial M23.20-●
anterior horn M23.21-●
posterior horn M23.22-●
specified NEC M23.23-●
retained —*see* Derangement, knee, meniscus, specified NEC
specified NEC M23.30-●
lateral M23.30-●
anterior horn M23.34-●
posterior horn M23.35-●
specified NEC M23.36-●
medial M23.30-●
anterior horn M23.31-●
posterior horn M23.32-●
specified NEC M23.33-●
old M23.8X-●
specified NEC —*see* subcategory M23.8
low back NEC —*see* Dorsopathy, specified NEC
meniscus —*see* Derangement, knee, meniscus
mental —*see* Psychosis
patella, specified NEC —*see* Disorder, patella, derangement NEC
semilunar cartilage (knee) —*see* Derangement, knee, meniscus, specified NEC
shoulder (internal) —*see* Derangement, joint, shoulder
Dercum's disease E88.2
Derealization (neurotic) F48.1
Dermal —*see* condition
Dermaphytid —*see* Dermatophytosis

- Dermatitis (eczematous) L3Ø.9
  - ab igne L59.Ø
  - acarine B88.Ø
  - actinic (due to sun) L57.8
    - other than from sun L59.8
  - allergic —*see* Dermatitis, contact, allergic
  - ambustionis, due to burn or scald —*see* Burn
  - amebic AØ6.7
  - ammonia L22
  - arsenical (ingested) L27.8
  - artefacta L98.1
    - psychogenic F54
  - atopic L2Ø.9
    - psychogenic F54
    - specified NEC L2Ø.89
  - autoimmune progesterone L3Ø.8
  - berlock, berloque L56.2
  - blastomycotic B4Ø.3
  - blister beetle L24.89
  - bullous, bullosa L13.9
    - mucosynechial, atrophic L12.1
    - seasonal L3Ø.8
    - specified NEC L13.8
  - calorica L59.Ø
    - due to burn or scald —*see* Burn
  - caterpillar L24.89
  - cercarial B65.3
  - combustionis L59.Ø
    - due to burn or scald —*see* Burn
  - congelationis T69.1
  - contact (occupational) L25.9
    - allergic L23.9
      - due to
        - adhesives L23.1
        - cement L23.5
        - chemical products NEC L23.5
        - chromium L23.Ø
        - cosmetics L23.2
        - dander (cat) (dog) L23.81
        - drugs in contact with skin L23.3
        - dyes L23.4
        - food in contact with skin L23.6
        - hair (cat) (dog) L23.81
        - insecticide L23.5
        - metals L23.Ø
        - nickel L23.Ø
        - plants, non-food L23.7
        - plastic L23.5
        - rubber L23.5
        - specified agent NEC L23.89
    - due to
      - cement L25.3
      - chemical products NEC L25.3
      - cosmetics L25.Ø
      - dander (cat) (dog) L23.81
      - drugs in contact with skin L25.1
      - dyes L25.2
      - food in contact with skin L25.4
      - hair (cat) (dog) L23.81
      - plants, non-food L25.5
      - specified agent NEC L25.8
    - irritant L24.9
      - due to
        - cement L24.5
        - chemical products NEC L24.5
        - cosmetics L24.3
        - detergents L24.Ø
        - drugs in contact with skin L24.4
        - food in contact with skin L24.6
        - oils and greases L24.1
        - plants, non-food L24.7
        - solvents L24.2
        - specified agent NEC L24.89
  - contusiformis L52
  - diabetic —*see* EØ8-E13 with .62Ø
  - diaper L22
  - diphtheritica A36.3
  - dry skin L85.3
  - due to
    - acetone (contact) (irritant) L24.2
    - acids (contact) (irritant) L24.5

- Dermatitis *(Continued)*
  - due to *(Continued)*
    - adhesive(s) (allergic) (contact) (plaster) L23.1
      - irritant L24.5
    - alcohol (irritant) (skin contact) (substances in category T51) L24.2
      - taken internally L27.8
    - alkalis (contact) (irritant) L24.5
    - arsenic (ingested) L27.8
    - carbon disulfide (contact) (irritant) L24.2
    - caustics (contact) (irritant) L24.5
    - cement (contact) L25.3
    - cereal (ingested) L27.2
    - chemical(s) NEC L25.3
      - taken internally L27.8
    - chlorocompounds L24.2
    - chromium (contact) (irritant) L24.81
    - coffee (ingested) L27.2
    - cold weather L3Ø.8
    - cosmetics (contact) L25.Ø
      - allergic L23.2
      - irritant L24.3
    - cyclohexanes L24.2
    - dander (cat) (dog) L23.81
    - Demodex species B88.Ø
    - Dermanyssus gallinae B88.Ø
    - detergents (contact) (irritant) L24.Ø
    - dichromate L24.81
    - drugs and medicaments (generalized) (internal use) L27.Ø
      - external —*see* Dermatitis, due to, drugs, in contact with skin
      - in contact with skin L25.1
        - allergic L23.3
        - irritant L24.4
      - localized skin eruption L27.1
      - specified substance —*see* Table of Drugs and Chemicals
    - dyes (contact) L25.2
      - allergic L23.4
      - irritant L24.89
    - epidermophytosis —*see* Dermatophytosis
    - esters L24.2
    - external irritant NEC L24.9
    - fish (ingested) L27.2
    - flour (ingested) L27.2
    - food (ingested) L27.2
      - in contact with skin L25.4
    - fruit (ingested) L27.2
    - furs (allergic) (contact) L23.81
    - glues —*see* Dermatitis, due to, adhesives
    - glycols L24.2
    - greases NEC (contact) (irritant) L24.1
    - hair (cat) (dog) L23.81
    - hot
      - objects and materials —*see* Burn
      - weather or places L59.Ø
    - hydrocarbons L24.2
    - infrared rays L59.8
    - ingestion, ingested substance L27.9
      - chemical NEC L27.8
      - drugs and medicaments —*see* Dermatitis, due to, drugs
      - food L27.2
      - specified NEC L27.8
    - insecticide in contact with skin L24.5
    - internal agent L27.9
      - drugs and medicaments (generalized) —*see* Dermatitis, due to, drugs
      - food L27.2
    - irradiation —*see* Dermatitis, due to, radioactive substance
    - ketones L24.2
    - lacquer tree (allergic) (contact) L23.7
    - light (sun) NEC L57.8
      - acute L56.8
      - other L59.8
    - Liponyssoides sanguineus B88.Ø
    - low temperature L3Ø.8
    - meat (ingested) L27.2

- Dermatitis *(Continued)*
  - due to *(Continued)*
    - metals, metal salts (contact) (irritant) L24.81
    - milk (ingested) L27.2
    - nickel (contact) (irritant) L24.81
    - nylon (contact) (irritant) L24.5
    - oils NEC (contact) (irritant) L24.1
    - paint solvent (contact) (irritant) L24.2
    - petroleum products (contact) (irritant) (substances in T52) L24.2
    - plants NEC (contact) L25.5
      - allergic L23.7
      - irritant L24.7
    - plasters (adhesive) (any) (allergic) (contact) L23.1
      - irritant L24.5
    - plastic (contact) L25.3
    - preservatives (contact) —*see* Dermatitis, due to, chemical, in contact with skin
    - primrose (allergic) (contact) L23.7
    - primula (allergic) (contact) L23.7
    - radiation L59.8
      - nonionizing (chronic exposure) L57.8
      - sun NEC L57.8
        - acute L56.8
    - radioactive substance L58.9
      - acute L58.Ø
      - chronic L58.1
    - radium L58.9
      - acute L58.Ø
      - chronic L58.1
    - ragweed (allergic) (contact) L23.7
    - Rhus (allergic) (contact) (diversiloba) (radicans) (toxicodendron) (venenata) (verniciflua) L23.7
    - rubber (contact) L24.5
    - Senecio jacobaea (allergic) (contact) L23.7
    - solvents (contact) (irritant) (substances in categories T52) L24.2
    - specified agent NEC (contact) L25.8
      - allergic L23.89
      - irritant L24.89
    - sunshine NEC L57.8
      - acute L56.8
    - tetrachlorethylene (contact) (irritant) L24.2
    - toluene (contact) (irritant) L24.2
    - turpentine (contact) L24.2
    - ultraviolet rays (sun NEC) (chronic exposure) L57.8
      - acute L56.8
    - vaccine or vaccination L27.Ø
      - specified substance —*see* Table of Drugs and Chemicals
    - varicose veins —*see* Varix, leg, with, inflammation
    - X-rays L58.9
      - acute L58.Ø
      - chronic L58.1
  - dyshydrotic L3Ø.1
  - dysmenorrheica N94.6
  - escharotica —*see* Burn
  - exfoliative, exfoliativa (generalized) L26
    - neonatorum LØØ
  - eyelid —*see also* Dermatosis, eyelid
    - allergic HØ1.119
      - left HØ1.116
        - lower HØ1.115
        - upper HØ1.114
      - right HØ1.113
        - lower HØ1.112
        - upper HØ1.111
    - contact —*see* Dermatitis, eyelid, allergic
    - due to
      - Demodex species B88.Ø
      - herpes (zoster) BØ2.39
        - simplex BØØ.59

Dermatitis *(Continued)*
- eyelid *(Continued)*
  - eczematous H01.139
    - left H01.136
      - lower H01.135
      - upper H01.134
    - right H01.133
      - lower H01.132
      - upper H01.131
- facta, factitia, factitial L98.1
  - psychogenic F54
- flexural NEC L20.82
- friction L30.4
- fungus B36.9
  - specified type NEC B36.8
- gangrenosa, gangrenous infantum L08.0
- harvest mite B88.0
- heat L59.0
- herpesviral, vesicular (ear) (lip) B00.1
- herpetiformis (bullous) (erythematous) (pustular) (vesicular) L13.0
  - juvenile L12.2
  - senile L12.0
- hiemalis L30.8
- hypostatic, hypostatica *—see* Varix, leg, with, inflammation
- infectious eczematoid L30.3
- infective L30.3
- irritant *—see* Dermatitis, contact, irritant
- Jacquet's (diaper dermatitis) L22
- Leptus B88.0
- lichenified NEC L28.0
- medicamentosa (generalized) (internal use) *—see* Dermatitis, due to drugs
- mite B88.0
- multiformis L13.0
  - juvenile L12.2
- napkin L22
- neurotica L13.0
- nummular L30.0
- papillaris capillitii L73.0
- pellagrous E52
- perioral L71.0
- photocontact L56.2
- polymorpha dolorosa L13.0
- pruriginosa L13.0
- pruritic NEC L30.8
- psychogenic F54
- purulent L08.0
- pustular
  - contagious B08.02
  - subcorneal L13.1
- pyococcal L08.0
- pyogenica L08.0
- repens L40.2
- Ritter's (exfoliativa) L00
- Schamberg's L81.7
- schistosome B65.3
- seasonal bullous L30.8
- seborrheic L21.9
  - infantile L21.1
  - specified NEC L21.8
- sensitization NOS L23.9
- septic L08.0
- solare L57.8
- specified NEC L30.8
- stasis I87.2
  - with
    - varicose ulcer *—see* Varix, leg, with ulcer, with inflammation
    - varicose veins *—see* Varix, leg, with, inflammation
  - due to postthrombotic syndrome *—see* Syndrome, postthrombotic
- suppurative L08.0
- traumatic NEC L30.4
- trophoneurotica L13.0
- ultraviolet (sun) (chronic exposure) L57.8
  - acute L56.8
- varicose *—see* Varix, leg, with, inflammation
- vegetans L10.1

Dermatitis *(Continued)*
- verrucosa B43.0
- vesicular, herpesviral B00.1

Dermatoarthritis, lipoid E78.81

Dermatochalasis, eyelid H02.839
- left H02.836
  - lower H02.835
  - upper H02.834
- right H02.833
  - lower H02.832
  - upper H02.831

Dermatofibroma (lenticulare) *—see* Neoplasm, skin, benign
- protuberans *—see* Neoplasm, skin, uncertain behavior

Dermatofibrosarcoma (pigmented) (protuberans) *—see* Neoplasm, skin, malignant

Dermatographia L50.3

Dermatolysis (exfoliativa) (congenital) Q82.8
- acquired L57.4
- eyelids *—see* Blepharochalasis
- palpebrarum *—see* Blepharochalasis
- senile L57.4

Dermatomegaly NEC Q82.8

Dermatomucosomyositis M33.10
- with
  - myopathy M33.12
  - respiratory involvement M33.11
  - specified organ involvement NEC M33.19

Dermatomycosis B36.9
- furfuracea B36.0
- specified type NEC B36.8

Dermatomyositis (acute) (chronic) *—see also* Dermatopolymyositis
- adult *—see also* Dermatomyositis, specified NEC M33.10
- in (due to) neoplastic disease *—see also* Neoplasm D49.9 *[M36.0]*
- juvenile M33.00
  - with
    - myopathy M33.02
    - respiratory involvement M33.01
    - specified organ involvement NEC M33.09
  - without myopathy M33.03
- specified NEC M33.10
  - with
    - myopathy M33.12
    - respiratory involvement M33.11
    - specified organ involvement NEC M33.19
  - without myopathy M33.13

Dermatoneuritis of children *—see* Poisoning, mercury

Dermatophilosis A48.8

Dermatophytid L30.2

Dermatophytide *—see* Dermatophytosis

Dermatophytosis (epidermophyton) (infection) (Microsporum) (tinea) (Trichophyton) B35.9
- beard B35.0
- body B35.4
- capitis B35.0
- corporis B35.4
- deep-seated B35.8
- disseminated B35.8
- foot B35.3
- granulomatous B35.8
- groin B35.6
- hand B35.2
- nail B35.1
- perianal (area) B35.6
- scalp B35.0
- specified NEC B35.8

Dermatopolymyositis M33.90
- with
  - myopathy M33.92
  - respiratory involvement M33.91
  - specified organ involvement NEC M33.99
- in neoplastic disease *—see also* Neoplasm D49.9 *[M36.0]*

Dermatopolymyositis *(Continued)*
- juvenile M33.00
  - with
    - myopathy M33.02
    - respiratory involvement M33.01
    - specified organ involvement NEC M33.09
- specified NEC M33.10
  - myopathy M33.12
  - respiratory involvement M33.11
  - specified organ involvement NEC M33.19
- without myopathy M33.93

Dermatopolyneuritis *—see* Poisoning, mercury

Dermatorrhexis (*see also* Syndrome, Ehlers-Danlos) Q79.60
- acquired L57.4

Dermatosclerosis *—see also* Scleroderma
- localized L94.0

Dermatosis L98.9
- Andrews' L08.89
- Bowen's *—see* Neoplasm, skin, in situ
- bullous L13.9
  - specified NEC L13.8
- exfoliativa L26
- eyelid (noninfectious)
  - dermatitis *—see* Dermatitis, eyelid
  - discoid lupus erythematosus *—see* Lupus, erythematosus, eyelid
  - xeroderma *—see* Xeroderma, acquired, eyelid
- factitial L98.1
- febrile neutrophilic L98.2
- gonococcal A54.89
- herpetiformis L13.0
  - juvenile L12.2
- linear IgA L13.8
- menstrual NEC L98.8
- neutrophilic, febrile L98.2
- occupational *—see* Dermatitis, contact
- papulosa nigra L82.1
- pigmentary L81.9
  - progressive L81.7
  - Schamberg's L81.7
- psychogenic F54
- purpuric, pigmented L81.7
- pustular, subcorneal L13.1
- transient acantholytic L11.1

Dermographia, dermographism L50.3

Dermoid (cyst) *—see also* Neoplasm, benign, by site
- with malignant transformation C56-●
- due to radiation (nonionizing) L57.8

Dermopathy
- infiltrative with thyrotoxicosis *—see* Thyrotoxicosis
- nephrogenic fibrosing L90.8

Dermophytosis *—see* Dermatophytosis

Descemetocele H18.73-●

Descemet's membrane *—see* condition

Descending *—see* condition

Descensus uteri *—see* Prolapse, uterus

Desert
- rheumatism B38.0
- sore *—see* Ulcer, skin

Desertion (newborn) *—see* Maltreatment

Desmoid (extra-abdominal) (tumor) *—see* Neoplasm, connective tissue, uncertain behavior
- abdominal D48.1

Despondency F32.9

Desquamation, skin R23.4

Destruction, destructive *—see also* Damage
- articular facet *—see also* Derangement, joint, specified type NEC
  - knee M23.8X-●
  - vertebra *—see* Spondylosis
- bone *—see also* Disorder, bone, specified type NEC
  - syphilitic A52.77
- joint *—see also* Derangement, joint, specified type NEC
  - sacroiliac M53.3
- rectal sphincter K62.89

Destruction, destructive *(Continued)*
septum (nasal) J34.89
tuberculous NEC —*see* Tuberculosis
tympanum, tympanic membrane (nontraumatic) —*see* Disorder, tympanic membrane, specified NEC
vertebral disc —*see* Degeneration, intervertebral disc
Destructiveness —*see also* Disorder, conduct
adjustment reaction —*see* Disorder, adjustment
Desultory labor O62.2
Detachment
cartilage —*see* Sprain
cervix, annular N88.8
complicating delivery O71.3
choroid (old) (postinfectional) (simple) (spontaneous) H31.40-●
hemorrhagic H31.41-●
serous H31.42-●
ligament —*see* Sprain
meniscus (knee) —*see also* Derangement, knee, meniscus, specified NEC
current injury —*see* Tear, meniscus
due to old tear or injury —*see* Derangement, knee, meniscus, due to old tear
retina (without retinal break) (serous) H33.2-●
with retinal:
break H33.00-●
giant H33.03-●
multiple H33.02-●
single H33.01-●
dialysis H33.04-●
pigment epithelium —*see* Degeneration, retina, separation of layers, pigment epithelium detachment
rhegmatogenous —*see* Detachment, retina, with retinal, break
specified NEC H33.8
total H33.05-●
traction H33.4-●
vitreous (body) H43.81
Detergent asthma J69.8
Deterioration
epileptic F06.8
general physical R53.81
heart, cardiac —*see* Degeneration, myocardial
mental —*see* Psychosis
myocardial, myocardium —*see* Degeneration, myocardial
senile (simple) R54
Deuteranomaly (anomalous trichromat) H53.53
Deuteranopia (complete) (incomplete) H53.53
Development
abnormal, bone Q79.9
arrested R62.50
bone —*see* Arrest, development or growth, bone
child R62.50
due to malnutrition E45
defective, congenital —*see also* Anomaly, by site
cauda equina Q06.3
left ventricle Q24.8
in hypoplastic left heart syndrome Q23.4
valve Q24.8
pulmonary Q22.3
delayed (*see also* Delay, development) R62.50
arithmetical skills F81.2
language (skills) (expressive) F80.1
learning skill F81.9
mixed skills F88
motor coordination F82
reading F81.0
specified learning skill NEC F81.89
speech F80.9
spelling F81.81
written expression F81.81
Development *(Continued)*
imperfect, congenital —*see also* Anomaly, by site
heart Q24.9
lungs Q33.6
incomplete
bronchial tree Q32.4
organ or site not listed —*see* Hypoplasia, by site
respiratory system Q34.9
sexual, precocious NEC E30.1
tardy, mental (*see also* Disability, intellectual) F79
Developmental —*see* condition
testing, infant or child —*see* Examination, child
Devergie's disease (pityriasis rubra pilaris) L44.0
Deviation (in)
conjugate palsy (eye) (spastic) H51.0
esophagus (acquired) K22.8
eye, skew H51.8
midline (jaw) (teeth) (dental arch) M26.29
specified site NEC —*see* Malposition
nasal septum J34.2
congenital Q67.4
opening and closing of the mandible M26.53
organ or site, congenital NEC —*see* Malposition, congenital
septum (nasal) (acquired) J34.2
congenital Q67.4
sexual F65.9
bestiality F65.89
erotomania F52.8
exhibitionism F65.2
fetishism, fetishistic F65.0
transvestism F65.1
frotteurism F65.81
masochism F65.51
multiple F65.89
necrophilia F65.89
nymphomania F52.8
pederosis F65.4
pedophilia F65.4
sadism, sadomasochism F65.52
satyriasis F52.8
specified type NEC F65.89
transvestism F64.1
voyeurism F65.3
teeth, midline M26.29
trachea J39.8
ureter, congenital Q62.61
Device
cerebral ventricle (communicating) in situ Z98.2
contraceptive —*see* Contraceptive, device
drainage, cerebrospinal fluid, in situ Z98.2
Devic's disease G36.0
Devil's
grip B33.0
pinches (purpura simplex) D69.2
Devitalized tooth K04.99
Devonshire colic —*see* Poisoning, lead
Dextraposition, aorta Q20.3
in tetralogy of Fallot Q21.3
Dextrinosis, limit (debrancher enzyme deficiency) E74.03
Dextrocardia (true) Q24.0
with
complete transposition of viscera Q89.3
situs inversus Q89.3
Dextrotransposition, aorta Q20.3
d-glycericacidemia E72.59
Dhat syndrome F48.8
Dhobi itch B35.6
Di George's syndrome D82.1
Di Guglielmo's disease C94.0-●
Diabetes, diabetic (mellitus) (sugar) E11.9
with
amyotrophy E11.44
arthropathy NEC E11.618
Diabetes, diabetic *(Continued)*
with *(Continued)*
autonomic (poly)neuropathy E11.43
cataract E11.36
Charcot's joints E11.610
chronic kidney disease E11.22
circulatory complication NEC E11.59
complication E11.8
specified NEC E11.69
dermatitis E11.620
foot ulcer E11.621
gangrene E11.52
gastroparalysis E11.43
gastroparesis E11.43
glomerulonephrosis, intracapillary E11.21
glomerulosclerosis, intercapillary E11.21
hyperglycemia E11.65
hyperosmolarity E11.00
with coma E11.01
hypoglycemia E11.649
with coma E11.641
ketoacidosis E11.10
with coma E11.11
kidney complications NEC E11.29
Kimmelsteil-Wilson disease E11.21
loss of protective sensation (LOPS) —*see* Diabetes, by type, with neuropathy
mononeuropathy E11.41
myasthenia E11.44
necrobiosis lipoidica E11.620
nephropathy E11.21
neuralgia E11.42
neurologic complication NEC E11.49
neuropathic arthropathy E11.610
neuropathy E11.40
ophthalmic complication NEC E11.39
oral complication NEC E11.638
osteomyelitis E11.69
periodontal disease E11.630
peripheral angiopathy E11.51
with gangrene E11.52
polyneuropathy E11.42
renal complication NEC E11.29
renal tubular degeneration E11.29
retinopathy E11.319
with macular edema E11.311
resolved following treatment E11.37
nonproliferative E11.329
with macular edema E11.321
mild E11.329
with macular edema E11.321
moderate E11.339
with macular edema E11.331
severe E11.349
with macular edema E11.341
proliferative E11.359
with
combined traction retinal detachment and rhegmatogenous retinal detachment E11.354
macular edema E11.351
stable proliferative diabetic retinopathy E11.355
traction retinal detachment involving the macula E11.352
traction retinal detachment not involving the macula E11.353
skin complication NEC E11.628
skin ulcer NEC E11.622
brittle —*see* Diabetes, type 1
bronzed E83.110
complicating pregnancy —*see* Pregnancy, complicated by, diabetes
dietary counseling and surveillance Z71.3
due to
autoimmune process —*see* Diabetes, type 1
immune mediated pancreatic islet beta-cell destruction —*see* Diabetes, type 1

Diabetes, diabetic *(Continued)*
  due to drug or chemical EØ9.9
    with
      amyotrophy EØ9.44
      arthropathy NEC EØ9.618
      autonomic (poly)neuropathy EØ9.43
      cataract EØ9.36
      Charcot's joints EØ9.61Ø
      chronic kidney disease EØ9.22
      circulatory complication NEC EØ9.59
      complication EØ9.8
        specified NEC EØ9.69
      dermatitis EØ9.62Ø
      foot ulcer EØ9.621
      gangrene EØ9.52
      gastroparalysis EØ9.43
      gastroparesis EØ9.43
      glomerulonephrosis, intracapillary EØ9.21
      glomerulosclerosis, intercapillary EØ9.21
      hyperglycemia EØ9.65
      hyperosmolarity EØ9.ØØ
        with coma EØ9.Ø1
      hypoglycemia EØ9.649
        with coma EØ9.641
      ketoacidosis EØ9.1Ø
        with coma EØ9.11
      kidney complications NEC EØ9.29
      Kimmelsteil-Wilson disease EØ9.21
      mononeuropathy EØ9.41
      myasthenia EØ9.44
      necrobiosis lipoidica EØ9.62Ø
      nephropathy EØ9.21
      neuralgia EØ9.42
      neurologic complication NEC EØ9.49
      neuropathic arthropathy EØ9.61Ø
      neuropathy EØ9.4Ø
      ophthalmic complication NEC EØ9.39
      oral complication NEC EØ9.638
      periodontal disease EØ9.63Ø
      peripheral angiopathy EØ9.51
        with gangrene EØ9.52
      polyneuropathy EØ9.42
      renal complication NEC EØ9.29
      renal tubular degeneration EØ9.29
      retinopathy EØ9.319
        with macular edema EØ9.311
          resolved following treatment EØ9.37
        nonproliferative EØ9.329
          with macular edema EØ9.321
          mild EØ9.329
            with macular edema EØ9.321
          moderate EØ9.339
            with macular edema EØ9.331
          severe EØ9.349
            with macular edema EØ9.341
        proliferative EØ9.359
          with
            combined traction retinal detachment and rhegmatogenous retinal detachment EØ9.354
            macular edema EØ9.351
            stable proliferative diabetic retinopathy EØ9.355
            traction retinal detachment involving the macula EØ9.352
            traction retinal detachment not involving the macula EØ9.353
      skin complication NEC EØ9.628
      skin ulcer NEC EØ9.622
  due to underlying condition EØ8.9
    with
      amyotrophy EØ8.44
      arthropathy NEC EØ8.618
      autonomic (poly)neuropathy EØ8.43
      cataract EØ8.36
      Charcot's joints EØ8.61Ø

Diabetes, diabetic *(Continued)*
  due to underlying condition *(Continued)*
    with *(Continued)*
      chronic kidney disease EØ8.22
      circulatory complication NEC EØ8.59
      complication EØ8.8
        specified NEC EØ8.69
      dermatitis EØ8.62Ø
      foot ulcer EØ8.621
      gangrene EØ8.52
      gastroparalysis EØ8.43
      gastroparesis EØ8.43
      glomerulonephrosis, intracapillary EØ8.21
      glomerulosclerosis, intercapillary EØ8.21
      hyperglycemia EØ8.69
      hyperosmolarity EØ8.ØØ
        with coma EØ8.Ø1
      hypoglycemia EØ8.649
        with coma EØ8.641
      ketoacidosis EØ8.1Ø
        with coma EØ8.11
      kidney complications NEC EØ8.29
      Kimmelsteil-WIlson disease EØ8.21
      mononeuropathy EØ8.41
      myasthenia EØ8.44
      necrobiosis lipoidica EØ8.62Ø
      nephropathy EØ8.21
      neuralgia EØ8.42
      neurologic complication NEC EØ8.49
      neuropathic arthropathy EØ8.61Ø
      neuropathy EØ8.4Ø
      ophthalmic complication NEC EØ8.39
      oral complication NEC EØ8.638
      periodontal disease EØ8.63Ø
      peripheral angiopathy EØ8.51
        with gangrene EØ8.52
      polyneuropathy EØ8.42
      renal complication NEC EØ8.29
      renal tubular degeneration EØ8.29
      retinopathy EØ8.319
        with macular edema EØ8.311
          resolved following treatment EØ8.37
        nonproliferative EØ8.329
          with macular edema EØ8.321
          mild EØ8.329
            with macular edema EØ8.321
          moderate EØ8.339
            with macular edema EØ8.331
          severe EØ8.349
            with macular edema EØ8.341
        proliferative EØ8.359
          with
            combined traction retinal detachment and rhegmatogenous retinal detachment EØ8.354
            macular edema EØ8.351
            stable proliferative diabetic retinopathy EØ8.355
            traction retinal detachment involving the macula EØ8.352
            traction retinal detachment not involving the macula EØ8.353
      skin complication NEC EØ8.628
      skin ulcer NEC EØ8.622
  gestational (in pregnancy) O24.419
    affecting newborn P7Ø.Ø
    diet-controlled O24.41Ø
    in childbirth O24.429
      diet-controlled O24.42Ø
      insulin (and diet) controlled O24.424
      oral drug controlled (antidiabetic) (hypoglycemic) O24.425
    insulin (and diet) controlled O24.414
    oral drug controlled (antidiabetic) (hypoglycemic) O24.415

Diabetes, diabetic *(Continued)*
  gestational (in pregnancy) *(Continued)*
    puerperal O24.439
      diet-controlled O24.43Ø
      insulin (and diet) controlled O24.434
      oral drug controlled (antidiabetic) (hypoglycemic) O24.435
  hepatogenous E13.9
  idiopathic —*see* Diabetes, type 1
  inadequately controlled — code to Diabetes, by type, with hyperglycemia
  insipidus E23.2
    nephrogenic N25.1
    pituitary E23.2
    vasopressin resistant N25.1
  insulin dependent — code to type of diabetes
  juvenile-onset —*see* Diabetes, type 1
  ketosis-prone —*see* Diabetes, type 1
  latent R73.Ø3
  neonatal (transient) P7Ø.2
  non-insulin dependent — code to type of diabetes
  out of control — code to Diabetes, by type, with hyperglycemia
  phosphate E83.39
  poorly controlled — code to Diabetes, by type, with hyperglycemia
  postpancreatectomy —*see* Diabetes, specified type NEC
  postprocedural —*see* Diabetes, specified type NEC
  secondary diabetes mellitus NEC —*see* Diabetes, specified type NEC
  specified type NEC E13.9
    with
      amyotrophy E13.44
      arthropathy NEC E13.618
      autonomic (poly)neuropathy E13.43
      cataract E13.36
      Charcot's joints E13.61Ø
      chronic kidney disease E13.22
      circulatory complication NEC E13.59
      complication E13.8
        specified NEC E13.69
      dermatitis E13.62Ø
      foot ulcer E13.621
      gangrene E13.52
      gastroparalysis E13.43
      gastroparesis E13.43
      glomerulonephrosis, intracapillary E13.21
      glomerulosclerosis, intercapillary E13.21
      hyperglycemia E13.65
      hyperosmolarity E13.ØØ
        with coma E13.Ø1
      hypoglycemia E13.649
        with coma E13.641
      ketoacidosis E13.1Ø
        with coma E13.11
      kidney complications NEC E13.29
      Kimmelsteil-Wilson disease E13.21
      mononeuropathy E13.41
      myasthenia E13.44
      necrobiosis lipoidica E13.62Ø
      nephropathy E13.21
      neuralgia E13.42
      neurologic complication NEC E13.49
      neuropathic arthropathy E13.61Ø
      neuropathy E13.4Ø
      ophthalmic complication NEC E13.39
      oral complication NEC E13.638
      periodontal disease E13.63Ø
      peripheral angiopathy E13.51
        with gangrene E13.52
      polyneuropathy E13.42
      renal complication NEC E13.29
      renal tubular degeneration E13.29
      retinopathy E13.319
        with macular edema E13.311
          resolved following treatment E13.37

Diabetes, diabetic *(Continued)*
  specified type NEC *(Continued)*
    with *(Continued)*
      retinopathy *(Continued)*
        nonproliferative E13.329
          with macular edema E13.321
          mild E13.329
            with macular edema E13.321
          moderate E13.339
            with macular edema E13.331
          severe E13.349
            with macular edema E13.341
        proliferative E13.359
          with
            combined traction retinal detachment and rhegmatogenous retinal detachment E13.354
            macular edema E13.351
            stable proliferative diabetic retinopathy E13.355
            traction retinal detachment involving the macula E13.352
            traction retinal detachment not involving the macula E13.353
      skin complication NEC E13.628
      skin ulcer NEC E13.622
  steroid-induced —*see* Diabetes, due to, drug or chemical
  type 1 E1Ø.9
    with
      amyotrophy E1Ø.44
      arthropathy NEC E1Ø.618
      autonomic (poly)neuropathy E1Ø.43
      cataract E1Ø.36
      Charcot's joints E1Ø.61Ø
      chronic kidney disease E1Ø.22
      circulatory complication NEC E1Ø.59
      complication E1Ø.8
        specified NEC E1Ø.69
      dermatitis E1Ø.62Ø
      foot ulcer E1Ø.621
      gangrene E1Ø.52
      gastroparalysis E1Ø.43
      gastroparesis E1Ø.43
      glomerulonephrosis, intracapillary E1Ø.21
      glomerulosclerosis, intercapillary E1Ø.21
      hyperglycemia E1Ø.65
      hypoglycemia E1Ø.649
        with coma E1Ø.641
      ketoacidosis E1Ø.1Ø
        with coma E1Ø.11
      kidney complications NEC E1Ø.29
      Kimmelsteil-Wilson disease E1Ø.21
      mononeuropathy E1Ø.41
      myasthenia E1Ø.44
      necrobiosis lipoidica E1Ø.62Ø
      nephropathy E1Ø.21
      neuralgia E1Ø.42
      neurologic complication NEC E1Ø.49
      neuropathic arthropathy E1Ø.61Ø
      neuropathy E1Ø.4Ø
      ophthalmic complication NEC E1Ø.39
      oral complication NEC E1Ø.638
      osteomyelitis E1Ø.69
      periodontal disease E1Ø.63Ø
      peripheral angiopathy E1Ø.51
        with gangrene E1Ø.52
      polyneuropathy E1Ø.42
      renal complication NEC E1Ø.29
      renal tubular degeneration E1Ø.29
      retinopathy E1Ø.319
        with macular edema E1Ø.311
          resolved following treatment E1Ø.37
        nonproliferative E1Ø.329
          with macular edema E1Ø.321
          mild E1Ø.329
            with macular edema E1Ø.321
          moderate E1Ø.339
            with macular edema E1Ø.331

Diabetes, diabetic *(Continued)*
  type 1 *(Continued)*
    with *(Continued)*
      retinopathy *(Continued)*
        nonproliferative *(Continued)*
          severe E1Ø.349
            with macular edema E1Ø.341
        proliferative E1Ø.359
          with
            combined traction retinal detachment and rhegmatogenous retinal detachment E13.354
            macular edema E13.351
            stable proliferative diabetic retinopathy E13.355
            traction retinal detachment involving the macula E13.352
            traction retinal detachment not involving the macula E13.353
      skin complication NEC E1Ø.628
      skin ulcer NEC E1Ø.622
  type 2 E11.9
    with
      amyotrophy E11.44
      arthropathy NEC E11.618
      autonomic (poly)neuropathy E11.43
      cataract E11.36
      Charcot's joints E11.61Ø
      chronic kidney disease E11.22
      circulatory complication NEC E11.59
      complication E11.8
        specified NEC E11.69
      dermatitis E11.62Ø
      foot ulcer E11.621
      gangrene E11.52
      gastroparalysis E11.43
      gastroparesis E11.43
      glomerulonephrosis, intracapillary E11.21
      glomerulosclerosis, intercapillary E11.21
      hyperglycemia E11.65
      hyperosmolarity E11.ØØ
        with coma E11.Ø1
      hypoglycemia E11.649
        with coma E11.641
      ketoacidosis E11.1Ø
        with coma E11.11
      kidney complications NEC E11.29
      Kimmelsteil-Wilson disease E11.21
      mononeuropathy E11.41
      myasthenia E11.44
      necrobiosis lipoidica E11.62Ø
      nephropathy E11.21
      neuralgia E11.42
      neurologic complication NEC E11.49
      neuropathic arthropathy E11.61Ø
      neuropathy E11.4Ø
      ophthalmic complication NEC E11.39
      oral complication NEC E11.638
      osteomyelitis E11.69
      periodontal disease E11.63Ø
      peripheral angiopathy E11.51
        with gangrene E11.52
      polyneuropathy E11.42
      renal complication NEC E11.29
      renal tubular degeneration E11.29
      retinopathy E11.319
        with macular edema E11.311
          resolved following treatment E11.37
        nonproliferative E11.329
          with macular edema E11.321
          mild E11.329
            with macular edema E11.321
          moderate E11.339
            with macular edema E11.331
          severe E11.349
            with macular edema E11.341
        proliferative E11.359
          with
            combined traction retinal detachment and rhegmatogenous retinal detachment E11.354

Diabetes, diabetic *(Continued)*
  type 2 *(Continued)*
    with *(Continued)*
      retinopathy *(Continued)*
        proliferative *(Continued)*
          with *(Continued)*
            macular edema E11.351
            stable proliferative diabetic retinopathy E11.355
            traction retinal detachment involving the macula E11.352
            traction retinal detachment not involving the macula E11.353
      skin complication NEC E11.628
      skin ulcer NEC E11.622
  uncontrolled
    meaning
      hyperglycemia —*see* Diabetes, by type, with, hyperglycemia
      hypoglycemia —*see* Diabetes, by type, with, hypoglycemia
Diacyclothrombopathia D69.1
Diagnosis deferred R69
Dialysis (intermittent) (treatment)
  noncompliance (with) Z91.15
  renal (hemodialysis) (peritoneal), status Z99.2
  retina, retinal —*see* Detachment, retina, with retinal, dialysis
Diamond-Blackfan anemia (congenital hypoplastic) D61.Ø1
Diamond-Gardener syndrome (autoerythrocyte sensitization) D69.2
Diaper rash L22
Diaphoresis (excessive) R61
Diaphragm —*see* condition
Diaphragmalgia RØ7.1
Diaphragmatitis, diaphragmitis J98.6
Diaphysial aclasis Q78.6
Diaphysitis —*see* Osteomyelitis, specified type NEC
Diarrhea, diarrheal (disease) (infantile) (inflammatory) R19.7
  achlorhydric K31.83
  allergic K52.29
    due to
      colitis —*see* Colitis, allergic
      enteritis —*see* Enteritis, allergic
  amebic —*see also* Amebiasis AØ6.Ø
    with abscess —*see* Abscess, amebic
    acute AØ6.Ø
    chronic AØ6.1
    nondysenteric AØ6.2
  bacillary —*see* Dysentery, bacillary
  balantidial AØ7.Ø
  cachectic NEC K52.89
  Chilomastix AØ7.8
  choleriformis AØØ.1
  chronic (noninfectious) K52.9
  coccidial AØ7.3
  Cochin-China K9Ø.1
    strongyloidiasis B78.Ø
  Dientamoeba AØ7.8
  dietetic —*see also* Diarrhea, allergic K52.29
  drug-induced K52.1
  due to
    bacteria AØ4.9
      specified NEC AØ4.8
    Campylobacter AØ4.5
    Capillaria philippinensis B81.1
    Clostridium difficile
      not specified as recurrent AØ4.72
      recurrent AØ4.71
    Clostridium perfringens (C) (F) AØ4.8
    Cryptosporidium AØ7.2
    drugs K52.1
    Escherichia coli AØ4.4
      enteroaggregative AØ4.4
      enterohemorrhagic AØ4.3
      enteroinvasive AØ4.2
      enteropathogenic AØ4.Ø
      enterotoxigenic AØ4.1
      specified NEC AØ4.4

- **Diarrhea, diarrheal** *(Continued)*
  - due to *(Continued)*
    - food hypersensitivity *—see also* Diarrhea, allergic K52.29
    - Necator americanus B76.1
    - S. japonicum B65.2
    - specified organism NEC A08.8
      - bacterial A04.8
      - viral A08.39
    - Staphylococcus A04.8
    - Trichuris trichiuria B79
    - virus *—see* Enteritis, viral
    - Yersinia enterocolitica A04.6
  - dysenteric A09
  - endemic A09
  - epidemic A09
  - flagellate A07.9
  - Flexner's (ulcerative) A03.1
  - functional K59.1
    - following gastrointestinal surgery K91.89
    - psychogenic F45.8
  - Giardia lamblia A07.1
  - giardial A07.1
  - hill K90.1
  - infectious A09
  - malarial *—see* Malaria
  - mite B88.0
  - mycotic NEC B49
  - neonatal (noninfectious) P78.3
  - nervous F45.8
  - neurogenic K59.1
  - noninfectious K52.9
  - postgastrectomy K91.1
  - postvagotomy K91.1
  - protozoal A07.9
    - specified NEC A07.8
  - psychogenic F45.8
  - specified
    - bacterium NEC A04.8
    - virus NEC A08.39
  - strongyloidiasis B78.0
  - toxic K52.1
  - trichomonal A07.8
  - tropical K90.1
  - tuberculous A18.32
  - viral *—see* Enteritis, viral
- **Diastasis**
  - cranial bones M84.88
    - congenital NEC Q75.8
  - joint (traumatic) *—see* Dislocation
  - muscle M62.00
    - ankle M62.07-●
    - congenital Q79.8
    - foot M62.07-●
    - forearm M62.03-●
    - hand M62.04-●
    - lower leg M62.06-●
    - pelvic region M62.05-●
    - shoulder region M62.01-●
    - specified site NEC M62.08
    - thigh M62.05-●
    - upper arm M62.02-●
  - recti (abdomen)
    - complicating delivery O71.89
    - congenital Q79.59
- **Diastema, tooth, teeth, fully erupted** M26.32
- **Diastematomyelia** Q06.2
- **Diataxia, cerebral** G80.4
- **Diathesis**
  - allergic *—see* History, allergy
  - bleeding (familial) D69.9
  - cystine (familial) E72.00
  - gouty *—see* Gout
  - hemorrhagic (familial) D69.9
    - newborn NEC P53
  - spasmophilic R29.0
- **Diaz's disease or osteochondrosis** (juvenile) (talus) *—see* Osteochondrosis, juvenile, tarsus
- **Dibothriocephalus, dibothriocephaliasis** (latus) (infection) (infestation) B70.0
  - larval B70.1
- **Dicephalus, dicephaly** Q89.4
- **Dichotomy, teeth** K00.2
- **Dichromat, dichromatopsia** (congenital) *—see* Deficiency, color vision
- **Dichuchwa** A65
- **Dicroceliasis** B66.2
- **Didelphia, didelphys** *—see* Double uterus
- **Didymytis** N45.1
  - with orchitis N45.3
- **Dietary**
  - inadequacy or deficiency E63.9
  - surveillance and counseling Z71.3
- **Dietl's crisis** N13.8
- **Dieulafoy lesion** (hemorrhagic)
  - duodenum K31.82
  - esophagus K22.8
  - intestine (colon) K63.81
  - stomach K31.82
- **Difficult, difficulty** (in)
  - acculturation Z60.3
  - feeding R63.3
    - newborn P92.9
      - breast P92.5
      - specified NEC P92.8
    - nonorganic (infant or child) F98.29
  - intubation, in anesthesia T88.4
  - mechanical, gastroduodenal stoma K91.89
    - causing obstruction *—see also* Obstruction, intestine, postoperative K91.30
  - micturition
    - need to immediately re-void R39.191
    - position dependent R39.192
    - specified NEC R39.198
  - reading (developmental) F81.0
    - secondary to emotional disorders F93.9
  - spelling (specific) F81.81
    - with reading disorder F81.89
    - due to inadequate teaching Z55.8
  - swallowing *—see* Dysphagia
  - walking R26.2
  - work
    - conditions NEC Z56.5
    - schedule Z56.3
- **Diffuse** *—see* condition
- **DiGeorge's syndrome** (thymic hypoplasia) D82.1
- **Digestive** *—see* condition
- **Dihydropyrimidine dehydrogenase disease** (DPD) E88.89
- **Diktyoma** *—see* Neoplasm, malignant, by site
- **Dilaceration, tooth** K00.4
- **Dilatation**
  - anus K59.8
    - venule *—see* Hemorrhoids
  - aorta (focal) (general) *—see* Ectasia, aorta
    - with aneurysm *—see* Aneurysm, aorta
    - congenital Q25.44
  - artery *—see* Aneurysm
  - bladder (sphincter) N32.89
    - congenital Q64.79
  - blood vessel I99.8
  - bronchial J47.9
    - with
      - exacerbation (acute) J47.1
      - lower respiratory infection J47.0
  - calyx (due to obstruction) *—see* Hydronephrosis
  - capillaries I78.8
  - cardiac (acute) (chronic) *—see also* Hypertrophy, cardiac
    - congenital Q24.8
      - valve NEC Q24.8
        - pulmonary Q22.3
    - valve *—see* Endocarditis
  - cavum septi pellucidi Q06.8
  - cervix (uteri) *—see also* Incompetency, cervix
    - incomplete, poor, slow complicating delivery O62.0
- **Dilatation** *(Continued)*
  - colon K59.39
    - congenital Q43.1
    - psychogenic F45.8
    - toxic K59.31
  - common duct (acquired) K83.8
    - congenital Q44.5
  - cystic duct (acquired) K82.8
    - congenital Q44.5
  - duct, mammary *—see* Ectasia, mammary duct
  - duodenum K59.8
  - esophagus K22.8
    - congenital Q39.5
    - due to achalasia K22.0
  - eustachian tube, congenital Q17.8
  - gallbladder K82.8
  - gastric *—see* Dilatation, stomach
  - heart (acute) (chronic) *—see also* Hypertrophy, cardiac
    - congenital Q24.8
    - valve *—see* Endocarditis
  - ileum K59.8
    - psychogenic F45.8
  - jejunum K59.8
    - psychogenic F45.8
  - kidney (calyx) (collecting structures) (cystic) (parenchyma) (pelvis) (idiopathic) N28.89
  - lacrimal passages or duct *—see* Disorder, lacrimal system, changes
  - lymphatic vessel I89.0
  - mammary duct *—see* Ectasia, mammary duct
  - Meckel's diverticulum (congenital) Q43.0
    - malignant *—see* Table of Neoplasms, small intestine, malignant
  - myocardium (acute) (chronic) *—see* Hypertrophy, cardiac organ or site, congenital NEC *—see* Distortion
  - pancreatic duct K86.89
  - pericardium *—see* Pericarditis
  - pharynx J39.2
  - prostate N42.89
  - pulmonary
    - artery (idiopathic) I28.8
    - valve, congenital Q22.3
  - pupil H57.04
  - rectum K59.39
  - saccule, congenital Q16.5
  - salivary gland (duct) K11.8
  - sphincter ani K62.89
  - stomach K31.89
    - acute K31.0
    - psychogenic F45.8
  - submaxillary duct K11.8
  - trachea, congenital Q32.1
  - ureter (idiopathic) N28.82
    - congenital Q62.2
    - due to obstruction N13.4
  - urethra (acquired) N36.8
  - vasomotor I73.9
  - vein I86.8
  - ventricular, ventricle (acute) (chronic) *—see also* Hypertrophy, cardiac
    - cerebral, congenital Q04.8
  - venule NEC I86.8
  - vesical orifice N32.89
- **Dilated, dilation** *—see* Dilatation
- **Diminished, diminution**
  - hearing (acuity) *—see* Deafness
  - sense or sensation (cold) (heat) (tactile) (vibratory) R20.8
  - vision NEC H54.7
  - vital capacity R94.2
- **Diminuta taenia** B71.0
- **Dimitri-Sturge-Weber disease** Q85.8
- **Dimple**
  - congenital sacral Q82.6
  - parasacral Q82.6
  - pilonidal or postanal *—see* Cyst, pilonidal

Dioctophyme renalis (infection) (infestation) B83.8
Dipetalonemiasis B74.4
Diphallus Q55.69
Diphtheria, diphtheritic (gangrenous) (hemorrhagic) A36.9
  carrier (suspected) Z22.2
  cutaneous A36.3
  faucial A36.0
  infection of wound A36.3
  laryngeal A36.2
  myocarditis A36.81
  nasal, anterior A36.89
  nasopharyngeal A36.1
  neurological complication A36.89
  pharyngeal A36.0
  specified site NEC A36.89
  tonsillar A36.0
Diphyllobothriasis (intestine) B70.0
  larval B70.1
Diplacusis H93.22-●
Diplegia (upper limbs) G83.0
  congenital (cerebral) G80.8
  facial G51.0
  lower limbs G82.20
  spastic G80.1
Diplococcus, diplococcal —*see* condition
Diplopia H53.2
Dipsomania F10.20
  with
    psychosis —*see* Psychosis, alcoholic
    remission F10.21
Dipylidiasis B71.1
DIRA (deficiency of interleukin 1 receptor antagonist) M04.8
Direction, teeth, abnormal, fully erupted M26.30
Dirofilariasis B74.8
Dirt-eating child F98.3
Disability, disabilities
  heart —*see* Disease, heart
  intellectual F79
    with
      autistic features F84.9
    mild (I.Q. 50-69) F70
    moderate (I.Q. 35-49) F71
    profound (I.Q. under 20) F73
    severe (I.Q. 20-34) F72
    specified level NEC F78
  knowledge acquisition F81.9
  learning F81.9
  limiting activities Z73.6
  spelling, specific F81.81
Disappearance of family member Z63.4
Disarticulation —*see* Amputation
  meaning traumatic amputation —*see* Amputation, traumatic
Discharge (from)
  abnormal finding in —*see* Abnormal, specimen
  breast (female) (male) N64.52
  diencephalic autonomic idiopathic —*see* Epilepsy, specified NEC
  ear —*see also* Otorrhea
    blood —*see* Otorrhagia
  excessive urine R35.8
  nipple N64.52
  penile R36.9
  postnasal R09.82
  prison, anxiety concerning Z65.2
  urethral R36.9
    without blood R36.0
    hematospermia R36.1
  vaginal N89.8
Discitis, diskitis M46.40
  cervical region M46.42
  cervicothoracic region M46.43
  lumbar region M46.46
  lumbosacral region M46.47
  multiple sites M46.49
  occipito-atlanto-axial region M46.41
Discitis, diskitis *(Continued)*
  pyogenic —*see* Infection, intervertebral disc, pyogenic
  sacrococcygeal region M46.48
  thoracic region M46.44
  thoracolumbar region M46.45
Discoid
  meniscus (congenital) Q68.6
  semilunar cartilage (congenital) —*see* Derangement, knee, meniscus, specified NEC
Discoloration
  nails L60.8
  teeth (posteruptive) K03.7
    during formation K00.8
Discomfort
  chest R07.89
  visual H53.14-●
Discontinuity, ossicles, ear H74.2-●
Discord (with)
  boss Z56.4
  classmates Z55.4
  counselor Z64.4
  employer Z56.4
  family Z63.8
  fellow employees Z56.4
  in-laws Z63.1
  landlord Z59.2
  lodgers Z59.2
  neighbors Z59.2
  probation officer Z64.4
  social worker Z64.4
  teachers Z55.4
  workmates Z56.4
Discordant connection
  atrioventricular (congenital) Q20.5
  ventriculoarterial Q20.3
Discrepancy
  centric occlusion maximum intercuspation M26.55
  leg length (acquired) —*see* Deformity, limb, unequal length
    congenital —*see* Defect, reduction, lower limb
  uterine size date O26.84-●
Discrimination
  ethnic Z60.5
  political Z60.5
  racial Z60.5
  religious Z60.5
  sex Z60.5
Disease, diseased —*see also* Syndrome
  absorbent system I87.8
  acid-peptic K30
  Acosta's T70.29
  Adams-Stokes (-Morgagni) (syncope with heart block) I45.9
  Addison's anemia (pernicious) D51.0
  adenoids (and tonsils) J35.9
  adrenal (capsule) (cortex) (gland) (medullary) E27.9
    hyperfunction E27.0
    specified NEC E27.8
  ainhum L94.6
  airway
    obstructive, chronic J44.9
      due to
        cotton dust J66.0
        specific organic dusts NEC J66.8
    reactive —*see* Asthma
  akamushi (scrub typhus) A75.3
  Albers-Schönberg (marble bones) Q78.2
  Albert's —*see* Tendinitis, Achilles
  alimentary canal K63.9
  alligator-skin Q80.9
    acquired L85.0
  alpha heavy chain C88.3
  alpine T70.29
  altitude T70.20
Disease, diseased *(Continued)*
  alveolar ridge
    edentulous K06.9
      specified NEC K06.8
  alveoli, teeth K08.9
  Alzheimer's G30.9 *[F02.80]*
    with behavioral disturbance G30.9 *[F02.81]*
    early onset G30.0 *[F02.80]*
      with behavioral disturbance G30.0 *[F02.81]*
    late onset G30.1 *[F02.80]*
      with behavioral disturbance G30.1 *[F02.81]*
    specified NEC G30.8 *[F02.80]*
      with behavioral disturbance G30.8 *[F02.81]*
  amyloid —*see* Amyloidosis
  Andersen's (glycogenosis IV) E74.09
  Andes T70.29
  Andrews' (bacterid) L08.89
  angiospastic I73.9
    cerebral G45.9
    vein I87.8
  anterior
    chamber H21.9
    horn cell G12.29
  antiglomerular basement membrane (anti-GBM) antibody M31.0
    tubulo-interstitial nephritis N12
  antral —*see* Sinusitis, maxillary
  anus K62.9
    specified NEC K62.89
  aorta (nonsyphilitic) I77.9
    syphilitic NEC A52.02
  aortic (heart) (valve) I35.9
    rheumatic I06.9
  Apollo B30.3
  aponeuroses —*see* Enthesopathy
  appendix K38.9
    specified NEC K38.8
  aqueous (chamber) H21.9
  Arnold-Chiari —*see* Arnold-Chiari disease
  arterial I77.9
    occlusive —*see* Occlusion, by site
      due to stricture or stenosis I77.1
    ▶peripheral I73.9
  arteriocardiorenal —*see* Hypertension, cardiorenal
  arteriolar (generalized) (obliterative) I77.9
  arteriorenal —*see* Hypertension, kidney
  arteriosclerotic —*see also* Arteriosclerosis
    cardiovascular —*see* Disease, heart, ischemic, atherosclerotic
    coronary (artery) —*see* Disease, heart, ischemic, atherosclerotic
    heart —*see* Disease, heart, ischemic, atherosclerotic
  artery I77.9
    cerebral I67.9
    coronary I25.10
      ➡with angina pectoris —*see* Arteriosclerosis, coronary (artery)
    ▶peripheral I73.9
  arthropod-borne NOS (viral) A94
    specified type NEC A93.8
  atticoantral, chronic H66.20
    left H66.22
      with right H66.23
    right H66.21
      with left H66.23
  auditory canal —*see* Disorder, ear, external
  auricle, ear NEC —*see* Disorder, pinna
  Australian X A83.4
  autoimmune (systemic) NOS M35.9
    hemolytic (cold type) (warm type) D59.1
      drug-induced D59.0
    thyroid E06.3
  autoinflammatory M04.9
    NOD2-associated M04.8
    specified type NEC M04.8
  aviator's —*see* Effect, adverse, high altitude
  Ayerza's (pulmonary artery sclerosis with pulmonary hypertension) I27.0

Disease, diseased *(Continued)*
Babington's (familial hemorrhagic telangiectasia) I78.0
bacterial A49.9
specified NEC A48.8
zoonotic A28.9
specified type NEC A28.8
Baelz's (cheilitis glandularis apostematosa) K13.0
bagasse J67.1
balloon —*see* Effect, adverse, high altitude
Bang's (brucella abortus) A23.1
Bannister's T78.3
barometer makers' —*see* Poisoning, mercury
Barraquer (-Simons') (progressive lipodystrophy) E88.1
Barrett's —*see* Barrett's, esophagus
Bartholin's gland N75.9
basal ganglia G25.9
degenerative G23.9
specified NEC G23.8
specified NEC G25.89
Basedow's (exophthalmic goiter) —*see* Hyperthyroidism, with, goiter (diffuse)
Bateman's B08.1
Batten-Steinert G71.11
Battey A31.0
Beard's (neurasthenia) F48.8
Becker
idiopathic mural endomyocardial I42.3
myotonia congenita G71.12
Begbie's (exophthalmic goiter) —*see* Hyperthyroidism, with, goiter (diffuse)
behavioral, organic F07.9
Beigel's (white piedra) B36.2
Benson's —*see* Deposit, crystalline
Bernard-Soulier (thrombopathy) D69.1
Bernhardt (-Roth) —*see* Mononeuropathy, lower limb, meralgia paresthetica
Biermer's (pernicious anemia) D51.0
bile duct (common) (hepatic) K83.9
with calculus, stones —*see* Calculus, bile duct
specified NEC K83.8
biliary (tract) K83.9
specified NEC K83.8
Billroth's —*see* Spina bifida
bird fancier's J67.2
black lung J60
bladder N32.9
in (due to)
schistosomiasis (bilharziasis) B65.0 *[N33]*
specified NEC N32.89
bleeder's D66
blood D75.9
forming organs D75.9
vessel I99.9
Bloodgood's —*see* Mastopathy, cystic
Bodechtel-Guttmann (subacute sclerosing panencephalitis) A81.1
bone —*see also* Disorder, bone
aluminum M83.4
fibrocystic NEC
jaw M27.49
bone-marrow D75.9
Borna A83.9
Bornholm (epidemic pleurodynia) B33.0
Bouchard's (myopathic dilatation of the stomach) K31.0
Bouillaud's (rheumatic heart disease) I01.9
Bourneville (-Brissaud) (tuberous sclerosis) Q85.1
Bouveret (-Hoffmann) (paroxysmal tachycardia) I47.9
bowel K63.9
functional K59.9
psychogenic F45.8
brain G93.9
arterial, artery I67.9
arteriosclerotic I67.2
congenital Q04.9

Disease, diseased *(Continued)*
brain *(Continued)*
degenerative —*see* Degeneration, brain
inflammatory —*see* Encephalitis
organic G93.9
arteriosclerotic I67.2
parasitic NEC B71.9 *[G94]*
senile NEC G31.1
specified NEC G93.89
breast (*see also* Disorder, breast) N64.9
cystic (chronic) —*see* Mastopathy, cystic
fibrocystic —*see* Mastopathy, cystic
Paget's
female, unspecified side C50.91- •
male, unspecified side C50.92- •
specified NEC N64.89
Breda's —*see* Yaws
Bretonneau's (diphtheritic malignant angina) A36.0
Bright's —*see* Nephritis
arteriosclerotic —*see* Hypertension, kidney
Brill's (recrudescent typhus) A75.1
Brill-Zinsser (recrudescent typhus) A75.1
Brion-Kayser —*see* Fever, paratyphoid
broad
beta E78.2
ligament (noninflammatory) N83.9
inflammatory —*see* Disease, pelvis, inflammatory
specified NEC N83.8
Brocq-Duhring (dermatitis herpetiformis) L13.0
Brocq's
meaning
dermatitis herpetiformis L13.0
prurigo L28.2
bronchopulmonary J98.4
bronchus NEC J98.09
bronze Addison's E27.1
tuberculous A18.7
budgerigar fancier's J67.2
Buerger's (thromboangiitis obliterans) I73.1
bullous L13.9
chronic of childhood L12.2
specified NEC L13.8
Bürger-Grütz (essential familial hyperlipemia) E78.3
bursa —*see* Bursopathy
caisson T70.3
California —*see* Coccidioidomycosis
capillaries I78.9
specified NEC I78.8
Carapata A68.0
cardiac —*see* Disease, heart
cardiopulmonary, chronic I27.9
cardiorenal (hepatic) (hypertensive) (vascular) —*see* Hypertension, cardiorenal
cardiovascular (atherosclerotic) I25.10
with angina pectoris —*see* Arteriosclerosis, coronary (artery),
congenital Q28.9
hypertensive —*see* Hypertension, heart
newborn P29.9
specified NEC P29.89
renal (hypertensive) —*see* Hypertension, cardiorenal
syphilitic (asymptomatic) A52.00
cartilage —*see* Disorder, cartilage
Castellani's A69.8
Castleman (unicentric) (multicentric) D47.Z2
HHV-8-associated —*see also* Herpesvirus, human, 8 D47.Z2
cat-scratch A28.1
Cavare's (familial periodic paralysis) G72.3
cecum K63.9
celiac (adult) (infantile) (with steatorrhea) K90.0
cellular tissue L98.9

Disease, diseased *(Continued)*
central core G71.2
cerebellar, cerebellum —*see* Disease, brain
cerebral —*see also* Disease, brain
degenerative —*see* Degeneration, brain
cerebrospinal G96.9
cerebrovascular I67.9
acute I67.89
embolic I63.4- •
thrombotic I63.3- •
arteriosclerotic I67.2
hereditary NEC I67.858
specified NEC I67.89
cervix (uteri) (noninflammatory) N88.9
inflammatory —*see* Cervicitis
specified NEC N88.8
Chabert's A22.9
Chandler's (osteochondritis dissecans, hip) —*see* Osteochondritis, dissecans, hip
Charlouis —*see* Yaws
Chédiak-Steinbrinck (-Higashi) (congenital gigantism of peroxidase granules) E70.330
chest J98.9
Chiari's (hepatic vein thrombosis) I82.0
Chicago B40.9
Chignon B36.8
chigo, chigoe B88.1
childhood granulomatous D71
Chinese liver fluke B66.1
chlamydial A74.9
specified NEC A74.89
cholecystic K82.9
choroid H31.9
specified NEC H31.8
Christmas D67
chronic bullous of childhood L12.2
chylomicron retention E78.3
ciliary body H21.9
specified NEC H21.89
circulatory (system) NEC I99.8
newborn P29.9
syphilitic A52.00
congenital A50.54
coagulation factor deficiency (congenital) —*see* Defect, coagulation
coccidioidal —*see* Coccidioidomycosis
cold
agglutinin or hemoglobinuria D59.1
paroxysmal D59.6
hemagglutinin (chronic) D59.1
collagen NOS (nonvascular) (vascular) M35.9
specified NEC M35.8
colon K63.9
functional K59.9
congenital Q43.2
ischemic —*see also* Ischemia, intestine, acute K55.039
colonic inflammatory bowel, unclassified (IBDU) K52.3
combined system —*see* Degeneration, combined
compressed air T70.3
Concato's (pericardial polyserositis) A19.9
nontubercular I31.1
pleural —*see* Pleurisy, with effusion
conjunctiva H11.9
chlamydial A74.0
specified NEC H11.89
viral B30.9
specified NEC B30.8
connective tissue, systemic (diffuse) M35.9
in (due to)
hypogammaglobulinemia D80.1 *[M36.8]*
ochronosis E70.29 *[M36.8]*
specified NEC M35.8
Conor and Bruch's (boutonneuse fever) A77.1
Cooper's —*see* Mastopathy, cystic
Cori's (glycogenosis III) E74.03
corkhandler's or corkworker's J67.3
cornea H18.9
specified NEC H18.89- •

Disease, diseased *(Continued)*
coronary (artery) —*see* Disease, heart, ischemic, atherosclerotic
congenital Q24.5
ostial, syphilitic (aortic) (mitral) (pulmonary) A52.03
corpus cavernosum N48.9
specified NEC N48.89
Cotugno's —*see* Sciatica
coxsackie (virus) NEC B34.1
cranial nerve NOS G52.9
Creutzfeldt-Jakob —*see* Creutzfeldt-Jakob disease or syndrome
Crocq's (acrocyanosis) I73.89
Crohn's —*see* Enteritis, regional
Curschmann G71.11
cystic
breast (chronic) —*see* Mastopathy, cystic
kidney, congenital Q61.9
liver, congenital Q44.6
lung J98.4
congenital Q33.0
cytomegalic inclusion (generalized) B25.9
with pneumonia B25.0
congenital P35.1
cytomegaloviral B25.9
specified NEC B25.8
Czerny's (periodic hydrarthrosis of the knee) —*see* Effusion, joint, knee
Daae (-Finsen) (epidemic pleurodynia) B33.0
Darling's —*see* Histoplasmosis capsulati
Débove's (splenomegaly) R16.1
deer fly —*see* Tularemia
Degos' I77.8
demyelinating, demyelinizating (nervous system) G37.9
multiple sclerosis G35
specified NEC G37.8
dense deposit —*see also* N00-N07 with fourth character .6 N05.6
deposition, hydroxyapatite —*see* Disease, hydroxyapatite deposition
de Quervain's (tendon sheath) M65.4
thyroid (subacute granulomatous thyroiditis) E06.1
Devergie's (pityriasis rubra pilaris) L44.0
Devic's G36.0
diaphorase deficiency D74.0
diaphragm J98.6
diarrheal, infectious NEC A09
digestive system K92.9
specified NEC K92.89
disc, degenerative —*see* Degeneration, intervertebral disc
discogenic —*see also* Displacement, intervertebral disc NEC
with myelopathy —*see* Disorder, disc, with, myelopathy
diverticular —*see* Diverticula
Dubois (thymus) A50.59 *[E35]*
Duchenne-Griesinger G71.01
Duchenne's
muscular dystrophy G71.01
pseudohypertrophy, muscles G71.01
ductless glands E34.9
Duhring's (dermatitis herpetiformis) L13.0
duodenum K31.9
specified NEC K31.89
Dupré's (meningism) R29.1
Dupuytren's (muscle contracture) M72.0
Durand-Nicholas-Favre (climatic bubo) A55
Duroziez's (congenital mitral stenosis) Q23.2
ear —*see* Disorder, ear
Eberth's —*see* Fever, typhoid
Ebola (virus) A98.4
Ebstein's heart Q22.5
Echinococcus —*see* Echinococcus
echovirus NEC B34.1
Eddowes' (brittle bones and blue sclera) Q78.0
edentulous (alveolar) ridge K06.9
specified NEC K06.8

Disease, diseased *(Continued)*
Edsall's T67.2
Eichstedt's (pityriasis versicolor) B36.0
Eisenmenger's (irreversible) I27.83
Ellis-van Creveld (chondroectodermal dysplasia) Q77.6
end stage renal (ESRD) N18.6
due to hypertension I12.0
endocrine glands or system NEC E34.9
endomyocardial (eosinophilic) I42.3
English (rickets) E55.0
enteroviral, enterovirus NEC B34.1
central nervous system NEC A88.8
epidemic B99.9
specified NEC B99.8
epididymis N50.9
Erb (-Landouzy) G71.02
Erdheim-Chester (ECD) E88.89
esophagus K22.9
functional K22.4
psychogenic F45.8
specified NEC K22.8
Eulenburg's (congenital paramyotonia) G71.19
eustachian tube —*see* Disorder, eustachian tube
external
auditory canal —*see* Disorder, ear, external
ear —*see* Disorder, ear, external
extrapyramidal G25.9
specified NEC G25.89
eye H57.9
anterior chamber H21.9
inflammatory NEC H57.89
muscle (external) —*see* Strabismus
specified NEC H57.89
syphilitic —*see* Oculopathy, syphilitic
eyeball H44.9
specified NEC H44.89
eyelid —*see* Disorder, eyelid
specified NEC —*see* Disorder, eyelid, specified type NEC
eyeworm of Africa B74.3
facial nerve (seventh) G51.9
newborn (birth injury) P11.3
Fahr (of brain) G23.8
Fahr Volhard (of kidney) I12.-●
fallopian tube (noninflammatory) N83.9
inflammatory —*see* Salpingo-oophoritis
specified NEC N83.8
familial periodic paralysis G72.3
Fanconi's (congenital pancytopenia) D61.09
fascia NEC —*see also* Disorder, muscle
inflammatory —*see* Myositis
specified NEC M62.89
Fauchard's (periodontitis) —*see* Periodontitis
Favre-Durand-Nicolas (climatic bubo) A55
Fede's K14.0
Feer's —*see* Poisoning, mercury
female pelvic inflammatory —*see also* Disease, pelvis, inflammatory N73.9
syphilitic (secondary) A51.42
tuberculous A18.17
Fernels' (aortic aneurysm) I71.9
fibrocaseous of lung —*see* Tuberculosis, pulmonary
fibrocystic —*see* Fibrocystic disease
Fiedler's (leptospiral jaundice) A27.0
fifth B08.3
file-cutter's —*see* Poisoning, lead
fish-skin Q80.9
acquired L85.0
Flajani (-Basedow) (exophthalmic goiter) —*see* Hyperthyroidism, with, goiter (diffuse)
flax-dresser's J66.1
fluke —*see* Infestation, fluke
foot and mouth B08.8
foot process N04.9
Forbes' (glycogenosis III) E74.03
Fordyce-Fox (apocrine miliaria) L75.2
Fordyce's (ectopic sebaceous glands) (mouth) Q38.6

Disease, diseased *(Continued)*
Forestier's (rhizomelic pseudopolyarthritis) M35.3
meaning ankylosing hyperostosis —*see* Hyperostosis, ankylosing
Fothergill's
neuralgia —*see* Neuralgia, trigeminal
scarlatina anginosa A38.9
Fournier (gangrene) N49.3
female N76.89
fourth B08.8
Fox (-Fordyce) (apocrine miliaria) L75.2
Francis' —*see* Tularemia
Franklin C88.2
Frei's (climatic bubo) A55
Friedreich's
combined systemic or ataxia G11.1
myoclonia G25.3
frontal sinus —*see* Sinusitis, frontal
fungus NEC B49
Gaisböck's (polycythemia hypertonica) D75.1
gallbladder K82.9
calculus —*see* Calculus, gallbladder
cholecystitis —*see* Cholecystitis
cholesterolosis K82.4
fistula —*see* Fistula, gallbladder
hydrops K82.1
obstruction —*see* Obstruction, gallbladder
perforation K82.2
specified NEC K82.8
gamma heavy chain C88.2
Gamna's (siderotic splenomegaly) D73.2
Gamstorp's (adynamia episodica hereditaria) G72.3
Gandy-Nanta (siderotic splenomegaly) D73.2
ganister J62.8
gastric —*see* Disease, stomach
gastroesophageal reflux (GERD) K21.9
with esophagitis K21.0
gastrointestinal (tract) K92.9
amyloid E85.4
functional K59.9
psychogenic F45.8
specified NEC K92.89
Gee (-Herter) (-Heubner) (-Thaysen) (nontropical sprue) K90.0
genital organs
female N94.9
male N50.9
Gerhardt's (erythromelalgia) I73.81
Gibert's (pityriasis rosea) L42
Gierke's (glycogenosis I) E74.01
Gilles de la Tourette's (motor-verbal tic) F95.2
gingiva K06.9
plaque induced K05.00
specified NEC K06.8
gland (lymph) I89.9
Glanzmann's (hereditary hemorrhagic thrombasthenia) D69.1
glass-blower's (cataract) —*see* Cataract, specified NEC
salivary gland hypertrophy K11.1
Glisson's —*see* Rickets
globe H44.9
specified NEC H44.89
glomerular —*see also* Glomerulonephritis
with edema —*see* Nephrosis
acute —*see* Nephritis, acute
chronic —*see* Nephritis, chronic
minimal change N05.0
rapidly progressive N01.9
glycogen storage E74.00
Andersen's E74.09
Cori's E74.03
Forbes' E74.03
generalized E74.00
glucose-6-phosphatase deficiency E74.01
heart E74.02 *[I43]*
hepatorenal E74.09
Hers' E74.09
liver and kidney E74.09

Disease, diseased *(Continued)*
glycogen storage *(Continued)*
McArdle's E74.04
muscle phosphofructokinase E74.09
myocardium E74.02 *[I43]*
Pompe's E74.02
Tauri's E74.09
type 0 E74.09
type I E74.01
type II E74.02
type III E74.03
type IV E74.09
type V E74.04
type VI-XI E74.09
Von Gierke's E74.01
Goldstein's (familial hemorrhagic telangiectasia) I78.0
gonococcal NOS A54.9
graft-versus-host (GVH) D89.813
acute D89.810
acute on chronic D89.812
chronic D89.811
grainhandler's J67.8
granulomatous (childhood) (chronic) D71
Graves' (exophthalmic goiter) —*see* Hyperthyroidism, with, goiter (diffuse)
Griesinger's —*see* Ancylostomiasis
Grisel's M43.6
Gruby's (tinea tonsurans) B35.0
Guillain-Barré G61.0
Guinon's (motor-verbal tic) F95.2
gum K06.9
gynecological N94.9
H (Hartnup's) E72.02
Haff —*see* Poisoning, mercury
Hageman (congenital factor XII deficiency) D68.2
hair (color) (shaft) L67.9
follicles L73.9
specified NEC L73.8
Hamman's (spontaneous mediastinal emphysema) J98.2
hand, foot and mouth B08.4
Hansen's —*see* Leprosy
Hantavirus, with pulmonary manifestations B33.4
with renal manifestations A98.5
Harada's H30.81-●
Hartnup (pellagra-cerebellar ataxia-renal aminoaciduria) E72.02
Hart's (pellagra-cerebellar ataxia-renal aminoaciduria) E72.02
Hashimoto's (struma lymphomatosa) E06.3
Hb —*see* Disease, hemoglobin
heart (organic) I51.9
with
pulmonary edema (acute) —*see also* Failure, ventricular, left I50.1
rheumatic fever (conditions in I00)
active I01.9
with chorea I02.0
specified NEC I01.8
inactive or quiescent (with chorea) I09.9
specified NEC I09.89
amyloid E85.4 *[I43]*
aortic (valve) I35.9
arteriosclerotic or sclerotic (senile) —*see* Disease, heart, ischemic, atherosclerotic
artery, arterial —*see* Disease, heart, ischemic, atherosclerotic
beer drinkers' I42.6
beriberi (wet) E51.12
black I27.0
congenital Q24.9
cyanotic Q24.9
specified NEC Q24.8
coronary —*see* Disease, heart, ischemic
cryptogenic I51.9

Disease, diseased *(Continued)*
heart *(Continued)*
fibroid —*see* Myocarditis
functional I51.89
psychogenic F45.8
glycogen storage E74.02 *[I43]*
gonococcal A54.83
hypertensive —*see* Hypertension, heart
hyperthyroid —*see also* Hyperthyroidism E05.90 *[I43]*
with thyroid storm E05.91 *[I43]*
ischemic (chronic or with a stated duration of over 4 weeks) I25.9
atherosclerotic (of) I25.10
with angina pectoris —*see* Arteriosclerosis, coronary (artery)
coronary artery bypass graft —*see* Arteriosclerosis, coronary (artery),
cardiomyopathy I25.5
diagnosed on ECG or other special investigation, but currently presenting no symptoms I25.6
silent I25.6
specified form NEC I25.89
kyphoscoliotic I27.1
meningococcal A39.50
endocarditis A39.51
myocarditis A39.52
pericarditis A39.53
mitral I05.9
specified NEC I05.8
muscular —*see* Degeneration, myocardial
psychogenic (functional) F45.8
pulmonary (chronic) I27.9
in schistosomiasis B65.9 *[I52]*
specified NEC I27.89
rheumatic (chronic) (inactive) (old) (quiescent) (with chorea) I09.9
active or acute I01.9
with chorea (acute) (rheumatic) (Sydenham's) I02.0
specified NEC I09.89
senile —*see* Myocarditis
syphilitic A52.06
aortic A52.03
aneurysm A52.01
congenital A50.54 *[I52]*
thyrotoxic —*see also* Thyrotoxicosis E05.90 *[I43]*
with thyroid storm E05.91 *[I43]*
valve, valvular (obstructive) (regurgitant) —*see also* Endocarditis
congenital NEC Q24.8
pulmonary Q22.3
vascular —*see* Disease, cardiovascular
heavy chain NEC C88.2
alpha C88.3
gamma C88.2
mu C88.2
Hebra's
pityriasis
maculata et circinata L42
rubra pilaris L44.0
prurigo L28.2
hematopoietic organs D75.9
hemoglobin or Hb
abnormal (mixed) NEC D58.2
with thalassemia D56.9
AS genotype D57.3
Bart's D56.0
C (Hb-C) D58.2
with other abnormal hemoglobin NEC D58.2
elliptocytosis D58.1
Hb-S D57.2-●
sickle-cell D57.2-●
thalassemia D56.8
Constant Spring D58.2
D (Hb-D) D58.2
E (Hb-E) D58.2

Disease, diseased *(Continued)*
hemoglobin or Hb *(Continued)*
E-beta thalassemia D56.5
elliptocytosis D58.1
H (Hb-H) (thalassemia) D56.0
with other abnormal hemoglobin NEC D56.9
Constant Spring D56.0
I thalassemia D56.9
M D74.0
S or SS D57.1
SC D57.2-●
SD D57.8-●
SE D57.8-●
spherocytosis D58.0
unstable, hemolytic D58.2
hemolytic (newborn) P55.9
autoimmune (cold type) (warm type) D59.1
drug-induced D59.0
due to or with
incompatibility
ABO (blood group) P55.1
blood (group) (Duffy) (K) (Kell) (Kidd) (Lewis) (M) (S) NEC P55.8
Rh (blood group) (factor) P55.0
Rh negative mother P55.0
specified type NEC P55.8
unstable hemoglobin D58.2
hemorrhagic D69.9
newborn P53
Henoch (-Schönlein) (purpura nervosa) D69.0
hepatic —*see* Disease, liver
hepatobiliary K83.9
toxic K71.9
hepatolenticular E83.01
heredodegenerative NEC
spinal cord G95.89
herpesviral, disseminated B00.7
Hers' (glycogenosis VI) E74.09
Herter (-Gee) (-Heubner) (nontropical sprue) K90.0
Heubner-Herter (nontropical sprue) K90.0
high fetal gene or hemoglobin thalassemia D56.9
Hildenbrand's —*see* Typhus
hip (joint) M25.9
congenital Q65.89
suppurative M00.9
tuberculous A18.02
His (-Werner) (trench fever) A79.0
Hodgson's I71.2
ruptured I71.1
Holla —*see* Spherocytosis
hookworm B76.9
specified NEC B76.8
host-versus-graft D89.813
acute D89.810
acute on chronic D89.812
chronic D89.811
human immunodeficiency virus (HIV) B20
Huntington's G10
with dementia G10 *[F02.80]*
Hutchinson's (cheiropompholyx) —*see* Hutchinson's disease
hyaline (diffuse) (generalized)
membrane (lung) (newborn) P22.0
adult J80
hydatid —*see* Echinococcus
hydroxyapatite deposition M11.00
ankle M11.07-●
elbow M11.02-●
foot joint M11.07-●
hand joint M11.04-●
hip M11.05-●
knee M11.06-●
multiple site M11.09
shoulder M11.01-●
vertebra M11.08
wrist M11.03-●
hyperkinetic —*see* Hyperkinesia
hypertensive —*see* Hypertension

Disease, diseased *(Continued)*
hypophysis E23.7
Iceland G93.3
I-cell E77.Ø
immune D89.9
immunoproliferative (malignant) C88.9
small intestinal C88.3
specified NEC C88.8
inclusion B25.9
salivary gland B25.9
infectious, infective B99.9
congenital P37.9
specified NEC P37.8
viral P35.9
specified type NEC P35.8
specified NEC B99.8
inflammatory
penis N48.29
abscess N48.21
cellulitis N48.22
prepuce N47.7
balanoposthitis N47.6
tubo-ovarian *—see* Salpingo-oophoritis
intervertebral disc *—see also* Disorder, disc
with myelopathy *—see* Disorder, disc, with, myelopathy
cervical, cervicothoracic *—see* Disorder, disc, cervical
with
myelopathy *—see* Disorder, disc, cervical, with myelopathy
neuritis, radiculitis or radiculopathy *—see* Disorder, disc, cervical, with neuritis
specified NEC *—see* Disorder, disc, cervical, specified type NEC
lumbar (with)
myelopathy M51.Ø6
neuritis, radiculitis, radiculopathy or sciatica M51.16
specified NEC M51.86
lumbosacral (with)
neuritis, radiculitis, radiculopathy or sciatica M51.17
specified NEC M51.87
specified NEC *—see* Disorder, disc, specified NEC
thoracic (with)
myelopathy M51.Ø4
neuritis, radiculitis or radiculopathy M51.14
specified NEC M51.84
thoracolumbar (with)
myelopathy M51.Ø5
neuritis, radiculitis or radiculopathy M51.15
specified NEC M51.85
intestine K63.9
functional K59.9
psychogenic F45.8
specified NEC K59.8
organic K63.9
protozoal AØ7.9
specified NEC K63.89
iris H21.9
specified NEC H21.89
iron metabolism or storage E83.1Ø
island (scrub typhus) A75.3
itai-itai *—see* Poisoning, cadmium
Jakob-Creutzfeldt *—see* Creutzfeldt-Jakob disease or syndrome
jaw M27.9
fibrocystic M27.49
specified NEC M27.8
jigger B88.1
joint *—see also* Disorder, joint
Charcot's *—see* Arthropathy, neuropathic (Charcot)
degenerative *—see* Osteoarthritis
multiple M15.9
spine *—see* Spondylosis

Disease, diseased *(Continued)*
joint *(Continued)*
hypertrophic *—see* Osteoarthritis
sacroiliac M53.3
specified NEC *—see* Disorder, joint, specified type NEC
spine NEC *—see* Dorsopathy
suppurative *—see* Arthritis, pyogenic or pyemic
Jourdain's (acute gingivitis) KØ5.ØØ
nonplaque induced KØ5.Ø1
plaque induced KØ5.ØØ
Kaschin-Beck (endemic polyarthritis) M12.1Ø
ankle M12.17-●
elbow M12.12-●
foot joint M12.17-●
hand joint M12.14-●
hip M12.15-●
knee M12.16-●
multiple site M12.19
shoulder M12.11-●
vertebra M12.18
wrist M12.13-●
Katayama B65.2
Kedani (scrub typhus) A75.3
Keshan E59
kidney (functional) (pelvis) N28.9
chronic N18.9
hypertensive *—see* Hypertension, kidney
stage 1 N18.1
stage 2 (mild) N18.2
stage 3 (moderate) N18.3
stage 4 (severe) N18.4
stage 5 N18.5
complicating pregnancy *—see* Pregnancy, complicated by, renal disease
cystic (congenital) Q61.9
diabetic *—see* EØ8-E13 with .22
fibrocystic (congenital) Q61.8
hypertensive *—see* Hypertension, kidney
in (due to)
schistosomiasis (bilharziasis) B65.9 *[N29]*
multicystic Q61.4
polycystic Q61.3
adult type Q61.2
childhood type NEC Q61.19
collecting duct dilatation Q61.11
Kimmelstiel (-Wilson) (intercapillary polycystic (congenital) glomerulosclerosis) *—see* EØ8-E13 with .21
Kimura D21.9
specified site (see Neoplasm, connective tissue benign)
Kinnier Wilson's (hepatolenticular degeneration) E83.Ø1
kissing *—see* Mononucleosis, infectious
Klebs' *—see also* Glomerulonephritis NØ5.-●
Klippel-Feil (brevicollis) Q76.1
Köhler-Pellegrini-Stieda (calcification, knee joint) *—see* Bursitis, tibial collateral
Kok Q89.8
König's (osteochondritis dissecans) *—see* Osteochondritis, dissecans
Korsakoff's (nonalcoholic) FØ4
alcoholic F1Ø.96
with dependence F1Ø.26
Kostmann's (infantile genetic agranulocytosis) D7Ø.Ø
kuru A81.81
Kyasanur Forest A98.2
labyrinth, ear *—see* Disorder, ear, inner
lacrimal system *—see* Disorder, lacrimal system
Lafora's *—see* Epilepsy, generalized, idiopathic
Lancereaux-Mathieu (leptospiral jaundice) A27.Ø
Landry's G61.Ø
Larrey-Weil (leptospiral jaundice) A27.Ø
larynx J38.7

Disease, diseased *(Continued)*
legionnaires' A48.1
nonpneumonic A48.2
Lenegre's I44.2
lens H27.9
specified NEC H27.8
Lev's (acquired complete heart block) I44.2
Lewy body (dementia) G31.83 *[FØ2.8Ø]*
with behavioral disturbance G31.83 *[FØ2.81]*
Lichtheim's (subacute combined sclerosis with pernicious anemia) D51.Ø
Lightwood's (renal tubular acidosis) N25.89
Lignac's (cystinosis) E72.Ø4
lip K13.Ø
lipid-storage E75.6
specified NEC E75.5
Lipschütz's N76.6
liver (chronic) (organic) K76.9
alcoholic (chronic) K7Ø.9
acute *—see* Disease, liver, alcoholic, hepatitis
cirrhosis K7Ø.3Ø
with ascites K7Ø.31
failure K7Ø.4Ø
with coma K7Ø.41
fatty liver K7Ø.Ø
fibrosis K7Ø.2
hepatitis K7Ø.1Ø
with ascites K7Ø.11
sclerosis K7Ø.2
cystic, congenital Q44.6
drug-induced (idiosyncratic) (toxic) (predictable) (unpredictable) *—see* Disease, liver, toxic
end stage K72.9Ø
due to hepatitis *—see* Hepatitis
fatty, nonalcoholic (NAFLD) K76.Ø
alcoholic K7Ø.Ø
fibrocystic (congenital) Q44.6
fluke
Chinese B66.1
oriental B66.1
sheep B66.3
gestational alloimmune (GALD) P78.84
glycogen storage E74.Ø9 *[K77]*
in (due to)
schistosomiasis (bilharziasis) B65.9 *[K77]*
inflammatory K75.9
alcoholic K7Ø.1
specified NEC K75.89
polycystic (congenital) Q44.6
toxic K71.9
with
cholestasis K71.Ø
cirrhosis (liver) K71.7
fibrosis (liver) K71.7
focal nodular hyperplasia K71.8
hepatic granuloma K71.8
hepatic necrosis K71.1Ø
with coma K71.11
hepatitis NEC K71.6
acute K71.2
chronic
active K71.5Ø
with ascites K71.51
lobular K71.4
persistent K71.3
lupoid K71.5Ø
with ascites K71.51
peliosis hepatis K71.8
veno-occlusive disease (VOD) of liver K71.8
veno-occlusive K76.5
Lobo's (keloid blastomycosis) B48.Ø
Lobstein's (brittle bones and blue sclera) Q78.Ø
Ludwig's (submaxillary cellulitis) K12.2
lumbosacral region M53.87
lung J98.4
black J6Ø
congenital Q33.9
cystic J98.4
congenital Q33.Ø

▶ New ➡ Revised ~~deleted~~ Deleted ● Use Additional Character(s)

Disease, diseased *(Continued)*
  lung *(Continued)*
    fibroid (chronic) —*see* Fibrosis, lung
    fluke B66.4
      oriental B66.4
    in
      amyloidosis E85.4 *[J99]*
      sarcoidosis D86.0
      Sjögren's syndrome M35.02
      systemic
        lupus erythematosus M32.13
        sclerosis M34.81
    interstitial J84.9
      of childhood, specified NEC J84.848
      respiratory bronchiolitis J84.115
      specified NEC J84.89
    obstructive (chronic) J43.9
      with
        acute
          bronchitis J44.0
          exacerbation NEC J44.1
          lower respiratory infection J44.0
        alveolitis, allergic J67.9
        asthma J44.9
        bronchiectasis J47.9
          with
            exacerbation (acute) J47.1
            lower respiratory infection J47.0
        bronchitis J44.9
          with
            exacerbation (acute) J44.1
            lower respiratory infection J44.0
        emphysema J43.9
        hypersensitivity pneumonitis J67.9
      decompensated J44.1
        with
          exacerbation (acute) J44.1
    polycystic J98.4
      congenital Q33.0
    rheumatoid (diffuse) (interstitial) —*see* Rheumatoid, lung
  Lutembacher's (atrial septal defect with mitral stenosis) Q21.1
  Lyme A69.20
  lymphatic (gland) (system) (channel) (vessel) I89.9
  lymphoproliferative D47.9
    specified NEC D47.Z9
    T-gamma D47.Z9
    X-linked D82.3
  Magitot's M27.2
  malarial —*see* Malaria
  malignant —*see also* Neoplasm, malignant, by site
  Manson's B65.1
  maple bark J67.6
  maple-syrup-urine E71.0
  Marburg (virus) A98.3
  Marion's (bladder neck obstruction) N32.0
  Marsh's (exophthalmic goiter) —*see* Hyperthyroidism, with, goiter (diffuse)
  mastoid (process) —*see* Disorder, ear, middle
  Mathieu's (leptospiral jaundice) A27.0
  Maxcy's A75.2
  McArdle (-Schmid-Pearson) (glycogenosis V) E74.04
  mediastinum J98.59
  medullary center (idiopathic) (respiratory) G93.89
  Meige's (chronic hereditary edema) Q82.0
  meningococcal —*see* Infection, meningococcal
  mental F99
    organic F09
  mesenchymal M35.9
  mesenteric embolic —*see also* Ischemia, intestine, acute K55.039
  metabolic, metabolism E88.9
    bilirubin E80.7
  metal-polisher's J62.8
  metastatic —*see also* Neoplasm, secondary, by site C79.9

Disease, diseased *(Continued)*
  microvascular — code to condition
  microvillus
    atrophy Q43.8
    inclusion (MVD) Q43.8
  middle ear —*see* Disorder, ear, middle
  Mikulicz' (dryness of mouth, absent or decreased lacrimation) K11.8
  Milroy's (chronic hereditary edema) Q82.0
  Minamata —*see* Poisoning, mercury
  minicore G71.2
  Minor's G95.19
  Minot's (hemorrhagic disease, newborn) P53
  Minot-von Willebrand-Jürgens (angiohemophilia) D68.0
  Mitchell's (erythromelalgia) I73.81
  mitral (valve) I05.9
    nonrheumatic I34.9
  mixed connective tissue M35.1
  moldy hay J67.0
  Monge's T70.29
  Morgagni-Adams-Stokes (syncope with heart block) I45.9
  Morgagni's (syndrome) (hyperostosis frontalis interna) M85.2
  Morton's (with metatarsalgia) —*see* Lesion, nerve, plantar
  Morvan's G60.8
  motor neuron (bulbar) (mixed type) (spinal) G12.20
    amyotrophic lateral sclerosis G12.21
    familial G12.24
    progressive bulbar palsy G12.22
    specified NEC G12.29
  moyamoya I67.5
  mu heavy chain disease C88.2
  multicore G71.2
  muscle —*see also* Disorder, muscle
    inflammatory —*see* Myositis
    ocular (external) —*see* Strabismus
  musculoskeletal system, soft tissue —*see also* Disorder, soft tissue
    specified NEC —*see* Disorder, soft tissue, specified type NEC
  mushroom workers' J67.5
  mycotic B49
  myelodysplastic, not classified C94.6
  myeloproliferative, not classified C94.6
    chronic D47.1
  myocardium, myocardial —*see also* Degeneration, myocardial I51.5
    primary (idiopathic) I42.9
  myoneural G70.9
  Naegeli's D69.1
  nails L60.9
    specified NEC L60.8
  Nairobi (sheep virus) A93.8
  nasal J34.9
  nemaline body G71.2
  nerve —*see* Disorder, nerve
  nervous system G98.8
    autonomic G90.9
    central G96.9
      specified NEC G96.8
    congenital Q07.9
    parasympathetic G90.9
    specified NEC G98.8
    sympathetic G90.9
    vegetative G90.9
  neuromuscular system G70.9
  Newcastle B30.8
  Nicolas (-Durand)-Favre (climatic bubo) A55
  nipple N64.9
    Paget's C50.01-●
      female C50.01-●
      male C50.02-●
  Nishimoto (-Takeuchi) I67.5
  nonarthropod-borne NOS (viral) B34.9
    enterovirus NEC B34.1
  nonautoimmune hemolytic D59.4
    drug-induced D59.2

Disease, diseased *(Continued)*
  Nonne-Milroy-Meige (chronic hereditary edema) Q82.0
  nose J34.9
  nucleus pulposus —*see* Disorder, disc
  nutritional E63.9
  oast-house-urine E72.19
    ocular
      herpesviral B00.50
      zoster B02.30
  obliterative vascular I77.1
  Ohara's —*see* Tularemia
  Opitz's (congestive splenomegaly) D73.2
  Oppenheim-Urbach (necrobiosis lipoidica diabeticorum) —*see* E08-E13 with .620
  optic nerve NEC —*see* Disorder, nerve, optic
    orbit —*see* Disorder, orbit
  Oriental liver fluke B66.1
  Oriental lung fluke B66.4
  Ormond's N13.5
  Oropouche virus A93.0
  Osler-Rendu (familial hemorrhagic telangiectasia) I78.0
  osteofibrocystic E21.0
  Otto's M24.7
  outer ear —*see* Disorder, ear, external
  ovary (noninflammatory) N83.9
    cystic N83.20-●
    inflammatory —*see* Salpingo-oophoritis
    polycystic E28.2
    specified NEC N83.8
  Owren's (congenital) —*see* Defect, coagulation
  pancreas K86.9
    cystic K86.2
    fibrocystic E84.9
    specified NEC K86.89
  panvalvular I08.9
    specified NEC I08.8
  parametrium (noninflammatory) N83.9
  parasitic B89
    cerebral NEC B71.9 *[G94]*
    intestinal NOS B82.9
    mouth B37.0
    skin NOS B88.9
    specified type —*see* Infestation
    tongue B37.0
  parathyroid (gland) E21.5
    specified NEC E21.4
  Parkinson's G20
  parodontal K05.6
  Parrot's (syphilitic osteochondritis) A50.02
  Parry's (exophthalmic goiter) —*see* Hyperthyroidism, with, goiter (diffuse)
  Parson's (exophthalmic goiter) —*see* Hyperthyroidism, with, goiter (diffuse)
  Paxton's (white piedra) B36.2
  pearl-worker's —*see* Osteomyelitis, specified type NEC
  Pellegrini-Stieda (calcification, knee joint) —*see* Bursitis, tibial collateral
  pelvis, pelvic
    female NOS N94.9
      specified NEC N94.89
    gonococcal (acute) (chronic) A54.24
    inflammatory (female) N73.9
      acute N73.0
      chlamydial A56.11
      chronic N73.1
      specified NEC N73.8
      syphilitic (secondary) A51.42
        late A52.76
      tuberculous A18.17
    organ, female N94.9
    peritoneum, female NEC N94.89
  penis N48.9
    inflammatory N48.29
      abscess N48.21
      cellulitis N48.22
    specified NEC N48.89

- Disease, diseased *(Continued)*
  - periapical tissues NOS KØ4.9Ø
  - periodontal KØ5.6
    - specified NEC KØ5.5
  - periosteum —*see* Disorder, bone, specified type NEC
  - peripheral
    - arterial I73.9
    - autonomic nervous system G9Ø.9
    - nerves —*see* Polyneuropathy
    - vascular NOS I73.9
  - peritoneum K66.9
    - pelvic, female NEC N94.89
    - specified NEC K66.8
  - persistent mucosal (middle ear) H66.2Ø
    - left H66.22
      - with right H66.23
    - right H66.21
      - with left H66.23
  - Petit's —*see* Hernia, abdomen, specified site NEC
  - pharynx J39.2
    - specified NEC J39.2
  - Phocas' —*see* Mastopathy, cystic
  - photochromogenic (acid-fast bacilli) (pulmonary) A31.Ø
    - nonpulmonary A31.9
  - Pick's G31.Ø1 *[FØ2.8Ø]*
    - with behavioral disturbance G31.Ø1 *[FØ2.81]*
    - brain G31.Ø1 *[FØ2.8Ø]*
      - with behavioral disturbance G31.Ø1 *[FØ2.81]*
    - of pericardium (pericardial pseudocirrhosis of liver) I31.1
  - pigeon fancier's J67.2
  - pineal gland E34.8
  - pink —*see* Poisoning, mercury
  - Pinkus' (lichen nitidus) L44.1
  - pinworm B8Ø
  - Piry virus A93.8
  - pituitary (gland) E23.7
  - pituitary-snuff-taker's J67.8
  - pleura (cavity) J94.9
    - specified NEC J94.8
  - pneumatic drill (hammer) T75.21
  - Pollitzer's (hidradenitis suppurativa) L73.2
  - polycystic
    - kidney or renal Q61.3
      - adult type Q61.2
      - childhood type NEC Q61.19
        - collecting duct dilatation Q61.11
    - liver or hepatic Q44.6
    - lung or pulmonary J98.4
      - congenital Q33.Ø
    - ovary, ovaries E28.2
    - spleen Q89.Ø9
  - polyethylene T84.Ø5- •
  - Pompe's (glycogenosis II) E74.Ø2
  - Posadas-Wernicke B38.9
  - Potain's (pulmonary edema) —*see* Edema, lung
  - prepuce N47.8
    - inflammatory N47.7
      - balanoposthitis N47.6
  - Pringle's (tuberous sclerosis) Q85.1
  - prion, central nervous system A81.9
    - specified NEC A81.89
  - prostate N42.9
    - specified NEC N42.89
  - protozoal B64
    - acanthamebiasis —*see* Acanthamebiasis
    - African trypanosomiasis —*see* African trypanosomiasis
    - babesiosis B6Ø.Ø
    - Chagas disease —*see* Chagas disease
    - intestine, intestinal AØ7.9
    - leishmaniasis —*see* Leishmaniasis
    - malaria —*see* Malaria
    - naegleriasis B6Ø.2

- Disease, diseased *(Continued)*
  - protozoal *(Continued)*
    - pneumocystosis B59
    - specified organism NEC B6Ø.8
    - toxoplasmosis —*see* Toxoplasmosis
  - pseudo-Hurler's E77.Ø
  - psychiatric F99
  - psychotic —*see* Psychosis
  - Puente's (simple glandular cheilitis) K13.Ø
  - puerperal —*see also* Puerperal O9Ø.89
  - pulmonary —*see also* Disease, lung
    - artery I28.9
    - chronic obstructive J44.9
      - with
        - acute bronchitis J44.Ø
        - exacerbation (acute) J44.1
        - lower respiratory infection (acute) J44.Ø
      - decompensated J44.1
        - with
          - exacerbation (acute) J44.1
    - heart I27.9
      - specified NEC I27.89
    - hypertensive (vascular) —*see also* Hypertension, pulmonary I27.2Ø
      - primary (idiopathic) I27.Ø
    - valve I37.9
      - rheumatic IØ9.89
  - pulp (dental) NOS KØ4.9Ø
  - pulseless M31.4
  - Putnam's (subacute combined sclerosis with pernicious anemia) D51.Ø
  - Pyle (-Cohn) (metaphyseal dysplasia) Q78.5
  - ragpicker's or ragsorter's A22.1
  - Raynaud's —*see* Raynaud's disease
  - reactive airway —*see* Asthma
  - Reclus' (cystic) —*see* Mastopathy, cystic
  - rectum K62.9
    - specified NEC K62.89
  - Refsum's (heredopathia atactica polyneuritiformis) G6Ø.1
  - renal (functional) (pelvis) —*see also* Disease, kidney N28.9
    - with
      - edema —*see* Nephrosis
      - glomerular lesion —*see* Glomerulonephritis
        - with edema —*see* Nephrosis
      - interstitial nephritis N12
    - acute N28.9
    - chronic —*see also* Disease, kidney, chronic N18.9
    - cystic, congenital Q61.9
    - diabetic —*see* EØ8-E13 with .22
    - end-stage (failure) N18.6
      - due to hypertension I12.Ø
    - fibrocystic (congenital) Q61.8
    - hypertensive —*see* Hypertension, kidney
    - lupus M32.14
    - phosphate-losing (tubular) N25.Ø
    - polycystic (congenital) Q61.3
      - adult type Q61.2
      - childhood type NEC Q61.19
        - collecting duct dilatation Q61.11
    - rapidly progressive NØ1.9
    - subacute NØ1.9
  - Rendu-Osler-Weber (familial hemorrhagic telangiectasia) I78.Ø
  - renovascular (arteriosclerotic) —*see* Hypertension, kidney
  - respiratory (tract) J98.9
    - acute or subacute NOS JØ6.9
      - due to
        - chemicals, gases, fumes or vapors (inhalation) J68.3
        - external agent J7Ø.9
          - specified NEC J7Ø.8
        - radiation J7Ø.Ø
        - smoke inhalation J7Ø.5
      - noninfectious J39.8

- Disease, diseased *(Continued)*
  - respiratory *(Continued)*
    - chronic NOS J98.9
      - due to
        - chemicals, gases, fumes or vapors J68.4
        - external agent J7Ø.9
          - specified NEC J7Ø.8
        - radiation J7Ø.1
      - newborn P27.9
        - specified NEC P27.8
    - due to
      - chemicals, gases, fumes or vapors J68.9
        - acute or subacute NEC J68.3
        - chronic J68.4
      - external agent J7Ø.9
        - specified NEC J7Ø.8
    - newborn P28.9
      - specified type NEC P28.89
    - upper J39.9
      - acute or subacute JØ6.9
      - noninfectious NEC J39.8
      - specified NEC J39.8
      - streptococcal JØ6.9
  - retina, retinal H35.9
    - Batten's or Batten-Mayou E75.4 *[H36]*
    - specified NEC H35.89
  - rheumatoid —*see* Arthritis, rheumatoid
  - rickettsial NOS A79.9
    - specified type NEC A79.89
  - Riga (-Fede) (cachectic aphthae) K14.Ø
  - Riggs' (compound periodontitis) —*see* Periodontitis
  - Ritter's LØØ
  - Rivalta's (cervicofacial actinomycosis) A42.2
  - Robles' (onchocerciasis) B73.Ø1
  - Roger's (congenital interventricular septal defect) Q21.Ø
  - Rosenthal's (factor XI deficiency) D68.1
  - Ross River B33.1
  - Rossbach's (hyperchlorhydria) K31.89
    - ▶psychogenic F45.8
  - Rotes Quérol —*see* Hyperostosis, ankylosing
  - Roth (-Bernhardt) —*see* Mononeuropathy, lower limb, meralgia paresthetica
  - Runeberg's (progressive pernicious anemia) D51.Ø
  - sacroiliac NEC M53.3
  - salivary gland or duct K11.9
    - inclusion B25.9
    - specified NEC K11.8
    - virus B25.9
  - sandworm B76.9
  - Schimmelbusch's —*see* Mastopathy, cystic
  - Schmorl's —*see* Schmorl's disease or nodes
  - Schönlein (-Henoch) (purpura rheumatica) D69.Ø
  - Schottmüller's —*see* Fever, paratyphoid
  - Schultz's (agranulocytosis) —*see* Agranulocytosis
  - Schwalbe-Ziehen-Oppenheim G24.1
  - Schwartz-Jampel G71.13
  - sclera H15.9
    - specified NEC H15.89
  - scrofulous (tuberculous) A18.2
  - scrotum N5Ø.9
  - sebaceous glands L73.9
  - semilunar cartilage, cystic —*see also* Derangement, knee, meniscus, cystic
  - seminal vesicle N5Ø.9
  - serum NEC —*see also* Reaction, serum T8Ø.69
  - sexually transmitted A64
    - anogenital
      - herpesviral infection —*see* Herpes, anogenital
      - warts A63.Ø
    - chancroid A57
    - chlamydial infection —*see* Chlamydia
    - gonorrhea —*see* Gonorrhea
    - granuloma inguinale A58
    - specified organism NEC A63.8

D

Disease, diseased *(Continued)*
sexually transmitted *(Continued)*
syphilis —*see* Syphilis
trichomoniasis —*see* Trichomoniasis
Sézary C84.1- ●
shimamushi (scrub typhus) A75.3
shipyard B30.0
sickle-cell D57.1
with crisis (vasoocclusive pain) D57.00
with
acute chest syndrome D57.01
splenic sequestration D57.02
elliptocytosis D57.8- ●
Hb-C D57.20
with crisis (vasoocclusive pain) D57.219
with
acute chest syndrome D57.211
splenic sequestration D57.212
without crisis D57.20
Hb-SD D57.80
with crisis D57.819
with
acute chest syndrome D57.811
splenic sequestration D57.812
Hb-SE D57.80
with crisis D57.819
with
acute chest syndrome D57.811
splenic sequestration D57.812
specified NEC D57.80
with crisis D57.819
with
acute chest syndrome D57.811
splenic sequestration D57.812
spherocytosis D57.80
with crisis D57.819
with
acute chest syndrome D57.811
splenic sequestration D57.812
thalassemia D57.40
with crisis (vasoocclusive pain) D57.419
with
acute chest syndrome D57.411
splenic sequestration D57.412
without crisis D57.40
silo-filler's J68.8
bronchitis J68.0
pneumonitis J68.0
pulmonary edema J68.1
simian B B00.4
Simons' (progressive lipodystrophy) E88.1
sin nombre virus B33.4
sinus —*see* Sinusitis
Sirkari's B55.0
sixth B08.20
due to human herpesvirus 6 B08.21
due to human herpesvirus 7 B08.22
skin L98.9
due to metabolic disorder NEC E88.9 *[L99]*
specified NEC L98.8
slim (HIV) B20
small vessel I73.9
Sneddon-Wilkinson (subcorneal pustular dermatosis) L13.1
South African creeping B88.0
spinal (cord) G95.9
congenital Q06.9
specified NEC G95.89
spine —*see also* Spondylopathy
joint —*see* Dorsopathy
tuberculous A18.01
spinocerebellar (hereditary) G11.9
specified NEC G11.8
spleen D73.9
amyloid E85.4 *[D77]*
organic D73.9
polycystic Q89.09
postinfectional D73.89
sponge-diver's —*see* Toxicity, venom, marine animal, sea anemone

Disease, diseased *(Continued)*
Startle Q89.8
Steinert's G71.11
Sticker's (erythema infectiosum) B08.3
Stieda's (calcification, knee joint) —*see* Bursitis, tibial collateral
Stokes' (exophthalmic goiter) —*see* Hyperthyroidism, with, goiter (diffuse)
Stokes-Adams (syncope with heart block) I45.9
stomach K31.9
functional, psychogenic F45.8
specified NEC K31.89
stonemason's J62.8
storage
glycogen —*see* Disease, glycogen storage
mucopolysaccharide —*see* Mucopolysaccharidosis
striatopallidal system NEC G25.89
Stuart-Prower (congenital factor X deficiency) D68.2
Stuart's (congenital factor X deficiency) D68.2
subcutaneous tissue —*see* Disease, skin
supporting structures of teeth K08.9
specified NEC K08.89
suprarenal (capsule) (gland) E27.9
hyperfunction E27.0
specified NEC E27.8
sweat glands L74.9
specified NEC L74.8
Sweeley-Klionsky E75.21
Swift (-Feer) —*see* Poisoning, mercury
swimming-pool granuloma A31.1
Sylvest's (epidemic pleurodynia) B33.0
sympathetic nervous system G90.9
synovium —*see* Disorder, synovium
syphilitic —*see* Syphilis
systemic tissue mast cell D47.02
tanapox (virus) B08.71
Tangier E78.6
Tarral-Besnier (pityriasis rubra pilaris) L44.0
Tauri's E74.09
tear duct —*see* Disorder, lacrimal system
tendon, tendinous —*see also* Disorder, tendon
nodular —*see* Trigger finger
terminal vessel I73.9
testis N50.9
thalassemia Hb-S —*see* Disease, sickle-cell, thalassemia
Thaysen-Gee (nontropical sprue) K90.0
Thomsen G71.12
throat J39.2
septic J02.0
thromboembolic —*see* Embolism
thymus (gland) E32.9
specified NEC E32.8
thyroid (gland) E07.9
heart —*see also* Hyperthyroidism E05.90 *[I43]*
with thyroid storm E05.91 *[I43]*
specified NEC E07.8
Tietze's M94.0
tongue K14.9
specified NEC K14.89
tonsils, tonsillar (and adenoids) J35.9
tooth, teeth K08.9
hard tissues K03.9
specified NEC K03.89
pulp NEC K04.99
specified NEC K08.89
Tourette's F95.2
trachea NEC J39.8
tricuspid I07.9
nonrheumatic I36.9
triglyceride-storage E75.5
trophoblastic —*see* Mole, hydatidiform
tsutsugamushi A75.3
tube (fallopian) (noninflammatory) N83.9
inflammatory —*see* Salpingitis
specified NEC N83.8
tuberculous NEC —*see* Tuberculosis

Disease, diseased *(Continued)*
tubo-ovarian (noninflammatory) N83.9
inflammatory —*see* Salpingo-oophoritis
specified NEC N83.8
tubotympanic, chronic —*see* Otitis, media, suppurative, chronic, tubotympanic
tubulo-interstitial N15.9
specified NEC N15.8
tympanum —*see* Disorder, tympanic membrane
Uhl's Q24.8
Underwood's (sclerema neonatorum) P83.0
Unverricht (-Lundborg) —*see* Epilepsy, generalized, idiopathic
Urbach-Oppenheim (necrobiosis lipoidica diabeticorum) —*see* E08-E13 with .620
ureter N28.9
in (due to)
schistosomiasis (bilharziasis) B65.0 *[N29]*
urethra N36.9
specified NEC N36.8
urinary (tract) N39.9
bladder N32.9
specified NEC N32.89
specified NEC N39.8
uterus (noninflammatory) N85.9
infective —*see* Endometritis
inflammatory —*see* Endometritis
specified NEC N85.8
uveal tract (anterior) H21.9
posterior H31.9
vagabond's B85.1
vagina, vaginal (noninflammatory) N89.9
inflammatory NEC N76.89
specified NEC N89.8
valve, valvular I38
multiple I08.9
specified NEC I08.8
van Creveld-von Gierke (glycogenosis I) E74.01
vas deferens N50.9
vascular I99.9
arteriosclerotic —*see* Arteriosclerosis
ciliary body NEC —*see* Disorder, iris, vascular
hypertensive —*see* Hypertension
iris NEC —*see* Disorder, iris, vascular
obliterative I77.1
peripheral I73.9
occlusive I99.8
peripheral (occlusive) I73.9
in diabetes mellitus —*see* E08-E13 with .51
vasomotor I73.9
vasospastic I73.9
vein I87.9
venereal —*see also* Disease, sexually transmitted A64
chlamydial NEC A56.8
anus A56.3
genitourinary NOS A56.2
pharynx A56.4
rectum A56.3
fifth A55
sixth A55
specified nature or type NEC A63.8
vertebra, vertebral —*see also* Spondylopathy
disc —*see* Disorder, disc
vibration —*see* Vibration, adverse effects
viral, virus —*see also* Disease, by type of virus B34.9
arbovirus NOS A94
arthropod-borne NOS A94
congenital P35.9
specified NEC P35.8
Hanta (with renal manifestations) (Dobrava) (Puumala) (Seoul) A98.5
with pulmonary manifestations (Andes) (Bayou) (Bermejo) (Black Creek Canal) (Choclo) (Juquitiba) (Laguna negra) (Lechiguanas) (New York) (Oran) (Sin nombre) B33.4

Disease, diseased *(Continued)*
viral, virus *(Continued)*
Hantaan (Korean hemorrhagic fever) A98.5
human immunodeficiency (HIV) B20
Kunjin A83.4
nonarthropod-borne NOS B34.9
Powassan A84.8
Rocio (encephalitis) A83.6
Sin nombre (Hantavirus) (cardio)-pulmonary syndrome B33.4
Tahyna B33.8
vesicular stomatitis A93.8
vitreous H43.9
specified NEC H43.89
vocal cord J38.3
Volkmann's, acquired T79.6
von Eulenburg's (congenital paramyotonia) G71.19
von Gierke's (glycogenosis I) E74.01
von Graefe's —*see* Strabismus, paralytic, ophthalmoplegia, progressive
von Willebrand (-Jürgens) (angiohemophilia) D68.0
Vrolik's (osteogenesis imperfecta) Q78.0
vulva (noninflammatory) N90.9
inflammatory NEC N76.89
specified NEC N90.89
Wallgren's (obstruction of splenic vein with collateral circulation) I87.8
Wassilieff's (leptospiral jaundice) A27.0
wasting NEC R64
due to malnutrition E41
Waterhouse-Friderichsen A39.1
Wegner's (syphilitic osteochondritis) A50.02
Weil's (leptospiral jaundice of lung) A27.0
Weir Mitchell's (erythromelalgia) I73.81
Werdnig-Hoffmann G12.0
Wermer's E31.21
Werner-His (trench fever) A79.0
Werner-Schultz (neutropenic splenomegaly) D73.81
Wernicke-Posadas B38.9
whipworm B79
white blood cells D72.9
specified NEC D72.89
white matter R90.82
white-spot, meaning lichen sclerosus et atrophicus L90.0
penis N48.0
vulva N90.4
Wilkie's K55.1
Wilkinson-Sneddon (subcorneal pustular dermatosis) L13.1
Willis' —*see* Diabetes
Wilson's (hepatolenticular degeneration) E83.01
woolsorter's A22.1
yaba monkey tumor B08.72
yaba pox (virus) B08.72
Zika virus A92.5
zoonotic, bacterial A28.9
congenital P35.4
specified type NEC A28.8
Disfigurement (due to scar) L90.5
Disgerminoma —*see* Dysgerminoma
DISH (diffuse idiopathic skeletal hyperostosis) —*see* Hyperostosis, ankylosing
Disinsertion, retina —*see* Detachment, retina
Dislocatable hip, congenital Q65.6
Dislocation (articular)
with fracture —*see* Fracture
acromioclavicular (joint) S43.10-●
with displacement
100%-200% S43.12-●
more than 200% S43.13-●
inferior S43.14-●
posterior S43.15-●
ankle S93.0-●
astragalus —*see* Dislocation, ankle
atlantoaxial S13.121
atlantooccipital S13.111

Dislocation *(Continued)*
atloidooccipital S13.111
breast bone S23.29
capsule, joint code by site under Dislocation
carpal (bone) —*see* Dislocation, wrist
carpometacarpal (joint) NEC S63.05-●
thumb S63.04-●
cartilage (joint) - code by site under Dislocation
cervical spine (vertebra) —*see* Dislocation, vertebra, cervical
chronic —*see* Dislocation, recurrent
clavicle —*see* Dislocation, acromioclavicular joint
coccyx S33.2
congenital NEC Q68.8
coracoid —*see* Dislocation, shoulder
costal cartilage S23.29
costochondral S23.29
cricoarytenoid articulation S13.29
cricothyroid articulation S13.29
dorsal vertebra —*see* Dislocation, vertebra, thoracic
ear ossicle —*see* Discontinuity, ossicles, ear
elbow S53.10-●
congenital Q68.8
pathological —*see* Dislocation, pathological NEC, elbow
radial head alone —*see* Dislocation, radial head
recurrent —*see* Dislocation, recurrent, elbow
traumatic S53.10-●
anterior S53.11-●
lateral S53.14-●
medial S53.13-●
posterior S53.12-●
specified type NEC S53.19-●
eye, nontraumatic —*see* Luxation, globe
eyeball, nontraumatic —*see* Luxation, globe
femur
distal end —*see* Dislocation, knee
proximal end —*see* Dislocation, hip
fibula
distal end —*see* Dislocation, ankle
proximal end —*see* Dislocation, knee
finger S63.25-●
index S63.25-●
interphalangeal S63.27-●
distal S63.29-●
index S63.29-●
little S63.29-●
middle S63.29-●
ring S63.29-●
index S63.27-●
little S63.27-●
middle S63.27-●
proximal S63.28-●
index S63.28-●
little S63.28-●
middle S63.28-●
ring S63.28-●
ring S63.27-●
little S63.25-●
metacarpophalangeal S63.26-●
index S63.26-●
little S63.26-●
middle S63.26-●
ring S63.26-●
middle S63.25-●
recurrent —*see* Dislocation, recurrent, finger
ring S63.25-●
thumb —*see* Dislocation, thumb
foot S93.30-●
recurrent —*see* Dislocation, recurrent, foot
specified site NEC S93.33-●
tarsal joint S93.31-●
tarsometatarsal joint S93.32-●
toe —*see* Dislocation, toe

Dislocation *(Continued)*
fracture —*see* Fracture
glenohumeral (joint) —*see* Dislocation, shoulder
glenoid —*see* Dislocation, shoulder
habitual —*see* Dislocation, recurrent
hip S73.00-●
anterior S73.03-●
obturator S73.02-●
central S73.04-●
congenital (total) Q65.2
bilateral Q65.1
partial Q65.5
bilateral Q65.4
unilateral Q65.3-●
unilateral Q65.0-●
developmental M24.85-●
pathological —*see* Dislocation, pathological NEC, hip
posterior S73.01-●
recurrent —*see* Dislocation, recurrent, hip
humerus, proximal end —*see* Dislocation, shoulder
incomplete —*see* Subluxation, by site
incus —*see* Discontinuity, ossicles, ear
infracoracoid —*see* Dislocation, shoulder
innominate (pubic junction) (sacral junction) S33.39
acetabulum —*see* Dislocation, hip
interphalangeal (joint(s))
finger S63.279
distal S63.29-●
index S63.29-●
little S63.29-●
middle S63.29-●
ring S63.29-●
index S63.27-●
little S63.27-●
middle S63.27-●
proximal S63.28-●
index S63.28-●
little S63.28-●
middle S63.28-●
ring S63.28-●
ring S63.27-●
foot or toe —*see* Dislocation, toe
thumb S63.12-●
jaw (cartilage) (meniscus) S03.0-●
joint prosthesis —*see* Complications, joint prosthesis, mechanical, displacement, by site
knee S83.106
cap —*see* Dislocation, patella
congenital Q68.2
old M23.8X-●
patella —*see* Dislocation, patella
pathological —*see* Dislocation, pathological NEC, knee
proximal tibia
anteriorly S83.11-●
laterally S83.14-●
medially S83.13-●
posteriorly S83.12-●
recurrent —*see also* Derangement, knee, specified NEC
specified type NEC S83.19-●
lacrimal gland H04.16-●
lens (complete) H27.10-●
anterior H27.12-●
congenital Q12.1
ocular implant —*see* Complications, intraocular lens
partial H27.11-●
posterior H27.13-●
traumatic S05.8X-●
ligament code by site under Dislocation
lumbar (vertebra) —*see* Dislocation, vertebra, lumbar

- Dislocation *(Continued)*
  - lumbosacral (vertebra) *—see also* Dislocation, vertebra, lumbar
    - congenital Q76.49
  - mandible S03.0- •
  - meniscus (knee) *—see* Tear, meniscus
    - other sites code by site under Dislocation
  - metacarpal (bone)
    - distal end *—see* Dislocation, finger
    - proximal end S63.06- •
  - metacarpophalangeal (joint)
    - finger S63.26- •
      - index S63.26- •
      - little S63.26- •
      - middle S63.26- •
      - ring S63.26- •
    - thumb S63.11- •
  - metatarsal (bone) *—see* Dislocation, foot
  - metatarsophalangeal (joint(s)) *—see* Dislocation, toe
  - midcarpal (joint) S63.03- •
  - midtarsal (joint) *—see* Dislocation, foot
  - neck S13.20
    - specified site NEC S13.29
    - vertebra *—see* Dislocation, vertebra, cervical
  - nose (septal cartilage) S03.1
  - occipitoatloid S13.111
  - old *—see* Derangement, joint, specified type NEC
  - ossicles, ear *—see* Discontinuity, ossicles, ear
  - partial *—see* Subluxation, by site
  - patella S83.006
    - congenital Q74.1
    - lateral S83.01- •
    - recurrent (nontraumatic) M22.0- •
      - incomplete M22.1- •
    - specified type NEC S83.09- •
  - pathological NEC M24.30
    - ankle M24.37- •
    - elbow M24.32- •
    - foot joint M24.37- •
    - hand joint M24.34- •
    - hip M24.35- •
    - knee M24.36- •
    - lumbosacral joint *—see* subcategory M53.2
    - pelvic region *—see* Dislocation, pathological, hip
    - sacroiliac *—see* subcategory M53.2
    - shoulder M24.31- •
    - wrist M24.33- •
  - pelvis NEC S33.30
    - specified NEC S33.39
  - phalanx
    - finger or hand *—see* Dislocation, finger
    - foot or toe *—see* Dislocation, toe
  - prosthesis, internal *—see* Complications, prosthetic device, by site, mechanical
  - radial head S53.006
    - anterior S53.01- •
    - posterior S53.02- •
    - specified type NEC S53.09- •
  - radiocarpal (joint) S63.02- •
  - radiohumeral (joint) *—see* Dislocation, radial head
  - radioulnar (joint)
    - distal S63.01- •
    - proximal *—see* Dislocation, elbow
  - radius
    - distal end *—see* Dislocation, wrist
    - proximal end *—see* Dislocation, radial head
  - recurrent M24.40
    - ankle M24.47- •
    - elbow M24.42- •
    - finger M24.44- •
    - foot joint M24.47- •
    - hand joint M24.44- •
    - hip M24.45- •
    - knee M24.46- •
      - patella *—see* Dislocation, patella, recurrent
- Dislocation *(Continued)*
  - recurrent *(Continued)*
    - patella *—see* Dislocation, patella, recurrent
    - sacroiliac *—see* subcategory M53.2
    - shoulder M24.41- •
    - toe M24.47- •
    - vertebra *—see also* subcategory M43.5
      - atlantoaxial M43.4
        - with myelopathy M43.3
    - wrist M24.43- •
  - rib (cartilage) S23.29
  - sacrococcygeal S33.2
  - sacroiliac (joint) (ligament) S33.2
    - congenital Q74.2
    - recurrent *—see* subcategory M53.2
  - sacrum S33.2
  - scaphoid (bone) (hand) (wrist) *—see* Dislocation, wrist
    - foot *—see* Dislocation, foot
  - scapula *—see* Dislocation, shoulder, girdle, scapula
  - semilunar cartilage, knee *—see* Tear, meniscus
  - septal cartilage (nose) S03.1
  - septum (nasal) (old) J34.2
  - sesamoid bone code by site under Dislocation
  - shoulder (blade) (ligament) (joint) (traumatic) S43.006
    - acromioclavicular *—see* Dislocation, acromioclavicular
    - chronic *—see* Dislocation, recurrent, shoulder
    - congenital Q68.8
    - girdle S43.30- •
      - scapula S43.31- •
      - specified site NEC S43.39- •
    - humerus S43.00- •
      - anterior S43.01- •
      - inferior S43.03- •
      - posterior S43.02- •
    - pathological *—see* Dislocation, pathological NEC, shoulder
    - recurrent *—see* Dislocation, recurrent, shoulder
    - specified type NEC S43.08- •
  - spine
    - cervical *—see* Dislocation, vertebra, cervical
    - congenital Q76.49
    - due to birth trauma P11.5
    - lumbar *—see* Dislocation, vertebra, lumbar
    - thoracic *—see* Dislocation, vertebra, thoracic
  - spontaneous *—see* Dislocation, pathological
  - sternoclavicular (joint) S43.206
    - anterior S43.21- •
    - posterior S43.22- •
  - sternum S23.29
  - subglenoid *—see* Dislocation, shoulder
  - symphysis pubis S33.4
  - talus *—see* Dislocation, ankle
  - tarsal (bone(s)) (joint(s)) *—see* Dislocation, foot
  - tarsometatarsal (joint(s)) *—see* Dislocation, foot
  - temporomandibular (joint) S03.0- •
  - thigh, proximal end *—see* Dislocation, hip
  - thorax S23.20
    - specified site NEC S23.29
    - vertebra *—see* Dislocation, vertebra
  - thumb S63.10- •
    - interphalangeal joint *—see* Dislocation, interphalangeal (joint), thumb
    - metacarpophalangeal joint *—see* Dislocation, metacarpophalangeal (joint), thumb
  - thyroid cartilage S13.29
  - tibia
    - distal end *—see* Dislocation, ankle
    - proximal end *—see* Dislocation, knee
  - tibiofibular (joint)
    - distal *—see* Dislocation, ankle
    - superior *—see* Dislocation, knee
- Dislocation *(Continued)*
  - toe(s) S93.106
    - great S93.10- •
      - interphalangeal joint S93.11- •
      - metatarsophalangeal joint S93.12- •
    - interphalangeal joint S93.119
    - lesser S93.106
      - interphalangeal joint S93.11- •
      - metatarsophalangeal joint S93.12- •
    - metatarsophalangeal joint S93.12- •
  - tooth S03.2
  - trachea S23.29
  - ulna
    - distal end S63.07- •
    - proximal end *—see* Dislocation, elbow
  - ulnohumeral (joint) *—see* Dislocation, elbow
  - vertebra (articular process) (body) (traumatic)
    - cervical S13.101
      - atlantoaxial joint S13.121
      - atlantooccipital joint S13.111
      - atloidooccipital joint S13.111
      - joint between
        - C0 and C1 S13.111
        - C1 and C2 S13.121
        - C2 and C3 S13.131
        - C3 and C4 S13.141
        - C4 and C5 S13.151
        - C5 and C6 S13.161
        - C6 and C7 S13.171
        - C7 and T1 S13.181
      - occipitoatloid joint S13.111
    - congenital Q76.49
    - lumbar S33.101
      - joint between
        - L1 and L2 S33.111
        - L2 and L3 S33.121
        - L3 and L4 S33.131
        - L4 and L5 S33.141
    - nontraumatic *—see* Displacement, intervertebral disc
    - partial *—see* Subluxation, by site
    - recurrent NEC *—see* subcategory M43.5
    - thoracic S23.101
      - joint between
        - T1 and T2 S23.111
        - T2 and T3 S23.121
        - T3 and T4 S23.123
        - T4 and T5 S23.131
        - T5 and T6 S23.133
        - T6 and T7 S23.141
        - T7 and T8 S23.143
        - T8 and T9 S23.151
        - T9 and T10 S23.153
        - T10 and T11 S23.161
        - T11 and T12 S23.163
        - T12 and L1 S23.171
  - wrist (carpal bone) S63.006
    - carpometacarpal joint *—see* Dislocation, carpometacarpal (joint)
    - distal radioulnar joint *—see* Dislocation, radioulnar (joint), distal
    - metacarpal bone, proximal *—see* Dislocation, metacarpal (bone), proximal end
    - midcarpal *—see* Dislocation, midcarpal (joint)
    - radiocarpal joint *—see* Dislocation, radiocarpal (joint)
    - recurrent *—see* Dislocation, recurrent, wrist
    - specified site NEC S63.09- •
    - ulna *—see* Dislocation, ulna, distal end
  - xiphoid cartilage S23.29
- Disorder (of) *—see also* Disease
  - acantholytic L11.9
    - specified NEC L11.8
  - acute
    - psychotic *—see* Psychosis, acute
    - stress F43.0

Disorder *(Continued)*
adjustment (grief) F43.20
with
anxiety F43.22
with depressed mood F43.23
conduct disturbance F43.24
with emotional disturbance F43.25
depressed mood F43.21
with anxiety F43.23
other specified symptom F43.29
adrenal (capsule) (gland) (medullary) E27.9
specified NEC E27.8
adrenogenital E25.9
drug-induced E25.8
iatrogenic E25.8
idiopathic E25.8
adult personality (and behavior) F69
specified NEC F68.8
affective (mood) —*see* Disorder, mood
aggressive, unsocialized F91.1
alcohol-related F10.99
with
amnestic disorder, persisting F10.96
anxiety disorder F10.980
dementia, persisting F10.97
intoxication F10.929
with delirium F10.921
uncomplicated F10.920
mood disorder F10.94
other specified F10.988
psychotic disorder F10.959
with
delusions F10.950
hallucinations F10.951
sexual dysfunction F10.981
sleep disorder F10.982
alcohol use
mild F10.10
with
alcohol-induced
anxiety disorder F10.180
bipolar and related disorder F10.14
depressive disorder F10.14
psychotic disorder F10.159
sexual dysfunction F10.181
sleep disorder F10.182
alcohol intoxication F10.129
delirium F10.121
in remission (early) (sustained) F10.11
moderate or severe F10.20
with
alcohol-induced
anxiety disorder F10.280
bipolar and related disorder F10.24
depressive disorder F10.24
major neurocognitive disorder, amnestic-confabulatory type F10.26
major neurocognitive disorder, nonamnestic-confabulatory type F10.27
mild neurocognitive disorder F10.288
psychotic disorder F10.259
sexual dysfunction F10.281
sleep disorder F10.282
alcohol intoxication F10.229
delirium F10.221
in remission (early) (sustained) F10.21
allergic —*see* Allergy
alveolar NEC J84.09
amino-acid
cystathioninuria E72.19
cystinosis E72.04
cystinuria E72.01
glycinuria E72.09
homocystinuria E72.11
metabolism —*see* Disturbance, metabolism, amino-acid
specified NEC E72.89
neonatal, transitory P74.8

Disorder *(Continued)*
amino-acid *(Continued)*
renal transport NEC E72.09
transport NEC E72.09
amnesic, amnestic
alcohol-induced F10.96
with dependence F10.26
due to (secondary to) general medical condition F04
psychoactive NEC-induced F19.96
with
abuse F19.16
dependence F19.26
sedative, hypnotic or anxiolytic-• induced F13.96
with dependence F13.26
amphetamine-type substance use
mild F15.10
in remission (early) (sustained) F15.11
moderate F15.20
in remission (early) (sustained) F15.21
severe F15.20
in remission (early) (sustained) F15.21
amphetamine (or other stimulant) use
mild
with
amphetamine (or other stimulant) -induced
anxiety disorder F15.180
bipolar and related disorder F15.14
depressive disorder F15.14
obsessive-compulsive and related disorder F15.188
psychotic disorder F15.159
sexual dysfunction F15.181
amphetamine, cocaine, or other stimulant intoxication
with perceptual disturbances F15.122
without perceptual disturbances F15.129
intoxication delirium F15.121
moderate or severe
with
amphetamine (or other stimulant) -induced
anxiety disorder F15.280
obsessive-compulsive and related disorder F15.288
sexual dysfunction F15.281
bipolar and related disorder F15.24
depressive disorder F15.24
psychotic disorder F15.259
amphetamine, cocaine, or other stimulant intoxication
with perceptual disturbances F15.222
without perceptual disturbances F15.229
intoxication delirium F15.221
anaerobic glycolysis with anemia D55.2
anxiety F41.9
due to (secondary to)
alcohol F10.980
in
abuse F10.180
dependence F10.280
amphetamine F15.980
in
abuse F15.180
dependence F15.280
anxiolytic F13.980
in
abuse F13.180
dependence F13.280
caffeine F15.980
in
abuse F15.180
dependence F15.280

Disorder *(Continued)*
anxiety *(Continued)*
due to *(Continued)*
cannabis F12.980
in
abuse F12.180
dependence F12.280
cocaine F14.980
in
abuse F14.180
dependence F14.180
general medical condition F06.4
hallucinogen F16.980
in
abuse F16.180
dependence F16.280
hypnotic F13.980
in
abuse F13.180
dependence F13.280
inhalant F18.980
in
abuse F18.180
dependence F18.280
phencyclidine F16.980
in
abuse F16.180
dependence F16.280
psychoactive substance NEC F19.980
in
abuse F19.180
dependence F19.280
sedative F13.980
in
abuse F13.180
dependence F13.280
volatile solvents F18.980
in
abuse F18.180
dependence F18.280
generalized F41.1
illness F45.21
mixed
with depression (mild) F41.8
specified NEC F41.3
organic F06.4
phobic F40.9
of childhood F40.8
specified NEC F41.8
aortic valve —*see* Endocarditis, aortic
aromatic amino-acid metabolism E70.9
specified NEC E70.8
arteriole NEC I77.89
artery NEC I77.89
articulation —*see* Disorder, joint
attachment (childhood)
disinhibited F94.2
reactive F94.1
attention-deficit hyperactivity (adolescent) (adult) (child) F98.8
combined
presentation F90.2
type F90.2
hyperactive
impulsive presentation F90.1
type F90.1
inattentive
presentation F90.0
type F90.0
specified type NEC F90.8
attention-deficit without hyperactivity (adolescent) (adult) (child) F90.0
auditory processing (central) H93.25
autism spectrum F84.0
autistic F84.0
autoimmune D89.89
autonomic nervous system G90.9
specified NEC G90.8
avoidant
child or adolescent F40.10
restrictive food intake F50.82

Disorder *(Continued)*
balance
acid-base E87.8
mixed E87.4
electrolyte E87.8
fluid NEC E87.8
behavioral (disruptive) —*see* Disorder, conduct
beta-amino-acid metabolism E72.89
bile acid and cholesterol metabolism E78.70
Barth syndrome E78.71
other specified E78.79
Smith-Lemli-Opitz syndrome E78.72
bilirubin excretion E80.6
binge eating F50.81
binocular
movement H51.9
convergence
excess H51.12
insufficiency H51.11
internuclear ophthalmoplegia —*see* Ophthalmoplegia, internuclear
palsy of conjugate gaze H51.0
specified type NEC H51.8
vision NEC —*see* Disorder, vision, binocular
bipolar (I) (type 1) F31.9
and related due to a known physiological condition
with
manic features F06.33
manic- or hypomanic-like episodes F06.33
mixed features F06.34
current (or most recent) episode
depressed F31.9
with psychotic features F31.5
without psychotic features F31.30
mild F31.31
moderate F31.32
severe (without psychotic features) F31.4
with psychotic features F31.5
hypomanic F31.0
manic F31.9
with psychotic features F31.2
without psychotic features F31.10
mild F31.11
moderate F31.12
severe (without psychotic features) F31.13
with psychotic features F31.2
mixed F31.60
mild F31.61
moderate F31.62
severe (without psychotic features) F31.63
with psychotic features F31.64
severe depression (without psychotic features) F31.4
with psychotic features F31.5
II (type 2) F31.81
in remission (currently) F31.70
in full remission
most recent episode
depressed F31.76
hypomanic F31.72
manic F31.74
mixed F31.78
in partial remission
most recent episode
depressed F31.75
hypomanic F31.71
manic F31.73
mixed F31.77
organic F06.30
single manic episode F30.9
mild F30.11
moderate F30.12
hhsevere (without psychotic symptoms) F30.13
with psychotic symptoms F30.2
specified NEC F31.89

Disorder *(Continued)*
bladder N32.9
functional NEC N31.9
in schistosomiasis B65.0 *[N33]*
specified NEC N32.89
bleeding D68.9
blood D75.9
in congenital early syphilis A50.09 *[D77]*
body dysmorphic F45.22
bone M89.9
continuity M84.9
specified type NEC M84.80
ankle M84.87-●
fibula M84.86-●
foot M84.87-●
hand M84.84-●
humerus M84.82-●
neck M84.88
pelvis M84.859
radius M84.83-●
rib M84.88
shoulder M84.81-●
skull M84.88
thigh M84.85-●
tibia M84.86-●
ulna M84.83-●
vertebra M84.88
density and structure M85.9
cyst —*see also* Cyst, bone, specified type NEC
aneurysmal —*see* Cyst, bone, aneurysmal
solitary —*see* Cyst, bone, solitary
diffuse idiopathic skeletal hyperostosis —*see* Hyperostosis, ankylosing
fibrous dysplasia (monostotic) —*see* Dysplasia, fibrous, bone
fluorosis —*see* Fluorosis, skeletal
hyperostosis of skull M85.2
osteitis condensans —*see* Osteitis, condensans
specified type NEC M85.8-●
ankle M85.87-●
foot M85.87-●
forearm M85.83-●
hand M85.84-●
lower leg M85.86-●
multiple sites M85.89
neck M85.88
rib M85.88
shoulder M85.81-●
skull M85.88
thigh M85.85-●
upper arm M85.82-●
vertebra M85.88
development and growth NEC M89.20
carpus M89.24-●
clavicle M89.21-●
femur M89.25-●
fibula M89.26-●
finger M89.24-●
humerus M89.22-●
ilium M89.259
ischium M89.259
metacarpus M89.24-●
metatarsus M89.27-●
multiple sites M89.29
neck M89.28
radius M89.23-●
rib M89.28
scapula M89.21-●
skull M89.28
tarsus M89.27-●
tibia M89.26-●
toe M89.27-●
ulna M89.23-●
vertebra M89.28
specified type NEC M89.8X-●
brachial plexus G54.0

Disorder *(Continued)*
branched-chain amino-acid metabolism E71.2
specified NEC E71.19
breast N64.9
agalactia —*see* Agalactia
associated with
lactation O92.70
specified NEC O92.79
pregnancy O92.20
specified NEC O92.29
puerperium O92.20
specified NEC O92.29
cracked nipple —*see* Cracked nipple
galactorrhea —*see* Galactorrhea
hypogalactia O92.4
lactation disorder NEC O92.79
mastitis —*see* Mastitis
nipple infection —*see* Infection, nipple
retracted nipple —*see* Retraction, nipple
specified type NEC N64.89
Briquet's F45.0
bullous, in diseases classified elsewhere L14
caffeine use
mild
with
caffeine-induced
anxiety disorder F15.180
sleep disorder F15.182
moderate or severe
with
caffeine-induced
anxiety disorder F15.280
sleep disorder F15.282
cannabis use
mild F12.10
with
cannabis-induced
anxiety disorder F12.180
psychotic disorder F12.159
sleep disorder F12.188
cannabis intoxication delirium F12.121
with perceptual disturbances F12.122
without perceptual disturbances F12.129
in remission (early) (sustained) F12.11
moderate or severe F12.20
with
cannabis-induced
anxiety disorder F12.280
psychotic disorder F12.259
sleep disorder F12.288
cannabis intoxication
with perceptual disturbances F12.222
without perceptual disturbances F12.229
delirium F12.221
in remission (early) (sustained) F12.21
carbohydrate
absorption, intestinal NEC E74.39
metabolism (congenital) E74.9
specified NEC E74.8
cardiac, functional I51.89
carnitine metabolism E71.40
cartilage M94.9
articular NEC —*see* Derangement, joint, articular cartilage
chondrocalcinosis —*see* Chondrocalcinosis
specified type NEC M94.8X-●
articular —*see* Derangement, joint, articular cartilage
multiple sites M94.8X0
catatonia (due to known physiological condition) (with another mental disorder) F06.1
catatonic
due to (secondary to) known physiological condition F06.1
organic F06.1

Disorder *(Continued)*
central auditory processing H93.25
cervical
region NEC M53.82
root (nerve) NEC G54.2
character NOS F6Ø.9
childhood disintegrative NEC F84.3
cholesterol and bile acid metabolism E78.7Ø
Barth syndrome E78.71
other specified E78.79
Smith-Lemli-Opitz syndrome E78.72
choroid H31.9
atrophy *—see* Atrophy, choroid
degeneration *—see* Degeneration, choroid
detachment *—see* Detachment, choroid
dystrophy *—see* Dystrophy, choroid
hemorrhage *—see* Hemorrhage, choroid
rupture *—see* Rupture, choroid
scar *—see* Scar, chorioretinal
solar retinopathy *—see* Retinopathy, solar
specified type NEC H31.8
ciliary body *—see* Disorder, iris
degeneration *—see* Degeneration, ciliary body
coagulation (factor) (*see also* Defect, coagulation) D68.9
newborn, transient P61.6
cocaine use
mild F14.1Ø
with
amphetamine, cocaine, or other stimulant intoxication
with perceptual disturbances F14.122
without perceptual disturbances F14.129
cocaine-induced
anxiety disorder F14.18Ø
bipolar and related disorder F14.14
depressive disorder F14.14
obsessive-compulsive and related disorder F14.188
psychotic disorder F14.159
sexual dysfunction F14.181
sleep disorder F14.182
cocaine intoxication delirium F14.121
in remission (early) (sustained) F14.11
moderate or severe F14.2Ø
with
amphetamine, cocaine, or other stimulant intoxication
with perceptual disturbances F14.222
without perceptual disturbances F14.229
cocaine-induced
anxiety disorder F14.28Ø
bipolar and related disorder F14.24
depressive disorder F14.24
obsessive-compulsive and related disorder F14.288
psychotic disorder F14.259
sexual dysfunction F14.281
sleep disorder F14.282
cocaine intoxication delirium F14.221
in remission (early) (sustained) F14.21
coccyx NEC M53.3
cognitive FØ9
due to (secondary to) general medical condition FØ9
persisting R41.89
due to
alcohol F1Ø.97
with dependence F1Ø.27
anxiolytics F13.97
with dependence F13.27
hypnotics F13.97
with dependence F13.27
sedatives F13.97
with dependence F13.27

Disorder *(Continued)*
cognitive *(Continued)*
persisting *(Continued)*
due to *(Continued)*
specified substance NEC F19.97
with
abuse F19.17
dependence F19.27
communication F8Ø.9
social pragmatic F8Ø.82
conduct (childhood) F91.9
adjustment reaction *—see* Disorder, adjustment
adolescent onset type F91.2
childhood onset type F91.1
compulsive F63.9
confined to family context F91.Ø
depressive F91.8
group type F91.2
hyperkinetic *—see* Disorder, attention-deficit hyperactivity
oppositional defiance F91.3
socialized F91.2
solitary aggressive type F91.1
specified NEC F91.8
unsocialized (aggressive) F91.1
conduction, heart I45.9
congenital glycosylation (CDG) E74.8
conjunctiva H11.9
infection *—see* Conjunctivitis
connective tissue, localized L94.9
specified NEC L94.8
conversion (functional neurological symptom disorder)
with
abnormal movement F44.4
anesthesia or sensory loss F44.6
attacks or seizures F44.5
mixed symptoms F44.7
special sensory symptoms F44.6
speech symptoms F44.4
swallowing symptoms F44.4
weakness or paralysis F44.4
convulsive (secondary) *—see* Convulsions
cornea H18.9
deformity *—see* Deformity, cornea
degeneration *—see* Degeneration, cornea
deposits *—see* Deposit, cornea
due to contact lens H18.82-●
specified as edema *—see* Edema, cornea
edema *—see* Edema, cornea
keratitis *—see* Keratitis
keratoconjunctivitis *—see* Keratoconjunctivitis
membrane change *—see* Change, corneal membrane
neovascularization *—see* Neovascularization, cornea
scar *—see* Opacity, cornea
specified type NEC H18.89-●
ulcer *—see* Ulcer, cornea
corpus cavernosum N48.9
cranial nerve *—see* Disorder, nerve, cranial
cyclothymic F34.Ø
defiant oppositional F91.3
delusional (persistent) (systematized) F22
induced F24
depersonalization F48.1
depressive F32.9
due to known physiological condition
with
depressive features FØ6.31
major depressive-like episode FØ6.32
mixed features FØ6.34
major F32.9
with psychotic symptoms F32.3
in remission (full) F32.5
partial F32.4
recurrent F33.9
with psychotic features F33.3

Disorder *(Continued)*
depressive *(Continued)*
major *(Continued)*
single episode F32.9
mild F32.Ø
moderate F32.1
severe (without psychotic symptoms) F32.2
with psychotic symptoms F32.3
organic FØ6.31
persistent F34.1
recurrent F33.9
current episode
mild F33.Ø
moderate F33.1
severe (without psychotic symptoms) F33.2
with psychotic symptoms F33.3
in remission F33.4Ø
full F33.42
partial F33.41
specified NEC F33.8
single episode *—see* Episode, depressive
specified NEC F32.89
developmental F89
arithmetical skills F81.2
coordination (motor) F82
expressive writing F81.81
language F8Ø.9
expressive F8Ø.1
mixed receptive and expressive F8Ø.2
receptive type F8Ø.2
specified NEC F8Ø.89
learning F81.9
arithmetical F81.2
reading F81.Ø
mixed F88
motor coordination or function F82
pervasive F84.9
specified NEC F84.8
phonological F8Ø.Ø
reading F81.Ø
scholastic skills *—see also* Disorder, learning
mixed F81.89
specified NEC F88
speech F8Ø.9
articulation F8Ø.Ø
specified NEC F8Ø.89
written expression F81.81
diaphragm J98.6
digestive (system) K92.9
newborn P78.9
specified NEC P78.89
postprocedural *—see* Complication, gastrointestinal
psychogenic F45.8
disc (intervertebral) M51.9
with
myelopathy
cervical region M5Ø.ØØ
cervicothoracic region M5Ø.Ø3
high cervical region M5Ø.Ø1
lumbar region M51.Ø6
mid-cervical region M5Ø.Ø2Ø
sacrococcygeal region M53.3
thoracic region M51.Ø4
thoracolumbar region M51.Ø5
radiculopathy
cervical region M5Ø.1Ø
cervicothoracic region M5Ø.13
high cervical region M5Ø.11
lumbar region M51.16
lumbosacral region M51.17
mid-cervical region M5Ø.12Ø
sacrococcygeal region M53.3
thoracic region M51.14
thoracolumbar region M51.15

Disorder (Continued)
disc (intervertebral) (Continued)
cervical M50.90
with
myelopathy M50.00
C2-C3 M50.01
C3-C4 M50.01
C4-C5 M50.021
C5-C6 M50.022
C6-C7 M50.023
C7-T1 M50.03
cervicothoracic region M50.03
high cervical region M50.01
mid-cervical region M50.020
neuritis, radiculitis or radiculopathy M50.10
C2-C3 M50.11
C3-C4 M50.11
C4-C5 M50.121
C5-C6 M50.122
C6-C7 M50.123
C7-T1 M50.13
cervicothoracic region M50.13
high cervical region M50.11
mid-cervical region M50.120
C2-C3 M50.91
C3-C4 M50.91
C4-C5 M50.921
C5-C6 M50.922
C6-C7 M50.923
C7-T1 M50.93
cervicothoracic region M50.93
degeneration M50.30
C2-C3 M50.31
C3-C4 M50.31
C4-C5 M50.321
C5-C6 M50.322
C6-C7 M50.323
C7-T1 M50.33
cervicothoracic region M50.33
high cervical region M50.31
mid-cervical region M50.320
displacement M50.20
C2-C3 M50.21
C3-C4 M50.21
C4-C5 M50.221
C5-C6 M50.222
C6-C7 M50.223
C7-T1 M50.23
cervicothoracic region M50.23
high cervical region M50.21
mid-cervical region M50.220
high cervical region M50.91
mid-cervical region M50.920
specified type NEC M50.80
C2-C3 M50.81
C3-C4 M50.81
C4-C5 M50.821
C5-C6 M50.822
C6-C7 M50.823
C7-T1 M50.83
cervicothoracic region M50.83
high cervical region M50.81
mid-cervical region M50.820
specified NEC
lumbar region M51.86
lumbosacral region M51.87
sacrococcygeal region M53.3
thoracic region M51.84
thoracolumbar region M51.85
disinhibited attachment (childhood) F94.2
disintegrative, childhood NEC F84.3
disruptive F91.9
mood dysregulation F34.81
specified NEC F91.8
disruptive behavior —*see* Disorder, conduct
dissocial personality F60.2
dissociative F44.9
affecting
motor function F44.4
and sensation F44.7

Disorder (Continued)
dissociative (Continued)
affecting (Continued)
sensation F44.6
and motor function F44.7
brief reactive F43.0
due to (secondary to) general medical condition F06.8
mixed F44.7
organic F06.8
other specified NEC F44.89
double heterozygous sickling —*see* Disease, sickle-cell
dream anxiety F51.5
drug induced hemorrhagic D68.32
drug related F19.99
abuse —*see* Abuse, drug
dependence —*see* Dependence, drug
dysmorphic body F45.22
dysthymic F34.1
ear H93.9-●
bleeding —*see* Otorrhagia
deafness —*see* Deafness
degenerative H93.09-●
discharge —*see* Otorrhea
external H61.9-●
auditory canal stenosis —*see* Stenosis, external ear canal
exostosis —*see* Exostosis, external ear canal
impacted cerumen —*see* Impaction, cerumen
otitis —*see* Otitis, externa
perichondritis —*see* Perichondritis, ear
pinna —*see* Disorder, pinna
specified type NEC H61.89-●
in diseases classified elsewhere H62.8X-●
inner H83.9-●
vestibular dysfunction —*see* Disorder, vestibular function
middle H74.9-●
adhesive H74.1-●
ossicle —*see* Abnormal, ear ossicles
polyp —*see* Polyp, ear (middle)
specified NEC, in diseases classified elsewhere H75.8-●
postprocedural —*see* Complications, ear, procedure
specified NEC, in diseases classified elsewhere H94.8-●
eating (adult) (psychogenic) F50.9
anorexia —*see* Anorexia
binge F50.81
bulimia F50.2
child F98.29
pica F98.3
rumination disorder F98.21
pica F50.89
childhood F98.3
electrolyte (balance) NEC E87.8
with
abortion —*see* Abortion by type complicated by specified condition NEC
ectopic pregnancy O08.5
molar pregnancy O08.5
acidosis (metabolic) (respiratory) E87.2
alkalosis (metabolic) (respiratory) E87.3
elimination, transepidermal L87.9
specified NEC L87.8
emotional (persistent) F34.9
of childhood F93.9
specified NEC F93.8
endocrine E34.9
postprocedural E89.89
specified NEC E89.89
erectile (male) (organic) —*see also* Dysfunction, sexual, male, erectile N52.9
nonorganic F52.21
erythematous —*see* Erythema

Disorder (Continued)
esophagus K22.9
functional K22.4
psychogenic F45.8
eustachian tube H69.9-●
infection —*see* Salpingitis, eustachian
obstruction —*see* Obstruction, eustachian tube
patulous —*see* Patulous, eustachian tube
specified NEC H69.8-●
exhibitionistic F65.2
extrapyramidal G25.9
in diseases classified elsewhere —*see* category G26
specified type NEC G25.89
eye H57.9
postprocedural —*see* Complication, postprocedural, eye
eyelid H02.9
cyst —*see* Cyst, eyelid
degenerative H02.70
chloasma —*see* Chloasma, eyelid
madarosis —*see* Madarosis
specified type NEC H02.79
vitiligo —*see* Vitiligo, eyelid
xanthelasma —*see* Xanthelasma
dermatochalasis —*see* Dermato-chalasis
edema —*see* Edema, eyelid
elephantiasis —*see* Elephantiasis, eyelid
foreign body, retained —*see* Foreign body, retained, eyelid
function H02.59
abnormal innervation syndrome —*see* Syndrome, abnormal innervation
blepharochalasis —*see* Blepharochalasis
blepharoclonus —*see* Blepharoclonus
blepharophimosis —*see* Blepharophimosis
blepharoptosis —*see* Blepharoptosis
lagophthalmos —*see* Lagophthalmos
lid retraction —*see* Retraction, lid
hypertrichosis —*see* Hypertrichosis, eyelid
specified type NEC H02.89
vascular H02.879
left H02.876
lower H02.875
upper H02.874
right H02.873
lower H02.872
upper H02.871
factitious
by proxy F68.A
imposed on another F68.A
imposed on self F68.10
with predominantly
psychological symptoms F68.11
with physical symptoms F68.13
physical symptoms F68.12
with psychological symptoms F68.13
factor, coagulation —*see* Defect, coagulation
fatty acid
metabolism E71.30
specified NEC E71.39
oxidation
LCAD E71.310
MCAD E71.311
SCAD E71.312
specified deficiency NEC E71.318
feeding (infant or child) —*see also* Disorder, eating R63.3-●
or eating disorder F50.9
specified NEC F50.9
feigned (with obvious motivation) Z76.5
without obvious motivation —*see* Disorder, factitious

Disorder *(Continued)*
  female
    hypoactive sexual desire F52.Ø
    orgasmic F52.31
    sexual interest/arousal F52.22
  fetishistic F65.Ø
  fibroblastic M72.9
    specified NEC M72.8
  fluency
    adult onset F98.5
    childhood onset F8Ø.81
    following
      cerebral infarction I69.323
      cerebrovascular disease I69.923
        specified disease NEC I69.823
      intracerebral hemorrhage I69.123
      nontraumatic intracranial hemorrhage NEC I69.223
      subarachnoid hemorrhage I69.Ø23
    in conditions classified elsewhere R47.82
  fluid balance E87.8
  follicular (skin) L73.9
    specified NEC L73.8
  frotteuristic F65.81
  fructose metabolism E74.1Ø
    essential fructosuria E74.11
    fructokinase deficiency E74.11
    fructose-1, 6-diphosphatase deficiency E74.19
    hereditary fructose intolerance E74.12
    other specified E74.19
  functional polymorphonuclear neutrophils D71
  gallbladder, biliary tract and pancreas in diseases classified elsewhere K87
  gambling F63.Ø
  gamma aminobutyric acid (GABA) metabolism E72.81
  gamma-glutamyl cycle E72.89
  gastric (functional) K31.9
    motility K3Ø
    psychogenic F45.8
    secretion K3Ø
  gastrointestinal (functional) NOS K92.9
    newborn P78.9
    psychogenic F45.8
  gender-identity or -role F64.9
    childhood F64.2
    effect on relationship F66
    of adolescence or adulthood F64.Ø
      nontranssexual F64.8
    specified NEC F64.8
    uncertainty F66
  genito-pelvic pain penetration F52.6
  genitourinary system
    female N94.9
    male N5Ø.9
    psychogenic F45.8
  globe H44.9
    degenerated condition H44.5Ø
      absolute glaucoma H44.51-●
      atrophy H44.52-●
      leucocoria H44.53-●
    degenerative H44.3Ø
      chalcosis H44.31-●
      myopia —*see also* Myopia, degenerative H44.2-●
      siderosis H44.32-●
      specified type NEC H44.39-●
    endophthalmitis —*see* Endophthalmitis
    foreign body, retained —*see* Foreign body, intraocular, old, retained
    hemophthalmos —*see* Hemophthalmos
    hypotony H44.4Ø
      due to
        ocular fistula H44.42-●
        specified disorder NEC H44.43-●
      flat anterior chamber H44.41-●
      primary H44.44-●
    luxation —*see* Luxation, globe
    specified type NEC H44.89

Disorder *(Continued)*
  glomerular (in) NØ5.9
    amyloidosis E85.4 *[NØ8]*
    cryoglobulinemia D89.1 *[NØ8]*
    disseminated intravascular coagulation D65 *[NØ8]*
    Fabry's disease E75.21 *[NØ8]*
    familial lecithin cholesterol acyltransferase deficiency E78.6 *[NØ8]*
    Goodpasture's syndrome M31.Ø
    hemolytic-uremic syndrome D59.3
    Henoch (-Schönlein) purpura D69.Ø *[NØ8]*
    malariae malaria B52.Ø
    microscopic polyangiitis M31.7 *[NØ8]*
    multiple myeloma C9Ø.Ø-● *[NØ8]*
    mumps B26.83
    schistosomiasis B65.9 *[NØ8]*
    sepsis NEC A41.-● *[NØ8]*
      streptococcal A4Ø.-● *[NØ8]*
    sickle-cell disorders D57.-● *[NØ8]*
    strongyloidiasis B78.9 *[NØ8]*
    subacute bacterial endocarditis I33.Ø *[NØ8]*
    syphilis A52.75
    systemic lupus erythematosus M32.14
    thrombotic thrombocytopenic purpura M31.1 *[NØ8]*
    Waldenström macroglobulinemia C88.Ø *[NØ8]*
    Wegener's granulomatosis M31.31
  gluconeogenesis E74.4
  glucosaminoglycan metabolism —*see* Disorder, metabolism, glucosaminoglycan
  glycine metabolism E72.5Ø
    d-glycericacidemia E72.59
    hyperhydroxyprolinemia E72.59
    hyperoxaluria R82.992
      primary E72.53
    hyperprolinemia E72.59
    non-ketotic hyperglycinemia E72.51
    oxalosis E72.53
    oxaluria E72.53
    sarcosinemia E72.59
    trimethylaminuria E72.52
  glycoprotein metabolism E77.9
    specified NEC E77.8
  habit (and impulse) F63.9
    involving sexual behavior NEC F65.9
    specified NEC F63.89
  hallucinogen use
    mild F16.1Ø
      with
        hallucinogen-induced
          anxiety disorder F16.18Ø
          bipolar and related disorder F16.14
          depressive disorder F16.14
          psychotic disorder F16.159
        hallucinogen intoxication delirium F16.121
        other hallucinogen intoxication F16.129
      in remission (early) (sustained) F16.11
    moderate or severe F16.2Ø
      with
        hallucinogen-induced
          anxiety disorder F16.28Ø
          bipolar and related disorder F16.24
          depressive disorder F16.24
          psychotic disorder F16.259
        hallucinogen intoxication delirium F16.221
        other hallucinogen intoxication F16.229
      in remission (early) (sustained) F16.21
  heart action I49.9
  hematological D75.9
    newborn (transient) P61.9
      specified NEC P61.8
  hematopoietic organs D75.9

Disorder *(Continued)*
  hemorrhagic NEC D69.9
    drug-induced D68.32
    due to
      extrinsic circulating anticoagulants D68.32
      increase in
        anti-IIa D68.32
        anti-Xa D68.32
      intrinsic
        circulating anticoagulants D68.318
        increase in
          antithrombin D68.318
          anti-VIIIa D68.318
          anti-IXa D68.318
          anti-XIa D68.318
    following childbirth O72.3
  hemostasis —*see* Defect, coagulation
  histidine metabolism E7Ø.4Ø
    histidinemia E7Ø.41
    other specified E7Ø.49
  hoarding F42.3
  hyperkinetic —*see* Disorder, attention-deficit hyperactivity
  hyperleucine-isoleucinemia E71.19
  hypervalinemia E71.19
  hypoactive sexual desire F52.Ø
  hypochondriacal F45.2Ø
    body dysmorphic F45.22
    neurosis F45.21
    other specified F45.29
  identity
    dissociative F44.81
    illness anxiety F45.21
    of childhood F93.8
  immune mechanism (immunity) D89.9
    specified type NEC D89.89
  impaired renal tubular function N25.9
    specified NEC N25.89
  impulse (control) F63.9
  inflammatory
    pelvic, in diseases classified elsewhere —*see* category N74
    penis N48.29
      abscess N48.21
      cellulitis N48.22
  inhalant use
    mild F18.1Ø
      with
        inhalant-induced
          anxiety disorder F18.18Ø
          depressive disorder F18.14
          major neurocognitive disorder F18.17
          mild neurocognitive disorder F18.188
          psychotic disorder F18.159
        inhalant intoxication F18.129
        inhalant intoxication delirium F18.121
      in remission (early) (sustained) F18.11
    moderate or severe F18.2Ø
      with
        inhalant-induced
          anxiety disorder F18.28Ø
          depressive disorder F18.24
          major neurocognitive disorder F18.27
          mild neurocognitive disorder F18.288
          psychotic disorder F18.259
        inhalant intoxication F18.229
        inhalant intoxication delirium F18.221
      in remission (early) (sustained) F18.21
  integument, newborn P83.9
    specified NEC P83.88
  intermittent explosive F63.81
  internal secretion pancreas —*see* Increased, secretion, pancreas, endocrine
  intestine, intestinal
    carbohydrate absorption NEC E74.39
      postoperative K91.2

Disorder *(Continued)*
intestine, intestinal *(Continued)*
functional NEC K59.9
postoperative K91.89
psychogenic F45.8
vascular K55.9
chronic K55.1
specified NEC K55.8
intraoperative (intraprocedural) *—see* Complications, intraoperative
involuntary emotional expression (IEED) F48.2
iris H21.9
adhesions *—see* Adhesions, iris
atrophy *—see* Atrophy, iris
chamber angle recession *—see* Recession, chamber angle
cyst *—see* Cyst, iris
degeneration *—see* Degeneration, iris
in diseases classified elsewhere H22
iridodialysis *—see* Iridodialysis
iridoschisis *—see* Iridoschisis
miotic pupillary cyst *—see* Cyst, pupillary
pupillary
abnormality *—see* Abnormality, pupillary
membrane *—see* Membrane, pupillary
specified type NEC H21.89
vascular NEC H21.1X- ●
iron metabolism E83.10
specified NEC E83.19
isovaleric acidemia E71.110
jaw, developmental M27.0
temporomandibular *—see also* Anomaly, dentofacial, temporomandibular joint M26.60- ●
joint M25.9
derangement *—see* Derangement, joint
effusion *—see* Effusion, joint
fistula *—see* Fistula, joint
hemarthrosis *—see* Hemarthrosis
instability *—see* Instability, joint
osteophyte *—see* Osteophyte
pain *—see* Pain, joint
psychogenic F45.8
specified type NEC M25.80
ankle M25.87- ●
elbow M25.82- ●
foot joint M25.87- ●
hand joint M25.84- ●
hip M25.85- ●
knee M25.86- ●
shoulder M25.81- ●
wrist M25.83- ●
stiffness *—see* Stiffness, joint
ketone metabolism E71.32
kidney N28.9
functional (tubular) N25.9
in
schistosomiasis B65.9 *[N29]*
tubular function N25.9
specified NEC N25.89
lacrimal system H04.9
changes H04.69
fistula *—see* Fistula, lacrimal
gland H04.19
atrophy *—see* Atrophy, lacrimal gland
cyst *—see* Cyst, lacrimal, gland
dacryops *—see* Dacryops
dislocation *—see* Dislocation, lacrimal gland
dry eye syndrome *—see* Syndrome, dry eye
infection *—see* Dacryoadenitis
granuloma *—see* Granuloma, lacrimal
inflammation *—see* Inflammation, lacrimal
obstruction *—see* Obstruction, lacrimal
specified NEC H04.89
lactation NEC O92.79
language (developmental) F80.9
expressive F80.1
mixed receptive and expressive F80.2
receptive F80.2

Disorder *(Continued)*
late luteal phase dysphoric N94.89
learning (specific) F81.9
acalculia R48.8
alexia R48.0
mathematics F81.2
reading F81.0
specified
with impairment in
mathematics F81.2
reading F81.0
written expression F81.81
specified NEC F81.89
spelling F81.81
written expression F81.81
lens H27.9
aphakia *—see* Aphakia
cataract *—see* Cataract
dislocation *—see* Dislocation, lens
specified type NEC H27.8
ligament M24.20
ankle M24.27- ●
attachment, spine *—see* Enthesopathy, spinal
elbow M24.22- ●
foot joint M24.27- ●
hand joint M24.24- ●
hip M24.25- ●
knee *—see* Derangement, knee, specified NEC
shoulder M24.21- ●
vertebra M24.28
wrist M24.23- ●
ligamentous attachments *—see also* Enthesopathy
spine *—see* Enthesopathy, spinal
lipid
metabolism, congenital E78.9
storage E75.6
specified NEC E75.5
lipoprotein
deficiency (familial) E78.6
metabolism E78.9
specified NEC E78.89
liver K76.9
malarial B54 *[K77]*
low back *—see also* Dorsopathy, specified NEC
lumbosacral
plexus G54.1
root (nerve) NEC G54.4
lung, interstitial, drug-induced J70.4
acute J70.2
chronic J70.3
lymphoproliferative, post-transplant (PTLD) D47.Z1
lysine and hydroxylysine metabolism E72.3
major neurocognitive *—see* Dementia, in (due to)
male
erectile (organic) *—see also* Dysfunction, sexual, male, erectile N52.9
nonorganic F52.21
hypoactive sexual desire F52.0
orgasmic F52.32
manic F30.9
organic F06.33
mast cell activation *—see* Activation, mast cell
mastoid *—see also* Disorder, ear, middle
postprocedural *—see* Complications, ear, procedure
meniscus *—see* Derangement, knee, meniscus
menopausal N95.9
specified NEC N95.8
menstrual N92.6
psychogenic F45.8
specified NEC N92.5
mental (or behavioral) (nonpsychotic) F99
due to (secondary to)
amphetamine
due to drug abuse *—see* Abuse, drug, stimulant

Disorder *(Continued)*
mental *(Continued)*
due to (secondary to) *(Continued)*
amphetamine *(Continued)*
due to drug dependence *—see* Dependence, drug, stimulant
brain disease, damage and dysfunction F09
caffeine use
due to drug abuse *—see* Abuse, drug, stimulant
due to drug dependence *—see* Dependence, drug, stimulant
cannabis use
due to drug abuse *—see* Abuse, drug, cannabis
due to drug dependence *—see* Dependence, drug, cannabis
general medical condition F09
sedative or hypnotic use
due to drug abuse *—see* Abuse, drug, sedative
due to drug dependence *—see* Dependence, drug, sedative
tobacco (nicotine) use *—see* Dependence, drug, nicotine
following organic brain damage F07.9
frontal lobe syndrome F07.0
personality change F07.0
postconcussional syndrome F07.81
specified NEC F07.89
infancy, childhood or adolescence F98.9
neurotic *—see* Neurosis
organic or symptomatic F09
presenile, psychotic F03
problem NEC
psychoneurotic *—see* Neurosis
psychotic *—see* Psychosis
puerperal F53.0
senile, psychotic NEC F03
metabolic, amino acid, transitory, newborn P74.8
metabolism NOS E88.9
amino-acid E72.9
aromatic E70.9
albinism *—see* Albinism
histidine E70.40
histidinemia E70.41
other specified E70.49
hyperphenylalaninemia E70.1
classical phenylketonuria E70.0
other specified E70.8
tryptophan E70.5
tyrosine E70.20
hypertyrosinemia E70.21
other specified E70.29
branched chain E71.2
3-methylglutaconic aciduria E71.111
hyperleucine-isoleucinemia E71.19
hypervalinemia E71.19
isovaleric acidemia E71.110
maple syrup urine disease E71.0
methylmalonic acidemia E71.120
organic aciduria NEC E71.118
other specified E71.19
proprionate NEC E71.128
proprionic acidemia E71.121
glycine E72.50
d-glycericacidemia E72.59
hyperhydroxyprolinemia E72.59
hyperoxaluria R82.992
primary E72.53
hyperprolinemia E72.59
non-ketotic hyperglycinemia E72.51
other specified E72.59
sarcosinemia E72.59
trimethylaminuria E72.52
hydroxylysine E72.3
lysine E72.3
ornithine E72.4

Disorder *(Continued)*
metabolism *(Continued)*
amino-acid *(Continued)*
other specified E72.89
beta-amino acid E72.89
gamma-glutamyl cycle E72.89
straight-chain E72.89
sulfur-bearing E72.10
homocystinuria E72.11
methylenetetrahydrofolate reductase deficiency E72.12
other specified E72.19
bile acid and cholesterol metabolism E78.70
bilirubin E80.7
specified NEC E80.6
calcium E83.50
hypercalcemia E83.52
hypocalcemia E83.51
other specified E83.59
carbohydrate E74.9
specified NEC E74.8
cholesterol and bile acid metabolism E78.70
congenital E88.9
copper E83.00
specified type NEC E83.09
Wilson's disease E83.01
cystinuria E72.01
fructose E74.10
galactose E74.20
glucosaminoglycan E76.9
mucopolysaccharidosis —*see* Mucopolysaccharidosis
specified NEC E76.8
glutamine E72.89
glycine E72.50
glycogen storage (hepatorenal) E74.09
glycoprotein E77.9
specified NEC E77.8
glycosaminoglycan E76.9
specified NEC E76.8
in labor and delivery O75.89
iron E83.10
isoleucine E71.19
leucine E71.19
lipoid E78.9
lipoprotein E78.9
specified NEC E78.89
magnesium E83.40
hypermagnesemia E83.41
hypomagnesemia E83.42
other specified E83.49
mineral E83.9
specified NEC E83.89
mitochondrial E88.40
MELAS syndrome E88.41
MERRF syndrome (myoclonic epilepsy associated with ragged-red fibers) E88.42
other specified E88.49
ornithine E72.4
phosphatases E83.30
phosphorus E83.30
acid phosphatase deficiency E83.39
hypophosphatasia E83.39
hypophosphatemia E83.39
familial E83.31
other specified E83.39
pseudovitamin D deficiency E83.32
plasma protein NEC E88.09
porphyrin —*see* Porphyria
postprocedural E89.89
specified NEC E89.89
purine E79.9
specified NEC E79.8
pyrimidine E79.9
specified NEC E79.8
pyruvate E74.4
serine E72.89
sodium E87.8
specified NEC E88.89

Disorder *(Continued)*
metabolism *(Continued)*
threonine E72.89
valine E71.19
zinc E83.2
methylmalonic acidemia E71.120
micturition NEC —*see also* Difficulty, micturition R39.198
feeling of incomplete emptying R39.14
hesitancy R39.11
poor stream R39.12
psychogenic F45.8
split stream R39.13
straining R39.16
urgency R39.15
mild neurocognitive G31.84
mitochondrial metabolism E88.40
mitral (valve) —*see* Endocarditis, mitral
mixed
anxiety and depressive F41.8
of scholastic skills (developmental) F81.89
receptive expressive language F80.2
mood F39
bipolar —*see* Disorder, bipolar
depressive —*see* Disorder, depressive
due to (secondary to)
alcohol F10.94
amphetamine F15.94
in
abuse F15.14
dependence F15.24
anxiolytic F13.94
in
abuse F13.14
dependence F13.24
cocaine F14.94
in
abuse F14.14
dependence F14.24
general medical condition F06.30
hallucinogen F16.94
in
abuse F16.14
dependence F16.24
hypnotic F13.94
in
abuse F13.14
dependence F13.24
inhalant F18.94
in
abuse F18.14
dependence F18.24
opioid F11.94
in
abuse F11.14
dependence F11.24
phencyclidine (PCP) F16.94
in
abuse F16.14
dependence F16.24
physiological condition F06.30
with
depressive features F06.31
major depressive-like episode F06.32
manic features F06.33
mixed features F06.34
psychoactive substance NEC F19.94
in
abuse F19.14
dependence F19.24
sedative F13.94
in
abuse F13.14
dependence F13.24
volatile solvents F18.94
in
abuse F18.14
dependence F18.24

Disorder *(Continued)*
mood *(Continued)*
manic episode F30.9
with psychotic symptoms F30.2
without psychotic symptoms F30.10
mild F30.11
moderate F30.12
severe F30.13
in remission (full) F30.4
partial F30.3
specified type NEC F30.8
organic F06.30
right hemisphere F07.89
persistent F34.9
cyclothymia F34.0
dysthymia F34.1
specified type NEC F34.89
recurrent F39
right hemisphere organic F07.89
movement G25.9
drug-induced G25.70
akathisia G25.71
specified NEC G25.79
hysterical F44.4
in diseases classified elsewhere —*see* category G26
periodic limb G47.61
sleep related G47.61
sleep related NEC G47.69
specified NEC G25.89
stereotyped F98.4
treatment-induced G25.9
multiple personality F44.81
muscle M62.9
attachment, spine —*see* Enthesopathy, spinal
in trichinellosis —*see* Trichinellosis, with muscle disorder
psychogenic F45.8
specified type NEC M62.89
tone, newborn P94.9
specified NEC P94.8
muscular
attachments —*see also* Enthesopathy
spine —*see* Enthesopathy, spinal
urethra N36.44
musculoskeletal system, soft tissue —*see* Disorder, soft tissue
postprocedural M96.89
psychogenic F45.8
myoneural G70.9
due to lead G70.1
specified NEC G70.89
toxic G70.1
myotonic NEC G71.19
nail, in diseases classified elsewhere L62
neck region NEC —*see* Dorsopathy, specified NEC
neonatal onset multisystemic inflammatory (NOMID) M04.2
nerve G58.9
abducent NEC —*see* Strabismus, paralytic, sixth nerve
accessory G52.8
acoustic —*see* subcategory H93.3
auditory —*see* subcategory H93.3
auriculotemporal G50.8
axillary G54.0
cerebral —*see* Disorder, nerve, cranial
cranial G52.9
eighth —*see* subcategory H93.3
eleventh G52.8
fifth G50.9
first G52.0
fourth NEC —*see* Strabismus, paralytic, fourth nerve
multiple G52.7
ninth G52.1
second NEC —*see* Disorder, nerve, optic
seventh NEC G51.8
sixth NEC —*see* Strabismus, paralytic, sixth nerve

Disorder *(Continued)*
nerve *(Continued)*
cranial *(Continued)*
specified NEC G52.8
tenth G52.2
third NEC —*see* Strabismus, paralytic, third nerve
twelfth G52.3
entrapment —*see* Neuropathy, entrapment
facial G51.9
specified NEC G51.8
femoral —*see* Lesion, nerve, femoral
glossopharyngeal NEC G52.1
hypoglossal G52.3
intercostal G58.Ø
lateral
cutaneous of thigh —*see* Mononeuropathy, lower limb, meralgia paresthetica
popliteal —*see* Lesion, nerve, popliteal
lower limb —*see* Mononeuropathy, lower limb
medial popliteal —*see* Lesion, nerve, popliteal, medial
median NEC —*see* Lesion, nerve, median
multiple G58.7
oculomotor NEC —*see* Strabismus, paralytic, third nerve
olfactory G52.Ø
optic NEC H47.Ø9-●
hemorrhage into sheath —*see* Hemorrhage, optic nerve
ischemic H47.Ø1-●
peroneal —*see* Lesion, nerve, popliteal
phrenic G58.8
plantar —*see* Lesion, nerve, plantar
pneumogastric G52.2
posterior tibial —*see* Syndrome, tarsal tunnel
radial —*see* Lesion, nerve, radial
recurrent laryngeal G52.2
root G54.9
cervical G54.2
lumbosacral G54.1
specified NEC G54.8
thoracic G54.3
sciatic NEC —*see* Lesion, nerve, sciatic
specified NEC G58.8
lower limb —*see* Mononeuropathy, lower limb, specified NEC
upper limb —*see* Mononeuropathy, upper limb, specified NEC
sympathetic G9Ø.9
tibial —*see* Lesion, nerve, popliteal, medial
trigeminal G5Ø.9
specified NEC G5Ø.8
trochlear NEC —*see* Strabismus, paralytic, fourth nerve
ulnar —*see* Lesion, nerve, ulnar
upper limb —*see* Mononeuropathy, upper limb
vagus G52.2
nervous system G98.8
autonomic (peripheral) G9Ø.9
specified NEC G9Ø.8
central G96.9
specified NEC G96.8
parasympathetic G9Ø.9
specified NEC G98.8
sympathetic G9Ø.9
vegetative G9Ø.9
neurocognitive R41.9
major
with
aggressive behavior FØ1.51
combative behavior FØ1.51
violent behavior FØ1.51
due to vascular disease, with behavioral disturbance FØ1.51
in (due to) (other diseases classified elsewhere) —*see also* Dementia, in (due to) FØ2.8Ø

Disorder *(Continued)*
neurocognitive *(Continued)*
major *(Continued)*
in *(Continued)*
with
aggressive behavior FØ2.81
combative behavior FØ2.81
violent behavior FØ2.81
without behavioral disturbance FØ1.5Ø
mild G31.84
neurodevelopmental F89
specified NEC F88
neurohypophysis NEC E23.3
neurological NEC R29.818
neuromuscular G7Ø.9
hereditary NEC G71.9
specified NEC G7Ø.89
toxic G7Ø.1
neurotic F48.9
specified NEC F48.8
neutrophil, polymorphonuclear D71
nicotine use —*see* Dependence, drug, nicotine
nightmare F51.5
non-rapid eye movement sleep arousal
sleep terror type F51.4
sleepwalking type F51.3
nose J34.9
specified NEC J34.89
obsessive-compulsive F42.9
and related disorder due to a known physiological condition FØ6.8
odontogenesis NOS KØØ.9
opioid use
with
opioid-induced psychotic disorder F11.959
with
delusions F11.95Ø
hallucinations F11.951
due to drug abuse —*see* Abuse, drug, opioid
due to drug dependence —*see* Dependence, drug, opioid
mild F11.1Ø
with
opioid-induced
anxiety disorder F11.188
depressive disorder F11.14
sexual dysfunction F11.181
opioid intoxication
with perceptual disturbances F11.122
delirium F11.121
without perceptual disturbances F11.129
in remission (early) (sustained) F11.11
moderate or severe F11.2Ø
with
opioid-induced
anxiety disorder F11.288
anxiety disorder F11.988
depressive disorder F11.24
depressive disorder F11.94
sexual dysfunction F11.281
sexual dysfunction F11.981
opioid intoxication
with perceptual disturbances F11.222
delirium F11.221
without perceptual disturbances F11.229
in remission (early) (sustained) F11.21
oppositional defiant F91.3
optic
chiasm H47.49
due to
inflammatory disorder H47.41
neoplasm H47.42
vascular disorder H47.43
disc H47.39-●
coloboma —*see* Coloboma, optic disc
drusen —*see* Drusen, optic disc
pseudopapilledema —*see* Pseudopapilledema

Disorder *(Continued)*
optic *(Continued)*
radiations —*see* Disorder, visual, pathway
tracts —*see* Disorder, visual, pathway
orbit HØ5.9
cyst —*see* Cyst, orbit
deformity —*see* Deformity, orbit
edema —*see* Edema, orbit
enophthalmos —*see* Enophthalmos
exophthalmos —*see* Exophthalmos
hemorrhage —*see* Hemorrhage, orbit
inflammation —*see* Inflammation, orbit
myopathy —*see* Myopathy, extraocular muscles
retained foreign body —*see* Foreign body, orbit, old
specified type NEC HØ5.89
organic
anxiety FØ6.4
catatonic FØ6.1
delusional FØ6.2
dissociative FØ6.8
emotionally labile (asthenic) FØ6.8
mood (affective) FØ6.3Ø
schizophrenia-like FØ6.2
orgasmic (female) F52.31
male F52.32
ornithine metabolism E72.4
overanxious F41.1
of childhood F93.8
pain
with related psychological factors F45.42
exclusively related to psychological factors F45.41
genito-pelvic penetration disorder F52.6
pancreatic internal secretion E16.9
specified NEC E16.8
panic F41.Ø
with agoraphobia F4Ø.Ø1
papulosquamous L44.9
in diseases classified elsewhere L45
specified NEC L44.8
paranoid F22
induced F24
shared F24
paraphilic F65.9
specified NEC F65.89
parathyroid (gland) E21.5
specified NEC E21.4
parietoalveolar NEC J84.Ø9
paroxysmal, mixed R56.9
patella M22.9-●
chondromalacia —*see* Chondromalacia, patella
derangement NEC M22.3X-●
recurrent
dislocation —*see* Dislocation, patella, recurrent
subluxation —*see* Dislocation, patella, recurrent, incomplete
specified NEC M22.8X-●
patellofemoral M22.2X-●
pedophilic F65.4
pentose phosphate pathway with anemia D55.1
perception, due to hallucinogens F16.983
in
abuse F16.183
dependence F16.283
peripheral nervous system NEC G64
peroxisomal E71.5Ø
biogenesis
neonatal adrenoleukodystrophy E71.511
specified disorder NEC E71.518
Zellweger syndrome E71.51Ø
rhizomelic chondrodysplasia punctata E71.54Ø
specified form NEC E71.548
group 1 E71.518
group 2 E71.53
group 3 E71.542

Disorder *(Continued)*
peroxisomal *(Continued)*
X-linked adrenoleukodystrophy E71.529
adolescent E71.521
adrenomyeloneuropathy E71.522
childhood E71.520
specified form NEC E71.528
Zellweger-like syndrome E71.541
persistent
(somatoform) pain F45.41
affective (mood) F34.9
personality —*see also* Personality F60.9
affective F34.0
aggressive F60.3
amoral F60.2
anankastic F60.5
antisocial F60.2
anxious F60.6
asocial F60.2
asthenic F60.7
avoidant F60.6
borderline F60.3
change (secondary) due to general medical condition F07.0
compulsive F60.5
cyclothymic F34.0
dependent (passive) F60.7
depressive F34.1
dissocial F60.2
emotional instability F60.3
expansive paranoid F60.0
explosive F60.3
following organic brain damage F07.9
histrionic F60.4
hyperthymic F34.0
hypothymic F34.1
hysterical F60.4
immature F60.89
inadequate F60.7
labile F60.3
mixed (nonspecific) F60.89
moral deficiency F60.2
narcissistic F60.81
negativistic F60.89
obsessional F60.5
obsessive (-compulsive) F60.5
organic F07.9
overconscientious F60.5
paranoid F60.0
passive (-dependent) F60.7
passive-aggressive F60.89
pathological NEC F60.9
pseudosocial F60.2
psychopathic F60.2
schizoid F60.1
schizotypal F21
self-defeating F60.7
specified NEC F60.89
type A F60.5
unstable (emotional) F60.3
pervasive, developmental F84.9
phencyclidine use
mild F16.10
with
phencyclidine-induced
anxiety disorder F16.180
bipolar and related disorder F16.14
depressive disorder F16.14
psychotic disorder F16.159
phencyclidine intoxication F16.129
phencyclidine intoxication delirium F16.121
in remission (early) (sustained) F16.11
moderate or severe F16.20
with
phencyclidine-induced
anxiety disorder F16.280
bipolar and related disorder F16.24
depressive disorder F16.24
psychotic disorder F16.259
phencyclidine intoxication F16.229

Disorder *(Continued)*
phencyclidine use *(Continued)*
moderate or severe *(Continued)*
with *(Continued)*
phencyclidine intoxication delirium F16.221
in remission (early) (sustained) F16.21
phobic anxiety, childhood F40.8
phosphate-losing tubular N25.0
pigmentation L81.9
choroid, congenital Q14.3
diminished melanin formation L81.6
iron L81.8
specified NEC L81.8
pinna (noninfective) H61.10- •
deformity, acquired H61.11- •
hematoma H61.12- •
perichondritis —*see* Perichondritis, ear
specified type NEC H61.19- •
pituitary gland E23.7
iatrogenic (postprocedural) E89.3
specified NEC E23.6
platelets D69.1
plexus G54.9
specified NEC G54.8
polymorphonuclear neutrophils D71
porphyrin metabolism —*see* Porphyria
postconcussional F07.81
posthallucinogen perception F16.983
in
abuse F16.183
dependence F16.283
postmenopausal N95.9
specified NEC N95.8
postprocedural (postoperative) —*see* Complications, postprocedural
post-transplant lymphoproliferative D47.z1
post-traumatic stress (PTSD) F43.10
acute F43.11
chronic F43.12
premenstrual dysphoric (PMDD) F32.81
prepuce N47.8
propionic acidemia E71.121
prostate N42.9
specified NEC N42.89
psychogenic NOS —*see also* condition F45.9
anxiety F41.8
appetite F50.9
asthenic F48.8
cardiovascular (system) F45.8
compulsive F42.8
cutaneous F54
depressive F32.9
digestive (system) F45.8
dysmenorrheic F45.8
dyspneic F45.8
endocrine (system) F54
eye NEC F45.8
feeding —*see* Disorder, eating
functional NEC F45.8
gastric F45.8
gastrointestinal (system) F45.8
genitourinary (system) F45.8
heart (function) (rhythm) F45.8
hyperventilatory F45.8
hypochondriacal —*see* Disorder, hypochondriacal
intestinal F45.8
joint F45.8
learning F81.9
limb F45.8
lymphatic (system) F45.8
menstrual F45.8
micturition F45.8
monoplegic NEC F44.4
motor F44.4
muscle F45.8
musculoskeletal F45.8
neurocirculatory F45.8
obsessive F42.8
occupational F48.8
organ or part of body NEC F45.8

Disorder *(Continued)*
psychogenic NOS *(Continued)*
paralytic NEC F44.4
phobic F40.9
physical NEC F45.8
rectal F45.8
respiratory (system) F45.8
rheumatic F45.8
sexual (function) F52.9
skin (allergic) (eczematous) F54
sleep F51.9
specified part of body NEC F45.8
stomach F45.8
psychological F99
associated with
disease classified elsewhere F54
sexual
development F66
relationship F66
uncertainty about gender identity F64.9
psychomotor NEC F44.4
hysterical F44.4
psychoneurotic —*see also* Neurosis
mixed NEC F48.8
psychophysiologic —*see* Disorder, somatoform
psychosexual F65.9
development F66
identity of childhood F64.2
psychosomatic NOS —*see* Disorder, somatoform
multiple F45.0
undifferentiated F45.1
psychotic —*see* Psychosis
transient (acute) F23
puberty E30.9
specified NEC E30.8
pulmonary (valve) —*see* Endocarditis, pulmonary
purine metabolism E79.9
pyrimidine metabolism E79.9
pyruvate metabolism E74.4
reactive attachment (childhood) F94.1
reading R48.0
developmental (specific) F81.0
receptive language F80.2
receptor, hormonal, peripheral —*see also* Syndrome, androgen insensitivity E34.50
recurrent brief depressive F33.8
reflex R29.2
refraction H52.7
aniseikonia H52.32
anisometropia H52.31
astigmatism —*see* Astigmatism
hypermetropia —*see* Hypermetropia
myopia —*see* Myopia
presbyopia H52.4
specified NEC H52.6
relationship F68.8
due to sexual orientation F66
REM sleep behavior G47.52
renal function, impaired (tubular) N25.9
resonance R49.9
specified NEC R49.8
respiratory function, impaired —*see also* Failure, respiration
postprocedural —*see* Complication, postoperative, respiratory system
psychogenic F45.8
retina H35.9
angioid streaks H35.33
changes in vascular appearance H35.01- •
degeneration —*see* Degeneration, retina
dystrophy (hereditary) —*see* Dystrophy, retina
edema H35.81
hemorrhage —*see* Hemorrhage, retina
ischemia H35.82
macular degeneration —*see* Degeneration, macula
microaneurysms H35.04- •
microvascular abnormality NEC H35.09

- Disorder *(Continued)*
  - retina *(Continued)*
    - neovascularization *—see* Neovascularization, retina
    - retinopathy *—see* Retinopathy
    - separation of layers H35.70
      - central serous chorioretinopathy H35.71- •
      - pigment epithelium detachment (serous) H35.72- •
        - hemorrhagic H35.73- •
    - specified type NEC H35.89
    - telangiectasis *—see* Telangiectasis, retina
    - vasculitis *—see* Vasculitis, retina
  - retroperitoneal K68.9
  - right hemisphere organic affective F07.89
  - rumination (infant or child) F98.21
  - sacrum, sacrococcygeal NEC M53.3
  - schizoaffective F25.9
    - bipolar type F25.0
    - depressive type F25.1
    - manic type F25.0
    - mixed type F25.0
    - specified NEC F25.8
  - schizoid of childhood F84.5
  - schizophrenia spectrum and other psychotic disorder F29
    - specified NEC F28
  - schizophreniform F20.81
    - brief F23
  - schizotypal (personality) F21
  - secretion, thyrocalcitonin E07.0
  - sedative, hypnotic, or anxiolytic use
    - mild F13.10
      - with
        - sedative, hypnotic, or anxiolytic-induced
          - anxiety disorder F13.180
          - bipolar and related disorder F13.14
          - depressive disorder F13.14
          - psychotic disorder F13.159
          - sexual dysfunction F13.181
        - sedative, hypnotic, or anxiolytic intoxication F13.129
        - sedative, hypnotic, or anxiolytic intoxication delirium F13.121
      - in remission (early) (sustained) F13.11
    - moderate or severe F13.20
      - with
        - sedative, hypnotic, or anxiolytic-induced
          - anxiety disorder F13.280
          - bipolar and related disorder F13.24
          - depressive disorder F13.24
          - major neurocognitive disorder F13.27
          - mild neurocognitive disorder F13.288
          - psychotic disorder F13.259
          - sexual dysfunction F13.281
        - sedative, hypnotic, or anxiolytic intoxication F13.229
        - sedative, hypnotic, or anxiolytic intoxication delirium F13.221
      - in remission (early) (sustained) F13.21
  - seizure *—see also* Epilepsy G40.909
    - intractable G40.919
      - with status epilepticus G40.911
  - semantic pragmatic F80.89
    - with autism F84.0
  - sense of smell R43.1
    - psychogenic F45.8
  - separation anxiety, of childhood F93.0
  - sexual
    - arousal, female F52.22
    - aversion F52.1
    - function, psychogenic F52.9
    - interest/arousal, female F52.22
    - masochism F65.51
    - maturation F66
    - nonorganic F52.9
    - preference *—see also* Deviation, sexual F65.9
      - fetishistic transvestism F65.1
    - relationship F66
    - sadism F65.52

- Disorder *(Continued)*
  - shyness, of childhood and adolescence F40.10
  - sibling rivalry F93.8
  - sickle-cell (sickling) (homozygous) *—see* Disease, sickle-cell
    - heterozygous D57.3
    - specified type NEC D57.8- •
    - trait D57.3
  - sinus (nasal) J34.9
    - specified NEC J34.89
  - skin L98.9
    - atrophic L90.9
      - specified NEC L90.8
    - granulomatous L92.9
      - specified NEC L92.8
    - hypertrophic L91.9
      - specified NEC L91.8
    - infiltrative NEC L98.6
    - newborn P83.9
      - specified NEC P83.88
    - picking F42.4
    - psychogenic (allergic) (eczematous) F54
  - sleep G47.9
    - breathing-related *—see* Apnea, sleep
    - circadian rhythm G47.20
      - advance sleep phase type G47.22
      - delayed sleep phase type G47.21
      - due to
        - alcohol
          - abuse F10.182
          - dependence F10.282
          - use F10.982
        - amphetamines
          - abuse F15.182
          - dependence F15.282
          - use F15.982
        - caffeine
          - abuse F15.182
          - dependence F15.282
          - use F15.982
        - cocaine
          - abuse F14.182
          - dependence F14.282
          - use F14.982
        - drug NEC
          - abuse F19.182
          - dependence F19.282
          - use F19.982
        - opioid
          - abuse F11.182
          - dependence F11.282
          - use F11.982
        - psychoactive substance NEC
          - abuse F19.182
          - dependence F19.282
          - use F19.982
        - sedative, hypnotic, or anxiolytic
          - abuse F13.182
          - dependence F13.282
          - use F13.982
        - stimulant NEC
          - abuse F15.182
          - dependence F15.282
          - use F15.982
      - free running type G47.24
      - in conditions classified elsewhere G47.27
      - irregular sleep wake type G47.23
      - jet lag type G47.25
      - non-24-hour sleep-wake type G47.24
      - shift work type G47.26
      - specified NEC G47.29
    - due to
      - alcohol
        - abuse F10.182
        - dependence F10.282
        - use F10.982
      - amphetamine
        - abuse F15.182
        - dependence F15.282
        - use F15.982

- Disorder *(Continued)*
  - sleep *(Continued)*
    - due to *(Continued)*
      - anxiolytic
        - abuse F13.182
        - dependence F13.282
        - use F13.982
      - caffeine
        - abuse F15.182
        - dependence F15.282
        - use F15.982
      - cocaine
        - abuse F14.182
        - dependence F14.282
        - use F14.982
      - drug NEC
        - abuse F19.182
        - dependence F19.282
        - use F19.982
      - hypnotic
        - abuse F13.182
        - dependence F13.282
        - use F13.982
      - opioid
        - abuse F11.182
        - dependence F11.282
        - use F11.982
      - psychoactive substance NEC
        - abuse F19.182
        - dependence F19.282
        - use F19.982
      - sedative
        - abuse F13.182
        - dependence F13.282
        - use F13.982
      - stimulant NEC
        - abuse F15.182
        - dependence F15.282
        - use F15.982
    - emotional F51.9
    - excessive somnolence *—see* Hypersomnia
    - hypersomnia type *—see* Hypersomnia
    - initiating or maintaining *—see* Insomnia
    - nightmares F51.5
    - nonorganic F51.9
      - specified NEC F51.8
    - parasomnia type G47.50
    - specified NEC G47.8
    - terrors F51.4
    - walking F51.3
  - sleep-wake pattern or schedule *—see also* Disorder, sleep, circadian rhythm G47.9
    - specified NEC G47.8
  - social
    - anxiety (of childhood) F40.10
      - generalized F40.11
    - functioning in childhood F94.9
      - specified NEC F94.8
    - pragmatic F80.82
  - soft tissue M79.9
    - ankle M79.9
    - due to use, overuse and pressure M70.90
      - ankle M70.97- •
      - bursitis *—see* Bursitis
      - foot M70.97- •
      - forearm M70.93- •
      - hand M70.94- •
      - lower leg M70.96- •
      - multiple sites M70.99
      - pelvic region M70.95- •
      - shoulder region M70.91- •
      - specified site NEC M70.98
      - specified type NEC M70.80
        - ankle M70.87- •
        - foot M70.87- •
        - forearm M70.83- •
        - hand M70.84- •
        - lower leg M70.86- •
        - multiple sites M70.89
        - pelvic region M70.85- •

Disorder *(Continued)*
soft tissue *(Continued)*
due to use, overuse and pressure *(Continued)*
specified type NEC *(Continued)*
shoulder region M70.81- •
specified site NEC M70.88
thigh M70.85- •
upper arm M70.82- •
thigh M70.95- •
upper arm M70.92- •
foot M79.9
forearm M79.9
hand M79.9
lower leg M79.9
multiple sites M79.9
occupational —*see* Disorder, soft tissue, due to use, overuse and pressure
pelvic region M79.9
shoulder region M79.9
specified type NEC M79.89
thigh M79.9
upper arm M79.9
somatic symptom F45.1
somatization F45.0
somatoform F45.9
pain (persistent) F45.41
somatization (multiple) (long-lasting) F45.0
specified NEC F45.8
undifferentiated F45.1
somnolence, excessive —*see* Hypersomnia
specific
arithmetical F81.2
developmental, of motor F82
reading F81.0
speech and language F80.9
spelling F81.81
written expression F81.81
speech R47.9
articulation (functional) (specific) F80.0
developmental F80.9
specified NEC R47.89
speech-sound F80.0
spelling (specific) F81.81
spine —*see also* Dorsopathy
ligamentous or muscular attachments, peripheral —*see* Enthesopathy, spinal
specified NEC —*see* Dorsopathy, specified NEC
stereotyped, habit or movement F98.4
stimulant use (other) (unspecified)
mild F15.10
in remission (early) (sustained) F15.11
moderate or severe F15.20
in remission (early) (sustained) F15.21
stomach (functional) —*see* Disorder, gastric
stress F43.9
acute F43.0
post-traumatic F43.10
acute F43.11
chronic F43.12
substance use (other) (unknown)
mild F19.10
with substance-induced
anxiety disorder F19.180
bipolar and related disorder F19.14
depressive disorder F19.14
major neurocognitive disorder F19.17
mild neurocognitive disorder F19.188
obsessive-compulsive and related disorder F19.188
sexual dysfunction F19.181
substance intoxication F19.129
substance intoxication delirium F19.121
moderate or severe F19.20
with substance-induced
anxiety disorder F19.280
bipolar and related disorder F19.24
depressive disorder F19.24
major neurocognitive disorder F19.27
mild neurocognitive disorder F19.288

Disorder *(Continued)*
substance use (other) (unknown) *(Continued)*
moderate or severe *(Continued)*
with substance-induced anxiety disorder*(Continued)*
obsessive-compulsive and related disorder F19.288
sexual dysfunction F19.281
in remission (early) (sustained) F19.21
substance intoxication F19.229
substance intoxication delirium F19.221
sulfur-bearing amino-acid metabolism E72.10
sweat gland (eccrine) L74.9
apocrine L75.9
specified NEC L75.8
specified NEC L74.8
synovium M67.90
acromioclavicular M67.91- •
ankle M67.97- •
elbow M67.92- •
foot M67.97- •
forearm M67.93- •
hand M67.94- •
hip M67.95- •
knee M67.96- •
multiple sites M67.99
rupture —*see* Rupture, synovium
shoulder M67.91- •
specified type NEC M67.80
acromioclavicular M67.81- •
ankle M67.87- •
elbow M67.82- •
foot M67.87- •
hand M67.84- •
hip M67.85- •
knee M67.86- •
multiple sites M67.89
wrist M67.83- •
synovitis —*see* Synovitis
upper arm M67.92- •
wrist M67.93- •
temperature regulation, newborn P81.9
specified NEC P81.8
temporomandibular joint M26.60- •
tendon M67.90
acromioclavicular M67.91- •
ankle M67.97- •
contracture —*see* Contracture, tendon
elbow M67.92- •
foot M67.97- •
forearm M67.93- •
hand M67.94- •
hip M67.95- •
knee M67.96- •
multiple sites M67.99
rupture —*see* Rupture, tendon
shoulder M67.91- •
specified type NEC M67.80
acromioclavicular M67.81- •
ankle M67.87- •
elbow M67.82- •
foot M67.87- •
hand M67.84- •
hip M67.85- •
knee M67.86- •
multiple sites M67.89
trunk M67.88
wrist M67.83- •
synovitis —*see* Synovitis
tendinitis —*see* Tendinitis
tenosynovitis —*see* Tenosynovitis
trunk M67.98
upper arm M67.92- •
wrist M67.93- •
thoracic root (nerve) NEC G54.3
thyrocalcitonin hypersecretion E07.0
thyroid (gland) E07.9
function NEC, neonatal, transitory P72.2
iodine-deficiency related E01.8
specified NEC E07.89
tic —*see* Tic

Disorder *(Continued)*
tobacco use
chewing tobacco (mild) (moderate) (severe)
in remission (early) (sustained) F17.221
cigarettes (mild) (moderate) (severe)
in remission (early) (sustained) F17.211
mild F17.200
in remission (early) (sustained) F17.201
moderate F17.200
in remission (early) (sustained) F17.201
severe F17.200
in remission (early) (sustained) F17.201
specified product NEC (mild) (moderate) (severe)
in remission (early) (sustained) F17.291
tooth K08.9
development K00.9
specified NEC K00.8
eruption K00.6
Tourette's F95.2
trance and possession F44.89
transvestic F65.1
trauma and stressor-related F43.9
other specified F43.8
tricuspid (valve) —*see* Endocarditis, tricuspid
tryptophan metabolism E70.5
tubular, phosphate-losing N25.0
tubulo-interstitial (in)
brucellosis A23.9 *[N16]*
cystinosis E72.04
diphtheria A36.84
glycogen storage disease E74.00 *[N16]*
leukemia NEC C95.9- • *[N16]*
lymphoma NEC C85.9- • *[N16]*
mixed cryoglobulinemia D89.1 *[N16]*
multiple myeloma C90.0- • *[N16]*
Salmonella infection A02.25
sarcoidosis D86.84
sepsis A41.9 *[N16]*
streptococcal A40.9 *[N16]*
systemic lupus erythematosus M32.15
toxoplasmosis B58.83
transplant rejection T86.91 *[N16]*
Wilson's disease E83.01 *[N16]*
tubulo-renal function, impaired N25.9
specified NEC N25.89
tympanic membrane H73.9- •
atrophy —*see* Atrophy, tympanic membrane
infection —*see* Myringitis
perforation —*see* Perforation, tympanum
specified NEC H73.89- •
unsocialized aggressive F91.1
urea cycle metabolism E72.20
argininemia E72.21
arginosuccinic aciduria E72.22
citrullinemia E72.23
ornithine transcarbamylase deficiency E72.4
other specified E72.29
ureter (in) N28.9
schistosomiasis B65.0 *[N29]*
tuberculosis A18.11
urethra N36.9
specified NEC N36.8
urinary system N39.9
specified NEC N39.8
valve, heart
aortic —*see* Endocarditis, aortic
mitral —*see* Endocarditis, mitral
pulmonary —*see* Endocarditis, pulmonary
rheumatic
aortic —*see* Endocarditis, aortic, rheumatic
mitral —*see* Endocarditis, mitral
pulmonary —*see* Endocarditis, pulmonary, rheumatic
tricuspid —*see* Endocarditis, tricuspid
tricuspid —*see* Endocarditis, tricuspid
vestibular function H81.9- •
specified NEC —*see* subcategory H81.8
in diseases classified elsewhere H82.- •
vertigo —*see* Vertigo

Disorder *(Continued)*
- vision, binocular H53.30
  - abnormal retinal correspondence H53.31
  - diplopia H53.2
  - fusion with defective stereopsis H53.32
  - simultaneous perception H53.33
  - suppression H53.34
- visual
  - cortex
    - blindness H47.619
      - left brain H47.612
      - right brain H47.611
    - due to
      - inflammatory disorder H47.629
        - left brain H47.622
        - right brain H47.621
      - neoplasm H47.639
        - left brain H47.632
        - right brain H47.631
      - vascular disorder H47.649
        - left brain H47.642
        - right brain H47.641
  - pathway H47.9
    - due to
      - inflammatory disorder H47.51- •
      - neoplasm H47.52- •
      - vascular disorder H47.53- •
    - optic chiasm —*see* Disorder, optic, chiasm
- vitreous body H43.9
  - crystalline deposits —*see* Deposit, crystalline
  - degeneration —*see* Degeneration, vitreous
  - hemorrhage —*see* Hemorrhage, vitreous
  - opacities —*see* Opacity, vitreous
  - prolapse —*see* Prolapse, vitreous
  - specified type NEC H43.89
- voice R49.9
  - specified type NEC R49.8
- volatile solvent use
  - due to drug abuse —*see* Abuse, drug, inhalant
  - due to drug dependence —*see* Dependence, drug, inhalant
- voyeuristic F65.3
- white blood cells D72.9
  - specified NEC D72.89
- withdrawing, child or adolescent F40.10

Disorientation R41.0

Displacement, displaced
- acquired traumatic of bone, cartilage, joint, tendon NEC —*see* Dislocation
- adrenal gland (congenital) Q89.1
- appendix, retrocecal (congenital) Q43.8
- auricle (congenital) Q17.4
- bladder (acquired) N32.89
  - congenital Q64.19
- brachial plexus (congenital) Q07.8
- brain stem, caudal (congenital) Q04.8
- canaliculus (lacrimalis), congenital Q10.6
- cardia through esophageal hiatus (congenital) Q40.1
- cerebellum, caudal (congenital) Q04.8
- cervix —*see* Malposition, uterus
- colon (congenital) Q43.3
- device, implant or graft —*see also* Complications, by site and type, mechanical T85.628
  - arterial graft NEC —*see* Complication, cardiovascular device, mechanical, vascular
  - breast (implant) T85.42
  - catheter NEC T85.628
    - dialysis (renal) T82.42
      - intraperitoneal T85.621
    - infusion NEC T82.524
      - spinal (epidural) (subdural) T85.620
    - urinary
      - cystostomy T83.020
      - Hopkins T83.028
      - ileostomy T83.028

Displacement, displaced *(Continued)*
- device, implant or graft *(Continued)*
  - catheter NEC *(Continued)*
    - urinary *(Continued)*
      - indwelling T83.021
      - nephrostomy T83.022
      - specified NEC T83.028
      - urostomy T83.028
  - electronic (electrode) (pulse generator) (stimulator) —*see* Complication, electronic stimulator
  - fixation, internal (orthopedic) NEC —*see* Complication, fixation device, mechanical
  - gastrointestinal —*see* Complications, prosthetic device, mechanical, gastrointestinal device
  - genital NEC T83.428
    - intrauterine contraceptive device (string) T83.32
    - penile prosthesis (cylinder) (implanted) (pump) (resevoir) T83.420
    - testicular prosthesis T83.421
  - heart NEC —*see* Complication, cardiovascular device, mechanical
  - joint prosthesis —*see* Complications, joint prosthesis, mechanical
  - ocular —*see* Complications, prosthetic device, mechanical, ocular device
  - orthopedic NEC —*see* Complication, orthopedic, device or graft, mechanical
  - specified NEC T85.628
  - urinary NEC T83.128
    - graft T83.22
    - sphincter, implanted T83.121
    - stent (ileal conduit) (nephroureteral) T83.123
    - ureteral indwelling T83.122
  - vascular NEC —*see* Complication, cardiovascular device, mechanical
  - ventricular intracranial shunt T85.02
- electronic stimulator
  - bone T84.320
  - cardiac —*see* Complications, cardiac device, electronic
  - nervous system —*see* Complication, prosthetic device, mechanical, electronic nervous system stimulator
  - urinary —*see* Complications, electronic stimulator, urinary
- esophageal mucosa into cardia of stomach, congenital Q39.8
- esophagus (acquired) K22.8
  - congenital Q39.8
- eyeball (acquired) (lateral) (old) —*see* Displacement, globe
  - congenital Q15.8
  - current —*see* Avulsion, eye
- fallopian tube (acquired) N83.4- •
  - congenital Q50.6
  - opening (congenital) Q50.6
- gallbladder (congenital) Q44.1
- gastric mucosa (congenital) Q40.2
- globe (acquired) (old) (lateral) H05.21- •
  - current —*see* Avulsion, eye
- heart (congenital) Q24.8
  - acquired I51.89
- hymen (upward) (congenital) Q52.4
- intervertebral disc NEC
  - with myelopathy —*see* Disorder, disc, with, myelopathy
  - cervical, cervicothoracic (with) M50.20
    - myelopathy —*see* Disorder, disc, cervical, with myelopathy
    - neuritis, radiculitis or radiculopathy —*see* Disorder, disc, cervical, with neuritis
  - due to trauma —*see* Dislocation, vertebra

Displacement, displaced *(Continued)*
- intervertebral disc NEC *(Continued)*
  - lumbar region M51.26
    - with
      - neuritis, radiculitis, radiculopathy or sciatica M51.16
  - lumbosacral region M51.27
    - with
      - myelopathy M51.07
      - neuritis, radiculitis, radiculopathy or sciatica M51.17
  - sacrococcygeal region M53.3
  - thoracic region M51.24
    - with
      - myelopathy M51.04
      - neuritis, radiculitis, radiculopathy M51.14
  - thoracolumbar region M51.25
    - with
      - myelopathy M51.05
      - neuritis, radiculitis, radiculopathy M51.15
- intrauterine device (string) T83.32
- kidney (acquired) N28.83
  - congenital Q63.2
- lachrymal, lacrimal apparatus or duct (congenital) Q10.6
- lens, congenital Q12.1
- macula (congenital) Q14.1
- Meckel's diverticulum Q43.0
  - malignant —*see* Table of Neoplasms, small intestine, malignant
- nail (congenital) Q84.6
  - acquired L60.8
- opening of Wharton's duct in mouth Q38.4
- organ or site, congenital NEC —*see* Malposition, congenital
- ovary (acquired) N83.4- •
  - congenital Q50.39
  - free in peritoneal cavity (congenital) Q50.39
  - into hernial sac N83.4- •
- oviduct (acquired) N83.4- •
  - congenital Q50.6
- parathyroid (gland) E21.4
- parotid gland (congenital) Q38.4
- punctum lacrimale (congenital) Q10.6
- sacro-iliac (joint) (congenital) Q74.2
  - current injury S33.2
  - old —*see* subcategory M53.2
- salivary gland (any) (congenital) Q38.4
- spleen (congenital) Q89.09
- stomach, congenital Q40.2
- sublingual duct Q38.4
- tongue (downward) (congenital) Q38.3
- tooth, teeth, fully erupted M26.30
  - horizontal M26.33
  - vertical M26.34
- trachea (congenital) Q32.1
- ureter or ureteric opening or orifice (congenital) Q62.62
- uterine opening of oviducts or fallopian tubes Q50.6
- uterus, uterine —*see* Malposition, uterus
- ventricular septum Q21.0
  - with rudimentary ventricle Q20.4

Disproportion
- between native and reconstructed breast N65.1
- fiber-type G71.2

Disruptio uteri —*see* Rupture, uterus

Disruption (of)
- ciliary body NEC H21.89
- closure of
  - cornea T81.31
  - craniotomy T81.32
  - fascia (muscular) (superficial) T81.32
  - internal organ or tissue T81.32
  - laceration (external) (internal) T81.33
  - ligament T81.32
  - mucosa T81.31
  - muscle or muscle flap T81.32

- **Disruption** *(Continued)*
  - closure of *(Continued)*
    - ribs or rib cage T81.32
    - skin and subcutaneous tissue (full-thickness) (superficial) T81.31
    - skull T81.32
    - sternum (sternotomy) T81.32
    - tendon T81.32
    - traumatic laceration (external) (internal) T81.33
  - family Z63.8
    - due to
      - absence of family member due to military deployment Z63.31
      - absence of family member NEC Z63.32
      - alcoholism and drug addiction in family Z63.72
      - bereavement Z63.4
      - death (assumed) or disappearance of family member Z63.4
      - divorce or separation Z63.5
      - drug addiction in family Z63.72
      - return of family member from military deployment (current or past conflict) Z63.71
      - stressful life events NEC Z63.79
  - iris NEC H21.89
  - ligament(s) —*see also* Sprain
    - knee
      - current injury —*see* Dislocation, knee
      - old (chronic) —*see* Derangement, knee, ligament, instability, chronic
      - spontaneous NEC —*see* Derangement, knee, disruption ligament
  - ossicular chain —*see* Discontinuity, ossicles, ear
  - pelvic ring (stable) S32.81Ø
    - unstable S32.811
  - traumatic injury wound repair T81.33
  - wound T81.3Ø
    - episiotomy O9Ø.1
    - operation T81.31
      - cesarean O9Ø.Ø
      - external operation wound (superficial) T81.31
      - internal operation wound (deep) T81.32
    - perineal (obstetric) O9Ø.1
  - traumatic injury repair T81.33
- **Dissatisfaction with**
  - employment Z56.9
  - school environment Z55.4
- **Dissecting** —*see* condition
- **Dissection**
  - aorta I71.ØØ
    - abdominal I71.Ø2
    - thoracic I71.Ø1
    - thoracoabdominal I71.Ø3
  - artery I77.7Ø
    - basilar (trunk) I77.75
    - carotid I77.71
    - cerebral (nonruptured) I67.Ø
      - ruptured —*see* Hemorrhage, intracranial, subarachnoid
    - coronary I25.42
    - extremity
      - lower I77.77
      - upper I77.76
    - iliac I77.72
    - precerebral
      - congenital (nonruptured) Q28.1
      - specified site NEC I77.75
    - renal I77.73
    - specified NEC I77.79
    - vertebral I77.74
  - precerebral artery, congenital (nonruptured) Q28.1
    - Heartland A93.8
  - traumatic —*see* Wound, open, by site
  - vascular I99.8
  - wound —*see* Wound, open
- **Disseminated** —*see* condition
- **Dissociation**
  - auriculoventricular or atrioventricular (AV) (any degree) (isorhythmic) I45.89
    - with heart block I44.2
  - interference I45.89
- **Dissociative reaction, state** F44.9
- **Dissolution, vertebra** —*see* Osteoporosis
- **Distension, distention**
  - abdomen R14.Ø
  - bladder N32.89
  - cecum K63.89
  - colon K63.89
  - gallbladder K82.8
  - intestine K63.89
  - kidney N28.89
  - liver K76.89
  - seminal vesicle N5Ø.89
  - stomach K31.89
    - acute K31.Ø
    - psychogenic F45.8
  - ureter —*see* Dilatation, ureter
  - uterus N85.8
- **Distoma hepaticum infestation** B66.3
- **Distomiasis** B66.9
  - bile passages B66.3
  - hemic B65.9
  - hepatic B66.3
    - due to Clonorchis sinensis B66.1
  - intestinal B66.5
  - liver B66.3
    - due to Clonorchis sinensis B66.1
  - lung B66.4
  - pulmonary B66.4
- **Distomolar** (fourth molar) KØØ.1
- **Disto-occlusion** (Division I) (Division II) M26.212
- **Distortion**(s) (congenital)
  - adrenal (gland) Q89.1
  - arm NEC Q68.8
  - bile duct or passage Q44.5
  - bladder Q64.79
  - brain QØ4.9
  - cervix (uteri) Q51.9
  - chest (wall) Q67.8
    - bones Q76.8
  - clavicle Q74.Ø
  - clitoris Q52.6
  - coccyx Q76.49
  - common duct Q44.5
  - coronary Q24.5
  - cystic duct Q44.5
  - ear (auricle) (external) Q17.3
    - inner Q16.5
    - middle Q16.4
      - ossicles Q16.3
  - endocrine NEC Q89.2
  - eustachian tube Q17.8
  - eye (adnexa) Q15.8
  - face bone(s) NEC Q75.8
  - fallopian tube Q5Ø.6
  - femur NEC Q68.8
  - fibula NEC Q68.8
  - finger(s) Q68.1
  - foot Q66.9-●
  - genitalia, genital organ(s)
    - female Q52.8
      - external Q52.79
      - internal NEC Q52.8
  - gyri QØ4.8
  - hand bone(s) Q68.1
  - heart (auricle) (ventricle) Q24.8
    - valve (cusp) Q24.8
  - hepatic duct Q44.5
  - humerus NEC Q68.8
  - hymen Q52.4
  - intrafamilial communications Z63.8
  - jaw NEC M26.89
  - labium (majus) (minus) Q52.79
  - leg NEC Q68.8
  - lens Q12.8
  - liver Q44.7
- **Distortion** *(Continued)*
  - lumbar spine Q76.49
    - with disproportion O33.8
      - causing obstructed labor O65.Ø
  - lumbosacral (joint) (region) Q76.49
    - kyphosis —*see* Kyphosis, congenital
    - lordosis —*see* Lordosis, congenital
  - nerve QØ7.8
  - nose Q3Ø.8
  - organ
    - of Corti Q16.5
    - or site not listed —*see* Anomaly, by site ossicles, ear Q16.3
  - oviduct Q5Ø.6
  - pancreas Q45.3
  - parathyroid (gland) Q89.2
  - pituitary (gland) Q89.2
  - radius NEC Q68.8
  - sacroiliac joint Q74.2
  - sacrum Q76.49
  - scapula Q74.Ø
  - shoulder girdle Q74.Ø
  - skull bone(s) NEC Q75.8
    - with
      - anencephalus QØØ.Ø
      - encephalocele —*see* Encephalocele
      - hydrocephalus QØ3.9
        - with spina bifida —*see* Spina bifida, with hydrocephalus
      - microcephaly QØ2
  - spinal cord QØ6.8
  - spine Q76.49
    - kyphosis —*see* Kyphosis, congenital
    - lordosis —*see* Lordosis, congenital
  - spleen Q89.Ø9
  - sternum NEC Q76.7
  - thorax (wall) Q67.8
    - bony Q76.8
  - thymus (gland) Q89.2
  - thyroid (gland) Q89.2
  - tibia NEC Q68.8
  - toe(s) Q66.9-●
  - tongue Q38.3
  - trachea (cartilage) Q32.1
  - ulna NEC Q68.8
  - ureter Q62.8
  - urethra Q64.79
    - causing obstruction Q64.39
  - uterus Q51.9
  - vagina Q52.4
  - vertebra Q76.49
    - kyphosis —*see* Kyphosis, congenital
    - lordosis —*see* Lordosis, congenital
  - visual —*see also* Disturbance, vision
    - shape and size H53.15
  - vulva Q52.79
  - wrist (bones) (joint) Q68.8
- **Distress**
  - abdomen —*see* Pain, abdominal
  - acute respiratory RØ6.Ø3
    - syndrome (adult) (child) J8Ø
  - epigastric R1Ø.13
  - fetal P84
    - complicating pregnancy —*see* Stress, fetal
  - gastrointestinal (functional) K3Ø
    - psychogenic F45.8
  - intestinal (functional) NOS K59.9
    - psychogenic F45.8
  - maternal, during labor and delivery O75.Ø
  - relationship, with spouse or intimate partner Z63.Ø
  - respiratory (adult) (child) RØ6.Ø3
    - newborn P22.9
      - specified NEC P22.8
    - orthopnea RØ6.Ø1
    - psychogenic F45.8
    - shortness of breath RØ6.Ø2
    - specified type NEC RØ6.Ø9
- **Distribution vessel, atypical** Q27.9
  - coronary artery Q24.5
  - precerebral Q28.1

Districhiasis L68.8
Disturbance(s) —*see also* Disease
absorption K90.9
calcium E58
carbohydrate K90.49
fat K90.49
pancreatic K90.3
protein K90.49
starch K90.49
vitamin —*see* Deficiency, vitamin
acid-base equilibrium E87.8
mixed E87.4
activity and attention (with hyperkinesis) —*see* Disorder, attention-deficit hyperactivity
amino acid transport E72.00
assimilation, food K90.9
auditory nerve, except deafness —*see* subcategory H93.3
behavior —*see* Disorder, conduct
blood clotting (mechanism) —*see also* Defect, coagulation D68.9
cerebral
nerve —*see* Disorder, nerve, cranial
status, newborn P91.9
specified NEC P91.88
circulatory I99.9
conduct —*see also* Disorder, conduct F91.9
adjustment reaction —*see* Disorder, adjustment
compulsive F63.9
disruptive F91.9
hyperkinetic —*see* Disorder, attention-deficit hyperactivity
socialized F91.2
specified NEC F91.8
unsocialized F91.1
coordination R27.8
cranial nerve —*see* Disorder, nerve, cranial
deep sensibility —*see* Disturbance, sensation
digestive K30
psychogenic F45.8
electrolyte —*see also* Imbalance, electrolyte
newborn, transitory P74.49
hyperammonemia P74.6
hyperchloremia P74.421
hyperchloremic metabolic acidosis P74.421
hypochloremia P74.422
potassium balance
hyperkalemia P74.31
hypokalemia P74.32
sodium balance
hypernatremia P74.21
hyponatremia P74.22
specified type NEC P74.49
emotions specific to childhood and adolescence F93.9
with
anxiety and fearfulness NEC F93.8
elective mutism F94.0
oppositional disorder F91.3
sensitivity (withdrawal) F40.10
shyness F40.10
social withdrawal F40.10
involving relationship problems F93.8
mixed F93.8
specified NEC F93.8
endocrine (gland) E34.9
neonatal, transitory P72.9
specified NEC P72.8
equilibrium R42
fructose metabolism E74.10
gait —*see* Gait
hysterical F44.4
psychogenic F44.4
gastrointestinal (functional) K30
psychogenic F45.8
habit, child F98.9
hearing, except deafness and tinnitus —*see* Abnormal, auditory perception

Disturbance *(Continued)*
heart, functional (conditions in I44-I50)
due to presence of (cardiac) prosthesis I97.19-●
postoperative I97.89
cardiac surgery —*see also* Infarct, myocardium, associated with revascularization procedure I97.19-●
hormones E34.9
innervation uterus (parasympathetic) (sympathetic) N85.8
keratinization NEC
gingiva K05.10
nonplaque induced K05.11
plaque induced K05.10
lip K13.0
oral (mucosa) (soft tissue) K13.29
tongue K13.29
learning (specific) —*see* Disorder, learning
memory —*see* Amnesia
mild, following organic brain damage F06.8
mental F99
associated with diseases classified elsewhere F54
metabolism E88.9
with
abortion —*see* Abortion, by type with other specified complication
ectopic pregnancy O08.5
molar pregnancy O08.5
amino-acid E72.9
aromatic E70.9
branched-chain E71.2
straight-chain E72.89
sulfur-bearing E72.10
ammonia E72.20
arginine E72.21
arginosuccinic acid E72.22
carbohydrate E74.9
cholesterol E78.9
citrulline E72.23
cystathionine E72.19
general E88.9
glutamine E72.89
histidine E70.40
homocystine E72.19
hydroxylysine E72.3
in labor or delivery O75.89
iron E83.10
lipoid E78.9
lysine E72.3
methionine E72.19
neonatal, transitory P74.9
calcium and magnesium P71.9
specified type NEC P71.8
carbohydrate metabolism P70.9
specified type NEC P70.8
specified NEC P74.8
ornithine E72.4
phosphate E83.39
sodium NEC E87.8
threonine E72.89
tryptophan E70.5
tyrosine E70.20
urea cycle E72.20
motor R29.2
nervous, functional R45.0
neuromuscular mechanism (eye), due to syphilis A52.15
nutritional E63.9
nail L60.3
ocular motion H51.9
psychogenic F45.8
oculogyric H51.8
psychogenic F45.8
oculomotor H51.9
psychogenic F45.8
olfactory nerve R43.1
optic nerve NEC —*see* Disorder, nerve, optic
oral epithelium, including tongue NEC K13.29

Disturbance *(Continued)*
perceptual due to
alcohol withdrawal F10.232
amphetamine intoxication F15.922
in
abuse F15.122
dependence F15.222
anxiolytic withdrawal F13.232
cannabis intoxication (acute) F12.922
in
abuse F12.122
dependence F12.222
cocaine intoxication (acute) F14.922
in
abuse F14.122
dependence F14.222
hypnotic withdrawal F13.232
opioid intoxication (acute) F11.922
in
abuse F11.122
dependence F11.222
phencyclidine intoxication (acute) F16.122
sedative withdrawal F13.232
personality (pattern) (trait) —*see also* Disorder, personality F60.9
following organic brain damage F07.9
polyglandular E31.9
specified NEC E31.8
potassium balance, newborn
hyperkalemia P74.31
hypokalemia P74.32
psychogenic F45.9
psychomotor F44.4
psychophysical visual H53.16
pupillary —*see* Anomaly, pupil, function
reflex R29.2
rhythm, heart I49.9
salivary secretion K11.7
sensation (cold) (heat) (localization) (tactile discrimination) (texture) (vibratory) NEC R20.9
hysterical F44.6
skin R20.9
anesthesia R20.0
hyperesthesia R20.3
hypoesthesia R20.1
paresthesia R20.2
specified type NEC R20.8
smell R43.9
and taste (mixed) R43.8
anosmia R43.0
parosmia R43.1
specified NEC R43.8
taste R43.9
and smell (mixed) R43.8
parageusia R43.2
specified NEC R43.8
sensory —*see* Disturbance, sensation
situational (transient) —*see also* Disorder, adjustment
acute F43.0
sleep G47.9
nonorganic origin F51.9
smell —*see* Disturbance, sensation, smell
sociopathic F60.2
sodium balance, newborn
hypernatremia P74.21
hyponatremia P74.22
speech R47.9
developmental F80.9
specified NEC R47.89
stomach (functional) K31.9
sympathetic (nerve) G90.9
taste —*see* Disturbance, sensation, taste
temperature
regulation, newborn P81.9
specified NEC P81.8
sense R20.8
hysterical F44.6

- **Disturbance** *(Continued)*
  - tooth
    - eruption K00.6
    - formation K00.4
    - structure, hereditary NEC K00.5
  - touch —*see* Disturbance, sensation
  - vascular I99.9
    - arteriosclerotic —*see* Arteriosclerosis
  - vasomotor I73.9
  - vasospastic I73.9
  - vision, visual H53.9
    - following
      - cerebral infarction I69.398
      - cerebrovascular disease I69.998
        - specified NEC I69.898
      - intracerebral hemorrhage I69.198
      - nontraumatic intracranial hemorrhage NEC I69.298
      - specified disease NEC I69.898
      - subarachnoid hemorrhage I69.098
    - psychophysical H53.16
    - specified NEC H53.8
    - subjective H53.10
      - day blindness H53.11
      - discomfort H53.14-●
      - distortions of shape and size H53.15
      - loss
        - sudden H53.13-●
        - transient H53.12-●
      - specified type NEC H53.19
  - voice R49.9
    - psychogenic F44.4
    - specified NEC R49.8
- **Diuresis** R35.8
- **Diver's palsy, paralysis or squeeze** T70.3
- **Diverticulitis** (acute) K57.92
  - bladder —*see* Cystitis
  - ileum —*see* Diverticulitis, intestine, small
  - intestine K57.92
    - with
      - abscess, perforation or peritonitis K57.80
        - with bleeding K57.81
      - bleeding K57.93
    - congenital Q43.8
    - large K57.32
      - with
        - abscess, perforation or peritonitis K57.20
          - with bleeding K57.21
        - bleeding K57.33
        - small intestine K57.52
          - with
            - abscess, perforation or peritonitis K57.40
              - with bleeding K57.41
            - bleeding K57.53
    - small K57.12
      - with
        - abscess, perforation or peritonitis K57.00
          - with bleeding K57.01
        - bleeding K57.13
        - large intestine K57.52
          - with
            - abscess, perforation or peritonitis K57.40
              - with bleeding K57.41
            - bleeding K57.53
- **Diverticulosis** K57.90
  - with bleeding K57.91
  - large intestine K57.30
    - with
      - bleeding K57.31
      - small intestine K57.50
        - with bleeding K57.51
  - small intestine K57.10
    - with
      - bleeding K57.11
      - large intestine K57.50
        - with bleeding K57.51
- **Diverticulum, diverticula** (multiple) K57.90
  - appendix (noninflammatory) K38.2
  - bladder (sphincter) N32.3
    - congenital Q64.6
  - bronchus (congenital) Q32.4
    - acquired J98.09
  - calyx, calyceal (kidney) N28.89
  - cardia (stomach) K31.4
  - cecum —*see* Diverticulosis, intestine, large
    - congenital Q43.8
  - colon —*see* Diverticulosis, intestine, large
    - congenital Q43.8
  - duodenum —*see* Diverticulosis, intestine, small
    - congenital Q43.8
  - epiphrenic (esophagus) K22.5
  - esophagus (congenital) Q39.6
    - acquired (epiphrenic) (pulsion) (traction) K22.5
  - eustachian tube —*see* Disorder, eustachian tube, specified NEC
  - fallopian tube N83.8
  - gastric K31.4
  - heart (congenital) Q24.8
  - ileum —*see* Diverticulosis, intestine, small
  - jejunum —*see* Diverticulosis, intestine, small
  - kidney (pelvis) (calyces) N28.89
    - with calculus —*see* Calculus, kidney
  - Meckel's (displaced) (hypertrophic) Q43.0
    - malignant —*see* Table of Neoplasms, small intestine, malignant
  - midthoracic K22.5
  - organ or site, congenital NEC —*see* Distortion
  - pericardium (congenital) (cyst) Q24.8
    - acquired I31.8
  - pharyngoesophageal (congenital) Q39.6
    - acquired K22.5
  - pharynx (congenital) Q38.7
  - rectosigmoid —*see* Diverticulosis, intestine, large
    - congenital Q43.8
  - rectum —*see* Diverticulosis, intestine, large
  - Rokitansky's K22.5
  - seminal vesicle N50.89
  - sigmoid —*see* Diverticulosis, intestine, large
    - congenital Q43.8
  - stomach (acquired) K31.4
    - congenital Q40.2
  - trachea (acquired) J39.8
  - ureter (acquired) N28.89
    - congenital Q62.8
  - ureterovesical orifice N28.89
  - urethra (acquired) N36.1
    - congenital Q64.79
  - ventricle, left (congenital) Q24.8
  - vesical N32.3
    - congenital Q64.6
  - Zenker's (esophagus) K22.5
- **Division**
  - cervix uteri (acquired) N88.8
  - glans penis Q55.69
  - labia minora (congenital) Q52.79
  - ligament (partial or complete) (current) —*see also* Sprain
    - with open wound —*see* Wound, open
  - muscle (partial or complete) (current) —*see also* Injury, muscle
    - with open wound —*see* Wound, open
  - nerve (traumatic) —*see* Injury, nerve
  - spinal cord —*see* Injury, spinal cord, by region
  - vein I87.8
- **Divorce, causing family disruption** Z63.5
- **Dix-Hallpike neurolabyrinthitis** —*see* Neuronitis, vestibular
- **Dizziness** R42
  - hysterical F44.89
  - psychogenic F45.8
- **DMAC** (disseminated mycobacterium avium-intracellulare complex) A31.2
- **DNR** (do not resuscitate) Z66
- **Doan-Wiseman syndrome** (primary splenic neutropenia) —*see* Agranulocytosis
- **Doehle-Heller aortitis** A52.02
- **Dog bite** —*see* Bite
- **Dohle body panmyelopathic syndrome** D72.0
- **Dolichocephaly** Q67.2
- **Dolichocolon** Q43.8
- **Dolichostenomelia** —*see* Syndrome, Marfan's
- **Donohue's syndrome** E34.8
- **Donor** (organ or tissue) Z52.9
  - blood (whole) Z52.000
    - autologous Z52.010
    - specified component (lymphocytes) (platelets) NEC Z52.008
      - autologous Z52.018
      - specified donor NEC Z52.098
    - specified donor NEC Z52.090
    - stem cells Z52.001
      - autologous Z52.011
      - specified donor NEC Z52.091
  - bone Z52.20
    - autologous Z52.21
    - marrow Z52.3
    - specified type NEC Z52.29
  - cornea Z52.5
  - egg (Oocyte) Z52.819
    - age 35 and over Z52.812
      - anonymous recipient Z52.812
      - designated recipient Z52.813
    - under age 35 Z52.810
      - anonymous recipient Z52.810
      - designated recipient Z52.811
  - kidney Z52.4
  - liver Z52.6
  - lung Z52.89
  - lymphocyte —*see* Donor, blood, specified components NEC
  - Oocyte —*see* Donor, egg
  - platelets Z52.008
  - potential, examination of Z00.5
  - semen Z52.89
  - skin Z52.10
    - autologous Z52.11
    - specified type NEC Z52.19
  - specified organ or tissue NEC Z52.89
  - sperm Z52.89
- **Donovanosis** A58
- **Dorsalgia** M54.9
  - psychogenic F45.41
  - specified NEC M54.89
- **Dorsopathy** M53.9
  - deforming M43.9
    - specified NEC —*see* subcategory M43.8
  - specified NEC M53.80
    - cervical region M53.82
    - cervicothoracic region M53.83
    - lumbar region M53.86
    - lumbosacral region M53.87
    - occipito-atlanto-axial region M53.81
    - sacrococcygeal region M53.88
    - thoracic region M53.84
    - thoracolumbar region M53.85
- **Double**
  - albumin E88.09
  - aortic arch Q25.45
  - auditory canal Q17.8
  - auricle (heart) Q20.8
  - bladder Q64.79
  - cervix Q51.820
    - with doubling of uterus (and vagina) Q51.10
      - with obstruction Q51.11
  - inlet ventricle Q20.4
  - kidney with double pelvis (renal) Q63.0
  - meatus urinarius Q64.75
  - monster Q89.4
  - outlet
    - left ventricle Q20.2
    - right ventricle Q20.1
  - pelvis (renal) with double ureter Q62.5
  - tongue Q38.3

Double *(Continued)*
ureter (one or both sides) Q62.5
with double pelvis (renal) Q62.5
urethra Q64.74
urinary meatus Q64.75
uterus Q51.2Ø
with
doubling of cervix (and vagina) Q51.1Ø
with obstruction Q51.11
complete Q51.21
in pregnancy or childbirth O34.Ø- •
causing obstructed labor O65.5
partial Q51.22
specified NEC Q51.28
vagina Q52.1Ø
with doubling of uterus (and cervix) Q51.1Ø
with obstruction Q51.11
vision H53.2
vulva Q52.79
Douglas' pouch, cul-de-sac —*see* condition
Down syndrome Q9Ø.9
meiotic nondisjunction Q9Ø.Ø
mitotic nondisjunction Q9Ø.1
mosaicism Q9Ø.1
translocation Q9Ø.2
DPD (dihydropyrimidine dehydrogenase deficiency) E88.89
Dracontiasis B72
Dracunculiasis, dracunculosis B72
Dream state, hysterical F44.89
Drepanocytic anemia —*see* Disease, sickle-cell
Dresbach's syndrome (elliptocytosis) D58.1
Dreschlera (hawaiiensis) (infection) B43.8
Dressler's syndrome I24.1
Drift, ulnar —*see* Deformity, limb, specified type NEC, forearm
Drinking (alcohol)
excessive, to excess NEC (without dependence) F1Ø.1Ø
habitual (continual) (without remission) F1Ø.2Ø
with remission F1Ø.21
Drip, postnasal (chronic) RØ9.82
due to
allergic rhinitis —*see* Rhinitis, allergic
common cold JØØ
gastroesophageal reflux —*see* Reflux, gastroesophageal
nasopharyngitis —*see* Nasopharyngitis
other known condition — code to condition
sinusitis —*see* Sinusitis
Droop
facial R29.81Ø
cerebrovascular disease I69.992
cerebral infarction I69.392
intracerebral hemorrhage I69.192
nontraumatic intracranial hemorrhage NEC I69.292
specified disease NEC I69.892
subarachnoid hemorrhage I69.Ø92
Drop (in)
attack NEC R55
finger —*see* Deformity, finger
foot —*see* Deformity, limb, foot, drop
hematocrit (precipitous) R71.Ø
hemoglobin R71.Ø
toe —*see* Deformity, toe, specified NEC
wrist —*see* Deformity, limb, wrist drop
Dropped heart beats I45.9
Dropsy, dropsical —*see also* Hydrops
abdomen R18.8
brain —*see* Hydrocephalus
cardiac, heart —*see* Failure, heart, congestive
gangrenous —*see* Gangrene
heart —*see* Failure, heart, congestive
kidney —*see* Nephrosis
lung —*see* Edema, lung
newborn due to isoimmunization P56.Ø
pericardium —*see* Pericarditis
Drowned, drowning (near) T75.1
Drowsiness R4Ø.Ø
Drug
abuse counseling and surveillance Z71.51
addiction —*see* Dependence
dependence —*see* Dependence
habit —*see* Dependence
harmful use —*see* Abuse, drug
induced fever R5Ø.2
overdose —*see* Table of Drugs and Chemicals, by drug, poisoning
poisoning —*see* Table of Drugs and Chemicals, by drug, poisoning
resistant organism infection —*see also* Resistant, organism, to, drug Z16.3Ø
therapy
long term (current) (prophylactic) —*see* Therapy, drug long-term (current) (prophylactic)
short term - omit code
wrong substance given or taken in error —*see* Table of Drugs and Chemicals, by drug, poisoning
Drunkenness (without dependence) F1Ø.129
acute in alcoholism F1Ø.229
chronic (without remission) F1Ø.2Ø
with remission F1Ø.21
pathological (without dependence) F1Ø.129
with dependence F1Ø.229
sleep F51.9
Drusen
macula (degenerative) (retina) —*see* Degeneration, macula, drusen
optic disc H47.32- •
Dry, dryness —*see also* condition
larynx J38.7
mouth R68.2
due to dehydration E86.Ø
nose J34.89
socket (teeth) M27.3
throat J39.2
DSAP L56.5
Duane's syndrome H5Ø.81- •
Dubin-Johnson disease or syndrome E8Ø.6
Dubois' disease (thymus gland) A5Ø.59 *[E35]*
Dubowitz' syndrome Q87.19
Duchenne-Aran muscular atrophy G12.21
Duchenne-Griesinger disease G71.Ø1
Duchenne's
disease or syndrome
motor neuron disease G12.22
muscular dystrophy G71.Ø1
locomotor ataxia (syphilitic) A52.11
paralysis
birth injury P14.Ø
due to or associated with
motor neuron disease G12.22
muscular dystrophy G71.Ø1
Ducrey's chancre A57
Duct, ductus —*see* condition
Duhring's disease (dermatitis herpetiformis) L13.Ø
Dullness, cardiac (decreased) (increased) RØ1.2
Dumb ague —*see* Malaria
Dumbness —*see* Aphasia
Dumdum fever B55.Ø
Dumping syndrome (postgastrectomy) K91.1
Duodenitis (nonspecific) (peptic) K29.8Ø
with bleeding K29.81
Duodenocholangitis —*see* Cholangitis
Duodenum, duodenal —*see* condition
Duplay's bursitis or periarthritis —*see* Tendinitis, calcific, shoulder
Duplication, duplex —*see also* Accessory
alimentary tract Q45.8
anus Q43.4
appendix (and cecum) Q43.4
biliary duct (any) Q44.5
bladder Q64.79
cecum (and appendix) Q43.4
cervix Q51.82Ø
Duplication, duplex *(Continued)*
chromosome NEC
with complex rearrangements NEC Q92.5
seen only at prometaphase Q92.8
cystic duct Q44.5
digestive organs Q45.8
esophagus Q39.8
frontonasal process Q75.8
intestine (large) (small) Q43.4
kidney Q63.Ø
liver Q44.7
pancreas Q45.3
penis Q55.69
respiratory organs NEC Q34.8
salivary duct Q38.4
spinal cord (incomplete) QØ6.2
stomach Q4Ø.2
Dupré's disease (meningism) R29.1
Dupuytren's contraction or disease M72.Ø
Durand-Nicolas-Favre disease A55
Durotomy (inadvertent) (incidental) G97.41
Duroziez's disease (congenital mitral stenosis) Q23.2
Dutton's relapsing fever (West African) A68.1
Dwarfism E34.3
achondroplastic Q77.4
congenital E34.3
constitutional E34.3
hypochondroplastic Q77.4
hypophyseal E23.Ø
infantile E34.3
Laron-type E34.3
Lorain (-Levi) type E23.Ø
metatropic Q77.8
nephrotic-glycosuric (with hypophosphatemic rickets) E72.Ø9
nutritional E45
pancreatic K86.89
pituitary E23.Ø
renal N25.Ø
thanatophoric Q77.1
Dyke-Young anemia (secondary) (symptomatic) D59.1
Dysacusis —*see* Abnormal, auditory perception
Dysadrenocortism E27.9
hyperfunction E27.Ø
Dysarthria R47.1
following
cerebral infarction I69.322
cerebrovascular disease I69.922
specified disease NEC I69.822
intracerebral hemorrhage I69.122
nontraumatic intracranial hemorrhage NEC I69.222
subarachnoid hemorrhage I69.Ø22
Dysautonomia (familial) G9Ø.1
Dysbarism T7Ø.3
Dysbasia R26.2
angiosclerotica intermittens I73.9
hysterical F44.4
lordotica (progressiva) G24.1
nonorganic origin F44.4
psychogenic F44.4
Dysbetalipoproteinemia (familial) E78.2
Dyscalculia R48.8
developmental F81.2
Dyschezia K59.ØØ
Dyschondroplasia (with hemangiomata) Q78.4
Dyschromia (skin) L81.9
Dyscollagenosis M35.9
Dyscranio-pygo-phalangy Q87.Ø
Dyscrasia
blood (with) D75.9
antepartum hemorrhage —*see* Hemorrhage, antepartum, with coagulation defect
intrapartum hemorrhage O67.Ø
newborn P61.9
specified type NEC P61.8
puerperal, postpartum O72.3
polyglandular, pluriglandular E31.9

Dysendocrinism E34.9
Dysentery, dysenteric (catarrhal) (diarrhea) (epidemic) (hemorrhagic) (infectious) (sporadic) (tropical) A09
- abscess, liver A06.4
- amebic —*see also* Amebiasis A06.0
  - with abscess —*see* Abscess, amebic
  - acute A06.0
  - chronic A06.1
- arthritis —*see also* category M01 A09
  - bacillary —*see also* category M01 A03.9
- bacillary A03.9
  - arthritis —*see also* category M01 A03.9
  - Boyd A03.2
  - Flexner A03.1
  - Schmitz (-Stutzer) A03.0
  - Shiga (-Kruse) A03.0
  - Shigella A03.9
    - boydii A03.2
    - dysenteriae A03.0
    - flexneri A03.1
    - group A A03.0
    - group B A03.1
    - group C A03.2
    - group D A03.3
    - sonnei A03.3
    - specified type NEC A03.8
  - Sonne A03.3
  - specified type NEC A03.8
- balantidial A07.0
- Balantidium coli A07.0
- Boyd's A03.2
- candidal B37.82
- Chilomastix A07.8
- Chinese A03.9
- coccidial A07.3
- Dientamoeba (fragilis) A07.8
- Embadomonas A07.8
- Entamoeba, entamebic —*see* Dysentery, amebic
- Flexner-Boyd A03.2
- Flexner's A03.1
- Giardia lamblia A07.1
- Hiss-Russell A03.1
- Lamblia A07.1
- leishmanial B55.0
- malarial —*see* Malaria
- metazoal B82.0
- monilial B37.82
- protozoal A07.9
- Salmonella A02.0
- schistosomal B65.1
- Schmitz (-Stutzer) A03.0
- Shiga (-Kruse) A03.0
- Shigella NOS —*see* Dysentery, bacillary
- Sonne A03.3
- strongyloidiasis B78.0
- trichomonal A07.8
- viral —*see also* Enteritis, viral A08.4

Dysequilibrium R42
Dysesthesia R20.8
- hysterical F44.6

Dysfibrinogenemia (congenital) D68.2
Dysfunction
- adrenal E27.9
  - hyperfunction E27.0
- autonomic
  - due to alcohol G31.2
  - somatoform F45.8
- bladder N31.9
  - neurogenic NOS —*see* Dysfunction, bladder, neuromuscular
  - neuromuscular NOS N31.9
    - atonic (motor) (sensory) N31.2
    - autonomous N31.2
    - flaccid N31.2
    - nonreflex N31.2
    - reflex N31.1
    - specified NEC N31.8
    - uninhibited N31.0
- bleeding, uterus N93.8

Dysfunction *(Continued)*
- cerebral G93.89
- colon K59.9
  - psychogenic F45.8
- colostomy K94.03
- cystic duct K82.8
- cystostomy (stoma) —*see* Complications, cystostomy
- ejaculatory N53.19
  - anejaculatory orgasm N53.13
  - painful N53.12
  - premature F52.4
  - retarded N53.11
- endocrine NOS E34.9
- endometrium N85.8
- enterostomy K94.13
- erectile —*see* Dysfunction, sexual, male, erectile
- gallbladder K82.8
- gastrostomy (stoma) K94.23
- gland, glandular NOS E34.9
  - meibomian, of eyelid -see Dysfunction, meibomian gland
- heart I51.89
- hemoglobin D75.89
- hepatic K76.89
- hypophysis E23.7
- hypothalamic NEC E23.3
- ileostomy (stoma) K94.13
- jejunostomy (stoma) K94.13
- kidney —*see* Disease, renal
- labyrinthine —*see* subcategory H83.2
- left ventricular, following sudden emotional stress I51.81
- liver K76.89
- male —*see* Dysfunction, sexual, male
- meibomian gland, of eyelid H02.889
  - left H02.886
    - lower H02.885
    - upper H02.884
    - upper and lower eyelids H02.88B
  - right H02.883
    - lower H02.882
    - upper H02.881
    - upper and lower eyelids H02.88A
- orgasmic (female) F52.31
  - male F52.32
- ovary E28.9
  - specified NEC E28.8
- papillary muscle I51.89
- parathyroid E21.4
- physiological NEC R68.89
  - psychogenic F59
- pineal gland E34.8
- pituitary (gland) E23.3
- platelets D69.1
- polyglandular E31.9
  - specified NEC E31.8
- psychophysiologic F59
- psychosexual F52.9
  - with
    - dyspareunia F52.6
    - premature ejaculation F52.4
    - vaginismus F52.5
- pylorus K31.9
- rectum K59.9
  - psychogenic F45.8
- reflex (sympathetic) —*see* Syndrome, pain, complex regional I
- segmental —*see* Dysfunction, somatic
- senile R54
- sexual (due to) R37
  - alcohol F10.981
  - amphetamine F15.981
    - in
      - abuse F15.181
      - dependence F15.281
  - anxiolytic F13.981
    - in
      - abuse F13.181
      - dependence F13.281

Dysfunction *(Continued)*
- sexual *(Continued)*
  - cocaine F14.981
    - in
      - abuse F14.181
      - dependence F14.281
  - excessive sexual drive F52.8
  - failure of genital response (male) F52.21
    - female F52.22
  - female N94.9
    - aversion F52.1
    - dyspareunia N94.10
      - psychogenic F52.6
    - frigidity F52.22
    - nymphomania F52.8
    - orgasmic F52.31
    - psychogenic F52.9
      - aversion F52.1
      - dyspareunia F52.6
      - frigidity F52.22
      - nymphomania F52.8
      - orgasmic F52.31
      - vaginismus F52.5
    - vaginismus N94.2
      - psychogenic F52.5
  - hypnotic F13.981
    - in
      - abuse F13.181
      - dependence F13.281
  - inhibited orgasm (female) F52.31
    - male F52.32
  - lack
    - of sexual enjoyment F52.1
    - or loss of sexual desire F52.0
  - male N53.9
    - anejaculatory orgasm N53.13
    - ejaculatory N53.19
      - painful N53.12
      - premature F52.4
      - retarded N53.11
    - erectile N52.9
      - drug induced N52.2
      - due to
        - disease classified elsewhere N52.1
        - drug N52.2
      - postoperative (postprocedural) N52.39
        - following
          - cryotherapy N52.37
          - interstitial seed therapy N52.36
          - prostate ablative therapy N52.37
          - prostatectomy N52.34
            - radical N52.31
          - radiation therapy N52.35
          - radical cystectomy N52.32
          - ultrasound ablative therapy N52.37
          - urethral surgery N52.33
      - psychogenic F52.21
      - specified cause NEC N52.8
      - vasculogenic
        - arterial insufficiency N52.01
          - with corporo-venous occlusive N52.03
        - corporo-venous occlusive N52.02
          - with arterial insufficiency N52.03
    - impotence —*see* Dysfunction, sexual, male, erectile
    - psychogenic F52.9
      - aversion F52.1
      - erectile F52.21
      - orgasmic F52.32
      - premature ejaculation F52.4
      - satyriasis F52.8
      - specified type NEC F52.8
    - specified type NEC N53.8
  - nonorganic F52.9
    - specified NEC F52.8
  - opioid F11.981
    - in
      - abuse F11.181
      - dependence F11.281

Dysfunction (Continued)
sexual (Continued)
orgasmic dysfunction (female) F52.31
male F52.32
premature ejaculation F52.4
psychoactive substances NEC F19.981
in
abuse F19.181
dependence F19.281
psychogenic F52.9
sedative F13.981
in
abuse F13.181
dependence F13.281
sexual aversion F52.1
vaginismus (nonorganic) (psychogenic) F52.5
sinoatrial node I49.5
somatic M99.09
abdomen M99.09
acromioclavicular M99.07
cervical region M99.01
cervicothoracic M99.01
costochondral M99.08
costovertebral M99.08
head region M99.00
hip M99.05
lower extremity M99.06
lumbar region M99.03
lumbosacral M99.03
occipitocervical M99.00
pelvic region M99.05
pubic M99.05
rib cage M99.08
sacral region M99.04
sacrococcygeal M99.04
sacroiliac M99.04
specified NEC M99.09
sternochondral M99.08
sternoclavicular M99.07
thoracic region M99.02
thoracolumbar M99.02
upper extremity M99.07
somatoform autonomic F45.8
stomach K31.89
psychogenic F45.8
suprarenal E27.9
hyperfunction E27.0
symbolic R48.9
specified type NEC R48.8
temporomandibular (joint) M26.69
joint-pain syndrome M26.62-●
testicular (endocrine) E29.9
specified NEC E29.8
thymus E32.9
thyroid E07.9
ureterostomy (stoma) —*see* Complications, stoma, urinary tract
urethrostomy (stoma) —*see* Complications, stoma, urinary tract
uterus, complicating delivery O62.9
hypertonic O62.4
hypotonic O62.2
primary O62.0
secondary O62.1
ventricular I51.9
with congestive heart failure —*see also* Failure, heart I50.9
left, reversible, following sudden emotional stress I51.81
Dysgenesis
gonadal (due to chromosomal anomaly) Q96.9
pure Q99.1
renal Q60.5
bilateral Q60.4
unilateral Q60.3
reticular D72.0
tidal platelet D69.3
Dysgerminoma
specified site —*see* Neoplasm, malignant, by site
Dysgerminoma (Continued)
unspecified site
female C56.9
male C62.90
Dysgeusia R43.2
Dysgraphia R27.8
Dyshidrosis, dysidrosis L30.1
Dyskaryotic cervical smear R87.619
Dyskeratosis L85.8
cervix —*see* Dysplasia, cervix
congenital Q82.8
uterus NEC N85.8
Dyskinesia G24.9
biliary (cystic duct or gallbladder) K82.8
drug induced
orofacial G24.01
esophagus K22.4
hysterical F44.4
intestinal K59.8
nonorganic origin F44.4
orofacial (idiopathic) G24.4
drug induced G24.01
psychogenic F44.4
subacute, drug induced G24.01
tardive G24.01
neuroleptic induced G24.01
trachea J39.8
tracheobronchial J98.09
Dyslalia (developmental) F80.0
Dyslexia R48.0
developmental F81.0
Dyslipidemia E78.5
depressed HDL cholesterol E78.6
elevated fasting triglycerides E78.1
Dysmaturity —*see also* Light for dates
pulmonary (newborn) (Wilson-Mikity) P27.0
Dysmenorrhea (essential) (exfoliative) N94.6
congestive (syndrome) N94.6
primary N94.4
psychogenic F45.8
secondary N94.5
Dysmetabolic syndrome X E88.81
Dysmetria R27.8
Dysmorphism (due to)
alcohol Q86.0
exogenous cause NEC Q86.8
hydantoin Q86.1
warfarin Q86.2
Dysmorphophobia (nondelusional) F45.22
delusional F22
Dysnomia R47.01
Dysorexia R63.0
psychogenic F50.89
Dysostosis
cleidocranial, cleidocranialis Q74.0
craniofacial Q75.1
Fairbank's (idiopathic familial generalized osteophytosis) Q78.9
mandibulofacial (incomplete) Q75.4
multiplex E76.01
oculomandibular Q75.5
Dyspareunia (female) N94.10
deep N94.12
male N53.12
nonorganic F52.6
psychogenic F52.6
secondary N94.19
specified NEC N94.19
superficial (introital) N94.11
Dyspepsia R10.13
atonic K30
functional (allergic) (congenital) (gastrointestinal) (occupational) (reflex) K30
intestinal K59.8
nervous F45.8
neurotic F45.8
psychogenic F45.8
Dysphagia R13.10
cervical R13.19
following
cerebral infarction I69.391
cerebrovascular disease I69.991
specified NEC I69.891
intracerebral hemorrhage I69.191
nontraumatic intracranial hemorrhage NEC I69.291
specified disease NEC I69.891
subarachnoid hemorrhage I69.091
functional (hysterical) F45.8
hysterical F45.8
nervous (hysterical) F45.8
neurogenic R13.19
oral phase R13.11
oropharyngeal phase R13.12
pharyngeal phase R13.13
pharyngoesophageal phase R13.14
psychogenic F45.8
sideropenic D50.1
spastica K22.4
specified NEC R13.19
Dysphagocytosis, congenital D71
Dysphasia R47.02
developmental
expressive type F80.1
receptive type F80.2
following
cerebrovascular disease I69.921
cerebral infarction I69.321
intracerebral hemorrhage I69.121
nontraumatic intracranial hemorrhage NEC I69.221
specified disease NEC I69.821
subarachnoid hemorrhage I69.021
Dysphonia R49.0
functional F44.4
hysterical F44.4
psychogenic F44.4
spastica J38.3
Dysphoria
gender F64.9
in
adolescence and adulthood F64.0
children F64.2
specified NEC F64.8
postpartal O90.6
Dyspituitarism E23.3
Dysplasia —*see also* Anomaly
acetabular, congenital Q65.89
alveolar capillary, with vein misalignment J84.843
anus (histologically confirmed) (mild) (moderate) K62.82
severe D01.3
arrhythmogenic right ventricular I42.8
arterial, fibromuscular I77.3
asphyxiating thoracic (congenital) Q77.2
brain Q07.9
bronchopulmonary, perinatal P27.1
cervix (uteri) N87.9
mild N87.0
moderate N87.1
severe D06.9
chondroectodermal Q77.6
colon D12.6
craniometaphyseal Q78.58
dentinal K00.5
diaphyseal, progressive Q78.3
dystrophic Q77.5
ectodermal (anhidrotic) (congenital) (hereditary) Q82.4
hydrotic Q82.8
epithelial, uterine cervix —*see* Dysplasia, cervix
eye (congenital) Q11.2
fibrous
bone NEC (monostotic) M85.00
ankle M85.07-●
foot M85.07-●

Dysplasia (Continued)
fibrous (Continued)
bone NEC (Continued)
forearm M85.03-●
hand M85.04-●
lower leg M85.06-●
multiple site M85.09
neck M85.08
rib M85.08
shoulder M85.01-●
skull M85.08
specified site NEC M85.08
thigh M85.05-●
toe M85.07-●
upper arm M85.02-●
vertebra M85.08
diaphyseal, progressive Q78.3
jaw M27.8
polyostotic Q78.1
florid osseous —see also Cyst, calcifying odontogenic
high grade, focal D12.6
hip, congenital Q65.89
joint, congenital Q74.8
kidney Q61.4
multicystic Q61.4
leg Q74.2
lung, congenital (not associated with short gestation) Q33.6
mammary (gland) (benign) N60.9-●
cyst (solitary) —see Cyst, breast
cystic —see Mastopathy, cystic
duct ectasia —see Ectasia, mammary duct
fibroadenosis —see Fibroadenosis, breast
fibrosclerosis —see Fibrosclerosis, breast
specified type NEC N60.8-●
metaphyseal Q78.5
muscle Q79.8
oculodentodigital Q87.0
periapical (cemental) (cemento-osseous) —see Cyst, calcifying odontogenic
periosteum —see Disorder, bone, specified type NEC
polyostotic fibrous Q78.1
prostate —see also Neoplasia, intraepithelial, prostate N42.30
severe D07.5
specified NEC N42.39
renal Q61.4
multicystic Q61.4
retinal, congenital Q14.1
right ventricular, arrhythmogenic I42.8
septo-optic Q04.4
skin L98.8
spinal cord Q06.1
spondyloepiphyseal Q77.7
thymic, with immunodeficiency D82.1
vagina N89.3
mild N89.0
moderate N89.1
severe NEC D07.2
vulva N90.3
mild N90.0
moderate N90.1
severe NEC D07.1
Dysplasminogenemia E88.02
Dyspnea (nocturnal) (paroxysmal) R06.00
asthmatic (bronchial) J45.909
with
bronchitis J45.909
with
exacerbation (acute) J45.901
status asthmaticus J45.902
chronic J44.9
exacerbation (acute) J45.901
status asthmaticus J45.902
cardiac —see Failure, ventricular, left
cardiac —see Failure, ventricular, left
functional F45.8
hyperventilation R06.4
hysterical F45.8
Dyspnea (Continued)
newborn P28.89
psychogenic F45.8
shortness of breath R06.02
specified type NEC R06.09
Dyspraxia R27.8
developmental (syndrome) F82
Dysproteinemia E88.09
Dysreflexia, autonomic G90.4
Dysrhythmia
cardiac I49.9
newborn
bradycardia P29.12
occurring before birth P03.819
before onset of labor P03.810
during labor P03.811
tachycardia P29.11
postoperative I97.89
cerebral or cortical —see Epilepsy
Dyssomnia —see Disorder, sleep
Dyssynergia
biliary K83.8
bladder sphincter N36.44
cerebellaris myoclonica (Hunt's ataxia) G11.1
Dysthymia F34.1
Dysthyroidism E07.9
Dystocia O66.9
affecting newborn P03.1
cervical (hypotonic) O62.2
affecting newborn P03.6
primary O62.0
secondary O62.1
contraction ring O62.4
fetal O66.9
abnormality NEC O66.3
conjoined twins O66.3
oversize O66.2
maternal O66.9
positional O64.9
shoulder (girdle) O66.0
causing obstructed labor O66.0
uterine NEC O62.4
Dystonia G24.9
cervical G24.3
deformans progressiva G24.1
drug induced NEC G24.09
acute G24.02
specified NEC G24.09
familial G24.1
idiopathic G24.1
familial G24.1
nonfamilial G24.2
orofacial G24.4
lenticularis G24.8
musculorum deformans G24.1
neuroleptic induced (acute) G24.02
orofacial (idiopathic) G24.4
oromandibular G24.4
due to drug G24.01
specified NEC G24.8
torsion (familial) (idiopathic) G24.1
acquired G24.8
genetic G24.1
symptomatic (nonfamilial) G24.2
Dystonic movements R25.8
Dystrophy, dystrophia
adiposogenital E23.6
autosomal recessive, childhood type, muscular dystrophy resembling Duchenne or Becker G71.01
Becker's type G71.01
cervical sympathetic G90.2
choroid (hereditary) H31.20
central areolar H31.22
choroideremia H31.21
gyrate atrophy H31.23
specified type NEC H31.29
cornea (hereditary) H18.50
endothelial H18.51
epithelial H18.52
Dystrophy, dystrophia (Continued)
cornea (Continued)
granular H18.53
lattice H18.54
macular H18.55
specified type NEC H18.59
Duchenne's type G71.01
due to malnutrition E45
Erb's G71.02
Fuchs' H18.51
Gower's muscular G71.01
hair L67.8
infantile neuraxonal G31.89
Landouzy-Déjérine G71.02
Leyden-Möbius G71.09
muscular G71.00
autosomal recessive, childhood type, muscular dystrophy resembling Duchenne or Becker G71.01
benign (Becker type) G71.01
scapuloperoneal with early contractures [Emery-Dreifuss] G71.09
congenital (hereditary) (progressive) (with specific morphological abnormalities of the muscle fiber) G71.09
myotonic G71.11
distal G71.09
Duchenne type G71.01
Emery-Dreifuss G71.09
Erb type G71.02
facioscapulohumeral G71.02
Gower's G71.01
hereditary (progressive) G71.09
Landouzy-Déjérine type G71.02
limb-girdle G71.09
myotonic G71.11
progressive (hereditary) G71.09
Charcot-Marie (-Tooth) type G60.0
pseudohypertrophic (infantile) G71.01
scapulohumeral G71.02
scapuloperoneal G71.09
severe (Duchenne type) G71.01
specified type NEC G71.09
myocardium, myocardial —see Degeneration, myocardial
nail L60.3
congenital Q84.6
nutritional E45
ocular G71.09
oculocerebrorenal E72.03
oculopharyngeal G71.09
ovarian N83.8
polyglandular E31.8
reflex (neuromuscular) (sympathetic) —see Syndrome, pain, complex regional I
retinal (hereditary) H35.50
in
lipid storage disorders E75.6 [H36]
systemic lipidoses E75.6 [H36]
involving
pigment epithelium H35.54
sensory area H35.53
pigmentary H35.52
vitreoretinal H35.51
Salzmann's nodular —see Degeneration, cornea, nodular
scapuloperoneal G71.09
skin NEC L98.8
sympathetic (reflex) —see Syndrome, pain, complex regional I
cervical G90.2
tapetoretinal H35.54
thoracic, asphyxiating Q77.2
unguium L60.3
congenital Q84.6
vitreoretinal H35.51
vulva N90.4
yellow (liver) —see Failure, hepatic
Dysuria R30.0
psychogenic F45.8

D

New Revised ~~deleted~~ Deleted ● Use Additional Character(s)

E

Eales' disease H35.06-●
Ear —*see also* condition
piercing Z41.3
tropical NEC B36.9 *[H62.40]*
in
aspergillosis B44.89
candidiasis B37.84
moniliasis B37.84
wax (impacted) H61.20
left H61.22
with right H61.23
right H61.21
with left H61.23
Earache —*see* subcategory H92.0
Early satiety R68.81
Eaton-Lambert syndrome—*see* Syndrome, Lambert-Eaton
Eberth's disease (typhoid fever) A01.00
Ebola virus disease A98.4
Ebstein's anomaly or syndrome (heart) Q22.5
Eccentro-osteochondrodysplasia E76.29
Ecchondroma —*see* Neoplasm, bone, benign
Ecchondrosis D48.0
Ecchymosis R58
conjunctiva —*see* Hemorrhage, conjunctiva
eye (traumatic) —*see* Contusion, eyeball
eyelid (traumatic) —*see* Contusion, eyelid
newborn P54.5
spontaneous R23.3
traumatic —*see* Contusion
Echinococciasis —*see* Echinococcus
Echinococcosis —*see* Echinococcus
Echinococcus (infection) B67.90
granulosus B67.4
bone B67.2
liver B67.0
lung B67.1
multiple sites B67.32
specified site NEC B67.39
thyroid B67.31
liver NOS B67.8
granulosus B67.0
multilocularis B67.5
lung NEC B67.99
granulosus B67.1
multilocularis B67.69
multilocularis B67.7
liver B67.5
multiple sites B67.61
specified site NEC B67.69
specified site NEC B67.99
granulosus B67.39
multilocularis B67.69
thyroid NEC B67.99
granulosus B67.31
multilocularis B67.69 *[E35]*
Echinorhynchiasis B83.8
Echinostomiasis B66.8
Echolalia R48.8
Echovirus, as cause of disease classified elsewhere B97.12
Eclampsia, eclamptic (coma) (convulsions) (delirium) (with hypertension) NEC O15.9
complicating
labor and delivery O15.1
postpartum O15.2
pregnancy O15.0-●
puerperium O15.2
Economic circumstances affecting care Z59.9
Economo's disease A85.8
Ectasia, ectasis
annuloaortic I35.8
aorta I77.819
with aneurysm —*see* Aneurysm, aorta
abdominal I77.811
thoracic I77.810
thoracoabdominal I77.812
breast —*see* Ectasia, mammary duct
capillary I78.8
cornea H18.71-●
Ectasia, ectasis *(Continued)*
gastric antral vascular (GAVE) K31.819
with hemorrhage K31.811
without hemorrhage K31.819
mammary duct N60.4-●
salivary gland (duct) K11.8
sclera —*see* Sclerectasia
Ecthyma L08.0
contagiosum B08.02
gangrenosum L08.0
infectiosum B08.02
Ectocardia Q24.8
Ectodermal dysplasia (anhidrotic) Q82.4
Ectodermosis erosiva pluriorificialis L51.1
Ectopic, ectopia (congenital)
abdominal viscera Q45.8
due to defect in anterior abdominal wall Q79.59
ACTH syndrome E24.3
adrenal gland Q89.1
anus Q43.5
atrial beats I49.1
beats I49.49
atrial I49.1
ventricular I49.3
bladder Q64.10
bone and cartilage in lung Q33.5
brain Q04.8
breast tissue Q83.8
cardiac Q24.8
cerebral Q04.8
cordis Q24.8
endometrium —*see* Endometriosis
gastric mucosa Q40.2
gestation —*see* Pregnancy, by site
heart Q24.8
hormone secretion NEC E34.2
kidney (crossed) (pelvis) Q63.2
lens, lentis Q12.1
mole —*see* Pregnancy, by site
organ or site NEC —*see* Malposition, congenital
pancreas Q45.3
pregnancy —*see* Pregnancy, ectopic
pupil —*see* Abnormality, pupillary
renal Q63.2
sebaceous glands of mouth Q38.6
spleen Q89.09
testis Q53.00
bilateral Q53.02
unilateral Q53.01
thyroid Q89.2
tissue in lung Q33.5
ureter Q62.63
ventricular beats I49.3
vesicae Q64.10
Ectromelia Q73.8
lower limb —*see* Defect, reduction, limb, lower, specified type NEC
upper limb —*see* Defect, reduction, limb, upper, specified type NEC
Ectropion H02.109
cervix N86
with cervicitis N72
congenital Q10.1
eyelid H02.109
cicatricial H02.119
left H02.116
lower H02.115
upper H02.114
right H02.113
lower H02.112
upper H02.111
congenital Q10.1
left H02.106
lower H02.105
upper H02.104
mechanical H02.129
left H02.126
lower H02.125
upper H02.124
Ectropion *(Continued)*
eyelid *(Continued)*
mechanical *(Continued)*
right H02.123
lower H02.122
upper H02.121
paralytic H02.159
left H02.156
lower H02.155
upper H02.154
right H02.153
lower H02.152
upper H02.151
right H02.103
lower H02.102
upper H02.101
senile H02.139
left H02.136
lower H02.135
upper H02.134
right H02.133
lower H02.132
upper H02.131
spastic H02.149
left H02.146
lower H02.145
upper H02.144
right H02.143
lower H02.142
upper H02.141
iris H21.89
lip (acquired) K13.0
congenital Q38.0
urethra N36.8
uvea H21.89
Eczema (acute) (chronic) (erythematous) (fissum) (rubrum) (squamous) (*see also* Dermatitis) L30.9
contact —*see* Dermatitis, contact
dyshydrotic L30.1
external ear —*see* Otitis, externa, acute, eczematoid
flexural L20.82
herpeticum B00.0
hypertrophicum L28.0
hypostatic —*see* Varix, leg, with, inflammation
impetiginous L01.1
infantile (due to any substance) L20.83
intertriginous L21.1
seborrheic L21.1
intertriginous NEC L30.4
infantile L21.1
intrinsic (allergic) L20.84
lichenified NEC L28.0
marginatum (hebrae) B35.6
pustular L30.3
stasis I87.2
with varicose veins —*see* Varix, leg, with, inflammation
vaccination, vaccinatum T88.1
varicose —*see* Varix, leg, with, inflammation
Eczematid L30.2
Eddowes (-Spurway) syndrome Q78.0
Edema, edematous (infectious) (pitting) (toxic) R60.9
with nephritis —*see* Nephrosis
allergic T78.3
amputation stump (surgical) (sequelae (late effect)) T87.89
angioneurotic (allergic) (any site) (with urticaria) T78.3
hereditary D84.1
angiospastic I73.9
Berlin's (traumatic) S05.8X-●
brain (cytotoxic) (vasogenic) G93.6
due to birth injury P11.0
newborn (anoxia or hypoxia) P52.4
birth injury P11.0
traumatic —*see* Injury, intracranial, cerebral edema
cardiac —*see* Failure, heart, congestive

Edema, edematous *(Continued)*
  cardiovascular —*see* Failure, heart, congestive
  cerebral —*see* Edema, brain
  cerebrospinal —*see* Edema, brain
  cervix (uteri) (acute) N88.8
    puerperal, postpartum O9Ø.89
  chronic hereditary Q82.Ø
  circumscribed, acute T78.3
    hereditary D84.1
  conjunctiva H11.42-●
  cornea H18.2-●
    idiopathic H18.22-●
    secondary H18.23-●
      due to contact lens H18.21-●
  due to
    lymphatic obstruction I89.Ø
    salt retention E87.Ø
  epiglottis —*see* Edema, glottis
  essential, acute T78.3
    hereditary D84.1
  extremities, lower —*see* Edema, legs
  eyelid NEC HØ2.849
    left HØ2.846
      lower HØ2.845
      upper HØ2.844
    right HØ2.843
      lower HØ2.842
      upper HØ2.841
  familial, hereditary Q82.Ø
  famine —*see* Malnutrition, severe
  generalized R6Ø.1
  glottis, glottic, glottidis (obstructive) (passive) J38.4
    allergic T78.3
      hereditary D84.1
  heart —*see* Failure, heart, congestive
  heat T67.7
  hereditary Q82.Ø
  inanition —*see* Malnutrition, severe
  intracranial G93.6
  iris H21.89
  joint —*see* Effusion, joint
  larynx —*see* Edema, glottis
  legs R6Ø.Ø
    due to venous obstruction I87.1
    hereditary Q82.Ø
  localized R6Ø.Ø
    due to venous obstruction I87.1
  lower limbs —*see* Edema, legs
  lung J81.1
    with heart condition or failure —*see* Failure, ventricular, left
    acute J81.Ø
    chemical (acute) J68.1
      chronic J68.1
    chronic J81.1
      due to
        chemicals, gases, fumes or vapors (inhalation) J68.1
        external agent J7Ø.9
          specified NEC J7Ø.8
        radiation J7Ø.1
    due to
      chemicals, fumes or vapors (inhalation) J68.1
      external agent J7Ø.9
        specified NEC J7Ø.8
      high altitude T7Ø.29
      near drowning T75.1
      radiation J7Ø.Ø
    meaning failure, left ventricle I5Ø.1
  lymphatic I89.Ø
    due to mastectomy I97.2
  macula H35.81
    cystoid, following cataract surgery —*see* Complications, postprocedural, following cataract surgery
    diabetic —*see* Diabetes, by type, with, retinopathy, with macular edema
  malignant —*see* Gangrene, gas
  Milroy's Q82.Ø

Edema, edematous *(Continued)*
  nasopharynx J39.2
  newborn P83.3Ø
    hydrops fetalis —*see* Hydrops, fetalis
    specified NEC P83.39
  nutritional —*see also* Malnutrition, severe
    with dyspigmentation, skin and hair E4Ø
  optic disc or nerve —*see* Papilledema
  orbit HØ5.22-●
  pancreas K86.89
  papilla, optic —*see* Papilledema
  penis N48.89
  periodic T78.3
    hereditary D84.1
  pharynx J39.2
  pulmonary —*see* Edema, lung
  Quincke's T78.3
    hereditary D84.1
  renal —*see* Nephrosis
  retina H35.81
    diabetic —*see* Diabetes, by type, with, retinopathy, with macular edema
  salt E87.Ø
  scrotum N5Ø.89
  seminal vesicle N5Ø.89
  spermatic cord N5Ø.89
  spinal (cord) (vascular) (nontraumatic) G95.19
  starvation —*see* Malnutrition, severe
  stasis —*see* Hypertension, venous, (chronic)
  subglottic —*see* Edema, glottis
  supraglottic —*see* Edema, glottis
  testis N44.8
  tunica vaginalis N5Ø.89
  vas deferens N5Ø.89
  vulva (acute) N9Ø.89
Edentulism —*see* Absence, teeth, acquired
Edsall's disease T67.2
Educational handicap Z55.9
  specified NEC Z55.8
Edward's syndrome —*see* Trisomy, 18
Effect, adverse
  abnormal gravitational (G) forces or states T75.81
  abuse —*see* Maltreatment
  air pressure T7Ø.9
    specified NEC T7Ø.8
  altitude (high) —*see* Effect, adverse, high altitude
  anesthesia —*see also* Anesthesia T88.59
    in labor and delivery O74.9
    local, toxic
      in labor and delivery O74.4-●
      in pregnancy NEC O29.3-●
      postpartum, puerperal O89.3
    postpartum, puerperal O89.9
    specified NEC T88.59
      in labor and delivery O74.8
      postpartum, puerperal O89.8
    spinal and epidural T88.59
      headache T88.59
        in labor and delivery O74.5
        postpartum, puerperal O89.4
      specified NEC
        in labor and delivery O74.6
        postpartum, puerperal O89.5
  antitoxin —*see* Complications, vaccination
  atmospheric pressure T7Ø.9
    due to explosion T7Ø.8
    high T7Ø.3
    low —*see* Effect, adverse, high altitude
    specified effect NEC T7Ø.8
  biological, correct substance properly administered —*see* Effect, adverse, drug
  blood (derivatives) (serum) (transfusion) —*see* Complications, transfusion
  chemical substance —*see* Table of Drugs and Chemicals
  cold (temperature) (weather) T69.9
    chilblains T69.1
    frostbite —*see* Frostbite
    specified effect NEC T69.8

Effect, adverse *(Continued)*
  drugs and medicaments T88.7
    specified drug —*see* Table of Drugs and Chemicals, by drug, adverse effect
    specified effect — code to condition
  electric current, electricity (shock) T75.4
    burn —*see* Burn
  exertion (excessive) T73.3
  exposure —*see* Exposure
  external cause NEC T75.89
  foodstuffs T78.1
    allergic reaction —*see* Allergy, food
      causing anaphylaxis —*see* Shock, anaphylactic, due to food
    noxious —*see* Poisoning, food, noxious
  gases, fumes, or vapors T59.9-●
    specified agent —*see* Table of Drugs and Chemicals
  glue (airplane) sniffing
    due to drug abuse —*see* Abuse, drug, inhalant
    due to drug dependence —*see* Dependence, drug, inhalant
  heat —*see* Heat
  high altitude NEC T7Ø.29
    anoxia T7Ø.29
    on
      ears T7Ø.Ø
      sinuses T7Ø.1
    polycythemia D75.1
  high pressure fluids T7Ø.4
  hot weather —*see* Heat
  hunger T73.Ø
  immersion, foot —*see* Immersion
  immunization —*see* Complications, vaccination
  immunological agents —*see* Complications, vaccination
  infrared (radiation) (rays) NOS T66
    dermatitis or eczema L59.8
  infusion —*see* Complications, infusion
  lack of care of infants —*see* Maltreatment, child
  lightning —*see* Lightning
  medical care T88.9
    specified NEC T88.8
  medicinal substance, correct, properly administered —*see* Effect, adverse, drug
  motion T75.3
  noise, on inner ear —*see* subcategory H83.3
  overheated places —*see* Heat
  psychosocial, of work environment Z56.5
  radiation (diagnostic) (infrared) (natural source) (therapeutic) (ultraviolet) (X-ray) NOS T66
    dermatitis or eczema —*see* Dermatitis, due to, radiation
    fibrosis of lung J7Ø.1
    pneumonitis J7Ø.Ø
    pulmonary manifestations
      acute J7Ø.Ø
      chronic J7Ø.1
    skin L59.9
  radioactive substance NOS
    dermatitis or eczema —*see* Radiodermatitis
  reduced temperature T69.9
    immersion foot or hand —*see* Immersion
    specified effect NEC T69.8
  serum NEC (*see also* Reaction, serum) T8Ø.69
  specified NEC T78.8
    external cause NEC T75.89
  strangulation —*see* Asphyxia, traumatic
  submersion T75.1
  thirst T73.1
  toxic —*see* Toxicity
  transfusion —*see* Complications, transfusion
  ultraviolet (radiation) (rays) NOS T66
    burn —*see* Burn
    dermatitis or eczema —*see* Dermatitis, due to, ultraviolet rays
      acute L56.8

E

Effect, adverse *(Continued)*
vaccine (any) *—see* Complications, vaccination
vibration *—see* Vibration, adverse effects
water pressure NEC T70.8
specified NEC T70.8
weightlessness T75.82
whole blood *—see* Complications, transfusion
work environment Z56.5
Effect(s) (of) (from) *—see* Effect, adverse NEC
Effects, late *—see* Sequelae
Effluvium
anagen L65.1
telogen L65.0
Effort syndrome (psychogenic) F45.8
Effusion
amniotic fluid *—see* Pregnancy, complicated by, prematue rupture of membranes
brain (serous) G93.6
bronchial *—see* Bronchitis
cerebral G93.6
cerebrospinal *—see also* Meningitis
vessel G93.6
chest *—see* Effusion, pleura
chylous, chyliform (pleura) J94.0
intracranial G93.6
joint M25.40
ankle M25.47-●
elbow M25.42-●
foot joint M25.47-●
hand joint M25.44-●
hip M25.45-●
knee M25.46-●
shoulder M25.41-●
specified joint NEC M25.48
wrist M25.43-●
malignant pleural J91.0
meninges *—see* Meningitis
pericardium, pericardial (noninflammatory) I31.3
acute *—see* Pericarditis, acute
peritoneal (chronic) R18.8
pleura, pleurisy, pleuritic, pleuropericardial J90
chylous, chyliform J94.0
due to systemic lupus erythematosis M32.13
in conditions classified elsewhere J91.8
influenzal *—see* Influenza, with, respiratory manifestations NEC
malignant J91.0
newborn P28.89
tuberculous NEC A15.6
primary (progressive) A15.7
spinal *—see* Meningitis
thorax, thoracic *—see* Effusion, pleura
Egg shell nails L60.3
congenital Q84.6
Egyptian splenomegaly B65.1
Ehlers-Danlos syndrome (*see also* Syndrome, Ehlers-Danlos) Q79.60
Ehrlichiosis A77.40
due to
E. chafeensis A77.41
E. sennetsu A79.81
specified organism NEC A77.49
Eichstedt's disease B36.0
Eisenmenger's
complex or syndrome I27.83
defect Q21.8
Ejaculation
delayed F52.32
painful N53.12
premature F52.4
retarded N53.11
retrograde N53.14
semen, painful N53.12
psychogenic F52.6
Ekbom's syndrome (restless legs) G25.81
Ekman's syndrome (brittle bones and blue sclera) Q78.0
Elastic skin Q82.8
acquired L57.4
Elastofibroma *—see* Neoplasm, connective tissue, benign
Elastoma (juvenile) Q82.8
Miescher's L87.2
Elastomyofibrosis I42.4
Elastosis
actinic, solar L57.8
atrophicans (senile) L57.4
perforans serpiginosa L87.2
senilis L57.4
Elbow *—see* condition
Electric current, electricity, effects (concussion) (fatal) (nonfatal) (shock) T75.4
burn *—see* Burn
Electric feet syndrome E53.8
Electrocution T75.4
from electroshock gun (taser) T75.4
Electrolyte imbalance E87.8
with
abortion *—see* Abortion by type, complicated by, electrolyte imbalance
ectopic pregnancy O08.5
molar pregnancy O08.5
Elephantiasis (nonfilarial) I89.0
arabicum *—see* Infestation, filarial
bancroftian B74.0
congenital (any site) (hereditary) Q82.0
due to
Brugia (malayi) B74.1
timori B74.2
mastectomy I97.2
Wuchereria (bancrofti) B74.0
eyelid H02.859
left H02.856
lower H02.855
upper H02.854
right H02.853
lower H02.852
upper H02.851
filarial, filariensis *—see* Infestation, filarial
glandular I89.0
graecorum A30.9
lymphangiectatic I89.0
lymphatic vessel I89.0
due to mastectomy I97.2
scrotum (nonfilarial) I89.0
streptococcal I89.0
surgical I97.89
postmastectomy I97.2
telangiectodes I89.0
vulva (nonfilarial) N90.89
Elevated, elevation
antibody titer R76.0
basal metabolic rate R94.8
blood pressure *—see also* Hypertension
reading (incidental) (isolated) (nonspecific), no diagnosis of hypertension R03.0
blood sugar R73.9
body temperature (of unknown origin) R50.9
C-reactive protein (CRP) R79.82
cancer antigen 125 [CA 125] R97.1
carcinoembryonic antigen [CEA] R97.0
cholesterol E78.00
with high triglycerides E78.2
conjugate, eye H51.0
diaphragm, congenital Q79.1
erythrocyte sedimentation rate R70.0
fasting glucose R73.01
fasting triglycerides E78.1
finding on laboratory examination *—see* Findings, abnormal, inconclusive, without diagnosis, by type of exam
GFR (glomerular filtration rate) *—see* Findings, abnormal, inconclusive, without diagnosis, by type of exam
glucose tolerance (oral) R73.02
immunoglobulin level R76.8
indoleacetic acid R82.5
lactic acid dehydrogenase (LDH) level R74.0
leukocytes D72.829
lipoprotein a (Lp(a)) level E78.41
Elevated, elevation *(Continued)*
liver function
study R94.5
test R79.89
alkaline phosphatase R74.8
aminotransferase R74.0
bilirubin R17
hepatic enzyme R74.8
lactate dehydrogenase R74.0
(Lp(a)) (lipoprotein(a)) E78.41
lymphocytes D72.820
prostate specific antigen [PSA] R97.20
Rh titer *—see* Complication(s), transfusion, incompatibility reaction, Rh (factor)
scapula, congenital Q74.0
sedimentation rate R70.0
SGOT R74.0
SGPT R74.0
transaminase level R74.0
triglycerides E78.1
with high cholesterol E78.2
tumor associated antigens [TAA] NEC R97.8
tumor specific antigens [TSA] NEC R97.8
urine level of
17-ketosteroids R82.5
catecholamine R82.5
indoleacetic acid R82.5
steroids R82.5
vanillylmandelic acid (VMA) R82.5
venous pressure I87.8
white blood cell count D72.829
specified NEC D72.828
Elliptocytosis (congenital) (hereditary) D58.1
Hb C (disease) D58.1
hemoglobin disease D58.1
sickle-cell (disease) D57.8-●
trait D57.3
Ellison-Zollinger syndrome E16.4
Ellis-van Creveld syndrome (chondroectodermal dysplasia) Q77.6
Elongated, elongation (congenital) *—see also* Distortion
bone Q79.9
cervix (uteri) Q51.828
acquired N88.4
hypertrophic N88.4
colon Q43.8
common bile duct Q44.5
cystic duct Q44.5
frenulum, penis Q55.69
labia minora (acquired) N90.69
ligamentum patellae Q74.1
petiolus (epiglottidis) Q31.8
tooth, teeth K00.2
uvula Q38.6
Eltor cholera A00.1
Emaciation (due to malnutrition) E41
Embadomoniasis A07.8
Embedded tooth, teeth K01.0
root only K08.3
Embolic *—see* condition
Embolism (multiple) (paradoxical) I74.9
air (any site) (traumatic) T79.0
following
abortion *—see* Abortion by type complicated by embolism
ectopic pregnancy O08.2
infusion, therapeutic injection or transfusion T80.0
molar pregnancy O08.2
procedure NEC
artery T81.719
mesenteric T81.710
renal T81.711
specified NEC T81.718
vein T81.72
in pregnancy, childbirth or puerperium *—see* Embolism, obstetric
amniotic fluid (pulmonary) *—see also* Embolism, obstetric
following
abortion *—see* Abortion by type complicated by embolism

E

Embolism *(Continued)*
amniotic fluid *(Continued)*
following *(Continued)*
ectopic pregnancy O08.2
molar pregnancy O08.2
aorta, aortic I74.10
abdominal I74.09
saddle I74.01
bifurcation I74.09
saddle I74.01
thoracic I74.11
artery I74.9
auditory, internal I65.8
basilar *—see* Occlusion, artery, basilar
carotid (common) (internal) *—see* Occlusion, artery, carotid
cerebellar (anterior inferior) (posterior inferior) (superior) I66.3
cerebral *—see* Occlusion, artery, cerebral
choroidal (anterior) I65.8
communicating posterior I65.8
coronary *—see also* Infarct, myocardium
not resulting in infarction I24.0
extremity I74.4
lower I74.3
upper I74.2
hypophyseal I65.8
iliac I74.5
limb I74.4
lower I74.3
upper I74.2
mesenteric (with gangrene) *—see also* Ischemia, intestine, acute K55.09
ophthalmic *—see* Occlusion, artery, retina
peripheral I74.4
pontine I65.8
precerebral *—see* Occlusion, artery, precerebral
pulmonary *—see* Embolism, pulmonary
renal N28.0
retinal *—see* Occlusion, artery, retina
septic I76
specified NEC I74.8
vertebral *—see* Occlusion, artery, vertebral
basilar (artery) I65.1
blood clot
following
abortion *—see* Abortion by type complicated by embolism
ectopic or molar pregnancy O08.2
in pregnancy, childbirth or puerperium *—see* Embolism, obstetric
brain *—see also* Occlusion, artery, cerebral
following
abortion *—see* Abortion by type complicated by embolism
ectopic or molar pregnancy O08.2
puerperal, postpartum, childbirth *—see* Embolism, obstetric
capillary I78.8
cardiac *—see also* Infarct, myocardium
not resulting in infarction I51.3
carotid (artery) (common) (internal) *—see* Occlusion, artery, carotid
cavernous sinus (venous) *—see* Embolism, intracranial venous sinus
cerebral *—see* Occlusion, artery, cerebral
cholesterol *—see* Atheroembolism
coronary (artery or vein) (systemic) *—see* Occlusion, coronary
due to device, implant or graft *—see also* Complications, by site and type, specified NEC
arterial graft NEC T82.818
breast (implant) T85.818
catheter NEC T85.818
dialysis (renal) T82.818
intraperitoneal T85.818
infusion NEC T82.818
spinal (epidural) (subdural) T85.810
urinary (indwelling) T83.81

Embolism *(Continued)*
due to device, implant or graft *(Continued)*
electronic (electrode) (pulse generator) (stimulator)
bone T84.81
cardiac T82.817
nervous system (brain) (peripheral nerve) (spinal) T85.810
urinary T83.81
fixation, internal (orthopedic) NEC T84.81
gastrointestinal (bile duct) (esophagus) T85.818
genital NEC T83.81
heart (graft) (valve) T82.817
joint prosthesis T84.81
ocular (corneal graft) (orbital implant) T85.818
orthopedic (bone graft) NEC T86.838
specified NEC T85.818
urinary (graft) NEC T83.81
vascular NEC T82.818
ventricular intracranial shunt T85.810
extremities
lower *—see* Embolism, vein, lower extremity
arterial I74.3
upper I74.2
eye H34.9
fat (cerebral) (pulmonary) (systemic) T79.1
complicating delivery *—see* Embolism, obstetric
following
abortion *—see* Abortion by type complicated by embolism
ectopic or molar pregnancy O08.2
following
abortion *—see* Abortion by type complicated by embolism
ectopic or molar pregnancy O08.2
infusion, therapeutic injection or transfusion
air T80.0
heart (fatty) *—see also* Infarct, myocardium
not resulting in infarction I51.3
hepatic (vein) I82.0
in pregnancy, childbirth or puerperium *—see* Embolism, obstetric
intestine (artery) (vein) (with gangrene) *—see also* Ischemia, intestine, acute K55.039
intracranial *—see also* Occlusion, artery, cerebral
venous sinus (any) G08
nonpyogenic I67.6
intraspinal venous sinuses or veins G08
nonpyogenic G95.19
kidney (artery) N28.0
lateral sinus (venous) *—see* Embolism, intracranial, venous sinus
leg *—see* Embolism, vein, lower extremity
arterial I74.3
longitudinal sinus (venous) *—see* Embolism, intracranial, venous sinus
lung (massive) *—see* Embolism, pulmonary
meninges I66.8
mesenteric (artery) (vein) (with gangrene) *—see also* Ischemia, intestine, acute K55.059
obstetric (in) (pulmonary)
childbirth O88.22
air O88.02
amniotic fluid O88.12
blood clot O88.22
fat O88.82
pyemic O88.32
septic O88.32
specified type NEC O88.82
pregnancy O88.21-●
air O88.01-●
amniotic fluid O88.11-●
blood clot O88.21-●
fat O88.81-●
pyemic O88.31-●
septic O88.31-●
specified type NEC O88.81-●

Embolism *(Continued)*
obstetric *(Continued)*
puerperal O88.23
air O88.03
amniotic fluid O88.13
blood clot O88.23
fat O88.83
pyemic O88.33
septic O88.33
specified type NEC O88.83
ophthalmic *—see* Occlusion, artery, retina
penis N48.81
peripheral artery NOS I74.4
pituitary E23.6
popliteal (artery) I74.3
portal (vein) I81
postoperative, postprocedural
artery T81.719
mesenteric T81.710
renal T81.711
specified NEC T81.718
vein T81.72
precerebral artery *—see* Occlusion, artery, precerebral
puerperal *—see* Embolism, obstetric
pulmonary (acute) (artery) (vein) I26.99
with acute cor pulmonale I26.09
chronic I27.82
following
abortion *—see* Abortion by type complicated by embolism
ectopic or molar pregnancy O08.2
healed or old Z86.711
in pregnancy, childbirth or puerperium *—see* Embolism, obstetric
▶ multiple subsegmental without acute cor pulmonale I26.94
personal history of Z86.711
saddle I26.92
with acute cor pulmonale I26.02
septic I26.90
with acute cor pulmonale I26.01
▶ single subsegmental without acute cor pulmonale I26.93
▶ subsegmental NOS I26.93
pyemic (multiple) I76
following
abortion *—see* Abortion by type complicated by embolism
ectopic or molar pregnancy O08.2
Hemophilus influenzae A41.3
pneumococcal A40.3
with pneumonia J13
puerperal, postpartum, childbirth (any organism) *—see* Embolism, obstetric
specified organism NEC A41.89
staphylococcal A41.2
streptococcal A40.9
renal (artery) N28.0
vein I82.3
retina, retinal *—see* Occlusion, artery, retina
saddle
abdominal aorta I74.01
pulmonary artery I26.92
with acute cor pulmonale I26.02
septic (arterial) I76
complicating abortion *—see* Abortion, by type, complicated by, embolism
sinus *—see* Embolism, intracranial, venous sinus
soap complicating abortion *—see* Abortion, by type, complicated by, embolism
spinal cord G95.19
pyogenic origin G06.1
spleen, splenic (artery) I74.8
upper extremity I74.2
vein (acute) I82.90
antecubital I82.61-●
chronic I82.71-●
axillary I82.A1-●
chronic I82.A2-●

E

Embolism (Continued)
vein (Continued)
basilic I82.61-●
chronic I82.71-●
brachial I82.62-●
chronic I82.72-●
brachiocephalic (innominate) I82.290
chronic I82.291
cephalic I82.61-●
chronic I82.71-●
chronic I82.91
deep (DVT) I82.40-●
calf I82.4Z-●
chronic I82.5Z-●
lower leg I82.4Z-●
chronic I82.5Z-●
thigh I82.4Y-●
chronic I82.5Y-●
upper leg I82.4Y
chronic I82.5y--●
femoral I82.41-●
chronic I82.51-●
iliac (iliofemoral) I82.42-●
chronic I82.52-●
innominate I82.290
chronic I82.291
internal jugular I82.C1-●
chronic I82.C2-●
lower extremity
deep I82.40-●
chronic I82.50-●
specified NEC I82.49-●
chronic NEC I82.59-●
distal
deep I82.4Z-●
proximal
deep I82.4Y-●
chronic I82.5Y-●
superficial I82.81-●
popliteal I82.43-●
chronic I82.53-●
radial I82.62-●
chronic I82.72-●
renal I82.3
saphenous (greater) (lesser) I82.81-●
specified NEC I82.890
chronic NEC I82.891
subclavian I82.B1-●
chronic I82.B2-●
thoracic NEC I82.290
chronic I82.291
tibial I82.44-●
chronic I82.54-●
ulnar I82.62-●
chronic I82.72-●
upper extremity I82.60-●
chronic I82.70-●
deep I82.62-●
chronic I82.72-●
superficial I82.61-●
chronic I82.71-●
vena cava
inferior (acute) I82.220
chronic I82.221
superior (acute) I82.210
chronic I82.211
venous sinus G08
vessels of brain —*see* Occlusion, artery, cerebral
Embolus —*see* Embolism
Embryoma —*see also* Neoplasm, uncertain behavior, by site
benign —*see* Neoplasm, benign, by site
kidney C64.-●
liver C22.0
malignant —*see also* Neoplasm, malignant, by site
kidney C64.-●
liver C22.0
testis C62.9-●
descended (scrotal) C62.1-●
undescended C62.0-●
Embryoma (Continued)
testis C62.9-●
descended (scrotal) C62.1-●
undescended C62.0-●
Embryonic
circulation Q28.9
heart Q28.9
vas deferens Q55.4
Embryopathia NOS Q89.9
Embryotoxon Q13.4
Emesis —*see* Vomiting
Emotional lability R45.86
Emotionality, pathological F60.3
Emotogenic disease —*see* Disorder, psychogenic
Emphysema (atrophic) (bullous) (chronic) (interlobular) (lung) (obstructive) (pulmonary) (senile) (vesicular) J43.9
cellular tissue (traumatic) T79.7
surgical T81.82
centrilobular J43.2
compensatory J98.3
congenital (interstitial) P25.0
conjunctiva H11.89
connective tissue (traumatic) T79.7
surgical T81.82
due to chemicals, gases, fumes or vapors J68.4
eyelid(s) —*see* Disorder, eyelid, specified type NEC
surgical T81.82
traumatic T79.7
interstitial J98.2
congenital P25.0
perinatal period P25.0
laminated tissue T79.7
surgical T81.82
mediastinal J98.2
newborn P25.2
orbit, orbital —*see* Disorder, orbit, specified type NEC
panacinar J43.1
panlobular J43.1
specified NEC J43.8
subcutaneous (traumatic) T79.7
nontraumatic J98.2
postprocedural T81.82
surgical T81.82
surgical T81.82
thymus (gland) (congenital) E32.8
traumatic (subcutaneous) T79.7
unilateral J43.0
Empty nest syndrome Z60.0
Empyema (acute) (chest) (double) (pleura) (supradiaphragmatic) (thorax) J86.9
with fistula J86.0
accessory sinus (chronic) —*see* Sinusitis
antrum (chronic) —*see* Sinusitis, maxillary
brain (any part) —*see* Abscess, brain
ethmoidal (chronic) (sinus) —*see* Sinusitis, ethmoidal
extradural —*see* Abscess, extradural
frontal (chronic) (sinus) —*see* Sinusitis, frontal
gallbladder K81.0
mastoid (process) (acute) —*see* Mastoiditis, acute
maxilla, maxillary M27.2
sinus (chronic) —*see* Sinusitis, maxillary
nasal sinus (chronic) —*see* Sinusitis
sinus (accessory) (chronic) (nasal) —*see* Sinusitis
sphenoidal (sinus) (chronic) —*see* Sinusitis, sphenoidal
subarachnoid —*see* Abscess, extradural
subdural —*see* Abscess, subdural
tuberculous A15.6
ureter —*see* Ureteritis
ventricular —*see* Abscess, brain
En coup de sabre lesion L94.1
Enamel pearls K00.2
Enameloma K00.2
Enanthema, viral B09
Encephalitis (chronic) (hemorrhagic) (idiopathic) (nonepidemic) (spurious) (subacute) G04.90
acute —*see also* Encephalitis, viral A86
disseminated G04.00
infectious G04.01
noninfectious G04.81
postimmunization (postvaccination) G04.02
postinfectious G04.01
inclusion body A85.8
necrotizing hemorrhagic G04.30
postimmunization G04.32
postinfectious G04.31
specified NEC G04.39
arboviral, arbovirus NEC A85.2
arthropod-borne NEC (viral) A85.2
Australian A83.4
California (virus) A83.5
Central European (tick-borne) A84.1
Czechoslovakian A84.1
Dawson's (inclusion body) A81.1
diffuse sclerosing A81.1
disseminated, acute G04.00
due to
cat scratch disease A28.1
human immunodeficiency virus (HIV) disease B20 *[G05.3]*
malaria —*see* Malaria
rickettsiosis —*see* Rickettsiosis
smallpox inoculation G04.02
typhus —*see* Typhus
Eastern equine A83.2
endemic (viral) A86
epidemic NEC (viral) A86
equine (acute) (infectious) (viral) A83.9
Eastern A83.2
Venezuelan A92.2
Western A83.1
Far Eastern (tick-borne) A84.0
following vaccination or other immunization procedure G04.02
herpes zoster B02.0
herpesviral B00.4
due to herpesvirus 6 B10.01
due to herpesvirus 7 B10.09
specified NEC B10.09
Ilheus (virus) A83.8
in (due to)
actinomycosis A42.82
adenovirus A85.1
African trypanosomiasis B56.9 *[G05.3]*
Chagas' disease (chronic) B57.42
cytomegalovirus B25.8
enterovirus A85.0
herpes (simplex) virus B00.4
due to herpesvirus 6 B10.01
due to herpesvirus 7 B10.09
specified NEC B10.09
infectious disease NEC B99 *[G05.3]*
influenza —*see* Influenza, with, encephalopathy
listeriosis A32.12
measles B05.0
mumps B26.2
naegleriasis B60.2
parasitic disease NEC B89 *[G05.3]*
poliovirus A80.9 *[G05.3]*
rubella B06.01
syphilis
congenital A50.42
late A52.14
systemic lupus erythematosus M32.19
toxoplasmosis (acquired) B58.2
congenital P37.1
tuberculosis A17.82
zoster B02.0

E

Encephalitis *(Continued)*
inclusion body A81.1
infectious (acute) (virus) NEC A86
Japanese (B type) A83.Ø
La Crosse A83.5
lead —*see* Poisoning, lead
lethargica (acute) (infectious) A85.8
louping ill A84.8
lupus erythematosus, systemic M32.19
lymphatica A87.2
Mengo A85.8
meningococcal A39.81
Murray Valley A83.4
otitic NEC H66.4Ø *[GØ5.3]*
parasitic NOS B71.9
periaxial G37.Ø
periaxialis (concentrica) (diffuse) G37.5
postchickenpox BØ1.11
postexanthematous NEC BØ9
postimmunization GØ4.Ø2
postinfectious NEC GØ4.Ø1
postmeasles BØ5.Ø
postvaccinal GØ4.Ø2
postvaricella BØ1.11
postviral NEC A86
Powassan A84.8
Rasmussen GØ4.81
Rio Bravo A85.8
Russian
autumnal A83.Ø
spring-summer (taiga) A84.Ø
saturnine —*see* Poisoning, lead
specified NEC GØ4.81
St. Louis A83.3
subacute sclerosing A81.1
summer A83.Ø
suppurative GØ4.81
tick-borne A84.9
Torula, torular (cryptococcal) B45.1
toxic NEC G92
trichinosis B75 *[GØ5.3]*
type
B A83.Ø
C A83.3
van Bogaert's A81.1
Venezuelan equine A92.2
Vienna A85.8
viral, virus A86
arthropod-borne NEC A85.2
mosquito-borne A83.9
Australian X disease A83.4
California virus A83.5
Eastern equine A83.2
Japanese (B type) A83.Ø
Murray Valley A83.4
specified NEC A83.8
St. Louis A83.3
type B A83.Ø
type C A83.3
Western equine A83.1
tick-borne A84.9
biundulant A84.1
central European A84.1
Czechoslovakian A84.1
diphasic meningoencephalitis A84.1
Far Eastern A84.Ø
Russian spring-summer (taiga) A84.Ø
specified NEC A84.8
specified type NEC A85.8
Western equine A83.1
Encephalocele QØ1.9
frontal QØ1.Ø
nasofrontal QØ1.1
occipital QØ1.2
specified NEC QØ1.8
Encephalocystocele —*see* Encephalocele
Encephaloduroarteriomyosynangiosis (EDAMS) I67.5
Encephalomalacia (brain) (cerebellar) (cerebral) —*see* Softening, brain
Encephalomeningitis —*see* Meningoencephalitis
Encephalomeningocele —*see* Encephalocele
Encephalomeningomyelitis —*see* Meningoencephalitis
Encephalomyelitis —*see also* Encephalitis GØ4.9Ø
acute disseminated GØ4.ØØ
infectious GØ4.Ø1
noninfectious GØ4.81
postimmunization GØ4.Ø2
postinfectious GØ4.Ø1
acute necrotizing hemorrhagic GØ4.3Ø
postimmunization GØ4.32
postinfectious GØ4.31
specified NEC GØ4.39
benign myalgic G93.3
equine A83.9
Eastern A83.2
Venezuelan A92.2
Western A83.1
in diseases classified elsewhere GØ5.3
myalgic, benign G93.3
postchickenpox BØ1.11
postinfectious NEC GØ4.Ø1
postmeasles BØ5.Ø
postvaccinal GØ4.Ø2
postvaricella BØ1.11
rubella BØ6.Ø1
specified NEC GØ4.81
Venezuelan equine A92.2
Encephalomyelocele —*see* Encephalocele
Encephalomyelomeningitis —*see* Meningoencephalitis
Encephalomyelopathy G96.9
Encephalomyeloradiculitis (acute) G61.Ø
Encephalomyeloradiculoneuritis (acute) (Guillain-Barré) G61.Ø
Encephalomyeloradiculopathy G96.9
Encephalopathia hyperbilirubinemica, newborn P57.9
due to isoimmunization (conditions in P55) P57.Ø
Encephalopathy (acute) G93.4Ø
acute necrotizing hemorrhagic GØ4.3Ø
postimmunization GØ4.32
postinfectious GØ4.31
specified NEC GØ4.39
alcoholic G31.2
anoxic —*see* Damage, brain, anoxic
arteriosclerotic I67.2
centrolobar progressive (Schilder) G37.Ø
congenital QØ7.9
degenerative, in specified disease NEC G32.89
due to
drugs (*see also* Table of Drugs and Chemicals) G92
demyelinating callosal G37.1
hepatic —*see* Failure, hepatic
hyperbilirubinemic, newborn P57.9
due to isoimmunization (conditions in P55) P57.Ø
hypertensive I67.4
hypoglycemic E16.2
hypoxic —*see* Damage, brain, anoxic
hypoxic ischemic P91.6Ø
mild P91.61
moderate P91.62
severe P91.63
in (due to) (with)
birth injury P11.1
hyperinsulinism E16.1 *[G94]*
influenza —*see* Influenza, with, encephalopathy
lack of vitamin (*see also* Deficiency, vitamin) E56.9 *[G32.89]*
neoplastic disease (*see also* Neoplasm) D49.9 *[G13.1]*
serum (*see also* Reaction, serum) T8Ø.69
syphilis A52.17
trauma (postconcussional) FØ7.81
current injury —*see* Injury, intracranial
vaccination GØ4.Ø2
Encephalopathy *(Continued)*
lead —*see* Poisoning, lead
metabolic G93.41
drug induced G92
toxic G92
myoclonic, early, symptomatic —*see* Epilepsy, generalized, specified NEC
necrotizing, subacute (Leigh) G31.82
neonatal P91.819
in diseases classified elsewhere P91.811
pellagrous E52 *[G32.89]*
portosystemic —*see* Failure, hepatic
postcontusional FØ7.81
current injury —*see* Injury, intracranial, diffuse
posthypoglycemic (coma) E16.1 *[G94]*
postradiation G93.89
saturnine —*see* Poisoning, lead
septic G93.41
specified NEC G93.49
spongioform, subacute (viral) A81.Ø9
toxic G92
metabolic G92
traumatic (postconcussional) FØ7.81
current injury —*see* Injury, intracranial
vitamin B deficiency NEC E53.9 *[G32.89]*
vitamin B1 E51.2
Wernicke's E51.2
Encephalorrhagia —*see* Hemorrhage, intracranial, intracerebral
Encephalosis, posttraumatic FØ7.81
Enchondroma —*see also* Neoplasm, bone, benign
Enchondromatosis (cartilaginous) (multiple) Q78.4
Encopresis R15.9
functional F98.1
nonorganic origin F98.1
psychogenic F98.1
Encounter (with health service) (for) Z76.89
adjustment and management (of)
breast implant Z45.81
implanted device NEC Z45.89
myringotomy device (stent) (tube) Z45.82
▶neurostimulator (brain) (gastric) (peripheral nerve) (sacral nerve) (spinal cord) (vagus nerve) Z45.42
administrative purpose only ZØ2.9
examination for
adoption ZØ2.82
armed forces ZØ2.3
disability determination ZØ2.71
driving license ZØ2.4
employment ZØ2.1
insurance ZØ2.6
medical certificate NEC ZØ2.79
paternity testing ZØ2.81
residential institution admission ZØ2.2
school admission ZØ2.Ø
sports ZØ2.5
specified reason NEC ZØ2.89
aftercare —*see* Aftercare
antenatal screening Z36.9
cervical length Z36.86
chromosomal anomalies Z36.Ø
congenital cardiac abnormalities Z36.83
elevated maternal serum alphafetoprotein level Z36.1
fetal growth retardation Z36.4
fetal lung maturity Z36.84
fetal macrosomia Z36.88
hydrops fetalis Z36.81
intrauterine growth restriction (IUGR)/small-for-dates Z36.4
isoimmunization Z36.5
large-for-dates Z36.88
malformations Z36.3
non-visualized anatomy on a previous scan Z36.2
nuchal translucency Z36.82

Encounter *(Continued)*
antenatal screening *(Continued)*
raised alphafetoprotein level Z36.1
risk of pre-term labor Z36.86
specified type NEC Z36.89
specified follow-up NEC Z36.2
specified genetic defects NEC Z36.8A
Streptococcus B Z36.85
suspected anomaly Z36.3
uncertain dates Z36.87
assisted reproductive fertility procedure cycle Z31.83
blood typing ZØ1.83
Rh typing ZØ1.83
breast augmentation or reduction Z41.1
breast implant exchange (different material) (different size) Z45.81
breast reconstruction following mastectomy Z42.1
check-up —*see* Examination
chemotherapy for neoplasm Z51.11
colonoscopy, screening Z12.11
counseling —*see* Counseling
delivery, full-term, uncomplicated O8Ø
cesarean, without indication O82
desensitization to allergens Z51.6
ear piercing Z41.3
examination —*see* Examination
expectant parent(s) (adoptive) pre-birth pediatrician visit Z76.81
fertility preservation procedure (prior to cancer therapy) (prior to removal of gonads) Z31.84
fitting (of) —*see* Fitting (and adjustment) (of)
genetic
counseling
nonprocreative Z71.83
procreative Z31.5
testing —*see* Test, genetic
hearing conservation and treatment ZØ1.12
immunotherapy for neoplasm Z51.12
in vitro fertilization cycle Z31.83
instruction (in)
child care (postpartal) (prenatal) Z32.3
childbirth Z32.2
natural family planning
procreative Z31.61
to avoid pregnancy Z3Ø.Ø2
insulin pump titration Z46.81
joint prosthesis insertion following prior explantation of joint prosthesis (staged procedure)
hip Z47.32
knee Z47.33
shoulder Z47.31
laboratory (as part of a general medical examination) ZØØ.ØØ
with abnormal findings ZØØ.Ø1
mental health services (for)
abuse NEC
perpetrator Z69.82
victim Z69.81
child abuse
nonparental
perpetrator Z69.Ø21
victim Z69.Ø2Ø
parental
perpetrator Z69.Ø11
victim Z69.Ø1Ø
child neglect
nonparental
perpetrator Z69.Ø21
victim Z69.Ø2Ø
parental
perpetrator Z69.Ø11
victim Z69.Ø1Ø
child psychological abuse
nonparental
perpetrator Z69.Ø21
victim Z69.Ø2Ø

Encounter *(Continued)*
mental health services *(Continued)*
child psychological abuse *(Continued)*
parental
perpetrator Z69.Ø11
victim Z69.Ø1Ø
child sexual abuse
nonparental
perpetrator Z69.Ø21
victim Z69.Ø2Ø
parental
perpetrator Z69.Ø11
victim Z69.Ø1Ø
non-spousal adult abuse
perpetrator Z69.82
victim Z69.81
spousal or partner
abuse
perpetrator Z69.12
victim Z69.11
neglect
perpetrator Z69.12
victim Z69.11
psychological abuse
perpetrator Z69.12
victim Z69.11
violence
perpetrator (physical) (sexual) Z69.12
victim (physical) Z69.11
sexual Z69.81
observation (for) (ruled out)
exposure to (suspected)
anthrax ZØ3.81Ø
biological agent NEC ZØ3.818
pediatrician visit, by expectant parent(s) (adoptive) Z76.81
placental sample (taken vaginally) —*see also* Encounter, antenatal screening Z36.9
plastic and reconstructive surgery following medical procedure or healed injury NEC Z42.8
pregnancy
supervision of —*see* Pregnancy, supervision of
test Z32.ØØ
result negative Z32.Ø2
result positive Z32.Ø1
procreative management and counseling for gestational carrier Z31.7
prophylactic measures Z29.9
antivenin Z29.12
fluoride administration Z29.3
immunotherapy for respiratory syncytial virus (RSV) Z29.11
rabies immune globin Z29.14
Rho (D) immune globulin Z29.13
specified NEC Z29.8
radiation therapy (antineoplastic) Z51.Ø
radiological (as part of a general medical examination) ZØØ.ØØ
with abnormal findings ZØØ.Ø1
reconstructive surgery following medical procedure or healed injury NEC Z42.8
removal (of) —*see also* Removal
artificial
arm Z44.ØØ- ●
complete Z44.Ø1- ●
partial Z44.Ø2- ●
eye Z44.2- ●
leg Z44.1Ø- ●
complete Z44.11- ●
partial Z44.12- ●
breast implant Z45.81
tissue expander (with or without synchronous insertion of permanent implant) Z45.81
device Z46.9
specified NEC Z46.89
external
fixation device — code to fracture with seventh character D

Encounter *(Continued)*
removal *(Continued)*
external *(Continued)*
prosthesis, prosthetic device Z44.9
breast Z44.3- ●
specified NEC Z44.8
implanted device NEC Z45.89
insulin pump Z46.81
internal fixation device Z47.2
myringotomy device (stent) (tube) Z45.82
nervous system device NEC Z46.2
brain neuropacemaker Z46.2
visual substitution device Z46.2
implanted Z45.31
non-vascular catheter Z46.82
orthodontic device Z46.4
stent
ureteral Z46.6
urinary device Z46.6
repeat cervical smear to confirm findings of recent normal smear following initial abnormal smear ZØ1.42
respirator [ventilator] use during power failure (Z99.12)
Rh typing ZØ1.83
screening —*see* Screening
specified NEC Z76.89
sterilization Z3Ø.2
suspected condition, ruled out
amniotic cavity and membrane ZØ3.71
cervical shortening ZØ3.75
fetal anomaly ZØ3.73
fetal growth ZØ3.74
maternal and fetal conditions NEC ZØ3.79
oligohydramnios ZØ3.71
placental problem ZØ3.72
polyhydramnios ZØ3.71
suspected exposure (to), ruled out
anthrax ZØ3.81Ø
biological agents NEC ZØ3.818
termination of pregnancy, elective Z33.2
testing —*see* Test
therapeutic drug level monitoring Z51.81
titration, insulin pump Z46.81
to determine fetal viability of pregnancy O36.8Ø
training
insulin pump Z46.81
X-ray of chest (as part of a general medical examination) ZØØ.ØØ)
with abnormal findings ZØØ.Ø1
Encystment —*see* Cyst
Endarteritis (bacterial, subacute) (infective) I77.6
brain I67.7
cerebral or cerebrospinal I67.7
deformans —*see* Arteriosclerosis
embolic —*see* Embolism
obliterans —*see also* Arteriosclerosis
pulmonary I28.8
pulmonary I28.8
retina —*see* Vasculitis, retina
senile —*see* Arteriosclerosis
syphilitic A52.Ø9
brain or cerebral A52.Ø4
congenital A5Ø.54 *[I79.8]*
tuberculous A18.89
Endemic —*see* condition
Endocarditis (chronic) (marantic) (nonbacterial) (thrombotic) (valvular) I38
with rheumatic fever (conditions in IØØ)
active —*see* Endocarditis, acute, rheumatic
inactive or quiescent (with chorea) IØ9.1
acute or subacute I33.9
infective I33.Ø
rheumatic (aortic) (mitral) (pulmonary) (tricuspid) IØ1.1
with chorea (acute) (rheumatic) (Sydenham's) IØ2.Ø

Endocarditis *(Continued)*
aortic (heart) (nonrheumatic) (valve) I35.8
with
mitral disease IØ8.Ø
with tricuspid (valve) disease IØ8.3
active or acute IØ1.1
with chorea (acute) (rheumatic) (Sydenham's) IØ2.Ø
rheumatic fever (conditions in IØØ)
active —*see* Endocarditis, acute, rheumatic
inactive or quiescent (with chorea) IØ6.9
tricuspid (valve) disease IØ8.2
with mitral (valve) disease IØ8.3
acute or subacute I33.9
arteriosclerotic I35.8
rheumatic IØ6.9
with mitral disease IØ8.Ø
with tricuspid (valve) disease IØ8.3
active or acute IØ1.1
with chorea (acute) (rheumatic) (Sydenham's) IØ2.Ø
active or acute IØ1.1
with chorea (acute) (rheumatic) (Sydenham's) IØ2.Ø
specified NEC IØ6.8
specified cause NEC I35.8
syphilitic A52.Ø3
arteriosclerotic I38
atypical verrucous (Libman-Sacks) M32.11
bacterial (acute) (any valve) (subacute) I33.Ø
candidal B37.6
congenital Q24.8
constrictive I33.Ø
Coxiella burnetii A78 *[I39]*
Coxsackie B33.21
due to
prosthetic cardiac valve T82.6
Q fever A78 *[I39]*
Serratia marcescens I33.Ø
typhoid (fever) AØ1.Ø2
gonococcal A54.83
infectious or infective (acute) (any valve) (subacute) I33.Ø
lenta (acute) (any valve) (subacute) I33.Ø
Libman-Sacks M32.11
listerial A32.82
Löffler's I42.3
malignant (acute) (any valve) (subacute) I33.Ø
meningococcal A39.51
mitral (chronic) (double) (fibroid) (heart) (inactive) (valve) (with chorea) IØ5.9
with
aortic (valve) disease IØ8.Ø
with tricuspid (valve) disease IØ8.3
active or acute IØ1.1
with chorea (acute) (rheumatic) (Sydenham's) IØ2.Ø
rheumatic fever (conditions in IØØ)
active —*see* Endocarditis, acute, rheumatic
inactive or quiescent (with chorea) IØ5.9
tricuspid (valve) disease IØ8.1
with aortic (valve) disease IØ8.3
active or acute IØ1.1
with chorea (acute) (rheumatic) (Sydenham's) IØ2.Ø
bacterial I33.Ø
arteriosclerotic I34.8
nonrheumatic I34.8
acute or subacute I33.9
specified NEC IØ5.8
monilial B37.6
multiple valves IØ8.9
specified disorders IØ8.8
mycotic (acute) (any valve) (subacute) I33.Ø
pneumococcal (acute) (any valve) (subacute) I33.Ø
pulmonary (chronic) (heart) (valve) I37.8

Endocarditis *(Continued)*
pulmonary *(Continued)*
with rheumatic fever (conditions in IØØ)
active —*see* Endocarditis, acute, rheumatic
inactive or quiescent (with chorea) IØ9.89
with aortic, mitral or tricuspid disease IØ8.8
acute or subacute I33.9
rheumatic IØ1.1
with chorea (acute) (rheumatic) (Sydenham's) IØ2.Ø
arteriosclerotic I37.8
congenital Q22.2
rheumatic (chronic) (inactive) (with chorea) IØ9.89
active or acute IØ1.1
with chorea (acute) (rheumatic) (Sydenham's) IØ2.Ø
syphilitic A52.Ø3
purulent (acute) (any valve) (subacute) I33.Ø
Q fever A78 *[I39]*
rheumatic (chronic) (inactive) (with chorea) IØ9.1
active or acute (aortic) (mitral) (pulmonary) (tricuspid) IØ1.1
with chorea (acute) (rheumatic) (Sydenham's) IØ2.Ø
rheumatoid —*see* Rheumatoid, carditis
septic (acute) (any valve) (subacute) I33.Ø
streptococcal (acute) (any valve) (subacute) I33.Ø
subacute —*see* Endocarditis, acute
suppurative (acute) (any valve) (subacute) I33.Ø
syphilitic A52.Ø3
toxic I33.9
tricuspid (chronic) (heart) (inactive) (rheumatic) (valve) (with chorea) IØ7.9
with
aortic (valve) disease IØ8.2
mitral (valve) disease IØ8.3
mitral (valve) disease IØ8.1
aortic (valve) disease IØ8.3
rheumatic fever (conditions in IØØ)
active —*see* Endocarditis, acute, rheumatic
inactive or quiescent (with chorea) IØ7.8
active or acute IØ1.1
with chorea (acute) (rheumatic) (Sydenham's) IØ2.Ø
arteriosclerotic I36.8
nonrheumatic I36.8
acute or subacute I33.9
specified cause, except rheumatic I36.8
tuberculous —*see* Tuberculosis, endocarditis
typhoid AØ1.Ø2
ulcerative (acute) (any valve) (subacute) I33.Ø
vegetative (acute) (any valve) (subacute) I33.Ø
verrucous (atypical) (nonbacterial) (nonrheumatic) M32.11
Endocardium, endocardial —*see also* condition
cushion defect Q21.2
Endocervicitis —*see also* Cervicitis
due to intrauterine (contraceptive) device T83.69
hyperplastic N72
Endocrine —*see* condition
Endocrinopathy, pluriglandular E31.9
Endodontic
overfill M27.52
underfill M27.53
Endodontitis KØ4.Ø1
irreversible KØ4.Ø2
reversible KØ4.Ø1
Endomastoiditis —*see* Mastoiditis
Endometrioma N8Ø.9
Endometriosis N8Ø.9
appendix N8Ø.5
bladder N8Ø.8

Endometriosis *(Continued)*
bowel N8Ø.5
broad ligament N8Ø.3
cervix N8Ø.Ø
colon N8Ø.5
cul-de-sac (Douglas') N8Ø.3
exocervix N8Ø.Ø
fallopian tube N8Ø.2
female genital organ NEC N8Ø.8
gallbladder N8Ø.8
in scar of skin N8Ø.6
internal N8Ø.Ø
intestine N8Ø.5
lung N8Ø.8
myometrium N8Ø.Ø
ovary N8Ø.1
parametrium N8Ø.3
pelvic peritoneum N8Ø.3
peritoneal (pelvic) N8Ø.3
rectovaginal septum N8Ø.4
rectum N8Ø.5
round ligament N8Ø.3
skin (scar) N8Ø.6
specified site NEC N8Ø.8
stromal D39.Ø
thorax N8Ø.8
umbilicus N8Ø.8
uterus (internal) N8Ø.Ø
vagina N8Ø.4
vulva N8Ø.8
Endometritis (decidual) (nonspecific) (purulent) (senile (atrophic) (suppurative) N71.9
with ectopic pregnancy OØ8.Ø
acute N71.Ø
blenorrhagic (gonococcal) (acute) (chronic) A54.24
cervix, cervical (with erosion or ectropion) —*see also* Cervicitis
hyperplastic N72
chlamydial A56.11
chronic N71.1
following
abortion —*see* Abortion by type complicated by genital infection
ectopic or molar pregnancy OØ8.Ø
gonococcal, gonorrheal (acute) (chronic) A54.24
hyperplastic —*see also* Hyperplasia, endometrial N85.ØØ- ●
cervix N72
puerperal, postpartum, childbirth O86.12
subacute N71.Ø
tuberculous A18.17
Endometrium —*see* condition
Endomyocardiopathy, South African I42.3
Endomyocarditis —*see* Endocarditis
Endomyofibrosis I42.3
Endomyometritis —*see* Endometritis
Endopericarditis —*see* Endocarditis
Endoperineuritis —*see* Disorder, nerve
Endophlebitis —*see* Phlebitis
Endophthalmia —*see* Endophthalmitis, purulent
Endophthalmitis (acute) (infective) (metastatic) (subacute) H44.ØØ9
bleb associated H59.4 —*see also* Bleb, inflammed (infected), postprocedural
gonorrheal A54.39
in (due to)
cysticercosis B69.1
onchocerciasis B73.Ø1
toxocariasis B83.Ø
panuveitis —*see* Panuveitis
parasitic H44.12- ●
purulent H44.ØØ- ●
panophthalmitis —*see* Panophthalmitis
vitreous abscess H44.Ø2- ●
specified NEC H44.19
sympathetic —*see* Uveitis, sympathetic
Endosalpingioma D28.2
Endosalpingiosis N94.89
Endosteitis —*see* Osteomyelitis

Endothelioma, bone —*see* Neoplasm, bone, malignant
Endotheliosis (hemorrhagic infectional) D69.8
Endotoxemia — code to condition
Endotrachelitis —*see* Cervicitis
Engelmann (-Camurati) **syndrome** Q78.3
English disease —*see* Rickets
Engman's disease L30.3
Engorgement
- breast N64.59
  - newborn P83.4
  - puerperal, postpartum O92.79
- lung (passive) —*see* Edema, lung
- pulmonary (passive) —*see* Edema, lung
- stomach K31.89
- venous, retina —*see* Occlusion, retina, vein, engorgement

Enlargement, enlarged —*see also* Hypertrophy
- adenoids J35.2
  - with tonsils J35.3
- alveolar ridge K08.89
  - congenital —*see* Anomaly, alveolar
- apertures of diaphragm (congenital) Q79.1
- gingival K06.1
- heart, cardiac —*see* Hypertrophy, cardiac
- labium majus, childhood asymmetric (CALME) N90.61
- lacrimal gland, chronic H04.03-●
- liver —*see* Hypertrophy, liver
- lymph gland or node R59.9
  - generalized R59.1
  - localized R59.0
- orbit H05.34-●
- organ or site, congenital NEC —*see* Anomaly, by site
- parathyroid (gland) E21.0
- pituitary fossa R93.0
- prostate N40.0
  - with lower urinary tract symptoms (LUTS) N40.1
  - without lower urinary tract symptoms (LUTS) N40.0
- sella turcica R93.0
- spleen —*see* Splenomegaly
- thymus (gland) (congenital) E32.0
- thyroid (gland) —*see* Goiter
- tongue K14.8
- tonsils J35.1
  - with adenoids J35.3
- uterus N85.2
- vestibular aqueduct Q16.5

Enophthalmos H05.40-●
- due to
  - orbital tissue atrophy H05.41-●
  - trauma or surgery H05.42-●

Enostosis M27.8
Entamebic, entamebiasis —*see* Amebiasis
Entanglement
- umbilical cord(s) O69.82
  - with compression O69.2
  - around neck (with compression) O69.81
    - with compression O69.1
    - without compression O69.81
  - of twins in monoamniotic sac O69.2
  - without compression O69.82

Enteralgia —*see* Pain, abdominal
Enteric —*see* condition
Enteritis (acute) (diarrheal) (hemorrhagic) (noninfective) K52.9
- adenovirus A08.2
- aertrycke infection A02.0
- allergic K52.29
  - with
    - eosinophilic gastritis or gastroenteritis K52.81
    - food protein-induced enterocolitis syndrome K52.21
    - food protein-induced enteropathy K52.22
    - FPIES K52.21

Enteritis *(Continued)*
- amebic (acute) A06.0
  - with abscess —*see* Abscess, amebic
  - chronic A06.1
    - with abscess —*see* Abscess, amebic
    - nondysenteric A06.2
  - nondysenteric A06.2
- astrovirus A08.32
- bacillary NOS A03.9
- bacterial A04.9
  - specified NEC A04.8
- calicivirus A08.31
- candidal B37.82
- Chilomastix A07.8
- choleriformis A00.1
- chronic (noninfectious) K52.9
  - ulcerative —*see* Colitis, ulcerative
- cicatrizing (chronic) —*see* Enteritis, regional, small intestine
- Clostridium
  - botulinum (food poisoning) A05.1
  - difficile
    - not specified as recurrent A04.72
    - recurrent A04.71
- coccidial A07.3
- coxsackie virus A08.39
- dietetic —*see also* Enteritis, allergic K52.29
- drug-induced K52.1
- due to
  - astrovirus A08.32
  - calicivirus A08.31
  - coxsackie virus A08.39
  - drugs K52.1
  - echovirus A08.39
  - enterovirus NEC A08.39
  - food hypersensitivity —*see also* Enteritis, allergic K52.29
  - infectious organism (bacterial) (viral) —*see* Enteritis, infectious
  - torovirus A08.39
  - Yersinia enterocolitica A04.6
- echovirus A08.39
- eltor A00.1
- enterovirus NEC A08.39
- eosinophilic K52.81
- epidemic (infectious) A09
- fulminant —*see also* Ischemia, intestine, acute K55.019
- gangrenous —*see* Enteritis, infectious
- giardial A07.1
- infectious NOS A09
  - due to
    - adenovirus A08.2
    - Aerobacter aerogenes A04.8
    - Arizona (bacillus) A02.0
    - bacteria NOS A04.9
      - specified NEC A04.8
    - Campylobacter A04.5
    - Clostridium difficile
      - not specified as recurrent A04.72
      - recurrent A04.71
    - Clostridium perfringens A04.8
    - Enterobacter aerogenes A04.8
    - enterovirus A08.39
    - Escherichia coli A04.4
      - enteroaggregative A04.4
      - enterohemorrhagic A04.3
      - enteroinvasive A04.2
      - enteropathogenic A04.0
      - enterotoxigenic A04.1
      - specified NEC A04.4
    - specified
      - bacteria NEC A04.8
      - virus NEC A08.39
    - Staphylococcus A04.8
    - virus NEC A08.4
      - specified type NEC A08.39
    - Yersinia enterocolitica A04.6
  - specified organism NEC A08.8
- influenzal —*see* Influenza, with, digestive manifestations

Enteritis *(Continued)*
- ischemic K55.9
  - acute —*see also* Ischemia, intestine, acute K55.019
  - chronic K55.1
- microsporidial A07.8
- mucomembranous, myxomembranous —*see* Syndrome, irritable bowel
- mucous —*see* Syndrome, irritable bowel
- necroticans A05.2
- necrotizing of newborn —*see* Enterocolitis, necrotizing, in newborn
- neurogenic —*see* Syndrome, irritable bowel
- newborn necrotizing —*see* Enterocolitis, necrotizing, in newborn
- noninfectious K52.9
- norovirus A08.11
- parasitic NEC B82.9
- paratyphoid (fever) —*see* Fever, paratyphoid
- protozoal A07.9
  - specified NEC A07.8
- radiation K52.0
- regional (of) K50.90
  - with
    - complication K50.919
      - abscess K50.914
      - fistula K50.913
      - intestinal obstruction K50.912
      - rectal bleeding K50.911
      - specified complication NEC K50.918
  - colon —*see* Enteritis, regional, large intestine
  - duodenum —*see* Enteritis, regional, small intestine
  - ileum —*see* Enteritis, regional, small intestine
  - jejunum —*see* Enteritis, regional, small intestine
  - large bowel —*see* Enteritis, regional, large intestine
  - large intestine (colon) (rectum) K50.10
    - with
      - complication K50.119
        - abscess K50.114
        - fistula K50.113
        - intestinal obstruction K50.112
        - rectal bleeding K50.111
        - small intestine (duodenum) (ileum) (jejunum) involvement K50.80
          - with
            - complication K50.819
              - abscess K50.814
              - fistula K50.813
              - intestinal obstruction K50.812
              - rectal bleeding K50.811
              - specified complication NEC K50.818
        - specified complication NEC K50.118
  - rectum —*see* Enteritis, regional, large intestine
  - small intestine (duodenum) (ileum) (jejunum) K50.00
    - with
      - complication K50.019
        - abscess K50.014
        - fistula K50.013
        - intestinal obstruction K50.012
        - large intestine (colon) (rectum) involvement K50.80
          - with
            - complication K50.819
              - abscess K50.814
              - fistula K50.813
              - intestinal obstruction K50.812
              - rectal bleeding K50.811
              - specified complication NEC K50.818
        - rectal bleeding K50.011
        - specified complication NEC K50.018
- rotaviral A08.0

- **Enteritis** *(Continued)*
  - Salmonella, salmonellosis (arizonae) (cholerae-suis) (enteritidis) (typhimurium) A02.0
  - segmental —*see* Enteritis, regional
  - septic A09
  - Shigella —*see* Infection, Shigella
  - small round structured NEC A08.19
  - spasmodic, spastic —*see* Syndrome, irritable bowel
  - staphylococcal A04.8
    - due to food A05.0
  - torovirus A08.39
  - toxic NEC K52.1
    - due to Clostridium difficile
      - not specified as recurrent A04.72
      - recurrent A04.71
  - trichomonal A07.8
  - tuberculous A18.32
  - typhosa A01.00
  - ulcerative (chronic) —*see* Colitis, ulcerative
  - viral A08.4
    - adenovirus A08.2
    - enterovirus A08.39
    - Rotavirus A08.0
    - small round structured NEC A08.19
    - specified NEC A08.39
    - virus specified NEC A08.39
- **Enterobiasis** B80
- **Enterobius vermicularis** (infection) (infestation) B80
- **Enterocele** —*see also* Hernia, abdomen
  - pelvic, pelvis (acquired) (congenital) N81.5
  - vagina, vaginal (acquired) (congenital) NEC N81.5
- **Enterocolitis** —*see also* Enteritis K52.9
  - due to Clostridium difficile
    - not specified as recurrent A04.72
    - recurrent A04.71
  - fulminant ischemic —*see also* Ischemia, intestine, acute K55.059
  - granulomatous —*see* Enteritis, regional
  - hemorrhagic (acute) —*see also* Ischemia, intestine, acute K55.059
    - chronic K55.1
  - infectious NEC A09
  - ischemic K55.9
  - necrotizing K55.30
    - with
      - perforation K55.33
      - pneumatosis K55.32
      - and perforation K55.33
    - due to Clostridium difficile
      - not specified as recurrent A04.72
      - recurrent A04.71
    - in non-newborn K55.30
      - stage 1 (without pneumatosis, without perforation) K55.31
      - stage 2 (with pneumatosis, without perforation) K55.32
      - stage 3 (with pneumatosis, with perforation) K55.33
    - in newborn P77.9
      - stage 1 (without pneumatosis, without perforation) P77.1
      - stage 2 (with pneumatosis, without perforation) P77.2
      - stage 3 (with pneumatosis, with perforation) P77.3
    - without pneumatosis or perforation K55.31
  - noninfectious K52.9
    - newborn —*see* Enterocolitis, necrotizing, in newborn
  - pseudomembranous (newborn)
    - not specified as recurrent A04.72
    - recurrent A04.71
  - radiation K52.0
    - newborn —*see* Enterocolitis, necrotizing, in newborn
  - ulcerative (chronic) —*see* Pancolitis, ulcerative (chronic)
- **Enterogastritis** —*see* Enteritis
- **Enteropathy** K63.9
  - celiac-gluten-sensitive K90.0
    - non-celiac K90.41
  - ➡food protein-induced K52.22
  - hemorrhagic, terminal —*see also* Ischemia, intestine, acute K55.059
  - protein-losing K90.49
- **Enteroperitonitis** —*see* Peritonitis
- **Enteroptosis** K63.4
- **Enterorrhagia** K92.2
- **Enterospasm** —*see also* Syndrome, irritable, bowel
  - psychogenic F45.8
- **Enterostenosis** —*see also* Obstruction, intestine, specified NEC K56.699
- **Enterostomy**
  - complication —*see* Complication, enterostomy
  - status Z93.4
- **Enterovirus, as cause of disease classified elsewhere** B97.10
  - coxsackievirus B97.11
  - echovirus B97.12
  - other specified B97.19
- ➡**Enthesopathy** (peripheral) M77.5-●
  - Achilles tendinitis —*see* Tendinitis, Achilles
  - ankle and tarsus M77.9
    - specified type NEC —*see* Enthesopathy, foot, specified type NEC
  - anterior tibial syndrome M76.81-●
  - calcaneal spur —*see* Spur, bone, calcaneal
  - elbow region M77.8
    - lateral epicondylitis —*see* Epicondylitis, lateral
    - medial epicondylitis —*see* Epicondylitis, medial
  - foot NEC M77.9
    - metatarsalgia —*see* Metatarsalgia
    - specified type NEC M77.5-●
  - forearm M77.9
  - gluteal tendinitis —*see* Tendinitis, gluteal
  - hand M77.9
  - hip —*see* Enthesopathy, lower limb, specified type NEC
  - iliac crest spur —*see* Spur, bone, iliac crest
  - iliotibial band syndrome —*see* Syndrome, iliotibial band
  - knee —*see* Enthesopathy, lower limb, lower leg, specified type NEC
  - lateral epicondylitis —*see* Epicondylitis, lateral
  - lower limb (excluding foot) M76.9
    - Achilles tendinitis —*see* Tendinitis, Achilles
    - ▶ankle and tarsus M77.5- [new]
      - ▶specified type NEC - *see* Enthesopathy, foot, specified type NEC
    - anterior tibial syndrome M76.81-●
    - gluteal tendinitis —*see* Tendinitis, gluteal
    - iliac crest spur —*see* Spur, bone, iliac crest
    - iliotibial band syndrome —*see* Syndrome, iliotibial band
    - patellar tendinitis —*see* Tendinitis, patellar
    - pelvic region —*see* Enthesopathy, lower limb, specified type NEC
    - peroneal tendinitis —*see* Tendinitis, peroneal
    - posterior tibial syndrome M76.82-●
    - psoas tendinitis —*see* Tendinitis, psoas
    - ~~shoulder M77.9~~
    - specified type NEC M76.89-●
    - tibial collateral bursitis —*see* Bursitis, tibial collateral
  - medial epicondylitis —*see* Epicondylitis, medial
  - multiple sites M77.9
  - patellar tendinitis —*see* Tendinitis, patellar
  - pelvis M77.9
  - periarthritis of wrist —*see* Periarthritis, wrist
  - peroneal tendinitis —*see* Tendinitis, peroneal
  - posterior tibial syndrome M76.82-●
  - psoas tendinitis —*see* Tendinitis, psoas
- **Enthesopathy** *(Continued)*
  - ▶shoulder M77.9
  - shoulder region —*see* Lesion, shoulder
  - specified site NEC M77.9
  - specified type NEC M77.8
  - spinal M46.00
    - cervical region M46.02
    - cervicothoracic region M46.03
    - lumbar region M46.06
    - lumbosacral region M46.07
    - multiple sites M46.09
    - occipito-atlanto-axial region M46.01
    - sacrococcygeal region M46.08
    - thoracic region M46.04
    - thoracolumbar region M46.05
  - tibial collateral bursitis —*see* Bursitis, tibial collateral
  - upper arm M77.9
  - wrist and carpus NEC M77.8
    - calcaneal spur —*see* Spur, bone, calcaneal
    - periarthritis of wrist —*see* Periarthritis, wrist
- **Entomophobia** F40.218
- **Entomophthoromycosis** B46.8
- **Entrance, air into vein** —*see* Embolism, air
- **Entrapment, nerve** —*see* Neuropathy, entrapment
- **Entropion** (eyelid) (paralytic) H02.009
  - cicatricial H02.019
    - left H02.016
      - lower H02.015
      - upper H02.014
    - right H02.013
      - lower H02.012
      - upper H02.011
  - congenital Q10.2
  - left H02.006
    - lower H02.005
    - upper H02.004
  - mechanical H02.029
    - left H02.026
      - lower H02.025
      - upper H02.024
    - right H02.023
      - lower H02.022
      - upper H02.021
  - right H02.003
    - lower H02.002
    - upper H02.001
  - senile H02.039
    - left H02.036
      - lower H02.035
      - upper H02.034
    - right H02.033
      - lower H02.032
      - upper H02.031
  - spastic H02.049
    - left H02.046
      - lower H02.045
      - upper H02.044
    - right H02.043
      - lower H02.042
      - upper H02.041
- **Enucleated eye** (traumatic, current) S05.7-●
- **Enuresis** R32
  - functional F98.0
  - habit disturbance F98.0
  - nocturnal N39.44
    - psychogenic F98.0
  - nonorganic origin F98.0
  - psychogenic F98.0
- **Eosinopenia** —*see* Agranulocytosis
- **Eosinophilia** (allergic) (hereditary) (idiopathic) (secondary) D72.1
  - with
    - angiolymphoid hyperplasia (ALHE) D18.01
  - infiltrative J82
  - Löffler's J82
  - peritoneal —*see* Peritonitis, eosinophilic
  - pulmonary NEC J82
  - tropical (pulmonary) J82

E

Eosinophilia-myalgia syndrome M35.8
Ependymitis (acute) (cerebral) (chronic) (granular) —*see* Encephalomyelitis
Ependymoblastoma
specified site —*see* Neoplasm, malignant, by site
unspecified site C71.9
Ependymoma (epithelial) (malignant)
anaplastic
specified site —*see* Neoplasm, malignant, by site
unspecified site C71.9
benign
specified site —*see* Neoplasm, benign, by site
unspecified site D33.2
myxopapillary D43.2
specified site —*see* Neoplasm, uncertain behavior, by site
unspecified site D43.2
papillary D43.2
specified site —*see* Neoplasm, uncertain behavior, by site
unspecified site D43.2
specified site —*see* Neoplasm, malignant, by site
unspecified site C71.9
Ependymopathy G93.89
Ephelis, ephelides L81.2
Epiblepharon (congenital) Q1Ø.3
Epicanthus, epicanthic fold (eyelid) (congenital) Q1Ø.3
Epicondylitis (elbow)
lateral M77.1-●
medial M77.Ø-●
Epicystitis —*see* Cystitis
Epidemic —*see* condition
Epidermidalization, cervix —*see* Dysplasia, cervix
Epidermis, epidermal —*see* condition
Epidermodysplasia verruciformis BØ7.8
Epidermolysis
bullosa (congenital) Q81.9
acquired L12.3Ø
drug-induced L12.31
specified cause NEC L12.35
dystrophica Q81.2
letalis Q81.1
simplex Q81.Ø
specified NEC Q81.8
necroticans combustiformis L51.2
due to drug —*see* Table of Drugs and Chemicals, by drug
Epidermophytid —*see* Dermatophytosis
Epidermophytosis (infected) —*see* Dermatophytosis
Epididymis —*see* condition
Epididymitis (acute) (nonvenereal) (recurrent) (residual) N45.1
with orchitis N45.3
blennorrhagic (gonococcal) A54.23
caseous (tuberculous) A18.15
chlamydial A56.19
filarial —*see also* Infestation, filarial B74.9 *[N51]*
gonococcal A54.23
syphilitic A52.76
tuberculous A18.15
Epididymo-orchitis —*see also* Epididymitis N45.3
Epidural —*see* condition
Epigastrium, epigastric —*see* condition
Epigastrocele —*see* Hernia, ventral
Epiglottis —*see* condition
Epiglottitis, epiglottiditis (acute) JØ5.1Ø
with obstruction JØ5.11
chronic J37.Ø
Epignathus Q89.4
Epilepsia partialis continua —*see also* Kozhevnikof's epilepsy G4Ø.1-●
Epilepsy, epileptic, epilepsia (attack) (cerebral) (convulsion) (fit) (seizure) G4Ø.9Ø9

Note: the following terms are to be considered equivalent to intractable: pharmacoresistant (pharmacologically resistant), treatment resistant, refractory (medically) and poorly controlled

with
complex partial seizures —*see* Epilepsy, localization-related, symptomatic, with complex partial seizures
grand mal seizures on awakening —*see* Epilepsy, generalized, specified NEC
myoclonic absences —*see* Epilepsy, generalized, specified NEC
myoclonic-astatic seizures —*see* Epilepsy, generalized, specified NEC
simple partial seizures —*see* Epilepsy, localization-related, symptomatic, with simple partial seizures
akinetic —*see* Epilepsy, generalized, specified NEC
benign childhood with centrotemporal EEG spikes —*see* Epilepsy, localization-related, idiopathic
benign myoclonic in infancy G4Ø.8Ø-●
Bravais-jacksonian —*see* Epilepsy, localization-related, symptomatic, with simple partial seizures
childhood
with occipital EEG paroxysms —*see* Epilepsy, localization-related, idiopathic
absence G4Ø.AØ9
intractable G4Ø.A19
with status epilepticus G4Ø.A11
without status epilepticus G4Ø.A19
not intractable G4Ø.AØ9
with status epilepticus G4Ø.AØ1
without status epilepticus G4Ø.AØ9
climacteric —*see* Epilepsy, specified NEC
cysticercosis B69.Ø
deterioration (mental) FØ6.8
due to syphilis A52.19
focal —*see* Epilepsy, localization-related, symptomatic, with simple partial seizures
generalized
idiopathic G4Ø.3Ø9
intractable G4Ø.319
with status epilepticus G4Ø.311
without status epilepticus G4Ø.319
not intractable G4Ø.3Ø9
with status epilepticus G4Ø.3Ø1
without status epilepticus G4Ø.3Ø9
specified NEC G4Ø.4Ø9
intractable G4Ø.419
with status epilepticus G4Ø.411
without status epilepticus G4Ø.419
not intractable G4Ø.4Ø9
with status epilepticus G4Ø.4Ø1
without status epilepticus G4Ø.4Ø9
impulsive petit mal —*see* Epilepsy, juvenile myoclonic
intractable G4Ø.919
with status epilepticus G4Ø.911
without status epilepticus G4Ø.919
juvenile absence G4Ø.AØ9
intractable G4Ø.A19
with status epilepticus G4Ø.A11
without status epilepticus G4Ø.A19
not intractable G4Ø.AØ9
with status epilepticus G4Ø.AØ1
without status epilepticus G4Ø.AØ9
juvenile myoclonic G4Ø.B11
intractable G4Ø.B19
with status epilepticus G4Ø.B11
without status epilepticus G4Ø.B19
Epilepsy, epileptic, epilepsia *(Continued)*
juvenile myoclonic *(Continued)*
not intractable G4Ø.BØ9
with status epilepticus G4Ø.BØ1
without status epilepticus G4Ø.BØ9
localization-related (focal) (partial)
idiopathic G4Ø.ØØ9
with seizures of localized onset G4Ø.ØØ9
intractable G4Ø.Ø19
with status epilepticus G4Ø.Ø11
without status epilepticus G4Ø.Ø19
not intractable G4Ø.ØØ9
with status epilepticus G4Ø.ØØ1
without status epilepticus G4Ø.ØØ9
symptomatic
with complex partial seizures G4Ø.2Ø9
intractable G4Ø.219
with status epilepticus G4Ø.211
without status epilepticus G4Ø.219
not intractable G4Ø.2Ø9
with status epilepticus G4Ø.2Ø1
without status epilepticus G4Ø.2Ø9
with simple partial seizures G4Ø.1Ø9
intractable G4Ø.119
with status epilepticus G4Ø.111
without status epilepticus G4Ø.119
not intractable G4Ø.1Ø9
with status epilepticus G4Ø.1Ø1
without status epilepticus G4Ø.1Ø9
myoclonus, myoclonic —*see* Epilepsy, generalized, specified NEC
progressive —*see* Epilepsy, generalized, idiopathic
not intractable G4Ø.9Ø9
with status epilepticus G4Ø.9Ø1
without status epilepticus G4Ø.9Ø9
on awakening —*see* Epilepsy, generalized, specified NEC
parasitic NOS B71.9 *[G94]*
partialis continua —*see also* Kozhevnikof's epilepsy G4Ø.1-●
peripheral —*see* Epilepsy, specified NEC
procursiva —*see* Epilepsy, localization-related, symptomatic, with simple partial seizures
progressive (familial) myoclonic —*see* Epilepsy, generalized, idiopathic
reflex —*see* Epilepsy, specified NEC
related to
alcohol G4Ø.5Ø9
not intractable G4Ø.5Ø9
with status epilepticus G4Ø.5Ø1
without status eplilepticus G4Ø.5Ø9
drugs G4Ø.5Ø9
not intractable G4Ø.5Ø9
with status epilepticus G4Ø.5Ø1
without status eplilepticus G4Ø.5Ø9
external causes G4Ø.5Ø9
not intractable G4Ø.5Ø9
with status epilepticus G4Ø.5Ø1
without status epilepticus G4Ø.5Ø9
hormonal changes G4Ø.5Ø9
not intractable G4Ø.5Ø9
with status epilepticus G4Ø.5Ø1
without status eplilepticus G4Ø.5Ø9
sleep deprivation G4Ø.5Ø9
not intractable G4Ø.5Ø9
with status epilepticus G4Ø.5Ø1
without status eplilepticus G4Ø.5Ø9
stress G4Ø.5Ø9
not intractable G4Ø.5Ø9
with status epilepticus G4Ø.5Ø1
without status eplilepticus G4Ø.5Ø9
somatomotor —*see* Epilepsy, localization-related, symptomatic, with simple partial seizures
somatosensory —*see* Epilepsy, localization-related, symptomatic, with simple partial seizures

E

Epilepsy, epileptic, epilepsia *(Continued)*
  spasms G4Ø.822
    intractable G4Ø.824
      with status epilepticus G4Ø.823
      without status epilepticus G4Ø.824
    not intractable G4Ø.822
      with status epilepticus G4Ø.821
      without status epilepticus G4Ø.822
  specified NEC G4Ø.8Ø2
    intractable G4Ø.8Ø4
      with status epilepticus G4Ø.8Ø3
      without status epilepticus G4Ø.8Ø4
    not intractable G4Ø.8Ø2
      with status epilepticus G4Ø.8Ø1
      without status epilepticus G4Ø.8Ø2
  syndromes
    generalized
      idiopathic G4Ø.3Ø9
        intractable G4Ø.319
          with status epilepticus G4Ø.311
          without status epilepticus G4Ø.319
        not intractable G4Ø.3Ø9
          with status epilepticus G4Ø.3Ø1
          without status epilepticus G4Ø.3Ø9
      specified NEC G4Ø.4Ø9
        intractable G4Ø.419
          with status epilepticus G4Ø.411
          without status epilepticus G4Ø.419
        not intractable G4Ø.4Ø9
          with status epilepticus G4Ø.4Ø1
          without status epilepticus G4Ø.4Ø9
    localization-related (focal) (partial)
      idiopathic G4Ø.ØØ9
        with seizures of localized onset G4Ø.ØØ9
          intractable G4Ø.Ø19
            with status epilepticus G4Ø.Ø11
            without status epilepticus G4Ø.Ø19
          not intractable G4Ø.ØØ9
            with status epilepticus G4Ø.ØØ1
            without status epilepticus G4Ø.ØØ9
      symptomatic
        with complex partial seizures G4Ø.2Ø9
          intractable G4Ø.219
            with status epilepticus G4Ø.211
            without status epilepticus G4Ø.219
          not intractable G4Ø.2Ø9
            with status epilepticus G4Ø.2Ø1
            without status epilepticus G4Ø.2Ø9
        with simple partial seizures G4Ø.1Ø9
          intractable G4Ø.119
            with status epilepticus G4Ø.111
            without status epilepticus G4Ø.119
          not intractable G4Ø.1Ø9
            with status epilepticus G4Ø.1Ø1
            without status epilepticus G4Ø.1Ø9
    specified NEC G4Ø.8Ø2
      intractable G4Ø.8Ø4
        with status epilepticus G4Ø.8Ø3
        without status epilepticus G4Ø.8Ø4
      not intractable G4Ø.8Ø2
        with status epilepticus G4Ø.8Ø1
        without status epilepticus G4Ø.8Ø2
  tonic (-clonic) —*see* Epilepsy, generalized, specified NEC
  twilight FØ5
  uncinate (gyrus) —*see* Epilepsy, localization-related, symptomatic, with complex partial seizures
  Unverricht (-Lundborg) (familial myoclonic) —*see* Epilepsy, generalized, idiopathic
  visceral —*see* Epilepsy, specified NEC
  visual —*see* Epilepsy, specified NEC
Epiloia Q85.1
Epimenorrhea N92.Ø
Epipharyngitis —*see* Nasopharyngitis
Epiphora HØ4.2Ø- ●
  due to
    excess lacrimation HØ4.21- ●
    insufficient drainage HØ4.22- ●
Epiphyseal arrest —*see* Arrest, epiphyseal
Epiphyseolysis, epiphysiolysis —*see* Osteochondropathy
Epiphysitis —*see also* Osteochondropathy
  juvenile M92.9
  syphilitic (congenital) A5Ø.Ø2
Epiplocele —*see* Hernia, abdomen
Epiploitis —*see* Peritonitis
Epiplosarcomphalocele —*see* Hernia, umbilicus
Episcleritis (suppurative) H15.1Ø- ●
  in (due to)
    syphilis A52.71
    tuberculosis A18.51
  nodular H15.12- ●
  periodica fugax H15.11- ●
    angioneurotic —*see* Edema, angioneurotic
  syphilitic (late) A52.71
  tuberculous A18.51
Episode
  affective, mixed F39
  depersonalization (in neurotic state) F48.1
  depressive F32.9
    major F32.9
      mild F32.Ø
      moderate F32.1
      severe (without psychotic symptoms) F32.2
        with psychotic symptoms F32.3
    recurrent F33.9
      brief F33.8
    specified NEC F32.89
  hypomanic F3Ø.8
  manic F3Ø.9
    with
      psychotic symptoms F3Ø.2
      remission (full) F3Ø.4
        partial F3Ø.3
    without psychotic symptoms F3Ø.1Ø
      mild F3Ø.11
      moderate F3Ø.12
      severe (without psychotic symptoms) F3Ø.13
        with psychotic symptoms F3Ø.2
    other specified F3Ø.8
    recurrent F31.89
  psychotic F23
    organic FØ6.8
  schizophrenic (acute) NEC, brief F23
Epispadias (female) (male) Q64.Ø
Episplenitis D73.89
Epistaxis (multiple) RØ4.Ø
  hereditary I78.Ø
  vicarious menstruation N94.89
Epithelioma (malignant) —*see also* Neoplasm, malignant, by site
  adenoides cysticum —*see* Neoplasm, skin, benign
  basal cell —*see* Neoplasm, skin, malignant
  benign —*see* Neoplasm, benign, by site
  Bowen's —*see* Neoplasm, skin, in situ
  calcifying, of Malherbe —*see* Neoplasm, skin, benign
  external site —*see* Neoplasm, skin, malignant
  intraepidermal, Jadassohn —*see* Neoplasm, skin, benign
  squamous cell —*see* Neoplasm, malignant, by site
Epitheliomatosis pigmented Q82.1
Epitheliopathy, multifocal placoid pigment H3Ø.14- ●
Epithelium, epithelial —*see* condition
Epituberculosis (with atelectasis) (allergic) A15.7
Eponychia Q84.6
Epstein's
  nephrosis or syndrome —*see* Nephrosis
  pearl KØ9.8
Epulis (gingiva) (fibrous) (giant cell) KØ6.8
Equinia A24.Ø
➠ **Equinovarus** (congenital) (talipes) Q66.Ø- ●
  acquired —*see* Deformity, limb, clubfoot
Equivalent
  convulsive (abdominal) —*see* Epilepsy, specified NEC
  epileptic (psychic) —*see* Epilepsy, localization-related, symptomatic, with complex partial seizures
Erb (-Duchenne) paralysis (birth injury) (newborn) P14.Ø
Erb's
  disease G71.Ø2
  palsy, paralysis (brachial) (birth) (newborn) P14.Ø
    spinal (spastic) syphilitic A52.17
  pseudohypertrophic muscular dystrophy G71.Ø2
Erb-Goldflam disease or syndrome G7Ø.ØØ
  with exacerbation (acute) G7Ø.Ø1
  in crisis G7Ø.Ø1
Erdheim's syndrome (acromegalic macrospondylitis) E22.Ø
Erection, painful (persistent) —*see* Priapism
Ergosterol deficiency (vitamin D) E55.9
  with
    adult osteomalacia M83.8
    rickets —*see* Rickets
Ergotism —*see also* Poisoning, food, noxious, plant
  from ergot used as drug (migraine therapy) —*see* Table of Drugs and Chemicals
Erosio interdigitalis blastomycetica B37.2
Erosion
  artery I77.2
    without rupture I77.89
  bone —*see* Disorder, bone, density and structure, specified NEC
  bronchus J98.Ø9
  cartilage (joint) —*see* Disorder, cartilage, specified type NEC
  cervix (uteri) (acquired) (chronic) (congenital) N86
    with cervicitis N72
  cornea (nontraumatic) —*see* Ulcer, cornea
    recurrent H18.83- ●
    traumatic —*see* Abrasion, cornea
  dental (idiopathic) (occupational) (due to diet, drugs or vomiting) KØ3.2
  duodenum, postpyloric —*see* Ulcer, duodenum
  esophagus K22.1Ø
    with bleeding K22.11
  gastric —*see* Ulcer, stomach
  gastrojejunal —*see* Ulcer, gastrojejunal
➠ implanted mesh —*see* Complications, prosthetic devise or implant, mesh
  intestine K63.3
  lymphatic vessel I89.8
  pylorus, pyloric (ulcer) —*see* Ulcer, stomach
  spine, aneurysmal A52.Ø9
  stomach —*see* Ulcer, stomach
  subcutaneous device pocket
    nervous system prosthetic device, implant, or graft T85.89Ø
    other internal prosthetic device, implant, or graft T85.898
  teeth (idiopathic) (occupational) (due to diet, drugs or vomiting) KØ3.2
  urethra N36.8
  uterus N85.8
Erotomania F52.8
Error
  metabolism, inborn —*see* Disorder, metabolism
  refractive —*see* Disorder, refraction
Eructation R14.2
  nervous or psychogenic F45.8
Eruption
  creeping B76.9
  drug (generalized) (taken internally) L27.Ø
    fixed L27.1
    in contact with skin —*see* Dermatitis, due to drugs
    localized L27.1

- Eruption *(Continued)*
  - Hutchinson, summer L56.4
  - Kaposi's varicelliform BØØ.Ø
  - napkin L22
  - polymorphous light (sun) L56.4
  - recalcitrant pustular L13.8
  - ringed R23.8
  - skin (nonspecific) R21
    - creeping (meaning hookworm) B76.9
    - due to inoculation/vaccination (generalized) —*see also* Dermatitis, due to, vaccine L27.Ø
      - localized L27.1
    - erysipeloid A26.Ø
    - feigned L98.1
    - Kaposi's varicelliform BØØ.Ø
    - lichenoid L28.Ø
    - meaning dermatitis —*see* Dermatitis
    - toxic NEC L53.Ø
  - tooth, teeth, abnormal (incomplete) (late) (premature) (sequence) KØØ.6
  - vesicular R23.8
- Erysipelas (gangrenous) (infantile) (newborn) (phlegmonous) (suppurative) A46
  - external ear A46 *[H62.4Ø]*
  - puerperal, postpartum O86.89
- Erysipeloid A26.9
  - cutaneous (Rosenbach's) A26.Ø
  - disseminated A26.8
  - sepsis A26.7
  - specified NEC A26.8
- Erythema, erythematous (infectional) (inflammation) L53.9
  - ab igne L59.Ø
  - annulare (centrifugum) (rheumaticum) L53.1
  - arthriticum epidemicum A25.1
  - brucellum —*see* Brucellosis
  - chronic figurate NEC L53.3
  - chronicum migrans (Borrelia burgdorferi) A69.2Ø
  - diaper L22
  - due to
    - chemical NEC L53.Ø
      - in contact with skin L24.5
    - drug (internal use) —*see* Dermatitis, due to, drugs
  - elevatum diutinum L95.1
  - endemic E52
  - epidemic, arthritic A25.1
  - figuratum perstans L53.3
  - gluteal L22
  - heat - code by site under Burn, first degree
  - ichthyosiforme congenitum bullous Q8Ø.3
  - in diseases classified elsewhere L54
  - induratum (nontuberculous) L52
    - tuberculous A18.4
  - infectiosum BØ8.3
  - intertrigo L3Ø.4
  - iris L51.9
  - marginatum L53.2
    - in (due to) acute rheumatic fever IØØ
  - medicamentosum —*see* Dermatitis, due to, drugs
  - migrans A26.Ø
    - chronicum A69.2Ø
    - tongue K14.1
  - multiforme (major) (minor) L51.9
    - bullous, bullosum L51.1
    - conjunctiva L51.1
    - nonbullous L51.Ø
    - pemphigoides L12.Ø
    - specified NEC L51.8
  - napkin L22
  - neonatorum P83.88
    - toxic P83.1
  - nodosum L52
    - tuberculous A18.4
  - palmar L53.8
  - pernio T69.1
  - rash, newborn P83.88
  - scarlatiniform (recurrent) (exfoliative) L53.8
- Erythema, erythematous *(Continued)*
  - solare L55.Ø
  - specified NEC L53.8
  - toxic, toxicum NEC L53.Ø
    - newborn P83.1
  - tuberculous (primary) A18.4
- Erythematous, erythematosus —*see* condition
- Erythermalgia (primary) I73.81
- Erythralgia I73.81
- Erythrasma LØ8.1
- Erythredema (polyneuropathy) —*see* Poisoning, mercury
- Erythremia (acute) C94.Ø-●
  - chronic D45
  - secondary D75.1
- Erythroblastopenia —*see also* Aplasia, red cell D6Ø.9
  - congenital D61.Ø1
- Erythroblastophthisis D61.Ø9
- Erythroblastosis (fetalis) (newborn) P55.9
  - due to
    - ABO (antibodies) (incompatibility) (isoimmunization) P55.1
    - Rh (antibodies) (incompatibility) (isoimmunization) P55.Ø
- Erythrocyanosis (crurum) I73.89
- Erythrocythemia —*see* Erythremia
- Erythrocytosis (megalosplenic) (secondary) D75.1
  - familial D75.Ø
  - oval, hereditary —*see* Elliptocytosis
  - secondary D75.1
  - stress D75.1
- Erythroderma (secondary) —*see also* Erythema L53.9
  - bullous ichthyosiform, congenital Q8Ø.3
  - desquamativum L21.1
  - ichthyosiform, congenital (bullous) Q8Ø.3
  - neonatorum P83.88
  - psoriaticum L4Ø.8
- Erythrodysesthesia, palmar plantar (PPE) L27.1
- Erythrogenesis imperfecta D61.Ø9
- Erythroleukemia C94.Ø-●
- Erythromelalgia I73.81
- Erythrophagocytosis D75.89
- Erythrophobia F4Ø.298
- Erythroplakia, oral epithelium, and tongue K13.29
- Erythroplasia (Queyrat) DØ7.4
  - specified site —*see* Neoplasm, skin, in situ
  - unspecified site DØ7.4
- Escherichia coli (E. coli), as cause of disease classified elsewhere B96.2Ø
  - non-O157 Shiga toxin-producing (with known O group) B96.22
  - non-Shiga toxin-producing B96.29
  - O157 with confirmation of Shiga toxin when H antigen is unknown, or is not H7 B96.21
  - O157:H- (nonmotile) with confirmation of Shiga toxin B96.21
  - O157:H7 with or without confirmation of Shiga toxin-production B96.21
  - Shiga toxin-producing (with unspecified O group) (STEC) B96.23
  - O157 B96.21
  - O157:H7 with or without confirmation of Shiga toxin-production B96.21
    - specified NEC B96.22
  - specified NEC B96.29
- Esophagismus K22.4
- Esophagitis (acute) (alkaline) (chemical) (chronic) (infectional) (necrotic) (peptic) (postoperative) K2Ø.9
  - candidal B37.81
  - due to gastrointestinal reflux disease K21.Ø
  - eosinophilic K2Ø.Ø
  - reflux K21.Ø
  - specified NEC K2Ø.8
  - tuberculous A18.83
  - ulcerative K22.1Ø
    - with bleeding K22.11
- Esophagocele K22.5
- Esophagomalacia K22.8
- Esophagospasm K22.4
- Esophagostenosis K22.2
- Esophagostomiasis B81.8
- Esophagotracheal —*see* condition
- Esophagus —*see* condition
- Esophoria H5Ø.51
  - convergence, excess H51.12
  - divergence, insufficiency H51.8
- Esotropia —*see* Strabismus, convergent concomitant
- Espundia B55.2
- Essential —*see* condition
- Esthesioneuroblastoma C3Ø.Ø
- Esthesioneurocytoma C3Ø.Ø
- Esthesioneuroepithelioma C3Ø.Ø
- Esthiomene A55
- Estivo-autumnal malaria (fever) B5Ø.9
- Estrangement (marital) Z63.5
  - parent-child NEC Z62.89Ø
- Estriasis —*see* Myiasis
- Ethanolism —*see* Alcoholism
- Etherism —*see* Dependence, drug, inhalant
- Ethmoid, ethmoidal —*see* condition
- Ethmoiditis (chronic) (nonpurulent) (purulent) —*see also* Sinusitis, ethmoidal
  - influenzal —*see* Influenza, with, respiratory manifestations NEC
  - Woakes' J33.1
- Ethylism —*see* Alcoholism
- Eulenburg's disease (congenital paramyotonia) G71.19
- Eumycetoma B47.Ø
- Eunuchoidism E29.1
  - hypogonadotropic E23.Ø
- European blastomycosis —*see* Cryptococcosis
- Eustachian —*see* condition
- Evaluation (for) (of)
  - development state
    - adolescent ZØØ.3
    - period of
      - delayed growth in childhood ZØØ.7Ø
        - with abnormal findings ZØØ.71
      - rapid growth in childhood ZØØ.2
    - puberty ZØØ.3
  - growth and developmental state (period of rapid growth) ZØØ.2
    - delayed growth ZØØ.7Ø
      - with abnormal findings ZØØ.71
  - mental health (status) ZØØ.8
    - requested by authority ZØ4.6
  - period of
    - delayed growth in childhood ZØØ.7Ø
      - with abnormal findings ZØØ.71
    - rapid growth in childhood ZØØ.2
  - suspected condition —*see* Observation
- Evans syndrome D69.41
- Event
  - apparent life threatening in newborn and infant (ALTE) R68.13
  - brief resolved unexplained event (BRUE) R68.13
- Eventration —*see also* Hernia, ventral
  - colon into chest —*see* Hernia, diaphragm
  - diaphragm (congenital) Q79.1
- Eversion
  - bladder N32.89
  - cervix (uteri) N86
    - with cervicitis N72
  - foot NEC —*see also* Deformity, valgus, ankle
    - congenital Q66.6
  - punctum lacrimale (postinfectional) (senile) HØ4.52-●
  - ureter (meatus) N28.89
  - urethra (meatus) N36.8
  - uterus N81.4
- Evidence
  - cytologic
    - of malignancy on anal smear R85.614
    - of malignancy on cervical smear R87.614
    - of malignancy on vaginal smear R87.624

Evisceration
  birth injury P15.8
  traumatic NEC
    eye —*see* Enucleated eye
Evulsion —*see* Avulsion
Ewing's sarcoma or tumor —*see* Neoplasm, bone, malignant
Examination (for) (following) (general) (of) (routine) ZØØ.ØØ
  with abnormal findings ZØØ.Ø1
  abuse, physical (alleged), ruled out
    adult ZØ4.71
    child ZØ4.72
  adolescent (development state) ZØØ.3
  alleged rape or sexual assault (victim), ruled out
    adult ZØ4.41
    child ZØ4.42
  allergy ZØ1.82
  annual (adult) (periodic) (physical) ZØØ.ØØ
    with abnormal findings ZØØ.Ø1
    gynecological ZØ1.419
      with abnormal findings ZØ1.411
  antibody response ZØ1.84
  blood —*see* Examination, laboratory
  blood pressure ZØ1.3Ø
    with abnormal findings ZØ1.31
  cancer staging —*see* Neoplasm, malignant, by site
  cervical Papanicolaou smear Z12.4
    as part of routine gynecological examination ZØ1.419
      with abnormal findings ZØ1.411
  child (over 28 days old) ZØØ.129
    with abnormal findings ZØØ.121
    under 28 days old —*see* Newborn, examination
  clinical research control or normal comparison (control) (participant) ZØØ.6
  contraceptive (drug) maintenance (routine) Z3Ø.8
    device (intrauterine) Z3Ø.431
  dental ZØ1.2Ø
    with abnormal findings ZØ1.21
  developmental —*see* Examination, child
  donor (potential) ZØØ.5
  ear ZØ1.1Ø
    with abnormal findings NEC ZØ1.118
  eye ZØ1.ØØ
    with abnormal findings ZØ1.Ø1
    ▶following failed vision screening ZØ1.Ø2Ø
      ▶with abnormal findings ZØ1.Ø21
  following
    accident NEC ZØ4.3
      transport ZØ4.1
      work ZØ4.2
    assault, alleged, ruled out
      adult ZØ4.71
      child ZØ4.72
    motor vehicle accident ZØ4.1
    treatment (for) ZØ9
      combined NEC ZØ9
        fracture ZØ9
        malignant neoplasm ZØ8
      malignant neoplasm ZØ8
      mental disorder ZØ9
      specified condition NEC ZØ9
  follow-up (routine) (following) ZØ9
    chemotherapy NEC ZØ9
      malignant neoplasm ZØ8
    fracture ZØ9
    malignant neoplasm ZØ8
    postpartum Z39.2
    psychotherapy ZØ9
    radiotherapy NEC ZØ9
      malignant neoplasm ZØ8
    surgery NEC ZØ9
      malignant neoplasm ZØ8
  forced sexual exploitation ZØ4.81
  forced labor exploitation ZØ4.82
Examination (*Continued*)
  gynecological ZØ1.419
    with abnormal findings ZØ1.411
    for contraceptive maintenance Z3Ø.8
  health —*see* Examination, medical
  hearing ZØ1.1Ø
    with abnormal findings NEC ZØ1.118
    infant or child (over 28 days old) ZØØ.129
      with abnormal findings ZØØ.121
    following failed hearing screening ZØ1.11Ø
  immunity status testing ZØ1.84
  laboratory (as part of a general medical examination) ZØØ.ØØ
    with abnormal findings ZØØ.Ø1
    preprocedural ZØ1.812
  lactating mother Z39.1
  medical (adult) (for) (of) ZØØ.ØØ
    with abnormal findings ZØØ.Ø1
    administrative purpose only ZØ2.9
      specified NEC ZØ2.89
    admission to
      armed forces ZØ2.3
      old age home ZØ2.2
      prison ZØ2.89
      residential institution ZØ2.2
      school ZØ2.Ø
        following illness or medical treatment ZØ2.Ø
      summer camp ZØ2.89
    adoption ZØ2.82
    blood alcohol or drug level ZØ2.83
    camp (summer) ZØ2.89
    clinical research, normal subject (control) (participant) ZØØ.6
    control subject in clinical research (normal comparison) (participant) ZØØ.6
    donor (potential) ZØØ.5
    driving license ZØ2.4
    general (adult) ZØØ.ØØ
      with abnormal findings ZØØ.Ø1
    immigration ZØ2.89
    insurance purposes ZØ2.6
    marriage ZØ2.89
    medicolegal reasons NEC ZØ4.89
    naturalization ZØ2.89
    participation in sport ZØ2.5
    paternity testing ZØ2.81
    population survey ZØØ.8
    pre-employment ZØ2.1
    pre-operative —*see* Examination, pre-procedural
    pre-procedural
      cardiovascular ZØ1.81Ø
      respiratory ZØ1.811
      specified NEC ZØ1.818
    preschool children
      for admission to school ZØ2.Ø
    prisoners
      for entrance into prison ZØ2.89
    recruitment for armed forces ZØ2.3
    specified NEC ZØØ.8
    sport competition ZØ2.5
  medicolegal reason NEC ZØ4.89
    forced sexual exploitation ZØ4.81
    forced labor exploitation ZØ4.82
  newborn —*see* Newborn, examination
  pelvic (annual) (periodic) ZØ1.419
    with abnormal findings ZØ1.411
  period of rapid growth in childhood ZØØ.2
  periodic (adult) (annual) (routine) ZØØ.ØØ
    with abnormal findings ZØØ.Ø1
  physical (adult) —*see also* Examination, medical ZØØ.ØØ
    sports ZØ2.5
  postpartum
    immediately after delivery Z39.Ø
    routine follow-up Z39.2
  pre-chemotherapy (antineoplastic) ZØ1.818
  prenatal (normal pregnancy) —*see also* Pregnancy, normal Z34.9-●
Examination (*Continued*)
  pre-procedural (pre-operative)
    cardiovascular ZØ1.81Ø
    laboratory ZØ1.812
    respiratory ZØ1.811
    specified NEC ZØ1.818
  prior to chemotherapy (antineoplastic) ZØ1.818
  psychiatric NEC ZØØ.8
    follow-up not needing further care ZØ9
    requested by authority ZØ4.6
  radiological (as part of a general medical examination) ZØØ.ØØ
    with abnormal findings ZØØ.Ø1
  repeat cervical smear to confirm findings of recent normal smear following initial abnormal smear ZØ1.42
  skin (hypersensitivity) ZØ1.82
  special —*see also* Examination, by type ZØ1.89
    specified type NEC ZØ1.89
  specified type or reason NEC ZØ4.89
  teeth ZØ1.2Ø
    with abnormal findings ZØ1.21
  urine —*see* Examination, laboratory
  vision ZØ1.ØØ
    with abnormal findings ZØ1.Ø1
    ▶following failed vision screening ZØ1.Ø2Ø
      ▶with abnormal findings ZØ1.Ø21
    infant or child (over 28 days old) ZØØ.129
      with abnormal findings ZØØ.121
Exanthem, exanthema —*see also* Rash
  with enteroviral vesicular stomatitis BØ8.4
  Boston A88.Ø
  epidemic with meningitis A88.Ø *[GØ2]*
  subitum BØ8.2Ø
    due to human herpesvirus 6 BØ8.21
    due to human herpesvirus 7 BØ8.22
  viral, virus BØ9
    specified type NEC BØ8.8
Excess, excessive, excessively
  alcohol level in blood R78.Ø
  androgen (ovarian) E28.1
  attrition, tooth, teeth KØ3.Ø
  carotene, carotin (dietary) E67.1
  cold, effects of T69.9
    specified effect NEC T69.8
  convergence H51.12
  crying
    in child, adolescent, or adult R45.83
    in infant R68.11
  development, breast N62
  divergence H51.8
  drinking (alcohol) NEC (without dependence) F1Ø.1Ø
    habitual (continual) (without remission) F1Ø.2Ø
  eating R63.2
  estrogen E28.Ø
  fat —*see also* Obesity
    in heart —*see* Degeneration, myocardial
    localized E65
  foreskin N47.8
  gas R14.Ø
  glucagon E16.3
  heat —*see* Heat
  intermaxillary vertical dimension of fully erupted teeth M26.37
  interocclusal distance of fully erupted teeth M26.37
  kalium E87.5
  large
    colon K59.39
      congenital Q43.8
    infant PØ8.Ø
    organ or site, congenital NEC —*see* Anomaly, by site
  long
    organ or site, congenital NEC —*see* Anomaly, by site
  menstruation (with regular cycle) N92.Ø
    with irregular cycle N92.1
  napping Z72.821
  natrium E87.Ø

Excess, excessive, excessively *(Continued)*
number of teeth KØØ.1
nutrient (dietary) NEC R63.2
potassium (K) E87.5
salivation K11.7
secretion —*see also* Hypersecretion
milk O92.6
sputum RØ9.3
sweat R61
sexual drive F52.8
short
organ or site, congenital NEC —*see* Anomaly, by site
umbilical cord in labor or delivery O69.3
skin L98.7
and subcutaneous tissue L98.7
eyelid (acquired) —*see* Blepharochalasis
congenital Q1Ø.3
sodium (Na) E87.Ø
spacing of fully erupted teeth M26.32
sputum RØ9.3
sweating R61
thirst R63.1
due to deprivation of water T73.1
tuberosity of jaw M26.Ø7
vitamin
A (dietary) E67.Ø
administered as drug (prolonged intake) —*see* Table of Drugs and Chemicals, vitamins, adverse effect
overdose or wrong substance given or taken —*see* Table of Drugs and Chemicals, vitamins, poisoning
D (dietary) E67.3
administered as drug (prolonged intake) —*see* Table of Drugs and Chemicals, vitamins, adverse effect
overdose or wrong substance given or taken —*see* Table of Drugs and Chemicals, vitamins, poisoning
weight
gain R63.5
loss R63.4
Excitability, abnormal, under minor stress (personality disorder) F6Ø.3
Excitation
anomalous atrioventricular I45.6
psychogenic F3Ø.8
reactive (from emotional stress, psychological trauma) F3Ø.8
Excitement
hypomanic F3Ø.8
manic F3Ø.9
mental, reactive (from emotional stress, psychological trauma) F3Ø.8
state, reactive (from emotional stress, psychological trauma) F3Ø.8
Excoriation (traumatic) —*see also* Abrasion
neurotic L98.1
skin picking disorder F42.4
Exfoliation
due to erythematous conditions according to extent of body surface involved L49.Ø
1Ø-19 percent of body surface L49.1
2Ø-29 percent of body surface L49.2
3Ø-39 percent of body surface L49.3
4Ø-49 percent of body surface L49.4
5Ø-59 percent of body surface L49.5
6Ø-69 percent of body surface L49.6
7Ø-79 percent of body surface L49.7
8Ø-89 percent of body surface L49.8
9Ø-99 percent of body surface L49.9
less than 1Ø percent of body surface L49.Ø
teeth, due to systemic causes KØ8.Ø
Exfoliative —*see* condition
Exhaustion, exhaustive (physical NEC) R53.83
battle F43.Ø
cardiac —*see* Failure, heart
delirium F43.Ø
Exhaustion, exhaustive *(Continued)*
due to
cold T69.8
excessive exertion T73.3
exposure T73.2
neurasthenia F48.8
heart —*see* Failure, heart
heat —*see also* Heat, exhaustion T67.5
due to
salt depletion T67.4
water depletion T67.3
maternal, complicating delivery O75.81
mental F48.8
myocardium, myocardial —*see* Failure, heart
nervous F48.8
old age R54
psychogenic F48.8
psychosis F43.Ø
senile R54
vital NEC Z73.Ø
Exhibitionism F65.2
Exocervicitis —*see* Cervicitis
Exomphalos Q79.2
meaning hernia —*see* Hernia, umbilicus
Exophoria H5Ø.52
convergence, insufficiency H51.11
divergence, excess H51.8
Exophthalmos HØ5.2-●
congenital Q15.8
constant NEC HØ5.24-●
displacement, globe —*see* Displacement, globe
due to thyrotoxicosis (hyperthyroidism) —*see* Hyperthyroidism, with, goiter (diffuse)
dysthyroid —*see* Hyperthyroidism, with, goiter (diffuse)
goiter —*see* Hyperthyroidism, with, goiter (diffuse)
intermittent NEC HØ5.25-●
malignant —*see* Hyperthyroidism, with, goiter (diffuse)
orbital
edema —*see* Edema, orbit
hemorrhage —*see* Hemorrhage, orbit
pulsating NEC HØ5.26-●
thyrotoxic, thyrotropic —*see* Hyperthyroidism, with, goiter (diffuse)
Exostosis —*see also* Disorder, bone
cartilaginous —*see* Neoplasm, bone, benign
congenital (multiple) Q78.6
external ear canal H61.81-●
gonococcal A54.49
jaw (bone) M27.8
multiple, congenital Q78.6
orbit HØ5.35-●
osteocartilaginous —*see* Neoplasm, bone, benign
syphilitic A52.77
Exotropia —*see* Strabismus, divergent concomitant
Explanation of
investigation finding Z71.2
medication Z71.89
Exposure (to) —*see also* Contact, with T75.89
acariasis Z2Ø.7
AIDS virus Z2Ø.6
air pollution Z77.11Ø
algae and algae toxins Z77.121
algae bloom Z77.121
anthrax Z2Ø.81Ø
aromatic amines Z77.Ø2Ø
aromatic (hazardous) compounds NEC Z77.Ø28
aromatic dyes NOS Z77.Ø28
arsenic Z77.Ø1Ø
asbestos Z77.Ø9Ø
bacterial disease NEC Z2Ø.818
benzene Z77.Ø21
blue-green algae bloom Z77.121
body fluids (potentially hazardous) Z77.21
brown tide Z77.121
Exposure *(Continued)*
chemicals (chiefly nonmedicinal) (hazardous) NEC Z77.Ø98
cholera Z2Ø.Ø9
chromium compounds Z77.Ø18
cold, effects of T69.9
specified effect NEC T69.8
communicable disease Z2Ø.9
bacterial NEC Z2Ø.818
specified NEC Z2Ø.89
viral NEC Z2Ø.828
Zika virus Z2Ø.821
cyanobacteria bloom Z77.121
disaster Z65.5
discrimination Z6Ø.5
dyes Z77.Ø98
effects of T73.9
environmental tobacco smoke (acute) (chronic) Z77.22
Escherichia coli (E. coli) Z2Ø.Ø1
exhaustion due to T73.2
fiberglass —*see* Table of Drugs and Chemicals, fiberglass
German measles Z2Ø.4
gonorrhea Z2Ø.2
hazardous metals NEC Z77.Ø18
hazardous substances NEC Z77.29
hazards in the physical environment NEC Z77.128
hazards to health NEC Z77.9
human immunodeficiency virus (HIV) Z2Ø.6
human T-lymphotropic virus type-1 (HTLV-1) Z2Ø.89
implanted
➡ mesh —*see* Complications, prosthetic device or implant, mesh
prosthetic materials NEC —*see* Complications, prosthetic materials NEC
infestation (parasitic) NEC Z2Ø.7
intestinal infectious disease NEC Z2Ø.Ø9
Escherichia coli (E. coli) Z2Ø.Ø1
lead Z77.Ø11
meningococcus Z2Ø.811
mold (toxic) Z77.12Ø
nickel dust Z77.Ø18
noise Z77.122
occupational
air contaminants NEC Z57.39
dust Z57.2
environmental tobacco smoke Z57.31
extreme temperature Z57.6
noise Z57.Ø
radiation Z57.1
risk factors Z57.9
specified NEC Z57.8
toxic agents (gases) (liquids) (solids) (vapors) in agriculture Z57.4
toxic agents (gases) (liquids) (solids) (vapors) in industry NEC Z57.5
vibration Z57.7
parasitic disease NEC Z2Ø.7
pediculosis Z2Ø.7
persecution Z6Ø.5
pfiesteria piscicida Z77.121
poliomyelitis Z2Ø.89
pollution
air Z77.11Ø
environmental NEC Z77.118
soil Z77.112
water Z77.111
polycyclic aromatic hydrocarbons Z77.Ø28
prenatal (drugs) (toxic chemicals) —*see* Newborn, affected by, noxious substances transmitted via placenta or breast milk
rabies Z2Ø.3
radiation, naturally occurring NEC Z77.123
radon Z77.123
red tide (Florida) Z77.121
rubella Z2Ø.4

E

Exposure *(Continued)*
  second hand tobacco smoke (acute) (chronic) Z77.22
    in the perinatal period P96.81
  sexually-transmitted disease Z20.2
  smallpox (laboratory) Z20.89
  syphilis Z20.2
  terrorism Z65.4
  torture Z65.4
  tuberculosis Z20.1
  uranium Z77.012
  varicella Z20.820
  venereal disease Z20.2
  viral disease NEC Z20.828
  war Z65.5
  water pollution Z77.111
    Zika virus Z20.821
Exsanguination —*see* Hemorrhage
Exstrophy
  abdominal contents Q45.8
  bladder Q64.10
    cloacal Q64.12
    specified type NEC Q64.19
    supravesical fissure Q64.11
Extensive —*see* condition
Extra —*see also* Accessory
  marker chromosomes (normal individual) Q92.61
    in abnormal individual Q92.62
  rib Q76.6
    cervical Q76.5
Extrasystoles (supraventricular) I49.49
  atrial I49.1
  auricular I49.1
  junctional I49.2
  ventricular I49.3
Extrauterine gestation or pregnancy —*see* Pregnancy, by site
Extravasation
  blood R58
  chyle into mesentery I89.8
  pelvicalyceal N13.8
  pyelosinus N13.8
  urine (from ureter) R39.0
  vesicant agent
    antineoplastic chemotherapy T80.810
    other agent NEC T80.818
Extremity —*see* condition, limb
Extrophy —*see* Exstrophy
Extroversion
  bladder Q64.19
  uterus N81.4
    complicating delivery O71.2
    postpartal (old) N81.4
Extruded tooth (teeth) M26.34
Extrusion
  breast implant (prosthetic) T85.42
  eye implant (globe) (ball) T85.328
  intervertebral disc —*see* Displacement, intervertebral disc
  ocular lens implant (prosthetic) —*see* Complications, intraocular lens
  vitreous —*see* Prolapse, vitreous
Exudate
  pleural —*see* Effusion, pleura
  retina H35.89
Exudative —*see* condition
Eye, eyeball, eyelid —*see* condition
Eyestrain —*see* Disturbance, vision, subjective
Eyeworm disease of Africa B74.3

E

F

- **Faber's syndrome** (achlorhydric anemia) D5Ø.9
- **Fabry** (-Anderson) **disease** E75.21
- **Faciocephalalgia, autonomic** —*see also* Neuropathy, peripheral, autonomic G9Ø.Ø9
- **Factor(s)**
  - psychic, associated with diseases classified elsewhere F54
  - psychological
    - affecting physical conditions F54
    - or behavioral
      - affecting general medical condition F54
      - associated with disorders or diseases classified elsewhere F54
- **Fahr disease** (of brain) G23.8
- **Fahr Volhard disease** (of kidney) I12.-●
- **Failure, failed**
  - abortion —*see* Abortion, attempted
  - aortic (valve) I35.8
    - rheumatic IØ6.8
  - attempted abortion —*see* Abortion, attempted
  - biventricular I5Ø.82
    - due to left heart failure I5Ø.814
  - bone marrow —*see* Anemia, aplastic
  - cardiac —*see* Failure, heart
  - cardiorenal (chronic) —*see* also Failure, renal, and Failure, heart I5Ø.9
    - hypertensive I13.2
  - cardiorespiratory (*see also* Failure, heart) RØ9.2
  - cardiovascular (chronic) —*see* Failure, heart
  - cerebrovascular I67.9
  - cervical dilatation in labor O62.Ø
  - circulation, circulatory (peripheral) R57.9
    - newborn P29.89
  - compensation —*see* Disease, heart
  - compliance with medical treatment or regimen —*see* Noncompliance
  - congestive —*see* Failure, heart, congestive
  - dental implant (endosseous) M27.69
    - due to
      - failure of dental prosthesis M27.63
      - lack of attached gingiva M27.62
      - occlusal trauma (poor prosthetic design) M27.62
      - parafunctional habits M27.62
      - periodontal infection (peri-implantitis) M27.62
      - poor oral hygiene M27.62
    - osseointegration M27.61
      - due to
        - complications of systemic disease M27.61
        - poor bone quality M27.61
      - iatrogenic M27.61
    - post-osseointegration
      - biological M27.62
      - due to complications of systemic disease M27.62
      - iatrogenic M27.62
      - mechanical M27.63
    - pre-integration M27.61
    - pre-osseointegration M27.61
    - specified NEC M27.69
  - descent of head (at term) of pregnancy (mother) O32.4
  - endosseous dental implant —*see* Failure, dental implant
  - engagement of head (term of pregnancy) (mother) O32.4
  - erection (penile) —*see also* Dysfunction, sexual, male, erectile N52.9
    - nonorganic F52.21
  - examination(s), anxiety concerning Z55.2
  - expansion terminal respiratory units (newborn) (primary) P28.Ø
  - forceps NOS (with subsequent cesarean delivery) O66.5

Failure, failed *(Continued)*
  - gain weight (child over 28 days old) R62.51
    - adult R62.7
    - newborn P92.6
  - genital response (male) F52.21
    - female F52.22
  - heart (acute) (senile) (sudden) I5Ø.9
    - with
      - acute pulmonary edema —*see* Failure, ventricular, left
      - decompensation —*see also* Failure, heart, by type as diastolic or systolic, acute and chronic I5Ø.9
      - dilatation —*see* Disease, heart
      - ▶hypertension —*see* Hypertension, heart
      - normal ejection fraction —*see* Failure, heart, diastolic
      - preserved ejection fraction —*see* Failure, heart, diastolic
      - reduced ejection fraction —*see* Failure, heart, systolic
    - arteriosclerotic I7Ø.9Ø
    - biventricular I5Ø.82
      - due to left heart failure I5Ø.814
    - combined left-right sided I5Ø.82
      - due to left heart failure I5Ø.814
    - compensated —*see also* Failure, heart, by type as diastolic or systolic, chronic I5Ø.9
    - complicating
      - anesthesia (general) (local) or other sedation
        - in labor and delivery O74.2
        - in pregnancy O29.12-●
        - postpartum, puerperal O89.1
      - delivery (cesarean) (instrumental) O75.4
    - congestive I5Ø.9
      - with rheumatic fever (conditions in IØØ)
        - active IØ1.8
        - inactive or quiescent (with chorea) IØ9.81
      - newborn P29.Ø
      - rheumatic (chronic) (inactive) (with chorea) IØ9.81
        - active or acute IØ1.8
          - with chorea IØ2.Ø
    - decompensated —*see also* Failure, heart, by type as diastolic or systolic, acute and chronic I5Ø.9
    - degenerative —*see* Degeneration, myocardial
    - diastolic (congestive) (left ventricular) I5Ø.3Ø
      - acute (congestive) I5Ø.31
        - and (on) chronic (congestive) I5Ø.33
      - chronic (congestive) I5Ø.32
        - and (on) acute (congestive) I5Ø.33
      - combined with systolic (congestive) I5Ø.4Ø
        - acute (congestive) I5Ø.41
          - and (on) chronic (congestive) I5Ø.43
        - chronic (congestive) I5Ø.42
          - and (on) acute (congestive) I5Ø.43
    - due to presence of cardiac prosthesis I97.13-●
    - end stage —*see also* Failure, heart, by type as diastolic or systolic, chronic I5Ø.84
    - following cardiac surgery I97.13-●
    - high output NOS I5Ø.83
    - hypertensive —*see* Hypertension, heart
    - left (ventricular) —*see also* Failure, ventricular, left
      - combined diastolic and systolic —*see* Failure, heart, diastolic, combined with systolic
      - diastolic —*see* Failure, heart, diastolic
      - systolic —*see* Failure, heart, systolic
    - low output (syndrome) NOS I5Ø.9
    - newborn P29.Ø
    - organic —*see* Disease, heart
    - peripartum O9Ø.3

Failure, failed *(Continued)*
  - heart *(Continued)*
    - postprocedural I97.13-●
    - rheumatic (chronic) (inactive) IØ9.9
    - right (isolated) (ventricular) I5Ø.81Ø
      - acute I5Ø.811
        - and (on) chronic I5Ø.813
      - chronic I5Ø.812
        - and acute I5Ø.813
      - secondary to left heart failure I5Ø.814
    - specified NEC I5Ø.89

> Note: heart failure stages A, B, C, and D are based on the American College of Cardiology and American Heart Association stages of heart failure, which complement and should not be confused with the New York Heart Association Classification of Heart Failure, into Class I, Class II, Class III, and Class IV

    - stage A Z91.89
    - stage B (see also Failure, heart, by type as diastolic or systolic) I5Ø.9
    - stage C (see also Failure, heart, by type as diastolic or systolic) I5Ø.9
    - stage D (see also Failure, heart, by type as diastolic or systolic, chronic) I5Ø.84
    - systolic (congestive) (left ventricular) I5Ø.2Ø
      - acute (congestive) I5Ø.21
        - and (on) chronic (congestive) I5Ø.23
      - chronic (congestive) I5Ø.22
        - and (on) acute (congestive) I5Ø.23
      - combined with diastolic (congestive) I5Ø.4Ø
        - acute (congestive) I5Ø.41
          - and (on) chronic (congestive) I5Ø.43
        - chronic (congestive) I5Ø.42
          - and (on) acute (congestive) I5Ø.43
    - thyrotoxic (see also Thyrotoxicosis) EØ5.9Ø [I43]
      - with
        - high output (see also Thyrotoxicosis) I5Ø.83
        - thyroid storm EØ5.91 [I43]
          - high output (see also Thyrotoxicosis) I5Ø.83
    - valvular —*see* Endocarditis
  - hepatic K72.9Ø
    - with coma K72.91
    - acute or subacute K72.ØØ
      - with coma K72.Ø1
      - due to drugs K71.1Ø
        - with coma K71.11
    - alcoholic (acute) (chronic) (subacute) K7Ø.4Ø
      - with coma K7Ø.41
    - chronic K72.1Ø
      - with coma K72.11
      - due to drugs (acute) (subacute) (chronic) K71.1Ø
        - with coma K71.11
    - due to drugs (acute) (subacute) (chronic) K71.1Ø
      - with coma K71.11
    - postprocedural K91.82
  - hepatorenal K76.7
  - induction (of labor) O61.9
    - abortion —*see* Abortion, attempted
    - by
      - oxytocic drugs O61.Ø
      - prostaglandins O61.Ø
    - instrumental O61.1
    - mechanical O61.1
    - medical O61.Ø
    - specified NEC O61.8
    - surgical O61.1

Failure, failed *(Continued)*
intubation during anesthesia T88.4
in pregnancy O29.6-●
labor and delivery O74.7
postpartum, puerperal O89.6
involution, thymus (gland) E32.Ø
kidney —*see also* Disease, kidney, chronic N19
acute —*see also* Failure, renal, acute N17.9-●
diabetic —*see* EØ8-E13 with .22
lactation (complete) O92.3
partial O92.4
Leydig's cell, adult E29.1
liver —*see* Failure, hepatic
menstruation at puberty N91.Ø
mitral IØ5.8
myocardial, myocardium —*see also* Failure, heart I5Ø.9
chronic —*see also* Failure, heart, congestive I5Ø.9
congestive —*see also* Failure, heart, congestive I5Ø.9
orgasm (female) (psychogenic) F52.31
male F52.32
ovarian (primary) E28.39
iatrogenic E89.4Ø
asymptomatic E89.4Ø
symptomatic E89.41
postprocedural (postablative) (postirradiation) (postsurgical) E89.4Ø
asymptomatic E89.4Ø
symptomatic E89.41
ovulation causing infertility N97.Ø
polyglandular, autoimmune E31.Ø
prosthetic joint implant —*see* Complications, joint prosthesis, mechanical, breakdown, by site
renal N19
with
tubular necrosis (acute) N17.Ø
acute N17.9
with
cortical necrosis N17.1
medullary necrosis N17.2
tubular necrosis N17.Ø
specified NEC N17.8
chronic N18.9
hypertensive —*see* Hypertension, kidney
congenital P96.Ø
end stage (chronic) N18.6
due to hypertension I12.Ø
following
abortion —*see* Abortion by type complicated by specified condition NEC
crushing T79.5
ectopic or molar pregnancy OØ8.4
labor and delivery (acute) O9Ø.4
hypertensive —*see* Hypertension, kidney
postprocedural N99.Ø
respiration, respiratory J96.9
with
hypercapnia J96.92
hypercarbia J96.Ø2
hypoxia J96.91
acute J96.ØØ
with
hypercapnia J96.Ø2
hypercarbia J96.92
hypoxia J96.Ø1
acute and (on) chronic J96.2Ø
with
hypercapnia J96.22
hypercarbia J96.22
hypoxia J96.21
center G93.89
chronic J96.1Ø
with
hypercapnia J96.12
hypercarbia J96.12
hypoxia J96.11

Failure, failed *(Continued)*
respiration, respiratory *(Continued)*
newborn P28.5
postprocedural (acute) J95.821
acute and chronic J95.822
rotation
cecum Q43.3
colon Q43.3
intestine Q43.3
kidney Q63.2
sedation (conscious) (moderate) during procedure T88.52
history of Z92.83
segmentation —*see also* Fusion
fingers —*see* Syndactylism, complex, fingers
vertebra Q76.49
with scoliosis Q76.3
seminiferous tubule, adult E29.1
senile (general) R54
sexual arousal (male) F52.21
female F52.22
testicular endocrine function E29.1
to thrive (child over 28 days old) R62.51
adult R62.7
newborn P92.6
transplant T86.92
bone T86.831
marrow T86.Ø2
cornea T86.841
heart T86.22
with lung(s) T86.32
intestine T86.851
kidney T86.12
liver T86.42
lung(s) T86.811
with heart T86.32
pancreas T86.891
skin (allograft) (autograft) T86.821
specified organ or tissue NEC T86.891
stem cell (peripheral blood) (umbilical cord) T86.5
trial of labor (with subsequent cesarean delivery) O66.4Ø
following previous cesarean delivery O66.41
tubal ligation N99.89
urinary —*see* Disease, kidney, chronic
vacuum extraction NOS (with subsequent cesarean delivery) O66.5
vasectomy N99.89
ventouse NOS (with subsequent cesarean delivery) O66.5
ventricular —*see also* Failure, heart I5Ø.9
left —*see also* Failure, heart, left I5Ø.1
with rheumatic fever (conditions in IØØ)
active IØ1.8
with chorea IØ2.Ø
inactive or quiescent (with chorea) IØ9.81
rheumatic (chronic) (inactive) (with chorea) IØ9.81
active or acute IØ1.8
with chorea IØ2.Ø
right —*see* Failure, heart, right
vital centers, newborn P91.88
Fainting (fit) R55
Fallen arches —*see* Deformity, limb, flat foot
Falling, falls (repeated) R29.6
any organ or part —*see* Prolapse
Fallopian
insufflation Z31.41
tube —*see* condition
Fallot's
pentalogy Q21.8
tetrad or tetralogy Q21.3
triad or trilogy Q22.3
False —*see also* condition
croup J38.5
joint —*see* Nonunion, fracture

False *(Continued)*
labor (pains) O47.9
at or after 37 completed weeks of gestation O47.1
before 37 completed weeks of gestation O47.Ø-●
passage, urethra (prostatic) N36.5
pregnancy F45.8
Family, familial —*see also* condition
disruption Z63.8
involving divorce or separation Z63.5
Li-Fraumeni (syndrome) Z15.Ø1
planning advice Z3Ø.Ø9
problem Z63.9
specified NEC Z63.8
retinoblastoma C69.2-●
Famine (effects of) T73.Ø
edema —*see* Malnutrition, severe
Fanconi (-de Toni)(-Debré) syndrome E72.Ø9
with cystinosis E72.Ø4
Fanconi's anemia (congenital pancytopenia) D61.Ø9
Farber's disease or syndrome E75.29
Farcy A24.Ø
Farmer's
lung J67.Ø
skin L57.8
Farsightedness —*see* Hypermetropia
Fascia —*see* condition
Fasciculation R25.3
Fasciitis M72.9
diffuse (eosinophilic) M35.4
infective M72.8
necrotizing M72.6
necrotizing M72.6
nodular M72.4
perirenal (with ureteral obstruction) N13.5
with infection N13.6
plantar M72.2
specified NEC M72.8
traumatic (old) M72.8
current - code by site under Sprain
Fascioliasis B66.3
Fasciolopsis, fasciolopsiasis (intestinal) B66.5
Fascioscapulohumeral myopathy G71.Ø2
Fast pulse RØØ.Ø
Fat
embolism —*see* Embolism, fat
excessive —*see also* Obesity
in heart —*see* Degeneration, myocardial
in stool R19.5
localized (pad) E65
heart —*see* Degeneration, myocardial
knee M79.4
retropatellar M79.4
necrosis
breast N64.1
mesentery K65.4
omentum K65.4
pad E65
knee M79.4
Fatigue R53.83
auditory deafness —*see* Deafness
chronic R53.82
combat F43.Ø
general R53.83
psychogenic F48.8
heat (transient) T67.6
muscle M62.89
myocardium —*see* Failure, heart
neoplasm-related R53.Ø
nervous, neurosis F48.8
operational F48.8
psychogenic (general) F48.8
senile R54
voice R49.8
Fatness —*see* Obesity

Fatty —*see also* condition
  apron E65
  degeneration —*see* Degeneration, fatty
  heart (enlarged) —*see* Degeneration, myocardial
  liver NEC K76.Ø
    alcoholic K7Ø.Ø
    nonalcoholic K76.Ø
  necrosis —*see* Degeneration, fatty
Fauces —*see* condition
Fauchard's disease (periodontitis) —*see* Periodontitis
Faucitis JØ2.9
Favism (anemia) D55.Ø
Favus —*see* Dermatophytosis
Fazio-Londe disease or syndrome G12.1
Fear complex or reaction F4Ø.9
Fear of —*see* Phobia
Feared complaint unfounded Z71.1
Febris, febrile —*see also* Fever
  flava —*see also* Fever, yellow A95.9
  melitensis A23.Ø
  pestis —*see* Plague
  recurrens —*see* Fever, relapsing
  rubra A38.9
Fecal
  incontinence R15.9
  smearing R15.1
  soiling R15.1
  urgency R15.2
Fecalith (impaction) K56.41
  appendix K38.1
  congenital P76.8
Fede's disease K14.Ø
Feeble rapid pulse due to shock following injury T79.4
Feeble-minded F7Ø
Feeding
  difficulties R63.3
  problem R63.3
    newborn P92.9
      specified NEC P92.8
    nonorganic (adult) —*see* Disorder, eating
Feeling (of)
  foreign body in throat RØ9.89
Feer's disease —*see* Poisoning, mercury
Feet —*see* condition
Feigned illness Z76.5
Feil-Klippel syndrome (brevicollis) Q76.1
Feinmesser's (hidrotic) ectodermal dysplasia Q82.4
Felinophobia F4Ø.218
Felon —*see also* Cellulitis, digit
  with lymphangitis —*see* Lymphangitis, acute, digit
Felty's syndrome MØ5.ØØ
  ankle MØ5.Ø7- •
  elbow MØ5.Ø2- •
  foot joint MØ5.Ø7- •
  hand joint MØ5.Ø4- •
  hip MØ5.Ø5- •
  knee MØ5.Ø6- •
  multiple site MØ5.Ø9
  shoulder MØ5.Ø1- •
  vertebra —*see* Spondylitis, ankylosing
  wrist MØ5.Ø3- •
Female genital cutting status —*see* Female genital mutilation status (FGM)
Female genital mutilation status (FGM) N9Ø.81Ø
  specified NEC N9Ø.818
  type I (clitorectomy status) N9Ø.811
  type II (clitorectomy with excision of labia minora status) N9Ø.812
  type III (infibulation status) N9Ø.813
  type IV N9Ø.818
Femur, femoral —*see* condition
Fenestration, fenestrated —*see also* Imperfect, closure
  aortico-pulmonary Q21.4
  cusps, heart valve NEC Q24.8
    pulmonary Q22.3
  pulmonic cusps Q22.3
Fernell's disease (aortic aneurysm) I71.9
Fertile eunuch syndrome E23.Ø
Fetid
  breath R19.6
  sweat L75.Ø
Fetishism F65.Ø
  transvestic F65.1
Fetus, fetal —*see also* condition
  alcohol syndrome (dysmorphic) Q86.Ø
  compressus O31.Ø- •
  hydantoin syndrome Q86.1
  lung tissue P28.Ø
  papyraceous O31.Ø- •
Fever (inanition) (of unknown origin) (persistent) (with chills) (with rigor) R5Ø.9
  abortus A23.1
  Aden (dengue) A9Ø
  African tick-borne A68.1
  American
    mountain (tick) A93.2
    spotted A77.Ø
  aphthous BØ8.8
  arbovirus, arboviral A94
    hemorrhagic A94
    specified NEC A93.8
  Argentinian hemorrhagic A96.Ø
  Assam B55.Ø
  Australian Q A78
  Bangkok hemorrhagic A91
  Barmah forest A92.8
  Bartonella A44.Ø
  bilious, hemoglobinuric B5Ø.8
  blackwater B5Ø.8
  blister BØØ.1
  Bolivian hemorrhagic A96.1
  Bonvale dam T73.3
  boutonneuse A77.1
  brain —*see* Encephalitis
  Brazilian purpuric A48.4
  breakbone A9Ø
  Bullis A77.Ø
  Bunyamwera A92.8
  Burdwan B55.Ø
  Bwamba A92.8
  Cameroon —*see* Malaria
  Canton A75.9
  catarrhal (acute) JØØ
    chronic J31.Ø
  cat-scratch A28.1
  Central Asian hemorrhagic A98.Ø
  cerebral —*see* Encephalitis
  cerebrospinal meningococcal A39.Ø
  Chagres B5Ø.9
  Chandipura A92.8
  Changuinola A93.1
  Charcot's (biliary) (hepatic) (intermittent) —*see* Calculus, bile duct
  Chikungunya (viral) (hemorrhagic) A92.Ø
  Chitral A93.1
  Colombo —*see* Fever, paratyphoid
  Colorado tick (virus) A93.2
  congestive (remittent) —*see* Malaria
  Congo virus A98.Ø
  continued malarial B5Ø.9
  Corsican —*see* Malaria
  Crimean-Congo hemorrhagic A98.Ø
  Cyprus —*see* Brucellosis
  dandy A9Ø
  deer fly —*see* Tularemia
  dengue (virus) A9Ø
    hemorrhagic A91
    sandfly A93.1
  desert B38.Ø
  drug induced R5Ø.2
Fever *(Continued)*
  due to
    conditions classified elsewhere R5Ø.81
    heat T67.Ø1
  enteric AØ1.ØØ
  enteroviral exanthematous (Boston exanthem) A88.Ø
  ephemeral (of unknown origin) R5Ø.9
  epidemic hemorrhagic A98.5
  erysipelatous —*see* Erysipelas
  estivo-autumnal (malarial) B5Ø.9
  famine A75.Ø
  five day A79.Ø
  following delivery O86.4
  Fort Bragg A27.89
  gastroenteric AØ1.ØØ
  gastromalarial —*see* Malaria
  Gibraltar —*see* Brucellosis
  glandular —*see* Mononucleosis, infectious
  Guama (viral) A92.8
  Haverhill A25.1
  hay (allergic) J3Ø.1
    with asthma (bronchial) J45.9Ø9
      with
        exacerbation (acute) J45.9Ø1
        status asthmaticus J45.9Ø2
    due to
      allergen other than pollen J3Ø.89
      pollen, any plant or tree J3Ø.1
  heat (effects) T67.Ø1
  hematuric, bilious B5Ø.8
  hemoglobinuric (malarial) (bilious) B5Ø.8
  hemorrhagic (arthropod-borne) NOS A94
    with renal syndrome A98.5
    arenaviral A96.9
      specified NEC A96.8
    Argentinian A96.Ø
    Bangkok A91
    Bolivian A96.1
    Central Asian A98.Ø
    Chikungunya A92.Ø
    Crimean-Congo A98.Ø
    dengue (virus) A91
    epidemic A98.5
    Junin (virus) A96.Ø
    Korean A98.5
    Kyasanur forest A98.2
    Machupo (virus) A96.1
    mite-borne A93.8
    mosquito-borne A92.8
    Omsk A98.1
    Philippine A91
    Russian A98.5
    Singapore A91
    Southeast Asia A91
    Thailand A91
    tick-borne NEC A93.8
    viral A99
      specified NEC A98.8
  hepatic —*see* Cholecystitis
  herpetic —*see* Herpes
  icterohemorrhagic A27.Ø
  Indiana A93.8
  infective B99.9
    specified NEC B99.8
  intermittent (bilious) —*see also* Malaria
    of unknown origin R5Ø.9
    pernicious B5Ø.9
  iodide R5Ø.2
  Japanese river A75.3
  jungle —*see also* Malaria
    yellow A95.Ø
  Junin (virus) hemorrhagic A96.Ø
  Katayama B65.2
  kedani A75.3
  Kenya (tick) A77.1
  Kew Garden A79.1
  Korean hemorrhagic A98.5
  Lassa A96.2
  Lone Star A77.Ø

F

Fever *(Continued)*
- Machupo (virus) hemorrhagic A96.1
- malaria, malarial —*see* Malaria
- Malta A23.9
- Marseilles A77.1
- marsh —*see* Malaria
- Mayaro (viral) A92.8
- Mediterranean —*see also* Brucellosis A23.9
  - familial MØ4.1
  - tick A77.1
- meningeal —*see* Meningitis
- Meuse A79.Ø
- Mexican A75.2
- mianeh A68.1
- miasmatic —*see* Malaria
- mosquito-borne (viral) A92.9
  - hemorrhagic A92.8
- mountain —*see also* Brucellosis
  - meaning Rocky Mountain spotted fever A77.Ø
  - tick (American) (Colorado) (viral) A93.2
- Mucambo (viral) A92.8
- mud A27.9
- Neapolitan —*see* Brucellosis
- neutropenic D7Ø.9
- newborn P81.9
  - environmental P81.Ø
- Nine-Mile A78
- non-exanthematous tick A93.2
- North Asian tick-borne A77.2
- Omsk hemorrhagic A98.1
- O'nyong-nyong (viral) A92.1
- Oropouche (viral) A93.Ø
- Oroya A44.Ø
- paludal —*see* Malaria
- Panama (malarial) B5Ø.9
- Pappataci A93.1
- paratyphoid AØ1.4
  - A AØ1.1
  - B AØ1.2
  - C AØ1.3
- parrot A7Ø
- periodic (Mediterranean) MØ4.1
- persistent (of unknown origin) R5Ø.9
- petechial A39.Ø
- pharyngoconjunctival B3Ø.2
- Philippine hemorrhagic A91
- phlebotomus A93.1
- Piry (virus) A93.8
- Pixuna (viral) A92.8
- Plasmodium ovale B53.Ø
- polioviral (nonparalytic) A8Ø.4
- Pontiac A48.2
- postimmunization R5Ø.83
- postoperative R5Ø.82
  - due to infection T81.4Ø
- posttransfusion R5Ø.84
- postvaccination R5Ø.83
- presenting with conditions classified elsewhere R5Ø.81
- pretibial A27.89
- puerperal O86.4
- Q A78
- quadrilateral A78
- quartan (malaria) B52.9
- Queensland (coastal) (tick) A77.3
- quintan A79.Ø
- rabbit —*see* Tularemia
- rat-bite A25.9
  - due to
    - Spirillum A25.Ø
    - Streptobacillus moniliformis A25.1
- recurrent —*see* Fever, relapsing
- relapsing (Borrelia) A68.9
  - Carter's (Asiatic) A68.1
  - Dutton's (West African) A68.1
  - Koch's A68.9
  - louse-borne A68.Ø
  - Novy's
    - louse-borne A68.Ø
    - tick-borne A68.1

Fever *(Continued)*
- relapsing (Borrelia) *(Continued)*
  - Obermeyer's (European) A68.Ø
  - tick-borne A68.1
- remittent (bilious) (congestive) (gastric) —*see* Malaria
- rheumatic (active) (acute) (chronic) (subacute) IØØ
  - with central nervous system involvement IØ2.9
  - active with heart involvement —*see* category IØ1
  - inactive or quiescent with
    - cardiac hypertrophy IØ9.89
    - carditis IØ9.9
    - endocarditis IØ9.1
      - aortic (valve) IØ6.9
        - with mitral (valve) disease IØ8.Ø
      - mitral (valve) IØ5.9
        - with aortic (valve) disease IØ8.Ø
      - pulmonary (valve) IØ9.89
      - tricuspid (valve) IØ7.8
    - heart disease NEC IØ9.89
    - heart failure (congestive) (conditions in category I5Ø.) IØ9.81
    - left ventricular failure (conditions in I5Ø.- I5Ø.4-) IØ9.81
    - myocarditis, myocardial degeneration (conditions in I51.4) IØ9.Ø
    - pancarditis IØ9.9
    - pericarditis IØ9.2
- Rift Valley (viral) A92.4
- Rocky Mountain spotted A77.Ø
- rose J3Ø.1
- Ross River B33.1
- Russian hemorrhagic A98.5
- San Joaquin (Valley) B38.Ø
- sandfly A93.1
- Sao Paulo A77.Ø
- scarlet A38.9
- seven day (leptospirosis) (autumnal) (Japanese) A27.89
  - dengue A9Ø
- shin-bone A79.Ø
- Singapore hemorrhagic A91
- solar A9Ø
- Songo A98.5
- sore BØØ.1
- South African tick-bite A68.1
- Southeast Asia hemorrhagic A91
- spinal —*see* Meningitis
- spirillary A25.Ø
- splenic —*see* Anthrax
- spotted A77.9
  - American A77.Ø
  - Brazilian A77.Ø
  - cerebrospinal meningitis A39.Ø
  - Colombian A77.Ø
  - due to Rickettsia
    - australis A77.3
    - conorii A77.1
    - rickettsii A77.Ø
    - sibirica A77.2
    - specified type NEC A77.8
  - Ehrlichiosis A77.4Ø
    - due to
      - E. chafeensis A77.41
      - specified organism NEC A77.49
  - Rocky Mountain A77.Ø
- steroid R5Ø.2
- streptobacillary A25.1
- subtertian B5Ø.9
- Sumatran mite A75.3
- sun A9Ø
- swamp A27.9
- swine AØ2.8
- sylvatic, yellow A95.Ø
- Tahyna B33.8
- tertian —*see* Malaria, tertian
- Thailand hemorrhagic A91
- ➠thermic T67.Ø1

Fever *(Continued)*
- three-day A93.1
- tick
  - American mountain A93.2
  - Colorado A93.2
  - Kemerovo A93.8
  - Mediterranean A77.1
  - mountain A93.2
  - nonexanthematous A93.2
  - Quaranfil A93.8
- tick-bite NEC A93.8
- tick-borne (hemorrhagic) NEC A93.8
- trench A79.Ø
- tsutsugamushi A75.3
- typhogastric AØ1.ØØ
- typhoid (abortive) (hemorrhagic) (intermittent) (malignant) AØ1.ØØ
  - complicated by
    - arthritis AØ1.Ø4
    - heart involvement AØ1.Ø2
    - meningitis AØ1.Ø1
    - osteomyelitis AØ1.Ø5
    - pneumonia AØ1.Ø3
    - specified NEC AØ1.Ø9
- typhomalarial —*see* Malaria
- typhus —*see* Typhus (fever)
- undulant —*see* Brucellosis
- unknown origin R5Ø.9
- uveoparotid D86.89
- valley B38.Ø
- Venezuelan equine A92.2
- vesicular stomatitis A93.8
- viral hemorrhagic —*see* Fever, hemorrhagic, by type of virus
- Volhynian A79.Ø
- Wesselsbron (viral) A92.8
- West
  - African B5Ø.8
  - Nile (viral) A92.3Ø
    - with
      - complications NEC A92.39
      - cranial nerve disorders A92.32
      - encephalitis A92.31
      - encephalomyelitis A92.31
      - neurologic manifestation NEC A92.32
      - optic neuritis A92.32
      - polyradiculitis A92.32
- Whitmore's —*see* Melioidosis
- Wolhynian A79.Ø
- worm B83.9
- yellow A95.9
  - jungle A95.Ø
  - sylvatic A95.Ø
  - urban A95.1
- Zika virus A92.5

Fibrillation
- atrial or auricular (established) I48.91
  - ➠chronic I48.2Ø
    - ▶persistent I48.19
  - paroxysmal I48.Ø
  - ➠permanent I48.21
  - ➠persistent (chronic) (NOS) (other) I48.19
    - ▶longstanding I48.11
- cardiac I49.8
- heart I49.8
- muscular M62.89
- ventricular I49.Ø1

Fibrin
- ball or bodies, pleural (sac) J94.1
- chamber, anterior (eye) (gelatinous exudate) —*see* Iridocyclitis, acute

Fibrinogenolysis —*see* Fibrinolysis

Fibrinogenopenia D68.8
- acquired D65
- congenital D68.2

Fibrinolysis (hemorrhagic) (acquired) D65
- antepartum hemorrhage —*see* Hemorrhage, antepartum, with coagulation defect
- following
  - abortion —*see* Abortion by type complicated by hemorrhage
  - ectopic or molar pregnancy OØ8.1

Fibrinolysis *(Continued)*
intrapartum O67.Ø
newborn, transient P6Ø
postpartum O72.3
Fibrinopenia (hereditary) D68.2
acquired D68.4
Fibrinopurulent —*see* condition
Fibrinous —*see* condition
Fibroadenoma
cellular intracanalicular D24-●
giant D24-●
intracanalicular
cellular D24-●
giant D24-●
specified site —*see* Neoplasm, benign, by site
unspecified site D24-●
juvenile D24-●
pericanalicular
specified site —*see* Neoplasm, benign, by site
unspecified site D24-●
phyllodes D24-●
prostate D29.1
specified site NEC —*see* Neoplasm, benign, by site
unspecified site D24-●
Fibroadenosis, breast (chronic) (cystic) (diffuse) (periodic) (segmental) N6Ø.2-●
Fibroangioma —*see also* Neoplasm, benign, by site
juvenile
specified site —*see* Neoplasm, benign, by site
unspecified site D1Ø.6
Fibrochondrosarcoma —*see* Neoplasm, cartilage, malignant
Fibrocystic
disease —*see also* Fibrosis, cystic
breast —*see* Mastopathy, cystic
jaw M27.49
kidney (congenital) Q61.8
liver Q44.6
pancreas E84.9
kidney (congenital) Q61.8
Fibrodysplasia ossificans progressiva —*see* Myositis, ossificans, progressiva
Fibroelastosis (cordis) (endocardial) (endomyocardial) I42.4
Fibroid (tumor) —*see also* Neoplasm, connective tissue, benign
disease, lung (chronic) —*see* Fibrosis, lung
heart (disease) —*see* Myocarditis
in pregnancy or childbirth O34.1-●
causing obstructed labor O65.5
induration, lung (chronic) —*see* Fibrosis, lung
lung —*see* Fibrosis, lung
pneumonia (chronic) —*see* Fibrosis, lung
uterus —*see also* Leiomyoma, uterus D25.9
Fibrolipoma —*see* Lipoma
Fibroliposarcoma —*see* Neoplasm, connective tissue, malignant
Fibroma —*see also* Neoplasm, connective tissue, benign
ameloblastic —*see* Cyst, calcifying odontogenic
bone (nonossifying) —*see* Disorder, bone, specified type NEC
ossifying —*see* Neoplasm, bone, benign
cementifying —*see* Neoplasm, bone, benign
chondromyxoid —*see* Neoplasm, bone, benign
desmoplastic —*see* Neoplasm, connective tissue, uncertain behavior
durum —*see* Neoplasm, connective tissue, benign
fascial —*see* Neoplasm, connective tissue, benign
invasive —*see* Neoplasm, connective tissue, uncertain behavior
molle —*see* Lipoma

Fibroma *(Continued)*
myxoid —*see* Neoplasm, connective tissue, benign
nasopharynx, nasopharyngeal (juvenile) D1Ø.6
nonosteogenic (nonossifying) —*see* Dysplasia, fibrous
odontogenic (central) —*see* Cyst, calcifying odontogenic
ossifying —*see* Neoplasm, bone, benign
periosteal —*see* Neoplasm, bone, benign
soft —*see* Lipoma
Fibromatosis M72.9
abdominal —*see* Neoplasm, connective tissue, uncertain behavior
aggressive —*see* Neoplasm, connective tissue, uncertain behavior
congenital generalized —*see* Neoplasm, connective tissue, uncertain behavior
Dupuytren's M72.Ø
gingival KØ6.1
palmar (fascial) M72.Ø
plantar (fascial) M72.2
pseudosarcomatous (proliferative) (subcutaneous) M72.4
retroperitoneal D48.3
specified NEC M72.8
Fibromyalgia M79.7
Fibromyoma —*see also* Neoplasm, connective tissue, benign
uterus (corpus) —*see also* Leiomyoma, uterus
in pregnancy or childbirth —*see* Fibroid, in pregnancy or childbirth
causing obstructed labor O65.5
Fibromyositis M79.7
Fibromyxolipoma D17.9
Fibromyxoma —*see* Neoplasm, connective tissue, benign
Fibromyxosarcoma —*see* Neoplasm, connective tissue, malignant
Fibro-odontoma, ameloblastic —*see* Cyst, calcifying odontogenic
Fibro-osteoma —*see* Neoplasm, bone, benign
Fibroplasia, retrolental H35.17
Fibropurulent —*see* condition
Fibrosarcoma —*see also* Neoplasm, connective tissue, malignant
ameloblastic C41.1
upper jaw (bone) C41.Ø
congenital —*see* Neoplasm, connective tissue, malignant
fascial —*see* Neoplasm, connective tissue, malignant
infantile —*see* Neoplasm, connective tissue, malignant
odontogenic C41.1
upper jaw (bone) C41.Ø
periosteal —*see* Neoplasm, bone, malignant
Fibrosclerosis
breast N6Ø.3-●
multifocal M35.5
penis (corpora cavernosa) N48.6
Fibrosis, fibrotic
adrenal (gland) E27.8
amnion O41.8X-●
anal papillae K62.89
arteriocapillary —*see* Arteriosclerosis
bladder N32.89
interstitial —*see* Cystitis, chronic, interstitial
localized submucosal —*see* Cystitis, chronic, interstitial
panmural —*see* Cystitis, chronic, interstitial
breast —*see* Fibrosclerosis, breast
capillary —*see also* Arteriosclerosis I7Ø.9Ø
lung (chronic) —*see* Fibrosis, lung
cardiac —*see* Myocarditis
cervix N88.8
chorion O41.8X-●
corpus cavernosum (sclerosing) N48.6
cystic (of pancreas) E84.9

Fibrosis, fibrotic *(Continued)*
cystic *(Continued)*
with
distal intestinal obstruction syndrome E84.19
fecal impaction E84.19
intestinal manifestations NEC E84.19
pulmonary manifestations E84.Ø
specified manifestations NEC E84.8
due to device, implant or graft —*see also* Complications, by site and type, specified NEC T85.828
arterial graft NEC T82.828
breast (implant) T85.828
catheter NEC T85.828
dialysis (renal) T82.828
intraperitoneal T85.828
infusion NEC T82.828
spinal (epidural) (subdural) T85.82Ø
urinary (indwelling) T83.82
electronic (electrode) (pulse generator) (stimulator)
bone T84.82
cardiac T82.827
nervous system (brain) (peripheral nerve) (spinal) T85.82Ø
urinary T83.82
fixation, internal (orthopedic) NEC T84.82
gastrointestinal (bile duct) (esophagus) T85.828
genital NEC T83.82
heart NEC T82.827
joint prosthesis T84.82
ocular (corneal graft) (orbital implant) NEC T85.828
orthopedic NEC T84.82
specified NEC T85.828
urinary NEC T83.82
vascular NEC T82.828
ventricular intracranial shunt T85.82Ø
ejaculatory duct N5Ø.89
endocardium —*see* Endocarditis
endomyocardial (tropical) I42.3
epididymis N5Ø.89
eye muscle —*see* Strabismus, mechanical
heart —*see* Myocarditis
hepatic —*see* Fibrosis, liver
hepatolienal (portal hypertension) K76.6
hepatosplenic (portal hypertension) K76.6
infrapatellar fat pad M79.4
intrascrotal N5Ø.89
kidney N26.9
liver K74.Ø
with sclerosis K74.2
alcoholic K7Ø.2
lung (atrophic) (chronic) (confluent) (massive) (perialveolar) (peribronchial) J84.1Ø
with
anthracosilicosis J6Ø
anthracosis J6Ø
asbestosis J61
bagassosis J67.1
bauxite J63.1
berylliosis J63.2
byssinosis J66.Ø
calcicosis J62.8
chalicosis J62.8
dust reticulation J64
farmer's lung J67.Ø
ganister disease J62.8
graphite J63.3
pneumoconiosis NOS J64
siderosis J63.4
silicosis J62.8
capillary J84.1Ø
congenital P27.8
diffuse (idiopathic) J84.1Ø
chemicals, gases, fumes or vapors (inhalation) J68.4

F

Fibrosis, fibrotic *(Continued)*
lung *(Continued)*
diffuse *(Continued)*
interstitial J84.10
acute J84.114
talc J62.0
following radiation J70.1
idiopathic J84.112
postinflammatory J84.10
silicotic J62.8
tuberculous —*see* Tuberculosis, pulmonary
lymphatic gland I89.8
median bar —*see* Hyperplasia, prostate
mediastinum (idiopathic) J98.59
meninges G96.19
myocardium, myocardial —*see* Myocarditis
ovary N83.8
oviduct N83.8
pancreas K86.89
penis NEC N48.6
pericardium I31.0
perineum, in pregnancy or childbirth O34.7-●
causing obstructed labor O65.5
pleura J94.1
popliteal fat pad M79.4
prostate (chronic) —*see* Hyperplasia, prostate
pulmonary —*see also* Fibrosis, lung J84.10
congenital P27.8
idiopathic J84.112
rectal sphincter K62.89
retroperitoneal, idiopathic (with ureteral obstruction) N13.5
with infection N13.6
sclerosing mesenteric (idiopathic) K65.4
scrotum N50.89
seminal vesicle N50.89
senile R54
skin L90.5
spermatic cord N50.89
spleen D73.89
in schistosomiasis (bilharziasis) B65.9 *[D77]*
subepidermal nodular —*see* Neoplasm, skin, benign
submucous (oral) (tongue) K13.5
testis N44.8
chronic, due to syphilis A52.76
thymus (gland) E32.8
tongue, submucous K13.5
tunica vaginalis N50.89
uterus (non-neoplastic) N85.8
vagina N89.8
valve, heart —*see* Endocarditis
vas deferens N50.89
vein I87.8
Fibrositis (periarticular) M79.7
nodular, chronic (Jaccoud's) (rheumatoid) —*see* Arthropathy, postrheumatic, chronic
Fibrothorax J94.1
Fibrotic —*see* Fibrosis
Fibrous —*see* condition
Fibroxanthoma —*see also* Neoplasm, connective tissue, benign
atypical —*see* Neoplasm, connective tissue, uncertain behavior
malignant —*see* Neoplasm, connective tissue, malignant
Fibroxanthosarcoma —*see* Neoplasm, connective tissue, malignant
Fiedler's
disease (icterohemorrhagic leptospirosis) A27.0
myocarditis (acute) I40.1
Fifth disease B08.3
venereal A55
Filaria, filarial, filariasis —*see* Infestation, filarial
Filatov's disease —*see* Mononucleosis, infectious
File-cutter's disease —*see* Poisoning, lead
Filling defect
biliary tract R93.2
bladder R93.41
duodenum R93.3
Filling defect *(Continued)*
gallbladder R93.2
gastrointestinal tract R93.3
intestine R93.3
kidney R93.42-●
stomach R93.3
ureter R93.41
urinary organs, specified NEC R93.49
Fimbrial cyst Q50.4
Financial problem affecting care NOS Z59.9
bankruptcy Z59.8
foreclosure on loan Z59.8
Findings, abnormal, inconclusive, without diagnosis —*see also* Abnormal
17-ketosteroids, elevated R82.5
acetonuria R82.4
alcohol in blood R78.0
anisocytosis R71.8
antenatal screening of mother O28.9
biochemical O28.1
chromosomal O28.5
cytological O28.2
genetic O28.5
hematological O28.0
radiological O28.4
specified NEC O28.8
ultrasonic O28.3
antibody titer, elevated R76.0
anticardiolipin antibody R76.0
antiphosphatidylglycerol antibody R76.0
antiphosphatidylinositol antibody R76.0
antiphosphatidylserine antibody R76.0
antiphospholipid antibody R76.0
bacteriuria R82.71
bicarbonate E87.8
bile in urine R82.2
blood sugar R73.09
high R73.9
low (transient) E16.2
body fluid or substance, specified NEC R88.8
casts, urine R82.998
catecholamines R82.5
cells, urine R82.998
chloride E87.8
cholesterol E78.9
high E78.00
with high triglycerides E78.2
chyluria R82.0
cloudy
dialysis effluent R88.0
urine R82.90
creatinine clearance R94.4
crystals, urine R82.998
culture
blood R78.81
positive —*see* Positive, culture
echocardiogram R93.1
electrolyte level, urinary R82.998
function study NEC R94.8
bladder R94.8
endocrine NEC R94.7
thyroid R94.6
kidney R94.4
liver R94.5
pancreas R94.8
placenta R94.8
pulmonary R94.2
spleen R94.8
gallbladder, nonvisualization R93.2
glucose (tolerance test) (non-fasting) R73.09
glycosuria R81
heart
shadow R93.1
sounds R01.2
hematinuria R82.3
hematocrit drop (precipitous) R71.0
hemoglobinuria R82.3
human papillomavirus (HPV) DNA test positive
cervix
high risk R87.810
low risk R87.820
Findings, abnormal, inconclusive, without diagnosis *(Continued)*
human papillomavirus (HPV) DNA test positive *(Continued)*
vagina
high risk R87.811
low risk R87.821
in blood (of substance not normally found in blood) R78.9
addictive drug NEC R78.4
alcohol (excessive level) R78.0
cocaine R78.2
hallucinogen R78.3
heavy metals (abnormal level) R78.79
lead R78.71
lithium (abnormal level) R78.89
opiate drug R78.1
psychotropic drug R78.5
specified substance NEC R78.89
steroid agent R78.6
indoleacetic acid, elevated R82.5
ketonuria R82.4
lactic acid dehydrogenase (LDH) R74.0
liver function test R79.89
mammogram NEC R92.8
calcification (calculus) R92.1
inconclusive result (due to dense breasts) R92.2
microcalcification R92.0
mediastinal shift R93.89
melanin, urine R82.998
myoglobinuria R82.1
neonatal screening P09
nonvisualization of gallbladder R93.2
odor of urine NOS R82.90
Papanicolaou cervix R87.619
non-atypical endometrial cells R87.618
pneumoencephalogram R93.0
poikilocytosis R71.8
potassium (deficiency) E87.6
excess E87.5
PPD R76.11
radiologic (X-ray) R93.89
abdomen R93.5
biliary tract R93.2
breast R92.8
gastrointestinal tract R93.3
genitourinary organs R93.89
head R93.0
inconclusive due to excess body fat of patient R93.9
intrathoracic organs NEC R93.1
▶musculoskeletal
▶limbs R93.6
▶other than limb R93.7
placenta R93.89
retroperitoneum R93.5
skin R93.89
skull R93.0
subcutaneous tissue R93.89
testis R93.81-●
red blood cell (count) (morphology) (sickling) (volume) R71.8
scan NEC R94.8
bladder R94.8
bone R94.8
kidney R94.4
liver R93.2
lung R94.2
pancreas R94.8
placental R94.8
spleen R94.8
thyroid R94.6
sedimentation rate, elevated R70.0
SGOT R74.0
SGPT R74.0
sodium (deficiency) E87.1
excess E87.0
specified body fluid NEC R88.8
stress test R94.39
thyroid (function) (metabolic rate) (scan) (uptake) R94.6

F

Findings, abnormal, inconclusive, without diagnosis *(Continued)*
transaminase (level) R74.0
triglycerides E78.9
high E78.1
with high cholesterol E78.2
tuberculin skin test (without active tuberculosis) R76.11
urine R82.90
acetone R82.4
bacteria R82.71
bile R82.2
casts or cells R82.998
chyle R82.0
culture positive R82.79
glucose R81
hemoglobin R82.3
ketone R82.4
sugar R81
vanillylmandelic acid (VMA), elevated R82.5
vectorcardiogram (VCG) R94.39
ventriculogram R93.0
white blood cell (count) (differential) (morphology) D72.9
xerography R92.8
Finger —*see* condition
Fire, Saint Anthony's —*see* Erysipelas
Fire-setting
pathological (compulsive) F63.1
Fish hook stomach K31.89
Fishmeal-worker's lung J67.8
Fissure, fissured
anus, anal K60.2
acute K60.0
chronic K60.1
congenital Q43.8
ear, lobule, congenital Q17.8
epiglottis (congenital) Q31.8
larynx J38.7
congenital Q31.8
lip K13.0
congenital —*see* Cleft, lip
nipple N64.0
associated with
lactation O92.13
pregnancy O92.11-●
puerperium O92.12
nose Q30.2
palate (congenital) —*see* Cleft, palate
skin R23.4
spine (congenital) —*see also* Spina bifida
with hydrocephalus —*see* Spina bifida, by site, with hydrocephalus
tongue (acquired) K14.5
congenital Q38.3
Fistula (cutaneous) L98.8
abdomen (wall) K63.2
bladder N32.2
intestine NEC K63.2
ureter N28.89
uterus N82.5
abdominorectal K63.2
abdominosigmoidal K63.2
abdominothoracic J86.0
abdominouterine N82.5
congenital Q51.7
abdominovesical N32.2
accessory sinuses —*see* Sinusitis
actinomycotic —*see* Actinomycosis
alveolar antrum —*see* Sinusitis, maxillary
alveolar process K04.6
anorectal K60.5
antrobuccal —*see* Sinusitis, maxillary
antrum —*see* Sinusitis, maxillary
anus, anal (recurrent) (infectional) K60.3
congenital Q43.6
with absence, atresia and stenosis Q42.2
tuberculous A18.32
aorta-duodenal I77.2
appendix, appendicular K38.3

Fistula *(Continued)*
arteriovenous (acquired) (nonruptured) I77.0
brain I67.1
congenital Q28.2
➡ruptured —*see* Fistula, arteriovenous, brain, ruptured
ruptured I60.8
▶intracerebral I61.8
▶intraparenchymal I61.8
▶intraventricular I61.5
▶subarachnoid I60.8
cerebral —*see* Fistula, arteriovenous, brain
congenital (peripheral) —*see also* Malformation, arteriovenous
brain Q28.2
➡ruptured —*see* Fistula, arteriovenous, brain, ruptured
coronary Q24.5
pulmonary Q25.72
coronary I25.41
congenital Q24.5
pulmonary I28.0
congenital Q25.72
surgically created (for dialysis) Z99.2
complication —*see* Complication, arteriovenous, fistula, surgically created
traumatic —*see* Injury, blood vessel
artery I77.2
aural (mastoid) —*see* Mastoiditis, chronic
auricle —*see also* Disorder, pinna, specified type NEC
congenital Q18.1
Bartholin's gland N82.8
bile duct (common) (hepatic) K83.3
with calculus, stones —*see* Calculus, bile duct
biliary (tract) —*see* Fistula, bile duct
bladder (sphincter) NEC —*see also* Fistula, vesico- N32.2
into seminal vesicle N32.2
bone —*see also* Disorder, bone, specified type NEC
with osteomyelitis, chronic —*see* Osteomyelitis, chronic, with draining sinus
brain G93.89
➡arteriovenous (acquired) (*see* Fistula, arteriovenous, brain) I67.1
congenital Q28.2
branchial (cleft) Q18.0
branchiogenous Q18.0
breast N61.0
puerperal, postpartum or gestational, due to mastitis (purulent) —*see* Mastitis, obstetric, purulent
bronchial J86.0
bronchocutaneous, bronchomediastinal, bronchopleural, bronchopleuromediastinal (infective) J86.0
tuberculous NEC A15.5
bronchoesophageal J86.0
congenital Q39.2
with atresia of esophagus Q39.1
bronchovisceral J86.0
buccal cavity (infective) K12.2
cecosigmoidal K63.2
cecum K63.2
cerebrospinal (fluid) G96.0
cervical, lateral Q18.1
cervicoaural Q18.1
cervicosigmoidal N82.4
cervicovesical N82.1
cervix N82.8
chest (wall) J86.0
cholecystenteric —*see* Fistula, gallbladder
cholecystocolic —*see* Fistula, gallbladder
cholecystocolonic —*see* Fistula, gallbladder
cholecystoduodenal —*see* Fistula, gallbladder
cholecystogastric —*see* Fistula, gallbladder
cholecystointestinal —*see* Fistula, gallbladder
choledochoduodenal —*see* Fistula, bile duct
cholocolic K82.3

Fistula *(Continued)*
coccyx —*see* Sinus, pilonidal
colon K63.2
colostomy K94.09
▶colovesical N32.1
common duct —*see* Fistula, bile duct
congenital, site not listed —*see* Anomaly, by site
coronary, arteriovenous I25.41
congenital Q24.5
costal region J86.0
cul-de-sac, Douglas' N82.8
cystic duct —*see also* Fistula, gallbladder
congenital Q44.5
dental K04.6
diaphragm J86.0
duodenum K31.6
ear (external) (canal) —*see* Disorder, ear, external, specified type NEC
enterocolic K63.2
enterocutaneous K63.2
enterouterine N82.4
congenital Q51.7
enterovaginal N82.4
congenital Q52.2
large intestine N82.3
small intestine N82.2
enterovesical N32.1
epididymis N50.89
tuberculous A18.15
esophagobronchial J86.0
congenital Q39.2
with atresia of esophagus Q39.1
esophagocutaneous K22.8
esophagopleural-cutaneous J86.0
esophagotracheal J86.0
congenital Q39.2
with atresia of esophagus Q39.1
esophagus K22.8
congenital Q39.2
with atresia of esophagus Q39.1
ethmoid —*see* Sinusitis, ethmoidal
eyeball (cornea) (sclera) —*see* Disorder, globe, hypotony
eyelid H01.8
fallopian tube, external N82.5
fecal K63.2
congenital Q43.6
from periapical abscess K04.6
frontal sinus —*see* Sinusitis, frontal
gallbladder K82.3
with calculus, cholelithiasis, stones —*see* Calculus, gallbladder
gastric K31.6
gastrocolic K31.6
congenital Q40.2
tuberculous A18.32
gastroenterocolic K31.6
gastroesophageal K31.6
gastrojejunal K31.6
gastrojejunocolic K31.6
genital tract (female) N82.9
specified NEC N82.8
to intestine NEC N82.4
to skin N82.5
hepatic artery-portal vein, congenital Q26.6
hepatopleural J86.0
hepatopulmonary J86.0
ileorectal or ileosigmoidal K63.2
ileovaginal N82.2
ileovesical N32.1
ileum K63.2
in ano K60.3
tuberculous A18.32
inner ear (labyrinth) —*see* subcategory H83.1
intestine NEC K63.2
intestinocolonic (abdominal) K63.2
intestinoureteral N28.89
intestinouterine N82.4
intestinovaginal N82.4
large intestine N82.3
small intestine N82.2

F

Fistula *(Continued)*
  intestinovesical N32.1
  ischiorectal (fossa) K61.39
  jejunum K63.2
  joint M25.1Ø
    ankle M25.17-●
    elbow M25.12-●
    foot joint M25.17-●
    hand joint M25.14-●
    hip M25.15-●
    knee M25.16-●
    shoulder M25.11-●
    specified joint NEC M25.18
    tuberculous —*see* Tuberculosis, joint
    vertebrae M25.18
    wrist M25.13-●
  kidney N28.89
  labium (majus) (minus) N82.8
  labyrinth —*see* subcategory H83.1
  lacrimal (gland) (sac) HØ4.61-●
  lacrimonasal duct —*see* Fistula, lacrimal
  laryngotracheal, congenital Q34.8
  larynx J38.7
  lip K13.Ø
    congenital Q38.Ø
  lumbar, tuberculous A18.Ø1
  lung J86.Ø
  lymphatic I89.8
  mammary (gland) N61.Ø
  mastoid (process) (region) —*see* Mastoiditis, chronic
  maxillary J32.Ø
  medial, face and neck Q18.8
  mediastinal J86.Ø
  mediastinobronchial J86.Ø
  mediastinocutaneous J86.Ø
  middle ear —*see* subcategory H74.8
  mouth K12.2
  nasal J34.89
    sinus —*see* Sinusitis
  nasopharynx J39.2
  nipple N64.Ø
  nose J34.89
  oral (cutaneous) K12.2
    maxillary J32.Ø
    nasal (with cleft palate) —*see* Cleft, palate
  orbit, orbital —*see* Disorder, orbit, specified type NEC
  oroantral J32.Ø
  oviduct, external N82.5
  palate (hard) M27.8
  pancreatic K86.89
  pancreaticoduodenal K86.89
  parotid (gland) K11.4
    region K12.2
  penis N48.89
  perianal K6Ø.3
  pericardium (pleura) (sac) —*see* Pericarditis
  pericecal K63.2
  perineorectal K6Ø.4 perineosigmoidal K63.2
  perineosigmoidal K63.2
  perineum, perineal (with urethral involvement) NEC N36.Ø
    tuberculous A18.13
    ureter N28.89
  perirectal K6Ø.4
    tuberculous A18.32
  peritoneum K65.9
  pharyngoesophageal J39.2
  pharynx J39.2
    branchial cleft (congenital) Q18.Ø
  pilonidal (infected) (rectum) —*see* Sinus, pilonidal
  pleura, pleural, pleurocutaneous, pleuroperitoneal J86.Ø
    tuberculous NEC A15.6
  pleuropericardial I31.8
  portal vein-hepatic artery, congenital Q26.6
  postauricular H7Ø.81-●
  postoperative, persistent T81.83
    specified site —*see* Fistula, by site

Fistula *(Continued)*
  preauricular (congenital) Q18.1
  prostate N42.89
  pulmonary J86.Ø
    arteriovenous I28.Ø
      congenital Q25.72
    tuberculous —*see* Tuberculosis, pulmonary
  pulmonoperitoneal J86.Ø
  rectolabial N82.4
  rectosigmoid (intercommunicating) K63.2
  rectoureteral N28.89
  rectourethral N36.Ø
    congenital Q64.73
  rectouterine N82.4
    congenital Q51.7
  rectovaginal N82.3
    congenital Q52.2
    tuberculous A18.18
  rectovesical N32.1
    congenital Q64.79
  rectovesicovaginal N82.3
  rectovulval N82.4
    congenital Q52.79
  rectum (to skin) K6Ø.4
    congenital Q43.6
      with absence, atresia and stenosis Q42.Ø
    tuberculous A18.32
  renal N28.89
  retroauricular —*see* Fistula, postauricular
  salivary duct or gland (any) K11.4
    congenital Q38.4
  scrotum (urinary) N5Ø.89
    tuberculous A18.15
  semicircular canals —*see* subcategory H83.1
  sigmoid K63.2
    to bladder N32.1
  sinus —*see* Sinusitis
  skin L98.8
    to genital tract (female) N82.5
  splenocolic D73.89
  stercoral K63.2
  stomach K31.6
  sublingual gland K11.4
  submandibular gland K11.4
  submaxillary (gland) K11.4
    region K12.2
  thoracic J86.Ø
    duct I89.8
  thoracoabdominal J86.Ø
  thoracogastric J86.Ø
  thoracointestinal J86.Ø
  thorax J86.Ø
  thyroglossal duct Q89.2
  thyroid EØ7.89
  trachea, congenital (external) (internal) Q32.1
  tracheoesophageal J86.Ø
    congenital Q39.2
      with atresia of esophagus Q39.1
    following tracheostomy J95.Ø4
  traumatic arteriovenous —*see* Injury, blood vessel, by site
  tuberculous - code by site under Tuberculosis
  typhoid AØ1.Ø9
  umbilicourinary Q64.8
  urachus, congenital Q64.4
  ureter (persistent) N28.89
  ureteroabdominal N28.89
  ureterorectal N28.89
  ureterosigmoido-abdominal N28.89
  ureterovaginal N82.1
  ureterovesical N32.2
  urethra N36.Ø
    congenital Q64.79
    tuberculous A18.13
  urethroperineal N36.Ø
  urethroperineovesical N32.2
  urethrorectal N36.Ø
    congenital Q64.73
  urethroscrotal N5Ø.89
  urethrovaginal N82.1
  urethrovesical N32.2

Fistula *(Continued)*
  urinary (tract) (persistent) (recurrent) N36.Ø
  uteroabdominal N82.5
    congenital Q51.7
  uteroenteric, uterointestinal N82.4
    congenital Q51.7
  uterorectal N82.4
    congenital Q51.7
  uteroureteric N82.1
  uterourethral Q51.7
  uterovaginal N82.8
  uterovesical N82.1
    congenital Q51.7
  uterus N82.8
  vagina (postpartal) (wall) N82.8
  vaginocutaneous (postpartal) N82.5
  vaginointestinal NEC N82.4
    large intestine N82.3
    small intestine N82.2
  vaginoperineal N82.5
  vasocutaneous, congenital Q55.7
  vesical NEC N32.2
  vesicoabdominal N32.2
  vesicocervicovaginal N82.1
  vesicocolic N32.1
  vesicocutaneous N32.2
  vesicoenteric N32.1
  vesicointestinal N32.1
  vesicometrorectal N82.4
  vesicoperineal N32.2
  vesicorectal N32.1
    congenital Q64.79
  vesicosigmoidal N32.1
  vesicosigmoidovaginal N82.3
  vesicoureteral N32.2
  vesicoureterovaginal N82.1
  vesicourethral N32.2
  vesicourethrorectal N32.1
  vesicouterine N82.1
    congenital Q51.7
  vesicovaginal N82.Ø
  vulvorectal N82.4
    congenital Q52.79
Fit R56.9
  epileptic —*see* Epilepsy
  fainting R55
  hysterical F44.5
  newborn P9Ø
Fitting (and adjustment) (of)
  artificial
    arm —*see* Admission, adjustment, artificial, arm
    breast Z44.3
    eye Z44.2
    leg —*see* Admission, adjustment, artificial, leg
  automatic implantable cardiac defibrillator (with synchronous cardiac pacemaker) Z45.Ø2
  brain neuropacemaker Z46.2
    implanted Z45.42
  cardiac defibrillator —*see* Fitting (and adjustment) (of), automatic implantable cardiac defibrillator
  catheter, non-vascular Z46.82
  colostomy belt Z46.89
  contact lenses Z46.Ø
  CRT-D (resynchronization therapy defibrillator) Z45.Ø2
  CRT-P (cardiac resynchronization therapy pacemaker) Z45.Ø18
    pulse generator Z45.Ø1Ø
  cystostomy device Z46.6
  defibrillator, cardiac —*see* Fitting (and adjustment) (of), automatic implantable cardiac defibrillator
  dentures Z46.3
  device NOS Z46.9
    abdominal Z46.89
    gastrointestinal NEC Z46.59
    implanted NEC Z45.89

Fitting *(Continued)*
device NOS *(Continued)*
nervous system Z46.2
implanted —*see* Admission, adjustment, device, implanted, nervous system
orthodontic Z46.4
orthoptic Z46.Ø
orthotic Z46.89
prosthetic (external) Z44.9
breast Z44.3
dental Z46.3
eye Z44.2
specified NEC Z44.8
specified NEC Z46.89
substitution
auditory Z46.2
implanted —*see* Admission, adjustment, device, implanted, hearing device
nervous system Z46.2
implanted —*see* Admission, adjustment, device, implanted, nervous system
visual Z46.2
implanted Z45.31
urinary Z46.6
gastric lap band Z46.51
gastrointestinal appliance NEC Z46.59
glasses (reading) Z46.Ø
hearing aid Z46.1
ileostomy device Z46.89
insulin pump Z46.81
intestinal appliance NEC Z46.89
myringotomy device (stent) (tube) Z45.82
neuropacemaker Z46.2
implanted Z45.42
non-vascular catheter Z46.82
orthodontic device Z46.4
orthopedic device (brace) (cast) (corset) (shoes) Z46.89
pacemaker (cardiac) (cardiac resynchronization therapy (CRT-P)) Z45.Ø18
nervous system (brain) (peripheral nerve) (spinal cord) Z46.2
implanted Z45.42
pulse generator Z45.Ø1Ø
portacath (port-a-cath) Z45.2
prosthesis (external) Z44.9
arm —*see* Admission, adjustment, artificial, arm
breast Z44.3
dental Z46.3
eye Z44.2
leg —*see* Admission, adjustment, artificial, leg
specified NEC Z44.8
spectacles Z46.Ø
wheelchair Z46.89
Fitzhugh-Curtis syndrome
due to
Chlamydia trachomatis A74.81
Neisseria gonorrhorea (gonococcal peritonitis) A54.85
Fitz's syndrome (acute hemorrhagic pancreatitis) —*see also* Pancreatitis, acute K85.8Ø
Fixation
joint —*see* Ankylosis
larynx J38.7
stapes —*see* Ankylosis, ear ossicles
deafness —*see* Deafness, conductive
uterus (acquired) —*see* Malposition, uterus
vocal cord J38.3
Flabby ridge KØ6.8
Flaccid —*see also* condition
palate, congenital Q38.5
Flail
chest S22.5- •
newborn (birth injury) P13.8
Flail *(Continued)*
joint (paralytic) M25.2Ø
ankle M25.27- •
elbow M25.22- •
foot joint M25.27- •
hand joint M25.24- •
hip M25.25- •
knee M25.26- •
shoulder M25.21- •
specified joint NEC M25.28
wrist M25.23- •
Flajani's disease —*see* Hyperthyroidism, with, goiter (diffuse)
Flap, liver K71.3
Flashbacks (residual to hallucinogen use) F16.283
Flat
chamber (eye) —*see* Disorder, globe, hypotony, flat anterior chamber
chest, congenital Q67.8
foot (acquired) (fixed type) (painful) (postural) —*see also* Deformity, limb, flat foot
congenital (rigid) (spastic (everted)) Q66.5- •
rachitic sequelae (late effect) E64.3
organ or site, congenital NEC —*see* Anomaly, by site
pelvis M95.5
with disproportion (fetopelvic) O33.Ø
causing obstructed labor O65.Ø
congenital Q74.2
Flatau-Schilder disease G37.Ø
Flatback syndrome M4Ø.3Ø
lumbar region M4Ø.36
lumbosacral region M4Ø.37
thoracolumbar region M4Ø.35
Flattening
head, femur M89.8X5
hip —*see* Coxa, plana
lip (congenital) Q18.8
nose (congenital) Q67.4
acquired M95.Ø
Flatulence R14.3
psychogenic F45.8
Flatus R14.3
vaginalis N89.8
Flax-dresser's disease J66.1
Flea bite —*see* Injury, bite, by site, superficial, insect
Flecks, glaucomatous (subcapsular) —*see* Cataract, complicated
Fleischer (-Kayser) ring (cornea) H18.Ø4- •
Fleshy mole OØ2.Ø
Flexibilitas cerea —*see* Catalepsy
Flexion
amputation stump (surgical) T87.89
cervix —*see* Malposition, uterus
contracture, joint —*see* Contraction, joint
deformity, joint —*see also* Deformity, limb, flexion M21.2Ø
hip, congenital Q65.89
uterus —*see also* Malposition, uterus
lateral —*see* Lateroversion, uterus
Flexner-Boyd dysentery AØ3.2
Flexner's dysentery AØ3.1
Flexure —*see* Flexion
Flint murmur (aortic insufficiency) I35.1
Floater, vitreous —*see* Opacity, vitreous
Floating
cartilage (joint) —*see also* Loose, body, joint
knee —*see* Derangement, knee, loose body
gallbladder, congenital Q44.1
kidney N28.89
congenital Q63.8
spleen D73.89
Flooding N92.Ø
Floor —*see* condition
Floppy
baby syndrome (nonspecific) P94.2
iris syndrome (intraoperative) (IFIS) H21.81
nonrheumatic mitral valve syndrome I34.1
Flu —*see also* Influenza
avian —*see also* Influenza, due to, identified novel influenza A virus JØ9.X2
bird —*see also* Influenza, due to, identified novel influenza A virus JØ9.X2
intestinal NEC AØ8.4
swine (viruses that normally cause infections in pigs) —*see also* Influenza, due to, identified novel influenza A virus JØ9.X2
Fluctuating blood pressure I99.8
Fluid
abdomen R18.8
chest J94.8
heart —*see* Failure, heart, congestive
joint —*see* Effusion, joint
loss (acute) E86.9
lung —*see* Edema, lung
overload E87.7Ø
specified NEC E87.79
peritoneal cavity R18.8
pleural cavity J94.8
retention R6Ø.9
Flukes NEC —*see also* Infestation, fluke
blood NEC —*see* Schistosomiasis
liver B66.3
Fluor (vaginalis) N89.8
trichomonal or due to Trichomonas (vaginalis) A59.ØØ
Fluorosis
dental KØØ.3
skeletal M85.1Ø
ankle M85.17- •
foot M85.17- •
forearm M85.13- •
hand M85.14- •
lower leg M85.16- •
multiple site M85.19
neck M85.18
rib M85.18
shoulder M85.11- •
skull M85.18
specified site NEC M85.18
thigh M85.15- •
toe M85.17- •
upper arm M85.12- •
vertebra M85.18
Flush syndrome E34.Ø
Flushing R23.2
menopausal N95.1
Flutter
atrial or auricular I48.92
atypical I48.4
type I I48.3
type II I48.4
typical I48.3
heart I49.8
atrial or auricular I48.92
atypical I48.4
type I I48.3
type II I48.4
typical I48.3
ventricular I49.Ø2
ventricular I49.Ø2
FNHTR (febrile nonhemolytic transfusion reaction) R5Ø.84
Fochier's abscess - code by site under Abscess
Focus, Assmann's —*see* Tuberculosis, pulmonary
Fogo selvagem L1Ø.3
Foix-Alajouanine syndrome G95.19
Fold, folds (anomalous) —*see also* Anomaly, by site
Descemet's membrane —*see* Change, corneal membrane, Descemet's, fold
epicanthic Q1Ø.3
heart Q24.8
Folie à deux F24
Follicle
cervix (nabothian) (ruptured) N88.8
graafian, ruptured, with hemorrhage N83.Ø- •
nabothian N88.8
Follicular —*see* condition

F

Folliculitis (superficial) L73.9
abscedens et suffodiens L66.3
cyst N83.Ø-●
decalvans L66.2
deep —*see* Furuncle, by site
gonococcal (acute) (chronic) A54.Ø1
keloid, keloidalis L73.Ø
pustular LØ1.Ø2
ulerythematosa reticulata L66.4
Folliculome lipidique
specified site —*see* Neoplasm, benign, by site
unspecified site
female D27.9
male D29.2Ø
Følling's disease E7Ø.Ø
Follow-up —*see* Examination, follow-up
Fong's syndrome (hereditary osteo-onychodysplasia) Q87.2
Food
allergy L27.2
asphyxia (from aspiration or inhalation) —*see* Foreign body, by site
choked on —*see* Foreign body, by site
deprivation T73.Ø
specified kind of food NEC E63.8
intoxication —*see* Poisoning, food
lack of T73.Ø
poisoning —*see* Poisoning, food
rejection NEC —*see* Disorder, eating
strangulation or suffocation —*see* Foreign body, by site
toxemia —*see* Poisoning, food
Foot —*see* condition
Foramen ovale (nonclosure) (patent) (persistent) Q21.1
Forbes' glycogen storage disease E74.Ø3
Fordyce-Fox disease L75.2
Fordyce's disease (mouth) Q38.6
Forearm —*see* condition
Foreign body
with
laceration —*see* Laceration, by site, with foreign body
puncture wound —*see* Puncture, by site, with foreign body
accidentally left following a procedure T81.5Ø9
aspiration T81.5Ø6
resulting in
adhesions T81.516
obstruction T81.526
perforation T81.536
specified complication NEC T81.596
cardiac catheterization T81.5Ø5
resulting in
acute reaction T81.6Ø
aseptic peritonitis T81.61
specified NEC T81.69
adhesions T81.515
obstruction T81.525
perforation T81.535
specified complication NEC T81.595
causing
acute reaction T81.6Ø
aseptic peritonitis T81.61
specified complication NEC T81.69
adhesions T81.519
aseptic peritonitis T81.61
obstruction T81.529
perforation T81.539
specified complication NEC T81.599
endoscopy T81.5Ø4
resulting in
adhesions T81.514
obstruction T81.524
perforation T81.534
specified complication NEC T81.594

Foreign body *(Continued)*
accidentally left following a procedure *(Continued)*
immunization T81.5Ø3
resulting in
adhesions T81.513
obstruction T81.523
perforation T81.533
specified complication NEC T81.593
infusion T81.5Ø1
resulting in
adhesions T81.511
obstruction T81.521
perforation T81.531
specified complication NEC T81.591
injection T81.5Ø3
resulting in
adhesions T81.513
obstruction T81.523
perforation T81.533
specified complication NEC T81.593
kidney dialysis T81.5Ø2
resulting in
adhesions T81.512
obstruction T81.522
perforation T81.532
specified complication NEC T81.592
packing removal T81.5Ø7
resulting in
acute reaction T81.6Ø
aseptic peritonitis T81.61
specified NEC T81.69
adhesions T81.517
obstruction T81.527
perforation T81.537
specified complication NEC T81.597
puncture T81.5Ø6
resulting in
adhesions T81.516
obstruction T81.526
perforation T81.536
specified complication NEC T81.596
specified procedure NEC T81.5Ø8
resulting in
acute reaction T81.6Ø
aseptic peritonitis T81.61
specified NEC T81.69
adhesions T81.518
obstruction T81.528
perforation T81.538
specified complication NEC T81.598
surgical operation T81.5ØØ
resulting in
acute reaction T81.6Ø
aseptic peritonitis T81.61
specified NEC T81.69
adhesions T81.51Ø
obstruction T81.52Ø
perforation T81.53Ø
specified complication NEC T81.59Ø
transfusion T81.5Ø1
resulting in
adhesions T81.511
obstruction T81.521
perforation T81.531
specified complication NEC T81.591
alimentary tract T18.9
anus T18.5
colon T18.4
esophagus —*see* Foreign body, esophagus
mouth T18.Ø
multiple sites T18.8
rectosigmoid (junction) T18.5
rectum T18.5
small intestine T18.3
specified site NEC T18.8
stomach T18.2
anterior chamber (eye) SØ5.5-●
auditory canal —*see* Foreign body, entering through orifice, ear

Foreign body *(Continued)*
bronchus T17.5Ø8
causing
asphyxiation T17.5ØØ
food (bone) (seed) T17.52Ø
gastric contents (vomitus) T17.51Ø
specified type NEC T17.59Ø
injury NEC T17.5Ø8
food (bone) (seed) T17.528
gastric contents (vomitus) T17.518
specified type NEC T17.598
canthus —*see* Foreign body, conjunctival sac
ciliary body (eye) SØ5.5-●
conjunctival sac T15.1-●
cornea T15.Ø-●
entering through orifice
accessory sinus T17.Ø
alimentary canal T18.9
multiple parts T18.8
specified part NEC T18.8
alveolar process T18.Ø
antrum (Highmore's) T17.Ø
anus T18.5
appendix T18.4
auditory canal —*see* Foreign body, entering through orifice, ear
auricle —*see* Foreign body, entering through orifice, ear
bladder T19.1
bronchioles —*see* Foreign body, respiratory tract, specified site NEC
bronchus (main) —*see* Foreign body, bronchus
buccal cavity T18.Ø
canthus (inner) —*see* Foreign body, conjunctival sac
cecum T18.4
cervix (canal) (uteri) T19.3
colon T18.4
conjunctival sac —*see* Foreign body, conjunctival sac
cornea —*see* Foreign body, cornea
digestive organ or tract NOS T18.9
multiple parts T18.8
specified part NEC T18.8
duodenum T18.3
ear (external) T16.-●
esophagus —*see* Foreign body, esophagus
eye (external) NOS T15.9-●
conjunctival sac —*see* Foreign body, conjunctival sac
cornea —*see* Foreign body, cornea
specified part NEC T15.8-●
eyeball —*see also* Foreign body, entering through orifice, eye, specified part NEC
with penetrating wound —*see* Puncture, eyeball
eyelid —*see also* Foreign body, conjunctival sac
with
laceration —*see* Laceration, eyelid, with foreign body
puncture —*see* Puncture, eyelid, with foreign body
superficial injury —*see* Foreign body, superficial, eyelid
gastrointestinal tract T18.9
multiple parts T18.8
specified part NEC T18.8
genitourinary tract T19.9
multiple parts T19.8
specified part NEC T19.8
globe —*see* Foreign body, entering through orifice, eyeball
gum T18.Ø
Highmore's antrum T17.Ø
hypopharynx —*see* Foreign body, pharynx
ileum T18.3
intestine (small) T18.3
large T18.4

- Foreign body *(Continued)*
  - entering through orifice *(Continued)*
    - lacrimal apparatus (punctum) —*see* Foreign body, entering through orifice, eye, specified part NEC
    - large intestine T18.4
    - larynx —*see* Foreign body, larynx
    - lung —*see* Foreign body, respiratory tract, specified site NEC
    - maxillary sinus T17.0
    - mouth T18.0
    - nasal sinus T17.0
    - nasopharynx —*see* Foreign body, pharynx
    - nose (passage) T17.1
    - nostril T17.1
    - oral cavity T18.0
    - palate T18.0
    - penis T19.4
    - pharynx —*see* Foreign body, pharynx
    - piriform sinus —*see* Foreign body, pharynx
    - rectosigmoid (junction) T18.5
    - rectum T18.5
    - respiratory tract —*see* Foreign body, respiratory tract
    - sinus (accessory) (frontal) (maxillary) (nasal) T17.0
      - piriform —*see* Foreign body, pharynx
    - small intestine T18.3
    - stomach T18.2
    - suffocation by —*see* Foreign body, by site
    - tear ducts or glands —*see* Foreign body, entering through orifice, eye, specified part NEC
    - throat —*see* Foreign body, pharynx
    - tongue T18.0
    - tonsil, tonsillar (fossa) —*see* Foreign body, pharynx
    - trachea —*see* Foreign body, trachea
    - ureter T19.8
    - urethra T19.0
    - uterus (any part) T19.3
    - vagina T19.2
    - vulva T19.2
  - esophagus T18.108
    - causing
      - injury NEC T18.108
        - food (bone) (seed) T18.128
        - gastric contents (vomitus) T18.118
        - specified type NEC T18.198
      - tracheal compression T18.100
        - food (bone) (seed) T18.120
        - gastric contents (vomitus) T18.110
        - specified type NEC T18.190
  - feeling of, in throat R09.89
  - fragment —*see* Retained, foreign body fragments (type of)
  - genitourinary tract T19.9
    - bladder T19.1
    - multiple parts T19.8
    - penis T19.4
    - specified site NEC T19.8
    - urethra T19.0
    - uterus T19.3
      - IUD Z97.5
    - vagina T19.2
      - contraceptive device Z97.5
    - vulva T19.2
  - granuloma (old) (soft tissue) —*see also* Granuloma, foreign body
    - skin L92.3
  - in
    - laceration —*see* Laceration, by site, with foreign body
    - puncture wound —*see* Puncture, by site, with foreign body
    - soft tissue (residual) M79.5
  - inadvertently left in operation wound —*see* Foreign body, accidentally left during a procedure
  - ingestion, ingested NOS T18.9
  - inhalation or inspiration —*see* Foreign body, by site
  - internal organ, not entering through a natural orifice - code as specific injury with foreign body
  - intraocular S05.5-●
    - old, retained (nonmagnetic) H44.70-●
      - anterior chamber H44.71-●
      - ciliary body H44.72-●
      - iris H44.72-●
      - lens H44.73-●
      - magnetic H44.60-●
        - anterior chamber H44.61-●
        - ciliary body H44.62-●
        - iris H44.62-●
        - lens H44.63-●
        - posterior wall H44.64-●
        - specified site NEC H44.69-●
        - vitreous body H44.65-●
      - posterior wall H44.74-●
      - specified site NEC H44.79-●
      - vitreous body H44.75-●
  - iris —*see* Foreign body, intraocular
  - lacrimal punctum —*see* Foreign body, entering through orifice, eye, specified part NEC
  - larynx T17.308
    - causing
      - asphyxiation T17.300
        - food (bone) (seed) T17.320
        - gastric contents (vomitus) T17.310
        - specified type NEC T17.390
      - injury NEC T17.308
        - food (bone) (seed) T17.328
        - gastric contents (vomitus) T17.318
        - specified type NEC T17.398
  - lens —*see* Foreign body, intraocular
  - ocular muscle S05.4-●
    - old, retained —*see* Foreign body, orbit, old
  - old or residual
    - soft tissue (residual) M79.5
  - operation wound, left accidentally —*see* Foreign body, accidentally left during a procedure
  - orbit S05.4-●
    - old, retained H05.5-●
  - pharynx T17.208
    - causing
      - asphyxiation T17.200
        - food (bone) (seed) T17.220
        - gastric contents (vomitus) T17.210
        - specified type NEC T17.290
      - injury NEC T17.208
        - food (bone) (seed) T17.228
        - gastric contents (vomitus) T17.218
        - specified type NEC T17.298
  - respiratory tract T17.908
    - bronchioles —*see* Foreign body, respiratory tract, specified site NEC
    - bronchus —*see* Foreign body, bronchus
    - causing
      - asphyxiation T17.900
        - food (bone) (seed) T17.920
        - gastric contents (vomitus) T17.910
        - specified type NEC T17.990
      - injury NEC T17.908
        - food (bone) (seed) T17.928
        - gastric contents (vomitus) T17.918
        - specified type NEC T17.998
    - larynx —*see* Foreign body, larynx
    - lung —*see* Foreign body, respiratory tract, specified site NEC
    - multiple parts —*see* Foreign body, respiratory tract, specified site NEC
    - nasal sinus T17.0
    - nasopharynx —*see* Foreign body, pharynx
    - nose T17.1
    - nostril T17.1
    - pharynx —*see* Foreign body, pharynx
    - specified site NEC T17.808
      - causing
        - asphyxiation T17.800
          - food (bone) (seed) T17.820
          - gastric contents (vomitus) T17.810
          - specified type NEC T17.890
        - injury NEC T17.808
          - food (bone) (seed) T17.828
          - gastric contents (vomitus) T17.818
          - specified type NEC T17.898
    - throat —*see* Foreign body, pharynx
    - trachea —*see* Foreign body, trachea
  - retained (old) (nonmagnetic) (in)
    - anterior chamber (eye) —*see* Foreign body, intraocular, old, retained, anterior chamber
      - magnetic —*see* Foreign body, intraocular, old, retained, magnetic, anterior chamber
    - ciliary body —*see* Foreign body, intraocular, old, retained, ciliary body
      - magnetic —*see* Foreign body, intraocular, old, retained, magnetic, ciliary body
    - eyelid H02.819
      - left H02.816
        - lower H02.815
        - upper H02.814
      - right H02.813
        - lower H02.812
        - upper H02.811
    - fragments —*see* Retained, foreign body fragments (type of)
    - globe —*see* Foreign body, intraocular, old, retained
      - magnetic —*see* Foreign body, intraocular, old, retained, magnetic
    - intraocular —*see* Foreign body, intraocular, old, retained
      - magnetic —*see* Foreign body, intraocular, old, retained, magnetic
    - iris —*see* Foreign body, intraocular, old, retained, iris
      - magnetic —*see* Foreign body, intraocular, old, retained, magnetic, iris
    - lens —*see* Foreign body, intraocular, old, retained, lens
      - magnetic —*see* Foreign body, intraocular, old, retained, magnetic, lens
    - muscle —*see* Foreign body, retained, soft tissue
    - orbit —*see* Foreign body, orbit, old
    - posterior wall of globe —*see* Foreign body, intraocular, old, retained, posterior wall
      - magnetic —*see* Foreign body, intraocular, old, retained, magnetic, posterior wall
    - retrobulbar —*see* Foreign body, orbit, old, retrobulbar
    - soft tissue M79.5
    - vitreous —*see* Foreign body, intraocular, old, retained, vitreous body
      - magnetic —*see* Foreign body, intraocular, old, retained, magnetic, vitreous body
  - retina S05.5-●
  - superficial, without open wound
    - abdomen, abdominal (wall) S30.851
    - alveolar process S00.552
    - ankle S90.55-●
    - antecubital space —*see* Foreign body, superficial, forearm
    - anus S30.857
    - arm (upper) S40.85-●
    - auditory canal —*see* Foreign body, superficial, ear
    - auricle —*see* Foreign body, superficial, ear
    - axilla —*see* Foreign body, superficial, arm
    - back, lower S30.850

F

Foreign body *(Continued)*
  superficial, without open wound *(Continued)*
    breast S20.15-●
    brow S00.85
    buttock S30.850
    calf *—see* Foreign body, superficial, leg
    canthus *—see* Foreign body, superficial, eyelid
    cheek S00.85
      internal S00.552
    chest wall *—see* Foreign body, superficial, thorax
    chin S00.85
    clitoris S30.854
    costal region *—see* Foreign body, superficial, thorax
    digit(s)
      foot *—see* Foreign body, superficial, toe
      hand *—see* Foreign body, superficial, finger
    ear S00.45-●
    elbow S50.35-●
    epididymis S30.853
    epigastric region S30.851
    epiglottis S10.15
    esophagus, cervical S10.15
    eyebrow *—see* Foreign body, superficial, eyelid
    eyelid S00.25-●
    face S00.85
    finger(s) S60.459
      index S60.45-●
      little S60.45-●
      middle S60.45-●
      ring S60.45-●
    flank S30.851
    foot (except toe(s) alone) S90.85-●
      toe *—see* Foreign body, superficial, toe
    forearm S50.85-●
      elbow only *—see* Foreign body, superficial, elbow
    forehead S00.85
    genital organs, external
      female S30.856
      male S30.855
    groin S30.851
    gum S00.552
    hand S60.55-●
    head S00.95
      ear *—see* Foreign body, superficial, ear
      eyelid *—see* Foreign body, superficial, eyelid
      lip S00.551
      nose S00.35
      oral cavity S00.552
      scalp S00.05
      specified site NEC S00.85
    heel *—see* Foreign body, superficial, foot
    hip S70.25-●
    inguinal region S30.851
    interscapular region S20.459
    jaw S00.85
    knee S80.25-●
    labium (majus) (minus) S30.854
    larynx S10.15
    leg (lower) S80.85-●
      knee *—see* Foreign body, superficial, knee
      upper *—see* Foreign body, superficial, thigh
    lip S00.551
    lower back S30.850
    lumbar region S30.850
    malar region S00.85
    mammary *—see* Foreign body, superficial, breast
    mastoid region S00.85
    mouth S00.552
    nail
      finger *—see* Foreign body, superficial, finger
      toe *—see* Foreign body, superficial, toe
    nape S10.85

Foreign body *(Continued)*
  superficial, without open wound *(Continued)*
    nasal S00.35
    neck S10.95
      specified site NEC S10.85
      throat S10.15
    nose S00.35
    occipital region S00.05
    oral cavity S00.552
    orbital region *—see* Foreign body, superficial, eyelid
    palate S00.552
    palm *—see* Foreign body, superficial, hand
    parietal region S00.05
    pelvis S30.850
    penis S30.852
    perineum
      female S30.854
      male S30.850
    periocular area *—see* Foreign body, superficial, eyelid
    phalanges
      finger *—see* Foreign body, superficial, finger
      toe *—see* Foreign body, superficial, toe
    pharynx S10.15
    pinna *—see* Foreign body, superficial, ear
    popliteal space *—see* Foreign body, superficial, knee
    prepuce S30.852
    pubic region S30.850
    pudendum
      female S30.856
      male S30.855
    sacral region S30.850
    scalp S00.05
    scapular region *—see* Foreign body, superficial, shoulder
    scrotum S30.853
    shin *—see* Foreign body, superficial, leg
    shoulder S40.25-●
    sternal region S20.359
    submaxillary region S00.85
    submental region S00.85
    subungual
      finger(s) *—see* Foreign body, superficial, finger
      toe(s) *—see* Foreign body, superficial, toe
    supraclavicular fossa S10.85
    supraorbital S00.85
    temple S00.85
    temporal region S00.85
    testis S30.853
    thigh S70.35-●
    thorax, thoracic (wall) S20.95
      back S20.45-●
      front S20.35-●
    throat S10.15
    thumb S60.35-●
    toe(s) (lesser) S90.456
      great S90.45-●
    tongue S00.552
    trachea S10.15
    tunica vaginalis S30.853
    tympanum, tympanic membrane *—see* Foreign body, superficial, ear
    uvula S00.552
    vagina S30.854
    vocal cords S10.15
    vulva S30.854
    wrist S60.85-●
  swallowed T18.9
  trachea T17.408
    causing
      asphyxiation T17.400
        food (bone) (seed) T17.420
        gastric contents (vomitus) T17.410
        specified type NEC T17.490
      injury NEC T17.408
        food (bone) (seed) T17.428
        gastric contents (vomitus) T17.418
        specified type NEC T17.498

Foreign body *(Continued)*
  type of fragment *—see* Retained, foreign body fragments (type of)
  vitreous (humor) S05.5-●
Forestier's disease (rhizomelic pseudopolyarthritis) M35.3-●
  meaning ankylosing hyperostosis *—see* Hyperostosis, ankylosing
Formation
  hyalin in cornea *—see* Degeneration, cornea
  sequestrum in bone (due to infection) *—see* Osteomyelitis, chronic
  valve
    colon, congenital Q43.8
    ureter (congenital) Q62.39
Formication R20.2
Fort Bragg fever A27.89
Fossa *—see also* condition
  pyriform *—see* condition
Foster-Kennedy syndrome H47.14-●
Fothergill's
  disease (trigeminal neuralgia) *—see also* Neuralgia, trigeminal
    scarlatina anginosa A38.9
Foul breath R19.6
Foundling Z76.1
Fournier disease or gangrene N49.3
  female N76.89
Fourth
  cranial nerve *—see* condition
  molar K00.1
Foville's (peduncular) disease or syndrome G46.3
Fox (-Fordyce) disease (apocrine miliaria) L75.2
➠ **FPIES (food protein-induced enterocolitis syndrome)** K52.21
Fracture, burst *—see* Fracture, traumatic, by site
Fracture, chronic *—see* Fracture, pathological, by site
Fracture, insufficiency *—see* Fracture, pathological, by site
Fracture, nontraumatic, NEC
  atypical
    femur M84.750-●
      complete
        oblique M84.759
          left side M84.758
          right side M84.757
        transverse M84.756
          left side M84.755
          right side M84.754
      incomplete M84.753
        left side M84.752
        right side M84.751
Fracture, pathological (pathologic) *—see also* Fracture, traumatic M84.40
  ankle M84.47-●
  carpus M84.44-●
  clavicle M84.41-●
  compression (not due to trauma) *—see also* Collapse, vertebra M48.50-●
  dental implant M27.63
  dental restorative material K08.539
    with loss of material K08.531
    without loss of material K08.530
  due to
    neoplastic disease NEC *—see also* Neoplasm M84.50
      ankle M84.57-●
      carpus M84.54-●
      clavicle M84.51-●
      femur M84.55-●
      fibula M84.56-●
      finger M84.54-●
      hip M84.559
      humerus M84.52-●
      ilium M84.550
      ischium M84.550
      metacarpus M84.54-●
      metatarsus M84.57-●
      neck M84.58
      pelvis M84.550
      radius M84.53-●

Fracture, pathological *(Continued)*
due to *(Continued)*
neoplastic disease NEC *(Continued)*
rib M84.58
scapula M84.51-●
skull M84.58
specified site NEC M84.58
tarsus M84.57-●
tibia M84.56-●
toe M84.57-●
ulna M84.53-●
vertebra M84.58
osteoporosis M8Ø.ØØ
disuse *—see* Osteoporosis, specified type NEC, with pathological fracture
drug-induced *—see* Osteoporosis, drug induced, with pathological fracture
idiopathic *—see* Osteoporosis, specified type NEC, with pathological fracture
postmenopausal *—see* Osteoporosis, postmenopausal, with pathological fracture
postoophorectomy *—see* Osteoporosis, postoophorectomy, with pathological fracture
postsurgical malabsorption *—see* Osteoporosis, specified type NEC, with pathological fracture
specified cause NEC *—see* Osteoporosis, specified type NEC, with pathological fracture
specified disease NEC M84.6Ø
ankle M84.67-●
carpus M84.64-●
clavicle M84.61-●
femur M84.65-●
fibula M84.66-●
finger M84.64-●
hip M84.65-●
humerus M84.62-●
ilium M84.65Ø
ischium M84.65Ø
metacarpus M84.64-●
metatarsus M84.67-●
neck M84.68
radius M84.63-●
rib M84.68
scapula M84.61-●
skull M84.68
tarsus M84.67-●
tibia M84.66-●
toe M84.67-●
ulna M84.63-●
vertebra M84.68
femur M84.45-●
fibula M84.46-●
finger M84.44-●
hip M84.459
humerus M84.42-●
ilium M84.454
ischium M84.454
joint prosthesis *—see* Complications, joint prosthesis, mechanical, breakdown, by site
periprosthetic *—see* Fracture, pathological, periprosthetic
metacarpus M84.44-●
metatarsus M84.47-●
neck M84.48
pelvis M84.454
periprosthetic M97.9
ankle M97.2-●
elbow M97.4-●
finger M97.8
hip M97.Ø-●
knee M97.1-●
other specified joint M97.8
shoulder M97.3-●
spinal joint M97.8
toe joint M97.8
wrist joint M97.8

Fracture, pathological *(Continued)*
radius M84.43-●
restorative material (dental) KØ8.539
with loss of material KØ8.531
without loss of material KØ8.53Ø
rib M84.48
scapula M84.41-●
skull M84.48
tarsus M84.47-●
tibia M84.46-●
toe M84.47-●
ulna M84.43-●
vertebra M84.48
Fracture, traumatic (abduction) (adduction) (separation) *—see also* Fracture, pathological T14.8
acetabulum S32.4Ø-●
column
anterior (displaced) (iliopubic) S32.43-●
nondisplaced S32.436
posterior (displaced) (ilioischial) S32.443
nondisplaced S32.44-●
dome (displaced) S32.48-●
nondisplaced S32.48
specified NEC S32.49-●
transverse (displaced) S32.45-●
with associated posterior wall fracture (displaced) S32.46-●
nondisplaced S32.46-●
nondisplaced S32.45-●
wall
anterior (displaced) S32.41-●
nondisplaced S32.41-●
medial (displaced) S32.47-●
nondisplaced S32.47-●
posterior (displaced) S32.42-●
with associated transverse fracture (displaced) S32.46-●
nondisplaced S32.46-●
nondisplaced S32.42-●
acromion *—see* Fracture, scapula, acromial process
ankle S82.899
bimalleolar (displaced) S82.84-●
nondisplaced S82.84-●
lateral malleolus only (displaced) S82.6-●
nondisplaced S82.6-●
medial malleolus (displaced) S82.5-●
associated with Maisonneuve's fracture *—see* Fracture, Maisonneuve's
nondisplaced S82.5-●
talus *—see* Fracture, tarsal, talus
trimalleolar (displaced) S82.85-●
nondisplaced S82.85-●
arm (upper) *—see also* Fracture, humerus, shaft
humerus *—see* Fracture, humerus
radius *—see* Fracture, radius
ulna *—see* Fracture, ulna
astragalus *—see* Fracture, tarsal, talus
atlas *—see* Fracture, neck, cervical vertebra, first
axis *—see* Fracture, neck, cervical vertebra, second
back *—see* Fracture, vertebra
Barton's *—see* Barton's fracture
base of skull *—see* Fracture, skull, base
basicervical (basal) (femoral) S72.Ø
Bennett's *—see* Bennett's fracture
bimalleolar *—see* Fracture, ankle, bimalleolar
blow-out SØ2.3-●
bone NEC T14.8
birth injury P13.9
following insertion of orthopedic implant, joint prosthesis or bone plate *—see* Fracture, following insertion of orthopedic implant, joint prosthesis or bone plate

Fracture, traumatic *(Continued)*
bone NEC *(Continued)*
in (due to) neoplastic disease NEC *—see* Fracture, pathological, due to, neoplastic disease
pathological (cause unknown) *—see* Fracture, pathological
breast bone *—see* Fracture, sternum
bucket handle (semilunar cartilage) *—see* Tear, meniscus
burst *—see* Fracture, traumatic, by site
calcaneus *—see* Fracture, tarsal, calcaneus
carpal bone(s) S62.1Ø-●
capitate (displaced) S62.13-●
nondisplaced S62.13-●
cuneiform *—see* Fracture, carpal bone, triquetrum
hamate (body) (displaced) S62.143
hook process (displaced) S62.15-●
nondisplaced S62.15-●
nondisplaced S62.14-●
larger multangular *—see* Fracture, carpal bones, trapezium
lunate (displaced) S62.12-●
nondisplaced S62.12-●
navicular S62.ØØ-●
distal pole (displaced) S62.Ø1-●
nondisplaced S62.Ø1-●
middle third (displaced) S62.Ø2-●
nondisplaced S62.Ø2-●
proximal third (displaced) S62.Ø3-●
nondisplaced S62.Ø3-●
volar tuberosity *—see* Fracture, carpal bones, navicular, distal pole
os magnum *—see* Fracture, carpal bones, capitate
pisiform (displaced) S62.16-●
nondisplaced S62.16-●
semilunar *—see* Fracture, carpal bones, lunate
smaller multangular *—see* Fracture, carpal bones, trapezoid
trapezium (displaced) S62.17-●
nondisplaced S62.17-●
trapezoid (displaced) S62.18-●
nondisplaced S62.18-●
triquetrum (displaced) S62.11-●
nondisplaced S62.11-●
unciform *—see* Fracture, carpal bones, hamate
cervical *—see* Fracture, vertebra, cervical
clavicle S42.ØØ-●
acromial end (displaced) S42.Ø3-●
nondisplaced S42.Ø3-●
birth injury P13.4
lateral end *—see* Fracture, clavicle, acromial end
shaft (displaced) S42.Ø2-●
nondisplaced S42.Ø2-●
sternal end (anterior) (displaced) S42.Ø1-●
nondisplaced S42.Ø1-●
posterior S42.Ø1-●
coccyx S32.2
collapsed *—see* Collapse, vertebra
collar bone *—see* Fracture, clavicle
Colles' *—see* Colles' fracture
coronoid process *—see* Fracture, ulna, upper end, coronoid process
corpus cavernosum penis S39.84Ø
costochondral cartilage S23.41
costochondral, costosternal junction *—see* Fracture, rib
cranium *—see* Fracture, skull
cricoid cartilage S12.8
cuboid (ankle) *—see* Fracture, tarsal, cuboid
cuneiform
foot *—see* Fracture, tarsal, cuneiform
wrist *—see* Fracture, carpal, triquetrum
delayed union *—see* Delay, union, fracture
dental restorative material KØ8.539
with loss of material KØ8.531
without loss of material KØ8.53Ø

F

Fracture, traumatic *(Continued)*
  due to
    birth injury —*see* Birth, injury, fracture
    osteoporosis —*see* Osteoporosis, with fracture
  Dupuytren's —*see* Fracture, ankle, lateral malleolus
  elbow S42.40- •
  ethmoid (bone) (sinus) —*see* Fracture, skull, base
  face bone S02.92
  fatigue —*see also* Fracture, stress
    vertebra M48.40
      cervical region M48.42
      cervicothoracic region M48.43
      lumbar region M48.46
      lumbosacral region M48.47
      occipito-atlanto-axial region M48.41
      sacrococcygeal region M48.48
      thoracic region M48.44
      thoracolumbar region M48.45
  femur, femoral S72.9- •
    basicervical (basal) S72.0
    birth injury P13.2
    capital epiphyseal S79.01- •
    condyles, epicondyles —*see* Fracture, femur, lower end
    distal end —*see* Fracture, femur, lower end
    epiphysis
      head —*see* Fracture, femur, upper end, epiphysis
      lower —*see* Fracture, femur, lower end, epiphysis
      upper —*see* Fracture, femur, upper end, epiphysis
    following insertion of implant, prosthesis or plate M96.66- •
    head —*see* Fracture, femur, upper end, head
    intertrochanteric —*see* Fracture, femur, trochanteric
    intratrochanteric —*see* Fracture, femur, trochanteric
    lower end S72.40- •
      condyle (displaced) S72.41- •
        lateral (displaced) S72.42- •
          nondisplaced S72.42- •
        medial (displaced) S72.43- •
          nondisplaced S72.43- •
        nondisplaced S72.41- •
      epiphysis (displaced) S72.44- •
        nondisplaced S72.44- •
      physeal S79.10- •
        Salter-Harris
          Type I S79.11- •
          Type II S79.12- •
          Type III S79.13- •
          Type IV S79.14- •
        specified NEC S79.19- •
      specified NEC S72.49- •
      supracondylar (displaced) S72.45- •
        with intracondylar extension (displaced) S72.46- •
          nondisplaced S72.46- •
        nondisplaced S72.45- •
      torus S72.47- •
    neck —*see* Fracture, femur, upper end, neck
    pertrochanteric —*see* Fracture, femur, trochanteric
    shaft (lower third) (middle third) (upper third) S72.30- •
      comminuted (displaced) S72.35- •
        nondisplaced S72.35- •
      oblique (displaced) S72.33- •
        nondisplaced S72.33- •
      segmental (displaced) S72.36- •
        nondisplaced S72.36- •
      specified NEC S72.39- •
      spiral (displaced) S72.34- •
        nondisplaced S72.34- •
      transverse (displaced) S72.32- •
        nondisplaced S72.32- •

Fracture, traumatic *(Continued)*
  femur, femoral *(Continued)*
    specified site NEC —*see* subcategory S72.8
    subcapital (displaced) S72.01- •
    subtrochanteric (region) (section) (displaced) S72.2- •
      nondisplaced S72.2- •
    transcervical —*see* Fracture, femur, midcervical
    transtrochanteric —*see* Fracture, femur, trochanteric
    trochanteric S72.10- •
      apophyseal (displaced) S72.13- •
        nondisplaced S72.13- •
      greater trochanter (displaced) S72.11- •
        nondisplaced S72.11- •
      intertrochanteric (displaced) S72.14- •
        nondisplaced S72.14- •
      lesser trochanter (displaced) S72.12- •
        nondisplaced S72.12- •
    upper end S72.00- •
      apophyseal (displaced) S72.13- •
        nondisplaced S72.13- •
      cervicotrochanteric —*see* Fracture, femur, upper end, neck, base
      epiphysis (displaced) S72.02- •
        nondisplaced S72.02- •
      head S72.05- •
        articular (displaced) S72.06- •
          nondisplaced S72.06- •
        specified NEC S72.09- •
      intertrochanteric (displaced) S72.14- •
        nondisplaced S72.14- •
      intracapsular S72.01- •
      midcervical (displaced) S72.03- •
        nondisplaced S72.03- •
      neck S72.00- •
        base (displaced) S72.04- •
          nondisplaced S72.04- •
        specified NEC S72.09- •
      pertrochanteric —*see* Fracture, femur, upper end, trochanteric
      physeal S79.00- •
        Salter-Harris type I S79.01- •
        specified NEC S79.09- •
      subcapital (displaced) S72.01- •
      subtrochanteric (displaced) S72.2- •
        nondisplaced S72.2- •
      transcervical —*see* Fracture, femur, upper end, midcervical
      trochanteric S72.10- •
        greater (displaced) S72.11- •
          nondisplaced S72.11- •
        lesser (displaced) S72.12- •
          nondisplaced S72.12- •
  fibula (shaft) (styloid) S82.40- •
    comminuted (displaced) S82.45- •
      nondisplaced S82.45- •
    following insertion of implant, prosthesis or plate M96.67- •
    involving ankle or malleolus —*see* Fracture, fibula, lateral malleolus
    lateral malleolus (displaced) S82.6- •
      nondisplaced S82.6- •
    lower end
      physeal S89.30- •
        Salter-Harris
          Type I S89.31- •
          Type II S89.32- •
        specified NEC S89.39- •
      specified NEC S82.83- •
      torus S82.82- •
    oblique (displaced) S82.43- •
      nondisplaced S82.43- •
    segmental (displaced) S82.46- •
      nondisplaced S82.46- •
    specified NEC S82.49- •
    spiral (displaced) S82.44- •
      nondisplaced S82.44- •
    transverse (displaced) S82.42- •
      nondisplaced S82.42- •

Fracture, traumatic *(Continued)*
  fibula (shaft) (styloid) *(Continued)*
    upper end
      physeal S89.20- •
        Salter-Harris
          Type I S89.21- •
          Type II S89.22- •
        specified NEC S89.29- •
      specified NEC S82.83- •
      torus S82.81- •
  finger (except thumb) S62.60- •
    distal phalanx (displaced) S62.63- •
      nondisplaced S62.66- •
    index S62.60- •
      distal phalanx (displaced) S62.63- •
        nondisplaced S62.66- •
      middle phalanx (displaced) S62.62- •
        nondisplaced S62.65- •
      proximal phalanx (displaced) S62.61- •
        nondisplaced S62.64- •
    little S62.60- •
      distal phalanx (displaced) S62.63- •
        nondisplaced S62.66- •
      middle phalanx (displaced) S62.62- •
        nondisplaced S62.65- •
      proximal phalanx (displaced) S62.61- •
        nondisplaced S62.64- •
    middle phalanx (displaced) S62.62- •
      nondisplaced S62.65- •
    middle S62.60- •
      distal phalanx (displaced) S62.63- •
        nondisplaced S62.66- •
      middle phalanx (displaced) S62.62- •
        nondisplaced S62.65- •
      proximal phalanx (displaced) S62.61- •
        nondisplaced S62.64- •
    proximal phalanx (displaced) S62.61- •
      nondisplaced S62.64- •
    ring S62.60- •
      distal phalanx (displaced) S62.63- •
        nondisplaced S62.66- •
      middle phalanx (displaced) S62.62- •
        nondisplaced S62.65- •
      proximal phalanx (displaced) S62.61- •
        nondisplaced S62.64- •
    thumb —*see* Fracture, thumb
  following insertion (intraoperative) (postoperative) of orthopedic implant, joint prosthesis or bone plate M96.69
    femur M96.66- •
    fibula M96.67- •
    humerus M96.62- •
    pelvis M96.65
    radius M96.63- •
    specified bone NEC M96.69
    tibia M96.67- •
    ulna M96.63- •
  foot S92.90- •
    astragalus —*see* Fracture, tarsal, talus
    calcaneus —*see* Fracture, tarsal, calcaneus
    cuboid —*see* Fracture, tarsal, cuboid
    cuneiform —*see* Fracture, tarsal, cuneiform
    metatarsal —*see* Fracture, metatarsal
    navicular —*see* Fracture, tarsal, navicular
    sesamoid S92.81- •
    specified NEC S92.81- •
    talus —*see* Fracture, tarsal, talus
    tarsal —*see* Fracture, tarsal
    toe —*see* Fracture, toe
  forearm S52.9- •
    radius —*see* Fracture, radius
    ulna —*see* Fracture, ulna
  fossa (anterior) (middle) (posterior) S02.19
  fragility —*see* Fracture, pathological, due to osteoporosis
  frontal (bone) (skull) S02.0
    sinus S02.19
  glenoid (cavity) (scapula) —*see* Fracture, scapula, glenoid cavity
  greenstick —*see* Fracture, by site
  hallux —*see* Fracture, toe, great

Fracture, traumatic (Continued)
hand S62.9-●
carpal —see Fracture, carpal bone
finger (except thumb) —see Fracture, finger
metacarpal —see Fracture, metacarpal
navicular (scaphoid) (hand) —see Fracture, carpal bone, navicular
thumb —see Fracture, thumb
healed or old
with complications - code by Nature of the complication
heel bone —see Fracture, tarsal, calcaneus
Hill-Sachs S42.29-●
hip —see Fracture, femur, neck
humerus S42.30-●
anatomical neck —see Fracture, humerus, upper end
articular process —see Fracture, humerus, lower end
capitellum —see Fracture, humerus, lower end, condyle, lateral
distal end —see Fracture, humerus, lower end
epiphysis
lower —see Fracture, humerus, lower end, physeal
upper —see Fracture, humerus, upper end, physeal
external condyle —see Fracture, humerus, lower end, condyle, lateral
following insertion of implant, prosthesis or plate M96.62-●
great tuberosity —see Fracture, humerus, upper end, greater tuberosity
intercondylar —see Fracture, humerus, lower end
internal epicondyle —see Fracture, humerus, lower end, epicondyle, medial
lesser tuberosity —see Fracture, humerus, upper end, lesser tuberosity
lower end S42.40-●
condyle
lateral (displaced) S42.45-●
nondisplaced S42.45-●
medial (displaced) S42.46-●
nondisplaced S42.46-●
epicondyle
lateral (displaced) S42.43-●
nondisplaced S42.43-●
medial (displaced) S42.44-●
incarcerated S42.44-●
nondisplaced S42.44-●
physeal S49.10-●
Salter-Harris
Type I S49.11-●
Type II S49.12-●
Type III S49.13-●
Type IV S49.14-●
specified NEC S49.19-●
specified NEC (displaced) S42.49-●
nondisplaced S42.49-●
supracondylar (simple) (displaced) S42.41-●
with intercondylar fracture —see Fracture, humerus, lower end
comminuted (displaced) S42.42-●
nondisplaced S42.42-●
nondisplaced S42.41-●
torus S42.48-●
transcondylar (displaced) S42.47-●
nondisplaced S42.47-●
proximal end —see Fracture, humerus, upper end
shaft S42.30-●
comminuted (displaced) S42.35-●
nondisplaced S42.35-●
greenstick S42.31-●
oblique (displaced) S42.33-●
nondisplaced S42.33-●
segmental (displaced) S42.36-●
nondisplaced S42.36-●
specified NEC S42.39-●

Fracture, traumatic (Continued)
humerus (Continued)
shaft (Continued)
spiral (displaced) S42.34-●
nondisplaced S42.34-●
transverse (displaced) S42.32-●
nondisplaced S42.32-●
supracondylar —see Fracture, humerus, lower end
surgical neck —see Fracture, humerus, upper end, surgical neck
trochlea —see Fracture, humerus, lower end, condyle, medial
tuberosity —see Fracture, humerus, upper end
upper end S42.20-●
anatomical neck —see Fracture, humerus, upper end, specified NEC
articular head —see Fracture, humerus, upper end, specified NEC
epiphysis —see Fracture, humerus, upper end, physeal
greater tuberosity (displaced) S42.25-●
nondisplaced S42.25-●
lesser tuberosity (displaced) S42.26-●
nondisplaced S42.26-●
physeal S49.00-●
Salter-Harris
Type I S49.01-●
Type II S49.02-●
Type III S49.03-●
Type IV S49.04-●
specified NEC S49.09-●
specified NEC (displaced) S42.29-●
nondisplaced S42.29-●
surgical neck (displaced) S42.21-●
four-part S42.24-●
nondisplaced S42.21-●
three-part S42.23-●
two-part (displaced) S42.22-●
nondisplaced S42.22-●
torus S42.27-●
transepiphyseal —see Fracture, humerus, upper end, physeal
hyoid bone S12.8
ilium S32.30-●
with disruption of pelvic ring —see Disruption, pelvic ring
avulsion (displaced) S32.31-●
nondisplaced S32.31-●
specified NEC S32.39-●
impaction, impacted - code as Fracture, by site
innominate bone —see Fracture, ilium
instep —see Fracture, foot
ischium S32.60-●
with disruption of pelvic ring —see Disruption, pelvic ring
avulsion (displaced) S32.61-●
nondisplaced S32.61-●
specified NEC S32.69-●
jaw (bone) (lower) —see Fracture, mandible
upper —see Fracture, maxilla
joint prosthesis —see Complications, joint prosthesis, mechanical, breakdown, by site
periprosthetic —see Fracture, traumatic, periprosthetic
knee cap —see Fracture, patella
larynx S12.8
late effects —see Sequelae, fracture
leg (lower) S82.9-●
ankle —see Fracture, ankle
femur —see Fracture, femur
fibula —see Fracture, fibula
malleolus —see Fracture, ankle
patella —see Fracture, patella
specified site NEC S82.89-●
tibia —see Fracture, tibia
lumbar spine —see Fracture, vertebra, lumbar
lumbosacral spine S32.9

Fracture, traumatic (Continued)
Maisonneuve's (displaced) S82.86-●
nondisplaced S82.86-●
malar bone —see also Fracture, maxilla S02.400
left side S02.40B
right side S02.40A
malleolus —see Fracture, ankle
malunion —see Fracture, by site
mandible (lower jawbone) S02.609
alveolus S02.67-●
angle (of jaw) S02.65-●
body, unspecified S02.600-●
left side S02.602
right side S02.601
condylar process S02.61-●
coronoid process S02.63-●
ramus, unspecified S02.64-●
specified site NEC S02.69
subcondylar process S02.62-●
symphysis S02.66
manubrium (sterni) S22.21
dissociation from sternum S22.23
march —see Fracture, traumatic, stress, by site
maxilla, maxillary (bone) (sinus) (superior) (upper jaw) S02.401
alveolus S02.42
inferior —see Fracture, mandible
LeFort I S02.411
LeFort II S02.412
LeFort III S02.413
left side S02.40D
right side S02.40C
metacarpal S62.309
base (displaced) S62.319
nondisplaced S62.349
fifth S62.30-●
base (displaced) S62.31-●
nondisplaced S62.34-●
neck (displaced) S62.33-●
nondisplaced S62.36-●
shaft (displaced) S62.32-●
nondisplaced S62.35-●
specified NEC S62.398
first S62.20-●
base NEC (displaced) S62.23-●
nondisplaced S62.23-●
Bennett's —see Bennett's fracture
neck (displaced) S62.25-●
nondisplaced S62.25-●
shaft (displaced) S62.24-●
nondisplaced S62.24-●
specified NEC S62.29-●
fourth S62.30-●
base (displaced) S62.31-●
nondisplaced S62.34-●
neck (displaced) S62.33-●
nondisplaced S62.36-●
shaft (displaced) S62.32-●
nondisplaced S62.35-●
specified NEC S62.39-●
neck (displaced) S62.33-●
nondisplaced S62.36-●
Rolando's —see Rolando's fracture
second S62.30-●
base (displaced) S62.31-●
nondisplaced S62.34-●
neck (displaced) S62.33-●
nondisplaced S62.36-●
shaft (displaced) S62.32-●
nondisplaced S62.35-●
specified NEC S62.39-●
shaft (displaced) S62.32-●
nondisplaced S62.35-●
specified NEC S62.399
third S62.30-●
base (displaced) S62.31-●
nondisplaced S62.34-●
neck (displaced) S62.33-●
nondisplaced S62.36-●
shaft (displaced) S62.32-●
nondisplaced S62.35-●
specified NEC S62.39-●

F

Fracture, traumatic *(Continued)*
  metastatic *—see* Fracture, pathological, due to, neoplastic disease *—see also* Neoplasm
  metatarsal bone S92.30-●
    fifth (displaced) S92.35-●
      nondisplaced S92.35-●
    first (displaced) S92.31-●
      nondisplaced S92.31-●
    fourth (displaced) S92.34-●
      nondisplaced S92.34-●
    physeal S99.10-●
      Salter-Harris
        Type I S99.11-●
        Type II S99.12-●
        Type III S99.13-●
        Type IV S99.14-●
      specified NEC S99.19-●
    second (displaced) S92.32-●
      nondisplaced S92.32-●
    third (displaced) S92.33-●
      nondisplaced S92.33-●
  Monteggia's *—see* Monteggia's fracture
  multiple
    hand (and wrist) NEC *—see* Fracture, by site
    ribs *—see* Fracture, rib, multiple
  nasal (bone(s)) S02.2
  navicular (scaphoid) (foot) *—see also* Fracture, tarsal, navicular
    hand *—see* Fracture, carpal, navicular
  neck S12.9
    cervical vertebra S12.9
      fifth (displaced) S12.400
        nondisplaced S12.401
        specified type NEC (displaced) S12.490
          nondisplaced S12.491
      first (displaced) S12.000
        burst (stable) S12.01
          unstable S12.02
        lateral mass (displaced) S12.040
          nondisplaced S12.041
        nondisplaced S12.001
        posterior arch (displaced) S12.030
          nondisplaced S12.031
        specified type NEC (displaced) S12.090
          nondisplaced S12.091
      fourth (displaced) S12.300
        nondisplaced S12.301
        specified type NEC (displaced) S12.390
          nondisplaced S12.391
      second (displaced) S12.100
        dens (anterior) (displaced) (type II) S12.110
          nondisplaced S12.112
          posterior S12.111
          specified type NEC (displaced) S12.120
            nondisplaced S12.121
        nondisplaced S12.101
        specified type NEC (displaced) S12.190
          nondisplaced S12.191
      seventh (displaced) S12.600
        nondisplaced S12.601
        specified type NEC (displaced) S12.690
          nondisplaced S12.691
      sixth (displaced) S12.500
        nondisplaced S12.501
        specified type NEC (displaced) S12.590
          nondisplaced S12.591
      third (displaced) S12.200
        nondisplaced S12.201
        specified type NEC (displaced) S12.290
          nondisplaced S12.291
    hyoid bone S12.8
    larynx S12.8

Fracture, traumatic *(Continued)*
  neck *(Continued)*
    specified site NEC S12.8
    thyroid cartilage S12.8
    trachea S12.8
  neoplastic NEC *—see* Fracture, pathological, due to, neoplastic disease
  neural arch *—see* Fracture, vertebra
  newborn *—see* Birth, injury, fracture
  nontraumatic *—see* Fracture, pathological
  nonunion *—see* Nonunion, fracture
  nose, nasal (bone) (septum) S02.2
  occiput *—see* Fracture, skull, base, occiput
  odontoid process *—see* Fracture, neck, cervical vertebra, second
  olecranon (process) (ulna) *—see* Fracture, ulna, upper end, olecranon process
  ➠orbit, orbital (bone) (region) S02.85
    floor (blow-out) S02.3-●
    ➠roof S02.12-●
    ▶wall S02.85
      ▶lateral S02.84-●
      ▶medial S02.83-●
  os
    calcis *—see* Fracture, tarsal, calcaneus
    magnum *—see* Fracture, carpal, capitate
    pubis *—see* Fracture, pubis
  palate S02.8-●
  parietal bone (skull) S02.0
  patella S82.00-●
    comminuted (displaced) S82.04-●
      nondisplaced S82.04-●
    longitudinal (displaced) S82.02-●
      nondisplaced S82.02-●
    osteochondral (displaced) S82.01-●
      nondisplaced S82.01-●
    specified NEC S82.09-●
    transverse (displaced) S82.03-●
      nondisplaced S82.03-●
  pedicle (of vertebral arch) *—see* Fracture, vertebra
  pelvis, pelvic (bone) S32.9
    acetabulum *—see* Fracture, acetabulum
    circle *—see* Disruption, pelvic ring
    following insertion of implant, prosthesis or plate M96.65
    ilium *—see* Fracture, ilium
    ischium *—see* Fracture, ischium
    multiple
      with disruption of pelvic ring (circle) *—see* Disruption, pelvic ring
      without disruption of pelvic ring (circle) S32.82
    pubis *—see* Fracture, pubis
    sacrum *—see* Fracture, sacrum
    specified site NEC S32.89
  periprosthetic, around internal prosthetic joint M97.9
    ankle M97.2-●
    elbow M97.4-●
    finger M97.8
    hip M97.0-●
    knee M97.1-●
    shoulder M97.3-●
    specified joint NEC M97.8
    spine M97.8
    toe M97.8
    wrist M97.8
  phalanx
    foot *—see* Fracture, toe
    hand *—see* Fracture, finger
  pisiform *—see* Fracture, carpal, pisiform
  pond *—see* Fracture, skull
  prosthetic device, internal *—see* Complications, prosthetic device, by site, mechanical
  pubis S32.50-●
    with disruption of pelvic ring *—see* Disruption, pelvic ring
    specified site NEC S32.59-●
    superior rim S32.59-●

Fracture, traumatic *(Continued)*
  radius S52.9-●
    distal end *—see* Fracture, radius, lower end
    following insertion of implant, prosthesis or plate M96.63-●
    head *—see* Fracture, radius, upper end, head
    lower end S52.50-●
      Barton's *—see* Barton's fracture
      Colles' *—see* Colles' fracture
      extraarticular NEC S52.55-●
      intraarticular NEC S52.57-●
      physeal S59.20-●
        Salter-Harris
          Type I S59.21-●
          Type II S59.22-●
          Type III S59.23-●
          Type IV S59.24-●
        specified NEC S59.29-●
      Smith's *—see* Smith's fracture
      specified NEC S52.59-●
      styloid process (displaced) S52.51-●
        nondisplaced S52.51-●
      torus S52.52-●
    neck *—see* Fracture, radius, upper end
    proximal end *—see* Fracture, radius, upper end
    shaft S52.30-●
      bent bone S52.38-●
      comminuted (displaced) S52.35-●
        nondisplaced S52.35-●
      Galeazzi's *—see* Galeazzi's fracture
      greenstick S52.31-●
      oblique (displaced) S52.33-●
        nondisplaced S52.33-●
      segmental (displaced) S52.36-●
        nondisplaced S52.36-●
      specified NEC S52.39-●
      spiral (displaced) S52.34-●
        nondisplaced S52.34-●
      transverse (displaced) S52.32-●
        nondisplaced S52.32-●
    upper end S52.10-●
      head (displaced) S52.12-●
        nondisplaced S52.12-●
      neck (displaced) S52.13-●
        nondisplaced S52.13-●
      physeal S59.10-●
        Salter-Harris
          Type I S59.11-●
          Type II S59.12-●
          Type III S59.13-●
          Type IV S59.14-●
        specified NEC S59.19-●
      specified NEC S52.18-●
      torus S52.11-●
  ramus
    inferior or superior, pubis *—see* Fracture, pubis
    mandible *—see* Fracture, mandible
  restorative material (dental) K08.539
    with loss of material K08.531
    without loss of material K08.530
  rib S22.3-●
    with flail chest *—see* Flail, chest
    multiple S22.4-●
      with flail chest *—see* Flail, chest
  root, tooth *—see* Fracture, tooth
  sacrum S32.10
    specified NEC S32.19
    Type
      1 S32.14
      2 S32.15
      3 S32.16
      4 S32.17
    Zone
      I S32.119
        displaced (minimally) S32.111
          severely S32.112
        nondisplaced S32.110

F

▶ New ➠ Revised ~~deleted~~ Deleted ● Use Additional Character(s)

Fracture, traumatic *(Continued)*
  sacrum *(Continued)*
    Zone *(Continued)*
      II S32.129
        displaced (minimally) S32.121
          severely S32.122
        nondisplaced S32.12Ø
      III S32.139
        displaced (minimally) S32.131
          severely S32.132
        nondisplaced S32.13Ø
  scaphoid (hand) *—see also* Fracture, carpal, navicular
    foot *—see* Fracture, tarsal, navicular
  scapula S42.1Ø- ●
    acromial process (displaced) S42.12- ●
      nondisplaced S42.12- ●
    body (displaced) S42.11- ●
      nondisplaced S42.11- ●
    coracoid process (displaced) S42.13- ●
      nondisplaced S42.13- ●
    glenoid cavity (displaced) S42.14- ●
      nondisplaced S42.14- ●
    neck (displaced) S42.15- ●
      nondisplaced S42.15- ●
    specified NEC S42.19- ●
  semilunar bone, wrist *—see* Fracture, carpal, lunate
  sequelae *—see* Sequelae, fracture
  sesamoid bone
    foot S92.81- ●
    hand *—see* Fracture, carpal
    other *—see* Fracture, traumatic, by site
  shepherd's *—see* Fracture, tarsal, talus
  shoulder (girdle) S42.9- ●
    blade *—see* Fracture, scapula
  sinus (ethmoid) (frontal) SØ2.19
  skull SØ2.91
    base SØ2.1Ø- ●
      occiput SØ2.119
        condyle SØ2.113
          type I SØ2.11Ø
            left side SØ2.11B
            right side SØ2.11A
          type II SØ2.111
            left side SØ2.11D
            right side SØ2.11C
          type III SØ2.112
            left side SØ2.11F
            right side SØ2.11E
          specified NEC SØ2.118
            left side SØ2.11H
            right side SØ2.11G
      specified NEC SØ2.19- ●
    birth injury P13.Ø
    frontal bone SØ2.Ø
    parietal bone SØ2.Ø
    specified site NEC SØ2.8
    temporal bone SØ2.19
    vault SØ2.Ø
  Smith's *—see* Smith's fracture
  sphenoid (bone) (sinus) SØ2.19
  spine *—see* Fracture, vertebra
  spinous process *—see* Fracture, vertebra
  spontaneous (cause unknown) *—see* Fracture, pathological
  stave (of thumb) *—see* Fracture, metacarpal, first
  sternum S22.2Ø
    with flail chest *—see* Flail, chest
    body S22.22
    manubrium S22.21
    xiphoid (process) S22.24
  stress M84.3Ø
    ankle M84.37- ●
    carpus M84.34- ●
    clavicle M84.31- ●
    femoral neck M84.359
    femur M84.35- ●
    fibula M84.36- ●
    finger M84.34- ●

Fracture, traumatic *(Continued)*
  stress *(Continued)*
    hip M84.359
    humerus M84.32- ●
    ilium M84.35Ø
    ischium M84.35Ø
    metacarpus M84.34- ●
    metatarsus M84.37- ●
    neck *—see* Fracture, fatigue, vertebra
    pelvis M84.35Ø
    radius M84.33- ●
    rib M84.38
    scapula M84.31- ●
    skull M84.38
    tarsus M84.37- ●
    tibia M84.36- ●
    toe M84.37- ●
    ulna M84.33- ●
    vertebra *—see* Fracture, fatigue, vertebra
  supracondylar, elbow *—see* Fracture, humerus, lower end, supracondylar
  symphysis pubis *—see* Fracture, pubis
  talus (ankle bone) *—see* Fracture, tarsal, talus
  tarsal bone(s) S92.2Ø- ●
    astragalus *—see* Fracture, tarsal, talus
    calcaneus S92.ØØ- ●
      anterior process (displaced) S92.Ø2- ●
        nondisplaced S92.Ø2- ●
      body (displaced) S92.Ø1- ●
        nondisplaced S92.Ø1- ●
      extraarticular NEC (displaced) S92.Ø5- ●
        nondisplaced S92.Ø5- ●
      intraarticular (displaced) S92.Ø6- ●
        nondisplaced S92.Ø6- ●
      physeal S99.ØØ- ●
        Salter-Harris
          Type I S99.Ø1- ●
          Type II S99.Ø2- ●
          Type III S99.Ø3- ●
          Type IV S99.Ø4- ●
        specified NEC S99.Ø9- ●
      tuberosity (displaced) S92.Ø4- ●
        avulsion (displaced) S92.Ø3- ●
          nondisplaced S92.Ø3- ●
        nondisplaced S92.Ø4- ●
    cuboid (displaced) S92.21- ●
      nondisplaced S92.21- ●
    cuneiform
      intermediate (displaced) S92.23- ●
        nondisplaced S92.23- ●
      lateral (displaced) S92.22- ●
        nondisplaced S92.22- ●
      medial (displaced) S92.24- ●
        nondisplaced S92.24- ●
    navicular (displaced) S92.25- ●
      nondisplaced S92.25- ●
    scaphoid *—see* Fracture, tarsal, navicular
    talus S92.1Ø- ●
      avulsion (displaced) S92.15- ●
        nondisplaced S92.15- ●
      body (displaced) S92.12- ●
        nondisplaced S92.12- ●
      dome (displaced) S92.14- ●
        nondisplaced S92.14- ●
      head (displaced) S92.12- ●
        nondisplaced S92.12- ●
      lateral process (displaced) S92.14- ●
        nondisplaced S92.14- ●
      neck (displaced) S92.11- ●
        nondisplaced S92.11- ●
      posterior process (displaced) S92.13- ●
        nondisplaced S92.13- ●
      specified NEC S92.19- ●
  temporal bone (styloid) SØ2.19
  thorax (bony) S22.9
    with flail chest *—see* Flail, chest
    rib S22.3- ●
      multiple S22.4- ●
        with flail chest *—see* Flail, chest

Fracture, traumatic *(Continued)*
  thorax *(Continued)*
    sternum S22.2Ø
      body S22.22
      manubrium S22.21
      xiphoid process S22.24
    vertebra (displaced) S22.ØØ9
      burst (stable) S22.ØØ1
        unstable S22.ØØ2
      eighth S22.Ø69
        burst (stable) S22.Ø61
          unstable S22.Ø62
        specified type NEC S22.Ø68
        wedge compression S22.Ø6Ø
      eleventh S22.Ø89
        burst (stable) S22.Ø81
          unstable S22.Ø82
        specified type NEC S22.Ø88
        wedge compression S22.Ø8Ø
      fifth S22.Ø59
        burst (stable) S22.Ø51
          unstable S22.Ø52
        specified type NEC S22.Ø58
        wedge compression S22.Ø5Ø
      first S22.Ø19
        burst (stable) S22.Ø11
          unstable S22.Ø12
        specified type NEC S22.Ø18
        wedge compression S22.Ø1Ø
      fourth S22.Ø49
        burst (stable) S22.Ø41
          unstable S22.Ø42
        specified type NEC S22.Ø48
        wedge compression S22.Ø4Ø
      ninth S22.Ø79
        burst (stable) S22.Ø71
          unstable S22.Ø72
        specified type NEC S22.Ø78
        wedge compression S22.Ø7Ø
      nondisplaced S22.ØØ1
      second S22.Ø29
        burst (stable) S22.Ø21
          unstable S22.Ø22
        specified type NEC S22.Ø28
        wedge compression S22.Ø2Ø
      seventh S22.Ø69
        burst (stable) S22.Ø61
          unstable S22.Ø62
        specified type NEC S22.Ø68
        wedge compression S22.Ø6Ø
      sixth S22.Ø59
        burst (stable) S22.Ø51
          unstable S22.Ø52
        specified type NEC S22.Ø58
        wedge compression S22.Ø5Ø
      specified type NEC S22.ØØ8
      tenth S22.Ø79
        burst (stable) S22.Ø71
          unstable S22.Ø72
        specified type NEC S22.Ø78
        wedge compression S22.Ø7Ø
      third S22.Ø39
        burst (stable) S22.Ø31
          unstable S22.Ø32
        specified type NEC S22.Ø38
        wedge compression S22.Ø3Ø
      twelfth S22.Ø89
        burst (stable) S22.Ø81
          unstable S22.Ø82
        specified type NEC S22.Ø88
        wedge compression S22.Ø8Ø
      wedge compression S22.ØØØ
  thumb S62.5Ø- ●
    distal phalanx (displaced) S62.52- ●
      nondisplaced S62.52- ●
    proximal phalanx (displaced) S62.51- ●
      nondisplaced S62.51- ●
  thyroid cartilage S12.8
  tibia (shaft) S82.2Ø- ●
    comminuted (displaced) S82.25- ●
      nondisplaced S82.25- ●

F

Fracture, traumatic *(Continued)*
tibia *(Continued)*
condyles —*see* Fracture, tibia, upper end
distal end —*see* Fracture, tibia, lower end
epiphysis
lower —*see* Fracture, tibia, lower end
upper —*see* Fracture, tibia, upper end
following insertion of implant, prosthesis or plate M96.67-●
head (involving knee joint) —*see* Fracture, tibia, upper end
intercondyloid eminence —*see* Fracture, tibia, upper end
involving ankle or malleolus —*see* Fracture, ankle, medial malleolus
lower end S82.30-●
physeal S89.10-●
Salter-Harris
Type I S89.11-●
Type II S89.12-●
Type III S89.13-●
Type IV S89.14-●
specified NEC S89.19-●
pilon (displaced) S82.87-●
nondisplaced S82.87-●
specified NEC S82.39-●
torus S82.31-●
malleolus —*see* Fracture, ankle, medial malleolus
oblique (displaced) S82.23-●
nondisplaced S82.23-●
pilon —*see* Fracture, tibia, lower end, pilon
proximal end —*see* Fracture, tibia, upper end
segmental (displaced) S82.26-●
nondisplaced S82.26-●
specified NEC S82.29-●
spine —*see* Fracture, tibia, upper end, spine
spiral (displaced) S82.24-●
nondisplaced S82.24-●
transverse (displaced) S82.22-●
nondisplaced S82.22-●
tuberosity —*see* Fracture, tibia, upper end, tuberosity
upper end S82.10-●
bicondylar (displaced) S82.14-●
nondisplaced S82.14-●
lateral condyle (displaced) S82.12-●
nondisplaced S82.12-●
medial condyle (displaced) S82.13-●
nondisplaced S82.13-●
physeal S89.00-●
Salter-Harris
Type I S89.01-●
Type II S89.02-●
Type III S89.03-●
Type IV S89.04-●
specified NEC S89.09-●
plateau —*see* Fracture, tibia, upper end, bicondylar
specified NEC S82.19-●
spine (displaced) S82.11-●
nondisplaced S82.11-●
torus S82.16-●
tuberosity (displaced) S82.15-●
nondisplaced S82.15-●
toe S92.91-●
great (displaced) S92.40-●
distal phalanx (displaced) S92.42-●
nondisplaced S92.42-●
nondisplaced S92.40-●
proximal phalanx (displaced) S92.41-●
nondisplaced S92.41-●
specified NEC S92.49-●
lesser (displaced) S92.50-●
distal phalanx (displaced) S92.53-●
nondisplaced S92.53-●
middle phalanx (displaced) S92.52-●
nondisplaced S92.52-●
nondisplaced S92.50-●

Fracture, traumatic *(Continued)*
toe *(Continued)*
lesser *(Continued)*
proximal phalanx (displaced) S92.51-●
nondisplaced S92.51-●
specified NEC S92.59-●
physeal
phalanx S99.20-●
Salter-Harris
Type I S99.21-●
Type II S99.22-●
Type III S99.23-●
Type IV S99.24-●
specified NEC S99.29-●
tooth (root) S02.5
trachea (cartilage) S12.8
transverse process —*see* Fracture, vertebra
trapezium or trapezoid bone —*see* Fracture, carpal
trimalleolar —*see* Fracture, ankle, trimalleolar
triquetrum (cuneiform of carpus) —*see* Fracture, carpal, triquetrum
trochanter —*see* Fracture, femur, trochanteric
tuberosity (external) —*see* Fracture, traumatic, by site
ulna (shaft) S52.20-●
bent bone S52.28-●
coronoid process —*see* Fracture, ulna, upper end, coronoid process
distal end —*see* Fracture, ulna, lower end
following insertion of implant, prosthesis or plate M96.63-●
head S52.60-●
lower end S52.60-●
physeal S59.00-●
Salter-Harris
Type I S59.01-●
Type II S59.02-●
Type III S59.03-●
Type IV S59.04-●
specified NEC S59.09-●
specified NEC S52.69-●
styloid process (displaced) S52.61-●
nondisplaced S52.61-●
torus S52.62-●
proximal end —*see* Fracture, ulna, upper end
shaft S52.20-●
comminuted (displaced) S52.25-●
nondisplaced S52.25-●
greenstick S52.21-●
Monteggia's —*see* Monteggia's fracture
oblique (displaced) S52.23-●
nondisplaced S52.23-●
segmental (displaced) S52.26-●
nondisplaced S52.26-●
specified NEC S52.29-●
spiral (displaced) S52.24-●
nondisplaced S52.24-●
transverse (displaced) S52.22-●
nondisplaced S52.22-●
upper end S52.00-●
coronoid process (displaced) S52.04-●
nondisplaced S52.04-●
olecranon process (displaced) S52.02-●
with intraarticular extension S52.03-●
nondisplaced S52.02-●
with intraarticular extension S52.03-●
specified NEC S52.09-●
torus S52.01-●
unciform —*see* Fracture, carpal, hamate
vault of skull S02.0
vertebra, vertebral (arch) (body) (column) (neural arch) (pedicle) (spinous process) (transverse process)
atlas —*see* Fracture, neck, cervical vertebra, first
axis —*see* Fracture, neck, cervical vertebra, second
cervical (teardrop) S12.9
axis —*see* Fracture, neck, cervical vertebra, second

Fracture, traumatic *(Continued)*
vertebra, vertebral *(Continued)*
cervical *(Continued)*
first (atlas) —*see* Fracture, neck, cervical vertebra, first
second (axis) —*see* Fracture, neck, cervical vertebra, second
chronic M84.48
coccyx S32.2
dorsal —*see* Fracture, thorax, vertebra
lumbar S32.009
burst (stable) S32.001
unstable S32.002
fifth S32.059
burst (stable) S32.051
unstable S32.052
specified type NEC S32.058
wedge compression S32.050
first S32.019
burst (stable) S32.011
unstable S32.012
specified type NEC S32.018
wedge compression S32.010
fourth S32.049
burst (stable) S32.041
unstable S32.042
specified type NEC S32.048
wedge compression S32.040
second S32.029
burst (stable) S32.021
unstable S32.022
specified type NEC S32.028
wedge compression S32.020
specified type NEC S32.008
third S32.039
burst (stable) S32.031
unstable S32.032
specified type NEC S32.038
wedge compression S32.030
wedge compression S32.000
metastatic —*see* Collapse, vertebra, in, specified disease NEC —*see also* Neoplasm
newborn (birth injury) P11.5
sacrum S32.10
specified NEC S32.19
Type
1 S32.14
2 S32.15
3 S32.16
4 S32.17
Zone
I S32.119
displaced (minimally) S32.111
severely S32.112
nondisplaced S32.110
II S32.129
displaced (minimally) S32.121
severely S32.122
nondisplaced S32.120
III S32.139
displaced (minimally) S32.131
severely S32.132
nondisplaced S32.130
thoracic —*see* Fracture, thorax, vertebra
vertex S02.0
vomer (bone) S02.2
wrist S62.10-●
carpal —*see* Fracture, carpal bone
navicular (scaphoid) (hand) —*see* Fracture, carpal, navicular
xiphisternum, xiphoid (process) S22.24
zygoma S02.442
left side S02.40F
right side S02.40E
Fragile, fragility
autosomal site Q95.5
bone, congenital (with blue sclera) Q78.0
capillary (hereditary) D69.8
hair L67.8
nails L60.3
non-sex chromosome site Q95.5
X chromosome Q99.2

Fragilitas
crinium L67.8
ossium (with blue sclerae) (hereditary) Q78.Ø
unguium L6Ø.3
congenital Q84.6
Fragments, cataract (lens), following cataract surgery H59.Ø2-●
retained foreign body *—see* Retained, foreign body fragments (type of)
Frailty (frail) R54
mental R41.81
Frambesia, frambesial (tropica) *—see also* Yaws
initial lesion or ulcer A66.Ø
primary A66.Ø
Frambeside
gummatous A66.4
of early yaws A66.2
Frambesioma A66.1
Franceschetti-Klein (-Wildervanck) **disease** or **syndrome** Q75.4
Francis' disease *—see* Tularemia
Franklin disease C88.2
Frank's essential thrombocytopenia D69.3
Fraser's syndrome Q87.Ø
Freckle(s) L81.2
malignant melanoma in *—see* Melanoma
melanotic (Hutchinson's) *—see* Melanoma, in situ
retinal D49.81
Frederickson's hyperlipoproteinemia, type
I and V E78.3
IIA E78.ØØ
IIB and III E78.2
IV E78.1
Freeman Sheldon syndrome Q87.Ø
Freezing *—see also* Effect, adverse, cold T69.9
Freiberg's disease (infraction of metatarsal head or osteochondrosis) *—see* Osteochondrosis, juvenile, metatarsus
Frei's disease A55
Fremitus, friction, cardiac RØ1.2
Frenum, frenulum
external os Q51.828
tongue (shortening) (congenital) Q38.1
Frequency micturition (nocturnal) R35.Ø
psychogenic F45.8
Frey's syndrome
auriculotemporal G5Ø.8
hyperhidrosis L74.52
Friction
burn *—see* Burn, by site
fremitus, cardiac RØ1.2
precordial RØ1.2
sounds, chest RØ9.89
Friderichsen-Waterhouse syndrome or **disease** A39.1
Friedländer's B (bacillus) NEC *—see also* condition A49.8
Friedreich's
ataxia G11.1
combined systemic disease G11.1
facial hemihypertrophy Q67.4
sclerosis (cerebellum) (spinal cord) G11.1
Frigidity F52.22
Fröhlich's syndrome E23.6
Frontal *—see also* condition
lobe syndrome FØ7.Ø
Frostbite (superficial) T33.9Ø
with
partial thickness skin loss *—see* Frostbite (superficial), by site
tissue necrosis T34.9Ø
abdominal wall T33.3
with tissue necrosis T34.3
ankle T33.81-●
with tissue necrosis T34.81-●
arm T33.4-●
with tissue necrosis T34.4-●
finger(s) *—see* Frostbite, finger
hand *—see* Frostbite, hand
wrist *—see* Frostbite, wrist
Frostbite *(Continued)*
ear T33.Ø1-●
with tissue necrosis T34.Ø1-●
face T33.Ø9
with tissue necrosis T34.Ø9
finger T33.53-●
with tissue necrosis T34.53-●
foot T33.82-●
with tissue necrosis T34.82-●
hand T33.52-●
with tissue necrosis T34.52-●
head T33.Ø9
with tissue necrosis T34.Ø9
ear *—see* Frostbite, ear
nose *—see* Frostbite, nose
hip (and thigh) T33.6-●
with tissue necrosis T34.6-●
knee T33.7-●
with tissue necrosis T34.7-●
leg T33.9-●
with tissue necrosis T34.9-●
ankle *—see* Frostbite, ankle
foot *—see* Frostbite, foot
knee *—see* Frostbite, knee
lower T33.7-●
with tissue necrosis T34.7-●
thigh *—see* Frostbite, hip
toe *—see* Frostbite, toe
limb
lower T33.99
with tissue necrosis T34.99
upper *—see* Frostbite, arm
neck T33.1
with tissue necrosis T34.1
nose T33.Ø2
with tissue necrosis T34.Ø2
pelvis T33.3
with tissue necrosis T34.3
specified site NEC T33.99
with tissue necrosis T34.99
thigh *—see* Frostbite, hip
thorax T33.2
with tissue necrosis T34.2
toes T33.83-●
with tissue necrosis T34.83-●
trunk T33.99
with tissue necrosis T34.99
wrist T33.51-●
with tissue necrosis T34.51-●
Frotteurism F65.81
Frozen *—see also* Effect, adverse, cold T69.9
pelvis (female) N94.89
male K66.8
shoulder *—see* Capsulitis, adhesive
Fructokinase deficiency E74.11
Fructose 1,6 diphosphatase deficiency E74.19
Fructosemia (benign) (essential) E74.12
Fructosuria (benign) (essential) E74.11
Fuchs'
black spot (myopic) *—see also* Myopia, degenerative H44.2-●
dystrophy (corneal endothelium) H18.51
heterochromic cyclitis *—see* Cyclitis, Fuchs' heterochromic
Fucosidosis E77.1
Fugue R68.89
dissociative F44.1
hysterical (dissociative) F44.1
postictal in epilepsy *—see* Epilepsy
reaction to exceptional stress (transient) F43.Ø
Fulminant, fulminating *—see* condition
Functional *—see also* condition
bleeding (uterus) N93.8
Functioning, intellectual, borderline R41.83
Fundus *—see* condition
Fungemia NOS B49
Fungus, fungous
cerebral G93.89
disease NOS B49
infection *—see* Infection, fungus
Funiculitis (acute) (chronic) (endemic) N49.1
gonococcal (acute) (chronic) A54.23
tuberculous A18.15
Funnel
breast (acquired) M95.4
congenital Q67.6
sequelae (late effect) of rickets E64.3
chest (acquired) M95.4
congenital Q67.6
sequelae (late effect) of rickets E64.3
pelvis (acquired) M95.5
with disproportion (fetopelvic) O33.3
causing obstructed labor O65.3
congenital Q74.2
FUO (fever of unknown origin) R5Ø.9
Furfur L21.Ø
microsporon B36.Ø
Furrier's lung J67.8
Furrowed K14.5
nail(s) (transverse) L6Ø.4
congenital Q84.6
tongue K14.5
congenital Q38.3
Furuncle LØ2.92
abdominal wall LØ2.221
ankle *—see* Furuncle, lower limb
antecubital space *—see* Furuncle, upper limb
anus K61.Ø
arm *—see* Furuncle, upper limb
auditory canal, external *—see* Abscess, ear, external
auricle (ear) *—see* Abscess, ear, external
axilla (region) LØ2.42-●
back (any part) LØ2.222
breast N61.1
buttock LØ2.32
cheek (external) LØ2.Ø2
chest wall LØ2.223
chin LØ2.Ø2
corpus cavernosum N48.21
ear, external *—see* Abscess, ear, external
external auditory canal *—see* Abscess, ear, external
eyelid *—see* Abscess, eyelid
face LØ2.Ø2
femoral (region) *—see* Furuncle, lower limb
finger *—see* Furuncle, hand
flank LØ2.221
foot LØ2.62-●
forehead LØ2.Ø2
gluteal (region) LØ2.32
groin LØ2.224
hand LØ2.52-●
head LØ2.821
face LØ2.Ø2
hip *—see* Furuncle, lower limb
kidney *—see* Abscess, kidney
knee *—see* Furuncle, lower limb
labium (majus) (minus) N76.4
lacrimal
gland *—see* Dacryoadenitis
passages (duct) (sac) *—see* Inflammation, lacrimal, passages, acute
leg (any part) *—see* Furuncle, lower limb
lower limb LØ2.42-●
malignant A22.Ø
mouth K12.2
navel LØ2.226
neck LØ2.12
nose J34.Ø
orbit, orbital *—see* Abscess, orbit
palmar (space) *—see* Furuncle, hand
partes posteriores LØ2.32
pectoral region LØ2.223
penis N48.21
perineum LØ2.225
pinna *—see* Abscess, ear, external
popliteal *—see* Furuncle, lower limb

Furuncle *(Continued)*
prepatellar *—see* Furuncle, lower limb
scalp LØ2.821
seminal vesicle N49.Ø
shoulder *—see* Furuncle, upper limb
specified site NEC LØ2.828
submandibular K12.2
temple (region) LØ2.Ø2
thumb *—see* Furuncle, hand
toe *—see* Furuncle, foot
trunk LØ2.229
abdominal wall LØ2.221
back LØ2.222
chest wall LØ2.223
groin LØ2.224
perineum LØ2.225
umbilicus LØ2.226
umbilicus LØ2.226
upper limb LØ2.42- ●
vulva N76.4
Furunculosis *—see* Furuncle
Fused *—see* Fusion, fused
Fusion, fused (congenital)
astragaloscaphoid Q74.2
atria Q21.1
auditory canal Q16.1
auricles, heart Q21.1
binocular with defective stereopsis H53.32
bone Q79.8
cervical spine M43.22

Fusion, fused *(Continued)*
choanal Q3Ø.Ø
commissure, mitral valve Q23.2
cusps, heart valve NEC Q24.8
mitral Q23.2
pulmonary Q22.1
tricuspid Q22.4
ear ossicles Q16.3
fingers Q7Ø.Ø- ●
hymen Q52.3
joint (acquired) *—see also* Ankylosis
congenital Q74.8
kidneys (incomplete) Q63.1
labium (majus) (minus) Q52.5
larynx and trachea Q34.8
limb, congenital Q74.8
lower Q74.2
upper Q74.Ø
lobes, lung Q33.8
lumbosacral (acquired) M43.27
arthrodesis status Z98.1
congenital Q76.49
postprocedural status Z98.1
nares, nose, nasal, nostril(s) Q3Ø.Ø
organ or site not listed *—see* Anomaly, by site
ossicles Q79.9
auditory Q16.3
pulmonic cusps Q22.1
ribs Q76.6

Fusion, fused *(Continued)*
sacroiliac (joint) (acquired) M43.28
arthrodesis status Z98.1
congenital Q74.2
postprocedural status Z98.1
spine (acquired) NEC M43.2Ø
arthrodesis status Z98.1
cervical region M43.22
cervicothoracic region M43.23
congenital Q76.49
lumbar M43.26
lumbosacral region M43.27
occipito-atlanto-axial region M43.21
postoperative status Z98.1
sacrococcygeal region M43.28
thoracic region M43.24
thoracolumbar region M43.25
sublingual duct with submaxillary duct at opening in mouth Q38.4
testes Q55.1
toes Q7Ø.2
tooth, teeth KØØ.2
trachea and esophagus Q39.8
twins Q89.4
vagina Q52.4
ventricles, heart Q21.Ø
vertebra (arch) *—see* Fusion, spine
vulva Q52.5
Fusospirillosis (mouth) (tongue) (tonsil) A69.1
Fussy baby R68.12

F

G

Gain in weight (abnormal) (excessive) —*see also* Weight, gain
Gaisböck's disease (polycythemia hypertonica) D75.1
Gait abnormality R26.9
  ataxic R26.Ø
  falling R29.6
  hysterical (ataxic) (staggering) F44.4
  paralytic R26.1
  spastic R26.1
  specified type NEC R26.89
  staggering R26.Ø
  unsteadiness R26.81
  walking difficulty NEC R26.2
Galactocele (breast) N64.89
  puerperal, postpartum O92.79
Galactokinase deficiency E74.29
Galactophoritis N61.Ø
  gestational, puerperal, postpartum O91.2- •
Galactorrhea O92.6
  not associated with childbirth N64.3
Galactosemia (classic) (congenital) E74.21
Galactosuria E74.29
Galacturia R82.Ø
  schistosomiasis (bilharziasis) B65.Ø
GALD (gestational alloimmune liver disease) P78.84
Galeazzi's fracture S52.37- •
Galen's vein —*see* condition
Galeophobia F4Ø.218
Gall duct —*see* condition
Gallbladder —*see also* condition
  acute K81.Ø
Gallop rhythm RØØ.8
Gallstone (colic) (cystic duct) (gallbladder) (impacted) (multiple) —*see also* Calculus, gallbladder
  with
    cholecystitis —*see* Calculus, gallbladder, with cholecystitis
  bile duct (common) (hepatic) —*see* Calculus, bile duct
  causing intestinal obstruction K56.3
  specified NEC K8Ø.8Ø
    with obstruction K8Ø.81
Gambling Z72.6
  pathological (compulsive) F63.Ø
Gammopathy (of undetermined significance [MGUS]) D47.2
  associated with lymphoplasmacytic dyscrasia D47.2
  monoclonal D47.2
  polyclonal D89.Ø
Gamna's disease (siderotic splenomegaly) D73.1
Gamophobia F4Ø.298
Gampsodactylia (congenital) Q66.7- •
Gamstorp's disease (adynamia episodica hereditaria) G72.3
Gandy-Nanta disease (siderotic splenomegaly) D73.1
Gang
  membership offenses Z72.81Ø
Gangliocytoma D36.1Ø
Ganglioglioma —*see* Neoplasm, uncertain behavior, by site
Ganglion (compound) (diffuse) (joint) (tendon (sheath)) M67.4Ø
  ankle M67.47- •
  foot M67.47- •
  forearm M67.43- •
  hand M67.44- •
  lower leg M67.46- •
  multiple sites M67.49
  of yaws (early) (late) A66.6
  pelvic region M67.45- •
  periosteal —*see* Periostitis
  shoulder region M67.41- •
  specified site NEC M67.48
Ganglion *(Continued)*
  thigh region M67.45- •
  tuberculous A18.Ø9
  upper arm M67.42- •
  wrist M67.43- •
Ganglioneuroblastoma —*see* Neoplasm, nerve, malignant
Ganglioneuroma D36.1Ø
  malignant —*see* Neoplasm, nerve, malignant
Ganglioneuromatosis D36.1Ø
Ganglionitis
  fifth nerve —*see* Neuralgia, trigeminal
  gasserian (postherpetic) (postzoster) BØ2.21
  geniculate G51.1
    newborn (birth injury) P11.3
    postherpetic, postzoster BØ2.21
  herpes zoster BØ2.21
  postherpetic geniculate BØ2.21
Gangliosidosis E75.1Ø
  GM1 E75.19
  GM2 E75.ØØ
    other specified E75.Ø9
    Sandhoff disease E75.Ø1
    Tay-Sachs disease E75.Ø2
  GM3 E75.19
  mucolipidosis IV E75.11
Gangosa A66.5
Gangrene, gangrenous (connective tissue) (dropsical) (dry) (moist) (skin) (ulcer) —*see also* Necrosis I96
  with diabetes (mellitus) —*see* Diabetes, gangrene
  abdomen (wall) I96
  alveolar M27.3
  appendix K35.8Ø
    with
      peritonitis, localized (*see also* Appendicitis) K35.31
  arteriosclerotic (general) (senile) —*see* Arteriosclerosis, extremities, with, gangrene
  auricle I96
  Bacillus welchii A48.Ø
  bladder (infectious) —*see* Cystitis, specified type NEC
  bowel, cecum, or colon —*see* Gangrene, intestine
  Clostridium perfringens or welchii A48.Ø
  cornea H18.89- •
  corpora cavernosa N48.29
    noninfective N48.89
  cutaneous, spreading I96
  decubital —*see* Ulcer, pressure, by site
  diabetic (any site) —*see* Diabetes, gangrene
  emphysematous —*see* Gangrene, gas
  epidemic —*see* Poisoning, food, noxious, plant
  epididymis (infectional) N45.1
  erysipelas —*see* Erysipelas
  extremity (lower) (upper) I96
  Fournier N49.3
    female N76.89
  fusospirochetal A69.Ø
  gallbladder —*see* Cholecystitis, acute
  gas (bacillus) A48.Ø
    following
      abortion —*see* Abortion by type complicated by infection
      ectopic or molar pregnancy OØ8.Ø
  glossitis K14.Ø
  hernia —*see* Hernia, by site, with gangrene
  intestine, intestinal (hemorrhagic) (massive) —*see also* Infarct, intestine K55.Ø69
    with
      mesenteric embolism —*see also* Infarct, intestine K55.Ø69
      obstruction —*see* Obstruction, intestine
  laryngitis JØ4.Ø
  limb (lower) (upper) I96
Gangrene, gangrenous *(Continued)*
  lung J85.Ø
    spirochetal A69.8
  lymphangitis I89.1
  Meleney's (synergistic) —*see* Ulcer, skin
  mesentery —*see also* Infarct, intestine K55.Ø69
    with
      embolism —*see also* Infarct, intestine K55.Ø69
      intestinal obstruction —*see* Obstruction, intestine
  mouth A69.Ø
  ovary —*see* Oophoritis
  pancreas —*see* Pancreatitis, acute
  penis N48.29
    noninfective N48.89
  perineum I96
  pharynx —*see also* Pharyngitis
    Vincent's A69.1
  presenile I73.1
  progressive synergistic —*see* Ulcer, skin
  pulmonary J85.Ø
  pulpal (dental) KØ4.1
  quinsy J36
  Raynaud's (symmetric gangrene) I73.Ø1
  retropharyngeal J39.2
  scrotum N49.3
    noninfective N5Ø.89
  senile (atherosclerotic) —*see* Arteriosclerosis, extremities, with, gangrene
  spermatic cord N49.1
    noninfective N5Ø.89
  spine I96
  spirochetal NEC A69.8
  spreading cutaneous I96
  stomatitis A69.Ø
  symmetrical I73.Ø1
  testis (infectional) N45.2
    noninfective N44.8
  throat —*see also* Pharyngitis
    diphtheritic A36.Ø
    Vincent's A69.1
  thyroid (gland) EØ7.89
  tooth (pulp) KØ4.1
  tuberculous NEC —*see* Tuberculosis
  tunica vaginalis N49.1
    noninfective N5Ø.89
  umbilicus I96
  uterus —*see* Endometritis
  uvulitis K12.2
  vas deferens N49.1
    noninfective N5Ø.89
  vulva N76.89
Ganister disease J62.8
Ganser's syndrome (hysterical) F44.89
Gardner-Diamond syndrome (autoerythrocyte sensitization) D69.2
Gargoylism E76.Ø1
Garré's disease, osteitis (sclerosing), **osteomyelitis** —*see* Osteomyelitis, specified type NEC
Garrod's pad, knuckle M72.1
Gartner's duct
  cyst Q52.4
  persistent Q5Ø.6
Gas R14.3
  asphyxiation, inhalation, poisoning, suffocation NEC —*see* Table of Drugs and Chemicals
  excessive R14.Ø
  gangrene A48.Ø
    following
      abortion —*see* Abortion by type complicated by infection
      ectopic or molar pregnancy OØ8.Ø
  on stomach R14.Ø
  pains R14.1
Gastralgia —*see also* Pain, abdominal
Gastrectasis K31.Ø
  psychogenic F45.8

Gastric —*see* condition
Gastrinoma
malignant
pancreas C25.4
specified site NEC —*see* Neoplasm, malignant, by site
unspecified site C25.4
specified site —*see* Neoplasm, uncertain behavior
unspecified site D37.9
Gastritis (simple) K29.70
with bleeding K29.71
acute (erosive) K29.00
with bleeding K29.01
alcoholic K29.20
with bleeding K29.21
allergic K29.60
with bleeding K29.61
atrophic (chronic) K29.40
with bleeding K29.41
chronic (antral) (fundal) K29.50
with bleeding K29.51
atrophic K29.40
with bleeding K29.41
superficial K29.30
with bleeding K29.31
dietary counseling and surveillance Z71.3
due to diet deficiency E63.9
eosinophilic K52.81
giant hypertrophic K29.60
with bleeding K29.61
granulomatous K29.60
with bleeding K29.61
hypertrophic (mucosa) K29.60
with bleeding K29.61
nervous F54
spastic K29.60
with bleeding K29.61
specified NEC K29.60
with bleeding K29.61
superficial chronic K29.30
with bleeding K29.31
tuberculous A18.83
viral NEC A08.4
Gastrocarcinoma —*see* Neoplasm, malignant, stomach
Gastrocolic —*see* condition
Gastrodisciasis, gastrodiscoidiasis B66.8
Gastroduodenitis K29.90
with bleeding K29.91
virus, viral A08.4
specified type NEC A08.39
Gastrodynia —*see* Pain, abdominal
Gastroenteritis (acute) (chronic) (noninfectious) (*see also* Enteritis) K52.9
allergic K52.29
with
eosinophilic gastritis or gastroenteritis K52.81
food protein-induced enterocolitis syndrome K52.21
food protein-induced enteropathy K52.22
dietetic —*see also* Gastroenteritis, allergic K52.29
drug-induced K52.1
due to
Cryptosporidium A07.2
drugs K52.1
food poisoning —*see* Intoxication, foodborne
radiation K52.0
eosinophilic K52.81
epidemic (infectious) A09
food hypersensitivity —*see also* Gastroenteritis, allergic K52.29
infectious —*see* Enteritis, infectious
influenzal —*see* Influenza, with gastroenteritis
noninfectious K52.9
specified NEC K52.89
rotaviral A08.0
Gastroenteritis *(Continued)*
Salmonella A02.0
toxic K52.1
viral NEC A08.4
acute infectious A08.39
type Norwalk A08.11
infantile (acute) A08.39
Norwalk agent A08.11
rotaviral A08.0
severe of infants A08.39
specified type NEC A08.39
Gastroenteropathy —*see also* Gastroenteritis K52.9
acute, due to Norovirus A08.11
acute, due to Norwalk agent A08.11
infectious A09
Gastroenteroptosis K63.4
Gastroesophageal laceration-hemorrhage syndrome K22.6
Gastrointestinal —*see* condition
Gastrojejunal —*see* condition
Gastrojejunitis —*see also* Enteritis K52.9
Gastrojejunocolic —*see* condition
Gastroliths K31.89
Gastromalacia K31.89
Gastroparalysis K31.84
diabetic —*see* Diabetes, gastroparalysis
Gastroparesis K31.84
diabetic —*see* Diabetes, by type, with gastroparesis
Gastropathy K31.9
congestive portal K31.89
erythematous K29.70
exudative K90.89
portal hypertensive K31.89
Gastroptosis K31.89
Gastrorrhagia K92.2
psychogenic F45.8
Gastroschisis (congenital) Q79.3
Gastrospasm (neurogenic) (reflex) K31.89
neurotic F45.8
psychogenic F45.8
Gastrostaxis —*see* Gastritis, with bleeding
Gastrostenosis K31.89
Gastrostomy
attention to Z43.1
status Z93.1
Gastrosuccorrhea (continuous) (intermittent) K31.89
neurotic F45.8
psychogenic F45.8
Gatophobia F40.218
Gaucher's disease or splenomegaly (adult) (infantile) E75.22
Gee (-Herter)(-Thaysen) **disease** (nontropical sprue) K90.0
Gélineau's syndrome G47.419
with cataplexy G47.411
Gemination, tooth, teeth K00.2
Gemistocytoma
specified site —*see* Neoplasm, malignant, by site
unspecified site C71.9
General, generalized —*see* condition
Genetic
carrier (status)
cystic fibrosis Z14.1
hemophilia A (asymptomatic) Z14.01
symptomatic Z14.02
specified NEC Z14.8
susceptibility to disease NEC Z15.89
malignant neoplasm Z15.09
breast Z15.01
endometrium Z15.04
ovary Z15.02
prostate Z15.03
specified NEC Z15.09
multiple endocrine neoplasia Z15.81
Genital —*see* condition
Genito-anorectal syndrome A55
Genitourinary system —*see* condition
Genu
congenital Q74.1
extrorsum (acquired) —*see also* Deformity, varus, knee
congenital Q74.1
sequelae (late effect) of rickets E64.3
introrsum (acquired) —*see also* Deformity, valgus, knee
congenital Q74.1
sequelae (late effect) of rickets E64.3
rachitic (old) E64.3
recurvatum (acquired) —*see also* Deformity, limb, specified type NEC, lower leg
congenital Q68.2
sequelae (late effect) of rickets E64.3
valgum (acquired) (knock-knee) M21.06- ●
congenital Q74.1
sequelae (late effect) of rickets E64.3
varum (acquired) (bowleg) M21.16- ●
congenital Q74.1
sequelae (late effect) of rickets E64.3
Geographic tongue K14.1
Geophagia —*see* Pica
Geotrichosis B48.3
stomatitis B48.3
Gephyrophobia F40.242
Gerbode defect Q21.0
GERD (gastroesophageal reflux disease) K21.9
Gerhardt's
disease (erythromelalgia) I73.81
syndrome (vocal cord paralysis) J38.00
bilateral J38.02
unilateral J38.01
German measles —*see also* Rubella
exposure to Z20.4
Germinoblastoma (diffuse) C85.9- ●
follicular C82.9- ●
Germinoma —*see* Neoplasm, malignant, by site
Gerontoxon —*see* Degeneration, cornea, senile
Gerstmann-Sträussler-Scheinker syndrome (GSS) A81.82
Gerstmann's syndrome R48.8
developmental F81.2
Gestation (period) —*see also* Pregnancy
ectopic —*see* Pregnancy, by site
multiple O30.9- ●
greater than quadruplets —*see* Pregnancy, multiple (gestation), specified NEC
specified NEC —*see* Pregnancy, multiple (gestation), specified NEC
Gestational
mammary abscess O91.11- ●
purulent mastitis O91.11- ●
subareolar abscess O91.11- ●
Ghon tubercle, primary infection A15.7
Ghost
teeth K00.4
vessels (cornea) H16.41- ●
Ghoul hand A66.3
Gianotti-Crosti disease L44.4
Giant
cell
epulis K06.8
peripheral granuloma K06.8
esophagus, congenital Q39.5
kidney, congenital Q63.3
urticaria T78.3
hereditary D84.1
Giardiasis A07.1
Gibert's disease or pityriasis L42
Giddiness R42
hysterical F44.89
psychogenic F45.8
Gierke's disease (glycogenosis I) E74.01
Gigantism (cerebral) (hypophyseal) (pituitary) E22.0
constitutional E34.4
Gilbert's disease or syndrome E80.4
Gilchrist's disease B40.9
Gilford-Hutchinson disease E34.8

Gilles de la Tourette's disease or syndrome (motor-verbal tic) F95.2
Gingivitis K05.10
acute (catarrhal) K05.00
necrotizing A69.1
nonplaque induced K05.01
plaque induced K05.00
chronic (desquamative) (hyperplastic) (simple marginal) (pregnancy associated) (ulcerative) K05.10
nonplaque induced K05.11
plaque induced K05.10
expulsiva —*see* Periodontitis
necrotizing ulcerative (acute) A69.1
pellagrous E52
acute necrotizing A69.1
Vincent's A69.1
Gingivoglossitis K14.0
Gingivopericementitis —*see* Periodontitis
Gingivosis —*see* Gingivitis, chronic
Gingivostomatitis K05.10
herpesviral B00.2
necrotizing ulcerative (acute) A69.1
Gland, glandular —*see* condition
Glanders A24.0
Glanzmann (-Naegeli) disease or thrombasthenia D69.1
Glasgow coma scale
total score
3-8 R40.243
9-12 R40.242
13-15 R40.241
Glass-blower's disease (cataract) —*see* Cataract, specified NEC
Glaucoma H40.9
with
increased episcleral venous pressure H40.81-●
pseudoexfoliation of lens —*see* Glaucoma, open angle, primary, capsular
absolute H44.51-●
angle-closure (primary) H40.20-●
acute (attack) (crisis) H40.21-●
chronic H40.22-●
intermittent H40.23-●
residual stage H40.24-●
borderline H40.00-●
capsular (with pseudoexfoliation of lens) —*see* Glaucoma, open angle, primary, capsular
childhood Q15.0
closed angle —*see* Glaucoma, angle-closure
congenital Q15.0
corticosteroid-induced —*see* Glaucoma, secondary, drugs
hypersecretion H40.82-●
in (due to)
amyloidosis E85.4 *[H42]*
aniridia Q13.1 *[H42]*
concussion of globe —*see* Glaucoma, secondary, trauma
dislocation of lens —*see* Glaucoma, secondary
disorder of lens NEC —*see* Glaucoma, secondary
drugs —*see* Glaucoma, secondary, drugs
endocrine disease NOS E34.9 *[H42]*
eye
inflammation —*see* Glaucoma, secondary, inflammation
trauma —*see* Glaucoma, secondary, trauma
hypermature cataract —*see* Glaucoma, secondary
iridocyclitis —*see* Glaucoma, secondary, inflammation
lens disorder —*see* Glaucoma, secondary,
Lowe's syndrome E72.03 *[H42]*
metabolic disease NOS E88.9 *[H42]*
ocular disorders NEC —*see* Glaucoma, secondary

Glaucoma *(Continued)*
in (due to) *(Continued)*
onchocerciasis B73.02
pupillary block —*see* Glaucoma, secondary
retinal vein occlusion —*see* Glaucoma, secondary
Rieger's anomaly Q13.81 *[H42]*
rubeosis of iris —*see* Glaucoma, secondary
tumor of globe —*see* Glaucoma, secondary
infantile Q15.0
low tension —*see* Glaucoma, open angle, primary, low-tension
malignant H40.83-●
narrow angle —*see* Glaucoma, angle-closure
newborn Q15.0
noncongestive (chronic) —*see* Glaucoma, open angle
nonobstructive —*see* Glaucoma, open angle
obstructive —*see also* Glaucoma, angle-closure
due to lens changes —*see* Glaucoma, secondary
open angle H40.10-●
primary H40.11-●
capsular (with pseudoexfoliation of lens) H40.14-●
low-tension H40.12-●
pigmentary H40.13-●
residual stage H40.15-●
phacolytic —*see* Glaucoma, secondary
pigmentary —*see* Glaucoma, open angle, primary, pigmentary
postinfectious —*see* Glaucoma, secondary, inflammation
secondary (to) H40.5-●
drugs H40.6-●
inflammation H40.4-●
trauma H40.3-●
simple (chronic) H40.11-●
simplex H40.11-●
specified type NEC H40.89
suspect H40.00-●
syphilitic A52.71
traumatic —*see also* Glaucoma, secondary, trauma
newborn (birth injury) P15.3
tuberculous A18.59
Glaucomatous flecks (subcapsular) —*see* Cataract, complicated
Glazed tongue K14.4
Gleet (gonococcal) A54.01
Glénard's disease K63.4
Glioblastoma (multiforme)
with sarcomatous component
specified site —*see* Neoplasm, malignant, by site
unspecified site C71.9
giant cell
specified site —*see* Neoplasm, malignant, by site
unspecified site C71.9
specified site —*see* Neoplasm, malignant, by site
unspecified site C71.9
Glioma (malignant)
astrocytic
specified site —*see* Neoplasm, malignant, by site
unspecified site C71.9
mixed
specified site —*see* Neoplasm, malignant, by site
unspecified site C71.9
nose Q30.8
specified site NEC —*see* Neoplasm, malignant, by site
subependymal D43.2
specified site —*see* Neoplasm, uncertain behavior, by site
unspecified site D43.2
unspecified site C71.9

Gliomatosis cerebri C71.0
Glioneuroma —*see* Neoplasm, uncertain behavior, by site
Gliosarcoma
specified site —*see* Neoplasm, malignant, by site
unspecified site C71.9
Gliosis (cerebral) G93.89
spinal G95.89
Glisson's disease —*see* Rickets
Globinuria R82.3
Globus (hystericus) F45.8
Glomangioma D18.00
intra-abdominal D18.03
intracranial D18.02
skin D18.01
specified site NEC D18.09
Glomangiomyoma D18.00
intra-abdominal D18.03
intracranial D18.02
skin D18.01
specified site NEC D18.09
Glomangiosarcoma —*see* Neoplasm, connective tissue, malignant
Glomerular
disease in syphilis A52.75
nephritis —*see* Glomerulonephritis
Glomerulitis —*see* Glomerulonephritis
Glomerulonephritis —*see also* Nephritis N05.9
with
edema —*see* Nephrosis
minimal change N05.0
minor glomerular abnormality N05.0
acute N00.9
chronic N03.9
crescentic (diffuse) NEC —*see also* N00-N07 with fourth character .7 N05.7
dense deposit —*see also* N00-N07 with fourth character .6 N05.6
diffuse
crescentic —*see also* N00-N07 with fourth character .7 N05.7
endocapillary proliferative —*see also* N00N07 with fourth character .4 N05.4
membranous —*see also* N00-N07 with fourth character .2 N05.2
mesangial proliferative —*see also* N00-N07 with fourth character .3 N05.3
mesangiocapillary —*see also* N00-N07 with fourth character .5 N05.5
sclerosing N18.9
endocapillary proliferative (diffuse) NEC —*see also* N00-N07 with fourth character .4 N05.4
extracapillary NEC —*see also* N00-N07 with fourth character .7 N05.7
focal (and segmental) —*see also* N00-N07 with fourth character .1 N05.1
hypocomplementemic —*see* Glomerulonephritis, membranoproliferative
IgA —*see* Nephropathy, IgA
immune complex (circulating) NEC N05.8
in (due to)
amyloidosis E85.4 *[N08]*
bilharziasis B65.9 *[N08]*
cryoglobulinemia D89.1 *[N08]*
defibrination syndrome D65 *[N08]*
diabetes mellitus —*see* Diabetes, glomerulosclerosis
disseminated intravascular coagulation D65 *[N08]*
Fabry (-Anderson) disease E75.21 *[N08]*
Goodpasture's syndrome M31.0
hemolytic-uremic syndrome D59.3
Henoch (-Schönlein) purpura D69.0 *[N08]*
lecithin cholesterol acyltransferase deficiency E78.6 *[N08]*

Glomerulonephritis *(Continued)*
- in *(Continued)*
  - microscopic polyangiitis M31.7 *[N08]*
  - multiple myeloma C90.0-● *[N08]*
  - Plasmodium malariae B52.0
  - schistosomiasis B65.9 *[N08]*
  - sepsis A41.9-● *[N08]*
    - streptococcal A40-● *[N08]*
  - sickle-cell disorders D57.-● *[N08]*
  - strongyloidiasis B78.9 *[N08]*
  - subacute bacterial endocarditis I33.0 *[N08]*
  - syphilis (late) congenital A50.59 *[N08]*
  - systemic lupus erythematosus M32.14
  - thrombotic thrombocytopenic purpura M31.1 *[N08]*
  - typhoid fever A01.09
  - Waldenström macroglobulinemia C88.0 *[N08]*
  - Wegener's granulomatosis M31.31
- latent or quiescent N03.9
- lobular, lobulonodular —*see* Glomerulonephritis, membranoproliferative
- membranoproliferative (diffuse) (type 1 or 3) —*see also* N00-N07 with fourth character .5 N05.5
  - dense deposit (type 2) NEC —*see also* N00-N07 with fourth character .6 N05.6
- membranous (diffuse) NEC —*see also* N00-N07 with fourth character .2 N05.2
- mesangial
  - IgA/IgG —*see* Nephropathy, IgA
  - proliferative (diffuse) NEC —*see also* N00-N07 with fourth character .3 N05.3
- mesangiocapillary (diffuse) NEC —*see also* N00-N07 with fourth character .5 N05.5
- necrotic, necrotizing NEC —*see also* N00-N07 with fourth character .8 N05.8
- nodular —*see* Glomerulonephritis, membranoproliferative
- poststreptococcal NEC N05.9
  - acute N00.9
  - chronic N03.9
  - rapidly progressive N01.9
- proliferative NEC —*see also* N00-N07 with fourth character .8 N05.8
  - diffuse (lupus) M32.14
- rapidly progressive N01.9
- sclerosing, diffuse N18.9
- specified pathology NEC —*see also* N00-N07 with fourth character .8 N05.8
- subacute N01.9

Glomerulopathy —*see* Glomerulonephritis

Glomerulosclerosis —*see also* Sclerosis, renal
- intercapillary (nodular) (with diabetes) —*see* Diabetes, glomerulosclerosis
- intracapillary —*see* Diabetes, glomerulosclerosis

Glossagra K14.6

Glossalgia K14.6

Glossitis (chronic superficial) (gangrenous) (Moeller's) K14.0
- areata exfoliativa K14.1
- atrophic K14.4
- benign migratory K14.1
- cortical superficial, sclerotic K14.0
- Hunter's D51.0
- interstitial, sclerous K14.0
- median rhomboid K14.2
- pellagrous E52
- superficial, chronic K14.0

Glossocele K14.8

Glossodynia K14.6
- exfoliativa K14.4

Glossoncus K14.8

Glossopathy K14.9

Glossophytia K14.3

Glossoplegia K14.8

Glossoptosis K14.8

Glossopyrosis K14.6

Glossotrichia K14.3

Glossy skin L90.8

Glottis —*see* condition

Glottitis —*see also* Laryngitis J04.0

Glucagonoma
- pancreas
  - benign D13.7
  - malignant C25.4
  - uncertain behavior D37.8
- specified site NEC
  - benign —*see* Neoplasm, benign, by site
  - malignant —*see* Neoplasm, malignant, by site
  - uncertain behavior —*see* Neoplasm, uncertain behavior, by site
- unspecified site
  - benign D13.7
  - malignant C25.4
  - uncertain behavior D37.8

Glucoglycinuria E72.51

Glucose-galactose malabsorption E74.39

Glue
- ear —*see* Otitis, media, nonsuppurative, chronic, mucoid
- sniffing (airplane) —*see* Abuse, drug, inhalant
  - dependence —*see* Dependence, drug, inhalant

Glutaric aciduria E72.3

Glycinemia E72.51

Glycinuria (renal) (with ketosis) E72.09

Glycogen
- infiltration —*see* Disease, glycogen storage
- storage disease —*see* Disease, glycogen storage

Glycogenosis (diffuse) (generalized) —*see also* Disease, glycogen storage
- cardiac E74.02 *[I43]*
- diabetic, secondary —*see* Diabetes, glycogenosis, secondary
- pulmonary interstitial J84.842

Glycopenia E16.2

Glycosuria R81
- renal E74.8

Gnathostoma spinigerum (infection) (infestation), **gnathostomiasis** (wandering swelling) B83.1

Goiter (plunging) (substernal) E04.9
- with
  - hyperthyroidism (recurrent) —*see* Hyperthyroidism, with, goiter
  - thyrotoxicosis —*see* Hyperthyroidism, with, goiter
- adenomatous —*see* Goiter, nodular
- cancerous C73
- congenital (nontoxic) E03.0
  - diffuse E03.0
  - parenchymatous E03.0
  - transitory, with normal functioning P72.0
- cystic E04.2
  - due to iodine-deficiency E01.1
- due to
  - enzyme defect in synthesis of thyroid hormone E07.1
  - iodine-deficiency (endemic) E01.2
- dyshormonogenetic (familial) E07.1
- endemic (iodine-deficiency) E01.2
  - diffuse E01.0
  - multinodular E01.1
- exophthalmic —*see* Hyperthyroidism, with, goiter
- iodine-deficiency (endemic) E01.2
  - diffuse E01.0
  - multinodular E01.1
  - nodular E01.1
- lingual Q89.2
- lymphadenoid E06.3
- malignant C73
- multinodular (cystic) (nontoxic) E04.2
  - toxic or with hyperthyroidism E05.20
    - with thyroid storm E05.21
- neonatal NEC P72.0
- nodular (nontoxic) (due to) E04.9
  - with
    - hyperthyroidism E05.20
      - with thyroid storm E05.21
    - thyrotoxicosis E05.20
      - with thyroid storm E05.21
  - endemic E01.1
  - iodine-deficiency E01.1
  - sporadic E04.9
  - toxic E05.20
    - with thyroid storm E05.21
- nontoxic E04.9
  - diffuse (colloid) E04.0
  - multinodular E04.2
  - simple E04.0
  - specified NEC E04.8
  - uninodular E04.1
- simple E04.0
- toxic —*see* Hyperthyroidism, with, goiter
- uninodular (nontoxic) E04.1
  - toxic or with hyperthyroidism E05.10
    - with thyroid storm E05.11

Goiter-deafness syndrome E07.1

Goldberg syndrome Q89.8

Goldberg-Maxwell syndrome E34.51

Goldblatt's hypertension or kidney I70.1

Goldenhar (-Gorlin) **syndrome** Q87.0

Goldflam-Erb disease or syndrome G70.00
- with exacerbation (acute) G70.01
- in crisis G70.01

Goldscheider's disease Q81.8

Goldstein's disease (familial hemorrhagic telangiectasia) I78.0

Golfer's elbow —*see* Epicondylitis, medial

Gonadoblastoma
- specified site —*see* Neoplasm, uncertain behavior, by site
- unspecified site
  - female D39.10
  - male D40.10

Gonecystitis —*see* Vesiculitis

Gongylonemiasis B83.8

Goniosynechiae —*see* Adhesions, iris, goniosynechiae

Gonococcemia A54.86

Gonococcus, gonococcal (disease) (infection) —*see also* condition A54.9
- anus A54.6
- bursa, bursitis A54.49
- conjunctiva, conjunctivitis (neonatorum) A54.31
- endocardium A54.83
- eye A54.30
  - conjunctivitis A54.31
  - iridocyclitis A54.32
  - keratitis A54.33
  - newborn A54.31
  - other specified A54.39
- fallopian tubes (acute) (chronic) A54.24
- genitourinary (organ) (system) (tract) (acute)
  - lower A54.00
    - with abscess (accessory gland) (periurethral) A54.1
  - upper —*see also* condition A54.29
- heart A54.83
- iridocyclitis A54.32
- joint A54.42
- lymphatic (gland) (node) A54.89
- meninges, meningitis A54.81
- musculoskeletal A54.40
  - arthritis A54.42
  - osteomyelitis A54.43
  - other specified A54.49
  - spondylopathy A54.41
- pelviperitonitis A54.24
- pelvis (acute) (chronic) A54.24

▶ New ⇒ Revised ~~deleted~~ Deleted ● Use Additional Character(s)

Gonococcus, gonococcal *(Continued)*
pharynx A54.5
proctitis A54.6
pyosalpinx (acute) (chronic) A54.24
rectum A54.6
skin A54.89
specified site NEC A54.89
tendon sheath A54.49
throat A54.5
urethra (acute) (chronic) A54.Ø1
with abscess (accessory gland) (periurethral) A54.1
vulva (acute) (chronic) A54.Ø2
Gonocytoma
specified site *—see* Neoplasm, uncertain behavior, by site
unspecified site
female D39.1Ø
male D4Ø.1Ø
Gonorrhea (acute) (chronic) A54.9
Bartholin's gland (acute) (chronic) (purulent) A54.Ø2
with abscess (accessory gland) (periurethral) A54.1
bladder A54.Ø1
cervix A54.Ø3
conjunctiva, conjunctivitis (neonatorum) A54.31
contact Z2Ø.2
Cowper's gland (with abscess) A54.1
exposure to Z2Ø.2
fallopian tube (acute) (chronic) A54.24
kidney (acute) (chronic) A54.21
lower genitourinary tract A54.ØØ
with abscess (accessory gland) (periurethral) A54.1
ovary (acute) (chronic) A54.24
pelvis (acute) (chronic) A54.24
female pelvic inflammatory disease A54.24
penis A54.Ø9
prostate (acute) (chronic) A54.22
seminal vesicle (acute) (chronic) A54.23
specified site not listed *—see also* Gonococcus A54.89
spermatic cord (acute) (chronic) A54.23
urethra A54.Ø1
with abscess (accessory gland) (periurethral) A54.1
vagina A54.Ø2
vas deferens (acute) (chronic) A54.23
vulva A54.Ø2
Goodall's disease AØ8.19
Goodpasture's syndrome M31.Ø
Gopalan's syndrome (burning feet) E53.Ø
Gorlin-Chaudry-Moss syndrome Q87.Ø
Gottron's papules L94.4
Gougerot's syndrome (trisymptomatic) L81.7
Gougerot-Blum syndrome (pigmented purpuric lichenoid dermatitis) L81.7
Gougerot-Carteaud disease or syndrome (confluent reticulate papillomatosis) L83
Gouley's syndrome (constrictive pericarditis) I31.1
Goundou A66.6
Gout, chronic (*see also* Gout, gouty) M1A.9-•
drug-induced M1A.2Ø
ankle M1A.27-•
elbow M1A.22-•
foot joint M1A.27-•
hand joint M1A.24-•
hip M1A.25-•
knee M1A.26-•
multiple site M1A.29-•
shoulder M1A.21-•
vertebrae M1A.28
wrist M1A.23-•
idiopathic M1A.ØØ
ankle M1A.Ø7-•
elbow M1A.Ø2-•
foot joint M1A.Ø7-•
hand joint M1A.Ø4-•
Gout, chronic *(Continued)*
idiopathic *(Continued)*
hip M1A.Ø5-•
knee M1A.Ø6-•
multiple site M1A.Ø9
shoulder M1A.Ø1-•
vertebrae M1A.Ø8
wrist M1A.Ø3-•
in (due to) renal impairment M1A.3Ø
ankle M1A.37-•
elbow M1A.32-•
foot joint M1A.37-•
hand joint M1A.34-•
hip M1A.35-•
knee M1A.36-•
multiple site M1A.39
shoulder M1A.31-•
vertebrae M1A.38
wrist M1A.33-•
lead-induced M1A.1Ø
ankle M1A.17-•
elbow M1A.12-•
foot joint M1A.17-•
hand joint M1A.14-•
hip M1A.15-•
knee M1A.16-•
multiple site M1A.19
shoulder M1A.11-•
vertebrae M1A.18
wrist M1A.13-•
primary *—see* Gout, chronic, idiopathic
saturnine *—see* Gout, chronic, lead-induced
secondary NEC M1A.4Ø
ankle M1A.47-•
elbow M1A.42-•
foot joint M1A.47-•
hand joint M1A.44-•
hip M1A.45-•
knee M1A.46-•
multiple site M1A.49
shoulder M1A.41-•
vertebrae M1A.48
wrist M1A.43-•
syphilitic *—see also* subcategory M14.8-• A52.77
tophi M1A.9
Gout, gouty (acute) (attack) (flare) *—see also* Gout, chronic M1Ø.9-•
drug-induced M1Ø.2Ø
ankle M1Ø.27-•
elbow M1Ø.22-•
foot joint M1Ø.27-•
hand joint M1Ø.24-•
hip M1Ø.25-•
knee M1Ø.26-•
multiple site M1Ø.29
shoulder M1Ø.21-•
vertebrae M1Ø.28
wrist M1Ø.23-•
idiopathic M1Ø.ØØ
ankle M1Ø.Ø7-•
elbow M1Ø.Ø2-•
foot joint M1Ø.Ø7-•
hand joint M1Ø.Ø4-•
hip M1Ø.Ø5-•
knee M1Ø.Ø6-•
multiple site M1Ø.Ø9
shoulder M1Ø.Ø1-•
vertebrae M1Ø.Ø8
wrist M1Ø.Ø3-•
in (due to) renal impairment M1Ø.3Ø
ankle M1Ø.37-•
elbow M1Ø.32-•
foot joint M1Ø.37-•
hand joint M1Ø.34-•
hip M1Ø.35-•
knee M1Ø.36-•
multiple site M1Ø.39
shoulder M1Ø.31-•
vertebrae M1Ø.38
wrist M1Ø.33-•
Gout, gouty *(Continued)*
lead-induced M1Ø.1Ø
ankle M1Ø.17-•
elbow M1Ø.12-•
foot joint M1Ø.17-•
hand joint M1Ø.14-•
hip M1Ø.15-•
knee M1Ø.16-•
multiple site M1Ø.19
shoulder M1Ø.11-•
vertebrae M1Ø.18
wrist M1Ø.13-•
primary *—see* Gout, idiopathic
saturnine *—see* Gout, lead-induced
secondary NEC M1Ø.4Ø
ankle M1Ø.47-•
elbow M1Ø.42-•
foot joint M1Ø.47-•
hand joint M1Ø.44-•
hip M1Ø.45-•
knee M1Ø.46-•
multiple site M1Ø.49
shoulder M1Ø.41-•
vertebrae M1Ø.48
wrist M1Ø.43-•
syphilitic *—see also* subcategory M14.8-• A52.77
tophi NEC *—see* Gout, chronic
Gower's
muscular dystrophy G71.Ø1
syndrome (vasovagal attack) R55
Gradenigo's syndrome *—see* Otitis, media, suppurative, acute
Graefe's disease *—see* Strabismus, paralytic, ophthalmoplegia, progressive
Graft-versus-host disease D89.813
acute D89.81Ø
acute on chronic D89.812
chronic D89.811
Grain mite (itch) B88.Ø
Grainhandler's disease or lung J67.8
Grand mal *—see* Epilepsy, generalized, specified NEC
Grand multipara status only (not pregnant) Z64.1
pregnant *—see* Pregnancy, complicated by, grand multiparity
Granite worker's lung J62.8
Granular *—see also* condition
inflammation, pharynx J31.2
kidney (contracting) *—see* Sclerosis, renal
liver K74.69
Granulation tissue (abnormal) (excessive) L92.9
postmastoidectomy cavity *—see* Complications, postmastoidectomy, granulation
Granulocytopenia (primary) (malignant) *—see* Agranulocytosis
Granuloma L92.9
abdomen K66.8
from residual foreign body L92.3
pyogenicum L98.Ø
actinic L57.5
annulare (perforating) L92.Ø
apical KØ4.5
aural *—see* Otitis, externa, specified NEC
beryllium (skin) L92.3
bone
eosinophilic C96.6
from residual foreign body *—see* Osteomyelitis, specified type NEC
lung C96.6
brain (any site) GØ6.Ø
schistosomiasis B65.9 *[GØ7]*
canaliculus lacrimalis *—see* Granuloma, lacrimal
candidal (cutaneous) B37.2
cerebral (any site) GØ6.Ø
coccidioidal (primary) (progressive) B38.7
lung B38.1
meninges B38.4

- Granuloma *(Continued)*
  - colon K63.89
  - conjunctiva H11.22-●
  - dental KØ4.5
  - ear, middle —*see* Cholesteatoma
  - eosinophilic C96.6
    - bone C96.6
    - lung C96.6
    - oral mucosa K13.4
    - skin L92.2
  - eyelid HØ1.8
  - facial (e) L92.2
  - foreign body (in soft tissue) NEC M6Ø.2Ø
    - ankle M6Ø.27-●
    - foot M6Ø.27-●
    - forearm M6Ø.23-●
    - hand M6Ø.24-●
    - in operation wound —*see* Foreign body, accidentally left during a procedure
    - lower leg M6Ø.26-●
    - pelvic region M6Ø.25-●
    - shoulder region M6Ø.21-●
    - skin L92.3
    - specified site NEC M6Ø.28
    - subcutaneous tissue L92.3
    - thigh M6Ø.25-●
    - upper arm M6Ø.22-●
  - gangraenescens M31.2
  - genito-inguinale A58
  - giant cell (central) (reparative) (jaw) M27.1
    - gingiva (peripheral) KØ6.8
  - gland (lymph) I88.8
  - hepatic NEC K75.3
    - in (due to)
      - berylliosis J63.2 *[K77]*
      - sarcoidosis D86.89
  - Hodgkin C81.9
  - ileum K63.89
  - infectious B99.9
    - specified NEC B99.8
  - inguinale (Donovan) (venereal) A58
  - intestine NEC K63.89
  - intracranial (any site) GØ6.Ø
  - intraspinal (any part) GØ6.1
  - iridocyclitis —*see* Iridocyclitis, chronic
  - jaw (bone) (central) M27.1
    - reparative giant cell M27.1
  - kidney —*see also* Infection, kidney N15.8
  - lacrimal HØ4.81-●
  - larynx J38.7
  - lethal midline (faciale (e)) M31.2
  - liver NEC —*see* Granuloma, hepatic
  - lung (infectious) —*see also* Fibrosis, lung
    - coccidioidal B38.1
    - eosinophilic C96.6
  - Majocchi's B35.8
  - malignant (facial (e)) M31.2
  - mandible (central) M27.1
  - midline (lethal) M31.2
  - monilial (cutaneous) B37.2
  - nasal sinus —*see* Sinusitis
  - operation wound T81.89
    - foreign body —*see* Foreign body, accidentally left during a procedure
    - stitch T81.89
    - talc —*see* Foreign body, accidentally left during a procedure
  - oral mucosa K13.4
  - orbit, orbital HØ5.11-●
  - paracoccidioidal B41.8
  - penis, venereal A58
  - periapical KØ4.5
  - peritoneum K66.8
    - due to ova of helminths NOS —*see also* Helminthiasis B83.9 *[K67]*
  - postmastoidectomy cavity —*see* Complications, postmastoidectomy, recurrent cholesteatoma
  - prostate N42.89
  - pudendi (ulcerating) A58
  - pulp, internal (tooth) KØ3.3
- Granuloma *(Continued)*
  - pyogenic, pyogenicum (of) (skin) L98.Ø
    - gingiva KØ6.8
    - maxillary alveolar ridge KØ4.5
    - oral mucosa K13.4
  - rectum K62.89
  - reticulohistiocytic D76.3
  - rubrum nasi L74.8
  - Schistosoma —*see* Schistosomiasis
  - septic (skin) L98.Ø
  - silica (skin) L92.3
  - sinus (accessory) (infective) (nasal) —*see* Sinusitis
  - skin L92.9
    - from residual foreign body L92.3
    - pyogenicum L98.Ø
  - spine
    - syphilitic (epidural) A52.19
    - tuberculous A18.Ø1
  - stitch (postoperative) T81.89
  - suppurative (skin) L98.Ø
  - swimming pool A31.1
  - talc —*see also* Granuloma, foreign body
    - in operation wound —*see* Foreign body, accidentally left during a procedure
  - telangiectaticum (skin) L98.Ø
  - tracheostomy J95.Ø9
  - trichophyticum B35.8
  - tropicum A66.4
  - umbilical P83.81
  - umbilicus P83.81
  - urethra N36.8
  - uveitis —*see* Iridocyclitis, chronic
  - vagina A58
  - venereum A58
  - vocal cord J38.3
- Granulomatosis L92.9
  - lymphoid C83.8-●
  - miliary (listerial) A32.89
  - necrotizing, respiratory M31.3Ø
  - progressive septic D71
  - specified NEC L92.8
  - Wegener's M31.3Ø
    - with renal involvement M31.31
- Granulomatous tissue (abnormal) (excessive) L92.9
- Granulosis rubra nasi L74.8
- Graphite fibrosis (of lung) J63.3
- Graphospasm F48.8
  - organic G25.89
- Grating scapula M89.8X1
- Gravel (urinary) —*see* Calculus, urinary
- Graves' disease —*see* Hyperthyroidism, with, goiter
- Gravis —*see* condition
- Grawitz tumor C64.-●
- Gray syndrome (newborn) P93.Ø
- Grayness, hair (premature) L67.1
  - congenital Q84.2
- Green sickness D5Ø.8
- Greenfield's disease
  - meaning
    - concentric sclerosis (encephalitis periaxialis concentrica) G37.5
    - metachromatic leukodystrophy E75.25
- Greenstick fracture - code as Fracture, by site
- Grey syndrome (newborn) P93.Ø
- Grief F43.21
  - prolonged F43.29
  - reaction —*see also* Disorder, adjustment F43.2Ø
- Griesinger's disease B76.Ø
- Grinder's lung or pneumoconiosis J62.8
- Grinding, teeth
  - psychogenic F45.8
  - sleep related G47.63
- Grip
  - Dabney's B33.Ø
  - devil's B33.Ø
- Grippe, grippal —*see also* Influenza
  - Balkan A78
  - summer, of Italy A93.1
- Grisel's disease M43.6
- Groin —*see* condition
- Grooved tongue K14.5
- Ground itch B76.9
- Grover's disease or syndrome L11.1
- Growing pains, children R29.898
- Growth (fungoid) (neoplastic) (new) —*see also* Neoplasm
  - adenoid (vegetative) J35.8
  - benign —*see* Neoplasm, benign, by site
  - malignant —*see* Neoplasm, malignant, by site
  - rapid, childhood ZØØ.2
  - secondary —*see* Neoplasm, secondary, by site
- Gruby's disease B35.Ø
- Gubler-Millard paralysis or syndrome G46.3
- Guerin-Stern syndrome Q74.3
- Guidance, insufficient anterior (occlusal) M26.54
- Guillain-Barré disease or syndrome G61.Ø
  - sequelae G65.Ø
- Guinea worms (infection) (infestation) B72
- Guinon's disease (motor-verbal tic) F95.2
- Gull's disease EØ3.4
- Gum —*see* condition
- Gumboil KØ4.7
  - with sinus KØ4.6
- Gumma (syphilitic) A52.79
  - artery A52.Ø9
    - cerebral A52.Ø4
  - bone A52.77
    - of yaws (late) A66.6
  - brain A52.19
  - cauda equina A52.19
  - central nervous system A52.3
  - ciliary body A52.71
  - congenital A5Ø.59
  - eyelid A52.71
  - heart A52.Ø6
  - intracranial A52.19
  - iris A52.71
  - kidney A52.75
  - larynx A52.73
  - leptomeninges A52.19
  - liver A52.74
  - meninges A52.19
  - myocardium A52.Ø6
  - nasopharynx A52.73
  - neurosyphilitic A52.3
  - nose A52.73
  - orbit A52.71
  - palate (soft) A52.79
  - penis A52.76
  - pericardium A52.Ø6
  - pharynx A52.73
  - pituitary A52.79
  - scrofulous (tuberculous) A18.4
  - skin A52.79
  - specified site NEC A52.79
  - spinal cord A52.19
  - tongue A52.79
  - tonsil A52.73
  - trachea A52.73
  - tuberculous A18.4
  - ulcerative due to yaws A66.4
  - ureter A52.75
  - yaws A66.4
    - bone A66.6
- Gunn's syndrome QØ7.8
- Gunshot wound —*see also* Wound, open
  - fracture - code as Fracture, by site
  - internal organs —*see* Injury, by site
- Gynandrism Q56.Ø
- Gynandroblastoma
  - specified site —*see* Neoplasm, uncertain behavior, by site
  - unspecified site
    - female D39.1Ø
    - male D4Ø.1Ø
- Gynecological examination (periodic) (routine) ZØ1.419
  - with abnormal findings ZØ1.411
- Gynecomastia N62
- Gynephobia F4Ø.291
- Gyrate scalp Q82.8

 ▶ New ➠ Revised ~~deleted~~ Deleted ● Use Additional Character(s)

H

H (Hartnup's) disease E72.Ø2
Haas' disease or osteochondrosis (juvenile) (head of humerus) —*see* Osteochondrosis, juvenile, humerus
Habit, habituation
  bad sleep Z72.821
  chorea F95.8
  disturbance, child F98.9
  drug —*see* Dependence, drug
  irregular sleep Z72.821
  laxative F55.2
  spasm —*see* Tic
  tic —*see* Tic
Haemophilus (H.) influenzae, as cause of disease classified elsewhere B96.3
Haff disease —*see* Poisoning, mercury
Hageman's factor defect, deficiency or disease D68.2
Haglund's disease or osteochondrosis (juvenile) (os tibiale externum) —*see* Osteochondrosis, juvenile, tarsus
Hailey-Hailey disease Q82.8
Hair —*see also* condition
  plucking F63.3
    in stereotyped movement disorder F98.4
  tourniquet syndrome —*see also* Constriction, external, by site
    finger S6Ø.44- •
    penis S3Ø.842
    thumb S6Ø.34- •
    toe S9Ø.44- •
Hairball in stomach T18.2
Hair-pulling, pathological (compulsive) F63.3
Hairy black tongue K14.3
Half vertebra Q76.49
Halitosis R19.6
Hallerman-Streiff syndrome Q87.Ø
Hallervorden-Spatz disease G23.Ø
Hallopeau's acrodermatitis or disease L4Ø.2
Hallucination R44.3
  auditory R44.Ø
  gustatory R44.2
  olfactory R44.2
  specified NEC R44.2
  tactile R44.2
  visual R44.1
Hallucinosis (chronic) F28
  alcoholic (acute) F1Ø.951
    in
      abuse F1Ø.151
      dependence F1Ø.251
  drug-induced F19.951
    cannabis F12.951
    cocaine F14.951
    hallucinogen F16.151
    in
      abuse F19.151
        cannabis F12.151
        cocaine F14.151
        hallucinogen F16.151
        inhalant F18.151
        opioid F11.151
        sedative, anxiolytic or hypnotic F13.151
        stimulant NEC F15.151
      dependence F19.251
        cannabis F12.251
        cocaine F14.251
        hallucinogen F16.251
        inhalant F18.251
        opioid F11.251
        sedative, anxiolytic or hypnotic F13.251
        stimulant NEC F15.251
    inhalant F18.951
    opioid F11.951
    sedative, anxiolytic or hypnotic F13.951
    stimulant NEC F15.951
  organic FØ6.Ø
Hallux
  deformity (acquired) NEC M2Ø.5X- •
  limitus M2Ø.5X- •
  malleus (acquired) NEC M2Ø.3- •
  rigidus (acquired) M2Ø.2- •
    congenital Q74.2
    sequelae (late effect) of rickets E64.3
  valgus (acquired) M2Ø.1- •
    congenital Q66.6
  varus (acquired) M2Ø.3- •
    congenital Q66.3- •
Halo, visual H53.19
Hamartoma, hamartoblastoma Q85.9
  epithelial (gingival), odontogenic, central or peripheral —*see* Cyst, calcifying odontogenic
Hamartosis Q85.9
Hamman-Rich syndrome J84.114
Hammer toe (acquired) NEC —*see also* Deformity, toe, hammer toe
  congenital Q66.89
  sequelae (late effect) of rickets E64.3
Hand —*see* condition
Hand-foot syndrome L27.1
Handicap, handicapped
  educational Z55.9
    specified NEC Z55.8
Hand-Schüller-Christian disease or syndrome C96.5
Hanging (asphyxia) (strangulation) (suffocation) —*see* Asphyxia, traumatic, due to mechanical threat
Hangnail —*see also* Cellulitis, digit
  with lymphangitis —*see* Lymphangitis, acute, digit
Hangover (alcohol) F1Ø.129
Hanhart's syndrome Q87.Ø
Hanot-Chauffard (-Troisier) syndrome E83.19
Hanot's cirrhosis or disease K74.3
Hansen's disease —*see* Leprosy
Hantaan virus disease (Korean hemorrhagic fever) A98.5
Hantavirus disease (with renal manifestations) (Dobrava) (Puumala) (Seoul) A98.5
  with pulmonary manifestations (Andes) (Bayou) (Bermejo) (Black Creek Canal) (Choclo) (Juquitiba) (Laguna negra) (Lechiguanas) (New York) (Oran) (Sin nombre) B33.4
Happy puppet syndrome Q93.59
Harada's disease or syndrome H3Ø.81- •
Hardening
  artery —*see* Arteriosclerosis
  brain G93.89
Harelip (complete) (incomplete) —*see* Cleft, lip
Harlequin (newborn) Q8Ø.4
Harley's disease D59.6
Harmful use (of)
  alcohol F1Ø.1Ø
  anxiolytics —*see* Abuse, drug, sedative
  cannabinoids —*see* Abuse, drug, cannabis
  cocaine —*see* Abuse, drug, cocaine
  drug —*see* Abuse, drug
  hallucinogens —*see* Abuse, drug, hallucinogen
  hypnotics —*see* Abuse, drug, sedative -
    opioids —*see* Abuse, drug, opioid
  PCP (phencyclidine) —*see* Abuse, drug, hallucinogen
  sedatives —*see* Abuse, drug, sedative
  stimulants NEC —*see* Abuse, drug, stimulant
Harris' lines —*see* Arrest, epiphyseal
Hartnup's disease E72.Ø2
Harvester's lung J67.Ø
Harvesting ovum for in vitro fertilization Z31.83
Hashimoto's disease or thyroiditis EØ6.3
Hashitoxicosis (transient) EØ6.3
Hassal-Henle bodies or warts (cornea) H18.49
Haut mal —*see* Epilepsy, generalized, specified NEC
Haverhill fever A25.1
Hay fever —*see also* Fever, hay J3Ø.1
Hayem-Widal syndrome D59.8
Haygarth's nodes M15.8
Haymaker's lung J67.Ø
Hb (abnormal)
  Bart's disease D56.Ø
  disease —*see* Disease, hemoglobin
  trait —*see* Trait
Head —*see* condition
Headache R51
  allergic NEC G44.89
  associated with sexual activity G44.82
  chronic daily R51
  cluster G44.ØØ9
    chronic G44.Ø29
      intractable G44.Ø21
      not intractable G44.Ø29
    episodic G44.Ø19
      intractable G44.Ø11
      not intractable G44.Ø19
    intractable G44.ØØ1
    not intractable G44.ØØ9
  cough (primary) G44.83
  daily chronic R51
  drug-induced NEC G44.4Ø
    intractable G44.41
    not intractable G44.4Ø
  exertional (primary) G44.84
  histamine G44.ØØ9
    intractable G44.ØØ1
    not intractable G44.ØØ9
  hypnic G44.81
  lumbar puncture G97.1
  medication overuse G44.4Ø
    intractable G44.41
    not intractable G44.4Ø
  menstrual —*see* Migraine, menstrual
  migraine (type) —*see also* Migraine G43.9Ø9
  nasal septum R51
  neuralgiform, short lasting unilateral, with conjunctival injection and tearing (SUNCT) G44.Ø59
    intractable G44.Ø51
    not intractable G44.Ø59
  new daily persistent (NDPH) G44.52
  orgasmic G44.82
  periodic syndromes in adults and children G43.CØ
    with refractory migraine G43.C1
    intractable G43.C1
    not intractable G43.CØ
    without refractory migraine G43.CØ
  postspinal puncture G97.1
  post-traumatic G44.3Ø9
    acute G44.319
      intractable G44.311
      not intractable G44.319
    chronic G44.329
      intractable G44.321
      not intractable G44.329
    intractable G44.3Ø1
    not intractable G44.3Ø9
  pre-menstrual —*see* Migraine, menstrual
  preorgasmic G44.82
  primary
    cough G44.83
    exertional G44.84
    stabbing G44.85
    thunderclap G44.53
  rebound G44.4Ø
    intractable G44.41
    not intractable G44.4Ø
  short lasting unilateral neuralgiform, with conjunctival injection and tearing (SUNCT) G44.Ø59
    intractable G44.Ø51
    not intractable G44.Ø59
  specified syndrome NEC G44.89

H

Headache *(Continued)*
spinal and epidural anesthesia - induced T88.59
in labor and delivery O74.5
in pregnancy O29.4-●
postpartum, puerperal O89.4
spinal fluid loss (from puncture) G97.1
stabbing (primary) G44.85
tension (-type) G44.209
chronic G44.229
intractable G44.221
not intractable G44.229
episodic G44.219
intractable G44.211
not intractable G44.219
intractable G44.201
not intractable G44.209
thunderclap (primary) G44.53
vascular NEC G44.1
Healthy
infant
accompanying sick mother Z76.3
receiving care Z76.2
person accompanying sick person Z76.3
Hearing examination Z01.10
with abnormal findings NEC Z01.118
infant or child (over 28 days old) Z00.129
with abnormal findings Z00.121
following failed hearing screening Z01.110
for hearing conservation and treatment Z01.12
Heart —*see* condition
Heart beat
abnormality R00.9
specified NEC R00.8
awareness R00.2
rapid R00.0
slow R00.1
Heartburn R12
psychogenic F45.8
Heartland virus disease A93.8
Heat (effects) T67.9
apoplexy T67.01
burn —*see also* Burn L55.9
collapse T67.1
cramps T67.2
dermatitis or eczema L59.0
edema T67.7
erythema - code by site under Burn, first degree
excessive T67.9
specified effect NEC T67.8
exhaustion T67.5
anhydrotic T67.3
due to
salt (and water) depletion T67.4
water depletion T67.3
with salt depletion T67.4
fatigue (transient) T67.6
fever T67.01
hyperpyrexia T67.01
prickly L74.0
prostration —*see* Heat, exhaustion
pyrexia T67.01
rash L74.0
specified effect NEC T67.8
stroke T67.01
▶exertional T67.02
▶specified NEC T67.09
sunburn —*see* Sunburn
syncope T67.1
Heavy-for-dates NEC (infant) (4000g to 4499g) P08.1
exceptionally (4500g or more) P08.0
Hebephrenia, hebephrenic (schizophrenia) F20.1
Heberden's disease or nodes (with arthropathy) M15.1
Hebra's
pityriasis L26
prurigo L28.2
Heel —*see* condition
Heerfordt's disease D86.89
Hegglin's anomaly or syndrome D72.0
Heilmeyer-Schoner disease D45
Heine-Medin disease A80.9
Heinz body anemia, congenital D58.2
Heliophobia F40.228
Heller's disease or syndrome F84.3
HELLP syndrome (hemolysis, elevated liver enzymes and low platelet count) O14.2-●
complicating
childbirth O14.24
puerperium O14.25
Helminthiasis —*see also* Infestation, helminth
Ancylostoma B76.0
intestinal B82.0
mixed types (types classifiable to more than one of the titles B65.0-B81.3 and B81.8) B81.4
specified type NEC B81.8
mixed types (intestinal) (types classifiable to more than one of the titles B65.0-B81.3 and B81.8) B81.4
Necator (americanus) B76.1
specified type NEC B83.8
Heloma L84
Hemangioblastoma —*see* Neoplasm, connective tissue, uncertain behavior
malignant —*see* Neoplasm, connective tissue, malignant
Hemangioendothelioma —*see also* Neoplasm, uncertain behavior, by site
benign D18.00
intra-abdominal D18.03
intracranial D18.02
skin D18.01
specified site NEC D18.09
bone (diffuse) —*see* Neoplasm, bone, malignant
epithelioid —*see also* Neoplasm, uncertain behavior, by site
malignant —*see* Neoplasm, malignant, by site
malignant —*see* Neoplasm, connective tissue, malignant
Hemangiofibroma —*see* Neoplasm, benign, by site
Hemangiolipoma —*see* Lipoma
Hemangioma D18.00
arteriovenous D18.00
intra-abdominal D18.03
intracranial D18.02
skin D18.01
specified site NEC D18.09
capillary I78.1
intra-abdominal D18.03
intracranial D18.02
skin D18.01
specified site NEC D18.09
cavernous D18.00
intra-abdominal D18.03
intracranial D18.02
skin D18.01
specified site NEC D18.09
epithelioid D18.00
intra-abdominal D18.03
intracranial D18.02
skin D18.01
specified site NEC D18.09
histiocytoid D18.00
intra-abdominal D18.03
intracranial D18.02
skin D18.01
specified site NEC D18.09
infantile D18.00
intra-abdominal D18.03
intracranial D18.02
skin D18.01
specified site NEC D18.09
intra-abdominal D18.03
intracranial D18.02
intramuscular D18.00
intra-abdominal D18.03
intracranial D18.02
skin D18.01
specified site NEC D18.09
Hemangioma *(Continued)*
intrathoracic structures D18.09
juvenile D18.00
malignant —*see* Neoplasm, connective tissue, malignant
plexiform D18.00
intra-abdominal D18.03
intracranial D18.02
skin D18.01
specified site NEC D18.09
racemose D18.00
intra-abdominal D18.03
intracranial D18.02
skin D18.01
specified site NEC D18.09
sclerosing —*see* Neoplasm, skin, benign
simplex D18.00
intra-abdominal D18.03
intracranial D18.02
skin D18.01
specified site NEC D18.09
skin D18.01
specified site NEC D18.09
venous D18.00
intra-abdominal D18.03
intracranial D18.02
skin D18.01
specified site NEC D18.09
verrucous keratotic D18.00
intra-abdominal D18.03
intracranial D18.02
skin D18.01
specified site NEC D18.09
Hemangiomatosis (systemic) I78.8
involving single site —*see* Hemangioma
Hemangiopericytoma —*see also* Neoplasm, connective tissue, uncertain behavior
benign —*see* Neoplasm, connective tissue, benign
malignant —*see* Neoplasm, connective tissue, malignant
Hemangiosarcoma —*see* Neoplasm, connective tissue, malignant
Hemarthrosis (nontraumatic) M25.00
ankle M25.07-●
elbow M25.02-●
foot joint M25.07-●
hand joint M25.04-●
hip M25.05-●
in hemophilic arthropathy —*see* Arthropathy, hemophilic
knee M25.06-●
shoulder M25.01-●
specified joint NEC M25.08
traumatic —*see* Sprain, by site
vertebrae M25.08
wrist M25.03-●
Hematemesis K92.0
with ulcer - code by site under Ulcer, with hemorrhage K27.4
newborn, neonatal P54.0
due to swallowed maternal blood P78.2
Hematidrosis L74.8
Hematinuria —*see also* Hemoglobinuria
malarial B50.8
Hematobilia K83.8
Hematocele
female NEC N94.89
with ectopic pregnancy O00.90
with intrauterine pregnancy O00.91
ovary N83.8
male N50.1
Hematochezia —*see also* Melena K92.1
Hematochyluria —*see also* Infestation, filarial
schistosomiasis (bilharziasis) B65.0
Hematocolpos (with hematometra or hematosalpinx) N89.7
Hematocornea —*see* Pigmentation, cornea, stromal
Hematogenous —*see* condition

Hematoma (traumatic) (skin surface intact) —*see also* Contusion
with
injury of internal organs —*see* Injury, by site
open wound —*see* Wound, open
amputation stump (surgical) (late) T87.89
aorta, dissecting I71.ØØ
abdominal I71.Ø2
thoracic I71.Ø1
thoracoabdominal I71.Ø3
aortic intramural —*see* Dissection, aorta
arterial (complicating trauma) —*see* Injury, blood vessel, by site
auricle —*see* Contusion, ear
nontraumatic —*see* Disorder, pinna, hematoma
birth injury NEC P15.8
brain (traumatic)
with
cerebral laceration or contusion (diffuse) —*see* Injury, intracranial, diffuse
focal —*see* Injury, intracranial, focal
cerebellar, traumatic SØ6.37-●
intracerebral, traumatic —*see* Injury, intracranial, intracerebral hemorrhage
newborn NEC P52.4
birth injury P1Ø.1
nontraumatic —*see* Hemorrhage, intracranial
subarachnoid, arachnoid, traumatic —*see* Injury, intracranial, subarachnoid hemorrhage
subdural, traumatic —*see* Injury, intracranial, subdural hemorrhage
breast (nontraumatic) N64.89
broad ligament (nontraumatic) N83.7
traumatic S37.892
cerebellar, traumatic SØ6.37-●
cerebral —*see* Hematoma, brain
cerebrum SØ6.36-●
left SØ6.35-●
right SØ6.34-●
cesarean delivery wound O9Ø.2
complicating delivery (perineal) (pelvic) (vagina) (vulva) O71.7
corpus cavernosum (nontraumatic) N48.89
epididymis (nontraumatic) N5Ø.1
epidural (traumatic) —*see* Injury, intracranial, epidural hemorrhage
spinal —*see* Injury, spinal cord, by region
episiotomy O9Ø.2
face, birth injury P15.4
genital organ NEC (nontraumatic)
female (nonobstetric) N94.89
traumatic S3Ø.2Ø2
male N5Ø.1
traumatic S3Ø.2Ø1
internal organs —*see* Injury, by site
intracerebral, traumatic —*see* Injury, intracranial, intracerebral hemorrhage
intraoperative —*see* Complications, intraoperative, hemorrhage
labia (nontraumatic) (nonobstetric) N9Ø.8
liver (subcapsular) (nontraumatic) K76.89
birth injury P15.Ø
mediastinum —*see* Injury, intrathoracic
mesosalpinx (nontraumatic) N83.7
traumatic S37.898
muscle - code by site under Contusion
nontraumatic
muscle M79.81
soft tissue M79.81
obstetrical surgical wound O9Ø.2
orbit, orbital (nontraumatic) —*see also* Hemorrhage, orbit
traumatic —*see* Contusion, orbit
pelvis (female) (nontraumatic) (nonobstetric) N94.89
obstetric O71.7
traumatic —*see* Injury, by site

Hematoma *(Continued)*
penis (nontraumatic) N48.89
birth injury P15.5
perianal (nontraumatic) K64.5
perineal S3Ø.23
complicating delivery O71.7
perirenal —*see* Injury, kidney
pinna —*see* Contusion, ear
nontraumatic —*see* Disorder, pinna, hematoma
placenta O43.89-●
postoperative (postprocedural) —*see* Complication, postprocedural, hematoma
retroperitoneal (nontraumatic) K66.1
traumatic S36.892
scrotum, superficial S3Ø.22
birth injury P15.5
seminal vesicle (nontraumatic) N5Ø.1
traumatic S37.892
spermatic cord (traumatic) S37.892
nontraumatic N5Ø.1
spinal (cord) (meninges) —*see also* Injury, spinal cord, by region
newborn (birth injury) P11.5
spleen D73.5
intraoperative —*see* Complications, intraoperative, hemorrhage, spleen
postprocedural (postoperative) —*see* Complications, postprocedural, hemorrhage, spleen
sternocleidomastoid, birth injury P15.2
sternomastoid, birth injury P15.2
subarachnoid (traumatic) —*see* Injury, intracranial, subarachnoid hemorrhage
newborn (nontraumatic) P52.5
due to birth injury P1Ø.3
nontraumatic —*see* Hemorrhage, intracranial, subarachnoid
subdural (traumatic) —*see* Injury, intracranial, subdural hemorrhage
newborn (localized) P52.8
birth injury P1Ø.Ø
nontraumatic —*see* Hemorrhage, intracranial, subdural
superficial, newborn P54.5
testis (nontraumatic) N5Ø.1
birth injury P15.5
tunica vaginalis (nontraumatic) N5Ø.1
umbilical cord, complicating delivery O69.5
uterine ligament (broad) (nontraumatic) N83.7
traumatic S37.892
vagina (ruptured) (nontraumatic) N89.8
complicating delivery O71.7
vas deferens (nontraumatic) N5Ø.1
traumatic S37.892
vitreous —*see* Hemorrhage, vitreous
vulva (nontraumatic) (nonobstetric) N9Ø.89
complicating delivery O71.7
newborn (birth injury) P15.5
Hematometra N85.7
with hematocolpos N89.7
Hematomyelia (central) G95.19
newborn (birth injury) P11.5
traumatic T14.8
Hematomyelitis GØ4.9Ø
Hematoperitoneum —*see* Hemoperitoneum
Hematophobia F4Ø.23Ø
Hematopneumothorax (*see* Hemothorax)
Hematopoiesis, cyclic D7Ø.4
Hematoporphyria —*see* Porphyria
Hematorachis, hematorrhachis G95.19
newborn (birth injury) P11.5
Hematosalpinx N83.6
with
hematocolpos N89.7
hematometra N85.7
with hematocolpos N89.7
infectional —*see* Salpingitis
Hematospermia R36.1

Hematothorax (*see* Hemothorax)
Hematuria R31.9
benign (familial) (of childhood) —*see also* Hematuria, idiopathic
essential microscopic R31.1
due to sulphonamide, sulfonamide —*see* Table of Drugs and Chemicals, by drug
endemic —*see also* Schistosomiasis B65.Ø
gross R31.Ø
idiopathic NØ2.9
with glomerular lesion
crescentic (diffuse) glomerulonephritis NØ2.7
dense deposit disease NØ2.6
endocapillary proliferative glomerulonephritis NØ2.4
focal and segmental hyalinosis or sclerosis NØ2.1
membranoproliferative (diffuse) NØ2.5
membranous (diffuse) NØ2.2
mesangial proliferative (diffuse) NØ2.3
mesangiocapillary (diffuse) NØ2.5
minor abnormality NØ2.Ø
proliferative NEC NØ2.8
specified pathology NEC NØ2.8
intermittent —*see* Hematuria, idiopathic
malarial B5Ø.8
microscopic NEC (with symptoms) R31.29
asymptomatic R31.21
benign essential R31.1
paroxysmal —*see also* Hematuria, idiopathic
nocturnal D59.5
persistent —*see* Hematuria, idiopathic
recurrent —*see* Hematuria, idiopathic
tropical —*see also* Schistosomiasis B65.Ø
tuberculous A18.13
Hemeralopia (day blindness) H53.11
vitamin A deficiency E5Ø.5
Hemi-akinesia R41.4
Hemianalgesia R2Ø.Ø
Hemianencephaly QØØ.Ø
Hemianesthesia R2Ø.Ø
Hemianopia, hemianopsia (heteronymous) H53.47
homonymous H53.46-●
syphilitic A52.71
Hemiathetosis R25.8
Hemiatrophy R68.89
cerebellar G31.9
face, facial, progressive (Romberg) G51.8
tongue K14.8
Hemiballism (us) G25.5
Hemicardia Q24.8
Hemicephalus, hemicephaly QØØ.Ø
Hemichorea G25.5
Hemicolitis, left —*see* Colitis, left sided
Hemicrania
congenital malformation QØØ.Ø
continua G44.51
meaning migraine —*see also* Migraine G43.9Ø9
paroxysmal G44.Ø39
chronic G44.Ø49
intractable G44.Ø41
not intractable G44.Ø49
episodic G44.Ø39
intractable G44.Ø31
not intractable G44.Ø39
intractable G44.Ø31
not intractable G44.Ø39
Hemidystrophy —*see* Hemiatrophy
Hemiectromelia Q73.8
Hemihypalgesia R2Ø.8
Hemihypesthesia R2Ø.1
Hemi-inattention R41.4
Hemimelia Q73.8
lower limb —*see* Defect, reduction, lower limb, specified type NEC
upper limb —*see* Defect, reduction, upper limb, specified type NEC
Hemiparalysis —*see* Hemiplegia
Hemiparesis —*see* Hemiplegia

H

Hemiparesthesia R2Ø.2
Hemiparkinsonism G2Ø
Hemiplegia G81.9-•
  alternans facialis G83.89
  ascending NEC G81.9Ø
    spinal G95.89
  congenital (cerebral) G8Ø.8
    spastic G8Ø.2
  embolic (current episode) I63.4-•
  flaccid G81.Ø-•
  following
    cerebrovascular disease I69.959
      cerebral infarction I69.35-•
      intracerebral hemorrhage I69.15-•
      nontraumatic intracranial hemorrhage NEC I69.25-•
      specified disease NEC I69.85-•
      stroke NOS I69.35-•
      subarachnoid hemorrhage I69.Ø5-•
  hysterical F44.4
  newborn NEC P91.88
    birth injury P11.9
  spastic G81.1-•
    congenital G8Ø.2
  thrombotic (current episode) I63.3-•
Hemisection, spinal cord —*see* Injury, spinal cord, by region
Hemispasm (facial) R25.2
Hemisporosis B48.8
Hemitremor R25.1
Hemivertebra Q76.49
  failure of segmentation with scoliosis Q76.3
  fusion with scoliosis Q76.3
Hemochromatosis E83.119
  with refractory anemia D46.1
  due to repeated red blood cell transfusion E83.111
  hereditary (primary) E83.11Ø
  neonatal P78.84
  primary E83.11Ø
  specified NEC E83.118
Hemoglobin —*see also* condition
  abnormal (disease) —*see* Disease, hemoglobin
  AS genotype D57.3
  Constant Spring D58.2
  E-beta thalassemia D56.5
  fetal, hereditary persistence (HPFH) D56.4
  H Constant Spring D56.Ø
  low NOS D64.9
  S (Hb S), heterozygous D57.3
Hemoglobinemia D59.9
  due to blood transfusion T8Ø.89
  paroxysmal D59.6
    nocturnal D59.5
Hemoglobinopathy (mixed) D58.2
  with thalassemia D56.8
  sickle-cell D57.1
    with thalassemia D57.4Ø
      with crisis (vasoocclusive pain) D57.419
        with
          acute chest syndrome D57.411
          splenic sequestration D57.412
      without crisis D57.4Ø
Hemoglobinuria R82.3
  with anemia, hemolytic, acquired (chronic) NEC D59.6
  cold (agglutinin) (paroxysmal) (with Raynaud's syndrome) D59.6
  due to exertion or hemolysis NEC D59.6
  intermittent D59.6
  malarial B5Ø.8
  march D59.6
  nocturnal (paroxysmal) D59.5
  paroxysmal (cold) D59.6
    nocturnal D59.5
Hemolymphangioma D18.1
Hemolysis
  intravascular
    with
      abortion —*see* Abortion, by type, complicated by, hemorrhage
      ectopic or molar pregnancy OØ8.1
Hemolysis *(Continued)*
  intravascular *(Continued)*
    with *(Continued)*
      hemorrhage
        antepartum —*see* Hemorrhage, antepartum, with coagulation defect
        intrapartum —*see also* Hemorrhage, complicating, delivery O67.Ø
    postpartum O72.3
  neonatal (excessive) P58.9
    specified NEC P58.8
Hemolytic —*see* condition
Hemopericardium I31.2
  following acute myocardial infarction (current complication) I23.Ø
  newborn P54.8
  traumatic —*see* Injury, heart, with hemopericardium
Hemoperitoneum K66.1
  infectional K65.9
  traumatic S36.899
    with open wound —*see* Wound, open, with penetration into peritoneal cavity
Hemophilia (classical) (familial) (hereditary) D66
  A D66
  B D67
  C D68.1
  acquired D68.311
  autoimmune D68.311
  calcipriva —*see also* Defect, coagulation D68.4
  nonfamilial —*see also* Defect, coagulation D68.4
  secondary D68.311
  vascular D68.Ø
Hemophthalmos H44.81-•
Hemopneumothorax —*see also* Hemothorax
  traumatic S27.2
Hemoptysis RØ4.2
  newborn P26.9
  tuberculous —*see* Tuberculosis, pulmonary
Hemorrhage, hemorrhagic (concealed) R58
  abdomen R58
  accidental antepartum —*see* Hemorrhage, antepartum
  acute idiopathic pulmonary, in infants RØ4.81
  adenoid J35.8
  adrenal (capsule) (gland) E27.49
    medulla E27.8
    newborn P54.4
  after delivery —*see* Hemorrhage, postpartum
  alveolar
    lung, newborn P26.8
    process KØ8.89
  alveolus KØ8.89
  amputation stump (surgical) T87.89
  anemia (chronic) D5Ø.Ø
    acute D62
  antepartum (with) O46.9Ø
    with coagulation defect O46.ØØ-•
      afibrinogenemia O46.Ø1-•
      disseminated intravascular coagulation O46.Ø2-•
      hypofibrinogenemia O46.Ø1-•
      specified defect NEC O46.Ø9-•
    before 2Ø weeks gestation O2Ø.9
      specified type NEC O2Ø.8
      threatened abortion O2Ø.Ø
    due to
      abruptio placenta —*see also* Abruptio placentae O45.9-•
      leiomyoma, uterus —*see* Hemorrhage, antepartum, specified cause NEC
      placenta previa O44.1-•
    specified cause NEC —*see* subcategory O46.8X-•
  anus (sphincter) K62.5
  apoplexy (stroke) —*see* Hemorrhage, intracranial, intracerebral
Hemorrhage, hemorrhagic *(Continued)*
  arachnoid —*see* Hemorrhage, intracranial, subarachnoid
  artery R58
    brain —*see* Hemorrhage, intracranial, intracerebral
  basilar (ganglion) I61.Ø
  bladder N32.89
  bowel K92.2
    newborn P54.3
  brain (miliary) (nontraumatic) —*see* Hemorrhage, intracranial, intracerebral
    due to
      birth injury P1Ø.1
      syphilis A52.Ø5
    epidural or extradural (traumatic) —*see* Injury, intracranial, epidural hemorrhage
    newborn P52.4
      birth injury P1Ø.1
    subarachnoid —*see* Hemorrhage, intracranial, subarachnoid
    subdural —*see* Hemorrhage, intracranial, subdural
  brainstem (nontraumatic) I61.3
    traumatic SØ6.38-•
  breast N64.59
  bronchial tube —*see* Hemorrhage, lung
  bronchopulmonary —*see* Hemorrhage, lung
  bronchus —*see* Hemorrhage, lung
  bulbar I61.5
  capillary I78.8
    primary D69.8
  cecum K92.2
  cerebellar, cerebellum (nontraumatic) I61.4
    newborn P52.6
    traumatic SØ6.37-•
  cerebral, cerebrum —*see also* Hemorrhage, intracranial, intracerebral
    lobe I61.1
    newborn (anoxic) P52.4
      birth injury P1Ø.1
  cerebromeningeal I61.8
  cerebrospinal —*see* Hemorrhage, intracranial, intracerebral
  cervix (uteri) (stump) NEC N88.8
  chamber, anterior (eye) —*see* Hyphema
  childbirth —*see* Hemorrhage, complicating, delivery
  choroid H31.3Ø-•
    expulsive H31.31-•
  ciliary body —*see* Hyphema
  cochlea —*see* subcategory H83.8
  colon K92.2
  complicating
    abortion —*see* Abortion, by type, complicated by, hemorrhage
    delivery O67.9
      associated with coagulation defect (afibrinogenemia) (DIC) (hyperfibrinolysis) O67.Ø
      specified cause NEC O67.8
    surgical procedure —*see* Hemorrhage, intraoperative
  conjunctiva H11.3-•
    newborn P54.8
  cord, newborn (stump) P51.9
  corpus luteum (ruptured) cyst N83.1-•
  cortical (brain) I61.1
  cranial —*see* Hemorrhage, intracranial
  cutaneous R23.3
    due to autosensitivity, erythrocyte D69.2
    newborn P54.5
  delayed
    following ectopic or molar pregnancy OØ8.1
    postpartum O72.2
  diathesis (familial) D69.9
  disease D69.9
    newborn P53
    specified type NEC D69.8

Hemorrhage, hemorrhagic *(Continued)*
due to or associated with
afibrinogenemia or other coagulation defect (conditions in categories D65-D69)
antepartum —*see* Hemorrhage, antepartum, with coagulation defect
intrapartum O67.Ø
dental implant M27.61
device, implant or graft —*see also* Complications, by site and type, specified NEC T85.838
arterial graft NEC T82.838
breast T85.838
catheter NEC T85.838
dialysis (renal) T82.838
intraperitoneal T85.838
infusion NEC T82.838
spinal (epidural) (subdural) T85.83Ø
urinary (indwelling) T83.83
electronic (electrode) (pulse generator) (stimulator)
bone T84.83
cardiac T82.837
nervous system (brain) (peripheral nerve) (spinal) T85.83Ø
urinary T83.83
fixation, internal (orthopedic) NEC T84.83
gastrointestinal (bile duct) (esophagus) T85.838
genital NEC T83.83
heart NEC T82.837
joint prosthesis T84.83
ocular (corneal graft) (orbital implant) NEC T85.838
orthopedic NEC T84.83
bone graft T86.838
specified NEC T85.838
urinary NEC T83.83
vascular NEC T82.838
ventricular intracranial shunt T85.838
duodenum, duodenal K92.2
ulcer —*see* Ulcer, duodenum, with hemorrhage
dura mater —*see* Hemorrhage, intracranial, subdural
endotracheal —*see* Hemorrhage, lung
epicranial subaponeurotic (massive), birth injury P12.2
epidural (traumatic) —*see also* Injury, intracranial, epidural hemorrhage
nontraumatic I62.1
esophagus K22.8
varix I85.Ø1
secondary I85.11
excessive, following ectopic gestation (subsequent episode) OØ8.1
extradural (traumatic) —*see* Injury, intracranial, epidural hemorrhage
birth injury P1Ø.8
newborn (anoxic) (nontraumatic) P52.8
nontraumatic I62.1
eye NEC H57.89
fundus —*see* Hemorrhage, retina
lid —*see* Disorder, eyelid, specified type NEC
fallopian tube N83.6
fibrinogenolysis —*see* Fibrinolysis
fibrinolytic (acquired) —*see* Fibrinolysis
from
ear (nontraumatic) —*see* Otorrhagia
tracheostomy stoma J95.Ø1
fundus, eye —*see* Hemorrhage, retina
funis —*see* Hemorrhage, umbilicus, cord
gastric —*see* Hemorrhage, stomach
gastroenteric K92.2
newborn P54.3
gastrointestinal (tract) K92.2
newborn P54.3
genital organ, male N5Ø.1

Hemorrhage, hemorrhagic *(Continued)*
genitourinary (tract) NOS R31.9
gingiva KØ6.8
globe (eye) —*see* Hemophthalmos
graafian follicle cyst (ruptured) N83.Ø-●
gum KØ6.8
heart I51.89
hypopharyngeal (throat) RØ4.1
intermenstrual (regular) N92.3
irregular N92.1
internal (organs) NEC R58
capsule I61.Ø
ear —*see* subcategory H83.8
newborn P54.8
intestine K92.2
newborn P54.3
intra-abdominal R58
intra-alveolar (lung), newborn P26.8
intracerebral (nontraumatic) —*see* Hemorrhage, intracranial, intracerebral
intracranial (nontraumatic) I62.9
birth injury P1Ø.9
epidural, nontraumatic I62.1
extradural, nontraumatic I62.1
intracerebral (nontraumatic) (in) I61.9
brain stem I61.3
cerebellum I61.4
hemisphere I61.2
cortical (superficial) I61.1
subcortical (deep) I61.Ø
intraoperative
during a nervous system procedure G97.31
during other procedure G97.32
intraventricular I61.5
multiple localized I61.6
newborn P52.4
birth injury P1Ø.1
postprocedural
following a nervous system procedure G97.51
following other procedure G97.52
specified NEC I61.8
superficial I61.1
traumatic (diffuse) —*see* Injury, intracranial, diffuse
focal —*see* Injury, intracranial, focal
newborn P52.9
specified NEC P52.8
subarachnoid (nontraumatic) (from) I6Ø.9
intracranial (cerebral) artery I6Ø.7
anterior communicating I6Ø.2
basilar I6Ø.4
carotid siphon and bifurcation I6Ø.Ø-●
communicating I6Ø.7
anterior I6Ø.2
posterior I6Ø.3-●
middle cerebral I6Ø.1-●
posterior communicating I6Ø.3-●
specified artery NEC I6Ø.6
vertebral I6Ø.5-●
newborn P52.5
birth injury P1Ø.3
specified NEC I6Ø.8
traumatic SØ6.6X-●
subdural (nontraumatic) I62.ØØ
acute I62.Ø1
birth injury P1Ø.Ø
chronic I62.Ø3
newborn (anoxic) (hypoxic) P52.8
birth injury P1Ø.Ø
spinal G95.19
subacute I62.Ø2
traumatic —*see* Injury, intracranial, subdural hemorrhage
traumatic —*see* Injury, intracranial, focal brain injury
intramedullary NEC G95.19

Hemorrhage, hemorrhagic *(Continued)*
intraocular —*see* Hemophthalmos
intraoperative, intraprocedural —*see* Complication, hemorrhage (hematoma), intraoperative (intraprocedural), by site
intrapartum —*see* Hemorrhage, complicating, delivery
intrapelvic
female N94.89
male K66.1
intraperitoneal K66.1
intrapontine I61.3
intraprocedural —*see* Complication, hemorrhage (hematoma), intraoperative (intraprocedural), by site
intrauterine N85.7
complicating delivery —*see also* Hemorrhage, complicating, delivery O67.9
postpartum —*see* Hemorrhage, postpartum
intraventricular I61.5
newborn (nontraumatic) —*see also* Newborn, affected by, hemorrhage P52.3
due to birth injury P1Ø.2
grade
1 P52.Ø
2 P52.1
3 P52.21
4 P52.22
intravesical N32.89
iris (postinfectional) (postinflammatory) (toxic) —*see* Hyphema
joint (nontraumatic) —*see* Hemarthrosis
kidney N28.89
knee (joint) (nontraumatic) —*see* Hemarthrosis, knee
labyrinth —*see* subcategory H83.8
lenticular striate artery I61.Ø
ligature, vessel —*see* Hemorrhage, postoperative
liver K76.89
lung RØ4.89
newborn P26.9
massive P26.1
specified NEC P26.8
tuberculous —*see* Tuberculosis, pulmonary
massive umbilical, newborn P51.Ø
mediastinum —*see* Hemorrhage, lung
medulla I61.3
membrane (brain) I6Ø.8
spinal cord —*see* Hemorrhage, spinal cord
meninges, meningeal (brain) (middle) I6Ø.8
spinal cord —*see* Hemorrhage, spinal cord
mesentery K66.1
metritis —*see* Endometritis
mouth K13.79
mucous membrane NEC R58
newborn P54.8
muscle M62.89
nail (subungual) L6Ø.8
nasal turbinate RØ4.Ø
newborn P54.8
navel, newborn P51.9
newborn P54.9
specified NEC P54.8
nipple N64.59
nose RØ4.Ø
newborn P54.8
omentum K66.1
optic nerve (sheath) H47.Ø2-●
orbit, orbital HØ5.23-●
ovary NEC N83.8
oviduct N83.6
pancreas K86.89
parathyroid (gland) (spontaneous) E21.4
parturition —*see* Hemorrhage, complicating, delivery
penis N48.89
pericardium, pericarditis I31.2
peritoneum, peritoneal K66.1
peritonsillar tissue J35.8
due to infection J36

Hemorrhage, hemorrhagic (Continued)
petechial R23.3
due to autosensitivity, erythrocyte D69.2
pituitary (gland) E23.6
pleura —see Hemorrhage, lung
polioencephalitis, superior E51.2
polymyositis —see Polymyositis
pons, pontine I61.3
posterior fossa (nontraumatic) I61.8
newborn P52.6
postmenopausal N95.Ø
postnasal RØ4.Ø
postoperative —see Complications, postprocedural, hemorrhage, by site
postpartum NEC (following delivery of placenta) O72.1
delayed or secondary O72.2
retained placenta O72.Ø
third stage O72.Ø
pregnancy —see Hemorrhage, antepartum
preretinal —see Hemorrhage, retina
prostate N42.1
puerperal —see Hemorrhage, postpartum
delayed or secondary O72.2
pulmonary RØ4.89
newborn P26.9
massive P26.1
specified NEC P26.8
tuberculous —see Tuberculosis, pulmonary
purpura (primary) D69.3
rectum (sphincter) K62.5
newborn P54.2
recurring, following initial hemorrhage at time of injury T79.2
renal N28.89
respiratory passage or tract RØ4.9
specified NEC RØ4.89
retina, retinal (vessels) H35.6-●
diabetic —see Diabetes, retinal, hemorrhage
retroperitoneal R58
scalp R58
scrotum N5Ø.1
secondary (nontraumatic) R58
following initial hemorrhage at time of injury T79.2
seminal vesicle N5Ø.1
skin R23.3
newborn P54.5
slipped umbilical ligature P51.8
spermatic cord N5Ø.1
spinal (cord) G95.19
newborn (birth injury) P11.5
spleen D73.5
intraoperative —see Complications, intraoperative, hemorrhage, spleen
postprocedural —see Complications, postprocedural, hemorrhage, spleen
stomach K92.2
newborn P54.3
ulcer —see Ulcer, stomach, with hemorrhage
subarachnoid (nontraumatic) —see Hemorrhage, intracranial, subarachnoid
subconjunctival —see also Hemorrhage, conjunctiva
birth injury P15.3
subcortical (brain) I61.Ø
subcutaneous R23.3
subdiaphragmatic R58
subdural (acute) (nontraumatic) —see Hemorrhage, intracranial, subdural
subependymal
newborn P52.Ø
with intraventricular extension P52.1
and intracerebral extension P52.22
subgaleal P12.2
subhyaloid —see Hemorrhage, retina
subperiosteal —see Disorder, bone, specified type NEC
subretinal —see Hemorrhage, retina
subtentorial —see Hemorrhage, intracranial, subdural

Hemorrhage, hemorrhagic (Continued)
subungual L6Ø.8
suprarenal (capsule) (gland) E27.49
newborn P54.4
tentorium (traumatic) NEC —see Hemorrhage, brain
newborn (birth injury) P1Ø.4
testis N5Ø.1
third stage (postpartum) O72.Ø
thorax —see Hemorrhage, lung
throat RØ4.1
thymus (gland) E32.8
thyroid (cyst) (gland) EØ7.89
tongue K14.8
tonsil J35.8
trachea —see Hemorrhage, lung
tracheobronchial RØ4.89
newborn P26.Ø
traumatic — code to specific injury
cerebellar —see Hemorrhage, brain
intracranial —see Hemorrhage, brain
recurring or secondary (following initial hemorrhage at time of injury) T79.2
tuberculous NEC —see also Tuberculosis, pulmonary A15.Ø
tunica vaginalis N5Ø.1
ulcer - code by site under Ulcer, with hemorrhage K27.4
umbilicus, umbilical
cord
after birth, newborn P51.9
complicating delivery O69.5
newborn P51.9
massive P51.Ø
slipped ligature P51.8
stump P51.9
urethra (idiopathic) N36.8
uterus, uterine (abnormal) N93.9
climacteric N92.4
complicating delivery —see Hemorrhage, complicating, delivery
dysfunctional or functional N93.8
intermenstrual (regular) N92.3
irregular N92.1
postmenopausal N95.Ø
postpartum —see Hemorrhage, postpartum
preclimacteric or premenopausal N92.4
prepubertal N93.8
pubertal N92.2
vagina (abnormal) N93.9
newborn P54.6
vas deferens N5Ø.1
vasa previa O69.4
ventricular I61.5
vesical N32.89
viscera NEC R58
newborn P54.8
vitreous (humor) (intraocular) H43.1-●
vulva N9Ø.89
Hemorrhoids (bleeding) (without mention of degree) K64.9
1st degree (grade/stage I) (without prolapse outside of anal canal) K64.Ø
2nd degree (grade/stage II) (that prolapse with straining but retract spontaneously) K64.1
3rd degree (grade/stage III) (that prolapse with straining and require manual replacement back inside anal canal) K64.2
4th degree (grade/stage IV) (with prolapsed tissue that cannot be manually replaced) K64.3
complicating
pregnancy O22.4
puerperium O87.2
external K64.4
with
thrombosis K64.5

Hemorrhoids (Continued)
internal (without mention of degree) K64.8
prolapsed K64.8
skin tags
anus K64.4
residual K64.4
specified NEC K64.8
strangulated —see also Hemorrhoids, by degree K64.8
thrombosed —see also Hemorrhoids, by degree K64.5
ulcerated —see also Hemorrhoids, by degree K64.8
Hemosalpinx N83.6
with
hematocolpos N89.7
hematometra N85.7
with hematocolpos N89.7
Hemosiderosis (dietary) E83.19
pulmonary, idiopathic E83.1 [J84.Ø3]
transfusion T8Ø.89
Hemothorax (bacterial) (nontuberculous) J94.2
newborn P54.8
traumatic S27.1
with pneumothorax S27.2
tuberculous NEC A15.6
Henoch (-Schönlein) disease or syndrome (purpura) D69.Ø
Henpue, henpuye A66.6
Hepar lobatum (syphilitic) A52.74
Hepatalgia K76.89
Hepatitis K75.9
acute B17.9
with coma K72.Ø1
with hepatic failure —see Failure, hepatic
alcoholic —see Hepatitis, alcoholic
infectious B15.9
non-viral K72.Ø
viral B17.9
alcoholic (acute) (chronic) K7Ø.1Ø
with ascites K7Ø.11
amebic —see Abscess, liver, amebic
anicteric (viral) —see Hepatitis, viral
antigen-associated (HAA) —see Hepatitis, B
Australia-antigen (positive) —see Hepatitis, B
autoimmune K75.4
B B19.1Ø
with hepatic coma B19.11
acute B16.9
with
delta-agent (coinfection) (without hepatic coma) B16.1
with hepatic coma B16.Ø
hepatic coma (without delta-agent coinfection) B16.2
chronic B18.1
with delta-agent B18.Ø
bacterial NEC K75.89
C (viral) B19.2Ø
with hepatic coma B19.21
acute B17.1Ø
with hepatic coma B17.11
chronic B18.2
catarrhal (acute) B15.9
with hepatic coma B15.Ø
cholangiolitic K75.89
cholestatic K75.89
chronic K73.9
active NEC K73.2
lobular NEC K73.1
persistent NEC K73.Ø
specified NEC K73.8
cytomegaloviral B25.1
due to ethanol (acute) (chronic) —see Hepatitis, alcoholic
epidemic B15.9
with hepatic coma B15.Ø
fulminant NEC (viral) —see Hepatitis, viral
granulomatous NEC K75.3
herpesviral BØØ.81

Hepatitis *(Continued)*
  history of
    B Z86.19
    C Z86.19
  homologous serum —*see* Hepatitis, viral, type B
  in (due to)
    mumps B26.81
    toxoplasmosis (acquired) B58.1
      congenital (active) P37.1 *[K77]*
  infectious, infective B15.9
    acute (subacute) B17.9
    chronic B18.9
  inoculation —*see* Hepatitis, viral, type B
  interstitial (chronic) K74.69
  lupoid NEC K75.2
  malignant NEC (with hepatic failure) K72.90
    with coma K72.91
  neonatal giant cell P59.29
  neonatal (idiopathic) (toxic) P59.29
  newborn P59.29
  postimmunization —*see* Hepatitis, viral, type B
  post-transfusion —*see* Hepatitis, viral, type B
  reactive, nonspecific K75.2
  serum —*see* Hepatitis, viral, type B
  specified type NEC
    with hepatic failure —*see* Failure, hepatic
  syphilitic (late) A52.74
    congenital (early) A50.08 *[K77]*
      late A50.59 *[K77]*
    secondary A51.45
  toxic —*see also* Disease, liver, toxic K71.6
  tuberculous A18.83
  viral, virus B19.9
    with hepatic coma B19.0
    acute B17.9
    chronic B18.9
      specified NEC B18.8
      type
        B B18.1
          with delta-agent B18.0
        C B18.2
    congenital P35.3
    coxsackie B33.8 *[K77]*
    cytomegalic inclusion B25.1
    in remission, any type — code to Hepatitis, chronic, by type
    non-A, non-B B17.8
    specified type NEC (with or without coma) B17.8
    type
      A B15.9
        with hepatic coma B15.0
      B B19.10
        with hepatic coma B19.11
        acute B16.9
          with
            delta-agent (coinfection) (without hepatic coma) B16.1
              with hepatic coma B16.0
            hepatic coma (without delta-agent coinfection) B16.2
        chronic B18.1
          with delta-agent B18.0
      C B19.20
        with hepatic coma B19.21
        acute B17.10
          with hepatic coma B17.11
        chronic B18.2
      E B17.2
      non-A, non-B B17.8
Hepatization lung (acute) —*see* Pneumonia, lobar
Hepatoblastoma C22.2
Hepatocarcinoma C22.0
Hepatocholangiocarcinoma C22.0
Hepatocholangioma, benign D13.4
Hepatocholangitis K75.89
Hepatolenticular degeneration E83.01
Hepatoma (malignant) C22.0
  benign D13.4
  embryonal C22.0
Hepatomegaly —*see also* Hypertrophy, liver
  with splenomegaly R16.2
  congenital Q44.7
  in mononucleosis
    gammaherpesviral B27.09
    infectious specified NEC B27.89
Hepatoptosis K76.89
Hepatorenal syndrome following labor and delivery O90.4
Hepatosis K76.89
Hepatosplenomegaly R16.2
  hyperlipemic (Bürger-Grütz type) E78.3 *[K77]*
Hereditary —*see* condition
Heredodegeneration, macular —*see* Dystrophy, retina
Heredopathia atactica polyneuritiformis G60.1
Heredosyphilis —*see* Syphilis, congenital
Herlitz' syndrome Q81.1
Hermansky-Pudlak syndrome E70.331
Hermaphrodite, hermaphroditism (true) Q56.0
  46,XX with streak gonads Q99.1
  46,XX/46,XY Q99.0
  46,XY with streak gonads Q99.1
  chimera 46,XX/46,XY Q99.0
Hernia, hernial (acquired) (recurrent) K46.9
  with
    gangrene —*see* Hernia, by site, with, gangrene
    incarceration —*see* Hernia, by site, with, obstruction
    irreducible —*see* Hernia, by site, with, obstruction
    obstruction —*see* Hernia, by site, with, obstruction
    strangulation —*see* Hernia, by site, with, obstruction
  abdomen, abdominal K46.9
    with
      gangrene (and obstruction) K46.1
      obstruction K46.0
    femoral —*see* Hernia, femoral
    incisional —*see* Hernia, incisional
    inguinal —*see* Hernia, inguinal
    specified site NEC K45.8
      with
        gangrene (and obstruction) K45.1
        obstruction K45.0
    umbilical —*see* Hernia, umbilical
    wall —*see* Hernia, ventral
  appendix —*see* Hernia, abdomen
  bladder (mucosa) (sphincter)
    congenital (female) (male) Q79.51
    female —*see* Cystocele
    male N32.89
  brain, congenital —*see* Encephalocele
  cartilage, vertebra —*see* Displacement, intervertebral disc
  cerebral, congenital —*see also* Encephalocele
    endaural Q01.8
  ciliary body (traumatic) S05.2-●
  colon —*see* Hernia, abdomen
  Cooper's —*see* Hernia, abdomen, specified site NEC
  crural —*see* Hernia, femoral
  diaphragm, diaphragmatic K44.9
    with
      gangrene (and obstruction) K44.1
      obstruction K44.0
    congenital Q79.0
  direct (inguinal) —*see* Hernia, inguinal
  diverticulum, intestine —*see* Hernia, abdomen
  double (inguinal) —*see* Hernia, inguinal, bilateral
  due to adhesions (with obstruction) K56.50
  epigastric —*see also* Hernia, ventral K43.9
  esophageal hiatus —*see* Hernia, hiatal
Hernia, hernial *(Continued)*
  external (inguinal) —*see* Hernia, inguinal
  fallopian tube N83.4-●
  fascia M62.89
  femoral K41.90
    with
      gangrene (and obstruction) K41.40
        not specified as recurrent K41.40
        recurrent K41.41
      obstruction K41.30
        not specified as recurrent K41.30
        recurrent K41.31
    bilateral K41.20
      with
        gangrene (and obstruction) K41.10
          not specified as recurrent K41.10
          recurrent K41.11
        obstruction K41.00
          not specified as recurrent K41.00
          recurrent K41.01
      not specified as recurrent K41.20
      recurrent K41.21
    not specified as recurrent K41.90
    recurrent K41.91
    unilateral K41.90
      with
        gangrene (and obstruction) K41.40
          not specified as recurrent K41.40
          recurrent K41.41
        obstruction K41.30
          not specified as recurrent K41.30
          recurrent K41.31
      not specified as recurrent K41.90
      recurrent K41.91
  foramen magnum G93.5
    congenital Q01.8
  funicular (umbilical) —*see also* Hernia, umbilicus
    spermatic (cord) —*see* Hernia, inguinal
  gastrointestinal tract —*see* Hernia, abdomen
  Hesselbach's —*see* Hernia, femoral, specified site NEC
  hiatal (esophageal) (sliding) K44.9
    with
      gangrene (and obstruction) K44.1
      obstruction K44.0
    congenital Q40.1
  hypogastric —*see* Hernia, ventral
  incarcerated —*see also* Hernia, by site, with obstruction
    with gangrene —*see* Hernia, by site, with gangrene
  incisional K43.92
    with
      gangrene (and obstruction) K43.1
      obstruction K43.0
  indirect (inguinal) —*see* Hernia, inguinal
  inguinal (direct) (external) (funicular) (indirect) (internal) (oblique) (scrotal) (sliding) K40.90
    with
      gangrene (and obstruction) K40.40
        not specified as recurrent K40.40
        recurrent K40.41
      obstruction K40.30
        not specified as recurrent K40.30
        recurrent K40.31
    bilateral K40.20
      with
        gangrene (and obstruction) K40.10
          not specified as recurrent K40.10
          recurrent K40.11
        obstruction K40.00
          not specified as recurrent K40.00
          recurrent K40.01
      not specified as recurrent K40.20
      recurrent K40.21
    not specified as recurrent K40.90
    recurrent K40.91

Hernia, hernial *(Continued)*
inguinal *(Continued)*
unilateral K4Ø.9Ø
with
gangrene (and obstruction) K4Ø.4Ø
not specified as recurrent K4Ø.4Ø
recurrent K4Ø.41
obstruction K4Ø.3Ø
not specified as recurrent K4Ø.3Ø
recurrent K4Ø.31
not specified as recurrent K4Ø.9Ø
recurrent K4Ø.91
internal *—see also* Hernia, abdomen
inguinal *—see* Hernia, inguinal
interstitial *—see* Hernia, abdomen
intervertebral cartilage or disc *—see* Displacement, intervertebral disc
intestine, intestinal *—see* Hernia, by site
intra-abdominal *—see* Hernia, abdomen
iris (traumatic) SØ5.2-●
irreducible *—see also* Hernia, by site, with obstruction
with gangrene *—see* Hernia, by site, with gangrene
ischiatic *—see* Hernia, abdomen, specified site NEC
ischiorectal *—see* Hernia, abdomen, specified site NEC
lens (traumatic) SØ5.2-●
linea (alba) (semilunaris) *—see* Hernia, ventral
Littre's *—see* Hernia, abdomen
lumbar *—see* Hernia, abdomen, specified site NEC
lung (subcutaneous) J98.4
mediastinum J98.59
mesenteric (internal) *—see* Hernia, abdomen
midline *—see* Hernia, ventral
muscle (sheath) M62.89
nucleus pulposus *—see* Displacement, intervertebral disc
oblique (inguinal) *—see* Hernia, inguinal
obstructive *—see also* Hernia, by site, with obstruction
with gangrene *—see* Hernia, by site, with gangrene
obturator *—see* Hernia, abdomen, specified site NEC
omental *—see* Hernia, abdomen
ovary N83.4-●
oviduct N83.4-●
paraesophageal *—see also* Hernia, diaphragm
congenital Q4Ø.1
parastomal K43.5
with
gangrene (and obstruction) K43.4
obstruction K43.3
paraumbilical *—see* Hernia, umbilicus
perineal *—see* Hernia, abdomen, specified site NEC
Petit's *—see* Hernia, abdomen, specified site NEC
postoperative *—see* Hernia, incisional
pregnant uterus *—see* Abnormal, uterus in pregnancy or childbirth
prevesical N32.89
properitoneal *—see* Hernia, abdomen, specified site NEC
pudendal *—see* Hernia, abdomen, specified site NEC
rectovaginal N81.6
retroperitoneal *—see* Hernia, abdomen, specified site NEC
Richter's *—see* Hernia, abdomen, with obstruction
Rieux's, Riex's *—see* Hernia, abdomen, specified site NEC
sac condition (adhesion) (dropsy) (inflammation) (laceration) (suppuration) - code by site under Hernia

Hernia, hernial *(Continued)*
sciatic *—see* Hernia, abdomen, specified site NEC
scrotum, scrotal *—see* Hernia, inguinal
sliding (inguinal) *—see also* Hernia, inguinal
hiatus *—see* Hernia, hiatal
spigelian *—see* Hernia, ventral
spinal *—see* Spina bifida
strangulated *—see also* Hernia, by site, with obstruction
with gangrene *—see* Hernia, by site, with gangrene
subxiphoid *—see* Hernia, ventral
supra-umbilicus *—see* Hernia, ventral
tendon *—see* Disorder, tendon, specified type NEC
Treitz's (fossa) *—see* Hernia, abdomen, specified site NEC
tunica vaginalis Q55.29
umbilicus, umbilical K42.9
with
gangrene (and obstruction) K42.1
obstruction K42.Ø
ureter N28.89
urethra, congenital Q64.79
urinary meatus, congenital Q64.79
uterus N81.4
pregnant *—see* Abnormal, uterus in pregnancy or childbirth
vaginal (anterior) (wall) *—see* Cystocele
Velpeau's *—see* Hernia, femoral
ventral K43.9
with
gangrene (and obstruction) K43.7
obstruction K43.6
incisional K43.2
with
gangrene (and obstruction) K43.1
obstruction K43.Ø
recurrent *—see* Hernia, incisional
specified NEC K43.9
with
gangrene (and obstruction) K43.7
obstruction K43.6
vesical
congenital (female) (male) Q79.51
female *—see* Cystocele
male N32.89
vitreous (into wound) SØ5.2-●
into anterior chamber *—see* Prolapse, vitreous
Herniation *—see also* Hernia
brain (stem) G93.5
cerebral G93.5
mediastinum J98.59
nucleus pulposus *—see* Displacement, intervertebral disc
Herpangina BØ8.5
Herpes, herpesvirus, herpetic BØØ.9
anogenital A6Ø.9
perianal skin A6Ø.1
rectum A6Ø.1
urogenital tract A6Ø.ØØ
cervix A6Ø.Ø3
male genital organ NEC A6Ø.Ø2
penis A6Ø.Ø1
specified site NEC A6Ø.Ø9
vagina A6Ø.Ø4
vulva A6Ø.Ø4
blepharitis (zoster) BØ2.39
simplex BØØ.59
circinatus B35.4
bullosus L12.Ø
conjunctivitis (simplex) BØØ.53
zoster BØ2.31
cornea BØ2.33
encephalitis BØØ.4
due to herpesvirus 6 B1Ø.Ø1
due to herpesvirus 7 B1Ø.Ø9
specified NEC B1Ø.Ø9

Herpes, herpesvirus, herpetic *(Continued)*
eye (zoster) BØ2.3Ø
simplex BØØ.5Ø
eyelid (zoster) BØ2.39
simplex BØØ.59
facialis BØØ.1
febrilis BØØ.1
geniculate ganglionitis BØ2.21
genital, genitalis A6Ø.ØØ
female A6Ø.Ø9
male A6Ø.Ø2
gestational, gestationis O26.4-●
gingivostomatitis BØØ.2
human BØØ.9
1 *—see* Herpes, simplex
2 *—see* Herpes, simplex
3 *—see* Varicella
4 *—see* Mononucleosis, Epstein-Barr (virus)
5 *—see* Disease, cytomegalic inclusion (generalized)
6
encephalitis B1Ø.Ø1
specified NEC B1Ø.81
7
encephalitis B1Ø.Ø9
specified NEC B1Ø.82
8 B1Ø.89
infection NEC B1Ø.89
Kaposi's sarcoma associated B1Ø.89
iridocyclitis (simplex) BØØ.51
zoster BØ2.32
iris (vesicular erythema multiforme) L51.9
iritis (simplex) BØØ.51
Kaposi's sarcoma associated B1Ø.89
keratitis (simplex) (dendritic) (disciform) (interstitial) BØØ.52
zoster (interstitial) BØ2.33
keratoconjunctivitis (simplex) BØØ.52
zoster BØ2.33
labialis BØØ.1
lip BØØ.1
meningitis (simplex) BØØ.3
zoster BØ2.1
ophthalmicus (zoster) NEC BØ2.3Ø
simplex BØØ.5Ø
penis A6Ø.Ø1
perianal skin A6Ø.1
pharyngitis, pharyngotonsillitis BØØ.2
rectum A6Ø.1
scrotum A6Ø.Ø2
sepsis BØØ.7
simplex BØØ.9
complicated NEC BØØ.89
congenital P35.2
conjunctivitis BØØ.53
external ear BØØ.1
eyelid BØØ.59
hepatitis BØØ.81
keratitis (interstitial) BØØ.52
myleitis BØØ.82
specified complication NEC BØØ.89
visceral BØØ.89
stomatitis BØØ.2
tonsurans B35.Ø
visceral BØØ.89
vulva A6Ø.Ø4
whitlow BØØ.89
zoster *—see also* condition BØ2.9
auricularis BØ2.21
complicated NEC BØ2.8
conjunctivitis BØ2.31
disseminated BØ2.7
encephalitis BØ2.Ø
eye(lid) BØ2.39
geniculate ganglionitis BØ2.21
keratitis (interstitial) BØ2.33
meningitis BØ2.1
myelitis BØ2.24
neuritis, neuralgia BØ2.29
ophthalmicus NEC BØ2.3Ø
oticus BØ2.21

Herpes, herpesvirus, herpetic *(Continued)*
zoster *(Continued)*
polyneuropathy B02.23
specified complication NEC B02.8
trigeminal neuralgia B02.22
Herpesvirus (human) —*see* Herpes
Herpetophobia F40.218
Herrick's anemia —*see* Disease, sickle-cell
Hers' disease E74.09
Herter-Gee syndrome K90.0
Herxheimer's reaction R68.89
Hesitancy
of micturition R39.11
urinary R39.11
Hesselbach's hernia —*see* Hernia, femoral, specified site NEC
Heterochromia (congenital) Q13.2
cataract —*see* Cataract, complicated
cyclitis (Fuchs) —*see* Cyclitis, Fuchs' heterochromic
hair L67.1
iritis —*see* Cyclitis, Fuchs' heterochromic
retained metallic foreign body (nonmagnetic) —*see* Foreign body, intraocular, old, retained
magnetic —*see* Foreign body, intraocular, old, retained, magnetic
uveitis —*see* Cyclitis, Fuchs' heterochromic
Heterophoria —*see* Strabismus, heterophoria
Heterophyes, heterophyiasis (small intestine) B66.8
Heterotopia, heterotopic —*see also* Malposition, congenital
cerebralis Q04.8
Heterotropia —*see* Strabismus
Heubner-Herter disease K90.0
Hexadactylism Q69.9
HGSIL (cytology finding) (high grade squamous intraepithelial lesion on cytologic smear) (Pap smear finding)
anus R85.613
cervix R87.613
biopsy (histology) finding — *see* Neoplasia, intraepithelial, cervix, grade II or grade III
vagina R87.623
biopsy (histology) finding — *see* Neoplasia, intraepithelial, vagina, grade II or grade III
Hibernoma —*see* Lipoma
Hiccup, hiccough R06.6
epidemic B33.0
psychogenic F45.8
Hidden penis (congenital) Q55.64
acquired N48.83
Hidradenitis (axillaris) (suppurative) L73.2
Hidradenoma (nodular) —*see also* Neoplasm, skin, benign
clear cell —*see* Neoplasm, skin, benign
papillary —*see* Neoplasm, skin, benign
Hidrocystoma —*see* Neoplasm, skin, benign
High
altitude effects T70.20
anoxia T70.29
on
ears T70.0
sinuses T70.1
polycythemia D75.1
arch
➠ foot Q66.7- ●
palate, congenital Q38.5
arterial tension —*see* Hypertension
basal metabolic rate R94.8
blood pressure —*see also* Hypertension
borderline R03.0
reading (incidental) (isolated) (nonspecific), without diagnosis of hypertension R03.0
cholesterol E78.00
with high triglycerides E78.2
diaphragm (congenital) Q79.1

High *(Continued)*
expressed emotional level within family Z63.8
head at term O32.4
palate, congenital Q38.5
risk
infant NEC Z76.2
sexual behavior (heterosexual) Z72.51
bisexual Z72.53
homosexual Z72.52
scrotal testis, testes
bilateral Q53.23
unilateral Q53.13
temperature (of unknown origin) R50.9
thoracic rib Q76.6
triglycerides E78.1
with high cholesterol E78.2
Hildenbrand's disease A75.0
Hilum —*see* condition
Hip —*see* condition
Hippel's disease Q85.8
Hippophobia F40.218
Hippus H57.09
Hirschsprung's disease or megacolon Q43.1
Hirsutism, hirsuties L68.0
Hirudiniasis
external B88.3
internal B83.4
Hiss-Russell dysentery A03.1
Histidinemia, histidinuria E70.41
Histiocytoma —*see also* Neoplasm, skin, benign
fibrous —*see also* Neoplasm, skin, benign
atypical —*see* Neoplasm, connective tissue, uncertain behavior
malignant —*see* Neoplasm, connective tissue, malignant
Histiocytosis D76.3
acute differentiated progressive C96.0
Langerhans' cell NEC C96.6
multifocal X
multisystemic (disseminated) C96.0
unisystemic C96.5
pulmonary, adult (adult PLCH) J84.82
unifocal (X) C96.6
lipid, lipoid D76.3
essential E75.29
malignant C96.A
mononuclear phagocytes NEC D76.1
Langerhans' cells C96.6
non-Langerhans cell D76.3
polyostotic sclerosing D76.3
sinus, with massive lymphadenopathy D76.3
syndrome NEC D76.3
X NEC C96.6
acute (progressive) C96.0
chronic C96.6
multifocal C96.5
multisystemic C96.0
unifocal C96.6
Histoplasmosis B39.9
with pneumonia NEC B39.2
African B39.5
American —*see* Histoplasmosis, capsulati
capsulati B39.4
disseminated B39.3
generalized B39.3
pulmonary B39.2
acute B39.0
chronic B39.1
Darling's B39.4
duboisii B39.5
lung NEC B39.2
History
family (of) —*see also* History, personal (of)
alcohol abuse Z81.1
allergy NEC Z84.89
anemia Z83.2
arthritis Z82.61
asthma Z82.5
blindness Z82.1
cardiac death (sudden) Z82.41
carrier of genetic disease Z84.81
chromosomal anomaly Z82.79

History *(Continued)*
family *(Continued)*
chronic
disabling disease NEC Z82.8
lower respiratory disease Z82.5
colonic polyps Z83.71
congenital malformations and deformations Z82.79
polycystic kidney Z82.71
consanguinity Z84.3
deafness Z82.2
diabetes mellitus Z83.3
disability NEC Z82.8
disease or disorder (of)
allergic NEC Z84.89
behavioral NEC Z81.8
blood and blood-forming organs Z83.2
cardiovascular NEC Z82.49
chronic disabling NEC Z82.8
digestive Z83.79
ear NEC Z83.52
~~elevated lipoprotein(a) (Lp(a)) Z83.430~~
▶ elevated lipoprotein (a) (Lp(a)) Z83.430
endocrine NEC Z83.49
eye NEC Z83.518
glaucoma Z83.511
familial hypercholesterolemia Z83.42
genitourinary NEC Z84.2
glaucoma Z83.511
hematological Z83.2
immune mechanism Z83.2
infectious NEC Z83.1
ischemic heart Z82.49
kidney Z84.1
lipoprotein metabolism Z83.438
mental NEC Z81.8
metabolic Z83.49
musculoskeletal NEC Z82.69
neurological NEC Z82.0
nutritional Z83.49
parasitic NEC Z83.1
psychiatric NEC Z81.8
respiratory NEC Z83.6
skin and subcutaneous tissue NEC Z84.0
specified NEC Z84.89
drug abuse NEC Z81.3
~~elevated lipoprotein(a) (Lp(a)) Z83.430~~
▶ elevated lipoprotein(a) (Lp (a)) Z83.430
epilepsy Z82.0
familial hypercholesterolemia Z83.42
genetic disease carrier Z84.81
glaucoma Z83.511
hearing loss Z82.2
human immunodeficiency virus (HIV) infection Z83.0
Huntington's chorea Z82.0
hyperlipidemia, familial combined Z83.438
intellectual disability Z81.0
leukemia Z80.6
lipidemia NEC Z83.438
malignant neoplasm (of) NOS Z80.9
bladder Z80.52
breast Z80.3
bronchus Z80.1
digestive organ Z80.0
gastrointestinal tract Z80.0
genital organ Z80.49
ovary Z80.41
prostate Z80.42
specified organ NEC Z80.49
testis Z80.43
hematopoietic NEC Z80.7
intrathoracic organ NEC Z80.2
kidney Z80.51
lung Z80.1
lymphatic NEC Z80.7
ovary Z80.41
prostate Z80.42
respiratory organ NEC Z80.2
specified site NEC Z80.8
testis Z80.43
trachea Z80.1

H

- History *(Continued)*
  - family *(Continued)*
    - malignant neoplasm *(Continued)*
      - urinary organ or tract Z80.59
        - bladder Z80.52
        - kidney Z80.51
    - mental
      - disorder NEC Z81.8
    - multiple endocrine neoplasia (MEN) syndrome Z83.41
    - osteoporosis Z82.62
    - polycystic kidney Z82.71
    - polyps (colon) Z83.71
    - psychiatric disorder Z81.8
    - psychoactive substance abuse NEC Z81.3
    - respiratory condition NEC Z83.6
      - asthma and other lower respiratory conditions Z82.5
    - self-harmful behavior Z81.8
    - SIDS (sudden infant death syndrome) Z84.82
    - skin condition Z84.0
    - specified condition NEC Z84.89
    - stroke (cerebrovascular) Z82.3
    - substance abuse NEC Z81.4
      - alcohol Z81.1
      - drug NEC Z81.3
      - psychoactive NEC Z81.3
      - tobacco Z81.2
    - sudden
      - cardiac death Z82.41
      - infant death syndrome (SIDS) Z84.82
    - tobacco abuse Z81.2
    - violence, violent behavior Z81.8
    - visual loss Z82.1
  - personal (of) —*see also* History, family (of)
    - abuse
      - adult Z91.419
        - forced labor or sexual exploitation Z91.42
        - physical and sexual Z91.410
        - psychological Z91.411
      - childhood Z62.819
        - forced labor or sexual exploitation in childhood Z62.813
        - physical Z62.810
        - psychological Z62.811
        - sexual Z62.810
    - alcohol dependence F10.21
    - allergy (to) Z88.9
      - analgesic agent NEC Z88.6
      - anesthetic Z88.4
      - antibiotic agent NEC Z88.1
      - anti-infective agent NEC Z88.3
      - contrast media Z91.041
      - drugs, medicaments and biological substances Z88.9
        - specified NEC Z88.8
      - food Z91.018
        - additives Z91.02
        - eggs Z91.012
        - milk products Z91.011
        - peanuts Z91.010
        - seafood Z91.013
        - specified food NEC Z91.018
      - insect Z91.038
        - bee Z91.030
      - latex Z91.040
      - medicinal agents Z88.9
        - specified NEC Z88.8
      - narcotic agent NEC Z88.5
      - nonmedicinal agents Z91.048
      - penicillin Z88.0
      - serum Z88.7
      - specified NEC Z91.09
      - sulfonamides Z88.2
      - vaccine Z88.7
    - anaphylactic shock Z87.892
    - anaphylaxis Z87.892
    - behavioral disorders Z86.59
    - benign carcinoid tumor Z86.012
- History *(Continued)*
  - personal *(Continued)*
    - benign neoplasm Z86.018
      - brain Z86.011
      - carcinoid Z86.012
      - colonic polyps Z86.010
    - brain injury (traumatic) Z87.820
    - breast implant removal Z98.86
    - calculi, renal Z87.442
    - cancer —*see* History, personal (of), malignant neoplasm (of)
    - cardiac arrest (death), successfully resuscitated Z86.74
    - cerebral infarction without residual deficit Z86.73
    - cervical dysplasia Z87.410
    - chemotherapy for neoplastic condition Z92.21
    - childhood abuse —*see* History, personal (of), abuse
    - cleft lip (corrected) Z87.730
    - cleft palate (corrected) Z87.730
    - collapsed vertebra (healed) Z87.311
      - due to osteoporosis Z87.310
    - combat and operational stress reaction Z86.51
    - congenital malformation (corrected) Z87.798
      - circulatory system (corrected) Z87.74
      - digestive system (corrected) NEC Z87.738
      - ear (corrected) Z87.721
      - eye (corrected) Z87.720
      - face and neck (corrected) Z87.790
      - genitourinary system (corrected) NEC Z87.718
      - heart (corrected) Z87.74
      - integument (corrected) Z87.76
      - limb(s) (corrected) Z87.76
      - musculoskeletal system (corrected) Z87.76
      - neck (corrected) Z87.790
      - nervous system (corrected) NEC Z87.728
      - respiratory system (corrected) Z87.75
      - sense organs (corrected) NEC Z87.728
      - specified NEC Z87.798
    - contraception Z92.0
    - deployment (military) Z91.82
    - diabetic foot ulcer Z86.31
    - disease or disorder (of) Z87.898
      - blood and blood-forming organs Z86.2
      - circulatory system Z86.79
        - specified condition NEC Z86.79
      - connective tissue NEC Z87.39
      - digestive system Z87.19
        - colonic polyp Z86.010
        - peptic ulcer disease Z87.11
        - specified condition NEC Z87.19
      - ear Z86.69
      - endocrine Z86.39
        - diabetic foot ulcer Z86.31
        - gestational diabetes Z86.32
        - specified type NEC Z86.39
      - eye Z86.69
      - genital (track) system NEC
        - female Z87.42
        - male Z87.438
      - hematological Z86.2
      - Hodgkin Z85.71
      - immune mechanism Z86.2
      - infectious Z86.19
        - malaria Z86.13
        - Methicillin resistant Staphylococcus aureus (MRSA) Z86.14
        - poliomyelitis Z86.12
        - specified NEC Z86.19
        - tuberculosis Z86.11
      - mental NEC Z86.59
      - metabolic Z86.39
        - diabetic foot ulcer Z86.31
        - gestational diabetes Z86.32
        - specified type NEC Z86.39
      - musculoskeletal NEC Z87.39
      - nervous system Z86.69
      - nutritional Z86.39
- History *(Continued)*
  - personal *(Continued)*
    - disease or disorder (of) *(Continued)*
      - parasitic Z86.19
      - respiratory system NEC Z87.09
      - sense organs Z86.69
      - skin Z87.2
      - specified site or type NEC Z87.898
      - subcutaneous tissue Z87.2
      - trophoblastic Z87.59
      - urinary system NEC Z87.448
    - drug dependence —*see* Dependence, drug, by type, in remission
    - drug therapy
      - antineoplastic chemotherapy Z92.21
      - estrogen Z92.23
      - immunosupression Z92.25
      - inhaled steroids Z92.240
      - monoclonal drug Z92.22
      - specified NEC Z92.29
      - steroid Z92.241
      - systemic steroids Z92.241
    - dysplasia
      - cervical (mild) (moderate) Z87.410
        - severe (grade III) Z86.001
      - prostatic Z87.430
      - ➠vaginal (mild) (moderate) Z87.411
        - ➠severe (grade III) Z86.002
      - vulvar (mild) (moderate) Z87.412
        - ➠severe (grade III) Z86.002
    - embolism (venous) Z86.718
      - pulmonary Z86.711
    - encephalitis Z86.61
    - estrogen therapy Z92.23
    - extracorporeal membrane oxygenation (ECMO) Z92.81
    - failed conscious sedation Z92.83
    - failed moderate sedation Z92.83
    - fall, falling Z91.81
    - forced labor or sexual exploitation Z91.42
      - in childhood Z62.813
    - fracture (healed)
      - fatigue Z87.312
      - fragility Z87.310
      - osteoporosis Z87.310
      - pathological NEC Z87.311
      - stress Z87.312
      - traumatic Z87.81
    - gestational diabetes Z86.32
    - hepatitis
      - B Z86.19
      - C Z86.19
    - Hodgkin disease Z85.71
    - hyperthermia, malignant Z88.4
    - hypospadias (corrected) Z87.710
    - hysterectomy Z90.710
    - immunosupression therapy Z92.25
    - in situ neoplasm
      - breast Z86.000
      - cervix uteri Z86.001
      - ▶digestive organs, specified NEC Z86.004
      - ▶esophagus Z86.003
      - ▶genital organs, specified NEC Z86.002
      - ▶melanoma Z86.006
      - ▶middle ear Z86.005
      - ▶oral cavity Z86.003
      - ▶respiratory system Z86.005
      - ▶skin Z86.007
      - specified NEC Z86.008
      - ▶stomach Z86.003
    - infection NEC Z86.19
      - central nervous system Z86.61
      - ▶latent tuberculosis Z86.15
      - Methicillin resistant Staphylococcus aureus (MRSA) Z86.14
      - urinary (tract) Z87.41
    - injury NEC Z87.828
    - in utero procedure during pregnancy Z98.870
    - in utero procedure while a fetus Z98.871
    - irradiation Z92.3
    - kidney stones Z87.442

H

History *(Continued)*
personal *(Continued)*
▶latent tuberculosis Z86.15
leukemia Z85.6
lymphoma (non-Hodgkin) Z85.72
malignant melanoma (skin) Z85.820
malignant neoplasm (of) Z85.9
accessory sinuses Z85.22
anus NEC Z85.048
carcinoid Z85.040
bladder Z85.51
bone Z85.830
brain Z85.841
breast Z85.3
bronchus NEC Z85.118
carcinoid Z85.110
carcinoid —*see* History, personal (of), malignant neoplasm, by site, carcinioid
cervix Z85.41
colon NEC Z85.038
carcinoid Z85.030
digestive organ Z85.00
specified NEC Z85.09
endocrine gland NEC Z85.858
epididymis Z85.48
esophagus Z85.01
eye Z85.840
gastrointestinal tract —*see* History, malignant neoplasm, digestive organ
genital organ
female Z85.40
specified NEC Z85.44
male Z85.45
specified NEC Z85.49
hematopoietic NEC Z85.79
intrathoracic organ Z85.20-●
kidney NEC Z85.528
carcinoid Z85.520
large intestine NEC Z85.038
carcinoid Z85.030
larynx Z85.21
liver Z85.05
lung NEC Z85.118
carcinoid Z85.110
mediastinum Z85.29
Merkel cell Z85.821
middle ear Z85.22
nasal cavities Z85.22
nervous system NEC Z85.848
oral cavity Z85.819
specified site NEC Z85.818
ovary Z85.43
pancreas Z85.07
pelvis Z85.53
pharynx Z85.819
specified site NEC Z85.818
pleura Z85.29
prostate Z85.46
rectosigmoid junction NEC Z85.048
carcinoid Z85.040
rectum NEC Z85.048
carcinoid Z85.040
respiratory organ Z85.20
sinuses, accessory Z85.22
skin NEC Z85.828
melanoma Z85.820
Merkel cell Z85.821
small intestine NEC Z85.068
carcinoid Z85.060
soft tissue Z85.831
specified site NEC Z85.89
stomach NEC Z85.028
carcinoid Z85.020
testis Z85.47
thymus NEC Z85.238
carcinoid Z85.230
thyroid Z85.850
tongue Z85.810
trachea Z85.12
ureter Z85.54

History *(Continued)*
personal *(Continued)*
malignant neoplasm (of) *(Continued)*
urinary organ or tract Z85.50
specified NEC Z85.59
uterus Z85.42
maltreatment Z91.89
medical treatment NEC Z92.89
➡melanoma Z85.820
▶in situ Z86.06
▶malignant (skin) Z85.820
meningitis Z86.61
mental disorder Z86.59
Merkel cell carcinoma (skin) Z85.821
Methicillin resistant Staphylococcus aureus (MRSA) Z86.14
military deployment Z91.82
military war, peacekeeping and humanitarian deployment (current or past conflict) Z91.82
myocardial infarction (old) I25.2
neglect (in)
adult Z91.412
childhood Z62.812
▶neoplasia
▶anal intraepithelial, III [AIN III] Z86.004
▶high-grade prostatic intraepithelial, III [HGPIN III] Z86.002
▶vaginal intraepithelial, III [VAIN III] Z86.002
▶vulvar intraepithelial, III [VIN III] Z86.002
neoplasm
benign Z86.018
brain Z86.011
colon polyp Z86.010
in situ
breast Z86.000
cervix uteri Z86.001
▶digestive organs, specified NEC Z86.004
▶esophagus Z86.003
▶genital organs, specified NEC Z86.002
▶melanoma Z86.006
▶middle ear Z86.005
▶oral cavity Z86.003
▶respiratory system Z86.005
▶skin Z86.007
specified NEC Z86.008
▶stomach Z86.003
malignant —*see* History of, malignant neoplasm
uncertain behavior Z86.03
nephrotic syndrome Z87.441
nicotine dependence Z87.891
noncompliance with medical treatment or regimen —*see* Noncompliance
nutritional deficiency Z86.39
obstetric complications Z87.59
childbirth Z87.59
pregnancy Z87.59
pre-term labor Z87.51
puerperium Z87.59
osteoporosis fractures Z87.31
parasuicide (attempt) Z91.5
physical trauma NEC Z87.828
self-harm or suicide attempt Z91.5
pneumonia (recurrent) Z87.01
poisoning NEC Z91.89
self-harm or suicide attempt Z91.5
poor personal hygiene Z91.89
preterm labor Z87.51
procedure during pregnancy Z98.870
procedure while a fetus Z98.871
prolonged reversible ischemic neurologic deficit (PRINO) Z86.73
prostatic dysplasia Z87.430
psychiatric disorder NEC Z87.89
psychological
abuse
adult Z91.411
child Z62.811
trauma, specified NEC Z91.49
radiation therapy Z92.3

History *(Continued)*
personal *(Continued)*
removal
implant
breast Z98.86
renal calculi Z87.442
respiratory condition NEC Z87.09
retained foreign body fully removed Z87.821
risk factors NEC Z91.89
self-harm Z91.5
self-poisoning attempt Z91.5
sex reassignment Z87.890
sleep-wake cycle problem Z72.821
specified NEC Z87.898
steroid therapy (systemic) Z92.241
inhaled Z92.240
stroke without residual deficits Z86.73
substance abuse NEC F10-F19
sudden cardiac arrest Z86.74
sudden cardiac death successfully resuscitated Z86.74
suicide attempt Z91.5
surgery NEC Z98.890
with uterine scar Z98.891
sex reassignment Z87.890
transplant —*see* Transplant
thrombophlebitis Z86.72
thrombosis (venous) Z86.718
pulmonary Z86.711
tobacco dependence Z87.891
transient ischemic attack (TIA) without residual deficits Z86.73
trauma (physical) NEC Z87.828
psychological NEC Z91.49
self-harm Z91.5
traumatic brain injury Z87.820
▶tuberculosis, latent infection Z86.15
unhealthy sleep-wake cycle Z72.821
unintended awareness under general anesthesia Z92.84
urinary (recurrent) (tract) infection(s) Z87.440
urinary calculi Z87.42
uterine scar from previous surgery Z98.891
vaginal dysplasia Z87.411
venous thrombosis or embolism Z86.718
pulmonary Z86.711
vulvar dysplasia Z87.412
His-Werner disease A79.0
HIV —*see also* Human, immunodeficiency virus B20
laboratory evidence (nonconclusive) R75
nonconclusive test (in infants) R75
positive, seropositive Z21
Hives (bold) —*see* Urticaria
Hoarseness R49.0
Hobo Z59.0
Hodgkin disease —*see* Lymphoma, Hodgkin
Hodgson's disease I71.2
ruptured I71.1
Hoffa-Kastert disease E88.89
Hoffa's disease E88.89
Hoffmann-Bouveret syndrome I47.9
Hoffmann's syndrome E03.9 *[G73.7]*
Hole (round)
macula H35.34-●
retina (without detachment) —*see* Break, retina, round hole
with detachment —*see* Detachment, retina, with retinal, break
Holiday relief care Z75.5
Hollenhorst's plaque —*see* Occlusion, artery, retina
➡**Hollow foot** (congenital) Q66.7-●
acquired —*see* Deformity, limb, foot, specified NEC
Holoprosencephaly Q04.2
Holt-Oram syndrome Q87.2
Homelessness Z59.0
Homesickness —*see* Disorder, adjustment
Homocystinemia, homocystinuria E72.11
Homogentisate 1,2-dioxygenase deficiency E70.29

H

Homologous serum hepatitis (prophylactic) (therapeutic) —*see* Hepatitis, viral, type B
Honeycomb lung J98.4
  congenital Q33.Ø
Hooded
  clitoris Q52.6
  penis Q55.69
Hookworm (disease) (infection) (infestation) B76.9
  with anemia B76.9 *[D63.8]*
  specified NEC B76.8
Hordeolum (eyelid) (externum) (recurrent) HØØ.Ø19
  internum HØØ.Ø29
    left HØØ.Ø26
      lower HØØ.Ø25
      upper HØØ.Ø24
    right HØØ.Ø23
      lower HØØ.Ø22
      upper HØØ.Ø21
  left HØØ.Ø16
    lower HØØ.Ø15
    upper HØØ.Ø14
  right HØØ.Ø13
    lower HØØ.Ø12
    upper HØØ.Ø11
Horn
  cutaneous L85.8
  nail L6Ø.2
    congenital Q84.6
Horner (-Claude Bernard) **syndrome** G9Ø.2
  traumatic —*see* Injury, nerve, cervical sympathetic
Horseshoe kidney (congenital) Q63.1
Horton's headache or neuralgia G44.Ø99
  intractable G44.Ø91
  not intractable G44.Ø99
Hospital hopper syndrome —*see* Disorder, factitious
Hospitalism in children —*see* Disorder, adjustment
Hostility R45.5
  towards child Z62.3
Hot flashes
  menopausal N95.1
Hourglass (contracture) —*see also* Contraction, hourglass
  stomach K31.89
    congenital Q4Ø.2
    stricture K31.2
Household, housing circumstance affecting care Z59.9
  specified NEC Z59.8
Housemaid's knee —*see* Bursitis, prepatellar
Hudson (-Stähli) **line** (cornea) —*see* Pigmentation, cornea, anterior
Human
  bite (open wound) —*see also* Bite
    intact skin surface —*see* Bite, superficial
  herpesvirus —*see* Herpes
  immunodeficiency virus (HIV) disease (infection) B2Ø
    asymptomatic status Z21
    contact Z2Ø.6
    counseling Z71.7
    dementia B2Ø *[FØ2.8Ø]*
      with behavioral disturbance B2Ø *[FØ2.81]*
    exposure to Z2Ø.6
    laboratory evidence R75
    type-2 (HIV 2) as cause of disease classified elsewhere B97.35
  papillomavirus (HPV)
    DNA test positive
      high risk
        cervix R87.81Ø
        vagina R87.811
      low risk
        cervix R87.82Ø
        vagina R87.821
    screening for Z11.51
Human *(Continued)*
  T-cell lymphotropic virus
    type-1 (HTLV-I) infection B33.3
      as cause of disease classified elsewhere B97.33
      carrier Z22.6
    type-2 (HTLV-II) as cause of disease classified elsewhere B97.34
Humidifier lung or pneumonitis J67.7
Humiliation (experience) **in childhood** Z62.898
Humpback (acquired) —*see* Kyphosis
Hunchback (acquired) —*see* Kyphosis
Hunger T73.Ø
  air, psychogenic F45.8
Hungry bone syndrome E83.81
Hunner's ulcer —*see* Cystitis, chronic, interstitial
Hunter's
  glossitis D51.Ø
  syndrome E76.1
Huntington's disease or chorea G1Ø
  with dementia G1Ø *[FØ2.8Ø]*
    with behavioral disturbance G1Ø *[FØ2.81]*
Hunt's
  disease or syndrome (herpetic geniculate ganglionitis) BØ2.21
    dyssynergia cerebellaris myoclonica G11.1
  neuralgia BØ2.21
Hurler (-Scheie) **disease or syndrome** E76.Ø2
Hurst's disease G36.1
Hurthle cell
  adenocarcinoma C73
  adenoma D34
  carcinoma C73
  tumor D34
Hutchinson-Boeck disease or syndrome —*see* Sarcoidosis
Hutchinson-Gilford disease or syndrome E34.8
Hutchinson's
  disease, meaning
    angioma serpiginosum L81.7
    pompholyx (cheiropompholyx) L3Ø.1
    prurigo estivalis L56.4
    summer eruption or summer prurigo L56.4
  melanotic freckle —*see* Melanoma, in situ
    malignant melanoma in —*see* Melanoma
  teeth or incisors (congenital syphilis) A5Ø.52
  triad (congenital syphilis) A5Ø.53
Hyalin plaque, sclera, senile H15.89
Hyaline membrane (disease) (lung) (pulmonary) (newborn) P22.Ø
Hyalinosis
  cutis (et mucosae) E78.89
  focal and segmental (glomerular) —*see also* NØØ-NØ7 with fourth character .1 NØ5.1
Hyalitis, hyalosis, asteroid —*see also* Deposit, crystalline
  syphilitic (late) A52.71
Hydatid
  cyst or tumor —*see* Echinococcus
  mole —*see* Hydatidiform mole
  Morgagni
    female Q5Ø.5
    male (epididymal) Q55.4
      testicular Q55.29
Hydatidiform mole (benign) (complicating pregnancy) (delivered) (undelivered) OØ1.9
  classical OØ1.Ø
  complete OØ1.Ø
  incomplete OØ1.1
  invasive D39.2
  malignant D39.2
  partial OØ1.1
Hydatidosis —*see* Echinococcus
Hydradenitis (axillaris) (suppurative) L73.2
Hydradenoma —*see* Hidradenoma
Hydramnios O4Ø.-●
Hydrancephaly, hydranencephaly QØ4.3
  with spina bifida —*see* Spina bifida, with hydrocephalus
Hydrargyrism NEC —*see* Poisoning, mercury
Hydrarthrosis —*see also* Effusion, joint
  gonococcal A54.42
Hydrarthrosis *(Continued)*
  intermittent M12.4Ø
    ankle M12.47-●
    elbow M12.42-●
    foot joint M12.47-●
    hand joint M12.44-●
    hip M12.45-●
    knee M12.46-●
    multiple site M12.49
    shoulder M12.41-●
    specified joint NEC M12.48
    wrist M12.43-●
  of yaws (early) (late) —*see also* subcategory M14.8-● A66.6
  syphilitic (late) A52.77
    congenital A5Ø.55 *[M12.8Ø]*
Hydremia D64.89
Hydrencephalocele (congenital) —*see* Encephalocele
Hydrencephalomeningocele (congenital) —*see* Encephalocele
Hydroa R23.8
  aestivale L56.4
  vacciniforme L56.4
Hydroadenitis (axillaris) (suppurative) L73.2
Hydrocalycosis —*see* Hydronephrosis
Hydrocele (spermatic cord) (testis) (tunica vaginalis) N43.3
  canal of Nuck N94.89
  communicating N43.2
    congenital P83.5
  congenital P83.5
  encysted N43.Ø
  female NEC N94.89
  infected N43.1
  newborn P83.5
  round ligament N94.89
  specified NEC N43.2
  spinalis —*see* Spina bifida
  vulva N9Ø.89
Hydrocephalus (acquired) (external) (internal) (malignant) (recurrent) G91.9
  aqueduct Sylvius stricture QØ3.Ø
  causing disproportion O33.6
    with obstructed labor O66.3
  communicating G91.Ø
  congenital (external) (internal) QØ3.9
    with spina bifida QØ5.4
      cervical QØ5.Ø
      dorsal QØ5.1
      lumbar QØ5.2
      lumbosacral QØ5.2
      sacral QØ5.3
      thoracic QØ5.1
      thoracolumbar QØ5.1
    specified NEC QØ3.8
  due to toxoplasmosis (congenital) P37.1
  foramen Magendie block (acquired) G91.1
    congenital —*see also* Hydrocephalus, congenital QØ3.1
  in (due to)
    infectious disease NEC B89 *[G91.4]*
    neoplastic disease NEC (*see also* Neoplasm) G91.4
    parasitic disease B89 *[G91.4]*
  newborn QØ3.9
    with spina bifida —*see* Spina bifida, with hydrocephalus
  noncommunicating G91.1
  normal pressure G91.2
    secondary G91.Ø
  obstructive G91.1
  otitic G93.2
  post-traumatic NEC G91.3
  secondary G91.4
    post-traumatic G91.3
  specified NEC G91.8
  syphilitic, congenital A5Ø.49
Hydrocolpos (congenital) N89.8
Hydrocystoma —*see* Neoplasm, skin, benign
Hydroencephalocele (congenital) —*see* Encephalocele

Hydroencephalomeningocele (congenital) —*see* Encephalocele
Hydrohematopneumothorax —*see* Hemothorax
Hydromeningitis —*see* Meningitis
Hydromeningocele (spinal) —*see also* Spina bifida
cranial —*see* Encephalocele
Hydrometra N85.8
Hydrometrocolpos N89.8
Hydromicrocephaly QØ2
Hydromphalos (since birth) Q45.8
Hydromyelia QØ6.4
Hydromyelocele —*see* Spina bifida
Hydronephrosis (atrophic) (early) (functionless) (intermittent) (primary) (secondary) NEC N13.3Ø
with
infection N13.6
obstruction (by) (of)
renal calculus N13.2
with infection N13.6
ureteral NEC N13.1
with infection N13.6
calculus N13.2
with infection N13.6
ureteropelvic junction (congenital) Q62.11
acquired N13.Ø
with infection N13.6
ureteral stricture NEC N13.1
with infection N13.6
congenital Q62.Ø
due to acquired occlusion of ureteropelvic junction N13.Ø
specified type NEC N13.39
tuberculous A18.11
Hydropericarditis —*see* Pericarditis
Hydropericardium —*see* Pericarditis
Hydroperitoneum R18.8
Hydrophobia —*see* Rabies
Hydrophthalmos Q15.Ø
Hydropneumohemothorax —*see* Hemothorax
Hydropneumopericarditis —*see* Pericarditis
Hydropneumopericardium —*see* Pericarditis
Hydropneumothorax J94.8
traumatic —*see* Injury, intrathoracic, lung
tuberculous NEC A15.6
Hydrops R6Ø.9
abdominis R18.8
articulorum intermittens —*see* Hydrarthrosis, intermittent
cardiac —*see* Failure, heart, congestive
causing obstructed labor (mother) O66.3
endolymphatic H81.Ø- •
fetal —*see* Pregnancy, complicated by, hydrops, fetalis
fetalis P83.2
due to
ABO isoimmunization P56.Ø
alpha thalassemia D56.Ø
hemolytic disease P56.9Ø
specified NEC P56.99
isoimmunization (ABO) (Rh) P56.Ø
other specified nonhemolytic disease NEC P83.2
Rh incompatibility P56.Ø
during pregnancy —*see* Pregnancy, complicated by, hydrops, fetalis
gallbladder K82.1
joint —*see* Effusion, joint
labyrinth H81.Ø
newborn (idiopathic) P83.2
due to
ABO isoimmunization P56.Ø
alpha thalassemia D56.Ø
hemolytic disease P56.9Ø
specified NEC P56.99
isoimmunization (ABO) (Rh) P56.Ø
Rh incompatibility P56.Ø
nutritional —*see* Malnutrition, severe
pericardium —*see* Pericarditis
pleura —*see* Hydrothorax
spermatic cord —*see* Hydrocele
Hydropyonephrosis N13.6
Hydrorachis QØ6.4
Hydrorrhea (nasal) J34.89
pregnancy —*see* Rupture, membranes, premature
Hydrosadenitis (axillaris) (suppurative) L73.2
Hydrosalpinx (fallopian tube) (follicularis) N7Ø.11
Hydrothorax (double) (pleura) J94.8
chylous (nonfilarial) I89.8
filarial —*see also* Infestation, filarial B74.9 *[J91.8]*
traumatic —*see* Injury, intrathoracic
tuberculous NEC (non primary) A15.6
Hydroureter —*see also* Hydronephrosis N13.4
with infection N13.6
congenital Q62.39
Hydroureteronephrosis —*see* Hydronephrosis
Hydrourethra N36.8
Hydroxykynureninuria E7Ø.8
Hydroxylysinemia E72.3
Hydroxyprolinemia E72.59
Hygiene, sleep
abuse Z72.821
inadequate Z72.821
poor Z72.821
Hygroma (congenital) (cystic) D18.1
praepatellare, prepatellar —*see* Bursitis, prepatellar
Hymen —*see* condition
Hymenolepis, hymenolepiasis (diminuta) (infection) (infestation) (nana) B71.Ø
Hypalgesia R2Ø.8
Hyperacidity (gastric) K31.89
psychogenic F45.8
Hyperactive, hyperactivity F9Ø.9
basal cell, uterine cervix —*see* Dysplasia, cervix
bowel sounds R19.12
cervix epithelial (basal) —*see* Dysplasia, cervix
child F9Ø.9
attention deficit —*see* Disorder, attention-deficit hyperactivity
detrusor muscle N32.81
gastrointestinal K31.89
psychogenic F45.8
nasal mucous membrane J34.3
stomach K31.89
thyroid (gland) —*see* Hyperthyroidism
Hyperacusis H93.23- •
Hyperadrenalism E27.5
Hyperadrenocorticism E24.9
congenital E25.Ø
iatrogenic E24.2
correct substance properly administered —*see* Table of Drugs and Chemicals, by drug, adverse effect
overdose or wrong substance given or taken —*see* Table of Drugs and Chemicals, by drug, poisoning
not associated with Cushing's syndrome E27.Ø
pituitary-dependent E24.Ø
Hyperaldosteronism E26.9
familial (type I) E26.Ø2
glucocorticoid-remediable E26.Ø2
primary (due to (bilateral) adrenal hyperplasia) E26.Ø9
primary NEC E26.Ø9
secondary E26.1
specified NEC E26.89
Hyperalgesia R2Ø.8
Hyperalimentation R63.2
carotene, carotin E67.1
specified NEC E67.8
vitamin
A E67.Ø
D E67.3
Hyperaminoaciduria
arginine E72.21
cystine E72.Ø1
lysine E72.3
ornithine E72.4
Hyperammonemia (congenital) E72.2Ø
Hyperazotemia —*see* Uremia
Hyperbetalipoproteinemia (familial) E78.ØØ
with prebetalipoproteinemia E78.2
Hyperbilirubinemia
constitutional E8Ø.6
familial conjugated E8Ø.6
neonatal (transient) —*see* Jaundice, newborn
Hypercalcemia, hypocalciuric, familial E83.52
Hypercalciuria, idiopathic R82.994
Hypercapnia RØ6.89
newborn P84
Hypercarotenemia (dietary) E67.1
Hypercementosis KØ3.4
Hyperchloremia E87.8
Hyperchlorhydria K31.89
neurotic F45.8
psychogenic F45.8
Hypercholesterinemia —*see* Hypercholesterolemia
Hypercholesterolemia (essential) (primary) (pure) E78.ØØ
with hyperglyceridemia, endogenous E78.2
dietary counseling and surveillance Z71.3
familial E78.Ø1
hereditary E78.Ø1
Hyperchylia gastrica, psychogenic F45.8
Hyperchylomicronemia (familial) (primary) E78.3
with hyperbetalipoproteinemia E78.3
Hypercoagulable (state) D68.59
activated protein C resistance D68.51
antithrombin (III) deficiency D68.59
factor V Leiden mutation D68.51
primary NEC D68.59
protein C deficiency D68.59
protein S deficiency D68.59
prothrombin gene mutation D68.52
secondary D68.69
specified NEC D68.69
Hypercoagulation (state) D68.59
Hypercorticalism, pituitary-dependent E24.Ø
Hypercorticosolism —*see* Cushing's, syndrome
Hypercorticosteronism E24.2
correct substance properly administered —*see* Table of Drugs and Chemicals, by drug, adverse effect
overdose or wrong substance given or taken —*see* Table of Drugs and Chemicals, by drug, poisoning
Hypercortisonism E24.2
correct substance properly administered —*see* Table of Drugs and Chemicals, by drug, adverse effect
overdose or wrong substance given or taken —*see* Table of Drugs and Chemicals, by drug, poisoning
Hyperekplexia Q89.8
Hyperelectrolytemia E87.8
Hyperemesis R11.1Ø
with nausea R11.2
gravidarum (mild) O21.Ø
with
carbohydrate depletion O21.1
dehydration O21.1
electrolyte imbalance O21.1
metabolic disturbance O21.1
severe (with metabolic disturbance) O21.1
projectile R11.12
psychogenic F45.8
Hyperemia (acute) (passive) R68.89
anal mucosa K62.89
bladder N32.89
cerebral I67.89
conjunctiva H11.43- •
ear internal, acute —*see* subcategory H83.Ø
enteric K59.8
eye —*see* Hyperemia, conjunctiva
eyelid (active) (passive) —*see* Disorder, eyelid, specified type NEC
intestine K59.8

H

Hyperemia *(Continued)*
  iris *—see* Disorder, iris, vascular
  kidney N28.89
  labyrinth *—see* subcategory H83.Ø
  liver (active) K76.89
  lung (passive) *—see* Edema, lung
  pulmonary (passive) *—see* Edema, lung
  renal N28.89
  retina H35.89
  stomach K31.89
Hyperesthesia (body surface) R2Ø.3
  larynx (reflex) J38.7
    hysterical F44.89
  pharynx (reflex) J39.2
    hysterical F44.89
Hyperestrogenism (drug-induced) (iatrogenic) E28.Ø
Hyperexplexia Q89.8
Hyperfibrinolysis *—see* Fibrinolysis
Hyperfructosemia E74.19
Hyperfunction
  adrenal cortex, not associated with Cushing's syndrome E27.Ø
    medulla E27.5
      adrenomedullary E27.5
    virilism E25.9
      congenital E25.Ø
  ovarian E28.8
  pancreas K86.89
  parathyroid (gland) E21.3
  pituitary (gland) (anterior) E22.9
    specified NEC E22.8
  polyglandular E31.1
  testicular E29.Ø
Hypergammaglobulinemia D89.2
  polyclonal D89.Ø
  Waldenström D89.Ø
Hypergastrinemia E16.4
Hyperglobulinemia R77.1
Hyperglycemia, hyperglycemic (transient) R73.9
  coma *—see* Diabetes, by type, with coma
  postpancreatectomy E89.1
Hyperglyceridemia (endogenous) (essential) (familial) (hereditary) (pure) E78.1
  mixed E78.3
Hyperglycinemia (non-ketotic) E72.51
Hypergonadism
  ovarian E28.8
  testicular (primary) (infantile) E29.Ø
Hyperheparinemia D68.32
Hyperhidrosis, hyperidrosis R61
  focal
    primary L74.519
      axilla L74.51Ø
      face L74.511
      palms L74.512
      soles L74.513
    secondary L74.52
  generalized R61
  localized
    primary L74.519
      axilla L74.51Ø
      face L74.511
      palms L74.512
      soles L74.513
    secondary L74.52
  psychogenic F45.8
  secondary R61
    focal L74.52
Hyperhistidinemia E7Ø.41
Hyperhomocysteinemia E72.11
Hyperhydroxyprolinemia E72.59
Hyperinsulinism (functional) E16.1
  with
    coma (hypoglycemic) E15
    encephalopathy E16.1 *[G94]*
  ectopic E16.1
  therapeutic misadventure (from administration of insulin) *—see* subcategory T38.3
Hyperkalemia E87.5
Hyperkeratosis *—see also* Keratosis L85.9
  cervix N88.Ø
  due to yaws (early) (late) (palmar or plantar) A66.3
  follicularis Q82.8
    penetrans (in cutem) L87.Ø
  palmoplantaris climacterica L85.1
  pinta A67.1
  senile (with pruritus) L57.Ø
  universalis congenita Q8Ø.8
  vocal cord J38.3
  vulva N9Ø.4
Hyperkinesia, hyperkinetic (disease) (reaction) (syndrome) (childhood) (adolescence) *— see also* Disorder, attention-deficit hyperactivity
  heart I51.89
Hyperleucine-isoleucinemia E71.19
Hyperlipemia, hyperlipidemia E78.5
  combined E78.2
    familial E78.49
  group
    A E78.ØØ
    B E78.1
    C E78.2
    D E78.3
  mixed E78.2
  specified NEC E78.49
Hyperlipidosis E75.6
  hereditary NEC E75.5
Hyperlipoproteinemia E78.5
  Fredrickson's type
    I E78.3
    IIa E78.ØØ
    IIb E78.2
    III E78.2
    IV E78.1
    V E78.3
  low-density-lipoprotein-type (LDL) E78.ØØ
  very-low-density-lipoprotein-type (VLDL) E78.1
Hyperlucent lung, unilateral J43.Ø
Hyperlysinemia E72.3
Hypermagnesemia E83.41
  neonatal P71.8
Hypermenorrhea N92.Ø
Hypermethioninemia E72.19
Hypermetropia (congenital) H52.Ø-●
Hypermobility, hypermotility
  cecum *—see* Syndrome, irritable bowel
  coccyx *—see* subcategory M53.2
  colon *—see* Syndrome, irritable bowel
    psychogenic F45.8
  ileum K58.9
  intestine *—see also* Syndrome, irritable bowel K58.9
    psychogenic F45.8
  meniscus (knee) *—see* Derangement, knee, meniscus
  scapula *—see* Instability, joint, shoulder
  stomach K31.89
    psychogenic F45.8
  syndrome M35.7
  urethra N36.41
    with intrinsic sphincter deficiency N36.43
Hypernasality R49.21
Hypernatremia E87.Ø
Hypernephroma C64.-●
Hyperopia *—see* Hypermetropia
Hyperorexia nervosa F5Ø.2
Hyperornithinemia E72.4
Hyperosmia R43.1
Hyperosmolality E87.Ø
Hyperostosis (monomelic) *—see also* Disorder, bone, density and structure, specified NEC
  ankylosing (spine) M48.1Ø
    cervical region M48.12
    cervicothoracic region M48.13
    lumbar region M48.16
    lumbosacral region M48.17
    multiple sites M48.19
    occipito-atlanto-axial region M48.11
Hyperostosis (monomelic) *(Continued)*
  ankylosing (spine) *(Continued)*
    sacrococcygeal region M48.18
    thoracic region M48.14
    thoracolumbar region M48.15
  cortical (skull) M85.2
    infantile M89.8X-●
  frontal, internal of skull M85.2
  interna frontalis M85.2
  skeletal, diffuse idiopathic *—see* Hyperostosis, ankylosing
  skull M85.2
    congenital Q75.8
  vertebral, ankylosing *—see* Hyperostosis, ankylosing
Hyperovarism E28.8
Hyperoxaluria (primary) R82.992
Hyperparathyroidism E21.3
  primary E21.Ø
  secondary (renal) N25.81
    non-renal E21.1
  specified NEC E21.2
  tertiary E21.2
Hyperpathia R2Ø.8
Hyperperistalsis R19.2
  psychogenic F45.8
Hyperpermeability, capillary I78.8
Hyperphagia R63.2
Hyperphenylalaninemia NEC E7Ø.1
Hyperphoria (alternating) H5Ø.53
Hyperphosphatemia E83.39
Hyperpiesis, hyperpiesia *—see* Hypertension
Hyperpigmentation *—see also* Pigmentation
  melanin NEC L81.4
  postinflammatory L81.Ø
Hyperpinealism E34.8
Hyperpituitarism E22.9
Hyperplasia, hyperplastic
  adenoids J35.2
  adrenal (capsule) (cortex) (gland) E27.8
    with
      sexual precocity (male) E25.9
        congenital E25.Ø
      virilism, adrenal E25.9
        congenital E25.Ø
      virilization (female) E25.9
        congenital E25.Ø
    congenital E25.Ø
      salt-losing E25.Ø
  adrenomedullary E27.5
  angiolymphoid, eosinophilia (ALHE) D18.Ø1
  appendix (lymphoid) K38.Ø
  artery, fibromuscular I77.3
  bone *—see also* Hypertrophy, bone
    marrow D75.89
  breast *—see also* Hypertrophy, breast
    ~~ductal (atypical) N6Ø.9-~~
  ▶atypical, atypia N6Ø.9-●
    ▶ductal N6Ø.9-●
    ▶lobular N6Ø.9-●
  C-cell, thyroid EØ7.Ø
  cementation (tooth) (teeth) KØ3.4
  cervical gland R59.Ø
  cervix (uteri) (basal cell) (endometrium) (polypoid) *—see also* Dysplasia, cervix
    congenital Q51.828
  clitoris, congenital Q52.6
  denture KØ6.2
  endocervicitis N72
  ➡endometrium, endometrial (adenomatous) (cystic) (glandular) (glandular-cystic) (polypoid) N85.ØØ
    with atypia N85.Ø2
  ▶benign N85.Ø1
    cervix *—see* Dysplasia, cervix
    complex (without atypia) N85.Ø1
    simple (without atypia) N85.Ø1
  epithelial L85.9
    focal, oral, including tongue K13.29
    nipple N62
    skin L85.9

Hyperplasia, hyperplastic *(Continued)*
  epithelial *(Continued)*
    tongue K13.29
    vaginal wall N89.3
  erythroid D75.89
  fibromuscular of artery (carotid) (renal) I77.3
  genital
    female NEC N94.89
    male N5Ø.89
  gingiva KØ6.1
  glandularis cystica uteri (interstitialis) —*see also* Hyperplasia, endometrial N85.ØØ- •
  gum KØ6.1
  hymen, congenital Q52.4
  irritative, edentulous (alveolar) KØ6.2
  jaw M26.Ø9
    alveolar M26.79
    lower M26.Ø3
      alveolar M26.72
    upper M26.Ø1
      alveolar M26.71
  kidney (congenital) Q63.3
  labia N9Ø.69
    epithelial N9Ø.3
  liver (congenital) Q44.7
    nodular, focal K76.89
  lymph gland or node R59.9
  mandible, mandibular M26.Ø3
    alveolar M26.72
    unilateral condylar M27.8
  maxilla, maxillary M26.Ø1
    alveolar M26.71
  myometrium, myometrial N85.2
  neuroendocrine cell, of infancy J84.841
  nose
    lymphoid J34.89
    polypoid J33.9
  oral mucosa (irritative) K13.6
  organ or site, congenital NEC —*see* Anomaly, by site
  ovary N83.8
  palate, papillary (irritative) K13.6
  pancreatic islet cells E16.9
    alpha E16.8
      with excess
        gastrin E16.4
        glucagon E16.3
    beta E16.1
  parathyroid (gland) E21.Ø
  pharynx (lymphoid) J39.2
  prostate (adenofibromatous) (nodular) N4Ø.Ø
    with lower urinary tract symptoms (LUTS) N4Ø.1
    without lower urinary tract symptoms (LUTS) N4Ø.Ø
  renal artery I77.89
  reticulo-endothelial (cell) D75.89
  salivary gland (any) K11.1
  Schimmelbusch's —*see* Mastopathy, cystic
  suprarenal capsule (gland) E27.8
  thymus (gland) (persistent) E32.Ø
  thyroid (gland) —*see* Goiter
  tonsils (faucial) (infective) (lingual) (lymphoid) J35.1
    with adenoids J35.3
  unilateral condylar M27.8
  uterus, uterine N85.2
    endometrium (glandular) —*see also* Hyperplasia, endometrial N85.ØØ- •
  vulva N9Ø.69
    epithelial N9Ø.3
Hyperpnea —*see* Hyperventilation
Hyperpotassemia E87.5
Hyperprebetalipoproteinemia (familial) E78.1
Hyperprolactinemia E22.1
Hyperprolinemia (type I) (type II) E72.59
Hyperproteinemia E88.Ø9
Hyperprothrombinemia, causing coagulation factor deficiency D68.4
Hyperpyrexia R5Ø.9
  heat (effects) T67.Ø1
  malignant, due to anesthetic T88.3
  rheumatic —*see* Fever, rheumatic
  unknown origin R5Ø.9
Hyper-reflexia R29.2
Hypersalivation K11.7
Hypersecretion
  ACTH (not associated with Cushing's syndrome) E27.Ø
    pituitary E24.Ø
  adrenaline E27.5
  adrenomedullary E27.5
  androgen (testicular) E29.Ø
    ovarian (drug-induced) (iatrogenic) E28.1
  calcitonin EØ7.Ø
  catecholamine E27.5
  corticoadrenal E24.9
  cortisol E24.9
  epinephrine E27.5
  estrogen E28.Ø
  gastric K31.89
    psychogenic F45.8
  gastrin E16.4
  glucagon E16.3
  hormone(s)
    ACTH (not associated with Cushing's syndrome) E27.Ø
      pituitary E24.Ø
    antidiuretic E22.2
    growth E22.Ø
    intestinal NEC E34.1
    ovarian androgen E28.1
    pituitary E22.9
    testicular E29.Ø
    thyroid stimulating EØ5.8Ø
      with thyroid storm EØ5.81
  insulin —*see* Hyperinsulinism
  lacrimal glands —*see* Epiphora
  medulloadrenal E27.5
  milk O92.6
  ovarian androgens E28.1
  salivary gland (any) K11.7
  thyrocalcitonin EØ7.Ø
  upper respiratory J39.8
Hypersegmentation, leukocytic, hereditary D72.Ø
Hypersensitive, hypersensitiveness, hypersensitivity —*see also* Allergy
  carotid sinus G9Ø.Ø1
  colon —*see* Irritable, colon
  drug T88.7
  gastrointestinal K52.29
    immediate K52.29
    psychogenic F45.8
  labyrinth —*see* subcategory H83.2
  pain R2Ø.8
  pneumonitis —*see* Pneumonitis, allergic
  reaction T78.4Ø
    upper respiratory tract NEC J39.3
Hypersomnia (organic) G47.1Ø
  due to
    alcohol
      abuse F1Ø.182
      dependence F1Ø.282
      use F1Ø.982
    amphetamines
      abuse F15.182
      dependence F15.282
      use F15.982
    caffeine
      abuse F15.182
      dependence F15.282
      use F15.982
    cocaine
      abuse F14.182
      dependence F14.282
      use F14.982
    drug NEC
      abuse F19.182
      dependence F19.282
      use F19.982
Hypersomnia *(Continued)*
  due to *(Continued)*
    medical condition G47.14
    mental disorder F51.13
    opioid
      abuse F11.182
      dependence F11.282
      use F11.982
    psychoactive substance NEC
      abuse F19.182
      dependence F19.282
      use F19.982
    sedative, hypnotic, or anxiolytic
      abuse F13.182
      dependence F13.282
      use F13.982
    stimulant NEC
      abuse F15.182
      dependence F15.282
      use F15.982
  idiopathic G47.11
    with long sleep time G47.11
    without long sleep time G47.12
  menstrual related G47.13
  nonorganic origin F51.11
    specified NEC F51.19
  not due to a substance or known physiological condition F51.11
    specified NEC F51.19
  primary F51.11
  recurrent G47.13
  specified NEC G47.19
Hypersplenia, hypersplenism D73.1
Hyperstimulation, ovaries (associated with induced ovulation) N98.1
Hypersusceptibility —*see* Allergy
Hypertelorism (ocular) (orbital) Q75.2
Hypertension, hypertensive (accelerated) (benign) (essential) (idiopathic) (malignant) (systemic) I1Ø
  with
    heart failure (congestive) I11.Ø
    heart involvement (conditions in I5Ø.-, I51.4-I51.9 due to hypertension) —*see* Hypertension, heart
    kidney involvement —*see* Hypertension, kidney
  benign, intracranial G93.2
  borderline RØ3.Ø
  cardiorenal (disease) I13.1Ø
    with heart failure I13.Ø
      with stage 1 through stage 4 chronic kidney disease I13.Ø
      with stage 5 or end stage renal disease I13.2
    without heart failure I13.1Ø
      with stage 1 through stage 4 chronic kidney disease I13.1Ø
      with stage 5 or end stage renal disease I13.11
  cardiovascular
    disease (arteriosclerotic) (sclerotic) —*see* Hypertension, heart
    renal (disease) —*see* Hypertension, cardiorenal
  chronic venous —*see* Hypertension, venous (chronic)
  complicating
    childbirth (labor) O16.4
      pre-existing O1Ø.92
        with
          heart disease O1Ø.12
            with renal disease O1Ø.32
          pre-eclampsia O11.4
          renal disease O1Ø.22
            with heart disease O1Ø.32
        essential O1Ø.Ø2
      secondary O1Ø.42
    pregnancy O16.- •
      with edema —*see also* Pre-eclampsia O14.9- •

Hypertension, hypertensive *(Continued)*
complicating *(Continued)*
pregnancy *(Continued)*
gestational (pregnancy induced) (without proteinuria) O13.-●
with proteinuria O14.9-●
mild pre-eclampsia O14.Ø-●
moderate pre-eclampsia O14.Ø-●
severe pre-eclampsia O14.1-●
with hemolysis, elevated liver enzymes and low platelet count (HELLP) O14.2-●
pre-existing O1Ø.91-●
with
heart disease O1Ø.11-●
with renal disease O1Ø.31-●
pre-eclampsia —*see* category O11
renal disease O1Ø.21-●
with heart disease O1Ø.31-●
essential O1Ø.Ø1-●
secondary O1Ø.41-●
transient O13.-●
puerperium pre-existing O16.5
pre-existing
with
heart disease O1Ø.13
with renal disease O1Ø.33
pre-eclampsia O11.5
renal disease O1Ø.23
with heart disease O1Ø.33
essential O1Ø.Ø3
pregnancy-induced O13.9
secondary O1Ø.43
crisis I16.9
due to
endocrine disorders I15.2
pheochromocytoma I15.2
renal disorders NEC I15.1
arterial I15.Ø
renovascular disorders I15.Ø
specified disease NEC I15.8
emergency I16.1
encephalopathy I67.4
gestational (without significant proteinuria) (pregnancy-induced) (transient) O13.-●
with significant proteinuria —*see* Pre-eclampsia
complicating
delivery O13.4
puerperium O13.5
Goldblatt's I7Ø.1
heart (disease) (conditions in I51.4-I51.9 due to hypertension) I11.9
with
heart failure (congestive) I11.Ø
kidney disease (chronic) —*see* Hypertension, cardiorenal
intracranial (benign) G93.2
kidney I12.9
with
heart disease —*see* Hypertension, cardiorenal
stage 1 through stage 4 chronic kidney disease I12.9
stage 5 chronic kidney disease (CKD) or end stage renal disease (ESRD) I12.Ø
lesser circulation I27.Ø
maternal O16.-●
newborn P29.2
pulmonary (persistent) P29.3Ø
ocular H4Ø.Ø5-●
pancreatic duct — code to underlying condition
with chronic pancreatitis K86.1
portal (due to chronic liver disease) (idiopathic) K76.6
gastropathy K31.89
in (due to) schistosomiasis (bilharziasis) B65.9 *[K77]*
postoperative I97.3
psychogenic F45.8
Hypertension, hypertensive *(Continued)*
pulmonary NEC I27.2Ø
with
cor pulmonale (chronic) I27.29
acute I26.Ø9
right heart ventricular strain/failure I27.29
acute I26.Ø9
right to left shunt related to congenital heart disease I27.83
unclear multifactorial mechanisms I27.29
arterial (associated) (drug-induced) (toxin-induced) I27.21
chronic thromboembolic I27.24
due to
hematologic disorders I27.29
left heart disease I27.22
lung diseases and hypoxia I27.23
metabolic disorders I27.29
specified systemic disorders NEC I27.29
group 1 (associated) (drug-induced) (toxin-induced) I27.21
group 2 I27.22
group 3 I27.23
group 4 I27.24
group 5 I27.29
of newborn (persistent) P29.3Ø
secondary
arterial I27.21
specified NEC I27.29
primary (idiopathic) I27.Ø
renal —*see* Hypertension, kidney
renovascular I15.Ø
secondary NEC I15.9
due to
endocrine disorders I15.2
pheochromocytoma I15.2
renal disorders NEC I15.1
arterial I15.Ø
renovascular disorders I15.Ø
specified NEC I15.8
transient RØ3.Ø
of pregnancy O13.●
urgency I16.Ø
venous (chronic)
due to
deep vein thrombosis —*see* Syndrome, postthrombotic
idiopathic I87.3Ø9
with
inflammation I87.32-●
with ulcer I87.33-●
specified complication NEC I87.39-●
ulcer I87.31-●
with inflammation I87.33-●
asymptomatic I87.3Ø-●
Hypertensive urgency —*see* Hypertension
Hyperthecosis ovary E28.8
Hyperthermia (of unknown origin) —*see also* Hyperpyrexia
malignant, due to anesthesia T88.3
newborn P81.9
environmental P81.Ø
Hyperthyroid (recurrent) —*see* Hyperthyroidism
Hyperthyroidism (latent) (pre-adult) (recurrent) EØ5.9Ø
with
goiter (diffuse) EØ5.ØØ
with thyroid storm EØ5.Ø1
nodular (multinodular) EØ5.2Ø
with thyroid storm EØ5.21
uninodular EØ5.1Ø
with thyroid storm EØ5.11
storm EØ5.91
due to ectopic thyroid tissue EØ5.3Ø
with thyroid storm EØ5.31
neonatal, transitory P72.1
specified NEC EØ5.8Ø
with thyroid storm EØ5.81
Hypertony, hypertonia, hypertonicity
bladder N31.8
congenital P94.1
Hypertony, hypertonia, hypertonicity *(Continued)*
stomach K31.89
psychogenic F45.8
uterus, uterine (contractions) (complicating delivery) O62.4
Hypertrichosis L68.9
congenital Q84.2
eyelid HØ2.869
left HØ2.866
lower HØ2.865
upper HØ2.864
right HØ2.863
lower HØ2.862
upper HØ2.861
lanuginosa Q84.2
acquired L68.1
localized L68.2
specified NEC L68.8
Hypertriglyceridemia, essential E78.1
Hypertrophy, hypertrophic
adenofibromatous, prostate —*see* Enlargement, enlarged, prostate
adenoids (infective) J35.2
with tonsils J35.3
adrenal cortex E27.8
alveolar process or ridge —*see* Anomaly, alveolar
anal papillae K62.89
artery I77.89
congenital NEC Q27.8
digestive system Q27.8
lower limb Q27.8
specified site NEC Q27.8
upper limb Q27.8
auricular —*see* Hypertrophy, cardiac
Bartholin's gland N75.8
bile duct (common) (hepatic) K83.8
bladder (sphincter) (trigone) N32.89
bone M89.3Ø
carpus M89.34-●
clavicle M89.31-●
femur M89.35-●
fibula M89.36-●
finger M89.34-●
humerus M89.32-●
ilium M89.359
ischium M89.359
metacarpus M89.34-●
metatarsus M89.37-●
multiple sites M89.39
neck M89.38
radius M89.33-●
rib M89.38
scapula M89.31-●
skull M89.38
tarsus M89.37-●
tibia M89.36-●
toe M89.37-●
ulna M89.33-●
vertebra M89.38
brain G93.89
breast N62
cystic —*see* Mastopathy, cystic
newborn P83.4
pubertal, massive N62
puerperal, postpartum —*see* Disorder, breast, specified type NEC
senile (parenchymatous) N62
cardiac (chronic) (idiopathic) I51.7
with rheumatic fever (conditions in IØØ)
active IØ1.8
inactive or quiescent (with chorea) IØ9.89
congenital NEC Q24.8
fatty —*see* Degeneration, myocardial
hypertensive —*see* Hypertension, heart
rheumatic (with chorea) IØ9.89
active or acute IØ1.8
with chorea IØ2.Ø
valve —*see* Endocarditis
cartilage —*see* Disorder, cartilage, specified type NEC

Hypertrophy, hypertrophic *(Continued)*
cecum —*see* Megacolon
cervix (uteri) N88.8
congenital Q51.828
elongation N88.4
clitoris (cirrhotic) N90.89
congenital Q52.6
colon —*see also* Megacolon
congenital Q43.2
conjunctiva, lymphoid H11.89
corpora cavernosa N48.89
cystic duct K82.8
duodenum K31.89
endometrium (glandular) —*see also* Hyperplasia, endometrial N85.00- •
cervix N88.8
epididymis N50.89
esophageal hiatus (congenital) Q79.1
with hernia —*see* Hernia, hiatal
eyelid —*see* Disorder, eyelid, specified type NEC
fat pad E65
knee (infrapatellar) (popliteal) (prepatellar) (retropatellar) M79.4
foot (congenital) Q74.2
frenulum, frenum (tongue) K14.8
lip K13.0
gallbladder K82.8
gastric mucosa K29.60
with bleeding K29.61
gland, glandular R59.9
generalized R59.1
localized R59.0
gum (mucous membrane) K06.1
heart (idiopathic) —*see also* Hypertrophy, cardiac
valve —*see also* Endocarditis I38
hemifacial Q67.4
hepatic —*see* Hypertrophy, liver
hiatus (esophageal) Q79.1
hilus gland R59.0
hymen, congenital Q52.4
ileum K63.89
intestine NEC K63.89
jejunum K63.89
kidney (compensatory) N28.81
congenital Q63.3
labium (majus) (minus) N90.60
ligament —*see* Disorder, ligament
lingual tonsil (infective) J35.1
with adenoids J35.3
lip K13.0
congenital Q18.6
liver R16.0
acute K76.89
cirrhotic —*see* Cirrhosis, liver
congenital Q44.7
fatty —*see* Fatty, liver
lymph, lymphatic gland R59.9
generalized R59.1
localized R59.0
tuberculous —*see* Tuberculosis, lymph gland
mammary gland —*see* Hypertrophy, breast
Meckel's diverticulum (congenital) Q43.0
malignant —*see* Table of Neoplasms, small intestine, malignant
median bar —*see* Hyperplasia, prostate
meibomian gland —*see* Chalazion
meniscus, knee, congenital Q74.1
metatarsal head —*see* Hypertrophy, bone, metatarsus
metatarsus —*see* Hypertrophy, bone, metatarsus
mucous membrane
alveolar ridge K06.2
gum K06.1
nose (turbinate) J34.3
muscle M62.89
muscular coat, artery I77.89
myocardium —*see also* Hypertrophy, cardiac
idiopathic I42.2

Hypertrophy, hypertrophic *(Continued)*
myometrium N85.2
nail L60.2
congenital Q84.5
nasal J34.89
alae J34.89
bone J34.89
cartilage J34.89
mucous membrane (septum) J34.3
sinus J34.89
turbinate J34.3
nasopharynx, lymphoid (infectional) (tissue) (wall) J35.2
nipple N62
organ or site, congenital NEC —*see* Anomaly, by site - ovary N83.8
palate (hard) M27.8
soft K13.79
pancreas, congenital Q45.3
parathyroid (gland) E21.0
parotid gland K11.1
penis N48.89
pharyngeal tonsil J35.2
pharynx J39.2
lymphoid (infectional) (tissue) (wall) J35.2
pituitary (anterior) (fossa) (gland) E23.6
prepuce (congenital) N47.8
female N90.89
prostate —*see* Enlargement, enlarged, prostate
congenital Q55.4
pseudomuscular G71.09
pylorus (adult) (muscle) (sphincter) K31.1
congenital or infantile Q40.0
rectal, rectum (sphincter) K62.89
rhinitis (turbinate) J31.0
salivary gland (any) K11.1
congenital Q38.4
scaphoid (tarsal) —*see* Hypertrophy, bone, tarsus
scar L91.0
scrotum N50.89
seminal vesicle N50.89
sigmoid —*see* Megacolon
skin L91.9
specified NEC L91.8
spermatic cord N50.89
spleen —*see* Splenomegaly
spondylitis —*see* Spondylosis
stomach K31.89
sublingual gland K11.1
submandibular gland K11.1
suprarenal cortex (gland) E27.8
synovial NEC M67.20
acromioclavicular M67.21- •
ankle M67.27- •
elbow M67.22- •
foot M67.27- •
hand M67.24- •
hip M67.25- •
knee M67.26- •
multiple sites M67.29
specified site NEC M67.28
wrist M67.23- •
tendon —*see* Disorder, tendon, specified type NEC
testis N44.8
congenital Q55.29
thymic, thymus (gland) (congenital) E32.0
thyroid (gland) —*see* Goiter
toe (congenital) Q74.2
acquired —*see also* Deformity, toe, specified NEC
tongue K14.8
congenital Q38.2
papillae (foliate) K14.3
tonsils (faucial) (infective) (lingual) (lymphoid) J35.1
with adenoids J35.3
tunica vaginalis N50.89
ureter N28.89
urethra N36.8

Hypertrophy, hypertrophic *(Continued)*
uterus N85.2
neck (with elongation) N88.4
puerperal O90.89
uvula K13.79
vagina N89.8
vas deferens N50.89
vein I87.8
ventricle, ventricular (heart) —*see also* Hypertrophy, cardiac
congenital Q24.8
in tetralogy of Fallot Q21.3
verumontanum N36.8
vocal cord J38.3
vulva N90.60
stasis (nonfilarial) N90.69
Hypertropia H50.2- •
Hypertyrosinemia E70.21
Hyperuricemia (asymptomatic) E79.0
Hyperuricosuria R82.993
Hypervalinemia E71.19
Hyperventilation (tetany) R06.4
hysterical F45.8
psychogenic F45.8
syndrome F45.8
Hypervitaminosis (dietary) NEC E67.8
A E67.0
administered as drug (prolonged intake) —*see* Table of Drugs and Chemicals, vitamins, adverse effect
overdose or wrong substance given or taken —*see* Table of Drugs and Chemicals, vitamins, poisoning
B6 E67.2
D E67.3
administered as drug (prolonged intake) —*see* Table of Drugs and Chemicals, vitamins, adverse effect
overdose or wrong substance given or taken —*see* Table of Drugs and Chemicals, vitamins, poisoning
K E67.8
administered as drug (prolonged intake) —*see* Table of Drugs and Chemicals, vitamins, adverse effect
overdose or wrong substance given or taken —*see* Table of Drugs and Chemicals, vitamins, poisoning
Hypervolemia E87.70
specified NEC E87.79
Hypesthesia R20.1
cornea —*see* Anesthesia, cornea
Hyphema H21.0- •
traumatic S05.1- •
Hypoacidity, gastric K31.89
psychogenic F45.8
Hypoadrenalism, hypoadrenia E27.40
primary E27.1
tuberculous A18.7
Hypoadrenocorticism E27.40
pituitary E23.0
primary E27.1
Hypoalbuminemia E88.09
Hypoaldosteronism E27.40
Hypoalphalipoproteinemia E78.6
Hypobarism T70.29
Hypobaropathy T70.29
Hypobetalipoproteinemia (familial) E78.6
Hypocalcemia E83.51
dietary E58
neonatal P71.1
due to cow's milk P71.0
phosphate-loading (newborn) P71.1
Hypochloremia E87.8
Hypochlorhydria K31.89
neurotic F45.8
psychogenic F45.8
Hypochondria, hypochondriac, hypochondriasis (reaction) F45.21
sleep F51.03
Hypochondrogenesis Q77.0

Hypochondroplasia Q77.4
Hypochromasia, blood cells D5Ø.8
Hypodontia —*see* Anodontia
Hypocitraturia R82.991
Hypoeosinophilia D72.89
Hypoesthesia R2Ø.1
Hypofibrinogenemia D68.8
acquired D65
congenital (hereditary) D68.2
Hypofunction
adrenocortical E27.4Ø
drug-induced E27.3
postprocedural E89.6
primary E27.1
adrenomedullary, postprocedural E89.6
cerebral R29.818
corticoadrenal NEC E27.4Ø
intestinal K59.8
labyrinth —*see* subcategory H83.2
ovary E28.39
pituitary (gland) (anterior) E23.Ø
testicular E29.1
postprocedural (postsurgical) (postirradiation) (iatrogenic) E89.5
Hypogalactia O92.4
Hypogammaglobulinemia —*see also* Agammaglobulinemia D8Ø.1
hereditary D8Ø.Ø
nonfamilial D8Ø.1
transient, of infancy D8Ø.7
Hypogenitalism (congenital) —*see* Hypogonadism
Hypoglossia Q38.3
Hypoglycemia (spontaneous) E16.2
coma E15
diabetic —*see* Diabetes, by type, with hypoglycemia, with coma
diabetic —*see* Diabetes, hypoglycemia
dietary counseling and surveillance Z71.3
drug-induced E16.Ø
with coma (nondiabetic) E15
due to insulin E16.Ø
with coma (nondiabetic) E15
therapeutic misadventure —*see* subcategory T38.3
functional, nonhyperinsulinemic E16.1
iatrogenic E16.Ø
with coma (nondiabetic) E15
in infant of diabetic mother P7Ø.1
gestational diabetes P7Ø.Ø
infantile E16.1
leucine-induced E71.19
neonatal (transitory) P7Ø.4
iatrogenic P7Ø.3
reactive (not drug-induced) E16.1
transitory neonatal P7Ø.4
Hypogonadism
female E28.39
hypogonadotropic E23.Ø
male E29.1
ovarian (primary) E28.39
pituitary E23.Ø
testicular (primary) E29.1
Hypohidrosis, hypoidrosis L74.4
Hypoinsulinemia, postprocedural E89.1
Hypokalemia E87.6
Hypoleukocytosis —*see* Agranulocytosis
Hypolipoproteinemia (alpha) (beta) E78.6
Hypomagnesemia E83.42
neonatal P71.2
Hypomania, hypomanic reaction F3Ø.8
Hypomenorrhea —*see* Oligomenorrhea
Hypometabolism R63.8
Hypomotility
gastrointestinal (tract) K31.89
psychogenic F45.8
intestine K59.8
psychogenic F45.8
stomach K31.89
psychogenic F45.8
Hyponasality R49.22
Hyponatremia E87.1
Hypo-osmolality E87.1
Hypo-ovarianism, hypo-ovarism E28.39
Hypoparathyroidism E2Ø.9
familial E2Ø.8
idiopathic E2Ø.Ø
neonatal, transitory P71.4
postprocedural E89.2
specified NEC E2Ø.8
Hypoperfusion (in)
newborn P96.89
Hypopharyngitis —*see* Laryngopharyngitis
Hypophoria H5Ø.53
Hypophosphatemia, hypophosphatasia (acquired) (congenital) (renal) E83.39
familial E83.31
Hypophyseal, hypophysis —*see also* condition
dwarfism E23.Ø
gigantism E22.Ø
Hypopiesis —*see* Hypotension
Hypopinealism E34.8
Hypopituitarism (juvenile) E23.Ø
drug-induced E23.1
due to
hypophysectomy E89.3
radiotherapy E89.3
iatrogenic NEC E23.1
postirradiation E89.3
postpartum O99.285
postprocedural E89.3
Hypoplasia, hypoplastic
adrenal (gland), congenital Q89.1
alimentary tract, congenital Q45.8
upper Q4Ø.8
anus, anal (canal) Q42.3
with fistula Q42.2
aorta, aortic Q25.42
ascending, in hypoplastic left heart syndrome Q23.4
valve Q23.1
in hypoplastic left heart syndrome Q23.4
areola, congenital Q83.8
arm (congenital) —*see* Defect, reduction, upper limb
artery (peripheral) Q27.8
brain (congenital) Q28.3
coronary Q24.5
digestive system Q27.8
lower limb Q27.8
pulmonary Q25.79
functional, unilateral J43.Ø
retinal (congenital) Q14.1
specified site NEC Q27.8
umbilical Q27.Ø
upper limb Q27.8
auditory canal Q17.8
causing impairment of hearing Q16.9
biliary duct or passage Q44.5
bone NOS Q79.9
face Q75.8
marrow D61.9
megakaryocytic D69.49
skull —*see* Hypoplasia, skull
brain QØ2
gyri QØ4.3
part of QØ4.3
breast (areola) N64.82
bronchus Q32.4
cardiac Q24.8
carpus —*see* Defect, reduction, upper limb, specified type NEC
cartilage hair Q78.8
cecum Q42.8
cementum KØØ.4
cephalic QØ2
cerebellum QØ4.3
cervix (uteri), congenital Q51.821
clavicle (congenital) Q74.Ø
coccyx Q76.49
colon Q42.9
specified NEC Q42.8
corpus callosum QØ4.Ø
cricoid cartilage Q31.2
Hypoplasia, hypoplastic *(Continued)*
digestive organ(s) or tract NEC Q45.8
upper (congenital) Q4Ø.8
ear (auricle) (lobe) Q17.2
middle Q16.4
enamel of teeth (neonatal) (postnatal) (prenatal) KØØ.4
endocrine (gland) NEC Q89.2
endometrium N85.8
epididymis (congenital) Q55.4
epiglottis Q31.2
erythroid, congenital D61.Ø1
esophagus (congenital) Q39.8
eustachian tube Q17.8
eye Q11.2
eyelid (congenital) Q1Ø.3
face Q18.8
bone(s) Q75.8
femur (congenital) —*see* Defect, reduction, lower limb, specified type NEC
fibula (congenital) —*see* Defect, reduction, lower limb, specified type NEC
finger (congenital) —*see* Defect, reduction, upper limb, specified type NEC
focal dermal Q82.8
foot —*see* Defect, reduction, lower limb, specified type NEC
gallbladder Q44.Ø
genitalia, genital organ(s)
female, congenital Q52.8
external Q52.79
internal NEC Q52.8
in adiposogenital dystrophy E23.6
glottis Q31.2
hair Q84.2
hand (congenital) —*see* Defect, reduction, upper limb, specified type NEC
heart Q24.8
humerus (congenital) —*see* Defect, reduction, upper limb, specified type NEC
intestine (small) Q41.9
large Q42.9
specified NEC Q42.8
jaw M26.Ø9
alveolar M26.79
lower M26.Ø4
alveolar M26.74
upper M26.Ø2
alveolar M26.73
kidney(s) Q6Ø.5
bilateral Q6Ø.4
unilateral Q6Ø.3
labium (majus) (minus), congenital Q52.79
larynx Q31.2
left heart syndrome Q23.4
leg (congenital) —*see* Defect, reduction, lower limb
limb Q73.8
lower (congenital) —*see* Defect, reduction, lower limb
upper (congenital) —*see* Defect, reduction, upper limb
liver Q44.7
lung (lobe) (not associated with short gestation) Q33.6
associated with immaturity, low birth weight, prematurity, or short gestation P28.Ø
mammary (areola), congenital Q83.8
mandible, mandibular M26.Ø4
alveolar M26.74
unilateral condylar M27.8
maxillary M26.Ø2
alveolar M26.73
medullary D61.9
megakaryocytic D69.49
metacarpus —*see* Defect, reduction, upper limb, specified type NEC
metatarsus —*see* Defect, reduction, lower limb, specified type NEC
muscle Q79.8

Hypoplasia, hypoplastic *(Continued)*
nail(s) Q84.6
nose, nasal Q30.1
optic nerve H47.03-•
osseous meatus (ear) Q17.8
ovary, congenital Q50.39
pancreas Q45.0
parathyroid (gland) Q89.2
parotid gland Q38.4
patella Q74.1
pelvis, pelvic girdle Q74.2
penis (congenital) Q55.62
peripheral vascular system Q27.8
digestive system Q27.8
lower limb Q27.8
specified site NEC Q27.8
upper limb Q27.8
pituitary (gland) (congenital) Q89.2
pulmonary (not associated with short gestation) Q33.6
artery, functional J43.0
associated with short gestation P28.0
radioulnar —*see* Defect, reduction, upper limb, specified type NEC
radius —*see* Defect, reduction, upper limb
rectum Q42.1
with fistula Q42.0
respiratory system NEC Q34.8
rib Q76.6
right heart syndrome Q22.6
sacrum Q76.49
scapula Q74.0
scrotum Q55.1
shoulder girdle Q74.0
skin Q82.8
skull (bone) Q75.8
with
anencephaly Q00.0
encephalocele —*see* Encephalocele
hydrocephalus Q03.9
with spina bifida —*see* Spina bifida, by site, with hydrocephalus
microcephaly Q02
spinal (cord) (ventral horn cell) Q06.1
spine Q76.49
sternum Q76.7
tarsus —*see* Defect, reduction, lower limb, specified type NEC
testis Q55.1
thymic, with immunodeficiency D82.1
thymus (gland) Q89.2
with immunodeficiency D82.1
thyroid (gland) E03.1
cartilage Q31.2
tibiofibular (congenital) —*see* Defect, reduction, lower limb, specified type NEC
toe —*see* Defect, reduction, lower limb, specified type NEC
tongue Q38.3
Turner's K00.4
ulna (congenital) —*see* Defect, reduction, upper limb
umbilical artery Q27.0
unilateral condylar M27.8
ureter Q62.8
uterus, congenital Q51.811
vagina Q52.4
vascular NEC peripheral Q27.8
brain Q28.3
digestive system Q27.8
lower limb Q27.8
specified site NEC Q27.8
upper limb Q27.8

Hypoplasia, hypoplastic *(Continued)*
vein(s) (peripheral) Q27.8
brain Q28.3
digestive system Q27.8
great Q26.8
lower limb Q27.8
specified site NEC Q27.8
upper limb Q27.8
vena cava (inferior) (superior) Q26.8
vertebra Q76.49
vulva, congenital Q52.79
zonule (ciliary) Q12.8
Hypoplasminogenemia E88.02
Hypopnea, obstructive sleep apnea G47.33
Hypopotassemia E87.6
Hypoproconvertinemia, congenital (hereditary) D68.2
Hypoproteinemia E77.8
Hypoprothrombinemia (congenital) (hereditary) (idiopathic) D68.2
acquired D68.4
newborn, transient P61.6
Hypoptyalism K11.7
Hypopyon (eye) (anterior chamber) —*see* Iridocyclitis, acute, hypopyon
Hypopyrexia R68.0
Hyporeflexia R29.2
Hyposecretion
ACTH E23.0
antidiuretic hormone E23.2
ovary E28.39
salivary gland (any) K11.7
vasopressin E23.2
Hyposegmentation, leukocytic, hereditary D72.0
Hyposiderinemia D50.9
Hypospadias Q54.9
balanic Q54.0
coronal Q54.0
glandular Q54.0
penile Q54.1
penoscrotal Q54.2
perineal Q54.3
specified NEC Q54.8
Hypospermatogenesis —*see* Oligospermia
Hyposplenism D73.0
Hypostasis pulmonary, passive —*see* Edema, lung
Hypostatic —*see* condition
Hyposthenuria N28.89
Hypotension (arterial) (constitutional) I95.9
chronic I95.89
drug-induced I95.2
due to (of) hemodialysis I95.3
iatrogenic I95.89
idiopathic (permanent) I95.0
intracranial, following ventricular shunting (ventriculostomy) G97.2
intra-dialytic I95.3
maternal, syndrome (following labor and delivery) O26.5-•
neurogenic, orthostatic G90.3
orthostatic (chronic) I95.1
due to drugs I95.2
neurogenic G90.3
postoperative I95.81
postural I95.1
specified NEC I95.89
Hypothermia (accidental) T68
due to anesthesia, anesthetic T88.51
low environmental temperature T68

Hypothermia *(Continued)*
neonatal P80.9
environmental (mild) NEC P80.8
mild P80.8
severe (chronic) (cold injury syndrome) P80.0
specified NEC P80.8
not associated with low environmental temperature R68.0
Hypothyroidism (acquired) E03.9
autoimmune —*see* Thyroiditis, autoimmune
congenital (without goiter) E03.1
with goiter (diffuse) E03.0
due to
exogenous substance NEC E03.2
iodine-deficiency, acquired E01.8
subclinical E02
irradiation therapy E89.0
medicament NEC E03.2
P-aminosalicylic acid (PAS) E03.2
phenylbutazone E03.2
resorcinol E03.2
sulfonamide E03.2
surgery E89.0
thiourea group drugs E03.2
iatrogenic NEC E03.2
iodine-deficiency (acquired) E01.8
congenital —*see* Syndrome, iodine-deficiency, congenital
subclinical E02
neonatal, transitory P72.2
postinfectious E03.3
postirradiation E89.0
postprocedural E89.0
postsurgical E89.0
specified NEC E03.8
subclinical, iodine-deficiency related E02
Hypotonia, hypotonicity, hypotony
bladder N31.2
congenital (benign) P94.2
eye —*see* Disorder, globe, hypotony
Hypotrichosis —*see* Alopecia
Hypotropia H50.2-•
Hypoventilation R06.89
congenital central alveolar G47.35
sleep related
idiopathic nonobstructive alveolar G47.34
in conditions classified elsewhere G47.36
Hypovitaminosis —*see* Deficiency, vitamin
Hypovolemia E86.1
surgical shock T81.19
traumatic (shock) T79.4
Hypoxemia R09.02
newborn P84
sleep related, in conditions classified elsewhere G47.36
Hypoxia —*see also* Anoxia R09.02
cerebral, during a procedure NEC G97.81
postprocedural NEC G97.82
intrauterine P84
myocardial —*see* Insufficiency, coronary
newborn P84
sleep-related G47.34
Hypsarhythmia —*see* Epilepsy, generalized, specified NEC
Hysteralgia, pregnant uterus O26.89-•
Hysteria, hysterical (conversion) (dissociative state) F44.9
anxiety F41.8
convulsions F44.5
psychosis, acute F44.9
Hysteroepilepsy F44.5

H

I

IBDU (colonic inflammatory bowel dissease unclassified) K52.3
Ichthyoparasitism due to Vandellia cirrhosa B88.8
Ichthyosis (congenital) Q8Ø.9
acquired L85.Ø
fetalis Q8Ø.4
hystrix Q8Ø.8
lamellar Q8Ø.2
lingual K13.29
palmaris and plantaris Q82.8
simplex Q8Ø.Ø
vera Q8Ø.8
vulgaris Q8Ø.Ø
X-linked Q8Ø.1
Ichthyotoxism —*see* Poisoning, fish
bacterial —*see* Intoxication, foodborne
Icteroanemia, hemolytic (acquired) D59.9
congenital —*see* Spherocytosis
Icterus —*see also* Jaundice
conjunctiva R17
gravis, newborn P55.Ø
hematogenous (acquired) D59.9
hemolytic (acquired) D59.9
congenital —*see* Spherocytosis
hemorrhagic (acute) (leptospiral) (spirochetal) A27.Ø
newborn P53
infectious B15.9
with hepatic coma B15.Ø
leptospiral A27.Ø
spirochetal A27.Ø
neonatorum —*see* Jaundice, newborn
newborn P59.9
spirochetal A27.Ø
➡ Ictus solaris, solis T67.Ø1
Ideation
homicidal R45.85Ø
suicidal R45.851
Identity disorder (child) F64.9
gender role F64.2
psychosexual F64.2
Idioglossia F8Ø.Ø
Idiopathic —*see* condition
Idiot, idiocy (congenital) F73
amaurotic (Bielschowsky(-Jansky)) (family) (infantile (late)) (juvenile (late)) (Vogt-Spielmeyer) E75.4
microcephalic QØ2
Id reaction (due to bacteria) L3Ø.2
IgE asthma J45.9Ø9
IIAC (idiopathic infantile arterial calcification) Q28.8
Ileitis (chronic) (noninfectious) —*see also* Enteritis K52.9
backwash —*see* Pancolitis, ulcerative (chronic)
infectious AØ9
regional (ulcerative) —*see* Enteritis, regional, small intestine
segmental —*see* Enteritis, regional
terminal (ulcerative) —*see* Enteritis, regional, small intestine
Ileocolitis —*see also* Enteritis K52.9
infectious AØ9
regional —*see* Enteritis, regional
ulcerative K51.Ø- ●
Ileostomy
attention to Z43.2
malfunctioning K94.13
status Z93.2
with complication —*see* Complications, enterostomy
Ileotyphus —*see* Typhoid
Ileum —*see* condition
Ileus (bowel) (colon) (inhibitory) (intestine) K56.7
adynamic K56.Ø
due to gallstone (in intestine) K56.3
duodenal (chronic) K31.5
Ileus *(Continued)*
gallstone K56.3
mechanical NEC —*see also* Obstruction, intestine, specified K56.699
meconium P76.Ø
in cystic fibrosis E84.11
meaning meconium plug (without cystic fibrosis) P76.Ø
myxedema K59.8
neurogenic K56.Ø
Hirschsprung's disease or megacolon Q43.1
newborn
due to meconium P76.Ø
in cystic fibrosis E84.11
meaning meconium plug (without cystic fibrosis) P76.Ø
transitory P76.1
obstructive —*see also* Obstruction, intestine, specified K56.699
paralytic K56.Ø
postoperative K91.89
Iliac —*see* condition
Iliotibial band syndrome M76.3- ●
Illiteracy Z55.Ø
Illness—*see also* Disease R69
manic-depressive —*see* Disorder, bipolar
Imbalance R26.89
autonomic G9Ø.8
constituents of food intake E63.1
electrolyte E87.8
with
abortion —*see* Abortion by type, complicated by, electrolyte imbalance
molar pregnancy OØ8.5
due to hyperemesis gravidarum O21.1
following ectopic or molar pregnancy OØ8.5
neonatal, transitory NEC P74.49
potassium
hyperkalemia P74.31
hypokalemia P74.32
sodium
hypernatremia P74.21
hyponatremia P74.22
endocrine E34.9
eye muscle NOS H5Ø.9
hormone E34.9
hysterical F44.4
labyrinth —*see* subcategory H83.2
posture R29.3
protein-energy —*see* Malnutrition
sympathetic G9Ø.8
Imbecile, imbecility (I.Q. 35-49) F71
Imbedding, intrauterine device T83.39
Imbibition, cholesterol (gallbladder) K82.4
Imbrication, teeth, fully erupted M26.3Ø
Imerslund (-Gräsbeck) syndrome D51.1
Immature —*see also* Immaturity
birth (less than 37 completed weeks) —*see* Preterm, newborn
extremely (less than 28 completed weeks) —*see* Immaturity, extreme
personality F6Ø.89
Immaturity (less than 37 completed weeks) —*see also* Preterm, newborn
extreme of newborn (less than 28 completed weeks of gestation) (less than 196 completed days of gestation) (unspecified weeks of gestation) PØ7.2Ø
gestational age
23 completed weeks (23 weeks, Ø days through 23 weeks, 6 days) PØ7.22
24 completed weeks (24 weeks, Ø days through 24 weeks, 6 days) PØ7.23
25 completed weeks (25 weeks, Ø days through 25 weeks, 6 days) PØ7.24
26 completed weeks (26 weeks, Ø days through 26 weeks, 6 days) PØ7.25
27 completed weeks (27 weeks, Ø days through 27 weeks, 6 days) PØ7.26
less than 23 completed weeks PØ7.21
Immaturity *(Continued)*
fetus or infant light-for-dates —*see* Light-for-dates
lung, newborn P28.Ø
organ or site NEC —*see* Hypoplasia
pulmonary, newborn P28.Ø
reaction F6Ø.89
sexual (female) (male), after puberty E3Ø.Ø
Immersion T75.1
foot T69.Ø2- ●
hand T69.Ø1- ●
Immobile, immobility
complete, due to severe physical disability or frailty R53.2
intestine K59.8
syndrome (paraplegic) M62.3
Immune reconstitution (inflammatory) syndrome [IRIS] D89.3
Immunization —*see also* Vaccination
ABO —*see* Incompatibility, ABO
in newborn P55.1
appropriate for age
child (over 28 days old) ZØØ.129
with abnormal findings ZØØ.121
complication —*see* Complications, vaccination
encounter for Z23
not done (not carried out) Z28.9
because (of)
acute illness of patient Z28.Ø1
allergy to vaccine (or component) Z28.Ø4
caregiver refusal Z28.82
chronic illness of patient Z28.Ø2
contraindication NEC Z28.Ø9
delay in delivery of vaccine Z28.83
group pressure Z28.1
guardian refusal Z28.82
immune compromised state of patient Z28.Ø3
lack of availability of vaccine Z28.83
manufacturer delay of vaccine Z28.83
parent refusal Z28.82
patient's belief Z28.1
patient had disease being vaccinated against Z28.81
patient refusal Z28.21
religious beliefs of patient Z28.1
specified reason NEC Z28.89
of patient Z28.29
unavailability of vaccine Z28.83
unspecified patient reason Z28.2Ø
Rh factor
affecting management of pregnancy NEC O36.Ø9- ●
anti-D antibody O36.Ø1- ●
from transfusion —*see* Complication(s), transfusion, incompatibility reaction, Rh (factor)
Immunocytoma C83.Ø- ●
Immunodeficiency D84.9
with
➡ adenosine-deaminase deficiency (*see also* Deficiency, adenosine deaminase) D81.3Ø
antibody defects D8Ø.9
specified type NEC D8Ø.8
hyperimmunoglobulinemia D8Ø.6
increased immunoglobulin M (IgM) D8Ø.5
major defect D82.9
specified type NEC D82.8
partial albinism D82.8
short-limbed stature D82.2
thrombocytopenia and eczema D82.Ø
antibody with
hyperimmunoglobulinemia D8Ø.6
near-normal immunoglobulins D8Ø.6
autosomal recessive, Swiss type D8Ø.Ø
combined D81.9
biotin-dependent carboxylase D81.819
biotinidase D81.81Ø
holocarboxylase synthetase D81.818
specified type NEC D81.818

- **Immunodeficiency** *(Continued)*
  - combined *(Continued)*
    - severe (SCID) D81.9
      - with
        - low or normal B-cell numbers D81.2
        - low T- and B-cell numbers D81.1
        - reticular dysgenesis D81.Ø
    - specified type NEC D81.89
  - common variable D83.9
    - with
      - abnormalities of B-cell numbers and function D83.Ø
      - autoantibodies to B- or T-cells D83.2
      - immunoregulatory T-cell disorders D83.1
    - specified type NEC D83.8
  - following hereditary defective response to Epstein-Barr virus (EBV) D82.3
  - selective, immunoglobulin
    - A (IgA) D8Ø.2
    - G (IgG) (subclasses) D8Ø.3
    - M (IgM) D8Ø.4
  - severe combined (SCID) D81.9
    - ▶due to adenosine deaminase deficiency D81.31
  - specified type NEC D84.8
  - X-linked, with increased IgM D8Ø.5
- **Immunotherapy** (encounter for)
  - antineoplastic Z51.12
- **Impaction, impacted**
  - bowel, colon, rectum —*see also* Impaction, fecal K56.49
    - by gallstone K56.3
  - calculus —*see* Calculus
  - cerumen (ear) (external) H61.2-●
  - cuspid —*see* Impaction, tooth
  - dental (same or adjacent tooth) KØ1.1
  - fecal, feces K56.41
  - fracture —*see* Fracture, by site
  - gallbladder —*see* Calculus, gallbladder
  - gallstone(s) —*see* Calculus, gallbladder
    - bile duct (common) (hepatic) —*see* Calculus, bile duct
    - cystic duct —*see* Calculus, gallbladder
    - in intestine, with obstruction (any part) K56.3
  - intestine (calculous) NEC —*see also* Impaction, fecal K56.49
    - gallstone, with ileus K56.3
  - intrauterine device (IUD) T83.39
  - molar —*see* Impaction, tooth
  - shoulder, causing obstructed labor O66.Ø
  - tooth, teeth KØ1.1
  - turbinate J34.89
- **Impaired, impairment** (function)
  - auditory discrimination —*see* Abnormal, auditory perception
  - cognitive, mild, so stated G31.84
  - dual sensory Z73.82
  - fasting glucose R73.Ø1
  - glucose tolerance (oral) R73.Ø2
  - hearing —*see* Deafness
  - heart —*see* Disease, heart
  - kidney N28.9
    - disorder resulting from N25.9
      - specified NEC N25.89
  - liver K72.9Ø
    - with coma K72.91
  - mastication KØ8.89
  - mild cognitive, so stated G31.84
  - mobility
    - ear ossicles —*see* Ankylosis, ear ossicles
    - requiring care provider Z74.Ø9
  - myocardium, myocardial —*see* Insufficiency, myocardial
  - rectal sphincter R19.8
  - renal (acute) (chronic) N28.9
    - disorder resulting from N25.9
      - specified NEC N25.89
  - vision NEC H54.7
    - both eyes H54.3
- **Impediment, speech** R47.9
  - psychogenic (childhood) F98.8
  - slurring R47.81
  - specified NEC R47.89
- **Impending**
  - coronary syndrome I2Ø.Ø
  - delirium tremens F1Ø.239
  - myocardial infarction I2Ø.Ø
- **Imperception auditory** (acquired) —*see also* Deafness
  - congenital H93.25
- **Imperfect**
  - aeration, lung (newborn) NEC —*see* Atelectasis
  - closure (congenital)
    - alimentary tract NEC Q45.8
      - lower Q43.8
      - upper Q4Ø.8
    - atrioventricular ostium Q21.2
    - atrium (secundum) Q21.1
    - branchial cleft NOS Q18.2
      - cyst Q18.Ø
      - fistula Q18.Ø
      - sinus Q18.Ø
    - choroid Q14.3
    - cricoid cartilage Q31.8
    - cusps, heart valve NEC Q24.8
      - pulmonary Q22.3
    - ductus
      - arteriosus Q25.Ø
      - Botalli Q25.Ø
    - ear drum (causing impairment of hearing) Q16.4
    - esophagus with communication to bronchus or trachea Q39.1
    - eyelid Q1Ø.3
    - foramen
      - botalli Q21.1
      - ovale Q21.1
    - genitalia, genital organ(s) or system
      - female Q52.8
        - external Q52.79
        - internal NEC Q52.8
      - male Q55.8
    - glottis Q31.8
    - interatrial ostium or septum Q21.1
    - interauricular ostium or septum Q21.1
    - interventricular ostium or septum Q21.Ø
    - larynx Q31.8
    - lip —*see* Cleft, lip
    - nasal septum Q3Ø.3
    - nose Q3Ø.2
    - omphalomesenteric duct Q43.Ø
    - optic nerve entry Q14.2
    - organ or site not listed —*see* Anomaly, by site
    - ostium
      - interatrial Q21.1
      - interauricular Q21.1
      - interventricular Q21.Ø
    - palate —*see* Cleft, palate
    - preauricular sinus Q18.1
    - retina Q14.1
    - roof of orbit Q75.8
    - sclera Q13.5
    - septum
      - aorticopulmonary Q21.4
      - atrial (secundum) Q21.1
      - between aorta and pulmonary artery Q21.4
      - heart Q21.9
      - interatrial (secundum) Q21.1
      - interauricular (secundum) Q21.1
      - interventricular Q21.Ø
        - in tetralogy of Fallot Q21.3
      - nasal Q3Ø.3
      - ventricular Q21.Ø
        - with pulmonary stenosis or atresia, dextraposition of aorta, and hypertrophy of right ventricle Q21.3
        - in tetralogy of Fallot Q21.3
- **Imperfect** *(Continued)*
  - closure *(Continued)*
    - skull Q75.Ø
      - with
        - anencephaly QØØ.Ø
        - encephalocele —*see* Encephalocele
        - hydrocephalus QØ3.9
          - with spina bifida —*see* Spina bifida, by site, with hydrocephalus
        - microcephaly QØ2
    - spine (with meningocele) —*see* Spina bifida
    - trachea Q32.1
    - tympanic membrane (causing impairment of hearing) Q16.4
    - uterus Q51.818
    - vitelline duct Q43.Ø
  - erection —*see* Dysfunction, sexual, male, erectile
  - fusion —*see* Imperfect, closure
  - inflation, lung (newborn) —*see* Atelectasis
  - posture R29.3
  - rotation, intestine Q43.3
  - septum, ventricular Q21.Ø
- **Imperfectly descended testis** —*see* Cryptorchid
- **Imperforate** (congenital) —*see also* Atresia
  - anus Q42.3
    - with fistula Q42.2
  - cervix (uteri) Q51.828
  - esophagus Q39.Ø
    - with tracheoesophageal fistula Q39.1
  - hymen Q52.3
  - jejunum Q41.1
  - pharynx Q38.8
  - rectum Q42.1
    - with fistula Q42.Ø
  - urethra Q64.39
  - vagina Q52.4
- **Impervious** (congenital) —*see also* Atresia
  - anus Q42.3
    - with fistula Q42.2
  - bile duct Q44.2
  - esophagus Q39.Ø
    - with tracheoesophageal fistula Q39.1
  - intestine (small) Q41.9
    - large Q42.9
      - specified NEC Q42.8
  - rectum Q42.1
    - with fistula Q42.Ø
  - ureter —*see* Atresia, ureter
  - urethra Q64.39
- **Impetiginization of dermatoses** LØ1.1
- **Impetigo** (any organism) (any site) (circinate) (contagiosa) (simplex) (vulgaris) LØ1.ØØ
  - Bockhart's LØ1.Ø2
  - bullous, bullosa LØ1.Ø3
  - external ear LØ1.ØØ *[H62.4Ø]*
  - follicularis LØ1.Ø2
  - furfuracea L3Ø.5
  - herpetiformis L4Ø.1
    - nonobstetrical L4Ø.1
  - neonatorum LØ1.Ø3
  - nonbullous LØ1.Ø1
  - specified type NEC LØ1.Ø9
  - ulcerative LØ1.Ø9
- **Impingement** (on teeth)
  - ▶joint —*see* Disorder, joint, specified type NEC
  - soft tissue
    - anterior M26.81
    - posterior M26.82
- **Implant, endometrial** N8Ø.9
- **Implantation**
  - anomalous —*see* Anomaly, by site
    - ureter Q62.63
  - cyst
    - external area or site (skin) NEC L72.Ø
    - iris —*see* Cyst, iris, implantation
    - vagina N89.8
    - vulva N9Ø.7
  - dermoid (cyst) —*see* Implantation, cyst

Impotence (sexual) N52.9
counseling Z7Ø.1
organic origin —*see also* Dysfunction, sexual, male, erectile N52.9
psychogenic F52.21
Impression, basilar Q75.8
Imprisonment, anxiety concerning Z65.1
Improper care (child) (newborn) —*see* Maltreatment
Improperly tied umbilical cord (causing hemorrhage) P51.8
Impulsiveness (impulsive) R45.87
Inability to swallow —*see* Aphagia
Inaccessible, inaccessibility
health care NEC Z75.3
due to
waiting period Z75.2
for admission to facility elsewhere Z75.1
other helping agencies Z75.4
Inactive —*see* condition
Inadequate, inadequacy
aesthetics of dental restoration KØ8.56
biologic, constitutional, functional, or social F6Ø.7
development
child R62.5Ø
genitalia
after puberty NEC E3Ø.Ø
congenital
female Q52.8
external Q52.79
internal Q52.8
male Q55.8
lungs Q33.6
associated with short gestation P28.Ø
organ or site not listed —*see* Anomaly, by site
diet (causing nutritional deficiency) E63.9
eating habits Z72.4
environment, household Z59.1
family support Z63.8
food (supply) NEC Z59.4
hunger effects T73.Ø
functional F6Ø.7
household care, due to
family member
handicapped or ill Z74.2
on vacation Z75.5
temporarily away from home Z74.2
technical defects in home Z59.1
temporary absence from home of person rendering care Z74.2
housing (heating) (space) Z59.1
income (financial) Z59.6
intrafamilial communication Z63.8
material resources Z59.9
mental —*see* Disability, intellectual
parental supervision or control of child Z62.Ø
personality F6Ø.7
pulmonary
function RØ6.89
newborn P28.5
ventilation, newborn P28.5
sample of cytologic smear
anus R85.615
cervix R87.615
vagina R87.625
social F6Ø.7
insurance Z59.7
skills NEC Z73.4
supervision of child by parent Z62.Ø
teaching affecting education Z55.8
welfare support Z59.7
Inanition R64
with edema —*see* Malnutrition, severe
due to
deprivation of food T73.Ø
malnutrition —*see* Malnutrition
fever R5Ø.9
Inappropriate
change in quantitative human chorionic gonadotropin (hCG) in early pregnancy OØ2.81
diet or eating habits Z72.4
level of quantitative human chorionic gonadotropin (hCG) for gestational age in early pregnancy OØ2.81
secretion
antidiuretic hormone (ADH) (excessive) E22.2
deficiency E23.2
pituitary (posterior) E22.2
Inattention at or after birth —*see* Neglect
Incarceration, incarcerated
enterocele K46.Ø
gangrenous K46.1
epiplocele K46.Ø
gangrenous K46.1
exomphalos K42.Ø
gangrenous K42.1
hernia —*see also* Hernia, by site, with obstruction
with gangrene —*see* Hernia, by site, with gangrene
iris, in wound —*see* Injury, eye, laceration, with prolapse
lens, in wound —*see* Injury, eye, laceration, with prolapse
omphalocele K42.Ø
prison, anxiety concerning Z65.1
rupture —*see* Hernia, by site
sarcoepiplocele K46.Ø
gangrenous K46.1
sarcoepiplomphalocele K42.Ø
with gangrene K42.1
uterus N85.8
gravid O34.51-●
causing obstructed labor O65.5
Incised wound
external —*see* Laceration
internal organs —*see* Injury, by site
Incision, incisional
hernia K43.2
with
gangrene (and obstruction) K43.1
obstruction K43.Ø
surgical, complication —*see* Complications, surgical procedure
traumatic
external —*see* Laceration
internal organs —*see* Injury, by site
Inclusion
azurophilic leukocytic D72.Ø
blennorrhea (neonatal) (newborn) P39.1
gallbladder in liver (congenital) Q44.1
Incompatibility
ABO
affecting management of pregnancy O36.11-●
anti-A sensitization O36.11-●
anti-B sensitization O36.19-●
specified NEC O36.19-●
infusion or transfusion reaction —*see* Complication(s), transfusion, incompatibility reaction, ABO
newborn P55.1
blood (group) (Duffy) (K) (Kell) (Kidd) (Lewis) (M) (S) NEC
affecting management of pregnancy O36.11-●
anti-A sensitization O36.11-●
anti-B sensitization O36.19-●
infusion or transfusion reaction T8Ø.89
newborn P55.8
divorce or estrangement Z63.5
Rh (blood group) (factor) Z31.82
affecting management of pregnancy NEC O36.Ø9-●
anti-D antibody O36.Ø1-●
Incompatibility *(Continued)*
Rh *(Continued)*
infusion or transfusion reaction —*see* Complication(s), transfusion, incompatibility reaction, Rh (factor)
newborn P55.Ø
rhesus —*see* Incompatibility, Rh
Incompetency, incompetent, incompetence
annular
aortic (valve) —*see* Insufficiency, aortic
mitral (valve) I34.Ø
pulmonary valve (heart) I37.1
aortic (valve) —*see* Insufficiency, aortic
cardiac valve —*see* Endocarditis
cervix, cervical (os) N88.3
in pregnancy O34.3-●
chronotropic I45.89
with
autonomic dysfunction G9Ø.8
ischemic heart disease I25.89
left ventricular dysfunction I51.89
sinus node dysfunction I49.8
esophagogastric (junction) (sphincter) K22.Ø
mitral (valve) —*see* Insufficiency, mitral
pelvic fundus N81.89
pubocervical tissue N81.82
pulmonary valve (heart) I37.1
congenital Q22.3
rectovaginal tissue N81.83
tricuspid (annular) (valve) —*see* Insufficiency, tricuspid
valvular —*see* Endocarditis
congenital Q24.8
vein, venous (saphenous) (varicose) —*see* Varix, leg
Incomplete —*see also* condition
bladder, emptying R33.9
defecation R15.Ø
expansion lungs (newborn) NEC —*see* Atelectasis
rotation, intestine Q43.3
Inconclusive
diagnostic imaging due to excess body fat of patient R93.9
findings on diagnostic imaging of breast NEC R92.8
mammogram (due to dense breasts) R92.2
Incontinence R32
anal sphincter R15.9
coital N39.491
feces R15.9
nonorganic origin F98.1
insensible (urinary) N39.42
overflow N39.49Ø
postural (urinary) N39.492
psychogenic F45.8
rectal R15.9
reflex N39.498
stress (female) (male) N39.3
and urge N39.46
urethral sphincter R32
urge N39.41
and stress (female) (male) N39.46
urine (urinary) R32
continuous N39.45
due to cognitive impairment, or severe physical disability or immobility R39.81
functional R39.81
insensible N39.42
mixed (stress and urge) N39.46
nocturnal N39.44
nonorganic origin F98.Ø
overflow N39.49Ø
post dribbling N39.43
postural N39.492
reflex N39.498
specified NEC N39.498
stress (female) (male) N39.3
and urge N39.46
total N39.498

- **Incontinence** *(Continued)*
  - urine *(Continued)*
    - unaware N39.42
    - urge N39.41
      - and stress (female) (male) N39.46
- **Incontinentia pigmenti** Q82.3
- **Incoordinate, incoordination**
  - esophageal-pharyngeal (newborn) —*see* Dysphagia
  - muscular R27.8
  - uterus (action) (contractions) (complicating delivery) O62.4
- **Increase, increased**
  - abnormal, in development R63.8
  - androgens (ovarian) E28.1
  - anticoagulants (antithrombin) (anti-VIIIa) (anti-IXa) (anti-Xa) (anti-XIa) —*see* Circulating anticoagulants
  - cold sense R20.8
  - estrogen E28.0
  - function
    - adrenal
      - cortex —*see* Cushing's, syndrome
      - medulla E27.5
    - pituitary (gland) (anterior) (lobe) E22.9
      - posterior E22.2
  - heat sense R20.8
  - intracranial pressure (benign) G93.2
  - permeability, capillaries I78.8
  - pressure, intracranial G93.2
  - secretion
    - gastrin E16.4
    - glucagon E16.3
    - pancreas, endocrine E16.9
      - growth hormone-releasing hormone E16.8
      - pancreatic polypeptide E16.8
      - somatostatin E16.8
      - vasoactive-intestinal polypeptide E16.8
  - sphericity, lens Q12.4
  - splenic activity D73.1
  - venous pressure I87.8
    - portal K76.6
- **Increta placenta** O43.22-●
- **Incrustation, cornea, foreign body** (lead) (zinc) —*see* Foreign body, cornea
- **Incyclophoria** H50.54
- **Incyclotropia** —*see* Cyclotropia
- **Indeterminate sex** Q56.4
- **India rubber skin** Q82.8
- **Indigestion** (acid) (bilious) (functional) K30
  - catarrhal K31.89
  - due to decomposed food NOS A05.9
  - nervous F45.8
  - psychogenic F45.8
- **Indirect** —*see* condition
- **Induratio penis plastica** N48.6
- **Induration, indurated**
  - brain G93.89
  - breast (fibrous) N64.51
    - puerperal, postpartum O92.29
  - broad ligament N83.8
  - chancre
    - anus A51.1
    - congenital A50.07
    - extragenital NEC A51.2
  - corpora cavernosa (penis) (plastic) N48.6
  - liver (chronic) K76.89
  - lung (black) (chronic) (fibroid) —*see also* Fibrosis, lung J84.10
    - essential brown J84.03
  - penile (plastic) N48.6
  - phlebitic —*see* Phlebitis
  - skin R23.4
- **Inebriety** (without dependence) —*see* Alcohol, intoxication
- **Inefficiency, kidney** N28.9
- **Inelasticity, skin** R23.4
- **Inequality, leg** (length) (acquired) —*see also* Deformity, limb, unequal length
  - congenital —*see* Defect, reduction, lower limb
  - lower leg —*see* Deformity, limb, unequal length
- **Inertia**
  - bladder (neurogenic) N31.2
  - stomach K31.89
    - psychogenic F45.8
  - uterus, uterine during labor O62.2
    - during latent phase of labor O62.0
    - primary O62.0
    - secondary O62.1
  - vesical (neurogenic) N31.2
- **Infancy, infantile, infantilism** —*see also* condition
  - celiac K90.0
  - genitalia, genitals (after puberty) E30.0
  - Herter's (nontropical sprue) K90.0
  - intestinal K90.0
  - Lorain E23.0
  - pancreatic K86.89
  - pelvis M95.5
    - with disproportion (fetopelvic) O33.1
      - causing obstructed labor O65.1
  - pituitary E23.0
  - renal N25.0
  - uterus —*see* Infantile, genitalia
- **Infant(s)** —*see also* Infancy
  - excessive crying R68.11
  - irritable child R68.12
  - lack of care —*see* Neglect
  - liveborn (singleton) Z38.2
    - born in hospital Z38.00
      - by cesarean Z38.01
    - born outside hospital Z38.1
    - multiple NEC Z38.8
      - born in hospital Z38.68
        - by cesarean Z38.69
      - born outside hospital Z38.7
    - quadruplet Z38.8
      - born in hospital Z38.63
        - by cesarean Z38.64
      - born outside hospital Z38.7
    - quintuplet Z38.8
      - born in hospital Z38.65
        - by cesarean Z38.66
      - born outside hospital Z38.7
    - triplet Z38.8
      - born in hospital Z38.61
        - by cesarean Z38.62
      - born outside hospital Z38.7
    - twin Z38.5
      - born in hospital Z38.30
        - by cesarean Z38.31
      - born outside hospital Z38.4
  - of diabetic mother (syndrome of) P70.1
    - gestational diabetes P70.0
- **Infantile** —*see also* condition
  - genitalia, genitals E30.0
  - os, uterine E30.0
  - penis E30.0
  - testis E29.1
  - uterus E30.0
- **Infantilism** —*see* Infancy
- **Infarct, infarction**
  - adrenal (capsule) (gland) E27.49
  - appendices epiploicae —*see also* Infarct, intestine K55.069
  - bowel —*see also* Infarct, intestine K55.069
  - brain (stem) —*see* Infarct, cerebral
  - breast N64.89
  - brewer's (kidney) N28.0
  - cardiac —*see* Infarct, myocardium
  - cerebellar —*see* Infarct, cerebral
  - ➠ cerebral (acute) (chronic) (*see also* Occlusion, artery cerebral or precerebral, with infarction) I63.9-●
    - aborted I63.9
    - cortical I63.9
    - due to
      - cerebral venous thrombosis, nonpyogenic I63.6
      - embolism
        - cerebral arteries I63.4-●
        - precerebral arteries I63.1-●

- **Infarct, infarction** *(Continued)*
  - cerebral *(Continued)*
    - due to *(Continued)*
      - occlusion NEC
        - cerebral arteries I63.5-●
        - precerebral arteries I63.2-●
        - small artery I63.81
      - stenosis NEC
        - cerebral arteries I63.5-●
        - precerebral arteries I63.2-●
        - small artery I63.81
      - thrombosis
        - cerebral artery I63.3-●
        - precerebral artery I63.0-●
    - intraoperative
      - during cardiac surgery I97.810
      - during other surgery I97.811
    - postprocedural
      - following cardiac surgery I97.820
      - following other surgery I97.821
    - specified NEC I63.89
  - colon (acute) (agnogenic) (embolic) (hemorrhagic) (nonocclusive) (nonthrombotic) (occlusive) (segmental) (thrombotic) (with gangrene) —*see also* Infarct, intestine K55.049
  - coronary artery —*see* Infarct, myocardium
  - embolic —*see* Embolism
  - fallopian tube N83.8
  - gallbladder K82.8
  - heart —*see* Infarct, myocardium
  - hepatic K76.3
  - hypophysis (anterior lobe) E23.6
  - impending (myocardium) I20.0
  - intestine (acute) (agnogenic) (embolic) (hemorrhagic) (nonocclusive) (nonthrombotic) (occlusive) (thrombotic) (with gangrene) K55.069
    - diffuse K55.062
    - focal K55.061
    - large K55.049
      - diffuse K55.042
      - focal K55.041
    - small K55.029
      - diffuse K55.022
      - focal K55.021
  - kidney N28.0
  - lacunar I63.81
  - liver K76.3
  - lung (embolic) (thrombotic) —*see* Embolism, pulmonary
  - lymph node I89.8
  - mesentery, mesenteric (embolic) (thrombotic) (with gangrene) —*see also* Infarct, intestine K55.069
  - muscle (ischemic) M62.20
    - ankle M62.27-●
    - foot M62.27-●
    - forearm M62.23-●
    - hand M62.24-●
    - lower leg M62.26-●
    - pelvic region M62.25-●
    - shoulder region M62.21-●
    - specified site NEC M62.28
    - thigh M62.25-●
    - upper arm M62.22-●
  - myocardium, myocardial (acute) (with stated duration of 4 weeks or less) I21.9
    - associated with revascularization procedure I21.A9
    - diagnosed on ECG, but presenting no symptoms I25.2
    - due to
      - demand ischemia I21.A1
      - ischemic imbalance I21.A1
    - healed or old I25.2
    - intraoperative —*see also* Infarct, myocardium, associated with revascularization procedure
      - during cardiac surgery I97.790
      - during other surgery I97.791

Infarct, infarction (Continued)
myocardium, myocardial (Continued)
non-Q wave I21.4
non-ST elevation (NSTEMI) I21.4
subsequent I22.2
nontransmural I21.4
past (diagnosed on ECG or other investigation, but currently presenting no symptoms) I25.2
postprocedural —see also Infarct, myocardium, associated with revascularization procedure
following cardiac surgery —see also Infarct, myocardium, type 4 or type 5 I97.190
following other surgery I97.191
Q wave —see also Infarct, myocardium, by site I21.3
secondary to
demand ischemia I21.A1
ischemic imbalance I21.A1
ST elevation (STEMI) I21.3
anterior (anteroapical) (anterolateral) (anteroseptal) (Q wave) (wall) I21.09
subsequent I22.0
inferior (diaphragmatic) (inferolateral) (inferoposterior) (wall) NEC I21.19
subsequent I22.1
inferoposterior transmural (Q wave) I21.11
involving
coronary artery of anterior wall NEC I21.09
coronary artery of inferior wall NEC I21.19
diagonal coronary artery I21.02
left anterior descending coronary artery I21.02
left circumflex coronary artery I21.21
left main coronary artery I21.01
oblique marginal coronary artery I21.21
right coronary artery I21.11
lateral (apical-lateral) (basal-lateral) (high) I21.29
subsequent I22.8
posterior (posterobasal) (posterolateral) (posteroseptal) (true) I21.29
subsequent I22.8
septal I21.29
subsequent I22.8
specified NEC I21.29
subsequent I22.8
subsequent I22.9
subsequent (recurrent) (reinfarction) I22.9
anterior (anteroapical) (anterolateral) (anteroseptal) (wall) I22.0
diaphragmatic (wall) I22.1
inferior (diaphragmatic) (inferolateral) (inferoposterior) (wall) I22.1
lateral (apical-lateral) (basal-lateral) (high) I22.8
non-ST elevation (NSTEMI) I22.2
posterior (posterobasal) (posterolateral) (posteroseptal) (true) I22.8
septal I22.8
specified NEC I22.8
ST elevation I22.9
anterior (anteroapical) (anterolateral) (anteroseptal) (wall) I22.0
inferior (diaphragmatic) (inferolateral) (inferoposterior) (wall) I22.1
specified NEC I22.8
subendocardial I22.2
transmural I22.9
anterior (anteroapical) (anterolateral) (anteroseptal) (wall) I22.0
diaphragmatic (wall) I22.1
inferior (diaphragmatic) (inferolateral) (inferoposterior) (wall) I22.1
lateral (apical-lateral) (basal-lateral) (high) I22.8
posterior (posterobasal) (posterolateral) (posteroseptal) (true) I22.8
specified NEC I22.8

Infarct, infarction (Continued)
myocardium, myocardial (Continued)
subsequent (Continued)
type 1 —see also Infarction, myocardial, subsequent, by site, or by ST elevation or non-ST elevation I22.9
type 2 I21.A1
type 3 I21.A9
type 4 I21.A9
type 5 I21.A9
syphilitic A52.06
transmural I21.9
anterior (anteroapical) (anterolateral) (anteroseptal) (Q wave) (wall) NEC I21.09
inferior (diaphragmatic) (inferolateral) (inferoposterior) (Q wave) (wall) NEC I21.19
inferoposterior (Q wave) I21.11
lateral (apical-lateral) (basal-lateral) (high) NEC I21.29
posterior (posterobasal) (posterolateral) (posteroseptal) (true) NEC I21.29
septal NEC I21.29
specified NEC I21.29
type 1 —see also Infarction, myocardial, by site, or by ST elevation or non-ST elevation I21.9
type 2 I21.A1
type 3 I21.A9
type 4 (a) (b) (c) I21.A9
type 5 I21.A9
nontransmural I21.4
omentum —see also Infarct, intestine K55.069
ovary N83.8
pancreas K86.89
papillary muscle —see Infarct, myocardium
parathyroid gland E21.4
pituitary (gland) E23.6
placenta O43.81-•
prostate N42.89
pulmonary (artery) (vein) (hemorrhagic) —see Embolism, pulmonary
renal (embolic) (thrombotic) N28.0
retina, retinal (artery) —see Occlusion, artery, retina
spinal (cord) (acute) (embolic) (nonembolic) G95.11
spleen D73.5
embolic or thrombotic I74.8
subendocardial (acute) (nontransmural) I21.4
suprarenal (capsule) (gland) E27.49
testis N50.1
thrombotic —see also Thrombosis
artery, arterial —see Embolism
thyroid (gland) E07.89
ventricle (heart) —see Infarct, myocardium
Infecting —see condition
Infection, infected, infective (opportunistic) B99.9
with
drug resistant organism —see Resistance (to), drug —see also specific organism
lymphangitis —see Lymphangitis
organ dysfunction (acute) R65.20
with septic shock R65.21
abscess (skin) - code by site under Abscess
Absidia —see Mucormycosis
Acanthamoeba —see Acanthamebiasis
Acanthocheilonema (perstans) (streptocerca) B74.4
accessory sinus (chronic) —see Sinusitis
achorion —see Dermatophytosis
Acremonium falciforme B47.0
acromioclavicular M00.9
Actinobacillus (actinomycetem-comitans) A28.8
mallei A24.0
muris A25.1
Actinomadura B47.1
Actinomyces (israelii) —see also Actinomycosis A42.9

Infection, infected, infective (Continued)
Actinomycetales —see Actinomycosis
actinomycotic NOS —see Actinomycosis
adenoid (and tonsil) J03.90
chronic J35.02
adenovirus NEC
as cause of disease classified elsewhere B97.0
unspecified nature or site B34.0
aerogenes capsulatus A48.0
aertrycke —see Infection, salmonella
alimentary canal NOS —see Enteritis, infectious
Allescheria boydii B48.2
Alternaria B48.8
alveolus, alveolar (process) K04.7
Ameba, amebic (histolytica) —see Amebiasis
amniotic fluid, sac or cavity O41.10-•
chorioamnionitis O41.12-•
placentitis O41.14-•
amputation stump (surgical) —see Complication, amputation stump, infection
Ancylostoma (duodenalis) B76.0
Anisakiasis, Anisakis larvae B81.0
anthrax —see Anthrax
antrum (chronic) —see Sinusitis, maxillary
anus, anal (papillae) (sphincter) K62.89
arbovirus (arbor virus) A94
specified type NEC A93.8
artificial insemination N98.0
Ascaris lumbricoides —see Ascariasis
Ascomycetes B47.0
Aspergillus (flavus) (fumigatus) (terreus) —see Aspergillosis
atypical
acid-fast (bacilli) —see Mycobacterium, atypical
mycobacteria —see Mycobacterium, atypical
virus A81.9
specified type NEC A81.89
auditory meatus (external) —see Otitis, externa, infective
auricle (ear) —see Otitis, externa, infective
axillary gland (lymph) L04.2
Bacillus A49.9
abortus A23.1
anthracis —see Anthrax
Ducrey's (any location) A57
Flexner's A03.1
Friedländer's NEC A49.8
gas (gangrene) A48.0
mallei A24.0
melitensis A23.0
paratyphoid, paratyphosus A01.4
A A01.1
B A01.2
C A01.3
Shiga (-Kruse) A03.0
suipestifer —see Infection, salmonella
swimming pool A31.1
typhosa A01.00
welchii —see Gangrene, gas
bacterial NOS A49.9
as cause of disease classified elsewhere B96.89
Bacteroides fragilis [B. fragilis] B96.6
Clostridium perfringens [C. perfringens] B96.7
Enterobacter sakazakii B96.89
Enterococcus B95.2
Escherichia coli [E. coli] (see also Escherichia coli) B96.20
Helicobacter pylori [H.pylori] B96.81
Hemophilus influenzae [H. influenzae] B96.3
Klebsiella pneumoniae [K. pneumoniae] B96.1
Mycoplasma pneumoniae [M. pneumoniae] B96.0
Proteus (mirabilis) (morganii) B96.4

Infection, infected, infective *(Continued)*
bacterial NOS *(Continued)*
as cause of disease classified elsewhere *(Continued)*
Pseudomonas (aeruginosa) (mallei) (pseudomallei) B96.5
Staphylococcus B95.8
aureus (methicillin susceptible) (MSSA) B95.61
methicillin resistant (MRSA) B95.62
specified NEC B95.7
Streptococcus B95.5
group A B95.Ø
group B B95.1
pneumoniae B95.3
specified NEC B95.4
Vibrio vulnificus B96.82
specified NEC A48.8
Bacterium
paratyphosum AØ1.4
A AØ1.1
B AØ1.2
C AØ1.3
typhosum AØ1.ØØ
Bacteroides NEC A49.8
fragilis, as cause of disease classified elsewhere B96.6
Balantidium coli AØ7.Ø
Bartholin's gland N75.8
Basidiobolus B46.8
bile duct (common) (hepatic) —*see* Cholangitis
bladder —*see* Cystitis
Blastomyces, blastomycotic —*see also* Blastomycosis
brasiliensis —*see* Paracoccidioidomycosis
dermatitidis —*see* Blastomycosis
European —*see* Cryptococcosis
Loboi B48.Ø
North American B4Ø.9
South American —*see* Paracoccidioidomycosis
bleb, postprocedure —*see* Blebitis
bone —*see* Osteomyelitis
Bordetella —*see* Whooping cough
Borrelia bergdorfi A69.2Ø
brain —*see also* Encephalitis GØ4.9Ø
membranes —*see* Meningitis
septic GØ6.Ø
meninges —*see* Meningitis, bacterial
branchial cyst Q18.Ø
breast —*see* Mastitis
bronchus —*see* Bronchitis
Brucella A23.9
abortus A23.1
canis A23.3
melitensis A23.Ø
mixed A23.8
specified NEC A23.8
suis A23.2
Brugia (malayi) B74.1
timori B74.2
bursa —*see* Bursitis, infective
buttocks (skin) LØ8.9
Campylobacter, intestinal AØ4.5
as cause of disease classified elsewhere B96.81
Candida (albicans) (tropicalis) —*see* Candidiasis
candiru B88.8
Capillaria (intestinal) B81.1
hepatica B83.8
philippinensis B81.1
cartilage —*see* Disorder, cartilage, specified type NEC
catheter-related bloodstream (CRBSI) T8Ø.211
cat liver fluke B66.Ø
cellulitis - code by site under Cellulitis
central line-associated T8Ø.219
bloodstream (CLABSI) T8Ø.211
specified NEC T8Ø.218

Infection, infected, infective *(Continued)*
Cephalosporium falciforme B47.Ø
cerebrospinal —*see* Meningitis
cervical gland (lymph) LØ4.Ø
cervix —*see* Cervicitis
cesarean delivery wound (puerperal) O86.ØØ
cestodes —*see* Infestation, cestodes
chest J22
Chilomastix (intestinal) AØ7.8
Chlamydia, chlamydial A74.9
anus A56.3
genitourinary tract A56.2
lower A56.ØØ
specified NEC A56.19
lymphogranuloma A55
pharynx A56.4
psittaci A7Ø
rectum A56.3
sexually transmitted NEC A56.8
cholera —*see* Cholera
Cladosporium
bantianum (brain abscess) B43.1
carrionii B43.Ø
castellanii B36.1
trichoides (brain abscess) B43.1
werneckii B36.1
Clonorchis (sinensis) (liver) B66.1
Clostridium NEC
bifermentans A48.Ø
botulinum (food poisoning) AØ5.1
infant A48.51
wound A48.52
difficile
as cause of disease classified elsewhere B96.89
foodborne (disease)
not specified as recurrent AØ4.72
recurrent AØ4.71
gas gangrene A48.Ø
necrotizing enterocolitis
not specified as recurrent AØ4.72
recurrent AØ4.71
sepsis A41.4
gas-forming NEC A48.Ø
histolyticum A48.Ø
novyi, causing gas gangrene A48.Ø
oedematiens A48.Ø
perfringens
as cause of disease classified elsewhere B96.7
due to food AØ5.2
foodborne (disease) AØ5.2
gas gangrene A48.Ø
sepsis A41.4
septicum, causing gas gangrene A48.Ø
sordellii, causing gas gangrene A48.Ø
welchii
as cause of disease classified elsewhere B96.7
foodborne (disease) AØ5.2
gas gangrene A48.Ø
necrotizing enteritis AØ5.2
sepsis A41.4
Coccidioides (immitis) —*see* Coccidioidomycosis
colon —*see* Enteritis, infectious
colostomy K94.Ø2
common duct —*see* Cholangitis
congenital P39.9
Candida (albicans) P37.5
cytomegalovirus P35.1
hepatitis, viral P35.3
herpes simplex P35.2
infectious or parasitic disease P37.9
specified NEC P37.8
listeriosis (disseminated) P37.2
malaria NEC P37.4
falciparum P37.3
Plasmodium falciparum P37.3
poliomyelitis P35.8
rubella P35.Ø

Infection, infected, infective *(Continued)*
congenital *(Continued)*
skin P39.4
toxoplasmosis (acute) (subacute) (chronic) P37.1
tuberculosis P37.Ø
urinary (tract) P39.3
vaccinia P35.8
virus P35.9
specified type NEC P35.8
Conidiobolus B46.8
coronavirus NEC B34.2
as cause of disease classified elsewhere B97.29
severe acute respiratory syndrome (SARS associated) B97.21
corpus luteum —*see* Salpingo-oophoritis
Corynebacterium diphtheriae —*see* Diphtheria
cotia virus BØ8.8
Coxiella burnetii A78
coxsackie —*see* Coxsackie
Cryptococcus neoformans —*see* Cryptococcosis
Cryptosporidium AØ7.2
Cunninghamella —*see* Mucormycosis
cyst —*see* Cyst
cystic duct —*see also* Cholecystitis K81.9
Cysticercus cellulosae —*see* Cysticercosis
cytomegalovirus, cytomegaloviral B25.9
congenital P35.1
maternal, maternal care for (suspected) damage to fetus O35.3
mononucleosis B27.1Ø
with
complication NEC B27.19
meningitis B27.12
polyneuropathy B27.11
delta-agent (acute), in hepatitis B carrier B17.Ø
dental (pulpal origin) KØ4.7
Deuteromycetes B47.Ø
Dicrocoelium dendriticum B66.2
Dipetalonema (perstans) (streptocerca) B74.4
diphtherial —*see* Diphtheria
Diphyllobothrium (adult) (latum) (pacificum) B7Ø.Ø
larval B7Ø.1
Diplogonoporus (grandis) B71.8
Dipylidium caninum B67.4
Dirofilaria B74.8
Dracunculus medinensis B72
Drechslera (hawaiiensis) B43.8
Ducrey Haemophilus (any location) A57
due to or resulting from
artificial insemination N98.Ø
central venous catheter T8Ø.219
bloodstream T8Ø.211
exit or insertion site T8Ø.212
localized T8Ø.212
port or reservoir T8Ø.212
specified NEC T8Ø.218
tunnel T8Ø.212
device, implant or graft —*see also* Complications, by site and type, infection or inflammation T85.79
arterial graft NEC T82.7
breast (implant) T85.79
catheter NEC T85.79
dialysis (renal) T82.7
intraperitoneal T85.71
infusion NEC T82.7
cranial T85.735
intrathecal T85.735
spinal (epidural) (subdural) T85.735
subarachnoid T85.735
urinary T83.518
cystostomy T83.51Ø
Hopkins T83.518
ileostomy T83.518
nephrostomy T83.512
specified NEC T83.518
urethral indwelling T83.511
urostomy T83.518

Infection, infected, infective *(Continued)*
  due to or resulting from *(Continued)*
    device, implant or graft *(Continued)*
      electronic (electrode) (pulse generator)
        (stimulator)
        bone T84.7
        cardiac T82.7
        nervous system T85.738
          brain T85.731
          cranial nerve T85.732
          gastric nerve T85.732
          generator pocket T85.734
          neurostimulator generator T85.734
          peripheral nerve T85.732
          sacral nerve T85.732
          spinal cord T85.733
          vagal nerve T85.732
        urinary T83.590
      fixation, internal (orthopedic) NEC —
        see Complication, fixation device,
        infection
      gastrointestinal (bile duct) (esophagus)
        T85.79
        neurostimulator electrode (lead)
          T85.732
      genital NEC T83.69
      heart NEC T82.7
        valve (prosthesis) T82.6
        graft T82.7
      joint prosthesis —*see* Complication, joint
        prosthesis, infection
      ocular (corneal graft) (orbital implant)
        NEC T85.79
      orthopedic NEC T84.7
      penile (cylinder) (pump) (resevoir) T83.61
      specified NEC T85.79
      testicular T83.62
      urinary NEC T83.598
        ileal conduit stent T83.593
        implanted neurostimulation T83.590
        implanted sphincter T83.591
        indwelling ureteral stent T83.592
        nephroureteral stent T83.593
        specified stent NEC T83.593
      vascular NEC T82.7
      ventricular intracranial (communicating)
        shunt T85.730
    Hickman catheter T80.219
      bloodstream T80.211
      localized T80.212
      specified NEC T80.218
    immunization or vaccination T88.0
    infusion, injection or transfusion NEC
      T80.29
      acute T80.22
    injury NEC - code by site under Wound,
      open
    peripherally inserted central catheter
      (PICC) T80.219
      bloodstream T80.211
      localized T80.212
      specified NEC T80.218
    portacath (port-a-cath) T80.219
      bloodstream T80.211
      localized T80.212
      specified NEC T80.218
    pulmonary artery catheter —*see* Infection,
      due to or resulting from, central
      venous catheter
    surgery T81.40
    Swan Ganz catheter —*see* Infection, due
      to or resulting from, central venous
      catheter
    triple lumen catheter T80.219
      bloodstream T80.211
      localized T80.212
      specified NEC T80.218
    umbilical venous catheter T80.219
      bloodstream T80.211
      localized T80.212
      specified NEC T80.218

Infection, infected, infective *(Continued)*
  during labor NEC O75.3
  ear (middle) —*see also* Otitis media
    external —*see* Otitis, externa, infective
    inner —*see* subcategory H83.0
  Eberthella typhosa A01.00
  Echinococcus —*see* Echinococcus
  echovirus
    as cause of disease classified elsewhere
      B97.12
    unspecified nature or site B34.1
  endocardium I33.0
  endocervix —*see* Cervicitis
  Entamoeba —*see* Amebiasis
  enteric —*see* Enteritis, infectious
  Enterobacter sakazakii B96.89
  Enterobius vermicularis B80
  enterostomy K94.12
  enterovirus B34.1
    as cause of disease classified elsewhere
      B97.10
      coxsackievirus B97.11
      echovirus B97.12
      specified NEC B97.19
  Entomophthora B46.8
  Epidermophyton —*see* Dermatophytosis
  epididymis —*see* Epididymitis
  episiotomy (puerperal) O86.09
  Erysipelothrix (insidiosa) (rhusiopathiae) —
    see Erysipeloid
  erythema infectiosum B08.3
  Escherichia (E.) coli NEC A49.8
    as cause of disease classified elsewhere —
      see also Escherichia coli B96.20
    congenital P39.8
      sepsis P36.4
    generalized A41.51
    intestinal —*see* Enteritis, infectious, due to,
      Escherichia coli
  ethmoidal (chronic) (sinus) —*see* Sinusitis,
    ethmoidal
  eustachian tube (ear) —*see* Salpingitis,
    eustachian
  external auditory canal (meatus) NEC —*see*
    Otitis, externa, infective
  eye (purulent) —*see* Endophthalmitis, purulent
  eyelid —*see* Inflammation, eyelid
  fallopian tube —*see* Salpingo-oophoritis
  Fasciola (gigantica) (hepatica) (indica) B66.3
  Fasciolopsis (buski) B66.5
  filarial —*see* Infestation, filarial
  finger (skin) L08.9
    nail L03.01-●
      fungus B35.1
  fish tapeworm B70.0
    larval B70.1
  flagellate, intestinal A07.9
  fluke —*see* Infestation, fluke
  focal
    teeth (pulpal origin) K04.7
    tonsils J35.01
  Fonsecaea (compactum) (pedrosoi) B43.0
  food —*see* Intoxication, foodborne
  foot (skin) L08.9
    dermatophytic fungus B35.3
  Francisella tularensis —*see* Tularemia
  frontal (sinus) (chronic) —*see* Sinusitis, frontal
  fungus NOS B49
    beard B35.0
    dermatophytic —*see* Dermatophytosis
    foot B35.3
    groin B35.6
    hand B35.2
    nail B35.1
    pathogenic to compromised host only B48.8
    perianal (area) B35.6
    scalp B35.0
    skin B36.9
      foot B35.3
      hand B35.2
      toenails B35.1

Infection, infected, infective *(Continued)*
  Fusarium B48.8
  gallbladder —*see* Cholecystitis
  gas bacillus —*see* Gangrene, gas
  gastrointestinal —*see* Enteritis, infectious
  generalized NEC —*see* Sepsis
  generator pocket, implanted electronic
    neurostimulator T85.734
  genital organ or tract
    female —*see* Disease, pelvis, inflammatory
    male N49.9
      multiple sites N49.8
      specified NEC N49.8
  Ghon tubercle, primary A15.7
  Giardia lamblia A07.1
  gingiva (chronic) K05.10
    acute K05.10
      nonplaque induced K05.01
      plaque induced K05.00
    nonplaque induced K05.11
    plaque induced K05.10
  glanders A24.0
  glenosporopsis B48.0
  Gnathostoma (spinigerum) B83.1
  Gongylonema B83.8
  gonococcal —*see* Gonococcus
  gram-negative bacilli NOS A49.9
  guinea worm B72
  gum (chronic) K05.10
    acute K05.00
      nonplaque induced K05.01
      plaque induced K05.00
    nonplaque induced K05.11
    plaque induced K05.10
  Haemophilus —*see* Infection, Hemophilus
  heart —*see* Carditis
  Helicobacter pylori A04.8
    as cause of disease classified elsewhere
      B96.81
  helminths B83.9
    intestinal B82.0
      mixed (types classifiable to more than
        one of the titles B65.0-B81.3 and
        B81.8) B81.4
      specified type NEC B81.8
    specified type NEC B83.8
  Hemophilus
    aegyptius, systemic A48.4
    ducrey (any location) A57
    generalized A41.3
    influenzae NEC A49.2
      as cause of disease classified elsewhere
        B96.3
  herpes (simplex) —*see also* Herpes
    congenital P35.2
    disseminated B00.7
    zoster B02.9
  herpesvirus, herpesviral —*see* Herpes
  Heterophyes (heterophyes) B66.8
  hip (joint) NEC M00.9
    due to internal joint prosthesis
      left T84.52
      right T84.51
    skin NEC L08.9
  Histoplasma —*see* Histoplasmosis
    American B39.4
    capsulatum B39.4
  hookworm B76.9
  human
    papilloma virus A63.0
    T-cell lymphotropic virus type-1 (HTLV-1)
      B33.3
  hydrocele N43.0
  Hymenolepis B71.0
  hypopharynx —*see* Pharyngitis
  inguinal (lymph) glands L04.1
    due to soft chancre A57
  intervertebral disc, pyogenic M46.30
    cervical region M46.32
    cervicothoracic region M46.33
    lumbar region M46.36

▶ New   ⇒ Revised   ~~deleted~~ Deleted   ● Use Additional Character(s)

Infection, infected, infective *(Continued)*
intervertebral disc, pyogenic *(Continued)*
lumbosacral region M46.37
multiple sites M46.39
occipito-atlanto-axial region M46.31
sacrococcygeal region M46.38
thoracic region M46.34
thoracolumbar region M46.35
intestine, intestinal —*see* Enteritis, infectious
specified NEC A08.8
intra-amniotic affecting newborn NEC P39.2
Isospora belli or hominis A07.3
Japanese B encephalitis A83.0
jaw (bone) (lower) (upper) M27.2
joint NEC M00.9
due to internal joint prosthesis T84.50
kidney (cortex) (hematogenous) N15.9
with calculus N20.0
with hydronephrosis N13.6
following ectopic gestation O08.83
pelvis and ureter (cystic) N28.85
puerperal (postpartum) O86.21
specified NEC N15.8
Klebsiella (K.) pneumoniae NEC A49.8
as cause of disease classified elsewhere B96.1
knee (joint) NEC M00.9
due to internal joint prosthesis
left T84.54
right T84.53
joint M00.9
skin L08.9
Koch's —*see* Tuberculosis
labia (majora) (minora) (acute) —*see* Vulvitis
lacrimal
gland —*see* Dacryoadenitis
passages (duct) (sac) —*see* Inflammation, lacrimal, passages
lancet fluke B66.2
larynx NEC J38.7
leg (skin) NOS L08.9
Legionella pneumophila A48.1
nonpneumonic A48.2
Leishmania —*see also* Leishmaniasis
aethiopica B55.1
braziliensis B55.2
chagasi B55.0
donovani B55.0
infantum B55.0
major B55.1
mexicana B55.1
tropica B55.1
lentivirus, as cause of disease classified elsewhere B97.31
Leptosphaeria senegalensis B47.0
Leptospira interrogans A27.9
autumnalis A27.89
canicola A27.89
hebdomadis A27.89
icterohaemorrhagiae A27.0
pomona A27.89
specified type NEC A27.89
leptospirochetal NEC —*see* Leptospirosis
Listeria monocytogenes —*see also* Listeriosis
congenital P37.2
Loa loa B74.3
with conjunctival infestation B74.3
eyelid B74.3
Loboa loboi B48.0
local, skin (staphylococcal) (streptococcal) L08.9
abscess - code by site under Abscess
cellulitis - code by site under Cellulitis
specified NEC L08.89
ulcer —*see* Ulcer, skin
Loefflerella mallei A24.0
lung —*see also* Pneumonia J18.9
atypical Mycobacterium A31.0
spirochetal A69.8
tuberculous —*see* Tuberculosis, pulmonary
virus —*see* Pneumonia, viral

Infection, infected, infective *(Continued)*
lymph gland —*see also* Lymphadenitis, acute
mesenteric I88.0
lymphoid tissue, base of tongue or posterior pharynx, NEC (chronic) J35.03
Madurella (grisea) (mycetomii) B47.0
major
following ectopic or molar pregnancy O08.0
puerperal, postpartum, childbirth O85
Malassezia furfur B36.0
Malleomyces
mallei A24.0
pseudomallei (whitmori) —*see* Melioidosis
mammary gland N61.0
Mansonella (ozzardi) (perstans) (streptocerca) B74.4
mastoid —*see* Mastoiditis
maxilla, maxillary M27.2
sinus (chronic) —*see* Sinusitis, maxillary
mediastinum J98.51
Medina (worm) B72
meibomian cyst or gland —*see* Hordeolum
meninges —*see* Meningitis, bacterial
meningococcal —*see also* condition A39.9
adrenals A39.1
brain A39.81
cerebrospinal A39.0
conjunctiva A39.89
endocardium A39.51
heart A39.50
endocardium A39.51
myocardium A39.52
pericardium A39.53
joint A39.83
meninges A39.0
meningococcemia A39.4
acute A39.2
chronic A39.3
myocardium A39.52
pericardium A39.53
retrobulbar neuritis A39.82
specified site NEC A39.89
mesenteric lymph nodes or glands NEC I88.0
Metagonimus B66.8
metatarsophalangeal M00.9
methicillin
resistant Staphylococcus aureus (MRSA) A49.02
susceptible Staphylococcus aureus (MSSA) A49.01
Microsporum, microsporic —*see* Dermatophytosis
mixed flora (bacterial) NEC A49.8
Monilia —*see* Candidiasis
Monosporium apiospermum B48.2
mouth, parasitic B37.0
Mucor —*see* Mucormycosis
muscle NEC —*see* Myositis, infective
mycelium NOS B49
mycetoma B47.9
actinomycotic NEC B47.1
mycotic NEC B47.0
Mycobacterium, mycobacterial —*see* Mycobacterium
Mycoplasma NEC A49.3
pneumoniae, as cause of disease classified elsewhere B96.0
mycotic NOS B49
pathogenic to compromised host only B48.8
skin NOS B36.9
myocardium NEC I40.0
nail (chronic)
with lymphangitis —*see* Lymphangitis, acute, digit
finger L03.01-●
fungus B35.1
ingrowing L60.0
toe L03.03-●
fungus B35.1

Infection, infected, infective *(Continued)*
nasal sinus (chronic) —*see* Sinusitis
nasopharynx —*see* Nasopharyngitis
navel L08.82
Necator americanus B76.1
Neisseria —*see* Gonococcus
Neotestudina rosatii B47.0
newborn P39.9
intra-amniotic NEC P39.2
skin P39.4
specified type NEC P39.8
nipple N61.0
associated with
lactation O91.03
pregnancy O91.01-●
puerperium O91.02
Nocardia —*see* Nocardiosis
obstetrical surgical wound (puerperal) O86.00
incisional site
deep O86.02
superficial O86.01
organ and space site O86.03
surgical site specified NEC O86.09
Oesophagostomum (apiostomum) B81.8
Oestrus ovis —*see* Myiasis
Oidium albicans B37.9
Onchocerca (volvulus) —*see* Onchocerciasis - oncovirus, as cause of disease classified elsewhere B97.32
operation wound T81.49
Opisthorchis (felineus) (viverrini) B66.0
orbit, orbital —*see* Inflammation, orbit
orthopoxvirus NEC B08.09
ovary —*see* Salpingo-oophoritis
Oxyuris vermicularis B80
pancreas (acute) —*see* Pancreatitis, acute
abscess —*see* Pancreatitis, acute
specified NEC —*see also* Pancreatitis, acute K85.80
papillomavirus, as cause of disease classified elsewhere B97.7
papovavirus NEC B34.4
Paracoccidioides brasiliensis —*see* Paracoccidioidomycosis
Paragonimus (westermani) B66.4
parainfluenza virus B34.8
parameningococcus NOS A39.9
parapoxvirus B08.60
specified NEC B08.69
parasitic B89
Parastrongylus
cantonensis B83.2
costaricensis B81.3
paratyphoid A01.4
Type A A01.1
Type B A01.2
Type C A01.3
paraurethral ducts N34.2
parotid gland —*see* Sialoadenitis
parvovirus NEC B34.3
as cause of disease classified elsewhere B97.6
Pasteurella NEC A28.0
multocida A28.0
pestis —*see* Plague
pseudotuberculosis A28.0
septica (cat bite) (dog bite) A28.0
tularensis —*see* Tularemia
pelvic, female —*see* Disease, pelvis, inflammatory
Penicillium (marneffei) B48.4
penis (glans) (retention) NEC N48.29
periapical K04.5
peridental, periodontal K05.20
generalized —*see* Periodontitis, aggressive, generalized
localized —*see* Periodontitis, aggressive, localized
perinatal period P39.9
specified type NEC P39.8
perineal repair (puerperal) O86.09

- **Infection, infected, infective** *(Continued)*
  - periorbital —*see* Inflammation, orbit
  - perirectal K62.89
  - perirenal —*see* Infection, kidney
  - peritoneal —*see* Peritonitis
  - periureteral N28.89
  - Petriellidium boydii B48.2
  - pharynx —*see also* Pharyngitis
    - coxsackievirus BØ8.5
    - posterior, lymphoid (chronic) J35.Ø3
  - Phialophora
    - gougerotii (subcutaneous abscess or cyst) B43.2
    - jeanselmei (subcutaneous abscess or cyst) B43.2
    - verrucosa (skin) B43.Ø
  - Piedraia hortae B36.3
  - pinta A67.9
    - intermediate A67.1
    - late A67.2
    - mixed A67.3
    - primary A67.Ø
  - pinworm B8Ø
  - pityrosporum furfur B36.Ø
  - pleuro-pneumonia-like organism (PPLO) NEC A49.3
    - as cause of disease classified elsewhere B96.Ø
  - pneumococcus, pneumococcal NEC A49.1
    - as cause of disease classified elsewhere B95.3
    - generalized (purulent) A4Ø.3
      - with pneumonia J13
  - Pneumocystis carinii (pneumonia) B59
  - Pneumocystis jiroveci (pneumonia) B59
  - port or reservoir T8Ø.212
  - postoperative T81.4Ø
  - postoperative wound T81.49
  - postprocedural T81.4Ø
    - surgical site
      - deep incisional T81.42
      - organ and space T81.43
      - specified NEC T81.49
      - superficial incisional T81.41
  - postvaccinal T88.Ø
  - prepuce NEC N47.7
    - with penile inflammation N47.6
  - prion —*see* Disease, prion, central nervous system
  - prostate (capsule) —*see* Prostatitis
  - Proteus (mirabilis) (morganii) (vulgaris) NEC A49.8
    - as cause of disease classified elsewhere B96.4
  - protozoal NEC B64
    - intestinal AØ7.9
      - specified NEC AØ7.8
    - specified NEC B6Ø.8
  - Pseudoallescheria boydii B48.2
  - Pseudomonas NEC A49.8
    - as cause of disease classified elsewhere B96.5
    - mallei A24.Ø
    - pneumonia J15.1
    - pseudomallei —*see* Melioidosis
  - puerperal O86.4
    - genitourinary tract NEC O86.89
    - major or generalized O85
    - minor O86.4
    - specified NEC O86.89
  - pulmonary —*see* Infection, lung
  - purulent —*see* Abscess
  - Pyrenochaeta romeroi B47.Ø
  - Q fever A78
  - rectum (sphincter) K62.89
  - renal —*see also* Infection, kidney
    - pelvis and ureter (cystic) N28.85
  - reovirus, as cause of disease classified elsewhere B97.5
  - respiratory (tract) NEC J98.8
    - acute J22
    - chronic J98.8

- **Infection, infected, infective** *(Continued)*
  - respiratory (tract) NEC *(Continued)*
    - influenzal (upper) (acute) —*see* Influenza, with, respiratory manifestations NEC
    - lower (acute) J22
      - chronic —*see* Bronchitis, chronic
    - rhinovirus JØØ
    - ~~syncytial virus, as cause of disease classified elsewhere B97.4~~
    - ▶syncytial virus (RSV) —*see* Infection, virus, respiratory syncytial (RSV)
    - upper (acute) NOS JØ6.9
      - chronic J39.8
      - streptococcal JØ6.9
      - viral NOS JØ6.9
        - ▶due to respiratory syncytial virus (RSV) JØ6.9 *[B97.1]*
  - resulting from
    - presence of internal prosthesis, implant, graft —*see* Complications, by site and type, infection
  - retortamoniasis AØ7.8
  - retroperitoneal NEC K68.9
  - retrovirus B33.3
    - as cause of disease classified elsewhere B97.3Ø
      - human
        - immunodeficiency, type 2 (HIV 2) B97.35
        - T-cell lymphotropic
          - type I (HTLV-I) B97.33
          - type II (HTLV-II) B97.34
      - lentivirus B97.31
      - oncovirus B97.32
      - specified NEC B97.39
  - Rhinosporidium (seeberi) B48.1
  - rhinovirus
    - as cause of disease classified elsewhere B97.89
    - unspecified nature or site B34.8
  - Rhizopus —*see* Mucormycosis
  - rickettsial NOS A79.9
  - roundworm (large) NEC B82.Ø
    - Ascariasis —*see also* Ascariasis B77.9
  - rubella —*see* Rubella
  - Saccharomyces —*see* Candidiasis
  - salivary duct or gland (any) —*see* Sialoadenitis
  - Salmonella (aertrycke) (arizonae) (callinarum) (cholerae-suis) (enteritidis) (suipestifer) (typhimurium) AØ2.9
    - with
      - (gastro) enteritis AØ2.Ø
      - sepsis AØ2.1
      - specified manifestation NEC AØ2.8
    - due to food (poisoning) AØ2.9
    - hirschfeldii AØ1.3
    - localized AØ2.2Ø
      - arthritis AØ2.23
      - meningitis AØ2.21
      - osteomyelitis AØ2.24
      - pneumonia AØ2.22
      - pyelonephritis AØ2.25
      - specified NEC AØ2.29
    - paratyphi AØ1.4
      - A AØ1.1
      - B AØ1.2
      - C AØ1.3
    - schottmuelleri AØ1.2
    - typhi, typhosa —*see* Typhoid
  - Sarcocystis AØ7.8
  - scabies B86
  - Schistosoma —*see* Infestation, Schistosoma
  - scrotum (acute) NEC N49.2
  - seminal vesicle —*see* Vesiculitis
  - septic
    - localized, skin —*see* Abscess
  - sheep liver fluke B66.3
  - Shigella AØ3.9
    - boydii AØ3.2
    - dysenteriae AØ3.Ø
    - flexneri AØ3.1

- **Infection, infected, infective** *(Continued)*
  - Shigella *(Continued)*
    - group
      - A AØ3.Ø
      - B AØ3.1
      - C AØ3.2
      - D AØ3.3
    - Schmitz (-Stutzer) AØ3.Ø
    - schmitzii AØ3.Ø
    - shigae AØ3.Ø
    - sonnei AØ3.3
    - specified NEC AØ3.8
  - shoulder (joint) NEC MØØ.9
    - due to internal joint prosthesis T84.59
    - skin NEC LØ8.9
  - sinus (accessory) (chronic) (nasal) —*see also* Sinusitis
    - pilonidal —*see* Sinus, pilonidal
    - skin NEC LØ8.89
  - Skene's duct or gland —*see* Urethritis
  - skin (local) (staphylococcal) (streptococcal) LØ8.9
    - abscess - code by site under Abscess
    - cellulitis - code by site under Cellulitis
    - due to fungus B36.9
      - specified type NEC B36.8
    - mycotic B36.9
      - specified type NEC B36.8
    - newborn P39.4
    - ulcer —*see* Ulcer, skin
  - slow virus A81.9
    - specified NEC A81.89
  - Sparganum (mansoni) (proliferum) (baxteri) B7Ø.1
  - specific —*see also* Syphilis
    - to perinatal period —*see* Infection, congenital
  - specified NEC B99.8
  - spermatic cord NEC N49.1
  - sphenoidal (sinus) —*see* Sinusitis, sphenoidal
  - spinal cord NOS —*see also* Myelitis GØ4.91
    - abscess GØ6.1
    - meninges —*see* Meningitis
    - streptococcal GØ4.89
  - Spirillum A25.Ø
  - spirochetal NOS A69.9
    - lung A69.8
    - specified NEC A69.8
  - Spirometra larvae B7Ø.1
  - spleen D73.89
  - Sporotrichum, Sporothrix (schenckii) —*see* Sporotrichosis
  - staphylococcal, unspecified site
    - aureus (methicillin susceptible) (MSSA) A49.Ø1
      - methicillin resistant (MRSA) A49.Ø2
    - as cause of disease classified elsewhere B95.8
      - aureus (methicillin susceptible) (MSSA) B95.61
        - methicillin resistant (MRSA) B95.62
      - specified NEC B95.7
    - food poisoning AØ5.Ø
    - generalized (purulent) A41.2
    - pneumonia —*see* Pneumonia, staphylococcal
  - Stellantchasmus falcatus B66.8
  - streptobacillus moniliformis A25.1
  - streptococcal NEC A49.1
    - as cause of disease classified elsewhere B95.5
    - B genitourinary complicating
      - childbirth O98.82
      - pregnancy O98.81-●
      - puerperium O98.83
    - congenital
      - sepsis P36.1Ø
        - group B P36.Ø
        - specified NEC P36.19
    - generalized (purulent) A4Ø.9

▶ New ➠ Revised ~~deleted~~ Deleted ● Use Additional Character(s)

- Infection, infected, infective *(Continued)*
  - Streptomyces B47.1
  - Strongyloides (stercoralis) —*see* Strongyloidiasis
  - stump (amputation) (surgical) —*see* Complication, amputation stump, infection
  - subcutaneous tissue, local L08.9
  - suipestifer —*see* Infection, salmonella
  - swimming pool bacillus A31.1
  - Taenia —*see* Infestation, Taenia
  - Taeniarhynchus saginatus B68.1
  - tapeworm —*see* Infestation, tapeworm
  - tendon (sheath) —*see* Tenosynovitis, infective NEC
  - Ternidens diminutus B81.8
  - testis —*see* Orchitis
  - threadworm B80
  - throat —*see* Pharyngitis
  - thyroglossal duct K14.8
  - toe (skin) L08.9
    - cellulitis L03.03-●
      - fungus B35.1
    - nail L03.03-●
      - fungus B35.1
  - tongue NEC K14.0
    - parasitic B37.0
  - tonsil (and adenoid) (faucial) (lingual) (pharyngeal) —*see* Tonsillitis
  - tooth, teeth K04.7
    - irreversible K04.02
    - periapical K04.7
    - peridental, periodontal K05.20
      - ➠generalized —*see* Periodontitis, aggressive, generalized
      - ➠localized —*see* Periodontitis, aggressive, localized
    - pulp K04.01
      - irreversible K04.02
      - reversible K04.01
  - TORCH —*see* Infection, congenital
    - without active infection P00.2
  - Torula histolytica —*see* Cryptococcosis
  - Toxocara (canis) (cati) (felis) B83.0
  - Toxoplasma gondii —*see* Toxoplasma
  - trachea, chronic J42
  - trematode NEC —*see* Infestation, fluke
  - trench fever A79.0
  - Treponema pallidum —*see* Syphilis
  - Trichinella (spiralis) B75
  - Trichomonas A59.9
    - cervix A59.09
    - intestine A07.8
    - prostate A59.02
    - specified site NEC A59.8
    - urethra A59.03
    - urogenitalis A59.00
    - vagina A59.01
    - vulva A59.01
  - Trichophyton, trichophytic —*see* Dermatophytosis
  - Trichosporon (beigelii) cutaneum B36.2
  - Trichostrongylus B81.2
  - Trichuris (trichiura) B79
  - Trombicula (irritans) B88.0
  - Trypanosoma
    - brucei
      - gambiense B56.0
      - rhodesiense B56.1
    - cruzi —*see* Chagas' disease
  - tubal —*see* Salpingo-oophoritis
  - ➠tuberculous
    - ▶latent (LTBI) Z22.7
    - ▶NEC —*see* Tuberculosis
  - tubo-ovarian —*see* Salpingo-oophoritis
  - tunica vaginalis N49.1
  - tunnel T80.212
  - tympanic membrane NEC —*see* Myringitis
  - typhoid (abortive) (ambulant) (bacillus) —*see* Typhoid
  - typhus A75.9
    - flea-borne A75.2
    - mite-borne A75.3
    - recrudescent A75.1
    - tick-borne A77.9
      - African A77.1
      - North Asian A77.2
  - umbilicus L08.82
  - ➠ureter —*see* Ureteritis
  - urethra —*see* Urethritis
  - urinary (tract) N39.0
    - bladder —*see* Cystitis
    - complicating
      - pregnancy O23.4-●
        - specified type NEC O23.3-●
    - kidney —*see* Infection, kidney
    - newborn P39.3
    - puerperal (postpartum) O86.20
    - tuberculous A18.13
    - urethra —*see* Urethritis
  - uterus, uterine —*see* Endometritis
  - vaccination T88.0
  - vaccinia not from vaccination B08.011
  - vagina (acute) —*see* Vaginitis
  - varicella B01.9
  - varicose veins —*see* Varix
  - vas deferens NEC N49.1
  - vesical —*see* Cystitis
  - Vibrio
    - cholerae A00.0
      - El Tor A00.1
    - parahaemolyticus (food poisoning) A05.3
    - vulnificus
      - as cause of disease classified elsewhere B96.82
      - foodborne intoxication A05.5
  - Vincent's (gum) (mouth) (tonsil) A69.1
  - virus, viral NOS B34.9
    - adenovirus
      - as cause of disease classified elsewhere B97.0
      - unspecified nature or site B34.0
    - arborvirus, arbovirus arthropod-borne A94
    - as cause of disease classified elsewhere B97.89
      - adenovirus B97.0
      - coronavirus B97.29
        - SARS-associated B97.21
      - coxsackievirus B97.11
      - echovirus B97.12
      - enterovirus B97.10
        - coxsackievirus B97.11
        - echovirus B97.12
        - specified NEC B97.19
      - human
        - immunodeficiency, type 2 (HIV 2) B97.35
        - metapneumovirus B97.81
        - T-cell lymphotropic,
          - type I (HTLV-I) B97.33
          - type II (HTLV-II) B97.34
      - papillomavirus B97.7
      - parvovirus B97.6
      - reovirus B97.5
      - ➠respiratory syncytial (RSV) —*see* Infection virus, respiratory syncytial (RSV)
      - retrovirus B97.30
        - human
          - immunodeficiency, type 2 (HIV 2) B97.35
          - T-cell lymphotropic,
            - type I (HTLV-I) B97.33
            - type II (HTLV-II) B97.34
        - lentivirus B97.31
        - oncovirus B97.32
        - specified NEC B97.39
      - specified NEC B97.89
    - central nervous system A89
      - atypical A81.9
        - specified NEC A81.89
      - enterovirus NEC A88.8
        - meningitis A87.0
      - slow virus A81.9
        - specified NEC A81.89
      - specified NEC A88.8
    - chest J98.8
    - cotia B08.8
    - coxsackie —*see also* Infection, coxsackie B34.1
      - as cause of disease classified elsewhere B97.11
    - ECHO
      - as cause of disease classified elsewhere B97.12
      - unspecified nature or site B34.1
    - encephalitis, tick-borne A84.9
    - enterovirus, as cause of disease classified elsewhere B97.10
      - coxsackievirus B97.11
      - echovirus B97.12
      - specified NEC B97.19
    - exanthem NOS B09
    - human metapneumovirus as cause of disease classified elsewhere B97.81
    - human papilloma as cause of disease classified elsewhere B97.7
    - intestine —*see* Enteritis, viral
    - ➠respiratory syncytial (RSV) —*see* Infection virus, respiratory syncytial (RSV)
      - ~~as cause of disease classified elsewhere B97.4~~
      - ▶bronchiolitis J21.0
      - ▶bronchitis J20.5
      - bronchopneumonia J12.1
      - ~~common cold syndrome J00~~
      - ~~nasopharyngitis (acute) J00~~
      - ▶otitis media H65.-● *[B97.4]*
      - ▶pneumonia J12.1
      - ▶upper respiratory infection J06.9 *[B97.4]*
    - rhinovirus
      - as cause of disease classified elsewhere B97.89
      - unspecified nature or site B34.8
    - slow A81.9
      - specified NEC A81.89
    - specified type NEC B33.8
      - as cause of disease classified elsewhere B97.89
      - unspecified nature or site B34.8
    - unspecified nature or site B34.9
    - West Nile —*see* Virus, West Nile
  - vulva (acute) —*see* Vulvitis
  - West Nile —*see* Virus, West Nile
  - whipworm B79
  - worms B83.9
    - specified type NEC B83.8
  - Wuchereria (bancrofti) B74.0
    - malayi B74.1
    - yatapoxvirus B08.70
      - specified NEC B08.79
  - yeast (*see also* Candidiasis) B37.9
  - yellow fever —*see* Fever, yellow
  - Yersinia
    - enterocolitica (intestinal) A04.6
    - pestis —*see* Plague
    - pseudotuberculosis A28.2
  - Zeis' gland —*see* Hordeolum
  - Zika virus A92.5
    - congenital P35.4
  - zoonotic bacterial NOS A28.9
  - Zopfia senegalensis B47.0
- Infective, infectious —*see* condition
- Infertility
  - female N97.9
    - age-related N97.8
    - associated with
      - anovulation N97.0
      - cervical (mucus) disease or anomaly N88.3

Infertility *(Continued)*
female *(Continued)*
associated with *(Continued)*
congenital anomaly
cervix N88.3
fallopian tube N97.1
uterus N97.2
vagina N97.8
dysmucorrhea N88.3
fallopian tube disease or anomaly N97.1
pituitary-hypothalamic origin E23.Ø
specified origin NEC N97.8
Stein-Leventhal syndrome E28.2
uterine disease or anomaly N97.2
vaginal disease or anomaly N97.8
due to
cervical anomaly N88.3
fallopian tube anomaly N97.1
ovarian failure E28.39
Stein-Leventhal syndrome E28.2
uterine anomaly N97.2
vaginal anomaly N97.8
nonimplantation N97.2
origin
cervical N88.3
tubal (block) (occlusion) (stenosis) N97.1
uterine N97.2
vaginal N97.8
male N46.9
azoospermia N46.Ø1
extratesticular cause N46.Ø29
drug therapy N46.Ø21
efferent duct obstruction N46.Ø23
infection N46.Ø22
radiation N46.Ø24
specified cause NEC N46.Ø29
systemic disease N46.Ø25
oligospermia N46.11
extratesticular cause N46.129
drug therapy N46.121
efferent duct obstruction N46.123
infection N46.122
radiation N46.124
specified cause NEC N46.129
systemic disease N46.125
specified type NEC N46.8
Infestation B88.9
Acanthocheilonema (perstans) (streptocerca) B74.4
Acariasis B88.Ø
demodex folliculorum B88.Ø
sarcoptes scabiei B86
trombiculae B88.Ø
Agamofilaria streptocerca B74.4
Ancylostoma, ankylostoma (braziliense) (caninum) (ceylanicum) (duodenale) B76.Ø
americanum B76.1
new world B76.1
Anisakis larvae, anisakiasis B81.Ø
arthropod NEC B88.2
Ascaris lumbricoides —*see* Ascariasis
Balantidium coli AØ7.Ø
beef tapeworm B68.1
Bothriocephalus (latus) B7Ø.Ø
larval B7Ø.1
broad tapeworm B7Ø.Ø
larval B7Ø.1
Brugia (malayi) B74.1
timori B74.2
candiru B88.8
Capillaria
hepatica B83.8
philippinensis B81.1
cat liver fluke B66.Ø
cestodes B71.9
diphyllobothrium —*see* Infestation, diphyllobothrium
dipylidiasis B71.1
hymenolepiasis B71.Ø
specified type NEC B71.8

Infestation *(Continued)*
chigger B88.Ø
chigo, chigoe B88.1
Clonorchis (sinensis) (liver) B66.1
coccidial AØ7.3
crab-lice B85.3
Cysticercus cellulosae —*see* Cysticercosis
Demodex (folliculorum) B88.Ø
Dermanyssus gallinae B88.Ø
Dermatobia (hominis) —*see* Myiasis
Dibothriocephalus (latus) B7Ø.Ø
larval B7Ø.1
Dicrocoelium dendriticum B66.2
Diphyllobothrium (adult) (latum) (intestinal) (pacificum) B7Ø.Ø
larval B7Ø.1
Diplogonoporus (grandis) B71.8
Dipylidium caninum B67.4
Distoma hepaticum B66.3
dog tapeworm B67.4
Dracunculus medinensis B72
dragon worm B72
dwarf tapeworm B71.Ø
Echinococcus —*see* Echinococcus
Echinostomum ilocanum B66.8
Entamoeba (histolytica) —*see* Infection, Ameba
Enterobius vermicularis B8Ø
eyelid
in (due to)
leishmaniasis B55.1
loiasis B74.3
onchocerciasis B73.Ø9
phthiriasis B85.3
parasitic NOS B89
eyeworm B74.3
Fasciola (gigantica) (hepatica) (indica) B66.3
Fasciolopsis (buski) (intestine) B66.5
filarial B74.9
bancroftian B74.Ø
conjunctiva B74.9
due to
Acanthocheilonema (perstans) (streptocerca) B74.4
Brugia (malayi) B74.1
timori B74.2
Dracunculus medinensis B72
guinea worm B72
loa loa B74.3
Mansonella (ozzardi) (perstans) (streptocerca) B74.4
Onchocerca volvulus B73.ØØ
eye B73.ØØ
eyelid B73.Ø9
Wuchereria (bancrofti) B74.Ø
Malayan B74.1
ozzardi B74.4
specified type NEC B74.8
fish tapeworm B7Ø.Ø
larval B7Ø.1
fluke B66.9
blood NOS —*see* Schistosomiasis
cat liver B66.Ø
intestinal B66.5
lancet B66.2
liver (sheep) B66.3
cat B66.Ø
Chinese B66.1
due to clonorchiasis B66.1
oriental B66.1
lung (oriental) B66.4
sheep liver B66.3
specified type NEC B66.8
fly larvae —*see* Myiasis
Gasterophilus (intestinalis) —*see* Myiasis
Gastrodiscoides hominis B66.8
Giardia lamblia AØ7.1
Gnathostoma (spinigerum) B83.1
Gongylonema B83.8
guinea worm B72
helminth B83.9

Infestation *(Continued)*
helminth *(Continued)*
angiostrongyliasis B83.2
intestinal B81.3
gnathostomiasis B83.1
hirudiniasis, internal B83.4
intestinal B82.Ø
angiostrongyliasis B81.3
anisakiasis B81.Ø
ascariasis —*see* Ascariasis
capillariasis B81.1
cysticercosis —*see* Cysticercosis
diphyllobothriasis —*see* Infestation, diphyllobothriasis
dracunculiasis B72
echinococcus —*see* Echinococcosis
enterobiasis B8Ø
filariasis —*see* Infestation, filarial
fluke —*see* Infestation, fluke
hookworm —*see* Infestation, hookworm
mixed (types classifiable to more than one of the titles B65.Ø-B81.3 and B81.8) B81.4
onchocerciasis —*see* Onchocerciasis
schistosomiasis —*see* Infestation, schistosoma
specified
cestode NEC —*see* Infestation, cestode
type NEC B81.8
strongyloidiasis —*see* Strongyloidiasis
taenia —*see* Infestation, taenia
trichinellosis B75
trichostrongyliasis B81.2
trichuriasis B79
specified type NEC B83.8
syngamiasis B83.3
visceral larva migrans B83.Ø
Heterophyes (heterophyes) B66.8
hookworm B76.9
ancylostomiasis B76.Ø
necatoriasis B76.1
specified type NEC B76.8
Hymenolepis (diminuta) (nana) B71.Ø
intestinal NEC B82.9
leeches (aquatic) (land) —*see* Hirudiniasis
Leishmania —*see* Leishmaniasis
lice, louse —*see* Infestation, Pediculus
Linguatula B88.8
Liponyssoides sanguineus B88.Ø
Loa loa B74.3
conjunctival B74.3
eyelid B74.3
louse —*see* Infestation, Pediculus
maggots —*see* Myiasis
Mansonella (ozzardi) (perstans) (streptocerca) B74.4
Medina (worm) B72
Metagonimus (yokogawai) B66.8
microfilaria streptocerca —*see* Onchocerciasis
eye B73.ØØ
eyelid B73.Ø9
mites B88.9
scabic B86
Monilia (albicans) —*see* Candidiasis
mouth B37.Ø
Necator americanus B76.1
nematode NEC (intestinal) B82.Ø
Ancylostoma B76.Ø
conjunctiva NEC B83.9
Enterobius vermicularis B8Ø
Gnathostoma spinigerum B83.1
physaloptera B8Ø
specified NEC B81.8
trichostrongylus B81.2
trichuris (trichuria) B79
Oesophagostomum (apiostomum) B81.8
Oestrus ovis —*see also* Myiasis B87.9
Onchocerca (volvulus) —*see* Onchocerciasis
Opisthorchis (felineus) (viverrini) B66.Ø
orbit, parasitic NOS B89
Oxyuris vermicularis B8Ø
Paragonimus (westermani) B66.4

Infestation *(Continued)*
parasite, parasitic B89
eyelid B89
intestinal NOS B82.9
mouth B37.Ø
skin B88.9
tongue B37.Ø
Parastrongylus
cantonensis B83.2
costaricensis B81.3
Pediculus B85.2
body B85.1
capitis (humanus) (any site) B85.Ø
corporis (humanus) (any site) B85.1
head B85.Ø
mixed (classifiable to more than one of the titles B85.Ø-B85.3) B85.4
pubis (any site) B85.3
Pentastoma B88.8
Phthirus (pubis) (any site) B85.3
with any infestation classifiable to B85.Ø-B85.2 B85.4
pinworm B8Ø
pork tapeworm (adult) B68.Ø
protozoal NEC B64
intestinal AØ7.9
specified NEC AØ7.8
specified NEC B6Ø.8
pubic, louse B85.3
rat tapeworm B71.Ø
red bug B88.Ø
roundworm (large) NEC B82.Ø
Ascariasis —*see also* Ascariasis B77.9
sandflea B88.1
Sarcoptes scabiei B86
scabies B86
Schistosoma B65.9
bovis B65.8
cercariae B65.3
haematobium B65.Ø
intercalatum B65.8
japonicum B65.2
mansoni B65.1
mattheei B65.8
mekongi B65.8
specified type NEC B65.8
spindale B65.8
screw worms —*see* Myiasis
skin NOS B88.9
Sparganum (mansoni) (proliferum) (baxteri) B7Ø.1
larval B7Ø.1
specified type NEC B88.8
Spirometra larvae B7Ø.1
Stellantchasmus falcatus B66.8
Strongyloides stercoralis —*see* Strongyloidiasis
Taenia B68.9
diminuta B71.Ø
echinococcus —*see* Echinococcus
mediocanellata B68.1
nana B71.Ø
saginata B68.1
solium (intestinal form) B68.Ø
larval form —*see* Cysticercosis
Taeniarhynchus saginatus B68.1
tapeworm B71.9
beef B68.1
broad B7Ø.Ø
larval B7Ø.1
dog B67.4
dwarf B71.Ø
fish B7Ø.Ø
larval B7Ø.1
pork B68.Ø
rat B71.Ø
Ternidens diminutus B81.8
Tetranychus molestissimus B88.Ø
threadworm B8Ø
tongue B37.Ø
Toxocara (canis) (cati) (felis) B83.Ø

Infestation *(Continued)*
trematode(s) NEC —*see* Infestation, fluke
Trichinella (spiralis) B75
Trichocephalus B79
Trichomonas —*see* Trichomoniasis
Trichostrongylus B81.2
Trichuris (trichiura) B79
Trombicula (irritans) B88.Ø
Tunga penetrans B88.1
Uncinaria americana B76.1
Vandellia cirrhosa B88.8
whipworm B79
worms B83.9
intestinal B82.Ø
Wuchereria (bancrofti) B74.Ø
Infiltrate, infiltration
amyloid (generalized) (localized) —*see* Amyloidosis
calcareous NEC R89.7
localized —*see* Degeneration, by site
calcium salt R89.7
cardiac
fatty —*see* Degeneration, myocardial
glycogenic E74.Ø2 *[I43]*
corneal —*see* Edema, cornea
eyelid —*see* Inflammation, eyelid
glycogen, glycogenic —*see* Disease, glycogen storage
heart, cardiac
fatty —*see* Degeneration, myocardial
glycogenic E74.Ø2 *[I43]*
inflammatory in vitreous H43.89
kidney N28.89
leukemic —*see* Leukemia
liver K76.89
fatty —*see* Fatty, liver NEC
glycogen —*see also* Disease, glycogen storage E74.Ø3 *[K77]*
lung R91.8
eosinophilic J82
lymphatic —*see also* Leukemia, lymphatic C91.9- ●
gland I88.9
muscle, fatty M62.89
myocardium, myocardial
fatty —*see* Degeneration, myocardial
glycogenic E74.Ø2 *[I43]*
on chest x-ray R91.8
pulmonary R91.8
with eosinophilia J82
skin (lymphocytic) L98.6
thymus (gland) (fatty) E32.8
urine R39.Ø
vesicant agent
antineoplastic chemotherapy T8Ø.81Ø
other agent NEC T8Ø.818
vitreous body H43.89
Infirmity R68.89
senile R54
Inflammation, inflamed, inflammatory (with exudation)
abducent (nerve) —*see* Strabismus, paralytic, sixth nerve
accessory sinus (chronic) —*see* Sinusitis
adrenal (gland) E27.8
alveoli, teeth M27.3
scorbutic E54
anal canal, anus K62.89
antrum (chronic) —*see* Sinusitis, maxillary
appendix —*see* Appendicitis
arachnoid —*see* Meningitis
areola N61.Ø
puerperal, postpartum or gestational —*see* Infection, nipple
areolar tissue NOS LØ8.9
artery —*see* Arteritis
auditory meatus (external) —*see* Otitis, externa
Bartholin's gland N75.8
bile duct (common) (hepatic) or passage —*see* Cholangitis

Inflammation, inflamed, inflammatory *(Continued)*
bladder —*see* Cystitis
bone —*see* Osteomyelitis
brain —*see also* Encephalitis
membrane —*see* Meningitis
breast N61.Ø
puerperal, postpartum, gestational —*see* Mastitis, obstetric
broad ligament —*see* Disease, pelvis, inflammatory
bronchi —*see* Bronchitis
catarrhal JØØ
cecum —*see* Appendicitis
cerebral —*see also* Encephalitis
membrane —*see* Meningitis
cerebrospinal
meningococcal A39.Ø
cervix (uteri) —*see* Cervicitis
chest J98.8
chorioretinal H3Ø.9- ●
cyclitis —*see* Cyclitis
disseminated H3Ø.1Ø- ●
generalized H3Ø.13- ●
peripheral H3Ø.12- ●
posterior pole H3Ø.11- ●
epitheliopathy —*see* Epitheliopathy
focal H3Ø.ØØ- ●
juxtapapillary H3Ø.Ø1- ●
macular H3Ø.Ø4- ●
paramacular —*see* Inflammation, chorioretinal, focal, macular
peripheral H3Ø.Ø3- ●
posterior pole H3Ø.Ø2- ●
specified type NEC H3Ø.89- ●
choroid —*see* Inflammation, chorioretinal
chronic, postmastoidectomy cavity —*see* Complications, postmastoidectomy, inflammation
colon —*see* Enteritis
connective tissue (diffuse) NEC —*see* Disorder, soft tissue, specified type NEC
cornea —*see* Keratitis
corpora cavernosa N48.29
cranial nerve —*see* Disorder, nerve, cranial
Douglas' cul-de-sac or pouch (chronic) N73.Ø
due to device, implant or graft —*see also* Complications, by site and type, infection or inflammation
arterial graft T82.7
breast (implant) T85.79
catheter T85.79
dialysis (renal) T82.7
intraperitoneal T85.71
infusion T82.7
cranial T85.735
intrathecal T85.735
spinal (epidural) (subdural) T85.735
subarachnoid T85.735
urinary T83.518
cystostomy T83.51Ø
Hopkins T83.518
ileostomy T83.518
nephrostomy T83.512
specified NEC T83.518
urethral indwelling T83.511
urostomy T83.518
electronic (electrode) (pulse generator) (stimulator)
bone T84.7
cardiac T82.7
nervous system T85.738
brain T85.731
cranial nerve T85.732
gastric nerve T85.732
neurostimulator generator T85.734
peripheral nerve T85.732
sacral nerve T85.732
spinal cord T85.733
vagal nerve T85.732
urinary T83.59Ø

Inflammation, inflamed, inflammatory *(Continued)*
due to device, implant or graft *(Continued)*
fixation, internal (orthopedic) NEC —*see* Complication, fixation device, infection
gastrointestinal (bile duct) (esophagus) T85.79
neurostimulator electrode (lead) T85.732
genital NEC T83.69
heart NEC T82.7
valve (prosthesis) T82.6
graft T82.7
joint prosthesis —*see* Complication, joint prosthesis, infection
ocular (corneal graft) (orbital implant) NEC T85.79
orthopedic NEC T84.7
penile (cylinder) (pump) (resevoir) T83.61
specified NEC T85.79
testicular T83.62
urinary NEC T83.598
ileal conduit stent T83.593
implanted neurostimulation T83.59Ø
implanted sphincter T83.591
indwelling ureteral stent T83.592
nephroureteral stent T83.593
specified stent NEC T83.593
vascular NEC T82.7
ventricular intracranial (communicating) shunt T85.73Ø
duodenum K29.8Ø
with bleeding K29.81
dura mater —*see* Meningitis
ear (middle) —*see also* Otitis, media
external —*see* Otitis, externa
inner —*see* subcategory H83.Ø
epididymis —*see* Epididymitis
esophagus K2Ø.9
ethmoidal (sinus) (chronic) —*see* Sinusitis, ethmoidal
eustachian tube (catarrhal) —*see* Salpingitis, eustachian
eyelid HØ1.9
abscess —*see* Abscess, eyelid
blepharitis —*see* Blepharitis
chalazion —*see* Chalazion
dermatosis (noninfectious) —*see* Dermatosis, eyelid
hordeolum —*see* Hordeolum
specified NEC HØ1.8
fallopian tube —*see* Salpingo-oophoritis
fascia —*see* Myositis
follicular, pharynx J31.2
frontal (sinus) (chronic) —*see* Sinusitis, frontal
gallbladder —*see* Cholecystitis
gastric —*see* Gastritis
gastrointestinal —*see* Enteritis
genital organ (internal) (diffuse)
female —*see* Disease, pelvis, inflammatory
male N49.9
multiple sites N49.8
specified NEC N49.8
gland (lymph) —*see* Lymphadenitis
glottis —*see* Laryngitis
granular, pharynx J31.2
gum KØ5.1Ø
nonplaque induced KØ5.11
plaque induced KØ5.1Ø
heart —*see* Carditis
hepatic duct —*see* Cholangitis
ileoanal (internal) pouch K91.85Ø
ileum —*see also* Enteritis
regional or terminal —*see* Enteritis, regional
intestinal pouch K91.85Ø
intestine (any part) —*see* Enteritis
jaw (acute) (bone) (chronic) (lower) (suppurative) (upper) M27.2
joint NEC —*see* Arthritis
sacroiliac M46.1
kidney —*see* Nephritis
Inflammation, inflamed, inflammatory *(Continued)*
knee (joint) M13.169
tuberculous A18.Ø2
labium (majus) (minus) —*see* Vulvitis
lacrimal
gland —*see* Dacryoadenitis
passages (duct) (sac) —*see also* Dacryocystitis
canaliculitis —*see* Canaliculitis, lacrimal
larynx —*see* Laryngitis
leg NOS LØ8.9
lip K13.Ø
liver (capsule) —*see also* Hepatitis
chronic K73.9
suppurative K75.Ø
lung (acute) —*see also* Pneumonia
chronic J98.4
lymphatic vessel —*see* Lymphangitis
lymph gland or node —*see* Lymphadenitis
maxilla, maxillary M27.2
sinus (chronic) —*see* Sinusitis, maxillary
membranes of brain or spinal cord —*see* Meningitis
meninges —*see* Meningitis
mouth K12.1
muscle —*see* Myositis
myocardium —*see* Myocarditis
nasal sinus (chronic) —*see* Sinusitis
nasopharynx —*see* Nasopharyngitis
navel LØ8.82
nerve NEC —*see* Neuralgia
nipple N61.Ø
puerperal, postpartum or gestational —*see* Infection, nipple
nose —*see* Rhinitis
oculomotor (nerve) —*see* Strabismus, paralytic, third nerve
optic nerve —*see* Neuritis, optic
orbit (chronic) HØ5.1Ø
acute HØ5.ØØ
abscess —*see* Abscess, orbit
cellulitis —*see* Cellulitis, orbit
osteomyelitis —*see* Osteomyelitis, orbit
periostitis —*see* Periostitis, orbital
tenonitis —*see* Tenonitis, eye
granuloma —*see* Granuloma, orbit
myositis —*see* Myositis, orbital
ovary —*see* Salpingo-oophoritis
oviduct —*see* Salpingo-oophoritis
pancreas (acute) —*see* Pancreatitis
parametrium N73.Ø
parotid region LØ8.9
pelvis, female —*see* Disease, pelvis, inflammatory
penis (corpora cavernosa) N48.29
perianal K62.89
pericardium —*see* Pericarditis
perineum (female) (male) LØ8.9
perirectal K62.89
peritoneum —*see* Peritonitis
periuterine —*see* Disease, pelvis, inflammatory
perivesical —*see* Cystitis
petrous bone (acute) (chronic) —*see* Petrositis
pharynx (acute) —*see* Pharyngitis
pia mater —*see* Meningitis
pleura —*see* Pleurisy
polyp, colon —*see also* Polyp, colon, inflammatory K51.4Ø
prostate —*see also* Prostatitis
specified type NEC N41.8
rectosigmoid —*see* Rectosigmoiditis
rectum —*see also* Proctitis K62.89
respiratory, upper —*see also* Infection, respiratory, upper JØ6.9
acute, due to radiation J7Ø.Ø
chronic, due to external agent —*see* condition, respiratory, chronic, due to
due to
chemicals, gases, fumes or vapors (inhalation) J68.2
radiation J7Ø.1
Inflammation, inflamed, inflammatory *(Continued)*
retina —*see* Chorioretinitis
retrocecal —*see* Appendicitis
retroperitoneal —*see* Peritonitis
salivary duct or gland (any) (suppurative) —*see* Sialoadenitis
scorbutic, alveoli, teeth E54
scrotum N49.2
seminal vesicle —*see* Vesiculitis
sigmoid —*see* Enteritis
sinus —*see* Sinusitis
Skene's duct or gland —*see* Urethritis
skin LØ8.9
spermatic cord N49.1
sphenoidal (sinus) —*see* Sinusitis, sphenoidal
spinal
cord —*see* Encephalitis
membrane —*see* Meningitis
nerve —*see* Disorder, nerve
spine —*see* Spondylopathy, inflammatory
spleen (capsule) D73.89
stomach —*see* Gastritis
subcutaneous tissue LØ8.9
suprarenal (gland) E27.8
synovial —*see* Tenosynovitis
tendon (sheath) NEC —*see* Tenosynovitis
testis —*see* Orchitis
throat (acute) —*see* Pharyngitis
thymus (gland) E32.8
thyroid (gland) —*see* Thyroiditis
tongue K14.Ø
tonsil —*see* Tonsillitis
trachea —*see* Tracheitis
trochlear (nerve) —*see* Strabismus, paralytic, fourth nerve
tubal —*see* Salpingo-oophoritis
tuberculous NEC —*see* Tuberculosis
tubo-ovarian —*see* Salpingo-oophoritis
tunica vaginalis N49.1
tympanic membrane —*see* Tympanitis
umbilicus, umbilical LØ8.82
uterine ligament —*see* Disease, pelvis, inflammatory
uterus (catarrhal) —*see* Endometritis
uveal tract (anterior) NOS —*see also* Iridocyclitis
posterior —*see* Chorioretinitis
vagina —*see* Vaginitis
vas deferens N49.1
vein —*see also* Phlebitis
intracranial or intraspinal (septic) GØ8
thrombotic I8Ø.9
leg —*see* Phlebitis, leg
lower extremity —*see* Phlebitis, leg
vocal cord J38.3
vulva —*see* Vulvitis
Wharton's duct (suppurative) —*see* Sialoadenitis
Inflation, lung, imperfect (newborn) —*see* Atelectasis
Influenza (bronchial) (epidemic) (respiratory (upper)) (unidentified influenza virus) J11.1
with
digestive manifestations J11.2
encephalopathy J11.81
enteritis J11.2
gastroenteritis J11.2
gastrointestinal manifestations J11.2
laryngitis J11.1
myocarditis J11.82
otitis media J11.83
pharyngitis J11.1
pneumonia J11.ØØ
specified type J11.Ø8
respiratory manifestations NEC J11.1
specified manifestation NEC J11.89
A/H5N1 —*see also* Influenza, due to, identified novel influenza A virus JØ9.X2
avian —*see also* Influenza, due to, identified novel influenza A virus JØ9.X2

Influenza *(Continued)*
bird —*see also* Influenza, due to, identified novel influenza A virus J09.X2
novel (2009) H1N1 influenza —*see also* Influenza, due to, identified influenza virus NEC J10.1
novel influenza A/H1N1 —*see also* Influenza, due to, identified influenza virus NEC J10.1
due to
avian (*see also* Influenza, due to, identified novel influenza A virus) J09.X2
identified influenza virus NEC J10.1
with
digestive manifestations J10.2
encephalopathy J10.81
enteritis J10.2
gastroenteritis J10.2
gastrointestinal manifestations J10.2
laryngitis J10.1
myocarditis J10.82
otitis media J10.83
pharyngitis J10.1
pneumonia (unspecified type) J10.00
with same identified influenza virus J10.01
specified type NEC J10.08
respiratory manifestations NEC J10.1
specified manifestation NEC J10.89
identified novel influenza A virus J09.X2
with
digestive manifestations J09.X3
encephalopathy J09.X9
enteritis J09.X3
gastroenteritis J09.X3
gastrointestinal manifestations J09.X3
laryngitis J09.X2
myocarditis J09.X9
otitis media J09.X9
pharyngitis J09.X2
pneumonia J09.X1
respiratory manifestations NEC J09.X2
specified manifestation NEC J09.X9
upper respiratory symptoms J09.X2
of other animal origin, not bird or swine (*see also* Influenza, due to, identified novel influenza A virus) J09.X2
swine (viruses that normally cause infections in pigs) —*see also* Influenza, due to, identified novel influenza A virus J09.X2
Influenza-like disease —*see* Influenza
Influenzal —*see* Influenza
Infraction, Freiberg's (metatarsal head) —*see* Osteochondrosis, juvenile, metatarsus
Infraeruption of tooth (teeth) M26.34
Infusion complication, misadventure, or reaction —*see* Complications, infusion
Ingestion
chemical —*see* Table of Drugs and Chemicals, by substance, poisoning
drug or medicament
correct substance properly administered —*see* Table of Drugs and Chemicals, by drug, adverse effect
overdose or wrong substance given or taken —*see* Table of Drugs and Chemicals, by drug, poisoning
foreign body —*see* Foreign body, alimentary tract
▶ multiple drug —*see* Table of Drugs and Chemicals, multiple
tularemia A21.3
Ingrowing
hair (beard) L73.1
nail (finger) (toe) L60.0
Inguinal —*see also* condition
testicle Q53.9
bilateral Q53.212
unilateral Q53.112
Inhalant-induced
anxiety disorder F18.980
depressive disorder F18.94

Inhalant-induced *(Continued)*
major neurocognitive disorder F18.97
mild neurocognitive disorder F18.988
psychotic disorder F18.959
Inhalation
anthrax A22.1
flame T27.3
food or foreign body —*see* Foreign body, by site
gases, fumes, or vapors NEC T59.9- •
specified agent —*see* Table of Drugs and Chemicals, by substance
liquid or vomitus —*see* Asphyxia
meconium (newborn) P24.00
with
with respiratory symptoms P24.01
pneumonia (pneumonitis) P24.01
mucus —*see* Asphyxia, mucus
oil or gasoline (causing suffocation) —*see* Foreign body, by site
smoke J70.5
due to chemicals, gases, fumes and vapors J68.9
steam —*see* Toxicity, vapors
stomach contents or secretions —*see* Foreign body, by site
due to anesthesia (general) (local) or other sedation T88.59
in labor and delivery O74.0
in pregnancy O29.01- •
postpartum, puerperal O89.01
Inhibition, orgasm
female F52.31
male F52.32
Inhibitor, systemic lupus erythematosus (presence of) D68.62
Iniencephalus, iniencephaly Q00.2
Injection, traumatic jet (air) (industrial) (water) (paint or dye) T70.4
Injury —*see also* specified injury type T14.90
abdomen, abdominal S39.91
blood vessel —*see* Injury, blood vessel, abdomen
cavity —*see* Injury, intra-abdominal
contusion S30.1
internal —*see* Injury, intra-abdominal
intra-abdominal organ —*see* Injury, intra-abdominal
nerve —*see* Injury, nerve, abdomen
open —*see* Wound, open, abdomen
specified NEC S39.81
superficial —*see* Injury, superficial, abdomen
Achilles tendon S86.00- •
laceration S86.02- •
specified type NEC S86.09- •
strain S86.01- •
acoustic, resulting in deafness —*see* Injury, nerve, acoustic
adrenal (gland) S37.819
contusion S37.812
laceration S37.813
specified type NEC S37.818
alveolar (process) S09.93
ankle S99.91- •
contusion —*see* Contusion, ankle
dislocation —*see* Dislocation, ankle
fracture —*see* Fracture, ankle
nerve —*see* Injury, nerve, ankle
open —*see* Wound, open, ankle
specified type NEC S99.81- •
sprain —*see* Sprain, ankle
superficial —*see* Injury, superficial, ankle
anterior chamber, eye —*see* Injury, eye, specified site NEC
anus —*see* Injury, abdomen
aorta (thoracic) S25.00
abdominal S35.00
laceration (minor) (superficial) S35.01
major S35.02
specified type NEC S35.09

Injury *(Continued)*
aorta (thoracic) *(Continued)*
laceration (minor) (superficial) S25.01
major S25.02
specified type NEC S25.09
arm (upper) S49.9- •
blood vessel —*see* Injury, blood vessel, arm
contusion —*see* Contusion, arm, upper
fracture —*see* Fracture, humerus
lower —*see* Injury, forearm
muscle —*see* Injury, muscle, shoulder
nerve —*see* Injury, nerve, arm
open —*see* Wound, open, arm
specified type NEC S49.8- •
superficial —*see* Injury, superficial, arm
artery (complicating trauma) —*see also* Injury, blood vessel, by site
cerebral or meningeal —*see* Injury, intracranial
auditory canal (external) (meatus) S09.91
auricle, auris, ear S09.91
axilla —*see* Injury, shoulder
back —*see* Injury, back, lower
bile duct S36.13
birth —*see also* Birth, injury P15.9
bladder (sphincter) S37.20
at delivery O71.5
contusion S37.22
laceration S37.23
obstetrical trauma O71.5
specified type NEC S37.29
blast (air) (hydraulic) (immersion) (underwater) NEC T14.8
acoustic nerve trauma —*see* Injury, nerve, acoustic
bladder —*see* Injury, bladder
brain —*see* Concussion
colon —*see* Injury, intestine, large, blast injury
ear (primary) S09.31- •
secondary S09.39- •
generalized T70.8
lung —*see* Injury, intrathoracic, lung, blast injury
multiple body organs T70.8
peritoneum S36.81
rectum S36.61
retroperitoneum S36.898
small intestine S36.419
duodenum S36.410
specified site NEC S36.418
specified
intra-abdominal organ NEC S36.898
pelvic organ NEC S37.899
blood vessel NEC T14.8
abdomen S35.9- •
aorta —*see* Injury, aorta, abdominal
celiac artery —*see* Injury, blood vessel, celiac artery
iliac vessel —*see* Injury, blood vessel, iliac
laceration S35.91
mesenteric vessel —*see* Injury, mesenteric
portal vein —*see* Injury, blood vessel, portal vein
renal vessel —*see* Injury, blood vessel, renal
specified vessel NEC S35.8X- •
splenic vessel —*see* Injury, blood vessel, splenic
vena cava —*see* Injury, vena cava, inferior
ankle —*see* Injury, blood vessel, foot
aorta (abdominal) (thoracic) —*see* Injury, aorta
arm (upper) NEC S45.90- •
forearm —*see* Injury, blood vessel, forearm
laceration S45.91- •
specified
site NEC S45.80- •
laceration S45.81- •
specified type NEC S45.89- •
type NEC S45.99- •

Injury *(Continued)*
  blood vessel NEC *(Continued)*
    arm (upper) NEC *(Continued)*
      superficial vein S45.3Ø-●
        laceration S45.31-●
        specified type NEC S45.39-●
    axillary
      artery S45.ØØ-●
        laceration S45.Ø1-●
        specified type NEC S45.Ø9-●
      vein S45.2Ø-●
        laceration S45.21-●
        specified type NEC S45.29-●
    azygos vein —*see* Injury, blood vessel, thoracic, specified site NEC
    brachial
      artery S45.1Ø-●
        laceration S45.11-●
        specified type NEC S45.19-●
      vein S45.2Ø-●
        laceration S45.219
        specified type NEC S45.29-●
    carotid artery (common) (external) (internal, extracranial) S15.ØØ-●
      internal, intracranial SØ6.8-●
      laceration (minor) (superficial) S15.Ø1-●
        major S15.Ø2-●
      specified type NEC S15.Ø9-●
    celiac artery S35.219
      branch S35.299
        laceration (minor) (superficial) S35.291
          major S35.292
        specified NEC S35.298
      laceration (minor) (superficial) S35.211
        major S35.212
      specified type NEC S35.218
    cerebral —*see* Injury, intracranial
    deep plantar —*see* Injury, blood vessel, plantar artery
    digital (hand) —*see* Injury, blood vessel, finger
    dorsal
      artery (foot) S95.ØØ-●
        laceration S95.Ø1-●
        specified type NEC S95.Ø9-●
      vein (foot) S95.2Ø-●
        laceration S95.21-●
        specified type NEC S95.29-●
    due to accidental laceration during procedure —*see* Laceration, accidental complicating surgery
    extremity —*see* Injury, blood vessel, limb
    femoral
      artery (common) (superficial) S75.ØØ-●
        laceration (minor) (superficial) S75.Ø1-●
          major S75.Ø2-●
        specified type NEC S75.Ø9-●
      vein (hip level) (thigh level) S75.1Ø-●
        laceration (minor) (superficial) S75.11-●
          major S75.12-●
        specified type NEC S75.19-●
    finger S65.5Ø-●
      index S65.5Ø-●
        laceration S65.51-●
        specified type NEC S65.59-●
      laceration S65.51-●
      little S65.5Ø-●
        laceration S65.51-●
        specified type NEC S65.59-●
      middle S65.5Ø-●
        laceration S65.51-●
        specified type NEC S65.59-●
      specified type NEC S65.59-●
      thumb —*see* Injury, blood vessel, thumb
    foot S95.9Ø-●
      dorsal
        artery —*see* Injury, blood vessel, dorsal, artery
        vein —*see* Injury, blood vessel, dorsal, vein

Injury *(Continued)*
  blood vessel NEC *(Continued)*
    foot *(Continued)*
      laceration S95.91-●
      plantar artery —*see* Injury, blood vessel, plantar artery
      specified
        site NEC S95.8Ø-●
          laceration S95.81-●
          specified type NEC S95.89-●
        specified type NEC S95.99-●
    forearm S55.9Ø-●
      laceration S55.91-●
      radial artery —*see* Injury, blood vessel, radial artery
      specified
        site NEC S55.8Ø-●
          laceration S55.81-●
          specified type NEC S55.89-●
        type NEC S55.99-●
      ulnar artery —*see* Injury, blood vessel, ulnar artery
      vein S55.2Ø-●
        laceration S55.21-●
        specified type NEC S55.29-●
    gastric
      artery —*see* Injury, mesenteric, artery, branch
      vein —*see* Injury, blood vessel, abdomen
    gastroduodenal artery —*see* Injury, mesenteric, artery, branch
    greater saphenous vein (lower leg level) S85.3Ø-●
      hip (and thigh) level S75.2Ø-●
        laceration (minor) (superficial) S75.21-●
          major S75.22-●
        specified type NEC S75.29-●
      laceration S85.31-●
      specified type NEC S85.39-●
    hand (level) S65.9Ø-●
      finger —*see* Injury, blood vessel, finger
      laceration S65.91-●
      palmar arch —*see* Injury, blood vessel, palmar arch
      radial artery —*see* Injury, blood vessel, radial artery, hand
      specified
        site NEC S65.8Ø-●
          laceration S65.81-●
          specified type NEC S65.89-●
        type NEC S65.99-●
      thumb —*see* Injury, blood vessel, thumb
      ulnar artery —*see* Injury, blood vessel, ulnar artery, hand
    head SØ9.Ø
      intracranial —*see* Injury, intracranial
      multiple SØ9.Ø
    hepatic
      artery —*see* Injury, mesenteric, artery
      vein —*see* Injury, vena cava, inferior
    hip S75.9Ø-●
      femoral artery —*see* Injury, blood vessel, femoral, artery
      femoral vein —*see* Injury, blood vessel, femoral, vein
      greater saphenous vein —*see* Injury, blood vessel, greater saphenous, hip level
      laceration S75.91-●
      specified
        site NEC S75.8Ø-●
          laceration S75.81-●
          specified type NEC S75.89-●
        type NEC S75.99-●
    hypogastric (artery) (vein) —*see* Injury, blood vessel, iliac
    iliac S35.5-●
      artery S35.51-●
      specified vessel NEC S35.5-●
      uterine vessel —*see* Injury, blood vessel, uterine
      vein S35.51-●

Injury *(Continued)*
  blood vessel NEC *(Continued)*
    innominate —*see* Injury, blood vessel, thoracic, innominate
    intercostal (artery) (vein) —*see* Injury, blood vessel, thoracic, intercostal
    jugular vein (external) S15.2Ø-●
      internal S15.3Ø-●
        laceration (minor) (superficial) S15.31-●
          major S15.32-●
        specified type NEC S15.39-●
      laceration (minor) (superficial) S15.21-●
        major S15.22-●
      specified type NEC S15.29-●
    leg (level) (lower) S85.9Ø-●
      greater saphenous —*see* Injury, blood vessel, greater saphenous
      laceration S85.91-●
      lesser saphenous —*see* Injury, blood vessel, lesser saphenous
      peroneal artery —*see* Injury, blood vessel, peroneal artery
      popliteal
        artery —*see* Injury, blood vessel, popliteal, artery
        vein —*see* Injury, blood vessel, popliteal, vein
      specified
        site NEC S85.8Ø-●
          laceration S85.81-●
          specified type NEC S85.89-●
        type NEC S85.99-●
      thigh —*see* Injury, blood vessel, hip
      tibial artery —*see* Injury, blood vessel, tibial artery
    lesser saphenous vein (lower leg level) S85.4Ø-●
      laceration S85.41-●
      specified type NEC S85.49-●
    limb
      lower —*see* Injury, blood vessel, leg
      upper —*see* Injury, blood vessel, arm
    lower back —*see* Injury, blood vessel, abdomen
      specified NEC —*see* Injury, blood vessel, abdomen, specified, site NEC
    mammary (artery) (vein) —*see* Injury, blood vessel, thoracic, specified site NEC
    mesenteric (inferior) (superior)
      artery —*see* Injury, mesenteric, artery
      vein —*see* Injury, mesenteric, vein
    neck S15.9
      specified site NEC S15.8
    ovarian (artery) (vein) —*see* subcategory S35.8
    palmar arch (superficial) S65.2Ø-●
      deep S65.3Ø-●
        laceration S65.31-●
        specified type NEC S65.39-●
      laceration S65.21-●
      specified type NEC S65.29-●
    pelvis —*see* Injury, blood vessel, abdomen
      specified NEC —*see* Injury, blood vessel, abdomen, specified, site NEC
    peroneal artery S85.2Ø-●
      laceration S85.21-●
      specified type NEC S85.29-●
    plantar artery (deep) (foot) S95.1Ø-●
      laceration S95.11-●
      specified type NEC S95.19-●
    popliteal
      artery S85.ØØ-●
        laceration S85.Ø1-●
        specified type NEC S85.Ø9-●
      vein S85.5Ø-●
        laceration S85.51-●
        specified type NEC S85.59-●
    portal vein S35.319
      laceration S35.311
      specified type NEC S35.318

- Injury *(Continued)*
  - blood vessel NEC *(Continued)*
    - precerebral —*see* Injury, blood vessel, neck
    - pulmonary (artery) (vein) —*see* Injury, blood vessel, thoracic, pulmonary
    - radial artery (forearm level) S55.10-●
      - hand and wrist (level) S65.10-●
        - laceration S65.11-●
        - specified type NEC S65.19-●
      - laceration S55.11-●
      - specified type NEC S55.19-●
    - renal
      - artery S35.40-●
        - laceration S35.41-●
        - specified NEC S35.49-●
      - vein S35.40-●
        - laceration S35.41-●
        - specified NEC S35.49-●
    - saphenous vein (greater) (lower leg level) —*see* Injury, blood vessel, greater saphenous
      - hip and thigh level —*see* Injury, blood vessel, greater saphenous, hip level
      - lesser —*see* Injury, blood vessel, lesser saphenous
    - shoulder
      - specified NEC —*see* Injury, blood vessel, arm, specified site NEC
      - superficial vein —*see* Injury, blood vessel, arm, superficial vein
    - specified NEC T14.8
    - splenic
      - artery —*see* Injury, blood vessel, celiac artery, branch
      - vein S35.329
        - laceration S35.321
        - specified NEC S35.328
    - subclavian —*see* Injury, blood vessel, thoracic, innominate
    - thigh —*see* Injury, blood vessel, hip
    - thoracic S25.90
      - aorta S25.00
        - laceration (minor) (superficial) S25.01
          - major S25.02
        - specified type NEC S25.09
      - azygos vein —*see* Injury, blood vessel, thoracic, specified, site NEC
      - innominate
        - artery S25.10-●
          - laceration (minor) (superficial) S25.11-●
            - major S25.12-●
          - specified type NEC S25.19-●
        - vein S25.30-●
          - laceration (minor) (superficial) S25.31-●
            - major S25.32-●
          - specified type NEC S25.39-●
      - intercostal S25.50-●
        - laceration S25.51-●
        - specified type NEC S25.59-●
      - laceration S25.91
      - mammary vessel —*see* Injury, blood vessel, thoracic, specified, site NEC
      - pulmonary S25.40-●
        - laceration (minor) (superficial) S25.41-●
          - major S25.42-●
        - specified type NEC S25.49-●
      - specified
        - site NEC S25.80-●
          - laceration S25.81-●
          - specified type NEC S25.89-●
        - type NEC S25.99
      - subclavian —*see* Injury, blood vessel, thoracic, innominate
      - vena cava (superior) S25.20
        - laceration (minor) (superficial) S25.21
          - major S25.22
        - specified type NEC S25.29

- Injury *(Continued)*
  - blood vessel NEC *(Continued)*
    - thumb S65.40-●
      - laceration S65.41-●
      - specified type NEC S65.49-●
    - tibial artery S85.10-●
      - anterior S85.13-●
        - laceration S85.14-●
        - specified injury NEC S85.15-●
      - laceration S85.11-●
      - posterior S85.16-●
        - laceration S85.17-●
        - specified injury NEC S85.18-●
      - specified injury NEC S85.12-●
    - ulnar artery (forearm level) S55.00-●
      - hand and wrist (level) S65.00-●
        - laceration S65.01-●
        - specified type NEC S65.09-●
      - laceration S55.01-●
      - specified type NEC S55.09-●
    - upper arm (level) —*see* Injury, blood vessel, arm
      - superficial vein —*see* Injury, blood vessel, arm, superficial vein
    - uterine S35.5-●
      - artery S35.53-●
      - vein S35.53-●
    - vena cava —*see* Injury, vena cava
    - vertebral artery S15.10-●
      - laceration (minor) (superficial) S15.11-●
        - major S15.12-●
      - specified type NEC S15.19-●
    - wrist (level) —*see* Injury, blood vessel, hand
  - brachial plexus S14.3
    - newborn P14.3
  - brain (traumatic) S06.9-●
    - diffuse (axonal) S06.2X-●
    - focal S06.30-●
  - brainstem S06.38-●
  - breast NOS S29.9
  - broad ligament —*see* Injury, pelvic organ, specified site NEC
  - bronchus, bronchi —*see* Injury, intrathoracic, bronchus
  - brow S09.90
  - buttock S39.92
  - canthus, eye S05.90
  - cardiac plexus —*see* Injury, nerve, thorax, sympathetic
  - cauda equina S34.3
  - cavernous sinus —*see* Injury, intracranial
  - cecum —*see* Injury, colon
  - celiac ganglion or plexus —*see* Injury, nerve, lumbosacral, sympathetic
  - cerebellum —*see* Injury, intracranial
  - cerebral —*see* Injury, intracranial
  - cervix (uteri) —*see* Injury, uterus
  - cheek (wall) S09.93
  - chest —*see* Injury, thorax
  - childbirth (newborn) —*see also* Birth, injury
    - maternal NEC O71.9
  - chin S09.93
  - choroid (eye) —*see* Injury, eye, specified site NEC
  - clitoris S39.94
  - coccyx —*see also* Injury, back, lower
    - complicating delivery O71.6
  - colon —*see* Injury, intestine, large
  - common bile duct —*see* Injury, liver
  - conjunctiva (superficial) —*see* Injury, eye, conjunctiva
  - conus medullaris —*see* Injury, spinal, sacral
  - cord
    - spermatic (pelvic region) S37.898
      - scrotal region S39.848
    - spinal —*see* Injury, spinal cord, by region
  - cornea —*see* Injury, eye, specified site NEC
    - abrasion —*see* Injury, eye, cornea, abrasion
  - cortex (cerebral) —*see also* Injury, intracranial
    - visual —*see* Injury, nerve, optic

- Injury *(Continued)*
  - costal region NEC S29.9
  - costochondral NEC S29.9
  - cranial
    - cavity —*see* Injury, intracranial
    - nerve —*see* Injury, nerve, cranial
  - crushing —*see* Crush
  - cutaneous sensory nerve
  - cystic duct —*see* Injury, liver
  - deep tissue —*see* Contusion, by site
    - meaning pressure ulcer —*see* Ulcer, pressure, unstageable, by site
  - delivery (newborn) P15.9
    - maternal NEC O71.9
  - Descemet's membrane —*see* Injury, eyeball, penetrating
  - diaphragm —*see* Injury, intrathoracic, diaphragm
  - duodenum —*see* Injury, intestine, small, duodenum
  - ear (auricle) (external) (canal) S09.91
    - abrasion —*see* Abrasion, ear
    - bite —*see* Bite, ear
    - blister —*see* Blister, ear
    - bruise —*see* Contusion, ear
    - contusion —*see* Contusion, ear
    - external constriction —*see* Constriction, external, ear
    - hematoma —*see* Hematoma, ear
    - inner —*see* Injury, ear, middle
    - laceration —*see* Laceration, ear
    - middle S09.30-●
      - blast —*see* Injury, blast, ear
      - specified NEC S09.39-●
    - puncture —*see* Puncture, ear
    - superficial —*see* Injury, superficial, ear
  - eighth cranial nerve (acoustic or auditory) —*see* Injury, nerve, acoustic
  - elbow S59.90-●
    - contusion —*see* Contusion, elbow
    - dislocation —*see* Dislocation, elbow
    - fracture —*see* Fracture, ulna, upper end
    - open —*see* Wound, open, elbow
    - specified NEC S59.80-●
    - sprain —*see* Sprain, elbow
    - superficial —*see* Injury, superficial, elbow
  - eleventh cranial nerve (accessory) —*see* Injury, nerve, accessory
  - epididymis S39.94
  - epigastric region S39.91
  - epiglottis NEC S19.89
  - esophageal plexus —*see* Injury, nerve, thorax, sympathetic
  - esophagus (thoracic part) —*see also* Injury, intrathoracic, esophagus
    - cervical NEC S19.85
  - eustachian tube S09.30-●
  - eye S05.9-●
    - avulsion S05.7-●
    - ball —*see* Injury, eyeball
    - conjunctiva S05.0-●
    - cornea
      - abrasion S05.0-●
    - laceration S05.3-●
      - with prolapse S05.2-●
    - lacrimal apparatus S05.8X-●
    - orbit penetration S05.4-●
    - specified site NEC S05.8X-●
  - eyeball S05.8X-●
    - contusion S05.1-●
    - penetrating S05.6-●
      - with
        - foreign body S05.5-●
        - prolapse or loss of intraocular tissue S05.2-●
      - without prolapse or loss of intraocular tissue S05.3-●
    - specified type NEC S05.8-●
  - eyebrow S09.93

- Injury *(Continued)*
  - eyelid S09.93
    - abrasion *—see* Abrasion, eyelid
    - contusion *—see* Contusion, eyelid
    - open *—see* Wound, open, eyelid
  - face S09.93
  - fallopian tube S37.509
    - bilateral S37.502
      - blast injury S37.512
      - contusion S37.522
      - laceration S37.532
      - specified type NEC S37.592
    - blast injury (primary) S37.519
      - bilateral S37.512
      - secondary *—see* Injury, fallopian tube, specified type NEC
      - unilateral S37.511
    - contusion S37.529
      - bilateral S37.522
      - unilateral S37.521
    - laceration S37.539
      - bilateral S37.532
      - unilateral S37.531
    - specified type NEC S37.599
      - bilateral S37.592
      - unilateral S37.591
    - unilateral S37.501
      - blast injury S37.511
      - contusion S37.521
      - laceration S37.531
      - specified type NEC S37.591
  - fascia *—see* Injury, muscle
  - fifth cranial nerve (trigeminal) *—see* Injury, nerve, trigeminal
  - finger (nail) S69.9- ●
    - blood vessel *—see* Injury, blood vessel, finger
    - contusion *—see* Contusion, finger
    - dislocation *—see* Dislocation, finger
    - fracture *—see* Fracture, finger
    - muscle *—see* Injury, muscle, finger
    - nerve *—see* Injury, nerve, digital, finger
    - open *—see* Wound, open, finger
    - specified NEC S69.8- ●
    - sprain *—see* Sprain, finger
    - superficial *—see* Injury, superficial, finger
  - first cranial nerve (olfactory) *—see* Injury, nerve, olfactory
  - flank *—see* Injury, abdomen
  - foot S99.92- ●
    - blood vessel *—see* Injury, blood vessel, foot
    - contusion *—see* Contusion, foot
    - dislocation *—see* Dislocation, foot
    - fracture *—see* Fracture, foot
    - muscle *—see* Injury, muscle, foot
    - open *—see* Wound, open, foot
    - specified type NEC S99.82- ●
    - sprain *—see* Sprain, foot
    - superficial *—see* Injury, superficial, foot
  - forceps NOS P15.9
  - forearm S59.91- ●
    - blood vessel *—see* Injury, blood vessel, forearm
    - contusion *—see* Contusion, forearm
    - fracture *—see* Fracture, forearm
    - muscle *—see* Injury, muscle, forearm
    - nerve *—see* Injury, nerve, forearm
    - open *—see* Wound, open, forearm
    - specified NEC S59.81- ●
    - superficial *—see* Injury, superficial, forearm
  - forehead S09.90
  - fourth cranial nerve (trochlear) *—see* Injury, nerve, trochlear
  - gallbladder S36.129
    - contusion S36.122
    - laceration S36.123
    - specified NEC S36.128
  - ganglion
    - celiac, coeliac *—see* Injury, nerve, lumbosacral, sympathetic
    - gasserian *—see* Injury, nerve, trigeminal

- Injury *(Continued)*
  - ganglion *(Continued)*
    - stellate *—see* Injury, nerve, thorax, sympathetic
    - thoracic sympathetic *—see* Injury, nerve, thorax, sympathetic
  - gasserian ganglion *—see* Injury, nerve, trigeminal
  - gastric artery *—see* Injury, blood vessel, celiac artery, branch
  - gastroduodenal artery *—see* Injury, blood vessel, celiac artery, branch
  - gastrointestinal tract *—see* Injury, intra-abdominal
    - with open wound into abdominal cavity *—see* Wound, open, with penetration into peritoneal cavity
    - colon *—see* Injury, intestine, large
    - rectum *—see* Injury, intestine, large, rectum
      - with open wound into abdominal cavity S36.61
    - small intestine *—see* Injury, intestine, small
    - specified site NEC *—see* Injury, intra-abdominal, specified, site NEC
    - stomach *—see* Injury, stomach
  - genital organ(s)
    - external S39.94
      - specified NEC S39.848
    - internal S37.90
      - fallopian tube *—see* Injury, fallopian tube
      - ovary *—see* Injury, ovary
      - prostate *—see* Injury, prostate
      - seminal vesicle *—see* Injury, pelvis, organ, specified site NEC
      - uterus *—see* Injury, uterus
      - vas deferens *—see* Injury, pelvis, organ, specified site NEC
    - obstetrical trauma O71.9
  - gland
    - lacrimal laceration *—see* Injury, eye, specified site NEC
    - salivary S09.93
    - thyroid NEC S19.84
  - globe (eye) S05.90
    - specified NEC S05.8X- ●
  - groin *—see* Injury, abdomen
  - gum S09.90
  - hand S69.9- ●
    - blood vessel *—see* Injury, blood vessel, hand
    - contusion *—see* Contusion, hand
    - fracture *—see* Fracture, hand
    - muscle *—see* Injury, muscle, hand
    - nerve *—see* Injury, nerve, hand
    - open *—see* Wound, open, hand
    - specified NEC S69.8- ●
    - sprain *—see* Sprain, hand
    - superficial *—see* Injury, superficial, hand
  - head S09.90
    - with loss of consciousness S06.9- ●
    - specified NEC S09.8- ●
  - heart S26.90
    - with hemopericardium S26.00
      - contusion S26.01
      - laceration (mild) S26.020
        - major S26.022
        - moderate S26.021
      - specified type NEC S26.09
    - without hemopericardium S26.10
      - contusion S26.11
      - laceration S26.12
      - specified type NEC S26.19
    - contusion S26.91
    - laceration S26.92
    - specified type NEC S26.99
  - heel *—see* Injury, foot
  - hepatic
    - artery *—see* Injury, blood vessel, celiac artery, branch
    - duct *—see* Injury, liver
    - vein *—see* Injury, vena cava, inferior

- Injury *(Continued)*
  - hip S79.91- ●
    - blood vessel *—see* Injury, blood vessel, hip
    - contusion *—see* Contusion, hip
    - dislocation *—see* Dislocation, hip
    - fracture *—see* Fracture, femur, neck
    - muscle *—see* Injury, muscle, hip
    - nerve *—see* Injury, nerve, hip
    - open *—see* Wound, open, hip
    - specified NEC S79.81- ●
    - sprain *—see* Sprain, hip
    - superficial *—see* Injury, superficial, hip
  - hymen S39.94
  - hypogastric
    - blood vessel *—see* Injury, blood vessel, iliac
    - plexus *—see* Injury, nerve, lumbosacral, sympathetic
  - ileum *—see* Injury, intestine, small
  - iliac region S39.91
  - instrumental (during surgery) *—see* Laceration, accidental complicating surgery
    - birth injury *—see* Birth, injury
    - nonsurgical *—see* Injury, by site
    - obstetrical O71.9
      - bladder O71.5
      - cervix O71.3
      - high vaginal O71.4
      - perineal NOS O70.9
      - urethra O71.5
      - uterus O71.5
        - with rupture or perforation O71.1
  - internal T14.8
    - aorta *—see* Injury, aorta
    - bladder (sphincter) *—see* Injury, bladder
      - with
        - ectopic or molar pregnancy O08.6
      - following ectopic or molar pregnancy O08.6
      - obstetrical trauma O71.5
    - bronchus, bronchi *—see* Injury, intrathoracic, bronchus
    - cecum *—see* Injury, intestine, large
    - cervix (uteri) *—see also* Injury, uterus
      - with ectopic or molar pregnancy O08.6
      - following ectopic or molar pregnancy O08.6
      - obstetrical trauma O71.3
    - chest *—see* Injury, intrathoracic
    - gastrointestinal tract *—see* Injury, intra-abdominal
    - heart *—see* Injury, heart
    - intestine NEC *—see* Injury, intestine
    - intrauterine *—see* Injury, uterus
    - mesentery *—see* Injury, intra-abdominal, specified, site NEC
    - pelvis, pelvic (organ) S37.90
      - following ectopic or molar pregnancy (subsequent episode) O08.6
      - obstetrical trauma NEC O71.5
        - rupture or perforation O71.1
      - specified NEC S39.83
    - rectum *—see* Injury, intestine, large, rectum
    - stomach *—see* Injury, stomach
    - ureter *—see* Injury, ureter
    - urethra (sphincter) following ectopic or molar pregnancy O08.6
    - uterus *—see* Injury, uterus
  - interscapular area *—see* Injury, thorax
  - intestine
    - large S36.509
      - ascending (right) S36.500
        - blast injury (primary) S36.510
          - secondary S36.590
        - contusion S36.520
        - laceration S36.530
        - specified type NEC S36.590

Injury *(Continued)*
intestine *(Continued)*
large *(Continued)*
blast injury (primary) S36.519
ascending (right) S36.510
descending (left) S36.512
rectum S36.61
sigmoid S36.513
specified site NEC S36.518
transverse S36.511
contusion S36.529
ascending (right) S36.520
descending (left) S36.522
rectum S36.62
sigmoid S36.523
specified site NEC S36.528
transverse S36.521
descending (left) S36.502
blast injury (primary) S36.512
secondary S36.592
contusion S36.522
laceration S36.532
specified type NEC S36.592
laceration S36.539
ascending (right) S36.530
descending (left) S36.532
rectum S36.63
sigmoid S36.533
specified site NEC S36.538
transverse S36.531
rectum S36.60
blast injury (primary) S36.61
secondary S36.69
contusion S36.62
laceration S36.63
specified type NEC S36.69
sigmoid S36.503
blast injury (primary) S36.513
secondary S36.593
contusion S36.523
laceration S36.533
specified type NEC S36.593
specified
site NEC S36.508
blast injury (primary) S36.518
secondary S36.598
contusion S36.528
laceration S36.538
specified type NEC S36.598
type NEC S36.599
ascending (right) S36.590
descending (left) S36.592
rectum S36.69
sigmoid S36.593
specified site NEC S36.598
transverse S36.591
transverse S36.501
blast injury (primary) S36.511
secondary S36.591
contusion S36.521
laceration S36.531
specified type NEC S36.591
small S36.409
blast injury (primary) S36.419
duodenum S36.410
secondary S36.499
duodenum S36.490
specified site NEC S36.498
specified site NEC S36.418
contusion S36.429
duodenum S36.420
specified site NEC S36.428
duodenum S36.400
blast injury (primary) S36.410
secondary S36.490
contusion S36.420
laceration S36.430
specified NEC S36.490
laceration S36.439
duodenum S36.430
specified site NEC S36.438

Injury *(Continued)*
intestine *(Continued)*
small *(Continued)*
specified
site NEC S36.408
type NEC S36.499
duodenum S36.490
specified site NEC S36.498
intra-abdominal S36.90
adrenal gland —*see* Injury, adrenal gland
bladder —*see* Injury, bladder
colon —*see* Injury, intestine, large
contusion S36.92
fallopian tube —*see* Injury, fallopian tube
gallbladder —*see* Injury, gallbladder
intestine —*see* Injury, intestine
kidney —*see* Injury, kidney
laceration S36.93
liver —*see* Injury, liver
ovary —*see* Injury, ovary
pancreas —*see* Injury, pancreas
pelvic NOS S37.90
peritoneum —*see* Injury, intra-abdominal, specified, site NEC
prostate —*see* Injury, prostate
rectum —*see* Injury, intestine, large, rectum
retroperitoneum —*see* Injury, intra-abdominal, specified, site NEC
seminal vesicle —*see* Injury, pelvis, organ, specified site NEC
small intestine —*see* Injury, intestine, small
specified
pelvic S37.90
specified
site NEC S37.899
specified type NEC S37.898
type NEC S37.99
site NEC S36.899
contusion S36.892
laceration S36.893
specified type NEC S36.898
type NEC S36.99
spleen —*see* Injury, spleen
stomach —*see* Injury, stomach
ureter —*see* Injury, ureter
urethra —*see* Injury, urethra
uterus —*see* Injury, uterus
vas deferens —*see* Injury, pelvis, organ, specified site NEC
intracranial (traumatic) S06.9-●
cerebellar hemorrhage, traumatic —*see* Injury, intracranial, focal
cerebral edema, traumatic S06.1X-●
diffuse S06.1X-●
focal S06.1X-●
diffuse (axonal) S06.2X-●
epidural hemorrhage (traumatic) S06.4X-●
focal brain injury S06.30-●
contusion —*see* Contusion, cerebral
laceration —*see* Laceration, cerebral
intracerebral hemorrhage, traumatic S06.36-●
left side S06.35-●
right side S06.34-●
subarachnoid hemorrhage, traumatic S06.6X-●
subdural hemorrhage, traumatic S06.5X-●
intraocular —*see* Injury, eyeball, penetrating
intrathoracic S27.9
bronchus S27.409
bilateral S27.402
blast injury (primary) S27.419
bilateral S27.412
secondary —*see* Injury, intrathoracic, bronchus, specified type NEC
unilateral S27.411
contusion S27.429
bilateral S27.422
unilateral S27.421
laceration S27.439
bilateral S27.432
unilateral S27.431

Injury *(Continued)*
intrathoracic *(Continued)*
bronchus *(Continued)*
specified type NEC S27.499
bilateral S27.492
unilateral S27.491
unilateral S27.401
diaphragm S27.809
contusion S27.802
laceration S27.803
specified type NEC S27.808
esophagus (thoracic) S27.819
contusion S27.812
laceration S27.813
specified type NEC S27.818
heart —*see* Injury, heart
hemopneumothorax S27.2
hemothorax S27.1
lung S27.309
aspiration J69.0
bilateral S27.302
blast injury (primary) S27.319
bilateral S27.312
secondary —*see* Injury, intrathoracic, lung, specified type NEC
unilateral S27.311
contusion S27.329
bilateral S27.322
unilateral S27.321
laceration S27.339
bilateral S27.332
unilateral S27.331
specified type NEC S27.399
bilateral S27.392
unilateral S27.391
unilateral S27.301
pleura S27.60
laceration S27.63
specified type NEC S27.69
pneumothorax S27.0
specified organ NEC S27.899
contusion S27.892
laceration S27.893
specified type NEC S27.898
thoracic duct —*see* Injury, intrathoracic, specified organ NEC
thymus gland —*see* Injury, intrathoracic, specified organ NEC
trachea, thoracic S27.50
blast (primary) S27.51
contusion S27.52
laceration S27.53
specified type NEC S27.59
iris —*see* Injury, eye, specified site NEC
penetrating —*see* Injury, eyeball, penetrating
jaw S09.93
jejunum —*see* Injury, intestine, small
joint NOS T14.8
old or residual —*see* Disorder, joint, specified type NEC
kidney S37.00-●
acute (nontraumatic) N17.9
contusion —*see* Contusion, kidney
laceration —*see* Laceration, kidney
specified NEC S37.09-●
knee S89.9-●
contusion —*see* Contusion, knee
dislocation —*see* Dislocation, knee
meniscus (lateral) (medial) —*see* Sprain, knee, specified site NEC
old injury or tear —*see* Derangement, knee, meniscus, due to old injury
open —*see* Wound, open, knee
specified NEC S89.8-●
sprain —*see* Sprain, knee
superficial —*see* Injury, superficial, knee
labium (majus) (minus) S39.94
labyrinth, ear S09.30-●
lacrimal apparatus, duct, gland, or sac —*see* Injury, eye, specified site NEC

Injury *(Continued)*
larynx NEC S19.81
leg (lower) S89.9- ●
blood vessel —*see* Injury, blood vessel, leg
contusion —*see* Contusion, leg
fracture —*see* Fracture, leg
muscle —*see* Injury, muscle, leg
nerve —*see* Injury, nerve, leg
open —*see* Wound, open, leg
specified NEC S89.8- ●
superficial —*see* Injury, superficial, leg
lens, eye —*see* Injury, eye, specified site NEC
penetrating —*see* Injury, eyeball, penetrating
limb NEC T14.8
lip S09.93
liver S36.119
contusion S36.112
laceration S36.113
major (stellate) S36.116
minor S36.114
moderate S36.115
specified NEC S36.118
lower back S39.92
specified NEC S39.82
lumbar, lumbosacral (region) S39.92
plexus —*see* Injury, lumbosacral plexus
lumbosacral plexus S34.4
lung —*see also* Injury, intrathoracic, lung
aspiration J69.0
transfusion-related (TRALI) J95.84
lymphatic thoracic duct —*see* Injury, intrathoracic, specified organ NEC
malar region S09.93
mastoid region S09.90
maxilla S09.93
mediastinum —*see* Injury, intrathoracic, specified organ NEC
membrane, brain —*see* Injury, intracranial
meningeal artery —*see* Injury, intracranial, subdural hemorrhage
meninges (cerebral) —*see* Injury, intracranial
mesenteric
artery
branch S35.299
laceration (minor) (superficial) S35.291
major S35.292
specified NEC S35.298
inferior S35.239
laceration (minor) (superficial) S35.231
major S35.232
specified NEC S35.238
superior S35.229
laceration (minor) (superficial) S35.221
major S35.222
specified NEC S35.228
plexus (inferior) (superior) —*see* Injury, nerve, lumbosacral, sympathetic
vein
inferior S35.349
laceration S35.341
specified NEC S35.348
superior S35.339
laceration S35.331
specified NEC S35.338
mesentery —*see* Injury, intra-abdominal, specified site NEC
mesosalpinx —*see* Injury, pelvic organ, specified site NEC
middle ear S09.30- ●
midthoracic region NOS S29.9
mouth S09.93
multiple NOS T07
muscle (and fascia) (and tendon)
abdomen S39.001
laceration S39.021
specified type NEC S39.091
strain S39.011
abductor
thumb, forearm level —*see* Injury, muscle, thumb, abductor

Injury *(Continued)*
muscle *(Continued)*
adductor
thigh S76.20- ●
laceration S76.22- ●
specified type NEC S76.29- ●
strain S76.21- ●
ankle —*see* Injury, muscle, foot
anterior muscle group, at leg level (lower) S86.20- ●
laceration S86.22- ●
specified type NEC S86.29- ●
strain S86.21- ●
arm (upper) —*see* Injury, muscle, shoulder
biceps (parts NEC) S46.20- ●
laceration S46.22- ●
long head S46.10- ●
laceration S46.12- ●
specified type NEC S46.19- ●
strain S46.11- ●
specified type NEC S46.29- ●
strain S46.21- ●
extensor
finger(s) (other than thumb) —*see* Injury, muscle, finger by site, extensor
forearm level, specified NEC —*see* Injury, muscle, forearm, extensor
thumb —*see* Injury, muscle, thumb, extensor
toe (large) (ankle level) (foot level) —*see* Injury, muscle, toe, extensor
finger
extensor (forearm level) S56.40- ●
hand level S66.309
laceration S66.329
specified type NEC S66.399
strain S66.319
laceration S56.429
specified type NEC S56.499
strain S56.419
flexor (forearm level) S56.10- ●
hand level S66.109
laceration S66.129
specified type NEC S66.199
strain S66.119
laceration S56.129
specified type NEC S56.199
strain S56.119
index
extensor (forearm level)
hand level S66.308
laceration S66.32- ●
specified type NEC S66.39- ●
strain S66.31- ●
specified type NEC S56.492- ●
flexor (forearm level)
hand level S66.108
laceration S66.12- ●
specified type NEC S66.19- ●
strain S66.11- ●
specified type NEC S56.19- ●
strain S56.11- ●
intrinsic S66.50- ●
laceration S66.52- ●
specified type NEC S66.59- ●
strain S66.51- ●
intrinsic S66.509
laceration S66.529
specified type NEC S66.599
strain S66.519
little
extensor (forearm level)
hand level S66.30- ●
laceration S66.32- ●
specified type NEC S66.39- ●
strain S66.31- ●
laceration S56.42- ●
specified type NEC S56.49- ●
strain S56.41- ●

Injury *(Continued)*
muscle *(Continued)*
finger *(Continued)*
little *(Continued)*
flexor (forearm level)
hand level S66.10- ●
laceration S66.12- ●
specified type NEC S66.19- ●
strain S66.11- ●
laceration S56.12- ●
specified type NEC S56.19- ●
strain S56.11- ●
intrinsic S66.50- ●
laceration S66.52- ●
specified type NEC S66.59- ●
strain S66.51- ●
middle
extensor (forearm level)
hand level S66.30- ●
laceration S66.32- ●
specified type NEC S66.39- ●
strain S66.31- ●
laceration S56.42- ●
specified type NEC S56.49- ●
strain S56.41- ●
flexor (forearm level)
hand level S66.10- ●
laceration S66.12- ●
specified type NEC S66.19- ●
strain S66.11- ●
laceration S56.12- ●
specified type NEC S56.19- ●
strain S56.11- ●
intrinsic S66.50- ●
laceration S66.52- ●
specified type NEC S66.59- ●
strain S66.51- ●
ring
extensor (forearm level)
hand level S66.30- ●
laceration S66.32- ●
specified type NEC S66.39- ●
strain S66.31- ●
laceration S56.42- ●
specified type NEC S56.49- ●
strain S56.41- ●
flexor (forearm level)
hand level S66.10- ●
laceration S66.12- ●
specified type NEC S66.19- ●
strain S66.11- ●
laceration S56.12- ●
specified type NEC S56.19- ●
strain S56.11- ●
intrinsic S66.50- ●
laceration S66.52- ●
specified type NEC S66.59- ●
strain S66.51- ●
flexor
finger(s) (other than thumb) — *see* Injury, muscle, finger
forearm level, specified NEC — *see* Injury, muscle, forearm, flexor
thumb —*see* Injury, muscle, thumb, flexor
toe (long) (ankle level) (foot level) —*see* Injury, muscle, toe, flexor
foot S96.90- ●
intrinsic S96.20- ●
laceration S96.22- ●
specified type NEC S96.29- ●
strain S96.21- ●
laceration S96.92- ●
long extensor, toe —*see* Injury, muscle, toe, extensor
long flexor, toe —*see* Injury, muscle, toe, flexor

Injury *(Continued)*
muscle *(Continued)*
foot *(Continued)*
specified
site NEC S96.80- •
laceration S96.82- •
specified type NEC S96.89- •
strain S96.81- •
type NEC S96.99- •
strain S96.91- •
forearm (level) S56.90- •
extensor S56.50- •
laceration S56.52- •
specified type NEC S56.59- •
strain S56.51- •
flexor S56.20- •
laceration S56.22- •
specified type NEC S56.29- •
strain S56.21- •
laceration S56.92- •
specified S56.99- •
site NEC S56.80- •
laceration S56.82- •
strain S56.81- •
type NEC S56.89- •
strain S56.91- •
hand (level) S66.90- •
laceration S66.92- •
specified
site NEC S66.80- •
laceration S66.82- •
specified type NEC S66.89- •
strain S66.81- •
type NEC S66.99- •
strain S66.91- •
head S09.10
laceration S09.12
specified type NEC S09.19
strain S09.11
hip NEC S76.00- •
laceration S76.02- •
specified type NEC S76.09- •
strain S76.01- •
intrinsic
ankle and foot level —*see* Injury, muscle, foot, intrinsic
finger (other than thumb) —*see* Injury, muscle, finger by site, intrinsic
foot (level) —*see* Injury, muscle, foot, intrinsic
thumb —*see* Injury, muscle, thumb, intrinsic
leg (level) (lower) S86.90- •
Achilles tendon —*see* Injury, Achilles tendon
anterior muscle group —*see* Injury, muscle, anterior muscle group
laceration S86.92- •
peroneal muscle group —*see* Injury, muscle, peroneal muscle group
posterior muscle group —*see* Injury, muscle, posterior muscle group, leg level
specified
site NEC S86.80- •
laceration S86.82- •
specified type NEC S86.89- •
strain S86.81- •
type NEC S86.99- •
strain S86.91- •
long
extensor toe, at ankle and foot level —*see* Injury, muscle, toe, extensor
flexor, toe, at ankle and foot level —*see* Injury, muscle, toe, flexor
head, biceps —*see* Injury, muscle, biceps, long head
lower back S39.002
laceration S39.022
specified type NEC S39.092
strain S39.012

Injury *(Continued)*
muscle *(Continued)*
neck (level) S16.9
laceration S16.2
specified type NEC S16.8
strain S16.1
pelvis S39.003
laceration S39.023
specified type NEC S39.093
strain S39.013
peroneal muscle group, at leg level (lower) S86.30- •
laceration S86.32- •
specified type NEC S86.39- •
strain S86.31- •
posterior muscle (group)
leg level (lower) S86.10- •
laceration S86.12- •
specified type NEC S86.19- •
strain S86.11- •
thigh level S76.30- •
laceration S76.32- •
specified type NEC S76.39- •
strain S76.31- •
quadriceps (thigh) S76.10- •
laceration S76.12- •
specified type NEC S76.19- •
strain S76.11- •
shoulder S46.90- •
laceration S46.92- •
rotator cuff —*see* Injury, rotator cuff
specified site NEC S46.80- •
laceration S46.82- •
specified type NEC S46.89- •
strain S46.81- •
specified type NEC S46.99- •
strain S46.91- •
thigh NEC (level) S76.90- •
adductor —*see* Injury, muscle, adductor, thigh
laceration S76.92- •
posterior muscle (group) —*see* Injury, muscle, posterior muscle, thigh level
quadriceps —*see* Injury, muscle, quadriceps
specified
site NEC S76.80- •
laceration S76.82- •
specified type NEC S76.89- •
strain S76.81- •
type NEC S76.99- •
strain S76.91- •
thorax (level) S29.009
back wall S29.002
front wall S29.001
laceration S29.029
back wall S29.022
front wall S29.021
specified type NEC S29.099
back wall S29.092
front wall S29.091
strain S29.019
back wall S29.012
front wall S29.011
thumb
abductor (forearm level) S56.30- •
laceration S56.32- •
specified type NEC S56.39- •
strain S56.31- •
extensor (forearm level) S56.30- •
hand level S66.20- •
laceration S66.22- •
specified type NEC S66.29- •
strain S66.21- •
laceration S56.32- •
specified type NEC S56.39- •
strain S56.31- •
flexor (forearm level) S56.00- •
hand level S66.00- •
laceration S66.02- •
specified type NEC S66.09- •
strain S66.01- •

Injury *(Continued)*
muscle *(Continued)*
thumb *(Continued)*
flexor *(Continued)*
laceration S56.02- •
specified type NEC S56.09- •
strain S56.01- •
wrist level —*see* Injury, muscle, thumb, flexor, hand level
intrinsic S66.40- •
laceration S66.42- •
specified type NEC S66.49- •
strain S66.41- •
toe —*see also* Injury, muscle, foot
extensor, long S96.10- •
laceration S96.12- •
specified type NEC S96.19- •
strain S96.11- •
flexor, long S96.00- •
laceration S96.02- •
specified type NEC S96.09- •
strain S96.01- •
triceps S46.30- •
laceration S46.32- •
specified type NEC S46.39- •
strain S46.31- •
wrist (and hand) level —*see* Injury, muscle, hand
musculocutaneous nerve —*see* Injury, nerve, musculocutaneous
myocardium —*see* Injury, heart
nape —*see* Injury, neck
nasal (septum) (sinus) S09.92
nasopharynx S09.92
neck S19.9
specified NEC S19.80
specified site NEC S19.89
nerve NEC T14.8
abdomen S34.9
peripheral S34.6
specified site NEC S34.8
abducens S04.4- •
contusion S04.4- •
laceration S04.4- •
specified type NEC S04.4- •
abducent —*see* Injury, nerve, abducens
accessory S04.7- •
contusion S04.7- •
laceration S04.7- •
specified type NEC S04.7- •
acoustic S04.6- •
contusion S04.6- •
laceration S04.6- •
specified type NEC S04.6- •
ankle S94.9- •
cutaneous sensory S94.3- •
specified site NEC —*see* subcategory S94.8
anterior crural, femoral —*see* Injury, nerve, femoral
arm (upper) S44.9- •
axillary —*see* Injury, nerve, axillary
cutaneous —*see* Injury, nerve, cutaneous, arm
median —*see* Injury, nerve, median, upper arm
musculocutaneous —*see* Injury, nerve, musculocutaneous
radial —*see* Injury, nerve, radial, upper arm
specified site NEC —*see* subcategory S44.8
ulnar —*see* Injury, nerve, ulnar, arm
auditory —*see* Injury, nerve, acoustic
axillary S44.3- •
brachial plexus —*see* Injury, brachial plexus
cervical sympathetic S14.5

- Injury *(Continued)*
  - nerve NEC *(Continued)*
    - cranial S04.9
      - contusion S04.9
      - eighth (acoustic or auditory) —*see* Injury, nerve, acoustic
      - eleventh (accessory) —*see* Injury, nerve, accessory
      - fifth (trigeminal) —*see* Injury, nerve, trigeminal
      - first (olfactory) —*see* Injury, nerve, olfactory
      - fourth (trochlear) —*see* Injury, nerve, trochlear
      - laceration S04.9
      - ninth (glossopharyngeal) —*see* Injury, nerve, glossopharyngeal
      - second (optic) —*see* Injury, nerve, optic
      - seventh (facial) —*see* Injury, nerve, facial
      - sixth (abducent) —*see* Injury, nerve, abducens
      - specified
        - nerve NEC S04.89-●
          - contusion S04.89-●
          - laceration S04.89-●
          - specified type NEC S04.89-●
        - type NEC S04.9
      - tenth (pneumogastric or vagus) —*see* Injury, nerve, vagus
      - third (oculomotor) —*see* Injury, nerve, oculomotor
      - twelfth (hypoglossal) —*see* Injury, nerve, hypoglossal
    - cutaneous sensory
      - ankle (level) S94.3-●
      - arm (upper) (level) S44.5-●
      - foot (level) —*see* Injury, nerve, cutaneous sensory, ankle
      - forearm (level) S54.3-●
      - hip (level) S74.2-●
      - leg (lower level) S84.2-●
      - shoulder (level) —*see* Injury, nerve, cutaneous sensory, arm
      - thigh (level) —*see* Injury, nerve, cutaneous sensory, hip
    - deep peroneal —*see* Injury, nerve, peroneal, foot
    - digital
      - finger S64.4-●
        - index S64.49-●
        - little S64.49-●
        - middle S64.49-●
        - ring S64.49-●
      - thumb S64.3-●
      - toe —*see* Injury, nerve, ankle, specified site NEC
    - eighth cranial (acoustic or auditory) —*see* Injury, nerve, acoustic
    - eleventh cranial (accessory) —*see* Injury, nerve, accessory
    - facial S04.5-●
      - contusion S04.5-●
      - laceration S04.5-●
      - newborn P11.3
      - specified type NEC S04.5-●
    - femoral (hip level) (thigh level) S74.1-●
    - fifth cranial (trigeminal) —*see* Injury, nerve, trigeminal
    - finger (digital) —*see* Injury, nerve, digital, finger
    - first cranial (olfactory) —*see* Injury, nerve, olfactory
    - foot S94.9-●
      - cutaneous sensory S94.3-●
      - deep peroneal S94.2-●
      - lateral plantar S94.0-●
      - medial plantar S94.1-●
      - specified site NEC —*see* subcategory S94.8
- Injury *(Continued)*
  - nerve NEC *(Continued)*
    - forearm (level) S54.9-●
      - cutaneous sensory —*see* Injury, nerve, cutaneous sensory, forearm
      - median —*see* Injury, nerve, median
      - radial —*see* Injury, nerve, radial
      - specified site NEC —*see* subcategory S54.8
      - ulnar —*see* Injury, nerve, ulnar
    - fourth cranial (trochlear) —*see* Injury, nerve, trochlear
    - glossopharyngeal S04.89-●
      - specified type NEC S04.89-●
    - hand S64.9-●
      - median —*see* Injury, nerve, median, hand
      - radial —*see* Injury, nerve, radial, hand
      - specified NEC —*see* subcategory S64.8
      - ulnar —*see* Injury, nerve, ulnar, hand
    - hip (level) S74.9-●
      - cutaneous sensory —*see* Injury, nerve, cutaneous sensory, hip
      - femoral —*see* Injury, nerve, femoral
      - sciatic —*see* Injury, nerve, sciatic
      - specified site NEC —*see* subcategory S74.8
    - hypoglossal S04.89-●
      - specified type NEC S04.89-●
    - lateral plantar S94.0-●
    - leg (lower) S84.9-●
      - cutaneous sensory —*see* Injury, nerve, cutaneous sensory, leg
      - peroneal —*see* Injury, nerve, peroneal
      - specified site NEC —*see* subcategory S84.8
      - tibial —*see* Injury, nerve, tibial
      - upper —*see* Injury, nerve, thigh
    - lower
      - back —*see* Injury, nerve, abdomen, specified site NEC
        - peripheral —*see* Injury, nerve, abdomen, peripheral
      - limb —*see* Injury, nerve, leg
    - lumbar plexus —*see* Injury, nerve, lumbosacral, sympathetic
    - lumbar spinal —*see* Injury, nerve, spinal, lumbar
    - lumbosacral
      - plexus —*see* Injury, nerve, lumbosacral, sympathetic
      - sympathetic S34.5
    - medial plantar S94.1-●
    - median (forearm level) S54.1-●
      - hand (level) S64.1-●
      - upper arm (level) S44.1-●
      - wrist (level) —*see* Injury, nerve, median, hand
    - musculocutaneous S44.4-●
    - musculospiral (upper arm level) —*see* Injury, nerve, radial, upper arm
    - neck S14.9
      - peripheral S14.4
      - specified site NEC S14.8
      - sympathetic S14.5
    - ninth cranial (glossopharyngeal) —*see* Injury, nerve, glossopharyngeal
    - oculomotor S04.1-●
      - contusion S04.1-●
      - laceration S04.1-●
      - specified type NEC S04.1-●
    - olfactory S04.81-●
      - specified type NEC S04.81-●
    - optic S04.01-●
      - contusion S04.01-●
      - laceration S04.01-●
      - specified type NEC S04.01-●
    - pelvic girdle —*see* Injury, nerve, hip
    - pelvis —*see* Injury, nerve, abdomen, specified site NEC
      - peripheral —*see* Injury, nerve, abdomen, peripheral
- Injury *(Continued)*
  - nerve NEC *(Continued)*
    - peripheral NEC T14.8
      - abdomen —*see* Injury, nerve, abdomen, peripheral
      - lower back —*see* Injury, nerve, abdomen, peripheral
      - neck —*see* Injury, nerve, neck, peripheral
      - pelvis —*see* Injury, nerve, abdomen, peripheral
      - specified NEC T14.8
    - peroneal (lower leg level) S84.1-●
      - foot S94.2-●
    - plexus
      - brachial —*see* Injury, brachial plexus
      - celiac, coeliac —*see* Injury, nerve, lumbosacral, sympathetic
      - mesenteric, inferior —*see* Injury, nerve, lumbosacral, sympathetic
      - sacral —*see* Injury, lumbosacral plexus
      - spinal
        - brachial —*see* Injury, brachial plexus
        - lumbosacral —*see* Injury, lumbosacral plexus
    - pneumogastric —*see* Injury, nerve, vagus
    - radial (forearm level) S54.2-●
      - hand (level) S64.2-●
      - upper arm (level) S44.2-●
      - wrist (level) —*see* Injury, nerve, radial, hand
    - root —*see* Injury, nerve, spinal, root
    - sacral plexus —*see* Injury, lumbosacral plexus
    - sacral spinal —*see* Injury, nerve, spinal, sacral
    - sciatic (hip level) (thigh level) S74.0-●
    - second cranial (optic) —*see* Injury, nerve, optic
    - seventh cranial (facial) —*see* Injury, nerve, facial
    - shoulder —*see* Injury, nerve, arm
    - sixth cranial (abducent) —*see* Injury, nerve, abducens
    - spinal
      - plexus —*see* Injury, nerve, plexus, spinal
      - root
        - cervical S14.2
        - dorsal S24.2
        - lumbar S34.21
        - sacral S34.22
        - thoracic —*see* Injury, nerve, spinal, root, dorsal
    - splanchnic —*see* Injury, nerve, lumbosacral, sympathetic
    - sympathetic NEC —*see* Injury, nerve, lumbosacral, sympathetic
      - cervical —*see* Injury, nerve, cervical sympathetic
    - tenth cranial (pneumogastric or vagus) —*see* Injury, nerve, vagus
    - thigh (level) —*see* Injury, nerve, hip
      - cutaneous sensory —*see* Injury, nerve, cutaneous sensory, hip
      - femoral —*see* Injury, nerve, femoral
      - sciatic —*see* Injury, nerve, sciatic
      - specified NEC —*see* Injury, nerve, hip
    - third cranial (oculomotor) —*see* Injury, nerve, oculomotor
    - thorax S24.9
      - peripheral S24.3
      - specified site NEC S24.8
      - sympathetic S24.4
    - thumb, digital —*see* Injury, nerve, digital, thumb
    - tibial (lower leg level) (posterior) S84.0-●
    - toe —*see* Injury, nerve, ankle
    - trigeminal S04.3-●
      - contusion S04.3-●
      - laceration S04.3-●
      - specified type NEC S04.3-●

Injury (Continued)
nerve NEC (Continued)
trochlear S04.2-●
contusion S04.2-●
laceration S04.2-●
specified type NEC S04.2-●
twelfth cranial (hypoglossal) —see Injury, nerve, hypoglossal
ulnar (forearm level) S54.0-●
arm (upper) (level) S44.0-●
hand (level) S64.0-●
wrist (level) —see Injury, nerve, ulnar, hand
vagus S04.89-●
specified type NEC S04.89-●
wrist (level) —see Injury, nerve, hand
ninth cranial nerve (glossopharyngeal) —see Injury, nerve, glossopharyngeal
nose (septum) S09.92
obstetrical O71.9
specified NEC O71.89
occipital (region) (scalp) S09.90
lobe —see Injury, intracranial
optic chiasm S04.02
optic radiation S04.03-●
optic tract and pathways S04.03-●
orbit, orbital (region) —see Injury, eye
penetrating (with foreign body) —see Injury, eye, orbit, penetrating
specified NEC —see Injury, eye, specified site NEC
ovary, ovarian S37.409
bilateral S37.402
contusion S37.422
laceration S37.432
specified type NEC S37.492
blood vessel —see Injury, blood vessel, ovarian
contusion S37.429
bilateral S37.422
unilateral S37.421
laceration S37.439
bilateral S37.432
unilateral S37.431
specified type NEC S37.499
bilateral S37.492
unilateral S37.491
unilateral S37.401
contusion S37.421
laceration S37.431
specified type NEC S37.491
palate (hard) (soft) S09.93
pancreas S36.209
body S36.201
contusion S36.221
laceration S36.231
major S36.261
minor S36.241
moderate S36.251
specified type NEC S36.291
contusion S36.229
head S36.200
contusion S36.220
laceration S36.230
major S36.260
minor S36.240
moderate S36.250
specified type NEC S36.290
laceration S36.239
major S36.269
minor S36.249
moderate S36.259
specified type NEC S36.299
tail S36.202
contusion S36.222
laceration S36.232
major S36.262
minor S36.242
moderate S36.252
specified type NEC S36.292

Injury (Continued)
parietal (region) (scalp) S09.90
lobe —see Injury, intracranial
patellar ligament (tendon) S76.10-●
laceration S76.12-●
specified NEC S76.19-●
strain S76.11-●
pelvis, pelvic (floor) S39.93
complicating delivery O70.1
joint or ligament, complicating delivery O71.6
organ S37.90
with ectopic or molar pregnancy O08.6
complication of abortion —see Abortion
contusion S37.92
following ectopic or molar pregnancy O08.6
laceration S37.93
obstetrical trauma NEC O71.5
specified
site NEC S37.899
contusion S37.892
laceration S37.893
specified type NEC S37.898
type NEC S37.99
specified NEC S39.83
penis S39.94
perineum S39.94
peritoneum S36.81
laceration S36.893
periurethral tissue —see Injury, urethra
complicating delivery O71.82
phalanges
foot —see Injury, foot
hand —see Injury, hand
pharynx NEC S19.85
pleura —see Injury, intrathoracic, pleura
plexus
brachial —see Injury, brachial plexus
cardiac —see Injury, nerve, thorax, sympathetic
celiac, coeliac —see Injury, nerve, lumbosacral, sympathetic
esophageal —see Injury, nerve, thorax, sympathetic
hypogastric —see Injury, nerve, lumbosacral, sympathetic
lumbar, lumbosacral —see Injury, lumbosacral plexus
mesenteric —see Injury, nerve, lumbosacral, sympathetic
pulmonary —see Injury, nerve, thorax, sympathetic
postcardiac surgery (syndrome) I97.0
prepuce S39.94
▶pressure
▶injury —see Ulcer, pressure, by site
prostate S37.829
contusion S37.822
laceration S37.823
specified type NEC S37.828
pubic region S39.94
pudendum S39.94
pulmonary plexus —see Injury, nerve, thorax, sympathetic
rectovaginal septum NEC S39.83
rectum —see Injury, intestine, large, rectum
retina —see Injury, eye, specified site NEC
penetrating —see Injury, eyeball, penetrating
retroperitoneal —see Injury, intra-abdominal, specified site NEC
rotator cuff (muscle(s)) (tendon(s)) S46.00-●
laceration S46.02-●
specified type NEC S46.09-●
strain S46.01-●
round ligament —see Injury, pelvic organ, specified site NEC
sacral plexus —see Injury, lumbosacral plexus
salivary duct or gland S09.93

Injury (Continued)
scalp S09.90
newborn (birth injury) P12.9
due to monitoring (electrode) (sampling incision) P12.4
specified NEC P12.89
caput succedaneum P12.81
scapular region —see Injury, shoulder
sclera —see Injury, eye, specified site NEC
penetrating —see Injury, eyeball, penetrating
scrotum S39.94
second cranial nerve (optic) —see Injury, nerve, optic
seminal vesicle —see Injury, pelvic organ, specified site NEC
seventh cranial nerve (facial) —see Injury, nerve, facial
shoulder S49.9-●
blood vessel —see Injury, blood vessel, arm
contusion —see Contusion, shoulder
dislocation —see Dislocation, shoulder
fracture —see Fracture, shoulder
muscle —see Injury, muscle, shoulder
nerve —see Injury, nerve, shoulder
open —see Wound, open, shoulder
specified type NEC S49.8-●
sprain —see Sprain, shoulder girdle
superficial —see Injury, superficial, shoulder
sinus
cavernous —see Injury, intracranial
nasal S09.92
sixth cranial nerve (abducent) —see Injury, nerve, abducens
skeleton, birth injury P13.9
specified part NEC P13.8
skin NEC T14.8
surface intact —see Injury, superficial
skull NEC S09.90
specified NEC T14.8
spermatic cord (pelvic region) S37.898
scrotal region S39.848
spinal (cord)
cervical (neck) S14.109
anterior cord syndrome S14.139
C1 level S14.131
C2 level S14.132
C3 level S14.133
C4 level S14.134
C5 level S14.135
C6 level S14.136
C7 level S14.137
C8 level S14.138
Brown-Séquard syndrome S14.149
C1 level S14.141
C2 level S14.142
C3 level S14.143
C4 level S14.144
C5 level S14.145
C6 level S14.146
C7 level S14.147
C8 level S14.148
C1 level S14.101
C2 level S14.102
C3 level S14.103
C4 level S14.104
C5 level S14.105
C6 level S14.106
C7 level S14.107
C8 level S14.108
central cord syndrome S14.129
C1 level S14.121
C2 level S14.122
C3 level S14.123
C4 level S14.124
C5 level S14.125
C6 level S14.126
C7 level S14.127
C8 level S14.128

Injury *(Continued)*
  spinal *(Continued)*
    cervical *(Continued)*
      complete lesion S14.119
        C1 level S14.111
        C2 level S14.112
        C3 level S14.113
        C4 level S14.114
        C5 level S14.115
        C6 level S14.116
        C7 level S14.117
        C8 level S14.118
      concussion S14.Ø
      edema S14.Ø
      incomplete lesion specified NEC S14.159
        C1 level S14.151
        C2 level S14.152
        C3 level S14.153
        C4 level S14.154
        C5 level S14.155
        C6 level S14.156
        C7 level S14.157
        C8 level S14.158
      posterior cord syndrome S14.159
        C1 level S14.151
        C2 level S14.152
        C3 level S14.153
        C4 level S14.154
        C5 level S14.155
        C6 level S14.156
        C7 level S14.157
        C8 level S14.158
    dorsal —*see* Injury, spinal, thoracic
    lumbar S34.1Ø9
      complete lesion S34.119
        L1 level S34.111
        L2 level S34.112
        L3 level S34.113
        L4 level S34.114
        L5 level S34.115
      concussion S34.Ø1
      edema S34.Ø1
      incomplete lesion S34.129
        L1 level S34.121
        L2 level S34.122
        L3 level S34.123
        L4 level S34.124
        L5 level S34.125
      L1 level S34.1Ø1
      L2 level S34.1Ø2
      L3 level S34.1Ø3
      L4 level S34.1Ø4
      L5 level S34.1Ø5
    nerve root NEC
      cervical —*see* Injury, nerve, spinal, root, cervical
      dorsal —*see* Injury, nerve, spinal, root, dorsal
      lumbar S34.21
      sacral S34.22
      thoracic —*see* Injury, nerve, spinal, root, dorsal
    plexus
      brachial —*see* Injury, brachial plexus
      lumbosacral —*see* Injury, lumbosacral plexus
    sacral S34.139
      complete lesion S34.131
      incomplete lesion S34.132
    thoracic S24.1Ø9
      anterior cord syndrome S24.139
        T1 level S24.131
        T2-T6 level S24.132
        T7-T1Ø level S24.133
        T11-T12 level S24.134
      Brown-Séquard syndrome S24.149
        T1 level S24.141
        T2-T6 level S24.142
        T7-T1Ø level S24.143
        T11-T12 level S24.144

Injury *(Continued)*
  spinal *(Continued)*
    thoracic *(Continued)*
      complete lesion S24.119
        T1 level S24.111
        T2-T6 level S24.112
        T7-T1Ø level S24.113
        T11-T12 level S24.114
      concussion S24.Ø
      edema S24.Ø
      incomplete lesion specified NEC S24.159
        T1 level S24.151
        T2-T6 level S24.152
        T7-T1Ø level S24.153
        T11-T12 level S24.154
      posterior cord syndrome S24.159
        T1 level S24.151
        T2-T6 level S24.152
        T7-T1Ø level S24.153
        T11-T12 level S24.154
      T1 level S24.1Ø1
      T2-T6 level S24.1Ø2
      T7-T1Ø level S24.1Ø3
      T11-T12 level S24.1Ø4
  splanchnic nerve —*see* Injury, nerve, lumbosacral, sympathetic
  spleen S36.ØØ
    contusion S36.Ø29
      major S36.Ø21
      minor S36.Ø2Ø
    laceration S36.Ø39
      major (massive) (stellate) S36.Ø32
      moderate S36.Ø31
      superficial (capsular) (minor) S36.Ø3Ø
    specified type NEC S36.Ø9
  splenic artery —*see* Injury, blood vessel, celiac artery, branch
  stellate ganglion —*see* Injury, nerve, thorax, sympathetic
  sternal region S29.9
  stomach S36.3Ø
    contusion S36.32
    laceration S36.33
    specified type NEC S36.39
  subconjunctival —*see* Injury, eye, conjunctiva
  subcutaneous NEC T14.8
  submaxillary region SØ9.93
  submental region SØ9.93
  subungual
    fingers —*see* Injury, hand
    toes —*see* Injury, foot
  superficial NEC T14.8
    abdomen, abdominal (wall) S3Ø.92
      abrasion S3Ø.811
      bite S3Ø.871
        insect S3Ø.861
      contusion S3Ø.1
      external constriction S3Ø.841
      foreign body S3Ø.851
    abrasion —*see* Abrasion, by site
    adnexa, eye NEC —*see* Injury, eye, specified site NEC
    alveolar process —*see* Injury, superficial, oral cavity
    ankle S9Ø.91-●
      abrasion —*see* Abrasion, ankle
      bite —*see* Bite, ankle
      blister —*see* Blister, ankle
      contusion —*see* Contusion, ankle
      external constriction —*see* Constriction, external, ankle
      foreign body —*see* Foreign body, superficial, ankle
    anus S3Ø.98
    arm (upper) S4Ø.92-●
      abrasion —*see* Abrasion, arm
      bite —*see* Bite, superficial, arm
      blister —*see* Blister, arm (upper)
      contusion —*see* Contusion, arm
      external constriction —*see* Constriction, external, arm

Injury *(Continued)*
  superficial NEC *(Continued)*
    arm *(Continued)*
      foreign body —*see* Foreign body, superficial, arm
    auditory canal (external) (meatus) —*see* Injury, superficial, ear
    auricle —*see* Injury, superficial, ear
    axilla —*see* Injury, superficial, arm
    back —*see also* Injury, superficial, thorax, back
      lower S3Ø.91
        abrasion S3Ø.81Ø
        contusion S3Ø.Ø
        external constriction S3Ø.84Ø
        superficial
          bite NEC S3Ø.87Ø
            insect S3Ø.86Ø
          foreign body S3Ø.85Ø
    bite NEC —*see* Bite, superficial NEC, by site
    blister —*see* Blister, by site
    breast S2Ø.1Ø-●
      abrasion —*see* Abrasion, breast
      bite —*see* Bite, superficial, breast
      contusion —*see* Contusion, breast
      external constriction —*see* Constriction, external, breast
      foreign body —*see* Foreign body, superficial, breast
    brow —*see* Injury, superficial, head, specified NEC
    buttock S3Ø.91
    calf —*see* Injury, superficial, leg
    canthus, eye —*see* Injury, superficial, periocular area
    cheek (external) —*see* Injury, superficial, head, specified NEC
      internal —*see* Injury, superficial, oral cavity
    chest wall —*see* Injury, superficial, thorax
    chin —*see* Injury, superficial, head NEC
    clitoris S3Ø.95
    conjunctiva —*see* Injury, eye, conjunctiva
      with foreign body (in conjunctival sac) —*see* Foreign body, conjunctival sac
    contusion —*see* Contusion, by site
    costal region —*see* Injury, superficial, thorax
    digit(s)
      hand —*see* Injury, superficial, finger
    ear (auricle) (canal) (external) SØØ.4Ø-●
      abrasion —*see* Abrasion, ear
      bite —*see* Bite, superficial, ear
      contusion —*see* Contusion, ear
      external constriction —*see* Constriction, external, ear
      foreign body —*see* Foreign body, superficial, ear
    elbow S5Ø.9Ø-●
      abrasion —*see* Abrasion, elbow
      bite —*see* Bite, superficial, elbow
      blister —*see* Blister, elbow
      contusion —*see* Contusion, elbow
      external constriction —*see* Constriction, external, elbow
      foreign body —*see* Foreign body, superficial, elbow
    epididymis S3Ø.94
    epigastric region S3Ø.92
    epiglottis —*see* Injury, superficial, throat
    esophagus
      cervical —*see* Injury, superficial, throat
    external constriction —*see* Constriction, external, by site
    extremity NEC T14.8
    eyeball NEC —*see* Injury, eye, specified site NEC
    eyebrow —*see* Injury, superficial, periocular area

Injury *(Continued)*
- superficial NEC *(Continued)*
  - eyelid S00.20- •
    - abrasion *—see* Abrasion, eyelid
    - bite *—see* Bite, superficial, eyelid
    - contusion *—see* Contusion, eyelid
    - external constriction *—see* Constriction, external, eyelid
    - foreign body *—see* Foreign body, superficial, eyelid
  - face NEC *—see* Injury, superficial, head, specified NEC
  - finger(s) S60.949
    - abrasion *—see* Abrasion, finger
    - bite *—see* Bite, superficial, finger
    - blister *—see* Blister, finger
    - contusion *—see* Contusion, finger
    - external constriction *—see* Constriction, external, finger
    - foreign body *—see* Foreign body, superficial, finger
    - index S60.94- •
    - insect bite *—see* Bite, by site, superficial, insect
    - little S60.94- •
    - middle S60.94- •
    - ring S60.94- •
  - flank S30.92
  - foot S90.92- •
    - abrasion *—see* Abrasion, foot
    - bite *—see* Bite, foot
    - blister *—see* Blister, foot
    - contusion *—see* Contusion, foot
    - external constriction *—see* Constriction, external, foot
    - foreign body *—see* Foreign body, superficial, foot
  - forearm S50.91- •
    - abrasion *—see* Abrasion, forearm
    - bite *—see* Bite, forearm, superficial
    - blister *—see* Blister, forearm
    - contusion *—see* Contusion, forearm
    - elbow only *—see* Injury, superficial, elbow
    - external constriction *—see* Constriction, external, forearm
    - foreign body *—see* Foreign body, superficial, forearm
  - forehead *—see* Injury, superficial, head NEC
  - foreign body *—see* Foreign body, superficial
  - genital organs, external
    - female S30.97
    - male S30.96
  - globe (eye) *—see* Injury, eye, specified site NEC
  - groin S30.92
  - gum *—see* Injury, superficial, oral cavity
  - hand S60.92- •
    - abrasion *—see* Abrasion, hand
    - bite *—see* Bite, superficial, hand
    - contusion *—see* Contusion, hand
    - external constriction *—see* Constriction, external, hand
    - foreign body *—see* Foreign body, superficial, hand
  - head S00.90
    - ear *—see* Injury, superficial, ear
    - eyelid *—see* Injury, superficial, eyelid
    - nose S00.30
    - oral cavity S00.502
    - scalp S00.00
    - specified site NEC S00.80
  - heel *—see* Injury, superficial, foot
  - hip S70.91- •
    - abrasion *—see* Abrasion, hip
    - bite *—see* Bite, superficial, hip
    - blister *—see* Blister, hip
    - contusion *—see* Contusion, hip

Injury *(Continued)*
- superficial NEC *(Continued)*
  - hip *(Continued)*
    - external constriction *—see* Constriction, external, hip
    - foreign body *—see* Foreign body, superficial, hip
  - iliac region *—see* Injury, superficial, abdomen
  - inguinal region *—see* Injury, superficial, abdomen
  - insect bite *—see* Bite, by site, superficial, insect
  - interscapular region *—see* Injury, superficial, thorax, back
  - jaw *—see* Injury, superficial, head, specified NEC
  - knee S80.91- •
    - abrasion *—see* Abrasion, knee
    - bite *—see* Bite, superficial, knee
    - blister *—see* Blister, knee
    - contusion *—see* Contusion, knee
    - external constriction *—see* Constriction, external, knee
    - foreign body *—see* Foreign body, superficial, knee
  - labium (majus) (minus) S30.95
  - lacrimal (apparatus) (gland) (sac) *—see* Injury, eye, specified site NEC
  - larynx *—see* Injury, superficial, throat
  - leg (lower) S80.92- •
    - abrasion *—see* Abrasion, leg
    - bite *—see* Bite, superficial, leg
    - contusion *—see* Contusion, leg
    - external constriction *—see* Constriction, external, leg
    - foreign body *—see* Foreign body, superficial, leg
    - knee *—see* Injury, superficial, knee
  - limb NEC T14.8
  - lip S00.501
  - lower back S30.91
  - lumbar region S30.91
  - malar region *—see* Injury, superficial, head, specified NEC
  - mammary *—see* Injury, superficial, breast
  - mastoid region *—see* Injury, superficial, head, specified NEC
  - mouth *—see* Injury, superficial, oral cavity
  - muscle NEC T14.8
  - nail NEC T14.8
    - finger *—see* Injury, superficial, finger
    - toe *—see* Injury, superficial, toe
  - nasal (septum) *—see* Injury, superficial, nose
  - neck S10.90
    - specified site NEC S10.80
  - nose (septum) S00.30
  - occipital region *—see* Injury, superficial, scalp
  - oral cavity S00.502
  - orbital region *—see* Injury, superficial, periocular area
  - palate *—see* Injury, superficial, oral cavity
  - palm *—see* Injury, superficial, hand
  - parietal region *—see* Injury, superficial, scalp
  - pelvis S30.91
    - girdle *—see* Injury, superficial, hip
  - penis S30.93
  - perineum
    - female S30.95
    - male S30.91
  - periocular area S00.20- •
    - abrasion *—see* Abrasion, eyelid
    - bite *—see* Bite, superficial, eyelid
    - contusion *—see* Contusion, eyelid
    - external constriction *—see* Constriction, external, eyelid
    - foreign body *—see* Foreign body, superficial, eyelid

Injury *(Continued)*
- superficial NEC *(Continued)*
  - phalanges
    - finger *—see* Injury, superficial, finger
    - toe *—see* Injury, superficial, toe
  - pharynx *—see* Injury, superficial, throat
  - pinna *—see* Injury, superficial, ear
  - popliteal space *—see* Injury, superficial, knee
  - prepuce S30.93
  - pubic region S30.91
  - pudendum
    - female S30.97
    - male S30.96
  - sacral region S30.91
  - scalp S00.00
  - scapular region *—see* Injury, superficial, shoulder
  - sclera *—see* Injury, eye, specified site NEC
  - scrotum S30.94
  - shin *—see* Injury, superficial, leg
  - shoulder S40.91- •
    - abrasion *—see* Abrasion, shoulder
    - bite *—see* Bite, superficial, shoulder
    - blister *—see* Blister, shoulder
    - contusion *—see* Contusion, shoulder
    - external constriction *—see* Constriction, external, shoulder
    - foreign body *—see* Foreign body, superficial, shoulder
  - skin NEC T14.8
  - sternal region *—see* Injury, superficial, thorax, front
  - subconjunctival *—see* Injury, eye, specified site NEC
  - subcutaneous NEC T14.8
  - submaxillary region *—see* Injury, superficial, head, specified NEC
  - submental region *—see* Injury, superficial, head, specified NEC
  - subungual
    - finger(s) *—see* Injury, superficial, finger
    - toe(s) *—see* Injury, superficial, toe
  - supraclavicular fossa *—see* Injury, superficial, neck
  - supraorbital *—see* Injury, superficial, head, specified NEC
  - temple *—see* Injury, superficial, head, specified NEC
  - temporal region *—see* Injury, superficial, head, specified NEC
  - testis S30.94
  - thigh S70.92- •
    - abrasion *—see* Abrasion, thigh
    - bite *—see* Bite, superficial, thigh
    - blister *—see* Blister, thigh
    - contusion *—see* Contusion, thigh
    - external constriction *—see* Constriction, external, thigh
    - foreign body *—see* Foreign body, superficial, thigh
  - thorax, thoracic (wall) S20.90
    - abrasion *—see* Abrasion, thorax
    - back S20.40- •
    - bite *—see* Bite, thorax, superficial
    - blister *—see* Blister, thorax
    - contusion *—see* Contusion, thorax
    - external constriction *—see* Constriction, external, thorax
    - foreign body *—see* Foreign body, superficial, thorax
    - front S20.30- •
  - throat S10.10
    - abrasion S10.11
    - bite S10.17
      - insect S10.16
    - blister S10.12
    - contusion S10.0
    - external constriction S10.14
    - foreign body S10.15

Injury *(Continued)*
superficial NEC *(Continued)*
thumb S6Ø.93-●
abrasion —*see* Abrasion, thumb
bite —*see* Bite, superficial, thumb
blister —*see* Blister, thumb
contusion —*see* Contusion, thumb
external constriction —*see* Constriction, external, thumb
foreign body —*see* Foreign body, superficial, thumb
insect bite —*see* Bite, by site, superficial, insect
specified type NEC S6Ø.39-●
toe(s) S9Ø.93-●
abrasion —*see* Abrasion, toe
bite —*see* Bite, toe
blister —*see* Blister, toe
contusion —*see* Contusion, toe
external constriction —*see* Constriction, external, toe
foreign body —*see* Foreign body, superficial, toe
great S9Ø.93-●
tongue —*see* Injury, superficial, oral cavity
tooth, teeth —*see* Injury, superficial, oral cavity
trachea S1Ø.1Ø
tunica vaginalis S3Ø.94
tympanum, tympanic membrane —*see* Injury, superficial, ear
uvula —*see* Injury, superficial, oral cavity
vagina S3Ø.95
vocal cords —*see* Injury, superficial, throat
vulva S3Ø.95
wrist S6Ø.91-●
supraclavicular region —*see* Injury, neck
supraorbital SØ9.93
suprarenal gland (multiple) —*see* Injury, adrenal
surgical complication (external or internal site) —*see* Laceration, accidental complicating surgery
temple SØ9.9Ø
temporal region SØ9.9Ø
tendon —*see also* Injury, muscle, by site
abdomen —*see* Injury, muscle, abdomen
Achilles —*see* Injury, Achilles tendon
lower back —*see* Injury, muscle, lower back
pelvic organs —*see* Injury, muscle, pelvis
tenth cranial nerve (pneumogastric or vagus) —*see* Injury, nerve, vagus
testis S39.94
thigh S79.92-●
blood vessel —*see* Injury, blood vessel, hip
contusion —*see* Contusion, thigh
fracture —*see* Fracture, femur
muscle —*see* Injury, muscle, thigh
nerve —*see* Injury, nerve, thigh
open —*see* Wound, open, thigh
specified NEC S79.82-●
superficial —*see* Injury, superficial, thigh
third cranial nerve (oculomotor) —*see* Injury, nerve, oculomotor
thorax, thoracic S29.9
blood vessel —*see* Injury, blood vessel, thorax
cavity —*see* Injury, intrathoracic
dislocation —*see* Dislocation, thorax
external (wall) S29.9
contusion —*see* Contusion, thorax
nerve —*see* Injury, nerve, thorax
open —*see* Wound, open, thorax
specified NEC S29.8
sprain —*see* Sprain, thorax
superficial —*see* Injury, superficial, thorax
fracture —*see* Fracture, thorax
internal —*see* Injury, intrathoracic

Injury *(Continued)*
thorax, thoracic *(Continued)*
intrathoracic organ —*see* Injury, intrathoracic
sympathetic ganglion —*see* Injury, nerve, thorax, sympathetic
throat —*see also* Injury, neck S19.9
thumb S69.9-●
blood vessel —*see* Injury, blood vessel, thumb
contusion —*see* Contusion, thumb
dislocation —*see* Dislocation, thumb
fracture —*see* Fracture, thumb
muscle —*see* Injury, muscle, thumb
nerve —*see* Injury, nerve, digital, thumb
open —*see* Wound, open, thumb
specified NEC S69.8-●
sprain —*see* Sprain, thumb
superficial —*see* Injury, superficial, thumb
thymus (gland) —*see* Injury, intrathoracic, specified organ NEC
thyroid (gland) NEC S19.84
toe S99.92-●
contusion —*see* Contusion, toe
dislocation —*see* Dislocation, toe
fracture —*see* Fracture, toe
muscle —*see* Injury, muscle, toe
open —*see* Wound, open, toe
specified type NEC S99.82-●
sprain —*see* Sprain, toe
superficial —*see* Injury, superficial, toe
tongue SØ9.93
tonsil SØ9.93
tooth SØ9.93
trachea (cervical) NEC S19.82
thoracic —*see* Injury, intrathoracic, trachea, thoracic
transfusion-related acute lung (TRALI) J95.84
tunica vaginalis S39.94
twelfth cranial nerve (hypoglossal) —*see* Injury, nerve, hypoglossal
ureter S37.1Ø
contusion S37.12
laceration S37.13
specified type NEC S37.19
urethra (sphincter) S37.3Ø
at delivery O71.5
contusion S37.32
laceration S37.33
specified type NEC S37.38
urinary organ S37.899
contusion S37.92
laceration S37.93
specified
site NEC S37.899
contusion S37.892
laceration S37.893
specified type NEC S37.898
type NEC S37.99
uterus, uterine S37.6Ø
with ectopic or molar pregnancy OØ8.6
blood vessel —*see* Injury, blood vessel, iliac
contusion S37.62
laceration S37.63
cervix at delivery O71.3
rupture associated with obstetrics —*see* Rupture, uterus
specified type NEC S37.69
uvula SØ9.93
vagina S39.93
abrasion S3Ø.814
bite S31.45
insect S3Ø.864
superficial NEC S3Ø.874
contusion S3Ø.23
crush S38.Ø3
during delivery —*see* Laceration, vagina, during delivery
external constriction S3Ø.844
insect bite S3Ø.864
laceration S31.41
with foreign body S31.42

Injury *(Continued)*
vagina *(Continued)*
open wound S31.4Ø
puncture S31.43
with foreign body S31.44
superficial S3Ø.95
foreign body S3Ø.854
vas deferens —*see* Injury, pelvic organ, specified site NEC
vascular NEC T14.8
vein —*see* Injury, blood vessel
vena cava (superior) S25.2Ø
inferior S35.1Ø
laceration (minor) (superficial) S35.11
major S35.12
specified type NEC S35.19
laceration (minor) (superficial) S25.21
major S25.22
specified type NEC S25.29
vesical (sphincter) —*see* Injury, bladder
visual cortex SØ4.Ø4-●
vitreous (humor) SØ5.9Ø
specified NEC SØ5.8X-●
vocal cord NEC S19.83
vulva S39.94
abrasion S3Ø.814
bite S31.45
insect S3Ø.864
superficial NEC S3Ø.874
contusion S3Ø.23
crush S38.Ø3
during delivery —*see* Laceration, perineum, female, during delivery
external constriction S3Ø.844
insect bite S3Ø.864
laceration S31.41
with foreign body S31.42
open wound S31.4Ø
puncture S31.43
with foreign body S31.44
superficial S3Ø.95
foreign body S3Ø.854
whiplash (cervical spine) S13.4
wrist S69.9-●
blood vessel —*see* Injury, blood vessel, hand
contusion —*see* Contusion, wrist
dislocation —*see* Dislocation, wrist
fracture —*see* Fracture, wrist
muscle —*see* Injury, muscle, hand
nerve —*see* Injury, nerve, hand
open —*see* Wound, open, wrist
specified NEC S69.8-●
sprain —*see* Sprain, wrist
superficial —*see* Injury, superficial, wrist
Inoculation —*see also* Vaccination
complication or reaction —*see* Complications, vaccination
Insanity, insane —*see also* Psychosis
adolescent —*see* Schizophrenia
confusional F28
acute or subacute FØ5
delusional F22
senile FØ3
Insect
bite —*see* Bite, by site, superficial, insect
venomous, poisoning NEC (by) —*see* Venom, arthropod
Insensitivity
adrenocorticotropin hormone (ACTH) E27.49
androgen E34.5Ø
complete E34.51
partial E34.52
Insertion
cord (umbilical) lateral or velamentous O43.12-●
intrauterine contraceptive device (encounter for) —*see* Intrauterine contraceptive device
➡ **Insolation** (sunstroke) T67.Ø1

Insomnia (organic) G47.ØØ
without objective findings F51.Ø2
adjustment F51.Ø2
adjustment disorder F51.Ø2
behavioral, of childhood Z73.819
combined type Z73.812
limit setting type Z73.811
sleep-onset association type Z73.81Ø
childhood Z73.819
chronic F51.Ø4
somatized tension F51.Ø4
conditioned F51.Ø4
due to
alcohol
abuse F1Ø.182
dependence F1Ø.282
use F1Ø.982
amphetamines
abuse F15.182
dependence F15.282
use F15.982
anxiety disorder F51.Ø5
caffeine
abuse F15.182
dependence F15.282
use F15.982
cocaine
abuse F14.182
dependence F14.282
use F14.982
depression F51.Ø5
drug NEC
abuse F19.182
dependence F19.282
use F19.982
medical condition G47.Ø1
mental disorder NEC F51.Ø5
opioid
abuse F11.182
dependence F11.282
use F11.982
psychoactive substance NEC
abuse F19.182
dependence F19.282
use F19.982
sedative, hypnotic, or anxiolytic
abuse F13.182
dependence F13.282
use F13.982
stimulant NEC
abuse F15.182
dependence F15.282
use F15.982
fatal familial (FFI) A81.83
idiopathic F51.Ø1
learned F51.3
nonorganic origin F51.Ø1
not due to a substance or known physiological condition F51.Ø1
specified NEC F51.Ø9
paradoxical F51.Ø3
primary F51.Ø1
psychiatric F51.Ø5
psychophysiologic F51.Ø4
related to psychopathology F51.Ø5
short-term F51.Ø2
specified NEC G47.Ø9
stress-related F51.Ø2
transient F51.Ø2
Inspiration
food or foreign body —*see* Foreign body, by site
mucus —*see* Asphyxia, mucus
Inspissated bile syndrome (newborn) P59.1
Instability
emotional (excessive) F6Ø.3
joint (post-traumatic) M25.3Ø
ankle M25.37-●
due to old ligament injury —*see* Disorder, ligament
elbow M25.32-●
Instability *(Continued)*
joint *(Continued)*
flail —*see* Flail, joint
foot M25.37-●
hand M25.34-●
hip M25.35-●
knee M25.36-●
lumbosacral —*see* subcategory M53.2
prosthesis —*see* Complications, joint prosthesis, mechanical, displacement, by site
sacroiliac —*see* subcategory M53.2
secondary to
old ligament injury —*see* Disorder, ligament
removal of joint prosthesis M96.89
shoulder (region) M25.31-●
spine —*see* subcategory M53.2
wrist M25.33-●
knee (chronic) M23.5-●
lumbosacral —*see* subcategory M53.2
nervous F48.8
personality (emotional) F6Ø.3
spine —*see* Instability, joint, spine
vasomotor R55
Institutional syndrome (childhood) F94.2
Institutionalization, affecting child Z62.22
disinhibited attachment F94.2
Insufficiency, insufficient
accommodation, old age H52.4
adrenal (gland) E27.4Ø
primary E27.1
adrenocortical E27.4Ø
drug-induced E27.3
iatrogenic E27.3
primary E27.1
anatomic crown height KØ8.89
anterior (occlusal) guidance M26.54
anus K62.89
aortic (valve) I35.1
with
mitral (valve) disease IØ8.Ø
with tricuspid (valve) disease IØ8.3
stenosis I35.2
tricuspid (valve) disease IØ8.2
with mitral (valve) disease IØ8.3
congenital Q23.1
rheumatic IØ6.1
with
mitral (valve) disease IØ8.Ø
with tricuspid (valve) disease IØ8.3
stenosis IØ6.2
with mitral (valve) disease IØ8.Ø
with tricuspid (valve) disease IØ8.3
tricuspid (valve) disease IØ8.2
with mitral (valve) disease IØ8.3
specified cause NEC I35.1
syphilitic A52.Ø3
arterial I77.1
basilar G45.Ø
carotid (hemispheric) G45.1
cerebral I67.81
coronary (acute or subacute) I24.8
mesenteric K55.1
peripheral I73.9
precerebral (multiple) (bilateral) G45.2
vertebral G45.Ø
arteriovenous I99.8
biliary K83.8
cardiac —*see also* Insufficiency, myocardial
due to presence of (cardiac) prosthesis I97.11-●
postprocedural I97.11-●
cardiorenal, hypertensive I13.2
cardiovascular —*see* Disease, cardiovascular
cerebrovascular (acute) I67.81
with transient focal neurological signs and symptoms G45.8
Insufficiency, insufficient *(Continued)*
circulatory NEC I99.8
newborn P29.89
clinical crown length KØ8.89
convergence H51.11
coronary (acute or subacute) I24.8
chronic or with a stated duration of over 4 weeks I25.89
corticoadrenal E27.4Ø
primary E27.1
dietary E63.9
divergence H51.8
food T73.Ø
gastroesophageal K22.8
gonadal
ovary E28.39
testis E29.1
heart —*see also* Insufficiency, myocardial
newborn P29.Ø
valve —*see* Endocarditis
hepatic —*see* Failure, hepatic
idiopathic autonomic G9Ø.Ø9
interocclusal distance of fully erupted teeth (ridge) M26.36
kidney N28.9
acute N28.9
chronic N18.9
lacrimal (secretion) HØ4.12-●
passages —*see* Stenosis, lacrimal
liver —*see* Failure, hepatic
lung —*see* Insufficiency, pulmonary
mental (congenital) —*see* Disability, intellectual
mesenteric K55.1
mitral (valve) I34.Ø
with
aortic valve disease IØ8.Ø
with tricuspid (valve) disease IØ8.3
obstruction or stenosis IØ5.2
with aortic valve disease IØ8.Ø
tricuspid (valve) disease IØ8.1
with aortic (valve) disease IØ8.3
congenital Q23.3
rheumatic IØ5.1
with
aortic valve disease IØ8.Ø
with tricuspid (valve) disease IØ8.3
obstruction or stenosis IØ5.2
with aortic valve disease IØ8.Ø
with tricuspid (valve) disease IØ8.3
tricuspid (valve) disease IØ8.1
with aortic (valve) disease IØ8.3
active or acute IØ1.1
with chorea, rheumatic (Sydenham's) IØ2.Ø
specified cause, except rheumatic I34.Ø
muscle —*see also* Disease, muscle
heart —*see* Insufficiency, myocardial
ocular NEC H5Ø.9
myocardial, myocardium (with arteriosclerosis) —*see also* Failure, heart I5Ø.9
with
rheumatic fever (conditions in IØØ) IØ9.Ø
active, acute or subacute IØ1.2
with chorea IØ2.Ø
inactive or quiescent (with chorea) IØ9.Ø
congenital Q24.8
hypertensive —*see* Hypertension, heart
newborn P29.Ø
rheumatic IØ9.Ø
active, acute, or subacute IØ1.2
syphilitic A52.Ø6
nourishment T73.Ø
pancreatic K86.89
exocrine K86.81
parathyroid (gland) E2Ø.9
peripheral vascular (arterial) I73.9
pituitary E23.Ø

- **Insufficiency, insufficient** *(Continued)*
  - placental (mother) O36.51-●
  - platelets D69.6
  - prenatal care affecting management of pregnancy OØ9.3-●
  - progressive pluriglandular E31.Ø
  - pulmonary J98.4
    - acute, following surgery (nonthoracic) J95.2
      - thoracic J95.1
    - chronic, following surgery J95.3
    - following
      - shock J98.4
      - trauma J98.4
    - newborn P28.89
    - valve I37.1
      - with stenosis I37.2
      - congenital Q22.2
      - rheumatic IØ9.89
        - with aortic, mitral or tricuspid (valve) disease IØ8.8
  - pyloric K31.89
  - renal (acute) N28.9
    - chronic N18.9
  - respiratory RØ6.89
    - newborn P28.5
  - rotation —*see* Malrotation
  - sleep syndrome F51.12
  - social insurance Z59.7
  - suprarenal E27.4Ø
    - primary E27.1
  - tarso-orbital fascia, congenital Q1Ø.3
  - testis E29.1
  - thyroid (gland) (acquired) EØ3.9
    - congenital EØ3.1
  - tricuspid (valve) (rheumatic) IØ7.1
    - with
      - aortic (valve) disease IØ8.2
        - with mitral (valve) disease IØ8.3
      - mitral (valve) disease IØ8.1
        - with aortic (valve) disease IØ8.3
      - obstruction or stenosis IØ7.2
        - with aortic (valve) disease IØ8.2
          - with mitral (valve) disease IØ8.3
    - congenital Q22.8
    - nonrheumatic I36.1
      - with stenosis I36.2
  - urethral sphincter R32
  - valve, valvular (heart) I38
    - aortic —*see* Insufficiency, aortic (valve)
    - mitral —*see* Insufficiency, mitral (valve)
    - pulmonary —*see* Insufficiency, pulmonary, valve
    - tricuspid —*see* Insufficiency, tricuspid (valve)
    - congenital Q24.8
  - vascular I99.8
    - intestine K55.9
      - acute —*see also* Ischemia, intestine, acute K55.Ø59
    - mesenteric K55.1
    - peripheral I73.9
    - renal —*see* Hypertension, kidney
  - velopharyngeal
    - acquired K13.79
    - congenital Q38.8
  - venous (chronic) (peripheral) I87.2
  - ventricular —*see* Insufficiency, myocardial
  - welfare support Z59.7
- **Insufflation, fallopian** Z31.41
- **Insular** —*see* condition
- **Insulinoma**
  - pancreas
    - benign D13.7
    - malignant C25.4
    - uncertain behavior D37.8
  - specified site
    - benign —*see* Neoplasm, by site, benign
    - malignant —*see* Neoplasm, by site, malignant
    - uncertain behavior —*see* Neoplasm, by site, uncertain behavior
- **Insulinoma** *(Continued)*
  - unspecified site
    - benign D13.7
    - malignant C25.4
    - uncertain behavior D37.8
- **Insuloma** —*see* Insulinoma
- **Interference**
  - balancing side M26.56
  - non-working side M26.56
- **Intermenstrual** —*see* condition
- **Intermittent** —*see* condition
- **Internal** —*see* condition
- **Interrogation**
  - cardiac defibrillator (automatic) (implantable) Z45.Ø2
  - cardiac pacemaker Z45.Ø18
  - cardiac (event) (loop) recorder Z45.Ø9
  - infusion pump (implanted) (intrathecal) Z45.1
  - neurostimulator Z46.2
- **Interruption**
  - aortic arch Q25.21
  - phase-shift, sleep cycle —*see* Disorder, sleep, circadian rhythm
  - sleep phase-shift, or 24 hour sleep-wake cycle —*see* Disorder, sleep, circadian rhythm
- **Interstitial** —*see* condition
- **Intertrigo** L3Ø.4
  - labialis K13.Ø
- **Intervertebral disc** —*see* condition
- **Intestine, intestinal** —*see* condition
- **Intolerance**
  - carbohydrate K9Ø.49
  - disaccharide, hereditary E73.Ø
  - fat NEC K9Ø.49
    - pancreatic K9Ø.3
  - food K9Ø.49
    - dietary counseling and surveillance Z71.3
  - fructose E74.1Ø
    - hereditary E74.12
  - glucose(-galactose) E74.39
  - gluten K9Ø.Ø1
  - lactose E73.9
    - specified NEC E73.8
  - lysine E72.3
  - milk NEC K9Ø.49
    - lactose E73.9
  - protein K9Ø.49
  - starch NEC K9Ø.49
  - sucrose (-isomaltose) E74.31
- **Intoxicated NEC** (without dependence) —*see* Alcohol, intoxication
- **Intoxication**
  - acid E87.2
  - alcoholic (acute) (without dependence) —*see* Alcohol, intoxication
  - alimentary canal K52.1
  - amphetamine (without dependence) —*see also* Abuse, drug, stimulant, with intoxication
    - ▶stimulant NEC F15.1Ø
      - ▶with
        - ▶anxiety disorder F15.18Ø
        - ▶intoxication F15.129
          - ▶with
            - ▶delirium F15.121
            - ▶perceptual disturbance F15.122
    - with dependence —*see* Dependence, drug, stimulant, with intoxication
  - anxiolytic (acute) (without dependence) —*see* Abuse, drug, sedative, with intoxication
    - with dependence —*see* Dependence, drug, sedative, with intoxication
  - caffeine F15.929
    - with dependence —*see* Dependence, drug, stimulant, with intoxication
  - cannabinoids (acute) (without dependence) —*see* Use, cannabis, with intoxication
    - with
      - abuse —*see* Abuse, drug, cannabis, with intoxication
- **Intoxication** *(Continued)*
  - cannabinoids *(Continued)*
    - with *(Continued)*
      - dependence —*see* Dependence, drug, cannabis, with intoxication
  - chemical —*see* Table of Drugs and Chemicals
    - via placenta or breast milk —*see* Absorption, chemical, through placenta
  - cocaine (acute) (without dependence) —*see* Abuse, drug, cocaine, with intoxication
    - with dependence —*see* Dependence, drug, cocaine, with intoxication
  - drug
    - acute (without dependence) —*see* Abuse, drug, by type with intoxication
      - with dependence —*see* Dependence, drug, by type with intoxication
    - addictive
      - via placenta or breast milk —*see* Absorption, drug, addictive, through placenta
    - newborn P93.8
      - gray baby syndrome P93.Ø
    - overdose or wrong substance given or taken —*see* Table of Drugs and Chemicals, by drug, poisoning
  - enteric K52.1
  - foodborne AØ5.9
    - bacterial AØ5.9
    - classical (Clostridium botulinum) AØ5.1
    - due to
      - Bacillus cereus AØ5.4
      - bacterium AØ5.9
        - specified NEC AØ5.8
      - Clostridium
        - botulinum AØ5.1
        - perfringens AØ5.2
        - welchii AØ5.2
      - Salmonella AØ2.9
        - with
          - (gastro) enteritis AØ2.Ø
          - localized infection(s) AØ2.2Ø
            - arthritis AØ2.23
            - meningitis AØ2.21
            - osteomyelitis AØ2.24
            - pneumonia AØ2.22
            - pyelonephritis AØ2.25
            - specified NEC AØ2.29
          - sepsis AØ2.1
          - specified manifestation NEC AØ2.8
      - Staphylococcus AØ5.Ø
      - Vibrio
        - parahaemolyticus AØ5.3
        - vulnificus AØ5.5
    - enterotoxin, staphylococcal AØ5.Ø
    - noxious —*see* Poisoning, food, noxious
  - gastrointestinal K52.1
  - hallucinogenic (without dependence) —*see* Abuse, drug, hallucinogen, with intoxication
    - with dependence —*see* Dependence, drug, hallucinogen, with intoxication
  - hypnotic (acute) (without dependence) —*see* Abuse, drug, sedative, with intoxication
    - with dependence —*see* Dependence, drug, sedative, with intoxication
  - inhalant (acute) (without dependence) —*see* Abuse, drug, inhalant, with intoxication
    - with dependence —*see* Dependence, drug, inhalant, with intoxication
  - meaning
    - inebriation —*see* category F1Ø
    - poisoning —*see* Table of Drugs and Chemicals
  - methyl alcohol (acute) (without dependence) —*see* Alcohol, intoxication
  - opioid (acute) (without dependence) —*see* Abuse, drug, opioid, with intoxication
    - with dependence —*see* Dependence, drug, opioid, with intoxication

Intoxication *(Continued)*
- pathologic NEC (without dependence) —*see* Alcohol, intoxication
- phencyclidine (without dependence) —*see* Abuse, drug, hallucinogen, with intoxication
  - with dependence —*see* Dependence, drug, hallucinogen, with intoxication
- potassium (K) E87.5
- psychoactive substance NEC (without dependence) —*see* Abuse, drug, psychoactive NEC, with intoxication
  - with dependence —*see* Dependence, drug, psychoactive NEC, with intoxication
- sedative (acute) (without dependence) —*see* Abuse, drug, sedative, with intoxication
  - with dependence —*see* Dependence, drug, sedative, with intoxication
- serum —*see also* Reaction, serum T8Ø.69
- uremic —*see* Uremia
- volatile solvents (acute) (without dependence) —*see* Abuse, drug, inhalant, with intoxication
  - with dependence —*see* Dependence, drug, inhalant, with intoxication
- water E87.79

Intraabdominal testis, testes
- bilateral Q53.211
- unilateral Q53.111

Intracranial —*see* condition

Intrahepatic gallbladder Q44.1

Intraligamentous —*see* condition

Intrathoracic —*see also* condition
- kidney Q63.2

Intrauterine contraceptive device
- checking Z3Ø.431
- in situ Z97.5
- insertion Z3Ø.43Ø
  - immediately following removal Z3Ø.433
- management Z3Ø.431
- reinsertion Z3Ø.433
- removal Z3Ø.432
- replacement Z3Ø.433
- retention in pregnancy O26.3-●

Intraventricular —*see* condition

Intrinsic deformity —*see* Deformity

Intubation, difficult or failed T88.4

Intumescence, lens (eye) (cataract) —*see* Cataract

Intussusception (bowel) (colon) (enteric) (ileocecal) (ileocolic) (intestine) (rectum) K56.1
- appendix K38.8
- congenital Q43.8
- ureter (with obstruction) N13.5

Invagination (bowel, colon, intestine or rectum) K56.1

Inversion
- albumin-globulin (A-G) ratio E88.Ø9
- bladder N32.89
- cecum —*see* Intussusception
- cervix N88.8
- chromosome in normal individual Q95.1
- circadian rhythm —*see* Disorder, sleep, circadian rhythm
- nipple N64.59
  - congenital Q83.8
  - gestational —*see* Retraction, nipple
  - puerperal, postpartum —*see* Retraction, nipple
- nyctohemeral rhythm —*see* Disorder, sleep, circadian rhythm
- optic papilla Q14.2
- organ or site, congenital NEC —*see* Anomaly, by site
- sleep rhythm —*see* Disorder, sleep, circadian rhythm
- testis (congenital) Q55.29
- uterus (chronic) (postinfectional) (postpartal, old) N85.5
  - postpartum O71.2
- vagina (posthysterectomy) N99.3
- ventricular Q2Ø.5

Investigation —*see also* Examination ZØ4.9
- clinical research subject (control) (normal comparison) (participant) ZØØ.6

Involuntary movement, abnormal R25.9

Involution, involutional —*see also* condition
- breast, cystic —*see* Dysplasia, mammary, specified type NEC
- depression (single episode) F32.89
  - recurrent episode F33.9
- melancholia (single episode) F32.89
  - recurrent episode F33.8
- ovary, senile —*see* Atrophy, ovary
- thymus failure E32.8

I.Q.
- under 2Ø F73
- 2Ø-34 F72
- 35-49 F71
- 5Ø-69 F7Ø

IRDS (type I) P22.Ø
- type II P22.1

Irideremia Q13.1

Iridis rubeosis —*see* Disorder, iris, vascular

Iridochoroiditis (panuveitis) —*see* Panuveitis

Iridocyclitis H2Ø.9-●
- acute H2Ø.Ø-●
  - hypopyon H2Ø.Ø5-●
  - primary H2Ø.Ø1-●
  - recurrent H2Ø.Ø2-●
  - secondary (noninfectious) H2Ø.Ø4-●
    - infectious H2Ø.Ø3-●
- chronic H2Ø.1-●
- due to allergy —*see* Iridocyclitis, acute, secondary
- endogenous —*see* Iridocyclitis, acute, primary
- Fuchs' —*see* Cyclitis, Fuchs' heterochromic
- gonococcal A54.32
- granulomatous —*see* Iridocyclitis, chronic
- herpes, herpetic (simplex) BØØ.51
  - zoster BØ2.32
- hypopyon —*see* Iridocyclitis, acute, hypopyon
- in (due to)
  - ankylosing spondylitis M45.9
  - gonococcal infection A54.32
  - herpes (simplex) virus BØØ.51
    - zoster BØ2.32
  - infectious disease NOS B99
  - parasitic disease NOS B89 *[H22]*
  - sarcoidosis D86.83
  - syphilis A51.43
  - tuberculosis A18.54
  - zoster BØ2.32
- lens-induced H2Ø.2-●
- nongranulomatous —*see* Iridocyclitis, acute
- recurrent —*see* Iridocyclitis, acute, recurrent
- rheumatic —*see* Iridocyclitis, chronic
- subacute —*see* Iridocyclitis, acute
- sympathetic —*see* Uveitis, sympathetic
- syphilitic (secondary) A51.43
- tuberculous (chronic) A18.54
- Vogt-Koyanagi H2Ø.82-●

Iridocyclochoroiditis (panuveitis) —*see* Panuveitis

Iridodialysis H21.53-●

Iridodonesis H21.89

Iridoplegia (complete) (partial) (reflex) H57.Ø9

Iridoschisis H21.25-●

Iris —*see also* condition
- bombé —*see* Membrane, pupillary

Iritis —*see also* Iridocyclitis
- chronic —*see* Iridocyclitis, chronic
- diabetic —*see* EØ8-E13 with .39
- due to
  - herpes simplex BØØ.51
  - leprosy A3Ø.9 *[H22]*
- gonococcal A54.32
- gouty —*see also* Gout, by type M1Ø.9 *[H22]*
- granulomatous —*see* Iridocyclitis, chronic
- lens induced —*see* Iridocyclitis, lens-induced
- papulosa (syphilitic) A52.71
- rheumatic —*see* Iridocyclitis, chronic

Iritis *(Continued)*
- syphilitic (secondary) A51.43
  - congenital (early) A5Ø.Ø1
  - late A52.71
- tuberculous A18.54

Iron —*see* condition

Iron-miner's lung J63.4

Irradiated enamel (tooth, teeth) KØ3.89

Irradiation effects, adverse T66

Irreducible, irreducibility —*see* condition

Irregular, irregularity
- action, heart I49.9
- alveolar process KØ8.89
- bleeding N92.6
- breathing RØ6.89
- contour of cornea (acquired) —*see* Deformity, cornea
  - congenital Q13.4
- contour, reconstructed breast N65.Ø
- dentin (in pulp) KØ4.3
- eye movements H55.89
  - nystagmus —*see* Nystagmus
  - saccadic H55.81
- labor O62.2
- menstruation (cause unknown) N92.6
- periods N92.6
- prostate N42.9
- pupil —*see* Abnormality, pupillary
- reconstructed breast N65.Ø
- respiratory RØ6.89
- septum (nasal) J34.2
- shape, organ or site, congenital NEC —*see* Distortion
- sleep-wake pattern (rhythm) G47.23

Irritable, irritability R45.4
- bladder N32.89
- bowel (syndrome) K58.9
  - with
    - constipation K58.1
    - diarrhea K58.Ø
  - mixed K58.2
  - psychogenic F45.8
  - specified NEC K58.8
- bronchial —*see* Bronchitis
- cerebral, in newborn P91.3
- colon —*see also* Irritable, bowel K58.9
  - with diarrhea K58.Ø
  - psychogenic F45.8
- duodenum K59.8
- heart (psychogenic) F45.8
- hip —*see* Derangement, joint, specified type NEC, hip
- ileum K59.8
- infant R68.12
- jejunum K59.8
- rectum K59.8
- stomach K31.89
  - psychogenic F45.8
- sympathetic G9Ø.8
- urethra N36.8

Irritation
- anus K62.89
- axillary nerve G54.Ø
- bladder N32.89
- brachial plexus G54.Ø
- bronchial —*see* Bronchitis
- cervical plexus G54.2
- cervix —*see* Cervicitis
- choroid, sympathetic —*see* Endophthalmitis
- cranial nerve —*see* Disorder, nerve, cranial
- gastric K31.89
  - psychogenic F45.8
- globe, sympathetic —*see* Uveitis, sympathetic
- labyrinth —*see* subcategory H83.2
- lumbosacral plexus G54.1
- meninges (traumatic) —*see* Injury, intracranial
  - nontraumatic —*see* Meningismus
- nerve —*see* Disorder, nerve
- nervous R45.Ø
- penis N48.89
- perineum NEC L29.3

Irritation *(Continued)*
peripheral autonomic nervous system G90.8
peritoneum —*see* Peritonitis
pharynx J39.2
plantar nerve —*see* Lesion, nerve, plantar
spinal (cord) (traumatic) —*see also* Injury, spinal cord, by region
nerve G58.9
root NEC —*see* Radiculopathy
nontraumatic —*see* Myelopathy
stomach K31.89
psychogenic F45.8
sympathetic nerve NEC G90.8
ulnar nerve —*see* Lesion, nerve, ulnar
vagina N89.8
Ischemia, ischemic I99.8
bowel (transient)
acute —*see also* Ischemia, intestine, acute K55.059
chronic K55.1
due to mesenteric artery insufficiency K55.1
brain —*see* Ischemia, cerebral
cardiac (*see* Disease, heart, ischemic)
cardiomyopathy I25.5
cerebral (chronic) (generalized) I67.82
arteriosclerotic I67.2
intermittent G45.9
newborn P91.0
recurrent focal G45.8
transient G45.9
colon chronic (due to mesenteric artery insufficiency) K55.1
coronary —*see* Disease, heart, ischemic
demand (coronary) —*see also* Angina I24.8
with myocardial infarction I21.A1
resulting in myocardial infarction I21.A1
heart (chronic or with a stated duration of over 4 weeks) I25.9
acute or with a stated duration of 4 weeks or less I24.9
subacute I24.9
infarction, muscle —*see* Infarct, muscle
intestine (large) (small) (transient) K55.9
acute K55.059
diffuse K55.052
focal K55.051
large K55.039
diffuse K55.032
focal K55.031
small K55.019
diffuse K55.012
focal K55.011
chronic K55.1
due to mesenteric artery insufficiency K55.1
kidney N28.0
Ischemia, ischemic *(Continued)*
mesenteric, acute —*see also* Ischemia, intestine, acute K55.059
muscle, traumatic T79.6
myocardium, myocardial (chronic or with a stated duration of over 4 weeks) I25.9
acute, without myocardial infarction I51.3
silent (asymptomatic) I25.6
transient of newborn P29.4
renal N28.0
retina, retinal —*see* Occlusion, artery, retina
small bowel
acute K55.019
diffuse K55.012
focal K55.011
chronic K55.1
due to mesenteric artery insufficiency K55.1
spinal cord G95.11
subendocardial —*see* Insufficiency, coronary
supply (coronary) —*see also* Angina I25.9
due to vasospasm I20.1
Ischial spine —*see* condition
Ischialgia —*see* Sciatica
Ischiopagus Q89.4
Ischium, ischial —*see* condition
Ischuria R34
Iselin's disease or osteochondrosis —*see* Osteochondrosis, juvenile, metatarsus
Islands of
parotid tissue in
lymph nodes Q38.6
neck structures Q38.6
submaxillary glands in
fascia Q38.6
lymph nodes Q38.6
neck muscles Q38.6
Islet cell tumor, pancreas D13.7
Isoimmunization NEC —*see also* Incompatibility
affecting management of pregnancy (ABO) (with hydrops fetalis) O36.11- ●
anti-A sensitization O36.11- ●
anti-B sensitization O36.19- ●
anti-c sensitization O36.09- ●
anti-C sensitization O36.09- ●
anti-e sensitization O36.09- ●
anti-E sensitization O36.09- ●
Rh NEC O36.09- ●
anti-D antibody O36.01- ●
specified NEC O36.19- ●
newborn P55.9
with
hydrops fetalis P56.0
kernicterus P57.0
ABO (blood groups) P55.1
Isoimmunization NEC *(Continued)*
newborn *(Continued)*
Rhesus (Rh) factor P55.0
specified type NEC P55.8
Isolation, isolated
dwelling Z59.8
family Z63.79
social Z60.4
Isoleucinosis E71.19
Isomerism atrial appendages (with asplenia or polysplenia) Q20.6
Isosporiasis, isosporosis A07.3
Isovaleric acidemia E71.110
Issue of
medical certificate Z02.79
for disability determination Z02.71
repeat prescription (appliance) (glasses) (medicinal substance, medicament, medicine) Z76.0
contraception —*see* Contraception
Itch, itching —*see also* Pruritus
baker's L23.6
barber's B35.0
bricklayer's L24.5
cheese B88.0
clam digger's B65.3
coolie B76.9
copra B88.0
dew B76.9
dhobi B35.6
filarial —*see* Infestation, filarial
grain B88.0
grocer's B88.0
ground B76.9
harvest B88.0
jock B35.6
Malabar B35.5
beard B35.0
foot B35.3
scalp B35.0
meaning scabies B86
Norwegian B86
perianal L29.0
poultrymen's B88.0
sarcoptic B86
scabies B86
scrub B88.0
straw B88.0
swimmer's B65.3
water B76.9
winter L29.8
Ivemark's syndrome (asplenia with congenital heart disease) Q89.01
Ivory bones Q78.2
Ixodiasis NEC B88.8

J

Jaccoud's syndrome —*see* Arthropathy, postrheumatic, chronic
Jackson's
- membrane Q43.3
- paralysis or syndrome G83.89
- veil Q43.3

Jacquet's dermatitis (diaper dermatitis) L22
Jadassohn-Pellizari's disease or anetoderma L90.2
Jadassohn's
- blue nevus —*see* Nevus
- intraepidermal epithelioma —*see* Neoplasm, skin, benign

Jaffe-Lichtenstein (-Uehlinger) **syndrome** —*see* Dysplasia, fibrous, bone NEC
Jakob-Creutzfeldt disease or syndrome —*see* Creutzfeldt-Jakob disease or syndrome
Jaksch-Luzet disease D64.89
Jamaican
- neuropathy G92
- paraplegic tropical ataxic-spastic syndrome G92

Janet's disease F48.8
Janiceps Q89.4
Jansky-Bielschowsky amaurotic idiocy E75.4
Japanese
- B-type encephalitis A83.0
- river fever A75.3

Jaundice (yellow) R17
- acholuric (familial) (splenomegalic) —*see also* Spherocytosis
  - acquired D59.8
- breast-milk (inhibitor) P59.3
- catarrhal (acute) B15.9
  - with hepatic coma B15.0
- cholestatic (benign) R17
- due to or associated with
  - delayed conjugation P59.8
    - associated with (due to) preterm delivery P59.0
  - preterm delivery P59.0
- epidemic (catarrhal) B15.9
  - with hepatic coma B15.0
  - leptospiral A27.0
  - spirochetal A27.0
- familial nonhemolytic (congenital) (Gilbert) E80.4
  - Crigler-Najjar E80.5
- febrile (acute) B15.9
  - with hepatic coma B15.0
  - leptospiral A27.0
  - spirochetal A27.0
- hematogenous D59.9
- hemolytic (acquired) D59.9
  - congenital —*see* Spherocytosis
- hemorrhagic (acute) (leptospiral) (spirochetal) A27.0
- infectious (acute) (subacute) B15.9
  - with hepatic coma B15.0
  - leptospiral A27.0
  - spirochetal A27.0
- leptospiral (hemorrhagic) A27.0
- malignant (without coma) K72.90
  - with coma K72.91
- neonatal —*see* Jaundice, newborn
- newborn P59.9
  - due to or associated with
    - ABO
      - antibodies P55.1
      - incompatibility, maternal/fetal P55.1
      - isoimmunization P55.1
    - absence or deficiency of enzyme system for bilirubin conjugation (congenital) P59.8
    - bleeding P58.1
    - breast milk inhibitors to conjugation P59.3
      - associated with preterm delivery P59.0
    - bruising P58.0
    - Crigler-Najjar syndrome E80.5
    - delayed conjugation P59.8
      - associated with preterm delivery P59.0
    - drugs or toxins
      - given to newborn P58.42
      - transmitted from mother P58.41
    - excessive hemolysis P58.9
      - due to
        - bleeding P58.1
        - bruising P58.0
        - drugs or toxins
          - given to newborn P58.42
          - transmitted from mother P58.41
        - infection P58.2
        - polycythemia P58.3
        - swallowed maternal blood P58.5
      - specified type NEC P58.8
    - galactosemia E74.21
    - Gilbert syndrome E80.4
    - hemolytic disease P55.9
      - ABO isoimmunization P55.1
      - Rh isoimmunization P55.0
      - specified NEC P55.8
    - hepatocellular damage P59.20
      - specified NEC P59.29
    - hereditary hemolytic anemia P58.8
    - hypothyroidism, congenital E03.1
    - incompatibility, maternal/fetal NOS P55.9
    - infection P58.2
    - inspissated bile syndrome P59.1
    - isoimmunization NOS P55.9
    - mucoviscidosis E84.9
    - polycythemia P58.3
    - preterm delivery P59.0
    - Rh
      - antibodies P55.0
      - incompatibility, maternal/fetal P55.0
      - isoimmunization P55.0
    - specified cause NEC P59.8
    - swallowed maternal blood P58.5
  - spherocytosis (congenital) D58.0
- nonhemolytic congenital familial (Gilbert) E80.4
- nuclear, newborn —*see also* Kernicterus of newborn P57.9
- obstructive —*see also* Obstruction, bile duct K83.1
- post-immunization —*see* Hepatitis, viral, type, B
- post-transfusion —*see* Hepatitis, viral, type, B
- regurgitation —*see also* Obstruction, bile duct K83.1
- serum (homologous) (prophylactic) (therapeutic) —*see* Hepatitis, viral, type, B
- spirochetal (hemorrhagic) A27.0
- symptomatic R17
  - newborn P59.9

Jaw —*see* condition
Jaw-winking phenomenon or syndrome Q07.8
Jealousy
- alcoholic F10.988
- childhood F93.8
- sibling F93.8

Jejunitis —*see* Enteritis
Jejunostomy status Z93.4
Jejunum, jejunal —*see* condition
Jensen's disease —*see* Inflammation, chorioretinal, focal, juxtapapillary
Jerks, myoclonic G25.3
Jervell-Lange-Nielsen syndrome I45.81
Jeune's disease Q77.2
Jigger disease B88.1
Job's syndrome (chronic granulomatous disease) D71
Joint —*see also* condition
- mice —*see* Loose, body, joint
  - knee M23.4-●

Jordan's anomaly or syndrome D72.0
Joseph-Diamond-Blackfan anemia (congenital hypoplastic) D61.01
Jungle yellow fever A95.0
Jüngling's disease —*see* Sarcoidosis
Juvenile —*see* condition

K

Kahler's disease C90.0- ●
Kakke E51.11
Kala-azar B55.0
Kallmann's syndrome E23.0
Kanner's syndrome (autism) —*see* Psychosis, childhood
Kaposi's
  dermatosis (xeroderma pigmentosum) Q82.1
  lichen ruber L44.0
    acuminatus L44.0
  sarcoma
    colon C46.4
    connective tissue C46.1
    gastrointestinal organ C46.4
    lung C46.5- ●
    lymph node (multiple) C46.3
    palate (hard) (soft) C46.2
    rectum C46.4
    skin (multiple sites) C46.0
    specified site NEC C46.7
    stomach C46.4
    unspecified site C46.9
  varicelliform eruption B00.0
    vaccinia T88.1
Kartagener's syndrome or triad (sinusitis, bronchiectasis, situs inversus) Q89.3
Karyotype
  with abnormality except iso (Xq) Q96.2
  45,X Q96.0
  46,X
    iso (Xq) Q96.1
  46,XX Q98.3
    with streak gonads Q50.32
    hermaphrodite (true) Q99.1
    male Q98.3
  46,XY
    with streak gonads Q56.1
    female Q97.3
    hermaphrodite (true) Q99.1
  47,XXX Q97.0
  47,XXY Q98.0
  47,XYY Q98.5
Kaschin-Beck disease —*see* Disease, Kaschin-Beck
Katayama's disease or fever B65.2
Kawasaki's syndrome M30.3
Kayser-Fleischer ring (cornea) (pseudosclerosis) H18.04- ●
Kaznelson's syndrome (congenital hypoplastic anemia) D61.01
Kearns-Sayre syndrome H49.81- ●
Kedani fever A75.3
Kelis L91.0
Kelly (-Patterson) syndrome (sideropenic dysphagia) D50.1
Keloid, cheloid L91.0
  acne L73.0
  Addison's L94.0
  cornea —*see* Opacity, cornea
  Hawkin's L91.0
  scar L91.0
Keloma L91.0
Kenya fever A77.1
Keratectasia —*see also* Ectasia, cornea
  congenital Q13.4
Keratinization of alveolar ridge mucosa
  excessive K13.23
  minimal K13.22
Keratinized residual ridge mucosa
  excessive K13.23
  minimal K13.22
Keratitis (nodular) (nonulcerative) (simple) (zonular) H16.9
  with ulceration (central) (marginal) (perforated) (ring) —*see* Ulcer, cornea
  actinic —*see* Photokeratitis
  arborescens (herpes simplex) B00.52
  areolar H16.11- ●
  bullosa H16.8
Keratitis *(Continued)*
  deep H16.309
    specified type NEC H16.399
  dendritic (a) (herpes simplex) B00.52
  disciform (is) (herpes simplex) B00.52
    varicella B01.81
  filamentary H16.12- ●
  gonococcal (congenital or prenatal) A54.33
  herpes, herpetic (simplex) B00.52
    zoster B02.33
  in (due to)
    acanthamebiasis B60.13
    adenovirus B30.0
    exanthema —*see also* Exanthem B09
    herpes (simplex) virus B00.52
    measles B05.81
    syphilis A50.31
    tuberculosis A18.52
    zoster B02.33
  interstitial (nonsyphilitic) H16.30- ●
    diffuse H16.32- ●
    herpes, herpetic (simplex) B00.52
      zoster B02.33
    sclerosing H16.33- ●
    specified type NEC H16.39- ●
    syphilitic (congenital) (late) A50.31
    tuberculous A18.52
  macular H16.11- ●
  nummular H16.11- ●
  oyster shuckers' H16.8
  parenchymatous —*see* Keratitis, interstitial
  petrificans H16.8
  postmeasles B05.81
  punctata
    leprosa A30.9 *[H16.14- ●]*
    syphilitic (profunda) A50.31
  punctate H16.14- ●
  purulent H16.8
  rosacea L71.8
  sclerosing H16.33- ●
  specified type NEC H16.8
  stellate H16.11- ●
  striate H16.11- ●
  superficial H16.10- ●
    with conjunctivitis —*see* Keratoconjunctivitis
    due to light —*see* Photokeratitis
  suppurative H16.8
  syphilitic (congenital) (prenatal) A50.31
  trachomatous A71.1
    sequelae B94.0
  tuberculous A18.52
  vesicular H16.8
  xerotic —*see also* Keratomalacia H16.8
    vitamin A deficiency E50.4
Keratoacanthoma L85.8
Keratocele —*see* Descemetocele
Keratoconjunctivitis H16.20- ●
  Acanthamoeba B60.13
  adenoviral B30.0
  epidemic B30.0
  exposure H16.21- ●
  herpes, herpetic (simplex) B00.52
    zoster B02.33
  in exanthema —*see also* Exanthem B09
  infectious B30.0
  lagophthalmic —*see* Keratoconjunctivitis, specified type NEC
  neurotrophic H16.23- ●
  phlyctenular H16.25- ●
  postmeasles B05.81
  shipyard B30.0
  sicca (Sjogren's) M35.0- ●
    not Sjogren's H16.22- ●
  specified type NEC H16.29- ●
  tuberculous (phlyctenular) A18.52
  vernal H16.26- ●
Keratoconus H18.60- ●
  congenital Q13.4
  stable H18.61- ●
  unstable H18.62- ●
Keratocyst (dental) (odontogenic) —*see* Cyst, calcifying odontogenic
Keratoderma, keratodermia (congenital) (palmaris et plantaris) (symmetrical) Q82.8
  acquired L85.1
    in diseases classified elsewhere L86
  climactericum L85.1
  gonococcal A54.89
  gonorrheal A54.89
  punctata L85.2
  Reiter's —*see* Reiter's disease
Keratodermatocele —*see* Descemetocele
Keratoglobus H18.79
  congenital Q15.8
    with glaucoma Q15.0
Keratohemia —*see* Pigmentation, cornea, stromal
Keratoiritis —*see also* Iridocyclitis
  syphilitic A50.39
  tuberculous A18.54
Keratoma L57.0
  palmaris and plantaris hereditarium Q82.8
  senile L57.0
Keratomalacia H18.44- ●
  vitamin A deficiency E50.4
Keratomegaly Q13.4
Keratomycosis B49
  nigrans, nigricans (palmaris) B36.1
Keratopathy H18.9
  band H18.42- ●
  bullous H18.1- ●
  bullous (aphakic), following cataract surgery H59.01- ●
Keratoscleritis, tuberculous A18.52
Keratosis L57.0
  actinic L57.0
  arsenical L85.8
  congenital, specified NEC Q80.8
  female genital NEC N94.89
  follicularis Q82.8
    acquired L11.0
    congenita Q82.8
    et parafollicularis in cutem penetrans L87.0
    spinulosa (decalvans) Q82.8
    vitamin A deficiency E50.8
  gonococcal A54.89
  male genital (external) N50.89
  nigricans L83
  obturans, external ear (canal) —*see* Cholesteatoma, external ear
  palmaris et plantaris (inherited) (symmetrical) Q82.8
    acquired L85.1
  penile N48.89
  pharynx J39.2
  pilaris, acquired L85.8
  punctata (palmaris et plantaris) L85.2
  scrotal N50.89
  seborrheic L82.1
    inflamed L82.0
  senile L57.0
  solar L57.0
  tonsillaris J35.8
  vagina N89.4
  vegetans Q82.8
  vitamin A deficiency E50.8
  vocal cord J38.3
Kerato-uveitis —*see* Iridocyclitis
Kerion (celsi) B35.0
Kernicterus of newborn (not due to isoimmunization) P57.9
  due to isoimmunization (conditions in P55.0-P55.9) P57.0
  specified type NEC P57.8
Kerunoparalysis T75.09
Keshan disease E59
Ketoacidosis E87.2
  diabetic —*see* Diabetes, by type, with ketoacidosis
Ketonuria R82.4

K

Ketosis NEC E88.89
  diabetic —*see* Diabetes, by type, with ketoacidosis
Kew Garden fever A79.1
Kidney —*see* condition
Kienböck's disease —*see also* Osteochondrosis, juvenile, hand, carpal lunate
  adult M93.1
Kimmelstiel (-Wilson) **disease** —*see* Diabetes, Kimmelstiel (-Wilson) disease
Kimura disease D21.9
  specified site (*see* Neoplasm, connective tissue benign)
Kink, kinking
  artery I77.1
  hair (acquired) L67.8
  ileum or intestine —*see* Obstruction, intestine
  Lane's —*see* Obstruction, intestine
  organ or site, congenital NEC —*see* Anomaly, by site
  ureter (pelvic junction) N13.5
    with
      hydronephrosis N13.1
        with infection N13.6
      pyelonephritis (chronic) N11.1
    congenital Q62.39
  vein(s) I87.8
    caval I87.1
    peripheral I87.1
Kinnier Wilson's disease (hepatolenticular degeneration) E83.01
Kissing spine M48.20
  cervical region M48.22
  cervicothoracic region M48.23
  lumbar region M48.26
  lumbosacral region M48.27
  occipito-atlanto-axial region M48.21
  thoracic region M48.24
  thoracolumbar region M48.25
Klatskin's tumor C24.0
Klauder's disease A26.8
Klebs' disease —*see also* Glomerulonephritis N05.- •
Klebsiella (K.) pneumoniae, as cause of disease classified elsewhere B96.1
Klein (e)-Levin syndrome G47.13
Kleptomania F63.2
Klinefelter's syndrome Q98.4
  karyotype 47,XXY Q98.0
  male with more than two X chromosomes Q98.1
Klippel-Feil deficiency, disease, or syndrome (brevicollis) Q76.1
Klippel's disease I67.2
Klippel-Trenaunay (-Weber) **syndrome** Q87.2
Klumpke (-Déjerine) **palsy, paralysis** (birth) (newborn) P14.1
Knee —*see* condition
Knock knee (acquired) M21.06- •
  congenital Q74.1
Knot(s)
  intestinal, syndrome (volvulus) K56.2
  surfer S89.8- •
  umbilical cord (true) O69.2
Knotting (of)
  hair L67.8
  intestine K56.2
Knuckle pad (Garrod's) M72.1
Koch's
  infection —*see* Tuberculosis
  relapsing fever A68.9
Koch-Weeks' conjunctivitis —*see* Conjunctivitis, acute, mucopurulent
Köebner's syndrome Q81.8
Köenig's disease (osteochondritis dissecans) —*see* Osteochondritis, dissecans
Köhler-Pellegrini-Steida disease or syndrome (calcification, knee joint) —*see* Bursitis, tibial collateral
Köhler's disease
  patellar —*see* Osteochondrosis, juvenile, patella
  tarsal navicular —*see* Osteochondrosis, juvenile, tarsus
Koilonychia L60.3
  congenital Q84.6
Kojevnikov's, epilepsy —*see* Kozhevnikof's epilepsy
Koplik's spots B05.9
Kopp's asthma E32.8
Korsakoff's (Wernicke) disease, psychosis or syndrome (alcoholic) F10.96
  with dependence F10.26
  drug-induced
    due to drug abuse —*see* Abuse, drug, by type, with amnestic disorder
    due to drug dependence —*see* Dependence, drug, by type, with amnestic disorder
  nonalcoholic F04
Korsakov's disease, psychosis or syndrome —*see* Korsakoff's disease
Korsakow's disease, psychosis or syndrome —*see* Korsakoff's disease
Kostmann's disease or syndrome (infantile genetic agranulocytosis) —*see* Agranulocytosis
Kozhevnikof's epilepsy G40.109
  intractable G40.119
    with status epilepticus G40.111
    without status epilepticus G40.119
  not intractable G40.109
    with status epilepticus G40.101
    without status epilepticus G40.109
Krabbe's
  disease E75.23
  syndrome, congenital muscle hypoplasia Q79.8
Kraepelin-Morel disease —*see* Schizophrenia
Kraft-Weber-Dimitri disease Q85.8
Kraurosis
  ani K62.89
  penis N48.0
Kraurosis *(Continued)*
  vagina N89.8
  vulva N90.4
Kreotoxism A05.9
Krukenberg's
  spindle —*see* Pigmentation, cornea, posterior
  tumor C79.6- •
Kufs' disease E75.4
Kugelberg-Welander disease G12.1
Kuhnt-Junius degeneration —*see also* Degeneration, macula H35.32- •
Kümmell's disease or spondylitis —*see* Spondylopathy, traumatic
Kupffer cell sarcoma C22.3
Kuru A81.81
Kussmaul's
  disease M30.0
  respiration E87.2
    in diabetic acidosis —*see* Diabetes, by type, with ketoacidosis
Kwashiorkor E40
  marasmic, marasmus type E42
Kyasanur Forest disease A98.2
Kyphoscoliosis, kyphoscoliotic (acquired) —*see also* Scoliosis M41.9
  congenital Q67.5
  heart (disease) I27.1
  sequelae of rickets E64.3
  tuberculous A18.01
Kyphosis, kyphotic (acquired) M40.209
  cervical region M40.202
  cervicothoracic region M40.203
  congenital Q76.419
    cervical region Q76.412
    cervicothoracic region Q76.413
    occipito-atlanto-axial region Q76.411
    thoracic region Q76.414
    thoracolumbar region Q76.415
  Morquio-Brailsford type (spinal) —*see also* subcategory M49.8 E76.219
  postlaminectomy M96.3
  postradiation therapy M96.2
  postural (adolescent) M40.00
    cervicothoracic region M40.03
    thoracic region M40.04
    thoracolumbar region M40.05
  secondary NEC M40.10
    cervical region M40.12
    cervicothoracic region M40.13
    thoracic region M40.14
    thoracolumbar region M40.15
  sequelae of rickets E64.3
  specified type NEC M40.299
    cervical region M40.292
    cervicothoracic region M40.293
    thoracic region M40.294
    thoracolumbar region M40.295
  syphilitic, congenital A50.56
  thoracic region M40.204
  thoracolumbar region M40.205
  tuberculous A18.01
Kyrle disease L87.0

K

L

Labia, labium —*see* condition
Labile
blood pressure R09.89
vasomotor system I73.9
Labioglossal paralysis G12.29
Labium leporinum —*see* Cleft, lip
Labor —*see* Delivery
Labored breathing —*see* Hyperventilation
Labyrinthitis (circumscribed) (destructive) (diffuse) (inner ear) (latent) (purulent) (suppurative) (*see also* subcategory) H83.0
syphilitic A52.79
Laceration
with abortion —*see* Abortion, by type, complicated by laceration of pelvic organs
abdomen, abdominal
wall S31.119
with
foreign body S31.129
penetration into peritoneal cavity S31.619
with foreign body S31.629
epigastric region S31.112
with
foreign body S31.122
penetration into peritoneal cavity S31.612
with foreign body S31.622
left
lower quadrant S31.114
with
foreign body S31.124
penetration into peritoneal cavity S31.614
with foreign body S31.624
upper quadrant S31.111
with
foreign body S31.121
penetration into peritoneal cavity S31.611
with foreign body S31.621
periumbilic region S31.115
with
foreign body S31.125
penetration into peritoneal cavity S31.615
with foreign body S31.625
right
lower quadrant S31.113
with
foreign body S31.123
penetration into peritoneal cavity S31.613
with foreign body S31.623
upper quadrant S31.110
with
foreign body S31.120
penetration into peritoneal cavity S31.610
with foreign body S31.620
accidental, complicating surgery —*see* Complications, surgical, accidental puncture or laceration
Achilles tendon S86.02-●
adrenal gland S37.813
alveolar (process) —*see* Laceration, oral cavity
ankle S91.01-●
with
foreign body S91.02-●
antecubital space —*see* Laceration, elbow
anus (sphincter) S31.831
with
ectopic or molar pregnancy O08.6
foreign body S31.832
complicating delivery —*see* Delivery, complicated, by, laceration, anus (sphincter)

Laceration *(Continued)*
anus *(Continued)*
following ectopic or molar pregnancy O08.6
nontraumatic, nonpuerperal —*see* Fissure, anus
arm (upper) S41.11-●
with foreign body S41.12-●
lower —*see* Laceration, forearm
auditory canal (external) (meatus) —*see* Laceration, ear
auricle, ear —*see* Laceration, ear
axilla —*see* Laceration, arm
back —*see also* Laceration, thorax, back
lower S31.010
with
foreign body S31.020
with penetration into retroperitoneal space S31.021
penetration into retroperitoneal space S31.011
bile duct S36.13
bladder S37.23
with ectopic or molar pregnancy O08.6
following ectopic or molar pregnancy O08.6
obstetrical trauma O71.5
blood vessel —*see* Injury, blood vessel
bowel —*see also* Laceration, intestine
with ectopic or molar pregnancy O08.6
complicating abortion —*see* Abortion, by type, complicated by, specified condition NEC
following ectopic or molar pregnancy O08.6
obstetrical trauma O71.5
brain (any part) (cortex) (diffuse) (membrane) —*see also* Injury, intracranial, diffuse
during birth P10.8
with hemorrhage P10.1
focal —*see* Injury, intracranial, focal brain injury
brainstem S06.38-●
breast S21.01-●
with foreign body S21.02-●
broad ligament S37.893
with ectopic or molar pregnancy O08.6
following ectopic or molar pregnancy O08.6
laceration syndrome N83.8
obstetrical trauma O71.6
syndrome (laceration) N83.8
buttock S31.801
with foreign body S31.802
left S31.821
with foreign body S31.822
right S31.811
with foreign body S31.812
calf —*see* Laceration, leg
canaliculus lacrimalis —*see* Laceration, eyelid
canthus, eye —*see* Laceration, eyelid
capsule, joint —*see* Sprain
causing eversion of cervix uteri (old) N86
central (perineal), complicating delivery O70.9
cerebellum, traumatic S06.37-●
cerebral S06.33-●
during birth P10.8
with hemorrhage P10.1
left side S06.32-●
right side S06.31-●
cervix (uteri)
with ectopic or molar pregnancy O08.6
following ectopic or molar pregnancy O08.6
nonpuerperal, nontraumatic N88.1
obstetrical trauma (current) O71.3
old (postpartal) N88.1
traumatic S37.63

Laceration *(Continued)*
cheek (external) S01.41-●
with foreign body S01.42-●
internal —*see* Laceration, oral cavity
chest wall —*see* Laceration, thorax
chin —*see* Laceration, head, specified site NEC
chordae tendinae NEC I51.1
concurrent with acute myocardial infarction —*see* Infarct, myocardium
following acute myocardial infarction (current complication) I23.4
clitoris —*see* Laceration, vulva
colon —*see* Laceration, intestine, large, colon
common bile duct S36.13
cortex (cerebral) —*see* Injury, intracranial, diffuse
costal region —*see* Laceration, thorax
cystic duct S36.13
diaphragm S27.803
digit(s)
foot —*see* Laceration, toe
hand —*see* Laceration, finger
duodenum S36.430
ear (canal) (external) S01.31-●
with foreign body S01.32-●
drum S09.2-●
elbow S51.01-●
with
foreign body S51.02-●
epididymis —*see* Laceration, testis
epigastric region —*see* Laceration, abdomen, wall, epigastric region
esophagus K22.8
traumatic
cervical S11.21
with foreign body S11.22
thoracic S27.813
eye (ball) S05.3-●
with prolapse or loss of intraocular tissue S05.2-●
penetrating S05.6-●
eyebrow —*see* Laceration, eyelid
eyelid S01.11-●
with foreign body S01.12-●
face NEC —*see* Laceration, head, specified site NEC
fallopian tube S37.539
bilateral S37.532
unilateral S37.531
finger(s) S61.219
with
damage to nail S61.319
with
foreign body S61.329
foreign body S61.229
index S61.218
with
damage to nail S61.318
with
foreign body S61.328
foreign body S61.228
left S61.211
with
damage to nail S61.311
with
foreign body S61.321
foreign body S61.221
right S61.210
with
damage to nail S61.310
with
foreign body S61.320
foreign body S61.220
little S61.218
with
damage to nail S61.318
with
foreign body S61.328
foreign body S61.228

Laceration (Continued)
finger (Continued)
little (Continued)
left S61.217
with
damage to nail S61.317
with
foreign body S61.327
foreign body S61.227
right S61.216
with
damage to nail S61.316
with
foreign body S61.326
foreign body S61.226
middle S61.218
with
damage to nail S61.318
with
foreign body S61.328
foreign body S61.228
left S61.213
with
damage to nail S61.313
with
foreign body S61.323
foreign body S61.223
right S61.212
with
damage to nail S61.312
with
foreign body S61.322
foreign body S61.222
ring S61.218
with
damage to nail S61.318
with
foreign body S61.328
foreign body S61.228
left S61.215
with
damage to nail S61.315
with
foreign body S61.325
foreign body S61.225
right S61.214
with
damage to nail S61.314
with
foreign body S61.324
foreign body S61.224
flank S31.119
with foreign body S31.129
foot (except toe(s) alone) S91.319
with foreign body S91.329
left S91.312
with foreign body S91.322
right S91.311
with foreign body S91.321
toe —*see* Laceration, toe
forearm S51.819
with
foreign body S51.829
elbow only —*see* Laceration, elbow
left S51.812
with
foreign body S51.822
right S51.811
with
foreign body S51.821
forehead SØ1.81
with foreign body SØ1.82
fourchette O7Ø.Ø
with ectopic or molar pregnancy OØ8.6
complicating delivery O7Ø.Ø
following ectopic or molar pregnancy OØ8.6
gallbladder S36.123

Laceration (Continued)
genital organs, external
female S31.512
with foreign body S31.522
vagina —*see* Laceration, vagina
vulva —*see* Laceration, vulva
male S31.511
with foreign body S31.521
penis —*see* Laceration, penis
scrotum —*see* Laceration, scrotum
testis —*see* Laceration, testis
groin —*see* Laceration, abdomen, wall
gum —*see* Laceration, oral cavity
hand S61.419
with
foreign body S61.429
finger —*see* Laceration, finger
left S61.412
with
foreign body S61.422
right S61.411
with
foreign body S61.421
thumb —*see* Laceration, thumb
head SØ1.91
with foreign body SØ1.92
cheek —*see* Laceration, cheek
ear —*see* Laceration, ear
eyelid —*see* Laceration, eyelid
lip —*see* Laceration, lip
nose —*see* Laceration, nose
oral cavity —*see* Laceration, oral cavity
scalp SØ1.Ø1
with foreign body SØ1.Ø2
specified site NEC SØ1.81
with foreign body SØ1.82
temporomandibular area —*see* Laceration, cheek
heart —*see* Injury, heart, laceration
heel —*see* Laceration, foot
hepatic duct S36.13
hip S71.Ø19
with foreign body S71.Ø29
left S71.Ø12
with foreign body S71.Ø22
right S71.Ø11
with foreign body S71.Ø21
hymen —*see* Laceration, vagina
hypochondrium —*see* Laceration, abdomen, wall
hypogastric region —*see* Laceration, abdomen, wall
ileum S36.438
inguinal region —*see* Laceration, abdomen, wall
instep —*see* Laceration, foot
internal organ —*see* Injury, by site
interscapular region —*see* Laceration, thorax, back
intestine
large
colon S36.539
ascending S36.53Ø
descending S36.532
sigmoid S36.533
specified site NEC S36.538
rectum S36.63
transverse S36.531
small S36.439
duodenum S36.43Ø
specified site NEC S36.438
intra-abdominal organ S36.93
intestine —*see* Laceration, intestine
liver —*see* Laceration, liver
pancreas —*see* Laceration, pancreas
peritoneum S36.81
specified site NEC S36.893
spleen —*see* Laceration, spleen
stomach —*see* Laceration, stomach

Laceration (Continued)
intracranial NEC —*see also* Injury, intracranial, diffuse
birth injury P1Ø.9
jaw —*see* Laceration, head, specified site NEC
jejunum S36.438
joint capsule —*see* Sprain, by site
kidney S37.Ø3- •
major (greater than 3 cm) (massive) (stellate) S37.Ø6- •
minor (less than 1 cm) S37.Ø4- •
moderate (1 to 3 cm) S37.Ø5- •
multiple S37.Ø6- •
knee S81.Ø1- •
with foreign body S81.Ø2- •
labium (majus) (minus) —*see* Laceration, vulva
lacrimal duct —*see* Laceration, eyelid
large intestine —*see* Laceration, intestine, large
larynx S11.Ø11
with foreign body S11.Ø12
leg (lower) S81.819
with foreign body S81.829
foot —*see* Laceration, foot
knee —*see* Laceration, knee
left S81.812
with foreign body S81.822
right S81.811
with foreign body S81.821
upper —*see* Laceration, thigh
ligament —*see* Sprain
lip SØ1.511
with foreign body SØ1.521
liver S36.113
major (stellate) S36.116
minor S36.114
moderate S36.115
loin —*see* Laceration, abdomen, wall
lower back —*see* Laceration, back, lower
lumbar region —*see* Laceration, back, lower
lung S27.339
bilateral S27.332
unilateral S27.331
malar region —*see* Laceration, head, specified site NEC
mammary —*see* Laceration, breast
mastoid region —*see* Laceration, head, specified site NEC
meninges —*see* Injury, intracranial, diffuse
meniscus —*see* Tear, meniscus
mesentery S36.893
mesosalpinx S37.893
mouth —*see* Laceration, oral cavity
muscle —*see* Injury, muscle, by site, laceration
nail
finger —*see* Laceration, finger, with damage to nail
toe —*see* Laceration, toe, with damage to nail
nasal (septum) (sinus) —*see* Laceration, nose
nasopharynx —*see* Laceration, head, specified site NEC
neck S11.91
with foreign body S11.92
involving
cervical esophagus S11.21
with foreign body S11.22
larynx —*see* Laceration, larynx
pharynx —*see* Laceration, pharynx
thyroid gland —*see* Laceration, thyroid gland
trachea —*see* Laceration, trachea
specified site NEC S11.81
with foreign body S11.82
nerve —*see* Injury, nerve
nose (septum) (sinus) SØ1.21
with foreign body SØ1.22
ocular NOS SØ5.3- •
adnexa NOS SØ1.11- •

L

Laceration *(Continued)*
  oral cavity SØ1.512
    with foreign body SØ1.522
  orbit (eye) —*see* Wound, open, ocular, orbit
  ovary S37.439
    bilateral S37.432
    unilateral S37.431
  palate —*see* Laceration, oral cavity
  palm —*see* Laceration, hand
  pancreas S36.239
    body S36.231
      major S36.261
      minor S36.241
      moderate S36.251
    head S36.23Ø
      major S36.26Ø
      minor S36.24Ø
      moderate S36.25Ø
    major S36.269
    minor S36.249
    moderate S36.259
    tail S36.232
      major S36.262
      minor S36.242
      moderate S36.252
  pelvic S31.Ø1Ø
    with
      foreign body S31.Ø2Ø
        penetration into retroperitoneal cavity S31.Ø21
      penetration into retroperitoneal cavity S31.Ø11
    floor —*see also* Laceration, back, lower
      with ectopic or molar pregnancy OØ8.6
      complicating delivery O7Ø.1
      following ectopic or molar pregnancy OØ8.6
      old (postpartal) N81.89
    organ S37.93
      with ectopic or molar pregnancy OØ8.6
      adrenal gland S37.813
      bladder S37.23
      fallopian tube —*see* Laceration, fallopian tube
      following ectopic or molar pregnancy OØ8.6
      kidney —*see* Laceration, kidney
      obstetrical trauma O71.5
      ovary —*see* Laceration, ovary
      prostate S37.823
      specified site NEC S37.893
      ureter S37.13
      urethra S37.33
      uterus S37.63
  penis S31.21
    with foreign body S31.22
  perineum
    female S31.41
      with
        ectopic or molar pregnancy OØ8.6
        foreign body S31.42
      during delivery O7Ø.9
        first degree O7Ø.Ø
        fourth degree O7Ø.3
        second degree O7Ø.1
        third degree —*see also* Delivery, complicated, by, laceration, perineum, third degree O7Ø.2Ø
      old (postpartal) N81.89
      postpartal N81.89
      secondary (postpartal) O9Ø.1
    male S31.119
      with foreign body S31.129
  periocular area (with or without lacrimal passages) —*see* Laceration, eyelid
  peritoneum S36.893
  periumbilic region —*see* Laceration, abdomen, wall, periumbilic

Laceration *(Continued)*
  periurethral tissue —*see* Laceration, urethra
  phalanges
    finger —*see* Laceration, finger
    toe —*see* Laceration, toe
  pharynx S11.21
    with foreign body S11.22
  pinna —*see* Laceration, ear
  popliteal space —*see* Laceration, knee
  prepuce —*see* Laceration, penis
  prostate S37.823
  pubic region S31.119
    with foreign body S31.129
  pudendum —*see* Laceration, genital organs, external
  rectovaginal septum —*see* Laceration, vagina
  rectum S36.63
  retroperitoneum S36.893
  round ligament S37.893
  sacral region —*see* Laceration, back, lower
  sacroiliac region —*see* Laceration, back, lower
  salivary gland —*see* Laceration, oral cavity
  scalp SØ1.Ø1
    with foreign body SØ1.Ø2
  scapular region —*see* Laceration, shoulder
  scrotum S31.31
    with foreign body S31.32
  seminal vesicle S37.893
  shin —*see* Laceration, leg
  shoulder S41.Ø19
    with foreign body S41.Ø29
    left S41.Ø12
      with foreign body S41.Ø22
    right S41.Ø11
      with foreign body S41.Ø21
  small intestine —*see* Laceration, intestine, small
  spermatic cord —*see* Laceration, testis
  spinal cord (meninges) —*see also* Injury, spinal cord, by region
    due to injury at birth P11.5
    newborn (birth injury) P11.5
  spleen S36.Ø39
    major (massive) (stellate) S36.Ø32
    moderate S36.Ø31
    superficial (minor) S36.Ø3Ø
  sternal region —*see* Laceration, thorax, front
  stomach S36.33
  submaxillary region —*see* Laceration, head, specified site NEC
  submental region —*see* Laceration, head, specified site NEC
  subungual
    finger(s) —*see* Laceration, finger, with damage to nail
    toe(s) —*see* Laceration, toe, with damage to nail
  suprarenal gland —*see* Laceration, adrenal gland
  temple, temporal region —*see* Laceration, head, specified site NEC
  temporomandibular area —*see* Laceration, cheek
  tendon —*see* Injury, muscle, by site, laceration
    Achilles S86.Ø2-●
  tentorium cerebelli —*see* Injury, intracranial, diffuse
  testis S31.31
    with foreign body S31.32
  thigh S71.11-●
    with foreign body S71.12-●
  thorax, thoracic (wall) S21.91
    with foreign body S21.92
      back S21.22-●
        with penetration into thoracic cavity S21.42-●
      front S21.12-●
        with penetration into thoracic cavity S21.32-●

Laceration *(Continued)*
  thorax, thoracic *(Continued)*
    back S21.21-●
      with
        foreign body S21.22-●
          with penetration into thoracic cavity S21.42-●
        penetration into thoracic cavity S21.41-●
    breast —*see* Laceration, breast
    front S21.11-●
      with
        foreign body S21.12-●
          with penetration into thoracic cavity S21.32-●
        penetration into thoracic cavity S21.31-●
  thumb S61.Ø19
    with
      damage to nail S61.119
        with
          foreign body S61.129
      foreign body S61.Ø29
    left S61.Ø12
      with
        damage to nail S61.112
          with
            foreign body S61.122
        foreign body S61.Ø22
    right S61.Ø11
      with
        damage to nail S61.111
          with
            foreign body S61.121
        foreign body S61.Ø21
  thyroid gland S11.11
    with foreign body S11.12
  toe(s) S91.119
    with
      damage to nail S91.219
        with
          foreign body S91.229
      foreign body S91.129
    great S91.113
      with
        damage to nail S91.213
          with
            foreign body S91.223
        foreign body S91.123
      left S91.112
        with
          damage to nail S91.212
            with
              foreign body S91.222
          foreign body S91.122
      right S91.111
        with
          damage to nail S91.211
            with
              foreign body S91.221
          foreign body S91.121
    lesser S91.116
      with
        damage to nail S91.216
          with
            foreign body S91.226
        foreign body S91.126
      left S91.115
        with
          damage to nail S91.215
            with
              foreign body S91.225
          foreign body S91.125
      right S91.114
        with
          damage to nail S91.214
            with
              foreign body S91.224
          foreign body S91.124
  tongue —*see* Laceration, oral cavity

Laceration (Continued)
trachea S11.021
with foreign body S11.022
tunica vaginalis —see Laceration, testis
tympanum, tympanic membrane —see Laceration, ear, drum
umbilical region S31.115
with foreign body S31.125
ureter S37.13
urethra S37.33
with or following ectopic or molar pregnancy O08.6
obstetrical trauma O71.5
urinary organ NEC S37.893
uterus S37.63
with ectopic or molar pregnancy O08.6
following ectopic or molar pregnancy O08.6
nonpuerperal, nontraumatic N85.8
obstetrical trauma NEC O71.81
old (postpartal) N85.8
uvula —see Laceration, oral cavity
vagina S31.41
with
ectopic or molar pregnancy O08.6
foreign body S31.42
during delivery O71.4
with perineal laceration —see Laceration, perineum, female, during delivery
following ectopic or molar pregnancy O08.6
nonpuerperal, nontraumatic N89.8
old (postpartal) N89.8
vas deferens S37.893
vesical —see Laceration, bladder
vocal cords S11.031
with foreign body S11.032
vulva S31.41
with
ectopic or molar pregnancy O08.6
foreign body S31.42
complicating delivery O70.0
following ectopic or molar pregnancy O08.6
nonpuerperal, nontraumatic N90.89
old (postpartal) N90.89
wrist S61.519
with
foreign body S61.529
left S61.512
with
foreign body S61.522
right S61.511
with
foreign body S61.521
Lack of
achievement in school Z55.3
adequate
food Z59.4
intermaxillary vertical dimension of fully erupted teeth M26.36
sleep Z72.820
appetite (see Anorexia) R63.0
awareness R41.9
care
in home Z74.2
of infant (at or after birth) T76.02
confirmed T74.02
cognitive functions R41.9
coordination R27.9
ataxia R27.0
specified type NEC R27.8
development (physiological) R62.50
failure to thrive (child over 28 days old) R62.51
adult R62.7
newborn P92.6
short stature R62.52
specified type NEC R62.59
energy R53.83
financial resources Z59.6
Lack of (Continued)
food T73.0
growth R62.52
heating Z59.1
housing (permanent) (temporary) Z59.0
adequate Z59.1
learning experiences in childhood Z62.898
leisure time (affecting life-style) Z73.2
material resources Z59.9
memory —see also Amnesia
mild, following organic brain damage F06.8
ovulation N97.0
parental supervision or control of child Z62.0
person able to render necessary care Z74.2
physical exercise Z72.3
play experience in childhood Z62.898
posterior occlusal support M26.57
relaxation (affecting life-style) Z73.2
sexual
desire F52.0
enjoyment F52.1
shelter Z59.0
sleep (adequate) Z72.820
supervision of child by parent Z62.0
support, posterior occlusal M26.57
water T73.1
Lacrimal —see condition
Lacrimation, abnormal —see Epiphora
Lacrimonasal duct —see condition
Lactation, lactating (breast) (puerperal, postpartum)
associated
cracked nipple O92.13
retracted nipple O92.03
defective O92.4
disorder NEC O92.79
excessive O92.6
failed (complete) O92.3
partial O92.4
mastitis NEC —see Mastitis, obstetric
mother (care and/or examination) Z39.1
nonpuerperal N64.3
Lacticemia, excessive E87.2
Lacunar skull Q75.8
Laennec's cirrhosis K70.30
with ascites K70.31
nonalcoholic K74.69
Lafora's disease —see Epilepsy, generalized, idiopathic
Lag, lid (nervous) —see Retraction, lid
Lagophthalmos (eyelid) (nervous) H02.209
bilateral, upper and lower eyelids H02.20C
cicatricial H02.219
bilateral, upper and lower eyelids H02.21C
left H02.216
lower H02.215
upper H02.214
upper and lower eyelids H02.21B
right H02.213
lower H02.212
upper H02.211
upper and lower eyelids H02.21A
keratoconjunctivitis —see Keratoconjunctivitis
left H02.206
lower H02.205
upper H02.204
upper and lower eyelids H02.20B
mechanical H02.229
bilateral, upper and lower eyelids H02.22C
left H02.226
lower H02.225
upper H02.224
upper and lower eyelids H02.22B
right H02.223
lower H02.222
upper H02.221
upper and lower eyelids H02.22A
Lagophthalmos (Continued)
paralytic H02.239
bilateral, upper and lower eyelids H02.23C
left H02.236
lower H02.235
upper H02.234
upper and lower eyelids H02.23B
right H02.233
lower H02.232
upper H02.231
upper and lower eyelids H02.23A
right H02.203
lower H02.202
upper H02.201
upper and lower eyelids H02.20A
Laki-Lorand factor deficiency —see Defect, coagulation, specified type NEC
Lalling F80.0
Lambert-Eaton syndrome —see Syndrome, Lambert-Eaton
Lambliasis, lambliosis A07.1
Landau-Kleffner syndrome —see Epilepsy, specified NEC
Landouzy-Déjérine dystrophy or facioscapulohumeral atrophy G71.02
Landouzy's disease (icterohemorrhagic leptospirosis) A27.0
Landry-Guillain-Barré, syndrome or paralysis G61.0
Landry's disease or paralysis G61.0
Lane's
band Q43.3
kink —see Obstruction, intestine
syndrome K90.2
Langdon Down's syndrome —see Trisomy, 21
Lapsed immunization schedule status Z28.3
Large
baby (regardless of gestational age) (4000g to 4499g) P08.1
ear, congenital Q17.1
physiological cup Q14.2
stature R68.89
Large-for-dates NEC (infant) (4000g to 4499g) P08.1
affecting management of pregnancy O36.6-•
exceptionally (4500g or more) P08.0
Larsen-Johansson disease orosteochondrosis —see Osteochondrosis, juvenile, patella
Larsen's syndrome (flattened facies and multiple congenital dislocations) Q74.8
Larva migrans
cutaneous B76.9
Ancylostoma B76.0
visceral B83.0
Laryngeal —see condition
Laryngismus (stridulus) J38.5
congenital P28.89
diphtheritic A36.2
Laryngitis (acute) (edematous) (fibrinous) (infective) (infiltrative) (malignant) (membranous) (phlegmonous) (pneumococcal) (pseudomembranous) (septic) (subglottic) (suppurative) (ulcerative) J04.0
with
influenza, flu, or grippe —see Influenza, with, laryngitis
tracheitis (acute) —see Laryngotracheitis
atrophic J37.0
catarrhal J37.0
chronic J37.0
with tracheitis (chronic) J37.1
diphtheritic A36.2
due to external agent —see Inflammation, respiratory, upper, due to
Hemophilus influenzae J04.0
H. influenzae J04.0
hypertrophic J37.0
influenzal —see Influenza, with, respiratory manifestations NEC

Laryngitis (Continued)
obstructive J05.0
sicca J37.0
spasmodic J05.0
acute J04.0
streptococcal J04.0
stridulous J05.0
syphilitic (late) A52.73
congenital A50.59 [J99]
early A50.03 [J99]
tuberculous A15.5
Vincent's A69.1
Laryngocele (congenital) (ventricular) Q31.3
Laryngofissure J38.7
congenital Q31.8
Laryngomalacia (congenital) Q31.5
Laryngopharyngitis (acute) J06.0
chronic J37.0
due to external agent —see Inflammation, respiratory, upper, due to
Laryngoplegia J38.00
bilateral J38.02
unilateral J38.01
Laryngoptosis J38.7
Laryngospasm J38.5
Laryngostenosis J38.6
Laryngotracheitis (acute) (Infectional) (infective) (viral) J04.2
atrophic J37.1
catarrhal J37.1
chronic J37.1
diphtheritic A36.2
due to external agent —see Inflammation, respiratory, upper, due to
Hemophilus influenzae J04.2
hypertrophic J37.1
influenzal —see Influenza, with, respiratory manifestations NEC
pachydermic J38.7
sicca J37.1
spasmodic J38.5
acute J05.0
streptococcal J04.2
stridulous J38.5
syphilitic (late) A52.73
congenital A50.59 [J99]
early A50.03 [J99]
tuberculous A15.5
Vincent's A69.1
Laryngotracheobronchitis —see Bronchitis
Larynx, laryngeal —see condition
Lassa fever A96.2
Lassitude —see Weakness
Late
talker R62.0
walker R62.0
Late effect(s) —see Sequelae
Latent —see condition
Laterocession —see Lateroversion
Lateroflexion —see Lateroversion
Lateroversion
cervix —see Lateroversion, uterus
uterus, uterine (cervix) (postinfectional) (postpartal, old) N85.4
congenital Q51.818
in pregnancy or childbirth O34.59-●
Lathyrism —see Poisoning, food, noxious, plant
Launois' syndrome (pituitary gigantism) E22.0
Launois-Bensaude adenolipomatosis E88.89
Laurence-Moon (-Bardet)-Biedl syndrome Q87.89
Lax, laxity —see also Relaxation
ligament (ous) —see also Disorder, ligament
familial M35.7
knee —see Derangement, knee
skin (acquired) L57.4
congenital Q82.8
Laxative habit F55.2
Lazy leukocyte syndrome D70.8
Lead miner's lung J63.6
Leak, leakage
air NEC J93.82
postprocedural J95.812
amniotic fluid —see Rupture, membranes, premature
blood (microscopic), fetal, into maternal circulation affecting management of pregnancy —see Pregnancy, complicated by
cerebrospinal fluid G96.0
from spinal (lumbar) puncture G97.0
device, implant or graft —see also Complications, by site and type, mechanical
arterial graft NEC —see Complication, cardiovascular device, mechanical, vascular
breast (implant) T85.43
catheter NEC T85.638
dialysis (renal) T82.43
intraperitoneal T85.631
infusion NEC T82.534
spinal (epidural) (subdural) T85.630
urinary T83.038
cystostomy T83.030
Hopkins T83.038
ileostomy T83.038
indwelling T83.031
nephrostomy T83.032
specified NEC T83.038
urostomy T83.038
gastrointestinal —see Complications, prosthetic device, mechanical, gastrointestinal device
genital NEC T83.498
penile prosthesis (cylinder) (implanted) (pump) (resevoir) T83.490
testicular prosthesis T83.491
heart NEC —see Complication, cardiovascular device, mechanical
joint prosthesis —see Complications, joint prosthesis, mechanical, specified NEC, by site
ocular NEC —see Complications, prosthetic device, mechanical, ocular device
orthopedic NEC —see Complication, orthopedic, device, mechanical
persistent air J93.82
specified NEC T85.638
urinary NEC —see also Complication, genitourinary, device, urinary, mechanical
graft T83.23
vascular NEC —see Complication, cardiovascular device, mechanical
ventricular intracranial shunt T85.03
urine —see Incontinence
Leaky heart —see Endocarditis
Learning defect (specific) F81.9
Leather bottle stomach C16.9
Leber's
congenital amaurosis H35.50
optic atrophy (hereditary) H47.22
Lederer's anemia D59.1
Leeches (external) —see Hirudiniasis
Leg —see condition
Legg (-Calvé)-Perthes disease, syndrome or osteochondrosis M91.1-●
Legionellosis A48.1
nonpneumonic A48.2
Legionnaires'
disease A48.1
nonpneumonic A48.2
pneumonia A48.1
Leigh's disease G31.82
Leiner's disease L21.1
Leiofibromyoma —see Leiomyoma
Leiomyoblastoma —see Neoplasm, connective tissue, benign
Leiomyofibroma —see also Neoplasm, connective tissue, benign
uterus (cervix) (corpus) D25.9
Leiomyoma —see also Neoplasm, connective tissue, benign
bizarre —see Neoplasm, connective tissue, benign
cellular —see Neoplasm, connective tissue, benign
epithelioid —see Neoplasm, connective tissue, benign
uterus (cervix) (corpus) D25.9
intramural D25.1
submucous D25.0
subserosal D25.2
vascular —see Neoplasm, connective tissue, benign
Leiomyoma, leiomyomatosis (intravascular) —see Neoplasm, connective tissue, uncertain behavior
Leiomyosarcoma —see also Neoplasm, connective tissue, malignant
epithelioid —see Neoplasm, connective tissue, malignant
myxoid —see Neoplasm, connective tissue, malignant
Leishmaniasis B55.9
American (mucocutaneous) B55.2
cutaneous B55.1
Asian Desert B55.1
Brazilian B55.2
cutaneous (any type) B55.1
dermal —see also Leishmaniasis, cutaneous
post-kala-azar B55.0
eyelid B55.1
infantile B55.0
Mediterranean B55.0
mucocutaneous (American) (New World) B55.2
naso-oral B55.2
nasopharyngeal B55.2
old world B55.1
tegumentaria diffusa B55.1
visceral B55.0
Leishmanoid, dermal —see also Leishmaniasis, cutaneous
post-kala-azar B55.0
Lenegre's disease I44.2
Lengthening, leg —see Deformity, limb, unequal length
Lennert's lymphoma —see Lymphoma, Lennert's
Lennox-Gastaut syndrome G40.812
intractable G40.814
with status epilepticus G40.813
without status epilepticus G40.814
not intractable G40.812
with status epilepticus G40.811
without status epilepticus G40.812
Lens —see condition
Lenticonus (anterior) (posterior) (congenital) Q12.8
Lenticular degeneration, progressive E83.01
Lentiglobus (posterior) (congenital) Q12.8
Lentigo (congenital) L81.4
maligna —see also Melanoma, in situ
melanoma —see Melanoma
Lentivirus, as cause of disease classified elsewhere B97.31
Leontiasis
ossium M85.2
syphilitic (late) A52.78
congenital A50.59
Lepothrix A48.8
Lepra —see Leprosy
Leprechaunism E34.8
Leprosy A30.-●
with muscle disorder A30.9 [M63.80]
ankle A30.9 [M63.87-●]
foot A30.9 [M63.87-●]
forearm A30.9 [M63.83-●]
hand A30.9 [M63.84-●]
lower leg A30.9 [M63.86-●]
multiple sites A30.9 [M63.89]

L

Leprosy *(Continued)*
with muscle disorder *(Continued)*
pelvic region A3Ø.9 *[M63.85-●]*
shoulder region A3Ø.9 *[M63.81-●]*
specified site NEC A3Ø.9 *[M63.88]*
thigh A3Ø.9 *[M63.85-●]*
upper arm A3Ø.9 *[M63.82-●]*
anesthetic A3Ø.9
BB A3Ø.3
BL A3Ø.4
borderline (infiltrated) (neuritic) A3Ø.3
lepromatous A3Ø.4
tuberculoid A3Ø.2
BT A3Ø.2
dimorphous (infiltrated) (neuritic) A3Ø.3
I A3Ø.Ø
indeterminate (macular) (neuritic) A3Ø.Ø
lepromatous (diffuse) (infiltrated) (macular) (neuritic) (nodular) A3Ø.5
LL A3Ø.5
macular (early) (neuritic) (simple) A3Ø.9
maculoanesthetic A3Ø.9
mixed A3Ø.3
neural A3Ø.9
nodular A3Ø.5
primary neuritic A3Ø.3
specified type NEC A3Ø.8
TT A3Ø.1
tuberculoid (major) (minor) A3Ø.1
Leptocytosis, hereditary D56.9
Leptomeningitis (chronic) (circumscribed) (hemorrhagic) (nonsuppurative) *—see* Meningitis
Leptomeningopathy G96.19
Leptospiral *—see* condition
Leptospirochetal *—see* condition
Leptospirosis A27.9
canicola A27.89
due to Leptospira interrogans serovar icterohaemorrhagiae A27.Ø
icterohemorrhagica A27.Ø
pomona A27.89
Weil's disease A27.Ø
Leptus dermatitis B88.Ø
Leriche's syndrome (aortic bifurcation occlusion) I74.Ø9
Leri's pleonosteosis Q78.8
Leri-Weill syndrome Q77.8
Lermoyez' syndrome *—see* Vertigo, peripheral NEC
Lesch-Nyhan syndrome E79.1
Leser-Trélat disease L82.1
inflamed L82.Ø
Lesion(s) (nontraumatic)
abducens nerve *—see* Strabismus, paralytic, sixth nerve
alveolar process KØ8.9
angiocentric immunoproliferative D47.Z9
anorectal K62.9
aortic (valve) I35.9
auditory nerve *—see* subcategory H93.3
basal ganglion G25.9
bile duct *—see* Disease, bile duct
biomechanical M99.9
specified type NEC M99.89
abdomen M99.89
acromioclavicular M99.87
cervical region M99.81
cervicothoracic M99.81
costochondral M99.88
costovertebral M99.88
head region M99.8Ø
hip M99.85
lower extremity M99.86
lumbar region M99.83
lumbosacral M99.83
occipitocervical M99.8Ø
pelvic region M99.85
pubic M99.85
rib cage M99.88
sacral region M99.84

Lesion *(Continued)*
biomechanical *(Continued)*
specified type NEC *(Continued)*
sacrococcygeal M99.84
sacroiliac M99.84
specified NEC M99.89
sternochondral M99.88
sternoclavicular M99.87
thoracic region M99.82
thoracolumbar M99.82
upper extremity M99.87
bladder N32.9
bone *—see* Disorder, bone
brachial plexus G54.Ø
brain G93.9
congenital QØ4.9
vascular I67.9
degenerative I67.9
hypertensive I67.4
buccal cavity K13.79
calcified *—see* Calcification
canthus *—see* Disorder, eyelid
carate *—see* Pinta, lesions
cardia K31.9
cardiac *—see also* Disease, heart I51.9
congenital Q24.9
valvular *—see* Endocarditis
cauda equina G83.4
cecum K63.9
cerebral *—see* Lesion, brain
cerebrovascular I67.9
degenerative I67.9
hypertensive I67.4
cervical (nerve) root NEC G54.2
chiasmal *—see* Disorder, optic, chiasm
chorda tympani G51.8
coin, lung R91.1
colon K63.9
combined periodontic - endodontic KØ5.5
congenital *—see* Anomaly, by site
conjunctiva H11.9
conus medullaris *—see* Injury, conus medullaris
coronary artery *—see* Ischemia, heart
cranial nerve G52.9
eighth *—see* Disorder, ear
eleventh G52.9
fifth G5Ø.9
first G52.Ø
fourth *—see* Strabismus, paralytic, fourth nerve
seventh G51.9
sixth *—see* Strabismus, paralytic, sixth nerve
tenth G52.2
twelfth G52.3
cystic *—see* Cyst
degenerative *—see* Degeneration
duodenum K31.9
edentulous (alveolar) ridge, associated with trauma, due to traumatic occlusion KØ6.2
en coup de sabre L94.1
eyelid *—see* Disorder, eyelid
gasserian ganglion G5Ø.8
gastric K31.9
gastroduodenal K31.9
gastrointestinal K63.9
gingiva, associated with trauma KØ6.2
glomerular
focal and segmental *—see also* NØØ-NØ7 with fourth character .1 NØ5.1
minimal change *—see also* NØØ-NØ7 with fourth character .Ø NØ5.Ø
heart (organic) *—see* Disease, heart
hyperchromic, due to pinta (carate) A67.1
hyperkeratotic *—see* Hyperkeratosis
hypothalamic E23.7
ileocecal K63.9
ileum K63.9
iliohypogastric nerve G57.8-●
inflammatory *—see* Inflammation
intestine K63.9

Lesion *(Continued)*
intracerebral *—see* Lesion, brain
intrachiasmal (optic) *—see* Disorder, optic, chiasm
intracranial, space-occupying R9Ø.Ø
joint *—see* Disorder, joint
sacroiliac (old) M53.3
keratotic *—see* Keratosis
kidney *—see* Disease, renal
laryngeal nerve (recurrent) G52.2
lip K13.Ø
liver K76.9
lumbosacral
plexus G54.1
root (nerve) NEC G54.4
lung (coin) R91.1
maxillary sinus J32.Ø
mitral IØ5.9
Morel-Lavallée *—see* Hematoma, by site
motor cortex NEC G93.89
mouth K13.79
nerve G58.9
femoral G57.2-●
median G56.1-●
carpal tunnel syndrome *—see* Syndrome, carpal tunnel
plantar G57.6-●
popliteal (lateral) G57.3-●
medial G57.4-●
radial G56.3-●
sciatic G57.Ø-●
spinal *—see* Injury, nerve, spinal
ulnar G56.2-●
nervous system, congenital QØ7.9
nonallopathic *—see* Lesion, biomechanical
nose (internal) J34.89
obstructive *—see* Obstruction
obturator nerve G57.8-●
oral mucosa K13.7Ø
organ or site NEC *—see* Disease, by site
osteolytic *—see* Osteolysis
peptic K27.9
periodontal, due to traumatic occlusion KØ5.5
pharynx J39.2
pigment, pigmented (skin) L81.9
pinta *—see* Pinta, lesions
polypoid *—see* Polyp
prechiasmal (optic) *—see* Disorder, optic, chiasm
primary *—see also* Syphilis, primary A51.Ø
carate A67.Ø
pinta A67.Ø
yaws A66.Ø
pulmonary J98.4
valve I37.9
pylorus K31.9
rectosigmoid K63.9
retina, retinal H35.9
sacroiliac (joint) (old) M53.3
salivary gland K11.9
benign lymphoepithelial K11.8
saphenous nerve G57.8-●
sciatic nerve G57.Ø-●
secondary *—see* Syphilis, secondary
shoulder (region) M75.9-●
specified NEC M75.8-●
sigmoid K63.9
sinus (accessory) (nasal) J34.89
skin L98.9
suppurative LØ8.Ø
SLAP S43.43-●
spinal cord G95.9
congenital QØ6.9
spleen D73.89
stomach K31.9
superior glenoid labrum S43.43-●
syphilitic *—see* Syphilis
tertiary *—see* Syphilis, tertiary
thoracic root (nerve) NEC G54.3
tonsillar fossa J35.9

Lesion (Continued)
tooth, teeth K08.9
white spot
chewing surface K02.51
pit and fissure surface K02.51
smooth surface K02.61
traumatic —see specific type of injury by site
tricuspid (valve) I07.9
nonrheumatic I36.9
trigeminal nerve G50.9
ulcerated or ulcerative —see Ulcer, skin
uterus N85.9
vagina N89.8
vulva N90.89
vagus nerve G52.2
valvular —see Endocarditis
vascular I99.9
affecting central nervous system I67.9
following trauma NEC T14.8
umbilical cord, complicating delivery O69.5
warty —see Verruca
white spot (tooth)
chewing surface K02.51
pit and fissure surface K02.51
smooth surface K02.61
Lethargic —see condition
Lethargy R53.83
Letterer-Siwe's disease C96.0
Leukemia, leukemic C95.9- ●
acute basophilic C94.8- ●
acute bilineal C95.0- ●
acute erythroid C94.0- ●
acute lymphoblastic C91.0- ●
acute megakaryoblastic C94.2- ●
acute megakaryocytic C94.2- ●
acute mixed lineage C95.0- ●
acute monoblastic (monoblastic/monocytic) C93.0- ●
acute monocytic (monoblastic/monocytic) C93.0- ●
acute myeloblastic (minimal differentiation) (with maturation) C92.0- ●
acute myeloid, NOS C92.0- ●
with
11q23-abnormality C92.6- ●
dysplasia of remaining hematopoesis and/or myelodysplastic disease in its history C92.A- ●
multilineage dysplasia C92.A- ●
variation of MLL-gene C92.6- ●
M6 (a)(b) C94.0- ●
M7 C94.2- ●
acute myelomonocytic C92.5- ●
acute promyelocytic C92.4- ●
adult T-cell (HTLV-1-associated) (acute variant) (chronic variant) (lymphomatoid variant) (smouldering variant) C91.5- ●
aggressive NK-cell C94.8- ●
AML (1/ETO) (M0) (M1) (M2) (without a FAB classification) C92.0- ●
AML M3 C92.4- ●
AML M4 (Eo with inv(16) or t(16;16)) C92.5- ●
AML M5 C93.0- ●
AML M5a C93.0- ●
AML M5b C93.0- ●
AML Me with t (15;17) and variants C92.4- ●
atypical chronic myeloid, BCR/ABL-negative C92.2- ●
biphenotypic acute C95.0- ●
blast cell C95.0- ●
Burkitt-type, mature B-cell C91.A- ●
chronic lymphocytic, of B-cell type C91.1- ●
chronic monocytic C93.1- ●
chronic myelogenous (Philadelphia chromosome (Ph1) positive) (t(9;22)) (q34;q11) (with crisis of blast cells) C92.1- ●
chronic myeloid, BCR/ABL-positive C92.1- ●
atypical, BCR/ABL-negative C92.2- ●
Leukemia, leukemic (Continued)
chronic myelomonocytic C93.1- ●
chronic neutrophilic D47.1
CMML (-1) (-2) (with eosinophilia) C93.1- ●
granulocytic —see also Category C92 C92.9- ●
hairy-cell C91.4- ●
juvenile myelomonocytic C93.3- ●
lymphoid C91.9- ●
specified NEC C91.Z- ●
mast cell C94.3- ●
mature B-cell, Burkitt-type C91.A- ●
monocytic (subacute) C93.9- ●
specified NEC C93.Z- ●
myelogenous —see also Category C92 C92.9- ●
myeloid C92.9- ●
specified NEC C92.Z- ●
plasma cell C90.1- ●
plasmacytic C90.1- ●
prolymphocytic
of B-cell type C91.3- ●
of T-cell type C91.6- ●
specified NEC C94.8- ●
stem cell, of unclear lineage C95.0- ●
subacute lymphocytic C91.9- ●
T-cell large granular lymphocytic C91.Z- ●
unspecified cell type C95.9- ●
acute C95.0- ●
chronic C95.1- ●
Leukemoid reaction —see also Reaction, leukemoid D72.823- ●
Leukoaraiosis (hypertensive) I67.81
Leukoariosis —see Leukoaraiosis
Leukocoria —see Disorder, globe, degenerated condition, leucocoria
Leukocytopenia D72.819
Leukocytosis D72.829
eosinophilic D72.1
Leukoderma, leukodermia NEC L81.5
syphilitic A51.39
late A52.79
Leukodystrophy E75.29
Leukoedema, oral epithelium K13.29
Leukoencephalitis G04.81
acute (subacute) hemorrhagic G36.1
postimmunization or postvaccinal G04.02
postinfectious G04.01
subacute sclerosing A81.1
van Bogaert's (sclerosing) A81.1
Leukoencephalopathy —see also Encephalopathy G93.49
Binswanger's I67.3
heroin vapor G92
metachromatic E75.25
multifocal (progressive) A81.2
postimmunization and postvaccinal G04.02
progressive multifocal A81.2
reversible, posterior G93.6
van Bogaert's (sclerosing) A81.1
vascular, progressive I67.3
Leukoerythroblastosis D75.9
Leukokeratosis —see also Leukoplakia
mouth K13.21
nicotina palati K13.24
oral mucosa K13.21
tongue K13.21
vocal cord J38.3
Leukokraurosis vulva (e) N90.4
Leukoma (cornea) —see also Opacity, cornea
adherent H17.0- ●
interfering with central vision —see Opacity, cornea, central
Leukomalacia, cerebral, newborn P91.2
periventricular P91.2
Leukomelanopathy, hereditary D72.0
Leukonychia (punctata) (striata) L60.8
congenital Q84.4
Leukopathia unguium L60.8
congenital Q84.4
Leukopenia D72.819
basophilic D72.818
chemotherapy (cancer) induced D70.1
congenital D70.0
cyclic D70.0
drug induced NEC D70.2
due to cytoreductive cancer chemotherapy D70.1
eosinophilic D72.818
familial D70.0
infantile genetic D70.0
malignant D70.9
periodic D70.0
transitory neonatal P61.5
Leukopenic —see condition
Leukoplakia
anus K62.89
bladder (postinfectional) N32.89
buccal K13.21
cervix (uteri) N88.0
esophagus K22.8
gingiva K13.21
hairy (oral mucosa) (tongue) K13.3
kidney (pelvis) N28.89
larynx J38.7
lip K13.21
mouth K13.21
oral epithelium, including tongue (mucosa) K13.21
palate K13.21
pelvis (kidney) N28.89
penis (infectional) N48.0
rectum K62.89
syphilitic (late) A52.79
tongue K13.21
ureter (postinfectional) N28.89
urethra (postinfectional) N36.8
uterus N85.8
vagina N89.4
vocal cord J38.3
vulva N90.4
Leukorrhea N89.8
due to Trichomonas (vaginalis) A59.00
trichomonal A59.00
Leukosarcoma C85.9
Levocardia (isolated) Q24.1
with situs inversus Q89.3
Levotransposition Q20.5
Lev's disease or syndrome (acquired complete heart block) I44.2
Levulosuria —see Fructosuria
Levurid L30.2
Lewy body (ies) (dementia) (disease) G31.83
Leyden-Moebius dystrophy G71.09
Leydig cell
carcinoma
specified site —see Neoplasm, malignant, by site
unspecified site
female C56.9- ●
male C62.9- ●
tumor
benign
specified site —see Neoplasm, benign, by site
unspecified site
female D27.- ●
male D29.2- ●
malignant
specified site —see Neoplasm, malignant, by site
unspecified site
female C56.- ●
male C62.9- ●
specified site —see Neoplasm, uncertain behavior, by site
unspecified site
female D39.1- ●
male D40.1- ●

L

- **Leydig-Sertoli cell tumor**
  - specified site —*see* Neoplasm, benign, by site
  - unspecified site
    - female D27.- •
    - male D29.2- •
- **LGSIL** (Low grade squamous intraepithelial lesion on cytologic smear of)
  - anus R85.612
  - cervix R87.612
  - vagina R87.622
- **Liar, pathologic** F60.2
- **Libido**
  - decreased R68.82
- **Libman-Sacks disease** M32.11
- **Lice** (infestation) B85.2
  - body (Pediculus corporis) B85.1
  - crab B85.3
  - head (Pediculus capitis) B85.0
  - mixed (classifiable to more than one of the titles B85.0-B85.3) B85.4
  - pubic (Phthirus pubis) B85.3
- **Lichen** L28.0
  - albus L90.0
    - penis N48.0
    - vulva N90.4
  - amyloidosis E85.4 *[L99]*
  - atrophicus L90.0
    - penis N48.0
    - vulva N90.4
  - congenital Q82.8
  - myxedematosus L98.5
  - nitidus L44.1
  - pilaris Q82.8
    - acquired L85.8
  - planopilaris L66.1
  - planus (chronicus) L43.9
    - annularis L43.8
    - bullous L43.1
    - follicular L66.1
    - hypertrophic L43.0
    - moniliformis L44.3
    - of Wilson L43.9
    - specified NEC L43.8
    - subacute (active) L43.3
    - tropicus L43.3
  - ruber
    - acuminatus L44.0
    - moniliformis L44.3
    - planus L43.9
  - sclerosus (et atrophicus) L90.0
    - penis N48.0
    - vulva N90.4
  - scrofulosus (primary) (tuberculous) A18.4
  - simplex (chronicus) (circumscriptus) L28.0
  - striatus L44.2
  - urticatus L28.2
- **Lichenification** L28.0
- **Lichenoides tuberculosis** (primary) A18.4
- ➠ **Lichtheim's disease or syndrome** D51.0
- **Lien migrans** D73.89
- **Ligament** —*see* condition
- **Light**
  - for gestational age —*see* Light for dates
  - headedness R42
- **Light-for-dates** (infant) P05.00
  - with weight of
    - 499 grams or less P05.01
    - 500-749 grams P05.02
    - 750-999 grams P05.03
    - 1000-1249 grams P05.04
    - 1250-1499 grams P05.05
    - 1500-1749 grams P05.06
    - 1750-1999 grams P05.07
    - 2000-2499 grams P05.08
    - 2500 grams and over P05.09
  - affecting management of pregnancy O36.59- •
  - and small-for-dates —*see* Small for dates
  - specified NEC P05.09
- **Lightning** (effects) (stroke) (struck by) T75.00
  - burn —*see* Burn
  - foot E53.8
  - shock T75.01
  - specified effect NEC T75.09
- **Lightwood-Albright syndrome** N25.89
- **Lightwood's disease or syndrome** (renal tubular acidosis) N25.89
- **Lignac** (-de Toni) (-Fanconi) (-Debré) **disease or syndrome** E72.09
  - with cystinosis E72.04
- **Ligneous thyroiditis** E06.5
- **Likoff's syndrome** I20.8
- **Limb** —*see* condition
- **Limbic epilepsy personality syndrome** F07.0
- **Limitation, limited**
  - activities due to disability Z73.6
  - cardiac reserve —*see* Disease, heart
  - eye muscle duction, traumatic —*see* Strabismus, mechanical
  - mandibular range of motion M26.52
- **Lindau** (-von Hippel) **disease** Q85.8
- **Line(s)**
  - Beau's L60.4
  - Harris' —*see* Arrest, epiphyseal
  - Hudson's (cornea) —*see* Pigmentation, cornea, anterior
  - Stähli's (cornea) —*see* Pigmentation, cornea, anterior
- **Linea corneae senilis** —*see* Change, cornea, senile
- **Lingua**
  - geographica K14.1
  - nigra (villosa) K14.3
  - plicata K14.5
  - tylosis K13.29
- **Lingual** —*see* condition
- **Linguatulosis** B88.8
- **Linitis** (gastric) **plastica** C16.9
- **Lip** —*see* condition
- **Lipedema** —*see* Edema
- **Lipemia** —*see also* Hyperlipidemia
  - retina, retinalis E78.3
- **Lipidosis** E75.6
  - cerebral (infantile) (juvenile) (late) E75.4
  - cerebroretinal E75.4
  - cerebroside E75.22
  - cholesterol (cerebral) E75.5
  - glycolipid E75.21
  - hepatosplenomegalic E78.3
  - sphingomyelin —*see* Niemann-Pick disease or syndrome
  - sulfatide E75.29
- **Lipoadenoma** —*see* Neoplasm, benign, by site
- **Lipoblastoma** —*see* Lipoma
- **Lipoblastomatosis** —*see* Lipoma
- **Lipochondrodystrophy** E76.01
- **Lipochrome histiocytosis** (familial) D71
- **Lipodermatosclerosis** —*see* Varix, leg, with, inflammation
  - ulcerated —*see* Varix, leg, with, ulcer, with inflammation by site
- **Lipodystrophia progressiva** E88.1
- **Lipodystrophy** (progressive) E88.1
  - insulin E88.1
  - intestinal K90.81
  - mesenteric K65.4
- **Lipofibroma** —*see* Lipoma
- **Lipofuscinosis, neuronal** (with ceroidosis) E75.4
- **Lipogranuloma, sclerosing** L92.8
- **Lipogranulomatosis** E78.89
- **Lipoid** —*see also* condition
  - histiocytosis D76.3
    - essential E75.29
  - nephrosis N04.9
  - proteinosis of Urbach E78.89
- **Lipoidemia** —*see* Hyperlipidemia
- **Lipoidosis** —*see* Lipidosis
- **Lipoma** D17.9
  - fetal D17.9
    - fat cell D17.9
  - infiltrating D17.9
  - intramuscular D17.9
  - pleomorphic D17.9
  - site classification
    - arms (skin) (subcutaneous) D17.2- •
    - connective tissue D17.30
      - intra-abdominal D17.5
      - intrathoracic D17.4
      - peritoneum D17.79
      - retroperitoneum D17.79
      - specified site NEC D17.39
      - spermatic cord D17.6
    - face (skin) (subcutaneous) D17.0
    - genitourinary organ NEC D17.72
    - head (skin) (subcutaneous) D17.0
    - intra-abdominal D17.5
    - intrathoracic D17.4
    - kidney D17.71
    - legs (skin) (subcutaneous) D17.2- •
    - neck (skin) (subcutaneous) D17.0
    - peritoneum D17.79
    - retroperitoneum D17.79
    - skin D17.30
      - specified site NEC D17.39
    - specified site NEC D17.79
    - spermatic cord D17.6
    - subcutaneous D17.30
      - specified site NEC D17.39
    - trunk (skin) (subcutaneous) D17.1
    - unspecified D17.9
  - spindle cell D17.9
- **Lipomatosis** E88.2
  - dolorosa (Dercum) E88.2
  - fetal —*see* Lipoma
  - Launois-Bensaude E88.89
- **Lipomyoma** —*see* Lipoma
- **Lipomyxoma** —*see* Lipoma
- **Lipomyxosarcoma** —*see* Neoplasm, connective tissue, malignant
- **Lipoprotein metabolism disorder** E78.9
- **Lipoproteinemia** E78.5
  - broad-beta E78.2
  - floating-beta E78.2
  - hyper-pre-beta E78.1
- **Liposarcoma** —*see also* Neoplasm, connective tissue, malignant
  - dedifferentiated —*see* Neoplasm, connective tissue, malignant
  - differentiated type —*see* Neoplasm, connective tissue, malignant
  - embryonal —*see* Neoplasm, connective tissue, malignant
  - mixed type —*see* Neoplasm, connective tissue, malignant
  - myxoid —*see* Neoplasm, connective tissue, malignant
  - pleomorphic —*see* Neoplasm, connective tissue, malignant
  - round cell —*see* Neoplasm, connective tissue, malignant
  - well differentiated type —*see* Neoplasm, connective tissue, malignant
- **Liposynovitis prepatellaris** E88.89
- **Lipping, cervix** N86
- **Lipschütz disease or ulcer** N76.6
- **Lipuria** R82.0
  - schistosomiasis (bilharziasis) B65.0
- **Lisping** F80.0
- **Lissauer's paralysis** A52.17
- **Lissencephalia, lissencephaly** Q04.3
- **Listeriosis, listerellosis** A32.9
  - congenital (disseminated) P37.2
  - cutaneous A32.0
  - neonatal, newborn (disseminated) P37.2
  - oculoglandular A32.81
  - specified NEC A32.89
- **Lithemia** E79.0
- **Lithiasis** —*see* Calculus

Lithosis J62.8
Lithuria R82.998
Litigation, anxiety concerning Z65.3
Little leaguer's elbow —*see* Epicondylitis, medial
Little's disease G80.9
Littre's
  gland —*see* condition
  hernia —*see* Hernia, abdomen
Littritis —*see* Urethritis
Livedo (annularis) (racemosa) (reticularis) R23.1
Liver —*see* condition
Living alone (problems with) Z60.2
  with handicapped person Z74.2
Lloyd's syndrome —*see* Adenomatosis, endocrine
Loa loa, loaiasis, loasis B74.3
Lobar —*see* condition
Lobomycosis B48.0
Lobo's disease B48.0
Lobotomy syndrome F07.0
Lobstein (-Ekman) disease or syndrome Q78.0
Lobster-claw hand Q71.6-•
Lobulation (congenital) —*see also* Anomaly, by site
  kidney, Q63.1
  liver, abnormal Q44.7
  spleen Q89.09
Lobule, lobular —*see* condition
Local, localized —*see* condition
Locked twins causing obstructed labor O66.1
Locked-in state G83.5
Locking
  joint —*see* Derangement, joint, specified type NEC
    knee —*see* Derangement, knee
Lockjaw —*see* Tetanus
Löffler's
  endocarditis I42.3
  eosinophilia J82
  pneumonia J82
  syndrome (eosinophilic pneumonitis) J82
Loiasis (with conjunctival infestation) (eyelid) B74.3
Lone Star fever A77.0
Long
  labor O63.9
    first stage O63.0
    second stage O63.1
  QT syndrome I45.81
Long-term (current) (prophylactic) drug therapy (use of)
  agents affecting estrogen receptors and estrogen levels NEC Z79.818
  anastrozole (Arimidex) Z79.811
  antibiotics Z79.2
    short-term use - omit code
  anticoagulants Z79.01
  anti-inflammatory, non-steroidal (NSAID) Z79.1
  antiplatelet Z79.02
  antithrombotics Z79.02
  aromatase inhibitors Z79.811
  aspirin Z79.82
  birth control pill or patch Z79.3
  bisphosphonates Z79.83
  contraceptive, oral Z79.3
  drug, specified NEC Z79.899
  estrogen receptor downregulators Z79.818
  Evista Z79.810
  exemestane (Aromasin) Z79.811
  Fareston Z79.810
  fulvestrant (Faslodex) Z79.818
  gonadotropin-releasing hormone (GnRH) agonist Z79.818
  goserelin acetate (Zoladex) Z79.818
  hormone replacement Z79.890
  insulin Z79.4
  letrozole (Femara) Z79.811
Long-term *(Continued)*
  leuprolide acetate (leuprorelin) (Lupron) Z79.818
  megestrol acetate (Megace) Z79.818
  methadone for pain management Z79.891
  Nolvadex Z79.810
  non-steroidal anti-inflammatories (NSAID) Z79.1
  opiate analgesic Z79.891
  oral
    antidiabetic Z79.84
    contraceptive Z79.3
    hypoglycemic Z79.84
  raloxifene (Evista) Z79.810
  selective estrogen receptor modulators (SERMs) Z79.810
  steroids
    inhaled Z79.51
    systemic Z79.52
  tamoxifen (Nolvadex) Z79.810
  toremifene (Fareston) Z79.810
Longitudinal stripes or grooves, nails L60.8
  congenital Q84.6
Loop
  intestine —*see* Volvulus
  vascular on papilla (optic) Q14.2
Loose —*see also* condition
  body
    joint M24.00
      ankle M24.07-•
      elbow M24.02-•
      hand M24.04-•
      hip M24.05-•
      knee M23.4-•
      shoulder (region) M24.01-•
      specified site NEC M24.08
      toe M24.07-•
      vertebra M24.08
      wrist M24.03-•
    knee M23.4-•
    sheath, tendon —*see* Disorder, tendon, specified type NEC
  cartilage —*see* Loose, body, joint
  skin and subcutaneous tissue (following bariatric surgery weight loss) (following dietary weight loss) L98.7
  tooth, teeth K08.89
Loosening
  aseptic
    joint prosthesis —*see* Complications, joint prosthesis, mechanical, loosening, by site
  epiphysis —*see* Osteochondropathy
  mechanical
    joint prosthesis —*see* Complications, joint prosthesis, mechanical, loosening, by site
Looser-Milkman (-Debray) syndrome M83.8
Lop ear (deformity) Q17.3
Lorain (-Levi) short stature syndrome E23.0
Lordosis M40.50
  acquired —*see* Lordosis, specified type NEC
  congenital Q76.429
    lumbar region Q76.426
    lumbosacral region Q76.427
    sacral region Q76.428
    sacrococcygeal region Q76.428
    thoracolumbar region Q76.425
  lumbar region M40.56
  lumbosacral region M40.57
  postsurgical M96.4
  postural —*see* Lordosis, specified type NEC
  rachitic (late effect) (sequelae) E64.3
  sequelae of rickets E64.3
  specified type NEC M40.40
    lumbar region M40.46
    lumbosacral region M40.47
    thoracolumbar region M40.45
  thoracolumbar region M40.55
  tuberculous A18.01
Loss (of)
  appetite (*see* Anorexia) R63.0
    hysterical F50.89
    nonorganic origin F50.89
    psychogenic F50.89
  blood —*see* Hemorrhage
  bone —*see* Loss, substance of, bone
  consciousness, transient R55
    traumatic —*see* Injury, intracranial
  control, sphincter, rectum R15.9
    nonorganic origin F98.1
  elasticity, skin R23.4
  family (member) in childhood Z62.898
  fluid (acute) E86.9
  function of labyrinth —*see* subcategory H83.2
  hair, nonscarring —*see* Alopecia
  hearing —*see also* Deafness
    central NOS H90.5
    conductive H90.2
      bilateral H90.0
      unilateral
        with
          restricted hearing on the contralateral side H90.A1-•
          unrestricted hearing on the contralateral side H90.1-•
    mixed conductive and sensorineural hearing loss H90.8
      bilateral H90.6
      unilateral
        with
          restricted hearing on the contralateral side H90.A3-•
          unrestricted hearing on the contralateral side H90.7-•
    neural NOS H90.5
    perceptive NOS H90.5
    sensorineural NOS H90.5
      bilateral H90.3
      unilateral
        with
          restricted hearing on the contralateral side H90.A2-•
          unrestricted hearing on the contralateral side H90.4-•
    sensory NOS H90.5
  height R29.890
  limb or member, traumatic, current —*see* Amputation, traumatic
  love relationship in childhood Z62.898
  memory —*see also* Amnesia
    mild, following organic brain damage F06.8
  mind —*see* Psychosis
  occlusal vertical dimension of fully erupted teeth M26.37
  organ or part —*see* Absence, by site, acquired
  ossicles, ear (partial) H74.32-•
  parent in childhood Z63.4
  pregnancy, recurrent N96
    without current pregnancy N96
    care in current pregnancy O26.2-•
  recurrent pregnancy —*see* Loss, pregnancy, recurrent
  self-esteem, in childhood Z62.898
  sense of
    smell —*see* Disturbance, sensation, smell
    taste —*see* Disturbance, sensation, taste
    touch R20.8
  sensory R44.9
    dissociative F44.6
  sexual desire F52.0
  sight (acquired) (complete) (congenital) —*see* Blindness
  substance of
    bone —*see* Disorder, bone, density and structure, specified NEC
      horizontal alveolar K06.3
    cartilage —*see* Disorder, cartilage, specified type NEC
      auricle (ear) —*see* Disorder, pinna, specified type NEC
    vitreous (humor) H15.89

L

Loss *(Continued)*
tooth, teeth —*see* Absence, teeth, acquired
vision, visual H54.7
both eyes H54.3
one eye H54.60
left (normal vision on right) H54.62
right (normal vision on left) H54.61
specified as blindness —*see* Blindness
subjective
sudden H53.13- ●
transient H53.12- ●
vitreous —*see* Prolapse, vitreous
voice —*see* Aphonia
weight (abnormal) (cause unknown) R63.4
Louis-Bar syndrome (ataxia-telangiectasia) G11.3
Louping ill (encephalitis) A84.8
Louse, lousiness —*see* Lice
Low
achiever, school Z55.3
back syndrome M54.5
basal metabolic rate R94.8
birthweight (2499 grams or less) P07.10
with weight of
1000-1249 grams P07.14
1250-1499 grams P07.15
1500-1749 grams P07.16
1750-1999 grams P07.17
2000-2499 grams P07.18
extreme (999 grams or less) P07.00
with weight of
499 grams or less P07.01
500-749 grams P07.02
750-999 grams P07.03
for gestational age —*see* Light for dates
blood pressure —*see also* Hypotension
reading (incidental) (isolated) (nonspecific) R03.1
cardiac reserve —*see* Disease, heart
function —*see also* Hypofunction
kidney N28.9
hematocrit D64.9
hemoglobin D64.9
income Z59.6
level of literacy Z55.0
lying
kidney N28.89
organ or site, congenital —*see* Malposition, congenital
output syndrome (cardiac) —*see* Failure, heart
platelets (blood) —*see* Thrombocytopenia
reserve, kidney N28.89
salt syndrome E87.1
self esteem R45.81
set ears Q17.4
vision H54.2X-
one eye (other eye normal) H54.50
left (normal vision on right) H54.52A-
other eye blind —*see* Blindness
right (normal vision on left) H54.511-
Low-density-lipoprotein-type (LDL) **hyperlipoproteinemia** E78.00
Lowe's syndrome E72.03
Lown-Ganong-Levine syndrome I45.6
LSD reaction (acute) (without dependence) F16.90
with dependence F16.20
L-shaped kidney Q63.8
▶ **LTBI** (lantent tuberculosis infection) Z22.7
Ludwig's angina or disease K12.2
Lues (venerea), **luetic** —*see* Syphilis
Luetscher's syndrome (dehydration) E86.0
Lumbago, lumbalgia M54.5
with sciatica M54.4- ●
due to intervertebral disc disorder M51.17
due to displacement, intervertebral disc M51.27
with sciatica M51.17
Lumbar —*see* condition
Lumbarization, vertebra, congenital Q76.49
Lumbermen's itch B88.0
Lump —*see also* Mass
breast N63.0
axillary tail
left N63.32
right N63.31
left
lower inner quadrant N63.24
lower outer quadrant N63.23
▶ overlapping quadrants N63.25
unspecified quadrant N63.20
upper inner quadrant N63.22
upper outer quadrant N63.21
right
lower inner quadrant N63.14
lower outer quadrant N63.13
▶ overlapping quadrants N63.15
unspecified quadrant N63.10
upper inner quadrant N63.12
upper outer quadrant N63.11
subareolar
left N63.42
right N63.41
Lunacy —*see* Psychosis
Lung —*see* condition
Lupoid (miliary) **of Boeck** D86.3
Lupus
anticoagulant D68.62
with
hemorrhagic disorder D68.312
hypercoagulable state D68.62
finding without diagnosis R76.0
discoid (local) L93.0
erythematosus (discoid) (local) L93.0
disseminated —*see* Lupus, erythematosus, systemic
eyelid H01.129
left H01.126
lower H01.125
upper H01.124
right H01.123
lower H01.122
upper H01.121
profundus L93.2
specified NEC L93.2
subacute cutaneous L93.1
systemic M32.9
with organ or system involvement M32.10
endocarditis M32.11
lung M32.13
pericarditis M32.12
renal (glomerular) M32.14
tubulo-interstitial M32.15
specified organ or system NEC M32.19
drug-induced M32.0
inhibitor (presence of) D68.62
with
hemorrhagic disorder D68.312
hypercoagulable state D68.62
finding without diagnosis R76.0
specified NEC M32.8
exedens A18.4
hydralazine M32.0
correct substance properly administered —*see* Table of Drugs and Chemicals, by drug, adverse effect
overdose or wrong substance given or taken —*see* Table of Drugs and Chemicals, by drug, poisoning
nephritis (chronic) M32.14
nontuberculous, not disseminated L93.0
panniculitis L93.2
pernio (Besnier) D86.3
systemic —*see* Lupus, erythematosus, systemic
tuberculous A18.4
eyelid A18.4
vulgaris A18.4
eyelid A18.4
Luteinoma D27.- ●
Lutembacher's disease or syndrome (atrial septal defect with mitral stenosis) Q21.1
Luteoma D27.- ●
Lutz (-Splendore-de Almeida) **disease** —*see* Paracoccidioidomycosis
Luxation —*see also* Dislocation
eyeball (nontraumatic) —*see* Luxation, globe
birth injury P15.3
globe, nontraumatic H44.82- ●
lacrimal gland —*see* Dislocation, lacrimal gland
lens (old) (partial) (spontaneous)
congenital Q12.1
syphilitic A50.39
Lycanthropy F22
Lyell's syndrome L51.2
due to drug L51.2
correct substance properly administered —*see* Table of Drugs and Chemicals, by drug, adverse effect
overdose or wrong substance given or taken —*see* Table of Drugs and Chemicals, by drug, poisoning
Lyme disease A69.20
Lymph
gland or node —*see* condition
scrotum —*see* Infestation, filarial
Lymphadenitis I88.9
with ectopic or molar pregnancy O08.0
acute L04.9
axilla L04.2
face L04.0
head L04.0
hip L04.3
limb
lower L04.3
upper L04.2
neck L04.0
shoulder L04.2
specified site NEC L04.8
trunk L04.1
anthracosis (occupational) J60
any site, except mesenteric I88.9
chronic I88.1
subacute I88.1
breast
gestational —*see* Mastitis, obstetric
puerperal, postpartum (nonpurulent) O91.22
chancroidal (congenital) A57
chronic I88.1
mesenteric I88.0
due to
Brugia (malayi) B74.1
timori B74.2
chlamydial lymphogranuloma A55
diphtheria (toxin) A36.89
lymphogranuloma venereum A55
Wuchereria bancrofti B74.0
following ectopic or molar pregnancy O08.0
gonorrheal A54.89
infective —*see* Lymphadenitis, acute
mesenteric (acute) (chronic) (nonspecific) (subacute) I88.0
due to Salmonella typhi A01.09
tuberculous A18.39
mycobacterial A31.8
purulent —*see* Lymphadenitis, acute
pyogenic —*see* Lymphadenitis, acute
regional, nonbacterial I88.8
septic —*see* Lymphadenitis, acute
subacute, unspecified site I88.1
suppurative —*see* Lymphadenitis, acute
syphilitic (early) (secondary) A51.49
late A52.79
tuberculous —*see* Tuberculosis, lymph gland
venereal (chlamydial) A55
Lymphadenoid goiter E06.3
Lymphadenopathy (generalized) R59.1
angioimmunoblastic, with dysproteinemia (AILD) C86.5

Lymphadenopathy *(Continued)*
due to toxoplasmosis (acquired) B58.89
congenital (acute) (subacute) (chronic) P37.1
localized R59.0
syphilitic (early) (secondary) A51.49
Lymphadenosis R59.1
Lymphangiectasis I89.0
conjunctiva H11.89
postinfectional I89.0
scrotum I89.0
Lymphangiectatic elephantiasis, nonfilarial I89.0
Lymphangioendothelioma D18.1
malignant —*see* Neoplasm, connective tissue, malignant
Lymphangioleiomyomatosis J84.81
Lymphangioma D18.1
capillary D18.1
cavernous D18.1
cystic D18.1
malignant —*see* Neoplasm, connective tissue, malignant
Lymphangiomyoma D18.1
Lymphangiomyomatosis J84.81
Lymphangiosarcoma —*see* Neoplasm, connective tissue, malignant
Lymphangitis I89.1
with
abscess - code by site under Abscess
cellulitis - code by site under Cellulitis
ectopic or molar pregnancy O08.0
acute L03.91
abdominal wall L03.321
ankle —*see* Lymphangitis, acute, lower limb
arm —*see* Lymphangitis, acute, upper limb
auricle (ear) —*see* Lymphangitis, acute, ear
axilla L03.12-●
back (any part) L03.322
buttock L03.327
cervical (meaning neck) L03.222
cheek (external) L03.212
chest wall L03.323
digit
finger —*see* Lymphangitis, acute, finger
toe —*see* Lymphangitis, acute, toe
ear (external) H60.1-●
external auditory canal —*see* Lymphangitis, acute, ear
eyelid —*see* Abscess, eyelid
face NEC L03.212
finger (intrathecal) (periosteal) (subcutaneous) (subcuticular) L03.02-●
foot —*see* Lymphangitis, acute, lower limb
gluteal (region) L03.327
groin L03.324
hand —*see* Lymphangitis, acute, upper limb
head NEC L03.891
face (any part, except ear, eye and nose) L03.212
heel —*see* Lymphangitis, acute, lower limb
hip —*see* Lymphangitis, acute, lower limb
jaw (region) L03.212
knee —*see* Lymphangitis, acute, lower limb
leg —*see* Lymphangitis, acute, lower limb
lower limb L03.12-●
toe —*see* Lymphangitis, acute, toe
navel L03.326
neck (region) L03.222
orbit, orbital —*see* Cellulitis, orbit
pectoral (region) L03.323
perineal, perineum L03.325
scalp (any part) L03.891
shoulder —*see* Lymphangitis, acute, upper limb
specified site NEC L03.898
thigh —*see* Lymphangitis, acute, lower limb

Lymphangitis *(Continued)*
acute *(Continued)*
thumb (intrathecal) (periosteal) (subcutaneous) (subcuticular) —*see* Lymphangitis, acute, finger
toe (intrathecal) (periosteal) (subcutaneous) (subcuticular) L03.04-●
trunk L03.329
abdominal wall L03.321
back (any part) L03.322
buttock L03.327
chest wall L03.323
groin L03.324
perineal, perineum L03.325
umbilicus L03.326
umbilicus L03.326
upper limb L03.12-●
axilla —*see* Lymphangitis, acute, axilla
finger —*see* Lymphangitis, acute, finger
thumb —*see* Lymphangitis, acute, finger
wrist —*see* Lymphangitis, acute, upper limb
breast
gestational —*see* Mastitis, obstetric
chancroidal A57
chronic (any site) I89.1
due to
Brugia (malayi) B74.1
timori B74.2
Wuchereria bancrofti B74.0
following ectopic or molar pregnancy O08.89
penis
acute N48.29
gonococcal (acute) (chronic) A54.09
puerperal, postpartum, childbirth O86.89
strumous, tuberculous A18.2
subacute (any site) I89.1
tuberculous —*see* Tuberculosis, lymph gland
Lymphatic (vessel) —*see* condition
Lymphatism E32.8
Lymphectasia I89.0
Lymphedema (acquired) —*see also* Elephantiasis
congenital Q82.0
hereditary (chronic) (idiopathic) Q82.0
postmastectomy I97.2
praecox I89.0
secondary I89.0
surgical NEC I97.89
postmastectomy (syndrome) I97.2
Lymphoblastic —*see* condition
Lymphoblastoma (diffuse) —*see* Lymphoma, lymphoblastic (diffuse)
giant follicular —*see* Lymphoma, lymphoblastic (diffuse)
macrofollicular —*see* Lymphoma, lymphoblastic (diffuse)
Lymphocele I89.8
Lymphocytic
chorioencephalitis (acute) (serous) A87.2
choriomeningitis (acute) (serous) A87.2
meningoencephalitis A87.2
Lymphocytoma, benign cutis L98.8
Lymphocytopenia D72.810
Lymphocytosis (symptomatic) D72.820
infectious (acute) B33.8
Lymphoepithelioma —*see* Neoplasm, malignant, by site
Lymphogranuloma (malignant) —*see also* Lymphoma, Hodgkin
chlamydial A55
inguinale A55
venereum (any site) (chlamydial) (with stricture of rectum) A55
Lymphogranulomatosis (malignant) —*see also* Lymphoma, Hodgkin
benign (Boeck's sarcoid) (Schaumann's) D86.1
Lymphohistiocytosis, hemophagocytic (familial) D76.1
Lymphoid —*see* condition

Lymphoma (of) (malignant) C85.90
adult T-cell (HTLV-1-associated) (acute variant) (chronic variant) (lymphomatoid variant) (smouldering variant) C91.5-●
anaplastic large cell
ALK-negative C84.7-●
ALK-positive C84.6-●
CD30-positive C84.6-●
primary cutaneous C86.6
angioimmunoblastic T-cell C86.5
BALT C88.4
B-cell C85.1-●
B-precursor C83.5-●
blastic NK-cell C86.4
blastic plasmacytoid dendritic cell neoplasm (BPDCN) C86.4
bronchial-associated lymphoid tissue [BALT-lymphoma] C88.4
Burkitt (atypical) C83.7-●
Burkitt-like C83.7-●
centrocytic C83.1-●
cutaneous follicle center C82.6-●
cutaneous T-cell C84.A-●
diffuse follicle center C82.5-●
diffuse large cell C83.3-●
anaplastic C83.3-●
B-cell C83.3-●
CD30-positive C83.3-●
centroblastic C83.3-●
immunoblastic C83.3-●
plasmablastic C83.3-●
subtype not specified C83.3-●
T-cell rich C83.3-●
enteropathy-type (associated) (intestinal) T-cell C86.2
extranodal marginal zone B-cell lymphoma of mucosa-associated lymphoid tissue [MALT-lymphoma] C88.4
extranodal NK/T-cell, nasal type C86.0
follicular C82.9-●
grade
I C82.0-●
II C82.1-●
III C82.2-●
IIIa C82.3-●
IIIb C82.4-●
specified NEC C82.8-●
hepatosplenic T-cell (alpha-beta) (gamma-delta) C86.1
histiocytic C85.9-●
true C96.A
Hodgkin C81.9
lymphocyte-rich (classical) C81.4-●
lymphocyte depleted (classical) C81.3-●
mixed cellularity (classical) C81.2-●
nodular sclerosis (classical) C81.1-●
specified NEC (classical) C81.7-●
lymphocyte-rich classical C81.4-●
lymphocyte depleted classical C81.3-●
mixed cellularity classical C81.2-●
nodular
lymphocyte predominant C81.0-●
sclerosis (classical) C81.1-●
intravascular large B-cell C83.8-●
Lennert's C84.4-●
lymphoblastic (diffuse) C83.5-●
lymphoblastic B-cell C83.5-●
lymphoblastic T-cell C83.5-●
lymphoepithelioid C84.4-●
lymphoplasmacytic C83.0-●
with IgM-production C88.0
MALT C88.4
mantle cell C83.1-●
mature T-cell NEC C84.4-●
mature T/NK-cell C84.9-●
specified NEC C84.Z-●
mediastinal (thymic) large B-cell C85.2-●
Mediterranean C88.3

L

Lymphoma *(Continued)*
mucosa-associated lymphoid tissue [MALT-lymphoma] C88.4
NK/T cell C84.9-●
nodal marginal zone C83.Ø-●
non-follicular (diffuse) C83.9-●
specified NEC C83.8-●
non-Hodgkin —*see also* Lymphoma, by type C85.9-●
specified NEC C85.8-●
non-leukemic variant of B-CLL C83.Ø-●
peripheral T-cell, not classified C84.4-●
primary cutaneous
anaplastic large cell C86.6
CD3Ø-positive large T-cell C86.6
primary effusion B-cell C83.8-●

Lymphoma *(Continued)*
SALT C88.4
skin-associated lymphoid tissue [SALT-lymphoma] C88.4
small cell B-cell C83.Ø-●
splenic marginal zone C83.Ø-●
subcutaneous panniculitis-like T-cell C86.3
T-precursor C83.5-●
true histiocytic C96.A
Lymphomatosis —*see* Lymphoma
Lymphopathia venereum, veneris A55
Lymphopenia D72.81Ø

Lymphoplasmacytic leukemia —*see* Leukemia, chronic lymphocytic, B-cell type
Lymphoproliferation, X-linked disease D82.3
Lymphoreticulosis, benign (of inoculation) A28.1
Lymphorrhea I89.8
Lymphosarcoma (diffuse) —*see also* Lymphoma C85.9-●
Lymphostasis I89.8
Lypemania —*see* Melancholia
Lysine and hydroxylysine metabolism disorder E72.3
Lyssa —*see* Rabies

L

M

Macacus ear Q17.3
Maceration, wet feet, tropical (syndrome) T69.02- •
MacLeod's syndrome J43.0
Macrocephalia, macrocephaly Q75.3
Macrocheilia, macrochilia (congenital)Q18.6
Macrocolon —see also Megacolon Q43.1
Macrocornea Q15.8
 with glaucoma Q15.0
Macrocytic —see condition
Macrocytosis D75.89
Macrodactylia, macrodactylism (fingers) (thumbs) Q74.0
 toes Q74.2
Macrodontia K00.2
Macrogenia M26.05
Macrogenitosomia (adrenal) (male) (praecox) E25.9
 congenital E25.0
Macroglobulinemia (idiopathic) (primary) C88.0
 monoclonal (essential) D47.2
 Waldenström C88.0
Macroglossia (congenital) Q38.2
 acquired K14.8
Macrognathia, macrognathism (congenital) (mandibular) (maxillary) M26.09
Macrogyria (congenital) Q04.8
Macrohydrocephalus —see Hydrocephalus
Macromastia —see Hypertrophy, breast
Macrophthalmos Q11.3
 in congenital glaucoma Q15.0
Macropsia H53.15
Macrosigmoid K59.39
 congenital Q43.2
Macrospondylitis, acromegalic E22.0
Macrostomia (congenital) Q18.4
Macrotia (external ear) (congenital) Q17.1
Macula
 cornea, corneal —see Opacity, cornea
 degeneration (atrophic) (exudative) (senile) —see also Degeneration, macula
  hereditary —see Dystrophy, retina
Maculae ceruleae — B85.1
Maculopathy, toxic —see Degeneration, macula, toxic
Madarosis (eyelid) H02.729
 left H02.726
  lower H02.725
  upper H02.724
 right H02.723
  lower H02.722
  upper H02.721
Madelung's
 deformity (radius) Q74.0
 disease
  radial deformity Q74.0
  symmetrical lipomas, neck E88.89
Madness —see Psychosis
Madura
 foot B47.9
  actinomycotic B47.1
  mycotic B47.0
Maduromycosis B47.0
Maffucci's syndrome Q78.4
Magnesium metabolism disorder —see Disorder, metabolism, magnesium
Main en griffe (acquired) —see also Deformity, limb, clawhand
 congenital Q74.0
Maintenance (encounter for)
 antineoplastic chemotherapy Z51.11
 antineoplastic radiation therapy Z51.0
 methadone F11.20
Majocchi's
 disease L81.7
 granuloma B35.8
Major —see condition
Malabar itch (any site) B35.5
Malabsorption K90.9
 calcium K90.89
 carbohydrate K90.49
 disaccharide E73.9
 fat K90.49
 galactose E74.20
 glucose(-galactose) E74.39
 intestinal K90.9
  specified NEC K90.89
 isomaltose E74.31
 lactose E73.9
 methionine E72.19
 monosaccharide E74.39
 postgastrectomy K91.2
 postsurgical K91.2
 protein K90.49
 starch K90.49
 sucrose E74.39
 syndrome K90.9
  postsurgical K91.2
Malacia, bone (adult) M83.9
 juvenile —see Rickets
Malacoplakia
 bladder N32.89
 pelvis (kidney) N28.89
 ureter N28.89
 urethra N36.8
Malacosteon, juvenile —see Rickets
Maladaptation —see Maladjustment
Maladie de Roger Q21.0
Maladjustment
 conjugal Z63.0
  involving divorce or estrangement Z63.5
 educational Z55.4
 family Z63.9
 marital Z63.0
  involving divorce or estrangement Z63.5
 occupational NEC Z56.89
 simple, adult —see Disorder, adjustment
 situational —see Disorder, adjustment
 social Z60.9
  due to
   acculturation difficulty Z60.3
   discrimination and persecution (perceived) Z60.5
   exclusion and isolation Z60.4
   life-cycle (phase of life) transition Z60.0
   rejection Z60.4
   specified reason NEC Z60.8
Malaise R53.81
Malakoplakia —see Malacoplakia
Malaria, malarial (fever) B54
 with
  blackwater fever B50.8
   hemoglobinuric (bilious) B50.8
  hemoglobinuria B50.8
 accidentally induced (therapeutically) - code by type under Malaria
 algid B50.9
 cerebral B50.0 *[G94]*
 clinically diagnosed (without parasitological confirmation) B54
 congenital NEC P37.4
  falciparum P37.3
 congestion, congestive B54
 continued (fever) B50.9
 estivo-autumnal B50.9
 falciparum B50.9
  with complications NEC B50.8
   cerebral B50.0 *[G94]*
  severe B50.8
 hemorrhagic B54
 malariae B52.9
  with
   complications NEC B52.8
   glomerular disorder B52.0
 malignant (tertian) —see Malaria, falciparum
 mixed infections — code to first listed type in B50-B53
 ovale B53.0
 parasitologically confirmed NEC B53.8
Malaria, malarial *(Continued)*
 pernicious, acute —see Malaria, falciparum
 Plasmodium (P.)
  falciparum NEC —see Malaria, falciparum
  malariae NEC B52.9
   with Plasmodium
    falciparum (and or vivax) —see Malaria, falciparum
    vivax —see also Malaria, vivax
     and falciparum —see Malaria, falciparum
  ovale B53.0
   with Plasmodium malariae —see also Malaria, malariae
    and vivax —see also Malaria, vivax
     and falciparum —see Malaria, falciparum
  simian B53.1
   with Plasmodium malariae —see also Malaria, malariae
    and vivax —see also Malaria, vivax
     and falciparum —see Malaria, falciparum
  vivax NEC B51.9
   with Plasmodium falciparum —see Malaria, falciparum
 quartan —see Malaria, malariae
 quotidian —see Malaria, falciparum
 recurrent B54
 remittent B54
 specified type NEC (parasitologically confirmed) B53.8
 spleen B54
 subtertian (fever) —see Malaria, falciparum
 tertian (benign) —see also Malaria, vivax
  malignant B50.9
 tropical B50.9
 typhoid B54
 vivax B51.9
  with
   complications NEC B51.8
   ruptured spleen B51.0
Malassez's disease (cystic) N50.89
Malassimilation K90.9
Mal de los pintos —see Pinta
Mal de mer T75.3
Maldescent, testis Q53.9
 bilateral Q53.20
  abdominal Q53.211
  perineal Q53.22
 unilateral Q53.10
  abdominal Q53.111
  perineal Q53.12
Maldevelopment —see also Anomaly
 brain Q07.9
 colon Q43.9
 hip Q74.2
  congenital dislocation Q65.2
   bilateral Q65.1
   unilateral Q65.0- •
 mastoid process Q75.8
 middle ear Q16.4
  except ossicles Q16.4
  ossicles Q16.3
 ossicles Q16.3
 spine Q76.49
 toe Q74.2
Male type pelvis Q74.2
 with disproportion (fetopelvic) O33.3
  causing obstructed labor O65.3
Malformation (congenital) —see also Anomaly
 adrenal gland Q89.1
 affecting multiple systems with skeletal changes NEC Q87.5
 alimentary tract Q45.9
  specified type NEC Q45.8
  upper Q40.9
   specified type NEC Q40.8
 aorta Q25.40
  absence Q25.41
  aneurysm, congenital Q25.43

M

Malformation *(Continued)*
aorta *(Continued)*
aplasia Q25.41
atresia Q25.29
aortic arch Q25.21
coarctation (preductal) (postductal) Q25.1
dilatation, congenital Q25.44
hypoplasia Q25.42
patent ductus arteriosus Q25.0
specified type NEC Q25.49
stenosis Q25.1
supravalvular Q25.3
aortic valve Q23.9
specified NEC Q23.8
arteriovenous, aneurysmatic (congenital) Q27.30
brain Q28.2
ruptured I60.8
intracerebral I61.8
intraparenchymal I61.8
intraventricular I61.5
subarachnoid I60.8
cerebral (*see* Malformation, arteriovenous, brain) Q28.2
peripheral Q27.30
congenital Q27.33
digestive system —*see* Angiodysplasia
lower limb Q27.32
other specified site Q27.39
renal vessel Q27.34
upper limb Q27.31
precerebral vessels (nonruptured) Q28.0
auricle
ear (congenital) Q17.3
acquired H61.119
left H61.112
with right H61.113
right H61.111
with left H61.113
bile duct Q44.5
bladder Q64.79
aplasia Q64.5
diverticulum Q64.6
exstrophy —*see* Exstrophy, bladder
neck obstruction Q64.31
bone Q79.9
face Q75.9
specified type NEC Q75.8
skull Q75.9
specified type NEC Q75.8
brain (multiple) Q04.9
arteriovenous Q28.2
specified type NEC Q04.8
branchial cleft Q18.2
breast Q83.9
specified type NEC Q83.8
broad ligament Q50.6
bronchus Q32.4
bursa Q79.9
cardiac
chambers Q20.9
specified type NEC Q20.8
septum Q21.9
specified type NEC Q21.8
cerebral Q04.9
vessels Q28.3
cervix uteri Q51.9
specified type NEC Q51.828
Chiari
Type I G93.5
Type II Q07.01
choroid (congenital) Q14.3
plexus Q07.8
circulatory system Q28.9
cochlea Q16.5
cornea Q13.4
coronary vessels Q24.5
corpus callosum (congenital) Q04.0
diaphragm Q79.1
digestive system NEC, specified type NEC Q45.8

Malformation *(Continued)*
dura Q07.9
brain Q04.9
spinal Q06.9
ear Q17.9
causing impairment of hearing Q16.9
external Q17.9
accessory auricle Q17.0
causing impairment of hearing Q16.9
absence of
auditory canal Q16.1
auricle Q16.0
macrotia Q17.1
microtia Q17.2
misplacement Q17.4
misshapen NEC Q17.3
prominence Q17.5
specified type NEC Q17.8
inner Q16.5
middle Q16.4
absence of eustachian tube Q16.2
ossicles (fusion) Q16.3
ossicles Q16.3
specified type NEC Q17.8
epididymis Q55.4
esophagus Q39.9
specified type NEC Q39.8
eye Q15.9
lid Q10.3
specified NEC Q15.8
fallopian tube Q50.6
genital organ —*see* Anomaly, genitalia
great
artery Q25.9
aorta —*see* Malformation, aorta
pulmonary artery —*see* Malformation, pulmonary, artery
specified type NEC Q25.8
vein Q26.9
anomalous
portal venous connection Q26.5
pulmonary venous connection Q26.4
partial Q26.3
total Q26.2
persistent left superior vena cava Q26.1
portal vein-hepatic artery fistula Q26.6
specified type NEC Q26.8
vena cava stenosis, congenital Q26.0
gum Q38.6
hair Q84.2
heart Q24.9
specified type NEC Q24.8
integument Q84.9
specified type NEC Q84.8
internal ear Q16.5
intestine Q43.9
specified type NEC Q43.8
iris Q13.2
joint Q74.9
ankle Q74.2
lumbosacral Q76.49
sacroiliac Q74.2
specified type NEC Q74.8
kidney Q63.9
accessory Q63.0
giant Q63.3
horseshoe Q63.1
hydronephrosis Q62.0
malposition Q63.2
specified type NEC Q63.8
lacrimal apparatus Q10.6
lingual Q38.3
lip Q38.0
liver Q44.7
lung Q33.9
meninges or membrane (congenital) Q07.9
cerebral Q04.8
spinal (cord) Q06.9
middle ear Q16.4
ossicles Q16.3
mitral valve Q23.9
specified NEC Q23.8

Malformation *(Continued)*
Mondini's (congenital) (malformation, cochlea) Q16.5
mouth (congenital) Q38.6
multiple types NEC Q89.7
musculoskeletal system Q79.9
myocardium Q24.8
nail Q84.6
nervous system (central) Q07.9
nose Q30.9
specified type NEC Q30.8
optic disc Q14.2
orbit Q10.7
ovary Q50.39
palate Q38.5
parathyroid gland Q89.2
pelvic organs or tissues NEC
in pregnancy or childbirth O34.8-•
causing obstructed labor O65.5
penis Q55.69
aplasia Q55.5
curvature (lateral) Q55.61
hypoplasia Q55.62
pericardium Q24.8
peripheral vascular system Q27.9
specified type NEC Q27.8
pharynx Q38.8
precerebral vessels Q28.1
prostate Q55.4
pulmonary
arteriovenous Q25.72
artery Q25.9
atresia Q25.5
specified type NEC Q25.79
stenosis Q25.6
valve Q22.3
renal artery Q27.2
respiratory system Q34.9
retina Q14.1
scrotum —*see* Malformation, testis and scrotum
seminal vesicles Q55.4
sense organs NEC Q07.9
skin Q82.9
specified NEC Q89.8
spinal
cord Q06.9
nerve root Q07.8
spine Q76.49
kyphosis —*see* Kyphosis, congenital
lordosis —*see* Lordosis, congenital
spleen Q89.09
stomach Q40.3
specified type NEC Q40.2
teeth, tooth K00.9
tendon Q79.9
testis and scrotum Q55.20
aplasia Q55.0
hypoplasia Q55.1
polyorchism Q55.21
retractile testis Q55.22
scrotal transposition Q55.23
specified NEC Q55.29
thorax, bony Q76.9
throat Q38.8
thyroid gland Q89.2
tongue (congenital) Q38.3
hypertrophy Q38.2
tie Q38.1
trachea Q32.1
tricuspid valve Q22.9
specified type NEC Q22.8
umbilical cord NEC (complicating delivery) O69.89
umbilicus Q89.9
ureter Q62.8
agenesis Q62.4
duplication Q62.5
malposition —*see* Malposition, congenital, ureter
obstructive defect —*see* Defect, obstructive, ureter
vesico-uretero-renal reflux Q62.7

M

Malformation *(Continued)*
urethra Q64.79
aplasia Q64.5
duplication Q64.74
posterior valves Q64.2
prolapse Q64.71
stricture Q64.32
urinary system Q64.9
uterus Q51.9
specified type NEC Q51.818
vagina Q52.4
vascular system, peripheral Q27.9
vas deferens Q55.4
atresia Q55.3
venous —*see* Anomaly, vein(s)
vulva Q52.70
Malfunction —*see also* Dysfunction
cardiac electronic device T82.119
electrode T82.110
pulse generator T82.111
specified type NEC T82.118
catheter device NEC T85.618
cystostomy T83.010
dialysis (renal) (vascular) T82.41
intraperitoneal T85.611
infusion NEC T82.514
cranial T85.610
epidural T85.610
intrathecal T85.610
spinal T85.610
subarachnoid T85.610
subdural T85.610
urinary —*see also* Breakdown, device, catheter T83.018
colostomy K94.03
valve K94.03
cystostomy (stoma) N99.512
catheter T83.010
enteric stoma K94.13
enterostomy K94.13
esophagostomy K94.33
gastroenteric K31.89
gastrostomy K94.23
ileostomy K94.13
valve K94.13
intrathecal infusion pump T85.615
jejunostomy K94.13
nervous system device, implant or graft, specified NEC T85.615
pacemaker —*see* Malfunction, cardiac electronic device
prosthetic device, internal —*see* Complications, prosthetic device, by site, mechanical
tracheostomy J95.03
urinary device NEC —*see* Complication, genitourinary, device, urinary, mechanical
valve
colostomy K94.03
heart T82.09
ileostomy K94.13
vascular graft or shunt NEC —*see* Complication, cardiovascular device, mechanical, vascular
ventricular (communicating shunt) T85.01
Malherbe's tumor —*see* Neoplasm, skin, benign
Malibu disease L98.8- ●
Malignancy —*see also* Neoplasm, malignant, by site
unspecified site (primary) C80.1
Malignant —*see* condition
Malingerer, malingering Z76.5
Mallet finger (acquired) —*see* Deformity, finger, mallet finger
congenital Q74.0
sequelae of rickets E64.3
Malleus A24.0
Mallory's bodies R89.7
Mallory-Weiss syndrome K22.6
Malnutrition E46
degree
first E44.1
mild (protein) E44.1
moderate (protein) E44.0
second E44.0
severe (protein-energy) E43
intermediate form E42
with
kwashiorkor (and marasmus) E42
marasmus E41
third E43
following gastrointestinal surgery K91.2
intrauterine
light-for-dates —*see* Light for dates
small-for-dates —*see* Small for dates
lack of care, or neglect (child) (infant) T76.02
confirmed T74.02
malignant E40
protein E46
calorie E46
mild E44.1
moderate E44.0
severe E43
intermediate form E42
with
kwashiorkor (and marasmus) E42
marasmus E41
energy E46
mild E44.1
moderate E44.0
severe E43
intermediate form E42
with
kwashiorkor (and marasmus) E42
marasmus E41
severe (protein-energy) E43
with
kwashiorkor (and marasmus) E42
marasmus E41
Malocclusion (teeth) M26.4
Angle's M26.219
class I M26.211
class II M26.212
class III M26.213
due to
abnormal swallowing M26.59
mouth breathing M26.59
tongue, lip or finger habits M26.59
temporomandibular (joint) M26.69
Malposition
cervix —*see* Malposition, uterus
congenital
adrenal (gland) Q89.1
alimentary tract Q45.8
lower Q43.8
upper Q40.8
aorta Q25.49
appendix Q43.8
arterial trunk Q20.0
artery (peripheral) Q27.8
coronary Q24.5
digestive system Q27.8
lower limb Q27.8
pulmonary Q25.79
specified site NEC Q27.8
upper limb Q27.8
auditory canal Q17.8
causing impairment of hearing Q16.9
auricle (ear) Q17.4
causing impairment of hearing Q16.9
cervical Q18.2
biliary duct or passage Q44.5
bladder (mucosa) —*see* Exstrophy, bladder
brachial plexus Q07.8
brain tissue Q04.8
breast Q83.8
bronchus Q32.4
Malposition *(Continued)*
congenital *(Continued)*
cecum Q43.8
clavicle Q74.0
colon Q43.8
digestive organ or tract NEC Q45.8
lower Q43.8
upper Q40.8
ear (auricle) (external) Q17.4
ossicles Q16.3
endocrine (gland) NEC Q89.2
epiglottis Q31.8
eustachian tube Q17.8
eye Q15.8
facial features Q18.8
fallopian tube Q50.6
finger(s) Q68.1
supernumerary Q69.0
foot Q66.9- ●
gallbladder Q44.1
gastrointestinal tract Q45.8
genitalia, genital organ(s) or tract
female Q52.8
external Q52.79
internal NEC Q52.8
male Q55.8
glottis Q31.8
hand Q68.1
heart Q24.8
dextrocardia Q24.0
with complete transposition of viscera Q89.3
hepatic duct Q44.5
hip (joint) Q65.89
intestine (large) (small) Q43.8
with anomalous adhesions, fixation or malrotation Q43.3
joint NEC Q68.8
kidney Q63.2
larynx Q31.8
limb Q68.8
lower Q68.8
upper Q68.8
liver Q44.7
lung (lobe) Q33.8
nail(s) Q84.6
nerve Q07.8
nervous system NEC Q07.8
nose, nasal (septum) Q30.8
organ or site not listed —*see* Anomaly, by site
ovary Q50.39
pancreas Q45.3
parathyroid (gland) Q89.2
patella Q74.1
peripheral vascular system Q27.8
pituitary (gland) Q89.2
respiratory organ or system NEC Q34.8
rib (cage) Q76.6
supernumerary in cervical region Q76.5
scapula Q74.0
shoulder Q74.0
spinal cord Q06.8
spleen Q89.09
sternum NEC Q76.7
stomach Q40.2
symphysis pubis Q74.2
thymus (gland) Q89.2
thyroid (gland) (tissue) Q89.2
cartilage Q31.8
toe(s) Q66.9- ●
supernumerary Q69.2
tongue Q38.3
trachea Q32.1
ureter Q62.60
deviation Q62.61
displacement Q62.62
ectopia Q62.63
specified type NEC Q62.69

Malposition *(Continued)*
congenital *(Continued)*
uterus Q51.818
vein(s) (peripheral) Q27.8
great Q26.8
vena cava (inferior) (superior) Q26.8
device, implant or graft —*see also* Complications, by site and type, mechanical T85.628
arterial graft NEC —*see* Complication, cardiovascular device, mechanical, vascular
breast (implant) T85.42
catheter NEC T85.628
cystostomy T83.020
dialysis (renal) T82.42
intraperitoneal T85.621
infusion NEC T82.524
spinal (epidural) (subdural) T85.620
urinary —*see also* Displacement, device, catheter, urinary T83.028
electronic (electrode) (pulse generator) (stimulator)
bone T84.320
cardiac T82.129
electrode T82.120
pulse generator T82.121
specified type NEC T82.128
nervous system —*see* Complication, prosthetic device, mechanical, electronic nervous system stimulator
urinary —*see* Complication, genitourinary, device, urinary, mechanical
fixation, internal (orthopedic) NEC —*see* Complication, fixation device, mechanical
gastrointestinal —*see* Complications, prosthetic device, mechanical, gastrointestinal device
genital NEC T83.428
intrauterine contraceptive device (string) T83.32
penile prosthesis (cylinder) (implanted) (pump) (resevoir) T83.420
testicular prosthesis T83.421
heart NEC —*see* Complication, cardiovascular device, mechanical
joint prosthesis —*see* Complication, joint prosthesis, mechanical
ocular NEC —*see* Complications, prosthetic device, mechanical, ocular device
orthopedic NEC —*see* Complication, orthopedic, device, mechanical
specified NEC T85.628
urinary NEC —*see also* Complication, genitourinary, device, urinary, mechanical
graft T83.22
vascular NEC —*see* Complication, cardiovascular device, mechanical
ventricular intracranial shunt T85.02
fetus —*see* Pregnancy, complicated by (management affected by), presentation, fetal
gallbladder K82.8
gastrointestinal tract, congenital Q45.8
heart, congenital NEC Q24.8
joint prosthesis —*see* Complications, joint prosthesis, mechanical, displacement, by site
stomach K31.89
congenital Q40.2
tooth, teeth, fully erupted M26.30
uterus (acute) (acquired) (adherent) (asymptomatic) (postinfectional) (postpartal, old) N85.4
anteflexion or anteversion N85.4
congenital Q51.818

Malposition *(Continued)*
uterus *(Continued)*
flexion N85.4
lateral —*see* Lateroversion, uterus
inversion N85.5
lateral (flexion) (version) —*see* Lateroversion, uterus
in pregnancy or childbirth —*see* subcategory O34.5
retroflexion or retroversion —*see* Retroversion, uterus
Malposture R29.3
Malrotation
cecum Q43.3
colon Q43.3
intestine Q43.3
kidney Q63.2
Malta fever —*see* Brucellosis
Maltreatment
adult
abandonment
confirmed T74.01
suspected T76.01
bullying
confirmed T74.31
suspected T76.31
confirmed T74.91
history of Z91.419
intimidation (through social media)
confirmed T74.31
suspected T76.31
neglect
confirmed T74.01
suspected T76.01
physical abuse
confirmed T74.11
suspected T76.11
psychological abuse
confirmed T74.31
history of Z91.411
suspected T76.31
sexual abuse
confirmed T74.21
suspected T76.21
suspected T76.91
child
abandonment
confirmed T74.02
suspected T76.02
bullying
confirmed T74.32
suspected T76.32
confirmed T74.92
history of —*see* History, personal (of), abuse
intimidation (through social media)
confirmed T74.32
suspected T76.32
neglect
confirmed T74.02
history of —*see* History, personal (of), abuse
suspected T76.02
physical abuse
confirmed T74.12
history of —*see* History, personal (of), abuse
suspected T76.12
psychological abuse
confirmed T74.32
history of —*see* History, personal (of), abuse
suspected T76.32
sexual abuse
confirmed T74.22
history of —*see* History, personal (of), abuse
suspected T76.22
suspected T76.92
personal history of Z91.89
Maltworker's lung J67.4

Malunion, fracture —*see* Fracture, by site
Mammillitis N61.0
puerperal, postpartum O91.02
Mammitis —*see* Mastitis
Mammogram (examination) Z12.39
routine Z12.31
Mammoplasia N62
Management (of)
bone conduction hearing device (implanted) Z45.320
cardiac pacemaker NEC Z45.018
cerebrospinal fluid drainage device Z45.41
cochlear device (implanted) Z45.321
contraceptive Z30.9
specified NEC Z30.8
implanted device Z45.9
specified NEC Z45.89
infusion pump Z45.1
procreative Z31.9
male factor infertility in female Z31.81
specified NEC Z31.89
prosthesis (external) —*see also* Fitting Z44.9
implanted Z45.9
specified NEC Z45.89
renal dialysis catheter Z49.01
vascular access device Z45.2
Mangled —*see* specified injury by site
Mania (monopolar) —*see also* Disorder, mood, manic episode
with psychotic symptoms F30.2
without psychotic symptoms F30.10
mild F30.11
moderate F30.12
severe F30.13
Bell's F30.8
chronic (recurrent) F31.89
hysterical F44.89
puerperal F30.8
recurrent F31.89
Manic depression F31.9
Manic-depressive insanity, psychosis, or syndrome —*see* Disorder, bipolar
Mannosidosis E77.1
Mansonelliasis, mansonellosis B74.4
Manson's
disease B65.1
schistosomiasis B65.1
Manual —*see* condition
Maple-bark-stripper's lung (disease) J67.6
Maple-syrup-urine disease E71.0
Marable's syndrome (celiac artery compression) I77.4
Marasmus E41
due to malnutrition E41
intestinal E41
nutritional E41
senile R54
tuberculous NEC —*see* Tuberculosis
Marble
bones Q78.2
skin R23.8
Marburg virus disease A98.3
March
fracture —*see* Fracture, traumatic, stress, by site
hemoglobinuria D59.6
Marchesani (-Weill) syndrome Q87.0
Marchiafava (-Bignami) syndrome or disease G37.1
Marchiafava-Micheli syndrome D59.5
Marcus Gunn's syndrome Q07.8
Marfan's syndrome —*see* Syndrome, Marfan's
Marie-Bamberger disease —*see* Osteoarthropathy, hypertrophic, specified NEC
Marie-Charcot-Tooth neuropathic muscular atrophy G60.0
Marie's
cerebellar ataxia (late-onset) G11.2
disease or syndrome (acromegaly) E22.0

M

Marie-Strümpell arthritis, disease or spondylitis —*see* Spondylitis, ankylosing
Marion's disease (bladder neck obstruction) N32.Ø
Marital conflict Z63.Ø
Mark
  port wine Q82.5
  raspberry Q82.5
  strawberry Q82.5
  stretch L9Ø.6
  tattoo L81.8
Marker heterochromatin —*see* Extra, marker chromosomes
Maroteaux-Lamy syndrome (mild) (severe) E76.29
Marrow (bone)
  arrest D61.9
  poor function D75.89
Marseilles fever A77.1
Marsh fever —*see* Malaria
Marshall's (hidrotic) ectodermal dysplasia Q82.4
Marsh's disease (exophthalmic goiter) EØ5.ØØ
  with storm EØ5.Ø1
Masculinization (female) with adrenal hyperplasia E25.9
  congenital E25.Ø
Masculinovoblastoma D27.-●
Masochism (sexual) F65.51
Mason's lung J62.8
Mass
  abdominal R19.ØØ
    epigastric R19.Ø6
    generalized R19.Ø7
    left lower quadrant R19.Ø4
    left upper quadrant R19.Ø2
    periumbilic R19.Ø5
    right lower quadrant R19.Ø3
    right upper quadrant R19.Ø1
    specified site NEC R19.Ø9
  breast —*see also* Lump, breast N63.Ø
  chest R22.2
  cystic —*see* Cyst
  ear H93.8-●
  head R22.Ø
  intra-abdominal (diffuse) (generalized) —*see* Mass, abdominal
  kidney N28.89
  liver R16.Ø
  localized (skin) R22.9
    chest R22.2
    head R22.Ø
    limb
      lower R22.4-●
      upper R22.3-●
    neck R22.1
    trunk R22.2
  lung R91.8
  malignant —*see* Neoplasm, malignant, by site
  neck R22.1
  pelvic (diffuse) (generalized) —*see* Mass, abdominal
  specified organ NEC —*see* Disease, by site
  splenic R16.1
  substernal thyroid —*see* Goiter
  superficial (localized) R22.9
  umbilical (diffuse) (generalized) R19.Ø9
Massive —*see* condition
Mast cell
  disease, systemic tissue D47.Ø2
  leukemia C94.3-●
  neoplasm
    malignant C96.2Ø
      specified type NEC C96.29
    of uncertain behavior NEC D47.Ø9
  sarcoma C96.22
  tumor D47.Ø9
Mastalgia N64.4
Masters-Allen syndrome N83.8
Mastitis (acute) (diffuse) (nonpuerperal) (subacute) N61.Ø
  with abscess N61.1
  chronic (cystic) —*see* Mastopathy, cystic
  cystic (Schimmelbusch's type) —*see* Mastopathy, cystic
  fibrocystic —*see* Mastopathy, cystic
  infective N61.Ø
    newborn P39.Ø
  interstitial, gestational or puerperal —*see* Mastitis, obstetric
  neonatal (noninfective) P83.4
    infective P39.Ø
  obstetric (interstitial) (nonpurulent)
    associated with
      lactation O91.23
      pregnancy O91.21-●
      puerperium O91.22
    purulent
      associated with
        lactation O91.13
        pregnancy O91.11-●
        puerperium O91.12
  periductal —*see* Ectasia, mammary duct
  phlegmonous —*see* Mastopathy, cystic
  plasma cell —*see* Ectasia, mammary duct
  without abscess N61.Ø
Mastocytoma (extracutaneous) D47.Ø9
  malignant C96.29
  solitary D47.Ø1
Mastocytosis D47.Ø9
  aggressive systemic C96.21
  cutaneous (diffuse) (maculopapular) D47.Ø1
    congenital Q82.2
    of neonatal onset Q82.2
    of newborn onset Q82.2
  indolent systemic D47.Ø2
  isolated bone marrow D47.Ø2
  malignant C96.29
  systemic (indolent) (smoldering)
    with an associated hematological non-mast cell lineage disease (SM-AHNMD) D47.Ø2
Mastodynia N64.4
Mastoid —*see* condition
Mastoidalgia —*see* subcategory H92.Ø
Mastoiditis (coalescent) (hemorrhagic) (suppurative) H7Ø.9-●
  acute, subacute H7Ø.ØØ-●
    complicated NEC H7Ø.Ø9-●
    subperiosteal H7Ø.Ø1-●
  chronic (necrotic) (recurrent) H7Ø.1-●
  in (due to)
    infectious disease NEC B99 *[H75.Ø-●]*
    parasitic disease NEC B89 *[H75.Ø-●]*
    tuberculosis A18.Ø3
  petrositis —*see* Petrositis
  postauricular fistula —*see* Fistula, postauricular
  specified NEC H7Ø.89-●
  tuberculous A18.Ø3
Mastopathy, mastopathia N64.9
  chronica cystica —*see* Mastopathy, cystic
  cystic (chronic) (diffuse) N6Ø.1
    with epithelial proliferation N6Ø.3-●
  diffuse cystic —*see* Mastopathy, cystic
  estrogenic, oestrogenica N64.89
  ovarian origin N64.89
Mastoplasia, mastoplastia N62
Masturbation (excessive) F98.8
Maternal care (for) —*see* Pregnancy (complicated by) (management affected by)
Matheiu's disease (leptospiral jaundice) A27.Ø
Mauclaire's disease or osteochondrosis —*see* Osteochondrosis, juvenile, hand, metacarpal
Maxcy's disease A75.2
Maxilla, maxillary —*see* condition
May (-Hegglin) anomaly or syndrome D72.Ø
McArdle (-Schmid)(-Pearson) disease (glycogen storage) E74.Ø4
McCune-Albright syndrome Q78.1
McQuarrie's syndrome (idiopathic familial hypoglycemia) E16.2
Meadow's syndrome Q86.1
Measles (black) (hemorrhagic) (suppressed) BØ5.9
  with
    complications NEC BØ5.89
    encephalitis BØ5.Ø
    intestinal complications BØ5.4
    keratitis (keratoconjunctivitis) BØ5.81
    meningitis BØ5.1
    otitis media BØ5.3
    pneumonia BØ5.2
  French —*see* Rubella
  German —*see* Rubella
  Liberty —*see* Rubella
Meatitis, urethral —*see* Urethritis
Meatus, meatal —*see* condition
Meat-wrappers' asthma J68.9
Meckel-Gruber syndrome Q61.9
Meckel's diverticulitis, diverticulum (displaced) (hypertrophic) Q43.Ø
Meconium
  ileus, newborn P76.Ø
    in cystic fibrosis E84.11
    meaning meconium plug (without cystic fibrosis) P76.Ø
  obstruction, newborn P76.Ø
    due to fecaliths P76.Ø
    in mucoviscidosis E84.11
  peritonitis P78.Ø
  plug syndrome (newborn) NEC P76.Ø
Median —*see also* condition
  arcuate ligament syndrome I77.4
  bar (prostate) (vesical orifice) —*see* Hyperplasia, prostate
  rhomboid glossitis K14.2
Mediastinal shift R93.89
Mediastinitis (acute) (chronic) J98.51
  syphilitic A52.73
  tuberculous A15.8
Mediastinopericarditis —*see also* Pericarditis
  acute I3Ø.9
  adhesive I31.Ø
  chronic I31.8
    rheumatic IØ9.2
Mediastinum, mediastinal —*see* condition
Medicine poisoning —*see* Table of Drugs and Chemicals, by drug, poisoning
Mediterranean
  fever —*see* Brucellosis
    familial MØ4.1
    tick A77.1
  kala-azar B55.Ø
  leishmaniasis B55.Ø
  tick fever A77.1
Medulla —*see* condition
Medullary cystic kidney Q61.5
Medullated fibers
  optic (nerve) Q14.8
  retina Q14.1
Medulloblastoma
  desmoplastic C71.6
  specified site —*see* Neoplasm, malignant, by site
  unspecified site C71.6
Medulloepithelioma —*see also* Neoplasm, malignant, by site
  teratoid —*see* Neoplasm, malignant, by site
Medullomyoblastoma
  specified site —*see* Neoplasm, malignant, by site
  unspecified site C71.6
Meekeren-Ehlers-Danlos syndrome —*see also* Syndrome, Ehlers-Danlos Q79.6
Megacolon (acquired) (functional) (not Hirschsprung's disease) (in) K59.39
  Chagas' disease B57.32
  congenital, congenitum (aganglionic) Q43.1
  Hirschsprung's (disease) Q43.1

M

Megacolon *(Continued)*
toxic NEC K59.31
due to Clostridium difficile
not specified as recurrent AØ4.72
recurrent AØ4.71
Megaesophagus (functional) K22.Ø
congenital Q39.5
in (due to) Chagas' disease B57.31
Megalencephaly QØ4.5
Megalerythema (epidemic) BØ8.3
Megaloappendix Q43.8
Megalocephalus, megalocephaly NEC Q75.3
Megalocornea Q15.8
with glaucoma Q15.Ø
Megalocytic anemia D53.1
Megalodactylia (fingers) (thumbs) (congenital) Q74.Ø
toes Q74.2
Megaloduodenum Q43.8
Megaloesophagus (functional) K22.Ø
congenital Q39.5
Megalogastria (acquired) K31.89
congenital Q4Ø.2
Megalophthalmos Q11.3
Megalopsia H53.15
Megalosplenia —*see* Splenomegaly
Megaloureter N28.82
congenital Q62.2
Megarectum K62.89
Megasigmoid K59.39
congenital Q43.2
Megaureter N28.82
congenital Q62.2
Megavitamin-B6 syndrome E67.2
Megrim —*see* Migraine
Meibomian
cyst, infected —*see* Hordeolum
gland —*see* condition
sty, stye —*see* Hordeolum
Meibomitis —*see* Hordeolum
Meige-Milroy disease (chronic hereditary edema) Q82.Ø
Meige's syndrome Q82.Ø
Melalgia, nutritional E53.8
Melancholia F32.9
climacteric (single episode) F32.89
recurrent episode F33.8
hypochondriac F45.29
intermittent (single episode) F32.89
recurrent episode F33.8
involutional (single episode) F32.89
recurrent episode F33.8
menopausal (single episode) F32.89
recurrent episode F33.8
puerperal F32.89
reactive (emotional stress or trauma) F32.3
recurrent F33.9
senile FØ3
stuporous (single episode) F32.89
recurrent episode F33.8
Melanemia R79.89
Melanoameloblastoma —*see* Neoplasm, bone, benign
Melanoblastoma —*see* Melanoma
Melanocarcinoma —*see* Melanoma
Melanocytoma, eyeball D31.9- •
Melanocytosis, neurocutaneous Q82.8
Melanoderma, melanodermia L81.4
Melanodontia, infantile KØ3.89
Melanodontoclasia KØ3.89
Melanoepithelioma —*see* Melanoma
Melanoma (malignant) C43.9
acral lentiginous, malignant —*see* Melanoma, skin, by site
amelanotic —*see* Melanoma, skin, by site
balloon cell —*see* Melanoma, skin, by site
benign —*see* Nevus
desmoplastic, malignant —*see* Melanoma, skin, by site
epithelioid cell —*see* Melanoma, skin, by site
with spindle cell, mixed —*see* Melanoma, skin, by site

Melanoma *(Continued)*
in
giant pigmented nevus —*see* Melanoma, skin, by site
Hutchinson's melanotic freckle —*see* Melanoma, skin, by site
junctional nevus —*see* Melanoma, skin, by site
precancerous melanosis —*see* Melanoma, skin, by site
in situ DØ3.9
abdominal wall DØ3.59
ala nasi DØ3.39
ankle DØ3.7- •
anus, anal (margin) (skin) DØ3.51
arm DØ3.6- •
auditory canal DØ3.2- •
auricle (ear) DØ3.2- •
auricular canal (external) DØ3.2- •
axilla, axillary fold DØ3.59
back DØ3.59
breast DØ3.52
brow DØ3.39
buttock DØ3.59
canthus (eye) DØ3.1- •
cheek (external) DØ3.39
chest wall DØ3.59
chin DØ3.39
choroid DØ3.8
conjunctiva DØ3.8
ear (external) DØ3.2- •
external meatus (ear) DØ3.2- •
eye DØ3.8
eyebrow DØ3.39
eyelid (lower) (upper) DØ3.1- •
face DØ3.3Ø
specified NEC DØ3.39
female genital organ (external) NEC DØ3.8
finger DØ3.6- •
flank DØ3.59
foot DØ3.7- •
forearm DØ3.6- •
forehead DØ3.39
foreskin DØ3.8
gluteal region DØ3.59
groin DØ3.59
hand DØ3.6- •
heel DØ3.7- •
helix DØ3.2- •
hip DØ3.7- •
interscapular region DØ3.59
iris DØ3.8
jaw DØ3.39
knee DØ3.7- •
labium (majus) (minus) DØ3.8
lacrimal gland DØ3.8
leg DØ3.7- •
lip (lower) (upper) DØ3.Ø
lower limb NEC DØ3.7- •
male genital organ (external) NEC DØ3.8
nail DØ3.9
finger DØ3.6- •
toe DØ3.7- •
neck DØ3.4
nose (external) DØ3.39
orbit DØ3.8
penis DØ3.8
perianal skin DØ3.51
perineum DØ3.51
pinna DØ3.2- •
popliteal fossa or space DØ3.7- •
prepuce DØ3.8
pudendum DØ3.8
retina DØ3.8
retrobulbar DØ3.8
scalp DØ3.4
scrotum DØ3.8
shoulder DØ3.6- •
specified site NEC DØ3.8
submammary fold DØ3.52
temple DØ3.39

Melanoma *(Continued)*
in situ *(Continued)*
thigh DØ3.7- •
toe DØ3.7- •
trunk NEC DØ3.59
umbilicus DØ3.59
upper limb NEC DØ3.6- •
vulva DØ3.8
juvenile —*see* Nevus
malignant, of soft parts except skin —*see* Neoplasm, connective tissue, malignant
metastatic
breast C79.81
genital organ C79.82
specified site NEC C79.89
neurotropic, malignant —*see* Melanoma, skin, by site
nodular —*see* Melanoma, skin, by site
regressing, malignant —*see* Melanoma, skin, by site
skin C43.9
abdominal wall C43.59
ala nasi C43.31
ankle C43.7- •
anus, anal (skin) C43.51
arm C43.6- •
auditory canal (external) C43.2- •
auricle (ear) C43.2- •
auricular canal (external) C43.2- •
axilla, axillary fold C43.59
back C43.59
breast (female) (male) C43.52
brow C43.39
buttock C43.59
canthus (eye) C43.1- •
cheek (external) C43.39
chest wall C43.59
chin C43.39
ear (external) C43.2- •
elbow C43.6- •
external meatus (ear) C43.2- •
eyebrow C43.39
eyelid (lower) (upper) C43.1- •
face C43.3Ø
specified NEC C43.39
female genital organ (external) NEC C51.9
finger C43.6- •
flank C43.59
foot C43.7- •
forearm C43.6- •
forehead C43.39
foreskin C6Ø.Ø
glabella C43.39
gluteal region C43.59
groin C43.59
hand C43.6- •
heel C43.7- •
helix C43.2- •
hip C43.7- •
interscapular region C43.59
jaw (external) C43.39
knee C43.7- •
labium C51.9
majus C51.Ø
minus C51.1
leg C43.7- •
lip (lower) (upper) C43.Ø
lower limb NEC C43.7- •
male genital organ (external) NEC C63.9
nail
finger C43.6- •
toe C43.7- •
nasolabial groove C43.39
nates C43.59
neck C43.4
nose (external) C43.31
overlapping site C43.8
palpebra C43.1- •
penis C6Ø.9
perianal skin C43.51
perineum C43.51

Melanoma *(Continued)*
  skin *(Continued)*
    pinna C43.2-•
    popliteal fossa or space C43.7-•
    prepuce C60.0
    pudendum C51.9
    scalp C43.4
    scrotum C63.2
    shoulder C43.6-•
    skin NEC C43.9
    submammary fold C43.52
    temple C43.39
    thigh C43.7-•
    toe C43.7-•
    trunk NEC C43.59
    umbilicus C43.59
    upper limb NEC C43.6-•
    vulva C51.9
      overlapping sites C51.8
  spindle cell
    with epithelioid, mixed —*see* Melanoma, skin, by site
    type A C69.4-•
    type B C69.4-•
  superficial spreading —*see* Melanoma, skin, by site
Melanosarcoma —*see also* Melanoma
  epithelioid cell —*see* Melanoma
Melanosis L81.4
  addisonian E27.1
    tuberculous A18.7
  adrenal E27.1
  colon K63.89
  conjunctiva —*see* Pigmentation, conjunctiva
    congenital Q13.89
  cornea (presenile) (senile) —*see also* Pigmentation, cornea
    congenital Q13.4
  eye NEC H57.89
    congenital Q15.8
  lenticularis progressiva Q82.1
  liver K76.89
  precancerous —*see also* Melanoma, in situ
    malignant melanoma in —*see* Melanoma
  Riehl's L81.4
  sclera H15.89
    congenital Q13.89
  suprarenal E27.1
  tar L81.4
  toxic L81.4
Melanuria R82.998
MELAS syndrome E88.41
Melasma L81.1
  adrenal (gland) E27.1
  suprarenal (gland) E27.1
Melena K92.1
  with ulcer - code by site under Ulcer, with hemorrhage K27.4
  due to swallowed maternal blood P78.2
  newborn, neonatal P54.1
    due to swallowed maternal blood P78.2
Meleney's
  gangrene (cutaneous) —*see* Ulcer, skin
  ulcer (chronic undermining) —*see* Ulcer, skin
Melioidosis A24.9
  acute A24.1
  chronic A24.2
  fulminating A24.1
  pneumonia A24.1
  pulmonary (chronic) A24.2
    acute A24.1
    subacute A24.2
  sepsis A24.1
  specified NEC A24.3
  subacute A24.2
Melitensis, febris A23.0
Melkersson (-Rosenthal) **syndrome** G51.2
Mellitus, diabetes —*see* Diabetes
Melorheostosis (bone) —*see* Disorder, bone, density and structure, specified NEC
Meloschisis Q18.4
Melotia Q17.4
Membrana
  capsularis lentis posterior Q13.89
  epipapillaris Q14.2
Membranacea placenta O43.19-•
Membranaceous uterus N85.8
Membrane(s), membranous —*see also* condition
  cyclitic —*see* Membrane, pupillary
  folds, congenital —*see* Web
  Jackson's Q43.3
  over face of newborn P28.9
  premature rupture —*see* Rupture, membranes, premature
  pupillary H21.4-•
    persistent Q13.89
  retained (with hemorrhage) (complicating delivery) O72.2
    without hemorrhage O73.1
  secondary cataract —*see* Cataract, secondary
  unruptured (causing asphyxia) —*see* Asphyxia, newborn
  vitreous —*see* Opacity, vitreous, membranes and strands
Membranitis —*see* Chorioamnionitis
Memory disturbance, lack or loss —*see also* Amnesia
  mild, following organic brain damage F06.8
Menadione deficiency E56.1
Menarche
  delayed E30.0
  precocious E30.1
Mendacity, pathologic F60.2
Mendelson's syndrome (due to anesthesia) J95.4
  in labor and delivery O74.0
  in pregnancy O29.01-•
  obstetric O74.0
  postpartum, puerperal O89.01
Ménétrier's disease or syndrome K29.60
  with bleeding K29.61
Ménière's disease, syndrome or vertigo H81.0-•
Meninges, meningeal —*see* condition
Meningioma —*see also* Neoplasm, meninges, benign
  angioblastic —*see* Neoplasm, meninges, benign
  angiomatous —*see* Neoplasm, meninges, benign
  endotheliomatous —*see* Neoplasm, meninges, benign
  fibroblastic —*see* Neoplasm, meninges, benign
  fibrous —*see* Neoplasm, meninges, benign
  hemangioblastic —*see* Neoplasm, meninges, benign
  hemangiopericytic —*see* Neoplasm, meninges, benign
  malignant —*see* Neoplasm, meninges, malignant
  meningiothelial —*see* Neoplasm, meninges, benign
  meningotheliomatous —*see* Neoplasm, meninges, benign
  mixed —*see* Neoplasm, meninges, benign
  multiple —*see* Neoplasm, meninges, uncertain behavior
  papillary —*see* Neoplasm, meninges, uncertain behavior
  psammomatous —*see* Neoplasm, meninges, benign
  syncytial —*see* Neoplasm, meninges, benign
  transitional —*see* Neoplasm, meninges, benign
Meningiomatosis (diffuse) —*see* Neoplasm, meninges, uncertain behavior
Meningism —*see* Meningismus
Meningismus (infectional) (pneumococcal) R29.1
  due to serum or vaccine R29.1
  influenzal —*see* Influenza, with, manifestations NEC
Meningitis (basal) (basic) (brain) (cerebral) (cervical) (congestive) (diffuse) (hemorrhagic) infantile) (membranous) (metastatic) (nonspecific) (pontine) (progressive) (simple) (spinal) (subacute) (sympathetic) (toxic) G03.9
  abacterial G03.0
  actinomycotic A42.81
  adenoviral A87.1
  arbovirus A87.8
  aseptic (acute) G03.0
  bacterial G00.9
    Escherichia coli (E. coli) G00.8
    Friedländer (bacillus) G00.8
    gram-negative G00.9
    H. influenzae G00.0
    Klebsiella G00.8
    pneumococcal G00.1
    specified organism NEC G00.8
    staphylococcal G00.3
    streptococcal (acute) G00.2
  benign recurrent (Mollaret) G03.2
  candidal B37.5
  caseous (tuberculous) A17.0
  cerebrospinal A39.0
  chronic NEC G03.1
  clear cerebrospinal fluid NEC G03.0
  coxsackievirus A87.0
  cryptococcal B45.1
  diplococcal (gram positive) A39.0
  echovirus A87.0
  enteroviral A87.0
  eosinophilic B83.2
  epidemic NEC A39.0
  Escherichia coli (E. coli) G00.8
  fibrinopurulent G00.9
    specified organism NEC G00.8
  Friedländer (bacillus) G00.8
  gonococcal A54.81
  gram-negative cocci G00.9
  gram-positive cocci G00.9
  Haemophilus (influenzae) G00.0
  H. influenzae G00.0
  in (due to)
    adenovirus A87.1
    African trypanosomiasis B56.9 *[G02]*
    anthrax A22.8
    bacterial disease NEC A48.8 *[G01]*
    Chagas' disease (chronic) B57.41
    chickenpox B01.0
    coccidioidomycosis B38.4
    Diplococcus pneumoniae G00.1
    enterovirus A87.0
    herpes (simplex) virus B00.3
      zoster B02.1
    infectious mononucleosis B27.92
    leptospirosis A27.81
    Listeria monocytogenes A32.11
    Lyme disease A69.21
    measles B05.1
    mumps (virus) B26.1
    neurosyphilis (late) A52.13
    parasitic disease NEC B89 *[G02]*
    poliovirus A80.9 *[G02]*
    preventive immunization, inoculation or vaccination G03.8
    rubella B06.02
    Salmonella infection A02.21
    specified cause NEC G03.8
    Streptococcal pneumoniae G00.1
    typhoid fever A01.01
    varicella B01.0
    viral disease NEC A87.8
    whooping cough A37.90
    zoster B02.1
  infectious G00.9
  influenzal (H. influenzae) G00.0
  Klebsiella G00.8
  leptospiral (aseptic) A27.81
  lymphocytic (acute) (benign) (serous) A87.2
  meningococcal A39.0

Meningitis (Continued)
Mima polymorpha G00.8
Mollaret (benign recurrent) G03.2
monilial B37.5
mycotic NEC B49 [G02]
Neisseria A39.0
nonbacterial G03.0
nonpyogenic NEC G03.0
ossificans G96.19
pneumococcal streptococcus pneumoniae G00.1
poliovirus A80.9 [G02]
postmeasles B05.1
purulent G00.9
specified organism NEC G00.8
pyogenic G00.9
specified organism NEC G00.8
Salmonella (arizonae) (Cholerae-Suis) (enteritidis) (typhimurium) A02.21
septic G00.9
specified organism NEC G00.8
serosa circumscripta NEC G03.0
serous NEC G93.2
specified organism NEC G00.8
sporotrichosis B42.81
staphylococcal G00.3
sterile G03.0
Streptococcal (acute) G00.2
pneumoniae G00.1
suppurative G00.9
specified organism NEC G00.8
syphilitic (late) (tertiary) A52.13
acute A51.41
congenital A50.41
secondary A51.41
Torula histolytica (cryptococcal) B45.1
traumatic (complication of injury) T79.8
tuberculous A17.0
typhoid A01.01
viral NEC A87.9
Yersinia pestis A20.3
Meningocele (spinal) —*see also* Spina bifida
with hydrocephalus —*see* Spina bifida, by site, with hydrocephalus
acquired (traumatic) G96.19
cerebral —*see* Encephalocele
Meningocerebritis —*see* Meningoencephalitis
Meningococcemia A39.4
acute A39.2
chronic A39.3
Meningococcus, meningococcal —*see also* condition A39.9
adrenalitis, hemorrhagic A39.1
carrier (suspected) of Z22.31
meningitis (cerebrospinal) A39.0
Meningoencephalitis —*see also* Encephalitis G04.90
acute NEC —*see also* Encephalitis, viral A86
bacterial NEC G04.2
California A83.5
diphasic A84.1
eosinophilic B83.2
epidemic A39.81
herpesviral, herpetic B00.4
due to herpesvirus 6 B10.01
due to herpesvirus 7 B10.09
specified NEC B10.09
in (due to)
blastomycosis NEC B40.81
diseases classified elsewhere G05.3
free-living amebae B60.2
Hemophilus influenzae (H. influenzae) G00.0
herpes B00.4
due to herpesvirus 6 B10.01
due to herpesvirus 7 B10.09
specified NEC B10.09
H. influenzae G00.0
Lyme disease A69.22
mercury —*see* subcategory T56.1
mumps B26.2
Meningoencephalitis (Continued)
in (due to) (Continued)
Naegleria (amebae) (organisms) (fowleri) B60.2
Parastrongylus cantonensis B83.2
toxoplasmosis (acquired) B58.2
congenital P37.1
infectious (acute) (viral) A86
influenzal (H. influenzae) G00.0
Listeria monocytogenes A32.12
lymphocytic (serous) A87.2
mumps B26.2
parasitic NEC B89 [G05.3]
pneumococcal G04.2
primary amebic B60.2
specific (syphilitic) A52.14
specified organism NEC G04.81
staphylococcal G04.2
streptococcal G04.2
syphilitic A52.14
toxic NEC G92
due to mercury —*see* subcategory T56.1
tuberculous A17.82
virus NEC A86
Meningoencephalocele —*see also* Encephalocele
syphilitic A52.19
congenital A50.49
Meningoencephalomyelitis —*see also* Meningoencephalitis
acute NEC (viral) A86
disseminated G04.00
postimmunization or postvaccination G04.02
postinfectious G04.01
due to
actinomycosis A42.82
Torula B45.1
Toxoplasma or toxoplasmosis (acquired) B58.2
congenital P37.1
postimmunization or postvaccination G04.02
Meningoencephalomyelopathy G96.9
Meningoencephalopathy G96.9
Meningomyelitis —*see also* Meningoencephalitis
bacterial NEC G04.2
blastomycotic NEC B40.81
cryptococcal B45.1
in diseases classified elsewhere G05.4
meningococcal A39.81
syphilitic A52.14
tuberculous A17.82
Meningomyelocele —*see also* Spina bifida
syphilitic A52.19
Meningomyeloneuritis —*see* Meningoencephalitis
Meningoradiculitis —*see* Meningitis
Meningovascular —*see* condition
Menkes' disease or syndrome E83.09
meaning maple-syrup-urine disease E71.0
Menometrorrhagia N92.1
Menopause, menopausal (asymptomatic) (state) Z78.0
arthritis (any site) NEC —*see* Arthritis, specified form NEC
bleeding N92.4
depression (single episode) F32.89
agitated (single episode) F32.2
recurrent episode F33.9
psychotic (single episode) F32.89
zrecurrent episode F33.8
recurrent episode F33.9
melancholia (single episode) F32.89
recurrent episode F33.8
paranoid state F22
premature E28.319
asymptomatic E28.319
postirradiation E89.40
postsurgical E89.40
Menopause, menopausal (Continued)
premature (Continued)
symptomatic E28.310
postirradiation E89.41
postsurgical E89.41
psychosis NEC F28
symptomatic N95.1
toxic polyarthritis NEC —*see* Arthritis, specified form NEC
Menorrhagia (primary) N92.0
climacteric N92.4
menopausal N92.4
menopausal N92.4
▶ perimenopausal N92.4
postclimacteric N95.0
postmenopausal N95.0
preclimacteric or premenopausal N92.4
pubertal (menses retained) N92.2
Menostaxis N92.0
Menses, retention N94.89
Menstrual —*see* Menstruation
Menstruation
absent —*see* Amenorrhea
anovulatory N97.0
cycle, irregular N92.6
delayed N91.0
disorder N93.9
psychogenic F45.8
during pregnancy O20.8
excessive (with regular cycle) N92.0
with irregular cycle N92.1
at puberty N92.2
frequent N92.0
infrequent —*see* Oligomenorrhea
irregular N92.6
specified NEC N92.5
latent N92.5
membranous N92.5
painful —*see also* Dysmenorrhea N94.6
primary N94.4
psychogenic F45.8
secondary N94.5
passage of clots N92.0
precocious E30.1
protracted N92.5
rare —*see* Oligomenorrhea
retained N94.89
retrograde N92.5
scanty —*see* Oligomenorrhea
suppression N94.89
vicarious (nasal) N94.89
Mental —*see also* condition
deficiency —*see* Disability, intellectual
deterioration —*see* Psychosis
disorder —*see* Disorder, mental
exhaustion F48.8
insufficiency (congenital) —*see* Disability, intellectual
observation without need for further medical care Z03.89
retardation —*see* Disability, intellectual
subnormality —*see* Disability, intellectual
upset —*see* Disorder, mental
Meralgia paresthetica G57.1- •
Mercurial —*see* condition
Mercurialism —*see* subcategory T56.1
MERRF syndrome (myoclonic epilepsy associated with ragged-red fiber) E88.42
Merkel cell tumor —*see* Carcinoma, Merkel cell
Merocele —*see* Hernia, femoral
Meromelia
lower limb —*see* Defect, reduction, lower limb
intercalary
femur —*see* Defect, reduction, lower limb, specified type NEC
tibiofibular (complete) (incomplete) —*see* Defect, reduction, lower limb
upper limb —*see* Defect, reduction, upper limb
intercalary, humeral, radioulnar —*see* Agenesis, arm, with hand present

M

- Merzbacher-Pelizaeus disease E75.29
- Mesaortitis —*see* Aortitis
- Mesarteritis —*see* Arteritis
- Mesencephalitis —*see* Encephalitis
- Mesenchymoma —*see also* Neoplasm, connective tissue, uncertain behavior
  - benign —*see* Neoplasm, connective tissue, benign
  - malignant —*see* Neoplasm, connective tissue, malignant
- Mesenteritis
  - retractile K65.4
  - sclerosing K65.4
- Mesentery, mesenteric —*see* condition
- Mesiodens, mesiodentes K00.1
- Mesio-occlusion M26.213
- Mesocolon —*see* condition
- Mesonephroma (malignant) —*see* Neoplasm, malignant, by site
  - benign —*see* Neoplasm, benign, by site
- Mesophlebitis —*see* Phlebitis
- Mesostromal dysgenesia Q13.89
- Mesothelioma (malignant) C45.9
  - benign
    - mesentery D19.1
    - mesocolon D19.1
    - omentum D19.1
    - peritoneum D19.1
    - pleura D19.0
    - specified site NEC D19.7
    - unspecified site D19.9
  - biphasic C45.9
    - benign
      - mesentery D19.1
      - mesocolon D19.1
      - omentum D19.1
      - peritoneum D19.1
      - pleura D19.0
      - specified site NEC D19.7
      - unspecified site D19.9
  - cystic D48.4
  - epithelioid C45.9
    - benign
      - mesentery D19.1
      - mesocolon D19.1
      - omentum D19.1
      - peritoneum D19.1
      - pleura D19.0
      - specified site NEC D19.7
      - unspecified site D19.9
  - fibrous C45.9
    - benign
      - mesentery D19.1
      - mesocolon D19.1
      - omentum D19.1
      - peritoneum D19.1
      - pleura D19.0
      - specified site NEC D19.7
      - unspecified site D19.9
  - site classification
    - liver C45.7
    - lung C45.7
    - mediastinum C45.7
    - mesentery C45.1
    - mesocolon C45.1
    - omentum C45.1
    - pericardium C45.2
    - peritoneum C45.1
    - pleura C45.0
      - parietal C45.0
    - retroperitoneum C45.7
    - specified site NEC C45.7
    - unspecified C45.9
- Metabolic syndrome E88.81
- Metagonimiasis B66.8
- Metagonimus infestation (intestine) B66.8
- Metal
  - pigmentation L81.8
  - polisher's disease J62.8
- Metamorphopsia H53.15
- Metaplasia
  - apocrine (breast) —*see* Dysplasia, mammary, specified type NEC
  - cervix (squamous) —*see* Dysplasia, cervix
  - endometrium (squamous) (uterus) N85.8
  - esophagus K22.7- •
  - kidney (pelvis) (squamous) N28.89
  - myelogenous D73.1
  - myeloid (agnogenic) (megakaryocytic) D73.1
  - spleen D73.1
  - squamous cell, bladder N32.89
- Metastasis, metastatic
  - abscess —*see* Abscess
  - calcification E83.59
  - cancer
    - from specified site —*see* Neoplasm, malignant, by site
    - to specified site —*see* Neoplasm, secondary, by site
  - deposits (in) —*see* Neoplasm, secondary, by site
  - disease (*see also* Neoplasm, secondary, by site) C79.9
  - spread (to) —*see* Neoplasm, secondary, by site
- Metastrongyliasis B83.8
- Metatarsalgia M77.4- •
  - anterior G57.6- •
  - Morton's G57.6- •
- Metatarsus, metatarsal —*see also* condition
  - adductus, congenital Q66.22- •
  - valgus (abductus), congenital Q66.6
  - varus (congenital) Q66.22- •
    - primus Q66.21- •
- Methadone use —*see* Use, opioid
- Methemoglobinemia D74.9
  - acquired (with sulfhemoglobinemia) D74.8
  - congenital D74.0
  - enzymatic (congenital) D74.0
  - Hb M disease D74.0
  - hereditary D74.0
  - toxic D74.8
- Methemoglobinuria —*see* Hemoglobinuria
- Methioninemia E72.19
- Methylmalonic acidemia E71.120
- Metritis (catarrhal) (hemorrhagic) (septic) (suppurative) —*see also* Endometritis
  - cervical —*see* Cervicitis
- Metropathia hemorrhagica N93.8
- Metroperitonitis —*see* Peritonitis, pelvic, female
- Metrorrhagia N92.1
  - climacteric N92.4
  - menopausal N92.4
  - ▶ perimenopausal N92.4
  - postpartum NEC (atonic) (following delivery of placenta) O72.1
    - delayed or secondary O72.2
  - preclimacteric or premenopausal N92.4
  - psychogenic F45.8
- Metrorrhexis —*see* Rupture, uterus
- Metrosalpingitis N70.91
- Metrostaxis N93.8
- Metrovaginitis —*see* Endometritis
- Meyer-Schwickerath and Weyers syndrome Q87.0
- Meynert's amentia (nonalcoholic) F04
  - alcoholic F10.96
    - with dependence F10.26
- Mibelli's disease (porokeratosis) Q82.8
- Mice, joint —*see* Loose, body, joint
  - knee M23.4
- Micrencephalon, micrencephaly Q02
- Microalbuminuria R80.9
- Microaneurysm, retinal —*see also* Disorder, retina, microaneurysms
  - diabetic —*see* E08-E13 with .31
- Microangiopathy (peripheral) I73.9
  - thrombotic M31.1
- Microcalcifications, breast R92.0
- Microcephalus, microcephalic, microcephaly Q02
  - due to toxoplasmosis (congenital) P37.1
- Microcheilia Q18.7
- Microcolon (congenital) Q43.8
- Microcornea (congenital) Q13.4
- Microcytic —*see* condition D57.40
- Microdeletions NEC Q93.88
- Microdontia K00.2
- Microdrepanocytosis D57.40
  - with crisis (vasoocclusive pain) D57.419
    - with
      - acute chest syndrome D57.411
      - splenic sequestration D57.412
- Microembolism
  - atherothrombotic —*see* Atheroembolism
  - retinal —*see* Occlusion, artery, retina
- Microencephalon Q02
- Microfilaria streptocerca infestation —*see* Onchocerciasis
- Microgastria (congenital) Q40.2
- Microgenia M26.06
- Microgenitalia, congenital
  - female Q52.8
  - male Q55.8
- Microglioma —*see* Lymphoma, non-Hodgkin, specified NEC
- Microglossia (congenital) Q38.3
- Micrognathia, micrognathism (congenital) (mandibular) (maxillary) M26.09
- Microgyria (congenital) Q04.3
- Microinfarct of heart —*see* Insufficiency, coronary
- Microlentia (congenital) Q12.8
- Microlithiasis, alveolar, pulmonary J84.02
- Micromastia N64.82
- Micromyelia (congenital) Q06.8
- Micropenis Q55.62
- Microphakia (congenital) Q12.8
- Microphthalmos, microphthalmia (congenital) Q11.2
  - due to toxoplasmosis P37.1
- Micropsia H53.15
- Microscopic polyangiitis (polyarteritis) M31.7
- Microsporidiosis B60.8
  - intestinal A07.8
- Microsporon furfur infestation B36.0
- Microsporosis —*see also* Dermatophytosis
  - nigra B36.1
- Microstomia (congenital) Q18.5
- Microtia (congenital) (external ear) Q17.2
- Microtropia H50.40
- Microvillus inclusion disease (MVD) (MVID) Q43.8
- Micturition
  - disorder NEC —*see also* Difficulty, micturition R39.198
    - psychogenic F45.8
  - frequency R35.0
    - psychogenic F45.8
  - hesitancy R39.11
  - incomplete emptying R39.14
  - nocturnal R35.1
  - painful R30.9
    - dysuria R30.0
    - psychogenic F45.8
    - tenesmus R30.1
  - poor stream R39.12
  - position dependent R39.192
  - split stream R39.13
  - straining R39.16
  - urgency R39.15
- Mid plane —*see* condition
- Middle
  - ear —*see* condition
  - lobe (right) syndrome J98.19
- Miescher's elastoma L87.2
- Mietens' syndrome Q87.2
- Migraine (idiopathic) G43.909
  - with refractory migraine G43.919
    - with status migrainosus G43.911
    - without status migrainosus G43.919

M

Migraine *(Continued)*
with aura (acute-onset) (prolonged) (typical) (without headache) G43.109
with refractory migraine G43.119
with status migrainosus G43.111
without status migrainosus G43.119
intractable G43.119
with status migrainosus G43.111
without status migrainosus G43.119
not intractable G43.109
with status migrainosus G43.101
without status migrainosus G43.109
persistent G43.509
with cerebral infarction G43.609
with refractory migraine G43.619
with status migrainosus G43.611
without status migrainosus G43.619
intractable G43.619
with status migrainosus G43.611
without status migrainosus G43.619
not intractable G43.609
with status migrainosus G43.601
without status migrainosus G43.609
without refractory migraine G43.609
with status migrainosus G43.601
without status migrainosus G43.609
without cerebral infarction G43.509
with refractory migraine G43.519
with status migrainosus G43.511
without status migrainosus G43.519
intractable G43.519
with status migrainosus G43.511
without status migrainosus G43.519
not intractable G43.509
with status migrainosus G43.501
without status migrainosus G43.509
without refractory migraine G43.509
with status migrainosus G43.501
without status migrainosus G43.509
without mention of refractory migraine G43.109
with status migrainosus G43.101
without status migrainosus G43.109
abdominal G43.D0
with refractory migraine G43.D1
intractable G43.D1
not intractable G43.D0
without refractory migraine G43.D0
basilar —*see* Migraine, with aura
classical —*see* Migraine, with aura
common —*see* Migraine, without aura
complicated G43.109
equivalents —*see* Migraine, with aura
familiar —*see* Migraine, hemiplegic
hemiplegic G43.409
with refractory migraine G43.419
with status migrainosus G43.411
without status migrainosus G43.419
intractable G43.419
with status migrainosus G43.411
without status migrainosus G43.419
not intractable G43.409
with status migrainosus G43.401
without status migrainosus G43.409
without refractory migraine G43.409
with status migrainosus G43.401
without status migrainosus G43.409
intractable G43.919
with status migrainosus G43.911
without status migrainosus G43.919
menstrual G43.829
with refractory migraine G43.839
with status migrainosus G43.831
without status migrainosus G43.839
intractable G43.839
with status migrainosus G43.831
without status migrainosus G43.839
not intractable G43.829
with status migrainosus G43.821
without status migrainosus G43.829
without refractory migraine G43.829
with status migrainosus G43.821
without status migrainosus G43.829

Migraine *(Continued)*
menstrually related —*see* Migraine, menstrual
not intractable G43.909
with status migrainosus G43.901
without status migrainosus G43.919
ophthalmoplegic G43.B0
with refractory migraine G43.B1
intractable G43.B1
not intractable G43.B0
without refractory migraine G43.B0
persistent aura (with, without) cerebral infarction —*see* Migraine, with aura, persistent
preceded or accompanied by transient focal neurological phenomena —*see* Migraine, with aura
pre-menstrual —*see* Migraine, menstrual
pure menstrual —*see* Migraine, menstrual
retinal —*see* Migraine, with aura
specified NEC G43.809
intractable G43.819
with status migrainosus G43.811
without status migrainosus G43.819
not intractable G43.809
with status migrainosus G43.801
without status migrainosus G43.809
sporadic —*see* Migraine, hemiplegic
transformed —*see* Migraine, without aura, chronic
triggered seizures —*see* Migraine, with aura
without aura G43.009
with refractory migraine G43.019
with status migrainosus G43.011
without status migrainosus G43.019
chronic G43.709
with refractory migraine G43.719
with status migrainosus G43.711
without status migrainosus G43.719
intractable
with status migrainosus G43.711
without status migrainosus G43.719
not intractable
with status migrainosus G43.701
without status migrainosus G43.709
without refractory migraine G43.709
with status migrainosus G43.701
without status migrainosus G43.709
intractable
with status migrainosus G43.011
without status migrainosus G43.019
not intractable
with status migrainosus G43.001
without status migrainosus G43.009
without mention of refractory migraine G43.009
with status migrainosus G43.001
without status migrainosus G43.009
without refractory migraine G43.909
with status migrainosus G43.901
without status migrainosus G43.919
Migrant, social Z59.0
Migration, anxiety concerning Z60.3
Migratory, migrating —*see also* condition
person Z59.0
testis Q55.29
Mikity-Wilson disease or syndrome P27.0
Mikulicz' disease or syndrome K11.8
Miliaria L74.3
alba L74.1
apocrine L75.2
crystallina L74.1
profunda L74.2
rubra L74.0
tropicalis L74.2
Miliary —*see* condition
Milium L72.0
colloid L57.8

Milk
crust L21.0
excessive secretion O92.6
poisoning —*see* Poisoning, food, noxious
retention O92.79
sickness —*see* Poisoning, food, noxious
spots I31.0
Milk-alkali disease or syndrome E83.52
Milk-leg (deep vessels) (nonpuerperal) —*see* Embolism, vein, lower extremity
complicating pregnancy O22.3-●
puerperal, postpartum, childbirth O87.1
Milkman's disease or syndrome M83.8
Milky urine —*see* Chyluria
Millard-Gubler (-Foville) paralysis or syndrome G46.3
Millar's asthma J38.5
Miller-Fisher syndrome G61.0
Mills' disease —*see* Hemiplegia
Millstone maker's pneumoconiosis J62.8
Milroy's disease (chronic hereditary edema) Q82.0
Minamata disease T56.1-●
Miners' asthma or lung J60
Minkowski-Chauffard syndrome —*see* Spherocytosis
Minor —*see* condition
Minor's disease (hematomyelia) G95.19
Minot's disease (hemorrhagic disease), newborn P53
Minot-von Willebrand-Jurgens disease or syndrome (angiohemophilia) D68.0
Minus (and plus) **hand** (intrinsic) —*see* Deformity, limb, specified type NEC, forearm
Miosis (pupil) H57.03
Mirizzi's syndrome (hepatic duct stenosis) K83.1
Mirror writing F81.0
Misadventure (of) (prophylactic) (therapeutic) —*see also* Complications T88.9
administration of insulin (by accident) —*see* subcategory T38.3
infusion —*see* Complications, infusion
local applications (of fomentations, plasters, etc.) T88.9
burn or scald —*see* Burn
specified NEC T88.8
medical care (early) (late) T88.9
adverse effect of drugs or chemicals —*see* Table of Drugs and Chemicals
medical care (early) (late)
burn or scald —*see* Burn
specified NEC T88.8
specified NEC T88.8
surgical procedure (early) (late) —*see* Complications, surgical procedure
transfusion —*see* Complications, transfusion
vaccination or other immunological procedure —*see* Complications, vaccination
Miscarriage O03.9
Misdirection, aqueous H40.83-●
Misperception, sleep state F51.02
Misplaced, misplacement
ear Q17.4
kidney (acquired) N28.89
congenital Q63.2
organ or site, congenital NEC —*see* Malposition, congenital
Missed
abortion O02.1
delivery O36.4
Missing —*see also* Absence
string of intrauterine contraceptive device T83.32
Misuse of drugs F19.99
Mitchell's disease (erythromelalgia) I73.81
Mite(s) (infestation) B88.9
diarrhea B88.0
grain (itch) B88.0
hair follicle (itch) B88.0
in sputum B88.0

M

Mitral —*see* condition
Mittelschmerz N94.Ø
Mixed —*see* condition
MMN (multifocal motor neuropathy) G61.82
MNGIE (Mitochondrial Neurogastrointestinal Encephalopathy) syndrome E88.49
Mobile, mobility
cecum Q43.3
excessive —*see* Hypermobility
gallbladder, congenital Q44.1
kidney N28.89
organ or site, congenital NEC —*see* Malposition, congenital
Mobitz heart block (atrioventricular) I44.1
Moebius, Möbius
disease (ophthalmoplegic migraine) —*see* Migraine, ophthalmoplegic
syndrome Q87.Ø
congenital oculofacial paralysis (with other anomalies) Q87.Ø
ophthalmoplegic migraine —*see* Migraine, ophthalmoplegic
Moeller's glossitis K14.Ø
Mohr's syndrome (Types I and II) Q87.Ø
Mola destruens D39.2
Molar pregnancy OØ2.Ø
Molarization of premolars KØØ.2
Molding, head (during birth) - omit code
Mole (pigmented) —*see also* Nevus
blood OØ2.Ø
Breus' OØ2.Ø
cancerous —*see* Melanoma
carneous OØ2.Ø
destructive D39.2
fleshy OØ2.Ø
hydatid, hydatidiform (benign) (complicating pregnancy) (delivered) (undelivered) OØ1.9
classical OØ1.Ø
complete OØ1.Ø
incomplete OØ1.1
invasive D39.2
malignant D39.2
partial OØ1.1
intrauterine OØ2.Ø
invasive (hydatidiform) D39.2
malignant
meaning
malignant hydatidiform mole D39.2
melanoma —*see* Melanoma
nonhydatidiform OØ2.Ø
nonpigmented —*see* Nevus
pregnancy NEC OØ2.Ø
skin —*see* Nevus
tubal OØØ.1Ø-
with intrauterine pregnancy OØØ.11-
vesicular —*see* Mole, hydatidiform
Molimen, molimina (menstrual) N94.3
Molluscum contagiosum (epitheliale) BØ8.1
Mönckeberg's arteriosclerosis, disease, or sclerosis —*see* Arteriosclerosis, extremities
Mondini's malformation (cochlea) Q16.5
Mondor's disease I8Ø.8
Monge's disease T7Ø.29
Monilethrix (congenital) Q84.1
Moniliasis —*see also* Candidiasis B37.9
neonatal P37.5
Monitoring (encounter for)
therapeutic drug level Z51.81
Monkey malaria B53.1
Monkeypox BØ4
Monoarthritis M13.1Ø
ankle M13.17- ●
elbow M13.12- ●
foot joint M13.17- ●
hand joint M13.14- ●
hip M13.15- ●
knee M13.16- ●
shoulder M13.11- ●
wrist M13.13- ●
Monoblastic —*see* condition
Monochromat (ism), **monochromatopsia** (acquired) (congenital) H53.51
Monocytic —*see* condition
Monocytopenia D72.818
Monocytosis (symptomatic) D72.821
Monomania —*see* Psychosis
Mononeuritis G58.9
cranial nerve —*see* Disorder, nerve, cranial
femoral nerve G57.2- ●
lateral
cutaneous nerve of thigh G57.1- ●
popliteal nerve G57.3- ●
lower limb G57.9- ●
specified nerve NEC G57.8- ●
medial popliteal nerve G57.4- ●
median nerve G56.1- ●
multiplex G58.7
plantar nerve G57.6- ●
posterior tibial nerve G57.5- ●
radial nerve G56.3- ●
sciatic nerve G57.Ø- ●
specified NEC G58.8
tibial nerve G57.4- ●
ulnar nerve G56.2- ●
upper limb G56.9- ●
specified nerve NEC G56.8- ●
vestibular —*see* subcategory H93.3
Mononeuropathy G58.9
carpal tunnel syndrome —*see* Syndrome, carpal tunnel
diabetic NEC —*see* EØ8-E13 with .41
femoral nerve —*see* Lesion, nerve, femoral
ilioinguinal nerve G57.8- ●
in diseases classified elsewhere —*see* category G59
intercostal G58.Ø
lower limb G57.9- ●
causalgia —*see* Causalgia, lower limb
femoral nerve —*see* Lesion, nerve, femoral
meralgia paresthetica G57.1- ●
plantar nerve —*see* Lesion, nerve, plantar
popliteal nerve —*see* Lesion, nerve, popliteal
sciatic nerve —*see* Lesion, nerve, sciatic
specified NEC G57.8- ●
tarsal tunnel syndrome —*see* Syndrome, tarsal tunnel
median nerve —*see* Lesion, nerve, median
multiplex G58.7
obturator nerve G57.8- ●
popliteal nerve —*see* Lesion, nerve, popliteal
radial nerve —*see* Lesion, nerve, radial
saphenous nerve G57.8- ●
specified NEC G58.8
tarsal tunnel syndrome —*see* Syndrome, tarsal tunnel
tuberculous A17.83
ulnar nerve —*see* Lesion, nerve, ulnar
upper limb G56.9- ●
carpal tunnel syndrome —*see* Syndrome, carpal tunnel
causalgia —*see* Causalgia
median nerve —*see* Lesion, nerve, median
radial nerve —*see* Lesion, nerve, radial
specified site NEC G56.8- ●
ulnar nerve —*see* Lesion, nerve, ulnar
Mononucleosis, infectious B27.9Ø
with
complication NEC B27.99
meningitis B27.92
polyneuropathy B27.91
cytomegaloviral B27.1Ø
with
complication NEC B27.19
meningitis B27.12
polyneuropathy B27.11
Epstein-Barr (virus) B27.ØØ
with
complication NEC B27.Ø9
meningitis B27.Ø2
polyneuropathy B27.Ø1
Mononucleosis, infectious *(Continued)*
gammaherpesviral B27.ØØ
with
complication NEC B27.Ø9
meningitis B27.Ø2
polyneuropathy B27.Ø1
specified NEC B27.8Ø
with
complication NEC B27.89
meningitis B27.82
polyneuropathy B27.81
Monoplegia G83.3- ●
congenital (cerebral) G8Ø.8
spastic G8Ø.1
embolic (current episode) I63.4- ●
following
cerebrovascular disease
cerebral infarction
lower limb I69.34- ●
upper limb I69.33- ●
intracerebral hemorrhage
lower limb I69.14- ●
upper limb I69.13- ●
lower limb I69.94- ●
nontraumatic intracranial hemorrhage NEC
lower limb I69.24- ●
upper limb I69.23- ●
specified disease NEC
lower limb I69.84- ●
upper limb I69.83- ●
stroke NOS
lower limb I69.34- ●
upper limb I69.33- ●
subarachnoid hemorrhage
lower limb I69.Ø4- ●
upper limb I69.Ø3- ●
upper limb I69.93- ●
hysterical (transient) F44.4
lower limb G83.1- ●
psychogenic (conversion reaction) F44.4
thrombotic (current episode) I63.3- ●
transient R29.818
upper limb G83.2- ●
Monorchism, monorchidism Q55.Ø
Monosomy —*see also* Deletion, chromosome Q93.9
specified NEC Q93.89
whole chromosome
meiotic nondisjunction Q93.Ø
mitotic nondisjunction Q93.1
mosaicism Q93.1
X Q96.9
Monster, monstrosity (single) Q89.7
acephalic QØØ.Ø
twin Q89.4
Monteggia's fracture (-dislocation) S52.27- ●
Mooren's ulcer (cornea) —*see* Ulcer, cornea, Mooren's
Moore's syndrome —*see* Epilepsy, specified NEC
Mooser-Neill reaction A75.2
Mooser's bodies A75.2
Morbidity not stated or unknown R69
Morbilli —*see* Measles
Morbus —*see also* Disease
angelicus, anglorum E55.Ø
Beigel B36.2
caducus —*see* Epilepsy
celiacus K9Ø.Ø
comitialis —*see* Epilepsy
cordis —*see also* Disease, heart I51.9
valvulorum —*see* Endocarditis
coxae senilis M16.9
tuberculous A18.Ø2
hemorrhagicus neonatorum P53
maculosus neonatorum P54.5
Morel (-Stewart)(-Morgagni) syndrome M85.2
Morel-Kraepelin disease —*see* Schizophrenia
Morel-Moore syndrome M85.2

M

Morgagni's
cyst, organ, hydatid, or appendage
female Q5Ø.5
male (epididymal) Q55.4
testicular Q55.29
syndrome M85.2
Morgagni-Stewart-Morel syndrome M85.2
Morgagni-Stokes-Adams syndrome I45.9
Morgagni-Turner (-Albright) **syndrome** Q96.9
Moria FØ7.Ø
Moron (I.Q. 5Ø-69) F7Ø
Morphea L94.Ø
Morphinism (without remission) F11.2Ø
with remission F11.21
Morphinomania (without remission) F11.2Ø
with remission F11.21
Morquio (-Ullrich)(-Brailsford) **disease or syndrome** —*see* Mucopolysaccharidosis
Mortification (dry) (moist) —*see* Gangrene
Morton's metatarsalgia (neuralgia)(neuroma) (syndrome) G57.6
Morvan's disease or syndrome G6Ø.8
Mosaicism, mosaic (autosomal) (chromosomal)
45,X/46,XX Q96.3
45,X/other cell lines NEC with abnormal sex chromosome Q96.4
sex chromosome
female Q97.8
lines with various numbers of X chromosomes Q97.2
male Q98.7
XY Q96.3
Moschowitz' disease M31.1
Mother yaw A66.Ø
Motion sickness (from travel, any vehicle) (from roundabouts or swings) T75.3
Mottled, mottling, teeth (enamel) (endemic) (nonendemic) KØØ.3
Mounier-Kuhn syndrome Q32.4
with bronchiectasis J47.9
exacerbation (acute) J47.1
lower respiratory infection J47.Ø
acquired J98.Ø9
with bronchiectasis J47.9
with
exacerbation (acute) J47.1
lower respiratory infection J47.Ø
Mountain
sickness T7Ø.29
with polycythemia , acquired (acute) D75.1
tick fever A93.2
Mouse, joint —*see* Loose, body, joint
knee M23.4-•
Mouth —*see* condition
Movable
coccyx —*see* subcategory M53.2
kidney N28.89
congenital Q63.8
spleen D73.89
Movements, dystonic R25.8
Moyamoya disease I67.5
MRSA (Methicillin resistant Staphylococcus aureus)
infection A49.Ø2
as the cause of diseases classified elsewhere B95.62
sepsis A41.Ø2
MSD (multiple sulfatase deficiency) E75.26
MSSA (Methicillin susceptible Staphylococcus aureus)
infection A49.Ø1
as the cause of diseases classified elsewhere B95.61
sepsis A41.Ø1
Mucha-Habermann disease L41.Ø
Mucinosis (cutaneous) (focal) (papular) (reticular erythematous) (skin) L98.5
oral K13.79
Mucocele
appendix K38.8
buccal cavity K13.79
Mucocele *(Continued)*
gallbladder K82.1
lacrimal sac, chronic HØ4.43-•
nasal sinus J34.1
nose J34.1
salivary gland (any) K11.6
sinus (accessory) (nasal) J34.1
turbinate (bone) (middle) (nasal) J34.1
uterus N85.8
Mucolipidosis
I E77.1
II, III E77.Ø
IV E75.11
Mucopolysaccharidosis E76.3
beta-gluduronidase deficiency E76.29
cardiopathy E76.3 *[I52]*
Hunter's syndrome E76.1
Hurler's syndrome E76.Ø1
Hurler-Scheie syndrome E76.Ø2
Maroteaux-Lamy syndrome E76.29
Morquio syndrome E76.219
A E76.21Ø
B E76.211
classic E76.21Ø
Sanfilippo syndrome E76.22
Scheie's syndrome E76.Ø3
specified NEC E76.29
type
I
Hurler's syndrome E76.Ø1
Hurler-Scheie syndrome E76.Ø2
Scheie's syndrome E76.Ø3
II E76.1
III E76.22
IV E76.219
IVA E76.21Ø
IVB E76.211
VI E76.29
VII E76.29
Mucormycosis B46.5
cutaneous B46.3
disseminated B46.4
gastrointestinal B46.2
generalized B46.4
pulmonary B46.Ø
rhinocerebral B46.1
skin B46.3
subcutaneous B46.3
Mucositis (ulcerative) K12.3Ø
due to drugs NEC K12.32
gastrointestinal K92.81
mouth (oral) (oropharyngeal) K12.3Ø
due to antineoplastic therapy K12.31
due to drugs NEC K12.32
due to radiation K12.33
specified NEC K12.39
viral K12.39
nasal J34.81
oral cavity —*see* Mucositis, mouth
oral soft tissues —*see* Mucositis, mouth
vagina and vulva N76.81
Mucositis necroticans agranulocytica —*see* Agranulocytosis
Mucous —*see also* condition
patches (syphilitic) A51.39
congenital A5Ø.Ø7
Mucoviscidosis E84.9
with meconium obstruction E84.11
Mucus
asphyxia or suffocation —*see* Asphyxia, mucus
in stool R19.5
plug —*see* Asphyxia, mucus
Muguet B37.Ø
Mulberry molars (congenital syphilis) A5Ø.52
Müllerian mixed tumor
specified site —*see* Neoplasm, malignant, by site
unspecified site C54.9
Multicystic kidney (development) Q61.4
Multiparity (grand) Z64.1
affecting management of pregnancy, labor and delivery (supervision only) OØ9.4-•
requiring contraceptive management —*see* Contraception
Multipartita placenta O43.19-•
Multiple, multiplex —*see also* condition
digits (congenital) Q69.9
endocrine neoplasia —*see* Neoplasia, endocrine, multiple [MEN}
personality F44.81
Mumps B26.9
arthritis B26.85
complication NEC B26.89
encephalitis B26.2
hepatitis B26.81
meningitis (aseptic) B26.1
meningoencephalitis B26.2
myocarditis B26.82
oophoritis B26.89
orchitis B26.Ø
pancreatitis B26.3
polyneuropathy B26.84
Mumu —*see also* Infestation, filarial B74.9 *[N51]*
Münchhausen's syndrome —*see* Disorder, factitious
Münchmeyer's syndrome —*see* Myositis, ossificans, progressiva
Mural —*see* condition
Murmur (cardiac) (heart) (organic) RØ1.1
abdominal R19.15
aortic (valve) —*see* Endocarditis, aortic
benign RØ1.Ø
diastolic —*see* Endocarditis
Flint I35.1
functional RØ1.Ø
Graham Steell I37.1
innocent RØ1.Ø
mitral (valve) —*see* Insufficiency, mitral
nonorganic RØ1.Ø
presystolic, mitral —*see* Insufficiency, mitral
pulmonic (valve) I37.8
systolic RØ1.1
tricuspid (valve) IØ7.9
valvular —*see* Endocarditis
Murri's disease (intermittent hemoglobinuria) D59.6
Muscle, muscular —*see also* condition
carnitine (palmityltransferase) deficiency E71.314
Musculoneuralgia —*see* Neuralgia
Mushroom-workers' (pickers') **disease or lung** J67.5
Mushrooming hip —*see* Derangement, joint, specified NEC, hip
Mutation(s)
factor V Leiden D68.51
surfactant, of lung J84.83
prothrombin gene D68.52
Mutism —*see also* Aphasia
deaf (acquired) (congenital) NEC H91.3
elective (adjustment reaction) (childhood) F94.Ø
hysterical F44.4
selective (childhood) F94.Ø
MVD (microvillus inclusion disease) Q43.8
MVID (microvillus inclusion disease) Q43.8
Myalgia M79.1Ø
auxiliary muscles, head and neck M79.12
epidemic (cervical) B33.Ø
mastication muscle M79.11
site specified NEC M79.18
traumatic NEC T14.8
Myasthenia G7Ø.9
congenital G7Ø.2
cordis —*see* Failure, heart
developmental G7Ø.2
gravis G7Ø.ØØ
with exacerbation (acute) G7Ø.Ø1
in crisis G7Ø.Ø1
neonatal, transient P94.Ø

M

Myasthenia *(Continued)*
gravis *(Continued)*
pseudoparalytica G70.00
with exacerbation (acute) G70.01
in crisis G70.01
stomach, psychogenic F45.8
syndrome
in
diabetes mellitus —*see* E08-E13 with .44
neoplastic disease —*see also* Neoplasm D49.9 *[G73.3]*
pernicious anemia D51.0 *[G73.3]*
thyrotoxicosis E05.90 *[G73.3]*
with thyroid storm E05.91 *[G73.3]*
Myasthenic M62.81
Mycelium infection B49
Mycetismus —*see* Poisoning, food, noxious, mushroom
Mycetoma B47.9
actinomycotic B47.1
bone (mycotic) B47.9 *[M90.80]*
eumycotic B47.0
foot B47.9
actinomycotic B47.1
mycotic B47.0
madurae NEC B47.9
mycotic B47.0
maduromycotic B47.0
mycotic B47.0
nocardial B47.1
Mycobacteriosis —*see* Mycobacterium
Mycobacterium, mycobacterial (infection) A31.9
anonymous A31.9
atypical A31.9
cutaneous A31.1
pulmonary A31.0
tuberculous —*see* Tuberculosis, pulmonary
specified site NEC A31.8
avium (intracellulare complex) A31.0
balnei A31.1
Battey A31.0
chelonei A31.8
cutaneous A31.1
extrapulmonary systemic A31.8
fortuitum A31.8
intracellulare (Battey bacillus) A31.0
kakaferifu A31.8
kansasii (yellow bacillus) A31.0
kasongo A31.8
leprae —*see also* Leprosy A30.9
luciflavum A31.1
marinum (M. balnei) A31.1
nonspecific —*see* Mycobacterium, atypical
pulmonary (atypical) A31.0
tuberculous —*see* Tuberculosis, pulmonary
scrofulaceum A31.8
simiae A31.8
systemic, extrapulmonary A31.8
szulgai A31.8
terrae A31.8
triviale A31.8
tuberculosis (human, bovine) —*see* Tuberculosis
ulcerans A31.1
xenopi A31.8
Mycoplasma (M.) **pneumoniae, as cause of disease classified elsewhere** B96.0
Mycosis, mycotic B49
cutaneous NEC B36.9
ear B36.9
in
aspergillosis B44.89
candidiasis B37.84
moniliasis B37.84
fungoides (extranodal) (solid organ) C84.0- ●
mouth B37.0
nails B35.1
opportunistic B48.8
skin NEC B36.9
Mycosis, mycotic *(Continued)*
specified NEC B48.8
stomatitis B37.0
vagina, vaginitis (candidal) B37.3
Mydriasis (pupil) H57.04
Myelatelia Q06.1
Myelinolysis, pontine, central G37.2
Myelitis (acute) (ascending) (childhood) (chronic) (descending) (diffuse) (disseminated) (idiopathic) (pressure) (progressive) (spinal cord) (subacute) —*see also* Encephalitis G04.91
herpes simplex B00.82
herpes zoster B02.24
in diseases classified elsewhere G05.4
necrotizing, subacute G37.4
optic neuritis in G36.0
postchickenpox B01.12
postherpetic B02.24
postimmunization G04.02
postinfectious NEC G04.89
postvaccinal G04.02
specified NEC G04.89
syphilitic (transverse) A52.14
toxic G92
transverse (in demyelinating diseases of central nervous system) G37.3
tuberculous A17.82
varicella B01.12
Myeloblastic —*see* condition
Myeloblastoma
granular cell —*see also* Neoplasm, connective tissue
malignant —*see* Neoplasm, connective tissue, malignant
tongue D10.1
Myelocele —*see* Spina bifida
Myelocystocele —*see* Spina bifida
Myelocytic —*see* condition
Myelodysplasia D46.9
specified NEC D46.Z
spinal cord (congenital) Q06.1
Myelodysplastic syndrome D46.9
with
5q deletion D46.C
isolated del (5q) chromosomal abnormality C46.C
specified NEC D46.Z
Myeloencephalitis —*see* Encephalitis
Myelofibrosis D75.81
with myeloid metaplasia D47.4
acute C94.4- ●
idiopathic (chronic) D47.4
primary D47.1
secondary D75.81
in myeloproliferative disease D47.4
Myelogenous —*see* condition
Myeloid —*see* condition
Myelokathexis D70.9
Myeloleukodystrophy E75.29
Myelolipoma —*see* Lipoma
Myeloma (multiple) C90.0- ●
monostotic C90.3
plasma cell C90.0- ●
plasma cell C90.0- ●
solitary —*see also* Plasmacytoma, solitary C90.3- ●
Myelomalacia G95.89
Myelomatosis C90.0- ●
Myelomeningitis —*see* Meningoencephalitis
Myelomeningocele (spinal cord) —*see* Spina bifida
Myelo-osteo-musculodysplasia hereditaria Q79.8
Myelopathic
anemia D64.89
muscle atrophy —*see* Atrophy, muscle, spinal
pain syndrome G89.0
Myelopathy (spinal cord) G95.9
drug-induced G95.89
in (due to)
degeneration or displacement, intervertebral disc NEC —*see* Disorder, disc, with, myelopathy
infection —*see* Encephalitis
intervertebral disc disorder —*see also* Disorder, disc, with, myelopathy
mercury —*see* subcategory T56.1
neoplastic disease —*see also* Neoplasm D49.9 *[G99.2]*
pernicious anemia D51.0 *[G99.2]*
spondylosis —*see* Spondylosis, with myelopathy NEC
necrotic (subacute) (vascular) G95.19
radiation-induced G95.89
spondylogenic NEC —*see* Spondylosis, with myelopathy NEC
toxic G95.89
transverse, acute G37.3
vascular G95.19
vitamin B12 E53.8 *[G32.0]*
Myelophthisis D61.82
Myeloradiculitis G04.91
Myeloradiculodysplasia (spinal) Q06.1
Myelosarcoma C92.3- ●
Myelosclerosis D75.89
with myeloid metaplasia D47.4
disseminated, of nervous system G35
megakaryocytic D47.4
with myeloid metaplasia D47.4
Myelosis
acute C92.0- ●
aleukemic C92.9- ●
chronic D47.1
erythremic (acute) C94.0- ●
megakaryocytic C94.2- ●
nonleukemic D72.828
subacute C92.9- ●
Myiasis (cavernous) B87.9
aural B87.4
creeping B87.0
cutaneous B87.0
dermal B87.0
ear (external) (middle) B87.4
eye B87.2
genitourinary B87.81
intestinal B87.82
laryngeal B87.3
nasopharyngeal B87.3
ocular B87.2
orbit B87.2
skin B87.0
specified site NEC B87.89
traumatic B87.1
wound B87.1
Myoadenoma, prostate —*see* Hyperplasia, prostate
Myoblastoma
granular cell —*see also* Neoplasm, connective tissue, benign
malignant —*see* Neoplasm, connective tissue, malignant
tongue D10.1
Myocardial —*see* condition
Myocardiopathy (congestive) (constrictive) (familial) (hypertrophic nonobstructive) (idiopathic) (infiltrative) (obstructive) (primary) (restrictive) (sporadic) —*see also* Cardiomyopathy I42.9
alcoholic I42.6
cobalt-beer I42.6
glycogen storage E74.02 *[I43]*
hypertrophic obstructive I42.1
in (due to)
beriberi E51.12
cardiac glycogenosis E74.02 *[I43]*
Friedreich's ataxia G11.1 *[I43]*
myotonia atrophica G71.11 *[I43]*
progressive muscular dystrophy G71.03 *[I43]*

M

Myocardiopathy *(Continued)*
obscure (African) I42.8
secondary I42.9
thyrotoxic E05.90 *[I43]*
with storm E05.91 *[I43]*
toxic NEC I42.7
Myocarditis (with arteriosclerosis) (chronic) (fibroid) (interstitial) (old) (progressive) (senile) I51.4
with
rheumatic fever (conditions in I00) I09.0
active —*see* Myocarditis, acute, rheumatic
inactive or quiescent (with chorea) I09.0
active I40.9
rheumatic I01.2
with chorea (acute) (rheumatic) (Sydenham's) I02.0
acute or subacute (interstitial) I40.9
due to
streptococcus (beta-hemolytic) I01.2
idiopathic I40.1
rheumatic I01.2
with chorea (acute) (rheumatic) (Sydenham's) I02.0
specified NEC I40.8
aseptic of newborn B33.22
bacterial (acute) I40.0
Coxsackie (virus) B33.22
diphtheritic A36.81
eosinophilic I40.1
epidemic of newborn (Coxsackie) B33.22
Fiedler's (acute) (isolated) I40.1
giant cell (acute) (subacute) I40.1
gonococcal A54.83
granulomatous (idiopathic) (isolated) (nonspecific) I40.1
hypertensive —*see* Hypertension, heart
idiopathic (granulomatous) I40.1
in (due to)
diphtheria A36.81
epidemic louse-borne typhus A75.0 *[I41]*
Lyme disease A69.29
sarcoidosis D86.85
scarlet fever A38.1
toxoplasmosis (acquired) B58.81
typhoid A01.02
typhus NEC A75.9 *[I41]*
infective I40.0
influenzal —*see* Influenza, with, myocarditis
isolated (acute) I40.1
meningococcal A39.52
mumps B26.82
nonrheumatic, active I40.9
parenchymatous I40.9
pneumococcal I40.0
rheumatic (chronic) (inactive) (with chorea) I09.0
active or acute I01.2
with chorea (acute) (rheumatic) (Sydenham's) I02.0
rheumatoid —*see* Rheumatoid, carditis
septic I40.0
staphylococcal I40.0
suppurative I40.0
syphilitic (chronic) A52.06
toxic I40.8
rheumatic —*see* Myocarditis, acute, rheumatic
tuberculous A18.84
typhoid A01.02
valvular —*see* Endocarditis
virus, viral I40.0
of newborn (Coxsackie) B33.22
Myocardium, myocardial —*see* condition
Myocardosis —*see* Cardiomyopathy
Myoclonus, myoclonic, myoclonia (familial) (essential) (multifocal) (simplex) G25.3
drug-induced G25.3
epilepsy —*see also* Epilepsy, generalized, specified NEC G40.4-•
familial (progressive) G25.3
Myoclonus, myoclonic, myoclonia *(Continued)*
epileptica G40.409
with status epilepticus G40.401
facial G51.3-•
familial progressive G25.3
Friedreich's G25.3
jerks G25.3
massive G25.3
palatal G25.3
pharyngeal G25.3
Myocytolysis I51.5
Myodiastasis —*see* Diastasis, muscle
Myoendocarditis —*see* Endocarditis
Myoepithelioma —*see* Neoplasm, benign, by site
Myofasciitis (acute) —*see* Myositis
Myofibroma —*see also* Neoplasm, connective tissue, benign
uterus (cervix) (corpus) —*see* Leiomyoma
Myofibromatosis D48.1
infantile Q89.8
Myofibrosis M62.89
heart —*see* Myocarditis
scapulohumeral —*see* Lesion, shoulder, specified NEC
Myofibrositis M79.7
scapulohumeral —*see* Lesion, shoulder, specified NEC
Myoglobulinuria, myoglobinuria (primary) R82.1
Myokymia, facial G51.4
Myolipoma —*see* Lipoma
Myoma —*see also* Neoplasm, connective tissue, benign
malignant —*see* Neoplasm, connective tissue, malignant
prostate D29.1
uterus (cervix) (corpus) —*see* Leiomyoma
Myomalacia M62.89
Myometritis —*see* Endometritis
Myometrium —*see* condition
Myonecrosis, clostridial A48.0
Myopathy G72.9
acute
necrotizing G72.81
quadriplegic G72.81
alcoholic G72.1
benign congenital G71.2
central core G71.2
centronuclear G71.2
congenital (benign) G71.2
critical illness G72.81
distal G71.09
drug-induced G72.0
endocrine NEC E34.9 *[G73.7]*
extraocular muscles H05.82-•
facioscapulohumeral G71.02
hereditary G71.9
specified NEC G71.8
immune NEC G72.49
in (due to)
Addison's disease E27.1 *[G73.7]*
alcohol G72.1
amyloidosis E85.0 *[G73.7]*
cretinism E00.9 *[G73.7]*
Cushing's syndrome E24.9 *[G73.7]*
drugs G72.0
endocrine disease NEC E34.9 *[G73.7]*
giant cell arteritis M31.6 *[G73.7]*
glycogen storage disease E74.00 *[G73.7]*
hyperadrenocorticism E24.9 *[G73.7]*
hyperparathyroidism NEC E21.3 *[G73.7]*
hypoparathyroidism E20.9 *[G73.7]*
hypopituitarism E23.0 *[G73.7]*
hypothyroidism E03.9 *[G73.7]*
infectious disease NEC B99 *[G73.7]*
lipid storage disease E75.6 *[G73.7]*
metabolic disease NEC E88.9 *[G73.7]*
myxedema E03.9 *[G73.7]*
parasitic disease NEC B89 *[G73.7]*
polyarteritis nodosa M30.0 *[G73.7]*
Myopathy *(Continued)*
in (due to) *(Continued)*
rheumatoid arthritis —*see* Rheumatoid, myopathy
sarcoidosis D86.87
scleroderma M34.82
sicca syndrome M35.03
Sjögren's syndrome M35.03
systemic lupus erythematosus M32.19
thyrotoxicosis (hyperthyroidism) E05.90 *[G73.7]*
with thyroid storm E05.91 *[G73.7]*
toxic agent NEC G72.2
inflammatory NEC G72.49
intensive care (ICU) G72.81
limb-girdle G71.09
mitochondrial NEC G71.3
myotubular G71.2
mytonic, proximal (PROMM) G71.11
nemaline G71.2
ocular G71.09
oculopharyngeal G71.09
of critical illness G72.81
primary G71.9
specified NEC G71.8
progressive NEC G72.89
proximal myotonic (PROMM) G71.11
rod G71.2
scapulohumeral G71.02
specified NEC G72.89
toxic G72.2
Myopericarditis —*see also* Pericarditis
chronic rheumatic I09.2
Myopia (axial) (congenital) H52.1-•
degenerative (malignant) H44.20
with
choroidal neovascularization H44.2A-•
foveoschisis H44.2D-•
macular hole H44.2B-•
retinal detachment H44.2C-•
specified maculopathy NEC H44.2E-•
bilateral H44.23
left eye H44.22
right eye H44.21
malignant —*see also* Myopia, degenerative H44.2-•
pernicious —*see also* Myopia, degenerative H44.2-•
progressive high (degenerative) —*see also* Myopia, degenerative H44.2-•
Myosarcoma —*see* Neoplasm, connective tissue, malignant
Myosis (pupil) H57.03
stromal (endolymphatic) D39.0
Myositis M60.9
clostridial A48.0
due to posture —*see* Myositis, specified type NEC
epidemic B33.0
fibrosa or fibrous (chronic), Volkmann's T79.6
foreign body granuloma —*see* Granuloma, foreign body
in (due to)
bilharziasis B65.9 *[M63.8-•]*
cysticercosis B69.81
leprosy A30.9 *[M63.8-•]*
mycosis B49 *[M63.8-•]*
sarcoidosis D86.87
schistosomiasis B65.9 *[M63.8-•]*
syphilis
late A52.78
secondary A51.49
toxoplasmosis (acquired) B58.82
trichinellosis B75 *[M63.8-•]*
tuberculosis A18.09
inclusion body [IBM] G72.41
infective M60.009
arm M60.002
left M60.001
right M60.000

M

Myositis (Continued)
infective (Continued)
leg M60.005
left M60.004
right M60.003
lower limb M60.005
ankle M60.07-●
foot M60.07-●
lower leg M60.06-●
thigh M60.05-●
toe M60.07-●
multiple sites M60.09
specified site NEC M60.08
upper limb M60.002
finger M60.04-●
forearm M60.03-●
hand M60.04-●
shoulder region M60.01-●
upper arm M60.02-●
interstitial M60.10
ankle M60.17-●
foot M60.17-●
forearm M60.13-●
hand M60.14-●
lower leg M60.16-●
multiple sites M60.19
shoulder region M60.11-●
specified site NEC M60.18
thigh M60.15-●
upper arm M60.12-●
mycotic B49 *[M63.8-●]*
ossificans or ossifying (circumscripta) —*see also* Ossification, muscle, specified NEC
in (due to)
burns M61.30
ankle M61.37-●
foot M61.37-●
forearm M61.33-●
hand M61.34-●
lower leg M61.36-●
multiple sites M61.39
pelvic region M61.35-●
shoulder region M61.31-●
specified site NEC M61.38
thigh M61.35-●
upper arm M61.32-●
quadriplegia or paraplegia M61.20
ankle M61.27-●
foot M61.27-●
forearm M61.23-●
hand M61.24-●
lower leg M61.26-●
multiple sites M61.29
pelvic region M61.25-●

Myositis (Continued)
ossificans or ossifying (Continued)
in (due to) (Continued)
quadriplegia or paraplegia (Continued)
shoulder region M61.21-●
specified site NEC M61.28
thigh M61.25-●
upper arm M61.22-●
progressiva M61.10
ankle M61.17-●
finger M61.14-●
foot M61.17-●
forearm M61.13-●
hand M61.14-●
lower leg M61.16-●
multiple sites M61.19
pelvic region M61.15-●
shoulder region M61.11-●
specified site NEC M61.18
thigh M61.15-●
toe M61.17-●
upper arm M61.12-●
traumatica M61.00
ankle M61.07-●
foot M61.07-●
forearm M61.03-●
hand M61.04-●
lower leg M61.06-●
multiple sites M61.09
pelvic region M61.05-●
shoulder region M61.01-●
specified site NEC M61.08
thigh M61.05-●
upper arm M61.02-●
purulent —*see* Myositis, infective
specified type NEC M60.80
ankle M60.87-●
foot M60.87-●
forearm M60.83-●
hand M60.84-●
lower leg M60.86-●
multiple sites M60.89
pelvic region M60.85-●
shoulder region M60.81-●
specified site NEC M60.88
thigh M60.85-●
upper arm M60.82-●
suppurative —*see* Myositis, infective
traumatic (old) —*see* Myositis, specified type NEC
Myospasia impulsiva F95.2
Myotonia (acquisita) (intermittens) M62.89
atrophica G71.11
chondrodystrophic G71.13

Myotonia (Continued)
congenita (acetazolamide responsive) (dominant) (recessive) G71.12
drug-induced G71.14
dystrophica G71.11
fluctuans G71.19
levior G71.12
permanens G71.19
symptomatic G71.19
Myotonic pupil —*see* Anomaly, pupil, function, tonic pupil
Myriapodiasis B88.2
Myringitis H73.2-●
with otitis media —*see* Otitis, media
acute H73.00-●
bullous H73.01-●
specified NEC H73.09-●
bullous —*see* Myringitis, acute, bullous
chronic H73.1-●
Mysophobia F40.228
Mytilotoxism —*see* Poisoning, fish
Myxadenitis labialis K13.0
Myxedema (adult) (idiocy) (infantile) (juvenile) —*see also* Hypothyroidism E03.9
circumscribed E05.90
with storm E05.91
coma E03.5
congenital E00.1
cutis L98.5
localized (pretibial) E05.90
with storm E05.91
papular L98.5
Myxochondrosarcoma —*see* Neoplasm, cartilage, malignant
Myxofibroma —*see* Neoplasm, connective tissue, benign
odontogenic —*see* Cyst, calcifying odontogenic
Myxofibrosarcoma —*see* Neoplasm, connective tissue, malignant
Myxolipoma D17.9
Myxoliposarcoma —*see* Neoplasm, connective tissue, malignant
Myxoma —*see also* Neoplasm, connective tissue, benign
nerve sheath —*see* Neoplasm, nerve, benign
odontogenic —*see* Cyst, calcifying odontogenic
Myxosarcoma —*see* Neoplasm, connective tissue, malignant

M

N

- Naegeli's
  - disease Q82.8
  - leukemia, monocytic C93.1-●
- Naegleriasis (with meningoencephalitis) B6Ø.2
- Naffziger's syndrome G54.Ø
- Naga sore —*see* Ulcer, skin
- Nägele's pelvis M95.5
  - with disproportion (fetopelvic) O33.Ø
    - causing obstructed labor O65.Ø
- Nail —*see also* condition
  - biting F98.8
  - patella syndrome Q87.2
- Nanism, nanosomia —*see* Dwarfism
- Nanophyetiasis B66.8
- Nanukayami A27.89
- Napkin rash L22
- Narcolepsy G47.419
  - with cataplexy G47.411
  - in conditions classified elsewhere G47.429
    - with cataplexy G47.421
- Narcosis RØ6.89
- Narcotism —*see* Dependence
- NARP (Neuropathy, Ataxia and Retinitis pigmentosa) syndrome E88.49
- Narrow
  - anterior chamber angle H4Ø.Ø3-●
  - gingival width (of periodontal soft tissue) KØ5.5
  - pelvis —*see* Contraction, pelvis
- Narrowing —*see also* Stenosis
  - artery I77.1
    - auditory, internal I65.8
    - basilar —*see* Occlusion, artery, basilar
    - carotid —*see* Occlusion, artery, carotid
    - cerebellar —*see* Occlusion, artery, cerebellar
    - cerebral —*see* Occlusion artery, cerebral
    - choroidal —*see* Occlusion, artery, precerebral, specified NEC
    - communicating posterior —*see* Occlusion, artery, precerebral, specified NEC
    - coronary —*see also* Disease, heart, ischemic, atherosclerotic
      - congenital Q24.5
        - syphilitic A5Ø.54 *[I52]*
      - due to syphilis NEC A52.Ø6
    - hypophyseal —*see* Occlusion, artery, precerebral, specified NEC
    - pontine —*see* Occlusion, artery, precerebral, specified NEC
    - precerebral —*see* Occlusion, artery, precerebral
    - vertebral —*see* Occlusion, artery, vertebral
  - auditory canal (external) —*see* Stenosis, external ear canal
  - eustachian tube —*see* Obstruction, eustachian tube
  - eyelid —*see* Disorder, eyelid function
  - larynx J38.6
  - mesenteric artery —*see also* Ischemia, intestine, acute K55.Ø59
  - palate M26.89
  - palpebral fissure —*see* Disorder, eyelid function
  - ureter N13.5
    - with infection N13.6
  - urethra —*see* Stricture, urethra
- Narrowness, abnormal, eyelid Q1Ø.3
- Nasal —*see* condition
- Nasolachrymal, nasolacrimal —*see* condition
- Nasopharyngeal —*see also* condition
  - pituitary gland Q89.2
  - torticollis M43.6
- Nasopharyngitis (acute) (infective) (streptococcal) (subacute) JØØ
  - chronic (suppurative) (ulcerative) J31.1
- Nasopharynx, nasopharyngeal —*see* condition
- Natal tooth, teeth KØØ.6
- Nausea (without vomiting) R11.Ø
  - with vomiting R11.2
  - gravidarum —*see* Hyperemesis, gravidarum
  - marina T75.3
  - navalis T75.3
- Navel —*see* condition
- Neapolitan fever —*see* Brucellosis
- Near drowning T75.1
- Nearsightedness —*see* Myopia
- Near-syncope R55
- Nebula, cornea —*see* Opacity, cornea
- Necator americanus infestation B76.1
- Necatoriasis B76.1
- Neck —*see* condition
- Necrobiosis R68.89
  - lipoidica NEC L92.1
    - with diabetes —*see* EØ8-E13 with .62Ø
- Necrolysis, toxic epidermal L51.2
  - due to drug
    - correct substance properly administered —*see* Table of Drugs and Chemicals, by drug, adverse effect
    - overdose or wrong substance given or taken —*see* Table of Drugs and Chemicals, by drug, poisoning
- Necrophilia F65.89
- Necrosis, necrotic (ischemic) —*see also* Gangrene
  - adrenal (capsule) (gland) E27.49
  - amputation stump (surgical) (late) T87.5Ø
    - arm T87.5-●
    - leg T87.5-●
  - antrum J32.Ø
  - aorta (hyaline) —*see also* Aneurysm, aorta
    - cystic medial —*see* Dissection, aorta
  - artery I77.5
  - bladder (aseptic) (sphincter) N32.89
  - bone —*see also* Osteonecrosis M87.9
    - aseptic or avascular —*see* Osteonecrosis
      - idiopathic M87.ØØ
    - ethmoid J32.2
    - jaw M27.2
    - tuberculous —*see* Tuberculosis, bone
  - brain I67.89
  - breast (aseptic) (fat) (segmental) N64.1
  - bronchus J98.Ø9
  - central nervous system NEC I67.89
  - cerebellar I67.89
  - cerebral I67.89
  - colon —*see also* Infarct, intestine K55.Ø49
  - cornea H18.89-●
  - cortical (acute) (renal) N17.1
  - cystic medial (aorta) —*see* Dissection, aorta
  - dental pulp KØ4.1
  - esophagus K22.8
  - ethmoid (bone) J32.2
  - eyelid —*see* Disorder, eyelid, degenerative
  - fat, fatty (generalized) —*see also* Disorder, soft tissue, specified type NEC
    - abdominal wall K65.4
    - breast (aseptic) (segmental) N64.1
    - localized —*see* Degeneration, by site, fatty
    - mesentery K65.4
    - omentum K65.4
    - pancreas K86.89
    - peritoneum K65.4
    - skin (subcutaneous), newborn P83.Ø
    - subcutaneous, due to birth injury P15.6
  - gallbladder —*see* Cholecystitis, acute
  - heart —*see* Infarct, myocardium
  - hip, aseptic or avascular —*see* Osteonecrosis, by type, femur
  - intestine (acute) (hemorrhagic) (massive) —*see also* Infarct, intestine K55.Ø69
  - jaw M27.2
  - kidney (bilateral) N28.Ø
    - acute N17.9
    - cortical (acute) (bilateral) N17.1
      - with ectopic or molar pregnancy OØ8.4
    - medullary (bilateral) (in acute renal failure) (papillary) N17.2
- Necrosis, necrotic *(Continued)*
  - kidney *(Continued)*
    - papillary (bilateral) (in acute renal failure) N17.2
    - tubular N17.Ø
      - with ectopic or molar pregnancy OØ8.4
      - complicating
        - abortion —*see* Abortion, by type, complicated by, tubular necrosis
        - ectopic or molar pregnancy OØ8.4
        - pregnancy —*see* Pregnancy, complicated by, diseases of, specified type or system NEC
      - following ectopic or molar pregnancy OØ8.4
      - traumatic T79.5
  - larynx J38.7
  - liver (with hepatic failure) (cell) —*see* Failure, hepatic
    - hemorrhagic, central K76.2
  - lung J85.Ø
  - lymphatic gland —*see* Lymphadenitis, acute
  - mammary gland (fat) (segmental) N64.1
  - mastoid (chronic) —*see* Mastoiditis, chronic
  - medullary (acute) (renal) N17.2
  - mesentery —*see also* Infarct, intestine K55.Ø69
    - fat K65.4
  - mitral valve —*see* Insufficiency, mitral
  - myocardium, myocardial —*see* Infarct, myocardium
  - nose J34.Ø
  - omentum (with mesenteric infarction) —*see also* Infarct, intestine K55.Ø69
    - fat K65.4
  - orbit, orbital —*see* Osteomyelitis, orbit
  - ossicles, ear —*see* Abnormal, ear ossicles
  - ovary N7Ø.92
  - pancreas (aseptic) (duct) (fat) K86.89
    - acute (infective) —*see* Pancreatitis, acute
    - infective —*see* Pancreatitis, acute
  - papillary (acute) (renal) N17.2
  - perineum N9Ø.89
  - peritoneum (with mesenteric infarction) —*see also* Infarct, intestine K55.Ø69
    - fat K65.4
  - pharynx JØ2.9
    - in granulocytopenia —*see* Neutropenia
    - Vincent's A69.1
  - phosphorus —*see* subcategory T54.2
  - pituitary (gland) E23.Ø
    - postpartum O99.285
    - Sheehan O99.285
  - pressure —*see* Ulcer, pressure, by site
  - pulmonary J85.Ø
  - pulp (dental) KØ4.1
  - radiation —*see* Necrosis, by site
  - radium —*see* Necrosis, by site
  - renal —*see* Necrosis, kidney
  - sclera H15.89
  - scrotum N5Ø.89
  - skin or subcutaneous tissue NEC I96
  - spine, spinal (column) —*see also* Osteonecrosis, by type, vertebra
    - cord G95.19
  - spleen D73.5
  - stomach K31.89
  - stomatitis (ulcerative) A69.Ø
  - subcutaneous fat, newborn P83.88
  - subendocardial (acute) I21.4
    - chronic I25.89
  - suprarenal (capsule) (gland) E27.49
  - testis N5Ø.89
  - thymus (gland) E32.8
  - tonsil J35.8
  - trachea J39.8
  - tuberculous NEC —*see* Tuberculosis
  - tubular (acute) (anoxic) (renal) (toxic) N17.Ø
    - postprocedural N99.Ø

Necrosis, necrotic *(Continued)*
vagina N89.8
vertebra —*see also* Osteonecrosis, by type, vertebra
tuberculous A18.01
vulva N90.89
X-ray —*see* Necrosis, by site
Necrospermia —*see* Infertility, male
Need (for)
care provider because (of)
assistance with personal care Z74.1
continuous supervision required Z74.3
impaired mobility Z74.09
no other household member able to render care Z74.2
specified reason NEC Z74.8
immunization —*see* Vaccination
vaccination —*see* Vaccination
Neglect
adult
confirmed T74.01
history of Z91.412
suspected T76.01
child (childhood)
confirmed T74.02
history of Z62.812
suspected T76.02
emotional, in childhood Z62.898
hemispatial R41.4
left-sided R41.4
sensory R41.4
visuospatial R41.4
Neisserian infection NEC —*see* Gonococcus
Nelaton's syndrome G60.8
Nelson's syndrome E24.1
Nematodiasis (intestinal) B82.0
Ancylostoma B76.0
Neonatal —*see also* Newborn
acne L70.4
bradycardia P29.12
screening, abnormal findings on P09
tachycardia P29.11
tooth, teeth K00.6
Neonatorum —*see* condition
Neoplasia
endocrine, multiple (MEN) E31.20
type I E31.21
type IIA E31.22
type IIB E31.23
intraepithelial (histologically confirmed)
anal (AIN) (histologically confirmed) K62.82
grade I K62.82
grade II K62.82
severe D01.3
cervical glandular (histologically confirmed) D06.9
cervix (uteri) (CIN) (histologically confirmed) N87.9
glandular D06.9
grade I N87.0
grade II N87.1
grade III (severe dysplasia) —*see also* Carcinoma, cervix uteri, in situ D06.9
prostate (histologically confirmed) (PIN) N42.31
grade I N42.31
grade II N42.31
grade III (severe dysplasia) D07.5
vagina (histologically confirmed) (VAIN) N89.3
grade I N89.0
grade II N89.1
grade III (severe dysplasia) D07.2
vulva (histologically confirmed) (VIN) N90.3
grade I N90.0
grade II N90.1
grade III (severe dysplasia) D07.1
Neoplasm, neoplastic —*see also* Table of Neoplasms
lipomatous, benign —*see* Lipoma
malignant mast cell C96.20
specified type NEC C96.29
mast cell, of uncertain behavior NEC D47.09
Neovascularization
ciliary body —*see* Disorder, iris, vascular
cornea H16.40-•
deep H16.44-•
ghost vessels —*see* Ghost, vessels
localized H16.43-•
pannus —*see* Pannus
iris —*see* Disorder, iris, vascular
retina H35.05-•
Nephralgia N23
Nephritis, nephritic (albuminuric) (azotemic) (congenital) (disseminated) (epithelial) (familial) (focal) (granulomatous) (hemorrhagic) (infantile) (nonsuppurative, excretory) (uremic) N05.9
with
dense deposit disease N05.6
diffuse
crescentic glomerulonephritis N05.7
endocapillary proliferative glomerulonephritis N05.4
membranous glomerulonephritis N05.2
mesangial proliferative glomerulonephritis N05.3
mesangiocapillary glomerulonephritis N05.5
edema —*see* Nephrosis
focal and segmental glomerular lesions N05.1
foot process disease N04.9
glomerular lesion
diffuse sclerosing N05.8
hypocomplementemic —*see* Nephritis, membranoproliferative
IgA —*see* Nephropathy, IgA
lobular, lobulonodular —*see* Nephritis, membranoproliferative
nodular —*see* Nephritis, membranoproliferative
lesion of
glomerulonephritis, proliferative N05.8
renal necrosis N05.9
minor glomerular abnormality N05.0
specified morphological changes NEC N05.8
acute N00.9
with
dense deposit disease N00.6
diffuse
crescentic glomerulonephritis N00.7
endocapillary proliferative glomerulonephritis N00.4
membranous glomerulonephritis N00.2
mesangial proliferative glomerulonephritis N00.3
mesangiocapillary glomerulonephritis N00.5
focal and segmental glomerular lesions N00.1
minor glomerular abnormality N00.0
specified morphological changes NEC N00.8
amyloid E85.4 *[N08]*
antiglomerular basement membrane (anti-GBM) antibody NEC
in Goodpasture's syndrome M31.0
antitubular basement membrane (tubulo-interstitial) NEC N12
toxic —*see* Nephropathy, toxic
arteriolar —*see* Hypertension, kidney
arteriosclerotic —*see* Hypertension, kidney
ascending —*see* Nephritis, tubulo-interstitial
atrophic N03.9
Nephritis, nephritic *(Continued)*
Balkan (endemic) N15.0
calculous, calculus —*see* Calculus, kidney
cardiac —*see* Hypertension, kidney
cardiovascular —*see* Hypertension, kidney
chronic N03.9
with
dense deposit disease N03.6
diffuse
crescentic glomerulonephritis N03.7
endocapillary proliferative glomerulonephritis N03.4
membranous glomerulonephritis N03.2
mesangial proliferative glomerulonephritis N03.3
mesangiocapillary glomerulonephritis N03.5
focal and segmental glomerular lesions N03.1
minor glomerular abnormality N03.0
specified morphological changes NEC N03.8
arteriosclerotic —*see* Hypertension, kidney
cirrhotic N26.9
complicating pregnancy O26.83-•
croupous N00.9
degenerative —*see* Nephrosis
diffuse sclerosing N05.8
due to
diabetes mellitus —*see* E08-E13 with .21
subacute bacterial endocarditis I33.0
systemic lupus erythematosus (chronic) M32.14
typhoid fever A01.09
gonococcal (acute) (chronic) A54.21
hypocomplementemic —*see* Nephritis, membranoproliferative
IgA —*see* Nephropathy, IgA
immune complex (circulating) NEC N05.8
infective —*see* Nephritis, tubulo-interstitial
interstitial —*see* Nephritis, tubulo-interstitial
lead N14.3
membranoproliferative (diffuse) (type 1 or 3) —*see also* N00-N07 with fourth character .5 N05.5
type 2 —*see also* N00-N07 with fourth character .6 N05.6
minimal change N05.0
necrotic, necrotizing NEC —*see also* N00-N07 with fourth character .8 N05.8
nephrotic —*see* Nephrosis
nodular —*see* Nephritis, membranoproliferative
polycystic Q61.3
adult type Q61.2
autosomal
dominant Q61.2
recessive NEC Q61.19
childhood type NEC Q61.19
infantile type NEC Q61.19
poststreptococcal N05.9
acute N00.9
chronic N03.9
rapidly progressive N01.9
proliferative NEC —*see also* N00-N07 with fourth character .8 N05.8
purulent —*see* Nephritis, tubulo-interstitial
rapidly progressive N01.9
with
dense deposit disease N01.6
diffuse
crescentic glomerulonephritis N01.7
endocapillary proliferative glomerulonephritis N01.4

Nephritis, nephritic (Continued)
rapidly progressive (Continued)
with (Continued)
diffuse (Continued)
membranous glomerulonephritis N01.2
mesangial proliferative glomerulonephritis N01.3
mesangiocapillary glomerulonephritis N01.5
focal and segmental glomerular lesions N01.1
minor glomerular abnormality N01.0
specified morphological changes NEC N01.8
salt losing or wasting NEC N28.89
saturnine N14.3
sclerosing, diffuse N05.8
septic —see Nephritis, tubulo-interstitial
specified pathology NEC —see also N00-N07
with fourth character .8 N05.8
subacute N01.9
suppurative —see Nephritis, tubulo-interstitial
syphilitic (late) A52.75
congenital A50.59 [N08]
early (secondary) A51.44
toxic —see Nephropathy, toxic
tubal, tubular —see Nephritis, tubulo-interstitial
tuberculous A18.11
tubulo-interstitial (in) N12
acute (infectious) N10
chronic (infectious) N11.9
nonobstructive N11.8
reflux-associated N11.0
obstructive N11.1
specified NEC N11.8
due to
brucellosis A23.9 [N16]
cryoglobulinemia D89.1 [N16]
glycogen storage disease E74.00 [N16]
Sjögren's syndrome M35.04
vascular —see Hypertension, kidney
war N00.9
Nephroblastoma (epithelial) (mesenchymal) C64-•
Nephrocalcinosis E83.59 [N29]
Nephrocystitis, pustular —see Nephritis, tubulo-interstitial
Nephrolithiasis (congenital) (pelvis) (recurrent) —see also Calculus, kidney
Nephroma C64-•
mesoblastic D41.0-•
Nephronephritis —see Nephrosis
Nephronophthisis Q61.5
Nephropathia epidemica A98.5
Nephropathy —see also Nephritis N28.9
with
edema —see Nephrosis
glomerular lesion —see Glomerulonephritis
amyloid, hereditary E85.0
analgesic N14.0
with medullary necrosis, acute N17.2
Balkan (endemic) N15.0
chemical —see Nephropathy, toxic
diabetic —see E08-E13 with .21
drug-induced N14.2
specified NEC N14.1
focal and segmental hyalinosis or sclerosis N02.1
heavy metal-induced N14.3
hereditary NEC N07.9
with
dense deposit disease N07.6
diffuse
crescentic glomerulonephritis N07.7
endocapillary proliferative glomerulonephritis N07.4
Nephropathy (Continued)
hereditary NEC (Continued)
with (Continued)
diffuse (Continued)
membranous glomerulonephritis N07.2
mesangial proliferative glomerulonephritis N07.3
mesangiocapillary glomerulonephritis N07.5
focal and segmental glomerular lesions N07.1
minor glomerular abnormality N07.0
specified morphological changes NEC N07.8
hypercalcemic N25.89
hypertensive —see Hypertension, kidney
hypokalemic (vacuolar) N25.89
IgA N02.8
with glomerular lesion N02.9
focal and segmental hyalinosis or sclerosis N02.1
membranoproliferative (diffuse) N02.5
membranous (diffuse) N02.2
mesangial proliferative (diffuse) N02.3
mesangiocapillary (diffuse) N02.5
proliferative NEC N02.8
specified pathology NEC N02.8
lead N14.3
membranoproliferative (diffuse) N02.5
membranous (diffuse) N02.2
mesangial (IgA/IgG) —see Nephropathy, IgA
proliferative (diffuse) N02.3
mesangiocapillary (diffuse) N02.5
obstructive N13.8
phenacetin N17.2
phosphate-losing N25.0
potassium depletion N25.89
pregnancy-related O26.83-•
proliferative NEC (see also N00-N07 with fourth character .8) N05.8
protein-losing N25.89
saturnine N14.3
sickle-cell D57.-• [N08]
toxic NEC N14.4
due to
drugs N14.2
analgesic N14.0
specified NEC N14.1
heavy metals N14.3
vasomotor N17.0
water-losing N25.89
Nephroptosis N28.83
Nephropyosis —see Abscess, kidney
Nephrorrhagia N28.89
Nephrosclerosis (arteriolar) (arteriosclerotic) (chronic) (hyaline) —see also Hypertension, kidney
hyperplastic —see Hypertension, kidney
senile N26.9
Nephrosis, nephrotic (Epstein's) (syndrome) (congenital) N04.9
with
foot process disease N04.9
glomerular lesion N04.1
hypocomplementemic N04.5
acute N04.9
anoxic —see Nephrosis, tubular
chemical —see Nephrosis, tubular
cholemic K76.7
diabetic —see E08-E13 with .21
Finnish type (congenital) Q89.8
hemoglobin N10
hemoglobinuric —see Nephrosis, tubular
in
amyloidosis E85.4 [N08]
diabetes mellitus —see E08-E13 with .21
epidemic hemorrhagic fever A98.5
malaria (malariae) B52.0
ischemic —see Nephrosis, tubular
lipoid N04.9
Nephrosis, nephrotic (Continued)
lower nephron —see Nephrosis, tubular
malarial (malariae) B52.0
minimal change N04.0
myoglobin N10
necrotizing —see Nephrosis, tubular
osmotic (sucrose) N25.89
radiation N04.9
syphilitic (late) A52.75
toxic —see Nephrosis, tubular
tubular (acute) N17.0
postprocedural N99.0
radiation N04.9
Nephrosonephritis, hemorrhagic (endemic) A98.5
Nephrostomy
attention to Z43.6
status Z93.6
Nerve —see also condition
injury —see Injury, nerve, by body site
Nerves R45.0
Nervous —see also condition R45.0
heart F45.8
stomach F45.8
tension R45.0
Nervousness R45.0
Nesidioblastoma
pancreas D13.7
specified site NEC —see Neoplasm, benign, by site
unspecified site D13.7
Nettleship's syndrome —see Urticaria pigmentosa
Neumann's disease or syndrome L10.1
Neuralgia, neuralgic (acute) M79.2
accessory (nerve) G52.8
acoustic (nerve) —see subcategory H93.3
auditory (nerve) —see subcategory H93.3
ciliary G44.009
intractable G44.001
not intractable G44.009
cranial
nerve —see also Disorder, nerve, cranial
fifth or trigeminal —see Neuralgia, trigeminal
postherpetic, postzoster B02.29
ear —see subcategory H92.0
facialis vera G51.1
Fothergill's —see Neuralgia, trigeminal
glossopharyngeal (nerve) G52.1
Horton's G44.099
intractable G44.091
not intractable G44.099
Hunt's B02.21
hypoglossal (nerve) G52.3
infraorbital —see Neuralgia, trigeminal
malarial —see Malaria
migrainous G44.009
intractable G44.001
not intractable G44.009
Morton's G57.6-•
nerve, cranial —see Disorder, nerve, cranial
nose G52.0
occipital M54.81
olfactory G52.0
penis N48.9
perineum R10.2
postherpetic NEC B02.29
trigeminal B02.22
pubic region R10.2
scrotum R10.2
Sluder's G44.89
specified nerve NEC G58.8
spermatic cord R10.2
sphenopalatine (ganglion) G90.09
trifacial —see Neuralgia, trigeminal
trigeminal G50.0
postherpetic, postzoster B02.22
vagus (nerve) G52.2
writer's F48.8
organic G25.89

N

Neurapraxia —*see* Injury, nerve
Neurasthenia F48.8
  cardiac F45.8
  gastric F45.8
  heart F45.8
Neurilemmoma —*see also* Neoplasm, nerve, benign
  acoustic (nerve) D33.3
  malignant —*see also* Neoplasm, nerve, malignant
    acoustic (nerve) C72.4
Neurilemmosarcoma —*see* Neoplasm, nerve, malignant
Neurinoma —*see* Neoplasm, nerve, benign
Neurinomatosis —*see* Neoplasm, nerve, uncertain behavior
Neuritis (rheumatoid) M79.2
  abducens (nerve) —*see* Strabismus, paralytic, sixth nerve
  accessory (nerve) G52.8
  acoustic (nerve) —*see also* subcategory H93.3
    in (due to)
      infectious disease NEC B99 *[H94.Ø-●]*
      parasitic disease NEC B89 *[H94.Ø-●]*
    syphilitic A52.15
  alcoholic G62.1
    with psychosis —*see* Psychosis, alcoholic
  amyloid, any site E85.4 *[G63]*
  auditory (nerve) —*see* subcategory H93.3
  brachial —*see* Radiculopathy
    due to displacement, intervertebral disc —*see* Disorder, disc, cervical, with neuritis
  cranial nerve
    due to Lyme disease A69.22
    eighth or acoustic or auditory —*see* subcategory H93.3
    eleventh or accessory G52.8
    fifth or trigeminal G51.Ø
    first or olfactory G52.Ø
    fourth or trochlear —*see* Strabismus, paralytic, fourth nerve
    second or optic —*see* Neuritis, optic
    seventh or facial G51.8
      newborn (birth injury) P11.3
    sixth or abducent —*see* Strabismus, paralytic, sixth nerve
    tenth or vagus G52.2
    third or oculomotor —*see* Strabismus, paralytic, third nerve
    twelfth or hypoglossal G52.3
  Déjérine-Sottas G6Ø.Ø
  diabetic (mononeuropathy) —*see* EØ8-E13 with .41
    polyneuropathy —*see* EØ8-E13 with .42
  due to
    beriberi E51.11
    displacement, prolapse or rupture, intervertebral disc —*see* Disorder, disc, with, radiculopathy
    herniation, nucleus pulposus M51.9 *[G55]*
  endemic E51.11
  facial G51.8
    newborn (birth injury) P11.3
  general —*see* Polyneuropathy
  geniculate ganglion G51.1
    due to herpes (zoster) BØ2.21
  gouty —*see also* Gout, by type M1Ø.9 *[G63]*
  hypoglossal (nerve) G52.3
  ilioinguinal (nerve) G57.9-●
  infectious (multiple) NEC G61.Ø
  interstitial hypertrophic progressive G6Ø.Ø
  lumbar M54.16
  lumbosacral M54.17
  multiple —*see also* Polyneuropathy
    endemic E51.11
    infective, acute G61.Ø
  multiplex endemica E51.11
  nerve root —*see* Radiculopathy
  oculomotor (nerve) —*see* Strabismus, paralytic, third nerve
Neuritis *(Continued)*
  olfactory nerve G52.Ø
  optic (nerve) (hereditary) (sympathetic) H46.9
    with demyelination G36.Ø
    in myelitis G36.Ø
    nutritional H46.2
    papillitis —*see* Papillitis, optic
    retrobulbar H46.1-●
    specified type NEC H46.8
    toxic H46.3
  peripheral (nerve) G62.9
    multiple —*see* Polyneuropathy
    single —*see* Mononeuritis
  pneumogastric (nerve) G52.2
  postherpetic, postzoster BØ2.29
  progressive hypertrophic interstitial G6Ø.Ø
  retrobulbar —*see also* Neuritis, optic, retrobulbar
    in (due to)
      late syphilis A52.15
      meningococcal infection A39.82
    meningococcal A39.82
    syphilitic A52.15
  sciatic (nerve) —*see also* Sciatica
    due to displacement of intervertebral disc —*see* Disorder, disc, with, radiculopathy
  serum —*see also* Reaction, serum T8Ø.69
  shoulder-girdle G54.5
  specified nerve NEC G58.8
  spinal (nerve) root —*see* Radiculopathy
  syphilitic A52.15
  thenar (median) G56.1-●
  thoracic M54.14
  toxic NEC G62.2
  trochlear (nerve) —*see* Strabismus, paralytic, fourth nerve
  vagus (nerve) G52.2
Neuroastrocytoma —*see* Neoplasm, uncertain behavior, by site
Neuroavitaminosis E56.9 *[G99.8]*
Neuroblastoma
  olfactory C3Ø.Ø
  specified site —*see* Neoplasm, malignant, by site
  unspecified site C74.9Ø
Neurochorioretinitis —*see* Chorioretinitis
Neurocirculatory asthenia F45.8
Neurocysticercosis B69.Ø
Neurocytoma —*see* Neoplasm, benign, by site
Neurodermatitis (circumscribed) (circumscripta) (local) L28.Ø
  atopic L2Ø.81
  diffuse (Brocq) L2Ø.81
  disseminated L2Ø.81
Neuroencephalomyelopathy, optic G36.Ø
Neuroepithelioma —*see also* Neoplasm, malignant, by site
  olfactory C3Ø.Ø
Neurofibroma —*see also* Neoplasm, nerve, benign
  melanotic —*see* Neoplasm, nerve, benign
  multiple —*see* Neurofibromatosis
  plexiform —*see* Neoplasm, nerve, benign
Neurofibromatosis (multiple) (nonmalignant) Q85.ØØ
  acoustic Q85.Ø2
  malignant —*see* Neoplasm, nerve, malignant
  specified NEC Q85.Ø9
  type 1 (von Recklinghausen) Q85.Ø1
  type 2 Q85.Ø2
Neurofibrosarcoma —*see* Neoplasm, nerve, malignant
Neurogenic —*see also* condition
  bladder —*see also* Dysfunction, bladder, neuromuscular N31.9
    cauda equina syndrome G83.4
  bowel NEC K59.2
  heart F45.8
Neuroglioma —*see* Neoplasm, uncertain behavior, by site
Neurolabyrinthitis (of Dix and Hallpike) —*see* Neuronitis, vestibular
Neurolathyrism —*see* Poisoning, food, noxious, plant
Neuroleprosy A3Ø.9
Neuroma —*see also* Neoplasm, nerve, benign
  acoustic (nerve) D33.3
  amputation (stump) (traumatic) (surgical complication) (late) T87.3-●
    arm T87.3-●
    leg T87.3-●
  digital (toe) G57.6-●
  interdigital G58.8
    lower limb toe G57.8-●
    upper limb G56.8-●
  intermetatarsal G57.8-●
  Morton's G57.6-●
  nonneoplastic
    arm G56.9-●
    leg G57.9-●
    lower extremity G57.9-●
    upper extremity G56.9-●
  optic (nerve) D33.3
  plantar G57.6-●
  plexiform —*see* Neoplasm, nerve, benign
  surgical (nonneoplastic)
    arm G56.9-●
    leg G57.9-●
    lower extremity G57.9-●
    upper extremity G56.9-●
Neuromyalgia —*see* Neuralgia
Neuromyasthenia (epidemic) (postinfectious) G93.3
Neuromyelitis G36.9
  ascending G61.Ø
  optica G36.Ø
Neuromyopathy G7Ø.9
  paraneoplastic D49.9 *[G13.Ø]*
Neuromyotonia (Isaacs) G71.19
Neuronevus —*see* Nevus
Neuronitis G58.9
  ascending (acute) G57.2-●
  vestibular H81.2-●
Neuroparalytic —*see* condition
Neuropathy, neuropathic G62.9
  acute motor G62.81
  alcoholic G62.1
    with psychosis —*see* Psychosis, alcoholic
  arm G56.9-●
  autonomic, peripheral —*see* Neuropathy, peripheral, autonomic
  axillary G56.9-●
  bladder N31.9
    atonic (motor) (sensory) N31.2
    autonomous N31.2
    flaccid N31.2
    nonreflex N31.2
    reflex N31.1
    uninhibited N31.Ø
  brachial plexus G54.Ø
  cervical plexus G54.2
  chronic
    progressive segmentally demyelinating G62.89
    relapsing demyelinating G62.89
  Déjérine-Sottas G6Ø.Ø
  diabetic —*see* EØ8-E13 with .4Ø
    mononeuropathy —*see* EØ8-E13 with .41
    polyneuropathy —*see* EØ8-E13 with .42
  entrapment G58.9
    iliohypogastric nerve G57.8-●
    ilioinguinal nerve G57.8-●
    lateral cutaneous nerve of thigh G57.1-●
    median nerve G56.Ø-●
    obturator nerve G57.8-●
    peroneal nerve G57.3-●
    posterior tibial nerve G57.5-●
    saphenous nerve G57.8-●
    ulnar nerve G56.2-●

N

Neuropathy, neuropathic *(Continued)*
  facial nerve G51.9
  hereditary G6Ø.9
    motor and sensory (types I-IV) G6Ø.Ø
    sensory G6Ø.8
    specified NEC G6Ø.8
  hypertrophic G6Ø.Ø
    Charcot-Marie-Tooth G6Ø.Ø
    Déjérine-Sottas G6Ø.Ø
    interstitial progressive G6Ø.Ø
    of infancy G6Ø.Ø
    Refsum G6Ø.1
  idiopathic G6Ø.9
    progressive G6Ø.3
    specified NEC G6Ø.8
  in association with hereditary ataxia G6Ø.2
  intercostal G58.Ø
  ischemic —*see* Disorder, nerve
  Jamaica (ginger) G62.2
  leg NEC G57.9-●
  lower extremity G57.9-●
  lumbar plexus G54.1
  median nerve G56.1-●
  motor and sensory —*see also* Polyneuropathy
    hereditary (types I-IV) G6Ø.Ø
  multifocal motor (MMN) G61.82
  multiple (acute) (chronic) —*see* Polyneuropathy
  optic (nerve) —*see also* Neuritis, optic
    ischemic H47.Ø1-●
  paraneoplastic (sensorial) (Denny Brown) D49.9 *[G13.Ø]*
  peripheral (nerve) —*see also* Polyneuropathy G62.9
    autonomic G9Ø.9
      idiopathic G9Ø.Ø9
      in (due to)
        amyloidosis E85.4 *[G99.Ø]*
        diabetes mellitus —*see* EØ8-E13 with .43
        endocrine disease NEC E34.9 *[G99.Ø]*
        gout M1Ø.ØØ *[G99.Ø]*
        hyperthyroidism EØ5.9Ø *[G99.Ø]*
          with thyroid storm EØ5.91 *[G99.Ø]*
        metabolic disease NEC E88.9 *[G99.Ø]*
    idiopathic G6Ø.9
      progressive G6Ø.3
    in (due to)
      antitetanus serum G62.Ø
      arsenic G62.2
      drugs NEC G62.Ø
      lead G62.2
      organophosphate compounds G62.2
      toxic agent NEC G62.2
  plantar nerves G57.6-●
  progressive
    hypertrophic interstitial G6Ø.Ø
    inflammatory G62.81
  radicular NEC —*see* Radiculopathy
  sacral plexus G54.1
  sciatic G57.Ø-●
  serum G61.1
  toxic NEC G62.2
  trigeminal sensory G5Ø.8
  ulnar nerve G56.2-●
  uremic N18.9 *[G63]*
  vitamin B12 E53.8 *[G63]*
    with anemia (pernicious) D51.Ø *[G63]*
      due to dietary deficiency D51.3 *[G63]*
Neurophthisis —*see also* Disorder, nerve
  peripheral, diabetic —*see* EØ8-E13 with .42
Neuroretinitis —*see* Chorioretinitis
Neuroretinopathy, hereditary optic H47.22
Neurosarcoma —*see* Neoplasm, nerve, malignant
Neurosclerosis —*see* Disorder, nerve
Neurosis, neurotic F48.9
  anankastic F42.8
  anxiety (state) F41.1
    panic type F41.Ø
  asthenic F48.8
  bladder F45.8
Neurosis, neurotic *(Continued)*
  cardiac (reflex) F45.8
  cardiovascular F45.8
  character F6Ø.9
  colon F45.8
  compensation F68.1Ø
  compulsive, compulsion F42.8
  conversion F44.9
  craft F48.8
  cutaneous F45.8
  depersonalization F48.1
  depressive (reaction) (type) F34.1
  environmental F48.8
  excoriation L98.1
  fatigue F48.8
  functional —*see* Disorder, somatoform
  gastric F45.8
  gastrointestinal F45.8
  heart F45.8
  hypochondriacal F45.21
  hysterical F44.9
  incoordination F45.8
    larynx F45.8
    vocal cord F45.8
  intestine F45.8
  larynx (sensory) F45.8
    hysterical F44.4
  mixed NEC F48.8
  musculoskeletal F45.8
  obsessional F42.8
  obsessive-compulsive F42.8
  occupational F48.8
  ocular NEC F45.8
  organ —*see* Disorder, somatoform
  pharynx F45.8
  phobic F4Ø.9
  posttraumatic (situational) F43.1Ø
    acute F43.11
    chronic F43.12
  psychasthenic (type) F48.8
  railroad F48.8
  rectum F45.8
  respiratory F45.8
  rumination F45.8
  sexual F65.9
  situational F48.8
  social F4Ø.1Ø
    generalized F4Ø.11
  specified type NEC F48.8
  state F48.9
    with depersonalization episode F48.1
  stomach F45.8
  traumatic F43.1Ø
    acute F43.11
    chronic F43.12
  vasomotor F45.8
  visceral F45.8
  war F48.8
Neurospongioblastosis diffusa Q85.1
Neurosyphilis (arrested) (early) (gumma) (late) (latent) (recurrent) (relapse) A52.3
  with ataxia (cerebellar) (locomotor) (spastic) (spinal) A52.19
  aneurysm (cerebral) A52.Ø5
  arachnoid (adhesive) A52.13
  arteritis (any artery) (cerebral) A52.Ø4
  asymptomatic A52.2
  congenital A5Ø.4Ø
  dura (mater) A52.13
  general paresis A52.17
  hemorrhagic A52.Ø5
  juvenile (asymptomatic) (meningeal) A5Ø.4Ø
  leptomeninges (aseptic) A52.13
  meningeal, meninges (adhesive) A52.13
  meningitis A52.13
  meningovascular (diffuse) A52.13
  optic atrophy A52.15
  parenchymatous (degenerative) A52.19
  paresis, paretic A52.17
    juvenile A5Ø.45
Neurosyphilis *(Continued)*
  remission in (sustained) A52.3
  serological (without symptoms) A52.2
  specified nature or site NEC A52.19
  tabes, tabetic (dorsalis) A52.11
    juvenile A5Ø.45
  taboparesis A52.17
    juvenile A5Ø.45
  thrombosis (cerebral) A52.Ø5
  vascular (cerebral) NEC A52.Ø5
Neurothekeoma —*see* Neoplasm, nerve, benign
Neurotic —*see* Neurosis
Neurotoxemia —*see* Toxemia
Neutroclusion M26.211
Neutropenia, neutropenic (chronic) (genetic) (idiopathic) (immune) (infantile) (malignant) (pernicious) (splenic) D7Ø.9
  congenital (primary) D7Ø.Ø
  cyclic D7Ø.4
  cytoreductive cancer chemotherapy sequela D7Ø.1
  drug-induced D7Ø.2
    due to cytoreductive cancer chemotherapy D7Ø.1
  due to infection D7Ø.3
  fever D7Ø.9
  neonatal, transitory (isoimmune) (maternal transfer) P61.5
  periodic D7Ø.4
  secondary (cyclic) (periodic) (splenic) D7Ø.4
    drug-induced D7Ø.2
      due to cytoreductive cancer chemotherapy D7Ø.1
  toxic D7Ø.8
Neutrophilia, hereditary giant D72.Ø
Nevocarcinoma —*see* Melanoma
Nevus D22.9
  achromic —*see* Neoplasm, skin, benign
  amelanotic —*see* Neoplasm, skin, benign
  angiomatous D18.ØØ
    intra-abdominal D18.Ø3
    intracranial D18.Ø2
    skin D18.Ø1
    specified site NEC D18.Ø9
  araneus I78.1
  balloon cell —*see* Neoplasm, skin, benign
  bathing trunk D48.5
  blue —*see* Neoplasm, skin, benign
    cellular —*see* Neoplasm, skin, benign
    giant —*see* Neoplasm, skin, benign
    Jadassohn's —*see* Neoplasm, skin, benign
    malignant —*see* Melanoma
  capillary D18.ØØ
    intra-abdominal D18.Ø3
    intracranial D18.Ø2
    skin D18.Ø1
    specified site NEC D18.Ø9
  cavernous D18.ØØ
    intra-abdominal D18.Ø3
    intracranial D18.Ø2
    skin D18.Ø1
    specified site NEC D18.Ø9
  cellular —*see* Neoplasm, skin, benign
    blue —*see* Neoplasm, skin, benign
  choroid D31.3-●
  comedonicus Q82.5
  conjunctiva D31.Ø-●
  dermal —*see* Neoplasm, skin, benign
    with epidermal nevus —*see* Neoplasm, skin, benign
  dysplastic —*see* Neoplasm, skin, benign
  eye D31.9-●
  flammeus Q82.5
  hemangiomatous D18.ØØ
    intra-abdominal D18.Ø3
    intracranial D18.Ø2
    skin D18.Ø1
    specified site NEC D18.Ø9
  iris D31.4-●
  lacrimal gland D31.5-●
  lymphatic D18.1

N

Nevus *(Continued)*
magnocellular
specified site —*see* Neoplasm, benign, by site
unspecified site D31.4Ø
malignant —*see* Melanoma
meaning hemangioma D18.ØØ
intra-abdominal D18.Ø3
intracranial D18.Ø2
skin D18.Ø1
specified site NEC D18.Ø9
mouth (mucosa) D1Ø.3Ø
specified site NEC D1Ø.39
white sponge Q38.6
multiplex Q85.1
non-neoplastic I78.1
oral mucosa D1Ø.3Ø
specified site NEC D1Ø.39
white sponge Q38.6
orbit D31.6- ●
pigmented
giant —*see also* Neoplasm, skin, uncertain behavior D48.5
malignant melanoma in —*see* Melanoma
portwine Q82.5
retina D31.2- ●
retrobulbar D31.6- ●
sanguineous Q82.5
senile I78.1
skin D22.9
abdominal wall D22.5
ala nasi D22.39
ankle D22.7- ●
anus, anal D22.5
arm D22.6- ●
auditory canal (external) D22.2- ●
auricle (ear) D22.2- ●
auricular canal (external) D22.2- ●
axilla, axillary fold D22.5
back D22.5
breast D22.5
brow D22.39
buttock D22.5
canthus (eye) D22.1- ●
cheek (external) D22.39
chest wall D22.5
chin D22.39
ear (external) D22.2- ●
external meatus (ear) D22.2- ●
eyebrow D22.39
eyelid (lower) (upper) D22.1- ●
face D22.3Ø
specified NEC D22.39
female genital organ (external) NEC D28.Ø
finger D22.6- ●
flank D22.5
foot D22.7- ●
forearm D22.6- ●
forehead D22.39
foreskin D29.Ø
genital organ (external) NEC
female D28.Ø
male D29.9
gluteal region D22.5
groin D22.5
hand D22.6- ●
heel D22.7- ●
helix D22.2- ●
hip D22.7- ●
interscapular region D22.5
jaw D22.39
knee D22.7- ●
labium (majus) (minus) D28.Ø
leg D22.7- ●
lip (lower) (upper) D22.Ø
lower limb D22.7- ●
male genital organ (external) D29.9
nail D22.9
finger D22.6- ●
toe D22.7- ●
nasolabial groove D22.39
nates D22.5

Nevus *(Continued)*
skin *(Continued)*
neck D22.4
nose (external) D22.39
palpebra D22.1- ●
penis D29.Ø
perianal skin D22.5
perineum D22.5
pinna D22.2- ●
popliteal fossa or space D22.7- ●
prepuce D29.Ø
pudendum D28.Ø
scalp D22.4
scrotum D29.4
shoulder D22.6- ●
submammary fold D22.5
temple D22.39
thigh D22.7- ●
toe D22.7- ●
trunk NEC D22.5
umbilicus D22.5
upper limb D22.6- ●
vulva D28.Ø
specified site NEC —*see* Neoplasm, benign, by site
spider I78.1
stellar I78.1
strawberry Q82.5
Sutton's benign D22.9
unius lateris Q82.5
Unna's Q82.5
vascular Q82.5
verrucous Q82.5
Newborn (infant) (liveborn) (singleton) Z38.2
abstinence syndrome P96.1
acne L7Ø.4
affected by
abnormalities of membranes PØ2.9
specified NEC PØ2.8
abruptio placenta PØ2.1
amino-acid metabolic disorder, transitory P74.8
amniocentesis (while in utero) PØØ.6
amnionitis PØ2.78
apparent life threatening event (ALTE) R68.13
bleeding (into)
cerebral cortex P52.22
germinal matrix P52.Ø
ventricles P52.1
breech delivery PØ3.Ø
cardiac arrest P29.81
cardiomyopathy I42.8
congenital I42.4
cerebral ischemia P91.Ø
Cesarean delivery PØ3.4
chemotherapy agents PØ4.11
chorioamnionitis PØ2.78
cocaine (crack) PØ4.41
complications of labor and delivery PØ3.9
specified NEC PØ3.89
compression of umbilical cord NEC PØ2.5
contracted pelvis PØ3.1
▶cyanosis P28.2
delivery PØ3.9
Cesarean PØ3.4
forceps PØ3.2
vacuum extractor PØ3.3
drugs of addiction PØ4.4Ø
cocaine PØ4.41
hallucinogens PØ4.42
specified drug NEC PØ4.49
entanglement (knot) in umbilical cord PØ2.5
environmental chemicals PØ4.6
fetal (intrauterine)
growth retardation PØ5.9
inflammatory response syndrome (FIRS) PØ2.7Ø
malnutrition not light or small for gestational age PØ5.2
FIRS (fetal inflammatory response syndrome) PØ2.7Ø

Newborn *(Continued)*
affected by *(Continued)*
forceps delivery PØ3.2
heart rate abnormalities
bradycardia P29.12
intrauterine PØ3.819
before onset of labor PØ3.81Ø
during labor PØ3.811
tachycardia P29.11
hemorrhage (antepartum) PØ2.1
cerebellar (nontraumatic) P52.6
intracerebral (nontraumatic) P52.4
intracranial (nontraumatic) P52.9
specified NEC P52.8
intraventricular (nontraumatic) P52.3
grade 1 P52.Ø
grade 2 P52.1
grade 3 P52.21
grade 4 P52.22
posterior fossa (nontraumatic) P52.6
subarachnoid (nontraumatic) P52.5
subependymal P52.Ø
with intracerebral extension P52.22
with intraventricular extension P52.1
with enlargment of ventricles P52.21
without intraventricular extension P52.Ø
hypoxic ischemic encephalopathy [HIE] P91.6Ø
mild P91.61
moderate P91.62
severe P91.63
induction of labor PØ3.89
intestinal perforation P78.Ø
intrauterine (fetal) blood loss P5Ø.9
due to (from)
cut end of co-twin cord P5Ø.5
hemorrhage into
co-twin P5Ø.3
maternal circulation P5Ø.4
placenta P5Ø.2
ruptured cord blood P5Ø.1
vasa previa P5Ø.Ø
specified NEC P5Ø.8
intrauterine (fetal) hemorrhage P5Ø.9
intrauterine (in utero) procedure P96.5
malpresentation (malposition) NEC PØ3.1
maternal (complication of) (use of)
alcohol PØ4.3
amphetamines PØ4.16
analgesia (maternal) PØ4.Ø
anesthesia (maternal) PØ4.Ø
anticonvulsants PØ4.13
antidepressants PØ4.15
antineoplastic chemotherapy PØ4.11
anxiolytics PØ4.1A
blood loss PØ2.1
cannabis PØ4.81
circulatory disease PØØ.3
condition PØØ.9
specified NEC PØØ.89
cytotoxic drugs PØ4.12
delivery PØ3.9
Cesarean PØ3.4
forceps PØ3.2
vacuum extractor PØ3.3
diabetes mellitus (pre-existing) P7Ø.1
disorder PØØ.9
specified NEC PØØ.89
drugs (addictive) (illegal) NEC PØ4.49
ectopic pregnancy PØ1.4
gestational diabetes P7Ø.Ø
hemorrhage PØ2.1
hypertensive disorder PØØ.Ø
incompetent cervix PØ1.Ø
infectious disease PØØ.2
injury PØØ.5
labor and delivery PØ3.9
malpresentation before labor PØ1.7
maternal death PØ1.6

Newborn (Continued)
affected by (Continued)
maternal (Continued)
medical procedure P00.7
medication P04.19
specified type NEC P04.18
multiple pregnancy P01.5
nutritional disorder P00.4
oligohydramnios P01.2
opiates P04.14
administered for procedures during pregnancy or labor and delivery P04.0
parasitic disease P00.2
periodontal disease P00.81
placenta previa P02.0
polyhydramnios P01.3
precipitate delivery P03.5
pregnancy P01.9
specified P01.8
premature rupture of membranes P01.1
renal disease P00.1
respiratory disease P00.3
sedative-hypnotics P04.17
surgical procedure P00.6
tranquilizers administered for procedures during pregnancy or labor and delivery P04.0
urinary tract disease P00.1
uterine contraction (abnormal) P03.6
meconium peritonitis P78.0
medication (legal) (maternal use) (prescribed) P04.19
membrane abnormalities P02.9
specified NEC P02.8
membranitis P02.78
methamphetamine(s) P04.49
mixed metabolic and respiratory acidosis P84
neonatal abstinence syndrome P96.1
noxious substances transmitted via placenta or breast milk P04.9
cannabis P04.81
specified NEC P04.89
nutritional supplements P04.5
placenta previa P02.0
placental
abnormality (functional) (morphological) P02.20
specified NEC P02.29
dysfunction P02.29
infarction P02.29
insufficiency P02.29
separation NEC P02.1
transfusion syndromes P02.3
placentitis P02.78
precipitate delivery P03.5
prolapsed cord P02.4
respiratory arrest P28.81
slow intrauterine growth P05.9
tobacco P04.2
twin to twin transplacental transfusion P02.3
umbilical cord (tightly) around neck P02.5
umbilical cord condition P02.60
short cord P02.69
specified NEC P02.69
uterine contractions (abnormal) P03.6
vasa previa P02.69
from intrauterine blood loss P50.0
apnea P28.4
obstructive P28.4
primary P28.3
sleep (central) (obstructive) (primary) P28.3
born in hospital Z38.00
by cesarean Z38.01
born outside hospital Z38.1
breast buds P96.89
breast engorgement P83.4
check-up *—see* Newborn, examination
convulsion P90
dehydration P74.1

Newborn (Continued)
examination
8 to 28 days old Z00.111
under 8 days old Z00.110
fever P81.9
environmentally-induced P81.0
hyperbilirubinemia P59.9
of prematurity P59.0
hypernatremia P74.21
hyponatremia P74.22
infection P39.9
candidal P37.5
specified NEC P39.8
urinary tract P39.3
jaundice P59.9
due to
breast milk inhibitor P59.3
hepatocellular damage P59.20
specified NEC P59.29
preterm delivery P59.0
of prematurity P59.0
specified NEC P59.8
late metabolic acidosis P74.0
mastitis P39.0
infective P39.0
noninfective P83.4
multiple born NEC Z38.8
born in hospital Z38.68
by cesarean Z38.69
born outside hospital Z38.7
omphalitis P38.9
with mild hemorrhage P38.1
without hemorrhage P38.9
post-term P08.21
prolonged gestation (over 42 completed weeks) P08.22
quadruplet Z38.8
born in hospital Z38.63
by cesarean Z38.64
born outside hospital Z38.7
quintuplet Z38.8
born in hospital Z38.65
by cesarean Z38.66
born outside hospital Z38.7
seizure P90
sepsis (congenital) P36.9
due to
anaerobes NEC P36.5
Escherichia coli P36.4
Staphylococcus P36.30
aureus P36.2
specified NEC P36.39
Streptococcus P36.10
group B P36.0
specified NEC P36.19
specified NEC P36.8
triplet Z38.8
born in hospital Z38.61
by cesarean Z38.62
born outside hospital Z38.7
twin Z38.5
born in hospital Z38.30
by cesarean Z38.31
born outside hospital Z38.4
vomiting P92.09
bilious P92.01
weight check Z00.111
Newcastle conjunctivitis or disease B30.8
Nezelof's syndrome (pure alymphocytosis) D81.4
Niacin (amide) deficiency E52
Nicolas (-Durand)-Favre disease A55
Nicotine *—see* Tobacco
Nicotinic acid deficiency E52
Niemann-Pick disease or syndrome E75.249
specified NEC E75.248
type
A E75.240
B E75.241
C E75.242
D E75.243

Night
blindness *—see* Blindness, night
sweats R61
terrors (child) F51.4
Nightmares (REM sleep type) F51.5
NIHSS (National Institutes of Health Stroke Scale) score R29.7-●
Nipple *—see* condition
Nisbet's chancre A57
Nishimoto (-Takeuchi) disease I67.5
Nitritoid crisis or reaction *—see* Crisis, nitritoid
Nitrosohemoglobinemia D74.8
Njovera A65
Nocardiosis, nocardiasis A43.9
cutaneous A43.1
lung A43.0
pneumonia A43.0
pulmonary A43.0
specified site NEC A43.8
Nocturia R35.1
psychogenic F45.8
Nocturnal *—see* condition
Nodal rhythm I49.8
Node(s) *—see also* Nodule
Bouchard's (with arthropathy) M15.2
Haygarth's M15.8
Heberden's (with arthropathy) M15.1
larynx J38.7
lymph *—see* condition
milker's B08.03
Osler's I33.0
Schmorl's *—see* Schmorl's disease
singer's J38.2
teacher's J38.2
tuberculous *—see* Tuberculosis, lymph gland
vocal cord J38.2
Nodule(s), nodular
actinomycotic *—see* Actinomycosis
breast NEC *—see also* Lump, breast N63.0
colloid (cystic), thyroid E04.1
cutaneous *—see* Swelling, localized
endometrial (stromal) D26.1
Haygarth's M15.8
inflammatory *—see* Inflammation
juxta-articular
syphilitic A52.77
yaws A66.7
larynx J38.7
lung, solitary (subsegmental branch of the bronchial tree) R91.1
multiple R91.8
milker's B08.03
prostate N40.2
with lower urinary tract symptoms (LUTS) N40.3
without lower urinary tract symptoms (LUTS) N40.2
pulmonary, solitary (subsegmental branch of the bronchial tree) R91.1
retrocardiac R09.89
rheumatoid M06.30
ankle M06.37-●
elbow M06.32-●
foot joint M06.37-●
hand joint M06.34-●
hip M06.35-●
knee M06.36-●
multiple site M06.39
shoulder M06.31-●
vertebra M06.38
wrist M06.33-●
scrotum (inflammatory) N49.2
singer's J38.2
solitary, lung (subsegmental branch of the bronchial tree) R91.1
multiple R91.8
subcutaneous *—see* Swelling, localized
teacher's J38.2

- Nodule(s), nodular *(Continued)*
  - thyroid (cold) (gland) (nontoxic) E04.1
    - with thyrotoxicosis E05.20
      - with thyroid storm E05.21
    - toxic or with hyperthyroidism E05.20
      - with thyroid storm E05.21
  - vocal cord J38.2
- Noma (gangrenous) (hospital) (infective) A69.0
  - auricle I96
  - mouth A69.0
  - pudendi N76.89
  - vulvae N76.89
- Nomad, nomadism Z59.0
- NOMID (neonatal onset multisystemic inflammatory disorder) M04.2
- Nonadherence to medical treatment Z91.19
- Nonautoimmune hemolytic anemia D59.4
  - drug-induced D59.2
- Nonclosure *—see also* Imperfect, closure
  - ductus arteriosus (Botallo's) Q25.0
  - foramen
    - botalli Q21.1
    - ovale Q21.1
- Noncompliance Z91.19
  - with
    - dialysis Z91.15
    - dietary regimen Z91.11
    - medical treatment Z91.19
    - medication regimen NEC Z91.14
      - underdosing *—see also* Table of Drugs and Chemicals, categories T36-T50, with final character 6 Z91.14
        - intentional NEC Z91.128
          - due to financial hardship of patient Z91.120
        - unintentional NEC Z91.138
          - due to patient's age related debility Z91.130
    - renal dialysis Z91.15
- Nondescent (congenital) *—see also* Malposition, congenital
  - cecum Q43.3
  - colon Q43.3
  - testicle Q53.9
    - bilateral Q53.20
      - abdominal Q53.211
      - perineal Q53.22
    - unilateral Q53.10
      - abdominal Q53.111
      - perineal Q53.12
- Nondevelopment
  - brain Q02
    - part of Q04.3
- Nondevelopment *(Continued)*
  - heart Q24.8
  - organ or site, congenital NEC *—see* Hypoplasia
- Nonengagement
  - head NEC O32.4
    - in labor, causing obstructed labor O64.8
- Nonexanthematous tick fever A93.2
- Nonexpansion, lung (newborn) P28.0
- Nonfunctioning
  - cystic duct *—see also* Disease, gallbladder K82.8
  - gallbladder *—see also* Disease, gallbladder K82.8
  - kidney N28.9
  - labyrinth *—see* subcategory H83.2
- Non-Hodgkin lymphoma NEC *—see* Lymphoma, non-Hodgkin
- Nonimplantation, ovum N97.2
- Noninsufflation, fallopian tube N97.1
- Non-ketotic hyperglycinemia E72.51
- Nonne-Milroy syndrome Q82.0
- Nonovulation N97.0
- Non-palpable testicle(s)
  - bilateral R39.84
  - unilateral R39.83
- Nonpatent fallopian tube N97.1
- Nonpneumatization, lung NEC P28.0
- Nonrotation *—see* Malrotation
- Nonsecretion, urine *—see* Anuria
- Nonunion
  - fracture *—see* Fracture, by site
  - joint, following fusion or arthrodesis M96.0
  - organ or site, congenital NEC *—see* Imperfect, closure
  - symphysis pubis, congenital Q74.2
- Nonvisualization, gallbladder R93.2
- Nonvital, nonvitalized tooth K04.99
- Non-working side interference M26.56
- Noonan's syndrome Q87.19
- Normocytic anemia (infectional) due to blood loss (chronic) D50.0
  - acute D62
- Norrie's disease (congenital) Q15.8
- North American blastomycosis B40.9
- Norwegian itch B86
- Nose, nasal *—see* condition
- Nosebleed R04.0
- Nose-picking F98.8
- Nosomania F45.21
- Nosophobia F45.22
- Nostalgia F43.20
- Notch of iris Q13.2
- Notching nose, congenital (tip) Q30.2
- Nothnagel's
  - syndrome *—see* Strabismus, paralytic, third nerve
  - vasomotor acroparesthesia I73.89
- Novy's relapsing fever A68.9
  - louse-borne A68.0
  - tick-borne A68.1
- Noxious
  - foodstuffs, poisoning by *—see* Poisoning, food, noxious, plant
  - substances transmitted through placenta or breast milk P04.9
- Nucleus pulposus *—see* condition
- Numbness R20.0
- Nuns' knee *—see* Bursitis, prepatellar
- Nursemaid's elbow S53.03- ●
- Nutcracker esophagus K22.4
- Nutmeg liver K76.1
- Nutrient element deficiency E61.9
  - specified NEC E61.8
- Nutrition deficient or insufficient *—see also* Malnutrition E46
  - due to
    - insufficient food T73.0
    - lack of
      - care (child) T76.02
        - adult T76.01
      - food T73.0
- Nutritional stunting E45
- Nyctalopia (night blindness) *—see* Blindness, night
- Nycturia R35.1
  - psychogenic F45.8
- Nymphomania F52.8
- Nystagmus H55.00
  - benign paroxysmal *—see* Vertigo, benign paroxysmal
  - central positional H81.4
  - congenital H55.01
  - dissociated H55.04
  - latent H55.02
  - miners' H55.09
  - positional
    - benign paroxysmal H81.4
    - central H81.4
  - specified form NEC H55.09
  - visual deprivation H55.03

O

Obermeyer's relapsing fever (European) A68.Ø
Obesity E66.9
with alveolar hypoventilation E66.2
adrenal E27.8
complicating
childbirth O99.214
pregnancy O99.21- ●
puerperium O99.215
constitutional E66.8
dietary counseling and surveillance Z71.3
drug-induced E66.1
due to
drug E66.1
excess calories E66.Ø9
morbid E66.Ø1
severe E66.Ø1
endocrine E66.8
endogenous E66.8
exogenous E66.Ø9
familial E66.8
glandular E66.8
hypothyroid —*see* Hypothyroidism
hypoventilation syndrome (OHS) E66.2
morbid E66.Ø1
with
alveolar hypoventilation E66.2
obesity hypoventilation syndrome (OHS) E66.2
due to excess calories E66.Ø1
nutritional E66.Ø9
pituitary E23.6
severe E66.Ø1
specified type NEC E66.8
Oblique —*see* condition
Obliteration
appendix (lumen) K38.8
artery I77.1
bile duct (noncalculous) K83.1
common duct (noncalculous) K83.1
cystic duct —*see* Obstruction, gallbladder
disease, arteriolar I77.1
endometrium N85.8
eye, anterior chamber —*see* Disorder, globe, hypotony
fallopian tube N97.1
lymphatic vessel I89.Ø
due to mastectomy I97.2
organ or site, congenital NEC —*see* Atresia, by site
ureter N13.5
with infection N13.6
urethra —*see* Stricture, urethra
vein I87.8
vestibule (oral) KØ8.89
Observation (following) (for) (without need for further medical care) ZØ4.9
accident NEC ZØ4.3
at work ZØ4.2
transport ZØ4.1
adverse effect of drug ZØ3.6
alleged rape or sexual assault (victim), ruled out
adult ZØ4.41
child ZØ4.42
criminal assault ZØ4.89
development state
adolescent ZØØ.3
period of rapid growth in childhood ZØØ.2
puberty ZØØ.3
disease, specified NEC ZØ3.89
following work accident ZØ4.2
forced sexual exploitation ZØ4.81
forced labor exploitation ZØ4.82
growth and development state —*see* Observation, development state
injuries (accidental) NEC —*see also* Observation, accident
Observation *(Continued)*
newborn (for)
suspected condition, related to exposure from the mother or birth process —*see* Newborn, affected by, maternal
ruled out ZØ5.9
cardiac ZØ5.Ø
connective tissue ZØ5.73
gastrointestinal ZØ5.5
genetic ZØ5.41
genitourinary ZØ5.6
immunologic ZØ5.43
infectious ZØ5.1
metabolic ZØ5.42
musculoskeletal ZØ5.72
neurological ZØ5.2
respiratory ZØ5.3
skin and subcutaneous tissue ZØ5.71
specified condition NEC ZØ5.8
postpartum
immediately after delivery Z39.Ø
routine follow-up Z39.2
pregnancy (normal) (without complication) Z34.9- ●
high risk OØ9.9- ●
suicide attempt, alleged NEC ZØ3.89
self-poisoning ZØ3.6
suspected, ruled out —*see also* Suspected condition, ruled out
abuse, physical
adult ZØ4.71
child ZØ4.72
accident at work ZØ4.2
adult battering victim ZØ4.71
child battering victim ZØ4.72
condition NEC ZØ3.89
newborn —*see also* Observation, newborn (for), suspected condition, ruled out ZØ5.9
drug poisoning or adverse effect ZØ3.6
exposure (to)
anthrax ZØ3.81Ø
biological agent NEC ZØ3.818
inflicted injury NEC ZØ4.89
suicide attempt, alleged ZØ3.89
self-poisoning ZØ3.6
toxic effects from ingested substance (drug) (poison) ZØ3.6
toxic effects from ingested substance (drug) (poison) ZØ3.6
Obsession, obsessional state F42.8
mixed thoughts and acts F42.2
Obsessive-compulsive neurosis or reaction F42.8
Obstetric embolism, septic —*see* Embolism, obstetric, septic
Obstetrical trauma (complicating delivery) O71.9
with or following ectopic or molar pregnancy OØ8.6
specified type NEC O71.89
Obstipation —*see* Constipation
Obstruction, obstructed, obstructive
airway J98.8
with
allergic alveolitis J67.9
asthma J45.9Ø9
with
exacerbation (acute) J45.9Ø1
status asthmaticus J45.9Ø2
bronchiectasis J47.9
with
exacerbation (acute) J47.1
lower respiratory infection J47.Ø
bronchitis (chronic) J44.9
emphysema J43.9
Obstruction, obstructed, obstructive *(Continued)*
airway *(Continued)*
chronic J44.9
with
allergic alveolitis —*see* Pneumonitis, hypersensitivity
bronchiectasis J47.9
with
exacerbation (acute) J47.1
lower respiratory infection J47.Ø
due to
foreign body —*see* Foreign body, by site, causing asphyxia
inhalation of fumes or vapors J68.9
laryngospasm J38.5
ampulla of Vater K83.1
aortic (heart) (valve) —*see* Stenosis, aortic
aortoiliac I74.Ø9
aqueduct of Sylvius G91.1
congenital QØ3.Ø
with spina bifida —*see* Spina bifida, by site, with hydrocephalus
Arnold-Chiari —*see* Arnold-Chiari disease
artery (*see also* Atherosclerosis, artery) I7Ø.9
basilar (complete) (partial) —*see* Occlusion, artery, basilar
carotid (complete) (partial) —*see* Occlusion, artery, carotid
cerebellar —*see* Occlusion, artery, cerebellar
cerebral (anterior) (middle) (posterior) —*see* Occlusion, artery, cerebral
precerebral —*see* Occlusion, artery, precerebral
renal N28.Ø
retinal NEC —*see* Occlusion, artery, retina
stent —*see* Restenosis, stent
vertebral (complete) (partial) —*see* Occlusion, artery, vertebral
band (intestinal) —*see also* Obstruction, intestine, specified NEC K56.699
bile duct or passage (common) (hepatic) (noncalculous) K83.1
with calculus K8Ø.51
congenital (causing jaundice) Q44.3
biliary (duct) (tract) K83.1
gallbladder K82.Ø
bladder-neck (acquired) N32.Ø
congenital Q64.31
due to hyperplasia (hypertrophy) of prostate —*see* Hyperplasia, prostate
bowel —*see* Obstruction, intestine
bronchus J98.Ø9
canal, ear —*see* Stenosis, external ear canal
cardia K22.2
caval veins (inferior) (superior) I87.1
cecum —*see* Obstruction, intestine
circulatory I99.8
colon —*see* Obstruction, intestine
common duct (noncalculous) K83.1
coronary (artery) —*see* Occlusion, coronary
cystic duct —*see also* Obstruction, gallbladder
with calculus K8Ø.21
device, implant or graft —*see also* Complications, by site and type, mechanical T85.698
arterial graft NEC —*see* Complication, cardiovascular device, mechanical, vascular
catheter NEC T85.628
cystostomy T83.Ø9Ø
dialysis (renal) T82.49
intraperitoneal T85.691
Hopkins T83.Ø98
ileostomy T83.Ø98
infusion NEC T82.594
spinal (epidural) (subdural) T85.69Ø
nephrostomy T83.Ø92
urethral indwelling T83.Ø91
urinary T83.Ø98
urostomy T83.Ø98

- **Obstruction, obstructed, obstructive** *(Continued)*
  - device, implant or graft *(Continued)*
    - due to infection T85.79
    - gastrointestinal —*see* Complications, prosthetic device, mechanical, gastrointestinal device
    - genital NEC T83.498
      - intrauterine contraceptive device T83.39
      - penile prosthesis (cylinder) (implanted) (pump) (resevoir) T83.49Ø
      - testicular prosthesis T83.491
    - heart NEC —*see* Complication, cardiovascular device, mechanical
    - joint prosthesis —*see* Complications, joint prosthesis, mechanical, specified NEC, by site
    - orthopedic NEC —*see* Complication, orthopedic, device, mechanical
    - specified NEC T85.628
    - urinary NEC —*see also* Complication, genitourinary, device, urinary, mechanical
      - graft T83.29
    - vascular NEC —*see* Complication, cardiovascular device, mechanical
    - ventricular intracranial shunt T85.Ø9
  - due to foreign body accidentally left in operative wound T81.529
  - duodenum K31.5
  - ejaculatory duct N5Ø.89
  - esophagus K22.2
  - eustachian tube (complete) (partial) H68.1Ø-●
    - cartilagenous (extrinsic) H68.13-●
      - intrinsic H68.12-●
    - osseous H68.11-●
  - fallopian tube (bilateral) N97.1
  - fecal K56.41
    - with hernia —*see* Hernia, by site, with obstruction
  - foramen of Monro (congenital) QØ3.8
    - with spina bifida —*see* Spina bifida, by site, with hydrocephalus
  - foreign body —*see* Foreign body
  - gallbladder K82.Ø
    - with calculus, stones K8Ø.21
    - congenital Q44.1
  - gastric outlet K31.1
  - gastrointestinal —*see* Obstruction, intestine
  - hepatic K76.89
    - duct (noncalculous) K83.1
  - hepatobiliary K83.1
  - ileum —*see* Obstruction, intestine
  - iliofemoral (artery) I74.5
  - intestine K56.6Ø9
    - complete K56.6Ø1
    - incomplete K56.6ØØ
    - partial K56.6ØØ
    - with
      - adhesions (intestinal) (peritoneal) K56.5Ø
        - complete K56.52
        - incomplete K56.51
        - partial K56.51
    - adynamic K56.Ø
    - by gallstone K56.3
    - congenital (small) Q41.9
      - large Q42.9
        - specified part NEC Q42.8
    - neurogenic K56.Ø
      - Hirschsprung's disease or megacolon Q43.1
    - newborn P76.9
      - due to
        - fecaliths P76.8
        - inspissated milk P76.2
        - meconium (plug) P76.Ø
          - in mucoviscidosis E84.11
      - specified NEC P76.8
    - postoperative K91.3Ø
      - complete K91.32
      - incomplete K91.31
      - partial K91.31

- **Obstruction, obstructed, obstructive** *(Continued)*
  - intestine *(Continued)*
    - reflex K56.Ø
    - specified NEC K56.699
      - complete K56.691
      - incomplete K56.69Ø
      - partial K56.69Ø
    - volvulus K56.2
  - intracardiac ball valve prosthesis T82.Ø9
  - jejunum —*see* Obstruction, intestine
  - joint prosthesis —*see* Complications, joint prosthesis, mechanical, specified NEC, by site
  - kidney (calices) N28.89
  - labor —*see* Delivery
  - lacrimal (passages) (duct)
    - by
      - dacryolith —*see* Dacryolith
      - stenosis —*see* Stenosis, lacrimal
    - congenital Q1Ø.5
    - neonatal HØ4.53-●
  - lacrimonasal duct —*see* Obstruction, lacrimal
  - lacteal, with steatorrhea K9Ø.2
  - laryngitis —*see* Laryngitis
  - larynx NEC J38.6
    - congenital Q31.8
  - lung J98.4
    - disease, chronic J44.9
  - lymphatic I89.Ø
  - meconium (plug)
    - newborn P76.Ø
      - due to fecaliths P76.Ø
      - in mucoviscidosis E84.11
  - mitral —*see* Stenosis, mitral
  - nasal J34.89
  - nasolacrimal duct —*see also* Obstruction, lacrimal
    - congenital Q1Ø.5
  - nasopharynx J39.2
  - nose J34.89
  - organ or site, congenital NEC —*see* Atresia, by site
  - pancreatic duct K86.89
  - parotid duct or gland K11.8
  - pelviureteral junction N13.5
    - with hydronephrosis N13.Ø
    - congenital Q62.39
  - pharynx J39.2
  - portal (circulation) (vein) I81
  - prostate —*see also* Hyperplasia, prostate
    - valve (urinary) N32.Ø
  - pulmonary valve (heart) I37.Ø
  - pyelonephritis (chronic) N11.1
  - pylorus
    - adult K31.1
    - congenital or infantile Q4Ø.Ø
  - rectosigmoid —*see* Obstruction, intestine
  - rectum K62.4
  - renal N28.89
    - outflow N13.8
    - pelvis, congenital Q62.39
  - respiratory J98.8
    - chronic J44.9
  - retinal (vessels) H34.9
  - salivary duct (any) K11.8
    - with calculus K11.5
  - sigmoid —*see* Obstruction, intestine
  - sinus (accessory) (nasal) J34.89
  - Stensen's duct K11.8
  - stomach NEC K31.89
    - acute K31.Ø
    - congenital Q4Ø.2
    - due to pylorospasm K31.3
  - submandibular duct K11.8
  - submaxillary gland K11.8
    - with calculus K11.5
  - thoracic duct I89.Ø
  - thrombotic —*see* Thrombosis
  - trachea J39.8

- **Obstruction, obstructed, obstructive** *(Continued)*
  - tracheostomy airway J95.Ø3
  - tricuspid (valve) —*see* Stenosis, tricuspid
  - upper respiratory, congenital Q34.8
  - ureter (functional) (pelvic junction) NEC N13.5
    - with
      - hydronephrosis N13.1
        - with infection N13.6
      - pyelonephritis (chronic) N11.1
    - congenital Q62.39
    - due to calculus —*see* Calculus, ureter
  - urethra NEC N36.8
    - congenital Q64.39
  - urinary (moderate) N13.9
    - due to hyperplasia (hypertrophy) of prostate —*see* Hyperplasia, prostate
    - organ or tract (lower) N13.9
    - prostatic valve N32.Ø
    - specified NEC N13.8
  - uropathy N13.9
  - uterus N85.8
  - vagina N89.5
  - valvular —*see* Endocarditis
  - vein, venous I87.1
    - caval (inferior) (superior) I87.1
    - thrombotic —*see* Thrombosis
  - vena cava (inferior) (superior) I87.1
  - vesical NEC N32.Ø
  - vesicourethral orifice N32.Ø
    - congenital Q64.31
  - vessel NEC I99.8
    - stent —*see* Restenosis, stent
- **Obturator** —*see* condition
- **Occlusal wear, teeth** KØ3.Ø
- **Occlusio pupillae** —*see* Membrane, pupillary
- **Occlusion, occluded**
  - anus K62.4
    - congenital Q42.3
      - with fistula Q42.2
  - aortoiliac (chronic) I74.Ø9
  - aqueduct of Sylvius G91.1
    - congenital QØ3.Ø
      - with spina bifida —*see* Spina bifida, by site, with hydrocephalus
  - artery —*see also* Atherosclerosis, artery I7Ø.9
    - auditory, internal I65.8
    - basilar I65.1
      - with
        - infarction I63.22
          - due to
            - embolism I63.12
            - thrombosis I63.Ø2
    - brain or cerebral I66.9
      - with infarction (due to) I63.5-●
        - embolism I63.4-●
        - thrombosis I63.3-●
    - carotid I65.2-●
      - with
        - infarction I63.23-●
          - due to
            - embolism I63.13-●
            - thrombosis I63.Ø3-●
    - cerebellar (anterior inferior) (posterior inferior) (superior) I66.3
      - with infarction I63.54-●
        - due to
          - embolism I63.44-●
          - thrombosis I63.34-●
    - cerebral I66.9
      - with infarction I63.5Ø
        - due to
          - embolism I63.4Ø
            - specified NEC I63.49
          - thrombosis I63.3Ø
            - specified NEC I63.39
      - anterior I66.1-●
        - with infarction I63.52-●
          - due to
            - embolism I63.42-●
            - thrombosis I63.32-●

- **Occlusion, occluded** *(Continued)*
  - artery *(Continued)*
    - cerebral *(Continued)*
      - middle I66.Ø-•
        - with infarction I63.51-•
          - due to
            - embolism I63.41-•
            - thrombosis I63.31-•
      - posterior I66.2-•
        - with infarction I63.53-•
          - due to
            - embolism I63.43-•
            - thrombosis I63.33-•
      - specified NEC I66.8
        - with infarction I63.59
          - due to
            - embolism I63.4-•
            - thrombosis I63.3-•
    - choroidal (anterior) —*see* Occlusion, artery, cerebral, specified NEC
    - communicating posterior —*see* Occlusion, artery, precerebral, specified NEC
    - complete
      - coronary I25.82
      - extremities I7Ø.92
    - coronary (acute) (thrombotic) (without myocardial infarction) I24.Ø
      - with myocardial infarction —*see* Infarction, myocardium
      - chronic total I25.82
      - complete I25.82
      - healed or old I25.2
      - total (chronic) I25.82
    - hypophyseal —*see* Occlusion, artery, precerebral, specified NEC
    - iliac I74.5
    - lower extremities due to stenosis or stricture I77.1
    - mesenteric (embolic) (thrombotic) —*see also* Infarct, intestine K55.Ø69
    - perforating —*see* Occlusion, artery, cerebral, specified NEC
    - peripheral I77.9
      - thrombotic or embolic I74.4
    - pontine —*see* Occlusion, artery, precerebral, specified NEC
    - precerebral I65.9
      - with infarction I63.2Ø
        - due to
          - embolism I63.1Ø
            - specified NEC I63.19
          - thrombosis I63.ØØ
            - specified NEC I63.Ø9
        - specified NEC I63.29
      - basilar —*see* Occlusion, artery, basilar
      - carotid —*see* Occlusion, artery, carotid
      - puerperal O88.23
      - specified NEC I65.8
        - with infarction I63.29
          - due to
            - embolism I63.19
            - thrombosis I63.Ø9
      - vertebral —*see* Occlusion, artery, vertebral
    - renal N28.Ø
    - retinal
      - branch H34.23-•
      - central H34.1-•
      - partial H34.21-•
      - transient H34.Ø-•
    - spinal —*see* Occlusion, artery, precerebral, vertebral
    - total (chronic)
      - coronary I25.82
      - extremities I7Ø.92
    - vertebral I65.Ø-•
      - with
        - infarction I63.21-•
          - due to
            - embolism I63.11-•
            - thrombosis I63.Ø1-•
- **Occlusion, occluded** *(Continued)*
  - basilar artery —*see* Occlusion, artery, basilar
  - bile duct (common) (hepatic) (noncalculous) K83.1
  - bowel —*see* Obstruction, intestine
  - carotid (artery) (common) (internal) —*see* Occlusion, artery, carotid
  - centric (of teeth) M26.59
    - maximum intercuspation discrepancy M26.55
  - cerebellar (artery) —*see* Occlusion, artery, cerebellar
  - cerebral (artery) —*see* Occlusion, artery, cerebral
  - cerebrovascular —*see also* Occlusion, artery, cerebral
    - with infarction I63.5-•
  - cervical canal —*see* Stricture, cervix
  - cervix (uteri) —*see* Stricture, cervix
  - choanal Q3Ø.Ø
  - choroidal (artery) —*see* Occlusion, artery, precerebral, specified NEC
  - colon —*see* Obstruction, intestine
  - communicating posterior artery —*see* Occlusion, artery, precerebral, specified NEC
  - coronary (artery) (vein) (thrombotic) —*see also* Infarct, myocardium
    - chronic total I25.82
    - healed or old I25.2
    - not resulting in infarction I24.Ø
    - total (chronic) I25.82
  - cystic duct —*see* Obstruction, gallbladder
  - embolic —*see* Embolism
  - fallopian tube N97.1
    - congenital Q5Ø.6
  - gallbladder —*see also* Obstruction, gallbladder
    - congenital (causing jaundice) Q44.1
  - gingiva, traumatic KØ6.2
  - hymen N89.6
    - congenital Q52.3
  - hypophyseal (artery) —*see* Occlusion, artery, precerebral, specified NEC
  - iliac artery I74.5
  - intestine —*see* Obstruction, intestine
  - lacrimal passages —*see* Obstruction, lacrimal
  - lung J98.4
  - lymph or lymphatic channel I89.Ø
  - mammary duct N64.89
  - mesenteric artery (embolic) (thrombotic) —*see also* Infarct, intestine K55.Ø69
  - nose J34.89
    - congenital Q3Ø.Ø
  - organ or site, congenital NEC —*see* Atresia, by site
  - oviduct N97.1
    - congenital Q5Ø.6
  - peripheral arteries
    - due to stricture or stenosis I77.1
    - upper extremity I74.2
  - pontine (artery) —*see* Occlusion, artery, precerebral, specified NEC
  - posterior lingual, of mandibular teeth M26.29
  - precerebral artery —*see* Occlusion, artery, precerebral
  - punctum lacrimale —*see* Obstruction, lacrimal
  - pupil —*see* Membrane, pupillary
  - pylorus, adult —*see also* Stricture, pylorus K31.1
  - renal artery N28.Ø
  - retina, retinal
    - artery —*see* Occlusion, artery, retinal
    - vein (central) H34.81-•
      - engorgement H34.82-•
      - tributary H34.83-•
    - vessels H34.9
  - spinal artery —*see* Occlusion, artery, precerebral, vertebral
  - teeth (mandibular) (posterior lingual) M26.29
- **Occlusion, occluded** *(Continued)*
  - thoracic duct I89.Ø
  - thrombotic —*see* Thrombosis, artery
  - traumatic
    - edentulous (alveolar) ridge KØ6.2
    - gingiva KØ6.2
    - periodontal KØ5.5
  - tubal N97.1
  - ureter (complete) (partial) N13.5
    - congenital Q62.1Ø
  - ureteropelvic junction N13.5
    - congenital Q62.11
  - ureterovesical orifice N13.5
    - congenital Q62.12
  - urethra —*see* Stricture, urethra
  - uterus N85.8
  - vagina N89.5
  - vascular NEC I99.8
  - vein —*see* Thrombosis
    - retinal —*see* Occlusion, retinal, vein
  - vena cava (inferior) (superior) —*see* Embolism, vena cava
  - ventricle (brain) NEC G91.1
  - vertebral (artery) —*see* Occlusion, artery, vertebral
  - vessel (blood) I99.8
  - vulva N9Ø.5
- **Occult**
  - blood in feces (stools) R19.5
- **Occupational**
  - problems NEC Z56.89
- **Ochlophobia** —*see* Agoraphobia
- **Ochronosis** (endogenous) E7Ø.29
- **Ocular muscle** —*see* condition
- **Oculogyric crisis or disturbance** H51.8
  - psychogenic F45.8
- **Oculomotor syndrome** H51.9
- **Oculopathy**
  - syphilitic NEC A52.71
    - congenital
      - early A5Ø.Ø1
      - late A5Ø.3Ø
    - early (secondary) A51.43
    - late A52.71
- **Oddi's sphincter spasm** K83.4
- **Odontalgia** KØ8.89
- **Odontoameloblastoma** —*see* Cyst, calcifying odontogenic
- **Odontoclasia** KØ3.89
- **Odontodysplasia, regional** KØØ.4
- **Odontogenesis imperfecta** KØØ.5
- **Odontoma** (ameloblastic) (complex) (compound) (fibroameloblastic) —*see* Cyst, calcifying odontogenic
- **Odontomyelitis** (closed) (open) KØ4.Ø1
  - irreversible KØ4.Ø2
  - reversible KØ4.Ø1
- **Odontorrhagia** KØ8.89
- **Odontosarcoma, ameloblastic** C41.1
  - upper jaw (bone) C41.Ø
- **Oestriasis** —*see* Myiasis
- **Oguchi's disease** H53.63
- **Ohara's disease** —*see* Tularemia
- **OHS** (obesity hypoventilation syndrome) E66.2
- **Oidiomycosis** —*see* Candidiasis
- **Oidium albicans infection** —*see* Candidiasis
- **Old** (previous) **myocardial infarction** I25.2
- **Old age** (without mention of debility) R54-•
  - dementia FØ3
- **Olfactory** —*see* condition
- **Oligemia** —*see* Anemia
- **Oligoastrocytoma**
  - specified site —*see* Neoplasm, malignant, by site
  - unspecified site C71.9
- **Oligocythemia** D64.9
- **Oligodendroblastoma**
  - specified site —*see* Neoplasm, malignant
  - unspecified site C71.9

Oligodendroglioma
anaplastic type
specified site —*see* Neoplasm, malignant, by site
unspecified site C71.9
specified site —*see* Neoplasm, malignant, by site
unspecified site C71.9
Oligodontia —*see* Anodontia
Oligoencephalon Q02
Oligohidrosis L74.4
Oligohydramnios O41.0-●
Oligohydrosis L74.4
Oligomenorrhea N91.5
primary N91.3
secondary N91.4
Oligophrenia —*see also* Disability, intellectual
phenylpyruvic E70.0
Oligospermia N46.11
due to
drug therapy N46.121
efferent duct obstruction N46.123
infection N46.122
radiation N46.124
specified cause NEC N46.129
systemic disease N46.125
Oligotrichia —*see* Alopecia
Oliguria R34
with, complicating or following ectopic or molar pregnancy O08.4
postprocedural N99.0
Ollier's disease Q78.4
Omenotocele —*see* Hernia, abdomen, specified site NEC
Omentitis —*see* Peritonitis
Omentum, omental —*see* condition
Omphalitis (congenital) (newborn) P38.9
with mild hemorrhage P38.1
without hemorrhage P38.9
not of newborn L08.82
tetanus A33
Omphalocele Q79.2
Omphalomesenteric duct, persistent Q43.0
Omphalorrhagia, newborn P51.9
Omsk hemorrhagic fever A98.1
Onanism (excessive) F98.8
Onchocerciasis, onchocercosis B73.1
with
eye disease B73.00
endophthalmitis B73.01
eyelid B73.09
glaucoma B73.02
specified NEC B73.09
eye NEC B73.00
eyelid B73.09
Oncocytoma —*see* Neoplasm, benign, by site
Oncovirus, as cause of disease classified elsewhere B97.32
Ondine's curse —*see* Apnea, sleep
Oneirophrenia F23
Onychauxis L60.2
congenital Q84.5
Onychia —*see also* Cellulitis, digit
with lymphangitis —*see* Lymphangitis, acute, digit
candidal B37.2
dermatophytic B35.1
Onychitis —*see also* Cellulitis, digit
with lymphangitis —*see* Lymphangitis, acute, digit
Onychocryptosis L60.0
Onychodystrophy L60.3
congenital Q84.6
Onychogryphosis, onychogryposis L60.2
Onycholysis L60.1
Onychomadesis L60.8
Onychomalacia L60.3
Onychomycosis (finger) (toe) B35.1
Onycho-osteodysplasia Q87.2
Onychophagia F98.8
Onychophosis L60.8
Onychoptosis L60.8
Onychorrhexis L60.3
congenital Q84.6
Onychoschizia L60.3
Onyxis (finger) (toe) L60.0
Onyxitis —*see also* Cellulitis, digit
with lymphangitis —*see* Lymphangitis, acute, digit
Oophoritis (cystic) (infectional) (interstitial) N70.92
with salpingitis N70.93
acute N70.02
with salpingitis N70.03
chronic N70.12
with salpingitis N70.13
complicating abortion —*see* Abortion, by type, complicated by, oophoritis
Oophorocele N83.4-●
Opacity, opacities
cornea H17.-●
central H17.1-●
congenital Q13.3
degenerative —*see* Degeneration, cornea
hereditary —*see* Dystrophy, cornea
inflammatory —*see* Keratitis
minor H17.81-●
peripheral H17.82-●
sequelae of trachoma (healed) B94.0
specified NEC H17.89
enamel (teeth) (fluoride) (nonfluoride) K00.3
lens —*see* Cataract
snowball —*see* Deposit, crystalline
vitreous (humor) NEC H43.39-●
congenital Q14.0
membranes and strands H43.31-●
Opalescent dentin (hereditary) K00.5
Open, opening
abnormal, organ or site, congenital —*see* Imperfect, closure
angle with
borderline
findings
high risk H40.02-●
low risk H40.01-●
intraocular pressure H40.00-●
cupping of discs H40.01-●
glaucoma (primary) —*see* Glaucoma, open angle
bite
anterior M26.220
posterior M26.221
false —*see* Imperfect, closure
margin on tooth restoration K08.51
restoration margins of tooth K08.51
wound —*see* Wound, open
Operational fatigue F48.8
Operative —*see* condition
Operculitis —*see* Periodontitis
Operculum —*see* Break, retina
Ophiasis L63.2
Ophthalmia —*see also* Conjunctivitis H10.9
actinic rays —*see* Photokeratitis
allergic (acute) —*see* Conjunctivitis, acute, atopic
blennorrhagic (gonococcal) (neonatorum) A54.31
diphtheritic A36.86
Egyptian A71.1
electrica —*see* Photokeratitis
gonococcal (neonatorum) A54.31
metastatic —*see* Endophthalmitis, purulent
migraine —*see* Migraine, ophthalmoplegic
neonatorum, newborn P39.1
gonococcal A54.31
nodosa H16.24-●
purulent —*see* Conjunctivitis, acute, mucopurulent
spring —*see* Conjunctivitis, acute, atopic
sympathetic —*see* Uveitis, sympathetic
Ophthalmitis —*see* Ophthalmia
Ophthalmocele (congenital) Q15.8
Ophthalmoneuromyelitis G36.0
Ophthalmoplegia —*see also* Strabismus, paralytic
anterior internuclear —*see* Ophthalmoplegia, internuclear
ataxia-areflexia G61.0
diabetic —*see* E08-E13 with .39
exophthalmic E05.00
with thyroid storm E05.01
external H49.88-●
progressive H49.4-●
with pigmentary retinopathy —*see* Kearns-Sayre syndrome
total H49.3-●
internal (complete) (total) H52.51-●
internuclear H51.2-●
migraine —*see* Migraine, ophthalmoplegic
Parinaud's H49.88-●
progressive external —*see* Ophthalmoplegia, external, progressive
supranuclear, progressive G23.1
total (external) —*see* Ophthalmoplegia, external, total
Opioid(s)
abuse —*see* Abuse, drug, opioids
dependence —*see* Dependence, drug, opioids
induced, without use disorder
anxiety disorder F11.988
delirium F11.921
depressive disorder F11.94
sexual dysfunction F11.981
sleep disorder F11.982
Opisthognathism M26.09
Opisthorchiasis (felineus) (viverrini) B66.0
Opitz' disease D73.2
Opiumism —*see* Dependence, drug, opioid
Oppenheim's disease G70.2
Oppenheim-Urbach disease (necrobiosis lipoidica diabeticorum) —*see* E08-E13 with .620
Optic nerve —*see* condition
Orbit —*see* condition
Orchioblastoma C62.9-●
Orchitis (gangrenous) (nonspecific) (septic) (suppurative) N45.2
blennorrhagic (gonococcal) (acute) (chronic) A54.23
chlamydial A56.19
filarial —*see also* Infestation, filarial B74.9 *[N51]*
gonococcal (acute) (chronic) A54.23
mumps B26.0
syphilitic A52.76
tuberculous A18.15
Orf (virus disease) B08.02
Organic —*see also* condition
brain syndrome F09
heart —*see* Disease, heart
mental disorder F09
psychosis F09
Orgasm
anejaculatory N53.13
Oriental
bilharziasis B65.2
schistosomiasis B65.2
Orifice —*see* condition
Origin of both great vessels from right ventricle Q20.1
Ormond's disease (with ureteral obstruction) N13.5
with infection N13.6
Ornithine metabolism disorder E72.4
Ornithinemia (Type I) (Type II) E72.4
Ornithosis A70
Orotaciduria, oroticaciduria (congenital) (hereditary) (pyrimidine deficiency) E79.8
anemia D53.0
Orthodontics
adjustment Z46.4
fitting Z46.4
Orthopnea R06.01

Orthopoxvirus B08.09
~~specified NEC B08.09~~
Os, uterus —*see* condition
Osgood-Schlatter disease or osteochondrosis —*see* Osteochondrosis, juvenile, tibia
Osler (-Weber)-Rendu disease I78.0
Osler's nodes I33.0
Osmidrosis L75.0
Osseous —*see* condition
Ossification
artery —*see* Arteriosclerosis
auricle (ear) —*see* Disorder, pinna, specified type NEC
bronchial J98.09
cardiac —*see* Degeneration, myocardial
cartilage (senile) —*see* Disorder, cartilage, specified type NEC
coronary (artery) —*see* Disease, heart, ischemic, atherosclerotic
diaphragm J98.6
ear, middle —*see* Otosclerosis
falx cerebri G96.19
fontanel, premature Q75.0
heart —*see also* Degeneration, myocardial
valve —*see* Endocarditis
larynx J38.7
ligament —*see* Disorder, tendon, specified type NEC
posterior longitudinal —*see* Spondylopathy, specified NEC
meninges (cerebral) (spinal) G96.19
multiple, eccentric centers —*see* Disorder, bone, development or growth
muscle —*see also* Calcification, muscle
due to burns —*see* Myositis, ossificans, in, burns
paralytic —*see* Myositis, ossificans, in, quadriplegia
progressive —*see* Myositis, ossificans, progressiva
specified NEC M61.50
ankle M61.57- ●
foot M61.57- ●
forearm M61.53- ●
hand M61.54- ●
lower leg M61.56- ●
multiple sites M61.59
pelvic region M61.55- ●
shoulder region M61.51- ●
specified site NEC M61.58
thigh M61.55- ●
upper arm M61.52- ●
traumatic —*see* Myositis, ossificans, traumatica
myocardium, myocardial —*see* Degeneration, myocardial
penis N48.89
periarticular —*see* Disorder, joint, specified type NEC
pinna —*see* Disorder, pinna, specified type NEC
rider's bone —*see* Ossification, muscle, specified NEC
sclera H15.89
subperiosteal, post-traumatic M89.8X- ●
tendon —*see* Disorder, tendon, specified type NEC
trachea J39.8
tympanic membrane —*see* Disorder, tympanic membrane, specified NEC
vitreous (humor) —*see* Deposit, crystalline
Osteitis —*see also* Osteomyelitis
alveolar M27.3
condensans M85.30
ankle M85.37- ●
foot M85.37- ●
forearm M85.33- ●
hand M85.34- ●
lower leg M85.36- ●
multiple site M85.39
Osteitis *(Continued)*
condensans *(Continued)*
neck M85.38
rib M85.38
shoulder M85.31- ●
skull M85.38
specified site NEC M85.38
thigh M85.35- ●
toe M85.37- ●
upper arm M85.32- ●
vertebra M85.38
deformans M88.9
in (due to)
malignant neoplasm of bone C41.9 *[M90.60]*
neoplastic disease —*see also* Neoplasm D49.9 *[M90.60]*
carpus D49.9 *[M90.64- ●]*
clavicle D49.9 *[M90.61- ●]*
femur D49.9 *[M90.65- ●]*
fibula D49.9 *[M90.66- ●]*
finger D49.9 *[M90.64- ●]*
humerus D49.9 *[M90.62- ●]*
ilium D49.9 *[M90.65- ●]*
ischium D49.9 *[M90.65- ●]*
metacarpus D49.9 *[M90.64- ●]*
metatarsus D49.9 *[M90.67- ●]*
multiple sites D49.9 *[M90.69]*
neck D49.9 *[M90.68]*
radius D49.9 *[M90.63- ●]*
rib D49.9 *[M90.68]*
scapula D49.9 *[M90.61- ●]*
skull D49.9 *[M90.68]*
tarsus D49.9 *[M90.67- ●]*
tibia D49.9 *[M90.66- ●]*
toe D49.9 *[M90.67- ●]*
ulna D49.9 *[M90.63- ●]*
vertebra D49.9 *[M90.68]*
skull M88.0
specified NEC —*see* Paget's disease, bone, by site
vertebra M88.1
due to yaws A66.6
fibrosa NEC —*see* Cyst, bone, by site
circumscripta —*see* Dysplasia, fibrous, bone NEC
cystica (generalisata) E21.0
disseminata Q78.1
osteoplastica E21.0
fragilitans Q78.0
Garr's (sclerosing) —*see* Osteomyelitis, specified type NEC
jaw (acute) (chronic) (lower) (suppurative) (upper) M27.2
parathyroid E21.0
petrous bone (acute) (chronic) —*see* Petrositis
sclerotic, nonsuppurative —*see* Osteomyelitis, specified type NEC
tuberculosa A18.09
cystica D86.89
multiplex cystoides D86.89
Osteoarthritis M19.90
ankle M19.07- ●
elbow M19.02- ●
foot joint M19.07- ●
generalized M15.9
erosive M15.4
primary M15.0
specified NEC M15.8
hand joint M19.04- ●
first carpometacarpal joint M18.9- ●
hip M16.1- ●
bilateral M16.0
due to hip dysplasia (unilateral) M16.3- ●
bilateral M16.2
interphalangeal
distal (Heberden) M15.1
proximal (Bouchard) M15.2
knee M17.1- ●
bilateral M17.0
Osteoarthritis *(Continued)*
post-traumatic NEC M19.92
ankle M19.17- ●
elbow M19.12- ●
foot joint M19.17- ●
hand joint M19.14- ●
first carpometacarpal joint M18.3- ●
bilateral M18.2
hip M16.5- ●
bilateral M16.4
knee M17.3- ●
bilateral M17.2
shoulder M19.11- ●
wrist M19.13- ●
primary M19.91
ankle M19.07- ●
elbow M19.02- ●
foot joint M19.07- ●
hand joint M19.04- ●
first carpometacarpal joint M18.1- ●
bilateral M18.0
hip M16.1- ●
bilateral M16.0
knee M17.1- ●
bilateral M17.0
▶ multiple sites M89.49
shoulder M19.01- ●
spine —*see* Spondylosis
wrist M19.03- ●
secondary M19.93
ankle M19.27- ●
elbow M19.22- ●
foot joint M19.27- ●
hand joint M19.24- ●
first carpometacarpal joint M18.5- ●
bilateral M18.4
hip M16.7
bilateral M16.6
knee M17.5
bilateral M17.4
multiple M15.3
shoulder M19.21- ●
spine —*see* Spondylosis
wrist M19.23- ●
shoulder M19.01- ●
spine —*see* Spondylosis
wrist M19.03- ●
Osteoarthropathy (hypertrophic) M19.90
ankle —*see* Osteoarthritis, primary, ankle
elbow —*see* Osteoarthritis, primary, elbow
foot joint —*see* Osteoarthritis, primary, foot
hand joint —*see* Osteoarthritis, primary, hand joint
knee joint —*see* Osteoarthritis, primary, knee
multiple site —*see* Osteoarthritis, primary, multiple joint
pulmonary —*see also* Osteoarthropathy, specified type NEC
hypertrophic —*see* Osteoarthropathy, hypertrophic, specified type NEC
secondary —*see* Osteoarthropathy, specified type NEC
secondary hypertrophic —*see* Osteoarthropathy, specified type NEC
shoulder —*see* Osteoarthritis, primary, shoulder
specified joint NEC —*see* Osteoarthritis, primary, specified joint NEC
specified type NEC M89.40
carpus M89.44- ●
clavicle M89.41- ●
femur M89.45- ●
fibula M89.46- ●
finger M89.44- ●
humerus M89.42- ●
ilium M89.459
ischium M89.459
metacarpus M89.44- ●
metatarsus M89.47- ●
multiple sites M89.49
neck M89.48
radius M89.43- ●

Osteoarthropathy *(Continued)*
specified type NEC *(Continued)*
rib M89.48
scapula M89.41-●
skull M89.48
tarsus M89.47-●
tibia M89.46-●
toe M89.47-●
ulna M89.43-●
vertebra M89.48
spine *—see* Spondylosis
wrist *—see* Osteoarthritis, primary, wrist
Osteoarthrosis (degenerative) (hypertrophic) (joint) *—see also* Osteoarthritis
deformans alkaptonurica E7Ø.29 *[M36.8]*
erosive M15.4
generalized M15.9
primary M15.Ø
polyarticular M15.9
spine *—see* Spondylosis
Osteoblastoma *—see* Neoplasm, bone, benign
aggressive *—see* Neoplasm, bone, uncertain behavior
Osteochondroarthrosis deformans endemica *—see* Disease, Kaschin-Beck
Osteochondritis *—see also* Osteochondropathy, by site
Brailsford's *—see* Osteochondrosis, juvenile, radius
dissecans M93.2Ø
ankle M93.27-●
elbow M93.22-●
foot M93.27-●
hand M93.24-●
hip M93.25-●
knee M93.26-●
multiple sites M93.29
shoulder joint M93.21-●
specified site NEC M93.28
wrist M93.23-●
juvenile M92.9
patellar *—see* Osteochondrosis, juvenile, patella
syphilitic (congenital) (early) A5Ø.Ø2 *[M9Ø.8Ø]*
ankle A5Ø.Ø2 *[M9Ø.87-●]*
elbow A5Ø.Ø2 *[M9Ø.82-●]*
foot A5Ø.Ø2 *[M9Ø.87-●]*
forearm A5Ø.Ø2 *[M9Ø.83-●]*
hand A5Ø.Ø2 *[M9Ø.84-●]*
hip A5Ø.Ø2 *[M9Ø.85-●]*
knee A5Ø.Ø2 *[M9Ø.86●-]*
multiple sites A5Ø.Ø2 *[M9Ø.89]*
shoulder joint A5Ø.Ø2 *[M9Ø.81-●]*
specified site NEC A5Ø.Ø2 *[M9Ø.88]*
Osteochondrodysplasia Q78.9
with defects of growth of tubular bones and spine Q77.9
specified NEC Q77.8
specified NEC Q78.8
Osteochondrodystrophy E78.9
Osteochondrolysis *—see* Osteochondritis, dissecans
Osteochondroma *—see* Neoplasm, bone, benign
Osteochondromatosis D48.Ø
syndrome Q78.4
Osteochondromyxosarcoma *—see* Neoplasm, bone, malignant
Osteochondropathy M93.9Ø
ankle M93.97-●
elbow M93.92-●
foot M93.97-●
hand M93.94-●
hip M93.95-●
Kienböck's disease of adults M93.1
knee M93.96-●
multiple joints M93.99
osteochondritis dissecans *—see* Osteochondritis, dissecans
osteochondrosis *—see* Osteochondrosis
shoulder region M93.91-●
Osteochondropathy *(Continued)*
slipped upper femoral epiphysis *—see* Slipped, epiphysis, upper femoral
specified joint NEC M93.98
specified type NEC M93.8Ø
ankle M93.87-●
elbow M93.82-●
foot M93.87-●
hand M93.84-●
hip M93.85-●
knee M93.86-●
multiple joints M93.89
shoulder region M93.81-●
specified joint NEC M93.88
wrist M93.83-●
syphilitic, congenital
early A5Ø.Ø2 *[M9Ø.8Ø]*
late A5Ø.56 *[M9Ø.8Ø]*
wrist M93.93-●
Osteochondrosarcoma *—see* Neoplasm, bone, malignant
Osteochondrosis *—see also* Osteochondropathy, by site
acetabulum (juvenile) M91.Ø
adult *—see* Osteochondropathy, specified type NEC, by site
astragalus (juvenile) *—see* Osteochondrosis, juvenile, tarsus
Blount's *—see* Osteochondrosis, juvenile, tibia
Buchanan's M91.Ø
Burns' *—see* Osteochondrosis, juvenile, ulna
calcaneus (juvenile) *—see* Osteochondrosis, juvenile, tarsus
capitular epiphysis (femur) (juvenile) *—see* Legg-Calvé-Perthes disease
carpal (juvenile) (lunate) (scaphoid) *—see* Osteochondrosis, juvenile, hand, carpal lunate
adult M93.1
coxae juvenilis *—see* Legg-Calvé-Perthes disease
deformans juvenilis, coxae *—see* Legg-Calvé-Perthes disease
Diaz's *—see* Osteochondrosis, juvenile, tarsus
dissecans (knee) (shoulder) *—see* Osteochondritis, dissecans
femoral capital epiphysis (juvenile) *—see* Legg-Calvé-Perthes disease
femur (head), juvenile *—see* Legg-Calvé-Perthes disease
fibula (juvenile) *—see* Osteochondrosis, juvenile, fibula
foot NEC (juvenile) M92.8
Freiberg's *—see* Osteochondrosis, juvenile, metatarsus
Haas' (juvenile) *—see* Osteochondrosis, juvenile, humerus
Haglund's *—see* Osteochondrosis, juvenile, tarsus
hip (juvenile) *—see* Legg-Calvé-Perthes disease
humerus (capitulum) (head) (juvenile) *—see* Osteochondrosis, juvenile, humerus
ilium, iliac crest (juvenile) M91.Ø
ischiopubic synchondrosis M91.Ø
Iselin's *—see* Osteochondrosis, juvenile, metatarsus
juvenile, juvenilis M92.9
after congenital dislocation of hip reduction *—see* Osteochondrosis, juvenile, hip, specified NEC
arm *—see* Osteochondrosis, juvenile, upper limb NEC
capitular epiphysis (femur) *—see* Legg-Calvé-Perthes disease
clavicle, sternal epiphysis *—see* Osteochondrosis, juvenile, upper limb NEC
coxae *—see* Legg-Calvé-Perthes disease
deformans M92.9
fibula M92.5-●
foot NEC M92.8
Osteochondrosis *(Continued)*
juvenile, juvenilis *(Continued)*
hand M92.2Ø-●
carpal lunate M92.21-●
metacarpal head M92.22-●
specified site NEC M92.29-●
head of femur *—see* Legg-Calvé-Perthes disease
hip and pelvis M91.9-●
coxa plana *—see* Coxa, plana
femoral head *—see* Legg-Calvé-Perthes disease
pelvis M91.Ø
pseudocoxalgia *—see* Pseudocoxalgia
specified NEC M91.8-●
humerus M92.Ø-●
limb
lower NEC M92.8
upper NEC *—see* Osteochondrosis, juvenile, upper limb NEC
medial cuneiform bone *—see* Osteochondrosis, juvenile, tarsus
metatarsus M92.7-●
patella M92.4-●
radius M92.1-●
specified site NEC M92.8
spine M42.ØØ
cervical region M42.Ø2
cervicothoracic region M42.Ø3
lumbar region M42.Ø6
lumbosacral region M42.Ø7
multiple sites M42.Ø9
occipito-atlanto-axial region M42.Ø1
sacrococcygeal region M42.Ø8
thoracic region M42.Ø4
thoracolumbar region M42.Ø5
tarsus M92.6-●
tibia M92.5-●
ulna M92.1-●
upper limb NEC M92.3-●
vertebra (body) (epiphyseal plates) (Calvé's) (Scheuermann's) *—see* Osteochondrosis, juvenile, spine
Kienböck's *—see* Osteochondrosis, juvenile, hand, carpal lunate
adult M93.1
Köhler's
patellar *—see* Osteochondrosis, juvenile, patella
tarsal navicular *—see* Osteochondrosis, juvenile, tarsus
Legg-Perthes (-Calvé's) (-Waldenström) *—see* Legg-Calvé-Perthes disease
limb
lower NEC (juvenile) M92.8
upper NEC (juvenile) *—see* Osteochondrosis, juvenile, upper limb NEC
lunate bone (carpal) (juvenile) *—see also* Osteochondrosis, juvenile, hand, carpal lunate
adult M93.1
Mauclaire's *—see* Osteochondrosis, juvenile, hand, metacarpal
metacarpal (head) (juvenile) *—see* Osteochondrosis, juvenile, hand, metacarpal
metatarsus (fifth) (head) (juvenile) (second) *—see* Osteochondrosis, juvenile, metatarsus
navicular (juvenile) *—see* Osteochondrosis, juvenile, tarsus
os
calcis (juvenile) *—see* Osteochondrosis, juvenile, tarsus
tibiale externum (juvenile) *—see* Osteochondrosis, juvenile, tarsus
Osgood-Schlatter *—see* Osteochondrosis, juvenile, tibia
Panner's *—see* Osteochondrosis, juvenile, humerus

Osteochondrosis *(Continued)*
patellar center (juvenile) (primary) (secondary) —*see* Osteochondrosis, juvenile, patella
pelvis (juvenile) M91.Ø
Pierson's M91.Ø
radius (head) (juvenile) —*see* Osteochondrosis, juvenile, radius
Scheuermann's —*see* Osteochondrosis, juvenile, spine
Sever's —*see* Osteochondrosis, juvenile, tarsus
Sinding-Larsen —*see* Osteochondrosis, juvenile, patella
spine M42.9
adult M42.1Ø
cervical region M42.12
cervicothoracic region M42.13
lumbar region M42.16
lumbosacral region M42.17
multiple sites M42.19
occipito-atlanto-axial region M42.11
sacrococcygeal region M42.18
thoracic region M42.14
thoracolumbar region M42.15
juvenile —*see* Osteochondrosis, juvenile, spine
symphysis pubis (juvenile) M91.Ø
syphilitic (congenital) A5Ø.Ø2
talus (juvenile) —*see* Osteochondrosis, juvenile, tarsus
tarsus (navicular) (juvenile) —*see* Osteochondrosis, juvenile, tarsus
tibia (proximal) (tubercle) (juvenile) —*see* Osteochondrosis, juvenile, tibia
tuberculous —*see* Tuberculosis, bone
ulna (lower) (juvenile) —*see* Osteochondrosis, juvenile, ulna
van Neck's M91.Ø
vertebral —*see* Osteochondrosis, spine
Osteoclastoma D48.Ø
malignant —*see* Neoplasm, bone, malignant
Osteodynia —*see* Disorder, bone, specified type NEC
Osteodystrophy Q78.9
azotemic N25.Ø
congenital Q78.9
parathyroid, secondary E21.1
renal N25.Ø
Osteofibroma —*see* Neoplasm, bone, benign
Osteofibrosarcoma —*see* Neoplasm, bone, malignant
Osteogenesis imperfecta Q78.Ø
Osteogenic —*see* condition
Osteolysis M89.5Ø
carpus M89.54- ●
clavicle M89.51- ●
femur M89.55- ●
fibula M89.56- ●
finger M89.54- ●
humerus M89.52- ●
ilium M89.559
ischium M89.559
joint prosthesis (periprosthetic) —*see* Complications, joint prosthesis, mechanical, periprosthetic, osteolysis, by site
metacarpus M89.54- ●
metatarsus M89.57- ●
multiple sites M89.59
neck M89.58
periprosthetic —*see* Complications, joint prosthesis, mechanical, periprosthetic, osteolysis, by site
radius M89.53- ●
rib M89.58
scapula M89.51- ●
skull M89.58

Osteolysis *(Continued)*
tarsus M89.57- ●
tibia M89.56- ●
toe M89.57- ●
ulna M89.53- ●
vertebra M89.58
Osteoma —*see also* Neoplasm, bone, benign
osteoid —*see also* Neoplasm, bone, benign
giant —*see* Neoplasm, bone, benign
Osteomalacia M83.9
adult M83.9
drug-induced NEC M83.5
due to
malabsorption (postsurgical) M83.2
malnutrition M83.3
specified NEC M83.8
aluminium-induced M83.4
infantile —*see* Rickets
juvenile —*see* Rickets
oncogenic E83.89
pelvis M83.8
puerperal M83.Ø
senile M83.1
vitamin-D-resistant in adults E83.31 *[M9Ø.8- ●]*
carpus E83.31 *[M9Ø.84- ●]*
clavicle E83.31 *[M9Ø.81- ●]*
femur E83.31 *[M9Ø.85- ●]*
fibula E83.31 *[M9Ø.86- ●]*
finger E83.31 *[M9Ø.84- ●]*
humerus E83.31 *[M9Ø.82- ●]*
ilium E83.31 *[M9Ø.859]*
ischium E83.31 *[M9Ø.859]*
metacarpus E83.31 *[M9Ø.84- ●]*
metatarsus E83.31 *[M9Ø.87- ●]*
multiple sites E83.31 *[M9Ø.89]*
neck E83.31 *[M9Ø.88]*
radius E83.31 *[M9Ø.83- ●]*
rib E83.31 *[M9Ø.88]*
scapula E83.31 *[M9Ø.819]*
skull E83.31 *[M9Ø.88]*
tarsus E83.31 *[M9Ø.879]*
tibia E83.31 *[M9Ø.869]*
toe E83.31 *[M9Ø.879]*
ulna E83.31 *[M9Ø.839]*
vertebra E83.31 *[M9Ø.88]*
Osteomyelitis (general) (infective) (localized) (neonatal) (purulent) (septic) (staphylococcal) (streptococcal) (suppurative) (with periostitis) M86.9
acute M86.1Ø
carpus M86.14- ●
clavicle M86.11- ●
femur M86.15- ●
fibula M86.16- ●
finger M86.14- ●
hematogenous M86.ØØ
carpus M86.Ø4- ●
clavicle M86.Ø1- ●
femur M86.Ø5- ●
fibula M86.Ø6- ●
finger M86.Ø4- ●
humerus M86.Ø2- ●
ilium M86.Ø59
ischium M86.Ø59
mandible M27.2
metacarpus M86.Ø4- ●
metatarsus M86.Ø7- ●
multiple sites M86.Ø9
neck M86.Ø8
orbit HØ5.Ø2- ●
petrous bone —*see* Petrositis
radius M86.Ø3- ●
rib M86.Ø8
scapula M86.Ø1- ●
skull M86.Ø8
tarsus M86.Ø7- ●
tibia M86.Ø6- ●
toe M86.Ø7- ●
ulna M86.Ø3- ●
vertebra —*see* Osteomyelitis, vertebra

Osteomyelitis *(Continued)*
acute *(Continued)*
humerus M86.12- ●
➡ ilium M86.18
➡ ischium M86.18
mandible M27.2
metacarpus M86.14- ●
metatarsus M86.17- ●
multiple sites M86.19
neck M86.18
orbit HØ5.Ø2- ●
petrous bone —*see* Petrositis
radius M86.13- ●
rib M86.18
scapula M86.11- ●
skull M86.18
tarsus M86.17- ●
tibia M86.16- ●
toe M86.17- ●
ulna M86.13- ●
vertebra —*see* Osteomyelitis, vertebra
chronic (or old) M86.6Ø
with draining sinus M86.4Ø
carpus M86.44- ●
clavicle M86.41- ●
femur M86.45- ●
fibula M86.46- ●
finger M86.44- ●
humerus M86.42- ●
ilium M86.459
ischium M86.459
mandible M27.2
metacarpus M86.44- ●
metatarsus M86.47- ●
multiple sites M86.49
neck M86.48
orbit HØ5.Ø2- ●
petrous bone —*see* Petrositis
radius M86.43- ●
rib M86.48
scapula M86.41- ●
skull M86.48
tarsus M86.47- ●
tibia M86.46- ●
toe M86.47- ●
ulna M86.43- ●
vertebra —*see* Osteomyelitis, vertebra
carpus M86.64- ●
clavicle M86.61- ●
femur M86.65- ●
fibula M86.66- ●
finger M86.64- ●
hematogenous NEC M86.5Ø
carpus M86.54- ●
clavicle M86.51- ●
femur M86.55- ●
fibula M86.56- ●
finger M86.54- ●
humerus M86.52- ●
ilium M86.559
ischium M86.559
mandible M27.2
metacarpus M86.54- ●
metatarsus M86.57- ●
multifocal M86.3Ø
carpus M86.34- ●
clavicle M86.31- ●
femur M86.35- ●
fibula M86.36- ●
finger M86.34- ●
humerus M86.32- ●
ilium M86.359
ischium M86.359
metacarpus M86.34- ●
metatarsus M86.37- ●
multiple sites M86.39
neck M86.38
radius M86.33- ●
rib M86.38
scapula M86.31- ●

Osteomyelitis *(Continued)*
chronic *(Continued)*
hematogenous NEC *(Continued)*
multifocal *(Continued)*
skull M86.38
tarsus M86.37-●
tibia M86.36-●
toe M86.37-●
ulna M86.33-●
vertebra —*see* Osteomyelitis, vertebra
multiple sites M86.59
neck M86.58
orbit HØ5.Ø2-●
petrous bone —*see* Petrositis
radius M86.53-●
rib M86.58
scapula M86.51-●
skull M86.58
tarsus M86.57-●
tibia M86.56-●
toe M86.57-●
ulna M86.53-●
vertebra —*see* Osteomyelitis, vertebra
humerus M86.62-●
ilium M86.659
ischium M86.659
mandible M27.2
metacarpus M86.64-●
metatarsus M86.67-●
multifocal —*see* Osteomyelitis, chronic, hematogenous, multifocal
multiple sites M86.69
neck M86.68
orbit HØ5.Ø2-●
petrous bone —*see* Petrositis
radius M86.63-●
rib M86.68
scapula M86.61-●
skull M86.68
tarsus M86.67-●
tibia M86.66-●
toe M86.67-●
ulna M86.63-●
vertebra —*see* Osteomyelitis, vertebra
echinococcal B67.2
Garr's —*see* Osteomyelitis, specified type NEC
in diabetes mellitus —*see* EØ8-E13 with .69
jaw (acute) (chronic) (lower) (neonatal) (suppurative) (upper) M27.2
nonsuppurating —*see* Osteomyelitis, specified type NEC
orbit HØ5.Ø2-●
petrous bone —*see* Petrositis
Salmonella (arizonae) (cholerae-suis) (enteritidis) (typhimurium) AØ2.24
sclerosing, nonsuppurative —*see* Osteomyelitis, specified type NEC
specified type NEC —*see also* subcategory M86.8X-●
mandible M27.2
orbit HØ5.Ø2-●
petrous bone —*see* Petrositis
vertebra —*see* Osteomyelitis, vertebra
subacute M86.2Ø
carpus M86.24-●
clavicle M86.21-●
femur M86.25-●
fibula M86.26-●
finger M86.24-●
humerus M86.22-●
mandible M27.2
metacarpus M86.24-●
metatarsus M86.27-●
multiple sites M86.29
neck M86.28
orbit HØ5.Ø2-●
petrous bone —*see* Petrositis
radius M86.23-●
rib M86.28
scapula M86.21-●

Osteomyelitis *(Continued)*
subacute *(Continued)*
skull M86.28
tarsus M86.27-●
tibia M86.26-●
toe M86.27-●
ulna M86.23-●
vertebra —*see* Osteomyelitis, vertebra
syphilitic A52.77
congenital (early) A5Ø.Ø2 *[M9Ø.8Ø]*
tuberculous —*see* Tuberculosis, bone
typhoid AØ1.Ø5
vertebra M46.2Ø
cervical region M46.22
cervicothoracic region M46.23
lumbar region M46.26
lumbosacral region M46.27
occipito-atlanto-axial region M46.21
sacrococcygeal region M46.28
thoracic region M46.24
thoracolumbar region M46.25
Osteomyelofibrosis D47.4
Osteomyelosclerosis D75.89
Osteonecrosis M87.9
due to
drugs —*see* Osteonecrosis, secondary, due to, drugs
trauma —*see* Osteonecrosis, secondary, due to, trauma
idiopathic aseptic M87.ØØ
ankle M87.Ø7-●
carpus M87.Ø3-●
clavicle M87.Ø1-●
femur M87.Ø5-●
fibula M87.Ø6-●
finger M87.Ø4-●
humerus M87.Ø2-●
ilium M87.Ø5Ø
ischium M87.Ø5Ø
metacarpus M87.Ø4-●
metatarsus M87.Ø7-●
multiple sites M87.Ø9
neck M87.Ø8
pelvis M87.Ø5Ø
radius M87.Ø3-●
rib M87.Ø8
scapula M87.Ø1-●
skull M87.Ø8
tarsus M87.Ø7-●
tibia M87.Ø6-●
toe M87.Ø7-●
ulna M87.Ø3-●
vertebra M87.Ø8
secondary NEC M87.3Ø
carpus M87.33-●
clavicle M87.31-●
due to
drugs M87.1Ø
carpus M87.13-●
clavicle M87.11-●
femur M87.15-●
fibula M87.16-●
finger M87.14-●
humerus M87.12-●
ilium M87.159
ischium M87.159
jaw M87.18Ø
metacarpus M87.14-●
metatarsus M87.17-●
multiple sites M87.19
neck M87.18
radius M87.13-●
rib M87.18
scapula M87.11-●
skull M87.18
tarsus M87.17-●
tibia M87.16-●
toe M87.17-●
ulna M87.13-●
vertebra M87.18

Osteonecrosis *(Continued)*
secondary NEC *(Continued)*
due to *(Continued)*
hemoglobinopathy NEC D58.2 *[M9Ø.5Ø]*
carpus D58.2 *[M9Ø.54-●]*
clavicle D58.2 *[M9Ø.51-●]*
femur D58.2 *[M9Ø.55-●]*
fibula D58.2 *[M9Ø.56-●]*
finger D58.2 *[M9Ø.54-●]*
humerus D58.2 *[M9Ø.52-●]*
ilium D58.2 *[M9Ø.55-●]*
ischium D58.2 *[M9Ø.55-●]*
metacarpus D58.2 *[M9Ø.54-●]*
metatarsus D58.2 *[M9Ø.57-●]*
multiple sites D58.2 *[M9Ø.58]*
neck D58.2 *[M9Ø.58]*
radius D58.2 *[M9Ø.53-●]*
rib D58.2 *[M9Ø.58]*
scapula D58.2 *[M9Ø.51-●]*
skull D58.2 *[M9Ø.58]*
tarsus D58.2 *[M9Ø.57-●]*
tibia D58.2 *[M9Ø.56-●]*
toe D58.2 *[M9Ø.57-●]*
ulna D58.2 *[M9Ø.53-●]*
vertebra D58.2 *[M9Ø.58]*
trauma (previous) M87.2Ø
carpus M87.23-●
clavicle M87.21-●
femur M87.25-●
fibula M87.26-●
finger M87.24-●
humerus M87.22-●
ilium M87.25-●
ischium M87.25-●
metacarpus M87.24-●
metatarsus M87.27-●
multiple sites M87.29
neck M87.28
radius M87.23-●
rib M87.28
scapula M87.21-●
skull M87.28
tarsus M87.27-●
tibia M87.26-●
toe M87.27-●
ulna M87.23-●
vertebra M87.28
femur M87.35-●
fibula M87.36-●
finger M87.34-●
humerus M87.32
ilium M87.35Ø
in
caisson disease T7Ø.3 *[M9Ø.5Ø]*
carpus T7Ø.3 *[M9Ø.54-●]*
clavicle T7Ø.3 *[M9Ø.51-●]*
femur T7Ø.3 *[M9Ø.55-●]*
fibula T7Ø.3 *[M9Ø.56-●]*
finger T7Ø.3 *[M9Ø.54-●]*
humerus T7Ø.3 *[M9Ø.52-●]*
ilium T7Ø.3 *[M9Ø.55-●]*
ischium T7Ø.3 *[M9Ø.55-●]*
metacarpus T7Ø.3 *[M9Ø.54-●]*
metatarsus T7Ø.3 *[M9Ø.57-●]*
multiple sites T7Ø.3 *[M9Ø.59]*
neck T7Ø.3 *[M9Ø.58]*
radius T7Ø.3 *[M9Ø.53-●]*
rib T7Ø.3 *[M9Ø.58]*
scapula T7Ø.3 *[M9Ø.51-●]*
skull T7Ø.3 *[M9Ø.58]*
tarsus T7Ø.3 *[M9Ø.57-●]*
tibia T7Ø.3 *[M9Ø.56-●]*
toe T7Ø.3 *[M9Ø.57-●]*
ulna T7Ø.3 *[M9Ø.53-●]*
vertebra T7Ø.3 *[M9Ø.58]*
ischium M87.35Ø
metacarpus M87.34-●
metatarsus M87.37-●
multiple site M87.39
neck M87.38

- **Osteonecrosis** *(Continued)*
  - secondary NEC *(Continued)*
    - radius M87.33-●
    - rib M87.38
    - scapula M87.319
    - skull M87.38
    - tarsus M87.379
    - tibia M87.366
    - toe M87.379
    - ulna M87.33-●
    - vertebra M87.38
  - specified type NEC M87.8Ø
    - carpus M87.83-●
    - clavicle M87.81-●
    - femur M87.85-●
    - fibula M87.86-●
    - finger M87.84-●
    - humerus M87.82-●
    - ilium M87.85-●
    - ischium M87.85-●
    - metacarpus M87.84-●
    - metatarsus M87.87-●
    - multiple sites M87.89
    - neck M87.88
    - radius M87.83-●
    - rib M87.88-●
    - scapula M87.81-●
    - skull M87.88
    - tarsus M87.87-●
    - tibia M87.86-●
    - toe M87.87-●
    - ulna M87.83-●
    - vertebra M87.88
- **Osteo-onycho-arthro-dysplasia** Q87.2
- **Osteo-onychodysplasia, hereditary** Q87.2
- **Osteopathia condensans disseminata** Q78.8
- **Osteopathy** *—see also* Osteomyelitis, Osteonecrosis, Osteoporosis
  - after poliomyelitis M89.6Ø
    - carpus M89.64-●
    - clavicle M89.61-●
    - femur M89.65-●
    - fibula M89.66-●
    - finger M89.64-●
    - humerus M89.62-●
    - ilium M89.659
    - ischium M89.659
    - metacarpus M89.64-●
    - metatarsus M89.67-●
    - multiple sites M89.69
    - neck M89.68
    - radius M89.63-●
    - rib M89.68
    - scapula M89.61-●
    - skull M89.68
    - tarsus M89.67-●
    - tibia M89.66-●
    - toe M89.67-●
    - ulna M89.63-●
    - vertebra M89.68
  - in (due to)
    - renal osteodystrophy N25.Ø
    - specified diseases classified elsewhere *— see* subcategory M9Ø.8
- **Osteopenia** M85.8-●
  - borderline M85.8-●
- **Osteoperiostitis** *—see* Osteomyelitis, specified type NEC
- **Osteopetrosis** (familial) Q78.2
- **Osteophyte** M25.7Ø
  - ankle M25.77-●
  - elbow M25.72-●
  - foot joint M25.77-●
  - hand joint M25.74-●
  - hip M25.75-●
  - knee M25.76-●
  - shoulder M25.71-●
  - spine M25.78
  - vertebrae M25.78
  - wrist M25.73-●
- **Osteopoikilosis** Q78.8
- **Osteoporosis** (female) (male) M81.Ø
  - with current pathological fracture M8Ø.ØØ
  - age-related M81.Ø
    - with current pathologic fracture M8Ø.ØØ
      - carpus M8Ø.Ø4-●
      - clavicle M8Ø.Ø1-●
      - fibula M8Ø.Ø6-●
      - finger M8Ø.Ø4-●
      - humerus M8Ø.Ø2-●
      - ilium M8Ø.Ø5-●
      - ischium M8Ø.Ø5-●
      - metacarpus M8Ø.Ø4-●
      - metatarsus M8Ø.Ø7-●
      - pelvis M8Ø.Ø5-●
      - radius M8Ø.Ø3-●
      - scapula M8Ø.Ø1-●
      - tarsus M8Ø.Ø7-●
      - tibia M8Ø.Ø6-●
      - toe M8Ø.Ø7-●
      - ulna M8Ø.Ø3-●
      - vertebra M8Ø.Ø8
  - disuse M81.8
    - with current pathological fracture M8Ø.8Ø
      - carpus M8Ø.84-●
      - clavicle M8Ø.81-●
      - fibula M8Ø.86-●
      - finger M8Ø.84-●
      - humerus M8Ø.82-●
      - ilium M8Ø.85-●
      - ischium M8Ø.85-●
      - metacarpus M8Ø.84-●
      - metatarsus M8Ø.87-●
      - pelvis M8Ø.85-●
      - radius M8Ø.83-●
      - scapula M8Ø.81-●
      - tarsus M8Ø.87-●
      - tibia M8Ø.86-●
      - toe M8Ø.87-●
      - ulna M8Ø.83-●
      - vertebra M8Ø.88
  - drug-induced *—see* Osteoporosis, specified type NEC
  - idiopathic *—see* Osteoporosis, specified type NEC
  - involutional *—see* Osteoporosis, age-related
  - Lequesne M81.6
  - localized M81.6
  - postmenopausal M81.Ø
    - with pathological fracture M8Ø.ØØ
      - carpus M8Ø.Ø4-●
      - clavicle M8Ø.Ø1-●
      - fibula M8Ø.Ø6-●
      - finger M8Ø.Ø4-●
      - humerus M8Ø.Ø2-●
      - ilium M8Ø.Ø5-●
      - ischium M8Ø.Ø5-●
      - metacarpus M8Ø.Ø4-●
      - metatarsus M8Ø.Ø7-●
      - pelvis M8Ø.Ø5-●
      - radius M8Ø.Ø3-●
      - scapula M8Ø.Ø1-●
      - tarsus M8Ø.Ø7-●
      - tibia M8Ø.Ø6-●
      - toe M8Ø.Ø7-●
      - ulna M8Ø.Ø3-●
      - vertebra M8Ø.Ø8
  - postoophorectomy *—see* Osteoporosis, specified type NEC
  - postsurgical malabsorption *—see* Osteoporosis, specified type NEC
  - post-traumatic *—see* Osteoporosis, specified type NEC
  - senile *—see* Osteoporosis, age-related
  - specified type NEC M81.8
    - with pathological fracture M8Ø.8Ø
      - carpus M8Ø.84-●
      - clavicle M8Ø.81-●
      - fibula M8Ø.86-●
      - finger M8Ø.84-●
      - humerus M8Ø.82-●
      - ilium M8Ø.85-●
- **Osteoporosis** *(Continued)*
  - specified type NEC *(Continued)*
    - with pathological fracture *(Continued)*
      - ischium M8Ø.85-●
      - metacarpus M8Ø.84-●
      - metatarsus M8Ø.87-●
      - pelvis M8Ø.85-●
      - radius M8Ø.83-●
      - scapula M8Ø.81-●
      - tarsus M8Ø.87-●
      - tibia M8Ø.86-●
      - toe M8Ø.87-●
      - ulna M8Ø.83-●
      - vertebra M8Ø.88
- **Osteopsathyrosis** (idiopathica) Q78.Ø
- **Osteoradionecrosis, jaw** (acute) (chronic) (lower) (suppurative) (upper) M27.2
- **Osteosarcoma** (any form) *—see* Neoplasm, bone, malignant
- **Osteosclerosis** Q78.2
  - acquired M85.8-●
  - congenita Q77.4
  - fragilitas (generalisata) Q78.2
  - myelofibrosis D75.81
- **Osteosclerotic anemia** D64.89
- **Osteosis**
  - cutis L94.2
  - renal fibrocystic N25.Ø
- **Österreicher-Turner syndrome** Q87.2
- **Ostium**
  - atrioventriculare commune Q21.2
  - primum (arteriosum) (defect) (persistent) Q21.2
  - secundum (arteriosum) (defect) (patent) (persistent) Q21.1
- **Ostrum-Furst syndrome** Q75.8
- **Otalgia** *—see* subcategory H92.Ø
- **Otitis** (acute) H66.9Ø
  - with effusion *—see also* Otitis, media, nonsuppurative
    - purulent *—see* Otitis, media, suppurative
  - adhesive *—see* subcategory H74.1
  - chronic *—see also* Otitis, media, chronic
    - with effusion *—see also* Otitis, media, nonsuppurative, chronic
  - externa H6Ø.9-●
    - abscess *—see* Abscess, ear, external
    - acute (noninfective) H6Ø.5Ø-●
      - actinic H6Ø.51-●
      - chemical H6Ø.52-●
      - contact H6Ø.53-●
      - eczematoid H6Ø.54-●
      - infective *—see* Otitis, externa, infective
      - reactive H6Ø.55-●
      - specified NEC H6Ø.59-●
    - cellulitis *—see* Cellulitis, ear
    - chronic H6Ø.6-●
    - diffuse *—see* Otitis, externa, infective, diffuse
    - hemorrhagic *—see* Otitis, externa, infective, hemorrhagic
    - in (due to)
      - aspergillosis B44.89
      - candidiasis B37.84
      - erysipelas A46 *[H62.4Ø]*
      - herpes (simplex) virus infection BØØ.1
        - zoster BØ2.8
      - impetigo LØ1.ØØ *[H62.4Ø]*
      - infectious disease NEC B99 *[H62.4-●]*
      - mycosis NEC B36.9 *[H62.4Ø]*
      - parasitic disease NEC B89 *[H62.4Ø]*
      - viral disease NEC B34.9 *[H62.4Ø]*
      - zoster BØ2.8
    - infective NEC H6Ø.39-●
      - abscess *—see* Abscess, ear, external
      - cellulitis *—see* Cellulitis, ear
      - diffuse H6Ø.31-●
      - hemorrhagic H6Ø.32-●
      - swimmer's ear *—see* Swimmer's, ear
    - malignant H6Ø.2-●

▶ New ➠ Revised ~~deleted~~ Deleted ● Use Additional Character(s)

Otitis *(Continued)*
externa *(Continued)*
mycotic NEC B36.9 *[H62.4Ø]*
in
aspergillosis B44.89
candidiasis B37.84
moniliasis B37.84
necrotizing —*see* Otitis, externa, malignant
Pseudomonas aeruginosa —*see* Otitis, externa, malignant
reactive —*see* Otitis, externa, acute, reactive
specified NEC —*see* subcategory H6Ø.8
tropical NEC B36.9 *[H62.4Ø]*
in
aspergillosis B44.89
candidiasis B37.84
moniliasis B37.84
insidiosa —*see* Otosclerosis
interna —*see* subcategory H83.Ø
media (hemorrhagic) (staphylococcal) (streptococcal) H66.9-●
with effusion (nonpurulent) —*see* Otitis, media, nonsuppurative
acute, subacute H66.9Ø
allergic —*see* Otitis, media, nonsuppurative, acute, allergic
exudative —*see* Otitis, media, suppurative, acute
mucoid —*see* Otitis, media, nonsuppurative, acute
necrotizing —*see also* Otitis, media, suppurative, acute
in
measles BØ5.3
scarlet fever A38.Ø
nonsuppurative NEC —*see* Otitis, media, nonsuppurative, acute
purulent —*see* Otitis, media, suppurative, acute
sanguinous —*see* Otitis, media, nonsuppurative, acute
secretory —*see* Otitis, media, nonsuppurative, acute, serous
seromucinous —*see* Otitis, media, nonsuppurative, acute
serous —*see* Otitis, media, nonsuppurative, acute, serous
suppurative —*see* Otitis, media, suppurative, acute
allergic —*see* Otitis, media, nonsuppurative
catarrhal —*see* Otitis, media, nonsuppurative
chronic H66.9Ø
with effusion (nonpurulent) —*see* Otitis, media, nonsuppurative, chronic
allergic —*see* Otitis, media, nonsuppurative, chronic, allergic
benign suppurative —*see* Otitis, media, suppurative, chronic, tubotympanic
catarrhal —*see* Otitis, media, nonsuppurative, chronic, serous
exudative —*see* Otitis, media, suppurative, chronic
mucinous —*see* Otitis, media, nonsuppurative, chronic, mucoid
mucoid —*see* Otitis, media, nonsuppurative, chronic, mucoid
nonsuppurative NEC —*see* Otitis, media, nonsuppurative, chronic
purulent —*see* Otitis, media, suppurative, chronic
secretory —*see* Otitis, media, nonsuppurative, chronic, mucoid
seromucinous —*see* Otitis, media, nonsuppurative, chronic
serous —*see* Otitis, media, nonsuppurative, chronic, serous
suppurative —*see* Otitis, media, suppurative, chronic

Otitis *(Continued)*
media *(Continued)*
chronic *(Continued)*
transudative —*see* Otitis, media, nonsuppurative, chronic, mucoid
exudative —*see* Otitis, media, nonsuppurative
in (due to) (with)
influenza —*see* Influenza, with, otitis media
measles BØ5.3
scarlet fever A38.Ø
tuberculosis A18.6
viral disease NEC B34.-● *[H67.-●]*
mucoid —*see* Otitis, media, nonsuppurative
nonsuppurative H65.9-●
acute or subacute NEC H65.19-●
allergic H65.11-●
recurrent H65.11-●
recurrent H65.19-●
secretory —*see* Otitis, media, nonsuppurative, serous
serous H65.Ø-●
recurrent H65.Ø-●
chronic H65.49-●
allergic H65.41-●
mucoid H65.3-●
serous H65.2-●
postmeasles BØ5.3
purulent —*see* Otitis, media, suppurative
secretory —*see* Otitis, media, nonsuppurative
seromucinous —*see* Otitis, media, nonsuppurative
serous —*see* Otitis, media, nonsuppurative
suppurative H66.4-●
acute H66.ØØ-●
with rupture of ear drum H66.Ø1-●
recurrent H66.ØØ-●
with rupture of ear drum H66.Ø1-●
chronic —*see also* subcategory H66.3
atticoantral H66.2-●
benign —*see* Otitis, media, suppurative, chronic, tubotympanic
tubotympanic H66.1-●
transudative —*see* Otitis, media, nonsuppurative
tuberculous A18.6
Otocephaly Q18.2
Otolith syndrome —*see* subcategory H81.8
Otomycosis (diffuse) NEC B36.9 *[H62.4Ø]*
in
aspergillosis B44.89
candidiasis B37.84
moniliasis B37.84
Otoporosis —*see* Otosclerosis
Otorrhagia (nontraumatic) H92.2-●
traumatic - code by Type of injury
Otorrhea H92.1-●
cerebrospinal G96.Ø
Otosclerosis (general) H8Ø.9-●
cochlear (endosteal) H8Ø.2-●
involving
otic capsule —*see* Otosclerosis, cochlear
oval window
nonobliterative H8Ø.Ø-●
obliterative H8Ø.1-●
round window —*see* Otosclerosis, cochlear
nonobliterative —*see* Otosclerosis, involving, oval window, nonobliterative
obliterative —*see* Otosclerosis, involving, oval window, obliterative
specified NEC H8Ø.8-●
Otospongiosis —*see* Otosclerosis
Otto's disease or pelvis M24.7
Outcome of delivery Z37.9
multiple births Z37.9
all liveborn Z37.5Ø
quadruplets Z37.52
quintuplets Z37.53

Outcome of delivery *(Continued)*
multiple births *(Continued)*
all liveborn *(Continued)*
sextuplets Z37.54
specified number NEC Z37.59
triplets Z37.51
all stillborn Z37.7
some liveborn Z37.6Ø
quadruplets Z37.62
quintuplets Z37.63
sextuplets Z37.64
specified number NEC Z37.69
triplets Z37.61
single NEC Z37.9
liveborn Z37.Ø
stillborn Z37.1
twins NEC Z37.9
both liveborn Z37.2
both stillborn Z37.4
one liveborn, one stillborn Z37.3
Outlet —*see* condition
Ovalocytosis (congenital) (hereditary) —*see* Elliptocytosis
Ovarian —*see* Condition
Ovariocele N83.4-●
Ovaritis (cystic) —*see* Oophoritis
Ovary, ovarian —*see also* condition
resistant syndrome E28.39
vein syndrome N13.8
Overactive —*see also* Hyperfunction
adrenal cortex NEC E27.Ø
bladder N32.81
hypothalamus E23.3
thyroid —*see* Hyperthyroidism
Overactivity R46.3
child —*see* Disorder, attention-deficit hyperactivity
Overbite (deep) (excessive) (horizontal) (vertical) M26.29
Overbreathing —*see* Hyperventilation
Overconscientious personality F6Ø.5
Overdevelopment —*see* Hypertrophy
Overdistension —*see* Distension
Overdose, overdosage (drug) —*see* Table of Drugs and Chemicals, by drug, poisoning
Overeating R63.2
nonorganic origin F5Ø.89
psychogenic F5Ø.89
Overexertion (effects) (exhaustion) T73.3
Overexposure (effects) T73.9
exhaustion T73.2
Overfeeding —*see* Overeating
newborn P92.4
Overfill, endodontic M27.52
Overgrowth, bone —*see* Hypertrophy, bone
Overhanging of dental restorative material (unrepairable) KØ8.52
Overheated (places) (effects) —*see* Heat
Overjet (excessive horizontal) M26.23
Overlaid, overlying (suffocation) —*see* Asphyxia, traumatic, due to mechanical threat
Overlap, excessive horizontal (teeth) M26.23
Overl apping toe (acquired) —*see also* Deformity, toe, specified NEC
congenital (fifth toe) Q66.89
Overload
circulatory, due to transfusion (blood) (blood components) (TACO) E87.71
fluid E87.7Ø
due to transfusion (blood) (blood components) E87.71
specified NEC E87.79
iron, due to repeated red blood cell transfusions E83.111
potassium (K) E87.5
sodium (Na) E87.Ø
Overnutrition —*see* Hyperalimentation
Overproduction —*see also* Hypersecretion
ACTH E27.Ø
catecholamine E27.5
growth hormone E22.Ø

Overprotection, child by parent Z62.1
Overriding
  aorta Q25.49
  finger (acquired) —*see* Deformity, finger
    congenital Q68.1
  toe (acquired) —*see also* Deformity, toe, specified NEC
    congenital Q66.89
Overstrained R53.83
  heart —*see* Hypertrophy, cardiac
Overuse, muscle NEC M70.8-●
Overweight E66.3
Overworked R53.83
Oviduct —*see* condition
Ovotestis Q56.0
Ovulation (cycle)
  failure or lack of N97.0
  pain N94.0
Ovum —*see* condition
Owren's disease or syndrome (parahemophilia) D68.2
Ox heart —*see* Hypertrophy, cardiac
Oxalosis E72.53
Oxaluria E72.53
Oxycephaly, oxycephalic Q75.0
  syphilitic, congenital A50.02
Oxyuriasis B80
Oxyuris vermicularis (infestation) B80
Ozena J31.0

P

Pachyderma, pachydermia L85.9
larynx (verrucosa) J38.7
Pachydermatocele (congenital) Q82.8
Pachydermoperiostosis —*see also* Osteoarthropathy, hypertrophic, specified type NEC
clubbed nail M89.40 *[L62]*
Pachygyria Q04.3
Pachymeningitis (adhesive) (basal) (brain) (cervical) (chronic) (circumscribed) (external) (fibrous) (hemorrhagic) (hypertrophic) (internal) (purulent) (spinal) (suppurative) —*see* Meningitis
Pachyonychia (congenital) Q84.5
Pacinian tumor —*see* Neoplasm, skin, benign
Pad, knuckle or Garrod's M72.1
Paget-Schroetter syndrome I82.890
Paget's disease
with infiltrating duct carcinoma —*see* Neoplasm, breast, malignant
bone M88.9
carpus M88.84-●
clavicle M88.81-●
femur M88.85-●
fibula M88.86-●
finger M88.84-●
humerus M88.82-●
ilium M88.85-●
in neoplastic disease —*see* Osteitis, deformans, in neoplastic disease
ischium M88.85-●
metacarpus M88.84-●
metatarsus M88.87-●
multiple sites M88.89
neck M88.88
radius M88.83-●
rib M88.88
scapula M88.81-●
skull M88.0
▶specified NEC M88.88
tarsus M88.87-●
tibia M88.86-●
toe M88.87-●
ulna M88.83-●
➠vertebra M88.1
breast (female) C50.01-●
male C50.02-●
extramammary —*see also* Neoplasm, skin, malignant
anus C21.0
margin C44.590
skin C44.590
intraductal carcinoma —*see* Neoplasm, breast, malignant
malignant —*see* Neoplasm, skin, malignant
breast (female) C50.01-●
male C50.02-●
unspecified site (female) C50.01-●
male C50.02-●
mammary —*see* Paget's disease, breast
nipple —*see* Paget's disease, breast
osteitis deformans —*see* Paget's disease, bone
Pain(s) —*see also* Painful R52
abdominal R10.9
colic R10.83
generalized R10.84
with acute abdomen R10.0
lower R10.30
left quadrant R10.32
pelvic or perineal R10.2
periumbilical R10.33
right quadrant R10.31
rebound —*see* Tenderness, abdominal, rebound
severe with abdominal rigidity R10.0
tenderness —*see* Tenderness, abdominal
upper R10.10
epigastric R10.13
left quadrant R10.12
right quadrant R10.11

Pain *(Continued)*
acute R52
due to trauma G89.11
neoplasm related G89.3
postprocedural NEC G89.18
post-thoracotomy G89.12
specified by site — code to Pain, by site
adnexa (uteri) R10.2
anginoid —*see* Pain, precordial
anus K62.89
arm —*see* Pain, limb, upper
axillary (axilla) M79.62-●
back (postural) M54.9
bladder R39.89
associated with micturition —*see* Micturition, painful
chronic R39.82
bone —*see* Disorder, bone, specified type NEC
breast N64.4
broad ligament R10.2
cancer associated (acute) (chronic) G89.3
cecum —*see* Pain, abdominal
cervicobrachial M53.1
chest (central) R07.9
anterior wall R07.89
atypical R07.89
ischemic I20.9
musculoskeletal R07.89
non-cardiac R07.89
on breathing R07.1
pleurodynia R07.81
precordial R07.2
wall (anterior) R07.89
chronic G89.29
associated with significant psychosocial dysfunction G89.4
due to trauma G89.21
neoplasm related G89.3
postoperative NEC G89.28
postprocedural NEC G89.28
post-thoracotomy G89.22
specified NEC G89.29
coccyx M53.3
colon —*see* Pain, abdominal
coronary —*see* Angina
costochondral R07.1
diaphragm R07.1
due to cancer G89.3
due to device, implant or graft —*see also* Complications, by site and type, specified NEC T85.848
arterial graft NEC T82.848
breast (implant) T85.848
catheter NEC T85.848
dialysis (renal) T82.848
intraperitoneal T85.848
infusion NEC T82.848
spinal (epidural) (subdural) T85.840
urinary (indwelling) T83.84
electronic (electrode) (pulse generator) (stimulator)
bone T84.84
cardiac T82.847
nervous system (brain) (peripheral nerve) (spinal) T85.840
urinary T83.84
fixation, internal (orthopedic) NEC T84.84
gastrointestinal (bile duct) (esophagus) T85.848
genital NEC T83.84
heart NEC T82.847
infusion NEC T85.848
joint prosthesis T84.84
ocular (corneal graft) (orbital implant) NEC T85.848
orthopedic NEC T84.84
specified NEC T85.848
urinary NEC T83.84
vascular NEC T82.848
ventricular intracranial shunt T85.840

Pain *(Continued)*
due to malignancy (primary) (secondary) G89.3
ear —*see* subcategory H92.0
epigastric, epigastrium R10.13
eye —*see* Pain, ocular
face, facial R51
atypical G50.1
female genital organs NEC N94.89
finger —*see* Pain, limb, upper
flank —*see* Pain, abdominal
foot —*see* Pain, limb, lower
gallbladder K82.9
gas (intestinal) R14.1
gastric —*see* Pain, abdominal
generalized NOS R52
genital organ
female N94.89
male N50.89
groin —*see* Pain, abdominal, lower
hand —*see* Pain, limb, upper
head —*see* Headache
heart —*see* Pain, precordial
infra-orbital —*see* Neuralgia, trigeminal
intercostal R07.82
intermenstrual N94.0
jaw R68.84
joint M25.50
ankle M25.57-●
elbow M25.52-●
finger M25.54-●
foot M25.57-●
hand M25.54-●
hip M25.55-●
knee M25.56-●
shoulder M25.51-●
toe M25.57-●
wrist M25.53-●
kidney N23
laryngeal R07.0
leg —*see* Pain, limb, lower
limb M79.609
lower M79.60-●
foot M79.67-●
lower leg M79.66-●
thigh M79.65-●
toe M79.67-●
upper M79.60-●
axilla M79.62-●
finger M79.64-●
forearm M79.63-●
hand M79.64-●
upper arm M79.62-●
loin M54.5
low back M54.5
lumbar region M54.5
mandibular R68.84
mastoid —*see* subcategory H92.0
maxilla R68.84
menstrual —*see also* Dysmenorrhea N94.6
metacarpophalangeal (joint) —*see* Pain, joint, hand
metatarsophalangeal (joint) —*see* Pain, joint, foot
mouth K13.79
muscle —*see* Myalgia
musculoskeletal —*see also* Pain, by site M79.18
myofascial M79.18
nasal J34.89
nasopharynx J39.2
neck NEC M54.2
nerve NEC —*see* Neuralgia
neuromuscular —*see* Neuralgia
nose J34.89
ocular H57.1-●
ophthalmic —*see* Pain, ocular
orbital region —*see* Pain, ocular
ovary N94.89
over heart —*see* Pain, precordial
ovulation N94.0
pelvic (female) R10.2

P

▶ New ➠ Revised ~~deleted~~ Deleted ● Use Additional Character(s)

- **Pain** *(Continued)*
  - penis N48.89
  - pericardial *—see* Pain, precordial
  - perineal, perineum R1Ø.2
  - pharynx J39.2
  - pleura, pleural, pleuritic RØ7.81
  - postoperative NOS G89.18
  - postprocedural NOS G89.18
  - post-thoracotomy G89.12
  - precordial (region) RØ7.2
  - premenstrual N94.3
  - psychogenic (persistent) (any site) F45.41
  - radicular (spinal) *—see* Radiculopathy
  - rectum K62.89
  - respiration RØ7.1
  - retrosternal RØ7.2
  - rheumatoid, muscular *—see* Myalgia
  - rib RØ7.81
  - root (spinal) *—see* Radiculopathy
  - round ligament (stretch) R1Ø.2
  - sacroiliac M53.3
  - sciatic *—see* Sciatica
  - scrotum N5Ø.82
  - seminal vesicle N5Ø.89
  - shoulder M25.51- ●
  - spermatic cord N5Ø.89
  - spinal root *—see* Radiculopathy
  - spine M54.9
    - cervical M54.2
    - low back M54.5
      - with sciatica M54.4- ●
    - thoracic M54.6
  - stomach *—see* Pain, abdominal
  - substernal RØ7.2
  - temporomandibular (joint) M26.62- ●
  - testis N5Ø.81- ●
  - thoracic spine M54.6
    - with radicular and visceral pain M54.14
  - throat RØ7.Ø
  - tibia *—see* Pain, limb, lower
  - toe *—see* Pain, limb, lower
  - tongue K14.6
  - tooth KØ8.89
  - trigeminal *—see* Neuralgia, trigeminal
  - tumor associated G89.3
  - ureter N23
  - urinary (organ) (system) N23
  - uterus NEC N94.89
  - vagina R1Ø.2
  - vertebrogenic (syndrome) M54.89
  - vesical R39.89
    - associated with micturition *—see* Micturition, painful
  - vulva R1Ø.2
- **Painful** *—see also* Pain
  - coitus
    - female N94.1Ø
    - male N53.12
    - psychogenic F52.6
  - ejaculation (semen) N53.12
    - psychogenic F52.6
  - erection *—see* Priapism
  - feet syndrome E53.8
  - joint replacement (hip) (knee) T84.84
  - menstruation *—see* Dysmenorrhea
    - psychogenic F45.8
  - micturition *—see* Micturition, painful
  - respiration RØ7.1
  - scar NEC L9Ø.5
  - wire sutures T81.89
- **Painter's colic** *—see* subcategory T56.Ø
- **Palate** *—see* condition
- **Palatoplegia** K13.79
- **Palatoschisis** *—see* Cleft, palate
- **Palilalia** R48.8
- **Palliative care** Z51.5
- **Pallor** R23.1
  - optic disc, temporal *—see* Atrophy, optic
- **Palmar** *—see also* condition
  - fascia *—see* condition
- **Palpable**
  - cecum K63.89
  - kidney N28.89
  - ovary N83.8
  - prostate N42.9
  - spleen *—see* Splenomegaly
- **Palpitations** (heart) RØØ.2
  - psychogenic F45.8
- **Palsy** *—see also* Paralysis G83.9
  - atrophic diffuse (progressive) G12.22
  - Bell's *—see also* Palsy, facial
    - newborn P11.3
  - brachial plexus NEC G54.Ø
    - newborn (birth injury) P14.3
  - brain *—see* Palsy, cerebral
  - bulbar (progressive) (chronic) G12.22
    - of childhood (Fazio-Londe) G12.1
    - pseudo NEC G12.29
    - supranuclear (progressive) G23.1
  - cerebral (congenital) G8Ø.9
    - ataxic G8Ø.4
    - athetoid G8Ø.3
    - choreathetoid G8Ø.3
    - diplegic G8Ø.8
      - spastic G8Ø.1
    - dyskinetic G8Ø.3
      - athetoid G8Ø.3
      - choreathetoid G8Ø.3
      - distonic G8Ø.3
    - dystonic G8Ø.3
    - hemiplegic G8Ø.8
      - spastic G8Ø.2
    - mixed G8Ø.8
    - monoplegic G8Ø.8
      - spastic G8Ø.1
    - paraplegic G8Ø.8
      - spastic G8Ø.1
    - quadriplegic G8Ø.8
      - spastic G8Ø.Ø
    - spastic G8Ø.1
      - diplegic G8Ø.1
      - hemiplegic G8Ø.2
      - monoplegic G8Ø.1
      - quadriplegic G8Ø.Ø
      - specified NEC G8Ø.1
      - tetrapelgic G8Ø.Ø
    - specified NEC G8Ø.8
    - syphilitic A52.12
      - congenital A5Ø.49
    - tetraplegic G8Ø.8
      - spastic G8Ø.Ø
  - cranial nerve *—see also* Disorder, nerve, cranial
    - multiple G52.7
      - in
        - infectious disease B99 *[G53]*
        - neoplastic disease *—see also* Neoplasm D49.9 *[G53]*
        - parasitic disease B89 *[G53]*
        - sarcoidosis D86.82
  - creeping G12.22
  - diver's T7Ø.3
  - Erb's P14.Ø
  - facial G51.Ø
    - newborn (birth injury) P11.3
  - glossopharyngeal G52.1
  - Klumpke (-Déjérine) P14.1
  - lead *—see* subcategory T56.Ø
  - median nerve (tardy) G56.1- ●
  - nerve G58.9
    - specified NEC G58.8
  - peroneal nerve (acute) (tardy) G57.3- ●
  - progressive supranuclear G23.1
  - pseudobulbar NEC G12.29
  - radial nerve (acute) G56.3- ●
  - seventh nerve *—see also* Palsy, facial
    - newborn P11.3
  - shaking *—see* Parkinsonism
  - spastic (cerebral) (spinal) G8Ø.1
  - ulnar nerve (tardy) G56.2- ●
  - wasting G12.29
- **Paludism** *—see* Malaria
- **Panangiitis** M3Ø.Ø
- **Panaris, panaritium** *—see also* Cellulitis, digit
  - with lymphangitis *—see* Lymphangitis, acute, digit
- **Panarteritis nodosa** M3Ø.Ø
  - brain or cerebral I67.7
- **Pancake heart** R93.1
  - with cor pulmonale (chronic) I27.81
- **Pancarditis** (acute) (chronic) I51.89
  - rheumatic IØ9.89
    - active or acute IØ1.8
- **Pancoast's syndrome or tumor** C34.1- ●
- **Pancolitis, ulcerative (chronic)** K51.ØØ
  - with
    - abscess K51.Ø14
    - complication K51.Ø19
    - fistula K51.Ø13
    - obstruction K51.Ø12
    - rectal bleeding K51.Ø11
    - specified complication NEC K51.Ø18
- **Pancreas, pancreatic** *—see* condition
- **Pancreatitis** (annular) (apoplectic) (calcareous) (edematous) (hemorrhagic) (malignant) (recurrent) (subacute) (suppurative) K85.9Ø
  - with necrosis (uninfected) K85.91
    - infected K85.92
  - acute (without necrosis or infection) K85.9Ø
    - with necrosis (uninfected) K85.91
      - infected K85.92
    - alcohol induced (without necrosis or infection) K85.2Ø
      - with necrosis (uninfected) K85.21
        - infected K85.22
    - biliary (without necrosis or infection) K85.1Ø
      - with necrosis (uninfected) K85.11
        - infected K85.12
    - drug induced (without necrosis or infection) K85.3Ø
      - with necrosis (uninfected) K85.31
        - infected K85.32
    - gallstone (without necrosis or infection) K85.1Ø
      - with necrosis (uninfected) K85.11
        - infected K85.12
    - idiopathic (without necrosis or infection) K85.ØØ
      - with necrosis (uninfected) K85.Ø1
        - infected K85.Ø2
    - specified NEC (without necrosis or infection) K85.8Ø
      - with necrosis (uninfected) K85.81
        - infected K85.82
  - chronic (infectious) K86.1
    - alcohol-induced K86.Ø
    - recurrent K86.1
    - relapsing K86.1
  - cystic (chronic) K86.1
  - cytomegaloviral B25.2
  - fibrous (chronic) K86.1
  - gallstone (without necrosis or infection) K85.1Ø
    - with necrosis (uninfected) K85.11
      - infected K85.12
  - gangrenous *—see* Pancreatitis, acute
  - interstitial (chronic) K86.1
    - acute *—see also* Pancreatitis, acute K85.8Ø
  - mumps B26.3
  - recurrent (chronic) K86.1
  - relapsing, chronic K86.1
  - syphilitic A52.74
- **Pancreatoblastoma** *—see* Neoplasm, pancreas, malignant
- **Pancreolithiasis** K86.89
- **Pancytolysis** D75.89

P

Pancytopenia (acquired) D61.818
with
malformations D61.Ø9
myelodysplastic syndrome —*see* Syndrome, myelodysplastic
antineoplastic chemotherapy induced D61.81Ø
congenital D61.Ø9
drug-induced NEC D61.811
PANDAS (pediatric autoimmune neuropsychiatric disorders associated with streptococcal infections syndrome) D89.89
Panencephalitis, subacute, sclerosing A81.1
Panhematopenia D61.9
congenital D61.Ø9
constitutional D61.Ø9
splenic, primary D73.1
Panhemocytopenia D61.9
congenital D61.Ø9
constitutional D61.Ø9
Panhypogonadism E29.1
Panhypopituitarism E23.Ø
prepubertal E23.Ø
Panic (attack) (state) F41.Ø
reaction to exceptional stress (transient) F43.Ø
Panmyelopathy, familial, constitutional D61.Ø9
Panmyelophthisis D61.82
congenital D61.Ø9
Panmyelosis (acute) (with myelofibrosis) C94.4-●
Panner's disease —*see* Osteochondrosis, juvenile, humerus
Panneuritis endemica E51.11
Panniculitis (nodular) (nonsuppurative) M79.3
back M54.ØØ
cervical region M54.Ø2
cervicothoracic region M54.Ø3
lumbar region M54.Ø6
lumbosacral region M54.Ø7
multiple sites M54.Ø9
occipito-atlanto-axial region M54.Ø1
sacrococcygeal region M54.Ø8
thoracic region M54.Ø4
thoracolumbar region M54.Ø5
lupus L93.2
mesenteric K65.4
neck M54.Ø2
cervicothoracic region M54.Ø3
occipito-atlanto-axial region M54.Ø1
relapsing M35.6
Panniculus adiposus (abdominal) E65
Pannus (allergic) (cornea) (degenerativus) (keratic) H16.42-●
abdominal (symptomatic) E65
trachomatosus, trachomatous (active) A71.1
Panophthalmitis H44.Ø1-●
Pansinusitis (chronic) (hyperplastic) (nonpurulent) (purulent) J32.4
acute JØ1.4Ø
recurrent JØ1.41
tuberculous A15.8
Panuveitis (sympathetic) H44.11-●
Panvalvular disease IØ8.9
specified NEC IØ8.8
PAPA (pyogenic arthritis, pyoderma gangrenosum, and acne syndrome) MØ4.8
Papanicolaou smear, cervix Z12.4
as part of routine gynecological examination ZØ1.419
with abnormal findings ZØ1.411
for suspected neoplasm Z12.4
nonspecific abnormal finding R87.619
routine ZØ1.419
with abnormal findings ZØ1.411
Papilledema (choked disc) H47.1Ø
associated with
decreased ocular pressure H47.12
increased intracranial pressure H47.11
retinal disorder H47.13
Foster-Kennedy syndrome H47.14-●
Papillitis H46.ØØ
anus K62.89
chronic lingual K14.4
necrotizing, kidney N17.2
optic H46.Ø-●
rectum K62.89
renal, necrotizing N17.2
tongue K14.Ø
Papilloma —*see also* Neoplasm, benign, by site
acuminatum (female) (male) (anogenital) A63.Ø
basal cell L82.1
inflamed L82.Ø
benign pinta (primary) A67.Ø
bladder (urinary) (transitional cell) D41.4
choroid plexus (lateral ventricle) (third ventricle) D33.Ø
anaplastic C71.5
fourth ventricle D33.1
malignant C71.5
renal pelvis (transitional cell) D41.1-●
benign D3Ø.1-●
Schneiderian
specified site —*see* Neoplasm, benign, by site
unspecified site D14.Ø
serous surface
borderline malignancy
specified site —*see* Neoplasm, uncertain behavior, by site
unspecified site D39.1Ø
specified site —*see* Neoplasm, benign, by site
unspecified site D27.9
transitional (cell)
bladder (urinary) D41.4
inverted type —*see* Neoplasm, uncertain behavior, by site
renal pelvis D41.1-●
ureter D41.2-●
ureter (transitional cell) D41.2-●
benign D3Ø.2-●
urothelial —*see* Neoplasm, uncertain behavior, by site
villous —*see* Neoplasm, uncertain behavior, by site
adenocarcinoma in —*see* Neoplasm, malignant, by site
in situ —*see* Neoplasm, in situ
yaws, plantar or palmar A66.1
Papillomata, multiple, of yaws A66.1
Papillomatosis —*see also* Neoplasm, benign, by site
confluent and reticulated L83
cystic, breast —*see* Mastopathy, cystic
ductal, breast —*see* Mastopathy, cystic
intraductal (diffuse) —*see* Neoplasm, benign, by site
subareolar duct D24-●
Papillomavirus, as cause of disease classified elsewhere B97.7
Papillon-Léage and Psaume syndrome Q87.Ø
Papule(s) R23.8
carate (primary) A67.Ø
fibrous, of nose D22.39
Gottron's L94.4
pinta (primary) A67.Ø
Papulosis
lymphomatoid C86.6
malignant I77.89
Papyraceous fetus O31.Ø-●
Para-albuminemia E88.Ø9
Paracephalus Q89.7
Parachute mitral valve Q23.2
Paracoccidioidomycosis B41.9
disseminated B41.7
generalized B41.7
mucocutaneous-lymphangitic B41.8
pulmonary B41.Ø
Paracoccidioidomycosis *(Continued)*
specified NEC B41.8
visceral B41.8
Paradentosis KØ5.4
Paraffinoma T88.8
Paraganglioma D44.7
adrenal D35.Ø-●
malignant C74.1-●
aortic body D44.7
malignant C75.5
carotid body D44.6
malignant C75.4
chromaffin —*see also* Neoplasm, benign, by site
malignant —*see* Neoplasm, malignant, by site
extra-adrenal D44.7
malignant C75.5
specified site —*see* Neoplasm, malignant, by site
unspecified site C75.5
specified site —*see* Neoplasm, uncertain behavior, by site
unspecified site D44.7
gangliocytic D13.2
specified site —*see* Neoplasm, benign, by site
unspecified site D13.2
glomus jugulare D44.7
malignant C75.5
jugular D44.7
malignant C75.5
specified site —*see* Neoplasm, malignant, by site
unspecified site C75.5
nonchromaffin D44.7
malignant C75.5
specified site —*see* Neoplasm, malignant, by site
unspecified site C75.5
specified site —*see* Neoplasm, uncertain behavior, by site
unspecified site D44.7
parasympathetic D44.7
specified site —*see* Neoplasm, uncertain behavior, by site
unspecified site D44.7
specified site —*see* Neoplasm, uncertain behavior, by site
sympathetic D44.7
specified site —*see* Neoplasm, uncertain behavior, by site
unspecified site D44.7
unspecified site D44.7
Parageusia R43.2
psychogenic F45.8
Paragonimiasis B66.4
Paragranuloma, Hodgkin —*see* Lymphoma, Hodgkin, specified NEC
Parahemophilia —*see also* Defect, coagulation D68.2
Parakeratosis R23.4
variegata L41.Ø
Paralysis, paralytic (complete) (incomplete) G83.9
with
syphilis A52.17
abducens, abducent (nerve) —*see* Strabismus, paralytic, sixth nerve
abductor, lower extremity G57.9-●
accessory nerve G52.8
accommodation —*see also* Paresis, of accommodation
hysterical F44.89
acoustic nerve (except Deafness) —*see* subcategory H93.3
agitans —*see also* Parkinsonism G2Ø
arteriosclerotic G21.4
alternating (oculomotor) G83.89
amyotrophic G12.21

P

 ▶ New ➠ Revised ~~deleted~~ Deleted ● Use Additional Character(s)

Paralysis, paralytic *(Continued)*
- ankle G57.9- ●
- anus (sphincter) K62.89
- arm *—see* Monoplegia, upper limb
- ascending (spinal), acute G61.0
- association G12.29
- asthenic bulbar G70.00
  - with exacerbation (acute) G70.01
  - in crisis G70.01
- ataxic (hereditary) G11.9
  - general (syphilitic) A52.17
- atrophic G58.9
  - infantile, acute *—see* Poliomyelitis, paralytic
  - progressive G12.22
  - spinal (acute) *—see* Poliomyelitis, paralytic
- axillary G54.0
- Babinski-Nageotte's G83.89
- Bell's G51.0
  - newborn P11.3
- Benedikt's G46.3
- birth injury P14.9
  - spinal cord P11.5
- bladder (neurogenic) (sphincter) N31.2
- bowel, colon or intestine K56.0
- brachial plexus G54.0
  - birth injury P14.3
  - newborn (birth injury) P14.3
- brain G83.9
  - diplegia G83.0
  - triplegia G83.89
- bronchial J98.09
- Brown-Séquard G83.81
- bulbar (chronic) (progressive) G12.22
  - infantile *—see* Poliomyelitis, paralytic
  - poliomyelitic *—see* Poliomyelitis, paralytic
  - pseudo G12.29
- bulbospinal G70.00
  - with exacerbation (acute) G70.01
  - in crisis G70.01
- cardiac *—see also* Failure, heart I50.9
- cerebrocerebellar, diplegic G80.1
- cervical
  - plexus G54.2
  - sympathetic G90.09
- Céstan-Chenais G46.3
- Charcot-Marie-Tooth type G60.0
- Clark's G80.9
- colon K56.0
- compressed air T70.3
- compression
  - arm G56.9- ●
  - leg G57.9- ●
  - lower extremity G57.9- ●
  - upper extremity G56.9- ●
- congenital (cerebral) *—see* Palsy, cerebral
- conjugate movement (gaze) (of eye) H51.0
  - cortical (nuclear) (supranuclear) H51.0
- cordis *—see* Failure, heart
- cranial or cerebral nerve G52.9
- creeping G12.22
- crossed leg G83.89
- crutch *—see* Injury, brachial plexus
- deglutition R13.0
  - hysterical F44.4
- dementia A52.17
- descending (spinal) NEC G12.29
- diaphragm (flaccid) J98.6
  - due to accidental dissection of phrenic nerve during procedure *—see* Puncture, accidental complicating surgery
- digestive organs NEC K59.8
- diplegic *—see* Diplegia
- divergence (nuclear) H51.8
- diver's T70.3
- Duchenne's
  - birth injury P14.0
  - due to or associated with
    - motor neuron disease G12.22
    - muscular dystrophy G71.01

Paralysis, paralytic *(Continued)*
- due to intracranial or spinal birth injury *—see* Palsy, cerebral
- embolic (current episode) I63.4- ●
- Erb (-Duchenne) (birth) (newborn) P14.0
- Erb's syphilitic spastic spinal A52.17
- esophagus K22.8
- eye muscle (extrinsic) H49.9
  - intrinsic *—see also* Paresis, of accommodation
- facial (nerve) G51.0
  - birth injury P11.3
  - congenital P11.3
  - following operation NEC *—see* Puncture, accidental complicating surgery
  - newborn (birth injury) P11.3
- familial (recurrent) (periodic) G72.3
  - spastic G11.4
- fauces J39.2
- finger G56.9- ●
- gait R26.1
- gastric nerve (nondiabetic) G52.2
- gaze, conjugate H51.0
- general (progressive) (syphilitic) A52.17
  - juvenile A50.45
- glottis J38.00
  - bilateral J38.02
  - unilateral J38.01
- gluteal G54.1
- Gubler (-Millard) G46.3
- hand *—see* Monoplegia, upper limb
- heart *—see* Arrest, cardiac
- hemiplegic *—see* Hemiplegia
- hyperkalemic periodic (familial) G72.3
- hypoglossal (nerve) G52.3
- hypokalemic periodic G72.3
- hysterical F44.4
- ileus K56.0
- infantile *—see also* Poliomyelitis, paralytic A80.30
  - bulbar *—see* Poliomyelitis, paralytic
  - cerebral *—see* Palsy, cerebral
  - spastic *—see* Palsy, cerebral, spastic
- infective *—see* Poliomyelitis, paralytic
- inferior nuclear G83.9
- internuclear *—see* Ophthalmoplegia, internuclear
- intestine K56.0
- iris H57.09
  - due to diphtheria (toxin) A36.89
- ischemic, Volkmann's (complicating trauma) T79.6
- Jackson's G83.89
- jake *—see* Poisoning, food, noxious, plant
- Jamaica ginger (jake) G62.2
- juvenile general A50.45
- Klumpke (-Déjérine) (birth) (newborn) P14.1
- labioglossal (laryngeal) (pharyngeal) G12.29
- Landry's G61.0
- laryngeal nerve (recurrent) (superior) (unilateral) J38.00
  - bilateral J38.02
  - unilateral J38.01
- larynx J38.00
  - bilateral J38.02
  - due to diphtheria (toxin) A36.2
  - unilateral J38.01
- lateral G12.23
- lead *—see* subcategory T56.0
- left side *—see* Hemiplegia
- leg G83.1- ●
  - both *—see* Paraplegia
  - crossed G83.89
  - hysterical F44.4
  - psychogenic F44.4
  - transient or transitory R29.818
    - traumatic NEC *—see* Injury, nerve, leg
- levator palpebrae superioris *—see* Blepharoptosis, paralytic
- limb *—see* Monoplegia
- lip K13.0

Paralysis, paralytic *(Continued)*
- Lissauer's A52.17
- lower limb *—see* Monoplegia, lower limb
  - both *—see* Paraplegia
- lung J98.4
- median nerve G56.1- ●
- medullary (tegmental) G83.89
- mesencephalic NEC G83.89
  - tegmental G83.89
- middle alternating G83.89
- Millard-Gubler-Foville G46.3
- monoplegic *—see* Monoplegia
- motor G83.9
- muscle, muscular NEC G72.89
  - due to nerve lesion G58.9
  - eye (extrinsic) H49.9
    - intrinsic *—see* Paresis, of accommodation
    - oblique *—see* Strabismus, paralytic, fourth nerve
  - iris sphincter H21.9
  - ischemic (Volkmann's) (complicating trauma) T79.6
  - progressive G12.21
  - ▶ progressive, spinal G12.25
  - pseudohypertrophic G71.02
  - ▶ spinal progressive G12.25
- musculocutaneous nerve G56.9- ●
- musculospiral G56.9- ●
- nerve *—see also* Disorder, nerve
  - abducent *—see* Strabismus, paralytic, sixth nerve
  - accessory G52.8
  - auditory (except Deafness) *—see* subcategory H93.3
  - birth injury P14.9
  - cranial or cerebral G52.9
  - facial G51.0
    - birth injury P11.3
    - congenital P11.3
    - newborn (birth injury) P11.3
  - fourth or trochlear *—see* Strabismus, paralytic, fourth nerve
  - newborn (birth injury) P14.9
  - oculomotor *—see* Strabismus, paralytic, third nerve
  - phrenic (birth injury) P14.2
  - radial G56.3- ●
  - seventh or facial G51.0
    - newborn (birth injury) P11.3
  - sixth or abducent *—see* Strabismus, paralytic, sixth nerve
  - syphilitic A52.15
  - third or oculomotor *—see* Strabismus, paralytic, third nerve
  - trigeminal G50.9
  - trochlear *—see* Strabismus, paralytic, fourth nerve
  - ulnar G56.2- ●
- normokalemic periodic G72.3
- ocular H49.9
  - alternating G83.89
- oculofacial, congenital (Moebius) Q87.0
- oculomotor (external bilateral) (nerve) *—see* Strabismus, paralytic, third nerve
- palate (soft) K13.79
- paratrigeminal G50.9
- periodic (familial) (hyperkalemic) (hypokalemic) (myotonic) (normokalemic) (potassium sensitive) (secondary) G72.3
- peripheral autonomic nervous system *—see* Neuropathy, peripheral, autonomic
- peroneal (nerve) G57.3- ●
- pharynx J39.2
- phrenic nerve G56.8- ●
- plantar nerve(s) G57.6- ●
- pneumogastric nerve G52.2
- poliomyelitis (current) *—see* Poliomyelitis, paralytic
- popliteal nerve G57.3- ●
- postepileptic transitory G83.84

P

Paralysis, paralytic *(Continued)*
progressive (atrophic) (bulbar) (spinal) G12.22
general A52.17
infantile acute *—see* Poliomyelitis, paralytic
supranuclear G23.1
pseudobulbar G12.29
pseudohypertrophic (muscle) G71.Ø9
psychogenic F44.4
quadriceps G57.9-•
quadriplegic *—see* Tetraplegia
radial nerve G56.3-•
rectus muscle (eye) H49.9
recurrent isolated sleep G47.53
respiratory (muscle) (system) (tract) RØ6.81
center NEC G93.89
congenital P28.89
newborn P28.89
right side *—see* Hemiplegia
saturnine *—see* subcategory T56.Ø
sciatic nerve G57.Ø-•
senile G83.9
shaking *—see* Parkinsonism
shoulder G56.9-•
sleep, recurrent isolated G47.53
spastic G83.9
cerebral *—see* Palsy, cerebral, spastic
congenital (cerebral) *—see* Palsy, cerebral, spastic
familial G11.4
hereditary G11.4
quadriplegic G8Ø.Ø
syphilitic (spinal) A52.17
sphincter, bladder *—see* Paralysis, bladder
spinal (cord) G83.9
accessory nerve G52.8
acute *—see* Poliomyelitis, paralytic
ascending acute G61.Ø
atrophic (acute) *—see also* Poliomyelitis, paralytic
spastic, syphilitic A52.17
congenital NEC *—see* Palsy, cerebral
hereditary G95.89
infantile *—see* Poliomyelitis, paralytic
progressive G12.21
▶ muscle G12.25
sequelae NEC G83.89
sternomastoid G52.8
stomach K31.84
diabetic *—see* Diabetes, by type, with gastroparesis
nerve G52.2
diabetic *—see* Diabetes, by type, with gastroparesis
stroke *—see* Infarct, brain
subcapsularis G56.8-•
supranuclear (progressive) G23.1
sympathetic G9Ø.8
cervical G9Ø.Ø9
nervous system *—see* Neuropathy, peripheral, autonomic
syndrome G83.9
specified NEC G83.89
syphilitic spastic spinal (Erb's) A52.17
thigh G57.9-•
throat J39.2
diphtheritic A36.Ø
muscle J39.2
thrombotic (current episode) I63.3-•
thumb G56.9-•
tick *—see* Toxicity, venom, arthropod, specified NEC
Todd's (postepileptic transitory paralysis) G83.84
toe G57.6-•
tongue K14.8
transient R29.5
arm or leg NEC R29.818
traumatic NEC *—see* Injury, nerve
trapezius G52.8
traumatic, transient NEC *—see* Injury, nerve

Paralysis, paralytic *(Continued)*
trembling *—see* Parkinsonism
triceps brachii G56.9-•
trigeminal nerve G5Ø.9
trochlear (nerve) *—see* Strabismus, paralytic, fourth nerve
ulnar nerve G56.2-•
upper limb *—see* Monoplegia, upper limb
uremic N18.9 *[G99.8]*
uveoparotitic D86.89
uvula K13.79
postdiphtheritic A36.Ø
vagus nerve G52.2
vasomotor NEC G9Ø.8
velum palati K13.79
vesical *—see* Paralysis, bladder
vestibular nerve (except Vertigo) *—see* subcategory H93.3
vocal cords J38.ØØ
bilateral J38.Ø2
unilateral J38.Ø1
Volkmann's (complicating trauma) T79.6
wasting G12.29
Weber's G46.3
wrist G56.9-•
Paramedial urethrovesical orifice Q64.79
Paramenia N92.6
Parametritis *—see also* Disease, pelvis, inflammatory N73.2
acute N73.Ø
complicating abortion *—see* Abortion, by type, complicated by, parametritis
Parametrium, parametric *—see* condition
Paramnesia *—see* Amnesia
Paramolar KØØ.1
Paramyloidosis E85.89
Paramyoclonus multiplex G25.3
Paramyotonia (congenita) G71.19
Parangi *—see* Yaws
Paranoia (querulans) F22
senile FØ3
Paranoid
dementia (senile) FØ3
praecox *—see* Schizophrenia
personality F6Ø.Ø
psychosis (climacteric) (involutional) (menopausal) F22
psychogenic (acute) F23
senile FØ3
reaction (acute) F23
chronic F22
schizophrenia F2Ø.Ø
state (climacteric) (involutional) (menopausal) (simple) F22
senile FØ3
tendencies F6Ø.Ø
traits F6Ø.Ø
trends F6Ø.Ø
type, psychopathic personality F6Ø.Ø
Paraparesis *—see* Paraplegia
Paraphasia R47.Ø2
Paraphilia F65.9
Paraphimosis (congenital) N47.2
chancroidal A57
Paraphrenia, paraphrenic (late) F22
schizophrenia F2Ø.Ø
Paraplegia (lower) G82.2Ø
ataxic *—see* Degeneration, combined, spinal cord
complete G82.21
congenital (cerebral) G8Ø.8
spastic G8Ø.1
familial spastic G11.4
functional (hysterical) F44.4
hereditary, spastic G11.4
hysterical F44.4
incomplete G82.22
Pott's A18.Ø1
psychogenic F44.4

Paraplegia *(Continued)*
spastic
Erb's spinal, syphilitic A52.17
hereditary G11.4
tropical GØ4.1
syphilitic (spastic) A52.17
traumatic
current injury - code to injury with seventh character A
sequela of previous injury - code to injury with seventh character S
tropical spastic GØ4.1
Parapoxvirus BØ8.6Ø
specified NEC BØ8.69
Paraproteinemia D89.2
benign (familial) D89.2
monoclonal D47.2
secondary to malignant disease D47.2
Parapsoriasis L41.9
en plaques L41.4
guttata L41.1
large plaque L41.4
retiform, retiformis L41.5
small plaque L41.3
specified NEC L41.8
varioliformis (acuta) L41.Ø
Parasitic *—see also* condition
disease NEC B89
stomatitis B37.Ø
sycosis (beard) (scalp) B35.Ø
twin Q89.4
Parasitism B89
intestinal B82.9
skin B88.9
specified *—see* Infestation
Parasitophobia F4Ø.218
Parasomnia G47.5Ø
due to
alcohol
abuse F1Ø.182
dependence F1Ø.282
use F1Ø.982
amphetamines
abuse F15.182
dependence F15.282
use F15.982
caffeine
abuse F15.182
dependence F15.282
use F15.982
cocaine
abuse F14.182
dependence F14.282
use F14.982
drug NEC
abuse F19.182
dependence F19.282
use F19.982
opioid
abuse F11.182
dependence F11.282
use F11.982
psychoactive substance NEC
abuse F19.182
dependence F19.282
use F19.982
sedative, hypnotic, or anxiolytic
abuse F13.182
dependence F13.282
use F13.982
stimulant NEC
abuse F15.182
dependence F15.282
use F15.982
in conditions classified elsewhere G47.54
nonorganic origin F51.8
organic G47.5Ø
specified NEC G47.59
Paraspadias Q54.9
Paraspasmus facialis G51.8

Parasuicide (attempt)
history of (personal) Z91.5
in family Z81.8
Parathyroid gland —*see* condition
Parathyroid tetany E2Ø.9
Paratrachoma A74.Ø
Paratyphilitis —*see* Appendicitis
Paratyphoid (fever) —*see* Fever, paratyphoid
Paratyphus —*see* Fever, paratyphoid
Paraurethral duct Q64.79
~~nonorganic origin F51.5~~
Paraurethritis —*see also* Urethritis
gonococcal (acute) (chronic) (with abscess) A54.1
Paravaccinia NEC BØ8.Ø4
Paravaginitis —*see* Vaginitis
Parencephalitis —*see also* Encephalitis
sequelae GØ9
Parent-child conflict —*see* Conflict, parent-child
estrangement NEC Z62.89Ø
Paresis —*see also* Paralysis
accommodation —*see* Paresis, of accommodation
Bernhardt's G57.1- •
bladder (sphincter) —*see also* Paralysis, bladder
tabetic A52.17
bowel, colon or intestine K56.Ø
extrinsic muscle, eye H49.9
general (progressive) (syphilitic) A52.17
juvenile A5Ø.45
heart —*see* Failure, heart
insane (syphilitic) A52.17
juvenile (general) A5Ø.45
of accommodation H52.52- •
peripheral progressive (idiopathic) G6Ø.3
pseudohypertrophic G71.Ø9
senile G83.9
syphilitic (general) A52.17
congenital A5Ø.45
vesical NEC N31.2
Paresthesia —*see also* Disturbance, sensation, skin R2Ø.2
Bernhardt G57.1- •
Paretic —*see* condition
Parinaud's
conjunctivitis H1Ø.89
oculoglandular syndrome H1Ø.89
ophthalmoplegia H49.88
Parkinsonism (idiopathic) (primary) G2Ø
with neurogenic orthostatic hypotension (symptomatic) G9Ø.3
arteriosclerotic G21.4
dementia G31.83 *[FØ2.8Ø]*
with behavioral disturbance G31.83 *[FØ2.81]*
due to
drugs NEC G21.19
neuroleptic G21.11
medication-induced NEC G21.19
neuroleptic induced G21.11
postencephalitic G21.3
secondary G21.9
due to
arteriosclerosis G21.4
drugs NEC G21.19
neuroleptic G21.11
encephalitis G21.3
external agents NEC G21.2
syphilis A52.19
specified NEC G21.8
syphilitic A52.19
treatment-induced NEC G21.19
vascular G21.4
Parkinson's disease, syndrome or tremor —*see* Parkinsonism
Parodontitis —*see* Periodontitis
Parodontosis KØ5.4
Paronychia —*see also* Cellulitis, digit
with lymphangitis —*see* Lymphangitis, acute, digit
candidal (chronic) B37.2
tuberculous (primary) A18.4
Parorexia (psychogenic) F5Ø.89
Parosmia R43.1
psychogenic F45.8
Parotid gland —*see* condition
Parotitis, parotiditis (allergic) (nonspecific toxic) (purulent) (septic) (suppurative) —*see also* Sialoadenitis
epidemic —*see* Mumps
infectious —*see* Mumps
postoperative K91.89
surgical K91.89
Parrot fever A7Ø
Parrot's disease (early congenital syphilitic pseudoparalysis) A5Ø.Ø2
Parry-Romberg syndrome G51.8
Parry's disease or syndrome EØ5.ØØ
with thyroid storm EØ5.Ø1
Pars planitis —*see* Cyclitis
Parsonage (-Aldren)-Turner syndrome G54.5
Parson's disease (exophthalmic goiter) EØ5.ØØ
with thyroid storm EØ5.Ø1
Particolored infant Q82.8
Parturition —*see* Delivery
Parulis KØ4.7
with sinus KØ4.6
Parvovirus, as cause of disease classified elsewhere B97.6
Pasini and Pierini's atrophoderma L9Ø.3
Passage
false, urethra N36.5
meconium (newborn) during delivery PØ3.82
of sounds or bougies —*see* Attention to, artificial, opening
Passive —*see* condition
smoking Z77.22
Pasteurella septica A28.Ø
Pasteurellosis —*see* Infection, Pasteurella
PAT (paroxysmal atrial tachycardia) I47.1
Patau's syndrome —*see* Trisomy, 13
Patches
mucous (syphilitic) A51.39
congenital A5Ø.Ø7
smokers' (mouth) K13.24
Patellar —*see* condition
Patent —*see also* Imperfect, closure
canal of Nuck Q52.4
cervix N88.3
ductus arteriosus or Botallo's Q25.Ø
foramen
botalli Q21.1
ovale Q21.1
interauricular septum Q21.1
interventricular septum Q21.Ø
omphalomesenteric duct Q43.Ø
os (uteri) —*see* Patent, cervix
ostium secundum Q21.1
urachus Q64.4
vitelline duct Q43.Ø
Paterson (-Brown)(-Kelly) syndrome or web D5Ø.1
Pathologic, pathological —*see also* condition
asphyxia RØ9.Ø1
fire-setting F63.1
gambling F63.Ø
ovum OØ2.Ø
resorption, tooth KØ3.3
stealing F63.2
Pathology (of) —*see* Disease
periradicular, associated with previous endodontic treatment NEC M27.59
Pattern, sleep-wake, irregular G47.23
Patulous —*see also* Imperfect, closure (congenital)
alimentary tract Q45.8
lower Q43.8
upper Q4Ø.8
eustachian tube H69.Ø- •
Pause, sinoatrial I49.5
Paxton's disease B36.2
Pearl(s)
enamel KØØ.2
Epstein's KØ9.8
Pearl-worker's disease —*see* Osteomyelitis, specified type NEC
Pectenosis K62.4
Pectoral —*see* condition
Pectus
carinatum (congenital) Q67.7
acquired M95.4
rachitic sequelae (late effect) E64.3
excavatum (congenital) Q67.6
acquired M95.4
rachitic sequelae (late effect) E64.3
recurvatum (congenital) Q67.6
Pedatrophia E41
Pederosis F65.4
Pediculosis (infestation) B85.2
capitis (head-louse) (any site) B85.Ø
corporis (body-louse) (any site) B85.1
eyelid B85.Ø
mixed (classifiable to more than one of the titles B85.Ø-B85.3) B85.4
pubis (pubic louse) (any site) B85.3
vestimenti B85.1
vulvae B85.3
Pediculus (infestation) —*see* Pediculosis
Pedophilia F65.4
Peg-shaped teeth KØØ.2
Pelade —*see* Alopecia, areata
Pelger-Huët anomaly or syndrome D72.Ø
Peliosis (rheumatica) D69.Ø
hepatis K76.4
with toxic liver disease K71.8
Pelizaeus-Merzbacher disease E75.29
Pellagra (alcoholic) (with polyneuropathy) E52
Pellagra-cerebellar-ataxia-renal aminoaciduria syndrome E72.Ø2
Pellegrini (-Stieda) disease or syndrome —*see* Bursitis, tibial collateral
Pellizzi's syndrome E34.8
Pel's crisis A52.11
Pelvic —*see also* condition
examination (periodic) (routine) ZØ1.419
with abnormal findings ZØ1.411
kidney, congenital Q63.2
Pelviolithiasis —*see* Calculus, kidney
Pelviperitonitis —*see also* Peritonitis, pelvic
gonococcal A54.24
puerperal O85
Pelvis —*see* condition or type
Pemphigoid L12.9
benign, mucous membrane L12.1
bullous L12.Ø
cicatricial L12.1
juvenile L12.2
ocular L12.1
specified NEC L12.8
Pemphigus L1Ø.9
benign familial (chronic) Q82.8
Brazilian L1Ø.3
circinatus L13.Ø
conjunctiva L12.1
drug-induced L1Ø.5
erythematosus L1Ø.4
foliaceous L1Ø.2
gangrenous —*see* Gangrene
neonatorum LØ1.Ø3
ocular L12.1
paraneoplastic L1Ø.81
specified NEC L1Ø.89
syphilitic (congenital) A5Ø.Ø6
vegetans L1Ø.1
vulgaris L1Ø.Ø
wildfire L1Ø.3
Pendred's syndrome EØ7.1
Pendulous
abdomen, in pregnancy —*see* Pregnancy, complicated by, abnormal, pelvic organs or tissues NEC
breast N64.89
Penetrating wound —*see also* Puncture
with internal injury —*see* Injury, by site
eyeball —*see* Puncture, eyeball

P

Penetrating wound *(Continued)*
orbit (with or without foreign body) —*see* Puncture, orbit
uterus by instrument with or following ectopic or molar pregnancy OØ8.6
Penicillosis B48.4
Penis —*see* condition
Penitis N48.29
Pentalogy of Fallot Q21.8
Pentasomy X syndrome Q97.1
Pentosuria (essential) E74.8
Percreta placenta O43.23- ●
Peregrinating patient —*see* Disorder, factitious
Perforation, perforated (nontraumatic) (of)
accidental during procedure (blood vessel) (nerve) (organ) —*see* Complication, accidental puncture or laceration
antrum —*see* Sinusitis, maxillary
appendix K35.22
with localized peritonitis K35.32
atrial septum, multiple Q21.1
attic, ear —*see* Perforation, tympanum, attic
bile duct (common) (hepatic) K83.2
cystic K82.2
bladder (urinary)
with or following ectopic or molar pregnancy OØ8.6
obstetrical trauma O71.5
traumatic S37.29
at delivery O71.5
bowel K63.1
with or following ectopic or molar pregnancy OØ8.6
newborn P78.Ø
obstetrical trauma O71.5
traumatic —*see* Laceration, intestine
broad ligament N83.8
with or following ectopic or molar pregnancy OØ8.6
obstetrical trauma O71.6
by
device, implant or graft —*see also* Complications, by site and type, mechanical T85.628
arterial graft NEC —*see* Complication, cardiovascular device, mechanical, vascular
breast (implant) T85.49
catheter NEC T85.698
cystostomy T83.Ø9Ø
dialysis (renal) T82.49
intraperitoneal T85.691
infusion NEC T82.594
spinal (epidural) (subdural) T85.69Ø
urinary —*see also* Complications, catheter, urinary T83.Ø98
electronic (electrode) (pulse generator) (stimulator)
bone T84.39Ø
cardiac T82.199
electrode T82.19Ø
pulse generator T82.191
specified type NEC T82.198
nervous system —*see* Complication, prosthetic device, mechanical, electronic nervous system stimulator
urinary —*see* Complication, genitourinary, device, urinary, mechanical
fixation, internal (orthopedic) NEC —*see* Complication, fixation device, mechanical
gastrointestinal —*see* Complications, prosthetic device, mechanical, gastrointestinal device
genital NEC T83.498
intrauterine contraceptive device T83.39
penile prosthesis T83.49Ø
heart NEC —*see* Complication, cardiovascular device, mechanical

Perforation, perforated *(Continued)*
by *(Continued)*
urinary *(Continued)*
joint prosthesis —*see* Complications, joint prosthesis, mechanical, specified NEC, by site
ocular NEC —*see* Complications, prosthetic device, mechanical, ocular device
orthopedic NEC —*see* Complication, orthopedic, device, mechanical
specified NEC T85.628
urinary NEC —*see also* Complication, genitourinary, device, urinary, mechanical
graft T83.29
vascular NEC —*see* Complication, cardiovascular device, mechanical
ventricular intracranial shunt T85.Ø9
foreign body left accidentally in operative wound T81.539
instrument (any) during a procedure, accidental —*see* Puncture, accidental complicating surgery
cecum K35.22
with localized peritonitis K35.32
cervix (uteri) N88.8
with or following ectopic or molar pregnancy OØ8.6
obstetrical trauma O71.3
colon K63.1
newborn P78.Ø
obstetrical trauma O71.5
traumatic —*see* Laceration, intestine, large
common duct (bile) K83.2
cornea (due to ulceration) —*see* Ulcer, cornea, perforated
cystic duct K82.2
diverticulum (intestine) K57.8Ø
with bleeding K57.81
large intestine K57.2Ø
with
bleeding K57.21
small intestine K57.4Ø
with bleeding K57.41
small intestine K57.ØØ
with
bleeding K57.Ø1
large intestine K57.4Ø
with bleeding K57.41
ear drum —*see* Perforation, tympanum
esophagus K22.3
ethmoidal sinus —*see* Sinusitis, ethmoidal
frontal sinus —*see* Sinusitis, frontal
gallbladder K82.2
heart valve —*see* Endocarditis
ileum K63.1
newborn P78.Ø
obstetrical trauma O71.5
traumatic —*see* Laceration, intestine, small
instrumental, surgical (accidental) (blood vessel) (nerve) (organ) —*see* Puncture, accidental complicating surgery
intestine NEC K63.1
with ectopic or molar pregnancy OØ8.6
newborn P78.Ø
obstetrical trauma O71.5
traumatic —*see* Laceration, intestine
ulcerative NEC K63.1
newborn P78.Ø
jejunum, jejunal K63.1
obstetrical trauma O71.5
traumatic —*see* Laceration, intestine, small
ulcer —*see* Ulcer, gastrojejunal, with perforation
joint prosthesis —*see* Complications, joint prosthesis, mechanical, specified NEC, by site
mastoid (antrum) (cell) —*see* Disorder, mastoid, specified NEC
maxillary sinus —*see* Sinusitis, maxillary

Perforation, perforated *(Continued)*
membrana tympani —*see* Perforation, tympanum
nasal
septum J34.89
congenital Q3Ø.3
syphilitic A52.73
sinus J34.89
congenital Q3Ø.8
due to sinusitis —*see* Sinusitis
palate —*see also* Cleft, palate Q35.9
syphilitic A52.79
palatine vault —*see also* Cleft, palate, hard Q35.1
syphilitic A52.79
congenital A5Ø.59
pars flaccida (ear drum) —*see* Perforation, tympanum, attic
pelvic
floor S31.Ø3Ø
with
ectopic or molar pregnancy OØ8.6
penetration into retroperitoneal space S31.Ø31
retained foreign body S31.Ø4Ø
with penetration into retroperitoneal space S31.Ø41
following ectopic or molar pregnancy OØ8.6
obstetrical trauma O7Ø.1
organ S37.99
adrenal gland S37.818
bladder —*see* Perforation, bladder
fallopian tube S37.599
bilateral S37.592
unilateral S37.591
kidney S37.Ø9- ●
obstetrical trauma O71.5
ovary S37.499
bilateral S37.492
unilateral S37.491
prostate S37.828
specified organ NEC S37.898
ureter —*see* Perforation, ureter
urethra —*see* Perforation, urethra
uterus —*see* Perforation, uterus
perineum —*see* Laceration, perineum
pharynx J39.2
rectum K63.1
newborn P78.Ø
obstetrical trauma O71.5
traumatic S36.63
root canal space due to endodontic treatment M27.51
sigmoid K63.1
newborn P78.Ø
obstetrical trauma O71.5
traumatic S36.533
sinus (accessory) (chronic) (nasal) J34.89
sphenoidal sinus —*see* Sinusitis, sphenoidal
surgical (accidental) (by instrument) (blood vessel) (nerve) (organ) —*see* Puncture, accidental complicating surgery
traumatic
external —*see* Puncture
eye —*see* Puncture, eyeball
internal organ —*see* Injury, by site
tympanum, tympanic (membrane) (persistent post-traumatic) (postinflammatory) H72.9- ●
attic H72.1- ●
multiple —*see* Perforation, tympanum, multiple
total —*see* Perforation, tympanum, total
central H72.Ø- ●
multiple —*see* Perforation, tympanum, multiple
total —*see* Perforation, tympanum, total
marginal NEC —*see* subcategory H72.2
multiple H72.81- ●
pars flaccida —*see* Perforation, tympanum, attic

- **Perforation, perforated** *(Continued)*
  - tympanum, tympanic *(Continued)*
    - total H72.82-●
    - traumatic, current episode S09.2-●
  - typhoid, gastrointestinal —*see* Typhoid
  - ulcer —*see* Ulcer, by site, with perforation
  - ureter N28.89
    - traumatic S37.19
  - urethra N36.8
    - with ectopic or molar pregnancy O08.6
    - following ectopic or molar pregnancy O08.6
    - obstetrical trauma O71.5
    - traumatic S37.39
      - at delivery O71.5
  - uterus
    - with ectopic or molar pregnancy O08.6
    - by intrauterine contraceptive device T83.39
    - following ectopic or molar pregnancy O08.6
    - obstetrical trauma O71.1
    - traumatic S37.69
      - obstetric O71.1
  - uvula K13.79
    - syphilitic A52.79
  - vagina
    - obstetrical trauma O71.4
    - other trauma - *see* Puncture, vagina
- **Periadenitis mucosa necrotica recurrens** K12.0
- **Periappendicitis** (acute) —*see* Appendicitis
- **Periarteritis nodosa** (disseminated) (infectious) (necrotizing) M30.0
- **Periarthritis** (joint) —*see also* Enthesopathy
  - Duplay's M75.0-●
  - gonococcal A54.42
  - humeroscapularis —*see* Capsulitis, adhesive
  - scapulohumeral —*see* Capsulitis, adhesive
  - shoulder —*see* Capsulitis, adhesive
  - wrist M77.2-●
- **Periarthrosis** (angioneural) —*see* Enthesopathy
- **Pericapsulitis, adhesive** (shoulder) —*see* Capsulitis, adhesive
- **Pericarditis** (with decompensation) (with effusion) I31.9
  - with rheumatic fever (conditions in I00)
    - active —*see* Pericarditis, rheumatic
    - inactive or quiescent I09.2
  - acute (hemorrhagic) (nonrheumatic) (Sicca) I30.9
    - with chorea (acute) (rheumatic) (Sydenham's) I02.0
    - benign I30.8
    - nonspecific I30.0
    - rheumatic I01.0
      - with chorea (acute) (Sydenham's) I02.0
  - adhesive or adherent (chronic) (external) (internal) I31.0
    - acute —*see* Pericarditis, acute
    - rheumatic I09.2
  - bacterial (acute) (subacute) (with serous or seropurulent effusion) I30.1
  - calcareous I31.1
  - cholesterol (chronic) I31.8
    - acute I30.9
  - chronic (nonrheumatic) I31.9
    - rheumatic I09.2
  - constrictive (chronic) I31.1
  - coxsackie B33.23
  - fibrinocaseous (tuberculous) A18.84
  - fibrinopurulent I30.1
  - fibrinous I30.8
  - fibrous I31.0
  - gonococcal A54.83
  - idiopathic I30.0
  - in systemic lupus erythematosus M32.12
  - infective I30.1
  - meningococcal A39.53
  - neoplastic (chronic) I31.8
    - acute I30.9
  - obliterans, obliterating I31.0
  - plastic I31.0
  - pneumococcal I30.1

- **Pericarditis** *(Continued)*
  - postinfarction I24.1
  - purulent I30.1
  - rheumatic (active) (acute) (with effusion) (with pneumonia) I01.0
    - with chorea (acute) (rheumatic) (Sydenham's) I02.0
    - chronic or inactive (with chorea) I09.2
  - rheumatoid —*see* Rheumatoid, carditis
  - septic I30.1
  - serofibrinous I30.8
  - staphylococcal I30.1
  - streptococcal I30.1
  - suppurative I30.1
  - syphilitic A52.06
  - tuberculous A18.84
  - uremic N18.9 *[I32]*
  - viral I30.1
- **Pericardium, pericardial** —*see* condition
- **Pericellulitis** —*see* Cellulitis
- **Pericementitis** (chronic) (suppurative) —*see also* Periodontitis
  - acute K05.20
    - ➡generalized —*see* Periodontitis, aggressive, generalized
    - ➡localized —*see* Periodontitis, aggressive, localized
- **Perichondritis**
  - auricle —*see* Perichondritis, ear
  - bronchus J98.09
  - ear (external) H61.00-●
    - acute H61.01-●
    - chronic H61.02-●
  - external auditory canal —*see* Perichondritis, ear
  - larynx J38.7
    - syphilitic A52.73
    - typhoid A01.09
  - nose J34.89
  - pinna —*see* Perichondritis, ear
  - trachea J39.8
- **Periclasia** K05.4
- **Pericoronitis** —*see* Periodontitis
- **Pericystitis** N30.90
  - with hematuria N30.91
- **Peridiverticulitis** (intestine) K57.92
  - cecum —*see* Diverticulitis, intestine, large
  - colon —*see* Diverticulitis, intestine, large
  - duodenum —*see* Diverticulitis, intestine, small
  - intestine —*see* Diverticulitis, intestine
  - jejunum —*see* Diverticulitis, intestine, small
  - rectosigmoid —*see* Diverticulitis, intestine, large
  - rectum —*see* Diverticulitis, intestine, large
  - sigmoid —*see* Diverticulitis, intestine, large
- **Periendocarditis** —*see* Endocarditis
- **Periepididymitis** N45.1
- **Perifolliculitis** L01.02
  - abscedens, caput, scalp L66.3
  - capitis, abscedens (et suffodiens) L66.3
  - superficial pustular L01.02
- **Perihepatitis** K65.8
- **Perilabyrinthitis** (acute) —*see* subcategory H83.0
- **Perimeningitis** —*see* Meningitis
- **Perimetritis** —*see* Endometritis
- **Perimetrosalpingitis** —*see* Salpingo-oophoritis
- **Perineocele** N81.81
- **Perinephric, perinephritic** —*see* condition
- **Perinephritis** —*see also* Infection, kidney
  - purulent —*see* Abscess, kidney
- **Perineum, perineal** —*see* condition
- **Perineuritis NEC** —*see* Neuralgia
- **Periodic** —*see* condition
- **Periodontitis** (chronic) (complex) (compound) (local) (simplex) K05.30
  - acute K05.20
    - generalized K05.229
      - moderate K05.222
      - severe K05.223
      - slight K05.221

- **Periodontitis** *(Continued)*
  - acute *(Continued)*
    - localized K05.219
      - moderate K05.212
      - severe K05.213
      - slight K05.211
  - apical K04.5
    - acute (pulpal origin) K04.4
  - generalized K05.329
    - moderate K05.322
    - severe K05.323
    - slight K05.321
  - localized K05.319
    - moderate K05.312
    - severe K05.313
    - slight K05.311
- **Periodontoclasia** K05.4
- **Periodontosis** (juvenile) K05.4
- **Periods** —*see also* Menstruation
  - heavy N92.0
  - irregular N92.6
  - shortened intervals (irregular) N92.1
- **Perionychia** —*see also* Cellulitis, digit
  - with lymphangitis —*see* Lymphangitis, acute, digit
- **Perioophoritis** —*see* Salpingo-oophoritis
- **Periorchitis** N45.2
- **Periosteum, periosteal** —*see* condition
- **Periostitis** (albuminosa) (circumscribed) (diffuse) (infective) (monomelic) —*see also* Osteomyelitis
  - alveolar M27.3
  - alveolodental M27.3
  - dental M27.3
  - gonorrheal A54.43
  - jaw (lower) (upper) M27.2
  - orbit H05.03-●
  - syphilitic A52.77
    - congenital (early) A50.02 *[M90.80]*
    - secondary A51.46
  - tuberculous —*see* Tuberculosis, bone
  - yaws (hypertrophic) (early) (late) A66.6 *[M90.80]*
- **Periostosis** (hyperplastic) —*see also* Disorder, bone, specified type NEC
  - with osteomyelitis —*see* Osteomyelitis, specified type NEC
- **Peripartum**
  - cardiomyopathy O90.3
- **Periphlebitis** —*see* Phlebitis
- **Periproctitis** K62.89
- **Periprostatitis** —*see* Prostatitis
- **Perirectal** —*see* condition
- **Perirenal** —*see* condition
- **Perisalpingitis** —*see* Salpingo-oophoritis
- **Perisplenitis** (infectional) D73.89
- **Peristalsis, visible or reversed** R19.2
- **Peritendinitis** —*see* Enthesopathy
- **Peritoneum, peritoneal** —*see* condition
- **Peritonitis** (adhesive) (bacterial) (fibrinous) (hemorrhagic) (idiopathic) (localized) (perforative) (primary) (with adhesions) (with effusion) K65.9
  - with or following
    - abscess K65.1
    - appendicitis
      - with perforation or rupture K35.32
      - generalized (*see also* Appendicitis) K35.20
      - localized (*see also* Appendicitis) K35.30
    - diverticular disease (intestine) K57.80
      - with bleeding K57.81
      - ectopic or molar pregnancy O08.0
      - large intestine K57.20
        - with
          - bleeding K57.21
          - small intestine K57.40
            - with bleeding K57.41
      - small intestine K57.00
        - with
          - bleeding K57.01
          - large intestine K57.40
            - with bleeding K57.41

P

- **Peritonitis** *(Continued)*
  - acute (generalized) K65.0
  - aseptic T81.61
  - bile, biliary K65.3
  - chemical T81.61
  - chlamydial A74.81
  - chronic proliferative K65.8
  - complicating abortion —*see* Abortion, by type, complicated by, pelvic peritonitis
  - congenital P78.1
  - diaphragmatic K65.0
  - diffuse K65.0
  - diphtheritic A36.89
  - disseminated K65.0
  - due to
    - bile K65.3
    - foreign
      - body or object accidentally left during a procedure (instrument) (sponge) (swab) T81.599
      - substance accidentally left during a procedure (chemical) (powder) (talc) T81.61
    - talc T81.61
    - urine K65.8
  - eosinophilic K65.8
    - acute K65.0
  - fibrocaseous (tuberculous) A18.31
  - fibropurulent K65.0
  - following ectopic or molar pregnancy O08.0
  - general (ized) K65.0
  - gonococcal A54.85
  - meconium (newborn) P78.0
  - neonatal P78.1
    - meconium P78.0
  - pancreatic K65.0
  - paroxysmal, familial E85.0
    - benign E85.0
  - pelvic
    - female N73.5
      - acute N73.3
      - chronic N73.4
        - with adhesions N73.6
    - male K65.0
  - periodic, familial E85.0
  - proliferative, chronic K65.8
  - puerperal, postpartum, childbirth O85
  - purulent K65.0
  - septic K65.0
  - specified NEC K65.8
  - spontaneous bacterial K65.2
  - subdiaphragmatic K65.0
  - subphrenic K65.0
  - suppurative K65.0
  - syphilitic A52.74
    - congenital (early) A50.08 *[K67]*
  - talc T81.61
  - tuberculous A18.31
  - urine K65.8
- **Peritonsillar** —*see* condition
- **Peritonsillitis** J36
- **Perityphlitis** K37
- **Periureteritis** N28.89
- **Periurethral** —*see* condition
- **Periurethritis** (gangrenous) —*see* Urethritis
- **Periuterine** —*see* condition
- **Perivaginitis** —*see* Vaginitis
- **Perivasculitis, retinal** H35.06- •
- **Perivasitis** (chronic) N49.1
- **Perivesiculitis** (seminal) —*see* Vesiculitis
- **Perlèche** NEC K13.0
  - due to
    - candidiasis B37.83
    - moniliasis B37.83
    - riboflavin deficiency E53.0
    - vitamin B2 (riboflavin) deficiency E53.0
- **Pernicious** —*see* condition
- **Pernio, perniosis** T69.1
- **Perpetrator** (of abuse) —*see* Index to External Causes of Injury, Perpetrator
- **Persecution**
  - delusion F22
  - social Z60.5
- **Perseveration** (tonic) R48.8
- **Persistence, persistent** (congenital)
  - anal membrane Q42.3
    - with fistula Q42.2
  - arteria stapedia Q16.3
  - atrioventricular canal Q21.2
  - branchial cleft NOS Q18.2
    - cyst Q18.0
    - fistula Q18.0
    - sinus Q18.0
  - bulbus cordis in left ventricle Q21.8
  - canal of Cloquet Q14.0
  - capsule (opaque) Q12.8
  - cilioretinal artery or vein Q14.8
  - cloaca Q43.7
  - communication —*see* Fistula, congenital
  - convolutions
    - aortic arch Q25.46
    - fallopian tube Q50.6
    - oviduct Q50.6
    - uterine tube Q50.6
  - double aortic arch Q25.45
  - ductus arteriosus (Botalli) Q25.0
  - fetal
    - circulation P29.38
    - form of cervix (uteri) Q51.828
    - hemoglobin, hereditary (HPFH) D56.4
  - foramen
    - Botalli Q21.1
    - ovale Q21.1
  - Gartner's duct Q52.4
  - hemoglobin, fetal (hereditary) (HPFH) D56.4
  - hyaloid
    - artery (generally incomplete) Q14.0
    - system Q14.8
  - hymen, in pregnancy or childbirth —*see* Pregnancy, complicated by, abnormal, vulva
  - lanugo Q84.2
  - left
    - posterior cardinal vein Q26.8
    - root with right arch of aorta Q25.49
    - superior vena cava Q26.1
  - Meckel's diverticulum Q43.0
    - malignant —*see* Table of Neoplasms, small intestine, malignant
  - mucosal disease (middle ear) —*see* Otitis, media, suppurative, chronic, tubotympanic
  - nail(s), anomalous Q84.6
  - omphalomesenteric duct Q43.0
  - organ or site not listed —*see* Anomaly, by site
  - ostium
    - atrioventriculare commune Q21.2
    - primum Q21.2
    - secundum Q21.1
  - ovarian rests in fallopian tube Q50.6
  - pancreatic tissue in intestinal tract Q43.8
  - primary (deciduous)
    - teeth K00.6
    - vitreous hyperplasia Q14.0
  - pupillary membrane Q13.89
  - rhesus (Rh)titer —*see* Complication(s), transfusion, incompatibility reaction, Rh (factor)
  - right aortic arch Q25.47
  - sinus
    - urogenitalis
      - female Q52.8
      - male Q55.8
    - venosus with imperfect incorporation in right auricle Q26.8
  - thymus (gland) (hyperplasia) E32.0
  - thyroglossal duct Q89.2
  - thyrolingual duct Q89.2
  - truncus arteriosus or communis Q20.0
  - tunica vasculosa lentis Q12.2
- **Persistence, persistent** *(Continued)*
  - umbilical sinus Q64.4
  - urachus Q64.4
  - vitelline duct Q43.0
- **Person** (with)
  - admitted for clinical research, as a control subject (normal comparison) (participant) Z00.6
  - awaiting admission to adequate facility elsewhere Z75.1
  - concern (normal) about sick person in family Z63.6
  - consulting on behalf of another Z71.0
  - feigning illness Z76.5
  - living (in)
    - without
      - adequate housing (heating) (space) Z59.1
      - housing (permanent) (temporary) Z59.0
      - person able to render necessary care Z74.2
      - shelter Z59.0
    - alone Z60.2
    - boarding school Z59.3
    - residential institution Z59.3
  - on waiting list Z75.1
  - sick or handicapped in family Z63.6
- **Personality** (disorder) F60.9
  - accentuation of traits (type A pattern) Z73.1
  - affective F34.0
  - aggressive F60.3
  - amoral F60.2
  - anacastic, anankastic F60.5
  - antisocial F60.2
  - anxious F60.6
  - asocial F60.2
  - asthenic F60.7
  - avoidant F60.6
  - borderline F60.3
  - change due to organic condition (enduring) F07.0
  - compulsive F60.5
  - cycloid F34.0
  - cyclothymic F34.0
  - dependent F60.7
  - depressive F34.1
  - dissocial F60.2
  - dual F44.81
  - eccentric F60.89
  - emotionally unstable F60.3
  - expansive paranoid F60.0
  - explosive F60.3
  - fanatic F60.0
  - haltlose type F60.89
  - histrionic F60.4
  - hyperthymic F34.0
  - hypothymic F34.1
  - hysterical F60.4
  - immature F60.89
  - inadequate F60.7
  - labile (emotional) F60.3
  - mixed (nonspecific) F60.89
  - morally defective F60.2
  - multiple F44.81
  - narcissistic F60.81
  - obsessional F60.5
  - obsessive (-compulsive) F60.5
  - organic F07.0
  - overconscientious F60.5
  - paranoid F60.0
  - passive (-dependent) F60.7
  - passive-aggressive F60.89
  - pathologic F60.9
  - pattern defect or disturbance F60.9
  - pseudopsychopathic (organic) F07.0
  - pseudoretarded (organic) F07.0
  - psychoinfantile F60.4
  - psychoneurotic NEC F60.89
  - psychopathic F60.2
  - querulant F60.0
  - sadistic F60.89
  - schizoid F60.1

Personality *(Continued)*
- ➠ self-defeating F6Ø.89
- sensitive paranoid F6Ø.Ø
- sociopathic (amoral) (antisocial) (asocial) (dissocial) F6Ø.2
- specified NEC F6Ø.89
- type A Z73.1
- unstable (emotional) F6Ø.3

Perthes' disease —*see* Legg-Calvé-Perthes disease
Pertussis (*see also* Whooping cough) A37.9Ø
Perversion, perverted
- appetite F5Ø.89
  - psychogenic F5Ø.89
- function
  - pituitary gland E23.2
    - posterior lobe E22.2
- sense of smell and taste R43.8
  - psychogenic F45.8
- sexual —*see* Deviation, sexual

Pervious, congenital —*see also* Imperfect, closure
- ductus arteriosus Q25.Ø

Pes (congenital) —*see also* Talipes
- acquired —*see also* Deformity, limb, foot, specified NEC
  - planus —*see* Deformity, limb, flat foot
- adductus Q66.89
- ➠ cavus Q66.7-●
- deformity NEC, acquired —*see* Deformity, limb, foot, specified NEC
- planus (acquired) (any degree) —*see also* Deformity, limb, flat foot
  - rachitic sequelae (late effect) E64.3
- valgus Q66.6

Pest, pestis —*see* Plague
Petechia, petechiae R23.3
- newborn P54.5

Petechial typhus A75.9
Peter's anomaly Q13.4
➠ **Petit mal seizure** —*see* Epilepsy, childhood, absence
Petit's hernia —*see* Hernia, abdomen, specified site NEC
Petrellidosis B48.2
Petrositis H7Ø.2Ø-●
- acute H7Ø.21-●
- chronic H7Ø.22-●

Peutz-Jeghers disease or syndrome Q85.8
Peyronie's disease N48.6
PFAPA (periodic fever, aphthous stomatitis, pharyngitis, and adenopathy syndrome) MØ4.8
Pfeiffer's disease —*see* Mononucleosis, infectious
Phagedena (dry) (moist) (sloughing) —*see also* Gangrene
- geometric L88
- penis N48.29
- tropical —*see* Ulcer, skin
- vulva N76.6

Phagedenic —*see* condition
Phakoma H35.89
Phakomatosis —*see also* specific eponymous syndromes Q85.9
- Bourneville's Q85.1
- specified NEC Q85.8

Phantom limb syndrome (without pain) G54.7
- with pain G54.6

Pharyngeal pouch syndrome D82.1
Pharyngitis (acute) (catarrhal) (gangrenous) (infective) (malignant) (membranous) (phlegmonous) (pseudomembranous) (simple) (subacute) (suppurative) (ulcerative) (viral) JØ2.9
- with influenza, flu, or grippe —*see* Influenza, with, pharyngitis
- aphthous BØ8.5
- atrophic J31.2
- chlamydial A56.4
- chronic (atrophic) (granular) (hypertrophic) J31.2
- coxsackievirus BØ8.5
- diphtheritic A36.Ø
- enteroviral vesicular BØ8.5
- follicular (chronic) J31.2
- fusospirochetal A69.1
- gonococcal A54.5
- granular (chronic) J31.2
- herpesviral BØØ.2
- hypertrophic J31.2
- infectional, chronic J31.2
- influenzal —*see* Influenza, with, respiratory manifestations NEC
- lymphonodular, acute (enteroviral) BØ8.8
- pneumococcal JØ2.8
- purulent JØ2.9
- putrid JØ2.9
- septic JØ2.Ø
- sicca J31.2
- specified organism NEC JØ2.8
- staphylococcal JØ2.8
- streptococcal JØ2.Ø
- syphilitic, congenital (early) A5Ø.Ø3
- tuberculous A15.8
- vesicular, enteroviral BØ8.5
- viral NEC JØ2.8

Pharyngoconjunctivitis, viral B3Ø.2
Pharyngolaryngitis (acute) JØ6.Ø
- chronic J37.Ø

Pharyngoplegia J39.2
Pharyngotonsillitis, herpesviral BØØ.2
Pharyngotracheitis, chronic J42
Pharynx, pharyngeal —*see* condition
Phencyclidine-induced
- anxiety disorder F16.98Ø
- bipolar and related disorder F16.94
- depressive disorder F16.94
- psychotic disorder F16.959

Phenomenon
- Arthus' —*see* Arthus' phenomenon
- jaw-winking QØ7.8
- lupus erythematosus (LE) cell M32.9
- Raynaud's (secondary) I73.ØØ
  - with gangrene I73.Ø1
- vasomotor R55
- vasospastic I73.9
- vasovagal R55
- Wenckebach's I44.1

Phenylketonuria E7Ø.1
- classical E7Ø.Ø
- maternal E7Ø.1

Pheochromoblastoma
- specified site —*see* Neoplasm, malignant, by site
- unspecified site C74.1Ø

Pheochromocytoma
- malignant
  - specified site —*see* Neoplasm, malignant, by site
  - unspecified site C74.1Ø
- specified site —*see* Neoplasm, benign, by site
- unspecified site D35.ØØ

Pheohyphomycosis —*see* Chromomycosis
Pheomycosis —*see* Chromomycosis
Phimosis (congenital) (due to infection) N47.1
- chancroidal A57

Phlebectasia —*see also* Varix
- congenital Q27.4

Phlebitis (infective) (pyemic) (septic) (suppurative) I8Ø.9
- antepartum —*see* Thrombophlebitis, antepartum
- blue —*see* Phlebitis, leg, deep
- breast, superficial I8Ø.8
- ▶ calf muscular vein (NOS) I8Ø.25-●
- cavernous (venous) sinus —*see* Phlebitis, intracranial (venous) sinus
- cerebral (venous) sinus —*see* Phlebitis, intracranial (venous) sinus
- chest wall, superficial I8Ø.8
- cranial (venous) sinus —*see* Phlebitis, intracranial (venous) sinus
- deep (vessels) —*see* Phlebitis, leg, deep
- due to implanted device —*see* Complications, by site and type, specified NEC
- during or resulting from a procedure T81.72
- femoral vein (superficial) I8Ø.1-●
- femoropopliteal vein I8Ø.Ø-●
- ▶ gastrocnemial vein I8Ø.25-●
- gestational —*see* Phlebopathy, gestational
- hepatic veins I8Ø.8
- ▶ iliac vein (common) (external) (internal) I8Ø.21-●
- iliofemoral —*see* Phlebitis, femoral vein
- intracranial (venous) sinus (any) GØ8
  - nonpyogenic I67.6
- intraspinal venous sinuses and veins GØ8
  - nonpyogenic G95.19
- lateral (venous) sinus —*see* Phlebitis, intracranial (venous) sinus
- leg I8Ø.3
  - antepartum —*see* Thrombophlebitis, antepartum
  - deep (vessels) NEC I8Ø.2Ø-●
    - iliac I8Ø.21-●
    - popliteal vein I8Ø.22-●
    - specified vessel NEC I8Ø.29-●
    - ➠ tibial vein (anterior) (posterior) I8Ø.23-●
  - femoral vein (superficial) I8Ø.1-●
  - superficial (vessels) I8Ø.Ø-●
- longitudinal sinus —*see* Phlebitis, intracranial (venous) sinus
- lower limb —*see* Phlebitis, leg
- migrans, migrating (superficial) I82.1
- pelvic
  - with ectopic or molar pregnancy OØ8.Ø
  - following ectopic or molar pregnancy OØ8.Ø
  - puerperal, postpartum O87.1
- ▶ peroneal vein I8Ø.24-●
- popliteal vein —*see* Phlebitis, leg, deep, popliteal
- portal (vein) K75.1
- postoperative T81.72
- pregnancy —*see* Thrombophlebitis, antepartum
- puerperal, postpartum, childbirth O87.Ø
  - deep O87.1
  - pelvic O87.1
  - superficial O87.Ø
- retina —*see* Vasculitis, retina
- saphenous (accessory) (great) (long) (small) —*see* Phlebitis, leg, superficial
- sinus (meninges) —*see* Phlebitis, intracranial (venous) sinus
- ▶ soleal vein I8Ø.25-●
- specified site NEC I8Ø.8
- syphilitic A52.Ø9
- tibial vein —*see* Phlebitis, leg, deep, tibial
- ulcerative I8Ø.9
  - leg —*see* Phlebitis, leg
- umbilicus I8Ø.8
- uterus (septic) —*see* Endometritis
- varicose (leg) (lower limb) —*see* Varix, leg, with, inflammation

Phlebofibrosis I87.8
Phleboliths I87.8
Phlebopathy
- gestational O22.9-●
- puerperal O87.9

Phlebosclerosis I87.8
Phlebothrombosis —*see also* Thrombosis
- antepartum —*see* Thrombophlebitis, antepartum
- pregnancy —*see* Thrombophlebitis, antepartum
- puerperal —*see* Thrombophlebitis, puerperal

Phlebotomus fever A93.1
Phlegmasia
- alba dolens O87.1
  - nonpuerperal —*see* Phlebitis, femoral vein
- cerulea dolens —*see* Phlebitis, leg, deep

Phlegmon —*see* Abscess
Phlegmonous —*see* condition

P

Phlyctenulosis (allergic) (keratoconjunctivitis) (nontuberculous) *—see also* Keratoconjunctivitis
cornea *—see* Keratoconjunctivitis
tuberculous A18.52
Phobia, phobic F40.9
animal F40.218
spiders F40.210
examination F40.298
reaction F40.9
simple F40.298
social F40.10
generalized F40.11
specific (isolated) F40.298
animal F40.218
spiders F40.210
blood F40.230
injection F40.231
injury F40.233
men F40.290
natural environment F40.228
thunderstorms F40.220
situational F40.248
bridges F40.242
closed in spaces F40.240
flying F40.243
heights F40.241
specified focus NEC F40.298
transfusion F40.231
women F40.291
specified NEC F40.8
medical care NEC F40.232
state F40.9
Phocas' disease *—see* Mastopathy, cystic
Phocomelia Q73.1
lower limb *—see* Agenesis, leg, with foot present
upper limb *—see* Agenesis, arm, with hand present
Phoria H50.50
Phosphate-losing tubular disorder N25.0
Phosphatemia E83.39
Phosphaturia E83.39
Photodermatitis (sun) L56.8
chronic L57.8
due to drug L56.8
light other than sun L59.8
Photokeratitis H16.13- •
Photophobia H53.14- •
Photophthalmia *—see* Photokeratitis
Photopsia H53.19
Photoretinitis *—see* Retinopathy, solar
Photosensitivity, photosensitization (sun) skin L56.8
light other than sun L59.8
Phrenitis *—see* Encephalitis
Phrynoderma (vitamin A deficiency) E50.8
Phthiriasis (pubis) B85.3
with any infestation classifiable to B85.0-B85.2 B85.4
Phthirus infestation *—see* Phthiriasis
Phthisis *—see also* Tuberculosis
bulbi (infectional) *—see* Disorder, globe, degenerated condition, atrophy
eyeball (due to infection) *—see* Disorder, globe, degenerated condition, atrophy
Phycomycosis *—see* Zygomycosis
Physalopteriasis B81.8
Physical restraint status Z78.1
Phytobezoar T18.9
intestine T18.3
stomach T18.2
Pian *—see* Yaws
Pianoma A66.1
Pica F50.89
in adults F50.89
infant or child F98.3
Picking, nose F98.8
Pick-Niemann disease *—see* Niemann-Pick disease or syndrome
Pick's
cerebral atrophy G31.01 *[F02.80]*
with behavioral disturbance G31.01 *[F02.81]*
disease or syndrome (brain) G31.01 *[F02.80]*
with behavioral disturbance G31.01 *[F02.81]*
brain G31.01 *[F02.80]*
with behavioral disturbance G31.01 *[F02.81]*
pericardium (pericardial pseudocirrhosis of liver) I31.1
syndrome
brain G31.01 *[F02.80]*
with behavioral disturbance G31.01 *[F02.81]*
of heart (pericardial pseudocirrhosis of liver) I31.1
Pickwickian syndrome E66.2
Piebaldism E70.39
Piedra (beard) (scalp) B36.8
black B36.3
white B36.2
Pierre Robin deformity or syndrome Q87.0
Pierson's disease or osteochondrosis M91.0
Pig-bel A05.2
Pigeon
breast or chest (acquired) M95.4
congenital Q67.7
rachitic sequelae (late effect) E64.3
breeder's disease or lung J67.2
fancier's disease or lung J67.2
toe *—see* Deformity, toe, specified NEC
Pigmentation (abnormal) (anomaly) L81.9
conjunctiva H11.13- •
cornea (anterior) H18.01- •
posterior H18.05- •
stromal H18.06- •
diminished melanin formation NEC L81.6
iron L81.8
lids, congenital Q82.8
limbus corneae *—see* Pigmentation, cornea
metals L81.8
optic papilla, congenital Q14.2
retina, congenital (grouped) (nevoid) Q14.1
scrotum, congenital Q82.8
tattoo L81.8
Piles *—see also* Hemorrhoids K64.9
Pili
annulati or torti (congenital) Q84.1
incarnati L73.1
Pill roller hand (intrinsic) *—see* Parkinsonism
Pilomatrixoma *—see* Neoplasm, skin, benign
malignant *—see* Neoplasm, skin, malignant
Pilonidal *—see* condition
Pimple R23.8
PIN *—see* Neoplasia, intraepithelial, prostate
Pinched nerve *—see* Neuropathy, entrapment
Pindborg tumor *—see* Cyst, calcifying odontogenic
Pineal body or gland *—see* condition
Pinealoblastoma C75.3
Pinealoma D44.5
malignant C75.3
Pineoblastoma C75.3
Pineocytoma D44.5
Pinguecula H11.15- •
Pingueculitis H10.81- •
Pinhole meatus *—see also* Stricture, urethra N35.919
Pink
disease *—see* subcategory T56.1
eye *—see* Conjunctivitis, acute, mucopurulent
Pinkus' disease (lichen nitidus) L44.1
Pinpoint
meatus *—see* Stricture, urethra
os (uteri) *—see* Stricture, cervix
Pins and needles R20.2
Pinta A67.9
cardiovascular lesions A67.2
chancre (primary) A67.0
Pinta *(Continued)*
erythematous plaques A67.1
hyperchromic lesions A67.1
hyperkeratosis A67.1
lesions A67.9
cardiovascular A67.2
hyperchromic A67.1
intermediate A67.1
late A67.2
mixed A67.3
primary A67.0
skin (achromic) (cicatricial) (dyschromic) A67.2
hyperchromic A67.1
mixed (achromic and hyperchromic) A67.3
papule (primary) A67.0
skin lesions (achromic) (cicatricial) (dyschromic) A67.2
hyperchromic A67.1
mixed (achromic and hyperchromic) A67.3
vitiligo A67.2
Pintids A67.1
Pinworm (disease) (infection) (infestation) B80
Piroplasmosis B60.0
Pistol wound *—see* Gunshot wound
Pitchers' elbow *—see* Derangement, joint, specified type NEC, elbow
Pithecoid pelvis Q74.2
with disproportion (fetopelvic) O33.0
causing obstructed labor O65.0
Pithiatism F48.8
Pitted *—see* Pitting
Pitting *—see also* Edema R60.9
lip R60.0
nail L60.8
teeth K00.4
Pituitary gland *—see* condition
Pituitary-snuff-taker's disease J67.8
Pityriasis (capitis) L21.0
alba L30.5
circinata (et maculata) L42
furfuracea L21.0
Hebra's L26
lichenoides L41.0
chronica L41.1
et varioliformis (acuta) L41.0
maculata (et circinata) L30.5
nigra B36.1
pilaris, Hebra's L44.0
rosea L42
rotunda L44.8
rubra (Hebra) pilaris L44.0
simplex L30.5
specified type NEC L30.5
streptogenes L30.5
versicolor (scrotal) B36.0
Placenta, placental *—see* Pregnancy, complicated by (care of) (management affected by), specified condition
Placentitis O41.14- •
Plagiocephaly Q67.3
Plague A20.9
abortive A20.8
ambulatory A20.8
asymptomatic A20.8
bubonic A20.0
cellulocutaneous A20.1
cutaneobubonic A20.1
lymphatic gland A20.0
meningitis A20.3
pharyngeal A20.8
pneumonic (primary) (secondary) A20.2
pulmonary, pulmonic A20.2
septicemic A20.7
tonsillar A20.8
septicemic A20.7
Planning, family
contraception Z30.9
procreation Z31.69

P

Plaque(s)
  artery, arterial —*see* Arteriosclerosis
  calcareous —*see* Calcification
  coronary, lipid rich I25.83
  epicardial I31.8
  erythematous, of pinta A67.1
  Hollenhorst's —*see* Occlusion, artery, retina
  lipid rich, coronary I25.83
  pleural (without asbestos) J92.9
    with asbestos J92.Ø
  tongue K13.29
Plasmacytoma C9Ø.3-•
  extramedullary C9Ø.2-•
  medullary C9Ø.Ø-•
  solitary C9Ø.3-•
Plasmacytopenia D72.818
Plasmacytosis D72.822
Plaster ulcer —*see* Ulcer, pressure, by site
Plateau iris syndrome (post-iridectomy) (postprocedural) (without glaucoma) H21.82
  with glaucoma H4Ø.22-•
Platybasia Q75.8
Platyonychia (congenital) Q84.6
  acquired L6Ø.8
Platypelloid pelvis M95.5
  with disproportion (fetopelvic) O33.Ø
    causing obstructed labor O65.Ø
  congenital Q74.2
Platyspondylisis Q76.49
Plaut (-Vincent) disease —*see also* Vincent's A69.1
Plethora R23.2
  newborn P61.1
Pleura, pleural —*see* condition
Pleuralgia RØ7.81
Pleurisy (acute) (adhesive) (chronic) (costal) (diaphragmatic) (double) (dry) (fibrinous) (fibrous) (interlobar) (latent) (plastic) (primary) (residual) (sicca) (sterile) (subacute) (unresolved) RØ9.1
  with
    adherent pleura J86.Ø
    effusion J9Ø
      chylous, chyliform J94.Ø
      tuberculous (non primary) A15.6
        primary (progressive) A15.7
    tuberculosis —*see* Pleurisy, tuberculous (non primary)
  encysted —*see* Pleurisy, with effusion
  exudative —*see* Pleurisy, with effusion
  fibrinopurulent, fibropurulent —*see* Pyothorax
  hemorrhagic —*see* Hemothorax
  pneumococcal J9Ø
  purulent —*see* Pyothorax
  septic —*see* Pyothorax
  serofibrinous —*see* Pleurisy, with effusion
  seropurulent —*see* Pyothorax
  serous —*see* Pleurisy, with effusion
  staphylococcal J86.9
  streptococcal J9Ø
  suppurative —*see* Pyothorax
  traumatic (post) (current) —*see* Injury, intrathoracic, pleura
  tuberculous (with effusion) (non primary) A15.6
    primary (progressive) A15.7
Pleuritis sicca —*see* Pleurisy
Pleurobronchopneumonia —*see* Pneumonia, broncho
Pleurodynia RØ7.81
  epidemic B33.Ø
  viral B33.Ø
Pleuropericarditis —*see also* Pericarditis
  acute I3Ø.9
Pleuropneumonia (acute) (bilateral) (double) (septic) —*see also* Pneumonia J18.8
  chronic —*see* Fibrosis, lung

Pleuro-pneumonia-like-organism (PPLO), as cause of disease classified elsewhere B96.Ø
Pleurorrhea —*see* Pleurisy, with effusion
Plexitis, brachial G54.Ø
Plica
  polonica B85.Ø
  syndrome, knee M67.5
  tonsil J35.8
Plicated tongue K14.5
Plug
  bronchus NEC J98.Ø9
  meconium (newborn) NEC syndrome P76.Ø
  mucus —*see* Asphyxia, mucus
Plumbism —*see* subcategory T56.Ø
Plummer's disease EØ5.2Ø
  with thyroid storm EØ5.21
Plummer-Vinson syndrome D5Ø.1
Pluricarential syndrome of infancy E4Ø
Plus (and minus) **hand** (intrinsic) —*see* Deformity, limb, specified type NEC, forearm
Pneumathemia —*see* Air, embolism
Pneumatic hammer (drill) **syndrome** T75.21
Pneumatocele (lung) J98.4
  intracranial G93.89
  tension J44.9
Pneumatosis
  cystoides intestinalis K63.89
  intestinalis K63.89
  peritonei K66.8
Pneumaturia R39.89
Pneumoblastoma —*see* Neoplasm, lung, malignant
Pneumocephalus G93.89
Pneumococcemia A4Ø.3
Pneumococcus, pneumococcal —*see* condition
Pneumoconiosis (due to) (inhalation of) J64
  with tuberculosis (any type in A15) J65
  aluminum J63.Ø
  asbestos J61
  bagasse, bagassosis J67.1
  bauxite J63.1
  beryllium J63.2
  coal miners' (simple) J6Ø
  coalworkers' (simple) J6Ø
  collier's J6Ø
  cotton dust J66.Ø
  diatomite (diatomaceous earth) J62.8
  dust
    inorganic NEC J63.6
    lime J62.8
    marble J62.8
    organic NEC J66.8
  fumes or vapors (from silo) J68.9
  graphite J63.3
  grinder's J62.8
  kaolin J62.8
  mica J62.8
  millstone maker's J62.8
  mineral fibers NEC J61
  miner's J6Ø
  moldy hay J67.Ø
  potter's J62.8
  rheumatoid —*see* Rheumatoid, lung
  sandblaster's J62.8
  silica, silicate NEC J62.8
    with carbon J6Ø
  stonemason's J62.8
  talc (dust) J62.Ø
Pneumocystis carinii pneumonia B59
Pneumocystis jiroveci (pneumonia) B59
Pneumocystosis (with pneumonia) B59
Pneumohemopericardium I31.2
Pneumohemothorax J94.2
  traumatic S27.2
Pneumohydropericardium —*see* Pericarditis
Pneumohydrothorax —*see* Hydrothorax
Pneumomediastinum J98.2
  congenital or perinatal P25.2
Pneumomycosis B49 *[J99]*

Pneumonia (acute) (double) (migratory) (purulent) (septic) (unresolved) J18.9
  with
    influenza —*see* Influenza, with, pneumonia
    lung abscess J85.1
      due to specified organism —*see* Pneumonia, in (due to)
  adenoviral J12.Ø
  adynamic J18.2
  alba A5Ø.Ø4
  allergic (eosinophilic) J82
  alveolar —*see* Pneumonia, lobar
  anaerobes J15.8
  anthrax A22.1
  apex, apical —*see* Pneumonia, lobar
  Ascaris B77.81
  aspiration J69.Ø
    due to
      aspiration of microorganisms
        bacterial J15.9
        viral J12.9
      food (regurgitated) J69.Ø
      gastric secretions J69.Ø
      milk (regurgitated) J69.Ø
      oils, essences J69.1
      solids, liquids NEC J69.8
      vomitus J69.Ø
    newborn P24.81
      amniotic fluid (clear) P24.11
      blood P24.21
      food (regurgitated) P24.31
      liquor (amnii) P24.11
      meconium P24.Ø1
      milk P24.31
      mucus P24.11
      specified NEC P24.81
      stomach contents P24.31
    postprocedural J95.4
  atypical NEC J18.9
  bacillus J15.9
    specified NEC J15.8
  bacterial J15.9
    specified NEC J15.8
  Bacteroides (fragilis) (oralis) (melaninogenicus) J15.8
  basal, basic, basilar —*see* Pneumonia, by type
  bronchiolitis obliterans organized (BOOP) J84.89
  broncho-, bronchial (confluent) (croupous) (diffuse) (disseminated) (hemorrhagic) (involving lobes) (lobar) (terminal) J18.Ø
    allergic (eosinophilic) J82
    aspiration —*see* Pneumonia, aspiration
    bacterial J15.9
      specified NEC J15.8
    chronic —*see* Fibrosis, lung
    diplococcal J13
    Eaton's agent J15.7
    Escherichia coli (E. coli) J15.5
    Friedländer's bacillus J15.Ø
    Hemophilus influenzae J14
    hypostatic J18.2
    inhalation —*see also* Pneumonia, aspiration
      due to fumes or vapors (chemical) J68.Ø
      of oils or essences J69.1
    Klebsiella (pneumoniae) J15.Ø
    lipid, lipoid J69.1
      endogenous J84.89
    Mycoplasma (pneumoniae) J15.7
    pleuro-pneumonia-like-organisms (PPLO) J15.7
    pneumococcal J13
    Proteus J15.6
    Pseudomonas J15.1
    Serratia marcescens J15.6
    specified organism NEC J16.8
    staphylococcal —*see* Pneumonia, staphylococcal
    streptococcal NEC J15.4
      group B J15.3
      pneumoniae J13
    viral, virus —*see* Pneumonia, viral

P

- Pneumonia *(Continued)*
  - Butyrivibrio (fibriosolvens) J15.8
  - Candida B37.1
  - caseous —*see* Tuberculosis, pulmonary
  - catarrhal —*see* Pneumonia, broncho
  - chlamydial J16.Ø
    - congenital P23.1
  - cholesterol J84.89
  - cirrhotic (chronic) —*see* Fibrosis, lung
  - Clostridium (haemolyticum) (novyi) J15.8
  - confluent —*see* Pneumonia, broncho
  - congenital (infective) P23.9
    - due to
      - bacterium NEC P23.6
      - Chlamydia P23.1
      - Escherichia coli P23.4
      - Haemophilus influenzae P23.6
      - infective organism NEC P23.8
      - Klebsiella pneumoniae P23.6
      - Mycoplasma P23.6
      - Pseudomonas P23.5
      - Staphylococcus P23.2
      - Streptococcus (except group B) P23.6
        - group B P23.3
      - viral agent P23.Ø
    - specified NEC P23.8
  - croupous —*see* Pneumonia, lobar
  - cryptogenic organizing J84.116
  - cytomegalic inclusion B25.Ø
  - cytomegaloviral B25.Ø
  - deglutition —*see* Pneumonia, aspiration
  - desquamative interstitial J84.117
  - diffuse —*see* Pneumonia, broncho
  - diplococcal, diplococcus (broncho-) (lobar) J13
  - disseminated (focal) —*see* Pneumonia, broncho
  - Eaton's agent J15.7
  - embolic, embolism —*see* Embolism, pulmonary
  - Enterobacter J15.6
  - eosinophilic J82
  - Escherichia coli (E. coli) J15.5
  - Eubacterium J15.8
  - fibrinous —*see* Pneumonia, lobar
  - fibroid, fibrous (chronic) —*see* Fibrosis, lung
  - Friedländer's bacillus J15.Ø
  - Fusobacterium (nucleatum) J15.8
  - gangrenous J85.Ø
  - giant cell (measles) BØ5.2
  - gonococcal A54.84
  - gram-negative bacteria NEC J15.6
    - anaerobic J15.8
  - Hemophilus influenzae (broncho) (lobar) J14
  - human metapneumovirus J12.3
  - hypostatic (broncho) (lobar) J18.2
  - in (due to)
    - actinomycosis A42.Ø
    - adenovirus J12.Ø
    - anthrax A22.1
    - ascariasis B77.81
    - aspergillosis B44.9
    - Bacillus anthracis A22.1
    - Bacterium anitratum J15.6
    - candidiasis B37.1
    - chickenpox BØ1.2
    - Chlamydia J16.Ø
      - neonatal P23.1
    - coccidioidomycosis B38.2
      - acute B38.Ø
      - chronic B38.1
    - cytomegalovirus disease B25.Ø
    - Diplococcus (pneumoniae) J13
    - Eaton's agent J15.7
    - Enterobacter J15.6
    - Escherichia coli (E. coli) J15.5
    - Friedländer's bacillus J15.Ø
    - fumes and vapors (chemical) (inhalation) J68.Ø
    - gonorrhea A54.84
    - Hemophilus influenzae (H. influenzae) J14

- Pneumonia *(Continued)*
  - in *(Continued)*
    - Herellea J15.6
    - histoplasmosis B39.2
      - acute B39.Ø
      - chronic B39.1
    - human metapneumovirus J12.3
    - Klebsiella (pneumoniae) J15.Ø
    - measles BØ5.2
    - Mycoplasma (pneumoniae) J15.7
    - nocardiosis, nocardiasis A43.Ø
    - ornithosis A7Ø
    - parainfluenza virus J12.2
    - pleuro-pneumonia-like-organism (PPLO) J15.7
    - pneumococcus J13
    - pneumocystosis (Pneumocystis carinii) (Pneumocystis jiroveci) B59
    - Proteus J15.6
    - Pseudomonas NEC J15.1
      - pseudomallei A24.1
    - psittacosis A7Ø
    - Q fever A78
    - respiratory syncytial virus (RSV) J12.1
    - rheumatic fever IØØ *[J17]*
    - rubella BØ6.81
    - Salmonella (infection) AØ2.22
      - typhi AØ1.Ø3
    - schistosomiasis B65.9 *[J17]*
    - Serratia marcescens J15.6
    - specified
      - bacterium NEC J15.8
      - organism NEC J16.8
    - spirochetal NEC A69.8
    - Staphylococcus J15.2Ø
      - aureus (methicillin susceptible) (MSSA) J15.211
        - methicillin resistant (MRSA) J15.212
      - specified NEC J15.29
    - Streptococcus J15.4
      - group B J15.3
      - pneumoniae J13
      - specified NEC J15.4
    - toxoplasmosis B58.3
    - tularemia A21.2
    - typhoid (fever) AØ1.Ø3
    - varicella BØ1.2
    - virus —*see* Pneumonia, viral
    - whooping cough A37.91
      - due to
        - Bordetella parapertussis A37.11
        - Bordetella pertussis A37.Ø1
        - specified NEC A37.81
    - Yersinia pestis A2Ø.2
  - inhalation of food or vomit —*see* Pneumonia, aspiration
  - interstitial J84.9
    - chronic J84.111
    - desquamative J84.117
    - due to
      - collagen vascular disease J84.17
      - known underlying cause J84.17
    - idiopathic NOS J84.111
    - in disease classified elsewhere J84.17
    - lymphocytic (due to collagen vascular disease) (in diseases classified elsewhere) J84.17
    - lymphoid J84.2
    - non-specific J84.89
      - due to
        - collagen vascular disease J84.17
        - known underlying cause J84.17
      - idiopathic J84.113
      - in diseases classified elsewhere J84.17
    - plasma cell B59
    - pseudomonas J15.1
    - usual J84.112
      - due to collagen vascular disease J84.17
      - idiopathic J84.112
      - in diseases classified elsewhere J84.17

- Pneumonia *(Continued)*
  - Klebsiella (pneumoniae) J15.Ø
  - lipid, lipoid (exogenous) J69.1
    - endogenous J84.89
  - lobar (disseminated) (double) (interstitial) J18.1
    - bacterial J15.9
      - specified NEC J15.8
    - chronic —*see* Fibrosis, lung
    - Escherichia coli (E. coli) J15.5
    - Friedländer's bacillus J15.Ø
    - Hemophilus influenzae J14
    - hypostatic J18.2
    - Klebsiella (pneumoniae) J15.Ø
    - pneumococcal J13
    - Proteus J15.6
    - Pseudomonas J15.1
    - specified organism NEC J16.8
    - staphylococcal —*see* Pneumonia, staphylococcal
    - streptococcal NEC J15.4
    - Streptococcus pneumoniae J13
    - viral, virus —*see* Pneumonia, viral
  - lobular —*see* Pneumonia, broncho
  - Löffler's J82
  - lymphoid interstitial J84.2
  - massive —*see* Pneumonia, lobar
  - meconium P24.Ø1
  - MRSA (Methicillin resistant Staphylococcus aureus) J15.212
  - MSSA (methicillin susceptible Staphylococcus aureus) J15.211
  - multilobar —*see* Pneumonia, by type
  - Mycoplasma (pneumoniae) J15.7
  - necrotic J85.Ø
  - neonatal P23.9
    - aspiration —*see* Aspiration, by substance, with pneumonia
  - nitrogen dioxide J68.Ø
  - organizing J84.89
    - due to
      - collagen vascular disease J84.17
      - known underlying cause J84.17
    - in diseases classified elsewhere J84.17
  - orthostatic J18.2
  - parainfluenza virus J12.2
  - parenchymatous —*see* Fibrosis, lung
  - passive J18.2
  - patchy —*see* Pneumonia, broncho
  - Peptococcus J15.8
  - Peptostreptococcus J15.8
  - plasma cell (of infants) B59
  - pleurolobar —*see* Pneumonia, lobar
  - pleuro-pneumonia-like organism (PPLO) J15.7
  - pneumococcal (broncho) (lobar) J13
  - Pneumocystis (carinii) (jiroveci) B59
  - postinfectional NEC B99 *[J17]*
  - postmeasles BØ5.2
  - Proteus J15.6
  - Pseudomonas J15.1
  - psittacosis A7Ø
  - radiation J7Ø.Ø
  - respiratory syncytial virus (RSV) J12.1
  - resulting from a procedure J95.89
  - rheumatic IØØ *[J17]*
  - Salmonella (arizonae) (cholerae-suis) (enteritidis) (typhimurium) AØ2.22
    - typhi AØ1.Ø3
    - typhoid fever AØ1.Ø3
  - SARS-associated coronavirus J12.81
  - segmented, segmental —*see* Pneumonia, broncho- •
  - Serratia marcescens J15.6
  - specified NEC J18.8
    - bacterium NEC J15.8
    - organism NEC J16.8
    - virus NEC J12.89
  - spirochetal NEC A69.8

Pneumonia *(Continued)*
  staphylococcal (broncho) (lobar) J15.2Ø
    aureus (methicillin susceptible) (MSSA) J15.211
      methicillin resistant (MRSA) J15.212
    specified NEC J15.29
  static, stasis J18.2
  streptococcal NEC (broncho) (lobar) J15.4
    group
      A J15.4
      B J15.3
      specified NEC J15.4
  Streptococcus pneumoniae J13
  syphilitic, congenital (early) A5Ø.Ø4
  traumatic (complication) (early) (secondary) T79.8
  tuberculous (any) —*see* Tuberculosis, pulmonary
  tularemic A21.2
  varicella BØ1.2
  Veillonella J15.8
  ventilator associated J95.851
  viral, virus (broncho) (interstitial) (lobar) J12.9
    adenoviral J12.Ø
    congenital P23.Ø
    human metapneumovirus J12.3
    parainfluenza J12.2
    ➧respiratory syncytial (RSV) J12.1
    SARS-associated coronavirus J12.81
    specified NEC J12.89
  white (congenital) A5Ø.Ø4
Pneumonic —*see* condition
Pneumonitis (acute) (primary) —*see also* Pneumonia
  air-conditioner J67.7
  allergic (due to) J67.9
    organic dust NEC J67.8
    red cedar dust J67.8
    sequoiosis J67.8
    wood dust J67.8
  aspiration J69.Ø
    due to
      anesthesia J95.4
        during
          labor and delivery O74.Ø
          pregnancy O29.Ø1-•
          puerperium O89.Ø1
      fumes or gases J68.Ø
    obstetric O74.Ø
  chemical (due to gases, fumes or vapors) (inhalation) J68.Ø
    due to anesthesia J95.4
  cholesterol J84.89
  chronic —*see* Fibrosis, lung
  congenital rubella P35.Ø
  crack (cocaine) J68.Ø
  due to
    beryllium J68.Ø
    cadmium J68.Ø
    crack (cocaine) J68.Ø
    detergent J69.8
    fluorocarbon-polymer J68.Ø
    food, vomit (aspiration) J69.Ø
    fumes or vapors J68.Ø
    gases, fumes or vapors (inhalation) J68.Ø
    inhalation
      blood J69.8
      essences J69.1
      food (regurgitated), milk, vomit J69.Ø
      oils, essences J69.1
      saliva J69.Ø
      solids, liquids NEC J69.8
    manganese J68.Ø
    nitrogen dioxide J68.Ø
    oils, essences J69.1
    solids, liquids NEC J69.8
    toxoplasmosis (acquired) B58.3
      congenital P37.1
    vanadium J68.Ø
    ventilator J95.851
  eosinophilic J82
  hypersensitivity J67.9
    air conditioner lung J67.7
    bagassosis J67.1
    bird fancier's lung J67.2
    farmer's lung J67.Ø
    maltworker's lung J67.4
    maple bark-stripper's lung J67.6
    mushroom worker's lung J67.5
    specified organic dust NEC J67.8
    suberosis J67.3
  interstitial (chronic) J84.89
    acute J84.114
    lymphoid J84.2
    non-specific J84.89
      idiopathic J84.113
  lymphoid, interstitial J84.2
  meconium P24.Ø1
  postanesthetic J95.4
    correct substance properly administered —*see* Table of Drugs and Chemcials, by drug, adverse effect
    in labor and delivery O74.Ø
    in pregnancy O29.Ø1-•
    obstetric O74.Ø
    overdose or wrong substance given or taken (by accident) —*see* Table of Drugs and Chemicals, by drug, poisoning
    postpartum, puerperal O89.Ø1
  postoperative J95.4
    obstetric O74.Ø
  radiation J7Ø.Ø
  rubella, congenital P35.Ø
  ventilation (air-conditioning) J67.7
  ventilator associated J95.851
  wood-dust J67.8
Pneumonoconiosis —*see* Pneumoconiosis
Pneumoparotid K11.8
Pneumopathy NEC J98.4
  alveolar J84.Ø9
  due to organic dust NEC J66.8
  parietoalveolar J84.Ø9
Pneumopericarditis —*see also* Pericarditis
  acute I3Ø.9
Pneumopericardium —*see also* Pericarditis
  congenital P25.3
  newborn P25.3
  traumatic (post) —*see* Injury, heart
Pneumophagia (psychogenic) F45.8
Pneumopleurisy, pneumopleuritis —*see also* Pneumonia J18.8
Pneumopyopericardium I3Ø.1
Pneumopyothorax —*see* Pyopneumothorax
  with fistula J86.Ø
Pneumorrhagia —*see also* Hemorrhage, lung
  tuberculous —*see* Tuberculosis, pulmonary
Pneumothorax NOS J93.9
  acute J93.83
  chronic J93.81
  congenital P25.1
  perinatal period P25.1
  postprocedural J95.811
  specified NEC J93.83
  spontaneous NOS J93.83
    newborn P25.1
    primary J93.11
    secondary J93.12
    tension J93.Ø
  tense valvular, infectional J93.Ø
  tension (spontaneous) J93.Ø
  traumatic S27.Ø
    with hemothorax S27.2
  tuberculous —*see* Tuberculosis, pulmonary
Podagra —*see also* Gout M1Ø.9
Podencephalus QØ1.9
Poikilocytosis R71.8
Poikiloderma L81.6
  Civatte's L57.3
  congenital Q82.8
  vasculare atrophicans L94.5
Poikilodermatomyositis M33.1Ø
  with
    myopathy M33.12
    respiratory involvement M33.11
    specified organ involvement NEC M33.19
Pointed ear (congenital) Q17.3
Poison ivy, oak, sumac or other plant dermatitis (allergic) (contact) L23.7
Poisoning (acute) —*see also* Table of Drugs and Chemicals
  algae and toxins T65.82-•
  Bacillus B (aertrycke) (cholerae (suis)) (paratyphosus) (suipestifer) AØ2.9
    botulinus AØ5.1
  bacterial toxins AØ5.9
  berries, noxious —*see* Poisoning, food, noxious, berries
  botulism AØ5.1
  ciguatera fish T61.Ø-•
  Clostridium botulinum AØ5.1
  death-cap (Amanita phalloides) (Amanita verna) —*see* Poisoning, food, noxious, mushrooms
  drug —*see* Table of Drugs and Chemicals, by drug, poisoning
  epidemic, fish (noxious) —*see* Poisoning, seafood
    bacterial AØ5.9
  fava bean D55.Ø
  fish (noxious) T61.9-•
    bacterial —*see* Intoxication, foodborne, by agent
    ciguatera fish —*see* Poisoning, ciguatera fish
    scombroid fish —*see* Poisoning, scombroid fish
    specified type NEC T61.77-•
  ➧food NEC AØ5.9
    bacterial —*see* Intoxication, foodborne, by agent
    due to
      Bacillus (aertrycke) (choleraesuis) (paratyphosus) (suipestifer) AØ2.9
        botulinus AØ5.1
      Clostridium (perfringens) (Welchii) AØ5.2
      salmonella (aertrycke) (callinarum) (choleraesuis) (enteritidis) (paratyphi) (suipestifer) AØ2.9
        with
          gastroenteritis AØ2.Ø
          sepsis AØ2.1
      staphylococcus AØ5.Ø
      Vibrio
        parahaemolyticus AØ5.3
        vulnificus AØ5.5
    noxious or naturally toxic T62.9-•
      berries —*see* subcategory T62.1-•
      fish —*see* Poisoning, seafood
      mushrooms —*see* subcategory T62.ØX-•
      plants NEC —*see* subcategory T62.2X-•
      seafood —*see* Poisoning, seafood
      specified NEC —*see* subcategory T62.8X-•
  ichthyotoxism —*see* Poisoning, seafood
  kreotoxism, food AØ5.9
  latex T65.81-•
  lead T56.Ø-•
  mushroom —*see* Poisoning, food, noxious, mushroom
  mussels —*see also* Poisoning, shellfish
    bacterial —*see* Intoxication, foodborne, by agent
  nicotine (tobacco) T65.2-•
  noxious foodstuffs —*see* Poisoning, food, noxious
  plants, noxious —*see* Poisoning, food, noxious, plants NEC
  ptomaine —*see* Poisoning, food
  radiation J7Ø.Ø

P

Poisoning *(Continued)*
Salmonella (arizonae) (cholerae-suis) (enteritidis) (typhimurium) A02.9
scombroid fish T61.1-●
seafood (noxious) T61.9-●
bacterial —*see* Intoxication, foodborne, by agent
fish —*see* Poisoning, fish
shellfish —*see* Poisoning, shellfish
specified NEC —*see* subcategory T61.8X-●
shellfish (amnesic) (azaspiracid) (diarrheic) (neurotoxic) (noxious) (paralytic) T61.78-●
bacterial —*see* Intoxication, foodborne, by agent
ciguatera mollusk —*see* Poisoning, ciguatera fish
specified substance NEC T65.891
Staphylococcus, food A05.0
tobacco (nicotine) T65.2-●
water E87.79
Poker spine —*see* Spondylitis, ankylosing
Poland syndrome Q79.8
Polioencephalitis (acute) (bulbar) A80.9
inferior G12.22
influenzal —*see* Influenza, with, encephalopathy
superior hemorrhagic (acute) (Wernicke's) E51.2
Wernicke's E51.2
Polioencephalomyelitis (acute) (anterior) A80.9
with beriberi E51.2
Polioencephalopathy, superior hemorrhagic E51.2
with
beriberi E51.11
pellagra E52
Poliomeningoencephalitis —*see* Meningoencephalitis
Poliomyelitis (acute) (anterior) (epidemic) A80.9
with paralysis (bulbar) —*see* Poliomyelitis, paralytic
abortive A80.4
ascending (progressive) —*see* Poliomyelitis, paralytic
bulbar (paralytic) —*see* Poliomyelitis, paralytic
congenital P35.8
nonepidemic A80.9
nonparalytic A80.4
paralytic A80.30
specified NEC A80.39
vaccine-associated A80.0
wild virus
imported A80.1
indigenous A80.2
spinal, acute A80.9
Poliosis (eyebrow) (eyelashes) L67.1
circumscripta, acquired L67.1
Pollakiuria R35.0
psychogenic F45.8
Pollinosis J30.1
Pollitzer's disease L73.2
Polyadenitis —*see also* Lymphadenitis
malignant A20.0
Polyalgia M79.89
Polyangiitis M30.0
microscopic M31.7
overlap syndrome M30.8
Polyarteritis
microscopic M31.7
nodosa M30.0
with lung involvement M30.1
juvenile M30.2
related condition NEC M30.8
Polyarthralgia —*see* Pain, joint
Polyarthritis, polyarthropathy —*see also* Arthritis M13.0
due to or associated with other specified conditions —*see* Arthritis

Polyarthritis, polyarthropathy *(Continued)*
epidemic (Australian) (with exanthema) B33.1
infective —*see* Arthritis, pyogenic or pyemic
inflammatory M06.4
juvenile (chronic) (seronegative) M08.3
migratory M13.8-●
rheumatic, acute —*see* Fever, rheumatic
Polyarthrosis M15.9
post-traumatic M15.3
primary M15.0
specified NEC M15.8
Polycarential syndrome of infancy E40
Polychondritis (atrophic) (chronic) —*see also* Disorder, cartilage, specified type NEC
relapsing M94.1
Polycoria Q13.2
Polycystic (disease)
degeneration, kidney Q61.3
autosomal dominant (adult type) Q61.2
autosomal recessive (infantile type) NEC Q61.19
kidney Q61.3
autosomal
dominant Q61.2
recessive NEC Q61.19
autosomal dominant (adult type) Q61.2
autosomal recessive (childhood type) NEC Q61.19
infantile type NEC Q61.19
liver Q44.6
lung J98.4
congenital Q33.0
ovary, ovaries E28.2
spleen Q89.09
Polycythemia (secondary) D75.1
acquired D75.1
benign (familial) D75.0
due to
donor twin P61.1
erythropoietin D75.1
fall in plasma volume D75.1
high altitude D75.1
maternal-fetal transfusion P61.1
stress D75.1
emotional D75.1
erythropoietin D75.1
familial (benign) D75.0
Gaisböck's (hypertonica) D75.1
high altitude D75.1
hypertonica D75.1
hypoxemic D75.1
neonatorum P61.1
nephrogenous D75.1
relative D75.1
secondary D75.1
spurious D75.1
stress D75.1
vera D45
Polycytosis cryptogenica D75.1
Polydactylism, polydactyly Q69.9
toes Q69.2
Polydipsia R63.1
Polydystrophy, pseudo-Hurler E77.0
Polyembryoma —*see* Neoplasm, malignant, by site
Polyglandular
deficiency E31.0
dyscrasia E31.9
dysfunction E31.9
syndrome E31.8
Polyhydramnios O40.-●
Polymastia Q83.1
Polymenorrhea N92.0
Polymyalgia M35.3
arteritica, giant cell M31.5
rheumatica M35.3
with giant cell arteritis M31.5

Polymyositis (acute) (chronic) (hemorrhagic) M33.20
with
myopathy M33.22
respiratory involvement M33.21
skin involvement —*see* Dermatopolymyositis
specified organ involvement NEC M33.29
ossificans (generalisata) (progressiva) —*see* Myositis, ossificans, progressiva
Polyneuritis, polyneuritic —*see also* Polyneuropathy
acute (post-)infective G61.0
alcoholic G62.1
cranialis G52.7
demyelinating, chronic inflammatory (CIDP) G61.81
diabetic —*see* Diabetes, polyneuropathy
diphtheritic A36.83
due to lack of vitamin NEC E56.9 *[G63]*
endemic E51.11
erythredema —*see* subcategory T56.1
febrile, acute G61.0
hereditary ataxic G60.1
idiopathic, acute G61.0
infective (acute) G61.0
inflammatory, chronic demyelinating (CIDP) G61.81
nutritional E63.9 *[G63]*
postinfective (acute) G61.0
specified NEC G62.89
Polyneuropathy (peripheral) G62.9
alcoholic G62.1
amyloid (Portuguese) E85.1 *[G63]*
transthyretin-related (ATTR) familial E85.1
arsenical E85.1 *[G63]*
critical illness G62.81
demyelinating, chronic inflammatory (CIDP) G61.81
diabetic —*see* Diabetes, polyneuropathy
drug-induced G62.0
hereditary G60.9
specified NEC G60.8
idiopathic G60.9
progressive G60.3
in (due to)
alcohol G62.1
sequelae G65.2
amyloidosis, familial (Portuguese) E85.1 *[G63]*
antitetanus serum G61.1
arsenic G62.2
sequelae G65.2
avitaminosis NEC E56.9 *[G63]*
beriberi E51.11
collagen vascular disease NEC M35.9 *[G63]*
deficiency (of)
B (-complex) vitamins E53.9 *[G63]*
vitamin B6 E53.1 *[G63]*
diabetes —*see* Diabetes, polyneuropathy
diphtheria A36.83
drug or medicament G62.0
correct substance properly administered —*see* Table of Drugs and Chemicals, by drug, adverse effect
overdose or wrong substance given or taken —*see* Table of Drugs and Chemicals, by drug, poisoning
endocrine disease NEC E34.9 *[G63]*
herpes zoster B02.23
hypoglycemia E16.2 *[G63]*
infectious
disease NEC B99 *[G63]*
mononucleosis B27.91
lack of vitamin NEC E56.9 *[G63]*
lead G62.2
sequelae G65.2
leprosy A30.9 *[G63]*
Lyme disease A69.22
metabolic disease NEC E88.9 *[G63]*

P

Polyneuropathy *(Continued)*
  in *(Continued)*
    microscopic polyangiitis M31.7 *[G63]*
    mumps B26.84
    neoplastic disease *—see also* Neoplasm D49.9 *[G63]*
    nutritional deficiency NEC E63.9 *[G63]*
    organophosphate compounds G62.2
      sequelae G65.2
    parasitic disease NEC B89 *[G63]*
    pellagra E52 *[G63]*
    polyarteritis nodosa M30.0
    porphyria E80.20 *[G63]*
    radiation G62.82
    rheumatoid arthritis *—see* Rheumatoid, polyneuropathy
    sarcoidosis D86.89
    serum G61.1
    syphilis (late) A52.15
      congenital A50.43
    systemic
      connective tissue disorder M35.9 *[G63]*
      lupus erythematosus M32.19
    toxic agent NEC G62.2
      sequelae G65.2
    transthyretin-related (ATTR) familial amyloid E85.1
      triorthocresyl phosphate G62.2
        sequelae G65.2
      tuberculosis A17.89
      uremia N18.9 [G63]
      vitamin B12 deficiency E53.8 [G63]
        with anemia (pernicious) D51.0 [G63]
          due to dietary deficiency D51.3 [G63]
      zoster B02.23
  inflammatory G61.9
    chronic demyelinating (CIDP) G61.81
    sequelae G65.1
    specified NEC G61.89
  lead G62.2
    sequelae G65.2
  nutritional NEC E63.9 *[G63]*
  postherpetic (zoster) B02.23
  progressive G60.3
  radiation-induced G62.82
  sensory (hereditary) (idiopathic) G60.8
  specified NEC G62.89
  syphilitic (late) A52.15
    congenital A50.43
Polyopia H53.8
Polyorchism, polyorchidism Q55.21
Polyosteoarthritis *—see also* Osteoarthritis, generalized M15.9-●
  post-traumatic M15.3
  specified NEC M15.8
Polyostotic fibrous dysplasia Q78.1
Polyotia Q17.0
Polyp, polypus
  accessory sinus J33.8
  adenocarcinoma in *—see* Neoplasm, malignant, by site
  adenocarcinoma in situ in *—see* Neoplasm, in situ, by site
  adenoid tissue J33.0
  adenomatous *—see also* Neoplasm, benign, by site
    adenocarcinoma in *—see* Neoplasm, malignant, by site
    adenocarcinoma in situ in *—see* Neoplasm, in situ, by site
    carcinoma in *—see* Neoplasm, malignant, by site
    carcinoma in situ in *—see* Neoplasm, in situ, by site
    multiple *—see* Neoplasm, benign
      adenocarcinoma in *—see* Neoplasm, malignant, by site
      adenocarcinoma in situ in *—see* Neoplasm, in situ, by site
  antrum J33.8

Polyp, polypus *(Continued)*
  anus, anal (canal) K62.0
  Bartholin's gland N84.3
  bladder D41.4
  carcinoma in *—see* Neoplasm, malignant, by site
  carcinoma in situ in *—see* Neoplasm, in situ, by site
  cecum D12.0
  cervix (uteri) N84.1
    in pregnancy or childbirth *—see* Pregnancy, complicated by, abnormal, cervix
    mucous N84.1
    nonneoplastic N84.1
  choanal J33.0
  cholesterol K82.4
  clitoris N84.3
  colon K63.5
    adenomatous D12.6
    ▶ascending D12.6
    ▶cecum D12.0
    ▶descending D12.4
    ~~ascending D12.2~~
    ~~cecum D12.0~~
    ~~descending D12.4~~
    inflammatory K51.40
      with
        abscess K51.414
        complication K51.419
          specified NEC K51.418
        fistula K51.413
        intestinal obstruction K51.412
        rectal bleeding K51.411
    sigmoid D12.5
    transverse D12.3
  corpus uteri N84.0
  dental K04.01
    irreversible K04.02
    reversible K04.01
  duodenum K31.7
  ear (middle) H74.4-●
  endometrium N84.0
  ethmoidal (sinus) J33.8
  fallopian tube N84.8
  female genital tract N84.9
    specified NEC N84.8
  frontal (sinus) J33.8
  gallbladder K82.4
  gingiva, gum K06.8
  ▶hyperplastic, (any site) K63.5
  labia, labium (majus) (minus) N84.3
  larynx (mucous) J38.1
    adenomatous D14.1
  malignant *—see* Neoplasm, malignant, by site
  maxillary (sinus) J33.8
  middle ear *—see* Polyp, ear (middle)
  myometrium N84.0
  nares
    anterior J33.9
    posterior J33.0
  nasal (mucous) J33.9
    cavity J33.0
    septum J33.0
  nasopharyngeal J33.0
  nose (mucous) J33.9
  oviduct N84.8
  pharynx J39.2
  placenta O90.89
  prostate *—see* Enlargement, enlarged, prostate
  pudenda, pudendum N84.3
  pulpal (dental) K04.01
    irreversible K04.02
    reversible K04.01
  rectum (nonadenomatous) K62.1
    adenomatous *—see* Polyp, adenomatous
  septum (nasal) J33.0
  sinus (accessory) (ethmoidal) (frontal) (maxillary) (sphenoidal) J33.8
  sphenoidal (sinus) J33.8
  stomach K31.7
    adenomatous D13.1

Polyp, polypus *(Continued)*
  tube, fallopian N84.8
  turbinate, mucous membrane J33.8
  umbilical, newborn P83.6
  ureter N28.89
  urethra N36.2
  uterus (body) (corpus) (mucous) N84.0
    cervix N84.1
    in pregnancy or childbirth *—see* Pregnancy, complicated by, tumor, uterus
  vagina N84.2
  vocal cord (mucous) J38.1
  vulva N84.3
Polyphagia R63.2
Polyploidy Q92.7
Polypoid *—see* condition
Polyposis *—see also* Polyp
  coli (adenomatous) D12.6
    adenocarcinoma in C18.9
    adenocarcinoma in situ in *—see* Neoplasm, in situ, by site
    carcinoma in C18.9
  colon (adenomatous) D12.6
  familial D12.6
    adenocarcinoma in situ in *—see* Neoplasm, in situ, by site
  intestinal (adenomatous) D12.6
  malignant lymphomatous C83.1
  multiple, adenomatous *—see also* Neoplasm, benign D36.9
Polyradiculitis *—see* Polyneuropathy
Polyradiculoneuropathy (acute) (postinfective) (segmentally demyelinating) G61.0
Polyserositis
  due to pericarditis I31.1
  pericardial I31.1
  periodic, familial E85.0
  tuberculous A19.9
    acute A19.1
    chronic A19.8
Polysplenia syndrome Q89.09
Polysyndactyly *—see also* Syndactylism, syndactyly Q70.4
Polytrichia L68.3
Polyunguia Q84.6
Polyuria R35.8
  nocturnal R35.1
  psychogenic F45.8
Pompe's disease (glycogen storage) E74.02
Pompholyx L30.1
Poncet's disease (tuberculous rheumatism) A18.09
Pond fracture *—see* Fracture, skull
Ponos B55.0
Pons, pontine *—see* condition
Poor
  aesthetic of existing restoration of tooth K08.56
  contractions, labor O62.2
  gingival margin to tooth restoration K08.51
  personal hygiene R46.0
  prenatal care, affecting management of pregnancy *—see* Pregnancy, complicated by, insufficient, prenatal care
  sucking reflex (newborn) R29.2
  urinary stream R39.12
  vision NEC H54.7
Poradenitis, nostras inguinalis or venerea A55
Porencephaly (congenital) (developmental) (true) Q04.6
  acquired G93.0
  nondevelopmental G93.0
  traumatic (post) F07.89
Porocephaliasis B88.8
Porokeratosis Q82.8
Poroma, eccrine *—see* Neoplasm, skin, benign
Porphyria (South African) E80.20
  acquired E80.20
  acute intermittent (hepatic) (Swedish) E80.21

P

Porphyria *(Continued)*
cutanea tarda (hereditary) (symptomatic) E80.1
due to drugs E80.20
correct substance properly administered — *see* Table of Drugs and Chemicals, by drug, adverse effect
overdose or wrong substance given or taken —*see* Table of Drugs and Chemicals, by drug, poisoning
erythropoietic (congenital) (hereditary) E80.0
hepatocutaneous type E80.1
secondary E80.20
toxic NEC E80.20
variegata E80.20
Porphyrinuria —*see* Porphyria
Porphyruria —*see* Porphyria
Portal —*see* condition
Port wine nevus, mark, or stain Q82.5
Posadas-Wernicke disease B38.9
Positive
culture (nonspecific)
blood R78.81
bronchial washings R84.5
cerebrospinal fluid R83.5
cervix uteri R87.5
nasal secretions R84.5
nipple discharge R89.5
nose R84.5
staphylococcus (Methicillin susceptible) Z22.321
Methicillin resistant Z22.322
peritoneal fluid R85.5
pleural fluid R84.5
prostatic secretions R86.5
saliva R85.5
seminal fluid R86.5
sputum R84.5
synovial fluid R89.5
throat scrapings R84.5
urine R82.79
vagina R87.5
vulva R87.5
wound secretions R89.5
PPD (skin test) R76.11
serology for syphilis A53.0
with signs or symptoms - code as Syphilis, by site and stage
false R76.8
skin test, tuberculin (without active tuberculosis) R76.11
test, human immunodeficiency virus (HIV) R75
VDRL A53.0
with signs or symptoms - code by site and stage under Syphilis A53.9
Wassermann reaction A53.0
Postcardiotomy syndrome I97.0
Postcaval ureter Q62.62
Postcholecystectomy syndrome K91.5
Postclimacteric bleeding N95.0
Postcommissurotomy syndrome I97.0
Postconcussional syndrome F07.81
Postcontusional syndrome F07.81
Postcricoid region —*see* condition
Post-dates (40-42 weeks) (pregnancy) (mother) O48.0
more than 42 weeks gestation O48.1
Postencephalitic syndrome F07.89
Posterior —*see* condition
Posterolateral sclerosis (spinal cord) —*see* Degeneration, combined
Postexanthematous —*see* condition
Postfebrile —*see* condition
Postgastrectomy dumping syndrome K91.1
Posthemiplegic chorea —*see* Monoplegia
Posthemorrhagic anemia (chronic) D50.0
acute D62
newborn P61.3
Postherpetic neuralgia (zoster) B02.29
trigeminal B02.22
Posthitis N47.7
Postimmunization complication or reaction — *see* Complications, vaccination
Postinfectious —*see* condition
Postlaminectomy syndrome NEC M96.1
Postleukotomy syndrome F07.0
Postmastectomy lymphedema (syndrome) I97.2
Postmaturity, postmature (over 42 weeks)
maternal (over 42 weeks gestation) O48.1
newborn P08.22
Postmeasles complication NEC —*see also* condition B05.89
Postmenopausal
endometrium (atrophic) N95.8
suppurative —*see also* Endometritis N71.9
osteoporosis —*see* Osteoporosis, postmenopausal
Postnasal drip R09.82
due to
allergic rhinitis —*see* Rhinitis, allergic
common cold J00
gastroesophageal reflux —*see* Reflux, gastroesophageal
nasopharyngitis —*see* Nasopharyngitis
other know condition — code to condition
sinusitis —*see* Sinusitis
Postnatal —*see* condition
Postoperative (postprocedural) —*see* Complication, postoperative
pneumothorax, therapeutic Z98.3
state NEC Z98.890
Postpancreatectomy hyperglycemia E89.1
Postpartum —*see* Puerperal
Postphlebitic syndrome —*see* Syndrome, postthrombotic
Postpolio (myelitic) syndrome G14
Postpoliomyelitic —*see also* condition
osteopathy —*see* Osteopathy, after poliomyelitis
Postprocedural —*see also* Postoperative
hypoinsulinemia E89.1
Postschizophrenic depression F32.89
Postsurgery status —*see also* Status (post)
pneumothorax, therapeutic Z98.3
Post-term (40-42 weeks) (pregnancy) (mother) O48.0
infant P08.21
more than 42 weeks gestation (mother) O48.1
Post-traumatic brain syndrome, nonpsychotic F07.81
Post-typhoid abscess A01.09
Postures, hysterical F44.2
Postvaccinal reaction or complication —*see* Complications, vaccination
Postvalvulotomy syndrome I97.0
Potain's
disease (pulmonary edema) —*see* Edema, lung
syndrome (gastrectasis with dyspepsia) K31.0
Potter's
asthma J62.8
facies Q60.6
lung J62.8
syndrome (with renal agenesis) Q60.6
Pott's
curvature (spinal) A18.01
disease or paraplegia A18.01
spinal curvature A18.01
tumor, puffy —*see* Osteomyelitis, specified type NEC
Pouch
bronchus Q32.4
Douglas' —*see* condition
esophagus, esophageal, congenital Q39.6
acquired K22.5
gastric K31.4
Hartmann's K82.8
pharynx, pharyngeal (congenital) Q38.7
Pouchitis K91.850
Poultrymen's itch B88.0
Poverty NEC Z59.6
extreme Z59.5
Poxvirus NEC B08.8
Prader-Willi syndrome Q87.11
Prader-Willi-like syndrome Q87.11
Preauricular appendage or tag Q17.0
Prebetalipoproteinemia (acquired) (essential) (familial) (hereditary) (primary) (secondary) E78.1
with chylomicronemia E78.3
Precipitate labor or delivery O62.3
Preclimacteric bleeding (menorrhagia) N92.4
Precocious
adrenarche E30.1
menarche E30.1
menstruation E30.1
pubarche E30.1
puberty E30.1
central E22.8
sexual development NEC E30.1
thelarche E30.8
Precocity, sexual (constitutional) (cryptogenic) (female) (idiopathic) (male) E30.1
with adrenal hyperplasia E25.9
congenital E25.0
Precordial pain R07.2
Predeciduous teeth K00.2
Prediabetes, prediabetic R73.03
complicating
pregnancy —*see* Pregnancy, complicated by, diseases of, specified type or system NEC
puerperium O99.89
Predislocation status of hip at birth Q65.6
Pre-eclampsia O14.9-●
with pre-existing hypertension —*see* Hypertension, complicating pregnancy, pre-existing, with, pre-eclampsia
complicating
childbirth O14.94
puerperium O14.95
mild O14.0-●
complicating
childbirth O14.04
puerperium O14.05
moderate O14.0-●
complicating
childbirth O14.04
puerperium O14.05
severe O14.1-●
with hemolysis, elevated liver enzymes and low platelet count (HELLP) O14.2-●
complicating
childbirth O14.24
puerperium O14.25
complicating
childbirth O14.14
puerperium O14.15
Pre-eruptive color change, teeth, tooth K00.8
Pre-excitation atrioventricular conduction I45.6
Preglaucoma H40.00-●
Pregnancy (single) (uterine) —*see also* Delivery and Puerperal

> Note: The Tabular must be reviewed for assignment of the appropriate character indicating the trimester of the pregnancy
>
> Note: The Tabular must be reviewed for assignment of appropriate seventh character for multiple gestation codes in Chapter 15

abdominal (ectopic) O00.00
with intrauterine pregnancy O00.01
with viable fetus O36.7-●
ampullar O00.10-●
with intrauterine pregnancy O00.11-●
biochemical O02.81
broad ligament O00.80
with intrauterine pregnancy O00.81
cervical O00.80
with intrauterine pregnancy O00.81

Pregnancy *(Continued)*
- chemical OØ2.81
- complicated NOS O26.9-●
- complicated by (care of) (management affected by)
  - abnormal, abnormality
    - cervix O34.4-●
      - causing obstructed labor O65.5
    - cord (umbilical) O69.9
    - fetal heart rate or rhythm O36.83-●
    - findings on antenatal screening of mother O28.9
      - biochemical O28.1
      - chromosomal O28.5
      - cytological O28.2
      - genetic O28.5
      - hematological O28.Ø
      - radiological O28.4
      - specified NEC O28.8
      - ultrasonic O28.3
    - glucose (tolerance) NEC O99.81Ø
    - pelvic organs O34.9-●
      - specified NEC O34.8-●
        - causing obstructed labor O65.5
    - pelvis (bony) (major) NEC O33.Ø
    - perineum O34.7-●
    - position
      - placenta O44.Ø-●
        - with hemorrhage O44.1-●
      - uterus O34.59-●
    - uterus O34.59-●
      - causing obstructed labor O65.5
      - congenital O34.Ø-●
    - vagina O34.6-●
      - causing obstructed labor O65.5
    - vulva O34.7-●
      - causing obstructed labor O65.5
  - abruptio placentae *—see* Abruptio placentae
  - abscess or cellulitis
    - bladder O23.1-●
    - breast O91.11-●
    - genital organ or tract O23.9-●
  - abuse
    - physical O9A.31-●
    - psychological O9A.51-●
    - sexual O9A.41-●
  - adverse effect anesthesia O29.9-●
    - aspiration pneumonitis O29.Ø1-●
    - cardiac arrest O29.11-●
    - cardiac complication NEC O29.19-●
    - cardiac failure O29.12-●
    - central nervous system complication NEC O29.29-●
    - cerebral anoxia O29.21-●
    - failed or difficult intubation O29.6-●
    - inhalation of stomach contents or secretions NOS O29.Ø1-●
    - local, toxic reaction O29.3X
    - Mendelson's syndrome O29.Ø1-●
    - pressure collapse of lung O29.Ø2-●
    - pulmonary complications NEC O29.Ø9-●
    - specified NEC O29.8X
    - spinal and epidural type NEC O29.5X
      - induced headache O29.4-●
  - albuminuria *—see also* Proteinuria, gestational O12.1-●
  - alcohol use O99.31-●
  - amnionitis O41.12-●
  - anaphylactoid syndrome of pregnancy O88.Ø1-●
  - anemia (conditions in D5Ø-D64) (pre-existing) O99.Ø1-●
    - complicating the puerperium O99.Ø3
  - antepartum hemorrhage O46.9-●
    - with coagulation defect *—see* Hemorrhage, antepartum, with coagulation defect
    - specified NEC O46.8X-●
  - appendicitis O99.61-●
  - atrophy (yellow) (acute) liver (subacute) O26.61-●

Pregnancy *(Continued)*
- complicated by *(Continued)*
  - bariatric surgery status O99.84-●
  - bicornis or bicornuate uterus O34.Ø-●
  - biliary tract problems O26.61-●
  - breech presentation O32.1
  - cardiovascular diseases (conditions in IØØ-IØ9, I2Ø-I52, I7Ø-I99) O99.41-●
  - cerebrovascular disorders (conditions in I6Ø-I69) O99.41-●
  - cervical shortening O26.87-●
  - cervicitis O23.51-●
  - chloasma (gravidarum) O26.89-●
  - cholecystitis O99.61-●
  - cholestasis (intrahepatic) O26.61-●
  - chorioamnionitis O41.12-●
  - circulatory system disorder (conditions in IØØ-IØ9, I2Ø-I99, O99.41-●)
  - compound presentation O32.6
  - conjoined twins O3Ø.Ø2-●
  - connective system disorders (conditions in MØØ-M99) O99.89
  - contracted pelvis (general) O33.1
    - inlet O33.2
    - outlet O33.3
  - convulsions (eclamptic) (uremic) *—see also* Eclampsia O15.9-●
  - cracked nipple O92.11-●
  - cystitis O23.1-●
  - cystocele O34.8-●
  - death of fetus (near term) O36.4
    - early pregnancy OØ2.1
    - of one fetus or more in multiple gestation O31.2-●
  - deciduitis O41.14-●
  - decreased fetal movement O36.81-●
  - dental problems O99.61-●
  - diabetes (mellitus) O24.91-●
    - gestational (pregnancy induced) *—see* Diabetes, gestational
    - pre-existing O24.31-●
      - specified NEC O24.81-●
      - type 1 O24.Ø1-●
      - type 2 O24.11-●
  - digestive system disorders (conditions in KØØ-K93) O99.61-●
  - diseases of *—see* Pregnancy, complicated by, specified body system disease
    - biliary tract O26.61-●
    - blood NEC (conditions in D65-D77) O99.11-●
    - liver O26.61-●
    - specified NEC O99.89
  - disorders of *—see* Pregnancy, complicated by, specified body system disorder
    - amniotic fluid and membranes O41.9-●
      - specified NEC O41.8X-●
    - biliary tract O26.61-●
    - ear and mastoid process (conditions in H6Ø-H95) O99.89
    - eye and adnexa (conditions in HØØ-H59) O99.89
    - liver O26.61-●
    - skin (conditions in LØØ-L99) O99.71-●
    - specified NEC O99.89
  - displacement, uterus NEC O34.59-●
    - causing obstructed labor O65.5
  - disproportion (due to) O33.9
    - fetal (ascites) (hydrops) (meningomyelocele) (sacral teratoma) (tumor) deformities NEC O33.7
    - generally contracted pelvis O33.1
    - hydrocephalic fetus O33.6
    - inlet contraction of pelvis O33.2
    - mixed maternal and fetal origin O33.4
    - specified NEC O33.8
  - double uterus O34.Ø-●
    - causing obstructed labor O65.5
  - drug use (conditions in F11-F19) O99.32-●

Pregnancy *(Continued)*
- complicated by *(Continued)*
  - eclampsia, eclamptic (coma) (convulsions) (delirium) (nephritis) (uremia) (*see also* Eclampsia) O15-●
  - ectopic pregnancy *—see* Pregnancy, ectopic
  - edema O12.Ø-●
    - with
      - gestational hypertension, mild *—see also* Pre-eclampsia O14.Ø-●
      - proteinuria O12.2-●
  - effusion, amniotic fluid *—see* Pregnancy, complicated by, premature rupture of membranes
  - elderly
    - multigravida OØ9.52-●
    - primigravida OØ9.51-●
  - embolism *—see also* Embolism, obstetric, pregnancy O88.-●
  - endocrine diseases NEC O99.28-●
  - endometritis O86.12
  - excessive weight gain O26.Ø-●
  - exhaustion O26.81-●
    - during labor and delivery O75.81
  - face presentation O32.3
  - failed induction of labor O61.9
  - failed or difficult intubation for anesthesia O29.6-●
    - instrumental O61.1
    - mechanical O61.1
    - medical O61.Ø
    - specified NEC O61.8
    - surgical O61.1
  - false labor (pains) O47.9
    - at or after 37 completed weeks of pregnancy O47.1
    - before 37 completed weeks of pregnancy O47.Ø-●
  - fatigue O26.81-●
    - during labor and delivery O75.81
  - fatty metamorphosis of liver O26.61-●
  - female genital mutilation O34.8-● *[N9Ø.81-●]*
  - fetal (maternal care for)
    - abnormality or damage O35.9
      - acid-base balance O68
      - specified type NEC O35.8
    - acidemia O68
    - acidosis O68
    - alkalosis O68
    - anemia and thrombocytopenia O36.82-●
    - anencephaly O35.Ø
    - ▶bradycardia O36.83-●
    - chromosomal abnormality (conditions in Q9Ø-Q99) O35.1
    - conjoined twins O3Ø.Ø2-●
    - damage from
      - amniocentesis O35.7
      - biopsy procedures O35.7
      - drug addiction O35.5
      - hematological investigation O35.7
      - intrauterine contraceptive device O35.7
      - maternal
        - alcohol addiction O35.4
        - cytomegalovirus infection O35.3
        - disease NEC O35.8
        - drug addiction O35.5
        - listeriosis O35.8
        - rubella O35.3
        - toxoplasmosis O35.8
        - viral infection O35.3
      - medical procedure NEC O35.7
      - radiation O35.6
    - death (near term) O36.4
      - early pregnancy OØ2.1
    - decreased movement O36.81-●
    - ▶depressed heart rate tones O36.83-●
    - disproportion due to deformity (fetal) O33.7
    - excessive growth (large for dates) O36.6-●
    - growth retardation O36.59-●
      - light for dates O36.59-●
      - small for dates O36.59-●

Pregnancy *(Continued)*
complicated by *(Continued)*
fetal *(Continued)*
heart rate irregularity (abnormal variability) (bradycardia) (decelerations) (tachycardia) O36.83- ●
hereditary disease O35.2
hydrocephalus O35.Ø
intrauterine death O36.4
non-reassuring heart rate or rhythm O36.83- ●
poor growth O36.59- ●
light for dates O36.59- ●
small for dates O36.59- ●
problem O36.9- ●
specified NEC O36.89- ●
reduction (elective) O31.3- ●
selective termination O31.3- ●
spina bifida O35.Ø
thrombocytopenia O36.82- ●
fibroid (tumor) (uterus) O34.1- ●
fissure of nipple O92.11- ●
gallstones O99.61- ●
gastric banding status O99.84- ●
gastric bypass status O99.84- ●
genital herpes (asymptomatic) (history of) (inactive) O98.3- ●
genital tract infection O23.9- ●
glomerular diseases (conditions in NØØ-NØ7) O26.83- ●
with hypertension, pre-existing —*see* Hypertension, complicating, pregnancy, pre-existing, with, renal disease
gonorrhea O98.21- ●
grand multiparity OØ9.4
habitual aborter —*see* Pregnancy, complicated by, recurrent pregnancy loss
HELLP syndrome (hemolysis, elevated liver enzymes and low platelet count) O14.2- ●
hemorrhage
antepartum —*see* Hemorrhage, antepartum
before 2Ø completed weeks gestation O2Ø.9
specified NEC O2Ø.8
due to premature separation, placenta —*see also* Abruptio placentae O45.9- ●
early O2Ø.9
specified NEC O2Ø.8
threatened abortion O2Ø.Ø
hemorrhoids O22.4- ●
hepatitis (viral) O98.41- ●
herniation of uterus O34.59- ●
high
head at term O32.4
risk —*see* Supervision (of) (for), high-risk
history of in utero procedure during previous pregnancy OØ9.82- ●
HIV O98.71- ●
human immunodeficiency virus (HIV) disease O98.71- ●
hydatidiform mole —*see also* Mole, hydatidiform OØ1.9- ●
hydramnios O4Ø.- ●
hydrocephalic fetus (disproportion) O33.6
hydrops
amnii O4Ø.- ●
fetalis O36.2- ●
associated with isoimmunization —*see also* Pregnancy, complicated by, isoimmunization O36.11- ●
hydrorrhea O42.9Ø
hyperemesis (gravidarum) (mild) —*see also* Hyperemesis, gravidarum O21.Ø- ●
hypertension —*see* Hypertension, complicating pregnancy

Pregnancy *(Continued)*
complicated by *(Continued)*
hypertensive
heart and renal disease, pre-existing —*see* Hypertension, complicating, pregnancy, pre-existing, with, heart disease, with renal disease
heart disease, pre-existing —*see* Hypertension, complicating, pregnancy, pre-existing, with, heart disease
renal disease, pre-existing —*see* Hypertension, complicating, pregnancy, pre-existing, with, renal disease
hypotension O26.5- ●
immune disorders NEC (conditions in D8Ø-D89) O99.11- ●
incarceration, uterus O34.51- ●
incompetent cervix O34.3- ●
inconclusive fetal viability O36.8Ø
infection(s) O98.91- ●
amniotic fluid or sac O41.1Ø- ●
bladder O23.1- ●
carrier state NEC O99.83Ø
streptococcus B O99.82Ø
genital organ or tract O23.9- ●
specified NEC O23.59- ●
genitourinary tract O23.9- ●
gonorrhea O98.21- ●
hepatitis (viral) O98.41- ●
HIV O98.71- ●
human immunodeficiency virus (HIV) O98.71- ●
kidney O23.Ø- ●
nipple O91.Ø1- ●
parasitic disease O98.91- ●
specified NEC O98.81- ●
protozoal disease O98.61- ●
sexually transmitted NEC O98.31- ●
specified type NEC O98.81- ●
syphilis O98.11- ●
tuberculosis O98.Ø1- ●
urethra O23.2- ●
urinary (tract) O23.4- ●
specified NEC O23.3- ●
viral disease O98.51- ●
injury or poisoning (conditions in SØØ-T88) O9A.21- ●
due to abuse
physical O9A.31- ●
psychological O9A.51- ●
sexual O9A.41- ●
insufficient
prenatal care OØ9.3- ●
weight gain O26.1- ●
insulin resistance O26.89
intrauterine fetal death (near term) O36.4
early pregnancy OØ2.1
multiple gestation (one fetus or more) O31.2- ●
isoimmunization O36.11- ●
anti-A sensitization O36.11- ●
anti-B sensitization O36.19- ●
Rh O36.Ø9- ●
anti-D antibody O36.Ø1- ●
specified NEC O36.19- ●
laceration of uterus NEC O71.81
malformation
placenta, placental (vessel) O43.1Ø- ●
specified NEC O43.19- ●
uterus (congenital) O34.Ø- ●
malnutrition (conditions in E4Ø-E46) O25.1- ●
maternal hypotension syndrome O26.5- ●
mental disorders (conditions in FØ1-FØ9, F2Ø-F99) O99.34- ●
alcohol use O99.31- ●
drug use O99.32- ●
smoking O99.33- ●
mentum presentation O32.3

Pregnancy *(Continued)*
complicated by *(Continued)*
metabolic disorders O99.28- ●
missed
abortion OØ2.1
delivery O36.4
multiple gestations O3Ø.9- ●
conjoined twins O3Ø.Ø2- ●
quadruplet —*see* Pregnancy, quadruplet
specified complication NEC O31.8X- ●
specified number of multiples NEC —*see* Pregnancy, multiple (gestation), specified NEC
triplet —*see* Pregnancy, triplet
twin —*see* Pregnancy, twin
musculoskeletal condition (conditions is MØØ-M99) O99.89
necrosis, liver (conditions in K72) O26.61- ●
neoplasm
benign
cervix O34.4- ●
corpus uteri O34.1- ●
uterus O34.1- ●
malignant O9A.11- ●
nephropathy NEC O26.83- ●
nervous system condition (conditions in GØØ-G99) O99.35- ●
nutritional diseases NEC O99.28- ●
obesity (pre-existing) O99.21- ●
obesity surgery status O99.84- ●
oblique lie or presentation O32.2
older mother —*see* Pregnancy, complicated by, elderly
oligohydramnios O41.Ø- ●
with premature rupture of membranes —*see also* Pregnancy, complicated by, premature rupture of membranes O42- ●
onset (spontaneous) of labor after 37 completed weeks of gestation but before 39 completed weeks gestation, with delivery by (planned) cesarean section O75.82
oophoritis O23.52- ●
overdose, drug —*see also* Table of Drugs and Chemicals, by drug, poisoning O9A.21- ●
oversize fetus O33.5
papyraceous fetus O31.Ø- ●
pelvic inflammatory disease O99.89
periodontal disease O99.61- ●
peripheral neuritis O26.82- ●
peritoneal (pelvic) adhesions O99.89
phlebitis O22.9- ●
phlebopathy O22.9- ●
phlebothrombosis (superficial) O22.2- ●
deep O22.3- ●
placenta accreta O43.21- ●
placenta increta O43.22- ●
placenta percreta O43.23- ●
placenta previa O44.Ø- ●
complete O44.Ø- ●
with hemorrhage O44.1- ●
marginal O44.2- ●
with hemorrhage O44.3- ●
partial O44.2- ●
with hemorrhage O44.3- ●
placental disorder O43.9- ●
specified NEC O43.89- ●
placental dysfunction O43.89- ●
placental infarction O43.81- ●
placental insufficiency O36.51- ●
placental transfusion syndromes
fetomaternal O43.Ø1- ●
fetus to fetus O43.Ø2- ●
maternofetal O43.Ø1- ●
placentitis O41.14- ●
pneumonia O99.51- ●
poisoning —*see also* Table of Drugs and Chemicals O9A.21- ●
polyhydramnios O4Ø- ●

P

Pregnancy (Continued)
complicated by (Continued)
polymorphic eruption of pregnancy O26.86
poor obstetric history NEC OØ9.29-•
postmaturity (post-term) (4Ø to 42 weeks) O48.Ø
more than 42 completed weeks gestation (prolonged) O48.1
pre-eclampsia O14.9-•
mild O14.Ø-•
moderate O14.Ø-•
severe O14.1-•
with hemolysis, elevated liver enzymes and low platelet count (HELLP) O14.2-•
premature labor —*see* Pregnancy, complicated by, preterm labor
premature rupture of membranes O42.9Ø
full-term, unspecified as to length of time between rupture and onset of labor O42.92
with onset of labor
within 24 hours O42.ØØ
at or after 37 weeks gestation, onset of labor within 24 hours of rupture O42.Ø2
pre-term (before 37 completed weeks of gestation) O42.Ø1-•
after 24 hours O42.1Ø
at or after 37 weeks gestation, onset of labor more than 24 hours following rupture O42.12
pre-term (before 37 completed weeks of gestation) O42.11-•
at or after 37 weeks gestation, unspecified as to length of time between rupture and onset of labor O42.92
pre-term (before 37 completed weeks of gestation) O42.91-•
premature separation of placenta —*see also* Abruptio placentae O45.9-•
presentation, fetal —*see* Delivery, complicated by, malposition
preterm delivery O6Ø.1Ø
preterm labor
with delivery O6Ø.1Ø
preterm O6Ø.1Ø
term O6Ø.2Ø
second trimester
with preterm delivery
second trimester O6Ø.12
third trimester O6Ø.13
with term delivery O6Ø.22
without delivery O6Ø.Ø2
third trimester
with term delivery O6Ø.23
with third trimester preterm delivery O6Ø.14
without delivery O6Ø.Ø3
without delivery O6Ø.ØØ
second trimester O6Ø.Ø2
third trimester O6Ø.Ø3
previous history of —*see* Pregnancy, supervision of, high-risk
prolapse, uterus O34.52-•
proteinuria (gestational) —*see also* Proteinuria, gestational O12.1-•
with edema O12.2-•
pruritic urticarial papules and plaques of pregnancy (PUPPP) O26.86
pruritus (neurogenic) O26.89-•
psychosis or psychoneurosis (puerperal) F53.1
ptyalism O26.89-•
PUPPP (pruritic urticarial papules and plaques of pregnancy) O26.86
pyelitis O23.Ø-•
recurrent pregnancy loss O26.2-•

Pregnancy (Continued)
complicated by (Continued)
renal disease or failure NEC O26.83-•
with secondary hypertension, pre-existing —*see* Hypertension, complicating, pregnancy, pre-existing, secondary
hypertensive, pre-existing —*see* Hypertension, complicating, pregnancy, pre-existing, with, renal disease
respiratory condition (conditions in JØØ-J99) O99.51-•
retained, retention
dead ovum OØ2.Ø
intrauterine contraceptive device O26.3-•
retroversion, uterus O34.53-•
Rh immunization, incompatibility or sensitization NEC O36.Ø9-•
anti-D antibody O36.Ø1-•
rupture
amnion (premature) —*see also* Pregnancy, complicated by, premature rupture of membranes O42-•
membranes (premature) —*see also* Pregnancy, complicated by, premature rupture of membranes O42-•
uterus (during labor) O71.1
before onset of labor O71.Ø-•
salivation (excessive) O26.89-•
salpingitis O23.52-•
salpingo-oophoritis O23.52-•
sepsis (conditions in A4Ø, A41) O98.81-•
size date discrepancy (uterine) O26.84-•
skin condition (conditions in LØØ-L99) O99.71-•
smoking (tobacco) O99.33-•
social problem OØ9.7-•
specified condition NEC O26.89-•
spotting O26.85-•
streptococcus group B (GBS) carrier state O99.82Ø
subluxation of symphysis (pubis) O26.71-•
syphilis (conditions in A5Ø-A53) O98.11-•
threatened
abortion O2Ø.Ø
labor O47.9
at or after 37 completed weeks of gestation O47.1
before 37 completed weeks of gestation O47.Ø-•
thrombophlebitis (superficial) O22.2-•
thrombosis O22.9-•
cerebral venous O22.5-•
cerebrovenous sinus O22.5-•
deep O22.3-•
tobacco use disorder (smoking) O99.33-•
torsion of uterus O34.59-•
toxemia O14.9-•
transverse lie or presentation O32.2
tuberculosis (conditions in A15-A19) O98.Ø1-•
tumor (benign)
cervix O34.4-•
malignant O9A.11-•
uterus O34.1-•
unstable lie O32.Ø
upper respiratory infection O99.51-•
urethritis O23.2-•
uterine size date discrepancy O26.84-•
vaginitis or vulvitis O23.59-•
varicose veins (lower extremities) O22.Ø-•
genitals O22.1-•
legs O22.Ø-•
perineal O22.1-•
vaginal or vulval O22.1-•
venereal disease NEC (conditions in A63.8) O98.31-•

Pregnancy (Continued)
complicated by (Continued)
venous disorders O22.9-•
specified NEC O22.8X-•
very young mother —*see* Pregnancy, complicated by, young mother
viral diseases (conditions in A8Ø-BØ9, B25-B34) O98.51-•
vomiting O21.9
due to diseases classified elsewhere O21.8
hyperemesis gravidarum (mild) —*see also* Hyperemesis, gravidarum O21.Ø-•
late (occurring after 2Ø weeks of gestation) O21.2
young mother
multigravida OØ9.62-•
primigravida OØ9.61-•
concealed OØ9.3-•
continuing following
elective fetal reduction of one or more fetus O31.3-•
intrauterine death of one or more fetus O31.2-•
spontaneous abortion of one or more fetus O31.1-•
cornual OØØ.8Ø
with intrauterine pregnancy OØØ.81
ectopic (ruptured) OØØ.9Ø
with intrauterine pregnancy OØØ.91
abdominal OØØ.ØØ
with
intrauterine pregnancy OØØ.Ø1
viable fetus O36.7-•
cervical OØØ.8Ø
with intrauterine pregnancy OØØ.81
complicated (by) OØ8.9
afibrinogenemia OØ8.1
cardiac arrest OØ8.81
chemical damage of pelvic organ(s) OØ8.6
circulatory collapse OØ8.3
defibrination syndrome OØ8.1
electrolyte imbalance OØ8.5
embolism (amniotic fluid) (blood clot) (pulmonary) (septic) OØ8.2
endometritis OØ8.Ø
genital tract and pelvic infection OØ8.Ø
hemorrhage (delayed) (excessive) OØ8.1
infection
genital tract or pelvic OØ8.Ø
kidney ØØ8.83
urinary tract OØ8.83
intravascular coagulation OØ8.1
laceration of pelvic organ(s) OØ8.6
metabolic disorder OØ8.5
oliguria OØ8.4
oophoritis OØ8.Ø
parametritis OØ8.Ø
pelvic peritonitis OØ8.Ø
perforation of pelvic organ(s) OØ8.6
renal failure or shutdown OØ8.4
salpingitis or salpingo-oophoritis OØ8.Ø
sepsis OØ8.82
shock OØ8.83
septic OØ8.82
specified condition NEC OØ8.89
tubular necrosis (renal) OØ8.4
uremia OØ8.4
urinary infection OØ8.83
venous complication NEC OØ8.7
embolism OØ8.2
cornual OØØ.8Ø
with intrauterine pregnancy OØØ.81
intraligamentous OØØ.8Ø
with intrauterine pregnancy OØØ.81

Pregnancy (Continued)
ectopic (Continued)
mural O00.80
with intrauterine pregnancy O00.81
ovarian O00.20-●
with intrauterine pregnancy O00.21-●
specified site NEC O00.80
with intrauterine pregnancy O00.81
tubal (ruptured) O00.10-●
with intrauterine pregnancy O00.11-●
examination (normal) Z34.9-●
first Z34.0-●
high-risk —see Pregnancy, supervision of, high-risk
specified Z34.8-●
extrauterine —see Pregnancy, ectopic
fallopian O00.10-●
with intrauterine pregnancy O00.11-●
false F45.8
gestational carrier Z33.3
heptachorionic, hepta-amniotic (septuplets) O30.83-●
hexachorionic, hexa-amniotic (sextuplets) O30.83-●
hidden O09.3-●
high-risk —see Pregnancy, supervision of, high-risk
incidental finding Z33.1
interstitial O00.80
with intrauterine pregnancy O00.81
intraligamentous O00.80
with intrauterine pregnancy O00.81
intramural O00.80
with intrauterine pregnancy O00.81
intraperitoneal O00.00
with intrauterine pregnancy O00.01
isthmian O00.10-●
with intrauterine pregnancy O00.11-●
mesometric (mural) O00.80
with intrauterine pregnancy O00.81
molar NEC O02.0
complicated (by) O08.9
afibrinogenemia O08.1
cardiac arrest O08.81
chemical damage of pelvic organ(s) O08.6
circulatory collapse O08.3
defibrination syndrome O08.1
electrolyte imbalance O08.5
embolism (amniotic fluid) (blood clot) (pulmonary) (septic) O08.2
endometritis O08.0
genital tract and pelvic infection O08.0
hemorrhage (delayed) (excessive) O08.1
infection
genital tract or pelvic O08.0
kidney O08.83
urinary tract O08.83
intravascular coagulation O08.1
laceration of pelvic organ(s) O08.6
metabolic disorder O08.5
oliguria O08.4
oophoritis O08.0
parametritis O08.0
pelvic peritonitis O08.0
perforation of pelvic organ(s) O08.6
renal failure or shutdown O08.4
salpingitis or salpingo-oophoritis O08.0
sepsis O08.82
shock O08.3
septic O08.82
specified condition NEC O08.89
tubular necrosis (renal) O08.4
uremia O08.4
urinary infection O08.83
venous complication NEC O08.7
embolism O08.2
hydatidiform —see also Mole, hydatidiform O01.9-●
multiple (gestation) O30.9-●
greater than quadruplets —see Pregnancy, multiple (gestation), specified NEC

Pregnancy (Continued)
multiple (gestation) (Continued)
specified NEC O30.80-●
with
two or more monoamniotic fetuses O30.82-●
two or more monochorionic fetuses O30.81-●
number of chorions and amnions are both equal to the number of fetuses O30.83-●
two or more monoamniotic fetuses O30.82-●
two or more monochorionic fetuses O30.81-●
unable to determine number of placenta and number of amniotic sacs O30.89-●
unspecified number of placenta and unspecified number of amniotic sacs O30.80-●
mural O00.80
with intrauterine pregnancy O00.81
normal (supervision of) Z34.9-●
first Z34.0-●
high-risk —see Pregnancy, supervision of, high-risk
specified Z34.8-●
ovarian O00.20-●
with intrauterine pregnancy O00.21-●
pentachorionic, penta-amniotic (quintuplets) O30.83-●
postmature (40 to 42 weeks) O48.0
more than 42 weeks gestation O48.1
post-term (40 to 42 weeks) O48.0
prenatal care only Z34.9-●
first Z34.0-●
high-risk —see Pregnancy, supervision of, high-risk
specified Z34.8-●
prolonged (more than 42 weeks gestation) O48.1
quadruplet O30.20-●
with
two or more monoamniotic fetuses O30.22-●
two or more monochorionic fetuses O30.21-●
quadrachorionic/quadra-amniotic O30.23-●
two or more monoamniotic fetuses O30.22-●
two or more monochorionic fetuses O30.21-●
unable to determine number of placenta and number of amniotic sacs O30.29-●
unspecified number of placenta and unspecified number of amniotic sacs O30.20-●
quintuplet —see Pregnancy, multiple (gestation), specified NEC
sextuplet —see Pregnancy, multiple (gestation), specified NEC
supervision of
concealed pregnancy O09.3-●
elderly mother
multigravida O09.52-●
primigravida O09.51-●
hidden pregnancy O09.3-●
high-risk O09.9-●
due to (history of)
ectopic pregnancy O09.1-●
elderly —see Pregnancy, supervision, elderly mother
grand multiparity O09.4
infertility O09.0-●
insufficient prenatal care O09.3-●
in utero procedure during previous pregnancy O09.82-●
in vitro fertilization O09.81-●
molar pregnancy O09.A-●
multiple previous pregnancies O09.4-●
older mother —see Pregnancy, supervision of, elderly mother

Pregnancy (Continued)
supervision of (Continued)
high-risk (Continued)
due to (Continued)
poor reproductive or obstetric history NEC O09.29-●
pre-term labor O09.21-●
previous
neonatal death O09.29-●
social problems O09.7-●
specified NEC O09.89-●
very young mother —see Pregnancy, supervision, young mother
resulting from in vitro fertilization O09.81-●
normal Z34.9-●
first Z34.0-●
specified NEC Z34.8-●
young mother
multigravida O09.62-●
primigravida O09.61-●
triplet O30.10-●
with
two or more monoamniotic fetuses O30.12-●
two or more monochorionic fetuses O30.11-●
trichorionic/triamniotic O30.13-●
two or more monoamniotic fetuses O30.12-●
two or more monochorionic fetuses O30.11-●
unable to determine number of placenta and number of amniotic sacs O30.19-●
unspecified number of placenta and unspecified number of amniotic sacs O30.10-●
tubal (with abortion) (with rupture) O00.10-●
with intrauterine pregnancy O00.11-●
twin O30.00-●
conjoined O30.02-●
dichorionic/diamniotic (two placenta, two amniotic sacs) O30.04-●
monochorionic/diamniotic (one placenta, two amniotic sacs) O30.03-●
monochorionic/monoamniotic (one placenta, one amniotic sac) O30.01-●
unable to determine number of placenta and number of amniotic sacs O30.09-●
unspecified number of placenta and unspecified number of amniotic sacs O30.00-●
unwanted Z64.0
weeks of gestation
8 weeks Z3A.08
9 weeks Z3A.09
10 weeks Z3A.10
11 weeks Z3A.11
12 weeks Z3A.12
13 weeks Z3A.13
14 weeks Z3A.14
15 weeks Z3A.15
16 weeks Z3A.16
17 weeks Z3A.17
18 weeks Z3A.18
19 weeks Z3A.19
20 weeks Z3A.20
21 weeks Z3A.21
22 weeks Z3A.22
23 weeks Z3A.23
24 weeks Z3A.24
25 weeks Z3A.25
26 weeks Z3A.26
27 weeks Z3A.27
28 weeks Z3A.28
29 weeks Z3A.29
30 weeks Z3A.30
31 weeks Z3A.31
32 weeks Z3A.32
33 weeks Z3A.33
34 weeks Z3A.34
35 weeks Z3A.35
36 weeks Z3A.36

Pregnancy (Continued)
weeks of gestation (Continued)
37 weeks Z3A.37
38 weeks Z3A.38
39 weeks Z3A.39
40 weeks Z3A.40
41 weeks Z3A.41
42 weeks Z3A.42
greater than 42 weeks Z3A.49
less than 8 weeks Z3A.01
not specified Z3A.00
Preiser's disease —see Osteonecrosis, secondary, due to, trauma, metacarpus
Pre-kwashiorkor —see Malnutrition, severe
Preleukemia (syndrome) D46.9
Preluxation, hip, congenital Q65.6
Premature —see also condition
adrenarche E27.0
aging E34.8
beats I49.40
atrial I49.1
auricular I49.1
supraventricular I49.1
birth NEC —see Preterm, newborn
closure, foramen ovale Q21.8
contraction
atrial I49.1
atrioventricular I49.49
auricular I49.1
auriculoventricular I49.2
heart (extrasystole) I49.49
junctional I49.2
ventricular I49.3
delivery —see also Pregnancy, complicated by, preterm labor O60.10
ejaculation F52.4
infant NEC —see Preterm, newborn
light-for-dates —see Light for dates
labor —see Pregnancy, complicated by, preterm labor
lungs P28.0
menopause E28.319
asymptomatic E28.319
symptomatic E28.310
newborn
extreme (less than 28 completed weeks) —see Immaturity, extreme
less than 37 completed weeks —see Preterm, newborn
puberty E30.1
rupture membranes or amnion —see Pregnancy, complicated by, premature rupture of membranes
senility E34.8
thelarche E30.8
ventricular systole I49.3
Prematurity NEC (less than 37 completed weeks) —see Preterm, newborn
extreme (less than 28 completed weeks) —see Immaturity, extreme
Premenstrual
dysphoric disorder (PMDD) F32.81
tension (syndrome) N94.3
Premolarization, cuspids K00.2
Prenatal
care, normal pregnancy —see Pregnancy, normal
screening of mother —see also Encounter, antenatal Z36.9
teeth K00.6
Preparatory care for subsequent treatment NEC
for dialysis Z49.01
peritoneal Z49.02
Prepartum —see condition
Preponderance, left or right ventricular I51.7
Prepuce —see condition
PRES (posterior reversible encephalopathy syndrome) I67.83
Presbycardia R54
Presbycusis, presbyacusia H91.1- •
Presbyesophagus K22.8
Presbyophrenia F03
Presbyopia H52.4
Prescription of contraceptives (initial) Z30.019
barrier Z30.018
diaphragm Z30.018
emergency (postcoital) Z30.012
implantable subdermal Z30.017
injectable Z30.013
intrauterine contraceptive device Z30.014
pills Z30.011
postcoital (emergency) Z30.012
repeat Z30.40
barrier Z30.49
diaphragm Z30.49
implantable subdermal Z30.46
injectable Z30.42
pills Z30.41
specified type NEC Z30.49
transdermal patch hormonal Z30.45
vaginal ring hormonal Z30.44
specified type NEC Z30.018
transdermal patch hormonal Z30.016
vaginal ring hormonal Z30.015
Presence (of)
ankle-joint implant (functional) (prosthesis) Z96.66- •
aortocoronary (bypass) graft Z95.1
arterial-venous shunt (dialysis) Z99.2
artificial
eye (globe) Z97.0
heart (fully implantable) (mechanical) Z95.812
valve Z95.2
larynx Z96.3
lens (intraocular) Z96.1
limb (complete) (partial) Z97.1- •
arm Z97.1- •
bilateral Z97.15
leg Z97.1- •
bilateral Z97.16
audiological implant (functional) Z96.29
bladder implant (functional) Z96.0
bone
conduction hearing device Z96.29
implant (functional) NEC Z96.7
joint (prosthesis) —see Presence, joint implant
cardiac
defibrillator (functional) (with synchronous cardiac pacemaker)Z95.810
implant or graft Z95.9
specified type NEC Z95.818
pacemaker Z95.0
resynchronization therapy
defibrillator Z95.810
pacemaker Z95.0
cerebrospinal fluid drainage device Z98.2
cochlear implant (functional) Z96.21
contact lens (es) Z97.3
coronary artery graft or prosthesis Z95.5
CRT-D (cardiac resynchronization therapy defibrillator) Z95.810
CRT-P (cardiac resynchronization therapy pacemaker) Z95.0
cardioverter-defibrillator (ICD) Z95.810
CSF shunt Z98.2
dental prosthesis device Z97.2
dentures Z97.2
device (external) NEC Z97.8
cardiac NEC Z95.818
heart assist Z95.811
implanted (functional) Z96.9
specified NEC Z96.89
prosthetic Z97.8
ear implant Z96.20
cochlear implant Z96.21
myringotomy tube Z96.22
specified type NEC Z96.29
elbow-joint implant (functional) (prosthesis) Z96.62- •
endocrine implant (functional) NEC Z96.49
Presence (Continued)
eustachian tube stent or device (functional) Z96.29
external hearing-aid or device Z97.4
finger-joint implant (functional) (prosthetic) Z96.69- •
functional implant Z96.9
specified NEC Z96.89
graft
cardiac NEC Z95.818
vascular NEC Z95.828
hearing-aid or device (external) Z97.4
implant (bone) (cochlear) (functional) Z96.21
heart assist device Z95.811
heart valve implant (functional) Z95.2
prosthetic Z95.2
specified type NEC Z95.4
xenogenic Z95.3
hip-joint implant (functional) (prosthesis) Z96.64- •
ICD (cardioverter-defibrillator) Z95.810
implanted device (artificial) (functional) (prosthetic) Z96.9
automatic cardiac defibrillator (with synchronous cardiac pacemaker) Z95.810
cardiac pacemaker Z95.0
cochlear Z96.21
dental Z96.5
heart Z95.812
heart valve Z95.2
prosthetic Z95.2
specified NEC Z95.4
xenogenic Z95.3
insulin pump Z96.41
intraocular lens Z96.1
joint Z96.60
ankle Z96.66- •
elbow Z96.62- •
finger Z96.69- •
hip Z96.64- •
knee Z96.65- •
shoulder Z96.61- •
specified NEC Z96.698
wrist Z96.63- •
larynx Z96.3
myringotomy tube Z96.22
otological Z96.20
cochlear Z96.21
eustachian stent Z96.29
myringotomy Z96.22
specified NEC Z96.29
stapes Z96.29
skin Z96.81
skull plate Z96.7
specified NEC Z96.89
urogenital Z96.0
insulin pump (functional) Z96.41
intestinal bypass or anastomosis Z98.0
intraocular lens (functional) Z96.1
intrauterine contraceptive device (IUD) Z97.5
intravascular implant (functional) (prosthetic) NEC Z95.9
coronary artery Z95.5
defibrillator (with synchronous cardiac pacemaker) Z95.810
peripheral vessel (with angioplasty) Z95.820
joint implant (prosthetic) (any) Z96.60
ankle —see Presence, ankle joint implant
elbow —see Presence, elbow joint implant
finger —see Presence, finger joint implant
hip —see Presence, hip joint implant
knee —see Presence, knee joint implant
shoulder —see Presence, shoulder joint implant
specified joint NEC Z96.698
wrist —see Presence, wrist joint implant
knee-joint implant (functional) (prosthesis) Z96.65- •
laryngeal implant (functional) Z96.3
mandibular implant (dental) Z96.5

Presence *(Continued)*
  myringotomy tube(s) Z96.22
  ▶neurostimulator (brain) (gastric) (peripheral nerve) (sacral nerve) (spinal cord) (vagus nerve) Z96.82
  orthopedic-joint implant (prosthetic) (any) —*see* Presence, joint implant
  otological implant (functional) Z96.29
  shoulder-joint implant (functional) (prosthesis) Z96.61-●
  skull-plate implant Z96.7
  spectacles Z97.3
  stapes implant (functional) Z96.29
  systemic lupus erythematosus [SLE] inhibitor D68.62
  tendon implant (functional) (graft) Z96.7
  tooth root(s) implant Z96.5
  ureteral stent Z96.Ø
  urethral stent Z96.Ø
  urogenital implant (functional) Z96.Ø
  vascular implant or device Z95.9
    access port device Z95.828
    specified type NEC Z95.828
  wrist-joint implant (functional) (prosthesis) Z96.63-●
Presenile —*see also* condition
  dementia FØ3
  premature aging E34.8
Presentation, fetal —*see* Delivery, complicated by, malposition
Prespondylolisthesis (congenital) Q76.2
Pressure
  area, skin —*see* Ulcer, pressure, by site
  brachial plexus G54.Ø
  brain G93.5
    injury at birth NEC P11.1
  cerebral —*see* Pressure, brain
  chest RØ7.89
  cone, tentorial G93.5
  hyposystolic —*see also* Hypotension
    incidental reading, without diagnosis of hypotension RØ3.1
  increased
    intracranial (benign) G93.2
      injury at birth P11.Ø
    intraocular H4Ø.Ø5-●
  ▶injury —*see* Ulcer, pressure, by site
  lumbosacral plexus G54.1
  mediastinum J98.59
  necrosis (chronic) —*see* Ulcer, pressure, by site
  parental, inappropriate (excessive) Z62.6
  sore (chronic) —*see* Ulcer, pressure, by site
  spinal cord G95.2Ø
  ulcer (chronic) —*see* Ulcer, pressure, by site
  venous, increased I87.8
Pre-syncope R55
Preterm
  delivery (*see also* Pregnancy, complicated by, preterm labor) O6Ø.1Ø
  labor —*see* Pregnancy, complicated by, preterm labor
  newborn (infant) PØ7.3Ø
    gestational age
      28 completed weeks (28 weeks, Ø days through 28 weeks, 6 days) PØ7.31
      29 completed weeks (29 weeks, Ø days through 29 weeks, 6 days) PØ7.32
      3Ø completed weeks (3Ø weeks, Ø days through 3Ø weeks, 6 days) PØ7.33
      31 completed weeks (31 weeks, Ø days through 31 weeks, 6 days) PØ7.34
      32 completed weeks (32 weeks, Ø days through 32 weeks, 6 days) PØ7.35
      33 completed weeks (33 weeks, Ø days through 33 weeks, 6 days) PØ7.36
      34 completed weeks (34 weeks, Ø days through 34 weeks, 6 days) PØ7.37
      35 completed weeks (35 weeks, Ø days through 35 weeks, 6 days) PØ7.38
      36 completed weeks (36 weeks, Ø days through 36 weeks, 6 days) PØ7.39
Previa
  placenta (total) (without hemorrhage) O44.Ø-●
    with hemorrhage O44.1-●
    complete O44.Ø-●
      with hemorrhage O44.1-●
    low —*see also* Delivery, complicated, by, placenta, low O44.4-●
      with hemorrhage O44.5-●
    marginal O44.2-●
      with hemorrhage O44.3-●
    partial O44.2-●
      with hemorrhage O44.3-●
  vasa O69.4
Priapism N48.3Ø
  due to
    disease classified elsewhere N48.32
    drug N48.33
    specified cause NEC N48.39
    trauma N48.31
Prickling sensation (skin) R2Ø.2
Prickly heat L74.Ø
Primary —*see* condition
Primigravida
  elderly, affecting management of pregnancy, labor and delivery (supervision only) —*see* Pregnancy, complicated by, elderly, primigravida
  older, affecting management of pregnancy, labor and delivery (supervision only) —*see* Pregnancy, complicated by, elderly, primigravida
  very young, affecting management of pregnancy, labor and delivery (supervision only) —*see* Pregnancy, complicated by, young mother, primigravida
Primipara
  elderly, affecting management of pregnancy, labor and delivery (supervision only) —*see* Pregnancy, complicated by, elderly, primigravida
  older, affecting management of pregnancy, labor and delivery (supervision only) —*see* Pregnancy, complicated by, elderly, primigravida
  very young, affecting management of pregnancy, labor and delivery (supervision only) —*see* Pregnancy, complicated by, young mother, primigravida
➠**Primus varus** (bilateral) Q66.21-●
PRIND (Prolonged reversible ischemic neurologic deficit) I63.9
Pringle's disease (tuberous sclerosis)Q85.1
Prinzmetal angina I2Ø.1
Prizefighter ear —*see* Cauliflower ear
Problem (with) (related to)
  academic Z55.8
  acculturation Z6Ø.3
  adjustment (to)
    change of job Z56.1
    life-cycle transition Z6Ø.Ø
    pension Z6Ø.Ø
    retirement Z6Ø.Ø
  adopted child Z62.821
  alcoholism in family Z63.72
  atypical parenting situation Z62.9
  bankruptcy Z59.8
  behavioral (adult) F69
    drug seeking Z76.5
  birth of sibling affecting child Z62.898
  care (of)
    provider dependency Z74.9
      specified NEC Z74.8
    sick or handicapped person in family or household Z63.6
  child
    abuse (affecting the child) —*see* Maltreatment, child
    custody or support proceedings Z65.3
Problem *(Continued)*
  child *(Continued)*
    in care of non-parental family member Z62.21
    in foster care Z62.21
    in welfare custody Z62.21
    living in orphanage or group home Z62.22
  child-rearing Z62.9
    specified NEC Z62.898
  communication (developmental) F8Ø.9
  conflict or discord (with)
    boss Z56.4
    classmates Z55.4
    counselor Z64.4
    employer Z56.4
    family Z63.9
      specified NEC Z63.8
    probation officer Z64.4
    social worker Z64.4
    teachers Z55.4
    workmates Z56.4
  conviction in legal proceedings Z65.Ø
    with imprisonment Z65.1
  counselor Z64.4
  creditors Z59.8
  digestive K92.9
  drug addict in family Z63.72
  ear —*see* Disorder, ear
  economic Z59.9
    affecting care Z59.9
    specified NEC Z59.8
  education Z55.9
    specified NEC Z55.8
  employment Z56.9
    change of job Z56.1
    discord Z56.4
    environment Z56.5
    sexual harassment Z56.81
    specified NEC Z56.89
    stress NEC Z56.6
    stressful schedule Z56.3
    threat of job loss Z56.2
    unemployment Z56.Ø
  enuresis, child F98.Ø
  eye H57.9
  failed examinations (school) Z55.2
  falling Z91.81
  family —*see also* Disruption, family Z63.9-●
    specified NEC Z63.8
  feeding (elderly) (infant) R63.3
    newborn P92.9
      breast P92.5
      overfeeding P92.4
      slow P92.2
      specified NEC P92.8
      underfeeding P92.3
    nonorganic F5Ø.89
  finance Z59.9
    specified NEC Z59.8
  foreclosure on loan Z59.8
  foster child Z62.822
  frightening experience(s) in childhood Z62.898
  genital NEC
    female N94.9
    male N5Ø.9
  health care Z75.9
    specified NEC Z75.8
  hearing —*see* Deafness
  homelessness Z59.Ø
  housing Z59.9
    inadequate Z59.1
    isolated Z59.8
    specified NEC Z59.8
  identity (of childhood) F93.8
  illegitimate pregnancy (unwanted) Z64.Ø
  illiteracy Z55.Ø
  impaired mobility Z74.Ø9
  imprisonment or incarceration Z65.1
  inadequate teaching affecting education Z55.8

Problem *(Continued)*
- inappropriate (excessive) parental pressure Z62.6
- influencing health status NEC Z78.9
- in-law Z63.1
- institutionalization, affecting child Z62.22
- intrafamilial communication Z63.8
- jealousy, child F93.8
- landlord Z59.2
- language (developmental) F80.9
- learning (developmental) F81.9
- legal Z65.3
  - conviction without imprisonment Z65.0
  - imprisonment Z65.1
  - release from prison Z65.2
- life-management Z73.9
  - specified NEC Z73.89
- life-style Z72.9
  - gambling Z72.6
  - high-risk sexual behavior (heterosexual) Z72.51
    - bisexual Z72.53
    - homosexual Z72.52
  - inappropriate eating habits Z72.4
  - self-damaging behavior NEC Z72.89
  - specified NEC Z72.89
  - tobacco use Z72.0
- literacy Z55.9
  - low level Z55.0
  - specified NEC Z55.8
- living alone Z60.2
- lodgers Z59.2
- loss of love relationship in childhood Z62.898
- marital Z63.0
  - involving
    - divorce Z63.5
    - estrangement Z63.5
    - gender identity F66
- mastication K08.89
- medical
  - care, within family Z63.6
  - facilities Z75.9
    - specified NEC Z75.8
- mental F48.9
- multiparity Z64.1
- negative life events in childhood Z62.9
  - altered pattern of family relationships Z62.898
  - frightening experience Z62.898
  - loss of
    - love relationship Z62.898
    - self-esteem Z62.898
  - physical abuse (alleged) —*see* Maltreatment, child
  - removal from home Z62.29
  - specified event NEC Z62.898
- neighbor Z59.2
- neurological NEC R29.818
- new step-parent affecting child Z62.898
- none (feared complaint unfounded) Z71.1
- occupational NEC Z56.89
- parent-child —*see* Conflict, parent-child
- personal hygiene Z91.89
- personality F69
- phase-of-life transition, adjustment Z60.0
- presence of sick or disabled person in family or household Z63.79
  - needing care Z63.6
- primary support group (family) Z63.9
  - specified NEC Z63.8
- probation officer Z64.4
- psychiatric F99
- psychosexual (development) F66
- psychosocial Z65.9
  - religious or spiritual Z65.8
  - specified NEC Z65.8
- relationship Z63.9
  - childhood F93.8
- release from prison Z65.2
  - religious or spiritual Z65.8

Problem *(Continued)*
- removal from home affecting child Z62.29
- seeking and accepting known hazardous and harmful
  - behavioral or psychological interventions Z65.8
  - chemical, nutritional or physical interventions Z65.8
- sexual function (nonorganic) F52.9
- sight H54.7
- sleep disorder, child F51.9
- smell —*see* Disturbance, sensation, smell
- social
  - environment Z60.9
    - specified NEC Z60.8
  - exclusion and rejection Z60.4
  - worker Z64.4
- speech R47.9
  - developmental F80.9
  - specified NEC R47.89
- swallowing —*see* Dysphagia
- taste —*see* Disturbance, sensation, taste
- tic, child F95.0
- underachievement in school Z55.3
- unemployment Z56.0
  - threatened Z56.2
- unwanted pregnancy Z64.0
- upbringing Z62.9
  - specified NEC Z62.898
- urinary N39.9
- voice production R47.89
- work schedule (stressful) Z56.3

Procedure (surgical)
- converted
  - arthroscopic to open Z53.33
  - laparoscopic to open Z53.31
  - specified procedure NEC to open Z53.39
  - thoracoscopic to open Z53.32
- for purpose other than remedying health state Z41.9
  - specified NEC Z41.8
- not done Z53.9
  - because of
    - administrative reasons Z53.8
    - contraindication Z53.09
      - smoking Z53.01
    - patient's decision Z53.20
      - for reasons of belief or group pressure Z53.1
      - left against medical advice (AMA) Z53.21
      - specified reason NEC Z53.29
    - specified reason NEC Z53.8

Procidentia (uteri) N81.3

Proctalgia K62.89
- fugax K59.4
- spasmodic K59.4

Proctitis K62.89
- amebic (acute) A06.0
- chlamydial A56.3
- gonococcal A54.6
- granulomatous —*see* Enteritis, regional, large intestine
- herpetic A60.1
- radiation K62.7
- tuberculous A18.32
- ulcerative (chronic) K51.20
  - with
    - complication K51.219
      - abscess K51.214
      - fistula K51.213
      - obstruction K51.212
      - rectal bleeding K51.211
      - specified NEC K51.218

Proctocele
- female (without uterine prolapse) N81.6
  - with uterine prolapse N81.2
    - complete N81.3
- male K62.3

Proctocolitis
- food-induced eosinophilic K52.82
- food protein-induced K52.82
- milk protein-induced K52.82
- mucosal —*see* Rectosigmoiditis, ulcerative

Proctoptosis K62.3

Proctorrhagia K62.5

Proctosigmoiditis K63.89
- ulcerative (chronic) —*see* Rectosigmoiditis, ulcerative

Proctospasm K59.4
- psychogenic F45.8

Profichet's disease —*see* Disorder, soft tissue, specified type NEC

Progeria E34.8

Prognathism (mandibular) (maxillary) M26.19

Progonoma (melanotic) —*see* Neoplasm, benign, by site

Progressive —*see* condition

Prolactinoma
- specified site —*see* Neoplasm, benign, by site
- unspecified site D35.2

Prolapse, prolapsed
- anus, anal (canal) (sphincter) K62.2
- arm or hand O32.2
  - causing obstructed labor O64.4
- bladder (mucosa) (sphincter) (acquired)
  - congenital Q79.4
  - female —*see* Cystocele
  - male N32.89
- breast implant (prosthetic) T85.49
- cecostomy K94.09
- cecum K63.4
- cervix, cervical (hypertrophied) N81.2
  - anterior lip, obstructing labor O65.5
  - congenital Q51.828
  - postpartal, old N81.2
  - stump N81.85
- ciliary body (traumatic) —*see* Laceration, eye(ball), with prolapse or loss of interocular tissue
- colon (pedunculated) K63.4
- colostomy K94.09
- disc (intervertebral) —*see* Displacement, intervertebral disc
- eye implant (orbital) T85.398
  - lens (ocular) —*see* Complications, intraocular lens
- fallopian tube N83.4- •
- gastric (mucosa) K31.89
- genital, female N81.9
  - specified NEC N81.89
- globe, nontraumatic —*see* Luxation, globe
- ileostomy bud K94.19
- intervertebral disc —*see* Displacement, intervertebral disc
- intestine (small) K63.4
- iris (traumatic) —*see* Laceration, eye(ball), with prolapse or loss of interocular tissue
  - nontraumatic H21.89
- kidney N28.83
  - congenital Q63.2
- laryngeal muscles or ventricle J38.7
- liver K76.89
- meatus urinarius N36.8
- mitral (valve) I34.1
- ocular lens implant —*see* Complications, intraocular lens
- organ or site, congenital NEC —*see* Malposition, congenital
- ovary N83.4- •
- pelvic floor, female N81.89
- perineum, female N81.89
- rectum (mucosa) (sphincter) K62.3
  - due to trichuris trichuria B79
- spleen D73.89
- stomach K31.89
- umbilical cord
  - complicating delivery O69.0

P

Prolapse, prolapsed *(Continued)*
urachus, congenital Q64.4
ureter N28.89
with obstruction N13.5
with infection N13.6
ureterovesical orifice N28.89
urethra (acquired) (infected) (mucosa) N36.8
congenital Q64.71
urinary meatus N36.8
congenital Q64.72
uterovaginal N81.4
complete N81.3
incomplete N81.2
uterus (with prolapse of vagina) N81.4
complete N81.3
congenital Q51.818
first degree N81.2
in pregnancy or childbirth —*see* Pregnancy, complicated by, abnormal, uterus
incomplete N81.2
postpartal (old) N81.4
second degree N81.2
third degree N81.3
uveal (traumatic) —*see* Laceration, eye(ball), with prolapse or loss of interocular tissue
vagina (anterior) (wall) —*see* Cystocele
with prolapse of uterus N81.4
complete N81.3
incomplete N81.2
posterior wall N81.6
posthysterectomy N99.3
vitreous (humor) H43.Ø-●
in wound —*see* Laceration, eye(ball), with prolapse or loss of interocular tissue
womb —*see* Prolapse, uterus
Prolapsus, female N81.9
specified NEC N81.89
Proliferation(s)
primary cutaneous CD3Ø-positive large T-cell C86.6
prostate, atypical small acinar N42.32
Proliferative —*see* condition
Prolonged, prolongation (of)
bleeding (time) (idiopathic) R79.1
coagulation (time) R79.1
gestation (over 42 completed weeks)
mother O48.1
newborn PØ8.22
interval I44.Ø
labor O63.9
first stage O63.Ø
second stage O63.1
partial thromboplastin time (PTT) R79.1
pregnancy (more than 42 weeks gestation) O48.1
prothrombin time R79.1
QT interval R94.31
uterine contractions in labor O62.4
Prominence, prominent
with disproportion (fetopelvic) O33.Ø
causing obstructed labor O65.Ø
auricle (congenital) (ear) Q17.5
ischial spine or sacral promontory
nose (congenital) acquired M95.Ø
Promiscuity —*see* High, risk, sexual behavior
Pronation
ankle —*see* Deformity, limb, foot, specified NEC
foot —*see also* Deformity, limb, foot, specified NEC
congenital Q74.2
Prophylactic
administration of
antibiotics, long-term Z79.2
short-term use - omit code
drug —*see also* Long-term (current) drug therapy (use of) Z79.899-●
medication Z79.899
Prophylactic *(Continued)*
organ removal (for neoplasia management) Z4Ø.ØØ
breast Z4Ø.Ø1
fallopian tube(s) Z4Ø.Ø3
with ovary(s) Z4Ø.Ø2
ovary(s) Z4Ø.Ø2
specified site NEC Z4Ø.Ø9
surgery Z4Ø.9
for risk factors related to malignant neoplasm —*see* Prophylactic, organ removal
specified NEC Z4Ø.8
vaccination Z23
Propionic acidemia E71.121
Proptosis (ocular) —*see also* Exophthalmos
thyroid —*see* Hyperthyroidism, with goiter
Prosecution, anxiety concerning Z65.3
Prosopagnosia R48.3
Prostadynia N42.81
Prostate, prostatic —*see* condition
Prostatism —*see* Hyperplasia, prostate
Prostatitis (congestive) (suppurative) (with cystitis) N41.9
acute N41.Ø
cavitary N41.8
chronic N41.1
diverticular N41.8
due to Trichomonas (vaginalis) A59.Ø2
fibrous N41.1
gonococcal (acute) (chronic) A54.22
granulomatous N41.4
hypertrophic N41.1
subacute N41.1
trichomonal A59.Ø2
tuberculous A18.14
Prostatocystitis N41.3
Prostatorrhea N42.89
Prostatosis N42.82
Prostration R53.83
heat —*see also* Heat, exhaustion
anhydrotic T67.3
due to
salt (and water) depletion T67.4
water depletion T67.3
nervous F48.8
senile R54
Protanomaly (anomalous trichromat) H53.54
Protanopia (complete) (incomplete) H53.54
Protection (against) (from) —*see* Prophylactic
Protein
deficiency NEC —*see* Malnutrition
malnutrition —*see* Malnutrition
sickness —*see also* Reaction, serum T8Ø.69
Proteinemia R77.9
Proteinosis
alveolar (pulmonary) J84.Ø1
lipid or lipoid (of Urbach) E78.89
Proteinuria R8Ø.9
Bence Jones R8Ø.3
complicating pregnancy —*see* Proteinuria, gestational
gestational
complicating
childbirth O12.14
pregnancy O12.1-●
with edema O12.2-●
puerperium O12.15
idiopathic R8Ø.Ø
isolated R8Ø.Ø
with glomerular lesion NØ6.9
dense deposit disease NØ6.6
diffuse
crescentic glomerulonephritis NØ6.7
endocapillary proliferative glomerulonephritis NØ6.4
mesangiocapillary glomerulonephritis NØ6.5
focal and segmental hyalinosis or sclerosis NØ6.1
membranous (diffuse) NØ6.2
Proteinuria *(Continued)*
isolated *(Continued)*
with glomerular lesion *(Continued)*
mesangial proliferative (diffuse) NØ6.3
minimal change NØ6.Ø
specified pathology NEC NØ6.8
orthostatic R8Ø.2
with glomerular lesion —*see* Proteinuria, isolated, with glomerular lesion
persistent R8Ø.1
with glomerular lesion —*see* Proteinuria, isolated, with glomerular lesion
postural R8Ø.2
with glomerular lesion —*see* Proteinuria, isolated, with glomerular lesion
pre-eclamptic —*see* Pre-eclampsia
puerperal O12.15
specified type NEC R8Ø.8
Proteolysis, pathologic D65
Proteus (mirabilis) (morganii), as cause of disease classified elsewhere B96.4
Prothrombin gene mutation D68.52
Protoporphyria, erythropoietic E8Ø.Ø
Protozoal —*see also* condition
disease B64
specified NEC B6Ø.8
Protrusion, protrusio
acetabuli M24.7
acetabulum (into pelvis) M24.7
device, implant or graft —*see also* Complications, by site and type, mechanical T85.698
arterial graft NEC —*see* Complication, cardiovascular device, mechanical, vascular
breast (implant) T85.49
catheter NEC T85.698
cystostomy T83.Ø9Ø
dialysis (renal) T82.49
intraperitoneal T85.691
infusion NEC T82.594
spinal (epidural) (subdural) T85.69Ø
urinary —*see also* Complications, catheter, urinary T83.Ø98
electronic (electrode) (pulse generator) (stimulator)
bone T84.39Ø
nervous system —*see* Complication, prosthetic device, mechanical, electronic nervous system stimulator
fixation, internal (orthopedic) NEC —*see* Complication, fixation device, mechanical
gastrointestinal —*see* Complications, prosthetic device, mechanical, gastrointestinal device
genital NEC T83.498
intrauterine contraceptive device T83.39
penile prosthesis (cylinder) (implanted) (pump) (resevoir) T83.49Ø
testicular prosthesis T83.491
heart NEC —*see* Complication, cardiovascular device, mechanical
joint prosthesis —*see* Complications, joint prosthesis, mechanical, specified NEC, by site
ocular NEC —*see* Complications, prosthetic device, mechanical, ocular device
orthopedic NEC —*see* Complication, orthopedic, device, mechanical
specified NEC T85.628
urinary NEC —*see also* Complication, genitourinary, device, urinary, mechanical
graft T83.29
vascular NEC —*see* Complication, cardiovascular device, mechanical

P

Protrusion, protrusio *(Continued)*
device, implant or graft *(Continued)*
ventricular intracranial shunt T85.Ø9
intervertebral disc —*see* Displacement, intervertebral disc
joint prosthesis —*see* Complications, joint prosthesis, mechanical, specified NEC, by site
nucleus pulposus —*see* Displacement, intervertebral disc
Prune belly (syndrome) Q79.4
Prurigo (ferox) (gravis) (Hebrae) (Hebra's) (mitis) (simplex) L28.2
Besnier's L2Ø.Ø
estivalis L56.4
nodularis L28.1
psychogenic F45.8
Pruritus, pruritic (essential) L29.9
ani, anus L29.Ø
psychogenic F45.8
anogenital L29.3
psychogenic F45.8
due to onchocerca volvulus B73.1
gravidarum —*see* Pregnancy, complicated by, specified pregnancy-related condition NEC
hiemalis L29.8
neurogenic (any site) F45.8
perianal L29.Ø
psychogenic (any site) F45.8
scroti, scrotum L29.1
psychogenic F45.8
senile, senilis L29.8
specified NEC L29.8
psychogenic F45.8
Trichomonas A59.9
vulva, vulvae L29.2
psychogenic F45.8
Pseudarthrosis, pseudoarthrosis (bone) —*see* Nonunion, fracture
clavicle, congenital Q74.Ø
joint, following fusion or arthrodesis M96.Ø
Pseudoaneurysm —*see* Aneurysm
Pseudoangina (pectoris) —*see* Angina
Pseudoangioma I81
Pseudoarteriosus Q28.8
Pseudoarthrosis —*see* Pseudarthrosis
Pseudobulbar affect (PBA) F48.2
Pseudochromhidrosis L67.8
Pseudocirrhosis, liver, pericardial I31.1
Pseudocowpox BØ8.Ø3
Pseudocoxalgia M91.3-●
Pseudocroup J38.5
Pseudo-Cushing's syndrome, alcohol-induced E24.4
Pseudocyesis F45.8
Pseudocyst
lung J98.4
pancreas K86.3
retina —*see* Cyst, retina
Pseudoelephantiasis neuroarthritica Q82.Ø
Pseudoexfoliation, capsule (lens) —*see* Cataract, specified NEC
Pseudofolliculitis barbae L73.1
Pseudoglioma H44.89
Pseudohemophilia (Bernuth's) (hereditary) (type B) D68.Ø
Type A D69.8
vascular D69.8
Pseudohermaphroditism Q56.3
adrenal E25.8
female Q56.2
with adrenocortical disorder E25.8
without adrenocortical disorder Q56.2
adrenal (congenital) E25.Ø
unspecified E25.9
male Q56.1
with
adrenocortical disorder E25.8
androgen resistance E34.51
Pseudohermaphroditism *(Continued)*
male *(Continued)*
with *(Continued)*
cleft scrotum Q56.1
feminizing testis E34.51
5-alpha-reductase deficiency E29.1
without gonadal disorder Q56.1
adrenal E25.8
unspecified E25.9
Pseudo-Hurler's polydystrophy E77.Ø
Pseudohydrocephalus G93.2
Pseudohypertrophic muscular dystrophy (Erb's) G71.Ø2
Pseudohypertrophy, muscle G71.Ø9
Pseudohypoparathyroidism E2Ø.1
Pseudoinsomnia F51.Ø3
Pseudoleukemia, infantile D64.89
Pseudomembranous —*see* condition
Pseudomeningocele (cerebral) (infective) (post-traumatic) G96.19
postprocedural (spinal) G97.82
Pseudomenses (newborn) P54.6
Pseudomenstruation (newborn) P54.6
Pseudomonas
aeruginosa, as cause of disease classified elsewhere B96.5
mallei infection A24.Ø
as cause of disease classified elsewhere B96.5
pseudomallei, as cause of disease classified elsewhere B96.5
Pseudomyotonia G71.19
Pseudomyxoma peritonei C78.6
Pseudoneuritis, optic (nerve) (disc) (papilla), congenital Q14.2
Pseudo-obstruction intestine (acute) (chronic) (idiopathic) (intermittent secondary) (primary) K59.8
Pseudopapilledema H47.33-●
congenital Q14.2
Pseudoparalysis
arm or leg R29.818
atonic, congenital P94.2
Pseudopelade L66.Ø
Pseudophakia Z96.1
Pseudopolyarthritis, rhizomelic M35.3
Pseudopolycythemia D75.1
Pseudopseudohypoparathyroidism E2Ø.1
Pseudopterygium H11.81-●
Pseudoptosis (eyelid) —*see* Blepharochalasis
Pseudopuberty, precocious
female heterosexual E25.8
male isosexual E25.8
Pseudorickets (renal) N25.Ø
Pseudorubella BØ8.2Ø
Pseudosclerema, newborn P83.88
Pseudosclerosis (brain)
Jakob's —*see* Creutzfeldt-Jakob disease or syndrome
of Westphal (Strüümpell) E83.Ø1
spastic —*see* Creutzfeldt-Jakob disease or syndrome
Pseudotetanus —*see* Convulsions
Pseudotetany R29.Ø
hysterical F44.5
Pseudotruncus arteriosus Q25.49
Pseudotuberculosis A28.2
enterocolitis AØ4.8
pasteurella (infection) A28.Ø
Pseudotumor
cerebri G93.2
orbital HØ5.11-●
Pseudoxanthoma elasticum Q82.8
Psilosis (sprue) (tropical) K9Ø.1
nontropical K9Ø.Ø
Psittacosis A7Ø
Psoitis M6Ø.88
Psoriasis L4Ø.9
arthropathic L4Ø.5Ø
arthritis mutilans L4Ø.52
distal interphalangeal L4Ø.51
Psoriasis *(Continued)*
arthropathic *(Continued)*
juvenile L4Ø.54
other specified L4Ø.59
spondylitis L4Ø.53
buccal K13.29
flexural L4Ø.8
guttate L4Ø.4
mouth K13.29
nummular L4Ø.Ø
plaque L4Ø.Ø
psychogenic F54
pustular (generalized) L4Ø.1
palmaris et plantaris L4Ø.3
specified NEC L4Ø.8
vulgaris L4Ø.Ø
Psychasthenia F48.8
Psychiatric disorder or problem F99
Psychogenic —*see also* condition
factors associated with physical conditions F54
Psychological and behavioral factors affecting medical condition F59
Psychoneurosis, psychoneurotic —*see also* Neurosis
anxiety (state) F41.1
depersonalization F48.1
hypochondriacal F45.21
hysteria F44.9
neurasthenic F48.8
personality NEC F6Ø.89
Psychopathy, psychopathic
affectionless F94.2
autistic F84.5
constitution, post-traumatic FØ7.81
personality —*see* Disorder, personality
sexual —*see* Deviation, sexual
state F6Ø.2
Psychosexual identity disorder of childhood F64.2
Psychosis, psychotic F29
acute (transient) F23
hysterical F44.9
affective —*see* Disorder, mood
alcoholic F1Ø.959
with
abuse F1Ø.159
anxiety disorder F1Ø.98Ø
with
abuse F1Ø.18Ø
dependence F1Ø.28Ø
delirium tremens F1Ø.231
delusions F1Ø.95Ø
with
abuse F1Ø.15Ø
dependence F1Ø.25Ø
dementia F1Ø.97
with dependence F1Ø.27
dependence F1Ø.259
hallucinosis F1Ø.951
with
abuse F1Ø.151
dependence F1Ø.251
mood disorder F1Ø.94
with
abuse F1Ø.14
dependence F1Ø.24
paranoia F1Ø.95Ø
with
abuse F1Ø.15Ø
dependence F1Ø.25Ø
persisting amnesia F1Ø.96
with dependence F1Ø.26
amnestic confabulatory F1Ø.96
with dependence F1Ø.26
delirium tremens F1Ø.231
Korsakoff's, Korsakov's, Korsakow's F1Ø.26
paranoid type F1Ø.95Ø
with
abuse F1Ø.15Ø
dependence F1Ø.25Ø

P

Psychosis, psychotic *(Continued)*
anergastic —*see* Psychosis, organic
arteriosclerotic (simple type) (uncomplicated) F01.50
with behavioral disturbance F01.51
childhood F84.0
atypical F84.8
climacteric —*see* Psychosis, involutional
confusional F29
acute or subacute F05
reactive F23
cycloid F23
depressive —*see* Disorder, depressive
disintegrative (childhood) F84.3
drug-induced —*see* F11-F19 with .x59
paranoid and hallucinatory states —*see* F11-F19 with .x50 or .x51
due to or associated with
addiction, drug —*see* F11-F19 with .X59
dependence
alcohol F10.259
drug —*see* F11-F19 with .x59
epilepsy F06.8
Huntington's chorea F06.8
ischemia, cerebrovascular (generalized) F06.8
multiple sclerosis F06.8
physical disease F06.8
presenile dementia F03
senile dementia F03
vascular disease (arteriosclerotic) (cerebral) F01.50
with behavioral disturbance F01.51
epileptic F06.8
episode F23
due to or associated with physical condition F06.8
exhaustive F43.0
hallucinatory, chronic F28
hypomanic F30.8
hysterical (acute) F44.9
induced F24
infantile F84.0
atypical F84.8
infective (acute) (subacute) F05
involutional F28
depressive —*see* Disorder, depressive
melancholic —*see* Disorder, depressive
paranoid (state) F22
Korsakoff's, Korsakov's, Korsakow's (nonalcoholic) F04
alcoholic F10.96
in dependence F10.26
induced by other psychoactive substance —*see* categories F11-F19 with .x5x
mania, manic (single episode) F30.2
recurrent type F31.89
manic-depressive —*see* Disorder, bipolar
menopausal —*see* Psychosis, involutional
mixed schizophrenic and affective F25.8
multi-infarct (cerebrovascular) F01.50
with behavioral disturbance F01.51
nonorganic F29
specified NEC F28
organic F09
due to or associated with
arteriosclerosis (cerebral) —*see* Psychosis, arteriosclerotic
cerebrovascular disease, arteriosclerotic —*see* Psychosis, arteriosclerotic
childbirth —*see* Psychosis, puerperal
Creutzfeldt-Jakob disease or syndrome —*see* Creutzfeldt-Jakob disease or syndrome
dependence, alcohol F10.259
disease
alcoholic liver F10.259
brain, arteriosclerotic —*see* Psychosis, arteriosclerotic

Psychosis, psychotic *(Continued)*
organic *(Continued)*
due to or associated with *(Continued)*
disease *(Continued)*
cerebrovascular F01.50
with behavioral disturbance F01.51
Creutzfeldt-Jakob —*see* Creutzfeldt-Jakob disease or syndrome
endocrine or metabolic F06.8
acute or subacute F05
liver, alcoholic F10.259
epilepsy transient (acute) F05
infection
brain (intracranial) F06.8
acute or subacute F05
intoxication
alcoholic (acute) F10.259
drug F11-F19 with .x59
ischemia, cerebrovascular (generalized) —*see* Psychosis, arteriosclerotic
puerperium —*see* Psychosis, puerperal
trauma, brain (birth) (from electric current) (surgical) F06.8
acute or subacute F05
infective F06.8
acute or subacute F05
post-traumatic F06.8
acute or subacute F05
paranoiac F22
paranoid (climacteric) (involutional) (menopausal) F22
psychogenic (acute) F23
schizophrenic F20.0
senile F03
postpartum F53.1
presbyophrenic (type) F03
presenile F03
psychogenic (paranoid) F23
depressive F32.3
puerperal F53.1
specified type —*see* Psychosis, by type
reactive (brief) (transient) (emotional stress) (psychological trauma) F23
depressive F32.3
recurrent F33.3
excitative type F30.8
schizoaffective F25.9
depressive type F25.1
manic type F25.0
schizophrenia, schizophrenic —*see* Schizophrenia
schizophrenia-like, in epilepsy F06.2
schizophreniform F20.81
affective type F25.9
brief F23
confusional type F23
mixed type F25.0
senile NEC F03
depressed or paranoid type F03
simple deterioration F03
specified type — code to condition
shared F24
situational (reactive) F23
symbiotic (childhood) F84.3
symptomatic F09
Psychosomatic —*see* Disorder, psychosomatic
Psychosyndrome, organic F07.9
Psychotic episode due to or associated with physical condition F06.8
Pterygium (eye) H11.00- •
amyloid H11.01- •
central H11.02- •
colli Q18.3
double H11.03- •
peripheral
progressive H11.05- •
stationary H11.04- •
recurrent H11.06- •
Ptilosis (eyelid) —*see* Madarosis

Ptomaine (poisoning) —*see* Poisoning, food
Ptosis —*see also* Blepharoptosis
adiposa (false) —*see* Blepharoptosis
breast N64.81
brow H57.81- •
cecum K63.4
colon K63.4
congenital (eyelid) Q10.0
specified site NEC —*see* Anomaly, by site
eyebrow H57.81- •
eyelid —*see* Blepharoptosis
congenital Q10.0
gastric K31.89
intestine K63.4
kidney N28.83
liver K76.89
renal N28.83
splanchnic K63.4
spleen D73.89
stomach K31.89
viscera K63.4
PTP D69.51
Ptyalism (periodic) K11.7
hysterical F45.8
pregnancy —*see* Pregnancy, complicated by, specified pregnancy-related condition NEC
psychogenic F45.8
Ptyalolithiasis K11.5
Pubarche, precocious E30.1
Pubertas praecox E30.1
Puberty (development state) Z00.3
bleeding (excessive) N92.2
delayed E30.0
precocious (constitutional) (cryptogenic) (idiopathic) E30.1
central E22.8
due to
ovarian hyperfunction E28.1
estrogen E28.0
testicular hyperfunction E29.0
premature E30.1
due to
adrenal cortical hyperfunction E25.8
pineal tumor E34.8
pituitary (anterior) hyperfunction E22.8
Puckering, macula —*see* Degeneration, macula, puckering
Pudenda, pudendum —*see* condition
Puente's disease (simple glandular cheilitis) K13.0
Puerperal, puerperium (complicated by, complications)
abnormal glucose (tolerance test) O99.815
abscess
areola O91.02
associated with lactation O91.03
Bartholin's gland O86.19
breast O91.12
associated with lactation O91.13
cervix (uteri) O86.11
genital organ NEC O86.19
kidney O86.21
mammary O91.12
associated with lactation O91.13
nipple O91.02
associated with lactation O91.03
peritoneum O85
subareolar O91.12
associated with lactation O91.13
urinary tract —*see* Puerperal, infection, urinary
uterus O86.12
vagina (wall) O86.13
vaginorectal O86.13
vulvovaginal gland O86.13
adnexitis O86.19
afibrinogenemia, or other coagulation defect O72.3
albuminuria (acute) (subacute) —*see* Proteinuria, gestational

Puerperal, puerperium *(Continued)*
  alcohol use O99.315
  anemia O90.81
    pre-existing (pre-pregnancy) O99.03
  anesthetic death O89.8
  apoplexy O99.43
  bariatric surgery status O99.845
  blood disorder NEC O99.13
  blood dyscrasia O72.3
  cardiomyopathy O90.3
  cerebrovascular disorder (conditions in I60-I69) O99.43
  cervicitis O86.11
  circulatory system disorder O99.43
  coagulopathy (any) O99.13
    with hemorrhage O72.3
  complications O90.9
    specified NEC O90.89
  convulsions —*see* Eclampsia
  cystitis O86.22
  cystopyelitis O86.29
  delirium NEC F05
  diabetes O24.93
    gestational —*see* Puerperal, gestational diabetes
    pre-existing O24.33
      specified NEC O24.83
      type 1 O24.03
      type 2 O24.13
  digestive system disorder O99.63
  disease O90.9
    breast NEC O92.29
    cerebrovascular (acute) O99.43
    nonobstetric NEC O99.89
    tubo-ovarian O86.19
    Valsuani's O99.03
  disorder O90.9
    biliary tract O26.63
    lactation O92.70
    liver O26.63
    nonobstetric NEC O99.89
  disruption
    cesarean wound O90.0
    episiotomy wound O90.1
    perineal laceration wound O90.1
  drug use O99.325
  eclampsia (with pre-existing hypertension) O15.2
  embolism (pulmonary) (blood clot) —*see* Embolism, obstetric, puerperal
  endocrine, nutritional or metabolic disease NEC O99.285
  endophlebitis —*see* Puerperal, phlebitis
  endotrachelitis O86.11
  failure
    lactation (complete) O92.3
      partial O92.4
    renal, acute O90.4
  fever (of unknown origin) O86.4
    septic O85
  fissure, nipple O92.12
    associated with lactation O92.13
  fistula
    breast (due to mastitis) O91.12
      associated with lactation O91.13
    nipple O91.02
      associated with lactation O91.03
  galactophoritis O91.22
    associated with lactation O91.23
  galactorrhea O92.6
  gastric banding status O99.845
  gastric bypass status O99.845
  gastrointestinal disease NEC O99.63
  gestational
    diabetes O24.439
      diet controlled O24.430
      insulin (and diet) controlled O24.434
      oral drug controlled (antidiabetic) (hypoglycemic) O24.435
    edema O12.05
      with proteinuria O12.25
    proteinuria O12.15

Puerperal, puerperium *(Continued)*
  gonorrhea O98.23
  hematoma, subdural O99.43
  hemiplegia, cerebral O99.355-●
    due to cerebrovascular disorder O99.43
  hemorrhage O72.1
    brain O99.43
    bulbar O99.43
    cerebellar O99.43
    cerebral O99.43
    cortical O99.43
    delayed or secondary O72.2
    extradural O99.43
    internal capsule O99.43
    intracranial O99.43
    intrapontine O99.43
    meningeal O99.43
    pontine O99.43
    retained placenta O72.0
    subarachnoid O99.43
    subcortical O99.43
    subdural O99.43
    third stage O72.0
    uterine, delayed O72.2
    ventricular O99.43
  hemorrhoids O87.2
  hepatorenal syndrome O90.4
  hypertension —*see* Hypertension, complicating, puerperium
  hypertrophy, breast O92.29
  induration breast (fibrous) O92.29
  infection O86.4
    cervix O86.11
    generalized O85
    genital tract NEC O86.19
      obstetric surgical wound O86.09
    kidney (bacillus coli) O86.21
    maternal O98.93
      carrier state NEC O99.835
      gonorrhea O98.23
      human immunodeficiency virus (HIV) O98.73
      protozoal O98.63
      sexually transmitted NEC O98.33
      specified NEC O98.83
      streptococcus group B (GBS) carrier state O99.825
      syphilis O98.13
      tuberculosis O98.03
      viral hepatitis O98.43
      viral NEC O98.53
    nipple O91.02
      associated with lactation O91.03
    peritoneum O85
    renal O86.21
    specified NEC O86.89
    urinary (asymptomatic) (tract) NEC O86.20
      bladder O86.22
      kidney O86.21
      specified site NEC O86.29
      urethra O86.22
    vagina O86.13
    vein —*see* Puerperal, phlebitis
  ischemia, cerebral O99.43
  lymphangitis O86.89
    breast O91.22
      associated with lactation O91.23
  malignancy O9A.13
  malnutrition O25.3
  mammillitis O91.02
    associated with lactation O91.03
  mammitis O91.22
    associated with lactation O91.23
  mania F30.8
  mastitis O91.22
    associated with lactation O91.23
    purulent O91.12
      associated with lactation O91.13

Puerperal, puerperium *(Continued)*
  melancholia —*see* Disorder, depressive
  mental disorder NEC O99.345
  metroperitonitis O85
  metrorrhagia —*see* Hemorrhage, postpartum
  metrosalpingitis O86.19
  metrovaginitis O86.13
  milk leg O87.1
  monoplegia, cerebral O99.43
  mood disturbance O90.6
  necrosis, liver (acute) (subacute) (conditions in subcategory K72.0) O26.63
    with renal failure O90.4
  nervous system disorder O99.355
  neuritis O90.89
  obesity (pre-existing prior to pregnancy) O99.215
  obesity surgery status O99.845
  occlusion, precerebral artery O99.43
  paralysis
    bladder (sphincter) O90.89
    cerebral O99.43
  paralytic stroke O99.43
  parametritis O85
  paravaginitis O86.13
  pelviperitonitis O85
  perimetritis O86.12
  perimetrosalpingitis O86.19
  perinephritis O86.21
  periphlebitis —*see* Puerperal phlebitis
  peritoneal infection O85
  peritonitis (pelvic) O85
  perivaginitis O86.13
  phlebitis O87.0
    deep O87.1
    pelvic O87.1
    superficial O87.0
  phlebothrombosis, deep O87.1
  phlegmasia alba dolens O87.1
  placental polyp O90.89
  pneumonia, embolic —*see* Embolism, obstetric, puerperal
  pre-eclampsia —*see* Pre-eclampsia
  psychosis F53.1
  pyelitis O86.21
  pyelocystitis O86.29
  pyelonephritis O86.21
  pyelonephrosis O86.21
  pyemia O85
  pyocystitis O86.29
  pyohemia O85
  pyometra O86.12
  pyonephritis O86.21
  pyosalpingitis O86.19
  pyrexia (of unknown origin) O86.4
  renal
    disease NEC O90.89
    failure O90.4
  respiratory disease NEC O99.53
  retention
    decidua —*see* Retention, decidua
    placenta O72.0
    secundines —*see* Retention, secundines
  retrated nipple O92.02
  salpingo-ovaritis O86.19
  salpingoperitonitis O85
  secondary perineal tear O90.1
  sepsis O85
  sepsis (pelvic) O85
  septic thrombophlebitis O86.81
  skin disorder NEC O99.73
  specified condition NEC O99.89
  stroke O99.43
  subinvolution (uterus) O90.89
  subluxation of symphysis (pubis) O26.73
  suppuration —*see* Puerperal, abscess
  tetanus A34

P

- **Puerperal, puerperium** *(Continued)*
  - thelitis O91.Ø2
    - associated with lactation O91.Ø3
  - thrombocytopenia O72.3
  - thrombophlebitis (superficial) O87.Ø
    - deep O87.1
    - pelvic O87.1
    - septic O86.81
  - thrombosis (venous) *—see* Thrombosis, puerperal
  - thyroiditis O9Ø.5
  - toxemia (eclamptic) (pre-eclamptic) (with convulsions) O15.2
  - trauma, non-obstetric O9A.23
    - caused by abuse (physical) (suspected) O9A.33
      - confirmed O9A.33
      - psychological (suspected) O9A.53
        - confirmed O9A.53
      - sexual (suspected) O9A.43
        - confirmed O9A.43
  - uremia (due to renal failure) O9Ø.4
  - urethritis O86.22
  - vaginitis O86.13
  - varicose veins (legs) O87.4
    - vulva or perineum O87.8
  - venous O87.9
  - vulvitis O86.19
  - vulvovaginitis O86.13
  - white leg O87.1
- **Puerperium** *—see* Puerperal
- **Pulmolithiasis** J98.4
- **Pulmonary** *—see* condition
- **Pulpitis** (acute) (anachoretic) (chronic) (hyperplastic) (putrescent) (suppurative) (ulcerative) KØ4.Ø1
  - irreversible KØ4.Ø2
  - reversible KØ4.Ø1
- **Pulpless tooth** KØ4.99
- **Pulse**
  - alternating RØØ.8
  - bigeminal RØØ.8
  - fast RØØ.Ø
  - feeble, rapid due to shock following injury T79.4
  - rapid RØØ.Ø
  - weak RØ9.89
- **Pulsus alternans or trigeminus** RØØ.8
- **Punch drunk** FØ7.81
- **Punctum lacrimale occlusion** *—see* Obstruction, lacrimal
- **Puncture**
  - abdomen, abdominal
    - wall S31.139
      - with
        - foreign body S31.149
        - penetration into peritoneal cavity S31.639
          - with foreign body S31.649
      - epigastric region S31.132
        - with
          - foreign body S31.142
          - penetration into peritoneal cavity S31.632
            - with foreign body S31.642
      - left
        - lower quadrant S31.134
          - with
            - foreign body S31.144
            - penetration into peritoneal cavity S31.634
              - with foreign body S31.644
        - upper quadrant S31.131
          - with
            - foreign body S31.141
            - penetration into peritoneal cavity S31.631
              - with foreign body S31.641

- **Puncture** *(Continued)*
  - abdomen, abdominal *(Continued)*
    - wall *(Continued)*
      - periumbilic region S31.135
        - with
          - foreign body S31.145
          - penetration into peritoneal cavity S31.635
            - with foreign body S31.645
      - right
        - lower quadrant S31.133
          - with
            - foreign body S31.143
            - penetration into peritoneal cavity S31.633
              - with foreign body S31.643
        - upper quadrant S31.13Ø
          - with
            - foreign body S31.14Ø
            - penetration into peritoneal cavity S31.63Ø
              - with foreign body S31.64Ø
  - accidental, complicating surgery *—see* Complication, accidental puncture or laceration
  - alveolar (process) *—see* Puncture, oral cavity
  - ankle S91.Ø39
    - with
      - foreign body S91.Ø49
    - left S91.Ø32
      - with
        - foreign body S91.Ø42
    - right S91.Ø31
      - with
        - foreign body S91.Ø41
  - anus S31.833
    - with foreign body S31.834
  - arm (upper) S41.139
    - with foreign body S41.149
    - left S41.132
      - with foreign body S41.142
    - lower *—see* Puncture, forearm
    - right S41.131
      - with foreign body S41.141
  - auditory canal (external) (meatus) *—see* Puncture, ear
  - auricle, ear *—see* Puncture, ear
  - axilla *—see* Puncture, arm
  - back *—see also* Puncture, thorax, back
    - lower S31.Ø3Ø
      - with
        - foreign body S31.Ø4Ø
          - with penetration into retroperitoneal space S31.Ø41
        - penetration into retroperitoneal space S31.Ø31
  - bladder (traumatic) S37.29
    - nontraumatic N32.89
  - breast S21.Ø39
    - with foreign body S21.Ø49
    - left S21.Ø32
      - with foreign body S21.Ø42
    - right S21.Ø31
      - with foreign body S21.Ø41
  - buttock S31.8Ø3
    - with foreign body S31.8Ø4
    - left S31.823
      - with foreign body S31.824
    - right S31.813
      - with foreign body S31.814
  - by
    - device, implant or graft *—see* Complications, by site and type, mechanical
    - foreign body left accidentally in operative wound T81.539
    - instrument (any) during a procedure, accidental *—see* Puncture, accidental complicating surgery
  - calf *—see* Puncture, leg
  - canaliculus lacrimalis *—see* Puncture, eyelid

- **Puncture** *(Continued)*
  - canthus, eye *—see* Puncture, eyelid
  - cervical esophagus S11.23
    - with foreign body S11.24
  - cheek (external) SØ1.439
    - with foreign body SØ1.449
    - internal *—see* Puncture, oral cavity
    - left SØ1.432
      - with foreign body SØ1.442
    - right SØ1.431
      - with foreign body SØ1.441
  - chest wall *—see* Puncture, thorax
  - chin *—see* Puncture, head, specified site NEC
  - clitoris *—see* Puncture, vulva
  - costal region *—see* Puncture, thorax
  - digit(s)
    - foot *—see* Puncture, toe
    - hand *—see* Puncture, finger
  - ear (canal) (external) SØ1.339
    - with foreign body SØ1.349
    - drum SØ9.2- ●
    - left SØ1.332
      - with foreign body SØ1.342
    - right SØ1.331
      - with foreign body SØ1.341
  - elbow S51.Ø39
    - with
      - foreign body S51.Ø49
    - left S51.Ø32
      - with
        - foreign body S51.Ø42
    - right S51.Ø31
      - with
        - foreign body S51.Ø41
  - epididymis *—see* Puncture, testis
  - epigastric region *—see* Puncture, abdomen, wall, epigastric
  - epiglottis S11.83
    - with foreign body S11.84
  - esophagus
    - cervical S11.23
      - with foreign body S11.24
    - thoracic S27.818
  - eyeball SØ5.6- ●
    - with foreign body SØ5.5- ●
  - eyebrow *—see* Puncture, eyelid
  - eyelid SØ1.13- ●
    - with foreign body SØ1.14- ●
    - left SØ1.132
      - with foreign body SØ1.142
    - right SØ1.131
      - with foreign body SØ1.141
  - face NEC *—see* Puncture, head, specified site NEC
  - finger(s) S61.239
    - with
      - damage to nail S61.339
        - with
          - foreign body S61.349
      - foreign body S61.249
    - index S61.238
      - with
        - damage to nail S61.338
          - with
            - foreign body S61.348
        - foreign body S61.248
      - left S61.231
        - with
          - damage to nail S61.331
            - with
              - foreign body S61.341
          - foreign body S61.241
      - right S61.23Ø
        - with
          - damage to nail S61.33Ø
            - with
              - foreign body S61.34Ø
          - foreign body S61.24Ø
    - little S61.238
      - with
        - damage to nail S61.338

P

- Puncture *(Continued)*
  - finger *(Continued)*
    - with *(Continued)*
      - with *(Continued)*
        - damage to nail *(Continued)*
          - with
            - foreign body S61.348
        - foreign body S61.248
      - left S61.237
        - with
          - damage to nail S61.337
            - with
              - foreign body S61.347
          - foreign body S61.247
      - right S61.236
        - with
          - damage to nail S61.336
            - with
              - foreign body S61.346
          - foreign body S61.246
    - middle S61.238
      - with
        - damage to nail S61.338
          - with
            - foreign body S61.348
        - foreign body S61.248
      - left S61.233
        - with
          - damage to nail S61.333
            - with
              - foreign body S61.343
          - foreign body S61.243
      - right S61.232
        - with
          - damage to nail S61.332
            - with
              - foreign body S61.342
          - foreign body S61.242
    - ring S61.238
      - with
        - damage to nail S61.338
          - with
            - foreign body S61.348
        - foreign body S61.248
      - left S61.235
        - with
          - damage to nail S61.335
            - with
              - foreign body S61.345
          - foreign body S61.245
      - right S61.234
        - with
          - damage to nail S61.334
            - with
              - foreign body S61.344
          - foreign body S61.244
  - flank S31.139
    - with foreign body S31.149
  - foot (except toe(s) alone) S91.339
    - with foreign body S91.349
    - left S91.332
      - with foreign body S91.342
    - right S91.331
      - with foreign body S91.341
    - toe —*see* Puncture, toe
  - forearm S51.839
    - with
      - foreign body S51.849
    - elbow only —*see* Puncture, elbow
    - left S51.832
      - with
        - foreign body S51.842
    - right S51.831
      - with
        - foreign body S51.841
  - forehead —*see* Puncture, head, specified site NEC
  - genital organs, external
    - female S31.532
      - with foreign body S31.542
      - vagina —*see* Puncture, vagina
      - vulva —*see* Puncture, vulva
- Puncture *(Continued)*
  - genital organs, external *(Continued)*
    - male S31.531
      - with foreign body S31.541
      - penis —*see* Puncture, penis
      - scrotum —*see* Puncture, scrotum
      - testis —*see* Puncture, testis
  - groin —*see* Puncture, abdomen, wall
  - gum —*see* Puncture, oral cavity
  - hand S61.439
    - with
      - foreign body S61.449
    - finger —*see* Puncture, finger
    - left S61.432
      - with
        - foreign body S61.442
    - right S61.431
      - with
        - foreign body S61.441
    - thumb —*see* Puncture, thumb
  - head S01.93
    - with foreign body S01.94
    - cheek —*see* Puncture, cheek
    - ear —*see* Puncture, ear
    - eyelid —*see* Puncture, eyelid
    - lip —*see* Puncture, oral cavity
    - nose —*see* Puncture, nose
    - oral cavity —*see* Puncture, oral cavity
    - scalp S01.03
      - with foreign body S01.04
    - specified site NEC S01.83
      - with foreign body S01.84
    - temporomandibular area —*see* Puncture, cheek
  - heart S26.99
    - with hemopericardium S26.09
    - without hemopericardium S26.19
  - heel —*see* Puncture, foot
  - hip S71.039
    - with foreign body S71.049
    - left S71.032
      - with foreign body S71.042
    - right S71.031
      - with foreign body S71.041
  - hymen —*see* Puncture, vagina
  - hypochondrium —*see* Puncture, abdomen, wall
  - hypogastric region —*see* Puncture, abdomen, wall
  - inguinal region —*see* Puncture, abdomen, wall
  - instep —*see* Puncture, foot
  - internal organs —*see* Injury, by site
  - interscapular region —*see* Puncture, thorax, back
  - intestine
    - large
      - colon S36.599
        - ascending S36.590
        - descending S36.592
        - sigmoid S36.593
        - specified site NEC S36.598
        - transverse S36.591
      - rectum S36.69
    - small S36.499
      - duodenum S36.490
      - specified site NEC S36.498
  - intra-abdominal organ S36.99
    - gallbladder S36.128
    - intestine —*see* Puncture, intestine
    - liver S36.118
    - pancreas —*see* Puncture, pancreas
    - peritoneum S36.81
    - specified site NEC S36.898
    - spleen S36.09
    - stomach S36.39
  - jaw —*see* Puncture, head, specified site NEC
  - knee S81.039
    - with foreign body S81.049
    - left S81.032
      - with foreign body S81.042
- Puncture *(Continued)*
  - knee *(Continued)*
    - right S81.031
      - with foreign body S81.041
  - labium (majus) (minus) —*see* Puncture, vulva
  - lacrimal duct —*see* Puncture, eyelid
  - larynx S11.013
    - with foreign body S11.014
  - leg (lower) S81.839
    - with foreign body S81.849
    - foot —*see* Puncture, foot
    - knee —*see* Puncture, knee
    - left S81.832
      - with foreign body S81.842
    - right S81.831
      - with foreign body S81.841
    - upper —*see* Puncture, thigh
  - lip S01.531
    - with foreign body S01.541
  - loin —*see* Puncture, abdomen, wall
  - lower back —*see* Puncture, back, lower
  - lumbar region —*see* Puncture, back, lower
  - malar region —*see* Puncture, head, specified site NEC
  - mammary —*see* Puncture, breast
  - mastoid region —*see* Puncture, head, specified site NEC
  - mouth —*see* Puncture, oral cavity
  - nail
    - finger —*see* Puncture, finger, with damage to nail
    - toe —*see* Puncture, toe, with damage to nail
  - nasal (septum) (sinus) —*see* Puncture, nose
  - nasopharynx —*see* Puncture, head, specified site NEC
  - neck S11.93
    - with foreign body S11.94
    - involving
      - cervical esophagus —*see* Puncture, cervical esophagus
      - larynx —*see* Puncture, larynx
      - pharynx —*see* Puncture, pharynx
      - thyroid gland —*see* Puncture, thyroid gland
      - trachea —*see* Puncture, trachea
    - specified site NEC S11.83
      - with foreign body S11.84
  - nose (septum) (sinus) S01.23
    - with foreign body S01.24
  - ocular —*see* Puncture, eyeball - oral cavity S01.532
    - with foreign body S01.542
  - orbit S05.4- ●
  - palate —*see* Puncture, oral cavity
  - palm —*see* Puncture, hand
  - pancreas S36.299
    - body S36.291
    - head S36.290
    - tail S36.292
  - pelvis —*see* Puncture, back, lower
  - penis S31.23
    - with foreign body S31.24
  - perineum
    - female S31.43
      - with foreign body S31.44
    - male S31.139
      - with foreign body S31.149
  - periocular area (with or without lacrimal passages) —*see* Puncture, eyelid
  - phalanges
    - finger —*see* Puncture, finger
    - toe —*see* Puncture, toe
  - pharynx S11.23
    - with foreign body S11.24
  - pinna —*see* Puncture, ear
  - popliteal space —*see* Puncture, knee
  - prepuce —*see* Puncture, penis
  - pubic region S31.139
    - with foreign body S31.149

Puncture *(Continued)*
- pudendum —*see* Puncture, genital organs, external
- rectovaginal septum —*see* Puncture, vagina
- sacral region —*see* Puncture, back, lower
- sacroiliac region —*see* Puncture, back, lower
- salivary gland —*see* Puncture, oral cavity
- scalp S01.Ø3
  - with foreign body S01.Ø4
- scapular region —*see* Puncture, shoulder
- scrotum S31.33
  - with foreign body S31.34
- shin —*see* Puncture, leg
- shoulder S41.Ø39
  - with foreign body S41.Ø49
  - left S41.Ø32
    - with foreign body S41.Ø42
  - right S41.Ø31
    - with foreign body S41.Ø41
- spermatic cord —*see* Puncture, testis
- sternal region —*see* Puncture, thorax, front
- submaxillary region —*see* Puncture, head, specified site NEC
- submental region —*see* Puncture, head, specified site NEC
- subungual
  - finger(s) —*see* Puncture, finger, with damage to nail
  - toe —*see* Puncture, toe, with damage to nail
- supraclavicular fossa —*see* Puncture, neck, specified site NEC
- temple, temporal region —*see* Puncture, head, specified site NEC
- temporomandibular area —*see* Puncture, cheek
- testis S31.33
  - with foreign body S31.34
- thigh S71.139
  - with foreign body S71.149
  - left S71.132
    - with foreign body S71.142
  - right S71.131
    - with foreign body S71.141
- thorax, thoracic (wall) S21.93
  - with foreign body S21.94
  - back S21.23-●
    - with
      - foreign body S21.24-●
        - with penetration S21.44
      - penetration S21.43
  - breast —*see* Puncture, breast
  - front S21.13-●
    - with
      - foreign body S21.14-●
        - with penetration S21.34
      - penetration S21.33
- throat —*see* Puncture, neck
- thumb S61.Ø39
  - with
    - damage to nail S61.139
      - with
        - foreign body S61.149
    - foreign body S61.Ø49
  - left S61.Ø32
    - with
      - damage to nail S61.132
        - with
          - foreign body S61.142
      - foreign body S61.Ø42
  - right S61.Ø31
    - with
      - damage to nail S61.131
        - with
          - foreign body S61.141
      - foreign body S61.Ø41

Puncture *(Continued)*
- thyroid gland S11.13
  - with foreign body S11.14
- toe(s) S91.139
  - with
    - damage to nail S91.239
      - with
        - foreign body S91.249
    - foreign body S91.149
  - great S91.133
    - with
      - damage to nail S91.233
        - with
          - foreign body S91.243
      - foreign body S91.143
    - left S91.132
      - with
        - damage to nail S91.232
          - with
            - foreign body S91.242
        - foreign body S91.142
    - right S91.131
      - with
        - damage to nail S91.231
          - with
            - foreign body S91.241
        - foreign body S91.141
  - lesser S91.136
    - with
      - damage to nail S91.236
        - with
          - foreign body S91.246
      - foreign body S91.146
    - left S91.135
      - with
        - damage to nail S91.235
          - with
            - foreign body S91.245
        - foreign body S91.145
    - right S91.134
      - with
        - damage to nail S91.234
          - with
            - foreign body S91.244
        - foreign body S91.144
- tongue —*see* Puncture, oral cavity
- trachea S11.Ø23
  - with foreign body S11.Ø24
- tunica vaginalis —*see* Puncture, testis
- tympanum, tympanic membrane S09.2-●
- umbilical region S31.135
  - with foreign body S31.145
- uvula —*see* Puncture, oral cavity
- vagina S31.43
  - with foreign body S31.44
- vocal cords S11.Ø33
  - with foreign body S11.Ø34
- vulva S31.43
  - with foreign body S31.44
- wrist S61.539
  - with
    - foreign body S61.549
  - left S61.532
    - with
      - foreign body S61.542
  - right S61.531
    - with
      - foreign body S61.541

PUO (pyrexia of unknown origin) R5Ø.9

Pupillary membrane (persistent) Q13.89

Pupillotonia —*see* Anomaly, pupil, function, tonic pupil

Purpura D69.2
- abdominal D69.Ø
- allergic D69.Ø
- anaphylactoid D69.Ø
- annularis telangiectodes L81.7
- arthritic D69.Ø
- autoerythrocyte sensitization D69.2
- autoimmune D69.Ø

Purpura *(Continued)*
- bacterial D69.Ø
- Bateman's (senile) D69.2
- capillary fragility (hereditary) (idiopathic) D69.8
- cryoglobulinemic D89.1
- Devil's pinches D69.2
- fibrinolytic —*see* Fibrinolysis
- fulminans, fulminous D65
- gangrenous D65
- hemorrhagic, hemorrhagica D69.3
  - not due to thrombocytopenia D69.Ø
- Henoch (-Schönlein) (allergic) D69.Ø
- hypergammaglobulinemic (benign) (Waldenström's) D89.Ø
- idiopathic (thrombocytopenic) D69.3
  - nonthrombocytopenic D69.Ø
- immune thrombocytopenic D69.3
- infectious D69.Ø
- malignant D69.Ø
- neonatorum P54.5
- nervosa D69.Ø
- newborn P54.5
- nonthrombocytopenic D69.2
  - hemorrhagic D69.Ø
  - idiopathic D69.Ø
- nonthrombopenic D69.2
- peliosis rheumatica D69.Ø
- posttransfusion (post-transfusion) (from (fresh) whole blood or blood products) D69.51
- primary D69.49
- red cell membrane sensitivity D69.2
- rheumatica D69.Ø
- Schönlein (-Henoch) (allergic) D69.Ø
- scorbutic E54 *[D77]*
- senile D69.2
- simplex D69.2
- symptomatica D69.Ø
- telangiectasia annularis L81.7
- thrombocytopenic D69.49
  - congenital D69.42
  - hemorrhagic D69.3
  - hereditary D69.42
  - idiopathic D69.3
  - immune D69.3
  - neonatal, transitory P61.Ø
  - thrombotic M31.1
- thrombohemolytic —*see* Fibrinolysis
- thrombolytic —*see* Fibrinolysis
- thrombopenic D69.49
- thrombotic, thrombocytopenic M31.1
- toxic D69.Ø
- vascular D69.Ø
- visceral symptoms D69.Ø

Purpuric spots R23.3

Purulent —*see* condition

Pus
- in
  - stool R19.5
  - urine N39.Ø
- tube (rupture) —*see* Salpingo-oophoritis

Pustular rash LØ8.Ø

Pustule (nonmalignant) LØ8.9
- malignant A22.Ø

Pustulosis palmaris et plantaris L4Ø.3

Putnam (-Dana) **disease or syndrome** —*see* Degeneration, combined

Putrescent pulp (dental) KØ4.1

Pyarthritis, pyarthrosis —*see* Arthritis, pyogenic or pyemic
- tuberculous —*see* Tuberculosis, joint

Pyelectasis —*see* Hydronephrosis

Pyelitis (congenital) (uremic) —*see also* Pyelonephritis
- with
  - calculus —*see* category N2Ø
    - ➠ with hydronephrosis N13.6
  - contracted kidney N11.9

Pyelitis *(Continued)*
acute N1Ø
chronic N11.9
with calculus —*see* category N2Ø
with hydronephrosis N13.6
cystica N28.84
puerperal (postpartum) O86.21
tuberculous A18.11
Pyelocystitis —*see* Pyelonephritis
Pyelonephritis —*see also* Nephritis, tubulo-interstitial
with
calculus —*see* category N2Ø
with hydronephrosis N13.6
contracted kidney N11.9
acute N1Ø
calculous —*see* category N2Ø
with hydronephrosis N13.6
chronic N11.9
with calculus —*see* category N2Ø
with hydronephrosis N13.6
associated with ureteral obstruction or stricture N11.1
nonobstructive N11.8
with reflux (vesicoureteral) N11.Ø
obstructive N11.1
specified NEC N11.8
in (due to)
brucellosis A23.9 *[N16]*
cryoglobulinemia (mixed) D89.1 *[N16]*
cystinosis E72.Ø4
diphtheria A36.84
glycogen storage disease E74.Ø9 *[N16]*
leukemia NEC C95.9-● *[N16]*
lymphoma NEC C85.9Ø *[N16]*
multiple myeloma C9Ø.Ø-● *[N16]*
obstruction N11.1
Salmonella infection AØ2.25
sarcoidosis D86.84
sepsis A41.9 *[N16]*
Sjögren's disease M35.Ø4
toxoplasmosis B58.83
transplant rejection T86.91 *[N16]*
Wilson's disease E83.Ø1 *[N16]*
nonobstructive N12
with reflux (vesicoureteral) N11.Ø
chronic N11.8
syphilitic A52.75
Pyelonephrosis (obstructive) N11.1
chronic N11.9
Pyelophlebitis I8Ø.8
Pyeloureteritis cystica N28.85
Pyemia, pyemic (fever) (infection) (purulent) —*see also* Sepsis
joint —*see* Arthritis, pyogenic or pyemic
liver K75.1
pneumococcal A4Ø.3
portal K75.1
postvaccinal T88.Ø
puerperal, postpartum, childbirth O85
specified organism NEC A41.89
tuberculous —*see* Tuberculosis, miliary
Pygopagus Q89.4
Pyknoepilepsy (idiopathic) —*see* Pyknolepsy
Pyknolepsy G4Ø.AØ9
intractable G4Ø.A19
with status epilepticus G4Ø.A11
without status epilepticus G4Ø.A19
not intractable G4Ø.AØ9
with status epilepticus G4Ø.AØ1
without status epilepticus G4Ø.AØ9
Pylephlebitis K75.1
Pyle's syndrome Q78.5
Pylethrombophlebitis K75.1
Pylethrombosis K75.1
Pyloritis K29.9Ø
with bleeding K29.91
Pylorospasm (reflex) NEC K31.3
congenital or infantile Q4Ø.Ø
neurotic F45.8
newborn Q4Ø.Ø
psychogenic F45.8
Pylorus, pyloric —*see* condition
Pyoarthrosis —*see* Arthritis, pyogenic or pyemic
Pyocele
mastoid —*see* Mastoiditis, acute
sinus (accessory) —*see* Sinusitis
turbinate (bone) J32.9
urethra —*see also* Urethritis N34.Ø
Pyocolpos —*see* Vaginitis
Pyocystitis N3Ø.8Ø
with hematuria N3Ø.81
Pyoderma, pyodermia LØ8.Ø
gangrenosum L88
newborn P39.4
phagedenic L88
vegetans LØ8.81
Pyodermatitis LØ8.Ø
vegetans LØ8.81
Pyogenic —*see* condition
Pyohydronephrosis N13.6
Pyometra, pyometrium, pyometritis —*see* Endometritis
Pyomyositis (tropical) —*see* Myositis, infective
Pyonephritis N12
Pyonephrosis N13.6
tuberculous A18.11
Pyo-oophoritis —*see* Salpingo-oophoritis
Pyo-ovarium —*see* Salpingo-oophoritis
Pyopericarditis, pyopericardium I3Ø.1
Pyophlebitis —*see* Phlebitis
Pyopneumopericardium I3Ø.1
Pyopneumothorax (infective) J86.9
with fistula J86.Ø
tuberculous NEC A15.6
Pyosalpinx, pyosalpingitis —*see also* Salpingo-oophoritis
Pyothorax J86.9
with fistula J86.Ø
tuberculous NEC A15.6
Pyoureter N28.89
tuberculous A18.11
Pyramidopallidonigral syndrome G2Ø
Pyrexia (of unknown origin) R5Ø.9
atmospheric T67.Ø1
during labor NEC O75.2
heat T67.Ø1
newborn P81.9
environmentally-induced P81.Ø
persistent R5Ø.9
puerperal O86.4
Pyroglobulinemia NEC E88.Ø9
Pyromania F63.1
Pyrosis R12
Pyuria (bacterial) R82.81

P

Q

Q fever A78
  with pneumonia A78
Quadricuspid aortic valve Q23.8
Quadrilateral fever A78
Quadriparesis —*see* Quadriplegia
  meaning muscle weakness M62.81
Quadriplegia G82.5Ø-•
  complete
    C1-C4 level G82.51
    C5-C7 level G82.53
  congenital (cerebral) (spinal) G8Ø.8
    spastic G8Ø.Ø
Quadriplegia *(Continued)*
  embolic (current episode) I63.4-•
  functional R53.2
  incomplete
    C1-C4 level G82.52
    C5-C7 level G82.54
  thrombotic (current episode) I63.3-•
  traumatic — code to injury with seventh character S
    current episode —*see* Injury, spinal (cord), cervical
Quadruplet, pregnancy —*see* Pregnancy, quadruplet
Quarrelsomeness F6Ø.3
Queensland fever A77.3
Quervain's disease M65.4
  thyroid EØ6.1
Queyrat's erythroplasia DØ7.4
  penis DØ7.4
  specified site —*see* Neoplasm, skin, in situ
  unspecified site DØ7.4
Quincke's disease or edema T78.3
  hereditary D84.1
Quinsy (gangrenous) J36
Quintan fever A79.Ø
Quintuplet, pregnancy —*see* Pregnancy, quintuplet

R

Rabbit fever —*see* Tularemia
Rabies A82.9
  contact Z2Ø.3
  exposure to Z2Ø.3
  inoculation reaction —*see* Complications, vaccination
  sylvatic A82.Ø
  urban A82.1
Rachischisis —*see* Spina bifida
Rachitic —*see also* condition
  deformities of spine (late effect) (sequelae) E64.3
  pelvis (late effect) (sequelae) E64.3
    with disproportion (fetopelvic) O33.Ø
      causing obstructed labor O65.Ø
Rachitis, rachitism (acute) (tarda) —*see also* Rickets
  renalis N25.Ø
  sequelae E64.3
Radial nerve —*see* condition
Radiation
  burn —*see* Burn
  effects NOS T66
  sickness NOS T66
  therapy, encounter for Z51.Ø
Radiculitis (pressure) (vertebrogenic) —*see* Radiculopathy
Radiculomyelitis —*see also* Encephalitis
  toxic, due to
    Clostridium tetani A35
    Corynebacterium diphtheriae A36.82
Radiculopathy M54.1Ø
  cervical region M54.12
  cervicothoracic region M54.13
  due to
    disc disorder
      C3 M5Ø.11
      C4 M5Ø.11
      C5 M5Ø.121
      C6 M5Ø.122
      C7 M5Ø.123
      C8 M5Ø.13
    displacement of intervertebral disc —*see* Disorder, disc, with, radiculopathy
  leg M54.1-•
  lumbar region M54.16
  lumbosacral region M54.17
  occipito-atlanto-axial region M54.11
  postherpetic BØ2.29
  sacrococcygeal region M54.18
  syphilitic A52.11
  thoracic region (with visceral pain) M54.14
  thoracolumbar region M54.15
Radiodermal burns (acute, chronic, or occupational) —*see* Burn
Radiodermatitis L58.9
  acute L58.Ø
  chronic L58.1
Radiotherapy session Z51.Ø
RAEB (refractory anemia with excess blasts) D46.2-•
Rage, meaning rabies —*see* Rabies
Ragpicker's disease A22.1
Ragsorter's disease A22.1
Raillietiniasis B71.8
Railroad neurosis F48.8
Railway spine F48.8
Raised —*see also* Elevated
  antibody titer R76.Ø
Rake teeth, tooth M26.39
Rales RØ9.89
Ramifying renal pelvis Q63.8
Ramsay-Hunt disease or syndrome —*see also* Hunt's disease BØ2.21
  meaning dyssynergia cerebellaris myoclonica G11.1
Ranula K11.6
  congenital Q38.4
Rape
  adult
    confirmed T74.21
    suspected T76.21
  alleged, observation or examination, ruled out
    adult ZØ4.41
    child ZØ4.42
  child
    confirmed T74.22
    suspected T76.22
Rapid
  feeble pulse, due to shock, following injury T79.4
  heart (beat) RØØ.Ø
    psychogenic F45.8
  second stage (delivery) O62.3
  time-zone change syndrome G47.25
Rarefaction, bone —*see* Disorder, bone, density and structure, specified NEC
Rash (toxic) R21
  canker A38.9
  diaper L22
  drug (internal use) L27.Ø
    contact —*see also* Dermatitis, due to, drugs, external L25.1
  following immunization T88.1
  food —*see* Dermatitis, due to, food
  heat L74.Ø
  napkin (psoriasiform) L22
  nettle —*see* Urticaria
  pustular LØ8.Ø
  rose R21
    epidemic BØ6.9
  scarlet A38.9
  serum —*see also* Reaction, serum T8Ø.69
  wandering tongue K14.1
Rasmussen aneurysm —*see* Tuberculosis, pulmonary
Rasmussen encephalitis GØ4.81
Rat-bite fever A25.9
  due to Streptobacillus moniliformis A25.1
  spirochetal (morsus muris) A25.Ø
Rathke's pouch tumor D44.3
Raymond (-Céstan) syndrome I65.8
Raynaud's disease, phenomenon or syndrome (secondary) I73.ØØ
  with gangrene (symmetric) I73.Ø1
RDS (newborn) (type I) P22.Ø
  type II P22.1
Reaction —*see also* Disorder
  adaptation —*see* Disorder, adjustment
  adjustment (anxiety) (conduct disorder) (depressiveness) (distress) —*see* Disorder, adjustment
    with
      mutism, elective (child) (adolescent) F94.Ø
  adverse
    food (any) (ingested) NEC T78.1
      anaphylactic —*see* Shock, anaphylactic, due to food
  anaphylactoid —*see* Shock, anaphylactic
  affective —*see* Disorder, mood
  allergic —*see* Allergy
  anaphylactic —*see* Shock, anaphylactic
  anesthesia —*see* Anesthesia, complication
  antitoxin (prophylactic) (therapeutic) —*see* Complications, vaccination
  anxiety F41.1
  Arthus —*see* Arthus' phenomenon
  asthenic F48.8
  combat and operational stress F43.Ø
  compulsive F42.8
  conversion F44.9
  crisis, acute F43.Ø
  deoxyribonuclease (DNA) (DNase) hypersensitivity D69.2
  depressive (single episode) F32.9
    affective (single episode) F31.4
      recurrent episode F33.9
    neurotic F34.1
    psychoneurotic F34.1
Reaction *(Continued)*
  depressive *(Continued)*
    psychotic F32.3
    recurrent —*see* Disorder, depressive, recurrent
  dissociative F44.9
  drug NEC T88.7
    addictive —*see* Dependence, drug
      transmitted via placenta or breast milk —*see* Absorption, drug, addictive, through placenta
    allergic —*see* Allergy, drug
    lichenoid L43.2
    newborn P93.8
      gray baby syndrome P93.Ø
    overdose or poisoning (by accident) —*see* Table of Drugs and Chemicals, by drug, poisoning
    photoallergic L56.1
    phototoxic L56.Ø
    withdrawal —*see* Dependence, by drug, with, withdrawal
      infant of dependent mother P96.1
      newborn P96.1
    wrong substance given or taken (by accident) —*see* Table of Drugs and Chemicals, by drug, poisoning
  fear F4Ø.9
    child (abnormal) F93.8
  febrile nonhemolytic transfusion (FNHTR) R5Ø.84
  fluid loss, cerebrospinal G97.1
  foreign
    body NEC —*see* Granuloma, foreign body
      in operative wound (inadvertently left) —*see* Foreign body, accidentally left during a procedure
    substance accidentally left during a procedure (chemical) (powder) (talc) T81.6Ø
      aseptic peritonitis T81.61
      body or object (instrument) (sponge) (swab) —*see* Foreign body, accidentally left during a procedure
      specified reaction NEC T81.69
  grief —*see* Disorder, adjustment
  Herxheimer's R68.89
  hyperkinetic —*see* Hyperkinesia
  hypochondriacal F45.2Ø
  hypoglycemic, due to insulin E16.Ø
    with coma (diabetic) —*see* Diabetes, coma
      nondiabetic E15
    therapeutic misadventure —*see* subcategory T38.3
  hypomanic F3Ø.8
  hysterical F44.9
  immunization —*see* Complications, vaccination
  incompatibility
    ABO blood group (infusion) (transfusion) —*see* Complication(s), transfusion, incompatibility reaction, ABO
      delayed serologic T8Ø.39
    minor blood group (Duffy) (E) (K) (Kell) (Kidd) (Lewis) (M) (N) (P) (S) T8Ø.89
    Rh (factor) (infusion) (transfusion) —*see* Complication(s), transfusion, incompatibility reaction, Rh (factor)
  inflammatory —*see* Infection
  infusion —*see* Complications, infusion
  inoculation (immune serum) —*see* Complications, vaccination
  insulin T38.3-•
  involutional psychotic —*see* Disorder, depressive
  leukemoid D72.823
    basophilic D72.823
    lymphocytic D72.823
    monocytic D72.823
    myelocytic D72.823
    neutrophilic D72.823

R

Reaction *(Continued)*
- LSD (acute)
  - due to drug abuse —*see* Abuse, drug, hallucinogen
  - due to drug dependence —*see* Dependence, drug, hallucinogen
- lumbar puncture G97.1
- manic-depressive —*see* Disorder, bipolar
- neurasthenic F48.8
- neurogenic —*see* Neurosis
- neurotic F48.9
- neurotic-depressive F34.1
- nitritoid —*see* Crisis, nitritoid - obsessive-compulsive F42
- nonspecific
  - to
    - cell mediated immunity measurement of gamma interferon antigen response without active tuberculosis R76.12
    - QuantiFERON-TB test (QFT) without active tuberculosis R76.12
    - tuberculin test —*see also* Reaction, tuberculin skin test R76.11
- obsessive-compulsive F42.8
- organic, acute or subacute —*see* Delirium
- paranoid (acute) F23
  - chronic F22
  - senile F03
- passive dependency F60.7
- phobic F40.9
- post-traumatic stress, uncomplicated Z73.3
- psychogenic F99
- psychoneurotic —*see also* Neurosis
  - compulsive F42.8
  - depersonalization F48.1
  - depressive F34.1
  - hypochondriacal F45.20
  - neurasthenic F48.8
  - obsessive F42.8
- psychophysiologic —*see* Disorder, somatoform
- psychosomatic —*see* Disorder, somatoform
- psychotic —*see* Psychosis
- scarlet fever toxin —*see* Complications, vaccination
- schizophrenic F23
  - acute (brief) (undifferentiated) F23
  - latent F21
  - undifferentiated (acute) (brief) F23
- serological for syphilis —*see* Serology for syphilis
- serum T80.69
  - anaphylactic (immediate) —*see also* Shock, anaphylactic T80.59
  - specified reaction NEC
    - due to
      - administration of blood and blood products T80.61
      - immunization T80.62
      - serum specified NEC T80.69
      - vaccination T80.62
- situational —*see* Disorder, adjustment
- somatization —*see* Disorder, somatoform
- spinal puncture G97.1
- stress (severe) F43.9
  - acute (agitation) ("daze") (disorientation) (disturbance of consciousness) (flight reaction) (fugue) F43.0
  - specified NEC F43.8
- surgical procedure —*see* Complications, surgical procedure
- tetanus antitoxin —*see* Complications, vaccination
- toxic, to local anesthesia T81.59
  - in labor and delivery O74.4
  - in pregnancy O29.3X- ●
  - postpartum, puerperal O89.3
- toxin-antitoxin —*see* Complications, vaccination
- transfusion (blood) (bone marrow) (lymphocytes) (allergic) —*see* Complications, transfusion
- tuberculin skin test, abnormal R76.11
- vaccination (any) —*see* Complications, vaccination
- withdrawing, child or adolescent F93.8

Reactive airway disease —*see* Asthma

Reactive depression —*see* Reaction, depressive

Rearrangement
- chromosomal
  - balanced (in) Q95.9
    - abnormal individual (autosomal) Q95.2
      - non-sex (autosomal) chromosomes Q95.2
      - sex/non-sex chromosomes Q95.3
    - specified NEC Q95.8

Recalcitrant patient —*see* Noncompliance

Recanalization, thrombus —*see* Thrombosis

Recession, receding
- chamber angle (eye) H21.55- ●
- chin M26.09
- gingival (postinfective) (postoperative)
  - generalized K06.020
    - minimal K06.021
    - moderate K06.022
    - severe K06.023
  - localized K06.010
    - minimal K06.011
    - moderate K06.012
    - severe K06.013

Recklinghausen's disease Q85.01
- bones E21.0

Reclus' disease (cystic) —*see* Mastopathy, cystic

Recrudescent typhus (fever) A75.1

Recruitment, auditory H93.21- ●

Rectalgia K62.89

Rectitis K62.89

Rectocele
- female (without uterine prolapse) N81.6
  - with uterine prolapse N81.4
    - incomplete N81.2
- in pregnancy —*see* Pregnancy, complicated by, abnormal, pelvic organs or tissues NEC
- male K62.3

Rectosigmoid junction —*see* condition

Rectosigmoiditis K63.89
- ulcerative (chronic) K51.30
  - with
    - complication K51.319
      - abscess K51.314
      - fistula K51.313
      - obstruction K51.312
      - rectal bleeding K51.311
      - specified NEC K51.318

Rectourethral —*see* condition

Rectovaginal —*see* condition

Rectovesical —*see* condition

Rectum, rectal —*see* condition

Recurrent —*see* condition
- pregnancy loss —*see* Loss (of), pregnancy, recurrent

Red bugs B88.0

Red-cedar lung or pneumonitis J67.8

Red tide —*see also* Table of Drugs and Chemicals T65.82- ●

Reduced
- mobility Z74.09
- ventilatory or vital capacity R94.2

Redundant, redundancy
- anus (congenital) Q43.8
- clitoris N90.89
- colon (congenital) Q43.8
- foreskin (congenital) N47.8
- intestine (congenital) Q43.8
- labia N90.69
- organ or site, congenital NEC —*see* Accessory
- panniculus (abdominal) E65
- prepuce (congenital) N47.8

Redundant, redundancy *(Continued)*
- pylorus K31.89
- rectum (congenital) Q43.8
- scrotum N50.89
- sigmoid (congenital) Q43.8
- skin L98.7
  - and subcutaneous tissue L98.7
  - of face L57.4
    - eyelids —*see* Blepharochalasis
- stomach K31.89

Reduplication —*see* Duplication

Reflex R29.2
- hyperactive gag J39.2
- pupillary, abnormal —*see* Anomaly, pupil, function
- vasoconstriction I73.9
- vasovagal R55

Reflux K21.9
- acid K21.9
- esophageal K21.9
  - with esophagitis K21.0
  - newborn P78.83
- gastroesophageal K21.9
  - with esophagitis K21.0
- mitral —*see* Insufficiency, mitral
- ureteral —*see* Reflux, vesicoureteral
- vesicoureteral (with scarring) N13.70
  - with
    - nephropathy N13.729
      - with hydroureter N13.739
        - bilateral N13.732
        - unilateral N13.731
      - without hydroureter N13.729
        - bilateral N13.722
        - unilateral N13.721
      - bilateral N13.722
      - unilateral N13.721
    - pyelonephritis (chronic) N11.0
  - without nephropathy N13.71
  - congenital Q62.7

Reforming, artificial openings —*see* Attention to, artificial, opening

Refractive error —*see* Disorder, refraction

Refsum's disease or syndrome G60.1

Refusal of
- food, psychogenic F50.89
- treatment (because of) Z53.20
  - left against medical advice (AMA) Z53.21
  - patient's decision NEC Z53.29
  - reasons of belief or group pressure Z53.1

Regional —*see* condition

Regurgitation R11.10
- aortic (valve) —*see* Insufficiency, aortic
- food —*see also* Vomiting
  - with reswallowing —*see* Rumination
  - newborn P92.1
- gastric contents —*see* Vomiting
- heart —*see* Endocarditis
- mitral (valve) —*see* Insufficiency, mitral
  - congenital Q23.3
- myocardial —*see* Endocarditis
- pulmonary (valve) (heart) I37.1
  - congenital Q22.2
  - syphilitic A52.03
- tricuspid —*see* Insufficiency, tricuspid
- valve, valvular —*see* Endocarditis
  - congenital Q24.8
- vesicoureteral —*see* Reflux, vesicoureteral

Reichmann's disease or syndrome K31.89

Reifenstein syndrome E34.52

Reinsertion
- implantable subdermal contraceptive Z30.46
- intrauterine contraceptive device Z30.433

Reiter's disease, syndrome, or urethritis M02.30
- ankle M02.37- ●
- elbow M02.32- ●
- foot joint M02.37- ●
- hand joint M02.34- ●
- hip M02.35- ●
- knee M02.36- ●

Reiter's disease, syndrome, or urethritis *(Continued)*
multiple site M02.39
shoulder M02.31-•
vertebra M02.38
wrist M02.33-•
Rejection
food, psychogenic F50.89
transplant T86.91
bone T86.830
marrow T86.01
cornea T86.840
heart T86.21
with lung(s) T86.31
intestine T86.850
kidney T86.11
liver T86.41
lung(s) T86.810
with heart T86.31
organ (immune or nonimmune cause) T86.91
pancreas T86.890
skin (allograft) (autograft) T86.820
specified NEC T86.890
stem cell (peripheral blood) (umbilical cord) T86.5
Relapsing fever A68.9
Carter's (Asiatic) A68.1
Dutton's (West African) A68.1
Koch's A68.9
louse-borne (epidemic) A68.0
Novy's (American) A68.1
Obermeyers's (European) A68.0
Spirillum A68.9
tick-borne (endemic) A68.1
Relationship
occlusal
open anterior M26.220
open posterior M26.221
Relaxation
anus (sphincter) K62.89
psychogenic F45.8
arch (foot) —*see also* Deformity, limb, flat foot
back ligaments —*see* Instability, joint, spine
bladder (sphincter) N31.2
cardioesophageal K21.9
cervix —*see* Incompetency, cervix
diaphragm J98.6
joint (capsule) (ligament) (paralytic) —*see* Flail, joint
congenital NEC Q74.8
lumbosacral (joint) —*see* subcategory M53.2
pelvic floor N81.89
perineum N81.89
posture R29.3
rectum (sphincter) K62.89
sacroiliac (joint) —*see* subcategory M53.2
scrotum N50.89
urethra (sphincter) N36.44
vesical N31.2
Release from prison, anxiety concerning Z65.2
Remains
canal of Cloquet Q14.0
capsule (opaque) Q14.8
Remittent fever (malarial) B54
Remnant
canal of Cloquet Q14.0
capsule (opaque) Q14.8
cervix, cervical stump (acquired) (postoperative) N88.8
cystic duct, postcholecystectomy K91.5
fingernail L60.8
congenital Q84.6
meniscus, knee —*see* Derangement, knee, meniscus, specified NEC
thyroglossal duct Q89.2
tonsil J35.8
infected (chronic) J35.01
urachus Q64.4
Removal (from) (of)
artificial
arm Z44.00-•
complete Z44.01-•
partial Z44.02-•
eye Z44.2-•
leg Z44.10-•
complete Z44.11-•
partial Z44.12-•
breast implant Z45.81
cardiac pulse generator (battery) (end-of-life) Z45.010
catheter (urinary) (indwelling) Z46.6
from artificial opening —*see* Attention to, artificial, opening
non-vascular Z46.82
vascular NEC Z45.2
device Z46.9
contraceptive Z30.432
implantable subdermal Z30.46
implanted NEC Z45.89
specified NEC Z46.89
drains Z48.03
dressing (nonsurgical) Z48.00
surgical Z48.01
external
fixation device — code to fracture with seventh character D
prosthesis, prosthetic device Z44.9
breast Z44.3-•
specified NEC Z44.8
home in childhood (to foster home or institution) Z62.29
ileostomy Z43.2
insulin pump Z46.81
myringotomy device (stent) (tube) Z45.82
nervous system device NEC Z46.2
brain neuropacemaker Z46.2
visual substitution device Z46.2
implanted Z45.31
non-vascular catheter Z46.82
organ, prophylactic (for neoplasia management) —*see* Prophylactic, organ removal
orthodontic device Z46.4
staples Z48.02
stent
ureteral Z46.6
suture Z48.02
urinary device Z46.6
vascular access device or catheter Z45.2
Ren
arcuatus Q63.1
mobile, mobilis N28.89
congenital Q63.8
unguliformis Q63.1
Renal —*see* condition
Rendu-Osler-Weber disease or syndrome I78.0
Reninoma D41.0-•
Renon-Delille syndrome E23.3
Reovirus, as cause of disease classified elsewhere B97.5
Repeated falls NEC R29.6
Replaced chromosome by dicentric ring Q93.2
Replacement by artificial or mechanical device or prosthesis of
bladder Z96.0
blood vessel NEC Z95.828
bone NEC Z96.7
cochlea Z96.21
coronary artery Z95.5
eustachian tube Z96.29
eye globe Z97.0
heart Z95.812
valve Z95.2
prosthetic Z95.2
specified NEC Z95.4
xenogenic Z95.3
intestine Z96.89
joint Z96.60
hip —*see* Presence, hip joint implant
knee —*see* Presence, knee joint implant
specified site NEC Z96.698
Replacement by artificial or mechanical device or prosthesis of *(Continued)*
larynx Z96.3
lens Z96.1
limb(s) —*see* Presence, artificial, limb
mandible NEC (for tooth root implant(s)) Z96.5
organ NEC Z96.89
peripheral vessel NEC Z95.828
stapes Z96.29
teeth Z97.2
tendon Z96.7
tissue NEC Z96.89
tooth root(s) Z96.5
vessel NEC Z95.828
coronary (artery) Z95.5
Request for expert evidence Z04.89
Reserve, decreased or low
cardiac —*see* Disease, heart
kidney N28.89
Residual —*see also* condition
ovary syndrome N99.83
state, schizophrenic F20.5
urine R39.198
Resistance, resistant (to)
activated protein C D68.51
complicating pregnancy O26.89
insulin E88.81
organism(s)
to
drug Z16.30
aminoglycosides Z16.29
amoxicillin Z16.11
ampicillin Z16.11
antibiotic(s) Z16.20
multiple Z16.24
specified NEC Z16.29
antifungal Z16.32
antimicrobial (single) Z16.30
multiple Z16.35
specified NEC Z16.39
antimycobacterial (single) Z16.341
multiple Z16.342
antiparasitic Z16.31
antiviral Z16.33
beta lactam antibiotics Z16.10
specified NEC Z16.19
cephalosporins Z16.19
extended beta lactamase (ESBL) Z16.12
fluoroquinolones Z16.23
macrolides Z16.29
methicillin —*see* MRSA
multiple drugs (MDRO)
antibiotics Z16.24
antimicrobial Z16.35
antimycobacterials Z16.342
penicillins Z16.11
quinine (and related compounds) Z16.31
quinolones Z16.23
sulfonamides Z16.29
tetracyclines Z16.29
tuberculostatics (single) Z16.341
multiple Z16.342
vancomycin Z16.21
related antibiotics Z16.22
thyroid hormone E07.89
Resorption
dental (roots) K03.3
alveoli M26.79
teeth (external) (internal) (pathological) (roots) K03.3
Respiration
Cheyne-Stokes R06.3
decreased due to shock, following injury T79.4
disorder of, psychogenic F45.8
insufficient, or poor R06.89
newborn P28.5
painful R07.1
sighing, psychogenic F45.8
Respiratory —*see also* condition
distress syndrome (newborn) (type I) P22.0
type II P22.1

R

Respiratory *(Continued)*
  syncytial virus, as cause of disease classified elsewhere (*see also* Virus, respiratory syncytial (RSV)) B97.4
Respite care Z75.5
Response (drug)
  photoallergic L56.1
  phototoxic L56.Ø
Restenosis
  stent
    vascular
      end stent
        adjacent to stent —*see* Arteriosclerosis
        within the stent
          coronary T82.855
          peripheral T82.856
      in stent
        coronary vessel T82.855
        peripheral vessel T82.856
Restless legs (syndrome) G25.81
Restlessness R45.1
Restoration (of)
  dental
    aesthetically inadequate or displeasing KØ8.56
    defective KØ8.5Ø
      specified NEC KØ8.59
    failure of marginal integrity KØ8.51
    failure of periodontal anatomical intergrity KØ8.54
  organ continuity from previous sterilization (tuboplasty) (vasoplasty) Z31.Ø
    aftercare Z31.42
  tooth (existing)
    contours biologically incompatible with oral health KØ8.54
    open margins KØ8.51
    overhanging KØ8.52
    poor aesthetic KØ8.56
    poor gingival margins KØ8.51
  unsatisfactory, of tooth KØ8.5Ø
    specified NEC KØ8.59
Restorative material (dental)
  allergy to KØ8.55
  fractured KØ8.539
    with loss of material KØ8.531
    without loss of material KØ8.53Ø
  unrepairable overhanging of KØ8.52
Restriction of housing space Z59.1
Rests, ovarian, in fallopian tube Q5Ø.6
Restzustand (schizophrenic) F2Ø.5
Retained —*see also* Retention
  cholelithiasis following cholecystectomy K91.86
  foreign body fragments (type of) Z18.9
    acrylics Z18.2
    animal quill(s) or spines Z18.31
    cement Z18.83
    concrete Z18.83
    crystalline Z18.83
    depleted isotope Z18.Ø9
    depleted uranium Z18.Ø1
    diethylhexyl phthalates Z18.2
    glass Z18.81
    isocyanate Z18.2
    magnetic metal Z18.11
    metal Z18.1Ø
    nonmagnetic metal Z18.12
    nontherapeutic radioactive Z18.Ø9
    organic NEC Z18.39
    plastic Z18.2
    quill(s) (animal) Z18.31
    radioactive (nontherapeutic) NEC Z18.Ø9
    specified NEC Z18.89
    spine(s) (animal) Z18.31
    stone Z18.83
    tooth (teeth) Z18.32
    wood Z18.33
  fragments (type of) Z18.9
    acrylics Z18.2
    animal quill(s) or spines Z18.31
    cement Z18.83
Retained *(Continued)*
  fragments (type of) *(Continued)*
    concrete Z18.83
    crystalline Z18.83
    depleted isotope Z18.Ø9
    depleted uranium Z18.Ø1
    diethylhexyl phthalates Z18.2
    glass Z18.81
    isocyanate Z18.2
    magnetic metal Z18.11
    metal Z18.1Ø
    nonmagnectic metal Z18.12
    nontherapeutic radioactive Z18.Ø9
    organic NEC Z18.39
    plastic Z18.2
    quill(s) (animal) Z18.31
    radioactive (nontherapeutic) NEC Z18.Ø9
    specified NEC Z18.89
    spine(s) (animal) Z18.31
    stone Z18.83
    tooth (teeth) Z18.32
    wood Z18.33
  gallstones, following cholecystectomy K91.86
Retardation
  development, developmental, specific —*see* Disorder, developmental
  endochondral bone growth —*see* Disorder, bone, development or growth
  growth R62.5Ø
    due to malnutrition E45
  mental —*see* Disability, intellectual
  motor function, specific F82
  physical (child) R62.52
    due to malnutrition E45
  reading (specific) F81.Ø
  spelling (specific) (without reading disorder) F81.81
Retching —*see* Vomiting
Retention —*see also* Retained
  bladder —*see* Retention, urine
  carbon dioxide E87.2
  cholelithiasis following cholecystectomy K91.86
  cyst —*see* Cyst
  dead
    fetus (at or near term) (mother) O36.4
      early fetal death OØ2.1
    ovum OØ2.Ø
  decidua (fragments) (following delivery) (with hemorrhage) O72.2
    without hemorrhage O73.1
  deciduous tooth KØØ.6
  dental root KØ8.3
  fecal —*see* Constipation
  fetus
    dead O36.4
      early OØ2.1
  fluid R6Ø.9
  foreign body —*see also* Foreign body, retained
    current trauma - code as Foreign body, by site or type
  gallstones, following cholecystectomy K91.86
  gastric K31.89
  intrauterine contraceptive device, in pregnancy —*see* Pregnancy, complicated by, retention, intrauterine device
  membranes (complicating delivery) (with hemorrhage) O72.2
    with abortion —*see* Abortion, by type
    without hemorrhage O73.1
  meniscus —*see* Derangement, meniscus
  menses N94.89
  milk (puerperal, postpartum) O92.79
  nitrogen, extrarenal R39.2
  ovary syndrome N99.83
  placenta (total) (with hemorrhage) O72.Ø
    without hemorrhage O73.Ø
    portions or fragments (with hemorrhage) O72.2
      without hemorrhage O73.1
Retention *(Continued)*
  products of conception
    early pregnancy (dead fetus) OØ2.1
    following
      delivery (with hemorrhage) O72.2
        without hemorrhage O73.1
  secundines (following delivery) (with hemorrhage) O72.Ø
    without hemorrhage O73.Ø
    complicating puerperium (delayed hemorrhage) O72.2
    partial O72.2
      without hemorrhage O73.1
  smegma, clitoris N9Ø.89
  urine R33.9
    drug-induced R33.Ø
    due to hyperplasia (hypertrophy) of prostate —*see* Hyperplasia, prostate
    organic R33.8
      drug-induced R33.Ø
    psychogenic F45.8
    specified NEC R33.8
  water (in tissues) —*see* Edema
Reticular erythematous mucinosis L98.5
Reticulation, dust —*see* Pneumoconiosis
Reticulocytosis R7Ø.1
Reticuloendotheliosis
  acute infantile C96.Ø
  leukemic C91.4- •
  nonlipid C96.Ø
Reticulohistiocytoma (giant-cell) D76.3
Reticuloid, actinic L57.1
Reticulosis (skin)
  acute of infancy C96.Ø
  hemophagocytic, familial D76.1
  histiocytic medullary C96.A
  lipomelanotic I89.8
  malignant (midline) C86.Ø
  polymorphic C86.Ø
  Sézary —*see* Sézary disease
Retina, retinal —*see also* condition
  dark area D49.81
Retinitis —*see also* Inflammation, chorioretinal
  albuminurica N18.9 *[H32]*
  diabetic —*see* Diabetes, retinitis
  disciformis —*see* Degeneration, macula
  focal —*see* Inflammation, chorioretinal, focal
  gravidarum —*see* Pregnancy, complicated by, specified pregnancy-related condition NEC
  juxtapapillaris —*see* Inflammation, chorioretinal, focal, juxtapapillary
  luetic —*see* Retinitis, syphilitic
  pigmentosa H35.52
  proliferans —*see* Disorder, globe, degenerative, specified type NEC
  proliferating —*see* Disorder, globe, degenerative, specified type NEC
  renal N18.9 *[H32]*
  syphilitic (early) (secondary) A51.43
    central, recurrent A52.71
    congenital (early) A5Ø.Ø1 *[H32]*
    late A52.71
  tuberculous A18.53
Retinoblastoma C69.2- •
  differentiated C69.2- •
  undifferentiated C69.2- •
Retinochoroiditis —*see also* Inflammation, chorioretinal
  disseminated —*see* Inflammation, chorioretinal, disseminated
    syphilitic A52.71
  focal —*see* Inflammation, chorioretinal
  juxtapapillaris —*see* Inflammation, chorioretinal, focal, juxtapapillary
Retinopathy (background) H35.ØØ
  arteriosclerotic I7Ø.8 *[H35.Ø- •]*
  atherosclerotic I7Ø.8 *[H35.Ø- •]*
  central serous —*see* Chorioretinopathy, central serous
  Coats H35.Ø2- •

Retinopathy *(Continued)*
  diabetic —*see* Diabetes, retinopathy
  exudative H35.02-●
  hypertensive H35.03-●
  in (due to)
    diabetes —*see* Diabetes, retinopathy
    sickle-cell disorders D57.-● *[H36]*
  of prematurity H35.10-●
    stage 0 H35.11-●
    stage 1 H35.12-●
    stage 2 H35.13-●
    stage 3 H35.14-●
    stage 4 H35.15-●
    stage 5 H35.16-●
  pigmentary, congenital —*see* Dystrophy,
    retina
  proliferative NEC H35.2-●
    diabetic —*see* Diabetes, retinopathy,
      proliferative
    sickle-cell D57.-● *[H36]*
  solar H31.02-●
Retinoschisis H33.10-●
  congenital Q14.1
  specified type NEC H33.19-●
Retortamoniasis A07.8
Retractile testis Q55.22
Retraction
  cervix —*see* Retroversion, uterus
  drum (membrane) —*see* Disorder, tympanic
    membrane, specified NEC
  finger —*see* Deformity, finger
  lid H02.539
    left H02.536
      lower H02.535
      upper H02.534
    right H02.533
      lower H02.532
      upper H02.531
  lung J98.4
  mediastinum J98.59
  nipple N64.53
    associated with
      lactation O92.03
      pregnancy O92.01-●
      puerperium O92.02
    congenital Q83.8
  palmar fascia M72.0
  pleura —*see* Pleurisy
  ring, uterus (Bandl's) (pathological)
    O62.4
  sternum (congenital) Q76.7
    acquired M95.4
  uterus —*see* Retroversion, uterus
  valve (heart) —*see* Endocarditis
Retrobulbar —*see* condition
Retrocecal —*see* condition
Retrocession —*see* Retroversion
Retrodisplacement —*see* Retroversion
Retroflection, retroflexion —*see* Retroversion
Retrognathia, retrognathism (mandibular)
  (maxillary) M26.19
Retrograde menstruation N92.5
Retroperineal —*see* condition
Retroperitoneal —*see* condition
Retroperitonitis K68.9
Retropharyngeal —*see* condition
Retroplacental —*see* condition
Retroposition —*see* Retroversion
Retroprosthetic membrane T85.398
Retrosternal thyroid (congenital)
  Q89.2
Retroversion, retroverted
  cervix —*see* Retroversion, uterus
  female NEC —*see* Retroversion, uterus
  iris H21.89
  testis (congenital) Q55.29
  uterus (acquired) (acute) (any degree)
    (asymptomatic) (cervix) (postinfectional)
    (postpartal, old) N85.4
    congenital Q51.818
    in pregnancy O34.53-●

Retrovirus, as cause of disease classified
    elsewhere B97.30
  human
    immunodeficiency, type 2 (HIV 2) B97.35
    T-cell lymphotropic
      type I (HTLV-I) B97.33
      type II (HTLV-II) B97.34
  lentivirus B97.31
  oncovirus B97.32
  specified NEC B97.39
Retrusion, premaxilla (developmental) M26.09
Rett's disease or syndrome F84.2
Reverse peristalsis R19.2
Reye's syndrome G93.7
Rh (factor)
  hemolytic disease (newborn) P55.0
  incompatibility, immunization or sensitization
    affecting management of pregnancy NEC
      O36.09-●
    anti-D antibody O36.01-●
    newborn P55.0
    transfusion reaction —*see* Complication(s),
      transfusion, incompatibility reaction,
      Rh (factor)
  negative mother affecting newborn P55.0
  titer elevated —*see* Complication(s),
    transfusion, incompatibility reaction, Rh
    (factor)
  transfusion reaction —*see* Complication(s),
    transfusion, incompatibility reaction, Rh
    (factor)
Rhabdomyolysis (idiopathic) NEC M62.82
  traumatic T79.6
Rhabdomyoma —*see also* Neoplasm, connective
    tissue, benign
  adult —*see* Neoplasm, connective tissue, benign
  fetal —*see* Neoplasm, connective tissue, benign
  glycogenic —*see* Neoplasm, connective tissue,
    benign
Rhabdomyosarcoma (any type) —*see*
    Neoplasm, connective tissue, malignant
Rhabdosarcoma —*see* Rhabdomyosarcoma
Rhesus (factor) incompatibility —*see* Rh,
    incompatibility
Rheumatic (acute) (subacute)
  adherent pericardium I09.2
  chronic I09.89
  coronary arteritis I01.8
  degeneration, myocardium I09.0
  fever (acute) —*see* Fever, rheumatic
  heart —*see* Disease, heart, rheumatic
  myocardial degeneration —*see* Degeneration,
    myocardium
  myocarditis (chronic) (inactive) (with chorea)
    I09.0
    with chorea (acute) (rheumatic)
      (Sydenham's) I02.0
    active or acute I01.2
  pancarditis, acute I01.8
    with chorea (acute (rheumatic)
      Sydenham's) I02.0
  pericarditis (active) (acute) (with effusion)
    (with pneumonia) I01.0
    with chorea (acute) (rheumatic)
      (Sydenham's) I02.0
    chronic or inactive I09.2
  pneumonia I00 *[J17]*
  torticollis M43.6
  typhoid fever A01.09
Rheumatism (articular) (neuralgic)
    (nonarticular) M79.0
  gout —*see* Arthritis, rheumatoid
  intercostal, meaning Tietze's disease M94.0
  palindromic (any site) M12.30
    ankle M12.37-●
    elbow M12.32-●
    foot joint M12.37-●
    hand joint M12.34-●
    hip M12.35-●
    knee M12.36-●
    multiple site M12.39

Rheumatism *(Continued)*
  palindromic *(Continued)*
    shoulder M12.31-●
    specified joint NEC M12.38
    vertebrae M12.38
    wrist M12.33-●
  sciatic M54.4-●
Rheumatoid —*see also* condition
  arthritis —*see also* Arthritis, rheumatoid
    with involvement of organs NEC M05.60
      ankle M05.67-●
      elbow M05.62-●
      foot joint M05.67-●
      hand joint M05.64-●
      hip M05.65-●
      knee M05.66-●
      multiple site M05.69
      shoulder M05.61-●
      vertebra —*see* Spondylitis, ankylosing
      wrist M05.63-●
    seronegative —*see* Arthritis, rheumatoid,
      seronegative
    seropositive —*see* Arthritis, rheumatoid,
      seropositive
  carditis M05.30
    ankle M05.37-●
    elbow M05.32-●
    foot joint M05.37-●
    hand joint M05.34-●
    hip M05.35-●
    knee M05.36-●
    multiple site M05.39
    shoulder M05.31-●
    vertebra —*see* Spondylitis, ankylosing
    wrist M05.33-●
  endocarditis —*see* Rheumatoid, carditis
  lung (disease) M05.10
    ankle M05.17-●
    elbow M05.12-●
    foot joint M05.17-●
    hand joint M05.14-●
    hip M05.15-●
    knee M05.16-●
    multiple site M05.19
    shoulder M05.11-●
    vertebra —*see* Spondylitis, ankylosing
    wrist M05.13-●
  myocarditis —*see* Rheumatoid, carditis
  myopathy M05.40
    ankle M05.47-●
    elbow M05.42-●
    foot joint M05.47-●
    hand joint M05.44-●
    hip M05.45-●
    knee M05.46-●
    multiple site M05.49
    shoulder M05.41-●
    vertebra —*see* Spondylitis, ankylosing
    wrist M05.43-●
  pericarditis —*see* Rheumatoid, carditis
  polyarthritis —*see* Arthritis, rheumatoid
  polyneuropathy M05.50
    ankle M05.57-●
    elbow M05.52-●
    foot joint M05.57-●
    hand joint M05.54-●
    hip M05.55-●
    knee M05.56-●
    multiple site M05.59
    shoulder M05.51-●
    vertebra —*see* Spondylitis, ankylosing
    wrist M05.53-●
  vasculitis M05.20
    ankle M05.27-●
    elbow M05.22-●
    foot joint M05.27-●
    hand joint M05.24-●
    hip M05.25-●
    knee M05.26-●
    multiple site M05.29
    shoulder M05.21-●
    vertebra —*see* Spondylitis, ankylosing
    wrist M05.23-●

Rhinitis (atrophic) (catarrhal) (chronic) (croupous) (fibrinous) (granulomatous) (hyperplastic) (hypertrophic) (membranous) (obstructive) (purulent) (suppurative) (ulcerative) J31.Ø
with
sore throat —*see* Nasopharyngitis
acute JØØ
allergic J3Ø.9
with asthma J45.9Ø9
with
exacerbation (acute) J45.9Ø1
status asthmaticus J45.9Ø2
due to
food J3Ø.5
pollen J3Ø.1
nonseasonal J3Ø.89
perennial J3Ø.89
seasonal NEC J3Ø.2
specified NEC J3Ø.89
infective JØØ
pneumococcal JØØ
syphilitic A52.73
congenital A5Ø.Ø5 *[J99]*
tuberculous A15.8
vasomotor J3Ø.Ø
Rhinoantritis (chronic) —*see* Sinusitis, maxillary
Rhinodacryolith —*see* Dacryolith
Rhinolith (nasal sinus) J34.89
Rhinomegaly J34.89
Rhinopharyngitis (acute) (subacute) —*see also* Nasopharyngitis
chronic J31.1
destructive ulcerating A66.5
mutilans A66.5
Rhinophyma L71.1
Rhinorrhea J34.89
cerebrospinal (fluid) G96.Ø
paroxysmal —*see* Rhinitis, allergic
spasmodic —*see* Rhinitis, allergic
Rhinosalpingitis —*see* Salpingitis, eustachian
Rhinoscleroma A48.8
Rhinosporidiosis B48.1
Rhinovirus infection NEC B34.8
Rhizomelic chondrodysplasia punctata E71.54Ø
Rhythm
atrioventricular nodal I49.8
disorder I49.9
coronary sinus I49.8
ectopic I49.8
nodal I49.8
escape I49.9
heart, abnormal I49.9
idioventricular I44.2
nodal I49.8
sleep, inversion G47.2-●
nonorganic origin —*see* Disorder, sleep, circadian rhythm, psychogenic
Rhytidosis facialis L98.8
Rib —*see also* condition
cervical Q76.5
Riboflavin deficiency E53.Ø
Rice bodies —*see also* Loose, body, joint
knee M23.4-●
Richter syndrome —*see* Leukemia, chronic lymphocytic, B-cell type
Richter's hernia —*see* Hernia, abdomen, with obstruction
Ricinism —*see* Poisoning, food, noxious, plant
Rickets (active) (acute) (adolescent) (chest wall) (congenital) (current) (infantile) (intestinal) E55.Ø
adult —*see* Osteomalacia
celiac K9Ø.Ø
hypophosphatemic with nephrotic-glycosuric dwarfism E72.Ø9
inactive E64.3
kidney N25.Ø
renal N25.Ø
sequelae, any E64.3
vitamin-D-resistant E83.31 *[M9Ø.8Ø]*
Rickettsial disease A79.9
specified type NEC A79.89
Rickettsialpox (Rickettsia akari) A79.1
Rickettsiosis A79.9
due to
Ehrlichia sennetsu A79.81
Rickettsia akari (rickettsialpox) A79.1
specified type NEC A79.89
tick-borne A77.9
vesicular A79.1
Rider's bone —*see* Ossification, muscle, specified NEC
Ridge, alveolus —*see also* condition
flabby KØ6.8
Ridged ear, congenital Q17.3
Riedel's
lobe, liver Q44.7
struma, thyroiditis or disease EØ6.5
Rieger's anomaly or syndrome Q13.81
Riehl's melanosis L81.4
Rietti-Greppi-Micheli anemia D56.9
Rieux's hernia —*see* Hernia, abdomen, specified site NEC
Riga (-Fede) **disease** K14.Ø
Riggs' disease —*see* Periodontitis
Right aortic arch Q25.47
Right middle lobe syndrome J98.11
Rigid, rigidity —*see also* condition
abdominal R19.3Ø
with severe abdominal pain R1Ø.Ø
epigastric R19.36
generalized R19.37
left lower quadrant R19.34
left upper quadrant R19.32
periumbilic R19.35
right lower quadrant R19.33
right upper quadrant R19.31
articular, multiple, congenital Q68.8
cervix (uteri) in pregnancy —*see* Pregnancy, complicated by, abnormal, cervix
hymen (acquired) (congenital) N89.6
nuchal R29.1
pelvic floor in pregnancy —*see* Pregnancy, complicated by, abnormal, pelvic organs or tissues NEC
perineum or vulva in pregnancy —*see* Pregnancy, complicated by, abnormal, vulva
spine —*see* Dorsopathy, specified NEC
vagina in pregnancy —*see* Pregnancy, complicated by, abnormal, vagina
Rigors R68.89
with fever R5Ø.9
Riley-Day syndrome G9Ø.1
RIND (reversible ischemic neurologic deficit) I63.9
Ring(s)
aorta (vascular) Q25.45
Bandl's O62.4
contraction, complicating delivery O62.4
esophageal, lower (muscular) K22.2
Fleischer's (cornea) H18.Ø4-●
hymenal, tight (acquired) (congenital) N89.6
Kayser-Fleischer (cornea) H18.Ø4-●
retraction, uterus, pathological O62.4
Schatzki's (esophagus) (lower) K22.2
congenital Q39.3
Soemmerring's —*see* Cataract, secondary
vascular (congenital) Q25.8
aorta Q25.45
Ringed hair (congenital) Q84.1
Ringworm B35.9
beard B35.Ø
black dot B35.Ø
body B35.4
Burmese B35.5
corporeal B35.4
foot B35.3
groin B35.6
hand B35.2
honeycomb B35.Ø
nails B35.1
Ringworm *(Continued)*
perianal (area) B35.6
scalp B35.Ø
specified NEC B35.8
Tokelau B35.5
Rise, venous pressure I87.8
Rising, PSA following treatment for malignant neoplasm of prostate R97.21
Risk
for
dental caries Z91.849
high Z91.843
low Z91.841
moderate Z91.842
suicidal
meaning personal history of attempted suicide Z91.5
meaning suicidal ideation —*see* Ideation, suicidal
Ritter's disease LØØ
Rivalry, sibling Z62.891
Rivalta's disease A42.2
River blindness B73.Ø1
Robert's pelvis Q74.2
with disproportion (fetopelvic) O33.Ø
causing obstructed labor O65.Ø
Robin (-Pierre) **syndrome** Q87.Ø
Robinow-Silvermann-Smith syndrome Q87.19
Robinson's (hidrotic) **ectodermal dysplasia or syndrome** Q82.4
Robles' disease B73.Ø1
Rocky Mountain (spotted) **fever** A77.Ø
Roetheln —*see* Rubella
Roger's disease Q21.Ø
Rokitansky-Aschoff sinuses (gallbladder) K82.8
Rolando's fracture (displaced) S62.22-●
nondisplaced S62.22-●
Romano-Ward (prolonged QT interval) **syndrome** I45.81
Romberg's disease or syndrome G51.8
Roof, mouth —*see* condition
Rosacea L71.9
acne L71.9
keratitis L71.8
specified NEC L71.8
Rosary, rachitic E55.Ø
Rose
cold J3Ø.1
fever J3Ø.1
rash R21
epidemic BØ6.9
Rosenbach's erysipeloid A26.Ø
Rosenthal's disease or syndrome D68.1
Roseola BØ9
infantum BØ8.2Ø
due to human herpesvirus 6 BØ8.21
due to human herpesvirus 7 BØ8.22
Ross River disease or fever B33.1
Rossbach's disease K31.89
psychogenic F45.8
Rostan's asthma (cardiac) —*see* Failure, ventricular, left
Rotation
anomalous, incomplete or insufficient, intestine Q43.3
cecum (congenital) Q43.3
colon (congenital) Q43.3
spine, incomplete or insufficient —*see* Dorsopathy, deforming, specified NEC
tooth, teeth, fully erupted M26.35
vertebra, incomplete or insufficient —*see* Dorsopathy, deforming, specified NEC
Rotes Quérol disease or syndrome —*see* Hyperostosis, ankylosing
Roth (-Bernhardt) **disease or syndrome** —*see* Meralgia paraesthetica
Rothmund (-Thomson) **syndrome** Q82.8
Rotor's disease or syndrome E8Ø.6
Round
back (with wedging of vertebrae) —*see* Kyphosis
sequelae (late effect) of rickets E64.3

- **Round** *(Continued)*
  - worms (large) (infestation) NEC B82.0
    - Ascariasis *—see also* Ascariasis B77.9
- **Roussy-Lévy syndrome** G60.0
- **Rubella** (German measles) B06.9
  - complication NEC B06.09
    - neurological B06.00
  - congenital P35.0
  - contact Z20.4
  - exposure to Z20.4
  - maternal
    - care for (suspected) damage to fetus O35.3
    - manifest rubella in infant P35.0
    - suspected damage to fetus affecting management of pregnancy O35.3
  - specified complications NEC B06.89
- **Rubeola** (meaning measles) *—see* Measles
  - meaning rubella *—see* Rubella
- **Rubeosis, iris** *—see* Disorder, iris, vascular
- **Rubinstein-Taybi syndrome** Q87.2
- **Rudimentary** (congenital) *—see also* Agenesis
  - arm *—see* Defect, reduction, upper limb
  - bone Q79.9
  - cervix uteri Q51.828
  - eye Q11.2
  - lobule of ear Q17.3
  - patella Q74.1
  - respiratory organs in thoracopagus Q89.4
  - tracheal bronchus Q32.4
  - uterus Q51.818
    - in male Q56.1
  - vagina Q52.0
- **Ruled out condition** *—see* Observation, suspected
- **Rumination** R11.10
  - with nausea R11.2
  - disorder of infancy F98.21
  - neurotic F42.8
  - newborn P92.1
  - obsessional F42.8
  - psychogenic F42.8
- **Runeberg's disease** D51.0
- **Runny nose** R09.89
- **Rupia** (syphilitic) A51.39
  - congenital A50.06
  - tertiary A52.79
- **Rupture, ruptured**
  - abscess (spontaneous) - code by site under Abscess
  - aneurysm *—see* Aneurysm
  - anus (sphincter) *—see* Laceration, anus
  - aorta, aortic I71.8
    - abdominal I71.3
    - arch I71.1
    - ascending I71.1
    - descending I71.8
      - abdominal I71.3
      - thoracic I71.1
    - syphilitic A52.01
    - thoracoabdominal I71.5
    - thorax, thoracic I71.1
    - transverse I71.1
    - traumatic *—see* Injury, aorta, laceration, major
    - valve or cusp *—see also* Endocarditis, aortic I35.8
  - appendix (with peritonitis) (*see also* Appendicitis) K35.32
    - with localized peritonitis (*see also* Appendicitis) K35.32
  - arteriovenous fistula, brain *—see* Fistula, arteriovenous, brain, ruptured
  - artery I77.2
    - brain *—see* Hemorrhage, intracranial, intracerebral
    - coronary *—see* Infarct, myocardium
    - heart *—see* Infarct, myocardium
    - pulmonary I28.8
    - traumatic (complication) *—see* Injury, blood vessel
  - bile duct (common) (hepatic) K83.2
    - cystic K82.2
- **Rupture, ruptured** *(Continued)*
  - bladder (sphincter) (nontraumatic) (spontaneous) N32.89
    - following ectopic or molar pregnancy O08.6
    - obstetrical trauma O71.5
    - traumatic S37.29
  - blood vessel *—see also* Hemorrhage
    - brain *—see* Hemorrhage, intracranial, intracerebral
    - heart *—see* Infarct, myocardium
    - traumatic (complication) *—see* Injury, blood vessel, laceration, major, by site
  - bone *—see* Fracture
  - bowel (nontraumatic) K63.1
  - brain
    - aneurysm (congenital) *—see also* Hemorrhage, intracranial, subarachnoid
      - syphilitic A52.05
    - hemorrhagic *—see* Hemorrhage, intracranial, intracerebral
  - capillaries I78.8
  - cardiac (auricle) (ventricle) (wall) I23.3
    - with hemopericardium I23.0
    - infectional I40.9
    - traumatic *—see* Injury, heart
  - cartilage (articular) (current) *—see also* Sprain
    - knee S83.3-●
    - semilunar *—see* Tear, meniscus
  - cecum (with peritonitis) K65.0
    - with peritoneal abscess K35.33
    - traumatic S36.598
  - celiac artery, traumatic *—see* Injury, blood vessel, celiac artery, laceration, major
  - cerebral aneurysm (congenital) (*see* Hemorrhage, intracranial, subarachnoid)
  - cervix (uteri)
    - with ectopic or molar pregnancy O08.6
    - following ectopic or molar pregnancy O08.6
    - obstetrical trauma O71.3
    - traumatic S37.69
  - chordae tendineae NEC I51.1
    - concurrent with acute myocardial infarction *—see* Infarct, myocardium
    - following acute myocardial infarction (current complication) I23.4
  - choroid (direct) (indirect) (traumatic) H31.32-●
  - circle of Willis I60.6
  - colon (nontraumatic) K63.1
    - traumatic *—see* Injury, intestine, large
  - cornea (traumatic) *—see* Injury, eye, laceration
  - coronary (artery) (thrombotic) *—see* Infarct, myocardium
  - corpus luteum (infected) (ovary) N83.1-●
  - cyst *—see* Cyst
  - cystic duct K82.2
  - Descemet's membrane *—see* Change, corneal membrane, Descemet's, rupture
    - traumatic *—see* Injury, eye, laceration
  - diaphragm, traumatic *—see* Injury, intrathoracic, diaphragm
  - disc *—see* Rupture, intervertebral disc
  - diverticulum (intestine) K57.80
    - with bleeding K57.81
    - bladder N32.3
    - large intestine K57.20
      - with
        - bleeding K57.21
        - small intestine K57.40
          - with bleeding K57.41
    - small intestine K57.00
      - with
        - bleeding K57.01
        - large intestine K57.40
          - with bleeding K57.41
  - duodenal stump K31.89
  - ear drum (nontraumatic) *—see also* Perforation, tympanum
    - traumatic S09.2-●
      - due to blast injury *—see* Injury, blast, ear
  - esophagus K22.3
  - eye (without prolapse or loss of intraocular tissue) *—see* Injury, eye, laceration
- **Rupture, ruptured** *(Continued)*
  - fallopian tube NEC (nonobstetric) (nontraumatic) N83.8
    - due to pregnancy O00.10-●
      - with intrauterine pregnancy O00.11-●
  - fontanel P13.1
  - gallbladder K82.2
    - traumatic S36.128
  - gastric *—see also* Rupture, stomach
    - vessel K92.2
  - globe (eye) (traumatic) *—see* Injury, eye, laceration
  - graafian follicle (hematoma) N83.0-●
  - heart *—see* Rupture, cardiac
  - hymen (nontraumatic) (nonintentional) N89.8
  - internal organ, traumatic *—see* Injury, by site
  - intervertebral disc *—see* Displacement, intervertebral disc
    - traumatic *—see* Rupture, traumatic, intervertebral disc
  - intestine NEC (nontraumatic) K63.1
    - traumatic *—see* Injury, intestine
  - iris *—see also* Abnormality, pupillary
    - traumatic *—see* Injury, eye, laceration
  - joint capsule, traumatic *—see* Sprain
  - kidney (traumatic) S37.06-●
    - birth injury P15.8
    - nontraumatic N28.89
  - lacrimal duct (traumatic) *—see* Injury, eye, specified site NEC
  - lens (cataract) (traumatic) *—see* Cataract, traumatic
  - ligament, traumatic *—see* Rupture, traumatic, ligament, by site
  - liver S36.116
    - birth injury P15.0
  - lymphatic vessel I89.8
  - marginal sinus (placental) (with hemorrhage) *—see* Hemorrhage, antepartum, specified cause NEC
  - membrana tympani (nontraumatic) *—see* Perforation, tympanum
  - membranes (spontaneous)
    - artificial
      - delayed delivery following O75.5
    - delayed delivery following *—see* Pregnancy, complicated by, premature rupture of membranes
  - meningeal artery I60.8
  - meniscus (knee) *—see also* Tear, meniscus
    - old *—see* Derangement, meniscus
    - site other than knee - code as Sprain
  - mesenteric artery, traumatic *—see* Injury, mesenteric, artery, laceration, major
  - mesentery (nontraumatic) K66.8
    - traumatic *—see* Injury, intra-abdominal, specified, site NEC
  - mitral (valve) I34.8
  - muscle (traumatic) *—see also* Strain
    - diastasis *—see* Diastasis, muscle
    - nontraumatic M62.10
      - ankle M62.17-●
      - foot M62.17-●
      - forearm M62.13-●
      - hand M62.14-●
      - lower leg M62.16-●
      - pelvic region M62.15-●
      - shoulder region M62.11-●
      - specified site NEC M62.18
      - thigh M62.15-●
      - upper arm M62.12-●
    - traumatic *—see* Strain, by site
  - musculotendinous junction NEC, nontraumatic *—see* Rupture, tendon, spontaneous
  - mycotic aneurysm causing cerebral hemorrhage *—see* Hemorrhage, intracranial, subarachnoid
  - myocardium, myocardial *—see* Rupture, cardiac
    - traumatic *—see* Injury, heart
  - nontraumatic, meaning hernia *—see* Hernia
  - obstructed *—see* Hernia, by site, obstructed

Rupture, ruptured *(Continued)*
operation wound —*see* Disruption, wound, operation
ovary, ovarian N83.8
corpus luteum cyst N83.1-●
follicle (graafian) N83.Ø-●
oviduct (nonobstetric) (nontraumatic) N83.8
due to pregnancy OØØ.1Ø-●
with intrauterine pregnancy OØØ.11-●
pancreas (nontraumatic) K86.89
traumatic S36.299
papillary muscle NEC I51.2
following acute myocardial infarction (current complication) I23.5
pelvic
floor, complicating delivery O7Ø.1
organ NEC, obstetrical trauma O71.5
perineum (nonobstetric) (nontraumatic) N9Ø.89
complicating delivery —*see* Delivery, complicated, by, laceration, anus (sphincter)
postoperative wound —*see* Disruption, wound, operation
prostate (traumatic) S37.828
pulmonary
artery I28.8
valve (heart) I37.8
vein I28.8
vessel I28.8
pus tube —*see* Salpingitis
pyosalpinx —*see* Salpingitis
rectum (nontraumatic) K63.1
traumatic S36.69
retina, retinal (traumatic) (without detachment) —*see also* Break, retina
with detachment —*see* Detachment, retina, with retinal, break
rotator cuff (nontraumatic) M75.1Ø-●
complete M75.12-●
incomplete M75.11-●
sclera —*see* Injury, eye, laceration
sigmoid (nontraumatic) K63.1
traumatic S36.593
spinal cord —*see also* Injury, spinal cord, by region
due to injury at birth P11.5
newborn (birth injury) P11.5
spleen (traumatic) S36.Ø9
birth injury P15.1
congenital (birth injury) P15.1
due to P. vivax malaria B51.Ø
nontraumatic D73.5
spontaneous D73.5
splenic vein R58
traumatic —*see* Injury, blood vessel, splenic vein
stomach (nontraumatic) (spontaneous) K31.89
traumatic S36.39
supraspinatus (complete) (incomplete) (nontraumatic) —*see* Tear, rotator cuff
symphysis pubis
obstetric O71.6
traumatic S33.4
synovium (cyst) M66.1Ø
ankle M66.17-●
elbow M66.12-●
finger M66.14-●
foot M66.17-●
forearm M66.13-●
hand M66.14-●
pelvic region M66.15-●
shoulder region M66.11-●
specified site NEC M66.18
thigh M66.15-●
toe M66.17-●
upper arm M66.12-●
wrist M66.13-●
tendon (traumatic) —*see* Strain
nontraumatic (spontaneous) M66.9
ankle M66.87-●
extensor M66.2Ø
ankle M66.27-●
foot M66.27-●

Rupture, ruptured *(Continued)*
tendon *(Continued)*
nontraumatic *(Continued)*
extensor *(Continued)*
forearm M66.23-●
hand M66.24-●
lower leg M66.26-●
multiple sites M66.29
pelvic region M66.25-●
shoulder region M66.21-●
specified site NEC M66.28
thigh M66.25-●
upper arm M66.22-●
flexor M66.3Ø
ankle M66.37-●
foot M66.37-●
forearm M66.33-●
hand M66.34-●
lower leg M66.36-●
multiple sites M66.39
pelvic region M66.35-●
shoulder region M66.31-●
specified site NEC M66.38
thigh M66.35-●
upper arm M66.32-●
foot M66.87-●
forearm M66.83-●
hand M66.84-●
lower leg M66.86-●
multiple sites M66.89
pelvic region M66.85-●
shoulder region M66.81-●
specified
site NEC M66.88
tendon M66.8Ø
thigh M66.85-●
upper arm M66.82-●
thoracic duct I89.8
tonsil J35.8
traumatic
aorta —*see* Injury, aorta, laceration, major
diaphragm —*see* Injury, intrathoracic, diaphragm
external site —*see* Wound, open, by site
eye —*see* Injury, eye, laceration
internal organ —*see* Injury, by site
intervertebral disc
cervical S13.Ø
lumbar S33.Ø
thoracic S23.Ø
kidney S37.Ø6-●
ligament —*see also* Sprain
ankle —*see* Sprain, ankle
carpus —*see* Rupture, traumatic, ligament, wrist
collateral (hand) —*see* Rupture, traumatic, ligament, finger, collateral
finger (metacarpophalangeal) (interphalangeal) S63.4Ø-●
collateral S63.41-●
index S63.41-●
little S63.41-●
middle S63.41-●
ring S63.41-●
index S63.4Ø-●
little S63.4Ø-●
middle S63.4Ø-●
palmar S63.42-●
index S63.42-●
little S63.42-●
middle S63.42-●
ring S63.42-●
ring S63.4Ø-●
specified site NEC S63.499
index S63.49-●
little S63.49-●
middle S63.49-●
ring S63.49-●
volar plate S63.43-●
index S63.43-●
little S63.43-●
middle S63.43-●
ring S63.43-●

Rupture, ruptured *(Continued)*
traumatic *(Continued)*
ligament *(Continued)*
foot —*see* Sprain, foot
radial collateral S53.2-●
radiocarpal —*see* Rupture, traumatic, ligament, wrist, radiocarpal
ulnar collateral S53.3-●
ulnocarpal —*see* Rupture, traumatic, ligament, wrist, ulnocarpal
wrist S63.3Ø-●
collateral S63.31-●
radiocarpal S63.32-●
specified site NEC S63.39-●
ulnocarpal (palmar) S63.33-●
liver S36.116
membrana tympani —*see* Rupture, ear drum, traumatic
muscle or tendon —*see* Strain
myocardium —*see* Injury, heart
pancreas S36.299
rectum S36.69
sigmoid S36.593
spleen S36.Ø9
stomach S36.39
symphysis pubis S33.4
tympanum, tympanic (membrane) —*see* Rupture, ear drum, traumatic
ureter S37.19
uterus S37.69
vagina —*see* Injury, vagina
vena cava —*see* Injury, vena cava, laceration, major
tricuspid (heart) (valve) IØ7.8
tube, tubal (nonobstetric) (nontraumatic) N83.8
abscess —*see* Salpingitis
due to pregnancy OØØ.1Ø-●
with intrauterine pregnancy OØØ.11-●
tympanum, tympanic (membrane) (nontraumatic) —*see also* Perforation, tympanic membrane H72.9-●
traumatic —*see* Rupture, ear drum, traumatic
umbilical cord, complicating delivery O69.89
ureter (traumatic) S37.19
nontraumatic N28.89
urethra (nontraumatic) N36.8
with ectopic or molar pregnancy OØ8.6
following ectopic or molar pregnancy OØ8.6
obstetrical trauma O71.5
traumatic S37.39
uterosacral ligament (nonobstetric) (nontraumatic) N83.8
uterus (traumatic) S37.69
before labor O71.Ø-●
during or after labor O71.1
nonpuerperal, nontraumatic N85.8
pregnant (during labor) O71.1
before labor O71.Ø-●
vagina —*see* Injury, vagina
valve, valvular (heart) —*see* Endocarditis
varicose vein —*see* Varix
varix —*see* Varix
vena cava R58
traumatic —*see* Injury, vena cava, laceration, major
vesical (urinary) N32.89
vessel (blood) R58
pulmonary I28.8
traumatic —*see* Injury, blood vessel
viscus R19.8
vulva complicating delivery O7Ø.Ø
Russell-Silver syndrome Q87.19
Russian spring-summer type encephalitis A84.Ø
Rust's disease (tuberculous cervical spondylitis) A18.Ø1
Ruvalcaba-Myhre-Smith syndrome E71.44Ø
Rytand-Lipsitch syndrome I44.2

R

S

Saber, sabre shin or tibia (syphilitic) A50.56 *[M90.8-•]*
Sac lacrimal —*see* condition
Saccharomyces infection B37.9
Saccharopinuria E72.3
Saccular —*see* condition
Sacculation
aorta (nonsyphilitic) —*see* Aneurysm, aorta
bladder N32.3
intralaryngeal (congenital) (ventricular) Q31.3
larynx (congenital) (ventricular) Q31.3
organ or site, congenital —*see* Distortion
pregnant uterus —*see* Pregnancy, complicated by, abnormal, uterus
ureter N28.89
urethra N36.1
vesical N32.3
Sachs' amaurotic familial idiocy or disease E75.02
Sachs-Tay disease E75.02
Sacks-Libman disease M32.11
Sacralgia M53.3
Sacralization Q76.49
Sacrodynia M53.3
Sacroiliac joint —*see* condition
Sacroiliitis NEC M46.1
Sacrum —*see* condition
Saddle
back —*see* Lordosis
embolus
abdominal aorta I74.01
pulmonary artery I26.92
with acute cor pulmonale I26.02
injury — code to condition
nose M95.0
due to syphilis A50.57
Sadism (sexual) F65.52
Sadness, postpartal O90.6
Sadomasochism F65.50
Saemisch's ulcer (cornea) —*see* Ulcer, cornea, central
Sagging
skin and subcutaneous tissue (following bariatric surgery weight loss) (following dietary weight loss) L98.7
Sahib disease B55.0
Sailors' skin L57.8
Saint
Anthony's fire —*see* Erysipelas
triad —*see* Hernia, diaphragm
Vitus' dance —*see* Chorea, Sydenham's
Salaam
attack(s) —*see* Epilepsy, spasms
tic R25.8
Salicylism
abuse F55.8
overdose or wrong substance given —*see* Table of Drugs and Chemicals, by drug, poisoning
Salivary duct or gland —*see* condition
Salivation, excessive K11.7
Salmonella —*see* Infection, Salmonella
Salmonellosis A02.0
Salpingitis (catarrhal) (fallopian tube) (nodular) (pseudofollicular) (purulent) (septic) N70.91
with oophoritis N70.93
acute N70.01
with oophoritis N70.03
chlamydial A56.11
chronic N70.11
with oophoritis N70.13
complicating abortion —*see* Abortion, by type, complicated by, salpingitis
ear —*see* Salpingitis, eustachian
eustachian (tube) H68.00-•
acute H68.01-•
chronic H68.02-•
Salpingitis *(Continued)*
follicularis N70.11
with oophoritis N70.13
gonococcal (acute) (chronic) A54.24
interstitial, chronic N70.11
with oophoritis N70.13
isthmica nodosa N70.11
with oophoritis N70.13
specific (gonococcal) (acute) (chronic) A54.24
tuberculous (acute) (chronic) A18.17
venereal (gonococcal) (acute) (chronic) A54.24
Salpingocele N83.4-•
Salpingo-oophoritis (catarrhal) (purulent) (ruptured) (septic) (suppurative) N70.93
acute N70.03
with ectopic or molar pregnancy O08.0
following ectopic or molar pregnancy O08.0
gonococcal A54.24
chronic N70.13
following ectopic or molar pregnancy O08.0
gonococcal (acute) (chronic) A54.24
puerperal O86.19
specific (gonococcal) (acute) (chronic) A54.24
subacute N70.03
tuberculous (acute) (chronic) A18.17
venereal (gonococcal) (acute) (chronic) A54.24
Salpingo-ovaritis —*see* Salpingo-oophoritis
Salpingoperitonitis —*see* Salpingo-oophoritis
Salzmann's nodular dystrophy —*see* Degeneration, cornea, nodular
Sampson's cyst or tumor N80.1
San Joaquin (Valley) **fever** B38.0
Sandblaster's asthma, lung or pneumoconiosis J62.8
Sander's disease (paranoia) F22
Sandfly fever A93.1
Sandhoff's disease E75.01
Sanfilippo (Type B) (Type C) (Type D) **syndrome** E76.22
Sanger-Brown ataxia G11.2
Sao Paulo fever or typhus A77.0
Saponification, mesenteric K65.8
Sarcocele (benign)
syphilitic A52.76
congenital A50.59
Sarcocystosis A07.8
Sarcoepiplocele —*see* Hernia
Sarcoepiplomphalocele Q79.2
Sarcoid —*see also* Sarcoidosis
arthropathy D86.86
Boeck's D86.9
Darier-Roussy D86.3
iridocyclitis D86.83
meningitis D86.81
myocarditis D86.85
myositis D86.87
pyelonephritis D86.84
Spiegler-Fendt L08.89
Sarcoidosis D86.9
with
cranial nerve palsies D86.82
hepatic granuloma D86.89
polyarthritis D86.86
tubulo-interstitial nephropathy D86.84
combined sites NEC D86.89
lung D86.0
and lymph nodes D86.2
lymph nodes D86.1
and lung D86.2
meninges D86.81
skin D86.3
specified type NEC D86.89
Sarcoma (of) —*see also* Neoplasm, connective tissue, malignant
alveolar soft part —*see* Neoplasm, connective tissue, malignant
ameloblastic C41.1
upper jaw (bone) C41.0
botryoid —*see* Neoplasm, connective tissue, malignant
Sarcoma *(Continued)*
botryoides —*see* Neoplasm, connective tissue, malignant
cerebellar C71.6
circumscribed (arachnoidal) C71.6
circumscribed (arachnoidal) cerebellar C71.6
clear cell —*see also* Neoplasm, connective tissue, malignant
kidney C64.-•
dendritic cells (accessory cells) C96.4
embryonal —*see* Neoplasm, connective tissue, malignant
endometrial (stromal) C54.1
isthmus C54.0
epithelioid (cell) —*see* Neoplasm, connective tissue, malignant
Ewing's —*see* Neoplasm, bone, malignant
follicular dendritic cell C96.4
germinoblastic (diffuse) —*see* Lymphoma, diffuse, large cell
follicular —*see* Lymphoma, follicular, specified NEC
giant cell (except of bone) —*see also* Neoplasm, connective tissue, malignant
bone —*see* Neoplasm, bone, malignant
glomoid —*see* Neoplasm, connective tissue, malignant
granulocytic C92.3-•
hemangioendothelial —*see* Neoplasm, connective tissue, malignant
hemorrhagic, multiple —*see* Sarcoma, Kaposi's
histiocytic C96.A
Hodgkin —*see* Lymphoma, Hodgkin
immunoblastic (diffuse) —*see* Lymphoma, diffuse large cell
interdigitating dendritic cell C96.4
Kaposi's
colon C46.4
connective tissue C46.1
gastrointestinal organ C46.4
lung C46.5-•
lymph node(s) C46.3
palate (hard) (soft) C46.2
rectum C46.4
skin C46.0
specified site NEC C46.7
stomach C46.4
unspecified site C46.9
Kupffer cell C22.3
Langerhans cell C96.4
leptomeningeal —*see* Neoplasm, meninges, malignant
liver NEC C22.4
lymphangioendothelial —*see* Neoplasm, connective tissue, malignant
lymphoblastic —*see* Lymphoma, lymphoblastic (diffuse)
lymphocytic —*see* Lymphoma, small cell B-cell
mast cell C96.22
melanotic —*see* Melanoma
meningeal —*see* Neoplasm, meninges, malignant
meningothelial —*see* Neoplasm, meninges, malignant
mesenchymal —*see also* Neoplasm, connective tissue, malignant
mixed —*see* Neoplasm, connective tissue, malignant
mesothelial —*see* Mesothelioma
monstrocellular
specified site —*see* Neoplasm, malignant, by site
unspecified site C71.9
myeloid C92.3-•
neurogenic —*see* Neoplasm, nerve, malignant
odontogenic C41.1
upper jaw (bone) C41.0

S

Sarcoma (Continued)
osteoblastic —see Neoplasm, bone, malignant
osteogenic —see also Neoplasm, bone, malignant
juxtacortical —see Neoplasm, bone, malignant
periosteal —see Neoplasm, bone, malignant
periosteal —see also Neoplasm, bone, malignant
osteogenic —see Neoplasm, bone, malignant
pleomorphic cell —see Neoplasm, connective tissue, malignant
reticulum cell (diffuse) —see Lymphoma, diffuse large cell
nodular —see Lymphoma, follicular
pleomorphic cell type —see Lymphoma, diffuse large cell
rhabdoid —see Neoplasm, malignant, by site
round cell —see Neoplasm, connective tissue, malignant
small cell —see Neoplasm, connective tissue, malignant
soft tissue —see Neoplasm, connective tissue, malignant
spindle cell —see Neoplasm, connective tissue, malignant
stromal (endometrial) C54.1
isthmus C54.Ø
synovial —see also Neoplasm, connective tissue, malignant
biphasic —see Neoplasm, connective tissue, malignant
epithelioid cell —see Neoplasm, connective tissue, malignant
spindle cell —see Neoplasm, connective tissue, malignant
Sarcomatosis
meningeal —see Neoplasm, meninges, malignant
specified site NEC —see Neoplasm, connective tissue, malignant
unspecified site C8Ø.1
Sarcopenia (age-related) M62.84
Sarcosinemia E72.59
Sarcosporidiosis (intestinal) AØ7.8
Satiety, early R68.81
Saturnine —see condition
Saturnism
overdose or wrong substance given or taken —see Table of Drugs and Chemicals, by drug, poisoning
Satyriasis F52.8
Sauriasis —see Ichthyosis
SBE (subacute bacterial endocarditis) I33.Ø
Scabies (any site) B86
Scabs R23.4
Scaglietti-Dagnini syndrome E22.Ø
Scald —see Burn
Scalenus anticus (anterior) syndrome G54.Ø
Scales R23.4
Scaling, skin R23.4
Scalp —see condition
Scapegoating affecting child Z62.3
Scaphocephaly Q75.Ø
Scapulalgia M89.8X1
Scapulohumeral myopathy G71.Ø2
Scar, scarring —see also Cicatrix L9Ø.5
adherent L9Ø.5
atrophic L9Ø.5
cervix
in pregnancy or childbirth —see Pregnancy, complicated by, abnormal cervix
cheloid L91.Ø
chorioretinal H31.ØØ-●
posterior pole macula H31.Ø1-●
postsurgical H59.81-●
solar retinopathy H31.Ø2-●
specified type NEC H31.Ø9-●

Scar, scarring (Continued)
choroid —see Scar, chorioretinal
conjunctiva H11.24-●
cornea H17.9
xerophthalmic —see also Opacity, cornea
vitamin A deficiency E5Ø.6
duodenum, obstructive K31.5
hypertrophic L91.Ø
keloid L91.Ø
labia N9Ø.89
lung (base) J98.4
macula —see Scar, chorioretinal, posterior pole
muscle M62.89
myocardium, myocardial I25.2
painful L9Ø.5
posterior pole (eye) —see Scar, chorioretinal, posterior pole
retina —see Scar, chorioretinal
trachea J39.8
transmural uterine, in pregnancy O34.29
uterus N85.8
in pregnancy O34.29
vagina N89.8
postoperative N99.2
vulva N9Ø.89
Scarabiasis B88.2
Scarlatina (anginosa) (maligna) A38.9
myocarditis (acute) A38.1
old —see Myocarditis
otitis media A38.Ø
ulcerosa A38.8
Scarlet fever (albuminuria) (angina) A38.9
Schamberg's disease (progressive pigmentary dermatosis) L81.7
Schatzki's ring (acquired) (esophagus) (lower) K22.2
congenital Q39.3
Schaufenster krankheit I2Ø.8
Schaumann's
benign lymphogranulomatosis D86.1
disease or syndrome —see Sarcoidosis
Scheie's syndrome E76.Ø3
Schenck's disease B42.1
Scheuermann's disease or osteochondrosis —see Osteochondrosis, juvenile, spine
Schilder (-Flatau) disease G37.Ø
Schilling-type monocytic leukemia C93.Ø-●
Schimmelbusch's disease, cystic mastitis, or hyperplasia —see Mastopathy, cystic
Schistosoma infestation —see Infestation, Schistosoma
Schistosomiasis B65.9
with muscle disorder B65.9 [M63.8Ø]
ankle B65.9 [M63.87-●]
foot B65.9 [M63.87-●]
forearm B65.9 [M63.83-●]
hand B65.9 [M63.84-●]
lower leg B65.9 [M63.86-●]
multiple sites B65.9 [M63.89]
pelvic region B65.9 [M63.85-●]
shoulder region B65.9 [M63.81-●]
specified site NEC B65.9 [M63.88]
thigh B65.9 [M63.85-●]
upper arm B65.9 [M63.82-●]
Asiatic B65.2
bladder B65.Ø
chestermani B65.8
colon B65.1
cutaneous B65.3
due to
S. haematobium B65.Ø
S. japonicum B65.2
S. mansoni B65.1
S. mattheii B65.8
Eastern B65.2
genitourinary tract B65.Ø
intestinal B65.1
lung NEC B65.9 [J99]
pneumonia B65.9 [J17]
Manson's (intestinal) B65.1

Schistosomiasis (Continued)
oriental B65.2
pulmonary NEC B65.9 [J99]
pneumonia B65.9
Schistosoma
haematobium B65.Ø
japonicum B65.2
mansoni B65.1
specified type NEC B65.8
urinary B65.Ø
vesical B65.Ø
Schizencephaly QØ4.6
Schizoaffective psychosis F25.9
Schizodontia KØØ.2
Schizoid personality F6Ø.1
Schizophrenia, schizophrenic F2Ø.9
acute (brief) (undifferentiated) F23
atypical (form) F2Ø.3
borderline F21
catalepsy F2Ø.2
catatonic (type) (excited) (withdrawn) F2Ø.2
cenesthopathic, cenesthesiopathic F2Ø.89
childhood type F84.5
chronic undifferentiated F2Ø.5
cyclic F25.Ø
disorganized (type) F2Ø.1
flexibilitas cerea F2Ø.2
hebephrenic (type) F2Ø.1
incipient F21
latent F21
negative type F2Ø.5
paranoid (type) F2Ø.Ø
paraphrenic F2Ø.Ø
post-psychotic depression F32.89
prepsychotic F21
prodromal F21
pseudoneurotic F21
pseudopsychopathic F21
reaction F23
residual (state) (type) F2Ø.5
restzustand F2Ø.5
schizoaffective (type) —see Psychosis, schizoaffective
simple (type) F2Ø.89
simplex F2Ø.89
specified type NEC F2Ø.89
spectrum and other psychotic disorder F29
specified NEC F28
stupor F2Ø.2
syndrome of childhood F84.5
undifferentiated (type) F2Ø.3
chronic F2Ø.5
Schizothymia (persistent) F6Ø.1
Schlatter-Osgood disease or osteochondrosis —see Osteochondrosis, juvenile, tibia
Schlatter's tibia —see Osteochondrosis, juvenile, tibia
Schmidt's syndrome (polyglandular, autoimmune) E31.Ø
Schmincke's carcinoma or tumor —see Neoplasm, nasopharynx, malignant
Schmitz (-Stutzer) dysentery AØ3.Ø
Schmorl's disease or nodes
lumbar region M51.46
lumbosacral region M51.47
sacrococcygeal region M53.3
thoracic region M51.44
thoracolumbar region M51.45
Schneiderian
papilloma —see Neoplasm, nasopharynx benign
specified site —see Neoplasm, benign, by site
unspecified site D14.Ø
specified site —see Neoplasm, malignant, by site
unspecified site C3Ø.Ø
Scholte's syndrome (malignant carcinoid) E34.Ø
Scholz (-Bielchowsky-Henneberg) disease or syndrome E75.25
Schönlein (-Henoch) disease or purpura (primary) (rheumatic) D69.Ø

S

- **Schottmuller's disease** A01.4
- **Schroeder's syndrome** (endocrine hypertensive) E27.Ø
- **Schüller-Christian disease or syndrome** C96.5
- **Schultze's type acroparesthesia, simple** I73.89
- **Schultz's disease or syndrome** —*see* Agranulocytosis
- **Schwalbe-Ziehen-Oppenheim disease** G24.1
- **Schwannoma** —*see also* Neoplasm, nerve, benign
  - malignant —*see also* Neoplasm, nerve, malignant
    - with rhabdomyoblastic differentiation —*see* Neoplasm, nerve, malignant
  - melanocytic —*see* Neoplasm, nerve, benign
  - pigmented —*see* Neoplasm, nerve, benign
- **Schwannomatosis** Q85.Ø3
- **Schwartz (-Jampel) syndrome** G71.13
- **Schwartz-Bartter syndrome** E22.2
- **Schweniger-Buzzi anetoderma** L9Ø.1
- **Sciatic** —*see* condition
- **Sciatica** (infective)
  - with lumbago M54.4-●
    - due to intervertebral disc disorder —*see* Disorder, disc, with, radiculopathy
  - due to displacement of intervertebral disc (with lumbago) —*see* Disorder, disc, with, radiculopathy
  - wallet M54.3-●
- **Scimitar syndrome** Q26.8
- **Sclera** —*see* condition
- **Sclerectasia** H15.84-●
- **Scleredema**
  - adultorum —*see* Sclerosis, systemic
  - Buschke's —*see* Sclerosis, systemic
  - newborn P83.Ø
- **Sclerema** (adiposum) (edematosum) (neonatorum) (newborn) P83.Ø
  - adultorum —*see* Sclerosis, systemic
- **Scleriasis** —*see* Scleroderma
- **Scleritis** H15.ØØ-●
  - with corneal involvement H15.Ø4-●
  - anterior H15.Ø1-●
  - brawny H15.Ø2-●
  - in (due to) zoster BØ2.34
  - posterior H15.Ø3-●
  - specified type NEC H15.Ø9-●
  - syphilitic A52.71
  - tuberculous (nodular) A18.51
- **Sclerochoroiditis** H31.8
- **Scleroconjunctivitis** —*see* Scleritis
- **Sclerocystic ovary syndrome** E28.2
- **Sclerodactyly, sclerodactylia** L94.3
- **Scleroderma, sclerodermia** (acrosclerotic) (diffuse) (generalized) (progressive) (pulmonary) —*see also* Sclerosis, systemic M34.9-●
  - circumscribed L94.Ø
  - linear L94.1
  - localized L94.Ø
  - newborn P83.88
  - systemic M34.9
- **Sclerokeratitis** H16.8
  - tuberculous A18.52
- **Scleroma nasi** A48.8
- **Scleromalacia** (perforans) H15.Ø5-●
- **Scleromyxedema** L98.5
- **Sclérose en plaques** G35
- **Sclerosis, sclerotic**
  - adrenal (gland) E27.8
  - Alzheimer's —*see* Disease, Alzheimer's
  - amyotrophic (lateral) G12.21
  - aorta, aortic I7Ø.Ø
    - valve —*see* Endocarditis, aortic
  - artery, arterial, arteriolar, arteriovascular —*see* Arteriosclerosis
  - ascending multiple G35
  - brain (generalized) (lobular) G37.9
    - artery, arterial I67.2
    - diffuse G37.Ø
    - disseminated G35
- **Sclerosis, sclerotic** *(Continued)*
  - brain *(Continued)*
    - insular G35
    - Krabbe's E75.23
    - miliary G35
    - multiple G35
    - presenile (Alzheimer's) —*see* Disease, Alzheimer's, early onset
    - senile (arteriosclerotic) I67.2
    - stem, multiple G35
    - tuberous Q85.1
  - bulbar, multiple G35
  - bundle of His I44.39
  - cardiac —*see* Disease, heart, ischemic, atherosclerotic
  - cardiorenal —*see* Hypertension, cardiorenal
  - cardiovascular —*see also* Disease, cardiovascular
    - renal —*see* Hypertension, cardiorenal
  - cerebellar —*see* Sclerosis, brain
  - cerebral —*see* Sclerosis, brain
  - cerebrospinal (disseminated) (multiple) G35
  - cerebrovascular I67.2
  - choroid —*see* Degeneration, choroid
  - combined (spinal cord) —*see also* Degeneration, combined
    - multiple G35
  - concentric (Balo) G37.5
  - cornea —*see* Opacity, cornea
  - coronary (artery) I25.1Ø
    - with angina pectoris —*see* Arteriosclerosis, coronary (artery),
  - corpus cavernosum
    - female N9Ø.89
    - male N48.6
  - diffuse (brain) (spinal cord) G37.Ø
  - disseminated G35
  - dorsal G35
  - dorsolateral (spinal cord) —*see* Degeneration, combined
  - endometrium N85.5
  - extrapyramidal G25.9
  - eye, nuclear (senile) —*see* Cataract, senile, nuclear
  - focal and segmental (glomerular) —*see also* NØØ-NØ7 with fourth character .1 NØ5.1
  - Friedreich's (spinal cord) G11.1
  - funicular (spermatic cord) N5Ø.89
  - general (vascular) —*see* Arteriosclerosis
  - gland (lymphatic) I89.8
  - hepatic K74.1
    - alcoholic K7Ø.2
  - hereditary
    - cerebellar G11.9
    - spinal (Friedreich's ataxia) G11.1
  - hippocampal G93.81
  - insular G35
  - kidney —*see* Sclerosis, renal
  - larynx J38.7
  - lateral (amyotrophic) (descending) (spinal) G12.21
    - primary G12.23
  - lens, senile nuclear —*see* Cataract, senile, nuclear
  - liver K74.1
    - with fibrosis K74.2
      - alcoholic K7Ø.2
    - alcoholic K7Ø.2
    - cardiac K76.1
  - lung —*see* Fibrosis, lung
  - mastoid —*see* Mastoiditis, chronic
  - mesial temporal G93.81
  - mitral IØ5.8
  - Mönckeberg's (medial) —*see* Arteriosclerosis, extremities
  - multiple (brain stem) (cerebral) (generalized) (spinal cord) G35
  - myocardium, myocardial —*see* Disease, heart, ischemic, atherosclerotic
  - nuclear (senile), eye —*see* Cataract, senile, nuclear
- **Sclerosis, sclerotic** *(Continued)*
  - ovary N83.8
  - pancreas K86.89
  - penis N48.6
  - peripheral arteries —*see* Arteriosclerosis, extremities
  - plaques G35
  - pluriglandular E31.8
  - polyglandular E31.8
  - posterolateral (spinal cord) —*see* Degeneration, combined
  - presenile (Alzheimer's) —*see* Disease, Alzheimer's, early onset
  - primary, lateral G12.23
  - progressive, systemic M34.Ø
  - pulmonary —*see* Fibrosis, lung
    - artery I27.Ø
    - valve (heart) —*see* Endocarditis, pulmonary
  - renal N26.9
    - with
      - cystine storage disease E72.Ø9
      - hypertensive heart disease (conditions in I11) —*see* Hypertension, cardiorenal
    - arteriolar (hyaline) (hyperplastic) —*see* Hypertension, kidney
  - retina (senile) (vascular) H35.ØØ
  - senile (vascular) —*see* Arteriosclerosis
  - spinal (cord) (progressive) G95.89
    - ascending G61.Ø
    - combined —*see also* Degeneration, combined
      - multiple G35
      - syphilitic A52.11
    - disseminated G35
    - dorsolateral —*see* Degeneration, combined
    - hereditary (Friedreich's) (mixed form) G11.1
    - ➠lateral (amyotrophic) G12.21
      - ▶progressive G12.23
    - multiple G35
    - posterior (syphilitic) A52.11
  - stomach K31.89
  - subendocardial, congenital I42.4
  - systemic M34.9
    - with
      - lung involvement M34.81
      - myopathy M34.82
      - polyneuropathy M34.83
    - drug-induced M34.2
    - due to chemicals NEC M34.2
    - progressive M34.Ø
    - specified NEC M34.89
  - temporal (mesial) G93.81
  - tricuspid (heart) (valve) IØ7.8
  - tuberous (brain) Q85.1
  - tympanic membrane —*see* Disorder, tympanic membrane, specified NEC
  - valve, valvular (heart) —*see* Endocarditis
  - vascular —*see* Arteriosclerosis
  - vein I87.8
- **Scoliosis** (acquired) (postural) M41.9
  - adolescent (idiopathic) —*see* Scoliosis, idiopathic, adolescent
  - congenital Q67.5
    - due to bony malformation Q76.3
    - failure of segmentation (hemivertebra) Q76.3
    - hemivertebra fusion Q76.3
    - postural Q67.5
  - idiopathic M41.2Ø
    - adolescent M41.129
      - cervical region M41.122
      - cervicothoracic region M41.123
      - lumbar region M41.126
      - lumbosacral region M41.127
      - thoracic region M41.124
      - thoracolumbar region M41.125
    - cervical region M41.22
    - cervicothoracic region M41.23

Scoliosis *(Continued)*
idiopathic *(Continued)*
infantile M41.ØØ
cervical region M41.Ø2
cervicothoracic region M41.Ø3
lumbar region M41.Ø6
lumbosacral region M41.Ø7
sacrococcygeal region M41.Ø8
thoracic region M41.Ø4
thoracolumbar region M41.Ø5
juvenile M41.119
cervical region M41.112
cervicothoracic region M41.113
lumbar region M41.116
lumbosacral region M41.117
thoracic region M41.114
thoracolumbar region M41.115
lumbar region M41.26
lumbosacral region M41.27
thoracic region M41.24
thoracolumbar region M41.25
infantile —*see* Scoliosis, idiopathic, infantile
neuromuscular M41.4Ø
cervical region M41.42
cervicothoracic region M41.43
lumbar region M41.46
lumbosacral region M41.47
occipito-atlanto-axial region M41.41
thoracic region M41.44
thoracolumbar region M41.45
paralytic —*see* Scoliosis, neuromuscular
postradiation therapy M96.5
rachitic (late effect or sequelae) E64.3 *[M49.8Ø]*
cervical region E64.3 *[M49.82]*
cervicothoracic region E64.3 *[M49.83]*
lumbar region E64.3 *[M49.86]*
lumbosacral region E64.3 *[M49.87]*
multiple sites E64.3 *[M49.89]*
occipito-atlanto-axial region E64.3 *[M49.81]*
sacrococcygeal region E64.3 *[M49.88]*
thoracic region E64.3 *[M49.84]*
thoracolumbar region E64.3 *[M49.85]*
sciatic M54.4-●
secondary (to) NEC M41.5Ø
cerebral palsy, Friedreich's ataxia, poliomyelitis, neuromuscular disorders —*see* Scoliosis, neuromuscular
cervical region M41.52
cervicothoracic region M41.53
lumbar region M41.56
lumbosacral region M41.57
thoracic region M41.54
thoracolumbar region M41.55
specified form NEC M41.8Ø
cervical region M41.82
cervicothoracic region M41.83
lumbar region M41.86
lumbosacral region M41.87
thoracic region M41.84
thoracolumbar region M41.85
thoracogenic M41.3Ø
thoracic region M41.34
thoracolumbar region M41.35
tuberculous A18.Ø1
Scoliotic pelvis
with disproportion (fetopelvic) O33.Ø
causing obstructed labor O65.Ø
Scorbutus, scorbutic —*see also* Scurvy
anemia D53.2
Score, NIHSS (National Institutes of Health Stroke Scale) R29.7-●
Scotoma (arcuate) (Bjerrum) (central) (ring) —*see also* Defect, visual field, localized, scotoma
scintillating H53.19
Scratch —*see* Abrasion
Scratchy throat RØ9.89
Screening (for) Z13.9
alcoholism Z13.33
anemia Z13.Ø
anomaly, congenital Z13.89
antenatal, of mother —*see also* Encounter, antenatal Z36.9
arterial hypertension Z13.6
arthropod-borne viral disease NEC Z11.59
autism Z13.41
bacteriuria, asymptomatic Z13.89
specified NEC Z13.39
behavioral disorder Z13.3Ø
brain injury, traumatic Z13.85Ø
bronchitis, chronic Z13.83
brucellosis Z11.2
cardiovascular disorder Z13.6
cataract Z13.5
chlamydial diseases Z11.8
cholera Z11.Ø
chromosomal abnormalities (nonprocreative) NEC Z13.79
colonoscopy Z12.11
congenital
dislocation of hip Z13.89
eye disorder Z13.5
malformation or deformation Z13.89
contamination NEC Z13.88
cystic fibrosis Z13.228
dengue fever Z11.59
dental disorder Z13.84
depression (adult) (adolescent) (child) Z13.31
maternal Z13.32
perinatal Z13.32
developmental
delays Z13.4Ø
global (milestones) Z13.42
specified NEC Z13.49
handicap Z13.42
in early childhood Z13.42
diabetes mellitus Z13.1
diphtheria Z11.2
disability, intellectual Z13.39
disease or disorder Z13.9
bacterial NEC Z11.2
intestinal infectious Z11.Ø
respiratory tuberculosis Z11.1
behavioral Z13.3Ø
specified NEC Z13.39
developmental delays Z13.4Ø
global (milestones) Z13.42
specified NEC Z13.49
mental health and behavioral Z13.3Ø
specified NEC Z13.39
blood or blood-forming organ Z13.Ø
cardiovascular Z13.6
Chagas' Z11.6
chlamydial Z11.8
dental Z13.89
digestive tract NEC Z13.818
lower GI Z13.811
upper GI Z13.81Ø
ear Z13.5
endocrine Z13.29
eye Z13.5
genitourinary Z13.89
heart Z13.6
human immunodeficiency virus (HIV) infection Z11.4
immunity Z13.Ø
infection
intestinal Z11.Ø
specified NEC Z11.6
infectious Z11.9
metabolic Z13.228
neurological Z13.89
nutritional Z13.21
metabolic Z13.228
lipoid disorders Z13.22Ø
Screening *(Continued)*
disease or disorder *(Continued)*
protozoal Z11.6
intestinal Z11.Ø
respiratory Z13.83
rheumatic Z13.828
rickettsial Z11.8
sexually-transmitted NEC Z11.3
human immunodeficiency virus (HIV) Z11.4
sickle-cell (trait) Z13.Ø
skin Z13.89
specified NEC Z13.89
spirochetal Z11.8
thyroid Z13.29
vascular Z13.6
venereal Z11.3
viral NEC Z11.59
human immunodeficiency virus (HIV) Z11.4
intestinal Z11.Ø
elevated titer Z13.89
emphysema Z13.83
encephalitis, viral (mosquito- or tick-borne) Z11.59
exposure to contaminants (toxic) Z13.88
fever
dengue Z11.59
hemorrhagic Z11.59
yellow Z11.59
filariasis Z11.6
galactosemia Z13.228
gastrointestinal condition Z13.818
genetic (nonprocreative)- for procreative management —*see* Testing, genetic, for procreative management
disease carrier status (nonprocreative) Z13.71
specified NEC (nonprocreative) Z13.79
genitourinary condition Z13.89
glaucoma Z13.5
gonorrhea Z11.3
gout Z13.89
helminthiasis (intestinal) Z11.6
hematopoietic malignancy Z12.89
hemoglobinopathies NEC Z13.Ø
hemorrhagic fever Z11.59
Hodgkin disease Z12.89
human immunodeficiency virus (HIV) Z11.4
human papillomavirus Z11.51
hypertension Z13.6
infant or child (over 28 days old) ZØØ.129
with abnormal findings ZØØ.121
immunity disorders Z13.Ø
infection
mycotic Z11.8
parasitic Z11.8
ingestion of radioactive substance Z13.88
intellectual disability Z13.39
intestinal
helminthiasis Z11.6
infectious disease Z11.Ø
leishmaniasis Z11.6
leprosy Z11.2
leptospirosis Z11.8
leukemia Z12.89
lymphoma Z12.89
malaria Z11.6
malnutrition Z13.29
metabolic Z13.228
nutritional Z13.21
measles Z11.59
mental health disorder Z13.3Ø
specified NEC Z13.39
metabolic errors, inborn Z13.228
multiphasic Z13.89
musculoskeletal disorder Z13.828
osteoporosis Z13.82Ø
mycoses Z11.8

S

Screening *(Continued)*
myocardial infarction (acute) Z13.6
neoplasm (malignant) (of) Z12.9
bladder Z12.6
blood Z12.89
breast Z12.39
routine mammogram Z12.31
cervix Z12.4
colon Z12.11
genitourinary organs NEC Z12.79
bladder Z12.6
cervix Z12.4
ovary Z12.73
prostate Z12.5
testis Z12.71
vagina Z12.72
hematopoietic system Z12.89
intestinal tract Z12.1Ø
colon Z12.11
rectum Z12.12
small intestine Z12.13
lung Z12.2
lymph (glands) Z12.89
nervous system Z12.82
oral cavity Z12.81
prostate Z12.5
rectum Z12.12
respiratory organs Z12.2
skin Z12.83
small intestine Z12.13
specified site NEC Z12.89
stomach Z12.Ø
nephropathy Z13.89
nervous system disorders NEC Z13.858
neurological condition Z13.89
osteoporosis Z13.82Ø
parasitic infestation Z11.9
specified NEC Z11.8
phenylketonuria Z13.228
plague Z11.2
poisoning (chemical) (heavy metal) Z13.88
poliomyelitis Z11.59
postnatal, chromosomal abnormalities Z13.89
prenatal, of mother —*see also* Encounter, antenatal Z36.9
protozoal disease Z11.6
intestinal Z11.Ø
pulmonary tuberculosis Z11.1
radiation exposure Z13.88
respiratory condition Z13.83
respiratory tuberculosis Z11.1
rheumatoid arthritis Z13.828
rubella Z11.59
schistosomiasis Z11.6
sexually-transmitted disease NEC Z11.3
human immunodeficiency virus (HIV) Z11.4
sickle-cell disease or trait Z13.Ø
skin condition Z13.89
sleeping sickness Z11.6
special Z13.9
specified NEC Z13.89
syphilis Z11.3
tetanus Z11.2
trachoma Z11.8
traumatic brain injury Z13.85Ø
trypanosomiasis Z11.6
tuberculosis, respiratory Z11.1
▶ active Z11.1
▶ latent Z11.7
venereal disease Z11.3
viral encephalitis (mosquito- or tick-borne) Z11.59
whooping cough Z11.2
worms, intestinal Z11.6
yaws Z11.8
yellow fever Z11.59
Scrofula, scrofulosis (tuberculosis of cervical lymph glands) A18.2
Scrofulide (primary) (tuberculous) A18.4
Scrofuloderma, scrofulodermia (any site) (primary) A18.4
Scrofulosus lichen (primary) (tuberculous) A18.4
Scrofulous —*see* condition
Scrotal tongue K14.5
Scrotum —*see* condition
Scurvy, scorbutic E54
anemia D53.2
gum E54
infantile E54
rickets E55.Ø *[M9Ø.8Ø]*
Sealpox BØ8.62
Seasickness T75.3
Seatworm (infection) (infestation) B8Ø
Sebaceous —*see also* condition
cyst —*see* Cyst, sebaceous
Seborrhea, seborrheic L21.9
capillitii R23.8
capitis L21.Ø
dermatitis L21.9
infantile L21.1
eczema L21.9
infantile L21.1
sicca L21.Ø
➠ **Seckel's syndrome** Q87.19
Seclusion, pupil —*see* Membrane, pupillary
Second hand tobacco smoke exposure (acute) (chronic) Z77.22
in the perinatal period P96.81
Secondary
dentin (in pulp) KØ4.3
neoplasm, secondaries —*see* Table of Neoplasms, secondary
Secretion
antidiuretic hormone, inappropriate E22.2
catecholamine, by pheochromocytoma E27.5
hormone
antidiuretic, inappropriate (syndrome) E22.2
by
carcinoid tumor E34.Ø
pheochromocytoma E27.5
ectopic NEC E34.2
urinary
excessive R35.8
suppression R34
Section
nerve, traumatic —*see* Injury, nerve
Sedative, hypnotic, or anxiolytic-induced
anxiety disorder F13.98Ø
bipolar and related disorder F13.94
delirium F13.921
depressive disorder F13.94
major neurocognitive disorder F13.97
mild neurocognitive disorder F13.988
psychotic disorder F13.959
sexual dysfunction F13.981
sleep disorder F13.982
Segmentation, incomplete (congenital) —*see also* Fusion
bone NEC Q78.8
lumbosacral (joint) (vertebra) Q76.49
Seitelberger's syndrome (infantile neuraxonal dystrophy) G31.89
Seizure(s) —*see also* Convulsions R56.9
▶ absence G4Ø.A-●
akinetic —*see* Epilepsy, generalized, specified NEC
atonic —*see* Epilepsy, generalized, specified NEC
autonomic (hysterical) F44.5
convulsive —*see* Convulsions
cortical (focal) (motor) —*see* Epilepsy, localization-related, symptomatic, with simple partial seizures
disorder —*see also* Epilepsy G4Ø.9Ø9
due to stroke —*see* Sequelae (of), disease, cerebrovascular, by type, specified NEC
epileptic —*see* Epilepsy
febrile (simple) R56.ØØ
with status epilepticus G4Ø.9Ø1
complex (atypical) (complicated) R56.Ø1
with status epilepticus G4Ø.9Ø1
Seizure *(Continued)*
grand mal G4Ø.4Ø9
intractable G4Ø.419
with status epilepticus G4Ø.411
without status epilepticus G4Ø.419
not intractable G4Ø.4Ø9
with status epilepticus G4Ø.4Ø1
without status epilepticus G4Ø.4Ø9
heart —*see* Disease, heart
hysterical F44.5
intractable G4Ø.919
with status epilepticus G4Ø.911
Jacksonian (focal) (motor type) (sensory type) —*see* Epilepsy, localization-related, symptomatic, with simple partial seizures
newborn P9Ø
nonspecific epileptic
atonic —*see* Epilepsy, generalized, specified NEC
clonic —*see* Epilepsy, generalized, specified NEC
myoclonic —*see* Epilepsy, generalized, specified NEC
tonic —*see* Epilepsy, generalized, specified NEC
tonic-clonic —*see* Epilepsy, generalized, specified NEC
partial, developing into secondarily generalized seizures
complex —*see* Epilepsy, localization-related, symptomatic, with complex partial seizures
simple —*see* Epilepsy, localization-related, symptomatic, with simple partial seizures
➠ petit mal G4Ø.A-●
intractable G4Ø.419
with status epilepticus G4Ø.411
without status epilepticus G4Ø.419
not intractable G4Ø.4Ø9
with status epilepticus G4Ø.4Ø1
without status epilepticus G4Ø.4Ø9
post traumatic R56.1
recurrent G4Ø.9Ø9
specified NEC G4Ø.89
uncinate —*see* Epilepsy, localization-related, symptomatic, with complex partial seizures
Selenium deficiency, dietary E59
Self-damaging behavior (life-style) Z72.89
Self-harm (attempted)
history (personal) Z91.5
in family Z81.8
Self-mutilation (attempted)
history (personal) Z91.5
in family Z81.8
Self-poisoning
history (personal) Z91.5
in family Z81.8
observation following (alleged) attempt ZØ3.6
Semicoma R4Ø.1
Seminal vesiculitis N49.Ø
Seminoma C62.9-●
specified site —*see* Neoplasm, malignant, by site
Senear-Usher disease or syndrome L1Ø.4
Senectus R54
Senescence (without mention of psychosis) R54
Senile, senility —*see also* condition R41.81
with
acute confusional state FØ5
mental changes NOS FØ3
psychosis NEC —*see* Psychosis, senile
asthenia R54
cervix (atrophic) N88.8
debility R54
endometrium (atrophic) N85.8
fallopian tube (atrophic) —*see* Atrophy, fallopian tube
heart (failure) R54

- **Senile, senility** *(Continued)*
  - ovary (atrophic) —*see* Atrophy, ovary
  - premature E34.8
  - vagina, vaginitis (atrophic) N95.2
  - wart L82.1
- **Sensation**
  - burning (skin) R2Ø.8
    - tongue K14.6
  - loss of R2Ø.8
  - prickling (skin) R2Ø.2
  - tingling (skin) R2Ø.2
- **Sense loss**
  - smell —*see* Disturbance, sensation, smell
  - taste —*see* Disturbance, sensation, taste
  - touch R2Ø.8
- **Sensibility disturbance** (cortical) (deep) (vibratory) R2Ø.9
- **Sensitive, sensitivity** —*see also* Allergy
  - carotid sinus G9Ø.Ø1
  - child (excessive) F93.8
  - cold, autoimmune D59.1
  - dentin KØ3.89
  - gluten (non-celiac) K9Ø.41
  - latex Z91.Ø4Ø
  - methemoglobin D74.8
  - tuberculin, without clinical or radiological symptoms R76.11
  - visual
    - glare H53.71
    - impaired contrast H53.72
- **Sensitiver Beziehungswahn** F22
- **Sensitization, auto-erythrocytic** D69.2
- **Separation**
  - anxiety, abnormal (of childhood) F93.Ø
  - apophysis, traumatic - code as Fracture, by site
  - choroid —*see* Detachment, choroid
  - epiphysis, epiphyseal
    - nontraumatic —*see also* Osteochondropathy, specified type NEC
      - upper femoral —*see* Slipped, epiphysis, upper femoral
    - traumatic - code as Fracture, by site
  - fracture —*see* Fracture
  - infundibulum cardiac from right ventricle by a partition Q24.3
  - joint (traumatic) (current) - code by site under Dislocation
  - ▶muscle (nontraumatic) —*see* Diastasis, muscle
  - pubic bone, obstetrical trauma O71.6
  - retina, retinal —*see* Detachment, retina
  - symphysis pubis, obstetrical trauma O71.6
  - tracheal ring, incomplete, congenital Q32.1
- **Sepsis** (generalized) (unspecified organism) A41.9
  - with
    - organ dysfunction (acute) (multiple) R65.2Ø
      - with septic shock R65.21
  - actinomycotic A42.7
  - adrenal hemorrhage syndrome (meningococcal) A39.1
  - anaerobic A41.4
  - Bacillus anthracis A22.7
  - Brucella —*see also* Brucellosis A23.9
  - candidal B37.7
  - cryptogenic A41.9
  - due to device, implant or graft T85.79
    - arterial graft NEC T82.7
    - breast (implant) T85.79
    - catheter NEC T85.79
      - dialysis (renal) T82.7
        - intraperitoneal T85.71
      - infusion NEC T82.7
        - spinal (cranial) (epidural) (intrathecal) (spinal) (subarachnoid) (subdural) T85.735
      - urethral indwelling T83.511
      - urinary T83.518
    - ectopic or molar pregnancy OØ8.82
    - electronic (electrode) (pulse generator) (stimulator)
      - bone T84.7
      - cardiac T82.7
      - nervous system T85.738
        - brain T85.731
        - neurostimulator generator T85.734
        - peripheral nerve T85.732
        - spinal cord T85.733
      - urinary T83.59Ø
    - fixation, internal (orthopedic) —*see* Complication, fixation device, infection
    - gastrointestinal (bile duct) (esophagus) T85.79
      - neurostimulator electrode (lead) T85.732
    - genital T83.69
    - heart NEC T82.7
      - valve (prosthesis) T82.6
        - graft T82.7
    - joint prosthesis —*see* Complication, joint prosthesis, infection
    - ocular (corneal graft) (orbital implant) T85.79
    - orthopedic NEC T84.7
      - fixation device, internal —*see* Complication, fixation device, infection
    - specified NEC T85.79
    - vascular T82.7
    - ventricular intracranial (communicating) shunt T85.73Ø
  - during labor O75.3
  - Enterococcus A41.81
  - Erysipelothrix (rhusiopathiae) (erysipeloid) A26.7
  - Escherichia coli (E. coli) A41.5
  - extraintestinal yersiniosis A28.2
  - following
    - abortion (subsequent episode) OØ8.Ø
      - current episode —*see* Abortion
    - ectopic or molar pregnancy OØ8.82
    - immunization T88.Ø
    - infusion, therapeutic injection or transfusion NEC T8Ø.29
    - obstetrical procedure O86.Ø4
  - gangrenous A41.9
  - gonococcal A54.86
  - Gram-negative (organism) A41.5
    - anaerobic A41.4
  - Haemophilus influenzae A41.3
  - herpesviral BØØ.7
  - intra-abdominal K65.1
  - intraocular —*see* Endophthalmitis, purulent
  - Listeria monocytogenes A32.7
  - localized — code to specific localized infection
    - in operation wound T81.49
    - skin —*see* Abscess
  - malleus A24.Ø
  - melioidosis A24.1
  - meningeal —*see* Meningitis
  - meningococcal A39.4
    - acute A39.2
    - chronic A39.3
  - MSSA (Methicillin susceptible Staphylococcus aureus) A41.Ø1
  - newborn P36.9
    - due to
      - anaerobes NEC P36.5
      - Escherichia coli P36.4
      - Staphylococcus P36.3Ø
        - aureus P36.2
        - specified NEC P36.39
      - Streptococcus P36.1Ø
        - group B P36.Ø
        - specified NEC P36.19
    - specified NEC P36.8
  - Pasteurella multocida A28.Ø
  - pelvic, puerperal, postpartum, childbirth O85
  - pneumococcal A4Ø.3
  - postprocedural T81.44
  - puerperal, postpartum, childbirth (pelvic) O85
  - Salmonella (arizonae) (cholerae-suis) (enteritidis) (typhimurium) AØ2.1
  - severe R65.2Ø
    - with septic shock R65.21
  - Shigella (*see also* Dysentery, bacillary) AØ3.9
  - skin, localized —*see* Abscess
  - specified organism NEC A41.89
  - Staphylococcus, staphylococcal A41.2
    - aureus (methicillin susceptible) (MSSA) A41.Ø1
      - methicillin resistant (MRSA) A41.Ø2
    - coagulase-negative A41.1
    - specified NEC A41.1
  - Streptococcus, streptococcal A4Ø.9
    - agalactiae A4Ø.1
    - group
      - A A4Ø.Ø
      - B A4Ø.1
      - D A41.81
    - neonatal P36.1Ø
      - group B P36.Ø
      - specified NEC P36.19
    - pneumoniae A4Ø.3
    - pyogenes A4Ø.Ø
    - specified NEC A4Ø.8
  - tracheostomy stoma J95.Ø2
  - tularemic A21.7
  - umbilical, umbilical cord (newborn) —*see* Sepsis, newborn
  - Yersinia pestis A2Ø.7
- **Septate** —*see* Septum
- **Septic** —*see* condition
  - arm —*see* Cellulitis, upper limb
    - with lymphangitis —*see* Lymphangitis, acute, upper limb
  - embolus —*see* Embolism
  - finger —*see* Cellulitis, digit
    - with lymphangitis —*see* Lymphangitis, acute, digit
  - foot —*see* Cellulitis, lower limb
    - with lymphangitis —*see* Lymphangitis, acute, lower limb
  - gallbladder (acute) K81.Ø
  - hand —*see* Cellulitis, upper limb
    - with lymphangitis —*see* Lymphangitis, acute, upper limb
  - joint —*see* Arthritis, pyogenic or pyemic
  - leg —*see* Cellulitis, lower limb
    - with lymphangitis —*see* Lymphangitis, acute, lower limb
  - nail —*see also* Cellulitis, digit
    - with lymphangitis —*see* Lymphangitis, acute, digit
  - sore —*see also* Abscess
    - throat JØ2.Ø
      - streptococcal JØ2.Ø
  - spleen (acute) D73.89
  - teeth, tooth (pulpal origin) KØ4.4
  - throat —*see* Pharyngitis
  - thrombus —*see* Thrombosis
  - toe —*see* Cellulitis, digit
    - with lymphangitis —*see* Lymphangitis, acute, digit
  - tonsils, chronic J35.Ø1
    - with adenoiditis J35.Ø3
  - uterus —*see* Endometritis
- **Septicemia** A41.9
  - meaning sepsis —*see* Sepsis
- **Septum, septate** (congenital) —*see also* Anomaly, by site
  - anal Q42.3
    - with fistula Q42.2
  - aqueduct of Sylvius QØ3.Ø
    - with spina bifida —*see* Spina bifida, by site, with hydrocephalus
  - uterus (complete) (partial) Q51.2Ø
    - complete Q51.21
    - partial Q51.22
    - specified NEC Q51.28

S

Septum, septate *(Continued)*
vagina Q52.10
in pregnancy —*see* Pregnancy, complicated by, abnormal vagina
causing obstructed labor O65.5
longitudinal Q52.129
microperforate
left side Q52.124
right side Q52.123
nonobstruction Q52.120
obstructing Q52.129
left side Q52.122
right side Q52.121
transverse Q52.11
Sequelae (of) —*see also* condition
abscess, intracranial or intraspinal (conditions in G06) G09
amputation — code to injury with seventh character S
burn and corrosion — code to injury with seventh character S
calcium deficiency E64.8
cerebrovascular disease —*see* Sequelae, disease, cerebrovascular
childbirth O94
contusion — code to injury with seventh character S
corrosion —*see* Sequelae, burn and corrosion
crushing injury — code to injury with seventh character S
disease
cerebrovascular I69.90
alteration of sensation I69.998
aphasia I69.920
apraxia I69.990
ataxia I69.993
cognitive deficits I69.91
disturbance of vision I69.998
dysarthria I69.922
dysphagia I69.991
dysphasia I69.921
facial droop I69.992
facial weakness I69.992
fluency disorder I69.923
hemiplegia I69.95-●
hemorrhage
intracerebral —*see* Sequelae, hemorrhage, intracerebral
intracranial, nontraumatic NEC —*see* Sequelae, hemorrhage, intracranial, nontraumatic
subarachnoid —*see* Sequelae, hemorrhage, subarachnoid
language deficit I69.928
monoplegia
lower limb I69.94-●
upper limb I69.93-●
paralytic syndrome I69.96-●
specified effect NEC I69.998
specified type NEC I69.80
alteration of sensation I69.898
aphasia I69.820
apraxia I69.890
ataxia I69.893
cognitive deficits I69.81
disturbance of vision I69.898
dysarthria I69.822
dysphagia I69.891
dysphasia I69.821
facial droop I69.892
facial weakness I69.892
fluency disorder I69.823
hemiplegia I69.85-●
language deficit I69.828
monoplegia
lower limb I69.84-●
upper limb I69.83-●
paralytic syndrome I69.86-●
specified effect NEC I69.898
speech deficit I69.928
speech deficit I69.828
stroke NOS —*see* Sequelae, stroke NOS

Sequelae *(Continued)*
dislocation — code to injury with seventh character S
encephalitis or encephalomyelitis (conditions in G04) G09
in infectious disease NEC B94.8
viral B94.1
external cause — code to injury with seventh character S
foreign body entering natural orifice — code to injury with seventh character S
fracture — code to injury with seventh character S
frostbite — code to injury with seventh character S
Hansen's disease B92
hemorrhage
intracerebral I69.10
alteration of sensation I69.198
aphasia I69.120
apraxia I69.190
ataxia I69.193
cognitive deficits I69.11
disturbance of vision I69.198
dysarthria I69.122
dysphagia I69.191
dysphasia I69.121
facial droop I69.192
facial weakness I69.192
fluency disorder I69.123
hemiplegia I69.15-●
language deficit NEC I69.128
monoplegia
lower limb I69.14-●
upper limb I69.13-●
paralytic syndrome I69.16-●
specified effect NEC I69.198
speech deficit NEC I69.128
intracranial, nontraumatic NEC I69.20
alteration of sensation I69.298
aphasia I69.220
apraxia I69.290
ataxia I69.293
cognitive deficits I69.21
disturbance of vision I69.298
dysarthria I69.222
dysphagia I69.291
dysphasia I69.221
facial droop I69.292
facial weakness I69.292
fluency disorder I69.223
hemiplegia I69.25-●
language deficit NEC I69.228
monoplegia
lower limb I69.24-●
upper limb I69.23-●
paralytic syndrome I69.26-●
specified effect NEC I69.298
speech deficit NEC I69.228
subarachnoid I69.00
alteration of sensation I69.098
aphasia I69.020
apraxia I69.090
ataxia I69.093
cognitive deficits —*see* subcategory I69.01-●
disturbance of vision I69.098
dysarthria I69.022
dysphagia I69.091
dysphasia I69.021
facial droop I69.092
facial weakness I69.092
fluency disorder I69.023
hemiplegia I69.05-●
language deficit NEC I69.028
monoplegia
lower limb I69.04-●
upper limb I69.03-●
paralytic syndrome I69.06-●
specified effect NEC I69.098
speech deficit NEC I69.028

Sequelae *(Continued)*
hepatitis, viral B94.2
hyperalimentation E68
infarction
cerebral I69.30
alteration of sensation I69.398
aphasia I69.320
apraxia I69.390
ataxia I69.393
cognitive deficits I69.31
disturbance of vision I69.398
dysarthria I69.322
dysphagia I69.391
dysphasia I69.321
facial droop I69.392
facial weakness I69.392
fluency disorder I69.323
hemiplegia I69.35-●
language deficit NEC I69.328
monoplegia
lower limb I69.34-●
upper limb I69.33-●
paralytic syndrome I69.36-●
specified effect NEC I69.398
speech deficit NEC I69.328
infection, pyogenic, intracranial or intraspinal G09
infectious disease B94.9
specified NEC B94.8
injury — code to injury with seventh character S
leprosy B92
meningitis
bacterial (conditions in G00) G09
other or unspecified cause (conditions in G03) G09
muscle (and tendon) injury — code to injury with seventh character S
myelitis —*see* Sequelae, encephalitis
niacin deficiency E64.8
nutritional deficiency E64.9
specified NEC E64.8
obstetrical condition O94
parasitic disease B94.9
phlebitis or thrombophlebitis of intracranial or intraspinal venous sinuses and veins (conditions in G08) G09
poisoning — code to poisoning with seventh character S
nonmedicinal substance —*see* Sequelae, toxic effect, nonmedicinal substance
poliomyelitis (acute) B91
pregnancy O94
protein-energy malnutrition E64.0
puerperium O94
rickets E64.3
selenium deficiency E64.8
sprain and strain — code to injury with seventh character S
stroke NOS I69.30
alteration in sensation I69.398
aphasia I69.320
apraxia I69.390
ataxia I69.393
cognitive deficits I69.31
disturbance of vision I69.398
dysarthria I69.322
dysphagia I69.391
dysphasia I69.321
facial droop I69.392
facial weakness I69.392
hemiplegia I69.35-●
language deficit NEC I69.328
monoplegia
lower limb I69.34-●
upper limb I69.33-●
paralytic syndrome I69.36-●
specified effect NEC I69.398
speech deficit NEC I69.328
tendon and muscle injury — code to injury with seventh character S

S

Sequelae (Continued)
thiamine deficiency E64.8
trachoma B94.Ø
tuberculosis B9Ø.9
bones and joints B9Ø.2
central nervous system B9Ø.Ø
genitourinary B9Ø.1
pulmonary (respiratory) B9Ø.9
specified organs NEC B9Ø.8
viral
encephalitis B94.1
hepatitis B94.2
vitamin deficiency NEC E64.8
A E64.1
B E64.8
C E64.2
wound, open — code to injury with seventh character S
Sequestration —*see also* Sequestrum
disk —*see* Displacement, intervertebral disk
lung, congenital Q33.2
Sequestrum
bone —*see* Osteomyelitis, chronic
dental M27.2
jaw bone M27.2
orbit —*see* Osteomyelitis, orbit
sinus (accessory) (nasal) —*see* Sinusitis
Sequoiosis lung or pneumonitis J67.8
Serology for syphilis
doubtful
with signs or symptoms - code by site and stage under Syphilis
follow-up of latent syphilis —*see* Syphilis, latent
negative, with signs or symptoms — code by site and stage under Syphilis
positive A53.Ø
with signs or symptoms - code by site and stage under Syphilis
reactivated A53.Ø
Seroma —*see also* Hematoma
postprocedural —*see* Complication, postprocedural, seroma
traumatic, secondary and recurrent T79.2
Seropurulent —*see* condition
Serositis, multiple K65.8
pericardial I31.1
peritoneal K65.8
Serous —*see* condition
Sertoli cell
adenoma
specified site —*see* Neoplasm, benign, by site
unspecified site
female D27.9
male D29.2Ø
carcinoma
specified site —*see* Neoplasm, malignant, by site
unspecified site (male) C62.9-●
female C56.9
tumor
with lipid storage
specified site —*see* Neoplasm, benign, by site
unspecified site
female D27.9
male D29.2Ø
specified site —*see* Neoplasm, benign, by site
unspecified site
female D27.9
male D29.2Ø
Sertoli-Leydig cell tumor —*see* Neoplasm, benign, by site
specified site —*see* Neoplasm, benign, by site
unspecified site
female D27.9
male D29.2Ø
Serum
allergy, allergic reaction —*see also* Reaction, serum T8Ø.69
shock —*see also* Shock, anaphylactic T8Ø.59
arthritis —*see also* Reaction, serum T8Ø.69
complication or reaction NEC —*see also* Reaction, serum T8Ø.69
disease NEC —*see also* Reaction, serum T8Ø.69
hepatitis —*see also* Hepatitis, viral, type B carrier (suspected) of B18.1
intoxication —*see also* Reaction, serum T8Ø.69
neuritis —*see also* Reaction, serum T8Ø.69
neuropathy G61.1
poisoning NEC —*see also* Reaction, serum T8Ø.69
rash NEC —*see also* Reaction, serum T8Ø.69
reaction NEC —*see also* Reaction, serum T8Ø.69
sickness NEC —*see also* Reaction, serum T8Ø.69
urticaria —*see also* Reaction, serum T8Ø.69
Sesamoiditis M25.8-●
Sever's disease or osteochondrosis —*see* Osteochondrosis, juvenile, tarsus
Severe sepsis R65.2Ø
with septic shock R65.21
Sex
chromosome mosaics Q97.8
lines with various numbers of X chromosomes Q97.2
education Z7Ø.8
reassignment surgery status Z87.89Ø
Sextuplet pregnancy —*see* Pregnancy, sextuplet
Sexual
function, disorder of (psychogenic) F52.9
immaturity (female) (male) E3Ø.Ø
impotence (psychogenic) organic origin NEC —*see* Dysfunction, sexual, male
precocity (constitutional) (cryptogenic) (female) (idiopathic) (male) E3Ø.1
Sexuality, pathologic —*see* Deviation, sexual
Sézary disease C84.1-●
Shadow, lung R91.8
Shaking palsy or paralysis —*see* Parkinsonism
Shallowness, acetabulum —*see* Derangement, joint, specified type NEC, hip
Shaver's disease J63.1
Sheath (tendon) —*see* condition
Sheathing, retinal vessels H35.Ø1-●
Shedding
nail L6Ø.8
premature, primary (deciduous) teeth KØØ.6
Sheehan's disease or syndrome E23.Ø
Shelf, rectal K62.89
Shell teeth KØØ.5
Shellshock (current) F43.Ø
lasting state —*see* Disorder, post-traumatic stress
Shield kidney Q63.1
Shift
auditory threshold (temporary) H93.24-●
mediastinal R93.89
Shifting sleep-work schedule (affecting sleep) G47.26
Shiga (-Kruse) dysentery AØ3.Ø
Shiga's bacillus AØ3.Ø
Shigella (dysentery) —*see* Dysentery, bacillary
Shigellosis AØ3.9
Group A AØ3.Ø
Group B AØ3.1
Group C AØ3.2
Group D AØ3.3
Shin splints S86.89
Shingles —*see* Herpes, zoster
Shipyard disease or eye B3Ø.Ø
Shirodkar suture, in pregnancy —*see* Pregnancy, complicated by, incompetent cervix
Shock R57.9
with ectopic or molar pregnancy OØ8.3
adrenal (cortical) (Addisonian) E27.2
adverse food reaction (anaphylactic) —*see* Shock, anaphylactic, due to food
allergic —*see* Shock, anaphylactic
anaphylactic T78.2
chemical —*see* Table of Drugs and Chemicals
due to drug or medicinal substance
correct substance properly administered T88.6
overdose or wrong substance given or taken (by accident) —*see* Table of Drugs and Chemicals, by drug, poisoning
due to food (nonpoisonous) T78.ØØ
additives T78.Ø6
dairy products T78.Ø7
eggs T78.Ø8
fish T78.Ø3
shellfish T78.Ø2
fruit T78.Ø4
milk T78.Ø7
nuts T78.Ø5
multiple types T78.Ø5
peanuts T78.Ø1
peanuts T78.Ø1
seeds T78.Ø5
specified type NEC T78.Ø9
vegetable T78.Ø4
following sting(s) —*see* Venom
immunization T8Ø.52
serum T8Ø.59
blood and blood products T8Ø.51
immunization T8Ø.52
specified NEC T8Ø.59
vaccination T8Ø.52
anaphylactoid —*see* Shock, anaphylactic
anesthetic
correct substance properly administered T88.2
overdose or wrong substance given or taken —*see* Table of Drugs and Chemicals, by drug, poisoning
specified anesthetic —*see* Table of Drugs and Chemicals, by drug, poisoning
cardiogenic R57.Ø
chemical substance —*see* Table of Drugs and Chemicals
complicating ectopic or molar pregnancy OØ8.3
culture —*see* Disorder, adjustment
drug
due to correct substance properly administered T88.6
overdose or wrong substance given or taken (by accident) —*see* Table of Drugs and Chemicals, by drug, poisoning
during or after labor and delivery O75.1
electric T75.4
(taser) T75.4
endotoxic R65.21
postprocedural (resulting from a procedure, not elsewhere classified) T81.12
following
ectopic or molar pregnancy OØ8.3
injury (immediate) (delayed) T79.4
labor and delivery O75.1
food (anaphylactic) —*see* Shock, anaphylactic, due to food
from electroshock gun (taser) T75.4
gram-negative R65.21
postprocedural (resulting from a procedure, not elsewhere classified) T81.12
hematologic R57.8
hemorrhagic R57.8
surgery (intraoperative) (postoperative) T81.19
trauma T79.4

Shock *(Continued)*
  hypovolemic R57.1
    surgical T81.19
    traumatic T79.4
  insulin E15
    therapeutic misadventure *—see* subcategory T38.3
  kidney N17.Ø
    traumatic (following crushing) T79.5
  lightning T75.Ø1
  liver K72.ØØ
  lung J8Ø
  obstetric O75.1
    with ectopic or molar pregnancy OØ8.3
    following ectopic or molar pregnancy OØ8.3
  pleural (surgical) T81.19
    due to trauma T79.4
  postprocedural (postoperative) T81.1Ø
    with ectopic or molar pregnancy OØ8.3
    cardiogenic T81.11
    endotoxic T81.12
    following ectopic or molar pregnancy OØ8.3
    gram-negative T81.12
    hypovolemic T81.19
    septic T81.12
    specified type NEC T81.19
  psychic F43.Ø
  septic (due to severe sepsis) R65.21
  specified NEC R57.8
  surgical T81.1Ø
  taser gun (taser) T75.4
  therapeutic misadventure NEC T81.1Ø
  thyroxin
    overdose or wrong substance given or taken *—see* Table of Drugs and Chemicals, by drug, poisoning
  toxic, syndrome A48.3
  transfusion *—see* Complications, transfusion
  traumatic (immediate) (delayed) T79.4
Shoemaker's chest M95.4
Short, shortening, shortness
  arm (acquired) *—see also* Deformity, limb, unequal length
    congenital Q71.81- ●
    forearm *—see* Deformity, limb, unequal length
  bowel syndrome K91.2
  breath RØ6.Ø2
  cervical (complicating pregnancy) O26.87- ●
    non-gravid uterus N88.3
  common bile duct, congenital Q44.5
  cord (umbilical), complicating delivery O69.3
  cystic duct, congenital Q44.5
  esophagus (congenital) Q39.8
  femur (acquired) *—see* Deformity, limb, unequal length, femur
    congenital *—see* Defect, reduction, lower limb, longitudinal, femur
  frenum, frenulum, linguae (congenital) Q38.1
  hip (acquired) *—see also* Deformity, limb, unequal length
    congenital Q65.89
  leg (acquired) *—see also* Deformity, limb, unequal length
    congenital Q72.81- ●
    lower leg *—see also* Deformity, limb, unequal length
  limbed stature, with immunodeficiency D82.2
  lower limb (acquired) *—see also* Deformity, limb, unequal length
    congenital Q72.81- ●
  organ or site, congenital NEC *—see* Distortion
  palate, congenital Q38.5
  radius (acquired) *—see also* Deformity, limb, unequal length
    congenital *—see* Defect, reduction, upper limb, longitudinal, radius
  rib syndrome Q77.2
  stature (child) (hereditary) (idiopathic) NEC R62.52
    constitutional E34.3
    due to endocrine disorder E34.3
    Laron-type E34.3

Short, shortening, shortness *(Continued)*
  tendon *—see also* Contraction, tendon
    with contracture of joint *—see* Contraction, joint
    Achilles (acquired) M67.Ø- ●
      congenital Q66.89
    congenital Q79.8
  thigh (acquired) *—see also* Deformity, limb, unequal length, femur
    congenital *—see* Defect, reduction, lower limb, longitudinal, femur
  tibialis anterior (tendon) *—see* Contraction, tendon
  umbilical cord
    complicating delivery O69.3
  upper limb, congenital *—see* Defect, reduction, upper limb, specified type NEC
  urethra N36.8
  uvula, congenital Q38.5
  vagina (congenital) Q52.4
Shortsightedness *—see* Myopia
Shoshin (acute fulminating beriberi) E51.11
Shoulder *—see* condition
Shovel-shaped incisors KØØ.2
Shower, thromboembolic *—see* Embolism
Shunt
  arterial-venous (dialysis) Z99.2
  arteriovenous, pulmonary (acquired) I28.Ø
    congenital Q25.72
  cerebral ventricle (communicating) in situ Z98.2
  surgical, prosthetic, with complications *—see* Complications, cardiovascular, device or implant Shutdown, renal N28.9
Shutdown, renal N28.9
Shy-Drager syndrome G9Ø.3
Sialadenitis, sialadenosis (any gland) (chronic) (periodic) (suppurative) *—see* Sialoadenitis
Sialectasia K11.8
Sialidosis E77.1
Sialitis, silitis (any gland) (chronic) (suppurative) *—see* Sialoadenitis
Sialoadenitis (any gland) (periodic) (suppurative) K11.2Ø
  acute K11.21
    recurrent K11.22
  chronic K11.23
Sialoadenopathy K11.9
Sialoangitis *—see* Sialoadenitis
Sialodochitis (fibrinosa) *—see* Sialoadenitis
Sialodocholithiasis K11.5
Sialolithiasis K11.5
Sialometaplasia, necrotizing K11.8
Sialorrhea *—see also* Ptyalism
  periodic *—see* Sialoadenitis
Sialosis K11.7
Siamese twin Q89.4
Sibling rivalry Z62.891
Sicard's syndrome G52.7
Sicca syndrome M35.ØØ
  with
    keratoconjunctivitis M35.Ø1
    lung involvement M35.Ø2
    myopathy M35.Ø3
    renal tubulo-interstitial disorders M35.Ø4
  specified organ involvement NEC M35.Ø9
Sick R69
  or handicapped person in family Z63.79
    needing care at home Z63.6
  sinus (syndrome) I49.5
Sick-euthyroid syndrome EØ7.81
Sickle-cell
  anemia *—see* Disease, sickle-cell
  trait D57.3
Sicklemia *—see also* Disease, sickle-cell
  trait D57.3
Sickness
  air (travel) T75.3
  airplane T75.3
  alpine T7Ø.29

Sickness *(Continued)*
  altitude T7Ø.2Ø
  Andes T7Ø.29
  aviator's T7Ø.29
  balloon T7Ø.29
  car T75.3
  compressed air T7Ø.3
  decompression T7Ø.3
  green D5Ø.8
  milk *—see* Poisoning, food, noxious
  motion T75.3
  mountain T7Ø.29
    acute D75.1
  protein *—see also* Reaction, serum T8Ø.69
  radiation T66
  roundabout (motion) T75.3
  sea T75.3
  serum NEC *—see also* Reaction, serum T8Ø.69
  sleeping (African) B56.9
    by Trypanosoma B56.9
      brucei
        gambiense B56.Ø
        rhodesiense B56.1
    East African B56.1
    Gambian B56.Ø
    Rhodesian B56.1
    West African B56.Ø
  swing (motion) T75.3
  train (railway) (travel) T75.3
  travel (any vehicle) T75.3
Sideropenia *—see* Anemia, iron deficiency
Siderosilicosis J62.8
Siderosis (lung) J63.4
  eye (globe) *—see* Disorder, globe, degenerative, siderosis
Siemens' syndrome (ectodermal dysplasia) Q82.8
Sighing RØ6.89
  psychogenic F45.8
Sigmoid *—see also* condition
  flexure *—see* condition
  kidney Q63.1
Sigmoiditis *—see also* Enteritis K52.9
  infectious AØ9
  noninfectious K52.9
Silfverskiöld's syndrome Q78.9
Silicosiderosis J62.8
Silicosis, silicotic (simple) (complicated) J62.8
  with tuberculosis J65
Silicotuberculosis J65
Silo-fillers' disease J68.8
  bronchitis J68.Ø
  pneumonitis J68.Ø
  pulmonary edema J68.1
Silver's syndrome Q87.19
Simian malaria B53.1
Simmonds' cachexia or disease E23.Ø
Simons' disease or syndrome (progressive lipodystrophy) E88.1
Simple, simplex *—see* condition
Simulation, conscious (of illness) Z76.5
Simultanagnosia (asimultagnosia) R48.3
Sin Nombre virus disease (Hantavirus) (cardio)-pulmonary syndrome) B33.4
Sinding-Larsen disease or osteochondrosis *—see* Osteochondrosis, juvenile, patella
Singapore hemorrhagic fever A91
Singer's node or nodule J38.2
Single
  atrium Q21.2
  coronary artery Q24.5
  umbilical artery Q27.Ø
  ventricle Q2Ø.4
Singultus RØ6.6
  epidemicus B33.Ø
Sinus *—see also* Fistula
  abdominal K63.89
  arrest I45.5
  arrhythmia I49.8
  bradycardia RØØ.1
  branchial cleft (internal) (external) Q18.Ø
  coccygeal *—see* Sinus, pilonidal

S

Sinus *(Continued)*
  dental K04.6
  dermal (congenital) Q06.8
    with abscess Q06.8
    coccygeal, pilonidal —*see* Sinus, coccygeal
  infected, skin NEC L08.89
  marginal, ruptured or bleeding —*see* Hemorrhage, antepartum, specified cause NEC
  medial, face and neck Q18.8
  pause I45.5
  pericranii Q01.9
  pilonidal (infected) (rectum) L05.92
    with abscess L05.02
  preauricular Q18.1
  rectovaginal N82.3
  Rokitansky-Aschoff (gallbladder) K82.8
  sacrococcygeal (dermoid) (infected) —*see* Sinus, pilonidal
  tachycardia R00.0
    paroxysmal I47.1
  tarsi syndrome M25.57-●
  testis N50.89
  tract (postinfective) —*see* Fistula
  urachus Q64.4
Sinusitis (accessory) (chronic) (hyperplastic) (nasal) (nonpurulent) (purulent) J32.9
  acute J01.90
    ethmoidal J01.20
      recurrent J01.21
    frontal J01.10
      recurrent J01.11
    involving more than one sinus, other than pansinusitis J01.80
      recurrent J01.81
    maxillary J01.00
      recurrent J01.01
    pansinusitis J01.40
      recurrent J01.41
    recurrent J01.91
    specified NEC J01.80
      recurrent J01.81
    sphenoidal J01.30
      recurrent J01.31
  allergic —*see* Rhinitis, allergic
  due to high altitude T70.1
  ethmoidal J32.2
    acute J01.20
      recurrent J01.21
  frontal J32.1
    acute J01.10
      recurrent J01.11
  influenzal —*see* Influenza, with, respiratory manifestations NEC
  involving more than one sinus but not pansinusitis J32.8
    acute J01.80
      recurrent J01.81
  maxillary J32.0
    acute J01.00
      recurrent J01.01
  sphenoidal J32.3
    acute J01.30
      recurrent J01.31
  tuberculous, any sinus A15.8
Sinusitis-bronchiectasis-situs inversus (syndrome) (triad) Q89.3
Sipple's syndrome E31.22
Sirenomelia (syndrome) Q87.2
Siriasis T67.01
Sirkari's disease B55.0
Siti A65
Situation, psychiatric F99
Situational
  disturbance (transient) —*see* Disorder, adjustment
    acute F43.0
  maladjustment —*see* Disorder, adjustment
  reaction —*see* Disorder, adjustment
    acute F43.0
Situs inversus or transversus (abdominalis) (thoracis) Q89.3
Sixth disease B08.20
  due to human herpesvirus 6 B08.21
  due to human herpesvirus 7 B08.22
Sjögren-Larsson syndrome Q87.19
Sjögren's syndrome or disease —*see* Sicca syndrome
Skeletal —*see* condition
Skene's gland —*see* condition
Skenitis —*see* Urethritis
Skerljevo A65
Skevas-Zerfus disease —*see* Toxicity, venom, marine animal, sea anemone
Skin —*see also* condition
  clammy R23.1
  donor —*see* Donor, skin
  hidebound M35.9
Slate-dressers' or slate-miners' lung J62.8
Sleep
  apnea —*see* Apnea, sleep
  deprivation Z72.820
  disorder or disturbance G47.9
    child F51.9
    nonorganic origin F51.9
    specified NEC G47.8
  disturbance G47.9
    nonorganic origin F51.9
  drunkenness F51.9
  rhythm inversion G47.2-●
  terrors F51.4
  walking F51.3
    hysterical F44.89
Sleep hygiene
  abuse Z72.821
  inadequate Z72.821
  poor Z72.821
Sleeping sickness —*see* Sickness, sleeping
Sleeplessness —*see* Insomnia
  menopausal N95.11
Sleep-wake schedule disorder G47.20
Slim disease (in HIV infection) B20
Slipped, slipping
  epiphysis (traumatic) —*see also* Osteochondropathy, specified type NEC
    capital femoral (traumatic)
      acute (on chronic) S79.01-●
    current traumatic - code as Fracture, by site
    upper femoral (nontraumatic) M93.00-●
      acute M93.01-●
        on chronic M93.03-●
      chronic M93.02-●
  intervertebral disc —*see* Displacement, intervertebral disc
  ligature, umbilical P51.8
  patella —*see* Disorder, patella, derangement NEC
  rib M89.8X8
  sacroiliac joint —*see* subcategory M53.2
  tendon —*see* Disorder, tendon
  ulnar nerve, nontraumatic —*see* Lesion, nerve, ulnar
  vertebra NEC —*see* Spondylolisthesis
Slocumb's syndrome E27.0
Sloughing (multiple) (phagedena) (skin) —*see also* Gangrene
  abscess —*see* Abscess
  appendix K38.8
  fascia —*see* Disorder, soft tissue, specified type NEC
  scrotum N50.89
  tendon —*see* Disorder, tendon
  transplanted organ —*see* Rejection, transplant
  ulcer —*see* Ulcer, skin
Slow
  feeding, newborn P92.2
  flow syndrome, coronary I20.8
  heart(beat) R00.1
Slowing, urinary stream R39.198
Sluder's neuralgia (syndrome) G44.89
Slurred, slurring speech R47.81
Small (ness)
  for gestational age —*see* Small for dates
  introitus, vagina N89.6
  kidney (unknown cause) N27.9
    bilateral N27.1
    unilateral N27.0
  ovary (congenital) Q50.39
  pelvis
    with disproportion (fetopelvic) O33.1
      causing obstructed labor O65.1
  uterus N85.8
  white kidney N03.9
Small-and-light-for-dates —*see* Small for dates
Small-for-dates (infant) P05.10
  with weight of
    499 grams or less P05.11
    500-749 grams P05.12
    750-999 grams P05.13
    1000-1249 grams P05.14
    1250-1499 grams P05.15
    1500-1749 grams P05.16
    1750-1999 grams P05.17
    2000-2499 grams P05.18
    2500 grams and over P05.19
  specified NEC P05.19
Smallpox B03
Smearing, fecal R15.1
Smith-Lemli-Opitz syndrome E78.72
Smith's fracture S52.54-●
Smoker —*see* Dependence, drug, nicotine
Smoker's
  bronchitis J41.0
  cough J41.0
  palate K13.24
  throat J31.2
  tongue K13.24
Smoking
  passive Z77.22
Smothering spells R06.81
Snaggle teeth, tooth M26.39
Snapping
  finger —*see* Trigger finger
  hip —*see* Derangement, joint, specified type NEC, hip
    involving the iliotiblial band M76.3-●
  knee —*see* Derangement, knee
    involving the iliotiblial band M76.3-●
Sneddon-Wilkinson disease or syndrome (subcorneal pustular dermatosis) L13.1
Sneezing (intractable) R06.7
Sniffing
  cocaine
    abuse —*see* Abuse, drug, cocaine
    dependence —*see* Dependence, drug, cocaine
  gasoline
    abuse —*see* Abuse, drug, inhalant
    dependence —*see* Dependence, drug, inhalant
  glue (airplane)
    abuse —*see* Abuse, drug, inhalant
    drug dependence —*see* Dependence, drug, inhalant
Sniffles
  newborn P28.89
Snoring R06.83
Snow blindness —*see* Photokeratitis
Snuffles (non-syphilitic) R06.5
  newborn P28.89
  syphilitic (infant) A50.05 *[J99]*
Social
  exclusion Z60.4
    due to discrimination or persecution (perceived) Z60.5
  migrant Z59.0
    acculturation difficulty Z60.3
  rejection Z60.4
    due to discrimination or persecution Z60.5

S

Social *(Continued)*
role conflict NEC Z73.5
skills inadequacy NEC Z73.4
transplantation Z60.3
Sodoku A25.0
Soemmerring's ring —*see* Cataract, secondary
Soft —*see also* condition
nails L60.3
Softening
bone —*see* Osteomalacia
brain (necrotic) (progressive) G93.89
congenital Q04.8
embolic I63.4- ●
hemorrhagic —*see* Hemorrhage, intracranial, intracerebral
occlusive I63.5- ●
thrombotic I63.3- ●
cartilage M94.2- ●
patella M22.4- ●
cerebellar —*see* Softening, brain
cerebral —*see* Softening, brain
cerebrospinal —*see* Softening, brain
myocardial, heart —*see* Degeneration, myocardial
spinal cord G95.89
stomach K31.89
Soldier's
heart F45.8
patches I31.0
Solitary
cyst, kidney N28.1
kidney, congenital Q60.0
Solvent abuse —*see* Abuse, drug, inhalant
dependence —*see* Dependence, drug, inhalant
Somatization reaction, somatic reaction —*see* Disorder, somatoform
Somnambulism F51.3
hysterical F44.89
Somnolence R40.0
nonorganic origin F51.11
Sonne dysentery A03.3
Soor B37.0
Sore
bed —*see* Ulcer, pressure, by site
chiclero B55.1
Delhi B55.1
desert —*see* Ulcer, skin
eye H57.1- ●
Lahore B55.1
mouth K13.79
canker K12.0
muscle M79.10
Naga —*see* Ulcer, skin
of skin —*see* Ulcer, skin - oriental B55.1
pressure —*see* Ulcer, pressure, by site
skin L98.9
soft A57
throat (acute) —*see also* Pharyngitis
with influenza, flu, or grippe —*see* Influenza, with, respiratory manifestations NEC
chronic J31.2
coxsackie (virus) B08.5
diphtheritic A36.0
herpesviral B00.2
influenzal —*see* Influenza, with, respiratory manifestations NEC
septic J02.0
streptococcal (ulcerative) J02.0
viral NEC J02.8
coxsackie B08.5
tropical —*see* Ulcer, skin
veldt —*see* Ulcer, skin
Soto's syndrome (cerebral gigantism) Q87.3
South African cardiomyopathy syndrome I42.8
Southeast Asian hemorrhagic fever A91
Spacing
abnormal, tooth, teeth, fully erupted M26.30
excessive, tooth, fully erupted M26.32
Spade-like hand (congenital) Q68.1
Spading nail L60.8
congenital Q84.6
Spanish collar N47.1
Sparganosis B70.1
Spasm(s), spastic, spasticity —*see also* condition R25.2
accommodation —*see* Spasm, of accommodation
ampulla of Vater K83.4
anus, ani (sphincter) (reflex) K59.4
psychogenic F45.8
artery I73.9
cerebral G45.9
Bell's G51.3- ●
bladder (sphincter, external or internal) N32.89
psychogenic F45.8
bronchus, bronchiole J98.01
cardia K22.0
cardiac I20.1
carpopedal —*see* Tetany
cerebral (arteries) (vascular) G45.9
cervix, complicating delivery O62.4
ciliary body (of accommodation) —*see* Spasm, of accommodation
colon —*see also* Irritable, bowel K58.9
with diarrhea K58.0
psychogenic F45.8
common duct K83.8
compulsive —*see* Tic
conjugate H51.8
coronary (artery) I20.1
diaphragm (reflex) R06.6
epidemic B33.0
psychogenic F45.8
duodenum K59.8
epidemic diaphragmatic (transient) B33.0
esophagus (diffuse) K22.4
psychogenic F45.8
facial G51.3- ●
fallopian tube N83.8
gastrointestinal (tract) K31.89
psychogenic F45.8
glottis J38.5
hysterical F44.4
psychogenic F45.8
conversion reaction F44.4
reflex through recurrent laryngeal nerve J38.5
habit —*see* Tic
heart I20.1
hemifacial (clonic) G51.3- ●
hourglass —*see* Contraction, hourglass
hysterical F44.4
infantile —*see* Epilepsy, spasms
inferior oblique, eye H51.8
intestinal —*see also* Syndrome, irritable bowel K58.9
psychogenic F45.8
larynx, laryngeal J38.5
hysterical F44.4
psychogenic F45.8
conversion reaction F44.4
levator palpebrae superioris —*see* Disorder, eyelid function
muscle NEC M62.838
back M62.830
nerve, trigeminal G51.0
nervous F45.8
nodding F98.4
occupational F48.8
oculogyric H51.8
psychogenic F45.8
of accommodation H52.53- ●
ophthalmic artery —*see* Occlusion, artery, retina
perineal, female N94.89
peroneo-extensor —*see also* Deformity, limb, flat foot
pharynx (reflex) J39.2
hysterical F45.8
psychogenic F45.8
Spasm(s), spastic, spasticity *(Continued)*
psychogenic F45.8
pylorus NEC K31.3
adult hypertrophic K31.89
congenital or infantile Q40.0
psychogenic F45.8
rectum (sphincter) K59.4
psychogenic F45.8
retinal (artery) —*see* Occlusion, artery, retina
sigmoid —*see also* Syndrome, irritable bowel K58.9
psychogenic F45.8
sphincter of Oddi K83.4
stomach K31.89
neurotic F45.8
throat J39.2
hysterical F45.8
psychogenic F45.8
tic F95.9
chronic F95.1
transient of childhood F95.0
tongue K14.8
torsion (progressive) G24.1
trigeminal nerve —*see* Neuralgia, trigeminal
ureter N13.5
urethra (sphincter) N35.919
uterus N85.8
complicating labor O62.4
vagina N94.2
psychogenic F52.5
vascular I73.9
vasomotor I73.9
vein NEC I87.8
viscera —*see* Pain, abdominal
Spasmodic —*see* condition
Spasmophilia —*see* Tetany
Spasmus nutans F98.4
Spastic, spasticity —*see also* Spasm
child (cerebral) (congenital) (paralysis) G80.1
Speaker's throat R49.8
Specific, specified —*see* condition
Speech
defect, disorder, disturbance, impediment R47.9
psychogenic, in childhood and adolescence F98.8
slurring R47.81
specified NEC R47.89
Spencer's disease A08.19
Spens' syndrome (syncope with heart block) I45.9
Sperm counts (fertility testing) Z31.41
postvasectomy Z30.8
reversal Z31.42
Spermatic cord —*see* condition
Spermatocele N43.40
congenital Q55.4
multiple N43.42
single N43.41
Spermatocystitis N49.0
Spermatocytoma C62.9- ●
specified site —*see* Neoplasm, malignant, by site
Spermatorrhea N50.89
Sphacelus —*see* Gangrene
Sphenoidal —*see* condition
Sphenoiditis (chronic) —*see* Sinusitis, sphenoidal
Sphenopalatine ganglion neuralgia G90.09
Sphericity, increased, lens (congenital) Q12.4
Spherocytosis (congenital) (familial) (hereditary) D58.0
hemoglobin disease D58.0
sickle-cell (disease) D57.8- ●
Spherophakia Q12.4
Sphincter —*see* condition
Sphincteritis, sphincter of Oddi —*see* Cholangitis
Sphingolipidosis E75.3
specified NEC E75.29

S

Sphingomyelinosis E75.3
Spicule tooth KØØ.2
Spider
  bite —*see* Toxicity, venom, spider
  fingers —*see* Syndrome, Marfan's
  nevus I78.1
  toes —*see* Syndrome, Marfan's
  vascular I78.1
Spiegler-Fendt
  benign lymphocytoma L98.8
  sarcoid LØ8.89
Spielmeyer-Vogt disease E75.4
Spina bifida (aperta) QØ5.9
  with hydrocephalus NEC QØ5.4
  cervical QØ5.5
    with hydrocephalus QØ5.Ø
  dorsal QØ5.6
    with hydrocephalus QØ5.1
  lumbar QØ5.7
    with hydrocephalus QØ5.2
  lumbosacral QØ5.7
    with hydrocephalus QØ5.2
  occulta Q76.Ø
  sacral QØ5.8
    with hydrocephalus QØ5.3
  thoracic QØ5.6
    with hydrocephalus QØ5.1
  thoracolumbar QØ5.6
    with hydrocephalus QØ5.1
Spindle, Krukenberg's —*see* Pigmentation, cornea, posterior
Spine, spinal —*see* condition
Spiradenoma (eccrine) —*see* Neoplasm, skin, benign
Spirillosis A25.Ø
Spirillum
  minus A25.Ø
  obermeieri infection A68.Ø
Spirochetal —*see* condition
Spirochetosis A69.9
  arthritic, arthritica A69.9
  bronchopulmonary A69.8
  icterohemorrhagic A27.Ø
  lung A69.8
Spirometrosis B7Ø.1
Spitting blood —*see* Hemoptysis
Splanchnoptosis K63.4
Spleen, splenic —*see* condition
Splenectasis —*see* Splenomegaly
Splenitis (interstitial) (malignant) (nonspecific) D73.89
  malarial —*see also* Malaria B54 *[D77]*
  tuberculous A18.85
Splenocele D73.89
Splenomegaly, splenomegalia (Bengal) (cryptogenic) (idiopathic) (tropical) R16.1
  with hepatomegaly R16.2
  cirrhotic D73.2
  congenital Q89.Ø9
  congestive, chronic D73.2
  Egyptian B65.1
  Gaucher's E75.22
  malarial —*see also* Malaria B54 *[D77]*
  neutropenic D73.81
  Niemann-Pick —*see* Niemann-Pick disease or syndrome
  siderotic D73.2
  syphilitic A52.79
    congenital (early) A5Ø.Ø8 *[D77]*
Splenopathy D73.9
Splenoptosis D73.89
Splenosis D73.89
Splinter —*see* Foreign body, superficial, by site
Split, splitting
  foot Q72.7-●
  hand Q71.6
  heart sounds RØ1.2
  lip, congenital —*see* Cleft, lip
  nails L6Ø.3
  urinary stream R39.13
Spondylarthrosis —*see* Spondylosis
Spondylitis (chronic) —*see also* Spondylopathy, inflammatory
  ankylopoietica —*see* Spondylitis, ankylosing
  ankylosing (chronic) M45.9
    with lung involvement M45.9 *[J99]*
    cervical region M45.2
    cervicothoracic region M45.3
    juvenile MØ8.1
    lumbar region M45.6
    lumbosacral region M45.7
    multiple sites M45.Ø
    occipito-atlanto-axial region M45.1
    sacrococcygeal region M45.8
    thoracic region M45.4
    thoracolumbar region M45.5
  atrophic (ligamentous) —*see* Spondylitis, ankylosing
  deformans (chronic) —*see* Spondylosis
  gonococcal A54.41
  gouty —*see also* Gout, by type, vertebrae M1Ø.Ø8
  in (due to)
    brucellosis A23.9 *[M49.8Ø]*
      cervical region A23.9 *[M49.82]*
      cervicothoracic region A23.9 *[M49.83]*
      lumbar region A23.9 *[M49.86]*
      lumbosacral region A23.9 *[M49.87]*
      multiple sites A23.9 *[M49.89]*
      occipito-atlanto-axial region A23.9 *[M49.81]*
      sacrococcygeal region A23.9 *[M49.88]*
      thoracic region A23.9 *[M49.84]*
      thoracolumbar region A23.9 *[M49.85]*
    enterobacteria —*see also* subcategory M49.8 AØ4.9
    tuberculosis A18.Ø1
  infectious NEC —*see* Spondylopathy, infective
  juvenile ankylosing (chronic) MØ8.1
  Kümmell's —*see* Spondylopathy, traumatic
  Marie-Strümpell —*see* Spondylitis, ankylosing
  muscularis —*see* Spondylopathy, specified NEC
  psoriatic L4Ø.53
  rheumatoid —*see* Spondylitis, ankylosing
  rhizomelica —*see* Spondylitis, ankylosing
  sacroiliac NEC M46.1
  senescent, senile —*see* Spondylosis
  traumatic (chronic) or post-traumatic —*see* Spondylopathy, traumatic
  tuberculous A18.Ø1
  typhosa AØ1.Ø5
Spondylolisthesis (acquired) (degenerative) M43.1Ø
  with disproportion (fetopelvic) O33.Ø
    causing obstructed labor O65.Ø
  cervical region M43.12
  cervicothoracic region M43.13
  congenital Q76.2
  lumbar region M43.16
  lumbosacral region M43.17
  multiple sites M43.19
  occipito-atlanto-axial region M43.11
  sacrococcygeal region M43.18
  thoracic region M43.14
  thoracolumbar region M43.15
  traumatic (old) M43.1Ø
    acute
      fifth cervical (displaced) S12.43Ø
        nondisplaced S12.431
        specified type NEC (displaced) S12.45Ø
          nondisplaced S12.451
        type III S12.44
      fourth cervical (displaced) S12.33Ø
        nondisplaced S12.331
        specified type NEC (displaced) S12.35Ø
          nondisplaced S12.351
        type III S12.34
Spondylolisthesis *(Continued)*
  traumatic *(Continued)*
    acute *(Continued)*
      second cervical (displaced) S12.13Ø
        nondisplaced S12.131
        specified type NEC (displaced) S12.15Ø
          nondisplaced S12.151
        type III S12.14
      seventh cervical (displaced) S12.63Ø
        nondisplaced S12.631
        specified type NEC (displaced) S12.65Ø
          nondisplaced S12.651
        type III S12.64
      sixth cervical (displaced) S12.53Ø
        nondisplaced S12.531
        specified type NEC (displaced) S12.55Ø
          nondisplaced S12.551
        type III S12.54
      third cervical (displaced) S12.23Ø
        nondisplaced S12.231
        specified type NEC (displaced) S12.25Ø
          nondisplaced S12.251
        type III S12.24
Spondylolysis (acquired) M43.ØØ
  cervical region M43.Ø2
  cervicothoracic region M43.Ø3
  congenital Q76.2
  lumbar region M43.Ø6
  lumbosacral region M43.Ø7
    with disproportion (fetopelvic) O33.Ø
      causing obstructed labor O65.8
  multiple sites M43.Ø9
  occipito-atlanto-axial region M43.Ø1
  sacrococcygeal region M43.Ø8
  thoracic region M43.Ø4
  thoracolumbar region M43.Ø5
Spondylopathy M48.9
  infective NEC M46.5Ø
    cervical region M46.52
    cervicothoracic region M46.53
    lumbar region M46.56
    lumbosacral region M46.57
    multiple sites M46.59
    occipito-atlanto-axial region M46.51
    sacrococcygeal region M46.58
    thoracic region M46.54
    thoracolumbar region M46.55
  inflammatory M46.9Ø
    cervical region M46.92
    cervicothoracic region M46.93
    lumbar region M46.96
    lumbosacral region M46.97
    multiple sites M46.99
    occipito-atlanto-axial region M46.91
    sacrococcygeal region M46.98
    specified type NEC M46.8Ø
      cervical region M46.82
      cervicothoracic region M46.83
      lumbar region M46.86
      lumbosacral region M46.87
      multiple sites M46.89
      occipito-atlanto-axial region M46.81
      sacrococcygeal region M46.88
      thoracic region M46.84
      thoracolumbar region M46.85
    thoracic region M46.94
    thoracolumbar region M46.95
  neuropathic, in
    syringomyelia and syringobulbia G95.Ø
    tabes dorsalis A52.11
  specified NEC —*see* subcategory M48.8
  traumatic M48.3Ø
    cervical region M48.32
    cervicothoracic region M48.33
    lumbar region M48.36
    lumbosacral region M48.37
    occipito-atlanto-axial region M48.31

Spondylopathy *(Continued)*
  traumatic *(Continued)*
    sacrococcygeal region M48.38
    thoracic region M48.34
    thoracolumbar region M48.35
Spondylosis M47.9
  with
    disproportion (fetopelvic) O33.0
      causing obstructed labor O65.0
    myelopathy NEC M47.10
      cervical region M47.12
      cervicothoracic region M47.13
      lumbar region M47.16
      occipito-atlanto-axial region M47.11
      thoracic region M47.14
      thoracolumbar region M47.15
    radiculopathy M47.20
      cervical region M47.22
      cervicothoracic region M47.23
      lumbar region M47.26
      lumbosacral region M47.27
      occipito-atlanto-axial region M47.21
      sacrococcygeal region M47.28
      thoracic region M47.24
      thoracolumbar region M47.25
  without myelopathy or radiculopathy M47.819
    cervical region M47.812
    cervicothoracic region M47.813
    lumbar region M47.816
    lumbosacral region M47.817
    occipito-atlanto-axial region M47.811
    sacrococcygeal region M47.818
    thoracic region M47.814
    thoracolumbar region M47.815
  specified NEC M47.899
    cervical region M47.892
    cervicothoracic region M47.893
    lumbar region M47.896
    lumbosacral region M47.897
    occipito-atlanto-axial region M47.891
    sacrococcygeal region M47.898
    thoracic region M47.894
    thoracolumbar region M47.895
  traumatic —*see* Spondylopathy, traumatic
Sponge
  inadvertently left in operation wound —*see* Foreign body, accidentally left during a procedure
  kidney (medullary) Q61.5
Sponge-diver's disease —*see* Toxicity, venom, marine animal, sea anemone
Spongioblastoma (any type) —*see* Neoplasm, malignant, by site
  specified site —*see* Neoplasm, malignant, by site
  unspecified site C71.9
Spongioneuroblastoma —*see* Neoplasm, malignant, by site
Spontaneous —*see also* condition
  fracture (cause unknown) —*see* Fracture, pathological
Spoon nail L60.3
  congenital Q84.6
Sporadic —*see* condition
Sporothrix schenckii infection —*see* Sporotrichosis
Sporotrichosis B42.9
  arthritis B42.82
  disseminated B42.7
  generalized B42.7
  lymphocutaneous (fixed) (progressive) B42.1
  pulmonary B42.0
  specified NEC B42.89
Spots, spotting (in) (of)
  Bitot's —*see also* Pigmentation, conjunctiva
    in the young child E50.1
    vitamin A deficiency E50.1
Spots, spotting *(Continued)*
  café, au lait L81.3
  Cayenne pepper I78.1
  cotton wool, retina —*see* Occlusion, artery, retina
  de Morgan's (senile angiomas) I78.1
  Fuchs' black (myopic) —*see also* Myopia, degenerative H44.2-•
  intermenstrual (regular) N92.0
    irregular N92.1
  Koplik's B05.9
  liver L81.4
  pregnancy O26.85-•
  purpuric R23.3
  ruby I78.1
Spotted fever —*see* Fever, spotted N92.3
Sprain (joint) (ligament)
  acromioclavicular joint or ligament S43.5-•
  ankle S93.40-•
    calcaneofibular ligament S93.41-•
    deltoid ligament S93.42-•
    internal collateral ligament —*see* Sprain, ankle, specified ligament NEC
    specified ligament NEC S93.49-•
    talofibular ligament —*see* Sprain, ankle, specified ligament NEC
    tibiofibular ligament S93.43-•
  anterior longitudinal, cervical S13.4
  atlas, atlanto-axial, atlanto-occipital S13.4
  breast bone —*see* Sprain, sternum
  calcaneofibular —*see* Sprain, ankle
  carpal —*see* Sprain, wrist
  carpometacarpal —*see* Sprain, hand, specified site NEC
  cartilage
    costal S23.41
    semilunar (knee) —*see* Sprain, knee, specified site NEC
      with current tear —*see* Tear, meniscus
    thyroid region S13.5
    xiphoid —*see* Sprain, sternum
  cervical, cervicodorsal, cervicothoracic S13.4
  chondrosternal S23.421
  coracoclavicular S43.8-•
  coracohumeral S43.41-•
  coronary, knee —*see* Sprain, knee, specified site NEC
  costal cartilage S23.41
  cricoarytenoid articulation or ligament S13.5
  cricothyroid articulation S13.5
  cruciate, knee —*see* Sprain, knee, cruciate
  deltoid, ankle —*see* Sprain, ankle
  dorsal (spine) S23.3
  elbow S53.40-•
    radial collateral ligament S53.43-•
    radiohumeral S53.41-•
    rupture
      radial collateral ligament —*see* Rupture, traumatic, ligament, radial collateral
      ulnar collateral ligament —*see* Rupture, traumatic, ligament, ulnar collateral
    specified type NEC S53.49-•
    ulnar collateral ligament S53.44-•
    ulnohumeral S53.42-•
  femur, head —*see* Sprain, hip
  fibular collateral, knee —*see* Sprain, knee, collateral
  fibulocalcaneal —*see* Sprain, ankle
  finger(s) S63.61-•
    index S63.61-•
    interphalangeal (joint) S63.63-•
      index S63.63-•
      little S63.63-•
      middle S63.63-•
      ring S63.63-•
    little S63.61-•
    metacarpophalangeal (joint) S63.65-•
    middle S63.61-•
    ring S63.61-•
Sprain *(Continued)*
  finger(s) *(Continued)*
    specified site NEC S63.69-•
      index S63.69-•
      little S63.69-•
      middle S63.69-•
      ring S63.69-•
  foot S93.60-•
    specified ligament NEC S93.69-•
    tarsal ligament S93.61-•
    tarsometatarsal ligament S93.62-•
    toe —*see* Sprain, toe
  hand S63.9-•
    finger —*see* Sprain, finger
    specified site NEC —*see* subcategory S63.8
    thumb —*see* Sprain, thumb
  head S03.9
  hip S73.10-•
    iliofemoral ligament S73.11-•
    ischiocapsular (ligament) S73.12-•
    specified NEC S73.19-•
  iliofemoral —*see* Sprain, hip
  innominate
    acetabulum —*see* Sprain, hip
    sacral junction S33.6
  internal
    collateral, ankle —*see* Sprain, ankle
    semilunar cartilage —*see* Sprain, knee, specified site NEC
  interphalangeal
    finger —*see* Sprain, finger, interphalangeal (joint)
    toe —*see* Sprain, toe, interphalangeal joint
  ischiocapsular —*see* Sprain, hip
  ischiofemoral —*see* Sprain, hip
  jaw (articular disc) (cartilage) (meniscus) S03.4-•
    old M26.69
  knee S83.9-•
    collateral ligament S83.40-•
      lateral (fibular) S83.42-•
      medial (tibial) S83.41-•
    cruciate ligament S83.50-•
      anterior S83.51-•
      posterior S83.52-•
    lateral (fibular) collateral ligament S83.42-•
    medial (tibial) collateral ligament S83.41-•
    patellar ligament S76.11-•
    specified site NEC S83.8X-•
    superior tibiofibular joint (ligament) S83.6-•
  lateral collateral, knee —*see* Sprain, knee, collateral
  lumbar (spine) S33.5
  lumbosacral S33.9
  mandible (articular disc) S03.4-•
    old M26.69
  medial collateral, knee —*see* Sprain, knee, collateral
  meniscus
    jaw S03.4-•
      old M26.69
    knee —*see* Sprain, knee, specified site NEC
      with current tear —*see* Tear, meniscus
        old —*see* Derangement, knee, meniscus, due to old tear
    mandible S03.4-•
      old M26.69
  metacarpal (distal) (proximal) —*see* Sprain, hand, specified site NEC
  metacarpophalangeal —*see* Sprain, finger, metacarpophalangeal (joint)
  metatarsophalangeal —*see* Sprain, toe, metatarsophalangeal joint
  midcarpal —*see* Sprain, hand, specified site NEC
  midtarsal —*see* Sprain, foot, specified site NEC
  neck S13.9
    anterior longitudinal cervical ligament S13.4
    atlanto-axial joint S13.4

S

Sprain *(Continued)*
neck *(Continued)*
atlanto-occipital joint S13.4
cervical spine S13.4
cricoarytenoid ligament S13.5
cricothyroid ligament S13.5
specified site NEC S13.8
thyroid region (cartilage) S13.5
nose SØ3.8
orbicular, hip —*see* Sprain, hip
patella —*see* Sprain, knee, specified site NEC
patellar ligament S76.11- ●
pelvis NEC S33.8
phalanx
finger —*see* Sprain, finger
toe —*see* Sprain, toe
pubofemoral —*see* Sprain, hip
radiocarpal —*see* Sprain, wrist
radiohumeral —*see* Sprain, elbow
radius, collateral —*see* Rupture, traumatic, ligament, radial collateral
rib (cage) S23.41
rotator cuff (capsule) S43.42- ●
sacroiliac (region)
chronic or old —*see* subcategory M53.2
joint S33.6
scaphoid (hand) —*see* Sprain, hand, specified site NEC
scapula (r) —*see* Sprain, shoulder girdle, specified site NEC
semilunar cartilage (knee) —*see* Sprain, knee, specified site NEC
with current tear —*see* Tear, meniscus
old —*see* Derangement, knee, meniscus, due to old tear
shoulder joint S43.4Ø- ●
acromioclavicular joint (ligament) —*see* Sprain, acromioclavicular joint
blade —*see* Sprain, shoulder, girdle, specified site NEC
coracoclavicular joint (ligament) —*see* Sprain, coracoclavicular joint
coracohumeral ligament —*see* Sprain, coracohumeral joint
girdle S43.9- ●
specified site NEC S43.8- ●
rotator cuff —*see* Sprain, rotator cuff
specified site NEC S43.49- ●
sternoclavicular joint (ligament) —*see* Sprain, sternoclavicular joint
spine
cervical S13.4
lumbar S33.5
thoracic S23.3
sternoclavicular joint S43.6- ●
sternum S23.429
chondrosternal joint S23.421
specified site NEC S23.428
sternoclavicular (joint) (ligament) S23.42Ø
symphysis
jaw SØ3.4- ●
old M26.69
mandibular SØ3.4- ●
old M26.69
talofibular —*see* Sprain, ankle
tarsal —*see* Sprain, foot, specified site NEC
tarsometatarsal —*see* Sprain, foot, specified site NEC
temporomandibular SØ3.4- ●
old M26.69
thorax S23.9
ribs S23.41
specified site NEC S23.8
spine S23.3
sternum —*see* Sprain, sternum
thumb S63.6Ø- ●
interphalangeal (joint) S63.62- ●
metacarpophalangeal (joint) S63.64- ●
specified site NEC S63.68- ●
thyroid cartilage or region S13.5

Sprain *(Continued)*
tibia (proximal end) —*see* Sprain, knee, specified site NEC
tibial collateral, knee —*see* Sprain, knee, collateral
tibiofibular
distal —*see* Sprain, ankle
superior —*see* Sprain, knee, specified site NEC
toe(s) S93.5Ø- ●
great S93.5Ø- ●
interphalangeal joint S93.51- ●
great S93.51- ●
lesser S93.51- ●
lesser S93.5Ø- ●
metatarsophalangeal joint S93.52- ●
great S93.52- ●
lesser S93.52- ●
ulna, collateral —*see* Rupture, traumatic, ligament, ulnar collateral
ulnohumeral —*see* Sprain, elbow
wrist S63.5Ø- ●
carpal S63.51- ●
radiocarpal S63.52- ●
specified site NEC S63.59- ●
xiphoid cartilage —*see* Sprain, sternum
Sprengel's deformity (congenital) Q74.Ø
Sprue (tropical) K9Ø.1
celiac K9Ø.Ø
idiopathic K9Ø.49
meaning thrush B37.Ø
nontropical K9Ø.Ø
Spur, bone —*see also* Enthesopathy
calcaneal M77.3- ●
iliac crest M76.2- ●
nose (septum) J34.89
Spurway's syndrome Q78.Ø
Sputum
abnormal (amount) (color) (odor) (purulent) RØ9.3
blood-stained RØ4.2
excessive (cause unknown) RØ9.3
Squamous —*see also* condition
epithelium in
cervical canal (congenital) Q51.828
uterine mucosa (congenital) Q51.818
Squashed nose M95.Ø
congenital Q67.4
Squeeze, diver's T7Ø.3
Squint —*see also* Strabismus
accommodative —*see* Strabismus, convergent concomitant
SSADHD (succinic semialdehyde dehydrogenase deficiency) E72.81
St. Hubert's disease A82.9
Stab —*see also* Laceration
internal organs —*see* Injury, by site
Stafne's cyst or cavity M27.Ø
Staggering gait R26.Ø
hysterical F44.4
Staghorn calculus —*see* Calculus, kidney
Stähli's line (cornea) (pigment) —*see* Pigmentation, cornea, anterior
Stain, staining
meconium (newborn) P96.83
port wine Q82.5
tooth, teeth (hard tissues) (extrinsic) KØ3.6
due to
accretions KØ3.6
deposits (betel) (black) (green) (materia alba) (orange) (soft) (tobacco) KØ3.6
metals (copper) (silver) KØ3.7
nicotine KØ3.6
pulpal bleeding KØ3.7
tobacco KØ3.6
intrinsic KØØ.8
Stammering —*see also* Disorder, fluency F8Ø.81
Standstill
auricular I45.5
cardiac —*see* Arrest, cardiac
sinoatrial I45.5
ventricular —*see* Arrest, cardiac

Stannosis J63.5
Stanton's disease —*see* Melioidosis
Staphylitis (acute) (catarrhal) (chronic) (gangrenous) (membranous) (suppurative) (ulcerative) K12.2
Staphylococcal scalded skin syndrome LØØ
Staphylococcemia A41.2
Staphylococcus, staphylococcal —*see also* condition
as cause of disease classified elsewhere B95.8
aureus (methicillin susceptible) (MSSA) B95.61
methicillin resistant (MRSA) B95.62
specified NEC, as cause of disease classified elsewhere B95.7
Staphyloma (sclera)
cornea H18.72- ●
equatorial H15.81- ●
localized (anterior) H15.82- ●
posticum H15.83- ●
ring H15.85- ●
Stargardt's disease —*see* Dystrophy, retina
Starvation (inanition) (due to lack of food) T73.Ø
edema —*see* Malnutrition, severe
Stasis
bile (noncalculous) K83.1
bronchus J98.Ø9
with infection —*see* Bronchitis
cardiac —*see* Failure, heart, congestive
cecum K59.8
colon K59.8
dermatitis I87.2
with
varicose ulcer —*see* Varix, leg, with ulcer, with inflammation
varicose veins —*see* Varix, leg, with, inflammation
due to postthrombotic syndrome —*see* Syndrome, postthrombotic
duodenal K31.5
eczema —*see* Varix, leg, with, inflammation
edema —*see* Hypertension, venous (chronic), idiopathic
foot T69.Ø- ●
ileocecal coil K59.8
ileum K59.8
intestinal K59.8
jejunum K59.8
kidney N19
liver (cirrhotic) K76.1
lymphatic I89.8
pneumonia J18.2
pulmonary —*see* Edema, lung
rectal K59.8
renal N19
tubular N17.Ø
ulcer —*see* Varix, leg, with, ulcer
without varicose veins I87.2
urine —*see* Retention, urine
venous I87.8
State (of)
affective and paranoid, mixed, organic psychotic FØ6.8
agitated R45.1
acute reaction to stress F43.Ø
anxiety (neurotic) F41.1
apprehension F41.1
burn-out Z73.Ø
climacteric, female Z78.Ø
symptomatic N95.1
compulsive F42.8
mixed with obsessional thoughts F42.2
confusional (psychogenic) F44.89
acute —*see also* Delirium
with
arteriosclerotic dementia FØ1.5Ø
with behavioral disturbance FØ1.51
senility or dementia FØ5
alcoholic F1Ø.231

S

State *(Continued)*
confusional (psychogenic) *(Continued)*
epileptic F05
reactive (from emotional stress, psychological trauma) F44.89
subacute —*see* Delirium
convulsive —*see* Convulsions
crisis F43.0
depressive F32.9
neurotic F34.1
dissociative F44.9
emotional shock (stress) R45.7
hypercoagulation —*see* Hypercoagulable
locked-in G83.5
menopausal Z78.0
symptomatic N95.1
neurotic F48.9
with depersonalization F48.1
obsessional F42.8
oneiroid (schizophrenia-like) F23
organic
hallucinatory (nonalcoholic) F06.0
paranoid (-hallucinatory) F06.2
panic F41.0
paranoid F22
climacteric F22
involutional F22
menopausal F22
organic F06.2
senile F03
simple F22
persistent vegetative R40.3
phobic F40.9
postleukotomy F07.0
pregnant
gestational carrier Z33.3
incidental Z33.1
psychogenic, twilight F44.89
psychopathic (constitutional) F60.2
psychotic, organic —*see also* Psychosis, organic
mixed paranoid and affective F06.8
senile or presenile F03
transient NEC F06.8
with
depression F06.31
hallucinations F06.0
residual schizophrenic F20.5
restlessness R45.1
stress (emotional) R45.7
tension (mental) F48.9
specified NEC F48.8
transient organic psychotic NEC F06.8
depressive type F06.31
hallucinatory type F06.0
twilight
epileptic F05
psychogenic F44.89
vegetative, persistent R40.3
vital exhaustion Z73.0
withdrawal —*see* Withdrawal, state
Status (post) —*see also* Presence (of)
absence, epileptic —*see* Epilepsy, by type, with status epilepticus
administration of tPA (rtPA) in a different facility within the last 24 hours prior to admission to the current facility Z92.82
adrenalectomy (unilateral) (bilateral) E89.6
anastomosis Z98.0
anginosus I20.9
angioplasty (peripheral) Z98.62
with implant Z95.820
coronary artery Z98.61
with implant Z95.5
aortocoronary bypass Z95.1
arthrodesis Z98.1
artificial opening (of) Z93.9
gastrointestinal tract Z93.4
specified NEC Z93.8

Status *(Continued)*
artificial opening (of) *(Continued)*
urinary tract Z93.6
vagina Z93.8
asthmaticus —*see* Asthma, by type, with status asthmaticus
awaiting organ transplant Z76.82
bariatric surgery Z98.84
bed confinement Z74.01
bleb, filtering (vitreous), after glaucoma surgery Z98.83
breast implant Z98.82
removal Z98.86
cataract extraction Z98.4-•
cholecystectomy Z90.49
clitorectomy N90.811
with excision of labia minora N90.812
colectomy (complete) (partial) Z90.49
colonization —*see* Carrier (suspected) of
colostomy Z93.3
convulsivus idiopathicus —*see* Epilepsy, by type, with status epilepticus
coronary artery angioplasty —*see* Status, angioplasty, coronary artery
coronary artery bypass graft Z95.1
cystectomy (urinary bladder) Z90.6
cystostomy Z93.50
appendico-vesicostomy Z93.52
cutaneous Z93.51
specified NEC Z93.59
delinquent immunization Z28.3
dental Z98.818
crown Z98.811
fillings Z98.811
restoration Z98.811
sealant Z98.810
specified NEC Z98.818
deployment (current) (military) Z56.82
dialysis (hemodialysis) (peritoneal) Z99.2
do not resuscitate (DNR) Z66
donor —*see* Donor
embedded fragments —*see* Retained, foreign body fragments (type of)
embedded splinter —*see* Retained, foreign body fragments (type of)
enterostomy Z93.4
epileptic, epilepticus —*see also* Epilepsy, by type, with status epilepticus G40.901
estrogen receptor
negative Z17.1
positive Z17.0
female genital cutting —*see* Female genital mutilation status
female genital mutilation —*see* Female genital mutilation status
filtering (vitreous) bleb after glaucoma surgery Z98.83
gastrectomy (complete) (partial) Z90.3
gastric banding Z98.84
gastric bypass for obesity Z98.84
gastrostomy Z93.1
human immunodeficiency virus (HIV) infection, asymptomatic Z21
hysterectomy (complete) (total) Z90.710
partial (with remaining cervial stump) Z90.711
ileostomy Z93.2
implant
breast Z98.82
infibulation N90.813
intestinal bypass Z98.0
jejunostomy Z93.4
lapsed immunization schedule Z28.3
laryngectomy Z90.02
lymphaticus E32.8
malignancy
castrate resistant prostate Z19.2
hormone resistant Z19.2
hormone sensitive Z19.1
marmoratus G80.3
mastectomy (unilateral) (bilateral) Z90.1-•

Status *(Continued)*
military deployment status (current) Z56.82
in theater or in support of military war, peacekeeping and humanitarian operations Z56.82
nephrectomy (unilateral) (bilateral) Z90.5
nephrostomy Z93.6
obesity surgery Z98.84
oophorectomy
bilateral Z90.722
unilateral Z90.721
organ replacement
by artificial or mechanical device or prosthesis of
artery Z95.828
bladder Z96.0
blood vessel Z95.828
breast Z97.8
eye globe Z97.0
heart Z95.812
valve Z95.2
intestine Z97.8
joint Z96.60
hip —*see* Presence, hip joint implant
knee —*see* Presence, knee joint implant
specified site NEC Z96.698
kidney Z97.8
larynx Z96.3
lens Z96.1
limbs —*see* Presence, artificial, limb
liver Z97.8
lung Z97.8
pancreas Z97.8
by organ transplant (heterologous) (homologous) —*see* Transplant
pacemaker
brain Z96.89
cardiac Z95.0
specified NEC Z96.89
pancreatectomy Z90.410
complete Z90.410
partial Z90.411
total Z90.410
pneumonectomy (complete) (partial) Z90.2
pneumothorax, therapeutic Z98.3
postcommotio cerebri F07.81
postoperative (postprocedural) NEC Z98.890
breast implant Z98.82
dental Z98.818
crown Z98.811
fillings Z98.811
restoration Z98.811
sealant Z98.810
specified NEC Z98.818
pneumothorax, therapeutic Z98.3
uterine scar Z98.891
postpartum (routine follow-up) Z39.2
care immediately after delivery Z39.0
postsurgical (postprocedural) NEC Z98.890
pneumothorax, therapeutic Z98.3
pregnancy, incidental Z33.1
prosthesis coronary angioplasty Z95.5
pseudophakia Z96.1
renal dialysis (hemodialysis) (peritoneal) Z99.2
retained foreign body —*see* Retained, foreign body fragments (type of)
reversed jejunal transposition (for bypass Z98.0
salpingo-oophorectomy
bilateral Z90.722
unilateral Z90.721
sex reassignment surgery status Z87.890
shunt
arteriovenous (for dialysis) Z99.2
cerebrospinal fluid Z98.2
ventricular (communicating) (for drainage) Z98.2

S

Status *(Continued)*
splenectomy Z9Ø.81
thymicolymphaticus E32.8
thymicus E32.8
thymolymphaticus E32.8
thyroidectomy (hypothyroidism) E89.Ø
tooth (teeth) extraction —*see also* Absence, teeth, acquired KØ8.4Ø9
tPA (rtPA) administration in a different facility within the last 24 hours prior to admission to current facility Z92.82
tracheostomy Z93.Ø
transplant —*see* Transplant
organ removed Z98.85
tubal ligation Z98.51
underimmunization Z28.3
ureterostomy Z93.6
urethrostomy Z93.6
vagina, artificial Z93.8
vasectomy Z98.52
wheelchair confinement Z99.3
Stealing
child problem F91.8
in company with others Z72.81Ø
pathological (compulsive) F63.2
Steam burn —*see* Burn
Steatocystoma multiplex L72.2
Steatohepatitis (nonalcoholic) (NASH) K75.81
Steatoma L72.3
eyelid (cystic) —*see* Dermatosis, eyelid
infected —*see* Hordeolum
Steatorrhea (chronic) K9Ø.9
with lacteal obstruction K9Ø.2
idiopathic (adult) (infantile) K9Ø.9
pancreatic K9Ø.3
primary K9Ø.Ø
tropical K9Ø.1
Steatosis E88.89
heart —*see* Degeneration, myocardial
kidney N28.89
liver NEC K76.Ø
Steele-Richardson-Olszewski disease or syndrome G23.1
Steinbrocker's syndrome G9Ø.8
Steinert's disease G71.11
Stein-Leventhal syndrome E28.2
Stein's syndrome E28.2
STEMI —*see also* Infarct, myocardium, ST elevation I21.3
Stenocardia I2Ø.8
Stenocephaly Q75.8
Stenosis, stenotic (cicatricial) —*see also* Stricture
ampulla of Vater K83.1
anus, anal (canal) (sphincter) K62.4
and rectum K62.4
congenital Q42.3
with fistula Q42.2
aorta (ascending) (supraventricular) (congenital) Q25.1
arteriosclerotic I7Ø.Ø
calcified I7Ø.Ø
supravalvular Q25.3
aortic (valve) I35.Ø
with insufficiency I35.2
congenital Q23.Ø
rheumatic IØ6.Ø
with
incompetency, insufficiency or regurgitation IØ6.2
with mitral (valve) disease IØ8.Ø
with tricuspid (valve) disease IØ8.3
mitral (valve) disease IØ8.Ø
with tricuspid (valve) disease IØ8.3
tricuspid (valve) disease IØ8.2
with mitral (valve) disease IØ8.3
specified cause NEC I35.Ø
syphilitic A52.Ø3

Stenosis, stenotic *(Continued)*
aqueduct of Sylvius (congenital) QØ3.Ø
with spina bifida —*see* Spina bifida, by site, with hydrocephalus
acquired G91.1
artery NEC —*see also* Arteriosclerosis I77.1
celiac I77.4
cerebral —*see* Occlusion, artery, cerebral
extremities —*see* Arteriosclerosis, extremities
precerebral —*see* Occlusion, artery, precerebral
pulmonary (congenital) Q25.6
acquired I28.8
renal I7Ø.1
stent
coronary T82.855
peripheral T82.856
bile duct (common) (hepatic) K83.1
congenital Q44.3
bladder-neck (acquired) N32.Ø
congenital Q64.31
brain G93.89
bronchus J98.Ø9
congenital Q32.3
syphilitic A52.72
cardia (stomach) K22.2
congenital Q39.3
cardiovascular —*see* Disease, cardiovascular
caudal M48.Ø8
cervix, cervical (canal) N88.2
congenital Q51.828
in pregnancy or childbirth —*see* Pregnancy, complicated by, abnormal cervix
colon —*see also* Obstruction, intestine
congenital Q42.9
specified NEC Q42.8
colostomy K94.Ø3
common (bile) duct K83.1
congenital Q44.3
coronary (artery) —*see* Disease, heart, ischemic, atherosclerotic
cystic duct —*see* Obstruction, gallbladder
due to presence of device, implant or graft —*see also* Complications, by site and type, specified NEC T85.858
arterial graft NEC T82.858
breast (implant) T85.858
catheter T85.858
dialysis (renal) T82.858
intraperitoneal T85.858
infusion NEC T82.858
spinal (epidural) (subdural) T85.85Ø
urinary (indwelling) T83.85
fixation, internal (orthopedic) NEC T84.85
gastrointestinal (bile duct) (esophagus) T85.858
genital NEC T83.85
heart NEC T82.857
joint prosthesis T84.85
ocular (corneal graft) (orbital implant) NEC T85.858
orthopedic NEC T84.85
specified NEC T85.858
urinary NEC T83.85
vascular NEC T82.858
ventricular intracranial shunt T85.85Ø
duodenum K31.5
congenital Q41.Ø
ejaculatory duct NEC N5Ø.89
endocervical os —*see* Stenosis, cervix
enterostomy K94.13
esophagus K22.2
congenital Q39.3
syphilitic A52.79
congenital A5Ø.59 *[K23]*
eustachian tube —*see* Obstruction, eustachian tube

Stenosis, stenotic *(Continued)*
external ear canal (acquired) H61.3Ø- •
congenital Q16.1
due to
inflammation H61.32- •
trauma H61.31- •
postprocedural H95.81- •
specified cause NEC H61.39- •
gallbladder —*see* Obstruction, gallbladder
glottis J38.6
heart valve (congenital) Q24.8
aortic Q23.Ø
mitral Q23.2
pulmonary Q22.1
tricuspid Q22.4
hepatic duct K83.1
hymen N89.6
hypertrophic subaortic (idiopathic) I42.1
ileum —*see also* Obstruction, intestine, specified NEC K56.699
congenital Q41.2
infundibulum cardia Q24.3
intervertebral foramina —*see also* Lesion, biomechanical, specified NEC
connective tissue M99.79
abdomen M99.79
cervical region M99.71
cervicothoracic M99.71
head region M99.7Ø
lumbar region M99.73
lumbosacral M99.73
occipitocervical M99.7Ø
sacral region M99.74
sacrococcygeal M99.74
sacroiliac M99.74
specified NEC M99.79
thoracic region M99.72
thoracolumbar M99.72
disc M99.79
abdomen M99.79
cervical region M99.71
cervicothoracic M99.71
head region M99.7Ø
lower extremity M99.76
lumbar region M99.73
lumbosacral M99.73
occipitocervical M99.7Ø
pelvic M99.75
rib cage M99.78
sacral region M99.74
sacrococcygeal M99.74
sacroiliac M99.74
specified NEC M99.79
thoracic region M99.72
thoracolumbar M99.72
upper extremity M99.77
osseous M99.69
abdomen M99.69
cervical region M99.61
cervicothoracic M99.61
head region M99.6Ø
lower extremity M99.66
lumbar region M99.63
lumbosacral M99.63
occipitocervical M99.6Ø
pelvic M99.65
rib cage M99.68
sacral region M99.64
sacrococcygeal M99.64
sacroiliac M99.64
specified NEC M99.69
thoracic region M99.62
thoracolumbar M99.62
upper extremity M99.67
subluxation —*see* Stenosis, intervertebral foramina, osseous
intestine —*see also* Obstruction, intestine
congenital (small) Q41.9
large Q42.9
specified NEC Q42.8
specified NEC Q41.8

Stenosis, stenotic *(Continued)*
  jejunum —*see also* Obstruction, intestine, specified NEC K56.699
    congenital Q41.1
  lacrimal (passage)
    canaliculi H04.54- •
    congenital Q10.5
    duct H04.55- •
    punctum H04.56- •
    sac H04.57- •
  lacrimonasal duct —*see* Stenosis, lacrimal, duct
    congenital Q10.5
  larynx J38.6
    congenital NEC Q31.8
      subglottic Q31.1
    syphilitic A52.73
      congenital A50.59 *[J99]*
  mitral (chronic) (inactive) (valve) I05.0
    with
      aortic valve disease I08.0
      incompetency, insufficiency or regurgitation I05.2
    active or acute I01.1
      with rheumatic or Sydenham's chorea I02.0
    congenital Q23.2
    specified cause, except rheumatic I34.2
    syphilitic A52.03
  myocardium, myocardial —*see also* Degeneration, myocardial
    hypertrophic subaortic (idiopathic) I42.1
  nares (anterior) (posterior) J34.89
    congenital Q30.0
  nasal duct —*see also* Stenosis, lacrimal, duct
    congenital Q10.5
  nasolacrimal duct —*see also* Stenosis, lacrimal, duct
    congenital Q10.5
  neural canal —*see also* Lesion, biomechanical, specified NEC
    connective tissue M99.49
      abdomen M99.49
      cervical region M99.41
      cervicothoracic M99.41
      head region M99.40
      lower extremity M99.46
      lumbar region M99.43
      lumbosacral M99.43
      occipitocervical M99.40
      pelvic M99.45
      rib cage M99.48
      sacral region M99.44
      sacrococcygeal M99.44
      sacroiliac M99.44
      specified NEC M99.49
      thoracic region M99.42
      thoracolumbar M99.42
      upper extremity M99.47
    intervertebral disc M99.59
      abdomen M99.59
      cervical region M99.51
      cervicothoracic M99.51
      head region M99.50
      lower extremity M99.56
      lumbar region M99.53
      lumbosacral M99.53
      occipitocervical M99.50
      pelvic M99.55
      rib cage M99.58
      sacral region M99.54
      sacrococcygeal M99.54
      sacroiliac M99.54
      specified NEC M99.59
      thoracic region M99.52
      thoracolumbar M99.52
      upper extremity M99.57
    osseous M99.39
      abdomen M99.39
      cervical region M99.31
      cervicothoracic M99.31
      head region M99.30

Stenosis, stenotic *(Continued)*
  neural canal *(Continued)*
    osseous *(Continued)*
      lower extremity M99.36
      lumbar region M99.33
      lumbosacral M99.33
      occipitocervical M99.30
      pelvic M99.35
      rib cage M99.38
      sacral region M99.34
      sacrococcygeal M99.34
      sacroiliac M99.34
      specified NEC M99.39
      thoracic region M99.32
      thoracolumbar M99.32
      upper extremity M99.37
    subluxation M99.29
      cervical region M99.21
      cervicothoracic M99.21
      head region M99.20
      lower extremity M99.26
      lumbar region M99.23
      lumbosacral M99.23
      occipitocervical M99.20
      pelvic M99.25
      rib cage M99.28
      sacral region M99.24
      sacrococcygeal M99.24
      sacroiliac M99.24
      specified NEC M99.29
      thoracic region M99.22
      thoracolumbar M99.22
      upper extremity M99.27
  organ or site, congenital NEC —*see* Atresia, by site
  papilla of Vater K83.1
  pulmonary (artery) (congenital) Q25.6
    with ventricular septal defect, transposition of aorta, and hypertrophy of right ventricle Q21.3
    acquired I28.8
    in tetralogy of Fallot Q21.3
    infundibular Q24.3
    subvalvular Q24.3
    supravalvular Q25.6
    valve I37.0
      with insufficiency I37.2
      congenital Q22.1
      rheumatic I09.89
        with aortic, mitral or tricuspid (valve) disease I08.8
    vein, acquired I28.8
    vessel NEC I28.8
  pulmonic (congenital) Q22.1
    infundibular Q24.3
    subvalvular Q24.3
  pylorus (hypertrophic) (acquired) K31.1
    adult K31.1
    congenital Q40.0
    infantile Q40.0
  rectum (sphincter) —*see* Stricture, rectum
  renal artery I70.1
    congenital Q27.1
  salivary duct (any) K11.8
  sphincter of Oddi K83.1
  spinal M48.00
    cervical region M48.02
    cervicothoracic region M48.03
    lumbar region (NOS) (without neurogenic claudication) M48.061
      with neurogenic claudication M48.062
    lumbosacral region M48.07
    occipito-atlanto-axial region M48.01
    sacrococcygeal region M48.08
    thoracic region M48.04
    thoracolumbar region M48.05
  stent
    vascular
      end stent
        adjacent to stent —*see* Arteriosclerosis

Stenosis, stenotic *(Continued)*
  stent *(Continued)*
    vascular *(Continued)*
      end stent *(Continued)*
        within the stent
          coronary T82.855
          peripheral T82.856
      in stent
        coronary vessel T82.855
        peripheral vessel T82.856
  stomach, hourglass K31.2
  subaortic (congenital) Q24.4
    hypertrophic (idiopathic) I42.1
  subglottic J38.6
    congenital Q31.1
    postprocedural J95.5
  trachea J39.8
    congenital Q32.1
    syphilitic A52.73
    tuberculous NEC A15.5
  tracheostomy J95.03
  tricuspid (valve) I07.0
    with
      aortic (valve) disease I08.2
      incompetency, insufficiency or regurgitation I07.2
        with aortic (valve) disease I08.2
          with mitral (valve) disease I08.3
      mitral (valve) disease I08.1
        with aortic (valve) disease I08.3
    congenital Q22.4
    nonrheumatic I36.0
      with insufficiency I36.2
  tubal N97.1
  ureter —*see* Atresia, ureter
  ureteropelvic junction, congenital Q62.11
  ureterovesical orifice, congenital Q62.12
  urethra (valve) —*see also* Stricture, urethra
    congenital Q64.32
  urinary meatus, congenital Q64.33
  vagina N89.5
    congenital Q52.4
    in pregnancy —*see* Pregnancy, complicated by, abnormal vagina
      causing obstructed labor O65.5
  valve (cardiac) (heart) —*see also* Endocarditis I38
    congenital Q24.8
      aortic Q23.0
      mitral Q23.2
      pulmonary Q22.1
      tricuspid Q22.4
  vena cava (inferior) (superior) I87.1
    congenital Q26.0
  vesicourethral orifice Q64.31
  vulva N90.5
Stent jail T82.897
Stercolith (impaction) K56.41
  appendix K38.1
Stercoraceous, stercoral ulcer K63.3
  anus or rectum K62.6
Stereotypies NEC F98.4
Sterility —*see* Infertility
Sterilization —*see* Encounter (for), sterilization
Sternalgia —*see* Angina
Sternopagus Q89.4
Sternum bifidum Q76.7
Steroid
  effects (adverse) (adrenocortical) (iatrogenic)
    cushingoid E24.2
      correct substance properly administered —*see* Table of Drugs and Chemicals, by drug, adverse effect
      overdose or wrong substance given or taken —*see* Table of Drugs and Chemicals, by drug, poisoning

S

Steroid *(Continued)*
effects *(Continued)*
diabetes —*see* category EØ9
correct substance properly administered —*see* Table of Drugs and Chemicals, by drug, adverse effect
overdose or wrong substance given or taken —*see* Table of Drugs and Chemicals, by drug, poisoning
fever R5Ø.2
insufficiency E27.3
correct substance properly administered —*see* Table of Drugs and Chemicals, by drug, adverse effect
overdose or wrong substance given or taken —*see* Table of Drugs and Chemicals, by drug, poisoning
responder H4Ø.Ø4-●
Stevens-Johnson disease or syndrome L51.1
toxic epidermal necrolysis overlap L51.3
Stewart-Morel syndrome M85.2
Sticker's disease BØ8.3
Sticky eye —*see* Conjunctivitis, acute, mucopurulent
Stieda's disease —*see* Bursitis, tibial collateral
Stiff neck —*see* Torticollis
Stiff-man syndrome G25.82
Stiffness, joint NEC M25.6Ø-●
ankle M25.67-●
ankylosis —*see* Ankylosis, joint
contracture —*see* Contraction, joint
elbow M25.62-●
foot M25.67-●
hand M25.64-●
hip M25.65-●
knee M25.66-●
shoulder M25.61-●
wrist M25.63-●
Stigmata congenital syphilis A5Ø.59
Stillbirth P95
Still-Felty syndrome —*see* Felty's syndrome
Still's disease or syndrome (juvenile) MØ8.2Ø
adult-onset MØ6.1
ankle MØ8.27-●
elbow MØ8.22-●
foot joint MØ8.27-●
hand joint MØ8.24-●
hip MØ8.25-●
knee MØ8.26-●
multiple site MØ8.29
shoulder MØ8.21-●
vertebra MØ8.28
wrist MØ8.23-●
Stimulation, ovary E28.1
Sting (venomous) (with allergic or anaphylactic shock) —*see* Table of Drugs and Chemicals, by animal or substance, poisoning
Stippled epiphyses Q78.8
Stitch
abscess T81.41
burst (in operation wound) —*see* Disruption, wound, operation
Stokes-Adams disease or syndrome I45.9
Stokes' disease EØ5.ØØ
with thyroid storm EØ5.Ø1
Stokvis (-Talma) disease D74.8
Stoma malfunction
colostomy K94.Ø3
enterostomy K94.13
gastrostomy K94.23
ileostomy K94.13
tracheostomy J95.Ø3
Stomach —*see* condition
Stomatitis (denture) (ulcerative) K12.1
angular K13.Ø
due to dietary or vitamin deficiency E53.Ø
aphthous K12.Ø
bovine BØ8.61
Stomatitis *(Continued)*
candidal B37.Ø
catarrhal K12.1
diphtheritic A36.89
due to
dietary deficiency E53.Ø
thrush B37.Ø
vitamin deficiency
B group NEC E53.9
B2 (riboflavin) E53.Ø
epidemic BØ8.8
epizootic BØ8.8
follicular K12.1
gangrenous A69.Ø
Geotrichum B48.3
herpesviral, herpetic BØØ.2
herpetiformis K12.Ø
malignant K12.1
membranous acute K12.1
monilial B37.Ø
mycotic B37.Ø
necrotizing ulcerative A69.Ø
parasitic B37.Ø
septic K12.1
spirochetal A69.1
suppurative (acute) K12.2
ulceromembranous A69.1
vesicular K12.1
with exanthem (enteroviral) BØ8.4
virus disease A93.8
Vincent's A69.1
Stomatocytosis D58.8
Stomatomycosis B37.Ø
Stomatorrhagia K13.79
Stone(s) —*see also* Calculus
bladder (diverticulum) N21.Ø
cystine E72.Ø9
heart syndrome I5Ø.1
kidney N2Ø.Ø
prostate N42.Ø
pulpal (dental) KØ4.2
renal N2Ø.Ø
salivary gland or duct (any) K11.5
urethra (impacted) N21.1
urinary (duct) (impacted) (passage) N2Ø.9
bladder (diverticulum) N21.Ø
lower tract N21.9
specified NEC N21.8
xanthine E79.8 *[N22]*
Stonecutter's lung J62.8
Stonemason's asthma, disease, lung or pneumoconiosis J62.8
Stoppage
heart —*see* Arrest, cardiac
urine —*see* Retention, urine
Storm, thyroid —*see* Thyrotoxicosis
Strabismus (congenital) (nonparalytic) H5Ø.9
concomitant H5Ø.4Ø
convergent —*see* Strabismus, convergent concomitant
divergent —*see* Strabismus, divergent concomitant
convergent concomitant H5Ø.ØØ
accommodative component H5Ø.43
alternating H5Ø.Ø5
with
A pattern H5Ø.Ø6
specified nonconcomitances NEC H5Ø.Ø8
V pattern H5Ø.Ø7
monocular H5Ø.Ø1-●
with
A pattern H5Ø.Ø2-●
specified noncomitances NEC H5Ø.Ø4-●
V pattern H5Ø.Ø3-●
intermittent H5Ø.31-●
alternating H5Ø.32
Strabismus *(Continued)*
cyclotropia H5Ø.41
divergent concomitant H5Ø.1Ø
alternating H5Ø.15
with
A pattern H5Ø.16
specified noncomitances NEC H5Ø.18
V pattern H5Ø.17
monocular H5Ø.11-●
with
A pattern H5Ø.12-●
specified noncomitances NEC H5Ø.14-●
V pattern H5Ø.13-●
intermittent H5Ø.33-●
alternating H5Ø.34
Duane's syndrome H5Ø.81-●
due to adhesions, scars H5Ø.69
heterophoria H5Ø.5Ø
alternating H5Ø.55
cyclophoria H5Ø.54
esophoria H5Ø.51
exophoria H5Ø.52
vertical H5Ø.53
heterotropia H5Ø.4Ø
intermittent H5Ø.3Ø
hypertropia H5Ø.2-●
hypotropia —*see* Hypertropia
latent H5Ø.5Ø
mechanical H5Ø.6Ø
Brown's sheath syndrome H5Ø.61-●
specified type NEC H5Ø.69
monofixation syndrome H5Ø.42
paralytic H49.9
abducens nerve H49.2-●
fourth nerve H49.1-●
Kearns-Sayre syndrome H49.81-●
ophthalmoplegia (external)
progressive H49.4-●
with pigmentary retinopathy H49.81-●
total H49.3-●
sixth nerve H49.2-●
specified type NEC H49.88-●
third nerve H49.Ø-●
trochlear nerve H49.1-●
specified type NEC H5Ø.89
vertical H5Ø.2-●
Strain
back S39.Ø12
cervical S16.1
eye NEC —*see* Disturbance, vision, subjective
heart —*see* Disease, heart
low back S39.Ø12
mental NOS Z73.3
work-related Z56.6
muscle (tendon) —*see* Injury, muscle, by site, strain
neck S16.1
physical NOS Z73.3
work-related Z56.6
postural —*see also* Disorder, soft tissue, due to use
psychological NEC Z73.3
tendon —*see* Injury, muscle, by site, strain
Straining, on urination R39.16
Strand, vitreous —*see* Opacity, vitreous, membranes and strands
Strangulation, strangulated —*see also* Asphyxia, traumatic
appendix K38.8
bladder-neck N32.Ø
bowel or colon K56.2
food or foreign body —*see* Foreign body, by site
hemorrhoids —*see* Hemorrhoids, with complication
hernia —*see also* Hernia, by site, with obstruction
with gangrene —*see* Hernia, by site, with gangrene

S

Strangulation, strangulated *(Continued)*
intestine (large) (small) K56.2
with hernia —*see also* Hernia, by site, with obstruction
with gangrene —*see* Hernia, by site, with gangrene
mesentery K56.2
mucus —*see* Asphyxia, mucus
omentum K56.2
organ or site, congenital NEC —*see* Atresia, by site
ovary —*see* Torsion, ovary
penis N48.89
foreign body T19.4
rupture —*see* Hernia, by site, with obstruction
stomach due to hernia —*see also* Hernia, by site, with obstruction
with gangrene —*see* Hernia, by site, with gangrene
vesicourethral orifice N32.Ø
Strangury R3Ø.Ø
Straw itch B88.Ø
Strawberry
gallbladder K82.4
mark Q82.5
tongue (red) (white) K14.3
Streak(s)
macula, angioid H35.33
ovarian Q5Ø.32
Strephosymbolia F81.Ø
secondary to organic lesion R48.8
Streptobacillary fever A25.1
Streptobacillosis A25.1
Streptobacillus moniliformis A25.1
Streptococcus, streptococcal —*see also* condition
as cause of disease classified elsewhere B95.5
group
A, as cause of disease classified elsewhere B95.Ø
B, as cause of disease classified elsewhere B95.1
D, as cause of disease classified elsewhere B95.2
pneumoniae, as cause of disease classified elsewhere B95.3
specified NEC, as cause of disease classified elsewhere B95.4
Streptomycosis B47.1
Streptotrichosis A48.8
Stress F43.9
family —*see* Disruption, family
fetal P84
complicating pregnancy O77.9
due to drug administration O77.1
mental NEC Z73.3
work-related Z56.6
physical NEC Z73.3
work-related Z56.6
polycythemia D75.1
reaction —*see also* Reaction, stress F43.9
work schedule Z56.3
Stretching, nerve —*see* Injury, nerve
Striae albicantes, atrophicae or distensae (cutis) L9Ø.6
Stricture —*see also* Stenosis
ampulla of Vater K83.1
anus (sphincter) K62.4
congenital Q42.3
with fistula Q42.2
infantile Q42.3
with fistula Q42.2
aorta (ascending) (congenital) Q25.1
arteriosclerotic I7Ø.Ø
calcified I7Ø.Ø
supravalvular, congenital Q25.3
aortic (valve) —*see* Stenosis, aortic
aqueduct of Sylvius (congenital) QØ3.Ø
with spina bifida —*see* Spina bifida, by site, with hydrocephalus
acquired G91.1

Stricture *(Continued)*
artery I77.1
basilar —*see* Occlusion, artery, basilar
carotid —*see* Occlusion, artery, carotid
celiac I77.4
congenital (peripheral) Q27.8
cerebral Q28.3
coronary Q24.5
digestive system Q27.8
lower limb Q27.8
retinal Q14.1
specified site NEC Q27.8
umbilical Q27.Ø
upper limb Q27.8
coronary —*see* Disease, heart, ischemic, atherosclerotic
congenital Q24.5
precerebral —*see* Occlusion, artery, precerebral
pulmonary (congenital) Q25.6
acquired I28.8
renal I7Ø.1
vertebral —*see* Occlusion, artery, vertebral
auditory canal (external) (congenital)
acquired —*see* Stenosis, external ear canal
bile duct (common) (hepatic) K83.1
congenital Q44.3
postoperative K91.89
bladder N32.89
neck N32.Ø
bowel —*see* Obstruction, intestine
brain G93.89
bronchus J98.Ø9
congenital Q32.3
syphilitic A52.72
cardia (stomach) K22.2
congenital Q39.3
cardiac —*see also* Disease, heart
orifice (stomach) K22.2
cecum —*see* Obstruction, intestine
cervix, cervical (canal) N88.2
congenital Q51.828
in pregnancy —*see* Pregnancy, complicated by, abnormal cervix
causing obstructed labor O65.5
colon —*see also* Obstruction, intestine
congenital Q42.9
specified NEC Q42.8
colostomy K94.Ø3
common (bile) duct K83.1
coronary (artery) —*see* Disease, heart, ischemic, atherosclerotic
cystic duct —*see* Obstruction, gallbladder
digestive organs NEC, congenital Q45.8
duodenum K31.5
congenital Q41.Ø
ear canal (external) (congenital) Q16.1
acquired —*see* Stricture, auditory canal, acquired
ejaculatory duct N5Ø.89
enterostomy K94.13
esophagus K22.2
congenital Q39.3
syphilitic A52.79
congenital A5Ø.59 *[K23]*
eustachian tube —*see also* Obstruction, eustachian tube
congenital Q17.8
fallopian tube N97.1
gonococcal A54.24
tuberculous A18.17
gallbladder —*see* Obstruction, gallbladder
glottis J38.6
heart —*see also* Disease, heart
valve (*see also* Endocarditis) I38
aortic Q23.Ø
mitral Q23.2
pulmonary Q22.1
tricuspid Q22.4
hepatic duct K83.1
hourglass, of stomach K31.2

Stricture *(Continued)*
hymen N89.6
hypopharynx J39.2
ileum —*see also* Obstruction, intestine, specified NEC K56.699
congenital Q41.2
intestine —*see also* Obstruction, intestine
congenital (small) Q41.9
large Q42.9
specified NEC Q42.8
specified NEC Q41.8
ischemic K55.1
jejunum —*see also* Obstruction, intestine, specified NEC K56.699
congenital Q41.1
lacrimal passages —*see also* Stenosis, lacrimal
congenital Q1Ø.5
larynx J38.6
congenital NEC Q31.8
subglottic Q31.1
syphilitic A52.73
congenital A5Ø.59 *[J99]*
meatus
ear (congenital) Q16.1
acquired —*see* Stricture, auditory canal, acquired
osseous (ear) (congenital) Q16.1
acquired —*see* Stricture, auditory canal, acquired
urinarius —*see also* Stricture, urethra
congenital Q64.33
mitral (valve) —*see* Stenosis, mitral
myocardium, myocardial I51.5
hypertrophic subaortic (idiopathic) I42.1
nares (anterior) (posterior) J34.89
congenital Q3Ø.Ø
nasal duct —*see also* Stenosis, lacrimal, duct
congenital Q1Ø.5
nasolacrimal duct —*see also* Stenosis, lacrimal, duct
congenital Q1Ø.5
nasopharynx J39.2
syphilitic A52.73
nose J34.89
congenital Q3Ø.Ø
nostril (anterior) (posterior) J34.89
congenital Q3Ø.Ø
syphilitic A52.73
congenital A5Ø.59 *[J99]*
organ or site, congenital NEC —*see* Atresia, by site
os uteri —*see* Stricture, cervix
osseous meatus (ear) (congenital) Q16.1
acquired —*see* Stricture, auditory canal, acquired
oviduct —*see* Stricture, fallopian tube
pelviureteric junction (congenital) Q62.11
acquired, with hydronephrosis N13.Ø
penis, by foreign body T19.4
pharynx J39.2
prostate N42.89
pulmonary, pulmonic
artery (congenital) Q25.6
acquired I28.8
noncongenital I28.8
infundibulum (congenital) Q24.3
valve I37.Ø
congenital Q22.1
vein, acquired I28.8
vessel NEC I28.8
punctum lacrimale —*see also* Stenosis, lacrimal, punctum
congenital Q1Ø.5
pylorus (hypertrophic) K31.1
adult K31.1
congenital Q4Ø.Ø
infantile Q4Ø.Ø
rectosigmoid —*see also* Obstruction, intestine, specified NEC K56.699
rectum (sphincter) K62.4
congenital Q42.1
with fistula Q42.Ø

Stricture *(Continued)*
rectum *(Continued)*
due to
chlamydial lymphogranuloma A55
irradiation K91.89
lymphogranuloma venereum A55
gonococcal A54.6
inflammatory (chlamydial) A55
syphilitic A52.74
tuberculous A18.32
renal artery I70.1
congenital Q27.1
salivary duct or gland (any) K11.8
sigmoid (flexure) *—see* Obstruction, intestine
spermatic cord N50.89
stoma (following) (of)
colostomy K94.03
enterostomy K94.13
gastrostomy K94.23
ileostomy K94.13
tracheostomy J95.03
stomach K31.89
congenital Q40.2
hourglass K31.2
subaortic Q24.4
hypertrophic (acquired) (idiopathic) I42.1
subglottic J38.6
syphilitic NEC A52.79
trachea J39.8
congenital Q32.1
syphilitic A52.73
tuberculous NEC A15.5
tracheostomy J95.03
tricuspid (valve) *—see* Stenosis, tricuspid
tunica vaginalis N50.89
ureter (postoperative) N13.5
with
hydronephrosis N13.1
with infection N13.6
pyelonephritis (chronic) N11.1
congenital *—see* Atresia, ureter
tuberculous A18.11
ureteropelvic junction (congenital) Q62.11
acquired, with hydronephrosis N13.0
ureterovesical orifice N13.5
with infection N13.6
urethra (organic) (spasmodic) (*see also* Stricture, urethra, male N35.919
associated with schistosomiasis B65.0 *[N37]*
congenital Q64.39
valvular (posterior) Q64.2
due to
infection *—see* Stricture, urethra, postinfective
trauma *—see* Stricture, urethra, post-traumatic
female N35.92
gonococcal, gonorrheal A54.01
infective NEC *—see* Stricture, urethra, postinfective
late effect (sequelae) of injury *—see* Stricture, urethra, post-traumatic
male N35.919
anterior urethra N35.914
bulbous urethra N35.912
meatal N35.911
membranous urethra N35.913
overlapping sites N35.916
postcatheterization *—see* Stricture, urethra, postprocedural
postinfective NEC
female N35.12
male N35.119
anterior urethra N35.114
bulbous urethra N35.112
meatal N35.111
membranous urethra N35.113
overlapping sites N35.116
postobstetric N35.021
postoperative *—see* Stricture, urethra, postprocedural

Stricture *(Continued)*
urethra (organic) (spasmodic) *(Continued)*
postprocedural
female N99.12
male N99.114
anterior bulbous urethra N99.113
bulbous urethra N99.111
fossa navicularis N99.115
meatal N99.110
membranous urethra N99.112
overlapping sites N35.116
post-traumatic
female N35.028
due to childbirth N35.021
male N35.014
anterior urethra N35.013
bulbous urethra N35.011
meatal N35.010
membranous urethra N35.012
overlapping sites N35.016
sequela (late effect) of
childbirth N35.021
injury *—see* Stricture, urethra, post-traumatic
specified cause NEC
female N35.82
male N35.819
anterior urethra N35.814
bulbous urethra N35.812
meatal N35.811
membranous urethra N35.813
overlapping sites N35.816
syphilitic A52.76
traumatic *—see* Stricture, urethra, post-traumatic
valvular (posterior), congenital Q64.2
urinary meatus *—see* Stricture, urethra
uterus, uterine (synechiae) N85.6
os (external) (internal) *—see* Stricture, cervix
vagina (outlet) *—see* Stenosis, vagina
valve (cardiac) (heart) *—see also* Endocarditis
congenital
aortic Q23.0
mitral Q23.2
pulmonary Q22.1
tricuspid Q22.4
vas deferens N50.89
congenital Q55.4
vein I87.1
vena cava (inferior) (superior) NEC I87.1
congenital Q26.0
vesicourethral orifice N32.0
congenital Q64.31
vulva (acquired) N90.5
Stridor R06.1
congenital (larynx) P28.89
Stridulous *—see* condition
Stroke (apoplectic) (brain) (embolic) (ischemic) (paralytic) (thrombotic) I63.9
cryptogenic *—see also* infarction, cerebral I63.9
epileptic *—see* Epilepsy
➡ heat T67.01
▶ exertional T67.02
▶ specified NEC T67.09
in evolution I63.9
intraoperative
during cardiac surgery I97.810
during other surgery I97.811
lightning *—see* Lightning
meaning
cerebral hemorrhage — code to Hemorrhage, intracranial
cerebral infarction — code to Infarction, cerebral
postprocedural
following cardiac surgery I97.820
following other surgery I97.821
▶ sun T67.01
▶ specified NEC T67.09
unspecified (NOS) I63.9
Stromatosis, endometrial D39.0

Strongyloidiasis, strongyloidosis B78.9
cutaneous B78.1
disseminated B78.7
intestinal B78.0
Strophulus pruriginosus L28.2
Struck by lightning *—see* Lightning
Struma *—see also* Goiter
Hashimoto E06.3
lymphomatosa E06.3
nodosa (simplex) E04.9
endemic E01.2
multinodular E01.1
multinodular E04.2
iodine-deficiency related E01.1
toxic or with hyperthyroidism E05.20
with thyroid storm E05.21
multinodular E05.20
with thyroid storm E05.21
uninodular E05.10
with thyroid storm E05.11
toxicosa E05.20
with thyroid storm E05.21
multinodular E05.20
with thyroid storm E05.21
uninodular E05.10
with thyroid storm E05.11
uninodular E04.1
ovarii D27.-●
Riedel's E06.5
Strumipriva cachexia E03.4
Strümpell-Marie spine *—see* Spondylitis, ankylosing
Strümpell-Westphal pseudosclerosis E83.01
Stuart deficiency disease (factor X) D68.2
Stuart-Prower factor deficiency (factor X) D68.2
Student's elbow *—see* Bursitis, elbow, olecranon
Stump *—see* Amputation
Stunting, nutritional E45
Stupor (catatonic) R40.1
depressive (single episode) F32.89
recurrent episode F33.8
dissociative F44.2
manic F30.2
manic-depressive F31.89
psychogenic (anergic) F44.2
reaction to exceptional stress (transient) F43.0
Sturge (-Weber) (-Dimitri) (-Kalischer) **disease or syndrome** Q85.8
Stuttering F80.81
adult onset F98.5
childhood onset F80.81
following cerebrovascular disease — *see* Disorder, fluency, following cerebrovascular disease
in conditions classified elsewhere R47.82
Sty, stye (external) (internal) (meibomian) (zeisian) *—see* Hordeolum
Subacidity, gastric K31.89
psychogenic F45.8
Subacute *—see* condition
Subarachnoid *—see* condition
Subcortical *—see* condition
Subcostal syndrome, nerve compression *—see* Mononeuropathy, upper limb, specified site NEC
Subcutaneous, subcuticular *—see* condition
Subdural *—see* condition
Subendocardium *—see* condition
Subependymoma
specified site *—see* Neoplasm, uncertain behavior, by site
unspecified site D43.2
Suberosis J67.3
Subglossitis *—see* Glossitis
Subhemophilia D66
Subinvolution
breast (postlactational) (postpuerperal) N64.89
puerperal O90.89
uterus (chronic) (nonpuerperal) N85.3
puerperal O90.89
Sublingual *—see* condition

S

▶ New ➡ Revised ~~deleted~~ Deleted ● Use Additional Character(s)

Sublinguitis —*see* Sialoadenitis
Subluxatable hip Q65.6
Subluxation —*see also* Dislocation
acromioclavicular S43.11-●
ankle S93.0-●
atlantoaxial, recurrent M43.4
with myelopathy M43.3
carpometacarpal (joint) NEC S63.05-●
thumb S63.04-●
complex, vertebral —*see* Complex, subluxation
congenital —*see also* Malposition, congenital
hip —*see* Dislocation, hip, congenital, partial
joint (excluding hip)
lower limb Q68.8
shoulder Q68.8
upper limb Q68.8
elbow (traumatic) S53.10-●
anterior S53.11-●
lateral S53.14-●
medial S53.13-●
posterior S53.12-●
specified type NEC S53.19-●
finger S63.20-●
index S63.20-●
interphalangeal S63.22-●
distal S63.24-●
index S63.24-●
little S63.24-●
middle S63.24-●
ring S63.24-●
index S63.22-●
little S63.22-●
middle S63.22-●
proximal S63.23-●
index S63.23-●
little S63.23-●
middle S63.23-●
ring S63.23-●
ring S63.22-●
little S63.20-●
metacarpophalangeal S63.21-●
index S63.21-●
little S63.21-●
middle S63.21-●
ring S63.21-●
middle S63.20-●
ring S63.20-●
foot S93.30-●
specified site NEC S93.33-●
tarsal joint S93.31-●
tarsometatarsal joint S93.32-●
toe —*see* Subluxation, toe
hip S73.00-●
anterior S73.03-●
obturator S73.02-●
central S73.04-●
posterior S73.01-●
interphalangeal (joint)
finger S63.22-●
distal joint S63.24-●
index S63.24-●
little S63.24-●
middle S63.24-●
ring S63.24-●
index S63.22-●
little S63.22-●
middle S63.22-●
proximal joint S63.23-●
index S63.23-●
little S63.23-●
middle S63.23-●
ring S63.23-●
ring S63.22-●
thumb S63.12-●
toe S93.13-●
great S93.13-●
lesser S93.13-●
joint prosthesis —*see* Complications, joint prosthesis, mechanical, displacement, by site
Subluxation *(Continued)*
knee S83.10-●
cap —*see* Subluxation, patella
patella —*see* Subluxation, patella
proximal tibia
anteriorly S83.11-●
laterally S83.14-●
medially S83.13-●
posteriorly S83.12-●
specified type NEC S83.19-●
lens —*see* Dislocation, lens, partial
ligament, traumatic —*see* Sprain, by site
metacarpal (bone)
proximal end S63.06-●
metacarpophalangeal (joint)
finger S63.21-●
index S63.21-●
little S63.21-●
middle S63.21-●
ring S63.21-●
thumb S63.11-●
metatarsophalangeal joint S93.14-●
great toe S93.14-●
lesser toe S93.14-●
midcarpal (joint) S63.03-●
patella S83.00-●
lateral S83.01-●
recurrent (nontraumatic) —*see* Dislocation, patella, recurrent, incomplete
specified type NEC S83.09-●
pathological —*see* Dislocation, pathological
radial head S53.00-●
anterior S53.01-●
nursemaid's elbow S53.03-●
posterior S53.02-●
specified type NEC S53.09-●
radiocarpal (joint) S63.02-●
radioulnar (joint)
distal S63.01-●
proximal —*see* Subluxation, elbow
shoulder
congenital Q68.8
girdle S43.30-●
scapula S43.31-●
specified site NEC S43.39-●
traumatic S43.00-●
anterior S43.01-●
inferior S43.03-●
posterior S43.02-●
specified type NEC S43.08-●
sternoclavicular (joint) S43.20-●
anterior S43.21-●
posterior S43.22-●
symphysis (pubis)
thumb S63.103
interphalangeal joint —*see* Subluxation, interphalangeal (joint), thumb
metacarpophalangeal joint —*see* Subluxation, metacarpophalangeal (joint), thumb
toe(s) S93.10-●
great S93.10-●
interphalangeal joint S93.13-●
metatarsophalangeal joint S93.14-●
interphalangeal joint S93.13-●
lesser S93.10-●
interphalangeal joint S93.13-●
metatarsophalangeal joint S93.14-●
metatarsophalangeal joint S93.149
ulnohumeral joint —*see* Subluxation, elbow
vertebral
recurrent NEC —*see* subcategory M43.5
traumatic
cervical S13.100
atlantoaxial joint S13.120
atlantooccipital joint S13.110
atloidooccipital joint S13.110
Subluxation *(Continued)*
vertebral *(Continued)*
traumatic *(Continued)*
cervical *(Continued)*
joint between
C0 and C1 S13.110
C1 and C2 S13.120
C2 and C3 S13.130
C3 and C4 S13.140
C4 and C5 S13.150
C5 and C6 S13.160
C6 and C7 S13.170
C7 and T1 S13.180
occipitoatloid joint S13.110
lumbar S33.100
joint between
L1 and L2 S33.110
L2 and L3 S33.120
L3 and L4 S33.130
L4 and L5 S33.140
thoracic S23.100
joint between
T1 and T2 S23.110
T2 and T3 S23.120
T3 and T4 S23.122
T4 and T5 S23.130
T5 and T6 S23.132
T6 and T7 S23.140
T7 and T8 S23.142
T8 and T9 S23.150
T9 and T10 S23.152
T10 and T11 S23.160
T11 and T12 S23.162
T12 and L1 S23.170
ulna
distal end S63.07-●
proximal end —*see* Subluxation, elbow
wrist (carpal bone) S63.00-●
carpometacarpal joint —*see* Subluxation, carpometacarpal (joint)
distal radioulnar joint —*see* Subluxation, radioulnar (joint), distal
metacarpal bone, proximal —*see* Subluxation, metacarpal (bone), proximal end
midcarpal —*see* Subluxation, midcarpal (joint)
radiocarpal joint —*see* Subluxation, radiocarpal (joint)
recurrent —*see* Dislocation, recurrent, wrist
specified site NEC S63.09-●
ulna —*see* Subluxation, ulna, distal end
Submaxillary —*see* condition
Submersion (fatal) (nonfatal) T75.1
Submucous —*see* condition
Subnormal, subnormality
accommodation (old age) H52.4
mental —*see* Disability, intellectual
temperature (accidental) T68
Subphrenic —*see* condition
Subscapular nerve —*see* condition
Subseptus uterus Q51.28
Subsiding appendicitis K36
Substance (other psychoactive) **-induced**
anxiety disorder F19.980
bipolar and related disorder F19.94
delirium F19.921
depressive disorder F19.94
major neurocognitive disorder F19.97
mild neurocognitive disorder F19.988
obsessive-compulsive and related disorder F19.988
psychotic disorder F19.959
sexual dysfunction F19.981
sleep disorder F19.982
Substernal thyroid E04.9
congenital Q89.2
Substitution disorder F44.9
Subtentorial —*see* condition
Subthyroidism (acquired) —*see also* Hypothyroidism
congenital E03.1

- Succenturiate placenta O43.19- ●
- Sucking thumb, child (excessive) F98.8
- Sudamen, sudamina L74.1
- Sudanese kala-azar B55.Ø
- Sudden
  - hearing loss —*see* Deafness, sudden
  - heart failure —*see* Failure, heart
- Sudeck's atrophy, disease, or syndrome —*see* Algoneurodystrophy
- Suffocation —*see* Asphyxia, traumatic
- Sugar
  - blood
    - high (transient) R73.9
    - low (transient) E16.2
  - in urine R81
- Suicide, suicidal (attempted) T14.91
  - by poisoning —*see* Table of Drugs and Chemicals
  - history of (personal) Z91.5
    - in family Z81.8
  - ideation —*see* Ideation, suicidal
  - risk
    - meaning personal history of attempted suicide Z91.5
    - meaning suicidal ideation —*see* Ideation, suicidal
  - tendencies
    - meaning personal history of attempted suicide Z91.5
    - meaning suicidal ideation —*see* Ideation, suicidal
  - trauma —*see* nature of injury by site
- Suipestifer infection —*see* Infection, salmonella
- Sulfhemoglobinemia, sulphemoglobinemia (acquired) (with methemoglobinemia) D74.8
- Sumatran mite fever A75.3
- Summer —*see* condition
- Sunburn L55.9
  - due to
    - tanning bed (acute) L56.8
      - chronic L57.8
    - ultraviolet radiation (acute) L56.8
      - chronic L57.8
  - first degree L55.Ø
  - second degree L55.1
  - third degree L55.2
- SUNCT (short lasting unilateral neuralgiform headache with conjunctival injection and tearing) G44.Ø59
  - intractable G44.Ø51
  - not intractable G44.Ø59
- Sundowning FØ5
- Sunken acetabulum —*see* Derangement, joint, specified type NEC, hip
- ➡ Sunstroke T67.Ø1
  - ▶ specified NEC T67.Ø9
- Superfecundation —*see* Pregnancy, multiple
- Superfetation —*see* Pregnancy, multiple
- Superinvolution (uterus) N85.8
- Supernumerary (congenital)
  - aortic cusps Q23.8
  - auditory ossicles Q16.3
  - bone Q79.8
  - breast Q83.1
  - carpal bones Q74.Ø
  - cusps, heart valve NEC Q24.8
    - aortic Q23.8
    - mitral Q23.2
    - pulmonary Q22.3
  - digit(s) Q69.9
  - ear (lobule) Q17.Ø
  - fallopian tube Q5Ø.6
  - finger Q69.Ø
  - hymen Q52.4
  - kidney Q63.Ø
  - lacrimonasal duct Q1Ø.6
  - lobule (ear) Q17.Ø
  - mitral cusps Q23.2
  - muscle Q79.8
  - nipple(s) Q83.3
- Supernumerary *(Continued)*
  - organ or site not listed —*see* Accessory
  - ossicles, auditory Q16.3
  - ovary Q5Ø.31
  - oviduct Q5Ø.6
  - pulmonary, pulmonic cusps Q22.3
  - rib Q76.6
    - cervical or first (syndrome) Q76.5
  - roots (of teeth) KØØ.2
  - spleen Q89.Ø9
  - tarsal bones Q74.2
  - teeth KØØ.1
  - testis Q55.29
  - thumb Q69.1
  - toe Q69.2
  - uterus Q51.28
  - vagina Q52.1
  - vertebra Q76.49
- Supervision (of)
  - contraceptive —*see* Prescription, contraceptives
  - dietary (for) Z71.3
    - allergy (food) Z71.3
    - colitis Z71.3
    - diabetes mellitus Z71.3
    - food allergy or intolerance Z71.3
    - gastritis Z71.3
    - hypercholesterolemia Z71.3
    - hypoglycemia Z71.3
    - intolerance (food) Z71.3
    - obesity Z71.3
    - specified NEC Z71.3
  - healthy infant or child Z76.2
    - foundling Z76.1
  - high-risk pregnancy —*see* Pregnancy, complicated by, high, risk
  - lactation Z39.1
  - pregnancy —*see* Pregnancy, supervision of
- Supplemental teeth KØØ.1
- Suppression
  - binocular vision H53.34
  - lactation O92.5
  - menstruation N94.89
  - ovarian secretion E28.39
  - renal N28.9
  - urine, urinary secretion R34
- Suppuration, suppurative —*see also* condition
  - accessory sinus (chronic) —*see* Sinusitis
  - adrenal gland
  - antrum (chronic) —*see* Sinusitis, maxillary
  - bladder —*see* Cystitis
  - brain GØ6.Ø
    - sequelae GØ9
  - breast N61.1
    - puerperal, postpartum or gestational —*see* Mastitis, obstetric, purulent
  - dental periosteum M27.3
  - ear (middle) —*see also* Otitis, media
    - external NEC —*see* Otitis, externa, infective
    - internal —*see* subcategory H83.Ø
  - ethmoidal (chronic) (sinus) —*see* Sinusitis, ethmoidal
  - fallopian tube —*see* Salpingo-oophoritis
  - frontal (chronic) (sinus) —*see* Sinusitis, frontal
  - gallbladder (acute) K81.Ø
  - gum KØ5.2Ø
    - ➡ generalized —*see* Periodontitis, aggressive, generalized
    - ➡ localized —*see* Periodontitis, aggressive, localized
  - intracranial GØ6.Ø
  - joint —*see* Arthritis, pyogenic or pyemic
  - labyrinthine —*see* subcategory H83.Ø
  - lung —*see* Abscess, lung
  - mammary gland N61.1
    - puerperal, postpartum O91.12
      - associated with lactation O91.13
  - maxilla, maxillary M27.2
    - sinus (chronic) —*see* Sinusitis, maxillary
  - muscle —*see* Myositis, infective
  - nasal sinus (chronic) —*see* Sinusitis
- Suppuration, suppurative *(Continued)*
  - pancreas, acute —*see also* Pancreatitis, acute K85.8Ø
  - parotid gland —*see* Sialoadenitis
  - pelvis, pelvic
    - female —*see* Disease, pelvis, inflammatory
    - male K65.Ø
  - pericranial —*see* Osteomyelitis
  - salivary duct or gland (any) —*see* Sialoadenitis
  - sinus (accessory) (chronic) (nasal) —*see* Sinusitis
  - sphenoidal sinus (chronic) —*see* Sinusitis, sphenoidal
  - thymus (gland) E32.1
  - thyroid (gland) EØ6.Ø
  - tonsil —*see* Tonsillitis
  - uterus —*see* Endometritis
- Supraeruption of tooth (teeth) M26.34
- Supraglottitis JØ4.3Ø
  - with obstruction JØ4.31
- Suprarenal (gland) —*see* condition
- Suprascapular nerve —*see* condition
- Suprasellar —*see* condition
- Surfer's knots or nodules S89.8- ●
- Surgical
  - emphysema T81.82
  - procedures, complication or misadventure —*see* Complications, surgical procedures
  - shock T81.1Ø
- Surveillance (of) (for) —*see also* Observation
  - alcohol abuse Z71.41
  - contraceptive —*see* Prescription, contraceptives
  - dietary Z71.3
  - drug abuse Z71.51
- Susceptibility to disease, genetic Z15.89
  - malignant neoplasm Z15.Ø9
    - breast Z15.Ø1
    - endometrium Z15.Ø4
    - ovary Z15.Ø2
    - prostate Z15.Ø3
    - specified NEC Z15.Ø9
  - multiple endocrine neoplasia Z15.81
- Suspected condition, ruled out —*see also* Observation, suspected
  - amniotic cavity and membrane ZØ3.71
  - cervical shortening ZØ3.75
  - fetal anomaly ZØ3.73
  - fetal growth ZØ3.74
  - maternal and fetal conditions NEC ZØ3.79
  - newborn —*see also* Observation, newborn, suspected condition ruled out ZØ5.9
  - oligohydramnios ZØ3.71
  - placental problem ZØ3.72
  - polyhydramnios ZØ3.71
- Suspended uterus
  - in pregnancy or childbirth —*see* Pregnancy, complicated by, abnormal uterus
- Sutton's nevus D22.9
- Suture
  - burst (in operation wound) T81.31
    - external operation wound T81.31
    - internal operation wound T81.32
  - inadvertently left in operation wound —*see* Foreign body, accidentally left during a procedure
  - removal Z48.Ø2
- Swab inadvertently left in operation wound —*see* Foreign body, accidentally left during a procedure
- Swallowed, swallowing
  - difficulty —*see* Dysphagia
  - foreign body —*see* Foreign body, alimentary tract
- Swan-neck deformity (finger) —*see* Deformity, finger, swan-neck
- Swearing, compulsive F42.8
  - in Gilles de la Tourette's syndrome F95.2
- Sweat, sweats
  - fetid L75.Ø
  - night R61

S

- **Sweating, excessive** R61
- **Sweeley-Klionsky disease** E75.21
- **Sweet's disease or dermatosis** L98.2
- **Swelling (of)** R60.9
  - abdomen, abdominal (not referable to any particular organ) —*see* Mass, abdominal
  - ankle —*see* Effusion, joint, ankle
  - arm M79.89
    - forearm M79.89
  - breast —*see also* Lump, breast N63.0
  - Calabar B74.3
  - cervical gland R59.0
  - chest, localized R22.2
  - ear H93.8-•
  - extremity (lower) (upper) —*see* Disorder, soft tissue, specified type NEC
  - finger M79.89
  - foot M79.89
  - glands R59.9
    - generalized R59.1
    - localized R59.0
  - hand M79.89
  - head (localized) R22.0
  - inflammatory —*see* Inflammation
  - intra-abdominal —*see* Mass, abdominal
  - joint —*see* Effusion, joint
  - leg M79.89
    - lower M79.89
  - limb —*see* Disorder, soft tissue, specified type NEC
  - localized (skin) R22.9
    - chest R22.2
    - head R22.0
    - limb
      - lower —*see* Mass, localized, limb, lower
      - upper —*see* Mass, localized, limb, upper
    - neck R22.1
    - trunk R22.2
  - neck (localized) R22.1
  - pelvic —*see* Mass, abdominal
  - scrotum N50.89
  - splenic —*see* Splenomegaly
  - testis N50.89
  - toe M79.89
  - umbilical R19.09
  - wandering, due to Gnathostoma (spinigerum) B83.1
  - white —*see* Tuberculosis, arthritis
- **Swift (-Feer) disease**
  - overdose or wrong substance given or taken —*see* Table of Drugs and Chemicals, by drug, poisoning
- **Swimmer's**
  - cramp T75.1
  - ear H60.33-•
  - itch B65.3
- **Swimming in the head** R42
- **Swollen** —*see* Swelling
- **Swyer syndrome** Q99.1
- **Sycosis** L73.8
  - barbae (not parasitic) L73.8
  - contagiosa (mycotic) B35.0
  - lupoides L73.8
  - mycotic B35.0
  - parasitic B35.0
  - vulgaris L73.8
- **Sydenham's chorea** —*see* Chorea, Sydenham's
- **Sylvatic yellow fever** A95.0
- **Sylvest's disease** B33.0
- **Symblepharon** H11.23-•
  - congenital Q10.3
- **Symond's syndrome** G93.2
- **Sympathetic** —*see* condition
- **Sympatheticotonia** G90.8
- **Sympathicoblastoma**
  - specified site —*see* Neoplasm, malignant, by site
  - unspecified site C74.90
- **Sympathogonioma** —*see* Sympathicoblastoma
- **Symphalangy (fingers) (toes)** Q70.9
- **Symptoms NEC** R68.89
  - breast NEC N64.59
  - cold J00
  - development NEC R63.8
  - factitious, self-induced —*see* Disorder, factitious
  - genital organs, female R10.2
  - involving
    - abdomen NEC R19.8
    - appearance NEC R46.89
    - awareness R41.9
      - altered mental status R41.82
      - amnesia —*see* Amnesia
      - borderline intellectual functioning R41.83
      - coma —*see* Coma
      - disorientation R41.0
      - neurologic neglect syndrome R41.4
      - senile cognitive decline R41.81
      - specified symptom NEC R41.89
    - behavior NEC R46.89
    - cardiovascular system NEC R09.89
    - chest NEC R09.89
    - circulatory system NEC R09.89
    - cognitive functions R41.9
      - altered mental status R41.82
      - amnesia —*see* Amnesia
      - borderline intellectual functioning R41.83
      - coma —*see* Coma
      - disorientation R41.0
      - neurologic neglect syndrome R41.4
      - senile cognitive decline R41.81
      - specified symptom NEC R41.89
    - development NEC R62.50
    - digestive system NEC R19.8
    - emotional state NEC R45.89
      - emotional lability R45.86
    - food and fluid intake R63.8
    - general perceptions and sensations R44.9
      - specified NEC R44.8
    - musculoskeletal system R29.91
      - specified NEC R29.898
    - nervous system R29.90
      - specified NEC R29.818
    - pelvis NEC R19.8
    - respiratory system NEC R09.89
    - skin and integument R23.9
    - urinary system R39.9
  - menopausal N95.1
  - metabolism NEC R63.8
  - neurotic F48.8
  - of infancy R68.19
  - pelvis NEC, female R10.2
  - skin and integument NEC R23.9
  - subcutaneous tissue NEC R23.9
  - viral cold J00
- **Sympus** Q74.2
- **Syncephalus** Q89.4
- **Synchondrosis**
  - abnormal (congenital) Q78.8
  - ischiopubic M91.0
- **Synchysis (scintillans) (senile) (vitreous body)** H43.89
- **Syncope (near) (pre-)** R55
  - anginosa I20.8
  - bradycardia R00.1
  - cardiac R55
  - carotid sinus G90.01
  - due to spinal (lumbar) puncture G97.1
  - heart R55
  - heat T67.1
  - laryngeal R05
  - psychogenic F48.8
  - tussive R05
  - vasoconstriction R55
  - vasodepressor R55
  - vasomotor R55
  - vasovagal R55
- **Syndactylism, syndactyly** Q70.9
  - complex (with synostosis)
    - fingers Q70.0-•
    - toes Q70.2-•
  - simple (without synostosis)
    - fingers Q70.1-•
    - toes Q70.3-•
- **Syndrome** —*see also* Disease
  - 5q minus NOS D46.C
  - 48,XXXX Q97.1
  - 49,XXXXX Q97.1
  - abdominal
    - acute R10.0
    - muscle deficiency Q79.4
  - abnormal innervation H02.519
    - left H02.516
      - lower H02.515
      - upper H02.514
    - right H02.513
      - lower H02.512
      - upper H02.511
  - abstinence, neonatal P96.1
  - acid pulmonary aspiration, obstetric O74.0
  - acquired immunodeficiency —*see* Human, immunodeficiency virus (HIV) disease
  - acute abdominal R10.0
  - acute respiratory distress (adult) (child) J80
    - idiopathic J84.114
  - Adair-Dighton Q78.0
  - Adams-Stokes (-Morgagni) I45.9
  - adiposogenital E23.6
  - adrenal
    - hemorrhage (meningococcal) A39.1
    - meningococcic A39.1
  - adrenocortical —*see* Cushing's, syndrome
  - adrenogenital E25.9
    - congenital, associated with enzyme deficiency E25.0
  - afferent loop NEC K91.89
  - Alagille's Q44.7
  - alcohol withdrawal (without convulsions) —*see* Dependence, alcohol, with, withdrawal
  - Alder's D72.0
  - Aldrich (-Wiskott) D82.0
  - alien hand R41.4
  - Alport Q87.81
  - alveolar hypoventilation E66.2
  - alveolocapillary block J84.10
  - amnesic, amnestic (confabulatory) (due to) —*see* Disorder, amnesic
  - amyostatic (Wilson's disease) E83.01
  - androgen insensitivity E34.50
    - complete E34.51
    - partial E34.52
  - androgen resistance (*see also* Syndrome, androgen insensitivity) E34.50
  - Angelman Q93.51
  - anginal —*see* Angina
  - ankyloglossia superior Q38.1
  - anterior
    - chest wall R07.89
    - cord G83.82
    - spinal artery G95.19
      - compression M47.019
        - cervical region M47.012
        - cervicothoracic region M47.013
        - lumbar region M47.016
        - occipito-atlanto-axial region M47.011
        - thoracic region M47.014
        - thoracolumbar region M47.015
    - tibial M76.81-•
  - antibody deficiency D80.9
    - agammaglobulinemic D80.1
      - hereditary D80.0
    - congenital D80.0
    - hypogammaglobulinemic D80.1
      - hereditary D80.0
  - anticardiolipin (-antibody) D68.61
  - antidepressant discontinuation T43.205
  - antiphospholipid (-antibody) D68.61

Syndrome *(Continued)*
- aortic
  - arch M31.4
  - bifurcation I74.09
- aortomesenteric duodenum occlusion K31.5
- apical ballooning (transient left ventricular) I51.81
- arcuate ligament I77.4
- argentaffin, argintaffinoma E34.0
- Arnold-Chiari —*see* Arnold-Chiari disease
- Arrillaga-Ayerza I27.0
- arterial tortuosity Q87.82
- arteriovenous steal T82.898- ●
- Asherman's N85.6
- aspiration, of newborn —*see* Aspiration, by substance, with pneumonia
  - meconium P24.01
- ataxia-telangiectasia G11.3
- auriculotemporal G50.8
- autoerythrocyte sensitization (Gardner-Diamond) D69.2
- autoimmune lymphoproliferative [ALPS] D89.82
- autoimmune polyglandular E31.0
- autoinflammatory M04.9
  - specified type NEC M04.8
- autosomal —*see* Abnormal, autosomes
- Avellis' G46.8
- Ayerza (-Arrillaga) I27.0
- Babinski-Nageotte G83.89
- Bakwin-Krida Q78.5
- bare lymphocyte D81.6
- Barré-Guillain G61.0
- Barré-Liéou M53.0
- Barrett's —*see* Barrett's, esophagus
- Barsony-Polgar K22.4
- Barsony-Teschendorf K22.4
- Barth E78.71
- Bartter's E26.81
- basal cell nevus Q87.89
- Basedow's E05.00
  - with thyroid storm E05.01
- basilar artery G45.0
- Batten-Steinert G71.11
- battered
  - baby or child —*see* Maltreatment, child, physical abuse
  - spouse —*see* Maltreatment, adult, physical abuse
- Beals Q87.40
- Beau's I51.5
- Beck's I65.8
- Benedikt's G46.3
- Béquez César (-Steinbrinck-Chédiak-Higashi) D70.330
- Bernhardt-Roth —*see* Meralgia paresthetica
- Bernheim's —*see* Failure, heart, right
- big spleen D73.1
- bilateral polycystic ovarian E28.2
- Bing-Horton's —*see* Horton's headache
- Birt-Hogg-Dube syndrome Q87.89
- Björck (-Thorsen) E34.0
- black
  - lung J60
  - widow spider bite —*see* Toxicity, venom, spider, black widow
- Blackfan-Diamond D61.01
- Blau M04.8
- blind loop K90.2
  - congenital Q43.8
  - postsurgical K91.2
- blue sclera Q78.0
- blue toe I75.02- ●
- Boder-Sedgewick G11.3
- Boerhaave's K22.3
- Borjeson Forssman Lehmann Q89.8
- Bouillaud's I01.9
- Bourneville (-Pringle) Q85.1
- Bouveret (-Hoffman) I47.9
- brachial plexus G54.0
- bradycardia-tachycardia I49.5

Syndrome *(Continued)*
- brain (nonpsychotic) F09
  - with psychosis, psychotic reaction F09
  - acute or subacute —*see* Delirium
  - congenital —*see* Disability, intellectual
  - organic F09
    - post-traumatic (nonpsychotic) F07.81
      - psychotic F09
  - personality change F07.0
  - postcontusional F07.81
  - post-traumatic, nonpsychotic F07.81
  - psycho-organic F09
  - psychotic F06.8
- brain stem stroke G46.3
- Brandt's (acrodermatitis enteropathica) E83.2
- broad ligament laceration N83.8
- Brock's J98.11
- bronze baby P83.88
- Brown-Sequard G83.81
- Brugada I49.8
- bubbly lung P27.0
- Buchem's M85.2
- Budd-Chiari I82.0
- bulbar (progressive) G12.22
- Bürger-Grütz E78.3
- Burke's K86.89
- Burnett's (milk-alkali) E83.52
- burning feet E53.9
- Bywaters' T79.5
- Call-Fleming I67.841
- carbohydrate-deficient glycoprotein (CDGS) E77.8
- carcinogenic thrombophlebitis I82.1
- carcinoid E34.0
- cardiac asthma I50.1
- cardiacos negros I27.0
- cardiofaciocutaneous Q87.89
- cardiopulmonary-obesity E66.2
- cardiorenal —*see* Hypertension, cardiorenal
- cardiorespiratory distress (idiopathic), newborn P22.0
- cardiovascular renal —*see* Hypertension, cardiorenal
- carotid
  - artery (hemispheric) (internal) G45.1
  - body G90.01
  - sinus G90.01
- carpal tunnel G56.0- ●
- Cassidy (-Scholte) E34.0
- cat-cry Q93.4
- cat eye Q92.8
- cauda equina G83.4
- causalgia —*see* Causalgia
- celiac K90.0
  - artery compression I77.4
  - axis I77.4
- central pain G89.0
- cerebellar
  - hereditary G11.9
  - stroke G46.4
- cerebellomedullary malformation —*see* Spina bifida
- cerebral
  - artery
    - anterior G46.1
    - middle G46.0
    - posterior G46.2
  - gigantism E22.0
- cervical (root) M53.1
  - disc —*see* Disorder, disc, cervical, with neuritis
  - fusion Q76.1
  - posterior, sympathicus M53.0
  - rib Q76.5
  - sympathetic paralysis G90.2
- cervicobrachial (diffuse) M53.1
- cervicocranial M53.0
- cervicodorsal outlet G54.2
- cervicothoracic outlet G54.0
- Céstan (-Raymond) I65.8
- Charcot's (angina cruris) (intermittent claudication) I73.9

Syndrome *(Continued)*
- Charcot-Weiss-Baker G90.09
- CHARGE Q89.8
- Chédiak-Higashi (-Steinbrinck) E70.330
- chest wall R07.1
- Chiari's (hepatic vein thrombosis) I82.0
- Chilaiditi's Q43.3
- child maltreatment —*see* Maltreatment, child
- chondrocostal junction M94.0
- chondroectodermal dysplasia Q77.6
- chromosome 4 short arm deletion Q93.3
- chromosome 5 short arm deletion Q93.4
- chronic
  - infantile neurological, cutaneous and articular (CINCA) M04.2
  - pain G89.4
    - personality F68.8
- ▶ Churg-Strauss M30.1
- Clarke-Hadfield K86.89
- Clerambault's automatism G93.89
- Clouston's (hidrotic ectodermal dysplasia) Q82.4
- clumsiness, clumsy child F82
- cluster headache G44.009
  - intractable G44.001
  - not intractable G44.009
- Coffin-Lowry Q89.8
- cold injury (newborn) P80.0
- combined immunity deficiency D81.9
- compartment (deep) (posterior) (traumatic) T79.A0
  - abdomen T79.A3
  - lower extremity (hip, buttock, thigh, leg, foot, toes) T79.A2
  - nontraumatic
    - abdomen M79.A3
    - lower extremity (hip, buttock, thigh, leg, foot, toes) M79.A2- ●
    - specified site NEC M79.A9
    - upper extremity (shoulder, arm, forearm, wrist, hand, fingers) M79.A1- ●
  - postprocedural —*see* Syndrome compartment, nontraumatic
  - specified site NEC T79.A9
  - upper extremity (shoulder, arm, forearm, wrist, hand, fingers) T79.A1
- complex regional pain —*see* Syndrome, pain, complex regional
- compression T79.5
  - anterior spinal —*see* Syndrome, anterior, spinal artery, compression
  - cauda equina G83.4
  - celiac artery I77.4
  - vertebral artery M47.029
    - cervical region M47.022
    - occipito-atlanto-axial region M47.021
- concussion F07.81
- congenital
  - affecting multiple systems NEC Q87.89
  - central alveolar hypoventilation G47.35
  - facial diplegia Q87.0
  - muscular hypertrophy-cerebral Q87.89
  - oculo-auriculovertebral Q87.0
  - oculofacial diplegia (Moebius) Q87.0
  - rubella (manifest) P35.0
- congestion-fibrosis (pelvic), female N94.89
- congestive dysmenorrhea N94.6
- Conn's E26.01
- connective tissue M35.9
  - overlap NEC M35.1
- conus medullaris G95.81
- cord
  - anterior G83.82
  - posterior G83.83
- coronary
  - acute NEC I24.9
  - insufficiency or intermediate I20.0
  - slow flow I20.8
- Costen's (complex) M26.69
- costochondral junction M94.0
- costoclavicular G54.0

Syndrome (Continued)
costovertebral E22.Ø
Cowden Q85.8
craniovertebral M53.Ø
Creutzfeldt-Jakob —see Creutzfeldt-Jakob disease or syndrome
cri-du-chat Q93.4
crib death R99
cricopharyngeal —see Dysphagia
croup JØ5.Ø
CRPS I —see Syndrome, pain, complex regional I
crush T79.5
cubital tunnel —see Lesion, nerve, ulnar
Curschmann (-Batten) (-Steinert) G71.11
Cushing's E24.9
alcohol-induced E24.4
drug-induced E24.2
due to
alcohol
drugs E24.2
ectopic ACTH E24.3
overproduction of pituitary ACTH E24.Ø
overdose or wrong substance given or taken —see Table of Drugs and Chemicals, by drug, poisoning
pituitary-dependent E24.Ø
specified type NEC E24.8
cryopyrin-associated periodic MØ4.2
cryptophthalmos Q87.Ø
cystic duct stump K91.5
Dana-Putnam D51.Ø
Danbolt (-Cross) (acrodermatitis enteropathica) E83.2
Dandy-Walker QØ3.1
with spina bifida QØ7.Ø1
Danlos' (see also Syndrome, Ehlers-Danlos) Q79.6Ø
defibrination —see also Fibrinolysis
with
antepartum hemorrhage —see Hemorrhage, antepartum, with coagulation defect
intrapartum hemorrhage —see Hemorrhage, complicating, delivery
newborn P6Ø
postpartum O72.3
Degos' I77.8
Déjérine-Roussy G89.Ø
delayed sleep phase G47.21
demyelinating G37.9
dependence —see F1Ø-F19 with fourth character .2
depersonalization (-derealization) F48.1
De Quervain E34.51
de Toni-Fanconi (-Debré) E72.Ø9
with cystinosis E72.Ø4
diabetes mellitus-hypertension-nephrosis —see Diabetes, nephrosis
diabetes mellitus in newborn infant P7Ø.2
diabetes-nephrosis —see Diabetes, nephrosis
diabetic amyotrophy —see Diabetes, amyotrophy
dialysis associated steal T82.898-●
Diamond-Blackfan D61.Ø1
Diamond-Gardener D69.2
DIC (diffuse or disseminated intravascular coagulopathy) D65
di George's D82.1
Dighton's Q78.Ø
disequilibrium E87.8
Döhle body-panmyelopathic D72.Ø
dorsolateral medullary G46.4
double athetosis G8Ø.3
Down (see also Down syndrome) Q9Ø.9
Dresbach's (elliptocytosis) D58.1
Dressler's (postmyocardial infarction) I24.1
postcardiotomy I97.Ø
drug withdrawal, infant of dependent mother P96.1
dry eye HØ4.12-●

Syndrome (Continued)
due to abnormality
chromosomal Q99.9
sex
female phenotype Q97.9
male phenotype Q98.9
specified NEC Q99.8
dumping (postgastrectomy) K91.1
nonsurgical K31.89
Dupré's (meningism) R29.1
dysmetabolic X E88.81
dyspraxia, developmental F82
Eagle-Barrett Q79.4
Eaton-Lambert —see Syndrome, Lambert-Eaton
Ebstein's Q22.5
ectopic ACTH E24.3
eczema-thrombocytopenia D82.Ø
Eddowes' Q78.Ø
effort (psychogenic) F45.8
Ehlers-Danlos Q79.6Ø
classical (cEDS) (classical EDS) Q79.61
hypermobile (hEDS) (hypermobile EDS) Q79.62
specified NEC Q79.69
vascular (vascular EDS) (vEDS) Q79.63
Eisenmenger's I27.83
Ekman's Q78.Ø
electric feet E53.8
Ellis-van Creveld Q77.6
empty nest Z6Ø.Ø
endocrine-hypertensive E27.Ø
entrapment —see Neuropathy, entrapment
eosinophilia-myalgia M35.8
epileptic —see also Epilepsy, by type
absence G4Ø.AØ9
intractable G4Ø.A19
with status epilepticus G4Ø.A11
without status epilepticus G4Ø.A19
not intractable G4Ø.AØ9
with status epilepticus G4Ø.AØ1
without status epilepticus G4Ø.AØ9
Erdheim-Chester (ECD) E88.89
Erdheim's E22.Ø
erythrocyte fragmentation D59.4
Evans D69.41
exhaustion F48.8
extrapyramidal G25.9
specified NEC G25.89
eye retraction —see Strabismus
eyelid-malar-mandible Q87.Ø
Faber's D5Ø.9
facial pain, paroxysmal G5Ø.Ø
Fallot's Q21.3
familial cold autoinflammatory MØ4.2
familial eczema-thrombocytopenia (Wiskott-Aldrich) D82.Ø
Fanconi (-de Toni) (-Debré) E72.Ø9
with cystinosis E72.Ø4
Fanconi's (anemia) (congenital pancytopenia) D61.Ø9
fatigue
chronic R53.82
psychogenic F48.8
faulty bowel habit K59.39
Feil-Klippel (brevicollis) Q76.1
Felty's —see Felty's syndrome
fertile eunuch E23.Ø
fetal
alcohol (dysmorphic) Q86.Ø
hydantoin Q86.1
Fiedler's I4Ø.1
first arch Q87.Ø
fish odor E72.89
Fisher's G61.Ø
Fitzhugh-Curtis
due to
Chlamydia trachomatis A74.81
Neisseria gonorrhorea (gonococcal peritonitis) A54.85
Fitz's —see also Pancreatitis, acute K85.8Ø
Flajani (-Basedow) EØ5.ØØ
with thyroid storm EØ5.Ø1

Syndrome (Continued)
flatback —see Flatback syndrome
floppy
baby P94.2
iris (intraoeprative) (IFIS) H21.81
mitral valve I34.1
flush E34.Ø
Foix-Alajouanine G95.19
Fong's Q87.2
food protein-induced enterocolitis (FPIES) K52.21
foramen magnum G93.5
Foster-Kennedy H47.14-●
Foville's (peduncular) G46.3
fragile X Q99.2
Franceschetti Q75.4
Frey's
auriculotemporal G5Ø.8
hyperhidrosis L74.52
Friderichsen-Waterhouse A39.1
Froin's G95.89
frontal lobe FØ7.Ø
Fukuhara E88.49
functional
bowel K59.9
prepubertal castrate E29.1
Gaisböck's D75.1
ganglion (basal ganglia brain) G25.9
geniculi G51.1
Gardner-Diamond D69.2
gastroesophageal
junction K22.Ø
laceration-hemorrhage K22.6
gastrojejunal loop obstruction K91.89
Gee-Herter-Heubner K9Ø.Ø
Gelineau's G47.419
with cataplexy G47.411
genito-anorectal A55
Gerstmann-Sträussler-Scheinker (GSS) A81.82
Gianotti-Crosti L44.4
giant platelet (Bernard-Soulier) D69.1
Gilles de la Tourette's F95.2
Glass Q87.89
goiter-deafness EØ7.1
Goldberg Q89.8
Goldberg-Maxwell E34.51
Good's D83.8
Gopalan' (burning feet) E53.8
Gorlin's Q87.89
Gougerot-Blum L81.7
Gouley's I31.1
Gower's R55
gray or grey (newborn) P93.Ø
platelet D69.1
Gubler-Millard G46.3
Guillain-Barré (-Strohl) G61.Ø
gustatory sweating G5Ø.8
Hadfield-Clarke K86.89
hair tourniquet —see Constriction, external, by site
Hamman's J98.19
hand-foot L27.1
hand-shoulder G9Ø.8
hantavirus (cardio)-pulmonary (HPS) (HCPS) B33.4
happy puppet Q93.51
Harada's H3Ø.81-●
Hayem-Faber D5Ø.9
headache NEC G44.89
complicated NEC G44.59
Heberden's I2Ø.8
Hedinger's E34.Ø
Hegglin's D72.Ø
HELLP (hemolysis, elevated liver enzymes and low platelet count) O14.2-●
complicating
childbirth O14.24
puerperium O14.25
hemolytic-uremic D59.3
hemophagocytic, infection-associated D76.2
Henoch-Schönlein D69.Ø

S

Syndrome *(Continued)*
hepatic flexure K59.8
hepatopulmonary K76.81
hepatorenal K76.7
following delivery O90.4
postoperative or postprocedural K91.83
postpartum, puerperal O90.4
hepatourologic K76.7
Herter (-Gee) (nontropical sprue) K90.0
Heubner-Herter K90.0
Heyd's K76.7
Hilger's G90.09
histamine-like (fish poisoning) —*see* Poisoning, fish
histiocytic D76.3
histiocytosis NEC D76.3
HIV infection, acute B20
Hoffmann-Werdnig G12.0
Hollander-Simons E88.1
Hoppe-Goldflam G70.00
with exacerbation (acute) G70.01
in crisis G70.01
Horner's G90.2
hungry bone E83.81
hunterian glossitis D51.0
Hutchinson's triad A50.53
hyperabduction G54.0
hyperammonemia-hyperornithinemia-homocitrullinemia E72.4
hypereosinophilic (idiopathic) D72.1
hyperimmunoglobulin D M04.1
hyperimmunoglobulin E (IgE) D82.4
hyperkalemic E87.5
hyperkinetic —*see* Hyperkinesia
hypermobility M35.7
hypernatremia E87.0
hyperosmolarity E87.0
hyperperfusion G97.82
hypersplenic D73.1
hypertransfusion, newborn P61.1
hyperventilation F45.8
hyperviscosity (of serum)
polycythemic D75.1
sclerothymic D58.8
hypoglycemic (familial) (neonatal) E16.2
hypokalemic E87.6
hyponatremic E87.1
hypopituitarism E23.0
hypoplastic left-heart Q23.4
hypopotassemia E87.6
hyposmolality E87.1
hypotension, maternal O26.5- ●
hypothenar hammer I73.89
hypoventilation, obesity (OHS) E66.2
ICF (intravascular coagulation-fibrinolysis) D65
idiopathic
cardiorespiratory distress, newborn P22.0
nephrotic (infantile) N04.9
iliotibial band M76.3- ●
immobility, immobilization (paraplegic) M62.3
immune reconstitution D89.3
immune reconstitution inflammatory [IRIS] D89.3
immunity deficiency, combined D81.9
immunodeficiency
acquired —*see* Human, immunodeficiency virus (HIV) disease
combined D81.9
impending coronary I20.0
impingement, shoulder M75.4- ●
inappropriate secretion of antidiuretic hormone E22.2
infant
gestational diabetes P70.0
of diabetic mother P70.1
infantilism (pituitary) E23.0
inferior vena cava I87.1
inspissated bile (newborn) P59.1
institutional (childhood) F94.2
insufficient sleep F51.12
intermediate coronary (artery) I20.0

Syndrome *(Continued)*
interspinous ligament —*see* Spondylopathy, specified NEC
intestinal
carcinoid E34.0
knot K56.2
intravascular coagulation-fibrinolysis (ICF) D65
iodine-deficiency, congenital E00.9
type
mixed E00.2
myxedematous E00.1
neurological E00.0
IRDS (idiopathic respiratory distress, newborn) P22.0
irritable
bowel K58.9
with
constipation K58.1
diarrhea K58.0
mixed K58.2
psychogenic F45.8
specified NEC K58.8
heart (psychogenic) F45.8
weakness F48.8
ischemic
bowel (transient) K55.9
chronic K55.1
due to mesenteric artery insufficiency K55.1
steal T82.898
IVC (intravascular coagulopathy) D65
Ivemark's Q89.01
Jaccoud's —*see* Arthropathy, postrheumatic, chronic
Jackson's G83.89
Jakob-Creutzfeldt —*see* Creutzfeldt-Jakob disease or syndrome
jaw-winking Q07.8
Jervell-Lange-Nielsen I45.81
jet lag G47.25
Job's D71
Joseph-Diamond-Blackfan D61.01
jugular foramen G52.7
Kabuki Q89.8
Kanner's (autism) F84.0
Kartagener's Q89.3
Kelly's D50.1
Kimmelsteil-Wilson —*see* Diabetes, specified type, with Kimmelsteil-Wilson disease
Klein (e)-Levine G47.13
Klippel-Feil (brevicollis) Q76.1
Köhler-Pellegrini-Steida —*see* Bursitis, tibial collateral
König's K59.8
Korsakoff (-Wernicke) (nonalcoholic) F04
alcoholic F10.26
Kostmann's D70.0
Krabbe's congenital muscle hypoplasia Q79.8
labyrinthine —*see* subcategory H83.2
lacunar NEC G46.7
Lambert-Eaton G70.80
in
neoplastic disease G73.1
specified disease NEC G70.81
Landau-Kleffner —*see* Epilepsy, specified NEC
Larsen's Q74.8
lateral
cutaneous nerve of thigh G57.1- ●
medullary G46.4
Launois' E22.0
lazy
leukocyte D70.8
posture M62.3
Lemiere I80.8
Lennox-Gastaut G40.812
intractable G40.814
with status epilepticus G40.813
without status epilepticus G40.814
not intractable G40.812
with status epilepticus G40.811
without status epilepticus G40.812

Syndrome *(Continued)*
lenticular, progressive E83.01
Leopold-Levi's E05.90
Lev's I44.2
Li-Fraumeni Z15.01
Lichtheim's D51.0
Lightwood's N25.89
Lignac (de Toni) (-Fanconi) (-Debré) E72.09
with cystinosis E72.04
Likoff's I20.8
limbic epilepsy personality F07.0
liver-kidney K76.7
lobotomy F07.0
Loffler's J82
long arm 18 or 21 deletion Q93.89
long QT I45.81
Louis-Barré G11.3
low
atmospheric pressure T70.29
back M54.5
output (cardiac) I50.9
lower radicular, newborn (birth injury) P14.8
Luetscher's (dehydration) E86.0
Lupus anticoagulant D68.62
Lutembacher's Q21.1
macrophage activation D76.1
due to infection D76.2
magnesium-deficiency R29.0
Majeed M04.8
Mal de Debarquement R42
malabsorption K90.9
postsurgical K91.2
malformation, congenital, due to
alcohol Q86.0
exogenous cause NEC Q86.8
hydantoin Q86.1
warfarin Q86.2
malignant
carcinoid E34.0
neuroleptic G21.0
Mallory-Weiss K22.6
mandibulofacial dysostosis Q75.4
manic-depressive —*see* Disorder, bipolar
maple-syrup-urine E71.0
Marable's I77.4
Marfan's Q87.40
with
cardiovascular manifestations Q87.418
aortic dilation Q87.410
ocular manifestations Q87.42
skeletal manifestations Q87.43
Marie's (acromegaly) E22.0
mast cell activation —*see* Activation, mast cell
maternal hypotension —*see* Syndrome, hypotension, maternal
May (-Hegglin) D72.0
McArdle (-Schmidt) (-Pearson) E74.04
McQuarrie's E16.2
meconium plug (newborn) P76.0
median arcuate ligament I77.4
Meekeren-Ehlers-Danlos Q79.6
megavitamin-B6 E67.2
Meige G24.4
MELAS E88.41
Mendelson's O74.0
MERRF (myoclonic epilepsy associated with ragged-red fibers) E88.42
mesenteric
artery (superior) K55.1
vascular insufficiency K55.1
metabolic E88.81
metastatic carcinoid E34.0
micrognathia-glossoptosis Q87.0
midbrain NEC G93.89
middle lobe (lung) J98.19
middle radicular G54.0
migraine —*see also* Migraine G43.909- ●
Mikulicz' K11.8
milk-alkali E83.52
Millard-Gubler G46.3

Syndrome *(Continued)*
- Miller-Dieker Q93.88
- Miller-Fisher G61.Ø
- Minkowski-Chauffard D58.Ø
- Mirizzi's K83.1
- MNGIE (Mitochondrial Neurogastrointestinal Encephalopathy) E88.49
- Möbius, ophthalmoplegic migraine *—see* Migraine, ophthalmoplegic
- monofixation H5Ø.42
- Morel-Moore M85.2
- Morel-Morgagni M85.2
- Morgagni (-Morel) (-Stewart) M85.2
- Morgagni-Adams-Stokes I45.9
- Mounier-Kuhn Q32.4
  - with bronchiectasis J47.9
    - with
      - exacerbation (acute) J47.1
      - lower respiratory infection J47.Ø
  - acquired J98.Ø9
    - with bronchiectasis J47.9
      - with
        - exacerbation (acute) J47.1
        - lower respiratory infection J47.Ø
- Muckle-Wells MØ4.2
- mucocutaneous lymph node (acute febrile) (MCLS) M3Ø.3
- multiple endocrine neoplasia (MEN) *—see* Neoplasia, endocrine, multiple (MEN}
- multiple operations *—see* Disorder, factitious
- myasthenic G7Ø.9
  - in
    - diabetes mellitus *—see* Diabetes, amyotrophy
    - endocrine disease NEC E34.9 *[G73.3]*
    - neoplastic disease *—see also* Neoplasm D49.9 *[G73.3]*
    - thyrotoxicosis (hyperthyroidism) EØ5.9Ø *[G73.3]*
      - with thyroid storm EØ5.91 *[G73.3]*
- myelodysplastic D46.9
  - with
    - 5q deletion D46.C
    - isolated del (5q) chromosomal abnormality D46.C
  - lesions, low grade D46.2Ø
  - specified NEC D46.Z
- myelopathic pain G89.Ø
- myeloproliferative (chronic) D47.1
- myofascial pain M79.18
- Naffziger's G54.Ø
- nail patella Q87.2
- NARP (Neuropathy, Ataxia and Retinitis pigmentosa) E88.49
- neonatal abstinence P96.1
- nephritic *—see also* Nephritis
  - with edema *—see* Nephrosis
  - acute NØØ.9
  - chronic NØ3.9
  - rapidly progressive NØ1.9
- nephrotic (congenital) *—see also* Nephrosis NØ4.9
  - with
    - dense deposit disease NØ4.6
    - diffuse
      - crescentic glomerulonephritis NØ4.7
      - endocapillary proliferative glomerulonephritis NØ4.4
      - membranous glomerulonephritis NØ4.2
      - mesangial proliferative glomerulonephritis NØ4.3
      - mesangiocapillary glomerulonephritis NØ4.5
    - focal and segmental glomerular lesions NØ4.1
    - minor glomerular abnormality NØ4.Ø
    - specified morphological changes NEC NØ4.8
  - diabetic *—see* Diabetes, nephrosis

Syndrome *(Continued)*
- neurologic neglect R41.4
- Nezelof's D81.4
- Nonne-Milroy-Meige Q82.Ø
- Nothnagel's vasomotor acroparesthesia I73.89
- obesity hypoventilation (OHS) E66.2
- oculomotor H51.9
- ophthalmoplegia-cerebellar ataxia *—see* Strabismus, paralytic, third nerve
- oral allergy T78.1
- oral-facial-digital Q87.Ø
- organic
  - affective FØ6.3Ø
  - amnesic (not alcohol- or drug-induced) FØ4
  - brain FØ9
  - depressive FØ6.31
  - hallucinosis FØ6.Ø
  - personality FØ7.Ø
- Ormond's N13.5
- oro-facial-digital Q87.Ø
- os trigonum Q68.8
- Osler-Weber-Rendu I78.Ø
- osteoporosis-osteomalacia M83.8
- Osterreicher-Turner Q87.2
- otolith *—see* subcategory H81.8
- oto-palatal-digital Q87.Ø
- outlet (thoracic) G54.Ø
- ovary
  - polycystic E28.2
  - resistant E28.39
  - sclerocystic E28.2
- Owren's D68.2
- Paget-Schroetter I82.89Ø
- pain *—see also* Pain
  - complex regional I G9Ø.5Ø
    - lower limb G9Ø.52- •
    - specified site NEC G9Ø.59
    - upper limb G9Ø.51- •
  - complex regional II *—see* Causalgia
- painful
  - bruising D69.2
  - feet E53.8
  - prostate N42.81
- paralysis agitans *—see* Parkinsonism
- paralytic G83.9
  - specified NEC G83.89
- Parinaud's H51.Ø
- parkinsonian *—see* Parkinsonism
- Parkinson's *—see* Parkinsonism
- paroxysmal facial pain G5Ø.Ø
- Parry's EØ5.ØØ
  - with thyroid storm EØ5.Ø1
- Parsonage (-Aldren)-Turner G54.5
- patella clunk M25.86- •
- Paterson (-Brown) (-Kelly) D5Ø.1
- pectoral girdle I77.89
- pectoralis minor I77.89
- pediatric autoimmune neuropsychiatric disorders associated with streptococcal infections (PANDAS) D89.89
- Pelger-Huet D72.Ø
- pellagra-cerebellar ataxia-renal aminoaciduria E72.Ø2
- pellagroid E52
- Pellegrini-Stieda *—see* Bursitis, tibial collateral
- pelvic congestion-fibrosis, female N94.89
- penta X Q97.1
- peptic ulcer *—see* Ulcer, peptic
- perabduction I77.89
- periodic fever MØ4.1
- periodic fever, aphthous stomatitis, pharyngitis, and adenopathy [PFAPA] MØ4.8
- periodic headache, in adults and children *— see* Headache, periodic syndromes in adults and children
- periurethral fibrosis N13.5
- phantom limb (without pain) G54.7
  - with pain G54.6
- pharyngeal pouch D82.1
- Pick's *—see* Disease, Pick's
- Pickwickian E66.2

Syndrome *(Continued)*
- PIE (pulmonary infiltration with eosinophilia) J82
- pigmentary pallidal degeneration (progressive) G23.Ø
- pineal E34.8
- pituitary E22.Ø
- placental transfusion *—see* Pregnancy, complicated by, placental transfusion syndromes
- plantar fascia M72.2
- plateau iris (post-iridectomy) (postprocedural) H21.82
- Plummer-Vinson D5Ø.1
- pluricarential of infancy E4Ø
- plurideficiency E4Ø
- pluriglandular (compensatory) E31.8
  - autoimmune E31.Ø
- pneumatic hammer T75.21
- polyangiitis overlap M3Ø.8
- polycarential of infancy E4Ø
- polyglandular E31.8
  - autoimmune E31.Ø
- polysplenia Q89.Ø9
- pontine NEC G93.89
- popliteal
  - artery entrapment I77.89
  - ▶ post endometrial ablation N99.85
  - web Q87.89
- postcardiac injury
  - postcardiotomy I97.Ø
  - postmyocardial infarction I24.1
- postcardiotomy I97.Ø
- post chemoembolization — code to associated conditions
- postcholecystectomy K91.5
- postcommissurotomy I97.Ø
- postconcussional FØ7.81
- postcontusional FØ7.81
- postencephalitic FØ7.89
- posterior
  - cervical sympathetic M53.Ø
  - cord G83.83
  - fossa compression G93.5
  - reversible encephalopathy (PRES) I67.83
- postgastrectomy (dumping) K91.1
- postgastric surgery K91.1
- postinfarction I24.1
- postlaminectomy NEC M96.1
- postleukotomy FØ7.Ø
- postmastectomy lymphedema I97.2
- postmyocardial infarction I24.1
- postoperative NEC T81.9
  - blind loop K9Ø.2
- postpartum panhypopituitary (Sheehan) E23.Ø
- postpolio (myelitic) G14
- postthrombotic I87.ØØ9
  - with
    - inflammation I87.Ø2- •
      - with ulcer I87.Ø3- •
    - specified complication NEC I87.Ø9- •
    - ulcer I87.Ø1- •
      - with inflammation I87.Ø3- •
  - asymptomatic I87.ØØ- •
- postvagotomy K91.1
- postvalvulotomy I97.Ø
- postviral NEC G93.3
  - fatigue G93.3
- Potain's K31.Ø
- potassium intoxication E87.5
- ▶ Prader-Willi Q87.11
- ▶ Prader-Willi-like Q87.19
- precerebral artery (multiple) (bilateral) G45.2
- preinfarction I2Ø.Ø
- preleukemic D46.9
- premature senility E34.8
- ➠ premenstrual dysphoric F32.81
- premenstrual tension N94.3
- Prinzmetal-Massumi RØ7.1
- prune belly Q79.4

S

Syndrome *(Continued)*
- pseudocarpal tunnel (sublimis) *—see* Syndrome, carpal tunnel
- pseudoparalytica G7Ø.ØØ
  - with exacerbation (acute) G7Ø.Ø1
  - in crisis G7Ø.Ø1
- ➠ pseudo-Turner's Q87.19
- psycho-organic (nonpsychotic severity) FØ7.9
  - acute or subacute FØ5
  - depressive type FØ6.31
  - hallucinatory type FØ6.Ø
  - nonpsychotic severity FØ7.Ø
  - specified NEC FØ7.89
- pulmonary
  - arteriosclerosis I27.Ø
  - dysmaturity (Wilson-Mikity) P27.Ø
  - hypoperfusion (idiopathic) P22.Ø
  - renal (hemorrhagic) (Goodpasture's) M31.Ø
- pure
  - motor lacunar G46.5
  - sensory lacunar G46.6
- Putnam-Dana D51.Ø
- pyogenic arthritis, pyoderma gangrenosum, and acne [PAPA] MØ4.8
- pyramidopallidonigral G2Ø
- pyriformis *—see* Lesion, nerve, sciatic
- QT interval prolongation I45.81
- radicular NEC *—see* Radiculopathy
  - upper limbs, newborn (birth injury) P14.3
- rapid time-zone change G47.25
- Rasmussen GØ4.81
- Raymond (-Céstan) I65.8
- Raynaud's I73.ØØ
  - with gangrene I73.Ø1
- RDS (respiratory distress syndrome, newborn) P22.Ø
- reactive airways dysfunction J68.3
- Refsum's G6Ø.1
- Reifenstein E34.52
- renal glomerulohyalinosis-diabetic *—see* Diabetes, nephrosis
- Rendu-Osler-Weber I78.Ø
- residual ovary N99.83
- resistant ovary E28.39
- respiratory
  - distress
    - acute J8Ø
      - adult J8Ø
      - child J8Ø
      - idiopathic J84.114
    - newborn (idiopathic) (type I) P22.Ø
      - type II P22.1
- restless legs G25.81
- retinoblastoma (familial) C69.2
- retroperitoneal fibrosis N13.5
- retroviral seroconversion (acute) Z21
- Reye's G93.7
- Richter *—see* Leukemia, chronic lymphocytic, B-cell type
- Ridley's I5Ø.1
- right
  - heart, hypoplastic Q22.6
  - ➠ ventricular obstruction *—see* Failure, heart, right
- Romano-Ward (prolonged QT interval) I45.81
- rotator cuff, shoulder *—see also* Tear, rotator cuff M75.1Ø-●
- Rotes Quérol *—see* Hyperostosis, ankylosing
- Roth *—see* Meralgia paresthetica
- rubella (congenital) P35.Ø
- Ruvalcaba-Myhre-Smith E71.44Ø
- Rytand-Lipsitch I44.2
- salt
  - depletion E87.1
    - due to heat NEC T67.8
      - causing heat exhaustion or prostration T67.4
  - low E87.1
- salt-losing N28.89
- ▶ SATB2-associated Q87.89
- Scaglietti-Dagnini E22.Ø
- scalenus anticus (anterior) G54.Ø
- scapulocostal *—see* Mononeuropathy, upper limb, specified site NEC
- scapuloperoneal G71.Ø9
- schizophrenic, of childhood NEC F84.5
- Schnitzler D47.2
- Scholte's E34.Ø
- Schroeder's E27.Ø
- Schüller-Christian C96.5
- Schwachman's *—see* Syndrome, Shwachman's
- Schwartz (-Jampel) G71.13
- Schwartz-Bartter E22.2
- scimitar Q26.8
- sclerocystic ovary E28.2
- Seitelberger's G31.89
- septicemic adrenal hemorrhage A39.1
- seroconversion, retroviral (acute) Z21
- serous meningitis G93.2
- severe acute respiratory (SARS) J12.81
- shaken infant T74.4
- shock (traumatic) T79.4
  - kidney N17.Ø
    - following crush injury T79.5
  - toxic A48.3
- shock-lung J8Ø
- Shone's — code to specific anomalies
- short
  - bowel K91.2
  - rib Q77.2
- shoulder-hand *—see* Algoneurodystrophy
- Shwachman's D7Ø.4
- sicca *—see* Sicca syndrome
- sick
  - cell E87.1
  - sinus I49.5
- sick-euthyroid EØ7.81
- sideropenic D5Ø.1
- Siemens' ectodermal dysplasia Q82.4
- Silfverskiöld's Q78.9
- Simons' E88.1
- sinus tarsi M25.57-●
- sinusitis-bronchiectasis-situs inversus Q89.3
- Sipple's E31.22
- sirenomelia Q87.2
- Slocumb's E27.Ø
- slow flow, coronary I2Ø.8
- Sluder's G44.89
- Smith-Magenis Q93.88
- Sneddon-Wilkinson L13.1
- Sotos' Q87.3
- South African cardiomyopathy I42.8
- spasmodic
  - upward movement, eyes H51.8
  - winking F95.8
- Spen's I45.9
- splenic
  - agenesis Q89.Ø1
  - flexure K59.8
  - neutropenia D73.81
- Spurway's Q78.Ø
- staphylococcal scalded skin LØØ
- steal
  - arteriovenous T82.898-●
  - ischemic T82.898-●
  - subclavian G45.8
- Stein-Leventhal E28.2
- Stein's E28.2
- Stevens-Johnson syndrome L51.1
  - toxic epidermal necrolysis overlap L51.3
- Stewart-Morel M85.2
- Stickler Q89.8
- stiff baby Q89.8
- stiff man G25.82
- Still-Felty *—see* Felty's syndrome
- Stokes (-Adams) I45.9
- stone heart I5Ø.1
- straight back, congenital Q76.49
- subclavian steal G45.8
- subcoracoid-pectoralis minor G54.Ø
- subcostal nerve compression I77.89
- subphrenic interposition Q43.3
- superior
  - cerebellar artery I63.89
  - mesenteric artery K55.1
  - semi-circular canal dehiscence H83.8X-●
  - vena cava I87.1
- supine hypotensive (maternal) *—see* Syndrome, hypotension, maternal
- suprarenal cortical E27.Ø
- supraspinatus *—see also* Tear, rotator cuff M75.1Ø-●
- Susac G93.49
- swallowed blood P78.2
- sweat retention L74.Ø
- Swyer Q99.1
- Symond's G93.2
- sympathetic
  - cervical paralysis G9Ø.2
  - pelvic, female N94.89
- systemic inflammatory response (SIRS), of non-infectious origin (without organ dysfunction) R65.1Ø
  - with acute organ dysfunction R65.11
- tachycardia-bradycardia I49.5
- takotsubo I51.81
- TAR (thrombocytopenia with absent radius) Q87.2
- tarsal tunnel G57.5-●
- teething KØØ.7
- tegmental G93.89
- telangiectasic-pigmentation-cataract Q82.8
- temporal pyramidal apex *—see* Otitis, media, suppurative, acute
- temporomandibular joint-pain-dysfunction M26.62-●
- Terry's *—see also* Myopia, degenerative H44.2-●
- testicular feminization *—see also* Syndrome, androgen insensitivity E34.51
- thalamic pain (hyperesthetic) G89.Ø
- thoracic outlet (compression) G54.Ø
- Thorson-Björck E34.Ø
- thrombocytopenia with absent radius (TAR) Q87.2
- thyroid-adrenocortical insufficiency E31.Ø
- tibial
  - anterior M76.81-●
  - posterior M76.82-●
- Tietze's M94.Ø
- time-zone (rapid) G47.25
- Toni-Fanconi E72.Ø9
  - with cystinosis E72.Ø4
- Touraine's Q79.8
- tourniquet *—see* Constriction, external, by site
- toxic shock A48.3
- transient left ventricular apical ballooning I51.81
- traumatic vasospastic T75.22
- Treacher Collins Q75.4
- triple X, female Q97.Ø
- trisomy Q92.9
  - 13 Q91.7
    - meiotic nondisjunction Q91.4
    - mitotic nondisjunction Q91.5
    - mosaicism Q91.5
    - translocation Q91.6
  - 18 Q91.3
    - meiotic nondisjunction Q91.Ø
    - mitotic nondisjunction Q91.1
    - mosaicism Q91.1
    - translocation Q91.2
  - 2Ø (q)(p) Q92.8
  - 21 Q9Ø.9
    - meiotic nondisjunction Q9Ø.Ø
    - mitotic nondisjunction Q9Ø.1
    - mosaicism Q9Ø.1
    - translocation Q9Ø.2
  - 22 Q92.8
- tropical wet feet T69.Ø-●
- Trousseau's I82.1

S

Syndrome *(Continued)*
tumor lysis (following antineoplastic chemotherapy) (spontaneous) NEC E88.3
tumor necrosis factor receptor associated periodic (TRAPS) M04.1
Twiddler's (due to)
automatic implantable defibrillator T82.198
cardiac pacemaker T82.198
Unverricht (-Lundborg) —*see* Epilepsy, generalized, idiopathic
upward gaze H51.8
uremia, chronic —*see also* Disease, kidney, chronic N18.9
urethral N34.3
urethro-oculo-articular —*see* Reiter's disease
urohepatic K76.7
vago-hypoglossal G52.7
van Buchem's M85.2
van der Hoeve's Q78.0
vascular NEC in cerebrovascular disease G46.8
vasoconstriction, reversible cerebrovascular I67.841
vasomotor I73.9
vasospastic (traumatic) T75.22
vasovagal R55
VATER Q87.2
velo-cardio-facial Q93.81
vena cava (inferior) (superior) (obstruction) I87.1
vertebral
artery G45.0
compression —*see* Syndrome, anterior, spinal artery, compression
steal G45.0
vertebro-basilar artery G45.0
vertebrogenic (pain) M54.89
vertiginous —*see* Disorder, vestibular function
Vinson-Plummer D50.1
virus B34.9
visceral larva migrans B83.0
visual disorientation H53.8
vitamin B6 deficiency E53.1
vitreal corneal H59.01-●
vitreous (touch) H59.01-●
Vogt-Koyanagi H20.82-●
Volkmann's T79.6
von Schroetter's I82.890
von Willebrand (-Jürgen) D68.0
Waldenström-Kjellberg D50.1
Wallenberg's G46.3
water retention E87.79
Waterhouse (-Friderichsen) A39.1
Weber-Gubler G46.3
Weber-Leyden G46.3
Weber's G46.3
Wegener's M31.30
with
kidney involvement M31.31
lung involvement M31.30
with kidney involvement M31.31
Weingarten's (tropical eosinophilia) J82
Weiss-Baker G90.09
Werdnig-Hoffman G12.0
Wermer's E31.21
Werner's E34.8
Wernicke-Korsakoff (nonalcoholic) F04
alcoholic F10.26
West's —*see* Epilepsy, spasms
Westphal-Strümpell E83.01
wet
feet (maceration) (tropical) T69.0-●
lung, newborn P22.1
whiplash S13.4
whistling face Q87.0
Wilkie's K55.1
Wilkinson-Sneddon L13.1
Willebrand (-Jürgens) D68.0

Syndrome *(Continued)*
Williams Q93.82
Wilson's (hepatolenticular degeneration) E83.01
Wiskott-Aldrich D82.0
withdrawal —*see* Withdrawal, state
drug
infant of dependent mother P96.1
therapeutic use, newborn P96.2
Woakes' (ethmoiditis) J33.1
Wright's (hyperabduction) G54.0
X I20.9
XXXX Q97.1
XXXXX Q97.1
XXXXY Q98.1
XXY Q98.0
Yao M04.8
yellow nail L60.5
Zahorsky's B08.5
Zellweger syndrome E71.510
Zellweger-like syndrome E71.541
Synechia (anterior) (iris) (posterior) (pupil) —*see also* Adhesions, iris
intra-uterine (traumatic) N85.6
Synesthesia R20.8
Syngamiasis, syngamosis B83.3
Synodontia K00.2
Synorchidism, synorchism Q55.1
Synostosis (congenital) Q78.8
astragalo-scaphoid Q74.2
radioulnar Q74.0
Synovial sarcoma —*see* Neoplasm, connective tissue, malignant
Synovioma (malignant) —*see also* Neoplasm, connective tissue, malignant
benign —*see* Neoplasm, connective tissue, benign
Synoviosarcoma —*see* Neoplasm, connective tissue, malignant
Synovitis —*see also* Tenosynovitis M65.9
crepitant
hand M70.0-●
wrist M70.03-●
gonococcal A54.49
gouty —*see* Gout
in (due to)
crystals M65.8-●
gonorrhea A54.49
syphilis (late) A52.78
use, overuse, pressure —*see* Disorder, soft tissue, due to use
infective NEC —*see* Tenosynovitis, infective NEC
specified NEC —*see* Tenosynovitis, specified type NEC
syphilitic A52.78
congenital (early) A50.02
toxic —*see* Synovitis, transient
transient M67.3-●
ankle M67.37-●
elbow M67.32-●
foot joint M67.37-●
hand joint M67.34-●
hip M67.35-●
knee M67.36-●
multiple site M67.39
pelvic region M67.35-●
shoulder M67.31-●
specified joint NEC M67.38
wrist M67.33-●
traumatic, current —*see* Sprain
tuberculous —*see* Tuberculosis, synovitis
villonodular (pigmented) M12.2-●
ankle M12.27-●
elbow M12.22-●
foot joint M12.27-●
hand joint M12.24-●
hip M12.25-●
knee M12.26-●
multiple site M12.29
pelvic region M12.25-●
shoulder M12.21-●
specified joint NEC M12.28

Synovitis *(Continued)*
villonodular (pigmented) *(Continued)*
vertebrae M12.28
wrist M12.23-●
Syphilid A51.39
congenital A50.06
newborn A50.06
tubercular (late) A52.79
Syphilis, syphilitic (acquired) A53.9
abdomen (late) A52.79
acoustic nerve A52.15
adenopathy (secondary) A51.49
adrenal (gland) (with cortical hypofunction) A52.79
age under 2 years NOS —*see also* Syphilis, congenital, early
acquired A51.9
alopecia (secondary) A51.32
anemia (late) A52.79 *[D63.8]*
aneurysm (aorta) (ruptured) A52.01
central nervous system A52.05
congenital A50.54 *[I79.0]*
anus (late) A52.74
primary A51.1
secondary A51.39
aorta (arch) (abdominal) (thoracic) A52.02
aneurysm A52.01
aortic (insufficiency) (regurgitation) (stenosis)A52.03
aneurysm A52.01
arachnoid (adhesive) (cerebral) (spinal) A52.13
asymptomatic —*see* Syphilis, latent
ataxia (locomotor) A52.11
atrophoderma maculatum A51.39
auricular fibrillation A52.06
bladder (late) A52.76
bone A52.77
secondary A51.46
brain A52.17
breast (late) A52.79
bronchus (late) A52.72
bubo (primary) A51.0
bulbar palsy A52.19
bursa (late) A52.78
cardiac decompensation A52.06
cardiovascular A52.00
central nervous system (late) (recurrent) (relapse) (tertiary) A52.3
with
ataxia A52.11
general paralysis A52.17
juvenile A50.45
paresis (general) A52.17
juvenile A50.45
tabes (dorsalis) A52.11
juvenile A50.45
taboparesis A52.17
juvenile A50.45
aneurysm A52.05
congenital A50.40
juvenile A50.40
remission in (sustained) A52.3
serology doubtful, negative, or positive A52.3
specified nature or site NEC A52.19
vascular A52.05
cerebral A52.17
meningovascular A52.13
nerves (multiple palsies) A52.15
sclerosis A52.17
thrombosis A52.05
cerebrospinal (tabetic type) A52.12
cerebrovascular A52.05
cervix (late) A52.76
chancre (multiple) A51.0
extragenital A51.2
Rollet's A51.0
Charcot's joint A52.16
chorioretinitis A51.43
congenital A50.01
late A52.71
prenatal A50.01

S

Syphilis, syphilitic *(Continued)*
  choroiditis *—see* Syphilitic chorioretinitis
  choroidoretinitis *—see* Syphilitic chorioretinitis
  ciliary body (secondary) A51.43
    late A52.71
  colon (late) A52.74
  combined spinal sclerosis A52.11
  condyloma (latum) A51.31
  congenital A5Ø.9
    with
      paresis (general) A5Ø.45
      tabes (dorsalis) A5Ø.45
      taboparesis A5Ø.45
    chorioretinitis, choroiditis A5Ø.Ø1 *[H32]*
    early, or less than 2 years after birth NEC A5Ø.2
      with manifestations *—see* Syphilis, congenital, early, symptomatic
      latent (without manifestations) A5Ø.1
        negative spinal fluid test A5Ø.1
        serology positive A5Ø.1
      symptomatic A5Ø.Ø9
        cutaneous A5Ø.Ø6
        mucocutaneous A5Ø.Ø7
        oculopathy A5Ø.Ø1
        osteochondropathy A5Ø.Ø2
        pharyngitis A5Ø.Ø3
        pneumonia A5Ø.Ø4
        rhinitis A5Ø.Ø5
        visceral A5Ø.Ø8
    interstitial keratitis A5Ø.31
    juvenile neurosyphilis A5Ø.45
    late, or 2 years or more after birth NEC A5Ø.7
      chorioretinitis, choroiditis A5Ø.32
      interstitial keratitis A5Ø.31
      juvenile neurosyphilis A5Ø.45
      latent (without manifestations) A5Ø.6
        negative spinal fluid test A5Ø.6
        serology positive A5Ø.6
      symptomatic or with manifestations NEC A5Ø.59
        arthropathy A5Ø.55
        cardiovascular A5Ø.54
        Clutton's joints A5Ø.51
        Hutchinson's teeth A5Ø.52
        Hutchinson's triad A5Ø.53
        osteochondropathy A5Ø.56
        saddle nose A5Ø.57
  conjugal A53.9
    tabes A52.11
  conjunctiva (late) A52.71
  contact Z2Ø.2
  cord bladder A52.19
  cornea, late A52.71
  coronary (artery) (sclerosis) A52.Ø6
  coryza, congenital A5Ø.Ø5
  cranial nerve A52.15
    multiple palsies A52.15
  cutaneous *—see* Syphilis, skin
  dacryocystitis (late) A52.71
  degeneration, spinal cord A52.12
  dementia paralytica A52.17
    juvenilis A5Ø.45
  destruction of bone A52.77
  dilatation, aorta A52.Ø1
  due to blood transfusion A53.9
  dura mater A52.13
  ear A52.79
    inner A52.79
      nerve (eighth) A52.15
      neurorecurrence A52.15
  early A51.9
    cardiovascular A52.ØØ
    central nervous system A52.3
    latent (without manifestations) (less than 2 years after infection) A51.5
      negative spinal fluid test A51.5
      serological relapse after treatment A51.5
      serology positive A51.5

Syphilis, syphilitic *(Continued)*
  early *(Continued)*
    relapse (treated, untreated) A51.9
    skin A51.39
    symptomatic A51.9
      extragenital chancre A51.2
      primary, except extragenital chancre A51.Ø
      secondary *—see also* Syphilis, secondary A51.39
        relapse (treated, untreated) A51.49
    ulcer A51.39
  eighth nerve (neuritis) A52.15
  endemic A65
  endocarditis A52.Ø3
    aortic A52.Ø3
    pulmonary A52.Ø3
  epididymis (late) A52.76
  epiglottis (late) A52.73
  epiphysitis (congenital) (early) A5Ø.Ø2
  episcleritis (late) A52.71
  esophagus A52.79
  eustachian tube A52.73
  exposure to Z2Ø.2
  eye A52.71
  eyelid (late) (with gumma) A52.71
  fallopian tube (late) A52.76
  fracture A52.77
  gallbladder (late) A52.74
  gastric (polyposis) (late) A52.74
  general A53.9
    paralysis A52.17
      juvenile A5Ø.45
  genital (primary) A51.Ø
  glaucoma A52.71
  gumma NEC A52.79
    cardiovascular system A52.ØØ
    central nervous system A52.3
    congenital A5Ø.59
  heart (block) (decompensation) (disease) (failure) A52.Ø6 *[I52]*
    valve NEC A52.Ø3
  hemianesthesia A52.19
  hemianopsia A52.71
  hemiparesis A52.17
  hemiplegia A52.17
  hepatic artery A52.Ø9
  hepatis A52.74
  hepatomegaly, congenital A5Ø.Ø8
  hereditaria tarda *—see* Syphilis, congenital, late
  hereditary *—see* Syphilis, congenital
  Hutchinson's teeth A5Ø.52
  hyalitis A52.71
  inactive *—see* Syphilis, latent
  infantum *—see* Syphilis, congenital
  inherited *—see* Syphilis, congenital
  internal ear A52.79
  intestine (late) A52.74
  iris, iritis (secondary) A51.43
    late A52.71
  joint (late) A52.77
  keratitis (congenital) (interstitial) (late) A5Ø.31
  kidney (late) A52.75
  lacrimal passages (late) A52.71
  larynx (late) A52.73
  late A52.9
    cardiovascular A52.ØØ
    central nervous system A52.3
    kidney A52.75
    latent or 2 years or more after infection (without manifestations) A52.8
      negative spinal fluid test A52.8
      serology positive A52.8
    paresis A52.17
    specified site NEC A52.79
    symptomatic or with manifestations A52.79
    tabes A52.11
  latent A53.Ø
    with signs or symptoms - code by site and stage under Syphilis

Syphilis, syphilitic *(Continued)*
  latent *(Continued)*
    central nervous system A52.2
    date of infection unspecified A53.Ø
    early, or less than 2 years after infection A51.5
    follow-up of latent syphilis A53.Ø
      date of infection unspecified A53.Ø
      late, or 2 years or more after infection A52.8
    late, or 2 years or more after infection A52.8
    positive serology (only finding) A53.Ø
      date of infection unspecified A53.Ø
      early, or less than 2 years after infection A51.5
      late, or 2 years or more after infection A52.8
  lens (late) A52.71
  leukoderma A51.39
    late A52.79
  lienitis A52.79
  lip A51.39
    chancre (primary) A51.2
    late A52.79
  Lissauer's paralysis A52.17
  liver A52.74
  locomotor ataxia A52.11
  lung A52.72
  lymph gland (early) (secondary) A51.49
    late A52.79
  lymphadenitis (secondary) A51.49
  macular atrophy of skin A51.39
    striated A52.79
  mediastinum (late) A52.73
  meninges (adhesive) (brain) (spinal cord) A52.13
  meningitis A52.13
    acute (secondary) A51.41
    congenital A5Ø.41
  meningoencephalitis A52.14
  meningovascular A52.13
    congenital A5Ø.41
  mesarteritis A52.Ø9
    brain A52.Ø4
  middle ear A52.77
  mitral stenosis A52.Ø3
  monoplegia A52.17
  mouth (secondary) A51.39
    late A52.79
  mucocutaneous (secondary) A51.39
    late A52.79
  mucous
    membrane (secondary) A51.39
      late A52.79
    patches A51.39
      congenital A5Ø.Ø7
  mulberry molars A5Ø.52
  muscle A52.78
  myocardium A52.Ø6
  nasal sinus (late) A52.73
  neonatorum *—see* Syphilis, congenital
  nephrotic syndrome (secondary) A51.44
  nerve palsy (any cranial nerve) A52.15
    multiple A52.15
  nervous system, central A52.3
  neuritis A52.15
    acoustic A52.15
  neurorecidive of retina A52.19
  neuroretinitis A52.19
  newborn *—see* Syphilis, congenital
  nodular superficial (late) A52.79
  nonvenereal A65
  nose (late) A52.73
    saddle back deformity A5Ø.57
  occlusive arterial disease A52.Ø9
  oculopathy A52.71
  ophthalmic (late) A52.71
  optic nerve (atrophy) (neuritis) (papilla) A52.15

Syphilis, syphilitic *(Continued)*
orbit (late) A52.71
organic A53.9
osseous (late) A52.77
osteochondritis (congenital) (early) A50.02 *[M90.80]*
osteoporosis A52.77
ovary (late) A52.76
oviduct (late) A52.76
palate (late) A52.79
pancreas (late) A52.74
paralysis A52.17
general A52.17
juvenile A50.45
paresis (general) A52.17
juvenile A50.45
paresthesia A52.19
Parkinson's disease or syndrome A52.19
paroxysmal tachycardia A52.06
pemphigus (congenital) A50.06
penis (chancre) A51.0
late A52.76
pericardium A52.06
perichondritis, larynx (late) A52.73
periosteum (late) A52.77
congenital (early) A50.02 *[M90.80]*
early (secondary) A51.46
peripheral nerve A52.79
petrous bone (late) A52.77
pharynx (late) A52.73
secondary A51.39
pituitary (gland) A52.79
pleura (late) A52.73
pneumonia, white A50.04
pontine lesion A52.17
portal vein A52.09
primary A51.0
anal A51.1
and secondary —*see* Syphilis, secondary
central nervous system A52.3
extragenital chancre NEC A51.2
fingers A51.2
genital A51.0
lip A51.2
specified site NEC A51.2
tonsils A51.2
prostate (late) A52.76
ptosis (eyelid) A52.71
pulmonary (late) A52.72
artery A52.09
pyelonephritis (late) A52.75
recently acquired, symptomatic A51.9
rectum (late) A52.74
respiratory tract (late) A52.73
retina, late A52.71
retrobulbar neuritis A52.15
salpingitis A52.76
sclera (late) A52.71
sclerosis
cerebral A52.17
coronary A52.06
multiple A52.11
scotoma (central) A52.71
scrotum (late) A52.76

Syphilis, syphilitic *(Continued)*
secondary (and primary) A51.49
adenopathy A51.49
anus A51.39
bone A51.46
chorioretinitis, choroiditis A51.43
hepatitis A51.45
liver A51.45
lymphadenitis A51.49
meningitis (acute) A51.41
mouth A51.39
mucous membranes A51.39
periosteum, periostitis A51.46
pharynx A51.39
relapse (treated, untreated) A51.49
skin A51.39
specified form NEC A51.49
tonsil A51.39
ulcer A51.39
viscera NEC A51.49
vulva A51.39
seminal vesicle (late) A52.76
seronegative with signs or symptoms - code by site and stage under Syphilis
seropositive
with signs or symptoms - code by site and stage under Syphilis
follow-up of latent syphilis —*see* Syphilis, latent
only finding —*see* Syphilis, latent
seventh nerve (paralysis) A52.15
sinus, sinusitis (late) A52.73
skeletal system A52.77
skin (with ulceration) (early) (secondary) A51.39
late or tertiary A52.79
small intestine A52.74
spastic spinal paralysis A52.17
spermatic cord (late) A52.76
spinal (cord) A52.12
spleen A52.79
splenomegaly A52.79
spondylitis A52.77
staphyloma A52.71
stigmata (congenital) A50.59
stomach A52.74
synovium A52.78
tabes dorsalis (late) A52.11
juvenile A50.45
tabetic type A52.11
juvenile A50.45
taboparesis A52.17
juvenile A50.45
tachycardia A52.06
tendon (late) A52.78
tertiary A52.9
with symptoms NEC A52.79
cardiovascular A52.00
central nervous system A52.3
multiple NEC A52.79
specified site NEC A52.79
testis A52.76
thorax A52.73
throat A52.73

Syphilis, syphilitic *(Continued)*
thymus (gland) (late) A52.79
thyroid (late) A52.79
tongue (late) A52.79
tonsil (lingual) (late) A52.73
primary A51.2
secondary A51.39
trachea (late) A52.73
tunica vaginalis (late) A52.76
ulcer (any site) (early) (secondary) A51.39
late A52.79
perforating A52.79
foot A52.11
urethra (late) A52.76
urogenital (late) A52.76
uterus (late) A52.76
uveal tract (secondary) A51.43
late A52.71
uveitis (secondary) A51.43
late A52.71
uvula (late) (perforated) A52.79
vagina A51.0
late A52.76
valvulitis NEC A52.03
vascular A52.00
brain (cerebral) A52.05
ventriculi A52.74
vesicae urinariae (late) A52.76
viscera (abdominal) (late) A52.74
secondary A51.49
vitreous (opacities) (late) A52.71
hemorrhage A52.71
vulva A51.0
late A52.76
secondary A51.39
Syphiloma A52.79
cardiovascular system A52.00
central nervous system A52.3
circulatory system A52.00
congenital A50.59
Syphilophobia F45.29
Syringadenoma —*see also* Neoplasm, skin, benign
papillary —*see* Neoplasm, skin, benign
Syringobulbia G95.0
Syringocystadenoma —*see* Neoplasm, skin, benign
papillary —*see* Neoplasm, skin, benign
Syringoma —*see also* Neoplasm, skin, benign
chondroid —*see* Neoplasm, skin, benign
Syringomyelia G95.0
Syringomyelitis —*see* Encephalitis
Syringomyelocele —*see* Spina bifida
Syringopontia G95.0
System, systemic —*see also* condition
disease, combined —*see* Degeneration, combined
inflammatory response syndrome (SIRS) of non-infectious origin (without organ dysfunction) R65.10
with acute organ dysfunction R65.11
lupus erythematosus M32.9
inhibitor present D68.62

T

- **Tabacism, tabacosis, tabagism** —*see also* Poisoning, tobacco
  - meaning dependence (without remission) F17.200
    - with
      - disorder F17.299
        - in remission F17.211
        - specified disorder NEC F17.298
        - withdrawal F17.203
- **Tabardillo** A75.9
  - flea-borne A75.2
  - louse-borne A75.0
- **Tabes, tabetic** A52.10
  - with
    - central nervous system syphilis A52.10
    - Charcot's joint A52.16
    - cord bladder A52.19
    - crisis, viscera (any) A52.19
    - paralysis, general A52.17
    - paresis (general) A52.17
    - perforating ulcer (foot) A52.19
  - arthropathy (Charcot) A52.16
  - bladder A52.19
  - bone A52.11
  - cerebrospinal A52.12
  - congenital A50.45
  - conjugal A52.10
  - dorsalis A52.11
    - juvenile A50.49
  - juvenile A50.49
  - latent A52.19
  - mesenterica A18.39
  - paralysis, insane, general A52.17
  - spasmodic A52.17
  - syphilis (cerebrospinal) A52.12
- **Taboparalysis** A52.17
- **Taboparesis** (remission) A52.17
  - juvenile A50.45
- **TAC** (trigeminal autonomic cephalgia) NEC G44.099
  - intractable G44.091
  - not intractable G44.099
- **Tache noir** S60.22-●
- **Tachyalimentation** K91.2
- **Tachyarrhythmia, tachyrhythmia** —*see* Tachycardia
- **Tachycardia** R00.0
  - atrial (paroxysmal) I47.1
  - auricular I47.1
  - AV nodal re-entry (re-entrant) I47.1
  - junctional (paroxysmal) I47.1
  - newborn P29.11
  - nodal (paroxysmal) I47.1
  - non-paroxysmal AV nodal I45.89
  - paroxysmal (sustained) (nonsustained) I47.9
    - with sinus bradycardia I49.5
    - atrial (PAT) I47.1
    - atrioventricular (AV) (re-entrant) I47.1
      - psychogenic F54
    - junctional I47.1
      - ectopic I47.1
    - nodal I47.1
    - psychogenic (atrial) (supraventricular) (ventricular) F54
    - supraventricular (sustained) I47.1
      - psychogenic F54
    - ventricular I47.2
      - psychogenic F54
  - psychogenic F45.8
  - sick sinus I49.5
  - sinoauricular NOS R00.0
    - paroxysmal I47.1
  - sinus [sinusal] NOS R00.0
    - paroxysmal I47.1
  - supraventricular I47.1
  - ventricular (paroxysmal) (sustained) I47.2
    - psychogenic F54
- **Tachygastria** K31.89
- **Tachypnea** R06.82
  - hysterical F45.8
  - newborn (idiopathic) (transitory) P22.1
  - psychogenic F45.8
  - transitory, of newborn P22.1
- **TACO** (transfusion associated circulatory overload) E87.71
- **Taenia** (infection) (infestation) B68.9
  - diminuta B71.0
  - echinococcal infestation B67.90
  - mediocanellata B68.1
  - nana B71.0
  - saginata B68.1
  - solium (intestinal form) B68.0
    - larval form —*see* Cysticercosis
- **Taeniasis** (intestine) —*see* Taenia
- **Tag** (hypertrophied skin) (infected) L91.8
  - adenoid J35.8
  - anus K64.4
  - hemorrhoidal K64.4
  - hymen N89.8
  - perineal N90.89
  - preauricular Q17.0
  - sentinel K64.4
  - skin L91.8
    - accessory (congenital) Q82.8
    - anus K64.4
    - congenital Q82.8
    - preauricular Q17.0
  - tonsil J35.8
  - urethra, urethral N36.8
  - vulva N90.89
- **Tahyna fever** B33.8
- **Takahara's disease** E80.3
- **Takayasu's disease or syndrome** M31.4
- **Talcosis** (pulmonary) J62.0
- **Talipes** (congenital) Q66.89
  - acquired, planus —*see* Deformity, limb, flat foot
  - asymmetric Q66.89
  - calcaneovalgus Q66.4-●
  - calcaneovarus Q66.1-●
  - calcaneus Q66.89
  - cavus Q66.7-●
  - equinovalgus Q66.6
  - equinovarus Q66.0-●
  - equinus Q66.89
  - percavus Q66.7-●
  - planovalgus Q66.6
  - planus (acquired) (any degree) —*see also* Deformity, limb, flat foot
    - congenital Q66.5-●
    - due to rickets (sequelae) E64.3
  - valgus Q66.6
  - varus Q66.3-●
- **Tall stature, constitutional** E34.4
- **Talma's disease** M62.89
- **Talon noir** S90.3-●
  - hand S60.22-●
  - heel S90.3-●
  - toe S90.1-●
- **Tamponade, heart** I31.4
- **Tanapox** (virus disease) B08.71
- **Tangier disease** E78.6
- **Tantrum, child problem** F91.8
- **Tapeworm** (infection) (infestation) —*see* Infestation, tapeworm
- **Tapia's syndrome** G52.7
- **TAR** (thrombocytopenia with absent radius) **syndrome** Q87.2
- **Tarral-Besnier disease** L44.0
- **Tarsal tunnel syndrome** —*see* Syndrome, tarsal tunnel
- **Tarsalgia** —*see* Pain, limb, lower
- **Tarsitis** (eyelid) H01.8
  - syphilitic A52.71
  - tuberculous A18.4
- **Tartar** (teeth) (dental calculus) K03.6
- **Tattoo** (mark) L81.8
- **Tauri's disease** E74.09
- **Taurodontism** K00.2
- **Taussig-Bing syndrome** Q20.1
- **Taybi's syndrome** Q87.2
- **Tay-Sachs amaurotic familial idiocy or disease** E75.02
- **TBI** (traumatic brain injury) S06.9
- **Teacher's node or nodule** J38.2
- **Tear, torn** (traumatic) —*see also* Laceration
  - with abortion —*see* Abortion
  - annular fibrosis M51.35
  - anus, anal (sphincter) S31.831
    - complicating delivery
      - with third degree perineal laceration —*see also* Delivery, complicated, by, laceration, perineum, third degree O70.20
        - with mucosa O70.3
      - without third degree perineal laceration O70.4
    - nontraumatic (healed) (old) K62.81
  - articular cartilage, old —*see* Derangement, joint, articular cartilage, by site
  - bladder
    - with ectopic or molar pregnancy O08.6
    - following ectopic or molar pregnancy O08.6
    - obstetrical O71.5
    - traumatic —*see* Injury, bladder
  - bowel
    - with ectopic or molar pregnancy O08.6
    - following ectopic or molar pregnancy O08.6
    - obstetrical trauma O71.5
  - broad ligament
    - with ectopic or molar pregnancy O08.6
    - following ectopic or molar pregnancy O08.6
    - obstetrical trauma O71.6
  - bucket handle (knee) (meniscus) —*see* Tear, meniscus
  - capsule, joint —*see* Sprain
  - cartilage —*see also* Sprain
    - articular, old —*see* Derangement, joint, articular cartilage, by site
  - cervix
    - with ectopic or molar pregnancy O08.6
    - following ectopic or molar pregnancy O08.6
    - obstetrical trauma (current) O71.3
    - old N88.1
    - traumatic —*see* Injury, uterus
  - dural G97.41
    - nontraumatic G96.11
  - internal organ —*see* Injury, by site
  - knee cartilage
    - articular (current) S83.3-●
    - old —*see* Derangement, knee, meniscus, due to old tear
  - ligament —*see* Sprain
  - meniscus (knee) (current injury) S83.209
    - bucket-handle S83.20-●
    - lateral
      - bucket-handle S83.25-●
      - complex S83.27-●
      - peripheral S83.26-●
      - specified type NEC S83.28-●
    - medial
      - bucket-handle S83.21-●
      - complex S83.23-●
      - peripheral S83.22-●
      - specified type NEC S83.24-●
    - old —*see* Derangement, knee, meniscus, due to old tear
    - site other than knee - code as Sprain
    - specified type NEC S83.20-●
  - muscle —*see* Strain
  - pelvic
    - floor, complicating delivery O70.1
    - organ NEC, obstetrical trauma O71.5
      - with ectopic or molar pregnancy O08.6
      - following ectopic or molar pregnancy O08.6
  - perineal, secondary O90.1

Tear, torn *(Continued)*
periurethral tissue, obstetrical trauma O71.82
with ectopic or molar pregnancy O08.6
following ectopic or molar pregnancy O08.6
rectovaginal septum *—see* Laceration, vagina
retina, retinal (without detachment) (horseshoe) *—see also* Break, retina, horseshoe
with detachment *—see* Detachment, retina, with retinal, break
rotator cuff (nontraumatic) M75.10-●
complete M75.12-●
incomplete M75.11-●
traumatic S46.01-●
capsule S43.42-●
semilunar cartilage, knee *—see* Tear, meniscus
supraspinatus (complete) (incomplete) (nontraumatic) *—see also* Tear, rotator cuff M75.10-●
tendon *—see* Strain
tentorial, at birth P10.4
umbilical cord
complicating delivery O69.89
urethra
with ectopic or molar pregnancy O08.6
following ectopic or molar pregnancy O08.6
obstetrical trauma O71.5
uterus *—see* Injury, uterus
vagina *—see* Laceration, vagina
vessel, from catheter *—see* Puncture, accidental complicating surgery
vulva, complicating delivery O70.0
Tear-stone *—see* Dacryolith
Teeth *—see also* condition
grinding
psychogenic F45.8
sleep related G47.63
Teething (syndrome) K00.7
Telangiectasia, telangiectasis (verrucous) I78.1
ataxic (cerebellar) (Louis-Bar) G11.3
familial I78.0
hemorrhagic, hereditary (congenital) (senile) I78.0
hereditary, hemorrhagic (congenital) (senile) I78.0
juxtafoveal H35.07-●
macular H35.07-●
macularis eruptiva perstans D47.01
parafoveal H35.07-●
retinal (idiopathic) (juxtafoveal) (macular) (parafoveal) H35.07-●
spider I78.1
Telephone scatologia F65.89
Telescoped bowel or intestine K56.1
congenital Q43.8
Temperature
body, high (of unknown origin) R50.9
cold, trauma from T69.9
newborn P80.0
specified effect NEC T69.8
Temple *—see* condition
Temporal *—see* condition
Temporomandibular joint pain-dysfunction syndrome M26.62-●
Temporosphenoidal *—see* condition
Tendency
bleeding *—see* Defect, coagulation
suicide
meaning personal history of attempted suicide Z91.5
meaning suicidal ideation *—see* Ideation, suicidal
to fall R29.6
Tenderness, abdominal R10.819
epigastric R10.816
generalized R10.817
left lower quadrant R10.814
left upper quadrant R10.812
periumbilic R10.815
Tenderness, abdominal *(Continued)*
rebound R10.829
epigastric R10.826
generalized R10.827
left lower quadrant R10.824
left upper quadrant R10.822
periumbilic R10.825
right lower quadrant R10.823
right upper quadrant R10.821
right lower quadrant R10.813
right upper quadrant R10.811
Tendinitis, tendonitis *—see also* Enthesopathy
Achilles M76.6-●
adhesive *—see* Tenosynovitis, specified type NEC
shoulder *—see* Capsulitis, adhesive
bicipital M75.2-●
calcific M65.2-●
ankle M65.27-●
foot M65.27-●
forearm M65.23-●
hand M65.24-●
lower leg M65.26-●
multiple sites M65.29
pelvic region M65.25-●
shoulder M75.3-●
specified site NEC M65.28
thigh M65.25-●
upper arm M65.22-●
due to use, overuse, pressure *—see also* Disorder, soft tissue, due to use
specified NEC *—see* Disorder, soft tissue, due to use, specified NEC
gluteal M76.0-●
patellar M76.5-●
peroneal M76.7-●
psoas M76.1-●
tibial (posterior) M76.82-●
anterior M76.81-●
trochanteric *—see* Bursitis, hip, trochanteric
Tendon *—see* condition
Tendosynovitis *—see* Tenosynovitis
Tenesmus (rectal) R19.8
vesical R30.1
Tennis elbow *—see* Epicondylitis, lateral
Tenonitis *—see also* Tenosynovitis
eye (capsule) H05.04-●
Tenontosynovitis *—see* Tenosynovitis
Tenontothecitis *—see* Tenosynovitis
Tenophyte *—see* Disorder, synovium, specified type NEC
Tenosynovitis *—see also* Synovitis M65.9
adhesive *—see* Tenosynovitis, specified type NEC
shoulder *—see* Capsulitis, adhesive
bicipital (calcifying) *—see* Tendinitis, bicipital
gonococcal A54.49
in (due to)
crystals M65.8-●
gonorrhea A54.49
syphilis (late) A52.78
use, overuse, pressure *—see also* Disorder, soft tissue, due to use
specified NEC *—see* Disorder, soft tissue, due to use, specified NEC
infective NEC M65.1-●
ankle M65.17-●
foot M65.17-●
forearm M65.13-●
hand M65.14-●
lower leg M65.16-●
multiple sites M65.19
pelvic region M65.15-●
shoulder region M65.11-●
specified site NEC M65.18
thigh M65.15-●
upper arm M65.12-●
radial styloid M65.4
shoulder region M65.81-●
adhesive *—see* Capsulitis, adhesive
Tenosynovitis *(Continued)*
specified type NEC M65.88-●
ankle M65.87-●
foot M65.87-●
forearm M65.83-●
hand M65.84-●
lower leg M65.86-●
multiple sites M65.89
pelvic region M65.85-●
shoulder region M65.81-●
specified site NEC M65.88
thigh M65.85-●
upper arm M65.82-●
tuberculous *—see* Tuberculosis, tenosynovitis
Tenovaginitis *—see* Tenosynovitis
Tension
arterial, high *—see also* Hypertension
without diagnosis of hypertension R03.0
headache G44.209
intractable G44.201
not intractable G44.209
nervous R45.0
pneumothorax J93.0
premenstrual N94.3
state (mental) F48.9
Tentorium *—see* condition
Teratencephalus Q89.8
Teratism Q89.7
Teratoblastoma (malignant) *—see* Neoplasm, malignant, by site
Teratocarcinoma *—see also* Neoplasm, malignant, by site
liver C22.7
Teratoma (solid) *—see also* Neoplasm, uncertain behavior, by site
with embryonal carcinoma, mixed *—see* Neoplasm, malignant, by site
with malignant transformation *—see* Neoplasm, malignant, by site
adult (cystic) *—see* Neoplasm, benign, by site
benign *—see* Neoplasm, benign, by site
combined with choriocarcinoma *—see* Neoplasm, malignant, by site
cystic (adult) *—see* Neoplasm, benign, by site
differentiated *—see* Neoplasm, benign, by site
embryonal *—see also* Neoplasm, malignant, by site
liver C22.7
immature *—see* Neoplasm, malignant, by site
liver C22.7
adult, benign, cystic, differentiated type or mature D13.4
malignant *—see also* Neoplasm, malignant, by site
anaplastic *—see* Neoplasm, malignant, by site
intermediate *—see* Neoplasm, malignant, by site
specified site *—see* Neoplasm, malignant, by site
unspecified site C62.90
undifferentiated *—see* Neoplasm, malignant, by site
mature *—see* Neoplasm, uncertain behavior, by site
malignant *—see* Neoplasm, by site, malignant, by site
ovary D27.-●
embryonal, immature or malignant C56-●
solid *—see* Neoplasm, uncertain behavior, by site
testis C62.9-●
adult, benign, cystic, differentiated type or mature D29.2-●
scrotal C62.1-●
undescended C62.0-●
Termination
anomalous *—see also* Malposition, congenital
right pulmonary vein Q26.3
pregnancy, elective Z33.2
Ternidens diminutus infestation B81.8
Ternidensiasis B81.8

Terror(s) night (child) F51.4
Terrorism, victim of Z65.4
Terry's syndrome —*see also* Myopia, degenerative H44.2- ●
Tertiary —*see* condition
Test, tests, testing (for)
adequacy (for dialysis)
hemodialysis Z49.31
peritoneal Z49.32
blood pressure Z01.30
abnormal reading —*see* Blood, pressure
blood typing Z01.83
Rh typing Z01.83
blood-alcohol Z04.89
positive —*see* Findings, abnormal, in blood
blood-drug Z04.89
positive —*see* Findings, abnormal, in blood
cardiac pulse generator (battery) Z45.010
fertility Z31.41
genetic
disease carrier status for procreative management
female Z31.430
male Z31.440
male partner of patient with recurrent pregnancy loss Z31.441
procreative management NEC
female Z31.438
male Z31.448
hearing Z01.10
with abnormal findings NEC Z01.118
infant or child (over 28 days old) Z00.129
with abnormal findings Z00.121
HIV (human immunodeficiency virus)
nonconclusive (in infants) R75
positive Z21
seropositive Z21
immunity status Z01.84
intelligence NEC Z01.89
laboratory (as part of a general medical examination) Z00.00
with abnormal finding Z00.01
for medicolegal reason NEC Z04.89
male partner of patient with recurrent pregnancy loss Z31.441
Mantoux (for tuberculosis) Z11.1
abnormal result R76.11
pregnancy, positive first pregnancy —*see* Pregnancy, normal, first
procreative Z31.49
fertility Z31.41
skin, diagnostic
allergy Z01.82
special screening examination —*see* Screening, by name of disease
Mantoux Z11.1
tuberculin Z11.1
specified NEC Z01.89
tuberculin Z11.1
abnormal result R76.11
vision Z01.00
with abnormal findings Z01.01
▶ following failed vision screening Z01.020
▶ with abnormal findings Z01.021
infant or child (over 28 days old) Z00.129
with abnormal findings Z00.121
Wassermann Z11.3
positive —*see* Serology for syphilis, positive
Testicle, testicular, testis —*see also* condition
feminization syndrome —*see also* Syndrome, androgen insensitivity E34.51
migrans Q55.29
Tetanus, tetanic (cephalic) (convulsions) A35
with
abortion A34
ectopic or molar pregnancy O08.0
following ectopic or molar pregnancy O08.0
inoculation reaction (due to serum) —*see* Complications, vaccination
neonatorum A33
obstetrical A34
puerperal, postpartum, childbirth A34
Tetany (due to) R29.0
alkalosis E87.3
associated with rickets E55.0
convulsions R29.0
hysterical F44.5
functional (hysterical) F44.5
hyperkinetic R29.0
hysterical F44.5
hyperpnea R06.4
hysterical F44.5
psychogenic F45.8
hyperventilation —*see also* Hyperventilation R06.4
hysterical F44.5
neonatal (without calcium or magnesium deficiency) P71.3
parathyroid (gland) E20.9
parathyroprival E89.2
post- (para)thyroidectomy E89.2
postoperative E89.2
pseudotetany R29.0
psychogenic (conversion reaction) F44.5
Tetralogy of Fallot Q21.3
Tetraplegia (chronic) —*see also* Quadriplegia G82.50- ●
Thailand hemorrhagic fever A91
Thalassanemia —*see* Thalassemia
Thalassemia (anemia) (disease) D56.9
with other hemoglobinopathy D56.8
alpha (major) (severe) (triple gene defect) D56.0
minor D56.3
silent carrier D56.3
trait D56.3
beta (severe) D56.1
homozygous D56.1
major D56.1
minor D56.3
trait D56.3
delta-beta (homozygous) D56.2
minor D56.3
trait D56.3
dominant D56.8
hemoglobin
C D56.8
E-beta D56.5
intermedia D56.1
major D56.1
minor D56.3
mixed D56.8
sickle-cell —*see* Disease, sickle-cell, thalassemia
specified type NEC D56.8
trait D56.3
variants D56.8
Thanatophoric dwarfism or short stature Q77.1
Thaysen-Gee disease (nontropical sprue) K90.0
Thaysen's disease K90.0
Thecoma D27- ●
luteinized D27- ●
malignant C56- ●
Thelarche, premature E30.8
Thelaziasis B83.8
Thelitis N61.0
puerperal, postpartum or gestational —*see* Infection, nipple
Therapeutic —*see* condition
Therapy
drug, long-term (current) (prophylactic)
agents affecting estrogen receptors and estrogen levels NEC Z79.818
anastrozole (Arimidex) Z79.811
antibiotics Z79.2
short-term use - omit code
anticoagulants Z79.01
anti-inflammatory Z79.1
antiplatelet Z79.02
antithrombotics Z79.02
aromatase inhibitors Z79.811
aspirin Z79.82
birth control pill or patch Z79.3
Therapy *(Continued)*
drug, long-term *(Continued)*
bisphosphonates Z79.83
contraceptive, oral Z79.3
drug, specified NEC Z79.899
estrogen receptor downregulators Z79.818
Evista Z79.810
exemestane (Aromasin) Z79.811
Fareston Z79.810
fulvestrant (Faslodex) Z79.818
gonadotropin-releasing hormone (GnRH) agonist Z79.818
goserelin acetate (Zoladex) Z79.818
hormone replacement Z79.890
insulin Z79.4
letrozole (Femara) Z79.811
leuprolide acetate (leuprorelin) (Lupron) Z79.818
megestrol acetate (Megace) Z79.818
methadone
for pain management Z79.891
maintenance therapy F11.20
Nolvadex Z79.810
opiate analgesic Z79.891
oral contraceptive Z79.3
raloxifene (Evista) Z79.810
selective estrogen receptor modulators (SERMs) Z79.810
short term - omit code
steroids
inhaled Z79.51
systemic Z79.52
tamoxifen (Nolvadex) Z79.810
toremifene (Fareston) Z79.810
Thermic —*see* condition
Thermography (abnormal) —*see also* Abnormal, diagnostic imaging R93.89
breast R92.8
➡ **Thermoplegia** T67.01
Thesaurismosis, glycogen —*see* Disease, glycogen storage
Thiamin deficiency E51.9
specified NEC E51.8
Thiaminic deficiency with beriberi E51.11
Thibierge-Weissenbach syndrome —*see* Sclerosis, systemic
Thickening
bone —*see* Hypertrophy, bone
breast N64.59
endometrium R93.89
epidermal L85.9
specified NEC L85.8
hymen N89.6
larynx J38.7
nail L60.2
congenital Q84.5
periosteal —*see* Hypertrophy, bone
pleura J92.9
with asbestos J92.0
skin R23.4
subepiglottic J38.7
tongue K14.8
valve, heart —*see* Endocarditis
Thigh —*see* condition
Thinning vertebra —*see* Spondylopathy, specified NEC
Thirst, excessive R63.1
due to deprivation of water T73.1
Thomsen disease G71.12
Thoracic —*see also* condition
kidney Q63.2
outlet syndrome G54.0
Thoracogastroschisis (congenital) Q79.8
Thoracopagus Q89.4
Thorax —*see* condition
Thorn's syndrome N28.89
Thorson-Björck syndrome E34.0
Threadworm (infection) (infestation) B80

Threatened
  abortion O2Ø.Ø
    with subsequent abortion OØ3.9
  job loss, anxiety concerning Z56.2
  labor (without delivery) O47.9
    at or after 37 completed weeks of gestation O47.1
    before 37 completed weeks of gestation O47.Ø-●
  loss of job, anxiety concerning Z56.2
  miscarriage O2Ø.Ø
  unemployment, anxiety concerning Z56.2
Three-day fever A93.1
Threshers' lung J67.Ø
Thrix annulata (congenital) Q84.1
Throat —*see* condition
Thrombasthenia (Glanzmann) (hemorrhagic) (hereditary) D69.1
Thromboangiitis I73.1
  obliterans (general) I73.1
    cerebral I67.89
    vessels
      brain I67.89
      spinal cord I67.89
Thromboarteritis —*see* Arteritis
Thromboasthenia (Glanzmann) (hemorrhagic) (hereditary) D69.1
Thrombocytasthenia (Glanzmann) D69.1
Thrombocythemia (essential) (hemorrhagic) (idiopathic) (primary) D47.3
Thrombocytopathy (dystrophic) (granulopenic) D69.1
Thrombocytopenia, thrombocytopenic D69.6
  with absent radius (TAR) Q87.2
  congenital D69.42
  dilutional D69.59
  due to
    drugs D69.59
    extracorporeal circulation of blood D69.59
    (massive)blood transfusion D69.59
    platelet alloimmunization D69.59
  essential D69.3
  heparin induced (HIT) D75.82
  hereditary D69.42
  idiopathic D69.3
  neonatal, transitory P61.Ø
    due to
      exchange transfusion P61.Ø
      idiopathic maternal thrombocytopenia P61.Ø
      isoimmunization P61.Ø
  primary NEC D69.49
    idiopathic D69.3
  puerperal, postpartum O72.3
  secondary D69.59
  transient neonatal P61.Ø
Thrombocytosis, essential D47.3
  primary D47.3
Thromboembolism —*see* Embolism
Thrombopathy (Bernard-Soulier) D69.1
  constitutional D68.Ø
  Willebrand-Jurgens D68.Ø
Thrombopenia —*see* Thrombocytopenia
Thrombophilia D68.59
  primary NEC D68.59
  secondary NEC D68.69
  specified NEC D68.69
Thrombophlebitis I8Ø.9
  antepartum O22.2-●
    deep O22.3-●
    superficial O22.2-●
  ▶calf muscular vein (NOS) I8Ø.25-●
  cavernous (venous) sinus GØ8
    complicating pregnancy O22.5-●
    nonpyogenic I67.6
  cerebral (sinus) (vein) GØ8
    nonpyogenic I67.6
    sequelae GØ9
  due to implanted device —*see* Complications, by site and type, specified NEC
  during or resulting from a procedure NEC T81.72
Thrombophlebitis *(Continued)*
  femoral vein (superficial) I8Ø.1-●
  femoropopliteal vein I8Ø.Ø-●
  ▶gastrocnemial vein I8Ø.25-●
  hepatic (vein) I8Ø.8
  idiopathic, recurrent I82.1
  ▶iliac vein (common) (external) (internal) I8Ø.21-●
  iliofemoral I8Ø.1-●
  intracranial venous sinus (any) GØ8
    nonpyogenic I67.6
    sequelae GØ9
  intraspinal venous sinuses and veins GØ8
    nonpyogenic G95.19
  lateral (venous) sinus GØ8
    nonpyogenic I67.6
  leg I8Ø.3
    superficial I8Ø.Ø-●
  longitudinal (venous) sinus GØ8
    nonpyogenic I67.6
  lower extremity I8Ø.299
  migrans, migrating I82.1
  pelvic
    with ectopic or molar pregnancy OØ8.Ø
    following ectopic or molar pregnancy OØ8.Ø
    puerperal O87.1
  ▶peroneal vein I8Ø.24-●
  popliteal vein —*see* Phlebitis, leg, deep, popliteal
  portal (vein) K75.1
  postoperative T81.72
  pregnancy —*see* Thrombophlebitis, antepartum
  puerperal, postpartum, childbirth O87.Ø
    deep O87.1
    pelvic O87.1
    septic O86.81
    superficial O87.Ø
  saphenous (greater) (lesser) I8Ø.Ø-●
  sinus (intracranial) GØ8
    nonpyogenic I67.6
  ▶soleal vein I8Ø.25-●
  specified site NEC I8Ø.8
  ➡tibial vein (anterior) (posterior) I8Ø.23-●
Thrombosis, thrombotic (bland) (multiple) (progressive) (silent) (vessel) I82.9Ø
  anal K64.5
  antepartum —*see* Thrombophlebitis, antepartum
  aorta, aortic I74.1Ø
    abdominal I74.Ø9
      saddle I74.Ø1
    bifurcation I74.Ø9
    saddle I74.Ø1
    specified site NEC I74.19
    terminal I74.Ø9
    thoracic I74.11
    valve —*see* Endocarditis, aortic
  apoplexy I63.3-●
  artery, arteries (postinfectional) I74.9
    auditory, internal —*see* Occlusion, artery, precerebral, specified NEC
    basilar —*see* Occlusion, artery, basilar
    carotid (common) (internal) —*see* Occlusion, artery, carotid
    cerebellar (anterior inferior) (posterior inferior) (superior) —*see* Occlusion, artery, cerebellar
    cerebral —*see* Occlusion, artery, cerebral
    choroidal (anterior) —*see* Occlusion, artery, precerebral, specified NEC
    communicating, posterior —*see* Occlusion, artery, precerebral, specified NEC
    coronary —*see also* Infarct, myocardium
      not resulting in infarction I24.Ø
    hepatic I74.8
    hypophyseal —*see* Occlusion, artery, precerebral, specified NEC
    iliac I74.5
    limb I74.4
      lower I74.3
      upper I74.2
Thrombosis, thrombotic *(Continued)*
  artery, arteries *(Continued)*
    meningeal, anterior or posterior —*see* Occlusion, artery, cerebral, specified NEC
    mesenteric (with gangrene) —*see also* Infarct, intestine K55.Ø69
    ophthalmic —*see* Occlusion, artery, retina
    pontine —*see* Occlusion, artery, precerebral, specified NEC
    precerebral —*see* Occlusion, artery, precerebral
    pulmonary (iatrogenic) —*see* Embolism, pulmonary
    renal N28.Ø
    retinal —*see* Occlusion, artery, retina
    spinal, anterior or posterior G95.11
    traumatic NEC T14.8
    vertebral —*see* Occlusion, artery, vertebral
  atrium, auricular —*see also* Infarct, myocardium
    following acute myocardial infarction (current complication) I23.6
    not resulting in infarction I51.3
    old I51.3
  basilar (artery) —*see* Occlusion, artery, basilar
  brain (artery) (stem) —*see also* Occlusion, artery, cerebral
    due to syphilis A52.Ø5
    puerperal O99.43
    sinus —*see* Thrombosis, intracranial venous sinus
  capillary I78.8
  cardiac —*see also* Infarct, myocardium
    not resulting in infarction I51.3
    valve —*see* Endocarditis
    old I51.3
  carotid (artery) (common) (internal) —*see* Occlusion, artery, carotid
  cavernous (venous) sinus —*see* Thrombosis, intracranial venous sinus
  cerebellar artery (anterior inferior) (posterior inferior) (superior) I66.3
  cerebral (artery) —*see* Occlusion, artery, cerebral
  cerebrovenous sinus —*see also* Thrombosis, intracranial venous sinus
    puerperium O87.3
  chronic I82.91
  coronary (artery) (vein) —*see also* Infarct, myocardium
    not resulting in infarction I24.Ø
  corpus cavernosum N48.89
  cortical I66.9
  deep —*see* Embolism, vein, lower extremity
  due to device, implant or graft —*see also* Complications, by site and type, specified NEC T85.868
    arterial graft NEC T82.868
    breast (implant) T85.868
    catheter NEC T85.868
      dialysis (renal) T82.868
        intraperitoneal T85.868
      infusion NEC T82.868
        spinal (epidural) (subdural) T85.86Ø
      urinary (indwelling) T83.86
    electronic (electrode) (pulse generator) (stimulator)
      bone T84.86
      cardiac T82.867
      nervous system (brain) (peripheral nerve) (spinal) T85.86Ø
      urinary T83.86
    fixation, internal (orthopedic) NEC T84.86
    gastrointestinal (bile duct) (esophagus) T85.868
    genital NEC T83.86
    heart T82.867
    joint prosthesis T84.86
    ocular (corneal graft) (orbital implant) NEC T85.868
    orthopedic NEC T84.86

Thrombosis, thrombotic *(Continued)*
due to device, implant or graft *(Continued)*
specified NEC T85.868
urinary NEC T83.86
vascular NEC T82.868
ventricular intracranial shunt T85.860
during the puerperium —*see* Thrombosis, puerperal
endocardial —*see also* Infarct, myocardium
not resulting in infarction I51.3
eye —*see* Occlusion, retina
genital organ
female NEC N94.89
pregnancy —*see* Thrombophlebitis, antepartum
male N50.1
gestational —*see* Phlebopathy, gestational
heart (chamber) —*see also* Infarct, myocardium
not resulting in infarction I51.3
old I51.3
hepatic (vein) I82.0
artery I74.8
history (of) Z86.718
intestine (with gangrene) —*see also* Infarct, intestine K55.069
intracardiac NEC (apical) (atrial) (auricular) (ventricular) (old) I51.3
intracranial (arterial) I66.9
venous sinus (any) G08
nonpyogenic origin I67.6
puerperium O87.3
intramural —*see also* Infarct, myocardium
not resulting in infarction I51.3
old I51.3
intraspinal venous sinuses and veins G08
nonpyogenic G95.19
kidney (artery) N28.0
lateral (venous) sinus —*see* Thrombosis, intracranial venous sinus
leg —*see* Thrombosis, vein, lower extremity
arterial I74.3
liver (venous) I82.0
artery I74.8
portal vein I81
longitudinal (venous) sinus —*see* Thrombosis, intracranial venous sinus
lower limb —*see* Thrombosis, vein, lower extremity
lung (iatrogenic) (postoperative) —*see* Embolism, pulmonary
meninges (brain) (arterial) I66.8
mesenteric (artery) (with gangrene) —*see also* Infarct, intestine K55.069
vein (inferior) (superior) K55.0
mitral I34.8
mural —*see also* Infarct, myocardium
due to syphilis A52.06
not resulting in infarction I51.3
old I51.3
omentum (with gangrene) —*see also* Infarct, intestine K55.069
ophthalmic —*see* Occlusion, retina
pampiniform plexus (male) N50.1
parietal —*see also* Infarct, myocardium
not resulting in infarction I24.0
penis, superficial vein N48.81
perianal venous K64.5
peripheral arteries I74.4
upper I74.2
personal history (of) Z86.718
portal I81
due to syphilis A52.09
precerebral artery —*see* Occlusion, artery, precerebral
puerperal, postpartum O87.0
brain (artery) O99.43
venous (sinus) O87.3
cardiac O99.43
cerebral (artery) O99.43
venous (sinus) O87.3
superficial O87.0

Thrombosis, thrombotic *(Continued)*
pulmonary (artery) (iatrogenic) (postoperative) (vein) —*see* Embolism, pulmonary
renal (artery) N28.0
vein I82.3
resulting from presence of device, implant or graft —*see* Complications, by site and type, specified NEC
retina, retinal —*see* Occlusion, retina
scrotum N50.1
seminal vesicle N50.1
sigmoid (venous) sinus —*see* Thrombosis, intracranial venous sinus
sinus, intracranial (any) —*see* Thrombosis, intracranial venous sinus
specified site NEC I82.890
chronic I82.891
spermatic cord N50.1
spinal cord (arterial) G95.11
due to syphilis A52.09
pyogenic origin G06.1
spleen, splenic D73.5
artery I74.8
testis N50.1
traumatic NEC T14.8
tricuspid I07.8
tumor —*see* Neoplasm, by site
tunica vaginalis N50.1
umbilical cord (vessels), complicating delivery O69.5
vas deferens N50.1
vein (acute) I82.90
antecubital I82.61- ●
chronic I82.71- ●
axillary I82.A1- ●
chronic I82.A2- ●
basilic I82.61- ●
chronic I82.71- ●
brachial I82.62- ●
chronic I82.72- ●
brachiocephalic (innominate) I82.290
chronic I82.291
cerebral, nonpyogenic I67.6
cephalic I82.61- ●
chronic I82.71- ●
chronic I82.91
deep (DVT) I82.40- ●
calf I82.4Z- ●
chronic I82.5Z- ●
lower leg I82.4Z- ●
chronic I82.5Z- ●
thigh I82.4Y- ●
chronic I82.5Y- ●
upper leg I82.4Y
chronic I82.5y- ●
femoral I82.41- ●
chronic I82.51- ●
iliac (iliofemoral) I82.42- ●
chronic I82.52- ●
innominate I82.290
chronic I82.291
internal jugular I82.C1- ●
chronic I82.C2- ●
lower extremity
deep I82.40- ●
chronic I82.50- ●
specified NEC I82.49- ●
chronic NEC I82.59- ●
distal
deep I82.4Z- ●
proximal
deep I82.4Y- ●
chronic I82.5Y- ●
superficial I82.81- ●
perianal K64.5
popliteal I82.43- ●
chronic I82.53- ●
radial I82.62- ●
chronic I82.72- ●
renal I82.3

Thrombosis, thrombotic *(Continued)*
vein *(Continued)*
saphenous (greater) (lesser) I82.81- ●
specified NEC I82.890
chronic NEC I82.891
subclavian I82.B1- ●
chronic I82.B2- ●
thoracic NEC I82.290
chronic I82.291
tibial I82.44- ●
chronic I82.54- ●
ulnar I82.62- ●
chronic I82.72- ●
upper extremity I82.60- ●
chronic I82.70- ●
deep I82.62- ●
chronic I82.72- ●
superficial I82.61- ●
chronic I82.71- ●
vena cava
inferior I82.220
chronic I82.221
superior I82.210
chronic I82.211
venous, perianal K64.5
ventricle —*see also* Infarct, myocardium
following acute myocardial infarction (current complication) I23.6
not resulting in infarction I24.0
old I51.3
Thrombus —*see* Thrombosis
Thrush —*see also* Candidiasis
newborn P37.5
oral B37.0
vaginal B37.3
Thumb —*see also* condition
sucking (child problem) F98.8
Thymitis E32.8
Thymoma (benign) D15.0
malignant C37
Thymus, thymic (gland) —*see* condition
Thyrocele —*see* Goiter
Thyroglossal —*see also* condition
cyst Q89.2
duct, persistent Q89.2
Thyroid (gland) (body) —*see also* condition
hormone resistance E07.89
lingual Q89.2
nodule (cystic) (nontoxic) (single) E04.1
Thyroiditis E06.9
acute (nonsuppurative) (pyogenic) (suppurative) E06.0
autoimmune E06.3
chronic (nonspecific) (sclerosing) E06.5
with thyrotoxicosis, transient E06.2
fibrous E06.5
lymphadenoid E06.3
lymphocytic E06.3
lymphoid E06.3
de Quervain's E06.1
drug-induced E06.4
fibrous (chronic) E06.5
giant-cell (follicular) E06.1
granulomatous (de Quervain) (subacute) E06.1
Hashimoto's (struma lymphomatosa) E06.3
iatrogenic E06.4
ligneous E06.5
lymphocytic (chronic) E06.3
lymphoid E06.3
lymphomatous E06.3
nonsuppurative E06.1
postpartum, puerperal O90.5
pseudotuberculous E06.1
pyogenic E06.0
radiation E06.4
Riedel's E06.5
subacute (granulomatous) E06.1
suppurative E06.0
tuberculous A18.81
viral E06.1
woody E06.5

T

- **Thyrolingual duct, persistent** Q89.2
- **Thyromegaly** EØ1.Ø
- **Thyrotoxic**
  - crisis *—see* Thyrotoxicosis
  - heart disease or failure *—see also* Thyrotoxicosis EØ5.9Ø *[I43]*
    - with thyroid storm EØ5.91 *[I43]*
  - storm *—see* Thyrotoxicosis
- **Thyrotoxicosis** (recurrent) EØ5.9Ø
  - with
    - goiter (diffuse) EØ5.ØØ
      - with thyroid storm EØ5.Ø1
      - adenomatous uninodular EØ5.1Ø
        - with thyroid storm EØ5.11
      - multinodular EØ5.2Ø
        - with thyroid storm EØ5.21
      - nodular EØ5.2Ø
        - with thyroid storm EØ5.21
      - uninodular EØ5.1Ø
        - with thyroid storm EØ5.11
    - infiltrative
      - dermopathy EØ5.ØØ
        - with thyroid storm EØ5.Ø1
      - ophthalmopathy EØ5.ØØ
        - with thyroid storm EØ5.Ø1
    - single thyroid nodule EØ5.1Ø
      - with thyroid storm EØ5.11
    - thyroid storm EØ5.91
  - due to
    - ectopic thyroid nodule or tissue EØ5.3Ø
      - with thyroid storm EØ5.31
    - ingestion of (excessive) thyroid material EØ5.4Ø
      - with thyroid storm EØ5.41
    - overproduction of thyroid-stimulating hormone EØ5.8Ø
      - with thyroid storm EØ5.81
    - specified cause NEC EØ5.8Ø
      - with thyroid storm EØ5.81
  - factitia EØ5.4Ø
    - with thyroid storm EØ5.41
  - heart *—see also* Failure, heart, high-output EØ5.9Ø *[I43]*
    - with thyroid storm *—see also* Failure, heart, high-output EØ5.91 *[I43]*
    - failure *—see also* Failure, heart, high-output EØ5.9Ø *[I43]*
  - neonatal (transient) P72.1
  - transient with chronic thyroiditis EØ6.2
- **Tibia vara** *—see* Osteochondrosis, juvenile, tibia
- **Tic** (disorder) F95.9
  - breathing F95.8
  - child problem F95.Ø
  - compulsive F95.1
  - de la Tourette F95.2
  - degenerative (generalized) (localized) G25.69
    - facial G25.69
  - disorder
    - chronic
      - motor F95.1
      - vocal F95.1
    - combined vocal and multiple motor F95.2
    - transient F95.Ø
  - douloureux G5Ø.Ø
    - atypical G5Ø.1
    - postherpetic, postzoster BØ2.22
  - drug-induced G25.61
  - eyelid F95.8
  - habit F95.9
    - chronic F95.1
    - transient of childhood F95.Ø
  - lid, transient of childhood F95.Ø
  - motor-verbal F95.2
  - occupational F48.8
  - orbicularis F95.8
    - transient of childhood F95.Ø
  - organic origin G25.69
  - postchoreic G25.69
  - provisional F95.Ø
  - psychogenic, compulsive F95.1
  - salaam R25.8
- **Tic** *(Continued)*
  - spasm (motor or vocal) F95.9
    - chronic F95.1
    - transient of childhood F95.Ø
  - specified NEC F95.8
- **Tick-borne** *—see* condition
- **Tietze's disease or syndrome** M94.Ø
- **Tight, tightness**
  - anus K62.89
  - chest RØ7.89
  - fascia (lata) M62.89
  - foreskin (congenital) N47.1
  - hymen, hymenal ring N89.6
  - introitus (acquired) (congenital) N89.6
  - rectal sphincter K62.89
  - tendon *—see* Short, tendon
  - urethral sphincter N35.919
- **Tilting vertebra** *—see* Dorsopathy, deforming, specified NEC
- **Timidity, child** F93.8
- **Tin-miner's lung** J63.5
- **Tinea** (intersecta) (tarsi) B35.9
  - amiantacea L44.8
  - asbestina B35.Ø
  - barbae B35.Ø
  - beard B35.Ø
  - black dot B35.Ø
  - blanca B36.2
  - capitis B35.Ø
  - corporis B35.4
  - cruris B35.6
  - flava B36.Ø
  - foot B35.3
  - furfuracea B36.Ø
  - imbricata (Tokelau) B35.5
  - kerion B35.Ø
  - manuum B35.2
  - microsporic *—see* Dermatophytosis
  - nigra B36.1
  - nodosa *—see* Piedra
  - pedis B35.3
  - scalp B35.Ø
  - specified NEC B35.8
  - sycosis B35.Ø
  - tonsurans B35.Ø
  - trichophytic *—see* Dermatophytosis
  - unguium B35.1
  - versicolor B36.Ø
- **Tingling sensation** (skin) R2Ø.2
- **Tinnitus NOS** H93.1- ●
  - audible H93.1- ●
  - aurium H93.1- ●
  - pulsatile H93.A- ●
  - subjective H93.1- ●
- **Tipped tooth** (teeth) M26.33
- **Tipping**
  - pelvis M95.5
    - with disproportion (fetopelvic) O33.Ø
      - causing obstructed labor O65.Ø
  - tooth (teeth), fully erupted M26.33
- **Tiredness** R53.83
- **Tissue** *—see* condition
- **Tobacco** (nicotine)
  - abuse *—see* Tobacco, use
  - dependence *—see* Dependence, drug, nicotine
  - harmful use Z72.Ø
  - heart *—see* Tobacco, toxic effect
  - maternal use, affecting newborn PØ4.2
  - toxic effect *—see* Table of Drugs and Chemicals, by substance, poisoning
    - chewing tobacco *—see* Table of Drugs and Chemicals, by substance, poisoning
    - cigarettes *—see* Table of Drugs and Chemicals, by substance, poisoning
  - use Z72.Ø
    - complicating
      - childbirth O99.334
      - pregnancy O99.33- ●
      - puerperium O99.335
    - counseling and surveillance Z71.6
    - history Z87.891
- **Tobacco** *(Continued)*
  - withdrawal state *—see also* Dependence, drug, nicotine F17.2Ø3
- **Tocopherol deficiency** E56.Ø
- **Todd's**
  - cirrhosis K74.3
  - paralysis (postepileptic) (transitory) G83.84
- **Toe** *—see* condition
- **Toilet, artificial opening** *—see* Attention to, artificial, opening
- **Tokelau** (ringworm) B35.5
- **Tollwut** *—see* Rabies
- **Tommaselli's disease** R31.9
  - correct substance properly administered *—see* Table of Drugs and Chemicals, by drug, adverse effect
  - overdose or wrong substance given or taken *—see* Table of Drugs and Chemicals, by drug, poisoning
- **Tongue** *—see also* condition
  - tie Q38.1
- **Tonic pupil** *—see* Anomaly, pupil, function, tonic pupil
- **Toni-Fanconi syndrome** (cystinosis) E72.Ø9
  - with cystinosis E72.Ø4
- **Tonsil** *—see* condition
- **Tonsillitis** (acute) (catarrhal) (croupous) (follicular) (gangrenous) (infective) (lacunar) (lingual) (malignant) (membranous) (parenchymatous) (phlegmonous) (pseudomembranous) (purulent) (septic) (subacute) (suppurative) (toxic) (ulcerative) (vesicular) (viral) JØ3.9Ø
  - chronic J35.Ø1
    - with adenoiditis J35.Ø3
  - diphtheritic A36.Ø
  - hypertrophic J35.Ø1
    - with adenoiditis J35.Ø3
  - recurrent JØ3.91
  - specified organism NEC JØ3.8Ø
    - recurrent JØ3.81
  - staphylococcal JØ3.8Ø
    - recurrent JØ3.81
  - streptococcal JØ3.ØØ
    - recurrent JØ3.Ø1
  - tuberculous A15.8
  - Vincent's A69.1
- **Tooth, teeth** *—see* condition
- **Toothache** KØ8.89
- **Topagnosis** R2Ø.8
- **Tophi** *—see* Gout, chronic
- **TORCH infection** *—see* Infection, congenital
  - without active infection PØØ.2
- **Torn** *—see* Tear
- **Tornwaldt's cyst or disease** J39.2
- **Torsion**
  - accessory tube *—see* Torsion, fallopian tube
  - adnexa (female) *—see* Torsion, fallopian tube
  - aorta, acquired I77.1
  - appendix epididymis N44.Ø4
  - appendix testis N44.Ø3
  - bile duct (common) (hepatic) K83.8
    - congenital Q44.5
  - bowel, colon or intestine K56.2
  - cervix *—see* Malposition, uterus
  - cystic duct K82.8
  - dystonia *—see* Dystonia, torsion
  - epididymis (appendix) N44.Ø4
  - fallopian tube N83.52- ●
    - with ovary N83.53
  - gallbladder K82.8
    - congenital Q44.1
  - hydatid of Morgagni
    - female N83.52- ●
    - male N44.Ø3
  - kidney (pedicle) (leading to infarction) N28.Ø
  - Meckel's diverticulum (congenital) Q43.Ø
    - malignant *—see* Table of Neoplasms, small intestine, malignant
  - mesentery K56.2
  - omentum K56.2

Torsion *(Continued)*
- organ or site, congenital NEC —*see* Anomaly, by site
- ovary (pedicle) N83.51-●
  - with fallopian tube N83.53
  - congenital Q5Ø.2
- oviduct —*see* Torsion, fallopian tube
- penis (acquired) N48.82
  - congenital Q55.63
- spasm —*see* Dystonia, torsion
- spermatic cord N44.Ø2
  - extravaginal N44.Ø1
  - intravaginal N44.Ø2
- spleen D73.5
- testis, testicle N44.ØØ
  - appendix N44.Ø3
- tibia —*see* Deformity, limb, specified type NEC, lower leg
- uterus —*see* Malposition, uterus

Torticollis (intermittent) (spastic) M43.6
- congenital (sternomastoid) Q68.Ø
- due to birth injury P15.8
- hysterical F44.4
- ocular R29.891
- psychogenic F45.8
  - conversion reaction F44.4
- rheumatic M43.6
- rheumatoid MØ6.88
- spasmodic G24.3
- traumatic, current S13.4

Tortipelvis G24.1

Tortuous
- aortic arch Q25.46
- artery I77.1
- organ or site, congenital NEC —*see* Distortion
- retinal vessel, congenital Q14.1
- ureter N13.8
- urethra N36.8
- vein —*see* Varix

Torture, victim of Z65.4

Torula, torular (histolytica) (infection) —*see* Cryptococcosis

Torulosis —*see* Cryptococcosis

Torus (mandibularis) (palatinus) M27.Ø
- fracture —*see* Fracture, by site, torus

Touraine's syndrome Q79.8

Tourette's syndrome F95.2

Tourniquet syndrome —*see* Constriction, external, by site

Tower skull Q75.Ø
- with exophthalmos Q87.Ø

Toxemia R68.89
- bacterial —*see* Sepsis
- burn —*see* Burn
- eclamptic (with pre-existing hypertension) —*see* Eclampsia
- erysipelatous —*see* Erysipelas
- fatigue R68.89
- food —*see* Poisoning, food
- gastrointestinal K52.1
- intestinal K52.1
- kidney —*see* Uremia
- malarial —*see* Malaria
- myocardial —*see* Myocarditis, toxic
- of pregnancy —*see* Pre-eclampsia
- pre-eclamptic —*see* Pre-eclampsia
- small intestine K52.1
- staphylococcal, due to food AØ5.Ø
- stasis R68.89
- uremic —*see* Uremia
- urinary —*see* Uremia

Toxemica cerebropathia psychica (nonalcoholic) FØ4
- alcoholic —*see* Alcohol, amnestic disorder

Toxic (poisoning) —*see also* condition T65.91
- effect —*see* Table of Drugs and Chemicals, by substance, poisoning
- shock syndrome A48.3
- thyroid (gland) —*see* Thyrotoxicosis

Toxicemia —*see* Toxemia

Toxicity —*see* Table of Drugs and Chemicals, by substance, poisoning

Toxic *(Continued)*
- fava bean D55.Ø
- food, noxious —*see* Poisoning, food
- from drug or nonmedicinal substance —*see* Table of Drugs and Chemicals, by drug

Toxicosis —*see also* Toxemia
- capillary, hemorrhagic D69.Ø

Toxinfection, gastrointestinal K52.1

Toxocariasis B83.Ø

Toxoplasma, toxoplasmosis (acquired) B58.9
- with
  - hepatitis B58.1
  - meningoencephalitis B58.2
  - ocular involvement B58.ØØ
  - other organ involvement B58.89
  - pneumonia, pneumonitis B58.3
- congenital (acute) (subacute) (chronic) P37.1
- maternal, manifest toxoplasmosis in infant (acute) (subacute) (chronic) P37.1

tPA (rtPA) administation in a different facility within the last 24 hours prior to admission to current facility Z92.82

Trabeculation, bladder N32.89

Trachea —*see* condition

Tracheitis (catarrhal) (infantile) (membranous) (plastic) (septal) (suppurative) (viral) JØ4.1Ø
- with
  - bronchitis (15 years of age and above) J4Ø
    - acute or subacute —*see* Bronchitis, acute
    - chronic J42
    - tuberculous NEC A15.5
    - under 15 years of age J2Ø.9
  - laryngitis (acute) JØ4.2
    - chronic J37.1
    - tuberculous NEC A15.5
- acute JØ4.1Ø
  - with obstruction JØ4.11
- chronic J42
  - with
    - bronchitis (chronic) J42
    - laryngitis (chronic) J37.1
- diphtheritic (membranous) A36.89
- due to external agent —*see* Inflammation, respiratory, upper, due to
- syphilitic A52.73
- tuberculous A15.5

Trachelitis (nonvenereal) —*see* Cervicitis

Tracheobronchial —*see* condition

Tracheobronchitis (15 years of age and above) —*see also* Bronchitis
- due to
  - Bordetella bronchiseptica A37.8Ø
    - with pneumonia A37.81
  - Francisella tularensis A21.8

Tracheobronchomegaly Q32.4
- with bronchiectasis J47.9
  - with
    - exacerbation (acute) J47.1
    - lower respiratory infection J47.Ø
- acquired J98.Ø9
  - with bronchiectasis J47.9
    - with
      - exacerbation (acute) J47.1
      - lower respiratory infection J47.Ø

Tracheobronchopneumonitis —*see* Pneumonia, broncho-●

Tracheocele (external) (internal) J39.8
- congenital Q32.1

Tracheomalacia J39.8
- congenital Q32.Ø

Tracheopharyngitis (acute) JØ6.9
- chronic J42
- due to external agent —*see* Inflammation, respiratory, upper, due to

Tracheostenosis J39.8

Tracheostomy
- complication —*see* Complication, tracheostomy
- status Z93.Ø
  - attention to Z43.Ø
  - malfunctioning J95.Ø3

Trachoma, trachomatous A71.9
- active (stage) A71.1
- contraction of conjunctiva A71.1
- dubium A71.Ø
- healed or sequelae B94.Ø
- initial (stage) A71.Ø
- pannus A71.1
- Türck's J37.Ø

Traction, vitreomacular H43.82-●

Train sickness T75.3

Trait(s)
- Hb-S D57.3
- hemoglobin
  - abnormal NEC D58.2
    - with thalassemia D56.3
  - C —*see* Disease, hemoglobin C
  - S (Hb-S) D57.3
- Lepore D56.3
- personality, accentuated Z73.1
- sickle-cell D57.3
  - with elliptocytosis or spherocytosis D57.3
- type A personality Z73.1

Tramp Z59.Ø

Trance R41.89
- hysterical F44.89

Transaminasemia R74.Ø

Transection
- abdomen (partial) S38.3
- aorta (incomplete) —*see also* Injury, aorta
  - complete —*see* Injury, aorta, laceration, major
- carotid artery (incomplete) —*see also* Injury, blood vessel, carotid, laceration
  - complete —*see* Injury, blood vessel, carotid, laceration, major
- celiac artery (incomplete) S35.211
  - branch (incomplete) S35.291
    - complete S35.292
  - complete S35.212
- innominate
  - artery (incomplete) —*see also* Injury, blood vessel, thoracic, innominate, artery, laceration
    - complete —*see* Injury, blood vessel, thoracic, innominate, artery, laceration, major
  - vein (incomplete) —*see also* Injury, blood vessel, thoracic, innominate, vein, laceration
    - complete —*see* Injury, blood vessel, thoracic, innominate, vein, laceration, major
- jugular vein (external) (incomplete) —*see also* Injury, blood vessel, jugular vein, laceration
  - complete —*see* Injury, blood vessel, jugular vein, laceration, major
  - internal (incomplete) —*see also* Injury, blood vessel, jugular vein, internal, laceration
    - complete —*see* Injury, blood vessel, jugular vein, internal, laceration, major
- mesenteric artery (incomplete) —*see also* Injury, mesenteric, artery, laceration
  - complete —*see* Injury, mesenteric artery, laceration, major
- pulmonary vessel (incomplete) —*see also* Injury, blood vessel, thoracic, pulmonary, laceration
  - complete —*see* Injury, blood vessel, thoracic, pulmonary, laceration, major
- subclavian —*see* Transection, innominate
- vena cava (incomplete) —*see also* Injury, vena cava
  - complete —*see* Injury, vena cava, laceration, major
- vertebral artery (incomplete) —*see also* Injury, blood vessel, vertebral, laceration
  - complete —*see* Injury, blood vessel, vertebral, laceration, major

T

Transfusion
associated (red blood cell) hemochromatosis E83.111
blood
ABO incompatible *—see* Complication(s), transfusion, incompatibility reaction, ABO
minor blood group (Duffy) (E) (K) (Kell) (Kidd) (Lewis) (M) (N) (P) (S) T8Ø.89
reaction or complication *—see* Complications, transfusion
fetomaternal (mother) *—see* Pregnancy, complicated by, placenta, transfusion syndrome
maternofetal (mother) *—see* Pregnancy, complicated by, placenta, transfusion syndrome
placental (syndrome) (mother) *—see* Pregnancy, complicated by, placenta, transfusion syndrome
reaction (adverse) *—see* Complications, transfusion
related acute lung injury (TRALI) J95.84
twin-to-twin *—see* Pregnancy, complicated by, placenta, transfusion syndrome, fetus to fetus
Transient (meaning homeless) *—see also* condition Z59.Ø
Translocation
balanced autosomal Q95.9
in normal individual Q95.Ø
chromosomes NEC Q99.8
balanced and insertion in normal individual Q95.Ø
Down's syndrome Q9Ø.2
trisomy
13 Q91.6
18 Q91.2
21 Q9Ø.2
Translucency, iris *—see* Degeneration, iris
Transmission of chemical substances through the placenta *—see* Absorption, chemical, through placenta
Transparency, lung, unilateral J43.Ø
Transplant (ed) (status) Z94.9
awaiting organ Z76.82
bone Z94.6
marrow Z94.81
candidate Z76.82
complication *—see* Complication, transplant
cornea Z94.7
heart Z94.1
and lung(s) Z94.3
valve Z95.2
prosthetic Z95.2
specified NEC Z95.4
xenogenic Z95.3
intestine Z94.82
kidney Z94.Ø
liver Z94.4
lung(s) Z94.2
and heart Z94.3
organ (failure) (infection) (rejection)Z94.9
removal status Z98.85
pancreas Z94.83
skin Z94.5
social Z6Ø.3
specified organ or tissue NEC Z94.89
stem cells Z94.84
tissue Z94.9
Transplants, ovarian, endometrial N8Ø.1
Transposed *—see* Transposition
Transposition (congenital) *—see also* Malposition, congenital
abdominal viscera Q89.3
aorta (dextra) Q2Ø.3
appendix Q43.8
colon Q43.8
corrected Q2Ø.5
great vessels (complete) (partial) Q2Ø.3
Transposition *(Continued)*
heart Q24.Ø
with complete transposition of viscera Q89.3
intestine (large) (small) Q43.8
reversed jejunal (for bypass) (status) Z98.Ø
scrotum Q55.23
stomach Q4Ø.2
with general transposition of viscera Q89.3
tooth, teeth, fully erupted M26.3Ø
vessels, great (complete) (partial) Q2Ø.3
viscera (abdominal) (thoracic) Q89.3
Transsexualism F64.Ø
Transverse *—see also* condition
arrest (deep), in labor O64.Ø
lie (mother) O32.2
causing obstructed labor O64.8
Transvestism, transvestitism (dual-role) F64.1
fetishistic F65.1
Trapped placenta (with hemorrhage) O72.Ø
without hemorrhage O73.Ø
TRAPS (tumor necrosis factor receptor associated periodic syndrome) MØ4.1
Trauma, traumatism *—see also* Injury
acoustic *—see* subcategory H83.3
birth *—see* Birth, injury
complicating ectopic or molar pregnancy OØ8.6
during delivery O71.9
following ectopic or molar pregnancy OØ8.6
obstetric O71.9
specified NEC O71.89
occlusal
primary KØ8.81
secondary KØ8.82
Traumatic *—see also* condition
brain injury SØ6.9
Treacher Collins syndrome Q75.4
Treitz's hernia *—see* Hernia, abdomen, specified site NEC
Trematode infestation *—see* Infestation, fluke
Trematodiasis *—see* Infestation, fluke
Trembling paralysis *—see* Parkinsonism
Tremor(s) R25.1
drug induced G25.1
essential (benign) G25.Ø
familial G25.Ø
hereditary G25.Ø
hysterical F44.4
intention G25.2
medication induced postural G25.1
mercurial *—see* subcategory T56.1
Parkinson's *—see* Parkinsonism
psychogenic (conversion reaction) F44.4
senilis R54
specified type NEC G25.2
Trench
fever A79.Ø
foot *—see* Immersion, foot
mouth A69.1
Treponema pallidum infection *—see* Syphilis
Treponematosis
due to
T. pallidum *—see* Syphilis
T. pertenue *—see* Yaws
Triad
Hutchinson's (congenital syphilis) A5Ø.53
Kartagener's Q89.3
Saint's *—see* Hernia, diaphragm
Trichiasis (eyelid) HØ2.Ø59
with entropion *—see* Entropion
left HØ2.Ø56
lower HØ2.Ø55
upper HØ2.Ø54
right HØ2.Ø53
lower HØ2.Ø52
upper HØ2.Ø51
Trichinella spiralis (infection) (infestation) B75
Trichinellosis, trichiniasis, trichinelliasis, trichinosis B75
with muscle disorder B75 *[M63.8Ø]*
ankle B75 *[M63.87-●]*
foot B75 *[M63.87-●]*
forearm B75 *[M63.83-●]*
hand B75 *[M63.84-●]*
lower leg B75 *[M63.86-●]*
multiple sites B75 *[M63.89]*
pelvic region B75 *[M63.85-●]*
shoulder region B75 *[M63.81-●]*
specified site NEC B75 *[M63.88]*
thigh B75 *[M63.85-●]*
upper arm B75 *[M63.82-●]*
Trichobezoar T18.9
intestine T18.3
stomach T18.2
Trichocephaliasis, trichocephalosis B79
Trichocephalus infestation B79
Trichoclasis L67.8
Trichoepithelioma *—see also* Neoplasm, skin, benign
malignant *—see* Neoplasm, skin, malignant
Trichofolliculoma *—see* Neoplasm, skin, benign
Tricholemmoma *—see* Neoplasm, skin, benign
Trichomoniasis A59.9
bladder A59.Ø3
cervix A59.Ø9
intestinal AØ7.8
prostate A59.Ø2
seminal vesicles A59.Ø9
specified site NEC A59.8
urethra A59.Ø3
urogenitalis A59.ØØ
vagina A59.Ø1
vulva A59.Ø1
Trichomycosis
axillaris A48.8
nodosa, nodularis B36.8
Trichonodosis L67.8
Trichophytid, trichophyton infection *—see* Dermatophytosis
Trichophytobezoar T18.9
intestine T18.3
stomach T18.2
Trichophytosis *—see* Dermatophytosis
Trichoptilosis L67.8
Trichorrhexis (nodosa) (invaginata) L67.Ø
Trichosis axillaris A48.8
Trichosporosis nodosa B36.2
Trichostasis spinulosa (congenital) Q84.1
Trichostrongyliasis, trichostrongylosis (small intestine) B81.2
Trichostrongylus infection B81.2
Trichotillomania F63.3
Trichromat, trichromatopsia, anomalous (congenital) H53.55
Trichuriasis B79
Trichuris trichiura (infection) (infestation) (any site) B79
Tricuspid (valve) *—see* condition
Trifid *—see also* Accessory
kidney (pelvis) Q63.8
tongue Q38.3
Trigeminal neuralgia *—see* Neuralgia, trigeminal
Trigeminy RØØ.8
Trigger finger (acquired) M65.3Ø
congenital Q74.Ø
index finger M65.32-●
little finger M65.35-●
middle finger M65.33-●
ring finger M65.34-●
thumb M65.31-●
Trigonitis (bladder) (chronic) (pseudomembranous) N3Ø.3Ø
with hematuria N3Ø.31
Trigonocephaly Q75.Ø
Trilocular heart *—see* Cor triloculare

Trimethylaminuria E72.52
Tripartite placenta O43.19-●
Triphalangeal thumb Q74.Ø
Triple —*see also* Accessory
  kidneys Q63.Ø
  uteri Q51.818
  X, female Q97.Ø
Triplegia G83.89
  congenital G8Ø.8
Triplet (newborn) —*see also* Newborn, triplet
  complicating pregnancy —*see* Pregnancy, triplet
Triplication —*see* Accessory
Triploidy Q92.7
Trismus R25.2
  neonatorum A33
  newborn A33
Trisomy (syndrome) Q92.9
  13 (partial) Q91.7
    meiotic nondisjunction Q91.4
    mitotic nondisjunction Q91.5
    mosaicism Q91.5
    translocation Q91.6
  18 (partial) Q91.3
    meiotic nondisjunction Q91.Ø
    mitotic nondisjunction Q91.1
    mosaicism Q91.1
    translocation Q91.2
  2Ø Q92.8
  21 (partial) Q9Ø.9
    meiotic nondisjunction Q9Ø.Ø
    mitotic nondisjunction Q9Ø.1
    mosaicism Q9Ø.1
    translocation Q9Ø.2
  22 Q92.8
  autosomes Q92.9
  chromosome specified NEC Q92.8
    partial Q92.2
      due to unbalanced translocation Q92.5
    specified NEC Q92.8
    whole (nonsex chromosome)
      meiotic nondisjunction Q92.Ø
      mitotic nondisjunction Q92.1
      mosaicism Q92.1
  due to
    dicentrics —*see* Extra, marker chromosomes
    extra rings —*see* Extra, marker chromosomes
    isochromosomes —*see* Extra, marker chromosomes
  specified NEC Q92.8
  whole chromosome Q92.9
    meiotic nondisjunction Q92.Ø
    mitotic nondisjunction Q92.1
    mosaicism Q92.1
    partial Q92.9
    specified NEC Q92.8
Tritanomaly, tritanopia H53.55
Trombiculosis, trombiculiasis, trombidiosis B88.Ø
Trophedema (congenital) (hereditary) Q82.Ø
Trophoblastic disease —*see also* Mole, hydatidiform OØ1.9
Tropholymphedema Q82.Ø
Trophoneurosis NEC G96.8
  disseminated M34.9
Tropical —*see* condition
Trouble —*see also* Disease
  heart —*see* Disease, heart
  kidney —*see* Disease, renal
  nervous R45.Ø
  sinus —*see* Sinusitis
Trousseau's syndrome (thrombophlebitis migrans) I82.1
Truancy, childhood
  from school Z72.81Ø
Truncus
  arteriosus (persistent) Q2Ø.Ø
  communis Q2Ø.Ø
Trunk —*see* condition
Trypanosomiasis
  African B56.9
    by Trypanosoma brucei
      gambiense B56.Ø
      rhodesiense B56.1
  American —*see* Chagas' disease
  Brazilian —*see* Chagas' disease
  by Trypanosoma
    brucei gambiense B56.Ø
    brucei rhodesiense B56.1
    cruzi —*see* Chagas' disease
  gambiensis, Gambian B56.Ø
  rhodesiensis, Rhodesian B56.1
  South American —*see* Chagas' disease
  where
    African trypanosomiasis is prevalent B56.9
    Chagas' disease is prevalent B57.2
T-shaped incisors KØØ.2
Tsutsugamushi (disease) (fever) A75.3
Tube, tubal, tubular —*see* condition
Tubercle —*see also* Tuberculosis
  brain, solitary A17.81
  Darwin's Q17.8
  Ghon, primary infection A15.7
Tuberculid, tuberculide (indurating, subcutaneous) (lichenoid) (miliary) (papulonecrotic) (primary) (skin) A18.4
Tuberculoma —*see also* Tuberculosis
  brain A17.81
  meninges (cerebral) (spinal) A17.1
  spinal cord A17.81
Tuberculosis, tubercular, tuberculous (calcification) (calcified) (caseous) (chromogenic acid-fast bacilli) (degeneration) (fibrocaseous) (fistula) (interstitial) (isolated circumscribed lesions) (necrosis) (parenchymatous) (ulcerative) A15.9
  with pneumoconiosis (any condition in J6Ø-J64) J65
  abdomen (lymph gland) A18.39
  abscess (respiratory) A15.9
    bone A18.Ø3
      hip A18.Ø2
      knee A18.Ø2
      sacrum A18.Ø1
      specified site NEC A18.Ø3
      spinal A18.Ø1
      vertebra A18.Ø1
    brain A17.81
    breast A18.89
    Cowper's gland A18.15
    dura (mater) (cerebral) (spinal) A17.81
    epidural (cerebral) (spinal) A17.81
    female pelvis A18.17
    frontal sinus A15.8
    genital organs NEC A18.1Ø
    genitourinary A18.1Ø
    gland (lymphatic) —*see* Tuberculosis, lymph gland
    hip A18.Ø2
    intestine A18.32
    ischiorectal A18.32
    joint NEC A18.Ø2
      hip A18.Ø2
      knee A18.Ø2
      specified NEC A18.Ø2
      vertebral A18.Ø1
    kidney A18.11
    knee A18.Ø2
    ➡ latent Z22.7
    lumbar (spine) A18.Ø1
    lung —*see* Tuberculosis, pulmonary
    meninges (cerebral) (spinal) A17.Ø
    muscle A18.Ø9
    perianal (fistula) A18.32
    perinephritic A18.11
    perirectal A18.32
    rectum A18.32
    retropharyngeal A15.8
    sacrum A18.Ø1
Tuberculosis, tubercular, tuberculous *(Continued)*
  abscess *(Continued)*
    scrofulous A18.2
    scrotum A18.15
    skin (primary) A18.4
    spinal cord A17.81
    spine or vertebra (column) A18.Ø1
    subdiaphragmatic A18.31
    testis A18.15
    urinary A18.13
    uterus A18.17
  accessory sinus —*see* Tuberculosis, sinus
  Addison's disease A18.7
  adenitis —*see* Tuberculosis, lymph gland
  adenoids A15.8
  adenopathy —*see* Tuberculosis, lymph gland
  adherent pericardium A18.84
  adnexa (uteri) A18.17
  adrenal (capsule) (gland) A18.7
  alimentary canal A18.32
  anemia A18.89
  ankle (joint) (bone) A18.Ø2
  anus A18.32
  apex, apical —*see* Tuberculosis, pulmonary
  appendicitis, appendix A18.32
  arachnoid A17.Ø
  artery, arteritis A18.89
    cerebral A18.89
  arthritis (chronic) (synovial) A18.Ø2
    spine or vertebra (column) A18.Ø1
  articular —*see* Tuberculosis, joint
  ascites A18.31
  asthma —*see* Tuberculosis, pulmonary
  axilla, axillary (gland) A18.2
  bladder A18.12
  bone A18.Ø3
    hip A18.Ø2
    knee A18.Ø2
    limb NEC A18.Ø3
    sacrum A18.Ø1
    spine or vertebral column A18.Ø1
  bowel (miliary) A18.32
  brain A17.81
  breast A18.89
  broad ligament A18.17
  bronchi, bronchial, bronchus A15.5
    ectasia, ectasis (bronchiectasis) —*see* Tuberculosis, pulmonary
    fistula A15.5
      primary (progressive) A15.7
    gland or node A15.4
      primary (progressive) A15.7
    lymph gland or node A15.4
      primary (progressive) A15.7
  bronchiectasis —*see* Tuberculosis, pulmonary
  bronchitis A15.5
  bronchopleural A15.6
  bronchopneumonia, bronchopneumonic —*see* Tuberculosis, pulmonary
  bronchorrhagia A15.5
  bronchotracheal A15.5
  bronze disease A18.7
  buccal cavity A18.83
  bulbourethral gland A18.15
  bursa A18.Ø9
  cachexia A15.9
  cardiomyopathy A18.84
  caries —*see* Tuberculosis, bone
  cartilage A18.Ø2
    intervertebral A18.Ø1
  catarrhal —*see* Tuberculosis, respiratory
  cecum A18.32
  cellulitis (primary) A18.4
  cerebellum A17.81
  cerebral, cerebrum A17.81
  cerebrospinal A17.81
    meninges A17.Ø
  cervical (lymph gland or node) A18.2
  cervicitis, cervix (uteri) A18.16
  chest —*see* Tuberculosis, respiratory

Tuberculosis, tubercular, tuberculous *(Continued)*
  chorioretinitis A18.53
  choroid, choroiditis A18.53
  ciliary body A18.54
  colitis A18.32
  collier's J65
  colliquativa (primary) A18.4
  colon A18.32
  complex, primary A15.7
  congenital P37.Ø
  conjunctiva A18.59
  connective tissue (systemic) A18.89
  contact Z2Ø.1
  cornea (ulcer) A18.52
  Cowper's gland A18.15
  coxae A18.Ø2
  coxalgia A18.Ø2
  cul-de-sac of Douglas A18.17
  curvature, spine A18.Ø1
  cutis (colliquativa) (primary) A18.4
  cyst, ovary A18.18
  cystitis A18.12
  dactylitis A18.Ø3
  diarrhea A18.32
  diffuse —*see* Tuberculosis, miliary
  digestive tract A18.32
  disseminated —*see* Tuberculosis, miliary
  duodenum A18.32
  dura (mater) (cerebral) (spinal) A17.Ø
    abscess (cerebral) (spinal) A17.81
  dysentery A18.32
  ear (inner) (middle) A18.6
    bone A18.Ø3
    external (primary) A18.4
    skin (primary) A18.4
  elbow A18.Ø2
  emphysema —*see* Tuberculosis, pulmonary
  empyema A15.6
  encephalitis A17.82
  endarteritis A18.89
  endocarditis A18.84
    aortic A18.84
    mitral A18.84
    pulmonary A18.84
    tricuspid A18.84
  endocrine glands NEC A18.82
  endometrium A18.17
  enteric, enterica, enteritis A18.32
  enterocolitis A18.32
  epididymis, epididymitis A18.15
  epidural abscess (cerebral) (spinal) A17.81
  epiglottis A15.5
  episcleritis A18.51
  erythema (induratum) (nodosum) (primary) A18.4
  esophagus A18.83
  eustachian tube A18.6
  exposure (to) Z2Ø.1
  exudative —*see* Tuberculosis, pulmonary
  eye A18.5Ø
  eyelid (primary) (lupus) A18.4
  fallopian tube (acute) (chronic) A18.17
  fascia A18.Ø9
  fauces A15.8
  female pelvic inflammatory disease A18.17
  finger A18.Ø3
  first infection A15.7
  gallbladder A18.83
  ganglion A18.Ø9
  gastritis A18.83
  gastrocolic fistula A18.32
  gastroenteritis A18.32
  gastrointestinal tract A18.32
  general, generalized —*see* Tuberculosis, miliary
  genital organs A18.1Ø
  genitourinary A18.1Ø
  genu A18.Ø2
  glandula suprarenalis A18.7
  glandular, general A18.2

Tuberculosis, tubercular, tuberculous *(Continued)*
  glottis A15.5
  grinder's J65
  gum A18.83
  hand A18.Ø3
  heart A18.84
  hematogenous —*see* Tuberculosis, miliary
  hemoptysis —*see* Tuberculosis, pulmonary
  hemorrhage NEC —*see* Tuberculosis, pulmonary
  hemothorax A15.6
  hepatitis A18.83
  hilar lymph nodes A15.4
    primary (progressive) A15.7
  hip (joint) (disease) (bone) A18.Ø2
  hydropneumothorax A15.6
  hydrothorax A15.6
  hypoadrenalism A18.7
  hypopharynx A15.8
  ileocecal (hyperplastic) A18.32
  ileocolitis A18.32
  ileum A18.32
  iliac spine (superior) A18.Ø3
  immunological findings only A15.7
  indurativa (primary) A18.4
  infantile A15.7
  infection A15.9
    without clinical manifestations A15.7
  infraclavicular gland A18.2
  inguinal gland A18.2
  inguinalis A18.2
  intestine (any part) A18.32
  iridocyclitis A18.54
  iris, iritis A18.54
  ischiorectal A18.32
  jaw A18.Ø3
  jejunum A18.32
  joint A18.Ø2
    vertebral A18.Ø1
  keratitis (interstitial) A18.52
  keratoconjunctivitis A18.52
  kidney A18.11
  knee (joint) A18.Ø2
  kyphosis, kyphoscoliosis A18.Ø1
  laryngitis A15.5
  larynx A15.5
  latent Z22.7
  leptomeninges, leptomeningitis (cerebral) (spinal) A17.Ø
  lichenoides (primary) A18.4
  linguae A18.83
  lip A18.83
  liver A18.83
  lordosis A18.Ø1
  lung —*see* Tuberculosis, pulmonary
  lupus vulgaris A18.4
  lymph gland or node (peripheral) A18.2
    abdomen A18.39
    bronchial A15.4
      primary (progressive) A15.7
    cervical A18.2
    hilar A15.4
      primary (progressive) A15.7
    intrathoracic A15.4
      primary (progressive) A15.7
    mediastinal A15.4
      primary (progressive) A15.7
    mesenteric A18.39
    retroperitoneal A18.39
    tracheobronchial A15.4
      primary (progressive) A15.7
  lymphadenitis —*see* Tuberculosis, lymph gland
  lymphangitis —*see* Tuberculosis, lymph gland
  lymphatic (gland) (vessel) —*see* Tuberculosis, lymph gland
  mammary gland A18.89
  marasmus A15.9
  mastoiditis A18.Ø3

Tuberculosis, tubercular, tuberculous *(Continued)*
  mediastinal lymph gland or node A15.4
    primary (progressive) A15.7
  mediastinitis A15.8
    primary (progressive) A15.7
  mediastinum A15.8
    primary (progressive) A15.7
  medulla A17.81
  melanosis, Addisonian A18.7
  meninges, meningitis (basilar) (cerebral) (cerebrospinal) (spinal) A17.Ø
  meningoencephalitis A17.82
  mesentery, mesenteric (gland or node) A18.39
  miliary A19.9
    acute A19.2
      multiple sites A19.1
      single specified site A19.Ø
    chronic A19.8
    specified NEC A19.8
  millstone makers' J65
  miner's J65
  molder's J65
  mouth A18.83
  multiple A19.9
    acute A19.1
    chronic A19.8
  muscle A18.Ø9
  myelitis A17.82
  myocardium, myocarditis A18.84
  nasal (passage) (sinus) A15.8
  nasopharynx A15.8
  neck gland A18.2
  nephritis A18.11
  nerve (mononeuropathy) A17.83
  nervous system A17.9
  nose (septum) A15.8
  ocular A18.5Ø
  omentum A18.31
  oophoritis (acute) (chronic) A18.17
  optic (nerve trunk) (papilla) A18.59
  orbit A18.59
  orchitis A18.15
  organ, specified NEC A18.89
  osseous —*see* Tuberculosis, bone
  osteitis —*see* Tuberculosis, bone
  osteomyelitis —*see* Tuberculosis, bone
  otitis media A18.6
  ovary, ovaritis (acute) (chronic) A18.17
  oviduct (acute) (chronic) A18.17
  pachymeningitis A17.Ø
  palate (soft) A18.83
  pancreas A18.83
  papulonecrotic (a) (primary) A18.4
  parathyroid glands A18.82
  paronychia (primary) A18.4
  parotid gland or region A18.83
  pelvis (bony) A18.Ø3
  penis A18.15
  peribronchitis A15.5
  pericardium, pericarditis A18.84
  perichondritis, larynx A15.5
  periostitis —*see* Tuberculosis, bone
  perirectal fistula A18.32
  peritoneum NEC A18.31
  peritonitis A18.31
  pharynx, pharyngitis A15.8
  phlyctenulosis (keratoconjunctivitis) A18.52
  phthisis NEC —*see* Tuberculosis, pulmonary
  pituitary gland A18.82
  pleura, pleural, pleurisy, pleuritis (fibrinous) (obliterative) (purulent) (simple plastic) (with effusion) A15.6
    primary (progressive) A15.7
  pneumonia, pneumonic —*see* Tuberculosis, pulmonary
  pneumothorax (spontaneous) (tense valvular) —*see* Tuberculosis, pulmonary
  polyneuropathy A17.89

Tuberculosis, tubercular, tuberculous (Continued)
polyserositis A19.9
acute A19.1
chronic A19.8
potter's J65
prepuce A18.15
primary (complex) A15.7
proctitis A18.32
prostate, prostatitis A18.14
pulmonalis —*see* Tuberculosis, pulmonary
pulmonary (cavitated) (fibrotic) (infiltrative) (nodular) A15.Ø
childhood type or first infection A15.7
primary (complex) A15.7
pyelitis A18.11
pyelonephritis A18.11
pyemia —*see* Tuberculosis, miliary
pyonephrosis A18.11
pyopneumothorax A15.6
pyothorax A15.6
rectum (fistula) (with abscess) A18.32
reinfection stage —*see* Tuberculosis, pulmonary
renal A18.11
renis A18.11
respiratory A15.9
primary A15.7
specified site NEC A15.8
retina, retinitis A18.53
retroperitoneal (lymph gland or node) A18.39
rheumatism NEC A18.Ø9
rhinitis A15.8
sacroiliac (joint) A18.Ø1
sacrum A18.Ø1
salivary gland A18.83
salpingitis (acute) (chronic) A18.17
sandblaster's J65
sclera A18.51
scoliosis A18.Ø1
scrofulous A18.2
scrotum A18.15
seminal tract or vesicle A18.15
senile A15.9
septic —*see* Tuberculosis, miliary
shoulder (joint) A18.Ø2
blade A18.Ø3
sigmoid A18.32
sinus (any nasal) A15.8
bone A18.Ø3
epididymis A18.15
skeletal NEC A18.Ø3
skin (any site) (primary) A18.4
small intestine A18.32
soft palate A18.83
spermatic cord A18.15
spine, spinal (column) A18.Ø1
cord A17.81
medulla A17.81
membrane A17.Ø
meninges A17.Ø
spleen, splenitis A18.85
spondylitis A18.Ø1
sternoclavicular joint A18.Ø2
stomach A18.83
stonemason's J65
subcutaneous tissue (cellular) (primary) A18.4
subcutis (primary) A18.4
subdeltoid bursa A18.83
submaxillary (region) A18.83
supraclavicular gland A18.2
suprarenal (capsule) (gland) A18.7
swelling, joint —*see also* category MØ1 (*see also* Tuberculosis, joint) A18.Ø2
symphysis pubis A18.Ø2
synovitis A18.Ø9
articular A18.Ø2
spine or vertebra A18.Ø1
systemic —*see* Tuberculosis, miliary

Tuberculosis, tubercular, tuberculous (Continued)
tarsitis A18.4
tendon (sheath) —*see* Tuberculosis, tenosynovitis
tenosynovitis A18.Ø9
spine or vertebra A18.Ø1
testis A18.15
throat A15.8
thymus gland A18.82
thyroid gland A18.81
tongue A18.83
tonsil, tonsillitis A15.8
trachea, tracheal A15.5
lymph gland or node A15.4
primary (progressive) A15.7
tracheobronchial A15.5
lymph gland or node A15.4
primary (progressive) A15.7
tubal (acute) (chronic) A18.17
tunica vaginalis A18.15
ulcer (skin) (primary) A18.4
bowel or intestine A18.32
specified NEC - code under Tuberculosis, by site
unspecified site A15.9
ureter A18.11
urethra, urethral (gland) A18.13
urinary organ or tract A18.13
uterus A18.17
uveal tract A18.54
uvula A18.83
vagina A18.18
vas deferens A18.15
verruca, verrucosa (cutis) (primary) A18.4
vertebra (column) A18.Ø1
vesiculitis A18.15
vulva A18.18
wrist (joint) A18.Ø2
Tuberculum
Carabelli —*see* Note at KØØ.2
occlusal —*see* Note at KØØ.2
paramolare KØØ.2
Tuberosity, enitre maxillary M26.Ø7
Tuberous sclerosis (brain) Q85.1
Tubo-ovarian —*see* condition
Tuboplasty, after previous sterilization Z31.Ø
aftercare Z31.42
Tubotympanitis, catarrhal (chronic) —*see* Otitis, media, nonsuppurative, chronic, serous
Tularemia A21.9
with
conjunctivitis A21.1
pneumonia A21.2
abdominal A21.3
bronchopneumonic A21.2
conjunctivitis A21.1
cryptogenic A21.3
enteric A21.3
gastrointestinal A21.3
generalized A21.7
ingestion A21.3
intestinal A21.3
oculoglandular A21.1
ophthalmic A21.1
pneumonia (any), pneumonic A21.2
pulmonary A21.2
sepsis A21.7
specified NEC A21.8
typhoidal A21.7
ulceroglandular A21.Ø
Tularensis conjunctivitis A21.1
Tumefaction —*see also* Swelling
liver —*see* Hypertrophy, liver
Tumor —*see also* Neoplasm, unspecified behavior, by site
acinar cell —*see* Neoplasm, uncertain behavior, by site
acinic cell —*see* Neoplasm, uncertain behavior, by site

Tumor (Continued)
adenocarcinoid —*see* Neoplasm, malignant, by site
adenomatoid —*see also* Neoplasm, benign, by site
odontogenic —*see* Cyst, calcifying odontogenic
adnexal (skin) —*see* Neoplasm, skin, benign, by site
adrenal
cortical (benign) D35.Ø- •
malignant C74.Ø- •
rest —*see* Neoplasm, benign, by site
alpha-cell
malignant
pancreas C25.4
specified site NEC —*see* Neoplasm, malignant, by site
unspecified site C25.4
pancreas D13.7
specified site NEC —*see* Neoplasm, benign, by site
unspecified site D13.7
aneurysmal —*see* Aneurysm
aortic body D44.7
malignant C75.5
Askin's —*see* Neoplasm, connective tissue, malignant
basal cell —*see also* Neoplasm, skin, uncertain behavior D48.5
Bednar —*see* Neoplasm, skin, malignant
benign (unclassified) —*see* Neoplasm, benign, by site
beta-cell
malignant
pancreas C25.4
specified site NEC —*see* Neoplasm, malignant, by site
unspecified site C25.4
pancreas D13.7
specified site NEC —*see* Neoplasm, benign, by site
unspecified site D13.7
Brenner D27.9
borderline malignancy D39.1- •
malignant C56- •
proliferating D39.1
bronchial alveolar, intravascular D38.1
Brooke's —*see* Neoplasm, skin, benign
brown fat —*see* Lipoma
Burkitt —*see* Lymphoma, Burkitt
calcifying epithelial odontogenic —*see* Cyst, calcifying odontogenic
➡ carcinoid D3A.ØØ
benign D3A.ØØ
appendix D3A.Ø2Ø
ascending colon D3A.Ø22
bronchus (lung) D3A.Ø9Ø
cecum D3A.Ø21
colon D3A.Ø29
descending colon D3A.Ø24
duodenum D3A.Ø1Ø
foregut NOS D3A.Ø94
hindgut NOS D3A.Ø96
ileum D3A.Ø12
jejunum D3A.Ø11
kidney D3A.Ø93
large intestine D3A.Ø29
lung (bronchus) D3A.Ø9Ø
midgut NOS D3A.Ø95
rectum D3A.Ø26
sigmoid colon D3A.Ø25
small intestine D3A.Ø19
specified NEC D3A.Ø98
stomach D3A.Ø92
thymus D3A.Ø91
transverse colon D3A.Ø23
malignant C7A.ØØ
appendix C7A.Ø2Ø
ascending colon C7A.Ø22
bronchus (lung) C7A.Ø9Ø

Tumor (Continued)
carcinoid (Continued)
malignant (Continued)
cecum C7A.Ø21
colon C7A.Ø29
descending colon C7A.Ø24
duodenum C7A.Ø1Ø
foregut NOS C7A.Ø94
hindgut NOS C7A.Ø96
ileum C7A.Ø12
jejunum C7A.Ø11
kidney C7A.Ø93
large intestine C7A.Ø29
lung (bronchus) C7A.Ø9Ø
midgut NOS C7A.Ø95
rectum C7A.Ø26
sigmoid colon C7A.Ø25
small intestine C7A.Ø19
specified NEC C7A.Ø98
stomach C7A.Ø92
thymus C7A.Ø91
transverse colon C7A.Ø23
mesentary metastasis C7B.Ø4
secondary C7B.ØØ
bone C7B.Ø3
distant lymph nodes C7B.Ø1
liver C7B.Ø2
peritoneum C7B.Ø4
specified NEC C7B.Ø9
carotid body D44.6
malignant C75.4
cells —*see also* Neoplasm, unspecified behavior, by site
benign —*see* Neoplasm, benign, by site
malignant —*see* Neoplasm, malignant, by site
uncertain whether benign or malignant —*see* Neoplasm, uncertain behavior, by site
cervix, in pregnancy or childbirth —*see* Pregnancy, complicated by, tumor, cervix
chondromatous giant cell —*see* Neoplasm, bone, benign
chromaffin —*see also* Neoplasm, benign, by site
malignant —*see* Neoplasm, malignant, by site
Cock's peculiar L72.3
Codman's —*see* Neoplasm, bone, benign
dentigerous, mixed —*see* Cyst, calcifying odontogenic
dermoid —*see* Neoplasm, benign, by site
with malignant transformation C56-●
desmoid (extra-abdominal) —*see also* Neoplasm, connective tissue, uncertain behavior
abdominal —*see* Neoplasm, connective tissue, uncertain behavior
embolus —*see* Neoplasm, secondary, by site
embryonal (mixed) —*see also* Neoplasm, uncertain behavior, by site
liver C22.7
endodermal sinus
specified site —*see* Neoplasm, malignant, by site
unspecified site
female C56.-●
male C62.9Ø
epithelial
benign —*see* Neoplasm, benign, by site
malignant —*see* Neoplasm, malignant, by site
Ewing's —*see* Neoplasm, bone, malignant, by site
fatty —*see* Lipoma
fibroid —*see* Leiomyoma

Tumor (Continued)
G cell
malignant
pancreas C25.4
specified site NEC —*see* Neoplasm, malignant, by site
unspecified site C25.4
specified site —*see* Neoplasm, uncertain behavior, by site
unspecified site D37.8
germ cell —*see also* Neoplasm, malignant, by site
mixed —*see* Neoplasm, malignant, by site
ghost cell, odontogenic —*see* Cyst, calcifying odontogenic
giant cell —*see also* Neoplasm, uncertain behavior, by site
bone D48.Ø
malignant —*see* Neoplasm, bone, malignant
chondromatous —*see* Neoplasm, bone, benign
malignant —*see* Neoplasm, malignant, by site
soft parts —*see* Neoplasm, connective tissue, uncertain behavior
malignant —*see* Neoplasm, connective tissue, malignant
glomus D18.ØØ
intra-abdominal D18.Ø3
intracranial D18.Ø2
jugulare D44.7
malignant C75.5
skin D18.Ø1
specified site NEC D18.Ø9
gonadal stromal —*see* Neoplasm, uncertain behavior, by site
granular cell —*see also* Neoplasm, connective tissue, benign
malignant —*see* Neoplasm, connective tissue, malignant
granulosa cell D39.1-●
juvenile D39.1-●
malignant C56-●
granulosa cell-theca cell D39.1-●
malignant C56-●
Grawitz's C64-●
hemorrhoidal —*see* Hemorrhoids
hilar cell D27-●
hilus cell D27-●
Hurthle cell (benign) D34
malignant C73
hydatid —*see* Echinococcus
hypernephroid —*see also* Neoplasm, uncertain behavior, by site
interstitial cell —*see also* Neoplasm, uncertain behavior, by site
benign —*see* Neoplasm, benign, by site
malignant —*see* Neoplasm, malignant, by site
intravascular bronchial alveolar D38.1
islet cell —*see* Neoplasm, benign, by site
malignant —*see* Neoplasm, malignant, by site
pancreas C25.4
specified site NEC —*see* Neoplasm, malignant, by site
unspecified site C25.4
pancreas D13.7
specified site NEC —*see* Neoplasm, benign, by site
unspecified site D13.7
juxtaglomerular D41.Ø-●
Klatskin's C24.Ø
Krukenberg's C79.6-●
Leydig cell —*see* Neoplasm, uncertain behavior, by site
benign —*see* Neoplasm, benign, by site
specified site —*see* Neoplasm, benign, by site

Tumor (Continued)
Leydig cell (Continued)
benign (Continued)
unspecified site
female D27.9
male D29.2Ø
malignant —*see* Neoplasm, malignant, by site
specified site —*see* Neoplasm, malignant, by site
unspecified site
female C56.9
male C62.9Ø
specified site —*see* Neoplasm, uncertain behavior, by site
unspecified site
female D39.1Ø
male D4Ø.1Ø
lipid cell, ovary D27-●
lipoid cell, ovary D27-●
malignant —*see also* Neoplasm, malignant, by site C8Ø.1
fusiform cell (type) C8Ø.1
giant cell (type) C8Ø.1
localized, plasma cell —*see* Plasmacytoma, solitary
mixed NEC C8Ø.1
small cell (type) C8Ø.1
spindle cell (type) C8Ø.1
unclassified C8Ø.1
mast cell D47.Ø9
melanotic, neuroectodermal —*see* Neoplasm, benign, by site
Merkel cell —*see* Carcinoma, Merkel cell
mesenchymal
malignant —*see* Neoplasm, connective tissue, malignant
mixed —*see* Neoplasm, connective tissue, uncertain behavior
mesodermal, mixed —*see also* Neoplasm, malignant, by site
liver C22.4
mesonephric —*see also* Neoplasm, uncertain behavior, by site
malignant —*see* Neoplasm, malignant, by site
metastatic
from specified site —*see* Neoplasm, malignant, by site
of specified site —*see* Neoplasm, malignant, by site
to specified site —*see* Neoplasm, secondary, by site
mixed NEC —*see also* Neoplasm, benign, by site
malignant —*see* Neoplasm, malignant, by site
mucinous of low malignant potential
specified site —*see* Neoplasm, malignant, by site
unspecified site C56.9
mucocarcinoid
specified site —*see* Neoplasm, malignant, by site
unspecified site C18.1
mucoepidermoid —*see* Neoplasm, uncertain behavior, by site
Müllerian, mixed
specified site —*see* Neoplasm, malignant, by site
unspecified site C54.9
myoepithelial —*see* Neoplasm, benign, by site
neuroectodermal (peripheral) —*see* Neoplasm, malignant, by site
primitive
specified site —*see* Neoplasm, malignant, by site
unspecified site C71.9

T

- Tumor *(Continued)*
  - neuroendocrine D3A.8
    - malignant poorly differentiated C7A.1
    - secondary NEC C7B.8
    - specified NEC C7A.8
  - neurogenic olfactory C3Ø.Ø
  - nonencapsulated sclerosing C73
  - odontogenic (adenomatoid) (benign) (calcifying epithelial) (keratocystic) (squamous) —*see* Cyst, calcifying odontogenic
    - malignant C41.1
      - upper jaw (bone) C41.Ø
  - ovarian stromal D39.1- ●
  - ovary, in pregnancy —*see* Pregnancy, complicated by
  - pacinian —*see* Neoplasm, skin, benign
  - Pancoast's —*see* Pancoast's syndrome
  - papillary —*see also* Papilloma
    - cystic D37.9
    - mucinous of low malignant potential C56- ●
      - specified site —*see* Neoplasm, malignant, by site
      - unspecified site C56.9
    - serous of low malignant potential
      - specified site —*see* Neoplasm, malignant, by site
      - unspecified site C56.9
  - pelvic, in pregnancy or childbirth —*see* Pregnancy, complicated by
  - phantom F45.8
  - phyllodes D48.6- ●
    - benign D24- ●
    - malignant —*see* Neoplasm, breast, malignant
  - Pindborg —*see* Cyst, calcifying odontogenic
  - placental site trophoblastic D39.2
  - plasma cell (malignant) (localized) —*see* Plasmacytoma, solitary
  - polyvesicular vitelline
    - specified site —*see* Neoplasm, malignant, by site
    - unspecified site
      - female C56.9
      - male C62.9Ø
  - Pott's puffy —*see* Osteomyelitis, specified NEC
  - Rathke's pouch D44.3
  - retinal anlage —*see* Neoplasm, benign, by site
  - salivary gland type, mixed —*see* Neoplasm, salivary gland, benign
    - malignant —*see* Neoplasm, salivary gland, malignant
  - Sampson's N8Ø.1
  - Schmincke's —*see* Neoplasm, nasopharynx, malignant
  - sclerosing stromal D27- ●
  - sebaceous —*see* Cyst, sebaceous
  - secondary —*see* Neoplasm, secondary, by site
    - carcinoid C7B.ØØ
      - bone C7B.Ø3
      - distant lymph nodes C7B.Ø1
      - liver C7B.Ø2
      - peritoneum C7B.Ø4
      - specified NEC C7B.Ø9
    - neuroendocrine NEC C7B.8
  - serous of low malignant potential
    - specified site —*see* Neoplasm, malignant, by site
    - unspecified site C56.9
  - Sertoli cell —*see* Neoplasm, benign, by site
    - with lipid storage
      - specified site —*see* Neoplasm, benign, by site
      - unspecified site
        - female D27.9
        - male D29.2Ø
    - specified site —*see* Neoplasm, benign, by site
    - unspecified site
      - female D27.9
      - male D29.2Ø
  - Sertoli-Leydig cell —*see* Neoplasm, benign, by site
    - specified site —*see* Neoplasm, benign, by site
    - unspecified site
      - female D27.9
      - male D29.2Ø
  - sex cord(-stromal) —*see* Neoplasm, uncertain behavior, by site
    - with annular tubules D39.1- ●
  - skin appendage —*see* Neoplasm, skin, benign
  - smooth muscle —*see* Neoplasm, connective tissue, uncertain behavior
  - soft tissue
    - benign —*see* Neoplasm, connective tissue, benign
    - malignant —*see* Neoplasm, connective tissue, malignant
  - sternomastoid (congenital) Q68.Ø
  - stromal
    - endometrial D39.Ø
    - gastric D48.1
      - benign D21.4
      - malignant C16.9
      - uncertain behavior D48.1
    - gastrointestinal C49.A- ●
      - benign D21.4
      - esophagus C49.A1
      - large intestine C49.A4
      - malignant C49.AØ
        - colon C49.A4
        - duodenum C49.A3
        - esophagus C49.A1
        - ileum C49.A3
        - jejunum C49.A3
        - Meckel diverticulum C49.A3
        - large intestine C49.A4
        - omentum C49.A9
        - peritoneum C49.A9
        - rectum C49.A5
        - small intestine C49.A3
        - specified site NEC C49.A9
        - stomach C49.A2
      - rectum C49.A5
      - small intestine C49.A3
      - specified site NEC C49.A9
      - stomach C49.A2
      - uncertain behavior D48.1
    - intestine
      - benign D21.4
      - malignant
        - large C49.A4
        - small C49.A3
      - uncertain behavior D48.1
    - ovarian D39.1- ●
    - stomach C49.A2
      - benign D21.4
      - malignant C49.A2
      - uncertain behavior D48.1
  - sweat gland —*see also* Neoplasm, skin, uncertain behavior
    - benign —*see* Neoplasm, skin, benign
    - malignant —*see* Neoplasm, skin, malignant
  - syphilitic, brain A52.17
  - testicular D4Ø.1Ø
  - testicular stromal D4Ø.1- ●
  - theca cell D27.- ●
  - theca cell-granulosa cell D39.1- ●
  - Triton, malignant —*see* Neoplasm, nerve, malignant
  - trophoblastic, placental site D39.2
  - turban D23.4
  - uterus (body), in pregnancy or childbirth —*see* Pregnancy, complicated by, tumor, uterus
  - vagina, in pregnancy or childbirth —*see* Pregnancy, complicated by
  - varicose —*see* Varix
  - von Recklinghausen's —*see* Neurofibromatosis
  - vulva or perineum, in pregnancy or childbirth —*see* Pregnancy, complicated by
    - causing obstructed labor O65.5
  - Warthin's —*see* Neoplasm, salivary gland, benign
  - Wilms' C64- ●
  - yolk sac —*see* Neoplasm, malignant, by site
    - specified site —*see* Neoplasm, malignant, by site
    - unspecified site
      - female C56.9
      - male C62.9Ø
- Tumor lysis syndrome (following antineoplastic chemotherapy) (spontaneous) NEC E88.3
- Tumorlet —*see* Neoplasm, uncertain behavior, by site
- Tungiasis B88.1
- Tunica vasculosa lentis Q12.2
- Turban tumor D23.4
- Türck's trachoma J37.Ø
- Turner-Kieser syndrome Q87.2
- ➠ Turner-like syndrome Q87.19
- Turner's
  - hypoplasia (tooth) KØØ.4
  - syndrome Q96.9
    - specified NEC Q96.8
  - tooth KØØ.4
- Turner-Ullrich syndrome Q96.9
- Tussis convulsiva —*see* Whooping cough
- Twiddler's syndrome (due to)
  - automatic implantable defibrillator T82.198
  - cardiac pacemaker T82.198
- Twilight state
  - epileptic FØ5
  - psychogenic F44.89
- Twin (newborn) —*see also* Newborn, twin
  - conjoined Q89.4
  - pregnancy —*see* Pregnancy, twin
- Twinning, teeth KØØ.2
- Twist, twisted
  - bowel, colon or intestine K56.2
  - hair (congenital) Q84.1
  - mesentery K56.2
  - omentum K56.2
  - organ or site, congenital NEC —*see* Anomaly, by site
  - ovarian pedicle —*see* Torsion, ovary
- Twitching R25.3
- Tylosis (acquired) L84
  - buccalis K13.29
  - linguae K13.29
  - palmaris et plantaris (congenital) (inherited) Q82.8
    - acquired L85.1
- Tympanism R14.Ø
- Tympanites (abdominal) (intestinal) R14.Ø
- Tympanitis —*see* Myringitis
- Tympanosclerosis —*see* subcategory H74.Ø
- Tympanum —*see* condition
- Tympany
  - abdomen R14.Ø
  - chest RØ9.89
- Type A behavior pattern Z73.1
- Typhlitis —*see* Appendicitis
- Typhoenteritis —*see* Typhoid
- Typhoid (abortive) (ambulant) (any site) (clinical) (fever) (hemorrhagic) (infection) (intermittent) (malignant) (rheumatic) (Widal negative) AØ1.ØØ
  - with pneumonia AØ1.Ø3
  - abdominal AØ1.Ø9
  - arthritis AØ1.Ø4
  - carrier (suspected) of Z22.Ø
  - cholecystitis (current) AØ1.Ø9
  - endocarditis AØ1.Ø2
  - heart involvement AØ1.Ø2

T

Typhoid *(Continued)*
inoculation reaction —*see* Complications, vaccination
meningitis A01.01
mesenteric lymph nodes A01.09
myocarditis A01.02
osteomyelitis A01.05
perichondritis, larynx A01.09
pneumonia A01.03
specified NEC A01.09
spine A01.05
ulcer (perforating) A01.09
Typhomalaria (fever) —*see* Malaria
Typhomania A01.00
Typhoperitonitis A01.09
Typhus (fever) A75.9
abdominal, abdominalis —*see* Typhoid
African tick A77.1
amarillic A95.9
brain A75.9 *[G94]*

Typhus *(Continued)*
cerebral A75.9 *[G94]*
classical A75.0
due to Rickettsia
prowazekii A75.0
recrudescent A75.1
tsutsugamushi A75.3
typhi A75.2
endemic (flea-borne) A75.2
epidemic (louse-borne) A75.0
exanthematic NEC A75.0
exanthematicus SAI A75.0
brillii SAI A75.1
mexicanus SAI A75.2
typhus murinus A75.2
flea-borne A75.2
India tick A77.1
Kenya (tick) A77.1
louse-borne A75.0
Mexican A75.2

Typhus *(Continued)*
mite-borne A75.3
murine A75.2
North Asian tick-borne A77.2
petechial A75.9
Queensland tick A77.3
rat A75.2
recrudescent A75.1
recurrens —*see* Fever, relapsing
Sao Paulo A77.0
scrub (China) (India) (Malaysia) (New Guinea) A75.3
shop (of Malaysia) A75.2
Siberian tick A77.2
tick-borne A77.9
tropical (mite-borne) A75.3
Tyrosinemia E70.21
newborn, transitory P74.5
Tyrosinosis E70.21
Tyrosinuria E70.29

U

- Uhl's anomaly or disease Q24.8
- Ulcer, ulcerated, ulcerating, ulceration, ulcerative
  - alveolar process M27.3
  - amebic (intestine) AØ6.1
    - skin AØ6.7
  - anastomotic —*see* Ulcer, gastrojejunal
  - anorectal K62.6
  - antral —*see* Ulcer, stomach
  - anus (sphincter) (solitary) K62.6
  - aorta —*see* Aneurysm
  - aphthous (oral) (recurrent) K12.Ø
    - genital organ(s)
      - female N76.6
      - male N5Ø.89
  - artery I77.2
  - atrophic —*see* Ulcer, skin
    - decubitus —*see* Ulcer, pressure, by site
  - back L98.429
    - with
      - bone involvement without evidence of necrosis L98.426
      - bone necrosis L98.424
      - exposed fat layer L98.422
      - muscle involvement without evidence of necrosis L98.425
      - muscle necrosis L98.423
      - skin breakdown only L98.421
      - specified severity NEC L98.428
  - Barrett's (esophagus) K22.1Ø
    - with bleeding K22.11
  - bile duct (common) (hepatic) K83.8
  - bladder (solitary) (sphincter) NEC N32.89
    - bilharzial B65.9 *[N33]*
    - in schistosomiasis (bilharzial) B65.9 *[N33]*
    - submucosal —*see* Cystitis, interstitial
    - tuberculous A18.12
  - bleeding K27.4
  - bone —*see* Osteomyelitis, specified type NEC
  - bowel —*see* Ulcer, intestine
  - breast N61.1
  - bronchus J98.Ø9
  - buccal (cavity) (traumatic) K12.1
  - Buruli A31.1
  - buttock L98.419
    - with
      - bone involvement without evidence of necrosis L98.416
      - bone necrosis L98.414
      - exposed fat layer L98.412
      - muscle involvement without evidence of necrosis L98.415
      - muscle necrosis L98.413
      - skin breakdown only L98.411
      - specified severity NEC L98.418
  - cancerous —*see* Neoplasm, malignant, by site
  - cardia K22.1Ø
    - with bleeding K22.11
  - cardioesophageal (peptic) K22.1Ø
    - with bleeding K22.11
  - cecum —*see* Ulcer, intestine
  - cervix (uteri) (decubitus) (trophic) N86
    - with cervicitis N72
  - chancroidal A57
  - chiclero B55.1
  - chronic (cause unknown) —*see* Ulcer, skin
  - Cochin-China B55.1
  - colon —*see* Ulcer, intestine
  - conjunctiva H1Ø.89
  - cornea H16.ØØ-●
    - with hypopyon H16.Ø3-●
    - central H16.Ø1-●
    - dendritic (herpes simplex) BØØ.52
    - marginal H16.Ø4-●
    - Mooren's H16.Ø5-●
    - mycotic H16.Ø6-●
    - perforated H16.Ø7-●
    - ring H16.Ø2-●
    - tuberculous (phlyctenular) A18.52

Ulcer, ulcerated, ulcerating, ulceration, ulcerative *(Continued)*

  - corpus cavernosum (chronic) N48.5
  - crural —*see* Ulcer, lower limb
  - Curling's —*see* Ulcer, peptic, acute
  - Cushing's —*see* Ulcer, peptic, acute
  - cystic duct K82.8
  - cystitis (interstitial) —*see* Cystitis, interstitial
  - decubitus —*see* Ulcer, pressure, by site
  - dendritic, cornea (herpes simplex) BØØ.52
  - diabetes, diabetic —*see* Diabetes, ulcer
  - Dieulafoy's K25.Ø
  - due to
    - infection NEC —*see* Ulcer, skin
    - radiation NEC L59.8
    - trophic disturbance (any region) —*see* Ulcer, skin
    - X-ray L58.1
  - duodenum, duodenal (eroded) (peptic) K26.9
    - with
      - hemorrhage K26.4
        - and perforation K26.6
      - perforation K26.5
    - acute K26.3
      - with
        - hemorrhage K26.Ø
          - and perforation K26.2
        - perforation K26.1
    - chronic K26.7
      - with
        - hemorrhage K26.4
          - and perforation K26.6
        - perforation K26.5
  - dysenteric AØ9
  - elusive —*see* Cystitis, interstitial
  - endocarditis (acute) (chronic) (subacute) I28.8
  - epiglottis J38.7
  - esophagus (peptic) K22.1Ø
    - with bleeding K22.11
    - due to
      - aspirin K22.1Ø
        - with bleeding K22.11
      - gastrointestinal reflux disease K21.Ø
      - ingestion of chemical or medicament K22.1Ø
        - with bleeding K22.11
    - fungal K22.1Ø
      - with bleeding K22.11
    - infective K22.1Ø
      - with bleeding K22.11
    - varicose —*see* Varix, esophagus
  - eyelid (region) HØ1.8
  - fauces J39.2
  - Fenwick (-Hunner) (solitary) —*see* Cystitis, interstitial
  - fistulous —*see* Ulcer, skin
  - foot (indolent) (trophic) —*see* Ulcer, lower limb
  - frambesial, initial A66.Ø
  - frenum (tongue) K14.Ø
  - gallbladder or duct K82.8
  - gangrenous —*see* Gangrene
  - gastric —*see* Ulcer, stomach
  - gastrocolic —*see* Ulcer, gastrojejunal
  - gastroduodenal —*see* Ulcer, peptic
  - gastroesophageal —*see* Ulcer, stomach
  - gastrointestinal —*see* Ulcer, gastrojejunal
  - gastrojejunal (peptic) K28.9
    - with
      - hemorrhage K28.4
        - and perforation K28.6
      - perforation K28.5
    - acute K28.3
      - with
        - hemorrhage K28.Ø
          - and perforation K28.2
        - perforation K28.1
    - chronic K28.7
      - with
        - hemorrhage K28.4
          - and perforation K28.6
        - perforation K28.5

Ulcer, ulcerated, ulcerating, ulceration, ulcerative *(Continued)*

  - gastrojejunocolic —*see* Ulcer, gastrojejunal
  - gingiva KØ6.8
  - gingivitis KØ5.1Ø
    - nonplaque induced KØ5.11
    - plaque induced KØ5.1Ø
  - glottis J38.7
  - granuloma of pudenda A58
  - gum KØ6.8
  - gumma, due to yaws A66.4
  - heel —*see* Ulcer, lower limb
  - hemorrhoid —*see also* Hemorrhoids, by degree K64.8
  - Hunner's —*see* Cystitis, interstitial
  - hypopharynx J39.2
  - hypopyon (chronic) (subacute) —*see* Ulcer, cornea, with hypopyon
  - hypostaticum —*see* Ulcer, varicose
  - ileum —*see* Ulcer, intestine
  - intestine, intestinal K63.3
    - with perforation K63.1
    - amebic AØ6.1
    - duodenal —*see* Ulcer, duodenum
    - granulocytopenic (with hemorrhage) —*see* Neutropenia
    - marginal —*see* Ulcer, gastrojejunal
    - perforating K63.1
      - newborn P78.Ø
    - primary, small intestine K63.3
    - rectum K62.6
    - stercoraceous, stercoral K63.3
    - tuberculous A18.32
    - typhoid (fever) —*see* Typhoid
    - varicose I86.8
  - jejunum, jejunal —*see* Ulcer, gastrojejunal
  - keratitis —*see* Ulcer, cornea
  - knee —*see* Ulcer, lower limb
  - labium (majus) (minus) N76.6
  - laryngitis —*see* Laryngitis
  - larynx (aphthous) (contact) J38.7
    - diphtheritic A36.2
  - leg —*see* Ulcer, lower limb
  - lip K13.Ø
  - Lipschütz's N76.6
  - lower limb (atrophic) (chronic) (neurogenic) (perforating) (pyogenic) (trophic) (tropical) L97.9Ø9
    - with
      - bone involvement without evidence of necrosis L97.9Ø6
      - bone necrosis L97.9Ø4
      - exposed fat layer L97.9Ø2
      - muscle involvement without evidence of necrosis L97.9Ø5
      - muscle necrosis L97.9Ø3
      - skin breakdown only L97.9Ø1
      - specified severity NEC L97.9Ø8
    - ankle L97.3Ø9
      - with
        - bone involvement without evidence of necrosis L97.3Ø6
        - bone necrosis L97.3Ø4
        - exposed fat layer L97.3Ø2
        - muscle involvement without evidence of necrosis L97.3Ø5
        - muscle necrosis L97.3Ø3
        - skin breakdown only L97.3Ø1
        - specified severity NEC L97.3Ø8
      - left L97.329
        - with
          - bone involvement without evidence of necrosis L97.326
          - bone necrosis L97.324
          - exposed fat layer L97.322
          - muscle involvement without evidence of necrosis L97.325
          - muscle necrosis L97.323
          - skin breakdown only L97.321
          - specified severity NEC L97.328

U

- Ulcer, ulcerated, ulcerating, ulceration, ulcerative *(Continued)*
  - lower limb *(Continued)*
    - ankle *(Continued)*
      - right L97.319
        - with
          - bone involvement without evidence of necrosis L97.316
          - bone necrosis L97.314
          - exposed fat layer L97.312
          - muscle involvement without evidence of necrosis L97.315
          - muscle necrosis L97.313
          - skin breakdown only L97.311
          - specified severity NEC L97.318
    - calf L97.209
      - with
        - bone involvement without evidence of necrosis L97.206
        - bone necrosis L97.204
        - exposed fat layer L97.202
        - muscle involvement without evidence of necrosis L97.205
        - muscle necrosis L97.203
        - skin breakdown only L97.201
        - specified severity NEC L97.208
      - left L97.229
        - with
          - bone involvement without evidence of necrosis L97.226
          - bone necrosis L97.224
          - exposed fat layer L97.222
          - muscle involvement without evidence of necrosis L97.225
          - muscle necrosis L97.223
          - skin breakdown only L97.221
          - specified severity NEC L97.228
      - right L97.219
        - with
          - bone involvement without evidence of necrosis L97.216
          - bone necrosis L97.214
          - exposed fat layer L97.212
          - muscle involvement without evidence of necrosis L97.215
          - muscle necrosis L97.213
          - skin breakdown only L97.211
          - specified severity NEC L97.218
    - decubitus —*see* Ulcer, pressure, by site
    - foot specified NEC L97.509
      - with
        - bone involvement without evidence of necrosis L97.506
        - bone necrosis L97.504
        - exposed fat layer L97.502
        - muscle involvement without evidence of necrosis L97.505
        - muscle necrosis L97.503
        - skin breakdown only L97.501
        - specified severity NEC L97.508
      - left L97.529
        - with
          - bone involvement without evidence of necrosis L97.526
          - bone necrosis L97.524
          - exposed fat layer L97.522
          - muscle involvement without evidence of necrosis L97.525
          - muscle necrosis L97.523
          - skin breakdown only L97.521
          - specified severity NEC L97.528
      - right L97.519
        - with
          - bone involvement without evidence of necrosis L97.516
          - bone necrosis L97.514
          - exposed fat layer L97.512
          - muscle involvement without evidence of necrosis L97.515
          - muscle necrosis L97.513
          - skin breakdown only L97.511
          - specified severity NEC L97.518

- Ulcer, ulcerated, ulcerating, ulceration, ulcerative *(Continued)*
  - lower limb *(Continued)*
    - heel L97.409
      - with
        - bone involvement without evidence of necrosis L97.406
        - bone necrosis L97.404
        - exposed fat layer L97.402
        - muscle involvement without evidence of necrosis L97.405
        - muscle necrosis L97.403
        - skin breakdown only L97.401
        - specified severity NEC L97.408
      - left L97.429
        - with
          - bone involvement without evidence of necrosis L97.426
          - bone necrosis L97.424
          - exposed fat layer L97.422
          - muscle involvement without evidence of necrosis L97.425
          - muscle necrosis L97.423
          - skin breakdown only L97.421
          - specified severity NEC L97.428
      - right L97.419
        - with
          - bone involvement without evidence of necrosis L97.416
          - bone necrosis L97.414
          - exposed fat layer L97.412
          - muscle involvement without evidence of necrosis L97.415
          - muscle necrosis L97.413
          - skin breakdown only L97.411
          - specified severity NEC L97.418
    - left L97.929
      - with
        - bone involvement without evidence of necrosis L97.926
        - bone necrosis L97.924
        - exposed fat layer L97.922
        - muscle involvement without evidence of necrosis L97.925
        - muscle necrosis L97.923
        - skin breakdown only L97.921
        - specified severity NEC L97.928
    - lower leg NOS L97.909
      - with
        - bone involvement without evidence of necrosis L97.906
        - bone necrosis L97.904
        - exposed fat layer L97.902
        - muscle involvement without evidence of necrosis L97.905
        - muscle necrosis L97.903
        - skin breakdown only L97.901
        - specified severity NEC L97.908
      - left L97.929
        - with
          - bone involvement without evidence of necrosis L97.926
          - bone necrosis L97.924
          - exposed fat layer L97.922
          - muscle involvement without evidence of necrosis L97.925
          - muscle necrosis L97.923
          - skin breakdown only L97.921
          - specified severity NEC L97.928
      - right L97.919
        - with
          - bone involvement without evidence of necrosis L97.916
          - bone necrosis L97.914
          - exposed fat layer L97.912
          - muscle involvement without evidence of necrosis L97.915
          - muscle necrosis L97.913
          - skin breakdown only L97.911
          - specified severity NEC L97.918
      - specified site NEC L97.809

- Ulcer, ulcerated, ulcerating, ulceration, ulcerative *(Continued)*
  - lower limb *(Continued)*
    - lower leg NOS *(Continued)*
      - specified site NEC *(Continued)*
        - with
          - bone involvement without evidence of necrosis L97.806
          - bone necrosis L97.804
          - exposed fat layer L97.802
          - muscle involvement without evidence of necrosis L97.805
          - muscle necrosis L97.803
          - skin breakdown only L97.801
          - specified severity NEC L97.808
        - left L97.829
          - with
            - bone involvement without evidence of necrosis L97.826
            - bone necrosis L97.824
            - exposed fat layer L97.822
            - muscle involvement without evidence of necrosis L97.825
            - muscle necrosis L97.823
            - skin breakdown only L97.821
            - specified severity NEC L97.828
        - right L97.819
          - with
            - bone involvement without evidence of necrosis L97.816
            - bone necrosis L97.814
            - exposed fat layer L97.812
            - muscle involvement without evidence of necrosis L97.815
            - muscle necrosis L97.813
            - skin breakdown only L97.811
            - specified severity NEC L97.818
    - midfoot L97.409
      - with
        - bone involvement without evidence of necrosis L97.406
        - bone necrosis L97.404
        - exposed fat layer L97.402
        - muscle involvement without evidence of necrosis L97.405
        - muscle necrosis L97.403
        - skin breakdown only L97.401
        - specified severity NEC L97.408
      - left L97.429
        - with
          - bone involvement without evidence of necrosis L97.426
          - bone necrosis L97.424
          - exposed fat layer L97.422
          - muscle involvement without evidence of necrosis L97.425
          - muscle necrosis L97.423
          - skin breakdown only L97.421
          - specified severity NEC L97.428
      - right L97.419
        - with
          - bone involvement without evidence of necrosis L97.416
          - bone necrosis L97.414
          - exposed fat layer L97.412
          - muscle involvement without evidence of necrosis L97.415
          - muscle necrosis L97.413
          - skin breakdown only L97.411
          - specified severity NEC L97.418
    - right L97.919
      - with
        - bone involvement without evidence of necrosis L97.916
        - bone necrosis L97.914
        - exposed fat layer L97.912
        - muscle involvement without evidence of necrosis L97.915
        - muscle necrosis L97.913
        - skin breakdown only L97.911
        - specified severity NEC L97.918

Ulcer, ulcerated, ulcerating, ulceration, ulcerative *(Continued)*
lower limb *(Continued)*
thigh L97.109
with
bone involvement without evidence of necrosis L97.106
bone necrosis L97.104
exposed fat layer L97.102
muscle involvement without evidence of necrosis L97.105
muscle necrosis L97.103
skin breakdown only L97.101
specified severity NEC L97.108
left L97.129
with
bone involvement without evidence of necrosis L97.126
bone necrosis L97.124
exposed fat layer L97.122
muscle involvement without evidence of necrosis L97.125
muscle necrosis L97.123
skin breakdown only L97.121
specified severity NEC L97.128
right L97.119
with
bone involvement without evidence of necrosis L97.116
bone necrosis L97.114
exposed fat layer L97.112
muscle involvement without evidence of necrosis L97.115
muscle necrosis L97.113
skin breakdown only L97.111
specified severity NEC L97.118
toe L97.509
with
bone involvement without evidence of necrosis L97.506
bone necrosis L97.504
exposed fat layer L97.502
muscle involvement without evidence of necrosis L97.505
muscle necrosis L97.503
skin breakdown only L97.501
specified severity NEC L97.508
left L97.529
with
bone involvement without evidence of necrosis L97.526
bone necrosis L97.524
exposed fat layer L97.522
muscle involvement without evidence of necrosis L97.525
muscle necrosis L97.523
skin breakdown only L97.521
specified severity NEC L97.528
right L97.519
with
bone involvement without evidence of necrosis L97.516
bone necrosis L97.514
exposed fat layer L97.512
muscle involvement without evidence of necrosis L97.515
muscle necrosis L97.513
skin breakdown only L97.511
specified severity NEC L97.518
leprous A30.1
syphilitic A52.19
varicose *—see* Varix, leg, with, ulcer
luetic *—see* Ulcer, syphilitic
lung J98.4
tuberculous *—see* Tuberculosis, pulmonary
malignant *—see* Neoplasm, malignant, by site
marginal NEC *—see* Ulcer, gastrojejunal
meatus (urinarius) N34.2
Meckel's diverticulum Q43.0
malignant *—see* Table of Neoplasms, small intestine, malignant

Ulcer, ulcerated, ulcerating, ulceration, ulcerative *(Continued)*
Meleney's (chronic undermining) *—see* Ulcer, skin
Mooren's (cornea) *—see* Ulcer, cornea, Mooren's
mycobacterial (skin) A31.1
nasopharynx J39.2
neck, uterus N86
neurogenic NEC *—see* Ulcer, skin
nose, nasal (passage) (infective) (septum) J34.0
skin *—see* Ulcer, skin
spirochetal A69.8
varicose (bleeding) I86.8
oral mucosa (traumatic) K12.1
palate (soft) K12.1
penis (chronic) N48.5
peptic (site unspecified) K27.9
with
hemorrhage K27.4
and perforation K27.6
perforation K27.5
acute K27.3
with
hemorrhage K27.0
and perforation K27.2
perforation K27.1
chronic K27.7
with
hemorrhage K27.4
and perforation K27.6
perforation K27.5
esophagus K22.10
with bleeding K22.11
newborn P78.82
perforating K27.5
skin *—see* Ulcer, skin
peritonsillar J35.8
phagedenic (tropical) *—see* Ulcer, skin
pharynx J39.2
phlebitis *—see* Phlebitis
plaster *—see* Ulcer, pressure, by site
popliteal space *—see* Ulcer, lower limb
postpyloric *—see* Ulcer, duodenum
prepuce N47.7
prepyloric *—see* Ulcer, stomach
pressure (pressure area) L89.9- •
ankle L89.5- •
back L89.1- •
buttock L89.3- •
coccyx L89.15- •
contiguous site of back, buttock, hip L89.4- •
elbow L89.0- •
face L89.81- •
head L89.81- •
heel L89.6- •
hip L89.2- •
sacral region (tailbone) L89.15- •
specified site NEC L89.89- •
stage 1 (healing) (pre-ulcer skin changes limited to persistent focal edema)
ankle L89.5- •
back L89.1- •
buttock L89.3- •
coccyx L89.15- •
contiguous site of back, buttock, hip L89.4- •
elbow L89.0- •
face L89.81- •
head L89.81- •
heel L89.6- •
hip L89.2- •
sacral region (tailbone) L89.15- •
specified site NEC L89.89- •
stage 2 (healing) (abrasion, blister, partial thickness skin loss involving epidermis and/or dermis)
ankle L89.5- •
back L89.1- •
buttock L89.3- •

Ulcer, ulcerated, ulcerating, ulceration, ulcerative *(Continued)*
pressure *(Continued)*
stage 2 *(Continued)*
coccyx L89.15- •
contiguous site of back, buttock, hip L89.4- •
elbow L89.0- •
face L89.81- •
head L89.81- •
heel L89.6- •
hip L89.2- •
sacral region (tailbone) L89.15- •
specified site NEC L89.89- •
stage 3 (healing) (full thickness skin loss involving damage or necrosis of subcutaneous tissue)
ankle L89.5- •
back L89.1- •
buttock L89.3- •
coccyx L89.15- •
contiguous site of back, buttock, hip L89.4- •
elbow L89.0- •
face L89.81- •
head L89.81- •
heel L89.6- •
hip L89.2- •
sacral region (tailbone) L89.15- •
specified site NEC L89.89- •
stage 4 (healing) (necrosis of soft tissues through to underlying muscle, tendon, or bone)
ankle L89.5- •
back L89.1- •
buttock L89.3- •
coccyx L89.15- •
contiguous site of back, buttock, hip L89.4- •
elbow L89.0- •
face L89.81- •
head L89.81- •
heel L89.6- •
hip L89.2- •
sacral region (tailbone) L89.15- •
specified site NEC L89.89- •
unspecified stage
ankle L89.5- •
back L89.1- •
buttock L89.3- •
coccyx L89.15- •
contiguous site of back, buttock, hip L89.4- •
elbow L89.0- •
face L89.81- •
head L89.81- •
heel L89.6- •
hip L89.2- •
sacral region (tailbone) L89.15- •
specified site NEC L89.89- •
unstageable
ankle L89.5- •
back L89.1- •
buttock L89.3- •
coccyx L89.15- •
contiguous site of back, buttock, hip L89.4- •
elbow L89.0- •
face L89.81- •
head L89.81- •
heel L89.6- •
hip L89.2- •
sacral region (tailbone) L89.15- •
specified site NEC L89.89- •
primary of intestine K63.3
with perforation K63.1
prostate N41.9
pyloric *—see* Ulcer, stomach
rectosigmoid K63.3
with perforation K63.1
rectum (sphincter) (solitary) K62.6
stercoraceous, stercoral K62.6

Ulcer, ulcerated, ulcerating, ulceration, ulcerative *(Continued)*
retina *—see* Inflammation, chorioretinal
rodent *—see also* Neoplasm, skin, malignant
sclera *—see* Scleritis
scrofulous (tuberculous) A18.2
scrotum N5Ø.89
tuberculous A18.15
varicose I86.1
seminal vesicle N5Ø.89
sigmoid *—see* Ulcer, intestine
skin (atrophic) (chronic) (neurogenic) (non-healing) (perforating) (pyogenic) (trophic) (tropical) L98.499
with gangrene *—see* Gangrene
amebic AØ6.7
back *—see* Ulcer, back
buttock *—see* Ulcer, buttock
decubitus *—see* Ulcer, pressure
lower limb *—see* Ulcer, lower limb
mycobacterial A31.1
specified site NEC L98.499
with
bone involvement without evidence of necrosis L98.496
bone necrosis L98.494
exposed fat layer L98.492
muscle involvement without evidence of necrosis L98.495
muscle necrosis L98.493
skin breakdown only L98.491
specified severity NEC L98.498
tuberculous (primary) A18.4
varicose *—see* Ulcer, varicose
sloughing *—see* Ulcer, skin
solitary, anus or rectum (sphincter) K62.6
sore throat JØ2.9
streptococcal JØ2.Ø
spermatic cord N5Ø.89
spine (tuberculous) A18.Ø1
stasis (venous) *—see* Varix, leg, with, ulcer
without varicose veins I87.2
stercoraceous, stercoral K63.3
with perforation K63.1
anus or rectum K62.6
stoma, stomal *—see* Ulcer, gastrojejunal
stomach (eroded) (peptic) (round) K25.9
with
hemorrhage K25.4
and perforation K25.6
perforation K25.5
acute K25.3
with
hemorrhage K25.Ø
and perforation K25.2
perforation K25.1
chronic K25.7
with
hemorrhage K25.4
and perforation K25.6
perforation K25.5
stomal *—see* Ulcer, gastrojejunal
stomatitis K12.1
stress *—see* Ulcer, peptic
strumous (tuberculous) A18.2
submucosal, bladder *—see* Cystitis, interstitial
syphilitic (any site) (early) (secondary) A51.39
late A52.79
perforating A52.79
foot A52.11
testis N5Ø.89
thigh *—see* Ulcer, lower limb
throat J39.2
diphtheritic A36.Ø
toe *—see* Ulcer, lower limb
tongue (traumatic) K14.Ø
tonsil J35.8
diphtheritic A36.Ø
trachea J39.8
trophic *—see* Ulcer, skin

Ulcer, ulcerated, ulcerating, ulceration, ulcerative *(Continued)*
tropical *—see* Ulcer, skin
tuberculous *—see* Tuberculosis, ulcer
tunica vaginalis N5Ø.89
turbinate J34.89
typhoid (perforating) *—see* Typhoid
unspecified site *—see* Ulcer, skin
urethra (meatus) *—see* Urethritis
uterus N85.8
cervix N86
with cervicitis N72
neck N86
with cervicitis N72
vagina N76.5
in Behçet's disease M35.2 *[N77.Ø]*
pessary N89.8
valve, heart I33.Ø
varicose (lower limb, any part) *—see also* Varix, leg, with, ulcer
broad ligament I86.2
esophagus *—see* Varix, esophagus
inflamed or infected *—see* Varix, leg, with ulcer, with inflammation
nasal septum I86.8
perineum I86.3
scrotum I86.1
specified site NEC I86.8
sublingual I86.Ø
vulva I86.3
vas deferens N5Ø.89
vulva (acute) (infectional) N76.6
in (due to)
Behçet's disease M35.2 *[N77.Ø]*
herpesviral (herpes simplex) infection A6Ø.Ø4
tuberculosis A18.18
vulvobuccal, recurring N76.6
X-ray L58.1
yaws A66.4
Ulcerosa scarlatina A38.8
Ulcus *—see also* Ulcer
cutis tuberculosum A18.4
duodeni *—see* Ulcer, duodenum
durum (syphilitic) A51.Ø
extragenital A51.2
gastrojejunale *—see* Ulcer, gastrojejunal
hypostaticum *—see* Ulcer, varicose
molle (cutis) (skin) A57
serpens corneae *—see* Ulcer, cornea, central
ventriculi *—see* Ulcer, stomach
Ulegyria QØ4.8
Ulerythema
ophryogenes, congenital Q84.2
sycosiforme L73.8
Ullrich(-Bonnevie)(-Turner) syndrome *—see also* Turner's syndrome Q87.19
Ullrich-Feichtiger syndrome Q87.Ø
Ulnar *—see* condition
Ulorrhagia, ulorrhea KØ6.8
Umbilicus, umbilical *—see* condition
Unacceptable
contours of tooth KØ8.54
morphology of tooth KØ8.54
Unavailability (of)
bed at medical facility Z75.1
health service-related agencies Z75.4
medical facilities (at) Z75.3
due to
investigation by social service agency Z75.2
lack of services at home Z75.Ø
remoteness from facility Z75.3
waiting list Z75.1
home Z75.Ø
outpatient clinic Z75.3
schooling Z55.1
social service agencies Z75.4
Uncinaria americana infestation B76.1
Uncinariasis B76.9
Uncongenial work Z56.5

Unconscious (ness) *—see* Coma
Underachievement in school Z55.3
Underdevelopment *—see also* Undeveloped
nose Q3Ø.1
sexual E3Ø.Ø
Underdosing *—see also* Table of Drugs and Chemicals, categories T36-T5Ø, with final character 6 Z91.14
intentional NEC Z91.128
due to financial hardship of patient Z91.12Ø
unintentional NEC Z91.138
due to patient's age related debility Z91.13Ø
Underfeeding, newborn P92.3
Underfill, endodontic M27.53
Underimmunization status Z28.3
Undernourishment *—see* Malnutrition
Undernutrition *—see* Malnutrition
Under observation *—see* Observation
Underweight R63.6
for gestational age *—see* Light for dates
Underwood's disease P83.Ø
Undescended *—see also* Malposition, congenital
cecum Q43.3
colon Q43.3
testicle *—see* Cryptorchid
Undeveloped, undevelopment *—see also* Hypoplasia
brain (congenital) QØ2
cerebral (congenital) QØ2
heart Q24.8
lung Q33.6
testis E29.1
uterus E3Ø.Ø
Undiagnosed (disease) R69
Undulant fever *—see* Brucellosis
Unemployment, anxiety concerning Z56.Ø
threatened Z56.2
Unequal length (acquired) (limb) *—see also* Deformity, limb, unequal length
leg *—see also* Deformity, limb, unequal length
congenital Q72.9- •
Unextracted dental root KØ8.3
Unguis incarnatus L6Ø.Ø
Unhappiness R45.2
Unicornate uterus Q51.4
in pregnancy or childbirth O34.ØØ
Unilateral *—see also* condition
development, breast N64.89
organ or site, congenital NEC *—see* Agenesis, by site
Unilocular heart Q2Ø.8
Union, abnormal *—see also* Fusion
larynx and trachea Q34.8
Universal mesentery Q43.3
Unrepairable overhanging of dental restorative materials KØ8.52
Unsatisfactory
restoration of tooth KØ8.5Ø
specified NEC KØ8.59
sample of cytologic smear
anus R85.615
cervix R87.615
vagina R87.625
surroundings Z59.1
work Z56.5
Unsoundness of mind *—see* Psychosis
Unstable
back NEC *—see* Instability, joint, spine
hip (congenital) Q65.6
acquired *—see* Derangement, joint, specified type NEC, hip
joint *—see* Instability, joint
secondary to removal of joint prosthesis M96.89
lie (mother) O32.Ø
lumbosacral joint (congenital) *—see* subcategory M53.2
~~acquired —see subcategory M53.2~~
sacroiliac *—see* subcategory M53.2
spine NEC *—see* Instability, joint, spine
Unsteadiness on feet R26.81

Untruthfulness, child problem F91.8
Unverricht(-Lundborg) disease or epilepsy — *see* Epilepsy, generalized, idiopathic
Unwanted pregnancy Z64.Ø
Upbringing, institutional Z62.22
away from parents NEC Z62.29
in care of non-parental family member Z62.21
in foster care Z62.21
in orphanage or group home Z62.22
in welfare custody Z62.21
Upper respiratory —*see* condition
Upset
gastric K3Ø
gastrointestinal K3Ø
psychogenic F45.8
intestinal (large) (small) K59.9
psychogenic F45.8
menstruation N93.9
mental F48.9
stomach K3Ø
psychogenic F45.8
Urachus —*see also* condition
patent or persistent Q64.4
Urbach-Oppenheim disease (necrobiosis lipoidica diabeticorum) —*see* EØ8-E13 with .62Ø
Urbach's lipoid proteinosis E78.89
Urbach-Wiethe disease E78.89
Urban yellow fever A95.1
Urea
blood, high —*see* Uremia
cycle metabolism disorder —*see* Disorder, urea cycle metabolism
Uremia, uremic N19
with
ectopic or molar pregnancy OØ8.4
polyneuropathy N18.9 *[G63]*
chronic NOS —*see also* Disease, kidney, chronic N18.9
due to hypertension —*see* Hypertensive, kidney
complicating
ectopic or molar pregnancy OØ8.4
congenital P96.Ø
extrarenal R39.2
following ectopic or molar pregnancy OØ8.4
newborn P96.Ø
prerenal R39.2
Ureter, ureteral —*see* condition
Ureteralgia N23
Ureterectasis —*see* Hydroureter
Ureteritis N28.89
cystica N28.86
due to calculus N2Ø.1
with calculus, kidney N2Ø.2
with hydronephrosis N13.2
gonococcal (acute) (chronic) A54.21
nonspecific N28.89
Ureterocele N28.89
congenital (orthotopic) Q62.31
ectopic Q62.32
Ureterolith, ureterolithiasis —*see* Calculus, ureter
Ureterostomy
attention to Z43.6
status Z93.6
Urethra, urethral —*see* condition
Urethralgia R39.89
Urethritis (anterior) (posterior) N34.2
calculous N21.1
candidal B37.41
chlamydial A56.Ø1
diplococcal (gonococcal) A54.Ø1
with abscess (accessory gland) (periurethral) A54.1
gonococcal A54.Ø1
with abscess (accessory gland) (periurethral) A54.1
Urethritis *(Continued)*
nongonococcal N34.1
Reiter's —*see* Reiter's disease
nonspecific N34.1
nonvenereal N34.1
postmenopausal N34.2
puerperal O86.22
Reiter's —*see* Reiter's disease
specified NEC N34.2
trichomonal or due to Trichomonas (vaginalis) A59.Ø3
Urethrocele N81.Ø
with
cystocele —*see* Cystocele
prolapse of uterus —*see* Prolapse, uterus
Urethrolithiasis (with colic or infection) N21.1
Urethrorectal —*see* condition
Urethrorrhagia N36.8
Urethrorrhea R36.9
Urethrostomy
attention to Z43.6
status Z93.6
Urethrotrigonitis —*see* Trigonitis
Urethrovaginal —*see* condition
Urgency
fecal R15.2
hypertensive —*see* Hypertension
urinary N39.15
Urhidrosis, uridrosis L74.8
Uric acid in blood (increased) E79.Ø
Uricacidemia (asymptomatic) E79.Ø
Uricemia (asymptomatic) E79.Ø
Uricosuria R82.998
Urinary —*see* condition
Urination
frequent R35.Ø
painful R3Ø.9
Urine
blood in —*see* Hematuria
discharge, excessive R35.8
enuresis, nonorganic origin F98.Ø
extravasation R39.Ø
frequency R35.Ø
incontinence R32
nonorganic origin F98.Ø
intermittent stream R39.198
pus in N39.Ø
retention or stasis R33.9
organic R33.8
drug-induced R33.Ø
psychogenic F45.8
secretion
deficient R34
excessive R35.8
frequency R35.Ø
stream
intermittent R39.198
slowing R39.198
splitting R39.13
weak R39.12
Urinemia —*see* Uremia
Urinoma, urethra N36.8
Uroarthritis, infectious (Reiter's) —*see* Reiter's disease
Urodialysis R34
Urolithiasis —*see* Calculus, urinary
Uronephrosis —*see* Hydronephrosis
Uropathy N39.9
obstructive N13.9
specified NEC N13.8
reflux N13.9
specified NEC N13.8
vesicoureteral reflux-associated —*see* Reflux, vesicoureteral
Urosepsis — code to condition
Urticaria L5Ø.9
with angioneurotic edema T78.3
hereditary D84.1
allergic L5Ø.Ø
cholinergic L5Ø.5
chronic L5Ø.8
Urticaria *(Continued)*
cold, familial L5Ø.2
contact L5Ø.6
dermatographic L5Ø.3
due to
cold or heat L5Ø.2
drugs L5Ø.Ø
food L5Ø.Ø
inhalants L5Ø.Ø
plants L5Ø.6
serum —*see also* Reaction, serum T8Ø.69
factitial L5Ø.3
familial cold MØ4.2
giant T78.3
hereditary D84.1
gigantea T78.3
idiopathic L5Ø.1
larynx T78.3
hereditary D84.1
neonatorum P83.88
nonallergic L5Ø.1
papulosa (Hebra) L28.2
pigmentosa D47.Ø1
congenital Q82.2
of neonatal onset Q82.2
of newborn onset Q82.2
recurrent periodic L5Ø.8
serum —*see also* Reaction, serum T8Ø.69
solar L56.3
specified type NEC L5Ø.8
thermal (cold) (heat) L5Ø.2
vibratory L5Ø.4
xanthelasmoidea —*see* Urticaria pigmentosa
Use (of)
alcohol Z72.89
with
intoxication F1Ø.929
sleep disorder F1Ø.982
harmful —*see* Abuse, alcohol
amphetamines —*see* Use, stimulant NEC
caffeine —*see* Use, stimulant NEC
cannabis F12.9Ø
with
anxiety disorder F12.98Ø
intoxication F12.929
with
delirium F12.921
perceptual disturbance F12.922
uncomplicated F12.92Ø
other specified disorder F12.988
psychosis F12.959
delusions F12.95Ø
hallucinations F12.951
unspecified disorder F12.99
withdrawal F12.93
cocaine F14.9Ø
with
anxiety disorder F14.98Ø
intoxication F14.929
with
delirium F14.921
perceptual disturbance F14.922
uncomplicated F14.92Ø
other specified disorder F14.988
psychosis F14.959
delusions F14.95Ø
hallucinations F14.951
sexual dysfunction F14.981
sleep disorder F14.982
unspecified disorder F14.99
harmful —*see* Abuse, drug, cocaine
drug(s) NEC F19.9Ø
with sleep disorder F19.982
harmful —*see* Abuse, drug, by type
hallucinogen NEC F16.9Ø
with
anxiety disorder F16.98Ø
intoxication F16.929
with
delirium F16.921
uncomplicated F16.92Ø

Use (Continued)
hallucinogen NEC (Continued)
with (Continued)
mood disorder F16.94
other specified disorder F16.988
perception disorder (flashbacks) F16.983
psychosis F16.959
delusions F16.950
hallucinations F16.951
unspecified disorder F16.99
harmful —see Abuse, drug, hallucinogen NEC
inhalants F18.90
with
anxiety disorder F18.980
intoxication F18.929
with delirium F18.921
uncomplicated F18.920
mood disorder F18.94
other specified disorder F18.988
persisting dementia F18.97
psychosis F18.959
delusions F18.950
hallucinations F18.951
unspecified disorder F18.99
harmful —see Abuse, drug, inhalant
methadone —see Use, opioid
nonprescribed drugs F19.90
harmful —see Abuse, non-psychoactive substance
opioid F11.90
with
disorder F11.99
mood F11.94
sleep F11.982
specified type NEC F11.988
intoxication F11.929
with
delirium F11.921
perceptual disturbance F11.922
uncomplicated F11.920
withdrawal F11.93
harmful —see Abuse, drug, opioid
patent medicines F19.90
harmful —see Abuse, non-psychoactive substance
psychoactive drug NEC F19.90
with
anxiety disorder F19.980

Use (Continued)
psychoactive drug NEC (Continued)
with (Continued)
intoxication F19.929
with
delirium F19.921
perceptual disturbance F19.922
uncomplicated F19.920
mood disorder F19.94
other specified disorder F19.988
persisting
amnestic disorder F19.96
dementia F19.97
psychosis F19.959
delusions F19.950
hallucinations F19.951
sexual dysfunction F19.981
sleep disorder F19.982
unspecified disorder F19.99
withdrawal F19.939
with
delirium F19.931
perceptual disturbance F19.932
uncomplicated F19.930
harmful —see Abuse, drug NEC, psychoactive NEC
sedative, hypnotic, or anxiolytic F13.90
with
anxiety disorder F13.980
intoxication F13.929
with
delirium F13.921
uncomplicated F13.920
other specified disorder F13.988
persisting
amnestic disorder F13.96
dementia F13.97
psychosis F13.959
delusions F13.950
hallucinations F13.951
sexual dysfunction F13.981
sleep disorder F13.982
unspecified disorder F13.99
harmful —see Abuse, drug, sedative, hypnotic, or anxiolytic
stimulant NEC F15.90
with
anxiety disorder F15.980
intoxication F15.929
with
delirium F15.921
perceptual disturbance F15.922
uncomplicated F15.920

Use (Continued)
stimulant NEC (Continued)
with (Continued)
mood disorder F15.94
other specified disorder F15.988
psychosis F15.959
delusions F15.950
hallucinations F15.951
sexual dysfunction F15.981
sleep disorder F15.982
unspecified disorder F15.99
withdrawal F15.93
harmful —see Abuse, drug, stimulant NEC
tobacco Z72.0
with dependence —see Dependence, drug, nicotine
volatile solvents —see also Use, inhalant F18.90
harmful —see Abuse, drug, inhalant
Usher-Senear disease or syndrome L10.4
Uta B55.1
Uteromegaly N85.2
Uterovaginal —see condition
Uterovesical —see condition
Uveal —see condition
Uveitis (anterior) —see also Iridocyclitis
acute —see Iridocyclitis, acute
chronic —see Iridocyclitis, chronic
due to toxoplasmosis (acquired) B58.09
congenital P37.1
granulomatous —see Iridocyclitis, chronic
heterochromic —see Cyclitis, Fuchs' heterochromic
lens-induced —see Iridocyclitis, lens-induced
posterior —see Chorioretinitis
sympathetic H44.13-●
syphilitic (secondary) A51.43
congenital (early) A50.01
late A52.71
tuberculous A18.54
Uveoencephalitis —see Inflammation, chorioretinal
Uveokeratitis —see Iridocyclitis
Uveoparotitis D86.89
Uvula —see condition
Uvulitis (acute) (catarrhal) (chronic) (membranous) (suppurative) (ulcerative) K12.2

U

V

Vaccination (prophylactic)
complication or reaction —*see* Complications, vaccination
delayed Z28.9
encounter for Z23
not done —*see* Immunization, not done, because (of)
Vaccinia (generalized) (localized) T88.1
without vaccination BØ8.Ø11
congenital P35.8
Vacuum, in sinus (accessory) (nasal) J34.89
Vagabond, vagabondage Z59.Ø
Vagabond's disease B85.1
Vagina, vaginal —*see* condition
Vaginalitis (tunica) (testis) N49.1
Vaginismus (reflex) N94.2
functional F52.5
nonorganic F52.5
psychogenic F52.5
secondary N94.2
Vaginitis (acute) (circumscribed) (diffuse) (emphysematous) (nonvenereal) (ulcerative) N76.Ø
with ectopic or molar pregnancy OØ8.Ø
amebic AØ6.82
atrophic, postmenopausal N95.2
bacterial N76.Ø
blennorrhagic (gonococcal) A54.Ø2
candidal B37.3
chlamydial A56.Ø2
chronic N76.1
due to Trichomonas (vaginalis) A59.Ø1
following ectopic or molar pregnancy OØ8.Ø
gonococcal A54.Ø2
with abscess (accessory gland) (periurethral) A54.1
granuloma A58
in (due to)
candidiasis B37.3
herpesviral (herpes simplex) infection A6Ø.Ø4
pinworm infection B8Ø *[N77.1]*
monilial B37.3
mycotic (candidal) B37.3
postmenopausal atrophic N95.2
puerperal (postpartum) O86.13
senile (atrophic) N95.2
subacute or chronic N76.1
syphilitic (early) A51.Ø
late A52.76
trichomonal A59.Ø1
tuberculous A18.18
Vaginosis —*see* Vaginitis
Vagotonia G52.2
Vagrancy Z59.Ø
VAIN —*see* Neoplasia, intraepithelial, vagina
Vallecula —*see* condition
Valley fever B38.Ø
Valsuani's disease —*see* Anemia, obstetric
Valve, valvular (formation) —*see also* condition
cerebral ventricle (communicating) in situ Z98.2
cervix, internal os Q51.828
congenital NEC —*see* Atresia, by site
ureter (pelvic junction) (vesical orifice) Q62.39
urethra (congenital) (posterior) Q64.2
Valvulitis (chronic) —*see* Endocarditis
Valvulopathy —*see* Endocarditis
Van Bogaert's leukoencephalopathy (sclerosing) (subacute) A81.1
Van Bogaert-Scherer-Epstein disease or syndrome E75.5
Van Buchem's syndrome M85.2
Van Creveld-von Gierke disease E74.Ø1
Van der Hoeve (-de Kleyn) syndrome Q78.Ø
Van der Woude's syndrome Q38.Ø
Van Neck's disease or osteochondrosis M91.Ø
Vanishing lung J44.9
Vapor asphyxia or suffocation T59.9
specified agent —*see* Table of Drugs and Chemicals
Variance, lethal ball, prosthetic heart valve T82.Ø9
Variants, thalassemic D56.8
Variations in hair color L67.1
Varicella BØ1.9
with
complications NEC BØ1.89
encephalitis BØ1.11
encephalomyelitis BØ1.11
meningitis BØ1.Ø
myelitis BØ1.12
pneumonia BØ1.2
congenital P35.8
Varices —*see* Varix
Varicocele (scrotum) (thrombosed) I86.1
ovary I86.2
perineum I86.3
spermatic cord (ulcerated) I86.1
Varicose
aneurysm (ruptured) I77.Ø
dermatitis —*see* Varix, leg, with, inflammation
eczema —*see* Varix, leg, with, inflammation
phlebitis —*see* Varix, with, inflammation
tumor —*see* Varix
ulcer (lower limb, any part) —*see also* Varix, leg, with, ulcer
anus —*see also* Hemorrhoids K64.8
esophagus —*see* Varix, esophagus
inflamed or infected —*see* Varix, leg, with ulcer, with inflammation
nasal septum I86.8
perineum I86.3
scrotum I86.1
specified site NEC I86.8
vein —*see* Varix
vessel —*see* Varix, leg
Varicosis, varicosities, varicosity —*see* Varix
Variola (major) (minor) BØ3
Varioloid BØ3
Varix (lower limb) I83.9Ø
with
bleeding I83.899
edema I83.899
inflammation I83.1Ø
with ulcer (venous) I83.2Ø9
pain I83.819
rupture I83.899
specified complication NEC I83.899
stasis dermatitis I83.1Ø
with ulcer (venous) I83.2Ø9
swelling I83.899
ulcer I83.ØØ9
with inflammation I83.2Ø9
aneurysmal I77.Ø
asymptomatic I83.9- ●
bladder I86.2
broad ligament I86.2
complicating
childbirth (lower extremity) O87.4
anus or rectum O87.2
genital (vagina, vulva or perineum) O87.8
pregnancy (lower extremity) O22.Ø- ●
anus or rectum O22.4- ●
genital (vagina, vulva or perineum) O22.1- ●
puerperium (lower extremity) O87.4
anus or rectum O87.2
genital (vagina, vulva, perineum) O87.8
congenital (any site) Q27.8
esophagus (idiopathic) (primary) (ulcerated) I85.ØØ
bleeding I85.Ø1
congenital Q27.8
in (due to)
alcoholic liver disease I85.1Ø
bleeding I85.11
cirrhosis of liver I85.1Ø
bleeding I85.11
Varix *(Continued)*
esophagus *(Continued)*
in *(Continued)*
portal hypertension I85.1Ø
bleeding I85.11
schistosomiasis I85.1Ø
bleeding I85.11
toxic liver disease I85.1Ø
bleeding I85.11
secondary I85.1Ø
bleeding I85.11
gastric I86.4
inflamed or infected I83.1Ø
ulcerated I83.2Ø9
labia (majora) I86.3
leg (asymptomatic) I83.9Ø
with
edema I83.899
inflammation I83.1Ø
with ulcer —*see* Varix, leg, with, ulcer, with inflammation by site
pain I83.819
specified complication NEC I83.899
swelling I83.899
ulcer I83.ØØ9
with inflammation I83.2Ø9
ankle I83.ØØ3
with inflammation I83.2Ø3
calf I83.ØØ2
with inflammation I83.2Ø2
foot NEC I83.ØØ5
with inflammation I83.2Ø5
heel I83.ØØ4
with inflammation I83.2Ø4
lower leg NEC I83.ØØ8
with inflammation I83.2Ø8
midfoot I83.ØØ4
with inflammation I83.2Ø4
thigh I83.ØØ1
with inflammation I83.2Ø1
bilateral (asymptomatic) I83.93
with
edema I83.893
pain I83.813
specified complication NEC I83.893
swelling I83.893
ulcer I83.Ø- ●
with inflammation I83.2Ø9
left (asymptomatic) I83.92
with
edema I83.892
inflammation I83.12
with ulcer —*see* Varix, leg, with, ulcer, with inflammation by site
pain I83.812
specified complication NEC I83.892
swelling I83.892
ulcer I83.Ø29
with inflammation I83.229
ankle I83.Ø23
with inflammation I83.223
calf I83.Ø22
with inflammation I83.222
foot NEC I83.Ø25
with inflammation I83.225
heel I83.Ø24
with inflammation I83.224
lower leg NEC I83.Ø28
with inflammation I83.228
midfoot I83.Ø24
with inflammation I83.224
thigh I83.Ø21
with inflammation I83.221
right (asymptomatic) I83.91
with
edema I83.891
inflammation I83.11
with ulcer —*see* Varix, leg, with, ulcer, with inflammation by site

Varix *(Continued)*
leg *(Continued)*
right *(Continued)*
with *(Continued)*
pain I83.811
specified complication NEC I83.891
swelling I83.891
ulcer I83.019
with inflammation I83.219
ankle I83.013
with inflammation I83.213
calf I83.012
with inflammation I83.212
foot NEC I83.015
with inflammation I83.215
heel I83.014
with inflammation I83.214
lower leg NEC I83.018
with inflammation I83.218
midfoot I83.014
with inflammation I83.214
thigh I83.011
with inflammation I83.211
nasal septum I86.8
orbit I86.8
congenital Q27.8
ovary I86.2
papillary I78.1
pelvis I86.2
perineum I86.3
pharynx I86.8
placenta O43.89- •
renal papilla I86.8
retina H35.09
scrotum (ulcerated) I86.1
sigmoid colon I86.8
specified site NEC I86.8
spinal (cord) (vessels) I86.8
spleen, splenic (vein) (with phlebolith) I86.8
stomach I86.4
sublingual I86.0
ulcerated I83.009
inflamed or infected I83.209
uterine ligament I86.2
vagina I86.8
vocal cord I86.8
vulva I86.3
Vas deferens —*see* condition
Vas deferentitis N49.1
Vasa previa O69.4
hemorrhage from, affecting newborn P50.0
Vascular —*see also* condition
loop on optic papilla Q14.2
spasm I73.9
spider I78.1
Vascularization, cornea —*see* Neovascularization, cornea
Vasculitis I77.6
allergic D69.0
cryoglobulinemic D89.1
disseminated I77.6
hypocomplementemic M31.8
kidney I77.89
livedoid L95.0
nodular L95.8
retina H35.06- •
rheumatic —*see* Fever, rheumatic
rheumatoid —*see* Rheumatoid, vasculitis
skin (limited to) L95.9
specified NEC L95.8
systemic M31.8
Vasculopathy, necrotizing M31.9
cardiac allograft T86.290
specified NEC M31.8
Vasitis (nodosa) N49.1
tuberculous A18.15
Vasodilation I73.9
Vasomotor —*see* condition
Vasoplasty, after previous sterilization Z31.0
aftercare Z31.42
Vasospasm (vasoconstriction) I73.9
cerebral (cerebrovascular) (artery) I67.848
reversible I67.841
coronary I20.1
nerve
arm —*see* Mononeuropathy, upper limb
brachial plexus G54.0
cervical plexus G54.2
leg —*see* Mononeuropathy, lower limb
peripheral NOS I73.9
retina (artery) —*see* Occlusion, artery, retina
Vasospastic —*see* condition
Vasovagal attack (paroxysmal) R55
psychogenic F45.8
VATER syndrome Q87.2
Vater's ampulla —*see* condition
Vegetation, vegetative
adenoid (nasal fossa) J35.8
endocarditis (acute) (any valve) (subacute) I33.0
heart (mycotic) (valve) I33.0
Veil
Jackson's Q43.3
Vein, venous —*see* condition
Veldt sore —*see* Ulcer, skin
Velpeau's hernia —*see* Hernia, femoral
Venereal
bubo A55
disease A64
granuloma inguinale A58
lymphogranuloma (Durand-Nicolas-Favre) A55
Venofibrosis I87.8
Venom, venomous —*see* Table of Drugs and Chemicals, by animal or substance, poisoning
Venous —*see* condition
Ventilator lung, newborn P27.8
Ventral —*see* condition
Ventricle, ventricular —*see also* condition
escape I49.3
inversion Q20.5
Ventriculitis (cerebral) —*see also* Encephalitis G04.90
Ventriculostomy status Z98.2
Vernet's syndrome G52.7
Verneuil's disease (syphilitic bursitis) A52.78
Verruca (due to HPV) (filiformis) (simplex) (viral) (vulgaris) B07.9
acuminata A63.0
necrogenica (primary) (tuberculosa) A18.4
plana B07.8
plantaris B07.0
seborrheica L82.1
inflamed L82.0
senile (seborrheic) L82.1
inflamed L82.0
tuberculosa (primary) A18.4
venereal A63.0
Verrucosities —*see* Verruca
Verruga peruana, peruviana A44.1
Version
with extraction
cervix —*see* Malposition, uterus
uterus (postinfectional) (postpartal, old) —*see* Malposition, uterus
Vertebra, vertebral —*see* condition
Vertical talus (congenital) Q66.80
left foot Q66.82
right foot Q66.81
Vertigo R42
auditory —*see* Vertigo, aural
aural H81.31- •
benign paroxysmal (positional) H81.1- •
central (origin) H81.4
cerebral H81.4
Dix and Hallpike (epidemic) —*see* Neuronitis, vestibular
due to infrasound T75.23
Vertigo *(Continued)*
epidemic A88.1
Dix and Hallpike —*see* Neuronitis, vestibular
Pedersen's —*see* Neuronitis, vestibular
vestibular neuronitis —*see* Neuronitis, vestibular
hysterical F44.89
infrasound T75.23
labyrinthine —*see* subcategory H81.0
laryngeal R05
malignant positional H81.4
Ménière's —*see* subcategory H81.40
menopausal N95.11
otogenic —*see* Vertigo, aural
paroxysmal positional, benign —*see* Vertigo, benign paroxysmal
Pedersen's (epidemic) —*see* Neuronitis, vestibular
peripheral NEC H81.39- •
positional
benign paroxysmal —*see* Vertigo, benign paroxysmal
malignant H81.4
Very-low-density-lipoprotein-type (VLDL) hyperlipoproteinemia E78.1
Vesania —*see* Psychosis
Vesical —*see* condition
Vesicle
cutaneous R23.8
seminal —*see* condition
skin R23.8
Vesicocolic —*see* condition
Vesicoperineal —*see* condition
Vesicorectal —*see* condition
Vesicourethrorectal —*see* condition
Vesicovaginal —*see* condition
Vesicular —*see* condition
Vesiculitis (seminal) N49.0
amebic A06.82
gonorrheal (acute) (chronic) A54.23
trichomonal A59.09
tuberculous A18.15
Vestibulitis (ear) —*see also* subcategory H83.0
nose (external) J34.89
vulvar N94.810
Vestibulopathy, acute peripheral (recurrent) —*see* Neuronitis, vestibular
Vestige, vestigial —*see also* Persistence
branchial Q18.0
structures in vitreous Q14.0
Vibration
adverse effects T75.20
pneumatic hammer syndrome T75.21
specified effect NEC T75.29
vasospastic syndrome T75.22
vertigo from infrasound T75.23
exposure (occupational) Z57.7
vertigo T75.23
Vibriosis A28.9
Victim (of)
crime Z65.4
disaster Z65.5
terrorism Z65.4
torture Z65.4
war Z65.5
Vidal's disease L28.0
Villaret's syndrome G52.7
Villous —*see* condition
VIN —*see* Neoplasia, intraepithelial, vulva
Vincent's infection (angina) (gingivitis) A69.1
stomatitis NEC A69.1
Vinson-Plummer syndrome D50.1
Violence, physical R45.6
Viosterol deficiency —*see* Deficiency, calciferol
Vipoma —*see* Neoplasm, malignant, by site
Viremia B34.9
Virilism (adrenal) E25.9
congenital E25.0
Virilization (female) (suprarenal) E25.9
congenital E25.0
isosexual E28.2

V

Virulent bubo A57
Virus, viral —*see also* condition
  as cause of disease classified elsewhere B97.89
    ▶respiratory syncytial virus (RSV) —*see* Virus, infection, respiratory syncytial (RSV)
  cytomegalovirus B25.9
  human immunodeficiency (HIV) —*see* Human, immunodeficiency virus (HIV) disease
  infection —*see* Infection, virus
▶respiratory syncytial (RSV)
  ▶as cause of disease classified elsewhere B97.4
  ▶bronchiolitis J21.0
  ▶bronchitis J20.5
  ▶bronchopneumonia J12.1
  ▶otitis media H65-● *[B97.4]*
  ▶pneumonia J12.1
  ▶upper respiratory infection J06.9 *[B97.4]*
  specified NEC B34.8
  swine influenza (viruses that normally cause infections in pigs) —*see also* Influenza, due to, identified novel influenza A virus J09.X2
  West Nile (fever) A92.30
    with
      complications NEC A92.39
      cranial nerve disorders A92.32
      encephalitis A92.31
      encephalomyelitis A92.31
      neurologic manifestation NEC A92.32
      optic neuritis A92.32
      polyradiculitis A92.32
Viscera, visceral —*see* condition
Visceroptosis K63.4
Visible peristalsis R19.2
Vision, visual
  binocular, suppression H53.34
  blurred, blurring H53.8
    hysterical F44.6
  defect, defective NEC H54.7
  disorientation (syndrome) H53.8
  disturbance H53.9
    hysterical F44.6
  double H53.2
  examination Z01.00
    with abnormal findings Z01.01
    ▶following failed vision screening Z01.020
      ▶with abnormal findings Z01.021
  field, limitation (defect) —*see* Defect, visual field
  hallucinations R44.1
  halos H53.19
  loss —*see* Loss, vision
    sudden —*see* Disturbance, vision, subjective, loss, sudden
  low (both eyes) —*see* Low, vision
  perception, simultaneous without fusion H53.33
Vitality, lack or want of R53.83
  newborn P96.89
Vitamin deficiency —*see* Deficiency, vitamin
Vitelline duct, persistent Q43.0
Vitiligo L80
  eyelid H02.739
    left H02.736
      lower H02.735
      upper H02.734
    right H02.733
      lower H02.732
      upper H02.731
  pinta A67.2
  vulva N90.89
Vitreal corneal syndrome H59.01-●
Vitreoretinopathy, proliferative —*see also* Retinopathy, proliferative
  with retinal detachment —*see* Detachment, retina, traction
Vitreous —*see also* condition
  touch syndrome —*see* Complication, postprocedural, following cataract surgery
Vocal cord —*see* condition
Vogt-Koyanagi syndrome H20.82-●
Vogt's disease or syndrome G80.3
Vogt-Spielmeyer amaurotic idiocy or disease E75.4
Voice
  change R49.9
    specified NEC R49.8
  loss —*see* Aphonia
Volhynian fever A79.0
Volkmann's ischemic contracture or paralysis (complicating trauma) T79.6
Volvulus (bowel) (colon) (intestine) K56.2
  with perforation K56.2
  congenital Q43.8
  duodenum K31.5
  fallopian tube —*see* Torsion, fallopian tube
  oviduct —*see* Torsion, fallopian tube
  stomach (due to absence of gastrocolic ligament) K31.89
Vomiting R11.10
  with nausea R11.2
  without nausea R11.11
  asphyxia —*see* Foreign body, by site, causing asphyxia, gastric contents
  bilious (cause unknown) R11.14
    following gastro-intestinal surgery K91.0
    in newborn P92.01
  blood —*see* Hematemesis
  causing asphyxia, choking, or suffocation —*see* Foreign body, by site
  ➠cyclical, in migraine G43.A0
    with refractory migraine G43.A1
    intractable G43.A1
    not intractable G43.A0
    psychogenic F50.89
    without refractory migraine G43.A0
  ▶cyclical syndrome NOS (unrelated to migraine) R53.1
    ▶persistent R11.15
Vomiting *(Continued)*
  fecal mater R11.13
  following gastrointestinal surgery K91.0
    psychogenic F50.89
  functional K31.89
  hysterical F50.89
  nervous F50.89
  neurotic F50.89
  newborn NEC P92.09
    bilious P92.01
  periodic R11.10
    psychogenic F50.89
  projectile R11.12
  psychogenic F50.89
  uremic —*see* Uremia
Vomito negro —*see* Fever, yellow
Von Bezold's abscess —*see* Mastoiditis, acute
Von Economo-Cruchet disease A85.8
Von Eulenburg's disease G71.19
Von Gierke's disease E74.01
Von Hippel (-Lindau) disease or syndrome Q85.8
Von Jaksch's anemia or disease D64.89
Von Recklinghausen
  disease (neurofibromatosis) Q85.01
    bones E21.0
Von Schroetter's syndrome I82.890
Von Willebrand (-Jurgens)(-Minot) disease or syndrome D68.0
Von Zumbusch's disease L40.1
Voyeurism F65.3
Vrolik's disease Q78.0
Vulva —*see* condition
Vulvismus N94.2
Vulvitis (acute) (allergic) (atrophic) (hypertrophic) (intertriginous) (senile) N76.2
  with ectopic or molar pregnancy O08.0
  adhesive, congenital Q52.79
  blennorrhagic (gonococcal) A54.02
  candidal B37.3
  chlamydial A56.02
  due to Haemophilus ducreyi A57
  following ectopic or molar pregnancy O08.0
  gonococcal A54.02
    with abscess (accessory gland) (periurethral) A54.1
  herpesviral A60.04
  leukoplakic N90.4
  monilial B37.3
  puerperal (postpartum) O86.19
  subacute or chronic N76.3
  syphilitic (early) A51.0
    late A52.76
  trichomonal A59.01
  tuberculous A18.18
Vulvodynia N94.819
  specified NEC N94.818
Vulvorectal —*see* condition
Vulvovaginitis (acute) —*see* Vaginitis

W

Waiting list, person on Z75.1
  for organ transplant Z76.82
  undergoing social agency investigation Z75.2
Waldenström
  hypergammaglobulinemia D89.Ø
  syndrome or macroglobulinemia C88.Ø
Waldenström-Kjellberg syndrome D5Ø.1
Walking
  difficulty R26.2
    psychogenic F44.4
  sleep F51.3
    hysterical F44.89
Wall, abdominal —*see* condition
Wallenberg's disease or syndrome G46.3
Wallgren's disease I87.8
Wandering
  gallbladder, congenital Q44.1
  in diseases classified elsewhere Z91.83
  kidney, congenital Q63.8
  organ or site, congenital NEC —*see* Malposition, congenital, by site
  pacemaker (heart) I49.8
  spleen D73.89
War neurosis F48.8
Wart (due to HPV) (filiform) (infectious) (viral) BØ7.9
  anogenital region (venereal) A63.Ø
  common BØ7.8
  external genital organs (venereal) A63.Ø
  flat BØ7.8
  Hassal-Henle's (of cornea) H18.49
  Peruvian A44.1
  plantar BØ7.Ø
  prosector (tuberculous) A18.4
  seborrheic L82.1
    inflamed L82.Ø
  senile (seborrheic) L82.1
    inflamed L82.Ø
  tuberculous A18.4
  venereal A63.Ø
Warthin's tumor —*see* Neoplasm, salivary gland, benign
Wassilieff's disease A27.Ø
Wasting
  disease R64
    due to malnutrition E41
  extreme (due to malnutrition) E41
  muscle NEC —*see* Atrophy, muscle
Water
  clefts (senile cataract) —*see* Cataract, senile, incipient
  deprivation of T73.1
  intoxication E87.79
  itch B76.9
  lack of T73.1
  loading E87.7Ø
  on
    brain —*see* Hydrocephalus
    chest J94.8
  poisoning E87.79
Waterbrash R12
Waterhouse(-Friderichsen) syndrome or disease (meningococcal) A39.1
Water-losing nephritis N25.89
Watermelon stomach K31.819
  with hemorrhage K31.811
  without hemorrhage K31.819
Watsoniasis B66.8
Wax in ear —*see* Impaction, cerumen
Weak, weakening, weakness (generalized) R53.1
  arches (acquired) —*see also* Deformity, limb, flat foot
  bladder (sphincter) R32
Weak, weakening, weakness *(Continued)*
  facial R29.81Ø
    following
      cerebrovascular disease I69.992
        cerebral infarction I69.392
        intracerebral hemorrhage I69.192
        nontraumatic intracranial hemorrhage NEC I69.292
        specified disease NEC I69.892
        stroke I69.392
        subarachnoid hemorrhage I69.Ø92
  foot (double) —*see also* Weak, arches
  heart, cardiac —*see* Failure, heart
  mind F7Ø
  muscle M62.81
  myocardium —*see* Failure, heart
  newborn P96.89
  pelvic fundus N81.89
  pubocervical tissue N81.82
  rectovaginal tissue N81.83
  senile R54
  urinary stream R39.12
  valvular —*see* Endocarditis
Wear, worn (with normal or routine use)
  articular bearing surface of internal joint prosthesis —*see* Complications, joint prosthesis, mechanical, wear of articular bearing surfaces, by site
  device, implant or graft —*see* Complications, by site, mechanical complication
  tooth, teeth (approximal) (hard tissues) (interproximal) (occlusal) KØ3.Ø
Weather, weathered
  effects of
    cold T69.9
      specified effect NEC T69.8
    hot —*see* Heat
  skin L57.8
Weaver's syndrome Q87.3
Web, webbed (congenital)
  duodenal Q43.8
  esophagus Q39.4
  fingers Q7Ø.1
  larynx (glottic) (subglottic) Q31.Ø
  neck (pterygium colli) Q18.3
  Paterson-Kelly D5Ø.1
  popliteal syndrome Q87.89
  toes Q7Ø.3
Weber-Christian disease M35.6
Weber-Cockayne syndrome (epidermolysis bullosa) Q81.8
Weber-Gubler syndrome G46.3
Weber-Leyden syndrome G46.3
Weber-Osler syndrome I78.Ø
Weber's paralysis or syndrome G46.3
Wedge-shaped or wedging vertebra —*see* Collapse, vertebra NEC
Wegener's granulomatosis or syndrome M31.3Ø
  with
    kidney involvement M31.31
    lung involvement M31.3Ø
      with kidney involvement M31.31
Wegner's disease A5Ø.Ø2
Weight
  1ØØØ-2499 grams at birth (low) —*see* Low, birthweight
  999 grams or less at birth (extremely low) —*see* Low, birthweight, extreme
  and length below 1Øth percentile for gestational age PØ5.1-●
  below but length above 1Øth percentile for gestational age PØ5.Ø-●
  gain (abnormal) (excessive) R63.5
    in pregnancy —*see* Pregnancy, complicated by, excessive weight gain
      low —*see* Pregnancy, complicated by, insufficient, weight gain
  loss (abnormal) (cause unknown) R63.4
Weightlessness (effect of) T75.82
Weil (l)-Marchesani syndrome Q87.19
Weil's disease A27.Ø
Weingarten's syndrome J82
Weir Mitchell's disease I73.81
Weiss-Baker syndrome G9Ø.Ø9
Wells' disease L98.3
Wen —*see* Cyst, sebaceous
Wenckebach's block or phenomenon I44.1
Werdnig-Hoffmann syndrome (muscular atrophy) G12.Ø
Werlhof's disease D69.3
Werner-His disease A79.Ø
Wermer's disease or syndrome E31.21
Werner's disease or syndrome E34.8
Wernicke-Korsakoff's syndrome or psychosis (alcoholic) F1Ø.96
  with dependence F1Ø.26
  drug-induced
    due to drug abuse —*see* Abuse, drug, by type, with amnestic disorder
    due to drug dependence —*see* Dependence, drug, by type, with amnestic disorder
  nonalcoholic FØ4
Wernicke-Posadas disease B38.9
Wernicke's
  developmental aphasia F8Ø.2
  disease or syndrome E51.2
  encephalopathy E51.2
  polioencephalitis, superior E51.2
West African fever B5Ø.8
Westphal-Strümpell syndrome E83.Ø1
West's syndrome —*see* Epilepsy, spasms
Wet
  feet, tropical (maceration) (syndrome) —*see* Immersion, foot
  lung (syndrome), newborn P22.1
Wharton's duct —*see* condition
Wheal —*see* Urticaria
Wheezing RØ6.2
Whiplash injury S13.4
Whipple's disease —*see also* subcategory M14.8-● K9Ø.81
Whipworm (disease) (infection) (infestation) B79
Whistling face Q87.Ø
White —*see also* condition
  kidney, small NØ3.9
  leg, puerperal, postpartum, childbirth O87.1
  mouth B37.Ø
  patches of mouth K13.29
  spot lesions, teeth
    chewing surface KØ2.51
    pit and fissure surface KØ2.51
    smooth surface KØ2.61
Whitehead L7Ø.Ø
Whitlow —*see also* Cellulitis, digit
  with lymphangitis —*see* Lymphangitis, acute, digit
  herpesviral BØØ.89
Whitmore's disease or fever —*see* Melioidosis
Whooping cough A37.9Ø
  with pneumonia A37.91
    due to Bordetella
      bronchiseptica A37.81
      parapertussis A37.11
      pertussis A37.Ø1
    specified organism NEC A37.81
  due to
    Bordetella
      bronchiseptica A37.8Ø
        with pneumonia A37.81
      parapertussis A37.1Ø
        with pneumonia A37.11
      pertussis A37.ØØ
        with pneumonia A37.Ø1
      specified NEC A37.8Ø
        with pneumonia A37.81
Wichman's asthma J38.5
Wide cranial sutures, newborn P96.3

W

Widening aorta —*see* Ectasia, aorta
with aneurysm —*see* Aneurysm, aorta
Wilkie's disease or syndrome K55.1
Wilkinson-Sneddon disease or syndrome L13.1
Willebrand (-Jürgens) thrombopathy D68.Ø
Williams syndrome Q93.82
Willige-Hunt disease or syndrome G23.1
Wilms' tumor C64-•
Wilson-Mikity syndrome P27.Ø
Wilson's
disease or syndrome E83.Ø1
hepatolenticular degeneration E83.Ø1
lichen ruber L43.9
Window —*see also* Imperfect, closure
aorticopulmonary Q21.4
Winter —*see* condition
Wiskott-Aldrich syndrome D82.Ø
Withdrawal state —*see also* Dependence, drug by type, with withdrawal
alcohol
with perceptual disturbances F1Ø.232
without perceptual disturbances F1Ø.239
caffeine F15.93
cannabis F12.23
newborn
correct therapeutic substance properly administered P96.2
infant of dependent mother P96.1
therapeutic substance, neonatal P96.2
Witts' anemia D5Ø.8
Witzelsucht FØ7.Ø
Woakes' ethmoiditis or syndrome J33.1
Wolff-Hirschorn syndrome Q93.3
Wolff-Parkinson-White syndrome I45.6
Wolhynian fever A79.Ø
Wolman's disease E75.5
Wood lung or pneumonitis J67.8
Woolly, wooly hair (congenital) (nevus) Q84.1
Woolsorter's disease A22.1
Word
blindness (congenital) (developmental) F81.Ø
deafness (congenital) (developmental) H93.25
Worm(s) (infection) (infestation) —*see also* Infestation, helminth
guinea B72
in intestine NEC B82.Ø
Worm-eaten soles A66.3
Worn out —*see* Exhaustion
cardiac
defibrillator (with synchronous cardiac pacemaker) Z45.Ø2
pacemaker
battery Z45.Ø1Ø
lead Z45.Ø18
device, implant or graft —*see* Complications, by site, mechanical
Worried well Z71.1
Worries R45.82
Wound check Z48.Ø-•
due to injury - code to Injury, by site, using appropriate seventh character for subsequent encounter
Wound, open T14.8-•
abdomen, abdominal
wall S31.1Ø9
with penetration into peritoneal cavity S31.6Ø9
bite —*see* Bite, abdomen, wall
epigastric region S31.1Ø2
with penetration into peritoneal cavity S31.6Ø2
bite —*see* Bite, abdomen, wall, epigastric region
laceration —*see* Laceration, abdomen, wall, epigastric region
puncture —*see* Puncture, abdomen, wall, epigastric region
Wound, open *(Continued)*
abdomen, abdominal *(Continued)*
wall *(Continued)*
laceration —*see* Laceration, abdomen, wall
left
lower quadrant S31.1Ø4
with penetration into peritoneal cavity S31.6Ø4
bite —*see* Bite, abdomen, wall, left, lower quadrant
laceration —*see* Laceration, abdomen, wall, left, lower quadrant
puncture —*see* Puncture, abdomen, wall, left, lower quadrant
upper quadrant S31.1Ø1
with penetration into peritoneal cavity S31.6Ø1
bite —*see* Bite, abdomen, wall, left, upper quadrant
laceration —*see* Laceration, abdomen, wall, left, upper quadrant
puncture —*see* Puncture, abdomen, wall, left, upper quadrant
periumbilic region S31.1Ø5
with penetration into peritoneal cavity S31.6Ø5
bite —*see* Bite, abdomen, wall, periumbilic region
laceration —*see* Laceration, abdomen, wall, periumbilic region
puncture —*see* Puncture, abdomen, wall, periumbilic region
puncture —*see* Puncture, abdomen, wall
right
lower quadrant S31.1Ø3
with penetration into peritoneal cavity S31.6Ø3
bite —*see* Bite, abdomen, wall, right, lower quadrant
laceration —*see* Laceration, abdomen, wall, right, lower quadrant
puncture —*see* Puncture, abdomen, wall, right, lower quadrant
upper quadrant S31.1ØØ
with penetration into peritoneal cavity S31.6ØØ
bite —*see* Bite, abdomen, wall, right, upper quadrant
laceration —*see* Laceration, abdomen, wall, right, upper quadrant
puncture —*see* Puncture, abdomen, wall, right, upper quadrant
alveolar (process) —*see* Wound, open, oral cavity
ankle S91.ØØ-•
bite —*see* Bite, ankle
laceration —*see* Laceration, ankle
puncture —*see* Puncture, ankle
antecubital space —*see* Wound, open, elbow
anterior chamber, eye —*see* Wound, open, ocular
anus S31.839
bite S31.835
laceration —*see* Laceration, anus
puncture —*see* Puncture, anus
arm (upper) S41.1Ø-•
with amputation —*see* Amputation, traumatic, arm
bite —*see* Bite, arm
forearm —*see* Wound, open, forearm
laceration —*see* Laceration, arm
puncture —*see* Puncture, arm
auditory canal (external) (meatus) —*see* Wound, open, ear
auricle, ear —*see* Wound, open, ear
axilla —*see* Wound, open, arm
Wound, open *(Continued)*
back —*see also* Wound, open, thorax, back
lower S31.ØØØ
with penetration into retroperitoneal space S31.ØØ1
bite —*see* Bite, back, lower
laceration —*see* Laceration, back, lower
puncture —*see* Puncture, back, lower
bite —*see* Bite
blood vessel —*see* Injury, blood vessel
breast S21.ØØ-•
with amputation —*see* Amputation, traumatic, breast
bite —*see* Bite, breast
laceration —*see* Laceration, breast
puncture —*see* Puncture, breast
buttock S31.8Ø9
bite —*see* Bite, buttock
laceration —*see* Laceration, buttock
left S31.829
puncture —*see* Puncture, buttock
right S31.819
calf —*see* Wound, open, leg
canaliculus lacrimalis —*see* Wound, open, eyelid
canthus, eye —*see* Wound, open, eyelid
cervical esophagus S11.2Ø
bite S11.25
laceration —*see* Laceration, esophagus, traumatic, cervical
puncture —*see* Puncture, cervical esophagus
cheek (external) SØ1.4Ø-•
bite —*see* Bite, cheek
internal —*see* Wound, open, oral cavity
laceration —*see* Laceration, cheek
puncture —*see* Puncture, cheek
chest wall —*see* Wound, open, thorax
chin —*see* Wound, open, head, specified site NEC
choroid —*see* Wound, open, ocular
ciliary body (eye) —*see* Wound, open, ocular
clitoris S31.4Ø
with amputation —*see* Amputation, traumatic, clitoris
bite S31.45
laceration —*see* Laceration, vulva
puncture —*see* Puncture, vulva
conjunctiva —*see* Wound, open, ocular
cornea —*see* Wound, open, ocular
costal region —*see* Wound, open, thorax
Descemet's membrane —*see* Wound, open, ocular
digit(s)
foot —*see* Wound, open, toe
hand —*see* Wound, open, finger
ear (canal) (external) SØ1.3Ø-•
with amputation —*see* Amputation, traumatic, ear
bite —*see* Bite, ear
drum SØ9.2-•
laceration —*see* Laceration, ear
puncture —*see* Puncture, ear
elbow S51.ØØ-•
bite —*see* Bite, elbow
laceration —*see* Laceration, elbow
puncture —*see* Puncture, elbow
epididymis —*see* Wound, open, testis
epigastric region S31.1Ø2
with penetration into peritoneal cavity S31.6Ø2
bite —*see* Bite, abdomen, wall, epigastric region
laceration —*see* Laceration, abdomen, wall, epigastric region
puncture —*see* Puncture, abdomen, wall, epigastric region
epiglottis —*see* Wound, open, neck, specified site NEC

W

Wound, open *(Continued)*
esophagus (thoracic) S27.819
cervical *—see* Wound, open, cervical esophagus
laceration S27.813
specified type NEC S27.818
eye *—see* Wound, open, ocular
eyeball *—see* Wound, open, ocular
eyebrow *—see* Wound, open, eyelid
eyelid S01.10- •
bite *—see* Bite, eyelid
laceration *—see* Laceration, eyelid
puncture *—see* Puncture, eyelid
face NEC *—see* Wound, open, head, specified site NEC
finger(s) S61.209
with
amputation *—see* Amputation, traumatic, finger
damage to nail S61.309
bite *—see* Bite, finger
index S61.208
with
damage to nail S61.308
left S61.201
with
damage to nail S61.301
right S61.200
with
damage to nail S61.300
laceration *—see* Laceration, finger
little S61.208
with
damage to nail S61.308
left S61.207
with damage to nail S61.307
right S61.206
with damage to nail S61.306
middle S61.208
with
damage to nail S61.308
left S61.203
with damage to nail S61.303
right S61.202
with damage to nail S61.302
puncture *—see* Puncture, finger
ring S61.208
with
damage to nail S61.308
left S61.205
with damage to nail S61.305
right S61.204
with damage to nail S61.304
flank *—see* Wound, open, abdomen, wall
foot (except toe(s) alone) S91.30- •
with amputation *—see* Amputation, traumatic, foot
bite *—see* Bite, foot
laceration *—see* Laceration, foot
puncture *—see* Puncture, foot
toe *—see* Wound, open, toe
forearm S51.80- •
with
amputation *—see* Amputation, traumatic, forearm
bite *—see* Bite, forearm
elbow only *—see* Wound, open, elbow
laceration *—see* Laceration, forearm
puncture *—see* Puncture, forearm
forehead *—see* Wound, open, head, specified site NEC
genital organs, external
with amputation *—see* Amputation, traumatic, genital organs
bite *—see* Bite, genital organ
female S31.502
vagina S31.40
vulva S31.40
laceration *—see* Laceration, genital organ

Wound, open *(Continued)*
genital organs, external *(Continued)*
male S31.501
penis S31.20
scrotum S31.30
testes S31.30
puncture *—see* Puncture, genital organ
globe (eye) *—see* Wound, open, ocular
groin *—see* Wound, open, abdomen, wall
gum *—see* Wound, open, oral cavity
hand S61.40- •
with
amputation *—see* Amputation, traumatic, hand
bite *—see* Bite, hand
finger(s) *—see* Wound, open, finger
laceration *—see* Laceration, hand
puncture *—see* Puncture, hand
thumb *—see* Wound, open, thumb
head S01.90
bite *—see* Bite, head
cheek *—see* Wound, open, cheek
ear *—see* Wound, open, ear
eyelid *—see* Wound, open, eyelid
laceration *—see* Laceration, head
lip *—see* Wound, open, lip
nose S01.20
oral cavity *—see* Wound, open, oral cavity
puncture *—see* Puncture, head
scalp *—see* Wound, open, scalp
specified site NEC S01.80
temporomandibular area *—see* Wound, open, cheek
heel *—see* Wound, open, foot
hip S71.00- •
with amputation *—see* Amputation, traumatic, hip
bite *—see* Bite, hip
laceration *—see* Laceration, hip
puncture *—see* Puncture, hip
hymen S31.40
bite *—see* Bite, vulva
laceration *—see* Laceration, vagina
puncture *—see* Puncture, vagina
hypochondrium S31.109
bite *—see* Bite, hypochondrium
laceration *—see* Laceration, hypochondrium
puncture *—see* Puncture, hypochondrium
hypogastric region S31.109
bite *—see* Bite, hypogastric region
laceration *—see* Laceration, hypogastric region
puncture *—see* Puncture, hypogastric region
iliac (region) *—see* Wound, open, inguinal region
inguinal region S31.109
bite *—see* Bite, abdomen, wall, lower quadrant
laceration *—see* Laceration, inguinal region
puncture *—see* Puncture, inguinal region
instep *—see* Wound, open, foot
interscapular region *—see* Wound, open, thorax, back
intraocular *—see* Wound, open, ocular
iris *—see* Wound, open, ocular
jaw *—see* Wound, open, head, specified site NEC
knee S81.00- •
bite *—see* Bite, knee
laceration *—see* Laceration, knee
puncture *—see* Puncture, knee
labium (majus) (minus) *—see* Wound, open, vulva
laceration *—see* Laceration, by site
lacrimal duct *—see* Wound, open, eyelid

Wound, open *(Continued)*
larynx S11.019
bite *—see* Bite, larynx
laceration *—see* Laceration, larynx
puncture *—see* Puncture, larynx
left
lower quadrant S31.104
with penetration into peritoneal cavity S31.604
bite *—see* Bite, abdomen, wall, left, lower quadrant
laceration *—see* Laceration, abdomen, wall, left, lower quadrant
puncture *—see* Puncture, abdomen, wall, left, lower quadrant
upper quadrant S31.101
with penetration into peritoneal cavity S31.601
bite *—see* Bite, abdomen, wall, left, upper quadrant
laceration *—see* Laceration, abdomen, wall, left, upper quadrant
puncture *—see* Puncture, abdomen, wall, left, upper quadrant
leg (lower) S81.80- •
with amputation *—see* Amputation, traumatic, leg
ankle *—see* Wound, open, ankle
bite *—see* Bite, leg
foot *—see* Wound, open, foot
knee *—see* Wound, open, knee
laceration *—see* Laceration, leg
puncture *—see* Puncture, leg
toe *—see* Wound, open, toe
upper *—see* Wound, open, thigh
lip S01.501
bite *—see* Bite, lip
laceration *—see* Laceration, lip
puncture *—see* Puncture, lip
loin S31.109
bite *—see* Bite, abdomen, wall
laceration *—see* Laceration, loin
puncture *—see* Puncture, loin
lower back *—see* Wound, open, back, lower
lumbar region *—see* Wound, open, back, lower
malar region *—see* Wound, open, head, specified site NEC
mammary *—see* Wound, open, breast
mastoid region *—see* Wound, open, head, specified site NEC
mouth *—see* Wound, open, oral cavity
nail
finger *—see* Wound, open, finger, with damage to nail
toe *—see* Wound, open, toe, with damage to nail
nape (neck) *—see* Wound, open, neck
nasal (septum) (sinus) *—see* Wound, open, nose
nasopharynx *—see* Wound, open, head, specified site NEC
neck S11.90
bite *—see* Bite, neck
involving
cervical esophagus S11.20
larynx *—see* Wound, open, larynx
pharynx S11.20
thyroid S11.10
trachea (cervical) S11.029
bite *—see* Bite, trachea
laceration S11.021
with foreign body S11.022
puncture S11.023
with foreign body S11.024
laceration *—see* Laceration, neck
puncture *—see* Puncture, neck
specified site NEC S11.80
specified type NEC S11.89

W

Wound, open *(Continued)*
nose (septum) (sinus) SØ1.2Ø
with amputation —*see* Amputation, traumatic, nose
bite —*see* Bite, nose
laceration —*see* Laceration, nose
puncture —*see* Puncture, nose
ocular SØ5.9Ø
avulsion (traumatic enucleation) SØ5.7-●
eyeball SØ5.6-●
with foreign body SØ5.5-●
eyelid —*see* Wound, open, eyelid
laceration and rupture SØ5.3-●
with prolapse or loss of intraocular tissue SØ5.2-●
orbit (penetrating) (with or without foreign body) SØ5.4-●
periocular area —*see* Wound, open, eyelid
specified NEC SØ5.8X-●
oral cavity SØ1.5Ø2
bite SØ1.552
laceration —*see* Laceration, oral cavity
puncture —*see* Puncture, oral cavity
orbit —*see* Wound, open, ocular, orbit
palate —*see* Wound, open, oral cavity
palm —*see* Wound, open, hand
pelvis, pelvic —*see also* Wound, open, back, lower
girdle —*see* Wound, open, hip
penetrating —*see* Puncture, by site
penis S31.2Ø
with amputation —*see* Amputation, traumatic, penis
bite S31.25
laceration —*see* Laceration, penis
puncture —*see* Puncture, penis
perineum
bite —*see* Bite, perineum
female S31.5Ø2
laceration —*see* Laceration, perineum
male S31.5Ø1
puncture —*see* Puncture, perineum
periocular area (with or without lacrimal passages) —*see* Wound, open, eyelid
periumbilic region S31.1Ø5
with penetration into peritoneal cavity S31.6Ø5
bite —*see* Bite, abdomen, wall, periumbilic region
laceration —*see* Laceration, abdomen, wall, periumbilic region
puncture —*see* Puncture, abdomen, wall, periumbilic region
phalanges
finger —*see* Wound, open, finger
toe —*see* Wound, open, toe
pharynx S11.2Ø
pinna —*see* Wound, open, ear
popliteal space —*see* Wound, open, knee
prepuce —*see* Wound, open, penis
pubic region —*see* Wound, open, back, lower
pudendum —*see* Wound, open, genital organs, external
puncture wound —*see* Puncture
rectovaginal septum —*see* Wound, open, vagina
right
lower quadrant S31.1Ø3
with penetration into peritoneal cavity S31.6Ø3
bite —*see* Bite, abdomen, wall, right, lower quadrant
laceration —*see* Laceration, abdomen, wall, right, lower quadrant
puncture —*see* Puncture, abdomen, wall, right, lower quadrant
upper quadrant S31.1ØØ
with penetration into peritoneal cavity S31.6ØØ

Wound, open *(Continued)*
right *(Continued)*
upper quadrant *(Continued)*
bite —*see* Bite, abdomen, wall, right, upper quadrant
laceration —*see* Laceration, abdomen, wall, right, upper quadrant
puncture —*see* Puncture, abdomen, wall, right, upper quadrant
sacral region —*see* Wound, open, back, lower
sacroiliac region —*see* Wound, open, back, lower
salivary gland —*see* Wound, open, oral cavity
scalp SØ1.ØØ
bite SØ1.Ø5
laceration —*see* Laceration, scalp
puncture —*see* Puncture, scalp
scalpel, newborn (birth injury) P15.8
scapular region —*see* Wound, open, shoulder
sclera —*see* Wound, open, ocular
scrotum S31.3Ø
with amputation —*see* Amputation, traumatic, scrotum
bite S31.35
laceration —*see* Laceration, scrotum
puncture —*see* Puncture, scrotum
shin —*see* Wound, open, leg
shoulder S41.ØØ-●
with amputation —*see* Amputation, traumatic, arm
bite —*see* Bite, shoulder
laceration —*see* Laceration, shoulder
puncture —*see* Puncture, shoulder
skin NOS T14.8
spermatic cord —*see* Wound, open, testis
sternal region —*see* Wound, open, thorax, front wall
submaxillary region —*see* Wound, open, head, specified site NEC
submental region —*see* Wound, open, head, specified site NEC
subungual
finger(s) —*see* Wound, open, finger
toe(s) —*see* Wound, open, toe
supraclavicular region —*see* Wound, open, neck, specified site NEC
temple, temporal region —*see* Wound, open, head, specified site NEC
temporomandibular area —*see* Wound, open, cheek
testis S31.3Ø
with amputation —*see* Amputation, traumatic, testes
bite S31.35
laceration —*see* Laceration, testis
puncture —*see* Puncture, testis
thigh S71.1Ø-●
with amputation —*see* Amputation, traumatic, hip
bite —*see* Bite, thigh
laceration —*see* Laceration, thigh
puncture —*see* Puncture, thigh
thorax, thoracic (wall) S21.9Ø
back S21.2Ø-●
with penetration S21.4Ø
bite —*see* Bite, thorax
breast —*see* Wound, open, breast
front S21.1Ø-●
with penetration S21.3Ø
laceration —*see* Laceration, thorax
puncture —*see* Puncture, thorax
throat —*see* Wound, open, neck
thumb S61.ØØ9
with
amputation —*see* Amputation, traumatic, thumb
damage to nail S61.1Ø9
bite —*see* Bite, thumb
laceration —*see* Laceration, thumb

Wound, open *(Continued)*
thumb *(Continued)*
left S61.ØØ2
with
damage to nail S61.1Ø2
puncture —*see* Puncture, thumb
right S61.ØØ1
with
damage to nail S61.1Ø1
thyroid (gland) —*see* Wound, open, neck, thyroid
toe(s) S91.1Ø9
with
amputation —*see* Amputation, traumatic, toe
damage to nail S91.2Ø9
bite —*see* Bite, toe
great S91.1Ø3
with
damage to nail S91.2Ø3
left S91.1Ø2
with
damage to nail S91.2Ø2
right S91.1Ø1
with
damage to nail S91.2Ø1
laceration —*see* Laceration, toe
lesser S91.1Ø6
with
damage to nail S91.2Ø6
left S91.1Ø5
with
damage to nail S91.2Ø5
right S91.1Ø4
with
damage to nail S91.2Ø4
puncture —*see* Puncture, toe
tongue —*see* Wound, open, oral cavity
trachea (cervical region) —*see* Wound, open, neck, trachea
tunica vaginalis —*see* Wound, open, testis
tympanum, tympanic membrane SØ9.2-●
laceration —*see* Laceration, ear, drum
puncture —*see* Puncture, tympanum
umbilical region —*see* Wound, open, abdomen, wall, periumbilic region
uvula —*see* Wound, open, oral cavity
vagina S31.4Ø
bite S31.45
laceration —*see* Laceration, vagina
puncture —*see* Puncture, vagina
vitreous (humor) —*see* Wound, open, ocular
vocal cord S11.Ø39
bite —*see* Bite, vocal cord
laceration S11.Ø31
with foreign body S11.Ø32
puncture S11.Ø33
with foreign body S11.Ø34
vulva S31.4Ø
with amputation —*see* Amputation, traumatic, vulva
bite S31.45
laceration —*see* Laceration, vulva
puncture —*see* Puncture, vulva
wrist S61.5Ø-●
bite —*see* Bite, wrist
laceration —*see* Laceration, wrist
puncture —*see* Puncture, wrist
Wound, superficial —*see* Injury (*see also* specified injury type)
Wright's syndrome G54.Ø
Wrist —*see* condition
Wrong drug (by accident) (given in error) —*see* Table of Drugs and Chemicals, by drug, poisoning
Wry neck —*see* Torticollis
Wuchereria (bancrofti) infestation B74.Ø
Wuchereriasis B74.Ø
Wuchernde Struma Langhans C73

X

Xanthelasma (eyelid) (palpebrarum) HØ2.6Ø
  left HØ2.66
    lower HØ2.65
    upper HØ2.64
  right HØ2.63
    lower HØ2.62
    upper HØ2.61
Xanthelasmatosis (essential) E78.2
Xanthinuria, hereditary E79.8
Xanthoastrocytoma
  specified site —*see* Neoplasm, malignant, by site
  unspecified site C71.9
Xanthofibroma —*see* Neoplasm, connective tissue, benign
Xanthogranuloma D76.3
Xanthoma(s), xanthomatosis (primary) (familial) (hereditary) E75.5
  with
    hyperlipoproteinemia
      Type I E78.3
      Type III E78.2
      Type IV E78.1
      Type V E78.3
  bone (generalisata) C96.5
  cerebrotendinous E75.5
  cutaneotendinous E75.5

Xanthoma(s), xanthomatosis *(Continued)*
  disseminatum (skin) E78.2
  eruptive E78.2
  hypercholesterinemic E78.ØØ
  hypercholesterolemic E78.ØØ
  hyperlipidemic E78.5
  joint E75.5
  multiple (skin) E78.2
  tendon (sheath) E75.5
  tuberosum E78.2
  tuberous E78.2
  tubo-eruptive E78.2
  verrucous, oral mucosa K13.4
Xanthosis R23.8
Xenophobia F4Ø.1Ø
Xeroderma —*see also* Ichthyosis
  acquired L85.Ø
    eyelid HØ1.149
      left HØ1.146
        lower HØ1.145
        upper HØ1.144
      right HØ1.143
        lower HØ1.142
        upper HØ1.141
  pigmentosum Q82.1
  vitamin A deficiency E5Ø.8
Xerophthalmia (vitamin A deficiency) E5Ø.7
  unrelated to vitamin A deficiency —*see* Keratoconjunctivitis

Xerosis
  conjunctiva H11.14-●
    with Bitot's spots —*see also* Pigmentation, conjunctiva
      vitamin A deficiency E5Ø.1
    vitamin A deficiency E5Ø.Ø
  cornea H18.89-●
    with ulceration —*see* Ulcer, cornea
      vitamin A deficiency E5Ø.3
    vitamin A deficiency E5Ø.2
  cutis L85.3
  skin L85.3
Xerostomia K11.7
Xiphopagus Q89.4
XO syndrome Q96.9
X-ray (of)
  abnormal findings —*see* Abnormal, diagnostic imaging
  breast (mammogram) (routine) Z12.31
  chest
    routine (as part of a general medical examination) ZØØ.ØØ
      with abnormal findings ZØØ.Ø1
  routine (as part of a general medical examination) ZØØ.ØØ
    with abnormal findings ZØØ.Ø1
XXXXY syndrome Q98.1
XXY syndrome Q98.Ø

Y

Yaba pox virus disease B08.72
Yatapoxvirus B08.70
  specified NEC B08.79
Yawning R06.89
  psychogenic F45.8
Yaws A66.9
  bone lesions A66.6
  butter A66.1
  chancre A66.0
  cutaneous, less than five years after infection A66.2
  early (cutaneous) (macular) (maculopapular) (micropapular) (papular) A66.2
    frambeside A66.2
    skin lesions NEC A66.2
  eyelid A66.2
  ganglion A66.6
  gangosis, gangosa A66.5
  gumma, gummata A66.4
    bone A66.6
  gummatous
    frambeside A66.4
    osteitis A66.6
    periostitis A66.6
  hydrarthrosis —*see also* subcategory M14.8- • A66.6
  hyperkeratosis (early) (late) A66.3
Yaws *(Continued)*
  initial lesions A66.0
  joint lesions —*see also* subcategory M14.8- • A66.6
  juxta-articular nodules A66.7
  late nodular (ulcerated) A66.4
  latent (without clinical manifestations) (with positive serology) A66.8
  mother A66.0
  mucosal A66.7
  multiple papillomata A66.1
  nodular, late (ulcerated) A66.4
  osteitis A66.6
  papilloma, plantar or palmar A66.1
  periostitis (hypertrophic) A66.6
  specified NEC A66.7
  ulcers A66.4
  wet crab A66.1
Yeast infection —*see also* Candidiasis B37.9
Yellow
  atrophy (liver) —*see* Failure, hepatic
  fever —*see* Fever, yellow
  jack —*see* Fever, yellow
  jaundice —*see* Jaundice
  nail syndrome L60.5
Yersiniosis —*see also* Infection, Yersinia
  extraintestinal A28.2
  intestinal A04.6

Z

Zahorsky's syndrome (herpangina) B08.5
➡ Zellweger's syndrome E71.510
Zenker's diverticulum (esophagus) K22.5
Ziehen-Oppenheim disease G24.1
Zieve's syndrome K70.0
Zika NOS A92.5
  congenital P35.4
Zinc
  deficiency, dietary E60
  metabolism disorder E83.2
Zollinger-Ellison syndrome E16.4
Zona —*see* Herpes, zoster
Zoophobia F40.218
Zoster (herpes) —*see* Herpes, zoster
Zygomycosis B46.9
  specified NEC B46.8
Zymotic —*see* condition

Y, Z

ICD-10-CM Table of Neoplasms

The list below gives the code numbers for neoplasms by anatomical site. For each site there are six possible code numbers according to whether the neoplasm in question is malignant, benign, in situ, of uncertain behavior, or of unspecified nature. The description of the neoplasm will often indicate which of the six columns is appropriate; e.g., malignant melanoma of skin, benign fibroadenoma of breast, carcinoma in situ of cervix uteri.

Where such descriptors are not present, the remainder of the Index should be consulted where guidance is given to the appropriate column for each morphological (histological) variety listed; e.g., Mesonephroma — *see Neoplasm, malignant;* Embryoma — *see also Neoplasm, uncertain behavior;* Disease, Bowen's — *see Neoplasm, skin, in situ.* However, the guidance in the Index can be overridden if one of the descriptors mentioned above is present; e.g., malignant adenoma of colon is coded to C18.9 and not to D12.6 as the adjective "Malignant" overrides the Index entry 'Adenoma — *see also Neoplasm, benign.*'

Codes listed with a dash -, following the code have a required additional character for laterality. The Tablular must be reviewed for the complete code.

	Malignant Primary	Malignant Secondary	Ca in situ	Benign	Uncertain Behavior	Unspecified Behavior
Neoplasm, neoplastic	C8Ø.1	C79.9	DØ9.9	D36.9	D48.9	D49.9
abdomen, abdominal	C76.2	C79.8-●	DØ9.8	D36.7	D48.7	D49.89
cavity	C76.2	C79.8-●	DØ9.8	D36.7	D48.7	D49.89
organ	C76.2	C79.8-●	DØ9.8	D36.7	D48.7	D49.89
viscera	C76.2	C79.8-●	DØ9.8	D36.7	D48.7	D49.89
wall — *see also Neoplasm, abdomen, wall, skin*	C44.5Ø9	C79.2-●	DØ4.5	D23.5	D48.5	D49.2
connective tissue	C49.4	C79.8-●	—	D21.4	D48.1	D49.2
skin	C44.5Ø9					
basal cell carcinoma	C44.519	—	—	—	—	—
specified type NEC	C44.599	—	—	—	—	—
squamous cell carcinoma	C44.529	—	—	—	—	—
abdominopelvic	C76.8	C79.8-●	—	D36.7	D48.7	D49.89
accessory sinus — *see Neoplasm, sinus*						
acoustic nerve	C72.4-●	C79.49	—	D33.3	D43.3	D49.7
adenoid (pharynx) (tissue)	C11.1	C79.89	DØØ.Ø8	D1Ø.6	D37.Ø5	D49.Ø
adipose tissue — *see also Neoplasm, connective tissue*	C49.4	C79.89	—	D21.9	D48.1	D49.2
adnexa (uterine)	C57.4	C79.89	DØ7.39	D28.7	D39.8	D49.59
adrenal	C74.9-●	C79.7-●	DØ9.3	D35.Ø-●	D44.1-●	D49.7
capsule	C74.9-●	C79.7-●	DØ9.3	D35.Ø-●	D44.1-●	D49.7
cortex	C74.Ø-●	C79.7-●	DØ9.3	D35.Ø-●	D44.1-●	D49.7
gland	C74.9-●	C79.7-●	DØ9.3	D35.Ø-●	D44.1-●	D49.7
medulla	C74.1-●	C79.7-●	DØ9.3	D35.Ø-●	D44.1-●	D49.7
ala nasi (external) — *see also Neoplasm, skin, nose*	C44.3Ø1	C79.2	DØ4.39	D23.39	D48.5	D49.2

	Malignant Primary	Malignant Secondary	Ca in situ	Benign	Uncertain Behavior	Unspecified Behavior
alimentary canal or tract NEC	C26.9	C78.8Ø	DØ1.9	D13.9	D37.9	D49.Ø
alveolar	CØ3.9	C79.89	DØØ.Ø3	D1Ø.39	D37.Ø9	D49.Ø
mucosa	CØ3.9	C79.89	DØØ.Ø3	D1Ø.39	D37.Ø9	D49.Ø
lower	CØ3.1	C79.89	DØØ.Ø3	D1Ø.39	D37.Ø9	D49.Ø
upper	CØ3.Ø	C79.89	DØØ.Ø3	D1Ø.39	D37.Ø9	D49.Ø
ridge or process	C41.1	C79.51	—	D16.5-●	D48.Ø	D49.2
carcinoma	CØ3.9	C79.8-●	—	—	—	—
lower	CØ3.1	C79.8-●	—	—	—	—
upper	CØ3.Ø	C79.8-●	—	—	—	—
lower	C41.1	C79.51	—	D16.5-●	D48.Ø	D49.2
mucosa	CØ3.9	C79.89	DØØ.Ø3	D1Ø.39	D37.Ø9	D49.Ø
lower	CØ3.1	C79.89	DØØ.Ø3	D1Ø.39	D37.Ø9	D49.Ø
upper	CØ3.Ø	C79.89	DØØ.Ø3	D1Ø.39	D37.Ø9	D49.Ø
upper	C41.Ø	C79.51	—	D16.4-●	D48.Ø	D49.2
sulcus	CØ6.1	C79.89	DØØ.Ø2	D1Ø.39	D37.Ø9	D49.Ø
alveolus	CØ3.9	C79.89	DØØ.Ø3	D1Ø.39	D37.Ø9	D49.Ø
lower	CØ3.1	C79.89	DØØ.Ø3	D1Ø.39	D37.Ø9	D49.Ø
upper	CØ3.Ø	C79.89	DØØ.Ø3	D1Ø.39	D37.Ø9	D49.Ø
ampulla of Vater	C24.1	C78.89	DØ1.5	D13.5	D37.6	D49.Ø
ankle NEC	C76.5-●	C79.89	DØ4.7-●	D36.7	D48.7	D49.89
anorectum, anorectal (junction)	C21.8	C78.5	DØ1.3	D12.9	D37.8	D49.Ø
antecubital fossa or space	C76.4-●	C79.89	DØ4.6-●	D36.7	D48.7	D49.89
antrum (Highmore) (maxillary)	C31.Ø	C78.39	DØ2.3	D14.Ø	D38.5	D49.1
pyloric	C16.3	C78.89	DØØ.2	D13.1	D37.1	D49.Ø
tympanicum	C3Ø.1	C78.39	DØ2.3	D14.Ø	D38.5	D49.1
anus, anal	C21.Ø	C78.5	DØ1.3	D12.9	D37.8	D49.Ø
canal	C21.1	C78.5	DØ1.3	D12.9	D37.8	D49.Ø
cloacogenic zone	C21.2	C78.5	DØ1.3	D12.9	D37.8	D49.Ø
margin — *see also Neoplasm, anus, skin*	C44.5ØØ	C79.2	DØ4.5	D23.5	D48.5	D49.2
overlapping lesion with rectosigmoid junction or rectum	C21.8	—	—	—	—	—
skin	C44.5ØØ	C79.2	DØ4.5	D23.5	D48.5	D49.2
basal cell carcinoma	C44.51Ø	—	—	—	—	—
specified type NEC	C44.59Ø	—	—	—	—	—
squamous cell carcinoma	C44.52Ø	—	—	—	—	—
sphincter	C21.1	C78.5	DØ1.3	D12.9	D37.8	D49.Ø
aorta (thoracic)	C49.3	C79.89	—	D21.3	D48.1	D49.2
abdominal	C49.4	C79.89	—	D21.4	D48.1	D49.2
aortic body	C75.5	C79.89	—	D35.6	D44.7	D49.7
aponeurosis	C49.9	C79.89	—	D21.9	D48.1	D49.2
palmar	C49.1-●	C79.89	—	D21.1-●	D48.1	D49.2
plantar	C49.2-●	C79.89	—	D21.2-●	D48.1	D49.2

	Malignant Primary	Malignant Secondary	Ca in situ	Benign	Uncertain Behavior	Unspecified Behavior
appendix	C18.1	C78.5	D01.0	D12.1	D37.3	D49.0
arachnoid	C70.9	C79.49	—	D32.9	D42.9	D49.7
cerebral	C70.0	C79.32	—	D32.0	D42.0	D49.7
spinal	C70.1	C79.49	—	D32.1	D42.1	D49.7
areola	C50.0-•	C79.81	D05.-•	D24.-•	D48.6-•	D49.3
arm NEC	C76.4-•	C79.89	D04.6-•	D36.7	D48.7	D49.89
artery — *see Neoplasm, connective tissue*						
aryepiglottic fold	C13.1	C79.89	D00.08	D10.7	D37.05	D49.0
hypopharyngeal aspect	C13.1	C79.89	D00.08	D10.7	D37.05	D49.0
laryngeal aspect	C32.1	C78.39	D02.0	D14.1	D38.0	D49.1
marginal zone	C13.1	C79.89	D00.08	D10.7	D37.05	D49.0
arytenoid (cartilage)	C32.3	C78.39	D02.0	D14.1	D38.0	D49.1
fold — *see Neoplasm, aryepiglottic*						
associated with transplanted organ	C80.2	—	—	—	—	—
atlas	C41.2	C79.51	—	D16.6	D48.0	D49.2
atrium, cardiac	C38.0	C79.89	—	D15.1	D48.7	D49.89
auditory						
canal (external) (skin)	C44.20-•	C79.2	D04.2-•	D23.2-•	D48.5	D49.2
internal	C30.1	C78.39	D02.3	D14.0	D38.5	D49.1
nerve	C72.4-•	C79.49	—	D33.3	D43.3	D49.7
tube	C30.1	C78.39	D02.3	D14.0	D38.5	D49.1
opening	C11.2	C79.89	D00.08	D10.6	D37.05	D49.0
auricle, ear — *see also Neoplasm, skin, ear*	C44.20-•	C79.2	D04.2-•	D23.2-•	D48.5	D49.2
auricular canal (external) — *see also Neoplasm, skin, ear*	C44.20-•	C79.2	D04.2-•	D23.2-•	D48.5	D49.2
internal	C30.1	C78.39	D02.3	D14.0	D38.5	D49.2
autonomic nerve or nervous system NEC *(see Neoplasm, nerve, peripheral)*						
axilla, axillary	C76.1	C79.89	D09.8	D36.7	D48.7	D49.89
fold — *see also Neoplasm, skin, trunk*	C44.509	C79.2	D04.5	D23.5	D48.5	D49.2
back NEC	C76.8	C79.89	D04.5	D36.7	D48.7	D49.89
Bartholin's gland	C51.0	C79.82	D07.1	D28.0	D39.8	D49.59
basal ganglia	C71.0	C79.31	—	D33.0	D43.0	D49.6
basis pedunculi	C71.7	C79.31	—	D33.1	D43.1	D49.6
bile or biliary (tract)	C24.9	C78.89	D01.5	D13.5	D37.6	D49.0
canaliculi (biliferi) (intrahepatic)	C22.1	C78.7	D01.5	D13.4	D37.6	D49.0
canals, interlobular	C22.1	C78.89	D01.5	D13.4	D37.6	D49.0

	Malignant Primary	Malignant Secondary	Ca in situ	Benign	Uncertain Behavior	Unspecified Behavior
bile or biliary *(Continued)*						
duct or passage (common) (cystic) (extrahepatic)	C24.0	C78.89	D01.5	D13.5	D37.6	D49.0
interlobular	C22.1	C78.89	D01.5	D13.4	D37.6	D49.0
intrahepatic	C22.1	C78.7	D01.5	D13.4	D37.6	D49.0
and extrahepatic	C24.8	C78.89	D01.5	D13.5	D37.6	D49.0
bladder (urinary)	C67.9	C79.11	D09.0	D30.3	D41.4	D49.4
dome	C67.1	C79.11	D09.0	D30.3	D41.4	D49.4
neck	C67.5	C79.11	D09.0	D30.3	D41.4	D49.4
orifice	C67.9	C79.11	D09.0	D30.3	D41.4	D49.4
ureteric	C67.6	C79.11	D09.0	D30.3	D41.4	D49.4
urethral	C67.5	C79.11	D09.0	D30.3	D41.4	D49.4
overlapping lesion	C67.8	—	—	—	—	—
sphincter	C67.8	C79.11	D09.0	D30.3	D41.4	D49.4
trigone	C67.0	C79.11	D09.0	D30.3	D41.4	D49.4
urachus	C67.7	C79.11	D09.0	D30.3	D41.4	D49.4
wall	C67.9	C79.11	D09.0	D30.3	D41.4	D49.4
anterior	C67.3	C79.11	D09.0	D30.3	D41.4	D49.4
lateral	C67.2	C79.11	D09.0	D30.3	D41.4	D49.4
posterior	C67.4	C79.11	D09.0	D30.3	D41.4	D49.4
blood vessel — *see Neoplasm, connective tissue*						
bone (periosteum)	C41.9	C79.51	—	D16.9-•	D48.0	D49.2
acetabulum	C41.4	C79.51	—	D16.8-•	D48.0	D49.2
ankle	C40.3-•	C79.51	—	D16.3-•	—	—
arm NEC	C40.0-•	C79.51	—	D16.0-•	—	—
astragalus	C40.3-•	C79.51	—	D16.3-•	—	—
atlas	C41.2	C79.51	—	D16.6-•	D48.0	D49.2
axis	C41.2	C79.51	—	D16.6-•	D48.0	D49.2
back NEC	C41.2	C79.51	—	D16.6-•	D48.0	D49.2
calcaneus	C40.3-•	C79.51	—	D16.3-•	—	—
calvarium	C41.0	C79.51	—	D16.4-•	D48.0	D49.2
carpus (any)	C40.1-•	C79.51	—	D16.1-•	—	—
cartilage NEC	C41.9	C79.51	—	D16.9-•	D48.0	D49.2
clavicle	C41.3	C79.51	—	D16.7-•	D48.0	D49.2
clivus	C41.0	C79.51	—	D16.4-•	D48.0	D49.2
coccygeal vertebra	C41.4	C79.51	—	D16.8-•	D48.0	D49.2
coccyx	C41.4	C79.51	—	D16.8-•	D48.0	D49.2
costal cartilage	C41.3	C79.51	—	D16.7-•	D48.0	D49.2
costovertebral joint	C41.3	C79.51	—	D16.7-•	D48.0	D49.2
cranial	C41.0	C79.51	—	D16.4-•	D48.0	D49.2
cuboid	C40.3-•	C79.51	—	D16.3-•	—	—
cuneiform	C41.9	C79.51	—	D16.9-•	D48.0	D49.2
elbow	C40.0-•	C79.51	—	D16.0-•	—	—

	Malignant Primary	Malignant Secondary	Ca in situ	Benign	Uncertain Behavior	Unspecified Behavior
bone *(Continued)*						
ethmoid (labyrinth)	C41.Ø	C79.51	—	D16.4-•	D48.Ø	D49.2
face	C41.Ø	C79.51	—	D16.4-•	D48.Ø	D49.2
femur (any part)	C40.2-•	C79.51	—	D16.2-•	—	—
fibula (any part)	C40.2-•	C79.51	—	D16.2-•	—	—
finger (any)	C40.1-•	C79.51	—	D16.1-•	—	—
foot	C40.3-•	C79.51	—	D16.3-•	—	—
forearm	C40.Ø-•	C79.51	—	D16.Ø-•	—	—
frontal	C41.Ø	C79.51	—	D16.4-•	D48.Ø	D49.2
hand	C40.1-•	C79.51	—	D16.1-•	—	—
heel	C40.3-•	C79.51	—	D16.3-•	—	—
hip	C41.4	C79.51	—	D16.8-•	D48.Ø	D49.2
humerus (any part)	C40.Ø-•	C79.51	—	D16.Ø-•	—	—
hyoid	C41.Ø	C79.51	—	D16.4-•	D48.Ø	D49.2
ilium	C41.4	C79.51	—	D16.8-•	D48.Ø	D49.2
innominate	C41.4	C79.51	—	D16.8-•	D48.Ø	D49.2
intervertebral cartilage or disc	C41.2	C79.51	—	D16.6-•	D48.Ø	D49.2
ischium	C41.4	C79.51	—	D16.8-•	D48.Ø	D49.2
jaw (lower)	C41.1	C79.51	—	D16.5-•	D48.Ø	D49.2
knee	C40.2-•	C79.51	—	D16.2-•	—	—
leg NEC	C40.2-•	C79.51	—	D16.2-•	—	—
limb NEC	C40.9-•	C79.51	—	D16.9-•	—	—
lower (long bones)	C40.2-•	C79.51	—	D16.2-•	—	—
short bones	C40.3-•	C79.51	—	D16.3-•	—	—
upper (long bones)	C40.Ø-•	C79.51	—	D16.Ø-•	—	—
short bones	C40.1-•	C79.51	—	D16.1-•	—	—
malar	C41.Ø	C79.51	—	D16.4-•	D48.Ø	D49.2
mandible	C41.1	C79.51	—	D16.5-•	D48.Ø	D49.2
marrow NEC (any bone)	C96.9	C79.52	—	—	D47.9	D49.89
mastoid	C41.Ø	C79.51	—	D16.4-•	D48.Ø	D49.2
maxilla, maxillary (superior)	C41.Ø	C79.51	—	D16.4-•	D48.Ø	D49.2
inferior	C41.1	C79.51	—	D16.5-•	D48.Ø	D49.2
metacarpus (any)	C40.1-•	C79.51	—	D16.1-•	—	—
metatarsus (any)	C40.3-•	C79.51	—	D16.3-•	—	—
overlapping sites	C40.8-•	—	—	—	—	—
navicular						
ankle	C40.3-•	C79.51	—	—	—	—
hand	C40.1-•	C79.51	—	—	—	—
nose, nasal	C41.Ø	C79.51	—	D16.4-•	D48.Ø	D49.2
occipital	C41.Ø	C79.51	—	D16.4-•	D48.Ø	D49.2
orbit	C41.Ø	C79.51	—	D16.4-•	D48.Ø	D49.2
parietal	C41.Ø	C79.51	—	D16.4-•	D48.Ø	D49.2
patella	C40.2-•	C79.51	—	—	—	—
pelvic	C41.4	C79.51	—	D16.8	D48.Ø	D49.2

	Malignant Primary	Malignant Secondary	Ca in situ	Benign	Uncertain Behavior	Unspecified Behavior
bone *(Continued)*						
phalanges						
foot	C40.3-•	C79.51	—	—	—	—
hand	C40.1-•	C79.51	—	—	—	—
pubic	C41.4	C79.51	—	D16.8	D48.Ø	D49.2
radius (any part)	C40.Ø-•	C79.51	—	D16.Ø-•	—	—
rib	C41.3	C79.51	—	D16.7	D48.Ø	D49.2
sacral vertebra	C41.4	C79.51	—	D16.8	D48.Ø	D49.2
sacrum	C41.4	C79.51	—	D16.8	D48.Ø	D49.2
scaphoid	—	—	—	—	—	—
of ankle	C40.3-•	C79.51	—	—	—	—
of hand	C40.1-•	C79.51	—	—	—	—
scapula (any part)	C40.Ø-•	C79.51	—	D16.Ø-•	—	—
sella turcica	C41.Ø	C79.51	—	D16.4-•	D48.Ø	D49.2
shoulder	C40.Ø-•	C79.51	—	D16.Ø-•	—	—
skull	C41.Ø	C79.51	—	D16.4-•	D48.Ø	D49.2
sphenoid	C41.Ø	C79.51	—	D16.4-•	D48.Ø	D49.2
spine, spinal (column)	C41.2	C79.51	—	D16.6	D48.Ø	D49.2
coccyx	C41.4	C79.51	—	D16.8	D48.Ø	D49.2
sacrum	C41.4	C79.51	—	D16.8	D48.Ø	D49.2
sternum	C41.3	C79.51	—	D16.7	D48.Ø	D49.2
tarsus (any)	C40.3-•	C79.51	—	—	—	—
temporal	C41.Ø	C79.51	—	D16.4-•	D48.Ø	D49.2
thumb	C40.1-•	C79.51	—	—	—	—
tibia (any part)	C40.2-•	C79.51	—	—	—	—
toe (any)	C40.3-•	C79.51	—	—	—	—
trapezium	C40.1-•	C79.51	—	—	—	—
trapezoid	C40.1-•	C79.51	—	—	—	—
turbinate	C41.Ø	C79.51	—	D16.4-•	D48.Ø	D49.2
ulna (any part)	C40.Ø-•	C79.51	—	D16.Ø-•	—	—
unciform	C40.1-•	C79.51	—	—	—	—
vertebra (column)	C41.2	C79.51	—	D16.6	D48.Ø	D49.2
coccyx	C41.4	C79.51	—	D16.8	D48.Ø	D49.2
sacrum	C41.4	C79.51	—	D16.8	D48.Ø	D49.2
vomer	C41.Ø	C79.51	—	D16.4-•	D48.Ø	D49.2
wrist	C40.1-•	C79.51	—	—	—	—
xiphoid process	C41.3	C79.51	—	D16.7	D48.Ø	D49.2
zygomatic	C41.Ø	C79.51	—	D16.4-•	D48.Ø	D49.2
book-leaf (mouth)	CØ6.89	C79.89	DØØ.ØØ	D1Ø.39	D37.Ø9	D49.Ø
bowel — *see Neoplasm, intestine*						
brachial plexus	C47.1-•	C79.89	—	D36.12	D48.2	D49.2
brain NEC	C71.9	C79.31	—	D33.2	D43.2	D49.6
basal ganglia	C71.Ø	C79.31	—	D33.Ø	D43.Ø	D49.6
cerebellopontine angle	C71.6	C79.31	—	D33.1	D43.1	D49.6

	Malignant Primary	Malignant Secondary	Ca in situ	Benign	Uncertain Behavior	Unspecified Behavior
brain NEC *(Continued)*						
cerebellum NOS	C71.6	C79.31	—	D33.1	D43.1	D49.6
cerebrum	C71.Ø	C79.31	—	D33.Ø	D43.Ø	D49.6
choroid plexus	C71.7	C79.31	—	D33.1	D43.1	D49.6
corpus callosum	C71.8	C79.31	—	D33.2	D43.2	D49.6
corpus striatum	C71.Ø	C79.31	—	D33.Ø	D43.Ø	D49.6
cortex (cerebral)	C71.Ø	C79.31	—	D33.Ø	D43.Ø	D49.6
frontal lobe	C71.1	C79.31	—	D33.Ø	D43.Ø	D49.6
globus pallidus	C71.Ø	C79.31	—	D33.Ø	D43.Ø	D49.6
hippocampus	C71.2	C79.31	—	D33.Ø	D43.Ø	D49.6
hypothalamus	C71.Ø	C79.31	—	D33.Ø	D43.Ø	D49.6
internal capsule	C71.Ø	C79.31	—	D33.Ø	D43.Ø	D49.6
medulla oblongata	C71.7	C79.31	—	D33.1	D43.1	D49.6
meninges	C70.0	C79.32	—	D32.Ø	D42.Ø	D49.7
midbrain	C71.7	C79.31	—	D33.1	D43.1	D49.6
occipital lobe	C71.4	C79.31	—	D33.Ø	D43.Ø	D49.6
overlapping lesion	C71.8	C79.31	—	—	—	—
parietal lobe	C71.3	C79.31	—	D33.Ø	D43.Ø	D49.6
peduncle	C71.7	C79.31	—	D33.1	D43.1	D49.6
pons	C71.7	C79.31	—	D33.1	D43.1	D49.6
stem	C71.7	C79.31	—	D33.1	D43.1	D49.6
tapetum	C71.8	C79.31	—	D33.2	D43.2	D49.6
temporal lobe	C71.2	C79.31	—	D33.Ø	D43.Ø	D49.6
thalamus	C71.Ø	C79.31	—	D33.Ø	D43.Ø	D49.6
uncus	C71.2	C79.31	—	D33.Ø	D43.Ø	D49.6
ventricle (floor)	C71.5	C79.31	—	D33.Ø	D43.Ø	D49.6
fourth	C71.7	C79.31	—	D33.1	D43.1	D49.6
branchial (cleft) (cyst) (vestiges)	C1Ø.4	C79.89	DØØ.Ø8	D1Ø.5	D37.Ø5	D49.Ø
breast (connective tissue) (glandular tissue) (soft parts)	C5Ø.9-●	C79.81	DØ5.-●	D24.-●	D48.6-●	D49.3
areola	C5Ø.Ø-●	C79.81	DØ5.-●	D24.-●	D48.6-●	D49.3
axillary tail	C5Ø.6-●	C79.81	DØ5.-●	D24.-●	D48.6-●	D49.3
central portion	C5Ø.1-●	C79.81	DØ5.-●	D24.-●	D48.6-●	D49.3
inner	C5Ø.8-●	C79.81	DØ5.-●	D24.-●	D48.6-●	D49.3
lower	C5Ø.8-●	C79.81	DØ5.-●	D24.-●	D48.6-●	D49.3
lower-inner quadrant	C5Ø.3-●	C79.81	DØ5.-●	D24.-●	D48.6-●	D49.3
lower-outer quadrant	C5Ø.5-●	C79.81	DØ5.-●	D24.-●	D48.6-●	D49.3
mastectomy site (skin) — *see also Neoplasm, breast, skin*	C44.5Ø1	C79.2	—	—	—	—
specified as breast tissue	C5Ø.8-●	C79.81	—	—	—	—
midline	C5Ø.8-●	C79.81	DØ5.-●	D24.-●	D48.6-●	D49.3
nipple	C5Ø.Ø-●	C79.81	DØ5.-●	D24.-●	D48.6-●	D49.3
outer	C5Ø.8-●	C79.81	DØ5.-●	D24.-●	D48.6-●	D49.3
overlapping lesion	C5Ø.8-●	—	—	—	—	—

	Malignant Primary	Malignant Secondary	Ca in situ	Benign	Uncertain Behavior	Unspecified Behavior
breast *(Continued)*						
skin	C44.5Ø1	C79.2	DØ4.5	D23.5	D48.5	D49.2
basal cell carcinoma	C44.511	—	—	—	—	—
specified type NEC	C44.591	—	—	—	—	—
squamous cell carcinoma	C44.521	—	—	—	—	—
tail (axillary)	C5Ø.6-●	C79.81	DØ5.-●	D24.-●	D48.6-●	D49.3
upper	C5Ø.8-●	C79.81	DØ5.-●	D24.-●	D48.6-●	D49.3
upper-inner quadrant	C5Ø.2-●	C79.81	DØ5.-●	D24.-●	D48.6-●	D49.3
upper-outer quadrant	C5Ø.4-●	C79.81	DØ5.-●	D24.-●	D48.6-●	D49.3
broad ligament	C57.1	C79.82	DØ7.39	D28.2	D39.8	D49.59
bronchiogenic, bronchogenic (lung)	C34.9-●	C78.Ø-●	DØ2.2-●	D14.3-●	D38.1	D49.1
bronchiole	C34.9-●	C78.Ø-●	DØ2.2-●	D14.3-●	D38.1	D49.1
bronchus	C34.9-●	C78.Ø-●	DØ2.2-●	D14.3-●	D38.1	D49.1
carina	C34.Ø-●	C78.Ø-●	DØ2.2-●	D14.3-●	D38.1	D49.1
lower lobe of lung	C34.3-●	C78.Ø-●	DØ2.2-●	D14.3-●	D38.1	D49.1
main	C34.Ø-●	C78.Ø-●	DØ2.2-●	D14.3-●	D38.1	D49.1
middle lobe of lung	C34.2	C78.Ø-●	DØ2.21	D14.31	D38.1	D49.1
overlapping lesion	C34.8-●	—	—	—	—	—
upper lobe of lung	C34.1-●	C78.Ø-●	DØ2.2-●	D14.3-●	D38.1	D49.1
brow	C44.3Ø9	C79.2	DØ4.39	D23.39	D48.5	D49.2
basal cell carcinoma	C44.319	—	—	—	—	—
specified type NEC	C44.399	—	—	—	—	—
squamous cell carcinoma	C44.329	—	—	—	—	—
buccal (cavity)	CØ6.9	C79.89	DØØ.ØØ	D1Ø.39	D37.Ø9	D49.Ø
commissure	CØ6.Ø	C79.89	DØØ.Ø2	D1Ø.39	D37.Ø9	D49.Ø
groove (lower) (upper)	CØ6.1	C79.89	DØØ.Ø2	D1Ø.39	D37.Ø9	D49.Ø
mucosa	CØ6.Ø	C79.89	DØØ.Ø2	D1Ø.39	D37.Ø9	D49.Ø
sulcus (lower) (upper)	CØ6.1	C79.89	DØØ.Ø2	D1Ø.39	D37.Ø9	D49.Ø
bulbourethral gland	C68.Ø	C79.19	DØ9.19	D3Ø.4	D41.3	D49.59
bursa — *see Neoplasm, connective tissue*						
buttock NEC	C76.3	C79.89	DØ4.5	D36.7	D48.7	D49.89
calf	C76.5-●	C79.89	DØ4.7-●	D36.7	D48.7	D49.89
calvarium	C41.Ø	C79.51	—	D16.4-●	D48.Ø	D49.2
calyx, renal	C65.-●	C79.Ø-●	DØ9.19	D3Ø.1-●	D41.1-●	D49.51-●
canal						
anal	C21.1	C78.5	DØ1.3	D12.9	D37.8	D49.Ø
auditory (external) — *see also Neoplasm, skin, ear*	C44.2Ø-●	C79.2	DØ4.2-●	D23.2-●	D48.5	D49.2
auricular (external) — *see also Neoplasm, skin, ear*	C44.2Ø-●	C79.2	DØ4.2-●	D23.2-●	D48.5	D49.2
canaliculi, biliary (biliferi) (intrahepatic)	C22.1	C78.7	DØ1.5	D13.4	D37.6	D49.Ø

TABLE OF NEOPLASMS

◄ New ◄ Revised ~~deleted~~ Deleted ● Use Additional Character(s)

	Malignant Primary	Malignant Secondary	Ca in situ	Benign	Uncertain Behavior	Unspecified Behavior
canthus (eye) (inner) (outer)	C44.1Ø-•	C79.2	DØ4.1-•	D23.1-•	D48.5	D49.2
basal cell carcinoma	C44.11-•	—	—	—	—	—
sebaceous cell	C44.13-•	—	—	—	—	—
specified type NEC	C44.19-•	—	—	—	—	—
squamous cell carcinoma	C44.12-•	—	—	—	—	—
capillary — *see Neoplasm, connective tissue*						
caput coli	C18.Ø	C78.5	DØ1.Ø	D12.Ø	D37.4	D49.Ø
carcinoid — *see Tumor, carcinoid*						
cardia (gastric)	C16.Ø	C78.89	DØØ.2	D13.1	D37.1	D49.Ø
cardiac orifice (stomach)	C16.Ø	C78.89	DØØ.2	D13.1	D37.1	D49.Ø
cardio-esophageal junction	C16.Ø	C78.89	DØØ.2	D13.1	D37.1	D49.Ø
cardio-esophagus	C16.Ø	C78.89	DØØ.2	D13.1	D37.1	D49.Ø
carina (bronchus)	C34.Ø-•	C78.Ø-•	DØ2.2-•	D14.3-•	D38.1	D49.1
carotid (artery)	C49.Ø	C79.89	—	D21.Ø	D48.1	D49.2
body	C75.4	C79.89	—	D35.5	D44.6	D49.7
carpus (any bone)	C4Ø.1-•	C79.51	—	D16.1-•	—	—
cartilage (articular) (joint) NEC — *see also Neoplasm, bone*	C41.9	C79.51	—	D16.9-•	D48.Ø	D49.2
arytenoid	C32.3	C78.39	DØ2.Ø	D14.1	D38.Ø	D49.1
auricular	C49.Ø	C79.89	—	D21.Ø	D48.1	D49.2
bronchi	C34.Ø-•	C78.39	—	D14.3-•	D38.1	D49.1
costal	C41.3	C79.51	—	D16.7	D48.Ø	D49.2
cricoid	C32.3	C78.39	DØ2.Ø	D14.1	D38.Ø	D49.1
cuneiform	C32.3	C78.39	DØ2.Ø	D14.1	D38.Ø	D49.1
ear (external)	C49.Ø	C79.89	—	D21.Ø	D48.1	D49.2
ensiform	C41.3	C79.51	—	D16.7	D48.Ø	D49.2
epiglottis	C32.1	C78.39	DØ2.Ø	D14.1	D38.Ø	D49.1
anterior surface	C1Ø.1	C79.89	DØØ.Ø8	D1Ø.5	D37.Ø5	D49.Ø
eyelid	C49.Ø	C79.89	—	D21.Ø	D48.1	D49.2
intervertebral	C41.2	C79.51	—	D16.6	D48.Ø	D49.2
larynx, laryngeal	C32.3	C78.39	DØ2.Ø	D14.1	D38.Ø	D49.1
nose, nasal	C3Ø.Ø	C78.39	DØ2.3	D14.Ø	D38.5	D49.1
pinna	C49.Ø	C79.89	—	D21.Ø	D48.1	D49.2
rib	C41.3	C79.51	—	D16.7	D48.Ø	D49.2
semilunar (knee)	C4Ø.2-•	C79.51	—	D16.2-•	D48.Ø	D49.2
thyroid	C32.3	C78.39	DØ2.Ø	D14.1	D38.Ø	D49.1
trachea	C33	C78.39	DØ2.1	D14.2	D38.1	D49.1
cauda equina	C72.1	C79.49	—	D33.4	D43.4	D49.7
cavity						
buccal	CØ6.9	C79.89	DØØ.ØØ	D1Ø.3Ø	D37.Ø9	D49.Ø
nasal	C3Ø.Ø	C78.39	DØ2.3	D14.Ø	D38.5	D49.1
oral	CØ6.9	C79.89	DØØ.ØØ	D1Ø.3Ø	D37.Ø9	D49.Ø
cavity *(Continued)*						
peritoneal	C48.2	C78.6	—	D2Ø.1	D48.4	D49.Ø
tympanic	C3Ø.1	C78.39	DØ2.3	D14.Ø	D38.5	D49.1
cecum	C18.Ø	C78.5	DØ1.Ø	D12.Ø	D37.4	D49.Ø
central nervous system	C72.9	C79.4Ø	—	—	—	—
cerebellopontine (angle)	C71.6	C79.31	—	D33.1	D43.1	D49.6
cerebellum, cerebellar	C71.6	C79.31	—	D33.1	D43.1	D49.6
cerebrum, cerebra (cortex) (hemisphere) (white matter)	C71.Ø	C79.31	—	D33.Ø	D43.Ø	D49.6
meninges	C7Ø.Ø	C79.32	—	D32.Ø	D42.Ø	D49.7
peduncle	C71.7	C79.31	—	D33.1	D43.1	D49.6
ventricle	C71.5	C79.31	—	D33.Ø	D43.Ø	D49.6
fourth	C71.7	C79.31	—	D33.1	D43.1	D49.6
cervical region	C76.Ø	C79.89	DØ9.8	D36.7	D48.7	D49.89
cervix (cervical) (uteri) (uterus)	C53.9	C79.82	DØ6.9	D26.Ø	D39.Ø	D49.59
canal	C53.Ø	C79.82	DØ6.Ø	D26.Ø	D39.Ø	D49.59
endocervix (canal) (gland)	C53.Ø	C79.82	DØ6.Ø	D26.Ø	D39.Ø	D49.59
exocervix	C53.1	C79.82	DØ6.1	D26.Ø	D39.Ø	D49.59
external os	C53.1	C79.82	DØ6.1	D26.Ø	D39.Ø	D49.59
internal os	C53.Ø	C79.82	DØ6.Ø	D26.Ø	D39.Ø	D49.59
nabothian gland	C53.Ø	C79.82	DØ6.Ø	D26.Ø	D39.Ø	D49.59
overlapping lesion	C53.8	—	—	—	—	—
squamocolumnar junction	C53.8	C79.82	DØ6.7	D26.Ø	D39.Ø	D49.59
stump	C53.8	C79.82	DØ6.7	D26.Ø	D39.Ø	D49.59
cheek	C76.Ø	C79.89	DØ9.8	D36.7	D48.7	D49.89
external	C44.3Ø9	C79.2	DØ4.39	D23.39	D48.5	D49.2
basal cell carcinoma	C44.319	—	—	—	—	—
specified type NEC	C44.399	—	—	—	—	—
squamous cell carcinoma	C44.329	—	—	—	—	—
inner aspect	CØ6.Ø	C79.89	DØØ.Ø2	D1Ø.39	D37.Ø9	D49.Ø
internal	CØ6.Ø	C79.89	DØØ.Ø2	D1Ø.39	D37.Ø9	D49.Ø
mucosa	CØ6.Ø	C79.89	DØØ.Ø2	D1Ø.39	D37.Ø9	D49.Ø
chest (wall) NEC	C76.1	C79.89	DØ9.8	D36.7	D48.7	D49.89
chiasma opticum	C72.3-•	C79.49	—	D33.3	D43.3	D49.7
chin	C44.3Ø9	C79.2	DØ4.39	D23.39	D48.5	D49.2
basal cell carcinoma	C44.319	—	—	—	—	—
specified type NEC	C44.399	—	—	—	—	—
squamous cell carcinoma	C44.329	—	—	—	—	—
choana	C11.3	C79.89	DØØ.Ø8	D1Ø.6	D37.Ø5	D49.Ø
cholangiole	C22.1	C78.89	DØ1.5	D13.4	D37.6	D49.Ø
choledochal duct	C24.Ø	C78.89	DØ1.5	D13.5	D37.6	D49.Ø
choroid	C69.3-•	C79.49	DØ9.2-•	D31.3-•	D48.7	D49.81
plexus	C71.5	C79.31	—	D33.Ø	D43.Ø	D49.6
ciliary body	C69.4-•	C79.49	DØ9.2-•	D31.4-•	D48.7	D49.89

	Malignant Primary	Malignant Secondary	Ca in situ	Benign	Uncertain Behavior	Unspecified Behavior
clavicle	C41.3	C79.51	—	D16.7	D48.Ø	D49.2
clitoris	C51.2	C79.82	DØ7.1	D28.Ø	D39.8	D49.59
clivus	C41.Ø	C79.51	—	D16.4-•	D48.Ø	D49.2
cloacogenic zone	C21.2	C78.5	DØ1.3	D12.9	D37.8	D49.Ø
coccygeal						
body or glomus	C49.5	C79.89	—	D21.5	D48.1	D49.2
vertebra	C41.4	C79.51	—	D16.8	D48.Ø	D49.2
coccyx	C41.4	C79.51	—	D16.8	D48.Ø	D49.2
colon — *see also Neoplasm, intestine, large*	C18.9	C78.5	—	—	—	—
with rectum	C19	C78.5	DØ1.1	D12.7	D37.5	D49.Ø
column, spinal — *see Neoplasm, spine*						
columnella — *see also Neoplasm, skin, face*	C44.39Ø	C79.2	DØ4.39	D23.39	D48.5	D49.2
commissure						
labial, lip	CØØ.6	C79.89	DØØ.Ø1	D1Ø.39	D37.Ø1	D49.Ø
laryngeal	C32.Ø	C78.39	DØ2.Ø	D14.1	D38.Ø	D49.1
common (bile) duct	C24.Ø	C78.89	DØ1.5	D13.5	D37.6	D49.Ø
concha — *see also Neoplasm, skin, ear*	C44.2Ø-•	C79.2	DØ4.2-•	D23.2-•	D48.5	D49.2
nose	C3Ø.Ø	C78.39	DØ2.3	D14.Ø	D38.5	D49.1
conjunctiva	C69.Ø-•	C79.49	DØ9.2-•	D31.Ø-•	D48.7	D49.89
connective tissue NEC	C49.9	C79.89	—	D21.9	D48.1	D49.2
Note: For neoplasms of connective tissue (blood vessel, bursa, fascia, ligament, muscle, peripheral nerves, sympathetic and parasympathetic nerves and ganglia, synovia, tendon, etc.) or of morphological types that indicate connective tissue, code according to the list under "Neoplasm, connective tissue." For sites that do not appear in this list, code to neoplasm of that site; e.g., fibrosarcoma, pancreas (C25.9)						
Note: Morphological types that indicate connective tissue appear in their proper place in the alphabetic index with the instruction "*see Neoplasm, connective tissue ....*"						
abdomen	C49.4	C79.89	—	D21.4	D48.1	D49.2
abdominal wall	C49.4	C79.89	—	D21.4	D48.1	D49.2
ankle	C49.2-•	C79.89	—	D21.2-•	D48.1	D49.2
antecubital fossa or space	C49.1-•	C79.89	—	D21.1-•	D48.1	D49.2
arm	C49.1-•	C79.89	—	D21.1-•	D48.1	D49.2
auricle (ear)	C49.Ø	C79.89	—	D21.Ø	D48.1	D49.2
axilla	C49.3	C79.89	—	D21.3	D48.1	D49.2
back	C49.6	C79.89	—	D21.6	D48.1	D49.2
breast — *see Neoplasm, breast*						
buttock	C49.5	C79.89	—	D21.5	D48.1	D49.2
calf	C49.2-•	C79.89	—	D21.2-•	D48.1	D49.2
cervical region	C49.Ø	C79.89	—	D21.Ø	D48.1	D49.2

	Malignant Primary	Malignant Secondary	Ca in situ	Benign	Uncertain Behavior	Unspecified Behavior
connective tissue NEC *(Continued)*						
cheek	C49.Ø	C79.89	—	D21.Ø	D48.1	D49.2
chest (wall)	C49.3	C79.89	—	D21.3	D48.1	D49.2
chin	C49.Ø	C79.89	—	D21.Ø	D48.1	D49.2
diaphragm	C49.3	C79.89	—	D21.3	D48.1	D49.2
ear (external)	C49.Ø	C79.89	—	D21.Ø	D48.1	D49.2
elbow	C49.1-•	C79.89	—	D21.1-•	D48.1	D49.2
extrarectal	C49.5	C79.89	—	D21.5	D48.1	D49.2
extremity	C49.9	C79.89	—	D21.9	D48.1	D49.2
lower	C49.2-•	C79.89	—	D21.2-•	D48.1	D49.2
upper	C49.1-•	C79.89	—	D21.1-•	D48.1	D49.2
eyelid	C49.Ø	C79.89	—	D21.Ø	D48.1	D49.2
face	C49.Ø	C79.89	—	D21.Ø	D48.1	D49.2
finger	C49.1-•	C79.89	—	D21.1-•	D48.1	D49.2
flank	C49.6	C79.89	—	D21.6	D48.1	D49.2
foot	C49.2-•	C79.89	—	D21.2-•	D48.1	D49.2
forearm	C49.1-•	C79.89	—	D21.1-•	D48.1	D49.2
forehead	C49.Ø	C79.89	—	D21.Ø	D48.1	D49.2
gastric	C49.4	C79.89	—	D21.4	D48.1	D49.2
gastrointestinal	C49.4	C79.89	—	D21.4	D48.1	D49.2
gluteal region	C49.5	C79.89	—	D21.5	D48.1	D49.2
great vessels NEC	C49.3	C79.89	—	D21.3	D48.1	D49.2
groin	C49.5	C79.89	—	D21.5	D48.1	D49.2
hand	C49.1-•	C79.89	—	D21.1-•	D48.1	D49.2
head	C49.Ø	C79.89	—	D21.Ø	D48.1	D49.2
heel	C49.2-•	C79.89	—	D21.2-•	D48.1	D49.2
hip	C49.2-•	C79.89	—	D21.2-•	D48.1	D49.2
hypochondrium	C49.4	C79.89	—	D21.4	D48.1	D49.2
iliopsoas muscle	C49.5	C79.89	—	D21.5	D48.1	D49.2
infraclavicular region	C49.3	C79.89	—	D21.3	D48.1	D49.2
inguinal (canal) (region)	C49.5	C79.89	—	D21.5	D48.1	D49.2
intestinal	C49.4	C79.89	—	D21.4	D48.1	D49.2
intrathoracic	C49.3	C79.89	—	D21.3	D48.1	D49.2
ischiorectal fossa	C49.5	C79.89	—	D21.5	D48.1	D49.2
jaw	CØ3.9	C79.89	DØØ.Ø3	D1Ø.39	D48.1	D49.Ø
knee	C49.2-•	C79.89	—	D21.2-•	D48.1	D49.2
leg	C49.2-•	C79.89	—	D21.2-•	D48.1	D49.2
limb NEC	C49.9	C79.89	—	D21.9	D48.1	D49.2
lower	C49.2-•	C79.89	—	D21.2-•	D48.1	D49.2
upper	C49.1-•	C79.89	—	D21.1-•	D48.1	D49.2
nates	C49.5	C79.89	—	D21.5	D48.1	D49.2
neck	C49.Ø	C79.89	—	D21.Ø	D48.1	D49.2
orbit	C69.6-•	C79.49	DØ9.2-•	D31.6-•	D48.1	D49.89
overlapping lesion	C49.8	—	—	—	—	—

	Malignant Primary	Malignant Secondary	Ca in situ	Benign	Uncertain Behavior	Unspecified Behavior
connective tissue NEC *(Continued)*						
pararectal	C49.5	C79.89	—	D21.5	D48.1	D49.2
para-urethral	C49.5	C79.89	—	D21.5	D48.1	D49.2
paravaginal	C49.5	C79.89	—	D21.5	D48.1	D49.2
pelvis (floor)	C49.5	C79.89	—	D21.5	D48.1	D49.2
pelvo-abdominal	C49.8	C79.89	—	D21.6	D48.1	D49.2
perineum	C49.5	C79.89	—	D21.5	D48.1	D49.2
perirectal (tissue)	C49.5	C79.89	—	D21.5	D48.1	D49.2
periurethral (tissue)	C49.5	C79.89	—	D21.5	D48.1	D49.2
popliteal fossa or space	C49.2-●	C79.89	—	D21.2-●	D48.1	D49.2
presacral	C49.5	C79.89	—	D21.5	D48.1	D49.2
psoas muscle	C49.4	C79.89	—	D21.4	D48.1	D49.2
pterygoid fossa	C49.0	C79.89	—	D21.0	D48.1	D49.2
rectovaginal septum or wall	C49.5	C79.89	—	D21.5	D48.1	D49.2
rectovesical	C49.5	C79.89	—	D21.5	D48.1	D49.2
retroperitoneum	C48.0	C78.6	—	D20.0	D48.3	D49.0
sacrococcygeal region	C49.5	C79.89	—	D21.5	D48.1	D49.2
scalp	C49.0	C79.89	—	D21.0	D48.1	D49.2
scapular region	C49.3	C79.89	—	D21.3	D48.1	D49.2
shoulder	C49.1-●	C79.89	—	D21.1-●	D48.1	D49.2
skin (dermis) NEC—*see also Neoplasm, skin, by site*	C44.90	C79.2	D04.9	D23.9	D48.5	D49.2
stomach	C49.4	C79.89	—	D21.4	D48.1	D49.2
submental	C49.0	C79.89	—	D21.0	D48.1	D49.2
supraclavicular region	C49.0	C79.89	—	D21.0	D48.1	D49.2
temple	C49.0	C79.89	—	D21.0	D48.1	D49.2
temporal region	C49.0	C79.89	—	D21.0	D48.1	D49.2
thigh	C49.2-●	C79.89	—	D21.2-●	D48.1	D49.2
thoracic (duct) (wall)	C49.3	C79.89	—	D21.3	D48.1	D49.2
thorax	C49.3	C79.89	—	D21.3	D48.1	D49.2
thumb	C49.1-●	C79.89	—	D21.1-●	D48.1	D49.2
toe	C49.2-●	C79.89	—	D21.2-●	D48.1	D49.2
trunk	C49.6	C79.89	—	D21.6	D48.1	D49.2
umbilicus	C49.4	C79.89	—	D21.4	D48.1	D49.2
vesicorectal	C49.5	C79.89	—	D21.5	D48.1	D49.2
wrist	C49.1-●	C79.89	—	D21.1-●	D48.1	D49.2
conus medullaris	C72.0	C79.49	—	D33.4	D43.4	D49.7
cord (true) (vocal)	C32.0	C78.39	D02.0	D14.1	D38.0	D49.1
false	C32.1	C78.39	D02.0	D14.1	D38.0	D49.1
spermatic	C63.1-●	C79.82	D07.69	D29.8	D40.8	D49.59
spinal (cervical) (lumbar) (thoracic)	C72.0	C79.49	—	D33.4	D43.4	D49.7
cornea (limbus)	C69.1-●	C79.49	D09.2-●	D31.1-●	D48.7	D49.89
corpus						

	Malignant Primary	Malignant Secondary	Ca in situ	Benign	Uncertain Behavior	Unspecified Behavior
corpus *(Continued)*						
albicans	C56.-●	C79.6-●	D07.39	D27.-●	D39.1-●	D49.59
callosum, brain	C71.0	C79.31	—	D33.2	D43.2	D49.6
cavernosum	C60.2	C79.82	D07.4	D29.0	D40.8	D49.59
gastric	C16.2	C78.89	D00.2	D13.1	D37.1	D49.0
overlapping sites	C54.8	—	—	—	—	—
penis	C60.2	C79.82	D07.4	D29.0	D40.8	D49.59
striatum, cerebrum	C71.0	C79.31	—	D33.0	D43.0	D49.6
uteri	C54.9	C79.82	D07.0	D26.1	D39.0	D49.59
isthmus	C54.0	C79.82	D07.0	D26.1	D39.0	D49.59
cortex						
adrenal	C74.0-●	C79.7-●	D09.3	D35.0-●	D44.1-●	D49.7
cerebral	C71.0	C79.31	—	D33.0	D43.0	D49.6
costal cartilage	C41.3	C79.51	—	D16.7	D48.0	D49.2
costovertebral joint	C41.3	C79.51	—	D16.7	D48.0	D49.2
Cowper's gland	C68.0	C79.19	D09.19	D30.4	D41.3	D49.59
cranial (fossa, any)	C71.9	C79.31	—	D33.2	D43.2	D49.6
meninges	C70.0	C79.32	—	D32.0	D42.0	D49.7
nerve	C72.50	C79.49	—	D33.3	D43.3	D49.7
specified NEC	C72.59	C79.49	—	D33.3	D43.3	D49.7
craniobuccal pouch	C75.2	C79.89	D09.3	D35.2	D44.3	D49.7
craniopharyngeal (duct) (pouch)	C75.2	C79.89	D09.3	D35.3	D44.4	D49.7
cricoid	C13.0	C79.89	D00.08	D10.7	D37.05	D49.0
cartilage	C32.3	C78.39	D02.0	D14.1	D38.0	D49.1
cricopharynx	C13.0	C79.89	D00.08	D10.7	D37.05	D49.0
crypt of Morgagni	C21.8	C78.5	D01.3	D12.9	D37.8	D49.0
crystalline lens	C69.4-●	C79.49	D09.2-●	D31.4-●	D48.7	D49.89
cul-de-sac (Douglas')	C48.1	C78.6	—	D20.1	D48.4	D49.0
cuneiform cartilage	C32.3	C78.39	D02.0	D14.1	D38.0	D49.1
cutaneous—*see Neoplasm, skin*						
cutis—*see Neoplasm, skin*						
cystic (bile) duct (common)	C24.0	C78.89	D01.5	D13.5	D37.6	D49.0
dermis—*see Neoplasm, skin*						
diaphragm	C49.3	C79.89	—	D21.3	D48.1	D49.2
digestive organs, system, tube, or tract NEC	C26.9	C78.89	D01.9	D13.9	D37.9	D49.0
disc, intervertebral	C41.2	C79.51	—	D16.6	D48.0	D49.2
disease, generalized	C80.0	—	—	—	—	—
disseminated	C80.0	—	—	—	—	—
Douglas' cul-de-sac or pouch	C48.1	C78.6	—	D20.1	D48.4	D49.0
duodenojejunal junction	C17.8	C78.4	D01.49	D13.39	D37.2	D49.0
duodenum	C17.0	C78.4	D01.49	D13.2	D37.2	D49.0

	Malignant Primary	Malignant Secondary	Ca in situ	Benign	Uncertain Behavior	Unspecified Behavior
dura (cranial) (mater)	C7Ø.9	C79.49	—	D32.9	D42.9	D49.7
cerebral	C7Ø.Ø	C79.32	—	D32.Ø	D42.Ø	D49.7
spinal	C7Ø.1	C79.49	—	D32.1	D42.1	D49.7
ear (external)—*see also Neoplasm, skin, ear*	C44.2Ø-•	C79.2	DØ4.2-•	D23.2-•	D48.5	D49.2
auricle or auris—*see also Neoplasm, skin, ear*	C44.2Ø-•	C79.2	DØ4.2-•	D23.2-•	D48.5	D49.2
canal, external—*see also Neoplasm, skin, ear*	C44.2Ø-•	C79.2	DØ4.2-•	D23.2-•	D48.5	D49.2
cartilage	C49.Ø	C79.89	—	D21.Ø	D48.1	D49.2
external meatus—*see also Neoplasm, skin, ear*	C44.2Ø-•	C79.2	DØ4.2-•	D23.2-•	D48.5	D49.2
inner	C3Ø.1	C78.39	DØ2.3	D14.Ø	D38.5	D49.1
lobule—*see also Neoplasm, skin, ear*	C44.2Ø-•	C79.2	DØ4.2-•	D23.2-•	D48.5	D49.2
middle	C3Ø.1	C78.39	DØ2.3	D14.Ø	D38.5	D49.1
overlapping lesion with accessory sinuses	C31.8	—	—	—	—	—
skin	C44.2Ø-•	C79.2	DØ4.2-•	D23.2-•	D48.5	D49.2
basal cell carcinoma	C44.21-•	—	—	—	—	—
specified type NEC	C44.29-•	—	—	—	—	—
squamous cell carcinoma	C44.22-•	—	—	—	—	—
earlobe	C44.2Ø-•	C79.2	DØ4.2-•	D23.2-•	D48.5	D49.2
basal cell carcinoma	C44.21-•	—	—	—	—	—
specified type NEC	C44.29-•	—	—	—	—	—
squamous cell carcinoma	C44.22-•	—	—	—	—	—
ejaculatory duct	C63.7	C79.82	DØ7.69	D29.8	D4Ø.8	D49.59
elbow NEC	C76.4-•	C79.89	DØ4.6-•	D36.7	D48.7	D49.89
endocardium	C38.Ø	C79.89	—	D15.1	D48.7	D49.89
endocervix (canal) (gland)	C53.Ø	C79.82	DØ6.Ø	D26.Ø	D39.Ø	D49.59
endocrine gland NEC	C75.9	C79.89	DØ9.3	D35.9	D44.9	D49.7
pluriglandular	C75.8	C79.89	DØ9.3	D35.7	D44.9	D49.7
endometrium (gland) (stroma)	C54.1	C79.82	DØ7.Ø	D26.1	D39.Ø	D49.59
ensiform cartilage	C41.3	C79.51	—	D16.7	D48.Ø	D49.2
enteric—*see Neoplasm, intestine*						
ependyma (brain)	C71.5	C79.31	—	D33.Ø	D43.Ø	D49.6
fourth ventricle	C71.7	C79.31	—	D33.1	D43.1	D49.6
epicardium	C38.Ø	C79.89	—	D15.1	D48.7	D49.89
epididymis	C63.Ø-•	C79.82	DØ7.69	D29.3-•	D4Ø.8	D49.59
epidural	C72.9	C79.49	—	D33.9	D43.9	D49.7
epiglottis	C32.1	C78.39	DØ2.Ø	D14.1	D38.Ø	D49.1
anterior aspect or surface	C1Ø.1	C79.89	DØØ.Ø8	D1Ø.5	D37.Ø5	D49.Ø
cartilage	C32.3	C78.39	DØ2.Ø	D14.1	D38.Ø	D49.1
free border (margin)	C1Ø.1	C79.89	DØØ.Ø8	D1Ø.5	D37.Ø5	D49.Ø
junctional region	C1Ø.8	C79.89	DØØ.Ø8	D1Ø.5	D37.Ø5	D49.Ø
posterior (laryngeal) surface	C32.1	C78.39	DØ2.Ø	D14.1	D38.Ø	D49.1
suprahyoid portion	C32.1	C78.39	DØ2.Ø	D14.1	D38.Ø	D49.1
esophagogastric junction	C16.Ø	C78.89	DØØ.2	D13.1	D37.1	D49.Ø
esophagus	C15.9	C78.89	DØØ.1	D13.Ø	D37.8	D49.Ø
abdominal	C15.5	C78.89	DØØ.1	D13.Ø	D37.8	D49.Ø
cervical	C15.3	C78.89	DØØ.1	D13.Ø	D37.8	D49.Ø
distal (third)	C15.5	C78.89	DØØ.1	D13.Ø	D37.8	D49.Ø
lower (third)	C15.5	C78.89	DØØ.1	D13.Ø	D37.8	D49.Ø
middle (third)	C15.4	C78.89	DØØ.1	D13.Ø	D37.8	D49.Ø
overlapping lesion	C15.8	—	—	—	—	—
proximal (third)	C15.3	C78.89	DØØ.1	D13.Ø	D37.8	D49.Ø
thoracic	C15.4	C78.89	DØØ.1	D13.Ø	D37.8	D49.Ø
upper (third)	C15.3	C78.89	DØØ.1	D13.Ø	D37.8	D49.Ø
ethmoid (sinus)	C31.1	C78.39	DØ2.3	D14.Ø	D38.5	D49.1
bone or labyrinth	C41.Ø	C79.51	—	D16.4-•	D48.Ø	D49.2
eustachian tube	C3Ø.1	C78.39	DØ2.3	D14.Ø	D38.5	D49.1
exocervix	C53.1	C79.82	DØ6.1	D26.Ø	D39.Ø	D49.59
external						
meatus (ear)—*see also Neoplasm, skin, ear*	C44.2Ø-•	C79.2	DØ4.2-•	D23.2-•	D48.5	D49.2
os, cervix uteri	C53.1	C79.82	DØ6.1	D26.Ø	D39.Ø	D49.59
extradural	C72.9	C79.49	—	D33.9	D43.9	D49.7
extrahepatic (bile) duct	C24.Ø	C78.89	DØ1.5	D13.5	D37.6	D49.Ø
overlapping lesion with gallbladder	C24.8	—	—	—	—	—
extraocular muscle	C69.6-•	C79.49	DØ9.2-•	D31.6-•	D48.7	D49.89
extrarectal	C76.3	C79.89	DØ9.8	D36.7	D48.7	D49.89
extremity	C76.8	C79.89	DØ4.8	D36.7	D48.7	D49.89
lower	C76.5-•	C79.89	DØ4.7-•	D36.7	D48.7	D49.89
upper	C76.4-•	C79.89	DØ4.6-•	D36.7	D48.7	D49.89
eye NEC	C69.9-•	C79.49	DØ9.2	D31.9	D48.7	D49.89
overlapping sites	C69.8	—	—	—	—	—
eyeball	C69.9-•	C79.49	DØ9.2-•	D31.9-•	D48.7	D49.89
eyebrow	C44.3Ø9	C79.2	DØ4.39	D23.39	D48.5	D49.2
basal cell carcinoma	C44.319	—	—	—	—	—
specified type NEC	C44.399	—	—	—	—	—
squamous cell carcinoma	C44.329	—	—	—	—	—
eyelid (lower) (skin) (upper)	C44.1Ø-•	—	—	—	—	—
basal cell carcinoma	C44.11-•	—	—	—	—	—
cartilage	C49.Ø	C79.89	—	D21.Ø	D48.1	D49.2
sebaceous cell	C44.13-•	—	—	—	—	—
specified type NEC	C44.19-•	—	—	—	—	—
squamous cell carcinoma	C44.12-•	—	—	—	—	—

New · Revised · ~~deleted~~ Deleted · • Use Additional Character(s)

	Malignant Primary	Malignant Secondary	Ca in situ	Benign	Uncertain Behavior	Unspecified Behavior
face NEC	C76.Ø	C79.89	DØ4.39	D36.7	D48.7	D49.89
fallopian tube (accessory)	C57.Ø-•	C79.82	DØ7.39	D28.2	D39.8	D49.59
falx (cerebella) (cerebri)	C7Ø.Ø	C79.32	—	D32.Ø	D42.Ø	D49.7
fascia — *see also Neoplasm, connective tissue*						
palmar	C49.1-•	C79.89	—	D21.1-•	D48.1	D49.2
plantar	C49.2-•	C79.89	—	D21.2-•	D48.1	D49.2
fatty tissue — *see Neoplasm, connective tissue*						
fauces, faucial NEC	C1Ø.9	C79.89	DØØ.Ø8	D1Ø.5	D37.Ø5	D49.Ø
pillars	CØ9.1	C79.89	DØØ.Ø8	D1Ø.5	D37.Ø5	D49.Ø
tonsil	CØ9.9	C79.89	DØØ.Ø8	D1Ø.4	D37.Ø5	D49.Ø
femur (any part)	C4Ø.2-•	—	—	D16.2-•	—	—
fetal membrane	C58	C79.82	DØ7.Ø	D26.7	D39.2	D49.59
fibrous tissue — *see Neoplasm, connective tissue*						
fibula (any part)	C4Ø.2-•	C79.51	—	D16.2-•	—	—
filum terminale	C72.Ø	C79.49	—	D33.4	D43.4	D49.7
finger NEC	C76.4-•	C79.89	DØ4.6-•	D36.7	D48.7	D49.89
flank NEC	C76.8	C79.89	DØ4.5	D36.7	D48.7	D49.89
follicle, nabothian	C53.Ø	C79.82	DØ6.Ø	D26.Ø	D39.Ø	D49.59
foot NEC	C76.5-•	C79.89	DØ4.7-•	D36.7	D48.7	D49.89
forearm NEC	C76.4-•	C79.89	DØ4.6-•	D36.7	D48.7	D49.89
forehead (skin)	C44.3Ø9	C79.2	DØ4.39	D23.39	D48.5	D49.2
basal cell carcinoma	C44.319	—	—	—	—	—
specified type NEC	C44.399	—	—	—	—	—
squamous cell carcinoma	C44.329	—	—	—	—	—
foreskin	C6Ø.Ø	C79.82	DØ7.4	D29.Ø	D4Ø.8	D49.59
fornix						
pharyngeal	C11.3	C79.89	DØØ.Ø8	D1Ø.6	D37.Ø5	D49.Ø
vagina	C52	C79.82	DØ7.2	D28.1	D39.8	D49.59
fossa (of)						
anterior (cranial)	C71.9	C79.31	—	D33.2	D43.2	D49.6
cranial	C71.9	C79.31	—	D33.2	D43.2	D49.6
ischiorectal	C76.3	C79.89	DØ9.8	D36.7	D48.7	D49.89
middle (cranial)	C71.9	C79.31	—	D33.2	D43.2	D49.6
piriform	C12	C79.89	DØØ.Ø8	D1Ø.7	D37.Ø5	D49.Ø
pituitary	C75.1	C79.89	DØ9.3	D35.2	D44.3	D49.7
posterior (cranial)	C71.9	C79.31	—	D33.2	D43.2	D49.6
pterygoid	C49.Ø	C79.89	—	D21.Ø	D48.1	D49.2
pyriform	C12	C79.89	DØØ.Ø8	D1Ø.7	D37.Ø5	D49.Ø
Rosenmuller	C11.2	C79.89	DØØ.Ø8	D1Ø.6	D37.Ø5	D49.Ø
tonsillar	CØ9.Ø	C79.89	DØØ.Ø8	D1Ø.5	D37.Ø5	D49.Ø
fourchette	C51.9	C79.82	DØ7.1	D28.Ø	D39.8	D49.59

	Malignant Primary	Malignant Secondary	Ca in situ	Benign	Uncertain Behavior	Unspecified Behavior
frenulum						
labii — *see Neoplasm, lip, internal*						
linguae	CØ2.2	C79.89	DØØ.Ø7	D1Ø.1	D37.Ø2	D49.Ø
frontal						
bone	C41.Ø	C79.51	—	D16.4-•	D48.Ø	D49.2
lobe, brain	C71.1	C79.31	—	D33.Ø	D43.Ø	D49.6
pole	C71.1	C79.31	—	D33.Ø	D43.Ø	D49.6
sinus	C31.2	C78.39	DØ2.3	D14.Ø	D38.5	D49.1
fundus						
stomach	C16.1	C78.89	DØØ.2	D13.1	D37.1	D49.Ø
uterus	C54.3	C79.82	DØ7.Ø	D26.1	D39.Ø	D49.59
gall duct (extrahepatic)	C24.Ø	C78.89	DØ1.5	D13.5	D37.6	D49.Ø
intrahepatic	C22.1	C78.7	DØ1.5	D13.4	D37.6	D49.Ø
gallbladder	C23	C78.89	DØ1.5	D13.5	D37.6	D49.Ø
overlapping lesion with extrahepatic bile ducts	C24.8	—	—	—	—	—
ganglia — *see also Neoplasm, nerve, peripheral*	C47.9	C79.89	—	D36.1Ø	D48.2	D49.2
basal	C71.Ø	C79.31	—	D33.Ø	D43.Ø	D49.6
cranial nerve	C72.5Ø	C79.49	—	D33.3	D43.3	D49.7
Gartner's duct	C52	C79.82	DØ7.2	D28.1	D39.8	D49.59
gastric — *see Neoplasm, stomach*						
gastrocolic	C26.9	C78.89	DØ1.9	D13.9	D37.9	D49.Ø
gastroesophageal junction	C16.Ø	C78.89	DØØ.2	D13.1	D37.1	D49.Ø
gastrointestinal (tract) NEC	C26.9	C78.89	DØ1.9	D13.9	D37.9	D49.Ø
generalized	C8Ø.Ø	—	—	—	—	—
genital organ or tract						
female NEC	C57.9	C79.82	DØ7.3Ø	D28.9	D39.9	D49.59
overlapping lesion	C57.8	—	—	—	—	—
specified site NEC	C57.7	C79.82	DØ7.39	D28.7	D39.8	D49.59
male NEC	C63.9	C79.82	DØ7.6Ø	D29.9	D4Ø.9	D49.59
overlapping lesion	C63.8	—	—	—	—	—
specified site NEC	C63.7	C79.82	DØ7.69	D29.8	D4Ø.8	D49.59
genitourinary tract						
female	C57.9	C79.82	DØ7.3Ø	D28.9	D39.9	D49.59
male	C63.9	C79.82	DØ7.6Ø	D29.9	D4Ø.9	D49.59
gingiva (alveolar) (marginal)	CØ3.9	C79.89	DØØ.Ø3	D1Ø.39	D37.Ø9	D49.Ø
lower	CØ3.1	C79.89	DØØ.Ø3	D1Ø.39	D37.Ø9	D49.Ø
mandibular	CØ3.1	C79.89	DØØ.Ø3	D1Ø.39	D37.Ø9	D49.Ø
maxillary	CØ3.Ø	C79.89	DØØ.Ø3	D1Ø.39	D37.Ø9	D49.Ø
upper	CØ3.Ø	C79.89	DØØ.Ø3	D1Ø.39	D37.Ø9	D49.Ø

	Malignant Primary	Malignant Secondary	Ca in situ	Benign	Uncertain Behavior	Unspecified Behavior
gland, glandular (lymphatic) (system) — *see also Neoplasm, lymph gland*						
endocrine NEC	C75.9	C79.89	DØ9.3	D35.9	D44.9	D49.7
salivary — *see Neoplasm, salivary gland*						
glans penis	C6Ø.1	C79.82	DØ7.4	D29.Ø	D4Ø.8	D49.59
globus pallidus	C71.Ø	C79.31	—	D33.Ø	D43.Ø	D49.6
glomus						
coccygeal	C49.5	C79.89	—	D21.5	D48.1	D49.2
jugularis	C75.5	C79.89	—	D35.6	D44.7	D49.7
glosso-epiglottic fold(s)	C1Ø.1	C79.89	DØØ.Ø8	D1Ø.5	D37.Ø5	D49.Ø
glossopalatine fold	CØ9.1	C79.89	DØØ.Ø8	D1Ø.5	D37.Ø5	D49.Ø
glossopharyngeal sulcus	CØ9.Ø	C79.89	DØØ.Ø8	D1Ø.5	D37.Ø5	D49.Ø
glottis	C32.Ø	C78.39	DØ2.Ø	D14.1	D38.Ø	D49.1
gluteal region	C76.3	C79.89	DØ4.5	D36.7	D48.7	D49.89
great vessels NEC	C49.3	C79.89	—	D21.3	D48.1	D49.2
groin NEC	C76.3	C79.89	DØ4.5	D36.7	D48.7	D49.89
gum	CØ3.9	C79.89	DØØ.Ø3	D1Ø.39	D37.Ø9	D49.Ø
lower	CØ3.1	C79.89	DØØ.Ø3	D1Ø.39	D37.Ø9	D49.Ø
upper	CØ3.Ø	C79.89	DØØ.Ø3	D1Ø.39	D37.Ø9	D49.Ø
hand NEC	C76.4-•	C79.89	DØ4.6-•	D36.7	D48.7	D49.89
head NEC	C76.Ø	C79.89	DØ4.4	D36.7	D48.7	D49.89
heart	C38.Ø	C79.89	—	D15.1	D48.7	D49.89
heel NEC	C76.5-•	C79.89	DØ4.7-•	D36.7	D48.7	D49.89
helix — *see also Neoplasm, skin, ear*	C44.2Ø-•	C79.2	DØ4.2-•	D23.2-•	D48.5	D49.2
hematopoietic, hemopoietic tissue NEC	C96.9	—	—	—	—	—
specified NEC	C96.Z	—	—	—	—	—
hemisphere, cerebral	C71.Ø	C79.31	—	D33.Ø	D43.Ø	D49.6
hemorrhoidal zone	C21.1	C78.5	DØ1.3	D12.9	D37.8	D49.Ø
hepatic — *see also Index to disease, by histology*	C22.9	C78.7	DØ1.5	D13.4	D37.6	D49.Ø
duct (bile)	C24.Ø	C78.89	DØ1.5	D13.5	D37.6	D49.Ø
flexure (colon)	C18.3	C78.5	DØ1.Ø	D12.3	D37.4	D49.Ø
primary	C22.8	C78.7	DØ1.5	D13.4	D37.6	D49.Ø
hepatobiliary	C24.9	C79.89	DØ1.5	D13.5	D37.6	D49.Ø
hepatoblastoma	C22.2	C78.7	DØ1.5	D13.4	D37.6	D49.Ø
hepatoma	C22.Ø	C78.7	DØ1.5	D13.4	D37.6	D49.Ø
hilus of lung	C34.Ø-•	C78.Ø-•	DØ2.2-•	D14.3-•	D38.1	D49.1
hip NEC	C76.5-•	C79.89	DØ4.7-•	D36.7	D48.7	D49.89
hippocampus, brain	C71.2	C79.31	—	D33.Ø	D43.Ø	D49.6
humerus (any part)	C4Ø.Ø-•	C79.51	—	D16.Ø-•	—	—
hymen	C52	C79.82	DØ7.2	D28.1	D39.8	D49.59
hypopharynx, hypopharyngeal NEC	C13.9	C79.89	DØØ.Ø8	D1Ø.7	D37.Ø5	D49.Ø
overlapping lesion	C13.8	—	—	—	—	—
postcricoid region	C13.Ø	C79.89	DØØ.Ø8	D1Ø.7	D37.Ø5	D49.Ø
posterior wall	C13.2	C79.89	DØØ.Ø8	D1Ø.7	D37.Ø5	D49.Ø
pyriform fossa (sinus)	C12	C79.89	DØØ.Ø8	D1Ø.7	D37.Ø5	D49.Ø
hypophysis	C75.1	C79.89	DØ9.3	D35.2	D44.3	D49.7
hypothalamus	C71.Ø	C79.31	—	D33.Ø	D43.Ø	D49.6
ileocecum, ileocecal (coil) (junction) (valve)	C18.Ø	C78.5	DØ1.Ø	D12.Ø	D37.4	D49.Ø
ileum	C17.2	C78.4	DØ1.49	D13.39	D37.2	D49.Ø
ilium	C41.4	C79.51	—	D16.8	D48.Ø	D49.2
immunoproliferative NEC	C88.9	—	—	—	—	—
infraclavicular (region)	C76.1	C79.89	DØ4.5	D36.7	D48.7	D49.89
inguinal (region)	C76.3	C79.89	DØ4.5	D36.7	D48.7	D49.89
insula	C71.Ø	C79.31	—	D33.Ø	D43.Ø	D49.6
insular tissue (pancreas)	C25.4	C78.89	DØ1.7	D13.7	D37.8	D49.Ø
brain	C71.Ø	C79.31	—	D33.Ø	D43.Ø	D49.6
interarytenoid fold	C13.1	C79.89	DØØ.Ø8	D1Ø.7	D37.Ø5	D49.Ø
hypopharyngeal aspect	C13.1	C79.89	DØØ.Ø8	D1Ø.7	D37.Ø5	D49.Ø
laryngeal aspect	C32.1	C78.39	DØ2.Ø	D14.1	D38.Ø	D49.1
marginal zone	C13.1	C79.89	DØØ.Ø8	D1Ø.7	D37.Ø5	D49.Ø
interdental papillae	CØ3.9	C79.89	DØØ.Ø3	D1Ø.39	D37.Ø9	D49.Ø
lower	CØ3.1	C79.89	DØØ.Ø3	D1Ø.39	D37.Ø9	D49.Ø
upper	CØ3.Ø	C79.89	DØØ.Ø3	D1Ø.39	D37.Ø9	D49.Ø
internal						
capsule	C71.Ø	C79.31	—	D33.Ø	D43.Ø	D49.6
os (cervix)	C53.Ø	C79.82	DØ6.Ø	D26.Ø	D39.Ø	D49.59
intervertebral cartilage or disc	C41.2	C79.51	—	D16.6	D48.Ø	D49.2
intestine, intestinal	C26.Ø	C78.8Ø	DØ1.4Ø	D13.9	D37.8	D49.Ø
large	C18.9	C78.5	DØ1.Ø	D12.6	D37.4	D49.Ø
appendix	C18.1	C78.5	DØ1.Ø	D12.1	D37.3	D49.Ø
caput coli	C18.Ø	C78.5	DØ1.Ø	D12.Ø	D37.4	D49.Ø
cecum	C18.Ø	C78.5	DØ1.Ø	D12.Ø	D37.4	D49.Ø
colon	C18.9	C78.5	DØ1.Ø	D12.6	D37.4	D49.Ø
and rectum	C19	C78.5	DØ1.1	D12.7	D37.5	D49.Ø
ascending	C18.2	C78.5	DØ1.Ø	D12.2	D37.4	D49.Ø
caput	C18.Ø	C78.5	DØ1.Ø	D12.Ø	D37.4	D49.Ø
descending	C18.6	C78.5	DØ1.Ø	D12.4	D37.4	D49.Ø
distal	C18.6	C78.5	DØ1.Ø	D12.4	D37.4	D49.Ø
left	C18.6	C78.5	DØ1.Ø	D12.4	D37.4	D49.Ø
overlapping lesion	C18.8	—	—	—	—	—
pelvic	C18.7	C78.5	DØ1.Ø	D12.5	D37.4	D49.Ø
right	C18.2	C78.5	DØ1.Ø	D12.2	D37.4	D49.Ø

	Malignant Primary	Malignant Secondary	Ca in situ	Benign	Uncertain Behavior	Unspecified Behavior
intestine, intestinal *(Continued)*						
large *(Continued)*						
colon *(Continued)*						
sigmoid (flexure)	C18.7	C78.5	DØ1.Ø	D12.5	D37.4	D49.Ø
transverse	C18.4	C78.5	DØ1.Ø	D12.3	D37.4	D49.Ø
hepatic flexure	C18.3	C78.5	DØ1.Ø	D12.3	D37.4	D49.Ø
ileocecum, ileocecal (coil) (valve)	C18.Ø	C78.5	DØ1.Ø	D12.Ø	D37.4	D49.Ø
overlapping lesion	C18.8	—	—	—	—	—
sigmoid flexure (lower) (upper)	C18.7	C78.5	DØ1.Ø	D12.5	D37.4	D49.Ø
splenic flexure	C18.5	C78.5	DØ1.Ø	D12.3	D37.4	D49.Ø
small	C17.9	C78.4	DØ1.4Ø	D13.3Ø	D37.2	D49.Ø
duodenum	C17.Ø	C78.4	DØ1.49	D13.2	D37.2	D49.Ø
ileum	C17.2	C78.4	DØ1.49	D13.39	D37.2	D49.Ø
jejunum	C17.1	C78.4	DØ1.49	D13.39	D37.2	D49.Ø
overlapping lesion	C17.8	—	—	—	—	—
tract NEC	C26.Ø	C78.89	DØ1.4Ø	D13.9	D37.8	D49.Ø
intra-abdominal	C76.2	C79.89	DØ9.8	D36.7	D48.7	D49.89
intracranial NEC	C71.9	C79.31	—	D33.2	D43.2	D49.6
intrahepatic (bile) duct	C22.1	C78.7	DØ1.5	D13.4	D37.6	D49.Ø
intraocular	C69.9-●	C79.49	DØ9.2-●	D31.9-●	D48.7	D49.89
intraorbital	C69.6-●	C79.49	DØ9.2-●	D31.6-●	D48.7	D49.89
intrasellar	C75.1	C79.89	DØ9.3	D35.2	D44.3	D49.7
intrathoracic (cavity) (organs)	C76.1	C79.89	DØ9.8	D15.9	D48.7	D49.89
specified NEC	C76.1	C79.89	DØ9.8	D15.7	—	—
iris	C69.4-●	C79.49	DØ9.2-●	D31.4-●	D48.7	D49.89
ischiorectal (fossa)	C76.3	C79.89	DØ9.8	D36.7	D48.7	D49.89
ischium	C41.4	C79.51	—	D16.8	D48.Ø	D49.2
island of Reil	C71.Ø	C79.31	—	D33.Ø	D43.Ø	D49.6
islands or islets of Langerhans	C25.4	C78.89	DØ1.7	D13.7	D37.8	D49.Ø
isthmus uteri	C54.Ø	C79.82	DØ7.Ø	D26.1	D39.Ø	D49.59
jaw	C76.Ø	C79.89	DØ9.8	D36.7	D48.7	D49.89
bone	C41.1	C79.51	—	D16.5-●	D48.Ø	D49.2
lower	C41.1	C79.51	—	D16.5-●	—	—
upper	C41.Ø	C79.51	—	D16.4-●	—	—
carcinoma (any type) (lower) (upper)	C76.Ø	C79.89	—	—	—	—
skin—*see also Neoplasm, skin, face*	C44.309	C79.2	DØ4.39	D23.39	D48.5	D49.2
soft tissues	CØ3.9	C79.89	DØØ.Ø3	D1Ø.39	D37.Ø9	D49.Ø
lower	CØ3.1	C79.89	DØØ.Ø3	D1Ø.39	D37.Ø9	D49.Ø
upper	CØ3.Ø	C79.89	DØØ.Ø3	D1Ø.39	D37.Ø9	D49.Ø
jejunum	C17.1	C78.4	DØ1.49	D13.39	D37.2	D49.Ø

	Malignant Primary	Malignant Secondary	Ca in situ	Benign	Uncertain Behavior	Unspecified Behavior
joint NEC—*see also Neoplasm, bone*	C41.9	C79.51	—	D16.9-●	D48.Ø	D49.2
acromioclavicular	C4Ø.Ø-●	C79.51	—	D16.Ø-●	—	—
bursa or synovial membrane—*see Neoplasm, connective tissue*						
costovertebral	C41.3	C79.51	—	D16.7	D48.Ø	D49.2
sternocostal	C41.3	C79.51	—	D16.7	D48.Ø	D49.2
temporomandibular	C41.1	C79.51	—	D16.5-●	D48.Ø	D49.2
junction						
anorectal	C21.8	C78.5	DØ1.3	D12.9	D37.8	D49.Ø
cardioesophageal	C16.Ø	C78.89	DØØ.2	D13.1	D37.1	D49.Ø
esophagogastric	C16.Ø	C78.89	DØØ.2	D13.1	D37.1	D49.Ø
gastroesophageal	C16.Ø	C78.89	DØØ.2	D13.1	D37.1	D49.Ø
hard and soft palate	CØ5.9	C79.89	DØØ.ØØ	D1Ø.39	D37.Ø9	D49.Ø
ileocecal	C18.Ø	C78.5	DØ1.Ø	D12.Ø	D37.4	D49.Ø
pelvirectal	C19	C78.5	DØ1.1	D12.7	D37.5	D49.Ø
pelviureteric	C65.-●	C79.Ø-●	DØ9.19	D3Ø.1-●	D41.1-●	D49.59
rectosigmoid	C19	C78.5	DØ1.1	D12.7	D37.5	D49.Ø
squamocolumnar, of cervix	C53.8	C79.82	DØ6.7	D26.Ø	D39.Ø	D49.59
Kaposi's sarcoma—*see Kaposi's, sarcoma*						
kidney (parenchymal)	C64.-●	C79.Ø-●	DØ9.19	D3Ø.Ø-●	D41.Ø-●	D49.51-●
calyx	C65.-●	C79.Ø-●	DØ9.19	D3Ø.1-●	D41.1-●	D49.51-●
hilus	C65.-●	C79.Ø-●	DØ9.19	D3Ø.1-●	D41.1-●	D49.51-●
pelvis	C65.-●	C79.Ø-●	DØ9.19	D3Ø.1-●	D41.1-●	D49.51-●
knee NEC	C76.5-●	C79.89	DØ4.7-●	D36.7	D48.7	D49.89
labia (skin)	C51.9	C79.82	DØ7.1	D28.Ø	D39.8	D49.59
majora	C51.Ø	C79.82	DØ7.1	D28.Ø	D39.8	D49.59
minora	C51.1	C79.82	DØ7.1	D28.Ø	D39.8	D49.59
labial—*see also Neoplasm, lip*	CØØ.9	C79.89	DØØ.Ø1	D1Ø.Ø	D37.Ø1	D49.Ø
sulcus (lower) (upper)	CØ6.1	C79.89	DØØ.Ø2	D1Ø.39	D37.Ø9	D49.Ø
labium (skin)	C51.9	C79.82	DØ7.1	D28.Ø	D39.8	D49.59
majus	C51.Ø	C79.82	DØ7.1	D28.Ø	D39.8	D49.59
minus	C51.1	C79.82	DØ7.1	D28.Ø	D39.8	D49.59
lacrimal						
canaliculi	C69.5-●	C79.49	DØ9.2-●	D31.5-●	D48.7	D49.89
duct (nasal)	C69.5-●	C79.49	DØ9.2-●	D31.5-●	D48.7	D49.89
gland	C69.5-●	C79.49	DØ9.2-●	D31.5-●	D48.7	D49.89
punctum	C69.5-●	C79.49	DØ9.2-●	D31.5-●	D48.7	D49.89
sac	C69.5-●	C79.49	DØ9.2-●	D31.5-●	D48.7	D49.89
Langerhans, islands or islets	C25.4	C78.89	DØ1.7	D13.7	D37.8	D49.Ø
laryngopharynx	C13.9	C79.89	DØØ.Ø8	D1Ø.7	D37.Ø5	D49.Ø

	Malignant Primary	Malignant Secondary	Ca in situ	Benign	Uncertain Behavior	Unspecified Behavior
larynx, laryngeal NEC	C32.9	C78.39	DØ2.Ø	D14.1	D38.Ø	D49.1
aryepiglottic fold	C32.1	C78.39	DØ2.Ø	D14.1	D38.Ø	D49.1
cartilage (arytenoid) (cricoid) (cuneiform) (thyroid)	C32.3	C78.39	DØ2.Ø	D14.1	D38.Ø	D49.1
commissure (anterior) (posterior)	C32.Ø	C78.39	DØ2.Ø	D14.1	D38.Ø	D49.1
extrinsic NEC	C32.1	C78.39	DØ2.Ø	D14.1	D38.Ø	D49.1
meaning hypopharynx	C13.9	C79.89	DØØ.Ø8	D1Ø.7	D37.Ø5	D49.Ø
interarytenoid fold	C32.1	C78.39	DØ2.Ø	D14.1	D38.Ø	D49.1
intrinsic	C32.Ø	C78.39	DØ2.Ø	D14.1	D38.Ø	D49.1
overlapping lesion	C32.8	—	—	—	—	—
ventricular band	C32.1	C78.39	DØ2.Ø	D14.1	D38.Ø	D49.1
leg NEC	C76.5-•	C79.89	DØ4.7-•	D36.7	D48.7	D49.89
lens, crystalline	C69.4-•	C79.49	DØ9.2-•	D31.4-•	D48.7	D49.89
lid (lower) (upper)	C44.1Ø-•	C79.2	DØ4.1-•	D23.1-•	D48.5	D49.2
basal cell carcinoma	C44.11-•	—	—	—	—	—
sebaceous cell	C44.13-•	—	—	—	—	—
specified type NEC	C44.19-•	—	—	—	—	—
squamous cell carcinoma	C44.12-•	—	—	—	—	—
ligament — *see also Neoplasm, connective tissue*						
broad	C57.1	C79.82	DØ7.39	D28.2	D39.8	D49.59
Mackenrodt's	C57.7	C79.82	DØ7.39	D28.7	D39.8	D49.59
non-uterine — *see Neoplasm, connective tissue*						
round	C57.2	C79.82	—	D28.2	D39.8	D49.59
sacro-uterine	C57.3	C79.82	—	D28.2	D39.8	D49.59
uterine	C57.3	C79.82	—	D28.2	D39.8	D49.59
utero-ovarian	C57.7	C79.82	DØ7.39	D28.2	D39.8	D49.59
uterosacral	C57.3	C79.82	—	D28.2	D39.8	D49.59
limb	C76.8	C79.89	DØ4.8	D36.7	D48.7	D49.89
lower	C76.5-•	C79.89	DØ4.7-•	D36.7	D48.7	D49.89
upper	C76.4-•	C79.89	DØ4.6-•	D36.7	D48.7	D49.89
limbus of cornea	C69.1-•	C79.49	DØ9.2-•	D31.1-•	D48.7	D49.89
lingual NEC — *see also Neoplasm, tongue*	CØ2.9	C79.89	DØØ.Ø7	D1Ø.1	D37.Ø2	D49.Ø
lingula, lung	C34.1-•	C78.Ø-•	DØ2.2-•	D14.3-•	D38.1	D49.1
lip	CØØ.9	C79.89	DØØ.Ø1	D1Ø.Ø	D37.Ø1	D49.Ø
buccal aspect — *see Neoplasm, lip, internal*						
commissure	CØØ.6	C79.89	DØØ.Ø1	D1Ø.Ø	D37.Ø1	D49.Ø
external	CØØ.2	C79.89	DØØ.Ø1	D1Ø.Ø	D37.Ø1	D49.Ø
lower	CØØ.1	C79.89	DØØ.Ø1	D1Ø.Ø	D37.Ø1	D49.Ø
upper	CØØ.Ø	C79.89	DØØ.Ø1	D1Ø.Ø	D37.Ø1	D49.Ø
frenulum — *see Neoplasm, lip, internal*						
lip *(Continued)*						
inner aspect — *see Neoplasm, lip, internal*						
internal	CØØ.5	C79.89	DØØ.Ø1	D1Ø.Ø	D37.Ø1	D49.Ø
lower	CØØ.4	C79.89	DØØ.Ø1	D1Ø.Ø	D37.Ø1	D49.Ø
upper	CØØ.3	C79.89	DØØ.Ø1	D1Ø.Ø	D37.Ø1	D49.Ø
lipstick area	CØØ.2	C79.89	DØØ.Ø1	D1Ø.Ø	D37.Ø1	D49.Ø
lower	CØØ.1	C79.89	DØØ.Ø1	D1Ø.Ø	D37.Ø1	D49.Ø
upper	CØØ.Ø	C79.89	DØØ.Ø1	D1Ø.Ø	D37.Ø1	D49.Ø
lower	CØØ.1	C79.89	DØØ.Ø1	D1Ø.Ø	D37.Ø1	D49.Ø
internal	CØØ.4	C79.89	DØØ.Ø1	D1Ø.Ø	D37.Ø1	D49.Ø
mucosa — *see Neoplasm, lip, internal*						
oral aspect — *see Neoplasm, lip, internal*						
overlapping lesion	CØØ.8	—	—	—	—	—
with oral cavity or pharynx	C14.8	—	—	—	—	—
skin (commissure) (lower) (upper)	C44.ØØ	C79.2	DØ4.Ø	D23.Ø	D48.5	D49.2
basal cell carcinoma	C44.Ø1	—	—	—	—	—
specified type NEC	C44.Ø9	—	—	—	—	—
squamous cell carcinoma	C44.Ø2	—	—	—	—	—
upper	CØØ.Ø	C79.89	DØØ.Ø1	D1Ø.Ø	D37.Ø1	D49.Ø
internal	CØØ.3	C79.89	DØØ.Ø1	D1Ø.Ø	D37.Ø1	D49.Ø
vermilion border	CØØ.2	C79.89	DØØ.Ø1	D1Ø.Ø	D37.Ø1	D49.Ø
lower	CØØ.1	C79.89	DØØ.Ø1	D1Ø.Ø	D37.Ø1	D49.Ø
upper	CØØ.Ø	C79.89	DØØ.Ø1	D1Ø.Ø	D37.Ø1	D49.Ø
lipomatous — *see Lipoma, by site*						
liver — *see also Index to disease, by histology*	C22.9	C78.7	DØ1.5	D13.4	D37.6	D49.Ø
primary	C22.8	C78.7	DØ1.5	D13.4	D37.6	D49.Ø
lumbosacral plexus	C47.5	C79.89	—	D36.16	D48.2	D49.2
lung	C34.9-•	C78.Ø-•	DØ2.2-•	D14.3-•	D38.1	D49.1
azygos lobe	C34.1-•	C78.Ø-•	DØ2.2-•	D14.3-•	D38.1	D49.1
carina	C34.Ø-•	C78.Ø-•	DØ2.2-•	D14.3-•	D38.1	D49.1
hilus	C34.Ø-•	C78.Ø-•	DØ2.2-•	D14.3-•	D38.1	D49.1
linqula	C34.1-•	C78.Ø-•	DØ2.2-•	D14.3-•	D38.1	D49.1
lobe NEC	C34.9-•	C78.Ø-•	DØ2.2-•	D14.3-•	D38.1	D49.1
lower lobe	C34.3-•	C78.Ø-•	DØ2.2-•	D14.3-•	D38.1	D49.1
main bronchus	C34.Ø-•	C78.Ø-•	DØ2.2-•	D14.3-•	D38.1	D49.1
mesothelioma — *see Mesothelioma*						
middle lobe	C34.2	C78.Ø-•	DØ2.21	D14.31	D38.1	D49.1
overlapping lesion	C34.8-•	—	—	—	—	—
upper lobe	C34.1-•	C78.Ø-•	DØ2.2-•	D14.3-•	D38.1	D49.1

	Malignant Primary	Malignant Secondary	Ca in situ	Benign	Uncertain Behavior	Unspecified Behavior
lymph, lymphatic channel NEC	C49.9	C79.89	—	D21.9	D48.1	D49.2
gland (secondary)	—	C77.9	—	D36.0	D48.7	D49.89
abdominal	—	C77.2	—	D36.0	D48.7	D49.89
aortic	—	C77.2	—	D36.0	D48.7	D49.89
arm	—	C77.3	—	D36.0	D48.7	D49.89
auricular (anterior) (posterior)	—	C77.0	—	D36.0	D48.7	D49.89
axilla, axillary	—	C77.3	—	D36.0	D48.7	D49.89
brachial	—	C77.3	—	D36.0	D48.7	D49.89
bronchial	—	C77.1	—	D36.0	D48.7	D49.89
bronchopulmonary	—	C77.1	—	D36.0	D48.7	D49.89
celiac	—	C77.2	—	D36.0	D48.7	D49.89
cervical	—	C77.0	—	D36.0	D48.7	D49.89
cervicofacial	—	C77.0	—	D36.0	D48.7	D49.89
Cloquet	—	C77.4	—	D36.0	D48.7	D49.89
colic	—	C77.2	—	D36.0	D48.7	D49.89
common duct	—	C77.2	—	D36.0	D48.7	D49.89
cubital	—	C77.3	—	D36.0	D48.7	D49.89
diaphragmatic	—	C77.1	—	D36.0	D48.7	D49.89
epigastric, inferior	—	C77.1	—	D36.0	D48.7	D49.89
epitrochlear	—	C77.3	—	D36.0	D48.7	D49.89
esophageal	—	C77.1	—	D36.0	D48.7	D49.89
face	—	C77.0	—	D36.0	D48.7	D49.89
femoral	—	C77.4	—	D36.0	D48.7	D49.89
gastric	—	C77.2	—	D36.0	D48.7	D49.89
groin	—	C77.4	—	D36.0	D48.7	D49.89
head	—	C77.0	—	D36.0	D48.7	D49.89
hepatic	—	C77.2	—	D36.0	D48.7	D49.89
hilar (pulmonary)	—	C77.1	—	D36.0	D48.7	D49.89
splenic	—	C77.2	—	D36.0	D48.7	D49.89
hypogastric	—	C77.5	—	D36.0	D48.7	D49.89
ileocolic	—	C77.2	—	D36.0	D48.7	D49.89
iliac	—	C77.5	—	D36.0	D48.7	D49.89
infraclavicular	—	C77.3	—	D36.0	D48.7	D49.89
inguina, inguinal	—	C77.4	—	D36.0	D48.7	D49.89
innominate	—	C77.1	—	D36.0	D48.7	D49.89
intercostal	—	C77.1	—	D36.0	D48.7	D49.89
intestinal	—	C77.2	—	D36.0	D48.7	D49.89
intrabdominal	—	C77.2	—	D36.0	D48.7	D49.89
intrapelvic	—	C77.5	—	D36.0	D48.7	D49.89
intrathoracic	—	C77.1	—	D36.0	D48.7	D49.89
jugular	—	C77.0	—	D36.0	D48.7	D49.89
leg	—	C77.4	—	D36.0	D48.7	D49.89
limb						
lower	—	C77.4	—	D36.0	D48.7	D49.89
upper	—	C77.3	—	D36.0	D48.7	D49.89
lymph, lymphatic channel NEC *(Continued)*						
gland *(Continued)*						
lower limb	—	C77.4	—	D36.0	D48.7	D49.89
lumbar	—	C77.2	—	D36.0	D48.7	D49.89
mandibular	—	C77.0	—	D36.0	D48.7	D49.89
mediastinal	—	C77.1	—	D36.0	D48.7	D49.89
mesenteric (inferior) (superior)	—	C77.2	—	D36.0	D48.7	D49.89
midcolic	—	C77.2	—	D36.0	D48.7	D49.89
multiple sites in categories C77.0 - C77.5	—	C77.8	—	D36.0	D48.7	D49.89
neck	—	C77.0	—	D36.0	D48.7	D49.89
obturator	—	C77.5	—	D36.0	D48.7	D49.89
occipital	—	C77.0	—	D36.0	D48.7	D49.89
pancreatic	—	C77.2	—	D36.0	D48.7	D49.89
para-aortic	—	C77.2	—	D36.0	D48.7	D49.89
paracervical	—	C77.5	—	D36.0	D48.7	D49.89
parametrial	—	C77.5	—	D36.0	D48.7	D49.89
parasternal	—	C77.1	—	D36.0	D48.7	D49.89
parotid	—	C77.0	—	D36.0	D48.7	D49.89
pectoral	—	C77.3	—	D36.0	D48.7	D49.89
pelvic	—	C77.5	—	D36.0	D48.7	D49.89
peri-aortic	—	C77.2	—	D36.0	D48.7	D49.89
peripancreatic	—	C77.2	—	D36.0	D48.7	D49.89
popliteal	—	C77.4	—	D36.0	D48.7	D49.89
porta hepatis	—	C77.2	—	D36.0	D48.7	D49.89
portal	—	C77.2	—	D36.0	D48.7	D49.89
preauricular	—	C77.0	—	D36.0	D48.7	D49.89
prelaryngeal	—	C77.0	—	D36.0	D48.7	D49.89
presymphysial	—	C77.5	—	D36.0	D48.7	D49.89
pretracheal	—	C77.0	—	D36.0	D48.7	D49.89
primary (any site) NEC	C96.9	—	—	—	—	—
pulmonary (hiler)	—	C77.1	—	D36.0	D48.7	D49.89
pyloric	—	C77.2	—	D36.0	D48.7	D49.89
retroperitoneal	—	C77.2	—	D36.0	D48.7	D49.89
retropharyngeal	—	C77.0	—	D36.0	D48.7	D49.89
Rosenmuller's	—	C77.4	—	D36.0	D48.7	D49.89
sacral	—	C77.5	—	D36.0	D48.7	D49.89
scalene	—	C77.0	—	D36.0	D48.7	D49.89
site NEC	—	C77.9	—	D36.0	D48.7	D49.89
splenic (hilar)	—	C77.2	—	D36.0	D48.7	D49.89
subclavicular	—	C77.3	—	D36.0	D48.7	D49.89
subinguinal	—	C77.4	—	D36.0	D48.7	D49.89

TABLE OF NEOPLASMS

	Malignant Primary	Malignant Secondary	Ca in situ	Benign	Uncertain Behavior	Unspecified Behavior
lymph, lymphatic channel NEC *(Continued)*						
gland *(Continued)*						
sublingual	—	C77.Ø	—	D36.Ø	D48.7	D49.89
submandibular	—	C77.Ø	—	D36.Ø	D48.7	D49.89
submaxillary	—	C77.Ø	—	D36.Ø	D48.7	D49.89
submental	—	C77.Ø	—	D36.Ø	D48.7	D49.89
subscapular	—	C77.3	—	D36.Ø	D48.7	D49.89
supraclavicular	—	C77.Ø	—	D36.Ø	D48.7	D49.89
thoracic	—	C77.1	—	D36.Ø	D48.7	D49.89
tibial	—	C77.4	—	D36.Ø	D48.7	D49.89
tracheal	—	C77.1	—	D36.Ø	D48.7	D49.89
tracheobronchial	—	C77.1	—	D36.Ø	D48.7	D49.89
upper limb	—	C77.3	—	D36.Ø	D48.7	D49.89
Virchow's	—	C77.Ø	—	D36.Ø	D48.7	D49.89
node — *see also Neoplasm, lymph gland*						
primary NEC	C96.9	—	—	—	—	—
vessel — *see also Neoplasm, connective tissue*	C49.9	C79.89	—	D21.9	D48.1	D49.2
Mackenrodt's ligament	C57.7	C79.82	DØ7.39	D28.7	D39.8	D49.59
malar	C41.Ø	C79.51	—	D16.4-•	D48.Ø	D49.2
region — *see Neoplasm, cheek*						
mammary gland — *see Neoplasm, breast*						
mandible	C41.1	C79.51	—	D16.5-•	D48.Ø	D49.2
alveolar						
mucosa (carcinoma)	CØ3.1	C79.89	DØØ.03	D1Ø.39	D37.Ø9	D49.Ø
ridge or process	C41.1	C79.51	—	D16.5-•	D48.Ø	D49.2
marrow (bone) NEC	C96.9	C79.52	—	—	D47.9	D49.89
mastectomy site (skin) — *see also Neoplasm, breast, skin*	C44.5Ø1	C79.2	—	—	—	—
specified as breast tissue	C5Ø.8-•	C79.81	—	—	—	—
mastoid (air cells) (antrum) (cavity)	C3Ø.1	C78.39	DØ2.3	D14.Ø	D38.5	D49.1
bone or process	C41.Ø	C79.51	—	D16.4-•	D48.Ø	D49.2
maxilla, maxillary (superior)	C41.Ø	C79.51	—	D16.4-•	D48.Ø	D49.2
alveolar						
mucosa	CØ3.Ø	C79.89	DØØ.Ø3	D1Ø.39	D37.Ø9	D49.Ø
ridge or process (carcinoma)	C41.Ø	C79.51	—	D16.4-•	D48.Ø	D49.2
antrum	C31.Ø	C78.39	DØ2.3	D14.Ø	D38.5	D49.1
carcinoma	CØ3.Ø	C79.51	—	—	—	—
inferior — *see Neoplasm, mandible*						
sinus	C31.Ø	C78.39	DØ2.3	D14.Ø	D38.5	D49.1
meatus external (ear) — *see also Neoplasm, skin, ear*	C44.2Ø-•	C79.2	DØ4.2-•	D23.2-•	D48.5	D49.2
Meckel diverticulum, malignant	C17.3	C78.4	DØ1.49	D13.39	D37.2	D49.Ø
mediastinum, mediastinal	C38.3	C78.1	—	D15.2	D38.3	D49.89
anterior	C38.1	C78.1	—	D15.2	D38.3	D49.89
posterior	C38.2	C78.1	—	D15.2	D38.3	D49.89
medulla						
adrenal	C74.1-•	C79.7-•	DØ9.3	D35.Ø-•	D44.1-•	D49.7
oblongata	C71.7	C79.31	—	D33.1	D43.1	D49.6
meibomian gland	C44.1Ø-•	C79.2	DØ4.1-•	D23.1-•	D48.5	D49.2
basal cell carcinoma	C44.11-•	—	—	—	—	—
sebaceous cell	C44.13-•	—	—	—	—	—
specified type NEC	C44.19-•	—	—	—	—	—
squamous cell carcinoma	C44.12-•	—	—	—	—	—
melanoma — *see Melanoma*						
meninges	C7Ø.9	C79.49	—	D32.9	D42.9	D49.7
brain	C7Ø.Ø	C79.32	—	D32.Ø	D42.Ø	D49.7
cerebral	C7Ø.Ø	C79.32	—	D32.Ø	D42.Ø	D49.7
crainial	C7Ø.Ø	C79.32	—	D32.Ø	D42.Ø	D49.7
intracranial	C7Ø.Ø	C79.32	—	D32.Ø	D42.Ø	D49.7
spinal (cord)	C7Ø.1	C79.49	—	D32.1	D42.1	D49.7
meniscus, knee joint (lateral) (medial)	C4Ø.2-•	C79.51	—	D16.2-•	D48.Ø	D49.2
Merkel cell — *see Carcinoma, Merkel cell*						
mesentery, mesenteric	C48.1	C78.6	—	D2Ø.1	D48.4	D49.Ø
mesoappendix	C48.1	C78.6	—	D2Ø.1	D48.4	D49.Ø
mesocolon	C48.1	C78.6	—	D2Ø.1	D48.4	D49.Ø
mesopharynx — *see Neoplasm, oropharynx*						
mesosalpinx	C57.1	C79.82	DØ7.39	D28.2	D39.8	D49.59
mesothelial tissue — *see Mesothelioma*						
mesothelioma — *see Mesothelioma*						
mesovarium	C57.1	C79.82	DØ7.39	D28.2	D39.8	D49.59
metacarpus (any bone)	C4Ø.1-•	C79.51	—	D16.1-•	—	—
metastatic NEC — *see also Neoplasm, by site, secondary*	—	C79.9	—	—	—	—
metatarsus (any bone)	C4Ø.3-•	C79.51	—	D16.3-•	—	—
midbrain	C71.7	C79.31	—	D33.1	D43.1	D49.6
milk duct — *see Neoplasm, breast*						
mons						
pubis	C51.9	C79.82	DØ7.1	D28.Ø	D39.8	D49.59
veneris	C51.9	C79.82	DØ7.1	D28.Ø	D39.8	D49.59

	Malignant Primary	Malignant Secondary	Ca in situ	Benign	Uncertain Behavior	Unspecified Behavior
motor tract	C72.9	C79.49	—	D33.9	D43.9	D49.7
brain	C71.9	C79.31	—	D33.2	D43.2	D49.6
cauda equina	C72.1	C79.49	—	D33.4	D43.4	D49.7
spinal	C72.0	C79.49	—	D33.4	D43.4	D49.7
mouth	C06.9	C79.89	D00.00	D10.30	D37.09	D49.0
book-leaf	C06.89	C79.89	—	—	—	—
floor	C04.9	C79.89	D00.06	D10.2	D37.09	D49.0
anterior portion	C04.0	C79.89	D00.06	D10.2	D37.09	D49.0
lateral portion	C04.1	C79.89	D00.06	D10.2	D37.09	D49.0
overlapping lesion	C04.8	—	—	—	—	—
overlapping NEC	C06.80	—	—	—	—	—
roof	C05.9	C79.89	D00.00	D10.39	D37.09	D49.0
specified part NEC	C06.89	C79.89	D00.00	D10.39	D37.09	D49.0
vestibule	C06.1	C79.89	D00.00	D10.39	D37.09	D49.0
mucosa						
alveolar (ridge or process)	C03.9	C79.89	D00.03	D10.39	D37.09	D49.0
lower	C03.1	C79.89	D00.03	D10.39	D37.09	D49.0
upper	C03.0	C79.89	D00.03	D10.39	D37.09	D49.0
buccal	C06.0	C79.89	D00.02	D10.39	D37.09	D49.0
cheek	C06.0	C79.89	D00.02	D10.39	D37.09	D49.0
lip — *see Neoplasm, lip, internal*						
nasal	C30.0	C78.39	D02.3	D14.0	D38.5	D49.1
oral	C06.0	C79.89	D00.02	D10.39	D37.09	D49.0
Mullerian duct						
female	C57.7	C79.82	D07.39	D28.7	D39.8	D49.59
male	C63.7	C79.82	D07.69	D29.8	D40.8	D49.59
muscle — *see also Neoplasm, connective tissue*						
extraocular	C69.6-•	C79.49	D09.2-•	D31.6-•	D48.7	D49.89
myocardium	C38.0	C79.89	—	D15.1	D48.7	D49.89
myometrium	C54.2	C79.82	D07.0	D26.1	D39.0	D49.59
myopericardium	C38.0	C79.89	—	D15.1	D48.7	D49.89
nabothian gland (follicle)	C53.0	C79.82	D06.0	D26.0	D39.0	D49.59
nail — *see also Neoplasm, skin, limb*	C44.90	C79.2	D04.9	D23.9	D48.5	D49.2
finger — *see also Neoplasm, skin, limb, upper*	C44.60-•	C79.2	D04.6-•	D23.6-•	D48.5	D49.2
toe — *see also Neoplasm, skin, limb, lower*	C44.70-•	C79.2	D04.7-•	D23.7-•	D48.5	D49.2
nares, naris (anterior) (posterior)	C30.0	C78.39	D02.3	D14.0	D38.5	D49.1
nasal — *see Neoplasm, nose*						
nasolabial groove — *see also Neoplasm, skin, face*	C44.309	C79.2	D04.39	D23.39	D48.5	D49.2
nasolacrimal duct	C69.5-•	C79.49	D09.2-•	D31.5-•	D48.7	D49.89

	Malignant Primary	Malignant Secondary	Ca in situ	Benign	Uncertain Behavior	Unspecified Behavior
nasopharynx, nasopharyngeal	C11.9	C79.89	D00.08	D10.6	D37.05	D49.0
floor	C11.3	C79.89	D00.08	D10.6	D37.05	D49.0
overlapping lesion	C11.8	—	—	—	—	—
roof	C11.0	C79.89	D00.08	D10.6	D37.05	D49.0
wall	C11.9	C79.89	D00.08	D10.6	D37.05	D49.0
anterior	C11.3	C79.89	D00.08	D10.6	D37.05	D49.0
lateral	C11.2	C79.89	D00.08	D10.6	D37.05	D49.0
posterior	C11.1	C79.89	D00.08	D10.6	D37.05	D49.0
superior	C11.0	C79.89	D00.08	D10.6	D37.05	D49.0
nates — *see also Neoplasm, skin, trunk*	C44.509	C79.2	D04.5	D23.5	D48.5	D49.2
neck NEC	C76.0	C79.89	D09.8	D36.7	D48.7	D49.89
skin	C44.40	—	—	—	—	—
basal cell carcinoma	C44.41	—	—	—	—	—
specified type NEC	C44.49	—	—	—	—	—
squamous cell carcinoma	C44.42	—	—	—	—	—
nerve (ganglion)	C47.9	C79.89	—	D36.10	D48.2	D49.2
abducens	C72.59	C79.49	—	D33.3	D43.3	D49.7
accessory (spinal)	C72.59	C79.49	—	D33.3	D43.3	D49.7
acoustic	C72.4-•	C79.49	—	D33.3	D43.3	D49.7
auditory	C72.4-•	C79.49	—	D33.3	D43.3	D49.7
autonomic NEC — *see also Neoplasm, nerve, peripheral*	C47.9	C79.89	—	D36.10	D48.2	D49.2
brachial	C47.1-•	C79.89	—	D36.12	D48.2	D49.2
cranial	C72.50	C79.49	—	D33.3	D43.3	D49.7
specified NEC	C72.59	C79.49	—	D33.3	D43.3	D49.7
facial	C72.59	C79.49	—	D33.3	D43.3	D49.7
femoral	C47.2-•	C79.89	—	D36.13	D48.2	D49.2
ganglion NEC — *see also Neoplasm, nerve, peripheral*	C47.9	C79.89	—	D36.10	D48.2	D49.2
glossopharyngeal	C72.59	C79.49	—	D33.3	D43.3	D49.7
hypoglossal	C72.59	C79.49	—	D33.3	D43.3	D49.7
intercostal	C47.3	C79.89	—	D36.14	D48.2	D49.2
lumbar	C47.6	C79.89	—	D36.17	D48.2	D49.2
median	C47.1-•	C79.89	—	D36.12	D48.2	D49.2
obturator	C47.2-•	C79.89	—	D36.13	D48.2	D49.2
oculomotor	C72.59	C79.49	—	D33.3	D43.3	D49.7
olfactory	C47.2-•	C79.49	—	D33.3	D43.3	D49.7
optic	C72.3-•	C79.49	—	D33.3	D43.3	D49.7
parasympathetic NEC	C47.9	C79.89	—	D36.10	D48.2	D49.2
peripheral NEC	C47.9	C79.89	—	D36.10	D48.2	D49.2
abdomen	C47.4	C79.89	—	D36.15	D48.2	D49.2
abdominal wall	C47.4	C79.89	—	D36.15	D48.2	D49.2

	Malignant Primary	Malignant Secondary	Ca in situ	Benign	Uncertain Behavior	Unspecified Behavior
nerve *(Continued)*						
peripheral NEC *(Continued)*						
ankle	C47.2-●	C79.89	—	D36.13	D48.2	D49.2
antecubital fossa or space	C47.1-●	C79.89	—	D36.12	D48.2	D49.2
arm	C47.1-●	C79.89	—	D36.12	D48.2	D49.2
auricle (ear)	C47.0	C79.89	—	D36.11	D48.2	D49.2
axilla	C47.3	C79.89	—	D36.12	D48.2	D49.2
back	C47.6	C79.89	—	D36.17	D48.2	D49.2
buttock	C47.5	C79.89	—	D36.16	D48.2	D49.2
calf	C47.2-●	C79.89	—	D36.13	D48.2	D49.2
cervical region	C47.0	C79.89	—	D36.11	D48.2	D49.2
cheek	C47.0	C79.89	—	D36.11	D48.2	D49.2
chest (wall)	C47.3	C79.89	—	D36.14	D48.2	D49.2
chin	C47.0	C79.89	—	D36.11	D48.2	D49.2
ear (external)	C47.0	C79.89	—	D36.11	D48.2	D49.2
elbow	C47.1-●	C79.89	—	D36.12	D48.2	D49.2
extrarectal	C47.5	C79.89	—	D36.16	D48.2	D49.2
extremity	C47.9	C79.89	—	D36.10	D48.2	D49.2
lower	C47.2-●	C79.89	—	D36.13	D48.2	D49.2
upper	C47.1-●	C79.89	—	D36.12	D48.2	D49.2
eyelid	C47.0	C79.89	—	D36.11	D48.2	D49.2
face	C47.0	C79.89	—	D36.11	D48.2	D49.2
finger	C47.1-●	C79.89	—	D36.12	D48.2	D49.2
flank	C47.6	C79.89	—	D36.17	D48.2	D49.2
foot	C47.2-●	C79.89	—	D36.13	D48.2	D49.2
forearm	C47.1-●	C79.89	—	D36.12	D48.2	D49.2
forehead	C47.0	C79.89	—	D36.11	D48.2	D49.2
gluteal region	C47.5	C79.89	—	D36.16	D48.2	D49.2
groin	C47.5	C79.89	—	D36.16	D48.2	D49.2
hand	C47.1-●	C79.89	—	D36.12	D48.2	D49.2
head	C47.0	C79.89	—	D36.11	D48.2	D49.2
heel	C47.2-●	C79.89	—	D36.13	D48.2	D49.2
hip	C47.2-●	C79.89	—	D36.13	D48.2	D49.2
infraclavicular region	C47.3	C79.89	—	D36.14	D48.2	D49.2
inguinal (canal) (region)	C47.5	C79.89	—	D36.16	D48.2	D49.2
intrathoracic	C47.3	C79.89	—	D36.14	D48.2	D49.2
ischiorectal fossa	C47.5	C79.89	—	D36.16	D48.2	D49.2
knee	C47.2-●	C79.89	—	D36.13	D48.2	D49.2
leg	C47.2-●	C79.89	—	D36.13	D48.2	D49.2
limb NEC	C47.9	C79.89	—	D36.10	D48.2	D49.2
lower	C47.2-●	C79.89	—	D36.13	D48.2	D49.2
upper	C47.1-●	C79.89	—	D36.12	D48.2	D49.2
nates	C47.5	C79.89	—	D36.16	D48.2	D49.2
neck	C47.0	C79.89	—	D36.11	D48.2	D49.2

	Malignant Primary	Malignant Secondary	Ca in situ	Benign	Uncertain Behavior	Unspecified Behavior
nerve *(Continued)*						
peripheral NEC *(Continued)*						
orbit	C69.6-●	C79.49	—	D31.6-●	D48.7	D49.2
pararectal	C47.5	C79.89	—	D36.16	D48.2	D49.2
paraurethral	C47.5	C79.89	—	D36.16	D48.2	D49.2
paravaginal	C47.5	C79.89	—	D36.16	D48.2	D49.2
pelvis (floor)	C47.5	C79.89	—	D36.16	D48.2	D49.2
pelvoabdominal	C47.8	C79.89	—	D36.17	D48.2	D49.2
perineum	C47.5	C79.89	—	D36.16	D48.2	D49.2
perirectal (tissue)	C47.5	C79.89	—	D36.16	D48.2	D49.2
periurethral (tissue)	C47.5	C79.89	—	D36.16	D48.2	D49.2
popliteal fossa or space	C47.2-●	C79.89	—	D36.13	D48.2	D49.2
presacral	C47.5	C79.89	—	D36.16	D48.2	D49.2
pterygoid fossa	C47.0	C79.89	—	D36.11	D48.2	D49.2
rectovaginal septum or wall	C47.5	C79.89	—	D36.16	D48.2	D49.2
rectovesical	C47.5	C79.89	—	D36.16	D48.2	D49.2
sacrococcygeal region	C47.5	C79.89	—	D36.16	D48.2	D49.2
scalp	C47.0	C79.89	—	D36.11	D48.2	D49.2
scapular region	C47.3	C79.89	—	D36.14	D48.2	D49.2
shoulder	C47.1-●	C79.89	—	D36.12	D48.2	D49.2
submental	C47.0	C79.89	—	D36.11	D48.2	D49.2
supraclavicular region	C47.0	C79.89	—	D36.11	D48.2	D49.2
temple	C47.0	C79.89	—	D36.11	D48.2	D49.2
temporal region	C47.0	C79.89	—	D36.11	D48.2	D49.2
thigh	C47.2-●	C79.89	—	D36.13	D48.2	D49.2
thoracic (duct) (wall)	C47.3	C79.89	—	D36.14	D48.2	D49.2
thorax	C47.3	C79.89	—	D36.14	D48.2	D49.2
thumb	C47.1-●	C79.89	—	D36.12	D48.2	D49.2
toe	C47.2-●	C79.89	—	D36.13	D48.2	D49.2
trunk	C47.6	C79.89	—	D36.17	D48.2	D49.2
umbilicus	C47.4	C79.89	—	D36.15	D48.2	D49.2
vesicorectal	C47.5	C79.89	—	D36.16	D48.2	D49.2
wrist	C47.1-●	C79.89	—	D36.12	D48.2	D49.2
radial	C47.1-●	C79.89	—	D36.12	D48.2	D49.2
sacral	C47.5	C79.89	—	D36.16	D48.2	D49.2
sciatic	C47.2-●	C79.89	—	D36.13	D48.2	D49.2
spinal NEC	C47.9	C79.89	—	D36.10	D48.2	D49.2
accessory	C72.59	C79.49	—	D33.3	D43.3	D49.7
sympathetic NEC — *see also Neoplasm, nerve, peripheral*	C47.9	C79.89	—	D36.10	D48.2	D49.2
trigeminal	C72.59	C79.49	—	D33.3	D43.3	D49.7
trochlear	C72.59	C79.49	—	D33.3	D43.3	D49.7
ulnar	C47.1-●	C79.89	—	D36.12	D48.2	D49.2
vagus	C72.59	C79.49	—	D33.3	D43.3	D49.7

◄ New   Revised   ~~deleted~~ Deleted   ● Use Additional Character(s)

	Malignant Primary	Malignant Secondary	Ca in situ	Benign	Uncertain Behavior	Unspecified Behavior
nervous system (central)	C72.9	C79.40	—	D33.9	D43.9	D49.7
autonomic — *see Neoplasm, nerve, peripheral*						
parasympathetic — *see Neoplasm, nerve, peripheral*						
specified site NEC	—	C79.49	—	D33.7	D43.8	—
sympathetic — *see Neoplasm, nerve, peripheral*						
nevus — *see Nevus*						
nipple	C50.0-•	C79.81	D05.-•	D24.-•	—	—
nose, nasal	C76.0	C79.89	D09.8	D36.7	D48.7	D49.89
ala (external) (nasi) — *see also Neoplasm, nose, skin*	C44.301	C79.2	D04.39	D23.39	D48.5	D49.2
bone	C41.0	C79.51	—	D16.4-•	D48.0	D49.2
cartilage	C30.0	C78.39	D02.3	D14.0	D38.5	D49.1
cavity	C30.0	C78.39	D02.3	D14.0	D38.5	D49.1
choana	C11.3	C79.89	D00.08	D10.6	D37.05	D49.0
external (skin) — *see also Neoplasm, nose, skin*	C44.301	C79.2	D04.39	D23.39	D48.5	D49.2
fossa	C30.0	C78.39	D02.3	D14.0	D38.5	D49.1
internal	C30.0	C78.39	D02.3	D14.0	D38.5	D49.1
mucosa	C30.0	C78.39	D02.3	D14.0	D38.5	D49.1
septum	C30.0	C78.39	D02.3	D14.0	D38.5	D49.1
posterior margin	C11.3	C79.89	D00.08	D10.6	D37.05	D49.0
sinus — *see Neoplasm, sinus*						
skin	C44.301	C79.2	D04.39	D23.39	D48.5	D49.2
basal cell carcinoma	C44.311	—	—	—	—	—
specified type NEC	C44.391	—	—	—	—	—
squamous cell carcinoma	C44.321	—	—	—	—	—
turbinate (mucosa)	C30.0	C78.39	D02.3	D14.0	D38.5	D49.1
bone	C41.0	C79.51	—	D16.4-•	D48.0	D49.2
vestibule	C30.0	C78.39	D02.3	D14.0	D38.5	D49.1
nostril	C30.0	C78.39	D02.3	D14.0	D38.5	D49.1
nucleus pulposus	C41.2	C79.51	—	D16.6	D48.0	D49.2
occipital						
bone	C41.0	C79.51	—	D16.4-•	D48.0	D49.2
lobe or pole, brain	C71.4	C79.31	—	D33.0	D43.0	D49.6
odontogenic — *see Neoplasm, jaw bone*						
olfactory nerve or bulb	C72.2-•	C79.49	—	D33.3	D43.3	D49.7
olive (brain)	C71.7	C79.31	—	D33.1	D43.1	D49.6
omentum	C48.1	C78.6	—	D20.1	D48.4	D49.0
operculum (brain)	C71.0	C79.31	—	D33.0	D43.0	D49.6
optic nerve, chiasm, or tract	C72.3-•	C79.49	—	D33.3	D43.3	D49.7

	Malignant Primary	Malignant Secondary	Ca in situ	Benign	Uncertain Behavior	Unspecified Behavior
oral (cavity)	C06.9	C79.89	D00.00	D10.30	D37.09	D49.0
ill-defined	C14.8	C79.89	D00.00	D10.30	D37.09	D49.0
mucosa	C06.0	C79.89	D00.02	D10.39	D37.09	D49.0
orbit	C69.6-•	C79.49	D09.2-•	D31.6-•	D48.7	D49.89
autonomic nerve	C69.6-•	C79.49	—	D31.6-•	D48.7	D49.2
bone	C41.0	C79.51	—	D16.4-•	D48.0	D49.2
eye	C69.6-•	C79.49	D09.2-•	D31.6-•	D48.7	D49.89
peripheral nerves	C69.6-•	C79.49	—	D31.6-•	D48.7	D49.2
soft parts	C69.6-•	C79.49	D09.2-•	D31.6-•	D48.7	D49.89
organ of Zuckerkandl	C75.5	C79.89	—	D35.6	D44.7	D49.7
oropharynx	C10.9	C79.89	D00.08	D10.5	D37.05	D49.0
branchial cleft (vestige)	C10.4	C79.89	D00.08	D10.5	D37.05	D49.0
junctional region	C10.8	C79.89	D00.08	D10.5	D37.05	D49.0
lateral wall	C10.2	C79.89	D00.08	D10.5	D37.05	D49.0
overlapping lesion	C10.8	—	—	—	—	—
pillars or fauces	C09.1	C79.89	D00.08	D10.5	D37.05	D49.0
posterior wall	C10.3	C79.89	D00.08	D10.5	D37.05	D49.0
vallecula	C10.0	C79.89	D00.08	D10.5	D37.05	D49.0
os						
external	C53.1	C79.82	D06.1	D26.0	D39.0	D49.59
internal	C53.0	C79.82	D06.0	D26.0	D39.0	D49.59
ovary	C56.-•	C79.6-•	D07.39	D27.-•	D39.1-•	D49.59
oviduct	C57.0-•	C79.82	D07.39	D28.2	D39.8	D49.59
palate	C05.9	C79.89	D00.00	D10.39	D37.09	D49.0
hard	C05.0	C79.89	D00.05	D10.39	D37.09	D49.0
junction of hard and soft palate	C05.9	C79.89	D00.00	D10.39	D37.09	D49.0
overlapping lesions	C05.8	—	—	—	—	—
soft	C05.1	C79.89	D00.04	D10.39	D37.09	D49.0
nasopharyngeal surface	C11.3	C79.89	D00.08	D10.6	D37.05	D49.0
posterior surface	C11.3	C79.89	D00.08	D10.6	D37.05	D49.0
superior surface	C11.3	C79.89	D00.08	D10.6	D37.05	D49.0
palatoglossal arch	C09.1	C79.89	D00.00	D10.5	D37.09	D49.0
palatopharyngeal arch	C09.1	C79.89	D00.00	D10.5	D37.09	D49.0
pallium	C71.0	C79.31	—	D33.0	D43.0	D49.6
palpebra	C44.10-•	C79.2	D04.1-•	D23.1-•	D48.5	D49.2
basal cell carcinoma	C44.11-•	—	—	—	—	—
sebaceous cell	C44.13-•	—	—	—	—	—
specified type NEC	C44.19-•	—	—	—	—	—
squamous cell carcinoma	C44.12-•	—	—	—	—	—
pancreas	C25.9	C78.89	D01.7	D13.6	D37.8	D49.0
body	C25.1	C78.89	D01.7	D13.6	D37.8	D49.0
duct (of Santorini) (of Wirsung)	C25.3	C78.89	D01.7	D13.6	D37.8	D49.0
ectopic tissue	C25.7	C78.89	—	D13.6	D37.8	D49.0
head	C25.0	C78.89	D01.7	D13.6	D37.8	D49.0

	Malignant Primary	Malignant Secondary	Ca in situ	Benign	Uncertain Behavior	Unspecified Behavior
pancreas *(Continued)*						
islet cells	C25.4	C78.89	D01.7	D13.7	D37.8	D49.0
neck	C25.7	C78.89	D01.7	D13.6	D37.8	D49.0
overlapping lesion	C25.8	—	—	—	—	—
tail	C25.2	C78.89	D01.7	D13.6	D37.8	D49.0
para-aortic body	C75.5	C79.89	—	D35.6	D44.7	D49.7
paraganglion NEC	C75.5	C79.89	—	D35.6	D44.7	D49.7
parametrium	C57.3	C79.82	—	D28.2	D39.8	D49.59
paranephric	C48.0	C78.6	—	D20.0	D48.3	D49.0
pararectal	C76.3	C79.89	—	D36.7	D48.7	D49.89
parasagittal (region)	C76.0	C79.89	D09.8	D36.7	D48.7	D49.89
parasellar	C72.9	C79.49	—	D33.9	D43.8	D49.7
parathyroid (gland)	C75.0	C79.89	D09.3	D35.1	D44.2	D49.7
paraurethral	C76.3	C79.89	—	D36.7	D48.7	D49.89
gland	C68.1	C79.19	D09.19	D30.8	D41.8	D49.59
paravaginal	C76.3	C79.89	—	D36.7	D48.7	D49.89
parenchyma, kidney	C64.-•	C79.0-•	D09.19	D30.0-•	D41.0-•	D49.51-•
parietal						
bone	C41.0	C79.51	—	D16.4-•	D48.0	D49.2
lobe, brain	C71.3	C79.31	—	D33.0	D43.0	D49.6
paroophoron	C57.1	C79.82	D07.39	D28.2	D39.8	D49.59
parotid (duct) (gland)	C07	C79.89	D00.00	D11.0	D37.030	D49.0
parovarium	C57.1	C79.82	D07.39	D28.2	D39.8	D49.59
patella	C40.20	C79.51	—	—	—	—
peduncle, cerebral	C71.7	C79.31	—	D33.1	D43.1	D49.6
pelvirectal junction	C19	C78.5	D01.1	D12.7	D37.5	D49.0
pelvis, pelvic	C76.3	C79.89	D09.8	D36.7	D48.7	D49.89
bone	C41.4	C79.51	—	D16.8	D48.0	D49.2
floor	C76.3	C79.89	D09.8	D36.7	D48.7	D49.89
renal	C65.-•	C79.0-•	D09.19	D30.1-•	D41.1-•	D49.51-•
viscera	C76.3	C79.89	D09.8	D36.7	D48.7	D49.89
wall	C76.3	C79.89	D09.8	D36.7	D48.7	D49.89
pelvo-abdominal	C76.8	C79.89	D09.8	D36.7	D48.7	D49.89
penis	C60.9	C79.82	D07.4	D29.0	D40.8	D49.59
body	C60.2	C79.82	D07.4	D29.0	D40.8	D49.59
corpus (cavernosum)	C60.2	C79.82	D07.4	D29.0	D40.8	D49.59
glans	C60.1	C79.82	D07.4	D29.0	D40.8	D49.59
overlapping sites	C60.8	—	—	—	—	—
skin NEC	C60.9	C79.82	D07.4	D29.0	D40.8	D49.59
periadrenal (tissue)	C48.0	C78.6	—	D20.0	D48.3	D49.0
perianal (skin) — *see also Neoplasm, anus, skin*	C44.500	C79.2	D04.5	D23.5	D48.5	D49.2
pericardium	C38.0	C79.89	—	D15.1	D48.7	D49.89
perinephric	C48.0	C78.6	—	D20.0	D48.3	D49.0
perineum	C76.3	C79.89	D09.8	D36.7	D48.7	D49.89
periodontal tissue NEC	C03.9	C79.89	D00.03	D10.39	D37.09	D49.0
periosteum — *see Neoplasm, bone*						
peripancreatic	C48.0	C78.6	—	D20.0	D48.3	D49.0
peripheral nerve NEC	C47.9	C79.89	—	D36.10	D48.2	D49.2
perirectal (tissue)	C76.3	C79.89	—	D36.7	D48.7	D49.89
perirenal (tissue)	C48.0	C78.6	—	D20.0	D48.3	D49.0
peritoneum, peritoneal (cavity)	C48.2	C78.6	—	D20.1	D48.4	D49.0
benign mesothelial tissue — *see Mesothelioma, benign*						
overlapping lesion	C48.8	—	—	—	—	—
with digestive organs	C26.9	—	—	—	—	—
parietal	C48.1	C78.6	—	D20.1	D48.4	D49.0
pelvic	C48.1	C78.6	—	D20.1	D48.4	D49.0
specified part NEC	C48.1	C78.6	—	D20.1	D48.4	D49.0
peritonsillar (tissue)	C76.0	C79.89	D09.8	D36.7	D48.7	D49.89
periurethral tissue	C76.3	C79.89	—	D36.7	D48.7	D49.89
phalanges						
foot	C40.3-•	C79.51	—	D16.3-•	—	—
hand	C40.1-•	C79.51	—	D16.1-•	—	—
pharynx, pharyngeal	C14.0	C79.89	D00.08	D10.9	D37.05	D49.0
bursa	C11.1	C79.89	D00.08	D10.6	D37.05	D49.0
fornix	C11.3	C79.89	D00.08	D10.6	D37.05	D49.0
recess	C11.2	C79.89	D00.08	D10.6	D37.05	D49.0
region	C14.0	C79.89	D00.08	D10.9	D37.05	D49.0
tonsil	C11.1	C79.89	D00.08	D10.6	D37.05	D49.0
wall (lateral) (posterior)	C14.0	C79.89	D00.08	D10.9	D37.05	D49.0
pia mater	C70.9	C79.40	—	D32.9	D42.9	D49.7
cerebral	C70.0	C79.32	—	D32.0	D42.0	D49.7
cranial	C70.0	C79.32	—	D32.0	D42.0	D49.7
spinal	C70.1	C79.49	—	D32.1	D42.1	D49.7
pillars of fauces	C09.1	C79.89	D00.08	D10.5	D37.05	D49.0
pineal (body) (gland)	C75.3	C79.89	D09.3	D35.4	D44.5	D49.7
pinna (ear) NEC — *see also Neoplasm, skin, ear*	C44.20-•	C79.2	D04.2-•	D23.2-•	D48.5	D49.2
piriform fossa or sinus	C12	C79.89	D00.08	D10.7	D37.05	D49.0
pituitary (body) (fossa) (gland) (lobe)	C75.1	C79.89	D09.3	D35.2	D44.3	D49.7
placenta	C58	C79.82	D07.0	D26.7	D39.2	D49.59
pleura, pleural (cavity)	C38.4	C78.2	—	D19.0	D38.2	D49.1
overlapping lesion with heart or mediastinum	C38.8	—	—	—	—	—
parietal	C38.4	C78.2	—	D19.0	D38.2	D49.1
visceral	C38.4	C78.2	—	D19.0	D38.2	D49.1

New Revised ~~deleted~~ Deleted • Use Additional Character(s)

TABLE OF NEOPLASMS

	Malignant Primary	Malignant Secondary	Ca in situ	Benign	Uncertain Behavior	Unspecified Behavior
plexus						
brachial	C47.1-•	C79.89	—	D36.12	D48.2	D49.2
cervical	C47.Ø	C79.89	—	D36.11	D48.2	D49.2
choroid	C71.5	C79.31	—	D33.Ø	D43.Ø	D49.6
lumbosacral	C47.5	C79.89	—	D36.16	D48.2	D49.2
sacral	C47.5	C79.89	—	D36.16	D48.2	D49.2
pluriendocrine	C75.8	C79.89	DØ9.3	D35.7	D44.9	D49.7
pole						
frontal	C71.1	C79.31	—	D33.Ø	D43.Ø	D49.6
occipital	C71.4	C79.31	—	D33.Ø	D43.Ø	D49.6
pons (varolii)	C71.7	C79.31	—	D33.1	D43.1	D49.6
popliteal fossa or space	C76.5-•	C79.89	DØ4.7-•	D36.7	D48.7	D49.89
postcricoid (region)	C13.Ø	C79.89	DØØ.Ø8	D1Ø.7	D37.Ø5	D49.Ø
posterior fossa (cranial)	C71.9	C79.31	—	D33.2	D43.2	D49.6
postnasal space	C11.9	C79.89	DØØ.Ø8	D1Ø.6	D37.Ø5	D49.Ø
prepuce	C6Ø.Ø	C79.82	DØ7.4	D29.Ø	D4Ø.8	D49.59
prepylorus	C16.4	C78.89	DØØ.2	D13.1	D37.1	D49.Ø
presacral (region)	C76.3	C79.89	—	D36.7	D48.7	D49.89
prostate (gland)	C61	C79.82	DØ7.5	D29.1	D4Ø.Ø	D49.59
utricle	C68.Ø	C79.19	DØ9.19	D3Ø.4	D41.3	D49.59
pterygoid fossa	C49.Ø	C79.89	—	D21.Ø	D48.1	D49.2
pubic bone	C41.4	C79.51	—	D16.8	D48.Ø	D49.2
pudenda, pudendum (female)	C51.9	C79.82	DØ7.1	D28.Ø	D39.8	D49.59
pulmonary — *see also Neoplasm, lung*	C34.9-•	C78.Ø-•	DØ2.2-•	D14.3-•	D38.1	D49.1
putamen	C71.Ø	C79.31	—	D33.Ø	D43.Ø	D49.6
pyloric						
antrum	C16.3	C78.89	DØØ.2	D13.1	D37.1	D49.Ø
canal	C16.4	C78.89	DØØ.2	D13.1	D37.1	D49.Ø
pylorus	C16.4	C78.89	DØØ.2	D13.1	D37.1	D49.Ø
pyramid (brain)	C71.7	C79.31	—	D33.1	D43.1	D49.6
pyriform fossa or sinus	C12	C79.89	DØØ.Ø8	D1Ø.7	D37.Ø5	D49.Ø
radius (any part)	C4Ø.Ø-•	C79.51	—	D16.Ø-•	—	—
Rathke's pouch	C75.1	C79.89	DØ9.3	D35.2	D44.3	D49.7
rectosigmoid (junction)	C19	C78.5	DØ1.1	D12.7	D37.5	D49.Ø
overlapping lesion with anus or rectum	C21.8	—	—	—	—	—
rectouterine pouch	C48.1	C78.6	—	D2Ø.1	D48.4	D49.Ø
rectovaginal septum or wall	C76.3	C79.89	DØ9.8	D36.7	D48.7	D49.89
rectovesical septum	C76.3	C79.89	DØ9.8	D36.7	D48.7	D49.89
rectum (ampulla)	C2Ø	C78.5	DØ1.2	D12.8	D37.5	D49.Ø
and colon	C19	C78.5	DØ1.1	D12.7	D37.5	D49.Ø
overlapping lesion with anus or rectosigmoid junction	C21.8	—	—	—	—	—

	Malignant Primary	Malignant Secondary	Ca in situ	Benign	Uncertain Behavior	Unspecified Behavior
renal	C64.-•	C79.Ø-•	DØ9.19	D3Ø.Ø-•	D41.Ø-•	D49.51-•
calyx	C65.-•	C79.Ø-•	DØ9.19	D3Ø.1-•	D41.1-•	D49.51-•
hilus	C65.-•	C79.Ø-•	DØ9.19	D3Ø.1-•	D41.1-•	D49.51-•
parenchyma	C64.-•	C79.Ø-•	DØ9.19	D3Ø.Ø-•	D41.Ø-•	D49.51-•
pelvis	C65.-•	C79.Ø-•	DØ9.19	D3Ø.1-•	D41.1-•	D49.51-•
respiratory						
organs or system NEC	C39.9	C78.3Ø	DØ2.4	D14.4	D38.6	D49.1
tract NEC	C39.9	C78.3Ø	DØ2.4	D14.4	D38.5	D49.1
upper	C39.Ø	C78.3Ø	DØ2.4	D14.4	D38.5	D49.1
retina	C69.2-•	C79.49	DØ9.2-•	D31.2-•	D48.7	D49.81
retrobulbar	C69.6-•	C79.49	—	D31.6-•	D48.7	D49.89
retrocecal	C48.Ø	C78.6	—	D2Ø.Ø	D48.3	D49.Ø
retromolar (area) (triangle) (trigone)	CØ6.2	C79.89	DØØ.ØØ	D1Ø.39	D37.Ø9	D49.Ø
retro-orbital	C76.Ø	C79.89	DØ9.8	D36.7	D48.7	D49.89
retroperitoneal (space) (tissue)	C48.Ø	C78.6	—	D2Ø.Ø	D48.3	D49.Ø
retroperitoneum	C48.Ø	C78.6	—	D2Ø.Ø	D48.3	D49.Ø
retropharyngeal	C14.Ø	C79.89	DØØ.Ø8	D1Ø.9	D37.Ø5	D49.Ø
retrovesical (septum)	C76.3	C79.89	DØ9.8	D36.7	D48.7	D49.89
rhinencephalon	C71.Ø	C79.31	—	D33.Ø	D43.Ø	D49.6
rib	C41.3	C79.51	—	D16.7	D48.Ø	D49.2
Rosenmuller's fossa	C11.2	C79.89	DØØ.Ø8	D1Ø.6	D37.Ø5	D49.Ø
round ligament	C57.2	C79.82	—	D28.2	D39.8	D49.59
sacrococcyx, sacrococcygeal	C41.4	C79.51	—	D16.8	D48.Ø	D49.2
region	C76.3	C79.89	DØ9.8	D36.7	D48.7	D49.89
sacrouterine ligament	C57.3	C79.82	—	D28.2	D39.8	D49.59
sacrum, sacral (vertebra)	C41.4	C79.51	—	D16.8	D48.Ø	D49.2
salivary gland or duct (major)	CØ8.9	C79.89	DØØ.ØØ	D11.9	D37.Ø39	D49.Ø
minor NEC	CØ6.9	C79.89	DØØ.ØØ	D1Ø.39	D37.Ø4	D49.Ø
overlapping lesion	CØ8.9	—	—	—	—	—
parotid	CØ7	C79.89	DØØ.ØØ	D11.Ø	D37.Ø3Ø	D49.Ø
pluriglandular	CØ8.9	C79.89	DØØ.ØØ	D11.9	D37.Ø39	D49.Ø
sublingual	CØ8.1	C79.89	DØØ.ØØ	D11.7	D37.Ø31	D49.Ø
submandibular	CØ8.Ø	C79.89	DØØ.ØØ	D11.7	D37.Ø32	D49.Ø
submaxillary	CØ8.Ø	C79.89	DØØ.ØØ	D11.7	D37.Ø32	D49.Ø
salpinx (uterine)	C57.Ø-•	C79.82	DØ7.39	D28.2	D39.8	D49.59
Santorini's duct	C25.3	C78.89	DØ1.7	D13.6	D37.8	D49.Ø
scalp	C44.4Ø	C79.2	DØ4.4	D23.4	D48.5	D49.2
basal cell carcinoma	C44.41	—	—	—	—	—
specified type NEC	C44.49	—	—	—	—	—
squamous cell carcinoma	C44.42	—	—	—	—	—
scapula (any part)	C4Ø.Ø-•	C79.51	—	D16.Ø-•	—	—
scapular region	C76.1	C79.89	DØ9.8	D36.7	D48.7	D49.89

	Malignant Primary	Malignant Secondary	Ca in situ	Benign	Uncertain Behavior	Unspecified Behavior
scar NEC—*see also Neoplasm, skin, by site*	C44.90	C79.2	D04.9	D23.9	D48.5	D49.2
sciatic nerve	C47.2-•	C79.89	—	D36.13	D48.2	D49.2
sclera	C69.4-•	C79.49	D09.2-•	D31.4-•	D48.7	D49.89
scrotum (skin)	C63.2	C79.82	D07.61	D29.4	D40.8	D49.59
sebaceous gland—*see Neoplasm, skin*						
sella turcica	C75.1	C79.89	D09.3	D35.2	D44.3	D49.7
bone	C41.0	C79.51	—	D16.4-•	D48.0	D49.2
semilunar cartilage (knee)	C40.2-•	C79.51	—	D16.2-•	D48.0	D49.2
seminal vesicle	C63.7	C79.82	D07.69	D29.8	D40.8	D49.59
septum						
nasal	C30.0	C78.39	D02.3	D14.0	D38.5	D49.1
posterior margin	C11.3	C79.89	D00.08	D10.6	D37.05	D49.0
rectovaginal	C76.3	C79.89	D09.8	D36.7	D48.7	D49.89
rectovesical	C76.3	C79.89	D09.8	D36.7	D48.7	D49.89
urethrovaginal	C57.9	C79.82	D07.30	D28.9	D39.9	D49.59
vesicovaginal	C57.9	C79.82	D07.30	D28.9	D39.9	D49.59
shoulder NEC	C76.4-•	C79.89	D04.6-•	D36.7	D48.7	D49.89
sigmoid flexure (lower) (upper)	C18.7	C78.5	D01.0	D12.5	D37.4	D49.0
sinus (accessory)	C31.9	C78.39	D02.3	D14.0	D38.5	D49.1
bone (any)	C41.0	C79.51	—	D16.4-•	D48.0	D49.2
ethmoidal	C31.1	C78.39	D02.3	D14.0	D38.5	D49.1
frontal	C31.2	C78.39	D02.3	D14.0	D38.5	D49.1
maxillary	C31.0	C78.39	D02.3	D14.0	D38.5	D49.1
nasal, paranasal NEC	C31.9	C78.39	D02.3	D14.0	D38.5	D49.1
overlapping lesion	C31.8	—	—	—	—	—
pyriform	C12	C79.89	D00.08	D10.7	D37.05	D49.0
sphenoid	C31.3	C78.39	D02.3	D14.0	D38.5	D49.1
skeleton, skeletal NEC	C41.9	C79.51	—	D16.9-•	D48.0	D49.2
Skene's gland	C68.1	C79.19	D09.19	D30.8	D41.8	D49.59
skin NOS	C44.90	C79.2	D04.9	D23.9	D48.5	D49.2
abdominal wall	C44.509	C79.2	D04.5	D23.5	D48.5	D49.2
basal cell carcinoma	C44.519	—	—	—	—	—
specified type NEC	C44.599	—	—	—	—	—
squamous cell carcinoma	C44.529	—	—	—	—	—
ala nasi—*see also Neoplasm, nose, skin*	C44.301	C79.2	D04.39	D23.39	D48.5	D49.2
ankle—*see also Neoplasm, skin, limb, lower*	C44.70-•	C79.2	D04.7-•	D23.7-•	D48.5	D49.2
antecubital space—*see also Neoplasm, skin, limb, upper*	C44.60-•	C79.2	D04.6-•	D23.6-•	D48.5	D49.2

	Malignant Primary	Malignant Secondary	Ca in situ	Benign	Uncertain Behavior	Unspecified Behavior
skin NOS *(Continued)*						
anus	C44.500	C79.2	D04.5	D23.5	D48.5	D49.2
basal cell carcinoma	C44.510	—	—	—	—	—
specified type NEC	C44.590	—	—	—	—	—
squamous cell carcinoma	C44.520	—	—	—	—	—
arm—*see also Neoplasm, skin, limb, upper*	C44.60-•	C79.2	D04.6-•	D23.6-•	D48.5	D49.2
auditory canal (external)—*see also Neoplasm, skin, ear*	C44.20-•	C79.2	D04.2-•	D23.2-•	D48.5	D49.2
auricle (ear)—*see also Neoplasm, skin, ear*	C44.20-•	C79.2	D04.2-•	D23.2-•	D48.5	D49.2
auricular canal (external)—*see also Neoplasm, skin, ear*	C44.20-•	C79.2	D04.2-•	D23.2-•	D48.5	D49.2
axilla, axillary fold—*see also Neoplasm, skin, trunk*	C44.509	C79.2	D04.5	D23.5	D48.5	D49.2
back—*see also Neoplasm, skin, trunk*	C44.509	C79.2	D04.5	D23.5	D48.5	D49.2
basal cell carcinoma	C44.91					
breast	C44.501	C79.2	D04.5	D23.5	D48.5	D49.2
basal cell carcinoma	C44.511	—	—	—	—	—
specified type NEC	C44.591	—	—	—	—	—
squamous cell carcinoma	C44.521	—	—	—	—	—
brow—*see also Neoplasm, skin, face*	C44.309	C79.2	D04.39	D23.39	D48.5	D49.2
buttock—*see also Neoplasm, skin, trunk*	C44.509	C79.2	D04.5	D23.5	D48.5	D49.2
calf—*see also Neoplasm, skin, limb, lower*	C44.70-•	C79.2	D04.7-•	D23.7-•	D48.5	D49.2
canthus (eye) (inner) (outer)	C44.10-•	C79.2	D04.1-•	D23.1-•	D48.5	D49.2
basal cell carcinoma	C44.11-•	—	—	—	—	—
sebaceous cell	C44.13-•	—	—	—	—	—
specified type NEC	C44.19-•	—	—	—	—	—
squamous cell carcinoma	C44.12-•	—	—	—	—	—
cervical region—*see also Neoplasm, skin, neck*	C44.40	C79.2	D04.4	D23.4	D48.5	D49.2
cheek (external)—*see also Neoplasm, skin, face*	C44.309	C79.2	D04.39	D23.39	D48.5	D49.2
chest (wall)—*see also Neoplasm, skin, trunk*	C44.509	C79.2	D04.5	D23.5	D48.5	D49.2
chin—*see also Neoplasm, skin, face*	C44.309	C79.2	D04.39	D23.39	D48.5	D49.2
clavicular area—*see also Neoplasm, skin, trunk*	C44.509	C79.2	D04.5	D23.5	D48.5	D49.2
clitoris	C51.2	C79.82	D07.1	D28.0	D39.8	D49.59

TABLE OF NEOPLASMS

	Malignant Primary	Malignant Secondary	Ca in situ	Benign	Uncertain Behavior	Unspecified Behavior
skin NOS *(Continued)*						
columnella — *see also Neoplasm, skin, face*	C44.309	C79.2	D04.39	D23.39	D48.5	D49.2
concha — *see also Neoplasm, skin, ear*	C44.20-●	C79.2	D04.2-●	D23.2-●	D48.5	D49.2
ear (external)	C44.20-●	C79.2	D04.2-●	D23.2-●	D48.5	D49.2
basal cell carcinoma	C44.21-●	—	—	—	—	—
specified type NEC	C44.29-●	—	—	—	—	—
squamous cell carcinoma	C44.22-●	—	—	—	—	—
elbow — *see also Neoplasm, skin, limb, upper*	C44.60-●	C79.2	D04.6-●	D23.6-●	D48.5	D49.2
eyebrow — *see also Neoplasm, skin, face*	C44.309	C79.2	D04.39	D23.39	D48.5	D49.2
eyelid	C44.10-●	C79.2	D04.1-●	D23.1-●	D48.5	D49.2
basal cell carcinoma	C44.11-●	—	—	—	—	—
sebaceous cell	C44.13-●	—	—	—	—	—
specified type NEC	C44.19-●	—	—	—	—	—
squamous cell carcinoma	C44.12-●	—	—	—	—	—
face NOS	C44.300	C79.2	D04.30	D23.30	D48.5	D49.2
basal cell carcinoma	C44.310	—	—	—	—	—
specified type NEC	C44.390	—	—	—	—	—
squamous cell carcinoma	C44.320	—	—	—	—	—
female genital organs (external)	C51.9	C79.82	D07.1	D28.0	D39.8	D49.59
clitoris	C51.2	C79.82	D07.1	D28.0	D39.8	D49.59
labium NEC	C51.9	C79.82	D07.1	D28.0	D39.8	D49.59
majus	C51.0	C79.82	D07.1	D28.0	D39.8	D49.59
minus	C51.1	C79.82	D07.1	D28.0	D39.8	D49.59
pudendum	C51.9	C79.82	D07.1	D28.0	D39.8	D49.59
vulva	C51.9	C79.82	D07.1	D28.0	D39.8	D49.59
finger — *see also Neoplasm, skin, limb, upper*	C44.60-●	C79.2	D04.6-●	D23.6-●	D48.5	D49.2
flank — *see also Neoplasm, skin, trunk*	C44.509	C79.2	D04.5	D23.5	D48.5	D49.2
foot — *see also Neoplasm, skin, limb, lower*	C44.70-●	C79.2	D04.7-●	D23.7-●	D48.5	D49.2
forearm — *see also Neoplasm, skin, limb, upper*	C44.60-●	C79.2	D04.6-●	D23.6-●	D48.5	D49.2
forehead — *see also Neoplasm, skin, face*	C44.309	C79.2	D04.39	D23.39	D48.5	D49.2
glabella — *see also Neoplasm, skin, face*	C44.309	C79.2	D04.39	D23.39	D48.5	D49.2
gluteal region — *see also Neoplasm, skin, trunk*	C44.509	C79.2	D04.5	D23.5	D48.5	D49.2
groin — *see also Neoplasm, skin, trunk*	C44.509	C79.2	D04.5	D23.5	D48.5	D49.2

	Malignant Primary	Malignant Secondary	Ca in situ	Benign	Uncertain Behavior	Unspecified Behavior
skin NOS *(Continued)*						
hand — *see also Neoplasm, skin, limb, upper*	C44.60-●	C79.2	D04.6-●	D23.6-●	D48.5	D49.2
head NEC — *see also Neoplasm, skin, scalp*	C44.40	C79.2	D04.4	D23.4	D48.5	D49.2
heel — *see also Neoplasm, skin, limb, lower*	C44.70-●	C79.2	D04.7-●	D23.7-●	D48.5	D49.2
helix — *see also Neoplasm, skin, ear*	C44.20-●	C79.2	D04.2-●	D23.2-●	D48.5	D49.2
hip — *see also Neoplasm, skin, limb, lower*	C44.70-●	C79.2	D04.7-●	D23.7-●	D48.5	D49.2
infraclavicular region — *see also Neoplasm, skin, trunk*	C44.509	C79.2	D04.5	D23.5	D48.5	D49.2
inguinal region — *see also Neoplasm, skin, trunk*	C44.509	C79.2	D04.5	D23.5	D48.5	D49.2
jaw — *see also Neoplasm, skin, face*	C44.309	C79.2	D04.39	D23.39	D48.5	D49.2
Kaposi's sarcoma — *see Kaposi's, sarcoma, skin*						
knee — *see also Neoplasm, skin, limb, lower*	C44.70-●	C79.2	D04.7-●	D23.7-●	D48.5	D49.2
labia						
majora	C51.0	C79.82	D07.1	D28.0	D39.8	D49.59
minora	C51.1	C79.82	D07.1	D28.0	D39.8	D49.59
leg — *see also Neoplasm, skin, limb, lower*	C44.70-●	C79.2	D04.7-●	D23.7-●	D48.5	D49.2
lid (lower) (upper)	C44.10-●	C79.2	D04.1-●	D23.1-●	D48.5	D49.2
basal cell carcinoma	C44.11-●	—	—	—	—	—
sebaceous cell	C44.13-●	—	—	—	—	—
specified type NEC	C44.19-●	—	—	—	—	—
squamous cell carcinoma	C44.12-●	—	—	—	—	—
limb NEC	C44.90	C79.2	D04.9	D23.9	D48.5	D49.2
basal cell carcinoma	C44.91					
lower	C44.70-●	C79.2	D04.7-●	D23.7-●	D48.5	D49.2
basal cell carcinoma	C44.71-●	—	—	—	—	—
specified type NEC	C44.79-●	—	—	—	—	—
squamous cell carcinoma	C44.72-●	—	—	—	—	—
upper	C44.60-●	C79.2	D04.6-●	D23.6-●	D48.5	D49.2
basal cell carcinoma	C44.61-●	—	—	—	—	—
specified type NEC	C44.69-●	—	—	—	—	—
squamous cell carcinoma	C44.62-●	—	—	—	—	—
lip (lower) (upper)	C44.00	C79.2	D04.0	D23.0	D48.5	D49.2
basal cell carcinoma	C44.01	—	—	—	—	—
specified type NEC	C44.09	—	—	—	—	—
squamous cell carcinoma	C44.02	—	—	—	—	—

	Malignant Primary	Malignant Secondary	Ca in situ	Benign	Uncertain Behavior	Unspecified Behavior
skin NOS *(Continued)*						
male genital organs	C63.9	C79.82	D07.60	D29.9	D40.8	D49.59
penis	C60.9	C79.82	D07.4	D29.0	D40.8	D49.59
prepuce	C60.0	C79.82	D07.4	D29.0	D40.8	D49.59
scrotum	C63.2	C79.82	D07.61	D29.4	D40.8	D49.59
mastectomy site (skin)—*see also Neoplasm, skin, breast*	C44.501	C79.2	—	—	—	—
specified as breast tissue	C50.8-●	C79.81	—	—	—	—
meatus, acoustic (external)—*see also Neoplasm, skin, ear*	C44.20-●	C79.2	D04.2-●	D23.2-●	D48.5	D49.2
melanotic—*see Melanoma*						
Merkel cell—*see Carcinoma, Merkel cell*						
nates—*see also Neoplasm, skin, trunk*	C44.509	C79.2	D04.5	D23.5	D48.5	D49.2
neck	C44.40	C79.2	D04.4	D23.4	D48.5	D49.2
basal cell carcinoma	C44.41	—	—	—	—	—
specified type NEC	C44.49	—	—	—	—	—
squamous cell carcinoma	C44.42	—	—	—	—	—
nevus—*see Nevus, skin*						
nose (external)—*see also Neoplasm, nose, skin*	C44.301	C79.2	D04.39	D23.39	D48.5	D49.2
overlapping lesion	C44.80	—	—	—	—	—
basal cell carcinoma	C44.81	—	—	—	—	—
specified type NEC	C44.89	—	—	—	—	—
squamous cell carcinoma	C44.82	—	—	—	—	—
palm—*see also Neoplasm, skin, limb, upper*	C44.60-●	C79.2	D04.6-●	D23.6-●	D48.5	D49.2
palpebra	C44.10-●	C79.2	D04.1-●	D23.1-●	D48.5	D49.2
basal cell carcinoma	C44.11-●	—	—	—	—	—
sebaceous cell	C44.13-●	—	—	—	—	—
specified type NEC	C44.19-●	—	—	—	—	—
squamous cell carcinoma	C44.12-●	—	—	—	—	—
penis NEC	C60.9	C79.82	D07.4	D29.0	D40.8	D49.59
perianal—*see also Neoplasm, skin, anus*	C44.500	C79.2	D04.5	D23.5	D48.5	D49.2
perineum—*see also Neoplasm, skin, anus*	C44.500	C79.2	D04.5	D23.5	D48.5	D49.2
pinna—*see also Neoplasm, skin, ear*	C44.20-●	C79.2	D04.2-●	D23.2-●	D48.5	D49.2
plantar—*see also Neoplasm, skin, limb, lower*	C44.70-●	C79.2	D04.7-●	D23.7-●	D48.5	D49.2
popliteal fossa or space—*see also Neoplasm, skin, limb, lower*	C44.70-●	C79.2	D04.7-●	D23.7-●	D48.5	D49.2
skin NOS *(Continued)*						
prepuce	C60.0	C79.82	D07.4	D29.0	D40.8	D49.59
pubes—*see also Neoplasm, skin, trunk*	C44.509	C79.2	D04.5	D23.5	D48.5	D49.2
sacrococcygeal region—*see also Neoplasm, skin, trunk*	C44.509	C79.2	D04.5	D23.5	D48.5	D49.2
scalp	C44.40	C79.2	D04.4	D23.4	D48.5	D49.2
basal cell carcinoma	C44.41	—	—	—	—	—
specified type NEC	C44.49	—	—	—	—	—
squamous cell carcinoma	C44.42	—	—	—	—	—
scapular region—*see also Neoplasm, skin, trunk*	C44.509	C79.2	D04.5	D23.5	D48.5	D49.2
scrotum	C63.2	C79.82	D07.61	D29.4	D40.8	D49.59
shoulder—*see also Neoplasm, skin, limb, upper*	C44.60-●	C79.2	D04.6-●	D23.6-●	D48.5	D49.2
sole (foot)—*see also Neoplasm, skin, limb, lower*	C44.70-●	C79.2	D04.7-●	D23.7-●	D48.5	D49.2
specified sites NEC	C44.80	C79.2	D04.8	D23.9	D48.5	D49.2
basal cell carcinoma	C44.81	—	—	—	—	—
specified type NEC	C44.89	—	—	—	—	—
squamous cell carcinoma	C44.82	—	—	—	—	—
specified type NEC	C44.99	—	—	—	—	—
squamous cell carcinoma	C44.92	—	—	—	—	—
submammary fold—*see also Neoplasm, skin, trunk*	C44.509	C79.2	D04.5	D23.5	D48.5	D49.2
supraclavicular region—*see also Neoplasm, skin, neck*	C44.40	C79.2	D04.4	D23.4	D48.5	D49.2
temple—*see also Neoplasm, skin, face*	C44.309	C79.2	D04.39	D23.39	D48.5	D49.2
thigh—*see also Neoplasm, skin, limb, lower*	C44.70-●	C79.2	D04.7-●	D23.7-●	D48.5	D49.2
thoracic wall—*see also Neoplasm, skin, trunk*	C44.509	C79.2	D04.5	D23.5	D48.5	D49.2
thumb—*see also Neoplasm, skin, limb, upper*	C44.60-●	C79.2	D04.6-●	D23.6-●	D48.5	D49.2
toe—*see also Neoplasm, skin, limb, lower*	C44.70-●	C79.2	D04.7-●	D23.7-●	D48.5	D49.2
tragus—*see also Neoplasm, skin, ear*	C44.20-●	C79.2	D04.2-●	D23.2-●	D48.5	D49.2
trunk	C44.509	C79.2	D04.5	D23.5	D48.5	D49.2
basal cell carcinoma	C44.519	—	—	—	—	—
specified type NEC	C44.599	—	—	—	—	—
squamous cell carcinoma	C44.529	—	—	—	—	—
umbilicus—*see also Neoplasm, skin, trunk*	C44.509	C79.2	D04.5	D23.5	D48.5	D49.2

New Revised ~~deleted~~ Deleted ● Use Additional Character(s)

	Malignant Primary	Malignant Secondary	Ca in situ	Benign	Uncertain Behavior	Unspecified Behavior
skin NOS *(Continued)*						
vulva	C51.9	C79.82	DØ7.1	D28.Ø	D39.8	D49.59
overlapping lesion	C51.8	—	—	—	—	—
wrist—*see also Neoplasm, skin, limb, upper*	C44.6Ø-•	C79.2	DØ4.6-•	D23.6-•	D48.5	D49.2
skull	C41.Ø	C79.51	—	D16.4-•	D48.Ø	D49.2
soft parts or tissues—*see Neoplasm, connective tissue*						
specified site NEC	C76.8	C79.89	DØ9.8	D36.7	D48.7	D49.89
spermatic cord	C63.1-•	C79.82	DØ7.69	D29.8	D4Ø.8	D49.59
sphenoid	C31.3	C78.39	DØ2.3	D14.Ø	D38.5	D49.1
bone	C41.Ø	C79.51	—	D16.4-•	D48.Ø	D49.2
sinus	C31.3	C78.39	DØ2.3	D14.Ø	D38.5	D49.1
sphincter						
anal	C21.1	C78.5	DØ1.3	D12.9	D37.8	D49.Ø
of Oddi	C24.Ø	C78.89	DØ1.5	D13.5	D37.6	D49.Ø
spine, spinal (column)	C41.2	C79.51	—	D16.6	D48.Ø	D49.2
bulb	C71.7	C79.31	—	D33.1	D43.1	D49.6
coccyx	C41.4	C79.51	—	D16.8	D48.Ø	D49.2
cord (cervical) (lumbar) (sacral) (thoracic)	C72.Ø	C79.49	—	D33.4	D43.4	D49.7
dura mater	C7Ø.1	C79.49	—	D32.1	D42.1	D49.7
lumbosacral	C41.2	C79.51	—	D16.6	D48.Ø	D49.2
marrow NEC	C96.9	C79.52	—	—	D47.9	D49.89
membrane	C7Ø.1	C79.49	—	D32.1	D42.1	D49.7
meninges	C7Ø.1	C79.49	—	D32.1	D42.1	D49.7
nerve (root)	C47.9	C79.89	—	D36.1Ø	D48.2	D49.2
pia mater	C7Ø.1	C79.49	—	D32.1	D42.1	D49.7
root	C47.9	C79.89	—	D36.1Ø	D48.2	D49.2
sacrum	C41.4	C79.51	—	D16.8	D48.Ø	D49.2
spleen, splenic NEC	C26.1	C78.89	DØ1.7	D13.9	D37.8	D49.Ø
flexure (colon)	C18.5	C78.5	DØ1.Ø	D12.3	D37.4	D49.Ø
stem, brain	C71.7	C79.31	—	D33.1	D43.1	D49.6
Stensen's duct	CØ7	C79.89	DØØ.ØØ	D11.Ø	D37.Ø3Ø	D49.Ø
sternum	C41.3	C79.51	—	D16.7	D48.Ø	D49.2
stomach	C16.9	C78.89	DØØ.2	D13.1	D37.1	D49.Ø
antrum (pyloric)	C16.3	C78.89	DØØ.2	D13.1	D37.1	D49.Ø
body	C16.2	C78.89	DØØ.2	D13.1	D37.1	D49.Ø
cardia	C16.Ø	C78.89	DØØ.2	D13.1	D37.1	D49.Ø
cardiac orifice	C16.Ø	C78.89	DØØ.2	D13.1	D37.1	D49.Ø
corpus	C16.2	C78.89	DØØ.2	D13.1	D37.1	D49.Ø
fundus	C16.1	C78.89	DØØ.2	D13.1	D37.1	D49.Ø
greater curvature NEC	C16.6	C78.89	DØØ.2	D13.1	D37.1	D49.Ø
lesser curvature NEC	C16.5	C78.89	DØØ.2	D13.1	D37.1	D49.Ø

	Malignant Primary	Malignant Secondary	Ca in situ	Benign	Uncertain Behavior	Unspecified Behavior
stomach *(Continued)*						
overlapping lesion	C16.8	—	—	—	—	—
prepylorus	C16.4	C78.89	DØØ.2	D13.1	D37.1	D49.Ø
pylorus	C16.4	C78.89	DØØ.2	D13.1	D37.1	D49.Ø
wall NEC	C16.9	C78.89	DØØ.2	D13.1	D37.1	D49.Ø
anterior NEC	C16.8	C78.89	DØØ.2	D13.1	D37.1	D49.Ø
posterior NEC	C16.8	C78.89	DØØ.2	D13.1	D37.1	D49.Ø
stroma, endometrial	C54.1	C79.82	DØ7.Ø	D26.1	D39.Ø	D49.59
stump, cervical	C53.8	C79.82	DØ6.7	D26.Ø	D39.Ø	D49.59
subcutaneous (nodule) (tissue) NEC—*see Neoplasm, connective tissue*						
subdural	C7Ø.9	C79.32	—	D32.9	D42.9	D49.7
subglottis, subglottic	C32.2	C78.39	DØ2.Ø	D14.1	D38.Ø	D49.1
sublingual	CØ4.9	C79.89	DØØ.Ø6	D1Ø.2	D37.Ø9	D49.Ø
gland or duct	CØ8.1	C79.89	DØØ.ØØ	D11.7	D37.Ø31	D49.Ø
submandibular gland	CØ8.Ø	C79.89	DØØ.ØØ	D11.7	D37.Ø32	D49.Ø
submaxillary gland or duct	CØ8.Ø	C79.89	DØØ.ØØ	D11.7	D37.Ø32	D49.Ø
submental	C76.Ø	C79.89	DØ9.8	D36.7	D48.7	D49.89
subpleural	C34.9-•	C78.Ø-•	DØ2.2-•	D14.3-•	D38.1	D49.1
substernal	C38.1	C78.1	—	D15.2	D38.3	D49.89
sudoriferous, sudoriparous gland, site unspecified	C44.9Ø	C79.2	DØ4.9	D23.9	D48.5	D49.2
specified site—*see Neoplasm, skin*						
supraclavicular region	C76.Ø	C79.89	DØ9.8	D36.7	D48.7	D49.89
supraglottis	C32.1	C78.39	DØ2.Ø	D14.1	D38.Ø	D49.1
suprarenal	C74.9-•	C79.7-•	DØ9.3	D35.Ø-•	D44.1-•	D49.7
capsule	C74.9-•	C79.7-•	DØ9.3	D35.Ø-•	D44.1-•	D49.7
cortex	C74.Ø-•	C79.7-•	DØ9.3	D35.Ø-•	D44.1-•	D49.7
gland	C74.9-•	C79.7-•	DØ9.3	D35.Ø-•	D44.1-•	D49.7
medulla	C74.1-•	C79.7-•	DØ9.3	D35.Ø-•	D44.1-•	D49.7
suprasellar (region)	C71.9	C79.31	—	D33.2	D43.2	D49.6
supratentorial (brain) NEC	C71.Ø	C79.31	—	D33.Ø	D43.Ø	D49.6
sweat gland (apocrine) (eccrine), site unspecified	C44.9Ø	C79.2	DØ4.9	D23.9	D48.5	D49.2
specified site—*see Neoplasm, skin*						
sympathetic nerve or nervous system NEC	C47.9	C79.89	—	D36.1Ø	D48.2	D49.2
symphysis pubis	C41.4	C79.51	—	D16.8	D48.Ø	D49.2
synovial membrane—*see Neoplasm, connective tissue*						
tapetum, brain	C71.8	C79.31	—	D33.2	D43.2	D49.6

	Malignant Primary	Malignant Secondary	Ca in situ	Benign	Uncertain Behavior	Unspecified Behavior
tarsus (any bone)	C40.3-●	C79.51	—	D16.3-●	—	—
temple (skin) — *see also Neoplasm, skin, face*	C44.309	C79.2	D04.39	D23.39	D48.5	D49.2
temporal						
bone	C41.0	C79.51	—	D16.4-●	D48.0	D49.2
lobe or pole	C71.2	C79.31	—	D33.0	D43.0	D49.6
region	C76.0	C79.89	D09.8	D36.7	D48.7	D49.89
skin — *see also Neoplasm, skin, face*	C44.309	C79.2	D04.39	D23.39	D48.5	D49.2
tendon (sheath) — *see Neoplasm, connective tissue*						
tentorium (cerebelli)	C70.0	C79.32	—	D32.0	D42.0	D49.7
testis, testes	C62.9-●	C79.82	D07.69	D29.2-●	D40.1-●	D49.59
descended	C62.1-●	C79.82	D07.69	D29.2-●	D40.1-●	D49.59
ectopic	C62.0-●	C79.82	D07.69	D29.2-●	D40.1-●	D49.59
retained	C62.0-●	C79.82	D07.69	D29.2-●	D40.1-●	D49.59
scrotal	C62.1-●	C79.82	D07.69	D29.2-●	D40.1-●	D49.59
undescended	C62.0-●	C79.82	D07.69	D29.2-●	D40.1-●	D49.59
unspecified whether descended or undescended	C62.9-●	C79.82	D07.69	D29.2-●	D40.1-●	D49.59
thalamus	C71.0	C79.31	—	D33.0	D43.0	D49.6
thigh NEC	C76.5-●	C79.89	D04.7-●	D36.7	D48.7	D49.89
thorax, thoracic (cavity) (organs NEC)	C76.1	C79.89	D09.8	D36.7	D48.7	D49.89
duct	C49.3	C79.89	—	D21.3	D48.1	D49.2
wall NEC	C76.1	C79.89	D09.8	D36.7	D48.7	D49.89
throat	C14.0	C79.89	D00.08	D10.9	D37.05	D49.0
thumb NEC	C76.4-●	C79.89	D04.6-●	D36.7	D48.7	D49.89
thymus (gland)	C37	C79.89	D09.3	D15.0	D38.4	D49.89
thyroglossal duct	C73	C79.89	D09.3	D34	D44.0	D49.7
thyroid (gland)	C73	C79.89	D09.3	D34	D44.0	D49.7
cartilage	C32.3	C78.39	D02.0	D14.1	D38.0	D49.1
tibia (any part)	C40.2-●	C79.51	—	D16.2-●	—	—
toe NEC	C76.5-●	C79.89	D04.7-●	D36.7	D48.7	D49.89
tongue	C02.9	C79.89	D00.07	D10.1	D37.02	D49.0
anterior (two-thirds) NEC	C02.3	C79.89	D00.07	D10.1	D37.02	D49.0
dorsal surface	C02.0	C79.89	D00.07	D10.1	D37.02	D49.0
ventral surface	C02.2	C79.89	D00.07	D10.1	D37.02	D49.0
base (dorsal surface)	C01	C79.89	D00.07	D10.1	D37.02	D49.0
border (lateral)	C02.1	C79.89	D00.07	D10.1	D37.02	D49.0
dorsal surface NEC	C02.0	C79.89	D00.07	D10.1	D37.02	D49.0
fixed part NEC	C01	C79.89	D00.07	D10.1	D37.02	D49.0
foreamen cecum	C02.0	C79.89	D00.07	D10.1	D37.02	D49.0
frenulum linguae	C02.2	C79.89	D00.07	D10.1	D37.02	D49.0

	Malignant Primary	Malignant Secondary	Ca in situ	Benign	Uncertain Behavior	Unspecified Behavior
tongue *(Continued)*						
junctional zone	C02.8	C79.89	D00.07	D10.1	D37.02	D49.0
margin (lateral)	C02.1	C79.89	D00.07	D10.1	D37.02	D49.0
midline NEC	C02.0	C79.89	D00.07	D10.1	D37.02	D49.0
mobile part NEC	C02.3	C79.89	D00.07	D10.1	D37.02	D49.0
overlapping lesion	C02.8	—	—	—	—	—
posterior (third)	C01	C79.89	D00.07	D10.1	D37.02	D49.0
root	C01	C79.89	D00.07	D10.1	D37.02	D49.0
surface (dorsal)	C02.0	C79.89	D00.07	D10.1	D37.02	D49.0
base	C01	C79.89	D00.07	D10.1	D37.02	D49.0
ventral	C02.2	C79.89	D00.07	D10.1	D37.02	D49.0
tip	C02.1	C79.89	D00.07	D10.1	D37.02	D49.0
tonsil	C02.4	C79.89	D00.07	D10.1	D37.02	D49.0
tonsil	C09.9	C79.89	D00.08	D10.4	D37.05	D49.0
fauces, faucial	C09.9	C79.89	D00.08	D10.4	D37.05	D49.0
lingual	C02.4	C79.89	D00.07	D10.1	D37.02	D49.0
overlapping sites	C09.8	—	—	—	—	—
palatine	C09.9	C79.89	D00.08	D10.4	D37.05	D49.0
pharyngeal	C11.1	C79.89	D00.08	D10.6	D37.05	D49.0
pillar (anterior) (posterior)	C09.1	C79.89	D00.08	D10.5	D37.05	D49.0
tonsillar fossa	C09.0	C79.89	D00.08	D10.5	D37.05	D49.0
tooth socket NEC	C03.9	C79.89	D00.03	D10.39	D37.09	D49.0
trachea (cartilage) (mucosa)	C33	C78.39	D02.1	D14.2	D38.1	D49.1
overlapping lesion with bronchus or lung	C34.8-●	—	—	—	—	—
tracheobronchial	C34.8-●	C78.39	D02.1	D14.2	D38.1	D49.1
overlapping lesion with lung	C34.8-●	—	—	—	—	—
tragus — *see also Neoplasm, skin, ear*	C44.20-●	C79.2	D04.2-●	D23.2-●	D48.5	D49.2
trunk NEC	C76.8	C79.89	D04.5	D36.7	D48.7	D49.89
tubo-ovarian	C57.8	C79.82	D07.39	D28.7	D39.8	D49.59
tunica vaginalis	C63.7	C79.82	D07.69	D29.8	D40.8	D49.59
turbinate (bone)	C41.0	C79.51	—	D16.4-●	D48.0	D49.2
nasal	C30.0	C78.39	D02.3	D14.0	D38.5	D49.1
tympanic cavity	C30.1	C78.39	D02.3	D14.0	D38.5	D49.1
ulna (any part)	C40.0-●	C79.51	—	D16.0-●	—	—
umbilicus, umbilical — *see also Neoplasm, skin, trunk*	C44.509	C79.2	D04.5	D23.5	D48.5	D49.2
uncus, brain	C71.2	C79.31	—	D33.0	D43.0	D49.6
unknown site or unspecified	C80.1	C79.9	D09.9	D36.9	D48.9	D49.9
urachus	C67.7	C79.11	D09.0	D30.3	D41.4	D49.4
ureter, ureteral	C66.-●	C79.19	D09.19	D30.2-●	D41.2-●	D49.59
orifice (bladder)	C67.6	C79.11	D09.0	D30.3	D41.4	D49.4
ureter-bladder (junction)	C67.6	C79.11	D09.0	D30.3	D41.4	D49.4

TABLE OF NEOPLASMS

New Revised ~~deleted~~ Deleted ● Use Additional Character(s)

	Malignant Primary	Malignant Secondary	Ca in situ	Benign	Uncertain Behavior	Unspecified Behavior
urethra, urethral (gland)	C68.Ø	C79.19	DØ9.19	D3Ø.4	D41.3	D49.59
orifice, internal	C67.5	C79.11	DØ9.Ø	D3Ø.3	D41.4	D49.4
urethrovaginal (septum)	C57.9	C79.82	DØ7.3Ø	D28.9	D39.8	D49.59
urinary organ or system	C68.9	C79.1Ø	DØ9.1Ø	D3Ø.9	D41.9	D49.59
bladder — *see Neoplasm, bladder*						
overlapping lesion	C68.8	—	—	—	—	—
specified sites NEC	C68.8	C79.19	DØ9.19	D3Ø.8	D41.8	D49.59
utero-ovarian	C57.8	C79.82	DØ7.39	D28.7	D39.8	D49.59
ligament	C57.1	C79.82	DØ7.39	D28.2	D39.8	D49.59
uterosacral ligament	C57.3	C79.82	—	D28.2	D39.8	D49.59
uterus, uteri, uterine	C55	C79.82	DØ7.Ø	D26.9	D39.Ø	D49.59
adnexa NEC	C57.4	C79.82	DØ7.39	D28.7	D39.8	D49.59
body	C54.9	C79.82	DØ7.Ø	D26.1	D39.Ø	D49.59
cervix	C53.9	C79.82	DØ6.9	D26.Ø	D39.Ø	D49.59
cornu	C54.9	C79.82	DØ7.Ø	D26.1	D39.Ø	D49.59
corpus	C54.9	C79.82	DØ7.Ø	D26.1	D39.Ø	D49.59
endocervix (canal) (gland)	C53.Ø	C79.82	DØ6.Ø	D26.Ø	D39.Ø	D49.59
endometrium	C54.1	C79.82	DØ7.Ø	D26.1	D39.Ø	D49.59
exocervix	C53.1	C79.82	DØ6.1	D26.Ø	D39.Ø	D49.59
external os	C53.1	C79.82	DØ6.1	D26.Ø	D39.Ø	D49.59
fundus	C54.3	C79.82	DØ7.Ø	D26.1	D39.Ø	D49.59
internal os	C53.Ø	C79.82	DØ6.Ø	D26.Ø	D39.Ø	D49.59
isthmus	C54.Ø	C79.82	DØ7.Ø	D26.1	D39.Ø	D49.59
ligament	C57.3	C79.82	—	D28.2	D39.8	D49.59
broad	C57.1	C79.82	DØ7.39	D28.2	D39.8	D49.59
round	C57.2	C79.82	—	D28.2	D39.8	D49.59
lower segment	C54.Ø	C79.82	DØ7.Ø	D26.1	D39.Ø	D49.59
myometrium	C54.2	C79.82	DØ7.Ø	D26.1	D39.Ø	D49.59
overlapping sites	C54.8	—	—	—	—	—
squamocolumnar junction	C53.8	C79.82	DØ6.7	D26.Ø	D39.Ø	D49.59
tube	C57.Ø-•	C79.82	DØ7.39	D28.2	D39.8	D49.59
utricle, prostatic	C68.Ø	C79.19	DØ9.19	D3Ø.4	D41.3	D49.59
uveal tract	C69.4-•	C79.49	DØ9.2-•	D31.4-•	D48.7	D49.89
uvula	CØ5.2	C79.89	DØØ.Ø4	D1Ø.39	D37.Ø9	D49.Ø
vagina, vaginal (fornix) (vault) (wall)	C52	C79.82	DØ7.2	D28.1	D39.8	D49.59
vaginovesical	C57.9	C79.82	DØ7.3Ø	D28.9	D39.9	D49.59
septum	C57.9	C79.82	DØ7.3Ø	D28.9	D39.9	D49.59
vallecula (epigiottis)	C1Ø.Ø	C79.89	DØØ.Ø8	D1Ø.5	D37.Ø5	D49.Ø
vas deferens	C63.1-•	C79.82	DØ7.69	D29.8	D4Ø.8	D49.59
vascular — *see Neoplasm, connective tissue*						

	Malignant Primary	Malignant Secondary	Ca in situ	Benign	Uncertain Behavior	Unspecified Behavior
Vater's ampulla	C24.1	C78.89	DØ1.5	D13.5	D37.6	D49.Ø
vein, venous — *see Neoplasm, connective tissue*						
vena cava (abdominal) (inferior)	C49.4	C79.89	—	D21.4	D48.1	D49.2
superior	C49.3	C79.89	—	D21.3	D48.1	D49.2
ventricle (cerebral) (floor) (lateral) (third)	C71.5	C79.31	—	D33.Ø	D43.Ø	D49.6
cardiac (left) (right)	C38.Ø	C79.89	—	D15.1	D48.7	D49.89
fourth	C71.7	C79.31	—	D33.1	D43.1	D49.6
ventricular band of larynx	C32.1	C78.39	DØ2.Ø	D14.1	D38.Ø	D49.1
ventriculus — *see Neoplasm, stomach*						
vermillion border — *see Neoplasm, lip*						
vermis, cerebellum	C71.6	C79.31	—	D33.1	D43.1	D49.6
vertebra (column)	C41.2	C79.51	—	D16.6	D48.Ø	D49.2
coccyx	C41.4	C79.51	—	D16.8-•	D48.Ø	D49.2
marrow NEC	C96.9	C79.52	—	—	D47.9	D49.89
sacrum	C41.4	C79.51	—	D16.8-•	D48.Ø	D49.2
vesical — *see Neoplasm, bladder*						
vesicle, seminal	C63.7	C79.82	DØ7.69	D29.8	D4Ø.8	D49.59
vesicocervical tissue	C57.9	C79.82	DØ7.3Ø	D28.9	D39.9	D49.59
vesicorectal	C76.3	C79.82	DØ9.8	D36.7	D48.7	D49.89
vesicovaginal	C57.9	C79.82	DØ7.3Ø	D28.9	D39.9	D49.59
septum	C57.9	C79.82	DØ7.3Ø	D28.9	D39.8	D49.59
vessel (blood) — *see Neoplasm, connective tissue*						
vestibular gland, greater	C51.Ø	C79.82	DØ7.1	D28.Ø	D39.8	D49.59
vestibule						
mouth	CØ6.1	C79.89	DØØ.ØØ	D1Ø.39	D37.Ø9	D49.Ø
nose	C3Ø.Ø	C78.39	DØ2.3	D14.Ø	D38.5	D49.1
Virchow's gland	C77.Ø	C77.Ø	—	D36.Ø	D48.7	D49.89
viscera NEC	C76.8	C79.89	DØ9.8	D36.7	D48.7	D49.89
vocal cords (true)	C32.Ø	C78.39	DØ2.Ø	D14.1	D38.Ø	D49.1
false	C32.1	C78.39	DØ2.Ø	D14.1	D38.Ø	D49.1
vomer	C41.Ø	C79.51	—	D16.4-•	D48.Ø	D49.2
vulva	C51.9	C79.82	DØ7.1	D28.Ø	D39.8	D49.59
vulvovaginal gland	C51.Ø	C79.82	DØ7.1	D28.Ø	D39.8	D49.59
Waldeyer's ring	C14.2	C79.89	DØØ.Ø8	D1Ø.9	D37.Ø5	D49.Ø
Wharton's duct	CØ8.Ø	C79.89	DØØ.ØØ	D11.7	D37.Ø32	D49.Ø
white matter (central) (cerebral)	C71.Ø	C79.31	—	D33.Ø	D43.Ø	D49.6
windpipe	C33	C78.39	DØ2.1	D14.2	D38.1	D49.1

	Malignant Primary	Malignant Secondary	Ca in situ	Benign	Uncertain Behavior	Unspecified Behavior
Wirsung's duct	C25.3	C78.89	DØ1.7	D13.6	D37.8	D49.Ø
wolffian (body) (duct)						
female	C57.7	C79.82	DØ7.39	D28.7	D39.8	D49.59
male	C63.7	C79.82	DØ7.69	D29.8	D4Ø.8	D49.59
womb — *see Neoplasm, uterus*						
wrist NEC	C76.4-●	C79.89	DØ4.6-●	D36.7	D48.7	D49.89
xiphoid process	C41.3	C79.51	—	D16.7	D48.Ø	D49.2
Zuckerkandl organ	C75.5	C79.89	—	D35.6	D44.7	D49.7

◄ New ⇐ Revised ~~deleted~~ Deleted ● Use Additional Character(s)

ICD-10-CM Table of Drugs and Chemicals

Substance	External Cause (T-Code)					
	Poisoning, Accidental (Unintentional)	Poisoning, Intentional Self-Harm	Poisoning, Assault	Poisoning, Undetermined	Adverse Effect	Underdosing
#						
1-propanol	T51.3X1	T51.3X2	T51.3X3	T51.3X4	—	—
2-propanol	T51.2X1	T51.2X2	T51.2X3	T51.2X4	—	—
2,4-D (dichlorophen-oxyacetic acid)	T6Ø.3X1	T6Ø.3X2	T6Ø.3X3	T6Ø.3X4	—	—
2,4-toluene diisocyanate	T65.ØX1	T65.ØX2	T65.ØX3	T65.ØX4	—	—
2,4,5-T (trichloro-phenoxyacetic acid)	T6Ø.1X1	T6Ø.1X2	T6Ø.1X3	T6Ø.1X4	—	—
3,4-methylenedioxy-methamphetamine	T43.641	T43.642	T43.643	T43.644	—	—
14-hydroxydihydro-morphinone	T4Ø.2X1	T4Ø.2X2	T4Ø.2X3	T4Ø.2X4	T4Ø.2X5	T4Ø.2X6
A						
ABOB	T37.5X1	T37.5X2	T37.5X3	T37.5X4	T37.5X5	T37.5X6
Abrine	T62.2X1	T62.2X2	T62.2X3	T62.2X4	—	—
Abrus (seed)	T62.2X1	T62.2X2	T62.2X3	T62.2X4	—	—
Absinthe	T51.ØX1	T51.ØX2	T51.ØX3	T51.ØX4	—	—
beverage	T51.ØX1	T51.ØX2	T51.ØX3	T51.ØX4	—	—
Acaricide	T6Ø.8X1	T6Ø.8X2	T6Ø.8X3	T6Ø.8X4	—	—
Acebutolol	T44.7X1	T44.7X2	T44.7X3	T44.7X4	T44.7X5	T44.7X6
Acecarbromal	T42.6X1	T42.6X2	T42.6X3	T42.6X4	T42.6X5	T42.6X6
Aceclidine	T44.1X1	T44.1X2	T44.1X3	T44.1X4	T44.1X5	T44.1X6
Acedapsone	T37.ØX1	T37.ØX2	T37.ØX3	T37.ØX4	T37.ØX5	T37.ØX6
Acefylline piperazine	T48.6X1	T48.6X2	T48.6X3	T48.6X4	T48.6X5	T48.6X6
Acemorphan	T4Ø.2X1	T4Ø.2X2	T4Ø.2X3	T4Ø.2X4	T4Ø.2X5	T4Ø.2X6
Acenocoumarin	T45.511	T45.512	T45.513	T45.514	T45.515	T45.516
Acenocoumarol	T45.511	T45.512	T45.513	T45.514	T45.515	T45.516
Acepifylline	T48.6X1	T48.6X2	T48.6X3	T48.6X4	T48.6X5	T48.6X6
Acepromazine	T43.3X1	T43.3X2	T43.3X3	T43.3X4	T43.3X5	T43.3X6
Acesulfamethoxypyridazine	T37.ØX1	T37.ØX2	T37.ØX3	T37.ØX4	T37.ØX5	T37.ØX6
Acetal	T52.8X1	T52.8X2	T52.8X3	T52.8X4	—	—
Acetaldehyde (vapor)	T52.8X1	T52.8X2	T52.8X3	T52.8X4	—	—
liquid	T65.891	T65.892	T65.893	T65.894	—	—
P-Acetamidophenol	T39.1X1	T39.1X2	T39.1X3	T39.1X4	T39.1X5	T39.1X6
Acetaminophen	T39.1X1	T39.1X2	T39.1X3	T39.1X4	T39.1X5	T39.1X6
Acetaminosalol	T39.1X1	T39.1X2	T39.1X3	T39.1X4	T39.1X5	T39.1X6
Acetanilide	T39.1X1	T39.1X2	T39.1X3	T39.1X4	T39.1X5	T39.1X6
Acetarsol	T37.3X1	T37.3X2	T37.3X3	T37.3X4	T37.3X5	T37.3X6
Acetazolamide	T5Ø.2X1	T5Ø.2X2	T5Ø.2X3	T5Ø.2X4	T5Ø.2X5	T5Ø.2X6
Acetiamine	T45.2X1	T45.2X2	T45.2X3	T45.2X4	T45.2X5	T45.2X6
Acetic						
acid	T54.2X1	T54.2X2	T54.2X3	T54.2X4	—	—
with sodium acetate (ointment)	T49.3X1	T49.3X2	T49.3X3	T49.3X4	T49.3X5	T49.3X6
Acetic *(Continued)*						
acid *(Continued)*						
ester (solvent) (vapor)	T52.8X1	T52.8X2	T52.8X3	T52.8X4	—	—
irrigating solution	T5Ø.3X1	T5Ø.3X2	T5Ø.3X3	T5Ø.3X4	T5Ø.3X5	T5Ø.3X6
medicinal (lotion)	T49.2X1	T49.2X2	T49.2X3	T49.2X4	T49.2X5	T49.2X6
anhydride	T65.891	T65.892	T65.893	T65.894	—	—
ether (vapor)	T52.8X1	T52.8X2	T52.8X3	T52.8X4	—	—
Acetohexamide	T38.3X1	T38.3X2	T38.3X3	T38.3X4	T38.3X5	T38.3X6
Acetohydroxamic acid	T5Ø.991	T5Ø.992	T5Ø.993	T5Ø.994	T5Ø.995	T5Ø.996
Acetomenaphthone	T45.7X1	T45.7X2	T45.7X3	T45.7X4	T45.7X5	T45.7X6
Acetomorphine	T4Ø.1X1	T4Ø.1X2	T4Ø.1X3	T4Ø.1X4	—	—
Acetone (oils)	T52.4X1	T52.4X2	T52.4X3	T52.4X4	—	—
chlorinated	T52.4X1	T52.4X2	T52.4X3	T52.4X4	—	—
vapor	T52.4X1	T52.4X2	T52.4X3	T52.4X4	—	—
Acetonitrile	T52.8X1	T52.8X2	T52.8X3	T52.8X4	—	—
Acetophenazine	T43.3X1	T43.3X2	T43.3X3	T43.3X4	T43.3X5	T43.3X6
Acetophenetedin	T39.1X1	T39.1X2	T39.1X3	T39.1X4	T39.1X5	T39.1X6
Acetophenone	T52.4X1	T52.4X2	T52.4X3	T52.4X4	—	—
Acetorphine	T4Ø.2X1	T4Ø.2X2	T4Ø.2X3	T4Ø.2X4	—	—
Acetosulfone (sodium)	T37.1X1	T37.1X2	T37.1X3	T37.1X4	T37.1X5	T37.1X6
Acetrizoate (sodium)	T5Ø.8X1	T5Ø.8X2	T5Ø.8X3	T5Ø.8X4	T5Ø.8X5	T5Ø.8X6
Acetylcarbromal	T42.6X1	T42.6X2	T42.6X3	T42.6X4	T42.6X5	T42.6X6
Acetrizoic acid	T5Ø.8X1	T5Ø.8X2	T5Ø.8X3	T5Ø.8X4	T5Ø.8X5	T5Ø.8X6
Acetyl						
bromide	T53.6X1	T53.6X2	T53.6X3	T53.6X4	—	—
chloride	T53.6X1	T53.6X2	T53.6X3	T53.6X4	—	—
Acetylcholine						
chloride	T44.1X1	T44.1X2	T44.1X3	T44.1X4	T44.1X5	T44.1X6
derivative	T44.1X1	T44.1X2	T44.1X3	T44.1X4	T44.1X5	T44.1X6
Acetylcysteine	T48.4X1	T48.4X2	T48.4X3	T48.4X4	T48.4X5	T48.4X6
Acetyldigitoxin	T46.ØX1	T46.ØX2	T46.ØX3	T46.ØX4	T46.ØX5	T46.ØX6
Acetyldigoxin	T46.ØX1	T46.ØX2	T46.ØX3	T46.ØX4	T46.ØX5	T46.ØX6
Acetyldihydrocodeine	T4Ø.2X1	T4Ø.2X2	T4Ø.2X3	T4Ø.2X4	—	—
Acetyldihydrocodeinone	T4Ø.2X1	T4Ø.2X2	T4Ø.2X3	T4Ø.2X4	—	—
Acetylene (gas)	T59.891	T59.892	T59.893	T59.894	—	—
dichloride	T53.6X1	T53.6X2	T53.6X3	T53.6X4	—	—
incomplete combustion of	T58.11	T58.12	T58.13	T58.14	—	—
industrial	T59.891	T59.892	T59.893	T59.894	—	—
tetrachloride	T53.6X1	T53.6X2	T53.6X3	T53.6X4	—	—
vapor	T53.6X1	T53.6X2	T53.6X3	T53.6X4	—	—
Acetylphenylhydrazine	T39.8X1	T39.8X2	T39.8X3	T39.8X4	T39.8X5	T39.8X6
Acetylpheneturide	T42.6X1	T42.6X2	T42.6X3	T42.6X4	T42.6X5	T42.6X6

		External Cause (T-Code)				
Substance	**Poisoning, Accidental (Unintentional)**	**Poisoning, Intentional Self-Harm**	**Poisoning, Assault**	**Poisoning, Undetermined**	**Adverse Effect**	**Underdosing**
Acetylsalicylic acid (salts)	T39.Ø11	T39.Ø12	T39.Ø13	T39.Ø14	T39.Ø15	T39.Ø16
enteric coated	T39.Ø11	T39.Ø12	T39.Ø13	T39.Ø14	T39.Ø15	T39.Ø16
Acetylsulfamethoxypyridazine	T37.ØX1	T37.ØX2	T37.ØX3	T37.ØX4	T37.ØX5	T37.ØX6
Achromycin	T36.4X1	T36.4X2	T36.4X3	T36.4X4	T36.4X5	T36.4X6
ophthalmic preparation	T49.5X1	T49.5X2	T49.5X3	T49.5X4	T49.5X5	T49.5X6
topical NEC	T49.ØX1	T49.ØX2	T49.ØX3	T49.ØX4	T49.ØX5	T49.ØX6
Aciclovir	T37.5X1	T37.5X2	T37.5X3	T37.5X4	T37.5X5	T37.5X6
Acid (corrosive) NEC	T54.2X1	T54.2X2	T54.2X3	T54.2X4	—	—
Acidifying agent NEC	T5Ø.9Ø1	T5Ø.9Ø2	T5Ø.9Ø3	T5Ø.9Ø4	T5Ø.9Ø5	T5Ø.9Ø6
Acipimox	T46.6X1	T46.6X2	T46.6X3	T46.6X4	T46.6X5	T46.6X6
Acitretin	T5Ø.991	T5Ø.992	T5Ø.993	T5Ø.994	T5Ø.995	T5Ø.996
Aclarubicin	T45.1X1	T45.1X2	T45.1X3	T45.1X4	T45.1X5	T45.1X6
Aclatonium napadisilate	T48.1X1	T48.1X2	T48.1X3	T48.1X4	T48.1X5	T48.1X6
Aconite (wild)	T46.991	T46.992	T46.993	T46.994	T46.995	T46.996
Aconitine	T46.991	T46.992	T46.993	T46.994	T46.995	T46.996
Aconitum ferox	T46.991	T46.992	T46.993	T46.994	T46.995	T46.996
Acridine	T65.6X1	T65.6X2	T65.6X3	T65.6X4	—	—
vapor	T59.891	T59.892	T59.893	T59.894	—	—
Acriflavine	T37.91	T37.92	T37.93	T37.94	T37.95	T37.96
Acriflavinium chloride	T49.ØX1	T49.ØX2	T49.ØX3	T49.ØX4	T49.ØX5	T49.ØX6
Acrinol	T49.ØX1	T49.ØX2	T49.ØX3	T49.ØX4	T49.ØX5	T49.ØX6
Acrisorcin	T49.ØX1	T49.ØX2	T49.ØX3	T49.ØX4	T49.ØX5	T49.ØX6
Acrivastine	T45.ØX1	T45.ØX2	T45.ØX3	T45.ØX4	T45.ØX5	T45.ØX6
Acrolein (gas)	T59.891	T59.892	T59.893	T59.894	—	—
liquid	T54.1X1	T54.1X2	T54.1X3	T54.1X4	—	—
Acrylamide	T65.891	T65.892	T65.893	T65.894	—	—
Acrylic resin	T49.3X1	T49.3X2	T49.3X3	T49.3X4	T49.3X5	T49.3X6
Acrylonitrile	T65.891	T65.892	T65.893	T65.894	—	—
Actaea spicata	T62.2X1	T62.2X2	T62.2X3	T62.2X4	—	—
berry	T62.1X1	T62.1X2	T62.1X3	T62.1X4	—	—
Acterol	T37.3X1	T37.3X2	T37.3X3	T37.3X4	T37.3X5	T37.3X6
ACTH	T38.811	T38.812	T38.813	T38.814	T38.815	T38.816
Actinomycin C	T45.1X1	T45.1X2	T45.1X3	T45.1X4	T45.1X5	T45.1X6
Actinomycin D	T45.1X1	T45.1X2	T45.1X3	T45.1X4	T45.1X5	T45.1X6
Activated charcoal — *see also Charcoal, medicinal*	T47.6X1	T47.6X2	T47.6X3	T47.6X4	T47.6X5	T47.6X6
Acyclovir	T37.5X1	T37.5X2	T37.5X3	T37.5X4	T37.5X5	T37.5X6
Adenine	T45.2X1	T45.2X2	T45.2X3	T45.2X4	T45.2X5	T45.2X6
arabinoside	T37.5X1	T37.5X2	T37.5X3	T37.5X4	T37.5X5	T37.5X6
Adenosine (phosphate)	T46.2X1	T46.2X2	T46.2X3	T46.2X4	T46.2X5	T46.2X6
ADH	T38.891	T38.892	T38.893	T38.894	T38.895	T38.896
Adhesive NEC	T65.891	T65.892	T65.893	T65.894	—	—

		External Cause (T-Code)				
Substance	**Poisoning, Accidental (Unintentional)**	**Poisoning, Intentional Self-Harm**	**Poisoning, Assault**	**Poisoning, Undetermined**	**Adverse Effect**	**Underdosing**
Adicillin	T36.ØX1	T36.ØX2	T36.ØX3	T36.ØX4	T36.ØX5	T36.ØX6
Adiphenine	T44.3X1	T44.3X2	T44.3X3	T44.3X4	T44.3X5	T44.3X6
Adipiodone	T5Ø.8X1	T5Ø.8X2	T5Ø.8X3	T5Ø.8X4	T5Ø.8X5	T5Ø.8X6
Adjunct, pharmaceutical	T5Ø.9Ø1	T5Ø.9Ø2	T5Ø.9Ø3	T5Ø.9Ø4	T5Ø.9Ø5	T5Ø.9Ø6
Adrenal (extract, cortex or medulla) (glucocorticoids) (hormones) (mineralo corticoids)	T38.ØX1	T38.ØX2	T38.ØX3	T38.ØX4	T38.ØX5	T38.ØX6
ENT agent	T49.6X1	T49.6X2	T49.6X3	T49.6X4	T49.6X5	T49.6X6
ophthalmic preparation	T49.5X1	T49.5X2	T49.5X3	T49.5X4	T49.5X5	T49.5X6
topical NEC	T49.ØX1	T49.ØX2	T49.ØX3	T49.ØX4	T49.ØX5	T49.ØX6
Adrenaline	T44.5X1	T44.5X2	T44.5X3	T44.5X4	T44.5X5	T44.5X6
Adrenalin — *see Adrenaline*						
Adrenergic NEC	T44.9Ø1	T44.9Ø2	T44.9Ø3	T44.9Ø4	T44.9Ø5	T44.9Ø6
blocking agent NEC	T44.8X1	T44.8X2	T44.8X3	T44.8X4	T44.8X5	T44.8X6
beta, heart	T44.7X1	T44.7X2	T44.7X3	T44.7X4	T44.7X5	T44.7X6
specified NEC	T44.991	T44.992	T44.993	T44.994	T44.995	T44.996
Adrenochrome						
(mono) semicarbazone	T46.991	T46.992	T46.993	T46.994	T46.995	T46.996
derivative	T46.991	T46.992	T46.993	T46.994	T46.995	T46.996
Adrenocorticotrophic hormone	T38.811	T38.812	T38.813	T38.814	T38.815	T38.816
Adrenocorticotrophin	T38.811	T38.812	T38.813	T38.814	T38.815	T38.816
Adriamycin	T45.1X1	T45.1X2	T45.1X3	T45.1X4	T45.1X5	T45.1X6
Aerosol spray NEC	T65.91	T65.92	T65.93	T65.94	—	—
Aerosporin	T36.8X1	T36.8X2	T36.8X3	T36.8X4	T36.8X5	T36.8X6
ENT agent	T49.6X1	T49.6X2	T49.6X3	T49.6X4	T49.6X5	T49.6X6
ophthalmic preparation	T49.5X1	T49.5X2	T49.5X3	T49.5X4	T49.5X5	T49.5X6
topical NEC	T49.ØX1	T49.ØX2	T49.ØX3	T49.ØX4	T49.ØX5	T49.ØX6
Aethusa cynapium	T62.2X1	T62.2X2	T62.2X3	T62.2X4	—	—
Afghanistan black	T4Ø.7X1	T4Ø.7X2	T4Ø.7X3	T4Ø.7X4	T4Ø.7X5	T4Ø.7X6
Aflatoxin	T64.Ø1	T64.Ø2	T64.Ø3	T64.Ø4	—	—
Afloqualone	T42.8X1	T42.8X2	T42.8X3	T42.8X4	T42.8X5	T42.8X6
African boxwood	T62.2X1	T62.2X2	T62.2X3	T62.2X4	—	—
Agar	T47.4X1	T47.4X2	T47.4X3	T47.4X4	T47.4X5	T47.4X6
Agonist						
predominantly						
alpha-adrenoreceptor	T44.4X1	T44.4X2	T44.4X3	T44.4X4	T44.4X5	T44.4X6
beta-adrenoreceptor	T44.5X1	T44.5X2	T44.5X3	T44.5X4	T44.5X5	T44.5X6
Agricultural agent NEC	T65.91	T65.92	T65.93	T65.94	—	—
Agrypnal	T42.3X1	T42.3X2	T42.3X3	T42.3X4	T42.3X5	T42.3X6
AHLG	T5Ø.Z11	T5Ø.Z12	T5Ø.Z13	T5Ø.Z14	T5Ø.Z15	T5Ø.Z16
Air contaminant(s), source/type NOS	T65.91	T65.92	T65.93	T65.94	—	—

New Revised ~~deleted~~ Deleted

Substance	External Cause (T-Code)					
	Poisoning, Accidental (Unintentional)	Poisoning, Intentional Self-Harm	Poisoning, Assault	Poisoning, Undetermined	Adverse Effect	Underdosing
Ajmaline	T46.2X1	T46.2X2	T46.2X3	T46.2X4	T46.2X5	T46.2X6
Akritoin	T37.8X1	T37.8X2	T37.8X3	T37.8X4	T37.8X5	T37.8X6
Akee	T62.1X1	T62.1X2	T62.1X3	T62.1X4	—	—
Akrinol	T49.ØX1	T49.ØX2	T49.ØX3	T49.ØX4	T49.ØX5	T49.ØX6
Alacepril	T46.4X1	T46.4X2	T46.4X3	T46.4X4	T46.4X5	T46.4X6
Alantolactone	T37.4X1	T37.4X2	T37.4X3	T37.4X4	T37.4X5	T37.4X6
Albamycin	T36.8X1	T36.8X2	T36.8X3	T36.8X4	T36.8X5	T36.8X6
Albendazole	T37.4X1	T37.4X2	T37.4X3	T37.4X4	T37.4X5	T37.4X6
Albumin						
bovine	T45.8X1	T45.8X2	T45.8X3	T45.8X4	T45.8X5	T45.8X6
human serum	T45.8X1	T45.8X2	T45.8X3	T45.8X4	T45.8X5	T45.8X6
salt-poor	T45.8X1	T45.8X2	T45.8X3	T45.8X4	T45.8X5	T45.8X6
normal human serum	T45.8X1	T45.8X2	T45.8X3	T45.8X4	T45.8X5	T45.8X6
Albuterol	T48.6X1	T48.6X2	T48.6X3	T48.6X4	T48.6X5	T48.6X6
Albutoin	T42.ØX1	T42.ØX2	T42.ØX3	T42.ØX4	T42.ØX5	T42.ØX6
Alclometasone	T49.ØX1	T49.ØX2	T49.ØX3	T49.ØX4	T49.ØX5	T49.ØX6
Alcohol	T51.91	T51.92	T51.93	T51.94	—	—
absolute	T51.ØX1	T51.ØX2	T51.ØX3	T51.ØX4	—	—
beverage	T51.ØX1	T51.ØX2	T51.ØX3	T51.ØX4	—	—
allyl	T51.8X1	T51.8X2	T51.8X3	T51.8X4	—	—
amyl	T51.3X1	T51.3X2	T51.3X3	T51.3X4	—	—
antifreeze	T51.1X1	T51.1X2	T51.1X3	T51.1X4	—	—
beverage	T51.ØX1	T51.ØX2	T51.ØX3	T51.ØX4	—	—
butyl	T51.3X1	T51.3X2	T51.3X3	T51.3X4	—	—
dehydrated	T51.ØX1	T51.ØX2	T51.ØX3	T51.ØX4	—	—
beverage	T51.ØX1	T51.ØX2	T51.ØX3	T51.ØX4	—	—
denatured	T51.ØX1	T51.ØX2	T51.ØX3	T51.ØX4	—	—
deterrent NEC	T5Ø.6X1	T5Ø.6X2	T5Ø.6X3	T5Ø.6X4	T5Ø.6X5	T5Ø.6X6
diagnostic (gastric function)	T5Ø.8X1	T5Ø.8X2	T5Ø.8X3	T5Ø.8X4	T5Ø.8X5	T5Ø.8X6
ethyl	T51.ØX1	T51.ØX2	T51.ØX3	T51.ØX4	—	—
beverage	T51.ØX1	T51.ØX2	T51.ØX3	T51.ØX4	—	—
grain	T51.ØX1	T51.ØX2	T51.ØX3	T51.ØX4	—	—
beverage	T51.ØX1	T51.ØX2	T51.ØX3	T51.ØX4	—	—
industrial	T51.ØX1	T51.ØX2	T51.ØX3	T51.ØX4	—	—
isopropyl	T51.2X1	T51.2X2	T51.2X3	T51.2X4	—	—
methyl	T51.1X1	T51.1X2	T51.1X3	T51.1X4	—	—
preparation for consumption	T51.ØX1	T51.ØX2	T51.ØX3	T51.ØX4	—	—
propyl	T51.3X1	T51.3X2	T51.3X3	T51.3X4	—	—
secondary	T51.2X1	T51.2X2	T51.2X3	T51.2X4	—	—
radiator	T51.1X1	T51.1X2	T51.1X3	T51.1X4	—	—
rubbing	T51.2X1	T51.2X2	T51.2X3	T51.2X4	—	—
specified type NEC	T51.8X1	T51.8X2	T51.8X3	T51.8X4	—	—
Alcohol *(Continued)*						
surgical	T51.ØX1	T51.ØX2	T51.ØX3	T51.ØX4	—	—
vapor (from any type of Alcohol)	T59.891	T59.892	T59.893	T59.894	—	—
wood	T51.1X1	T51.1X2	T51.1X3	T51.1X4	—	—
Alcuronium (chloride)	T48.1X1	T48.1X2	T48.1X3	T48.1X4	T48.1X5	T48.1X6
Aldactone	T5Ø.ØX1	T5Ø.ØX2	T5Ø.ØX3	T5Ø.ØX4	T5Ø.ØX5	T5Ø.ØX6
Aldesulfone sodium	T37.1X1	T37.1X2	T37.1X3	T37.1X4	T37.1X5	T37.1X6
Aldicarb	T6Ø.ØX1	T6Ø.ØX2	T6Ø.ØX3	T6Ø.ØX4	—	—
Aldomet	T46.5X1	T46.5X2	T46.5X3	T46.5X4	T46.5X5	T46.5X6
Aldosterone	T5Ø.ØX1	T5Ø.ØX2	T5Ø.ØX3	T5Ø.ØX4	T5Ø.ØX5	T5Ø.ØX6
Aldrin (dust)	T6Ø.1X1	T6Ø.1X2	T6Ø.1X3	T6Ø.1X4	—	—
Aleve — *see Naproxen*						
Alexitol sodium	T47.1X1	T47.1X2	T47.1X3	T47.1X4	T47.1X5	T47.1X6
Alfacalcidol	T45.2X1	T45.2X2	T45.2X3	T45.2X4	T45.2X5	T45.2X6
Alfadolone	T41.1X1	T41.1X2	T41.1X3	T41.1X4	T41.1X5	T41.1X6
Alfaxalone	T41.1X1	T41.1X2	T41.1X3	T41.1X4	T41.1X5	T41.1X6
Alfentanil	T4Ø.4X1	T4Ø.4X2	T4Ø.4X3	T4Ø.4X4	T4Ø.4X5	T4Ø.4X6
Alfuzosin (hydrochloride)	T44.8X1	T44.8X2	T44.8X3	T44.8X4	T44.8X5	T44.8X6
Algae (harmful) (toxin)	T65.821	T65.822	T65.823	T65.824	—	—
Algeldrate	T47.1X1	T47.1X2	T47.1X3	T47.1X4	T47.1X5	T47.1X6
Algin	T47.8X1	T47.8X2	T47.8X3	T47.8X4	T47.8X5	T47.8X6
Alglucerase	T45.3X1	T45.3X2	T45.3X3	T45.3X4	T45.3X5	T45.3X6
Alidase	T45.3X1	T45.3X2	T45.3X3	T45.3X4	T45.3X5	T45.3X6
Alimemazine	T43.3X1	T43.3X2	T43.3X3	T43.3X4	T43.3X5	T43.3X6
Aliphatic thiocyanates	T65.ØX1	T65.ØX2	T65.ØX3	T65.ØX4	—	—
Alizapride	T45.ØX1	T45.ØX2	T45.ØX3	T45.ØX4	T45.ØX5	T45.ØX6
Alkali (caustic)	T54.3X1	T54.3X2	T54.3X3	T54.3X4	—	—
Alkalizing agent NEC	T5Ø.9Ø1	T5Ø.9Ø2	T5Ø.9Ø3	T5Ø.9Ø4	T5Ø.9Ø5	T5Ø.9Ø6
Alkaline antiseptic solution (aromatic)	T49.6X1	T49.6X2	T49.6X3	T49.6X4	T49.6X5	T49.6X6
Alkalinizing agents (medicinal)	T5Ø.9Ø1	T5Ø.9Ø2	T5Ø.9Ø3	T5Ø.9Ø4	T5Ø.9Ø5	T5Ø.9Ø6
Alka-seltzer	T39.Ø11	T39.Ø12	T39.Ø13	T39.Ø14	T39.Ø15	T39.Ø16
Alkavervir	T46.5X1	T46.5X2	T46.5X3	T46.5X4	T46.5X5	T46.5X6
Alkonium (bromide)	T49.ØX1	T49.ØX2	T49.ØX3	T49.ØX4	T49.ØX5	T49.ØX6
Alkylating drug NEC	T45.1X1	T45.1X2	T45.1X3	T45.1X4	T45.1X5	T45.1X6
antimyeloproliferative	T45.1X1	T45.1X2	T45.1X3	T45.1X4	T45.1X5	T45.1X6
lymphatic	T45.1X1	T45.1X2	T45.1X3	T45.1X4	T45.1X5	T45.1X6
Alkylisocyanate	T65.ØX1	T65.ØX2	T65.ØX3	T65.ØX4	—	—
Allantoin	T49.411	T49.412	T49.413	T49.414	T49.415	T49.416
Allegron	T43.ØX1	T43.ØX2	T43.ØX3	T43.ØX4	T43.ØX5	T43.ØX6
Allethrin	T49.ØX1	T49.ØX2	T49.ØX3	T49.ØX4	T49.ØX5	T49.ØX6
Allobarbital	T42.3X1	T42.3X2	T42.3X3	T42.3X4	T42.3X5	T42.3X6

	External Cause (T-Code)					
Substance	Poisoning, Accidental (Unintentional)	Poisoning, Intentional Self-Harm	Poisoning, Assault	Poisoning, Undetermined	Adverse Effect	Underdosing
Allopurinol	T50.4X1	T50.4X2	T50.4X3	T50.4X4	T50.4X5	T50.4X6
Allyl						
alcohol	T51.8X1	T51.8X2	T51.8X3	T51.8X4	—	—
disulfide	T46.6X1	T46.6X2	T46.6X3	T46.6X4	T46.6X5	T46.6X6
Allylestrenol	T38.5X1	T38.5X2	T38.5X3	T38.5X4	T38.5X5	T38.5X6
Allylisopropylacetylurea	T42.6X1	T42.6X2	T42.6X3	T42.6X4	T42.6X5	T42.6X6
Allylisopropylmalonylurea	T42.3X1	T42.3X2	T42.3X3	T42.3X4	T42.3X5	T42.3X6
Allylthiourea	T49.3X1	T49.3X2	T49.3X3	T49.3X4	T49.3X5	T49.3X6
Allyltribromide	T42.6X1	T42.6X2	T42.6X3	T42.6X4	T42.6X5	T42.6X6
Allypropymal	T42.3X1	T42.3X2	T42.3X3	T42.3X4	T42.3X5	T42.3X6
Almagate	T47.1X1	T47.1X2	T47.1X3	T47.1X4	T47.1X5	T47.1X6
Almasilate	T47.1X1	T47.1X2	T47.1X3	T47.1X4	T47.1X5	T47.1X6
Almitrine	T50.7X1	T50.7X2	T50.7X3	T50.7X4	T50.7X5	T50.7X6
Aloes	T47.2X1	T47.2X2	T47.2X3	T47.2X4	T47.2X5	T47.2X6
Aloglutamol	T47.1X1	T47.1X2	T47.1X3	T47.1X4	T47.1X5	T47.1X6
Aloin	T47.2X1	T47.2X2	T47.2X3	T47.2X4	T47.2X5	T47.2X6
Aloxidone	T42.2X1	T42.2X2	T42.2X3	T42.2X4	T42.2X5	T42.2X6
Alpha						
acetyldigoxin	T46.0X1	T46.0X2	T46.0X3	T46.0X4	T46.0X5	T46.0X6
adrenergic blocking drug	T44.6X1	T44.6X2	T44.6X3	T44.6X4	T44.6X5	T44.6X6
amylase	T45.3X1	T45.3X2	T45.3X3	T45.3X4	T45.3X5	T45.3X6
tocoferol (acetate)	T45.2X1	T45.2X2	T45.2X3	T45.2X4	T45.2X5	T45.2X6
tocopherol	T45.2X1	T45.2X2	T45.2X3	T45.2X4	T45.2X5	T45.2X6
Alphadolone	T41.1X1	T41.1X2	T41.1X3	T41.1X4	T41.1X5	T41.1X6
Alphaprodine	T40.4X1	T40.4X2	T40.4X3	T40.4X4	T40.4X5	T40.4X6
Alphaxalone	T41.1X1	T41.1X2	T41.1X3	T41.1X4	T41.1X5	T41.1X6
Alprazolam	T42.4X1	T42.4X2	T42.4X3	T42.4X4	T42.4X5	T42.4X6
Alprenolol	T44.7X1	T44.7X2	T44.7X3	T44.7X4	T44.7X5	T44.7X6
Alprostadil	T46.7X1	T46.7X2	T46.7X3	T46.7X4	T46.7X5	T46.7X6
Alsactide	T38.811	T38.812	T38.813	T38.814	T38.815	T38.816
Alseroxylon	T46.5X1	T46.5X2	T46.5X3	T46.5X4	T46.5X5	T46.5X6
Alteplase	T45.611	T45.612	T45.613	T45.614	T45.615	T45.616
Altizide	T50.2X1	T50.2X2	T50.2X3	T50.2X4	T50.2X5	T50.2X6
Altretamine	T45.1X1	T45.1X2	T45.1X3	T45.1X4	T45.1X5	T45.1X6
Alum (medicinal)	T49.4X1	T49.4X2	T49.4X3	T49.4X4	T49.4X5	T49.4X6
nonmedicinal (ammonium) (potassium)	T56.891	T56.892	T56.893	T56.894	—	—
Aluminium, aluminum						
acetate	T49.2X1	T49.2X2	T49.2X3	T49.2X4	T49.2X5	T49.2X6
solution	T49.0X1	T49.0X2	T49.0X3	T49.0X4	T49.0X5	T49.0X6
aspirin	T39.011	T39.012	T39.013	T39.014	T39.015	T39.016
bis (acetylsalicylate)	T39.011	T39.012	T39.013	T39.014	T39.015	T39.016

	External Cause (T-Code)					
Substance	Poisoning, Accidental (Unintentional)	Poisoning, Intentional Self-Harm	Poisoning, Assault	Poisoning, Undetermined	Adverse Effect	Underdosing
Aluminium, aluminum *(Continued)*						
carbonate (gel, basic)	T47.1X1	T47.1X2	T47.1X3	T47.1X4	T47.1X5	T47.1X6
chlorhydroxide-complex	T47.1X1	T47.1X2	T47.1X3	T47.1X4	T47.1X5	T47.1X6
chloride	T49.2X1	T49.2X2	T49.2X3	T49.2X4	T49.2X5	T49.2X6
clofibrate	T46.6X1	T46.6X2	T46.6X3	T46.6X4	T46.6X5	T46.6X6
diacetate	T49.2X1	T49.2X2	T49.2X3	T49.2X4	T49.2X5	T49.2X6
glycinate	T47.1X1	T47.1X2	T47.1X3	T47.1X4	T47.1X5	T47.1X6
hydroxide (gel)	T47.1X1	T47.1X2	T47.1X3	T47.1X4	T47.1X5	T47.1X6
hydroxide-magnesium carb. gel	T47.1X1	T47.1X2	T47.1X3	T47.1X4	T47.1X5	T47.1X6
magnesium silicate	T47.1X1	T47.1X2	T47.1X3	T47.1X4	T47.1X5	T47.1X6
nicotinate	T46.7X1	T46.7X2	T46.7X3	T46.7X4	T46.7X5	T46.7X6
ointment (surgical) (topical)	T49.3X1	T49.3X2	T49.3X3	T49.3X4	T49.3X5	T49.3X6
phosphate	T47.1X1	T47.1X2	T47.1X3	T47.1X4	T47.1X5	T47.1X6
salicylate	T39.091	T39.092	T39.093	T39.094	T39.095	T39.096
silicate	T47.1X1	T47.1X2	T47.1X3	T47.1X4	T47.1X5	T47.1X6
sodium silicate	T47.1X1	T47.1X2	T47.1X3	T47.1X4	T47.1X5	T47.1X6
subacetate	T49.2X1	T49.2X2	T49.2X3	T49.2X4	T49.2X5	T49.2X6
sulfate	T49.0X1	T49.0X2	T49.0X3	T49.0X4	T49.0X5	T49.0X6
tannate	T47.6X1	T47.6X2	T47.6X3	T47.6X4	T47.6X5	T47.6X6
topical NEC	T49.3X1	T49.3X2	T49.3X3	T49.3X4	T49.3X5	T49.3X6
Alurate	T42.3X1	T42.3X2	T42.3X3	T42.3X4	T42.3X5	T42.3X6
Alverine	T44.3X1	T44.3X2	T44.3X3	T44.3X4	T44.3X5	T44.3X6
Alvodine	T40.2X1	T40.2X2	T40.2X3	T40.2X4	T40.2X5	T40.2X6
Amanita phalloides	T62.0X1	T62.0X2	T62.0X3	T62.0X4	—	—
Amanitine	T62.0X1	T62.0X2	T62.0X3	T62.0X4	—	—
Amantadine	T42.8X1	T42.8X2	T42.8X3	T42.8X4	T42.8X5	T42.8X6
Ambazone	T49.6X1	T49.6X2	T49.6X3	T49.6X4	T49.6X5	T49.6X6
Ambenonium (chloride)	T44.0X1	T44.0X2	T44.0X3	T44.0X4	T44.0X5	T44.0X6
Ambroxol	T48.4X1	T48.4X2	T48.4X3	T48.4X4	T48.4X5	T48.4X6
Ambuphylline	T48.6X1	T48.6X2	T48.6X3	T48.6X4	T48.6X5	T48.6X6
Ambutonium bromide	T44.3X1	T44.3X2	T44.3X3	T44.3X4	T44.3X5	T44.3X6
Amcinonide	T49.0X1	T49.0X2	T49.0X3	T49.0X4	T49.0X5	T49.0X6
Amdinocilline	T36.0X1	T36.0X2	T36.0X3	T36.0X4	T36.0X5	T36.0X6
Ametazole	T50.8X1	T50.8X2	T50.8X3	T50.8X4	T50.8X5	T50.8X6
Amethocaine	T41.3X1	T41.3X2	T41.3X3	T41.3X4	T41.3X5	T41.3X6
regional	T41.3X1	T41.3X2	T41.3X3	T41.3X4	T41.3X5	T41.3X6
spinal	T41.3X1	T41.3X2	T41.3X3	T41.3X4	T41.3X5	T41.3X6
Amethopterin	T45.1X1	T45.1X2	T45.1X3	T45.1X4	T45.1X5	T45.1X6
Amezinium metilsulfate	T44.991	T44.992	T44.993	T44.994	T44.995	T44.996
Amfebutamone	T43.291	T43.292	T43.293	T43.294	T43.295	T43.296
Amfepramone	T50.5X1	T50.5X2	T50.5X3	T50.5X4	T50.5X5	T50.5X6

New Revised ~~deleted~~ Deleted

Substance	Poisoning, Accidental (Unintentional)	Poisoning, Intentional Self-Harm	Poisoning, Assault	Poisoning, Undetermined	Adverse Effect	Underdosing
	External Cause (T-Code)					
Amfetamine	T43.621	T43.622	T43.623	T43.624	T43.625	T43.626
Amfetaminil	T43.621	T43.622	T43.623	T43.624	T43.625	T43.626
Amfomycin	T36.8X1	T36.8X2	T36.8X3	T36.8X4	T36.8X5	T36.8X6
Amidefrine mesilate	T48.5X1	T48.5X2	T48.5X3	T48.5X4	T48.5X5	T48.5X6
Amidone	T4Ø.3X1	T4Ø.3X2	T4Ø.3X3	T4Ø.3X4	T4Ø.3X5	T4Ø.3X6
Amidopyrine	T39.2X1	T39.2X2	T39.2X3	T39.2X4	T39.2X5	T39.2X6
Amidotrizoate	T5Ø.8X1	T5Ø.8X2	T5Ø.8X3	T5Ø.8X4	T5Ø.8X5	T5Ø.8X6
Amiflamine	T43.1X1	T43.1X2	T43.1X3	T43.1X4	T43.1X5	T43.1X6
Amikacin	T36.5X1	T36.5X2	T36.5X3	T36.5X4	T36.5X5	T36.5X6
Amikhelline	T46.3X1	T46.3X2	T46.3X3	T46.3X4	T46.3X5	T46.3X6
Amiloride	T5Ø.2X1	T5Ø.2X2	T5Ø.2X3	T5Ø.2X4	T5Ø.2X5	T5Ø.2X6
Aminacrine	T49.ØX1	T49.ØX2	T49.ØX3	T49.ØX4	T49.ØX5	T49.ØX6
Amineptine	T43.Ø11	T43.Ø12	T43.Ø13	T43.Ø14	T43.Ø15	T43.Ø16
Aminitrozole	T37.3X1	T37.3X2	T37.3X3	T37.3X4	T37.3X5	T37.3X6
Aminoacetic acid (derivatives)	T5Ø.3X1	T5Ø.3X2	T5Ø.3X3	T5Ø.3X4	T5Ø.3X5	T5Ø.3X6
Amino acids	T5Ø.3X1	T5Ø.3X2	T5Ø.3X3	T5Ø.3X4	T5Ø.3X5	T5Ø.3X6
Aminoacridine	T49.ØX1	T49.ØX2	T49.ØX3	T49.ØX4	T49.ØX5	T49.ØX6
Aminobenzoic acid (-p)	T49.3X1	T49.3X2	T49.3X3	T49.3X4	T49.3X5	T49.3X6
4-Aminobutyric acid	T43.8X1	T43.8X2	T43.8X3	T43.8X4	T43.8X5	T43.8X6
Aminocaproic acid	T45.621	T45.622	T45.623	T45.624	T45.625	T45.626
Aminofenazone	T39.2X1	T39.2X2	T39.2X3	T39.2X4	T39.2X5	T39.2X6
Aminoethylisothiourium	T45.8X1	T45.8X2	T45.8X3	T45.8X4	T45.8X5	T45.8X6
Aminoglutethimide	T45.1X1	T45.1X2	T45.1X3	T45.1X4	T45.1X5	T45.1X6
Aminohippuric acid	T5Ø.8X1	T5Ø.8X2	T5Ø.8X3	T5Ø.8X4	T5Ø.8X5	T5Ø.8X6
Aminomethylbenzoic acid	T45.691	T45.692	T45.693	T45.694	T45.695	T45.696
Aminometradine	T5Ø.2X1	T5Ø.2X2	T5Ø.2X3	T5Ø.2X4	T5Ø.2X5	T5Ø.2X6
Aminopentamide	T44.3X1	T44.3X2	T44.3X3	T44.3X4	T44.3X5	T44.3X6
Aminophenazone	T39.2X1	T39.2X2	T39.2X3	T39.2X4	T39.2X5	T39.2X6
Aminophenol	T54.ØX1	T54.ØX2	T54.ØX3	T54.ØX4	—	—
4-Aminophenol derivatives	T39.1X1	T39.1X2	T39.1X3	T39.1X4	T39.1X5	T39.1X6
Aminophenylpyridone	T43.591	T43.592	T43.593	T43.594	T43.595	T43.596
Aminophylline	T48.6X1	T48.6X2	T48.6X3	T48.6X4	T48.6X5	T48.6X6
Aminopterin sodium	T45.1X1	T45.1X2	T45.1X3	T45.1X4	T45.1X5	T45.1X6
Aminopyrine	T39.2X1	T39.2X2	T39.2X3	T39.2X4	T39.2X5	T39.2X6
8-Aminoquinoline drugs	T37.2X1	T37.2X2	T37.2X3	T37.2X4	T37.2X5	T37.2X6
Aminorex	T5Ø.5X1	T5Ø.5X2	T5Ø.5X3	T5Ø.5X4	T5Ø.5X5	T5Ø.5X6
Aminosalicylic acid	T37.1X1	T37.1X2	T37.1X3	T37.1X4	T37.1X5	T37.1X6
Aminosalylum	T37.1X1	T37.1X2	T37.1X3	T37.1X4	T37.1X5	T37.1X6
Amiodarone	T46.2X1	T46.2X2	T46.2X3	T46.2X4	T46.2X5	T46.2X6
Amiphenazole	T5Ø.7X1	T5Ø.7X2	T5Ø.7X3	T5Ø.7X4	T5Ø.7X5	T5Ø.7X6
Amiquinsin	T46.5X1	T46.5X2	T46.5X3	T46.5X4	T46.5X5	T46.5X6
Amisometradine	T5Ø.2X1	T5Ø.2X2	T5Ø.2X3	T5Ø.2X4	T5Ø.2X5	T5Ø.2X6
Amisulpride	T43.591	T43.592	T43.593	T43.594	T43.595	T43.596
Amitriptyline	T43.Ø21	T43.Ø22	T43.Ø23	T43.Ø24	T43.Ø25	T43.Ø26
Amitriptylinoxide	T43.Ø21	T43.Ø22	T43.Ø23	T43.Ø24	T43.Ø25	T43.Ø26
Amlexanox	T48.6X1	T48.6X2	T48.6X3	T48.6X4	T48.6X5	T48.6X6
Ammonia (fumes) (gas) (vapor)	T59.891	T59.892	T59.893	T59.894	—	—
aromatic spirit	T48.991	T48.992	T48.993	T48.994	T48.995	T48.996
liquid (household)	T54.3X1	T54.3X2	T54.3X3	T54.3X4	—	—
Ammoniated mercury	T49.ØX1	T49.ØX2	T49.ØX3	T49.ØX4	T49.ØX5	T49.ØX6
Ammonium						
acid tartrate	T49.5X1	T49.5X2	T49.5X3	T49.5X4	T49.5X5	T49.5X6
bromide	T42.6X1	T42.6X2	T42.6X3	T42.6X4	T42.6X5	T42.6X6
carbonate	T54.3X1	T54.3X2	T54.3X3	T54.3X4	—	—
chloride	T5Ø.991	T5Ø.992	T5Ø.993	T5Ø.994	T5Ø.995	T5Ø.996
expectorant	T48.4X1	T48.4X2	T48.4X3	T48.4X4	T48.4X5	T48.4X6
compounds (household) NEC	T54.3X1	T54.3X2	T54.3X3	T54.3X4	—	—
fumes (any usage)	T59.891	T59.892	T59.893	T59.894	—	—
industrial	T54.3X1	T54.3X2	T54.3X3	T54.3X4	—	—
ichthyosulronate	T49.4X1	T49.4X2	T49.4X3	T49.4X4	T49.4X5	T49.4X6
mandelate	T37.91	T37.92	T37.93	T37.94	T37.95	T37.96
sulfamate	T6Ø.3X1	T6Ø.3X2	T6Ø.3X3	T6Ø.3X4	—	—
sulfonate resin	T47.8X1	T47.8X2	T47.8X3	T47.8X4	T47.8X5	T47.8X6
Amobarbital (sodium)	T42.3X1	T42.3X2	T42.3X3	T42.3X4	T42.3X5	T42.3X6
Amodiaquine	T37.2X1	T37.2X2	T37.2X3	T37.2X4	T37.2X5	T37.2X6
Amopyroquin(e)	T37.2X1	T37.2X2	T37.2X3	T37.2X4	T37.2X5	T37.2X6
Amoxapine	T43.Ø11	T43.Ø12	T43.Ø13	T43.Ø14	T43.Ø15	T43.Ø16
Amoxicillin	T36.ØX1	T36.ØX2	T36.ØX3	T36.ØX4	T36.ØX5	T36.ØX6
Amperozide	T43.591	T43.592	T43.593	T43.594	T43.595	T43.596
Amphenidone	T43.591	T43.592	T43.593	T43.594	T43.595	T43.596
Amphetamine NEC	T43.621	T43.622	T43.623	T43.624	T43.625	T43.626
Amphomycin	T36.8X1	T36.8X2	T36.8X3	T36.8X4	T36.8X5	T36.8X6
Amphotalide	T37.4X1	T37.4X2	T37.4X3	T37.4X4	T37.4X5	T37.4X6
Amphotericin B	T36.7X1	T36.7X2	T36.7X3	T36.7X4	T36.7X5	T36.7X6
topical	T49.ØX1	T49.ØX2	T49.ØX3	T49.ØX4	T49.ØX5	T49.ØX6
Ampicillin	T36.ØX1	T36.ØX2	T36.ØX3	T36.ØX4	T36.ØX5	T36.ØX6
Amprotropine	T44.3X1	T44.3X2	T44.3X3	T44.3X4	T44.3X5	T44.3X6
Amsacrine	T45.1X1	T45.1X2	T45.1X3	T45.1X4	T45.1X5	T45.1X6
Amygdaline	T62.2X1	T62.2X2	T62.2X3	T62.2X4	—	—
Amyl						
acetate	T52.8X1	T52.8X2	T52.8X3	T52.8X4	—	—
vapor	T59.891	T59.892	T59.893	T59.894	—	—
alcohol	T51.3X1	T51.3X2	T51.3X3	T51.3X4	—	—
chloride	T53.6X1	T53.6X2	T53.6X3	T53.6X4	—	—

Substance	External Cause (T-Code)					
	Poisoning, Accidental (Unintentional)	Poisoning, Intentional Self-Harm	Poisoning, Assault	Poisoning, Undetermined	Adverse Effect	Underdosing
Amyl *(Continued)*						
formate	T52.8X1	T52.8X2	T52.8X3	T52.8X4	—	—
nitrite	T46.3X1	T46.3X2	T46.3X3	T46.3X4	T46.3X5	T46.3X6
propionate	T65.891	T65.892	T65.893	T65.894	—	—
Amylase	T47.5X1	T47.5X2	T47.5X3	T47.5X4	T47.5X5	T47.5X6
Amyleine, regional	T41.3X1	T41.3X2	T41.3X3	T41.3X4	T41.3X5	T41.3X6
Amylene						
dichloride	T53.6X1	T53.6X2	T53.6X3	T53.6X4	—	—
hydrate	T51.3X1	T51.3X2	T51.3X3	T51.3X4	—	—
Amylmetacresol	T49.6X1	T49.6X2	T49.6X3	T49.6X4	T49.6X5	T49.6X6
Amylobarbitone	T42.3X1	T42.3X2	T42.3X3	T42.3X4	T42.3X5	T42.3X6
Amylocaine, regional	T41.3X1	T41.3X2	T41.3X3	T41.3X4	T41.3X5	T41.3X6
infiltration (subcutaneous)	T41.3X1	T41.3X2	T41.3X3	T41.3X4	T41.3X5	T41.3X6
nerve block (peripheral) (plexus)	T41.3X1	T41.3X2	T41.3X3	T41.3X4	T41.3X5	T41.3X6
spinal	T41.3X1	T41.3X2	T41.3X3	T41.3X4	T41.3X5	T41.3X6
topical (surface)	T41.3X1	T41.3X2	T41.3X3	T41.3X4	T41.3X5	T41.3X6
Amylopectin	T47.6X1	T47.6X2	T47.6X3	T47.6X4	T47.6X5	T47.6X6
Amytal (sodium)	T42.3X1	T42.3X2	T42.3X3	T42.3X4	T42.3X5	T42.3X6
Anabolic steroid	T38.7X1	T38.7X2	T38.7X3	T38.7X4	T38.7X5	T38.7X6
Analeptic NEC	T5Ø.7X1	T5Ø.7X2	T5Ø.7X3	T5Ø.7X4	T5Ø.7X5	T5Ø.7X6
Analgesic	T39.91	T39.92	T39.93	T39.94	T39.95	T39.96
anti-inflammatory NEC	T39.91	T39.92	T39.93	T39.94	T39.95	T39.96
propionic acid derivative	T39.311	T39.312	T39.313	T39.314	T39.315	T39.316
antirheumatic NEC	T39.4X1	T39.4X2	T39.4X3	T39.4X4	T39.4X5	T39.4X6
aromatic NEC	T39.1X1	T39.1X2	T39.1X3	T39.1X4	T39.1X5	T39.1X6
narcotic NEC	T4Ø.6Ø1	T4Ø.6Ø2	T4Ø.6Ø3	T4Ø.6Ø4	T4Ø.6Ø5	T4Ø.6Ø6
combination	T4Ø.6Ø1	T4Ø.6Ø2	T4Ø.6Ø3	T4Ø.6Ø4	T4Ø.6Ø5	T4Ø.6Ø6
obstetric	T4Ø.6Ø1	T4Ø.6Ø2	T4Ø.6Ø3	T4Ø.6Ø4	T4Ø.6Ø5	T4Ø.6Ø6
non-narcotic NEC	T39.91	T39.92	T39.93	T39.94	T39.95	T39.96
combination	T39.91	T39.92	T39.93	T39.94	T39.95	T39.96
pyrazole	T39.2X1	T39.2X2	T39.2X3	T39.2X4	T39.2X5	T39.2X6
specified NEC	T39.8X1	T39.8X2	T39.8X3	T39.8X4	T39.8X5	T39.8X6
Analgin	T39.2X1	T39.2X2	T39.2X3	T39.2X4	T39.2X5	T39.2X6
Anamirta cocculus	T62.1X1	T62.1X2	T62.1X3	T62.1X4	—	—
Ancillin	T36.ØX1	T36.ØX2	T36.ØX3	T36.ØX4	T36.ØX5	T36.ØX6
Ancrod	T45.691	T45.692	T45.693	T45.694	T45.695	T45.696
Androgen	T38.7X1	T38.7X2	T38.7X3	T38.7X4	T38.7X5	T38.7X6
Androgen-estrogen mixture	T38.7X1	T38.7X2	T38.7X3	T38.7X4	T38.7X5	T38.7X6
Androstalone	T38.7X1	T38.7X2	T38.7X3	T38.7X4	T38.7X5	T38.7X6
Androstanolone	T38.7X1	T38.7X2	T38.7X3	T38.7X4	T38.7X5	T38.7X6
Androsterone	T38.7X1	T38.7X2	T38.7X3	T38.7X4	T38.7X5	T38.7X6

Substance	External Cause (T-Code)					
	Poisoning, Accidental (Unintentional)	Poisoning, Intentional Self-Harm	Poisoning, Assault	Poisoning, Undetermined	Adverse Effect	Underdosing
Anemone pulsatilla	T62.2X1	T62.2X2	T62.2X3	T62.2X4	—	—
Anesthesia						
caudal	T41.3X1	T41.3X2	T41.3X3	T41.3X4	T41.3X5	T41.3X6
endotracheal	T41.ØX1	T41.ØX2	T41.ØX3	T41.ØX4	T41.ØX5	T41.ØX6
epidural	T41.3X1	T41.3X2	T41.3X3	T41.3X4	T41.3X5	T41.3X6
inhalation	T41.ØX1	T41.ØX2	T41.ØX3	T41.ØX4	T41.ØX5	T41.ØX6
local	T41.3X1	T41.3X2	T41.3X3	T41.3X4	T41.3X5	T41.3X6
mucosal	T41.3X1	T41.3X2	T41.3X3	T41.3X4	T41.3X5	T41.3X6
muscle relaxation	T48.1X1	T48.1X2	T48.1X3	T48.1X4	T48.1X5	T48.1X6
nerve blocking	T41.3X1	T41.3X2	T41.3X3	T41.3X4	T41.3X5	T41.3X6
plexus blocking	T41.3X1	T41.3X2	T41.3X3	T41.3X4	T41.3X5	T41.3X6
potentiated	T41.2Ø1	T41.2Ø2	T41.2Ø3	T41.2Ø4	T41.2Ø5	T41.2Ø6
rectal	T41.2Ø1	T41.2Ø2	T41.2Ø3	T41.2Ø4	T41.2Ø5	T41.2Ø6
general	T41.2Ø1	T41.2Ø2	T41.2Ø3	T41.2Ø4	T41.2Ø5	T41.2Ø6
local	T41.3X1	T41.3X2	T41.3X3	T41.3X4	T41.3X5	T41.3X6
regional	T41.3X1	T41.3X2	T41.3X3	T41.3X4	T41.3X5	T41.3X6
surface	T41.3X1	T41.3X2	T41.3X3	T41.3X4	T41.3X5	T41.3X6
Anesthetic NEC — *see also Anesthesia*	T41.41	T41.42	T41.43	T41.44	T41.45	T41.46
with muscle relaxant	T41.2Ø1	T41.2Ø2	T41.2Ø3	T41.2Ø4	T41.2Ø5	T41.2Ø6
general	T41.2Ø1	T41.2Ø2	T41.2Ø3	T41.2Ø4	T41.2Ø5	T41.2Ø6
local	T41.3X1	T41.3X2	T41.3X3	T41.3X4	T41.3X5	T41.3X6
gaseous NEC	T41.ØX1	T41.ØX2	T41.ØX3	T41.ØX4	T41.ØX5	T41.ØX6
general NEC	T41.2Ø1	T41.2Ø2	T41.2Ø3	T41.2Ø4	T41.2Ø5	T41.2Ø6
halogenated hydrocarbon derivatives NEC	T41.ØX1	T41.ØX2	T41.ØX3	T41.ØX4	T41.ØX5	T41.ØX6
infiltration NEC	T41.3X1	T41.3X2	T41.3X3	T41.3X4	T41.3X5	T41.3X6
intravenous NEC	T41.1X1	T41.1X2	T41.1X3	T41.1X4	T41.1X5	T41.1X6
local NEC	T41.3X1	T41.3X2	T41.3X3	T41.3X4	T41.3X5	T41.3X6
rectal	T41.2Ø1	T41.2Ø2	T41.2Ø3	T41.2Ø4	T41.2Ø5	T41.2Ø6
general	T41.2Ø1	T41.2Ø2	T41.2Ø3	T41.2Ø4	T41.2Ø5	T41.2Ø6
local	T41.3X1	T41.3X2	T41.3X3	T41.3X4	T41.3X5	T41.3X6
regional NEC	T41.3X1	T41.3X2	T41.3X3	T41.3X4	T41.3X5	T41.3X6
spinal NEC	T41.3X1	T41.3X2	T41.3X3	T41.3X4	T41.3X5	T41.3X6
thiobarbiturate	T41.1X1	T41.1X2	T41.1X3	T41.1X4	T41.1X5	T41.1X6
topical	T41.3X1	T41.3X2	T41.3X3	T41.3X4	T41.3X5	T41.3X6
Aneurine	T45.2X1	T45.2X2	T45.2X3	T45.2X4	T45.2X5	T45.2X6
Angio-Conray	T5Ø.8X1	T5Ø.8X2	T5Ø.8X3	T5Ø.8X4	T5Ø.8X5	T5Ø.8X6
Angiotensin	T44.5X1	T44.5X2	T44.5X3	T44.5X4	T44.5X5	T44.5X6
Angiotensinamide	T44.991	T44.992	T44.993	T44.994	T44.995	T44.996
Anhydrohydroxy-progesterone	T38.5X1	T38.5X2	T38.5X3	T38.5X4	T38.5X5	T38.5X6
Anhydron	T5Ø.2X1	T5Ø.2X2	T5Ø.2X3	T5Ø.2X4	T5Ø.2X5	T5Ø.2X6
Anileridine	T4Ø.4X1	T4Ø.4X2	T4Ø.4X3	T4Ø.4X4	T4Ø.4X5	T4Ø.4X6

Substance	Poisoning, Accidental (Unintentional)	Poisoning, Intentional Self-Harm	Poisoning, Assault	Poisoning, Undetermined	Adverse Effect	Underdosing
	External Cause (T-Code)					
Aniline (dye) (liquid)	T65.3X1	T65.3X2	T65.3X3	T65.3X4	—	—
analgesic	T39.1X1	T39.1X2	T39.1X3	T39.1X4	T39.1X5	T39.1X6
derivatives, therapeutic NEC	T39.1X1	T39.1X2	T39.1X3	T39.1X4	T39.1X5	T39.1X6
vapor	T65.3X1	T65.3X2	T65.3X3	T65.3X4	—	—
Anise oil	T47.5X1	T47.5X2	T47.5X3	T47.5X4	T47.5X5	T47.5X6
Aniscoropine	T44.3X1	T44.3X2	T44.3X3	T44.3X4	T44.3X5	T44.3X6
Anisidine	T65.3X1	T65.3X2	T65.3X3	T65.3X4	—	—
Anisindione	T45.511	T45.512	T45.513	T45.514	T45.515	T45.516
Anisotropine methyl-bromide	T44.3X1	T44.3X2	T44.3X3	T44.3X4	T44.3X5	T44.3X6
Anistreplase	T45.611	T45.612	T45.613	T45.614	T45.615	T45.616
Anorexiant (central)	T50.5X1	T50.5X2	T50.5X3	T50.5X4	T50.5X5	T50.5X6
Anorexic agents	T50.5X1	T50.5X2	T50.5X3	T50.5X4	T50.5X5	T50.5X6
Ansamycin	T36.6X1	T36.6X2	T36.6X3	T36.6X4	T36.6X5	T36.6X6
Ant (bite) (sting)	T63.421	T63.422	T63.423	T63.424	—	—
Antabuse	T50.6X1	T50.6X2	T50.6X3	T50.6X4	T50.6X5	T50.6X6
Ant poison — *see Insecticide*						
Antacid NEC	T47.1X1	T47.1X2	T47.1X3	T47.1X4	T47.1X5	T47.1X6
Antagonist						
Aldosterone	T50.0X1	T50.0X2	T50.0X3	T50.0X4	T50.0X5	T50.0X6
alpha-adrenoreceptor	T44.6X1	T44.6X2	T44.6X3	T44.6X4	T44.6X5	T44.6X6
anticoagulant	T45.7X1	T45.7X2	T45.7X3	T45.7X4	T45.7X5	T45.7X6
beta-adrenoreceptor	T44.7X1	T44.7X2	T44.7X3	T44.7X4	T44.7X5	T44.7X6
extrapyramidal NEC	T44.3X1	T44.3X2	T44.3X3	T44.3X4	T44.3X5	T44.3X6
folic acid	T45.1X1	T45.1X2	T45.1X3	T45.1X4	T45.1X5	T45.1X6
H2 receptor	T47.0X1	T47.0X2	T47.0X3	T47.0X4	T47.0X5	T47.0X6
heavy metal	T45.8X1	T45.8X2	T45.8X3	T45.8X4	T45.8X5	T45.8X6
narcotic analgesic	T50.7X1	T50.7X2	T50.7X3	T50.7X4	T50.7X5	T50.7X6
opiate	T50.7X1	T50.7X2	T50.7X3	T50.7X4	T50.7X5	T50.7X6
pyrimidine	T45.1X1	T45.1X2	T45.1X3	T45.1X4	T45.1X5	T45.1X6
serotonin	T46.5X1	T46.5X2	T46.5X3	T46.5X4	T46.5X5	T46.5X6
Antazolin(e)	T45.0X1	T45.0X2	T45.0X3	T45.0X4	T45.0X5	T45.0X6
Anterior pituitary hormone NEC	T38.811	T38.812	T38.813	T38.814	T38.815	T38.816
Anthelmintic NEC	T37.4X1	T37.4X2	T37.4X3	T37.4X4	T37.4X5	T37.4X6
Anthiolimine	T37.4X1	T37.4X2	T37.4X3	T37.4X4	T37.4X5	T37.4X6
Anthralin	T49.4X1	T49.4X2	T49.4X3	T49.4X4	T49.4X5	T49.4X6
Anthramycin	T45.1X1	T45.1X2	T45.1X3	T45.1X4	T45.1X5	T45.1X6
Antiadrenergic NEC	T44.8X1	T44.8X2	T44.8X3	T44.8X4	T44.8X5	T44.8X6
Antiallergic NEC	T45.0X1	T45.0X2	T45.0X3	T45.0X4	T45.0X5	T45.0X6
Anti-anemic (drug) (preparation)	T45.8X1	T45.8X2	T45.8X3	T45.8X4	T45.8X5	T45.8X6
Antiandrogen NEC	T38.6X1	T38.6X2	T38.6X3	T38.6X4	T38.6X5	T38.6X6
Antianxiety drug NEC	T43.501	T43.502	T43.503	T43.504	T43.505	T43.506
Antiaris toxicaria	T65.891	T65.892	T65.893	T65.894	—	—
Antiarteriosclerotic drug	T46.6X1	T46.6X2	T46.6X3	T46.6X4	T46.6X5	T46.6X6
Antiasthmatic drug NEC	T48.6X1	T48.6X2	T48.6X3	T48.6X4	T48.6X5	T48.6X6
Antibiotic NEC	T36.91	T36.92	T36.93	T36.94	T36.95	T36.96
aminoglycoside	T36.5X1	T36.5X2	T36.5X3	T36.5X4	T36.5X5	T36.5X6
anticancer	T45.1X1	T45.1X2	T45.1X3	T45.1X4	T45.1X5	T45.1X6
antifungal	T36.7X1	T36.7X2	T36.7X3	T36.7X4	T36.7X5	T36.7X6
antimycobacterial	T36.5X1	T36.5X2	T36.5X3	T36.5X4	T36.5X5	T36.5X6
antineoplastic	T45.1X1	T45.1X2	T45.1X3	T45.1X4	T45.1X5	T45.1X6
cephalosporin (group)	T36.1X1	T36.1X2	T36.1X3	T36.1X4	T36.1X5	T36.1X6
chloramphenicol (group)	T36.2X1	T36.2X2	T36.2X3	T36.2X4	T36.2X5	T36.2X6
ENT	T49.6X1	T49.6X2	T49.6X3	T49.6X4	T49.6X5	T49.6X6
eye	T49.5X1	T49.5X2	T49.5X3	T49.5X4	T49.5X5	T49.5X6
fungicidal (local)	T49.0X1	T49.0X2	T49.0X3	T49.0X4	T49.0X5	T49.0X6
intestinal	T36.8X1	T36.8X2	T36.8X3	T36.8X4	T36.8X5	T36.8X6
b-lactam NEC	T36.1X1	T36.1X2	T36.1X3	T36.1X4	T36.1X5	T36.1X6
local	T49.0X1	T49.0X2	T49.0X3	T49.0X4	T49.0X5	T49.0X6
macrolides	T36.3X1	T36.3X2	T36.3X3	T36.3X4	T36.3X5	T36.3X6
polypeptide	T36.8X1	T36.8X2	T36.8X3	T36.8X4	T36.8X5	T36.8X6
specified NEC	T36.8X1	T36.8X2	T36.8X3	T36.8X4	T36.8X5	T36.8X6
tetracycline (group)	T36.4X1	T36.4X2	T36.4X3	T36.4X4	T36.4X5	T36.4X6
throat	T49.6X1	T49.6X2	T49.6X3	T49.6X4	T49.6X5	T49.6X6
Anticancer agents NEC	T45.1X1	T45.1X2	T45.1X3	T45.1X4	T45.1X5	T45.1X6
Anticholesterolemic drug NEC	T46.6X1	T46.6X2	T46.6X3	T46.6X4	T46.6X5	T46.6X6
Anticholinergic NEC	T44.3X1	T44.3X2	T44.3X3	T44.3X4	T44.3X5	T44.3X6
Anticholinesterase	T44.0X1	T44.0X2	T44.0X3	T44.0X4	T44.0X5	T44.0X6
organophosphorus	T44.0X1	T44.0X2	T44.0X3	T44.0X4	T44.0X5	T44.0X6
insecticide	T60.0X1	T60.0X2	T60.0X3	T60.0X4	—	—
nerve gas	T59.891	T59.892	T59.893	T59.894	—	—
reversible	T44.0X1	T44.0X2	T44.0X3	T44.0X4	T44.0X5	T44.0X6
ophthalmological	T49.5X1	T49.5X2	T49.5X3	T49.5X4	T49.5X5	T49.5X6
Anticoagulant NEC	T45.511	T45.512	T45.513	T45.514	T45.515	T45.516
Antagonist	T45.7X1	T45.7X2	T45.7X3	T45.7X4	T45.7X5	T45.7X6
Anti-common-cold drug NEC	T48.5X1	T48.5X2	T48.5X3	T48.5X4	T48.5X5	T48.5X6
Anticonvulsant	T42.71	T42.72	T42.73	T42.74	T42.75	T42.76
barbiturate	T42.3X1	T42.3X2	T42.3X3	T42.3X4	T42.3X5	T42.3X6
combination (with barbiturate)	T42.3X1	T42.3X2	T42.3X3	T42.3X4	T42.3X5	T42.3X6
hydantoin	T42.0X1	T42.0X2	T42.0X3	T42.0X4	T42.0X5	T42.0X6
hypnotic NEC	T42.6X1	T42.6X2	T42.6X3	T42.6X4	T42.6X5	T42.6X6
oxazolidinedione	T42.2X1	T42.2X2	T42.2X3	T42.2X4	T42.2X5	T42.2X6
pyrimidinedione	T42.6X1	T42.6X2	T42.6X3	T42.6X4	T42.6X5	T42.6X6
specified NEC	T42.6X1	T42.6X2	T42.6X3	T42.6X4	T42.6X5	T42.6X6
succinimide	T42.2X1	T42.2X2	T42.2X3	T42.2X4	T42.2X5	T42.2X6

		External Cause (T-Code)				
Substance	Poisoning, Accidental (Unintentional)	Poisoning, Intentional Self-Harm	Poisoning, Assault	Poisoning, Undetermined	Adverse Effect	Underdosing
Anti-D immunoglobulin (human)	T50.Z11	T50.Z12	T50.Z13	T50.Z14	T50.Z15	T50.Z16
Antidepressant NEC	T43.201	T43.202	T43.203	T43.204	T43.205	T43.206
monoamine oxidase inhibitor	T43.1X1	T43.1X2	T43.1X3	T43.1X4	T43.1X5	T43.1X6
selective serotonin norepinephrine reuptake inhibitor	T43.211	T43.212	T43.213	T43.214	T43.215	T43.216
selective serotonin reuptake inhibitor	T43.221	T43.222	T43.223	T43.224	T43.225	T43.226
specified NEC	T43.291	T43.292	T43.293	T43.294	T43.295	T43.296
tetracyclic	T43.021	T43.022	T43.023	T43.024	T43.025	T43.026
triazolopyridine	T43.221	T43.222	T43.223	T43.224	T43.225	T43.226
tricyclic	T43.011	T43.012	T43.013	T43.014	T43.015	T43.016
Antidiabetic NEC	T38.3X1	T38.3X2	T38.3X3	T38.3X4	T38.3X5	T38.3X6
biguanide	T38.3X1	T38.3X2	T38.3X3	T38.3X4	T38.3X5	T38.3X6
and sulfonyl combined	T38.3X1	T38.3X2	T38.3X3	T38.3X4	T38.3X5	T38.3X6
combined	T38.3X1	T38.3X2	T38.3X3	T38.3X4	T38.3X5	T38.3X6
sulfonylurea	T38.3X1	T38.3X2	T38.3X3	T38.3X4	T38.3X5	T38.3X6
Antidiarrheal drug NEC	T47.6X1	T47.6X2	T47.6X3	T47.6X4	T47.6X5	T47.6X6
absorbent	T47.6X1	T47.6X2	T47.6X3	T47.6X4	T47.6X5	T47.6X6
Antidiphtheria serum	T50.Z11	T50.Z12	T50.Z13	T50.Z14	T50.Z15	T50.Z16
Antidiuretic hormone	T38.891	T38.892	T38.893	T38.894	T38.895	T38.896
Antidote NEC	T50.6X1	T50.6X2	T50.6X3	T50.6X4	T50.6X5	T50.6X6
heavy metal	T45.8X1	T45.8X2	T45.8X3	T45.8X4	T45.8X5	T45.8X6
Antidysrhythmic NEC	T46.2X1	T46.2X2	T46.2X3	T46.2X4	T46.2X5	T46.2X6
Antiemetic drug	T45.0X1	T45.0X2	T45.0X3	T45.0X4	T45.0X5	T45.0X6
Antiepilepsy agent	T42.71	T42.72	T42.73	T42.74	T42.75	T42.76
combination	T42.5X1	T42.5X2	T42.5X3	T42.5X4	T42.5X5	T42.5X6
mixed	T42.5X1	T42.5X2	T42.5X3	T42.5X4	T42.5X5	T42.5X6
specified, NEC	T42.6X1	T42.6X2	T42.6X3	T42.6X4	T42.6X5	T42.6X6
Antiestrogen NEC	T38.6X1	T38.6X2	T38.6X3	T38.6X4	T38.6X5	T38.6X6
Antifertility pill	T38.4X1	T38.4X2	T38.4X3	T38.4X4	T38.4X5	T38.4X6
Antifibrinolytic drug	T45.621	T45.622	T45.623	T45.624	T45.625	T45.626
Antifilarial drug	T37.4X1	T37.4X2	T37.4X3	T37.4X4	T37.4X5	T37.4X6
Antiflatulent	T47.5X1	T47.5X2	T47.5X3	T47.5X4	T47.5X5	T47.5X6
Antifreeze	T65.91	T65.92	T65.93	T65.94	—	—
alcohol	T51.1X1	T51.1X2	T51.1X3	T51.1X4	—	—
ethylene glycol	T51.8X1	T51.8X2	T51.8X3	T51.8X4	—	—
Antifungal						
antibiotic (systemic)	T36.7X1	T36.7X2	T36.7X3	T36.7X4	T36.7X5	T36.7X6
anti-infective NEC	T37.91	T37.92	T37.93	T37.94	T37.95	T37.96
disinfectant, local	T49.0X1	T49.0X2	T49.0X3	T49.0X4	T49.0X5	T49.0X6
nonmedicinal (spray)	T60.3X1	T60.3X2	T60.3X3	T60.3X4	—	—
topical	T49.0X1	T49.0X2	T49.0X3	T49.0X4	T49.0X5	T49.0X6

		External Cause (T-Code)				
Substance	Poisoning, Accidental (Unintentional)	Poisoning, Intentional Self-Harm	Poisoning, Assault	Poisoning, Undetermined	Adverse Effect	Underdosing
Anti-gastric-secretion drug NEC	T47.1X1	T47.1X2	T47.1X3	T47.1X4	T47.1X5	T47.1X6
Antigonadotrophin NEC	T38.6X1	T38.6X2	T38.6X3	T38.6X4	T38.6X5	T38.6X6
Antihallucinogen	T43.501	T43.502	T43.503	T43.504	T43.505	T43.506
Antihelmintics	T37.4X1	T37.4X2	T37.4X3	T37.4X4	T37.4X5	T37.4X6
Antihemophilic						
factor	T45.8X1	T45.8X2	T45.8X3	T45.8X4	T45.8X5	T45.8X6
fraction	T45.8X1	T45.8X2	T45.8X3	T45.8X4	T45.8X5	T45.8X6
globulin concentrate	T45.7X1	T45.7X2	T45.7X3	T45.7X4	T45.7X5	T45.7X6
human plasma	T45.8X1	T45.8X2	T45.8X3	T45.8X4	T45.8X5	T45.8X6
plasma, dried	T45.7X1	T45.7X2	T45.7X3	T45.7X4	T45.7X5	T45.7X6
Antihemorrhoidal preparation	T49.2X1	T49.2X2	T49.2X3	T49.2X4	T49.2X5	T49.2X6
Antiheparin drug	T45.7X1	T45.7X2	T45.7X3	T45.7X4	T45.7X5	T45.7X6
Antihistamine	T45.0X1	T45.0X2	T45.0X3	T45.0X4	T45.0X5	T45.0X6
Antihookworm drug	T37.4X1	T37.4X2	T37.4X3	T37.4X4	T37.4X5	T37.4X6
Anti-human lymphocytic globulin	T50.Z11	T50.Z12	T50.Z13	T50.Z14	T50.Z15	T50.Z16
Antihyperlipidemic drug	T46.6X1	T46.6X2	T46.6X3	T46.6X4	T46.6X5	T46.6X6
Antihypertensive drug NEC	T46.5X1	T46.5X2	T46.5X3	T46.5X4	T46.5X5	T46.5X6
Anti-infective NEC	T37.91	T37.92	T37.93	T37.94	T37.95	T37.96
anthelmintic	T37.4X1	T37.4X2	T37.4X3	T37.4X4	T37.4X5	T37.4X6
antibiotics	T36.91	T36.92	T36.93	T36.94	T36.95	T36.96
specified NEC	T36.8X1	T36.8X2	T36.8X3	T36.8X4	T36.8X5	T36.8X6
antimalarial	T37.2X1	T37.2X2	T37.2X3	T37.2X4	T37.2X5	T37.2X6
antimycobacterial NEC	T37.1X1	T37.1X2	T37.1X3	T37.1X4	T37.1X5	T37.1X6
antibiotics	T36.5X1	T36.5X2	T36.5X3	T36.5X4	T36.5X5	T36.5X6
antiprotozoal NEC	T37.3X1	T37.3X2	T37.3X3	T37.3X4	T37.3X5	T37.3X6
blood	T37.2X1	T37.2X2	T37.2X3	T37.2X4	T37.2X5	T37.2X6
antiviral	T37.5X1	T37.5X2	T37.5X3	T37.5X4	T37.5X5	T37.5X6
arsenical	T37.8X1	T37.8X2	T37.8X3	T37.8X4	T37.8X5	T37.8X6
bismuth, local	T49.0X1	T49.0X2	T49.0X3	T49.0X4	T49.0X5	T49.0X6
ENT	T49.6X1	T49.6X2	T49.6X3	T49.6X4	T49.6X5	T49.6X6
eye NEC	T49.5X1	T49.5X2	T49.5X3	T49.5X4	T49.5X5	T49.5X6
heavy metals NEC	T37.8X1	T37.8X2	T37.8X3	T37.8X4	T37.8X5	T37.8X6
local NEC	T49.0X1	T49.0X2	T49.0X3	T49.0X4	T49.0X5	T49.0X6
specified NEC	T49.0X1	T49.0X2	T49.0X3	T49.0X4	T49.0X5	T49.0X6
mixed	T37.91	T37.92	T37.93	T37.94	T37.95	T37.96
ophthalmic preparation	T49.5X1	T49.5X2	T49.5X3	T49.5X4	T49.5X5	T49.5X6
topical NEC	T49.0X1	T49.0X2	T49.0X3	T49.0X4	T49.0X5	T49.0X6
Anti-inflammatory drug NEC	T49.0X1	T49.0X2	T49.0X3	T49.0X4	T49.0X5	T49.0X6
local	T49.0X1	T49.0X2	T49.0X3	T49.0X4	T49.0X5	T49.0X6
nonsteroidal NEC	T39.391	T39.392	T39.393	T39.394	T39.395	T39.396
propionic acid derivative	T39.311	T39.312	T39.313	T39.314	T39.315	T39.316
specified NEC	T39.391	T39.392	T39.393	T39.394	T39.395	T39.396

Substance	External Cause (T-Code) Poisoning, Accidental (Unintentional)	Poisoning, Intentional Self-Harm	Poisoning, Assault	Poisoning, Undetermined	Adverse Effect	Underdosing
Antikaluretic	T5Ø.3X1	T5Ø.3X2	T5Ø.3X3	T5Ø.3X4	T5Ø.3X5	T5Ø.3X6
Antiknock (tetraethyl lead)	T56.ØX1	T56.ØX2	T56.ØX3	T56.ØX4	—	—
Antilipemic drug NEC	T46.6X1	T46.6X2	T46.6X3	T46.6X4	T46.6X5	T46.6X6
Antimalarial	T37.2X1	T37.2X2	T37.2X3	T37.2X4	T37.2X5	T37.2X6
prophylactic NEC	T37.2X1	T37.2X2	T37.2X3	T37.2X4	T37.2X5	T37.2X6
pyrimidine derivative	T37.2X1	T37.2X2	T37.2X3	T37.2X4	T37.2X5	T37.2X6
Antimetabolite	T45.1X1	T45.1X2	T45.1X3	T45.1X4	T45.1X5	T45.1X6
Antimitotic agent	T45.1X1	T45.1X2	T45.1X3	T45.1X4	T45.1X5	T45.1X6
Antimony (compounds) (vapor) NEC	T56.891	T56.892	T56.893	T56.894	—	—
anti-infectives	T37.8X1	T37.8X2	T37.8X3	T37.8X4	T37.8X5	T37.8X6
dimercaptosuccinate	T37.3X1	T37.3X2	T37.3X3	T37.3X4	T37.3X5	T37.3X6
hydride	T56.891	T56.892	T56.893	T56.894	—	—
pesticide (vapor)	T6Ø.8X1	T6Ø.8X2	T6Ø.8X3	T6Ø.8X4	—	—
potassium (sodium) tartrate	T37.8X1	T37.8X2	T37.8X3	T37.8X4	T37.8X5	T37.8X6
sodium dimercaptosuccinate	T37.3X1	T37.3X2	T37.3X3	T37.3X4	T37.3X5	T37.3X6
tartrated	T37.8X1	T37.8X2	T37.8X3	T37.8X4	T37.8X5	T37.8X6
Antimuscarinic NEC	T44.3X1	T44.3X2	T44.3X3	T44.3X4	T44.3X5	T44.3X6
Antimycobacterial drug NEC	T37.1X1	T37.1X2	T37.1X3	T37.1X4	T37.1X5	T37.1X6
antibiotics	T36.5X1	T36.5X2	T36.5X3	T36.5X4	T36.5X5	T36.5X6
combination	T37.1X1	T37.1X2	T37.1X3	T37.1X4	T37.1X5	T37.1X6
Antinausea drug	T45.ØX1	T45.ØX2	T45.ØX3	T45.ØX4	T45.ØX5	T45.ØX6
Antinematode drug	T37.4X1	T37.4X2	T37.4X3	T37.4X4	T37.4X5	T37.4X6
Antineoplastic NEC	T45.1X1	T45.1X2	T45.1X3	T45.1X4	T45.1X5	T45.1X6
alkaloidal	T45.1X1	T45.1X2	T45.1X3	T45.1X4	T45.1X5	T45.1X6
antibiotics	T45.1X1	T45.1X2	T45.1X3	T45.1X4	T45.1X5	T45.1X6
combination	T45.1X1	T45.1X2	T45.1X3	T45.1X4	T45.1X5	T45.1X6
estrogen	T38.5X1	T38.5X2	T38.5X3	T38.5X4	T38.5X5	T38.5X6
steroid	T38.7X1	T38.7X2	T38.7X3	T38.7X4	T38.7X5	T38.7X6
Antiparasitic drug (systemic)	T37.91	T37.92	T37.93	T37.94	T37.95	T37.96
local	T49.ØX1	T49.ØX2	T49.ØX3	T49.ØX4	T49.ØX5	T49.ØX6
specified NEC	T37.8X1	T37.8X2	T37.8X3	T37.8X4	T37.8X5	T37.8X6
Antiparkinsonism drug NEC	T42.8X1	T42.8X2	T42.8X3	T42.8X4	T42.8X5	T42.8X6
Antiperspirant NEC	T49.2X1	T49.2X2	T49.2X3	T49.2X4	T49.2X5	T49.2X6
Antiphlogistic NEC	T39.4X1	T39.4X2	T39.4X3	T39.4X4	T39.4X5	T39.4X6
Antiplatyhelmintic drug	T37.4X1	T37.4X2	T37.4X3	T37.4X4	T37.4X5	T37.4X6
Antiprotozoal drug NEC	T37.3X1	T37.3X2	T37.3X3	T37.3X4	T37.3X5	T37.3X6
blood	T37.2X1	T37.2X2	T37.2X3	T37.2X4	T37.2X5	T37.2X6
local	T49.ØX1	T49.ØX2	T49.ØX3	T49.ØX4	T49.ØX5	T49.ØX6
Antipruritic drug NEC	T49.1X1	T49.1X2	T49.1X3	T49.1X4	T49.1X5	T49.1X6
Antipsychotic drug	T43.5Ø1	T43.5Ø2	T43.5Ø3	T43.5Ø4	T43.5Ø5	T43.5Ø6
specified NEC	T43.591	T43.592	T43.593	T43.594	T43.595	T43.596

Substance	External Cause (T-Code) Poisoning, Accidental (Unintentional)	Poisoning, Intentional Self-Harm	Poisoning, Assault	Poisoning, Undetermined	Adverse Effect	Underdosing
Antipyretic	T39.91	T39.92	T39.93	T39.94	T39.95	T39.96
specified NEC	T39.8X1	T39.8X2	T39.8X3	T39.8X4	T39.8X5	T39.8X6
Antipyrine	T39.2X1	T39.2X2	T39.2X3	T39.2X4	T39.2X5	T39.2X6
Antirabies hyperimmune serum	T5Ø.Z11	T5Ø.Z12	T5Ø.Z13	T5Ø.Z14	T5Ø.Z15	T5Ø.Z16
Antirheumatic NEC	T39.4X1	T39.4X2	T39.4X3	T39.4X4	T39.4X5	T39.4X6
Antirigidity drug NEC	T42.8X1	T42.8X2	T42.8X3	T42.8X4	T42.8X5	T42.8X6
Antischistosomal drug	T37.4X1	T37.4X2	T37.4X3	T37.4X4	T37.4X5	T37.4X6
Antiscorpion sera	T5Ø.Z11	T5Ø.Z12	T5Ø.Z13	T5Ø.Z14	T5Ø.Z15	T5Ø.Z16
Antiseborrheics	T49.4X1	T49.4X2	T49.4X3	T49.4X4	T49.4X5	T49.4X6
Antiseptics (external) (medicinal)	T49.ØX1	T49.ØX2	T49.ØX3	T49.ØX4	T49.ØX5	T49.ØX6
Antistine	T45.ØX1	T45.ØX2	T45.ØX3	T45.ØX4	T45.ØX5	T45.ØX6
Antitapeworm drug	T37.4X1	T37.4X2	T37.4X3	T37.4X4	T37.4X5	T37.4X6
Antitetanus immunoglobulin	T5Ø.Z11	T5Ø.Z12	T5Ø.Z13	T5Ø.Z14	T5Ø.Z15	T5Ø.Z16
Antithrombotic	T45.521	T45.522	T45.523	T45.524	T45.525	T45.526
Antithyroid drug NEC	T38.2X1	T38.2X2	T38.2X3	T38.2X4	T38.2X5	T38.2X6
Antitoxin	T5Ø.Z11	T5Ø.Z12	T5Ø.Z13	T5Ø.Z14	T5Ø.Z15	T5Ø.Z16
diphtheria	T5Ø.Z11	T5Ø.Z12	T5Ø.Z13	T5Ø.Z14	T5Ø.Z15	T5Ø.Z16
gas gangrene	T5Ø.Z11	T5Ø.Z12	T5Ø.Z13	T5Ø.Z14	T5Ø.Z15	T5Ø.Z16
tetanus	T5Ø.Z11	T5Ø.Z12	T5Ø.Z13	T5Ø.Z14	T5Ø.Z15	T5Ø.Z16
Antitoxin, any	T5Ø.9Ø1	T5Ø.9Ø2	T5Ø.9Ø3	T5Ø.9Ø4	T5Ø.9Ø5	T5Ø.9Ø6
Antitrichomonal drug	T37.3X1	T37.3X2	T37.3X3	T37.3X4	T37.3X5	T37.3X6
Antituberculars	T37.1X1	T37.1X2	T37.1X3	T37.1X4	T37.1X5	T37.1X6
antibiotics	T36.5X1	T36.5X2	T36.5X3	T36.5X4	T36.5X5	T36.5X6
Antitussive NEC	T48.3X1	T48.3X2	T48.3X3	T48.3X4	T48.3X5	T48.3X6
codeine mixture	T4Ø.2X1	T4Ø.2X2	T4Ø.2X3	T4Ø.2X4	T4Ø.2X5	T4Ø.2X6
opiate	T4Ø.2X1	T4Ø.2X2	T4Ø.2X3	T4Ø.2X4	T4Ø.2X5	T4Ø.2X6
Antivaricose drug	T46.8X1	T46.8X2	T46.8X3	T46.8X4	T46.8X5	T46.8X6
Antivenin, antivenom (sera)	T5Ø.Z11	T5Ø.Z12	T5Ø.Z13	T5Ø.Z14	T5Ø.Z15	T5Ø.Z16
crotaline	T5Ø.Z11	T5Ø.Z12	T5Ø.Z13	T5Ø.Z14	T5Ø.Z15	T5Ø.Z16
spider bite	T5Ø.Z11	T5Ø.Z12	T5Ø.Z13	T5Ø.Z14	T5Ø.Z15	T5Ø.Z16
Antivertigo drug	T45.ØX1	T45.ØX2	T45.ØX3	T45.ØX4	T45.ØX5	T45.ØX6
Antiviral drug NEC	T37.5X1	T37.5X2	T37.5X3	T37.5X4	T37.5X5	T37.5X6
eye	T49.5X1	T49.5X2	T49.5X3	T49.5X4	T49.5X5	T49.5X6
Antiwhipworm drug	T37.4X1	T37.4X2	T37.4X3	T37.4X4	T37.4X5	T37.4X6
Ant poisons — *see Pesticides*						
Antrol — *see also by specific chemical substance*	T6Ø.91	T6Ø.92	T6Ø.93	T6Ø.94	—	—
fungicide	T6Ø.91	T6Ø.92	T6Ø.93	T6Ø.94	—	—
ANTU (alpha naphthylthiourea)	T6Ø.4X1	T6Ø.4X2	T6Ø.4X3	T6Ø.4X4	—	—
Apalcillin	T36.ØX1	T36.ØX2	T36.ØX3	T36.ØX4	T36.ØX5	T36.ØX6
APC	T48.5X1	T48.5X2	T48.5X3	T48.5X4	T48.5X5	T48.5X6
Aplonidine	T44.4X1	T44.4X2	T44.4X3	T44.4X4	T44.4X5	T44.4X6
Apomorphine	T47.7X1	T47.7X2	T47.7X3	T47.7X4	T47.7X5	T47.7X6

Substance	External Cause (T-Code): Poisoning, Accidental (Unintentional)	Poisoning, Intentional Self-Harm	Poisoning, Assault	Poisoning, Undetermined	Adverse Effect	Underdosing
Appetite depressants, central	T5Ø.5X1	T5Ø.5X2	T5Ø.5X3	T5Ø.5X4	T5Ø.5X5	T5Ø.5X6
Apraclonidine (hydrochloride)	T44.4X1	T44.4X2	T44.4X3	T44.4X4	T44.4X5	T44.4X6
Apresoline	T46.5X1	T46.5X2	T46.5X3	T46.5X4	T46.5X5	T46.5X6
Aprindine	T46.2X1	T46.2X2	T46.2X3	T46.2X4	T46.2X5	T46.2X6
Aprobarbital	T42.3X1	T42.3X2	T42.3X3	T42.3X4	T42.3X5	T42.3X6
Apronalide	T42.6X1	T42.6X2	T42.6X3	T42.6X4	T42.6X5	T42.6X6
Aprotinin	T45.621	T45.622	T45.623	T45.624	T45.625	T45.626
Aptocaine	T41.3X1	T41.3X2	T41.3X3	T41.3X4	T41.3X5	T41.3X6
Aqua fortis	T54.2X1	T54.2X2	T54.2X3	T54.2X4	—	—
Ara-A	T37.5X1	T37.5X2	T37.5X3	T37.5X4	T37.5X5	T37.5X6
Ara-C	T45.1X1	T45.1X2	T45.1X3	T45.1X4	T45.1X5	T45.1X6
Arachis oil	T49.3X1	T49.3X2	T49.3X3	T49.3X4	T49.3X5	T49.3X6
cathartic	T47.4X1	T47.4X2	T47.4X3	T47.4X4	T47.4X5	T47.4X6
Aralen	T37.2X1	T37.2X2	T37.2X3	T37.2X4	T37.2X5	T37.2X6
Arecoline	T44.1X1	T44.1X2	T44.1X3	T44.1X4	T44.1X5	T44.1X6
Arginine	T5Ø.991	T5Ø.992	T5Ø.993	T5Ø.994	T5Ø.995	T5Ø.996
glutamate	T5Ø.991	T5Ø.992	T5Ø.993	T5Ø.994	T5Ø.995	T5Ø.996
Argyrol	T49.ØX1	T49.ØX2	T49.ØX3	T49.ØX4	T49.ØX5	T49.ØX6
ENT agent	T49.6X1	T49.6X2	T49.6X3	T49.6X4	T49.6X5	T49.6X6
ophthalmic preparation	T49.5X1	T49.5X2	T49.5X3	T49.5X4	T49.5X5	T49.5X6
Aristocort	T38.ØX1	T38.ØX2	T38.ØX3	T38.ØX4	T38.ØX5	T38.ØX6
ENT agent	T49.6X1	T49.6X2	T49.6X3	T49.6X4	T49.6X5	T49.6X6
ophthalmic preparation	T49.5X1	T49.5X2	T49.5X3	T49.5X4	T49.5X5	T49.5X6
topical NEC	T49.ØX1	T49.ØX2	T49.ØX3	T49.ØX4	T49.ØX5	T49.ØX6
Aromatics, corrosive	T54.1X1	T54.1X2	T54.1X3	T54.1X4	—	—
disinfectants	T54.1X1	T54.1X2	T54.1X3	T54.1X4	—	—
Arsenate of lead	T57.ØX1	T57.ØX2	T57.ØX3	T57.ØX4	—	—
herbicide	T57.ØX1	T57.ØX2	T57.ØX3	T57.ØX4	—	—
Arsenic, arsenicals (compounds) (dust) (vapor) NEC	T57.ØX1	T57.ØX2	T57.ØX3	T57.ØX4	—	—
anti-infectives	T37.8X1	T37.8X2	T37.8X3	T37.8X4	T37.8X5	T37.8X6
pesticide (dust) (fumes)	T57.ØX1	T57.ØX2	T57.ØX3	T57.ØX4	—	—
Arsine (gas)	T57.ØX1	T57.ØX2	T57.ØX3	T57.ØX4	—	—
Arsphenamine (silver)	T37.8X1	T37.8X2	T37.8X3	T37.8X4	T37.8X5	T37.8X6
Arsthinol	T37.3X1	T37.3X2	T37.3X3	T37.3X4	T37.3X5	T37.3X6
Artane	T44.3X1	T44.3X2	T44.3X3	T44.3X4	T44.3X5	T44.3X6
Arthropod (venomous) NEC	T63.481	T63.482	T63.483	T63.484	—	—
Articaine	T41.3X1	T41.3X2	T41.3X3	T41.3X4	T41.3X5	T41.3X6
Asbestos	T57.8X1	T57.8X2	T57.8X3	T57.8X4	—	—
Ascaridole	T37.4X1	T37.4X2	T37.4X3	T37.4X4	T37.4X5	T37.4X6
Ascorbic acid	T45.2X1	T45.2X2	T45.2X3	T45.2X4	T45.2X5	T45.2X6
Asiaticoside	T49.ØX1	T49.ØX2	T49.ØX3	T49.ØX4	T49.ØX5	T49.ØX6

Substance	External Cause (T-Code): Poisoning, Accidental (Unintentional)	Poisoning, Intentional Self-Harm	Poisoning, Assault	Poisoning, Undetermined	Adverse Effect	Underdosing
Asparaginase	T45.1X1	T45.1X2	T45.1X3	T45.1X4	T45.1X5	T45.1X6
Aspidium (oleoresin)	T37.4X1	T37.4X2	T37.4X3	T37.4X4	T37.4X5	T37.4X6
Aspirin (aluminum) (soluble)	T39.Ø11	T39.Ø12	T39.Ø13	T39.Ø14	T39.Ø15	T39.Ø16
Aspoxicillin	T36.ØX1	T36.ØX2	T36.ØX3	T36.ØX4	T36.ØX5	T36.ØX6
Astemizole	T45.ØX1	T45.ØX2	T45.ØX3	T45.ØX4	T45.ØX5	T45.ØX6
Astringent (local)	T49.2X1	T49.2X2	T49.2X3	T49.2X4	T49.2X5	T49.2X6
specified NEC	T49.2X1	T49.2X2	T49.2X3	T49.2X4	T49.2X5	T49.2X6
Astromicin	T36.5X1	T36.5X2	T36.5X3	T36.5X4	T36.5X5	T36.5X6
Ataractic drug NEC	T43.5Ø1	T43.5Ø2	T43.5Ø3	T43.5Ø4	T43.5Ø5	T43.5Ø6
Atenolol	T44.7X1	T44.7X2	T44.7X3	T44.7X4	T44.7X5	T44.7X6
Atonia drug, intestinal	T47.4X1	T47.4X2	T47.4X3	T47.4X4	T47.4X5	T47.4X6
Atophan	T5Ø.4X1	T5Ø.4X2	T5Ø.4X3	T5Ø.4X4	T5Ø.4X5	T5Ø.4X6
Atracurium besilate	T48.1X1	T48.1X2	T48.1X3	T48.1X4	T48.1X5	T48.1X6
Atropine	T44.3X1	T44.3X2	T44.3X3	T44.3X4	T44.3X5	T44.3X6
derivative	T44.3X1	T44.3X2	T44.3X3	T44.3X4	T44.3X5	T44.3X6
methonitrate	T44.3X1	T44.3X2	T44.3X3	T44.3X4	T44.3X5	T44.3X6
Attapulgite	T47.6X1	T47.6X2	T47.6X3	T47.6X4	T47.6X5	T47.6X6
Attenuvax	T5Ø.991	T5Ø.992	T5Ø.993	T5Ø.994	T5Ø.995	T5Ø.996
Auramine	T65.891	T65.892	T65.893	T65.894	—	—
dye	T65.6X1	T65.6X2	T65.6X3	T65.6X4	—	—
fungicide	T6Ø.3X1	T6Ø.3X2	T6Ø.3X3	T6Ø.3X4	—	—
Auranofin	T39.4X1	T39.4X2	T39.4X3	T39.4X4	T39.4X5	T39.4X6
Aurantiin	T46.991	T46.992	T46.993	T46.994	T46.995	T46.996
Aureomycin	T36.4X1	T36.4X2	T36.4X3	T36.4X4	T36.4X5	T36.4X6
ophthalmic preparation	T49.5X1	T49.5X2	T49.5X3	T49.5X4	T49.5X5	T49.5X6
topical NEC	T49.ØX1	T49.ØX2	T49.ØX3	T49.ØX4	T49.ØX5	T49.ØX6
Aurothioglucose	T39.4X1	T39.4X2	T39.4X3	T39.4X4	T39.4X5	T39.4X6
Aurothioglycanide	T39.4X1	T39.4X2	T39.4X3	T39.4X4	T39.4X5	T39.4X6
Aurothiomalate sodium	T39.4X1	T39.4X2	T39.4X3	T39.4X4	T39.4X5	T39.4X6
Aurotioprol	T39.4X1	T39.4X2	T39.4X3	T39.4X4	T39.4X5	T39.4X6
Automobile fuel	T52.ØX1	T52.ØX2	T52.ØX3	T52.ØX4	—	—
Autonomic nervous system agent NEC	T44.9Ø1	T44.9Ø2	T44.9Ø3	T44.9Ø4	T44.9Ø5	T44.9Ø6
Avlosulfon	T37.1X1	T37.1X2	T37.1X3	T37.1X4	T37.1X5	T37.1X6
Avomine	T42.6X1	T42.6X2	T42.6X3	T42.6X4	T42.6X5	T42.6X6
Axerophthol	T45.2X1	T45.2X2	T45.2X3	T45.2X4	T45.2X5	T45.2X6
Azacitidine	T45.1X1	T45.1X2	T45.1X3	T45.1X4	T45.1X5	T45.1X6
Azacyclonol	T43.591	T43.592	T43.593	T43.594	T43.595	T43.596
Azadirachta	T6Ø.2X1	T6Ø.2X2	T6Ø.2X3	T6Ø.2X4	—	—
Azanidazole	T37.3X1	T37.3X2	T37.3X3	T37.3X4	T37.3X5	T37.3X6
Azapetine	T46.7X1	T46.7X2	T46.7X3	T46.7X4	T46.7X5	T46.7X6
Azapropazone	T39.2X1	T39.2X2	T39.2X3	T39.2X4	T39.2X5	T39.2X6

◀ New   Revised   ~~deleted~~ Deleted

Substance	External Cause (T-Code)					
	Poisoning, Accidental (Unintentional)	Poisoning, Intentional Self-Harm	Poisoning, Assault	Poisoning, Undetermined	Adverse Effect	Underdosing
Azaribine	T45.1X1	T45.1X2	T45.1X3	T45.1X4	T45.1X5	T45.1X6
Azaserine	T45.1X1	T45.1X2	T45.1X3	T45.1X4	T45.1X5	T45.1X6
Azatadine	T45.ØX1	T45.ØX2	T45.ØX3	T45.ØX4	T45.ØX5	T45.ØX6
Azatepa	T45.1X1	T45.1X2	T45.1X3	T45.1X4	T45.1X5	T45.1X6
Azathioprine	T45.1X1	T45.1X2	T45.1X3	T45.1X4	T45.1X5	T45.1X6
Azelaic acid	T49.ØX1	T49.ØX2	T49.ØX3	T49.ØX4	T49.ØX5	T49.ØX6
Azelastine	T45.ØX1	T45.ØX2	T45.ØX3	T45.ØX4	T45.ØX5	T45.ØX6
Azidocillin	T36.ØX1	T36.ØX2	T36.ØX3	T36.ØX4	T36.ØX5	T36.ØX6
Azidothymidine	T37.5X1	T37.5X2	T37.5X3	T37.5X4	T37.5X5	T37.5X6
Azinphos (ethyl) (methyl)	T6Ø.ØX1	T6Ø.ØX2	T6Ø.ØX3	T6Ø.ØX4	—	—
Aziridine (chelating)	T54.1X1	T54.1X2	T54.1X3	T54.1X4	—	—
Azithromycin	T36.3X1	T36.3X2	T36.3X3	T36.3X4	T36.3X5	T36.3X6
Azlocillin	T36.Ø1	T36.Ø2	T36.Ø3	T36.Ø4	T36.Ø5	T36.Ø6
Azobenzene smoke	T65.3X1	T65.3X2	T65.3X3	T65.3X4	—	—
acaricide	T6Ø.8X1	T6Ø.8X2	T6Ø.8X3	T6Ø.8X4	—	—
Azosulfamide	T37.ØX1	T37.ØX2	T37.ØX3	T37.ØX4	T37.ØX5	T37.ØX6
AZT	T37.5X1	T37.5X2	T37.5X3	T37.5X4	T37.5X5	T37.5X6
Aztreonam	T36.1X1	T36.1X2	T36.1X3	T36.1X4	T36.1X5	T36.1X6
Azulfidine	T37.ØX1	T37.ØX2	T37.ØX3	T37.ØX4	T37.ØX5	T37.ØX6
Azuresin	T5Ø.8X1	T5Ø.8X2	T5Ø.8X3	T5Ø.8X4	T5Ø.8X5	T5Ø.8X6
B						
Bacampicillin	T36.ØX1	T36.ØX2	T36.ØX3	T36.ØX4	T36.ØX5	T36.ØX6
Bacillus						
lactobacillus	T47.8X1	T47.8X2	T47.8X3	T47.8X4	T47.8X5	T47.8X6
subtilis	T47.6X1	T47.6X2	T47.6X3	T47.6X4	T47.6X5	T47.6X6
Bacimycin	T49.ØX1	T49.ØX2	T49.ØX3	T49.ØX4	T49.ØX5	T49.ØX6
ophthalmic preparation	T49.5X1	T49.5X2	T49.5X3	T49.5X4	T49.5X5	T49.5X6
Bacitracin zinc	T49.ØX1	T49.ØX2	T49.ØX3	T49.ØX4	T49.ØX5	T49.ØX6
with neomycin	T49.ØX1	T49.ØX2	T49.ØX3	T49.ØX4	T49.ØX5	T49.ØX6
ENT agent	T49.6X1	T49.6X2	T49.6X3	T49.6X4	T49.6X5	T49.6X6
ophthalmic preparation	T49.5X1	T49.5X2	T49.5X3	T49.5X4	T49.5X5	T49.5X6
topical NEC	T49.ØX1	T49.ØX2	T49.ØX3	T49.ØX4	T49.ØX5	T49.ØX6
Baclofen	T42.8X1	T42.8X2	T42.8X3	T42.8X4	T42.8X5	T42.8X6
Baking soda	T5Ø.991	T5Ø.992	T5Ø.993	T5Ø.994	T5Ø.995	T5Ø.996
BAL	T45.8X1	T45.8X2	T45.8X3	T45.8X4	T45.8X5	T45.8X6
Bambuterol	T48.6X1	T48.6X2	T48.6X3	T48.6X4	T48.6X5	T48.6X6
Bamethan (sulfate)	T46.7X1	T46.7X2	T46.7X3	T46.7X4	T46.7X5	T46.7X6
Bamifylline	T48.6X1	T48.6X2	T48.6X3	T48.6X4	T48.6X5	T48.6X6
Bamipine	T45.ØX1	T45.ØX2	T45.ØX3	T45.ØX4	T45.ØX5	T45.ØX6
Baneberry — *see Actaea spicata*						
Banewort — *see Belladonna*						

Substance	External Cause (T-Code)					
	Poisoning, Accidental (Unintentional)	Poisoning, Intentional Self-Harm	Poisoning, Assault	Poisoning, Undetermined	Adverse Effect	Underdosing
Barbenyl	T42.3X1	T42.3X2	T42.3X3	T42.3X4	T42.3X5	T42.3X6
Barbexaclone	T42.6X1	T42.6X2	T42.6X3	T42.6X4	T42.6X5	T42.6X6
Barbital	T42.3X1	T42.3X2	T42.3X3	T42.3X4	T42.3X5	T42.3X6
sodium	T42.3X1	T42.3X2	T42.3X3	T42.3X4	T42.3X5	T42.3X6
Barbitone	T42.3X1	T42.3X2	T42.3X3	T42.3X4	T42.3X5	T42.3X6
Barbiturate NEC	T42.3X1	T42.3X2	T42.3X3	T42.3X4	T42.3X5	T42.3X6
with tranquilizer	T42.3X1	T42.3X2	T42.3X3	T42.3X4	T42.3X5	T42.3X6
anesthetic (intravenous)	T41.1X1	T41.1X2	T41.1X3	T41.1X4	T41.1X5	T41.1X6
Barium (carbonate) (chloride) (sulfite)	T57.8X1	T57.8X2	T57.8X3	T57.8X4	—	—
diagnostic agent	T5Ø.8X1	T5Ø.8X2	T5Ø.8X3	T5Ø.8X4	T5Ø.8X5	T5Ø.8X6
pesticide	T6Ø.4X1	T6Ø.4X2	T6Ø.4X3	T6Ø.4X4	—	—
rodenticide	T6Ø.4X1	T6Ø.4X2	T6Ø.4X3	T6Ø.4X4	—	—
sulfate (medicinal)	T5Ø.8X1	T5Ø.8X2	T5Ø.8X3	T5Ø.8X4	T5Ø.8X5	T5Ø.8X6
Barrier cream	T49.3X1	T49.3X2	T49.3X3	T49.3X4	T49.3X5	T49.3X6
Basic fuchsin	T49.ØX1	T49.ØX2	T49.ØX3	T49.ØX4	T49.ØX5	T49.ØX6
Battery acid or fluid	T54.2X1	T54.2X2	T54.2X3	T54.2X4	—	—
Bay rum	T51.8X1	T51.8X2	T51.8X3	T51.8X4	—	—
BCG (vaccine)	T5Ø.A91	T5Ø.A92	T5Ø.A93	T5Ø.A94	T5Ø.A95	T5Ø.A96
BCNU	T45.1X1	T45.1X2	T45.1X3	T45.1X4	T45.1X5	T45.1X6
Bearsfoot	T62.2X1	T62.2X2	T62.2X3	T62.2X4	—	—
Beclamide	T42.6X1	T42.6X2	T42.6X3	T42.6X4	T42.6X5	T42.6X6
Beclomethasone	T44.5X1	T44.5X2	T44.5X3	T44.5X4	T44.5X5	T44.5X6
Bee (sting) (venom)	T63.441	T63.442	T63.443	T63.444	—	—
Befunolol	T49.5X1	T49.5X2	T49.5X3	T49.5X4	T49.5X5	T49.5X6
Bekanamycin	T36.5X1	T36.5X2	T36.5X3	T36.5X4	T36.5X5	T36.5X6
Belladonna — *see also Nightshade*						
alkaloids	T44.3X1	T44.3X2	T44.3X3	T44.3X4	T44.3X5	T44.3X6
extract	T44.3X1	T44.3X2	T44.3X3	T44.3X4	T44.3X5	T44.3X6
herb	T44.3X1	T44.3X2	T44.3X3	T44.3X4	T44.3X5	T44.3X6
Bemegride	T5Ø.7X1	T5Ø.7X2	T5Ø.7X3	T5Ø.7X4	T5Ø.7X5	T5Ø.7X6
Benactyzine	T44.3X1	T44.3X2	T44.3X3	T44.3X4	T44.3X5	T44.3X6
Benadryl	T45.ØX1	T45.ØX2	T45.ØX3	T45.ØX4	T45.ØX5	T45.ØX6
Benaprizine	T44.3X1	T44.3X2	T44.3X3	T44.3X4	T44.3X5	T44.3X6
Benazepril	T46.4X1	T46.4X2	T46.4X3	T46.4X4	T46.4X5	T46.4X6
Bencyclane	T46.7X1	T46.7X2	T46.7X3	T46.7X4	T46.7X5	T46.7X6
Bendazol	T46.3X1	T46.3X2	T46.3X3	T46.3X4	T46.3X5	T46.3X6
Bendrofluazide	T5Ø.2X1	T5Ø.2X2	T5Ø.2X3	T5Ø.2X4	T5Ø.2X5	T5Ø.2X6
Bendroflumethiazide	T5Ø.2X1	T5Ø.2X2	T5Ø.2X3	T5Ø.2X4	T5Ø.2X5	T5Ø.2X6
Benemid	T5Ø.4X1	T5Ø.4X2	T5Ø.4X3	T5Ø.4X4	T5Ø.4X5	T5Ø.4X6
Benethamine penicillin	T36.ØX1	T36.ØX2	T36.ØX3	T36.ØX4	T36.ØX5	T36.ØX6
Benisone	T49.ØX1	T49.ØX2	T49.ØX3	T49.ØX4	T49.ØX5	T49.ØX6

Substance	External Cause (T-Code): Poisoning, Accidental (Unintentional)	Poisoning, Intentional Self-Harm	Poisoning, Assault	Poisoning, Undetermined	Adverse Effect	Underdosing
Benexate	T47.1X1	T47.1X2	T47.1X3	T47.1X4	T47.1X5	T47.1X6
Benfluorex	T46.6X1	T46.6X2	T46.6X3	T46.6X4	T46.6X5	T46.6X6
Benfotiamine	T45.2X1	T45.2X2	T45.2X3	T45.2X4	T45.2X5	T45.2X6
Benomyl	T60.0X1	T60.0X2	T60.0X3	T60.0X4	—	—
Benoquin	T49.8X1	T49.8X2	T49.8X3	T49.8X4	T49.8X5	T49.8X6
Benoxinate	T41.3X1	T41.3X2	T41.3X3	T41.3X4	T41.3X5	T41.3X6
Benperidol	T43.4X1	T43.4X2	T43.4X3	T43.4X4	T43.4X5	T43.4X6
Benproperine	T48.3X1	T48.3X2	T48.3X3	T48.3X4	T48.3X5	T48.3X6
Benserazide	T42.8X1	T42.8X2	T42.8X3	T42.8X4	T42.8X5	T42.8X6
Bentazepam	T42.4X1	T42.4X2	T42.4X3	T42.4X4	T42.4X5	T42.4X6
Bentiromide	T50.8X1	T50.8X2	T50.8X3	T50.8X4	T50.8X5	T50.8X6
Bentonite	T49.3X1	T49.3X2	T49.3X3	T49.3X4	T49.3X5	T49.3X6
Benzalbutyramide	T46.6X1	T46.6X2	T46.6X3	T46.6X4	T46.6X5	T46.6X6
Benzalkonium (chloride)	T49.0X1	T49.0X2	T49.0X3	T49.0X4	T49.0X5	T49.0X6
ophthalmic preparation	T49.5X1	T49.5X2	T49.5X3	T49.5X4	T49.5X5	T49.5X6
Benzamine	T41.3X1	T41.3X2	T41.3X3	T41.3X4	T41.3X5	T41.3X6
lactate	T49.1X1	T49.1X2	T49.1X3	T49.1X4	T49.1X5	T49.1X6
Benzamidosalicylate (calcium)	T37.1X1	T37.1X2	T37.1X3	T37.1X4	T37.1X5	T37.1X6
Benzamphetamine	T50.5X1	T50.5X2	T50.5X3	T50.5X4	T50.5X5	T50.5X6
Benzapril hydrochloride	T46.5X1	T46.5X2	T46.5X3	T46.5X4	T46.5X5	T46.5X6
Benzathine benzylpenicillin	T36.0X1	T36.0X2	T36.0X3	T36.0X4	T36.0X5	T36.0X6
Benzathine penicillin	T36.0X1	T36.0X2	T36.0X3	T36.0X4	T36.0X5	T36.0X6
Benzatropine	T42.8X1	T42.8X2	T42.8X3	T42.8X4	T42.8X5	T42.8X6
Benzbromarone	T50.4X1	T50.4X2	T50.4X3	T50.4X4	T50.4X5	T50.4X6
Benzcarbimine	T45.1X1	T45.1X2	T45.1X3	T45.1X4	T45.1X5	T45.1X6
Benzedrex	T44.991	T44.992	T44.993	T44.994	T44.995	T44.996
Benzedrine (amphetamine)	T43.621	T43.622	T43.623	T43.624	T43.625	T43.626
Benzenamine	T65.3X1	T65.3X2	T65.3X3	T65.3X4	—	—
Benzene	T52.1X1	T52.1X2	T52.1X3	T52.1X4	—	—
homologues (acetyl) (dimethyl) (methyl) (solvent)	T52.2X1	T52.2X2	T52.2X3	T52.2X4	—	—
Benzethonium (chloride)	T49.0X1	T49.0X2	T49.0X3	T49.0X4	T49.0X5	T49.0X6
Benzfetamine	T50.5X1	T50.5X2	T50.5X3	T50.5X4	T50.5X5	T50.5X6
Benzhexol	T44.3X1	T44.3X2	T44.3X3	T44.3X4	T44.3X5	T44.3X6
Benzhydramine (chloride)	T45.0X1	T45.0X2	T45.0X3	T45.0X4	T45.0X5	T45.0X6
Benzidine	T65.891	T65.892	T65.893	T65.894	—	—
Benzilonium bromide	T44.3X1	T44.3X2	T44.3X3	T44.3X4	T44.3X5	T44.3X6
Benzimidazole	T60.3X1	T60.3X2	T60.3X3	T60.3X4	—	—
Benzin(e) — *see Ligroin*						
Benziodarone	T46.3X1	T46.3X2	T46.3X3	T46.3X4	T46.3X5	T46.3X6
Benznidazole	T37.3X1	T37.3X2	T37.3X3	T37.3X4	T37.3X5	T37.3X6
Benzocaine	T41.3X1	T41.3X2	T41.3X3	T41.3X4	T41.3X5	T41.3X6
Benzoctamine	T43.0X1	T43.0X2	T43.0X3	T43.0X4	T43.0X5	T43.0X6
Benzodiapin	T42.4X1	T42.4X2	T42.4X3	T42.4X4	T42.4X5	T42.4X6
Benzodiazepine NEC	T42.4X1	T42.4X2	T42.4X3	T42.4X4	T42.4X5	T42.4X6
Benzoic acid	T49.0X1	T49.0X2	T49.0X3	T49.0X4	T49.0X5	T49.0X6
with salicylic acid	T49.0X1	T49.0X2	T49.0X3	T49.0X4	T49.0X5	T49.0X6
Benzoin (tincture)	T48.5X1	T48.5X2	T48.5X3	T48.5X4	T48.5X5	T48.5X6
Benzol (benzene)	T52.1X1	T52.1X2	T52.1X3	T52.1X4	—	—
vapor	T52.0X1	T52.0X2	T52.0X3	T52.0X4	—	—
Benzomorphan	T40.2X1	T40.2X2	T40.2X3	T40.2X4	T40.2X5	T40.2X6
Benzonatate	T48.3X1	T48.3X2	T48.3X3	T48.3X4	T48.3X5	T48.3X6
Benzophenones	T49.3X1	T49.3X2	T49.3X3	T49.3X4	T49.3X5	T49.3X6
Benzopyrone	T46.991	T46.992	T46.993	T46.994	T46.995	T46.996
Benzothiadiazides	T50.2X1	T50.2X2	T50.2X3	T50.2X4	T50.2X5	T50.2X6
Benzoxonium chloride	T49.0X1	T49.0X2	T49.0X3	T49.0X4	T49.0X5	T49.0X6
Benzoyl peroxide	T49.0X1	T49.0X2	T49.0X3	T49.0X4	T49.0X5	T49.0X6
Benzoylpas calcium	T37.1X1	T37.1X2	T37.1X3	T37.1X4	T37.1X5	T37.1X6
Benzperidin	T43.591	T43.592	T43.593	T43.594	T43.595	T43.596
Benzperidol	T43.591	T43.592	T43.593	T43.594	T43.595	T43.596
Benzphetamine	T50.5X1	T50.5X2	T50.5X3	T50.5X4	T50.5X5	T50.5X6
Benzpyrinium bromide	T44.1X1	T44.1X2	T44.1X3	T44.1X4	T44.1X5	T44.1X6
Benzquinamide	T45.0X1	T45.0X2	T45.0X3	T45.0X4	T45.0X5	T45.0X6
Benzthiazide	T50.2X1	T50.2X2	T50.2X3	T50.2X4	T50.2X5	T50.2X6
Benztropine						
anticholinergic	T44.3X1	T44.3X2	T44.3X3	T44.3X4	T44.3X5	T44.3X6
antiparkinson	T42.8X1	T42.8X2	T42.8X3	T42.8X4	T42.8X5	T42.8X6
Benzydamine	T49.0X1	T49.0X2	T49.0X3	T49.0X4	T49.0X5	T49.0X6
Benzyl						
acetate	T52.8X1	T52.8X2	T52.8X3	T52.8X4	—	—
alcohol	T49.0X1	T49.0X2	T49.0X3	T49.0X4	T49.0X5	T49.0X6
benzoate	T49.0X1	T49.0X2	T49.0X3	T49.0X4	T49.0X5	T49.0X6
Benzoic acid	T49.0X1	T49.0X2	T49.0X3	T49.0X4	T49.0X5	T49.0X6
morphine	T40.2X1	T40.2X2	T40.2X3	T40.2X4	—	—
nicotinate	T46.6X1	T46.6X2	T46.6X3	T46.6X4	T46.6X5	T46.6X6
penicillin	T36.0X1	T36.0X2	T36.0X3	T36.0X4	T36.0X5	T36.0X6
Benzylhydrochlorthia-zide	T50.2X1	T50.2X2	T50.2X3	T50.2X4	T50.2X5	T50.2X6
Benzylpenicillin	T36.0X1	T36.0X2	T36.0X3	T36.0X4	T36.0X5	T36.0X6
Benzylthiouracil	T38.2X1	T38.2X2	T38.2X3	T38.2X4	T38.2X5	T38.2X6
Bephenium hydroxy-naphthoate	T37.4X1	T37.4X2	T37.4X3	T37.4X4	T37.4X5	T37.4X6
Bepridil	T46.1X1	T46.1X2	T46.1X3	T46.1X4	T46.1X5	T46.1X6
Bergamot oil	T65.891	T65.892	T65.893	T65.894	—	—
Bergapten	T50.991	T50.992	T50.993	T50.994	T50.995	T50.996
Berries, poisonous	T62.1X1	T62.1X2	T62.1X3	T62.1X4	—	—

Substance	External Cause (T-Code)					
	Poisoning, Accidental (Unintentional)	Poisoning, Intentional Self-Harm	Poisoning, Assault	Poisoning, Undetermined	Adverse Effect	Underdosing
Beryllium (compounds)	T56.7X1	T56.7X2	T56.7X3	T56.7X4	—	—
b-acetyldigoxin	T46.0X1	T46.0X2	T46.0X3	T46.0X4	T46.0X5	T46.0X6
beta adrenergic blocking agent, heart	T44.7X1	T44.7X2	T44.7X3	T44.7X4	T44.7X5	T44.7X6
b-benzalbutyramide	T46.6X1	T46.6X2	T46.6X3	T46.6X4	T46.6X5	T46.6X6
Betacarotene	T45.2X1	T45.2X2	T45.2X3	T45.2X4	T45.2X5	T45.2X6
b-eucaine	T49.1X1	T49.1X2	T49.1X3	T49.1X4	T49.1X5	T49.1X6
Beta-Chlor	T42.6X1	T42.6X2	T42.6X3	T42.6X4	T42.6X5	T42.6X6
b-galactosidase	T47.5X1	T47.5X2	T47.5X3	T47.5X4	T47.5X5	T47.5X6
Betahistine	T46.7X1	T46.7X2	T46.7X3	T46.7X4	T46.7X5	T46.7X6
Betaine	T47.5X1	T47.5X2	T47.5X3	T47.5X4	T47.5X5	T47.5X6
Betamethasone	T49.0X1	T49.0X2	T49.0X3	T49.0X4	T49.0X5	T49.0X6
topical	T49.0X1	T49.0X2	T49.0X3	T49.0X4	T49.0X5	T49.0X6
Betamicin	T36.8X1	T36.8X2	T36.8X3	T36.8X4	T36.8X5	T36.8X6
Betanidine	T46.5X1	T46.5X2	T46.5X3	T46.5X4	T46.5X5	T46.5X6
b-sitosterol(s)	T46.6X1	T46.6X2	T46.6X3	T46.6X4	T46.6X5	T46.6X6
Betaxolol	T44.7X1	T44.7X2	T44.7X3	T44.7X4	T44.7X5	T44.7X6
Betazole	T50.8X1	T50.8X2	T50.8X3	T50.8X4	T50.8X5	T50.8X6
Bethanechol	T44.1X1	T44.1X2	T44.1X3	T44.1X4	T44.1X5	T44.1X6
chloride	T44.1X1	T44.1X2	T44.1X3	T44.1X4	T44.1X5	T44.1X6
Bethanidine	T46.5X1	T46.5X2	T46.5X3	T46.5X4	T46.5X5	T46.5X6
Betoxycaine	T41.3X1	T41.3X2	T41.3X3	T41.3X4	T41.3X5	T41.3X6
Betula oil	T49.3X1	T49.3X2	T49.3X3	T49.3X4	T49.3X5	T49.3X6
Bevantolol	T44.7X1	T44.7X2	T44.7X3	T44.7X4	T44.7X5	T44.7X6
Bevonium metilsulfate	T44.3X1	T44.3X2	T44.3X3	T44.3X4	T44.3X5	T44.3X6
Bezafibrate	T46.6X1	T46.6X2	T46.6X3	T46.6X4	T46.6X5	T46.6X6
Bezitramide	T40.4X1	T40.4X2	T40.4X3	T40.4X4	T40.4X5	T40.4X6
BHA	T50.991	T50.992	T50.993	T50.994	T50.995	T50.996
Bhang	T40.7X1	T40.7X2	T40.7X3	T40.7X4	T40.7X5	T40.7X6
BHC (medicinal)	T49.0X1	T49.0X2	T49.0X3	T49.0X4	T49.0X5	T49.0X6
nonmedicinal (vapor)	T53.6X1	T53.6X2	T53.6X3	T53.6X4	—	—
Bialamicol	T37.3X1	T37.3X2	T37.3X3	T37.3X4	T37.3X5	T37.3X6
Bibenzonium bromide	T48.3X1	T48.3X2	T48.3X3	T48.3X4	T48.3X5	T48.3X6
Bibrocathol	T49.5X1	T49.5X2	T49.5X3	T49.5X4	T49.5X5	T49.5X6
Bichloride of mercury — *see Mercury, chloride*						
Bichromates (calcium) (potassium) (sodium) (crystals)	T57.8X1	T57.8X2	T57.8X3	T57.8X4	—	—
fumes	T56.2X1	T56.2X2	T56.2X3	T56.2X4	—	—
Biclotymol	T49.6X1	T49.6X2	T49.6X3	T49.6X4	T49.6X5	T49.6X6
Bicucculine	T50.7X1	T50.7X2	T50.7X3	T50.7X4	T50.7X5	T50.7X6
Bifemelane	T43.291	T43.292	T43.293	T43.294	T43.295	T43.296
Biguanide derivatives, oral	T38.3X1	T38.3X2	T38.3X3	T38.3X4	T38.3X5	T38.3X6

Substance	External Cause (T-Code)					
	Poisoning, Accidental (Unintentional)	Poisoning, Intentional Self-Harm	Poisoning, Assault	Poisoning, Undetermined	Adverse Effect	Underdosing
Biligrafin	T50.8X1	T50.8X2	T50.8X3	T50.8X4	T50.8X5	T50.8X6
Bile salts	T47.5X1	T47.5X2	T47.5X3	T47.5X4	T47.5X5	T47.5X6
Bilopaque	T50.8X1	T50.8X2	T50.8X3	T50.8X4	T50.8X5	T50.8X6
Binifibrate	T46.6X1	T46.6X2	T46.6X3	T46.6X4	T46.6X5	T46.6X6
Binitrobenzol	T65.3X1	T65.3X2	T65.3X3	T65.3X4	—	—
Bioflavonoid(s)	T46.991	T46.992	T46.993	T46.994	T46.995	T46.996
Biological substance NEC	T50.901	T50.902	T50.903	T50.904	T50.905	T50.906
Biotin	T45.2X1	T45.2X2	T45.2X3	T45.2X4	T45.2X5	T45.2X6
Biperiden	T44.3X1	T44.3X2	T44.3X3	T44.3X4	T44.3X5	T44.3X6
Bisacodyl	T47.2X1	T47.2X2	T47.2X3	T47.2X4	T47.2X5	T47.2X6
Bisbentiamine	T45.2X1	T45.2X2	T45.2X3	T45.2X4	T45.2X5	T45.2X6
Bisbutiamine	T45.2X1	T45.2X2	T45.2X3	T45.2X4	T45.2X5	T45.2X6
Bisdequalinium (salts) (diacetate)	T49.6X1	T49.6X2	T49.6X3	T49.6X4	T49.6X5	T49.6X6
Bishydroxycoumarin	T45.511	T45.512	T45.513	T45.514	T45.515	T45.516
Bismarsen	T37.8X1	T37.8X2	T37.8X3	T37.8X4	T37.8X5	T37.8X6
Bismuth salts	T47.6X1	T47.6X2	T47.6X3	T47.6X4	T47.6X5	T47.6X6
aluminate	T47.1X1	T47.1X2	T47.1X3	T47.1X4	T47.1X5	T47.1X6
anti-infectives	T37.8X1	T37.8X2	T37.8X3	T37.8X4	T37.8X5	T37.8X6
formic iodide	T49.0X1	T49.0X2	T49.0X3	T49.0X4	T49.0X5	T49.0X6
glycolylarsenate	T49.0X1	T49.0X2	T49.0X3	T49.0X4	T49.0X5	T49.0X6
nonmedicinal (compounds) NEC	T65.91	T65.92	T65.93	T65.94	—	—
subcarbonate	T47.6X1	T47.6X2	T47.6X3	T47.6X4	T47.6X5	T47.6X6
subsalicylate	T37.8X1	T37.8X2	T37.8X3	T37.8X4	T37.8X5	T37.8X6
sulfarsphenamine	T37.8X1	T37.8X2	T37.8X3	T37.8X4	T37.8X5	T37.8X6
Bisoprolol	T44.7X1	T44.7X2	T44.7X3	T44.7X4	T44.7X5	T44.7X6
Bisoxatin	T47.2X1	T47.2X2	T47.2X3	T47.2X4	T47.2X5	T47.2X6
Bisulepin (hydrochloride)	T45.0X1	T45.0X2	T45.0X3	T45.0X4	T45.0X5	T45.0X6
Bithionol	T37.8X1	T37.8X2	T37.8X3	T37.8X4	T37.8X5	T37.8X6
anthelminthic	T37.4X1	T37.4X2	T37.4X3	T37.4X4	T37.4X5	T37.4X6
Bitolterol	T48.6X1	T48.6X2	T48.6X3	T48.6X4	T48.6X5	T48.6X6
Bitoscanate	T37.4X1	T37.4X2	T37.4X3	T37.4X4	T37.4X5	T37.4X6
Bitter almond oil	T62.8X1	T62.8X2	T62.8X3	T62.8X4	—	—
Bittersweet	T62.2X1	T62.2X2	T62.2X3	T62.2X4	—	—
Black						
flag	T60.91	T60.92	T60.93	T60.94	—	—
henbane	T62.2X1	T62.2X2	T62.2X3	T62.2X4	—	—
leaf (40)	T60.91	T60.92	T60.93	T60.94	—	—
widow spider (bite)	T63.311	T63.312	T63.313	T63.314	—	—
antivenin	T50.Z11	T50.Z12	T50.Z13	T50.Z14	T50.Z15	T50.Z16
Blast furnace gas (carbon monoxide from)	T58.8X1	T58.8X2	T58.8X3	T58.8X4	—	—
Bleach	T54.91	T54.92	T54.93	T54.94	—	—

Substance	External Cause (T-Code)					
	Poisoning, Accidental (Unintentional)	Poisoning, Intentional Self-Harm	Poisoning, Assault	Poisoning, Undetermined	Adverse Effect	Underdosing
Bleaching agent (medicinal)	T49.4X1	T49.4X2	T49.4X3	T49.4X4	T49.4X5	T49.4X6
Bleomycin	T45.1X1	T45.1X2	T45.1X3	T45.1X4	T45.1X5	T45.1X6
Blockain	T41.3X1	T41.3X2	T41.3X3	T41.3X4	T41.3X5	T41.3X6
infiltration (subcutaneous)	T41.3X1	T41.3X2	T41.3X3	T41.3X4	T41.3X5	T41.3X6
nerve block (peripheral) (plexus)	T41.3X1	T41.3X2	T41.3X3	T41.3X4	T41.3X5	T41.3X6
topical (surface)	T41.3X1	T41.3X2	T41.3X3	T41.3X4	T41.3X5	T41.3X6
Blockers, calcium channel	T46.1X1	T46.1X2	T46.1X3	T46.1X4	T46.1X5	T46.1X6
Blood (derivatives) (natural) (plasma) (whole)	T45.8X1	T45.8X2	T45.8X3	T45.8X4	T45.8X5	T45.8X6
dried	T45.8X1	T45.8X2	T45.8X3	T45.8X4	T45.8X5	T45.8X6
drug affecting NEC	T45.91	T45.92	T45.93	T45.94	T45.95	T45.96
expander NEC	T45.8X1	T45.8X2	T45.8X3	T45.8X4	T45.8X5	T45.8X6
fraction NEC	T45.8X1	T45.8X2	T45.8X3	T45.8X4	T45.8X5	T45.8X6
substitute (macromolecular)	T45.8X1	T45.8X2	T45.8X3	T45.8X4	T45.8X5	T45.8X6
Blue velvet	T4Ø.2X1	T4Ø.2X2	T4Ø.2X3	T4Ø.2X4	—	—
Bone meal	T62.8X1	T62.8X2	T62.8X3	T62.8X4	—	—
Bonine	T45.ØX1	T45.ØX2	T45.ØX3	T45.ØX4	T45.ØX5	T45.ØX6
Bopindolol	T44.7X1	T44.7X2	T44.7X3	T44.7X4	T44.7X5	T44.7X6
Boracic acid	T49.ØX1	T49.ØX2	T49.ØX3	T49.ØX4	T49.ØX5	T49.ØX6
ENT agent	T49.6X1	T49.6X2	T49.6X3	T49.6X4	T49.6X5	T49.6X6
ophthalmic preparation	T49.5X1	T49.5X2	T49.5X3	T49.5X4	T49.5X5	T49.5X6
Borane complex	T57.8X1	T57.8X2	T57.8X3	T57.8X4	—	—
Borate(s)	T57.8X1	T57.8X2	T57.8X3	T57.8X4	—	—
buffer	T5Ø.991	T5Ø.992	T5Ø.993	T5Ø.994	T5Ø.995	T5Ø.996
cleanser	T54.91	T54.92	T54.93	T54.94	—	—
sodium	T57.8X1	T57.8X2	T57.8X3	T57.8X4	—	—
Borax (cleanser)	T54.91	T54.92	T54.93	T54.94	—	—
Bordeaux mixture	T6Ø.3X1	T6Ø.3X2	T6Ø.3X3	T6Ø.3X4	—	—
Boric acid	T49.ØX1	T49.ØX2	T49.ØX3	T49.ØX4	T49.ØX5	T49.ØX6
ENT agent	T49.6X1	T49.6X2	T49.6X3	T49.6X4	T49.6X5	T49.6X6
ophthalmic preparation	T49.5X1	T49.5X2	T49.5X3	T49.5X4	T49.5X5	T49.5X6
Bornaprine	T44.3X1	T44.3X2	T44.3X3	T44.3X4	T44.3X5	T44.3X6
Boron	T57.8X1	T57.8X2	T57.8X3	T57.8X4	—	—
hydride NEC	T57.8X1	T57.8X2	T57.8X3	T57.8X4	—	—
fumes or gas	T57.8X1	T57.8X2	T57.8X3	T57.8X4	—	—
trifluoride	T59.891	T59.892	T59.893	T59.894	—	—
Botox	T48.291	T48.292	T48.293	T48.294	T48.295	T48.296
Botulinus anti-toxin (type A, B)	T5Ø.Z11	T5Ø.Z12	T5Ø.Z13	T5Ø.Z14	T5Ø.Z15	T5Ø.Z16
Brake fluid vapor	T59.891	T59.892	T59.893	T59.894	—	—
Brallobarbital	T42.3X1	T42.3X2	T42.3X3	T42.3X4	T42.3X5	T42.3X6
Bran (wheat)	T47.4X1	T47.4X2	T47.4X3	T47.4X4	T47.4X5	T47.4X6
Brass (fumes)	T56.891	T56.892	T56.893	T56.894	—	—
Brasso	T52.ØX1	T52.ØX2	T52.ØX3	T52.ØX4	—	—
Bretylium tosilate	T46.2X1	T46.2X2	T46.2X3	T46.2X4	T46.2X5	T46.2X6
Brevital (sodium)	T41.1X1	T41.1X2	T41.1X3	T41.1X4	T41.1X5	T41.1X6
Brinase	T45.3X1	T45.3X2	T45.3X3	T45.3X4	T45.3X5	T45.3X6
British antilewisite	T45.8X1	T45.8X2	T45.8X3	T45.8X4	T45.8X5	T45.8X6
Brodifacoum	T6Ø.4X1	T6Ø.4X2	T6Ø.4X3	T6Ø.4X4	—	—
Bromal (hydrate)	T42.6X1	T42.6X2	T42.6X3	T42.6X4	T42.6X5	T42.6X6
Bromazepam	T42.4X1	T42.4X2	T42.4X3	T42.4X4	T42.4X5	T42.4X6
Bromazine	T45.ØX1	T45.ØX2	T45.ØX3	T45.ØX4	T45.ØX5	T45.ØX6
Brombenzylcyanide	T59.3X1	T59.3X2	T59.3X3	T59.3X4	—	—
Bromelains	T45.3X1	T45.3X2	T45.3X3	T45.3X4	T45.3X5	T45.3X6
Bromethalin	T6Ø.4X1	T6Ø.4X2	T6Ø.4X3	T6Ø.4X4	—	—
Bromhexine	T48.4X1	T48.4X2	T48.4X3	T48.4X4	T48.4X5	T48.4X6
Bromide salts	T42.6X1	T42.6X2	T42.6X3	T42.6X4	T42.6X5	T42.6X6
Bromindione	T45.511	T45.512	T45.513	T45.514	T45.515	T45.516
Bromine						
compounds (medicinal)	T42.6X1	T42.6X2	T42.6X3	T42.6X4	T42.6X5	T42.6X6
sedative	T42.6X1	T42.6X2	T42.6X3	T42.6X4	T42.6X5	T42.6X6
vapor	T59.891	T59.892	T59.893	T59.894	—	—
Bromisovalum	T42.6X1	T42.6X2	T42.6X3	T42.6X4	T42.6X5	T42.6X6
Bromisoval	T42.6X1	T42.6X2	T42.6X3	T42.6X4	T42.6X5	T42.6X6
Bromobenzylcyanide	T59.3X1	T59.3X2	T59.3X3	T59.3X4	—	—
Bromochlorosalicylani-lide	T49.ØX1	T49.ØX2	T49.ØX3	T49.ØX4	T49.ØX5	T49.ØX6
Bromocriptine	T42.8X1	T42.8X2	T42.8X3	T42.8X4	T42.8X5	T42.8X6
Bromodiphenhydramine	T45.ØX1	T45.ØX2	T45.ØX3	T45.ØX4	T45.ØX5	T45.ØX6
Bromoform	T42.6X1	T42.6X2	T42.6X3	T42.6X4	T42.6X5	T42.6X6
Bromophenol blue reagent	T5Ø.991	T5Ø.992	T5Ø.993	T5Ø.994	T5Ø.995	T5Ø.996
Bromopride	T47.8X1	T47.8X2	T47.8X3	T47.8X4	T47.8X5	T47.8X6
Bromosalicylchloranitide	T49.ØX1	T49.ØX2	T49.ØX3	T49.ØX4	T49.ØX5	T49.ØX6
Bromosalicylhydroxamic acid	T37.1X1	T37.1X2	T37.1X3	T37.1X4	T37.1X5	T37.1X6
Bromo-seltzer	T39.1X1	T39.1X2	T39.1X3	T39.1X4	T39.1X5	T39.1X6
Bromoxynil	T6Ø.3X1	T6Ø.3X2	T6Ø.3X3	T6Ø.3X4	—	—
Bromperidol	T43.4X1	T43.4X2	T43.4X3	T43.4X4	T43.4X5	T43.4X6
Brompheniramine	T45.ØX1	T45.ØX2	T45.ØX3	T45.ØX4	T45.ØX5	T45.ØX6
Bromsulfophthalein	T5Ø.8X1	T5Ø.8X2	T5Ø.8X3	T5Ø.8X4	T5Ø.8X5	T5Ø.8X6
Bromural	T42.6X1	T42.6X2	T42.6X3	T42.6X4	T42.6X5	T42.6X6
Bromvaletone	T42.6X1	T42.6X2	T42.6X3	T42.6X4	T42.6X5	T42.6X6
Bronchodilator NEC	T48.6X1	T48.6X2	T48.6X3	T48.6X4	T48.6X5	T48.6X6
Brotizolam	T42.4X1	T42.4X2	T42.4X3	T42.4X4	T42.4X5	T42.4X6
Brovincamine	T46.7X1	T46.7X2	T46.7X3	T46.7X4	T46.7X5	T46.7X6
Brown spider (bite) (venom)	T63.391	T63.392	T63.393	T63.394	—	—

TABLE OF DRUGS AND CHEMICALS

Substance	External Cause (T-Code)					
	Poisoning, Accidental (Unintentional)	Poisoning, Intentional Self-Harm	Poisoning, Assault	Poisoning, Undetermined	Adverse Effect	Underdosing
Brown recluse spider (bite) (venom)	T63.331	T63.332	T63.333	T63.334	—	—
Broxaterol	T48.6X1	T48.6X2	T48.6X3	T48.6X4	T48.6X5	T48.6X6
Broxuridine	T45.1X1	T45.1X2	T45.1X3	T45.1X4	T45.1X5	T45.1X6
Broxyquinoline	T37.8X1	T37.8X2	T37.8X3	T37.8X4	T37.8X5	T37.8X6
Bruceine	T48.291	T48.292	T48.293	T48.294	T48.295	T48.296
Brucia	T62.2X1	T62.2X2	T62.2X3	T62.2X4	—	—
Brucine	T65.1X1	T65.1X2	T65.1X3	T65.1X4	—	—
Brunswick green — *see Copper*						
Bruten — *see Ibuprofen*						
Bryonia	T47.2X1	T47.2X2	T47.2X3	T47.2X4	T47.2X5	T47.2X6
Buclizine	T45.ØX1	T45.ØX2	T45.ØX3	T45.ØX4	T45.ØX5	T45.ØX6
Buclosamide	T49.ØX1	T49.ØX2	T49.ØX3	T49.ØX4	T49.ØX5	T49.ØX6
Budesonide	T44.5X1	T44.5X2	T44.5X3	T44.5X4	T44.5X5	T44.5X6
Budralazine	T46.5X1	T46.5X2	T46.5X3	T46.5X4	T46.5X5	T46.5X6
Bufferin	T39.Ø11	T39.Ø12	T39.Ø13	T39.Ø14	T39.Ø15	T39.Ø16
Buflomedil	T46.7X1	T46.7X2	T46.7X3	T46.7X4	T46.7X5	T46.7X6
Buformin	T38.3X1	T38.3X2	T38.3X3	T38.3X4	T38.3X5	T38.3X6
Bufotenine	T40.991	T40.992	T40.993	T40.994	—	—
Bufrolin	T48.6X1	T48.6X2	T48.6X3	T48.6X4	T48.6X5	T48.6X6
Bufylline	T48.6X1	T48.6X2	T48.6X3	T48.6X4	T48.6X5	T48.6X6
Bulk filler	T50.5X1	T50.5X2	T50.5X3	T50.5X4	T50.5X5	T50.5X6
cathartic	T47.4X1	T47.4X2	T47.4X3	T47.4X4	T47.4X5	T47.4X6
Bumetanide	T50.1X1	T50.1X2	T50.1X3	T50.1X4	T50.1X5	T50.1X6
Bunaftine	T46.2X1	T46.2X2	T46.2X3	T46.2X4	T46.2X5	T46.2X6
Bunamiodyl	T50.8X1	T50.8X2	T50.8X3	T50.8X4	T50.8X5	T50.8X6
Bunazosin	T44.6X1	T44.6X2	T44.6X3	T44.6X4	T44.6X5	T44.6X6
Bunitrolol	T44.7X1	T44.7X2	T44.7X3	T44.7X4	T44.7X5	T44.7X6
Buphenine	T46.7X1	T46.7X2	T46.7X3	T46.7X4	T46.7X5	T46.7X6
Bupivacaine	T41.3X1	T41.3X2	T41.3X3	T41.3X4	T41.3X5	T41.3X6
infiltration (subcutaneous)	T41.3X1	T41.3X2	T41.3X3	T41.3X4	T41.3X5	T41.3X6
nerve block (peripheral) (plexus)	T41.3X1	T41.3X2	T41.3X3	T41.3X4	T41.3X5	T41.3X6
spinal	T41.3X1	T41.3X2	T41.3X3	T41.3X4	T41.3X5	T41.3X6
Bupranolol	T44.7X1	T44.7X2	T44.7X3	T44.7X4	T44.7X5	T44.7X6
Buprenorphine	T40.4X1	T40.4X2	T40.4X3	T40.4X4	T40.4X5	T40.4X6
Bupropion	T43.291	T43.292	T43.293	T43.294	T43.295	T43.296
Burimamide	T47.1X1	T47.1X2	T47.1X3	T47.1X4	T47.1X5	T47.1X6
Buserelin	T38.891	T38.892	T38.893	T38.894	T38.895	T38.896
Buspirone	T43.591	T43.592	T43.593	T43.594	T43.595	T43.596
Busulfan, busulphan	T45.1X1	T45.1X2	T45.1X3	T45.1X4	T45.1X5	T45.1X6
Butabarbital (sodium)	T42.3X1	T42.3X2	T42.3X3	T42.3X4	T42.3X5	T42.3X6
Butabarbitone	T42.3X1	T42.3X2	T42.3X3	T42.3X4	T42.3X5	T42.3X6

Substance	External Cause (T-Code)					
	Poisoning, Accidental (Unintentional)	Poisoning, Intentional Self-Harm	Poisoning, Assault	Poisoning, Undetermined	Adverse Effect	Underdosing
Butabarpal	T42.3X1	T42.3X2	T42.3X3	T42.3X4	T42.3X5	T42.3X6
Butacaine	T41.3X1	T41.3X2	T41.3X3	T41.3X4	T41.3X5	T41.3X6
Butalamine	T46.7X1	T46.7X2	T46.7X3	T46.7X4	T46.7X5	T46.7X6
Butalbital	T42.3X1	T42.3X2	T42.3X3	T42.3X4	T42.3X5	T42.3X6
Butallylonal	T42.3X1	T42.3X2	T42.3X3	T42.3X4	T42.3X5	T42.3X6
Butamben	T41.3X1	T41.3X2	T41.3X3	T41.3X4	T41.3X5	T41.3X6
Butamirate	T48.3X1	T48.3X2	T48.3X3	T48.3X4	T48.3X5	T48.3X6
Butane (distributed in mobile container)	T59.891	T59.892	T59.893	T59.894	—	—
distributed through pipes	T59.891	T59.892	T59.893	T59.894	—	—
incomplete combustion	T58.11	T58.12	T58.13	T58.14	—	—
Butanilicaine	T41.3X1	T41.3X2	T41.3X3	T41.3X4	T41.3X5	T41.3X6
Butanol	T51.3X1	T51.3X2	T51.3X3	T51.3X4	—	—
Butanone, 2-butanone	T52.4X1	T52.4X2	T52.4X3	T52.4X4	—	—
Butantrone	T49.4X1	T49.4X2	T49.4X3	T49.4X4	T49.4X5	T49.4X6
Butaperazine	T43.3X1	T43.3X2	T43.3X3	T43.3X4	T43.3X5	T43.3X6
Butazolidin	T39.2X1	T39.2X2	T39.2X3	T39.2X4	T39.2X5	T39.2X6
Butetamate	T48.6X1	T48.6X2	T48.6X3	T48.6X4	T48.6X5	T48.6X6
Butethal	T42.3X1	T42.3X2	T42.3X3	T42.3X4	T42.3X5	T42.3X6
Butethamate	T44.3X1	T44.3X2	T44.3X3	T44.3X4	T44.3X5	T44.3X6
Buthalitone (sodium)	T41.1X1	T41.1X2	T41.1X3	T41.1X4	T41.1X5	T41.1X6
Butisol (sodium)	T42.3X1	T42.3X2	T42.3X3	T42.3X4	T42.3X5	T42.3X6
Butizide	T50.2X1	T50.2X2	T50.2X3	T50.2X4	T50.2X5	T50.2X6
Butobarbital	T42.3X1	T42.3X2	T42.3X3	T42.3X4	T42.3X5	T42.3X6
sodium	T42.3X1	T42.3X2	T42.3X3	T42.3X4	T42.3X5	T42.3X6
Butobarbitone	T42.3X1	T42.3X2	T42.3X3	T42.3X4	T42.3X5	T42.3X6
Butoconazole (nitrate)	T49.ØX1	T49.ØX2	T49.ØX3	T49.ØX4	T49.ØX5	T49.ØX6
Butorphanol	T40.4X1	T40.4X2	T40.4X3	T40.4X4	T40.4X5	T40.4X6
Butriptyline	T43.Ø11	T43.Ø12	T43.Ø13	T43.Ø14	T43.Ø15	T43.Ø16
Butropium bromide	T44.3X1	T44.3X2	T44.3X3	T44.3X4	T44.3X5	T44.3X6
Buttercups	T62.2X1	T62.2X2	T62.2X3	T62.2X4	—	—
Butter of antimony — *see Antimony*						
Butyl						
acetate (secondary)	T52.8X1	T52.8X2	T52.8X3	T52.8X4	—	—
alcohol	T51.3X1	T51.3X2	T51.3X3	T51.3X4	—	—
aminobenzoate	T41.3X1	T41.3X2	T41.3X3	T41.3X4	T41.3X5	T41.3X6
butyrate	T52.8X1	T52.8X2	T52.8X3	T52.8X4	—	—
carbinol	T51.3X1	T51.3X2	T51.3X3	T51.3X4	—	—
carbitol	T52.3X1	T52.3X2	T52.3X3	T52.3X4	—	—
cellosolve	T52.3X1	T52.3X2	T52.3X3	T52.3X4	—	—
chloral (hydrate)	T42.6X1	T42.6X2	T42.6X3	T42.6X4	T42.6X5	T42.6X6
formate	T52.8X1	T52.8X2	T52.8X3	T52.8X4	—	—

Substance	External Cause (T-Code): Poisoning, Accidental (Unintentional)	Poisoning, Intentional Self-Harm	Poisoning, Assault	Poisoning, Undetermined	Adverse Effect	Underdosing
Butyl *(Continued)*						
lactate	T52.8X1	T52.8X2	T52.8X3	T52.8X4	—	—
propionate	T52.8X1	T52.8X2	T52.8X3	T52.8X4	—	—
scopolamine bromide	T44.3X1	T44.3X2	T44.3X3	T44.3X4	T44.3X5	T44.3X6
thiobarbital sodium	T41.1X1	T41.1X2	T41.1X3	T41.1X4	T41.1X5	T41.1X6
Butylated hydroxy-anisole	T50.991	T50.992	T50.993	T50.994	T50.995	T50.996
Butylchloral hydrate	T42.6X1	T42.6X2	T42.6X3	T42.6X4	T42.6X5	T42.6X6
Butyltoluene	T52.2X1	T52.2X2	T52.2X3	T52.2X4	—	—
Butyn	T41.3X1	T41.3X2	T41.3X3	T41.3X4	T41.3X5	T41.3X6
Butyrophenone (-based tranquilizers)	T43.4X1	T43.4X2	T43.4X3	T43.4X4	T43.4X5	T43.4X6
C						
Cabergoline	T42.8X1	T42.8X2	T42.8X3	T42.8X4	T42.8X5	T42.8X6
Cacodyl, cacodylic acid	T57.0X1	T57.0X2	T57.0X3	T57.0X4	—	—
Cactinomycin	T45.1X1	T45.1X2	T45.1X3	T45.1X4	T45.1X5	T45.1X6
Cade oil	T49.4X1	T49.4X2	T49.4X3	T49.4X4	T49.4X5	T49.4X6
Cadexomer iodine	T49.0X1	T49.0X2	T49.0X3	T49.0X4	T49.0X5	T49.0X6
Cadmium (chloride) (fumes) (oxide)	T56.3X1	T56.3X2	T56.3X3	T56.3X4	—	—
sulfide (medicinal) NEC	T49.4X1	T49.4X2	T49.4X3	T49.4X4	T49.4X5	T49.4X6
Cadralazine	T46.5X1	T46.5X2	T46.5X3	T46.5X4	T46.5X5	T46.5X6
Caffeine	T43.611	T43.612	T43.613	T43.614	T43.615	T43.616
Calabar bean	T62.2X1	T62.2X2	T62.2X3	T62.2X4	—	—
Caladium seguinum	T62.2X1	T62.2X2	T62.2X3	T62.2X4	—	—
Calamine (lotion)	T49.3X1	T49.3X2	T49.3X3	T49.3X4	T49.3X5	T49.3X6
Calcifediol	T45.2X1	T45.2X2	T45.2X3	T45.2X4	T45.2X5	T45.2X6
Calciferol	T45.2X1	T45.2X2	T45.2X3	T45.2X4	T45.2X5	T45.2X6
Calcitonin	T50.991	T50.992	T50.993	T50.994	T50.995	T50.996
Calcitriol	T45.2X1	T45.2X2	T45.2X3	T45.2X4	T45.2X5	T45.2X6
Calcium	T50.3X1	T50.3X2	T50.3X3	T50.3X4	T50.3X5	T50.3X6
actylsalicylate	T39.011	T39.012	T39.013	T39.014	T39.015	T39.016
benzamidosalicylate	T37.1X1	T37.1X2	T37.1X3	T37.1X4	T37.1X5	T37.1X6
bromide	T42.6X1	T42.6X2	T42.6X3	T42.6X4	T42.6X5	T42.6X6
bromolactobionate	T42.6X1	T42.6X2	T42.6X3	T42.6X4	T42.6X5	T42.6X6
carbaspirin	T39.011	T39.012	T39.013	T39.014	T39.015	T39.016
carbimide	T50.6X1	T50.6X2	T50.6X3	T50.6X4	T50.6X5	T50.6X6
carbonate	T47.1X1	T47.1X2	T47.1X3	T47.1X4	T47.1X5	T47.1X6
chloride	T50.991	T50.992	T50.993	T50.994	T50.995	T50.996
anhydrous	T50.991	T50.992	T50.993	T50.994	T50.995	T50.996
cyanide	T57.8X1	T57.8X2	T57.8X3	T57.8X4	—	—
dioctyl sulfosuccinate	T47.4X1	T47.4X2	T47.4X3	T47.4X4	T47.4X5	T47.4X6
disodium edathamil	T45.8X1	T45.8X2	T45.8X3	T45.8X4	T45.8X5	T45.8X6
Calcium *(Continued)*						
disodium edetate	T45.8X1	T45.8X2	T45.8X3	T45.8X4	T45.8X5	T45.8X6
dobesilate	T46.991	T46.992	T46.993	T46.994	T46.995	T46.996
EDTA	T45.8X1	T45.8X2	T45.8X3	T45.8X4	T45.8X5	T45.8X6
ferrous citrate	T45.4X1	T45.4X2	T45.4X3	T45.4X4	T45.4X5	T45.4X6
folinate	T45.8X1	T45.8X2	T45.8X3	T45.8X4	T45.8X5	T45.8X6
glubionate	T50.3X1	T50.3X2	T50.3X3	T50.3X4	T50.3X5	T50.3X6
gluconate	T50.3X1	T50.3X2	T50.3X3	T50.3X4	T50.3X5	T50.3X6
gluconogalactogluconate	T50.3X1	T50.3X2	T50.3X3	T50.3X4	T50.3X5	T50.3X6
hydrate, hydroxide	T54.3X1	T54.3X2	T54.3X3	T54.3X4	—	—
hypochlorite	T54.3X1	T54.3X2	T54.3X3	T54.3X4	—	—
iodide	T48.4X1	T48.4X2	T48.4X3	T48.4X4	T48.4X5	T48.4X6
ipodate	T50.8X1	T50.8X2	T50.8X3	T50.8X4	T50.8X5	T50.8X6
lactate	T50.3X1	T50.3X2	T50.3X3	T50.3X4	T50.3X5	T50.3X6
leucovorin	T45.8X1	T45.8X2	T45.8X3	T45.8X4	T45.8X5	T45.8X6
mandelate	T37.91	T37.92	T37.93	T37.94	T37.95	T37.96
oxide	T54.3X1	T54.3X2	T54.3X3	T54.3X4	—	—
pantothenate	T45.2X1	T45.2X2	T45.2X3	T45.2X4	T45.2X5	T45.2X6
phosphate	T50.3X1	T50.3X2	T50.3X3	T50.3X4	T50.3X5	T50.3X6
salicylate	T39.091	T39.092	T39.093	T39.094	T39.095	T39.096
salts	T50.3X1	T50.3X2	T50.3X3	T50.3X4	T50.3X5	T50.3X6
Calculus-dissolving drug	T50.991	T50.992	T50.993	T50.994	T50.995	T50.996
Calomel	T49.0X1	T49.0X2	T49.0X3	T49.0X4	T49.0X5	T49.0X6
Caloric agent	T50.3X1	T50.3X2	T50.3X3	T50.3X4	T50.3X5	T50.3X6
Calusterone	T38.7X1	T38.7X2	T38.7X3	T38.7X4	T38.7X5	T38.7X6
Camazepam	T42.4X1	T42.4X2	T42.4X3	T42.4X4	T42.4X5	T42.4X6
Camomile	T49.0X1	T49.0X2	T49.0X3	T49.0X4	T49.0X5	T49.0X6
Camoquin	T37.2X1	T37.2X2	T37.2X3	T37.2X4	T37.2X5	T37.2X6
Camphor						
insecticide	T60.2X1	T60.2X2	T60.2X3	T60.2X4	—	—
medicinal	T49.8X1	T49.8X2	T49.8X3	T49.8X4	T49.8X5	T49.8X6
Camylofin	T44.3X1	T44.3X2	T44.3X3	T44.3X4	T44.3X5	T44.3X6
Cancer chemotherapy drug regimen	T45.1X1	T45.1X2	T45.1X3	T45.1X4	T45.1X5	T45.1X6
Candeptin	T49.0X1	T49.0X2	T49.0X3	T49.0X4	T49.0X5	T49.0X6
Candicidin	T49.0X1	T49.0X2	T49.0X3	T49.0X4	T49.0X5	T49.0X6
Cannabinol	T40.7X1	T40.7X2	T40.7X3	T40.7X4	T40.7X5	T40.7X6
Cannabis (derivatives)	T40.7X1	T40.7X2	T40.7X3	T40.7X4	T40.7X5	T40.7X6
Canned heat	T51.1X1	T51.1X2	T51.1X3	T51.1X4	—	—
Canrenoic acid	T50.0X1	T50.0X2	T50.0X3	T50.0X4	T50.0X5	T50.0X6
Canrenone	T50.0X1	T50.0X2	T50.0X3	T50.0X4	T50.0X5	T50.0X6
Cantharides, cantharidin, cantharis	T49.8X1	T49.8X2	T49.8X3	T49.8X4	T49.8X5	T49.8X6

◀ New ◀ Revised ~~deleted~~ Deleted

Substance	External Cause (T-Code)					
	Poisoning, Accidental (Unintentional)	Poisoning, Intentional Self-Harm	Poisoning, Assault	Poisoning, Undetermined	Adverse Effect	Underdosing
Canthaxanthin	T5Ø.991	T5Ø.992	T5Ø.993	T5Ø.994	T5Ø.995	T5Ø.996
Capillary-active drug NEC	T46.9Ø1	T46.9Ø2	T46.9Ø3	T46.9Ø4	T46.9Ø5	T46.9Ø6
Capreomycin	T36.8X1	T36.8X2	T36.8X3	T36.8X4	T36.8X5	T36.8X6
Capsicum	T49.4X1	T49.4X2	T49.4X3	T49.4X4	T49.4X5	T49.4X6
Captafol	T6Ø.3X1	T6Ø.3X2	T6Ø.3X3	T6Ø.3X4	—	—
Captan	T6Ø.3X1	T6Ø.3X2	T6Ø.3X3	T6Ø.3X4	—	—
Captodiame, captodiamine	T43.591	T43.592	T43.593	T43.594	T43.595	T43.596
Captopril	T46.4X1	T46.4X2	T46.4X3	T46.4X4	T46.4X5	T46.4X6
Caramiphen	T44.3X1	T44.3X2	T44.3X3	T44.3X4	T44.3X5	T44.3X6
Carazolol	T44.7X1	T44.7X2	T44.7X3	T44.7X4	T44.7X5	T44.7X6
Carbachol	T44.1X1	T44.1X2	T44.1X3	T44.1X4	T44.1X5	T44.1X6
Carbacrylamine (resin)	T5Ø.3X1	T5Ø.3X2	T5Ø.3X3	T5Ø.3X4	T5Ø.3X5	T5Ø.3X6
Carbamate (insecticide)	T6Ø.ØX1	T6Ø.ØX2	T6Ø.ØX3	T6Ø.ØX4	—	—
Carbamate (sedative)	T42.6X1	T42.6X2	T42.6X3	T42.6X4	T42.6X5	T42.6X6
herbicide	T6Ø.ØX1	T6Ø.ØX2	T6Ø.ØX3	T6Ø.ØX4	—	—
insecticide	T6Ø.ØX1	T6Ø.ØX2	T6Ø.ØX3	T6Ø.ØX4	—	—
Carbamazepine	T42.1X1	T42.1X2	T42.1X3	T42.1X4	T42.1X5	T42.1X6
Carbamide	T47.3X1	T47.3X2	T47.3X3	T47.3X4	T47.3X5	T47.3X6
peroxide	T49.ØX1	T49.ØX2	T49.ØX3	T49.ØX4	T49.ØX5	T49.ØX6
topical	T49.8X1	T49.8X2	T49.8X3	T49.8X4	T49.8X5	T49.8X6
Carbamylcholine chloride	T44.1X1	T44.1X2	T44.1X3	T44.1X4	T44.1X5	T44.1X6
Carbaril	T6Ø.ØX1	T6Ø.ØX2	T6Ø.ØX3	T6Ø.ØX4	—	—
Carbarsone	T37.3X1	T37.3X2	T37.3X3	T37.3X4	T37.3X5	T37.3X6
Carbaryl	T6Ø.ØX1	T6Ø.ØX2	T6Ø.ØX3	T6Ø.ØX4	—	—
Carbaspirin	T39.Ø11	T39.Ø12	T39.Ø13	T39.Ø14	T39.Ø15	T39.Ø16
Carbazochrome (salicylate) (sodium sulfonate)	T49.4X1	T49.4X2	T49.4X3	T49.4X4	T49.4X5	T49.4X6
Carbenicillin	T36.ØX1	T36.ØX2	T36.ØX3	T36.ØX4	T36.ØX5	T36.ØX6
Carbenoxolone	T47.1X1	T47.1X2	T47.1X3	T47.1X4	T47.1X5	T47.1X6
Carbetapentane	T48.3X1	T48.3X2	T48.3X3	T48.3X4	T48.3X5	T48.3X6
Carbethyl salicylate	T39.Ø91	T39.Ø92	T39.Ø93	T39.Ø94	T39.Ø95	T39.Ø96
Carbidopa (with levodopa)	T42.8X1	T42.8X2	T42.8X3	T42.8X4	T42.8X5	T42.8X6
Carbimazole	T38.2X1	T38.2X2	T38.2X3	T38.2X4	T38.2X5	T38.2X6
Carbinol	T51.1X1	T51.1X2	T51.1X3	T51.1X4	—	—
Carbinoxamine	T45.ØX1	T45.ØX2	T45.ØX3	T45.ØX4	T45.ØX5	T45.ØX6
Carbiphene	T39.8X1	T39.8X2	T39.8X3	T39.8X4	T39.8X5	T39.8X6
Carbitol	T52.3X1	T52.3X2	T52.3X3	T52.3X4	—	—
Carbocaine	T41.3X1	T41.3X2	T41.3X3	T41.3X4	T41.3X5	T41.3X6
infiltration (subcutaneous)	T41.3X1	T41.3X2	T41.3X3	T41.3X4	T41.3X5	T41.3X6
nerve block (peripheral) (plexus)	T41.3X1	T41.3X2	T41.3X3	T41.3X4	T41.3X5	T41.3X6
topical (surface)	T41.3X1	T41.3X2	T41.3X3	T41.3X4	T41.3X5	T41.3X6
Carbo medicinalis	T47.6X1	T47.6X2	T47.6X3	T47.6X4	T47.6X5	T47.6X6

Substance	External Cause (T-Code)					
	Poisoning, Accidental (Unintentional)	Poisoning, Intentional Self-Harm	Poisoning, Assault	Poisoning, Undetermined	Adverse Effect	Underdosing
Carbomycin	T36.8X1	T36.8X2	T36.8X3	T36.8X4	T36.8X5	T36.8X6
Carbocisteine	T48.4X1	T48.4X2	T48.4X3	T48.4X4	T48.4X5	T48.4X6
Carbocromen	T46.3X1	T46.3X2	T46.3X3	T46.3X4	T46.3X5	T46.3X6
Carbol fuchsin	T49.ØX1	T49.ØX2	T49.ØX3	T49.ØX4	T49.ØX5	T49.ØX6
Carbolic acid — *see also Phenol*	T54.ØX1	T54.ØX2	T54.ØX3	T54.ØX4	—	—
Carbolonium (bromide)	T48.1X1	T48.1X2	T48.1X3	T48.1X4	T48.1X5	T48.1X6
Carbon						
bisulfide (liquid)	T65.4X1	T65.4X2	T65.4X3	T65.4X4	—	—
vapor	T65.4X1	T65.4X2	T65.4X3	T65.4X4	—	—
dioxide (gas)	T59.7X1	T59.7X2	T59.7X3	T59.7X4	—	—
medicinal	T41.5X1	T41.5X2	T41.5X3	T41.5X4	T41.5X5	T41.5X6
nonmedicinal	T59.7X1	T59.7X2	T59.7X3	T59.7X4	—	—
snow	T49.4X1	T49.4X2	T49.4X3	T49.4X4	T49.4X5	T49.4X6
disulfide (liquid)	T65.4X1	T65.4X2	T65.4X3	T65.4X4	—	—
vapor	T65.4X1	T65.4X2	T65.4X3	T65.4X4	—	—
monoxide (from incomplete combustion)	T58.91	T58.92	T58.93	T58.94	—	—
blast furnace gas	T58.8X1	T58.8X2	T58.8X3	T58.8X4	—	—
butane (distributed in mobile container)	T58.11	T58.12	T58.13	T58.14	—	—
distributed through pipes	T58.11	T58.12	T58.13	T58.14	—	—
charcoal fumes	T58.2X1	T58.2X2	T58.2X3	T58.2X4	—	—
coal	T58.2X1	T58.2X2	T58.2X3	T58.2X4		
coke (in domestic stoves, fireplaces)	T58.2X1	T58.2X2	T58.2X3	T58.2X4	—	—
gas (piped)	T58.11	T58.12	T58.13	T58.14	—	—
solid (in domestic stoves, fireplaces)	T58.2X1	T58.2X2	T58.2X3	T58.2X4	—	—
exhaust gas (motor) not in transit	T58.Ø1	T58.Ø2	T58.Ø3	T58.Ø4	—	—
combustion engine, any not in watercraft	T58.Ø1	T58.Ø2	T58.Ø3	T58.Ø4	—	—
farm tractor, not in transit	T58.Ø1	T58.Ø2	T58.Ø3	T58.Ø4	—	—
gas engine	T58.Ø1	T58.Ø2	T58.Ø3	T58.Ø4	—	—
motor pump	T58.Ø1	T58.Ø2	T58.Ø3	T58.Ø4	—	—
motor vehicle, not in transit	T58.Ø1	T58.Ø2	T58.Ø3	T58.Ø4	—	—
fuel (in domestic use)	T58.2X1	T58.2X2	T58.2X3	T58.2X4	—	—
gas (piped)	T58.11	T58.12	T58.13	T58.14	—	—
in mobile container	T58.11	T58.12	T58.13	T58.14	—	—
utility	T58.11	T58.12	T58.13	T58.14	—	—
in mobile container	T58.11	T58.12	T58.13	T58.14	—	—
piped (natural)	T58.11	T58.12	T58.13	T58.14	—	—

Substance	External Cause (T-Code) Poisoning, Accidental (Unintentional)	Poisoning, Intentional Self-Harm	Poisoning, Assault	Poisoning, Undetermined	Adverse Effect	Underdosing
Carbon *(Continued)*						
monoxide *(Continued)*						
illuminating gas	T58.11	T58.12	T58.13	T58.14	—	—
industrial fuels or gases, any	T58.8X1	T58.8X2	T58.8X3	T58.8X4	—	—
kerosene (in domestic stoves, fireplaces)	T58.2X1	T58.2X2	T58.2X3	T58.2X4	—	—
kiln gas or vapor	T58.8X1	T58.8X2	T58.8X3	T58.8X4	—	—
motor exhaust gas, not in transit	T58.Ø1	T58.Ø2	T58.Ø3	T58.Ø4	—	—
piped gas (manufactured) (natural)	T58.11	T58.12	T58.13	T58.14	—	—
producer gas	T58.8X1	T58.8X2	T58.8X3	T58.8X4	—	—
propane (distributed in mobile container)	T58.11	T58.12	T58.13	T58.14	—	—
distributed through pipes	T58.11	T58.12	T58.13	T58.14	—	—
specified source NEC	T58.8X1	T58.8X2	T58.8X3	T58.8X4	—	—
stove gas	T58.11	T58.12	T58.13	T58.14	—	—
piped	T58.11	T58.12	T58.13	T58.14	—	—
utility gas	T58.11	T58.12	T58.13	T58.14	—	—
piped	T58.11	T58.12	T58.13	T58.14	—	—
water gas	T58.11	T58.12	T58.13	T58.14	—	—
wood (in domestic stoves, fireplaces)	T58.2X1	T58.2X2	T58.2X3	T58.2X4	—	—
tetrachloride (vapor) NEC	T53.ØX1	T53.ØX2	T53.ØX3	T53.ØX4	—	—
liquid (cleansing agent) NEC	T53.ØX1	T53.ØX2	T53.ØX3	T53.ØX4	—	—
solvent	T53.ØX1	T53.ØX2	T53.ØX3	T53.ØX4	—	—
Carbonic acid gas	T59.7X1	T59.7X2	T59.7X3	T59.7X4	—	—
anhydrase inhibitor NEC	T5Ø.2X1	T5Ø.2X2	T5Ø.2X3	T5Ø.2X4	T5Ø.2X5	T5Ø.2X6
Carbophenothion	T6Ø.ØX1	T6Ø.ØX2	T6Ø.ØX3	T6Ø.ØX4	—	—
Carboplatin	T45.1X1	T45.1X2	T45.1X3	T45.1X4	T45.1X5	T45.1X6
Carboprost	T48.ØX1	T48.ØX2	T48.ØX3	T48.ØX4	T48.ØX5	T48.ØX6
Carboquone	T45.1X1	T45.1X2	T45.1X3	T45.1X4	T45.1X5	T45.1X6
Carbowax	T49.3X1	T49.3X2	T49.3X3	T49.3X4	T49.3X5	T49.3X6
Carboxymethyl-cellulose	T47.4X1	T47.4X2	T47.4X3	T47.4X4	T47.4X5	T47.4X6
S-Carboxymethyl-cysteine	T48.4X1	T48.4X2	T48.4X3	T48.4X4	T48.4X5	T48.4X6
Carbrital	T42.3X1	T42.3X2	T42.3X3	T42.3X4	T42.3X5	T42.3X6
Carbromal	T42.6X1	T42.6X2	T42.6X3	T42.6X4	T42.6X5	T42.6X6
Carbutamide	T38.3X1	T38.3X2	T38.3X3	T38.3X4	T38.3X5	T38.3X6
Carbuterol	T48.6X1	T48.6X2	T48.6X3	T48.6X4	T48.6X5	T48.6X6
Cardiac						
depressants	T46.2X1	T46.2X2	T46.2X3	T46.2X4	T46.2X5	T46.2X6
rhythm regulator	T46.2X1	T46.2X2	T46.2X3	T46.2X4	T46.2X5	T46.2X6
specified NEC	T46.2X1	T46.2X2	T46.2X3	T46.2X4	T46.2X5	T46.2X6

Substance	External Cause (T-Code) Poisoning, Accidental (Unintentional)	Poisoning, Intentional Self-Harm	Poisoning, Assault	Poisoning, Undetermined	Adverse Effect	Underdosing
Cardiografin	T5Ø.8X1	T5Ø.8X2	T5Ø.8X3	T5Ø.8X4	T5Ø.8X5	T5Ø.8X6
Cardio-green	T5Ø.8X1	T5Ø.8X2	T5Ø.8X3	T5Ø.8X4	T5Ø.8X5	T5Ø.8X6
Cardiotonic (glycoside) NEC	T46.ØX1	T46.ØX2	T46.ØX3	T46.ØX4	T46.ØX5	T46.ØX6
Cardiovascular drug NEC	T46.9Ø1	T46.9Ø2	T46.9Ø3	T46.9Ø4	T46.9Ø5	T46.9Ø6
Cardrase	T5Ø.2X1	T5Ø.2X2	T5Ø.2X3	T5Ø.2X4	T5Ø.2X5	T5Ø.2X6
Carfusin	T49.ØX1	T49.ØX2	T49.ØX3	T49.ØX4	T49.ØX5	T49.ØX6
Carfecillin	T36.ØX1	T36.ØX2	T36.ØX3	T36.ØX4	T36.ØX5	T36.ØX6
Carfenazine	T43.3X1	T43.3X2	T43.3X3	T43.3X4	T43.3X5	T43.3X6
Carindacillin	T36.ØX1	T36.ØX2	T36.ØX3	T36.ØX4	T36.ØX5	T36.ØX6
Carisoprodol	T42.8X1	T42.8X2	T42.8X3	T42.8X4	T42.8X5	T42.8X6
Carmellose	T47.4X1	T47.4X2	T47.4X3	T47.4X4	T47.4X5	T47.4X6
Carminative	T47.5X1	T47.5X2	T47.5X3	T47.5X4	T47.5X5	T47.5X6
Carmofur	T45.1X1	T45.1X2	T45.1X3	T45.1X4	T45.1X5	T45.1X6
Carmustine	T45.1X1	T45.1X2	T45.1X3	T45.1X4	T45.1X5	T45.1X6
Carotene	T45.2X1	T45.2X2	T45.2X3	T45.2X4	T45.2X5	T45.2X6
Carphenazine	T43.3X1	T43.3X2	T43.3X3	T43.3X4	T43.3X5	T43.3X6
Carpipramine	T42.4X1	T42.4X2	T42.4X3	T42.4X4	T42.4X5	T42.4X6
Carprofen	T39.311	T39.312	T39.313	T39.314	T39.315	T39.316
Carpronium chloride	T44.3X1	T44.3X2	T44.3X3	T44.3X4	T44.3X5	T44.3X6
Carrageenan	T47.8X1	T47.8X2	T47.8X3	T47.8X4	T47.8X5	T47.8X6
Carteolol	T44.7X1	T44.7X2	T44.7X3	T44.7X4	T44.7X5	T44.7X6
Carter's Little Pills	T47.2X1	T47.2X2	T47.2X3	T47.2X4	T47.2X5	T47.2X6
Cascara (sagrada)	T47.2X1	T47.2X2	T47.2X3	T47.2X4	T47.2X5	T47.2X6
Cassava	T62.2X1	T62.2X2	T62.2X3	T62.2X4	—	—
Castellani's paint	T49.ØX1	T49.ØX2	T49.ØX3	T49.ØX4	T49.ØX5	T49.ØX6
Castor						
bean	T62.2X1	T62.2X2	T62.2X3	T62.2X4	—	—
oil	T47.2X1	T47.2X2	T47.2X3	T47.2X4	T47.2X5	T47.2X6
Catalase	T45.3X1	T45.3X2	T45.3X3	T45.3X4	T45.3X5	T45.3X6
Caterpillar (sting)	T63.431	T63.432	T63.433	T63.434	—	—
Catha (edulis) (tea)	T43.691	T43.692	T43.693	T43.694	—	—
Cathartic NEC	T47.4X1	T47.4X2	T47.4X3	T47.4X4	T47.4X5	T47.4X6
anthacene derivative	T47.2X1	T47.2X2	T47.2X3	T47.2X4	T47.2X5	T47.2X6
bulk	T47.4X1	T47.4X2	T47.4X3	T47.4X4	T47.4X5	T47.4X6
contact	T47.2X1	T47.2X2	T47.2X3	T47.2X4	T47.2X5	T47.2X6
emollient NEC	T47.4X1	T47.4X2	T47.4X3	T47.4X4	T47.4X5	T47.4X6
irritant NEC	T47.2X1	T47.2X2	T47.2X3	T47.2X4	T47.2X5	T47.2X6
mucilage	T47.4X1	T47.4X2	T47.4X3	T47.4X4	T47.4X5	T47.4X6
saline	T47.3X1	T47.3X2	T47.3X3	T47.3X4	T47.3X5	T47.3X6
vegetable	T47.2X1	T47.2X2	T47.2X3	T47.2X4	T47.2X5	T47.2X6
Cathine	T5Ø.5X1	T5Ø.5X2	T5Ø.5X3	T5Ø.5X4	T5Ø.5X5	T5Ø.5X6
Cathomycin	T36.8X1	T36.8X2	T36.8X3	T36.8X4	T36.8X5	T36.8X6

Substance	External Cause (T-Code) Poisoning, Accidental (Unintentional)	Poisoning, Intentional Self-Harm	Poisoning, Assault	Poisoning, Undetermined	Adverse Effect	Underdosing
Cation exchange resin	T5Ø.3X1	T5Ø.3X2	T5Ø.3X3	T5Ø.3X4	T5Ø.3X5	T5Ø.3X6
Caustic(s) NEC	T54.91	T54.92	T54.93	T54.94	—	—
alkali	T54.3X1	T54.3X2	T54.3X3	T54.3X4	—	—
hydroxide	T54.3X1	T54.3X2	T54.3X3	T54.3X4	—	—
potash	T54.3X1	T54.3X2	T54.3X3	T54.3X4	—	—
soda	T54.3X1	T54.3X2	T54.3X3	T54.3X4	—	—
specified NEC	T54.91	T54.92	T54.93	T54.94	—	—
Ceepryn	T49.ØX1	T49.ØX2	T49.ØX3	T49.ØX4	T49.ØX5	T49.ØX6
ENT agent	T49.6X1	T49.6X2	T49.6X3	T49.6X4	T49.6X5	T49.6X6
lozenges	T49.6X1	T49.6X2	T49.6X3	T49.6X4	T49.6X5	T49.6X6
Cefacetrile	T36.1X1	T36.1X2	T36.1X3	T36.1X4	T36.1X5	T36.1X6
Cefaclor	T36.1X1	T36.1X2	T36.1X3	T36.1X4	T36.1X5	T36.1X6
Cefadroxil	T36.1X1	T36.1X2	T36.1X3	T36.1X4	T36.1X5	T36.1X6
Cefalexin	T36.1X1	T36.1X2	T36.1X3	T36.1X4	T36.1X5	T36.1X6
Cefaloglycin	T36.1X1	T36.1X2	T36.1X3	T36.1X4	T36.1X5	T36.1X6
Cefaloridine	T36.1X1	T36.1X2	T36.1X3	T36.1X4	T36.1X5	T36.1X6
Cefalosporins	T36.1X1	T36.1X2	T36.1X3	T36.1X4	T36.1X5	T36.1X6
Cefalotin	T36.1X1	T36.1X2	T36.1X3	T36.1X4	T36.1X5	T36.1X6
Cefamandole	T36.1X1	T36.1X2	T36.1X3	T36.1X4	T36.1X5	T36.1X6
Cefamycin antibiotic	T36.1X1	T36.1X2	T36.1X3	T36.1X4	T36.1X5	T36.1X6
Cefapirin	T36.1X1	T36.1X2	T36.1X3	T36.1X4	T36.1X5	T36.1X6
Cefatrizine	T36.1X1	T36.1X2	T36.1X3	T36.1X4	T36.1X5	T36.1X6
Cefazedone	T36.1X1	T36.1X2	T36.1X3	T36.1X4	T36.1X5	T36.1X6
Cefazolin	T36.1X1	T36.1X2	T36.1X3	T36.1X4	T36.1X5	T36.1X6
Cefbuperazone	T36.1X1	T36.1X2	T36.1X3	T36.1X4	T36.1X5	T36.1X6
Cefetamet	T36.1X1	T36.1X2	T36.1X3	T36.1X4	T36.1X5	T36.1X6
Cefixime	T36.1X1	T36.1X2	T36.1X3	T36.1X4	T36.1X5	T36.1X6
Cefmenoxime	T36.1X1	T36.1X2	T36.1X3	T36.1X4	T36.1X5	T36.1X6
Cefmetazole	T36.1X1	T36.1X2	T36.1X3	T36.1X4	T36.1X5	T36.1X6
Cefminox	T36.1X1	T36.1X2	T36.1X3	T36.1X4	T36.1X5	T36.1X6
Cefonicid	T36.1X1	T36.1X2	T36.1X3	T36.1X4	T36.1X5	T36.1X6
Cefoperazone	T36.1X1	T36.1X2	T36.1X3	T36.1X4	T36.1X5	T36.1X6
Ceforanide	T36.1X1	T36.1X2	T36.1X3	T36.1X4	T36.1X5	T36.1X6
Cefotaxime	T36.1X1	T36.1X2	T36.1X3	T36.1X4	T36.1X5	T36.1X6
Cefotetan	T36.1X1	T36.1X2	T36.1X3	T36.1X4	T36.1X5	T36.1X6
Cefotiam	T36.1X1	T36.1X2	T36.1X3	T36.1X4	T36.1X5	T36.1X6
Cefoxitin	T36.1X1	T36.1X2	T36.1X3	T36.1X4	T36.1X5	T36.1X6
Cefpimizole	T36.1X1	T36.1X2	T36.1X3	T36.1X4	T36.1X5	T36.1X6
Cefpiramide	T36.1X1	T36.1X2	T36.1X3	T36.1X4	T36.1X5	T36.1X6
Cefradine	T36.1X1	T36.1X2	T36.1X3	T36.1X4	T36.1X5	T36.1X6
Cefroxadine	T36.1X1	T36.1X2	T36.1X3	T36.1X4	T36.1X5	T36.1X6
Cefsulodin	T36.1X1	T36.1X2	T36.1X3	T36.1X4	T36.1X5	T36.1X6

Substance	External Cause (T-Code) Poisoning, Accidental (Unintentional)	Poisoning, Intentional Self-Harm	Poisoning, Assault	Poisoning, Undetermined	Adverse Effect	Underdosing
Ceftazidime	T36.1X1	T36.1X2	T36.1X3	T36.1X4	T36.1X5	T36.1X6
Cefteram	T36.1X1	T36.1X2	T36.1X3	T36.1X4	T36.1X5	T36.1X6
Ceftezole	T36.1X1	T36.1X2	T36.1X3	T36.1X4	T36.1X5	T36.1X6
Ceftizoxime	T36.1X1	T36.1X2	T36.1X3	T36.1X4	T36.1X5	T36.1X6
Ceftriaxone	T36.1X1	T36.1X2	T36.1X3	T36.1X4	T36.1X5	T36.1X6
Cefuroxime	T36.1X1	T36.1X2	T36.1X3	T36.1X4	T36.1X5	T36.1X6
Cefuzonam	T36.1X1	T36.1X2	T36.1X3	T36.1X4	T36.1X5	T36.1X6
Celestone	T38.ØX1	T38.ØX2	T38.ØX3	T38.ØX4	T38.ØX5	T38.ØX6
topical	T49.ØX1	T49.ØX2	T49.ØX3	T49.ØX4	T49.ØX5	T49.ØX6
Celiprolol	T44.7X1	T44.7X2	T44.7X3	T44.7X4	T44.7X5	T44.7X6
Cellosolve	T52.91	T52.92	T52.93	T52.94	—	—
Cell stimulants and proliferants	T49.8X1	T49.8X2	T49.8X3	T49.8X4	T49.8X5	T49.8X6
Cellulose						
cathartic	T47.4X1	T47.4X2	T47.4X3	T47.4X4	T47.4X5	T47.4X6
hydroxyethyl	T47.4X1	T47.4X2	T47.4X3	T47.4X4	T47.4X5	T47.4X6
nitrates (topical)	T49.3X1	T49.3X2	T49.3X3	T49.3X4	T49.3X5	T49.3X6
oxidized	T49.4X1	T49.4X2	T49.4X3	T49.4X4	T49.4X5	T49.4X6
Centipede (bite)	T63.411	T63.412	T63.413	T63.414	—	—
Central nervous system						
depressants	T42.71	T42.72	T42.73	T42.74	T42.75	T42.76
anesthetic (general) NEC	T41.2Ø1	T41.2Ø2	T41.2Ø3	T41.2Ø4	T41.2Ø5	T41.2Ø6
gases NEC	T41.ØX1	T41.ØX2	T41.ØX3	T41.ØX4	T41.ØX5	T41.ØX6
intravenous	T41.1X1	T41.1X2	T41.1X3	T41.1X4	T41.1X5	T41.1X6
barbiturates	T42.3X1	T42.3X2	T42.3X3	T42.3X4	T42.3X5	T42.3X6
benzodiazepines	T42.4X1	T42.4X2	T42.4X3	T42.4X4	T42.4X5	T42.4X6
bromides	T42.6X1	T42.6X2	T42.6X3	T42.6X4	T42.6X5	T42.6X6
cannabis sativa	T4Ø.7X1	T4Ø.7X2	T4Ø.7X3	T4Ø.7X4	T4Ø.7X5	T4Ø.7X6
chloral hydrate	T42.6X1	T42.6X2	T42.6X3	T42.6X4	T42.6X5	T42.6X6
ethanol	T51.ØX1	T51.ØX2	T51.ØX3	T51.ØX4	—	—
hallucinogenics	T4Ø.9Ø1	T4Ø.9Ø2	T4Ø.9Ø3	T4Ø.9Ø4	T4Ø.9Ø5	T4Ø.9Ø6
hypnotics	T42.71	T42.72	T42.73	T42.74	T42.75	T42.76
specified NEC	T42.6X1	T42.6X2	T42.6X3	T42.6X4	T42.6X5	T42.6X6
muscle relaxants	T42.8X1	T42.8X2	T42.8X3	T42.8X4	T42.8X5	T42.8X6
paraldehyde	T42.6X1	T42.6X2	T42.6X3	T42.6X4	T42.6X5	T42.6X6
sedatives; sedative-hypnotics	T42.71	T42.72	T42.73	T42.74	T42.75	T42.76
mixed NEC	T42.6X1	T42.6X2	T42.6X3	T42.6X4	T42.6X5	T42.6X6
specified NEC	T42.6X1	T42.6X2	T42.6X3	T42.6X4	T42.6X5	T42.6X6
muscle-tone depressants	T42.8X1	T42.8X2	T42.8X3	T42.8X4	T42.8X5	T42.8X6
stimulants	T43.6Ø1	T43.6Ø2	T43.6Ø3	T43.6Ø4	T43.6Ø5	T43.6Ø6
amphetamines	T43.621	T43.622	T43.623	T43.624	T43.625	T43.626
analeptics	T5Ø.7X1	T5Ø.7X2	T5Ø.7X3	T5Ø.7X4	T5Ø.7X5	T5Ø.7X6

Substance	Poisoning, Accidental (Unintentional)	Poisoning, Intentional Self-Harm	Poisoning, Assault	Poisoning, Undetermined	Adverse Effect	Underdosing
	External Cause (T-Code)					
Central nervous system *(Continued)*						
stimulants *(Continued)*						
antidepressants	T43.2Ø1	T43.2Ø2	T43.2Ø3	T43.2Ø4	T43.2Ø5	T43.2Ø6
opiate antagonists	T5Ø.7X1	T5Ø.7X2	T5Ø.7X3	T5Ø.7X4	T5Ø.7X5	T5Ø.7X6
specified NEC	T43.691	T43.692	T43.693	T43.694	T43.695	T43.696
Cephalexin	T36.1X1	T36.1X2	T36.1X3	T36.1X4	T36.1X5	T36.1X6
Cephaloglycin	T36.1X1	T36.1X2	T36.1X3	T36.1X4	T36.1X5	T36.1X6
Cephaloridine	T36.1X1	T36.1X2	T36.1X3	T36.1X4	T36.1X5	T36.1X6
Cephalosporins	T36.1X1	T36.1X2	T36.1X3	T36.1X4	T36.1X5	T36.1X6
N (adicillin)	T36.ØX1	T36.ØX2	T36.ØX3	T36.ØX4	T36.ØX5	T36.ØX6
Cephalothin	T36.1X1	T36.1X2	T36.1X3	T36.1X4	T36.1X5	T36.1X6
Cephalotin	T36.1X1	T36.1X2	T36.1X3	T36.1X4	T36.1X5	T36.1X6
Cephradine	T36.1X1	T36.1X2	T36.1X3	T36.1X4	T36.1X5	T36.1X6
Cerbera (odallam)	T62.2X1	T62.2X2	T62.2X3	T62.2X4	—	—
Cerberin	T46.ØX1	T46.ØX2	T46.ØX3	T46.ØX4	T46.ØX5	T46.ØX6
Cerebral stimulants	T43.6Ø1	T43.6Ø2	T43.6Ø3	T43.6Ø4	T43.6Ø5	T43.6Ø6
psychotherapeutic	T43.6Ø1	T43.6Ø2	T43.6Ø3	T43.6Ø4	T43.6Ø5	T43.6Ø6
specified NEC	T43.691	T43.692	T43.693	T43.694	T43.695	T43.696
Cerium oxalate	T45.ØX1	T45.ØX2	T45.ØX3	T45.ØX4	T45.ØX5	T45.ØX6
Cerous oxalate	T45.ØX1	T45.ØX2	T45.ØX3	T45.ØX4	T45.ØX5	T45.ØX6
Ceruletide	T5Ø.8X1	T5Ø.8X2	T5Ø.8X3	T5Ø.8X4	T5Ø.8X5	T5Ø.8X6
Cetalkonium (chloride)	T49.ØX1	T49.ØX2	T49.ØX3	T49.ØX4	T49.ØX5	T49.ØX6
Cethexonium chloride	T49.ØX1	T49.ØX2	T49.ØX3	T49.ØX4	T49.ØX5	T49.ØX6
Cetiedil	T46.7X1	T46.7X2	T46.7X3	T46.7X4	T46.7X5	T46.7X6
Cetirizine	T45.ØX1	T45.ØX2	T45.ØX3	T45.ØX4	T45.ØX5	T45.ØX6
Cetomacrogol	T5Ø.991	T5Ø.992	T5Ø.993	T5Ø.994	T5Ø.995	T5Ø.996
Cetotiamine	T45.2X1	T45.2X2	T45.2X3	T45.2X4	T45.2X5	T45.2X6
Cetoxime	T45.ØX1	T45.ØX2	T45.ØX3	T45.ØX4	T45.ØX5	T45.ØX6
Cetraxate	T47.1X1	T47.1X2	T47.1X3	T47.1X4	T47.1X5	T47.1X6
Cetrimide	T49.ØX1	T49.ØX2	T49.ØX3	T49.ØX4	T49.ØX5	T49.ØX6
Cetrimonium (bromide)	T49.ØX1	T49.ØX2	T49.ØX3	T49.ØX4	T49.ØX5	T49.ØX6
Cetylpyridinium chloride	T49.ØX1	T49.ØX2	T49.ØX3	T49.ØX4	T49.ØX5	T49.ØX6
ENT agent	T49.6X1	T49.6X2	T49.6X3	T49.6X4	T49.6X5	T49.6X6
lozenges	T49.6X1	T49.6X2	T49.6X3	T49.6X4	T49.6X5	T49.6X6
Cevadillasee Sabadilla						
Cevitamic acid	T45.2X1	T45.2X2	T45.2X3	T45.2X4	T45.2X5	T45.2X6
Chalk, precipitated	T47.1X1	T47.1X2	T47.1X3	T47.1X4	T47.1X5	T47.1X6
Chamomile	T49.ØX1	T49.ØX2	T49.ØX3	T49.ØX4	T49.ØX5	T49.ØX6
Ch'an su	T46.ØX1	T46.ØX2	T46.ØX3	T46.ØX4	T46.ØX5	T46.ØX6
Charcoal	T47.6X1	T47.6X2	T47.6X3	T47.6X4	T47.6X5	T47.6X6
activated — *see also Charcoal, medicinal*	T47.6X1	T47.6X2	T47.6X3	T47.6X4	T47.6X5	T47.6X6

Substance	Poisoning, Accidental (Unintentional)	Poisoning, Intentional Self-Harm	Poisoning, Assault	Poisoning, Undetermined	Adverse Effect	Underdosing
	External Cause (T-Code)					
Charcoal *(Continued)*						
fumes (Carbon monoxide)	T58.2X1	T58.2X2	T58.2X3	T58.2X4	—	—
industrial	T58.8X1	T58.8X2	T58.8X3	T58.8X4	—	—
medicinal (activated)	T47.6X1	T47.6X2	T47.6X3	T47.6X4	T47.6X5	T47.6X6
antidiarrheal	T47.6X1	T47.6X2	T47.6X3	T47.6X4	T47.6X5	T47.6X6
poison control	T47.8X1	T47.8X2	T47.8X3	T47.8X4	T47.8X5	T47.8X6
specified use other than for diarrhea	T47.8X1	T47.8X2	T47.8X3	T47.8X4	T47.8X5	T47.8X6
topical	T49.8X1	T49.8X2	T49.8X3	T49.8X4	T49.8X5	T49.8X6
Chaulmosulfone	T37.1X1	T37.1X2	T37.1X3	T37.1X4	T37.1X5	T37.1X6
Chelating agent NEC	T5Ø.6X1	T5Ø.6X2	T5Ø.6X3	T5Ø.6X4	T5Ø.6X5	T5Ø.6X6
Chelidonium majus	T62.2X1	T62.2X2	T62.2X3	T62.2X4	—	—
Chemical substance NEC	T65.91	T65.92	T65.93	T65.94	—	—
Chenodeoxycholic acid	T47.5X1	T47.5X2	T47.5X3	T47.5X4	T47.5X5	T47.5X6
Chenodiol	T47.5X1	T47.5X2	T47.5X3	T47.5X4	T47.5X5	T47.5X6
Chenopodium	T37.4X1	T37.4X2	T37.4X3	T37.4X4	T37.4X5	T37.4X6
Cherry laurel	T62.2X1	T62.2X2	T62.2X3	T62.2X4	—	—
Chinidin(e)	T46.2X1	T46.2X2	T46.2X3	T46.2X4	T46.2X5	T46.2X6
Chiniofon	T37.8X1	T37.8X2	T37.8X3	T37.8X4	T37.8X5	T37.8X6
Chlophedianol	T48.3X1	T48.3X2	T48.3X3	T48.3X4	T48.3X5	T48.3X6
Chloral	T42.6X1	T42.6X2	T42.6X3	T42.6X4	T42.6X5	T42.6X6
derivative	T42.6X1	T42.6X2	T42.6X3	T42.6X4	T42.6X5	T42.6X6
hydrate	T42.6X1	T42.6X2	T42.6X3	T42.6X4	T42.6X5	T42.6X6
Chloralamide	T42.6X1	T42.6X2	T42.6X3	T42.6X4	T42.6X5	T42.6X6
Chloralodol	T42.6X1	T42.6X2	T42.6X3	T42.6X4	T42.6X5	T42.6X6
Chloralose	T6Ø.4X1	T6Ø.4X2	T6Ø.4X3	T6Ø.4X4	—	—
Chlorambucil	T45.1X1	T45.1X2	T45.1X3	T45.1X4	T45.1X5	T45.1X6
Chloramine	T57.8X1	T57.8X2	T57.8X3	T57.8X4	—	—
T	T49.ØX1	T49.ØX2	T49.ØX3	T49.ØX4	T49.ØX5	T49.ØX6
topical	T49.ØX1	T49.ØX2	T49.ØX3	T49.ØX4	T49.ØX5	T49.ØX6
Chloramphenicol	T36.2X1	T36.2X2	T36.2X3	T36.2X4	T36.2X5	T36.2X6
ENT agent	T49.6X1	T49.6X2	T49.6X3	T49.6X4	T49.6X5	T49.6X6
ophthalmic preparation	T49.5X1	T49.5X2	T49.5X3	T49.5X4	T49.5X5	T49.5X6
topical NEC	T49.ØX1	T49.ØX2	T49.ØX3	T49.ØX4	T49.ØX5	T49.ØX6
Chlorate (potassium) (sodium) NEC	T6Ø.3X1	T6Ø.3X2	T6Ø.3X3	T6Ø.3X4	—	—
herbicide	T6Ø.3X1	T6Ø.3X2	T6Ø.3X3	T6Ø.3X4	—	—
Chlorazanil	T5Ø.2X1	T5Ø.2X2	T5Ø.2X3	T5Ø.2X4	T5Ø.2X5	T5Ø.2X6
Chlorbenzene, chlorbenzol	T53.7X1	T53.7X2	T53.7X3	T53.7X4	—	—
Chlorbenzoxamine	T44.3X1	T44.3X2	T44.3X3	T44.3X4	T44.3X5	T44.3X6
Chlorbutol	T42.6X1	T42.6X2	T42.6X3	T42.6X4	T42.6X5	T42.6X6
Chlorcyclizine	T45.ØX1	T45.ØX2	T45.ØX3	T45.ØX4	T45.ØX5	T45.ØX6

New Revised ~~deleted~~ Deleted

Substance	External Cause (T-Code) Poisoning, Accidental (Unintentional)	Poisoning, Intentional Self-Harm	Poisoning, Assault	Poisoning, Undetermined	Adverse Effect	Underdosing
Chlordan(e) (dust)	T60.1X1	T60.1X2	T60.1X3	T60.1X4	—	—
Chlordantoin	T49.ØX1	T49.ØX2	T49.ØX3	T49.ØX4	T49.ØX5	T49.ØX6
Chlordiazepoxide	T42.4X1	T42.4X2	T42.4X3	T42.4X4	T42.4X5	T42.4X6
Chlordiethyl benzamide	T49.3X1	T49.3X2	T49.3X3	T49.3X4	T49.3X5	T49.3X6
Chloresium	T49.8X1	T49.8X2	T49.8X3	T49.8X4	T49.8X5	T49.8X6
Chlorethiazol	T42.6X1	T42.6X2	T42.6X3	T42.6X4	T42.6X5	T42.6X6
Chlorethyl — *see Ethyl chloride*						
Chloretone	T42.6X1	T42.6X2	T42.6X3	T42.6X4	T42.6X5	T42.6X6
Chlorex	T53.6X1	T53.6X2	T53.6X3	T53.6X4	—	—
insecticide	T6Ø.1X1	T6Ø.1X2	T6Ø.1X3	T6Ø.1X4	—	—
Chlorfenvinphos	T6Ø.ØX1	T6Ø.ØX2	T6Ø.ØX3	T6Ø.ØX4	—	—
Chlorhexadol	T42.6X1	T42.6X2	T42.6X3	T42.6X4	T42.6X5	T42.6X6
Chlorhexamide	T45.1X1	T45.1X2	T45.1X3	T45.1X4	T45.1X5	T45.1X6
Chlorhexidine	T49.ØX1	T49.ØX2	T49.ØX3	T49.ØX4	T49.ØX5	T49.ØX6
Chlorhydroxyquinolin	T49.ØX1	T49.ØX2	T49.ØX3	T49.ØX4	T49.ØX5	T49.ØX6
Chloride of lime (bleach)	T54.3X1	T54.3X2	T54.3X3	T54.3X4	—	—
Chlorimipramine	T43.Ø11	T43.Ø12	T43.Ø13	T43.Ø14	T43.Ø15	T43.Ø16
Chlorinated						
camphene	T53.6X1	T53.6X2	T53.6X3	T53.6X4	—	—
diphenyl	T53.7X1	T53.7X2	T53.7X3	T53.7X4	—	—
hydrocarbons NEC	T53.91	T53.92	T53.93	T53.94	—	—
solvents	T53.91	T53.92	T53.93	T53.94	—	—
lime (bleach)	T54.3X1	T54.3X2	T54.3X3	T54.3X4	—	—
and boric acid solution	T49.ØX1	T49.ØX2	T49.ØX3	T49.ØX4	T49.ØX5	T49.ØX6
naphthalene (insecticide)	T6Ø.1X1	T6Ø.1X2	T6Ø.1X3	T6Ø.1X4	—	—
industrial (non-pesticide)	T53.7X1	T53.7X2	T53.7X3	T53.7X4	—	—
pesticide NEC	T6Ø.8X1	T6Ø.8X2	T6Ø.8X3	T6Ø.8X4	—	—
soda — *see also Sodium hypochlorite*						
solution	T49.ØX1	T49.ØX2	T49.ØX3	T49.ØX4	T49.ØX5	T49.ØX6
Chlorine (fumes) (gas)	T59.4X1	T59.4X2	T59.4X3	T59.4X4	—	—
bleach	T54.3X1	T54.3X2	T54.3X3	T54.3X4	—	—
compound gas NEC	T59.4X1	T59.4X2	T59.4X3	T59.4X4	—	—
disinfectant	T59.4X1	T59.4X2	T59.4X3	T59.4X4	—	—
releasing agents NEC	T59.4X1	T59.4X2	T59.4X3	T59.4X4	—	—
Chlorisondamine chloride	T46.991	T46.992	T46.993	T46.994	T46.995	T46.996
Chlormadinone	T38.5X1	T38.5X2	T38.5X3	T38.5X4	T38.5X5	T38.5X6
Chlormephos	T6Ø.ØX1	T6Ø.ØX2	T6Ø.ØX3	T6Ø.ØX4	—	—
Chlormerodrin	T5Ø.2X1	T5Ø.2X2	T5Ø.2X3	T5Ø.2X4	T5Ø.2X5	T5Ø.2X6
Chlormethiazole	T42.6X1	T42.6X2	T42.6X3	T42.6X4	T42.6X5	T42.6X6
Chlormethine	T45.1X1	T45.1X2	T45.1X3	T45.1X4	T45.1X5	T45.1X6
Chlormethylenecycline	T36.4X1	T36.4X2	T36.4X3	T36.4X4	T36.4X5	T36.4X6
Chlormezanone	T42.6X1	T42.6X2	T42.6X3	T42.6X4	T42.6X5	T42.6X6
Chloroacetic acid	T6Ø.3X1	T6Ø.3X2	T6Ø.3X3	T6Ø.3X4	—	—
Chloroacetone	T59.3X1	T59.3X2	T59.3X3	T59.3X4	—	—
Chloroacetophenone	T59.3X1	T59.3X2	T59.3X3	T59.3X4	—	—
Chloroaniline	T53.7X1	T53.7X2	T53.7X3	T53.7X4	—	—
Chlorobenzene, chlorobenzol	T53.7X1	T53.7X2	T53.7X3	T53.7X4	—	—
Chlorobromomethane (fire extinguisher)	T53.6X1	T53.6X2	T53.6X3	T53.6X4	—	—
Chlorobutanol	T49.ØX1	T49.ØX2	T49.ØX3	T49.ØX4	T49.ØX5	T49.ØX6
Chlorocresol	T49.ØX1	T49.ØX2	T49.ØX3	T49.ØX4	T49.ØX5	T49.ØX6
Chlorodehydro-methyltestosterone	T38.7X1	T38.7X2	T38.7X3	T38.7X4	T38.7X5	T38.7X6
Chlorodinitrobenzene	T53.7X1	T53.7X2	T53.7X3	T53.7X4	—	—
dust or vapor	T53.7X1	T53.7X2	T53.7X3	T53.7X4	—	—
Chlorodiphenyl	T53.7X1	T53.7X2	T53.7X3	T53.7X4	—	—
Chloroethane — *see Ethyl chloride*						
Chloroethylene	T53.6X1	T53.6X2	T53.6X3	T53.6X4	—	—
Chlorofluorocarbons	T53.5X1	T53.5X2	T53.5X3	T53.5X4	—	—
Chloroform (fumes) (vapor)	T53.1X1	T53.1X2	T53.1X3	T53.1X4	—	—
anesthetic	T41.ØX1	T41.ØX2	T41.ØX3	T41.ØX4	T41.ØX5	T41.ØX6
solvent	T53.1X1	T53.1X2	T53.1X3	T53.1X4	—	—
water, concentrated	T41.ØX1	T41.ØX2	T41.ØX3	T41.ØX4	T41.ØX5	T41.ØX6
Chloroguanide	T37.2X1	T37.2X2	T37.2X3	T37.2X4	T37.2X5	T37.2X6
Chloromycetin	T36.2X1	T36.2X2	T36.2X3	T36.2X4	T36.2X5	T36.2X6
ENT agent	T49.6X1	T49.6X2	T49.6X3	T49.6X4	T49.6X5	T49.6X6
ophthalmic preparation	T49.5X1	T49.5X2	T49.5X3	T49.5X4	T49.5X5	T49.5X6
otic solution	T49.6X1	T49.6X2	T49.6X3	T49.6X4	T49.6X5	T49.6X6
topical NEC	T49.ØX1	T49.ØX2	T49.ØX3	T49.ØX4	T49.ØX5	T49.ØX6
Chloronitrobenzene	T53.7X1	T53.7X2	T53.7X3	T53.7X4	—	—
dust or vapor	T53.7X1	T53.7X2	T53.7X3	T53.7X4	—	—
Chlorophacinone	T6Ø.4X1	T6Ø.4X2	T6Ø.4X3	T6Ø.4X4	—	—
Chlorophenol	T53.7X1	T53.7X2	T53.7X3	T53.7X4	—	—
Chlorophenothane	T6Ø.1X1	T6Ø.1X2	T6Ø.1X3	T6Ø.1X4	—	—
Chlorophyll	T5Ø.991	T5Ø.992	T5Ø.993	T5Ø.994	T5Ø.995	T5Ø.996
Chloropicrin (fumes)	T53.6X1	T53.6X2	T53.6X3	T53.6X4	—	—
fumigant	T6Ø.8X1	T6Ø.8X2	T6Ø.8X3	T6Ø.8X4	—	—
fungicide	T6Ø.3X1	T6Ø.3X2	T6Ø.3X3	T6Ø.3X4	—	—
pesticide	T6Ø.8X1	T6Ø.8X2	T6Ø.8X3	T6Ø.8X4	—	—
Chloroprocaine	T41.3X1	T41.3X2	T41.3X3	T41.3X4	T41.3X5	T41.3X6
infiltration (subcutaneous)	T41.3X1	T41.3X2	T41.3X3	T41.3X4	T41.3X5	T41.3X6
nerve block (peripheral) (plexus)	T41.3X1	T41.3X2	T41.3X3	T41.3X4	T41.3X5	T41.3X6
spinal	T41.3X1	T41.3X2	T41.3X3	T41.3X4	T41.3X5	T41.3X6

Substance	External Cause (T-Code)					
	Poisoning, Accidental (Unintentional)	Poisoning, Intentional Self-Harm	Poisoning, Assault	Poisoning, Undetermined	Adverse Effect	Underdosing
Chloroptic	T49.5X1	T49.5X2	T49.5X3	T49.5X4	T49.5X5	T49.5X6
Chloropurine	T45.1X1	T45.1X2	T45.1X3	T45.1X4	T45.1X5	T45.1X6
Chloropyramine	T45.ØX1	T45.ØX2	T45.ØX3	T45.ØX4	T45.ØX5	T45.ØX6
Chloropyrifos	T6Ø.ØX1	T6Ø.ØX2	T6Ø.ØX3	T6Ø.ØX4	—	—
Chloropyrilene	T45.ØX1	T45.ØX2	T45.ØX3	T45.ØX4	T45.ØX5	T45.ØX6
Chloroquine	T37.2X1	T37.2X2	T37.2X3	T37.2X4	T37.2X5	T37.2X6
Chlorothalonil	T6Ø.3X1	T6Ø.3X2	T6Ø.3X3	T6Ø.3X4	—	—
Chlorothen	T45.ØX1	T45.ØX2	T45.ØX3	T45.ØX4	T45.ØX5	T45.ØX6
Chlorothiazide	T5Ø.2X1	T5Ø.2X2	T5Ø.2X3	T5Ø.2X4	T5Ø.2X5	T5Ø.2X6
Chlorothymol	T49.4X1	T49.4X2	T49.4X3	T49.4X4	T49.4X5	T49.4X6
Chlorotrianisene	T38.5X1	T38.5X2	T38.5X3	T38.5X4	T38.5X5	T38.5X6
Chlorovinyldichloro-arsine, not in war	T57.ØX1	T57.ØX2	T57.ØX3	T57.ØX4	—	—
Chloroxine	T49.4X1	T49.4X2	T49.4X3	T49.4X4	T49.4X5	T49.4X6
Chloroxylenol	T49.ØX1	T49.ØX2	T49.ØX3	T49.ØX4	T49.ØX5	T49.ØX6
Chlorphenamine	T45.ØX1	T45.ØX2	T45.ØX3	T45.ØX4	T45.ØX5	T45.ØX6
Chlorphenesin	T42.8X1	T42.8X2	T42.8X3	T42.8X4	T42.8X5	T42.8X6
topical (antifungal)	T49.ØX1	T49.ØX2	T49.ØX3	T49.ØX4	T49.ØX5	T49.ØX6
Chlorpheniramine	T45.ØX1	T45.ØX2	T45.ØX3	T45.ØX4	T45.ØX5	T45.ØX6
Chlorphenoxamine	T45.ØX1	T45.ØX2	T45.ØX3	T45.ØX4	T45.ØX5	T45.ØX6
Chlorphentermine	T5Ø.5X1	T5Ø.5X2	T5Ø.5X3	T5Ø.5X4	T5Ø.5X5	T5Ø.5X6
Chlorprocaine — *see Chloroprocaine*						
Chlorproguanil	T37.2X1	T37.2X2	T37.2X3	T37.2X4	T37.2X5	T37.2X6
Chlorpromazine	T43.3X1	T43.3X2	T43.3X3	T43.3X4	T43.3X5	T43.3X6
Chlorpropamide	T38.3X1	T38.3X2	T38.3X3	T38.3X4	T38.3X5	T38.3X6
Chlorprothixene	T43.4X1	T43.4X2	T43.4X3	T43.4X4	T43.4X5	T43.4X6
Chlorquinaldol	T49.ØX1	T49.ØX2	T49.ØX3	T49.ØX4	T49.ØX5	T49.ØX6
Chlorquinol	T49.ØX1	T49.ØX2	T49.ØX3	T49.ØX4	T49.ØX5	T49.ØX6
Chlortalidone	T5Ø.2X1	T5Ø.2X2	T5Ø.2X3	T5Ø.2X4	T5Ø.2X5	T5Ø.2X6
Chlortetracycline	T36.4X1	T36.4X2	T36.4X3	T36.4X4	T36.4X5	T36.4X6
Chlorthalidone	T5Ø.2X1	T5Ø.2X2	T5Ø.2X3	T5Ø.2X4	T5Ø.2X5	T5Ø.2X6
Chlorthiophos	T6Ø.ØX1	T6Ø.ØX2	T6Ø.ØX3	T6Ø.ØX4	—	—
Chlorotrianisene	T38.5X1	T38.5X2	T38.5X3	T38.5X4	T38.5X5	T38.5X6
Chlor-Trimeton	T45.ØX1	T45.ØX2	T45.ØX3	T45.ØX4	T45.ØX5	T45.ØX6
Chlorthion	T6Ø.ØX1	T6Ø.ØX2	T6Ø.ØX3	T6Ø.ØX4	—	—
Chlorzoxazone	T42.8X1	T42.8X2	T42.8X3	T42.8X4	T42.8X5	T42.8X6
Choke damp	T59.7X1	T59.7X2	T59.7X3	T59.7X4	—	—
Cholagogues	T47.5X1	T47.5X2	T47.5X3	T47.5X4	T47.5X5	T47.5X6
Cholebrine	T5Ø.8X1	T5Ø.8X2	T5Ø.8X3	T5Ø.8X4	T5Ø.8X5	T5Ø.8X6
Cholecalciferol	T45.2X1	T45.2X2	T45.2X3	T45.2X4	T45.2X5	T45.2X6
Cholecystokinin	T5Ø.8X1	T5Ø.8X2	T5Ø.8X3	T5Ø.8X4	T5Ø.8X5	T5Ø.8X6
Cholera vaccine	T5Ø.A91	T5Ø.A92	T5Ø.A93	T5Ø.A94	T5Ø.A95	T5Ø.A96

Substance	External Cause (T-Code)					
	Poisoning, Accidental (Unintentional)	Poisoning, Intentional Self-Harm	Poisoning, Assault	Poisoning, Undetermined	Adverse Effect	Underdosing
Choleretic	T47.5X1	T47.5X2	T47.5X3	T47.5X4	T47.5X5	T47.5X6
Cholesterol-lowering agents	T46.6X1	T46.6X2	T46.6X3	T46.6X4	T46.6X5	T46.6X6
Cholestyramine (resin)	T46.6X1	T46.6X2	T46.6X3	T46.6X4	T46.6X5	T46.6X6
Cholic acid	T47.5X1	T47.5X2	T47.5X3	T47.5X4	T47.5X5	T47.5X6
Choline	T48.6X1	T48.6X2	T48.6X3	T48.6X4	T48.6X5	T48.6X6
chloride	T5Ø.991	T5Ø.992	T5Ø.993	T5Ø.994	T5Ø.995	T5Ø.996
dihydrogen citrate	T5Ø.991	T5Ø.992	T5Ø.993	T5Ø.994	T5Ø.995	T5Ø.996
salicylate	T39.Ø91	T39.Ø92	T39.Ø93	T39.Ø94	T39.Ø95	T39.Ø96
theophyllinate	T48.6X1	T48.6X2	T48.6X3	T48.6X4	T48.6X5	T48.6X6
Cholinergic (drug) NEC	T44.1X1	T44.1X2	T44.1X3	T44.1X4	T44.1X5	T44.1X6
muscle tone enhancer	T44.1X1	T44.1X2	T44.1X3	T44.1X4	T44.1X5	T44.1X6
organophosphorus	T44.ØX1	T44.ØX2	T44.ØX3	T44.ØX4	T44.ØX5	T44.ØX6
insecticide	T6Ø.ØX1	T6Ø.ØX2	T6Ø.ØX3	T6Ø.ØX4	—	—
nerve gas	T59.891	T59.892	T59.893	T59.894	—	—
trimethyl ammonium propanediol	T44.1X1	T44.1X2	T44.1X3	T44.1X4	T44.1X5	T44.1X6
Cholinesterase reactivator	T5Ø.6X1	T5Ø.6X2	T5Ø.6X3	T5Ø.6X4	T5Ø.6X5	T5Ø.6X6
Chlorografin	T5Ø.8X1	T5Ø.8X2	T5Ø.8X3	T5Ø.8X4	T5Ø.8X5	T5Ø.8X6
Chorionic gonadotropin	T38.891	T38.892	T38.893	T38.894	T38.895	T38.896
Chromate	T56.2X1	T56.2X2	T56.2X3	T56.2X4	—	—
dust or mist	T56.2X1	T56.2X2	T56.2X3	T56.2X4	—	—
lead — *see also Lead*	T56.ØX1	T56.ØX2	T56.ØX3	T56.ØX4	—	—
paint	T56.ØX1	T56.ØX2	T56.ØX3	T56.ØX4	—	—
Chromic						
acid	T56.2X1	T56.2X2	T56.2X3	T56.2X4	—	—
dust or mist	T56.2X1	T56.2X2	T56.2X3	T56.2X4	—	—
phosphate 32P	T45.1X1	T45.1X2	T45.1X3	T45.1X4	T45.1X5	T45.1X6
Chromium	T56.2X1	T56.2X2	T56.2X3	T56.2X4	—	—
compounds — *see Chromate*						
sesquioxide	T5Ø.8X1	T5Ø.8X2	T5Ø.8X3	T5Ø.8X4	T5Ø.8X5	T5Ø.8X6
Chromomycin A3	T45.1X1	T45.1X2	T45.1X3	T45.1X4	T45.1X5	T45.1X6
Chromonar	T46.3X1	T46.3X2	T46.3X3	T46.3X4	T46.3X5	T46.3X6
Chromyl chloride	T56.2X1	T56.2X2	T56.2X3	T56.2X4	—	—
Chrysarobin	T49.4X1	T49.4X2	T49.4X3	T49.4X4	T49.4X5	T49.4X6
Chrysazin	T47.2X1	T47.2X2	T47.2X3	T47.2X4	T47.2X5	T47.2X6
Chymar	T45.3X1	T45.3X2	T45.3X3	T45.3X4	T45.3X5	T45.3X6
ophthalmic preparation	T49.5X1	T49.5X2	T49.5X3	T49.5X4	T49.5X5	T49.5X6
Chymopapain	T45.3X1	T45.3X2	T45.3X3	T45.3X4	T45.3X5	T45.3X6
Chymotrypsin	T45.3X1	T45.3X2	T45.3X3	T45.3X4	T45.3X5	T45.3X6
ophthalmic preparation	T49.5X1	T49.5X2	T49.5X3	T49.5X4	T49.5X5	T49.5X6
Cianidanol	T5Ø.991	T5Ø.992	T5Ø.993	T5Ø.994	T5Ø.995	T5Ø.996
Cianopramine	T43.Ø11	T43.Ø12	T43.Ø13	T43.Ø14	T43.Ø15	T43.Ø16
Cibenzoline	T46.2X1	T46.2X2	T46.2X3	T46.2X4	T46.2X5	T46.2X6

Substance	Poisoning, Accidental (Unintentional)	Poisoning, Intentional Self-Harm	Poisoning, Assault	Poisoning, Undetermined	Adverse Effect	Underdosing
		External Cause (T-Code)				
Ciclacillin	T36.ØX1	T36.ØX2	T36.ØX3	T36.ØX4	T36.ØX5	T36.ØX6
Ciclobarbital — *see Hexobarbital*						
Ciclonicate	T46.7X1	T46.7X2	T46.7X3	T46.7X4	T46.7X5	T46.7X6
Ciclopirox (olamine)	T49.ØX1	T49.ØX2	T49.ØX3	T49.ØX4	T49.ØX5	T49.ØX6
Ciclosporin	T45.1X1	T45.1X2	T45.1X3	T45.1X4	T45.1X5	T45.1X6
Cicuta maculata or virosa	T62.2X1	T62.2X2	T62.2X3	T62.2X4	—	—
Cicutoxin	T62.2X1	T62.2X2	T62.2X3	T62.2X4	—	—
Cigarette lighter fluid	T52.ØX1	T52.ØX2	T52.ØX3	T52.ØX4	—	—
Cigarettes (tobacco)	T65.221	T65.222	T65.223	T65.224	—	—
Ciguatoxin	T61.Ø1	T61.Ø2	T61.Ø3	T61.Ø4	—	—
Cilazapril	T46.4X1	T46.4X2	T46.4X3	T46.4X4	T46.4X5	T46.4X6
Cimetidine	T47.ØX1	T47.ØX2	T47.ØX3	T47.ØX4	T47.ØX5	T47.ØX6
Cimetropium bromide	T44.3X1	T44.3X2	T44.3X3	T44.3X4	T44.3X5	T44.3X6
Cinchocaine	T41.3X1	T41.3X2	T41.3X3	T41.3X4	T41.3X5	T41.3X6
topical (surface)	T41.3X1	T41.3X2	T41.3X3	T41.3X4	T41.3X5	T41.3X6
Cinchona	T37.2X1	T37.2X2	T37.2X3	T37.2X4	T37.2X5	T37.2X6
Cinchonine alkaloids	T37.2X1	T37.2X2	T37.2X3	T37.2X4	T37.2X5	T37.2X6
Cinchophen	T5Ø.4X1	T5Ø.4X2	T5Ø.4X3	T5Ø.4X4	T5Ø.4X5	T5Ø.4X6
Cinepazide	T46.7X1	T46.7X2	T46.7X3	T46.7X4	T46.7X5	T46.7X6
Cinnamedrine	T48.5X1	T48.5X2	T48.5X3	T48.5X4	T48.5X5	T48.5X6
Cinnarizine	T45.ØX1	T45.ØX2	T45.ØX3	T45.ØX4	T45.ØX5	T45.ØX6
Cinoxacin	T37.8X1	T37.8X2	T37.8X3	T37.8X4	T37.8X5	T37.8X6
Ciprofibrate	T46.6X1	T46.6X2	T46.6X3	T46.6X4	T46.6X5	T46.6X6
Ciprofloxacin	T36.8X1	T36.8X2	T36.8X3	T36.8X4	T36.8X5	T36.8X6
Cisapride	T47.8X1	T47.8X2	T47.8X3	T47.8X4	T47.8X5	T47.8X6
Cisplatin	T45.1X1	T45.1X2	T45.1X3	T45.1X4	T45.1X5	T45.1X6
Citalopram	T43.221	T43.222	T43.223	T43.224	T43.225	T43.226
Citanest	T41.3X1	T41.3X2	T41.3X3	T41.3X4	T41.3X5	T41.3X6
infiltration (subcutaneous)	T41.3X1	T41.3X2	T41.3X3	T41.3X4	T41.3X5	T41.3X6
nerve block (peripheral) (plexus)	T41.3X1	T41.3X2	T41.3X3	T41.3X4	T41.3X5	T41.3X6
Citric acid	T47.5X1	T47.5X2	T47.5X3	T47.5X4	T47.5X5	T47.5X6
Citrovorum (factor)	T45.8X1	T45.8X2	T45.8X3	T45.8X4	T45.8X5	T45.8X6
Claviceps purpurea	T62.2X1	T62.2X2	T62.2X3	T62.2X4	—	—
Clavulanic acid	T36.1X1	T36.1X2	T36.1X3	T36.1X4	T36.1X5	T36.1X6
Cleaner, cleansing agent, type not specified	T65.891	T65.892	T65.893	T65.894	—	—
of paint or varnish	T52.91	T52.92	T52.93	T52.94	—	—
specified type NEC	T65.891	T65.892	T65.893	T65.894	—	—
Clebopride	T47.8X1	T47.8X2	T47.8X3	T47.8X4	T47.8X5	T47.8X6
Clefamide	T37.3X1	T37.3X2	T37.3X3	T37.3X4	T37.3X5	T37.3X6
Clemastine	T45.ØX1	T45.ØX2	T45.ØX3	T45.ØX4	T45.ØX5	T45.ØX6
Clematis vitalba	T62.2X1	T62.2X2	T62.2X3	T62.2X4	—	—

Substance	Poisoning, Accidental (Unintentional)	Poisoning, Intentional Self-Harm	Poisoning, Assault	Poisoning, Undetermined	Adverse Effect	Underdosing
		External Cause (T-Code)				
Clemizole	T45.ØX1	T45.ØX2	T45.ØX3	T45.ØX4	T45.ØX5	T45.ØX6
penicillin	T36.ØX1	T36.ØX2	T36.ØX3	T36.ØX4	T36.ØX5	T36.ØX6
Clenbuterol	T48.6X1	T48.6X2	T48.6X3	T48.6X4	T48.6X5	T48.6X6
Clidinium bromide	T44.3X1	T44.3X2	T44.3X3	T44.3X4	T44.3X5	T44.3X6
Clindamycin	T36.8X1	T36.8X2	T36.8X3	T36.8X4	T36.8X5	T36.8X6
Clinofibrate	T46.6X1	T46.6X2	T46.6X3	T46.6X4	T46.6X5	T46.6X6
Clioquinol	T37.8X1	T37.8X2	T37.8X3	T37.8X4	T37.8X5	T37.8X6
Cliradon	T4Ø.2X1	T4Ø.2X2	T4Ø.2X3	T4Ø.2X4	—	—
Clobazam	T42.4X1	T42.4X2	T42.4X3	T42.4X4	T42.4X5	T42.4X6
Clobenzorex	T5Ø.5X1	T5Ø.5X2	T5Ø.5X3	T5Ø.5X4	T5Ø.5X5	T5Ø.5X6
Clobetasol	T49.ØX1	T49.ØX2	T49.ØX3	T49.ØX4	T49.ØX5	T49.ØX6
Clobetasone	T49.ØX1	T49.ØX2	T49.ØX3	T49.ØX4	T49.ØX5	T49.ØX6
Clobutinol	T48.3X1	T48.3X2	T48.3X3	T48.3X4	T48.3X5	T48.3X6
Clocapramine	T43.ØX1	T43.ØX2	T43.ØX3	T43.ØX4	T43.ØX5	T43.ØX6
Clocortolone	T38.ØX1	T38.ØX2	T38.ØX3	T38.ØX4	T38.ØX5	T38.ØX6
Clodantoin	T49.ØX1	T49.ØX2	T49.ØX3	T49.ØX4	T49.ØX5	T49.ØX6
Clodronic acid	T5Ø.991	T5Ø.992	T5Ø.993	T5Ø.994	T5Ø.995	T5Ø.996
Clofazimine	T37.1X1	T37.1X2	T37.1X3	T37.1X4	T37.1X5	T37.1X6
Clofedanol	T48.3X1	T48.3X2	T48.3X3	T48.3X4	T48.3X5	T48.3X6
Clofenamide	T5Ø.2X1	T5Ø.2X2	T5Ø.2X3	T5Ø.2X4	T5Ø.2X5	T5Ø.2X6
Clofenotane	T49.ØX1	T49.ØX2	T49.ØX3	T49.ØX4	T49.ØX5	T49.ØX6
Clofezone	T39.2X1	T39.2X2	T39.2X3	T39.2X4	T39.2X5	T39.2X6
Clofibrate	T46.6X1	T46.6X2	T46.6X3	T46.6X4	T46.6X5	T46.6X6
Clofibride	T46.6X1	T46.6X2	T46.6X3	T46.6X4	T46.6X5	T46.6X6
Cloforex	T5Ø.5X1	T5Ø.5X2	T5Ø.5X3	T5Ø.5X4	T5Ø.5X5	T5Ø.5X6
Clomacran	T43.ØX1	T43.ØX2	T43.ØX3	T43.ØX4	T43.ØX5	T43.ØX6
Clomethiazole	T42.6X1	T42.6X2	T42.6X3	T42.6X4	T42.6X5	T42.6X6
Clometocillin	T36.ØX1	T36.ØX2	T36.ØX3	T36.ØX4	T36.ØX5	T36.ØX6
Clomifene	T38.5X1	T38.5X2	T38.5X3	T38.5X4	T38.5X5	T38.5X6
Clomiphene	T38.5X1	T38.5X2	T38.5X3	T38.5X4	T38.5X5	T38.5X6
Clomipramine	T43.Ø11	T43.Ø12	T43.Ø13	T43.Ø14	T43.Ø15	T43.Ø16
Clomocycline	T36.4X1	T36.4X2	T36.4X3	T36.4X4	T36.4X5	T36.4X6
Clonazepam	T42.4X1	T42.4X2	T42.4X3	T42.4X4	T42.4X5	T42.4X6
Clonidine	T46.5X1	T46.5X2	T46.5X3	T46.5X4	T46.5X5	T46.5X6
Clonixin	T39.8X1	T39.8X2	T39.8X3	T39.8X4	T39.8X5	T39.8X6
Clopamide	T5Ø.2X1	T5Ø.2X2	T5Ø.2X3	T5Ø.2X4	T5Ø.2X5	T5Ø.2X6
Clopenthixol	T43.4X1	T43.4X2	T43.4X3	T43.4X4	T43.4X5	T43.4X6
Cloperastine	T48.3X1	T48.3X2	T48.3X3	T48.3X4	T48.3X5	T48.3X6
Clophedianol	T48.3X1	T48.3X2	T48.3X3	T48.3X4	T48.3X5	T48.3X6
Cloponone	T36.2X1	T36.2X2	T36.2X3	T36.2X4	T36.2X5	T36.2X6
Cloprednol	T38.ØX1	T38.ØX2	T38.ØX3	T38.ØX4	T38.ØX5	T38.ØX6
Cloral betaine	T42.6X1	T42.6X2	T42.6X3	T42.6X4	T42.6X5	T42.6X6

		External Cause (T-Code)				
Substance	**Poisoning, Accidental (Unintentional)**	**Poisoning, Intentional Self-Harm**	**Poisoning, Assault**	**Poisoning, Undetermined**	**Adverse Effect**	**Underdosing**
Cloramfenicol	T36.2X1	T36.2X2	T36.2X3	T36.2X4	T36.2X5	T36.2X6
Clorazepate (dipotassium)	T42.4X1	T42.4X2	T42.4X3	T42.4X4	T42.4X5	T42.4X6
Clorexolone	T50.2X1	T50.2X2	T50.2X3	T50.2X4	T50.2X5	T50.2X6
Clorox (bleach)	T54.91	T54.92	T54.93	T54.94	—	—
Clorfenamine	T45.0X1	T45.0X2	T45.0X3	T45.0X4	T45.0X5	T45.0X6
Clorgiline	T43.1X1	T43.1X2	T43.1X3	T43.1X4	T43.1X5	T43.1X6
Clorotepine	T44.3X1	T44.3X2	T44.3X3	T44.3X4	T44.3X5	T44.3X6
Clorprenaline	T48.6X1	T48.6X2	T48.6X3	T48.6X4	T48.6X5	T48.6X6
Clortermine	T50.5X1	T50.5X2	T50.5X3	T50.5X4	T50.5X5	T50.5X6
Clotiapine	T43.591	T43.592	T43.593	T43.594	T43.595	T43.596
Clotiazepam	T42.4X1	T42.4X2	T42.4X3	T42.4X4	T42.4X5	T42.4X6
Clotibric acid	T46.6X1	T46.6X2	T46.6X3	T46.6X4	T46.6X5	T46.6X6
Clotrimazole	T49.0X1	T49.0X2	T49.0X3	T49.0X4	T49.0X5	T49.0X6
Cloxacillin	T36.0X1	T36.0X2	T36.0X3	T36.0X4	T36.0X5	T36.0X6
Cloxazolam	T42.4X1	T42.4X2	T42.4X3	T42.4X4	T42.4X5	T42.4X6
Cloxiquine	T49.0X1	T49.0X2	T49.0X3	T49.0X4	T49.0X5	T49.0X6
Clozapine	T42.4X1	T42.4X2	T42.4X3	T42.4X4	T42.4X5	T42.4X6
Coagulant NEC	T45.7X1	T45.7X2	T45.7X3	T45.7X4	T45.7X5	T45.7X6
Coal (carbon monoxide from) — *see also Carbon, monoxide, coal*	T58.2X1	T58.2X2	T58.2X3	T58.2X4	—	—
oil — *see Kerosene*						
tar	T49.1X1	T49.1X2	T49.1X3	T49.1X4	T49.1X5	T49.1X6
fumes	T59.891	T59.892	T59.893	T59.894	—	—
medicinal (ointment)	T49.4X1	T49.4X2	T49.4X3	T49.4X4	T49.4X5	T49.4X6
analgesics NEC	T39.2X1	T39.2X2	T39.2X3	T39.2X4	T39.2X5	T39.2X6
naphtha (solvent)	T52.0X1	T52.0X2	T52.0X3	T52.0X4		
Cobalamine	T45.2X1	T45.2X2	T45.2X3	T45.2X4	T45.2X5	T45.2X6
Cobalt (nonmedicinal) (fumes) (industrial)	T56.891	T56.892	T56.893	T56.894		
medicinal (trace) (chloride)	T45.8X1	T45.8X2	T45.8X3	T45.8X4	T45.8X5	T45.8X6
Cobra (venom)	T63.041	T63.042	T63.043	T63.044		
Coca (leaf)	T40.5X1	T40.5X2	T40.5X3	T40.5X4	T40.5X5	T40.5X6
Cocaine	T40.5X1	T40.5X2	T40.5X3	T40.5X4	T40.5X5	T40.5X6
topical anesthetic	T41.3X1	T41.3X2	T41.3X3	T41.3X4	T41.3X5	T41.3X6
Cocarboxylase	T45.3X1	T45.3X2	T45.3X3	T45.3X4	T45.3X5	T45.3X6
Coccidioidin	T50.8X1	T50.8X2	T50.8X3	T50.8X4	T50.8X5	T50.8X6
Cocculus indicus	T62.1X1	T62.1X2	T62.1X3	T62.1X4		
Cochineal	T65.6X1	T65.6X2	T65.6X3	T65.6X4		
medicinal products	T50.991	T50.992	T50.993	T50.994	T50.995	T50.996
Codeine	T40.2X1	T40.2X2	T40.2X3	T40.2X4	T40.2X5	T40.2X6
Cod-liver oil	T45.2X1	T45.2X2	T45.2X3	T45.2X4	T45.2X5	T45.2X6
Coenzyme A	T50.991	T50.992	T50.993	T50.994	T50.995	T50.996
Coffee	T62.8X1	T62.8X2	T62.8X3	T62.8X4	—	—
Cogalactoisomerase	T50.991	T50.992	T50.993	T50.994	T50.995	T50.996
Cogentin	T44.3X1	T44.3X2	T44.3X3	T44.3X4	T44.3X5	T44.3X6
Coke fumes or gas (carbon monoxide)	T58.2X1	T58.2X2	T58.2X3	T58.2X4	—	—
industrial use	T58.8X1	T58.8X2	T58.8X3	T58.8X4	—	—
Colace	T47.4X1	T47.4X2	T47.4X3	T47.4X4	T47.4X5	T47.4X6
Colaspase	T45.1X1	T45.1X2	T45.1X3	T45.1X4	T45.1X5	T45.1X6
Colchicine	T50.4X1	T50.4X2	T50.4X3	T50.4X4	T50.4X5	T50.4X6
Colchicum	T62.2X1	T62.2X2	T62.2X3	T62.2X4	—	—
Cold cream	T49.3X1	T49.3X2	T49.3X3	T49.3X4	T49.3X5	T49.3X6
Colecalciferol	T45.2X1	T45.2X2	T45.2X3	T45.2X4	T45.2X5	T45.2X6
Colestipol	T46.6X1	T46.6X2	T46.6X3	T46.6X4	T46.6X5	T46.6X6
Colestyramine	T46.6X1	T46.6X2	T46.6X3	T46.6X4	T46.6X5	T46.6X6
Colimycin	T36.8X1	T36.8X2	T36.8X3	T36.8X4	T36.8X5	T36.8X6
Colistimethate	T36.8X1	T36.8X2	T36.8X3	T36.8X4	T36.8X5	T36.8X6
Colistin	T36.8X1	T36.8X2	T36.8X3	T36.8X4	T36.8X5	T36.8X6
sulfate (eye preparation)	T49.5X1	T49.5X2	T49.5X3	T49.5X4	T49.5X5	T49.5X6
Collagen	T50.991	T50.992	T50.993	T50.994	T50.995	T50.996
Collagenase	T49.4X1	T49.4X2	T49.4X3	T49.4X4	T49.4X5	T49.4X6
Collodion	T49.3X1	T49.3X2	T49.3X3	T49.3X4	T49.3X5	T49.3X6
Colocynth	T47.2X1	T47.2X2	T47.2X3	T47.2X4	T47.2X5	T47.2X6
Colophony adhesive	T49.3X1	T49.3X2	T49.3X3	T49.3X4	T49.3X5	T49.3X6
Colorant — *see also Dye*	T50.991	T50.992	T50.993	T50.994	T50.995	T50.996
Coloring matter — *see Dye(s)*						
Combustion gas (after combustion) — *see Carbon, monoxide*						
prior to combustion	T59.891	T59.892	T59.893	T59.894	—	—
Compazine	T43.3X1	T43.3X2	T43.3X3	T43.3X4	T43.3X5	T43.3X6
Compound						
42 (warfarin)	T60.4X1	T60.4X2	T60.4X3	T60.4X4	—	—
269 (endrin)	T60.1X1	T60.1X2	T60.1X3	T60.1X4	—	—
497 (dieldrin)	T60.1X1	T60.1X2	T60.1X3	T60.1X4	—	—
1080 (sodium fluoroacetate)	T60.4X1	T60.4X2	T60.4X3	T60.4X4	—	—
3422 (parathion)	T60.0X1	T60.0X2	T60.0X3	T60.0X4	—	—
3911 (phorate)	T60.0X1	T60.0X2	T60.0X3	T60.0X4	—	—
3956 (toxaphene)	T60.1X1	T60.1X2	T60.1X3	T60.1X4	—	—
4049 (malathion)	T60.0X1	T60.0X2	T60.0X3	T60.0X4	—	—
4069 (malathion)	T60.0X1	T60.0X2	T60.0X3	T60.0X4	—	—
4124 (dicapthon)	T60.0X1	T60.0X2	T60.0X3	T60.0X4	—	—

Substance	External Cause (T-Code)					
	Poisoning, Accidental (Unintentional)	Poisoning, Intentional Self-Harm	Poisoning, Assault	Poisoning, Undetermined	Adverse Effect	Underdosing
Compound *(Continued)*						
E (cortisone)	T38.ØX1	T38.ØX2	T38.ØX3	T38.ØX4	T38.ØX5	T38.ØX6
F (hydrocortisone)	T38.ØX1	T38.ØX2	T38.ØX3	T38.ØX4	T38.ØX5	T38.ØX6
Congener, anabolic	T38.7X1	T38.7X2	T38.7X3	T38.7X4	T38.7X5	T38.7X6
Congo red	T5Ø.8X1	T5Ø.8X2	T5Ø.8X3	T5Ø.8X4	T5Ø.8X5	T5Ø.8X6
Coniine, conine	T62.2X1	T62.2X2	T62.2X3	T62.2X4	—	—
Conium (maculatum)	T62.2X1	T62.2X2	T62.2X3	T62.2X4	—	—
Conjugated estrogenic substances	T38.5X1	T38.5X2	T38.5X3	T38.5X4	T38.5X5	T38.5X6
Contac	T48.5X1	T48.5X2	T48.5X3	T48.5X4	T48.5X5	T48.5X6
Contact lens solution	T49.5X1	T49.5X2	T49.5X3	T49.5X4	T49.5X5	T49.5X6
Contraceptive (oral)	T38.4X1	T38.4X2	T38.4X3	T38.4X4	T38.4X5	T38.4X6
vaginal	T49.8X1	T49.8X2	T49.8X3	T49.8X4	T49.8X5	T49.8X6
Contrast medium, radiography	T5Ø.8X1	T5Ø.8X2	T5Ø.8X3	T5Ø.8X4	T5Ø.8X5	T5Ø.8X6
Convallaria glycosides	T46.ØX1	T46.ØX2	T46.ØX3	T46.ØX4	T46.ØX5	T46.ØX6
Convallaria majalis	T62.2X1	T62.2X2	T62.2X3	T62.2X4	—	—
berry	T62.1X1	T62.1X2	T62.1X3	T62.1X4	—	—
Copper (dust) (fumes) (nonmedicinal) NEC	T56.4X1	T56.4X2	T56.4X3	T56.4X4	—	—
arsenate, arsenite	T57.ØX1	T57.ØX2	T57.ØX3	T57.ØX4	—	—
insecticide	T6Ø.2X1	T6Ø.2X2	T6Ø.2X3	T6Ø.2X4	—	—
emetic	T47.7X1	T47.7X2	T47.7X3	T47.7X4	T47.7X5	T47.7X6
fungicide	T6Ø.3X1	T6Ø.3X2	T6Ø.3X3	T6Ø.3X4	—	—
gluconate	T49.ØX1	T49.ØX2	T49.ØX3	T49.ØX4	T49.ØX5	T49.ØX6
insecticide	T6Ø.2X1	T6Ø.2X2	T6Ø.2X3	T6Ø.2X4	—	—
medicinal (trace)	T45.8X1	T45.8X2	T45.8X3	T45.8X4	T45.8X5	T45.8X6
oleate	T49.ØX1	T49.ØX2	T49.ØX3	T49.ØX4	T49.ØX5	T49.ØX6
sulfate	T56.4X1	T56.4X2	T56.4X3	T56.4X4	—	—
cupric	T56.4X1	T56.4X2	T56.4X3	T56.4X4	—	—
fungicide	T6Ø.3X1	T6Ø.3X2	T6Ø.3X3	T6Ø.3X4	—	—
medicinal						
ear	T49.6X1	T49.6X2	T49.6X3	T49.6X4	T49.6X5	T49.6X6
emetic	T47.7X1	T47.7X2	T47.7X3	T47.7X4	T47.7X5	T47.7X6
eye	T49.5X1	T49.5X2	T49.5X3	T49.5X4	T49.5X5	T49.5X6
cuprous	T56.4X1	T56.4X2	T56.4X3	T56.4X4	—	—
fungicide	T6Ø.3X1	T6Ø.3X2	T6Ø.3X3	T6Ø.3X4	—	—
medicinal						
ear	T49.6X1	T49.6X2	T49.6X3	T49.6X4	T49.6X5	T49.6X6
emetic	T47.7X1	T47.7X2	T47.7X3	T47.7X4	T47.7X5	T47.7X6
eye	T49.5X1	T49.5X2	T49.5X3	T49.5X4	T49.5X5	T49.5X6
Copperhead snake (bite) (venom)	T63.Ø61	T63.Ø62	T63.Ø63	T63.Ø64	—	—
Coral (sting)	T63.691	T63.692	T63.693	T63.694	—	—
snake (bite) (venom)	T63.Ø21	T63.Ø22	T63.Ø23	T63.Ø24	—	—
Corbadrine	T49.6X1	T49.6X2	T49.6X3	T49.6X4	T49.6X5	T49.6X6
Cordran	T49.ØX1	T49.ØX2	T49.ØX3	T49.ØX4	T49.ØX5	T49.ØX6
Cordite	T65.891	T65.892	T65.893	T65.894	—	—
vapor	T59.891	T59.892	T59.893	T59.894	—	—
Corn cures	T49.4X1	T49.4X2	T49.4X3	T49.4X4	T49.4X5	T49.4X6
Cornhusker's lotion	T49.3X1	T49.3X2	T49.3X3	T49.3X4	T49.3X5	T49.3X6
Corn starch	T49.3X1	T49.3X2	T49.3X3	T49.3X4	T49.3X5	T49.3X6
Coronary vasodilator NEC	T46.3X1	T46.3X2	T46.3X3	T46.3X4	T46.3X5	T46.3X6
Corrosive NEC	T54.91	T54.92	T54.93	T54.94	—	—
acid NEC	T54.2X1	T54.2X2	T54.2X3	T54.2X4	—	—
aromatics	T54.1X1	T54.1X2	T54.1X3	T54.1X4	—	—
disinfectant	T54.1X1	T54.1X2	T54.1X3	T54.1X4	—	—
fumes NEC	T54.91	T54.92	T54.93	T54.94	—	—
specified NEC	T54.91	T54.92	T54.93	T54.94	—	—
sublimate	T56.1X1	T56.1X2	T56.1X3	T56.1X4	—	—
Cortate	T38.ØX1	T38.ØX2	T38.ØX3	T38.ØX4	T38.ØX5	T38.ØX6
Cort-Dome	T38.ØX1	T38.ØX2	T38.ØX3	T38.ØX4	T38.ØX5	T38.ØX6
ENT agent	T49.6X1	T49.6X2	T49.6X3	T49.6X4	T49.6X5	T49.6X6
ophthalmic preparation	T49.5X1	T49.5X2	T49.5X3	T49.5X4	T49.5X5	T49.5X6
topical NEC	T49.ØX1	T49.ØX2	T49.ØX3	T49.ØX4	T49.ØX5	T49.ØX6
Cortef	T38.ØX1	T38.ØX2	T38.ØX3	T38.ØX4	T38.ØX5	T38.ØX6
ENT agent	T49.6X1	T49.6X2	T49.6X3	T49.6X4	T49.6X5	T49.6X6
ophthalmic preparation	T49.5X1	T49.5X2	T49.5X3	T49.5X4	T49.5X5	T49.5X6
topical NEC	T49.ØX1	T49.ØX2	T49.ØX3	T49.ØX4	T49.ØX5	T49.ØX6
Corticosteroid	T38.ØX1	T38.ØX2	T38.ØX3	T38.ØX4	T38.ØX5	T38.ØX6
ENT agent	T49.6X1	T49.6X2	T49.6X3	T49.6X4	T49.6X5	T49.6X6
mineral	T5Ø.ØX1	T5Ø.ØX2	T5Ø.ØX3	T5Ø.ØX4	T5Ø.ØX5	T5Ø.ØX6
ophthalmic	T49.5X1	T49.5X2	T49.5X3	T49.5X4	T49.5X5	T49.5X6
topical NEC	T49.ØX1	T49.ØX2	T49.ØX3	T49.ØX4	T49.ØX5	T49.ØX6
Corticotropin	T38.811	T38.812	T38.813	T38.814	T38.815	T38.816
Cortisol	T49.ØX1	T49.ØX2	T49.ØX3	T49.ØX4	T49.ØX5	T49.ØX6
ENT agent	T49.6X1	T49.6X2	T49.6X3	T49.6X4	T49.6X5	T49.6X6
ophthalmic preparation	T49.5X1	T49.5X2	T49.5X3	T49.5X4	T49.5X5	T49.5X6
topical NEC	T49.ØX1	T49.ØX2	T49.ØX3	T49.ØX4	T49.ØX5	T49.ØX6
Cortisone (acetate)	T38.ØX1	T38.ØX2	T38.ØX3	T38.ØX4	T38.ØX5	T38.ØX6
ENT agent	T49.6X1	T49.6X2	T49.6X3	T49.6X4	T49.6X5	T49.6X6
ophthalmic preparation	T49.5X1	T49.5X2	T49.5X3	T49.5X4	T49.5X5	T49.5X6
topical NEC	T49.ØX1	T49.ØX2	T49.ØX3	T49.ØX4	T49.ØX5	T49.ØX6
Cortivazol	T38.ØX1	T38.ØX2	T38.ØX3	T38.ØX4	T38.ØX5	T38.ØX6
Cortogen	T38.ØX1	T38.ØX2	T38.ØX3	T38.ØX4	T38.ØX5	T38.ØX6
ENT agent	T49.6X1	T49.6X2	T49.6X3	T49.6X4	T49.6X5	T49.6X6
ophthalmic preparation	T49.5X1	T49.5X2	T49.5X3	T49.5X4	T49.5X5	T49.5X6

		External Cause (T-Code)				
Substance	Poisoning, Accidental (Unintentional)	Poisoning, Intentional Self-Harm	Poisoning, Assault	Poisoning, Undetermined	Adverse Effect	Underdosing
Cortone	T38.ØX1	T38.ØX2	T38.ØX3	T38.ØX4	T38.ØX5	T38.ØX6
ENT agent	T49.6X1	T49.6X2	T49.6X3	T49.6X4	T49.6X5	T49.6X6
ophthalmic preparation	T49.5X1	T49.5X2	T49.5X3	T49.5X4	T49.5X5	T49.5X6
Cortril	T38.ØX1	T38.ØX2	T38.ØX3	T38.ØX4	T38.ØX5	T38.ØX6
ENT agent	T49.6X1	T49.6X2	T49.6X3	T49.6X4	T49.6X5	T49.6X6
ophthalmic preparation	T49.5X1	T49.5X2	T49.5X3	T49.5X4	T49.5X5	T49.5X6
topical NEC	T49.ØX1	T49.ØX2	T49.ØX3	T49.ØX4	T49.ØX5	T49.ØX6
Corynebacterium parvum	T45.1X1	T45.1X2	T45.1X3	T45.1X4	T45.1X5	T45.1X6
Cosmetic preparation	T49.8X1	T49.8X2	T49.8X3	T49.8X4	T49.8X5	T49.8X6
Cosmetics	T49.8X1	T49.8X2	T49.8X3	T49.8X4	T49.8X5	T49.8X6
Cosyntropin	T38.811	T38.812	T38.813	T38.814	T38.815	T38.816
Cotarnine	T45.7X1	T45.7X2	T45.7X3	T45.7X4	T45.7X5	T45.7X6
Co-trimoxazole	T36.8X1	T36.8X2	T36.8X3	T36.8X4	T36.8X5	T36.8X6
Cottonseed oil	T49.3X1	T49.3X2	T49.3X3	T49.3X4	T49.3X5	T49.3X6
Cough mixture (syrup)	T48.4X1	T48.4X2	T48.4X3	T48.4X4	T48.4X5	T48.4X6
containing opiates	T4Ø.2X1	T4Ø.2X2	T4Ø.2X3	T4Ø.2X4	T4Ø.2X5	T4Ø.2X6
expectorants	T48.4X1	T48.4X2	T48.4X3	T48.4X4	T48.4X5	T48.4X6
Coumadin	T45.511	T45.512	T45.513	T45.514	T45.515	T45.516
rodenticide	T6Ø.4X1	T6Ø.4X2	T6Ø.4X3	T6Ø.4X4	—	—
Coumaphos	T6Ø.ØX1	T6Ø.ØX2	T6Ø.ØX3	T6Ø.ØX4	—	—
Coumarin	T45.511	T45.512	T45.513	T45.514	T45.515	T45.516
Coumetarol	T45.511	T45.512	T45.513	T45.514	T45.515	T45.516
Cowbane	T62.2X1	T62.2X2	T62.2X3	T62.2X4	—	—
Cozyme	T45.2X1	T45.2X2	T45.2X3	T45.2X4	T45.2X5	T45.2X6
Crack	T4Ø.5X1	T4Ø.5X2	T4Ø.5X3	T4Ø.5X4	—	—
Crataegus extract	T46.ØX1	T46.ØX2	T46.ØX3	T46.ØX4	T46.ØX5	T46.ØX6
Creolin	T54.1X1	T54.1X2	T54.1X3	T54.1X4	—	—
disinfectant	T54.1X1	T54.1X2	T54.1X3	T54.1X4	—	—
Creosol (compound)	T49.ØX1	T49.ØX2	T49.ØX3	T49.ØX4	T49.ØX5	T49.ØX6
Creosote (coal tar) (beechwood)	T49.ØX1	T49.ØX2	T49.ØX3	T49.ØX4	T49.ØX5	T49.ØX6
medicinal (expectorant)	T48.4X1	T48.4X2	T48.4X3	T48.4X4	T48.4X5	T48.4X6
syrup	T48.4X1	T48.4X2	T48.4X3	T48.4X4	T48.4X5	T48.4X6
Cresol(s)	T49.ØX1	T49.ØX2	T49.ØX3	T49.ØX4	T49.ØX5	T49.ØX6
and soap solution	T49.ØX1	T49.ØX2	T49.ØX3	T49.ØX4	T49.ØX5	T49.ØX6
Cresyl acetate	T49.ØX1	T49.ØX2	T49.ØX3	T49.ØX4	T49.ØX5	T49.ØX6
Cresylic acid	T49.ØX1	T49.ØX2	T49.ØX3	T49.ØX4	T49.ØX5	T49.ØX6
Crimidine	T6Ø.4X1	T6Ø.4X2	T6Ø.4X3	T6Ø.4X4	—	—
Croconazole	T37.8X1	T37.8X2	T37.8X3	T37.8X4	T37.8X5	T37.8X6
Cromoglicic acid	T48.6X1	T48.6X2	T48.6X3	T48.6X4	T48.6X5	T48.6X6
Cromolyn	T48.6X1	T48.6X2	T48.6X3	T48.6X4	T48.6X5	T48.6X6
Cromonar	T46.3X1	T46.3X2	T46.3X3	T46.3X4	T46.3X5	T46.3X6

		External Cause (T-Code)				
Substance	Poisoning, Accidental (Unintentional)	Poisoning, Intentional Self-Harm	Poisoning, Assault	Poisoning, Undetermined	Adverse Effect	Underdosing
Cropropamide	T39.8X1	T39.8X2	T39.8X3	T39.8X4	T39.8X5	T39.8X6
with crotethamide	T5Ø.7X1	T5Ø.7X2	T5Ø.7X3	T5Ø.7X4	T5Ø.7X5	T5Ø.7X6
Crotamiton	T49.ØX1	T49.ØX2	T49.ØX3	T49.ØX4	T49.ØX5	T49.ØX6
Crotethamide	T39.8X1	T39.8X2	T39.8X3	T39.8X4	T39.8X5	T39.8X6
with cropropamide	T5Ø.7X1	T5Ø.7X2	T5Ø.7X3	T5Ø.7X4	T5Ø.7X5	T5Ø.7X6
Croton (oil)	T47.2X1	T47.2X2	T47.2X3	T47.2X4	T47.2X5	T47.2X6
chloral	T42.6X1	T42.6X2	T42.6X3	T42.6X4	T42.6X5	T42.6X6
Crude oil	T52.ØX1	T52.ØX2	T52.ØX3	T52.ØX4	—	—
Cryogenine	T39.8X1	T39.8X2	T39.8X3	T39.8X4	T39.8X5	T39.8X6
Cryolite (vapor)	T6Ø.1X1	T6Ø.1X2	T6Ø.1X3	T6Ø.1X4	—	—
insecticide	T6Ø.1X1	T6Ø.1X2	T6Ø.1X3	T6Ø.1X4	—	—
Cryptenamine (tannates)	T46.5X1	T46.5X2	T46.5X3	T46.5X4	T46.5X5	T46.5X6
Crystal violet	T49.ØX1	T49.ØX2	T49.ØX3	T49.ØX4	T49.ØX5	T49.ØX6
Cuckoopint	T62.2X1	T62.2X2	T62.2X3	T62.2X4	—	—
Cumetharol	T45.511	T45.512	T45.513	T45.514	T45.515	T45.516
Cupric						
acetate	T6Ø.3X1	T6Ø.3X2	T6Ø.3X3	T6Ø.3X4	—	—
acetoarsenite	T57.ØX1	T57.ØX2	T57.ØX3	T57.ØX4	—	—
arsenate	T57.ØX1	T57.ØX2	T57.ØX3	T57.ØX4	—	—
gluconate	T49.ØX1	T49.ØX2	T49.ØX3	T49.ØX4	T49.ØX5	T49.ØX6
oleate	T49.ØX1	T49.ØX2	T49.ØX3	T49.ØX4	T49.ØX5	T49.ØX6
sulfate	T56.4X1	T56.4X2	T56.4X3	T56.4X4	—	—
Cuprous sulfate — *see also Copper sulfate*	T56.4X1	T56.4X2	T56.4X3	T56.4X4	—	—
Curare, curarine	T48.1X1	T48.1X2	T48.1X3	T48.1X4	T48.1X5	T48.1X6
Cyamemazine	T43.3X1	T43.3X2	T43.3X3	T43.3X4	T43.3X5	T43.3X6
Cyamopsis tetragono-loba	T46.6X1	T46.6X2	T46.6X3	T46.6X4	T46.6X5	T46.6X6
Cyanacetyl hydrazide	T37.1X1	T37.1X2	T37.1X3	T37.1X4	T37.1X5	T37.1X6
Cyanic acid (gas)	T59.891	T59.892	T59.893	T59.894	—	—
Cyanide(s) (compounds) (potassium) (sodium) NEC	T65.ØX1	T65.ØX2	T65.ØX3	T65.ØX4	—	—
dust or gas (inhalation) NEC	T57.3X1	T57.3X2	T57.3X3	T57.3X4	—	—
fumigant	T65.ØX1	T65.ØX2	T65.ØX3	T65.ØX4	—	—
hydrogen	T57.3X1	T57.3X2	T57.3X3	T57.3X4	—	—
mercuric — *see Mercury*						
pesticide (dust) (fumes)	T65.ØX1	T65.ØX2	T65.ØX3	T65.ØX4	—	—
Cyanoacrylate adhesive	T49.3X1	T49.3X2	T49.3X3	T49.3X4	T49.3X5	T49.3X6
Cyanocobalamin	T45.8X1	T45.8X2	T45.8X3	T45.8X4	T45.8X5	T45.8X6
Cyanogen (chloride) (gas) NEC	T59.891	T59.892	T59.893	T59.894	—	—
Cyclacillin	T36.ØX1	T36.ØX2	T36.ØX3	T36.ØX4	T36.ØX5	T36.ØX6
Cyclaine	T41.3X1	T41.3X2	T41.3X3	T41.3X4	T41.3X5	T41.3X6
Cyclamate	T5Ø.991	T5Ø.992	T5Ø.993	T5Ø.994	T5Ø.995	T5Ø.996

	External Cause (T-Code)					
Substance	Poisoning, Accidental (Unintentional)	Poisoning, Intentional Self-Harm	Poisoning, Assault	Poisoning, Undetermined	Adverse Effect	Underdosing
Cyclamen europaeum	T62.2X1	T62.2X2	T62.2X3	T62.2X4	—	—
Cyclandelate	T46.7X1	T46.7X2	T46.7X3	T46.7X4	T46.7X5	T46.7X6
Cyclazocine	T5Ø.7X1	T5Ø.7X2	T5Ø.7X3	T5Ø.7X4	T5Ø.7X5	T5Ø.7X6
Cyclizine	T45.ØX1	T45.ØX2	T45.ØX3	T45.ØX4	T45.ØX5	T45.ØX6
Cyclobarbital	T42.3X1	T42.3X2	T42.3X3	T42.3X4	T42.3X5	T42.3X6
Cyclobarbitone	T42.3X1	T42.3X2	T42.3X3	T42.3X4	T42.3X5	T42.3X6
Cyclobenzaprine	T48.1X1	T48.1X2	T48.1X3	T48.1X4	T48.1X5	T48.1X6
Cyclodrine	T44.3X1	T44.3X2	T44.3X3	T44.3X4	T44.3X5	T44.3X6
Cycloguanil embonate	T37.2X1	T37.2X2	T37.2X3	T37.2X4	T37.2X5	T37.2X6
Cycloheptadiene	T43.291	T43.292	T43.293	T43.294	T43.295	T43.296
Cyclohexane	T52.8X1	T52.8X2	T52.8X3	T52.8X4	—	—
Cyclohexanol	T51.8X1	T51.8X2	T51.8X3	T51.8X4	—	—
Cyclohexanone	T52.4X1	T52.4X2	T52.4X3	T52.4X4	—	—
Cycloheximide	T6Ø.3X1	T6Ø.3X2	T6Ø.3X3	T6Ø.3X4	—	—
Cyclohexyl acetate	T52.8X1	T52.8X2	T52.8X3	T52.8X4	—	—
Cycloleucin	T45.1X1	T45.1X2	T45.1X3	T45.1X4	T45.1X5	T45.1X6
Cyclomethycaine	T41.3X1	T41.3X2	T41.3X3	T41.3X4	T41.3X5	T41.3X6
Cyclopentamine	T44.4X1	T44.4X2	T44.4X3	T44.4X4	T44.4X5	T44.4X6
Cyclopenthiazide	T5Ø.2X1	T5Ø.2X2	T5Ø.2X3	T5Ø.2X4	T5Ø.2X5	T5Ø.2X6
Cyclopentolate	T44.3X1	T44.3X2	T44.3X3	T44.3X4	T44.3X5	T44.3X6
Cyclophosphamide	T45.1X1	T45.1X2	T45.1X3	T45.1X4	T45.1X5	T45.1X6
Cycloplegic drug	T49.5X1	T49.5X2	T49.5X3	T49.5X4	T49.5X5	T49.5X6
Cyclopropane	T41.291	T41.292	T41.293	T41.294	T41.295	T41.296
Cyclopyrabital	T39.8X1	T39.8X2	T39.8X3	T39.8X4	T39.8X5	T39.8X6
Cycloserine	T37.1X1	T37.1X2	T37.1X3	T37.1X4	T37.1X5	T37.1X6
Cyclosporin	T45.1X1	T45.1X2	T45.1X3	T45.1X4	T45.1X5	T45.1X6
Cyclothiazide	T5Ø.2X1	T5Ø.2X2	T5Ø.2X3	T5Ø.2X4	T5Ø.2X5	T5Ø.2X6
Cycrimine	T44.3X1	T44.3X2	T44.3X3	T44.3X4	T44.3X5	T44.3X6
Cyhalothrin	T6Ø.1X1	T6Ø.1X2	T6Ø.1X3	T6Ø.1X4	—	—
Cymarin	T46.ØX1	T46.ØX2	T46.ØX3	T46.ØX4	T46.ØX5	T46.ØX6
Cypermethrin	T6Ø.1X1	T6Ø.1X2	T6Ø.1X3	T6Ø.1X4	—	—
Cyphenothrin	T6Ø.2X1	T6Ø.2X2	T6Ø.2X3	T6Ø.2X4	—	—
Cyproheptadine	T45.ØX1	T45.ØX2	T45.ØX3	T45.ØX4	T45.ØX5	T45.ØX6
Cyprolidol	T43.291	T43.292	T43.293	T43.294	T43.295	T43.296
Cyproterone	T38.6X1	T38.6X2	T38.6X3	T38.6X4	T38.6X5	T38.6X6
Cysteamine	T5Ø.6X1	T5Ø.6X2	T5Ø.6X3	T5Ø.6X4	T5Ø.6X5	T5Ø.6X6
Cytarabine	T45.1X1	T45.1X2	T45.1X3	T45.1X4	T45.1X5	T45.1X6
Cytisus						
laburnum	T62.2X1	T62.2X2	T62.2X3	T62.2X4	—	—
scoparius	T62.2X1	T62.2X2	T62.2X3	T62.2X4	—	—
Cytochrome C	T47.5X1	T47.5X2	T47.5X3	T47.5X4	T47.5X5	T47.5X6
Cytomel	T38.1X1	T38.1X2	T38.1X3	T38.1X4	T38.1X5	T38.1X6
Cytosine arabinoside	T45.1X1	T45.1X2	T45.1X3	T45.1X4	T45.1X5	T45.1X6
Cytoxan	T45.1X1	T45.1X2	T45.1X3	T45.1X4	T45.1X5	T45.1X6
Cytozyme	T45.7X1	T45.7X2	T45.7X3	T45.7X4	T45.7X5	T45.7X6
2,4-D	T6Ø.3X1	T6Ø.3X2	T6Ø.3X3	T6Ø.3X4	—	—
D						
Dacarbazine	T45.1X1	T45.1X2	T45.1X3	T45.1X4	T45.1X5	T45.1X6
Dactinomycin	T45.1X1	T45.1X2	T45.1X3	T45.1X4	T45.1X5	T45.1X6
DADPS	T37.1X1	T37.1X2	T37.1X3	T37.1X4	T37.1X5	T37.1X6
Dakin's solution	T49.ØX1	T49.ØX2	T49.ØX3	T49.ØX4	T49.ØX5	T49.ØX6
Dalapon (sodium)	T6Ø.3X1	T6Ø.3X2	T6Ø.3X3	T6Ø.3X4	—	—
Dalmane	T42.4X1	T42.4X2	T42.4X3	T42.4X4	T42.4X5	T42.4X6
Danazol	T38.6X1	T38.6X2	T38.6X3	T38.6X4	T38.6X5	T38.6X6
Danilone	T45.511	T45.512	T45.513	T45.514	T45.515	T45.516
Danthron	T47.2X1	T47.2X2	T47.2X3	T47.2X4	T47.2X5	T47.2X6
Dantrolene	T42.8X1	T42.8X2	T42.8X3	T42.8X4	T42.8X5	T42.8X6
Dantron	T47.2X1	T47.2X2	T47.2X3	T47.2X4	T47.2X5	T47.2X6
Daphne (gnidium) (mezereum)	T62.2X1	T62.2X2	T62.2X3	T62.2X4	—	—
berry	T62.1X1	T62.1X2	T62.1X3	T62.1X4	—	—
Dapsone	T37.1X1	T37.1X2	T37.1X3	T37.1X4	T37.1X5	T37.1X6
Daraprim	T37.2X1	T37.2X2	T37.2X3	T37.2X4	T37.2X5	T37.2X6
Darnel	T62.2X1	T62.2X2	T62.2X3	T62.2X4	—	—
Darvon	T39.8X1	T39.8X2	T39.8X3	T39.8X4	T39.8X5	T39.8X6
Daunomycin	T45.1X1	T45.1X2	T45.1X3	T45.1X4	T45.1X5	T45.1X6
Daunorubicin	T45.1X1	T45.1X2	T45.1X3	T45.1X4	T45.1X5	T45.1X6
DBI	T38.3X1	T38.3X2	T38.3X3	T38.3X4	T38.3X5	T38.3X6
D-Con	T6Ø.91	T6Ø.92	T6Ø.93	T6Ø.94	—	—
insecticide	T6Ø.2X1	T6Ø.2X2	T6Ø.2X3	T6Ø.2X4	—	—
rodenticide	T6Ø.4X1	T6Ø.4X2	T6Ø.4X3	T6Ø.4X4	—	—
DDAVP	T38.891	T38.892	T38.893	T38.894	T38.895	T38.896
DDE (bis(chlorophenyl)-dichloroethylene)	T6Ø.2X1	T6Ø.2X2	T6Ø.2X3	T6Ø.2X4	—	—
DDS	T37.1X1	T37.1X2	T37.1X3	T37.1X4	T37.1X5	T37.1X6
DDT (dust)	T6Ø.1X1	T6Ø.1X2	T6Ø.1X3	T6Ø.1X4	—	—
Deadly nightshade — *see also Belladonna*	T62.2X1	T62.2X2	T62.2X3	T62.2X4	—	—
berry	T62.1X1	T62.1X2	T62.1X3	T62.1X4	—	—
Deamino-D-arginine vasopressin	T38.891	T38.892	T38.893	T38.894	T38.895	T38.896
Deanol (aceglumate)	T5Ø.991	T5Ø.992	T5Ø.993	T5Ø.994	T5Ø.995	T5Ø.996
Debrisoquine	T46.5X1	T46.5X2	T46.5X3	T46.5X4	T46.5X5	T46.5X6
Decaborane	T57.8X1	T57.8X2	T57.8X3	T57.8X4	—	—
fumes	T59.891	T59.892	T59.893	T59.894	—	—

Substance	Poisoning, Accidental (Unintentional)	Poisoning, Intentional Self-Harm	Poisoning, Assault	Poisoning, Undetermined	Adverse Effect	Underdosing
Decadron	T38.0X1	T38.0X2	T38.0X3	T38.0X4	T38.0X5	T38.0X6
ENT agent	T49.6X1	T49.6X2	T49.6X3	T49.6X4	T49.6X5	T49.6X6
ophthalmic preparation	T49.5X1	T49.5X2	T49.5X3	T49.5X4	T49.5X5	T49.5X6
topical NEC	T49.0X1	T49.0X2	T49.0X3	T49.0X4	T49.0X5	T49.0X6
Decahydronaphthalene	T52.8X1	T52.8X2	T52.8X3	T52.8X4	—	—
Decalin	T52.8X1	T52.8X2	T52.8X3	T52.8X4	—	—
Decamethonium (bromide)	T48.1X1	T48.1X2	T48.1X3	T48.1X4	T48.1X5	T48.1X6
Decholin	T47.5X1	T47.5X2	T47.5X3	T47.5X4	T47.5X5	T47.5X6
Declomycin	T36.4X1	T36.4X2	T36.4X3	T36.4X4	T36.4X5	T36.4X6
Decongestant, nasal (mucosa)	T48.5X1	T48.5X2	T48.5X3	T48.5X4	T48.5X5	T48.5X6
combination	T48.5X1	T48.5X2	T48.5X3	T48.5X4	T48.5X5	T48.5X6
Deet	T60.8X1	T60.8X2	T60.8X3	T60.8X4	—	—
Deferoxamine	T45.8X1	T45.8X2	T45.8X3	T45.8X4	T45.8X5	T45.8X6
Deflazacort	T38.0X1	T38.0X2	T38.0X3	T38.0X4	T38.0X5	T38.0X6
Deglycyrrhizinized extract of licorice	T48.4X1	T48.4X2	T48.4X3	T48.4X4	T48.4X5	T48.4X6
Dehydrocholic acid	T47.5X1	T47.5X2	T47.5X3	T47.5X4	T47.5X5	T47.5X6
Dehydroemetine	T37.3X1	T37.3X2	T37.3X3	T37.3X4	T37.3X5	T37.3X6
Dekalin	T52.8X1	T52.8X2	T52.8X3	T52.8X4	—	—
Delalutin	T38.5X1	T38.5X2	T38.5X3	T38.5X4	T38.5X5	T38.5X6
Delphinium	T62.2X1	T62.2X2	T62.2X3	T62.2X4	—	—
Deltasone	T38.0X1	T38.0X2	T38.0X3	T38.0X4	T38.0X5	T38.0X6
Deltra	T38.0X1	T38.0X2	T38.0X3	T38.0X4	T38.0X5	T38.0X6
Delvinal	T42.3X1	T42.3X2	T42.3X3	T42.3X4	T42.3X5	T42.3X6
Delorazepam	T42.4X1	T42.4X2	T42.4X3	T42.4X4	T42.4X5	T42.4X6
Deltamethrin	T60.1X1	T60.1X2	T60.1X3	T60.1X4	—	—
Demecarium (bromide)	T49.5X1	T49.5X2	T49.5X3	T49.5X4	T49.5X5	T49.5X6
Demeclocycline	T36.4X1	T36.4X2	T36.4X3	T36.4X4	T36.4X5	T36.4X6
Demecolcine	T45.1X1	T45.1X2	T45.1X3	T45.1X4	T45.1X5	T45.1X6
Demegestone	T38.5X1	T38.5X2	T38.5X3	T38.5X4	T38.5X5	T38.5X6
Demelanizing agents	T49.8X1	T49.8X2	T49.8X3	T49.8X4	T49.8X5	T49.8X6
Demephion -O and -S	T60.0X1	T60.0X2		T60.0X4	—	—
Demerol	T40.2X1	T40.2X2	T40.2X3	T40.2X4	T40.2X5	T40.2X6
Demethylchlortetracycline	T36.4X1	T36.4X2	T36.4X3	T36.4X4	T36.4X5	T36.4X6
Demethyltetracycline	T36.4X1	T36.4X2	T36.4X3	T36.4X4	T36.4X5	T36.4X6
Demeton -O and -S	T60.0X1	T60.0X2	T60.0X3	T60.0X4	—	—
Demulcent (external)	T49.3X1	T49.3X2	T49.3X3	T49.3X4	T49.3X5	T49.3X6
specified NEC	T49.3X1	T49.3X2	T49.3X3	T49.3X4	T49.3X5	T49.3X6
Demulen	T38.4X1	T38.4X2	T38.4X3	T38.4X4	T38.4X5	T38.4X6
Denatured alcohol	T51.0X1	T51.0X2	T51.0X3	T51.0X4	—	—
Dendrid	T49.5X1	T49.5X2	T49.5X3	T49.5X4	T49.5X5	T49.5X6
Dental drug, topical application NEC	T49.7X1	T49.7X2	T49.7X3	T49.7X4	T49.7X5	T49.7X6

Substance	Poisoning, Accidental (Unintentional)	Poisoning, Intentional Self-Harm	Poisoning, Assault	Poisoning, Undetermined	Adverse Effect	Underdosing
Dentifrice	T49.7X1	T49.7X2	T49.7X3	T49.7X4	T49.7X5	T49.7X6
Deodorant spray (feminine hygiene)	T49.8X1	T49.8X2	T49.8X3	T49.8X4	T49.8X5	T49.8X6
Deoxycortone	T50.0X1	T50.0X2	T50.0X3	T50.0X4	T50.0X5	T50.0X6
2-Deoxy-5-fluorouridine	T45.1X1	T45.1X2	T45.1X3	T45.1X4	T45.1X5	T45.1X6
5-Deoxy-5-fluorouridine	T45.1X1	T45.1X2	T45.1X3	T45.1X4	T45.1X5	T45.1X6
Deoxyribonuclease (pancreatic)	T45.3X1	T45.3X2	T45.3X3	T45.3X4	T45.3X5	T45.3X6
Depilatory	T49.4X1	T49.4X2	T49.4X3	T49.4X4	T49.4X5	T49.4X6
Deprenalin	T42.8X1	T42.8X2	T42.8X3	T42.8X4	T42.8X5	T42.8X6
Deprenyl	T42.8X1	T42.8X2	T42.8X3	T42.8X4	T42.8X5	T42.8X6
Depressant, appetite	T50.5X1	T50.5X2	T50.5X3	T50.5X4	T50.5X5	T50.5X6
Depressant						
appetite, central	T50.5X1	T50.5X2	T50.5X3	T50.5X4	T50.5X5	T50.5X6
cardiac	T46.2X1	T46.2X2	T46.2X3	T46.2X4	T46.2X5	T46.2X6
central nervous system (anesthetic) — see also Central nervous system, depressants	T42.71	T42.72	T42.73	T42.74	T42.75	T42.76
general anesthetic	T41.201	T41.202	T41.203	T41.204	T41.205	T41.206
muscle tone	T42.8X1	T42.8X2	T42.8X3	T42.8X4	T42.8X5	T42.8X6
muscle tone, central	T42.8X1	T42.8X2	T42.8X3	T42.8X4	T42.8X5	T42.8X6
psychotherapeutic	T43.501	T43.502	T43.503	T43.504	T43.505	T43.506
Deptropine	T45.0X1	T45.0X2	T45.0X3	T45.0X4	T45.0X5	T45.0X6
Dequalinium (chloride)	T49.0X1	T49.0X2	T49.0X3	T49.0X4	T49.0X5	T49.0X6
Derris root	T60.2X1	T60.2X2	T60.2X3	T60.2X4	—	—
Deserpidine	T43.011	T43.012	T43.013	T43.014	T43.015	T43.016
Desferrioxamine	T45.8X1	T45.8X2	T45.8X3	T45.8X4	T45.8X5	T45.8X6
Desipramine	T43.0X1	T43.0X2	T43.0X3	T43.0X4	T43.0X5	T43.0X6
Deslanoside	T46.0X1	T46.0X2	T46.0X3	T46.0X4	T46.0X5	T46.0X6
Desloughing agent	T49.4X1	T49.4X2	T49.4X3	T49.4X4	T49.4X5	T49.4X6
Desmethylimipramine	T43.011	T43.012	T43.013	T43.014	T43.015	T43.016
Desmopressin	T38.891	T38.892	T38.893	T38.894	T38.895	T38.896
Desocodeine	T40.2X1	T40.2X2	T40.2X3	T40.2X4	T40.2X5	T40.2X6
Desogestrel	T38.5X1	T38.5X2	T38.5X3	T38.5X4	T38.5X5	T38.5X6
Desomorphine	T40.2X1	T40.2X2	T40.2X3	T40.2X4	—	—
Desonide	T49.0X1	T49.0X2	T49.0X3	T49.0X4	T49.0X5	T49.0X6
Desoximetasone	T49.0X1	T49.0X2	T49.0X3	T49.0X4	T49.0X5	T49.0X6
Desoxycorticosteroid	T50.0X1	T50.0X2	T50.0X3	T50.0X4	T50.0X5	T50.0X6
Desoxycortone	T50.0X1	T50.0X2	T50.0X3	T50.0X4	T50.0X5	T50.0X6
Desoxyephedrine	T43.621	T43.622	T43.623	T43.624	T43.625	T43.626
Detaxtran	T46.6X1	T46.6X2	T46.6X3	T46.6X4	T46.6X5	T46.6X6
Detergent	T49.2X1	T49.2X2	T49.2X3	T49.2X4	T49.2X5	T49.2X6
external medication	T49.2X1	T49.2X2	T49.2X3	T49.2X4	T49.2X5	T49.2X6
local	T49.2X1	T49.2X2	T49.2X3	T49.2X4	T49.2X5	T49.2X6

◀ New   ◀ Revised   ~~deleted~~ Deleted

Substance	Poisoning, Accidental (Unintentional)	Poisoning, Intentional Self-Harm	Poisoning, Assault	Poisoning, Undetermined	Adverse Effect	Underdosing
Detergent *(Continued)*						
medicinal	T49.2X1	T49.2X2	T49.2X3	T49.2X4	T49.2X5	T49.2X6
nonmedicinal	T55.1X1	T55.1X2	T55.1X3	T55.1X4	—	—
specified NEC	T55.1X1	T55.1X2	T55.1X3	T55.1X4	T55.1X5	T55.1X6
Deterrent, alcohol	T50.6X1	T50.6X2	T50.6X3	T50.6X4	T50.6X5	T50.6X6
Detoxifying agent	T50.6X1	T50.6X2	T50.6X3	T50.6X4	T50.6X5	T50.6X6
Detrothyronine	T38.1X1	T38.1X2	T38.1X3	T38.1X4	T38.1X5	T38.1X6
Dettol (external medication)	T49.0X1	T49.0X2	T49.0X3	T49.0X4	T49.0X5	T49.0X6
Dexamethasone	T38.0X1	T38.0X2	T38.0X3	T38.0X4	T38.0X5	T38.0X6
ENT agent	T49.6X1	T49.6X2	T49.6X3	T49.6X4	T49.6X5	T49.6X6
ophthalmic preparation	T49.5X1	T49.5X2	T49.5X3	T49.5X4	T49.5X5	T49.5X6
topical NEC	T49.0X1	T49.0X2	T49.0X3	T49.0X4	T49.0X5	T49.0X6
Dexamfetamine	T43.621	T43.622	T43.623	T43.624	T43.625	T43.626
Dexamphetamine	T43.621	T43.622	T43.623	T43.624	T43.625	T43.626
Dexbrompheniramine	T45.0X1	T45.0X2	T45.0X3	T45.0X4	T45.0X5	T45.0X6
Dexchlorpheniramine	T45.0X1	T45.0X2	T45.0X3	T45.0X4	T45.0X5	T45.0X6
Dexedrine	T43.621	T43.622	T43.623	T43.624	T43.625	T43.626
Dexetimide	T44.3X1	T44.3X2	T44.3X3	T44.3X4	T44.3X5	T44.3X6
Dexfenfluramine	T50.5X1	T50.5X2	T50.5X3	T50.5X4	T50.5X5	T50.5X6
Dexpanthenol	T45.2X1	T45.2X2	T45.2X3	T45.2X4	T45.2X5	T45.2X6
Dextran (40) (70) (150)	T45.8X1	T45.8X2	T45.8X3	T45.8X4	T45.8X5	T45.8X6
Dextriferron	T45.4X1	T45.4X2	T45.4X3	T45.4X4	T45.4X5	T45.4X6
Dextroamphetamine	T43.621	T43.622	T43.623	T43.624	T43.625	T43.626
Dextro calcium pantothenate	T45.2X1	T45.2X2	T45.2X3	T45.2X4	T45.2X5	T45.2X6
Dextromethorphan	T48.3X1	T48.3X2	T48.3X3	T48.3X4	T48.3X5	T48.3X6
Dextromoramide	T40.4X1	T40.4X2	T40.4X3	T40.4X4	—	—
topical	T49.8X1	T49.8X2	T49.8X3	T49.8X4	T49.8X5	T49.8X6
Dextro pantothenyl alcohol	T45.2X1	T45.2X2	T45.2X3	T45.2X4	T45.2X5	T45.2X6
Dextropropoxyphene	T40.4X1	T40.4X2	T40.4X3	T40.4X4	T40.4X5	T40.4X6
Dextrorphan	T40.2X1	T40.2X2	T40.2X3	T40.2X4	T40.2X5	T40.2X6
Dextrose	T50.3X1	T50.3X2	T50.3X3	T50.3X4	T50.3X5	T50.3X6
concentrated solution, intravenous	T46.8X1	T46.8X2	T46.8X3	T46.8X4	T46.8X5	T46.8X6
Dextrothyroxin	T38.1X1	T38.1X2	T38.1X3	T38.1X4	T38.1X5	T38.1X6
Dextrothyroxine sodium	T38.1X1	T38.1X2	T38.1X3	T38.1X4	T38.1X5	T38.1X6
DFP	T44.0X1	T44.0X2	T44.0X3	T44.0X4	T44.0X5	T44.0X6
DHE	T37.3X1	T37.3X2	T37.3X3	T37.3X4	T37.3X5	T37.3X6
45	T46.5X1	T46.5X2	T46.5X3	T46.5X4	T46.5X5	T46.5X6
Diabinese	T38.3X1	T38.3X2	T38.3X3	T38.3X4	T38.3X5	T38.3X6
Diacetone alcohol	T52.4X1	T52.4X2	T52.4X3	T52.4X4	—	—
Diacetyl monoxime	T50.991	T50.992	T50.993	T50.994	—	—
Diacetylmorphine	T40.1X1	T40.1X2	T40.1X3	T40.1X4	—	—

Substance	Poisoning, Accidental (Unintentional)	Poisoning, Intentional Self-Harm	Poisoning, Assault	Poisoning, Undetermined	Adverse Effect	Underdosing
Diachylon plaster	T49.4X1	T49.4X2	T49.4X3	T49.4X4	T49.4X5	T49.4X6
Diaethylstilboestrolum	T38.5X1	T38.5X2	T38.5X3	T38.5X4	T38.5X5	T38.5X6
Diagnostic agent NEC	T50.8X1	T50.8X2	T50.8X3	T50.8X4	T50.8X5	T50.8X6
Dial (soap)	T49.2X1	T49.2X2	T49.2X3	T49.2X4	T49.2X5	T49.2X6
sedative	T42.3X1	T42.3X2	T42.3X3	T42.3X4	T42.3X5	T42.3X6
Dialkyl carbonate	T52.91	T52.92	T52.93	T52.94	—	—
Diallylbarbituric acid	T42.3X1	T42.3X2	T42.3X3	T42.3X4	T42.3X5	T42.3X6
Diallymal	T42.3X1	T42.3X2	T42.3X3	T42.3X4	T42.3X5	T42.3X6
Dialysis solution (intraperitoneal)	T50.3X1	T50.3X2	T50.3X3	T50.3X4	T50.3X5	T50.3X6
Diaminodiphenylsulfone	T37.1X1	T37.1X2	T37.1X3	T37.1X4	T37.1X5	T37.1X6
Diamorphine	T40.1X1	T40.1X2	T40.1X3	T40.1X4	—	—
Diamox	T50.2X1	T50.2X2	T50.2X3	T50.2X4	T50.2X5	T50.2X6
Diamthazole	T49.0X1	T49.0X2	T49.0X3	T49.0X4	T49.0X5	T49.0X6
Dianthone	T47.2X1	T47.2X2	T47.2X3	T47.2X4	T47.2X5	T47.2X6
Diaphenylsulfone	T37.0X1	T37.0X2	T37.0X3	T37.0X4	T37.0X5	T37.0X6
Diasone (sodium)	T37.1X1	T37.1X2	T37.1X3	T37.1X4	T37.1X5	T37.1X6
Diastase	T47.5X1	T47.5X2	T47.5X3	T47.5X4	T47.5X5	T47.5X6
Diatrizoate	T50.8X1	T50.8X2	T50.8X3	T50.8X4	T50.8X5	T50.8X6
Diazepam	T42.4X1	T42.4X2	T42.4X3	T42.4X4	T42.4X5	T42.4X6
Diazinon	T60.0X1	T60.0X2	T60.0X3	T60.0X4	—	—
Diazomethane (gas)	T59.891	T59.892	T59.893	T59.894	—	—
Diazoxide	T46.5X1	T46.5X2	T46.5X3	T46.5X4	T46.5X5	T46.5X6
Dibekacin	T36.5X1	T36.5X2	T36.5X3	T36.5X4	T36.5X5	T36.5X6
Dibenamine	T44.6X1	T44.6X2	T44.6X3	T44.6X4	T44.6X5	T44.6X6
Dibenzepin	T43.011	T43.012	T43.013	T43.014	T43.015	T43.016
Dibenzheptropine	T45.0X1	T45.0X2	T45.0X3	T45.0X4	T45.0X5	T45.0X6
Dibenzyline	T44.6X1	T44.6X2	T44.6X3	T44.6X4	T44.6X5	T44.6X6
Diborane (gas)	T59.891	T59.892	T59.893	T59.894	—	—
Dibromochloropropane	T60.8X1	T60.8X2	T60.8X3	T60.8X4	—	—
Dibromodulcitol	T45.1X1	T45.1X2	T45.1X3	T45.1X4	T45.1X5	T45.1X6
Dibromoethane	T53.6X1	T53.6X2	T53.6X3	T53.6X4	—	—
Dibromomannitol	T45.1X1	T45.1X2	T45.1X3	T45.1X4	T45.1X5	T45.1X6
Dibromopropamidine isethionate	T49.0X1	T49.0X2	T49.0X3	T49.0X4	T49.0X5	T49.0X6
Dibrompropamidine	T49.0X1	T49.0X2	T49.0X3	T49.0X4	T49.0X5	T49.0X6
Dibucaine	T41.3X1	T41.3X2	T41.3X3	T41.3X4	T41.3X5	T41.3X6
topical (surface)	T41.3X1	T41.3X2	T41.3X3	T41.3X4	T41.3X5	T41.3X6
Dibunate sodium	T48.3X1	T48.3X2	T48.3X3	T48.3X4	T48.3X5	T48.3X6
Dibutoline sulfate	T44.3X1	T44.3X2	T44.3X3	T44.3X4	T44.3X5	T44.3X6
Dicamba	T60.3X1	T60.3X2	T60.3X3	T60.3X4	—	—
Dicapthon	T60.0X1	T60.0X2	T60.0X3	T60.0X4	—	—
Dichlobenil	T60.3X1	T60.3X2	T60.3X3	T60.3X4	—	—
Dichlone	T60.3X1	T60.3X2	T60.3X3	T60.3X4	—	—

◀ New ◀ Revised ~~deleted~~ Deleted

Substance	External Cause (T-Code)					
	Poisoning, Accidental (Unintentional)	Poisoning, Intentional Self-Harm	Poisoning, Assault	Poisoning, Undetermined	Adverse Effect	Underdosing
Dichloralphenozone	T42.6X1	T42.6X2	T42.6X3	T42.6X4	T42.6X5	T42.6X6
Dichlorbenzidine	T65.3X1	T65.3X2	T65.3X3	T65.3X4	—	—
Dichlorhydrin	T52.8X1	T52.8X2	T52.8X3	T52.8X4	—	—
Dichlorhydroxyquinoline	T37.8X1	T37.8X2	T37.8X3	T37.8X4	T37.8X5	T37.8X6
Dichlorobenzene	T53.7X1	T53.7X2	T53.7X3	T53.7X4	—	—
Dichlorobenzyl alcohol	T49.6X1	T49.6X2	T49.6X3	T49.6X4	T49.6X5	T49.6X6
Dichlorodifluoromethane	T53.5X1	T53.5X2	T53.5X3	T53.5X4	—	—
Dichloroethane	T52.8X1	T52.8X2	T52.8X3	T52.8X4	—	—
Sym-Dichloroethyl ether	T53.6X1	T53.6X2	T53.6X3	T53.6X4	—	—
Dichloroethyl sulfide, not in war	T59.891	T59.892	T59.893	T59.894	—	—
Dichloroethylene	T53.6X1	T53.6X2	T53.6X3	T53.6X4	—	—
Dichloroformoxine, not in war	T59.891	T59.892	T59.893	T59.894	—	—
Dichlorohydrin, alpha-dichlorohydrin	T52.8X1	T52.8X2	T52.8X3	T52.8X4	—	—
Dichloromethane (solvent)	T53.4X1	T53.4X2	T53.4X3	T53.4X4	—	—
vapor	T53.4X1	T53.4X2	T53.4X3	T53.4X4	—	—
Dichloronaphthoquinone	T60.3X1	T60.3X2	T60.3X3	T60.3X4	—	—
Dichlorophen	T37.4X1	T37.4X2	T37.4X3	T37.4X4	T37.4X5	T37.4X6
2,4-Dichlorophenoxy-acetic acid	T60.3X1	T60.3X2	T60.3X3	T60.3X4	—	—
Dichloropropene	T60.3X1	T60.3X2	T60.3X3	T60.3X4	—	—
Dichloropropionic acid	T60.3X1	T60.3X2	T60.3X3	T60.3X4	—	—
Dichlorphenamide	T50.2X1	T50.2X2	T50.2X3	T50.2X4	T50.2X5	T50.2X6
Dichlorvos	T60.0X1	T60.0X2	T60.0X3	T60.0X4	—	—
Diclofenac	T39.391	T39.392	T39.393	T39.394	T39.395	T39.396
Diclofenamide	T50.2X1	T50.2X2	T50.2X3	T50.2X4	T50.2X5	T50.2X6
Diclofensine	T43.291	T43.292	T43.293	T43.294	T43.295	T43.296
Diclonixine	T39.8X1	T39.8X2	T39.8X3	T39.8X4	T39.8X5	T39.8X6
Dicloxacillin	T36.0X1	T36.0X2	T36.0X3	T36.0X4	T36.0X5	T36.0X6
Dicophane	T49.0X1	T49.0X2	T49.0X3	T49.0X4	T49.0X5	T49.0X6
Dicoumarol, dicoumarin, dicumarol	T45.511	T45.512	T45.513	T45.514	T45.515	T45.516
Dicrotophos	T60.0X1	T60.0X2	T60.0X3	T60.0X4	—	—
Dicyanogen (gas)	T65.0X1	T65.0X2	T65.0X3	T65.0X4	—	—
Dicyclomine	T44.3X1	T44.3X2	T44.3X3	T44.3X4	T44.3X5	T44.3X6
Dicycloverine	T44.3X1	T44.3X2	T44.3X3	T44.3X4	T44.3X5	T44.3X6
Dideoxycytidine	T37.5X1	T37.5X2	T37.5X3	T37.5X4	T37.5X5	T37.5X6
Dideoxyinosine	T37.5X1	T37.5X2	T37.5X3	T37.5X4	T37.5X5	T37.5X6
Dieldrin (vapor)	T60.1X1	T60.1X2	T60.1X3	T60.1X4	—	—
Diemal	T42.3X1	T42.3X2	T42.3X3	T42.3X4	T42.3X5	T42.3X6
Dienestrol	T38.5X1	T38.5X2	T38.5X3	T38.5X4	T38.5X5	T38.5X6
Dienoestrol	T38.5X1	T38.5X2	T38.5X3	T38.5X4	T38.5X5	T38.5X6
Dietetic drug NEC	T50.901	T50.902	T50.903	T50.904	T50.905	T50.906
Diethazine	T42.8X1	T42.8X2	T42.8X3	T42.8X4	T42.8X5	T42.8X6

Substance	External Cause (T-Code)					
	Poisoning, Accidental (Unintentional)	Poisoning, Intentional Self-Harm	Poisoning, Assault	Poisoning, Undetermined	Adverse Effect	Underdosing
Diethyl						
barbituric acid	T42.3X1	T42.3X2	T42.3X3	T42.3X4	T42.3X5	T42.3X6
carbamazine	T37.4X1	T37.4X2	T37.4X3	T37.4X4	T37.4X5	T37.4X6
carbinol	T51.3X1	T51.3X2	T51.3X3	T51.3X4	—	—
carbonate	T52.8X1	T52.8X2	T52.8X3	T52.8X4	—	—
ether (vapor) — see also Ether	T41.0X1	T41.0X2	T41.0X3	T41.0X4	T41.0X5	T41.0X6
oxide	T52.8X1	T52.8X2	T52.8X3	T52.8X4	—	—
propion	T50.5X1	T50.5X2	T50.5X3	T50.5X4	T50.5X5	T50.5X6
stilbestrol	T38.5X1	T38.5X2	T38.5X3	T38.5X4	T38.5X5	T38.5X6
toluamide (nonmedicinal)	T60.8X1	T60.8X2	T60.8X3	T60.8X4	—	—
medicinal	T49.3X1	T49.3X2	T49.3X3	T49.3X4	T49.3X5	T49.3X6
Diethylcarbamazine	T37.4X1	T37.4X2	T37.4X3	T37.4X4	T37.4X5	T37.4X6
Diethylene						
dioxide	T52.8X1	T52.8X2	T52.8X3	T52.8X4		
glycol (monoacetate) (monobutyl ether) (monoethyl ether)	T52.3X1	T52.3X2	T52.3X3	T52.3X4		—
Diethylhexylphthalate	T65.891	T65.892	T65.893	T65.894	—	—
Diethylpropion	T50.5X1	T50.5X2	T50.5X3	T50.5X4	T50.5X5	T50.5X6
Diethylstilbestrol	T38.5X1	T38.5X2	T38.5X3	T38.5X4	T38.5X5	T38.5X6
Diethylstilboestrol	T38.5X1	T38.5X2	T38.5X3	T38.5X4	T38.5X5	T38.5X6
Diethylsulfone-diethylmethane	T42.6X1	T42.6X2	T42.6X3	T42.6X4	T42.6X5	T42.6X6
Diethyltoluamide	T49.0X1	T49.0X2	T49.0X3	T49.0X4	T49.0X5	T49.0X6
Diethyltryptamine (DET)	T40.991	T40.992	T40.993	T40.994	—	—
Difebarbamate	T42.3X1	T42.3X2	T42.3X3	T42.3X4	T42.3X5	T42.3X6
Difencloxazine	T40.2X1	T40.2X2	T40.2X3	T40.2X4	T40.2X5	T40.2X6
Difenidol	T45.0X1	T45.0X2	T45.0X3	T45.0X4	T45.0X5	T45.0X6
Difenoxin	T47.6X1	T47.6X2	T47.6X3	T47.6X4	T47.6X5	T47.6X6
Difetarsone	T37.3X1	T37.3X2	T37.3X3	T37.3X4	T37.3X5	T37.3X6
Diffusin	T45.3X1	T45.3X2	T45.3X3	T45.3X4	T45.3X5	T45.3X6
Diflorasone	T49.0X1	T49.0X2	T49.0X3	T49.0X4	T49.0X5	T49.0X6
Diflubenzuron	T60.1X1	T60.1X2	T60.1X3	T60.1X4	—	—
Diflos	T44.0X1	T44.0X2	T44.0X3	T44.0X4	T44.0X5	T44.0X6
Diflucortolone	T49.0X1	T49.0X2	T49.0X3	T49.0X4	T49.0X5	T49.0X6
Diflunisal	T39.091	T39.092	T39.093	T39.094	T39.095	T39.096
Difluoromethyldopa	T42.8X1	T42.8X2	T42.8X3	T42.8X4	T42.8X5	T42.8X6
Difluorophate	T44.0X1	T44.0X2	T44.0X3	T44.0X4	T44.0X5	T44.0X6
Digestant NEC	T47.5X1	T47.5X2	T47.5X3	T47.5X4	T47.5X5	T47.5X6
Digitalin(e)	T46.0X1	T46.0X2	T46.0X3	T46.0X4	T46.0X5	T46.0X6
Digitalis (leaf) (glycoside)	T46.0X1	T46.0X2	T46.0X3	T46.0X4	T46.0X5	T46.0X6
lanata	T46.0X1	T46.0X2	T46.0X3	T46.0X4	T46.0X5	T46.0X6
purpurea	T46.0X1	T46.0X2	T46.0X3	T46.0X4	T46.0X5	T46.0X6
Digitoxin	T46.0X1	T46.0X2	T46.0X3	T46.0X4	T46.0X5	T46.0X6

◀ New ◀ Revised ~~deleted~~ Deleted

Substance	Poisoning, Accidental (Unintentional)	Poisoning, Intentional Self-Harm	Poisoning, Assault	Poisoning, Undetermined	Adverse Effect	Underdosing
	External Cause (T-Code)					
Digitoxose	T46.0X1	T46.0X2	T46.0X3	T46.0X4	T46.0X5	T46.0X6
Digoxin	T46.0X1	T46.0X2	T46.0X3	T46.0X4	T46.0X5	T46.0X6
Digoxine	T46.0X1	T46.0X2	T46.0X3	T46.0X4	T46.0X5	T46.0X6
Dihydralazine	T46.5X1	T46.5X2	T46.5X3	T46.5X4	T46.5X5	T46.5X6
Dihydrazine	T46.5X1	T46.5X2	T46.5X3	T46.5X4	T46.5X5	T46.5X6
Dihydrocodeinone	T40.2X1	T40.2X2	T40.2X3	T40.2X4	T40.2X5	T40.2X6
Dihydroergocornine	T46.7X1	T46.7X2	T46.7X3	T46.7X4	T46.7X5	T46.7X6
Dihydroergocristine (mesilate)	T46.7X1	T46.7X2	T46.7X3	T46.7X4	T46.7X5	T46.7X6
Dihydroergokryptine	T46.7X1	T46.7X2	T46.7X3	T46.7X4	T46.7X5	T46.7X6
Dihydroergotamine	T46.5X1	T46.5X2	T46.5X3	T46.5X4	T46.5X5	T46.5X6
Dihydroergotoxine	T46.7X1	T46.7X2	T46.7X3	T46.7X4	T46.7X5	T46.7X6
mesilate	T46.7X1	T46.7X2	T46.7X3	T46.7X4	T46.7X5	T46.7X6
Dihydrohydroxycodein-one	T40.2X1	T40.2X2	T40.2X3	T40.2X4	T40.2X5	T40.2X6
Dihydrohydroxymorphinone	T40.2X1	T40.2X2	T40.2X3	T40.2X4	T40.2X5	T40.2X6
Dihydroisocodeine	T40.2X1	T40.2X2	T40.2X3	T40.2X4	T40.2X5	T40.2X6
Dihydromorphine	T40.2X1	T40.2X2	T40.2X3	T40.2X4	—	—
Dihydromorphinone	T40.2X1	T40.2X2	T40.2X3	T40.2X4	T40.2X5	T40.2X6
Dihydrostreptomycin	T36.5X1	T36.5X2	T36.5X3	T36.5X4	T36.5X5	T36.5X6
Dihydrotachysterol	T45.2X1	T45.2X2	T45.2X3	T45.2X4	T45.2X5	T45.2X6
Dihydroxyaluminum aminoacetate	T47.1X1	T47.1X2	T47.1X3	T47.1X4	T47.1X5	T47.1X6
Dihydroxyaluminum sodium carbonate	T47.1X1	T47.1X2	T47.1X3	T47.1X4	T47.1X5	T47.1X6
Dihydroxyanthraquinone	T47.2X1	T47.2X2	T47.2X3	T47.2X4	T47.2X5	T47.2X6
Dihydroxycodeinone	T40.2X1	T40.2X2	T40.2X3	T40.2X4	T40.2X5	T40.2X6
Dihydroxypropyl theophylline	T50.2X1	T50.2X2	T50.2X3	T50.2X4	T50.2X5	T50.2X6
Diiodohydroxyquin	T37.8X1	T37.8X2	T37.8X3	T37.8X4	T37.8X5	T37.8X6
topical	T49.0X1	T49.0X2	T49.0X3	T49.0X4	T49.0X5	T49.0X6
Diiodohydroxyquinoline	T37.8X1	T37.8X2	T37.8X3	T37.8X4	T37.8X5	T37.8X6
Diiodotyrosine	T38.2X1	T38.2X2	T38.2X3	T38.2X4	T38.2X5	T38.2X6
Diisopromine	T44.3X1	T44.3X2	T44.3X3	T44.3X4	T44.3X5	T44.3X6
Diisopropylamine	T46.3X1	T46.3X2	T46.3X3	T46.3X4	T46.3X5	T46.3X6
Diisopropylfluorophosphonate	T44.0X1	T44.0X2	T44.0X3	T44.0X4	T44.0X5	T44.0X6
Dilantin	T42.0X1	T42.0X2	T42.0X3	T42.0X4	T42.0X5	T42.0X6
Dilaudid	T40.2X1	T40.2X2	T40.2X3	T40.2X4	T40.2X5	T40.2X6
Dilazep	T46.3X1	T46.3X2	T46.3X3	T46.3X4	T46.3X5	T46.3X6
Dill	T47.5X1	T47.5X2	T47.5X3	T47.5X4	T47.5X5	T47.5X6
Diloxanide	T37.3X1	T37.3X2	T37.3X3	T37.3X4	T37.3X5	T37.3X6
Diltiazem	T46.1X1	T46.1X2	T46.1X3	T46.1X4	T46.1X5	T46.1X6
Dimazole	T49.0X1	T49.0X2	T49.0X3	T49.0X4	T49.0X5	T49.0X6
Dimefline	T50.7X1	T50.7X2	T50.7X3	T50.7X4	T50.7X5	T50.7X6
Dimefox	T60.0X1	T60.0X2	T60.0X3	T60.0X4	—	—

Substance	Poisoning, Accidental (Unintentional)	Poisoning, Intentional Self-Harm	Poisoning, Assault	Poisoning, Undetermined	Adverse Effect	Underdosing
	External Cause (T-Code)					
Dimemorfan	T48.3X1	T48.3X2	T48.3X3	T48.3X4	T48.3X5	T48.3X6
Dimenhydrinate	T45.0X1	T45.0X2	T45.0X3	T45.0X4	T45.0X5	T45.0X6
Dimercaprol (British anti-lewisite)	T45.8X1	T45.8X2	T45.8X3	T45.8X4	T45.8X5	T45.8X6
Dimercaptopropanol	T45.8X1	T45.8X2	T45.8X3	T45.8X4	T45.8X5	T45.8X6
Dimestrol	T38.5X1	T38.5X2	T38.5X3	T38.5X4	T38.5X5	T38.5X6
Dimetane	T45.0X1	T45.0X2	T45.0X3	T45.0X4	T45.0X5	T45.0X6
Dimethicone	T47.1X1	T47.1X2	T47.1X3	T47.1X4	T47.1X5	T47.1X6
Dimethindene	T45.0X1	T45.0X2	T45.0X3	T45.0X4	T45.0X5	T45.0X6
Dimethisoquin	T49.1X1	T49.1X2	T49.1X3	T49.1X4	T49.1X5	T49.1X6
Dimethisterone	T38.5X1	T38.5X2	T38.5X3	T38.5X4	T38.5X5	T38.5X6
Dimethoate	T60.0X1	T60.0X2	T60.0X3	T60.0X4	—	—
Dimethocaine	T41.3X1	T41.3X2	T41.3X3	T41.3X4	T41.3X5	T41.3X6
Dimethoxanate	T48.3X1	T48.3X2	T48.3X3	T48.3X4	T48.3X5	T48.3X6
Dimethyl						
arsine, arsinic acid	T57.0X1	T57.0X2	T57.0X3	T57.0X4	—	—
carbinol	T51.2X1	T51.2X2	T51.2X3	T51.2X4	—	—
carbonate	T52.8X1	T52.8X2	T52.8X3	T52.8X4	—	—
diguanide	T38.3X1	T38.3X2	T38.3X3	T38.3X4	T38.3X5	T38.3X6
ketone	T52.4X1	T52.4X2	T52.4X3	T52.4X4	—	—
vapor	T52.4X1	T52.4X2	T52.4X3	T52.4X4	—	—
meperidine	T40.2X1	T40.2X2	T40.2X3	T40.2X4	T40.2X5	T40.2X6
parathion	T60.0X1	T60.0X2	T60.0X3	T60.0X4	—	—
phthlate	T49.3X1	T49.3X2	T49.3X3	T49.3X4	T49.3X5	T49.3X6
polysiloxane	T47.8X1	T47.8X2	T47.8X3	T47.8X4	T47.8X5	T47.8X6
sulfate (fumes)	T59.891	T59.892	T59.893	T59.894	—	—
liquid	T65.891	T65.892	T65.893	T65.894	—	—
sulfoxide (nonmedicinal)	T52.8X1	T52.8X2	T52.8X3	T52.8X4	—	—
medicinal	T49.4X1	T49.4X2	T49.4X3	T49.4X4	T49.4X5	T49.4X6
tryptamine	T40.991	T40.992	T40.993	T40.994	—	—
tubocurarine	T48.1X1	T48.1X2	T48.1X3	T48.1X4	T48.1X5	T48.1X6
Dimethylamine sulfate	T49.4X1	T49.4X2	T49.4X3	T49.4X4	T49.4X5	T49.4X6
Dimethylformamide	T52.8X1	T52.8X2	T52.8X3	T52.8X4	—	—
Dimethyltubocurarinium chloride	T48.1X1	T48.1X2	T48.1X3	T48.1X4	T48.1X5	T48.1X6
Dimeticone	T47.1X1	T47.1X2	T47.1X3	T47.1X4	T47.1X5	T47.1X6
Dimetilan	T60.0X1	T60.0X2	T60.0X3	T60.0X4	—	—
Dimetindene	T45.0X1	T45.0X2	T45.0X3	T45.0X4	T45.0X5	T45.0X6
Dimetotiazine	T43.3X1	T43.3X2	T43.3X3	T43.3X4	T43.3X5	T43.3X6
Dimorpholamine	T50.7X1	T50.7X2	T50.7X3	T50.7X4	T50.7X5	T50.7X6
Dimoxyline	T46.3X1	T46.3X2	T46.3X3	T46.3X4	T46.3X5	T46.3X6
Dinitrobenzene	T65.3X1	T65.3X2	T65.3X3	T65.3X4	—	—
vapor	T59.891	T59.892	T59.893	T59.894	—	—

	External Cause (T-Code)					
Substance	Poisoning, Accidental (Unintentional)	Poisoning, Intentional Self-Harm	Poisoning, Assault	Poisoning, Undetermined	Adverse Effect	Underdosing
Dinitrobenzol	T65.3X1	T65.3X2	T65.3X3	T65.3X4	—	—
vapor	T59.891	T59.892	T59.893	T59.894	—	—
Dinitrobutylphenol	T65.3X1	T65.3X2	T65.3X3	T65.3X4	—	—
Dinitro (-ortho-)cresol (pesticide) (spray)	T65.3X1	T65.3X2	T65.3X3	T65.3X4	—	—
Dinitrocyclohexylphenol	T65.3X1	T65.3X2	T65.3X3	T65.3X4	—	—
Dinitrophenol	T65.3X1	T65.3X2	T65.3X3	T65.3X4	—	—
Dinoprost	T48.ØX1	T48.ØX2	T48.ØX3	T48.ØX4	T48.ØX5	T48.ØX6
Dinoprostone	T48.ØX1	T48.ØX2	T48.ØX3	T48.ØX4	T48.ØX5	T48.ØX6
Dinoseb	T6Ø.3X1	T6Ø.3X2	T6Ø.3X3	T6Ø.3X4	—	—
Dioctyl sulfosuccinate (calcium) (sodium)	T47.4X1	T47.4X2	T47.4X3	T47.4X4	T47.4X5	T47.4X6
Diodone	T5Ø.8X1	T5Ø.8X2	T5Ø.8X3	T5Ø.8X4	T5Ø.8X5	T5Ø.8X6
Diodoquin	T37.8X1	T37.8X2	T37.8X3	T37.8X4	T37.8X5	T37.8X6
Dionin	T4Ø.2X1	T4Ø.2X2	T4Ø.2X3	T4Ø.2X4	T4Ø.2X5	T4Ø.2X6
Diosmin	T46.991	T46.992	T46.993	T46.994	T46.995	T46.996
Dioxane	T52.8X1	T52.8X2	T52.8X3	T52.8X4	—	—
Dioxathion	T6Ø.ØX1	T6Ø.ØX2	T6Ø.ØX3	T6Ø.ØX4	—	—
Dioxin	T53.7X1	T53.7X2	T53.7X3	T53.7X4	—	—
Dioxopromethazine	T43.3X1	T43.3X2	T43.3X3	T43.3X4	T43.3X5	T43.3X6
Dioxyline	T46.3X1	T46.3X2	T46.3X3	T46.3X4	T46.3X5	T46.3X6
Dipentene	T52.8X1	T52.8X2	T52.8X3	T52.8X4	—	—
Diperodon	T41.3X1	T41.3X2	T41.3X3	T41.3X4	T41.3X5	T41.3X6
Diphacinone	T6Ø.4X1	T6Ø.4X2	T6Ø.4X3	T6Ø.4X4	—	—
Diphemanil	T44.3X1	T44.3X2	T44.3X3	T44.3X4	T44.3X5	T44.3X6
metilsulfate	T44.3X1	T44.3X2	T44.3X3	T44.3X4	T44.3X5	T44.3X6
Diphenadione	T45.511	T45.512	T45.513	T45.514	T45.515	T45.516
rodenticide	T6Ø.4X1	T6Ø.4X2	T6Ø.4X3	T6Ø.4X4	—	—
Diphenhydramine	T45.ØX1	T45.ØX2	T45.ØX3	T45.ØX4	T45.ØX5	T45.ØX6
Diphenidol	T45.ØX1	T45.ØX2	T45.ØX3	T45.ØX4	T45.ØX5	T45.ØX6
Diphenoxylate	T47.6X1	T47.6X2	T47.6X3	T47.6X4	T47.6X5	T47.6X6
Diphenylamine	T65.3X1	T65.3X2	T65.3X3	T65.3X4	—	—
Diphenylbutazone	T39.2X1	T39.2X2	T39.2X3	T39.2X4	T39.2X5	T39.2X6
Diphenylchloroarsine, not in war	T57.ØX1	T57.ØX2	T57.ØX3	T57.ØX4	—	—
Diphenylhydantoin	T42.ØX1	T42.ØX2	T42.ØX3	T42.ØX4	T42.ØX5	T42.ØX6
Diphenylmethane dye	T52.1X1	T52.1X2	T52.1X3	T52.1X4	—	—
Diphenylpyraline	T45.ØX1	T45.ØX2	T45.ØX3	T45.ØX4	T45.ØX5	T45.ØX6
Diphtheria						
antitoxin	T5Ø.Z11	T5Ø.Z12	T5Ø.Z13	T5Ø.Z14	T5Ø.Z15	T5Ø.Z16
toxoid	T5Ø.A91	T5Ø.A92	T5Ø.A93	T5Ø.A94	T5Ø.A95	T5Ø.A96
with tetanus toxoid	T5Ø.A21	T5Ø.A22	T5Ø.A23	T5Ø.A24	T5Ø.A25	T5Ø.A26
with pertussis component	T5Ø.A11	T5Ø.A12	T5Ø.A13	T5Ø.A14	T5Ø.A15	T5Ø.A16

	External Cause (T-Code)					
Substance	Poisoning, Accidental (Unintentional)	Poisoning, Intentional Self-Harm	Poisoning, Assault	Poisoning, Undetermined	Adverse Effect	Underdosing
Diphtheria *(Continued)*						
vaccine (combination)	T5Ø.A91	T5Ø.A92	T5Ø.A93	T5Ø.A94	T5Ø.A95	T5Ø.A96
combination						
including pertussis	T5Ø.A11	T5Ø.A12	T5Ø.A13	T5Ø.A14	T5Ø.A15	T5Ø.A16
without pertussis	T5Ø.A21	T5Ø.A22	T5Ø.A23	T5Ø.A24	T5Ø.A25	T5Ø.A26
Diphylline	T5Ø.2X1	T5Ø.2X2	T5Ø.2X3	T5Ø.2X4	T5Ø.2X5	T5Ø.2X6
Dipipanone	T4Ø.4X1	T4Ø.4X2	T4Ø.4X3	T4Ø.4X4	—	—
Dipivefrine	T49.5X1	T49.5X2	T49.5X3	T49.5X4	T49.5X5	T49.5X6
Diplovax	T5Ø.B91	T5Ø.B92	T5Ø.B93	T5Ø.B94	T5Ø.B95	T5Ø.B96
Diprophylline	T5Ø.2X1	T5Ø.2X2	T5Ø.2X3	T5Ø.2X4	T5Ø.2X5	T5Ø.2X6
Dipropyline	T48.291	T48.292	T48.293	T48.294	T48.295	T48.296
Dipyridamole	T46.3X1	T46.3X2	T46.3X3	T46.3X4	T46.3X5	T46.3X6
Dipyrone	T39.2X1	T39.2X2	T39.2X3	T39.2X4	T39.2X5	T39.2X6
Diquat (dibromide)	T6Ø.3X1	T6Ø.3X2	T6Ø.3X3	T6Ø.3X4	—	—
Disinfectant	T65.891	T65.892	T65.893	T65.894	—	—
alkaline	T54.3X1	T54.3X2	T54.3X3	T54.3X4	—	—
aromatic	T54.1X1	T54.1X2	T54.1X3	T54.1X4	—	—
intestinal	T37.8X1	T37.8X2	T37.8X3	T37.8X4	T37.8X5	T37.8X6
Disipal	T42.8X1	T42.8X2	T42.8X3	T42.8X4	T42.8X5	T42.8X6
Disodium edetate	T5Ø.6X1	T5Ø.6X2	T5Ø.6X3	T5Ø.6X4	T5Ø.6X5	T5Ø.6X6
Disoprofol	T41.291	T41.292	T41.293	T41.294	T41.295	T41.296
Disopyramide	T46.2X1	T46.2X2	T46.2X3	T46.2X4	T46.2X5	T46.2X6
Distigmine (bromide)	T44.ØX1	T44.ØX2	T44.ØX3	T44.ØX4	T44.ØX5	T44.ØX6
Disulfamide	T5Ø.2X1	T5Ø.2X2	T5Ø.2X3	T5Ø.2X4	T5Ø.2X5	T5Ø.2X6
Disulfanilamide	T37.ØX1	T37.ØX2	T37.ØX3	T37.ØX4	T37.ØX5	T37.ØX6
Disulfiram	T5Ø.6X1	T5Ø.6X2	T5Ø.6X3	T5Ø.6X4	T5Ø.6X5	T5Ø.6X6
Disulfoton	T6Ø.ØX1	T6Ø.ØX2	T6Ø.ØX3	T6Ø.ØX4	—	—
Dithiazanine iodide	T37.4X1	T37.4X2	T37.4X3	T37.4X4	T37.4X5	T37.4X6
Dithiocarbamate	T6Ø.ØX1	T6Ø.ØX2	T6Ø.ØX3	T6Ø.ØX4	—	—
Dithranol	T49.4X1	T49.4X2	T49.4X3	T49.4X4	T49.4X5	T49.4X6
Diucardin	T5Ø.2X1	T5Ø.2X2	T5Ø.2X3	T5Ø.2X4	T5Ø.2X5	T5Ø.2X6
Diupres	T5Ø.2X1	T5Ø.2X2	T5Ø.2X3	T5Ø.2X4	T5Ø.2X5	T5Ø.2X6
Diuretic NEC	T5Ø.2X1	T5Ø.2X2	T5Ø.2X3	T5Ø.2X4	T5Ø.2X5	T5Ø.2X6
benzothiadiazine	T5Ø.2X1	T5Ø.2X2	T5Ø.2X3	T5Ø.2X4	T5Ø.2X5	T5Ø.2X6
carbonic acid anhydrase inhibitors	T5Ø.2X1	T5Ø.2X2	T5Ø.2X3	T5Ø.2X4	T5Ø.2X5	T5Ø.2X6
furfuryl NEC	T5Ø.2X1	T5Ø.2X2	T5Ø.2X3	T5Ø.2X4	T5Ø.2X5	T5Ø.2X6
loop (high-ceiling)	T5Ø.1X1	T5Ø.1X2	T5Ø.1X3	T5Ø.1X4	T5Ø.1X5	T5Ø.1X6
mercurial NEC	T5Ø.2X1	T5Ø.2X2	T5Ø.2X3	T5Ø.2X4	T5Ø.2X5	T5Ø.2X6
osmotic	T5Ø.2X1	T5Ø.2X2	T5Ø.2X3	T5Ø.2X4	T5Ø.2X5	T5Ø.2X6
purine NEC	T5Ø.2X1	T5Ø.2X2	T5Ø.2X3	T5Ø.2X4	T5Ø.2X5	T5Ø.2X6
saluretic NEC	T5Ø.2X1	T5Ø.2X2	T5Ø.2X3	T5Ø.2X4	T5Ø.2X5	T5Ø.2X6

◀ New ▮ Revised ~~deleted~~ Deleted

	External Cause (T-Code)					
Substance	Poisoning, Accidental (Unintentional)	Poisoning, Intentional Self-Harm	Poisoning, Assault	Poisoning, Undetermined	Adverse Effect	Underdosing
Diuretic NEC *(Continued)*						
sulfonamide	T5Ø.2X1	T5Ø.2X2	T5Ø.2X3	T5Ø.2X4	T5Ø.2X5	T5Ø.2X6
thiazide NEC	T5Ø.2X1	T5Ø.2X2	T5Ø.2X3	T5Ø.2X4	T5Ø.2X5	T5Ø.2X6
xanthine	T5Ø.2X1	T5Ø.2X2	T5Ø.2X3	T5Ø.2X4	T5Ø.2X5	T5Ø.2X6
Diurgin	T5Ø.2X1	T5Ø.2X2	T5Ø.2X3	T5Ø.2X4	T5Ø.2X5	T5Ø.2X6
Diuril	T5Ø.2X1	T5Ø.2X2	T5Ø.2X3	T5Ø.2X4	T5Ø.2X5	T5Ø.2X6
Diuron	T6Ø.3X1	T6Ø.3X2	T6Ø.3X3	T6Ø.3X4	—	—
Divalproex	T42.6X1	T42.6X2	T42.6X3	T42.6X4	T42.6X5	T42.6X6
Divinyl ether	T41.ØX1	T41.ØX2	T41.ØX3	T41.ØX4	T41.ØX5	T41.ØX6
Dixanthogen	T49.ØX1	T49.ØX2	T49.ØX3	T49.ØX4	T49.ØX5	T49.ØX6
Dixyrazine	T43.3X1	T43.3X2	T43.3X3	T43.3X4	T43.3X5	T43.3X6
D-lysergic acid diethylamide	T4Ø.8X1	T4Ø.8X2	T4Ø.8X3	T4Ø.8X4	—	—
DMCT	T36.4X1	T36.4X2	T36.4X3	T36.4X4	T36.4X5	T36.4X6
DMSO — *see Dimethyl sulfoxide*						
DNBP	T6Ø.3X1	T6Ø.3X2	T6Ø.3X3	T6Ø.3X4	—	—
DNOC	T65.3X1	T65.3X2	T65.3X3	T65.3X4	—	—
DOCA	T38.ØX1	T38.ØX2	T38.ØX3	T38.ØX4	T38.ØX5	T38.ØX6
Dobutamine	T44.5X1	T44.5X2	T44.5X3	T44.5X4	T44.5X5	T44.5X6
Docusate sodium	T47.4X1	T47.4X2	T47.4X3	T47.4X4	T47.4X5	T47.4X6
Dodicin	T49.ØX1	T49.ØX2	T49.ØX3	T49.ØX4	T49.ØX5	T49.ØX6
Dofamium chloride	T49.ØX1	T49.ØX2	T49.ØX3	T49.ØX4	T49.ØX5	T49.ØX6
Dolophine	T4Ø.3X1	T4Ø.3X2	T4Ø.3X3	T4Ø.3X4	T4Ø.3X5	T4Ø.3X6
Doloxene	T39.8X1	T39.8X2	T39.8X3	T39.8X4	T39.8X5	T39.8X6
Domestic gas (after combustion) — *see Gas, utility*						
prior to combustion	T59.891	T59.892	T59.893	T59.894	—	—
Domiodol	T48.4X1	T48.4X2	T48.4X3	T48.4X4	T48.4X5	T48.4X6
Domiphen (bromide)	T49.ØX1	T49.ØX2	T49.ØX3	T49.ØX4	T49.ØX5	T49.ØX6
Domperidone	T45.ØX1	T45.ØX2	T45.ØX3	T45.ØX4	T45.ØX5	T45.ØX6
Dopa	T42.8X1	T42.8X2	T42.8X3	T42.8X4	T42.8X5	T42.8X6
Dopamine	T44.991	T44.992	T44.993	T44.994	T44.995	T44.996
Doriden	T42.6X1	T42.6X2	T42.6X3	T42.6X4	T42.6X5	T42.6X6
Dormiral	T42.3X1	T42.3X2	T42.3X3	T42.3X4	T42.3X5	T42.3X6
Dormison	T42.6X1	T42.6X2	T42.6X3	T42.6X4	T42.6X5	T42.6X6
Dornase	T48.4X1	T48.4X2	T48.4X3	T48.4X4	T48.4X5	T48.4X6
Dorsacaine	T41.3X1	T41.3X2	T41.3X3	T41.3X4	T41.3X5	T41.3X6
Dosulepin	T43.Ø11	T43.Ø12	T43.Ø13	T43.Ø14	T43.Ø15	T43.Ø16
Dothiepin	T43.Ø11	T43.Ø12	T43.Ø13	T43.Ø14	T43.Ø15	T43.Ø16
Doxantrazole	T48.6X1	T48.6X2	T48.6X3	T48.6X4	T48.6X5	T48.6X6
Doxapram	T5Ø.7X1	T5Ø.7X2	T5Ø.7X3	T5Ø.7X4	T5Ø.7X5	T5Ø.7X6
Doxazosin	T44.6X1	T44.6X2	T44.6X3	T44.6X4	T44.6X5	T44.6X6
Doxepin	T43.Ø11	T43.Ø12	T43.Ø13	T43.Ø14	T43.Ø15	T43.Ø16

	External Cause (T-Code)					
Substance	Poisoning, Accidental (Unintentional)	Poisoning, Intentional Self-Harm	Poisoning, Assault	Poisoning, Undetermined	Adverse Effect	Underdosing
Doxifluridine	T45.1X1	T45.1X2	T45.1X3	T45.1X4	T45.1X5	T45.1X6
Doxorubicin	T45.1X1	T45.1X2	T45.1X3	T45.1X4	T45.1X5	T45.1X6
Doxycycline	T36.4X1	T36.4X2	T36.4X3	T36.4X4	T36.4X5	T36.4X6
Doxylamine	T45.ØX1	T45.ØX2	T45.ØX3	T45.ØX4	T45.ØX5	T45.ØX6
Dramamine	T45.ØX1	T45.ØX2	T45.ØX3	T45.ØX4	T45.ØX5	T45.ØX6
Drano (drain cleaner)	T54.3X1	T54.3X2	T54.3X3	T54.3X4	—	—
Dressing, live pulp	T49.7X1	T49.7X2	T49.7X3	T49.7X4	T49.7X5	T49.7X6
Drocode	T4Ø.2X1	T4Ø.2X2	T4Ø.2X3	T4Ø.2X4	T4Ø.2X5	T4Ø.2X6
Dromoran	T4Ø.2X1	T4Ø.2X2	T4Ø.2X3	T4Ø.2X4	T4Ø.2X5	T4Ø.2X6
Dromostanolone	T38.7X1	T38.7X2	T38.7X3	T38.7X4	T38.7X5	T38.7X6
Dronabinol	T4Ø.7X1	T4Ø.7X2	T4Ø.7X3	T4Ø.7X4	T4Ø.7X5	T4Ø.7X6
Droperidol	T43.591	T43.592	T43.593	T43.594	T43.595	T43.596
Dropropizine	T48.3X1	T48.3X2	T48.3X3	T48.3X4	T48.3X5	T48.3X6
Drostanolone	T38.7X1	T38.7X2	T38.7X3	T38.7X4	T38.7X5	T38.7X6
Drotaverine	T44.3X1	T44.3X2	T44.3X3	T44.3X4	T44.3X5	T44.3X6
Drotrecogin alfa	T45.511	T45.512	T45.513	T45.514	T45.515	T45.516
Drug NEC	T5Ø.9Ø1	T5Ø.9Ø2	T5Ø.9Ø3	T5Ø.9Ø4	T5Ø.9Ø5	T5Ø.9Ø6
specified NEC	T5Ø.991	T5Ø.992	T5Ø.993	T5Ø.994	T5Ø.995	T5Ø.996
DTIC	T45.1X1	T45.1X2	T45.1X3	T45.1X4	T45.1X5	T45.1X6
Duboisine	T44.3X1	T44.3X2	T44.3X3	T44.3X4	T44.3X5	T44.3X6
Dulcolax	T47.2X1	T47.2X2	T47.2X3	T47.2X4	T47.2X5	T47.2X6
Duponol (C) (EP)	T49.2X1	T49.2X2	T49.2X3	T49.2X4	T49.2X5	T49.2X6
Durabolin	T38.7X1	T38.7X2	T38.7X3	T38.7X4	T38.7X5	T38.7X6
Dyclone	T41.3X1	T41.3X2	T41.3X3	T41.3X4	T41.3X5	T41.3X6
Dyclonine	T41.3X1	T41.3X2	T41.3X3	T41.3X4	T41.3X5	T41.3X6
Dydrogesterone	T38.5X1	T38.5X2	T38.5X3	T38.5X4	T38.5X5	T38.5X6
Dye NEC	T65.6X1	T65.6X2	T65.6X3	T65.6X4	—	—
antiseptic	T49.ØX1	T49.ØX2	T49.ØX3	T49.ØX4	T49.ØX5	T49.ØX6
diagnostic agents	T5Ø.8X1	T5Ø.8X2	T5Ø.8X3	T5Ø.8X4	T5Ø.8X5	T5Ø.8X6
pharmaceutical NEC	T5Ø.9Ø1	T5Ø.9Ø2	T5Ø.9Ø3	T5Ø.9Ø4	T5Ø.9Ø5	T5Ø.9Ø6
Dyflos	T44.ØX1	T44.ØX2	T44.ØX3	T44.ØX4	T44.ØX5	T44.ØX6
Dymelor	T38.3X1	T38.3X2	T38.3X3	T38.3X4	T38.3X5	T38.3X6
Dynamite	T65.3X1	T65.3X2	T65.3X3	T65.3X4	—	—
fumes	T59.891	T59.892	T59.893	T59.894	—	—
Dyphylline	T44.3X1	T44.3X2	T44.3X3	T44.3X4	T44.3X5	T44.3X6
E						
Ear drug NEC	T49.6X1	T49.6X2	T49.6X3	T49.6X4	T49.6X5	T49.6X6
Ear preparations	T49.6X1	T49.6X2	T49.6X3	T49.6X4	T49.6X5	T49.6X6
Econazole	T49.ØX1	T49.ØX2	T49.ØX3	T49.ØX4	T49.ØX5	T49.ØX6
Ecothiopate iodide	T49.5X1	T49.5X2	T49.5X3	T49.5X4	T49.5X5	T49.5X6
Echothiophate, echothiopate, ecothiopate	T49.5X1	T49.5X2	T49.5X3	T49.5X4	T49.5X5	T49.5X6

Substance	Poisoning, Accidental (Unintentional)	Poisoning, Intentional Self-Harm	Poisoning, Assault	Poisoning, Undetermined	Adverse Effect	Underdosing
Ecstasy	T43.641	T43.642	T43.643	T43.644	—	—
Ectylurea	T42.6X1	T42.6X2	T42.6X3	T42.6X4	T42.6X5	T42.6X6
Edathamil disodium	T45.8X1	T45.8X2	T45.8X3	T45.8X4	T45.8X5	T45.8X6
Edecrin	T50.1X1	T50.1X2	T50.1X3	T50.1X4	T50.1X5	T50.1X6
Edetate, disodium (calcium)	T45.8X1	T45.8X2	T45.8X3	T45.8X4	T45.8X5	T45.8X6
Edoxudine	T49.5X1	T49.5X2	T49.5X3	T49.5X4	T49.5X5	T49.5X6
Edrophonium	T44.0X1	T44.0X2	T44.0X3	T44.0X4	T44.0X5	T44.0X6
chloride	T44.0X1	T44.0X2	T44.0X3	T44.0X4	T44.0X5	T44.0X6
EDTA	T50.6X1	T50.6X2	T50.6X3	T50.6X4	T50.6X5	T50.6X6
Eflornithine	T37.2X1	T37.2X2	T37.2X3	T37.2X4	T37.2X5	T37.2X6
Efloxate	T46.3X1	T46.3X2	T46.3X3	T46.3X4	T46.3X5	T46.3X6
Elase	T49.8X1	T49.8X2	T49.8X3	T49.8X4	T49.8X5	T49.8X6
Elastase	T47.5X1	T47.5X2	T47.5X3	T47.5X4	T47.5X5	T47.5X6
Elaterium	T47.2X1	T47.2X2	T47.2X3	T47.2X4	T47.2X5	T47.2X6
Elcatonin	T50.991	T50.992	T50.993	T50.994	T50.995	T50.996
Elder	T62.2X1	T62.2X2	T62.2X3	T62.2X4	—	—
berry (unripe)	T62.1X1	T62.1X2	T62.1X3	T62.1X4	—	—
Electrolyte balance drug	T50.3X1	T50.3X2	T50.3X3	T50.3X4	T50.3X5	T50.3X6
Electrolytes NEC	T50.3X1	T50.3X2	T50.3X3	T50.3X4	T50.3X5	T50.3X6
Electrolytic agent NEC	T50.3X1	T50.3X2	T50.3X3	T50.3X4	T50.3X5	T50.3X6
Elemental diet	T50.901	T50.902	T50.903	T50.904	T50.905	T50.906
Elliptinium acetate	T45.1X1	T45.1X2	T45.1X3	T45.1X4	T45.1X5	T45.1X6
Embramine	T45.0X1	T45.0X2	T45.0X3	T45.0X4	T45.0X5	T45.0X6
Emepronium (salts)	T44.3X1	T44.3X2	T44.3X3	T44.3X4	T44.3X5	T44.3X6
bromide	T44.3X1	T44.3X2	T44.3X3	T44.3X4	T44.3X5	T44.3X6
Emetic NEC	T47.7X1	T47.7X2	T47.7X3	T47.7X4	T47.7X5	T47.7X6
Emetine	T37.3X1	T37.3X2	T37.3X3	T37.3X4	T37.3X5	T37.3X6
Emollient NEC	T49.3X1	T49.3X2	T49.3X3	T49.3X4	T49.3X5	T49.3X6
Emorfazone	T39.8X1	T39.8X2	T39.8X3	T39.8X4	T39.8X5	T39.8X6
Emylcamate	T43.591	T43.592	T43.593	T43.594	T43.595	T43.596
Enalapril	T46.4X1	T46.4X2	T46.4X3	T46.4X4	T46.4X5	T46.4X6
Enalaprilat	T46.4X1	T46.4X2	T46.4X3	T46.4X4	T46.4X5	T46.4X6
Encainide	T46.2X1	T46.2X2	T46.2X3	T46.2X4	T46.2X5	T46.2X6
Endocaine	T41.3X1	T41.3X2	T41.3X3	T41.3X4	T41.3X5	T41.3X6
Endosulfan	T60.2X1	T60.2X2	T60.2X3	T60.2X4	—	—
Endothall	T60.3X1	T60.3X2	T60.3X3	T60.3X4	—	—
Endralazine	T46.5X1	T46.5X2	T46.5X3	T46.5X4	T46.5X5	T46.5X6
Endrin	T60.1X1	T60.1X2	T60.1X3	T60.1X4	—	—
Enflurane	T41.0X1	T41.0X2	T41.0X3	T41.0X4	T41.0X5	T41.0X6
Enhexymal	T42.3X1	T42.3X2	T42.3X3	T42.3X4	T42.3X5	T42.3X6
Enocitabine	T45.1X1	T45.1X2	T45.1X3	T45.1X4	T45.1X5	T45.1X6
Enovid	T38.4X1	T38.4X2	T38.4X3	T38.4X4	T38.4X5	T38.4X6

Substance	Poisoning, Accidental (Unintentional)	Poisoning, Intentional Self-Harm	Poisoning, Assault	Poisoning, Undetermined	Adverse Effect	Underdosing
Enoxacin	T36.8X1	T36.8X2	T36.8X3	T36.8X4	T36.8X5	T36.8X6
Enoxaparin (sodium)	T45.511	T45.512	T45.513	T45.514	T45.515	T45.516
Enpiprazole	T43.591	T43.592	T43.593	T43.594	T43.595	T43.596
Enprofylline	T48.6X1	T48.6X2	T48.6X3	T48.6X4	T48.6X5	T48.6X6
Enprostil	T47.1X1	T47.1X2	T47.1X3	T47.1X4	T47.1X5	T47.1X6
ENT preparations (anti-infectives)	T49.6X1	T49.6X2	T49.6X3	T49.6X4	T49.6X5	T49.6X6
Enviomycin	T36.8X1	T36.8X2	T36.8X3	T36.8X4	T36.8X5	T36.8X6
Enzodase	T45.3X1	T45.3X2	T45.3X3	T45.3X4	T45.3X5	T45.3X6
Enzyme NEC	T45.3X1	T45.3X2	T45.3X3	T45.3X4	T45.3X5	T45.3X6
depolymerizing	T49.8X1	T49.8X2	T49.8X3	T49.8X4	T49.8X5	T49.8X6
fibrolytic	T45.3X1	T45.3X2	T45.3X3	T45.3X4	T45.3X5	T45.3X6
gastric	T47.5X1	T47.5X2	T47.5X3	T47.5X4	T47.5X5	T47.5X6
intestinal	T47.5X1	T47.5X2	T47.5X3	T47.5X4	T47.5X5	T47.5X6
local action	T49.4X1	T49.4X2	T49.4X3	T49.4X4	T49.4X5	T49.4X6
proteolytic	T49.4X1	T49.4X2	T49.4X3	T49.4X4	T49.4X5	T49.4X6
thrombolytic	T45.3X1	T45.3X2	T45.3X3	T45.3X4	T45.3X5	T45.3X6
EPAB	T41.3X1	T41.3X2	T41.3X3	T41.3X4	T41.3X5	T41.3X6
Epanutin	T42.0X1	T42.0X2	T42.0X3	T42.0X4	T42.0X5	T42.0X6
Ephedra	T44.991	T44.992	T44.993	T44.994	T44.995	T44.996
Ephedrine	T44.991	T44.992	T44.993	T44.994	T44.995	T44.996
Epichlorhydrin, epichlorohydrin	T52.8X1	T52.8X2	T52.8X3	T52.8X4	—	—
Epicillin	T36.0X1	T36.0X2	T36.0X3	T36.0X4	T36.0X5	T36.0X6
Epiestriol	T38.5X1	T38.5X2	T38.5X3	T38.5X4	T38.5X5	T38.5X6
Epilim — see Sodium valproate						
Epimestrol	T38.5X1	T38.5X2	T38.5X3	T38.5X4	T38.5X5	T38.5X6
Epinephrine	T44.5X1	T44.5X2	T44.5X3	T44.5X4	T44.5X5	T44.5X6
Epirubicin	T45.1X1	T45.1X2	T45.1X3	T45.1X4	T45.1X5	T45.1X6
Epitiostanol	T38.7X1	T38.7X2	T38.7X3	T38.7X4	T38.7X5	T38.7X6
Epitizide	T50.2X1	T50.2X2	T50.2X3	T50.2X4	T50.2X5	T50.2X6
EPN	T60.0X1	T60.0X2	T60.0X3	T60.0X4	—	—
EPO	T45.8X1	T45.8X2	T45.8X3	T45.8X4	T45.8X5	T45.8X6
Epoetin alpha	T45.8X1	T45.8X2	T45.8X3	T45.8X4	T45.8X5	T45.8X6
Epomediol	T50.991	T50.992	T50.993	T50.994	T50.995	T50.996
Epoprostenol	T45.521	T45.522	T45.523	T45.524	T45.525	T45.526
Epoxy resin	T65.891	T65.892	T65.893	T65.894	—	—
Eprazinone	T48.4X1	T48.4X2	T48.4X3	T48.4X4	T48.4X5	T48.4X6
Epsilon amino-caproic acid	T45.621	T45.622	T45.623	T45.624	T45.625	T45.626
Epsom salt	T47.3X1	T47.3X2	T47.3X3	T47.3X4	T47.3X5	T47.3X6
Eptazocine	T40.4X1	T40.4X2	T40.4X3	T40.4X4	T40.4X5	T40.4X6
Equanil	T43.591	T43.592	T43.593	T43.594	T43.595	T43.596
Equisetum	T62.2X1	T62.2X2	T62.2X3	T62.2X4	—	—
diuretic	T50.2X1	T50.2X2	T50.2X3	T50.2X4	T50.2X5	T50.2X6

◀ New　◀ Revised　~~deleted~~ Deleted

Substance	External Cause (T-Code) Poisoning, Accidental (Unintentional)	Poisoning, Intentional Self-Harm	Poisoning, Assault	Poisoning, Undetermined	Adverse Effect	Underdosing
Ergobasine	T48.ØX1	T48.ØX2	T48.ØX3	T48.ØX4	T48.ØX5	T48.ØX6
Ergocalciferol	T45.2X1	T45.2X2	T45.2X3	T45.2X4	T45.2X5	T45.2X6
Ergoloid mesylates	T46.7X1	T46.7X2	T46.7X3	T46.7X4	T46.7X5	T46.7X6
Ergometrine	T48.ØX1	T48.ØX2	T48.ØX3	T48.ØX4	T48.ØX5	T48.ØX6
Ergonovine	T48.ØX1	T48.ØX2	T48.ØX3	T48.ØX4	T48.ØX5	T48.ØX6
Ergot NEC	T64.81	T64.82	T64.83	T64.84	—	—
- derivative	T48.ØX1	T48.ØX2	T48.ØX3	T48.ØX4	T48.ØX5	T48.ØX6
- medicinal (alkaloids)	T48.ØX1	T48.ØX2	T48.ØX3	T48.ØX4	T48.ØX5	T48.ØX6
- prepared	T48.ØX1	T48.ØX2	T48.ØX3	T48.ØX4	T48.ØX5	T48.ØX6
Ergotamine	T46.5X1	T46.5X2	T46.5X3	T46.5X4	T46.5X5	T46.5X6
Ergotocine	T48.ØX1	T48.ØX2	T48.ØX3	T48.ØX4	T48.ØX5	T48.ØX6
Ergotrate	T48.ØX1	T48.ØX2	T48.ØX3	T48.ØX4	T48.ØX5	T48.ØX6
Eritrityl tetranitrate	T46.3X1	T46.3X2	T46.3X3	T46.3X4	T46.3X5	T46.3X6
Erythrityl tetranitrate	T46.3X1	T46.3X2	T46.3X3	T46.3X4	T46.3X5	T46.3X6
Erythrol tetranitrate	T46.3X1	T46.3X2	T46.3X3	T46.3X4	T46.3X5	T46.3X6
Erythromycin (salts)	T36.3X1	T36.3X2	T36.3X3	T36.3X4	T36.3X5	T36.3X6
- ophthalmic preparation	T49.5X1	T49.5X2	T49.5X3	T49.5X4	T49.5X5	T49.5X6
- topical NEC	T49.ØX1	T49.ØX2	T49.ØX3	T49.ØX4	T49.ØX5	T49.ØX6
Erythropoietin	T45.8X1	T45.8X2	T45.8X3	T45.8X4	T45.8X5	T45.8X6
- human	T45.8X1	T45.8X2	T45.8X3	T45.8X4	T45.8X5	T45.8X6
Escin	T46.991	T46.992	T46.993	T46.994	T46.995	T46.996
Esculin	T45.2X1	T45.2X2	T45.2X3	T45.2X4	T45.2X5	T45.2X6
Esculoside	T45.2X1	T45.2X2	T45.2X3	T45.2X4	T45.2X5	T45.2X6
ESDT (ether-soluble tar distillate)	T49.1X1	T49.1X2	T49.1X3	T49.1X4	T49.1X5	T49.1X6
Eserine	T49.5X1	T49.5X2	T49.5X3	T49.5X4	T49.5X5	T49.5X6
Esflurbiprofen	T39.311	T39.312	T39.313	T39.314	T39.315	T39.316
Eskabarb	T42.3X1	T42.3X2	T42.3X3	T42.3X4	T42.3X5	T42.3X6
Eskalith	T43.8X1	T43.8X2	T43.8X3	T43.8X4	T43.8X5	T43.8X6
Esmolol	T44.7X1	T44.7X2	T44.7X3	T44.7X4	T44.7X5	T44.7X6
Estanozolol	T38.7X1	T38.7X2	T38.7X3	T38.7X4	T38.7X5	T38.7X6
Estazolam	T42.4X1	T42.4X2	T42.4X3	T42.4X4	T42.4X5	T42.4X6
Estradiol	T38.5X1	T38.5X2	T38.5X3	T38.5X4	T38.5X5	T38.5X6
- with testosterone	T38.7X1	T38.7X2	T38.7X3	T38.7X4	T38.7X5	T38.7X6
- benzoate	T38.5X1	T38.5X2	T38.5X3	T38.5X4	T38.5X5	T38.5X6
Estramustine	T45.1X1	T45.1X2	T45.1X3	T45.1X4	T45.1X5	T45.1X6
Estriol	T38.5X1	T38.5X2	T38.5X3	T38.5X4	T38.5X5	T38.5X6
Estrogen	T38.5X1	T38.5X2	T38.5X3	T38.5X4	T38.5X5	T38.5X6
- with progesterone	T38.5X1	T38.5X2	T38.5X3	T38.5X4	T38.5X5	T38.5X6
- conjugated	T38.5X1	T38.5X2	T38.5X3	T38.5X4	T38.5X5	T38.5X6
Estrone	T38.5X1	T38.5X2	T38.5X3	T38.5X4	T38.5X5	T38.5X6
Estropipate	T38.5X1	T38.5X2	T38.5X3	T38.5X4	T38.5X5	T38.5X6

Substance	External Cause (T-Code) Poisoning, Accidental (Unintentional)	Poisoning, Intentional Self-Harm	Poisoning, Assault	Poisoning, Undetermined	Adverse Effect	Underdosing
Etacrynate sodium	T5Ø.1X1	T5Ø.1X2	T5Ø.1X3	T5Ø.1X4	T5Ø.1X5	T5Ø.1X6
Etacrynic acid	T5Ø.1X1	T5Ø.1X2	T5Ø.1X3	T5Ø.1X4	T5Ø.1X5	T5Ø.1X6
Etafedrine	T48.6X1	T48.6X2	T48.6X3	T48.6X4	T48.6X5	T48.6X6
Etafenone	T46.3X1	T46.3X2	T46.3X3	T46.3X4	T46.3X5	T46.3X6
Etambutol	T37.1X1	T37.1X2	T37.1X3	T37.1X4	T37.1X5	T37.1X6
Etamiphyllin	T48.6X1	T48.6X2	T48.6X3	T48.6X4	T48.6X5	T48.6X6
Etamivan	T5Ø.7X1	T5Ø.7X2	T5Ø.7X3	T5Ø.7X4	T5Ø.7X5	T5Ø.7X6
Etamsylate	T45.7X1	T45.7X2	T45.7X3	T45.7X4	T45.7X5	T45.7X6
Etebenecid	T5Ø.4X1	T5Ø.4X2	T5Ø.4X3	T5Ø.4X4	T5Ø.4X5	T5Ø.4X6
Ethacridine	T49.ØX1	T49.ØX2	T49.ØX3	T49.ØX4	T49.ØX5	T49.ØX6
Ethacrynic acid	T5Ø.1X1	T5Ø.1X2	T5Ø.1X3	T5Ø.1X4	T5Ø.1X5	T5Ø.1X6
Ethadione	T42.2X1	T42.2X2	T42.2X3	T42.2X4	T42.2X5	T42.2X6
Ethambutol	T37.1X1	T37.1X2	T37.1X3	T37.1X4	T37.1X5	T37.1X6
Ethamide	T5Ø.2X1	T5Ø.2X2	T5Ø.2X3	T5Ø.2X4	T5Ø.2X5	T5Ø.2X6
Ethamivan	T5Ø.7X1	T5Ø.7X2	T5Ø.7X3	T5Ø.7X4	T5Ø.7X5	T5Ø.7X6
Ethamsylate	T45.7X1	T45.7X2	T45.7X3	T45.7X4	T45.7X5	T45.7X6
Ethanol	T51.ØX1	T51.ØX2	T51.ØX3	T51.ØX4	—	—
- beverage	T51.ØX1	T51.ØX2	T51.ØX3	T51.ØX4	—	—
Ethanolamine oleate	T46.8X1	T46.8X2	T46.8X3	T46.8X4	T46.8X5	T46.8X6
Ethaverine	T44.3X1	T44.3X2	T44.3X3	T44.3X4	T44.3X5	T44.3X6
Ethchlorvynol	T42.6X1	T42.6X2	T42.6X3	T42.6X4	T42.6X5	T42.6X6
Ethebenecid	T5Ø.4X1	T5Ø.4X2	T5Ø.4X3	T5Ø.4X4	T5Ø.4X5	T5Ø.4X6
Ether (vapor)	T41.ØX1	T41.ØX2	T41.ØX3	T41.ØX4	T41.ØX5	T41.ØX6
- anesthetic	T41.ØX1	T41.ØX2	T41.ØX3	T41.ØX4	T41.ØX5	T41.ØX6
- divinyl	T41.ØX1	T41.ØX2	T41.ØX3	T41.ØX4	T41.ØX5	T41.ØX6
- ethyl (medicinal)	T41.ØX1	T41.ØX2	T41.ØX3	T41.ØX4	T41.ØX5	T41.ØX6
- - nonmedicinal	T52.8X1	T52.8X2	T52.8X3	T52.8X4	—	—
- petroleum — *see Ligroin*						
- solvent	T52.8X1	T52.8X2	T52.8X3	T52.8X4	—	—
Ethiazide	T5Ø.2X1	T5Ø.2X2	T5Ø.2X3	T5Ø.2X4	T5Ø.2X5	T5Ø.2X6
Ethidium chloride (vapor)	T59.891	T59.892	T59.893	T59.894	—	—
Ethinamate	T42.6X1	T42.6X2	T42.6X3	T42.6X4	T42.6X5	T42.6X6
Ethinylestradiol, ethinyloestradiol	T38.5X1	T38.5X2	T38.5X3	T38.5X4	T38.5X5	T38.5X6
- with						
- - levonorgestrel	T38.4X1	T38.4X2	T38.4X3	T38.4X4	T38.4X5	T38.4X6
- - norethisterone	T38.4X1	T38.4X2	T38.4X3	T38.4X4	T38.4X5	T38.4X6
Ethiodized oil (131 I)	T5Ø.8X1	T5Ø.8X2	T5Ø.8X3	T5Ø.8X4	T5Ø.8X5	T5Ø.8X6
Ethion	T6Ø.ØX1	T6Ø.ØX2	T6Ø.ØX3	T6Ø.ØX4	—	—
Ethionamide	T37.1X1	T37.1X2	T37.1X3	T37.1X4	T37.1X5	T37.1X6
Ethioniamide	T37.1X1	T37.1X2	T37.1X3	T37.1X4	T37.1X5	T37.1X6
Ethisterone	T38.5X1	T38.5X2	T38.5X3	T38.5X4	T38.5X5	T38.5X6
Ethobral	T42.3X1	T42.3X2	T42.3X3	T42.3X4	T42.3X5	T42.3X6

Substance	External Cause (T-Code)					
	Poisoning, Accidental (Unintentional)	Poisoning, Intentional Self-Harm	Poisoning, Assault	Poisoning, Undetermined	Adverse Effect	Underdosing
Ethocaine (infiltration) (topical)	T41.3X1	T41.3X2	T41.3X3	T41.3X4	T41.3X5	T41.3X6
nerve block (peripheral) (plexus)	T41.3X1	T41.3X2	T41.3X3	T41.3X4	T41.3X5	T41.3X6
spinal	T41.3X1	T41.3X2	T41.3X3	T41.3X4	T41.3X5	T41.3X6
Ethoheptazine	T4Ø.4X1	T4Ø.4X2	T4Ø.4X3	T4Ø.4X4	T4Ø.4X5	T4Ø.4X6
Ethopropazine	T44.3X1	T44.3X2	T44.3X3	T44.3X4	T44.3X5	T44.3X6
Ethosuximide	T42.2X1	T42.2X2	T42.2X3	T42.2X4	T42.2X5	T42.2X6
Ethotoin	T42.ØX1	T42.ØX2	T42.ØX3	T42.ØX4	T42.ØX5	T42.ØX6
Ethoxazene	T37.91	T37.92	T37.93	T37.94	T37.95	T37.96
Ethoxazorutoside	T46.991	T46.992	T46.993	T46.994	T46.995	T46.996
2-Ethoxyethanol	T52.3X1	T52.3X2	T52.3X3	T52.3X4	—	—
Ethoxzolamide	T5Ø.2X1	T5Ø.2X2	T5Ø.2X3	T5Ø.2X4	T5Ø.2X5	T5Ø.2X6
Ethyl						
acetate	T52.8X1	T52.8X2	T52.8X3	T52.8X4	—	—
alcohol	T51.ØX1	T51.ØX2	T51.ØX3	T51.ØX4	—	—
beverage	T51.ØX1	T51.ØX2	T51.ØX3	T51.ØX4	—	—
aldehyde (vapor)	T59.891	T59.892	T59.893	T59.894	—	—
liquid	T52.8X1	T52.8X2	T52.8X3	T52.8X4	—	—
aminobenzoate	T41.3X1	T41.3X2	T41.3X3	T41.3X4	T41.3X5	T41.3X6
aminophenothiazine	T43.3X1	T43.3X2	T43.3X3	T43.3X4	T43.3X5	T43.3X6
benzoate	T52.8X1	T52.8X2	T52.8X3	T52.8X4	—	—
biscoumacetate	T45.511	T45.512	T45.513	T45.514	T45.515	T45.516
bromide (anesthetic)	T41.ØX1	T41.ØX2	T41.ØX3	T41.ØX4	T41.ØX5	T41.ØX6
carbamate	T45.1X1	T45.1X2	T45.1X3	T45.1X4	T45.1X5	T45.1X6
carbinol	T51.3X1	T51.3X2	T51.3X3	T51.3X4	—	—
carbonate	T52.8X1	T52.8X2	T52.8X3	T52.8X4	—	—
chaulmoograte	T37.1X1	T37.1X2	T37.1X3	T37.1X4	T37.1X5	T37.1X6
chloride (anesthetic)	T41.ØX1	T41.ØX2	T41.ØX3	T41.ØX4	T41.ØX5	T41.ØX6
anesthetic (local)	T41.3X1	T41.3X2	T41.3X3	T41.3X4	T41.3X5	T41.3X6
inhaled	T41.ØX1	T41.ØX2	T41.ØX3	T41.ØX4	T41.ØX5	T41.ØX6
local	T49.4X1	T49.4X2	T49.4X3	T49.4X4	T49.4X5	T49.4X6
solvent	T53.6X1	T53.6X2	T53.6X3	T53.6X4	—	—
dibunate	T48.3X1	T48.3X2	T48.3X3	T48.3X4	T48.3X5	T48.3X6
dichloroarsine (vapor)	T57.ØX1	T57.ØX2	T57.ØX3	T57.ØX4	—	—
estranol	T38.7X1	T38.7X2	T38.7X3	T38.7X4	T38.7X5	T38.7X6
ether—*see also* Ether	T52.8X1	T52.8X2	T52.8X3	T52.8X4	—	—
formate NEC (solvent)	T52.ØX1	T52.ØX2	T52.ØX3	T52.ØX4	—	—
fumarate	T49.4X1	T49.4X2	T49.4X3	T49.4X4	T49.4X5	T49.4X6
hydroxyisobutyrate NEC (solvent)	T52.8X1	T52.8X2	T52.8X3	T52.8X4	—	—
iodoacetate	T59.3X1	T59.3X2	T59.3X3	T59.3X4	—	—
lactate NEC (solvent)	T52.8X1	T52.8X2	T52.8X3	T52.8X4	—	—
loflazepate	T42.4X1	T42.4X2	T42.4X3	T42.4X4	T42.4X5	T42.4X6
Ethyl *(Continued)*						
mercuric chloride	T56.1X1	T56.1X2	T56.1X3	T56.1X4	—	—
methylcarbinol	T51.8X1	T51.8X2	T51.8X3	T51.8X4	—	—
morphine	T4Ø.2X1	T4Ø.2X2	T4Ø.2X3	T4Ø.2X4	T4Ø.2X5	T4Ø.2X6
noradrenaline	T48.6X1	T48.6X2	T48.6X3	T48.6X4	T48.6X5	T48.6X6
oxybutyrate NEC (solvent)	T52.8X1	T52.8X2	T52.8X3	T52.8X4	—	—
Ethylene (gas)	T59.891	T59.892	T59.893	T59.894	—	—
anesthetic (general)	T41.ØX1	T41.ØX2	T41.ØX3	T41.ØX4	T41.ØX5	T41.ØX6
chlorohydrin	T52.8X1	T52.8X2	T52.8X3	T52.8X4	—	—
vapor	T53.6X1	T53.6X2	T53.6X3	T53.6X4	—	—
dichloride	T52.8X1	T52.8X2	T52.8X3	T52.8X4	—	—
vapor	T53.6X1	T53.6X2	T53.6X3	T53.6X4	—	—
dinitrate	T52.3X1	T52.3X2	T52.3X3	T52.3X4	—	—
glycol(s)	T52.8X1	T52.8X2	T52.8X3	T52.8X4	—	—
dinitrate	T52.3X1	T52.3X2	T52.3X3	T52.3X4	—	—
monobutyl ether	T52.3X1	T52.3X2	T52.3X3	T52.3X4	—	—
imine	T54.1X1	T54.1X2	T54.1X3	T54.1X4	—	—
oxide (fumigant) (nonmedicinal)	T59.891	T59.892	T59.893	T59.894	—	—
medicinal	T49.ØX1	T49.ØX2	T49.ØX3	T49.ØX4	T49.ØX5	T49.ØX6
Ethylenediamine theophylline	T48.6X1	T48.6X2	T48.6X3	T48.6X4	T48.6X5	T48.6X6
Ethylenediaminetetra-acetic acid	T5Ø.6X1	T5Ø.6X2	T5Ø.6X3	T5Ø.6X4	T5Ø.6X5	T5Ø.6X6
Ethylenedinitrilotetra-acetate	T5Ø.6X1	T5Ø.6X2	T5Ø.6X3	T5Ø.6X4	T5Ø.6X5	T5Ø.6X6
Ethylestrenol	T38.7X1	T38.7X2	T38.7X3	T38.7X4	T38.7X5	T38.7X6
Ethylhydroxycellulose	T47.4X1	T47.4X2	T47.4X3	T47.4X4	T47.4X5	T47.4X6
Ethylidene						
chloride NEC	T53.6X1	T53.6X2	T53.6X3	T53.6X4	—	—
diacetate	T6Ø.3X1	T6Ø.3X2	T6Ø.3X3	T6Ø.3X4	—	—
dicoumarin	T45.511	T45.512	T45.513	T45.514	T45.515	T45.516
dicoumarol	T45.511	T45.512	T45.513	T45.514	T45.515	T45.516
diethyl ether	T52.ØX1	T52.ØX2	T52.ØX3	T52.ØX4	—	—
Ethylmorphine	T4Ø.2X1	T4Ø.2X2	T4Ø.2X3	T4Ø.2X4	T4Ø.2X5	T4Ø.2X6
Ethylnorepinephrine	T48.6X1	T48.6X2	T48.6X3	T48.6X4	T48.6X5	T48.6X6
Ethylparachlorophen-oxyisobutyrate	T46.6X1	T46.6X2	T46.6X3	T46.6X4	T46.6X5	T46.6X6
Ethynodiol	T38.4X1	T38.4X2	T38.4X3	T38.4X4	T38.4X5	T38.4X6
with mestranol diacetate	T38.4X1	T38.4X2	T38.4X3	T38.4X4	T38.4X5	T38.4X6
Etidocaine	T41.3X1	T41.3X2	T41.3X3	T41.3X4	T41.3X5	T41.3X6
infiltration (subcutaneous)	T41.3X1	T41.3X2	T41.3X3	T41.3X4	T41.3X5	T41.3X6
nerve (peripheral) (plexus)	T41.3X1	T41.3X2	T41.3X3	T41.3X4	T41.3X5	T41.3X6
Etidronate	T5Ø.991	T5Ø.992	T5Ø.993	T5Ø.994	T5Ø.995	T5Ø.996
Etidronic acid (disodium salt)	T5Ø.991	T5Ø.992	T5Ø.993	T5Ø.994	T5Ø.995	T5Ø.996
Etifoxine	T42.6X1	T42.6X2	T42.6X3	T42.6X4	T42.6X5	T42.6X6

New Revised ~~deleted~~ Deleted

		External Cause (T-Code)				
Substance	Poisoning, Accidental (Unintentional)	Poisoning, Intentional Self-Harm	Poisoning, Assault	Poisoning, Undetermined	Adverse Effect	Underdosing
Etilefrine	T44.4X1	T44.4X2	T44.4X3	T44.4X4	T44.4X5	T44.4X6
Etilfen	T42.3X1	T42.3X2	T42.3X3	T42.3X4	T42.3X5	T42.3X6
Etinodiol	T38.4X1	T38.4X2	T38.4X3	T38.4X4	T38.4X5	T38.4X6
Etiroxate	T46.6X1	T46.6X2	T46.6X3	T46.6X4	T46.6X5	T46.6X6
Etizolam	T42.4X1	T42.4X2	T42.4X3	T42.4X4	T42.4X5	T42.4X6
Etodolac	T39.391	T39.392	T39.393	T39.394	T39.395	T39.396
Etofamide	T37.3X1	T37.3X2	T37.3X3	T37.3X4	T37.3X5	T37.3X6
Etofibrate	T46.6X1	T46.6X2	T46.6X3	T46.6X4	T46.6X5	T46.6X6
Etofylline	T46.7X1	T46.7X2	T46.7X3	T46.7X4	T46.7X5	T46.7X6
clofibrate	T46.6X1	T46.6X2	T46.6X3	T46.6X4	T46.6X5	T46.6X6
Etoglucid	T45.1X1	T45.1X2	T45.1X3	T45.1X4	T45.1X5	T45.1X6
Etomidate	T41.1X1	T41.1X2	T41.1X3	T41.1X4	T41.1X5	T41.1X6
Etomide	T39.8X1	T39.8X2	T39.8X3	T39.8X4	T39.8X5	T39.8X6
Etomidoline	T44.3X1	T44.3X2	T44.3X3	T44.3X4	T44.3X5	T44.3X6
Etoposide	T45.1X1	T45.1X2	T45.1X3	T45.1X4	T45.1X5	T45.1X6
Etorphine	T40.2X1	T40.2X2	T40.2X3	T40.2X4	T40.2X5	T40.2X6
Etoval	T42.3X1	T42.3X2	T42.3X3	T42.3X4	T42.3X5	T42.3X6
Etozolin	T50.1X1	T50.1X2	T50.1X3	T50.1X4	T50.1X5	T50.1X6
Etretinate	T50.991	T50.992	T50.993	T50.994	T50.995	T50.996
Etryptamine	T43.691	T43.692	T43.693	T43.694	T43.695	T43.696
Etybenzatropine	T44.3X1	T44.3X2	T44.3X3	T44.3X4	T44.3X5	T44.3X6
Etynodiol	T38.4X1	T38.4X2	T38.4X3	T38.4X4	T38.4X5	T38.4X6
Eucaine	T41.3X1	T41.3X2	T41.3X3	T41.3X4	T41.3X5	T41.3X6
Eucalyptus oil	T49.7X1	T49.7X2	T49.7X3	T49.7X4	T49.7X5	T49.7X6
Eucatropine	T49.5X1	T49.5X2	T49.5X3	T49.5X4	T49.5X5	T49.5X6
Eucodal	T40.2X1	T40.2X2	T40.2X3	T40.2X4	T40.2X5	T40.2X6
Euneryl	T42.3X1	T42.3X2	T42.3X3	T42.3X4	T42.3X5	T42.3X6
Euphthalmine	T44.3X1	T44.3X2	T44.3X3	T44.3X4	T44.3X5	T44.3X6
Eurax	T49.0X1	T49.0X2	T49.0X3	T49.0X4	T49.0X5	T49.0X6
Euresol	T49.4X1	T49.4X2	T49.4X3	T49.4X4	T49.4X5	T49.4X6
Euthroid	T38.1X1	T38.1X2	T38.1X3	T38.1X4	T38.1X5	T38.1X6
Evans blue	T50.8X1	T50.8X2	T50.8X3	T50.8X4	T50.8X5	T50.8X6
Evipal	T42.3X1	T42.3X2	T42.3X3	T42.3X4	T42.3X5	T42.3X6
sodium	T41.1X1	T41.1X2	T41.1X3	T41.1X4	T41.1X5	T41.1X6
Evipan	T42.3X1	T42.3X2	T42.3X3	T42.3X4	T42.3X5	T42.3X6
sodium	T41.1X1	T41.1X2	T41.1X3	T41.1X4	T41.1X5	T41.1X6
Exalamide	T49.0X1	T49.0X2	T49.0X3	T49.0X4	T49.0X5	T49.0X6
Exalgin	T39.1X1	T39.1X2	T39.1X3	T39.1X4	T39.1X5	T39.1X6
Excipients, pharmaceutical	T50.901	T50.902	T50.903	T50.904	T50.905	T50.906
Exhaust gas (engine) (motor vehicle)	T58.01	T58.02	T58.03	T58.04	—	—
Ex-Lax (phenolphthalein)	T47.2X1	T47.2X2	T47.2X3	T47.2X4	T47.2X5	T47.2X6
Expectorant NEC	T48.4X1	T48.4X2	T48.4X3	T48.4X4	T48.4X5	T48.4X6
Extended insulin zinc suspension	T38.3X1	T38.3X2	T38.3X3	T38.3X4	T38.3X5	T38.3X6
External medications (skin) (mucous membrane)	T49.91	T49.92	T49.93	T49.94	T49.95	T49.96
dental agent	T49.7X1	T49.7X2	T49.7X3	T49.7X4	T49.7X5	T49.7X6
ENT agent	T49.6X1	T49.6X2	T49.6X3	T49.6X4	T49.6X5	T49.6X6
ophthalmic preparation	T49.5X1	T49.5X2	T49.5X3	T49.5X4	T49.5X5	T49.5X6
specified NEC	T49.8X1	T49.8X2	T49.8X3	T49.8X4	T49.8X5	T49.8X6
Extrapyramidal antagonist NEC	T44.3X1	T44.3X2	T44.3X3	T44.3X4	T44.3X5	T44.3X6
Eye agents (anti-infective)	T49.5X1	T49.5X2	T49.5X3	T49.5X4	T49.5X5	T49.5X6
Eye drug NEC	T49.5X1	T49.5X2	T49.5X3	T49.5X4	T49.5X5	T49.5X6
F						
FAC (fluorouracil + doxorubicin + cyclophosphamide)	T45.1X1	T45.1X2	T45.1X3	T45.1X4	T45.1X5	T45.1X6
Factor						
I (fibrinogen)	T45.8X1	T45.8X2	T45.8X3	T45.8X4	T45.8X5	T45.8X6
III (thromboplastin)	T45.8X1	T45.8X2	T45.8X3	T45.8X4	T45.8X5	T45.8X6
VIII (antihemophilic Factor) (Concentrate)	T45.8X1	T45.8X2	T45.8X3	T45.8X4	T45.8X5	T45.8X6
IX complex	T45.7X1	T45.7X2	T45.7X3	T45.7X4	T45.7X5	T45.7X6
human	T45.8X1	T45.8X2	T45.8X3	T45.8X4	T45.8X5	T45.8X6
Famotidine	T47.0X1	T47.0X2	T47.0X3	T47.0X4	T47.0X5	T47.0X6
Fat suspension, intravenous	T50.991	T50.992	T50.993	T50.994	T50.995	T50.996
Fazadinium bromide	T48.1X1	T48.1X2	T48.1X3	T48.1X4	T48.1X5	T48.1X6
Febarbamate	T42.3X1	T42.3X2	T42.3X3	T42.3X4	T42.3X5	T42.3X6
Fecal softener	T47.4X1	T47.4X2	T47.4X3	T47.4X4	T47.4X5	T47.4X6
Fedrilate	T48.3X1	T48.3X2	T48.3X3	T48.3X4	T48.3X5	T48.3X6
Felodipine	T46.1X1	T46.1X2	T46.1X3	T46.1X4	T46.1X5	T46.1X6
Felypressin	T38.891	T38.892	T38.893	T38.894	T38.895	T38.896
Femoxetine	T43.221	T43.222	T43.223	T43.224	T43.225	T43.226
Fenalcomine	T46.3X1	T46.3X2	T46.3X3	T46.3X4	T46.3X5	T46.3X6
Fenamisal	T37.1X1	T37.1X2	T37.1X3	T37.1X4	T37.1X5	T37.1X6
Fenazone	T39.2X1	T39.2X2	T39.2X3	T39.2X4	T39.2X5	T39.2X6
Fenbendazole	T37.4X1	T37.4X2	T37.4X3	T37.4X4	T37.4X5	T37.4X6
Fenbutrazate	T50.5X1	T50.5X2	T50.5X3	T50.5X4	T50.5X5	T50.5X6
Fencamfamine	T43.691	T43.692	T43.693	T43.694	T43.695	T43.696
Fendiline	T46.1X1	T46.1X2	T46.1X3	T46.1X4	T46.1X5	T46.1X6
Fenetylline	T43.691	T43.692	T43.693	T43.694	T43.695	T43.696
Fenflumizole	T39.391	T39.392	T39.393	T39.394	T39.395	T39.396
Fenfluramine	T50.5X1	T50.5X2	T50.5X3	T50.5X4	T50.5X5	T50.5X6
Fenobarbital	T42.3X1	T42.3X2	T42.3X3	T42.3X4	T42.3X5	T42.3X6
Fenofibrate	T46.6X1	T46.6X2	T46.6X3	T46.6X4	T46.6X5	T46.6X6
Fenoprofen	T39.311	T39.312	T39.313	T39.314	T39.315	T39.316
Fenoterol	T48.6X1	T48.6X2	T48.6X3	T48.6X4	T48.6X5	T48.6X6

Substance	External Cause (T-Code) Poisoning, Accidental (Unintentional)	Poisoning, Intentional Self-Harm	Poisoning, Assault	Poisoning, Undetermined	Adverse Effect	Underdosing
Fenoverine	T44.3X1	T44.3X2	T44.3X3	T44.3X4	T44.3X5	T44.3X6
Fenoxazoline	T48.5X1	T48.5X2	T48.5X3	T48.5X4	T48.5X5	T48.5X6
Fenproporex	T50.5X1	T50.5X2	T50.5X3	T50.5X4	T50.5X5	T50.5X6
Fenquizone	T50.2X1	T50.2X2	T50.2X3	T50.2X4	T50.2X5	T50.2X6
Fentanyl	T40.4X1	T40.4X2	T40.4X3	T40.4X4	T40.4X5	T40.4X6
Fentazin	T43.3X1	T43.3X2	T43.3X3	T43.3X4	T43.3X5	T43.3X6
Fenthion	T60.0X1	T60.0X2	T60.0X3	T60.0X4	—	—
Fenticlor	T49.0X1	T49.0X2	T49.0X3	T49.0X4	T49.0X5	T49.0X6
Fenylbutazone	T39.2X1	T39.2X2	T39.2X3	T39.2X4	T39.2X5	T39.2X6
Feprazone	T39.2X1	T39.2X2	T39.2X3	T39.2X4	T39.2X5	T39.2X6
Fer de lance (bite) (venom)	T63.061	T63.062	T63.063	T63.064	—	—
Ferric — *see also Iron*						
chloride	T45.4X1	T45.4X2	T45.4X3	T45.4X4	T45.4X5	T45.4X6
citrate	T45.4X1	T45.4X2	T45.4X3	T45.4X4	T45.4X5	T45.4X6
hydroxide						
colloidal	T45.4X1	T45.4X2	T45.4X3	T45.4X4	T45.4X5	T45.4X6
polymaltose	T45.4X1	T45.4X2	T45.4X3	T45.4X4	T45.4X5	T45.4X6
pyrophosphate	T45.4X1	T45.4X2	T45.4X3	T45.4X4	T45.4X5	T45.4X6
Ferritin	T45.4X1	T45.4X2	T45.4X3	T45.4X4	T45.4X5	T45.4X6
Ferrocholinate	T45.4X1	T45.4X2	T45.4X3	T45.4X4	T45.4X5	T45.4X6
Ferrodextrane	T45.4X1	T45.4X2	T45.4X3	T45.4X4	T45.4X5	T45.4X6
Ferropolimaler	T45.4X1	T45.4X2	T45.4X3	T45.4X4	T45.4X5	T45.4X6
Ferrous — *see also Iron*						
phosphate	T45.4X1	T45.4X2	T45.4X3	T45.4X4	T45.4X5	T45.4X6
salt	T45.4X1	T45.4X2	T45.4X3	T45.4X4	T45.4X5	T45.4X6
with folic acid	T45.4X1	T45.4X2	T45.4X3	T45.4X4	T45.4X5	T45.4X6
Ferrous fumerate, gluconate, lactate, salt NEC, sulfate (medicinal)	T45.4X1	T45.4X2	T45.4X3	T45.4X4	T45.4X5	T45.4X6
Ferrovanadium (fumes)	T59.891	T59.892	T59.893	T59.894	—	—
Ferrum — *see Iron*						
Fertilizers NEC	T65.891	T65.892	T65.893	T65.894	—	—
with herbicide mixture	T60.3X1	T60.3X2	T60.3X3	T60.3X4	—	—
Fetoxilate	T47.6X1	T47.6X2	T47.6X3	T47.6X4	T47.6X5	T47.6X6
Fiber, dietary	T47.4X1	T47.4X2	T47.4X3	T47.4X4	T47.4X5	T47.4X6
Fibrinogen (human)	T45.8X1	T45.8X2	T45.8X3	T45.8X4	T45.8X5	T45.8X6
Fibrinolysin (human)	T45.691	T45.692	T45.693	T45.694	T45.695	T45.696
Fibrinolysis						
affecting drug	T45.601	T45.602	T45.603	T45.604	T45.605	T45.606
inhibitor NEC	T45.621	T45.622	T45.623	T45.624	T45.625	T45.626
Fibrinolytic drug	T45.611	T45.612	T45.613	T45.614	T45.615	T45.616
Filix mas	T37.4X1	T37.4X2	T37.4X3	T37.4X4	T37.4X5	T37.4X6
Filtering cream	T49.3X1	T49.3X2	T49.3X3	T49.3X4	T49.3X5	T49.3X6

Substance	External Cause (T-Code) Poisoning, Accidental (Unintentional)	Poisoning, Intentional Self-Harm	Poisoning, Assault	Poisoning, Undetermined	Adverse Effect	Underdosing
Fiorinal	T39.011	T39.012	T39.013	T39.014	T39.015	T39.016
Firedamp	T59.891	T59.892	T59.893	T59.894	—	—
Fish, noxious, nonbacterial	T61.91	T61.92	T61.93	T61.94	—	—
ciguatera	T61.01	T61.02	T61.03	T61.04	—	—
scombroid	T61.11	T61.12	T61.13	T61.14	—	—
shell	T61.781	T61.782	T61.783	T61.784	—	—
specified NEC	T61.771	T61.772	T61.773	T61.774	—	—
Flagyl	T37.3X1	T37.3X2	T37.3X3	T37.3X4	T37.3X5	T37.3X6
Flavine adenine dinucleotide	T45.2X1	T45.2X2	T45.2X3	T45.2X4	T45.2X5	T45.2X6
Flavodic acid	T46.991	T46.992	T46.993	T46.994	T46.995	T46.996
Flavoxate	T44.3X1	T44.3X2	T44.3X3	T44.3X4	T44.3X5	T44.3X6
Flaxedil	T48.1X1	T48.1X2	T48.1X3	T48.1X4	T48.1X5	T48.1X6
Flaxseed (medicinal)	T49.3X1	T49.3X2	T49.3X3	T49.3X4	T49.3X5	T49.3X6
Flecainide	T46.2X1	T46.2X2	T46.2X3	T46.2X4	T46.2X5	T46.2X6
Fleroxacin	T36.8X1	T36.8X2	T36.8X3	T36.8X4	T36.8X5	T36.8X6
Floctafenine	T39.8X1	T39.8X2	T39.8X3	T39.8X4	T39.8X5	T39.8X6
Flomax	T44.6X1	T44.6X2	T44.6X3	T44.6X4	T44.6X5	T44.6X6
Flomoxef	T36.1X1	T36.1X2	T36.1X3	T36.1X4	T36.1X5	T36.1X6
Flopropione	T44.3X1	T44.3X2	T44.3X3	T44.3X4	T44.3X5	T44.3X6
Florantyrone	T47.5X1	T47.5X2	T47.5X3	T47.5X4	T47.5X5	T47.5X6
Floraquin	T37.8X1	T37.8X2	T37.8X3	T37.8X4	T37.8X5	T37.8X6
Florinef	T38.0X1	T38.0X2	T38.0X3	T38.0X4	T38.0X5	T38.0X6
ENT agent	T49.6X1	T49.6X2	T49.6X3	T49.6X4	T49.6X5	T49.6X6
ophthalmic preparation	T49.5X1	T49.5X2	T49.5X3	T49.5X4	T49.5X5	T49.5X6
topical NEC	T49.0X1	T49.0X2	T49.0X3	T49.0X4	T49.0X5	T49.0X6
Flowers of sulfur	T49.4X1	T49.4X2	T49.4X3	T49.4X4	T49.4X5	T49.4X6
Floxuridine	T45.1X1	T45.1X2	T45.1X3	T45.1X4	T45.1X5	T45.1X6
Fluanisone	T43.4X1	T43.4X2	T43.4X3	T43.4X4	T43.4X5	T43.4X6
Flubendazole	T37.4X1	T37.4X2	T37.4X3	T37.4X4	T37.4X5	T37.4X6
Fluclorolone acetonide	T49.0X1	T49.0X2	T49.0X3	T49.0X4	T49.0X5	T49.0X6
Flucloxacillin	T36.0X1	T36.0X2	T36.0X3	T36.0X4	T36.0X5	T36.0X6
Fluconazole	T37.8X1	T37.8X2	T37.8X3	T37.8X4	T37.8X5	T37.8X6
Flucytosine	T37.8X1	T37.8X2	T37.8X3	T37.8X4	T37.8X5	T37.8X6
Fludeoxyglucose (18F)	T50.8X1	T50.8X2	T50.8X3	T50.8X4	T50.8X5	T50.8X6
Fludiazepam	T42.4X1	T42.4X2	T42.4X3	T42.4X4	T42.4X5	T42.4X6
Fludrocortisone	T50.0X1	T50.0X2	T50.0X3	T50.0X4	T50.0X5	T50.0X6
ENT agent	T49.6X1	T49.6X2	T49.6X3	T49.6X4	T49.6X5	T49.6X6
ophthalmic preparation	T49.5X1	T49.5X2	T49.5X3	T49.5X4	T49.5X5	T49.5X6
topical NEC	T49.0X1	T49.0X2	T49.0X3	T49.0X4	T49.0X5	T49.0X6
Fludroxycortide	T49.0X1	T49.0X2	T49.0X3	T49.0X4	T49.0X5	T49.0X6
Flufenamic acid	T39.391	T39.392	T39.393	T39.394	T39.395	T39.396
Fluindione	T45.511	T45.512	T45.513	T45.514	T45.515	T45.516

New Revised ~~deleted~~ Deleted

Substance	External Cause (T-Code)					
	Poisoning, Accidental (Unintentional)	Poisoning, Intentional Self-Harm	Poisoning, Assault	Poisoning, Undetermined	Adverse Effect	Underdosing
Flumequine	T37.8X1	T37.8X2	T37.8X3	T37.8X4	T37.8X5	T37.8X6
Flumethasone	T49.0X1	T49.0X2	T49.0X3	T49.0X4	T49.0X5	T49.0X6
Flumethiazide	T50.2X1	T50.2X2	T50.2X3	T50.2X4	T50.2X5	T50.2X6
Flumidin	T37.5X1	T37.5X2	T37.5X3	T37.5X4	T37.5X5	T37.5X6
Flunarizine	T46.7X1	T46.7X2	T46.7X3	T46.7X4	T46.7X5	T46.7X6
Flunidazole	T37.8X1	T37.8X2	T37.8X3	T37.8X4	T37.8X5	T37.8X6
Flunisolide	T48.6X1	T48.6X2	T48.6X3	T48.6X4	T48.6X5	T48.6X6
Flunitrazepam	T42.4X1	T42.4X2	T42.4X3	T42.4X4	T42.4X5	T42.4X6
Fluocinolone (acetonide)	T49.0X1	T49.0X2	T49.0X3	T49.0X4	T49.0X5	T49.0X6
Fluocinonide	T49.0X1	T49.0X2	T49.0X3	T49.0X4	T49.0X5	T49.0X6
Fluocortin (butyl)	T49.0X1	T49.0X2	T49.0X3	T49.0X4	T49.0X5	T49.0X6
Fluocortolone	T49.0X1	T49.0X2	T49.0X3	T49.0X4	T49.0X5	T49.0X6
Fluohydrocortisone	T38.0X1	T38.0X2	T38.0X3	T38.0X4	T38.0X5	T38.0X6
ENT agent	T49.6X1	T49.6X2	T49.6X3	T49.6X4	T49.6X5	T49.6X6
ophthalmic preparation	T49.5X1	T49.5X2	T49.5X3	T49.5X4	T49.5X5	T49.5X6
topical NEC	T49.0X1	T49.0X2	T49.0X3	T49.0X4	T49.0X5	T49.0X6
Fluonid	T49.0X1	T49.0X2	T49.0X3	T49.0X4	T49.0X5	T49.0X6
Fluopromazine	T43.3X1	T43.3X2	T43.3X3	T43.3X4	T43.3X5	T43.3X6
Fluoroacetate	T60.8X1	T60.8X2	T60.8X3	T60.8X4	—	—
Fluorescein	T50.8X1	T50.8X2	T50.8X3	T50.8X4	T50.8X5	T50.8X6
Fluorhydrocortisone	T50.0X1	T50.0X2	T50.0X3	T50.0X4	T50.0X5	T50.0X6
Fluoride (nonmedicinal) (pesticide) (sodium) NEC	T60.8X1	T60.8X2	T60.8X3	T60.8X4	—	—
hydrogen—*see Hydrofluoric acid*						
medicinal NEC	T50.991	T50.992	T50.993	T50.994	T50.995	T50.996
dental use	T49.7X1	T49.7X2	T49.7X3	T49.7X4	T49.7X5	T49.7X6
not pesticide NEC	T54.91	T54.92	T54.93	T54.94	—	—
stannous	T49.7X1	T49.7X2	T49.7X3	T49.7X4	T49.7X5	T49.7X6
Fluorinated corticosteroids	T38.0X1	T38.0X2	T38.0X3	T38.0X4	T38.0X5	T38.0X6
Fluorine (gas)	T59.5X1	T59.5X2	T59.5X3	T59.5X4	—	—
salt—*see Fluoride(s)*						
Fluoristan	T49.7X1	T49.7X2	T49.7X3	T49.7X4	T49.7X5	T49.7X6
Fluormetholone	T49.0X1	T49.0X2	T49.0X3	T49.0X4	T49.0X5	T49.0X6
Fluoroacetate	T60.8X1	T60.8X2	T60.8X3	T60.8X4	—	—
Fluorocarbon monomer	T53.6X1	T53.6X2	T53.6X3	T53.6X4	—	—
Fluorocytosine	T37.8X1	T37.8X2	T37.8X3	T37.8X4	T37.8X5	T37.8X6
Fluorodeoxyuridine	T45.1X1	T45.1X2	T45.1X3	T45.1X4	T45.1X5	T45.1X6
Fluorometholone	T49.0X1	T49.0X2	T49.0X3	T49.0X4	T49.0X5	T49.0X6
ophthalmic preparation	T49.5X1	T49.5X2	T49.5X3	T49.5X4	T49.5X5	T49.5X6
Fluorophosphate insecticide	T60.0X1	T60.0X2	T60.0X3	T60.0X4	—	—
Fluorosol	T46.3X1	T46.3X2	T46.3X3	T46.3X4	T46.3X5	T46.3X6
Fluorouracil	T45.1X1	T45.1X2	T45.1X3	T45.1X4	T45.1X5	T45.1X6
Fluorphenylalanine	T49.5X1	T49.5X2	T49.5X3	T49.5X4	T49.5X5	T49.5X6
Fluothane	T41.0X1	T41.0X2	T41.0X3	T41.0X4	T41.0X5	T41.0X6
Fluoxetine	T43.221	T43.222	T43.223	T43.224	T43.225	T43.226
Fluoxymesterone	T38.7X1	T38.7X2	T38.7X3	T38.7X4	T38.7X5	T38.7X6
Flupenthixol	T43.4X1	T43.4X2	T43.4X3	T43.4X4	T43.4X5	T43.4X6
Flupentixol	T43.4X1	T43.4X2	T43.4X3	T43.4X4	T43.4X5	T43.4X6
Fluphenazine	T43.3X1	T43.3X2	T43.3X3	T43.3X4	T43.3X5	T43.3X6
Fluprednidene	T49.0X1	T49.0X2	T49.0X3	T49.0X4	T49.0X5	T49.0X6
Fluprednisolone	T38.0X1	T38.0X2	T38.0X3	T38.0X4	T38.0X5	T38.0X6
Fluradoline	T39.8X1	T39.8X2	T39.8X3	T39.8X4	T39.8X5	T39.8X6
Flurandrenolide	T49.0X1	T49.0X2	T49.0X3	T49.0X4	T49.0X5	T49.0X6
Flurandrenolone	T49.0X1	T49.0X2	T49.0X3	T49.0X4	T49.0X5	T49.0X6
Flurazepam	T42.4X1	T42.4X2	T42.4X3	T42.4X4	T42.4X5	T42.4X6
Flurbiprofen	T39.311	T39.312	T39.313	T39.314	T39.315	T39.316
Flurobate	T49.0X1	T49.0X2	T49.0X3	T49.0X4	T49.0X5	T49.0X6
Flurotyl	T43.291	T43.292	T43.293	T43.294	T43.295	T43.296
Fluroxene	T41.0X1	T41.0X2	T41.0X3	T41.0X4	T41.0X5	T41.0X6
Fluspirilene	T43.591	T43.592	T43.593	T43.594	T43.595	T43.596
Flutamide	T38.6X1	T38.6X2	T38.6X3	T38.6X4	T38.6X5	T38.6X6
Flutazolam	T42.4X1	T42.4X2	T42.4X3	T42.4X4	T42.4X5	T42.4X6
Fluticasone propionate	T38.0X1	T38.0X2	T38.0X3	T38.0X4	T38.0X5	T38.0X6
Flutoprazepam	T42.4X1	T42.4X2	T42.4X3	T42.4X4	T42.4X5	T42.4X6
Flutropium bromide	T48.6X1	T48.6X2	T48.6X3	T48.6X4	T48.6X5	T48.6X6
Fluvoxamine	T43.221	T43.222	T43.223	T43.224	T43.225	T43.226
Folacin	T45.8X1	T45.8X2	T45.8X3	T45.8X4	T45.8X5	T45.8X6
Folic acid	T45.8X1	T45.8X2	T45.8X3	T45.8X4	T45.8X5	T45.8X6
with ferrous salt	T45.2X1	T45.2X2	T45.2X3	T45.2X4	T45.2X5	T45.2X6
antagonist	T45.1X1	T45.1X2	T45.1X3	T45.1X4	T45.1X5	T45.1X6
Folinic acid	T45.8X1	T45.8X2	T45.8X3	T45.8X4	T45.8X5	T45.8X6
Folium stramoniae	T48.6X1	T48.6X2	T48.6X3	T48.6X4	T48.6X5	T48.6X6
Follicle-stimulating hormone, human	T38.811	T38.812	T38.813	T38.814	T38.815	T38.816
Folpet	T60.3X1	T60.3X2	T60.3X3	T60.3X4	—	—
Fominoben	T48.3X1	T48.3X2	T48.3X3	T48.3X4	T48.3X5	T48.3X6
Food, foodstuffs, noxious, nonbacterial, NEC	T62.91	T62.92	T62.93	T62.94	—	—
berries	T62.1X1	T62.1X2	T62.1X3	T62.1X4	—	—
fish—*see also Fish*	T61.91	T61.92	T61.93	T61.94	—	—
mushrooms	T62.0X1	T62.0X2	T62.0X3	T62.0X4	—	—
plants	T62.2X1	T62.2X2	T62.2X3	T62.2X4	—	—
seafood	T61.91	T61.92	T61.93	T61.94	—	—
specified NEC	T61.8X1	T61.8X2	T61.8X3	T61.8X4	—	—
seeds	T62.2X1	T62.2X2	T62.2X3	T62.2X4	—	—

Substance	Poisoning, Accidental (Unintentional)	Poisoning, Intentional Self-Harm	Poisoning, Assault	Poisoning, Undetermined	Adverse Effect	Underdosing
	External Cause (T-Code)					
Food, foodstuffs, noxious, nonbacterial, NEC *(Continued)*						
shellfish	T61.781	T61.782	T61.783	T61.784	—	—
specified NEC	T62.8X1	T62.8X2	T62.8X3	T62.8X4	—	—
Fool's parsley	T62.2X1	T62.2X2	T62.2X3	T62.2X4	—	—
Formaldehyde (solution), gas or vapor	T59.2X1	T59.2X2	T59.2X3	T59.2X4	—	—
fungicide	T6Ø.3X1	T6Ø.3X2	T6Ø.3X3	T6Ø.3X4	—	—
Formalin	T59.2X1	T59.2X2	T59.2X3	T59.2X4	—	—
fungicide	T6Ø.3X1	T6Ø.3X2	T6Ø.3X3	T6Ø.3X4	—	—
vapor	T59.2X1	T59.2X2	T59.2X3	T59.2X4	—	—
Formic acid	T54.2X1	T54.2X2	T54.2X3	T54.2X4	—	—
vapor	T59.891	T59.892	T59.893	T59.894	—	—
Foscarnet sodium	T37.5X1	T37.5X2	T37.5X3	T37.5X4	T37.5X5	T37.5X6
Fosfestrol	T38.5X1	T38.5X2	T38.5X3	T38.5X4	T38.5X5	T38.5X6
Fosfomycin	T36.8X1	T36.8X2	T36.8X3	T36.8X4	T36.8X5	T36.8X6
Fosfonet sodium	T37.5X1	T37.5X2	T37.5X3	T37.5X4	T37.5X5	T37.5X6
Fosinopril	T46.4X1	T46.4X2	T46.4X3	T46.4X4	T46.4X5	T46.4X6
sodium	T46.4X1	T46.4X2	T46.4X3	T46.4X4	T46.4X5	T46.4X6
Fowler's solution	T57.ØX1	T57.ØX2	T57.ØX3	T57.ØX4	—	—
Foxglove	T62.2X1	T62.2X2	T62.2X3	T62.2X4	—	—
Framycetin	T36.5X1	T36.5X2	T36.5X3	T36.5X4	T36.5X5	T36.5X6
Frangula	T47.2X1	T47.2X2	T47.2X3	T47.2X4	T47.2X5	T47.2X6
extract	T47.2X1	T47.2X2	T47.2X3	T47.2X4	T47.2X5	T47.2X6
Frei antigen	T5Ø.8X1	T5Ø.8X2	T5Ø.8X3	T5Ø.8X4	T5Ø.8X5	T5Ø.8X6
Freon	T53.5X1	T53.5X2	T53.5X3	T53.5X4	—	—
Fructose	T5Ø.3X1	T5Ø.3X2	T5Ø.3X3	T5Ø.3X4	T5Ø.3X5	T5Ø.3X6
Frusemide	T5Ø.1X1	T5Ø.1X2	T5Ø.1X3	T5Ø.1X4	T5Ø.1X5	T5Ø.1X6
FSH	T38.811	T38.812	T38.813	T38.814	T38.815	T38.816
Ftorafur	T45.1X1	T45.1X2	T45.1X3	T45.1X4	T45.1X5	T45.1X6
Fuel						
automobile	T52.ØX1	T52.ØX2	T52.ØX3	T52.ØX4	—	—
exhaust gas, not in transit	T58.Ø1	T58.Ø2	T58.Ø3	T58.Ø4	—	—
vapor NEC	T52.ØX1	T52.ØX2	T52.ØX3	T52.ØX4	—	—
gas (domestic use) — *see also Carbon, monoxide, fuel, utility*	T59.891	T59.892	T59.893	T59.894	—	—
utility	T59.891	T59.892	T59.893	T59.894	—	—
in mobile container	T59.891	T59.892	T59.893	T59.894	—	—
incomplete combustion of — *see Carbon, monoxide, fuel, utility*						
piped (natural)	T59.891	T59.892	T59.893	T59.894	—	—
industrial, incomplete combustion	T58.8X1	T58.8X2	T58.8X3	T58.8X4	—	—

Substance	Poisoning, Accidental (Unintentional)	Poisoning, Intentional Self-Harm	Poisoning, Assault	Poisoning, Undetermined	Adverse Effect	Underdosing
	External Cause (T-Code)					
Fugillin	T36.8X1	T36.8X2	T36.8X3	T36.8X4	T36.8X5	T36.8X6
Fulminate of mercury	T56.1X1	T56.1X2	T56.1X3	T56.1X4	—	—
Fulvicin	T36.7X1	T36.7X2	T36.7X3	T36.7X4	T36.7X5	T36.7X6
Fumadil	T36.8X1	T36.8X2	T36.8X3	T36.8X4	T36.8X5	T36.8X6
Fumagillin	T36.8X1	T36.8X2	T36.8X3	T36.8X4	T36.8X5	T36.8X6
Fumaric acid	T49.4X1	T49.4X2	T49.4X3	T49.4X4	T49.4X5	T49.4X6
Fumes (from)	T59.91	T59.92	T59.93	T59.94	—	—
carbon monoxide — *see Carbon, monoxide*						
charcoal (domestic use) — *see Charcoal, fumes*						
chloroform — *see Chloroform*						
coke (in domestic stoves, fireplaces) — *see Coke, fumes*						
corrosive NEC	T54.91	T54.92	T54.93	T54.94	—	—
ether — *see Ether*						
freons	T53.5X1	T53.5X2	T53.5X3	T53.5X4	—	—
hydrocarbons	T59.891	T59.892	T59.893	T59.894	—	—
petroleum (liquefied)	T59.891	T59.892	T59.893	T59.894	—	—
distributed through pipes (pure or mixed with air)	T59.891	T59.892	T59.893	T59.894	—	—
lead — *see Lead*						
metal — *see Metals, or the specified metal*						
nitrogen dioxide	T59.ØX1	T59.ØX2	T59.ØX3	T59.ØX4	—	—
pesticides — *see Pesticides*						
petroleum (liquefied)	T59.891	T59.892	T59.893	T59.894	—	—
distributed through pipes (pure or mixed with air)	T59.891	T59.892	T59.893	T59.894	—	—
polyester	T59.891	T59.892	T59.893	T59.894	—	—
specified source NEC — *see also substance specified*	T59.891	T59.892	T59.893	T59.894	—	—
sulfur dioxide	T59.1X1	T59.1X2	T59.1X3	T59.1X4	—	—
Fumigant NEC	T6Ø.91	T6Ø.92	T6Ø.93	T6Ø.94	—	—
Fungi, noxious, used as food	T62.ØX1	T62.ØX2	T62.ØX3	T62.ØX4	—	—
Fungicide NEC (nonmedicinal)	T6Ø.3X1	T6Ø.3X2	T6Ø.3X3	T6Ø.3X4	—	—
Fungizone	T36.7X1	T36.7X2	T36.7X3	T36.7X4	T36.7X5	T36.7X6
topical	T49.ØX1	T49.ØX2	T49.ØX3	T49.ØX4	T49.ØX5	T49.ØX6
Furacin	T49.ØX1	T49.ØX2	T49.ØX3	T49.ØX4	T49.ØX5	T49.ØX6
Furadantin	T37.91	T37.92	T37.93	T37.94	T37.95	T37.96
Furazolidone	T37.8X1	T37.8X2	T37.8X3	T37.8X4	T37.8X5	T37.8X6
Furazolium chloride	T49.ØX1	T49.ØX2	T49.ØX3	T49.ØX4	T49.ØX5	T49.ØX6
Furfural	T52.8X1	T52.8X2	T52.8X3	T52.8X4	—	—

Substance	External Cause (T-Code) Poisoning, Accidental (Unintentional)	Poisoning, Intentional Self-Harm	Poisoning, Assault	Poisoning, Undetermined	Adverse Effect	Underdosing
Furnace (coal burning) (domestic), gas from industrial	T58.2X1	T58.2X2	T58.2X3	T58.2X4	—	—
industrial	T58.8X1	T58.8X2	T58.8X3	T58.8X4	—	—
Furniture polish	T65.891	T65.892	T65.893	T65.894	—	—
Furosemide	T50.1X1	T50.1X2	T50.1X3	T50.1X4	T50.1X5	T50.1X6
Furoxone	T37.91	T37.92	T37.93	T37.94	T37.95	T37.96
Fursultiamine	T45.2X1	T45.2X2	T45.2X3	T45.2X4	T45.2X5	T45.2X6
Fusafungine	T36.8X1	T36.8X2	T36.8X3	T36.8X4	T36.8X5	T36.8X6
Fusel oil (any) (amyl) (butyl) (propyl), vapor	T51.3X1	T51.3X2	T51.3X3	T51.3X4	—	—
Fusidate (ethanolamine) (sodium)	T36.8X1	T36.8X2	T36.8X3	T36.8X4	T36.8X5	T36.8X6
Fusidic acid	T36.8X1	T36.8X2	T36.8X3	T36.8X4	T36.8X5	T36.8X6
Fytic acid, nonasodium	T50.6X1	T50.6X2	T50.6X3	T50.6X4	T50.6X5	T50.6X6
G						
GABA	T43.8X1	T43.8X2	T43.8X3	T43.8X4	T43.8X5	T43.8X6
Gadopentetic acid	T50.8X1	T50.8X2	T50.8X3	T50.8X4	T50.8X5	T50.8X6
Galactose	T50.3X1	T50.3X2	T50.3X3	T50.3X4	T50.3X5	T50.3X6
b-Galactosidase	T47.5X1	T47.5X2	T47.5X3	T47.5X4	T47.5X5	T47.5X6
Galantamine	T44.0X1	T44.0X2	T44.0X3	T44.0X4	T44.0X5	T44.0X6
Gallamine (triethiodide)	T48.1X1	T48.1X2	T48.1X3	T48.1X4	T48.1X5	T48.1X6
Gallium citrate	T50.991	T50.992	T50.993	T50.994	T50.995	T50.996
Gallopamil	T46.1X1	T46.1X2	T46.1X3	T46.1X4	T46.1X5	T46.1X6
Gamboge	T47.2X1	T47.2X2	T47.2X3	T47.2X4	T47.2X5	T47.2X6
Gamimune	T50.Z11	T50.Z12	T50.Z13	T50.Z14	T50.Z15	T50.Z16
Gamma-aminobutyric acid	T43.8X1	T43.8X2	T43.8X3	T43.8X4	T43.8X5	T43.8X6
Gamma-benzene hexachloride (medicinal)	T49.0X1	T49.0X2	T49.0X3	T49.0X4	T49.0X5	T49.0X6
nonmedicinal, vapor	T53.6X1	T53.6X2	T53.6X3	T53.6X4	—	—
Gamma-BHC (medicinal) — *see also Gamma-benzene hexachloride*	T49.0X1	T49.0X2	T49.0X3	T49.0X4	T49.0X5	T49.0X6
Gamma globulin	T50.Z11	T50.Z12	T50.Z13	T50.Z14	T50.Z15	T50.Z16
Gamulin	T50.Z11	T50.Z12	T50.Z13	T50.Z14	T50.Z15	T50.Z16
Ganciclovir (sodium)	T37.5X1	T37.5X2	T37.5X3	T37.5X4	T37.5X5	T37.5X6
Ganglionic blocking drug NEC	T44.2X1	T44.2X2	T44.2X3	T44.2X4	T44.2X5	T44.2X6
specified NEC	T44.2X1	T44.2X2	T44.2X3	T44.2X4	T44.2X5	T44.2X6
Ganja	T40.7X1	T40.7X2	T40.7X3	T40.7X4	T40.7X5	T40.7X6
Garamycin	T36.5X1	T36.5X2	T36.5X3	T36.5X4	T36.5X5	T36.5X6
ophthalmic preparation	T49.5X1	T49.5X2	T49.5X3	T49.5X4	T49.5X5	T49.5X6
topical NEC	T49.0X1	T49.0X2	T49.0X3	T49.0X4	T49.0X5	T49.0X6
Gardenal	T42.3X1	T42.3X2	T42.3X3	T42.3X4	T42.3X5	T42.3X6
Gardepanyl	T42.3X1	T42.3X2	T42.3X3	T42.3X4	T42.3X5	T42.3X6

Substance	External Cause (T-Code) Poisoning, Accidental (Unintentional)	Poisoning, Intentional Self-Harm	Poisoning, Assault	Poisoning, Undetermined	Adverse Effect	Underdosing
Gas NEC	T59.91	T59.92	T59.93	T59.94	—	—
acetylene	T59.891	T59.892	T59.893	T59.894	—	—
incomplete combustion of	T58.11	T58.12	T58.13	T58.14	—	—
air contaminants, source or type not specified	T59.91	T59.92	T59.93	T59.94	—	—
anesthetic	T41.0X1	T41.0X2	T41.0X3	T41.0X4	T41.0X5	T41.0X6
blast furnace	T58.8X1	T58.8X2	T58.8X3	T58.8X4	—	—
butane — see Butane						
carbon monoxide — see Carbon, monoxide						
chlorine	T59.4X1	T59.4X2	T59.4X3	T59.4X4	—	—
coal	T58.2X1	T58.2X2	T58.2X3	T58.2X4	—	—
cyanide	T57.3X1	T57.3X2	T57.3X3	T57.3X4	—	—
dicyanogen	T65.0X1	T65.0X2	T65.0X3	T65.0X4	—	—
domestic — see Domestic gas	T57.91	T57.92	T57.93	T57.94	—	—
exhaust	T57.91	T57.92	T57.93	T57.94	—	—
from utility (for cooking, heating, or lighting) (after combustion) — see Carbon, monoxide, fuel, utility						
prior to combustion	T59.891	T59.892	T59.893	T59.894	—	—
from wood or coal-burning stove or fireplace	T57.91	T57.92	T57.93	T57.94	—	—
fuel (domestic use) (after combustion) — see also Carbon, monoxide, fuel	T57.91	T57.92	T57.93	T57.94	—	—
industrial use	T58.8X1	T58.8X2	T58.8X3	T58.8X4	—	—
prior to combustion	T59.891	T59.892	T59.893	T59.894	—	—
utility	T59.891	T59.892	T59.893	T59.894	—	—
in mobile container	T59.891	T59.892	T59.893	T59.894	—	—
incomplete combustion of — see Carbon, monoxide, fuel, utility						
piped (natural)	T59.891	T59.892	T59.893	T59.894	—	—
garage	T58.01	T58.02	T58.03	T58.04	—	—
hydrocarbon NEC	T59.891	T59.892	T59.893	T59.894	—	—
incomplete combustion of — see Carbon, monoxide, fuel, utility						
liquefied — see Butane						
piped	T59.891	T59.892	T59.893	T59.894	—	—
hydrocyanic acid	T65.0X1	T65.0X2	T65.0X3	T65.0X4	—	—

Substance	External Cause (T-Code)					
	Poisoning, Accidental (Unintentional)	Poisoning, Intentional Self-Harm	Poisoning, Assault	Poisoning, Undetermined	Adverse Effect	Underdosing
Gas NEC (Continued)						
illuminating (after combustion)	T58.11	T58.12	T58.13	T58.14	—	—
prior to combustion	T59.891	T59.892	T59.893	T59.894	—	—
incomplete combustion, any — see Carbon, monoxide						
kiln	T58.8X1	T58.8X2	T58.8X3	T58.8X4	—	—
lacrimogenic	T59.3X1	T59.3X2	T59.3X3	T59.3X4	—	—
liquefied petroleum — see Butane						
marsh	T59.891	T59.892	T59.893	T59.894	—	—
motor exhaust, not in transit	T58.01	T58.02	T58.03	T58.04	—	—
mustard, not in war	T59.891	T59.892	T59.893	T59.894	—	—
natural	T59.891	T59.892	T59.893	T59.894	—	—
nerve, not in war	T59.91	T59.92	T59.93	T59.94	—	—
oil	T52.0X1	T52.0X2	T52.0X3	T52.0X4	—	—
petroleum (liquefied) (distributed in mobile containers)	T59.891	T59.892	T59.893	T59.894	—	—
piped (pure or mixed with air)	T59.891	T59.892	T59.893	T59.894	—	—
piped (manufactured) (natural) NEC	T59.891	T59.892	T59.893	T59.894	—	—
producer	T58.8X1	T58.8X2	T58.8X3	T58.8X4	—	—
propane — see Propane						
refrigerant (chlorofluoro-carbon)	T53.5X1	T53.5X2	T53.5X3	T53.5X4	—	—
not chlorofluoro-carbon	T59.891	T59.892	T59.893	T59.894	—	—
sewer	T59.91	T59.92	T59.93	T59.94	—	—
specified source NEC	T59.91	T59.92	T59.93	T59.94	—	—
stove (after combustion)	T58.11	T58.12	T58.13	T58.14	—	—
tear	T59.3X1	T59.3X2	T59.3X3	T59.3X4	—	—
therapeutic	T41.5X1	T41.5X2	T41.5X3	T41.5X4	T41.5X5	T41.5X6
utility (for cooking, heating, or lighting) (piped) NEC	T59.891	T59.892	T59.893	T59.894	—	—
in mobile container	T59.891	T59.892	T59.893	T59.894	—	—
incomplete combustion of — see Carbon, monoxide, fuel, utilty						
piped (natural)	T59.891	T59.892	T59.893	T59.894	—	—
water	T58.11	T58.12	T58.13	T58.14	—	—
incomplete combustion of — see Carbon, monoxide, fuel, utility						

Substance	External Cause (T-Code)					
	Poisoning, Accidental (Unintentional)	Poisoning, Intentional Self-Harm	Poisoning, Assault	Poisoning, Undetermined	Adverse Effect	Underdosing
Gaseous substance — see Gas						
Gasoline	T52.0X1	T52.0X2	T52.0X3	T52.0X4	—	—
vapor	T52.0X1	T52.0X2	T52.0X3	T52.0X4	—	—
Gastric enzymes	T47.5X1	T47.5X2	T47.5X3	T47.5X4	T47.5X5	T47.5X6
Gastrografin	T50.8X1	T50.8X2	T50.8X3	T50.8X4	T50.8X5	T50.8X6
Gastrointestinal drug	T47.91	T47.92	T47.93	T47.94	T47.95	T47.96
biological	T47.8X1	T47.8X2	T47.8X3	T47.8X4	T47.8X5	T47.8X6
specified NEC	T47.8X1	T47.8X2	T47.8X3	T47.8X4	T47.8X5	T47.8X6
Gaultheria procumbens	T62.2X1	T62.2X2	T62.2X3	T62.2X4	—	—
Gelatin (intravenous)	T45.8X1	T45.8X2	T45.8X3	T45.8X4	T45.8X5	T45.8X6
absorbable (sponge)	T45.7X1	T45.7X2	T45.7X3	T45.7X4	T45.7X5	T45.7X6
Gefarnate	T44.3X1	T44.3X2	T44.3X3	T44.3X4	T44.3X5	T44.3X6
Gelfilm	T49.8X1	T49.8X2	T49.8X3	T49.8X4	T49.8X5	T49.8X6
Gelfoam	T45.7X1	T45.7X2	T45.7X3	T45.7X4	T45.7X5	T45.7X6
Gelsemine	T50.991	T50.992	T50.993	T50.994	T50.995	T50.996
Gelsemium (sempervirens)	T62.2X1	T62.2X2	T62.2X3	T62.2X4	—	—
Gemeprost	T48.0X1	T48.0X2	T48.0X3	T48.0X4	T48.0X5	T48.0X6
Gemfibrozil	T46.6X1	T46.6X2	T46.6X3	T46.6X4	T46.6X5	T46.6X6
Gemonil	T42.3X1	T42.3X2	T42.3X3	T42.3X4	T42.3X5	T42.3X6
Gentamicin	T36.5X1	T36.5X2	T36.5X3	T36.5X4	T36.5X5	T36.5X6
ophthalmic preparation	T49.5X1	T49.5X2	T49.5X3	T49.5X4	T49.5X5	T49.5X6
topical NEC	T49.0X1	T49.0X2	T49.0X3	T49.0X4	T49.0X5	T49.0X6
Gentian	T47.5X1	T47.5X2	T47.5X3	T47.5X4	T47.5X5	T47.5X6
violet	T49.0X1	T49.0X2	T49.0X3	T49.0X4	T49.0X5	T49.0X6
Gepefrine	T44.4X1	T44.4X2	T44.4X3	T44.4X4	T44.4X5	T44.4X6
Gestonorone caproate	T38.5X1	T38.5X2	T38.5X3	T38.5X4	T38.5X5	T38.5X6
Gexane	T49.0X1	T49.0X2	T49.0X3	T49.0X4	T49.0X5	T49.0X6
Gila monster (venom)	T63.111	T63.112	T63.113	T63.114	—	—
Ginger	T47.5X1	T47.5X2	T47.5X3	T47.5X4	T47.5X5	T47.5X6
Jamaica — see Jamaica, ginger						
Gitalin	T46.0X1	T46.0X2	T46.0X3	T46.0X4	T46.0X5	T46.0X6
amorphous	T46.0X1	T46.0X2	T46.0X3	T46.0X4	T46.0X5	T46.0X6
Gitaloxin	T46.0X1	T46.0X2	T46.0X3	T46.0X4	T46.0X5	T46.0X6
Gitoxin	T46.0X1	T46.0X2	T46.0X3	T46.0X4	T46.0X5	T46.0X6
Glafenine	T39.8X1	T39.8X2	T39.8X3	T39.8X4	T39.8X5	T39.8X6
Glandular extract (medicinal) NEC	T50.Z91	T50.Z92	T50.Z93	T50.Z94	T50.Z95	T50.Z96
Glaucarubin	T37.3X1	T37.3X2	T37.3X3	T37.3X4	T37.3X5	T37.3X6
Glibenclamide	T38.3X1	T38.3X2	T38.3X3	T38.3X4	T38.3X5	T38.3X6
Glibornuride	T38.3X1	T38.3X2	T38.3X3	T38.3X4	T38.3X5	T38.3X6
Gliclazide	T38.3X1	T38.3X2	T38.3X3	T38.3X4	T38.3X5	T38.3X6
Glimidine	T38.3X1	T38.3X2	T38.3X3	T38.3X4	T38.3X5	T38.3X6

◀ New ◀ Revised ~~deleted~~ Deleted

Substance	Poisoning, Accidental (Unintentional)	Poisoning, Intentional Self-Harm	Poisoning, Assault	Poisoning, Undetermined	Adverse Effect	Underdosing
	External Cause (T-Code)					
Glipizide	T38.3X1	T38.3X2	T38.3X3	T38.3X4	T38.3X5	T38.3X6
Gliquidone	T38.3X1	T38.3X2	T38.3X3	T38.3X4	T38.3X5	T38.3X6
Glisolamide	T38.3X1	T38.3X2	T38.3X3	T38.3X4	T38.3X5	T38.3X6
Glisoxepide	T38.3X1	T38.3X2	T38.3X3	T38.3X4	T38.3X5	T38.3X6
Globin zinc insulin	T38.3X1	T38.3X2	T38.3X3	T38.3X4	T38.3X5	T38.3X6
Globulin						
antilymphocytic	T50.Z11	T50.Z12	T50.Z13	T50.Z14	T50.Z15	T50.Z16
antirhesus	T50.Z11	T50.Z12	T50.Z13	T50.Z14	T50.Z15	T50.Z16
antivenin	T50.Z11	T50.Z12	T50.Z13	T50.Z14	T50.Z15	T50.Z16
antiviral	T50.Z11	T50.Z12	T50.Z13	T50.Z14	T50.Z15	T50.Z16
Glucagon	T38.3X1	T38.3X2	T38.3X3	T38.3X4	T38.3X5	T38.3X6
Glucocorticoids	T38.0X1	T38.0X2	T38.0X3	T38.0X4	T38.0X5	T38.0X6
Glucocorticosteroid	T38.0X1	T38.0X2	T38.0X3	T38.0X4	T38.0X5	T38.0X6
Gluconic acid	T50.991	T50.992	T50.993	T50.994	T50.995	T50.996
Glucosamine sulfate	T39.4X1	T39.4X2	T39.4X3	T39.4X4	T39.4X5	T39.4X6
Glucose	T50.3X1	T50.3X2	T50.3X3	T50.3X4	T50.3X5	T50.3X6
with sodium chloride	T50.3X1	T50.3X2	T50.3X3	T50.3X4	T50.3X5	T50.3X6
Glucosulfone sodium	T37.1X1	T37.1X2	T37.1X3	T37.1X4	T37.1X5	T37.1X6
Glucurolactone	T47.8X1	T47.8X2	T47.8X3	T47.8X4	T47.8X5	T47.8X6
Glue NEC	T52.8X1	T52.8X2	T52.8X3	T52.8X4	—	—
Glutamic acid	T47.5X1	T47.5X2	T47.5X3	T47.5X4	T47.5X5	T47.5X6
Glutaral (medicinal)	T49.0X1	T49.0X2	T49.0X3	T49.0X4	T49.0X5	T49.0X6
nonmedicinal	T65.891	T65.892	T65.893	T65.894	—	—
Glutaraldehyde (nonmedicinal)	T65.891	T65.892	T65.893	T65.894	—	—
medicinal	T49.0X1	T49.0X2	T49.0X3	T49.0X4	T49.0X5	T49.0X6
Glutathione	T50.6X1	T50.6X2	T50.6X3	T50.6X4	T50.6X5	T50.6X6
Glutethimide	T42.6X1	T42.6X2	T42.6X3	T42.6X4	T42.6X5	T42.6X6
Glyburide	T38.3X1	T38.3X2	T38.3X3	T38.3X4	T38.3X5	T38.3X6
Glycerin	T47.4X1	T47.4X2	T47.4X3	T47.4X4	T47.4X5	T47.4X6
Glycerol	T47.4X1	T47.4X2	T47.4X3	T47.4X4	T47.4X5	T47.4X6
borax	T49.6X1	T49.6X2	T49.6X3	T49.6X4	T49.6X5	T49.6X6
intravenous	T50.3X1	T50.3X2	T50.3X3	T50.3X4	T50.3X5	T50.3X6
iodinated	T48.4X1	T48.4X2	T48.4X3	T48.4X4	T48.4X5	T48.4X6
Glycerophosphate	T50.991	T50.992	T50.993	T50.994	T50.995	T50.996
Glyceryl						
gualacolate	T48.4X1	T48.4X2	T48.4X3	T48.4X4	T48.4X5	T48.4X6
nitrate	T46.3X1	T46.3X2	T46.3X3	T46.3X4	T46.3X5	T46.3X6
triacetate (topical)	T49.0X1	T49.0X2	T49.0X3	T49.0X4	T49.0X5	T49.0X6
trinitrate	T46.3X1	T46.3X2	T46.3X3	T46.3X4	T46.3X5	T46.3X6
Glycine	T50.3X1	T50.3X2	T50.3X3	T50.3X4	T50.3X5	T50.3X6
Glyclopyramide	T38.3X1	T38.3X2	T38.3X3	T38.3X4	T38.3X5	T38.3X6
Glycobiarsol	T37.3X1	T37.3X2	T37.3X3	T37.3X4	T37.3X5	T37.3X6

Substance	Poisoning, Accidental (Unintentional)	Poisoning, Intentional Self-Harm	Poisoning, Assault	Poisoning, Undetermined	Adverse Effect	Underdosing
	External Cause (T-Code)					
Glycols (ether)	T52.3X1	T52.3X2	T52.3X3	T52.3X4	—	—
Glyconiazide	T37.1X1	T37.1X2	T37.1X3	T37.1X4	T37.1X5	T37.1X6
Glycopyrrolate	T44.3X1	T44.3X2	T44.3X3	T44.3X4	T44.3X5	T44.3X6
Glycopyrronium	T44.3X1	T44.3X2	T44.3X3	T44.3X4	T44.3X5	T44.3X6
bromide	T44.3X1	T44.3X2	T44.3X3	T44.3X4	T44.3X5	T44.3X6
Glycoside, cardiac (stimulant)	T46.0X1	T46.0X2	T46.0X3	T46.0X4	T46.0X5	T46.0X6
Glycyclamide	T38.3X1	T38.3X2	T38.3X3	T38.3X4	T38.3X5	T38.3X6
Glycyrrhiza extract	T48.4X1	T48.4X2	T48.4X3	T48.4X4	T48.4X5	T48.4X6
Glycyrrhizic acid	T48.4X1	T48.4X2	T48.4X3	T48.4X4	T48.4X5	T48.4X6
Glycyrrhizinate potassium	T48.4X1	T48.4X2	T48.4X3	T48.4X4	T48.4X5	T48.4X6
Glymidine sodium	T38.3X1	T38.3X2	T38.3X3	T38.3X4	T38.3X5	T38.3X6
Glyphosate	T60.3X1	T60.3X2	T60.3X3	T60.3X4	—	—
Glyphylline	T48.6X1	T48.6X2	T48.6X3	T48.6X4	T48.6X5	T48.6X6
Gold						
colloidal (198Au)	T45.1X1	T45.1X2	T45.1X3	T45.1X4	T45.1X5	T45.1X6
salts	T39.4X1	T39.4X2	T39.4X3	T39.4X4	T39.4X5	T39.4X6
Golden sulfide of antimony	T56.891	T56.892	T56.893	T56.894	—	—
Goldylocks	T62.2X1	T62.2X2	T62.2X3	T62.2X4	—	—
Gonadal tissue extract	T38.901	T38.902	T38.903	T38.904	T38.905	T38.906
female	T38.5X1	T38.5X2	T38.5X3	T38.5X4	T38.5X5	T38.5X6
male	T38.7X1	T38.7X2	T38.7X3	T38.7X4	T38.7X5	T38.7X6
Gonadorelin	T38.891	T38.892	T38.893	T38.894	T38.895	T38.896
Gonadotropin	T38.891	T38.892	T38.893	T38.894	T38.895	T38.896
chorionic	T38.891	T38.892	T38.893	T38.894	T38.895	T38.896
pituitary	T38.811	T38.812	T38.813	T38.814	T38.815	T38.816
Goserelin	T45.1X1	T45.1X2	T45.1X3	T45.1X4	T45.1X5	T45.1X6
Grain alcohol	T51.0X1	T51.0X2	T51.0X3	T51.0X4	—	—
Gramicidin	T49.0X1	T49.0X2	T49.0X3	T49.0X4	T49.0X5	T49.0X6
Granisetron	T45.0X1	T45.0X2	T45.0X3	T45.0X4	T45.0X5	T45.0X6
Gratiola officinalis	T62.2X1	T62.2X2	T62.2X3	T62.2X4	—	—
Grease	T65.891	T65.892	T65.893	T65.894	—	—
Green hellebore	T62.2X1	T62.2X2	T62.2X3	T62.2X4	—	—
Green soap	T49.2X1	T49.2X2	T49.2X3	T49.2X4	T49.2X5	T49.2X6
Grifulvin	T36.7X1	T36.7X2	T36.7X3	T36.7X4	T36.7X5	T36.7X6
Griseofulvin	T36.7X1	T36.7X2	T36.7X3	T36.7X4	T36.7X5	T36.7X6
Growth hormone	T38.811	T38.812	T38.813	T38.814	T38.815	T38.816
Guaiacol derivatives	T48.4X1	T48.4X2	T48.4X3	T48.4X4	T48.4X5	T48.4X6
Guaiac reagent	T50.991	T50.992	T50.993	T50.994	T50.995	T50.996
Guaifenesin	T48.4X1	T48.4X2	T48.4X3	T48.4X4	T48.4X5	T48.4X6
Guaimesal	T48.4X1	T48.4X2	T48.4X3	T48.4X4	T48.4X5	T48.4X6
Guaiphenesin	T48.4X1	T48.4X2	T48.4X3	T48.4X4	T48.4X5	T48.4X6
Guamecycline	T36.4X1	T36.4X2	T36.4X3	T36.4X4	T36.4X5	T36.4X6

Substance	External Cause (T-Code)					
	Poisoning, Accidental (Unintentional)	Poisoning, Intentional Self-Harm	Poisoning, Assault	Poisoning, Undetermined	Adverse Effect	Underdosing
Guanabenz	T46.5X1	T46.5X2	T46.5X3	T46.5X4	T46.5X5	T46.5X6
Guanacline	T46.5X1	T46.5X2	T46.5X3	T46.5X4	T46.5X5	T46.5X6
Guanadrel	T46.5X1	T46.5X2	T46.5X3	T46.5X4	T46.5X5	T46.5X6
Guanatol	T37.2X1	T37.2X2	T37.2X3	T37.2X4	T37.2X5	T37.2X6
Guanethidine	T46.5X1	T46.5X2	T46.5X3	T46.5X4	T46.5X5	T46.5X6
Guanfacine	T46.5X1	T46.5X2	T46.5X3	T46.5X4	T46.5X5	T46.5X6
Guano	T65.891	T65.892	T65.893	T65.894	—	—
Guanochlor	T46.5X1	T46.5X2	T46.5X3	T46.5X4	T46.5X5	T46.5X6
Guanoclor	T46.5X1	T46.5X2	T46.5X3	T46.5X4	T46.5X5	T46.5X6
Guanoctine	T46.5X1	T46.5X2	T46.5X3	T46.5X4	T46.5X5	T46.5X6
Guanoxabenz	T46.5X1	T46.5X2	T46.5X3	T46.5X4	T46.5X5	T46.5X6
Guanoxan	T46.5X1	T46.5X2	T46.5X3	T46.5X4	T46.5X5	T46.5X6
Guar gum (medicinal)	T46.6X1	T46.6X2	T46.6X3	T46.6X4	T46.6X5	T46.6X6
H						
Hachimycin	T36.7X1	T36.7X2	T36.7X3	T36.7X4	T36.7X5	T36.7X6
Hair						
dye	T49.4X1	T49.4X2	T49.4X3	T49.4X4	T49.4X5	T49.4X6
preparation NEC	T49.4X1	T49.4X2	T49.4X3	T49.4X4	T49.4X5	T49.4X6
Halazepam	T42.4X1	T42.4X2	T42.4X3	T42.4X4	T42.4X5	T42.4X6
Halcinolone	T49.ØX1	T49.ØX2	T49.ØX3	T49.ØX4	T49.ØX5	T49.ØX6
Halcinonide	T49.ØX1	T49.ØX2	T49.ØX3	T49.ØX4	T49.ØX5	T49.ØX6
Halethazole	T49.ØX1	T49.ØX2	T49.ØX3	T49.ØX4	T49.ØX5	T49.ØX6
Hallucinogen NOS	T4Ø.9Ø1	T4Ø.9Ø2	T4Ø.9Ø3	T4Ø.9Ø4	T4Ø.9Ø5	T4Ø.9Ø6
specified NEC	T4Ø.991	T4Ø.992	T4Ø.993	T4Ø.994	T4Ø.995	T4Ø.996
Halofantrine	T37.2X1	T37.2X2	T37.2X3	T37.2X4	T37.2X5	T37.2X6
Halofenate	T46.6X1	T46.6X2	T46.6X3	T46.6X4	T46.6X5	T46.6X6
Halometasone	T49.ØX1	T49.ØX2	T49.ØX3	T49.ØX4	T49.ØX5	T49.ØX6
Haloperidol	T43.4X1	T43.4X2	T43.4X3	T43.4X4	T43.4X5	T43.4X6
Haloprogin	T49.ØX1	T49.ØX2	T49.ØX3	T49.ØX4	T49.ØX5	T49.ØX6
Halotex	T49.ØX1	T49.ØX2	T49.ØX3	T49.ØX4	T49.ØX5	T49.ØX6
Halothane	T41.ØX1	T41.ØX2	T41.ØX3	T41.ØX4	T41.ØX5	T41.ØX6
Haloxazolam	T42.4X1	T42.4X2	T42.4X3	T42.4X4	T42.4X5	T42.4X6
Halquinols	T49.ØX1	T49.ØX2	T49.ØX3	T49.ØX4	T49.ØX5	T49.ØX6
Hamamelis	T49.2X1	T49.2X2	T49.2X3	T49.2X4	T49.2X5	T49.2X6
Haptendextran	T45.8X1	T45.8X2	T45.8X3	T45.8X4	T45.8X5	T45.8X6
Harmonyl	T46.5X1	T46.5X2	T46.5X3	T46.5X4	T46.5X5	T46.5X6
Hartmann's solution	T5Ø.3X1	T5Ø.3X2	T5Ø.3X3	T5Ø.3X4	T5Ø.3X5	T5Ø.3X6
Hashish	T4Ø.7X1	T4Ø.7X2	T4Ø.7X3	T4Ø.7X4	T4Ø.7X5	T4Ø.7X6
Hawaiian Woodrose seeds	T4Ø.991	T4Ø.992	T4Ø.993	T4Ø.994	—	—
HCB	T6Ø.3X1	T6Ø.3X2	T6Ø.3X3	T6Ø.3X4	—	—
HCH	T53.6X1	T53.6X2	T53.6X3	T53.6X4	—	—
medicinal	T49.ØX1	T49.ØX2	T49.ØX3	T49.ØX4	T49.ØX5	T49.ØX6
HCN	T57.3X1	T57.3X2	T57.3X3	T57.3X4	—	—
Headache cures, drugs, powders NEC	T5Ø.9Ø1	T5Ø.9Ø2	T5Ø.9Ø3	T5Ø.9Ø4	T5Ø.9Ø5	T5Ø.9Ø6
Heavenly Blue (morning glory)	T4Ø.991	T4Ø.992	T4Ø.993	T4Ø.994	—	—
Heavy metal antidote	T45.8X1	T45.8X2	T45.8X3	T45.8X4	T45.8X5	T45.8X6
Hedaquinium	T49.ØX1	T49.ØX2	T49.ØX3	T49.ØX4	T49.ØX5	T49.ØX6
Hedge hyssop	T62.2X1	T62.2X2	T62.2X3	T62.2X4	—	—
Heet	T49.8X1	T49.8X2	T49.8X3	T49.8X4	T49.8X5	T49.8X6
Helium	T48.991	T48.992	T48.993	T48.994	T48.995	T48.996
Helenin	T37.4X1	T37.4X2	T37.4X3	T37.4X4	T37.4X5	T37.4X6
Hellebore (black) (green) (white)	T62.2X1	T62.2X2	T62.2X3	T62.2X4	—	—
Helium (nonmedicinal) NEC	T59.891	T59.892	T59.893	T59.894	—	—
medicinal	T48.991	T48.992	T48.993	T48.994	T48.995	T48.996
Hematin	T45.8X1	T45.8X2	T45.8X3	T45.8X4	T45.8X5	T45.8X6
Hematinic preparation	T45.8X1	T45.8X2	T45.8X3	T45.8X4	T45.8X5	T45.8X6
Hemlock	T62.2X1	T62.2X2	T62.2X3	T62.2X4	—	—
Hemostatic	T45.621	T45.622	T45.623	T45.624	T45.625	T45.626
drug, systemic	T45.621	T45.622	T45.623	T45.624	T45.625	T45.626
Hemostyptic	T49.4X1	T49.4X2	T49.4X3	T49.4X4	T49.4X5	T49.4X6
Henbane	T62.2X1	T62.2X2	T62.2X3	T62.2X4	—	—
Heparin (sodium)	T45.511	T45.512	T45.513	T45.514	T45.515	T45.516
action reverser	T45.7X1	T45.7X2	T45.7X3	T45.7X4	T45.7X5	T45.7X6
Heparin-fraction	T45.511	T45.512	T45.513	T45.514	T45.515	T45.516
Heparinoid (systemic)	T45.511	T45.512	T45.513	T45.514	T45.515	T45.516
Hepatic secretion stimulant	T47.8X1	T47.8X2	T47.8X3	T47.8X4	T47.8X5	T47.8X6
Hepatitis B						
immune globulin	T5Ø.Z11	T5Ø.Z12	T5Ø.Z13	T5Ø.Z14	T5Ø.Z15	T5Ø.Z16
vaccine	T5Ø.B91	T5Ø.B92	T5Ø.B93	T5Ø.B94	T5Ø.B95	T5Ø.B96
Hepronicate	T46.7X1	T46.7X2	T46.7X3	T46.7X4	T46.7X5	T46.7X6
Heptabarb	T42.3X1	T42.3X2	T42.3X3	T42.3X4	T42.3X5	T42.3X6
Heptabarbitone	T42.3X1	T42.3X2	T42.3X3	T42.3X4	T42.3X5	T42.3X6
Heptabarbital	T42.3X1	T42.3X2	T42.3X3	T42.3X4	T42.3X5	T42.3X6
Heptachlor	T6Ø.1X1	T6Ø.1X2	T6Ø.1X3	T6Ø.1X4	—	—
Heptalgin	T4Ø.2X1	T4Ø.2X2	T4Ø.2X3	T4Ø.2X4	T4Ø.2X5	T4Ø.2X6
Heptaminol	T46.3X1	T46.3X2	T46.3X3	T46.3X4	T46.3X5	T46.3X6
Herbicide NEC	T6Ø.3X1	T6Ø.3X2	T6Ø.3X3	T6Ø.3X4	—	—
Heroin	T4Ø.1X1	T4Ø.1X2	T4Ø.1X3	T4Ø.1X4	—	—
Herplex	T49.5X1	T49.5X2	T49.5X3	T49.5X4	T49.5X5	T49.5X6
HES	T45.8X1	T45.8X2	T45.8X3	T45.8X4	T45.8X5	T45.8X6
Hesperidin	T46.991	T46.992	T46.993	T46.994	T46.995	T46.996
Hetacillin	T36.ØX1	T36.ØX2	T36.ØX3	T36.ØX4	T36.ØX5	T36.ØX6

◀ New ◀ Revised ~~deleted~~ Deleted

Substance	Poisoning, Accidental (Unintentional)	Poisoning, Intentional Self-Harm	Poisoning, Assault	Poisoning, Undetermined	Adverse Effect	Underdosing
	External Cause (T-Code)					
Hetastarch	T45.8X1	T45.8X2	T45.8X3	T45.8X4	T45.8X5	T45.8X6
HETP	T6Ø.ØX1	T6Ø.ØX2	T6Ø.ØX3	T6Ø.ØX4	—	—
Hexachlorobenzene (vapor)	T6Ø.3X1	T6Ø.3X2	T6Ø.3X3	T6Ø.3X4	—	—
Hexachlorocyclohexane	T53.6X1	T53.6X2	T53.6X3	T53.6X4	—	—
Hexachlorophene	T49.ØX1	T49.ØX2	T49.ØX3	T49.ØX4	T49.ØX5	T49.ØX6
Hexadiline	T46.3X1	T46.3X2	T46.3X3	T46.3X4	T46.3X5	T46.3X6
Hexadimethrine (bromide)	T45.7X1	T45.7X2	T45.7X3	T45.7X4	T45.7X5	T45.7X6
Hexadylamine	T46.3X1	T46.3X2	T46.3X3	T46.3X4	T46.3X5	T46.3X6
Hexaethyl tetraphosphate	T6Ø.ØX1	T6Ø.ØX2	T6Ø.ØX3	T6Ø.ØX4	—	—
Hexafluorenium bromide	T48.1X1	T48.1X2	T48.1X3	T48.1X4	T48.1X5	T48.1X6
Hexafluorodiethyl ether	T43.291	T43.292	T43.293	T43.294	T43.295	T43.296
Hexafluronium (bromide)	T48.1X1	T48.1X2	T48.1X3	T48.1X4	T48.1X5	T48.1X6
Hexahydrobenzol	T52.8X1	T52.8X2	T52.8X3	T52.8X4	—	—
Hexahydrocresol(s)	T51.8X1	T51.8X2	T51.8X3	T51.8X4	—	—
arsenide	T57.ØX1	T57.ØX2	T57.ØX3	T57.ØX4	—	—
arseniurated	T57.ØX1	T57.ØX2	T57.ØX3	T57.ØX4	—	—
cyanide	T57.3X1	T57.3X2	T57.3X3	T57.3X4	—	—
gas	T59.891	T59.892	T59.893	T59.894	—	—
Fluoride (liquid)	T57.8X1	T57.8X2	T57.8X3	T57.8X4	—	—
vapor	T59.891	T59.892	T59.893	T59.894	—	—
phophorated	T6Ø.ØX1	T6Ø.ØX2	T6Ø.ØX3	T6Ø.ØX4	—	—
sulfate	T57.8X1	T57.8X2	T57.8X3	T57.8X4	—	—
sulfide (gas)	T59.6X1	T59.6X2	T59.6X3	T59.6X4	—	—
arseniurated	T57.ØX1	T57.ØX2	T57.ØX3	T57.ØX4	—	—
sulfurated	T57.8X1	T57.8X2	T57.8X3	T57.8X4	—	—
Hexahydrophenol	T51.8X1	T51.8X2	T51.8X3	T51.8X4	—	—
Hexa-germ	T49.2X1	T49.2X2	T49.2X3	T49.2X4	T49.2X5	T49.2X6
Hexalen	T51.8X1	T51.8X2	T51.8X3	T51.8X4	—	—
Hexamethonium bromide	T44.2X1	T44.2X2	T44.2X3	T44.2X4	T44.2X5	T44.2X6
Hexamethylene	T52.8X1	T52.8X2	T52.8X3	T52.8X4	—	—
Hexamethylmelamine	T45.1X1	T45.1X2	T45.1X3	T45.1X4	T45.1X5	T45.1X6
Hexamidine	T49.ØX1	T49.ØX2	T49.ØX3	T49.ØX4	T49.ØX5	T49.ØX6
Hexamine (mandelate)	T37.8X1	T37.8X2	T37.8X3	T37.8X4	T37.8X5	T37.8X6
Hexanone, 2-hexanone	T52.4X1	T52.4X2	T52.4X3	T52.4X4	—	—
Hexanuorenium	T48.1X1	T48.1X2	T48.1X3	T48.1X4	T48.1X5	T48.1X6
Hexapropymate	T42.6X1	T42.6X2	T42.6X3	T42.6X4	T42.6X5	T42.6X6
Hexasonium iodide	T44.3X1	T44.3X2	T44.3X3	T44.3X4	T44.3X5	T44.3X6
Hexcarbacholine bromide	T48.1X1	T48.1X2	T48.1X3	T48.1X4	T48.1X5	T48.1X6
Hexemal	T42.3X1	T42.3X2	T42.3X3	T42.3X4	T42.3X5	T42.3X6
Hexestrol	T38.5X1	T38.5X2	T38.5X3	T38.5X4	T38.5X5	T38.5X6
Hexethal (sodium)	T42.3X1	T42.3X2	T42.3X3	T42.3X4	T42.3X5	T42.3X6
Hexetidine	T37.8X1	T37.8X2	T37.8X3	T37.8X4	T37.8X5	T37.8X6
Hexobarbital	T42.3X1	T42.3X2	T42.3X3	T42.3X4	T42.3X5	T42.3X6
rectal	T41.291	T41.292	T41.293	T41.294	T41.295	T41.296
sodium	T41.1X1	T41.1X2	T41.1X3	T41.1X4	T41.1X5	T41.1X6
Hexobendine	T46.3X1	T46.3X2	T46.3X3	T46.3X4	T46.3X5	T46.3X6
Hexocyclium	T44.3X1	T44.3X2	T44.3X3	T44.3X4	T44.3X5	T44.3X6
metilsulfate	T44.3X1	T44.3X2	T44.3X3	T44.3X4	T44.3X5	T44.3X6
Hexoestrol	T38.5X1	T38.5X2	T38.5X3	T38.5X4	T38.5X5	T38.5X6
Hexone	T52.4X1	T52.4X2	T52.4X3	T52.4X4	—	—
Hexoprenaline	T48.6X1	T48.6X2	T48.6X3	T48.6X4	T48.6X5	T48.6X6
Hexylcaine	T41.3X1	T41.3X2	T41.3X3	T41.3X4	T41.3X5	T41.3X6
Hexylresorcinol	T52.2X1	T52.2X2	T52.2X3	T52.2X4	—	—
HGH (human growth hormone)	T38.811	T38.812	T38.813	T38.814	T38.815	T38.816
Hinkle's pills	T47.2X1	T47.2X2	T47.2X3	T47.2X4	T47.2X5	T47.2X6
Histalog	T5Ø.8X1	T5Ø.8X2	T5Ø.8X3	T5Ø.8X4	T5Ø.8X5	T5Ø.8X6
Histamine (phosphate)	T5Ø.8X1	T5Ø.8X2	T5Ø.8X3	T5Ø.8X4	T5Ø.8X5	T5Ø.8X6
Histoplasmin	T5Ø.8X1	T5Ø.8X2	T5Ø.8X3	T5Ø.8X4	T5Ø.8X5	T5Ø.8X6
Holly berries	T62.2X1	T62.2X2	T62.2X3	T62.2X4	—	—
Homatropine	T44.3X1	T44.3X2	T44.3X3	T44.3X4	T44.3X5	T44.3X6
methylbromide	T44.3X1	T44.3X2	T44.3X3	T44.3X4	T44.3X5	T44.3X6
Homochlorcyclizine	T45.ØX1	T45.ØX2	T45.ØX3	T45.ØX4	T45.ØX5	T45.ØX6
Homosalate	T49.3X1	T49.3X2	T49.3X3	T49.3X4	T49.3X5	T49.3X6
Homo-tet	T5Ø.Z11	T5Ø.Z12	T5Ø.Z13	T5Ø.Z14	T5Ø.Z15	T5Ø.Z16
Hormone	T38.8Ø1	T38.8Ø2	T38.8Ø3	T38.8Ø4	T38.8Ø5	T38.8Ø6
adrenal cortical steroids	T38.ØX1	T38.ØX2	T38.ØX3	T38.ØX4	T38.ØX5	T38.ØX6
androgenic	T38.7X1	T38.7X2	T38.7X3	T38.7X4	T38.7X5	T38.7X6
anterior pituitary NEC	T38.811	T38.812	T38.813	T38.814	T38.815	T38.816
antidiabetic agents	T38.3X1	T38.3X2	T38.3X3	T38.3X4	T38.3X5	T38.3X6
antidiuretic	T38.891	T38.892	T38.893	T38.894	T38.895	T38.896
cancer therapy	T45.1X1	T45.1X2	T45.1X3	T45.1X4	T45.1X5	T45.1X6
follicle stimulating	T38.811	T38.812	T38.813	T38.814	T38.815	T38.816
gonadotropic	T38.891	T38.892	T38.893	T38.894	T38.895	T38.896
pituitary	T38.811	T38.812	T38.813	T38.814	T38.815	T38.816
growth	T38.811	T38.812	T38.813	T38.814	T38.815	T38.816
luteinizing	T38.811	T38.812	T38.813	T38.814	T38.815	T38.816
ovarian	T38.5X1	T38.5X2	T38.5X3	T38.5X4	T38.5X5	T38.5X6
oxytocic	T48.ØX1	T48.ØX2	T48.ØX3	T48.ØX4	T48.ØX5	T48.ØX6
parathyroid (derivatives)	T5Ø.991	T5Ø.992	T5Ø.993	T5Ø.994	T5Ø.995	T5Ø.996
pituitary (posterior) NEC	T38.891	T38.892	T38.893	T38.894	T38.895	T38.896
anterior	T38.811	T38.812	T38.813	T38.814	T38.815	T38.816
specified, NEC	T38.891	T38.892	T38.893	T38.894	T38.895	T38.896
thyroid	T38.1X1	T38.1X2	T38.1X3	T38.1X4	T38.1X5	T38.1X6
Hornet (sting)	T63.451	T63.452	T63.453	T63.454	—	—

Substance	Poisoning, Accidental (Unintentional)	Poisoning, Intentional Self-Harm	Poisoning, Assault	Poisoning, Undetermined	Adverse Effect	Underdosing
	External Cause (T-Code)					
Horse anti-human lymphocytic serum	T5Ø.Z11	T5Ø.Z12	T5Ø.Z13	T5Ø.Z14	T5Ø.Z15	T5Ø.Z16
Horticulture agent NEC	T65.91	T65.92	T65.93	T65.94	—	—
with pesticide	T6Ø.91	T6Ø.92	T6Ø.93	T6Ø.94	—	—
Human						
albumin	T45.8X1	T45.8X2	T45.8X3	T45.8X4	T45.8X5	T45.8X6
growth hormone (HGH)	T38.811	T38.812	T38.813	T38.814	T38.815	T38.816
immune serum	T5Ø.Z11	T5Ø.Z12	T5Ø.Z13	T5Ø.Z14	T5Ø.Z15	T5Ø.Z16
Hyaluronidase	T45.3X1	T45.3X2	T45.3X3	T45.3X4	T45.3X5	T45.3X6
Hyazyme	T45.3X1	T45.3X2	T45.3X3	T45.3X4	T45.3X5	T45.3X6
Hycodan	T4Ø.2X1	T4Ø.2X2	T4Ø.2X3	T4Ø.2X4	T4Ø.2X5	T4Ø.2X6
Hydantoin derivative NEC	T42.ØX1	T42.ØX2	T42.ØX3	T42.ØX4	T42.ØX5	T42.ØX6
Hydeltra	T38.ØX1	T38.ØX2	T38.ØX3	T38.ØX4	T38.ØX5	T38.ØX6
Hydergine	T44.6X1	T44.6X2	T44.6X3	T44.6X4	T44.6X5	T44.6X6
Hydrabamine penicillin	T36.ØX1	T36.ØX2	T36.ØX3	T36.ØX4	T36.ØX5	T36.ØX6
Hydralazine	T46.5X1	T46.5X2	T46.5X3	T46.5X4	T46.5X5	T46.5X6
Hydrargaphen	T49.ØX1	T49.ØX2	T49.ØX3	T49.ØX4	T49.ØX5	T49.ØX6
Hydrargyri amino-chloridum	T49.ØX1	T49.ØX2	T49.ØX3	T49.ØX4	T49.ØX5	T49.ØX6
Hydrastine	T48.291	T48.292	T48.293	T48.294	T48.295	T48.296
Hydrazine	T54.1X1	T54.1X2	T54.1X3	T54.1X4	—	—
monoamine oxidase inhibitors	T43.1X1	T43.1X2	T43.1X3	T43.1X4	T43.1X5	T43.1X6
Hydrazoic acid, azides	T54.2X1	T54.2X2	T54.2X3	T54.2X4	—	—
Hydriodic acid	T48.4X1	T48.4X2	T48.4X3	T48.4X4	T48.4X5	T48.4X6
Hydrocarbon gas	T59.891	T59.892	T59.893	T59.894	—	—
incomplete combustion of— *see Carbon, monoxide, fuel, utility*						
liquefied (mobile container)	T59.891	T59.892	T59.893	T59.894	—	—
piped (natural)	T59.891	T59.892	T59.893	T59.894	—	—
Hydrochloric acid (liquid)	T54.2X1	T54.2X2	T54.2X3	T54.2X4	—	—
medicinal (digestant)	T47.5X1	T47.5X2	T47.5X3	T47.5X4	T47.5X5	T47.5X6
vapor	T59.891	T59.892	T59.893	T59.894	—	—
Hydrochlorothiazide	T5Ø.2X1	T5Ø.2X2	T5Ø.2X3	T5Ø.2X4	T5Ø.2X5	T5Ø.2X6
Hydrocodone	T4Ø.2X1	T4Ø.2X2	T4Ø.2X3	T4Ø.2X4	T4Ø.2X5	T4Ø.2X6
Hydrocortisone (derivatives)	T38.ØX1	T38.ØX2	T38.ØX3	T38.ØX4	T38.ØX5	T38.ØX6
aceponate	T49.ØX1	T49.ØX2	T49.ØX3	T49.ØX4	T49.ØX5	T49.ØX6
ENT agent	T49.6X1	T49.6X2	T49.6X3	T49.6X4	T49.6X5	T49.6X6
ophthalmic preparation	T49.5X1	T49.5X2	T49.5X3	T49.5X4	T49.5X5	T49.5X6
topical NEC	T49.ØX1	T49.ØX2	T49.ØX3	T49.ØX4	T49.ØX5	T49.ØX6
Hydrocortone	T38.ØX1	T38.ØX2	T38.ØX3	T38.ØX4	T38.ØX5	T38.ØX6
ENT agent	T49.6X1	T49.6X2	T49.6X3	T49.6X4	T49.6X5	T49.6X6
ophthalmic preparation	T49.5X1	T49.5X2	T49.5X3	T49.5X4	T49.5X5	T49.5X6
topical NEC	T49.ØX1	T49.ØX2	T49.ØX3	T49.ØX4	T49.ØX5	T49.ØX6

Substance	Poisoning, Accidental (Unintentional)	Poisoning, Intentional Self-Harm	Poisoning, Assault	Poisoning, Undetermined	Adverse Effect	Underdosing
	External Cause (T-Code)					
Hydrocyanic acid (liquid)	T57.3X1	T57.3X2	T57.3X3	T57.3X4	—	—
gas	T65.ØX1	T65.ØX2	T65.ØX3	T65.ØX4	—	—
Hydroflumethiazide	T5Ø.2X1	T5Ø.2X2	T5Ø.2X3	T5Ø.2X4	T5Ø.2X5	T5Ø.2X6
Hydrofluoric acid (liquid)	T54.2X1	T54.2X2	T54.2X3	T54.2X4	—	—
vapor	T59.891	T59.892	T59.893	T59.894	—	—
Hydrogen	T59.891	T59.892	T59.893	T59.894	—	—
arsenide	T57.ØX1	T57.ØX2	T57.ØX3	T57.ØX4	—	—
arseniureted	T57.ØX1	T57.ØX2	T57.ØX3	T57.ØX4	—	—
chloride	T57.8X1	T57.8X2	T57.8X3	T57.8X4	—	—
cyanide (salts)	T57.3X1	T57.3X2	T57.3X3	T57.3X4	—	—
gas	T57.3X1	T57.3X2	T57.3X3	T57.3X4	—	—
Fluoride	T59.5X1	T59.5X2	T59.5X3	T59.5X4	—	—
vapor	T59.5X1	T59.5X2	T59.5X3	T59.5X4	—	—
peroxide	T49.ØX1	T49.ØX2	T49.ØX3	T49.ØX4	T49.ØX5	T49.ØX6
phosphureted	T57.1X1	T57.1X2	T57.1X3	T57.1X4	—	—
sulfide	T59.6X1	T59.6X2	T59.6X3	T59.6X4	—	—
arseniureted	T57.ØX1	T57.ØX2	T57.ØX3	T57.ØX4	—	—
sulfureted	T59.6X1	T59.6X2	T59.6X3	T59.6X4	—	—
Hydromethylpyridine	T46.7X1	T46.7X2	T46.7X3	T46.7X4	T46.7X5	T46.7X6
Hydromorphinol	T4Ø.2X1	T4Ø.2X2	T4Ø.2X3	T4Ø.2X4	—	—
Hydromorphinone	T4Ø.2X1	T4Ø.2X2	T4Ø.2X3	T4Ø.2X4	T4Ø.2X5	T4Ø.2X6
Hydromorphone	T4Ø.2X1	T4Ø.2X2	T4Ø.2X3	T4Ø.2X4	T4Ø.2X5	T4Ø.2X6
Hydromox	T5Ø.2X1	T5Ø.2X2	T5Ø.2X3	T5Ø.2X4	T5Ø.2X5	T5Ø.2X6
Hydrophilic lotion	T49.3X1	T49.3X2	T49.3X3	T49.3X4	T49.3X5	T49.3X6
Hydroquinidine	T46.2X1	T46.2X2	T46.2X3	T46.2X4	T46.2X5	T46.2X6
Hydroquinone	T52.2X1	T52.2X2	T52.2X3	T52.2X4	—	—
vapor	T59.891	T59.892	T59.893	T59.894	—	—
Hydrosulfuric acid (gas)	T59.6X1	T59.6X2	T59.6X3	T59.6X4	—	—
Hydrotalcite	T47.1X1	T47.1X2	T47.1X3	T47.1X4	T47.1X5	T47.1X6
Hydrous wool fat	T49.3X1	T49.3X2	T49.3X3	T49.3X4	T49.3X5	T49.3X6
Hydroxide, caustic	T54.3X1	T54.3X2	T54.3X3	T54.3X4	—	—
Hydroxocobalamin	T45.8X1	T45.8X2	T45.8X3	T45.8X4	T45.8X5	T45.8X6
Hydroxyamphetamine	T49.5X1	T49.5X2	T49.5X3	T49.5X4	T49.5X5	T49.5X6
Hydroxycarbamide	T45.1X1	T45.1X2	T45.1X3	T45.1X4	T45.1X5	T45.1X6
Hydroxychloroquine	T37.8X1	T37.8X2	T37.8X3	T37.8X4	T37.8X5	T37.8X6
Hydroxydihydrocodeinone	T4Ø.2X1	T4Ø.2X2	T4Ø.2X3	T4Ø.2X4	T4Ø.2X5	T4Ø.2X6
Hydroxyestrone	T38.5X1	T38.5X2	T38.5X3	T38.5X4	T38.5X5	T38.5X6
Hydroxyethyl starch	T45.8X1	T45.8X2	T45.8X3	T45.8X4	T45.8X5	T45.8X6
Hydroxymethylpentanone	T52.4X1	T52.4X2	T52.4X3	T52.4X4	—	—
Hydroxyphenamate	T43.591	T43.592	T43.593	T43.594	T43.595	T43.596
Hydroxyphenylbutazone	T39.2X1	T39.2X2	T39.2X3	T39.2X4	T39.2X5	T39.2X6

◀ New ◀ Revised ~~deleted~~ Deleted

Substance	External Cause (T-Code) Poisoning, Accidental (Unintentional)	Poisoning, Intentional Self-Harm	Poisoning, Assault	Poisoning, Undetermined	Adverse Effect	Underdosing
Hydroxyprogesterone	T38.5X1	T38.5X2	T38.5X3	T38.5X4	T38.5X5	T38.5X6
caproate	T38.5X1	T38.5X2	T38.5X3	T38.5X4	T38.5X5	T38.5X6
Hydroxyquinoline (derivatives) NEC	T37.8X1	T37.8X2	T37.8X3	T37.8X4	T37.8X5	T37.8X6
Hydroxystilbamidine	T37.3X1	T37.3X2	T37.3X3	T37.3X4	T37.3X5	T37.3X6
Hydroxytoluene (nonmedicinal)	T54.ØX1	T54.ØX2	T54.ØX3	T54.ØX4	—	—
medicinal	T49.ØX1	T49.ØX2	T49.ØX3	T49.ØX4	T49.ØX5	T49.ØX6
Hydroxyurea	T45.1X1	T45.1X2	T45.1X3	T45.1X4	T45.1X5	T45.1X6
Hydroxyzine	T43.591	T43.592	T43.593	T43.594	T43.595	T43.596
Hyoscine	T44.3X1	T44.3X2	T44.3X3	T44.3X4	T44.3X5	T44.3X6
Hyoscyamine	T44.3X1	T44.3X2	T44.3X3	T44.3X4	T44.3X5	T44.3X6
Hyoscyamus	T44.3X1	T44.3X2	T44.3X3	T44.3X4	T44.3X5	T44.3X6
dry extract	T44.3X1	T44.3X2	T44.3X3	T44.3X4	T44.3X5	T44.3X6
Hypaque	T5Ø.8X1	T5Ø.8X2	T5Ø.8X3	T5Ø.8X4	T5Ø.8X5	T5Ø.8X6
Hypertussis	T5Ø.Z11	T5Ø.Z12	T5Ø.Z13	T5Ø.Z14	T5Ø.Z15	T5Ø.Z16
Hypnotic	T42.71	T42.72	T42.73	T42.74	T42.75	T42.76
anticonvulsant	T42.71	T42.72	T42.73	T42.74	T42.75	T42.76
specified NEC	T42.6X1	T42.6X2	T42.6X3	T42.6X4	T42.6X5	T42.6X6
Hypochlorite	T49.ØX1	T49.ØX2	T49.ØX3	T49.ØX4	T49.ØX5	T49.ØX6
Hypophysis, posterior	T38.891	T38.892	T38.893	T38.894	T38.895	T38.896
Hypotensive NEC	T46.5X1	T46.5X2	T46.5X3	T46.5X4	T46.5X5	T46.5X6
Hypromellose	T49.5X1	T49.5X2	T49.5X3	T49.5X4	T49.5X5	T49.5X6
I						
Ibacitabine	T37.5X1	T37.5X2	T37.5X3	T37.5X4	T37.5X5	T37.5X6
Ibopamine	T44.991	T44.992	T44.993	T44.994	T44.995	T44.996
Ibufenac	T39.311	T39.312	T39.313	T39.314	T39.315	T39.316
Ibuprofen	T39.311	T39.312	T39.313	T39.314	T39.315	T39.316
Ibuproxam	T39.311	T39.312	T39.313	T39.314	T39.315	T39.316
Ibuterol	T48.6X1	T48.6X2	T48.6X3	T48.6X4	T48.6X5	T48.6X6
Ichthammol	T49.ØX1	T49.ØX2	T49.ØX3	T49.ØX4	T49.ØX5	T49.ØX6
Ichthyol	T49.4X1	T49.4X2	T49.4X3	T49.4X4	T49.4X5	T49.4X6
Idarubicin	T45.1X1	T45.1X2	T45.1X3	T45.1X4	T45.1X5	T45.1X6
Idrocilamide	T42.8X1	T42.8X2	T42.8X3	T42.8X4	T42.8X5	T42.8X6
Ifenprodil	T46.7X1	T46.7X2	T46.7X3	T46.7X4	T46.7X5	T46.7X6
Ifosfamide	T45.1X1	T45.1X2	T45.1X3	T45.1X4	T45.1X5	T45.1X6
Iletin	T38.3X1	T38.3X2	T38.3X3	T38.3X4	T38.3X5	T38.3X6
Ilex	T62.2X1	T62.2X2	T62.2X3	T62.2X4	—	—
Illuminating gas (after combustion)	T58.11	T58.12	T58.13	T58.14	—	—
prior to combustion	T59.891	T59.892	T59.893	T59.894	—	—
Ilopan	T45.2X1	T45.2X2	T45.2X3	T45.2X4	T45.2X5	T45.2X6
Iloprost	T46.7X1	T46.7X2	T46.7X3	T46.7X4	T46.7X5	T46.7X6
Ilotycin	T36.3X1	T36.3X2	T36.3X3	T36.3X4	T36.3X5	T36.3X6
ophthalmic preparation	T49.5X1	T49.5X2	T49.5X3	T49.5X4	T49.5X5	T49.5X6
topical NEC	T49.ØX1	T49.ØX2	T49.ØX3	T49.ØX4	T49.ØX5	T49.ØX6
Imidazole-4-carboxamide	T45.1X1	T45.1X2	T45.1X3	T45.1X4	T45.1X5	T45.1X6
Imipenem	T36.ØX1	T36.ØX2	T36.ØX3	T36.ØX4	T36.ØX5	T36.ØX6
Imipramine	T43.Ø11	T43.Ø12	T43.Ø13	T43.Ø14	T43.Ø15	T43.Ø16
Iminostilbene	T42.1X1	T42.1X2	T42.1X3	T42.1X4	T42.1X5	T42.1X6
Immu-G	T5Ø.Z11	T5Ø.Z12	T5Ø.Z13	T5Ø.Z14	T5Ø.Z15	T5Ø.Z16
Immuglobin	T5Ø.Z11	T5Ø.Z12	T5Ø.Z13	T5Ø.Z14	T5Ø.Z15	T5Ø.Z16
Immune						
globulin	T5Ø.Z11	T5Ø.Z12	T5Ø.Z13	T5Ø.Z14	T5Ø.Z15	T5Ø.Z16
serum globulin	T5Ø.Z11	T5Ø.Z12	T5Ø.Z13	T5Ø.Z14	T5Ø.Z15	T5Ø.Z16
Immunoglobin human (intravenous) (normal)	T5Ø.Z11	T5Ø.Z12	T5Ø.Z13	T5Ø.Z14	T5Ø.Z15	T5Ø.Z16
unmodified	T5Ø.Z11	T5Ø.Z12	T5Ø.Z13	T5Ø.Z14	T5Ø.Z15	T5Ø.Z16
Immunosuppressive drug	T45.1X1	T45.1X2	T45.1X3	T45.1X4	T45.1X5	T45.1X6
Immu-tetanus	T5Ø.Z11	T5Ø.Z12	T5Ø.Z13	T5Ø.Z14	T5Ø.Z15	T5Ø.Z16
Indalpine	T43.221	T43.222	T43.223	T43.224	T43.225	T43.226
Indanazoline	T48.5X1	T48.5X2	T48.5X3	T48.5X4	T48.5X5	T48.5X6
Indandione (derivatives)	T45.511	T45.512	T45.513	T45.514	T45.515	T45.516
Indapamide	T46.5X1	T46.5X2	T46.5X3	T46.5X4	T46.5X5	T46.5X6
Indendione (derivatives)	T45.511	T45.512	T45.513	T45.514	T45.515	T45.516
Indenolol	T44.7X1	T44.7X2	T44.7X3	T44.7X4	T44.7X5	T44.7X6
Inderal	T44.7X1	T44.7X2	T44.7X3	T44.7X4	T44.7X5	T44.7X6
Indian						
hemp	T4Ø.7X1	T4Ø.7X2	T4Ø.7X3	T4Ø.7X4	T4Ø.7X5	T4Ø.7X6
tobacco	T62.2X1	T62.2X2	T62.2X3	T62.2X4	—	—
Indigo carmine	T5Ø.8X1	T5Ø.8X2	T5Ø.8X3	T5Ø.8X4	T5Ø.8X5	T5Ø.8X6
Indobufen	T45.521	T45.522	T45.523	T45.524	T45.525	T45.526
Indocin	T39.2X1	T39.2X2	T39.2X3	T39.2X4	T39.2X5	T39.2X6
Indocyanine green	T5Ø.8X1	T5Ø.8X2	T5Ø.8X3	T5Ø.8X4	T5Ø.8X5	T5Ø.8X6
Indometacin	T39.391	T39.392	T39.393	T39.394	T39.395	T39.396
Indomethacin	T39.391	T39.392	T39.393	T39.394	T39.395	T39.396
farnesil	T39.4X1	T39.4X2	T39.4X3	T39.4X4	T39.4X5	T39.4X6
Indoramin	T44.6X1	T44.6X2	T44.6X3	T44.6X4	T44.6X5	T44.6X6
Industrial						
alcohol	T51.ØX1	T51.ØX2	T51.ØX3	T51.ØX4	—	—
fumes	T59.891	T59.892	T59.893	T59.894	—	—
solvents (fumes) (vapors)	T52.91	T52.92	T52.93	T52.94	—	—
Influenza vaccine	T5Ø.B91	T5Ø.B92	T5Ø.B93	T5Ø.B94	T5Ø.B95	T5Ø.B96
Ingested substance NEC	T65.91	T65.92	T65.93	T65.94	—	—
INH	T37.1X1	T37.1X2	T37.1X3	T37.1X4	T37.1X5	T37.1X6

Substance	Poisoning, Accidental (Unintentional)	External Cause (T-Code) Poisoning, Intentional Self-Harm	Poisoning, Assault	Poisoning, Undetermined	Adverse Effect	Underdosing
Inhalation, gas (noxious) — *see Gas*						
Inhibitor						
angiotensin-converting enzyme	T46.4X1	T46.4X2	T46.4X3	T46.4X4	T46.4X5	T46.4X6
carbonic anhydrase	T50.2X1	T50.2X2	T50.2X3	T50.2X4	T50.2X5	T50.2X6
fibrinolysis	T45.621	T45.622	T45.623	T45.624	T45.625	T45.626
monoamine oxidase NEC	T43.1X1	T43.1X2	T43.1X3	T43.1X4	T43.1X5	T43.1X6
hydrazine	T43.1X1	T43.1X2	T43.1X3	T43.1X4	T43.1X5	T43.1X6
postsynaptic	T43.8X1	T43.8X2	T43.8X3	T43.8X4	T43.8X5	T43.8X6
prothrombin synthesis	T45.511	T45.512	T45.513	T45.514	T45.515	T45.516
Ink	T65.891	T65.892	T65.893	T65.894	—	—
Inorganic substance NEC	T57.91	T57.92	T57.93	T57.94	—	—
Inosine pranobex	T37.5X1	T37.5X2	T37.5X3	T37.5X4	T37.5X5	T37.5X6
Inositol	T50.991	T50.992	T50.993	T50.994	T50.995	T50.996
nicotinate	T46.7X1	T46.7X2	T46.7X3	T46.7X4	T46.7X5	T46.7X6
Inproquone	T45.1X1	T45.1X2	T45.1X3	T45.1X4	T45.1X5	T45.1X6
Insect (sting), venomous	T63.481	T63.482	T63.483	T63.484	—	—
ant	T63.421	T63.422	T63.423	T63.424	—	—
bee	T63.441	T63.442	T63.443	T63.444	—	—
caterpillar	T63.431	T63.432	T63.433	T63.434	—	—
hornet	T63.451	T63.452	T63.453	T63.454	—	—
wasp	T63.461	T63.462	T63.463	T63.464	—	—
Insecticide NEC	T60.91	T60.92	T60.93	T60.94	—	—
carbamate	T60.0X1	T60.0X2	T60.0X3	T60.0X4	—	—
chlorinated	T60.1X1	T60.1X2	T60.1X3	T60.1X4	—	—
mixed	T60.91	T60.92	T60.93	T60.94	—	—
organochlorine	T60.1X1	T60.1X2	T60.1X3	T60.1X4	—	—
organophosphorus	T60.0X1	T60.0X2	T60.0X3	T60.0X4	—	—
Insular tissue extract	T38.3X1	T38.3X2	T38.3X3	T38.3X4	T38.3X5	T38.3X6
Insulin (amorphous) (globin) (isophane) (Lente) (NPH) (Semilente) (Ultralente)	T38.3X1	T38.3X2	T38.3X3	T38.3X4	T38.3X5	T38.3X6
defalan	T38.3X1	T38.3X2	T38.3X3	T38.3X4	T38.3X5	T38.3X6
human	T38.3X1	T38.3X2	T38.3X3	T38.3X4	T38.3X5	T38.3X6
injection, soluble	T38.3X1	T38.3X2	T38.3X3	T38.3X4	T38.3X5	T38.3X6
biphasic	T38.3X1	T38.3X2	T38.3X3	T38.3X4	T38.3X5	T38.3X6
intermediate acting	T38.3X1	T38.3X2	T38.3X3	T38.3X4	T38.3X5	T38.3X6
protamine zinc	T38.3X1	T38.3X2	T38.3X3	T38.3X4	T38.3X5	T38.3X6
slow acting	T38.3X1	T38.3X2	T38.3X3	T38.3X4	T38.3X5	T38.3X6
zinc						
protamine injection	T38.3X1	T38.3X2	T38.3X3	T38.3X4	T38.3X5	T38.3X6
suspension (amorphous) (crystalline)	T38.3X1	T38.3X2	T38.3X3	T38.3X4	T38.3X5	T38.3X6
Interferon (alpha) (beta) (gamma)	T37.5X1	T37.5X2	T37.5X3	T37.5X4	T37.5X5	T37.5X6
Intestinal motility control drug	T47.6X1	T47.6X2	T47.6X3	T47.6X4	T47.6X5	T47.6X6
biological	T47.8X1	T47.8X2	T47.8X3	T47.8X4	T47.8X5	T47.8X6
Intranarcon	T41.1X1	T41.1X2	T41.1X3	T41.1X4	T41.1X5	T41.1X6
Intravenous						
amino acids	T50.991	T50.992	T50.993	T50.994	T50.995	T50.996
fat suspension	T50.991	T50.992	T50.993	T50.994	T50.995	T50.996
Inulin	T50.8X1	T50.8X2	T50.8X3	T50.8X4	T50.8X5	T50.8X6
Invert sugar	T50.3X1	T50.3X2	T50.3X3	T50.3X4	T50.3X5	T50.3X6
Inza — *see Naproxen*						
Iobenzamic acid	T50.8X1	T50.8X2	T50.8X3	T50.8X4	T50.8X5	T50.8X6
Iocarmic acid	T50.8X1	T50.8X2	T50.8X3	T50.8X4	T50.8X5	T50.8X6
Iocetamic acid	T50.8X1	T50.8X2	T50.8X3	T50.8X4	T50.8X5	T50.8X6
Iodamide	T50.8X1	T50.8X2	T50.8X3	T50.8X4	T50.8X5	T50.8X6
Iodide NEC — *see also Iodine*	T49.0X1	T49.0X2	T49.0X3	T49.0X4	T49.0X5	T49.0X6
mercury (ointment)	T49.0X1	T49.0X2	T49.0X3	T49.0X4	T49.0X5	T49.0X6
methylate	T49.0X1	T49.0X2	T49.0X3	T49.0X4	T49.0X5	T49.0X6
potassium (expectorant) NEC	T48.4X1	T48.4X2	T48.4X3	T48.4X4	T48.4X5	T48.4X6
Iodinated						
contrast medium	T50.8X1	T50.8X2	T50.8X3	T50.8X4	T50.8X5	T50.8X6
glycerol	T48.4X1	T48.4X2	T48.4X3	T48.4X4	T48.4X5	T48.4X6
human serum albumin (131I)	T50.8X1	T50.8X2	T50.8X3	T50.8X4	T50.8X5	T50.8X6
Iodine (antiseptic, external) (tincture) NEC	T49.0X1	T49.0X2	T49.0X3	T49.0X4	T49.0X5	T49.0X6
125 — *see also Radiation sickness, and Exposure to radioactivce isotopes*	T50.8X1	T50.8X2	T50.8X3	T50.8X4	T50.8X5	T50.8X6
therapeutic	T50.991	T50.992	T50.993	T50.994	T50.995	T50.996
131 — *see also Radiation sickness, and Exposure to radioactivce isotopes*	T50.8X1	T50.8X2	T50.8X3	T50.8X4	T50.8X5	T50.8X6
therapeutic	T38.2X1	T38.2X2	T38.2X3	T38.2X4	T38.2X5	T38.2X6
diagnostic	T50.8X1	T50.8X2	T50.8X3	T50.8X4	T50.8X5	T50.8X6
for thyroid conditions (antithyroid)	T38.2X1	T38.2X2	T38.2X3	T38.2X4	T38.2X5	T38.2X6
solution	T49.0X1	T49.0X2	T49.0X3	T49.0X4	T49.0X5	T49.0X6
vapor	T59.891	T59.892	T59.893	T59.894	—	—
Iodipamide	T50.8X1	T50.8X2	T50.8X3	T50.8X4	T50.8X5	T50.8X6
Iodized (poppy seed) oil	T50.8X1	T50.8X2	T50.8X3	T50.8X4	T50.8X5	T50.8X6
Iodobismitol	T37.8X1	T37.8X2	T37.8X3	T37.8X4	T37.8X5	T37.8X6
Iodochlorhydroxyquin	T37.8X1	T37.8X2	T37.8X3	T37.8X4	T37.8X5	T37.8X6
topical	T49.0X1	T49.0X2	T49.0X3	T49.0X4	T49.0X5	T49.0X6
Iodochlorhydroxyquino-line	T37.8X1	T37.8X2	T37.8X3	T37.8X4	T37.8X5	T37.8X6
Iodocholesterol (131I)	T50.8X1	T50.8X2	T50.8X3	T50.8X4	T50.8X5	T50.8X6

◀ New ◀ Revised ~~deleted~~ Deleted

Substance	External Cause (T-Code)					
	Poisoning, Accidental (Unintentional)	Poisoning, Intentional Self-Harm	Poisoning, Assault	Poisoning, Undetermined	Adverse Effect	Underdosing
Iodoform	T49.0X1	T49.0X2	T49.0X3	T49.0X4	T49.0X5	T49.0X6
Iodohippuric acid	T50.8X1	T50.8X2	T50.8X3	T50.8X4	T50.8X5	T50.8X6
Iodopanoic acid	T50.8X1	T50.8X2	T50.8X3	T50.8X4	T50.8X5	T50.8X6
Iodophthalein (sodium)	T50.8X1	T50.8X2	T50.8X3	T50.8X4	T50.8X5	T50.8X6
Iodopyracet	T50.8X1	T50.8X2	T50.8X3	T50.8X4	T50.8X5	T50.8X6
Iodoquinol	T37.8X1	T37.8X2	T37.8X3	T37.8X4	T37.8X5	T37.8X6
Iodoxamic acid	T50.8X1	T50.8X2	T50.8X3	T50.8X4	T50.8X5	T50.8X6
Iofendylate	T50.8X1	T50.8X2	T50.8X3	T50.8X4	T50.8X5	T50.8X6
Ioglycamic acid	T50.8X1	T50.8X2	T50.8X3	T50.8X4	T50.8X5	T50.8X6
Iohexol	T50.8X1	T50.8X2	T50.8X3	T50.8X4	T50.8X5	T50.8X6
Ion exchange resin						
anion	T47.8X1	T47.8X2	T47.8X3	T47.8X4	T47.8X5	T47.8X6
cation	T50.3X1	T50.3X2	T50.3X3	T50.3X4	T50.3X5	T50.3X6
cholestyramine	T46.6X1	T46.6X2	T46.6X3	T46.6X4	T46.6X5	T46.6X6
intestinal	T47.8X1	T47.8X2	T47.8X3	T47.8X4	T47.8X5	T47.8X6
Iopamidol	T50.8X1	T50.8X2	T50.8X3	T50.8X4	T50.8X5	T50.8X6
Iopanoic acid	T50.8X1	T50.8X2	T50.8X3	T50.8X4	T50.8X5	T50.8X6
Iophenoic acid	T50.8X1	T50.8X2	T50.8X3	T50.8X4	T50.8X5	T50.8X6
Iopodate, sodium	T50.8X1	T50.8X2	T50.8X3	T50.8X4	T50.8X5	T50.8X6
Iopodic acid	T50.8X1	T50.8X2	T50.8X3	T50.8X4	T50.8X5	T50.8X6
Iopromide	T50.8X1	T50.8X2	T50.8X3	T50.8X4	T50.8X5	T50.8X6
Iopydol	T50.8X1	T50.8X2	T50.8X3	T50.8X4	T50.8X5	T50.8X6
Iotalamic acid	T50.8X1	T50.8X2	T50.8X3	T50.8X4	T50.8X5	T50.8X6
Iothalamate	T50.8X1	T50.8X2	T50.8X3	T50.8X4	T50.8X5	T50.8X6
Iothiouracil	T38.2X1	T38.2X2	T38.2X3	T38.2X4	T38.2X5	T38.2X6
Iotrol	T50.8X1	T50.8X2	T50.8X3	T50.8X4	T50.8X5	T50.8X6
Iotrolan	T50.8X1	T50.8X2	T50.8X3	T50.8X4	T50.8X5	T50.8X6
Iotroxate	T50.8X1	T50.8X2	T50.8X3	T50.8X4	T50.8X5	T50.8X6
Iotroxic acid	T50.8X1	T50.8X2	T50.8X3	T50.8X4	T50.8X5	T50.8X6
Ioversol	T50.8X1	T50.8X2	T50.8X3	T50.8X4	T50.8X5	T50.8X6
Ioxaglate	T50.8X1	T50.8X2	T50.8X3	T50.8X4	T50.8X5	T50.8X6
Ioxaglic acid	T50.8X1	T50.8X2	T50.8X3	T50.8X4	T50.8X5	T50.8X6
Ioxitalamic acid	T50.8X1	T50.8X2	T50.8X3	T50.8X4	T50.8X5	T50.8X6
Ipecac	T47.7X1	T47.7X2	T47.7X3	T47.7X4	T47.7X5	T47.7X6
Ipecacuanha	T48.4X1	T48.4X2	T48.4X3	T48.4X4	T48.4X5	T48.4X6
Ipodate, calcium	T50.8X1	T50.8X2	T50.8X3	T50.8X4	T50.8X5	T50.8X6
Ipral	T42.3X1	T42.3X2	T42.3X3	T42.3X4	T42.3X5	T42.3X6
Ipratropium (bromide)	T48.6X1	T48.6X2	T48.6X3	T48.6X4	T48.6X5	T48.6X6
Ipriflavone	T46.3X1	T46.3X2	T46.3X3	T46.3X4	T46.3X5	T46.3X6
Iprindole	T43.011	T43.012	T43.013	T43.014	T43.015	T43.016
Iproclozide	T43.1X1	T43.1X2	T43.1X3	T43.1X4	T43.1X5	T43.1X6
Iprofenin	T50.8X1	T50.8X2	T50.8X3	T50.8X4	T50.8X5	T50.8X6

Substance	External Cause (T-Code)					
	Poisoning, Accidental (Unintentional)	Poisoning, Intentional Self-Harm	Poisoning, Assault	Poisoning, Undetermined	Adverse Effect	Underdosing
Iproheptine	T49.2X1	T49.2X2	T49.2X3	T49.2X4	T49.2X5	T49.2X6
Iproniazid	T43.1X1	T43.1X2	T43.1X3	T43.1X4	T43.1X5	T43.1X6
Iproplatin	T45.1X1	T45.1X2	T45.1X3	T45.1X4	T45.1X5	T45.1X6
Iproveratril	T46.1X1	T46.1X2	T46.1X3	T46.1X4	T46.1X5	T46.1X6
Iron (compounds) (medicinal) NEC	T45.4X1	T45.4X2	T45.4X3	T45.4X4	T45.4X5	T45.4X6
ammonium	T45.4X1	T45.4X2	T45.4X3	T45.4X4	T45.4X5	T45.4X6
dextran injection	T45.4X1	T45.4X2	T45.4X3	T45.4X4	T45.4X5	T45.4X6
nonmedicinal	T56.891	T56.892	T56.893	T56.894	—	—
salts	T45.4X1	T45.4X2	T45.4X3	T45.4X4	T45.4X5	T45.4X6
sorbitex	T45.4X1	T45.4X2	T45.4X3	T45.4X4	T45.4X5	T45.4X6
sorbitol citric acid complex	T45.4X1	T45.4X2	T45.4X3	T45.4X4	T45.4X5	T45.4X6
Irrigating fluid (vaginal)	T49.8X1	T49.8X2	T49.8X3	T49.8X4	T49.8X5	T49.8X6
eye	T49.5X1	T49.5X2	T49.5X3	T49.5X4	T49.5X5	T49.5X6
Isepamicin	T36.5X1	T36.5X2	T36.5X3	T36.5X4	T36.5X5	T36.5X6
Isoaminile (citrate)	T48.3X1	T48.3X2	T48.3X3	T48.3X4	T48.3X5	T48.3X6
Isoamyl nitrite	T46.3X1	T46.3X2	T46.3X3	T46.3X4	T46.3X5	T46.3X6
Isobenzan	T60.1X1	T60.1X2	T60.1X3	T60.1X4	—	—
Isobutyl acetate	T52.8X1	T52.8X2	T52.8X3	T52.8X4	—	—
Isocarboxazid	T43.1X1	T43.1X2	T43.1X3	T43.1X4	T43.1X5	T43.1X6
Isoconazole	T49.0X1	T49.0X2	T49.0X3	T49.0X4	T49.0X5	T49.0X6
Isocyanate	T65.0X1	T65.0X2	T65.0X3	T65.0X4	—	—
Isoephedrine	T44.991	T44.992	T44.993	T44.994	T44.995	T44.996
Isoetarine	T48.6X1	T48.6X2	T48.6X3	T48.6X4	T48.6X5	T48.6X6
Isoethadione	T42.2X1	T42.2X2	T42.2X3	T42.2X4	T42.2X5	T42.2X6
Isoetharine	T44.5X1	T44.5X2	T44.5X3	T44.5X4	T44.5X5	T44.5X6
Isoflurane	T41.0X1	T41.0X2	T41.0X3	T41.0X4	T41.0X5	T41.0X6
Isoflurophate	T44.0X1	T44.0X2	T44.0X3	T44.0X4	T44.0X5	T44.0X6
Isomaltose, ferric complex	T45.4X1	T45.4X2	T45.4X3	T45.4X4	T45.4X5	T45.4X6
Isometheptene	T44.3X1	T44.3X2	T44.3X3	T44.3X4	T44.3X5	T44.3X6
Isoniazid	T37.1X1	T37.1X2	T37.1X3	T37.1X4	T37.1X5	T37.1X6
with						
rifampicin	T36.6X1	T36.6X2	T36.6X3	T36.6X4	T36.6X5	T36.6X6
thioacetazone	T37.1X1	T37.1X2	T37.1X3	T37.1X4	T37.1X5	T37.1X6
Isonicotinic acid hydrazide	T37.1X1	T37.1X2	T37.1X3	T37.1X4	T37.1X5	T37.1X6
Isonipecaine	T40.4X1	T40.4X2	T40.4X3	T40.4X4	T40.4X5	T40.4X6
Isopentaquine	T37.2X1	T37.2X2	T37.2X3	T37.2X4	T37.2X5	T37.2X6
Isophane insulin	T38.3X1	T38.3X2	T38.3X3	T38.3X4	T38.3X5	T38.3X6
Isophorone	T65.891	T65.892	T65.893	T65.894	—	—
Isophosphamide	T45.1X1	T45.1X2	T45.1X3	T45.1X4	T45.1X5	T45.1X6
Isopregnenone	T38.5X1	T38.5X2	T38.5X3	T38.5X4	T38.5X5	T38.5X6
Isoprenaline	T48.6X1	T48.6X2	T48.6X3	T48.6X4	T48.6X5	T48.6X6
Isopromethazine	T43.3X1	T43.3X2	T43.3X3	T43.3X4	T43.3X5	T43.3X6

TABLE OF DRUGS AND CHEMICALS

	External Cause (T-Code)					
Substance	Poisoning, Accidental (Unintentional)	Poisoning, Intentional Self-Harm	Poisoning, Assault	Poisoning, Undetermined	Adverse Effect	Underdosing
Isopropamide	T44.3X1	T44.3X2	T44.3X3	T44.3X4	T44.3X5	T44.3X6
iodide	T44.3X1	T44.3X2	T44.3X3	T44.3X4	T44.3X5	T44.3X6
Isopropanol	T51.2X1	T51.2X2	T51.2X3	T51.2X4	—	—
Isopropyl						
acetate	T52.8X1	T52.8X2	T52.8X3	T52.8X4	—	—
alcohol	T51.2X1	T51.2X2	T51.2X3	T51.2X4	—	—
medicinal	T49.4X1	T49.4X2	T49.4X3	T49.4X4	T49.4X5	T49.4X6
ether	T52.8X1	T52.8X2	T52.8X3	T52.8X4	—	—
Isopropylaminophena-zone	T39.2X1	T39.2X2	T39.2X3	T39.2X4	T39.2X5	T39.2X6
Isoproterenol	T48.6X1	T48.6X2	T48.6X3	T48.6X4	T48.6X5	T48.6X6
Isosorbide dinitrate	T46.3X1	T46.3X2	T46.3X3	T46.3X4	T46.3X5	T46.3X6
Isothipendyl	T45.0X1	T45.0X2	T45.0X3	T45.0X4	T45.0X5	T45.0X6
Isotretinoin	T50.991	T50.992	T50.993	T50.994	T50.995	T50.996
Isoxazolyl penicillin	T36.0X1	T36.0X2	T36.0X3	T36.0X4	T36.0X5	T36.0X6
Isoxicam	T39.391	T39.392	T39.393	T39.394	T39.395	T39.396
Isoxsuprine	T46.7X1	T46.7X2	T46.7X3	T46.7X4	T46.7X5	T46.7X6
Ispagula	T47.4X1	T47.4X2	T47.4X3	T47.4X4	T47.4X5	T47.4X6
husk	T47.4X1	T47.4X2	T47.4X3	T47.4X4	T47.4X5	T47.4X6
Isradipine	T46.1X1	T46.1X2	T46.1X3	T46.1X4	T46.1X5	T46.1X6
I-thyroxine sodium	T38.1X1	T38.1X2	T38.1X3	T38.1X4	T38.1X5	T38.1X6
Itraconazole	T37.8X1	T37.8X2	T37.8X3	T37.8X4	T37.8X5	T37.8X6
Itramin tosilate	T46.3X1	T46.3X2	T46.3X3	T46.3X4	T46.3X5	T46.3X6
Ivermectin	T37.4X1	T37.4X2	T37.4X3	T37.4X4	T37.4X5	T37.4X6
Izoniazid	T37.1X1	T37.1X2	T37.1X3	T37.1X4	T37.1X5	T37.1X6
with thioacetazone	T37.1X1	T37.1X2	T37.1X3	T37.1X4	T37.1X5	T37.1X6
J						
Jalap	T47.2X1	T47.2X2	T47.2X3	T47.2X4	T47.2X5	T47.2X6
Jamaica						
dogwood (bark)	T39.8X1	T39.8X2	T39.8X3	T39.8X4	T39.8X5	T39.8X6
ginger	T65.891	T65.892	T65.893	T65.894	—	—
root	T62.2X1	T62.2X2	T62.2X3	T62.2X4	—	—
Jatropha	T62.2X1	T62.2X2	T62.2X3	T62.2X4	—	—
curcas	T62.2X1	T62.2X2	T62.2X3	T62.2X4	—	—
Jectofer	T45.4X1	T45.4X2	T45.4X3	T45.4X4	T45.4X5	T45.4X6
Jellyfish (sting)	T63.621	T63.622	T63.623	T63.624	—	—
Jequirity (bean)	T62.2X1	T62.2X2	T62.2X3	T62.2X4	—	—
Jimson weed (stramonium)	T62.2X1	T62.2X2	T62.2X3	T62.2X4	—	—
seeds	T62.2X1	T62.2X2	T62.2X3	T62.2X4	—	—
Josamycin	T36.3X1	T36.3X2	T36.3X3	T36.3X4	T36.3X5	T36.3X6
Juniper tar	T49.1X1	T49.1X2	T49.1X3	T49.1X4	T49.1X5	T49.1X6
K						
Kallidinogenase	T46.7X1	T46.7X2	T46.7X3	T46.7X4	T46.7X5	T46.7X6
Kallikrein	T46.7X1	T46.7X2	T46.7X3	T46.7X4	T46.7X5	T46.7X6
Kanamycin	T36.5X1	T36.5X2	T36.5X3	T36.5X4	T36.5X5	T36.5X6
Kantrex	T36.5X1	T36.5X2	T36.5X3	T36.5X4	T36.5X5	T36.5X6
Kaolin	T47.6X1	T47.6X2	T47.6X3	T47.6X4	T47.6X5	T47.6X6
light	T47.6X1	T47.6X2	T47.6X3	T47.6X4	T47.6X5	T47.6X6
Karaya (gum)	T47.4X1	T47.4X2	T47.4X3	T47.4X4	T47.4X5	T47.4X6
Kebuzone	T39.2X1	T39.2X2	T39.2X3	T39.2X4	T39.2X5	T39.2X6
Kelevan	T60.1X1	T60.1X2	T60.1X3	T60.1X4	—	—
Kemithal	T41.1X1	T41.1X2	T41.1X3	T41.1X4	T41.1X5	T41.1X6
Kenacort	T38.0X1	T38.0X2	T38.0X3	T38.0X4	T38.0X5	T38.0X6
Keratolytic drug NEC	T49.4X1	T49.4X2	T49.4X3	T49.4X4	T49.4X5	T49.4X6
anthracene	T49.4X1	T49.4X2	T49.4X3	T49.4X4	T49.4X5	T49.4X6
Keratoplastic NEC	T49.4X1	T49.4X2	T49.4X3	T49.4X4	T49.4X5	T49.4X6
Kerosene, kerosine (fuel) (solvent) NEC	T52.0X1	T52.0X2	T52.0X3	T52.0X4	—	—
insecticide	T52.0X1	T52.0X2	T52.0X3	T52.0X4	—	—
vapor	T52.0X1	T52.0X2	T52.0X3	T52.0X4	—	—
Ketamine	T41.291	T41.292	T41.293	T41.294	T41.295	T41.296
Ketazolam	T42.4X1	T42.4X2	T42.4X3	T42.4X4	T42.4X5	T42.4X6
Ketazon	T39.2X1	T39.2X2	T39.2X3	T39.2X4	T39.2X5	T39.2X6
Ketobemidone	T40.4X1	T40.4X2	T40.4X3	T40.4X4	—	—
Ketoconazole	T49.0X1	T49.0X2	T49.0X3	T49.0X4	T49.0X5	T49.0X6
Ketols	T52.4X1	T52.4X2	T52.4X3	T52.4X4	—	—
Ketone oils	T52.4X1	T52.4X2	T52.4X3	T52.4X4	—	—
Ketoprofen	T39.311	T39.312	T39.313	T39.314	T39.315	T39.316
Ketorolac	T39.8X1	T39.8X2	T39.8X3	T39.8X4	T39.8X5	T39.8X6
Ketotifen	T45.0X1	T45.0X2	T45.0X3	T45.0X4	T45.0X5	T45.0X6
Khat	T43.691	T43.692	T43.693	T43.694	—	—
Khellin	T46.3X1	T46.3X2	T46.3X3	T46.3X4	T46.3X5	T46.3X6
Khelloside	T46.3X1	T46.3X2	T46.3X3	T46.3X4	T46.3X5	T46.3X6
Kiln gas or vapor (carbon monoxide)	T58.8X1	T58.8X2	T58.8X3	T58.8X4	—	—
Kitasamycin	T36.3X1	T36.3X2	T36.3X3	T36.3X4	T36.3X5	T36.3X6
Konsyl	T47.4X1	T47.4X2	T47.4X3	T47.4X4	T47.4X5	T47.4X6
Kosam seed	T62.2X1	T62.2X2	T62.2X3	T62.2X4	—	—
Krait (venom)	T63.091	T63.092	T63.093	T63.094	—	—
Kwell (insecticide)	T60.1X1	T60.1X2	T60.1X3	T60.1X4	—	—
anti-infective (topical)	T49.0X1	T49.0X2	T49.0X3	T49.0X4	T49.0X5	T49.0X6

New Revised ~~deleted~~ Deleted

Substance	Poisoning, Accidental (Unintentional)	Poisoning, Intentional Self-Harm	Poisoning, Assault	Poisoning, Undetermined	Adverse Effect	Underdosing
	External Cause (T-Code)					
L						
Labetalol	T44.8X1	T44.8X2	T44.8X3	T44.8X4	T44.8X5	T44.8X6
Laburnum (seeds)	T62.2X1	T62.2X2	T62.2X3	T62.2X4	—	—
leaves	T62.2X1	T62.2X2	T62.2X3	T62.2X4	—	—
Lachesine	T49.5X1	T49.5X2	T49.5X3	T49.5X4	T49.5X5	T49.5X6
Lacidipine	T46.5X1	T46.5X2	T46.5X3	T46.5X4	T46.5X5	T46.5X6
Lacquer	T65.6X1	T65.6X2	T65.6X3	T65.6X4	—	—
Lacrimogenic gas	T59.3X1	T59.3X2	T59.3X3	T59.3X4	—	—
Lactated potassic saline	T5Ø.3X1	T5Ø.3X2	T5Ø.3X3	T5Ø.3X4	T5Ø.3X5	T5Ø.3X6
Lactic acid	T49.8X1	T49.8X2	T49.8X3	T49.8X4	T49.8X5	T49.8X6
Lactobacillus						
acidophilus	T47.6X1	T47.6X2	T47.6X3	T47.6X4	T47.6X5	T47.6X6
compound	T47.6X1	T47.6X2	T47.6X3	T47.6X4	T47.6X5	T47.6X6
bifidus, lyophilized	T47.6X1	T47.6X2	T47.6X3	T47.6X4	T47.6X5	T47.6X6
bulgaricus	T47.6X1	T47.6X2	T47.6X3	T47.6X4	T47.6X5	T47.6X6
sporogenes	T47.6X1	T47.6X2	T47.6X3	T47.6X4	T47.6X5	T47.6X6
Lactoflavin	T45.2X1	T45.2X2	T45.2X3	T45.2X4	T45.2X5	T45.2X6
Lactose (as excipient)	T5Ø.9Ø1	T5Ø.9Ø2	T5Ø.9Ø3	T5Ø.9Ø4	T5Ø.9Ø5	T5Ø.9Ø6
Lactuca (virosa) (extract)	T42.6X1	T42.6X2	T42.6X3	T42.6X4	T42.6X5	T42.6X6
Lactucarium	T42.6X1	T42.6X2	T42.6X3	T42.6X4	T42.6X5	T42.6X6
Lactulose	T47.3X1	T47.3X2	T47.3X3	T47.3X4	T47.3X5	T47.3X6
Laevo — *see* *Levo-*						
Lanatosides	T46.ØX1	T46.ØX2	T46.ØX3	T46.ØX4	T46.ØX5	T46.ØX6
Lanolin	T49.3X1	T49.3X2	T49.3X3	T49.3X4	T49.3X5	T49.3X6
Largactil	T43.3X1	T43.3X2	T43.3X3	T43.3X4	T43.3X5	T43.3X6
Larkspur	T62.2X1	T62.2X2	T62.2X3	T62.2X4	—	—
Laroxyl	T43.Ø11	T43.Ø12	T43.Ø13	T43.Ø14	T43.Ø15	T43.Ø16
Lassar's paste	T49.4X1	T49.4X2	T49.4X3	T49.4X4	T49.4X5	T49.4X6
Lasix	T5Ø.1X1	T5Ø.1X2	T5Ø.1X3	T5Ø.1X4	T5Ø.1X5	T5Ø.1X6
Latamoxef	T36.1X1	T36.1X2	T36.1X3	T36.1X4	T36.1X5	T36.1X6
Latex	T65.811	T65.812	T65.813	T65.814	—	—
Lathyrus (seed)	T62.2X1	T62.2X2	T62.2X3	T62.2X4	—	—
Laudanum	T4Ø.ØX1	T4Ø.ØX2	T4Ø.ØX3	T4Ø.ØX4	T4Ø.ØX5	T4Ø.ØX6
Laudexium	T48.1X1	T48.1X2	T48.1X3	T48.1X4	T48.1X5	T48.1X6
Laughing gas	T41.ØX1	T41.ØX2	T41.ØX3	T41.ØX4	T41.ØX5	T41.ØX6
Laurel, black or cherry	T62.2X1	T62.2X2	T62.2X3	T62.2X4	—	—
Laurolinium	T49.ØX1	T49.ØX2	T49.ØX3	T49.ØX4	T49.ØX5	T49.ØX6
Lauryl sulfoacetate	T49.2X1	T49.2X2	T49.2X3	T49.2X4	T49.2X5	T49.2X6

Substance	Poisoning, Accidental (Unintentional)	Poisoning, Intentional Self-Harm	Poisoning, Assault	Poisoning, Undetermined	Adverse Effect	Underdosing
	External Cause (T-Code)					
Laxative NEC	T47.4X1	T47.4X2	T47.4X3	T47.4X4	T47.4X5	T47.4X6
osmotic	T47.3X1	T47.3X2	T47.3X3	T47.3X4	T47.3X5	T47.3X6
saline	T47.3X1	T47.3X2	T47.3X3	T47.3X4	T47.3X5	T47.3X6
stimulant	T47.2X1	T47.2X2	T47.2X3	T47.2X4	T47.2X5	T47.2X6
L-dopa	T42.8X1	T42.8X2	T42.8X3	T42.8X4	T42.8X5	T42.8X6
Lead (dust) (fumes) (vapor) NEC	T56.ØX1	T56.ØX2	T56.ØX3	T56.ØX4	—	—
acetate	T49.2X1	T49.2X2	T49.2X3	T49.2X4	T49.2X5	T49.2X6
alkyl (fuel additive)	T56.ØX1	T56.ØX2	T56.ØX3	T56.ØX4	—	—
anti-infectives	T37.8X1	T37.8X2	T37.8X3	T37.8X4	T37.8X5	T37.8X6
antiknock compound (tetraethyl)	T56.ØX1	T56.ØX2	T56.ØX3	T56.ØX4	—	—
arsenate, arsenite (dust) (herbicide) (insecticide) (vapor)	T57.ØX1	T57.ØX2	T57.ØX3	T57.ØX4	—	—
carbonate	T56.ØX1	T56.ØX2	T56.ØX3	T56.ØX4	—	—
paint	T56.ØX1	T56.ØX2	T56.ØX3	T56.ØX4	—	—
chromate	T56.ØX1	T56.ØX2	T56.ØX3	T56.ØX4	—	—
paint	T56.ØX1	T56.ØX2	T56.ØX3	T56.ØX4	—	—
dioxide	T56.ØX1	T56.ØX2	T56.ØX3	T56.ØX4	—	—
inorganic	T56.ØX1	T56.ØX2	T56.ØX3	T56.ØX4	—	—
iodide	T56.ØX1	T56.ØX2	T56.ØX3	T56.ØX4	—	—
pigment (paint)	T56.ØX1	T56.ØX2	T56.ØX3	T56.ØX4	—	—
monoxide (dust)	T56.ØX1	T56.ØX2	T56.ØX3	T56.ØX4	—	—
paint	T56.ØX1	T56.ØX2	T56.ØX3	T56.ØX4	—	—
organic	T56.ØX1	T56.ØX2	T56.ØX3	T56.ØX4	—	—
oxide	T56.ØX1	T56.ØX2	T56.ØX3	T56.ØX4	—	—
paint	T56.ØX1	T56.ØX2	T56.ØX3	T56.ØX4	—	—
paint	T56.ØX1	T56.ØX2	T56.ØX3	T56.ØX4	—	—
salts	T56.ØX1	T56.ØX2	T56.ØX3	T56.ØX4	—	—
specified compound NEC	T56.ØX1	T56.ØX2	T56.ØX3	T56.ØX4	—	—
tetra-ethyl	T56.ØX1	T56.ØX2	T56.ØX3	T56.ØX4	—	—
Lebanese red	T4Ø.7X1	T4Ø.7X2	T4Ø.7X3	T4Ø.7X4	T4Ø.7X5	T4Ø.7X6
Lefetamine	T39.8X1	T39.8X2	T39.8X3	T39.8X4	T39.8X5	T39.8X6
Lenperone	T43.4X1	T43.4X2	T43.4X3	T43.4X4	T43.4X5	T43.4X6
Lente lietin (insulin)	T38.3X1	T38.3X2	T38.3X3	T38.3X4	T38.3X5	T38.3X6
Leptazol	T5Ø.7X1	T5Ø.7X2	T5Ø.7X3	T5Ø.7X4	T5Ø.7X5	T5Ø.7X6
Leptophos	T6Ø.ØX1	T6Ø.ØX2	T6Ø.ØX3	T6Ø.ØX4	—	—
Leritine	T4Ø.2X1	T4Ø.2X2	T4Ø.2X3	T4Ø.2X4	T4Ø.2X5	T4Ø.2X6
Letosteine	T48.4X1	T48.4X2	T48.4X3	T48.4X4	T48.4X5	T48.4X6
Letter	T38.1X1	T38.1X2	T38.1X3	T38.1X4	T38.1X5	T38.1X6
Lettuce opium	T42.6X1	T42.6X2	T42.6X3	T42.6X4	T42.6X5	T42.6X6
Leucinocaine	T41.3X1	T41.3X2	T41.3X3	T41.3X4	T41.3X5	T41.3X6

Substance	External Cause (T-Code)					
	Poisoning, Accidental (Unintentional)	Poisoning, Intentional Self-Harm	Poisoning, Assault	Poisoning, Undetermined	Adverse Effect	Underdosing
Leucocianidol	T46.991	T46.992	T46.993	T46.994	T46.995	T46.996
Leucovorin (factor)	T45.8X1	T45.8X2	T45.8X3	T45.8X4	T45.8X5	T45.8X6
Leukeran	T45.1X1	T45.1X2	T45.1X3	T45.1X4	T45.1X5	T45.1X6
Leuprolide	T38.891	T38.892	T38.893	T38.894	T38.895	T38.896
Levalbuterol	T48.6X1	T48.6X2	T48.6X3	T48.6X4	T48.6X5	T48.6X6
Levallorphan	T5Ø.7X1	T5Ø.7X2	T5Ø.7X3	T5Ø.7X4	T5Ø.7X5	T5Ø.7X6
Levamisole	T37.4X1	T37.4X2	T37.4X3	T37.4X4	T37.4X5	T37.4X6
Levanil	T42.6X1	T42.6X2	T42.6X3	T42.6X4	T42.6X5	T42.6X6
Levarterenol	T44.4X1	T44.4X2	T44.4X3	T44.4X4	T44.4X5	T44.4X6
Levdropropizine	T48.3X1	T48.3X2	T48.3X3	T48.3X4	T48.3X5	T48.3X6
Levobunolol	T49.5X1	T49.5X2	T49.5X3	T49.5X4	T49.5X5	T49.5X6
Levocabastine (hydrochloride)	T45.ØX1	T45.ØX2	T45.ØX3	T45.ØX4	T45.ØX5	T45.ØX6
Levocarnitine	T5Ø.991	T5Ø.992	T5Ø.993	T5Ø.994	T5Ø.995	T5Ø.996
Levodopa	T42.8X1	T42.8X2	T42.8X3	T42.8X4	T42.8X5	T42.8X6
with carbidopa	T42.8X1	T42.8X2	T42.8X3	T42.8X4	T42.8X5	T42.8X6
Levo-dromoran	T4Ø.2X1	T4Ø.2X2	T4Ø.2X3	T4Ø.2X4	T4Ø.2X5	T4Ø.2X6
Levoglutamide	T5Ø.991	T5Ø.992	T5Ø.993	T5Ø.994	T5Ø.995	T5Ø.996
Levoid	T38.1X1	T38.1X2	T38.1X3	T38.1X4	T38.1X5	T38.1X6
Levo-iso-methadone	T4Ø.3X1	T4Ø.3X2	T4Ø.3X3	T4Ø.3X4	T4Ø.3X5	T4Ø.3X6
Levomepromazine	T43.3X1	T43.3X2	T43.3X3	T43.3X4	T43.3X5	T43.3X6
Levonordefrin	T49.6X1	T49.6X2	T49.6X3	T49.6X4	T49.6X5	T49.6X6
Levonorgestrel	T38.4X1	T38.4X2	T38.4X3	T38.4X4	T38.4X5	T38.4X6
with ethinylestradiol	T38.5X1	T38.5X2	T38.5X3	T38.5X4	T38.5X5	T38.5X6
Levopromazine	T43.3X1	T43.3X2	T43.3X3	T43.3X4	T43.3X5	T43.3X6
Levoprome	T42.6X1	T42.6X2	T42.6X3	T42.6X4	T42.6X5	T42.6X6
Levopropoxyphene	T4Ø.4X1	T4Ø.4X2	T4Ø.4X3	T4Ø.4X4	T4Ø.4X5	T4Ø.4X6
Levopropylhexedrine	T5Ø.5X1	T5Ø.5X2	T5Ø.5X3	T5Ø.5X4	T5Ø.5X5	T5Ø.5X6
Levoproxyphylline	T48.6X1	T48.6X2	T48.6X3	T48.6X4	T48.6X5	T48.6X6
Levorphanol	T4Ø.4X1	T4Ø.4X2	T4Ø.4X3	T4Ø.4X4	T4Ø.4X5	T4Ø.4X6
Levothyroxine	T38.1X1	T38.1X2	T38.1X3	T38.1X4	T38.1X5	T38.1X6
sodium	T38.1X1	T38.1X2	T38.1X3	T38.1X4	T38.1X5	T38.1X6
Levsin	T44.3X1	T44.3X2	T44.3X3	T44.3X4	T44.3X5	T44.3X6
Levulose	T5Ø.3X1	T5Ø.3X2	T5Ø.3X3	T5Ø.3X4	T5Ø.3X5	T5Ø.3X6
Lewisite (gas), not in war	T57.ØX1	T57.ØX2	T57.ØX3	T57.ØX4	—	—
Librium	T42.4X1	T42.4X2	T42.4X3	T42.4X4	T42.4X5	T42.4X6
Lidex	T49.ØX1	T49.ØX2	T49.ØX3	T49.ØX4	T49.ØX5	T49.ØX6
Lidocaine	T41.3X1	T41.3X2	T41.3X3	T41.3X4	T41.3X5	T41.3X6
regional	T41.3X1	T41.3X2	T41.3X3	T41.3X4	T41.3X5	T41.3X6
spinal	T41.3X1	T41.3X2	T41.3X3	T41.3X4	T41.3X5	T41.3X6
Lidofenin	T5Ø.8X1	T5Ø.8X2	T5Ø.8X3	T5Ø.8X4	T5Ø.8X5	T5Ø.8X6
Lidoflazine	T46.1X1	T46.1X2	T46.1X3	T46.1X4	T46.1X5	T46.1X6
Lighter fluid	T52.ØX1	T52.ØX2	T52.ØX3	T52.ØX4	—	—
Lignin hemicellulose	T47.6X1	T47.6X2	T47.6X3	T47.6X4	T47.6X5	T47.6X6
Lignocaine	T41.3X1	T41.3X2	T41.3X3	T41.3X4	T41.3X5	T41.3X6
regional	T41.3X1	T41.3X2	T41.3X3	T41.3X4	T41.3X5	T41.3X6
spinal	T41.3X1	T41.3X2	T41.3X3	T41.3X4	T41.3X5	T41.3X6
Ligroin(e) (solvent)	T52.ØX1	T52.ØX2	T52.ØX3	T52.ØX4	—	—
vapor	T59.891	T59.892	T59.893	T59.894	—	—
Ligustrum vulgare	T62.2X1	T62.2X2	T62.2X3	T62.2X4	—	—
Lily of the valley	T62.2X1	T62.2X2	T62.2X3	T62.2X4	—	—
Lime (chloride)	T54.3X1	T54.3X2	T54.3X3	T54.3X4	—	—
Limonene	T52.8X1	T52.8X2	T52.8X3	T52.8X4	—	—
Lincomycin	T36.8X1	T36.8X2	T36.8X3	T36.8X4	T36.8X5	T36.8X6
Lindane (insecticide) (nonmedicinal) (vapor)	T53.6X1	T53.6X2	T53.6X3	T53.6X4	—	—
medicinal	T49.ØX1	T49.ØX2	T49.ØX3	T49.ØX4	T49.ØX5	T49.ØX6
Liniments NEC	T49.91	T49.92	T49.93	T49.94	T49.95	T49.96
Linoleic acid	T46.6X1	T46.6X2	T46.6X3	T46.6X4	T46.6X5	T46.6X6
Linolenic acid	T46.6X1	T46.6X2	T46.6X3	T46.6X4	T46.6X5	T46.6X6
Linseed	T47.4X1	T47.4X2	T47.4X3	T47.4X4	T47.4X5	T47.4X6
Liothyronine	T38.1X1	T38.1X2	T38.1X3	T38.1X4	T38.1X5	T38.1X6
Liotrix	T38.1X1	T38.1X2	T38.1X3	T38.1X4	T38.1X5	T38.1X6
Lipancreatin	T47.5X1	T47.5X2	T47.5X3	T47.5X4	T47.5X5	T47.5X6
Lipo-alprostadil	T46.7X1	T46.7X2	T46.7X3	T46.7X4	T46.7X5	T46.7X6
Lipo-Lutin	T38.5X1	T38.5X2	T38.5X3	T38.5X4	T38.5X5	T38.5X6
Lipotropic drug NEC	T5Ø.9Ø1	T5Ø.9Ø2	T5Ø.9Ø3	T5Ø.9Ø4	T5Ø.9Ø5	T5Ø.9Ø6
Liquefied petroleum gases	T59.891	T59.892	T59.893	T59.894	—	—
piped (pure or mixed with air)	T59.891	T59.892	T59.893	T59.894	—	—
Liquid						
paraffin	T47.4X1	T47.4X2	T47.4X3	T47.4X4	T47.4X5	T47.4X6
petrolatum	T47.4X1	T47.4X2	T47.4X3	T47.4X4	T47.4X5	T47.4X6
topical	T49.3X1	T49.3X2	T49.3X3	T49.3X4	T49.3X5	T49.3X6
specified NEC	T65.891	T65.892	T65.893	T65.894	—	—
substance	T65.91	T65.92	T65.93	T65.94	—	—
Liquor creosolis compositus	T65.891	T65.892	T65.893	T65.894	—	—
Liquorice	T48.4X1	T48.4X2	T48.4X3	T48.4X4	T48.4X5	T48.4X6
extract	T47.8X1	T47.8X2	T47.8X3	T47.8X4	T47.8X5	T47.8X6
Lirugen	T5Ø.991	T5Ø.992	T5Ø.993	T5Ø.994	T5Ø.995	T5Ø.996
Lisinopril	T46.4X1	T46.4X2	T46.4X3	T46.4X4	T46.4X5	T46.4X6
Lisuride	T42.8X1	T42.8X2	T42.8X3	T42.8X4	T42.8X5	T42.8X6
Lithane	T43.8X1	T43.8X2	T43.8X3	T43.8X4	T43.8X5	T43.8X6
Lithium	T56.891	T56.892	T56.893	T56.894	—	—
gluconate	T43.591	T43.592	T43.593	T43.594	T43.595	T43.596
salts (carbonate)	T43.591	T43.592	T43.593	T43.594	T43.595	T43.596

◀ New ◀ Revised ~~deleted~~ Deleted

Substance	Poisoning, Accidental (Unintentional)	Poisoning, Intentional Self-Harm	Poisoning, Assault	Poisoning, Undetermined	Adverse Effect	Underdosing
	External Cause (T-Code)					
Lithonate	T43.8X1	T43.8X2	T43.8X3	T43.8X4	T43.8X5	T43.8X6
Liver						
extract	T45.8X1	T45.8X2	T45.8X3	T45.8X4	T45.8X5	T45.8X6
for parenteral use	T45.8X1	T45.8X2	T45.8X3	T45.8X4	T45.8X5	T45.8X6
fraction 1	T45.8X1	T45.8X2	T45.8X3	T45.8X4	T45.8X5	T45.8X6
hydrolysate	T45.8X1	T45.8X2	T45.8X3	T45.8X4	T45.8X5	T45.8X6
Lizard (bite) (venom)	T63.121	T63.122	T63.123	T63.124	—	—
LMD	T45.8X1	T45.8X2	T45.8X3	T45.8X4	T45.8X5	T45.8X6
Lobelia	T62.2X1	T62.2X2	T62.2X3	T62.2X4	—	—
Lobeline	T5Ø.7X1	T5Ø.7X2	T5Ø.7X3	T5Ø.7X4	T5Ø.7X5	T5Ø.7X6
Local action drug NEC	T49.8X1	T49.8X2	T49.8X3	T49.8X4	T49.8X5	T49.8X6
Locorten	T49.ØX1	T49.ØX2	T49.ØX3	T49.ØX4	T49.ØX5	T49.ØX6
Lofepramine	T43.Ø11	T43.Ø12	T43.Ø13	T43.Ø14	T43.Ø15	T43.Ø16
Lolium temulentum	T62.2X1	T62.2X2	T62.2X3	T62.2X4	—	—
Lomotil	T47.6X1	T47.6X2	T47.6X3	T47.6X4	T47.6X5	T47.6X6
Lomustine	T45.1X1	T45.1X2	T45.1X3	T45.1X4	T45.1X5	T45.1X6
Lonidamine	T45.1X1	T45.1X2	T45.1X3	T45.1X4	T45.1X5	T45.1X6
Loperamide	T47.6X1	T47.6X2	T47.6X3	T47.6X4	T47.6X5	T47.6X6
Loprazolam	T42.4X1	T42.4X2	T42.4X3	T42.4X4	T42.4X5	T42.4X6
Lorajmine	T46.2X1	T46.2X2	T46.2X3	T46.2X4	T46.2X5	T46.2X6
Loratidine	T45.ØX1	T45.ØX2	T45.ØX3	T45.ØX4	T45.ØX5	T45.ØX6
Lorazepam	T42.4X1	T42.4X2	T42.4X3	T42.4X4	T42.4X5	T42.4X6
Lorcainide	T46.2X1	T46.2X2	T46.2X3	T46.2X4	T46.2X5	T46.2X6
Lormetazepam	T42.4X1	T42.4X2	T42.4X3	T42.4X4	T42.4X5	T42.4X6
Lotions NEC	T49.91	T49.92	T49.93	T49.94	T49.95	T49.96
Lotusate	T42.3X1	T42.3X2	T42.3X3	T42.3X4	T42.3X5	T42.3X6
Lovastatin	T46.6X1	T46.6X2	T46.6X3	T46.6X4	T46.6X5	T46.6X6
Loxapine	T43.591	T43.592	T43.593	T43.594	T43.595	T43.596
Lowila	T49.2X1	T49.2X2	T49.2X3	T49.2X4	T49.2X5	T49.2X6
Lozenges (throat)	T49.6X1	T49.6X2	T49.6X3	T49.6X4	T49.6X5	T49.6X6
LSD	T4Ø.8X1	T4Ø.8X2	T4Ø.8X3	T4Ø.8X4	—	—
L-Tryptophan — *see Amino acid*						
Lubricant, eye	T49.5X1	T49.5X2	T49.5X3	T49.5X4	T49.5X5	T49.5X6
Lubricating oil NEC	T52.ØX1	T52.ØX2	T52.ØX3	T52.ØX4	—	—
Lucanthone	T37.4X1	T37.4X2	T37.4X3	T37.4X4	T37.4X5	T37.4X6
Luminal	T42.3X1	T42.3X2	T42.3X3	T42.3X4	T42.3X5	T42.3X6
Lung irritant (gas) NEC	T59.91	T59.92	T59.93	T59.94	—	—
Luteinizing hormone	T38.811	T38.812	T38.813	T38.814	T38.815	T38.816
Lutocylol	T38.5X1	T38.5X2	T38.5X3	T38.5X4	T38.5X5	T38.5X6
Lutromone	T38.5X1	T38.5X2	T38.5X3	T38.5X4	T38.5X5	T38.5X6
Lututrin	T48.291	T48.292	T48.293	T48.294	T48.295	T48.296
Lye (Concentrated)	T54.3X1	T54.3X2	T54.3X3	T54.3X4	—	—

Substance	Poisoning, Accidental (Unintentional)	Poisoning, Intentional Self-Harm	Poisoning, Assault	Poisoning, Undetermined	Adverse Effect	Underdosing
	External Cause (T-Code)					
Lygranum (skin test)	T5Ø.8X1	T5Ø.8X2	T5Ø.8X3	T5Ø.8X4	T5Ø.8X5	T5Ø.8X6
Lymecycline	T36.4X1	T36.4X2	T36.4X3	T36.4X4	T36.4X5	T36.4X6
Lymphogranuloma venereum antigen	T5Ø.8X1	T5Ø.8X2	T5Ø.8X3	T5Ø.8X4	T5Ø.8X5	T5Ø.8X6
Lynestrenol	T38.4X1	T38.4X2	T38.4X3	T38.4X4	T38.4X5	T38.4X6
Lypressin	T38.891	T38.892	T38.893	T38.894	T38.895	T38.896
Lyovac Sodium Edecrin	T5Ø.1X1	T5Ø.1X2	T5Ø.1X3	T5Ø.1X4	T5Ø.1X5	T5Ø.1X6
Lysergic acid diethylamide	T4Ø.8X1	T4Ø.8X2	T4Ø.8X3	T4Ø.8X4	—	—
Lysergide	T4Ø.8X1	T4Ø.8X2	T4Ø.8X3	T4Ø.8X4	—	—
Lysine vasopressin	T38.891	T38.892	T38.893	T38.894	T38.895	T38.896
Lysol	T54.1X1	T54.1X2	T54.1X3	T54.1X4	—	—
Lysozyme	T49.ØX1	T49.ØX2	T49.ØX3	T49.ØX4	T49.ØX5	T49.ØX6
Lytta (vitatta)	T49.8X1	T49.8X2	T49.8X3	T49.8X4	T49.8X5	T49.8X6
M						
Mace	T59.3X1	T59.3X2	T59.3X3	T59.3X4	—	—
Macrogol	T5Ø.991	T5Ø.992	T5Ø.993	T5Ø.994	T5Ø.995	T5Ø.996
Macrolide						
anabolic drug	T38.7X1	T38.7X2	T38.7X3	T38.7X4	T38.7X5	T38.7X6
antibiotic	T36.3X1	T36.3X2	T36.3X3	T36.3X4	T36.3X5	T36.3X6
Mafenide	T49.ØX1	T49.ØX2	T49.ØX3	T49.ØX4	T49.ØX5	T49.ØX6
Magaldrate	T47.1X1	T47.1X2	T47.1X3	T47.1X4	T47.1X5	T47.1X6
Magic mushroom	T4Ø.991	T4Ø.992	T4Ø.993	T4Ø.994	—	—
Magnamycin	T36.8X1	T36.8X2	T36.8X3	T36.8X4	T36.8X5	T36.8X6
Magnesia magma	T47.1X1	T47.1X2	T47.1X3	T47.1X4	T47.1X5	T47.1X6
Magnesium NEC	T56.891	T56.892	T56.893	T56.894	—	—
carbonate	T47.1X1	T47.1X2	T47.1X3	T47.1X4	T47.1X5	T47.1X6
citrate	T47.4X1	T47.4X2	T47.4X3	T47.4X4	T47.4X5	T47.4X6
hydroxide	T47.1X1	T47.1X2	T47.1X3	T47.1X4	T47.1X5	T47.1X6
oxide	T47.1X1	T47.1X2	T47.1X3	T47.1X4	T47.1X5	T47.1X6
peroxide	T49.ØX1	T49.ØX2	T49.ØX3	T49.ØX4	T49.ØX5	T49.ØX6
salicylate	T39.Ø91	T39.Ø92	T39.Ø93	T39.Ø94	T39.Ø95	T39.Ø96
silicofluoride	T5Ø.3X1	T5Ø.3X2	T5Ø.3X3	T5Ø.3X4	T5Ø.3X5	T5Ø.3X6
sulfate	T47.4X1	T47.4X2	T47.4X3	T47.4X4	T47.4X5	T47.4X6
thiosulfate	T45.ØX1	T45.ØX2	T45.ØX3	T45.ØX4	T45.ØX5	T45.ØX6
trisilicate	T47.1X1	T47.1X2	T47.1X3	T47.1X4	T47.1X5	T47.1X6
Malathion (medicinal)	T49.ØX1	T49.ØX2	T49.ØX3	T49.ØX4	T49.ØX5	T49.ØX6
insecticide	T6Ø.ØX1	T6Ø.ØX2	T6Ø.ØX3	T6Ø.ØX4	—	—
Male fern extract	T37.4X1	T37.4X2	T37.4X3	T37.4X4	T37.4X5	T37.4X6
M-AMSA	T45.1X1	T45.1X2	T45.1X3	T45.1X4	T45.1X5	T45.1X6
Mandelic acid	T37.8X1	T37.8X2	T37.8X3	T37.8X4	T37.8X5	T37.8X6
Manganese (dioxide) (salts)	T57.2X1	T57.2X2	T57.2X3	T57.2X4	—	—
medicinal	T5Ø.991	T5Ø.992	T5Ø.993	T5Ø.994	T5Ø.995	T5Ø.996

	External Cause (T-Code)					
Substance	Poisoning, Accidental (Unintentional)	Poisoning, Intentional Self-Harm	Poisoning, Assault	Poisoning, Undetermined	Adverse Effect	Underdosing
Mannitol	T47.3X1	T47.3X2	T47.3X3	T47.3X4	T47.3X5	T47.3X6
hexanitrate	T46.3X1	T46.3X2	T46.3X3	T46.3X4	T46.3X5	T46.3X6
Mannomustine	T45.1X1	T45.1X2	T45.1X3	T45.1X4	T45.1X5	T45.1X6
MAO inhibitors	T43.1X1	T43.1X2	T43.1X3	T43.1X4	T43.1X5	T43.1X6
Mapharsen	T37.8X1	T37.8X2	T37.8X3	T37.8X4	T37.8X5	T37.8X6
Maphenide	T49.0X1	T49.0X2	T49.0X3	T49.0X4	T49.0X5	T49.0X6
Maprotiline	T43.021	T43.022	T43.023	T43.024	T43.025	T43.026
Marcaine	T41.3X1	T41.3X2	T41.3X3	T41.3X4	T41.3X5	T41.3X6
infiltration (subcutaneous)	T41.3X1	T41.3X2	T41.3X3	T41.3X4	T41.3X5	T41.3X6
nerve block (peripheral) (plexus)	T41.3X1	T41.3X2	T41.3X3	T41.3X4	T41.3X5	T41.3X6
Marezine	T45.0X1	T45.0X2	T45.0X3	T45.0X4	T45.0X5	T45.0X6
Marihuana	T40.7X1	T40.7X2	T40.7X3	T40.7X4	T40.7X5	T40.7X6
Marijuana	T40.7X1	T40.7X2	T40.7X3	T40.7X4	T40.7X5	T40.7X6
Marine (sting)	T63.691	T63.692	T63.693	T63.694	—	—
animals (sting)	T63.691	T63.692	T63.693	T63.694	—	—
plants (sting)	T63.711	T63.712	T63.713	T63.714	—	—
Marplan	T43.1X1	T43.1X2	T43.1X3	T43.1X4	T43.1X5	T43.1X6
Marsh gas	T59.891	T59.892	T59.893	T59.894	—	—
Marsilid	T43.1X1	T43.1X2	T43.1X3	T43.1X4	T43.1X5	T43.1X6
Matulane	T45.1X1	T45.1X2	T45.1X3	T45.1X4	T45.1X5	T45.1X6
Mazindol	T50.5X1	T50.5X2	T50.5X3	T50.5X4	T50.5X5	T50.5X6
MCPA	T60.3X1	T60.3X2	T60.3X3	T60.3X4	—	—
MDMA	T43.641	T43.642	T43.643	T43.644	—	—
Meadow saffron	T62.2X1	T62.2X2	T62.2X3	T62.2X4	—	—
Measles virus vaccine (attenuated)	T50.B91	T50.B92	T50.B93	T50.B94	T50.B95	T50.B96
Meat, noxious	T62.8X1	T62.8X2	T62.8X3	T62.8X4	—	—
Meballymal	T42.3X1	T42.3X2	T42.3X3	T42.3X4	T42.3X5	T42.3X6
Mebanazine	T43.1X1	T43.1X2	T43.1X3	T43.1X4	T43.1X5	T43.1X6
Mebaral	T42.3X1	T42.3X2	T42.3X3	T42.3X4	T42.3X5	T42.3X6
Mebendazole	T37.4X1	T37.4X2	T37.4X3	T37.4X4	T37.4X5	T37.4X6
Mebeverine	T44.3X1	T44.3X2	T44.3X3	T44.3X4	T44.3X5	T44.3X6
Mebhydrolin	T45.0X1	T45.0X2	T45.0X3	T45.0X4	T45.0X5	T45.0X6
Mebumal	T42.3X1	T42.3X2	T42.3X3	T42.3X4	T42.3X5	T42.3X6
Mebutamate	T43.591	T43.592	T43.593	T43.594	T43.595	T43.596
Mecamylamine	T44.2X1	T44.2X2	T44.2X3	T44.2X4	T44.2X5	T44.2X6
Mechlorethamine	T45.1X1	T45.1X2	T45.1X3	T45.1X4	T45.1X5	T45.1X6
Mecillinam	T36.0X1	T36.0X2	T36.0X3	T36.0X4	T36.0X5	T36.0X6
Meclizine (hydrochloride)	T45.0X1	T45.0X2	T45.0X3	T45.0X4	T45.0X5	T45.0X6
Meclocycline	T36.4X1	T36.4X2	T36.4X3	T36.4X4	T36.4X5	T36.4X6
Meclofenamate	T39.391	T39.392	T39.393	T39.394	T39.395	T39.396
Meclofenamic acid	T39.391	T39.392	T39.393	T39.394	T39.395	T39.396
Meclofenoxate	T43.691	T43.692	T43.693	T43.694	T43.695	T43.696
Meclozine	T45.0X1	T45.0X2	T45.0X3	T45.0X4	T45.0X5	T45.0X6
Mecobalamin	T45.8X1	T45.8X2	T45.8X3	T45.8X4	T45.8X5	T45.8X6
Mecoprop	T60.3X1	T60.3X2	T60.3X3	T60.3X4	—	—
Mecrilate	T49.3X1	T49.3X2	T49.3X3	T49.3X4	T49.3X5	T49.3X6
Mecysteine	T48.4X1	T48.4X2	T48.4X3	T48.4X4	T48.4X5	T48.4X6
Medazepam	T42.4X1	T42.4X2	T42.4X3	T42.4X4	T42.4X5	T42.4X6
Medicament NEC	T50.901	T50.902	T50.903	T50.904	T50.905	T50.906
Medinal	T42.3X1	T42.3X2	T42.3X3	T42.3X4	T42.3X5	T42.3X6
Medomin	T42.3X1	T42.3X2	T42.3X3	T42.3X4	T42.3X5	T42.3X6
Medrogestone	T38.5X1	T38.5X2	T38.5X3	T38.5X4	T38.5X5	T38.5X6
Medroxalol	T44.8X1	T44.8X2	T44.8X3	T44.8X4	T44.8X5	T44.8X6
Medroxyprogesterone acetate (depot)	T38.5X1	T38.5X2	T38.5X3	T38.5X4	T38.5X5	T38.5X6
Medrysone	T49.0X1	T49.0X2	T49.0X3	T49.0X4	T49.0X5	T49.0X6
Mefenamic acid	T39.391	T39.392	T39.393	T39.394	T39.395	T39.396
Mefenorex	T50.5X1	T50.5X2	T50.5X3	T50.5X4	T50.5X5	T50.5X6
Mefloquine	T37.2X1	T37.2X2	T37.2X3	T37.2X4	T37.2X5	T37.2X6
Mefruside	T50.2X1	T50.2X2	T50.2X3	T50.2X4	T50.2X5	T50.2X6
Megahallucinogen	T40.901	T40.902	T40.903	T40.904	T40.905	T40.906
Megestrol	T38.5X1	T38.5X2	T38.5X3	T38.5X4	T38.5X5	T38.5X6
Meglumine						
antimoniate	T37.8X1	T37.8X2	T37.8X3	T37.8X4	T37.8X5	T37.8X6
diatrizoate	T50.8X1	T50.8X2	T50.8X3	T50.8X4	T50.8X5	T50.8X6
iodipamide	T50.8X1	T50.8X2	T50.8X3	T50.8X4	T50.8X5	T50.8X6
iotroxate	T50.8X1	T50.8X2	T50.8X3	T50.8X4	T50.8X5	T50.8X6
MEK (methyl ethyl ketone)	T52.4X1	T52.4X2	T52.4X3	T52.4X4	—	—
Meladrazine	T44.3X1	T44.3X2	T44.3X3	T44.3X4	T44.3X5	T44.3X6
Meladinin	T49.3X1	T49.3X2	T49.3X3	T49.3X4	T49.3X5	T49.3X6
Melaleuca alternifolia oil	T49.0X1	T49.0X2	T49.0X3	T49.0X4	T49.0X5	T49.0X6
Melanizing agents	T49.3X1	T49.3X2	T49.3X3	T49.3X4	T49.3X5	T49.3X6
Melanocyte-stimulating hormone	T38.891	T38.892	T38.893	T38.894	T38.895	T38.896
Melarsonyl potassium	T37.3X1	T37.3X2	T37.3X3	T37.3X4	T37.3X5	T37.3X6
Melarsoprol	T37.3X1	T37.3X2	T37.3X3	T37.3X4	T37.3X5	T37.3X6
Melia azedarach	T62.2X1	T62.2X2	T62.2X3	T62.2X4	—	—
Melitracen	T43.011	T43.012	T43.013	T43.014	T43.015	T43.016
Mellaril	T43.3X1	T43.3X2	T43.3X3	T43.3X4	T43.3X5	T43.3X6
Meloxine	T49.3X1	T49.3X2	T49.3X3	T49.3X4	T49.3X5	T49.3X6
Melperone	T43.4X1	T43.4X2	T43.4X3	T43.4X4	T43.4X5	T43.4X6
Melphalan	T45.1X1	T45.1X2	T45.1X3	T45.1X4	T45.1X5	T45.1X6
Memantine	T43.8X1	T43.8X2	T43.8X3	T43.8X4	T43.8X5	T43.8X6

New Revised ~~deleted~~ Deleted

Substance	External Cause (T-Code) Poisoning, Accidental (Unintentional)	Poisoning, Intentional Self-Harm	Poisoning, Assault	Poisoning, Undetermined	Adverse Effect	Underdosing
Menadiol	T45.7X1	T45.7X2	T45.7X3	T45.7X4	T45.7X5	T45.7X6
sodium sulfate	T45.7X1	T45.7X2	T45.7X3	T45.7X4	T45.7X5	T45.7X6
Menadione	T45.7X1	T45.7X2	T45.7X3	T45.7X4	T45.7X5	T45.7X6
sodium bisulfite	T45.7X1	T45.7X2	T45.7X3	T45.7X4	T45.7X5	T45.7X6
Menaphthone	T45.7X1	T45.7X2	T45.7X3	T45.7X4	T45.7X5	T45.7X6
Menaquinone	T45.7X1	T45.7X2	T45.7X3	T45.7X4	T45.7X5	T45.7X6
Menatetrenone	T45.7X1	T45.7X2	T45.7X3	T45.7X4	T45.7X5	T45.7X6
Meningococcal vaccine	T5Ø.A91	T5Ø.A92	T5Ø.A93	T5Ø.A94	T5Ø.A95	T5Ø.A96
Menningovax (-AC) (-C)	T5Ø.A91	T5Ø.A92	T5Ø.A93	T5Ø.A94	T5Ø.A95	T5Ø.A96
Menotropins	T38.811	T38.812	T38.813	T38.814	T38.815	T38.816
Menthol	T48.5X1	T48.5X2	T48.5X3	T48.5X4	T48.5X5	T48.5X6
Mepacrine	T37.2X1	T37.2X2	T37.2X3	T37.2X4	T37.2X5	T37.2X6
Meparfynol	T42.6X1	T42.6X2	T42.6X3	T42.6X4	T42.6X5	T42.6X6
Mepartricin	T36.7X1	T36.7X2	T36.7X3	T36.7X4	T36.7X5	T36.7X6
Mepazine	T43.3X1	T43.3X2	T43.3X3	T43.3X4	T43.3X5	T43.3X6
Mepenzolate	T44.3X1	T44.3X2	T44.3X3	T44.3X4	T44.3X5	T44.3X6
bromide	T44.3X1	T44.3X2	T44.3X3	T44.3X4	T44.3X5	T44.3X6
Meperidine	T4Ø.4X1	T4Ø.4X2	T4Ø.4X3	T4Ø.4X4	T4Ø.4X5	T4Ø.4X6
Mephebarbital	T42.3X1	T42.3X2	T42.3X3	T42.3X4	T42.3X5	T42.3X6
Mephenamin(e)	T42.8X1	T42.8X2	T42.8X3	T42.8X4	T42.8X5	T42.8X6
Mephenesin	T42.8X1	T42.8X2	T42.8X3	T42.8X4	T42.8X5	T42.8X6
Mephenhydramine	T45.ØX1	T45.ØX2	T45.ØX3	T45.ØX4	T45.ØX5	T45.ØX6
Mephenoxalone	T42.8X1	T42.8X2	T42.8X3	T42.8X4	T42.8X5	T42.8X6
Mephentermine	T44.991	T44.992	T44.993	T44.994	T44.995	T44.996
Mephenytoin	T42.ØX1	T42.ØX2	T42.ØX3	T42.ØX4	T42.ØX5	T42.ØX6
with phenobarbital	T42.3X1	T42.3X2	T42.3X3	T42.3X4	T42.3X5	T42.3X6
Mephobarbital	T42.3X1	T42.3X2	T42.3X3	T42.3X4	T42.3X5	T42.3X6
Mephosfolan	T6Ø.ØX1	T6Ø.ØX2	T6Ø.ØX3	T6Ø.ØX4	—	—
Mepindolol	T44.7X1	T44.7X2	T44.7X3	T44.7X4	T44.7X5	T44.7X6
Mepiperphenidol	T44.3X1	T44.3X2	T44.3X3	T44.3X4	T44.3X5	T44.3X6
Mepitiostane	T38.7X1	T38.7X2	T38.7X3	T38.7X4	T38.7X5	T38.7X6
Mepivacaine	T41.3X1	T41.3X2	T41.3X3	T41.3X4	T41.3X5	T41.3X6
epidural	T41.3X1	T41.3X2	T41.3X3	T41.3X4	T41.3X5	T41.3X6
Meprednisone	T38.ØX1	T38.ØX2	T38.ØX3	T38.ØX4	T38.ØX5	T38.ØX6
Meprobam	T43.591	T43.592	T43.593	T43.594	T43.595	T43.596
Meprobamate	T43.591	T43.592	T43.593	T43.594	T43.595	T43.596
Meproscillarin	T46.ØX1	T46.ØX2	T46.ØX3	T46.ØX4	T46.ØX5	T46.ØX6
Meprylcaine	T41.3X1	T41.3X2	T41.3X3	T41.3X4	T41.3X5	T41.3X6
Meptazinol	T39.8X1	T39.8X2	T39.8X3	T39.8X4	T39.8X5	T39.8X6
Mepyramine	T45.ØX1	T45.ØX2	T45.ØX3	T45.ØX4	T45.ØX5	T45.ØX6
Mequitazine	T43.3X1	T43.3X2	T43.3X3	T43.3X4	T43.3X5	T43.3X6
Meralluride	T5Ø.2X1	T5Ø.2X2	T5Ø.2X3	T5Ø.2X4	T5Ø.2X5	T5Ø.2X6

Substance	External Cause (T-Code) Poisoning, Accidental (Unintentional)	Poisoning, Intentional Self-Harm	Poisoning, Assault	Poisoning, Undetermined	Adverse Effect	Underdosing
Merbaphen	T5Ø.2X1	T5Ø.2X2	T5Ø.2X3	T5Ø.2X4	T5Ø.2X5	T5Ø.2X6
Merbromin	T49.ØX1	T49.ØX2	T49.ØX3	T49.ØX4	T49.ØX5	T49.ØX6
Mercaptobenzothiazole salts	T49.ØX1	T49.ØX2	T49.ØX3	T49.ØX4	T49.ØX5	T49.ØX6
Mercaptomerin	T5Ø.2X1	T5Ø.2X2	T5Ø.2X3	T5Ø.2X4	T5Ø.2X5	T5Ø.2X6
Mercaptopurine	T45.1X1	T45.1X2	T45.1X3	T45.1X4	T45.1X5	T45.1X6
Mercumatilin	T5Ø.2X1	T5Ø.2X2	T5Ø.2X3	T5Ø.2X4	T5Ø.2X5	T5Ø.2X6
Mercuramide	T5Ø.2X1	T5Ø.2X2	T5Ø.2X3	T5Ø.2X4	T5Ø.2X5	T5Ø.2X6
Mercurochrome	T49.ØX1	T49.ØX2	T49.ØX3	T49.ØX4	T49.ØX5	T49.ØX6
Mercurophylline	T5Ø.2X1	T5Ø.2X2	T5Ø.2X3	T5Ø.2X4	T5Ø.2X5	T5Ø.2X6
Mercury, mercurial, mercuric, mercurous (compounds) (cyanide) (fumes) (nonmedicinal) (vapor) NEC	T56.1X1	T56.1X2	T56.1X3	T56.1X4	—	—
ammoniated	T49.ØX1	T49.ØX2	T49.ØX3	T49.ØX4	T49.ØX5	T49.ØX6
anti-infective						
local	T49.ØX1	T49.ØX2	T49.ØX3	T49.ØX4	T49.ØX5	T49.ØX6
systemic	T37.8X1	T37.8X2	T37.8X3	T37.8X4	T37.8X5	T37.8X6
topical	T49.ØX1	T49.ØX2	T49.ØX3	T49.ØX4	T49.ØX5	T49.ØX6
chloride (ammoniated)	T49.ØX1	T49.ØX2	T49.ØX3	T49.ØX4	T49.ØX5	T49.ØX6
fungicide	T56.1X1	T56.1X2	T56.1X3	T56.1X4	—	—
diuretic NEC	T5Ø.2X1	T5Ø.2X2	T5Ø.2X3	T5Ø.2X4	T5Ø.2X5	T5Ø.2X6
fungicide	T56.1X1	T56.1X2	T56.1X3	T56.1X4	—	—
organic (fungicide)	T56.1X1	T56.1X2	T56.1X3	T56.1X4	—	—
oxide, yellow	T49.ØX1	T49.ØX2	T49.ØX3	T49.ØX4	T49.ØX5	T49.ØX6
Mersalyl	T5Ø.2X1	T5Ø.2X2	T5Ø.2X3	T5Ø.2X4	T5Ø.2X5	T5Ø.2X6
Merthiolate	T49.ØX1	T49.ØX2	T49.ØX3	T49.ØX4	T49.ØX5	T49.ØX6
ophthalmic preparation	T49.5X1	T49.5X2	T49.5X3	T49.5X4	T49.5X5	T49.5X6
Meruvax	T5Ø.B91	T5Ø.B92	T5Ø.B93	T5Ø.B94	T5Ø.B95	T5Ø.B96
Mesalazine	T47.8X1	T47.8X2	T47.8X3	T47.8X4	T47.8X5	T47.8X6
Mescal buttons	T4Ø.991	T4Ø.992	T4Ø.993	T4Ø.994	—	—
Mescaline	T4Ø.991	T4Ø.992	T4Ø.993	T4Ø.994	—	—
Mesna	T48.4X1	T48.4X2	T48.4X3	T48.4X4	T48.4X5	T48.4X6
Mesoglycan	T46.6X1	T46.6X2	T46.6X3	T46.6X4	T46.6X5	T46.6X6
Mesoridazine	T43.3X1	T43.3X2	T43.3X3	T43.3X4	T43.3X5	T43.3X6
Mestanolone	T38.7X1	T38.7X2	T38.7X3	T38.7X4	T38.7X5	T38.7X6
Mesterolone	T38.7X1	T38.7X2	T38.7X3	T38.7X4	T38.7X5	T38.7X6
Mestranol	T38.5X1	T38.5X2	T38.5X3	T38.5X4	T38.5X5	T38.5X6
Mesulergine	T42.8X1	T42.8X2	T42.8X3	T42.8X4	T42.8X5	T42.8X6
Mesulfen	T49.ØX1	T49.ØX2	T49.ØX3	T49.ØX4	T49.ØX5	T49.ØX6
Mesuximide	T42.2X1	T42.2X2	T42.2X3	T42.2X4	T42.2X5	T42.2X6
Metabutethamine	T41.3X1	T41.3X2	T41.3X3	T41.3X4	T41.3X5	T41.3X6
Metactesylacetate	T49.ØX1	T49.ØX2	T49.ØX3	T49.ØX4	T49.ØX5	T49.ØX6

	External Cause (T-Code)					
Substance	Poisoning, Accidental (Unintentional)	Poisoning, Intentional Self-Harm	Poisoning, Assault	Poisoning, Undetermined	Adverse Effect	Underdosing
Metacycline	T36.4X1	T36.4X2	T36.4X3	T36.4X4	T36.4X5	T36.4X6
Metaldehyde (snail killer) NEC	T60.8X1	T60.8X2	T60.8X3	T60.8X4	—	—
Metals (heavy) (nonmedicinal)	T56.91	T56.92	T56.93	T56.94	—	—
dust, fumes, or vapor NEC	T56.91	T56.92	T56.93	T56.94	—	—
light NEC	T56.91	T56.92	T56.93	T56.94	—	—
dust, fumes, or vapor NEC	T56.91	T56.92	T56.93	T56.94	—	—
specified NEC	T56.891	T56.892	T56.893	T56.894	—	—
thallium	T56.811	T56.812	T56.813	T56.814	—	—
Metamfetamine	T43.621	T43.622	T43.623	T43.624	T43.625	T43.626
Metamizole sodium	T39.2X1	T39.2X2	T39.2X3	T39.2X4	T39.2X5	T39.2X6
Metampicillin	T36.0X1	T36.0X2	T36.0X3	T36.0X4	T36.0X5	T36.0X6
Metamucil	T47.4X1	T47.4X2	T47.4X3	T47.4X4	T47.4X5	T47.4X6
Metaphen	T49.0X1	T49.0X2	T49.0X3	T49.0X4	T49.0X5	T49.0X6
Metandienone	T38.7X1	T38.7X2	T38.7X3	T38.7X4	T38.7X5	T38.7X6
Metandrostenolone	T38.7X1	T38.7X2	T38.7X3	T38.7X4	T38.7X5	T38.7X6
Metaphos	T60.0X1	T60.0X2	T60.0X3	T60.0X4	—	—
Metapramine	T43.011	T43.012	T43.013	T43.014	T43.015	T43.016
Metaproterenol	T48.291	T48.292	T48.293	T48.294	T48.295	T48.296
Metaraminol	T44.4X1	T44.4X2	T44.4X3	T44.4X4	T44.4X5	T44.4X6
Metaxalone	T42.8X1	T42.8X2	T42.8X3	T42.8X4	T42.8X5	T42.8X6
Metenolone	T38.7X1	T38.7X2	T38.7X3	T38.7X4	T38.7X5	T38.7X6
Metergoline	T42.8X1	T42.8X2	T42.8X3	T42.8X4	T42.8X5	T42.8X6
Metescufylline	T46.991	T46.992	T46.993	T46.994	T46.995	T46.996
Metetoin	T42.0X1	T42.0X2	T42.0X3	T42.0X4	T42.0X5	T42.0X6
Metformin	T38.3X1	T38.3X2	T38.3X3	T38.3X4	T38.3X5	T38.3X6
Methacholine	T44.1X1	T44.1X2	T44.1X3	T44.1X4	T44.1X5	T44.1X6
Methacycline	T36.4X1	T36.4X2	T36.4X3	T36.4X4	T36.4X5	T36.4X6
Methadone	T40.3X1	T40.3X2	T40.3X3	T40.3X4	T40.3X5	T40.3X6
Methallenestril	T38.5X1	T38.5X2	T38.5X3	T38.5X4	T38.5X5	T38.5X6
Methallenoestril	T38.5X1	T38.5X2	T38.5X3	T38.5X4	T38.5X5	T38.5X6
Methamphetamine	T43.621	T43.622	T43.623	T43.624	T43.625	T43.626
Methampyrone	T39.2X1	T39.2X2	T39.2X3	T39.2X4	T39.2X5	T39.2X6
Methandienone	T38.7X1	T38.7X2	T38.7X3	T38.7X4	T38.7X5	T38.7X6
Methandriol	T38.7X1	T38.7X2	T38.7X3	T38.7X4	T38.7X5	T38.7X6
Methandrostenolone	T38.7X1	T38.7X2	T38.7X3	T38.7X4	T38.7X5	T38.7X6
Methane	T59.891	T59.892	T59.893	T59.894	—	—
Methanethiol	T59.891	T59.892	T59.893	T59.894	—	—
Methaniazide	T37.1X1	T37.1X2	T37.1X3	T37.1X4	T37.1X5	T37.1X6
Methanol (vapor)	T51.1X1	T51.1X2	T51.1X3	T51.1X4	—	—
Methantheline	T44.3X1	T44.3X2	T44.3X3	T44.3X4	T44.3X5	T44.3X6
Methanthelinium bromide	T44.3X1	T44.3X2	T44.3X3	T44.3X4	T44.3X5	T44.3X6
Methaphenilene	T45.0X1	T45.0X2	T45.0X3	T45.0X4	T45.0X5	T45.0X6
Methapyrilene	T45.0X1	T45.0X2	T45.0X3	T45.0X4	T45.0X5	T45.0X6
Methaqualone (compound)	T42.6X1	T42.6X2	T42.6X3	T42.6X4	T42.6X5	T42.6X6
Metharbital	T42.3X1	T42.3X2	T42.3X3	T42.3X4	T42.3X5	T42.3X6
Methazolamide	T50.2X1	T50.2X2	T50.2X3	T50.2X4	T50.2X5	T50.2X6
Methdilazine	T43.3X1	T43.3X2	T43.3X3	T43.3X4	T43.3X5	T43.3X6
Methedrine	T43.621	T43.622	T43.623	T43.624	T43.625	T43.626
Methenamine (mandelate)	T37.8X1	T37.8X2	T37.8X3	T37.8X4	T37.8X5	T37.8X6
Methenolone	T38.7X1	T38.7X2	T38.7X3	T38.7X4	T38.7X5	T38.7X6
Methergine	T48.0X1	T48.0X2	T48.0X3	T48.0X4	T48.0X5	T48.0X6
Methetoin	T42.0X1	T42.0X2	T42.0X3	T42.0X4	T42.0X5	T42.0X6
Methiacil	T38.2X1	T38.2X2	T38.2X3	T38.2X4	T38.2X5	T38.2X6
Methicillin	T36.0X1	T36.0X2	T36.0X3	T36.0X4	T36.0X5	T36.0X6
Methimazole	T38.2X1	T38.2X2	T38.2X3	T38.2X4	T38.2X5	T38.2X6
Methiodal sodium	T50.8X1	T50.8X2	T50.8X3	T50.8X4	T50.8X5	T50.8X6
Methionine	T50.991	T50.992	T50.993	T50.994	T50.995	T50.996
Methisazone	T37.5X1	T37.5X2	T37.5X3	T37.5X4	T37.5X5	T37.5X6
Methisoprinol	T37.5X1	T37.5X2	T37.5X3	T37.5X4	T37.5X5	T37.5X6
Methitural	T42.3X1	T42.3X2	T42.3X3	T42.3X4	T42.3X5	T42.3X6
Methixene	T44.3X1	T44.3X2	T44.3X3	T44.3X4	T44.3X5	T44.3X6
Methobarbital, methobarbitone	T42.3X1	T42.3X2	T42.3X3	T42.3X4	T42.3X5	T42.3X6
Methocarbamol	T42.8X1	T42.8X2	T42.8X3	T42.8X4	T42.8X5	T42.8X6
skeletal muscle relaxant	T48.1X1	T48.1X2	T48.1X3	T48.1X4	T48.1X5	T48.1X6
Methohexital	T41.1X1	T41.1X2	T41.1X3	T41.1X4	T41.1X5	T41.1X6
Methohexitone	T41.1X1	T41.1X2	T41.1X3	T41.1X4	T41.1X5	T41.1X6
Methoin	T42.0X1	T42.0X2	T42.0X3	T42.0X4	T42.0X5	T42.0X6
Methopholine	T39.8X1	T39.8X2	T39.8X3	T39.8X4	T39.8X5	T39.8X6
Methopromazine	T43.3X1	T43.3X2	T43.3X3	T43.3X4	T43.3X5	T43.3X6
Methorate	T48.3X1	T48.3X2	T48.3X3	T48.3X4	T48.3X5	T48.3X6
Methoserpidine	T46.5X1	T46.5X2	T46.5X3	T46.5X4	T46.5X5	T46.5X6
Methotrexate	T45.1X1	T45.1X2	T45.1X3	T45.1X4	T45.1X5	T45.1X6
Methotrimeprazine	T43.3X1	T43.3X2	T43.3X3	T43.3X4	T43.3X5	T43.3X6
Methoxa-Dome	T49.3X1	T49.3X2	T49.3X3	T49.3X4	T49.3X5	T49.3X6
Methoxamine	T44.4X1	T44.4X2	T44.4X3	T44.4X4	T44.4X5	T44.4X6
Methoxsalen	T50.991	T50.992	T50.993	T50.994	T50.995	T50.996
Methoxyaniline	T65.3X1	T65.3X2	T65.3X3	T65.3X4	—	—
Methoxybenzyl penicillin	T36.0X1	T36.0X2	T36.0X3	T36.0X4	T36.0X5	T36.0X6
Methoxychlor	T53.7X1	T53.7X2	T53.7X3	T53.7X4	—	—
Methoxy-DDT	T53.7X1	T53.7X2	T53.7X3	T53.7X4	—	—
2-Methoxyethanol	T52.3X1	T52.3X2	T52.3X3	T52.3X4	—	—
Methoxyflurane	T41.0X1	T41.0X2	T41.0X3	T41.0X4	T41.0X5	T41.0X6
Methoxyphenamine	T48.6X1	T48.6X2	T48.6X3	T48.6X4	T48.6X5	T48.6X6
Methoxypromazine	T43.3X1	T43.3X2	T43.3X3	T43.3X4	T43.3X5	T43.3X6

◄ New ▮ Revised ~~deleted~~ Deleted

	External Cause (T-Code)					
Substance	**Poisoning, Accidental (Unintentional)**	**Poisoning, Intentional Self-Harm**	**Poisoning, Assault**	**Poisoning, Undetermined**	**Adverse Effect**	**Underdosing**
5-Methoxypsoralen (5-MOP)	T5Ø.991	T5Ø.992	T5Ø.993	T5Ø.994	T5Ø.995	T5Ø.996
8-Methoxypsoralen (8-MOP)	T5Ø.991	T5Ø.992	T5Ø.993	T5Ø.994	T5Ø.995	T5Ø.996
Methscopolamine bromide	T44.3X1	T44.3X2	T44.3X3	T44.3X4	T44.3X5	T44.3X6
Methsuximide	T42.2X1	T42.2X2	T42.2X3	T42.2X4	T42.2X5	T42.2X6
Methyclothiazide	T5Ø.2X1	T5Ø.2X2	T5Ø.2X3	T5Ø.2X4	T5Ø.2X5	T5Ø.2X6
Methyl						
acetate	T52.4X1	T52.4X2	T52.4X3	T52.4X4	—	—
acetone	T52.4X1	T52.4X2	T52.4X3	T52.4X4	—	—
acrylate	T65.891	T65.892	T65.893	T65.894	—	—
alcohol	T51.1X1	T51.1X2	T51.1X3	T51.1X4	—	—
aminophenol	T65.3X1	T65.3X2	T65.3X3	T65.3X4	—	—
amphetamine	T43.621	T43.622	T43.623	T43.624	T43.625	T43.626
androstanolone	T38.7X1	T38.7X2	T38.7X3	T38.7X4	T38.7X5	T38.7X6
atropine	T44.3X1	T44.3X2	T44.3X3	T44.3X4	T44.3X5	T44.3X6
benzene	T52.2X1	T52.2X2	T52.2X3	T52.2X4	—	—
benzoate	T52.8X1	T52.8X2	T52.8X3	T52.8X4	—	—
benzol	T52.2X1	T52.2X2	T52.2X3	T52.2X4	—	—
bromide (gas)	T59.891	T59.892	T59.893	T59.894	—	—
fumigant	T6Ø.8X1	T6Ø.8X2	T6Ø.8X3	T6Ø.8X4	—	—
butanol	T51.3X1	T51.3X2	T51.3X3	T51.3X4	—	—
carbinol	T51.1X1	T51.1X2	T51.1X3	T51.1X4	—	—
carbonate	T52.8X1	T52.8X2	T52.8X3	T52.8X4	—	—
CCNU	T45.1X1	T45.1X2	T45.1X3	T45.1X4	T45.1X5	T45.1X6
cellosolve	T52.91	T52.92	T52.93	T52.94	—	—
cellulose	T47.4X1	T47.4X2	T47.4X3	T47.4X4	T47.4X5	T47.4X6
chloride (gas)	T59.891	T59.892	T59.893	T59.894	—	—
chloroformate	T59.3X1	T59.3X2	T59.3X3	T59.3X4	—	—
cyclohexane	T52.8X1	T52.8X2	T52.8X3	T52.8X4	—	—
cyclohexanol	T51.8X1	T51.8X2	T51.8X3	T51.8X4	—	—
cyclohexanone	T52.8X1	T52.8X2	T52.8X3	T52.8X4	—	—
cyclohexyl acetate	T52.8X1	T52.8X2	T52.8X3	T52.8X4	—	—
demeton	T6Ø.ØX1	T6Ø.ØX2	T6Ø.ØX3	T6Ø.ØX4	—	—
dihydromorphinone	T4Ø.2X1	T4Ø.2X2	T4Ø.2X3	T4Ø.2X4	T4Ø.2X5	T4Ø.2X6
ergometrine	T48.ØX1	T48.ØX2	T48.ØX3	T48.ØX4	T48.ØX5	T48.ØX6
ergonovine	T48.ØX1	T48.ØX2	T48.ØX3	T48.ØX4	T48.ØX5	T48.ØX6
ethyl ketone	T52.4X1	T52.4X2	T52.4X3	T52.4X4	—	—
glucamine antimonate	T37.8X1	T37.8X2	T37.8X3	T37.8X4	T37.8X5	T37.8X6
hydrazine	T65.891	T65.892	T65.893	T65.894	—	—
iodide	T65.891	T65.892	T65.893	T65.894	—	—
isobutyl ketone	T52.4X1	T52.4X2	T52.4X3	T52.4X4	—	—
isothiocyanate	T6Ø.3X1	T6Ø.3X2	T6Ø.3X3	T6Ø.3X4	—	—
mercaptan	T59.891	T59.892	T59.893	T59.894	—	—

	External Cause (T-Code)					
Substance	**Poisoning, Accidental (Unintentional)**	**Poisoning, Intentional Self-Harm**	**Poisoning, Assault**	**Poisoning, Undetermined**	**Adverse Effect**	**Underdosing**
Methyl *(Continued)*						
morphine NEC	T4Ø.2X1	T4Ø.2X2	T4Ø.2X3	T4Ø.2X4	T4Ø.2X5	T4Ø.2X6
nicotinate	T49.4X1	T49.4X2	T49.4X3	T49.4X4	T49.4X5	T49.4X6
paraben	T49.ØX1	T49.ØX2	T49.ØX3	T49.ØX4	T49.ØX5	T49.ØX6
parafynol	T42.6X1	T42.6X2	T42.6X3	T42.6X4	T42.6X5	T42.6X6
parathion	T6Ø.ØX1	T6Ø.ØX2	T6Ø.ØX3	T6Ø.ØX4	—	—
peridol	T43.4X1	T43.4X2	T43.4X3	T43.4X4	T43.4X5	T43.4X6
phenidate	T43.631	T43.632	T43.633	T43.634	T43.635	T43.636
prednisolone	T38.ØX1	T38.ØX2	T38.ØX3	T38.ØX4	T38.ØX5	T38.ØX6
ENT agent	T49.6X1	T49.6X2	T49.6X3	T49.6X4	T49.6X5	T49.6X6
ophthalmic preparation	T49.5X1	T49.5X2	T49.5X3	T49.5X4	T49.5X5	T49.5X6
topical NEC	T49.ØX1	T49.ØX2	T49.ØX3	T49.ØX4	T49.ØX5	T49.ØX6
propylcarbinol	T51.3X1	T51.3X2	T51.3X3	T51.3X4	—	—
rosaniline NEC	T49.ØX1	T49.ØX2	T49.ØX3	T49.ØX4	T49.ØX5	T49.ØX6
salicylate	T49.2X1	T49.2X2	T49.2X3	T49.2X4	T49.2X5	T49.2X6
sulfate (fumes)	T59.891	T59.892	T59.893	T59.894	—	—
liquid	T52.8X1	T52.8X2	T52.8X3	T52.8X4	—	—
sulfonal	T42.6X1	T42.6X2	T42.6X3	T42.6X4	T42.6X5	T42.6X6
testosterone	T38.7X1	T38.7X2	T38.7X3	T38.7X4	T38.7X5	T38.7X6
thiouracil	T38.2X1	T38.2X2	T38.2X3	T38.2X4	T38.2X5	T38.2X6
Methylamphetamine	T43.621	T43.622	T43.623	T43.624	T43.625	T43.626
Methylated spirit	T51.1X1	T51.1X2	T51.1X3	T51.1X4	—	—
Methylatropine nitrate	T44.3X1	T44.3X2	T44.3X3	T44.3X4	T44.3X5	T44.3X6
Methylbenactyzium bromide	T44.3X1	T44.3X2	T44.3X3	T44.3X4	T44.3X5	T44.3X6
Methylbenzethonium chloride	T49.ØX1	T49.ØX2	T49.ØX3	T49.ØX4	T49.ØX5	T49.ØX6
Methylcellulose	T47.4X1	T47.4X2	T47.4X3	T47.4X4	T47.4X5	T47.4X6
laxative	T47.4X1	T47.4X2	T47.4X3	T47.4X4	T47.4X5	T47.4X6
Methylchlorophenoxy-acetic acid	T6Ø.3X1	T6Ø.3X2	T6Ø.3X3	T6Ø.3X4	—	—
Methyldopa	T46.5X1	T46.5X2	T46.5X3	T46.5X4	T46.5X5	T46.5X6
Methyldopate	T46.5X1	T46.5X2	T46.5X3	T46.5X4	T46.5X5	T46.5X6
Methylene						
blue	T5Ø.6X1	T5Ø.6X2	T5Ø.6X3	T5Ø.6X4	T5Ø.6X5	T5Ø.6X6
chloride or dichloride (solvent) NEC	T53.4X1	T53.4X2	T53.4X3	T53.4X4	—	—
Methylenedioxyamphet-amine	T43.621	T43.622	T43.623	T43.624	T43.625	T43.626
Methylenedioxymethamphetamine	T43.641	T43.642	T43.643	T43.644	—	—
Methylergometrine	T48.ØX1	T48.ØX2	T48.ØX3	T48.ØX4	T48.ØX5	T48.ØX6
Methylergonovine	T48.ØX1	T48.ØX2	T48.ØX3	T48.ØX4	T48.ØX5	T48.ØX6
Methylestrenolone	T38.5X1	T38.5X2	T38.5X3	T38.5X4	T38.5X5	T38.5X6
Methylethyl cellulose	T5Ø.991	T5Ø.992	T5Ø.993	T5Ø.994	T5Ø.995	T5Ø.996
Methylhexabital	T42.3X1	T42.3X2	T42.3X3	T42.3X4	T42.3X5	T42.3X6
Methylmorphine	T4Ø.2X1	T4Ø.2X2	T4Ø.2X3	T4Ø.2X4	T4Ø.2X5	T4Ø.2X6

Substance	Poisoning, Accidental (Unintentional)	Poisoning, Intentional Self-Harm	Poisoning, Assault	Poisoning, Undetermined	Adverse Effect	Underdosing
		External Cause (T-Code)				
Methylparaben (ophthalmic)	T49.5X1	T49.5X2	T49.5X3	T49.5X4	T49.5X5	T49.5X6
Methylparafynol	T42.6X1	T42.6X2	T42.6X3	T42.6X4	T42.6X5	T42.6X6
Methylpentynol, methylpenthynol	T42.6X1	T42.6X2	T42.6X3	T42.6X4	T42.6X5	T42.6X6
Methylphenidate	T43.631	T43.632	T43.633	T43.634	T43.635	T43.636
Methylphenobarbital	T42.3X1	T42.3X2	T42.3X3	T42.3X4	T42.3X5	T42.3X6
Methylpolysiloxane	T47.1X1	T47.1X2	T47.1X3	T47.1X4	T47.1X5	T47.1X6
Methylprednisolone — *see Methyl, prednisolone*						
Methylrosaniline	T49.0X1	T49.0X2	T49.0X3	T49.0X4	T49.0X5	T49.0X6
Methylrosanilinium chloride	T49.0X1	T49.0X2	T49.0X3	T49.0X4	T49.0X5	T49.0X6
Methyltestosterone	T38.7X1	T38.7X2	T38.7X3	T38.7X4	T38.7X5	T38.7X6
Methylthionine chloride	T50.6X1	T50.6X2	T50.6X3	T50.6X4	T50.6X5	T50.6X6
Methylthioninium chloride	T50.6X1	T50.6X2	T50.6X3	T50.6X4	T50.6X5	T50.6X6
Methylthiouracil	T38.2X1	T38.2X2	T38.2X3	T38.2X4	T38.2X5	T38.2X6
Methyprylon	T42.6X1	T42.6X2	T42.6X3	T42.6X4	T42.6X5	T42.6X6
Methysergide	T46.5X1	T46.5X2	T46.5X3	T46.5X4	T46.5X5	T46.5X6
Metiamide	T47.1X1	T47.1X2	T47.1X3	T47.1X4	T47.1X5	T47.1X6
Meticillin	T36.0X1	T36.0X2	T36.0X3	T36.0X4	T36.0X5	T36.0X6
Meticrane	T50.2X1	T50.2X2	T50.2X3	T50.2X4	T50.2X5	T50.2X6
Metildigoxin	T46.0X1	T46.0X2	T46.0X3	T46.0X4	T46.0X5	T46.0X6
Metipranolol	T49.5X1	T49.5X2	T49.5X3	T49.5X4	T49.5X5	T49.5X6
Metirosine	T46.5X1	T46.5X2	T46.5X3	T46.5X4	T46.5X5	T46.5X6
Metisazone	T37.5X1	T37.5X2	T37.5X3	T37.5X4	T37.5X5	T37.5X6
Metixene	T44.3X1	T44.3X2	T44.3X3	T44.3X4	T44.3X5	T44.3X6
Metizoline	T48.5X1	T48.5X2	T48.5X3	T48.5X4	T48.5X5	T48.5X6
Metoclopramide	T45.0X1	T45.0X2	T45.0X3	T45.0X4	T45.0X5	T45.0X6
Metofenazate	T43.3X1	T43.3X2	T43.3X3	T43.3X4	T43.3X5	T43.3X6
Metofoline	T39.8X1	T39.8X2	T39.8X3	T39.8X4	T39.8X5	T39.8X6
Metolazone	T50.2X1	T50.2X2	T50.2X3	T50.2X4	T50.2X5	T50.2X6
Metopon	T40.2X1	T40.2X2	T40.2X3	T40.2X4	T40.2X5	T40.2X6
Metoprine	T45.1X1	T45.1X2	T45.1X3	T45.1X4	T45.1X5	T45.1X6
Metoprolol	T44.7X1	T44.7X2	T44.7X3	T44.7X4	T44.7X5	T44.7X6
Metrifonate	T60.0X1	T60.0X2	T60.0X3	T60.0X4	—	—
Metrizamide	T50.8X1	T50.8X2	T50.8X3	T50.8X4	T50.8X5	T50.8X6
Metrizoic acid	T50.8X1	T50.8X2	T50.8X3	T50.8X4	T50.8X5	T50.8X6
Metronidazole	T37.8X1	T37.8X2	T37.8X3	T37.8X4	T37.8X5	T37.8X6
Metycaine	T41.3X1	T41.3X2	T41.3X3	T41.3X4	T41.3X5	T41.3X6
infiltration (subcutaneous)	T41.3X1	T41.3X2	T41.3X3	T41.3X4	T41.3X5	T41.3X6
nerve block (peripheral) (plexus)	T41.3X1	T41.3X2	T41.3X3	T41.3X4	T41.3X5	T41.3X6
topical (surface)	T41.3X1	T41.3X2	T41.3X3	T41.3X4	T41.3X5	T41.3X6
Metyrapone	T50.8X1	T50.8X2	T50.8X3	T50.8X4	T50.8X5	T50.8X6
Mevinphos	T60.0X1	T60.0X2	T60.0X3	T60.0X4	—	—

Substance	Poisoning, Accidental (Unintentional)	Poisoning, Intentional Self-Harm	Poisoning, Assault	Poisoning, Undetermined	Adverse Effect	Underdosing
		External Cause (T-Code)				
Mexazolam	T42.4X1	T42.4X2	T42.4X3	T42.4X4	T42.4X5	T42.4X6
Mexenone	T49.3X1	T49.3X2	T49.3X3	T49.3X4	T49.3X5	T49.3X6
Mexiletine	T46.2X1	T46.2X2	T46.2X3	T46.2X4	T46.2X5	T46.2X6
Mezereon	T62.2X1	T62.2X2	T62.2X3	T62.2X4	—	—
berries	T62.1X1	T62.1X2	T62.1X3	T62.1X4	—	—
Mezlocillin	T36.0X1	T36.0X2	T36.0X3	T36.0X4	T36.0X5	T36.0X6
Mianserin	T43.021	T43.022	T43.023	T43.024	T43.025	T43.026
Micatin	T49.0X1	T49.0X2	T49.0X3	T49.0X4	T49.0X5	T49.0X6
Miconazole	T49.0X1	T49.0X2	T49.0X3	T49.0X4	T49.0X5	T49.0X6
Micronomicin	T36.5X1	T36.5X2	T36.5X3	T36.5X4	T36.5X5	T36.5X6
Midazolam	T42.4X1	T42.4X2	T42.4X3	T42.4X4	T42.4X5	T42.4X6
Midecamycin	T36.3X1	T36.3X2	T36.3X3	T36.3X4	T36.3X5	T36.3X6
Mifepristone	T38.6X1	T38.6X2	T38.6X3	T38.6X4	T38.6X5	T38.6X6
Milk of magnesia	T47.1X1	T47.1X2	T47.1X3	T47.1X4	T47.1X5	T47.1X6
Millipede (tropical) (venomous)	T63.411	T63.412	T63.413	T63.414	—	—
Miltown	T43.591	T43.592	T43.593	T43.594	T43.595	T43.596
Milverine	T44.3X1	T44.3X2	T44.3X3	T44.3X4	T44.3X5	T44.3X6
Minaprine	T43.291	T43.292	T43.293	T43.294	T43.295	T43.296
Minaxolone	T41.291	T41.292	T41.293	T41.294	T41.295	T41.296
Mineral						
acids	T54.2X1	T54.2X2	T54.2X3	T54.2X4	—	—
oil (laxative) (medicinal)	T47.4X1	T47.4X2	T47.4X3	T47.4X4	T47.4X5	T47.4X6
emulsion	T47.2X1	T47.2X2	T47.2X3	T47.2X4	T47.2X5	T47.2X6
nonmedicinal	T52.0X1	T52.0X2	T52.0X3	T52.0X4	—	—
topical	T49.3X1	T49.3X2	T49.3X3	T49.3X4	T49.3X5	T49.3X6
salt NEC	T50.3X1	T50.3X2	T50.3X3	T50.3X4	T50.3X5	T50.3X6
spirits	T52.0X1	T52.0X2	T52.0X3	T52.0X4	—	—
Mineralocorticosteroid	T50.0X1	T50.0X2	T50.0X3	T50.0X4	T50.0X5	T50.0X6
Minocycline	T36.4X1	T36.4X2	T36.4X3	T36.4X4	T36.4X5	T36.4X6
Minoxidil	T46.7X1	T46.7X2	T46.7X3	T46.7X4	T46.7X5	T46.7X6
Miokamycin	T36.3X1	T36.3X2	T36.3X3	T36.3X4	T36.3X5	T36.3X6
Miotic drug	T49.5X1	T49.5X2	T49.5X3	T49.5X4	T49.5X5	T49.5X6
Mipafox	T60.0X1	T60.0X2	T60.0X3	T60.0X4	—	—
Mirex	T60.1X1	T60.1X2	T60.1X3	T60.1X4	—	—
Mirtazapine	T43.021	T43.022	T43.023	T43.024	T43.025	T43.026
Misonidazole	T37.3X1	T37.3X2	T37.3X3	T37.3X4	T37.3X5	T37.3X6
Misoprostol	T47.1X1	T47.1X2	T47.1X3	T47.1X4	T47.1X5	T47.1X6
Mithramycin	T45.1X1	T45.1X2	T45.1X3	T45.1X4	T45.1X5	T45.1X6
Mitobronitol	T45.1X1	T45.1X2	T45.1X3	T45.1X4	T45.1X5	T45.1X6
Mitoguazone	T45.1X1	T45.1X2	T45.1X3	T45.1X4	T45.1X5	T45.1X6
Mitolactol	T45.1X1	T45.1X2	T45.1X3	T45.1X4	T45.1X5	T45.1X6
Mitomycin	T45.1X1	T45.1X2	T45.1X3	T45.1X4	T45.1X5	T45.1X6

◀ New   Revised   ~~deleted~~ Deleted

Substance	Poisoning, Accidental (Unintentional)	Poisoning, Intentional Self-Harm	Poisoning, Assault	Poisoning, Undetermined	Adverse Effect	Underdosing
	External Cause (T-Code)					
Mitopodozide	T45.1X1	T45.1X2	T45.1X3	T45.1X4	T45.1X5	T45.1X6
Mitotane	T45.1X1	T45.1X2	T45.1X3	T45.1X4	T45.1X5	T45.1X6
Mitoxantrone	T45.1X1	T45.1X2	T45.1X3	T45.1X4	T45.1X5	T45.1X6
Mivacurium chloride	T48.1X1	T48.1X2	T48.1X3	T48.1X4	T48.1X5	T48.1X6
Miyari bacteria	T47.6X1	T47.6X2	T47.6X3	T47.6X4	T47.6X5	T47.6X6
Moclobemide	T43.1X1	T43.1X2	T43.1X3	T43.1X4	T43.1X5	T43.1X6
Moderil	T46.5X1	T46.5X2	T46.5X3	T46.5X4	T46.5X5	T46.5X6
Mofebutazone	T39.2X1	T39.2X2	T39.2X3	T39.2X4	T39.2X5	T39.2X6
Mogadon — *see Nitrazepam*						
Molindone	T43.591	T43.592	T43.593	T43.594	T43.595	T43.596
Molsidomine	T46.3X1	T46.3X2	T46.3X3	T46.3X4	T46.3X5	T46.3X6
Mometasone	T49.ØX1	T49.ØX2	T49.ØX3	T49.ØX4	T49.ØX5	T49.ØX6
Monistat	T49.ØX1	T49.ØX2	T49.ØX3	T49.ØX4	T49.ØX5	T49.ØX6
Monkshood	T62.2X1	T62.2X2	T62.2X3	T62.2X4	—	—
Monoamine oxidase inhibitor NEC	T43.1X1	T43.1X2	T43.1X3	T43.1X4	T43.1X5	T43.1X6
hydrazine	T43.1X1	T43.1X2	T43.1X3	T43.1X4	T43.1X5	T43.1X6
Monobenzone	T49.4X1	T49.4X2	T49.4X3	T49.4X4	T49.4X5	T49.4X6
Monochloroacetic acid	T6Ø.3X1	T6Ø.3X2	T6Ø.3X3	T6Ø.3X4	—	—
Monochlorobenzene	T53.7X1	T53.7X2	T53.7X3	T53.7X4	—	—
Monoethanolamine	T46.8X1	T46.8X2	T46.8X3	T46.8X4	T46.8X5	T46.8X6
oleate	T46.8X1	T46.8X2	T46.8X3	T46.8X4	T46.8X5	T46.8X6
Monooctanoin	T5Ø.991	T5Ø.992	T5Ø.993	T5Ø.994	T5Ø.995	T5Ø.996
Monophenylbutazone	T39.2X1	T39.2X2	T39.2X3	T39.2X4	T39.2X5	T39.2X6
Monosodium glutamate	T65.891	T65.892	T65.893	T65.894	—	—
Monosulfiram	T49.ØX1	T49.ØX2	T49.ØX3	T49.ØX4	T49.ØX5	T49.ØX6
Monoxide, carbon — *see Carbon, monoxide*	T57.91	T57.92	T57.93	T57.94	—	—
Monoxidine hydrochloride	T46.1X1	T46.1X2	T46.1X3	T46.1X4	T46.1X5	T46.1X6
Monuron	T6Ø.3X1	T6Ø.3X2	T6Ø.3X3	T6Ø.3X4	—	—
Moperone	T43.4X1	T43.4X2	T43.4X3	T43.4X4	T43.4X5	T43.4X6
Mopidamol	T45.1X1	T45.1X2	T45.1X3	T45.1X4	T45.1X5	T45.1X6
MOPP (mechlorethamine + vincristine + prednisone + procarbazine)	T45.1X1	T45.1X2	T45.1X3	T45.1X4	T45.1X5	T45.1X6
Morfin	T4Ø.2X1	T4Ø.2X2	T4Ø.2X3	T4Ø.2X4	T4Ø.2X5	T4Ø.2X6
Morinamide	T37.1X1	T37.1X2	T37.1X3	T37.1X4	T37.1X5	T37.1X6
Morning glory seeds	T4Ø.991	T4Ø.992	T4Ø.993	T4Ø.994	—	—
Moroxydine	T37.5X1	T37.5X2	T37.5X3	T37.5X4	T37.5X5	T37.5X6
Morphazinamide	T37.1X1	T37.1X2	T37.1X3	T37.1X4	T37.1X5	T37.1X6
Morphine	T4Ø.2X1	T4Ø.2X2	T4Ø.2X3	T4Ø.2X4	T4Ø.2X5	T4Ø.2X6
antagonist	T5Ø.7X1	T5Ø.7X2	T5Ø.7X3	T5Ø.7X4	T5Ø.7X5	T5Ø.7X6
Morpholinylethylmorphine	T4Ø.2X1	T4Ø.2X2	T4Ø.2X3	T4Ø.2X4	—	—
Morsuximide	T42.2X1	T42.2X2	T42.2X3	T42.2X4	T42.2X5	T42.2X6
Mosapramine	T43.591	T43.592	T43.593	T43.594	T43.595	T43.596
Moth balls — *see also Pesticides*	T6Ø.2X1	T6Ø.2X2	T6Ø.2X3	T6Ø.2X4	—	—
naphthalene	T6Ø.2X1	T6Ø.2X2	T6Ø.2X3	T6Ø.2X4	—	—
paradichlorobenzene	T6Ø.1X1	T6Ø.1X2	T6Ø.1X3	T6Ø.1X4	—	—
Motor exhaust gas	T58.Ø1	T58.Ø2	T58.Ø3	T58.Ø4	—	—
Mouthwash (antiseptic) (zinc chloride)	T49.6X1	T49.6X2	T49.6X3	T49.6X4	T49.6X5	T49.6X6
Moxastine	T45.ØX1	T45.ØX2	T45.ØX3	T45.ØX4	T45.ØX5	T45.ØX6
Moxaverine	T44.3X1	T44.3X2	T44.3X3	T44.3X4	T44.3X5	T44.3X6
Moxifensine	T43.291	T43.292	T43.293	T43.294	T43.295	T43.296
Moxisylyte	T46.7X1	T46.7X2	T46.7X3	T46.7X4	T46.7X5	T46.7X6
Mucilage, plant	T47.4X1	T47.4X2	T47.4X3	T47.4X4	T47.4X5	T47.4X6
Mucolytic drug	T48.4X1	T48.4X2	T48.4X3	T48.4X4	T48.4X5	T48.4X6
Mucomyst	T48.4X1	T48.4X2	T48.4X3	T48.4X4	T48.4X5	T48.4X6
Mucous membrane agents (external)	T49.91	T49.92	T49.93	T49.94	T49.95	T49.96
specified NEC	T49.8X1	T49.8X2	T49.8X3	T49.8X4	T49.8X5	T49.8X6
Multiple unspecified drugs, medicaments and biological substances	T5Ø.911	T5Ø.912	T5Ø.913	T5Ø.914	T5Ø.915	T5Ø.916 ◀
Mumps						
immune globulin (human)	T5Ø.Z11	T5Ø.Z12	T5Ø.Z13	T5Ø.Z14	T5Ø.Z15	T5Ø.Z16
skin test antigen	T5Ø.8X1	T5Ø.8X2	T5Ø.8X3	T5Ø.8X4	T5Ø.8X5	T5Ø.8X6
vaccine	T5Ø.B91	T5Ø.B92	T5Ø.B93	T5Ø.B94	T5Ø.B95	T5Ø.B96
Mumpsvax	T5Ø.B91	T5Ø.B92	T5Ø.B93	T5Ø.B94	T5Ø.B95	T5Ø.B96
Mupirocin	T49.ØX1	T49.ØX2	T49.ØX3	T49.ØX4	T49.ØX5	T49.ØX6
Muriatic acid — *see Hydrochloric acid*						
Muromonab-CD3	T45.1X1	T45.1X2	T45.1X3	T45.1X4	T45.1X5	T45.1X6
Muscle relaxant — *see Relaxant, muscle*						
Muscle-action drug NEC	T48.2Ø1	T48.2Ø2	T48.2Ø3	T48.2Ø4	T48.2Ø5	T48.2Ø6
Muscle affecting agents NEC	T48.2Ø1	T48.2Ø2	T48.2Ø3	T48.2Ø4	T48.2Ø5	T48.2Ø6
oxytocic	T48.ØX1	T48.ØX2	T48.ØX3	T48.ØX4	T48.ØX5	T48.ØX6
relaxants	T48.2Ø1	T48.2Ø2	T48.2Ø3	T48.2Ø4	T48.2Ø5	T48.2Ø6
central nervous system	T42.8X1	T42.8X2	T42.8X3	T42.8X4	T42.8X5	T42.8X6
skeletal	T48.1X1	T48.1X2	T48.1X3	T48.1X4	T48.1X5	T48.1X6
smooth	T44.3X1	T44.3X2	T44.3X3	T44.3X4	T44.3X5	T44.3X6
Muscle-tone depressant, central NEC	T42.8X1	T42.8X2	T42.8X3	T42.8X4	T42.8X5	T42.8X6
specified NEC	T42.8X1	T42.8X2	T42.8X3	T42.8X4	T42.8X5	T42.8X6
Mushroom, noxious	T62.ØX1	T62.ØX2	T62.ØX3	T62.ØX4	—	—
Mussel, noxious	T61.781	T61.782	T61.783	T61.784	—	—

Substance	External Cause (T-Code)					
	Poisoning, Accidental (Unintentional)	Poisoning, Intentional Self-Harm	Poisoning, Assault	Poisoning, Undetermined	Adverse Effect	Underdosing
Mustard (emetic)	T47.7X1	T47.7X2	T47.7X3	T47.7X4	T47.7X5	T47.7X6
black	T47.7X1	T47.7X2	T47.7X3	T47.7X4	T47.7X5	T47.7X6
gas, not in war	T59.91	T59.92	T59.93	T59.94	—	—
nitrogen	T45.1X1	T45.1X2	T45.1X3	T45.1X4	T45.1X5	T45.1X6
Mustine	T45.1X1	T45.1X2	T45.1X3	T45.1X4	T45.1X5	T45.1X6
M-vac	T45.1X1	T45.1X2	T45.1X3	T45.1X4	T45.1X5	T45.1X6
Mycifradin	T36.5X1	T36.5X2	T36.5X3	T36.5X4	T36.5X5	T36.5X6
topical	T49.ØX1	T49.ØX2	T49.ØX3	T49.ØX4	T49.ØX5	T49.ØX6
Mycitracin	T36.8X1	T36.8X2	T36.8X3	T36.8X4	T36.8X5	T36.8X6
ophthalmic preparation	T49.5X1	T49.5X2	T49.5X3	T49.5X4	T49.5X5	T49.5X6
Mycostatin	T36.7X1	T36.7X2	T36.7X3	T36.7X4	T36.7X5	T36.7X6
topical	T49.ØX1	T49.ØX2	T49.ØX3	T49.ØX4	T49.ØX5	T49.ØX6
Mycotoxins	T64.81	T64.82	T64.83	T64.84	—	—
aflatoxin	T64.Ø1	T64.Ø2	T64.Ø3	T64.Ø4	—	—
specified NEC	T64.81	T64.82	T64.83	T64.84	—	—
Mydriacyl	T44.3X1	T44.3X2	T44.3X3	T44.3X4	T44.3X5	T44.3X6
Mydriatic drug	T49.5X1	T49.5X2	T49.5X3	T49.5X4	T49.5X5	T49.5X6
Myelobromal	T45.1X1	T45.1X2	T45.1X3	T45.1X4	T45.1X5	T45.1X6
Myleran	T45.1X1	T45.1X2	T45.1X3	T45.1X4	T45.1X5	T45.1X6
Myochrysin(e)	T39.2X1	T39.2X2	T39.2X3	T39.2X4	T39.2X5	T39.2X6
Myoneural blocking agents	T48.1X1	T48.1X2	T48.1X3	T48.1X4	T48.1X5	T48.1X6
Myralact	T49.ØX1	T49.ØX2	T49.ØX3	T49.ØX4	T49.ØX5	T49.ØX6
Myristica fragrans	T62.2X1	T62.2X2	T62.2X3	T62.2X4	—	—
Myristicin	T65.891	T65.892	T65.893	T65.894	—	—
Mysoline	T42.3X1	T42.3X2	T42.3X3	T42.3X4	T42.3X5	T42.3X6
N						
Nabilone	T4Ø.7X1	T4Ø.7X2	T4Ø.7X3	T4Ø.7X4	T4Ø.7X5	T4Ø.7X6
Nabumetone	T39.391	T39.392	T39.393	T39.394	T39.395	T39.396
Nadolol	T44.7X1	T44.7X2	T44.7X3	T44.7X4	T44.7X5	T44.7X6
Nafcillin	T36.ØX1	T36.ØX2	T36.ØX3	T36.ØX4	T36.ØX5	T36.ØX6
Nafoxidine	T38.6X1	T38.6X2	T38.6X3	T38.6X4	T38.6X5	T38.6X6
Naftazone	T46.991	T46.992	T46.993	T46.994	T46.995	T46.996
Naftidrofuryl (oxalate)	T46.7X1	T46.7X2	T46.7X3	T46.7X4	T46.7X5	T46.7X6
Naftifine	T49.ØX1	T49.ØX2	T49.ØX3	T49.ØX4	T49.ØX5	T49.ØX6
Nail polish remover	T52.91	T52.92	T52.93	T52.94	—	—
Nalbuphine	T4Ø.4X1	T4Ø.4X2	T4Ø.4X3	T4Ø.4X4	T4Ø.4X5	T4Ø.4X6
Naled	T6Ø.ØX1	T6Ø.ØX2	T6Ø.ØX3	T6Ø.ØX4	—	—
Nalidixic acid	T37.8X1	T37.8X2	T37.8X3	T37.8X4	T37.8X5	T37.8X6
Nalorphine	T5Ø.7X1	T5Ø.7X2	T5Ø.7X3	T5Ø.7X4	T5Ø.7X5	T5Ø.7X6
Naloxone	T5Ø.7X1	T5Ø.7X2	T5Ø.7X3	T5Ø.7X4	T5Ø.7X5	T5Ø.7X6
Naltrexone	T5Ø.7X1	T5Ø.7X2	T5Ø.7X3	T5Ø.7X4	T5Ø.7X5	T5Ø.7X6
Namenda	T43.8X1	T43.8X2	T43.8X3	T43.8X4	T43.8X5	T43.8X6
Nandrolone	T38.7X1	T38.7X2	T38.7X3	T38.7X4	T38.7X5	T38.7X6
Naphazoline	T48.5X1	T48.5X2	T48.5X3	T48.5X4	T48.5X5	T48.5X6
Naphtha (painters') (petroleum)	T52.ØX1	T52.ØX2	T52.ØX3	T52.ØX4	—	—
solvent	T52.ØX1	T52.ØX2	T52.ØX3	T52.ØX4	—	—
vapor	T52.ØX1	T52.ØX2	T52.ØX3	T52.ØX4	—	—
Naphthalene (non-chlorinated)	T6Ø.2X1	T6Ø.2X2	T6Ø.2X3	T6Ø.2X4	—	—
chlorinated	T6Ø.1X1	T6Ø.1X2	T6Ø.1X3	T6Ø.1X4	—	—
vapor	T6Ø.1X1	T6Ø.1X2	T6Ø.1X3	T6Ø.1X4	—	—
insecticide or moth repellent	T6Ø.2X1	T6Ø.2X2	T6Ø.2X3	T6Ø.2X4	—	—
chlorinated	T6Ø.1X1	T6Ø.1X2	T6Ø.1X3	T6Ø.1X4	—	—
vapor	T6Ø.2X1	T6Ø.2X2	T6Ø.2X3	T6Ø.2X4	—	—
chlorinated	T6Ø.1X1	T6Ø.1X2	T6Ø.1X3	T6Ø.1X4	—	—
Naphthol	T65.891	T65.892	T65.893	T65.894	—	—
Naphthylamine	T65.891	T65.892	T65.893	T65.894	—	—
Naphthylthiourea (ANTU)	T6Ø.4X1	T6Ø.4X2	T6Ø.4X3	T6Ø.4X4	—	—
Naprosyn — *see Naproxen*						
Naproxen	T39.311	T39.312	T39.313	T39.314	T39.315	T39.316
Narcotic (drug)	T4Ø.6Ø1	T4Ø.6Ø2	T4Ø.6Ø3	T4Ø.6Ø4	T4Ø.6Ø5	T4Ø.6Ø6
analgesic NEC	T4Ø.6Ø1	T4Ø.6Ø2	T4Ø.6Ø3	T4Ø.6Ø4	T4Ø.6Ø5	T4Ø.6Ø6
antagonist	T5Ø.7X1	T5Ø.7X2	T5Ø.7X3	T5Ø.7X4	T5Ø.7X5	T5Ø.7X6
specified NEC	T4Ø.691	T4Ø.692	T4Ø.693	T4Ø.694	T4Ø.695	T4Ø.696
synthetic	T4Ø.4X1	T4Ø.4X2	T4Ø.4X3	T4Ø.4X4	T4Ø.4X5	T4Ø.4X6
Narcotine	T48.3X1	T48.3X2	T48.3X3	T48.3X4	T48.3X5	T48.3X6
Nardil	T43.1X1	T43.1X2	T43.1X3	T43.1X4	T43.1X5	T43.1X6
Nasal drug NEC	T49.6X1	T49.6X2	T49.6X3	T49.6X4	T49.6X5	T49.6X6
Natamycin	T49.ØX1	T49.ØX2	T49.ØX3	T49.ØX4	T49.ØX5	T49.ØX6
Natrium cyanide — *see Cyanide(s)*						
Natural gas	T59.891	T59.892	T59.893	T59.894	—	—
incomplete combustion	T57.91	T57.92	T57.93	T57.94	—	—
Natural						
blood (product)	T45.8X1	T45.8X2	T45.8X3	T45.8X4	T45.8X5	T45.8X6
gas (piped)	T59.891	T59.892	T59.893	T59.894	—	—
incomplete combustion	T58.11	T58.12	T58.13	T58.14	—	—
Nealbarbital	T42.3X1	T42.3X2	T42.3X3	T42.3X4	T42.3X5	T42.3X6
Nectadon	T48.3X1	T48.3X2	T48.3X3	T48.3X4	T48.3X5	T48.3X6
Nedocromil	T48.6X1	T48.6X2	T48.6X3	T48.6X4	T48.6X5	T48.6X6
Nefopam	T39.8X1	T39.8X2	T39.8X3	T39.8X4	T39.8X5	T39.8X6
Nematocyst (sting)	T63.691	T63.692	T63.693	T63.694	—	—
Nembutal	T42.3X1	T42.3X2	T42.3X3	T42.3X4	T42.3X5	T42.3X6
Nemonapride	T43.591	T43.592	T43.593	T43.594	T43.595	T43.596
Neoarsphenamine	T37.8X1	T37.8X2	T37.8X3	T37.8X4	T37.8X5	T37.8X6

New Revised ~~deleted~~ Deleted

Substance	External Cause (T-Code) Poisoning, Accidental (Unintentional)	Poisoning, Intentional Self-Harm	Poisoning, Assault	Poisoning, Undetermined	Adverse Effect	Underdosing
Neocinchophen	T5Ø.4X1	T5Ø.4X2	T5Ø.4X3	T5Ø.4X4	T5Ø.4X5	T5Ø.4X6
Neomycin (derivatives)	T36.5X1	T36.5X2	T36.5X3	T36.5X4	T36.5X5	T36.5X6
with						
bacitracin	T49.ØX1	T49.ØX2	T49.ØX3	T49.ØX4	T49.ØX5	T49.ØX6
neostigmine	T44.ØX1	T44.ØX2	T44.ØX3	T44.ØX4	T44.ØX5	T44.ØX6
ENT agent	T49.6X1	T49.6X2	T49.6X3	T49.6X4	T49.6X5	T49.6X6
ophthalmic preparation	T49.5X1	T49.5X2	T49.5X3	T49.5X4	T49.5X5	T49.5X6
topical NEC	T49.ØX1	T49.ØX2	T49.ØX3	T49.ØX4	T49.ØX5	T49.ØX6
Neonal	T42.3X1	T42.3X2	T42.3X3	T42.3X4	T42.3X5	T42.3X6
Neoprontosil	T37.ØX1	T37.ØX2	T37.ØX3	T37.ØX4	T37.ØX5	T37.ØX6
Neosalvarsan	T37.8X1	T37.8X2	T37.8X3	T37.8X4	T37.8X5	T37.8X6
Neosilversalvarsan	T37.8X1	T37.8X2	T37.8X3	T37.8X4	T37.8X5	T37.8X6
Neosporin	T36.8X1	T36.8X2	T36.8X3	T36.8X4	T36.8X5	T36.8X6
ENT agent	T49.6X1	T49.6X2	T49.6X3	T49.6X4	T49.6X5	T49.6X6
opthalmic preparation	T49.5X1	T49.5X2	T49.5X3	T49.5X4	T49.5X5	T49.5X6
topical NEC	T49.ØX1	T49.ØX2	T49.ØX3	T49.ØX4	T49.ØX5	T49.ØX6
Neostigmine bromide	T44.ØX1	T44.ØX2	T44.ØX3	T44.ØX4	T44.ØX5	T44.ØX6
Neraval	T42.3X1	T42.3X2	T42.3X3	T42.3X4	T42.3X5	T42.3X6
Neravan	T42.3X1	T42.3X2	T42.3X3	T42.3X4	T42.3X5	T42.3X6
Nerium oleander	T62.2X1	T62.2X2	T62.2X3	T62.2X4	—	—
Nerve gas, not in war	T59.91	T59.92	T59.93	T59.94	—	—
Nesacaine	T41.3X1	T41.3X2	T41.3X3	T41.3X4	T41.3X5	T41.3X6
infiltration (subcutaneous)	T41.3X1	T41.3X2	T41.3X3	T41.3X4	T41.3X5	T41.3X6
nerve block (peripheral) (plexus)	T41.3X1	T41.3X2	T41.3X3	T41.3X4	T41.3X5	T41.3X6
Netilmicin	T36.5X1	T36.5X2	T36.5X3	T36.5X4	T36.5X5	T36.5X6
Neurobarb	T42.3X1	T42.3X2	T42.3X3	T42.3X4	T42.3X5	T42.3X6
Neuroleptic drug NEC	T43.5Ø1	T43.5Ø2	T43.5Ø3	T43.5Ø4	T43.5Ø5	T43.5Ø6
Neuromuscular blocking drug	T48.1X1	T48.1X2	T48.1X3	T48.1X4	T48.1X5	T48.1X6
Neutral insulin injection	T38.3X1	T38.3X2	T38.3X3	T38.3X4	T38.3X5	T38.3X6
Neutral spirits	T51.ØX1	T51.ØX2	T51.ØX3	T51.ØX4	—	—
beverage	T51.ØX1	T51.ØX2	T51.ØX3	T51.ØX4	—	—
Niacin	T46.7X1	T46.7X2	T46.7X3	T46.7X4	T46.7X5	T46.7X6
Niacinamide	T45.2X1	T45.2X2	T45.2X3	T45.2X4	T45.2X5	T45.2X6
Nialamide	T43.1X1	T43.1X2	T43.1X3	T43.1X4	T43.1X5	T43.1X6
Niaprazine	T42.6X1	T42.6X2	T42.6X3	T42.6X4	T42.6X5	T42.6X6
Nicametate	T46.7X1	T46.7X2	T46.7X3	T46.7X4	T46.7X5	T46.7X6
Nicardipine	T46.1X1	T46.1X2	T46.1X3	T46.1X4	T46.1X5	T46.1X6
Nicergoline	T46.7X1	T46.7X2	T46.7X3	T46.7X4	T46.7X5	T46.7X6
Nickel (carbonyl) (tetra-carbonyl) (fumes) (vapor)	T56.891	T56.892	T56.893	T56.894	—	—
Nickelocene	T56.891	T56.892	T56.893	T56.894	—	—
Niclosamide	T37.4X1	T37.4X2	T37.4X3	T37.4X4	T37.4X5	T37.4X6
Nicofuranose	T46.7X1	T46.7X2	T46.7X3	T46.7X4	T46.7X5	T46.7X6
Nicomorphine	T4Ø.2X1	T4Ø.2X2	T4Ø.2X3	T4Ø.2X4	—	—
Nicorandil	T46.3X1	T46.3X2	T46.3X3	T46.3X4	T46.3X5	T46.3X6
Nicotiana (plant)	T62.2X1	T62.2X2	T62.2X3	T62.2X4	—	—
Nicotinamide	T45.2X1	T45.2X2	T45.2X3	T45.2X4	T45.2X5	T45.2X6
Nicotine (insecticide) (spray) (sulfate) NEC	T6Ø.2X1	T6Ø.2X2	T6Ø.2X3	T6Ø.2X4	—	—
from tobacco	T65.291	T65.292	T65.293	T65.294	—	—
cigarettes	T65.221	T65.222	T65.223	T65.224	—	—
not insecticide	T65.291	T65.292	T65.293	T65.294	—	—
Nicotinic acid	T46.7X1	T46.7X2	T46.7X3	T46.7X4	T46.7X5	T46.7X6
Nicotinyl alcohol	T46.7X1	T46.7X2	T46.7X3	T46.7X4	T46.7X5	T46.7X6
Nicoumalone	T45.511	T45.512	T45.513	T45.514	T45.515	T45.516
Nifedipine	T46.1X1	T46.1X2	T46.1X3	T46.1X4	T46.1X5	T46.1X6
Nifenazone	T39.2X1	T39.2X2	T39.2X3	T39.2X4	T39.2X5	T39.2X6
Nifuraldezone	T37.91	T37.92	T37.93	T37.94	T37.95	T37.96
Nifuratel	T37.8X1	T37.8X2	T37.8X3	T37.8X4	T37.8X5	T37.8X6
Nifurtimox	T37.3X1	T37.3X2	T37.3X3	T37.3X4	T37.3X5	T37.3X6
Nifurtoinol	T37.8X1	T37.8X2	T37.8X3	T37.8X4	T37.8X5	T37.8X6
Nightshade, deadly (solanum)—*see also Belladonna*	T62.2X1	T62.2X2	T62.2X3	T62.2X4	—	—
berry	T62.1X1	T62.1X2	T62.1X3	T62.1X4	—	—
Nikethamide	T5Ø.7X1	T5Ø.7X2	T5Ø.7X3	T5Ø.7X4	T5Ø.7X5	T5Ø.7X6
Nilstat	T36.7X1	T36.7X2	T36.7X3	T36.7X4	T36.7X5	T36.7X6
topical	T49.ØX1	T49.ØX2	T49.ØX3	T49.ØX4	T49.ØX5	T49.ØX6
Nilutamide	T38.6X1	T38.6X2	T38.6X3	T38.6X4	T38.6X5	T38.6X6
Nimesulide	T39.391	T39.392	T39.393	T39.394	T39.395	T39.396
Nimetazepam	T42.4X1	T42.4X2	T42.4X3	T42.4X4	T42.4X5	T42.4X6
Nimodipine	T46.1X1	T46.1X2	T46.1X3	T46.1X4	T46.1X5	T46.1X6
Nimorazole	T37.3X1	T37.3X2	T37.3X3	T37.3X4	T37.3X5	T37.3X6
Nimustine	T45.1X1	T45.1X2	T45.1X3	T45.1X4	T45.1X5	T45.1X6
Niridazole	T37.4X1	T37.4X2	T37.4X3	T37.4X4	T37.4X5	T37.4X6
Nisentil	T4Ø.2X1	T4Ø.2X2	T4Ø.2X3	T4Ø.2X4	T4Ø.2X5	T4Ø.2X6
Nisoldipine	T46.1X1	T46.1X2	T46.1X3	T46.1X4	T46.1X5	T46.1X6
Nitramine	T65.3X1	T65.3X2	T65.3X3	T65.3X4	—	—
Nitrate, organic	T46.3X1	T46.3X2	T46.3X3	T46.3X4	T46.3X5	T46.3X6
Nitrazepam	T42.4X1	T42.4X2	T42.4X3	T42.4X4	T42.4X5	T42.4X6
Nitrefazole	T5Ø.6X1	T5Ø.6X2	T5Ø.6X3	T5Ø.6X4	T5Ø.6X5	T5Ø.6X6
Nitrendipine	T46.1X1	T46.1X2	T46.1X3	T46.1X4	T46.1X5	T46.1X6

	External Cause (T-Code)					
Substance	**Poisoning, Accidental (Unintentional)**	**Poisoning, Intentional Self-Harm**	**Poisoning, Assault**	**Poisoning, Undetermined**	**Adverse Effect**	**Underdosing**
Nitric						
acid (liquid)	T54.2X1	T54.2X2	T54.2X3	T54.2X4	—	—
vapor	T59.891	T59.892	T59.893	T59.894	—	—
oxide (gas)	T59.0X1	T59.0X2	T59.0X3	T59.0X4	—	—
Nitrimidazine	T37.3X1	T37.3X2	T37.3X3	T37.3X4	T37.3X5	T37.3X6
Nitrite, amyl (medicinal) (vapor)	T46.3X1	T46.3X2	T46.3X3	T46.3X4	T46.3X5	T46.3X6
Nitroaniline	T65.3X1	T65.3X2	T65.3X3	T65.3X4	—	—
vapor	T59.891	T59.892	T59.893	T59.894	—	—
Nitrobenzene, nitrobenzol	T65.3X1	T65.3X2	T65.3X3	T65.3X4	—	—
vapor	T65.3X1	T65.3X2	T65.3X3	T65.3X4	—	—
Nitrocellulose	T65.891	T65.892	T65.893	T65.894	—	—
lacquer	T65.891	T65.892	T65.893	T65.894	—	—
Nitrodiphenyl	T65.3X1	T65.3X2	T65.3X3	T65.3X4	—	—
Nitrofural	T49.0X1	T49.0X2	T49.0X3	T49.0X4	T49.0X5	T49.0X6
Nitrofurantoin	T37.8X1	T37.8X2	T37.8X3	T37.8X4	T37.8X5	T37.8X6
Nitrofurazone	T49.0X1	T49.0X2	T49.0X3	T49.0X4	T49.0X5	T49.0X6
Nitrogen	T59.0X1	T59.0X2	T59.0X3	T59.0X4	—	—
mustard	T45.1X1	T45.1X2	T45.1X3	T45.1X4	T45.1X5	T45.1X6
Nitroglycerin, nitro-glycerol (medicinal)	T46.3X1	T46.3X2	T46.3X3	T46.3X4	T46.3X5	T46.3X6
nonmedicinal	T65.5X1	T65.5X2	T65.5X3	T65.5X4	—	—
fumes	T65.5X1	T65.5X2	T65.5X3	T65.5X4	—	—
Nitroglycol	T52.3X1	T52.3X2	T52.3X3	T52.3X4	—	—
Nitrohydrochloric acid	T54.2X1	T54.2X2	T54.2X3	T54.2X4	—	—
Nitromersol	T49.0X1	T49.0X2	T49.0X3	T49.0X4	T49.0X5	T49.0X6
Nitronaphthalene	T65.891	T65.892	T65.893	T65.894	—	—
Nitrophenol	T54.0X1	T54.0X2	T54.0X3	T54.0X4	—	—
Nitropropane	T52.8X1	T52.8X2	T52.8X3	T52.8X4	—	—
Nitroprusside	T46.5X1	T46.5X2	T46.5X3	T46.5X4	T46.5X5	T46.5X6
Nitrosodimethylamine	T65.3X1	T65.3X2	T65.3X3	T65.3X4	—	—
Nitrothiazol	T37.4X1	T37.4X2	T37.4X3	T37.4X4	T37.4X5	T37.4X6
Nitrotoluene, nitrotoluol	T65.3X1	T65.3X2	T65.3X3	T65.3X4	—	—
vapor	T65.3X1	T65.3X2	T65.3X3	T65.3X4	—	—
Nitrous						
acid (liquid)	T54.2X1	T54.2X2	T54.2X3	T54.2X4	—	—
fumes	T59.891	T59.892	T59.893	T59.894	—	—
ether spirit	T46.3X1	T46.3X2	T46.3X3	T46.3X4	T46.3X5	T46.3X6
oxide	T41.0X1	T41.0X2	T41.0X3	T41.0X4	T41.0X5	T41.0X6
Nitroxoline	T37.8X1	T37.8X2	T37.8X3	T37.8X4	T37.8X5	T37.8X6
Nitrozone	T49.0X1	T49.0X2	T49.0X3	T49.0X4	T49.0X5	T49.0X6
Nizatidine	T47.0X1	T47.0X2	T47.0X3	T47.0X4	T47.0X5	T47.0X6
Nizofenone	T43.8X1	T43.8X2	T43.8X3	T43.8X4	T43.8X5	T43.8X6
Noctec	T42.6X1	T42.6X2	T42.6X3	T42.6X4	T42.6X5	T42.6X6
Noludar	T42.6X1	T42.6X2	T42.6X3	T42.6X4	T42.6X5	T42.6X6
Noptil	T42.3X1	T42.3X2	T42.3X3	T42.3X4	T42.3X5	T42.3X6
Nomegestrol	T38.5X1	T38.5X2	T38.5X3	T38.5X4	T38.5X5	T38.5X6
Nomifensine	T43.291	T43.292	T43.293	T43.294	T43.295	T43.296
Nonoxinol	T49.8X1	T49.8X2	T49.8X3	T49.8X4	T49.8X5	T49.8X6
Nonylphenoxy (polyethoxy-ethanol)	T49.8X1	T49.8X2	T49.8X3	T49.8X4	T49.8X5	T49.8X6
Noptil	T42.3X1	T42.3X2	T42.3X3	T42.3X4	T42.3X5	T42.3X6
Noradrenaline	T44.4X1	T44.4X2	T44.4X3	T44.4X4	T44.4X5	T44.4X6
Noramidopyrine	T39.2X1	T39.2X2	T39.2X3	T39.2X4	T39.2X5	T39.2X6
methanesulfonate sodium	T39.2X1	T39.2X2	T39.2X3	T39.2X4	T39.2X5	T39.2X6
Norbormide	T60.4X1	T60.4X2	T60.4X3	T60.4X4	—	—
Nordazepam	T42.4X1	T42.4X2	T42.4X3	T42.4X4	T42.4X5	T42.4X6
Norepinephrine	T44.4X1	T44.4X2	T44.4X3	T44.4X4	T44.4X5	T44.4X6
Norethandrolone	T38.7X1	T38.7X2	T38.7X3	T38.7X4	T38.7X5	T38.7X6
Norethindrone	T38.4X1	T38.4X2	T38.4X3	T38.4X4	T38.4X5	T38.4X6
Norethisterone (acetate) (enantate)	T38.4X1	T38.4X2	T38.4X3	T38.4X4	T38.4X5	T38.4X6
with ethinylestradiol	T38.5X1	T38.5X2	T38.5X3	T38.5X4	T38.5X5	T38.5X6
Noretynodrel	T38.5X1	T38.5X2	T38.5X3	T38.5X4	T38.5X5	T38.5X6
Norfenefrine	T44.4X1	T44.4X2	T44.4X3	T44.4X4	T44.4X5	T44.4X6
Norfloxacin	T36.8X1	T36.8X2	T36.8X3	T36.8X4	T36.8X5	T36.8X6
Norgestrel	T38.4X1	T38.4X2	T38.4X3	T38.4X4	T38.4X5	T38.4X6
Norgestrienone	T38.4X1	T38.4X2	T38.4X3	T38.4X4	T38.4X5	T38.4X6
Norlestrin	T38.4X1	T38.4X2	T38.4X3	T38.4X4	T38.4X5	T38.4X6
Norlutin	T38.4X1	T38.4X2	T38.4X3	T38.4X4	T38.4X5	T38.4X6
Normal serum albumin (human), salt-poor	T45.8X1	T45.8X2	T45.8X3	T45.8X4	T45.8X5	T45.8X6
Normethandrone	T38.5X1	T38.5X2	T38.5X3	T38.5X4	T38.5X5	T38.5X6
Normison — *see Benzodiazepines*						
Normorphine	T40.2X1	T40.2X2	T40.2X3	T40.2X4	—	—
Norpseudoephedrine	T50.5X1	T50.5X2	T50.5X3	T50.5X4	T50.5X5	T50.5X6
Nortestosterone (furanpropionate)	T38.7X1	T38.7X2	T38.7X3	T38.7X4	T38.7X5	T38.7X6
Nortriptyline	T43.011	T43.012	T43.013	T43.014	T43.015	T43.016
Noscapine	T48.3X1	T48.3X2	T48.3X3	T48.3X4	T48.3X5	T48.3X6
Nose preparations	T49.6X1	T49.6X2	T49.6X3	T49.6X4	T49.6X5	T49.6X6
Novobiocin	T36.5X1	T36.5X2	T36.5X3	T36.5X4	T36.5X5	T36.5X6
Novocain (infiltration) (topical)	T41.3X1	T41.3X2	T41.3X3	T41.3X4	T41.3X5	T41.3X6
nerve block (peripheral) (plexus)	T41.3X1	T41.3X2	T41.3X3	T41.3X4	T41.3X5	T41.3X6
spinal	T41.3X1	T41.3X2	T41.3X3	T41.3X4	T41.3X5	T41.3X6

◀ New   Revised   ~~deleted~~ Deleted

Substance	Poisoning, Accidental (Unintentional)	Poisoning, Intentional Self-Harm	Poisoning, Assault	Poisoning, Undetermined	Adverse Effect	Underdosing
	External Cause (T-Code)					
Noxious foodstuff	T62.91	T62.92	T62.93	T62.94	—	—
specified NEC	T62.8X1	T62.8X2	T62.8X3	T62.8X4	—	—
Noxiptiline	T43.Ø11	T43.Ø12	T43.Ø13	T43.Ø14	T43.Ø15	T43.Ø16
Noxytiolin	T49.ØX1	T49.ØX2	T49.ØX3	T49.ØX4	T49.ØX5	T49.ØX6
NPH Iletin (insulin)	T38.3X1	T38.3X2	T38.3X3	T38.3X4	T38.3X5	T38.3X6
Numorphan	T4Ø.2X1	T4Ø.2X2	T4Ø.2X3	T4Ø.2X4	T4Ø.2X5	T4Ø.2X6
Nunol	T42.3X1	T42.3X2	T42.3X3	T42.3X4	T42.3X5	T42.3X6
Nupercaine (spinal anesthetic)	T41.3X1	T41.3X2	T41.3X3	T41.3X4	T41.3X5	T41.3X6
topical (surface)	T41.3X1	T41.3X2	T41.3X3	T41.3X4	T41.3X5	T41.3X6
Nutmeg oil (liniment)	T49.3X1	T49.3X2	T49.3X3	T49.3X4	T49.3X5	T49.3X6
Nutritional supplement	T5Ø.9Ø1	T5Ø.9Ø2	T5Ø.9Ø3	T5Ø.9Ø4	T5Ø.9Ø5	T5Ø.9Ø6
Nux vomica	T65.1X1	T65.1X2	T65.1X3	T65.1X4	—	—
Nydrazid	T37.1X1	T37.1X2	T37.1X3	T37.1X4	T37.1X5	T37.1X6
Nylidrin	T46.7X1	T46.7X2	T46.7X3	T46.7X4	T46.7X5	T46.7X6
Nystatin	T36.7X1	T36.7X2	T36.7X3	T36.7X4	T36.7X5	T36.7X6
topical	T49.ØX1	T49.ØX2	T49.ØX3	T49.ØX4	T49.ØX5	T49.ØX6
Nytol	T45.ØX1	T45.ØX2	T45.ØX3	T45.ØX4	T45.ØX5	T45.ØX6
O						
Obidoxime chloride	T5Ø.6X1	T5Ø.6X2	T5Ø.6X3	T5Ø.6X4	T5Ø.6X5	T5Ø.6X6
Octafonium (chloride)	T49.3X1	T49.3X2	T49.3X3	T49.3X4	T49.3X5	T49.3X6
Octamethyl pyrophosphoramide	T6Ø.ØX1	T6Ø.ØX2	T6Ø.ØX3	T6Ø.ØX4	—	—
Octanoin	T5Ø.991	T5Ø.992	T5Ø.993	T5Ø.994	T5Ø.995	T5Ø.996
Octatropine methylbromide	T44.3X1	T44.3X2	T44.3X3	T44.3X4	T44.3X5	T44.3X6
Octotiamine	T45.2X1	T45.2X2	T45.2X3	T45.2X4	T45.2X5	T45.2X6
Octoxinol (9)	T49.8X1	T49.8X2	T49.8X3	T49.8X4	T49.8X5	T49.8X6
Octreotide	T38.991	T38.992	T38.993	T38.994	T38.995	T38.996
Octyl nitrite	T46.3X1	T46.3X2	T46.3X3	T46.3X4	T46.3X5	T46.3X6
Oestradiol	T38.5X1	T38.5X2	T38.5X3	T38.5X4	T38.5X5	T38.5X6
Oestriol	T38.5X1	T38.5X2	T38.5X3	T38.5X4	T38.5X5	T38.5X6
Oestrogen	T38.5X1	T38.5X2	T38.5X3	T38.5X4	T38.5X5	T38.5X6
Oestrone	T38.5X1	T38.5X2	T38.5X3	T38.5X4	T38.5X5	T38.5X6
Ofloxacin	T36.8X1	T36.8X2	T36.8X3	T36.8X4	T36.8X5	T36.8X6
Oil (of)	T65.891	T65.892	T65.893	T65.894	—	—
bitter almond	T62.8X1	T62.8X2	T62.8X3	T62.8X4	—	—
cloves	T49.7X1	T49.7X2	T49.7X3	T49.7X4	T49.7X5	T49.7X6
colors	T65.6X1	T65.6X2	T65.6X3	T65.6X4	—	—
fumes	T59.891	T59.892	T59.893	T59.894	—	—
lubricating	T52.ØX1	T52.ØX2	T52.ØX3	T52.ØX4	—	—
Niobe	T52.8X1	T52.8X2	T52.8X3	T52.8X4	—	—

Substance	Poisoning, Accidental (Unintentional)	Poisoning, Intentional Self-Harm	Poisoning, Assault	Poisoning, Undetermined	Adverse Effect	Underdosing
	External Cause (T-Code)					
Oil (of) *(Continued)*						
vitriol (liquid)	T54.2X1	T54.2X2	T54.2X3	T54.2X4	—	—
fumes	T54.2X1	T54.2X2	T54.2X3	T54.2X4	—	—
wintergreen (bitter) NEC	T49.3X1	T49.3X2	T49.3X3	T49.3X4	T49.3X5	T49.3X6
Oily preparation (for skin)	T49.3X1	T49.3X2	T49.3X3	T49.3X4	T49.3X5	T49.3X6
Ointment NEC	T49.3X1	T49.3X2	T49.3X3	T49.3X4	T49.3X5	T49.3X6
Olanzapine	T43.591	T43.592	T43.593	T43.594	T43.595	T43.596
Oleander	T62.2X1	T62.2X2	T62.2X3	T62.2X4	—	—
Oleandomycin	T36.3X1	T36.3X2	T36.3X3	T36.3X4	T36.3X5	T36.3X6
Oleandrin	T46.ØX1	T46.ØX2	T46.ØX3	T46.ØX4	T46.ØX5	T46.ØX6
Oleic acid	T46.6X1	T46.6X2	T46.6X3	T46.6X4	T46.6X5	T46.6X6
Oleovitamin A	T45.2X1	T45.2X2	T45.2X3	T45.2X4	T45.2X5	T45.2X6
Oleum ricini	T47.2X1	T47.2X2	T47.2X3	T47.2X4	T47.2X5	T47.2X6
Olive oil (medicinal) NEC	T47.4X1	T47.4X2	T47.4X3	T47.4X4	T47.4X5	T47.4X6
Olivomycin	T45.1X1	T45.1X2	T45.1X3	T45.1X4	T45.1X5	T45.1X6
Olsalazine	T47.8X1	T47.8X2	T47.8X3	T47.8X4	T47.8X5	T47.8X6
Omeprazole	T47.1X1	T47.1X2	T47.1X3	T47.1X4	T47.1X5	T47.1X6
OMPA	T6Ø.ØX1	T6Ø.ØX2	T6Ø.ØX3	T6Ø.ØX4	—	—
Ondansetron	T45.ØX1	T45.ØX2	T45.ØX3	T45.ØX4	T45.ØX5	T45.ØX6
Oncovin	T45.1X1	T45.1X2	T45.1X3	T45.1X4	T45.1X5	T45.1X6
Ophthaine	T41.3X1	T41.3X2	T41.3X3	T41.3X4	T41.3X5	T41.3X6
Ophthetic	T41.3X1	T41.3X2	T41.3X3	T41.3X4	T41.3X5	T41.3X6
Opiate NEC	T4Ø.6Ø1	T4Ø.6Ø2	T4Ø.6Ø3	T4Ø.6Ø4	T4Ø.6Ø5	T4Ø.6Ø6
antagonists	T5Ø.7X1	T5Ø.7X2	T5Ø.7X3	T5Ø.7X4	T5Ø.7X5	T5Ø.7X6
Opioid NEC	T4Ø.2X1	T4Ø.2X2	T4Ø.2X3	T4Ø.2X4	T4Ø.2X5	T4Ø.2X6
Opipramol	T43.Ø11	T43.Ø12	T43.Ø13	T43.Ø14	T43.Ø15	T43.Ø16
Opium alkaloids (total)	T4Ø.ØX1	T4Ø.ØX2	T4Ø.ØX3	T4Ø.ØX4	T4Ø.ØX5	T4Ø.ØX6
standardized powdered	T4Ø.ØX1	T4Ø.ØX2	T4Ø.ØX3	T4Ø.ØX4	T4Ø.ØX5	T4Ø.ØX6
tincture (camphorated)	T4Ø.ØX1	T4Ø.ØX2	T4Ø.ØX3	T4Ø.ØX4	T4Ø.ØX5	T4Ø.ØX6
Oracon	T38.4X1	T38.4X2	T38.4X3	T38.4X4	T38.4X5	T38.4X6
Oragrafin	T5Ø.8X1	T5Ø.8X2	T5Ø.8X3	T5Ø.8X4	T5Ø.8X5	T5Ø.8X6
Oral contraceptives	T38.4X1	T38.4X2	T38.4X3	T38.4X4	T38.4X5	T38.4X6
Oral rehydration salts	T5Ø.3X1	T5Ø.3X2	T5Ø.3X3	T5Ø.3X4	T5Ø.3X5	T5Ø.3X6
Orazamide	T5Ø.991	T5Ø.992	T5Ø.993	T5Ø.994	T5Ø.995	T5Ø.996
Orciprenaline	T48.291	T48.292	T48.293	T48.294	T48.295	T48.296
Organidin	T48.4X1	T48.4X2	T48.4X3	T48.4X4	T48.4X5	T48.4X6
Organonitrate NEC	T46.3X1	T46.3X2	T46.3X3	T46.3X4	T46.3X5	T46.3X6
Organophosphates	T6Ø.ØX1	T6Ø.ØX2	T6Ø.ØX3	T6Ø.ØX4	—	—
Orimune	T5Ø.B91	T5Ø.B92	T5Ø.B93	T5Ø.B94	T5Ø.B95	T5Ø.B96
Orinase	T38.3X1	T38.3X2	T38.3X3	T38.3X4	T38.3X5	T38.3X6
Ormeloxifene	T38.6X1	T38.6X2	T38.6X3	T38.6X4	T38.6X5	T38.6X6

Substance	Poisoning, Accidental (Unintentional)	Poisoning, Intentional Self-Harm	Poisoning, Assault	Poisoning, Undetermined	Adverse Effect	Underdosing
	External Cause (T-Code)					
Ornidazole	T37.3X1	T37.3X2	T37.3X3	T37.3X4	T37.3X5	T37.3X6
Ornithine aspartate	T5Ø.991	T5Ø.992	T5Ø.993	T5Ø.994	T5Ø.995	T5Ø.996
Ornoprostil	T47.1X1	T47.1X2	T47.1X3	T47.1X4	T47.1X5	T47.1X6
Orphenadrine (hydrochloride)	T42.8X1	T42.8X2	T42.8X3	T42.8X4	T42.8X5	T42.8X6
Ortal (sodium)	T42.3X1	T42.3X2	T42.3X3	T42.3X4	T42.3X5	T42.3X6
Orthoboric acid	T49.ØX1	T49.ØX2	T49.ØX3	T49.ØX4	T49.ØX5	T49.ØX6
ENT agent	T49.6X1	T49.6X2	T49.6X3	T49.6X4	T49.6X5	T49.6X6
ophthalmic preparation	T49.5X1	T49.5X2	T49.5X3	T49.5X4	T49.5X5	T49.5X6
Orthocaine	T41.3X1	T41.3X2	T41.3X3	T41.3X4	T41.3X5	T41.3X6
Orthodichlorobenzene	T53.7X1	T53.7X2	T53.7X3	T53.7X4	—	—
Ortho-Novum	T38.4X1	T38.4X2	T38.4X3	T38.4X4	T38.4X5	T38.4X6
Orthotolidine (reagent)	T54.2X1	T54.2X2	T54.2X3	T54.2X4	—	—
Osmic acid (liquid)	T54.2X1	T54.2X2	T54.2X3	T54.2X4	—	—
fumes	T54.2X1	T54.2X2	T54.2X3	T54.2X4	—	—
Osmotic diuretics	T5Ø.2X1	T5Ø.2X2	T5Ø.2X3	T5Ø.2X4	T5Ø.2X5	T5Ø.2X6
Otilonium bromide	T44.3X1	T44.3X2	T44.3X3	T44.3X4	T44.3X5	T44.3X6
Otorhinolaryngological drug NEC	T49.6X1	T49.6X2	T49.6X3	T49.6X4	T49.6X5	T49.6X6
Ouabain(e)	T46.ØX1	T46.ØX2	T46.ØX3	T46.ØX4	T46.ØX5	T46.ØX6
Ovarian						
hormone	T38.5X1	T38.5X2	T38.5X3	T38.5X4	T38.5X5	T38.5X6
stimulant	T38.5X1	T38.5X2	T38.5X3	T38.5X4	T38.5X5	T38.5X6
Ovral	T38.4X1	T38.4X2	T38.4X3	T38.4X4	T38.4X5	T38.4X6
Ovulen	T38.4X1	T38.4X2	T38.4X3	T38.4X4	T38.4X5	T38.4X6
Oxacillin	T36.ØX1	T36.ØX2	T36.ØX3	T36.ØX4	T36.ØX5	T36.ØX6
Oxalic acid	T54.2X1	T54.2X2	T54.2X3	T54.2X4	—	—
ammonium salt	T5Ø.991	T5Ø.992	T5Ø.993	T5Ø.994	T5Ø.995	T5Ø.996
Oxamniquine	T37.4X1	T37.4X2	T37.4X3	T37.4X4	T37.4X5	T37.4X6
Oxanamide	T43.591	T43.592	T43.593	T43.594	T43.595	T43.596
Oxandrolone	T38.7X1	T38.7X2	T38.7X3	T38.7X4	T38.7X5	T38.7X6
Oxantel	T37.4X1	T37.4X2	T37.4X3	T37.4X4	T37.4X5	T37.4X6
Oxapium iodide	T44.3X1	T44.3X2	T44.3X3	T44.3X4	T44.3X5	T44.3X6
Oxaprotiline	T43.Ø21	T43.Ø22	T43.Ø23	T43.Ø24	T43.Ø25	T43.Ø26
Oxaprozin	T39.311	T39.312	T39.313	T39.314	T39.315	T39.316
Oxatomide	T45.ØX1	T45.ØX2	T45.ØX3	T45.ØX4	T45.ØX5	T45.ØX6
Oxazepam	T42.4X1	T42.4X2	T42.4X3	T42.4X4	T42.4X5	T42.4X6
Oxazimedrine	T5Ø.5X1	T5Ø.5X2	T5Ø.5X3	T5Ø.5X4	T5Ø.5X5	T5Ø.5X6
Oxazolam	T42.4X1	T42.4X2	T42.4X3	T42.4X4	T42.4X5	T42.4X6
Oxazolidine derivatives	T42.2X1	T42.2X2	T42.2X3	T42.2X4	T42.2X5	T42.2X6
Oxazolidinedione (derivative)	T42.2X1	T42.2X2	T42.2X3	T42.2X4	T42.2X5	T42.2X6
Ox bile extract	T47.5X1	T47.5X2	T47.5X3	T47.5X4	T47.5X5	T47.5X6
Oxcarbazepine	T42.1X1	T42.1X2	T42.1X3	T42.1X4	T42.1X5	T42.1X6
Oxedrine	T44.4X1	T44.4X2	T44.4X3	T44.4X4	T44.4X5	T44.4X6

Substance	Poisoning, Accidental (Unintentional)	Poisoning, Intentional Self-Harm	Poisoning, Assault	Poisoning, Undetermined	Adverse Effect	Underdosing
	External Cause (T-Code)					
Oxeladin (citrate)	T48.3X1	T48.3X2	T48.3X3	T48.3X4	T48.3X5	T48.3X6
Oxendolone	T38.5X1	T38.5X2	T38.5X3	T38.5X4	T38.5X5	T38.5X6
Oxetacaine	T41.3X1	T41.3X2	T41.3X3	T41.3X4	T41.3X5	T41.3X6
Oxethazine	T41.3X1	T41.3X2	T41.3X3	T41.3X4	T41.3X5	T41.3X6
Oxetorone	T39.8X1	T39.8X2	T39.8X3	T39.8X4	T39.8X5	T39.8X6
Oxiconazole	T49.ØX1	T49.ØX2	T49.ØX3	T49.ØX4	T49.ØX5	T49.ØX6
Oxidizing agent NEC	T54.91	T54.92	T54.93	T54.94	—	—
Oxipurinol	T5Ø.4X1	T5Ø.4X2	T5Ø.4X3	T5Ø.4X4	T5Ø.4X5	T5Ø.4X6
Oxitriptan	T43.291	T43.292	T43.293	T43.294	T43.295	T43.296
Oxitropium bromide	T48.6X1	T48.6X2	T48.6X3	T48.6X4	T48.6X5	T48.6X6
Oxodipine	T46.1X1	T46.1X2	T46.1X3	T46.1X4	T46.1X5	T46.1X6
Oxolamine	T48.3X1	T48.3X2	T48.3X3	T48.3X4	T48.3X5	T48.3X6
Oxolinic acid	T37.8X1	T37.8X2	T37.8X3	T37.8X4	T37.8X5	T37.8X6
Oxomemazine	T43.3X1	T43.3X2	T43.3X3	T43.3X4	T43.3X5	T43.3X6
Oxophenarsine	T37.3X1	T37.3X2	T37.3X3	T37.3X4	T37.3X5	T37.3X6
Oxprenolol	T44.7X1	T44.7X2	T44.7X3	T44.7X4	T44.7X5	T44.7X6
Oxsoralen	T49.3X1	T49.3X2	T49.3X3	T49.3X4	T49.3X5	T49.3X6
Oxtriphylline	T48.6X1	T48.6X2	T48.6X3	T48.6X4	T48.6X5	T48.6X6
Oxybate sodium	T41.291	T41.292	T41.293	T41.294	T41.295	T41.296
Oxybuprocaine	T41.3X1	T41.3X2	T41.3X3	T41.3X4	T41.3X5	T41.3X6
Oxybutynin	T44.3X1	T44.3X2	T44.3X3	T44.3X4	T44.3X5	T44.3X6
Oxychlorosene	T49.ØX1	T49.ØX2	T49.ØX3	T49.ØX4	T49.ØX5	T49.ØX6
Oxycodone	T4Ø.2X1	T4Ø.2X2	T4Ø.2X3	T4Ø.2X4	T4Ø.2X5	T4Ø.2X6
Oxyfedrine	T46.3X1	T46.3X2	T46.3X3	T46.3X4	T46.3X5	T46.3X6
Oxygen	T41.5X1	T41.5X2	T41.5X3	T41.5X4	T41.5X5	T41.5X6
Oxylone	T49.ØX1	T49.ØX2	T49.ØX3	T49.ØX4	T49.ØX5	T49.ØX6
ophthalmic preparation	T49.5X1	T49.5X2	T49.5X3	T49.5X4	T49.5X5	T49.5X6
Oxymesterone	T38.7X1	T38.7X2	T38.7X3	T38.7X4	T38.7X5	T38.7X6
Oxymetazoline	T48.5X1	T48.5X2	T48.5X3	T48.5X4	T48.5X5	T48.5X6
Oxymetholone	T38.7X1	T38.7X2	T38.7X3	T38.7X4	T38.7X5	T38.7X6
Oxymorphone	T4Ø.2X1	T4Ø.2X2	T4Ø.2X3	T4Ø.2X4	T4Ø.2X5	T4Ø.2X6
Oxypertine	T43.591	T43.592	T43.593	T43.594	T43.595	T43.596
Oxyphenbutazone	T39.2X1	T39.2X2	T39.2X3	T39.2X4	T39.2X5	T39.2X6
Oxyphencyclimine	T44.3X1	T44.3X2	T44.3X3	T44.3X4	T44.3X5	T44.3X6
Oxyphenisatine	T47.2X1	T47.2X2	T47.2X3	T47.2X4	T47.2X5	T47.2X6
Oxyphenonium bromide	T44.3X1	T44.3X2	T44.3X3	T44.3X4	T44.3X5	T44.3X6
Oxypolygelatin	T45.8X1	T45.8X2	T45.8X3	T45.8X4	T45.8X5	T45.8X6
Oxyquinoline (derivatives)	T37.8X1	T37.8X2	T37.8X3	T37.8X4	T37.8X5	T37.8X6
Oxytetracycline	T36.4X1	T36.4X2	T36.4X3	T36.4X4	T36.4X5	T36.4X6
Oxytocic drug NEC	T48.ØX1	T48.ØX2	T48.ØX3	T48.ØX4	T48.ØX5	T48.ØX6
Oxytocin (synthetic)	T48.ØX1	T48.ØX2	T48.ØX3	T48.ØX4	T48.ØX5	T48.ØX6
Ozone	T59.891	T59.892	T59.893	T59.894	—	—

Substance	Poisoning, Accidental (Unintentional)	Poisoning, Intentional Self-Harm	Poisoning, Assault	Poisoning, Undetermined	Adverse Effect	Underdosing
	External Cause (T-Code)					
P						
PABA	T49.3X1	T49.3X2	T49.3X3	T49.3X4	T49.3X5	T49.3X6
Packed red cells	T45.8X1	T45.8X2	T45.8X3	T45.8X4	T45.8X5	T45.8X6
Padimate	T49.3X1	T49.3X2	T49.3X3	T49.3X4	T49.3X5	T49.3X6
Paint NEC	T65.6X1	T65.6X2	T65.6X3	T65.6X4	—	—
cleaner	T52.91	T52.92	T52.93	T52.94	—	—
fumes NEC	T59.891	T59.892	T59.893	T59.894	—	—
lead (fumes)	T56.0X1	T56.0X2	T56.0X3	T56.0X4	—	—
solvent NEC	T52.8X1	T52.8X2	T52.8X3	T52.8X4	—	—
stripper	T52.8X1	T52.8X2	T52.8X3	T52.8X4	—	—
Palfium	T40.2X1	T40.2X2	T40.2X3	T40.2X4	—	—
Palm kernel oil	T50.991	T50.992	T50.993	T50.994	T50.995	T50.996
Paludrine	T37.2X1	T37.2X2	T37.2X3	T37.2X4	T37.2X5	T37.2X6
PAM (pralidoxime)	T50.6X1	T50.6X2	T50.6X3	T50.6X4	T50.6X5	T50.6X6
Pamaquine (naphthoute)	T37.2X1	T37.2X2	T37.2X3	T37.2X4	T37.2X5	T37.2X6
Panadol	T39.1X1	T39.1X2	T39.1X3	T39.1X4	T39.1X5	T39.1X6
Pancreatic						
digestive secretion stimulant	T47.8X1	T47.8X2	T47.8X3	T47.8X4	T47.8X5	T47.8X6
dornase	T45.3X1	T45.3X2	T45.3X3	T45.3X4	T45.3X5	T45.3X6
Pancreatin	T47.5X1	T47.5X2	T47.5X3	T47.5X4	T47.5X5	T47.5X6
Pancrelipase	T47.5X1	T47.5X2	T47.5X3	T47.5X4	T47.5X5	T47.5X6
Pancuronium (bromide)	T48.1X1	T48.1X2	T48.1X3	T48.1X4	T48.1X5	T48.1X6
Pangamic acid	T45.2X1	T45.2X2	T45.2X3	T45.2X4	T45.2X5	T45.2X6
Panthenol	T45.2X1	T45.2X2	T45.2X3	T45.2X4	T45.2X5	T45.2X6
topical	T49.8X1	T49.8X2	T49.8X3	T49.8X4	T49.8X5	T49.8X6
Pantopon	T40.0X1	T40.0X2	T40.0X3	T40.0X4	T40.0X5	T40.0X6
Pantothenic acid	T45.2X1	T45.2X2	T45.2X3	T45.2X4	T45.2X5	T45.2X6
Panwarfin	T45.511	T45.512	T45.513	T45.514	T45.515	T45.516
Papain	T47.5X1	T47.5X2	T47.5X3	T47.5X4	T47.5X5	T47.5X6
digestant	T47.5X1	T47.5X2	T47.5X3	T47.5X4	T47.5X5	T47.5X6
Papaveretum	T40.0X1	T40.0X2	T40.0X3	T40.0X4	T40.0X5	T40.0X6
Papaverine	T44.3X1	T44.3X2	T44.3X3	T44.3X4	T44.3X5	T44.3X6
Para-acetamidophenol	T39.1X1	T39.1X2	T39.1X3	T39.1X4	T39.1X5	T39.1X6
Para-aminobenzoic acid	T49.3X1	T49.3X2	T49.3X3	T49.3X4	T49.3X5	T49.3X6
Para-aminophenol derivatives	T39.1X1	T39.1X2	T39.1X3	T39.1X4	T39.1X5	T39.1X6
Para-aminosalicylic acid	T37.1X1	T37.1X2	T37.1X3	T37.1X4	T37.1X5	T37.1X6
Paracetaldehyde	T42.6X1	T42.6X2	T42.6X3	T42.6X4	T42.6X5	T42.6X6
Paracetamol	T39.1X1	T39.1X2	T39.1X3	T39.1X4	T39.1X5	T39.1X6
Parachlorophenol (camphorated)	T49.0X1	T49.0X2	T49.0X3	T49.0X4	T49.0X5	T49.0X6
Paracodin	T40.2X1	T40.2X2	T40.2X3	T40.2X4	T40.2X5	T40.2X6
Paradione	T42.2X1	T42.2X2	T42.2X3	T42.2X4	T42.2X5	T42.2X6

Substance	Poisoning, Accidental (Unintentional)	Poisoning, Intentional Self-Harm	Poisoning, Assault	Poisoning, Undetermined	Adverse Effect	Underdosing
	External Cause (T-Code)					
Paraffin(s) (wax)	T52.0X1	T52.0X2	T52.0X3	T52.0X4	—	—
liquid (medicinal)	T47.4X1	T47.4X2	T47.4X3	T47.4X4	T47.4X5	T47.4X6
nonmedicinal	T52.0X1	T52.0X2	T52.0X3	T52.0X4	—	—
Paraformaldehyde	T60.3X1	T60.3X2	T60.3X3	T60.3X4	—	—
Paraldehyde	T42.6X1	T42.6X2	T42.6X3	T42.6X4	T42.6X5	T42.6X6
Paramethadione	T42.2X1	T42.2X2	T42.2X3	T42.2X4	T42.2X5	T42.2X6
Paramethasone	T38.0X1	T38.0X2	T38.0X3	T38.0X4	T38.0X5	T38.0X6
acetate	T49.0X1	T49.0X2	T49.0X3	T49.0X4	T49.0X5	T49.0X6
Paraoxon	T60.0X1	T60.0X2	T60.0X3	T60.0X4	—	—
Paraquat	T60.3X1	T60.3X2	T60.3X3	T60.3X4	—	—
Parasympatholytic NEC	T44.3X1	T44.3X2	T44.3X3	T44.3X4	T44.3X5	T44.3X6
Parasympathomimetic drug NEC	T44.1X1	T44.1X2	T44.1X3	T44.1X4	T44.1X5	T44.1X6
Parathion	T60.0X1	T60.0X2	T60.0X3	T60.0X4	—	—
Parathormone	T50.991	T50.992	T50.993	T50.994	T50.995	T50.996
Parathyroid extract	T50.991	T50.992	T50.993	T50.994	T50.995	T50.996
Paratyphoid vaccine	T50.A91	T50.A92	T50.A93	T50.A94	T50.A95	T50.A96
Paredrine	T44.4X1	T44.4X2	T44.4X3	T44.4X4	T44.4X5	T44.4X6
Paregoric	T40.0X1	T40.0X2	T40.0X3	T40.0X4	T40.0X5	T40.0X6
Pargyline	T46.5X1	T46.5X2	T46.5X3	T46.5X4	T46.5X5	T46.5X6
Paris green	T57.0X1	T57.0X2	T57.0X3	T57.0X4	—	—
insecticide	T57.0X1	T57.0X2	T57.0X3	T57.0X4	—	—
Parnate	T43.1X1	T43.1X2	T43.1X3	T43.1X4	T43.1X5	T43.1X6
Paromomycin	T36.5X1	T36.5X2	T36.5X3	T36.5X4	T36.5X5	T36.5X6
Paroxypropione	T45.1X1	T45.1X2	T45.1X3	T45.1X4	T45.1X5	T45.1X6
Parzone	T40.2X1	T40.2X2	T40.2X3	T40.2X4	T40.2X5	T40.2X6
PAS	T37.1X1	T37.1X2	T37.1X3	T37.1X4	T37.1X5	T37.1X6
Pasiniazid	T37.1X1	T37.1X2	T37.1X3	T37.1X4	T37.1X5	T37.1X6
PBB (polybrominated biphenyls)	T65.891	T65.892	T65.893	T65.894	—	—
PCB	T65.891	T65.892	T65.893	T65.894	—	—
PCP						
meaning pentachlorophenol	T60.1X1	T60.1X2	T60.1X3	T60.1X4	—	—
fungicide	T60.3X1	T60.3X2	T60.3X3	T60.3X4	—	—
herbicide	T60.3X1	T60.3X2	T60.3X3	T60.3X4	—	—
insecticide	T60.1X1	T60.1X2	T60.1X3	T60.1X4	—	—
meaning phencyclidine	T40.991	T40.992	T40.993	T40.994	—	—
Peach kernel oil (emulsion)	T47.4X1	T47.4X2	T47.4X3	T47.4X4	T47.4X5	T47.4X6
Peanut oil (emulsion) NEC	T47.4X1	T47.4X2	T47.4X3	T47.4X4	T47.4X5	T47.4X6
topical	T49.3X1	T49.3X2	T49.3X3	T49.3X4	T49.3X5	T49.3X6
Pearly Gates (morning glory seeds)	T40.991	T40.992	T40.993	T40.994	—	—
Pecazine	T43.3X1	T43.3X2	T43.3X3	T43.3X4	T43.3X5	T43.3X6
Pectin	T47.6X1	T47.6X2	T47.6X3	T47.6X4	T47.6X5	T47.6X6

	External Cause (T-Code)					
Substance	Poisoning, Accidental (Unintentional)	Poisoning, Intentional Self-Harm	Poisoning, Assault	Poisoning, Undetermined	Adverse Effect	Underdosing
Pefloxacin	T37.8X1	T37.8X2	T37.8X3	T37.8X4	T37.8X5	T37.8X6
Pegademase, bovine	T5Ø.Z91	T5Ø.Z92	T5Ø.Z93	T5Ø.Z94	T5Ø.Z95	T5Ø.Z96
Pelletierine tannate	T37.4X1	T37.4X2	T37.4X3	T37.4X4	T37.4X5	T37.4X6
Pemirolast (potassium)	T48.6X1	T48.6X2	T48.6X3	T48.6X4	T48.6X5	T48.6X6
Pemoline	T5Ø.7X1	T5Ø.7X2	T5Ø.7X3	T5Ø.7X4	T5Ø.7X5	T5Ø.7X6
Pempidine	T44.2X1	T44.2X2	T44.2X3	T44.2X4	T44.2X5	T44.2X6
Penamecillin	T36.ØX1	T36.ØX2	T36.ØX3	T36.ØX4	T36.ØX5	T36.ØX6
Penbutolol	T44.7X1	T44.7X2	T44.7X3	T44.7X4	T44.7X5	T44.7X6
Penethamate	T36.ØX1	T36.ØX2	T36.ØX3	T36.ØX4	T36.ØX5	T36.ØX6
Penfluridol	T43.591	T43.592	T43.593	T43.594	T43.595	T43.596
Penflutizide	T5Ø.2X1	T5Ø.2X2	T5Ø.2X3	T5Ø.2X4	T5Ø.2X5	T5Ø.2X6
Pengitoxin	T46.ØX1	T46.ØX2	T46.ØX3	T46.ØX4	T46.ØX5	T46.ØX6
Penicillamine	T5Ø.6X1	T5Ø.6X2	T5Ø.6X3	T5Ø.6X4	T5Ø.6X5	T5Ø.6X6
Penicillin (any)	T36.ØX1	T36.ØX2	T36.ØX3	T36.ØX4	T36.ØX5	T36.ØX6
Penicillinase	T45.3X1	T45.3X2	T45.3X3	T45.3X4	T45.3X5	T45.3X6
Penicilloyl polylysine	T5Ø.8X1	T5Ø.8X2	T5Ø.8X3	T5Ø.8X4	T5Ø.8X5	T5Ø.8X6
Penimepicycline	T36.4X1	T36.4X2	T36.4X3	T36.4X4	T36.4X5	T36.4X6
Pentachloroethane	T53.6X1	T53.6X2	T53.6X3	T53.6X4	—	—
Pentachloronaphthalene	T53.7X1	T53.7X2	T53.7X3	T53.7X4	—	—
Pentachlorophenol (pesticide)	T6Ø.1X1	T6Ø.1X2	T6Ø.1X3	T6Ø.1X4	—	—
fungicide	T6Ø.3X1	T6Ø.3X2	T6Ø.3X3	T6Ø.3X4	—	—
herbicide	T6Ø.3X1	T6Ø.3X2	T6Ø.3X3	T6Ø.3X4	—	—
insecticide	T6Ø.1X1	T6Ø.1X2	T6Ø.1X3	T6Ø.1X4	—	—
Pentaerythritol tetranitrate	T46.3X1	T46.3X2	T46.3X3	T46.3X4	T46.3X5	T46.3X6
Pentaerythritol	T46.3X1	T46.3X2	T46.3X3	T46.3X4	T46.3X5	T46.3X6
chloral	T42.6X1	T42.6X2	T42.6X3	T42.6X4	T42.6X5	T42.6X6
tetranitrate NEC	T46.3X1	T46.3X2	T46.3X3	T46.3X4	T46.3X5	T46.3X6
Pentagastrin	T5Ø.8X1	T5Ø.8X2	T5Ø.8X3	T5Ø.8X4	T5Ø.8X5	T5Ø.8X6
Pentalin	T53.6X1	T53.6X2	T53.6X3	T53.6X4	—	—
Pentamethonium bromide	T44.2X1	T44.2X2	T44.2X3	T44.2X4	T44.2X5	T44.2X6
Pentamidine	T37.3X1	T37.3X2	T37.3X3	T37.3X4	T37.3X5	T37.3X6
Pentanol	T51.3X1	T51.3X2	T51.3X3	T51.3X4	—	—
Pentapyrrolinium (bitartrate)	T44.2X1	T44.2X2	T44.2X3	T44.2X4	T44.2X5	T44.2X6
Pentaquine	T37.2X1	T37.2X2	T37.2X3	T37.2X4	T37.2X5	T37.2X6
Pentazocine	T4Ø.4X1	T4Ø.4X2	T4Ø.4X3	T4Ø.4X4	T4Ø.4X5	T4Ø.4X6
Pentetrazole	T5Ø.7X1	T5Ø.7X2	T5Ø.7X3	T5Ø.7X4	T5Ø.7X5	T5Ø.7X6
Penthienate bromide	T44.3X1	T44.3X2	T44.3X3	T44.3X4	T44.3X5	T44.3X6
Pentifylline	T46.7X1	T46.7X2	T46.7X3	T46.7X4	T46.7X5	T46.7X6
Pentobarbital	T42.3X1	T42.3X2	T42.3X3	T42.3X4	T42.3X5	T42.3X6
sodium	T42.3X1	T42.3X2	T42.3X3	T42.3X4	T42.3X5	T42.3X6
Pentobarbitone	T42.3X1	T42.3X2	T42.3X3	T42.3X4	T42.3X5	T42.3X6
Pentolonium tartrate	T44.2X1	T44.2X2	T44.2X3	T44.2X4	T44.2X5	T44.2X6
Pentosan polysulfate (sodium)	T39.8X1	T39.8X2	T39.8X3	T39.8X4	T39.8X5	T39.8X6
Pentostatin	T45.1X1	T45.1X2	T45.1X3	T45.1X4	T45.1X5	T45.1X6
Pentothal	T41.1X1	T41.1X2	T41.1X3	T41.1X4	T41.1X5	T41.1X6
Pentoxifylline	T46.7X1	T46.7X2	T46.7X3	T46.7X4	T46.7X5	T46.7X6
Pentoxyverine	T48.3X1	T48.3X2	T48.3X3	T48.3X4	T48.3X5	T48.3X6
Pentrinat	T46.3X1	T46.3X2	T46.3X3	T46.3X4	T46.3X5	T46.3X6
Pentylenetetrazole	T5Ø.7X1	T5Ø.7X2	T5Ø.7X3	T5Ø.7X4	T5Ø.7X5	T5Ø.7X6
Pentylsalicylamide	T37.1X1	T37.1X2	T37.1X3	T37.1X4	T37.1X5	T37.1X6
Pentymal	T42.3X1	T42.3X2	T42.3X3	T42.3X4	T42.3X5	T42.3X6
Peplomycin	T45.1X1	T45.1X2	T45.1X3	T45.1X4	T45.1X5	T45.1X6
Peppermint (oil)	T47.5X1	T47.5X2	T47.5X3	T47.5X4	T47.5X5	T47.5X6
Pepsin	T47.5X1	T47.5X2	T47.5X3	T47.5X4	T47.5X5	T47.5X6
digestant	T47.5X1	T47.5X2	T47.5X3	T47.5X4	T47.5X5	T47.5X6
Pepstatin	T47.1X1	T47.1X2	T47.1X3	T47.1X4	T47.1X5	T47.1X6
Peptavlon	T5Ø.8X1	T5Ø.8X2	T5Ø.8X3	T5Ø.8X4	T5Ø.8X5	T5Ø.8X6
Perazine	T43.3X1	T43.3X2	T43.3X3	T43.3X4	T43.3X5	T43.3X6
Percaine (spinal)	T41.3X1	T41.3X2	T41.3X3	T41.3X4	T41.3X5	T41.3X6
topical (surface)	T41.3X1	T41.3X2	T41.3X3	T41.3X4	T41.3X5	T41.3X6
Perchloroethylene	T53.3X1	T53.3X2	T53.3X3	T53.3X4	—	—
medicinal	T37.4X1	T37.4X2	T37.4X3	T37.4X4	T37.4X5	T37.4X6
vapor	T53.3X1	T53.3X2	T53.3X3	T53.3X4	—	—
Percodan	T4Ø.2X1	T4Ø.2X2	T4Ø.2X3	T4Ø.2X4	T4Ø.2X5	T4Ø.2X6
Percogesic — *see also* *Acetaminophen*	T45.ØX1	T45.ØX2	T45.ØX3	T45.ØX4	T45.ØX5	T45.ØX6
Percorten	T38.ØX1	T38.ØX2	T38.ØX3	T38.ØX4	T38.ØX5	T38.ØX6
Pergolide	T42.8X1	T42.8X2	T42.8X3	T42.8X4	T42.8X5	T42.8X6
Pergonal	T38.811	T38.812	T38.813	T38.814	T38.815	T38.816
Perhexilene	T46.3X1	T46.3X2	T46.3X3	T46.3X4	T46.3X5	T46.3X6
Perhexiline (maleate)	T46.3X1	T46.3X2	T46.3X3	T46.3X4	T46.3X5	T46.3X6
Periactin	T45.ØX1	T45.ØX2	T45.ØX3	T45.ØX4	T45.ØX5	T45.ØX6
Periciazine	T43.3X1	T43.3X2	T43.3X3	T43.3X4	T43.3X5	T43.3X6
Periclor	T42.6X1	T42.6X2	T42.6X3	T42.6X4	T42.6X5	T42.6X6
Perindopril	T46.4X1	T46.4X2	T46.4X3	T46.4X4	T46.4X5	T46.4X6
Perisoxal	T39.8X1	T39.8X2	T39.8X3	T39.8X4	T39.8X5	T39.8X6
Peritrate	T46.3X1	T46.3X2	T46.3X3	T46.3X4	T46.3X5	T46.3X6
Peritoneal dialysis solution	T5Ø.3X1	T5Ø.3X2	T5Ø.3X3	T5Ø.3X4	T5Ø.3X5	T5Ø.3X6
Perlapine	T42.4X1	T42.4X2	T42.4X3	T42.4X4	T42.4X5	T42.4X6
Permanganate	T65.891	T65.892	T65.893	T65.894	—	—
Permethrin	T6Ø.1X1	T6Ø.1X2	T6Ø.1X3	T6Ø.1X4	—	—
Pernocton	T42.3X1	T42.3X2	T42.3X3	T42.3X4	T42.3X5	T42.3X6
Pernoston	T42.3X1	T42.3X2	T42.3X3	T42.3X4	T42.3X5	T42.3X6
Peronine	T4Ø.2X1	T4Ø.2X2	T4Ø.2X3	T4Ø.2X4	—	—
Perphenazine	T43.3X1	T43.3X2	T43.3X3	T43.3X4	T43.3X5	T43.3X6

◀ New ◀ Revised ~~deleted~~ Deleted

Substance	External Cause (T-Code)					
	Poisoning, Accidental (Unintentional)	Poisoning, Intentional Self-Harm	Poisoning, Assault	Poisoning, Undetermined	Adverse Effect	Underdosing
Pertofrane	T43.Ø11	T43.Ø12	T43.Ø13	T43.Ø14	T43.Ø15	T43.Ø16
Pertussis						
immune serum (human)	T5Ø.Z11	T5Ø.Z12	T5Ø.Z13	T5Ø.Z14	T5Ø.Z15	T5Ø.Z16
vaccine (with diphtheria toxoid) (with tetanus toxoid)	T5Ø.A11	T5Ø.A12	T5Ø.A13	T5Ø.A14	T5Ø.A15	T5Ø.A16
Peruvian balsam	T49.ØX1	T49.ØX2	T49.ØX3	T49.ØX4	T49.ØX5	T49.ØX6
Peruvoside	T46.ØX1	T46.ØX2	T46.ØX3	T46.ØX4	T46.ØX5	T46.ØX6
Pesticide (dust) (fumes) (vapor) NEC	T6Ø.91	T6Ø.92	T6Ø.93	T6Ø.94	—	—
arsenic	T57.ØX1	T57.ØX2	T57.ØX3	T57.ØX4	—	—
chlorinated	T6Ø.1X1	T6Ø.1X2	T6Ø.1X3	T6Ø.1X4	—	—
cyanide	T65.ØX1	T65.ØX2	T65.ØX3	T65.ØX4	—	—
kerosene	T52.ØX1	T52.ØX2	T52.ØX3	T52.ØX4	—	—
mixture (of compounds)	T6Ø.91	T6Ø.92	T6Ø.93	T6Ø.94	—	—
naphthalene	T6Ø.2X1	T6Ø.2X2	T6Ø.2X3	T6Ø.2X4	—	—
organochlorine (compounds)	T6Ø.1X1	T6Ø.1X2	T6Ø.1X3	T6Ø.1X4	—	—
petroleum (distillate) (products) NEC	T6Ø.8X1	T6Ø.8X2	T6Ø.8X3	T6Ø.8X4	—	—
specified ingredient NEC	T6Ø.8X1	T6Ø.8X2	T6Ø.8X3	T6Ø.8X4	—	—
strychnine	T65.1X1	T65.1X2	T65.1X3	T65.1X4	—	—
thallium	T6Ø.4X1	T6Ø.4X2	T6Ø.4X3	T6Ø.4X4	—	—
Pethidine	T4Ø.4X1	T4Ø.4X2	T4Ø.4X3	T4Ø.4X4	T4Ø.4X5	T4Ø.4X6
Petrichloral	T42.6X1	T42.6X2	T42.6X3	T42.6X4	T42.6X5	T42.6X6
Petrol	T52.ØX1	T52.ØX2	T52.ØX3	T52.ØX4	—	—
vapor	T52.ØX1	T52.ØX2	T52.ØX3	T52.ØX4	—	—
Petrolatum	T49.3X1	T49.3X2	T49.3X3	T49.3X4	T49.3X5	T49.3X6
hydrophilic	T49.3X1	T49.3X2	T49.3X3	T49.3X4	T49.3X5	T49.3X6
liquid	T47.4X1	T47.4X2	T47.4X3	T47.4X4	T47.4X5	T47.4X6
topical	T49.3X1	T49.3X2	T49.3X3	T49.3X4	T49.3X5	T49.3X6
nonmedicinal	T52.ØX1	T52.ØX2	T52.ØX3	T52.ØX4	—	—
red veterinary	T49.3X1	T49.3X2	T49.3X3	T49.3X4	T49.3X5	T49.3X6
white	T49.3X1	T49.3X2	T49.3X3	T49.3X4	T49.3X5	T49.3X6
Petroleum (products) NEC	T52.ØX1	T52.ØX2	T52.ØX3	T52.ØX4	—	—
benzine(s) — *see Ligroin*						
ether — *see Ligroin*						
jelly — *see Petrolatum*						
naphtha — *see Ligroin*						
pesticide	T6Ø.8X1	T6Ø.8X2	T6Ø.8X3	T6Ø.8X4	—	—
solids	T52.ØX1	T52.ØX2	T52.ØX3	T52.ØX4	—	—
solvents	T52.ØX1	T52.ØX2	T52.ØX3	T52.ØX4	—	—
vapor	T52.ØX1	T52.ØX2	T52.ØX3	T52.ØX4	—	—
Peyote	T4Ø.991	T4Ø.992	T4Ø.993	T4Ø.994	—	—
Phanodorm, phanodorn	T42.3X1	T42.3X2	T42.3X3	T42.3X4	T42.3X5	T42.3X6

Substance	External Cause (T-Code)					
	Poisoning, Accidental (Unintentional)	Poisoning, Intentional Self-Harm	Poisoning, Assault	Poisoning, Undetermined	Adverse Effect	Underdosing
Phanquinone	T37.3X1	T37.3X2	T37.3X3	T37.3X4	T37.3X5	T37.3X6
Phanquone	T37.3X1	T37.3X2	T37.3X3	T37.3X4	T37.3X5	T37.3X6
Pharmaceutical						
adjunct NEC	T5Ø.9Ø1	T5Ø.9Ø2	T5Ø.9Ø3	T5Ø.9Ø4	T5Ø.9Ø5	T5Ø.9Ø6
excipient NEC	T5Ø.9Ø1	T5Ø.9Ø2	T5Ø.9Ø3	T5Ø.9Ø4	T5Ø.9Ø5	T5Ø.9Ø6
sweetener	T5Ø.9Ø1	T5Ø.9Ø2	T5Ø.9Ø3	T5Ø.9Ø4	T5Ø.9Ø5	T5Ø.9Ø6
viscous agent	T5Ø.9Ø1	T5Ø.9Ø2	T5Ø.9Ø3	T5Ø.9Ø4	T5Ø.9Ø5	T5Ø.9Ø6
Phemitone	T42.3X1	T42.3X2	T42.3X3	T42.3X4	T42.3X5	T42.3X6
Phenacaine	T41.3X1	T41.3X2	T41.3X3	T41.3X4	T41.3X5	T41.3X6
Phenacemide	T42.6X1	T42.6X2	T42.6X3	T42.6X4	T42.6X5	T42.6X6
Phenacetin	T39.1X1	T39.1X2	T39.1X3	T39.1X4	T39.1X5	T39.1X6
Phenadoxone	T4Ø.2X1	T4Ø.2X2	T4Ø.2X3	T4Ø.2X4	—	—
Phenaglycodol	T43.591	T43.592	T43.593	T43.594	T43.595	T43.596
Phenantoin	T42.ØX1	T42.ØX2	T42.ØX3	T42.ØX4	T42.ØX5	T42.ØX6
Phenaphthazine reagent	T5Ø.991	T5Ø.992	T5Ø.993	T5Ø.994	T5Ø.995	T5Ø.996
Phenazocine	T4Ø.4X1	T4Ø.4X2	T4Ø.4X3	T4Ø.4X4	T4Ø.4X5	T4Ø.4X6
Phenazone	T39.2X1	T39.2X2	T39.2X3	T39.2X4	T39.2X5	T39.2X6
Phenazopyridine	T39.8X1	T39.8X2	T39.8X3	T39.8X4	T39.8X5	T39.8X6
Phenbenicillin	T36.ØX1	T36.ØX2	T36.ØX3	T36.ØX4	T36.ØX5	T36.ØX6
Phenbutrazate	T5Ø.5X1	T5Ø.5X2	T5Ø.5X3	T5Ø.5X4	T5Ø.5X5	T5Ø.5X6
Phencyclidine	T4Ø.991	T4Ø.992	T4Ø.993	T4Ø.994	T4Ø.995	T4Ø.996
Phendimetrazine	T5Ø.5X1	T5Ø.5X2	T5Ø.5X3	T5Ø.5X4	T5Ø.5X5	T5Ø.5X6
Phenelzine	T43.1X1	T43.1X2	T43.1X3	T43.1X4	T43.1X5	T43.1X6
Phenemal	T42.3X1	T42.3X2	T42.3X3	T42.3X4	T42.3X5	T42.3X6
Phenergan	T42.6X1	T42.6X2	T42.6X3	T42.6X4	T42.6X5	T42.6X6
Pheneticillin	T36.ØX1	T36.ØX2	T36.ØX3	T36.ØX4	T36.ØX5	T36.ØX6
Pheneturide	T42.6X1	T42.6X2	T42.6X3	T42.6X4	T42.6X5	T42.6X6
Phenformin	T38.3X1	T38.3X2	T38.3X3	T38.3X4	T38.3X5	T38.3X6
Phenglutarimide	T44.3X1	T44.3X2	T44.3X3	T44.3X4	T44.3X5	T44.3X6
Phenicarbazide	T39.8X1	T39.8X2	T39.8X3	T39.8X4	T39.8X5	T39.8X6
Phenindamine	T45.ØX1	T45.ØX2	T45.ØX3	T45.ØX4	T45.ØX5	T45.ØX6
Phenindione	T45.511	T45.512	T45.513	T45.514	T45.515	T45.516
Pheniprazine	T43.1X1	T43.1X2	T43.1X3	T43.1X4	T43.1X5	T43.1X6
Pheniramine	T45.ØX1	T45.ØX2	T45.ØX3	T45.ØX4	T45.ØX5	T45.ØX6
Phenisatin	T47.2X1	T47.2X2	T47.2X3	T47.2X4	T47.2X5	T47.2X6
Phenmetrazine	T5Ø.5X1	T5Ø.5X2	T5Ø.5X3	T5Ø.5X4	T5Ø.5X5	T5Ø.5X6
Phenobal	T42.3X1	T42.3X2	T42.3X3	T42.3X4	T42.3X5	T42.3X6
Phenobarbital	T42.3X1	T42.3X2	T42.3X3	T42.3X4	T42.3X5	T42.3X6
with						
mephenytoin	T42.3X1	T42.3X2	T42.3X3	T42.3X4	T42.3X5	T42.3X6
phenytoin	T42.3X1	T42.3X2	T42.3X3	T42.3X4	T42.3X5	T42.3X6
sodium	T42.3X1	T42.3X2	T42.3X3	T42.3X4	T42.3X5	T42.3X6

Substance	Poisoning, Accidental (Unintentional)	Poisoning, Intentional Self-Harm	Poisoning, Assault	Poisoning, Undetermined	Adverse Effect	Underdosing
	External Cause (T-Code)					
Phenobarbitone	T42.3X1	T42.3X2	T42.3X3	T42.3X4	T42.3X5	T42.3X6
Phenobutiodil	T50.8X1	T50.8X2	T50.8X3	T50.8X4	T50.8X5	T50.8X6
Phenoctide	T49.0X1	T49.0X2	T49.0X3	T49.0X4	T49.0X5	T49.0X6
Phenol	T49.0X1	T49.0X2	T49.0X3	T49.0X4	T49.0X5	T49.0X6
disinfectant	T54.0X1	T54.0X2	T54.0X3	T54.0X4	—	—
in oil injection	T46.8X1	T46.8X2	T46.8X3	T46.8X4	T46.8X5	T46.8X6
medicinal	T49.1X1	T49.1X2	T49.1X3	T49.1X4	T49.1X5	T49.1X6
nonmedicinal NEC	T54.0X1	T54.0X2	T54.0X3	T54.0X4	—	—
pesticide	T60.8X1	T60.8X2	T60.8X3	T60.8X4	—	—
red	T50.8X1	T50.8X2	T50.8X3	T50.8X4	T50.8X5	T50.8X6
Phenolic preparation	T49.1X1	T49.1X2	T49.1X3	T49.1X4	T49.1X5	T49.1X6
Phenolphthalein	T47.2X1	T47.2X2	T47.2X3	T47.2X4	T47.2X5	T47.2X6
Phenolsulfonphthalein	T50.8X1	T50.8X2	T50.8X3	T50.8X4	T50.8X5	T50.8X6
Phenomorphan	T40.2X1	T40.2X2	T40.2X3	T40.2X4	—	—
Phenonyl	T42.3X1	T42.3X2	T42.3X3	T42.3X4	T42.3X5	T42.3X6
Phenoperidine	T40.4X1	T40.4X2	T40.4X3	T40.4X4	—	—
Phenopyrazone	T46.991	T46.992	T46.993	T46.994	T46.995	T46.996
Phenoquin	T50.4X1	T50.4X2	T50.4X3	T50.4X4	T50.4X5	T50.4X6
Phenothiazine (psychotropic) NEC	T43.3X1	T43.3X2	T43.3X3	T43.3X4	T43.3X5	T43.3X6
insecticide	T60.2X1	T60.2X2	T60.2X3	T60.2X4	—	—
Phenothrin	T49.0X1	T49.0X2	T49.0X3	T49.0X4	T49.0X5	T49.0X6
Phenoxybenzamine	T46.7X1	T46.7X2	T46.7X3	T46.7X4	T46.7X5	T46.7X6
Phenoxyethanol	T49.0X1	T49.0X2	T49.0X3	T49.0X4	T49.0X5	T49.0X6
Phenoxymethyl penicillin	T36.0X1	T36.0X2	T36.0X3	T36.0X4	T36.0X5	T36.0X6
Phenprobamate	T42.8X1	T42.8X2	T42.8X3	T42.8X4	T42.8X5	T42.8X6
Phenprocoumon	T45.511	T45.512	T45.513	T45.514	T45.515	T45.516
Phensuximide	T42.2X1	T42.2X2	T42.2X3	T42.2X4	T42.2X5	T42.2X6
Phentermine	T50.5X1	T50.5X2	T50.5X3	T50.5X4	T50.5X5	T50.5X6
Phenthicillin	T36.0X1	T36.0X2	T36.0X3	T36.0X4	T36.0X5	T36.0X6
Phentolamine	T46.7X1	T46.7X2	T46.7X3	T46.7X4	T46.7X5	T46.7X6
Phenyl						
butazone	T39.2X1	T39.2X2	T39.2X3	T39.2X4	T39.2X5	T39.2X6
enediamine	T65.3X1	T65.3X2	T65.3X3	T65.3X4	—	—
hydrazine	T65.3X1	T65.3X2	T65.3X3	T65.3X4	—	—
antineoplastic	T45.1X1	T45.1X2	T45.1X3	T45.1X4	T45.1X5	T45.1X6
mercuric compounds — *see Mercury*						
salicylate	T49.3X1	T49.3X2	T49.3X3	T49.3X4	T49.3X5	T49.3X6
Phenylalanine mustard	T45.1X1	T45.1X2	T45.1X3	T45.1X4	T45.1X5	T45.1X6
Phenylbutazone	T39.2X1	T39.2X2	T39.2X3	T39.2X4	T39.2X5	T39.2X6
Phenylenediamine	T65.3X1	T65.3X2	T65.3X3	T65.3X4	—	—
Phenylephrine	T44.4X1	T44.4X2	T44.4X3	T44.4X4	T44.4X5	T44.4X6

Substance	Poisoning, Accidental (Unintentional)	Poisoning, Intentional Self-Harm	Poisoning, Assault	Poisoning, Undetermined	Adverse Effect	Underdosing
	External Cause (T-Code)					
Phenylethylbiguanide	T38.3X1	T38.3X2	T38.3X3	T38.3X4	T38.3X5	T38.3X6
Phenylmercuric						
acetate	T49.0X1	T49.0X2	T49.0X3	T49.0X4	T49.0X5	T49.0X6
borate	T49.0X1	T49.0X2	T49.0X3	T49.0X4	T49.0X5	T49.0X6
nitrate	T49.0X1	T49.0X2	T49.0X3	T49.0X4	T49.0X5	T49.0X6
Phenylmethylbarbitone	T42.3X1	T42.3X2	T42.3X3	T42.3X4	T42.3X5	T42.3X6
Phenylpropanol	T47.5X1	T47.5X2	T47.5X3	T47.5X4	T47.5X5	T47.5X6
Phenylpropanolamine	T44.991	T44.992	T44.993	T44.994	T44.995	T44.996
Phenylsulfthion	T60.0X1	T60.0X2	T60.0X3	T60.0X4	—	—
Phenyltoloxamine	T45.0X1	T45.0X2	T45.0X3	T45.0X4	T45.0X5	T45.0X6
Phenyramidol, phenyramidon	T39.8X1	T39.8X2	T39.8X3	T39.8X4	T39.8X5	T39.8X6
Phenytoin	T42.0X1	T42.0X2	T42.0X3	T42.0X4	T42.0X5	T42.0X6
with Phenobarbital	T42.3X1	T42.3X2	T42.3X3	T42.3X4	T42.3X5	T42.3X6
pHisoHex	T49.2X1	T49.2X2	T49.2X3	T49.2X4	T49.2X5	T49.2X6
Pholcodine	T48.3X1	T48.3X2	T48.3X3	T48.3X4	T48.3X5	T48.3X6
Pholedrine	T46.991	T46.992	T46.993	T46.994	T46.995	T46.996
Phorate	T60.0X1	T60.0X2	T60.0X3	T60.0X4	—	—
Phosdrin	T60.0X1	T60.0X2	T60.0X3	T60.0X4	—	—
Phosfolan	T60.0X1	T60.0X2	T60.0X3	T60.0X4	—	—
Phosgene (gas)	T59.891	T59.892	T59.893	T59.894	—	—
Phosphamidon	T60.0X1	T60.0X2	T60.0X3	T60.0X4	—	—
Phosphate	T65.891	T65.892	T65.893	T65.894	—	—
laxative	T47.4X1	T47.4X2	T47.4X3	T47.4X4	T47.4X5	T47.4X6
organic	T60.0X1	T60.0X2	T60.0X3	T60.0X4	—	—
solvent	T52.91	T52.92	T52.93	T52.94	—	—
tricresyl	T65.891	T65.892	T65.893	T65.894	—	—
Phosphine	T57.1X1	T57.1X2	T57.1X3	T57.1X4	—	—
fumigant	T57.1X1	T57.1X2	T57.1X3	T57.1X4	—	—
Phospholine	T49.5X1	T49.5X2	T49.5X3	T49.5X4	T49.5X5	T49.5X6
Phosphoric acid	T54.2X1	T54.2X2	T54.2X3	T54.2X4	—	—
Phosphorus (compound) NEC	T57.1X1	T57.1X2	T57.1X3	T57.1X4	—	—
pesticide	T60.0X1	T60.0X2	T60.0X3	T60.0X4	—	—
Phthalates	T65.891	T65.892	T65.893	T65.894	—	—
Phthalic anhydride	T65.891	T65.892	T65.893	T65.894	—	—
Phthalimidoglutarimide	T42.6X1	T42.6X2	T42.6X3	T42.6X4	T42.6X5	T42.6X6
Phthalylsulfathiazole	T37.0X1	T37.0X2	T37.0X3	T37.0X4	T37.0X5	T37.0X6
Phylloquinone	T45.7X1	T45.7X2	T45.7X3	T45.7X4	T45.7X5	T45.7X6
Physeptone	T40.3X1	T40.3X2	T40.3X3	T40.3X4	T40.3X5	T40.3X6
Physostigma venenosum	T62.2X1	T62.2X2	T62.2X3	T62.2X4	—	—
Physostigmine	T49.5X1	T49.5X2	T49.5X3	T49.5X4	T49.5X5	T49.5X6
Phytolacca decandra	T62.2X1	T62.2X2	T62.2X3	T62.2X4	—	—
berries	T62.1X1	T62.1X2	T62.1X3	T62.1X4	—	—

Substance	Poisoning, Accidental (Unintentional)	Poisoning, Intentional Self-Harm	Poisoning, Assault	Poisoning, Undetermined	Adverse Effect	Underdosing
	External Cause (T-Code)					
Phytomenadione	T45.7X1	T45.7X2	T45.7X3	T45.7X4	T45.7X5	T45.7X6
Phytonadione	T45.7X1	T45.7X2	T45.7X3	T45.7X4	T45.7X5	T45.7X6
Picoperine	T48.3X1	T48.3X2	T48.3X3	T48.3X4	T48.3X5	T48.3X6
Picosulfate (sodium)	T47.2X1	T47.2X2	T47.2X3	T47.2X4	T47.2X5	T47.2X6
Picric (acid)	T54.2X1	T54.2X2	T54.2X3	T54.2X4	—	—
Picrotoxin	T5Ø.7X1	T5Ø.7X2	T5Ø.7X3	T5Ø.7X4	T5Ø.7X5	T5Ø.7X6
Piketoprofen	T49.ØX1	T49.ØX2	T49.ØX3	T49.ØX4	T49.ØX5	T49.ØX6
Pilocarpine	T44.1X1	T44.1X2	T44.1X3	T44.1X4	T44.1X5	T44.1X6
Pilocarpus (jaborandi) extract	T44.1X1	T44.1X2	T44.1X3	T44.1X4	T44.1X5	T44.1X6
Pilsicainide (hydrochloride)	T46.2X1	T46.2X2	T46.2X3	T46.2X4	T46.2X5	T46.2X6
Pimaricin	T36.7X1	T36.7X2	T36.7X3	T36.7X4	T36.7X5	T36.7X6
Pimeclone	T5Ø.7X1	T5Ø.7X2	T5Ø.7X3	T5Ø.7X4	T5Ø.7X5	T5Ø.7X6
Pimelic ketone	T52.8X1	T52.8X2	T52.8X3	T52.8X4	—	—
Pimethixene	T45.ØX1	T45.ØX2	T45.ØX3	T45.ØX4	T45.ØX5	T45.ØX6
Piminodine	T4Ø.2X1	T4Ø.2X2	T4Ø.2X3	T4Ø.2X4	T4Ø.2X5	T4Ø.2X6
Pimozide	T43.591	T43.592	T43.593	T43.594	T43.595	T43.596
Pinacidil	T46.5X1	T46.5X2	T46.5X3	T46.5X4	T46.5X5	T46.5X6
Pinaverium bromide	T44.3X1	T44.3X2	T44.3X3	T44.3X4	T44.3X5	T44.3X6
Pinazepam	T42.4X1	T42.4X2	T42.4X3	T42.4X4	T42.4X5	T42.4X6
Pindolol	T44.7X1	T44.7X2	T44.7X3	T44.7X4	T44.7X5	T44.7X6
Pindone	T6Ø.4X1	T6Ø.4X2	T6Ø.4X3	T6Ø.4X4	—	—
Pine oil (disinfectant)	T65.891	T65.892	T65.893	T65.894	—	—
Pinkroot	T37.4X1	T37.4X2	T37.4X3	T37.4X4	T37.4X5	T37.4X6
Pipadone	T4Ø.2X1	T4Ø.2X2	T4Ø.2X3	T4Ø.2X4	—	—
Pipamazine	T45.ØX1	T45.ØX2	T45.ØX3	T45.ØX4	T45.ØX5	T45.ØX6
Pipamperone	T43.4X1	T43.4X2	T43.4X3	T43.4X4	T43.4X5	T43.4X6
Pipazetate	T48.3X1	T48.3X2	T48.3X3	T48.3X4	T48.3X5	T48.3X6
Pipemidic acid	T37.8X1	T37.8X2	T37.8X3	T37.8X4	T37.8X5	T37.8X6
Pipenzolate bromide	T44.3X1	T44.3X2	T44.3X3	T44.3X4	T44.3X5	T44.3X6
Piperacetazine	T43.3X1	T43.3X2	T43.3X3	T43.3X4	T43.3X5	T43.3X6
Piperacillin	T36.ØX1	T36.ØX2	T36.ØX3	T36.ØX4	T36.ØX5	T36.ØX6
Piperazine	T37.4X1	T37.4X2	T37.4X3	T37.4X4	T37.4X5	T37.4X6
estrone sulfate	T38.5X1	T38.5X2	T38.5X3	T38.5X4	T38.5X5	T38.5X6
Piper cubeba	T62.2X1	T62.2X2	T62.2X3	T62.2X4	—	—
Piperidione	T48.3X1	T48.3X2	T48.3X3	T48.3X4	—	—
Piperidolate	T44.3X1	T44.3X2	T44.3X3	T44.3X4	T44.3X5	T44.3X6
Piperocaine	T41.3X1	T41.3X2	T41.3X3	T41.3X4	T41.3X5	T41.3X6
infiltration (subcutaneous)	T41.3X1	T41.3X2	T41.3X3	T41.3X4	T41.3X5	T41.3X6
nerve block (peripheral) (plexus)	T41.3X1	T41.3X2	T41.3X3	T41.3X4	T41.3X5	T41.3X6
topical (surface)	T41.3X1	T41.3X2	T41.3X3	T41.3X4	T41.3X5	T41.3X6
Piperonyl butoxide	T6Ø.8X1	T6Ø.8X2	T6Ø.8X3	T6Ø.8X4	—	—
Pipethanate	T44.3X1	T44.3X2	T44.3X3	T44.3X4	T44.3X5	T44.3X6
Pipobroman	T45.1X1	T45.1X2	T45.1X3	T45.1X4	T45.1X5	T45.1X6
Pipofezine	T43.ØX1	T43.ØX2	T43.ØX3	T43.ØX4	T43.ØX5	T43.ØX6
Pipotiazine	T43.3X1	T43.3X2	T43.3X3	T43.3X4	T43.3X5	T43.3X6
Pipoxizine	T45.ØX1	T45.ØX2	T45.ØX3	T45.ØX4	T45.ØX5	T45.ØX6
Pipradrol	T43.691	T43.692	T43.693	T43.694	T43.695	T43.696
Piprinhydrinate	T45.ØX1	T45.ØX2	T45.ØX3	T45.ØX4	T45.ØX5	T45.ØX6
Pirarubicin	T45.1X1	T45.1X2	T45.1X3	T45.1X4	T45.1X5	T45.1X6
Pirazinamide	T37.1X1	T37.1X2	T37.1X3	T37.1X4	T37.1X5	T37.1X6
Pirbuterol	T48.6X1	T48.6X2	T48.6X3	T48.6X4	T48.6X5	T48.6X6
Pirenzepine	T47.1X1	T47.1X2	T47.1X3	T47.1X4	T47.1X5	T47.1X6
Piretanide	T5Ø.1X1	T5Ø.1X2	T5Ø.1X3	T5Ø.1X4	T5Ø.1X5	T5Ø.1X6
Piribedil	T42.8X1	T42.8X2	T42.8X3	T42.8X4	T42.8X5	T42.8X6
Piridoxilate	T46.3X1	T46.3X2	T46.3X3	T46.3X4	T46.3X5	T46.3X6
Piritramide	T4Ø.4X1	T4Ø.4X2	T4Ø.4X3	T4Ø.4X4	—	—
Pirlindole	T43.ØX1	T43.ØX2	T43.ØX3	T43.ØX4	T43.ØX5	T43.ØX6
Piromidic acid	T37.8X1	T37.8X2	T37.8X3	T37.8X4	T37.8X5	T37.8X6
Piroxicam	T39.391	T39.392	T39.393	T39.394	T39.395	T39.396
beta-cyclodextrin complex	T39.8X1	T39.8X2	T39.8X3	T39.8X4	T39.8X5	T39.8X6
Pirozadil	T46.6X1	T46.6X2	T46.6X3	T46.6X4	T46.6X5	T46.6X6
Piscidia (bark) (erythrina)	T39.8X1	T39.8X2	T39.8X3	T39.8X4	T39.8X5	T39.8X6
Pitch	T65.891	T65.892	T65.893	T65.894	—	—
Pitkin's solution	T41.3X1	T41.3X2	T41.3X3	T41.3X4	T41.3X5	T41.3X6
Pitocin	T48.ØX1	T48.ØX2	T48.ØX3	T48.ØX4	T48.ØX5	T48.ØX6
Pitressin (tannate)	T38.891	T38.892	T38.893	T38.894	T38.895	T38.896
Pituitary extracts (posterior)	T38.891	T38.892	T38.893	T38.894	T38.895	T38.896
anterior	T38.811	T38.812	T38.813	T38.814	T38.815	T38.816
Pituitrin	T38.891	T38.892	T38.893	T38.894	T38.895	T38.896
Pivampicillin	T36.ØX1	T36.ØX2	T36.ØX3	T36.ØX4	T36.ØX5	T36.ØX6
Pivmecillinam	T36.ØX1	T36.ØX2	T36.ØX3	T36.ØX4	T36.ØX5	T36.ØX6
Placental hormone	T38.891	T38.892	T38.893	T38.894	T38.895	T38.896
Placidyl	T42.6X1	T42.6X2	T42.6X3	T42.6X4	T42.6X5	T42.6X6
Plague vaccine	T5Ø.A91	T5Ø.A92	T5Ø.A93	T5Ø.A94	T5Ø.A95	T5Ø.A96
Plant						
food or fertilizer NEC	T65.891	T65.892	T65.893	T65.894	—	—
containing herbicide	T6Ø.3X1	T6Ø.3X2	T6Ø.3X3	T6Ø.3X4	—	—
noxious, used as food	T62.2X1	T62.2X2	T62.2X3	T62.2X4	—	—
berries	T62.1X1	T62.1X2	T62.1X3	T62.1X4	—	—
seeds	T62.2X1	T62.2X2	T62.2X3	T62.2X4	—	—
specified type NEC	T62.2X1	T62.2X2	T62.2X3	T62.2X4	—	—
Plasma	T45.8X1	T45.8X2	T45.8X3	T45.8X4	T45.8X5	T45.8X6
expander NEC	T45.8X1	T45.8X2	T45.8X3	T45.8X4	T45.8X5	T45.8X6
protein fraction (human)	T45.8X1	T45.8X2	T45.8X3	T45.8X4	T45.8X5	T45.8X6

Substance	External Cause (T-Code) Poisoning, Accidental (Unintentional)	Poisoning, Intentional Self-Harm	Poisoning, Assault	Poisoning, Undetermined	Adverse Effect	Underdosing
Plasmanate	T45.8X1	T45.8X2	T45.8X3	T45.8X4	T45.8X5	T45.8X6
Plasminogen (tissue) activator	T45.611	T45.612	T45.613	T45.614	T45.615	T45.616
Plaster dressing	T49.3X1	T49.3X2	T49.3X3	T49.3X4	T49.3X5	T49.3X6
Plastic dressing	T49.3X1	T49.3X2	T49.3X3	T49.3X4	T49.3X5	T49.3X6
Plegicil	T43.3X1	T43.3X2	T43.3X3	T43.3X4	T43.3X5	T43.3X6
Plicamycin	T45.1X1	T45.1X2	T45.1X3	T45.1X4	T45.1X5	T45.1X6
Podophyllotoxin	T49.8X1	T49.8X2	T49.8X3	T49.8X4	T49.8X5	T49.8X6
Podophyllum (resin)	T49.4X1	T49.4X2	T49.4X3	T49.4X4	T49.4X5	T49.4X6
Poison NEC	T65.91	T65.92	T65.93	T65.94	—	—
Poisonous berries	T62.1X1	T62.1X2	T62.1X3	T62.1X4	—	—
Pokeweed (any part)	T62.2X1	T62.2X2	T62.2X3	T62.2X4	—	—
Poldine metilsulfate	T44.3X1	T44.3X2	T44.3X3	T44.3X4	T44.3X5	T44.3X6
Polidexide (sulfate)	T46.6X1	T46.6X2	T46.6X3	T46.6X4	T46.6X5	T46.6X6
Polidocanol	T46.8X1	T46.8X2	T46.8X3	T46.8X4	T46.8X5	T46.8X6
Poliomyelitis vaccine	T5Ø.B91	T5Ø.B92	T5Ø.B93	T5Ø.B94	T5Ø.B95	T5Ø.B96
Polish (car) (floor) (furniture) (metal) (porcelain) (silver)	T65.891	T65.892	T65.893	T65.894	—	—
abrasive	T65.891	T65.892	T65.893	T65.894	—	—
porcelain	T65.891	T65.892	T65.893	T65.894	—	—
Poloxalkol	T47.4X1	T47.4X2	T47.4X3	T47.4X4	T47.4X5	T47.4X6
Poloxamer	T47.4X1	T47.4X2	T47.4X3	T47.4X4	T47.4X5	T47.4X6
Polyaminostyrene resins	T5Ø.3X1	T5Ø.3X2	T5Ø.3X3	T5Ø.3X4	T5Ø.3X5	T5Ø.3X6
Polycarbophil	T47.4X1	T47.4X2	T47.4X3	T47.4X4	T47.4X5	T47.4X6
Polychlorinated biphenyl	T65.891	T65.892	T65.893	T65.894	—	—
Polycycline	T36.4X1	T36.4X2	T36.4X3	T36.4X4	T36.4X5	T36.4X6
Polyester fumes	T59.891	T59.892	T59.893	T59.894	—	—
Polyester resin hardener	T52.91	T52.92	T52.93	T52.94	—	—
fumes	T59.891	T59.892	T59.893	T59.894	—	—
Polyestradiol phosphate	T38.5X1	T38.5X2	T38.5X3	T38.5X4	T38.5X5	T38.5X6
Polyethanolamine alkyl sulfate	T49.2X1	T49.2X2	T49.2X3	T49.2X4	T49.2X5	T49.2X6
Polyethylene adhesive	T49.3X1	T49.3X2	T49.3X3	T49.3X4	T49.3X5	T49.3X6
Polyferose	T45.4X1	T45.4X2	T45.4X3	T45.4X4	T45.4X5	T45.4X6
Polygeline	T45.8X1	T45.8X2	T45.8X3	T45.8X4	T45.8X5	T45.8X6
Polymyxin	T36.8X1	T36.8X2	T36.8X3	T36.8X4	T36.8X5	T36.8X6
B	T36.8X1	T36.8X2	T36.8X3	T36.8X4	T36.8X5	T36.8X6
ENT agent	T49.6X1	T49.6X2	T49.6X3	T49.6X4	T49.6X5	T49.6X6
ophthalmic preparation	T49.5X1	T49.5X2	T49.5X3	T49.5X4	T49.5X5	T49.5X6
topical NEC	T49.ØX1	T49.ØX2	T49.ØX3	T49.ØX4	T49.ØX5	T49.ØX6
E sulfate (eye preparation)	T49.5X1	T49.5X2	T49.5X3	T49.5X4	T49.5X5	T49.5X6
Polynoxylin	T49.ØX1	T49.ØX2	T49.ØX3	T49.ØX4	T49.ØX5	T49.ØX6
Polyoestradiol phosphate	T38.5X1	T38.5X2	T38.5X3	T38.5X4	T38.5X5	T38.5X6
Polyoxymethyleneurea	T49.ØX1	T49.ØX2	T49.ØX3	T49.ØX4	T49.ØX5	T49.ØX6

Substance	External Cause (T-Code) Poisoning, Accidental (Unintentional)	Poisoning, Intentional Self-Harm	Poisoning, Assault	Poisoning, Undetermined	Adverse Effect	Underdosing
Polysilane	T47.8X1	T47.8X2	T47.8X3	T47.8X4	T47.8X5	T47.8X6
Polytetrafluoroethylene (inhaled)	T59.891	T59.892	T59.893	T59.894	—	—
Polythiazide	T5Ø.2X1	T5Ø.2X2	T5Ø.2X3	T5Ø.2X4	T5Ø.2X5	T5Ø.2X6
Polyvidone	T45.8X1	T45.8X2	T45.8X3	T45.8X4	T45.8X5	T45.8X6
Polyvinylpyrrolidone	T45.8X1	T45.8X2	T45.8X3	T45.8X4	T45.8X5	T45.8X6
Pontocaine (hydrochloride) (infiltration) (topical)	T41.3X1	T41.3X2	T41.3X3	T41.3X4	T41.3X5	T41.3X6
nerve block (peripheral) (plexus)	T41.3X1	T41.3X2	T41.3X3	T41.3X4	T41.3X5	T41.3X6
spinal	T41.3X1	T41.3X2	T41.3X3	T41.3X4	T41.3X5	T41.3X6
Porfiromycin	T45.1X1	T45.1X2	T45.1X3	T45.1X4	T45.1X5	T45.1X6
Posterior pituitary hormone NEC	T38.891	T38.892	T38.893	T38.894	T38.895	T38.896
Pot	T4Ø.7X1	T4Ø.7X2	T4Ø.7X3	T4Ø.7X4	T4Ø.7X5	T4Ø.7X6
Potash (caustic)	T54.3X1	T54.3X2	T54.3X3	T54.3X4	—	—
Potassic saline injection (lactated)	T5Ø.3X1	T5Ø.3X2	T5Ø.3X3	T5Ø.3X4	T5Ø.3X5	T5Ø.3X6
Potassium (salts) NEC	T5Ø.3X1	T5Ø.3X2	T5Ø.3X3	T5Ø.3X4	T5Ø.3X5	T5Ø.3X6
aminobenzoate	T45.8X1	T45.8X2	T45.8X3	T45.8X4	T45.8X5	T45.8X6
aminosalicylate	T37.1X1	T37.1X2	T37.1X3	T37.1X4	T37.1X5	T37.1X6
antimony 'tartrate'	T37.8X1	T37.8X2	T37.8X3	T37.8X4	T37.8X5	T37.8X6
arsenite (solution)	T57.ØX1	T57.ØX2	T57.ØX3	T57.ØX4	—	—
bichromate	T56.2X1	T56.2X2	T56.2X3	T56.2X4	—	—
bisulfate	T47.3X1	T47.3X2	T47.3X3	T47.3X4	T47.3X5	T47.3X6
bromide	T42.6X1	T42.6X2	T42.6X3	T42.6X4	T42.6X5	T42.6X6
canrenoate	T5Ø.ØX1	T5Ø.ØX2	T5Ø.ØX3	T5Ø.ØX4	T5Ø.ØX5	T5Ø.ØX6
carbonate	T54.3X1	T54.3X2	T54.3X3	T54.3X4	—	—
chlorate NEC	T65.891	T65.892	T65.893	T65.894	—	—
chloride	T5Ø.3X1	T5Ø.3X2	T5Ø.3X3	T5Ø.3X4	T5Ø.3X5	T5Ø.3X6
citrate	T5Ø.991	T5Ø.992	T5Ø.993	T5Ø.994	T5Ø.995	T5Ø.996
cyanide	T65.ØX1	T65.ØX2	T65.ØX3	T65.ØX4	—	—
ferric hexacyanoferrate (medicinal)	T5Ø.6X1	T5Ø.6X2	T5Ø.6X3	T5Ø.6X4	T5Ø.6X5	T5Ø.6X6
nonmedicinal	T65.891	T65.892	T65.893	T65.894	—	—
Fluoride	T57.8X1	T57.8X2	T57.8X3	T57.8X4	—	—
glucaldrate	T47.1X1	T47.1X2	T47.1X3	T47.1X4	T47.1X5	T47.1X6
hydroxide	T54.3X1	T54.3X2	T54.3X3	T54.3X4	—	—
iodate	T49.ØX1	T49.ØX2	T49.ØX3	T49.ØX4	T49.ØX5	T49.ØX6
iodide	T48.4X1	T48.4X2	T48.4X3	T48.4X4	T48.4X5	T48.4X6
nitrate	T57.8X1	T57.8X2	T57.8X3	T57.8X4	—	—
oxalate	T65.891	T65.892	T65.893	T65.894	—	—
perchlorate (nonmedicinal) NEC	T65.891	T65.892	T65.893	T65.894	—	—
antithyroid	T38.2X1	T38.2X2	T38.2X3	T38.2X4	T38.2X5	T38.2X6
medicinal	T38.2X1	T38.2X2	T38.2X3	T38.2X4	T38.2X5	T38.2X6

Substance	Poisoning, Accidental (Unintentional)	Poisoning, Intentional Self-Harm	Poisoning, Assault	Poisoning, Undetermined	Adverse Effect	Underdosing
	External Cause (T-Code)					
Permanganate (nonmedicinal)	T65.891	T65.892	T65.893	T65.894	—	—
medicinal	T49.0X1	T49.0X2	T49.0X3	T49.0X4	T49.0X5	T49.0X6
sulfate	T47.2X1	T47.2X2	T47.2X3	T47.2X4	T47.2X5	T47.2X6
Potassium-removing resin	T50.3X1	T50.3X2	T50.3X3	T50.3X4	T50.3X5	T50.3X6
Potassium-retaining drug	T50.3X1	T50.3X2	T50.3X3	T50.3X4	T50.3X5	T50.3X6
Povidone	T45.8X1	T45.8X2	T45.8X3	T45.8X4	T45.8X5	T45.8X6
iodine	T49.0X1	T49.0X2	T49.0X3	T49.0X4	T49.0X5	T49.0X6
Practolol	T44.7X1	T44.7X2	T44.7X3	T44.7X4	T44.7X5	T44.7X6
Prajmalium bitartrate	T46.2X1	T46.2X2	T46.2X3	T46.2X4	T46.2X5	T46.2X6
Pralidoxime (iodide)	T50.6X1	T50.6X2	T50.6X3	T50.6X4	T50.6X5	T50.6X6
chloride	T50.6X1	T50.6X2	T50.6X3	T50.6X4	T50.6X5	T50.6X6
Pramiverine	T44.3X1	T44.3X2	T44.3X3	T44.3X4	T44.3X5	T44.3X6
Pramocaine	T49.1X1	T49.1X2	T49.1X3	T49.1X4	T49.1X5	T49.1X6
Pramoxine	T49.1X1	T49.1X2	T49.1X3	T49.1X4	T49.1X5	T49.1X6
Prasterone	T38.7X1	T38.7X2	T38.7X3	T38.7X4	T38.7X5	T38.7X6
Pravastatin	T46.6X1	T46.6X2	T46.6X3	T46.6X4	T46.6X5	T46.6X6
Prazepam	T42.4X1	T42.4X2	T42.4X3	T42.4X4	T42.4X5	T42.4X6
Praziquantel	T37.4X1	T37.4X2	T37.4X3	T37.4X4	T37.4X5	T37.4X6
Prazitone	T43.291	T43.292	T43.293	T43.294	T43.295	T43.296
Prazosin	T44.6X1	T44.6X2	T44.6X3	T44.6X4	T44.6X5	T44.6X6
Prednicarbate	T49.0X1	T49.0X2	T49.0X3	T49.0X4	T49.0X5	T49.0X6
Prednimustine	T45.1X1	T45.1X2	T45.1X3	T45.1X4	T45.1X5	T45.1X6
Prednisolone	T38.0X1	T38.0X2	T38.0X3	T38.0X4	T38.0X5	T38.0X6
ENT agent	T49.6X1	T49.6X2	T49.6X3	T49.6X4	T49.6X5	T49.6X6
ophthalmic preparation	T49.5X1	T49.5X2	T49.5X3	T49.5X4	T49.5X5	T49.5X6
steaglate	T49.0X1	T49.0X2	T49.0X3	T49.0X4	T49.0X5	T49.0X6
topical NEC	T49.0X1	T49.0X2	T49.0X3	T49.0X4	T49.0X5	T49.0X6
Prednisone	T38.0X1	T38.0X2	T38.0X3	T38.0X4	T38.0X5	T38.0X6
Prednylidene	T38.0X1	T38.0X2	T38.0X3	T38.0X4	T38.0X5	T38.0X6
Pregnandiol	T38.5X1	T38.5X2	T38.5X3	T38.5X4	T38.5X5	T38.5X6
Pregneninolone	T38.5X1	T38.5X2	T38.5X3	T38.5X4	T38.5X5	T38.5X6
Preludin	T43.691	T43.692	T43.693	T43.694	T43.695	T43.696
Premarin	T38.5X1	T38.5X2	T38.5X3	T38.5X4	T38.5X5	T38.5X6
Premedication anesthetic	T41.201	T41.202	T41.203	T41.204	T41.205	T41.206
Prenalterol	T44.5X1	T44.5X2	T44.5X3	T44.5X4	T44.5X5	T44.5X6
Prenoxdiazine	T48.3X1	T48.3X2	T48.3X3	T48.3X4	T48.3X5	T48.3X6
Prenylamine	T46.3X1	T46.3X2	T46.3X3	T46.3X4	T46.3X5	T46.3X6
Preparation, local	T49.4X1	T49.4X2	T49.4X3	T49.4X4	T49.4X5	T49.4X6
Preparation H	T49.8X1	T49.8X2	T49.8X3	T49.8X4	T49.8X5	T49.8X6
Preservative (nonmedicinal)	T65.891	T65.892	T65.893	T65.894	—	—
medicinal	T50.901	T50.902	T50.903	T50.904	T50.905	T50.906
wood	T60.91	T60.92	T60.93	T60.94	—	—

Substance	Poisoning, Accidental (Unintentional)	Poisoning, Intentional Self-Harm	Poisoning, Assault	Poisoning, Undetermined	Adverse Effect	Underdosing
	External Cause (T-Code)					
Prethcamide	T50.7X1	T50.7X2	T50.7X3	T50.7X4	T50.7X5	T50.7X6
Pride of China	T62.2X1	T62.2X2	T62.2X3	T62.2X4	—	—
Pridinol	T44.3X1	T44.3X2	T44.3X3	T44.3X4	T44.3X5	T44.3X6
Prifinium bromide	T44.3X1	T44.3X2	T44.3X3	T44.3X4	T44.3X5	T44.3X6
Prilocaine	T41.3X1	T41.3X2	T41.3X3	T41.3X4	T41.3X5	T41.3X6
infiltration (subcutaneous)	T41.3X1	T41.3X2	T41.3X3	T41.3X4	T41.3X5	T41.3X6
nerve block (peripheral) (plexus)	T41.3X1	T41.3X2	T41.3X3	T41.3X4	T41.3X5	T41.3X6
regional	T41.3X1	T41.3X2	T41.3X3	T41.3X4	T41.3X5	T41.3X6
Primaquine	T37.2X1	T37.2X2	T37.2X3	T37.2X4	T37.2X5	T37.2X6
Primidone	T42.6X1	T42.6X2	T42.6X3	T42.6X4	T42.6X5	T42.6X6
Primula (veris)	T62.2X1	T62.2X2	T62.2X3	T62.2X4	—	—
Prinadol	T40.2X1	T40.2X2	T40.2X3	T40.2X4	T40.2X5	T40.2X6
Priscol, Priscoline	T44.6X1	T44.6X2	T44.6X3	T44.6X4	T44.6X5	T44.6X6
Pristinamycin	T36.3X1	T36.3X2	T36.3X3	T36.3X4	T36.3X5	T36.3X6
Privet	T62.2X1	T62.2X2	T62.2X3	T62.2X4	—	—
berries	T62.1X1	T62.1X2	T62.1X3	T62.1X4	—	—
Privine	T44.4X1	T44.4X2	T44.4X3	T44.4X4	T44.4X5	T44.4X6
Pro-Banthine	T44.3X1	T44.3X2	T44.3X3	T44.3X4	T44.3X5	T44.3X6
Probarbital	T42.3X1	T42.3X2	T42.3X3	T42.3X4	T42.3X5	T42.3X6
Probenecid	T50.4X1	T50.4X2	T50.4X3	T50.4X4	T50.4X5	T50.4X6
Probucol	T46.6X1	T46.6X2	T46.6X3	T46.6X4	T46.6X5	T46.6X6
Procainamide	T46.2X1	T46.2X2	T46.2X3	T46.2X4	T46.2X5	T46.2X6
Procaine	T41.3X1	T41.3X2	T41.3X3	T41.3X4	T41.3X5	T41.3X6
benzylpenicillin	T36.0X1	T36.0X2	T36.0X3	T36.0X4	T36.0X5	T36.0X6
nerve block (periphreal) (plexus)	T41.3X1	T41.3X2	T41.3X3	T41.3X4	T41.3X5	T41.3X6
penicillin G	T36.0X1	T36.0X2	T36.0X3	T36.0X4	T36.0X5	T36.0X6
regional	T41.3X1	T41.3X2	T41.3X3	T41.3X4	T41.3X5	T41.3X6
spinal	T41.3X1	T41.3X2	T41.3X3	T41.3X4	T41.3X5	T41.3X6
Procalmidol	T43.591	T43.592	T43.593	T43.594	T43.595	T43.596
Procarbazine	T45.1X1	T45.1X2	T45.1X3	T45.1X4	T45.1X5	T45.1X6
Procaterol	T44.5X1	T44.5X2	T44.5X3	T44.5X4	T44.5X5	T44.5X6
Prochlorperazine	T43.3X1	T43.3X2	T43.3X3	T43.3X4	T43.3X5	T43.3X6
Procyclidine	T44.3X1	T44.3X2	T44.3X3	T44.3X4	T44.3X5	T44.3X6
Producer gas	T58.8X1	T58.8X2	T58.8X3	T58.8X4	—	—
Profadol	T40.4X1	T40.4X2	T40.4X3	T40.4X4	T40.4X5	T40.4X6
Profenamine	T44.3X1	T44.3X2	T44.3X3	T44.3X4	T44.3X5	T44.3X6
Profenil	T44.3X1	T44.3X2	T44.3X3	T44.3X4	T44.3X5	T44.3X6
Proflavine	T49.0X1	T49.0X2	T49.0X3	T49.0X4	T49.0X5	T49.0X6
Progabide	T42.6X1	T42.6X2	T42.6X3	T42.6X4	T42.6X5	T42.6X6
Progestin	T38.5X1	T38.5X2	T38.5X3	T38.5X4	T38.5X5	T38.5X6
oral contraceptive	T38.4X1	T38.4X2	T38.4X3	T38.4X4	T38.4X5	T38.4X6

Substance	Poisoning, Accidental (Unintentional)	Poisoning, Intentional Self-Harm	Poisoning, Assault	Poisoning, Undetermined	Adverse Effect	Underdosing
	External Cause (T-Code)					
Progesterone	T38.5X1	T38.5X2	T38.5X3	T38.5X4	T38.5X5	T38.5X6
Progestogen NEC	T38.5X1	T38.5X2	T38.5X3	T38.5X4	T38.5X5	T38.5X6
Progestone	T38.5X1	T38.5X2	T38.5X3	T38.5X4	T38.5X5	T38.5X6
Proglumide	T47.1X1	T47.1X2	T47.1X3	T47.1X4	T47.1X5	T47.1X6
Proguanil	T37.2X1	T37.2X2	T37.2X3	T37.2X4	T37.2X5	T37.2X6
Prolactin	T38.811	T38.812	T38.813	T38.814	T38.815	T38.816
Prolintane	T43.691	T43.692	T43.693	T43.694	T43.695	T43.696
Proloid	T38.1X1	T38.1X2	T38.1X3	T38.1X4	T38.1X5	T38.1X6
Proluton	T38.5X1	T38.5X2	T38.5X3	T38.5X4	T38.5X5	T38.5X6
Promacetin	T37.1X1	T37.1X2	T37.1X3	T37.1X4	T37.1X5	T37.1X6
Promazine	T43.3X1	T43.3X2	T43.3X3	T43.3X4	T43.3X5	T43.3X6
Promedol	T4Ø.2X1	T4Ø.2X2	T4Ø.2X3	T4Ø.2X4	—	—
Promegestone	T38.5X1	T38.5X2	T38.5X3	T38.5X4	T38.5X5	T38.5X6
Promethazine (teoclate)	T43.3X1	T43.3X2	T43.3X3	T43.3X4	T43.3X5	T43.3X6
Promin	T37.1X1	T37.1X2	T37.1X3	T37.1X4	T37.1X5	T37.1X6
Pronase	T45.3X1	T45.3X2	T45.3X3	T45.3X4	T45.3X5	T45.3X6
Pronestyl (hydrochloride)	T46.2X1	T46.2X2	T46.2X3	T46.2X4	T46.2X5	T46.2X6
Pronetalol	T44.7X1	T44.7X2	T44.7X3	T44.7X4	T44.7X5	T44.7X6
Prontosil	T37.ØX1	T37.ØX2	T37.ØX3	T37.ØX4	T37.ØX5	T37.ØX6
Propachlor	T6Ø.3X1	T6Ø.3X2	T6Ø.3X3	T6Ø.3X4	—	—
Propafenone	T46.2X1	T46.2X2	T46.2X3	T46.2X4	T46.2X5	T46.2X6
Propallylonal	T42.3X1	T42.3X2	T42.3X3	T42.3X4	T42.3X5	T42.3X6
Propamidine	T49.ØX1	T49.ØX2	T49.ØX3	T49.ØX4	T49.ØX5	T49.ØX6
Propane (distributed in mobile container)	T59.891	T59.892	T59.893	T59.894	—	—
distributed through pipes	T59.891	T59.892	T59.893	T59.894	—	—
incomplete combustion	T57.11	T57.12	T57.13	T57.14	—	—
Propanidid	T41.291	T41.292	T41.293	T41.294	T41.295	T41.296
Propanil	T6Ø.3X1	T6Ø.3X2	T6Ø.3X3	T6Ø.3X4	—	—
1-Propanol	T51.3X1	T51.3X2	T51.3X3	T51.3X4	—	—
2-Propanol	T51.2X1	T51.2X2	T51.2X3	T51.2X4	—	—
Propantheline	T44.3X1	T44.3X2	T44.3X3	T44.3X4	T44.3X5	T44.3X6
bromide	T44.3X1	T44.3X2	T44.3X3	T44.3X4	T44.3X5	T44.3X6
Proparacaine	T41.3X1	T41.3X2	T41.3X3	T41.3X4	T41.3X5	T41.3X6
Propatylnitrate	T46.3X1	T46.3X2	T46.3X3	T46.3X4	T46.3X5	T46.3X6
Propicillin	T36.ØX1	T36.ØX2	T36.ØX3	T36.ØX4	T36.ØX5	T36.ØX6
Propiolactone	T49.ØX1	T49.ØX2	T49.ØX3	T49.ØX4	T49.ØX5	T49.ØX6
Propiomazine	T45.ØX1	T45.ØX2	T45.ØX3	T45.ØX4	T45.ØX5	T45.ØX6
Propionaldehyde (medicinal)	T42.6X1	T42.6X2	T42.6X3	T42.6X4	T42.6X5	T42.6X6
Propionate (calcium) (sodium)	T49.ØX1	T49.ØX2	T49.ØX3	T49.ØX4	T49.ØX5	T49.ØX6
Propion gel	T49.ØX1	T49.ØX2	T49.ØX3	T49.ØX4	T49.ØX5	T49.ØX6
Propitocaine	T41.3X1	T41.3X2	T41.3X3	T41.3X4	T41.3X5	T41.3X6
infiltration (subcutaneous)	T41.3X1	T41.3X2	T41.3X3	T41.3X4	T41.3X5	T41.3X6
nerve block (peripheral) (plexus)	T41.3X1	T41.3X2	T41.3X3	T41.3X4	T41.3X5	T41.3X6
Propofol	T41.291	T41.292	T41.293	T41.294	T41.295	T41.296
Propoxur	T6Ø.ØX1	T6Ø.ØX2	T6Ø.ØX3	T6Ø.ØX4	—	—
Propoxycaine	T41.3X1	T41.3X2	T41.3X3	T41.3X4	T41.3X5	T41.3X6
infiltration (subcutaneous)	T41.3X1	T41.3X2	T41.3X3	T41.3X4	T41.3X5	T41.3X6
nerve block (peripheral) (plexus)	T41.3X1	T41.3X2	T41.3X3	T41.3X4	T41.3X5	T41.3X6
topical (surface)	T41.3X1	T41.3X2	T41.3X3	T41.3X4	T41.3X5	T41.3X6
Propoxyphene	T4Ø.4X1	T4Ø.4X2	T4Ø.4X3	T4Ø.4X4	T4Ø.4X5	T4Ø.4X6
Propranolol	T44.7X1	T44.7X2	T44.7X3	T44.7X4	T44.7X5	T44.7X6
Propyl						
alcohol	T51.3X1	T51.3X2	T51.3X3	T51.3X4	—	—
carbinol	T51.3X1	T51.3X2	T51.3X3	T51.3X4	—	—
hexadrine	T44.4X1	T44.4X2	T44.4X3	T44.4X4	T44.4X5	T44.4X6
iodone	T5Ø.8X1	T5Ø.8X2	T5Ø.8X3	T5Ø.8X4	T5Ø.8X5	T5Ø.8X6
thiouracil	T38.2X1	T38.2X2	T38.2X3	T38.2X4	T38.2X5	T38.2X6
Propylaminophenothiazine	T43.3X1	T43.3X2	T43.3X3	T43.3X4	T43.3X5	T43.3X6
Propylene	T59.891	T59.892	T59.893	T59.894	—	—
Propylhexedrine	T48.5X1	T48.5X2	T48.5X3	T48.5X4	T48.5X5	T48.5X6
Propyliodone	T5Ø.8X1	T5Ø.8X2	T5Ø.8X3	T5Ø.8X4	T5Ø.8X5	T5Ø.8X6
Propylthiouracil	T38.2X1	T38.2X2	T38.2X3	T38.2X4	T38.2X5	T38.2X6
Propylparaben (ophthalmic)	T49.5X1	T49.5X2	T49.5X3	T49.5X4	T49.5X5	T49.5X6
Propyphenazone	T39.2X1	T39.2X2	T39.2X3	T39.2X4	T39.2X5	T39.2X6
Proquazone	T39.391	T39.392	T39.393	T39.394	T39.395	T39.396
Proscillaridin	T46.ØX1	T46.ØX2	T46.ØX3	T46.ØX4	T46.ØX5	T46.ØX6
Prostacyclin	T45.521	T45.522	T45.523	T45.524	T45.525	T45.526
Prostaglandin (I2)	T45.521	T45.522	T45.523	T45.524	T45.525	T45.526
E1	T46.7X1	T46.7X2	T46.7X3	T46.7X4	T46.7X5	T46.7X6
E2	T48.ØX1	T48.ØX2	T48.ØX3	T48.ØX4	T48.ØX5	T48.ØX6
F2 alpha	T48.ØX1	T48.ØX2	T48.ØX3	T48.ØX4	T48.ØX5	T48.ØX6
Prostigmin	T44.ØX1	T44.ØX2	T44.ØX3	T44.ØX4	T44.ØX5	T44.ØX6
Prosultiamine	T45.2X1	T45.2X2	T45.2X3	T45.2X4	T45.2X5	T45.2X6
Protamine sulfate	T45.7X1	T45.7X2	T45.7X3	T45.7X4	T45.7X5	T45.7X6
zinc insulin	T38.3X1	T38.3X2	T38.3X3	T38.3X4	T38.3X5	T38.3X6
Protease	T47.5X1	T47.5X2	T47.5X3	T47.5X4	T47.5X5	T47.5X6
Protectant, skin NEC	T49.3X1	T49.3X2	T49.3X3	T49.3X4	T49.3X5	T49.3X6
Protein hydrolysate	T5Ø.991	T5Ø.992	T5Ø.993	T5Ø.994	T5Ø.995	T5Ø.996
Prothiaden — *see Dothiepin hydrochloride*						
Prothionamide	T37.1X1	T37.1X2	T37.1X3	T37.1X4	T37.1X5	T37.1X6

		External Cause (T-Code)				
Substance	**Poisoning, Accidental (Unintentional)**	**Poisoning, Intentional Self-Harm**	**Poisoning, Assault**	**Poisoning, Undetermined**	**Adverse Effect**	**Underdosing**
Prothipendyl	T43.591	T43.592	T43.593	T43.594	T43.595	T43.596
Prothoate	T60.0X1	T60.0X2	T60.0X3	T60.0X4	—	—
Prothrombin						
activator	T45.7X1	T45.7X2	T45.7X3	T45.7X4	T45.7X5	T45.7X6
synthesis inhibitor	T45.511	T45.512	T45.513	T45.514	T45.515	T45.516
Protionamide	T37.1X1	T37.1X2	T37.1X3	T37.1X4	T37.1X5	T37.1X6
Protirelin	T38.891	T38.892	T38.893	T38.894	T38.895	T38.896
Protokylol	T48.6X1	T48.6X2	T48.6X3	T48.6X4	T48.6X5	T48.6X6
Protopam	T50.6X1	T50.6X2	T50.6X3	T50.6X4	T50.6X5	T50.6X6
Protoveratrine(s) (A) (B)	T46.5X1	T46.5X2	T46.5X3	T46.5X4	T46.5X5	T46.5X6
Protriptyline	T43.011	T43.012	T43.013	T43.014	T43.015	T43.016
Provera	T38.5X1	T38.5X2	T38.5X3	T38.5X4	T38.5X5	T38.5X6
Provitamin A	T45.2X1	T45.2X2	T45.2X3	T45.2X4	T45.2X5	T45.2X6
Proxibarbal	T42.3X1	T42.3X2	T42.3X3	T42.3X4	T42.3X5	T42.3X6
Proxymetacaine	T41.3X1	T41.3X2	T41.3X3	T41.3X4	T41.3X5	T41.3X6
Proxyphylline	T48.6X1	T48.6X2	T48.6X3	T48.6X4	T48.6X5	T48.6X6
Prozac — *see Fluoxetine hydrochloride*						
Prunus						
laurocerasus	T62.2X1	T62.2X2	T62.2X3	T62.2X4	—	—
virginiana	T62.2X1	T62.2X2	T62.2X3	T62.2X4	—	—
Prussian blue						
commercial	T65.891	T65.892	T65.893	T65.894	—	—
therapeutic	T50.6X1	T50.6X2	T50.6X3	T50.6X4	T50.6X5	T50.6X6
Prussic acid	T65.0X1	T65.0X2	T65.0X3	T65.0X4	—	—
vapor	T57.3X1	T57.3X2	T57.3X3	T57.3X4	—	—
Pseudoephedrine	T44.991	T44.992	T44.993	T44.994	T44.995	T44.996
Psilocin	T40.991	T40.992	T40.993	T40.994	—	—
Psilocybin	T40.991	T40.992	T40.993	T40.994	—	—
Psilocybine	T40.991	T40.992	T40.993	T40.994	—	—
Psoralene (nonmedicinal)	T65.891	T65.892	T65.893	T65.894	—	—
Psoralens (medicinal)	T50.991	T50.992	T50.993	T50.994	T50.995	T50.996
PSP (phenolsulfonphthalein)	T50.8X1	T50.8X2	T50.8X3	T50.8X4	T50.8X5	T50.8X6
Psychodysleptic drug NOS	T40.901	T40.902	T40.903	T40.904	T40.905	T40.906
specified NEC	T40.991	T40.992	T40.993	T40.994	T40.995	T40.996
Psychostimulant	T43.601	T43.602	T43.603	T43.604	T43.605	T43.606
amphetamine	T43.621	T43.622	T43.623	T43.624	T43.625	T43.626
caffeine	T43.611	T43.612	T43.613	T43.614	T43.615	T43.616
methylphenidate	T43.631	T43.632	T43.633	T43.634	T43.635	T43.636
specified NEC	T43.691	T43.692	T43.693	T43.694	T43.695	T43.696
Psychotherapeutic drug NEC	T43.91	T43.92	T43.93	T43.94	T43.95	T43.96
antidepressants — *see also Antidepressant*	T43.201	T43.202	T43.203	T43.204	T43.205	T43.206
Psychotherapeutic drug NEC *(Continued)*						
specified NEC	T43.8X1	T43.8X2	T43.8X3	T43.8X4	T43.8X5	T43.8X6
tranquilizers NEC	T43.501	T43.502	T43.503	T43.504	T43.505	T43.506
Psychotomimetic agents	T40.901	T40.902	T40.903	T40.904	T40.905	T40.906
Psychotropic drug NEC	T43.91	T43.92	T43.93	T43.94	T43.95	T43.96
specified NEC	T43.8X1	T43.8X2	T43.8X3	T43.8X4	T43.8X5	T43.8X6
Psyllium hydrophilic mucilloid	T47.4X1	T47.4X2	T47.4X3	T47.4X4	T47.4X5	T47.4X6
Pteroylglutamic acid	T45.8X1	T45.8X2	T45.8X3	T45.8X4	T45.8X5	T45.8X6
Pteroyltriglutamate	T45.1X1	T45.1X2	T45.1X3	T45.1X4	T45.1X5	T45.1X6
PTFE — *see Polytetrafluoroethylene*						
Pulp						
devitalizing paste	T49.7X1	T49.7X2	T49.7X3	T49.7X4	T49.7X5	T49.7X6
dressing	T49.7X1	T49.7X2	T49.7X3	T49.7X4	T49.7X5	T49.7X6
Pulsatilla	T62.2X1	T62.2X2	T62.2X3	T62.2X4	—	—
Pumpkin seed extract	T37.4X1	T37.4X2	T37.4X3	T37.4X4	T37.4X5	T37.4X6
Purex (bleach)	T54.91	T54.92	T54.93	T54.94	—	—
Purgative NEC — *see also Cathartic*	T47.4X1	T47.4X2	T47.4X3	T47.4X4	T47.4X5	T47.4X6
Purine analogue (antineoplastic)	T45.1X1	T45.1X2	T45.1X3	T45.1X4	T45.1X5	T45.1X6
Purine diuretics	T50.2X1	T50.2X2	T50.2X3	T50.2X4	T50.2X5	T50.2X6
Purinethol	T45.1X1	T45.1X2	T45.1X3	T45.1X4	T45.1X5	T45.1X6
PVP	T45.8X1	T45.8X2	T45.8X3	T45.8X4	T45.8X5	T45.8X6
Pyrabital	T39.8X1	T39.8X2	T39.8X3	T39.8X4	T39.8X5	T39.8X6
Pyramidon	T39.2X1	T39.2X2	T39.2X3	T39.2X4	T39.2X5	T39.2X6
Pyrantel	T37.4X1	T37.4X2	T37.4X3	T37.4X4	T37.4X5	T37.4X6
Pyrathiazine	T45.0X1	T45.0X2	T45.0X3	T45.0X4	T45.0X5	T45.0X6
Pyrazinamide	T37.1X1	T37.1X2	T37.1X3	T37.1X4	T37.1X5	T37.1X6
Pyrazinoic acid (amide)	T37.1X1	T37.1X2	T37.1X3	T37.1X4	T37.1X5	T37.1X6
Pyrazole (derivatives)	T39.2X1	T39.2X2	T39.2X3	T39.2X4	T39.2X5	T39.2X6
Pyrazolone analgesic NEC	T39.2X1	T39.2X2	T39.2X3	T39.2X4	T39.2X5	T39.2X6
Pyrethrin, pyrethrum (nonmedicinal)	T60.2X1	T60.2X2	T60.2X3	T60.2X4	—	—
Pyrethrum extract	T49.0X1	T49.0X2	T49.0X3	T49.0X4	T49.0X5	T49.0X6
Pyribenzamine	T45.0X1	T45.0X2	T45.0X3	T45.0X4	T45.0X5	T45.0X6
Pyridine	T52.8X1	T52.8X2	T52.8X3	T52.8X4	—	—
aldoxime methiodide	T50.6X1	T50.6X2	T50.6X3	T50.6X4	T50.6X5	T50.6X6
aldoxime methyl chloride	T50.6X1	T50.6X2	T50.6X3	T50.6X4	T50.6X5	T50.6X6
vapor	T59.891	T59.892	T59.893	T59.894	—	—
Pyridium	T39.8X1	T39.8X2	T39.8X3	T39.8X4	T39.8X5	T39.8X6
Pyridostigmine bromide	T44.0X1	T44.0X2	T44.0X3	T44.0X4	T44.0X5	T44.0X6
Pyridoxal phosphate	T45.2X1	T45.2X2	T45.2X3	T45.2X4	T45.2X5	T45.2X6

	External Cause (T-Code)					
Substance	Poisoning, Accidental (Unintentional)	Poisoning, Intentional Self-Harm	Poisoning, Assault	Poisoning, Undetermined	Adverse Effect	Underdosing
Pyridoxine	T45.2X1	T45.2X2	T45.2X3	T45.2X4	T45.2X5	T45.2X6
Pyrilamine	T45.ØX1	T45.ØX2	T45.ØX3	T45.ØX4	T45.ØX5	T45.ØX6
Pyrimethamine	T37.2X1	T37.2X2	T37.2X3	T37.2X4	T37.2X5	T37.2X6
with sulfadoxine	T37.2X1	T37.2X2	T37.2X3	T37.2X4	T37.2X5	T37.2X6
Pyrimidine antagonist	T45.1X1	T45.1X2	T45.1X3	T45.1X4	T45.1X5	T45.1X6
Pyriminil	T6Ø.4X1	T6Ø.4X2	T6Ø.4X3	T6Ø.4X4	—	—
Pyrithione zinc	T49.4X1	T49.4X2	T49.4X3	T49.4X4	T49.4X5	T49.4X6
Pyrithyldione	T42.6X1	T42.6X2	T42.6X3	T42.6X4	T42.6X5	T42.6X6
Pyrogallic acid	T49.ØX1	T49.ØX2	T49.ØX3	T49.ØX4	T49.ØX5	T49.ØX6
Pyrogallol	T49.ØX1	T49.ØX2	T49.ØX3	T49.ØX4	T49.ØX5	T49.ØX6
Pyroxylin	T49.3X1	T49.3X2	T49.3X3	T49.3X4	T49.3X5	T49.3X6
Pyrrobutamine	T45.ØX1	T45.ØX2	T45.ØX3	T45.ØX4	T45.ØX5	T45.ØX6
Pyrrolizidine alkaloids	T62.8X1	T62.8X2	T62.8X3	T62.8X4	—	—
Pyrvinium chloride	T37.4X1	T37.4X2	T37.4X3	T37.4X4	T37.4X5	T37.4X6
PZI	T38.3X1	T38.3X2	T38.3X3	T38.3X4	T38.3X5	T38.3X6
Q						
Quaalude	T42.6X1	T42.6X2	T42.6X3	T42.6X4	T42.6X5	T42.6X6
Quarternary ammonium						
anti-infective	T49.ØX1	T49.ØX2	T49.ØX3	T49.ØX4	T49.ØX5	T49.ØX6
ganglion blocking	T44.2X1	T44.2X2	T44.2X3	T44.2X4	T44.2X5	T44.2X6
parasympatholytic	T44.3X1	T44.3X2	T44.3X3	T44.3X4	T44.3X5	T44.3X6
Quazepam	T42.4X1	T42.4X2	T42.4X3	T42.4X4	T42.4X5	T42.4X6
Quicklime	T54.3X1	T54.3X2	T54.3X3	T54.3X4	—	—
Quillaja extract	T48.4X1	T48.4X2	T48.4X3	T48.4X4	T48.4X5	T48.4X6
Quinacrine	T37.2X1	T37.2X2	T37.2X3	T37.2X4	T37.2X5	T37.2X6
Quinaglute	T46.2X1	T46.2X2	T46.2X3	T46.2X4	T46.2X5	T46.2X6
Quinalbarbital	T42.3X1	T42.3X2	T42.3X3	T42.3X4	T42.3X5	T42.3X6
Quinalbarbitone sodium	T42.3X1	T42.3X2	T42.3X3	T42.3X4	T42.3X5	T42.3X6
Quinalphos	T6Ø.ØX1	T6Ø.ØX2	T6Ø.ØX3	T6Ø.ØX4	—	—
Quinapril	T46.4X1	T46.4X2	T46.4X3	T46.4X4	T46.4X5	T46.4X6
Quinestradiol	T38.5X1	T38.5X2	T38.5X3	T38.5X4	T38.5X5	T38.5X6
Quinestradol	T38.5X1	T38.5X2	T38.5X3	T38.5X4	T38.5X5	T38.5X6
Quinestrol	T38.5X1	T38.5X2	T38.5X3	T38.5X4	T38.5X5	T38.5X6
Quinethazone	T5Ø.2X1	T5Ø.2X2	T5Ø.2X3	T5Ø.2X4	T5Ø.2X5	T5Ø.2X6
Quingestanol	T38.4X1	T38.4X2	T38.4X3	T38.4X4	T38.4X5	T38.4X6
Quinidine	T46.2X1	T46.2X2	T46.2X3	T46.2X4	T46.2X5	T46.2X6
Quinine	T37.2X1	T37.2X2	T37.2X3	T37.2X4	T37.2X5	T37.2X6
Quiniobine	T37.8X1	T37.8X2	T37.8X3	T37.8X4	T37.8X5	T37.8X6
Quinisocaine	T49.1X1	T49.1X2	T49.1X3	T49.1X4	T49.1X5	T49.1X6
Quinocide	T37.2X1	T37.2X2	T37.2X3	T37.2X4	T37.2X5	T37.2X6
Quinoline (derivatives) NEC	T37.8X1	T37.8X2	T37.8X3	T37.8X4	T37.8X5	T37.8X6

	External Cause (T-Code)					
Substance	Poisoning, Accidental (Unintentional)	Poisoning, Intentional Self-Harm	Poisoning, Assault	Poisoning, Undetermined	Adverse Effect	Underdosing
Quinupramine	T43.Ø11	T43.Ø12	T43.Ø13	T43.Ø14	T43.Ø15	T43.Ø16
Quotane	T41.3X1	T41.3X2	T41.3X3	T41.3X4	T41.3X5	T41.3X6
R						
Rabies						
immune globulin (human)	T5Ø.Z11	T5Ø.Z12	T5Ø.Z13	T5Ø.Z14	T5Ø.Z15	T5Ø.Z16
vaccine	T5Ø.B91	T5Ø.B92	T5Ø.B93	T5Ø.B94	T5Ø.B95	T5Ø.B96
Racemoramide	T4Ø.2X1	T4Ø.2X2	T4Ø.2X3	T4Ø.2X4	—	—
Racemorphan	T4Ø.2X1	T4Ø.2X2	T4Ø.2X3	T4Ø.2X4	T4Ø.2X5	T4Ø.2X6
Racepinefrin	T44.5X1	T44.5X2	T44.5X3	T44.5X4	T44.5X5	T44.5X6
Raclopride	T43.591	T43.592	T43.593	T43.594	T43.595	T43.596
Radiator alcohol	T51.1X1	T51.1X2	T51.1X3	T51.1X4	—	—
Radioactive drug NEC	T5Ø.8X1	T5Ø.8X2	T5Ø.8X3	T5Ø.8X4	T5Ø.8X5	T5Ø.8X6
Radio-opaque (drugs) (materials)	T5Ø.8X1	T5Ø.8X2	T5Ø.8X3	T5Ø.8X4	T5Ø.8X5	T5Ø.8X6
Ramifenazone	T39.2X1	T39.2X2	T39.2X3	T39.2X4	T39.2X5	T39.2X6
Ramipril	T46.4X1	T46.4X2	T46.4X3	T46.4X4	T46.4X5	T46.4X6
Ranitidine	T47.ØX1	T47.ØX2	T47.ØX3	T47.ØX4	T47.ØX5	T47.ØX6
Ranunculus	T62.2X1	T62.2X2	T62.2X3	T62.2X4	—	—
Rat poison NEC	T6Ø.4X1	T6Ø.4X2	T6Ø.4X3	T6Ø.4X4	—	—
Rattlesnake (venom)	T63.Ø11	T63.Ø12	T63.Ø13	T63.Ø14	—	—
Raubasine	T46.7X1	T46.7X2	T46.7X3	T46.7X4	T46.7X5	T46.7X6
Raudixin	T46.5X1	T46.5X2	T46.5X3	T46.5X4	T46.5X5	T46.5X6
Rautensin	T46.5X1	T46.5X2	T46.5X3	T46.5X4	T46.5X5	T46.5X6
Rautina	T46.5X1	T46.5X2	T46.5X3	T46.5X4	T46.5X5	T46.5X6
Rautotal	T46.5X1	T46.5X2	T46.5X3	T46.5X4	T46.5X5	T46.5X6
Rauwiloid	T46.5X1	T46.5X2	T46.5X3	T46.5X4	T46.5X5	T46.5X6
Rauwoldin	T46.5X1	T46.5X2	T46.5X3	T46.5X4	T46.5X5	T46.5X6
Rauwolfia (alkaloids)	T46.5X1	T46.5X2	T46.5X3	T46.5X4	T46.5X5	T46.5X6
Razoxane	T45.1X1	T45.1X2	T45.1X3	T45.1X4	T45.1X5	T45.1X6
Realgar	T57.ØX1	T57.ØX2	T57.ØX3	T57.ØX4	—	—
Recombinant (R) — *see specific protein*						
Red blood cells, packed	T45.8X1	T45.8X2	T45.8X3	T45.8X4	T45.8X5	T45.8X6
Red squill (scilliroside)	T6Ø.4X1	T6Ø.4X2	T6Ø.4X3	T6Ø.4X4	—	—
Reducing agent, industrial NEC	T65.891	T65.892	T65.893	T65.894	—	—
Refrigerant gas (chlorofluoro-carbon)	T53.5X1	T53.5X2	T53.5X3	T53.5X4	—	—
not chlorofluoro-carbon	T59.891	T59.892	T59.893	T59.894	—	—
Regroton	T5Ø.2X1	T5Ø.2X2	T5Ø.2X3	T5Ø.2X4	T5Ø.2X5	T5Ø.2X6
Rehydration salts (oral)	T5Ø.3X1	T5Ø.3X2	T5Ø.3X3	T5Ø.3X4	T5Ø.3X5	T5Ø.3X6
Rela	T42.8X1	T42.8X2	T42.8X3	T42.8X4	T42.8X5	T42.8X6

	External Cause (T-Code)					
Substance	Poisoning, Accidental (Unintentional)	Poisoning, Intentional Self-Harm	Poisoning, Assault	Poisoning, Undetermined	Adverse Effect	Underdosing
Relaxant, muscle						
anesthetic	T48.1X1	T48.1X2	T48.1X3	T48.1X4	T48.1X5	T48.1X6
central nervous system	T42.8X1	T42.8X2	T42.8X3	T42.8X4	T42.8X5	T42.8X6
skeletal NEC	T48.1X1	T48.1X2	T48.1X3	T48.1X4	T48.1X5	T48.1X6
smooth NEC	T44.3X1	T44.3X2	T44.3X3	T44.3X4	T44.3X5	T44.3X6
Remoxipride	T43.591	T43.592	T43.593	T43.594	T43.595	T43.596
Renese	T50.2X1	T50.2X2	T50.2X3	T50.2X4	T50.2X5	T50.2X6
Renografin	T50.8X1	T50.8X2	T50.8X3	T50.8X4	T50.8X5	T50.8X6
Replacement solution	T50.3X1	T50.3X2	T50.3X3	T50.3X4	T50.3X5	T50.3X6
Reproterol	T48.6X1	T48.6X2	T48.6X3	T48.6X4	T48.6X5	T48.6X6
Rescinnamine	T46.5X1	T46.5X2	T46.5X3	T46.5X4	T46.5X5	T46.5X6
Reserpin(e)	T46.5X1	T46.5X2	T46.5X3	T46.5X4	T46.5X5	T46.5X6
Resorcin, resorcinol (nonmedicinal)	T65.891	T65.892	T65.893	T65.894	—	—
medicinal	T49.4X1	T49.4X2	T49.4X3	T49.4X4	T49.4X5	T49.4X6
Respaire	T48.4X1	T48.4X2	T48.4X3	T48.4X4	T48.4X5	T48.4X6
Respiratory drug NEC	T48.901	T48.902	T48.903	T48.904	T48.905	T48.906
antiasthmatic NEC	T48.6X1	T48.6X2	T48.6X3	T48.6X4	T48.6X5	T48.6X6
anti-common-cold NEC	T48.5X1	T48.5X2	T48.5X3	T48.5X4	T48.5X5	T48.5X6
expectorant NEC	T48.4X1	T48.4X2	T48.4X3	T48.4X4	T48.4X5	T48.4X6
stimulant	T48.901	T48.902	T48.903	T48.904	T48.905	T48.906
Retinoic acid	T49.0X1	T49.0X2	T49.0X3	T49.0X4	T49.0X5	T49.0X6
Retinol	T45.2X1	T45.2X2	T45.2X3	T45.2X4	T45.2X5	T45.2X6
Rh (D) immune globulin (human)	T50.Z11	T50.Z12	T50.Z13	T50.Z14	T50.Z15	T50.Z16
Rhodine	T39.011	T39.012	T39.013	T39.014	T39.015	T39.016
RhoGAM	T50.Z11	T50.Z12	T50.Z13	T50.Z14	T50.Z15	T50.Z16
Rhubarb						
dry extract	T47.2X1	T47.2X2	T47.2X3	T47.2X4	T47.2X5	T47.2X6
tincture, compound	T47.2X1	T47.2X2	T47.2X3	T47.2X4	T47.2X5	T47.2X6
Ribavirin	T37.5X1	T37.5X2	T37.5X3	T37.5X4	T37.5X5	T37.5X6
Riboflavin	T45.2X1	T45.2X2	T45.2X3	T45.2X4	T45.2X5	T45.2X6
Ribostamycin	T36.5X1	T36.5X2	T36.5X3	T36.5X4	T36.5X5	T36.5X6
Ricin	T62.2X1	T62.2X2	T62.2X3	T62.2X4	—	—
Ricinus communis	T62.2X1	T62.2X2	T62.2X3	T62.2X4	—	—
Rickettsial vaccine NEC	T50.A91	T50.A92	T50.A93	T50.A94	T50.A95	T50.A96
Rifabutin	T36.6X1	T36.6X2	T36.6X3	T36.6X4	T36.6X5	T36.6X6
Rifamide	T36.6X1	T36.6X2	T36.6X3	T36.6X4	T36.6X5	T36.6X6
Rifampicin	T36.6X1	T36.6X2	T36.6X3	T36.6X4	T36.6X5	T36.6X6
with isoniazid	T37.1X1	T37.1X2	T37.1X3	T37.1X4	T37.1X5	T37.1X6
Rifampin	T36.6X1	T36.6X2	T36.6X3	T36.6X4	T36.6X5	T36.6X6
Rifamycin	T36.6X1	T36.6X2	T36.6X3	T36.6X4	T36.6X5	T36.6X6
Rifaximin	T36.6X1	T36.6X2	T36.6X3	T36.6X4	T36.6X5	T36.6X6

	External Cause (T-Code)					
Substance	Poisoning, Accidental (Unintentional)	Poisoning, Intentional Self-Harm	Poisoning, Assault	Poisoning, Undetermined	Adverse Effect	Underdosing
Rimantadine	T37.5X1	T37.5X2	T37.5X3	T37.5X4	T37.5X5	T37.5X6
Rimazolium metilsulfate	T39.8X1	T39.8X2	T39.8X3	T39.8X4	T39.8X5	T39.8X6
Rimifon	T37.1X1	T37.1X2	T37.1X3	T37.1X4	T37.1X5	T37.1X6
Rimiterol	T48.6X1	T48.6X2	T48.6X3	T48.6X4	T48.6X5	T48.6X6
Ringer (lactate) solution	T50.3X1	T50.3X2	T50.3X3	T50.3X4	T50.3X5	T50.3X6
Ristocetin	T36.8X1	T36.8X2	T36.8X3	T36.8X4	T36.8X5	T36.8X6
Ritalin	T43.631	T43.632	T43.633	T43.634	T43.635	T43.636
Ritodrine	T44.5X1	T44.5X2	T44.5X3	T44.5X4	T44.5X5	T44.5X6
Roach killer — *see Insecticide*						
Rociverine	T44.3X1	T44.3X2	T44.3X3	T44.3X4	T44.3X5	T44.3X6
Rocky Mountain spotted fever vaccine	T50.A91	T50.A92	T50.A93	T50.A94	T50.A95	T50.A96
Rodenticide NEC	T60.4X1	T60.4X2	T60.4X3	T60.4X4	—	—
Rohypnol	T42.4X1	T42.4X2	T42.4X3	T42.4X4	T42.4X5	T42.4X6
Rokitamycin	T36.3X1	T36.3X2	T36.3X3	T36.3X4	T36.3X5	T36.3X6
Rolaids	T47.1X1	T47.1X2	T47.1X3	T47.1X4	T47.1X5	T47.1X6
Rolitetracycline	T36.4X1	T36.4X2	T36.4X3	T36.4X4	T36.4X5	T36.4X6
Romilar	T48.3X1	T48.3X2	T48.3X3	T48.3X4	T48.3X5	T48.3X6
Ronifibrate	T46.6X1	T46.6X2	T46.6X3	T46.6X4	T46.6X5	T46.6X6
Rosaprostol	T47.1X1	T47.1X2	T47.1X3	T47.1X4	T47.1X5	T47.1X6
Rose bengal sodium (131I)	T50.8X1	T50.8X2	T50.8X3	T50.8X4	T50.8X5	T50.8X6
Rose water ointment	T49.3X1	T49.3X2	T49.3X3	T49.3X4	T49.3X5	T49.3X6
Rosoxacin	T37.8X1	T37.8X2	T37.8X3	T37.8X4	T37.8X5	T37.8X6
Rotenone	T60.2X1	T60.2X2	T60.2X3	T60.2X4	—	—
Rotoxamine	T45.0X1	T45.0X2	T45.0X3	T45.0X4	T45.0X5	T45.0X6
Rough-on-rats	T60.4X1	T60.4X2	T60.4X3	T60.4X4	—	—
Roxatidine	T47.0X1	T47.0X2	T47.0X3	T47.0X4	T47.0X5	T47.0X6
Roxithromycin	T36.3X1	T36.3X2	T36.3X3	T36.3X4	T36.3X5	T36.3X6
Rt-PA	T45.611	T45.612	T45.613	T45.614	T45.615	T45.616
Rubbing alcohol	T51.2X1	T51.2X2	T51.2X3	T51.2X4	—	—
Rubefacient	T49.4X1	T49.4X2	T49.4X3	T49.4X4	T49.4X5	T49.4X6
Rubella vaccine	T50.B91	T50.B92	T50.B93	T50.B94	T50.B95	T50.B96
Rubelogen	T50.B91	T50.B92	T50.B93	T50.B94	T50.B95	T50.B96
Rubeovax	T50.991	T50.992	T50.993	T50.994	T50.995	T50.996
Rubidium chloride Rb82	T50.8X1	T50.8X2	T50.8X3	T50.8X4	T50.8X5	T50.8X6
Rubidomycin	T45.1X1	T45.1X2	T45.1X3	T45.1X4	T45.1X5	T45.1X6
Rue	T62.2X1	T62.2X2	T62.2X3	T62.2X4	—	—
Rufocromomycin	T45.1X1	T45.1X2	T45.1X3	T45.1X4	T45.1X5	T45.1X6
Russel's viper venin	T45.7X1	T45.7X2	T45.7X3	T45.7X4	T45.7X5	T45.7X6
Ruta (graveolens)	T62.2X1	T62.2X2	T62.2X3	T62.2X4	—	—
Rutinum	T46.991	T46.992	T46.993	T46.994	T46.995	T46.996
Rutoside	T46.991	T46.992	T46.993	T46.994	T46.995	T46.996

Substance	External Cause (T-Code): Poisoning, Accidental (Unintentional)	Poisoning, Intentional Self-Harm	Poisoning, Assault	Poisoning, Undetermined	Adverse Effect	Underdosing
S						
Sabadilla (plant)	T62.2X1	T62.2X2	T62.2X3	T62.2X4	—	—
pesticide	T60.2X1	T60.2X2	T60.2X3	T60.2X4	—	—
Saccharated iron oxide	T45.8X1	T45.8X2	T45.8X3	T45.8X4	T45.8X5	T45.8X6
Saccharin	T50.901	T50.902	T50.903	T50.904	T50.905	T50.906
Saccharomyces boulardii	T47.6X1	T47.6X2	T47.6X3	T47.6X4	T47.6X5	T47.6X6
Safflower oil	T46.6X1	T46.6X2	T46.6X3	T46.6X4	T46.6X5	T46.6X6
Safrazine	T43.1X1	T43.1X2	T43.1X3	T43.1X4	T43.1X5	T43.1X6
Salazosulfapyridine	T37.0X1	T37.0X2	T37.0X3	T37.0X4	T37.0X5	T37.0X6
Salbutamol	T48.6X1	T48.6X2	T48.6X3	T48.6X4	T48.6X5	T48.6X6
Salicylamide	T39.091	T39.092	T39.093	T39.094	T39.095	T39.096
Salicylate NEC	T39.091	T39.092	T39.093	T39.094	T39.095	T39.096
methyl	T49.3X1	T49.3X2	T49.3X3	T49.3X4	T49.3X5	T49.3X6
theobromine calcium	T50.2X1	T50.2X2	T50.2X3	T50.2X4	T50.2X5	T50.2X6
Salicylazosulfapyridine	T37.0X1	T37.0X2	T37.0X3	T37.0X4	T37.0X5	T37.0X6
Salicylhydroxamic acid	T49.0X1	T49.0X2	T49.0X3	T49.0X4	T49.0X5	T49.0X6
Salicylic acid	T49.4X1	T49.4X2	T49.4X3	T49.4X4	T49.4X5	T49.4X6
with benzoic acid	T49.4X1	T49.4X2	T49.4X3	T49.4X4	T49.4X5	T49.4X6
congeners	T39.091	T39.092	T39.093	T39.094	T39.095	T39.096
derivative	T39.091	T39.092	T39.093	T39.094	T39.095	T39.096
salts	T39.091	T39.092	T39.093	T39.094	T39.095	T39.096
Salinazid	T37.1X1	T37.1X2	T37.1X3	T37.1X4	T37.1X5	T37.1X6
Salmeterol	T48.6X1	T48.6X2	T48.6X3	T48.6X4	T48.6X5	T48.6X6
Salol	T49.3X1	T49.3X2	T49.3X3	T49.3X4	T49.3X5	T49.3X6
Salsalate	T39.091	T39.092	T39.093	T39.094	T39.095	T39.096
Salt substitute	T50.901	T50.902	T50.903	T50.904	T50.905	T50.906
Salt-replacing drug	T50.901	T50.902	T50.903	T50.904	T50.905	T50.906
Salt-retaining mineralocorticoid	T50.0X1	T50.0X2	T50.0X3	T50.0X4	T50.0X5	T50.0X6
Saluretic NEC	T50.2X1	T50.2X2	T50.2X3	T50.2X4	T50.2X5	T50.2X6
Saluron	T50.2X1	T50.2X2	T50.2X3	T50.2X4	T50.2X5	T50.2X6
Salvarsan 606 (neosilver) (silver)	T37.8X1	T37.8X2	T37.8X3	T37.8X4	T37.8X5	T37.8X6
Sambucus canadensis	T62.2X1	T62.2X2	T62.2X3	T62.2X4	—	—
berry	T62.1X1	T62.1X2	T62.1X3	T62.1X4	—	—
Sandril	T46.5X1	T46.5X2	T46.5X3	T46.5X4	T46.5X5	T46.5X6
Sanguinaria canadensis	T62.2X1	T62.2X2	T62.2X3	T62.2X4	—	—
Saniflush (cleaner)	T54.2X1	T54.2X2	T54.2X3	T54.2X4	—	—
Santonin	T37.4X1	T37.4X2	T37.4X3	T37.4X4	T37.4X5	T37.4X6
Santyl	T49.8X1	T49.8X2	T49.8X3	T49.8X4	T49.8X5	T49.8X6
Saralasin	T46.5X1	T46.5X2	T46.5X3	T46.5X4	T46.5X5	T46.5X6
Sarcolysin	T45.1X1	T45.1X2	T45.1X3	T45.1X4	T45.1X5	T45.1X6
Sarkomycin	T45.1X1	T45.1X2	T45.1X3	T45.1X4	T45.1X5	T45.1X6
Saroten	T43.011	T43.012	T43.013	T43.014	T43.015	T43.016

Substance	External Cause (T-Code): Poisoning, Accidental (Unintentional)	Poisoning, Intentional Self-Harm	Poisoning, Assault	Poisoning, Undetermined	Adverse Effect	Underdosing
Saturnine — *see Lead*						
Savin (oil)	T49.4X1	T49.4X2	T49.4X3	T49.4X4	T49.4X5	T49.4X6
Scammony	T47.2X1	T47.2X2	T47.2X3	T47.2X4	T47.2X5	T47.2X6
Scarlet red	T49.8X1	T49.8X2	T49.8X3	T49.8X4	T49.8X5	T49.8X6
Scheele's green	T57.0X1	T57.0X2	T57.0X3	T57.0X4	—	—
insecticide	T57.0X1	T57.0X2	T57.0X3	T57.0X4	—	—
Schizontozide (blood) (tissue)	T37.2X1	T37.2X2	T37.2X3	T37.2X4	T37.2X5	T37.2X6
Schradan	T60.0X1	T60.0X2	T60.0X3	T60.0X4	—	—
Schweinfurth green	T57.0X1	T57.0X2	T57.0X3	T57.0X4	—	—
insecticide	T57.0X1	T57.0X2	T57.0X3	T57.0X4	—	—
Scilla, rat poison	T60.4X1	T60.4X2	T60.4X3	T60.4X4	—	—
Scillaren	T60.4X1	T60.4X2	T60.4X3	T60.4X4	—	—
Sclerosing agent	T46.8X1	T46.8X2	T46.8X3	T46.8X4	T46.8X5	T46.8X6
Scombrotoxin	T61.11	T61.12	T61.13	T61.14	—	—
Scopolamine	T44.3X1	T44.3X2	T44.3X3	T44.3X4	T44.3X5	T44.3X6
Scopolia extract	T44.3X1	T44.3X2	T44.3X3	T44.3X4	T44.3X5	T44.3X6
Scouring powder	T65.891	T65.892	T65.893	T65.894	—	—
Sea						
anemone (sting)	T63.631	T63.632	T63.633	T63.634	—	—
cucumber (sting)	T63.691	T63.692	T63.693	T63.694	—	—
snake (bite) (venom)	T63.091	T63.092	T63.093	T63.094	—	—
urchin spine (puncture)	T63.691	T63.692	T63.693	T63.694	—	—
Seafood	T61.91	T61.92	T61.93	T61.94	—	—
specified NEC	T61.8X1	T61.8X2	T61.8X3	T61.8X4	—	—
Secbutabarbital	T42.3X1	T42.3X2	T42.3X3	T42.3X4	T42.3X5	T42.3X6
Secbutabarbitone	T42.3X1	T42.3X2	T42.3X3	T42.3X4	T42.3X5	T42.3X6
Secnidazole	T37.3X1	T37.3X2	T37.3X3	T37.3X4	T37.3X5	T37.3X6
Secobarbital	T42.3X1	T42.3X2	T42.3X3	T42.3X4	T42.3X5	T42.3X6
Seconal	T42.3X1	T42.3X2	T42.3X3	T42.3X4	T42.3X5	T42.3X6
Secretin	T50.8X1	T50.8X2	T50.8X3	T50.8X4	T50.8X5	T50.8X6
Sedative NEC	T42.71	T42.72	T42.73	T42.74	T42.75	T42.76
mixed NEC	T42.6X1	T42.6X2	T42.6X3	T42.6X4	T42.6X5	T42.6X6
Sedormid	T42.6X1	T42.6X2	T42.6X3	T42.6X4	T42.6X5	T42.6X6
Seed disinfectant or dressing	T60.8X1	T60.8X2	T60.8X3	T60.8X4	—	—
Seeds (poisonous)	T62.2X1	T62.2X2	T62.2X3	T62.2X4	—	—
Selegiline	T42.8X1	T42.8X2	T42.8X3	T42.8X4	T42.8X5	T42.8X6
Selenium NEC	T56.891	T56.892	T56.893	T56.894	—	—
disulfide or sulfide	T49.4X1	T49.4X2	T49.4X3	T49.4X4	T49.4X5	T49.4X6
fumes	T59.891	T59.892	T59.893	T59.894	—	—
sulfide	T49.4X1	T49.4X2	T49.4X3	T49.4X4	T49.4X5	T49.4X6
Selenomethionine (75Se)	T50.8X1	T50.8X2	T50.8X3	T50.8X4	T50.8X5	T50.8X6
Selsun	T49.4X1	T49.4X2	T49.4X3	T49.4X4	T49.4X5	T49.4X6

New Revised ~~deleted~~ Deleted

Substance	Poisoning, Accidental (Unintentional)	Poisoning, Intentional Self-Harm	Poisoning, Assault	Poisoning, Undetermined	Adverse Effect	Underdosing
	External Cause (T-Code)					
Semustine	T45.1X1	T45.1X2	T45.1X3	T45.1X4	T45.1X5	T45.1X6
Senega syrup	T48.4X1	T48.4X2	T48.4X3	T48.4X4	T48.4X5	T48.4X6
Senna	T47.2X1	T47.2X2	T47.2X3	T47.2X4	T47.2X5	T47.2X6
Sennoside A+B	T47.2X1	T47.2X2	T47.2X3	T47.2X4	T47.2X5	T47.2X6
Septisol	T49.2X1	T49.2X2	T49.2X3	T49.2X4	T49.2X5	T49.2X6
Seractide	T38.811	T38.812	T38.813	T38.814	T38.815	T38.816
Serax	T42.4X1	T42.4X2	T42.4X3	T42.4X4	T42.4X5	T42.4X6
Serenesil	T42.6X1	T42.6X2	T42.6X3	T42.6X4	T42.6X5	T42.6X6
Serenium (hydrochloride)	T37.91	T37.92	T37.93	T37.94	T37.95	T37.96
Serepax — *see Oxazepam*						
Sermorelin	T38.891	T38.892	T38.893	T38.894	T38.895	T38.896
Sernyl	T41.1X1	T41.1X2	T41.1X3	T41.1X4	T41.1X5	T41.1X6
Serotonin	T50.991	T50.992	T50.993	T50.994	T50.995	T50.996
Serpasil	T46.5X1	T46.5X2	T46.5X3	T46.5X4	T46.5X5	T46.5X6
Serrapeptase	T45.3X1	T45.3X2	T45.3X3	T45.3X4	T45.3X5	T45.3X6
Serum						
antibotulinus	T50.Z11	T50.Z12	T50.Z13	T50.Z14	T50.Z15	T50.Z16
anticytotoxic	T50.Z11	T50.Z12	T50.Z13	T50.Z14	T50.Z15	T50.Z16
antidiphtheria	T50.Z11	T50.Z12	T50.Z13	T50.Z14	T50.Z15	T50.Z16
antimeningococcus	T50.Z11	T50.Z12	T50.Z13	T50.Z14	T50.Z15	T50.Z16
anti-Rh	T50.Z11	T50.Z12	T50.Z13	T50.Z14	T50.Z15	T50.Z16
anti-snake-bite	T50.Z11	T50.Z12	T50.Z13	T50.Z14	T50.Z15	T50.Z16
antitetanic	T50.Z11	T50.Z12	T50.Z13	T50.Z14	T50.Z15	T50.Z16
antitoxic	T50.Z11	T50.Z12	T50.Z13	T50.Z14	T50.Z15	T50.Z16
complement (inhibitor)	T45.8X1	T45.8X2	T45.8X3	T45.8X4	T45.8X5	T45.8X6
convalescent	T50.Z11	T50.Z12	T50.Z13	T50.Z14	T50.Z15	T50.Z16
hemolytic complement	T45.8X1	T45.8X2	T45.8X3	T45.8X4	T45.8X5	T45.8X6
immune (human)	T50.Z11	T50.Z12	T50.Z13	T50.Z14	T50.Z15	T50.Z16
protective NEC	T50.Z11	T50.Z12	T50.Z13	T50.Z14	T50.Z15	T50.Z16
Setastine	T45.0X1	T45.0X2	T45.0X3	T45.0X4	T45.0X5	T45.0X6
Setoperone	T43.591	T43.592	T43.593	T43.594	T43.595	T43.596
Sewer gas	T59.91	T59.92	T59.93	T59.94	—	—
Shampoo	T55.0X1	T55.0X2	T55.0X3	T55.0X4	—	—
Shellfish, noxious, nonbacterial	T61.781	T61.782	T61.783	T61.784	—	—
Sildenafil	T46.7X1	T46.7X2	T46.7X3	T46.7X4	T46.7X5	T46.7X6
Silibinin	T50.991	T50.992	T50.993	T50.994	T50.995	T50.996
Silicone NEC	T65.891	T65.892	T65.893	T65.894	—	—
medicinal	T49.3X1	T49.3X2	T49.3X3	T49.3X4	T49.3X5	T49.3X6
Silvadene	T49.0X1	T49.0X2	T49.0X3	T49.0X4	T49.0X5	T49.0X6
Silver	T49.0X1	T49.0X2	T49.0X3	T49.0X4	T49.0X5	T49.0X6
anti-infectives	T49.0X1	T49.0X2	T49.0X3	T49.0X4	T49.0X5	T49.0X6
arsphenamine	T37.8X1	T37.8X2	T37.8X3	T37.8X4	T37.8X5	T37.8X6

Substance	Poisoning, Accidental (Unintentional)	Poisoning, Intentional Self-Harm	Poisoning, Assault	Poisoning, Undetermined	Adverse Effect	Underdosing
	External Cause (T-Code)					
Silver *(Continued)*						
colloidal	T49.0X1	T49.0X2	T49.0X3	T49.0X4	T49.0X5	T49.0X6
nitrate	T49.0X1	T49.0X2	T49.0X3	T49.0X4	T49.0X5	T49.0X6
ophthalmic preparation	T49.5X1	T49.5X2	T49.5X3	T49.5X4	T49.5X5	T49.5X6
toughened (keratolytic)	T49.4X1	T49.4X2	T49.4X3	T49.4X4	T49.4X5	T49.4X6
nonmedicinal (dust)	T56.891	T56.892	T56.893	T56.894	—	—
protein	T49.5X1	T49.5X2	T49.5X3	T49.5X4	T49.5X5	T49.5X6
salvarsan	T37.8X1	T37.8X2	T37.8X3	T37.8X4	T37.8X5	T37.8X6
sulfadiazine	T49.4X1	T49.4X2	T49.4X3	T49.4X4	T49.4X5	T49.4X6
Silymarin	T50.991	T50.992	T50.993	T50.994	T50.995	T50.996
Simaldrate	T47.1X1	T47.1X2	T47.1X3	T47.1X4	T47.1X5	T47.1X6
Simazine	T60.3X1	T60.3X2	T60.3X3	T60.3X4	—	—
Simethicone	T47.1X1	T47.1X2	T47.1X3	T47.1X4	T47.1X5	T47.1X6
Simfibrate	T46.6X1	T46.6X2	T46.6X3	T46.6X4	T46.6X5	T46.6X6
Simvastatin	T46.6X1	T46.6X2	T46.6X3	T46.6X4	T46.6X5	T46.6X6
Sincalide	T50.8X1	T50.8X2	T50.8X3	T50.8X4	T50.8X5	T50.8X6
Sinequan	T43.011	T43.012	T43.013	T43.014	T43.015	T43.016
Singoserp	T46.5X1	T46.5X2	T46.5X3	T46.5X4	T46.5X5	T46.5X6
Sintrom	T45.511	T45.512	T45.513	T45.514	T45.515	T45.516
Sisomicin	T36.5X1	T36.5X2	T36.5X3	T36.5X4	T36.5X5	T36.5X6
Sitosterols	T46.6X1	T46.6X2	T46.6X3	T46.6X4	T46.6X5	T46.6X6
Skeletal muscle relaxants	T48.1X1	T48.1X2	T48.1X3	T48.1X4	T48.1X5	T48.1X6
Skin						
agents (external)	T49.91	T49.92	T49.93	T49.94	T49.95	T49.96
specified NEC	T49.8X1	T49.8X2	T49.8X3	T49.8X4	T49.8X5	T49.8X6
test antigen	T50.8X1	T50.8X2	T50.8X3	T50.8X4	T50.8X5	T50.8X6
Sleep-eze	T45.0X1	T45.0X2	T45.0X3	T45.0X4	T45.0X5	T45.0X6
Sleeping draught, pill	T42.71	T42.72	T42.73	T42.74	T42.75	T42.76
Smallpox vaccine	T50.B11	T50.B12	T50.B13	T50.B14	T50.B15	T50.B16
Smelter fumes NEC	T56.91	T56.92	T56.93	T56.94	—	—
Smog	T59.1X1	T59.1X2	T59.1X3	T59.1X4	—	—
Smoke NEC	T59.811	T59.812	T59.813	T59.814	—	—
Smooth muscle relaxant	T44.3X1	T44.3X2	T44.3X3	T44.3X4	T44.3X5	T44.3X6
Snail killer NEC	T60.8X1	T60.8X2	T60.8X3	T60.8X4	—	—
Snake venom or bite	T63.001	T63.002	T63.003	T63.004	—	—
hemocoagulase	T45.7X1	T45.7X2	T45.7X3	T45.7X4	T45.7X5	T45.7X6
Snuff	T65.211	T65.212	T65.213	T65.214	—	—
Soap (powder) (product)	T55.0X1	T55.0X2	T55.0X3	T55.0X4	—	—
enema	T47.4X1	T47.4X2	T47.4X3	T47.4X4	T47.4X5	T47.4X6
medicinal, soft	T49.2X1	T49.2X2	T49.2X3	T49.2X4	T49.2X5	T49.2X6
superfatted	T49.2X1	T49.2X2	T49.2X3	T49.2X4	T49.2X5	T49.2X6
Sobrerol	T48.4X1	T48.4X2	T48.4X3	T48.4X4	T48.4X5	T48.4X6

Substance	Poisoning, Accidental (Unintentional)	Poisoning, Intentional Self-Harm	Poisoning, Assault	Poisoning, Undetermined	Adverse Effect	Underdosing
	External Cause (T-Code)					
Soda (caustic)	T54.3X1	T54.3X2	T54.3X3	T54.3X4	—	—
bicarb	T47.1X1	T47.1X2	T47.1X3	T47.1X4	T47.1X5	T47.1X6
chlorinated — *see Sodium, hypochlorite*						
Sodium						
acetosulfone	T37.1X1	T37.1X2	T37.1X3	T37.1X4	T37.1X5	T37.1X6
acetrizoate	T5Ø.8X1	T5Ø.8X2	T5Ø.8X3	T5Ø.8X4	T5Ø.8X5	T5Ø.8X6
acid phosphate	T5Ø.3X1	T5Ø.3X2	T5Ø.3X3	T5Ø.3X4	T5Ø.3X5	T5Ø.3X6
alginate	T47.8X1	T47.8X2	T47.8X3	T47.8X4	T47.8X5	T47.8X6
amidotrizoate	T5Ø.8X1	T5Ø.8X2	T5Ø.8X3	T5Ø.8X4	T5Ø.8X5	T5Ø.8X6
aminopterin	T45.1X1	T45.1X2	T45.1X3	T45.1X4	T45.1X5	T45.1X6
amylosulfate	T47.8X1	T47.8X2	T47.8X3	T47.8X4	T47.8X5	T47.8X6
amytal	T42.3X1	T42.3X2	T42.3X3	T42.3X4	T42.3X5	T42.3X6
antimony gluconate	T37.3X1	T37.3X2	T37.3X3	T37.3X4	T37.3X5	T37.3X6
arsenate	T57.ØX1	T57.ØX2	T57.ØX3	T57.ØX4	—	—
aurothiomalate	T39.4X1	T39.4X2	T39.4X3	T39.4X4	T39.4X5	T39.4X6
aurothiosulfate	T39.4X1	T39.4X2	T39.4X3	T39.4X4	T39.4X5	T39.4X6
barbiturate	T42.3X1	T42.3X2	T42.3X3	T42.3X4	T42.3X5	T42.3X6
basic phosphate	T47.4X1	T47.4X2	T47.4X3	T47.4X4	T47.4X5	T47.4X6
bicarbonate	T47.1X1	T47.1X2	T47.1X3	T47.1X4	T47.1X5	T47.1X6
bichromate	T57.8X1	T57.8X2	T57.8X3	T57.8X4	—	—
biphosphate	T5Ø.3X1	T5Ø.3X2	T5Ø.3X3	T5Ø.3X4	T5Ø.3X5	T5Ø.3X6
bisulfate	T65.891	T65.892	T65.893	T65.894	—	—
borate						
cleanser	T57.8X1	T57.8X2	T57.8X3	T57.8X4	—	—
eye	T49.5X1	T49.5X2	T49.5X3	T49.5X4	T49.5X5	T49.5X6
therapeutic	T49.8X1	T49.8X2	T49.8X3	T49.8X4	T49.8X5	T49.8X6
bromide	T42.6X1	T42.6X2	T42.6X3	T42.6X4	T42.6X5	T42.6X6
cacodylate (nonmedicinal) NEC	T5Ø.8X1	T5Ø.8X2	T5Ø.8X3	T5Ø.8X4	T5Ø.8X5	T5Ø.8X6
anti-infective	T37.8X1	T37.8X2	T37.8X3	T37.8X4	T37.8X5	T37.8X6
herbicide	T6Ø.3X1	T6Ø.3X2	T6Ø.3X3	T6Ø.3X4	—	—
calcium edetate	T45.8X1	T45.8X2	T45.8X3	T45.8X4	T45.8X5	T45.8X6
carbonate NEC	T54.3X1	T54.3X2	T54.3X3	T54.3X4	—	—
chlorate NEC	T65.891	T65.892	T65.893	T65.894	—	—
herbicide	T54.91	T54.92	T54.93	T54.94	—	—
chloride	T5Ø.3X1	T5Ø.3X2	T5Ø.3X3	T5Ø.3X4	T5Ø.3X5	T5Ø.3X6
with glucose	T5Ø.3X1	T5Ø.3X2	T5Ø.3X3	T5Ø.3X4	T5Ø.3X5	T5Ø.3X6
chromate	T65.891	T65.892	T65.893	T65.894	—	—
citrate	T5Ø.991	T5Ø.992	T5Ø.993	T5Ø.994	T5Ø.995	T5Ø.996
cromoglicate	T48.6X1	T48.6X2	T48.6X3	T48.6X4	T48.6X5	T48.6X6
cyanide	T65.ØX1	T65.ØX2	T65.ØX3	T65.ØX4	—	—
cyclamate	T5Ø.3X1	T5Ø.3X2	T5Ø.3X3	T5Ø.3X4	T5Ø.3X5	T5Ø.3X6
Sodium *(Continued)*						
dehydrocholate	T45.8X1	T45.8X2	T45.8X3	T45.8X4	T45.8X5	T45.8X6
diatrizoate	T5Ø.8X1	T5Ø.8X2	T5Ø.8X3	T5Ø.8X4	T5Ø.8X5	T5Ø.8X6
dibunate	T48.4X1	T48.4X2	T48.4X3	T48.4X4	T48.4X5	T48.4X6
dioctyl sulfosuccinate	T47.4X1	T47.4X2	T47.4X3	T47.4X4	T47.4X5	T47.4X6
dipantoyl ferrate	T45.8X1	T45.8X2	T45.8X3	T45.8X4	T45.8X5	T45.8X6
edetate	T45.8X1	T45.8X2	T45.8X3	T45.8X4	T45.8X5	T45.8X6
ethacrynate	T5Ø.1X1	T5Ø.1X2	T5Ø.1X3	T5Ø.1X4	T5Ø.1X5	T5Ø.1X6
feredetate	T45.8X1	T45.8X2	T45.8X3	T45.8X4	T45.8X5	T45.8X6
Fluoride — *see Fluoride*						
fluoroacetate (dust) (pesticide)	T6Ø.4X1	T6Ø.4X2	T6Ø.4X3	T6Ø.4X4	—	—
free salt	T5Ø.3X1	T5Ø.3X2	T5Ø.3X3	T5Ø.3X4	T5Ø.3X5	T5Ø.3X6
fusidate	T36.8X1	T36.8X2	T36.8X3	T36.8X4	T36.8X5	T36.8X6
glucaldrate	T47.1X1	T47.1X2	T47.1X3	T47.1X4	T47.1X5	T47.1X6
glucosulfone	T37.1X1	T37.1X2	T37.1X3	T37.1X4	T37.1X5	T37.1X6
glutamate	T45.8X1	T45.8X2	T45.8X3	T45.8X4	T45.8X5	T45.8X6
hydrogen carbonate	T5Ø.3X1	T5Ø.3X2	T5Ø.3X3	T5Ø.3X4	T5Ø.3X5	T5Ø.3X6
hydroxide	T54.3X1	T54.3X2	T54.3X3	T54.3X4	—	—
hypochlorite (bleach) NEC	T54.3X1	T54.3X2	T54.3X3	T54.3X4	—	—
disinfectant	T54.3X1	T54.3X2	T54.3X3	T54.3X4	—	—
medicinal (anti-infective) (external)	T49.ØX1	T49.ØX2	T49.ØX3	T49.ØX4	T49.ØX5	T49.ØX6
vapor	T54.3X1	T54.3X2	T54.3X3	T54.3X4	—	—
hyposulfite	T49.ØX1	T49.ØX2	T49.ØX3	T49.ØX4	T49.ØX5	T49.ØX6
indigotin disulfonate	T5Ø.8X1	T5Ø.8X2	T5Ø.8X3	T5Ø.8X4	T5Ø.8X5	T5Ø.8X6
iodide	T5Ø.991	T5Ø.992	T5Ø.993	T5Ø.994	T5Ø.995	T5Ø.996
I-131	T5Ø.8X1	T5Ø.8X2	T5Ø.8X3	T5Ø.8X4	T5Ø.8X5	T5Ø.8X6
therapeutic	T38.2X1	T38.2X2	T38.2X3	T38.2X4	T38.2X5	T38.2X6
iodohippurate (131I)	T5Ø.8X1	T5Ø.8X2	T5Ø.8X3	T5Ø.8X4	T5Ø.8X5	T5Ø.8X6
iopodate	T5Ø.8X1	T5Ø.8X2	T5Ø.8X3	T5Ø.8X4	T5Ø.8X5	T5Ø.8X6
iothalamate	T5Ø.8X1	T5Ø.8X2	T5Ø.8X3	T5Ø.8X4	T5Ø.8X5	T5Ø.8X6
iron edetate	T45.4X1	T45.4X2	T45.4X3	T45.4X4	T45.4X5	T45.4X6
lactate (compound solution)	T45.8X1	T45.8X2	T45.8X3	T45.8X4	T45.8X5	T45.8X6
lauryl (sulfate)	T49.2X1	T49.2X2	T49.2X3	T49.2X4	T49.2X5	T49.2X6
(L)-triiodothyronine	T38.1X1	T38.1X2	T38.1X3	T38.1X4	T38.1X5	T38.1X6
magnesium citrate	T5Ø.991	T5Ø.992	T5Ø.993	T5Ø.994	T5Ø.995	T5Ø.996
mersalate	T5Ø.2X1	T5Ø.2X2	T5Ø.2X3	T5Ø.2X4	T5Ø.2X5	T5Ø.2X6
metasilicate	T65.891	T65.892	T65.893	T65.894	—	—
metrizoate	T5Ø.8X1	T5Ø.8X2	T5Ø.8X3	T5Ø.8X4	T5Ø.8X5	T5Ø.8X6
monofluoroacetate (pesticide)	T6Ø.1X1	T6Ø.1X2	T6Ø.1X3	T6Ø.1X4	—	—
morrhuate	T46.8X1	T46.8X2	T46.8X3	T46.8X4	T46.8X5	T46.8X6
nafcillin	T36.ØX1	T36.ØX2	T36.ØX3	T36.ØX4	T36.ØX5	T36.ØX6

Substance	External Cause (T-Code)					
	Poisoning, Accidental (Unintentional)	Poisoning, Intentional Self-Harm	Poisoning, Assault	Poisoning, Undetermined	Adverse Effect	Underdosing
Sodium *(Continued)*						
nitrate (oxidizing agent)	T65.891	T65.892	T65.893	T65.894	—	—
nitrite	T50.6X1	T50.6X2	T50.6X3	T50.6X4	T50.6X5	T50.6X6
nitroferricyanide	T46.5X1	T46.5X2	T46.5X3	T46.5X4	T46.5X5	T46.5X6
nitroprusside	T46.5X1	T46.5X2	T46.5X3	T46.5X4	T46.5X5	T46.5X6
oxalate	T65.891	T65.892	T65.893	T65.894	—	—
oxide/peroxide	T65.891	T65.892	T65.893	T65.894	—	—
oxybate	T41.291	T41.292	T41.293	T41.294	T41.295	T41.296
para-aminohippurate	T50.8X1	T50.8X2	T50.8X3	T50.8X4	T50.8X5	T50.8X6
perborate (nonmedicinal) NEC	T65.891	T65.892	T65.893	T65.894	—	—
medicinal	T49.0X1	T49.0X2	T49.0X3	T49.0X4	T49.0X5	T49.0X6
soap	T55.0X1	T55.0X2	T55.0X3	T55.0X4	—	—
percarbonate — *see Sodium, perborate*						
pertechnetate Tc99m	T50.8X1	T50.8X2	T50.8X3	T50.8X4	T50.8X5	T50.8X6
phosphate						
cellulose	T45.8X1	T45.8X2	T45.8X3	T45.8X4	T45.8X5	T45.8X6
dibasic	T47.2X1	T47.2X2	T47.2X3	T47.2X4	T47.2X5	T47.2X6
monobasic	T47.2X1	T47.2X2	T47.2X3	T47.2X4	T47.2X5	T47.2X6
phytate	T50.6X1	T50.6X2	T50.6X3	T50.6X4	T50.6X5	T50.6X6
picosulfate	T47.2X1	T47.2X2	T47.2X3	T47.2X4	T47.2X5	T47.2X6
polyhydroxyaluminium monocarbonate	T47.1X1	T47.1X2	T47.1X3	T47.1X4	T47.1X5	T47.1X6
polystyrene sulfonate	T50.3X1	T50.3X2	T50.3X3	T50.3X4	T50.3X5	T50.3X6
propionate	T49.0X1	T49.0X2	T49.0X3	T49.0X4	T49.0X5	T49.0X6
propyl hydroxybenzoate	T50.991	T50.992	T50.993	T50.994	T50.995	T50.996
psylliate	T46.8X1	T46.8X2	T46.8X3	T46.8X4	T46.8X5	T46.8X6
removing resins	T50.3X1	T50.3X2	T50.3X3	T50.3X4	T50.3X5	T50.3X6
salicylate	T39.091	T39.092	T39.093	T39.094	T39.095	T39.096
salt NEC	T50.3X1	T50.3X2	T50.3X3	T50.3X4	T50.3X5	T50.3X6
selenate	T60.2X1	T60.2X2	T60.2X3	T60.2X4	—	—
stibogluconate	T37.3X1	T37.3X2	T37.3X3	T37.3X4	T37.3X5	T37.3X6
sulfate	T47.4X1	T47.4X2	T47.4X3	T47.4X4	T47.4X5	T47.4X6
sulfoxone	T37.1X1	T37.1X2	T37.1X3	T37.1X4	T37.1X5	T37.1X6
tetradecyl sulfate	T46.8X1	T46.8X2	T46.8X3	T46.8X4	T46.8X5	T46.8X6
thiopental	T41.1X1	T41.1X2	T41.1X3	T41.1X4	T41.1X5	T41.1X6
thiosalicylate	T39.091	T39.092	T39.093	T39.094	T39.095	T39.096
thiosulfate	T50.6X1	T50.6X2	T50.6X3	T50.6X4	T50.6X5	T50.6X6
tolbutamide	T38.3X1	T38.3X2	T38.3X3	T38.3X4	T38.3X5	T38.3X6
l-triiodothyronine	T38.1X1	T38.1X2	T38.1X3	T38.1X4	T38.1X5	T38.1X6
tyropanoate	T50.8X1	T50.8X2	T50.8X3	T50.8X4	T50.8X5	T50.8X6
valproate	T42.6X1	T42.6X2	T42.6X3	T42.6X4	T42.6X5	T42.6X6
versenate	T50.6X1	T50.6X2	T50.6X3	T50.6X4	T50.6X5	T50.6X6
Sodium-free salt	T50.901	T50.902	T50.903	T50.904	T50.905	T50.906
Sodium-removing resin	T50.3X1	T50.3X2	T50.3X3	T50.3X4	T50.3X5	T50.3X6
Soft soap	T55.0X1	T55.0X2	T55.0X3	T55.0X4	—	—
Solanine	T62.2X1	T62.2X2	T62.2X3	T62.2X4	—	—
berries	T62.1X1	T62.1X2	T62.1X3	T62.1X4	—	—
Solanum dulcamara	T62.2X1	T62.2X2	T62.2X3	T62.2X4	—	—
berries	T62.1X1	T62.1X2	T62.1X3	T62.1X4	—	—
Solapsone	T37.1X1	T37.1X2	T37.1X3	T37.1X4	T37.1X5	T37.1X6
Solar lotion	T49.3X1	T49.3X2	T49.3X3	T49.3X4	T49.3X5	T49.3X6
Solasulfone	T37.1X1	T37.1X2	T37.1X3	T37.1X4	T37.1X5	T37.1X6
Soldering fluid	T65.891	T65.892	T65.893	T65.894	—	—
Solid substance	T65.91	T65.92	T65.93	T65.94	—	—
specified NEC	T65.891	T65.892	T65.893	T65.894	—	—
Solvent, industrial NEC	T52.91	T52.92	T52.93	T52.94	—	—
naphtha	T52.0X1	T52.0X2	T52.0X3	T52.0X4	—	—
petroleum	T52.0X1	T52.0X2	T52.0X3	T52.0X4	—	—
specified NEC	T52.8X1	T52.8X2	T52.8X3	T52.8X4	—	—
Soma	T42.8X1	T42.8X2	T42.8X3	T42.8X4	T42.8X5	T42.8X6
Somatorelin	T38.891	T38.892	T38.893	T38.894	T38.895	T38.896
Somatostatin	T38.991	T38.992	T38.993	T38.994	T38.995	T38.996
Somatotropin	T38.811	T38.812	T38.813	T38.814	T38.815	T38.816
Somatrem	T38.811	T38.812	T38.813	T38.814	T38.815	T38.816
Somatropin	T38.811	T38.812	T38.813	T38.814	T38.815	T38.816
Sominex	T45.0X1	T45.0X2	T45.0X3	T45.0X4	T45.0X5	T45.0X6
Somnos	T42.6X1	T42.6X2	T42.6X3	T42.6X4	T42.6X5	T42.6X6
Somonal	T42.3X1	T42.3X2	T42.3X3	T42.3X4	T42.3X5	T42.3X6
Soneryl	T42.3X1	T42.3X2	T42.3X3	T42.3X4	T42.3X5	T42.3X6
Soothing syrup	T50.901	T50.902	T50.903	T50.904	T50.905	T50.906
Sopor	T42.6X1	T42.6X2	T42.6X3	T42.6X4	T42.6X5	T42.6X6
Soporific	T42.71	T42.72	T42.73	T42.74	T42.75	T42.76
Soporific drug	T42.71	T42.72	T42.73	T42.74	T42.75	T42.76
specified type NEC	T42.6X1	T42.6X2	T42.6X3	T42.6X4	T42.6X5	T42.6X6
Sorbide nitrate	T46.3X1	T46.3X2	T46.3X3	T46.3X4	T46.3X5	T46.3X6
Sorbitol	T47.4X1	T47.4X2	T47.4X3	T47.4X4	T47.4X5	T47.4X6
Sotalol	T44.7X1	T44.7X2	T44.7X3	T44.7X4	T44.7X5	T44.7X6
Sotradecol	T46.8X1	T46.8X2	T46.8X3	T46.8X4	T46.8X5	T46.8X6
Soysterol	T46.6X1	T46.6X2	T46.6X3	T46.6X4	T46.6X5	T46.6X6
Spacoline	T44.3X1	T44.3X2	T44.3X3	T44.3X4	T44.3X5	T44.3X6
Spanish fly	T49.8X1	T49.8X2	T49.8X3	T49.8X4	T49.8X5	T49.8X6
Sparine	T43.3X1	T43.3X2	T43.3X3	T43.3X4	T43.3X5	T43.3X6
Sparteine	T48.0X1	T48.0X2	T48.0X3	T48.0X4	T48.0X5	T48.0X6

Substance	Poisoning, Accidental (Unintentional)	Poisoning, Intentional Self-Harm	Poisoning, Assault	Poisoning, Undetermined	Adverse Effect	Underdosing
	External Cause (T-Code)					
Spasmolytic						
anticholinergics	T44.3X1	T44.3X2	T44.3X3	T44.3X4	T44.3X5	T44.3X6
autonomic	T44.3X1	T44.3X2	T44.3X3	T44.3X4	T44.3X5	T44.3X6
bronchial NEC	T48.6X1	T48.6X2	T48.6X3	T48.6X4	T48.6X5	T48.6X6
quaternary ammonium	T44.3X1	T44.3X2	T44.3X3	T44.3X4	T44.3X5	T44.3X6
skeletal muscle NEC	T48.1X1	T48.1X2	T48.1X3	T48.1X4	T48.1X5	T48.1X6
Spectinomycin	T36.5X1	T36.5X2	T36.5X3	T36.5X4	T36.5X5	T36.5X6
Speed	T43.621	T43.622	T43.623	T43.624	T43.625	T43.626
Spermicide	T49.8X1	T49.8X2	T49.8X3	T49.8X4	T49.8X5	T49.8X6
Spider (bite) (venom)	T63.391	T63.392	T63.393	T63.394	—	—
antivenin	T50.Z11	T50.Z12	T50.Z13	T50.Z14	T50.Z15	T50.Z16
Spigelia (root)	T37.4X1	T37.4X2	T37.4X3	T37.4X4	T37.4X5	T37.4X6
Spindle inactivator	T50.4X1	T50.4X2	T50.4X3	T50.4X4	T50.4X5	T50.4X6
Spiperone	T43.4X1	T43.4X2	T43.4X3	T43.4X4	T43.4X5	T43.4X6
Spiramycin	T36.3X1	T36.3X2	T36.3X3	T36.3X4	T36.3X5	T36.3X6
Spirapril	T46.4X1	T46.4X2	T46.4X3	T46.4X4	T46.4X5	T46.4X6
Spirilene	T43.591	T43.592	T43.593	T43.594	T43.595	T43.596
Spirit(s) (neutral) NEC	T51.ØX1	T51.ØX2	T51.ØX3	T51.ØX4	—	—
beverage	T51.ØX1	T51.ØX2	T51.ØX3	T51.ØX4	—	—
industrial	T51.ØX1	T51.ØX2	T51.ØX3	T51.ØX4	—	—
mineral	T52.ØX1	T52.ØX2	T52.ØX3	T52.ØX4	—	—
of salt — *see Hydrochloric acid*						
surgical	T51.ØX1	T51.ØX2	T51.ØX3	T51.ØX4	—	—
Spironolactone	T50.ØX1	T50.ØX2	T50.ØX3	T50.ØX4	T50.ØX5	T50.ØX6
Spiroperidol	T43.4X1	T43.4X2	T43.4X3	T43.4X4	T43.4X5	T43.4X6
Sponge, absorbable (gelatin)	T45.7X1	T45.7X2	T45.7X3	T45.7X4	T45.7X5	T45.7X6
Sporostacin	T49.ØX1	T49.ØX2	T49.ØX3	T49.ØX4	T49.ØX5	T49.ØX6
Spray (aerosol)	T65.91	T65.92	T65.93	T65.94	—	—
cosmetic	T65.891	T65.892	T65.893	T65.894	—	—
medicinal NEC	T50.901	T50.902	T50.903	T50.904	T50.905	T50.906
pesticides — *see Pesticides*						
specified content — *see specific substance*						
Spurge flax	T62.2X1	T62.2X2	T62.2X3	T62.2X4	—	—
Spurges	T62.2X1	T62.2X2	T62.2X3	T62.2X4	—	—
Sputum viscosity-lowering drug	T48.4X1	T48.4X2	T48.4X3	T48.4X4	T48.4X5	T48.4X6
Squill	T46.ØX1	T46.ØX2	T46.ØX3	T46.ØX4	T46.ØX5	T46.ØX6
rat poison	T60.4X1	T60.4X2	T60.4X3	T60.4X4	—	—
Squirting cucumber (cathartic)	T47.2X1	T47.2X2	T47.2X3	T47.2X4	T47.2X5	T47.2X6
Stains	T65.6X1	T65.6X2	T65.6X3	T65.6X4	—	—
Stannous fluoride	T49.7X1	T49.7X2	T49.7X3	T49.7X4	T49.7X5	T49.7X6
Stanolone	T38.7X1	T38.7X2	T38.7X3	T38.7X4	T38.7X5	T38.7X6

Substance	Poisoning, Accidental (Unintentional)	Poisoning, Intentional Self-Harm	Poisoning, Assault	Poisoning, Undetermined	Adverse Effect	Underdosing
	External Cause (T-Code)					
Stanozolol	T38.7X1	T38.7X2	T38.7X3	T38.7X4	T38.7X5	T38.7X6
Staphisagria or stavesacre (pediculicide)	T49.ØX1	T49.ØX2	T49.ØX3	T49.ØX4	T49.ØX5	T49.ØX6
Starch	T50.901	T50.902	T50.903	T50.904	T50.905	T50.906
Stelazine	T43.3X1	T43.3X2	T43.3X3	T43.3X4	T43.3X5	T43.3X6
Stemetil	T43.3X1	T43.3X2	T43.3X3	T43.3X4	T43.3X5	T43.3X6
Stepronin	T48.4X1	T48.4X2	T48.4X3	T48.4X4	T48.4X5	T48.4X6
Sterculia	T47.4X1	T47.4X2	T47.4X3	T47.4X4	T47.4X5	T47.4X6
Sternutator gas	T59.891	T59.892	T59.893	T59.894	—	—
Steroid	T38.ØX1	T38.ØX2	T38.ØX3	T38.ØX4	T38.ØX5	T38.ØX6
anabolic	T38.7X1	T38.7X2	T38.7X3	T38.7X4	T38.7X5	T38.7X6
androgenic	T38.7X1	T38.7X2	T38.7X3	T38.7X4	T38.7X5	T38.7X6
antineoplastic, hormone	T38.7X1	T38.7X2	T38.7X3	T38.7X4	T38.7X5	T38.7X6
estrogen	T38.5X1	T38.5X2	T38.5X3	T38.5X4	T38.5X5	T38.5X6
ENT agent	T49.6X1	T49.6X2	T49.6X3	T49.6X4	T49.6X5	T49.6X6
ophthalmic preparation	T49.5X1	T49.5X2	T49.5X3	T49.5X4	T49.5X5	T49.5X6
topical NEC	T49.ØX1	T49.ØX2	T49.ØX3	T49.ØX4	T49.ØX5	T49.ØX6
Stibine	T56.891	T56.892	T56.893	T56.894	—	—
Stibogluconate	T37.3X1	T37.3X2	T37.3X3	T37.3X4	T37.3X5	T37.3X6
Stibophen	T37.4X1	T37.4X2	T37.4X3	T37.4X4	T37.4X5	T37.4X6
Stilbamidine (isetionate)	T37.3X1	T37.3X2	T37.3X3	T37.3X4	T37.3X5	T37.3X6
Stilbestrol	T38.5X1	T38.5X2	T38.5X3	T38.5X4	T38.5X5	T38.5X6
Stilboestrol	T38.5X1	T38.5X2	T38.5X3	T38.5X4	T38.5X5	T38.5X6
Stimulant						
central nervous system — *see also Psychostimulant*	T43.601	T43.602	T43.603	T43.604	T43.605	T43.606
analeptics	T50.7X1	T50.7X2	T50.7X3	T50.7X4	T50.7X5	T50.7X6
opiate antagonist	T50.7X1	T50.7X2	T50.7X3	T50.7X4	T50.7X5	T50.7X6
psychotherapeutic NEC — *see also Psychotherapeutic drug*	T43.601	T43.602	T43.603	T43.604	T43.605	T43.606
specified NEC	T43.691	T43.692	T43.693	T43.694	T43.695	T43.696
respiratory	T48.901	T48.902	T48.903	T48.904	T48.905	T48.906
Stone-dissolving drug	T50.901	T50.902	T50.903	T50.904	T50.905	T50.906
Storage battery (cells) (acid)	T54.2X1	T54.2X2	T54.2X3	T54.2X4	—	—
Stovaine	T41.3X1	T41.3X2	T41.3X3	T41.3X4	T41.3X5	T41.3X6
infiltration (subcutaneous)	T41.3X1	T41.3X2	T41.3X3	T41.3X4	T41.3X5	T41.3X6
nerve block (peripheral) (plexus)	T41.3X1	T41.3X2	T41.3X3	T41.3X4	T41.3X5	T41.3X6
spinal	T41.3X1	T41.3X2	T41.3X3	T41.3X4	T41.3X5	T41.3X6
topical (surface)	T41.3X1	T41.3X2	T41.3X3	T41.3X4	T41.3X5	T41.3X6
Stovarsal	T37.8X1	T37.8X2	T37.8X3	T37.8X4	T37.8X5	T37.8X6
Stove gas — *see Gas, stove*	T57.91	T57.92	T57.93	T57.94	—	—

	External Cause (T-Code)					
Substance	**Poisoning, Accidental (Unintentional)**	**Poisoning, Intentional Self-Harm**	**Poisoning, Assault**	**Poisoning, Undetermined**	**Adverse Effect**	**Underdosing**
Stoxil	T49.5X1	T49.5X2	T49.5X3	T49.5X4	T49.5X5	T49.5X6
Stramonium	T48.6X1	T48.6X2	T48.6X3	T48.6X4	T48.6X5	T48.6X6
natural state	T62.2X1	T62.2X2	T62.2X3	T62.2X4	—	—
Streptodornase	T45.3X1	T45.3X2	T45.3X3	T45.3X4	T45.3X5	T45.3X6
Streptoduocin	T36.5X1	T36.5X2	T36.5X3	T36.5X4	T36.5X5	T36.5X6
Streptokinase	T45.611	T45.612	T45.613	T45.614	T45.615	T45.616
Streptomycin (derivative)	T36.5X1	T36.5X2	T36.5X3	T36.5X4	T36.5X5	T36.5X6
Streptonivicin	T36.5X1	T36.5X2	T36.5X3	T36.5X4	T36.5X5	T36.5X6
Streptovarycin	T36.5X1	T36.5X2	T36.5X3	T36.5X4	T36.5X5	T36.5X6
Streptozocin	T45.1X1	T45.1X2	T45.1X3	T45.1X4	T45.1X5	T45.1X6
Streptozotocin	T45.1X1	T45.1X2	T45.1X3	T45.1X4	T45.1X5	T45.1X6
Stripper (paint) (solvent)	T52.8X1	T52.8X2	T52.8X3	T52.8X4	—	—
Strobane	T6Ø.1X1	T6Ø.1X2	T6Ø.1X3	T6Ø.1X4	—	—
Strofantina	T46.ØX1	T46.ØX2	T46.ØX3	T46.ØX4	T46.ØX5	T46.ØX6
Strophanthin (g) (k)	T46.ØX1	T46.ØX2	T46.ØX3	T46.ØX4	T46.ØX5	T46.ØX6
Strophanthus	T46.ØX1	T46.ØX2	T46.ØX3	T46.ØX4	T46.ØX5	T46.ØX6
Strophantin	T46.ØX1	T46.ØX2	T46.ØX3	T46.ØX4	T46.ØX5	T46.ØX6
Strophantin-g	T46.ØX1	T46.ØX2	T46.ØX3	T46.ØX4	T46.ØX5	T46.ØX6
Strychnine (nonmedicinal) (pesticide) (salts)	T65.1X1	T65.1X2	T65.1X3	T65.1X4	—	—
medicinal	T48.291	T48.292	T48.293	T48.294	T48.295	T48.296
Strychnos (ignatii) — *see Strychnine*						
Styramate	T42.8X1	T42.8X2	T42.8X3	T42.8X4	T42.8X5	T42.8X6
Styrene	T65.891	T65.892	T65.893	T65.894	—	—
Succinimide, antiepileptic or anticonvulsant	T42.2X1	T42.2X2	T42.2X3	T42.2X4	T42.2X5	T42.2X6
mercuric — *see Mercury*						
Succinylcholine	T48.1X1	T48.1X2	T48.1X3	T48.1X4	T48.1X5	T48.1X6
Succinylsulfathiazole	T37.ØX1	T37.ØX2	T37.ØX3	T37.ØX4	T37.ØX5	T37.ØX6
Sucralfate	T47.1X1	T47.1X2	T47.1X3	T47.1X4	T47.1X5	T47.1X6
Sucrose	T5Ø.3X1	T5Ø.3X2	T5Ø.3X3	T5Ø.3X4	T5Ø.3X5	T5Ø.3X6
Sufentanil	T4Ø.4X1	T4Ø.4X2	T4Ø.4X3	T4Ø.4X4	T4Ø.4X5	T4Ø.4X6
Sulbactam	T36.ØX1	T36.ØX2	T36.ØX3	T36.ØX4	T36.ØX5	T36.ØX6
Sulbenicillin	T36.ØX1	T36.ØX2	T36.ØX3	T36.ØX4	T36.ØX5	T36.ØX6
Sulbentine	T49.ØX1	T49.ØX2	T49.ØX3	T49.ØX4	T49.ØX5	T49.ØX6
Sulfacetamide	T49.ØX1	T49.ØX2	T49.ØX3	T49.ØX4	T49.ØX5	T49.ØX6
ophthalmic preparation	T49.5X1	T49.5X2	T49.5X3	T49.5X4	T49.5X5	T49.5X6
Sulfachlorpyridazine	T37.ØX1	T37.ØX2	T37.ØX3	T37.ØX4	T37.ØX5	T37.ØX6
Sulfacitine	T37.ØX1	T37.ØX2	T37.ØX3	T37.ØX4	T37.ØX5	T37.ØX6
Sulfadiasulfone sodium	T37.ØX1	T37.ØX2	T37.ØX3	T37.ØX4	T37.ØX5	T37.ØX6
Sulfadiazine	T37.ØX1	T37.ØX2	T37.ØX3	T37.ØX4	T37.ØX5	T37.ØX6
silver (topical)	T49.ØX1	T49.ØX2	T49.ØX3	T49.ØX4	T49.ØX5	T49.ØX6
Sulfadimethoxine	T37.ØX1	T37.ØX2	T37.ØX3	T37.ØX4	T37.ØX5	T37.ØX6
Sulfadimidine	T37.ØX1	T37.ØX2	T37.ØX3	T37.ØX4	T37.ØX5	T37.ØX6
Sulfadoxine	T37.ØX1	T37.ØX2	T37.ØX3	T37.ØX4	T37.ØX5	T37.ØX6
with pyrimethamine	T37.2X1	T37.2X2	T37.2X3	T37.2X4	T37.2X5	T37.2X6
Sulfaethidole	T37.ØX1	T37.ØX2	T37.ØX3	T37.ØX4	T37.ØX5	T37.ØX6
Sulfafurazole	T37.ØX1	T37.ØX2	T37.ØX3	T37.ØX4	T37.ØX5	T37.ØX6
Sulfaguanidine	T37.ØX1	T37.ØX2	T37.ØX3	T37.ØX4	T37.ØX5	T37.ØX6
Sulfalene	T37.ØX1	T37.ØX2	T37.ØX3	T37.ØX4	T37.ØX5	T37.ØX6
Sulfaloxate	T37.ØX1	T37.ØX2	T37.ØX3	T37.ØX4	T37.ØX5	T37.ØX6
Sulfaloxic acid	T37.ØX1	T37.ØX2	T37.ØX3	T37.ØX4	T37.ØX5	T37.ØX6
Sulfamazone	T39.2X1	T39.2X2	T39.2X3	T39.2X4	T39.2X5	T39.2X6
Sulfamerazine	T37.ØX1	T37.ØX2	T37.ØX3	T37.ØX4	T37.ØX5	T37.ØX6
Sulfameter	T37.ØX1	T37.ØX2	T37.ØX3	T37.ØX4	T37.ØX5	T37.ØX6
Sulfamethazine	T37.ØX1	T37.ØX2	T37.ØX3	T37.ØX4	T37.ØX5	T37.ØX6
Sulfamethizole	T37.ØX1	T37.ØX2	T37.ØX3	T37.ØX4	T37.ØX5	T37.ØX6
Sulfamethoxazole	T37.ØX1	T37.ØX2	T37.ØX3	T37.ØX4	T37.ØX5	T37.ØX6
with trimethoprim	T36.8X1	T36.8X2	T36.8X3	T36.8X4	T36.8X5	T36.8X6
Sulfamethoxydiazine	T37.ØX1	T37.ØX2	T37.ØX3	T37.ØX4	T37.ØX5	T37.ØX6
Sulfamethoxypyridazine	T37.ØX1	T37.ØX2	T37.ØX3	T37.ØX4	T37.ØX5	T37.ØX6
Sulfamethylthiazole	T37.ØX1	T37.ØX2	T37.ØX3	T37.ØX4	T37.ØX5	T37.ØX6
Sulfametoxydiazine	T37.ØX1	T37.ØX2	T37.ØX3	T37.ØX4	T37.ØX5	T37.ØX6
Sulfamidopyrine	T39.2X1	T39.2X2	T39.2X3	T39.2X4	T39.2X5	T39.2X6
Sulfamonomethoxine	T37.ØX1	T37.ØX2	T37.ØX3	T37.ØX4	T37.ØX5	T37.ØX6
Sulfamoxole	T37.ØX1	T37.ØX2	T37.ØX3	T37.ØX4	T37.ØX5	T37.ØX6
Sulfamylon	T49.ØX1	T49.ØX2	T49.ØX3	T49.ØX4	T49.ØX5	T49.ØX6
Sulfan blue (diagnostic dye)	T5Ø.8X1	T5Ø.8X2	T5Ø.8X3	T5Ø.8X4	T5Ø.8X5	T5Ø.8X6
Sulfanilamide	T37.ØX1	T37.ØX2	T37.ØX3	T37.ØX4	T37.ØX5	T37.ØX6
Sulfanilylguanidine	T37.ØX1	T37.ØX2	T37.ØX3	T37.ØX4	T37.ØX5	T37.ØX6
Sulfaperin	T37.ØX1	T37.ØX2	T37.ØX3	T37.ØX4	T37.ØX5	T37.ØX6
Sulfaphenazole	T37.ØX1	T37.ØX2	T37.ØX3	T37.ØX4	T37.ØX5	T37.ØX6
Sulfaphenylthiazole	T37.ØX1	T37.ØX2	T37.ØX3	T37.ØX4	T37.ØX5	T37.ØX6
Sulfaproxyline	T37.ØX1	T37.ØX2	T37.ØX3	T37.ØX4	T37.ØX5	T37.ØX6
Sulfapyridine	T37.ØX1	T37.ØX2	T37.ØX3	T37.ØX4	T37.ØX5	T37.ØX6
Sulfapyrimidine	T37.ØX1	T37.ØX2	T37.ØX3	T37.ØX4	T37.ØX5	T37.ØX6
Sulfarsphenamine	T37.8X1	T37.8X2	T37.8X3	T37.8X4	T37.8X5	T37.8X6
Sulfasalazine	T37.ØX1	T37.ØX2	T37.ØX3	T37.ØX4	T37.ØX5	T37.ØX6
Sulfasuxidine	T37.ØX1	T37.ØX2	T37.ØX3	T37.ØX4	T37.ØX5	T37.ØX6
Sulfasymazine	T37.ØX1	T37.ØX2	T37.ØX3	T37.ØX4	T37.ØX5	T37.ØX6
Sulfated amylopectin	T47.8X1	T47.8X2	T47.8X3	T47.8X4	T47.8X5	T47.8X6
Sulfathiazole	T37.ØX1	T37.ØX2	T37.ØX3	T37.ØX4	T37.ØX5	T37.ØX6
Sulfatostearate	T49.2X1	T49.2X2	T49.2X3	T49.2X4	T49.2X5	T49.2X6
Sulfinpyrazone	T5Ø.4X1	T5Ø.4X2	T5Ø.4X3	T5Ø.4X4	T5Ø.4X5	T5Ø.4X6

Substance	Poisoning, Accidental (Unintentional)	Poisoning, Intentional Self-Harm	Poisoning, Assault	Poisoning, Undetermined	Adverse Effect	Underdosing
	External Cause (T-Code)					
Sulfiram	T49.ØX1	T49.ØX2	T49.ØX3	T49.ØX4	T49.ØX5	T49.ØX6
Sulfisomidine	T37.ØX1	T37.ØX2	T37.ØX3	T37.ØX4	T37.ØX5	T37.ØX6
Sulfisoxazole	T37.ØX1	T37.ØX2	T37.ØX3	T37.ØX4	T37.ØX5	T37.ØX6
ophthalmic preparation	T49.5X1	T49.5X2	T49.5X3	T49.5X4	T49.5X5	T49.5X6
Sulfobromophthalein (sodium)	T5Ø.8X1	T5Ø.8X2	T5Ø.8X3	T5Ø.8X4	T5Ø.8X5	T5Ø.8X6
Sulfobromphthalein	T5Ø.8X1	T5Ø.8X2	T5Ø.8X3	T5Ø.8X4	T5Ø.8X5	T5Ø.8X6
Sulfogaiacol	T48.4X1	T48.4X2	T48.4X3	T48.4X4	T48.4X5	T48.4X6
Sulfomyxin	T36.8X1	T36.8X2	T36.8X3	T36.8X4	T36.8X5	T36.8X6
Sulfonal	T42.6X1	T42.6X2	T42.6X3	T42.6X4	T42.6X5	T42.6X6
Sulfonamide NEC	T37.ØX1	T37.ØX2	T37.ØX3	T37.ØX4	T37.ØX5	T37.ØX6
eye	T49.5X1	T49.5X2	T49.5X3	T49.5X4	T49.5X5	T49.5X6
Sulfonazide	T37.1X1	T37.1X2	T37.1X3	T37.1X4	T37.1X5	T37.1X6
Sulfones	T37.1X1	T37.1X2	T37.1X3	T37.1X4	T37.1X5	T37.1X6
Sulfonethylmethane	T42.6X1	T42.6X2	T42.6X3	T42.6X4	T42.6X5	T42.6X6
Sulfonmethane	T42.6X1	T42.6X2	T42.6X3	T42.6X4	T42.6X5	T42.6X6
Sulfonphthal, sulfonphthol	T5Ø.8X1	T5Ø.8X2	T5Ø.8X3	T5Ø.8X4	T5Ø.8X5	T5Ø.8X6
Sulfonylurea derivatives, oral	T38.3X1	T38.3X2	T38.3X3	T38.3X4	T38.3X5	T38.3X6
Sulforidazine	T43.3X1	T43.3X2	T43.3X3	T43.3X4	T43.3X5	T43.3X6
Sulfoxone	T37.1X1	T37.1X2	T37.1X3	T37.1X4	T37.1X5	T37.1X6
Sulfur, sulfurated, sulfuric, sulfurous, sulfuryl (compounds NEC) (medicinal)	T49.4X1	T49.4X2	T49.4X3	T49.4X4	T49.4X5	T49.4X6
acid	T54.2X1	T54.2X2	T54.2X3	T54.2X4	—	—
dioxide (gas)	T59.1X1	T59.1X2	T59.1X3	T59.1X4	—	—
ether — *see Ether(s)*						
hydrogen	T59.6X1	T59.6X2	T59.6X3	T59.6X4	—	—
medicinal (keratolytic) (ointment) NEC	T49.4X1	T49.4X2	T49.4X3	T49.4X4	T49.4X5	T49.4X6
ointment	T49.ØX1	T49.ØX2	T49.ØX3	T49.ØX4	T49.ØX5	T49.ØX6
pesticide (vapor)	T6Ø.91	T6Ø.92	T6Ø.93	T6Ø.94	—	—
vapor NEC	T59.891	T59.892	T59.893	T59.894	—	—
Sulfuric acid	T54.2X1	T54.2X2	T54.2X3	T54.2X4	—	—
Sulglicotide	T47.1X1	T47.1X2	T47.1X3	T47.1X4	T47.1X5	T47.1X6
Sulindac	T39.391	T39.392	T39.393	T39.394	T39.395	T39.396
Sulisatin	T47.2X1	T47.2X2	T47.2X3	T47.2X4	T47.2X5	T47.2X6
Sulisobenzone	T49.3X1	T49.3X2	T49.3X3	T49.3X4	T49.3X5	T49.3X6
Sulkowitch's reagent	T5Ø.8X1	T5Ø.8X2	T5Ø.8X3	T5Ø.8X4	T5Ø.8X5	T5Ø.8X6
Sulmetozine	T44.3X1	T44.3X2	T44.3X3	T44.3X4	T44.3X5	T44.3X6
Suloctidil	T46.7X1	T46.7X2	T46.7X3	T46.7X4	T46.7X5	T46.7X6
Sulph — *see also Sulf-*						
Sulphadiazine	T37.ØX1	T37.ØX2	T37.ØX3	T37.ØX4	T37.ØX5	T37.ØX6

Substance	Poisoning, Accidental (Unintentional)	Poisoning, Intentional Self-Harm	Poisoning, Assault	Poisoning, Undetermined	Adverse Effect	Underdosing
	External Cause (T-Code)					
Sulphadimethoxine	T37.ØX1	T37.ØX2	T37.ØX3	T37.ØX4	T37.ØX5	T37.ØX6
Sulphadimidine	T37.ØX1	T37.ØX2	T37.ØX3	T37.ØX4	T37.ØX5	T37.ØX6
Sulphadione	T37.1X1	T37.1X2	T37.1X3	T37.1X4	T37.1X5	T37.1X6
Sulphafurazole	T37.ØX1	T37.ØX2	T37.ØX3	T37.ØX4	T37.ØX5	T37.ØX6
Sulphamethizole	T37.ØX1	T37.ØX2	T37.ØX3	T37.ØX4	T37.ØX5	T37.ØX6
Sulphamethoxazole	T37.ØX1	T37.ØX2	T37.ØX3	T37.ØX4	T37.ØX5	T37.ØX6
Sulphan blue	T5Ø.8X1	T5Ø.8X2	T5Ø.8X3	T5Ø.8X4	T5Ø.8X5	T5Ø.8X6
Sulphaphenazole	T37.ØX1	T37.ØX2	T37.ØX3	T37.ØX4	T37.ØX5	T37.ØX6
Sulphapyridine	T37.ØX1	T37.ØX2	T37.ØX3	T37.ØX4	T37.ØX5	T37.ØX6
Sulphasalazine	T37.ØX1	T37.ØX2	T37.ØX3	T37.ØX4	T37.ØX5	T37.ØX6
Sulphinpyrazone	T5Ø.4X1	T5Ø.4X2	T5Ø.4X3	T5Ø.4X4	T5Ø.4X5	T5Ø.4X6
Sulpiride	T43.591	T43.592	T43.593	T43.594	T43.595	T43.596
Sulprostone	T48.ØX1	T48.ØX2	T48.ØX3	T48.ØX4	T48.ØX5	T48.ØX6
Sulpyrine	T39.2X1	T39.2X2	T39.2X3	T39.2X4	T39.2X5	T39.2X6
Sultamicillin	T36.ØX1	T36.ØX2	T36.ØX3	T36.ØX4	T36.ØX5	T36.ØX6
Sulthiame	T42.6X1	T42.6X2	T42.6X3	T42.6X4	T42.6X5	T42.6X6
Sultiame	T42.6X1	T42.6X2	T42.6X3	T42.6X4	T42.6X5	T42.6X6
Sultopride	T43.591	T43.592	T43.593	T43.594	T43.595	T43.596
Sumatriptan	T39.8X1	T39.8X2	T39.8X3	T39.8X4	T39.8X5	T39.8X6
Sunflower seed oil	T46.6X1	T46.6X2	T46.6X3	T46.6X4	T46.6X5	T46.6X6
Superinone	T48.4X1	T48.4X2	T48.4X3	T48.4X4	T48.4X5	T48.4X6
Suprofen	T39.311	T39.312	T39.313	T39.314	T39.315	T39.316
Suramin (sodium)	T37.4X1	T37.4X2	T37.4X3	T37.4X4	T37.4X5	T37.4X6
Surfacaine	T41.3X1	T41.3X2	T41.3X3	T41.3X4	T41.3X5	T41.3X6
Surital	T41.1X1	T41.1X2	T41.1X3	T41.1X4	T41.1X5	T41.1X6
Sutilains	T45.3X1	T45.3X2	T45.3X3	T45.3X4	T45.3X5	T45.3X6
Suxamethonium (chloride)	T48.1X1	T48.1X2	T48.1X3	T48.1X4	T48.1X5	T48.1X6
Suxethonium (chloride)	T48.1X1	T48.1X2	T48.1X3	T48.1X4	T48.1X5	T48.1X6
Suxibuzone	T39.2X1	T39.2X2	T39.2X3	T39.2X4	T39.2X5	T39.2X6
Sweet oil (birch)	T49.3X1	T49.3X2	T49.3X3	T49.3X4	T49.3X5	T49.3X6
Sweet niter spirit	T46.3X1	T46.3X2	T46.3X3	T46.3X4	T46.3X5	T46.3X6
Sweetener	T5Ø.9Ø1	T5Ø.9Ø2	T5Ø.9Ø3	T5Ø.9Ø4	T5Ø.9Ø5	T5Ø.9Ø6
Sym-dichloroethyl ether	T53.6X1	T53.6X2	T53.6X3	T53.6X4	—	—
Sympatholytic NEC	T44.8X1	T44.8X2	T44.8X3	T44.8X4	T44.8X5	T44.8X6
haloalkylamine	T44.8X1	T44.8X2	T44.8X3	T44.8X4	T44.8X5	T44.8X6
Sympathomimetic NEC	T44.9Ø1	T44.9Ø2	T44.9Ø3	T44.9Ø4	T44.9Ø5	T44.9Ø6
anti-common-cold	T48.5X1	T48.5X2	T48.5X3	T48.5X4	T48.5X5	T48.5X6
bronchodilator	T48.6X1	T48.6X2	T48.6X3	T48.6X4	T48.6X5	T48.6X6
specified NEC	T44.991	T44.992	T44.993	T44.994	T44.995	T44.996
Synagis	T5Ø.B91	T5Ø.B92	T5Ø.B93	T5Ø.B94	T5Ø.B95	T5Ø.B96
Synalar	T49.ØX1	T49.ØX2	T49.ØX3	T49.ØX4	T49.ØX5	T49.ØX6
Synthroid	T38.1X1	T38.1X2	T38.1X3	T38.1X4	T38.1X5	T38.1X6

Substance	Poisoning, Accidental (Unintentional)	Poisoning, Intentional Self-Harm	Poisoning, Assault	Poisoning, Undetermined	Adverse Effect	Underdosing
Syntocinon	T48.ØX1	T48.ØX2	T48.ØX3	T48.ØX4	T48.ØX5	T48.ØX6
Syrosingopine	T46.5X1	T46.5X2	T46.5X3	T46.5X4	T46.5X5	T46.5X6
Systemic drug	T45.91	T45.92	T45.93	T45.94	T45.95	T45.96
specified NEC	T45.8X1	T45.8X2	T45.8X3	T45.8X4	T45.8X5	T45.8X6
2,4,5-T	T6Ø.3X1	T6Ø.3X2	T6Ø.3X3	T6Ø.3X4	—	—
T						
Tablets — *see also specified substance*	T5Ø.9Ø1	T5Ø.9Ø2	T5Ø.9Ø3	T5Ø.9Ø4	T5Ø.9Ø5	T5Ø.9Ø6
Tace	T38.5X1	T38.5X2	T38.5X3	T38.5X4	T38.5X5	T38.5X6
Tacrine	T44.ØX1	T44.ØX2	T44.ØX3	T44.ØX4	T44.ØX5	T44.ØX6
Tadalafil	T46.7X1	T46.7X2	T46.7X3	T46.7X4	T46.7X5	T46.7X6
Talampicillin	T36.ØX1	T36.ØX2	T36.ØX3	T36.ØX4	T36.ØX5	T36.ØX6
Talbutal	T42.3X1	T42.3X2	T42.3X3	T42.3X4	T42.3X5	T42.3X6
Talc powder	T49.3X1	T49.3X2	T49.3X3	T49.3X4	T49.3X5	T49.3X6
Talcum	T49.3X1	T49.3X2	T49.3X3	T49.3X4	T49.3X5	T49.3X6
Taleranol	T38.6X1	T38.6X2	T38.6X3	T38.6X4	T38.6X5	T38.6X6
Tamoxifen	T38.6X1	T38.6X2	T38.6X3	T38.6X4	T38.6X5	T38.6X6
Tamsulosin	T44.6X1	T44.6X2	T44.6X3	T44.6X4	T44.6X5	T44.6X6
Tandearil, tanderil	T39.2X1	T39.2X2	T39.2X3	T39.2X4	T39.2X5	T39.2X6
Tannic acid	T49.2X1	T49.2X2	T49.2X3	T49.2X4	T49.2X5	T49.2X6
medicinal (astringent)	T49.2X1	T49.2X2	T49.2X3	T49.2X4	T49.2X5	T49.2X6
Tannin — *see Tannic acid*						
Tansy	T62.2X1	T62.2X2	T62.2X3	T62.2X4	—	—
TAO	T36.3X1	T36.3X2	T36.3X3	T36.3X4	T36.3X5	T36.3X6
Tapazole	T38.2X1	T38.2X2	T38.2X3	T38.2X4	T38.2X5	T38.2X6
Tar NEC	T52.ØX1	T52.ØX2	T52.ØX3	T52.ØX4	—	—
camphor	T6Ø.1X1	T6Ø.1X2	T6Ø.1X3	T6Ø.1X4	—	—
distillate	T49.1X1	T49.1X2	T49.1X3	T49.1X4	T49.1X5	T49.1X6
fumes	T59.891	T59.892	T59.893	T59.894	—	—
medicinal	T49.1X1	T49.1X2	T49.1X3	T49.1X4	T49.1X5	T49.1X6
ointment	T49.1X1	T49.1X2	T49.1X3	T49.1X4	T49.1X5	T49.1X6
Taractan	T43.591	T43.592	T43.593	T43.594	T43.595	T43.596
Tarantula (venomous)	T63.321	T63.322	T63.323	T63.324	—	—
Tartar emetic	T37.8X1	T37.8X2	T37.8X3	T37.8X4	T37.8X5	T37.8X6
Tartaric acid	T65.891	T65.892	T65.893	T65.894	—	—
Tartrated antimony (anti-infective)	T37.8X1	T37.8X2	T37.8X3	T37.8X4	T37.8X5	T37.8X6
Tartrate, laxative	T47.4X1	T47.4X2	T47.4X3	T47.4X4	T47.4X5	T47.4X6
Tauromustine	T45.1X1	T45.1X2	T45.1X3	T45.1X4	T45.1X5	T45.1X6
TCA — *see Trichloroacetic acid*						
TCDD	T53.7X1	T53.7X2	T53.7X3	T53.7X4	—	—
TDI (vapor)	T65.ØX1	T65.ØX2	T65.ØX3	T65.ØX4	—	—
Tear						
gas	T59.3X1	T59.3X2	T59.3X3	T59.3X4	—	—
solution	T49.5X1	T49.5X2	T49.5X3	T49.5X4	T49.5X5	T49.5X6
Teclothiazide	T5Ø.2X1	T5Ø.2X2	T5Ø.2X3	T5Ø.2X4	T5Ø.2X5	T5Ø.2X6
Teclozan	T37.3X1	T37.3X2	T37.3X3	T37.3X4	T37.3X5	T37.3X6
Tegafur	T45.1X1	T45.1X2	T45.1X3	T45.1X4	T45.1X5	T45.1X6
Tegretol	T42.1X1	T42.1X2	T42.1X3	T42.1X4	T42.1X5	T42.1X6
Teicoplanin	T36.8X1	T36.8X2	T36.8X3	T36.8X4	T36.8X5	T36.8X6
Telepaque	T5Ø.8X1	T5Ø.8X2	T5Ø.8X3	T5Ø.8X4	T5Ø.8X5	T5Ø.8X6
Tellurium	T56.891	T56.892	T56.893	T56.894	—	—
fumes	T56.891	T56.892	T56.893	T56.894	—	—
TEM	T45.1X1	T45.1X2	T45.1X3	T45.1X4	T45.1X5	T45.1X6
Temazepam	T42.4X1	T42.4X2	T42.4X3	T42.4X4	T42.4X5	T42.4X6
Temocillin	T36.ØX1	T36.ØX2	T36.ØX3	T36.ØX4	T36.ØX5	T36.ØX6
Tenamfetamine	T43.621	T43.622	T43.623	T43.624	T43.625	T43.626
Teniposide	T45.1X1	T45.1X2	T45.1X3	T45.1X4	T45.1X5	T45.1X6
Tenitramine	T46.3X1	T46.3X2	T46.3X3	T46.3X4	T46.3X5	T46.3X6
Tenoglicin	T48.4X1	T48.4X2	T48.4X3	T48.4X4	T48.4X5	T48.4X6
Tenonitrozole	T37.3X1	T37.3X2	T37.3X3	T37.3X4	T37.3X5	T37.3X6
Tenoxicam	T39.391	T39.392	T39.393	T39.394	T39.395	T39.396
TEPA	T45.1X1	T45.1X2	T45.1X3	T45.1X4	T45.1X5	T45.1X6
TEPP	T6Ø.ØX1	T6Ø.ØX2	T6Ø.ØX3	T6Ø.ØX4	—	—
Teprotide	T46.5X1	T46.5X2	T46.5X3	T46.5X4	T46.5X5	T46.5X6
Terazosin	T44.6X1	T44.6X2	T44.6X3	T44.6X4	T44.6X5	T44.6X6
Terbufos	T6Ø.ØX1	T6Ø.ØX2	T6Ø.ØX3	T6Ø.ØX4	—	—
Terbutaline	T48.6X1	T48.6X2	T48.6X3	T48.6X4	T48.6X5	T48.6X6
Terconazole	T49.ØX1	T49.ØX2	T49.ØX3	T49.ØX4	T49.ØX5	T49.ØX6
Terfenadine	T45.ØX1	T45.ØX2	T45.ØX3	T45.ØX4	T45.ØX5	T45.ØX6
Teriparatide (acetate)	T5Ø.991	T5Ø.992	T5Ø.993	T5Ø.994	T5Ø.995	T5Ø.996
Terizidone	T37.1X1	T37.1X2	T37.1X3	T37.1X4	T37.1X5	T37.1X6
Terlipressin	T38.891	T38.892	T38.893	T38.894	T38.895	T38.896
Terodiline	T46.3X1	T46.3X2	T46.3X3	T46.3X4	T46.3X5	T46.3X6
Teroxalene	T37.4X1	T37.4X2	T37.4X3	T37.4X4	T37.4X5	T37.4X6
Terpin(cis) hydrate	T48.4X1	T48.4X2	T48.4X3	T48.4X4	T48.4X5	T48.4X6
Terramycin	T36.4X1	T36.4X2	T36.4X3	T36.4X4	T36.4X5	T36.4X6
Tertatolol	T44.7X1	T44.7X2	T44.7X3	T44.7X4	T44.7X5	T44.7X6
Tessalon	T48.3X1	T48.3X2	T48.3X3	T48.3X4	T48.3X5	T48.3X6
Testolactone	T38.7X1	T38.7X2	T38.7X3	T38.7X4	T38.7X5	T38.7X6
Testosterone	T38.7X1	T38.7X2	T38.7X3	T38.7X4	T38.7X5	T38.7X6
Tetanus toxoid or vaccine	T5Ø.A91	T5Ø.A92	T5Ø.A93	T5Ø.A94	T5Ø.A95	T5Ø.A96
antitoxin	T5Ø.Z11	T5Ø.Z12	T5Ø.Z13	T5Ø.Z14	T5Ø.Z15	T5Ø.Z16
immune globulin (human)	T5Ø.Z11	T5Ø.Z12	T5Ø.Z13	T5Ø.Z14	T5Ø.Z15	T5Ø.Z16

(Column group header: External Cause (T-Code))

Substance	Poisoning, Accidental (Unintentional)	Poisoning, Intentional Self-Harm	Poisoning, Assault	Poisoning, Undetermined	Adverse Effect	Underdosing
	External Cause (T-Code)					
Tetanus toxoid or vaccine *(Continued)*						
toxoid	T5Ø.A91	T5Ø.A92	T5Ø.A93	T5Ø.A94	T5Ø.A95	T5Ø.A96
with diphtheria toxoid	T5Ø.A21	T5Ø.A22	T5Ø.A23	T5Ø.A24	T5Ø.A25	T5Ø.A26
with pertussis	T5Ø.A11	T5Ø.A12	T5Ø.A13	T5Ø.A14	T5Ø.A15	T5Ø.A16
Tetrabenazine	T43.591	T43.592	T43.593	T43.594	T43.595	T43.596
Tetracaine	T41.3X1	T41.3X2	T41.3X3	T41.3X4	T41.3X5	T41.3X6
nerve block (peripheral) (plexus)	T41.3X1	T41.3X2	T41.3X3	T41.3X4	T41.3X5	T41.3X6
regional	T41.3X1	T41.3X2	T41.3X3	T41.3X4	T41.3X5	T41.3X6
spinal	T41.3X1	T41.3X2	T41.3X3	T41.3X4	T41.3X5	T41.3X6
Tetrachlorethylene — *see Tetrachloroethylene*						
Tetrachlormethiazide	T5Ø.2X1	T5Ø.2X2	T5Ø.2X3	T5Ø.2X4	T5Ø.2X5	T5Ø.2X6
2,3,7,8-Tetrachlorodibenzo-p-dioxin	T53.7X1	T53.7X2	T53.7X3	T53.7X4	—	—
Tetrachloroethane	T53.6X1	T53.6X2	T53.6X3	T53.6X4	—	—
vapor	T53.6X1	T53.6X2	T53.6X3	T53.6X4	—	—
paint or varnish	T53.6X1	T53.6X2	T53.6X3	T53.6X4	—	—
Tetrachloroethylene (liquid)	T53.3X1	T53.3X2	T53.3X3	T53.3X4	—	—
medicinal	T37.4X1	T37.4X2	T37.4X3	T37.4X4	T37.4X5	T37.4X6
vapor	T53.3X1	T53.3X2	T53.3X3	T53.3X4	—	—
Tetrachloromethane — *see Carbon tetrachloride*						
Tetracosactide	T38.811	T38.812	T38.813	T38.814	T38.815	T38.816
Tetracosactrin	T38.811	T38.812	T38.813	T38.814	T38.815	T38.816
Tetracycline	T36.4X1	T36.4X2	T36.4X3	T36.4X4	T36.4X5	T36.4X6
ophthalmic preparation	T49.5X1	T49.5X2	T49.5X3	T49.5X4	T49.5X5	T49.5X6
topical NEC	T49.ØX1	T49.ØX2	T49.ØX3	T49.ØX4	T49.ØX5	T49.ØX6
Tetradifon	T6Ø.8X1	T6Ø.8X2	T6Ø.8X3	T6Ø.8X4	—	—
Tetradotoxin	T61.771	T61.772	T61.773	T61.774	—	—
Tetraethyl						
lead	T56.ØX1	T56.ØX2	T56.ØX3	T56.ØX4	—	—
pyrophosphate	T6Ø.ØX1	T6Ø.ØX2	T6Ø.ØX3	T6Ø.ØX4	—	—
Tetraethylammonium chloride	T44.2X1	T44.2X2	T44.2X3	T44.2X4	T44.2X5	T44.2X6
Tetraethylthiuram disulfide	T5Ø.6X1	T5Ø.6X2	T5Ø.6X3	T5Ø.6X4	T5Ø.6X5	T5Ø.6X6
Tetrahydroaminoacridine	T44.ØX1	T44.ØX2	T44.ØX3	T44.ØX4	T44.ØX5	T44.ØX6
Tetrahydrocannabinol	T4Ø.7X1	T4Ø.7X2	T4Ø.7X3	T4Ø.7X4	T4Ø.7X5	T4Ø.7X6
Tetrahydrofuran	T52.8X1	T52.8X2	T52.8X3	T52.8X4	—	—
Tetrahydronaphthalene	T52.8X1	T52.8X2	T52.8X3	T52.8X4	—	—
Tetrahydrozoline	T49.5X1	T49.5X2	T49.5X3	T49.5X4	T49.5X5	T49.5X6
Tetralin	T52.8X1	T52.8X2	T52.8X3	T52.8X4	—	—
Tetramethrin	T6Ø.2X1	T6Ø.2X2	T6Ø.2X3	T6Ø.2X4	—	—

Substance	Poisoning, Accidental (Unintentional)	Poisoning, Intentional Self-Harm	Poisoning, Assault	Poisoning, Undetermined	Adverse Effect	Underdosing
	External Cause (T-Code)					
Tetramethylthiuram (disulfide) NEC	T6Ø.3X1	T6Ø.3X2	T6Ø.3X3	T6Ø.3X4	—	—
medicinal	T49.ØX1	T49.ØX2	T49.ØX3	T49.ØX4	T49.ØX5	T49.ØX6
Tetramisole	T37.4X1	T37.4X2	T37.4X3	T37.4X4	T37.4X5	T37.4X6
Tetranicotinoyl fructose	T46.7X1	T46.7X2	T46.7X3	T46.7X4	T46.7X5	T46.7X6
Tetronal	T42.6X1	T42.6X2	T42.6X3	T42.6X4	T42.6X5	T42.6X6
Tetrazepam	T42.4X1	T42.4X2	T42.4X3	T42.4X4	T42.4X5	T42.4X6
Tetryl	T65.3X1	T65.3X2	T65.3X3	T65.3X4	—	—
Tetrylammonium chloride	T44.2X1	T44.2X2	T44.2X3	T44.2X4	T44.2X5	T44.2X6
Tetryzoline	T49.5X1	T49.5X2	T49.5X3	T49.5X4	T49.5X5	T49.5X6
Thalidomide	T45.1X1	T45.1X2	T45.1X3	T45.1X4	T45.1X5	T45.1X6
Thallium (compounds) (dust) NEC	T56.811	T56.812	T56.813	T56.814	—	—
pesticide	T6Ø.4X1	T6Ø.4X2	T6Ø.4X3	T6Ø.4X4	—	—
THC	T4Ø.7X1	T4Ø.7X2	T4Ø.7X3	T4Ø.7X4	T4Ø.7X5	T4Ø.7X6
Thebacon	T48.3X1	T48.3X2	T48.3X3	T48.3X4	T48.3X5	T48.3X6
Thebaine	T4Ø.2X1	T4Ø.2X2	T4Ø.2X3	T4Ø.2X4	T4Ø.2X5	T4Ø.2X6
Thenoic acid	T49.6X1	T49.6X2	T49.6X3	T49.6X4	T49.6X5	T49.6X6
Thenyldiamine	T45.ØX1	T45.ØX2	T45.ØX3	T45.ØX4	T45.ØX5	T45.ØX6
Theobromine (calcium salicylate)	T48.6X1	T48.6X2	T48.6X3	T48.6X4	T48.6X5	T48.6X6
sodium salicylate	T48.6X1	T48.6X2	T48.6X3	T48.6X4	T48.6X5	T48.6X6
Theophyllamine	T48.6X1	T48.6X2	T48.6X3	T48.6X4	T48.6X5	T48.6X6
Theophylline	T48.6X1	T48.6X2	T48.6X3	T48.6X4	T48.6X5	T48.6X6
aminobenzoic acid	T48.6X1	T48.6X2	T48.6X3	T48.6X4	T48.6X5	T48.6X6
ethylenediamine	T48.6X1	T48.6X2	T48.6X3	T48.6X4	T48.6X5	T48.6X6
piperazine p-amino-benzoate	T48.6X1	T48.6X2	T48.6X3	T48.6X4	T48.6X5	T48.6X6
Thiabendazole	T37.4X1	T37.4X2	T37.4X3	T37.4X4	T37.4X5	T37.4X6
Thialbarbital	T41.1X1	T41.1X2	T41.1X3	T41.1X4	T41.1X5	T41.1X6
Thiamazole	T38.2X1	T38.2X2	T38.2X3	T38.2X4	T38.2X5	T38.2X6
Thiambutosine	T37.1X1	T37.1X2	T37.1X3	T37.1X4	T37.1X5	T37.1X6
Thiamine	T45.2X1	T45.2X2	T45.2X3	T45.2X4	T45.2X5	T45.2X6
Thiamphenicol	T36.2X1	T36.2X2	T36.2X3	T36.2X4	T36.2X5	T36.2X6
Thiamylal	T41.1X1	T41.1X2	T41.1X3	T41.1X4	T41.1X5	T41.1X6
sodium	T41.1X1	T41.1X2	T41.1X3	T41.1X4	T41.1X5	T41.1X6
Thiazesim	T43.291	T43.292	T43.293	T43.294	T43.295	T43.296
Thiazides (diuretics)	T5Ø.2X1	T5Ø.2X2	T5Ø.2X3	T5Ø.2X4	T5Ø.2X5	T5Ø.2X6
Thiazinamium metilsulfate	T43.3X1	T43.3X2	T43.3X3	T43.3X4	T43.3X5	T43.3X6
Thiethylperazine	T43.3X1	T43.3X2	T43.3X3	T43.3X4	T43.3X5	T43.3X6
Thimerosal	T49.ØX1	T49.ØX2	T49.ØX3	T49.ØX4	T49.ØX5	T49.ØX6
ophthalmic preparation	T49.5X1	T49.5X2	T49.5X3	T49.5X4	T49.5X5	T49.5X6
Thioacetazone	T37.1X1	T37.1X2	T37.1X3	T37.1X4	T37.1X5	T37.1X6
with isoniazid	T37.1X1	T37.1X2	T37.1X3	T37.1X4	T37.1X5	T37.1X6
Thiobarbital sodium	T41.1X1	T41.1X2	T41.1X3	T41.1X4	T41.1X5	T41.1X6

◀ New ◀ Revised ~~deleted~~ Deleted

Substance	External Cause (T-Code)					
	Poisoning, Accidental (Unintentional)	Poisoning, Intentional Self-Harm	Poisoning, Assault	Poisoning, Undetermined	Adverse Effect	Underdosing
Thiobarbiturate anesthetic	T41.1X1	T41.1X2	T41.1X3	T41.1X4	T41.1X5	T41.1X6
Thiobismol	T37.8X1	T37.8X2	T37.8X3	T37.8X4	T37.8X5	T37.8X6
Thiobutabarbital sodium	T41.1X1	T41.1X2	T41.1X3	T41.1X4	T41.1X5	T41.1X6
Thiocarbamate (insecticide)	T6Ø.ØX1	T6Ø.ØX2	T6Ø.ØX3	T6Ø.ØX4	—	—
Thiocarbamide	T38.2X1	T38.2X2	T38.2X3	T38.2X4	T38.2X5	T38.2X6
Thiocarbarsone	T37.8X1	T37.8X2	T37.8X3	T37.8X4	T37.8X5	T37.8X6
Thiocarlide	T37.1X1	T37.1X2	T37.1X3	T37.1X4	T37.1X5	T37.1X6
Thioctamide	T5Ø.991	T5Ø.992	T5Ø.993	T5Ø.994	T5Ø.995	T5Ø.996
Thioctic acid	T5Ø.991	T5Ø.992	T5Ø.993	T5Ø.994	T5Ø.995	T5Ø.996
Thiofos	T6Ø.ØX1	T6Ø.ØX2	T6Ø.ØX3	T6Ø.ØX4	—	—
Thioglycolate	T49.4X1	T49.4X2	T49.4X3	T49.4X4	T49.4X5	T49.4X6
Thioglycolic acid	T65.891	T65.892	T65.893	T65.894	—	—
Thioguanine	T45.1X1	T45.1X2	T45.1X3	T45.1X4	T45.1X5	T45.1X6
Thiomercaptomerin	T5Ø.2X1	T5Ø.2X2	T5Ø.2X3	T5Ø.2X4	T5Ø.2X5	T5Ø.2X6
Thiomerin	T5Ø.2X1	T5Ø.2X2	T5Ø.2X3	T5Ø.2X4	T5Ø.2X5	T5Ø.2X6
Thiomersal	T49.ØX1	T49.ØX2	T49.ØX3	T49.ØX4	T49.ØX5	T49.ØX6
Thionazin	T6Ø.ØX1	T6Ø.ØX2	T6Ø.ØX3	T6Ø.ØX4	—	—
Thiopental (sodium)	T41.1X1	T41.1X2	T41.1X3	T41.1X4	T41.1X5	T41.1X6
Thiopentone (sodium)	T41.1X1	T41.1X2	T41.1X3	T41.1X4	T41.1X5	T41.1X6
Thiopropazate	T43.3X1	T43.3X2	T43.3X3	T43.3X4	T43.3X5	T43.3X6
Thioproperazine	T43.3X1	T43.3X2	T43.3X3	T43.3X4	T43.3X5	T43.3X6
Thioridazine	T43.3X1	T43.3X2	T43.3X3	T43.3X4	T43.3X5	T43.3X6
Thiosinamine	T49.3X1	T49.3X2	T49.3X3	T49.3X4	T49.3X5	T49.3X6
Thiotepa	T45.1X1	T45.1X2	T45.1X3	T45.1X4	T45.1X5	T45.1X6
Thiothixene	T43.4X1	T43.4X2	T43.4X3	T43.4X4	T43.4X5	T43.4X6
Thiouracil (benzyl) (methyl) (propyl)	T38.2X1	T38.2X2	T38.2X3	T38.2X4	T38.2X5	T38.2X6
Thiourea	T38.2X1	T38.2X2	T38.2X3	T38.2X4	T38.2X5	T38.2X6
Thiphenamil	T44.3X1	T44.3X2	T44.3X3	T44.3X4	T44.3X5	T44.3X6
Thiram	T6Ø.3X1	T6Ø.3X2	T6Ø.3X3	T6Ø.3X4	—	—
medicinal	T49.2X1	T49.2X2	T49.2X3	T49.2X4	T49.2X5	T49.2X6
Thonzylamine (systemic)	T45.ØX1	T45.ØX2	T45.ØX3	T45.ØX4	T45.ØX5	T45.ØX6
mucosal decongestant	T48.5X1	T48.5X2	T48.5X3	T48.5X4	T48.5X5	T48.5X6
Thorazine	T43.3X1	T43.3X2	T43.3X3	T43.3X4	T43.3X5	T43.3X6
Thorium dioxide suspension	T5Ø.8X1	T5Ø.8X2	T5Ø.8X3	T5Ø.8X4	T5Ø.8X5	T5Ø.8X6
Thornapple	T62.2X1	T62.2X2	T62.2X3	T62.2X4	—	—
Throat drug NEC	T49.6X1	T49.6X2	T49.6X3	T49.6X4	T49.6X5	T49.6X6
Thrombin	T45.7X1	T45.7X2	T45.7X3	T45.7X4	T45.7X5	T45.7X6
Thrombolysin	T45.611	T45.612	T45.613	T45.614	T45.615	T45.616
Thromboplastin	T45.7X1	T45.7X2	T45.7X3	T45.7X4	T45.7X5	T45.7X6
Thurfyl nicotinate	T46.7X1	T46.7X2	T46.7X3	T46.7X4	T46.7X5	T46.7X6
Thymol	T49.ØX1	T49.ØX2	T49.ØX3	T49.ØX4	T49.ØX5	T49.ØX6
Thymopentin	T37.5X1	T37.5X2	T37.5X3	T37.5X4	T37.5X5	T37.5X6
Thymoxamine	T46.7X1	T46.7X2	T46.7X3	T46.7X4	T46.7X5	T46.7X6
Thymus extract	T38.891	T38.892	T38.893	T38.894	T38.895	T38.896
Thyreotrophic hormone	T38.811	T38.812	T38.813	T38.814	T38.815	T38.816
Thyroglobulin	T38.1X1	T38.1X2	T38.1X3	T38.1X4	T38.1X5	T38.1X6
Thyroid (hormone)	T38.1X1	T38.1X2	T38.1X3	T38.1X4	T38.1X5	T38.1X6
Thyrolar	T38.1X1	T38.1X2	T38.1X3	T38.1X4	T38.1X5	T38.1X6
Thyrotrophin	T38.811	T38.812	T38.813	T38.814	T38.815	T38.816
Thyrotropic hormone	T38.811	T38.812	T38.813	T38.814	T38.815	T38.816
Thyroxine	T38.1X1	T38.1X2	T38.1X3	T38.1X4	T38.1X5	T38.1X6
Tiabendazole	T37.4X1	T37.4X2	T37.4X3	T37.4X4	T37.4X5	T37.4X6
Tiamizide	T5Ø.2X1	T5Ø.2X2	T5Ø.2X3	T5Ø.2X4	T5Ø.2X5	T5Ø.2X6
Tianeptine	T43.291	T43.292	T43.293	T43.294	T43.295	T43.296
Tiapamil	T46.1X1	T46.1X2	T46.1X3	T46.1X4	T46.1X5	T46.1X6
Tiapride	T43.591	T43.592	T43.593	T43.594	T43.595	T43.596
Tiaprofenic acid	T39.311	T39.312	T39.313	T39.314	T39.315	T39.316
Tiaramide	T39.8X1	T39.8X2	T39.8X3	T39.8X4	T39.8X5	T39.8X6
Ticarcillin	T36.ØX1	T36.ØX2	T36.ØX3	T36.ØX4	T36.ØX5	T36.ØX6
Ticlatone	T49.ØX1	T49.ØX2	T49.ØX3	T49.ØX4	T49.ØX5	T49.ØX6
Ticlopidine	T45.521	T45.522	T45.523	T45.524	T45.525	T45.526
Ticrynafen	T5Ø.1X1	T5Ø.1X2	T5Ø.1X3	T5Ø.1X4	T5Ø.1X5	T5Ø.1X6
Tidiacic	T5Ø.991	T5Ø.992	T5Ø.993	T5Ø.994	T5Ø.995	T5Ø.996
Tiemonium	T44.3X1	T44.3X2	T44.3X3	T44.3X4	T44.3X5	T44.3X6
iodide	T44.3X1	T44.3X2	T44.3X3	T44.3X4	T44.3X5	T44.3X6
Tienilic acid	T5Ø.1X1	T5Ø.1X2	T5Ø.1X3	T5Ø.1X4	T5Ø.1X5	T5Ø.1X6
Tifenamil	T44.3X1	T44.3X2	T44.3X3	T44.3X4	T44.3X5	T44.3X6
Tigan	T45.ØX1	T45.ØX2	T45.ØX3	T45.ØX4	T45.ØX5	T45.ØX6
Tigloidine	T44.3X1	T44.3X2	T44.3X3	T44.3X4	T44.3X5	T44.3X6
Tilactase	T47.5X1	T47.5X2	T47.5X3	T47.5X4	T47.5X5	T47.5X6
Tiletamine	T41.291	T41.292	T41.293	T41.294	T41.295	T41.296
Tilidine	T4Ø.4X1	T4Ø.4X2	T4Ø.4X3	T4Ø.4X4	—	—
Timepidium bromide	T44.3X1	T44.3X2	T44.3X3	T44.3X4	T44.3X5	T44.3X6
Timiperone	T43.4X1	T43.4X2	T43.4X3	T43.4X4	T43.4X5	T43.4X6
Timolol	T44.7X1	T44.7X2	T44.7X3	T44.7X4	T44.7X5	T44.7X6
Tin (chloride) (dust) (oxide) NEC	T56.6X1	T56.6X2	T56.6X3	T56.6X4	—	—
anti-infectives	T37.8X1	T37.8X2	T37.8X3	T37.8X4	T37.8X5	T37.8X6
Tincture, iodine — *see Iodine*						
Tindal	T43.3X1	T43.3X2	T43.3X3	T43.3X4	T43.3X5	T43.3X6
Tinidazole	T37.3X1	T37.3X2	T37.3X3	T37.3X4	T37.3X5	T37.3X6
Tinoridine	T39.8X1	T39.8X2	T39.8X3	T39.8X4	T39.8X5	T39.8X6
Tiocarlide	T37.1X1	T37.1X2	T37.1X3	T37.1X4	T37.1X5	T37.1X6
Tioclomarol	T45.511	T45.512	T45.513	T45.514	T45.515	T45.516

Substance	Poisoning, Accidental (Unintentional)	External Cause (T-Code)				
		Poisoning, Intentional Self-Harm	Poisoning, Assault	Poisoning, Undetermined	Adverse Effect	Underdosing
Tioconazole	T49.0X1	T49.0X2	T49.0X3	T49.0X4	T49.0X5	T49.0X6
Tioguanine	T45.1X1	T45.1X2	T45.1X3	T45.1X4	T45.1X5	T45.1X6
Tiopronin	T50.991	T50.992	T50.993	T50.994	T50.995	T50.996
Tiotixene	T43.4X1	T43.4X2	T43.4X3	T43.4X4	T43.4X5	T43.4X6
Tioxolone	T49.4X1	T49.4X2	T49.4X3	T49.4X4	T49.4X5	T49.4X6
Tipepidine	T48.3X1	T48.3X2	T48.3X3	T48.3X4	T48.3X5	T48.3X6
Tiquizium bromide	T44.3X1	T44.3X2	T44.3X3	T44.3X4	T44.3X5	T44.3X6
Tiratricol	T38.1X1	T38.1X2	T38.1X3	T38.1X4	T38.1X5	T38.1X6
Tisopurine	T50.4X1	T50.4X2	T50.4X3	T50.4X4	T50.4X5	T50.4X6
Titanium (compounds) (vapor)	T56.891	T56.892	T56.893	T56.894	—	—
dioxide	T49.3X1	T49.3X2	T49.3X3	T49.3X4	T49.3X5	T49.3X6
ointment	T49.3X1	T49.3X2	T49.3X3	T49.3X4	T49.3X5	T49.3X6
oxide	T49.3X1	T49.3X2	T49.3X3	T49.3X4	T49.3X5	T49.3X6
tetrachloride	T56.891	T56.892	T56.893	T56.894	—	—
Titanocene	T56.891	T56.892	T56.893	T56.894	—	—
Titroid	T38.1X1	T38.1X2	T38.1X3	T38.1X4	T38.1X5	T38.1X6
Tizanidine	T42.8X1	T42.8X2	T42.8X3	T42.8X4	T42.8X5	T42.8X6
TMTD	T60.3X1	T60.3X2	T60.3X3	T60.3X4	—	—
TNT (fumes)	T65.3X1	T65.3X2	T65.3X3	T65.3X4	—	—
Toadstool	T62.0X1	T62.0X2	T62.0X3	T62.0X4	—	—
Tobacco NEC	T65.291	T65.292	T65.293	T65.294	—	—
cigarettes	T65.221	T65.222	T65.223	T65.224	—	—
Indian	T62.2X1	T62.2X2	T62.2X3	T62.2X4	—	—
smoke, second-hand	T65.221	T65.222	T65.223	T65.224	—	—
Tobramycin	T36.5X1	T36.5X2	T36.5X3	T36.5X4	T36.5X5	T36.5X6
Tocainide	T46.2X1	T46.2X2	T46.2X3	T46.2X4	T46.2X5	T46.2X6
Tocoferol	T45.2X1	T45.2X2	T45.2X3	T45.2X4	T45.2X5	T45.2X6
Tocopherol	T45.2X1	T45.2X2	T45.2X3	T45.2X4	T45.2X5	T45.2X6
acetate	T45.2X1	T45.2X2	T45.2X3	T45.2X4	T45.2X5	T45.2X6
Tocosamine	T48.0X1	T48.0X2	T48.0X3	T48.0X4	T48.0X5	T48.0X6
Todralazine	T46.5X1	T46.5X2	T46.5X3	T46.5X4	T46.5X5	T46.5X6
Tofisopam	T42.4X1	T42.4X2	T42.4X3	T42.4X4	T42.4X5	T42.4X6
Tofranil	T43.011	T43.012	T43.013	T43.014	T43.015	T43.016
Toilet deodorizer	T65.891	T65.892	T65.893	T65.894	—	—
Tolamolol	T44.7X1	T44.7X2	T44.7X3	T44.7X4	T44.7X5	T44.7X6
Tolazamide	T38.3X1	T38.3X2	T38.3X3	T38.3X4	T38.3X5	T38.3X6
Tolazoline	T46.7X1	T46.7X2	T46.7X3	T46.7X4	T46.7X5	T46.7X6
Tolbutamide (sodium)	T38.3X1	T38.3X2	T38.3X3	T38.3X4	T38.3X5	T38.3X6
Tolciclate	T49.0X1	T49.0X2	T49.0X3	T49.0X4	T49.0X5	T49.0X6
Tolmetin	T39.391	T39.392	T39.393	T39.394	T39.395	T39.396
Tolnaftate	T49.0X1	T49.0X2	T49.0X3	T49.0X4	T49.0X5	T49.0X6
Tolonidine	T46.5X1	T46.5X2	T46.5X3	T46.5X4	T46.5X5	T46.5X6

Substance	Poisoning, Accidental (Unintentional)	External Cause (T-Code)				
		Poisoning, Intentional Self-Harm	Poisoning, Assault	Poisoning, Undetermined	Adverse Effect	Underdosing
Toloxatone	T42.6X1	T42.6X2	T42.6X3	T42.6X4	T42.6X5	T42.6X6
Tolperisone	T44.3X1	T44.3X2	T44.3X3	T44.3X4	T44.3X5	T44.3X6
Tolserol	T42.8X1	T42.8X2	T42.8X3	T42.8X4	T42.8X5	T42.8X6
Toluene (liquid)	T52.2X1	T52.2X2	T52.2X3	T52.2X4	—	—
diisocyanate	T65.0X1	T65.0X2	T65.0X3	T65.0X4	—	—
Toluidine	T65.891	T65.892	T65.893	T65.894	—	—
vapor	T59.891	T59.892	T59.893	T59.894	—	—
Toluol (liquid)	T52.2X1	T52.2X2	T52.2X3	T52.2X4	—	—
vapor	T52.2X1	T52.2X2	T52.2X3	T52.2X4	—	—
Toluylenediamine	T65.3X1	T65.3X2	T65.3X3	T65.3X4	—	—
Tolylene-2,4-diisocyanate	T65.0X1	T65.0X2	T65.0X3	T65.0X4	—	—
Tonic NEC	T50.901	T50.902	T50.903	T50.904	T50.905	T50.906
Topical action drug NEC	T49.91	T49.92	T49.93	T49.94	T49.95	T49.96
ear, nose or throat	T49.6X1	T49.6X2	T49.6X3	T49.6X4	T49.6X5	T49.6X6
eye	T49.5X1	T49.5X2	T49.5X3	T49.5X4	T49.5X5	T49.5X6
skin	T49.91	T49.92	T49.93	T49.94	T49.95	T49.96
specified NEC	T49.8X1	T49.8X2	T49.8X3	T49.8X4	T49.8X5	T49.8X6
Toquizine	T44.3X1	T44.3X2	T44.3X3	T44.3X4	T44.3X5	T44.3X6
Toremifene	T38.6X1	T38.6X2	T38.6X3	T38.6X4	T38.6X5	T38.6X6
Tosylchloramide sodium	T49.8X1	T49.8X2	T49.8X3	T49.8X4	T49.8X5	T49.8X6
Toxaphene (dust) (spray)	T60.1X1	T60.1X2	T60.1X3	T60.1X4	—	—
Toxin, diphtheria (Schick Test)	T50.8X1	T50.8X2	T50.8X3	T50.8X4	T50.8X5	T50.8X6
Toxoid						
combined	T50.A21	T50.A22	T50.A23	T50.A24	T50.A25	T50.A26
diphtheria	T50.A91	T50.A92	T50.A93	T50.A94	T50.A95	T50.A96
tetanus	T50.A91	T50.A92	T50.A93	T50.A94	T50.A95	T50.A96
Trace element NEC	T45.8X1	T45.8X2	T45.8X3	T45.8X4	T45.8X5	T45.8X6
Tractor fuel NEC	T52.0X1	T52.0X2	T52.0X3	T52.0X4	—	—
Tragacanth	T50.991	T50.992	T50.993	T50.994	T50.995	T50.996
Tramadol	T40.4X1	T40.4X2	T40.4X3	T40.4X4	T40.4X5	T40.4X6
Tramazoline	T48.5X1	T48.5X2	T48.5X3	T48.5X4	T48.5X5	T48.5X6
Tranexamic acid	T45.621	T45.622	T45.623	T45.624	T45.625	T45.626
Tranilast	T45.0X1	T45.0X2	T45.0X3	T45.0X4	T45.0X5	T45.0X6
Tranquilizer NEC	T43.501	T43.502	T43.503	T43.504	T43.505	T43.506
with hypnotic or sedative	T42.6X1	T42.6X2	T42.6X3	T42.6X4	T42.6X5	T42.6X6
benzodiazepine NEC	T42.4X1	T42.4X2	T42.4X3	T42.4X4	T42.4X5	T42.4X6
butyrophenone NEC	T43.4X1	T43.4X2	T43.4X3	T43.4X4	T43.4X5	T43.4X6
carbamate	T43.591	T43.592	T43.593	T43.594	T43.595	T43.596
dimethylamine	T43.3X1	T43.3X2	T43.3X3	T43.3X4	T43.3X5	T43.3X6
ethylamine	T43.3X1	T43.3X2	T43.3X3	T43.3X4	T43.3X5	T43.3X6
hydroxyzine	T43.591	T43.592	T43.593	T43.594	T43.595	T43.596
major NEC	T43.501	T43.502	T43.503	T43.504	T43.505	T43.506

Substance	External Cause (T-Code)					
	Poisoning, Accidental (Unintentional)	Poisoning, Intentional Self-Harm	Poisoning, Assault	Poisoning, Undetermined	Adverse Effect	Underdosing
Tranquilizer NEC *(Continued)*						
penothiazine NEC	T43.3X1	T43.3X2	T43.3X3	T43.3X4	T43.3X5	T43.3X6
phenothiazine-based	T43.3X1	T43.3X2	T43.3X3	T43.3X4	T43.3X5	T43.3X6
piperazine NEC	T43.3X1	T43.3X2	T43.3X3	T43.3X4	T43.3X5	T43.3X6
piperidine	T43.3X1	T43.3X2	T43.3X3	T43.3X4	T43.3X5	T43.3X6
propylamine	T43.3X1	T43.3X2	T43.3X3	T43.3X4	T43.3X5	T43.3X6
specified NEC	T43.591	T43.592	T43.593	T43.594	T43.595	T43.596
thioxanthene NEC	T43.591	T43.592	T43.593	T43.594	T43.595	T43.596
Tranxene	T42.4X1	T42.4X2	T42.4X3	T42.4X4	T42.4X5	T42.4X6
Tranylcypromine	T43.1X1	T43.1X2	T43.1X3	T43.1X4	T43.1X5	T43.1X6
Trapidil	T46.3X1	T46.3X2	T46.3X3	T46.3X4	T46.3X5	T46.3X6
Trasentine	T44.3X1	T44.3X2	T44.3X3	T44.3X4	T44.3X5	T44.3X6
Travert	T5Ø.3X1	T5Ø.3X2	T5Ø.3X3	T5Ø.3X4	T5Ø.3X5	T5Ø.3X6
Trazodone	T43.211	T43.212	T43.213	T43.214	T43.215	T43.216
Trecator	T37.1X1	T37.1X2	T37.1X3	T37.1X4	T37.1X5	T37.1X6
Treosulfan	T45.1X1	T45.1X2	T45.1X3	T45.1X4	T45.1X5	T45.1X6
Tretamine	T45.1X1	T45.1X2	T45.1X3	T45.1X4	T45.1X5	T45.1X6
Tretinoin	T49.ØX1	T49.ØX2	T49.ØX3	T49.ØX4	T49.ØX5	T49.ØX6
Tretoquinol	T48.6X1	T48.6X2	T48.6X3	T48.6X4	T48.6X5	T48.6X6
Triacetin	T49.ØX1	T49.ØX2	T49.ØX3	T49.ØX4	T49.ØX5	T49.ØX6
Triacetoxyanthracene	T49.4X1	T49.4X2	T49.4X3	T49.4X4	T49.4X5	T49.4X6
Triacetyloleandomycin	T36.3X1	T36.3X2	T36.3X3	T36.3X4	T36.3X5	T36.3X6
Triamcinolone	T38.ØX1	T38.ØX2	T38.ØX3	T38.ØX4	T38.ØX5	T38.ØX6
ENT agent	T49.6X1	T49.6X2	T49.6X3	T49.6X4	T49.6X5	T49.6X6
hexacetonide	T49.ØX1	T49.ØX2	T49.ØX3	T49.ØX4	T49.ØX5	T49.ØX6
ophthalmic preparation	T49.5X1	T49.5X2	T49.5X3	T49.5X4	T49.5X5	T49.5X6
topical NEC	T49.ØX1	T49.ØX2	T49.ØX3	T49.ØX4	T49.ØX5	T49.ØX6
Triampyzine	T44.3X1	T44.3X2	T44.3X3	T44.3X4	T44.3X5	T44.3X6
Triamterene	T5Ø.2X1	T5Ø.2X2	T5Ø.2X3	T5Ø.2X4	T5Ø.2X5	T5Ø.2X6
Triazine (herbicide)	T6Ø.3X1	T6Ø.3X2	T6Ø.3X3	T6Ø.3X4	—	—
Triaziquone	T45.1X1	T45.1X2	T45.1X3	T45.1X4	T45.1X5	T45.1X6
Triazolam	T42.4X1	T42.4X2	T42.4X3	T42.4X4	T42.4X5	T42.4X6
Triazole (herbicide)	T6Ø.3X1	T6Ø.3X2	T6Ø.3X3	T6Ø.3X4	—	—
Tribenoside	T46.991	T46.992	T46.993	T46.994	T46.995	T46.996
Tribromacetaldehyde	T42.6X1	T42.6X2	T42.6X3	T42.6X4	T42.6X5	T42.6X6
Tribromoethanol, rectal	T41.291	T41.292	T41.293	T41.294	T41.295	T41.296
Tribromomethane	T42.6X1	T42.6X2	T42.6X3	T42.6X4	T42.6X5	T42.6X6
Trichlorethane	T53.2X1	T53.2X2	T53.2X3	T53.2X4	—	—
Trichlorethylene	T53.2X1	T53.2X2	T53.2X3	T53.2X4	—	—
Trichlorfon	T6Ø.ØX1	T6Ø.ØX2	T6Ø.ØX3	T6Ø.ØX4	—	—
Trichlormethiazide	T5Ø.2X1	T5Ø.2X2	T5Ø.2X3	T5Ø.2X4	T5Ø.2X5	T5Ø.2X6
Trichlormethine	T45.1X1	T45.1X2	T45.1X3	T45.1X4	T45.1X5	T45.1X6

Substance	External Cause (T-Code)					
	Poisoning, Accidental (Unintentional)	Poisoning, Intentional Self-Harm	Poisoning, Assault	Poisoning, Undetermined	Adverse Effect	Underdosing
Trichloroacetic acid, Trichloracetic acid	T54.2X1	T54.2X2	T54.2X3	T54.2X4	—	—
medicinal	T49.4X1	T49.4X2	T49.4X3	T49.4X4	T49.4X5	T49.4X6
Trichloroethane	T53.2X1	T53.2X2	T53.2X3	T53.2X4	—	—
Trichloroethanol	T42.6X1	T42.6X2	T42.6X3	T42.6X4	T42.6X5	T42.6X6
Trichloroethylene (liquid) (vapor)	T53.2X1	T53.2X2	T53.2X3	T53.2X4	—	—
anesthetic (gas)	T41.ØX1	T41.ØX2	T41.ØX3	T41.ØX4	T41.ØX5	T41.ØX6
vapor NEC	T53.2X1	T53.2X2	T53.2X3	T53.2X4	—	—
Trichloroethyl phosphate	T42.6X1	T42.6X2	T42.6X3	T42.6X4	T42.6X5	T42.6X6
Trichlorofluoromethane NEC	T53.5X1	T53.5X2	T53.5X3	T53.5X4	—	—
Trichloronate	T6Ø.ØX1	T6Ø.ØX2	T6Ø.ØX3	T6Ø.ØX4	—	—
2,4,5-Trichlorophen-oxyacetic acid	T6Ø.3X1	T6Ø.3X2	T6Ø.3X3	T6Ø.3X4	—	—
Trichloropropane	T53.6X1	T53.6X2	T53.6X3	T53.6X4	—	—
Trichlorotriethylamine	T45.1X1	T45.1X2	T45.1X3	T45.1X4	T45.1X5	T45.1X6
Trichomonacides NEC	T37.3X1	T37.3X2	T37.3X3	T37.3X4	T37.3X5	T37.3X6
Trichomycin	T36.7X1	T36.7X2	T36.7X3	T36.7X4	T36.7X5	T36.7X6
Triclobisonium chloride	T49.ØX1	T49.ØX2	T49.ØX3	T49.ØX4	T49.ØX5	T49.ØX6
Triclocarban	T49.ØX1	T49.ØX2	T49.ØX3	T49.ØX4	T49.ØX5	T49.ØX6
Triclofos	T42.6X1	T42.6X2	T42.6X3	T42.6X4	T42.6X5	T42.6X6
Triclosan	T49.ØX1	T49.ØX2	T49.ØX3	T49.ØX4	T49.ØX5	T49.ØX6
Tricresyl phosphate	T65.891	T65.892	T65.893	T65.894	—	—
solvent	T52.91	T52.92	T52.93	T52.94	—	—
Tricyclamol chloride	T44.3X1	T44.3X2	T44.3X3	T44.3X4	T44.3X5	T44.3X6
Tridesilon	T49.ØX1	T49.ØX2	T49.ØX3	T49.ØX4	T49.ØX5	T49.ØX6
Tridihexethyl iodide	T44.3X1	T44.3X2	T44.3X3	T44.3X4	T44.3X5	T44.3X6
Tridione	T42.2X1	T42.2X2	T42.2X3	T42.2X4	T42.2X5	T42.2X6
Trientine	T45.8X1	T45.8X2	T45.8X3	T45.8X4	T45.8X5	T45.8X6
Triethanolamine NEC	T54.3X1	T54.3X2	T54.3X3	T54.3X4	—	—
detergent	T54.3X1	T54.3X2	T54.3X3	T54.3X4	—	—
trinitrate (biphosphate)	T46.3X1	T46.3X2	T46.3X3	T46.3X4	T46.3X5	T46.3X6
Triethanomelamine	T45.1X1	T45.1X2	T45.1X3	T45.1X4	T45.1X5	T45.1X6
Triethylenemelamine	T45.1X1	T45.1X2	T45.1X3	T45.1X4	T45.1X5	T45.1X6
Triethylenephosphoramide	T45.1X1	T45.1X2	T45.1X3	T45.1X4	T45.1X5	T45.1X6
Triethylenethiophosphoramide	T45.1X1	T45.1X2	T45.1X3	T45.1X4	T45.1X5	T45.1X6
Trifluoperazine	T43.3X1	T43.3X2	T43.3X3	T43.3X4	T43.3X5	T43.3X6
Trifluoroethyl vinyl ether	T41.ØX1	T41.ØX2	T41.ØX3	T41.ØX4	T41.ØX5	T41.ØX6
Trifluperidol	T43.4X1	T43.4X2	T43.4X3	T43.4X4	T43.4X5	T43.4X6
Triflupromazine	T43.3X1	T43.3X2	T43.3X3	T43.3X4	T43.3X5	T43.3X6
Trifluridine	T37.5X1	T37.5X2	T37.5X3	T37.5X4	T37.5X5	T37.5X6
Triflusal	T45.521	T45.522	T45.523	T45.524	T45.525	T45.526
Trihexyphenidyl	T44.3X1	T44.3X2	T44.3X3	T44.3X4	T44.3X5	T44.3X6
Triiodothyronine	T38.1X1	T38.1X2	T38.1X3	T38.1X4	T38.1X5	T38.1X6

Substance	External Cause (T-Code) Poisoning, Accidental (Unintentional)	Poisoning, Intentional Self-Harm	Poisoning, Assault	Poisoning, Undetermined	Adverse Effect	Underdosing
Trilene	T41.ØX1	T41.ØX2	T41.ØX3	T41.ØX4	T41.ØX5	T41.ØX6
Trilostane	T38.991	T38.992	T38.993	T38.994	T38.995	T38.996
Trimebutine	T44.3X1	T44.3X2	T44.3X3	T44.3X4	T44.3X5	T44.3X6
Trimecaine	T41.3X1	T41.3X2	T41.3X3	T41.3X4	T41.3X5	T41.3X6
Trimeprazine (tartrate)	T44.3X1	T44.3X2	T44.3X3	T44.3X4	T44.3X5	T44.3X6
Trimetaphan camsilate	T44.2X1	T44.2X2	T44.2X3	T44.2X4	T44.2X5	T44.2X6
Trimetazidine	T46.7X1	T46.7X2	T46.7X3	T46.7X4	T46.7X5	T46.7X6
Trimethadione	T42.2X1	T42.2X2	T42.2X3	T42.2X4	T42.2X5	T42.2X6
Trimethaphan	T44.2X1	T44.2X2	T44.2X3	T44.2X4	T44.2X5	T44.2X6
Trimethidinium	T44.2X1	T44.2X2	T44.2X3	T44.2X4	T44.2X5	T44.2X6
Trimethobenzamide	T45.ØX1	T45.ØX2	T45.ØX3	T45.ØX4	T45.ØX5	T45.ØX6
Trimethoprim	T37.8X1	T37.8X2	T37.8X3	T37.8X4	T37.8X5	T37.8X6
with sulfamethoxazole	T36.8X1	T36.8X2	T36.8X3	T36.8X4	T36.8X5	T36.8X6
Trimethylcarbinol	T51.3X1	T51.3X2	T51.3X3	T51.3X4	—	—
Trimethylpsoralen	T49.3X1	T49.3X2	T49.3X3	T49.3X4	T49.3X5	T49.3X6
Trimeton	T45.ØX1	T45.ØX2	T45.ØX3	T45.ØX4	T45.ØX5	T45.ØX6
Trimetrexate	T45.1X1	T45.1X2	T45.1X3	T45.1X4	T45.1X5	T45.1X6
Trimipramine	T43.Ø11	T43.Ø12	T43.Ø13	T43.Ø14	T43.Ø15	T43.Ø16
Trimustine	T45.1X1	T45.1X2	T45.1X3	T45.1X4	T45.1X5	T45.1X6
Trinitrine	T46.3X1	T46.3X2	T46.3X3	T46.3X4	T46.3X5	T46.3X6
Trinitrobenzol	T65.3X1	T65.3X2	T65.3X3	T65.3X4	—	—
Trinitrophenol	T65.3X1	T65.3X2	T65.3X3	T65.3X4	—	—
Trinitrotoluene (fumes)	T65.3X1	T65.3X2	T65.3X3	T65.3X4	—	—
Trional	T42.6X1	T42.6X2	T42.6X3	T42.6X4	T42.6X5	T42.6X6
Triorthocresyl phosphate	T65.891	T65.892	T65.893	T65.894	—	—
Trioxide of arsenic	T57.ØX1	T57.ØX2	T57.ØX3	T57.ØX4	—	—
Trioxysalen	T49.4X1	T49.4X2	T49.4X3	T49.4X4	T49.4X5	T49.4X6
Tripamide	T5Ø.2X1	T5Ø.2X2	T5Ø.2X3	T5Ø.2X4	T5Ø.2X5	T5Ø.2X6
Triparanol	T46.6X1	T46.6X2	T46.6X3	T46.6X4	T46.6X5	T46.6X6
Tripelennamine	T45.ØX1	T45.ØX2	T45.ØX3	T45.ØX4	T45.ØX5	T45.ØX6
Triperiden	T44.3X1	T44.3X2	T44.3X3	T44.3X4	T44.3X5	T44.3X6
Triperidol	T43.4X1	T43.4X2	T43.4X3	T43.4X4	T43.4X5	T43.4X6
Triphenylphosphate	T65.891	T65.892	T65.893	T65.894	—	—
Triple						
bromides	T42.6X1	T42.6X2	T42.6X3	T42.6X4	T42.6X5	T42.6X6
carbonate	T47.1X1	T47.1X2	T47.1X3	T47.1X4	T47.1X5	T47.1X6
vaccine						
DPT	T5Ø.A11	T5Ø.A12	T5Ø.A13	T5Ø.A14	T5Ø.A15	T5Ø.A16
including pertussis	T5Ø.A11	T5Ø.A12	T5Ø.A13	T5Ø.A14	T5Ø.A15	T5Ø.A16
MMR	T5Ø.B91	T5Ø.B92	—	—	—	—
Triprolidine	T45.ØX1	T45.ØX2	T45.ØX3	T45.ØX4	T45.ØX5	T45.ØX6
Trisodium hydrogen edetate	T5Ø.6X1	T5Ø.6X2	T5Ø.6X3	T5Ø.6X4	T5Ø.6X5	T5Ø.6X6

Substance	External Cause (T-Code) Poisoning, Accidental (Unintentional)	Poisoning, Intentional Self-Harm	Poisoning, Assault	Poisoning, Undetermined	Adverse Effect	Underdosing
Trisoralen	T49.3X1	T49.3X2	T49.3X3	T49.3X4	T49.3X5	T49.3X6
Trisulfapyrimidines	T37.ØX1	T37.ØX2	T37.ØX3	T37.ØX4	T37.ØX5	T37.ØX6
Trithiozine	T44.3X1	T44.3X2	T44.3X3	T44.3X4	T44.3X5	T44.3X6
Tritiozine	T44.3X1	T44.3X2	T44.3X3	T44.3X4	T44.3X5	T44.3X6
Tritoqualine	T45.ØX1	T45.ØX2	T45.ØX3	T45.ØX4	T45.ØX5	T45.ØX6
Trofosfamide	T45.1X1	T45.1X2	T45.1X3	T45.1X4	T45.1X5	T45.1X6
Troleandomycin	T36.3X1	T36.3X2	T36.3X3	T36.3X4	T36.3X5	T36.3X6
Trolnitrate (phosphate)	T46.3X1	T46.3X2	T46.3X3	T46.3X4	T46.3X5	T46.3X6
Tromantadine	T37.5X1	T37.5X2	T37.5X3	T37.5X4	T37.5X5	T37.5X6
Trometamol	T5Ø.2X1	T5Ø.2X2	T5Ø.2X3	T5Ø.2X4	T5Ø.2X5	T5Ø.2X6
Tromethamine	T5Ø.2X1	T5Ø.2X2	T5Ø.2X3	T5Ø.2X4	T5Ø.2X5	T5Ø.2X6
Tronothane	T41.3X1	T41.3X2	T41.3X3	T41.3X4	T41.3X5	T41.3X6
Tropacine	T44.3X1	T44.3X2	T44.3X3	T44.3X4	T44.3X5	T44.3X6
Tropatepine	T44.3X1	T44.3X2	T44.3X3	T44.3X4	T44.3X5	T44.3X6
Tropicamide	T44.3X1	T44.3X2	T44.3X3	T44.3X4	T44.3X5	T44.3X6
Trospium chloride	T44.3X1	T44.3X2	T44.3X3	T44.3X4	T44.3X5	T44.3X6
Troxerutin	T46.991	T46.992	T46.993	T46.994	T46.995	T46.996
Troxidone	T42.2X1	T42.2X2	T42.2X3	T42.2X4	T42.2X5	T42.2X6
Tryparsamide	T37.3X1	T37.3X2	T37.3X3	T37.3X4	T37.3X5	T37.3X6
Trypsin	T45.3X1	T45.3X2	T45.3X3	T45.3X4	T45.3X5	T45.3X6
Tryptizol	T43.Ø11	T43.Ø12	T43.Ø13	T43.Ø14	T43.Ø15	T43.Ø16
TSH	T38.811	T38.812	T38.813	T38.814	T38.815	T38.816
Tuaminoheptane	T48.5X1	T48.5X2	T48.5X3	T48.5X4	T48.5X5	T48.5X6
Tuberculin, purified protein derivative (PPD)	T5Ø.8X1	T5Ø.8X2	T5Ø.8X3	T5Ø.8X4	T5Ø.8X5	T5Ø.8X6
Tubocurare	T48.1X1	T48.1X2	T48.1X3	T48.1X4	T48.1X5	T48.1X6
Tubocurarine (chloride)	T48.1X1	T48.1X2	T48.1X3	T48.1X4	T48.1X5	T48.1X6
Tulobuterol	T48.6X1	T48.6X2	T48.6X3	T48.6X4	T48.6X5	T48.6X6
Turpentine (spirits of)	T52.8X1	T52.8X2	T52.8X3	T52.8X4	—	—
vapor	T52.8X1	T52.8X2	T52.8X3	T52.8X4	—	—
Tybamate	T43.591	T43.592	T43.593	T43.594	T43.595	T43.596
Tyloxapol	T48.4X1	T48.4X2	T48.4X3	T48.4X4	T48.4X5	T48.4X6
Tymazoline	T48.5X1	T48.5X2	T48.5X3	T48.5X4	T48.5X5	T48.5X6
Typhoid-paratyphoid vaccine	T5Ø.A91	T5Ø.A92	T5Ø.A93	T5Ø.A94	T5Ø.A95	T5Ø.A96
Typhus vaccine	T5Ø.A91	T5Ø.A92	T5Ø.A93	T5Ø.A94	T5Ø.A95	T5Ø.A96
Tyropanoate	T5Ø.8X1	T5Ø.8X2	T5Ø.8X3	T5Ø.8X4	T5Ø.8X5	T5Ø.8X6
Tyrothricin	T49.6X1	T49.6X2	T49.6X3	T49.6X4	T49.6X5	T49.6X6
ENT agent	T49.6X1	T49.6X2	T49.6X3	T49.6X4	T49.6X5	T49.6X6
ophthalmic preparation	T49.5X1	T49.5X2	T49.5X3	T49.5X4	T49.5X5	T49.5X6
U						
Ufenamate	T39.391	T39.392	T39.393	T39.394	T39.395	T39.396
Ultraviolet light protectant	T49.3X1	T49.3X2	T49.3X3	T49.3X4	T49.3X5	T49.3X6

◀ New ◀ Revised ~~deleted~~ Deleted

Substance	External Cause (T-Code) Poisoning, Accidental (Unintentional)	Poisoning, Intentional Self-Harm	Poisoning, Assault	Poisoning, Undetermined	Adverse Effect	Underdosing
Undecenoic acid	T49.ØX1	T49.ØX2	T49.ØX3	T49.ØX4	T49.ØX5	T49.ØX6
Undecoylium	T49.ØX1	T49.ØX2	T49.ØX3	T49.ØX4	T49.ØX5	T49.ØX6
Undecylenic acid (derivatives)	T49.ØX1	T49.ØX2	T49.ØX3	T49.ØX4	T49.ØX5	T49.ØX6
Unna's boot	T49.3X1	T49.3X2	T49.3X3	T49.3X4	T49.3X5	T49.3X6
Unsaturated fatty acid	T46.6X1	T46.6X2	T46.6X3	T46.6X4	T46.6X5	T46.6X6
Uracil mustard	T45.1X1	T45.1X2	T45.1X3	T45.1X4	T45.1X5	T45.1X6
Uramustine	T45.1X1	T45.1X2	T45.1X3	T45.1X4	T45.1X5	T45.1X6
Urapidil	T46.5X1	T46.5X2	T46.5X3	T46.5X4	T46.5X5	T46.5X6
Urari	T48.1X1	T48.1X2	T48.1X3	T48.1X4	T48.1X5	T48.1X6
Urate oxidase	T5Ø.4X1	T5Ø.4X2	T5Ø.4X3	T5Ø.4X4	T5Ø.4X5	T5Ø.4X6
Urea	T47.3X1	T47.3X2	T47.3X3	T47.3X4	T47.3X5	T47.3X6
peroxide	T49.ØX1	T49.ØX2	T49.ØX3	T49.ØX4	T49.ØX5	T49.ØX6
stibamine	T37.4X1	T37.4X2	T37.4X3	T37.4X4	T37.4X5	T37.4X6
topical	T49.8X1	T49.8X2	T49.8X3	T49.8X4	T49.8X5	T49.8X6
Urethane	T45.1X1	T45.1X2	T45.1X3	T45.1X4	T45.1X5	T45.1X6
Urginea (maritima) (scilla) — *see Squill*						
Uric acid metabolism drug NEC	T5Ø.4X1	T5Ø.4X2	T5Ø.4X3	T5Ø.4X4	T5Ø.4X5	T5Ø.4X6
Uricosuric agent	T5Ø.4X1	T5Ø.4X2	T5Ø.4X3	T5Ø.4X4	T5Ø.4X5	T5Ø.4X6
Urinary anti-infective	T37.8X1	T37.8X2	T37.8X3	T37.8X4	T37.8X5	T37.8X6
Urofollitropin	T38.811	T38.812	T38.813	T38.814	T38.815	T38.816
Urokinase	T45.611	T45.612	T45.613	T45.614	T45.615	T45.616
Urokon	T5Ø.8X1	T5Ø.8X2	T5Ø.8X3	T5Ø.8X4	T5Ø.8X5	T5Ø.8X6
Ursodeoxycholic acid	T5Ø.991	T5Ø.992	T5Ø.993	T5Ø.994	T5Ø.995	T5Ø.996
Ursodiol	T5Ø.991	T5Ø.992	T5Ø.993	T5Ø.994	T5Ø.995	T5Ø.996
Urtica	T62.2X1	T62.2X2	T62.2X3	T62.2X4	—	—
Utility gas — *see Gas, utility*						
V						
Vaccine NEC	T5Ø.Z91	T5Ø.Z92	T5Ø.Z93	T5Ø.Z94	T5Ø.Z95	T5Ø.Z96
antineoplastic	T5Ø.Z91	T5Ø.Z92	T5Ø.Z93	T5Ø.Z94	T5Ø.Z95	T5Ø.Z96
bacterial NEC	T5Ø.A91	T5Ø.A92	T5Ø.A93	T5Ø.A94	T5Ø.A95	T5Ø.A96
with						
other bacterial component	T5Ø.A91	T5Ø.A92	T5Ø.A93	T5Ø.A94	T5Ø.A95	T5Ø.A96
pertussis component	T5Ø.A91	T5Ø.A92	T5Ø.A93	T5Ø.A94	T5Ø.A95	T5Ø.A96
viral-rickettsial component	T5Ø.A91	T5Ø.A92	T5Ø.A93	T5Ø.A94	T5Ø.A95	T5Ø.A96
mixed NEC	T5Ø.A91	T5Ø.A92	T5Ø.A93	T5Ø.A94	T5Ø.A95	T5Ø.A96
BCG	T5Ø.A91	T5Ø.A92	T5Ø.A93	T5Ø.A94	T5Ø.A95	T5Ø.A96
cholera	T5Ø.A91	T5Ø.A92	T5Ø.A93	T5Ø.A94	T5Ø.A95	T5Ø.A96
diphtheria	T5Ø.A91	T5Ø.A92	T5Ø.A93	T5Ø.A94	T5Ø.A95	T5Ø.A96
with tetanus	T5Ø.A21	T5Ø.A22	T5Ø.A23	T5Ø.A24	T5Ø.A25	T5Ø.A26
and pertussis	T5Ø.A11	T5Ø.A12	T5Ø.A13	T5Ø.A14	T5Ø.A15	T5Ø.A16
Vaccine NEC *(Continued)*						
influenza	T5Ø.B91	T5Ø.B92	T5Ø.B93	T5Ø.B94	T5Ø.B95	T5Ø.B96
measles	T5Ø.B91	T5Ø.B92	T5Ø.B93	T5Ø.B94	T5Ø.B95	T5Ø.B96
with mumps and rubella	T5Ø.B91	T5Ø.B92	T5Ø.B93	T5Ø.B94	T5Ø.B95	T5Ø.B96
meningococcal	T5Ø.A91	T5Ø.A92	T5Ø.A93	T5Ø.A94	T5Ø.A95	T5Ø.A96
mumps	T5Ø.B91	T5Ø.B92	T5Ø.B93	T5Ø.B94	T5Ø.B95	T5Ø.B96
paratyphoid	T5Ø.A91	T5Ø.A92	T5Ø.A93	T5Ø.A94	T5Ø.A95	T5Ø.A96
pertussis	T5Ø.A11	T5Ø.A12	T5Ø.A13	T5Ø.A14	T5Ø.A15	T5Ø.A16
with diphtheria	T5Ø.A11	T5Ø.A12	T5Ø.A13	T5Ø.A14	T5Ø.A15	T5Ø.A16
and tetanus	T5Ø.A11	T5Ø.A12	T5Ø.A13	T5Ø.A14	T5Ø.A15	T5Ø.A16
plague	T5Ø.A91	T5Ø.A92	T5Ø.A93	T5Ø.A94	T5Ø.A95	T5Ø.A96
poliomyelitis	T5Ø.B91	T5Ø.B92	T5Ø.B93	T5Ø.B94	T5Ø.B95	T5Ø.B96
poliovirus	T5Ø.B91	T5Ø.B92	T5Ø.B93	T5Ø.B94	T5Ø.B95	T5Ø.B96
rabies	T5Ø.B91	T5Ø.B92	T5Ø.B93	T5Ø.B94	T5Ø.B95	T5Ø.B96
respiratory syncytial virus	T5Ø.B91	T5Ø.B92	T5Ø.B93	T5Ø.B94	T5Ø.B95	T5Ø.B96
rickettsial NEC	T5Ø.A91	T5Ø.A92	T5Ø.A93	T5Ø.A94	T5Ø.A95	T5Ø.A96
with						
bacterial component	T5Ø.A21	T5Ø.A22	T5Ø.A23	T5Ø.A24	T5Ø.A25	T5Ø.A26
Rocky Mountain spotted fever	T5Ø.A91	T5Ø.A92	T5Ø.A93	T5Ø.A94	T5Ø.A95	T5Ø.A96
rubella	T5Ø.B91	T5Ø.B92	T5Ø.B93	T5Ø.B94	T5Ø.B95	T5Ø.B96
sabin oral	T5Ø.B91	T5Ø.B92	T5Ø.B93	T5Ø.B94	T5Ø.B95	T5Ø.B96
smallpox	T5Ø.B11	T5Ø.B12	T5Ø.B13	T5Ø.B14	T5Ø.B15	T5Ø.B16
TAB	T5Ø.A91	T5Ø.A92	T5Ø.A93	T5Ø.A94	T5Ø.A95	T5Ø.A96
tetanus	T5Ø.A91	T5Ø.A92	T5Ø.A93	T5Ø.A94	T5Ø.A95	T5Ø.A96
typhoid	T5Ø.A91	T5Ø.A92	T5Ø.A93	T5Ø.A94	T5Ø.A95	T5Ø.A96
typhus	T5Ø.A91	T5Ø.A92	T5Ø.A93	T5Ø.A94	T5Ø.A95	T5Ø.A96
viral NEC	T5Ø.B91	T5Ø.B92	T5Ø.B93	T5Ø.B94	T5Ø.B95	T5Ø.B96
yellow fever	T5Ø.B91	T5Ø.B92	T5Ø.B93	T5Ø.B94	T5Ø.B95	T5Ø.B96
Vaccinia immune globulin	T5Ø.Z11	T5Ø.Z12	T5Ø.Z13	T5Ø.Z14	T5Ø.Z15	T5Ø.Z16
Vaginal contraceptives	T49.8X1	T49.8X2	T49.8X3	T49.8X4	T49.8X5	T49.8X6
Valerian						
root	T42.6X1	T42.6X2	T42.6X3	T42.6X4	T42.6X5	T42.6X6
tincture	T42.6X1	T42.6X2	T42.6X3	T42.6X4	T42.6X5	T42.6X6
Valethamate bromide	T44.3X1	T44.3X2	T44.3X3	T44.3X4	T44.3X5	T44.3X6
Valisone	T49.ØX1	T49.ØX2	T49.ØX3	T49.ØX4	T49.ØX5	T49.ØX6
Valium	T42.4X1	T42.4X2	T42.4X3	T42.4X4	T42.4X5	T42.4X6
Valmid	T42.6X1	T42.6X2	T42.6X3	T42.6X4	T42.6X5	T42.6X6
Valnoctamide	T42.6X1	T42.6X2	T42.6X3	T42.6X4	T42.6X5	T42.6X6
Valproate (sodium)	T42.6X1	T42.6X2	T42.6X3	T42.6X4	T42.6X5	T42.6X6
Valproic acid	T42.6X1	T42.6X2	T42.6X3	T42.6X4	T42.6X5	T42.6X6
Valpromide	T42.6X1	T42.6X2	T42.6X3	T42.6X4	T42.6X5	T42.6X6
Vanadium	T56.891	T56.892	T56.893	T56.894	—	—

Substance	Poisoning, Accidental (Unintentional)	Poisoning, Intentional Self-Harm	Poisoning, Assault	Poisoning, Undetermined	Adverse Effect	Underdosing
	External Cause (T-Code)					
Vancomycin	T36.8X1	T36.8X2	T36.8X3	T36.8X4	T36.8X5	T36.8X6
Vapor—*see also Gas*	T59.91	T59.92	T59.93	T59.94	—	—
kiln (carbon monoxide)	T58.8X1	T58.8X2	T58.8X3	T58.8X4	—	—
lead—*see Lead*						
specified source NEC	T59.891	T59.892	T59.893	T59.894	—	—
Vardenafil	T46.7X1	T46.7X2	T46.7X3	T46.7X4	T46.7X5	T46.7X6
Varicose reduction drug	T46.8X1	T46.8X2	T46.8X3	T46.8X4	T46.8X5	T46.8X6
Varnish	T65.4X1	T65.4X2	T65.4X3	T65.4X4	—	—
cleaner	T52.91	T52.92	T52.93	T52.94	—	—
Vaseline	T49.3X1	T49.3X2	T49.3X3	T49.3X4	T49.3X5	T49.3X6
Vasodilan	T46.7X1	T46.7X2	T46.7X3	T46.7X4	T46.7X5	T46.7X6
Vasodilator						
coronary NEC	T46.3X1	T46.3X2	T46.3X3	T46.3X4	T46.3X5	T46.3X6
peripheral NEC	T46.7X1	T46.7X2	T46.7X3	T46.7X4	T46.7X5	T46.7X6
Vasopressin	T38.891	T38.892	T38.893	T38.894	T38.895	T38.896
Vasopressor drugs	T38.891	T38.892	T38.893	T38.894	T38.895	T38.896
Vecuronium bromide	T48.1X1	T48.1X2	T48.1X3	T48.1X4	T48.1X5	T48.1X6
Vegetable extract, astringent	T49.2X1	T49.2X2	T49.2X3	T49.2X4	T49.2X5	T49.2X6
Venlafaxine	T43.211	T43.212	T43.213	T43.214	T43.215	T43.216
Venom, venomous (bite) (sting)	T63.91	T63.92	T63.93	T63.94	—	—
amphibian NEC	T63.831	T63.832	T63.833	T63.834	—	—
animal NEC	T63.891	T63.892	T63.893	T63.894	—	—
ant	T63.421	T63.422	T63.423	T63.424	—	—
arthropod NEC	T63.481	T63.482	T63.483	T63.484	—	—
bee	T63.441	T63.442	T63.443	T63.444	—	—
centipede	T63.411	T63.412	T63.413	T63.414	—	—
fish	T63.591	T63.592	T63.593	T63.594	—	—
frog	T63.811	T63.812	T63.813	T63.814	—	—
hornet	T63.451	T63.452	T63.453	T63.454	—	—
insect NEC	T63.481	T63.482	T63.483	T63.484	—	—
lizard	T63.121	T63.122	T63.123	T63.124	—	—
marine						
animals	T63.691	T63.692	T63.693	T63.694	—	—
bluebottle	T63.611	T63.612	T63.613	T63.614	—	—
jellyfish NEC	T63.621	T63.622	T63.623	T63.624	—	—
Portugese Man-o-war	T63.611	T63.612	T63.613	T63.614	—	—
sea anemone	T63.631	T63.632	T63.633	T63.634	—	—
specified NEC	T63.691	T63.692	T63.693	T63.694	—	—
fish	T63.591	T63.592	T63.593	T63.594	—	—
plants	T63.711	T63.712	T63.713	T63.714	—	—
sting ray	T63.511	T63.512	T63.513	T63.514	—	—
Venom, venomous *(Continued)*						
millipede (tropical)	T63.411	T63.412	T63.413	T63.414	—	—
plant NEC	T63.791	T63.792	T63.793	T63.794	—	—
marine	T63.711	T63.712	T63.713	T63.714	—	—
reptile	T63.191	T63.192	T63.193	T63.194	—	—
gila monster	T63.111	T63.112	T63.113	T63.114	—	—
lizard NEC	T63.121	T63.122	T63.123	T63.124	—	—
scorpion	T63.2X1	T63.2X2	T63.2X3	T63.2X4	—	—
snake	T63.001	T63.002	T63.003	T63.004	—	—
African NEC	T63.081	T63.082	T63.083	T63.084	—	—
American (North) (South) NEC	T63.061	T63.062	T63.063	T63.064	—	—
Asian	T63.081	T63.082	T63.083	T63.084	—	—
Australian	T63.071	T63.072	T63.073	T63.074	—	—
cobra	T63.041	T63.042	T63.043	T63.044	—	—
coral snake	T63.021	T63.022	T63.023	T63.024	—	—
rattlesnake	T63.011	T63.012	T63.013	T63.014	—	—
specified NEC	T63.091	T63.092	T63.093	T63.094	—	—
taipan	T63.031	T63.032	T63.033	T63.034	—	—
specified NEC	T63.891	T63.892	T63.893	T63.894	—	—
spider	T63.301	T63.302	T63.303	T63.304	—	—
black widow	T63.311	T63.312	T63.313	T63.314	—	—
brown recluse	T63.331	T63.332	T63.333	T63.334	—	—
specified NEC	T63.391	T63.392	T63.393	T63.394	—	—
tarantula	T63.321	T63.322	T63.323	T63.324	—	—
sting ray	T63.511	T63.512	T63.513	T63.514	—	—
toad	T63.821	T63.822	T63.823	T63.824	—	—
wasp	T63.461	T63.462	T63.463	T63.464	—	—
Venous sclerosing drug NEC	T46.8X1	T46.8X2	T46.8X3	T46.8X4	T46.8X5	T46.8X6
Ventolin—*see Albuterol*						
Verapamil	T46.1X1	T46.1X2	T46.1X3	T46.1X4	T46.1X5	T46.1X6
Veramon	T42.3X1	T42.3X2	T42.3X3	T42.3X4	T42.3X5	T42.3X6
Veratrine	T46.5X1	T46.5X2	T46.5X3	T46.5X4	T46.5X5	T46.5X6
Veratrum						
album	T62.2X1	T62.2X2	T62.2X3	T62.2X4	—	—
alkaloids	T46.5X1	T46.5X2	T46.5X3	T46.5X4	T46.5X5	T46.5X6
viride	T62.2X1	T62.2X2	T62.2X3	T62.2X4	—	—
Verdigris	T60.3X1	T60.3X2	T60.3X3	T60.3X4	—	—
Veronal	T42.3X1	T42.3X2	T42.3X3	T42.3X4	T42.3X5	T42.3X6
Veroxil	T37.4X1	T37.4X2	T37.4X3	T37.4X4	T37.4X5	T37.4X6
Versenate	T50.6X1	T50.6X2	T50.6X3	T50.6X4	T50.6X5	T50.6X6

TABLE OF DRUGS AND CHEMICALS

New Revised ~~deleted~~ Deleted

Substance	External Cause (T-Code) Poisoning, Accidental (Unintentional)	Poisoning, Intentional Self-Harm	Poisoning, Assault	Poisoning, Undetermined	Adverse Effect	Underdosing
Versidyne	T39.8X1	T39.8X2	T39.8X3	T39.8X4	T39.8X5	T39.8X6
Vetrabutine	T48.0X1	T48.0X2	T48.0X3	T48.0X4	T48.0X5	T48.0X6
Vidarabine	T37.5X1	T37.5X2	T37.5X3	T37.5X4	T37.5X5	T37.5X6
Vienna						
green	T57.0X1	T57.0X2	T57.0X3	T57.0X4	—	—
insecticide	T60.2X1	T60.2X2	T60.2X3	T60.2X4	—	—
red	T57.0X1	T57.0X2	T57.0X3	T57.0X4	—	—
pharmaceutical dye	T50.991	T50.992	T50.993	T50.994	T50.995	T50.996
Vigabatrin	T42.6X1	T42.6X2	T42.6X3	T42.6X4	T42.6X5	T42.6X6
Viloxazine	T43.291	T43.292	T43.293	T43.294	T43.295	T43.296
Viminol	T39.8X1	T39.8X2	T39.8X3	T39.8X4	T39.8X5	T39.8X6
Vinbarbital, vinbarbitone	T42.3X1	T42.3X2	T42.3X3	T42.3X4	T42.3X5	T42.3X6
Vinblastine	T45.1X1	T45.1X2	T45.1X3	T45.1X4	T45.1X5	T45.1X6
Vinburnine	T46.7X1	T46.7X2	T46.7X3	T46.7X4	T46.7X5	T46.7X6
Vincamine	T45.1X1	T45.1X2	T45.1X3	T45.1X4	T45.1X5	T45.1X6
Vincristine	T45.1X1	T45.1X2	T45.1X3	T45.1X4	T45.1X5	T45.1X6
Vindesine	T45.1X1	T45.1X2	T45.1X3	T45.1X4	T45.1X5	T45.1X6
Vinesthene, vinethene	T41.0X1	T41.0X2	T41.0X3	T41.0X4	T41.0X5	T41.0X6
Vinorelbine tartrate	T45.1X1	T45.1X2	T45.1X3	T45.1X4	T45.1X5	T45.1X6
Vinpocetine	T46.7X1	T46.7X2	T46.7X3	T46.7X4	T46.7X5	T46.7X6
Vinyl						
acetate	T65.891	T65.892	T65.893	T65.894	—	—
bital	T42.3X1	T42.3X2	T42.3X3	T42.3X4	T42.3X5	T42.3X6
bromide	T65.891	T65.892	T65.893	T65.894	—	—
chloride	T59.891	T59.892	T59.893	T59.894	—	—
ether	T41.0X1	T41.0X2	T41.0X3	T41.0X4	T41.0X5	T41.0X6
Vinylbital	T42.3X1	T42.3X2	T42.3X3	T42.3X4	T42.3X5	T42.3X6
Vinylidene chloride	T65.891	T65.892	T65.893	T65.894	—	—
Vioform	T37.8X1	T37.8X2	T37.8X3	T37.8X4	T37.8X5	T37.8X6
topical	T49.0X1	T49.0X2	T49.0X3	T49.0X4	T49.0X5	T49.0X6
Viomycin	T36.8X1	T36.8X2	T36.8X3	T36.8X4	T36.8X5	T36.8X6
Viosterol	T45.2X1	T45.2X2	T45.2X3	T45.2X4	T45.2X5	T45.2X6
Viper (venom)	T63.091	T63.092	T63.093	T63.094	—	—
Viprynium	T37.4X1	T37.4X2	T37.4X3	T37.4X4	T37.4X5	T37.4X6
Viquidil	T46.7X1	T46.7X2	T46.7X3	T46.7X4	T46.7X5	T46.7X6
Viral vaccine NEC	T50.B91	T50.B92	T50.B93	T50.B94	T50.B95	T50.B96
Virginiamycin	T36.8X1	T36.8X2	T36.8X3	T36.8X4	T36.8X5	T36.8X6
Virugon	T37.5X1	T37.5X2	T37.5X3	T37.5X4	T37.5X5	T37.5X6
Viscous agent	T50.901	T50.902	T50.903	T50.904	T50.905	T50.906
Visine	T49.5X1	T49.5X2	T49.5X3	T49.5X4	T49.5X5	T49.5X6
Visnadine	T46.3X1	T46.3X2	T46.3X3	T46.3X4	T46.3X5	T46.3X6

Substance	External Cause (T-Code) Poisoning, Accidental (Unintentional)	Poisoning, Intentional Self-Harm	Poisoning, Assault	Poisoning, Undetermined	Adverse Effect	Underdosing
Vitamin NEC	T45.2X1	T45.2X2	T45.2X3	T45.2X4	T45.2X5	T45.2X6
A	T45.2X1	T45.2X2	T45.2X3	T45.2X4	T45.2X5	T45.2X6
B NEC	T45.2X1	T45.2X2	T45.2X3	T45.2X4	T45.2X5	T45.2X6
nicotinic acid	T46.7X1	T46.7X2	T46.7X3	T46.7X4	T46.7X5	T46.7X6
B1	T45.2X1	T45.2X2	T45.2X3	T45.2X4	T45.2X5	T45.2X6
B2	T45.2X1	T45.2X2	T45.2X3	T45.2X4	T45.2X5	T45.2X6
B6	T45.2X1	T45.2X2	T45.2X3	T45.2X4	T45.2X5	T45.2X6
B12	T45.2X1	T45.2X2	T45.2X3	T45.2X4	T45.2X5	T45.2X6
B15	T45.2X1	T45.2X2	T45.2X3	T45.2X4	T45.2X5	T45.2X6
C	T45.2X1	T45.2X2	T45.2X3	T45.2X4	T45.2X5	T45.2X6
D	T45.2X1	T45.2X2	T45.2X3	T45.2X4	T45.2X5	T45.2X6
D2	T45.2X1	T45.2X2	T45.2X3	T45.2X4	T45.2X5	T45.2X6
D3	T45.2X1	T45.2X2	T45.2X3	T45.2X4	T45.2X5	T45.2X6
E	T45.2X1	T45.2X2	T45.2X3	T45.2X4	T45.2X5	T45.2X6
E acetate	T45.2X1	T45.2X2	T45.2X3	T45.2X4	T45.2X5	T45.2X6
hematopoietic	T45.8X1	T45.8X2	T45.8X3	T45.8X4	T45.8X5	T45.8X6
K NEC	T45.7X1	T45.7X2	T45.7X3	T45.7X4	T45.7X5	T45.7X6
K1	T45.7X1	T45.7X2	T45.7X3	T45.7X4	T45.7X5	T45.7X6
K2	T45.7X1	T45.7X2	T45.7X3	T45.7X4	T45.7X5	T45.7X6
PP	T45.2X1	T45.2X2	T45.2X3	T45.2X4	T45.2X5	T45.2X6
ulceroprotectant	T47.1X1	T47.1X2	T47.1X3	T47.1X4	T47.1X5	T47.1X6
Vleminckx's solution	T49.4X1	T49.4X2	T49.4X3	T49.4X4	T49.4X5	T49.4X6
Voltaren — *see Diclofenac sodium*						
W						
Warfarin	T45.511	T45.512	T45.513	T45.514	T45.515	T45.516
rodenticide	T60.4X1	T60.4X2	T60.4X3	T60.4X4	—	—
sodium	T45.511	T45.512	T45.513	T45.514	T45.515	T45.516
Wasp (sting)	T63.461	T63.462	T63.463	T63.464	—	—
Water						
balance drug	T50.3X1	T50.3X2	T50.3X3	T50.3X4	T50.3X5	T50.3X6
distilled	T50.3X1	T50.3X2	T50.3X3	T50.3X4	T50.3X5	T50.3X6
gas — *see Gas, water*						
incomplete combustion of — *see Carbon, monoxide, fuel, utility*						
hemlock	T62.2X1	T62.2X2	T62.2X3	T62.2X4	—	—
moccasin (venom)	T63.061	T63.062	T63.063	T63.064	—	—
purified	T50.3X1	T50.3X2	T50.3X3	T50.3X4	T50.3X5	T50.3X6
Wax (paraffin) (petroleum)	T52.0X1	T52.0X2	T52.0X3	T52.0X4	—	—
automobile	T65.891	T65.892	T65.893	T65.894	—	—
floor	T52.0X1	T52.0X2	T52.0X3	T52.0X4	—	—

Substance	Poisoning, Accidental (Unintentional)	Poisoning, Intentional Self-Harm	Poisoning, Assault	Poisoning, Undetermined	Adverse Effect	Underdosing
	External Cause (T-Code)					
Weed killers NEC	T6Ø.3X1	T6Ø.3X2	T6Ø.3X3	T6Ø.3X4	—	—
Welldorm	T42.6X1	T42.6X2	T42.6X3	T42.6X4	T42.6X5	T42.6X6
White						
arsenic	T57.ØX1	T57.ØX2	T57.ØX3	T57.ØX4	—	—
hellebore	T62.2X1	T62.2X2	T62.2X3	T62.2X4	—	—
lotion (keratolytic)	T49.4X1	T49.4X2	T49.4X3	T49.4X4	T49.4X5	T49.4X6
spirit	T52.ØX1	T52.ØX2	T52.ØX3	T52.ØX4	—	—
Whitewash	T65.891	T65.892	T65.893	T65.894	—	—
Whole blood (human)	T45.8X1	T45.8X2	T45.8X3	T45.8X4	T45.8X5	T45.8X6
Wild						
black cherry	T62.2X1	T62.2X2	T62.2X3	T62.2X4	—	—
poisonous plants NEC	T62.2X1	T62.2X2	T62.2X3	T62.2X4	—	—
Window cleaning fluid	T65.891	T65.892	T65.893	T65.894	—	—
Wintergreen (oil)	T49.3X1	T49.3X2	T49.3X3	T49.3X4	T49.3X5	T49.3X6
Wisterine	T62.2X1	T62.2X2	T62.2X3	T62.2X4	—	—
Witch hazel	T49.2X1	T49.2X2	T49.2X3	T49.2X4	T49.2X5	T49.2X6
Wood alcohol or spirit	T51.1X1	T51.1X2	T51.1X3	T51.1X4	—	—
Wool fat (hydrous)	T49.3X1	T49.3X2	T49.3X3	T49.3X4	T49.3X5	T49.3X6
Woorali	T48.1X1	T48.1X2	T48.1X3	T48.1X4	T48.1X5	T48.1X6
Wormseed, American	T37.4X1	T37.4X2	T37.4X3	T37.4X4	T37.4X5	T37.4X6
X						
Xamoterol	T44.5X1	T44.5X2	T44.5X3	T44.5X4	T44.5X5	T44.5X6
Xanthine diuretics	T5Ø.2X1	T5Ø.2X2	T5Ø.2X3	T5Ø.2X4	T5Ø.2X5	T5Ø.2X6
Xanthinol nicotinate	T46.7X1	T46.7X2	T46.7X3	T46.7X4	T46.7X5	T46.7X6
Xanthotoxin	T49.3X1	T49.3X2	T49.3X3	T49.3X4	T49.3X5	T49.3X6
Xantinol nicotinate	T46.7X1	T46.7X2	T46.7X3	T46.7X4	T46.7X5	T46.7X6
Xantocillin	T36.ØX1	T36.ØX2	T36.ØX3	T36.ØX4	T36.ØX5	T36.ØX6
Xenon (127Xe) (133Xe)	T5Ø.8X1	T5Ø.8X2	T5Ø.8X3	T5Ø.8X4	T5Ø.8X5	T5Ø.8X6
Xenysalate	T49.4X1	T49.4X2	T49.4X3	T49.4X4	T49.4X5	T49.4X6
Xibornol	T37.8X1	T37.8X2	T37.8X3	T37.8X4	T37.8X5	T37.8X6
Xigris	T45.511	T45.512	T45.513	T45.514	T45.515	T45.516
Xipamide	T5Ø.2X1	T5Ø.2X2	T5Ø.2X3	T5Ø.2X4	T5Ø.2X5	T5Ø.2X6
Xylene (vapor)	T52.2X1	T52.2X2	T52.2X3	T52.2X4	—	—
Xylocaine (infiltration) (topical)	T41.3X1	T41.3X2	T41.3X3	T41.3X4	T41.3X5	T41.3X6
nerve block (peripheral) (plexus)	T41.3X1	T41.3X2	T41.3X3	T41.3X4	T41.3X5	T41.3X6
spinal	T41.3X1	T41.3X2	T41.3X3	T41.3X4	T41.3X5	T41.3X6
Xylol (vapor)	T52.2X1	T52.2X2	T52.2X3	T52.2X4	—	—
Xylometazoline	T48.5X1	T48.5X2	T48.5X3	T48.5X4	T48.5X5	T48.5X6

Substance	Poisoning, Accidental (Unintentional)	Poisoning, Intentional Self-Harm	Poisoning, Assault	Poisoning, Undetermined	Adverse Effect	Underdosing
	External Cause (T-Code)					
Y						
Yeast	T45.2X1	T45.2X2	T45.2X3	T45.2X4	T45.2X5	T45.2X6
dried	T45.2X1	T45.2X2	T45.2X3	T45.2X4	T45.2X5	T45.2X6
Yellow						
fever vaccine	T5Ø.B91	T5Ø.B92	T5Ø.B93	T5Ø.B94	T5Ø.B95	T5Ø.B96
jasmine	T62.2X1	T62.2X2	T62.2X3	T62.2X4	—	—
phenolphthalein	T47.2X1	T47.2X2	T47.2X3	T47.2X4	T47.2X5	T47.2X6
Yew	T62.2X1	T62.2X2	T62.2X3	T62.2X4	—	—
Yohimbic acid	T4Ø.991	T4Ø.992	T4Ø.993	T4Ø.994	T4Ø.995	T4Ø.996
Z						
Zactane	T39.8X1	T39.8X2	T39.8X3	T39.8X4	T39.8X5	T39.8X6
Zalcitabine	T37.5X1	T37.5X2	T37.5X3	T37.5X4	T37.5X5	T37.5X6
Zaroxolyn	T5Ø.2X1	T5Ø.2X2	T5Ø.2X3	T5Ø.2X4	T5Ø.2X5	T5Ø.2X6
Zephiran (topical)	T49.ØX1	T49.ØX2	T49.ØX3	T49.ØX4	T49.ØX5	T49.ØX6
ophthalmic preparation	T49.5X1	T49.5X2	T49.5X3	T49.5X4	T49.5X5	T49.5X6
Zeranol	T38.7X1	T38.7X2	T38.7X3	T38.7X4	T38.7X5	T38.7X6
Zerone	T51.1X1	T51.1X2	T51.1X3	T51.1X4	—	—
Zidovudine	T37.5X1	T37.5X2	T37.5X3	T37.5X4	T37.5X5	T37.5X6
Zimeldine	T43.221	T43.222	T43.223	T43.224	T43.225	T43.226
Zinc (compounds) (fumes) (vapor) NEC	T56.5X1	T56.5X2	T56.5X3	T56.5X4	—	—
anti-infectives	T49.ØX1	T49.ØX2	T49.ØX3	T49.ØX4	T49.ØX5	T49.ØX6
antivaricose	T46.8X1	T46.8X2	T46.8X3	T46.8X4	T46.8X5	T46.8X6
bacitracin	T49.ØX1	T49.ØX2	T49.ØX3	T49.ØX4	T49.ØX5	T49.ØX6
chloride (mouthwash)	T49.6X1	T49.6X2	T49.6X3	T49.6X4	T49.6X5	T49.6X6
chromate	T56.5X1	T56.5X2	T56.5X3	T56.5X4	—	—
gelatin	T49.3X1	T49.3X2	T49.3X3	T49.3X4	T49.3X5	T49.3X6
oxide	T49.3X1	T49.3X2	T49.3X3	T49.3X4	T49.3X5	T49.3X6
plaster	T49.3X1	T49.3X2	T49.3X3	T49.3X4	T49.3X5	T49.3X6
peroxide	T49.ØX1	T49.ØX2	T49.ØX3	T49.ØX4	T49.ØX5	T49.ØX6
pesticides	T56.5X1	T56.5X2	T56.5X3	T56.5X4	—	—
phosphide	T6Ø.4X1	T6Ø.4X2	T6Ø.4X3	T6Ø.4X4	—	—
pyrithionate	T49.4X1	T49.4X2	T49.4X3	T49.4X4	T49.4X5	T49.4X6
stearate	T49.3X1	T49.3X2	T49.3X3	T49.3X4	T49.3X5	T49.3X6
sulfate	T49.5X1	T49.5X2	T49.5X3	T49.5X4	T49.5X5	T49.5X6
ENT agent	T49.6X1	T49.6X2	T49.6X3	T49.6X4	T49.6X5	T49.6X6
ophthalmic solution	T49.5X1	T49.5X2	T49.5X3	T49.5X4	T49.5X5	T49.5X6
topical NEC	T49.ØX1	T49.ØX2	T49.ØX3	T49.ØX4	T49.ØX5	T49.ØX6
undecylenate	T49.ØX1	T49.ØX2	T49.ØX3	T49.ØX4	T49.ØX5	T49.ØX6

Substance	Poisoning, Accidental (Unintentional)	Poisoning, Intentional Self-Harm	Poisoning, Assault	Poisoning, Undetermined	Adverse Effect	Underdosing
Zineb	T60.ØX1	T60.ØX2	T60.ØX3	T60.ØX4	—	—
Zinostatin	T45.1X1	T45.1X2	T45.1X3	T45.1X4	T45.1X5	T45.1X6
Zipeprol	T48.3X1	T48.3X2	T48.3X3	T48.3X4	T48.3X5	T48.3X6
Zofenopril	T46.4X1	T46.4X2	T46.4X3	T46.4X4	T46.4X5	T46.4X6
Zolpidem	T42.6X1	T42.6X2	T42.6X3	T42.6X4	T42.6X5	T42.6X6
Zomepirac	T39.391	T39.392	T39.393	T39.394	T39.395	T39.396
Zopiclone	T42.6X1	T42.6X2	T42.6X3	T42.6X4	T42.6X5	T42.6X6
Zorubicin	T45.1X1	T45.1X2	T45.1X3	T45.1X4	T45.1X5	T45.1X6
Zotepine	T43.591	T43.592	T43.593	T43.594	T43.595	T43.596
Zovant	T45.511	T45.512	T45.513	T45.514	T45.515	T45.516
Zoxazolamine	T42.8X1	T42.8X2	T42.8X3	T42.8X4	T42.8X5	T42.8X6
Zuclopenthixol	T43.4X1	T43.4X2	T43.4X3	T43.4X4	T43.4X5	T43.4X6
Zygadenus (venenosus)	T62.2X1	T62.2X2	T62.2X3	T62.2X4	—	—
Zyprexa	T43.591	T43.592	T43.593	T43.594	T43.595	T43.596

External Cause (T-Code)

External Cause of Injuries Index

A

- **Abandonment** (causing exposure to weather conditions) (with intent to injure or kill) NEC X58
- **Abuse** (adult) (child) (mental) (physical) (sexual) X58
- **Accident** (to) X58
  - aircraft (in transit) (powered) —*see also* Accident, transport, aircraft
    - due to, caused by cataclysm —*see* Forces of nature, by type
  - animal-drawn vehicle —*see* Accident, transport, animal-drawn vehicle occupant
  - animal-rider —*see* Accident, transport, animal-rider
  - automobile —*see* Accident, transport, car occupant
  - bare foot water skiier V94.4
  - boat, boating —*see also* Accident, watercraft
    - striking swimmer
      - powered V94.11
      - unpowered V94.12
  - bus —*see* Accident, transport, bus occupant
  - cable car, not on rails V98.Ø
    - on rails —*see* Accident, transport, streetcar occupant
  - car —*see* Accident, transport, car occupant
  - caused by, due to
    - animal NEC W64
    - chain hoist W24.Ø
    - cold (excessive) —*see* Exposure, cold
    - corrosive liquid, substance —*see* Table of Drugs and Chemicals
    - cutting or piercing instrument —*see* Contact, with, by type of instrument
    - drive belt W24.Ø
    - electric
      - current —*see* Exposure, electric current
      - motor —*see also* Contact, with, by type of machine W31.3
        - current (of) W86.8
    - environmental factor NEC X58
    - explosive material —*see* Explosion
    - fire, flames —*see* Exposure, fire
    - firearm missile —*see* Discharge, firearm by type
    - heat (excessive) —*see* Heat
    - hot —*see* Contact, with, hot
    - ignition —*see* Ignition
    - lifting device W24.Ø
    - lightning —*see* subcategory T75.Ø
      - causing fire —*see* Exposure, fire
    - machine, machinery —*see* Contact, with, by type of machine
    - natural factor NEC X58
    - pulley (block) W24.Ø
    - radiation —*see* Radiation
    - steam X13.1
      - inhalation X13.Ø
      - pipe X16
    - thunderbolt —*see* subcategory T75.Ø
      - causing fire —*see* Exposure, fire
    - transmission device W24.1
  - coach —*see* Accident, transport, bus occupant
  - coal car —*see* Accident, transport, industrial vehicle occupant
  - diving —*see also* Fall, into, water
    - with
      - drowning or submersion —*see* Drowning
  - forklift —*see* Accident, transport, industrial vehicle occupant
  - heavy transport vehicle NOS —*see* Accident, transport, truck occupant
  - ice yacht V98.2

Accident *(Continued)*
  - in
    - medical, surgical procedure
      - as, or due to misadventure —*see* Misadventure
      - causing an abnormal reaction or later complication without mention of misadventure —*see also* Complication of or following, by type of procedure Y84.9
  - land yacht V98.1
  - late effect of —*see* WØØ-X58 with 7th character S
  - logging car —*see* Accident, transport, industrial vehicle occupant
  - machine, machinery —*see also* Contact, with, by type of machine
    - on board watercraft V93.69
      - explosion —*see* Explosion, in, watercraft
      - fire —*see* Burn, on board watercraft
      - powered craft V93.63
        - ferry boat V93.61
        - fishing boat V93.62
        - jet ski V93.63
        - liner V93.61
        - merchant ship V93.6Ø
        - passenger ship V93.61
        - sailboat V93.64
  - mine tram —*see* Accident, transport, industrial vehicle occupant
  - mobility scooter (motorized) —*see* Accident, transport, pedestrian, conveyance, specified type NEC
  - motor scooter —*see* Accident, transport, motorcyclist
  - motor vehicle NOS (traffic) —*see also* Accident, transport V89.2
    - nontraffic V89.Ø
    - three-wheeled NOS —*see* Accident, transport, three-wheeled motor vehicle occupant
  - motorcycle NOS —*see* Accident, transport, motorcyclist
  - nonmotor vehicle NOS (nontraffic) —*see also* Accident, transport V89.1
    - traffic NOS V89.3
  - nontraffic (victim's mode of transport NOS) V88.9
    - collision (between) V88.7
      - bus and truck V88.5
      - car and:
        - bus V88.3
        - pickup V88.2
        - three-wheeled motor vehicle V88.Ø
        - train V88.6
        - truck V88.4
        - two-wheeled motor vehicle V88.Ø
        - van V88.2
      - specified vehicle NEC and:
        - three-wheeled motor vehicle V88.1
        - two-wheeled motor vehicle V88.1
    - known mode of transport —*see* Accident, transport, by type of vehicle
    - noncollision V88.8
  - on board watercraft V93.89
    - powered craft V93.83
      - ferry boat V93.81
      - fishing boat V93.82
      - jet ski V93.83
      - liner V93.81
      - merchant ship V93.8Ø
      - passenger ship V93.81
    - unpowered craft V93.88
      - canoe V93.85
      - inflatable V93.86
        - in tow
          - recreational V94.31
          - specified NEC V94.32
      - kayak V93.85

Accident *(Continued)*
  - on board watercraft *(Continued)*
    - unpowered craft *(Continued)*
      - sailboat V93.84
      - surf-board V93.88
      - water skis V93.87
      - windsurfer V93.88
  - parachutist V97.29
    - entangled in object V97.21
    - injured on landing V97.22
  - pedal cycle —*see* Accident, transport, pedal cyclist
  - pedestrian (on foot)
    - with
      - another pedestrian W51
        - with fall WØ3
          - due to ice or snow WØØ.Ø
        - on pedestrian conveyance NEC VØØ.Ø9
      - roller skater (in-line) VØØ.Ø1
      - skate boarder VØØ.Ø2
      - transport vehicle —*see* Accident, transport
    - on pedestrian conveyance —*see* Accident, transport, pedestrian, conveyance
  - pick-up truck or van —*see* Accident, transport, pickup truck occupant
  - quarry truck —*see* Accident, transport, industrial vehicle occupant
  - railway vehicle (any) (in motion) —*see* Accident, transport, railway vehicle occupant
    - due to cataclysm —*see* Forces of nature, by type
  - scooter (non-motorized) —*see* Accident, transport, pedestrian, conveyance, scooter
  - sequelae of —*see* WØØ-X58 with 7th character S
  - skateboard —*see* Accident, transport, pedestrian, conveyance, skateboard
  - ski (ing) —*see* Accident, transport, pedestrian, conveyance
    - lift V98.3
  - specified cause NEC X58
  - streetcar —*see* Accident, transport, streetcar occupant
  - traffic (victim's mode of transport NOS) V87.9
    - collision (between) V87.7
      - bus and truck V87.5
      - car and:
        - bus V87.3
        - pickup V87.2
        - three-wheeled motor vehicle V87.Ø
        - train V87.6
        - truck V87.4
        - two-wheeled motor vehicle V87.Ø
        - van V87.2
      - ➡specified vehicle NEC V86.39
        - ▶and
          - ▶three-wheeled motor vehicle V87.1
          - ▶two-wheeled motor vehicle V87.1
        - ▶driver V86.Ø9
        - ▶person on outside V86.29
        - ▶passenger V86.19
        - ~~three-wheeled motor vehicle V87.1~~
        - ~~two-wheeled motor vehicle V87.1~~
        - ▶while boarding or alighting V86.49
    - known mode of transport —*see* Accident, transport, by type of vehicle
    - noncollision V87.8
  - transport (involving injury to) V99
    - 18 wheeler —*see* Accident, transport, truck occupant
    - agricultural vehicle occupant (nontraffic) V84.9
      - driver V84.5
      - hanger-on V84.7
      - passenger V84.6

- **Accident** *(Continued)*
  - transport *(Continued)*
    - agricultural vehicle occupant *(Continued)*
      - traffic V84.3
        - driver V84.0
        - hanger-on V84.2
        - passenger V84.1
      - while boarding or alighting V84.4
    - aircraft NEC V97.89
      - military NEC V97.818
        - with civilian aircraft V97.810
        - civilian injured by V97.811
      - occupant injured (in)
        - nonpowered craft accident V96.9
          - balloon V96.00
            - collision V96.03
            - crash V96.01
            - explosion V96.05
            - fire V96.04
            - forced landing V96.02
            - specified type NEC V96.09
          - glider V96.20
            - collision V96.23
            - crash V96.21
            - explosion V96.25
            - fire V96.24
            - forced landing V96.22
            - specified type NEC V96.29
          - hang glider V96.10
            - collision V96.13
            - crash V96.11
            - explosion V96.15
            - fire V96.14
            - forced landing V96.12
            - specified type NEC V96.19
          - specified craft NEC V96.8
        - powered craft accident V95.9
          - fixed wing NEC
            - commercial V95.30
              - collision V95.33
              - crash V95.31
              - explosion V95.35
              - fire V95.34
              - forced landing V95.32
              - specified type NEC V95.39
            - private V95.20
              - collision V95.23
              - crash V95.21
              - explosion V95.25
              - fire V95.24
              - forced landing V95.22
              - specified type NEC V95.29
          - glider V95.10
            - collision V95.13
            - crash V95.11
            - explosion V95.15
            - fire V95.14
            - forced landing V95.12
            - specified type NEC V95.19
          - helicopter V95.00
            - collision V95.03
            - crash V95.01
            - explosion V95.05
            - fire V95.04
            - forced landing V95.02
            - specified type NEC V95.09
          - spacecraft V95.40
            - collision V95.43
            - crash V95.41
            - explosion V95.45
            - fire V95.44
            - forced landing V95.42
            - specified type NEC V95.49
          - specified craft NEC V95.8
          - ultralight V95.10
            - collision V95.13
            - crash V95.11
            - explosion V95.15
            - fire V95.14
            - forced landing V95.12
            - specified type NEC V95.19

- **Accident** *(Continued)*
  - transport *(Continued)*
    - aircraft NEC *(Continued)*
      - occupant injured *(Continued)*
        - specified accident NEC V97.0
        - while boarding or alighting V97.1
      - person (injured by)
        - falling from, in or on aircraft V97.0
        - machinery on aircraft V97.89
        - on ground with aircraft involvement V97.39
        - rotating propeller V97.32
        - struck by object falling from aircraft V97.31
        - sucked into aircraft jet V97.33
        - while boarding or alighting aircraft V97.1
    - airport (battery-powered) passenger vehicle —*see* Accident, transport, industrial vehicle occupant
    - all-terrain vehicle occupant (nontraffic) V86.95
      - driver V86.55
      - dune buggy —*see* Accident, transport, dune buggy occupant
      - hanger-on V86.75
      - passenger V86.65
      - snowmobile —*see* Accident, transport, snowmobile occupant
      - specified type NEC V86.99
        - ▶driver V86.59
        - ▶passenger V86.69
        - ▶person on outside V86.79
      - traffic V86.35
        - driver V86.05
        - hanger-on V86.25
        - passenger V86.15
      - while boarding or alighting V86.45
    - ambulance occupant (traffic) V86.31
      - driver V86.01
      - hanger-on V86.21
      - nontraffic V86.91
        - driver V86.51
        - hanger-on V86.71
        - passenger V86.61
      - passenger V86.11
      - while boarding or alighting V86.41
    - animal-drawn vehicle occupant (in) V80.929
      - collision (with)
        - animal V80.12
          - being ridden V80.711
        - animal-drawn vehicle V80.721
        - bus V80.42
        - car V80.42
        - fixed or stationary object V80.82
        - military vehicle V80.920
        - nonmotor vehicle V80.791
        - pedal cycle V80.22
        - pedestrian V80.12
        - pickup V80.42
        - railway train or vehicle V80.62
        - specified motor vehicle NEC V80.52
        - streetcar V80.731
        - truck V80.42
        - two-or three-wheeled motor vehicle V80.32
        - van V80.42
      - noncollision V80.02
      - specified circumstance NEC V80. 928
    - animal-rider V80.919
      - collision (with)
        - animal V80.11
          - being ridden V80.710
        - animal-drawn vehicle V80.720
        - bus V80.41
        - car V80.41
        - fixed or stationary object V80.81
        - military vehicle V80.910
        - nonmotor vehicle V80.790
        - pedal cycle V80.21
        - pedestrian V80.11
        - pickup V80.41

- **Accident** *(Continued)*
  - transport *(Continued)*
    - animal-rider *(Continued)*
      - collision *(Continued)*
        - railway train or vehicle V80.61
        - specified motor vehicle NEC V80.51
        - streetcar V80.730
        - truck V80.41
        - two- or three-wheeled motor vehicle V80.31
        - van V80.41
      - noncollision V80.018
        - specified as horse rider V80.010
      - specified circumstance NEC V80.918
    - armored car —*see* Accident, transport, truck occupant
    - battery-powered truck (baggage) (mail) —*see* Accident, transport, industrial vehicle occupant
    - bus occupant V79.9
      - collision (with)
        - animal (traffic) V70.9
          - being ridden (traffic) V76.9
            - nontraffic V76.3
            - while boarding or alighting V76.4
          - nontraffic V70.3
          - while boarding or alighting V70.4
        - animal-drawn vehicle (traffic) V76.9
          - nontraffic V76.3
          - while boarding or alighting V76.4
        - bus (traffic) V74.9
          - nontraffic V74.3
          - while boarding or alighting V74.4
        - car (traffic) V73.9
          - nontraffic V73.3
          - while boarding or alighting V73.4
        - motor vehicle NOS (traffic) V79.60
          - nontraffic V79.20
          - specified type NEC (traffic) V79.69
            - nontraffic V79.29
        - pedal cycle (traffic) V71.9
          - nontraffic V71.3
          - while boarding or alighting V71.4
        - pickup truck (traffic) V73.9
          - nontraffic V73.3
          - while boarding or alighting V73.4
        - railway vehicle (traffic) V75.9
          - nontraffic V75.3
          - while boarding or alighting V75.4
        - specified vehicle NEC (traffic) V76.9
          - nontraffic V76.3
          - while boarding or alighting V76.4
        - stationary object (traffic) V77.9
          - nontraffic V77.3
          - while boarding or alighting V77.4
        - streetcar (traffic) V76.9
          - nontraffic V76.3
          - while boarding or alighting V76.4
        - three wheeled motor vehicle (traffic) V72.9
          - nontraffic V72.3
          - while boarding or alighting V72.4
        - truck (traffic) V74.9
          - nontraffic V74.3
          - while boarding or alighting V74.4
        - two wheeled motor vehicle (traffic) V72.9
          - nontraffic V72.3
          - while boarding or alighting V72.4
        - van (traffic) V73.9
          - nontraffic V73.3
          - while boarding or alighting V73.4
      - driver
        - collision (with)
          - animal (traffic) V70.5
            - being ridden (traffic) V76.5
              - nontraffic V76.0
            - nontraffic V70.0
          - animal-drawn vehicle (traffic) V76.5
            - nontraffic V76.0
          - bus (traffic) V74.5
            - nontraffic V74.0

A

- Accident *(Continued)*
  - transport *(Continued)*
    - bus occupant *(Continued)*
      - driver *(Continued)*
        - collision *(Continued)*
          - car (traffic) V73.5
            - nontraffic V73.0
          - motor vehicle NOS (traffic) V79.40
            - nontraffic V79.00
            - specified type NEC (traffic) V79.49
              - nontraffic V79.09
          - pedal cycle (traffic) V71.5
            - nontraffic V71.0
          - pickup truck (traffic) V73.5
            - nontraffic V73.0
          - railway vehicle (traffic) V75.5
            - nontraffic V75.0
          - specified vehicle NEC (traffic) V76.5
            - nontraffic V76.0
          - stationary object (traffic) V77.5
            - nontraffic V77.0
          - streetcar (traffic) V76.5
            - nontraffic V76.0
          - three wheeled motor vehicle (traffic) V72.5
            - nontraffic V72.0
          - truck (traffic) V74.5
            - nontraffic V74.0
          - two wheeled motor vehicle (traffic) V72.5
            - nontraffic V72.0
          - van (traffic) V73.5
            - nontraffic V73.0
        - noncollision accident (traffic) V78.5
          - nontraffic V78.0
      - hanger-on
        - collision (with)
          - animal (traffic) V70.7
            - being ridden (traffic) V76.7
              - nontraffic V76.2
            - nontraffic V70.2
          - animal-drawn vehicle (traffic) V76.7
            - nontraffic V76.2
          - bus (traffic) V74.7
            - nontraffic V74.2
          - car (traffic) V73.7
            - nontraffic V73.2
          - pedal cycle (traffic) V71.7
            - nontraffic V71.2
          - pickup truck (traffic) V73.7
            - nontraffic V73.2
          - railway vehicle (traffic) V75.7
            - nontraffic V75.2
          - specified vehicle NEC (traffic) V76.7
            - nontraffic V76.2
          - stationary object (traffic) V77.7
            - nontraffic V77.2
          - streetcar (traffic) V76.7
            - nontraffic V76.2
          - three wheeled motor vehicle (traffic) V72.7
            - nontraffic V72.2
          - truck (traffic) V74.7
            - nontraffic V74.2
          - two wheeled motor vehicle (traffic) V72.7
            - nontraffic V72.2
          - van (traffic) V73.7
            - nontraffic V73.2
        - noncollision accident (traffic) V78.7
          - nontraffic V78.2
      - noncollision accident (traffic) V78.9
        - nontraffic V78.3
        - while boarding or alighting V78.4
      - nontraffic V79.3
      - passenger
        - collision (with)
          - animal (traffic) V70.6
            - being ridden (traffic) V76.6
              - nontraffic V76.1
            - nontraffic V70.1

- Accident *(Continued)*
  - transport *(Continued)*
    - bus occupant *(Continued)*
      - passenger *(Continued)*
        - collision *(Continued)*
          - animal-drawn vehicle (traffic) V76.6
            - nontraffic V76.1
          - bus (traffic) V74.6
            - nontraffic V74.1
          - car (traffic) V73.6
            - nontraffic V73.1
          - motor vehicle NOS (traffic) V79.50
            - nontraffic V79.10
            - specified type NEC (traffic) V79.59
              - nontraffic V79.19
          - pedal cycle (traffic) V71.6
            - nontraffic V71.1
          - pickup truck (traffic) V73.6
            - nontraffic V73.1
          - railway vehicle (traffic) V75.6
            - nontraffic V75.1
          - specified vehicle NEC (traffic) V76.6
            - nontraffic V76.1
          - stationary object (traffic) V77.6
            - nontraffic V77.1
          - streetcar (traffic) V76.6
            - nontraffic V76.1
          - three wheeled motor vehicle (traffic) V72.6
            - nontraffic V72.1
          - truck (traffic) V74.6
            - nontraffic V74.1
          - two wheeled motor vehicle (traffic) V72.6
            - nontraffic V72.1
          - van (traffic) V73.6
            - nontraffic V73.1
        - noncollision accident (traffic) V78.6
          - nontraffic V78.1
      - specified type NEC V79.88
        - military vehicle V79.81
    - cable car, not on rails V98.0
      - on rails —*see* Accident, transport, streetcar occupant
    - car occupant V49.9
      - ambulance occupant —*see* Accident, transport, ambulance occupant
      - collision (with)
        - animal (traffic) V40.9
          - being ridden (traffic) V46.9
            - nontraffic V46.3
            - while boarding or alighting V46.4
          - nontraffic V40.3
          - while boarding or alighting V40.4
        - animal-drawn vehicle (traffic) V46.9
          - nontraffic V46.3
          - while boarding or alighting V46.4
        - bus (traffic) V44.9
          - nontraffic V44.3
          - while boarding or alighting V44.4
        - car (traffic) V43.92
          - nontraffic V43.32
          - while boarding or alighting V43.42
        - motor vehicle NOS (traffic) V49.60
          - nontraffic V49.20
          - specified type NEC (traffic) V49.69
            - nontraffic V49.29
        - pedal cycle (traffic) V41.9
          - nontraffic V41.3
          - while boarding or alighting V41.4
        - pickup truck (traffic) V43.93
          - nontraffic V43.33
          - while boarding or alighting V43.43
        - railway vehicle (traffic) V45.9
          - nontraffic V45.3
          - while boarding or alighting V45.4
        - specified vehicle NEC (traffic) V46.9
          - nontraffic V46.3
          - while boarding or alighting V46.4

- Accident *(Continued)*
  - transport *(Continued)*
    - car occupant *(Continued)*
      - collision *(Continued)*
        - sport utility vehicle (traffic) V43.91
          - nontraffic V43.31
          - while boarding or alighting V43.41
        - stationary object (traffic) V47.9
          - nontraffic V47.3
          - while boarding or alighting V47.4
        - streetcar (traffic) V46.9
          - nontraffic V46.3
          - while boarding or alighting V46.4
        - three wheeled motor vehicle (traffic) V42.9
          - nontraffic V42.3
          - while boarding or alighting V42.4
        - truck (traffic) V44.9
          - nontraffic V44.3
          - while boarding or alighting V44.4
        - two wheeled motor vehicle (traffic) V42.9
          - nontraffic V42.3
          - while boarding or alighting V42.4
        - van (traffic) V43.94
          - nontraffic V43.34
          - while boarding or alighting V43.44
      - driver
        - collision (with)
          - animal (traffic) V40.5
            - being ridden (traffic) V46.5
              - nontraffic V46.0
            - nontraffic V40.0
          - animal-drawn vehicle (traffic) V46.5
            - nontraffic V46.0
          - bus (traffic) V44.5
            - nontraffic V44.0
          - car (traffic) V43.52
            - nontraffic V43.02
          - motor vehicle NOS (traffic) V49.40
            - nontraffic V49.00
            - specified type NEC (traffic) V49.49
              - nontraffic V49.09
          - pedal cycle (traffic) V41.5
            - nontraffic V41.0
          - pickup truck (traffic) V43.53
            - nontraffic V43.03
          - railway vehicle (traffic) V45.5
            - nontraffic V45.0
          - specified vehicle NEC (traffic) V46.5
            - nontraffic V46.0
          - sport utility vehicle (traffic) V43.51
            - nontraffic V43.01
          - stationary object (traffic) V47.5
            - nontraffic V47.0
          - streetcar (traffic) V46.5
            - nontraffic V46.0
          - three wheeled motor vehicle (traffic) V42.5
            - nontraffic V42.0
          - truck (traffic) V44.5
            - nontraffic V44.0
          - two wheeled motor vehicle (traffic) V42.5
            - nontraffic V42.0
          - van (traffic) V43.54
            - nontraffic V43.04
        - noncollision accident (traffic) V48.5
          - nontraffic V48.0
      - hanger-on
        - collision (with)
          - animal (traffic) V40.7
            - being ridden (traffic) V46.7
              - nontraffic V46.2
            - nontraffic V40.2
          - animal-drawn vehicle (traffic) V46.7
            - nontraffic V46.2
          - bus (traffic) V44.7
            - nontraffic V44.2

A

Accident *(Continued)*
  transport *(Continued)*
    car occupant *(Continued)*
      hanger-on *(Continued)*
        collision *(Continued)*
          car (traffic) V43.72
            nontraffic V43.22
          pedal cycle (traffic) V41.7
            nontraffic V41.2
          pickup truck (traffic) V43.73
            nontraffic V43.23
          railway vehicle (traffic) V45.7
            nontraffic V45.2
          specified vehicle NEC (traffic) V46.7
            nontraffic V46.2
          sport utility vehicle (traffic) V43.71
            nontraffic V43.21
          stationary object (traffic) V47.7
            nontraffic V47.2
          streetcar (traffic) V46.7
            nontraffic V46.2
          three wheeled motor vehicle (traffic) V42.7
            nontraffic V42.2
          truck (traffic) V44.7
            nontraffic V44.2
          two wheeled motor vehicle (traffic) V42.7
            nontraffic V42.2
          van (traffic) V43.74
            nontraffic V43.24
        noncollision accident (traffic) V48.7
          nontraffic V48.2
      noncollision accident (traffic) V48.9
        nontraffic V48.3
        while boarding or alighting V48.4
      nontraffic V49.3
      passenger
        collision (with)
          animal (traffic) V40.6
            being ridden (traffic) V46.6
              nontraffic V46.1
            nontraffic V40.1
          animal-drawn vehicle (traffic) V46.6
            nontraffic V46.1
          bus (traffic) V44.6
            nontraffic V44.1
          car (traffic) V43.62
            nontraffic V43.12
          motor vehicle NOS (traffic) V49.50
            nontraffic V49.10
            specified type NEC (traffic) V49.59
              nontraffic V49.19
          pedal cycle (traffic) V41.6
            nontraffic V41.1
          pickup truck (traffic) V43.63
            nontraffic V43.13
          railway vehicle (traffic) V45.6
            nontraffic V45.1
          specified vehicle NEC (traffic) V46.6
            nontraffic V46.1
          sport utility vehicle (traffic) V43.61
            nontraffic V43.11
          stationary object (traffic) V47.6
            nontraffic V47.1
          streetcar (traffic) V46.6
            nontraffic V46.1
          three wheeled motor vehicle (traffic) V42.6
            nontraffic V42.1
          truck (traffic) V44.6
            nontraffic V44.1
          two wheeled motor vehicle (traffic) V42.6
            nontraffic V42.1
          van (traffic) V43.64
            nontraffic V43.14
        noncollision accident (traffic) V48.6
          nontraffic V48.1
      specified type NEC V49.88
        military vehicle V49.81

Accident *(Continued)*
  transport *(Continued)*
    coal car —*see* Accident, transport, industrial vehicle occupant
    construction vehicle occupant (nontraffic) V85.9
      driver V85.5
      hanger-on V85.7
      passenger V85.6
      traffic V85.3
        driver V85.0
        hanger-on V85.2
        passenger V85.1
      while boarding or alighting V85.4
    dirt bike rider (nontraffic) V86.96
      driver V86.56
      hanger-on V86.76
      passenger V86.66
      traffic V86.36
        driver V86.06
        hanger-on V86.26
        passenger V86.16
      while boarding or alighting V86.46
    due to cataclysm —*see* Forces of nature, by type
    dune buggy occupant (nontraffic) V86.93
      driver V86.53
      hanger-on V86.73
      passenger V86.63
      traffic V86.33
        driver V86.03
        hanger-on V86.23
        passenger V86.13
      while boarding or alighting V86.43
    forklift —*see* Accident, transport, industrial vehicle occupant
    go cart —*see* Accident, transport, all-terrain vehicle occupant
    golf cart —*see* Accident, transport, all-terrain vehicle occupant
    heavy transport vehicle occupant —*see* Accident, transport, truck occupant
    ice yacht V98.2
    industrial vehicle occupant (nontraffic) V83.9
      driver V83.5
      hanger-on V83.7
      passenger V83.6
      traffic V83.3
        driver V83.0
        hanger-on V83.2
        passenger V83.1
      while boarding or alighting V83.4
    interurban electric car —*see* Accident, transport, streetcar
    land yacht V98.1
    logging car —*see* Accident, transport, industrial vehicle occupant
    military vehicle occupant (traffic) V86.34
      driver V86.04
      hanger-on V86.24
      nontraffic V86.94
        driver V86.54
        hanger-on V86.74
        passenger V86.64
      passenger V86.14
      while boarding or alighting V86.44
    mine tram —*see* Accident, transport, industrial vehicle occupant
    motor vehicle NEC occupant (traffic) V89.2
    motorcoach —*see* Accident, transport, bus occupant
    motor/cross bike rider —*see also* Accident, transport, dirt bike rider V86.96
    motorcyclist V29.9
      collision (with)
        animal (traffic) V20.9
          being ridden (traffic) V26.9
            nontraffic V26.2
            while boarding or alighting V26.3
          nontraffic V20.2
          while boarding or alighting V20.3

Accident *(Continued)*
  transport *(Continued)*
    motorcyclist *(Continued)*
      collision *(Continued)*
        animal-drawn vehicle (traffic) V26.9
          nontraffic V26.2
          while boarding or alighting V26.3
        bus (traffic) V24.9
          nontraffic V24.2
          while boarding or alighting V24.3
        car (traffic) V23.9
          nontraffic V23.2
          while boarding or alighting V23.3
        motor vehicle NOS (traffic) V29.60
          nontraffic V29.20
          specified type NEC (traffic) V29.69
            nontraffic V29.29
        pedal cycle (traffic) V21.9
          nontraffic V21.2
          while boarding or alighting V21.3
        pickup truck (traffic) V23.9
          nontraffic V23.2
          while boarding or alighting V23.3
        railway vehicle (traffic) V25.9
          nontraffic V25.2
          while boarding or alighting V25.3
        specified vehicle NEC (traffic) V26.9
          nontraffic V26.2
          while boarding or alighting V26.3
        stationary object (traffic) V27.9
          nontraffic V27.2
          while boarding or alighting V27.3
        streetcar (traffic) V26.9
          nontraffic V26.2
          while boarding or alighting V26.3
        three wheeled motor vehicle (traffic) V22.9
          nontraffic V22.2
          while boarding or alighting V22.3
        truck (traffic) V24.9
          nontraffic V24.2
          while boarding or alighting V24.3
        two wheeled motor vehicle (traffic) V22.9
          nontraffic V22.2
          while boarding or alighting V22.3
        van (traffic) V23.9
          nontraffic V23.2
          while boarding or alighting V23.3
      driver
        collision (with)
          animal (traffic) V20.4
            being ridden (traffic) V26.4
              nontraffic V26.0
            nontraffic V20.0
          animal-drawn vehicle (traffic) V26.4
            nontraffic V26.0
          bus (traffic) V24.4
            nontraffic V24.0
          car (traffic) V23.4
            nontraffic V23.0
          motor vehicle NOS (traffic) V29.40
            nontraffic V29.00
            specified type NEC (traffic) V29.49
              nontraffic V29.09
          pedal cycle (traffic) V21.4
            nontraffic V21.0
          pickup truck (traffic) V23.4
            nontraffic V23.0
          railway vehicle (traffic) V25.4
            nontraffic V25.0
          specified vehicle NEC (traffic) V26.4
            nontraffic V26.0
          stationary object (traffic) V27.4
            nontraffic V27.0
          streetcar (traffic) V26.4
            nontraffic V26.0
          three wheeled motor vehicle (traffic) V22.4
            nontraffic V22.0

A

- Accident *(Continued)*
  - transport *(Continued)*
    - motorcyclist *(Continued)*
      - driver *(Continued)*
        - collision *(Continued)*
          - truck (traffic) V24.4
            - nontraffic V24.Ø
          - two wheeled motor vehicle (traffic) V22.4
            - nontraffic V22.Ø
          - van (traffic) V23.4
            - nontraffic V23.Ø
        - noncollision accident (traffic) V28.4
          - nontraffic V28.Ø
      - noncollision accident (traffic) V28.9
        - nontraffic V28.2
        - while boarding or alighting V28.3
      - nontraffic V29.3
      - passenger
        - collision (with)
          - animal (traffic) V2Ø.5
            - being ridden (traffic) V26.5
              - nontraffic V26.1
            - nontraffic V2Ø.1
          - animal-drawn vehicle (traffic) V26.5
            - nontraffic V26.1
          - bus (traffic) V24.5
            - nontraffic V24.1
          - car (traffic) V23.5
            - nontraffic V23.1
          - motor vehicle NOS (traffic) V29.5Ø
            - nontraffic V29.1Ø
            - specified type NEC (traffic) V29.59
              - nontraffic V29.19
          - pedal cycle (traffic) V21.5
            - nontraffic V21.1
          - pickup truck (traffic) V23.5
            - nontraffic V23.1
          - railway vehicle (traffic) V25.5
            - nontraffic V25.1
          - specified vehicle NEC (traffic) V26.5
            - nontraffic V26.1
          - stationary object (traffic) V27.5
            - nontraffic V27.1
          - streetcar (traffic) V26.5
            - nontraffic V26.1
          - three wheeled motor vehicle (traffic) V22.5
            - nontraffic V22.1
          - truck (traffic) V24.5
            - nontraffic V24.1
          - two wheeled motor vehicle (traffic) V22.5
            - nontraffic V22.1
          - van (traffic) V23.5
            - nontraffic V23.1
        - noncollision accident (traffic) V28.5
          - nontraffic V28.1
      - specified type NEC V29.88
        - military vehicle V29.81
    - occupant (of)
      - aircraft (powered) V95.9
        - fixed wing
          - commercial *—see* Accident, transport, aircraft, occupant, powered, fixed wing, commercial
          - private *—see* Accident, transport, aircraft, occupant, powered, fixed wing, private
        - nonpowered V96.9
        - specified NEC V95.8
      - airport battery-powered vehicle *—see* Accident, transport, industrial vehicle occupant
      - all-terrain vehicle (ATV) *—see* Accident, transport, all-terrain vehicle occupant
      - animal-drawn vehicle *—see* Accident, transport, animal-drawn vehicle occupant

- Accident *(Continued)*
  - transport *(Continued)*
    - occupant *(Continued)*
      - automobile *—see* Accident, transport, car occupant
      - balloon V96.ØØ
      - battery-powered vehicle *—see* Accident, transport, industrial vehicle occupant
      - bicycle *—see* Accident, transport, pedal cyclist
        - motorized *—see* Accident, transport, motorcycle rider
      - boat NEC *—see* Accident, watercraft
      - bulldozer *—see* Accident, transport, construction vehicle occupant
      - bus *—see* Accident, transport, bus occupant
      - cable car (on rails) *—see also* Accident, transport, streetcar occupant
        - not on rails V98.Ø
      - car *—see also* Accident, transport, car occupant
        - cable (on rails) *—see also* Accident, transport, streetcar occupant
          - not on rails V98.Ø
      - coach *—see* Accident, transport, bus occupant
      - coal-car *—see* Accident, transport, industrial vehicle occupant
      - digger *—see* Accident, transport, construction vehicle occupant
      - dump truck *—see* Accident, transport, construction vehicle occupant
      - earth-leveler *—see* Accident, transport, construction vehicle occupant
      - farm machinery (self-propelled) *—see* Accident, transport, agricultural vehicle occupant
      - forklift *—see* Accident, transport, industrial vehicle occupant
      - glider (unpowered) V96.2Ø
        - hang V96.1Ø
        - powered (microlight) (ultralight) *—see* Accident, transport, aircraft, occupant, powered, glider
      - glider (unpowered) NEC V96.2Ø
      - hang-glider V96.1Ø
      - harvester *—see* Accident, transport, agricultural vehicle occupant
      - heavy (transport) vehicle *—see* Accident, transport, truck occupant
      - helicopter *—see* Accident, transport, aircraft, occupant, helicopter
      - ice-yacht V98.2
      - kite (carrying person) V96.8
      - land-yacht V98.1
      - logging car *—see* Accident, transport, industrial vehicle occupant
      - mechanical shovel *—see* Accident, transport, construction vehicle occupant
      - microlight *—see* Accident, transport, aircraft, occupant, powered, glider
      - minibus *—see* Accident, transport, pickup truck occupant
      - minivan *—see* Accident, transport, pickup truck occupant
      - moped *—see* Accident, transport, motorcycle
      - motor scooter *—see* Accident, transport, motorcycle
      - motorcycle (with sidecar) *—see* Accident, transport, motorcycle
      - off-road motor-vehicle *—see also* Accident, transport, all-terrain vehicle occupant V86.99
      - pedal cycle *—see also* Accident, transport, pedal cyclist
      - pick-up (truck) *—see* Accident, transport, pickup truck occupant

- Accident *(Continued)*
  - transport *(Continued)*
    - occupant *(Continued)*
      - railway (train) (vehicle) (subterranean) (elevated) *—see* Accident, transport, railway vehicle occupant
      - rickshaw *—see* Accident, transport, pedal cycle
        - pedal driven *—see* Accident, transport, pedal cyclist
      - road-roller *—see* Accident, transport, construction vehicle occupant
      - ship NOS V94.9
      - ski-lift (chair) (gondola) V98.3
      - snowmobile *—see* Accident, transport, snowmobile occupant
      - spacecraft, spaceship *—see* Accident, transport, aircraft, occupant, spacecraft
      - sport utility vehicle *—see* Accident, transport, pickup truck occupant
      - streetcar (interurban) (operating on public street or highway) *—see* Accident, transport, streetcar occupant
      - SUV *—see* Accident, transport, pickup truck occupant
      - téléférique V98.Ø
      - three-wheeled vehicle (motorized) *—see also* Accident, transport, three-wheeled motor vehicle occupant
        - nonmotorized *—see* Accident, transport, pedal cycle
      - tractor (farm) (and trailer) *—see* Accident, transport, agricultural vehicle occupant
      - train *—see* Accident, transport, railway vehicle occupant
      - tram *—see* Accident, transport, streetcar occupant
        - in mine or quarry *—see* Accident, transport, industrial vehicle occupant
      - tricycle *—see* Accident, transport, pedal cycle
        - motorized *—see* Accident, transport, three-wheeled motor vehicle
      - trolley *—see* Accident, transport, streetcar occupant
        - in mine or quarry *—see* Accident, transport, industrial vehicle occupant
      - tub, in mine or quarry *—see* Accident, transport, industrial vehicle occupant
      - ultralight *—see* Accident, transport, aircraft, occupant, powered, glider
      - van *—see* Accident, transport, van occupant
      - vehicle NEC V89.9
        - heavy transport *—see* Accident, transport, truck occupant
        - motor (traffic) NEC V89.2
          - nontraffic NEC V89.Ø
      - watercraft NOS V94.9
        - causing drowning *—see* Drowning, resulting from accident to boat
    - off-road motor-vehicle *—see also* Accident, transport, all-terrain vehicle occupant V86.99
    - parachutist V97.29
      - after accident to aircraft *—see* Accident, transport, aircraft
      - entangled in object V97.21
      - injured on landing V97.22
    - pedal cyclist V19.9
      - collision (with)
        - animal (traffic) V1Ø.9
          - being ridden (traffic) V16.9
            - nontraffic V16.2
            - while boarding or alighting V16.3

A

- Accident *(Continued)*
  - transport *(Continued)*
    - pedal cyclist *(Continued)*
      - collision *(Continued)*
        - animal (traffic) V10.9 *(Continued)*
          - nontraffic V10.2
          - while boarding or alighting V10.3
        - animal-drawn vehicle (traffic) V16.9
          - nontraffic V16.2
          - while boarding or alighting V16.3
        - bus (traffic) V14.9
          - nontraffic V14.2
          - while boarding or alighting V14.3
        - car (traffic) V13.9
          - nontraffic V13.2
          - while boarding or alighting V13.3
        - motor vehicle NOS (traffic) V19.60
          - nontraffic V19.20
          - specified type NEC (traffic) V19.69
            - nontraffic V19.29
        - pedal cycle (traffic) V11.9
          - nontraffic V11.2
          - while boarding or alighting V11.3
        - pickup truck (traffic) V13.9
          - nontraffic V13.2
          - while boarding or alighting V13.3
        - railway vehicle (traffic) V15.9
          - nontraffic V15.2
          - while boarding or alighting V15.3
        - specified vehicle NEC (traffic) V16.9
          - nontraffic V16.2
          - while boarding or alighting V16.3
        - stationary object (traffic) V17.9
          - nontraffic V17.2
          - while boarding or alighting V17.3
        - streetcar (traffic) V16.9
          - nontraffic V16.2
          - while boarding or alighting V16.3
        - three wheeled motor vehicle (traffic) V12.9
          - nontraffic V12.2
          - while boarding or alighting V12.3
        - truck (traffic) V14.9
          - nontraffic V14.2
          - while boarding or alighting V14.3
        - two wheeled motor vehicle (traffic) V12.9
          - nontraffic V12.2
          - while boarding or alighting V12.3
        - van (traffic) V13.9
          - nontraffic V13.2
          - while boarding or alighting V13.3
      - driver
        - collision (with)
          - animal (traffic) V10.4
            - being ridden (traffic) V16.4
              - nontraffic V16.0
            - nontraffic V10.0
          - animal-drawn vehicle (traffic) V16.4
            - nontraffic V16.0
          - bus (traffic) V14.4
            - nontraffic V14.0
          - car (traffic) V13.4
            - nontraffic V13.0
          - motor vehicle NOS (traffic) V19.40
            - nontraffic V19.00
            - specified type NEC (traffic) V19.49
              - nontraffic V19.09
          - pedal cycle (traffic) V11.4
            - nontraffic V11.0
          - pickup truck (traffic) V13.4
            - nontraffic V13.0
          - railway vehicle (traffic) V15.4
            - nontraffic V15.0
          - specified vehicle NEC (traffic) V16.4
            - nontraffic V16.0
          - stationary object (traffic) V17.4
            - nontraffic V17.0
          - streetcar (traffic) V16.4
            - nontraffic V16.0
          - three wheeled motor vehicle (traffic) V12.4
            - nontraffic V12.0

- Accident *(Continued)*
  - transport *(Continued)*
    - pedal cyclist *(Continued)*
      - driver *(Continued)*
        - collision *(Continued)*
          - truck (traffic) V14.4
            - nontraffic V14.0
          - two wheeled motor vehicle (traffic) V12.4
            - nontraffic V12.0
          - van (traffic) V13.4
            - nontraffic V13.0
        - noncollision accident (traffic) V18.4
          - nontraffic V18.0
      - noncollision accident (traffic) V18.9
        - nontraffic V18.2
        - while boarding or alighting V18.3
      - nontraffic V19.3
      - passenger
        - collision (with)
          - animal (traffic) V10.5
            - being ridden (traffic) V16.5
              - nontraffic V16.1
            - nontraffic V10.1
          - animal-drawn vehicle (traffic) V16.5
            - nontraffic V16.1
          - bus (traffic) V14.5
            - nontraffic V14.1
          - car (traffic) V13.5
            - nontraffic V13.1
          - motor vehicle NOS (traffic) V19.50
            - nontraffic V19.10
            - specified type NEC (traffic) V19.59
              - nontraffic V19.19
          - pedal cycle (traffic) V11.5
            - nontraffic V11.1
          - pickup truck (traffic) V13.5
            - nontraffic V13.1
          - railway vehicle (traffic) V15.5
            - nontraffic V15.1
          - specified vehicle NEC (traffic) V16.5
            - nontraffic V16.1
          - stationary object (traffic) V17.5
            - nontraffic V17.1
          - streetcar (traffic) V16.5
            - nontraffic V16.1
          - three wheeled motor vehicle (traffic) V12.5
            - nontraffic V12.1
          - truck (traffic) V14.5
            - nontraffic V14.1
          - two wheeled motor vehicle (traffic) V12.5
            - nontraffic V12.1
          - van (traffic) V13.5
            - nontraffic V13.1
        - noncollision accident (traffic) V18.5
          - nontraffic V18.1
      - specified type NEC V19.88
        - military vehicle V19.81
    - pedestrian
      - conveyance (occupant) V09.9
        - baby stroller V00.828
          - collision (with) V09.9
            - animal being ridden or animal drawn vehicle V06.99
              - nontraffic V06.09
              - traffic V06.19
            - bus or heavy transport V04.99
              - nontraffic V04.09
              - traffic V04.19
            - car V03.99
              - nontraffic V03.09
              - traffic V03.19
            - pedal cycle V01.99
              - nontraffic V01.09
              - traffic V01.19
            - pick-up truck or van V03.99
              - nontraffic V03.09
              - traffic V03.19

- Accident *(Continued)*
  - transport *(Continued)*
    - pedestrian *(Continued)*
      - conveyance *(Continued)*
        - babystroller *(Continued)*
          - collision *(Continued)*
            - railway (train) (vehicle) V05.99
              - nontraffic V05.09
              - traffic V05.19
            - stationary object V00.822
            - streetcar V06.99
              - nontraffic V06.09
              - traffic V06.19
            - two- or three-wheeled motor vehicle V02.99
              - nontraffic V02.09
              - traffic V02.19
            - vehicle V09.9
              - animal-drawn V06.99
                - nontraffic V06.09
                - traffic V06.19
              - motor
                - nontraffic V09.00
                - traffic V09.20
          - fall V00.821
          - nontraffic V09.1
            - involving motor vehicle NEC V09.00
          - traffic V09.3
            - involving motor vehicle NEC V09.20
        - flat-bottomed NEC V00.388
          - collision (with) V09.9
            - animal being ridden or animal drawn vehicle V06.99
              - nontraffic V06.09
              - traffic V06.19
            - bus or heavy transport V04.99
              - nontraffic V04.09
              - traffic V04.19
            - car V03.99
              - nontraffic V03.09
              - traffic V03.19
            - pedal cycle V01.99
              - nontraffic V01.09
              - traffic V01.19
            - pick-up truck or van V03.99
              - nontraffic V03.09
              - traffic V03.19
            - railway (train) (vehicle) V05.99
              - nontraffic V05.09
              - traffic V05.19
            - stationary object V00.382
            - streetcar V06.99
              - nontraffic V06.09
              - traffic V06.19
            - two-or three-wheeled motor vehicle V02.99
              - nontraffic V02.09
              - traffic V02.19
            - vehicle V09.9
              - animal-drawn V06.99
                - nontraffic V06.09
                - traffic V06.19
              - motor
                - nontraffic V09.00
                - traffic V09.20
          - fall V00.381
          - nontraffic V09.1
            - involving motor vehicle NEC V09.00
          - snow
            - board —*see* Accident, transport, pedestrian, conveyance, snow board
            - ski —*see* Accident, transport, pedestrian, conveyance, skis (snow)
          - traffic V09.3
            - involving motor vehicle NEC V09.20

A

Accident *(Continued)*
  transport *(Continued)*
    pedestrian *(Continued)*
      conveyance *(Continued)*
        gliding type NEC V00.288
          collision (with) V09.9
            animal being ridden or animal
              drawn vehicle V06.99
              nontraffic V06.09
              traffic V06.19
            bus or heavy transport
              V04.99
              nontraffic V04.09
              traffic V04.19
            car V03.99
              nontraffic V03.09
              traffic V03.19
            pedal cycle V01.99
              nontraffic V01.09
              traffic V01.19
            pick-up truck or van V03.99
              nontraffic V03.09
              traffic V03.19
            railway (train) (vehicle) V05.99
              nontraffic V05.09
              traffic V05.19
            stationary object V00.282
            streetcar V06.99
              nontraffic V06.09
              traffic V06.19
            two- or three-wheeled motor
              vehicle V02.99
              nontraffic V02.09
              traffic V02.19
            vehicle V09.9
              animal-drawn V06.99
                nontraffic V06.09
                traffic V06.19
              motor
                nontraffic V09.00
                traffic V09.20
          fall V00.281
          heelies —*see* Accident, transport,
            pedestrian, conveyance,
            heelies
          ice skate —*see* Accident, transport,
            pedestrian, conveyance, ice
            skate
          nontraffic V09.1
            involving motor vehicle NEC
              V09.00
          sled —*see* Accident, transport,
            pedestrian, conveyance, sled
          traffic V09.3
            involving motor vehicle NEC
              V09.20
          wheelies —*see* Accident,
            transport, pedestrian,
            conveyance, heelies
        heelies V00.158
          colliding with stationary object
            V00.152
          fall V00.151
        ice skates V00.218
          collision (with) V09.9
            animal being ridden or animal
              drawn vehicle V06.99
              nontraffic V06.09
              traffic V06.19
            bus or heavy transport V04.99
              nontraffic V04.09
              traffic V04.19
            car V03.99
              nontraffic V03.09
              traffic V03.19
            pedal cycle V01.99
              nontraffic V01.09
              traffic V01.19
            pick-up truck or van V03.99
              nontraffic V03.09
              traffic V03.19

Accident *(Continued)*
  transport *(Continued)*
    pedestrian *(Continued)*
      conveyance *(Continued)*
        ice skates *(Continued)*
          collision *(Continued)*
            railway (train) (vehicle)
              V05.99
              nontraffic V05.09
              traffic V05.19
            stationary object V00.212
            streetcar V06.99
              nontraffic V06.09
              traffic V06.19
            two- or three-wheeled motor
              vehicle V02.99
              nontraffic V02.09
              traffic V02.19
            vehicle V09.9
              animal-drawn V06.99
                nontraffic V06.09
                traffic V06.19
              motor
                nontraffic V09.00
                traffic V09.20
          fall V00.211
          nontraffic V09.1
            involving motor vehicle NEC
              V09.00
          traffic V09.3
            involving motor vehicle NEC
              V09.20
        motorized mobility scooter
          V00.838
          collision with stationary object
            V00.832
          fall from V00.831
        nontraffic V09.1
          involving motor vehicle
            V09.00
           military V09.01
           specified type NEC V09.09
        roller skates (non in-line) V00.128
          collision (with) V09.9
            animal being ridden or animal
              drawn vehicle V06.91
              nontraffic V06.01
              traffic V06.11
            bus or heavy transport
              V04.91
              nontraffic V04.01
              traffic V04.11
            car V03.91
              nontraffic V03.01
              traffic V03.11
            pedal cycle V01.91
              nontraffic V01.01
              traffic V01.11
            pick-up truck or van V03.91
              nontraffic V03.01
              traffic V03.11
            railway (train) (vehicle)
              V05.91
              nontraffic V05.01
              traffic V05.11
            stationary object V00.122
            streetcar V06.91
              nontraffic V06.01
              traffic V06.11
            two- or three-wheeled motor
              vehicle V02.91
              nontraffic V02.01
              traffic V02.11
            vehicle V09.9
              animal-drawn V06.91
                nontraffic V06.01
                traffic V06.11
              motor
                nontraffic V09.00
                traffic V09.20
          fall V00.121

Accident *(Continued)*
  transport *(Continued)*
    pedestrian *(Continued)*
      conveyance *(Continued)*
        roller skates *(Continued)*
          in-line V00.118
            collision —*see also* Accident,
              transport, pedestrian,
              conveyance occupant, roller
              skates, collision
              with stationary object
                V00.112
            fall V00.111
            nontraffic V09.1
             involving motor vehicle NEC
              V09.00
            traffic V09.3
             involving motor vehicle NEC
              V09.20
        rolling shoes V00.158
          colliding with stationary object
            V00.152
          fall V00.151
        rolling type NEC V00.188
          collision (with) V09.9
            animal being ridden or animal
              drawn vehicle V06.99
              nontraffic V06.09
              traffic V06.19
            bus or heavy transport V04.99
              nontraffic V04.09
              traffic V04.19
            car V03.99
              nontraffic V03.09
              traffic V03.19
            pedal cycle V01.99
              nontraffic V01.09
              traffic V01.19
            pick-up truck or van V03.99
              nontraffic V03.09
              traffic V03.19
            railway (train) (vehicle)
              V05.99
              nontraffic V05.09
              traffic V05.19
            stationary object V00.182
            streetcar V06.99
              nontraffic V06.09
              traffic V06.19
            two- or three-wheeled motor
              vehicle V02.99
              nontraffic V02.09
              traffic V02.19
            vehicle V09.9
              animal-drawn V06.99
                nontraffic V06.09
                traffic V06.19
              motor
                nontraffic V09.00
                traffic V09.20
          fall V00.181
        in-line roller skate —*see* Accident,
          transport, pedestrian,
          conveyance, roller skate,
          in-line
        nontraffic V09.1
          involving motor vehicle NEC
            V09.00
        roller skate —*see* Accident,
          transport, pedestrian,
          conveyance, roller skate
        scooter (non-motorized) —
          see Accident, transport,
          pedestrian, conveyance,
          scooter
        skateboard —*see* Accident,
          transport, pedestrian,
          conveyance, skateboard
        traffic V09.3
          involving motor vehicle NEC
            V09.20

▷ New   ⇨ Revised   ~~deleted~~ Deleted   ● Use Additional Character(s)

- **Accident** *(Continued)*
  - transport *(Continued)*
    - pedestrian *(Continued)*
      - conveyance *(Continued)*
        - scooter (non-motorized) V00.148
          - collision (with) V09.9
            - animal being ridden or animal drawn vehicle V06.99
              - nontraffic V06.09
              - traffic V06.19
            - bus or heavy transport V04.99
              - nontraffic V04.09
              - traffic V04.19
            - car V03.99
              - nontraffic V03.09
              - traffic V03.19
            - pedal cycle V01.99
              - nontraffic V01.09
              - traffic V01.19
            - pick-up truck or van V03.99
              - nontraffic V03.09
              - traffic V03.19
            - railway (train) (vehicle) V05.99
              - nontraffic V05.09
              - traffic V05.19
            - stationary object V00.142
            - streetcar V06.99
              - nontraffic V06.09
              - traffic V06.19
            - two- or three-wheeled motor vehicle V02.99
              - nontraffic V02.09
              - traffic V02.19
            - vehicle V09.9
              - animal-drawn V06.99
                - nontraffic V06.09
                - traffic V06.19
              - motor
                - nontraffic V09.00
                - traffic V09.20
          - fall V00.141
          - nontraffic V09.1
            - involving motor vehicle NEC V09.00
          - traffic V09.3
            - involving motor vehicle NEC V09.20
        - skate board V00.138
          - collision (with) V09.9
            - animal being ridden or animal drawn vehicle V06.92
              - nontraffic V06.02
              - traffic V06.12
            - bus or heavy transport V04.92
              - nontraffic V04.02
              - traffic V04.12
            - car V03.92
              - nontraffic V03.02
              - traffic V03.12
            - pedal cycle V01.92
              - nontraffic V01.02
              - traffic V01.12
            - pick-up truck or van V03.92
              - nontraffic V03.02
              - traffic V03.12
            - railway (train) (vehicle) V05.92
              - nontraffic V05.02
              - traffic V05.12
            - stationary object V00.132
            - streetcar V06.92
              - nontraffic V06.02
              - traffic V06.12
            - two- or three-wheeled motor vehicle V02.92
              - nontraffic V02.02
              - traffic V02.12

- **Accident** *(Continued)*
  - transport *(Continued)*
    - pedestrian *(Continued)*
      - conveyance *(Continued)*
        - skate board *(Continued)*
          - collision *(Continued)*
            - vehicle V09.9
              - animal-drawn V06.92
                - nontraffic V06.02
                - traffic V06.12
              - motor
                - nontraffic V09.00
                - traffic V09.20
          - fall V00.131
          - nontraffic V09.1
            - involving motor vehicle NEC V09.00
          - traffic V09.3
            - involving motor vehicle NEC V09.20
        - skis (snow) V00.328
          - collision (with) V09.9
            - animal being ridden or animal drawn vehicle V06.99
              - nontraffic V06.09
              - traffic V06.19
            - bus or heavy transport V04.99
              - nontraffic V04.09
              - traffic V04.19
            - car V03.99
              - nontraffic V03.09
              - traffic V03.19
            - pedal cycle V01.99
              - nontraffic V01.09
              - traffic V01.19
            - pick-up truck or van V03.99
              - nontraffic V03.09
              - traffic V03.19
            - railway (train) (vehicle) V05.99
              - nontraffic V05.09
              - traffic V05.19
            - stationary object V00.322
            - streetcar V06.99
              - nontraffic V06.09
              - traffic V06.19
            - two- or three-wheeled motor vehicle V02.99
              - nontraffic V02.09
              - traffic V02.19
            - vehicle V09.9
              - animal-drawn V06.99
                - nontraffic V06.09
                - traffic V06.19
              - motor
                - nontraffic V09.00
                - traffic V09.20
          - fall V00.321
          - nontraffic V09.1
            - involving motor vehicle NEC V09.00
          - traffic V09.3
            - involving motor vehicle NEC V09.20
        - sled V00.228
          - collision (with) V09.9
            - animal being ridden or animal drawn vehicle V06.99
              - nontraffic V06.09
              - traffic V06.19
            - bus or heavy transport V04.99
              - nontraffic V04.09
              - traffic V04.19
            - car V03.99
              - nontraffic V03.09
              - traffic V03.19
            - pedal cycle V01.99
              - nontraffic V01.09
              - traffic V01.19
            - pick-up truck or van V03.99
              - nontraffic V03.09
              - traffic V03.19

- **Accident** *(Continued)*
  - transport *(Continued)*
    - pedestrian *(Continued)*
      - conveyance *(Continued)*
        - sled *(Continued)*
          - collision *(Continued)*
            - railway (train) (vehicle) V05.99
              - nontraffic V05.09
              - traffic V05.19
            - stationary object V00.222
            - streetcar V06.99
              - nontraffic V06.09
              - traffic V06.19
            - two- or three-wheeled motor vehicle V02.99
              - nontraffic V02.09
              - traffic V02.19
            - vehicle V09.9
              - animal-drawn V06.99
                - nontraffic V06.09
                - traffic V06.19
              - motor
                - nontraffic V09.00
                - traffic V09.20
          - fall V00.221
          - nontraffic V09.1
            - involving motor vehicle NEC V09.00
          - traffic V09.3
            - involving motor vehicle NEC V09.20
        - snow board V00.318
          - collision (with) V09.9
            - animal being ridden or animal drawn vehicle V06.99
              - nontraffic V06.09
              - traffic V06.19
            - bus or heavy transport V04.99
              - nontraffic V04.09
              - traffic V04.19
            - car V03.99
              - nontraffic V03.09
              - traffic V03.19
            - pedal cycle V01.99
              - nontraffic V01.09
              - traffic V01.19
            - pick-up truck or van V03.99
              - nontraffic V03.09
              - traffic V03.19
            - railway (train) (vehicle) V05.99
              - nontraffic V05.09
              - traffic V05.19
            - stationary object V00.312
            - streetcar V06.99
              - nontraffic V06.09
              - traffic V06.19
            - two- or three-wheeled motor vehicle V02.99
              - nontraffic V02.09
              - traffic V02.19
            - vehicle V09.9
              - animal-drawn V06.99
                - nontraffic V06.09
                - traffic V06.19
              - motor
                - nontraffic V09.00
                - traffic V09.20
          - fall V00.311
          - nontraffic V09.1
            - involving motor vehicle NEC V09.00
          - traffic V09.3
            - involving motor vehicle NEC V09.20
        - specified type NEC V00.898
          - collision (with) V09.9
            - animal being ridden or animal drawn vehicle V06.99
              - nontraffic V06.09
              - traffic V06.19

A

- Accident *(Continued)*
  - transport *(Continued)*
    - pedestrian *(Continued)*
      - conveyance *(Continued)*
        - specified type NEC *(Continued)*
          - collision *(Continued)*
            - bus or heavy transport V04.99
              - nontraffic V04.09
              - traffic V04.19
            - car V03.99
              - nontraffic V03.09
              - traffic V03.19
            - pedal cycle V01.99
              - nontraffic V01.09
              - traffic V01.19
            - pick-up truck or van V03.99
              - nontraffic V03.09
              - traffic V03.19
            - railway (train) (vehicle) V05.99
              - nontraffic V05.09
              - traffic V05.19
            - stationary object V00.892
            - streetcar V06.99
              - nontraffic V06.09
              - traffic V06.19
            - two- or three-wheeled motor vehicle V02.99
              - nontraffic V02.09
              - traffic V02.19
            - vehicle V09.9
              - animal-drawn V06.99
                - nontraffic V06.09
                - traffic V06.19
              - motor
                - nontraffic V09.00
                - traffic V09.20
          - fall V00.891
          - nontraffic V09.1
            - involving motor vehicle NEC V09.00
          - traffic V09.3
            - involving motor vehicle NEC V09.20
        - traffic V09.3
          - involving motor vehicle V09.20
            - military V09.21
            - specified type NEC V09.29
        - wheelchair (powered) V00.818
          - collision (with) V09.9
            - animal being ridden or animal drawn vehicle V06.99
              - nontraffic V06.09
              - traffic V06.19
            - bus or heavy transport V04.99
              - nontraffic V04.09
              - traffic V04.19
            - car V03.99
              - nontraffic V03.09
              - traffic V03.19
            - pedal cycle V01.99
              - nontraffic V01.09
              - traffic V01.19
            - pick-up truck or van V03.99
              - nontraffic V03.09
              - traffic V03.19
            - railway (train) (vehicle) V05.99
              - nontraffic V05.09
              - traffic V05.19
            - stationary object V00.812
            - streetcar V06.99
              - nontraffic V06.09
              - traffic V06.19
            - two- or three-wheeled motor vehicle V02.99
              - nontraffic V02.09
              - traffic V02.19

- Accident *(Continued)*
  - transport *(Continued)*
    - pedestrian *(Continued)*
      - conveyance *(Continued)*
        - wheelchair *(Continued)*
          - collision *(Continued)*
            - vehicle V09.9
              - animal-drawn V06.99
                - nontraffic V06.09
                - traffic V06.19
              - motor
                - nontraffic V09.00
                - traffic V09.20
          - fall V00.811
          - nontraffic V09.1
            - involving motor vehicle NEC V09.00
          - traffic V09.3
            - involving motor vehicle NEC V09.20
        - wheeled shoe V00.158
          - colliding with stationary object V00.152
          - fall V00.151
      - on foot —*see also* Accident, pedestrian
        - collision (with)
          - animal being ridden or animal drawn vehicle V06.90
            - nontraffic V06.00
            - traffic V06.10
          - bus or heavy transport V04.90
            - nontraffic V04.00
            - traffic V04.10
          - car V03.90
            - nontraffic V03.00
            - traffic V03.10
          - pedal cycle V01.90
            - nontraffic V01.00
            - traffic V01.10
          - pick-up truck or van V03.90
            - nontraffic V03.00
            - traffic V03.10
          - railway (train) (vehicle) V05.90
            - nontraffic V05.00
            - traffic V05.10
          - streetcar V06.90
            - nontraffic V06.00
            - traffic V06.10
          - two- or three-wheeled motor vehicle V02.90
            - nontraffic V02.00
            - traffic V02.10
          - vehicle V09.9
            - animal-drawn V06.90
              - nontraffic V06.00
              - traffic V06.10
            - motor
              - nontraffic V09.00
              - traffic V09.20
        - nontraffic V09.1
          - involving motor vehicle V09.00
            - military V09.01
            - specified type NEC V09.09
        - traffic V09.3
          - involving motor vehicle V09.20
            - military V09.21
            - specified type NEC V09.29
    - person NEC (unknown way or transportation) V99
      - collision (between)
        - bus (with)
          - heavy transport vehicle (traffic) V87.5
            - nontraffic V88.5
        - car (with)
          - nontraffic V88.5
          - bus (traffic) V87.3
            - nontraffic V88.3
          - heavy transport vehicle (traffic) V87.4
            - nontraffic V88.4

- Accident *(Continued)*
  - transport *(Continued)*
    - person NEC *(Continued)*
      - collision *(Continued)*
        - car *(Continued)*
          - pick-up truck or van (traffic) V87.2
            - nontraffic V88.2
          - train or railway vehicle (traffic) V87.6
            - nontraffic V88.6
          - two- or three-wheeled motor vehicle (traffic) V87.0
            - nontraffic V88.0
        - motor vehicle (traffic) NEC V87.7
          - nontraffic V88.7
        - two- or three-wheeled vehicle (with) (traffic)
          - motor vehicle NEC V87.1
            - nontraffic V88.1
      - nonmotor vehicle (collision) (noncollision) (traffic) V87.9
        - nontraffic V88.9
    - pickup truck occupant V59.9
      - collision (with)
        - animal (traffic) V50.9
          - being ridden (traffic) V56.9
            - nontraffic V56.3
            - while boarding or alighting V56.4
          - nontraffic V50.3
          - while boarding or alighting V50.4
        - animal-drawn vehicle (traffic) V56.9
          - nontraffic V56.3
          - while boarding or alighting V56.4
        - bus (traffic) V54.9
          - nontraffic V54.3
          - while boarding or alighting V54.4
        - car (traffic) V53.9
          - nontraffic V53.3
          - while boarding or alighting V53.4
        - motor vehicle NOS (traffic) V59.60
          - nontraffic V59.20
          - specified type NEC (traffic) V59.69
            - nontraffic V59.29
        - pedal cycle (traffic) V51.9
          - nontraffic V51.3
          - while boarding or alighting V51.4
        - pickup truck (traffic) V53.9
          - nontraffic V53.3
          - while boarding or alighting V53.4
        - railway vehicle (traffic) V55.9
          - nontraffic V55.3
          - while boarding or alighting V55.4
        - specified vehicle NEC (traffic) V56.9
          - nontraffic V56.3
          - while boarding or alighting V56.4
        - stationary object (traffic) V57.9
          - nontraffic V57.3
          - while boarding or alighting V57.4
        - streetcar (traffic) V56.9
          - nontraffic V56.3
          - while boarding or alighting V56.4
        - three wheeled motor vehicle (traffic) V52.9
          - nontraffic V52.3
          - while boarding or alighting V52.4
        - truck (traffic) V54.9
          - nontraffic V54.3
          - while boarding or alighting V54.4
        - two wheeled motor vehicle (traffic) V52.9
          - nontraffic V52.3
          - while boarding or alighting V52.4
        - van (traffic) V53.9
          - nontraffic V53.3
          - while boarding or alighting V53.4
      - driver
        - collision (with)
          - animal (traffic) V50.5
            - being ridden (traffic) V56.5
              - nontraffic V56.0
            - nontraffic V50.0

A

- Accident *(Continued)*
  - transport *(Continued)*
    - pickup truck occupant *(Continued)*
      - driver *(Continued)*
        - collision *(Continued)*
          - animal-drawn vehicle (traffic) V56.5
            - nontraffic V56.0
          - bus (traffic) V54.5
            - nontraffic V54.0
          - car (traffic) V53.5
            - nontraffic V53.0
          - motor vehicle NOS (traffic) V59.40
            - nontraffic V59.00
            - specified type NEC (traffic) V59.49
              - nontraffic V59.09
          - pedal cycle (traffic) V51.5
            - nontraffic V51.0
          - pickup truck (traffic) V53.5
            - nontraffic V53.0
          - railway vehicle (traffic) V55.5
            - nontraffic V55.0
          - specified vehicle NEC (traffic) V56.5
            - nontraffic V56.0
          - stationary object (traffic) V57.5
            - nontraffic V57.0
          - streetcar (traffic) V56.5
            - nontraffic V56.0
          - three wheeled motor vehicle (traffic) V52.5
            - nontraffic V52.0
          - truck (traffic) V54.5
            - nontraffic V54.0
          - two wheeled motor vehicle (traffic) V52.5
            - nontraffic V52.0
          - van (traffic) V53.5
            - nontraffic V53.0
        - noncollision accident (traffic) V58.5
          - nontraffic V58.0
      - hanger-on
        - collision (with)
          - animal (traffic) V50.7
            - being ridden (traffic) V56.7
              - nontraffic V56.2
            - nontraffic V50.2
          - animal-drawn vehicle (traffic) V56.7
            - nontraffic V56.2
          - bus (traffic) V54.7
            - nontraffic V54.2
          - car (traffic) V53.7
            - nontraffic V53.2
          - pedal cycle (traffic) V51.7
            - nontraffic V51.2
          - pickup truck (traffic) V53.7
            - nontraffic V53.2
          - railway vehicle (traffic) V55.7
            - nontraffic V55.2
          - specified vehicle NEC (traffic) V56.7
            - nontraffic V56.2
          - stationary object (traffic) V57.7
            - nontraffic V57.2
          - streetcar (traffic) V56.7
            - nontraffic V56.2
          - three wheeled motor vehicle (traffic) V52.7
            - nontraffic V52.2
          - truck (traffic) V54.7
            - nontraffic V54.2
          - two wheeled motor vehicle (traffic) V52.7
            - nontraffic V52.2
          - van (traffic) V53.7
            - nontraffic V53.2
        - noncollision accident (traffic) V58.7
          - nontraffic V58.2
      - noncollision accident (traffic) V58.9
        - nontraffic V58.3
        - while boarding or alighting V58.4
      - nontraffic V59.3

- Accident *(Continued)*
  - transport *(Continued)*
    - pickup truck occupant *(Continued)*
      - passenger
        - collision (with)
          - animal (traffic) V50.6
            - being ridden (traffic) V56.6
              - nontraffic V56.1
            - nontraffic V50.1
          - animal-drawn vehicle (traffic) V56.6
            - nontraffic V56.1
          - bus (traffic) V54.6
            - nontraffic V54.1
          - car (traffic) V53.6
            - nontraffic V53.1
          - motor vehicle NOS (traffic) V59.50
            - nontraffic V59.10
            - specified type NEC (traffic) V59.59
              - nontraffic V59.19
          - pedal cycle (traffic) V51.6
            - nontraffic V51.1
          - pickup truck (traffic) V53.6
            - nontraffic V53.1
          - railway vehicle (traffic) V55.6
            - nontraffic V55.1
          - specified vehicle NEC (traffic) V56.6
            - nontraffic V56.1
          - stationary object (traffic) V57.6
            - nontraffic V57.1
          - streetcar (traffic) V56.6
            - nontraffic V56.1
          - three wheeled motor vehicle (traffic) V52.6
            - nontraffic V52.1
          - truck (traffic) V54.6
            - nontraffic V54.1
          - two wheeled motor vehicle (traffic) V52.6
            - nontraffic V52.1
          - van (traffic) V53.6
            - nontraffic V53.1
        - noncollision accident (traffic) V58.6
          - nontraffic V58.1
      - specified type NEC V59.88
        - military vehicle V59.81
    - quarry truck *—see* Accident, transport, industrial vehicle occupant
    - race car *—see* Accident, transport, motor vehicle NEC occupant
    - railway vehicle occupant V81.9
      - collision (with) V81.3
        - motor vehicle (non-military) (traffic) V81.1
          - military V81.83
          - nontraffic V81.0
        - rolling stock V81.2
        - specified object NEC V81.3
      - during derailment V81.7
        - with antecedent collision *—see* Accident, transport, railway vehicle occupant, collision
      - explosion V81.81
      - fall (in railway vehicle) V81.5
        - during derailment V81.7
          - with antecedent collision *—see* Accident, transport, railway vehicle occupant, collision
        - from railway vehicle V81.6
          - during derailment V81.7
            - with antecedent collision *—see* Accident, transport, railway vehicle occupant, collision
        - while boarding or alighting V81.4
      - fire V81.81
      - object falling onto train V81.82
      - specified type NEC V81.89
      - while boarding or alighting V81.4
    - ski lift V98.3

- Accident *(Continued)*
  - transport *(Continued)*
    - snowmobile occupant (nontraffic) V86.92
      - driver V86.52
      - hanger-on V86.72
      - passenger V86.62
      - traffic V86.32
        - driver V86.02
        - hanger-on V86.22
        - passenger V86.12
      - while boarding or alighting V86.42
    - specified NEC V98.8
    - sport utility vehicle occupant *—see also* Accident, transport, pickup truck occupant
    - streetcar occupant V82.9
      - collision (with) V82.3
        - motor vehicle (traffic) V82.1
          - nontraffic V82.0
        - rolling stock V82.2
      - during derailment V82.7
        - with antecedent collision *—see* Accident, transport, streetcar occupant, collision
      - fall (in streetcar) V82.5
        - during derailment V82.7
          - with antecedent collision *—see* Accident, transport, streetcar occupant, collision
        - from streetcar V82.6
          - during derailment V82.7
            - with antecedent collision *—see* Accident, transport, streetcar occupant, collision
          - while boarding or alighting V82.4
        - while boarding or alighting V82.4
      - specified type NEC V82.8
      - while boarding or alighting V82.4
    - three-wheeled motor vehicle occupant V39.9
      - collision (with)
        - animal (traffic) V30.9
          - being ridden (traffic) V36.9
            - nontraffic V36.3
            - while boarding or alighting V36.4
          - nontraffic V30.3
          - while boarding or alighting V30.4
        - animal-drawn vehicle (traffic) V36.9
          - nontraffic V36.3
          - while boarding or alighting V36.4
        - bus (traffic) V34.9
          - nontraffic V34.3
          - while boarding or alighting V34.4
        - car (traffic) V33.9
          - nontraffic V33.3
          - while boarding or alighting V33.4
        - motor vehicle NOS (traffic) V39.60
          - nontraffic V39.20
          - specified type NEC (traffic) V39.69
            - nontraffic V39.29
        - pedal cycle (traffic) V31.9
          - nontraffic V31.3
          - while boarding or alighting V31.4
        - pickup truck (traffic) V33.9
          - nontraffic V33.3
          - while boarding or alighting V33.4
        - railway vehicle (traffic) V35.9
          - nontraffic V35.3
          - while boarding or alighting V35.4

A

- **Accident** *(Continued)*
  - transport *(Continued)*
    - three-wheeled motor vehicle occupant *(Continued)*
      - collision *(Continued)*
        - specified vehicle NEC (traffic) V36.9
          - nontraffic V36.3
          - while boarding or alighting V36.4
        - stationary object (traffic) V37.9
          - nontraffic V37.3
          - while boarding or alighting V37.4
        - streetcar (traffic) V36.9
          - nontraffic V36.3
          - while boarding or alighting V36.4
        - three wheeled motor vehicle (traffic) V32.9
          - nontraffic V32.3
          - while boarding or alighting V32.4
        - truck (traffic) V34.9
          - nontraffic V34.3
          - while boarding or alighting V34.4
        - two wheeled motor vehicle (traffic) V32.9
          - nontraffic V32.3
          - while boarding or alighting V32.4
        - van (traffic) V33.9
          - nontraffic V33.3
          - while boarding or alighting V33.4
      - driver
        - collision (with)
          - animal (traffic) V30.5
            - being ridden (traffic) V36.5
              - nontraffic V36.0
            - nontraffic V30.0
          - animal-drawn vehicle (traffic) V36.5
            - nontraffic V36.0
          - bus (traffic) V34.5
            - nontraffic V34.0
          - car (traffic) V33.5
            - nontraffic V33.0
          - motor vehicle NOS (traffic) V39.40
            - nontraffic V39.00
            - specified type NEC (traffic) V39.49
              - nontraffic V39.09
          - pedal cycle (traffic) V31.5
            - nontraffic V31.0
          - pickup truck (traffic) V33.5
            - nontraffic V33.0
          - railway vehicle (traffic) V35.5
            - nontraffic V35.0
          - specified vehicle NEC (traffic) V36.5
            - nontraffic V36.0
          - stationary object (traffic) V37.5
            - nontraffic V37.0
          - streetcar (traffic) V36.5
            - nontraffic V36.0
          - three wheeled motor vehicle (traffic) V32.5
            - nontraffic V32.0
          - truck (traffic) V34.5
            - nontraffic V34.0
          - two wheeled motor vehicle (traffic) V32.5
            - nontraffic V32.0
          - van (traffic) V33.5
            - nontraffic V33.0
        - noncollision accident (traffic) V38.5
          - nontraffic V38.0
      - hanger-on
        - collision (with)
          - animal (traffic) V30.7
            - being ridden (traffic) V36.7
              - nontraffic V36.2
            - nontraffic V30.2
          - animal-drawn vehicle (traffic) V36.7
            - nontraffic V36.2
          - bus (traffic) V34.7
            - nontraffic V34.2
          - car (traffic) V33.7
            - nontraffic V33.2

- **Accident** *(Continued)*
  - transport *(Continued)*
    - three-wheeled motor vehicle occupant *(Continued)*
      - hanger-on *(Continued)*
        - collision *(Continued)*
          - pedal cycle (traffic) V31.7
            - nontraffic V31.2
          - pickup truck (traffic) V33.7
            - nontraffic V33.2
          - railway vehicle (traffic) V35.7
            - nontraffic V35.2
          - specified vehicle NEC (traffic) V36.7
            - nontraffic V36.2
          - stationary object (traffic) V37.7
            - nontraffic V37.2
          - streetcar (traffic) V36.7
            - nontraffic V36.2
          - three wheeled motor vehicle (traffic) V32.7
            - nontraffic V32.2
          - truck (traffic) V34.7
            - nontraffic V34.2
          - two wheeled motor vehicle (traffic) V32.7
            - nontraffic V32.2
          - van (traffic) V33.7
            - nontraffic V33.2
        - noncollision accident (traffic) V38.7
          - nontraffic V38.2
      - noncollision accident (traffic) V38.9
        - nontraffic V38.3
        - while boarding or alighting V38.4
      - nontraffic V39.3
      - passenger
        - collision (with)
          - animal (traffic) V30.6
            - being ridden (traffic) V36.6
              - nontraffic V36.1
            - nontraffic V30.1
          - animal-drawn vehicle (traffic) V36.6
            - nontraffic V36.1
          - bus (traffic) V34.6
            - nontraffic V34.1
          - car (traffic) V33.6
            - nontraffic V33.1
          - motor vehicle NOS (traffic) V39.50
            - nontraffic V39.10
            - specified type NEC (traffic) V39.59
              - nontraffic V39.19
          - pedal cycle (traffic) V31.6
            - nontraffic V31.1
          - pickup truck (traffic) V33.6
            - nontraffic V33.1
          - railway vehicle (traffic) V35.6
            - nontraffic V35.1
          - specified vehicle NEC (traffic) V36.6
            - nontraffic V36.1
          - stationary object (traffic) V37.6
            - nontraffic V37.1
          - streetcar (traffic) V36.6
            - nontraffic V36.1
          - three wheeled motor vehicle (traffic) V32.6
            - nontraffic V32.1
          - truck (traffic) V34.6
            - nontraffic V34.1
          - two wheeled motor vehicle (traffic) V32.6
            - nontraffic V32.1
          - van (traffic) V33.6
            - nontraffic V33.1
        - noncollision accident (traffic) V38.6
          - nontraffic V38.1
      - specified type NEC V39.89
        - military vehicle V39.81
    - tractor (farm) (and trailer) *—see* Accident, transport, agricultural vehicle occupant

- **Accident** *(Continued)*
  - transport *(Continued)*
    - tram *—see* Accident, transport, streetcar
      - in mine or quarry *—see* Accident, transport, industrial vehicle occupant
    - trolley *—see* Accident, transport, streetcar
      - in mine or quarry *—see* Accident, transport, industrial vehicle occupant
    - truck (heavy) occupant V69.9
      - collision (with)
        - animal (traffic) V60.9
          - being ridden (traffic) V66.9
            - nontraffic V66.3
            - while boarding or alighting V66.4
          - nontraffic V60.3
          - while boarding or alighting V60.4
        - animal-drawn vehicle (traffic) V66.9
          - nontraffic V66.3
          - while boarding or alighting V66.4
        - bus (traffic) V64.9
          - nontraffic V64.3
          - while boarding or alighting V64.4
        - car (traffic) V63.9
          - nontraffic V63.3
          - while boarding or alighting V63.4
        - motor vehicle NOS (traffic) V69.60
          - nontraffic V69.20
          - specified type NEC (traffic) V69.69
            - nontraffic V69.29
        - pedal cycle (traffic) V61.9
          - nontraffic V61.3
          - while boarding or alighting V61.4
        - pickup truck (traffic) V63.9
          - nontraffic V63.3
          - while boarding or alighting V63.4
        - railway vehicle (traffic) V65.9
          - nontraffic V65.3
          - while boarding or alighting V65.4
        - specified vehicle NEC (traffic) V66.9
          - nontraffic V66.3
          - while boarding or alighting V66.4
        - stationary object (traffic) V67.9
          - nontraffic V67.3
          - while boarding or alighting V67.4
        - streetcar (traffic) V66.9
          - nontraffic V66.3
          - while boarding or alighting V66.4
        - three wheeled motor vehicle (traffic) V62.9
          - nontraffic V62.3
          - while boarding or alighting V62.4
        - truck (traffic) V64.9
          - nontraffic V64.3
          - while boarding or alighting V64.4
        - two wheeled motor vehicle (traffic) V62.9
          - nontraffic V62.3
          - while boarding or alighting V62.4
        - van (traffic) V63.9
          - nontraffic V63.3
          - while boarding or alighting V63.4
      - driver
        - collision (with)
          - animal (traffic) V60.5
            - being ridden (traffic) V66.5
              - nontraffic V66.0
            - nontraffic V60.0
          - animal-drawn vehicle (traffic) V66.5
            - nontraffic V66.0
          - bus (traffic) V64.5
            - nontraffic V64.0
          - car (traffic) V63.5
            - nontraffic V63.0
          - motor vehicle NOS (traffic) V69.40
            - nontraffic V69.00
            - specified type NEC (traffic) V69.49
              - nontraffic V69.09

A

Accident *(Continued)*
transport *(Continued)*
truck occupant *(Continued)*
driver *(Continued)*
collision *(Continued)*
pedal cycle (traffic) V61.5
nontraffic V61.0
pickup truck (traffic) V63.5
nontraffic V63.0
railway vehicle (traffic) V65.5
nontraffic V65.0
specified vehicle NEC (traffic) V66.5
nontraffic V66.0
stationary object (traffic) V67.5
nontraffic V67.0
streetcar (traffic) V66.5
nontraffic V66.0
three wheeled motor vehicle (traffic) V62.5
nontraffic V62.0
truck (traffic) V64.5
nontraffic V64.0
two wheeled motor vehicle (traffic) V62.5
nontraffic V62.0
van (traffic) V63.5
nontraffic V63.0
noncollision accident (traffic) V68.5
nontraffic V68.0
dump —*see* Accident, transport, construction vehicle occupant
hanger-on
collision (with)
animal (traffic) V60.7
being ridden (traffic) V66.7
nontraffic V66.2
nontraffic V60.2
animal-drawn vehicle (traffic) V66.7
nontraffic V66.2
bus (traffic) V64.7
nontraffic V64.2
car (traffic) V63.7
nontraffic V63.2
pedal cycle (traffic) V61.7
nontraffic V61.2
pickup truck (traffic) V63.7
nontraffic V63.2
railway vehicle (traffic) V65.7
nontraffic V65.2
specified vehicle NEC (traffic) V66.7
nontraffic V66.2
stationary object (traffic) V67.7
nontraffic V67.2
streetcar (traffic) V66.7
nontraffic V66.2
three wheeled motor vehicle (traffic) V62.7
nontraffic V62.2
truck (traffic) V64.7
nontraffic V64.2
two wheeled motor vehicle (traffic) V62.7
nontraffic V62.2
van (traffic) V63.7
nontraffic V63.2
noncollision accident (traffic) V68.7
nontraffic V68.2
noncollision accident (traffic) V68.9
nontraffic V68.3
while boarding or alighting V68.4
nontraffic V69.3
passenger
collision (with)
animal (traffic) V60.6
being ridden (traffic) V66.6
nontraffic V66.1
nontraffic V60.1
animal-drawn vehicle (traffic) V66.6
nontraffic V66.1
bus (traffic) V64.6
nontraffic V64.1

Accident *(Continued)*
transport *(Continued)*
truck occupant *(Continued)*
passenger *(Continued)*
collision *(Continued)*
car (traffic) V63.6
nontraffic V63.1
motor vehicle NOS (traffic) V69.50
nontraffic V69.10
specified type NEC (traffic) V69.59
nontraffic V69.19
pedal cycle (traffic) V61.6
nontraffic V61.1
pickup truck (traffic) V63.6
nontraffic V63.1
railway vehicle (traffic) V65.6
nontraffic V65.1
specified vehicle NEC (traffic) V66.6
nontraffic V66.1
stationary object (traffic) V67.6
nontraffic V67.1
streetcar (traffic) V66.6
nontraffic V66.1
three wheeled motor vehicle (traffic) V62.6
nontraffic V62.1
truck (traffic) V64.6
nontraffic V64.1
two wheeled motor vehicle (traffic) V62.6
nontraffic V62.1
van (traffic) V63.6
nontraffic V63.1
noncollision accident (traffic) V68.6
nontraffic V68.1
pickup —*see* Accident, transport, pickup truck occupant
specified type NEC V69.88
military vehicle V69.81
van occupant V59.9
collision (with)
animal (traffic) V50.9
being ridden (traffic) V56.9
nontraffic V56.3
while boarding or alighting V56.4
nontraffic V50.3
while boarding or alighting V50.4
animal-drawn vehicle (traffic) V56.9
nontraffic V56.3
while boarding or alighting V56.4
bus (traffic) V54.9
nontraffic V54.3
while boarding or alighting V54.4
car (traffic) V53.9
nontraffic V53.3
while boarding or alighting V53.4
motor vehicle NOS (traffic) V59.60
nontraffic V59.20
specified type NEC (traffic) V59.69
nontraffic V59.29
pedal cycle (traffic) V51.9
nontraffic V51.3
while boarding or alighting V51.4
pickup truck (traffic) V53.9
nontraffic V53.3
while boarding or alighting V53.4
railway vehicle (traffic) V55.9
nontraffic V55.3
while boarding or alighting V55.4
specified vehicle NEC (traffic) V56.9
nontraffic V56.3
while boarding or alighting V56.4
stationary object (traffic) V57.9
nontraffic V57.3
while boarding or alighting V57.4
streetcar (traffic) V56.9
nontraffic V56.3
while boarding or alighting V56.4

Accident *(Continued)*
transport *(Continued)*
van occupant *(Continued)*
collision *(Continued)*
three wheeled motor vehicle (traffic) V52.9
nontraffic V52.3
while boarding or alighting V52.4
truck (traffic) V54.9
nontraffic V54.3
while boarding or alighting V54.4
two wheeled motor vehicle (traffic) V52.9
nontraffic V52.3
while boarding or alighting V52.4
van (traffic) V53.9
nontraffic V53.3
while boarding or alighting V53.4
driver
collision (with)
animal (traffic) V50.5
being ridden (traffic) V56.5
nontraffic V56.0
nontraffic V50.0
animal-drawn vehicle (traffic) V56.5
nontraffic V56.0
bus (traffic) V54.5
nontraffic V54.0
car (traffic) V53.5
nontraffic V53.0
motor vehicle NOS (traffic) V59.40
nontraffic V59.00
specified type NEC (traffic) V59.49
nontraffic V59.09
pedal cycle (traffic) V51.5
nontraffic V51.0
pickup truck (traffic) V53.5
nontraffic V53.0
railway vehicle (traffic) V55.5
nontraffic V55.0
specified vehicle NEC (traffic) V56.5
nontraffic V56.0
stationary object (traffic) V57.5
nontraffic V57.0
streetcar (traffic) V56.5
nontraffic V56.0
three wheeled motor vehicle (traffic) V52.5
nontraffic V52.0
truck (traffic) V54.5
nontraffic V54.0
two wheeled motor vehicle (traffic) V52.5
nontraffic V52.0
van (traffic) V53.5
nontraffic V53.0
noncollision accident (traffic) V58.5
nontraffic V58.0
hanger-on
collision (with)
animal (traffic) V50.7
being ridden (traffic) V56.7
nontraffic V56.2
nontraffic V50.2
animal-drawn vehicle (traffic) V56.7
nontraffic V56.2
bus (traffic) V54.7
nontraffic V54.2
car (traffic) V53.7
nontraffic V53.2
pedal cycle (traffic) V51.7
nontraffic V51.2
pickup truck (traffic) V53.7
nontraffic V53.2
railway vehicle (traffic) V55.7
nontraffic V55.2
specified vehicle NEC (traffic) V56.7
nontraffic V56.2
stationary object (traffic) V57.7
nontraffic V57.2

A

- **Accident** *(Continued)*
  - transport *(Continued)*
    - van occupant *(Continued)*
      - hanger-on *(Continued)*
        - collision *(Continued)*
          - streetcar (traffic) V56.7
            - nontraffic V56.2
          - three wheeled motor vehicle (traffic) V52.7
            - nontraffic V52.2
          - truck (traffic) V54.7
            - nontraffic V54.2
          - two wheeled motor vehicle (traffic) V52.7
            - nontraffic V52.2
          - van (traffic) V53.7
            - nontraffic V53.2
        - noncollision accident (traffic) V58.7
          - nontraffic V58.2
      - noncollision accident (traffic) V58.9
        - nontraffic V58.3
        - while boarding or alighting V58.4
      - nontraffic V59.3
      - passenger
        - collision (with)
          - animal (traffic) V50.6
            - being ridden (traffic) V56.6
              - nontraffic V56.1
            - nontraffic V50.1
          - animal-drawn vehicle (traffic) V56.6
            - nontraffic V56.1
          - bus (traffic) V54.6
            - nontraffic V54.1
          - car (traffic) V53.6
            - nontraffic V53.1
          - motor vehicle NOS (traffic) V59.50
            - nontraffic V59.10
            - specified type NEC (traffic) V59.59
              - nontraffic V59.19
          - pedal cycle (traffic) V51.6
            - nontraffic V51.1
          - pickup truck (traffic) V53.6
            - nontraffic V53.1
          - railway vehicle (traffic) V55.6
            - nontraffic V55.1
          - specified vehicle NEC (traffic) V56.6
            - nontraffic V56.1
          - stationary object (traffic) V57.6
            - nontraffic V57.1
          - streetcar (traffic) V56.6
            - nontraffic V56.1
          - three wheeled motor vehicle (traffic) V52.6
            - nontraffic V52.1
          - truck (traffic) V54.6
            - nontraffic V54.1
          - two wheeled motor vehicle (traffic) V52.6
            - nontraffic V52.1
          - van (traffic) V53.6
            - nontraffic V53.1
        - noncollision accident (traffic) V58.6
          - nontraffic V58.1
      - specified type NEC V59.88
        - military vehicle V59.81
    - watercraft occupant —*see* Accident, watercraft
  - vehicle NEC V89.9
    - animal-drawn NEC —*see* Accident, transport, animal-drawn vehicle occupant
    - special
      - agricultural —*see* Accident, transport, agricultural vehicle occupant
      - construction —*see* Accident, transport, construction vehicle occupant
      - industrial —*see* Accident, transport, industrial vehicle occupant
    - three-wheeled NEC (motorized) —*see* Accident, transport, three-wheeled motor vehicle occupant
- **Accident** *(Continued)*
  - watercraft V94.9
    - causing
      - drowning —*see* Drowning, due to, accident to, watercraft
      - injury NEC V91.89
        - crushed between craft and object V91.19
          - powered craft V91.13
            - ferry boat V91.11
            - fishing boat V91.12
            - jet ski V91.13
            - liner V91.11
            - merchant ship V91.10
            - passenger ship V91.11
          - unpowered craft V91.18
            - canoe V91.15
            - inflatable V91.16
            - kayak V91.15
            - sailboat V91.14
            - surf-board V91.18
            - windsurfer V91.18
        - fall on board V91.29
          - powered craft V91.23
            - ferry boat V91.21
            - fishing boat V91.22
            - jet ski V91.23
            - liner V91.21
            - merchant ship V91.20
            - passenger ship V91.21
          - unpowered craft
            - canoe V91.25
            - inflatable V91.26
            - kayak V91.25
            - sailboat V91.24
        - fire on board causing burn V91.09
          - powered craft V91.03
            - ferry boat V91.01
            - fishing boat V91.02
            - jet ski V91.03
            - liner V91.01
            - merchant ship V91.00
            - passenger ship V91.01
          - unpowered craft V91.08
            - canoe V91.05
            - inflatable V91.06
            - kayak V91.05
            - sailboat V91.04
            - surf-board V91.08
            - water skis V91.07
            - windsurfer V91.08
        - hit by falling object V91.39
          - powered craft V91.33
            - ferry boat V91.31
            - fishing boat V91.32
            - jet skis V91.33
            - liner V91.31
            - merchant ship V91.30
            - passenger ship V91.31
          - unpowered craft V91.38
            - canoe V91.35
            - inflatable V91.36
            - kayak V91.35
            - sailboat V91.34
            - surf-board V91.38
            - water skis V91.37
            - windsurfer V91.38
        - specified type NEC V91.89
          - powered craft V91.83
            - ferry boat V91.81
            - fishing boat V91.82
            - jet ski V91.83
            - liner V91.81
            - merchant ship V91.80
            - passenger ship V91.81
          - unpowered craft V91.88
            - canoe V91.85
            - inflatable V91.86
            - kayak V91.85
            - sailboat V91.84
            - surf-board V91.88
- **Accident** *(Continued)*
  - watercraft *(Continued)*
    - causing *(Continued)*
      - injury NEC *(Continued)*
        - specified type NEC *(Continued)*
          - unpowered craft *(Continued)*
            - water skis V91.87
            - windsurfer V91.88
    - due to, caused by cataclysm —*see* Forces of nature, by type
    - military NEC V94.818
      - with civilian watercraft V94.810
      - civilian in water injured by V94.811
    - nonpowered, struck by
      - nonpowered vessel V94.22
      - powered vessel V94.21
    - specified type NEC V94.89
    - striking swimmer
      - powered V94.11
      - unpowered V94.12
- **Acid throwing** (assault) Y08.89
- **Activity** (involving) (of victim at time of event) Y93.9
  - aerobic and step exercise (class) Y93.A3
  - alpine skiing Y93.23
  - animal care NEC Y93.K9
  - arts and handcrafts NEC Y93.D9
  - athletics NEC Y93.79
  - athletics played as a team or group NEC Y93.69
  - athletics played individually NEC Y93.59
  - baking Y93.G3
  - ballet Y93.41
  - barbells Y93.B3
  - BASE (Building, Antenna, Span, Earth) jumping Y93.33
  - baseball Y93.64
  - basketball Y93.67
  - bathing (personal) Y93.E1
  - beach volleyball Y93.68
  - bike riding Y93.55
  - blackout game Y93.85
  - boogie boarding Y93.18
  - bowling Y93.54
  - boxing Y93.71
  - brass instrument playing Y93.J4
  - building construction Y93.H3
  - bungee jumping Y93.34
  - calisthenics Y93.A2
  - canoeing (in calm and turbulent water) Y93.16
  - capture the flag Y93.6A
  - cardiorespiratory exercise NEC Y93.A9
  - caregiving (providing) NEC Y93.F9
    - bathing Y93.F1
    - lifting Y93.F2
  - cellular
    - communication device Y93.C2
    - telephone Y93.C2
  - challenge course Y93.A5
  - cheerleading Y93.45
  - choking game Y93.85
  - circuit training Y93.A4
  - cleaning
    - floor Y93.E5
  - climbing NEC Y93.39
    - mountain Y93.31
    - rock Y93.31
    - wall Y93.31
  - clothing care and maintenance NEC Y93.E9
  - combatives Y93.75
  - computer
    - keyboarding Y93.C1
    - technology NEC Y93.C9
  - confidence course Y93.A5
  - construction (building) Y93.H3
  - cooking and baking Y93.G3
  - cool down exercises Y93.A2
  - cricket Y93.69
  - crocheting Y93.D1
  - cross country skiing Y93.24
  - dancing (all types) Y93.41

A

Activity *(Continued)*
- digging
  - dirt Y93.H1
- dirt digging Y93.H1
- dishwashing Y93.G1
- diving (platform) (springboard) Y93.12
  - underwater Y93.15
- dodge ball Y93.6A
- downhill skiing Y93.23
- drum playing Y93.J2
- dumbbells Y93.B3
- electronic
  - devices NEC Y93.C9
    - hand held interactive Y93.C2
  - game playing (using) (with)
    - interactive device Y93.C2
    - keyboard or other stationary device Y93.C1
- elliptical machine Y93.A1
- exercise(s)
  - machines ((primarily) for)
    - cardiorespiratory conditioning Y93.A1
    - muscle strengthening Y93.B1
  - muscle strengthening (non-machine) NEC Y93.B9
- external motion NEC Y93.I9
  - rollercoaster Y93.I1
- fainting game Y93.85
- field hockey Y93.65
- figure skating (pairs) (singles) Y93.21
- flag football Y93.62
- floor mopping and cleaning Y93.E5
- food preparation and clean up Y93.G1
- football (American) NOS Y93.61
  - flag Y93.62
  - tackle Y93.61
  - touch Y93.62
- four square Y93.6A
- free weights Y93.B3
- frisbee (ultimate) Y93.74
- furniture
  - building Y93.D3
  - finishing Y93.D3
  - repair Y93.D3
- game playing (electronic)
  - using interactive device Y93.C2
  - using keyboard or other stationary device Y93.C1
- gardening Y93.H2
- golf Y93.53
- grass drills Y93.A6
- grilling and smoking food Y93.G2
- grooming and shearing an animal Y93.K3
- guerilla drills Y93.A6
- gymnastics (rhythmic) Y93.43
- hand held interactive electronic device Y93.C2
- handball Y93.73
- handcrafts NEC Y93.D9
- hang gliding Y93.35
- hiking (on level or elevated terrain) Y93.Ø1
- hockey (ice) Y93.22
  - field Y93.65
- horseback riding Y93.52
- household (interior) maintenance NEC Y93.E9
- ice NEC Y93.29
  - dancing Y93.21
  - hockey Y93.22
  - skating Y93.21
- inline roller skating Y93.51
- ironing Y93.E4
- judo Y93.75
- jumping (off) NEC Y93.39
  - BASE (Building, Antenna, Span, Earth) Y93.33
  - bungee Y93.34
  - jacks Y93.A2
  - rope Y93.56
- jumping jacks Y93.A2
- jumping rope Y93.56
- karate Y93.75

Activity *(Continued)*
- kayaking (in calm and turbulent water) Y93.16
- keyboarding (computer) Y93.C1
- kickball Y93.6A
- knitting Y93.D1
- lacrosse Y93.65
- land maintenance NEC Y93.H9
- landscaping Y93.H2
- laundry Y93.E2
- machines (exercise)
  - primarily for cardiorespiratory conditioning Y93.A1
  - primarily for muscle strengthening Y93.B1
- maintenance
  - exterior building NEC Y93.H9
  - household (interior) NEC Y93.E9
  - land Y93.H9
  - property Y93.H9
- marching (on level or elevated terrain) Y93.Ø1
- martial arts Y93.75
- microwave oven Y93.G3
- milking an animal Y93.K2
- mopping (floor) Y93.E5
- mountain climbing Y93.31
- muscle strengthening
  - exercises (non-machine) NEC Y93.B9
  - machines Y93.B1
- musical keyboard (electronic) playing Y93.J1
- nordic skiing Y93.24
- obstacle course Y93.A5
- oven (microwave) Y93.G3
- packing up and unpacking in moving to a new residence Y93.E6
- parasailing Y93.19
- pass out game Y93.85
- percussion instrument playing NEC Y93.J2
- personal
  - bathing and showering Y93.E1
  - hygiene NEC Y93.E8
  - showering Y93.E1
- physical games generally associated with school recess, summer camp and children Y93.6A
- physical training NEC Y93.A9
- piano playing Y93.J1
- pilates Y93.B4
- platform diving Y93.12
- playing musical instrument
  - brass instrument Y93.J4
  - drum Y93.J2
  - musical keyboard (electronic) Y93.J1
  - percussion instrument NEC Y93.J2
  - piano Y93.J1
  - string instrument Y93.J3
  - winds instrument Y93.J4
- property maintenance
  - exterior NEC Y93.H9
  - interior NEC Y93.E9
- pruning (garden and lawn) Y93.H2
- pull-ups Y93.B2
- push-ups Y93.B2
- racquetball Y93.73
- rafting (in calm and turbulent water) Y93.16
- raking (leaves) Y93.H1
- rappelling Y93.32
- refereeing a sports activity Y93.81
- residential relocation Y93.E6
- rhythmic gymnastics Y93.43
- rhythmic movement NEC Y93.49
- riding
  - horseback Y93.52
  - rollercoaster Y93.I1
- rock climbing Y93.31
- roller skating (inline) Y93.51
- rollercoaster riding Y93.I1
- rough housing and horseplay Y93.83
- rowing (in calm and turbulent water) Y93.16
- rugby Y93.63
- SCUBA diving Y93.15
- sewing Y93.D2

Activity *(Continued)*
- shoveling Y93.H1
  - dirt Y93.H1
  - snow Y93.H1
- showering (personal) Y93.E1
- sit-ups Y93.B2
- skateboarding Y93.51
- skating (ice) Y93.21
  - roller Y93.51
- skiing (alpine) (downhill) Y93.23
  - cross country Y93.24
  - nordic Y93.24
  - water Y93.17
- sledding (snow) Y93.23
- sleeping (sleep) Y93.84
- smoking and grilling food Y93.G2
- snorkeling Y93.15
- snow NEC Y93.29
  - boarding Y93.23
  - shoveling Y93.H1
  - sledding Y93.23
  - tubing Y93.23
- soccer Y93.66
- softball Y93.64
- specified NEC Y93.89
- spectator at an event Y93.82
- sports NEC Y93.79
  - sports played as a team or group NEC Y93.69
  - sports played individually NEC Y93.59
- springboard diving Y93.12
- squash Y93.73
- stationary bike Y93.A1
- step (stepping) exercise (class) Y93.A3
- stepper machine Y93.A1
- stove Y93.G3
- string instrument playing Y93.J3
- surfing Y93.18
  - wind Y93.18
- swimming Y93.11
- tackle football Y93.61
- tap dancing Y93.41
- tennis Y93.73
- tobogganing Y93.23
- touch football Y93.62
- track and field events (non-running) Y93.57
  - running Y93.Ø2
- trampoline Y93.44
- treadmill Y93.A1
- trimming shrubs Y93.H2
- tubing (in calm and turbulent water) Y93.16
  - snow Y93.23
- ultimate frisbee Y93.74
- underwater diving Y93.15
- unpacking in moving to a new residence Y93.E6
- use of stove, oven and microwave oven Y93.G3
- vacuuming Y93.E3
- volleyball (beach) (court) Y93.68
- wake boarding Y93.17
- walking (on level or elevated terrain) Y93.Ø1
  - an animal Y93.K1
- walking an animal Y93.K1
- wall climbing Y93.31
- warm up and cool down exercises Y93.A2
- water NEC Y93.19
  - aerobics Y93.14
  - craft NEC Y93.19
  - exercise Y93.14
  - polo Y93.13
  - skiing Y93.17
  - sliding Y93.18
  - survival training and testing Y93.19
- weeding (garden and lawn) Y93.H2
- wind instrument playing Y93.J4
- windsurfing Y93.18
- wrestling Y93.72
- yoga Y93.42

Adverse effect of drugs —*see* Table of Drugs and Chemicals

Aerosinusitis —*see* Air, pressure
After-effect, late —*see* Sequelae
Air
- blast in war operations —*see* War operations, air blast
- pressure
  - change, rapid
    - during
      - ascent W94.29
        - while (in) (surfacing from)
          - aircraft W94.23
          - deep water diving W94.21
          - underground W94.22
      - descent W94.39
        - in
          - aircraft W94.31
          - water W94.32
  - high, prolonged W94.Ø
  - low, prolonged W94.12
    - due to residence or long visit at high altitude W94.11

Alpine sickness W94.11
Altitude sickness W94.11
Anaphylactic shock, anaphylaxis —*see* Table of Drugs and Chemicals
Andes disease W94.11
Arachnidism, arachnoidism X58
Arson (with intent to injure or kill) X97
Asphyxia, asphyxiation
- by
  - food (bone) (seed) —*see* categories T17 and T18
  - gas —*see also* Table of Drugs and Chemicals
    - legal
      - execution —*see* Legal, intervention, gas
      - intervention —*see* Legal, intervention, gas
- from
  - fire —*see also* Exposure, fire
    - in war operations —*see* War operations, fire
  - ignition —*see* Ignition
  - vomitus T17.81
- in war operations —*see* War operations, restriction of airway

Aspiration
- food (any type) (into respiratory tract) (with asphyxia, obstruction respiratory tract, suffocation) —*see* categories T17 and T18
- foreign body —*see* Foreign body, aspiration
- vomitus (with asphyxia, obstruction respiratory tract, suffocation) T17.81

Assassination (attempt) —*see* Assault
Assault (homicidal) (by) (in) YØ9
- arson X97
- bite (of human being) YØ4.1
- bodily force YØ4.8
  - bite YØ4.1
  - bumping into YØ4.2
  - sexual —*see* subcategories T74.Ø, T76.Ø
  - unarmed fight YØ4.Ø

Assault *(Continued)*
- bomb X96.9
  - antipersonnel X96.Ø
  - fertilizer X96.3
  - gasoline X96.1
  - letter X96.2
  - petrol X96.1
  - pipe X96.3
  - specified NEC X96.8
- brawl (hand) (fists) (foot) (unarmed) YØ4.Ø
- burning, burns (by fire) NEC X97
  - acid YØ8.89
  - caustic, corrosive substance YØ8.89
  - chemical from swallowing caustic, corrosive substance —*see* Table of Drugs and Chemicals
  - cigarette(s) X97
  - hot object X98.9
    - fluid NEC X98.2
    - household appliance X98.3
    - specified NEC X98.8
    - steam X98.Ø
    - tap water X98.1
    - vapors X98.Ø
  - scalding —*see* Assault, burning
  - steam X98.Ø
  - vitriol YØ8.89
- caustic, corrosive substance (gas) YØ8.89
- crashing of
  - aircraft YØ8.81
  - motor vehicle YØ3.8
    - pushed in front of YØ2.Ø
    - run over YØ3.Ø
    - specified NEC YØ3.8
- cutting or piercing instrument X99.9
  - dagger X99.2
  - glass X99.Ø
  - knife X99.1
  - specified NEC X99.8
  - sword X99.2
- dagger X99.2
- drowning (in) X92.9
  - bathtub X92.Ø
  - natural water X92.3
  - specified NEC X92.8
  - swimming pool X92.1
    - following fall X92.2
- dynamite X96.8
- explosive(s) (material) X96.9
- fight (hand) (fists) (foot) (unarmed) YØ4.Ø
  - with weapon —*see* Assault, by type of weapon
- fire X97
- firearm X95.9
  - airgun X95.Ø1
  - handgun X93
  - hunting rifle X94.1
  - larger X94.9
    - specified NEC X94.8
  - machine gun X94.2
  - shotgun X94.Ø
  - specified NEC X95.8

Assault *(Continued)*
- from high place YØ1
- gunshot (wound) NEC —*see* Assault, firearm, by type
- incendiary device X97
- injury YØ9
  - to child due to criminal abortion attempt NEC YØ8.89
- knife X99.1
- late effect of —*see* X92-YØ8 with 7th character S
- placing before moving object NEC YØ2.8
  - motor vehicle YØ2.Ø
- poisoning —*see* categories T36-T65 with 7th character S
- puncture, any part of body —*see* Assault, cutting or piercing instrument
- pushing
  - before moving object NEC YØ2.8
    - motor vehicle YØ2.Ø
    - subway train YØ2.1
    - train YØ2.1
- rape T74.2- ●
- scalding —*see* Assault, burning
- sequelae of —*see* X92-YØ8 with 7th character S
- sexual (by bodily force) T74.2- ●
- shooting —*see* Assault, firearm
- specified means NEC YØ8.89
- stab, any part of body —*see* Assault, cutting or piercing instrument
- steam X98.Ø
- striking against
  - other person YØ4.2
  - sports equipment YØ8.Ø9
    - baseball bat YØ8.Ø2
    - hockey stick YØ8.Ø1
- struck by
  - sports equipment YØ8.Ø9
    - baseball bat YØ8.Ø2
    - hockey stick YØ8.Ø1
- submersion —*see* Assault, drowning
- violence YØ9
- weapon YØ9
  - blunt YØØ
  - cutting or piercing —*see* Assault, cutting or piercing instrument
  - firearm —*see* Assault, firearm
- wound YØ9
  - cutting —*see* Assault, cutting or piercing instrument
  - gunshot —*see* Assault, firearm
  - knife X99.1
  - piercing —*see* Assault, cutting or piercing instrument
  - puncture —*see* Assault, cutting or piercing instrument
  - stab —*see* Assault, cutting or piercing instrument

Attack by mammals NEC W55.89
Avalanche —*see* Landslide
Aviator's disease —*see* Air, pressure

B

Barotitis, barodontalgia, barosinusitis, barotrauma (otitic) (sinus) —*see* Air, pressure
Battered (baby) (child) (person) (syndrome) X58
Bayonet wound W26.1
- in
  - legal intervention —*see* Legal, intervention, sharp object, bayonet
  - war operations —*see* War operations, combat
- stated as undetermined whether accidental or intentional Y28.8
- suicide (attempt) X78.2

Bean in nose —*see* categories T17 and T18
Bed set on fire NEC —*see* Exposure, fire, uncontrolled, building, bed
Beheading (by guillotine)
- homicide X99.9
- legal execution —*see* Legal, intervention

Bending, injury in (prolonged) (static) X5Ø.1
Bends —*see* Air, pressure, change
Bite, bitten by
- alligator W58.Ø1
- arthropod (nonvenomous) NEC W57
- bull W55.21
- cat W55.Ø1
- cow W55.21
- crocodile W58.11
- dog W54.Ø
- goat W55.31
- hoof stock NEC W55.31
- horse W55.11
- human being (accidentally) W5Ø.3
  - with intent to injure or kill YØ4.1
  - as, or caused by, a crowd or human stampede (with fall) W52
  - assault YØ4.1
  - homicide (attempt) YØ4.1
  - in
    - fight YØ4.1
- insect (nonvenomous) W57
- lizard (nonvenomous) W59.Ø1
- mammal NEC W55.81
  - marine W56.31
- marine animal (nonvenomous) W56.81
- millipede W57
- moray eel W56.51
- mouse W53.Ø1
- person(s) (accidentally) W5Ø.3
  - with intent to injure or kill YØ4.1
  - as, or caused by, a crowd or human stampede (with fall) W52
  - assault YØ4.1
  - homicide (attempt) YØ4.1
  - in
    - fight YØ4.1
- pig W55.41
- raccoon W55.51
- rat W53.11
- reptile W59.81
  - lizard W59.Ø1
  - snake W59.11
  - turtle W59.21
    - terrestrial W59.81
- rodent W53.81
  - mouse W53.Ø1
  - rat W53.11
  - specified NEC W53.81
  - squirrel W53.21
- shark W56.41
- sheep W55.31
- snake (nonvenomous) W59.11
- spider (nonvenomous) W57
- squirrel W53.21

Blast (air) in war operations —*see* War operations, blast
Blizzard X37.2
Blood alcohol level Y9Ø.9
- 2Ø-39mg/1ØØml Y9Ø.1
- 4Ø-59mg/1ØØml Y9Ø.2
- 6Ø-79mg/1ØØml Y9Ø.3
- 8Ø-99mg/1ØØml Y9Ø.4
- 1ØØ-119mg/1ØØml Y9Ø.5
- 12Ø-199mg/1ØØml Y9Ø.6
- 2ØØ-239mg/1ØØml Y9Ø.7
- less than 2Ømg/1ØØml Y9Ø.Ø
- presence in blood, level not specified Y9Ø.9

Blow X58
- by law-enforcing agent, police (on duty) —*see* Legal, intervention, manhandling
  - blunt object —*see* Legal, intervention, blunt object

Blowing up —*see* Explosion
Brawl (hand) (fists) (foot) YØ4.Ø
Breakage (accidental) (part of)
- ladder (causing fall) W11
- scaffolding (causing fall) W12

Broken
- glass, contact with —*see* Contact, with, glass
- power line (causing electric shock) W85

Bumping against, into (accidentally)
- object NEC W22.8
  - with fall —*see* Fall, due to, bumping against, object
  - caused by crowd or human stampede (with fall) W52
  - sports equipment W21.9
- person(s) W51
  - with fall WØ3
    - due to ice or snow WØØ.Ø
  - assault YØ4.2
  - caused by, a crowd or human stampede (with fall) W52
  - homicide (attempt) YØ4.2
- sports equipment W21.9

Burn, burned, burning (accidental) (by) (from) (on)
- acid NEC —*see* Table of Drugs and Chemicals
- bed linen —*see* Exposure, fire, uncontrolled, in building, bed
- blowtorch XØ8.8
  - with ignition of clothing NEC XØ6.2
    - nightwear XØ5
- bonfire, campfire (controlled) —*see also* Exposure, fire, controlled, not in building
  - uncontrolled —*see* Exposure, fire, uncontrolled, not in building
- candle XØ8.8
  - with ignition of clothing NEC XØ6.2
    - nightwear XØ5
- caustic liquid, substance (external) (internal) NEC —*see* Table of Drugs and Chemicals
- chemical (external) (internal) —*see also* Table of Drugs and Chemicals
  - in war operations —*see* War operations, fire
- cigar(s) or cigarette(s) XØ8.8
  - with ignition of clothing NEC XØ6.2
    - nightwear XØ5
- clothes, clothing NEC (from controlled fire) XØ6.2
  - with conflagration —*see* Exposure, fire, uncontrolled, building
    - not in building or structure —*see* Exposure, fire, uncontrolled, not in building
- cooker (hot) X15.8
  - stated as undetermined whether accidental or intentional Y27.3
  - suicide (attempt) X77.3
- electric blanket X16
- engine (hot) X17
- fire, flames —*see* Exposure, fire
- flare, Very pistol —*see* Discharge, firearm NEC

Burn, burned, burning *(Continued)*
- heat
  - from appliance (electrical) (household) X15.8
    - cooker X15.8
    - hotplate X15.2
    - kettle X15.8
    - light bulb X15.8
    - saucepan X15.3
    - skillet X15.3
    - stated as undetermined whether accidental or intentional Y27.3
    - stove X15.Ø
    - suicide (attempt) X77.3
    - toaster X15.1
  - in local application or packing during medical or surgical procedure Y63.5
- heating
  - appliance, radiator or pipe X16
- homicide (attempt) —*see* Assault, burning
- hot
  - air X14.1
  - cooker X15.8
  - drink X1Ø.Ø
  - engine X17
  - fat X1Ø.2
  - fluid NEC X12
  - food X1Ø.1
  - gases X14.1
  - heating appliance X16
  - household appliance NEC X15.8
  - kettle X15.8
  - liquid NEC X12
  - machinery X17
  - metal (molten) (liquid) NEC X18
  - object (not producing fire or flames) NEC X19
  - oil (cooking) X1Ø.2
  - pipe(s) X16
  - radiator X16
  - saucepan (glass) (metal) X15.3
  - stove (kitchen) X15.Ø
  - substance NEC X19
    - caustic or corrosive NEC —*see* Table of Drugs and Chemicals
  - toaster X15.1
  - tool X17
  - vapor X13.1
  - water (tap) —*see* Contact, with, hot, tap water
- hotplate X15.2
  - suicide (attempt) X77.3
- ignition —*see* Ignition
- in war operations —*see* War operations, fire
- inflicted by other person X97
  - by hot objects, hot vapor, and steam —*see* Assault, burning, hot object
- internal, from swallowed caustic, corrosive liquid, substance —*see* Table of Drugs and Chemicals
- iron (hot) X15.8
  - stated as undetermined whether accidental or intentional Y27.3
  - suicide (attempt) X77.3
- kettle (hot) X15.8
  - stated as undetermined whether accidental or intentional Y27.3
  - suicide (attempt) X77.3
- lamp (flame) XØ8.8
  - with ignition of clothing NEC XØ6.2
    - nightwear XØ5
- lighter (cigar) (cigarette) XØ8.8
  - with ignition of clothing NEC XØ6.2
    - nightwear XØ5
- lightning —*see* subcategory T75.Ø
  - causing fire —*see* Exposure, fire
- liquid (boiling) (hot) NEC X12
  - stated as undetermined whether accidental or intentional Y27.2
  - suicide (attempt) X77.2

B

Burn, burned, burning *(Continued)*
local application of externally applied substance in medical or surgical care Y63.5
machinery (hot) X17
matches X08.8
with ignition of clothing NEC X06.2
nightwear X05
mattress —*see* Exposure, fire, uncontrolled, building, bed
medicament, externally applied Y63.5
metal (hot) (liquid) (molten) NEC X18
nightwear (nightclothes, nightdress, gown, pajamas, robe) X05
object (hot) NEC X19
on board watercraft
due to
accident to watercraft V91.09
powered craft V91.03
ferry boat V91.01
fishing boat V91.02
jet ski V91.03
liner V91.01
merchant ship V91.00
passenger ship V91.01
unpowered craft V91.08
canoe V91.05
inflatable V91.06
kayak V91.05
sailboat V91.04
surf-board V91.08
water skis V91.07
windsurfer V91.08
fire on board V93.09
ferry boat V93.01
fishing boat V93.02
jet ski V93.03
liner V93.01
merchant ship V93.00
passenger ship V93.01
powered craft NEC V93.03
sailboat V93.04

Burn, burned, burning *(Continued)*
on board watercraft *(Continued)*
due to *(Continued)*
specified heat source NEC on board V93.19
ferry boat V93.11
fishing boat V93.12
jet ski V93.13
liner V93.11
merchant ship V93.10
passenger ship V93.11
powered craft NEC V93.13
sailboat V93.14
pipe (hot) X16
smoking X08.8
with ignition of clothing NEC X06.2
nightwear X05
powder —*see* Powder burn
radiator (hot) X16
saucepan (hot) (glass) (metal) X15.3
stated as undetermined whether accidental or intentional Y27.3
suicide (attempt) X77.3
self-inflicted X76
stated as undetermined whether accidental or intentional Y26
stated as undetermined whether accidental or intentional Y27.0
steam X13.1
pipe X16
stated as undetermined whether accidental or intentional Y27.8
stated as undetermined whether accidental or intentional Y27.0
suicide (attempt) X77.0
stove (hot) (kitchen) X15.0
stated as undetermined whether accidental or intentional Y27.3
suicide (attempt) X77.3

Burn, burned, burning *(Continued)*
substance (hot) NEC X19
boiling X12
stated as undetermined whether accidental or intentional Y27.2
suicide (attempt) X77.2
molten (metal) X18
suicide (attempt) NEC X76
hot
household appliance X77.3
object X77.9
stated as undetermined whether accidental or intentional Y27.0
therapeutic misadventure
heat in local application or packing during medical or surgical procedure Y63.5
overdose of radiation Y63.2
toaster (hot) X15.1
stated as undetermined whether accidental or intentional Y27.3
suicide (attempt) X77.3
tool (hot) X17
torch, welding X08.8
with ignition of clothing NEC X06.2
nightwear X05
trash fire (controlled) —*see* Exposure, fire, controlled, not in building
uncontrolled —*see* Exposure, fire, uncontrolled, not in building
vapor (hot) X13.1
stated as undetermined whether accidental or intentional Y27.0
suicide (attempt) X77.0
Very pistol —*see* Discharge, firearm NEC
Butted by animal W55.82
bull W55.22
cow W55.22
goat W55.32
horse W55.12
pig W55.42
sheep W55.32

B

C

- **Caisson disease** —*see* Air, pressure, change
- **Campfire** (exposure to) (controlled) —*see also* Exposure, fire, controlled, not in building
  - uncontrolled —*see* Exposure, fire, uncontrolled, not in building
- **Capital punishment** (any means) —*see* Legal, intervention
- **Car sickness** T75.3
- **Casualty** (not due to war) NEC X58
  - war —*see* War operations
- **Cat**
  - bite W55.Ø1
  - scratch W55.Ø3
- **Cataclysm, cataclysmic** (any injury) NEC —*see* Forces of nature
- **Catching fire** —*see* Exposure, fire
- **Caught**
  - between
    - folding object W23.Ø
    - objects (moving) (stationary and moving) W23.Ø
      - and machinery —*see* Contact, with, by type of machine
      - stationary W23.1
    - sliding door and door frame W23.Ø
  - by, in
    - machinery (moving parts of) —*see* Contact, with, by type of machine
    - washing-machine wringer W23.Ø
  - under packing crate (due to losing grip) W23.1
- **Cave-in** caused by cataclysmic earth surface movement or eruption —*see* Landslide
- **Change(s) in air pressure** —*see* Air, pressure, change
- **Choked, choking** (on) (any object except food or vomitus)
  - food (bone) (seed) —*see* categories T17 and T18
  - vomitus T17.81-●
- **Civil insurrection** —*see* War operations
- **Cloudburst** (any injury) X37.8
- **Cold, exposure to** (accidental) (excessive) (extreme) (natural) (place) NEC —*see* Exposure, cold
- **Collapse**
  - building W2Ø.1
    - burning (uncontrolled fire) XØØ.2
  - dam or man-made structure (causing earth movement) X36.Ø
  - machinery —*see* Contact, with, by type of machine
  - structure W2Ø.1
    - burning (uncontrolled fire) XØØ.2
- **Collision** (accidental) NEC —*see also* Accident, transport V89.9
  - pedestrian W51
    - with fall WØ3
      - due to ice or snow WØØ.Ø
      - involving pedestrian conveyance —*see* Accident, transport, pedestrian, conveyance
    - and
      - crowd or human stampede (with fall) W52
      - object W22.8
        - with fall —*see* Fall, due to, bumping against, object
  - person(s) —*see* Collision, pedestrian
  - transport vehicle NEC V89.9
    - and
      - avalanche, fallen or not moving —*see* Accident, transport
        - falling or moving —*see* Landslide
      - landslide, fallen or not moving —*see* Accident, transport
        - falling or moving —*see* Landslide

Collision NEC *(Continued)*
  - transport vehicle NEC *(Continued)*
    - due to cataclysm —*see* Forces of nature, by type
    - intentional, purposeful suicide (attempt) —*see* Suicide, collision
- **Combustion, spontaneous** —*see* Ignition
- **Complication** (delayed) of or following (medical or surgical procedure) Y84.9
  - with misadventure —*see* Misadventure
  - amputation of limb(s) Y83.5
  - anastomosis (arteriovenous) (blood vessel) (gastrojejunal) (tendon) (natural or artificial material) Y83.2
  - aspiration (of fluid) Y84.4
    - tissue Y84.8
  - biopsy Y84.8
  - blood
    - sampling Y84.7
    - transfusion
      - procedure Y84.8
  - bypass Y83.2
  - catheterization (urinary) Y84.6
    - cardiac Y84.Ø
  - colostomy Y83.3
  - cystostomy Y83.3
  - dialysis (kidney) Y84.1
  - drug —*see* Table of Drugs and Chemicals
  - due to misadventure —*see* Misadventure
  - duodenostomy Y83.3
  - electroshock therapy Y84.3
  - external stoma, creation of Y83.3
  - formation of external stoma Y83.3
  - gastrostomy Y83.3
  - graft Y83.2
  - hypothermia (medically-induced) Y84.8
  - implant, implantation (of)
    - artificial
      - internal device (cardiac pacemaker) (electrodes in brain) (heart valve prosthesis) (orthopedic) Y83.1
      - material or tissue (for anastomosis or bypass) Y83.2
        - with creation of external stoma Y83.3
    - natural tissues (for anastomosis or bypass) Y83.2
      - with creation of external stoma Y83.3
  - infusion
    - procedure Y84.8
  - injection —*see* Table of Drugs and Chemicals
    - procedure Y84.8
  - insertion of gastric or duodenal sound Y84.5
  - insulin-shock therapy Y84.3
  - paracentesis (abdominal) (thoracic) (aspirative) Y84.4
  - procedures other than surgical operation —*see* Complication of or following, by type of procedure
  - radiological procedure or therapy Y84.2
  - removal of organ (partial) (total) NEC Y83.6
  - sampling
    - blood Y84.7
    - fluid NEC Y84.4
    - tissue Y84.8
  - shock therapy Y84.3
  - surgical operation NEC —*see also* Complication of or following, by type of operation Y83.9
    - reconstructive NEC Y83.4
      - with
        - anastomosis, bypass or graft Y83.2
        - formation of external stoma Y83.3
    - specified NEC Y83.8
  - transfusion —*see also* Table of Drugs and Chemicals
    - procedure Y84.8
  - transplant, transplantation (heart) (kidney) (liver) (whole organ, any) Y83.Ø
    - partial organ Y83.4
  - ureterostomy Y83.3

Complication of or following *(Continued)*
  - vaccination —*see also* Table of Drugs and Chemicals
    - procedure Y84.8
- **Compression**
  - divers' squeeze —*see* Air, pressure, change
  - trachea by
    - food (lodged in esophagus) —*see* categories T17 and T18
    - vomitus (lodged in esophagus) T17.81-●
- **Conflagration** —*see* Exposure, fire, uncontrolled
- **Constriction** (external)
  - hair W49.Ø1
  - jewelry W49.Ø4
  - ring W49.Ø4
  - rubber band W49.Ø3
  - specified item NEC W49.Ø9
  - string W49.Ø2
  - thread W49.Ø2
- **Contact** (accidental)
  - with
    - abrasive wheel (metalworking) W31.1
    - alligator W58.Ø9
      - bite W58.Ø1
      - crushing W58.Ø3
      - strike W58.Ø2
    - amphibian W62.9
      - frog W62.Ø
      - toad W62.1
    - animal (nonvenomous) NEC W64
      - marine W56.89
        - bite W56.81
        - dolphin —*see* Contact, with, dolphin
        - fish NEC —*see* Contact, with, fish
        - mammal —*see* Contact, with, mammal, marine
        - orca —*see* Contact, with, orca
        - sea lion —*see* Contact, with, sea lion
        - shark —*see* Contact, with, shark
        - strike W56.82
    - animate mechanical force NEC W64
    - arrow W21.89
      - not thrown, projected or falling W45.8
    - arthropods (nonvenomous) W57
    - axe W27.Ø
    - band-saw (industrial) W31.2
    - bayonet —*see* Bayonet wound
    - bee(s) X58
    - bench-saw (industrial) W31.2
    - bird W61.99
      - bite W61.91
      - chicken —*see* Contact, with, chicken
      - duck —*see* Contact, with, duck
      - goose —*see* Contact, with, goose
      - macaw —*see* Contact, with, macaw
      - parrot —*see* Contact, with, parrot
      - psittacine —*see* Contact, with, psittacine
      - strike W61.92
      - turkey —*see* Contact, with, turkey
    - blender W29.Ø
    - boiling water X12
      - stated as undetermined whether accidental or intentional Y27.2
      - suicide (attempt) X77.2
    - bore, earth-drilling or mining (land) (seabed) W31.Ø
    - buffalo —*see* Contact, with, hoof stock NEC
    - bull W55.29
      - bite W55.21
      - gored W55.22
      - strike W55.22
    - bumper cars W31.81
    - camel —*see* Contact, with, hoof stock NEC
    - can
      - lid W26.8
      - opener W27.4
        - powered W29.Ø
    - cat W55.Ø9
      - bite W55.Ø1
      - scratch W55.Ø3
    - caterpillar (venomous) X58

C

Contact *(Continued)*
with *(Continued)*
centipede (venomous) X58
chain
hoist W24.0
agricultural operations W30.89
saw W29.3
chicken W61.39
peck W61.33
strike W61.32
chisel W27.0
circular saw W31.2
cobra X58
combine (harvester) W30.0
conveyer belt W24.1
cooker (hot) X15.8
stated as undetermined whether accidental or intentional Y27.3
suicide (attempt) X77.3
coral X58
cotton gin W31.82
cow W55.29
bite W55.21
strike W55.22
crane W24.0
agricultural operations W30.89
crocodile W58.19
bite W58.11
crushing W58.13
strike W58.12
dagger W26.1
stated as undetermined whether accidental or intentional Y28.2
suicide (attempt) X78.2
dairy equipment W31.82
dart W21.89
not thrown, projected or falling W45.8
deer —*see* Contact, with, hoof stock NEC
derrick W24.0
agricultural operations W30.89
hay W30.2
dog W54.8
bite W54.0
strike W54.1
dolphin W56.09
bite W56.01
strike W56.02
donkey —*see* Contact, with, hoof stock NEC
drill (powered) W29.8
earth (land) (seabed) W31.0
nonpowered W27.8
drive belt W24.0
agricultural operations W30.89
dry ice —*see* Exposure, cold, man-made
dryer (clothes) (powered) (spin) W29.2
duck W61.69
bite W61.61
strike W61.62
earth(-)
drilling machine (industrial) W31.0
scraping machine in stationary use W31.83
edge of stiff paper W26.2
electric
beater W29.0
blanket X16
fan W29.2
commercial W31.82
knife W29.1
mixer W29.0
elevator (building) W24.0
agricultural operations W30.89
grain W30.3
engine(s), hot NEC X17
excavating machine W31.0
farm machine W30.9
feces —*see* Contact, with, by type of animal
fer de lance X58

Contact *(Continued)*
with *(Continued)*
fish W56.59
bite W56.51
shark —*see* Contact, with, shark
strike W56.52
flying horses W31.81
forging (metalworking) machine W31.1
fork W27.4
forklift (truck) W24.0
agricultural operations W30.89
frog W62.0
garden
cultivator (powered) W29.3
riding W30.89
fork W27.1
gas turbine W31.3
Gila monster X58
giraffe —*see* Contact, with, hoof stock NEC
glass (sharp) (broken) W25
with subsequent fall W18.02
assault X99.0
due to fall —*see* Fall, by type
stated as undetermined whether accidental or intentional Y28.0
suicide (attempt) X78.0
goat W55.39
bite W55.31
strike W55.32
goose W61.59
bite W61.51
strike W61.52
hand
saw W27.0
tool (not powered) NEC W27.8
powered W29.8
harvester W30.0
hay-derrick W30.2
heat NEC X19
from appliance (electrical) (household) —*see* Contact, with, hot, household appliance
heating appliance X16
heating
appliance (hot) X16
pad (electric) X16
hedge-trimmer (powered) W29.3
hoe W27.1
hoist (chain) (shaft) NEC W24.0
agricultural W30.89
hoof stock NEC W55.39
bite W55.31
strike W55.32
hornet(s) X58
horse W55.19
bite W55.11
strike W55.12
hot
air X14.1
inhalation X14.0
cooker X15.8
drinks X10.0
engine X17
fats X10.2
fluids NEC X12
assault X98.2
suicide (attempt) X77.2
undetermined whether accidental or intentional Y27.2
food X10.1
gases X14.1
inhalation X14.0
heating appliance X16
household appliance X15.8
assault X98.3
cooker X15.8
hotplate X15.2
kettle X15.8
light bulb X15.8

Contact *(Continued)*
with *(Continued)*
hot *(Continued)*
household appliance *(Continued)*
object NEC X19
assault X98.8
stated as undetermined whether accidental or intentional Y27.9
suicide (attempt) X77.8
saucepan X15.3
skillet X15.3
stated as undetermined whether accidental or intentional Y27.3
stove X15.0
suicide (attempt) X77.3
toaster X15.1
kettle X15.8
light bulb X15.8
liquid NEC —*see also* Burn X12
drinks X10.0
stated as undetermined whether accidental or intentional Y27.2
suicide (attempt) X77.2
tap water X11.8
stated as undetermined whether accidental or intentional Y27.1
suicide (attempt) X77.1
machinery X17
metal (molten) (liquid) NEC X18
object (not producing fire or flames) NEC X19
oil (cooking) X10.2
pipe X16
plate X15.2
radiator X16
saucepan (glass) (metal) X15.3
skillet X15.3
stove (kitchen) X15.0
substance NEC X19
tap-water X11.8
assault X98.1
heated on stove X12
stated as undetermined whether accidental or intentional Y27.2
suicide (attempt) X77.2
in bathtub X11.0
running X11.1
stated as undetermined whether accidental or intentional Y27.1
suicide (attempt) X77.1
toaster X15.1
tool X17
vapors X13.1
inhalation X13.0
water (tap) X11.8
boiling X12
stated as undetermined whether accidental or intentional Y27.2
suicide (attempt) X77.2
heated on stove X12
stated as undetermined whether accidental or intentional Y27.2
suicide (attempt) X77.2
in bathtub X11.0
running X11.1
stated as undetermined whether accidental or intentional Y27.1
suicide (attempt) X77.1
hotplate X15.2
ice-pick W27.4
insect (nonvenomous) NEC W57
kettle (hot) X15.8
knife W26.0
assault X99.1
electric W29.1
stated as undetermined whether accidental or intentional Y28.1
suicide (attempt) X78.1
lathe (metalworking) W31.1
turnings W45.8
woodworking W31.2

C

- **Contact** *(Continued)*
  - with *(Continued)*
    - lawnmower (powered) (ridden) W28
      - causing electrocution W86.8
        - suicide (attempt) X83.1
      - unpowered W27.1
    - lift, lifting (devices) W24.0
      - agricultural operations W30.89
      - shaft W24.0
    - liquefied gas —*see* Exposure, cold, man-made
    - liquid air, hydrogen, nitrogen —*see* Exposure, cold, man-made
    - lizard (nonvenomous) W59.09
      - bite W59.01
      - strike W59.02
    - llama —*see* Contact, with, hoof stock NEC
    - macaw W61.19
      - bite W61.11
      - strike W61.12
    - machine, machinery W31.9
      - abrasive wheel W31.1
      - agricultural including animal-powered W30.9
        - combine harvester W30.0
        - grain storage elevator W30.3
        - hay derrick W30.2
        - power take-off device W30.1
        - reaper W30.0
        - specified NEC W30.89
        - thresher W30.0
        - transport vehicle, stationary W30.81
      - band saw W31.2
      - bench saw W31.2
      - circular saw W31.2
      - commercial NEC W31.82
      - drilling, metal (industrial) W31.1
      - earth-drilling W31.0
      - earthmoving or scraping W31.89
      - excavating W31.89
      - forging machine W31.1
      - gas turbine W31.3
      - hot X17
      - internal combustion engine W31.3
      - land drill W31.0
      - lathe W31.1
      - lifting (devices) W24.0
      - metal drill W31.1
      - metalworking (industrial) W31.1
      - milling, metal W31.1
      - mining W31.0
      - molding W31.2
      - overhead plane W31.2
      - power press, metal W31.1
      - prime mover W31.3
      - printing W31.89
      - radial saw W31.2
      - recreational W31.81
      - roller-coaster W31.81
      - rolling mill, metal W31.1
      - sander W31.2
      - seabed drill W31.0
      - shaft
        - hoist W31.0
        - lift W31.0
      - specified NEC W31.89
      - spinning W31.89
      - steam engine W31.3
      - transmission W24.1
      - undercutter W31.0
      - water driven turbine W31.3
      - weaving W31.89
      - woodworking or forming (industrial) W31.2
    - mammal (feces) (urine) W55.89
      - bull —*see* Contact, with, bull
      - cat —*see* Contact, with, cat
      - cow —*see* Contact, with, cow
      - goat —*see* Contact, with, goat
      - hoof stock —*see* Contact, with, hoof stock

- **Contact** *(Continued)*
  - with *(Continued)*
    - mammal *(Continued)*
      - horse —*see* Contact, with, horse
      - marine W56.39
        - dolphin —*see* Contact, with, dolphin
        - orca —*see* Contact, with, orca
        - sea lion —*see* Contact, with, sea lion
        - specified NEC W56.39
          - bite W56.31
          - strike W56.32
      - pig —*see* Contact, with, pig
      - raccoon —*see* Contact, with, raccoon
      - rodent —*see* Contact, with, rodent
      - sheep —*see* Contact, with, sheep
      - specified NEC W55.89
        - bite W55.81
        - strike W55.82
    - marine
      - animal W56.89
        - bite W56.81
        - dolphin —*see* Contact, with, dolphin
        - fish NEC —*see* Contact, with, fish
        - mammal —*see* Contact, with, mammal, marine
        - orca —*see* Contact, with, orca
        - sea lion —*see* Contact, with, sea lion
        - shark —*see* Contact, with, shark
        - strike W56.82
    - meat
      - grinder (domestic) W29.0
        - industrial W31.82
        - nonpowered W27.4
      - slicer (domestic) W29.0
        - industrial W31.82
    - merry go round W31.81
    - metal, (hot) (liquid) (molten) NEC X18
    - millipede W57
    - nail W45.0
      - gun W29.4
    - needle (sewing) W27.3
      - hypodermic W46.0
        - contaminated W46.1
    - object (blunt) NEC
      - hot NEC X19
      - legal intervention —*see* Legal, intervention, blunt object
      - sharp NEC W45.8
        - inflicted by other person NEC W45.8
          - stated as
            - intentional homicide (attempt) —*see* Assault, cutting or piercing instrument
        - legal intervention —*see* Legal, intervention, sharp object
        - self-inflicted X78.9
    - orca W56.29
      - bite W56.21
      - strike W56.22
    - overhead plane W31.2
    - paper (as sharp object) W26.2
    - paper-cutter W27.5
    - parrot W61.09
      - bite W61.01
      - strike W61.02
    - pig W55.49
      - bite W55.41
      - strike W55.42
    - pipe, hot X16
    - pitchfork W27.1
    - plane (metal) (wood) W27.0
      - overhead W31.2
    - plant thorns, spines, sharp leaves or other mechanisms W60
    - powered
      - garden cultivator W29.3
      - household appliance, implement, or machine W29.8
      - saw (industrial) W31.2
        - hand W29.8
    - printing machine W31.89

- **Contact** *(Continued)*
  - with *(Continued)*
    - psittacine bird W61.29
      - bite W61.21
      - macaw —*see* Contact, with, macaw
      - parrot —*see* Contact, with, parrot
      - strike W61.22
    - pulley (block) (transmission) W24.0
      - agricultural operations W30.89
    - raccoon W55.59
      - bite W55.51
      - strike W55.52
    - radial-saw (industrial) W31.2
    - radiator (hot) X16
    - rake W27.1
    - rattlesnake X58
    - reaper W30.0
    - reptile W59.89
      - lizard —*see* Contact, with, lizard
      - snake —*see* Contact, with, snake
      - specified NEC W59.89
        - bite W59.81
        - crushing W59.83
        - strike W59.82
      - turtle —*see* Contact, with, turtle
    - rivet gun (powered) W29.4
    - road scraper —*see* Accident, transport, construction vehicle
    - rodent (feces) (urine) W53.89
      - bite W53.81
      - mouse W53.09
        - bite W53.01
      - rat W53.19
        - bite W53.11
      - specified NEC W53.89
        - bite W53.81
      - squirrel W53.29
        - bite W53.21
    - roller coaster W31.81
    - rope NEC W24.0
      - agricultural operations W30.89
    - saliva —*see* Contact, with, by type of animal
    - sander W29.8
      - industrial W31.2
    - saucepan (hot) (glass) (metal) X15.3
    - saw W27.0
      - band (industrial) W31.2
      - bench (industrial) W31.2
      - chain W29.3
      - hand W27.0
    - sawing machine, metal W31.1
    - scissors W27.2
    - scorpion X58
    - screwdriver W27.0
      - powered W29.8
    - sea
      - anemone, cucumber or urchin (spine) X58
      - lion W56.19
        - bite W56.11
        - strike W56.12
    - serpent —*see* Contact, with, snake, by type
    - sewing-machine (electric) (powered) W29.2
      - not powered W27.8
    - shaft (hoist) (lift) (transmission) NEC W24.0
      - agricultural W30.89
    - shark W56.49
      - bite W56.41
      - strike W56.42
    - sharp object(s) W26.9
      - specified NEC W26.8
    - shears (hand) W27.2
      - powered (industrial) W31.1
        - domestic W29.2
    - sheep W55.39
      - bite W55.31
      - strike W55.32
    - shovel W27.8
      - steam —*see* Accident, transport, construction vehicle

C

Contact *(Continued)*
with *(Continued)*
snake (nonvenomous) W59.19
bite W59.11
crushing W59.13
strike W59.12
spade W27.1
spider (venomous) X58
spin-drier W29.2
spinning machine W31.89
splinter W45.8
sports equipment W21.9
staple gun (powered) W29.8
steam X13.1
engine W31.3
inhalation X13.0
pipe X16
shovel W31.89
stove (hot) (kitchen) X15.0
substance, hot NEC X19
molten (metal) X18
sword W26.1
assault X99.2
stated as undetermined whether accidental or intentional Y28.2
suicide (attempt) X78.2
tarantula X58
thresher W30.0
tin can lid W26.8
toad W62.1
toaster (hot) X15.1
tool W27.8
hand (not powered) W27.8
auger W27.0
axe W27.0
can opener W27.4
chisel W27.0
fork W27.4
garden W27.1
handsaw W27.0
hoe W27.1
ice-pick W27.4
kitchen utensil W27.4
manual
lawn mower W27.1
sewing machine W27.8
meat grinder W27.4
needle (sewing) W27.3
hypodermic W46.0
contaminated W46.1
paper cutter W27.5
pitchfork W27.1
rake W27.1
scissors W27.2
screwdriver W27.0
specified NEC W27.8
workbench W27.0
hot X17
powered W29.8
blender W29.0
commercial W31.82
can opener W29.0
commercial W31.82
chainsaw W29.3
clothes dryer W29.2
commercial W31.82
dishwasher W29.2
commercial W31.82
edger W29.3
electric fan W29.2
commercial W31.82
electric knife W29.1
food processor W29.0
commercial W31.82
garbage disposal W29.0
commercial W31.82

Contact *(Continued)*
with *(Continued)*
tool *(Continued)*
powered *(Continued)*
garden tool W29.3
hedge trimmer W29.3
ice maker W29.0
commercial W31.82
kitchen appliance W29.0
commercial W31.82
lawn mower W28
meat grinder W29.0
commercial W31.82
mixer W29.0
commercial W31.82
rototiller W29.3
sewing machine W29.2
commercial W31.82
washing machine W29.2
commercial W31.82
transmission device (belt, cable, chain, gear, pinion, shaft) W24.1
agricultural operations W30.89
turbine (gas) (water-driven) W31.3
turkey W61.49
peck W61.43
strike W61.42
turtle (nonvenomous) W59.29
bite W59.21
strike W59.22
terrestrial W59.89
bite W59.81
crushing W59.83
strike W59.82
under-cutter W31.0
urine —*see* Contact, with, by type of animal
vehicle
agricultural use (transport) —*see* Accident, transport, agricultural vehicle
not on public highway W30.81
industrial use (transport) —*see* Accident, transport, industrial vehicle
not on public highway W31.83
off-road use (transport) —*see* Accident, transport, all-terrain or off-road vehicle
not on public highway W31.83
special construction use (transport) —*see* Accident, transport, construction vehicle
not on public highway W31.83
venomous
animal X58
arthropods X58
lizard X58
marine animal NEC X58
marine plant NEC X58
millipedes (tropical) X58
plant(s) X58
snake X58
spider X58
viper X58
washing-machine (powered) W29.2
wasp X58
weaving-machine W31.89
winch W24.0
agricultural operations W30.89
wire NEC W24.0
agricultural operations W30.89
wood slivers W45.8
yellow jacket X58
zebra —*see* Contact, with, hoof stock NEC
pressure X50.9
stress X50.9
Coup de soleil X32

Crash
aircraft (in transit) (powered) V95.9
balloon V96.01
fixed wing NEC (private) V95.21
commercial V95.31
glider V96.21
hang V96.11
powered V95.11
helicopter V95.01
in war operations —*see* War operations, destruction of aircraft
microlight V95.11
nonpowered V96.9
specified NEC V96.8
powered NEC V95.8
stated as
homicide (attempt) Y08.81
suicide (attempt) X83.0
ultralight V95.11
spacecraft V95.41
transport vehicle NEC —*see also* Accident, transport V89.9
homicide (attempt) Y03.8
motor NEC (traffic) V89.2
homicide (attempt) Y03.8
suicide (attempt) —*see* Suicide, collision
Cruelty (mental) (physical) (sexual) X58
Crushed (accidentally) X58
between objects (moving) (stationary and moving) W23.0
stationary W23.1
by
alligator W58.03
avalanche NEC —*see* Landslide
cave-in W20.0
caused by cataclysmic earth surface movement —*see* Landslide
crocodile W58.13
crowd or human stampede W52
falling
aircraft V97.39
in war operations —*see* War operations, destruction of aircraft
earth, material W20.0
caused by cataclysmic earth surface movement —*see* Landslide
object NEC W20.8
landslide NEC —*see* Landslide
lizard (nonvenomous) W59.09
machinery —*see* Contact, with, by type of machine
reptile NEC W59.89
snake (nonvenomous) W59.13
in
machinery —*see* Contact, with, by type of machine
Cut, cutting (any part of body) (accidental) —*see also* Contact, with, by object or machine
during medical or surgical treatment as misadventure —*see* Index to Diseases and Injuries, Complications
homicide (attempt) —*see* Assault, cutting or piercing instrument
inflicted by other person —*see* Assault, cutting or piercing instrument
legal
execution —*see* Legal, intervention
intervention —*see* Legal, intervention, sharp object
machine NEC —*see also* Contact, with, by type of machine W31.9
self-inflicted —*see* Suicide, cutting or piercing instrument
suicide (attempt) —*see* Suicide, cutting or piercing instrument
Cyclone (any injury) X37.1

D

- **Decapitation** (accidental circumstances)
  - NEC X58
  - homicide X99.9
  - legal execution —*see* Legal, intervention
- **Dehydration from lack of water** X58
- **Deprivation** X58
- **Derailment** (accidental)
  - railway (rolling stock) (train) (vehicle) (without antecedent collision) V81.7
    - with antecedent collision —*see* Accident, transport, railway vehicle occupant
  - streetcar (without antecedent collision) V82.7
    - with antecedent collision —*see* Accident, transport, streetcar occupant
- **Descent**
  - parachute (voluntary) (without accident to aircraft) V97.29
    - due to accident to aircraft —*see* Accident, transport, aircraft
- **Desertion** X58
- **Destitution** X58
- **Disability, late effect or sequela of injury** —*see* Sequelae
- **Discharge** (accidental)
  - airgun W34.010
    - assault X95.01
    - homicide (attempt) X95.01
    - stated as undetermined whether accidental or intentional Y24.0
    - suicide (attempt) X74.01
  - BB gun —*see* Discharge, airgun
  - firearm (accidental) W34.00
    - assault X95.9
    - handgun (pistol) (revolver) W32.0
      - assault X93
      - homicide (attempt) X93
      - legal intervention —*see* Legal, intervention, firearm, handgun
      - stated as undetermined whether accidental or intentional Y22
      - suicide (attempt) X72
    - homicide (attempt) X95.9
    - hunting rifle W33.02
      - assault X94.1
      - homicide (attempt) X94.1
      - legal intervention
        - injuring
          - bystander Y35.032
          - law enforcement personnel Y35.031
          - suspect Y35.033
          - ▶unspecified person Y35.039
      - stated as undetermined whether accidental or intentional Y23.1
      - suicide (attempt) X73.1
    - larger W33.00
      - assault X94.9
      - homicide (attempt) X94.9
      - hunting rifle —*see* Discharge, firearm, hunting rifle
      - legal intervention —*see* Legal, intervention, firearm by type of firearm
      - machine gun —*see* Discharge, firearm, machine gun
      - shotgun —*see* Discharge, firearm, shotgun
      - specified NEC W33.09
        - assault X94.8
        - homicide (attempt) X94.8
        - legal intervention
          - injuring
            - bystander Y35.092
            - law enforcement personnel Y35.091
            - suspect Y35.093
            - ▶unspecified person Y35.099
        - stated as undetermined whether accidental or intentional Y23.8
        - suicide (attempt) X73.8

Discharge *(Continued)*
- firearm *(Continued)*
  - larger *(Continued)*
    - stated as undetermined whether accidental or intentional Y23.9
    - suicide (attempt) X73.9
  - legal intervention
    - injuring
      - bystander Y35.002
      - law enforcement personnel Y35.001
      - suspect Y35.03
      - ▶unspecified person Y35.009
    - using rubber bullet
      - injuring
        - bystander Y35.042
        - law enforcement personnel Y35.041
        - suspect Y35.043
        - ▶unspecified person Y35.049
  - machine gun W33.03
    - assault X94.2
    - homicide (attempt) X94.2
    - legal intervention —*see* Legal, intervention, firearm, machine gun
    - stated as undetermined whether accidental or intentional Y23.3
    - suicide (attempt) X73.2
  - pellet gun —*see* Discharge, airgun
  - shotgun W33.01
    - assault X94.0
    - homicide (attempt) X94.0
    - legal intervention —*see* Legal, intervention, firearm, specified NEC
    - stated as undetermined whether accidental or intentional Y23.0
    - suicide (attempt) X73.0
  - specified NEC W34.09
    - assault X95.8
    - homicide (attempt) X95.8
    - legal intervention —*see* Legal, intervention, firearm, specified NEC
    - stated as undetermined whether accidental or intentional Y24.8
    - suicide (attempt) X74.8
  - stated as undetermined whether accidental or intentional Y24.9
  - suicide (attempt) X74.9
  - Very pistol W34.09
    - assault X95.8
    - homicide (attempt) X95.8
    - stated as undetermined whether accidental or intentional Y24.8
    - suicide (attempt) X74.8
- firework(s) W39
  - stated as undetermined whether accidental or intentional Y25
- gas-operated gun NEC W34.018
  - airgun —*see* Discharge, airgun
  - assault X95.09
  - homicide (attempt) X95.09
  - paintball gun —*see* Discharge, paintball gun
  - stated as undetermined whether accidental or intentional Y24.8
  - suicide (attempt) X74.09
- gun NEC —*see also* Discharge, firearm NEC
  - air —*see* Discharge, airgun
  - BB —*see* Discharge, airgun
  - for single hand use —*see* Discharge, firearm, handgun
  - hand —*see* Discharge, firearm, handgun
  - machine —*see* Discharge, firearm, machine gun
  - other specified —*see* Discharge, firearm NEC
  - paintball —*see* Discharge, paintball gun
  - pellet —*see* Discharge, airgun
- handgun —*see* Discharge, firearm, handgun
- machine gun —*see* Discharge, firearm, machine gun
- paintball gun W34.011
  - assault X95.02
  - homicide (attempt) X95.02

Discharge *(Continued)*
- paintball gun *(Continued)*
  - stated as undetermined whether accidental or intentional Y24.8
  - suicide (attempt) X74.02
- pistol —*see* Discharge, firearm, handgun
  - flare —*see* Discharge, firearm, Very pistol
  - pellet —*see* Discharge, airgun
  - Very —*see* Discharge, firearm, Very pistol
- revolver —*see* Discharge, firearm, handgun
- rifle (hunting) —*see* Discharge, firearm, hunting rifle
- shotgun —*see* Discharge, firearm, shotgun
- spring-operated gun NEC W34.018
  - assault X95.09
  - homicide (attempt) X95.09
  - stated as undetermined whether accidental or intentional Y24.8
  - suicide (attempt) X74.09

- **Disease**
  - Andes W94.11
  - aviator's —*see* Air, pressure
  - range W94.11
- **Diver's disease, palsy, paralysis, squeeze** —*see* Air, pressure
- **Diving** (into water) —*see* Accident, diving
- **Dog bite** W54.0
- **Dragged by transport vehicle NEC** —*see also* Accident, transport V09.9
- **Drinking poison** (accidental) —*see* Table of Drugs and Chemicals
- **Dropped** (accidentally) **while being carried or supported by other person** W04
- **Drowning** (accidental) W74
  - assault X92.9
  - due to
    - accident (to)
      - machinery —*see* Contact, with, by type of machine
      - watercraft V90.89
        - burning V90.29
          - powered V90.23
            - fishing boat V90.22
            - jet ski V90.23
            - merchant ship V90.20
            - passenger ship V90.21
          - unpowered V90.28
            - canoe V90.25
            - inflatable V90.26
            - kayak V90.25
            - sailboat V90.24
            - water skis V90.27
        - crushed V90.39
          - powered V90.33
            - fishing boat V90.32
            - jet ski V90.33
            - merchant ship V90.30
            - passenger ship V90.31
          - unpowered V90.38
            - canoe V90.35
            - inflatable V90.36
            - kayak V90.35
            - sailboat V90.34
            - water skis V90.37
        - overturning V90.09
          - powered V90.03
            - fishing boat V90.02
            - jet ski V90.03
            - merchant ship V90.00
            - passenger ship V90.01
          - unpowered V90.08
            - canoe V90.05
            - inflatable V90.06
            - kayak V90.05
            - sailboat V90.04
        - sinking V90.19
          - powered V90.13
            - fishing boat V90.12
            - jet ski V90.13
            - merchant ship V90.10
            - passenger ship V90.11

D

- Drowning *(Continued)*
  - due to *(Continued)*
    - accident *(Continued)*
      - watercraft *(Continued)*
        - sinking *(Continued)*
          - unpowered V9Ø.18
            - canoe V9Ø.15
            - inflatable V9Ø.16
            - kayak V9Ø.15
            - sailboat V9Ø.14
        - specified type NEC V9Ø.89
          - powered V9Ø.83
            - fishing boat V9Ø.82
            - jet ski V9Ø.83
            - merchant ship V9Ø.8Ø
            - passenger ship V9Ø.81
          - unpowered V9Ø.88
            - canoe V9Ø.85
            - inflatable V9Ø.86
            - kayak V9Ø.85
            - sailboat V9Ø.84
            - water skis V9Ø.87
    - avalanche —*see* Landslide
    - cataclysmic
      - earth surface movement NEC —*see* Forces of nature, earth movement
      - storm —*see* Forces of nature, cataclysmic storm
    - cloudburst X37.8
    - cyclone X37.1
    - fall overboard (from) V92.Ø9
      - powered craft V92.Ø3
        - ferry boat V92.Ø1
        - fishing boat V92.Ø2
        - jet ski V92.Ø3
        - liner V92.Ø1
        - merchant ship V92.ØØ
        - passenger ship V92.Ø1
      - resulting from
        - accident to watercraft —*see* Drowning, due to, accident to, watercraft
        - being washed overboard (from) V92.29
          - powered craft V92.23
            - ferry boat V92.21
            - fishing boat V92.22
            - jet ski V92.23
            - liner V92.21
            - merchant ship V92.2Ø
            - passenger ship V92.21
          - unpowered craft V92.28
            - canoe V92.25
            - inflatable V92.26
            - kayak V92.25
            - sailboat V92.24
            - surf-board V92.28
            - water skis V92.27
            - windsurfer V92.28
        - motion of watercraft V92.19
          - powered craft V92.13
            - ferry boat V92.11
            - fishing boat V92.12
            - jet ski V92.13
            - liner V92.11
            - merchant ship V92.1Ø
            - passenger ship V92.11
          - unpowered craft
            - canoe V92.15
            - inflatable V92.16
            - kayak V92.15
            - sailboat V92.14
      - unpowered craft V92.Ø8
        - canoe V92.Ø5
        - inflatable V92.Ø6
        - kayak V92.Ø5

- Drowning *(Continued)*
  - due to *(Continued)*
    - fall overboard *(Continued)*
      - unpowered craft *(Continued)*
        - sailboat V92.Ø4
        - surf-board V92.Ø8
        - water skis V92.Ø7
        - windsurfer V92.Ø8
    - hurricane X37.Ø
    - jumping into water from watercraft (involved in accident) —*see also* Drowning, due to, accident to, watercraft
      - without accident to or on watercraft W16.711
    - tidal wave NEC —*see* Forces of nature, tidal wave
    - torrential rain X37.8
  - following
    - fall
      - into
        - bathtub W16.211
        - bucket W16.221
        - fountain —*see* Drowning, following, fall, into, water, specified NEC
        - quarry —*see* Drowning, following, fall, into, water, specified NEC
        - reservoir —*see* Drowning, following, fall, into, water, specified NEC
        - swimming-pool W16.Ø11
          - stated as undetermined whether accidental or intentional Y21.3
          - striking
            - bottom W16.Ø21
            - wall W16.Ø31
          - suicide (attempt) X71.2
        - water NOS W16.41
          - natural (lake) (open sea) (river) (stream) (pond) W16.111
            - striking
              - bottom W16.121
              - side W16.131
          - specified NEC W16.311
            - striking
              - bottom W16.321
              - wall W16.331
      - overboard NEC —*see* Drowning, due to, fall overboard
    - jump or dive
      - from boat W16.711
        - striking bottom W16.721
      - into
        - fountain —*see* Drowning, following, jump or dive, into, water, specified NEC
        - quarry —*see* Drowning, following, jump or dive, into, water, specified NEC
        - reservoir —*see* Drowning, following, jump or dive, into, water, specified NEC
        - swimming-pool W16.511
          - striking
            - bottom W16.521
            - wall W16.531
          - suicide (attempt) X71.2
        - water NOS W16.91
          - natural (lake) (open sea) (river) (stream) (pond) W16.611
          - specified NEC W16.811
            - striking
              - bottom W16.821
              - wall W16.831
          - striking bottom W16.621

- Drowning *(Continued)*
  - homicide (attempt) X92.9
  - in
    - bathtub (accidental) W65
      - assault X92.Ø
      - following fall W16.211
        - stated as undetermined whether accidental or intentional Y21.1
      - stated as undetermined whether accidental or intentional Y21.Ø
      - suicide (attempt) X71.Ø
    - lake —*see* Drowning, in, natural water
    - natural water (lake) (open sea) (river) (stream) (pond) W69
      - assault X92.3
      - following
        - dive or jump W16.611
          - striking bottom W16.621
        - fall W16.111
          - striking
            - bottom W16.121
            - side W16.131
      - stated as undetermined whether accidental or intentional Y21.4
      - suicide (attempt) X71.3
    - quarry —*see* Drowning, in, specified place NEC
    - quenching tank —*see* Drowning, in, specified place NEC
    - reservoir —*see* Drowning, in, specified place NEC
    - river —*see* Drowning, in, natural water
    - sea —*see* Drowning, in, natural water
    - specified place NEC W73
      - assault X92.8
      - following
        - dive or jump W16.811
          - striking
            - bottom W16.821
            - wall W16.831
        - fall W16.311
          - striking
            - bottom W16.321
            - wall W16.331
      - stated as undetermined whether accidental or intentional Y21.8
      - suicide (attempt) X71.8
    - stream —*see* Drowning, in, natural water
    - swimming-pool W67
      - assault X92.1
        - following fall X92.2
      - following
        - dive or jump W16.511
          - striking
            - bottom W16.521
            - wall W16.531
        - fall W16.Ø11
          - striking
            - bottom W16.Ø21
            - wall W16.Ø31
      - stated as undetermined whether accidental or intentional Y21.2
        - following fall Y21.3
      - suicide (attempt) X71.1
        - following fall X71.2
    - war operations —*see* War operations, restriction of airway
  - resulting from accident to watercraft —*see* Drowning, due to, accident, watercraft
  - self-inflicted X71.9
  - stated as undetermined whether accidental or intentional Y21.9
  - suicide (attempt) X71.9

D

E

- **Earth** (surface) movement NEC —*see* Forces of nature, earth movement
- **Earth falling** (on) W2Ø.Ø
  - caused by cataclysmic earth surface movement or eruption —*see* Landslide
- **Earthquake** (any injury) X34
- **Effect(s)** (adverse) of
  - air pressure (any) —*see* Air, pressure
  - cold, excessive (exposure to) —*see* Exposure, cold
  - heat (excessive) —*see* Heat
  - hot place (weather) —*see* Heat
  - insolation X3Ø
  - late —*see* Sequelae
  - motion —*see* Motion
  - nuclear explosion or weapon in war operations —*see* War operations, nuclear weapon
  - radiation —*see* Radiation
  - travel —*see* Travel
- **Electric shock** (accidental) (by) (in) —*see* Exposure, electric current
- **Electrocution** (accidental) —*see* Exposure, electric current
- **Endotracheal tube wrongly placed during anesthetic procedure** Y65.3
- **Entanglement**
  - in
    - bed linen, causing suffocation —*see* category T71
    - wheel of pedal cycle V19.88
- **Entry of foreign body or material** —*see* Foreign body
- **Environmental pollution related condition** —*see* Z57
- **Execution, legal** (any method) —*see* Legal, intervention
- **Exhaustion**
  - cold —*see* Exposure, cold
  - due to excessive exertion —*see also* Overexertion X5Ø.9
  - heat —*see* Heat
- **Explosion** (accidental) (of) (with secondary fire) W4Ø.9
  - acetylene W4Ø.1
  - aerosol can W36.1
  - air tank (compressed) (in machinery) W36.2
  - aircraft (in transit) (powered) NEC V95.9
    - balloon V96.Ø5
    - fixed wing NEC (private) V95.25
      - commercial V95.35
    - glider V96.25
      - hang V96.15
      - powered V95.15
    - helicopter V95.Ø5
    - in war operations —*see* War operations, destruction of aircraft
    - microlight V95.15
    - nonpowered V96.9
      - specified NEC V96.8
    - powered NEC V95.8
    - stated as
      - homicide (attempt) YØ3.8
      - suicide (attempt) X83.Ø
    - ultralight V95.15
  - anesthetic gas in operating room W4Ø.1
  - antipersonnel bomb W4Ø.8
    - assault X96.Ø
    - homicide (attempt) X96.Ø
    - suicide (attempt) X75
  - assault X96.9
  - bicycle tire W37.Ø
  - blasting (cap) (materials) W4Ø.Ø
  - boiler (machinery), not on transport vehicle W35
    - on watercraft —*see* Explosion, in, watercraft
  - butane W4Ø.1
  - caused by other person X96.9
  - coal gas W4Ø.1

- **Explosion** *(Continued)*
  - detonator W4Ø.Ø
  - dump (munitions) W4Ø.8
  - dynamite W4Ø.Ø
    - in
      - assault X96.8
      - homicide (attempt) X96.8
      - legal intervention
        - injuring
          - bystander Y35.112
          - law enforcement personnel Y35.111
          - suspect Y35.113
          - ▶unspecified person Y35.119
      - suicide (attempt) X75
  - explosive (material) W4Ø.9
    - gas W4Ø.1
    - in blasting operation W4Ø.Ø
    - specified NEC W4Ø.8
      - in
        - assault X96.8
        - homicide (attempt) X96.8
        - legal intervention
          - injuring
            - bystander Y35.192
            - law enforcement personnel Y35.191
            - suspect Y35.193
            - ▶unspecified person Y35.199
        - suicide (attempt) X75
  - factory (munitions) W4Ø.8
  - fertilizer bomb W4Ø.8
    - assault X96.3
    - homicide (attempt) X96.3
    - suicide (attempt) X75
  - fire-damp W4Ø.1
  - firearm (parts) NEC W34.19
    - airgun W34.11Ø
    - BB gun W34.11Ø
    - gas, air or spring-operated gun NEC W34.118
    - handgun W32.1
    - hunting rifle W33.12
    - larger firearm W33.1Ø
      - specified NEC W33.19
    - machine gun W33.13
    - paintball gun W34.111
    - pellet gun W34.11Ø
    - shotgun W33.11
    - Very pistol [flare] W34.19
  - fireworks W39
  - gas (coal) (explosive) W4Ø.1
    - cylinder W36.9
      - aerosol can W36.1
      - air tank W36.2
      - pressurized W36.3
      - specified NEC W36.8
  - gasoline (fumes) (tank) not in moving motor vehicle W4Ø.1
    - bomb W4Ø.8
      - assault X96.1
      - homicide (attempt) X96.1
      - suicide (attempt) X75
    - in motor vehicle —*see* Accident, transport, by type of vehicle
  - grain store W4Ø.8
  - grenade W4Ø.8
    - in
      - assault X96.8
      - homicide (attempt) X96.8
      - legal intervention
        - injuring
          - bystander Y35.192
          - law enforcement personnel Y35.191
          - suspect Y35.193
          - ▶unspecified person Y35.199
      - suicide (attempt) X75
  - handgun (parts) —*see* Explosion, firearm, handgun (parts)
  - homicide (attempt) X96.9
    - antipersonnel bomb —*see* Explosion, antipersonnel bomb
    - fertilizer bomb —*see* Explosion, fertilizer bomb

- **Explosion** *(Continued)*
  - homicide *(Continued)*
    - gasoline bomb —*see* Explosion, gasoline bomb
    - letter bomb —*see* Explosion, letter bomb
    - pipe bomb —*see* Explosion, pipe bomb
    - specified NEC X96.8
  - hose, pressurized W37.8
  - hot water heater, tank (in machinery) W35
    - on watercraft —*see* Explosion, in, watercraft
  - in, on
    - dump W4Ø.8
    - factory W4Ø.8
    - mine (of explosive gases) NEC W4Ø.1
    - watercraft V93.59
      - powered craft V93.53
        - ferry boat V93.51
        - fishing boat V93.52
        - jet ski V93.53
        - liner V93.51
        - merchant ship V93.5Ø
        - passenger ship V93.51
        - sailboat V93.54
  - letter bomb W4Ø.8
    - assault X96.2
    - homicide (attempt) X96.2
    - suicide (attempt) X75
  - machinery —*see also* Contact, with, by type of machine
    - on board watercraft —*see* Explosion, in, watercraft
    - pressure vessel —*see* Explosion, by type of vessel
  - methane W4Ø.1
  - mine W4Ø.1
  - missile NEC W4Ø.8
  - mortar bomb W4Ø.8
    - in
      - assault X96.8
      - homicide (attempt) X96.8
      - legal intervention
        - injuring
          - bystander Y35.192
          - law enforcement personnel Y35.191
          - suspect Y35.193
          - ▶unspecified person Y35.199
      - suicide (attempt) X75
  - munitions (dump) (factory) W4Ø.8
  - pipe, pressurized W37.8
    - bomb W4Ø.8
      - assault X96.4
      - homicide (attempt) X96.4
      - suicide (attempt) X75
  - pressure, pressurized
    - cooker W38
    - gas tank (in machinery) W36.3
    - hose W37.8
    - pipe W37.8
    - specified device NEC W38
    - tire W37.8
      - bicycle W37.Ø
    - vessel (in machinery) W38
  - propane W4Ø.1
  - self-inflicted X75
  - shell (artillery) NEC W4Ø.8
    - during war operations —*see* War operations, explosion
    - in
      - legal intervention
        - injuring
          - bystander Y35.122
          - law enforcement personnel Y35.121
          - suspect Y35.123
          - ▶unspecified person Y35.129
      - war —*see* War operations, explosion
  - spacecraft V95.45
  - stated as undetermined whether accidental or intentional Y25
  - steam or water lines (in machinery) W37.8
  - stove W4Ø.9
  - suicide (attempt) X75

E

- **Explosion** *(Continued)*
  - tire, pressurized W37.8
    - bicycle W37.Ø
  - undetermined whether accidental or intentional Y25
  - vehicle tire NEC W37.8
    - bicycle W37.Ø
  - war operations —*see* War operations, explosion
- **Exposure** (to) X58
  - air pressure change —*see* Air, pressure
  - cold (accidental) (excessive) (extreme) (natural) (place) X31
    - assault YØ8.89
    - due to
      - man-made conditions W93.8
        - dry ice (contact) W93.Ø1
          - inhalation W93.Ø2
        - liquid air (contact) (hydrogen) (nitrogen) W93.11
          - inhalation W93.12
        - refrigeration unit (deep freeze) W93.2
        - suicide (attempt) X83.2
      - weather (conditions) X31
    - homicide (attempt) YØ8.89
    - self-inflicted X83.2
  - due to abandonment or neglect X58
  - electric current W86.8
    - appliance (faulty) W86.8
      - domestic W86.Ø
    - caused by other person YØ8.89
    - conductor (faulty) W86.1
    - control apparatus (faulty) W86.1
    - electric power generating plant, distribution station W86.1
    - electroshock gun —*see* Exposure, electric current, taser
    - high-voltage cable W85
    - homicide (attempt) YØ8.89
    - legal execution —*see* Legal, intervention, specified means NEC
    - lightning —*see* subcategory T75.Ø
    - live rail W86.8
    - misadventure in medical or surgical procedure in electroshock therapy Y63.4
    - motor (electric) (faulty) W86.8
      - domestic W86.Ø
    - self-inflicted X83.1
    - specified NEC W86.8
      - domestic W86.Ø
    - stun gun —*see* Exposure, electric current, taser
    - suicide (attempt) X83.1
    - taser W86.8
      - assault YØ8.89
      - legal intervention —*see* category Y35
      - self-harm (intentional) X83.8
      - undetermined intent Y33
    - third rail W86.8
    - transformer (faulty) W86.1
    - transmission lines W85
  - environmental tobacco smoke X58
  - excessive
    - cold —*see* Exposure, cold
    - heat (natural) NEC X3Ø
      - man-made W92
  - factor(s) NOS X58
    - environmental NEC X58
      - man-made NEC W99
      - natural NEC —*see* Forces of nature
    - specified NEC X58
  - fire, flames (accidental) XØ8.8
    - assault X97
    - campfire —*see* Exposure, fire, controlled, not in building
    - controlled (in)
      - with ignition (of) clothing —*see also* Ignition, clothes XØ6.2
        - nightwear XØ5
- **Exposure** *(Continued)*
  - fire, flames *(Continued)*
    - controlled *(Continued)*
      - bonfire —*see* Exposure, fire, controlled, not in building
      - brazier (in building or structure) —*see also* Exposure, fire, controlled, building
        - not in building or structure —*see* Exposure, fire, controlled, not in building
      - building or structure XØ2.Ø
        - with
          - fall from building XØ2.3
          - from building XØ2.5
          - injury due to building collapse XØ2.2
          - smoke inhalation XØ2.1
        - hit by object from building XØ2.4
        - specified mode of injury NEC XØ2.8
      - fireplace, furnace or stove —*see* Exposure, fire, controlled, building
      - not in building or structure XØ3.Ø
        - with
          - fall XØ3.3
          - smoke inhalation XØ3.1
        - hit by object XØ3.4
        - specified mode of injury NEC XØ3.8
      - trash —*see* Exposure, fire, controlled, not in building
    - fireplace —*see* Exposure, fire, controlled, building
    - fittings or furniture (in building or structure) (uncontrolled) —*see* Exposure, fire, uncontrolled, building
    - forest (uncontrolled) —*see* Exposure, fire, uncontrolled, not in building
    - grass (uncontrolled) —*see* Exposure, fire, uncontrolled, not in building
    - hay (uncontrolled) —*see* Exposure, fire, uncontrolled, not in building
    - homicide (attempt) X97
    - ignition of highly flammable material XØ4
    - in, of, on, starting in
      - machinery —*see* Contact, with, by type of machine
      - motor vehicle (in motion) —*see also* Accident, transport, occupant by type of vehicle V87.8
        - with collision —*see* Collision
      - railway rolling stock, train, vehicle V81.81
        - with collision —*see* Accident, transport, railway vehicle occupant
      - street car (in motion) V82.8
        - with collision —*see* Accident, transport, streetcar occupant
      - transport vehicle NEC —*see also* Accident, transport
        - with collision —*see* Collision
      - war operations —*see also* War operations, fire
        - from nuclear explosion —*see* War operations, nuclear weapons
      - watercraft (in transit) (not in transit) V91.Ø9
        - localized —*see* Burn, on board watercraft, due to, fire on board
        - powered craft V91.Ø3
          - ferry boat V91.Ø1
          - fishing boat V91.Ø2
          - jet skis V91.Ø3
          - liner V91.Ø1
          - merchant ship V91.ØØ
          - passenger ship V91.Ø1
        - unpowered craft V91.Ø8
          - canoe V91.Ø5
          - inflatable V91.Ø6
          - kayak V91.Ø5
          - sailboat V91.Ø4
- **Exposure** *(Continued)*
  - fire, flames *(Continued)*
    - in, of, on, starting in *(Continued)*
      - watercraft *(Continued)*
        - unpowered craft *(Continued)*
          - surf-board V91.Ø8
          - waterskis V91.Ø7
          - windsurfer V91.Ø8
    - lumber (uncontrolled) —*see* Exposure, fire, uncontrolled, not in building
    - mine (uncontrolled) —*see* Exposure, fire, uncontrolled, not in building
    - prairie (uncontrolled) —*see* Exposure, fire, uncontrolled, not in building
    - resulting from
      - explosion —*see* Explosion
      - lightning XØ8.8
    - self-inflicted X76
    - specified NEC XØ8.8
    - started by other person X97
    - stated as undetermined whether accidental or intentional Y26
    - stove —*see* Exposure, fire, controlled, building
    - suicide (attempt) X76
    - tunnel (uncontrolled) —*see* Exposure, fire, uncontrolled, not in building
    - uncontrolled
      - in building or structure XØØ.Ø
        - with
          - fall from building XØØ.3
          - injury due to building collapse XØØ.2
          - jump from building XØØ.5
          - smoke inhalation XØØ.1
        - bed XØ8.ØØ
          - due to
            - cigarette XØ8.Ø1
            - specified material NEC XØ8.Ø9
        - furniture NEC XØ8.2Ø
          - due to
            - cigarette XØ8.21
            - specified material NEC XØ8.29
        - hit by object from building XØØ.4
        - sofa XØ8.1Ø
          - due to
            - cigarette XØ8.11
            - specified material NEC XØ8.19
        - specified mode of injury NEC XØØ.8
      - not in building or structure (any) XØ1.Ø
        - with
          - fall XØ1.3
          - smoke inhalation XØ1.1
        - hit by object XØ1.4
        - specified mode of injury NEC XØ1.8
    - undetermined whether accidental or intentional Y26
  - forces of nature NEC —*see* Forces of nature
  - G-forces (abnormal) W49.9
  - gravitational forces (abnormal) W49.9
  - heat (natural) NEC —*see* Heat
  - high-pressure jet (hydraulic) (pneumatic) W49.9
  - hydraulic jet W49.9
  - inanimate mechanical force W49.9
  - jet, high-pressure (hydraulic) (pneumatic) W49.9
  - lightning —*see* subcategory T75.Ø
    - causing fire —*see* Exposure, fire
  - mechanical forces NEC W49.9
    - animate NEC W64
    - inanimate NEC W49.9
  - noise W42.9
    - supersonic W42.Ø
  - noxious substance —*see* Table of Drugs and Chemicals
  - pneumatic jet W49.9

E

Exposure *(Continued)*
prolonged in deep-freeze unit or refrigerator W93.2
radiation —*see* Radiation
smoke —*see also* Exposure, fire
tobacco, second hand Z77.22
specified factors NEC X58
sunlight X32
man-made (sun lamp) W89.8
tanning bed W89.1
supersonic waves W42.Ø
transmission line(s), electric W85
vibration W49.9

Exposure *(Continued)*
waves
infrasound W49.9
sound W42.9
supersonic W42.Ø
weather NEC —*see* Forces of nature

External cause status Y99.9
child assisting in compensated work for family Y99.8
civilian activity done for financial or other compensation Y99.Ø
civilian activity done for income or pay Y99.Ø

External cause status *(Continued)*
family member assisting in compensated work for other family member Y99.8
hobby not done for income Y99.8
leisure activity Y99.8
military activity Y99.1
off-duty activity of military personnel Y99.8
recreation or sport not for income or while a student Y99.8
specified NEC Y99.8
student activity Y99.8
volunteer activity Y99.2

F

Factors, supplemental
  alcohol
    blood level
      less than 20mg/100ml Y90.0
      presence in blood, level not specified Y90.9
      20-39mg/100ml Y90.1
      40-59mg/100ml Y90.2
      60-79mg/100ml Y90.3
      80-99mg/100ml Y90.4
      100-119mg/100ml Y90.5
      120-199mg/100ml Y90.6
      200-239mg/100ml Y90.7
      240mg/100ml or more Y90.8
    presence in blood, but level not specified Y90.9
  environmental-pollution-related condition —*see* Z57
  nosocomial condition Y95
  work-related condition Y99.0
Failure
  in suture or ligature during surgical procedure Y65.2
  mechanical, of instrument or apparatus (any) (during any medical or surgical procedure) Y65.8
  sterile precautions (during medical and surgical care) —*see* Misadventure, failure, sterile precautions, by type of procedure
  to
    introduce tube or instrument Y65.4
      endotracheal tube during anesthesia Y65.3
    make curve (transport vehicle) NEC —*see* Accident, transport
    remove tube or instrument Y65.4
Fall, falling (accidental) W19
  building W20.1
    burning (uncontrolled fire) X00.3
  down
    embankment W17.81
    escalator W10.0
    hill W17.81
    ladder W11
    ramp W10.2
    stairs, steps W10.9
  due to
    bumping against
      object W18.00
        sharp glass W18.02
        specified NEC W18.09
        sports equipment W18.01
      person W03
        due to ice or snow W00.0
        on pedestrian conveyance —*see* Accident, transport, pedestrian, conveyance
    collision with another person W03
      due to ice or snow W00.0
      involving pedestrian conveyance —*see* Accident, transport, pedestrian, conveyance
    grocery cart tipping over W17.82
    ice or snow W00.9
      from one level to another W00.2
        on stairs or steps W00.1
      involving pedestrian conveyance —*see* Accident, transport, pedestrian, conveyance
      on same level W00.0
    slipping (on moving sidewalk) W01.0
      with subsequent striking against object W01.10
        furniture W01.190
        sharp object W01.119
          glass W01.110
          power tool or machine W01.111
          specified NEC W01.118
        specified NEC W01.198

Fall, falling *(Continued)*
  due to *(Continued)*
    striking against
      object W18.00
        sharp glass W18.02
        specified NEC W18.09
        sports equipment W18.01
      person W03
        due to ice or snow W00.0
        on pedestrian conveyance —*see* Accident, transport, pedestrian, conveyance
  earth (with asphyxia or suffocation (by pressure)) —*see* Earth, falling
  from, off, out of
    aircraft NEC (with accident to aircraft NEC) V97.0
      while boarding or alighting V97.1
    balcony W13.0
    bed W06
    boat, ship, watercraft NEC (with drowning or submersion) —*see* Drowning, due to, fall overboard
      with hitting bottom or object V94.0
    bridge W13.1
    building W13.9
      burning (uncontrolled fire) X00.3
    cavity W17.2
    chair W07
    cherry picker W17.89
    cliff W15
    dock W17.4
    embankment W17.81
    escalator W10.0
    flagpole W13.8
    furniture NEC W08
    grocery cart W17.82
    haystack W17.89
    high place NEC W17.89
      stated as undetermined whether accidental or intentional Y30
    hole W17.2
    incline W10.2
    ladder W11
    lifting device W17.89
    machine, machinery —*see also* Contact, with, by type of machine
      not in operation W17.89
    manhole W17.1
    mobile elevated work platform [MEWP] W17.89
    motorized mobility scooter W05.2
    one level to another NEC W17.89
      intentional, purposeful, suicide (attempt) X80
      stated as undetermined whether accidental or intentional Y30
    pit W17.2
    playground equipment W09.8
      jungle gym W09.2
      slide W09.0
      swing W09.1
    quarry W17.89
    railing W13.9
    ramp W10.2
    roof W13.2
    scaffolding W12
    scooter (nonmotorized) W05.1
      motorized mobility W05.2
    sky lift W17.89
    stairs, steps W10.9
      curb W10.1
      due to ice or snow W00.1
      escalator W10.0
      incline W10.2
      ramp W10.2
      sidewalk curb W10.1
      specified NEC W10.8
    stepladder W11
    storm drain W17.1

Fall, falling *(Continued)*
  from, off, out of *(Continued)*
    streetcar NEC V82.6
      with antecedent collision —*see* Accident, transport, streetcar occupant
      while boarding or alighting V82.4
    structure NEC W13.8
      burning (uncontrolled fire) X00.3
    table W08
    toilet W18.11
      with subsequent striking against object W18.12
    train NEC V81.6
      during derailment (without antecedent collision) V81.7
        with antecedent collision —*see* Accident, transport, railway vehicle occupant
      while boarding or alighting V81.4
    transport vehicle after collision —*see* Accident, transport, by type of vehicle, collision
    tree W14
    vehicle (in motion) NEC —*see also* Accident, transport V89.9
      motor NEC —*see also* Accident, transport, occupant, by type of vehicle V87.8
      stationary W17.89
        while boarding or alighting —*see* Accident, transport, by type of vehicle, while boarding or alighting
    viaduct W13.8
    wall W13.8
    watercraft —*see also* Drowning, due to, fall overboard
      with hitting bottom or object V94.0
    well W17.0
    wheelchair, non-moving W05.0
      powered —*see* Accident, transport, pedestrian, conveyance occupant, specified type NEC
    window W13.4
  in, on
    aircraft NEC V97.0
      with accident to aircraft V97.0
      while boarding or alighting V97.1
    bathtub (empty) W18.2
      filled W16.212
        causing drowning W16.211
    escalator W10.0
    incline W10.2
    ladder W11
    machine, machinery —*see* Contact, with, by type of machine
    object, edged, pointed or sharp (with cut) —*see* Fall, by type
    playground equipment W09.8
      jungle gym W09.2
      slide W09.0
      swing W09.1
    ramp W10.2
    scaffolding W12
    shower W18.2
      causing drowning W16.211
    staircase, stairs, steps W10.9
      curb W10.1
      due to ice or snow W00.1
      escalator W10.0
      incline W10.2
      specified NEC W10.8
    streetcar (without antecedent collision) V82.5
      with antecedent collision —*see* Accident, transport, streetcar occupant
      while boarding or alighting V82.4

Fall, falling *(Continued)*
in, on *(Continued)*
train (without antecedent collision) V81.5
with antecedent collision —*see* Accident, transport, railway vehicle occupant
during derailment (without antecedent collision) V81.7
with antecedent collision —*see* Accident, transport, railway vehicle occupant
while boarding or alighting V81.4
transport vehicle after collision —*see* Accident, transport, by type of vehicle, collision
watercraft V93.39
due to
accident to craft V91.29
powered craft V91.23
ferry boat V91.21
fishing boat V91.22
jet ski V91.23
liner V91.21
merchant ship V91.2Ø
passenger ship V91.21
unpowered craft
canoe V91.25
inflatable V91.26
kayak V91.25
sailboat V91.24
powered craft V93.33
ferry boat V93.31
fishing boat V93.32
jet ski V93.33
liner V93.31
merchant ship V93.3Ø
passenger ship V93.31
unpowered craft V93.38
canoe V93.35
inflatable V93.36
kayak V93.35
sailboat V93.34
surf-board V93.38
windsurfer V93.38
into
cavity W17.2
dock W17.4
fire —*see* Exposure, fire, by type
haystack W17.89
hole W17.2
manhole W17.1
moving part of machinery —*see* Contact, with, by type of machine
ocean —*see* Fall, into, water
opening in surface NEC W17.89
pit W17.2
pond —*see* Fall, into, water
quarry W17.89
river —*see* Fall, into, water
shaft W17.89
storm drain W17.1
stream —*see* Fall, into, water
swimming pool —*see also* Fall, into, water, in, swimming pool
empty W17.3
tank W17.89
water W16.42
causing drowning W16.41
from watercraft —*see* Drowning, due to, fall overboard
hitting diving board W21.4
in
bathtub W16.212
causing drowning W16.211
bucket W16.222
causing drowning W16.221
natural body of water W16.112
causing drowning W16.111
striking
bottom W16.122
causing drowning W16.121

Fall, falling *(Continued)*
into *(Continued)*
water *(Continued)*
in *(Continued)*
natural body of water *(Continued)*
striking *(Continued)*
side W16.132
causing drowning W16.131
specified water NEC W16.312
causing drowning W16.311
striking
bottom W16.322
causing drowning W16.321
wall W16.332
causing drowning W16.331
swimming pool W16.Ø12
causing drowning W16.Ø11
striking
bottom W16.Ø22
causing drowning W16.Ø21
wall W16.Ø32
causing drowning W16.Ø31
utility bucket W16.222
causing drowning W16.221
well W17.Ø
involving
bed WØ6
chair WØ7
furniture NEC WØ8
glass —*see* Fall, by type
playground equipment WØ9.8
jungle gym WØ9.2
slide WØ9.Ø
swing WØ9.1
roller blades —*see* Accident, transport, pedestrian, conveyance
skateboard(s) —*see* Accident, transport, pedestrian, conveyance
skates (ice) (in line) (roller) —*see* Accident, transport, pedestrian, conveyance
skis —*see* Accident, transport, pedestrian, conveyance
table WØ8
wheelchair, non-moving WØ5.Ø
powered —*see* Accident, transport, pedestrian, conveyance, specified type NEC
object —*see* Struck by, object, falling
off
toilet W18.11
with subsequent striking against object W18.12
on same level W18.3Ø
due to
specified NEC W18.39
stepping on an object W18.31
out of
bed WØ6
building NEC W13.8
chair WØ7
furniture NEC WØ8
wheelchair, non-moving WØ5.Ø
powered —*see* Accident, transport, pedestrian, conveyance, specified type NEC
window W13.4
over
animal WØ1.Ø
cliff W15
embankment W17.81
small object WØ1.Ø
rock W2Ø.8
same level W18.3Ø
from
being crushed, pushed, or stepped on by a crowd or human stampede W52
collision, pushing, shoving, by or with other person WØ3
slipping, stumbling, tripping WØ1.Ø

Fall, falling *(Continued)*
same level *(Continued)*
involving ice or snow WØØ.Ø
involving skates (ice) (roller), skateboard, skis —*see* Accident, transport, pedestrian, conveyance
snowslide (avalanche) —*see* Landslide
stone W2Ø.8
structure W2Ø.1
burning (uncontrolled fire) XØØ.3
through
bridge W13.1
floor W13.3
roof W13.2
wall W13.8
window W13.4
timber W2Ø.8
tree (caused by lightning) W2Ø.8
while being carried or supported by other person(s) WØ4
Fallen on by
animal (not being ridden) NEC W55.89
Felo-de-se —*see* Suicide
Fight (hand) (fists) (foot) —*see* Assault, fight
Fire (accidental) —*see* Exposure, fire
Firearm discharge —*see* Discharge, firearm
Fireball effects from nuclear explosion in war operations —*see* War operations, nuclear weapons
Fireworks (explosion) W39
Flash burns from explosion —*see* Explosion
Flood (any injury) (caused by) X38
collapse of man-made structure causing earth movement X36.Ø
tidal wave —*see* Forces of nature, tidal wave
Food (any type) in
air passages (with asphyxia, obstruction, or suffocation) —*see* categories T17 and T18
alimentary tract causing asphyxia (due to compression of trachea) —*see* categories T17 and T18
Forces of nature X39.8
avalanche X36.1
causing transport accident —*see* Accident, transport, by type of vehicle
blizzard X37.2
cataclysmic storm X37.9
with flood X38
blizzard X37.2
cloudburst X37.8
cyclone X37.1
dust storm X37.3
hurricane X37.Ø
specified storm NEC X37.8
storm surge X37.Ø
tornado X37.1
twister X37.1
typhoon X37.Ø
cloudburst X37.8
cold (natural) X31
cyclone X37.1
dam collapse causing earth movement X36.Ø
dust storm X37.3
earth movement X36.1
caused by dam or structure collapse X36.Ø
earthquake X34
earthquake X34
flood (caused by) X38
dam collapse X36.Ø
tidal wave —*see* Forces of nature, tidal wave
heat (natural) X3Ø
hurricane X37.Ø
landslide X36.1
causing transport accident —*see* Accident, transport, by type of vehicle
lightning —*see* subcategory T75.Ø
causing fire —*see* Exposure, fire
mudslide X36.1
causing transport accident —*see* Accident, transport, by type of vehicle

F

Forces of nature *(Continued)*
radiation (natural) X39.Ø8
radon X39.Ø1
radon X39.Ø1
specified force NEC X39.8
storm surge X37.Ø
structure collapse causing earth movement X36.Ø
sunlight X32
tidal wave X37.41
due to
earthquake X37.41
landslide X37.43
storm X37.42
volcanic eruption X37.41
tornado X37.1
tsunami X37.41
twister X37.1
typhoon X37.Ø
volcanic eruption X35
Foreign body
aspiration —*see* Index to Diseases and Injuries, Foreign body, respitory tract
embedded in skin W45
entering through skin W45.8
can lid W26.2
nail W45.Ø
paper W26.2
specified NEC 45.8
splinter W45.8
Forest fire (exposure to) —*see* Exposure, fire, uncontrolled, not in building
Found injured X58
from exposure (to) —*see* Exposure
on
highway, road(way), street V89.9
railway right of way V81.9
Fracture (circumstances unknown or unspecified) X58
due to specified cause NEC X58
Freezing —*see* Exposure, cold
Frostbite X31
due to man-made conditions —*see* Exposure, cold, man-made
Frozen —*see* Exposure, cold

G

Gored by bull W55.22
Gunshot wound W34.ØØ

H

Hailstones, injured by X39.8
Hanged herself or himself —*see* Hanging, self-inflicted
Hanging (accidental) —*see also* category T71
legal execution —*see* Legal, intervention, specified means NEC
Heat (effects of) (excessive) X3Ø
due to
man-made conditions W92
on board watercraft V93.29
fishing boat V93.22
merchant ship V93.2Ø
passenger ship V93.21
sailboat V93.24
specified powered craft NEC V93.23
weather (conditions) X3Ø
from
electric heating apparatus causing burning X16
nuclear explosion in war operations —*see* War operations, nuclear weapons
inappropriate in local application or packing in medical or surgical procedure Y63.5
Hemorrhage
delayed following medical or surgical treatment without mention of misadventure —*see* Index to Diseases and Injuries, Complication(s)
during medical or surgical treatment as misadventure —*see* Index to Diseases and Injuries, Complication(s)
High
altitude (effects) —*see* Air, pressure, low
level of radioactivity, effects —*see* Radiation
pressure (effects) —*see* Air, pressure, high
temperature, effects —*see* Heat
Hit, hitting (accidental) by —*see* Struck by
Hitting against —*see* Striking against
Homicide (attempt) (justifiable) —*see* Assault
Hot
place, effects —*see also* Heat
weather, effects X3Ø
House fire (uncontrolled) —*see* Exposure, fire, uncontrolled, building
Humidity, causing problem X39.8
Hunger X58
Hurricane (any injury) X37.Ø
Hypobarism, hypobaropathy —*see* Air, pressure, low

I

- **Ictus**
  - caloris —*see also* Heat
  - solaris X3Ø
- **Ignition** (accidental) —*see also* Exposure, fire X08.8
  - anesthetic gas in operating room W4Ø.1
  - apparel XØ6.2
    - from highly flammable material XØ4
    - nightwear XØ5
  - bed linen (sheets) (spreads) (pillows) (mattress) —*see* Exposure, fire, uncontrolled, building, bed
  - benzine XØ4
  - clothes, clothing NEC (from controlled fire) XØ6.2
    - from
      - highly flammable material XØ4
  - ether XØ4
    - in operating room W4Ø.1
  - explosive material —*see* Explosion
  - gasoline XØ4
  - jewelry (plastic) (any) XØ6.Ø
  - kerosene XØ4
  - material
    - explosive —*see* Explosion
    - highly flammable with secondary explosion XØ4
  - nightwear XØ5
  - paraffin XØ4
  - petrol XØ4
- **Immersion** (accidental) —*see also* Drowning
  - hand or foot due to cold (excessive) X31
- **Implantation of quills of porcupine** W55.89
- **Inanition** (from) (hunger) X58
  - thirst X58.8
- **Inappropriate operation performed**
  - correct operation on wrong side or body part (wrong side) (wrong site) Y65.53
  - operation intended for another patient done on wrong patient Y65.52
  - wrong operation performed on correct patient Y65.51
- **Inattention after, at birth** (homicidal intent) (infanticidal intent) X58
- **Incident, adverse**
  - device
    - anesthesiology Y7Ø.8
      - accessory Y7Ø.2
      - diagnostic Y7Ø.Ø
      - miscellaneous Y7Ø.8
      - monitoring Y7Ø.Ø
      - prosthetic Y7Ø.2
      - rehabilitative Y7Ø.1
      - surgical Y7Ø.3
      - therapeutic Y7Ø.1
    - cardiovascular Y71.8
      - accessory Y71.2
      - diagnostic Y71.Ø
      - miscellaneous Y71.8
      - monitoring Y71.Ø
      - prosthetic Y71.2
      - rehabilitative Y71.1
      - surgical Y71.3
      - therapeutic Y71.1
    - gastroenterology Y73.8
      - accessory Y73.2
      - diagnostic Y73.Ø
      - miscellaneous Y73.8
      - monitoring Y73.Ø
      - prosthetic Y73.2
      - rehabilitative Y73.1
      - surgical Y73.3
      - therapeutic Y73.1
    - general
      - hospital Y74.8
        - accessory Y74.2
        - diagnostic Y74.Ø

- **Incident, adverse** *(Continued)*
  - device *(Continued)*
    - general *(Continued)*
      - hospital *(Continued)*
        - miscellaneous Y74.8
        - monitoring Y74.Ø
        - prosthetic Y74.2
        - rehabilitative Y74.1
        - surgical Y74.3
        - therapeutic Y74.1
      - surgical Y81.8
        - accessory Y81.2
        - diagnostic Y81.Ø
        - miscellaneous Y81.8
        - monitoring Y81.Ø
        - prosthetic Y81.2
        - rehabilitative Y81.1
        - surgical Y81.3
        - therapeutic Y81.1
    - gynecological Y76.8
      - accessory Y76.2
      - diagnostic Y76.Ø
      - miscellaneous Y76.8
      - monitoring Y76.Ø
      - prosthetic Y76.2
      - rehabilitative Y76.1
      - surgical Y76.3
      - therapeutic Y76.1
    - medical Y82.9
      - specified type NEC Y82.8
    - neurological Y75.8
      - accessory Y75.2
      - diagnostic Y75.Ø
      - miscellaneous Y75.8
      - monitoring Y75.Ø
      - prosthetic Y75.2
      - rehabilitative Y75.1
      - surgical Y75.3
      - therapeutic Y75.1
    - obstetrical Y76.8
      - accessory Y76.2
      - diagnostic Y76.Ø
      - miscellaneous Y76.8
      - monitoring Y76.Ø
      - prosthetic Y76.2
      - rehabilitative Y76.1
      - surgical Y76.3
      - therapeutic Y76.1
    - ophthalmic Y77.8
      - accessory Y77.2
      - diagnostic Y77.Ø
      - miscellaneous Y77.8
      - monitoring Y77.Ø
      - prosthetic Y77.2
      - rehabilitative Y77.1
      - surgical Y77.3
      - therapeutic Y77.1
    - orthopedic Y79.8
      - accessory Y79.2
      - diagnostic Y79.Ø
      - miscellaneous Y79.8
      - monitoring Y79.Ø
      - prosthetic Y79.2
      - rehabilitative Y79.1
      - surgical Y79.3
      - therapeutic Y79.1
    - otorhinolaryngological Y72.8
      - accessory Y72.2
      - diagnostic Y72.Ø
      - miscellaneous Y72.8
      - monitoring Y72.Ø
      - prosthetic Y72.2
      - rehabilitative Y72.1
      - surgical Y72.3
      - therapeutic Y72.1
    - personal use Y74.8
      - accessory Y74.2
      - diagnostic Y74.Ø
      - miscellaneous Y74.8
      - monitoring Y74.Ø
      - prosthetic Y74.2

- **Incident, adverse** *(Continued)*
  - device *(Continued)*
    - personal use *(Continued)*
      - rehabilitative Y74.1
      - surgical Y74.3
      - therapeutic Y74.1
    - physical medicine Y8Ø.8
      - accessory Y8Ø.2
      - diagnostic Y8Ø.Ø
      - miscellaneous Y8Ø.8
      - monitoring Y8Ø.Ø
      - prosthetic Y8Ø.2
      - rehabilitative Y8Ø.1
      - surgical Y8Ø.3
      - therapeutic Y8Ø.1
    - plastic surgical Y81.8
      - accessory Y81.2
      - diagnostic Y81.Ø
      - miscellaneous Y81.8
      - monitoring Y81.Ø
      - prosthetic Y81.2
      - rehabilitative Y81.1
      - surgical Y81.3
      - therapeutic Y81.1
    - radiological Y78.8
      - accessory Y78.2
      - diagnostic Y78.Ø
      - miscellaneous Y78.8
      - monitoring Y78.Ø
      - prosthetic Y78.2
      - rehabilitative Y78.1
      - surgical Y78.3
      - therapeutic Y78.1
    - urology Y73.8
      - accessory Y73.2
      - diagnostic Y73.Ø
      - miscellaneous Y73.8
      - monitoring Y73.Ø
      - prosthetic Y73.2
      - rehabilitative Y73.1
      - surgical Y73.3
      - therapeutic Y73.1
- **Incineration** (accidental) —*see* Exposure, fire
- **Infanticide** —*see* Assault
- **Infrasound waves** (causing injury) W49.9
- **Ingestion**
  - foreign body (causing injury) (with obstruction) —*see* Foreign body, alimentary canal
  - poisonous
    - plant(s) X58
    - substance NEC —*see* Table of Drugs and Chemicals
- **Inhalation**
  - excessively cold substance, man-made —*see* Exposure, cold, man-made
  - food (any type) (into respiratory tract) (with asphyxia, obstruction respiratory tract, suffocation) —*see* categories T17 and T18
  - foreign body —*see* Foreign body, aspiration
  - gastric contents (with asphyxia, obstruction respiratory passage, suffocation) T17.81- ●
  - hot air or gases X14.Ø
  - liquid air, hydrogen, nitrogen W93.12
    - suicide (attempt) X83.2
  - steam X13.Ø
    - assault X98.Ø
    - stated as undetermined whether accidental or intentional Y27.Ø
    - suicide (attempt) X77.Ø
  - toxic gas —*see* Table of Drugs and Chemicals
  - vomitus (with asphyxia, obstruction respiratory passage, suffocation) T17.81- ●
- **Injury, injured** (accidental(ly)) NOS X58
  - by, caused by, from
    - assault —*see* Assault
    - law-enforcing agent, police, in course of legal intervention —*see* Legal intervention
    - suicide (attempt) X83.8

Injury, injured NOS *(Continued)*
- due to, in
  - civil insurrection —*see* War operations
  - fight —*see also* Assault, fight Y04.0
  - war operations —*see* War operations
- homicide —*see also* Assault Y09
- inflicted (by)
  - in course of arrest (attempted), suppression of disturbance, maintenance of order, by law-enforcing agents —*see* Legal intervention

Injury, injured NOS *(Continued)*
- inflicted *(Continued)*
  - other person
    - stated as
      - accidental X58
      - intentional, homicide (attempt) —*see* Assault
      - undetermined whether accidental or intentional Y33
- purposely (inflicted) by other person(s) —*see* Assault
- self-inflicted X83.8
  - stated as accidental X58
- specified cause NEC X58

Injury, injured NOS *(Continued)*
- undetermined whether accidental or intentional Y33

Insolation, effects X30
Insufficient nourishment X58
Interruption of respiration (by)
- food (lodged in esophagus) —*see* categories T17 and T18
- vomitus (lodged in esophagus) T17.81- ●

Intervention, legal —*see* Legal intervention
Intoxication
- drug —*see* Table of Drugs and Chemicals
- poison —*see* Table of Drugs and Chemicals

J

Jammed (accidentally)
- between objects (moving) (stationary and moving) W23.0
  - stationary W23.1

Jumped, jumping
- before moving object NEC X81.8
  - motor vehicle X81.0
  - subway train X81.1
  - train X81.1
  - undetermined whether accidental or intentional Y31
- from
  - boat (into water) voluntarily, without accident (to or on boat) W16.712
    - with
      - accident to or on boat —*see* Accident, watercraft
      - drowning or submersion W16.711
        - suicide (attempt) X71.3

Jumped, jumping *(Continued)*
- from *(Continued)*
  - boat voluntarily, without accident *(Continued)*
    - striking bottom W16.722
      - causing drowning W16.721
  - building —*see also* Jumped, from, high place W13.9
    - burning (uncontrolled fire) X00.5
  - high place NEC W17.89
    - suicide (attempt) X80
    - undetermined whether accidental or intentional Y30
  - structure —*see also* Jumped, from, high place W13.9
    - burning (uncontrolled fire) X00.5
- into water W16.92
  - causing drowning W16.91
  - from, off watercraft —*see* Jumped, from, boat

Jumped, jumping *(Continued)*
- into water *(Continued)*
  - in
    - natural body W16.612
      - causing drowning W16.611
      - striking bottom W16.622
        - causing drowning W16.621
    - specified place NEC W16.812
      - causing drowning W16.811
      - striking
        - bottom W16.822
          - causing drowning W16.821
        - wall W16.832
          - causing drowning W16.831
    - swimming pool W16.512
      - causing drowning W16.511
      - striking
        - bottom W16.522
          - causing drowning W16.521
        - wall W16.532
          - causing drowning W16.531
  - suicide (attempt) X71.3

K

Kicked by
- animal NEC W55.82
- person(s) (accidentally) W50.1
  - with intent to injure or kill Y04.0
  - as, or caused by, a crowd or human stampede (with fall) W52
  - assault Y04.0
  - homicide (attempt) Y04.0
  - in
    - fight Y04.0
    - legal intervention
      - injuring
        - bystander Y35.812
        - law enforcement personnel Y35.811
        - suspect Y35.813
        - ▶unspecified person Y35.819

Kicking
- against
  - object W22.8
    - sports equipment W21.9
    - stationary W22.09
      - sports equipment W21.89
  - person —*see* Striking against, person
  - sports equipment W21.9
- carpet stretcher with knee X50.3

Killed, killing (accidentally) **NOS** —*see also* Injury X58
- in
  - action —*see* War operations
  - brawl, fight (hand) (fists) (foot) Y04.0
    - by weapon —*see also* Assault
      - cutting, piercing —*see* Assault, cutting or piercing instrument
      - firearm —*see* Discharge, firearm, by type, homicide

Killed, killing NOS *(Continued)*
- self
  - stated as
    - accident NOS X58
    - suicide —*see* Suicide
    - undetermined whether accidental or intentional Y33

Kneeling (prolonged) (static) X50.1
Knocked down (accidentally) (by) **NOS** X58
- animal (not being ridden) NEC —*see also* Struck by, by type of animal
- crowd or human stampede W52
- person W51
  - in brawl, fight Y04.0
- transport vehicle NEC —*see also* Accident, transport V09.9

L

- **Laceration NEC** —*see* Injury
- **Lack of**
  - care (helpless person) (infant) (newborn) X58
  - food except as result of abandonment or neglect X58
    - due to abandonment or neglect X58
  - water except as result of transport accident X58
    - due to transport accident —*see* Accident, transport, by type
    - helpless person, infant, newborn X58
- **Landslide** (falling on transport vehicle) X36.1
  - caused by collapse of man-made structure X36.Ø
- **Late effect** —*see* Sequelae
- **Legal**
  - execution (any method) —*see* Legal, intervention
  - intervention (by)
    - baton —*see* Legal, intervention, blunt object, baton
    - bayonet —*see* Legal, intervention, sharp object, bayonet
    - blow —*see* Legal, intervention, manhandling
    - blunt object
      - baton
        - injuring
          - bystander Y35.312
          - law enforcement personnel Y35.311
          - suspect Y35.313
          - ▶unspecified person Y35.319
      - injuring
        - bystander Y35.3Ø2
        - law enforcement personnel Y35.3Ø1
        - suspect Y35.3Ø3
        - ▶unspecified person Y35.3Ø9
      - specified NEC
        - injuring
          - bystander Y35.392
          - law enforcement personnel Y35.391
          - suspect Y35.393
          - ▶unspecified person Y35.399
      - stave
        - injuring
          - bystander Y35.392
          - law enforcement personnel Y35.391
          - suspect Y35.393
          - ▶unspecified person Y35.399
    - bomb —*see* Legal, intervention, explosive
    - ▶conducted energy device
      - ▶injuring
        - ▶bystander Y35.832
        - ▶law enforcement personnel Y35.831
        - ▶suspect Y35.833
        - ▶unspecified person Y35.839
    - cutting or piercing instrument —*see* Legal, intervention, sharp object
    - dynamite —*see* Legal, intervention, explosive, dynamite
    - ▶electroshock device (taser)
      - ▶injuring
        - ▶bystander Y35.832
        - ▶law enforcement personnel Y35.831
        - ▶suspect Y35.833
        - ▶unspecified person Y35.839
    - explosive(s)
      - dynamite
        - injuring
          - bystander Y35.112
          - law enforcement personnel Y35.111
          - suspect Y35.113
          - ▶unspecified person Y35.119
      - grenade
        - injuring
          - bystander Y35.192
          - law enforcement personnel Y35.191
          - suspect Y35.193
          - ▶unspecified person Y35.199

Legal *(Continued)*
- intervention *(Continued)*
  - explosive *(Continued)*
    - injuring
      - bystander Y35.1Ø2
      - law enforcement personnel Y35.1Ø1
      - suspect Y35.1Ø3
      - ▶unspecified person Y35.1Ø9
    - mortar bomb
      - injuring
        - bystander Y35.192
        - law enforcement personnel Y35.191
        - suspect Y35.193
        - ▶unspecified person Y35.199
    - shell
      - injuring
        - bystander Y35.122
        - law enforcement personnel Y35.121
        - suspect Y35.123
        - ▶unspecified person Y35.129
    - specified NEC
      - injuring
        - bystander Y35.192
        - law enforcement personnel Y35.191
        - suspect Y35.193
        - ▶unspecified person Y35.199
  - firearm(s) (discharge)
    - handgun
      - injuring
        - bystander Y35.Ø22
        - law enforcement personnel Y35.Ø21
        - suspect Y35.Ø23
        - ▶unspecified person Y35.Ø29
    - injuring
      - bystander Y35.ØØ2
      - law enforcement personnel Y35.ØØ1
      - suspect Y35.ØØ3
      - ▶unspecified person Y35.ØØ9
    - machine gun
      - injuring
        - bystander Y35.Ø12
        - law enforcement personnel Y35.Ø11
        - suspect Y35.Ø13
        - ▶unspecified person Y35.Ø19
    - rifle pellet
      - injuring
        - bystander Y35.Ø32
        - law enforcement personnel Y35.Ø31
        - suspect Y35.Ø33
        - ▶unspecified person Y35.Ø39
    - rubber bullet
      - injuring
        - bystander Y35.Ø42
        - law enforcement personnel Y35.Ø41
        - suspect Y35.Ø43
        - ▶unspecified person Y35.Ø49
    - shotgun —*see* Legal, intervention, firearm, specified NEC
    - specified NEC
      - injuring
        - bystander Y35.Ø92
        - law enforcement personnel Y35.Ø91
        - suspect Y35.Ø93
        - ▶unspecified person Y35.Ø99
  - gas (asphyxiation) (poisoning)
    - injuring
      - bystander Y35.2Ø2
      - law enforcement personnel Y35.2Ø1
      - suspect Y35.2Ø3
      - ▶unspecified person Y35.2Ø9
    - specified NEC
      - injuring
        - bystander Y35.292
        - law enforcement personnel Y35.291
        - suspect Y35.293
        - ▶unspecified person Y35.299
    - tear gas
      - injuring
        - bystander Y35.212
        - law enforcement personnel Y35.211
        - suspect Y35.213
        - ▶unspecified person Y35.219

Legal *(Continued)*
- intervention *(Continued)*
  - grenade —*see* Legal, intervention, explosive, grenade
  - injuring
    - bystander Y35.92
    - law enforcement personnel Y35.91
    - suspect Y35.93
    - ▶unspecified person Y35.99
  - late effect (of) —*see* with 7th character S Y35
  - manhandling
    - injuring
      - bystander Y35.812
      - law enforcement personnel Y35.811
      - suspect Y35.813
      - ▶unspecified person Y35.819
  - sequelae (of) —*see* with 7th character S Y35
  - sharp objects
    - bayonet
      - injuring
        - bystander Y35.412
        - law enforcement personnel Y35.411
        - suspect Y35.413
        - ▶unspecified person Y35.419
    - injuring
      - bystander Y35.4Ø2
      - law enforcement personnel Y35.4Ø1
      - suspect Y35.4Ø3
      - ▶unspecified person Y35.4Ø9
    - specified NEC
      - injuring
        - bystander Y35.492
        - law enforcement personnel Y35.491
        - suspect Y35.493
        - ▶unspecified person Y35.499
  - specified means NEC
    - injuring
      - bystander Y35.892
      - law enforcement personnel Y35.891
      - suspect Y35.893
  - stabbing —*see* Legal, intervention, sharp object
  - stave —*see* Legal, intervention, blunt object, stave
  - ▶stun gun
    - ▶injuring
      - ▶bystander Y35.832
      - ▶law enforcement personnel Y35.831
      - ▶suspect Y35.833
      - ▶unspecified person Y35.839
  - ▶taser
    - ▶injuring
    - ▶bystander Y35.832
    - ▶law enforcement personnel Y35.831
    - ▶suspect Y35.833
    - ▶unspecified person Y35.839
  - tear gas —*see* Legal, intervention, gas, tear gas
  - truncheon —*see* Legal, intervention, blunt object, stave
- **Lifting** —*see also* Overexertion
  - heavy objects X5Ø.Ø
  - weights X5Ø.Ø
- **Lightning** (shock) (stroke) (struck by) —*see* subcategory T75.Ø
  - causing fire —*see* Exposure, fire
- **Loss of control** (transport vehicle) NEC —*see* Accident, transport
- **Lost at sea NOS** —*see* Drowning, due to, fall overboard
- **Low**
  - pressure (effects) —*see* Air, pressure, low
  - temperature (effects) —*see* Exposure, cold
- **Lying before train, vehicle or other moving object** X81.8
  - subway train X81.1
  - train X81.1
  - undetermined whether accidental or intentional Y31
- **Lynching** —*see* Assault

L

M

- **Malfunction** (mechanism or component) (of)
  - firearm
    - airgun W34.1Ø
    - BB gun W34.11Ø
    - gas, air or spring-operated gun NEC W34.118
    - handgun W32.1
    - hunting rifle W33.12
    - larger firearm W33.1Ø
      - specified NEC W33.19
    - machine gun W33.13
    - paintball gun W34.111
    - pellet gun W34.11Ø
    - shotgun W33.11
    - specified NEC W34.19
    - Very pistol [flare] W34.19
  - handgun —*see* Malfunction, firearm, handgun
- **Maltreatment** —*see* Perpetrator
- **Mangled** (accidentally) NOS X58
- **Manhandling** (in brawl, fight) YØ4.Ø
  - legal intervention —*see* Legal, intervention, manhandling
- **Manslaughter** (nonaccidental) —*see* Assault
- **Mauled by animal NEC** W55.89
- **Medical procedure, complication of** (delayed or as an abnormal reaction without mention of misadventure) —*see* Complication of or following, by specified type of procedure
  - due to or as a result of misadventure —*see* Misadventure
- **Melting** (due to fire) —*see also* Exposure, fire
  - apparel NEC XØ6.3
  - clothes, clothing NEC XØ6.3
    - nightwear XØ5
  - fittings or furniture (burning building) (uncontrolled fire) XØØ.8
  - nightwear XØ5
  - plastic jewelry XØ6.1
- **Mental cruelty** X58
- **Military operations** (injuries to military and civilians occuring during peacetime on military property and during routine military exercises and operations) (by) (from) (involving) Y37.9Ø-•
  - air blast Y37.2Ø-•
  - aircraft
    - destruction —*see* Military operations, destruction of aircraft
  - airway restriction —*see* Military operations, restriction of airways
  - asphyxiation —*see* Military operations, restriction of airways
  - biological weapons Y37.6X-•
  - blast Y37.2Ø-•
  - blast fragments Y37.2Ø-•
  - blast wave Y37.2Ø-•
  - blast wind Y37.2Ø-•
  - bomb Y37.2Ø-•
    - dirty Y37.5Ø-•
    - gasoline Y37.31-•
    - incendiary Y37.31-•
    - petrol Y37.31-•
  - bullet Y37.43-•
    - incendiary Y37.32-•
    - rubber Y37.41-•
  - chemical weapons Y37.7X-•
  - combat
    - hand to hand (unarmed) combat Y37.44-•
    - using blunt or piercing object Y37.45-•
  - conflagration —*see* Military operations, fire
  - conventional warfare NEC Y37.49-•
  - depth-charge Y37.Ø1-•
  - destruction of aircraft Y37.1Ø-•
    - due to
      - air to air missile Y37.11-•
      - collision with other aircraft Y37.12-•

Military operations *(Continued)*
  - destruction of aircraft *(Continued)*
    - due to *(Continued)*
      - detonation (accidental) of onboard munitions and explosives Y37.14-•
      - enemy fire or explosives Y37.11-•
      - explosive placed on aircraft Y37.11-•
      - onboard fire Y37.13-•
      - rocket propelled grenade [RPG] Y37.11-•
      - small arms fire Y37.11-•
      - surface to air missile Y37.11-•
    - specified NEC Y37.19-•
  - detonation (accidental) of
    - onboard marine weapons Y37.Ø5-•
    - own munitions or munitions launch device Y37.24-•
  - dirty bomb Y37.5Ø-•
  - explosion (of) Y37.2Ø-•
    - aerial bomb Y37.21-•
    - bomb NOS —*see also* Military operations, bomb(s) Y37.2Ø-•
    - fragments Y37.2Ø-•
    - grenade Y37.29-•
    - guided missile Y37.22-•
    - improvised explosive device [IED] (person-borne) (roadside) (vehicle-borne) Y37.23-•
    - land mine Y37.29-•
    - marine mine (at sea) (in harbor) Y37.Ø2-•
    - marine weapon Y37.ØØ-•
      - specified NEC Y37.Ø9-•
    - own munitions or munitions launch device (accidental) Y37.24-•
    - sea-based artillery shell Y37.Ø3-•
    - specified NEC Y37.29-•
    - torpedo Y37.Ø4-•
  - fire Y37.3Ø-•
    - specified NEC Y37.39-•
  - firearms
    - discharge Y37.43-•
    - pellets Y37.42-•
  - flamethrower Y37.33-•
  - fragments (from) (of)
    - improvised explosive device [IED] (person-borne) (roadside) (vehicle-borne) Y37.26-•
    - munitions Y37.25-•
    - specified NEC Y37.29-•
    - weapons Y37.27-•
  - friendly fire Y37.92-•
  - hand to hand (unarmed) combat Y37.44-•
  - hot substances —*see* Military operations, fire
  - incendiary bullet Y37.32-•
  - nuclear weapon (effects of) Y37.5Ø-•
    - acute radiation exposure Y37.54-•
    - blast pressure Y37.51-•
    - direct blast Y37.51-•
    - direct heat Y37.53-•
    - fallout exposure Y37.54-•
    - fireball Y37.53-•
    - indirect blast (struck or crushed by blast debris) (being thrown by blast) Y37.52-•
    - ionizing radiation (immediate exposure) Y37.54-•
    - nuclear radiation Y37.54-•
    - radiation
      - ionizing (immediate exposure) Y37.54-•
      - nuclear Y37.54-•
      - thermal Y37.53-•
    - secondary effects Y37.54-•
    - specified NEC Y37.59-•
    - thermal radiation Y37.53-•
  - restriction of air (airway)
    - intentional Y37.46-•
    - unintentional Y37.47-•
  - rubber bullets Y37.41-•
  - shrapnel NOS Y37.29-•
  - suffocation —*see* Military operations, restriction of airways
  - unconventional warfare NEC Y37.7X-•

Military operations *(Continued)*
  - underwater blast NOS Y37.ØØ-•
  - warfare
    - conventional NEC Y37.49-•
    - unconventional NEC Y37.7X-•
  - weapon of mass destruction [WMD] Y37.91-•
  - weapons
    - biological weapons Y37.6X-•
    - chemical Y37.7X-•
    - nuclear (effects of) Y37.5Ø-•
      - acute radiation exposure Y37.54-•
      - blast pressure Y37.51-•
      - direct blast Y37.51-•
      - direct heat Y37.53-•
      - fallout exposure Y37.54-•
      - fireball Y37.53-•
      - radiation
        - ionizing (immediate exposure) Y37.54-•
        - nuclear Y37.54-•
        - thermal Y37.53-•
      - secondary effects Y37.54-•
      - specified NEC Y37.59-•
    - of mass destruction [WMD] Y37.91-•
- **Misadventure(s) to patient(s) during surgical or medical care** Y69
  - contaminated medical or biological substance (blood, drug, fluid) Y64.9
    - administered (by) NEC Y64.9
      - immunization Y64.1
      - infusion Y64.Ø
      - injection Y64.1
      - specified means NEC Y64.8
      - transfusion Y64.Ø
      - vaccination Y64.1
  - excessive amount of blood or other fluid during transfusion or infusion Y63.Ø
  - failure
    - in dosage Y63.9
      - electroshock therapy Y63.4
      - inappropriate temperature (too hot or too cold) in local application and packing Y63.5
      - infusion
        - excessive amount of fluid Y63.Ø
        - incorrect dilution of fluid Y63.1
      - insulin-shock therapy Y63.4
      - nonadministration of necessary drug or biological substance Y63.6
      - overdose —*see* Table of Drugs and Chemicals
        - radiation, in therapy Y63.2
      - radiation
        - overdose Y63.2
      - specified procedure NEC Y63.8
      - transfusion
        - excessive amount of blood Y63.Ø
    - mechanical, of instrument or apparatus (any) (during any procedure) Y65.8
    - sterile precautions (during procedure) Y62.9
      - aspiration of fluid or tissue (by puncture or catheterization, except heart) Y62.6
      - biopsy (except needle aspiration) Y62.8
        - needle (aspirating) Y62.6
      - blood sampling Y62.6
      - catheterization Y62.6
        - heart Y62.5
      - dialysis (kidney) Y62.2
      - endoscopic examination Y62.4
      - enema Y62.8
      - immunization Y62.3
      - infusion Y62.1
      - injection Y62.3
      - needle biopsy Y62.6
      - paracentesis (abdominal) (thoracic) Y62.6
      - perfusion Y62.2

M

Misadventure(s) to patient(s) during surgical or medical care *(Continued)*
- failure *(Continued)*
  - sterile precautions *(Continued)*
    - puncture (lumbar) Y62.6
    - removal of catheter or packing Y62.8
    - specified procedure NEC Y62.8
    - surgical operation Y62.Ø
    - transfusion Y62.1
    - vaccination Y62.3
  - suture or ligature during surgical procedure Y65.2
  - to introduce or to remove tube or instrument —*see* Failure, to
- hemorrhage —*see* Index to Diseases and Injuries, Complication(s)
- inadvertent exposure of patient to radiation Y63.3
- inappropriate
  - operation performed —*see* Inappropriate operation performed
  - temperature (too hot or too cold) in local application or packing Y63.5
- infusion —*see also* Misadventure, by type, infusion Y69
  - excessive amount of fluid Y63.Ø
  - incorrect dilution of fluid Y63.1
  - wrong fluid Y65.1
- mismatched blood in transfusion Y65.Ø
- nonadministration of necessary drug or biological substance Y63.6
- overdose —*see* Table of Drugs and Chemicals
  - radiation (in therapy) Y63.2
- perforation —*see* Index to Diseases and Injuries, Complication(s)
- performance of inappropriate operation —*see* Inappropriate operation performed
- puncture —*see* Index to Diseases and Injuries, Complication(s)
- specified type NEC Y65.8
  - failure
    - suture or ligature during surgical operation Y65.2
    - to introduce or to remove tube or instrument —*see* Failure, to
  - infusion of wrong fluid Y65.1
  - performance of inappropriate operation —*see* Inappropriate operation performed
  - transfusion of mismatched blood Y65.Ø
  - wrong
    - fluid in infusion Y65.1
    - placement of endotracheal tube during anesthetic procedure Y65.3
- transfusion —*see* Misadventure, by type, transfusion
  - excessive amount of blood Y63.Ø
  - mismatched blood Y65.Ø
- wrong
  - drug given in error —*see* Table of Drugs and Chemicals
  - fluid in infusion Y65.1
  - placement of endotracheal tube during anesthetic procedure Y65.3

Mismatched blood in transfusion Y65.Ø

Motion sickness T75.3

Mountain sickness W94.11

Mudslide (of cataclysmic nature) —*see* Landslide

Murder (attempt) —*see* Assault

N

Nail
- contact with W45.Ø
  - gun W29.4
- embedded in skin W45.Ø

Neglect (criminal) (homicidal intent) X58

Noise (causing injury) (pollution) W42.9
- supersonic W42.Ø

Nonadministration (of)
- drug or biological substance (necessary) Y63.6
- surgical and medical care Y66

Nosocomial condition Y95

O

Object
- falling
  - from, in, on, hitting
    - machinery —*see* Contact, with, by type of machine
- set in motion by
  - accidental explosion or rupture of pressure vessel W38
  - firearm —*see* Discharge, firearm, by type
  - machine (ry) —*see* Contact, with, by type of machine

Overdose (drug) —*see* Table of Drugs and Chemicals
- radiation Y63.2

Overexertion X5Ø.9
- from
  - prolonged static or awkward postures X5Ø.1
  - repetitive movements X5Ø.3
  - specified strenuous movements or postures NEC X5Ø.9
  - strenuous movement or load X5Ø.Ø

Overexposure (accidental) (to)
- cold —*see also* Exposure, cold X31
  - due to man-made conditions —*see* Exposure, cold, man-made
- heat —*see also* Heat X3Ø
- radiation —*see* Radiation
- radioactivity W88.Ø
- sun (sunburn) X32
- weather NEC —*see* Forces of nature
- wind NEC —*see* Forces of nature

Overheated —*see* Heat

Overturning (accidental)
- machinery —*see* Contact, with, by type of machine
- transport vehicle NEC —*see also* Accident, transport V89.9
- watercraft (causing drowning, submersion) —*see also* Drowning, due to, accident to, watercraft, overturning
  - causing injury except drowning or submersion —*see* Accident, watercraft, causing, injury NEC

M, N, & O

P

- Parachute descent (voluntary) (without accident to aircraft) V97.29
  - due to accident to aircraft —*see* Accident, transport, aircraft
- Pecked by bird W61.99
- Perforation during medical or surgical treatment as misadventure —*see* Index to Diseases and Injuries, Complication(s)
- Perpetrator, perpetration, of assault, maltreatment and neglect (by) YØ7.9
  - boyfriend YØ7.Ø3
  - brother YØ7.41Ø
    - stepbrother YØ7.435
  - coach YØ7.53
  - cousin
    - female YØ7.491
    - male YØ7.49Ø
  - daycare provider YØ7.519
    - at-home
      - adult care YØ7.512
      - childcare YØ7.51Ø
    - care center
      - adult care YØ7.513
      - childcare YØ7.511
  - family member NEC YØ7.499
  - father YØ7.11
    - adoptive YØ7.13
    - foster YØ7.42Ø
    - stepfather YØ7.43Ø
  - foster father YØ7.42Ø
  - foster mother YØ7.421
  - girl friend YØ7.Ø4
  - healthcare provider YØ7.529
    - mental health YØ7.521
    - specified NEC YØ7.528
  - husband YØ7.Ø1
  - instructor YØ7.53
  - mother YØ7.12
    - adoptive YØ7.14
    - foster YØ7.421
    - stepmother YØ7.433
  - nonfamily member YØ7.5Ø
    - specified NEC YØ7.59
  - nurse YØ7.528
  - occupational therapist YØ7.528
  - partner of parent
    - female YØ7.434
    - male YØ7.432
  - physical therapist YØ7.528
  - sister YØ7.411
  - speech therapist YØ7.528
  - stepbrother YØ7.435
  - stepfather YØ7.43Ø
  - stepmother YØ7.433
  - stepsister YØ7.436
  - teacher YØ7.53
  - wife YØ7.Ø2
- Piercing —*see* Contact, with, by type of object or machine
- Pinched
  - between objects (moving) (stationary and moving) W23.Ø
    - stationary W23.1
- Pinned under machine (ry) —*see* Contact, with, by type of machine
- Place of occurrence Y92.9
  - abandoned house Y92.89
  - airplane Y92.813
  - airport Y92.52Ø
  - ambulatory health services establishment NEC Y92.538
  - ambulatory surgery center Y92.53Ø
  - amusement park Y92.831
  - apartment (co-op) —*see* Place of occurrence, residence, apartment
  - assembly hall Y92.29
  - bank Y92.51Ø
  - barn Y92.71
  - baseball field Y92.32Ø

Place of occurrence *(Continued)*

  - basketball court Y92.31Ø
  - beach Y92.832
  - boarding house —*see* Place of occurrence, residence, boarding house
  - boat Y92.814
  - bowling alley Y92.39
  - bridge Y92.89
  - building under construction Y92.61
  - bus Y92.811
    - station Y92.521
  - cafe Y92.511
  - campsite Y92.833
  - campus —*see* Place of occurrence, school
  - canal Y92.89
  - car Y92.81Ø
  - casino Y92.59
  - children's home —*see* Place of occurrence, residence, institutional, orphanage
  - church Y92.22
  - cinema Y92.26
  - clubhouse Y92.29
  - coal pit Y92.64
  - college (community) Y92.214
  - condominium —*see* Place of occurrence, residence, apartment
  - construction area —*see* Place of occurrence, industrial and construction area
  - convalescent home —*see* Place of occurrence, residence, institutional, nursing home
  - court-house Y92.24Ø
  - cricket ground Y92.328
  - cultural building Y92.258
    - art gallery Y92.25Ø
    - museum Y92.251
    - music hall Y92.252
    - opera house Y92.253
    - specified NEC Y92.258
    - theater Y92.254
  - dancehall Y92.252
  - day nursery Y92.21Ø
  - dentist office Y92.531
  - derelict house Y92.89
  - desert Y92.82Ø
  - dock NOS Y92.89
  - dockyard Y92.62
  - doctor's office Y92.531
  - dormitory —*see* Place of occurrence, residence, institutional, school dormitory
  - dry dock Y92.62
  - factory (building) (premises) Y92.63
  - farm (land under cultivation) (outbuildings) Y92.79
    - barn Y92.71
    - chicken coop Y92.72
    - field Y92.73
    - hen house Y92.72
    - house —*see* Place of occurrence, residence, house
    - orchard Y92.74
    - specified NEC Y92.79
  - football field Y92.321
  - forest Y92.821
  - freeway Y92.411
  - gallery Y92.25Ø
  - garage (commercial) Y92.59
    - boarding house Y92.Ø44
    - military base Y92.135
    - mobile home Y92.Ø25
    - nursing home Y92.124
    - orphanage Y92.114
    - private house Y92.Ø15
    - reform school Y92.155
  - gas station Y92.524
  - gasworks Y92.69
  - golf course Y92.39
  - gravel pit Y92.64
  - grocery Y92.512
  - gymnasium Y92.39
  - handball court Y92.318
  - harbor Y92.89

Place of occurrence *(Continued)*

  - harness racing course Y92.39
  - healthcare provider office Y92.531
  - highway (interstate) Y92.411
  - hill Y92.828
  - hockey rink Y92.33Ø
  - home —*see* Place of occurrence, residence
  - hospice —*see* Place of occurrence, residence, institutional, nursing home
  - hospital Y92.239
    - cafeteria Y92.233
    - corridor Y92.232
    - operating room Y92.234
    - patient
      - bathroom Y92.231
      - room Y92.23Ø
    - specified NEC Y92.238
  - hotel Y92.59
  - house —*see also* Place of occurrence, residence
    - abandoned Y92.89
    - under construction Y92.61
  - industrial and construction area (yard) Y92.69
    - building under construction Y92.61
    - dock Y92.62
    - dry dock Y92.62
    - factory Y92.63
    - gasworks Y92.69
    - mine Y92.64
    - oil rig Y92.65
    - pit Y92.64
    - power station Y92.69
    - shipyard Y92.62
    - specified NEC Y92.69
    - tunnel under construction Y92.69
    - workshop Y92.69
  - kindergarten Y92.211
  - lacrosse field Y92.328
  - lake Y92.828
  - library Y92.241
  - mall Y92.59
  - market Y92.512
  - marsh Y92.828
  - military
    - base —*see* Place of occurrence, residence, institutional, military base
    - training ground Y92.84
  - mine Y92.64
  - mosque Y92.22
  - motel Y92.59
  - motorway (interstate) Y92.411
  - mountain Y92.828
  - movie-house Y92.26
  - museum Y92.251
  - music-hall Y92.252
  - not applicable Y92.9
  - nuclear power station Y92.69
  - nursing home —*see* Place of occurrence, residence, institutional, nursing home
  - office building Y92.59
  - offshore installation Y92.65
  - oil rig Y92.65
  - old people's home —*see* Place of occurrence, residence, institutional, specified NEC
  - opera-house Y92.253
  - orphanage —*see* Place of occurrence, residence, institutional, orphanage
  - outpatient surgery center Y92.53Ø
  - park (public) Y92.83Ø
    - amusement Y92.831
  - parking garage Y92.89
    - lot Y92.481
  - pavement Y92.48Ø
  - physician office Y92.531
  - polo field Y92.328
  - pond Y92.828
  - post office Y92.242
  - power station Y92.69
  - prairie Y92.828
  - prison —*see* Place of occurrence, residence, institutional, prison

- Place of occurrence *(Continued)*
  - public
    - administration building Y92.248
      - city hall Y92.243
      - courthouse Y92.240
      - library Y92.241
      - post office Y92.242
      - specified NEC Y92.248
    - building NEC Y92.29
    - hall Y92.29
    - place NOS Y92.89
  - race course Y92.39
  - radio station Y92.59
  - railway line (bridge) Y92.85
  - ranch (outbuildings) —*see* Place of occurrence, farm
  - recreation area Y92.838
    - amusement park Y92.831
    - beach Y92.832
    - campsite Y92.833
    - park (public) Y92.830
    - seashore Y92.832
    - specified NEC Y92.838
  - reform school —*see* Place of occurrence, residence, institutional, reform school
  - religious institution Y92.22
  - residence (non-institutional) (private) Y92.009
    - apartment Y92.039
      - bathroom Y92.031
      - bedroom Y92.032
      - kitchen Y92.030
      - specified NEC Y92.038
    - bathroom Y92.002
    - bedroom Y92.003
    - boarding house Y92.049
      - bathroom Y92.041
      - bedroom Y92.042
      - driveway Y92.043
      - garage Y92.044
      - garden Y92.046
      - kitchen Y92.040
      - specified NEC Y92.048
      - swimming pool Y92.045
      - yard Y92.046
    - dining room Y92.001
    - garden Y92.007
    - home Y92.009
    - house, single family Y92.019
      - bathroom Y92.012
      - bedroom Y92.013
      - dining room Y92.011
      - driveway Y92.014
      - garage Y92.015
      - garden Y92.017
      - kitchen Y92.010
      - specified NEC Y92.018
      - swimming pool Y92.016
      - yard Y92.017
    - institutional Y92.10
      - children's home —*see* Place of occurrence, residence, institutional, orphanage
      - hospice —*see* Place of occurrence, residence, institutional, nursing home
      - military base Y92.139
        - barracks Y92.133
        - garage Y92.135
        - garden Y92.137
        - kitchen Y92.130
        - mess hall Y92.131
        - specified NEC Y92.138
        - swimming pool Y92.136
        - yard Y92.137
      - nursing home Y92.129
        - bathroom Y92.121
        - bedroom Y92.122
        - driveway Y92.123
        - garage Y92.124
        - garden Y92.126
        - kitchen Y92.120

- Place of occurrence *(Continued)*
  - residence *(Continued)*
    - institutional *(Continued)*
      - nursing home *(Continued)*
        - specified NEC Y92.128
        - swimming pool Y92.125
        - yard Y92.126
      - orphanage Y92.119
        - bathroom Y92.111
        - bedroom Y92.112
        - driveway Y92.113
        - garage Y92.114
        - garden Y92.116
        - kitchen Y92.110
        - specified NEC Y92.118
        - swimming pool Y92.115
        - yard Y92.116
      - prison Y92.149
        - bathroom Y92.142
        - cell Y92.143
        - courtyard Y92.147
        - dining room Y92.141
        - kitchen Y92.140
        - specified NEC Y92.148
        - swimming pool Y92.146
      - reform school Y92.159
        - bathroom Y92.152
        - bedroom Y92.153
        - dining room Y92.151
        - driveway Y92.154
        - garage Y92.155
        - garden Y92.157
        - kitchen Y92.150
        - specified NEC Y92.158
        - swimming pool Y92.156
        - yard Y92.157
      - school dormitory Y92.169
        - bathroom Y92.162
        - bedroom Y92.163
        - dining room Y92.161
        - kitchen Y92.160
        - specified NEC Y92.168
      - specified NEC Y92.199
        - bathroom Y92.192
        - bedroom Y92.193
        - dining room Y92.191
        - driveway Y92.194
        - garage Y92.195
        - garden Y92.197
        - kitchen Y92.190
        - specified NEC Y92.198
        - swimming pool Y92.196
        - yard Y92.197
    - kitchen Y92.000
    - mobile home Y92.029
      - bathroom Y92.022
      - bedroom Y92.023
      - dining room Y92.021
      - driveway Y92.024
      - garage Y92.025
      - garden Y92.027
      - kitchen Y92.020
      - specified NEC Y92.028
      - swimming pool Y92.026
      - yard Y92.027
    - specified place in residence NEC Y92.008
    - specified residence type NEC Y92.099
      - bathroom Y92.091
      - bedroom Y92.092
      - driveway Y92.093
      - garage Y92.094
      - garden Y92.096
      - kitchen Y92.090
      - specified NEC Y92.098
      - swimming pool Y92.095
      - yard Y92.096
  - restaurant Y92.511
  - riding school Y92.39
  - river Y92.828
  - road Y92.410
  - rodeo ring Y92.39

- Place of occurrence *(Continued)*
  - rugby field Y92.328
  - same day surgery center Y92.530
  - sand pit Y92.64
  - school (private) (public) (state) Y92.219
    - college Y92.214
    - daycare center Y92.210
    - elementary school Y92.211
    - high school Y92.213
    - kindergarten Y92.211
    - middle school Y92.212
    - specified NEC Y92.218
    - trace school Y92.215
    - university Y92.214
    - vocational school Y92.215
  - sea (shore) Y92.832
  - senior citizen center Y92.29
  - service area
    - airport Y92.520
    - bus station Y92.521
    - gas station Y92.524
    - highway rest stop Y92.523
    - railway station Y92.522
  - shipyard Y92.62
  - shop(commercial) Y92.513
  - sidewalk Y92.480
  - silo Y92.79
  - skating rink (roller) Y92.331
    - ice Y92.330
  - slaughter house Y92.86
  - soccer field Y92.322
  - specified place NEC Y92.89
  - sports area Y92.39
    - athletic
      - court Y92.318
        - basketball Y92.310
        - specified NEC Y92.318
        - squash Y92.311
        - tennis Y92.312
      - field Y92.328
        - baseball Y92.320
        - cricket ground Y92.328
        - football Y92.321
        - hockey Y92.328
        - soccer Y92.322
        - specified NEC Y92.328
    - golf course Y92.39
    - gymnasium Y92.39
    - riding school Y92.39
    - skating rink (roller) Y92.331
      - ice Y92.330
    - stadium Y92.39
    - swimming pool Y92.34
  - squash court Y92.311
  - stadium Y92.39
  - steeplechasing course Y92.39
  - store Y92.512
  - stream Y92.828
  - street and highway Y92.410
    - bike path Y92.482
    - freeway Y92.411
    - highway ramp Y92.415
    - interstate highway Y92.411
    - local residential or business street Y92.414
    - motorway Y92.411
    - parking lot Y92.481
    - parkway Y92.412
    - sidewalk Y92.480
    - specified NEC Y92.488
    - state road Y92.413
  - subway car Y92.816
  - supermarket Y92.512
  - swamp Y92.828
  - swimming pool (public) Y92.34
    - private (at) Y92.095
      - boarding house Y92.045
      - military base Y92.136
      - mobile home Y92.026
      - nursing home Y92.125
      - orphanage Y92.115

P

- Place of occurrence *(Continued)*
  - swimming pool *(Continued)*
    - private *(Continued)*
      - prison Y92.146
      - reform school Y92.156
      - single family residence Y92.Ø16
  - synagogue Y92.22
  - television station Y92.59
  - tennis court Y92.312
  - theater Y92.254
  - trade area Y92.59
    - bank Y92.51Ø
    - cafe Y92.511
    - casino Y92.59
    - garage Y92.59
    - hotel Y92.59
    - market Y92.512
    - office building Y92.59
    - radio station Y92.59
    - restaurant Y92.511
    - shop Y92.513
    - shopping mall Y92.59
    - store Y92.512
    - supermarket Y92.512
    - television station Y92.59
    - warehouse Y92.59
  - trailer park, residential —*see* Place of occurrence, residence, mobile home
  - trailer site NOS Y92.89
  - train Y92.815
    - station Y92.522
  - truck Y92.812
  - tunnel under construction Y92. 69
  - university Y92.214
  - urgent (health) care center Y92.532
  - vehicle (transport) Y92.818
    - airplane Y92.813
    - boat Y92.814
    - bus Y92.811
    - car Y92.81Ø
    - specified NEC Y92.818
    - subway car Y92.816
    - train Y92.815
    - truck Y92.812
  - warehouse Y92.59
  - water reservoir Y92.89
  - wilderness area Y92.828
    - desert Y92.82Ø
    - forest Y92.821
    - marsh Y92.828
    - mountain Y92.828
    - prairie Y92.828
    - specified NEC Y92.828
    - swamp Y92.828
  - workshop Y92.69
  - yard, private Y92.Ø96
    - boarding house Y92.Ø46
    - mobile home Y92.Ø27
    - single family house Y92.Ø17

- Place of occurrence *(Continued)*
  - youth center Y92.29
  - zoo (zoological garden) Y92.834
- **Plumbism** —*see* Table of Drugs and Chemicals, lead
- **Poisoning** (accidental) (by) —*see also* Table of Drugs and Chemicals
  - by plant, thorns, spines, sharp leaves or other mechanisms NEC X58
  - carbon monoxide
    - generated by
      - motor vehicle —*see* Accident, transport
      - watercraft (in transit) (not in transit) V93.89
        - ferry boat V93.81
        - fishing boat V93.82
        - jet skis V93.83
        - liner V93.81
        - merchant ship V93.8Ø
        - passenger ship V93.81
        - powered craft NEC V93.83
  - caused by injection of poisons into skin by plant thorns, spines, sharp leaves X58
    - marine or sea plants (venomous) X58
  - exhaust gas
    - generated by
      - motor vehicle —*see* Accident, transport
      - watercraft (in transit) (not in transit) V93.89
        - ferry boat V93.81
        - fishing boat V93.82
        - jet skis V93.83
        - liner V93.81
        - merchant ship V93.8Ø
        - passenger ship V93.81
        - powered craft NEC V93.83
  - fumes or smoke due to
    - explosion —*see also* Explosion W4Ø.9
    - fire —*see* Exposure, fire
    - ignition —*see* Ignition
  - gas
    - in legal intervention —*see* Legal, intervention, gas
    - legal execution —*see* Legal, intervention, gas
  - in war operations —*see* War operations
  - legal
  - execution —*see* Legal, intervention, gas
    - intervention
      - by gas —*see* Legal, intervention, gas
      - other specified means —*see* Legal, intervention, specified means NEC
- **Powder burn** (by) (from)
  - airgun W34.11Ø
  - BB gun W34.11Ø
  - firearm NEC W34.19
  - gas, air or spring-operated gun NEC W34.118
  - handgun W32.1
  - hunting rifle W33.12

- Powder burn *(Continued)*
  - larger firearm W33.1Ø
    - specified NEC W33.19
  - machine gun W33.13
  - paintball gun W34.111
  - pellet gun W34.11Ø
  - shotgun W33.11
  - Very pistol [flare] W34.19
- **Premature cessation** (of) **surgical and medical care** Y66
- **Privation** (food) (water) X58
- **Procedure** (operation)
  - correct, on wrong side or body part (wrong side) (wrong site) Y65.53
  - intended for another patient done on wrong patient Y65.52
  - performed on patient not scheduled for surgery Y65.52
  - performed on wrong patient Y65.52
  - wrong, performed on correct patient Y65.51
- **Prolonged**
  - sitting in transport vehicle —*see* Travel, by type of vehicle
  - stay in
    - high altitude as cause of anoxia, barodontalgia, barotitis or hypoxia W94.11
    - weightless environment X52
- **Pulling, excessive** —*see also* Overexertion X5Ø.9
- **Puncture, puncturing** —*see also* Contact, with, by type of object or machine
  - by
    - plant thorns, spines, sharp leaves or other mechanisms NEC W6Ø
  - during medical or surgical treatment as misadventure —*see* Index to Diseases and Injuries, Complication(s)
- **Pushed, pushing** (accidental) (injury in)
  - by other person(s) (accidental) W51
    - with fall WØ3
      - due to ice or snow WØØ.Ø
    - as, or caused by, a crowd or human stampede (with fall) W52
    - before moving object NEC YØ2.8
      - motor vehicle YØ2.Ø
      - subway train YØ2.1
      - train YØ2.1
    - from
      - high place NEC
        - in accidental circumstances W17.89
        - stated as
          - intentional, homicide (attempt) YØ1
          - undetermined whether accidental or intentional Y3Ø
      - transport vehicle NEC —*see also* Accident, transport V89.9
        - stated as
          - intentional, homicide (attempt) YØ8.89
      - overexertion X5Ø.9

P

R

Radiation (exposure to)
- arc lamps W89.Ø
- atomic power plant (malfunction) NEC W88.1
- complication of or abnormal reaction to medical radiotherapy Y84.2
- electromagnetic, ionizing W88.Ø
- gamma rays W88.1
- in
  - war operations (from or following nuclear explosion) —*see also* War operations
- inadvertent exposure of patient (receiving test or therapy) Y63.3
- infrared (heaters and lamps) W9Ø.1
  - excessive heat from W92
- ionized, ionizing (particles, artificially accelerated)
  - radioisotopes W88.1
  - specified NEC W88.8
  - x-rays W88.Ø
- isotopes, radioactive —*see* Radiation, radioactive isotopes
- laser(s) W9Ø.2
  - in war operations —*see* War operations
  - misadventure in medical care Y63.2
- light sources (man-made visible and ultraviolet) W89.9
  - natural X32
  - specified NEC W89.8
  - tanning bed W89.1
  - welding light W89.Ø
- man-made visible light W89.9
  - specified NEC W89.8
  - tanning bed W89.1
  - welding light W89.Ø
- microwave W9Ø.8
- misadventure in medical or surgical procedure Y63.2
- natural NEC X39.Ø8
  - radon X39.Ø1
- overdose (in medical or surgical procedure) Y63.2
- radar W9Ø.Ø
- radioactive isotopes (any) W88.1
  - atomic power plant malfunction W88.1
  - misadventure in medical or surgical treatment Y63.2
- radiofrequency W9Ø.Ø
- radium NEC W88.1
- sun X32
- ultraviolet (light) (man-made) W89.9
  - natural X32
  - specified NEC W89.8
  - tanning bed W89.1
  - welding light W89.Ø
- welding arc, torch, or light W89.Ø
  - excessive heat from W92
- x-rays (hard) (soft) W88.Ø

Range disease W94.11

Rape (attempted) T74.2-•

Rat bite W53.11

Reaching (prolonged) (static) X5Ø.1

Reaction, abnormal to medical procedure —*see also* Complication of or following, by type of procedure Y84.9
- with misadventure —*see* Misadventure
- biologicals —*see* Table of Drugs and Chemicals
- drugs —*see* Table of Drugs and Chemicals
- vaccine —*see* Table of Drugs and Chemicals

Recoil
- airgun W34.11Ø
- BB gun W34.11Ø
- firearm NEC W34.19
- gas, air or spring-operated gun NEC W34.118
- handgun W32.1
- hunting rifle W33.12
- larger firearm W33.1Ø
  - specified NEC W33.19
- machine gun W33.13
- paintball gun W34.111
- pellet W34.11Ø
- shotgun W33.11
- Very pistol [flare] W34.19

Reduction in
- atmospheric pressure —*see* Air, pressure, change

Rock falling on or hitting (accidentally) (person) W2Ø.8
- in cave-in W2Ø.Ø

Run over (accidentally) (by)
- animal (not being ridden) NEC W55.89
- machinery —*see* Contact, with, by specified type of machine
- transport vehicle NEC —*see also* Accident, transport VØ9.9
  - intentional homicide (attempt) YØ3.Ø
  - motor NEC VØ9.2Ø
    - intentional homicide (attempt) YØ3.Ø

Running
- before moving object X81.8
  - motor vehicle X81.Ø

Running off, away
- animal (being ridden) —*see also* Accident, transport V8Ø.918
  - not being ridden W55.89
- animal-drawn vehicle NEC —*see also* Accident, transport V8Ø.928
- highway, road(way), street
  - transport vehicle NEC —*see also* Accident, transport V89.9

Rupture pressurized devices —*see* Explosion, by type of device

R

S

- **Saturnism** —*see* Table of Drugs and Chemicals, lead
- **Scald, scalding** (accidental) (by) (from) (in) X19
  - air (hot) X14.1
  - gases (hot) X14.1
  - homicide (attempt) —*see* Assault, burning, hot object
  - inflicted by other person
    - stated as intentional, homicide (attempt) —*see* Assault, burning, hot object
  - liquid (boiling) (hot) NEC X12
    - stated as undetermined whether accidental or intentional Y27.2
    - suicide (attempt) X77.2
  - local application of externally applied substance in medical or surgical care Y63.5
  - metal (molten) (liquid) (hot) NEC X18
  - self-inflicted X77.9
  - stated as undetermined whether accidental or intentional Y27.8
  - steam X13.1
    - assault X98.Ø
    - stated as undetermined whether accidental or intentional Y27.Ø
    - suicide (attempt) X77.Ø
  - suicide (attempt) X77.9
  - vapor (hot) X13.1
    - assault X98.Ø
    - stated as undetermined whether accidental or intentional Y27.Ø
    - suicide (attempt) X77.Ø
- **Scratched by**
  - cat W55.Ø3
  - person(s) (accidentally) W5Ø.4
    - with intent to injure or kill YØ4.Ø
    - as, or caused by, a crowd or human stampede (with fall) W52
    - assault YØ4.Ø
    - homicide (attempt) YØ4.Ø
    - in
      - fight YØ4.Ø
      - legal intervention
        - injuring
          - bystander Y35.892
          - law enforcement personnel Y35.891
          - suspect Y35.893
- **Seasickness** T75.3
- **Self-harm NEC** —*see also* External cause by type, undetermined whether accidental or intentional
  - intentional —*see* Suicide
  - poisoning NEC —*see* Table of drugs and biologicals, accident
- **Self-inflicted** (injury) NEC —*see also* External cause by type, undetermined whether accidental or intentional
  - intentional —*see* Suicide
  - poisoning NEC —*see* Table of drugs and biologicals, accident
- **Sequelae** (of)
  - accident NEC —*see* WØØ-X58 with 7th character S
  - assault (homicidal) (any means) —*see* X92-YØ8 with 7th character S
  - homicide, attempt (any means) —*see* X92-YØ8 with 7th character S
  - injury undetermined whether accidentally or purposely inflicted —*see* Y21-Y33 with 7th character S
  - intentional self-harm (classifiable to X71-X83) —*see* X71-X83 with 7th character S
  - legal intervention (*see* with 7th character S Y35)
  - motor vehicle accident —*see* VØØ-V99 with 7th character S
  - suicide, attempt (any means) —*see* X71-X83 with 7th character S
- **Sequelae** *(Continued)*
  - transport accident —*see* VØØ-V99 with 7th character S
  - war operations —*see* War operations
- **Shock**
  - electric —*see* Exposure, electric current
  - from electric appliance (any) (faulty) W86.8
    - domestic W86.Ø
    - suicide (attempt) X83.1
- **Shooting, shot** (accidental (ly)) —*see also* Discharge, firearm, by type
  - herself or himself —*see* Discharge, firearm by type, self-inflicted
  - homicide (attempt) —*see* Discharge, firearm by type, homicide
  - in war operations —*see* War operations
  - inflicted by other person —*see* Discharge, firearm by type, homicide
    - accidental —*see* Discharge, firearm, by type of firearm
  - legal
    - execution —*see* Legal, intervention, firearm
    - intervention —*see* Legal, intervention, firearm
  - self-inflicted —*see* Discharge, firearm by type, suicide
    - accidental —*see* Discharge, firearm, by type of firearm
  - suicide (attempt) —*see* Discharge, firearm by type, suicide
- **Shoving** (accidentally) **by other person** —*see* Pushed, by other person
- **Sickness**
  - alpine W94.11
  - motion —*see* Motion
  - mountain W94.11
- **Sinking** (accidental)
  - watercraft (causing drowning, submersion) —*see also* Drowning, due to, accident to, watercraft, sinking
    - causing injury except drowning or submersion —*see* Accident, watercraft, causing, injury NEC
- **Siriasis** X32
- **Sitting** (prolonged) (static) X5Ø.1
- **Slashed wrists** —*see* Cut, self-inflicted
- **Slipping** (accidental) (on same level) (with fall) WØ1.Ø
  - without fall W18.4Ø
    - due to
      - specified NEC W18.49
      - stepping from one level to another W18.43
      - stepping into hole or opening W18.42
      - stepping on object W18.41
  - on
    - ice WØØ.Ø
      - with skates —*see* Accident, transport, pedestrian, conveyance
    - mud WØ1.Ø
    - oil WØ1.Ø
    - snow WØØ.Ø
      - with skis —*see* Accident, transport, pedestrian, conveyance
    - surface (slippery) (wet) NEC WØ1.Ø
- **Sliver, wood, contact with** W45.8
- **Smoldering** (due to fire) —*see* Exposure, fire
- **Sodomy** (attempted) **by force** T74.2-●
- **Sound waves** (causing injury) W42.9
  - supersonic W42.Ø
- **Splinter, contact with** W45.8
- **Stab, stabbing** —*see* Cut
- **Standing** (prolonged) (static) X5Ø.1
- **Starvation** X58
- **Status of external cause** Y99.9
  - child assisting in compensated work for family Y99.8
  - civilian activity done for financial or other compensation Y99.Ø
  - civilian activity done for income or pay Y99.Ø
- **Status of external cause** *(Continued)*
  - family member assisting in compensated work for other family member Y99.8
  - hobby not done for income Y99.8
  - leisure activity Y99.8
  - military activity Y99.1
  - off-duty activity of military personnel Y99.8
  - recreation or sport not for income or while a student Y99.8
  - specified NEC Y99.8
  - student activity Y99.8
  - volunteer activity Y99.2
- **Stepped on**
  - by
    - animal (not being ridden) NEC W55.89
    - crowd or human stampede W52
    - person W5Ø.Ø
- **Stepping on**
  - object W22.8
    - with fall W18.31
    - sports equipment W21.9
    - stationary W22.Ø9
      - sports equipment W21.89
  - person W51
    - by crowd or human stampede W52
  - sports equipment W21.9
- **Sting**
  - arthropod, nonvenomous W57
  - insect, nonvenomous W57
- **Storm** (cataclysmic) —*see* Forces of nature, cataclysmic storm
- **Straining, excessive** —*see also* Overexertion X5Ø.9
- **Strangling** —*see* Strangulation
- **Strangulation** (accidental) —*see* category T71
- **Strenuous movements** —*see also* Overexertion X5Ø.9
- **Striking against**
  - airbag (automobile) W22.1Ø
    - driver side W22.11
    - front passenger side W22.12
    - specified NEC W22.19
  - bottom when
    - diving or jumping into water (in) W16.822
      - causing drowning W16.821
      - from boat W16.722
        - causing drowning W16.721
      - natural body W16.622
        - causing drowning W16.821
      - swimming pool W16.522
        - causing drowning W16.521
    - falling into water (in) W16.322
      - causing drowning W16.321
      - fountain —*see* Striking against, bottom when, falling into water, specified NEC
      - natural body W16.122
        - causing drowning W16.121
      - reservoir —*see* Striking against, bottom when, falling into water, specified NEC
      - specified NEC W16.322
        - causing drowning W16.321
      - swimming pool W16.Ø22
        - causing drowning W16.Ø21
  - diving board (swimming-pool) W21.4
  - object W22.8
    - with
      - drowning or submersion —*see* Drowning
      - fall —*see* Fall, due to, bumping against, object
    - caused by crowd or human stampede (with fall) W52
    - furniture W22.Ø3
    - lamppost W22.Ø2
    - sports equipment W21.9
    - stationary W22.Ø9
      - sports equipment W21.89
    - wall W22.Ø1

S

▶ New ➡ Revised ~~deleted~~ Deleted ● Use Additional Character(s)

Striking against *(Continued)*
- person(s) W51
  - with fall WØ3
    - due to ice or snow WØØ.Ø
  - as, or caused by, a crowd or human stampede (with fall) W52
  - assault YØ4.2
  - homicide (attempt) YØ4.2
- sports equipment W21.9
- wall (when) W22.Ø1
  - diving or jumping into water (in) W16.832
    - causing drowning W16.831
    - swimming pool W16.532
      - causing drowning W16.531
  - falling into water (in) W16.332
    - causing drowning W16.331
    - fountain —*see* Striking against, wall when, falling into water, specified NEC
    - natural body W16.132
      - causing drowning W16.131
    - reservoir —*see* Striking against, wall when, falling into water, specified NEC
    - specified NEC W16.332
      - causing drowning W16.331
    - swimming pool W16.Ø32
      - causing drowning W16.Ø31
  - swimming pool (when) W22.Ø42
    - causing drowning W22.Ø41
    - diving or jumping into water W16.532
      - causing drowning W16.531
    - falling into water W16.Ø32
      - causing drowning W16.Ø31

Struck (accidentally) by
- airbag (automobile) W22.1Ø
  - driver side W22.11
  - front passenger side W22.12
  - specified NEC W22.19
- alligator W58.Ø2
- animal (not being ridden) NEC W55.89
- avalanche —*see* Landslide
- ball (hit) (thrown) W21.ØØ
  - assault YØ8.Ø9
  - baseball W21.Ø3
  - basketball W21.Ø5
  - football W21.Ø1
  - golf ball W21.Ø4
  - football W21.Ø1
  - soccer W21.Ø2
  - softball W21.Ø7
  - specified NEC W21.Ø9
  - volleyball W21.Ø6
- bat or racquet
  - baseball bat W21.11
    - assault YØ8.Ø2
  - golf club W21.13
    - assault YØ8.Ø9
  - specified NEC W21.19
    - assault YØ8.Ø9
  - tennis racquet W21.12
    - assault YØ8.Ø9
- bullet —*see also* Discharge, firearm by type
  - in war operations —*see* War operations
- crocodile W58.12
- dog W54.1
- flare, Very pistol —*see* Discharge, firearm NEC
- hailstones X39.8
- hockey (ice)
  - field
    - puck W21.221
    - stick W21.211
  - puck W21.22Ø
  - stick W21.21Ø
    - assault YØ8.Ø1
- landslide —*see* Landslide
- law-enforcement agent (on duty) —*see* Legal, intervention, manhandling
  - with blunt object —*see* Legal, intervention, blunt object

Struck by *(Continued)*
- lightning —*see* subcategory T75.Ø
  - causing fire —*see* Exposure, fire
- machine —*see* Contact, with, by type of machine
- mammal NEC W55.89
  - marine W56.32
- marine animal W56.82
- missile
  - firearm —*see* Discharge, firearm by type
  - in war operations —*see* War operations, missile
- object W22.8
  - blunt W22.8
    - assault YØØ
    - suicide (attempt) X79
    - undetermined whether accidental or intentional Y29
  - falling W2Ø.8
    - from, in, on
      - building W2Ø.1
        - burning (uncontrolled fire) XØØ.4
      - cataclysmic
        - earth surface movement NEC —*see* Landslide
        - storm —*see* Forces of nature, cataclysmic storm
      - cave-in W2Ø.Ø
      - earthquake X34
      - machine (in operation) —*see* Contact, with, by type of machine
      - structure W2Ø.1
        - burning XØØ.4
      - transport vehicle (in motion) —*see* Accident, transport, by type of vehicle
      - watercraft V93.49
        - due to
          - accident to craft V91.39
            - powered craft V91.33
              - ferry boat V91.31
              - fishing boat V91.32
              - jet ski V91.33
              - liner V91.31
              - merchant ship V91.3Ø
              - passenger ship V91.31
            - unpowered craft V91.38
              - canoe V91.35
              - inflatable V91.36
              - kayak V91.35
              - sailboat V91.34
              - surf-board V91.38
              - windsurfer V91.38
        - powered craft V93.43
          - ferry boat V93.41
          - fishing boat V93.42
          - jet ski V93.43
          - liner V93.41
          - merchant ship V93.4Ø
          - passenger ship V93.41
        - unpowered craft V93.48
          - sailboat V93.44
          - surf-board V93.48
          - windsurfer V93.48
  - moving NEC W2Ø.8
  - projected W2Ø.8
    - assault YØØ
    - in sports W21.9
      - assault YØ8.Ø9
      - ball W21.ØØ
        - baseball W21.Ø3
        - basketball W21.Ø5
        - football W21.Ø1
        - golf ball W21.Ø4
        - soccer W21.Ø2
        - softball W21.Ø7
        - specified NEC W21.Ø9
        - volleyball W21.Ø6
      - bat or racquet
        - baseball bat W21.11
          - assault YØ8.Ø2

Struck by *(Continued)*
- object *(Continued)*
  - projected *(Continued)*
    - in sports *(Continued)*
      - bat or racquet *(Continued)*
        - golf club W21.13
          - assault YØ8.Ø9-•
        - specified NEC W21.19
          - assault YØ8.Ø9
        - tennis racquet W21.12
          - assault YØ8.Ø9
      - hockey (ice)
        - field
          - puck W21.221
          - stick W21.211
        - puck W21.22Ø
        - stick W21.21Ø
          - assault YØ8.Ø1
      - specified NEC W21.89
  - set in motion by explosion —*see* Explosion
  - thrown W2Ø.8
    - assault YØØ
    - in sports W21.9
      - assault YØ8.Ø9
      - ball W21.ØØ
        - baseball W21.Ø3
        - basketball W21.Ø5
        - football W21.Ø1
        - golf ball W21.Ø4
        - soccer W21.Ø2
        - soft ball W21.Ø7
        - specified NEC W21.Ø9
        - volleyball W21.Ø6
      - bat or racquet
        - baseball bat W21.11
          - assault YØ8.Ø2
        - golf club W21.13
          - assault YØ8.Ø9
        - specified NEC W21.19
          - assault YØ8.Ø9
        - tennis racquet W21.12
          - assault YØ8.Ø9
      - hockey (ice)
        - field
          - puck W21.221
          - stick W21.211
        - puck W21.22Ø
        - stick W21.21Ø
          - assault YØ8.Ø1
      - specified NEC W21.89
- other person(s) W5Ø.Ø
  - with
    - blunt object W22.8
      - intentional, homicide (attempt) YØØ
      - sports equipment W21.9
      - undetermined whether accidental or intentional Y29
    - fall WØ3
      - due to ice or snow WØØ.Ø
  - as, or caused by, a crowd or human stampede (with fall) W52
  - assault YØ4.2
  - homicide (attempt) YØ4.2
  - in legal intervention
    - injuring
      - bystander Y35.812
      - law enforcement personnel Y35.811
      - suspect Y35.813
      - ▶unspecified person Y35.819
  - sports equipment W21.9
- police (on duty) —*see* Legal, intervention, manhandling
  - with blunt object —*see* Legal, intervention, blunt object
- sports equipment W21.9
  - assault YØ8.Ø9
  - ball W21.ØØ
    - baseball W21.Ø3
    - basketball W21.Ø5
    - football W21.Ø1
    - golf ball W21.Ø4
    - soccer W21.Ø2

S

- **Struck by** *(Continued)*
  - sports equipment *(Continued)*
    - ball *(Continued)*
      - soft ball W21.Ø7
      - specified NEC W21.Ø9
      - volleyball W21.Ø6
    - bat or racquet
      - baseball bat W21.11
        - assault YØ8.Ø2
      - golf club W21.13
        - assault YØ8.Ø9
      - specified NEC W21.19
      - tennis racquet W21.12
        - assault YØ8.Ø9
    - cleats (shoe) W21.31
    - foot wear NEC W21.39
    - football helmet W21.81
    - hockey (ice)
      - field
        - puck W21.221
        - stick W21.211
      - puck W21.22Ø
      - stick W21.21Ø
        - assault YØ8.Ø1
    - skate blades W21.32
    - specified NEC W21.89
      - assault YØ8.Ø9
  - thunderbolt —*see* subcategory T75.Ø
    - causing fire —*see* Exposure, fire
  - transport vehicle NEC —*see also* Accident, transport VØ9.9
    - intentional, homicide (attempt) YØ3.Ø
    - motor NEC —*see also* Accident, transport VØ9.2Ø
      - homicide YØ3.Ø
  - vehicle (transport) NEC —*see* Accident, transport, by type of vehicle
    - stationary (falling from jack, hydraulic lift, ramp) W2Ø.8
- **Stumbling**
  - without fall W18.4Ø
    - due to
      - specified NEC W18.49
      - stepping from one level to another W18.43
      - stepping into hole or opening W18.42
      - stepping on object W18.41
  - over
    - animal NEC WØ1.Ø
      - with fall W18.Ø9
    - carpet, rug or (small) object W22.8
      - with fall W18.Ø9
    - person W51
      - with fall WØ3
        - due to ice or snow WØØ.Ø
- **Submersion** (accidental) —*see* Drowning
- **Suffocation** (accidental) (by external means) (by pressure) (mechanical) —*see also* category T71
  - due to, by
    - avalanche —*see* Landslide
    - explosion —*see* Explosion
    - fire —*see* Exposure, fire
    - food, any type (aspiration) (ingestion) (inhalation) —*see* categories T17 and T18
    - ignition —*see* Ignition
    - landslide —*see* Landslide
    - machine (ry) —*see* Contact, with, by type of machine
    - vomitus (aspiration) (inhalation) T17.81-●
  - in
    - burning building XØØ.8
- **Suicide, suicidal** (attempted) (by) X83.8
  - blunt object X79
  - burning, burns X76
    - hot object X77.9
      - fluid NEC X77.2
      - household appliance X77.3
      - specified NEC X77.8
      - steam X77.Ø
      - tap water X77.1
      - vapors X77.Ø
  - caustic substance —*see* Table of Drugs and Chemicals
  - cold, extreme X83.2
  - collision of motor vehicle with
    - motor vehicle X82.Ø
    - specified NEC X82.8
    - train X82.1
    - tree X82.2
  - crashing of aircraft X83.Ø
  - cut (any part of body) X78.9
  - cutting or piercing instrument X78.9
    - dagger X78.2
    - glass X78.Ø
    - knife X78.1
    - specified NEC X78.8
    - sword X78.2
  - drowning (in) X71.9
    - bathtub X71.Ø
    - natural water X71.3
    - specified NEC X71.8
    - swimming pool X71.1
      - following fall X71.2
  - electrocution X83.1
  - explosive(s) (material) X75
  - fire, flames X76
  - firearm X74.9
    - airgun X74.Ø1
    - handgun X72
- **Suicide, suicidal** *(Continued)*
  - firearm *(Continued)*
    - hunting rifle X73.1
    - larger X73.9
      - specified NEC X73.8
    - machine gun X73.2
    - shotgun X73.Ø
    - specified NEC X74.8
  - hanging X83.8
  - hot object —*see* Suicide, burning, hot object
  - jumping
    - before moving object X81.8
      - motor vehicle X81.Ø
      - subway train X81.1
      - train X81.1
    - from high place X8Ø
  - late effect of attempt —*see* X71-X83 with 7th character S
  - lying before moving object, train, vehicle X81.8
  - poisoning —*see* Table of Drugs and Chemicals
  - puncture (any part of body) —*see* Suicide, cutting or piercing instrument
  - scald —*see* Suicide, burning, hot object
  - sequelae of attempt —*see* X71-X83 with 7th character S
  - sharp object (any) —*see* Suicide, cutting or piercing instrument
  - shooting —*see* Suicide, firearm
  - specified means NEC X83.8
  - stab (any part of body) —*see* Suicide, cutting or piercing instrument
  - steam, hot vapors X77.Ø
  - strangulation X83.8
  - submersion —*see* Suicide, drowning
  - suffocation X83.8
  - wound NEC X83.8
- **Sunstroke** X32
- **Supersonic waves** (causing injury) W42.Ø
- **Surgical procedure, complication of** (delayed or as an abnormal reaction without mention of misadventure) —*see also* Complication of or following, by type of procedure
  - due to or as a result of misadventure —*see* Misadventure
- **Swallowed, swallowing**
  - foreign body —*see* Foreign body, alimentary canal
  - poison —*see* Table of Drugs and Chemicals
  - substance
    - caustic or corrosive —*see* Table of Drugs and Chemicals
    - poisonous —*see* Table of Drugs and Chemicals

S

T

- **Tackle in sport** WØ3
- **Terrorism** (involving) Y38.8Ø
  - biological weapons Y38.6X-●
  - chemical weapons Y38.7X-●
  - conflagration Y38.3X-●
  - drowning and submersion Y38.89-●
  - explosion Y38.2X-●
    - destruction of aircraft Y38.1X-●
    - marine weapons Y38.ØX-●
  - fire Y38.3X-●
  - firearms Y38.4X-●
  - hot substances Y38.3X-●
  - lasers Y38.89-●
  - nuclear weapons Y38.5X-●
  - piercing or stabbing instruments Y38.89-●
  - secondary effects Y38.9X-●
  - specified method NEC Y38.89-●
  - suicide bomber Y38.81-●
- **Thirst** X58
- **Threat to breathing**
  - aspiration —*see* Aspiration
  - due to cave-in, falling earth or substance NEC —*see* category T71
- **Thrown** (accidentally)
  - against part (any) of or object in transport vehicle (in motion) NEC —*see also* Accident, transport

Thrown *(Continued)*
  - from
    - high place, homicide (attempt) YØ1
    - machinery —*see* Contact, with, by type of machine
    - transport vehicle NEC —*see also* Accident, transport V89.9
  - off —*see* Thrown, from
- **Thunderbolt** —*see* subcategory T75.Ø
  - causing fire —*see* Exposure, fire
- **Tidal wave** (any injury) **NEC** —*see* Forces of nature, tidal wave
- **Took**
  - overdose (drug) —*see* Table of Drugs and Chemicals
  - poison —*see* Table of Drugs and Chemicals
- **Tornado** (any injury) X37.1
- **Torrential rain** (any injury) X37.8
- **Torture** X58
- **Trampled by animal NEC** W55.89
- **Trapped** (accidentally)
  - between objects (moving) (stationary and moving) —*see* Caught
  - by part (any) of
    - motorcycle V29.88
    - pedal cycle V19.88
    - transport vehicle NEC —*see also* Accident, transport V89.9
- **Travel** (effects) (sickness) T75.3
- **Tree falling on or hitting** (accidentally) (person) W2Ø.8
- **Tripping**
  - without fall W18.4Ø
    - due to
      - specified NEC W18.49
      - stepping from one level to another W18.43
      - stepping into hole or opening W18.42
      - stepping on object W18.41
  - over
    - animal WØ1.Ø
      - with fall WØ1.Ø
    - carpet, rug or (small) object W22.8
      - with fall W18.Ø9
    - person W51
      - with fall WØ3
        - due to ice or snow WØØ.Ø
- **Twisted by person**(s) (accidentally) W5Ø.2
  - with intent to injure or kill YØ4.Ø
  - as, or caused by, a crowd or human stampede (with fall) W52
  - assault YØ4.Ø
  - homicide (attempt) YØ4.Ø
  - in
    - fight YØ4.Ø
    - legal intervention —*see* Legal, intervention, manhandling
- **Twisting** (prolonged) (static) X5Ø.1

U

- **Underdosing of necessary drugs, medicaments or biological substances** Y63.6
- **Undetermined intent** (contact) (exposure)
  - automobile collision Y32
  - blunt object Y29
  - drowning (submersion) (in) Y21.9
    - bathtub Y21.Ø
      - after fall Y21.1
    - natural water (lake) (ocean) (pond) (river) (stream) Y21.4
    - specified place NEC Y21.8
    - swimming pool Y21.2
      - after fall Y21.3
  - explosive material Y25
  - fall, jump or push from high place Y3Ø
  - falling, lying or running before moving object Y31
  - fire Y26

Undetermined intent *(Continued)*
  - firearm discharge Y24.9
    - airgun (BB) (pellet) Y24.Ø
    - handgun (pistol) (revolver) Y22
    - hunting rifle Y23.1
    - larger Y23.9
      - hunting rifle Y23.1
      - machine gun Y23.3
      - military Y23.2
      - shotgun Y23.Ø
      - specified type NEC Y23.8
    - machine gun Y23.3
    - military Y23.2
    - shotgun Y23.Ø
    - specified type NEC Y24.8
    - Very pistol Y24.8
  - hot object Y27.9
    - fluid NEC Y27.2
    - household appliance Y27.3
    - specified object NEC Y27.8

Undetermined intent *(Continued)*
  - hot object *(Continued)*
    - steam Y27.Ø
    - tap water Y27.1
    - vapor Y27.Ø
  - jump, fall or push from high place Y3Ø
  - lying, falling or running before moving object Y31
  - motor vehicle crash Y32
  - push, fall or jump from high place Y3Ø
  - running, falling or lying before moving object Y31
  - sharp object Y28.9
    - dagger Y28.2
    - glass Y28.Ø
    - knife Y28.1
    - specified object NEC Y28.8
    - sword Y28.2
  - smoke Y26
  - specified event NEC Y33
- **Use of hand as hammer** X5Ø.3

V

- **Vibration** (causing injury) W49.9
- **Victim** (of)
  - avalanche —*see* Landslide
  - earth movements NEC —*see* Forces of nature, earth movement
  - earthquake X34

Victim *(Continued)*
  - flood —*see* Flood
  - landslide —*see* Landslide
  - lightning —*see* subcategory T75.Ø
    - causing fire —*see* Exposure, fire
  - storm (cataclysmic) NEC —*see* Forces of nature, cataclysmic storm
  - volcanic eruption X35
- **Volcanic eruption** (any injury) X35
- **Vomitus, gastric contents in air passages** (with asphyxia, obstruction or suffocation) T17.81-●

W

- **Walked into stationary object** (any) W22.Ø9
  - furniture W22.Ø3
  - lamppost W22.Ø2
  - wall W22.Ø1
- **War operations** (injuries to military personnel and civilians during war, civil insurrection and peacekeeping missions) (by) (from) (involving) Y36.9Ø-●
  - after cessation of hostilities Y36.89-●
    - explosion (of)
      - bomb placed during war operations Y36.82-●
      - mine placed during war operations Y36.81-●
    - specified NEC Y36.88-●
  - air blast Y36.2Ø-●
  - aircraft
    - destruction —*see* War operations, destruction of aircraft
  - airway restriction —*see* War operations, restriction of airways
  - asphyxiation —*see* War operations, restriction of airways
  - biological weapons Y36.6X-●
  - blast Y36.2Ø-●
  - blast fragments Y36.2Ø-●
  - blast wave Y36.2Ø-●
  - blast wind Y36.2Ø-●
  - bomb Y36.2Ø-●
    - dirty Y36.5Ø-●
    - gasoline Y36.31-●
    - incendiary Y36.31-●
    - petrol Y36.31-●
  - bullet Y36.43-●
    - incendiary Y36.32-●
    - rubber Y36.41-●
  - chemical weapons Y36.7X-●
  - combat
    - hand to hand (unarmed) combat Y36.44-●
    - using blunt or piercing object Y36.45-●
  - conflagration —*see* War operations, fire
  - conventional warfare NEC Y36.49-●
  - depth-charge Y36.Ø1-●
  - destruction of aircraft Y36.1Ø-●
    - due to
      - air to air missile Y36.11-●
      - collision with other aircraft Y36.12-●
      - detonation (accidental) of onboard munitions and explosives Y36.14-●
      - enemy fire or explosives Y36.11-●
      - explosive placed on aircraft Y36.11-●
      - onboard fire Y36.13-●
      - rocket propelled grenade [RPG] Y36.11-●
      - small arms fire Y36.11-●
      - surface to air missile Y36.11-●
    - specified NEC Y36.19-●
  - detonation (accidental) of
    - onboard marine weapons Y36.Ø5-●
    - own munitions or munitions launch device Y36.24-●

War operations *(Continued)*
  - dirty bomb Y36.5Ø-●
  - explosion (of) Y36.2Ø-●
    - aerial bomb Y36.21-●
    - after cessation of hostilities
      - bomb placed during war operations Y36.82-●
      - mine placed during war operations Y36.81-●
    - bomb NOS —*see also* War operations, bomb(s) Y36.2Ø-●
    - fragments Y36.2Ø-●
    - grenade Y36.29-●
    - guided missile Y36.22-●
    - improvised explosive device [IED] (person-borne) (roadside) (vehicle-borne) Y36.23-●
    - land mine Y36.29-●
    - marine mine (at sea) (in harbor) Y36.Ø2-●
    - marine weapon Y36.ØØ-●
      - specified NEC Y36.Ø9-●
    - own munitions or munitions launch device (accidental) Y36.24-●
    - sea-based artillery shell Y36.Ø3-●
    - specified NEC Y36.29-●
    - torpedo Y36.Ø4-●
  - fire Y36.3Ø-●
    - specified NEC Y36.39-●
  - firearms
    - discharge Y36.43-●
    - pellets Y36.42-●
  - flamethrower Y36.33-●
  - fragments (from) (of)
    - improvised explosive device [IED] (person-borne) (roadside) (vehicle-borne) Y36.26-●
    - munitions Y36.25-●
    - specified NEC Y36.29-●
    - weapons Y36.27-●
  - friendly fire Y36.92
  - hand to hand (unarmed) combat Y36.44-●
  - hot substances —*see* War operations, fire
  - incendiary bullet Y36.32-●
  - nuclear weapon (effects of) Y36.5Ø-●
    - acute radiation exposure Y36.54-●
    - blast pressure Y36.51-●
    - direct blast Y36.51-●
    - direct heat Y36.53-●
    - fallout exposure Y36.54-●
    - fireball Y36.53-●
    - indirect blast (struck or crushed by blast debris) (being thrown by blast) Y36.52-●
    - ionizing radiation (immediate exposure) Y36.54-●
    - nuclear radiation Y36.54-●
    - radiation
      - ionizing (immediate exposure) Y36.54-●

War operations *(Continued)*
  - nuclear weapon *(Continued)*
    - radiation *(Continued)*
      - nuclear Y36.54-●
      - thermal Y36.53-●
    - secondary effects Y36.54-●
    - specified NEC Y36.59-●
    - thermal radiation Y36.53-●
  - restriction of air (airway)
    - intentional Y36.46-●
    - unintentional Y36.47-●
  - rubber bullets Y36.41-●
  - shrapnel NOS Y36.29-●
  - suffocation —*see* War operations, restriction of airways
  - unconventional warfare NEC Y36.7X-●
  - underwater blast NOS Y36.ØØ-●
  - warfare
    - conventional NEC Y36.49-●
    - unconventional NEC Y36.7X-●
  - weapon of mass destruction [WMD] Y36.91
  - weapons
    - biological weapons Y36.6X-●
    - chemical Y36.7X-●
    - nuclear (effects of) Y36.5Ø-●
      - acute radiation exposure Y36.54-●
      - blast pressure Y36.51-●
      - direct blast Y36.51-●
      - direct heat Y36.53-●
      - fallout exposure Y36.54-●
      - fireball Y36.53-●
      - radiation
        - ionizing (immediate exposure) Y36.54-●
        - nuclear Y36.54-●
        - thermal Y36.53-●
      - secondary effects Y36.54-●
      - specified NEC Y36.59-●
    - of mass destruction [WMD] Y36.91-●
- **Washed**
  - away by flood —*see* Flood
  - off road by storm (transport vehicle) —*see* Forces of nature, cataclysmic storm
- **Weather exposure NEC** —*see* Forces of nature
- **Weightlessness** (causing injury) (effects of) (in spacecraft, real or simulated) X52
- **Work related condition** Y99.Ø
- **Wound** (accidental) NEC —*see also* Injury X58
  - battle —*see also* War operations Y36.9Ø
  - gunshot —*see* Discharge, firearm by type
- **Wreck transport vehicle NEC** —*see also* Accident, transport V89.9
- **Wrong**
  - device implanted into correct surgical site Y65.51
  - fluid in infusion Y65.1
  - patient, procedure performed on Y65.52
  - procedure (operation) on correct patient Y65.51

PART III

ICD-10-CM Tabular List of Diseases and Injuries

CHAPTER 1

CERTAIN INFECTIOUS AND PARASITIC DISEASES (A00-B99)

OGCR Chapter-Specific Coding Guidelines

1. Chapter 1: Certain Infectious and Parasitic Diseases (A00-B99)

a. Human Immunodeficiency Virus (HIV) Infections

1) Code only confirmed cases

Code only confirmed cases of HIV infection/illness. This is an exception to the hospital inpatient guideline Section II, H.

In this context, "confirmation" does not require documentation of positive serology or culture for HIV; the provider's diagnostic statement that the patient is HIV positive, or has an HIV-related illness is sufficient.

2) Selection and sequencing of HIV codes

(a) Patient admitted for HIV-related condition

If a patient is admitted for an HIV-related condition, the principal diagnosis should be B20, Human immunodeficiency virus [HIV] disease followed by additional diagnosis codes for all reported HIV-related conditions.

(b) Patient with HIV disease admitted for unrelated condition

If a patient with HIV disease is admitted for an unrelated condition (such as a traumatic injury), the code for the unrelated condition (e.g., the nature of injury code) should be the principal diagnosis. Other diagnoses would be B20 followed by additional diagnosis codes for all reported HIV-related conditions.

(c) Whether the patient is newly diagnosed

Whether the patient is newly diagnosed or has had previous admissions/encounters for HIV conditions is irrelevant to the sequencing decision.

(d) Asymptomatic human immunodeficiency virus

Z21, Asymptomatic human immunodeficiency virus [HIV] infection status, is to be applied when the patient without any documentation of symptoms is listed as being "HIV positive," "known HIV," "HIV test positive," or similar terminology. Do not use this code if the term "AIDS" is used or if the patient is treated for any HIV-related illness or is described as having any condition(s) resulting from his/her HIV positive status; use B20 in these cases.

(e) Patients with inconclusive HIV serology

Patients with inconclusive HIV serology, but no definitive diagnosis or manifestations of the illness, may be assigned code R75, Inconclusive laboratory evidence of human immunodeficiency virus [HIV].

(f) Previously diagnosed HIV-related illness

Patients with any known prior diagnosis of an HIV-related illness should be coded to B20. Once a patient has developed an HIV-related illness, the patient should always be assigned code B20 on every subsequent admission/encounter. Patients previously diagnosed with any HIV illness (B20) should never be assigned to R75 or Z21, Asymptomatic human immunodeficiency virus [HIV] infection status.

(g) HIV Infection in Pregnancy, Childbirth and the Puerperium

During pregnancy, childbirth or the puerperium, a patient admitted (or presenting for a health care encounter) because of an HIV-related illness should receive a principal diagnosis code of O98.7-, Human immunodeficiency [HIV] disease complicating pregnancy, childbirth and the puerperium, followed by B20 and the code(s) for the HIV-related illness(es). Codes from Chapter 15 always take sequencing priority.

Patients with asymptomatic HIV infection status admitted (or presenting for a health care encounter) during pregnancy, childbirth, or the puerperium should receive codes of O98.7- and Z21.

(h) Encounters for testing for HIV

If a patient is being seen to determine his/her HIV status, use code Z11.4, Encounter for screening for human immunodeficiency virus [HIV]. Use additional codes for any associated high-risk behavior.

If a patient with signs or symptoms is being seen for HIV testing, code the signs and symptoms. An additional counseling code Z71.7, Human immunodeficiency virus [HIV] counseling, may be used if counseling is provided during the encounter for the test.

When a patient returns to be informed of his/her HIV test results and the test result is negative, use code Z71.7, Human immunodeficiency virus [HIV] counseling.

If the results are positive, see previous guidelines and assign codes as appropriate.

b. Infectious agents as the cause of diseases classified to other chapters

Certain infections are classified in chapters other than Chapter 1 and no organism is identified as part of the infection code. In these instances, it is necessary to use an additional code from Chapter 1 to identify the organism. A code from category B95, Streptococcus, Staphylococcus, and Enterococcus as the cause of diseases classified to other chapters, B96, Other bacterial agents as the cause of diseases classified to other chapters, or B97, Viral agents as the cause of diseases classified to other chapters, is to be used as an additional code to identify the organism. An instructional note will be found at the infection code advising that an additional organism code is required.

c. Infections resistant to antibiotics

Many bacterial infections are resistant to current antibiotics. It is necessary to identify all infections documented as antibiotic resistant. Assign a code from category Z16, Resistance to antimicrobial drugs, following the infection code only if the infection code does not identify drug resistance.

d. Sepsis, Severe Sepsis, and Septic Shock

1) Coding of Sepsis and Severe Sepsis

(a) Sepsis

For a diagnosis of sepsis, assign the appropriate code for the underlying systemic infection. If the type of infection or causal organism is not further specified, assign code A41.9, Sepsis, unspecified organism.

A code from subcategory R65.2, Severe sepsis, should not be assigned unless severe sepsis or an associated acute organ dysfunction is documented.

(i) Negative or inconclusive blood cultures and sepsis

Negative or inconclusive blood cultures do not preclude a diagnosis of sepsis in patients with clinical evidence of the condition, however, the provider should be queried.

(ii) Urosepsis

The term urosepsis is a nonspecific term. It is not to be considered synonymous with sepsis. It has no default code in the Alphabetic Index. Should a provider use this term, he/she must be queried for clarification.

(iii) Sepsis with organ dysfunction

If a patient has sepsis and associated acute organ dysfunction or multiple organ dysfunction (MOD), follow the instructions for coding severe sepsis.

(iv) Acute organ dysfunction that is not clearly associated with the sepsis

If a patient has sepsis and an acute organ dysfunction, but the medical record documentation indicates that the acute organ dysfunction is related to a medical condition other than the sepsis, do not assign a code from subcategory R65.2, Severe sepsis. An acute organ dysfunction must be associated with the sepsis in order to assign the severe sepsis code. If the documentation is not clear as to whether an acute organ dysfunction is related to the sepsis or another medical condition, query the provider.

(b) Severe sepsis

The coding of severe sepsis requires a minimum of 2 codes: first a code for the underlying systemic infection, followed by a code from subcategory R65.2, Severe sepsis. If the causal organism is not documented, assign code A41.9, Sepsis, unspecified organism, for the infection. Additional code(s) for the associated acute organ dysfunction are also required.

Due to the complex nature of severe sepsis, some cases may require querying the provider prior to assignment of the codes.

2) Septic shock

(a) Septic shock generally refers to circulatory failure associated with severe sepsis, and therefore, it represents a type of acute organ dysfunction.

For all cases of septic shock, the code for the systemic infection should be sequenced first, followed by code R65.21, Severe sepsis with septic shock or code T81.12, Postprocedural septic shock.

Any additional codes for the other acute organ dysfunctions should also be assigned. As noted in the sequencing instructions in the Tabular List, the code for septic shock cannot be assigned as a principal diagnosis.

3) Sequencing of severe sepsis

If severe sepsis is present on admission, and meets the definition of principal diagnosis, the underlying systemic infection should be assigned as principal diagnosis followed by the appropriate code from subcategory R65.2 as required by the sequencing rules in the Tabular List. A code from subcategory R65.2 can never be assigned as a principal diagnosis.

When severe sepsis develops during an encounter (it was not present on admission) the underlying systemic infection and the appropriate code from subcategory R65.2 should be assigned as secondary diagnoses.

Severe sepsis may be present on admission but the diagnosis may not be confirmed until sometime after admission. If the documentation is not clear whether severe sepsis was present on admission, the provider should be queried.

4) Sepsis and severe sepsis with a localized infection

If the reason for admission is both sepsis or severe sepsis and a localized infection, such as pneumonia or cellulitis, a code(s) for the underlying systemic infection should be assigned first and the code for the localized infection should be assigned as a secondary diagnosis. If the patient has severe sepsis, a code from subcategory R65.2 should also be assigned as a secondary diagnosis. If the patient is admitted with a localized infection, such as pneumonia, and sepsis/severe sepsis doesn't develop until after admission, the localized infection should be assigned first, followed by the appropriate sepsis/severe sepsis codes.

5) Sepsis due to a postprocedural infection

(a) Documentation of causal relationship

As with all postprocedural complications, code assignment is based on the provider's documentation of the relationship between the infection and the procedure.

(b) Sepsis due to a postprocedural infection

For infections following a procedure, a code from T81.4Ø, to T81.43. Infection following a procedure, or O86.ØØ to O86.Ø3, Infection of obstetric surgical wound, that identifies the site of the infection should be coded first, if known. Assign an additional code for sepsis following a procedure (T81.44) or sepsis following an obstetrical procedure (O86.Ø4). Use an additional code to identify the infectious agent. If the patient has severe sepsis the appropriate code from subcategory R65.2 should also be assigned with the additional code(s) for any acute organ dysfunction.

For infections following infusion, transfusion, therapeutic injection, or immunization, a code from subcategory T8Ø.2, Infections following infusion, transfusion, and therapeutic injection, or code T88.Ø-, Infection following immunization, should be coded first, followed by the code for the specific infection. If the patient has severe sepsis, the appropriate code from subcategory R65.2 should also be assigned, with the additional codes(s) for any acute organ dysfunction.

(c) Postprocedural infection and postprocedural septic shock

If a postprocedural infection has resulted in postprocedural septic shock, assign the codes indicated above for sepsis due to a postprocedural infection, followed by code T81.12-, Postprocedural septic shock. Do not assign code R65.21, Severe sepsis with septic shock. Additional code(s) should be assigned for any acute organ dysfunction.

6) Sepsis and severe sepsis associated with a noninfectious process (condition)

In some cases a noninfectious process (condition), such as trauma, may lead to an infection which can result in sepsis or severe sepsis. If sepsis or severe sepsis is documented as associated with a noninfectious condition, such as a burn or serious injury, and this condition meets the definition for principal diagnosis, the code for the noninfectious condition should be sequenced first, followed by the code for the resulting infection. If severe sepsis is present, a code from subcategory R65.2 should also be assigned with any associated organ dysfunction(s) codes. It is not necessary to assign a code from subcategory R65.1, Systemic inflammatory response syndrome (SIRS) of noninfectious origin, for these cases.

If the infection meets the definition of principal diagnosis it should be sequenced before the noninfectious condition. When both the associated noninfectious condition and the infection meet the definition of principal diagnosis either may be assigned as principal diagnosis.

Only one code from category R65, Symptoms and signs specifically associated with systemic inflammation and infection, should be assigned. Therefore, when a noninfectious condition leads to an infection resulting in severe sepsis, assign the appropriate code from subcategory R65.2, Severe sepsis. Do not additionally assign a code from subcategory R65.1, Systemic inflammatory response syndrome (SIRS) of noninfectious origin.

See Section I.C.18. SIRS due to non-infectious process

7) Sepsis and septic shock complicating abortion, pregnancy, childbirth, and the puerperium

See Section I.C.15. Sepsis and septic shock complicating abortion, pregnancy, childbirth and the puerperium

8) Newborn sepsis

See Section I.C.16. f. Bacterial sepsis of Newborn

e. Methicillin Resistant Staphylococcus aureus (MRSA) Conditions

1) Selection and sequencing of MRSA codes

(a) Combination codes for MRSA infection

When a patient is diagnosed with an infection that is due to methicillin resistant *Staphylococcus aureus* (MRSA), and that infection has a combination code that includes the causal organism (e.g., sepsis, pneumonia) assign the appropriate combination code for the condition (e.g., code A41.Ø2, Sepsis due to Methicillin resistant Staphylococcus aureus or code J15.212, Pneumonia due to Methicillin resistant Staphylococcus aureus). Do not assign code B95.62, Methicillin resistant Staphylococcus aureus infection as the cause of diseases classified elsewhere, as an additional code because the combination code includes the type of infection and the MRSA organism. Do not assign a code from subcategory Z16.11, Resistance to penicillins, as an additional diagnosis.

See Section C.1. for instructions on coding and sequencing of sepsis and severe sepsis.

(b) Other codes for MRSA infection

When there is documentation of a current infection (e.g., wound infection, stitch abscess, urinary tract infection) due to MRSA, and that infection does not have a combination code that includes the causal organism, assign the appropriate code to identify the condition along with code B95.62, Methicillin resistant Staphylococcus aureus infection as the cause of diseases classified elsewhere for the MRSA infection. Do not assign a code from subcategory Z16.11, Resistance to penicillins.

(c) Methicillin susceptible Staphylococcus aureus (MSSA) and MRSA colonization

The condition or state of being colonized or carrying MSSA or MRSA is called colonization or carriage, while an individual person is described as being colonized or being a carrier. Colonization means that MSSA or MSRA is present on or in the body without necessarily causing illness. A positive MRSA colonization test might be documented by the provider as "MRSA screen positive" or "MRSA nasal swab positive".

Assign code Z22.322, Carrier or suspected carrier of Methicillin resistant Staphylococcus aureus, for patients documented as having MRSA colonization. Assign code Z22.321, Carrier or suspected carrier of Methicillin susceptible Staphylococcus aureus, for patient documented as having MSSA colonization. Colonization is not necessarily indicative of a disease process or as the cause of a specific condition the patient may have unless documented as such by the provider.

(d) MRSA colonization and infection

If a patient is documented as having both MRSA colonization and infection during a hospital admission, code Z22.322, Carrier or suspected carrier of Methicillin resistant Staphylococcus aureus, and a code for the MRSA infection may both be assigned.

f. Zika virus infections

1) Code only confirmed cases

Code only a confirmed diagnosis of Zika virus (A92.5, Zika virus disease) as documented by the provider. This is an exception to the hospital inpatient guideline Section II, H.

In this context, "confirmation" does not require documentation of the type of test performed; the physician's diagnostic statement that the condition is confirmed is sufficient. This code should be assigned regardless of the stated mode of transmission.

If the provider documents "suspected", "possible" or "probable" Zika, do not assign code A92.5. Assign a code(s) explaining the reason for encounter (such as fever, rash, or joint pain) or Z2Ø.821, Contact with and (suspected) exposure to Zika virus.

CHAPTER 1

CERTAIN INFECTIOUS AND PARASITIC DISEASES (A00-B99)

Includes diseases generally recognized as communicable or transmissible

Use additional code to identify resistance to antimicrobial drugs (Z16.-)

Excludes1 certain localized infections - see body system-related chapters

Excludes2 carrier or suspected carrier of infectious disease (Z22.-)
infectious and parasitic diseases complicating pregnancy, childbirth and the puerperium (O98.-)
infectious and parasitic diseases specific to the perinatal period (P35-P39)
influenza and other acute respiratory infections (J00-J22)

This chapter contains the following blocks:

A00-A09	Intestinal infectious diseases
A15-A19	Tuberculosis
A20-A28	Certain zoonotic bacterial diseases
A30-A49	Other bacterial diseases
A50-A64	Infections with a predominantly sexual mode of transmission
A65-A69	Other spirochetal diseases
A70-A74	Other diseases caused by chlamydiae
A75-A79	Rickettsioses
A80-A89	Viral and prion infections of the central nervous system
A90-A99	Arthropod-borne viral fevers and viral hemorrhagic fevers
B00-B09	Viral infections characterized by skin and mucous membrane lesions
B10	Other human herpesviruses
B15-B19	Viral hepatitis
B20	Human immunodeficiency virus [HIV] disease
B25-B34	Other viral diseases
B35-B49	Mycoses
B50-B64	Protozoal diseases
B65-B83	Helminthiases
B85-B89	Pediculosis, acariasis and other infestations
B90-B94	Sequelae of infectious and parasitic diseases
B95-B97	Bacterial and viral infectious agents
B99	Other infectious diseases

INTESTINAL INFECTIOUS DISEASES (A00-A09)

A00 Cholera
A serious, often deadly, infectious disease of the small intestine

A00.0 Cholera due to Vibrio cholerae 01, biovar cholerae
Classical cholera

A00.1 Cholera due to Vibrio cholerae 01, biovar eltor
Cholera eltor

A00.9 Cholera, unspecified

A01 Typhoid and paratyphoid fevers
Caused by Salmonella typhi and Salmonella paratyphi A, B, and C bacteria

A01.0 Typhoid fever
Infection due to Salmonella typhi

A01.00 Typhoid fever, unspecified

A01.01 Typhoid meningitis

A01.02 Typhoid fever with heart involvement
Typhoid endocarditis
Typhoid myocarditis

A01.03 Typhoid pneumonia

A01.04 Typhoid arthritis

A01.05 Typhoid osteomyelitis

A01.09 Typhoid fever with other complications

A01.1 Paratyphoid fever A

A01.2 Paratyphoid fever B

A01.3 Paratyphoid fever C

A01.4 Paratyphoid fever, unspecified
Infection due to Salmonella paratyphi NOS

A02 Other salmonella infections

Includes infection or foodborne intoxication due to any Salmonella species other than S. typhi and S. paratyphi

A02.0 Salmonella enteritis
Salmonellosis

A02.1 Salmonella sepsis

A02.2 Localized salmonella infections

A02.20 Localized salmonella infection, unspecified
Specified in the documentation as localized, but unspecified as to type

A02.21 Salmonella meningitis
Specified as localized in the meninges

A02.22 Salmonella pneumonia
Specified as localized in the lungs

A02.23 Salmonella arthritis
Specified as localized in the joints

A02.24 Salmonella osteomyelitis
Specified as localized in bone

A02.25 Salmonella pyelonephritis
Salmonella tubulo-interstitial nephropathy

A02.29 Salmonella with other localized infection
Specified as localized (because it is still under localized heading) but does not assign into any of the above codes

A02.8 Other specified salmonella infections
Any specified salmonella infection which does NOT assign into any of the above codes (not specified as localized)

A02.9 Salmonella infection, unspecified
Unspecified in the documentation as to specific type of salmonella

A03 Shigellosis
An infectious disease caused by bacteria (Shigella)

A03.0 Shigellosis due to Shigella dysenteriae
Group A shigellosis [Shiga-Kruse dysentery]

A03.1 Shigellosis due to Shigella flexneri
Group B shigellosis

A03.2 Shigellosis due to Shigella boydii
Group C shigellosis

A03.3 Shigellosis due to Shigella sonnei
Group D shigellosis

A03.8 Other shigellosis

A03.9 Shigellosis, unspecified
Bacillary dysentery NOS

Item 1–1 Salmonella is a bacterium that lives in the intestines of fowl and mammals and can spread to humans through improper food preparation and cooking. Salmonellosis is an infection with the bacterium. Symptoms include diarrhea, fever, and abdominal cramps 12 to 72 hours after infection. The illness usually lasts 4 to 7 days, and most persons recover without treatment. The diarrhea may be so severe that the patient needs to be hospitalized. Patients with immunocompromised systems in chronic, ill health are more likely to have the infection invade their bloodstream with life-threatening results. For example, patients with sickle cell disease are more prone to salmonella osteomyelitis than others.

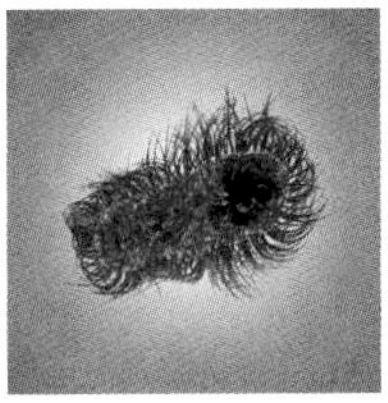

Figure 1-1 Electron micrograph of escherichia coli (E. coli) expressing P fimbriae. (Getty Image)

Item 1-2 ***Escherichia coli [E. coli]*** is a Gram-negative bacterium found in the intestinal tracts of humans and animals and is usually nonpathogenic. Pathogenic strains can cause diarrhea or pyogenic (pus-producing) infections. Can be a threat to food safety.

● A04 **Other bacterial intestinal infections**
Excludes1 bacterial foodborne intoxications, NEC (A05.-)
tuberculous enteritis (A18.32)

A04.0 **Enteropathogenic Escherichia coli infection**
Pertaining to or producing intestinal disease

A04.1 **Enterotoxigenic Escherichia coli infection**
Producing or containing intestinal toxin

A04.2 **Enteroinvasive Escherichia coli infection**
Capable of penetrating and spreading through intestinal mucosal epithelium

A04.3 **Enterohemorrhagic Escherichia coli infection**
Causing bloody diarrhea, resulting from microorganisms

A04.4 **Other intestinal Escherichia coli infections**
Escherichia coli enteritis NOS

A04.5 **Campylobacter enteritis**
Spiral shaped bacterium

A04.6 **Enteritis due to Yersinia enterocolitica**
Excludes1 extraintestinal yersiniosis (A28.2)
Transmitted by infected food/water and person-to-person contact, affecting intestinal tract

● A04.7 **Enterocolitis due to Clostridium difficile**
Foodborne intoxication by Clostridium difficile
Pseudomembraneous colitis
Marked by fibrinous deposit (false membrane) with enmeshed necrotic cells

A04.71 **Enterocolitis due to Clostridium difficile, recurrent**

A04.72 **Enterocolitis due to Clostridium difficile, not specified as recurrent**

A04.8 **Other specified bacterial intestinal infections**

A04.9 **Bacterial intestinal infection, unspecified**
Bacterial enteritis NOS

● A05 **Other bacterial foodborne intoxications, not elsewhere classified**
Excludes1 Clostridium difficile foodborne intoxication and infection (A04.7-)
Escherichia coli infection (A04.0-A04.4)
listeriosis (A32.-)
salmonella foodborne intoxication and infection (A02.-)
toxic effect of noxious foodstuffs (T61-T62)

A05.0 **Foodborne staphylococcal intoxication**

A05.1 **Botulism food poisoning**
Botulism NOS
Classical foodborne intoxication due to Clostridium botulinum
Excludes1 infant botulism (A48.51)
wound botulism (A48.52)

A05.2 **Foodborne Clostridium perfringens [Clostridium welchii] intoxication**
Type A causes gas gangrene and necrotizing colitis; major cause of food poisoning in humans
Enteritis necroticans
Pig-bel

A05.3 **Foodborne Vibrio parahaemolyticus intoxication**
Organism that survives only in high salt environment (halophilic), major cause of gastroenteritis due to consumption of raw or improperly cooked fish/seafood

A05.4 **Foodborne Bacillus cereus intoxication**
Spore-forming species commonly found in soil, causes food poisoning from formation of intestinal toxins in contaminated foods

A05.5 **Foodborne Vibrio vulnificus intoxication**
Species that survives in high salt environment (halophilic) with infection by eating raw seafood causes septicemia and cellulitis

A05.8 **Other specified bacterial foodborne intoxications**

A05.9 **Bacterial foodborne intoxication, unspecified**

● A06 **Amebiasis**
An intestinal illness caused by the microscopic parasite Entamoeba histolytica
Includes infection due to Entamoeba histolytica
Excludes1 other protozoal intestinal diseases (A07.-)
Excludes2 acanthamebiasis (B60.1-)
Naegleriasis (B60.2)

A06.0 **Acute amebic dysentery**
Acute amebiasis
Intestinal amebiasis NOS

A06.1 **Chronic intestinal amebiasis**

A06.2 **Amebic nondysenteric colitis**
Pertaining to single cell microorganism

A06.3 **Ameboma of intestine**
Tumorlike mass produced by localized inflammation often in intestine
Ameboma NOS

A06.4 **Amebic liver abscess**
Hepatic amebiasis

A06.5 **Amebic lung abscess**
Amebic abscess of lung (and liver)

A06.6 **Amebic brain abscess**
Amebic abscess of brain (and liver) (and lung)

A06.7 **Cutaneous amebiasis**

● A06.8 **Amebic infection of other sites**

A06.81 **Amebic cystitis**

A06.82 **Other amebic genitourinary infections**
Amebic balanitis
Amebic vesiculitis
Amebic vulvovaginitis

A06.89 **Other amebic infections**
Amebic appendicitis
Amebic splenic abscess

A06.9 **Amebiasis, unspecified**

CHAPTER 1 (A00-B99)

A07 Other protozoal intestinal diseases

A07.0 Balantidiasis
Balantidial dysentery
Infection by protozoa that may cause diarrhea and dysentery, with ulceration of colonic mucous membranes

A07.1 Giardiasis [lambliasis]
Common infection in small intestine spread by contaminated food, water, or direct person-to-person contact

A07.2 Cryptosporidiosis
Human infection with protozoa usually seen as self-limited diarrhea in those who work with cattle

A07.3 Isosporiasis
Human intestinal disease caused by protozoa
Infection due to Isospora belli and Isospora hominis
Intestinal coccidiosis
Isosporosis

A07.4 Cyclosporiasis
Infection by protozoa with most common species infecting humans being C cayetanensis

A07.8 Other specified protozoal intestinal diseases
Intestinal microsporidiosis
Intestinal trichomoniasis
Sarcocystosis
Sarcosporidiosis

A07.9 Protozoal intestinal disease, unspecified
Flagellate diarrhea
Protozoal colitis
Protozoal diarrhea
Protozoal dysentery

A08 Viral and other specified intestinal infections
Excludes1 influenza with involvement of gastrointestinal tract (J09.X3, J10.2, J11.2)

A08.0 Rotaviral enteritis

A08.1 Acute gastroenteropathy due to Norwalk agent and other small round viruses

A08.11 Acute gastroenteropathy due to Norwalk agent
Acute gastroenteropathy due to Norovirus
Acute gastroenteropathy due to Norwalk-like agent

A08.19 Acute gastroenteropathy due to other small round viruses
Acute gastroenteropathy due to small round virus [SRV] NOS

A08.2 Adenoviral enteritis

A08.3 Other viral enteritis

A08.31 Calicivirus enteritis

A08.32 Astrovirus enteritis

A08.39 Other viral enteritis
Coxsackie virus enteritis
Echovirus enteritis
Enterovirus enteritis NEC
Torovirus enteritis

A08.4 Viral intestinal infection, unspecified
Viral enteritis NOS
Viral gastroenteritis NOS
Viral gastroenteropathy NOS
Coding Clinic: 2016, Q3, P12

A08.8 Other specified intestinal infections

A09 Infectious gastroenteritis and colitis, unspecified
Infectious colitis NOS
Infectious enteritis NOS
Infectious gastroenteritis NOS
Excludes1 colitis NOS (K52.9)
diarrhea NOS (R19.7)
enteritis NOS (K52.9)
gastroenteritis NOS (K52.9)
noninfective gastroenteritis and colitis, unspecified (K52.9)

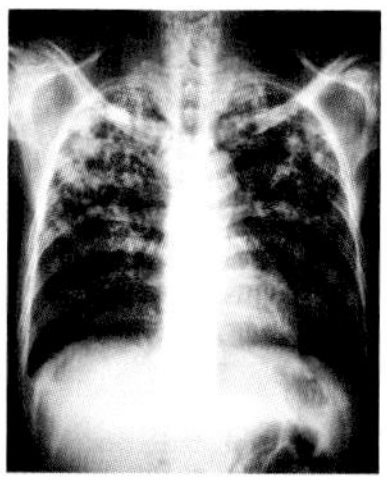

Figure 1-2 Far advanced bilateral pulmonary tuberculosis before and after 8 months of treatment with streptomycin, PAS, and isoniazid. (Getty Image)

Item 1-3 **Tuberculosis** is a common and deadly infectious disease caused by the *Mycobacterium tuberculosis* organism. The first tuberculosis infection is called the **primary infection** and most commonly attacks the lungs but can affect the central nervous system, lymphatic system, circulatory system, genitourinary system, bones, joints, and even the skin. A **Ghon** lesion is the **initial lesion.** A **secondary lesion** occurs when the tubercle bacilli are carried to other areas.

Item 1-4 Although it primarily affects the lungs, the bacteria ***Mycobacterium tuberculosis*** can travel from the pulmonary circulation to virtually any organ in the body, much as a cancer metastasizes to a secondary site. If the immune system becomes compromised by age or disease, what would otherwise be a self-limiting primary tuberculosis in the lungs will develop in other organs. These are known as extrapulmonary sites.

TUBERCULOSIS (A15-A19)

Includes infections due to Mycobacterium tuberculosis and Mycobacterium bovis
Excludes1 congenital tuberculosis (P37.0)
nonspecific reaction to test for tuberculosis without active tuberculosis (R76.1-)
pneumoconiosis associated with tuberculosis, any type in A15 (J65)
positive PPD (R76.11)
positive tuberculin skin test without active tuberculosis (R76.11)
sequelae of tuberculosis (B90.-)
silicotuberculosis (J65)

A15 Respiratory tuberculosis

A15.0 Tuberculosis of lung
Tuberculous bronchiectasis
Chronic dilatation of bronchi
Tuberculous fibrosis of lung
Tuberculous pneumonia
Tuberculous pneumothorax

A15.4 Tuberculosis of intrathoracic lymph nodes
Tuberculosis of hilar lymph nodes
Tuberculosis of mediastinal lymph nodes
Tuberculosis of tracheobronchial lymph nodes
Excludes1 tuberculosis specified as primary (A15.7)

A15.5 Tuberculosis of larynx, trachea and bronchus
Tuberculosis of bronchus
Tuberculosis of glottis
Tuberculosis of larynx
Tuberculosis of trachea

A15.6 Tuberculous pleurisy
Tuberculosis of pleura
Tuberculous empyema
Excludes1 primary respiratory tuberculosis (A15.7)

A15.7 Primary respiratory tuberculosis

A15.8 Other respiratory tuberculosis
Mediastinal tuberculosis
Nasopharyngeal tuberculosis
Tuberculosis of nose
Tuberculosis of sinus [any nasal]

A15.9 Respiratory tuberculosis unspecified

● **A17 Tuberculosis of nervous system**

A17.Ø Tuberculous meningitis
Tuberculosis of meninges (cerebral) (spinal)
Tuberculous leptomeningitis
Excludes1 tuberculous meningoencephalitis (A17.82)

A17.1 Meningeal tuberculoma
Tuberculoma of meninges (cerebral) (spinal)
Excludes2 tuberculoma of brain and spinal cord (A17.81)

● **A17.8 Other tuberculosis of nervous system**

A17.81 Tuberculoma of brain and spinal cord
Tuberculous abscess of brain and spinal cord

A17.82 Tuberculous meningoencephalitis
Inflammation of brain and meninges; AKA cerebromeningitis and encephalomeningitis
Tuberculous myelitis

A17.83 Tuberculous neuritis
Tuberculous mononeuropathy

A17.89 Other tuberculosis of nervous system
Tuberculous polyneuropathy

A17.9 Tuberculosis of nervous system, unspecified

● **A18 Tuberculosis of other organs**

● **A18.Ø Tuberculosis of bones and joints**

A18.Ø1 Tuberculosis of spine
Pott's disease or curvature of spine
Tuberculous arthritis
Tuberculous osteomyelitis of spine
Tuberculous spondylitis

A18.Ø2 Tuberculous arthritis of other joints
Tuberculosis of hip (joint)
Tuberculosis of knee (joint)

A18.Ø3 Tuberculosis of other bones
Tuberculous mastoiditis
Tuberculous osteomyelitis

A18.Ø9 Other musculoskeletal tuberculosis
Tuberculous myositis
Tuberculous synovitis
Tuberculous tenosynovitis

● **A18.1 Tuberculosis of genitourinary system**

A18.1Ø Tuberculosis of genitourinary system, unspecified

A18.11 Tuberculosis of kidney and ureter

A18.12 Tuberculosis of bladder

A18.13 Tuberculosis of other urinary organs
Tuberculous urethritis

A18.14 Tuberculosis of prostate ♂ A

A18.15 Tuberculosis of other male genital organs ♂

A18.16 Tuberculosis of cervix ♀

A18.17 Tuberculous female pelvic inflammatory disease ♀
Tuberculous endometritis
Tuberculous oophoritis and salpingitis
Oophoritis = inflammation of ovary
Salpingitis = inflammation of fallopian tube

A18.18 Tuberculosis of other female genital organs ♀
Tuberculous ulceration of vulva

A18.2 Tuberculous peripheral lymphadenopathy
Tuberculous adenitis
Excludes2 tuberculosis of bronchial and mediastinal lymph nodes (A15.4)
tuberculosis of mesenteric and retroperitoneal lymph nodes (A18.39)
tuberculous tracheobronchial adenopathy (A15.4)

● **A18.3 Tuberculosis of intestines, peritoneum and mesenteric glands**

A18.31 Tuberculous peritonitis
Tuberculous ascites

A18.32 Tuberculous enteritis
Tuberculosis of anus and rectum
Tuberculosis of intestine (large) (small)

A18.39 Retroperitoneal tuberculosis
Tuberculosis of mesenteric glands
Tuberculosis of retroperitoneal (lymph glands)

A18.4 Tuberculosis of skin and subcutaneous tissue
Erythema induratum, tuberculous
Lupus excedens
Lupus vulgaris NOS
Lupus vulgaris of eyelid
Cutaneous tuberculosis characterized by reddish brown plaque on skin surrounded by papules and nodules
Scrofuloderma
Type of cutaneous tuberculosis, with direct extension of tuberculosis into skin from underlying structures; AKA tuberculosis colliquativa
Tuberculosis of external ear
Excludes2 lupus erythematosus (L93.-)
~~lupus NOS (M32.9)~~
➠ systemic lupus erythematosus (M32.-)

● **A18.5 Tuberculosis of eye**
Excludes2 lupus vulgaris of eyelid (A18.4)

A18.5Ø Tuberculosis of eye, unspecified

A18.51 Tuberculous episcleritis
Inflammation of episclera and adjacent tissues

A18.52 Tuberculous keratitis
Tuberculous interstitial keratitis
Tuberculous keratoconjunctivitis (interstitial) (phlyctenular)
Inflammation of cornea and conjunctiva

A18.53 Tuberculous chorioretinitis
Inflammation of choroid and retina; retinochoroiditis

A18.54 Tuberculous iridocyclitis
Inflammation of iris and ciliary body

A18.59 Other tuberculosis of eye
Tuberculous conjunctivitis

A18.6 Tuberculosis of (inner) (middle) ear
Tuberculous otitis media
Excludes2 tuberculosis of external ear (A18.4)
tuberculous mastoiditis (A18.Ø3)

A18.7 Tuberculosis of adrenal glands
Tuberculous Addison's disease

● **A18.8 Tuberculosis of other specified organs**

A18.81 Tuberculosis of thyroid gland

A18.82 Tuberculosis of other endocrine glands
Tuberculosis of pituitary gland
Tuberculosis of thymus gland

A18.83 Tuberculosis of digestive tract organs, not elsewhere classified
Excludes1 tuberculosis of intestine (A18.32)

A18.84 Tuberculosis of heart
Tuberculous cardiomyopathy
Tuberculous endocarditis
Tuberculous myocarditis
Tuberculous pericarditis

A18.85 Tuberculosis of spleen

A18.89 Tuberculosis of other sites
Tuberculosis of muscle
Tuberculous cerebral arteritis

Item 1–5 Miliary tuberculosis can be a life-threatening condition. If a tuberculous lesion enters a blood vessel, immense dissemination of tuberculous organisms can occur if the immune system is weak. High-risk populations—children under 4 years of age, the elderly, or the immunocompromised—are particularly prone to this type of infection. The lesions will have a millet seedlike appearance on chest x-ray. Bronchial washings and biopsy may aid in diagnosis.

● **A19 Miliary tuberculosis**
Includes disseminated tuberculosis
generalized tuberculosis
tuberculous polyserositis

A19.0 **Acute miliary tuberculosis of a single specified site**
A19.1 **Acute miliary tuberculosis of multiple sites**
A19.2 **Acute miliary tuberculosis, unspecified**
A19.8 **Other miliary tuberculosis**
A19.9 **Miliary tuberculosis, unspecified**

CERTAIN ZOONOTIC BACTERIAL DISEASES (A20-A28)

● **A20 Plague**
Infectious disease caused by a Yersinia pestis bacterium, transmitted by a rodent flea bite or handling of infected animal
Includes infection due to Yersinia pestis

A20.0 **Bubonic plague**
A20.1 **Cellulocutaneous plague**
Skin and subcutaneous tissue plague
A20.2 **Pneumonic plague** HCC
A20.3 **Plague meningitis**
A20.7 **Septicemic plague** HCC
A20.8 **Other forms of plague**
Abortive plague
Asymptomatic plague
Pestis minor
Systemic bacterial disease
A20.9 **Plague, unspecified**

● **A21 Tularemia**
Caused by Francisella tularensis bacterium found in rodents, rabbits, and hares and transmitted to humans by contact with infected animal tissues or by ticks, biting flies, or mosquitoes
Includes deer-fly fever
infection due to Francisella tularensis
rabbit fever
Coding Clinic: 2016, Q4, P25

A21.0 **Ulceroglandular tularemia**
Most common form of tularemia in humans is painful, swollen, erythematous papule at point of inoculation that ruptures to form shallow ulcer
A21.1 **Oculoglandular tularemia**
Primary site of entry is conjunctival sac, results in granulomatous corneal lesions
Ophthalmic tularemia
A21.2 **Pulmonary tularemia** HCC
A21.3 **Gastrointestinal tularemia**
Abdominal tularemia
A21.7 **Generalized tularemia**
A21.8 **Other forms of tularemia**
A21.9 **Tularemia, unspecified**

● **A22 Anthrax**
An acute infectious disease caused by the spore-forming Bacillus anthracis; occurs in humans exposed to infected animals or tissue from infected animals
Includes infection due to Bacillus anthracis

A22.0 **Cutaneous anthrax**
Malignant carbuncle
Malignant pustule
A22.1 **Pulmonary anthrax** HCC
Inhalation anthrax
Ragpicker's disease
Woolsorter's disease
A22.2 **Gastrointestinal anthrax**
A22.7 **Anthrax sepsis** HCC
Infectious bacterial disease
A22.8 **Other forms of anthrax**
Anthrax meningitis
A22.9 **Anthrax, unspecified**

● **A23 Brucellosis**
Includes Malta fever
Mediterranean fever
undulant fever

A23.0 **Brucellosis due to Brucella melitensis**
Resulting in flu-like symptoms that may lead to chronic symptoms that include recurrent fevers, joint pain, and fatigue
A23.1 **Brucellosis due to Brucella abortus**
Most common cause of brucellosis in humans; AKA Bang bacillus
A23.2 **Brucellosis due to Brucella suis**
Species found primarily in pigs, rabbits, and reindeer
A23.3 **Brucellosis due to Brucella canis**
Species that causes respiratory tract infection in humans
A23.8 **Other brucellosis**
A23.9 **Brucellosis, unspecified**

● **A24 Glanders and melioidosis**
Infection, usually of rodents, which spreads to other animals and humans, caused by Burkholderia pseudomallei *through break in skin contaminated with infested soil or water*

A24.0 **Glanders**
Infection due to Pseudomonas mallei
Malleus
A24.1 **Acute and fulminating melioidosis**
Melioidosis pneumonia
Melioidosis sepsis
A24.2 **Subacute and chronic melioidosis**
A24.3 **Other melioidosis**
A24.9 **Melioidosis, unspecified**
Infection due to Pseudomonas pseudomallei NOS
Whitmore's disease

Item 1-6 Brucellosis: An infectious disease caused by the bacterium Brucella. Humans are infected by contact with contaminated animals or animal products. In humans brucellosis symptoms that are similar to the flu include fever, sweats, headaches, back pains, and physical weakness. Severe infections of the central nervous system or lining of the heart may occur. Brucellosis can also cause chronic symptoms that include recurrent fevers, joint pain, and fatigue.

● A25 **Rat-bite fevers**
RBF, infectious disease caused by Streptobacillus moniliformis or Spirillum minus.

A25.0 **Spirillosis**
Any disease condition caused by spirilla
Sodoku

A25.1 **Streptobacillosis**
Acute, febrile human illness caused by bacteria transmitted by rats in most cases, passed from rodent to human via rodent's urine or mucous secretions; AKA rat fever
Epidemic arthritic erythema
Haverhill fever
Streptobacillary rat-bite fever

A25.9 **Rat-bite fever, unspecified**

● A26 **Erysipeloid**
Infection with Erysipelothrix rhusiopathiae*, occurring often as occupational disease resulting from handling infected fish, shellfish, meat, or poultry*

A26.0 **Cutaneous erysipeloid**
Erythema migrans

A26.7 **Erysipelothrix sepsis**

A26.8 **Other forms of erysipeloid**

A26.9 **Erysipeloid, unspecified**

● A27 **Leptospirosis**
Occurs most commonly in the tropics

A27.0 **Leptospirosis icterohemorrhagica**
Leptospiral or spirochetal jaundice (hemorrhagic)
Weil's disease

● A27.8 **Other forms of leptospirosis**

A27.81 **Aseptic meningitis in leptospirosis**

A27.89 **Other forms of leptospirosis**

A27.9 **Leptospirosis, unspecified**

● A28 **Other zoonotic bacterial diseases, not elsewhere classified**

A28.0 **Pasteurellosis**
Infection of humans or other animals by species of Pasteurella

A28.1 **Cat-scratch disease**
Cat-scratch fever

A28.2 **Extraintestinal yersiniosis**
Infection from Yersinia enterocolitica*; AKA enteric yersiniosis, intestinal yersiniosis, Yersinia enteritis*

Excludes1 enteritis due to Yersinia enterocolitica (A04.6)
plague (A20.-)

A28.8 **Other specified zoonotic bacterial diseases, not elsewhere classified**

A28.9 **Zoonotic bacterial disease, unspecified**

OTHER BACTERIAL DISEASES (A30-A49)

● A30 **Leprosy [Hansen's disease]**
Chronic infectious disease attacking the skin, peripheral nerves, and mucous membranes

Includes infection due to Mycobacterium leprae

Excludes1 sequelae of leprosy (B92)

A30.0 **Indeterminate leprosy**
I leprosy

A30.1 **Tuberculoid leprosy**
TT leprosy

A30.2 **Borderline tuberculoid leprosy**
BT leprosy

A30.3 **Borderline leprosy**
BB leprosy

A30.4 **Borderline lepromatous leprosy**
BL leprosy

A30.5 **Lepromatous leprosy**
LL leprosy

A30.8 **Other forms of leprosy**

A30.9 **Leprosy, unspecified**

● A31 **Infection due to other mycobacteria**

Excludes2 leprosy (A30.-)
tuberculosis (A15-A19)

A31.0 **Pulmonary mycobacterial infection**
Infection due to Mycobacterium avium
Infection due to Mycobacterium intracellulare [Battey bacillus]
Infection due to Mycobacterium kansasii

A31.1 **Cutaneous mycobacterial infection**
Buruli ulcer
Infection due to Mycobacterium marinum
Infection due to Mycobacterium ulcerans

A31.2 **Disseminated mycobacterium avium-intracellulare complex (DMAC)**
MAC sepsis

A31.8 **Other mycobacterial infections**

A31.9 **Mycobacterial infection, unspecified**
Atypical mycobacterial infection NOS
Mycobacteriosis NOS

● A32 **Listeriosis**
Infection caused by Listeria monocytogenes

Includes listerial foodborne infection

Excludes1 neonatal (disseminated) listeriosis (P37.2)

A32.0 **Cutaneous listeriosis**

● A32.1 **Listerial meningitis and meningoencephalitis**

A32.11 **Listerial meningitis**

A32.12 **Listerial meningoencephalitis**

A32.7 **Listerial sepsis**

● A32.8 **Other forms of listeriosis**

A32.81 **Oculoglandular listeriosis**
Primary infection site is conjunctival sac, which if untreated may result in perforation of cornea and optic atrophy

A32.82 **Listerial endocarditis**
Exudative and proliferative inflammatory condition of endocardium caused by listeria bacteria

A32.89 **Other forms of listeriosis**
Listerial cerebral arteritis

A32.9 **Listeriosis, unspecified**

A33 **Tetanus neonatorum** N
Neonate = newborn

A34 **Obstetrical tetanus** ♀ M

A35 **Other tetanus**
Tetanus NOS

Excludes1 tetanus neonatorum (A33)
obstetrical tetanus (A34)

● A36 **Diphtheria**

A36.0 **Pharyngeal diphtheria**
Diphtheritic membranous angina
Tonsillar diphtheria

A36.1 **Nasopharyngeal diphtheria**

A36.2 **Laryngeal diphtheria**
Diphtheritic laryngotracheitis

A36.3 **Cutaneous diphtheria**

Excludes2 erythrasma (L08.1)

Item 1-7 Diphtheria: A highly contagious bacterial disease that results in the formation of an adherent membrane in the throat that may lead to suffocation. In its most poisonous form, it attacks the heart and lungs. It is spread by direct physical contact or breathing the aerosolized secretions of infected individuals. The exact location is specified in the codes.

CHAPTER 1 (A00-B99)

A36.8 Other diphtheria
- A36.81 Diphtheritic cardiomyopathy
  - Diphtheritic myocarditis
- A36.82 Diphtheritic radiculomyelitis
- A36.83 Diphtheritic polyneuritis
- A36.84 Diphtheritic tubulo-interstitial nephropathy
- A36.85 Diphtheritic cystitis
- A36.86 Diphtheritic conjunctivitis
- A36.89 Other diphtheritic complications
  - Diphtheritic peritonitis

A36.9 Diphtheria, unspecified

A37 Whooping cough

Pertussis is a highly contagious disease caused by the bacterium Bordetella pertussis and results in a whooping sounding cough.

A37.Ø Whooping cough due to Bordetella pertussis
- A37.ØØ Whooping cough due to Bordetella pertussis without pneumonia
- A37.Ø1 Whooping cough due to Bordetella pertussis with pneumonia

A37.1 Whooping cough due to Bordetella parapertussis
- A37.1Ø Whooping cough due to Bordetella parapertussis without pneumonia
- A37.11 Whooping cough due to Bordetella parapertussis with pneumonia

A37.8 Whooping cough due to other Bordetella species
- A37.8Ø Whooping cough due to other Bordetella species without pneumonia
- A37.81 Whooping cough due to other Bordetella species with pneumonia

A37.9 Whooping cough, unspecified species
- A37.9Ø Whooping cough, unspecified species without pneumonia
- A37.91 Whooping cough, unspecified species with pneumonia

A38 Scarlet fever

Most commonly caused by the bacteria Streptococcus pneumoniae and Neisseria meningitides

Includes scarlatina

Excludes2 streptococcal sore throat (JØ2.Ø)

- A38.Ø Scarlet fever with otitis media
- A38.1 Scarlet fever with myocarditis
- A38.8 Scarlet fever with other complications
- A38.9 Scarlet fever, uncomplicated
  - Scarlet fever, NOS

A39 Meningococcal infection

Most commonly caused by the bacteria Streptococcus pneumoniae and Neisseria meningitides

- A39.Ø Meningococcal meningitis
- A39.1 Waterhouse-Friderichsen syndrome
  - *Fulminating complication of meningococcemia*
  - Meningococcal hemorrhagic adrenalitis
  - Meningococcic adrenal syndrome
- A39.2 Acute meningococcemia
- A39.3 Chronic meningococcemia
- A39.4 Meningococcemia, unspecified

A39.5 Meningococcal heart disease
- A39.5Ø Meningococcal carditis, unspecified
- A39.51 Meningococcal endocarditis
- A39.52 Meningococcal myocarditis
- A39.53 Meningococcal pericarditis

A39.8 Other meningococcal infections
- A39.81 Meningococcal encephalitis
- A39.82 Meningococcal retrobulbar neuritis
  - *Optic neuritis in portion of optic nerve posterior to eyeball; AKA postocular optic neuritis*
- A39.83 Meningococcal arthritis
- A39.84 Postmeningococcal arthritis
- A39.89 Other meningococcal infections
  - Meningococcal conjunctivitis

A39.9 Meningococcal infection, unspecified
- Meningococcal disease NOS

A4Ø Streptococcal sepsis

Code first
- postprocedural streptococcal sepsis (T81.44)
- streptococcal sepsis during labor (O75.3)
- streptococcal sepsis following abortion or ectopic or molar pregnancy (OØ3-OØ7, OØ8.Ø)
- streptococcal sepsis following immunization (T88.Ø)
- streptococcal sepsis following infusion, transfusion or therapeutic injection (T8Ø.2-)

Excludes1
- neonatal (P36.Ø-P36.1)
- puerperal sepsis (O85)
- sepsis due to Streptococcus, group D (A41.81)

- A4Ø.Ø Sepsis due to streptococcus, group A
- A4Ø.1 Sepsis due to streptococcus, group B
  - Coding Clinic: 2Ø19, Q1, P14
- A4Ø.3 Sepsis due to Streptococcus pneumoniae
  - Pneumococcal sepsis
- A4Ø.8 Other streptococcal sepsis
- A4Ø.9 Streptococcal sepsis, unspecified

A41 Other sepsis

Code first
- postprocedural sepsis (T81.44)
- sepsis during labor (O75.3)
- sepsis following abortion, ectopic or molar pregnancy (OØ3-OØ7, OØ8.Ø)
- sepsis following immunization (T88.Ø)
- sepsis following infusion, transfusion or therapeutic injection (T8Ø.2-)

Excludes1
- bacteremia NOS (R78.81)
- neonatal (P36.-)
- puerperal sepsis (O85)
- streptococcal sepsis (A4Ø.-)

Excludes2
- sepsis (due to) (in) actinomycotic (A42.7)
- sepsis (due to) (in) anthrax (A22.7)
- sepsis (due to) (in) candidal (B37.7)
- sepsis (due to) (in) Erysipelothrix (A26.7)
- sepsis (due to) (in) extraintestinal yersiniosis (A28.2)
- sepsis (due to) (in) gonococcal (A54.86)
- sepsis (due to) (in) herpesviral (BØØ.7)
- sepsis (due to) (in) listerial (A32.7)
- sepsis (due to) (in) melioidosis (A24.1)
- sepsis (due to) (in) meningococcal (A39.2-A39.4)
- sepsis (due to) (in) plague (A2Ø.7)
- sepsis (due to) (in) tularemia (A21.7)
- toxic shock syndrome (A48.3)

Coding Clinic: 2Ø16, Q1, P39

A41.Ø Sepsis due to Staphylococcus aureus
- A41.Ø1 Sepsis due to Methicillin susceptible Staphylococcus aureus
  - MSSA sepsis
  - Staphylococcus aureus sepsis NOS
- A41.Ø2 Sepsis due to Methicillin resistant Staphylococcus aureus

CHAPTER 1 (AØØ-B99)

Item 1–8 Gas gangrene is a necrotizing subcutaneous infection that will cause tissue death. Patients with poor circulation (e.g., diabetes, peripheral nephropathy) will have low oxygen content in their tissues (hypoxia), which allows the Clostridium bacteria to flourish. Gas gangrene often occurs at the site of a surgical wound or trauma. Onset is sudden and dramatic. Treatment can include debridement, amputation, and/or hyperbaric oxygen treatments.

A41.1 **Sepsis due to other specified staphylococcus**
Coagulase negative staphylococcus sepsis
A41.2 **Sepsis due to unspecified staphylococcus**
A41.3 **Sepsis due to Hemophilus influenzae**
A41.4 **Sepsis due to anaerobes**
Excludes1 gas gangrene (A48.0)
A41.5 **Sepsis due to other Gram-negative organisms**
A41.50 **Gram-negative sepsis, unspecified**
Gram-negative sepsis NOS
A41.51 **Sepsis due to Escherichia coli [E. coli]**
Coding Clinic: 2018, Q1, P16
A41.52 **Sepsis due to Pseudomonas**
Pseudomonas aeroginosa
A41.53 **Sepsis due to Serratia**
A41.59 **Other Gram-negative sepsis**
Coding Clinic: 2019, Q1, P13
A41.8 **Other specified sepsis**
A41.81 **Sepsis due to Enterococcus**
A41.89 **Other specified sepsis**
Coding Clinic: 2016, Q3, P8-14
A41.9 **Sepsis, unspecified organism**
Septicemia NOS
Coding Clinic: 2018, Q4, P18

A42 **Actinomycosis**
Excludes1 actinomycetoma (B47.1)
A42.0 **Pulmonary actinomycosis**
A42.1 **Abdominal actinomycosis**
A42.2 **Cervicofacial actinomycosis**
A42.7 **Actinomycotic sepsis**
A42.8 **Other forms of actinomycosis**
A42.81 **Actinomycotic meningitis**
A42.82 **Actinomycotic encephalitis**
A42.89 **Other forms of actinomycosis**
A42.9 **Actinomycosis, unspecified**

A43 **Nocardiosis**
A43.0 **Pulmonary nocardiosis**
A43.1 **Cutaneous nocardiosis**
A43.8 **Other forms of nocardiosis**
A43.9 **Nocardiosis, unspecified**

A44 **Bartonellosis**
A44.0 **Systemic bartonellosis**
Oroya fever
A44.1 **Cutaneous and mucocutaneous bartonellosis**
Verruga peruana
A44.8 **Other forms of bartonellosis**
A44.9 **Bartonellosis, unspecified**

A46 **Erysipelas**
Excludes1 postpartum or puerperal erysipelas (O86.89)

A48 **Other bacterial diseases, not elsewhere classified**
Excludes1 actinomycetoma (B47.1)
A48.0 **Gas gangrene**
Clostridial cellulitis
Clostridial myonecrosis
Coding Clinic: 2017, Q4, P102
A48.1 **Legionnaires' disease**
A48.2 **Nonpneumonic Legionnaires' disease [Pontiac fever]**
A48.3 **Toxic shock syndrome**
Use additional code to identify the organism (B95, B96)
Excludes1 endotoxic shock NOS (R57.8)
sepsis NOS (A41.9)
A48.4 **Brazilian purpuric fever**
Systemic Hemophilus aegyptius infection
A48.5 **Other specified botulism**
Non-foodborne intoxication due to toxins of Clostridium botulinum [C. botulinum]
Excludes1 food poisoning due to toxins of Clostridium botulinum (A05.1)
A48.51 **Infant botulism** P
A48.52 **Wound botulism**
Non-foodborne botulism NOS
Use additional code for associated wound
A48.8 **Other specified bacterial diseases**

A49 **Bacterial infection of unspecified site**
Excludes1 bacterial agents as the cause of diseases classified elsewhere (B95-B96)
chlamydial infection NOS (A74.9)
meningococcal infection NOS (A39.9)
rickettsial infection NOS (A79.9)
spirochetal infection NOS (A69.9)
A49.0 **Staphylococcal infection, unspecified site**
A49.01 **Methicillin susceptible Staphylococcus aureus infection, unspecified site**
Methicillin susceptible Staphylococcus aureus (MSSA) infection
Staphylococcus aureus infection NOS
A49.02 **Methicillin resistant Staphylococcus aureus infection, unspecified site**
Methicillin resistant Staphylococcus aureus (MRSA) infection
A49.1 **Streptococcal infection, unspecified site**
A49.2 **Hemophilus influenzae infection, unspecified site**
Any of seven bacterium of genus Haemophilus
A49.3 **Mycoplasma infection, unspecified site**
Bacterium of class Mollicutes, unusual group of bacteria distinguished by absence of cell wall
A49.8 **Other bacterial infections of unspecified site**
A49.9 **Bacterial infection, unspecified**
Excludes1 bacteremia NOS (R78.81)

INFECTIONS WITH A PREDOMINANTLY SEXUAL MODE OF TRANSMISSION (A50-A64)

Excludes1 human immunodeficiency virus [HIV] disease (B20)
nonspecific and nongonococcal urethritis (N34.1)
Reiter's disease (M02.3-)

A50 **Congenital syphilis**
A50.0 **Early congenital syphilis, symptomatic**
Any congenital syphilitic condition specified as early or manifest less than two years after birth
A50.01 **Early congenital syphilitic oculopathy**
A50.02 **Early congenital syphilitic osteochondropathy**
A50.03 **Early congenital syphilitic pharyngitis**
Early congenital syphilitic laryngitis
A50.04 **Early congenital syphilitic pneumonia**
A50.05 **Early congenital syphilitic rhinitis**
A50.06 **Early cutaneous congenital syphilis**
A50.07 **Early mucocutaneous congenital syphilis**
A50.08 **Early visceral congenital syphilis**
A50.09 **Other early congenital syphilis, symptomatic**

CHAPTER 1 (A00-B99)

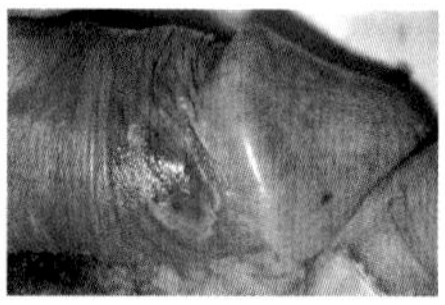

Figure 1-3 Chancre of primary syphilis. (From James WD, Berger TG, Elston DM: Andrews' Diseases of the Skin: Clinical Dermatology, Philadelphia, Saunders Elsevier, 2006)

Item 1-9 Syphilis, also known as lues, is the most serious of the venereal diseases caused by *Treponema pallidum*. The **primary** stage is characterized by an ulceration known as **chancre,** which usually appears on the genitals but can also develop on the anus, lips, tonsils, breasts, or fingers. Syphilis is easy to cure in its early stages. A single intramuscular injection of penicillin will usually cure a person who has had syphilis for less than a year.

The **secondary** stage is characterized by a rash that can affect any area of the body. **Latent** syphilis is divided into **early,** which is diagnosed within two years of infection, and **late,** which is diagnosed two years or more after infection. Additional doses of penicillin or another antibiotic are needed to treat someone who has had syphilis for longer than a year. For those allergic to penicillin, there are other antibiotic treatments. **Congenital** syphilis is also labeled **early** or **late** based on the time of diagnosis.

A5Ø.1 **Early congenital syphilis, latent**
Congenital syphilis without clinical manifestations, with positive serological reaction and negative spinal fluid test, less than two years after birth

A5Ø.2 **Early congenital syphilis, unspecified**
Congenital syphilis NOS less than two years after birth

● A5Ø.3 **Late congenital syphilitic oculopathy**
Excludes1 Hutchinson's triad (A5Ø.53)

A5Ø.3Ø **Late congenital syphilitic oculopathy, unspecified**

A5Ø.31 **Late congenital syphilitic interstitial keratitis**

A5Ø.32 **Late congenital syphilitic chorioretinitis**

A5Ø.39 **Other late congenital syphilitic oculopathy**

● A5Ø.4 **Late congenital neurosyphilis [juvenile neurosyphilis]**
Use additional code to identify any associated mental disorder
Excludes1 Hutchinson's triad (A5Ø.53)

A5Ø.4Ø **Late congenital neurosyphilis, unspecified**
Juvenile neurosyphilis NOS

A5Ø.41 **Late congenital syphilitic meningitis**

A5Ø.42 **Late congenital syphilitic encephalitis**

A5Ø.43 **Late congenital syphilitic polyneuropathy**

A5Ø.44 **Late congenital syphilitic optic nerve atrophy**

A5Ø.45 **Juvenile general paresis**
Dementia paralytica juvenilis
Juvenile tabetoparetic neurosyphilis

A5Ø.49 **Other late congenital neurosyphilis**
Juvenile tabes dorsalis

● A5Ø.5 **Other late congenital syphilis, symptomatic**
Any congenital syphilitic condition specified as late or manifest two years or more after birth

A5Ø.51 **Clutton's joints**

A5Ø.52 **Hutchinson's teeth**

A5Ø.53 **Hutchinson's triad**

A5Ø.54 **Late congenital cardiovascular syphilis**

A5Ø.55 **Late congenital syphilitic arthropathy** (HCC)

A5Ø.56 **Late congenital syphilitic osteochondropathy**

A5Ø.57 **Syphilitic saddle nose**

A5Ø.59 **Other late congenital syphilis, symptomatic**

A5Ø.6 **Late congenital syphilis, latent**
Congenital syphilis without clinical manifestations, with positive serological reaction and negative spinal fluid test, two years or more after birth.

A5Ø.7 **Late congenital syphilis, unspecified**
Congenital syphilis NOS two years or more after birth.

A5Ø.9 **Congenital syphilis, unspecified**

● A51 **Early syphilis**

A51.Ø **Primary genital syphilis**
Syphilitic chancre NOS

A51.1 **Primary anal syphilis**

A51.2 **Primary syphilis of other sites**

● A51.3 **Secondary syphilis of skin and mucous membranes**

A51.31 **Condyloma latum**

A51.32 **Syphilitic alopecia**

A51.39 **Other secondary syphilis of skin**
Syphilitic leukoderma
Syphilitic mucous patch
Excludes1 late syphilitic leukoderma (A52.79)

● A51.4 **Other secondary syphilis**

A51.41 **Secondary syphilitic meningitis**

A51.42 **Secondary syphilitic female pelvic disease** ♀

A51.43 **Secondary syphilitic oculopathy**
Secondary syphilitic chorioretinitis
Secondary syphilitic iridocyclitis, iritis
Secondary syphilitic uveitis

A51.44 **Secondary syphilitic nephritis**

A51.45 **Secondary syphilitic hepatitis**

A51.46 **Secondary syphilitic osteopathy**

A51.49 **Other secondary syphilitic conditions**
Secondary syphilitic lymphadenopathy
Secondary syphilitic myositis

A51.5 **Early syphilis, latent**
Syphilis (acquired) without clinical manifestations, with positive serological reaction and negative spinal fluid test, less than two years after infection.

A51.9 **Early syphilis, unspecified**

● A52 **Late syphilis**

● A52.Ø **Cardiovascular and cerebrovascular syphilis**

A52.ØØ **Cardiovascular syphilis, unspecified**

A52.Ø1 **Syphilitic aneurysm of aorta**

A52.Ø2 **Syphilitic aortitis**

A52.Ø3 **Syphilitic endocarditis**
Syphilitic aortic valve incompetence or stenosis
Syphilitic mitral valve stenosis
Syphilitic pulmonary valve regurgitation

A52.Ø4 **Syphilitic cerebral arteritis**

A52.Ø5 **Other cerebrovascular syphilis**
Syphilitic cerebral aneurysm (ruptured) (non-ruptured)
Syphilitic cerebral thrombosis

A52.Ø6 **Other syphilitic heart involvement**
Syphilitic coronary artery disease
Syphilitic myocarditis
Syphilitic pericarditis

A52.Ø9 **Other cardiovascular syphilis**

● A52.1 **Symptomatic neurosyphilis**

A52.1Ø **Symptomatic neurosyphilis, unspecified**

A52.11 **Tabes dorsalis**
Cognitive decline with progressive degeneration of posterior columns, roots, and ganglia of spinal cord, occur 15-2Ø years after initial infection of syphilis; AKA Duchenne disease
Locomotor ataxia (progressive)
Tabetic neurosyphilis

A52.12 **Other cerebrospinal syphilis**

A52.13 **Late syphilitic meningitis**

A52.14 **Late syphilitic encephalitis**

A52.15 **Late syphilitic neuropathy**
Late syphilitic acoustic neuritis
Late syphilitic optic (nerve) atrophy
Late syphilitic polyneuropathy
Late syphilitic retrobulbar neuritis

A52.16 **Charcôt's arthropathy (tabetic)**
Progressive musculoskeletal condition characterized by joint dislocation, fractures, and deformities, results in progressive destruction of bone and soft tissue of weight-bearing joints

A52.17 **General paresis**
Chronic meningoencephalitis results in loss of cortical function, or progressive dementia and generalized paralysis, occurring 1Ø-2Ø years after initial infection of syphilis; AKA Bayle disease, dementia paralytica, paralytic dementiaparetic neurosyphilis, syphilitic meningoencephalitis
Dementia paralytica

A52.19 **Other symptomatic neurosyphilis**
Syphilitic parkinsonism

A52.2 **Asymptomatic neurosyphilis**

A52.3 **Neurosyphilis, unspecified**
Gumma (syphilitic)
Destructive lesions of syphilis
Syphilis (late)
Syphiloma

● A52.7 **Other symptomatic late syphilis**

A52.71 **Late syphilitic oculopathy**
Late syphilitic chorioretinitis
Late syphilitic episcleritis

A52.72 **Syphilis of lung and bronchus**

A52.73 **Symptomatic late syphilis of other respiratory organs**

A52.74 **Syphilis of liver and other viscera**
Late syphilitic peritonitis

A52.75 **Syphilis of kidney and ureter**
Syphilitic glomerular disease

A52.76 **Other genitourinary symptomatic late syphilis** ♀
Late syphilitic female pelvic inflammatory disease

A52.77 **Syphilis of bone and joint**

A52.78 **Syphilis of other musculoskeletal tissue**
Late syphilitic bursitis
Syphilis [stage unspecified] of bursa
Syphilis [stage unspecified] of muscle
Syphilis [stage unspecified] of synovium
Syphilis [stage unspecified] of tendon

A52.79 **Other symptomatic late syphilis**
Late syphilitic leukoderma
Syphilis of adrenal gland
Syphilis of pituitary gland
Syphilis of thyroid gland
Syphilitic splenomegaly
Excludes1 syphilitic leukoderma (secondary) (A51.39)

A52.8 **Late syphilis, latent**
Syphilis (acquired) without clinical manifestations, with positive serological reaction and negative spinal fluid test, two years or more after infection

A52.9 **Late syphilis, unspecified**

● A53 **Other and unspecified syphilis**

A53.Ø **Latent syphilis, unspecified as early or late**
Latent syphilis NOS
Positive serological reaction for syphilis

A53.9 **Syphilis, unspecified**
Infection due to Treponema pallidum NOS
Syphilis (acquired) NOS
Excludes1 syphilis NOS under two years of age (A5Ø.2)

Item 1-10 An STD (sexually transmitted disease) caused by **Neisseria gonorrhoeae** that flourishes in the warm, moist areas of the reproductive tract. Untreated gonorrhea spreads to other parts of the body, causing inflammation of the testes or prostate or pelvic inflammatory disease (PID).

● A54 **Gonococcal infection**

● A54.Ø **Gonococcal infection of lower genitourinary tract without periurethral or accessory gland abscess**
Excludes1 gonococcal infection with genitourinary gland abscess (A54.1)
gonococcal infection with periurethral abscess (A54.1)

A54.ØØ **Gonococcal infection of lower genitourinary tract, unspecified**

A54.Ø1 **Gonococcal cystitis and urethritis, unspecified**

A54.Ø2 **Gonococcal vulvovaginitis, unspecified** ♀

A54.Ø3 **Gonococcal cervicitis, unspecified** ♀

A54.Ø9 **Other gonococcal infection of lower genitourinary tract**

A54.1 **Gonococcal infection of lower genitourinary tract with periurethral and accessory gland abscess**
Gonococcal Bartholin's gland abscess

● A54.2 **Gonococcal pelviperitonitis and other gonococcal genitourinary infection**

A54.21 **Gonococcal infection of kidney and ureter**

A54.22 **Gonococcal prostatitis** ♂

A54.23 **Gonococcal infection of other male genital organs** ♂
Gonococcal epididymitis
Gonococcal orchitis

A54.24 **Gonococcal female pelvic inflammatory disease** ♀
Gonococcal pelviperitonitis
Excludes1 gonococcal peritonitis (A54.85)

A54.29 **Other gonococcal genitourinary infections**

● A54.3 **Gonococcal infection of eye**

A54.3Ø **Gonococcal infection of eye, unspecified**

A54.31 **Gonococcal conjunctivitis**
Form of bacterial conjunctivitis contracted by newborns during delivery; AKA neonatal conjunctivitis
Ophthalmia neonatorum due to gonococcus

A54.32 **Gonococcal iridocyclitis**
Inflammation of iris and of ciliary body due to gonococcal infection

A54.33 **Gonococcal keratitis**
Inflammation of cornea due to gonococcal infection; AKA keratoconjunctivitis, keratopathy

A54.39 **Other gonococcal eye infection**
Gonococcal endophthalmia

● A54.4 **Gonococcal infection of musculoskeletal system**

A54.4Ø **Gonococcal infection of musculoskeletal system, unspecified**

A54.41 **Gonococcal spondylopathy**
Disorder of vertebrae due to gonococcal infection; AKA rachiopathy

A54.42 **Gonococcal arthritis**
Excludes2 gonococcal infection of spine (A54.41)

A54.43 **Gonococcal osteomyelitis**
Excludes2 gonococcal infection of spine (A54.41)

A54.49 **Gonococcal infection of other musculoskeletal tissue**
Gonococcal bursitis
Gonococcal myositis
Gonococcal synovitis
Gonococcal tenosynovitis

A54.5 Gonococcal pharyngitis
A54.6 Gonococcal infection of anus and rectum
● A54.8 Other gonococcal infections
A54.81 Gonococcal meningitis
A54.82 Gonococcal brain abscess
A54.83 Gonococcal heart infection
Gonococcal endocarditis
Gonococcal myocarditis
Gonococcal pericarditis
A54.84 Gonococcal pneumonia
A54.85 Gonococcal peritonitis
Excludes1 gonococcal pelviperitonitis (A54.24)
A54.86 Gonococcal sepsis
A54.89 Other gonococcal infections
Gonococcal keratoderma
Gonococcal lymphadenitis
A54.9 Gonococcal infection, unspecified

A55 Chlamydial lymphogranuloma (venereum)
Climatic or tropical bubo
Durand-Nicolas-Favre disease
Esthiomene
Lymphogranuloma inguinale

● A56 Other sexually transmitted chlamydial diseases
Includes sexually transmitted diseases due to Chlamydia trachomatis
Excludes1 neonatal chlamydial conjunctivitis (P39.1)
neonatal chlamydial pneumonia (P23.1)
Excludes2 chlamydial lymphogranuloma (A55)
conditions classified to A74.-
● A56.0 Chlamydial infection of lower genitourinary tract
A56.00 Chlamydial infection of lower genitourinary tract, unspecified
A56.01 Chlamydial cystitis and urethritis
A56.02 Chlamydial vulvovaginitis ♀
A56.09 Other chlamydial infection of lower genitourinary tract
Chlamydial cervicitis
● A56.1 Chlamydial infection of pelviperitoneum and other genitourinary organs
A56.11 Chlamydial female pelvic inflammatory disease ♀
A56.19 Other chlamydial genitourinary infection
Chlamydial epididymitis
Chlamydial orchitis
A56.2 Chlamydial infection of genitourinary tract, unspecified
A56.3 Chlamydial infection of anus and rectum
A56.4 Chlamydial infection of pharynx
A56.8 Sexually transmitted chlamydial infection of other sites

A57 Chancroid
Ulcus molle
Sexually transmitted infection caused by bacteria, Haemophilus ducreyi

A58 Granuloma inguinale
Chronic, progressive, ulcerative granulomatous disease
Donovanosis

● A59 Trichomoniasis
Excludes2 intestinal trichomoniasis (A07.8)
A common STD caused by a parasite, Trichomonas vaginalis
● A59.0 Urogenital trichomoniasis
A59.00 Urogenital trichomoniasis, unspecified
Fluor (vaginalis) due to Trichomonas
Leukorrhea (vaginalis) due to Trichomonas
A59.01 Trichomonal vulvovaginitis ♀
A59.02 Trichomonal prostatitis ♂
A59.03 Trichomonal cystitis and urethritis
A59.09 Other urogenital trichomoniasis
Common sexually transmitted disease (STD) caused by single-celled protozoan parasite; AKA trich
Trichomonas cervicitis
A59.8 Trichomoniasis of other sites
A59.9 Trichomoniasis, unspecified

● A60 Anogenital herpesviral [herpes simplex] infections
● A60.0 Herpesviral infection of genitalia and urogenital tract
A60.00 Herpesviral infection of urogenital system, unspecified
A60.01 Herpesviral infection of penis ♂
A60.02 Herpesviral infection of other male genital organs ♂
A60.03 Herpesviral cervicitis ♀
A60.04 Herpesviral vulvovaginitis ♀
Herpesviral [herpes simplex] ulceration
Herpesviral [herpes simplex] vaginitis
Herpesviral [herpes simplex] vulvitis
A60.09 Herpesviral infection of other urogenital tract
A60.1 Herpesviral infection of perianal skin and rectum
A60.9 Anogenital herpesviral infection, unspecified

● A63 Other predominantly sexually transmitted diseases, not elsewhere classified
Excludes2 molluscum contagiosum (B08.1)
papilloma of cervix (D26.0)
A63.0 Anogenital (venereal) warts
Anogenital warts due to (human) papillomavirus [HPV]
Condyloma acuminatum
A63.8 Other specified predominantly sexually transmitted diseases

A64 Unspecified sexually transmitted disease

OTHER SPIROCHETAL DISEASES (A65-A69)

Excludes2 leptospirosis (A27.-)
syphilis (A50-A53)

A65 Nonvenereal syphilis
Bejel
Endemic syphilis
Njovera

● A66 Yaws
Endemic, infectious, tropical disease caused by spirochete, spread by direct contact; AKA frambesia, framboesia, frambesia tropica
Includes bouba
frambesia (tropica)
pian
A66.0 Initial lesions of yaws
Chancre of yaws
Frambesia, initial or primary
Initial frambesial ulcer
Mother yaw
A66.1 Multiple papillomata and wet crab yaws
Frambesioma
Pianoma
Plantar or palmar papilloma of yaws
A66.2 Other early skin lesions of yaws
Cutaneous yaws, less than five years after infection
Early yaws (cutaneous)(macular)(maculopapular)(micropapular)(papular)
Frambeside of early yaws

A66.3 Hyperkeratosis of yaws
Hypertrophy of stratum corneum of skin in which there are small, hard, verrucous scales
Ghoul hand
Hyperkeratosis, palmar or plantar (early) (late) due to yaws
Worm-eaten soles

A66.4 Gummata and ulcers of yaws
Small, rubbery granuloma with necrotic center and inflamed characteristic of advanced stage of syphilis; AKA syphiloma
Gummatous frambeside
Nodular late yaws (ulcerated)

A66.5 Gangosa
Manifestation of yaws that develops in the soft palate and spreads eroding bone, cartilage, and soft tissue
Rhinopharyngitis mutilans

A66.6 Bone and joint lesions of yaws
Yaws ganglion
Yaws goundou
Yaws gumma, bone
Yaws gummatous osteitis or periostitis
Yaws hydrarthrosis
Yaws osteitis
Yaws periostitis (hypertrophic)

A66.7 Other manifestations of yaws
Juxta-articular nodules of yaws
Mucosal yaws

A66.8 Latent yaws
Yaws without clinical manifestations, with positive serology

A66.9 Yaws, unspecified

● **A67 Pinta [carate]**
Group of nonvenereal diseases caused by Treponema species

A67.Ø Primary lesions of pinta
Chancre (primary) of pinta
Papule (primary) of pinta

A67.1 Intermediate lesions of pinta
Erythematous plaques of pinta
Hyperchromic lesions of pinta
Hyperkeratosis of pinta
Pintids

A67.2 Late lesions of pinta
Achromic skin lesions of pinta
Cicatricial skin lesions of pinta
Dyschromic skin lesions of pinta

A67.3 Mixed lesions of pinta
Achromic with hyperchromic skin lesions of pinta [carate]

A67.9 Pinta, unspecified

● **A68 Relapsing fevers**
Includes recurrent fever
Excludes2 Lyme disease (A69.2-)

A68.Ø Louse-borne relapsing fever
Relapsing fever due to Borrelia recurrentis

A68.1 Tick-borne relapsing fever
Relapsing fever due to any Borrelia species other than Borrelia recurrentis

A68.9 Relapsing fever, unspecified

Item 1-11 Cancrum oris, also known as **noma** or **gangrenous stomatitis,** begins as an ulcer of the gingiva and results in a progressive gangrenous process.

● **A69 Other spirochetal infections**

A69.Ø Necrotizing ulcerative stomatitis
Cancrum oris
Fusospirochetal gangrene
Noma
Stomatitis gangrenosa

A69.1 Other Vincent's infections
Fusospirochetal pharyngitis
Necrotizing ulcerative (acute) gingivitis
Necrotizing ulcerative (acute) gingivostomatitis
Spirochetal stomatitis
Trench mouth
Vincent's angina
Vincent's gingivitis

● **A69.2 Lyme disease**
Erythema chronicum migrans due to Borrelia burgdorferi

A69.2Ø Lyme disease, unspecified

A69.21 Meningitis due to Lyme disease

A69.22 Other neurologic disorders in Lyme disease
Cranial neuritis
Meningoencephalitis
Polyneuropathy

A69.23 Arthritis due to Lyme disease

A69.29 Other conditions associated with Lyme disease
Myopericarditis due to Lyme disease
Coding Clinic: 2Ø16, Q3, P12

A69.8 Other specified spirochetal infections

A69.9 Spirochetal infection, unspecified

OTHER DISEASES CAUSED BY CHLAMYDIAE (A7Ø-A74)

Excludes1 sexually transmitted chlamydial diseases (A55-A56)

A7Ø Chlamydia psittaci infections
Ornithosis
Parrot fever
Psittacosis

● **A71 Trachoma**
Excludes1 sequelae of trachoma (B94.Ø)

A71.Ø Initial stage of trachoma
Trachoma dubium

A71.1 Active stage of trachoma
Granular conjunctivitis (trachomatous)
Trachomatous follicular conjunctivitis
Trachomatous pannus

A71.9 Trachoma, unspecified

● **A74 Other diseases caused by chlamydiae**
Excludes1 neonatal chlamydial conjunctivitis (P39.1)
neonatal chlamydial pneumonia (P23.1)
Reiter's disease (MØ2.3-)
sexually transmitted chlamydial diseases (A55-A56)
Excludes2 chlamydial pneumonia (J16.Ø)

A74.Ø Chlamydial conjunctivitis
Paratrachoma

● **A74.8 Other chlamydial diseases**

A74.81 Chlamydial peritonitis

A74.89 Other chlamydial diseases

A74.9 Chlamydial infection, unspecified
Chlamydiosis NOS

CHAPTER 1 (AØØ-B99)

Item 1–12 Rickettsioses are diseases spread from ticks, lice, fleas, or mites to humans.

Typhus is spread to humans chiefly by the fleas of rats.

Endemic identifies a disease as being present in low numbers of humans at all times, whereas **epidemic** identifies a disease as being present in high numbers of humans at a specific time. Morbidity (death) is higher in epidemic diseases.

Brill's disease, also known as **Brill-Zinsser disease,** is spread from human to human by body lice and also from the lice of flying squirrels. **Scrub typhus** is spread in the same ways as Brill's disease.

Malaria is spread to humans by mosquitoes.

RICKETTSIOSES (A75-A79)

● A75 Typhus fever
  Excludes1 rickettsiosis due to Ehrlichia sennetsu (A79.81)

A75.Ø **Epidemic louse-borne typhus fever due to Rickettsia prowazekii**
  Organisms transmitted between humans via louse
  Classical typhus (fever)
  Epidemic (louse-borne) typhus

A75.1 **Recrudescent typhus [Brill's disease]**
  Brill-Zinsser disease

A75.2 **Typhus fever due to Rickettsia typhi**
  Murine (flea-borne) typhus

A75.3 **Typhus fever due to Rickettsia tsutsugamushi**
  Scrub (mite-borne) typhus
  Tsutsugamushi fever

A75.9 **Typhus fever, unspecified**
  Typhus (fever) NOS

● A77 Spotted fever [tick-borne rickettsioses]

A77.Ø **Spotted fever due to Rickettsia rickettsii**
  Rocky Mountain spotted fever
  Sao Paulo fever

A77.1 **Spotted fever due to Rickettsia conorii**
  African tick typhus
  Boutonneuse fever
  India tick typhus
  Kenya tick typhus
  Marseilles fever
  Mediterranean tick fever

A77.2 **Spotted fever due to Rickettsia siberica**
  North Asian tick fever
  Siberian tick typhus

A77.3 **Spotted fever due to Rickettsia australis**
  Queensland tick typhus

● A77.4 **Ehrlichiosis**
  Type of tick-borne fever caused by bacteria infection
  Excludes1 Rickettsiosis due to Ehrlichia sennetsu (A79.81)

A77.4Ø **Ehrlichiosis, unspecified**

A77.41 **Ehrlichiosis chafeensis [E. chafeensis]**

A77.49 **Other ehrlichiosis**

A77.8 **Other spotted fevers**

A77.9 **Spotted fever, unspecified**
  Tick-borne typhus NOS

A78 Q fever
  Infection due to Coxiella burnetii
  Nine Mile fever
  Quadrilateral fever

● A79 Other rickettsioses

A79.Ø **Trench fever**
  Quintan fever
  Wolhynian fever

A79.1 **Rickettsialpox due to Rickettsia akari**
  Kew Garden fever
  Vesicular rickettsiosis

● A79.8 **Other specified rickettsioses**

A79.81 **Rickettsiosis due to Ehrlichia sennetsu**

A79.89 **Other specified rickettsioses**

A79.9 **Rickettsiosis, unspecified**
  Rickettsial infection NOS

Item 1–13 Acute Poliomyelitis: Also called infantile paralysis and is caused by the poliovirus, which enters the body orally and infects the intestinal wall and then enters the blood stream and central nervous system, causing muscle weakness and paralysis. This disease has been nearly eradicated with the polio vaccine.

VIRAL AND PRION INFECTIONS OF THE CENTRAL NERVOUS SYSTEM (A8Ø-A89)

Excludes1 postpolio syndrome (G14)
  sequelae of poliomyelitis (B91)
  sequelae of viral encephalitis (B94.1)

● A8Ø Acute poliomyelitis

A8Ø.Ø **Acute paralytic poliomyelitis, vaccine-associated**

A8Ø.1 **Acute paralytic poliomyelitis, wild virus, imported**

A8Ø.2 **Acute paralytic poliomyelitis, wild virus, indigenous**

● A8Ø.3 **Acute paralytic poliomyelitis, other and unspecified**

A8Ø.3Ø **Acute paralytic poliomyelitis, unspecified**

A8Ø.39 **Other acute paralytic poliomyelitis**

A8Ø.4 **Acute nonparalytic poliomyelitis**

A8Ø.9 **Acute poliomyelitis, unspecified**

● A81 Atypical virus infections of central nervous system
  Includes diseases of the central nervous system caused by prions
  Use additional code to identify:
  dementia with behavioral disturbance (FØ2.81)
  dementia without behavioral disturbance (FØ2.8Ø)

● A81.Ø **Creutzfeldt-Jakob disease**

A81.ØØ **Creutzfeldt-Jakob disease, unspecified**
  Jakob-Creutzfeldt disease, unspecified

A81.Ø1 **Variant Creutzfeldt-Jakob disease**
  vCJD

A81.Ø9 **Other Creutzfeldt-Jakob disease**
  CJD
  Familial Creutzfeldt-Jakob disease
  Iatrogenic Creutzfeldt-Jakob disease
  Sporadic Creutzfeldt-Jakob disease
  Subacute spongiform encephalopathy (with dementia)

A81.1 **Subacute sclerosing panencephalitis**
  Type of viral encephalitis that causes parenchymatous lesions in gray and white matter of brain
  Dawson's inclusion body encephalitis
  Van Bogaert's sclerosing leukoencephalopathy

A81.2 **Progressive multifocal leukoencephalopathy**
  Group of diseases affecting white matter of brain
  Multifocal leukoencephalopathy NOS

● A81.8 **Other atypical virus infections of central nervous system**

A81.81 **Kuru**

A81.82 **Gerstmann-Sträussler-Scheinker syndrome**
  GSS syndrome

A81.83 **Fatal familial insomnia**
  FFI

A81.89 **Other atypical virus infections of central nervous system**

A81.9 **Atypical virus infection of central nervous system, unspecified**
  Prion diseases of the central nervous system NOS

● A82 Rabies
  Viral disease affecting the central nervous system and transmitted from infected mammals to man

A82.Ø **Sylvatic rabies**

A82.1 **Urban rabies**

A82.9 **Rabies, unspecified**

Item 1-14 **Encephalitis** is an inflammation of the brain most often caused by a virus but may also be caused by a bacteria and most commonly transmitted by a mosquito. **Myelitis** is an inflammation of the spinal cord that may disrupt CNS function. Untreated myelitis may rapidly lead to permanent damage to the spinal cord. **Encephalomyelitis** is a general term for an inflammation of the brain and spinal cord.

● A83 Mosquito-borne viral encephalitis
Inflammation of the brain caused most commonly by Herpes Simplex virus
Includes mosquito-borne viral meningoencephalitis
Excludes2 Venezuelan equine encephalitis (A92.2)
West Nile fever (A92.3-)
West Nile virus (A92.3-)

A83.Ø **Japanese encephalitis**
A83.1 **Western equine encephalitis**
A83.2 **Eastern equine encephalitis**
A83.3 **St. Louis encephalitis**
A83.4 **Australian encephalitis**
Kunjin virus disease
A83.5 **California encephalitis**
California meningoencephalitis
La Crosse encephalitis
A83.6 **Rocio virus disease**
Mosquito-borne virus
A83.8 **Other mosquito-borne viral encephalitis**
A83.9 **Mosquito-borne viral encephalitis, unspecified**

● A84 Tick-borne viral encephalitis
Includes tick-borne viral meningoencephalitis

A84.Ø **Far Eastern tick-borne encephalitis [Russian spring-summer encephalitis]**
A84.1 **Central European tick-borne encephalitis**
A84.8 **Other tick-borne viral encephalitis**
Louping ill
Powassan virus disease
A84.9 **Tick-borne viral encephalitis, unspecified**

● A85 Other viral encephalitis, not elsewhere classified
Includes specified viral encephalomyelitis NEC
specified viral meningoencephalitis NEC
Excludes1 benign myalgic encephalomyelitis (G93.3)
encephalitis due to cytomegalovirus (B25.8)
encephalitis due to herpesvirus NEC (B1Ø.Ø-)
encephalitis due to herpesvirus [herpes simplex] (BØØ.4)
encephalitis due to measles virus (BØ5.Ø)
encephalitis due to mumps virus (B26.2)
encephalitis due to poliomyelitis virus (A8Ø.-)
encephalitis due to zoster (BØ2.Ø)
lymphocytic choriomeningitis (A87.2)

A85.Ø **Enteroviral encephalitis**
Enteroviral encephalomyelitis
A85.1 **Adenoviral encephalitis**
Adenoviral meningoencephalitis
A85.2 **Arthropod-borne viral encephalitis, unspecified**
Excludes1 West nile virus with encephalitis (A92.31)
A85.8 **Other specified viral encephalitis**
Encephalitis lethargica
Von Economo-Cruchet disease

A86 **Unspecified viral encephalitis**
Viral encephalomyelitis NOS
Viral meningoencephalitis NOS

● A87 Viral meningitis
Excludes1 meningitis due to herpesvirus [herpes simplex] (BØØ.3)
meningitis due to measles virus (BØ5.1)
meningitis due to mumps virus (B26.1)
meningitis due to poliomyelitis virus (A8Ø.-)
meningitis due to zoster (BØ2.1)

A87.Ø **Enteroviral meningitis**
Group of common viruses responsible for the majority of viral meningitis
Coxsackievirus meningitis
Echovirus meningitis
A87.1 **Adenoviral meningitis**
A87.2 **Lymphocytic choriomeningitis**
Lymphocytic meningoencephalitis
A87.8 **Other viral meningitis**
A87.9 **Viral meningitis, unspecified**

● A88 Other viral infections of central nervous system, not elsewhere classified
Excludes1 viral encephalitis NOS (A86)
viral meningitis NOS (A87.9)

A88.Ø **Enteroviral exanthematous fever [Boston exanthem]**
Infectious skin eruption
A88.1 **Epidemic vertigo**
A88.8 **Other specified viral infections of central nervous system**

A89 **Unspecified viral infection of central nervous system**

OGCR Section I. C.1.f.

Certain Infectious and Parasitic Diseases (AØØ-B99)

Zika virus infections

Code only confirmed cases

Code only a confirmed diagnosis of Zika virus (A92.5, Zika virus disease) as documented by the provider. This is an exception to the hospital inpatient guideline Section II, H.

In this context, "confirmation" does not require documentation of the type of test performed; the physician's diagnostic statement that the condition is confirmed is sufficient. This code should be assigned regardless of the stated mode of transmission.

If the provider documents "suspected", "possible" or "probable" Zika, do not assign code A92.5. Assign a code(s) explaining the reason for encounter (such as fever, rash, or joint pain) or Z2Ø.828, Contact with and (suspected) exposure to other viral communicable diseases.

ARTHROPOD-BORNE VIRAL FEVERS AND VIRAL HEMORRHAGIC FEVERS (A9Ø-A99)

A9Ø **Dengue fever [classical dengue]**
Acute, self-limited disease, characterized by fever, prostration, severe muscle pains, headache, rash, lymphadenopathy, and leukopenia, caused by dengue virus; AKA breakbone, dandy
Excludes1 dengue hemorrhagic fever (A91)
Coding Clinic: 2016, Q3, P13

A91 **Dengue hemorrhagic fever**
Serious follow-up to regular dengue, with symptoms of hemorrhage

● A92 Other mosquito-borne viral fevers
Excludes1 Ross River disease (B33.1)

A92.Ø **Chikungunya virus disease**
Transmitted by mosquitoes
Chikungunya (hemorrhagic) fever
A92.1 **O'nyong-nyong fever**
Acute, nonfatal febrile disease transmitted by mosquitoes, which clinically resembles dengue and chikungunya

A92.2 **Venezuelan equine fever**
Venezuelan equine encephalitis
Venezuelan equine encephalomyelitis virus disease

● A92.3 **West Nile virus infection**
West Nile fever

A92.30 **West Nile virus infection, unspecified**
West Nile fever NOS
West Nile fever without complications
West Nile virus NOS

A92.31 **West Nile virus infection with encephalitis**
West Nile encephalitis
West Nile encephalomyelitis
Coding Clinic: 2016, Q3, P13

A92.32 **West Nile virus infection with other neurologic manifestation**
Use additional code to specify the neurologic manifestation

A92.39 **West Nile virus infection with other complications**
Use additional code to specify the other conditions

A92.4 **Rift Valley fever**

A92.5 **Zika virus disease**
Zika virus fever
Zika virus infection
Zika NOS
Excludes1 congenital Zika virus disease (P35.4)
Coding Clinic: 2016, Q4, P4-7, 121

A92.8 **Other specified mosquito-borne viral fevers**

A92.9 **Mosquito-borne viral fever, unspecified**

● A93 Other arthropod-borne viral fevers, not elsewhere classified

A93.0 **Oropouche virus disease**
Tropical viral infection
Oropouche fever

A93.1 **Sandfly fever**
Pappataci fever
Phlebotomus fever

A93.2 **Colorado tick fever**

A93.8 **Other specified arthropod-borne viral fevers**
Piry virus disease
Vesicular stomatitis virus disease [Indiana fever]

A94 **Unspecified arthropod-borne viral fever**
Arboviral fever NOS
Arbovirus infection NOS

● A95 **Yellow fever**
Acute infectious disease transmitted by mosquitoes

A95.0 **Sylvatic yellow fever**
Jungle yellow fever

A95.1 **Urban yellow fever**

A95.9 **Yellow fever, unspecified**

● A96 **Arenaviral hemorrhagic fever**
Virus that causes various hemorrhagic fevers

A96.0 **Junin hemorrhagic fever**
Argentinian hemorrhagic fever

A96.1 **Machupo hemorrhagic fever**
Transmitted by contact with infected rodents
Bolivian hemorrhagic fever

A96.2 **Lassa fever**
Acute type of hemorrhagic fever caused by contact with disease carrying mouse or person

A96.8 **Other arenaviral hemorrhagic fevers**

A96.9 **Arenaviral hemorrhagic fever, unspecified**

● A98 **Other viral hemorrhagic fevers, not elsewhere classified**
Excludes1 chikungunya hemorrhagic fever (A92.0)
dengue hemorrhagic fever (A91)

A98.0 **Crimean-Congo hemorrhagic fever**
Virus transmitted by ticks and contact with blood, secretions, or fluids from infected humans or animals
Central Asian hemorrhagic fever

A98.1 **Omsk hemorrhagic fever**
Transmitted to humans by bites of infected ticks or contact with infected muskrats

A98.2 **Kyasanur Forest disease**
Transmitted via infected monkeys, voles, ticks

A98.3 **Marburg virus disease**
Rare, acute, often fatal type of hemorrhagic fever

A98.4 **Ebola virus disease**

A98.5 **Hemorrhagic fever with renal syndrome**
Epidemic hemorrhagic fever
Korean hemorrhagic fever
Russian hemorrhagic fever
Hantaan virus disease
Hantavirus disease with renal manifestations
Nephropathia epidemica
Songo fever
Excludes1 hantavirus (cardio)-pulmonary syndrome (B33.4)

A98.8 **Other specified viral hemorrhagic fevers**

A99 **Unspecified viral hemorrhagic fever**

VIRAL INFECTIONS CHARACTERIZED BY SKIN AND MUCOUS MEMBRANE LESIONS (B00-B09)

● B00 **Herpesviral [herpes simplex] infections**
Excludes1 congenital herpesviral infections (P35.2)
Excludes2 anogenital herpesviral infection (A60.-)
gammaherpesviral mononucleosis (B27.0-)
herpangina (B08.5)

B00.0 **Eczema herpeticum**
Cutaneous eruption caused by herpes simplex virus (HSV) type 1, HSV-2, coxsackievirus A16, or vaccinia virus
Kaposi's varicelliform eruption

B00.1 **Herpesviral vesicular dermatitis**
Vesicle formation; characteristics include formation of blisters and scabs on feet and legs
Herpes simplex facialis
Herpes simplex labialis
Herpes simplex otitis externa
Vesicular dermatitis of ear
Vesicular dermatitis of lip

B00.2 **Herpesviral gingivostomatitis and pharyngotonsillitis**
Inflammation involving both gingivae and oral mucosa
Herpesviral pharyngitis
Inflammation of pharynx and tonsils; AKA tonsillopharyngitis

B00.3 **Herpesviral meningitis**

B00.4 **Herpesviral encephalitis**
Herpesviral meningoencephalitis
Simian B disease
Excludes1 herpesviral encephalitis due to herpesvirus 6 and 7 (B10.01, B10.09)
non-simplex herpesviral encephalitis (B10.0-)

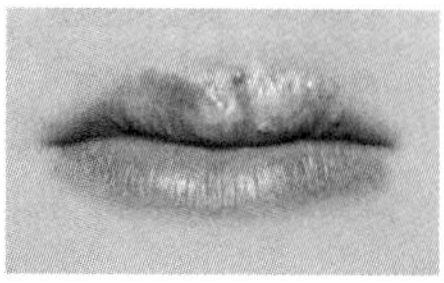

Figure 1-4 Primary herpes simplex in and around the mouth. The infection is usually acquired from siblings or parents and is readily transmitted to other direct contacts. (Getty Image)

Item 1-15 **Herpes** is a viral disease for which there is no cure. There are two types of the herpes simplex virus: **Type I** causes **cold sores** or **fever blisters,** and **Type II** causes **genital herpes.** The virus can be spread from a sore on the lips to the genitals or from the genitals to the lips.

● **B00.5** Herpesviral ocular disease
- **B00.50** **Herpesviral ocular disease, unspecified**
- **B00.51** **Herpesviral iridocyclitis**
  - Herpesviral iritis
  - Herpesviral uveitis, anterior
- **B00.52** **Herpesviral keratitis**
  - Herpesviral keratoconjunctivitis
- **B00.53** **Herpesviral conjunctivitis**
- **B00.59** **Other herpesviral disease of eye**
  - Herpesviral dermatitis of eyelid

B00.7 **Disseminated herpesviral disease**
- Herpesviral sepsis

● **B00.8** Other forms of herpesviral infections
- **B00.81** **Herpesviral hepatitis**
- **B00.82** **Herpes simplex myelitis**
- **B00.89** **Other herpesviral infection**
  - Herpesviral whitlow

B00.9 **Herpesviral infection, unspecified**
- Herpes simplex infection NOS

● **B01** Varicella [chickenpox]

Very contagious disease caused by the varicella zoster virus that results in an itchy outbreak of skin blisters (varicella). The same virus causes shingles (zoster).

B01.0 Varicella **meningitis**

● **B01.1** Varicella encephalitis, myelitis and encephalomyelitis
- Postchickenpox encephalitis, myelitis and encephalomyelitis
- **B01.11** **Varicella encephalitis and encephalomyelitis**
  - Postchickenpox encephalitis and encephalomyelitis
- **B01.12** **Varicella myelitis**
  - Postchickenpox myelitis

B01.2 Varicella **pneumonia**

● **B01.8** Varicella with other complications
- **B01.81** **Varicella keratitis**
- **B01.89** **Other varicella complications**

B01.9 **Varicella without complication**
- Varicella NOS

● **B02** Zoster [herpes zoster]

Includes shingles
zona

B02.0 Zoster **encephalitis**
- Zoster meningoencephalitis

B02.1 Zoster **meningitis**

● **B02.2** Zoster with other nervous system involvement

Coding Clinic: 2019, Q1, P18
- **B02.21** **Postherpetic geniculate ganglionitis**
- **B02.22** **Postherpetic trigeminal neuralgia**
- **B02.23** **Postherpetic polyneuropathy**
- **B02.24** **Postherpetic myelitis**
  - Herpes zoster myelitis
- **B02.29** **Other postherpetic nervous system involvement**
  - Postherpetic radiculopathy

Item 1-16 Zoster: Also known as ***shingles*** and is caused by the same virus as chickenpox. After exposure, the virus lies dormant in nerve tissue and is activated by factors including aging, stress, suppression of the immune system, and certain medication. It begins as a unilateral rash that leads to blisters and sores on the skin. It may involve the nerve pathways of the eye, forehead, nose, and eyelids and may be very painful with long-term systemic effects.

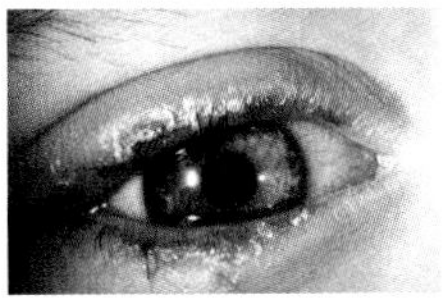

Figure 1-5 Photograph of eyelids with marginal blepharitis. (From Hoyt CS, Taylor D: Pediatric Ophthalmology and Strabismus, London, Elsevier Saunders, 2005)

Item 1-17 Blepharitis is a common condition in which the eyelid is swollen and yellow scaling and conjunctivitis develop. Usually the hair on the scalp and brow is involved.

● **B02.3** Zoster ocular disease
- **B02.30** Zoster ocular disease, **unspecified**
- **B02.31** Zoster **conjunctivitis**
- **B02.32** Zoster **iridocyclitis**
- **B02.33** Zoster **keratitis**
  - Herpes zoster keratoconjunctivitis
- **B02.34** Zoster **scleritis**
- **B02.39** **Other herpes zoster eye disease**
  - Zoster blepharitis

B02.7 **Disseminated zoster**

B02.8 **Zoster with other complications**
- Herpes zoster otitis externa

B02.9 **Zoster without complications**
- Zoster NOS

B03 Smallpox

Note: In 1980 the 33rd World Health Assembly declared that smallpox had been eradicated. The classification is maintained for surveillance purposes.

B04 Monkeypox

Disease occurring in captive monkeys and other mammals that may be transmitted to humans, clinically similar to smallpox

● **B05** Measles

Includes morbilli

Excludes1 subacute sclerosing panencephalitis (A81.1)

B05.0 Measles complicated by **encephalitis**
- Postmeasles encephalitis

B05.1 Measles complicated by **meningitis**
- Postmeasles meningitis

B05.2 Measles complicated by **pneumonia**
- Postmeasles pneumonia

B05.3 Measles complicated by **otitis media**
- Postmeasles otitis media

B05.4 Measles with **intestinal complications**

● **B05.8** Measles with other complications
- **B05.81** **Measles keratitis and keratoconjunctivitis**
- **B05.89** **Other measles complications**

B05.9 **Measles without complication**
- Measles NOS

● **B06** Rubella [German measles]

Excludes1 congenital rubella (P35.0)

● **B06.0** Rubella with neurological complications
- **B06.00** Rubella with neurological complication, **unspecified**
- **B06.01** Rubella **encephalitis**
  - Rubella meningoencephalitis
- **B06.02** Rubella **meningitis**
- **B06.09** **Other neurological complications of rubella**

● **B06.8** Rubella with other complications
- **B06.81** Rubella **pneumonia**
- **B06.82** Rubella **arthritis**
- **B06.89** **Other rubella complications**

B06.9 **Rubella without complication**
- Rubella NOS

B07 Viral warts

Includes verruca simplex
verruca vulgaris
viral warts due to human papillomavirus

Excludes2 anogenital (venereal) warts (A63.0)
papilloma of bladder (D41.4)
papilloma of cervix (D26.0)
papilloma larynx (D14.1)

B07.0 Plantar wart
Verruca plantaris

B07.8 Other viral warts
Common wart
Flat wart
Verruca plana

B07.9 Viral wart, unspecified

B08 Other viral infections characterized by skin and mucous membrane lesions, not elsewhere classified

Excludes1 vesicular stomatitis virus disease (A93.8)

B08.0 Other orthopoxvirus infections

Excludes2 monkeypox (B04)

B08.01 Cowpox and vaccinia not from vaccine

B08.010 Cowpox

B08.011 Vaccinia not from vaccine

Excludes1 vaccinia (from vaccination) (generalized) (T88.1)

B08.02 Orf virus disease
Contagious pustular dermatitis
Ecthyma contagiosum

B08.03 Pseudocowpox [milker's node]

B08.04 Paravaccinia, unspecified

B08.09 Other orthopoxvirus infections
Orthopoxvirus infection NOS

B08.1 Molluscum contagiosum
Various skin diseases characterized by soft, rounded, cutaneous lesions

B08.2 Exanthema subitum [sixth disease] Roseola infantum
Acute, short-lived high fever in infants and young children followed by a rash mainly on the trunk, caused by human herpesvirus 6

B08.20 Exanthema subitum [sixth disease], unspecified Roseola infantum, unspecified P

B08.21 Exanthema subitum [sixth disease] due to human herpesvirus 6 Roseola infantum due to human herpesvirus 6 P
Virus results in sudden rash; infection results in lifelong persistence

B08.22 Exanthema subitum [sixth disease] due to human herpesvirus 7 Roseola infantum due to human herpesvirus 7 P

B08.3 Erythema infectiosum [fifth disease]
Moderately contagious, epidemic disease in children caused by B19 virus; onset of rash that begins as redness of cheeks, later there is rash on trunk and limbs; when this fades, there may be central clearing that leaves lacelike pattern

B08.4 Enteroviral vesicular stomatitis with exanthem
Hand, foot and mouth disease
Check your documentation—this code is HAND, foot, and mouth disease. Code B08.8 is foot and mouth disease.

B08.5 Enteroviral vesicular pharyngitis
Herpangina

B08.6 Parapoxvirus infections

B08.60 Parapoxvirus infection, unspecified

B08.61 Bovine stomatitis

B08.62 Sealpox

B08.69 Other parapoxvirus infections

B08.7 Yatapoxvirus infections

B08.70 Yatapoxvirus infection, unspecified

B08.71 Tanapox virus disease

B08.72 Yaba pox virus disease
Yaba monkey tumor disease

B08.79 Other yatapoxvirus infections

B08.8 Other specified viral infections characterized by skin and mucous membrane lesions
Enteroviral lymphonodular pharyngitis
Foot-and-mouth disease
Check your documentation. Code B08.4 is for HAND, foot, and mouth disease.
Poxvirus NEC

B09 Unspecified viral infection characterized by skin and mucous membrane lesions
Viral enanthema NOS
Viral exanthema NOS

OTHER HUMAN HERPESVIRUSES (B10)

B10 Other human herpesviruses

Excludes2 cytomegalovirus (B25.9)
Epstein-Barr virus (B27.0-)
herpes NOS (B00.9)
herpes simplex (B00.-)
herpes zoster (B02.-)
human herpesvirus NOS (B00.-)
human herpesvirus 1 and 2 (B00.-)
human herpesvirus 3 (B01.-, B02.-)
human herpesvirus 4 (B27.0-)
human herpesvirus 5 (B25.-)
varicella (B01.-)
zoster (B02.-)

B10.0 Other human herpesvirus encephalitis

Excludes2 herpes encephalitis NOS (B00.4)
herpes simplex encephalitis (B00.4)
human herpesvirus encephalitis (B00.4)
simian B herpes virus encephalitis (B00.4)

B10.01 Human herpesvirus 6 encephalitis
Sudden rash or roseola

B10.09 Other human herpesvirus encephalitis
Human herpesvirus 7 encephalitis
Virus closely related to human herpesvirus 6, but not known to cause any disease

B10.8 Other human herpesvirus infection

B10.81 Human herpesvirus 6 infection
Causative agent of exanthema subitum that results in sudden rash

B10.82 Human herpesvirus 7 infection
Closely related to human herpesvirus 6, but not known cause any disease

B10.89 Other human herpesvirus infection
Human herpesvirus 8 infection
May be the cause of Kaposi sarcoma, a malignant tumor
Kaposi's sarcoma-associated herpesvirus infection

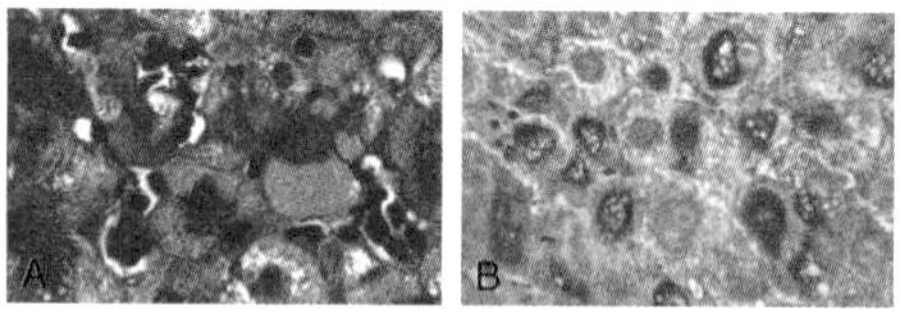

Figure 1-6 Hepatitis B viral infection. **A.** Liver parenchyma showing hepatocytes with diffuse granular cytoplasm, so-called ground glass hepatocytes (H&E). **B.** Immunoperoxidase stains from the same case, showing cytoplasmic inclusions of viral particles. (From Kumar: Robbins and Cotran: Pathologic Basis of Disease, ed 8, Saunders, An Imprint of Elsevier, 2009)

Item 1-18 Hepatitis A (HAV) was formerly called epidemic, infectious, short-incubation, or acute catarrhal jaundice hepatitis. The primary transmission mode is the oral–fecal route. **Hepatitis B (HBV)** was formerly called long-incubation period, serum, or homologous serum hepatitis. Transmission modes are through blood from infected persons and from body fluids of infected mother to neonate. **Hepatitis C (HCV),** caused by the hepatitis C virus, is primarily transfusion associated. **Hepatitis D (HDV),** also called delta hepatitis, is caused by the hepatitis D virus in patients formerly or currently infected with hepatitis B. **Hepatitis E (HEV)** is also called enterically transmitted non-A, non-B hepatitis. The primary transmission mode is the oral–fecal route, usually through contaminated water.

VIRAL HEPATITIS (B15-B19)

Excludes1 sequelae of viral hepatitis (B94.2)
Excludes2 cytomegaloviral hepatitis (B25.1)
herpesviral [herpes simplex] hepatitis (B00.81)

● **B15** Acute hepatitis A
- **B15.0** **Hepatitis A with hepatic coma**
- **B15.9** **Hepatitis A without hepatic coma**
  Hepatitis A (acute) (viral) NOS

● **B16** Acute hepatitis B
- **B16.0** **Acute hepatitis B with delta-agent with hepatic coma**
- **B16.1** **Acute hepatitis B with delta-agent without hepatic coma**
- **B16.2** **Acute hepatitis B without delta-agent with hepatic coma**
- **B16.9** **Acute hepatitis B without delta-agent and without hepatic coma**
  Hepatitis B (acute) (viral) NOS
  Coding Clinic: 2016, Q3, P13

● **B17** Other acute viral hepatitis
- **B17.0** **Acute delta-(super) infection of hepatitis B carrier**
- ● **B17.1** **Acute hepatitis C**
  - **B17.10** **Acute hepatitis C without hepatic coma**
    Acute hepatitis C NOS
  - **B17.11** **Acute hepatitis C with hepatic coma**
- **B17.2** **Acute hepatitis E**
- **B17.8** **Other specified acute viral hepatitis**
  Hepatitis non-A non-B (acute) (viral) NEC
- **B17.9** **Acute viral hepatitis, unspecified**
  Acute hepatitis NOS
  Acute infectious hepatitis NOS

● **B18** Chronic viral hepatitis
Includes Carrier of viral hepatitis
- **B18.0** **Chronic viral hepatitis B with delta-agent** HCC
- **B18.1** **Chronic viral hepatitis B without delta-agent** HCC
  Carrier of viral hepatitis B
  Chronic (viral) hepatitis B
- **B18.2** **Chronic viral hepatitis C** HCC
  Carrier of viral hepatitis C
  Coding Clinic: 2018, Q1, P4; 2017, Q1, P41
- **B18.8** **Other chronic viral hepatitis** HCC
  Carrier of other viral hepatitis
- **B18.9** **Chronic viral hepatitis, unspecified** HCC
  Carrier of unspecified viral hepatitis

● **B19** Unspecified viral hepatitis
- **B19.0** **Unspecified viral hepatitis with hepatic coma**
- ● **B19.1** **Unspecified viral hepatitis B**
  - **B19.10** **Unspecified viral hepatitis B without hepatic coma**
    Unspecified viral hepatitis B NOS
  - **B19.11** **Unspecified viral hepatitis B with hepatic coma**
- ● **B19.2** **Unspecified viral hepatitis C**
  - **B19.20** **Unspecified viral hepatitis C without hepatic coma**
    Viral hepatitis C NOS
  - **B19.21** **Unspecified viral hepatitis C with hepatic coma**
- **B19.9** **Unspecified viral hepatitis without hepatic coma**
  Viral hepatitis NOS

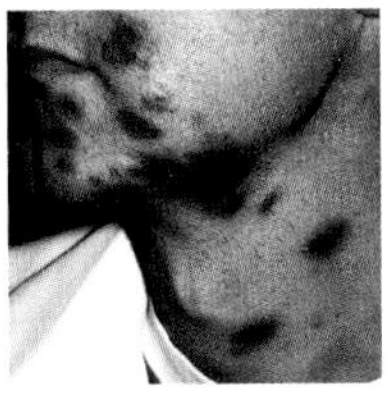

Figure 1-7 Kaposi's sarcoma. There are large confluent hyperpigmented patch-stage lesions with lymphedema. (From Kanski, JJ: Clinical Diagnosis in Ophthalmology, London, Elsevier Mosby, 2006)

Item 1-19 AIDS (acquired immune deficiency syndrome) is caused by **HIV** (human immunodeficiency virus). HIV affects certain white blood cells (T-4 lymphocytes) and destroys the ability of the cells to fight infections, making patients susceptible to a host of infectious diseases (e.g., ***Pneumocystis carinii pneumonia [PCP], Kaposi's sarcoma,*** and ***lymphoma).*** ***AIDS-related complex (ARC)*** is an early stage of AIDS in which tests for HIV are positive but the symptoms are mild.

OGCR Section I. C.1.a.

Certain Infectious and Parasitic Diseases (A00-B99)

a. Human Immunodeficiency Virus (HIV) Infections

1) Code only confirmed cases

Code only confirmed cases of HIV infection illness. This is an exception to the hospital inpatient guideline Section II, H.

In this context, "confirmation" does not require documentation of positive serology or culture for HIV; the provider's diagnostic statement that the patient is HIV positive or has an HIV-related illness is sufficient.

HUMAN IMMUNODEFICIENCY VIRUS [HIV] DISEASE (B20)

B20 Human immunodeficiency virus [HIV] disease HCC
Includes acquired immune deficiency syndrome [AIDS]
AIDS-related complex [ARC]
HIV infection, symptomatic

Code first Human immunodeficiency virus [HIV] disease complicating pregnancy, childbirth and the puerperium, if applicable (O98.7-)

Use additional code(s) to identify all manifestations of HIV infection

Excludes1 asymptomatic human immunodeficiency virus [HIV] infection status (Z21)
exposure to HIV virus (Z20.6)
inconclusive serologic evidence of HIV (R75)

Coding Clinic: 2019, Q1, P9-11

OTHER VIRAL DISEASES (B25-B34)

● **B25** Cytomegaloviral disease
AKA: HCMV or Human Herpesvirus 5 (HHV-5)
Excludes1 congenital cytomegalovirus infection (P35.1)
cytomegaloviral mononucleosis (B27.1-)
- **B25.0** **Cytomegaloviral pneumonitis** HCC
- **B25.1** **Cytomegaloviral hepatitis** HCC
- **B25.2** **Cytomegaloviral pancreatitis** HCC
- **B25.8** **Other cytomegaloviral diseases** HCC
  Cytomegaloviral encephalitis
- **B25.9** **Cytomegaloviral disease, unspecified** HCC

● **B26** Mumps
Includes epidemic parotitis
infectious parotitis
Acute, contagious, viral disease
- **B26.0** **Mumps orchitis** ♂
- **B26.1** **Mumps meningitis**
- **B26.2** **Mumps encephalitis**
- **B26.3** **Mumps pancreatitis**

CHAPTER 1 (A00-B99)

● B26.8 **Mumps with other complications**

B26.81 **Mumps hepatitis**

B26.82 **Mumps myocarditis**

B26.83 **Mumps nephritis**

B26.84 **Mumps polyneuropathy**

B26.85 **Mumps arthritis** (HCC)

B26.89 **Other mumps complications**

B26.9 **Mumps without complication**
Mumps NOS
Mumps parotitis NOS

● B27 **Infectious mononucleosis**
Includes glandular fever
monocytic angina
Pfeiffer's disease

● B27.Ø **Gammaherpesviral mononucleosis**
AKA: Pfeiffer's disease, infective mononucleosis
Mononucleosis due to Epstein-Barr virus

B27.ØØ **Gammaherpesviral mononucleosis without complication**
Infective mononucleosis

B27.Ø1 **Gammaherpesviral mononucleosis with polyneuropathy**

B27.Ø2 **Gammaherpesviral mononucleosis with meningitis**

B27.Ø9 **Gammaherpesviral mononucleosis with other complications**
Hepatomegaly in gammaherpesviral mononucleosis

● B27.1 **Cytomegaloviral mononucleosis**
Infectious disease resembling infectious mononucleosis

B27.1Ø **Cytomegaloviral mononucleosis without complications**

B27.11 **Cytomegaloviral mononucleosis with polyneuropathy**

B27.12 **Cytomegaloviral mononucleosis with meningitis**

B27.19 **Cytomegaloviral mononucleosis with other complication**
Hepatomegaly in cytomegaloviral mononucleosis

● B27.8 **Other infectious mononucleosis**

B27.8Ø **Other infectious mononucleosis without complication**

B27.81 **Other infectious mononucleosis with polyneuropathy**

B27.82 **Other infectious mononucleosis with meningitis**

B27.89 **Other infectious mononucleosis with other complication**
Hepatomegaly in other infectious mononucleosis

● B27.9 **Infectious mononucleosis, unspecified**

B27.9Ø **Infectious mononucleosis, unspecified without complication**

B27.91 **Infectious mononucleosis, unspecified with polyneuropathy**

B27.92 **Infectious mononucleosis, unspecified with meningitis**

B27.99 **Infectious mononucleosis, unspecified with other complication**
Hepatomegaly in unspecified infectious mononucleosis

● B3Ø **Viral conjunctivitis**
Excludes1 herpesviral [herpes simplex] ocular disease (BØØ.5)
ocular zoster (BØ2.3)

B3Ø.Ø **Keratoconjunctivitis due to adenovirus**
Epidemic keratoconjunctivitis
Shipyard eye

B3Ø.1 **Conjunctivitis due to adenovirus**
Acute adenoviral follicular conjunctivitis
Swimming-pool conjunctivitis

B3Ø.2 **Viral pharyngoconjunctivitis**

B3Ø.3 **Acute epidemic hemorrhagic conjunctivitis (enteroviral)**
Conjunctivitis due to coxsackievirus 24
Conjunctivitis due to enterovirus 7Ø
Hemorrhagic conjunctivitis (acute)(epidemic)

B3Ø.8 **Other viral conjunctivitis**
Newcastle conjunctivitis

B3Ø.9 **Viral conjunctivitis, unspecified**

● B33 **Other viral diseases, not elsewhere classified**

B33.Ø **Epidemic myalgia**
Acute infectious disease, caused by group A coxsackie viruses or other enteroviruses with symptoms that include sudden pain in chest or upper abdomen with fever
Bornholm disease

B33.1 **Ross River disease**
Epidemic polyarthritis and exanthema
Ross River fever

● B33.2 **Viral carditis**
Coxsackie (virus) carditis

B33.2Ø **Viral carditis, unspecified**

B33.21 **Viral endocarditis**

B33.22 **Viral myocarditis**

B33.23 **Viral pericarditis**

B33.24 **Viral cardiomyopathy** (HCC)

B33.3 **Retrovirus infections, not elsewhere classified**
Retrovirus infection NOS

B33.4 **Hantavirus (cardio)-pulmonary syndrome [HPS] [HCPS]**
Hantavirus disease with pulmonary manifestations
Sin nombre virus disease
Use additional code to identify any associated acute kidney failure (N17.9)
Excludes1 hantavirus disease with renal manifestations (A98.5)
hemorrhagic fever with renal manifestations (A98.5)

B33.8 **Other specified viral diseases**
Excludes1 anogenital human papillomavirus infection (A63.Ø)
viral warts due to human papillomavirus infection (BØ7)

● B34 **Viral infection of unspecified site**
Excludes1 anogenital human papillomavirus infection (A63.Ø)
cytomegaloviral disease NOS (B25.9)
herpesvirus [herpes simplex] infection NOS (BØØ.9)
retrovirus infection NOS (B33.3)
viral agents as the cause of diseases classified elsewhere (B97.-)
viral warts due to human papillomavirus infection (BØ7)

B34.Ø **Adenovirus infection, unspecified**

B34.1 **Enterovirus infection, unspecified**
Intestinal tract infection
Coxsackievirus infection NOS
Echovirus infection NOS

B34.2 **Coronavirus infection, unspecified**
Excludes1 pneumonia due to SARS-associated coronavirus (J12.81)

B34.3 Parvovirus infection, unspecified

B34.4 Papovavirus infection, unspecified

B34.8 Other viral infections of unspecified site

B34.9 Viral infection, unspecified
Viremia NOS
Coding Clinic: 2Ø16, Q3, P1Ø

MYCOSES (B35-B49)

Excludes2 hypersensitivity pneumonitis due to organic dust (J67.-)
mycosis fungoides (C84.Ø-)

● B35 Dermatophytosis
AKA tinea or ringworm
Includes favus
infections due to species of Epidermophyton, Micro-sporum and Trichophyton
tinea, any type except those in B36.-

B35.Ø Tinea barbae and tinea capitis
Beard ringworm
Kerion
Scalp ringworm
Sycosis, mycotic

B35.1 Tinea unguium
White patches or pits on surface or edges of nails, followed by infection under nail plate
Dermatophytic onychia
Dermatophytosis of nail
Onychomycosis
Ringworm of nails

B35.2 Tinea manuum
Tinea of hands
Dermatophytosis of hand
Hand ringworm

B35.3 Tinea pedis
Tinea affecting feet
Athlete's foot
Dermatophytosis of foot
Foot ringworm

B35.4 Tinea corporis
Infecting skin areas other than hands
Ringworm of the body

B35.5 Tinea imbricata
Chronic tropical tinea corporis; AKA Oriental ringworm, tinea inguinalis, tinea cruris
Tokelau

B35.6 Tinea cruris
In groin or perineal area, spreading to adjacent regions; AKA jock itch, eczema marginatum, ringworm of groin, or tinea inguinalis
Dhobi itch
Groin ringworm
Jock itch

B35.8 Other dermatophytoses
Disseminated dermatophytosis
Granulomatous dermatophytosis

B35.9 Dermatophytosis, unspecified
Ringworm NOS

● B36 Other superficial mycoses

B36.Ø Pityriasis versicolor
Common, chronic, symptomless disorder that includes macular patches of various sizes and shapes; AKA liver spots
Tinea flava
Tinea versicolor

B36.1 Tinea nigra
Minor fungal infection, with dark lesions, usually on skin of hands
Keratomycosis nigricans palmaris
Microsporosis nigra
Pityriasis nigra

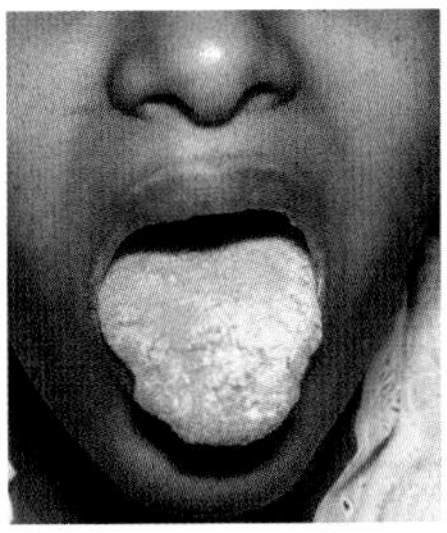

Figure 1-8 Oral candidiasis (thrush). (From James WD, Berger T, Elston D: Andrews' Diseases of the Skin: Clinical Dermatology, 11e, Saunders, 2011)

Item 1-20 Candidiasis, also called oidiomycosis or moniliasis, is a fungal infection. It most often appears on moist cutaneous areas of the body but can also be responsible for a variety of systemic infections such as endocarditis, meningitis, arthritis, and myositis. Antifungal medications cure most yeast infections.

B36.2 White piedra
White to light brown nodules on hair of beard, axilla, or groin; AKA trichosporosis
Tinea blanca

B36.3 Black piedra
Characterized by small black or brown nodules on shafts of scalp hair

B36.8 Other specified superficial mycoses

B36.9 Superficial mycosis, unspecified

● B37 Candidiasis
Includes candidosis
moniliasis
Excludes1 neonatal candidiasis (P37.5)

B37.Ø Candidal stomatitis
Oral thrush

B37.1 Pulmonary candidiasis
Candidal bronchitis
Candidal pneumonia

B37.2 Candidiasis of skin and nail
Candidal onychia
Candidal paronychia
Excludes2 diaper dermatitis (L22)

B37.3 Candidiasis of vulva and vagina ♀
Candidal vulvovaginitis
Monilial vulvovaginitis
Vaginal thrush

● B37.4 Candidiasis of other urogenital sites

B37.41 Candidal cystitis and urethritis

B37.42 Candidal balanitis ♂
Male condition only

B37.49 Other urogenital candidiasis
Candidal pyelonephritis

B37.5 Candidal meningitis

B37.6 Candidal endocarditis

B37.7 Candidal sepsis
Disseminated candidiasis systemic candidiasis

● B37.8 Candidiasis of other sites

B37.81 Candidal esophagitis

B37.82 Candidal enteritis
Candidal proctitis

B37.83 Candidal cheilitis
Inflammation affecting lip

B37.84 Candidal otitis externa
Inflammation of external auditory canal

B37.89 Other sites of candidiasis
Infection manifested by invasive candidiasis
Candidal osteomyelitis

B37.9 Candidiasis, unspecified
Thrush NOS

Item 1-21 Bird and bat droppings that fall into the soil give rise to a fungus that can spread airborne spores. When inhaled into the lungs, these spores divide and multiply into lesions. Histoplasmosis capsulatum takes three forms: primary (lodged in the lungs only), chronic (resembles TB), and disseminated (infection has moved to other organs). This is an opportunistic infection in immunosuppressed patients.

● B38 Coccidioidomycosis
Fungal disease; AKA coccidioidosis, coccidioidal granuloma, Posadas, or Posadas-Wernicke disease
B38.0 **Acute pulmonary** coccidioidomycosis
B38.1 **Chronic pulmonary** coccidioidomycosis
B38.2 **Pulmonary** coccidioidomycosis, **unspecified**
B38.3 **Cutaneous** coccidioidomycosis
B38.4 Coccidioidomycosis **meningitis**
B38.7 **Disseminated** coccidioidomycosis
Generalized coccidioidomycosis
● B38.8 Other forms of coccidioidomycosis
B38.81 **Prostatic** coccidioidomycosis ♂
B38.89 **Other forms** of coccidioidomycosis
B38.9 Coccidioidomycosis, **unspecified**

● B39 Histoplasmosis
Infection resulting from inhalation or ingestion of spores; AKA Darling disease
Code first associated AIDS (B20)
Use additional code for any associated manifestations, such as:
endocarditis (I39)
meningitis (G02)
pericarditis (I32)
retinitis (H32)
B39.0 **Acute pulmonary** histoplasmosis capsulati
B39.1 **Chronic pulmonary** histoplasmosis capsulati
B39.2 **Pulmonary** histoplasmosis capsulati, **unspecified**
B39.3 **Disseminated** histoplasmosis capsulati
Generalized histoplasmosis capsulati
B39.4 Histoplasmosis **capsulati, unspecified**
American histoplasmosis
B39.5 Histoplasmosis **duboisii**
African histoplasmosis
B39.9 Histoplasmosis, **unspecified**

● B40 Blastomycosis
Rare and potentially fatal infection caused by inhaling fungus found in moist soil in temperate climates.
Excludes1 Brazilian blastomycosis (B41.-)
keloidal blastomycosis (B48.0)
B40.0 **Acute pulmonary** blastomycosis
B40.1 **Chronic pulmonary** blastomycosis
B40.2 **Pulmonary** blastomycosis, **unspecified**
B40.3 **Cutaneous** blastomycosis
B40.7 **Disseminated** blastomycosis
Generalized blastomycosis
● B40.8 Other forms of blastomycosis
B40.81 **Blastomycotic meningoencephalitis**
Meningomyelitis due to blastomycosis
B40.89 **Other forms** of blastomycosis
B40.9 Blastomycosis, **unspecified**

● B41 Paracoccidioidomycosis
Fungal infection usually chronic that begins in lungs, spreads to mucocutaneous areas which may extend to skin, tonsils, gastrointestinal lymphatics, liver, and spleen; AKA Almeida or Lutz-Splendore-Almeida disease, Brazilian or South American blastomycosis, or paracoccidioidal granuloma
Includes Brazilian blastomycosis
Lutz' disease
B41.0 **Pulmonary** paracoccidioidomycosis
B41.7 **Disseminated** paracoccidioidomycosis
Generalized paracoccidioidomycosis
B41.8 **Other forms** of paracoccidioidomycosis
B41.9 Paracoccidioidomycosis, **unspecified**

● B42 Sporotrichosis
Chronic fungal infection with nodular lesions
B42.0 **Pulmonary** sporotrichosis
B42.1 **Lymphocutaneous** sporotrichosis
B42.7 **Disseminated** sporotrichosis
Generalized sporotrichosis
● B42.8 Other forms of sporotrichosis
B42.81 **Cerebral** sporotrichosis
Meningitis due to sporotrichosis
B42.82 **Sporotrichosis arthritis**
B42.89 **Other forms** of sporotrichosis
B42.9 Sporotrichosis, **unspecified**

● B43 Chromomycosis and pheomycotic abscess
Chronic fungal infection of skin, initiated at site of puncture affecting lower limb or foot (mossy foot)
B43.0 **Cutaneous** chromomycosis
Dermatitis verrucosa
B43.1 **Pheomycotic brain abscess**
Cerebral chromomycosis
B43.2 **Subcutaneous pheomycotic abscess and cyst**
B43.8 **Other forms** of chromomycosis
B43.9 Chromomycosis, **unspecified**

● B44 Aspergillosis
Infection marked by inflammatory lesions in skin, ear, orbit, nasal sinuses, lungs, and occasionally bones and meninges
Includes aspergilloma
B44.0 **Invasive pulmonary** aspergillosis
B44.1 **Other pulmonary** aspergillosis
B44.2 **Tonsillar** aspergillosis
B44.7 **Disseminated** aspergillosis
Generalized aspergillosis
● B44.8 Other forms of aspergillosis
B44.81 **Allergic bronchopulmonary** aspergillosis
B44.89 **Other forms** of aspergillosis
B44.9 Aspergillosis, **unspecified**

● B45 Cryptococcosis
Infection in the immunocompromised and fatal if left untreated; AKA torulosis, Buschke, or Busse-Buschke disease
B45.0 **Pulmonary** cryptococcosis
B45.1 **Cerebral** cryptococcosis
Cryptococcal meningitis
Cryptococcosis meningocerebralis
B45.2 **Cutaneous** cryptococcosis
B45.3 **Osseous** cryptococcosis
B45.7 **Disseminated** cryptococcosis
Generalized cryptococcosis
B45.8 **Other forms** of cryptococcosis
B45.9 Cryptococcosis, **unspecified**

● B46 Zygomycosis
Fungal infections including subcutaneous lesions and infection of sinuses, brain, or lungs
B46.0 **Pulmonary** mucormycosis
Fungal infection affecting lung
B46.1 **Rhinocerebral** mucormycosis
B46.2 **Gastrointestinal** mucormycosis
B46.3 **Cutaneous** mucormycosis
Subcutaneous mucormycosis
B46.4 **Disseminated** mucormycosis
Generalized mucormycosis
B46.5 Mucormycosis, **unspecified**
B46.8 **Other zygomycoses**
Entomophthoromycosis
B46.9 Zygomycosis, **unspecified**
Phycomycosis NOS

B47 Mycetoma
Slow progressive, destructive fungal infection of cutaneous and subcutaneous tissues, fascia, and bone, primarily seen in foot (Madura foot) or leg

B47.0 Eumycetoma
Madura foot, mycotic Maduromycosis

B47.1 Actinomycetoma

B47.9 Mycetoma, unspecified
Madura foot NOS

B48 Other mycoses, not elsewhere classified

B48.0 Lobomycosis
Infection with symptoms of red, smooth, hard cutaneous nodules resembling keloids
Keloidal blastomycosis
Lobo's disease

B48.1 Rhinosporidiosis
Chronic, localized granulomatous fungal infection, affecting mucocutaneous tissues, usually of nose characterized by polyps, papillomas, and wartlike lesions

B48.2 Allescheriasis
Fungal infection
Infection due to Pseudallescheria boydii
Excludes1 eumycetoma (B47.0)

B48.3 Geotrichosis
Fungal infection usually of bronchi, lungs, mouth, or intestinal tract
Geotrichum stomatitis

B48.4 Penicillosis
Fungal infection

B48.8 Other specified mycoses
Adiaspiromycosis
Infection of tissue and organs by Alternaria
Infection of tissue and organs by Drechslera
Infection of tissue and organs by Fusarium
Infection of tissue and organs by saprophytic fungi NEC

B49 Unspecified mycosis
Fungemia NOS

PROTOZOAL DISEASES (B50-B64)

Excludes1 amebiasis (A06.-)
other protozoal intestinal diseases (A07.-)

B50 Plasmodium falciparum malaria
Severe form of malaria that can be fatal
Includes mixed infections of Plasmodium falciparum with any other Plasmodium species

B50.0 Plasmodium falciparum malaria with cerebral complications
Cerebral malaria NOS

B50.8 Other severe and complicated Plasmodium falciparum malaria
Severe or complicated Plasmodium falciparum malaria NOS

B50.9 Plasmodium falciparum malaria, unspecified

B51 Plasmodium vivax malaria
Includes mixed infections of Plasmodium vivax with other Plasmodium species, except Plasmodium falciparum
Excludes1 plasmodium vivax with Plasmodium falciparum (B50.-)

B51.0 Plasmodium vivax malaria with rupture of spleen

B51.8 Plasmodium vivax malaria with other complications

B51.9 Plasmodium vivax malaria without complication
Plasmodium vivax malaria NOS

B52 Plasmodium malariae malaria
Causes fever that recurs at approximately three-day intervals (quartan fever), longer than two-day (tertian) intervals of other malarial parasites
Includes mixed infections of Plasmodium malariae with other Plasmodium species, except Plasmodium falciparum and Plasmodium vivax
Excludes1 plasmodium falciparum (B50.-)
plasmodium vivax (B51.-)

B52.0 Plasmodium malariae malaria with nephropathy

B52.8 Plasmodium malariae malaria with other complications

B52.9 Plasmodium malariae malaria without complication
Plasmodium malariae malaria NOS

B53 Other specified malaria

B53.0 Plasmodium ovale malaria
Least diagnosed type of malaria spread by female mosquitoes of rare species
Excludes1 plasmodium ovale with Plasmodium falciparum (B50.-)
plasmodium ovale with Plasmodium malariae (B52.-)
plasmodium ovale with Plasmodium vivax (B51.-)

B53.1 Malaria due to simian plasmodia
Malaria-like disease (parasite infection)
Excludes1 malaria due to simian plasmodia with Plasmodium falciparum (B50.-)
malaria due to simian plasmodia with Plasmodium malariae (B52.-)
malaria due to simian plasmodia with Plasmodium ovale (B53.0)
malaria due to simian plasmodia with Plasmodium vivax (B51.-)

B53.8 Other malaria, not elsewhere classified

B54 Unspecified malaria

B55 Leishmaniasis
Protozoal infection

B55.0 Visceral leishmaniasis
Kala-azar
Post-kala-azar dermal leishmaniasis

B55.1 Cutaneous leishmaniasis

B55.2 Mucocutaneous leishmaniasis

B55.9 Leishmaniasis, unspecified

B56 African trypanosomiasis
Human African trypanosomiasis (HAT) is transmitted by fly bites

B56.0 Gambiense trypanosomiasis
Infection due to Trypanosoma brucei gambiense
West African sleeping sickness

B56.1 Rhodesiense trypanosomiasis
East African sleeping sickness
Infection due to Trypanosoma brucei rhodesiense

B56.9 African trypanosomiasis, unspecified
Sleeping sickness NOS

B57 Chagas' disease
Tropical parasitic disease
Includes American trypanosomiasis
infection due to Trypanosoma cruzi

B57.0 Acute Chagas' disease with heart involvement
Acute Chagas' disease with myocarditis

B57.1 Acute Chagas' disease without heart involvement
Acute Chagas' disease NOS

B57.2 Chagas' disease (chronic) with heart involvement
American trypanosomiasis NOS
Chagas' disease (chronic) NOS
Chagas' disease (chronic) with myocarditis
Trypanosomiasis NOS

- B57.3 Chagas' disease (chronic) with digestive system involvement
  - B57.30 Chagas' disease with digestive system involvement, unspecified
  - B57.31 Megaesophagus in Chagas' disease
  - B57.32 Megacolon in Chagas' disease
  - B57.39 Other digestive system involvement in Chagas' disease
- B57.4 Chagas' disease (chronic) with nervous system involvement
  - B57.40 Chagas' disease with nervous system involvement, unspecified
  - B57.41 Meningitis in Chagas' disease
  - B57.42 Meningoencephalitis in Chagas' disease
  - B57.49 Other nervous system involvement in Chagas' disease
- B57.5 Chagas' disease (chronic) with other organ involvement

B58 Toxoplasmosis

Infection by protozoon transmitted in cysts in feces of cats

Includes infection due to Toxoplasma gondii

Excludes1 congenital toxoplasmosis (P37.1)

- B58.0 Toxoplasma oculopathy
  - B58.00 Toxoplasma oculopathy, unspecified
  - B58.01 Toxoplasma chorioretinitis
  - B58.09 Other toxoplasma oculopathy
    Toxoplasma uveitis
- B58.1 Toxoplasma hepatitis
- B58.2 Toxoplasma meningoencephalitis
- B58.3 Pulmonary toxoplasmosis
- B58.8 Toxoplasmosis with other organ involvement
  - B58.81 Toxoplasma myocarditis
  - B58.82 Toxoplasma myositis
  - B58.83 Toxoplasma tubulo-interstitial nephropathy
    Toxoplasma pyelonephritis
  - B58.89 Toxoplasmosis with other organ involvement
- B58.9 Toxoplasmosis, unspecified

B59 Pneumocystosis

Caused by fungus

Pneumonia due to Pneumocystis carinii
Pneumonia due to Pneumocystis jiroveci

B60 Other protozoal diseases, not elsewhere classified

Excludes1 cryptosporidiosis (A07.2)
intestinal microsporidiosis (A07.8)
isosporiasis (A07.3)

- B60.0 Babesiosis
  Tickborne disease caused by microscopic organisms
  Piroplasmosis
- B60.1 Acanthamebiasis
  - B60.10 Acanthamebiasis, unspecified
  - B60.11 Meningoencephalitis due to Acanthamoeba (culbertsoni)
  - B60.12 Conjunctivitis due to Acanthamoeba
  - B60.13 Keratoconjunctivitis due to Acanthamoeba
  - B60.19 Other acanthamebic disease
- B60.2 Naegleriasis
  Infection with microscopic organisms
  Primary amebic meningoencephalitis
- B60.8 Other specified protozoal diseases
  Microsporidiosis

B64 Unspecified protozoal disease

Item 1–22 Toxoplasmosis is caused by the protozoa **Toxoplasma gondii,** of which the house cat can be a host. Human infection occurs when contact is made with materials containing the pathogen, such as feces, contaminated soil, or ingestion of infected lamb, goat, or pork. Of the infected, very few have symptoms because a healthy person's immune system keeps the parasite from causing illness. When the immune system is compromised, symptoms may occur. Clinical symptoms include flu-like symptoms, but the disease progresses to include the eyes and the brain in babies.

HELMINTHIASES (B65-B83)

Diseases or infestations caused by parasitic worms

B65 Schistosomiasis [bilharziasis]

Infection with flukes (flat parasitic worms)

Includes snail fever

- B65.0 Schistosomiasis due to Schistosoma haematobium [urinary schistosomiasis]
- B65.1 Schistosomiasis due to Schistosoma mansoni [intestinal schistosomiasis]
- B65.2 Schistosomiasis due to Schistosoma japonicum
  Asiatic schistosomiasis
- B65.3 Cercarial dermatitis
  Swimmer's itch
- B65.8 Other schistosomiasis
  Infection due to Schistosoma intercalatum
  Infection due to Schistosoma mattheei
  Infection due to Schistosoma mekongi
- B65.9 Schistosomiasis, unspecified

B66 Other fluke infections

Trematode (parasitic worms)

- B66.0 Opisthorchiasis
  Infection due to cat liver fluke
  Infection due to Opisthorchis (felineus)(viverrini)
- B66.1 Clonorchiasis
  Chinese liver fluke disease
  Infection due to Clonorchis sinensis
  Oriental liver fluke disease
- B66.2 Dicroceliasis
  Liver fluke
  Infection due to Dicrocoelium dendriticum
  Lancet fluke infection
- B66.3 Fascioliasis
  Infection due to Fasciola gigantica
  Infection due to Fasciola hepatica
  Infection due to Fasciola indica
  Sheep liver fluke disease
- B66.4 Paragonimiasis
  Infection due to Paragonimus species
  Lung fluke disease
  Pulmonary distomiasis
- B66.5 Fasciolopsiasis
  Largest intestinal fluke in humans
  Infection due to Fasciolopsis buski
  Intestinal distomiasis
- B66.8 Other specified fluke infections
  Echinostomiasis
  Heterophyiasis
  Metagonimiasis
  Nanophyetiasis
  Watsoniasis
- B66.9 Fluke infection, unspecified

B67 Echinococcosis

Larval forms of tapeworms usually of liver or lungs

Includes hydatidosis

- B67.0 Echinococcus granulosus infection of liver
- B67.1 Echinococcus granulosus infection of lung
- B67.2 Echinococcus granulosus infection of bone
- B67.3 Echinococcus granulosus infection, other and multiple sites
  - B67.31 Echinococcus granulosus infection, thyroid gland
  - B67.32 Echinococcus granulosus infection, multiple sites
  - B67.39 Echinococcus granulosus infection, other sites
- B67.4 Echinococcus granulosus infection, unspecified
  Dog tapeworm (infection)

Item 1-23 Echinococcosis: Also known as hydatid disease; is caused by Echinococcus granulosus, E. multilocularis, and E. vogeli tapeworms; and is contracted from infected food. Found in southern South America, the Mediterranean, the Middle East, central Asia, and Africa and uncommon in the United States but has been reported in California, New Mexico, Arizona and Utah. The disease is treated with medication over a long course, as it is resistive.

B67.5 Echinococcus multilocularis infection of liver
● **B67.6 Echinococcus multilocularis infection, other and multiple sites**
B67.61 Echinococcus multilocularis infection, multiple sites
B67.69 Echinococcus multilocularis infection, other sites
B67.7 Echinococcus multilocularis infection, unspecified
B67.8 Echinococcosis, unspecified, of liver
● **B67.9 Echinococcosis, other and unspecified**
B67.90 Echinococcosis, unspecified
Echinococcosis NOS
B67.99 Other echinococcosis

● **B68 Taeniasis**
Intestinal tapeworm (cestode) infection from raw or undercooked meat of infected animal
Excludes1 cysticercosis (B69.-)
B68.0 Taenia solium taeniasis
Pork tapeworm (infection)
B68.1 Taenia saginata taeniasis
Beef tapeworm (infection)
Infection due to adult tapeworm Taenia saginata
B68.9 Taeniasis, unspecified

● **B69 Cysticercosis**
Systemic illness caused by the larvae of pork tapeworm
Includes cysticerciasis infection due to larval form of Taenia solium
B69.0 Cysticercosis of central nervous system
B69.1 Cysticercosis of eye
● **B69.8 Cysticercosis of other sites**
B69.81 Myositis in cysticercosis
B69.89 Cysticercosis of other sites
B69.9 Cysticercosis, unspecified

● **B70 Diphyllobothriasis and sparganosis**
Infection with tapeworms seen most often from inadequately cooked fish
B70.0 Diphyllobothriasis
Diphyllobothrium (adult) (latum) (pacificum) infection
Fish tapeworm (infection)
Excludes2 larval diphyllobothriasis (B70.1)
B70.1 Sparganosis
Infection with migrating tapeworm larvae, which invade subcutaneous tissues, causing inflammation and fibrosis that resembles cellulitis
Infection due to Sparganum (mansoni) (proliferum)
Infection due to Spirometra larva
Larval diphyllobothriasis
Spirometrosis

● **B71 Other cestode infections**
B71.0 Hymenolepiasis
Intestinal infestation with tapeworms
Dwarf tapeworm infection
Rat tapeworm (infection)
B71.1 Dipylidiasis
Infection with tapeworm common to dogs and cats and seen in children having close contact with infected pets
B71.8 Other specified cestode infections
Infection by the larval stage of a tapeworm, usually through fruit or vegetables
Coenurosis
B71.9 Cestode infection, unspecified
Tapeworm (infection) NOS

B72 Dracunculiasis
Infection with roundworms
Includes guinea worm infection
infection due to Dracunculus medinensis

● **B73 Onchocerciasis**
Infection with parasitic worm
Includes onchocerca volvulus infection
onchocercosis
river blindness
● **B73.0 Onchocerciasis with eye disease**
B73.00 Onchocerciasis with eye involvement, unspecified
B73.01 Onchocerciasis with endophthalmitis
B73.02 Onchocerciasis with glaucoma
B73.09 Onchocerciasis with other eye involvement
Infestation of eyelid due to onchocerciasis
B73.1 Onchocerciasis without eye disease

● **B74 Filariasis**
Infestation with slender threadlike worms
Excludes2 onchocerciasis (B73)
tropical (pulmonary) eosinophilia NOS (J82)
B74.0 Filariasis due to Wuchereria bancrofti
Bancroftian elephantiasis
Bancroftian filariasis
B74.1 Filariasis due to Brugia malayi
B74.2 Filariasis due to Brugia timori
B74.3 Loiasis
Infection with round worms growing in subcutaneous connective tissue
Calabar swelling
Eyeworm disease of Africa
Loa loa infection
B74.4 Mansonelliasis
Infection with filarial parasite
Infection due to Mansonella ozzardi
Infection due to Mansonella perstans
Infection due to Mansonella streptocerca
B74.8 Other filariases
Dirofilariasis
B74.9 Filariasis, unspecified

B75 Trichinellosis
Infestation with parasitic roundworms ingested in undercooked contaminated meat
Includes infection due to Trichinella species trichiniasis

● **B76 Hookworm diseases**
Occurs in hot, humid parts of world where larvae are soil borne, enter digestive tract through skin of feet/legs or in contaminated food/water; AKA ground itch
Includes uncinariasis
B76.0 Ancylostomiasis
Infection due to Ancylostoma species
B76.1 Necatoriasis
Infection due to Necator americanus
B76.8 Other hookworm diseases
B76.9 Hookworm disease, unspecified
Cutaneous larva migrans NOS

● **B77 Ascariasis**
Infection by roundworm in small intestine
Includes ascaridiasis
roundworm infection
B77.0 Ascariasis with intestinal complications
● **B77.8 Ascariasis with other complications**
B77.81 Ascariasis pneumonia
B77.89 Ascariasis with other complications
B77.9 Ascariasis, unspecified

CHAPTER 1 (A00-B99)

● **B78 Strongyloidiasis**
Infection with adult female roundworms
Excludes1 trichostrongyliasis (B81.2)
- **B78.0 Intestinal strongyloidiasis**
- **B78.1 Cutaneous strongyloidiasis**
- **B78.7 Disseminated strongyloidiasis**
- **B78.9 Strongyloidiasis, unspecified**

B79 Trichuriasis
Intestinal infection with roundworms
Includes trichocephaliasis
whipworm (disease)(infection)

B80 Enterobiasis
Intestinal infection with pinworms
Includes oxyuriasis
pinworm infection
threadworm infection

● **B81 Other intestinal helminthiases, not elsewhere classified**
Diseases or infestations caused by parasitic worms
Excludes1 angiostrongyliasis due to:
Angiostrongylus cantonensis (B83.2)
Parastrongylus cantonensis (B83.2)

B81.0 Anisakiasis
Roundworm infection via contaminated undercooked infected fish or marine mammals
Infection due to Anisakis larva

B81.1 Intestinal capillariasis
Infestation with of parasites (nematodes)
Capillariasis NOS
Infection due to Capillaria philippinensis
Excludes2 hepatic capillariasis (B83.8)

B81.2 Trichostrongyliasis

B81.3 Intestinal angiostrongyliasis
Angiostrongyliasis due to:
Angiostrongylus costaricensis (B83.2)
Parastrongylus costaricensis (B83.2)

B81.4 Mixed intestinal helminthiases
Infection due to intestinal helminths classified to more than one of the categories B65.0-B81.3 and B81.8
Mixed helminthiasis NOS

B81.8 Other specified intestinal helminthiases
Infection due to Oesophagostomum species [esophagostomiasis]
Infection due to Ternidens diminutus [ternidensiasis]

● **B82 Unspecified intestinal parasitism**

B82.0 Intestinal helminthiasis, unspecified
Infected with worms

B82.9 Intestinal parasitism, unspecified

● **B83 Other helminthiases**
Caused by parasitic worms
Excludes1 capillariasis NOS (B81.1)
Excludes2 intestinal capillariasis (B81.1)

B83.0 Visceral larva migrans
Prolonged migration of nematode larvae
Toxocariasis

B83.1 Gnathostomiasis
Infection with nematode occurring from ingested undercooked fish contaminated with larvae; larvae migrate to subcutaneous tissue or deeper tissues, results are abscesses
Wandering swelling

B83.2 Angiostrongyliasis due to Parastrongylus cantonensis
Nematode infection caused by eating contaminated raw snails, slugs, or paratenic hosts such as prawns or crabs; larval worms migrate to central nervous system resulting in eosinophilic meningitis
Eosinophilic meningoencephalitis due to Parastrongylus cantonensis
Excludes2 intestinal angiostrongyliasis (B81.3)

B83.3 Syngamiasis
Infestation with gapeworm from turkey, pheasant, guinea fowl, goose, and wild birds
Syngamosis

B83.4 Internal hirudiniasis
Infestation by leeches
Excludes2 external hirudiniasis (B88.3)

B83.8 Other specified helminthiases
Parasitic worm infestation
Acanthocephaliasis
Gongylonemiasis
Hepatic capillariasis
Metastrongyliasis
Thelaziasis

B83.9 Helminthiasis, unspecified
Worms NOS
Excludes1 intestinal helminthiasis NOS (B82.0)

PEDICULOSIS, ACARIASIS AND OTHER INFESTATIONS (B85-B89)

● **B85 Pediculosis and phthiriasis**
Infestation of lice

B85.0 Pediculosis due to Pediculus humanus capitis
Head-louse infestation

B85.1 Pediculosis due to Pediculus humanus corporis
Body-louse infestation

B85.2 Pediculosis, unspecified

B85.3 Phthiriasis
Crab or pubic lice
Infestation by crab-louse
Infestation by Phthirus pubis

B85.4 Mixed pediculosis and phthiriasis
Infestation classifiable to more than one of the categories B85.0-B85.3

B86 Scabies
Contagious dermatitis caused by mites
Sarcoptic itch

● **B87 Myiasis**
Infestation by fly maggots
Includes infestation by larva of flies

B87.0 Cutaneous myiasis
Creeping myiasis

B87.1 Wound myiasis
Traumatic myiasis

B87.2 Ocular myiasis

B87.3 Nasopharyngeal myiasis
Laryngeal myiasis

B87.4 Aural myiasis

● **B87.8 Myiasis of other sites**
- **B87.81 Genitourinary myiasis**
- **B87.82 Intestinal myiasis**
- **B87.89 Myiasis of other sites**

B87.9 Myiasis, unspecified

CHAPTER 1 (A00-B99)

B88 Other infestations

B88.0 Other acariasis
Acarine dermatitis
Dermatitis due to Demodex species
Dermatitis due to Dermanyssus gallinae
Dermatitis due to Liponyssoides sanguineus
Trombiculosis
Excludes2 scabies (B86)

B88.1 Tungiasis [sandflea infestation]
Inflammatory skin disease caused by infestation of fleas

B88.2 Other arthropod infestations
Scarabiasis

B88.3 External hirudiniasis
Leech infestation NOS
Excludes2 internal hirudiniasis (B83.4)

B88.8 Other specified infestations
Infection of topical fresh water fish parasite
Ichthyoparasitism due to Vandellia cirrhosa
Linguatulosis
Porocephaliasis

B88.9 Infestation, unspecified
Infestation (skin) NOS
Infestation by mites NOS
Skin parasites NOS

B89 Unspecified parasitic disease

SEQUELAE OF INFECTIOUS AND PARASITIC DISEASES (B90-B94)

Note: Categories B90-B94 are to be used to indicate conditions in categories A00-B89 as the cause of sequelae, which are themselves classified elsewhere. The 'sequelae' include conditions specified as such; they also include residuals of diseases classifiable to the above categories if there is evidence that the disease itself is no longer present. Codes from these categories are not to be used for chronic infections. Code chronic current infections to active infectious disease as appropriate.

Code first condition resulting from (sequela) the infectious or parasitic disease

B90 Sequelae of tuberculosis
Condition resulting from tuberculosis

B90.0 Sequelae of central nervous system tuberculosis

B90.1 Sequelae of genitourinary tuberculosis

B90.2 Sequelae of tuberculosis of bones and joints

B90.8 Sequelae of tuberculosis of other organs
Excludes2 sequelae of respiratory tuberculosis (B90.9)

B90.9 Sequelae of respiratory and unspecified tuberculosis
Sequelae of tuberculosis NOS

B91 Sequelae of poliomyelitis
Excludes1 postpolio syndrome (G14)

B92 Sequelae of leprosy

B94 Sequelae of other and unspecified infectious and parasitic diseases

B94.0 Sequelae of trachoma

B94.1 Sequelae of viral encephalitis

B94.2 Sequelae of viral hepatitis

B94.8 Sequelae of other specified infectious and parasitic diseases

B94.9 Sequelae of unspecified infectious and parasitic disease
Coding Clinic: 2017, Q4, P109

OGCR Section I.C.1.b.

Certain infectious and parasitic diseases

Infectious agents as the cause of diseases classified to other chapters

Certain infections are classified in chapters other than Chapter 1 and no organism is identified as part of the infection code. In these instances, it is necessary to use an additional code from Chapter 1 to identify the organism. A code from category B95, Streptococcus, Staphylococcus, and Enterococcus as the cause of diseases classified to other chapters, B96, Other bacterial agents as the cause of diseases classified to other chapters, or B97, Viral agents as the cause of diseases classified to other chapters, is to be used as an additional code to identify the organism. An instructional note will be found at the infection code advising that an additional organism code is required.

BACTERIAL AND VIRAL INFECTIOUS AGENTS (B95-B97)

Note: These categories are provided for use as supplementary or additional codes to identify the infectious agent(s) in diseases classified elsewhere.

Code the disease first, then the bacterium. Do not report codes from B95-B97 for sepsis.

B95 Streptococcus, Staphylococcus, and Enterococcus as the cause of diseases classified elsewhere

B95.0 Streptococcus, group A, as the cause of diseases classified elsewhere

B95.1 Streptococcus, group B, as the cause of diseases classified elsewhere
Coding Clinic: 2019, Q2, P9-10; 2018, Q4, P23

B95.2 Enterococcus as the cause of diseases classified elsewhere

B95.3 Streptococcus pneumoniae as the cause of diseases classified elsewhere

B95.4 Other streptococcus as the cause of diseases classified elsewhere

B95.5 Unspecified streptococcus as the cause of diseases classified elsewhere

B95.6 Staphylococcus aureus as the cause of diseases classified elsewhere

B95.61 Methicillin susceptible Staphylococcus aureus infection as the cause of diseases classified elsewhere
Methicillin susceptible Staphylococcus aureus (MSSA) infection as the cause of diseases classified elsewhere
Staphylococcus aureus infection NOS as the cause of diseases classified elsewhere

B95.62 Methicillin resistant Staphylococcus aureus infection as the cause of diseases classified elsewhere
Methicillin resistant staphylococcus aureus (MRSA) infection as the cause of diseases classified elsewhere
Coding Clinic: 2016, Q1, P13

B95.7 Other staphylococcus as the cause of diseases classified elsewhere

B95.8 Unspecified staphylococcus as the cause of diseases classified elsewhere

B96 Other bacterial agents as the cause of diseases classified elsewhere

B96.0 Mycoplasma pneumoniae [M. pneumoniae] as the cause of diseases classified elsewhere
Pleuro-pneumonia-like-organism [PPLO]

B96.1 Klebsiella pneumoniae [K. pneumoniae] as the cause of diseases classified elsewhere

CHAPTER 1 (A00-B99)

● B96.2 **Escherichia coli [E. coli] as the cause of diseases classified elsewhere**

B96.20 **Unspecified Escherichia coli [E. coli] as the cause of diseases classified elsewhere**
Escherichia coli [E. coli] NOS
Coding Clinic: 2018, Q4, P34; 2018, Q1, P16

B96.21 **Shiga toxin-producing Escherichia coli [E. coli] [STEC] O157 as the cause of diseases classified elsewhere**
E. coli O157:H- (nonmotile) with confirmation of Shiga toxin
E. coli O157 with confirmation of Shiga toxin when H antigen is unknown, or is not H7
O157:H7 Escherichia coli [E.coli] with or without confirmation of Shiga toxin-production
Shiga toxin-producing Escherichia coli [E.coli] O157:H7 with or without confirmation of Shiga toxin-production
STEC O157:H7 with or without confirmation of Shiga toxin-production

B96.22 **Other specified Shiga toxin-producing Escherichia coli [E. coli] [STEC] as the cause of diseases classified elsewhere**
Non-O157 Shiga toxin-producing Escherichia coli [E.coli]
Non-O157 Shiga toxin-producing Escherichia coli [E.coli] with known O group

B96.23 **Unspecified Shiga toxin-producing Escherichia coli [E. coli] [STEC] as the cause of diseases classified elsewhere**
Shiga toxin-producing Escherichia coli [E. coli] with unspecified O group
STEC NOS

B96.29 **Other Escherichia coli [E. coli] as the cause of diseases classified elsewhere**
Non-Shiga toxin-producing E. coli

B96.3 **Hemophilus influenzae [H. influenzae] as the cause of diseases classified elsewhere**

B96.4 **Proteus (mirabilis) (morganii) as the cause of diseases classified elsewhere**

B96.5 **Pseudomonas (aeruginosa) (mallei) (pseudomallei) as the cause of diseases classified elsewhere**
Coding Clinic: 2015, Q1, P18

B96.6 **Bacteroides fragilis [B. fragilis] as the cause of diseases classified elsewhere**

B96.7 **Clostridium perfringens [C. perfringens] as the cause of diseases classified elsewhere**

● B96.8 Other specified bacterial agents as the cause of diseases classified elsewhere

B96.81 **Helicobacter pylori [H. pylori] as the cause of diseases classified elsewhere**

B96.82 **Vibrio vulnificus as the cause of diseases classified elsewhere**

B96.89 **Other specified bacterial agents as the cause of diseases classified elsewhere**

● B97 Viral agents as the cause of diseases classified elsewhere

B97.0 **Adenovirus as the cause of diseases classified elsewhere**

● B97.1 **Enterovirus as the cause of diseases classified elsewhere**

B97.10 **Unspecified enterovirus as the cause of diseases classified elsewhere**

B97.11 **Coxsackievirus as the cause of diseases classified elsewhere**

B97.12 **Echovirus as the cause of diseases classified elsewhere**

B97.19 **Other enterovirus as the cause of diseases classified elsewhere**

Item 1-24 Retrovirus develops by copying its RNA, genetic materials, into the DNA, which then produces new virus particles. It is from the Retroviridae virus family. **Human T-cell lymphotropic virus, Type I (HTLV-I),** is also called human T-cell leukemia virus, Type I, and is a retrovirus thought to cause T-cell leukemia/lymphoma. **Human T-cell lymphotropic virus, Type II (HTLV-II),** is also called human T-cell leukemia virus, Type II, and is a retrovirus associated with hematologic disorders.

HIV-2 is one of the serotypes of HIV and is usually confined to West Africa, whereas **HIV-1** is found worldwide.

● B97.2 **Coronavirus as the cause of diseases classified elsewhere**

B97.21 **SARS-associated coronavirus as the cause of diseases classified elsewhere**
Excludes1 pneumonia due to SARS-associated coronavirus (J12.81)

B97.29 **Other coronavirus as the cause of diseases classified elsewhere**

● B97.3 **Retrovirus as the cause of diseases classified elsewhere**
Excludes1 human immunodeficiency virus [HIV] disease (B20)

B97.30 **Unspecified retrovirus as the cause of diseases classified elsewhere**

B97.31 **Lentivirus as the cause of diseases classified elsewhere**

B97.32 **Oncovirus as the cause of diseases classified elsewhere**

B97.33 **Human T-cell lymphotrophic virus, type I [HTLV-I] as the cause of diseases classified elsewhere**

B97.34 **Human T-cell lymphotrophic virus, type II [HTLV-II] as the cause of diseases classified elsewhere**

B97.35 **Human immunodeficiency virus, type 2 [HIV 2] as the cause of diseases classified elsewhere** HCC

B97.39 **Other retrovirus as the cause of diseases classified elsewhere**

B97.4 **Respiratory syncytial virus as the cause of diseases classified elsewhere**
▶RSV as the cause of diseases classified elsewhere
▶*Code first related disorders, such as:*
▶otitis media (H65.-)
▶upper respiratory infection (J06.9)
▶**Excludes2** acute bronchiolitis due to respiratory syncytial virus (RSV) (J21.0)
▶acute bronchitis due to respiratory syncytial virus (RSV) (J20.5)
▶respiratory syncytial virus (RSV) pneumonia (J12.1)

B97.5 **Reovirus as the cause of diseases classified elsewhere**

B97.6 **Parvovirus as the cause of diseases classified elsewhere**

B97.7 **Papillomavirus as the cause of diseases classified elsewhere**

● B97.8 **Other viral agents as the cause of diseases classified elsewhere**

B97.81 **Human metapneumovirus as the cause of diseases classified elsewhere**

B97.89 **Other viral agents as the cause of diseases classified elsewhere**
Coding Clinic: 2016, Q3, P8-10, 14

OTHER INFECTIOUS DISEASES (B99)

● B99 Other and unspecified infectious diseases

B99.8 **Other infectious disease**

B99.9 **Unspecified infectious disease**

CHAPTER 2

NEOPLASMS (CØØ-D49)

OGCR Chapter-Specific Coding Guidelines

2. **Chapter 2: Neoplasms (CØØ-D49)**

General guidelines

Chapter 2 of the ICD-10-CM contains the codes for most benign and all malignant neoplasms. Certain benign neoplasms, such as prostatic adenomas, may be found in the specific body system chapters. To properly code a neoplasm it is necessary to determine from the record if the neoplasm is benign, in-situ, malignant, or of uncertain histologic behavior. If malignant, any secondary (metastatic) sites should also be determined.

Primary malignant neoplasms overlapping site boundaries

A primary malignant neoplasm that overlaps two or more contiguous (next to each other) sites should be classified to the subcategory/code .8 ('overlapping lesion'), unless the combination is specifically indexed elsewhere. For multiple neoplasms of the same site that are not contiguous such as tumors in different quadrants of the same breast, codes for each site should be assigned.

Malignant neoplasm of ectopic tissue

Malignant neoplasms of ectopic tissue are to be coded to the site of origin mentioned, e.g., ectopic pancreatic malignant neoplasms involving the stomach are coded to malignant neoplasm of pancreas, unspecified (C25.9).

The neoplasm table in the Alphabetic Index should be referenced first. However, if the histological term is documented, that term should be referenced first, rather than going immediately to the Neoplasm Table, in order to determine which column in the Neoplasm Table is appropriate. For example, if the documentation indicates "adenoma," refer to the term in the Alphabetic Index to review the entries under this term and the instructional note to "see also neoplasm, by site, benign." The table provides the proper code based on the type of neoplasm and the site. It is important to select the proper column in the table that corresponds to the type of neoplasm. The Tabular List should then be referenced to verify that the correct code has been selected from the table and that a more specific site code does not exist.

See Section I.C.21. Factors influencing health status and contact with health services, Status, for information regarding Z15.Ø, codes for genetic susceptibility to cancer.

a. Treatment directed at the malignancy

If the treatment is directed at the malignancy, designate the malignancy as the principal diagnosis.

The only exception to this guideline is if a patient admission/encounter is solely for the administration of chemotherapy, immunotherapy or external beam radiation therapy, assign the appropriate Z51.— code as the first-listed or principal diagnosis, and the diagnosis or problem for which the service is being performed as a secondary diagnosis.

b. Treatment of secondary site

When a patient is admitted because of a primary neoplasm with metastasis and treatment is directed toward the secondary site only, the secondary neoplasm is designated as the principal diagnosis even though the primary malignancy is still present.

c. Coding and sequencing of complications

Coding and sequencing of complications associated with the malignancies or with the therapy thereof are subject to the following guidelines:

1) Anemia associated with malignancy

When admission/encounter is for management of an anemia associated with the malignancy, and the treatment is only for anemia, the appropriate code for the malignancy is sequenced as the principal or first-listed diagnosis followed by the appropriate code for the anemia (such as code D63.Ø, Anemia in neoplastic disease).

2) Anemia associated with chemotherapy, immunotherapy and radiation therapy

When the admission/encounter is for management of an anemia associated with an adverse effect of the administration of chemotherapy or immunotherapy and the only treatment is for the anemia, the anemia code is sequenced first followed by the appropriate codes for the neoplasm and the adverse effect (T45.1X5, Adverse effect of antineoplastic and immunosuppressive drugs).

When the admission/encounter is for management of an anemia associated with an adverse effect of radiotherapy, the anemia code should be sequenced first, followed by the appropriate neoplasm code and code Y84.2, Radiological procedure and radiotherapy as the cause of abnormal reaction of the patient, or of later complication, without mention of misadventure at the time of the procedure.

3) Management of dehydration due to the malignancy

When the admission/encounter is for management of dehydration due to the malignancy and only the dehydration is being treated (intravenous rehydration), the dehydration is sequenced first, followed by the code(s) for the malignancy.

4) Treatment of a complication resulting from a surgical procedure

When the admission/encounter is for treatment of a complication resulting from a surgical procedure, designate the complication as the principal or first-listed diagnosis if treatment is directed at resolving the complication.

d. Primary malignancy previously excised

When a primary malignancy has been previously excised or eradicated from its site and there is no further treatment directed to that site and there is no evidence of any existing primary malignancy at that site, a code from category Z85, Personal history of malignant neoplasm, should be used to indicate the former site of the malignancy. Any mention of extension, invasion, or metastasis to another site is coded as a secondary malignant neoplasm to that site. The secondary site may be the principal or first-listed with the Z85 code used as a secondary code.

e. Admissions/Encounters involving chemotherapy, immunotherapy and radiation therapy

1) Episode of care involves surgical removal of neoplasm

When an episode of care involves the surgical removal of a neoplasm, primary or secondary site, followed by adjunct chemotherapy or radiation treatment during the same episode of care, the code for the neoplasm should be assigned as principal or first-listed diagnosis.

2) Patient admission/encounter solely for administration of chemotherapy, immunotherapy and radiation therapy

If a patient admission/encounter is solely for the administration of chemotherapy, immunotherapy or external beam radiation therapy assign code Z51.Ø, Encounter for antineoplastic radiation therapy, or Z51.11, Encounter for antineoplastic chemotherapy, or Z51.12, Encounter for antineoplastic immunotherapy as the first-listed or principal diagnosis. If a patient receives more than one of these therapies during the same admission more than one of these codes may be assigned, in any sequence.

The malignancy for which the therapy is being administered should be assigned as a secondary diagnosis.

If a patient admission/encounter is for the insertion or implantation of radioactive elements (e.g., brachytherapy) the appropriate code for the malignancy is sequenced as the principal or first-listed diagnosis. Code Z51.Ø should not be assigned.

3) Patient admitted for radiation therapy, chemotherapy or immunotherapy and develops complications

When a patient is admitted for the purpose of external beam radiotherapy, immunotherapy or chemotherapy and develops complications such as uncontrolled nausea and vomiting or dehydration, the principal or first-listed diagnosis is Z51.Ø, Encounter for antineoplastic radiation therapy, or Z51.11, Encounter for antineoplastic chemotherapy, or Z51.12, Encounter for antineoplastic immunotherapy followed by any codes for the complications.

When a patient is admitted for the purpose of insertion or implantation of radioactive elements (e.g., brachytherapy) and develops complications such as uncontrolled nausea and vomiting or dehydration, the principal or first-listed diagnosis is the appropriate code for the malignancy followed by any codes for the complications.

f. Admission/encounter to determine extent of malignancy

When the reason for admission/encounter is to determine the extent of the malignancy, or for a procedure such as paracentesis or thoracentesis, the primary malignancy or appropriate metastatic site is designated as the principal or first-listed diagnosis, even though chemotherapy or radiotherapy is administered.

g. Symptoms, signs, and abnormal findings listed in Chapter 18 associated with neoplasms

Symptoms, signs, and ill-defined conditions listed in Chapter 18 characteristic of, or associated with, an existing primary or secondary site malignancy cannot be used to replace the malignancy as principal or first-listed diagnosis, regardless of the number of admissions or encounters for treatment and care of the neoplasm.

See Section I.C.21. Factors influencing health status and contact with health services, Encounter for prophylactic organ removal.

h. Admission/encounter for pain control/management

See Section I.C.6. for information on coding admission/encounter for pain control/management.

i. Malignancy in two or more noncontiguous sites

A patient may have more than one malignant tumor in the same organ. These tumors may represent different primaries or metastatic disease, depending on the site. Should the documentation be unclear, the provider should be queried as to the status of each tumor so that the correct codes can be assigned.

j. Disseminated malignant neoplasm, unspecified

Code C80.0, Disseminated malignant neoplasm, unspecified, is for use only in those cases where the patient has advanced metastatic disease and no known primary or secondary sites are specified. It should not be used in place of assigning codes for the primary site and all known secondary sites.

k. Malignant neoplasm without specification of site

Code C80.1, Malignant (primary) neoplasm, unspecified, equates to Cancer, unspecified. This code should only be used when no determination can be made as to the primary site of a malignancy. This code should rarely be used in the inpatient setting.

l. Sequencing of neoplasm codes

1) Encounter for treatment of primary malignancy

If the reason for the encounter is for treatment of a primary malignancy, assign the malignancy as the principal/first-listed diagnosis. The primary site is to be sequenced first, followed by any metastatic sites.

2) Encounter for treatment of secondary malignancy

When an encounter is for a primary malignancy with metastasis and treatment is directed toward the metastatic (secondary) site(s) only, the metastatic site(s) is designated as the principal/first-listed diagnosis. The primary malignancy is coded as an additional code.

3) Malignant neoplasm in a pregnant patient

When a pregnant woman has a malignant neoplasm, a code from subcategory O9A.1-, Malignant neoplasm complicating pregnancy, childbirth, and the puerperium, should be sequenced first, followed by the appropriate code from Chapter 2 to indicate the type of neoplasm.

4) Encounter for complication associated with a neoplasm

When an encounter is for management of a complication associated with a neoplasm, such as dehydration, and the treatment is only for the complication, the complication is coded first, followed by the appropriate code(s) for the neoplasm.

The exception to this guideline is anemia. When the admission/encounter is for management of an anemia associated with the malignancy, and the treatment is only for anemia, the appropriate code for the malignancy is sequenced as the principal or first-listed diagnosis followed by code D63.0, Anemia in neoplastic disease.

5) Complication from surgical procedure for treatment of a neoplasm

When an encounter is for treatment of a complication resulting from a surgical procedure performed for the treatment of the neoplasm, designate the complication as the principal/first-listed diagnosis. See guideline regarding the coding of a current malignancy versus personal history to determine if the code for the neoplasm should also be assigned.

6) Pathologic fracture due to a neoplasm

When an encounter is for a pathological fracture due to a neoplasm, and the focus of treatment is the fracture, a code from subcategory M84.5, Pathological fracture in neoplastic disease, should be sequenced first, followed by the code for the neoplasm.

If the focus of treatment is the neoplasm with an associated pathological fracture, the neoplasm code should be sequenced first, followed by a code from M84.5 for the pathological fracture.

m. Current malignancy versus personal history of malignancy

When a primary malignancy has been excised but further treatment, such as an additional surgery for the malignancy, radiation therapy or chemotherapy is directed to that site, the primary malignancy code should be used until treatment is completed.

When a primary malignancy has been previously excised or eradicated from its site, there is no further treatment (of the malignancy) directed to that site, and there is no evidence of any existing primary malignancy at that site, a code from category Z85, Personal history of malignant neoplasm, should be used to indicate the former site of the malignancy.

Subcategories Z85.0–Z85.7 should only be assigned for the former site of a primary malignancy, not the site of a secondary malignancy. Codes from subcategory Z85.8-, may be assigned for the former site(s) of either a primary or secondary malignancy included in this subcategory.

See Section I.C.21. Factors influencing health status and contact with health services, History (of)

n. Leukemia, Multiple Myeloma, and Malignant Plasma Cell Neoplasms in remission versus personal history

The categories for leukemia, and category C90, Multiple myeloma and malignant plasma cell neoplasms, have codes indicating whether or not the leukemia has achieved remission. There are also codes Z85.6, Personal history of leukemia, and Z85.79, Personal history of other malignant neoplasms of lymphoid, hematopoietic and related tissues. If the documentation is unclear, as to whether the leukemia has achieved remission, the provider should be queried.

See Section I.C.21. Factors influencing health status and contact with health services, History (of)

o. Aftercare following surgery for neoplasm

See Section I.C.21. Factors influencing health status and contact with health services, Aftercare

p. Follow-up care for completed treatment of a malignancy

See Section I.C.21. Factors influencing health status and contact with health services, Follow-up

q. Prophylactic organ removal for prevention of malignancy

See Section I.C. 21, Factors influencing health status and contact with health services, Prophylactic organ removal

r. Malignant neoplasm associated with transplanted organ

A malignant neoplasm of a transplanted organ should be coded as a transplant complication. Assign first the appropriate code from category T86.-, Complications of transplanted organs and tissue, followed by code C80.2, Malignant neoplasm associated with transplanted organ. Use an additional code for the specific malignancy.

Item 2-1 Neoplasm: Neo = new, plasm = growth, development, formation. This new growth (mass, tumor) can be malignant or benign, which is confirmed by the pathology report. Do not assign a code to a neoplasm until you review the pathology report. Certain CPT codes will specify benign or malignant lesion, so be certain the diagnosis code supports the procedure code.

CHAPTER 2

NEOPLASMS (C00-D49)

This chapter contains the following blocks:

C00-C14	Malignant neoplasms of lip, oral cavity and pharynx
C15-C26	Malignant neoplasms of digestive organs
C30-C39	Malignant neoplasms of respiratory and intrathoracic organs
C40-C41	Malignant neoplasms of bone and articular cartilage
C43-C44	Melanoma and other malignant neoplasms of skin
C45-C49	Malignant neoplasms of mesothelial and soft tissue
C50	Malignant neoplasms of breast
C51-C58	Malignant neoplasms of female genital organs
C60-C63	Malignant neoplasms of male genital organs
C64-C68	Malignant neoplasms of urinary tract
C69-C72	Malignant neoplasms of eye, brain and other parts of central nervous system
C73-C75	Malignant neoplasms of thyroid and other endocrine glands
C7A	Malignant neuroendocrine tumors
C7B	Secondary neuroendocrine tumors
C76-C80	Malignant neoplasms of ill-defined, other secondary and unspecified sites
C81-C96	Malignant neoplasms of lymphoid, hematopoietic and related tissue
D00-D09	In situ neoplasms
D10-D36	Benign neoplasms, except benign neuroendocrine tumors
D3A	Benign neuroendocrine tumors
D37-D48	Neoplasms of uncertain behavior, polycythemia vera and myelodysplastic syndromes
D49	Neoplasms of unspecified behavior

Notes: Functional activity

All neoplasms are classified in this chapter, whether they are functionally active or not. An additional code from Chapter 4 may be used, to identify functional activity associated with any neoplasm.

Morphology [Histology]

Chapter 2 classifies neoplasms primarily by site (topography), with broad groupings for behavior, malignant, in situ, benign, etc. The Table of Neoplasms should be used to identify the correct topography code. In a few cases, such as for malignant melanoma and certain neuroendocrine tumors, the morphology (histologic type) is included in the category and codes.

Primary malignant neoplasms overlapping site boundaries

A primary malignant neoplasm that overlaps two or more contiguous (next to each other) sites should be classified to the subcategory/code .8 ("overlapping lesion"), unless the combination is specifically indexed elsewhere. For multiple neoplasms of the same site that are not contiguous, such as tumors in different quadrants of the same breast, codes for each site should be assigned.

Malignant neoplasm of ectopic tissue

Malignant neoplasms of ectopic tissue are to be coded to the site mentioned, e.g., ectopic pancreatic malignant neoplasms are coded to pancreas, unspecified (C25.9).

MALIGNANT NEOPLASMS (C00-C96)

MALIGNANT NEOPLASMS, STATED OR PRESUMED TO BE PRIMARY (OF SPECIFIED SITES), AND CERTAIN SPECIFIED HISTOLOGIES, EXCEPT NEUROENDOCRINE, AND OF LYMPHOID, HEMATOPOIETIC AND RELATED TISSUE (C00-C75)

MALIGNANT NEOPLASMS OF LIP, ORAL CAVITY AND PHARYNX (C00-C14)

● **C00 Malignant neoplasm of lip**

Use additional code to identify:
- alcohol abuse and dependence (F10.-)
- history of tobacco dependence (Z87.891)
- tobacco dependence (F17.-)
- tobacco use (Z72.0)

Excludes1 malignant melanoma of lip (C43.0)
Merkel cell carcinoma of lip (C4A.0)
other and unspecified malignant neoplasm of skin of lip (C44.0-)

C00.0 Malignant neoplasm of external upper lip
Malignant neoplasm of lipstick area of upper lip
Malignant neoplasm of upper lip NOS
Malignant neoplasm of vermilion border of upper lip

C00.1 Malignant neoplasm of external lower lip
Malignant neoplasm of lower lip NOS
Malignant neoplasm of lipstick area of lower lip
Malignant neoplasm of vermilion border of lower lip

C00.2 Malignant neoplasm of external lip, unspecified
Malignant neoplasm of vermilion border of lip NOS

C00.3 Malignant neoplasm of upper lip, inner aspect
Malignant neoplasm of buccal aspect of upper lip
Malignant neoplasm of frenulum of upper lip
Malignant neoplasm of mucosa of upper lip
Malignant neoplasm of oral aspect of upper lip

C00.4 Malignant neoplasm of lower lip, inner aspect
Malignant neoplasm of buccal aspect of lower lip
Malignant neoplasm of frenulum of lower lip
Malignant neoplasm of mucosa of lower lip
Malignant neoplasm of oral aspect of lower lip

C00.5 Malignant neoplasm of lip, unspecified, inner aspect
Malignant neoplasm of buccal aspect of lip, unspecified
Malignant neoplasm of frenulum of lip, unspecified
Malignant neoplasm of mucosa of lip, unspecified
Malignant neoplasm of oral aspect of lip, unspecified

C00.6 Malignant neoplasm of commissure of lip, unspecified
Commissure: Site of union of corresponding parts

C00.8 Malignant neoplasm of overlapping sites of lip

C00.9 Malignant neoplasm of lip, unspecified

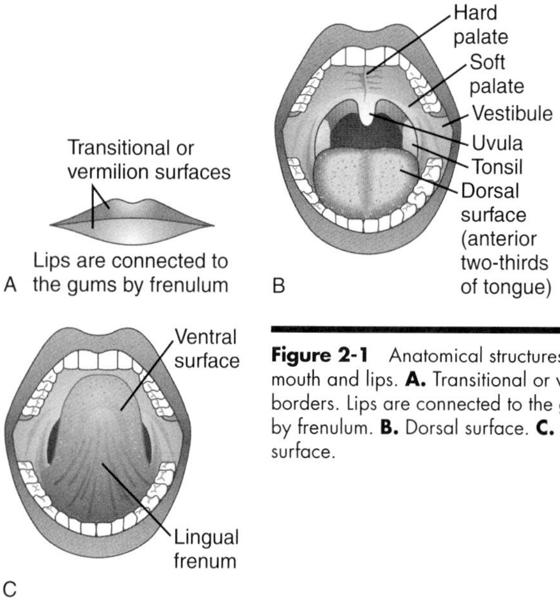

Figure 2-1 Anatomical structures of the mouth and lips. **A.** Transitional or vermilion borders. Lips are connected to the gums by frenulum. **B.** Dorsal surface. **C.** Ventral surface.

CØ1 Malignant neoplasm of base of tongue
Malignant neoplasm of dorsal surface of base of tongue
Malignant neoplasm of fixed part of tongue NOS
Malignant neoplasm of posterior third of tongue
Use additional code to identify:
alcohol abuse and dependence (F1Ø.-)
history of tobacco dependence (Z87.891)
tobacco dependence (F17.-)
tobacco use (Z72.Ø)

CØ2 Malignant neoplasm of other and unspecified parts of tongue
Use additional code to identify:
alcohol abuse and dependence (F1Ø.-)
history of tobacco dependence (Z87.891)
tobacco dependence (F17.-)
tobacco use (Z72.Ø)

CØ2.Ø Malignant neoplasm of dorsal surface of tongue
Malignant neoplasm of anterior two-thirds of tongue, dorsal surface
Excludes2 malignant neoplasm of dorsal surface of base of tongue (CØ1)

CØ2.1 Malignant neoplasm of border of tongue
Malignant neoplasm of tip of tongue

CØ2.2 Malignant neoplasm of ventral surface of tongue
Malignant neoplasm of anterior two-thirds of tongue, ventral surface
Malignant neoplasm of frenulum linguae

CØ2.3 Malignant neoplasm of anterior two-thirds of tongue, part unspecified
Malignant neoplasm of middle third of tongue NOS
Malignant neoplasm of mobile part of tongue NOS

CØ2.4 Malignant neoplasm of lingual tonsil
Lingual tonsil: Aggregation of lymph follicles at root of tongue
Excludes2 malignant neoplasm of tonsil NOS (CØ9.9)

CØ2.8 Malignant neoplasm of overlapping sites of tongue
Malignant neoplasm of two or more contiguous sites of tongue

CØ2.9 Malignant neoplasm of tongue, unspecified

CØ3 Malignant neoplasm of gum
Includes malignant neoplasm of alveolar (ridge) mucosa
malignant neoplasm of gingiva
Use additional code to identify:
alcohol abuse and dependence (F1Ø.-)
history of tobacco dependence (Z87.891)
tobacco dependence (F17.-)
tobacco use (Z72.Ø)
Excludes2 malignant odontogenic neoplasms (C41.Ø-C41.1)

CØ3.Ø Malignant neoplasm of upper gum

CØ3.1 Malignant neoplasm of lower gum

CØ3.9 Malignant neoplasm of gum, unspecified

CØ4 Malignant neoplasm of floor of mouth
Use additional code to identify:
alcohol abuse and dependence (F1Ø.-)
history of tobacco dependence (Z87.891)
tobacco dependence (F17.-)
tobacco use (Z72.Ø)

CØ4.Ø Malignant neoplasm of anterior floor of mouth
Malignant neoplasm of anterior to the premolar-canine junction

CØ4.1 Malignant neoplasm of lateral floor of mouth

CØ4.8 Malignant neoplasm of overlapping sites of floor of mouth

CØ4.9 Malignant neoplasm of floor of mouth, unspecified

CØ5 Malignant neoplasm of palate
Use additional code to identify:
alcohol abuse and dependence (F1Ø.-)
history of tobacco dependence (Z87.891)
tobacco dependence (F17.-)
tobacco use (Z72.Ø)
Excludes1 Kaposi's sarcoma of palate (C46.2)

CØ5.Ø Malignant neoplasm of hard palate

CØ5.1 Malignant neoplasm of soft palate
Excludes2 malignant neoplasm of nasopharyngeal surface of soft palate (C11.3)

CØ5.2 Malignant neoplasm of uvula

CØ5.8 Malignant neoplasm of overlapping sites of palate

CØ5.9 Malignant neoplasm of palate, unspecified
Malignant neoplasm of roof of mouth

CØ6 Malignant neoplasm of other and unspecified parts of mouth
Use additional code to identify:
alcohol abuse and dependence (F1Ø.-)
history of tobacco dependence (Z87.891)
tobacco dependence (F17.-)
tobacco use (Z72.Ø)

CØ6.Ø Malignant neoplasm of cheek mucosa
Malignant neoplasm of buccal mucosa NOS
Malignant neoplasm of internal cheek

CØ6.1 Malignant neoplasm of vestibule of mouth
Malignant neoplasm of buccal sulcus (upper) (lower)
Malignant neoplasm of labial sulcus (upper) (lower)

CØ6.2 Malignant neoplasm of retromolar area

CØ6.8 Malignant neoplasm of overlapping sites of other and unspecified parts of mouth

CØ6.8Ø Malignant neoplasm of overlapping sites of unspecified parts of mouth

CØ6.89 Malignant neoplasm of overlapping sites of other parts of mouth
'book leaf' neoplasm [ventral surface of tongue and floor of mouth]

CØ6.9 Malignant neoplasm of mouth, unspecified
Malignant neoplasm of minor salivary gland, unspecified site
Malignant neoplasm of oral cavity NOS

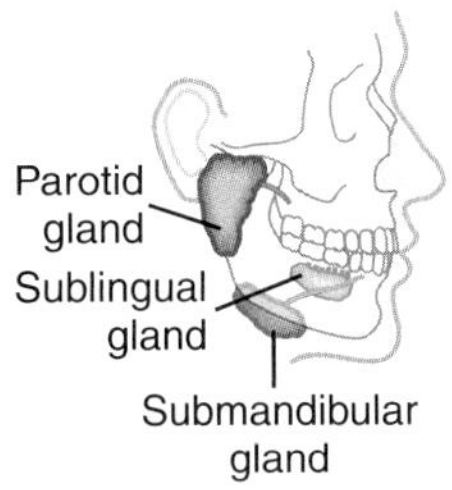

Figure 2-2 Major salivary glands.

C07 Malignant neoplasm of parotid gland
Use additional code to identify:
alcohol abuse and dependence (F10.-)
exposure to environmental tobacco smoke (Z77.22)
exposure to tobacco smoke in the perinatal period (P96.81)
history of tobacco dependence (Z87.891)
occupational exposure to environmental tobacco smoke (Z57.31)
tobacco dependence (F17.-)
tobacco use (Z72.0)

● C08 Malignant neoplasm of other and unspecified major salivary glands
Includes malignant neoplasm of salivary ducts
Use additional code to identify:
alcohol abuse and dependence (F10.-)
exposure to environmental tobacco smoke (Z77.22)
exposure to tobacco smoke in the perinatal period (P96.81)
history of tobacco dependence (Z87.891)
occupational exposure to environmental tobacco smoke (Z57.31)
tobacco dependence (F17.-)
tobacco use (Z72.0)
Excludes1 malignant neoplasms of specified minor salivary glands which are classified according to their anatomical location
Excludes2 malignant neoplasms of minor salivary glands NOS (C06.9)
malignant neoplasm of parotid gland (C07)

C08.0 Malignant neoplasm of submandibular gland
Malignant neoplasm of submaxillary gland

C08.1 Malignant neoplasm of sublingual gland

C08.9 Malignant neoplasm of major salivary gland, unspecified
Malignant neoplasm of salivary gland (major) NOS

★ **(See Plate 28 of the Anatomy Illustrations.)**

● C09 Malignant neoplasm of tonsil
Use additional code to identify:
alcohol abuse and dependence (F10.-)
exposure to environmental tobacco smoke (Z77.22)
exposure to tobacco smoke in the perinatal period (P96.81)
history of tobacco dependence (Z87.891)
occupational exposure to environmental tobacco smoke (Z57.31)
tobacco dependence (F17.-)
tobacco use (Z72.0)
Excludes2 malignant neoplasm of lingual tonsil (C02.4)
malignant neoplasm of pharyngeal tonsil (C11.1)

C09.0 Malignant neoplasm of tonsillar fossa
Surface of palatine (two masses of lymphatic tissue on sides of throat) tonsils

C09.1 Malignant neoplasm of tonsillar pillar (anterior) (posterior)
Extension from palatine (two masses of lymphatic tissue on sides of throat) tonsils

C09.8 Malignant neoplasm of overlapping sites of tonsil

C09.9 Malignant neoplasm of tonsil, unspecified
Malignant neoplasm of tonsil NOS
Malignant neoplasm of faucial tonsils
Malignant neoplasm of palatine tonsils

● C10 Malignant neoplasm of oropharynx
Area of throat at back of mouth
Use additional code to identify:
alcohol abuse and dependence (F10.-)
exposure to environmental tobacco smoke (Z77.22)
exposure to tobacco smoke in the perinatal period (P96.81)
history of tobacco dependence (Z87.891)
occupational exposure to environmental tobacco smoke (Z57.31)
tobacco dependence (F17.-)
tobacco use (Z72.0)
Excludes2 malignant neoplasm of tonsil (C09.-)

C10.0 Malignant neoplasm of vallecula
Vallecula, depression or furrow

C10.1 Malignant neoplasm of anterior surface of epiglottis
Malignant neoplasm of epiglottis, free border [margin]
Malignant neoplasm of glossoepiglottic fold(s)
Excludes2 malignant neoplasm of epiglottis (suprahyoid portion) NOS (C32.1)

C10.2 Malignant neoplasm of lateral wall of oropharynx

C10.3 Malignant neoplasm of posterior wall of oropharynx

C10.4 Malignant neoplasm of branchial cleft
Congenital slitlike openings formed between branchial arches pharyngeal groove
Malignant neoplasm of branchial cyst [site of neoplasm]

C10.8 Malignant neoplasm of overlapping sites of oropharynx
Malignant neoplasm of junctional region of oropharynx

C10.9 Malignant neoplasm of oropharynx, unspecified

● C11 Malignant neoplasm of nasopharynx
Use additional code to identify:
exposure to environmental tobacco smoke (Z77.22)
exposure to tobacco smoke in the perinatal period (P96.81)
history of tobacco dependence (Z87.891)
occupational exposure to environmental tobacco smoke (Z57.31)
tobacco dependence (F17.-)
tobacco use (Z72.0)

C11.0 Malignant neoplasm of superior wall of nasopharynx
Part of pharynx that lies above soft palate
Malignant neoplasm of roof of nasopharynx

C11.1 Malignant neoplasm of posterior wall of nasopharynx
Malignant neoplasm of adenoid
Malignant neoplasm of pharyngeal tonsil

C11.2 Malignant neoplasm of lateral wall of nasopharynx
Malignant neoplasm of fossa of Rosenmüller
Malignant neoplasm of opening of auditory tube
Malignant neoplasm of pharyngeal recess

C11.3 Malignant neoplasm of anterior wall of nasopharynx
Malignant neoplasm of floor of nasopharynx
Malignant neoplasm of nasopharyngeal (anterior) (posterior) surface of soft palate
Malignant neoplasm of posterior margin of nasal choana
Malignant neoplasm of posterior margin of nasal septum

C11.8 Malignant neoplasm of overlapping sites of nasopharynx

C11.9 Malignant neoplasm of nasopharynx, unspecified
Malignant neoplasm of nasopharyngeal wall NOS

C12 Malignant neoplasm of pyriform sinus
Malignant neoplasm of pyriform fossa
Use additional code to identify:
exposure to environmental tobacco smoke (Z77.22)
exposure to tobacco smoke in the perinatal period (P96.81)
history of tobacco dependence (Z87.891)
occupational exposure to environmental tobacco smoke (Z57.31)
tobacco dependence (F17.-)
tobacco use (Z72.0)

CHAPTER 2 (C00-D49)

C13 Malignant neoplasm of hypopharynx
Use additional code to identify:
exposure to environmental tobacco smoke (Z77.22)
exposure to tobacco smoke in the perinatal period (P96.81)
history of tobacco dependence (Z87.891)
occupational exposure to environmental tobacco smoke (Z57.31)
tobacco dependence (F17.-)
tobacco use (Z72.Ø)

Excludes2 malignant neoplasm of pyriform sinus (C12)

C13.Ø Malignant neoplasm of postcricoid region
Behind the cricoid cartilage of neck

C13.1 Malignant neoplasm of aryepiglottic fold, hypopharyngeal aspect
Arytenoepiglottic fold, triangular opening between side of epiglottis and apex of arytenoid cartilage
Malignant neoplasm of aryepiglottic fold, marginal zone
Malignant neoplasm of aryepiglottic fold NOS
Malignant neoplasm of interarytenoid fold, marginal zone
Malignant neoplasm of interarytenoid fold NOS
Excludes2 malignant neoplasm of aryepiglottic fold or interarytenoid fold, laryngeal aspect (C32.1)

C13.2 Malignant neoplasm of posterior wall of hypopharynx

C13.8 Malignant neoplasm of overlapping sites of hypopharynx

C13.9 Malignant neoplasm of hypopharynx, unspecified
Malignant neoplasm of hypopharyngeal wall NOS

C14 Malignant neoplasm of other and ill-defined sites in the lip, oral cavity and pharynx
Use additional code to identify:
alcohol abuse and dependence (F1Ø.-)
exposure to environmental tobacco smoke (Z77.22)
exposure to tobacco smoke in the perinatal period (P96.81)
history of tobacco dependence (Z87.891)
occupational exposure to environmental tobacco smoke (Z57.31)
tobacco dependence (F17.-)
tobacco use (Z72.Ø)

Excludes1 malignant neoplasm of oral cavity NOS (CØ6.9)

C14.Ø Malignant neoplasm of pharynx, unspecified

C14.2 Malignant neoplasm of Waldeyer's ring

C14.8 Malignant neoplasm of overlapping sites of lip, oral cavity and pharynx
Primary malignant neoplasm of two or more contiguous sites of lip, oral cavity and pharynx
Excludes1 'book leaf' neoplasm [ventral surface of tongue and floor of mouth] (CØ6.89)

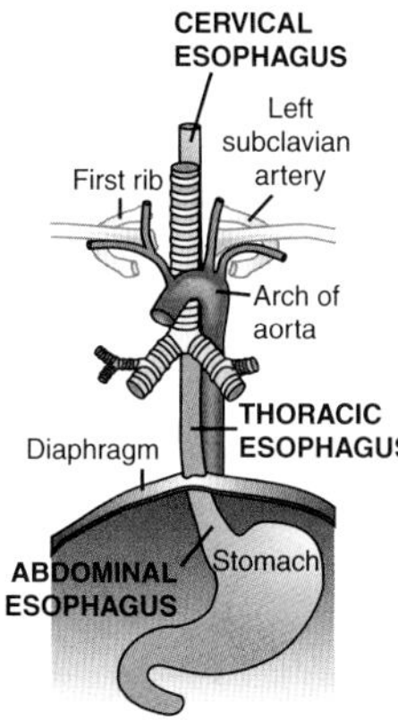

Figure 2-3 The esophagus is the muscular tube that connects the pharynx and the stomach. The 1Ø inch (25 cm) long esophagus is divided into three parts: **cervical, thoracic,** and **abdominal.**

MALIGNANT NEOPLASM OF DIGESTIVE ORGANS (C15-C26)

Excludes1 Kaposi's sarcoma of gastrointestinal sites (C46.4)

Excludes2 gastrointestinal stromal tumors (C49.A-)

C15 Malignant neoplasms of esophagus
Use additional code to identify:
alcohol abuse and dependence (F1Ø.-)

C15.3 Malignant neoplasm of upper third of esophagus

C15.4 Malignant neoplasm of middle third of esophagus

C15.5 Malignant neoplasm of lower third of esophagus
Excludes1 malignant neoplasm of cardio-esophageal junction (C16.Ø)

C15.8 Malignant neoplasm of overlapping sites of esophagus

C15.9 Malignant neoplasm of esophagus, unspecified

C16 Malignant neoplasm of stomach
Use additional code to identify:
alcohol abuse and dependence (F1Ø.-)

Excludes2 malignant carcinoid tumor of the stomach (C7A.Ø92)

C16.Ø Malignant neoplasm of cardia
Malignant neoplasm of cardiac orifice
Malignant neoplasm of cardio-esophageal junction
Malignant neoplasm of esophagus and stomach
Malignant neoplasm of gastro-esophageal junction

C16.1 Malignant neoplasm of fundus of stomach

C16.2 Malignant neoplasm of body of stomach

C16.3 Malignant neoplasm of pyloric antrum
Malignant neoplasm of gastric antrum

C16.4 Malignant neoplasm of pylorus
Malignant neoplasm of prepylorus
Malignant neoplasm of pyloric canal

C16.5 Malignant neoplasm of lesser curvature of stomach, unspecified
Malignant neoplasm of lesser curvature of stomach, not classifiable to C16.1-C16.4

C16.6 Malignant neoplasm of greater curvature of stomach, unspecified
Malignant neoplasm of greater curvature of stomach, not classifiable to C16.Ø-C16.4

C16.8 Malignant neoplasm of overlapping sites of stomach

C16.9 Malignant neoplasm of stomach, unspecified
Gastric cancer NOS

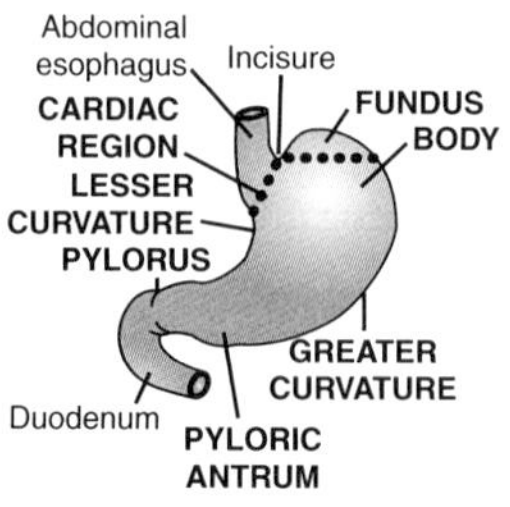

Figure 2-4 Parts of the stomach.

Item 2-2 The esophagus opens into the stomach through the **cardiac orifice,** also called the **cardioesophageal junction.** The **cardia** is adjacent to the cardiac orifice. The stomach widens into the **greater** and **lesser curvatures.** The **pyloric antrum** precedes the **pylorus,** which opens to the duodenum.

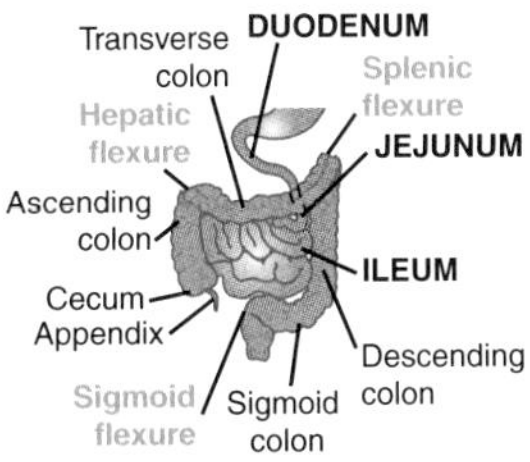

Figure 2-5 Small intestine and colon.

C17 Malignant neoplasm of small intestine

Excludes1 malignant carcinoid tumor of the small intestine (C7A.Ø1)

C17.Ø Malignant neoplasm of duodenum
First or proximal portion of small intestine, extending from pylorus to jejunum

C17.1 Malignant neoplasm of jejunum
Second section of small intestine, extending from duodenum to ileum

C17.2 Malignant neoplasm of ileum
Distal and longest portion of small intestine, extending from jejunum to cecum
Excludes1 malignant neoplasm of ileocecal valve (C18.Ø)

C17.3 Meckel's diverticulum, malignant
Appendage of ileum
Excludes1 Meckel's diverticulum, congenital (Q43.Ø)

C17.8 Malignant neoplasm of overlapping sites of small intestine

C17.9 Malignant neoplasm of small intestine, unspecified

C18 Malignant neoplasm of colon

Excludes1 malignant carcinoid tumors of the colon (C7A.Ø2)

C18.Ø Malignant neoplasm of cecum
First section of large intestine
Malignant neoplasm of ileocecal valve

C18.1 Malignant neoplasm of appendix
Blind ended tube connected to the cecum; AKA vermiform appendix

C18.2 Malignant neoplasm of ascending colon
Ascending colon is between cecum and right colic flexure

C18.3 Malignant neoplasm of hepatic flexure
A flexure is a bending in a structure or organ. Note the three flexures illustrated in Figure 2–5.

C18.4 Malignant neoplasm of transverse colon
Portion of colon that runs transversely across upper part of abdomen, between right and left colic flexures

C18.5 Malignant neoplasm of splenic flexure
Bend at junction of transverse and descending colon

C18.6 Malignant neoplasm of descending colon
Portion between left colic flexure and sigmoid colon at pelvic brim; AKA iliac colon

C18.7 Malignant neoplasm of sigmoid colon
S-shaped part of colon extending from pelvic brim to third segment of sacrum
Malignant neoplasm of sigmoid (flexure)
Excludes1 malignant neoplasm of rectosigmoid junction (C19)

C18.8 Malignant neoplasm of overlapping sites of colon

C18.9 Malignant neoplasm of colon, unspecified
Malignant neoplasm of large intestine NOS

C19 Malignant neoplasm of rectosigmoid junction
Malignant neoplasm of colon with rectum
Malignant neoplasm of rectosigmoid (colon)
Excludes1 malignant carcinoid tumors of the colon (C7A.Ø2-)

C2Ø Malignant neoplasm of rectum
Malignant neoplasm of rectal ampulla
Excludes1 malignant carcinoid tumor of the rectum (C7A.Ø26)

C21 Malignant neoplasm of anus and anal canal

Excludes2 malignant carcinoid tumors of the colon (C7A.Ø2-)
malignant melanoma of anal margin (C43.51)
malignant melanoma of anal skin (C43.51)
malignant melanoma of perianal skin (C43.51)
other and unspecified malignant neoplasm of anal margin (C44.5ØØ, C44.51Ø, C44.52Ø, C44.59Ø)
other and unspecified malignant neoplasm of anal skin (C44.5ØØ, C44.51Ø, C44.52Ø, C44.59Ø)
other and unspecified malignant neoplasm of perianal skin (C44.5ØØ, C44.51Ø, C44.52Ø, C44.59Ø)

C21.Ø Malignant neoplasm of anus, unspecified

C21.1 Malignant neoplasm of anal canal
Terminal part of large intestine
Malignant neoplasm of anal sphincter

C21.2 Malignant neoplasm of cloacogenic zone

C21.8 Malignant neoplasm of overlapping sites of rectum, anus and anal canal
Malignant neoplasm of anorectal junction
Malignant neoplasm of anorectum
Primary malignant neoplasm of two or more contiguous sites of rectum, anus and anal canal

C22 Malignant neoplasm of liver and intrahepatic bile ducts
Intrahepatic: Within liver

Use additional code to identify:
alcohol abuse and dependence (F1Ø.-)
hepatitis B (B16.-, B18.Ø-B18.1) hepatitis C (B17.1-, B18.2)

Excludes1 malignant neoplasm of biliary tract NOS (C24.9)
secondary malignant neoplasm of liver and intrahepatic bile duct (C78.7)

C22.Ø Liver cell carcinoma
Hepatocellular carcinoma
Hepatoma

C22.1 Intrahepatic bile duct carcinoma
Cholangiocarcinoma
Adenocarcinoma (cancer that originates in glandular tissue) arising from epithelium of intrahepatic bile ducts
Excludes1 malignant neoplasm of hepatic duct (C24.Ø)

C22.2 Hepatoblastoma
Malignant intrahepatic tumor

C22.3 Angiosarcoma of liver
Kupffer cell sarcoma

C22.4 Other sarcomas of liver

C22.7 Other specified carcinomas of liver

C22.8 Malignant neoplasm of liver, primary, unspecified as to type

C22.9 Malignant neoplasm of liver, not specified as primary or secondary

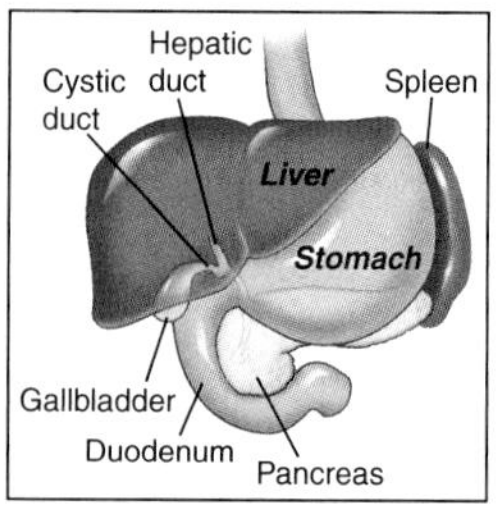

Figure 2-6 Diagram of liver, gallbladder, hepatic duct, pancreas, and spleen. (From Thibodeau and Patton: Anatomy and Physiology, ed 7, Mosby, 2010)

C23 **Malignant neoplasm of gallbladder**

● C24 **Malignant neoplasm of other and unspecified parts of biliary tract**

Excludes1 malignant neoplasm of intrahepatic bile duct (C22.1)

C24.Ø **Malignant neoplasm of extrahepatic bile duct**
Extrahepatic = outside the liver
Malignant neoplasm of biliary duct or passage NOS
Malignant neoplasm of common bile duct
Malignant neoplasm of cystic duct
Malignant neoplasm of hepatic duct

C24.1 **Malignant neoplasm of ampulla of Vater**
Union of pancreatic duct and common bile duct

C24.8 **Malignant neoplasm of overlapping sites of biliary tract**
Malignant neoplasm involving both intrahepatic and extrahepatic bile ducts
Primary malignant neoplasm of two or more contiguous sites of biliary tract

C24.9 **Malignant neoplasm of biliary tract, unspecified**

● C25 **Malignant neoplasm of pancreas**
Check documentation for specific site.
Code also exocrine pancreatic insufficiency (K86.81)
Use additional code to identify:
alcohol abuse and dependence (F1Ø.-)

C25.Ø **Malignant neoplasm of head of pancreas**

C25.1 **Malignant neoplasm of body of pancreas**
Coding Clinic: 2018, Q4, P4Ø

C25.2 **Malignant neoplasm of tail of pancreas**

C25.3 **Malignant neoplasm of pancreatic duct**

C25.4 **Malignant neoplasm of endocrine pancreas**
Malignant neoplasm of islets of Langerhans
That part of the pancreas that acts as endocrine gland and consists of islets of Langerhans
Use additional code to identify any functional activity.

C25.7 **Malignant neoplasm of other parts of pancreas**
Malignant neoplasm of neck of pancreas

C25.8 **Malignant neoplasm of overlapping sites of pancreas**

C25.9 **Malignant neoplasm of pancreas, unspecified**

Item 2-3 **Islets** of Langerhans (endocrine producing cells comprising 1% to 2% of the pancreatic mass) make and secrete hormones that regulate the body's production of insulin, glucagon, and stomach acid. Breakdown of the insulin-producing cells can cause diabetes mellitus. Islet cell tumors can be benign or malignant and include glucagonomas, insulinomas, gastrinomas, and neuroendocrine tumor. The neoplasm table must be consulted for the correct neoplasm code.

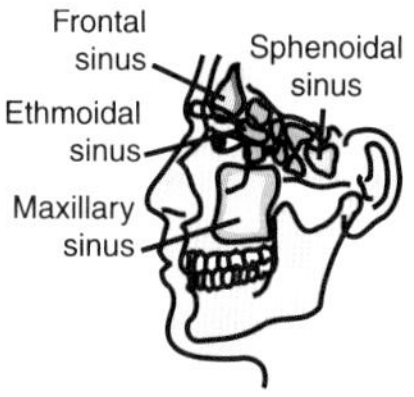

Figure 2-7 Paranasal sinuses. (From Buck CJ: Step-by-Step Medical Coding, ed 2016, St. Louis, Elsevier, 2016)

● C26 **Malignant neoplasm of other and ill-defined digestive organs**

Excludes1 malignant neoplasm of peritoneum and retroperitoneum (C48.-)

C26.Ø **Malignant neoplasm of intestinal tract, part unspecified**
Malignant neoplasm of intestine NOS

C26.1 **Malignant neoplasm of spleen**

Excludes1 Hodgkin lymphoma (C81.-)
non-Hodgkin lymphoma (C82-C85)

C26.9 **Malignant neoplasm of ill-defined sites within the digestive system**
Malignant neoplasm of alimentary canal or tract NOS
Malignant neoplasm of gastrointestinal tract NOS

Excludes1 malignant neoplasm of abdominal NOS (C76.2)
malignant neoplasm of intra-abdominal NOS (C76.2)

MALIGNANT NEOPLASMS OF RESPIRATORY AND INTRATHORACIC ORGANS (C3Ø-C39)

Includes malignant neoplasm of middle ear
Excludes1 mesothelioma (C45.-)

● C3Ø **Malignant neoplasm of nasal cavity and middle ear**

C3Ø.Ø **Malignant neoplasm of nasal cavity**
Malignant neoplasm of cartilage of nose
Malignant neoplasm of nasal concha
Malignant neoplasm of internal nose
Malignant neoplasm of septum of nose
Malignant neoplasm of vestibule of nose
Anterior part of nasal cavity

Excludes1 malignant neoplasm of nasal bone (C41.Ø)
malignant neoplasm of nose NOS (C76.Ø)
malignant neoplasm of olfactory bulb (C72.2-)
malignant neoplasm of posterior margin of nasal septum and choana (C11.3)
malignant melanoma of skin of nose (C43.31)
malignant neoplasm of turbinates (C41.Ø)
other and unspecified malignant neoplasm of skin of nose C44.3Ø1, C44.311, C44.321, C44.391)

C3Ø.1 **Malignant neoplasm of middle ear**
Malignant neoplasm of antrum tympanicum
Boney cavity or chamber
Malignant neoplasm of auditory tube
Malignant neoplasm of eustachian tube
Malignant neoplasm of inner ear
Malignant neoplasm of mastoid air cells
Malignant neoplasm of tympanic cavity

Excludes1 malignant neoplasm of auricular canal (external) (C43.2-, C44.2-)
malignant neoplasm of bone of ear (meatus) (C41.Ø)
malignant neoplasm of cartilage of ear (C49.Ø)
malignant melanoma of skin of (external) ear (C43.2-)
other and unspecified malignant neoplasm of skin of (external) ear (C44.2-)

● C31 **Malignant neoplasm of accessory sinuses**
Paired sinuses in bones of face

C31.Ø **Malignant neoplasm of maxillary sinus**
Malignant neoplasm of antrum (Highmore) (maxillary)

C31.1 **Malignant neoplasm of ethmoidal sinus**

C31.2 **Malignant neoplasm of frontal sinus**

C31.3 **Malignant neoplasm of sphenoid sinus**

C31.8 **Malignant neoplasm of overlapping sites of accessory sinuses**

C31.9 **Malignant neoplasm of accessory sinus, unspecified**

C32 Malignant neoplasm of larynx
Use additional code to identify:
alcohol abuse and dependence (F1Ø.-)
exposure to environmental tobacco smoke (Z77.22)
exposure to tobacco smoke in the perinatal period (P96.81)
history of tobacco dependence (Z87.891)
occupational exposure to environmental tobacco smoke (Z57.31)
tobacco dependence (F17.-)
tobacco use (Z72.Ø)

C32.Ø Malignant neoplasm of glottis
Vocal apparatus of larynx, consisting of true vocal cords (plicae vocales) and opening between them (rima glottidis)
Malignant neoplasm of intrinsic larynx
Malignant neoplasm of laryngeal commissure (anterior) (posterior)
Malignant neoplasm of vocal cord (true) NOS
True vocal cords ("lower vocal folds") produce vocalization when air from the lungs passes between them. Check your documentation. Code C32.1 is for malignant neoplasm of the false vocal cords.

C32.1 Malignant neoplasm of supraglottis
Area of pharynx above glottis
Malignant neoplasm of aryepiglottic fold or interarytenoid fold, laryngeal aspect
Malignant neoplasm of epiglottis (suprahyoid portion) NOS
Malignant neoplasm of extrinsic larynx
Malignant neoplasm of false vocal cord
False vocal cords ("upper vocal folds") are not involved in vocalization. Check your documentation. Code C32.Ø is for true vocal cords.
Malignant neoplasm of posterior (laryngeal) surface of epiglottis
Malignant neoplasm of ventricular bands

Excludes2 malignant neoplasm of anterior surface of epiglottis (C1Ø.1)
malignant neoplasm of aryepiglottic fold or interarytenoid fold, hypopharyngeal aspect (C13.1)
malignant neoplasm of aryepiglottic fold or interarytenoid fold, marginal zone (C13.1)
malignant neoplasm of aryepiglottic fold or interarytenoid fold NOS (C13.1)

C32.2 Malignant neoplasm of subglottis
Lowest part of larynx from just below vocal cords down to top of trachea

C32.3 Malignant neoplasm of laryngeal cartilage
Cartilages of larynx, including cricoid, thyroid, and epiglottic, and two each of arytenoid, corniculate, and cuneiform

C32.8 Malignant neoplasm of overlapping sites of larynx

C32.9 Malignant neoplasm of larynx, unspecified

C33 Malignant neoplasm of trachea
Use additional code to identify:
exposure to environmental tobacco smoke (Z77.22)
exposure to tobacco smoke in the perinatal period (P96.81)
history of tobacco dependence (Z87.891)
occupational exposure to environmental tobacco smoke (Z57.31)
tobacco dependence (F17.-)
tobacco use (Z72.Ø)

C34 Malignant neoplasm of bronchus and lung
Use additional code to identify:
exposure to environmental tobacco smoke (Z77.22)
exposure to tobacco smoke in the perinatal period (P96.81)
history of tobacco dependence (Z87.891)
occupational exposure to environmental tobacco smoke (Z57.31)
tobacco dependence (F17.-)
tobacco use (Z72.Ø)

Excludes1 Kaposi's sarcoma of lung (C46.5-)
malignant carcinoid tumor of the bronchus and lung (C7A.Ø9Ø)

C34.Ø Malignant neoplasm of main bronchus
Malignant neoplasm of carina
Ridgelike structure
Malignant neoplasm of hilus (of lung)
Anatomic depression or pit

C34.ØØ Malignant neoplasm of unspecified main bronchus

C34.Ø1 Malignant neoplasm of right main bronchus

C34.Ø2 Malignant neoplasm of left main bronchus

C34.1 Malignant neoplasm of upper lobe, bronchus or lung

C34.1Ø Malignant neoplasm of unspecified bronchus or lung

C34.11 Malignant neoplasm of upper lobe, right bronchus or lung

C34.12 Malignant neoplasm of upper lobe, left bronchus or lung

C34.2 Malignant neoplasm of middle lobe, bronchus or lung

C34.3 Malignant neoplasm of lower lobe, bronchus or lung

C34.3Ø Malignant neoplasm of lower lobe, unspecified bronchus or lung

C34.31 Malignant neoplasm of lower lobe, right bronchus or lung

C34.32 Malignant neoplasm of lower lobe, left bronchus or lung

C34.8 Malignant neoplasm of overlapping sites of bronchus and lung

C34.8Ø Malignant neoplasm of overlapping sites of unspecified bronchus and lung

C34.81 Malignant neoplasm of overlapping sites of right bronchus and lung

C34.82 Malignant neoplasm of overlapping sites of left bronchus and lung

C34.9 Malignant neoplasm of unspecified part of bronchus or lung

C34.9Ø Malignant neoplasm of unspecified part of unspecified bronchus or lung
Lung cancer NOS

C34.91 Malignant neoplasm of unspecified part of right bronchus or lung

C34.92 Malignant neoplasm of unspecified part of left bronchus or lung

C37 Malignant neoplasm of thymus
Excludes1 malignant carcinoid tumor of the thymus (C7A.Ø91)

CHAPTER 2 (CØØ-D49)

● C38 Malignant neoplasm of heart, mediastinum and pleura

Excludes1 mesothelioma (C45.-)

C38.Ø Malignant neoplasm of heart
Malignant neoplasm of pericardium
Excludes1 malignant neoplasm of great vessels (C49.3)

C38.1 Malignant neoplasm of anterior mediastinum

C38.2 Malignant neoplasm of posterior mediastinum

C38.3 Malignant neoplasm of mediastinum, part unspecified

C38.4 Malignant neoplasm of pleura

C38.8 Malignant neoplasm of overlapping sites of heart, mediastinum and pleura
Pleura are comprised of serous membrane that lines the thoracic cavity (parietal) and covers the lungs (visceral).

● C39 Malignant neoplasm of other and ill-defined sites in the respiratory system and intrathoracic organs
Intrathoracic: within thorax/chest

Use additional code to identify:
exposure to environmental tobacco smoke (Z77.22)
exposure to tobacco smoke in the perinatal period (P96.81)
history of tobacco dependence (Z87.891)
occupational exposure to environmental tobacco smoke (Z57.31)
tobacco dependence (F17.-)
tobacco use (Z72.Ø)

Excludes1 intrathoracic malignant neoplasm NOS (C76.1)
thoracic malignant neoplasm NOS (C76.1)

C39.Ø Malignant neoplasm of upper respiratory tract, part unspecified

C39.9 Malignant neoplasm of lower respiratory tract, part unspecified
Malignant neoplasm of respiratory tract NOS

MALIGNANT NEOPLASMS OF BONE AND ARTICULAR CARTILAGE (C4Ø-C41)

Includes malignant neoplasm of cartilage (articular) (joint)
malignant neoplasm of periosteum

Excludes1 malignant neoplasm of bone marrow NOS (C96.9)
malignant neoplasm of synovia (C49.-)

● C4Ø Malignant neoplasm of bone and articular cartilage of limbs

Use additional code to identify major osseous defect, if applicable (M89.7-)

● C4Ø.Ø Malignant neoplasm of scapula and long bones of upper limb

C4Ø.ØØ Malignant neoplasm of scapula and long bones of unspecified upper limb

C4Ø.Ø1 Malignant neoplasm of scapula and long bones of right upper limb

C4Ø.Ø2 Malignant neoplasm of scapula and long bones of left upper limb

● C4Ø.1 Malignant neoplasm of short bones of upper limb

C4Ø.1Ø Malignant neoplasm of short bones of unspecified upper limb

C4Ø.11 Malignant neoplasm of short bones of right upper limb

C4Ø.12 Malignant neoplasm of short bones of left upper limb

● C4Ø.2 Malignant neoplasm of long bones of lower limb

C4Ø.2Ø Malignant neoplasm of long bones of unspecified lower limb

C4Ø.21 Malignant neoplasm of long bones of right lower limb

C4Ø.22 Malignant neoplasm of long bones of left lower limb

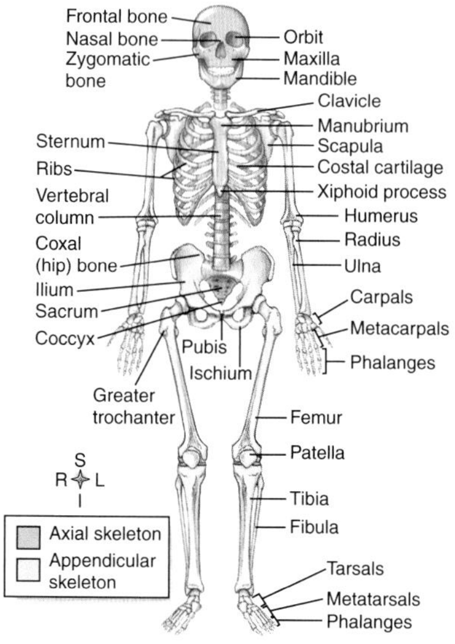

Figure 2-8 Diagram of skeleton of trunk and limbs with bones labeled. (From Thibodeau and Patton: Anatomy and Physiology, ed 7, Mosby, 2010)

● C4Ø.3 Malignant neoplasm of short bones of lower limb

C4Ø.3Ø Malignant neoplasm of short bones of unspecified lower limb

C4Ø.31 Malignant neoplasm of short bones of right lower limb

C4Ø.32 Malignant neoplasm of short bones of left lower limb

● C4Ø.8 Malignant neoplasm of overlapping sites of bone and articular cartilage of limb

C4Ø.8Ø Malignant neoplasm of overlapping sites of bone and articular cartilage of unspecified limb

C4Ø.81 Malignant neoplasm of overlapping sites of bone and articular cartilage of right limb

C4Ø.82 Malignant neoplasm of overlapping sites of bone and articular cartilage of left limb

● C4Ø.9 Malignant neoplasm of unspecified bones and articular cartilage of limb

C4Ø.9Ø Malignant neoplasm of unspecified bones and articular cartilage of unspecified limb

C4Ø.91 Malignant neoplasm of unspecified bones and articular cartilage of right limb

C4Ø.92 Malignant neoplasm of unspecified bones and articular cartilage of left limb

● C41 Malignant neoplasm of bone and articular cartilage of other and unspecified sites

Excludes1 malignant neoplasm of bones of limbs (C4Ø.-)
malignant neoplasm of cartilage of ear (C49.Ø)
malignant neoplasm of cartilage of eyelid (C49.Ø)
malignant neoplasm of cartilage of larynx (C32.3)
malignant neoplasm of cartilage of limbs (C4Ø.-)
malignant neoplasm of cartilage of nose (C3Ø.Ø)

C41.Ø Malignant neoplasm of bones of skull and face
Malignant neoplasm of maxilla (superior)
Malignant neoplasm of orbital bone
Excludes2 carcinoma, any type except intraosseous or odontogenic of:
maxillary sinus (C31.Ø)
upper jaw (CØ3.Ø)
malignant neoplasm of jaw bone (lower) (C41.1)

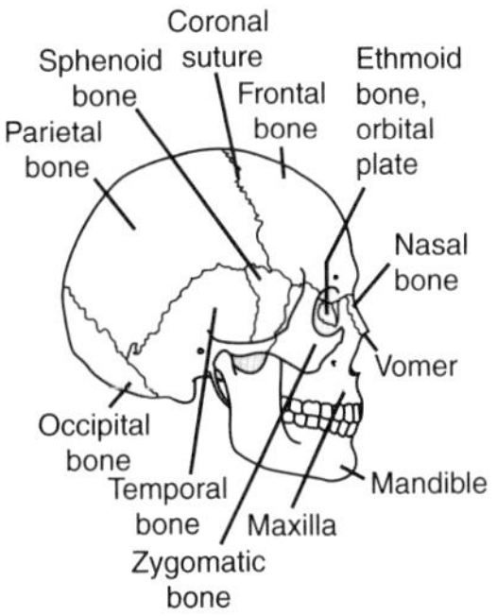

Figure 2-9 Bones of the skull.

C41.1 Malignant neoplasm of mandible
Malignant neoplasm of inferior maxilla
Malignant neoplasm of lower jaw bone
Excludes2 carcinoma, any type except intraosseous or odontogenic of:
jaw NOS (CØ3.9)
lower (CØ3.1)
malignant neoplasm of upper jaw bone (C41.Ø)

C41.2 Malignant neoplasm of vertebral column
Excludes1 malignant neoplasm of sacrum and coccyx (C41.4)

C41.3 Malignant neoplasm of ribs, sternum and clavicle

C41.4 Malignant neoplasm of pelvic bones, sacrum and coccyx

C41.9 Malignant neoplasm of bone and articular cartilage, unspecified

MELANOMA AND OTHER MALIGNANT NEOPLASMS OF SKIN (C43-C44)

C43 Malignant melanoma of skin
Excludes1 melanoma in situ (DØ3.-)
Excludes2 malignant melanoma of skin of genital organs (C51-C52, C6Ø.-, C63.-)
Merkel cell carcinoma (C4A.-)
sites other than skin-code to malignant neoplasm of the site

C43.Ø Malignant melanoma of lip
Excludes1 malignant neoplasm of vermilion border of lip (CØØ.Ø-CØØ.2)

C43.1 Malignant melanoma of eyelid, including canthus
Canthus: Either corner of eye where upper and lower eyelids meet

C43.10 Malignant melanoma of unspecified eyelid, including canthus

C43.11 Malignant melanoma of right eyelid, including canthus

C43.111 Malignant melanoma of right upper eyelid, including canthus

C43.112 Malignant melanoma of right lower eyelid, including canthus

C43.12 Malignant melanoma of left eyelid, including canthus

C43.121 Malignant melanoma of left upper eyelid, including canthus

C43.122 Malignant melanoma of left lower eyelid, including canthus

C43.2 Malignant melanoma of ear and external auricular canal

C43.2Ø Malignant melanoma of unspecified ear and external auricular canal

C43.21 Malignant melanoma of right ear and external auricular canal

C43.22 Malignant melanoma of left ear and external auricular canal

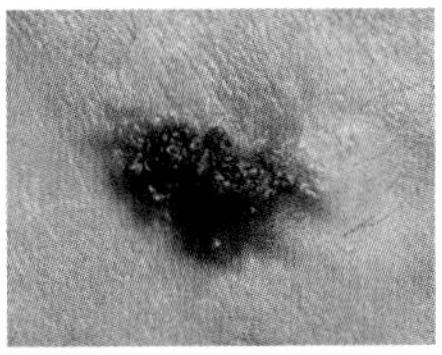

Figure 2-10 Malignant melanoma of skin. (Getty Image)

Item 2-4 Malignant melanoma is a serious form of skin cancer that affects the melanocytes (pigment-forming cells) and is caused by ultraviolet (UV) rays from the sun that damage skin. It is most commonly seen in the 4Ø- to 6Ø-year-olds with fair skin, blue or green eyes, and red or blond hair who sunburn easily.

Melanoma can spread very rapidly and is the most deadly form of skin cancer. It is less common than other types of skin cancer. The rate of melanoma is increasing and currently is the leading cause of death from skin disease.

C43.3 Malignant melanoma of other and unspecified parts of face

C43.3Ø Malignant melanoma of unspecified part of face

C43.31 Malignant melanoma of nose

C43.39 Malignant melanoma of other parts of face

C43.4 Malignant melanoma of scalp and neck

C43.5 Malignant melanoma of trunk
Excludes2 malignant neoplasm of anus NOS (C21.Ø)
malignant neoplasm of scrotum (C63.2)

C43.51 Malignant melanoma of anal skin
Malignant melanoma of anal margin
Malignant melanoma of perianal skin

C43.52 Malignant melanoma of skin of breast

C43.59 Malignant melanoma of other part of trunk

C43.6 Malignant melanoma of upper limb, including shoulder

C43.6Ø Malignant melanoma of upper limb, including shoulder, unspecified side

C43.61 Malignant melanoma of right upper limb, including shoulder

C43.62 Malignant melanoma of left upper limb, including shoulder

C43.7 Malignant melanoma of lower limb, including hip

C43.7Ø Malignant melanoma of unspecified lower limb, including hip

C43.71 Malignant melanoma of right lower limb, including hip

C43.72 Malignant melanoma of left lower limb, including hip

C43.8 Malignant melanoma of overlapping sites of skin

C43.9 Malignant melanoma of skin, unspecified
Malignant melanoma of unspecified site of skin
Melanoma (malignant) NOS

C4A Merkel cell carcinoma

C4A.Ø Merkel cell carcinoma of lip
Excludes1 malignant neoplasm of vermilion border of lip (CØØ.Ø-CØØ.2)

C4A.1 Merkel cell carcinoma of eyelid, including canthus

C4A.1Ø Merkel cell carcinoma of unspecified eyelid, including canthus

C4A.11 Merkel cell carcinoma of right eyelid, including canthus

C4A.111 Merkel cell carcinoma of right upper eyelid, including canthus

C4A.112 Merkel cell carcinoma of right lower eyelid, including canthus

C4A.12 Merkel cell carcinoma of left eyelid, including canthus

C4A.121 Merkel cell carcinoma of left upper eyelid, including canthus

C4A.122 Merkel cell carcinoma of left lower eyelid, including canthus

● C4A.2 Merkel cell carcinoma of **ear and external auricular canal**
C4A.20 Merkel cell carcinoma of **unspecified** ear and external auricular canal
C4A.21 Merkel cell carcinoma of **right** ear and external auricular canal
C4A.22 Merkel cell carcinoma of **left** ear and external auricular canal
● C4A.3 Merkel cell carcinoma of **other and unspecified parts** of face
C4A.30 Merkel cell carcinoma of **unspecified** part of face
C4A.31 Merkel cell carcinoma of **nose**
C4A.39 Merkel cell carcinoma of **other** parts of face
C4A.4 Merkel cell carcinoma of **scalp and neck**
● C4A.5 Merkel cell carcinoma of **trunk**
Excludes2 malignant neoplasm of anus NOS (C21.Ø)
malignant neoplasm of scrotum (C63.2)
C4A.51 Merkel cell carcinoma of **anal skin**
Merkel cell carcinoma of anal margin
Merkel cell carcinoma of perianal skin
C4A.52 Merkel cell carcinoma of **skin of breast**
C4A.59 Merkel cell carcinoma of **other** part of trunk
● C4A.6 Merkel cell carcinoma of **upper limb, including shoulder**
C4A.60 Merkel cell carcinoma of **unspecified** upper limb, including shoulder
C4A.61 Merkel cell carcinoma of **right** upper limb, including shoulder
C4A.62 Merkel cell carcinoma of **left** upper limb, including shoulder
● C4A.7 Merkel cell carcinoma of **lower limb, including hip**
C4A.70 Merkel cell carcinoma of **unspecified** lower limb, including hip
C4A.71 Merkel cell carcinoma of **right** lower limb, including hip
C4A.72 Merkel cell carcinoma of **left** lower limb, including hip
C4A.8 Merkel cell carcinoma of **overlapping sites**
C4A.9 Merkel cell carcinoma, **unspecified**
Merkel cell carcinoma of unspecified site
Merkel cell carcinoma NOS

● C44 Other and unspecified malignant neoplasm of **skin**
Includes malignant neoplasm of sebaceous glands
malignant neoplasm of sweat glands
Excludes1 Kaposi's sarcoma of skin (C46.Ø)
malignant melanoma of skin (C43.-)
malignant neoplasm of skin of genital organs (C51-C52, C6Ø.-, C63.2)
Merkel cell carcinoma (C4A.-)
● C44.Ø Other and unspecified malignant neoplasm of skin of lip
Excludes1 malignant neoplasm of lip (CØØ.-)
C44.ØØ **Unspecified** malignant neoplasm of skin of lip
C44.Ø1 **Basal cell** carcinoma of skin of lip
C44.Ø2 **Squamous cell** carcinoma of skin of lip
C44.Ø9 **Other** specified malignant neoplasm of skin of lip

● C44.1 Other and unspecified malignant neoplasm of skin of **eyelid, including canthus**
Excludes1 connective tissue of eyelid (C49.Ø)
● C44.1Ø **Unspecified** malignant neoplasm of skin of eyelid, including canthus
C44.1Ø1 Unspecified malignant neoplasm of skin of **unspecified** eyelid, including canthus
● C44.1Ø2 Unspecified malignant neoplasm of skin of **right** eyelid, including canthus
C44.1Ø21 Unspecified malignant neoplasm of skin of right upper eyelid, including canthus
C44.1Ø22 Unspecified malignant neoplasm of skin of right lower eyelid, including canthus
● C44.1Ø9 Unspecified malignant neoplasm of skin of **left** eyelid, including canthus
C44.1Ø91 Unspecified malignant neoplasm of skin of left upper eyelid, including canthus
C44.1Ø92 Unspecified malignant neoplasm of skin of left lower eyelid, including canthus
● C44.11 **Basal cell carcinoma** of skin of eyelid, including canthus
C44.111 Basal cell carcinoma of skin of **unspecified** eyelid, including canthus
● C44.112 Basal cell carcinoma of skin of **right** eyelid, including canthus
C44.1121 Basal cell carcinoma of skin of right upper eyelid, including canthus
C44.1122 Basal cell carcinoma of skin of right lower eyelid, including canthus
● C44.119 Basal cell carcinoma of skin of **left** eyelid, including canthus
C44.1191 Basal cell carcinoma of skin of left upper eyelid, including canthus
C44.1192 Basal cell carcinoma of skin of left lower eyelid, including canthus
● C44.12 **Squamous cell carcinoma** of skin of eyelid, including canthus
C44.121 Squamous cell carcinoma of skin of **unspecified** eyelid, including canthus
● C44.122 Squamous cell carcinoma of skin of **right** eyelid, including canthus
C44.1221 Squamous cell carcinoma of skin of right upper eyelid, including canthus
C44.1222 Squamous cell carcinoma of skin of right lower eyelid, including canthus
● C44.129 Squamous cell carcinoma of skin of **left** eyelid, including canthus
C44.1291 Squamous cell carcinoma of skin of left upper eyelid, including canthus
C44.1292 Squamous cell carcinoma of skin of left lower eyelid, including canthus

● C44.13 Sebaceous cell carcinoma of skin of eyelid, including canthus
- C44.131 Sebaceous cell carcinoma of skin of unspecified eyelid, including canthus
- ● C44.132 Sebaceous cell carcinoma of skin of right eyelid, including canthus
  - C44.1321 Sebaceous cell carcinoma of skin of right upper eyelid, including canthus
  - C44.1322 Sebaceous cell carcinoma of skin of right lower eyelid, including canthus
- ● C44.139 Sebaceous cell carcinoma of skin of left eyelid, including canthus
  - C44.1391 Sebaceous cell carcinoma of skin of left upper eyelid, including canthus
  - C44.1392 Sebaceous cell carcinoma of skin of left lower eyelid, including canthus

● C44.19 **Other specified** malignant neoplasm of skin of eyelid, including canthus
- C44.191 Other specified malignant neoplasm of skin of **unspecified** eyelid, including canthus
- ● C44.192 Other specified malignant neoplasm of skin of **right** eyelid, including canthus
  - C44.1921 Other specified malignant neoplasm of skin of right upper eyelid, including canthus
  - C44.1922 Other specified malignant neoplasm of skin of right lower eyelid, including canthus
- ● C44.199 Other specified malignant neoplasm of skin of **left** eyelid, including canthus
  - C44.1991 Other specified malignant neoplasm of skin of left upper eyelid, including canthus
  - C44.1992 Other specified malignant neoplasm of skin of left lower eyelid, including canthus

● C44.2 Other and unspecified malignant neoplasm of skin of **ear and external auricular canal**

Excludes1 connective tissue of ear (C49.Ø)

● C44.2Ø **Unspecified** malignant neoplasm of skin of ear and external auricular canal
- C44.2Ø1 Unspecified malignant neoplasm of skin of **unspecified** ear and external auricular canal
- C44.2Ø2 Unspecified malignant neoplasm of skin of **right** ear and external auricular canal
- C44.2Ø9 Unspecified malignant neoplasm of skin of **left** ear and external auricular canal

● C44.21 **Basal cell carcinoma** of skin of ear and external auricular canal
- C44.211 Basal cell carcinoma of skin of **unspecified** ear and external auricular canal
- C44.212 Basal cell carcinoma of skin of **right** ear and external auricular canal
- C44.219 Basal cell carcinoma of skin of **left** ear and external auricular canal

● C44.22 **Squamous cell carcinoma** of skin of ear and external auricular canal
- C44.221 Squamous cell carcinoma of skin of **unspecified** ear and external auricular canal
- C44.222 Squamous cell carcinoma of skin of **right** ear and external auricular canal
- C44.229 Squamous cell carcinoma of skin of **left** ear and external auricular canal

● C44.29 **Other specified** malignant neoplasm of skin of ear and external auricular canal
- C44.291 Other specified malignant neoplasm of skin of **unspecified** ear and external auricular canal
- C44.292 Other specified malignant neoplasm of skin of **right** ear and external auricular canal
- C44.299 Other specified malignant neoplasm of skin of **left** ear and external auricular canal

● C44.3 Other and unspecified malignant neoplasm of skin of **other and unspecified parts of face**

● C44.3Ø Unspecified malignant neoplasm of skin of other and unspecified parts of face
- C44.3ØØ Unspecified malignant neoplasm of skin of **unspecified** part of face
- C44.3Ø1 Unspecified malignant neoplasm of skin of **nose**
- C44.3Ø9 Unspecified malignant neoplasm of skin of **other parts of face**

● C44.31 **Basal cell carcinoma** of skin of other and unspecified parts of face
- C44.31Ø Basal cell carcinoma of skin of **unspecified** parts of face
- C44.311 Basal cell carcinoma of skin of **nose**
- C44.319 Basal cell carcinoma of skin of **other parts of face**
  Coding Clinic: 2017, Q1, P4

● C44.32 **Squamous cell carcinoma** of skin of other and unspecified parts of face
- C44.32Ø Squamous cell carcinoma of skin of **unspecified** parts of face
- C44.321 Squamous cell carcinoma of skin of **nose**
- C44.329 Squamous cell carcinoma of skin of **other parts of face**

● C44.39 Other specified malignant neoplasm of skin of **other and unspecified parts of face**
- C44.39Ø Other specified malignant neoplasm of skin of **unspecified** parts of face
- C44.391 Other specified malignant neoplasm of skin of **nose**
- C44.399 Other specified malignant neoplasm of skin of **other parts of face**

● C44.4 Other and unspecified malignant neoplasm of skin of **scalp and neck**
- C44.4Ø **Unspecified** malignant neoplasm of skin of scalp and neck
- C44.41 **Basal cell carcinoma** of skin of scalp and neck
- C44.42 **Squamous cell carcinoma** of skin of scalp and neck
- C44.49 **Other** specified malignant neoplasm of skin of scalp and neck

CHAPTER 2 (CØØ-D49)

● C44.5 Other and unspecified malignant neoplasm of skin of trunk
 Excludes1 anus NOS (C21.Ø)
 scrotum (C63.2)
 ● C44.50 **Unspecified** malignant neoplasm of skin of trunk
 C44.500 Unspecified malignant neoplasm of **anal skin**
 Unspecified malignant neoplasm of anal margin
 Unspecified malignant neoplasm of perianal skin
 C44.501 Unspecified malignant neoplasm of **skin of breast**
 C44.509 Unspecified malignant neoplasm of skin of **other** part of trunk
 ● C44.51 **Basal cell carcinoma** of skin of trunk
 C44.510 Basal cell carcinoma of **anal skin**
 Basal cell carcinoma of anal margin
 Basal cell carcinoma of perianal skin
 C44.511 Basal cell carcinoma of skin of **breast**
 C44.519 Basal cell carcinoma of skin of **other** part of trunk
 ● C44.52 **Squamous cell carcinoma** of skin of trunk
 C44.520 Squamous cell carcinoma of **anal skin**
 Squamous cell carcinoma of anal margin
 Squamous cell carcinoma of perianal skin
 C44.521 Squamous cell carcinoma of **skin of breast**
 C44.529 Squamous cell carcinoma of skin of **other** part of trunk
 ● C44.59 **Other** specified malignant neoplasm of skin of trunk
 C44.590 Other specified malignant neoplasm of **anal skin**
 Other specified malignant neoplasm of anal margin
 Other specified malignant neoplasm of perianal skin
 C44.591 Other specified malignant neoplasm of **skin of breast**
 C44.599 Other specified malignant neoplasm of skin of **other** part of trunk

● C44.6 Other and unspecified malignant neoplasm of skin of **upper limb, including shoulder**
 ● C44.60 **Unspecified** malignant neoplasm of skin of upper limb, including shoulder
 C44.601 Unspecified malignant neoplasm of skin of **unspecified** upper limb, including shoulder
 C44.602 Unspecified malignant neoplasm of skin of **right** upper limb, including shoulder
 C44.609 Unspecified malignant neoplasm of skin of **left** upper limb, including shoulder
 ● C44.61 **Basal cell carcinoma** of skin of upper limb, including shoulder
 C44.611 Basal cell carcinoma of skin of **unspecified** upper limb, including shoulder
 C44.612 Basal cell carcinoma of skin of **right** upper limb, including shoulder
 C44.619 Basal cell carcinoma of skin of **left** upper limb, including shoulder
 ● C44.62 **Squamous cell carcinoma** of skin of upper limb, including shoulder
 C44.621 Squamous cell carcinoma of skin of **unspecified** upper limb, including shoulder
 C44.622 Squamous cell carcinoma of skin of **right** upper limb, including shoulder
 C44.629 Squamous cell carcinoma of skin of **left** upper limb, including shoulder
 ● C44.69 **Other specified** malignant neoplasm of skin of upper limb, including shoulder
 C44.691 Other specified malignant neoplasm of skin of **unspecified** upper limb, including shoulder
 C44.692 Other specified malignant neoplasm of skin of **right** upper limb, including shoulder
 C44.699 Other specified malignant neoplasm of skin of **left** upper limb, including shoulder

● C44.7 Other and unspecified malignant neoplasm of skin of **lower limb, including hip**
 ● C44.70 **Unspecified** malignant neoplasm of skin of lower limb, including hip
 C44.701 Unspecified malignant neoplasm of skin of **unspecified** lower limb, including hip
 C44.702 Unspecified malignant neoplasm of skin of **right** lower limb, including hip
 C44.709 Unspecified malignant neoplasm of skin of **left** lower limb, including hip
 ● C44.71 **Basal cell carcinoma** of skin of lower limb, including hip
 C44.711 Basal cell carcinoma of skin of **unspecified** lower limb, including hip
 C44.712 Basal cell carcinoma of skin of **right** lower limb, including hip
 C44.719 Basal cell carcinoma of skin of **left** lower limb, including hip
 ● C44.72 **Squamous cell carcinoma** of skin of lower limb, including hip
 C44.721 Squamous cell carcinoma of skin of **unspecified** lower limb, including hip
 C44.722 Squamous cell carcinoma of skin of **right** lower limb, including hip
 C44.729 Squamous cell carcinoma of skin of **left** lower limb, including hip
 ● C44.79 **Other specified** malignant neoplasm of skin of lower limb, including hip
 C44.791 Other specified malignant neoplasm of skin of **unspecified** lower limb, including hip
 C44.792 Other specified malignant neoplasm of skin of **right** lower limb, including hip
 C44.799 Other specified malignant neoplasm of skin of **left** lower limb, including hip

● C44.8 Other and unspecified malignant neoplasm of **overlapping sites** of skin
 C44.80 **Unspecified** malignant neoplasm of overlapping sites of skin
 C44.81 **Basal cell carcinoma** of overlapping sites of skin
 C44.82 **Squamous cell carcinoma** of overlapping sites of skin
 C44.89 **Other** specified malignant neoplasm of overlapping sites of skin

● C44.9 **Other and unspecified malignant neoplasm of skin, unspecified**

C44.90 **Unspecified malignant neoplasm of skin, unspecified**
Malignant neoplasm of unspecified site of skin

C44.91 **Basal cell carcinoma of skin, unspecified**

C44.92 **Squamous cell carcinoma of skin, unspecified**

C44.99 **Other specified malignant neoplasm of skin, unspecified**

MALIGNANT NEOPLASMS OF MESOTHELIAL AND SOFT TISSUE (C45-C49)

● C45 **Mesothelioma**

Malignant cells develop in protective lining that covers internal organs (mesothelium) caused by exposure to asbestos

C45.0 **Mesothelioma of pleura**

Excludes1 other malignant neoplasm of pleura (C38.4)

Coding Clinic: 2017, Q2, P11

C45.1 **Mesothelioma of peritoneum**
Mesothelioma of cul-de-sac
Mesothelioma of mesentery
Mesothelioma of mesocolon
Mesothelioma of omentum
Mesothelioma of peritoneum (parietal) (pelvic)

Excludes1 other malignant neoplasm of soft tissue of peritoneum (C48.-)

C45.2 **Mesothelioma of pericardium**

Excludes1 other malignant neoplasm of pericardium (C38.0)

C45.7 **Mesothelioma of other sites**

C45.9 **Mesothelioma, unspecified**

● C46 **Kaposi's sarcoma**

Code first any human immunodeficiency virus [HIV] disease (B20)

C46.0 **Kaposi's sarcoma of skin**

C46.1 **Kaposi's sarcoma of soft tissue**
Kaposi's sarcoma of blood vessel
Kaposi's sarcoma of connective tissue
Kaposi's sarcoma of fascia
Kaposi's sarcoma of ligament
Kaposi's sarcoma of lymphatic(s) NEC
Kaposi's sarcoma of muscle

Excludes2 Kaposi's sarcoma of lymph glands and nodes (C46.3)

C46.2 **Kaposi's sarcoma of palate**

C46.3 **Kaposi's sarcoma of lymph nodes**

C46.4 **Kaposi's sarcoma of gastrointestinal sites**

● C46.5 **Kaposi's sarcoma of lung**

C46.50 **Kaposi's sarcoma of unspecified lung**

C46.51 **Kaposi's sarcoma of right lung**

C46.52 **Kaposi's sarcoma of left lung**

C46.7 **Kaposi's sarcoma of other sites**

C46.9 **Kaposi's sarcoma, unspecified**
Kaposi's sarcoma of unspecified site

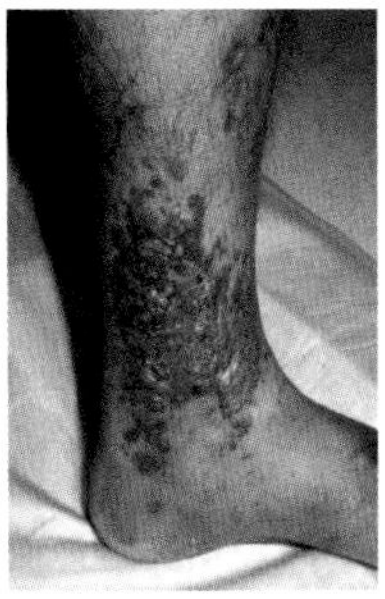

Figure 2-11 Kaposi's sarcoma. There are large confluent hyperpigmented patch-stage lesions with lymphedema. (From Goldman L, Ausiello D, Arend W, Armitage J, Clemmons D, Drazen J, Griggs R, et al: Cecil Medicine: Expert Consult, 23e, Saunders, 2007)

Item 2–5 **Kaposi's sarcoma** is a cancer that causes patches of abnormal tissue to grow under the skin; in the lining of the mouth, nose, and throat; or in other organs, often beginning and spreading to other organs. Patients who have had organ transplants or patients with AIDS are at high risk for this malignancy.

● C47 **Malignant neoplasm of peripheral nerves and autonomic nervous system**

Includes malignant neoplasm of sympathetic and parasympathetic nerves and ganglia

Excludes1 Kaposi's sarcoma of soft tissue (C46.1)

C47.0 **Malignant neoplasm of peripheral nerves of head, face and neck**

Excludes1 malignant neoplasm of peripheral nerves of orbit (C69.6-)

● C47.1 **Malignant neoplasm of peripheral nerves of upper limb, including shoulder**

C47.10 **Malignant neoplasm of peripheral nerves of unspecified upper limb, including shoulder**

C47.11 **Malignant neoplasm of peripheral nerves of right upper limb, including shoulder**

C47.12 **Malignant neoplasm of peripheral nerves of left upper limb, including shoulder**

● C47.2 **Malignant neoplasm of peripheral nerves of lower limb, including hip**

C47.20 **Malignant neoplasm of peripheral nerves of unspecified lower limb, including hip**

C47.21 **Malignant neoplasm of peripheral nerves of right lower limb, including hip**

C47.22 **Malignant neoplasm of peripheral nerves of left lower limb, including hip**

C47.3 **Malignant neoplasm of peripheral nerves of thorax**

C47.4 **Malignant neoplasm of peripheral nerves of abdomen**

C47.5 **Malignant neoplasm of peripheral nerves of pelvis**

C47.6 **Malignant neoplasm of peripheral nerves of trunk, unspecified**
Malignant neoplasm of peripheral nerves of unspecified part of trunk

C47.8 **Malignant neoplasm of overlapping sites of peripheral nerves and autonomic nervous system**

C47.9 **Malignant neoplasm of peripheral nerves and autonomic nervous system, unspecified**
Malignant neoplasm of unspecified site of peripheral nerves and autonomic nervous system

● C48 **Malignant neoplasm of retroperitoneum and peritoneum**

Excludes1 Kaposi's sarcoma of connective tissue (C46.1)
mesothelioma (C45.-)

C48.0 **Malignant neoplasm of retroperitoneum**
Behind/outside of peritoneum

C48.1 **Malignant neoplasm of specified parts of peritoneum**
Serous membrane lining abdominopelvic walls and covering viscera
Malignant neoplasm of cul-de-sac
Malignant neoplasm of mesentery
Malignant neoplasm of mesocolon
Malignant neoplasm of omentum
Malignant neoplasm of parietal peritoneum
Malignant neoplasm of pelvic peritoneum

C48.2 **Malignant neoplasm of peritoneum, unspecified**

C48.8 **Malignant neoplasm of overlapping sites of retroperitoneum and peritoneum**

CHAPTER 2 (C00-D49)

C49 Malignant neoplasm of other connective and soft tissue

Includes malignant neoplasm of blood vessel
malignant neoplasm of bursa
malignant neoplasm of cartilage
malignant neoplasm of fascia
malignant neoplasm of fat
malignant neoplasm of ligament, except uterine
malignant neoplasm of lymphatic vessel
malignant neoplasm of muscle
malignant neoplasm of synovia
malignant neoplasm of tendon (sheath)

Excludes1 malignant neoplasm of cartilage (of):
articular (C4Ø-C41)
larynx (C32.3)
nose (C3Ø.Ø)
malignant neoplasm of connective tissue of breast (C5Ø.-)

Excludes2 Kaposi's sarcoma of soft tissue (C46.1)
malignant neoplasm of heart (C38.Ø)
malignant neoplasm of peripheral nerves and autonomic nervous system (C47.-)
malignant neoplasm of peritoneum (C48.2)
malignant neoplasm of retroperitoneum (C48.Ø)
malignant neoplasm of uterine ligament (C57.3)
mesothelioma (C45.-)

C49.Ø Malignant neoplasm of connective and soft tissue of head, face and neck
Malignant neoplasm of connective tissue of ear
Malignant neoplasm of connective tissue of eyelid
Excludes1 connective tissue of orbit (C69.6-)

C49.1 Malignant neoplasm of connective and soft tissue of upper limb, including shoulder

C49.1Ø Malignant neoplasm of connective and soft tissue of unspecified upper limb, including shoulder

C49.11 Malignant neoplasm of connective and soft tissue of right upper limb, including shoulder

C49.12 Malignant neoplasm of connective and soft tissue of left upper limb, including shoulder

C49.2 Malignant neoplasm of connective and soft tissue of lower limb, including hip

C49.2Ø Malignant neoplasm of connective and soft tissue of unspecified lower limb, including hip

C49.21 Malignant neoplasm of connective and soft tissue of right lower limb, including hip

C49.22 Malignant neoplasm of connective and soft tissue of left lower limb, including hip

C49.3 Malignant neoplasm of connective and soft tissue of thorax
Malignant neoplasm of axilla
Malignant neoplasm of diaphragm
Malignant neoplasm of great vessels
Excludes1 malignant neoplasm of breast (C5Ø.-)
malignant neoplasm of heart (C38.Ø)
malignant neoplasm of mediastinum (C38.1-C38.3)
malignant neoplasm of thymus (C37)
Coding Clinic: 2015, Q3, P19

C49.4 Malignant neoplasm of connective and soft tissue of abdomen
Malignant neoplasm of abdominal wall
Malignant neoplasm of hypochondrium

C49.5 Malignant neoplasm of connective and soft tissue of pelvis
Malignant neoplasm of buttock
Malignant neoplasm of groin
Malignant neoplasm of perineum

C49.6 Malignant neoplasm of connective and soft tissue of trunk, unspecified
Malignant neoplasm of back NOS

C49.8 Malignant neoplasm of overlapping sites of connective and soft tissue
Primary malignant neoplasm of two or more contiguous sites of connective and soft tissue

C49.9 Malignant neoplasm of connective and soft tissue, unspecified

C49.A Gastrointestinal stromal tumor
Coding Clinic: 2016, Q4, P8

C49.AØ Gastrointestinal stromal tumor, unspecified site

C49.A1 Gastrointestinal stromal tumor of esophagus

C49.A2 Gastrointestinal stromal tumor of stomach

C49.A3 Gastrointestinal stromal tumor of small intestine

C49.A4 Gastrointestinal stromal tumor of large intestine

C49.A5 Gastrointestinal stromal tumor of rectum

C49.A9 Gastrointestinal stromal tumor of other sites

MALIGNANT NEOPLASMS OF BREAST (C5Ø)

C5Ø Malignant neoplasm of breast

Includes connective tissue of breast
Paget's disease of breast
Paget's disease of nipple
Intraductal carcinoma of breast characterized by eczema-like inflammatory skin changes

Use additional code to identify estrogen receptor status (Z17.Ø, Z17.1)

Excludes1 skin of breast (C44.5Ø1, C44.511, C44.521, C44.591)

C5Ø.Ø Malignant neoplasm of nipple and areola

C5Ø.Ø1 Malignant neoplasm of nipple and areola, female

C5Ø.Ø11 Malignant neoplasm of nipple and areola, right female breast ♀

C5Ø.Ø12 Malignant neoplasm of nipple and areola, left female breast ♀

C5Ø.Ø19 Malignant neoplasm of nipple and areola, unspecified female breast ♀

C5Ø.Ø2 Malignant neoplasm of nipple and areola, male

C5Ø.Ø21 Malignant neoplasm of nipple and areola, right male breast ♂

C5Ø.Ø22 Malignant neoplasm of nipple and areola, left male breast ♂

C5Ø.Ø29 Malignant neoplasm of nipple and areola, unspecified male breast ♂

C5Ø.1 Malignant neoplasm of central portion of breast

C5Ø.11 Malignant neoplasm of central portion of breast, female

C5Ø.111 Malignant neoplasm of central portion of right female breast ♀

C5Ø.112 Malignant neoplasm of central portion of left female breast ♀

C5Ø.119 Malignant neoplasm of central portion of unspecified female breast ♀

C5Ø.12 Malignant neoplasm of central portion of breast, male

C5Ø.121 Malignant neoplasm of central portion of right male breast ♂

C5Ø.122 Malignant neoplasm of central portion of left male breast ♂

C5Ø.129 Malignant neoplasm of central portion of unspecified male breast ♂

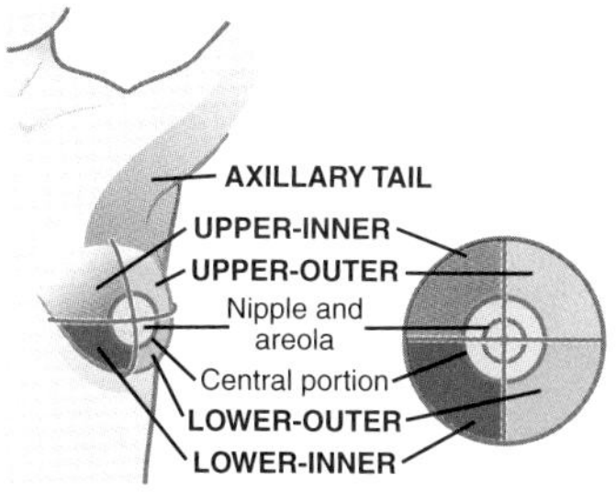

Figure 2-12 Female breast quadrants and axillary tail.

- C5Ø.2 Malignant neoplasm of **upper-inner quadrant** of breast
  - C5Ø.21 Malignant neoplasm of upper-inner quadrant of breast, **female**
    - C5Ø.211 Malignant neoplasm of upper-inner quadrant of **right** female breast ♀
    - C5Ø.212 Malignant neoplasm of upper-inner quadrant of **left** female breast ♀
    - C5Ø.219 Malignant neoplasm of upper-inner quadrant of **unspecified** female breast ♀
  - C5Ø.22 Malignant neoplasm of upper-inner quadrant of breast, **male**
    - C5Ø.221 Malignant neoplasm of upper-inner quadrant of **right** male breast ♂
    - C5Ø.222 Malignant neoplasm of upper-inner quadrant of **left** male breast ♂
    - C5Ø.229 Malignant neoplasm of upper-inner quadrant of **unspecified** male breast ♂
- C5Ø.3 Malignant neoplasm of **lower-inner quadrant** of breast
  - C5Ø.31 Malignant neoplasm of lower-inner quadrant of breast, **female**
    - C5Ø.311 Malignant neoplasm of lower-inner quadrant of **right** female breast ♀
    - C5Ø.312 Malignant neoplasm of lower-inner quadrant of **left** female breast ♀
    - C5Ø.319 Malignant neoplasm of lower-inner quadrant of **unspecified** female breast ♀
  - C5Ø.32 Malignant neoplasm of lower-inner quadrant of breast, **male**
    - C5Ø.321 Malignant neoplasm of lower-inner quadrant of **right** male breast ♂
    - C5Ø.322 Malignant neoplasm of lower-inner quadrant of **left** male breast ♂
    - C5Ø.329 Malignant neoplasm of lower-inner quadrant of **unspecified** male breast ♂
- C5Ø.4 Malignant neoplasm of **upper-outer quadrant** of breast
  - C5Ø.41 Malignant neoplasm of upper-outer quadrant of breast, **female**
    - C5Ø.411 Malignant neoplasm of upper-outer quadrant of **right** female breast ♀
    - C5Ø.412 Malignant neoplasm of upper-outer quadrant of **left** female breast ♀
    - C5Ø.419 Malignant neoplasm of upper-outer quadrant of **unspecified** female breast ♀
  - C5Ø.42 Malignant neoplasm of upper-outer quadrant of breast, **male**
    - C5Ø.421 Malignant neoplasm of upper-outer quadrant of **right** male breast ♂
    - C5Ø.422 Malignant neoplasm of upper-outer quadrant of **left** male breast ♂
    - C5Ø.429 Malignant neoplasm of upper-outer quadrant of **unspecified** male breast ♂
- C5Ø.5 Malignant neoplasm of **lower-outer quadrant** of breast
  - C5Ø.51 Malignant neoplasm of lower-outer quadrant of breast, **female**
    - C5Ø.511 Malignant neoplasm of lower-outer quadrant of **right** female breast ♀
    - C5Ø.512 Malignant neoplasm of lower-outer quadrant of **left** female breast ♀
    - C5Ø.519 Malignant neoplasm of lower-outer quadrant of **unspecified** female breast ♀
  - C5Ø.52 Malignant neoplasm of lower-outer quadrant of breast, **male**
    - C5Ø.521 Malignant neoplasm of lower-outer quadrant of **right** male breast ♂
    - C5Ø.522 Malignant neoplasm of lower-outer quadrant of **left** male breast ♂
    - C5Ø.529 Malignant neoplasm of lower-outer quadrant of **unspecified** male breast ♂
- C5Ø.6 Malignant neoplasm of **axillary tail** of breast
  - C5Ø.61 Malignant neoplasm of axillary tail of breast, **female**
    - C5Ø.611 Malignant neoplasm of axillary tail of **right** female breast ♀
    - C5Ø.612 Malignant neoplasm of axillary tail of **left** female breast ♀
    - C5Ø.619 Malignant neoplasm of axillary tail of **unspecified** female breast ♀
  - C5Ø.62 Malignant neoplasm of axillary tail of breast, **male**
    - C5Ø.621 Malignant neoplasm of axillary tail of **right** male breast ♂
    - C5Ø.622 Malignant neoplasm of axillary tail of **left** male breast ♂
    - C5Ø.629 Malignant neoplasm of axillary tail of **unspecified** male breast ♂
- C5Ø.8 Malignant neoplasm of **overlapping sites** of breast
  - C5Ø.81 Malignant neoplasm of overlapping sites of breast, **female**
    - C5Ø.811 Malignant neoplasm of overlapping sites of **right** female breast ♀
    - C5Ø.812 Malignant neoplasm of overlapping sites of **left** female breast ♀
    - C5Ø.819 Malignant neoplasm of overlapping sites of **unspecified** female breast ♀
  - C5Ø.82 Malignant neoplasm of overlapping sites of breast, **male**
    - C5Ø.821 Malignant neoplasm of overlapping sites of **right** male breast ♂
    - C5Ø.822 Malignant neoplasm of overlapping sites of **left** male breast ♂
    - C5Ø.829 Malignant neoplasm of overlapping sites of **unspecified** male breast ♂
- C5Ø.9 Malignant neoplasm of breast of **unspecified site**
  - C5Ø.91 Malignant neoplasm of breast of unspecified site, **female**
    - C5Ø.911 Malignant neoplasm of unspecified site of **right** female breast ♀
    - C5Ø.912 Malignant neoplasm of unspecified site of **left** female breast ♀
    - C5Ø.919 Malignant neoplasm of unspecified site of **unspecified** female breast ♀
  - C5Ø.92 Malignant neoplasm of breast of unspecified site, **male**
    - C5Ø.921 Malignant neoplasm of unspecified site of **right** male breast ♂
    - C5Ø.922 Malignant neoplasm of unspecified site of **left** male breast ♂
    - C5Ø.929 Malignant neoplasm of unspecified site of **unspecified** male breast ♂

MALIGNANT NEOPLASMS OF FEMALE GENITAL ORGANS (C51-C58)

Includes malignant neoplasm of skin of female genital organs

● C51 **Malignant neoplasm of vulva**
- **Excludes1** carcinoma in situ of vulva (DØ7.1)
- C51.Ø **Malignant neoplasm of labium majus** ♀
  - *Outer folds of skin external female genitalia*
  - Malignant neoplasm of Bartholin's [greater vestibular] gland
- C51.1 **Malignant neoplasm of labium minus** ♀
  - *Two inner folds surrounding vulva in female genitalia*
- C51.2 **Malignant neoplasm of clitoris** ♀
- C51.8 **Malignant neoplasm of overlapping sites of vulva** ♀
- C51.9 **Malignant neoplasm of vulva, unspecified** ♀
  - Malignant neoplasm of external female genitalia NOS
  - Malignant neoplasm of pudendum

C52 **Malignant neoplasm of vagina** ♀
- **Excludes1** carcinoma in situ of vagina (DØ7.2)

● C53 **Malignant neoplasm of cervix uteri**
- **Excludes1** carcinoma in situ of cervix uteri (DØ6.-)
- C53.Ø **Malignant neoplasm of endocervix** ♀
  - *Inside the cervix*
- C53.1 **Malignant neoplasm of exocervix** ♀
  - *Outside the cervix*
- C53.8 **Malignant neoplasm of overlapping sites of cervix uteri** ♀
- C53.9 **Malignant neoplasm of cervix uteri, unspecified** ♀**Coding Clinic: 2017, Q4, P103**

● C54 **Malignant neoplasm of corpus uteri**
- C54.Ø **Malignant neoplasm of isthmus uteri** ♀
  - *Constricted part of uterus between cervix and body*
  - Malignant neoplasm of lower uterine segment
- C54.1 **Malignant neoplasm of endometrium** ♀
  - *Lining of uterus*
- C54.2 **Malignant neoplasm of myometrium** ♀
  - *Middle layer of uterine wall consisting of smooth muscle supporting stromal and vascular tissue*
- C54.3 **Malignant neoplasm of fundus uteri** ♀
  - *Top rounded portion of uterus*
- C54.8 **Malignant neoplasm of overlapping sites of corpus uteri** ♀
  - *Main body of uterus*
- C54.9 **Malignant neoplasm of corpus uteri, unspecified** ♀

C55 **Malignant neoplasm of uterus, part unspecified** ♀

● C56 **Malignant neoplasm of ovary**
- Use additional code to identify any functional activity
- C56.1 **Malignant neoplasm of right ovary** ♀
- C56.2 **Malignant neoplasm of left ovary** ♀
- C56.9 **Malignant neoplasm of unspecified ovary** ♀

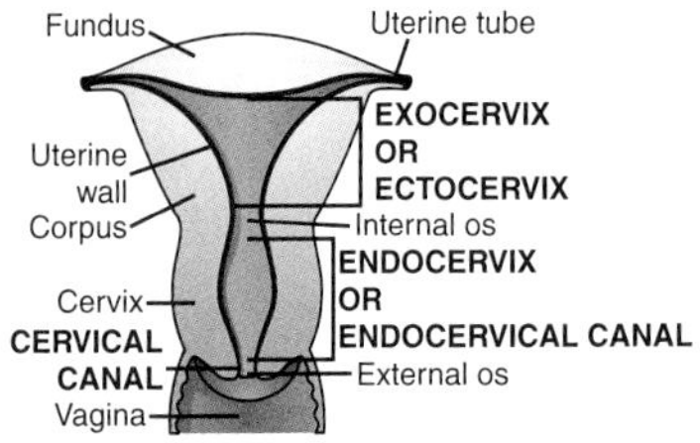

Figure 2-13 Cervix uteri.

● C57 **Malignant neoplasm of other and unspecified female genital organs**
- ● C57.Ø **Malignant neoplasm of fallopian tube**
  - Malignant neoplasm of oviduct
  - Malignant neoplasm of uterine tube
  - C57.ØØ **Malignant neoplasm of unspecified fallopian tube** ♀
  - C57.Ø1 **Malignant neoplasm of right fallopian tube** ♀
  - C57.Ø2 **Malignant neoplasm of left fallopian tube** ♀
- ● C57.1 **Malignant neoplasm of broad ligament**
  - C57.1Ø **Malignant neoplasm of unspecified broad ligament** ♀
  - C57.11 **Malignant neoplasm of right broad ligament** ♀
  - C57.12 **Malignant neoplasm of left broad ligament** ♀
- ● C57.2 **Malignant neoplasm of round ligament**
  - C57.2Ø **Malignant neoplasm of unspecified round ligament** ♀
  - C57.21 **Malignant neoplasm of right round ligament** ♀
  - C57.22 **Malignant neoplasm of left round ligament** ♀
- C57.3 **Malignant neoplasm of parametrium** ♀
  - Malignant neoplasm of uterine ligament NOS
- C57.4 **Malignant neoplasm of uterine adnexa, unspecified** ♀
- C57.7 **Malignant neoplasm of other specified female genital organs** ♀
  - Malignant neoplasm of wolffian body or duct
- C57.8 **Malignant neoplasm of overlapping sites of female genital organs** ♀
  - Primary malignant neoplasm of two or more contiguous sites of the female genital organs whose point of origin cannot be determined
  - Primary tubo-ovarian malignant neoplasm whose point of origin cannot be determined
  - Primary utero-ovarian malignant neoplasm whose point of origin cannot be determined
- C57.9 **Malignant neoplasm of female genital organ, unspecified** ♀
  - Malignant neoplasm of female genitourinary tract NOS

C58 **Malignant neoplasm of placenta** ♀ **M**
- **Includes** choriocarcinoma NOS
  - chorionepithelioma NOS
- **Excludes1** chorioadenoma (destruens) (D39.2)
  - hydatidiform mole NOS (OØ1.9)
  - invasive hydatidiform mole (D39.2)
  - male choriocarcinoma NOS (C62.9-)
  - malignant hydatidiform mole (D39.2)

MALIGNANT NEOPLASMS OF MALE GENITAL ORGANS (C6Ø-C63)

Includes malignant neoplasm of skin of male genital organs

● C6Ø **Malignant neoplasm of penis**
- C6Ø.Ø **Malignant neoplasm of prepuce** ♂
  - Malignant neoplasm of foreskin
- C6Ø.1 **Malignant neoplasm of glans penis** ♂
- C6Ø.2 **Malignant neoplasm of body of penis** ♂
  - Malignant neoplasm of corpus cavernosum
- C6Ø.8 **Malignant neoplasm of overlapping sites of penis** ♂
- C6Ø.9 **Malignant neoplasm of penis, unspecified** ♂
  - Malignant neoplasm of skin of penis NOS

C61 **Malignant neoplasm of prostate** ♂
- Use additional code to identify:
  - hormone sensitivity status (Z19.1-Z19.2)
  - rising PSA following treatment for malignant neoplasm of prostate (R97.21)
- **Excludes1** malignant neoplasm of seminal vesicle (C63.7)

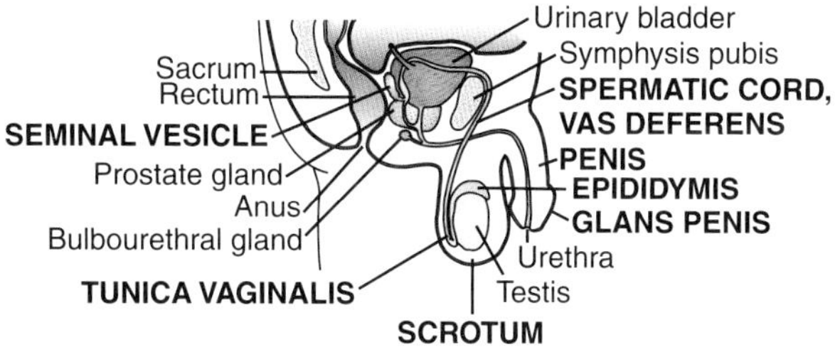

Figure 2-14 Penis and other male genital organs.

C62 Malignant neoplasm of testis
Use additional code to identify any functional activity.
- **C62.0 Malignant neoplasm of undescended testis**
  Malignant neoplasm of ectopic testis
  Malignant neoplasm of retained testis
  - C62.00 **Malignant neoplasm of unspecified undescended testis** ♂
  - C62.01 **Malignant neoplasm of undescended right testis** ♂
  - C62.02 **Malignant neoplasm of undescended left testis** ♂
- **C62.1 Malignant neoplasm of descended testis**
  Malignant neoplasm of scrotal testis
  - C62.10 **Malignant neoplasm of unspecified descended testis, unspecified side** ♂
  - C62.11 **Malignant neoplasm of descended right testis** ♂
  - C62.12 **Malignant neoplasm of descended left testis** ♂
- **C62.9 Malignant neoplasm of testis, unspecified whether descended or undescended**
  - C62.90 **Malignant neoplasm of unspecified testis, unspecified whether descended or undescended** ♂
    Malignant neoplasm of testis NOS
  - C62.91 **Malignant neoplasm of right testis, unspecified whether descended or undescended** ♂
  - C62.92 **Malignant neoplasm of left testis, unspecified whether descended or undescended** ♂

C63 Malignant neoplasm of other and unspecified male genital organs
- **C63.0 Malignant neoplasm of epididymis**
  - C63.00 **Malignant neoplasm of unspecified epididymis** ♂
  - C63.01 **Malignant neoplasm of right epididymis** ♂
  - C63.02 **Malignant neoplasm of left epididymis** ♂
- **C63.1 Malignant neoplasm of spermatic cord**
  - C63.10 **Malignant neoplasm of unspecified spermatic cord** ♂
  - C63.11 **Malignant neoplasm of right spermatic cord** ♂
  - C63.12 **Malignant neoplasm of left spermatic cord** ♂
- C63.2 **Malignant neoplasm of scrotum** ♂
  Malignant neoplasm of skin of scrotum
- C63.7 **Malignant neoplasm of other specified male genital organs** ♂
  Malignant neoplasm of seminal vesicle
  Malignant neoplasm of tunica vaginalis
- C63.8 **Malignant neoplasm of overlapping sites of male genital organs** ♂
  Primary malignant neoplasm of two or more contiguous sites of male genital organs whose point of origin cannot be determined
- C63.9 **Malignant neoplasm of male genital organ, unspecified** ♂
  Malignant neoplasm of male genitourinary tract NOS

MALIGNANT NEOPLASMS OF URINARY TRACT (C64-C68)

C64 Malignant neoplasm of kidney, except renal pelvis
Excludes1 malignant carcinoid tumor of the kidney (C7A.093)
malignant neoplasm of renal calyces (C65.-)
malignant neoplasm of renal pelvis (C65.-)
- C64.1 **Malignant neoplasm of right kidney, except renal pelvis**
- C64.2 **Malignant neoplasm of left kidney, except renal pelvis**
- C64.9 **Malignant neoplasm of unspecified kidney, except renal pelvis**

C65 Malignant neoplasm of renal pelvis
Includes malignant neoplasm of pelviureteric junction
malignant neoplasm of renal calyces
- C65.1 **Malignant neoplasm of right renal pelvis**
- C65.2 **Malignant neoplasm of left renal pelvis**
- C65.9 **Malignant neoplasm of unspecified renal pelvis**

C66 Malignant neoplasm of ureter
Excludes1 malignant neoplasm of ureteric orifice of bladder (C67.6)
- C66.1 **Malignant neoplasm of right ureter**
- C66.2 **Malignant neoplasm of left ureter**
- C66.9 **Malignant neoplasm of unspecified ureter**

C67 Malignant neoplasm of bladder
- C67.0 **Malignant neoplasm of trigone of bladder**
  Triangular area formed by three openings in the floor of urinary bladder
- C67.1 **Malignant neoplasm of dome of bladder**
  Vaulted roof
- C67.2 **Malignant neoplasm of lateral wall of bladder**
  Side walls
- C67.3 **Malignant neoplasm of anterior wall of bladder**
  Front wall
- C67.4 **Malignant neoplasm of posterior wall of bladder**
  Back wall
- C67.5 **Malignant neoplasm of bladder neck**
  Joining of bladder and urethra
  Malignant neoplasm of internal urethral orifice
- C67.6 **Malignant neoplasm of ureteric orifice**
  Opening from bladder to ureters
- C67.7 **Malignant neoplasm of urachus**
  Embryonic canal that connects the urinary bladder with the structure that forms the umbilical cord (allantois)
- C67.8 **Malignant neoplasm of overlapping sites of bladder**
- C67.9 **Malignant neoplasm of bladder, unspecified**
  Coding Clinic: 2017, Q1, P6; 2016, Q1, P19

C68 Malignant neoplasm of other and unspecified urinary organs
Excludes1 malignant neoplasm of female genitourinary tract NOS (C57.9)
malignant neoplasm of male genitourinary tract NOS (C63.9)
- C68.0 **Malignant neoplasm of urethra**
  Excludes1 malignant neoplasm of urethral orifice of bladder (C67.5)
- C68.1 **Malignant neoplasm of paraurethral glands**
  Group of glands of female urethra drained by paraurethral ducts; AKA Skene glands, female prostate
- C68.8 **Malignant neoplasm of overlapping sites of urinary organs**
  Primary malignant neoplasm of two or more contiguous sites of urinary organs whose point of origin cannot be determined
- C68.9 **Malignant neoplasm of urinary organ, unspecified**
  Malignant neoplasm of urinary system NOS

CHAPTER 2 (C00-D49)

MALIGNANT NEOPLASMS OF EYE, BRAIN AND OTHER PARTS OF CENTRAL NERVOUS SYSTEM (C69-C72)

C69 Malignant neoplasm of eye and adnexa
Excludes1 malignant neoplasm of connective tissue of eyelid (C49.Ø)
malignant neoplasm of eyelid (skin) (C43.1-, C44.1-)
malignant neoplasm of optic nerve (C72.3-)

C69.Ø Malignant neoplasm of conjunctiva
C69.ØØ Malignant neoplasm of **unspecified** conjunctiva
C69.Ø1 Malignant neoplasm of **right** conjunctiva
C69.Ø2 Malignant neoplasm of **left** conjunctiva

C69.1 Malignant neoplasm of cornea
C69.1Ø Malignant neoplasm of **unspecified** cornea
C69.11 Malignant neoplasm of **right** cornea
C69.12 Malignant neoplasm of **left** cornea

C69.2 Malignant neoplasm of retina
Excludes1 dark area on retina (D49.81)
neoplasm of unspecified behavior of retina and choroid (D49.81)
retinal freckle (D49.81)
C69.2Ø Malignant neoplasm of **unspecified** retina
C69.21 Malignant neoplasm of **right** retina
C69.22 Malignant neoplasm of **left** retina

C69.3 Malignant neoplasm of choroid
C69.3Ø Malignant neoplasm of **unspecified** choroid
C69.31 Malignant neoplasm of **right** choroid
C69.32 Malignant neoplasm of **left** choroid

C69.4 Malignant neoplasm of ciliary body
C69.4Ø Malignant neoplasm of **unspecified** ciliary body
C69.41 Malignant neoplasm of **right** ciliary body
C69.42 Malignant neoplasm of **left** ciliary body

C69.5 Malignant neoplasm of lacrimal gland and duct
Malignant neoplasm of lacrimal sac
Malignant neoplasm of nasolacrimal duct
C69.5Ø Malignant neoplasm of **unspecified** lacrimal gland and duct
C69.51 Malignant neoplasm of **right** lacrimal gland and duct
C69.52 Malignant neoplasm of **left** lacrimal gland and duct

C69.6 Malignant neoplasm of orbit
Malignant neoplasm of connective tissue of orbit
Malignant neoplasm of extraocular muscle
Malignant neoplasm of peripheral nerves of orbit
Malignant neoplasm of retrobulbar tissue
Malignant neoplasm of retro-ocular tissue
Excludes1 malignant neoplasm of orbital bone (C41.Ø)
C69.6Ø Malignant neoplasm of **unspecified** orbit
C69.61 Malignant neoplasm of **right** orbit
C69.62 Malignant neoplasm of **left** orbit

C69.8 Malignant neoplasm of overlapping sites of eye and adnexa
C69.8Ø Malignant neoplasm of overlapping sites of **unspecified** eye and adnexa
C69.81 Malignant neoplasm of overlapping sites of **right** eye and adnexa
C69.82 Malignant neoplasm of overlapping sites of **left** eye and adnexa

C69.9 Malignant neoplasm of unspecified site of eye
Malignant neoplasm of eyeball
C69.9Ø Malignant neoplasm of unspecified site of **unspecified** eye
C69.91 Malignant neoplasm of unspecified site of **right** eye
C69.92 Malignant neoplasm of unspecified site of **left** eye

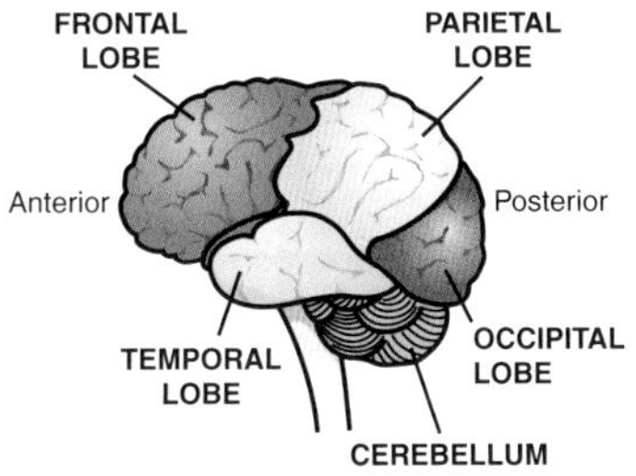

Figure 2-15 The brain.

C7Ø Malignant neoplasm of meninges
C7Ø.Ø Malignant neoplasm of **cerebral** meninges
C7Ø.1 Malignant neoplasm of **spinal** meninges
C7Ø.9 Malignant neoplasm of meninges, **unspecified**

C71 Malignant neoplasm of brain
Excludes1 malignant neoplasm of cranial nerves (C72.2-C72.5)
retrobulbar malignant neoplasm (C69.6-)
C71.Ø Malignant neoplasm of **cerebrum, except lobes and ventricles**
Malignant neoplasm of supratentorial NOS
C71.1 Malignant neoplasm of **frontal lobe**
C71.2 Malignant neoplasm of **temporal lobe**
C71.3 Malignant neoplasm of **parietal lobe**
C71.4 Malignant neoplasm of **occipital lobe**
C71.5 Malignant neoplasm of **cerebral ventricle**
Excludes1 malignant neoplasm of fourth cerebral ventricle (C71.7)
C71.6 Malignant neoplasm of **cerebellum**
C71.7 Malignant neoplasm of **brain stem**
Malignant neoplasm of fourth cerebral ventricle
Infratentorial malignant neoplasm NOS
C71.8 Malignant neoplasm of **overlapping sites of brain**
C71.9 Malignant neoplasm of **brain, unspecified**

C72 Malignant neoplasm of spinal cord, cranial nerves and other parts of central nervous system
Excludes1 malignant neoplasm of meninges (C7Ø.-)
malignant neoplasm of peripheral nerves and autonomic nervous system (C47.-)
C72.Ø Malignant neoplasm of **spinal cord**
C72.1 Malignant neoplasm of **cauda equina**
Lower end of spinal column

C72.2 Malignant neoplasm of olfactory nerve
Malignant neoplasm of olfactory bulb
C72.2Ø Malignant neoplasm of **unspecified** olfactory nerve
C72.21 Malignant neoplasm of **right** olfactory nerve
C72.22 Malignant neoplasm of **left** olfactory nerve

C72.3 Malignant neoplasm of optic nerve
C72.3Ø Malignant neoplasm of **unspecified** optic nerve
C72.31 Malignant neoplasm of **right** optic nerve
C72.32 Malignant neoplasm of **left** optic nerve

C72.4 Malignant neoplasm of acoustic nerve
C72.4Ø Malignant neoplasm of **unspecified** acoustic nerve
C72.41 Malignant neoplasm of **right** acoustic nerve
C72.42 Malignant neoplasm of **left** acoustic nerve

C72.5 Malignant neoplasm of other and unspecified cranial nerves

C72.50 **Malignant neoplasm of unspecified cranial nerve**
Malignant neoplasm of cranial nerve NOS

C72.59 **Malignant neoplasm of other cranial nerves**

C72.9 **Malignant neoplasm of central nervous system, unspecified**
Malignant neoplasm of unspecified site of central nervous system
Malignant neoplasm of nervous system NOS

MALIGNANT NEOPLASMS OF THYROID AND OTHER ENDOCRINE GLANDS (C73-C75)

C73 **Malignant neoplasm of thyroid gland**
Use additional code to identify any functional activity

C74 **Malignant neoplasm of adrenal gland**

C74.Ø **Malignant neoplasm of cortex of adrenal gland**

C74.ØØ **Malignant neoplasm of cortex of unspecified adrenal gland**

C74.Ø1 **Malignant neoplasm of cortex of right adrenal gland**

C74.Ø2 **Malignant neoplasm of cortex of left adrenal gland**

C74.1 **Malignant neoplasm of medulla of adrenal gland**
Pair of glands situated on top of or above each kidney ("suprarenal")

C74.10 **Malignant neoplasm of medulla of unspecified adrenal gland**

C74.11 **Malignant neoplasm of medulla of right adrenal gland**

C74.12 **Malignant neoplasm of medulla of left adrenal gland**

C74.9 **Malignant neoplasm of unspecified part of adrenal gland**

C74.90 **Malignant neoplasm of unspecified part of unspecified adrenal gland**

C74.91 **Malignant neoplasm of unspecified part of right adrenal gland**

C74.92 **Malignant neoplasm of unspecified part of left adrenal gland**

C75 **Malignant neoplasm of other endocrine glands and related structures**

Excludes1 malignant carcinoid tumors (C7A.Ø-)
malignant neoplasm of adrenal gland (C74.-)
malignant neoplasm of endocrine pancreas (C25.4)
malignant neoplasm of islets of Langerhans (C25.4)
malignant neoplasm of ovary (C56.-)
malignant neoplasm of testis (C62.-)
malignant neoplasm of thymus (C37)
malignant neoplasm of thyroid gland (C73)
malignant neuroendocrine tumors (C7A.-)

C75.Ø **Malignant neoplasm of parathyroid gland**

C75.1 **Malignant neoplasm of pituitary gland**

C75.2 **Malignant neoplasm of craniopharyngeal duct**

C75.3 **Malignant neoplasm of pineal gland**

C75.4 **Malignant neoplasm of carotid body**

C75.5 **Malignant neoplasm of aortic body and other paraganglia**

C75.8 **Malignant neoplasm with pluriglandular involvement, unspecified**

C75.9 **Malignant neoplasm of endocrine gland, unspecified**

MALIGNANT NEUROENDOCRINE TUMORS (C7A)

C7A **Malignant neuroendocrine tumors**
Code also any associated multiple endocrine neoplasia [MEN] syndromes (E31.2-)
Use additional code to identify any associated endocrine syndrome, such as:
carcinoid syndrome (E34.Ø)

Excludes2 malignant pancreatic islet cell tumors (C25.4)
Merkel cell carcinoma (C4A.-)

C7A.Ø **Malignant carcinoid tumors**

C7A.ØØ **Malignant carcinoid tumor of unspecified site**

C7A.Ø1 **Malignant carcinoid tumors of the small intestine**

C7A.Ø1Ø **Malignant carcinoid tumor of the duodenum**

C7A.Ø11 **Malignant carcinoid tumor of the jejunum**

C7A.Ø12 **Malignant carcinoid tumor of the ileum**

C7A.Ø19 **Malignant carcinoid tumor of the small intestine, unspecified portion**

C7A.Ø2 **Malignant carcinoid tumors of the appendix, large intestine, and rectum**

C7A.Ø2Ø **Malignant carcinoid tumor of the appendix**

C7A.Ø21 **Malignant carcinoid tumor of the cecum**

C7A.Ø22 **Malignant carcinoid tumor of the ascending colon**

C7A.Ø23 **Malignant carcinoid tumor of the transverse colon**

C7A.Ø24 **Malignant carcinoid tumor of the descending colon**

C7A.Ø25 **Malignant carcinoid tumor of the sigmoid colon**

C7A.Ø26 **Malignant carcinoid tumor of the rectum**

C7A.Ø29 **Malignant carcinoid tumor of the large intestine, unspecified portion**
Malignant carcinoid tumor of the colon NOS

C7A.Ø9 **Malignant carcinoid tumors of other sites**

C7A.Ø9Ø **Malignant carcinoid tumor of the bronchus and lung**

C7A.Ø91 **Malignant carcinoid tumor of the thymus**

C7A.Ø92 **Malignant carcinoid tumor of the stomach**

C7A.Ø93 **Malignant carcinoid tumor of the kidney**

C7A.Ø94 **Malignant carcinoid tumor of the foregut, unspecified**

C7A.Ø95 **Malignant carcinoid tumor of the midgut, unspecified**

C7A.Ø96 **Malignant carcinoid tumor of the hindgut, unspecified**

C7A.Ø98 **Malignant carcinoid tumors of other sites**

C7A.1 **Malignant poorly differentiated neuroendocrine tumors**
Malignant poorly differentiated neuroendocrine tumor NOS
Malignant poorly differentiated neuroendocrine carcinoma, any site
High grade neuroendocrine carcinoma, any site

C7A.8 **Other malignant neuroendocrine tumors**
Secondary neuroendocrine tumors (C7B)

SECONDARY NEUROENDOCRINE TUMORS (C7B)

● **C7B Secondary neuroendocrine tumors**
Use additional code to identify any functional activity

● **C7B.0 Secondary carcinoid tumors**
- **C7B.00 Secondary carcinoid tumors, unspecified site** HCC
- **C7B.01 Secondary carcinoid tumors of distant lymph nodes** HCC
- **C7B.02 Secondary carcinoid tumors of liver** HCC
- **C7B.03 Secondary carcinoid tumors of bone** HCC
- **C7B.04 Secondary carcinoid tumors of peritoneum** HCC
  Mesentary metastasis of carcinoid tumor
- **C7B.09 Secondary carcinoid tumors of other sites** HCC

C7B.1 Secondary Merkel cell carcinoma HCC
Merkel cell carcinoma nodal presentation
Merkel cell carcinoma visceral metastatic presentation

C7B.8 Other secondary neuroendocrine tumors HCC

MALIGNANT NEOPLASMS OF ILL-DEFINED, OTHER SECONDARY AND UNSPECIFIED SITES (C76-C80)

● **C76 Malignant neoplasm of other and ill-defined sites**
Excludes1 malignant neoplasm of female genitourinary tract NOS (C57.9)
malignant neoplasm of male genitourinary tract NOS (C63.9)
malignant neoplasm of lymphoid, hematopoietic and related tissue (C81-C96)
malignant neoplasm of skin (C44.-)
malignant neoplasm of unspecified site NOS (C80.1)

C76.0 Malignant neoplasm of head, face and neck HCC
Malignant neoplasm of cheek NOS
Malignant neoplasm of nose NOS

C76.1 Malignant neoplasm of thorax HCC
Intrathoracic malignant neoplasm NOS
Malignant neoplasm of axilla NOS
Thoracic malignant neoplasm NOS

C76.2 Malignant neoplasm of abdomen HCC

C76.3 Malignant neoplasm of pelvis HCC
Malignant neoplasm of groin NOS
Malignant neoplasm of sites overlapping systems within the pelvis
Rectovaginal (septum) malignant neoplasm
Between rectum and vagina
Rectovesical (septum) malignant neoplasm
Between rectum and urinary bladder; AKA vesicorectal

● **C76.4 Malignant neoplasm of upper limb**
- **C76.40 Malignant neoplasm of unspecified upper limb** HCC
- **C76.41 Malignant neoplasm of right upper limb** HCC
- **C76.42 Malignant neoplasm of left upper limb** HCC

● **C76.5 Malignant neoplasm of lower limb**
- **C76.50 Malignant neoplasm of unspecified lower limb** HCC
- **C76.51 Malignant neoplasm of right lower limb** HCC
- **C76.52 Malignant neoplasm of left lower limb** HCC

C76.8 Malignant neoplasm of other specified ill-defined sites HCC
Malignant neoplasm of overlapping ill-defined sites

● **C77 Secondary and unspecified malignant neoplasm of lymph nodes**
Excludes1 malignant neoplasm of lymph nodes, specified as primary (C81-C86, C88, C96.-)
mesentary metastasis of carcinoid tumor (C7B.04)
secondary carcinoid tumors of distant lymph nodes (C7B.01)

C77.0 Secondary and unspecified malignant neoplasm of lymph nodes of head, face and neck HCC
Secondary and unspecified malignant neoplasm of supraclavicular lymph nodes

C77.1 Secondary and unspecified malignant neoplasm of intrathoracic lymph nodes HCC

C77.2 Secondary and unspecified malignant neoplasm of intra-abdominal lymph nodes HCC

C77.3 Secondary and unspecified malignant neoplasm of axilla and upper limb lymph nodes HCC
Secondary and unspecified malignant neoplasm of pectoral lymph nodes

C77.4 Secondary and unspecified malignant neoplasm of inguinal and lower limb lymph nodes HCC

C77.5 Secondary and unspecified malignant neoplasm of intrapelvic lymph nodes HCC

C77.8 Secondary and unspecified malignant neoplasm of lymph nodes of multiple regions HCC

C77.9 Secondary and unspecified malignant neoplasm of lymph node, unspecified HCC

● **C78 Secondary malignant neoplasm of respiratory and digestive organs**
Excludes1 secondary carcinoid tumors of liver (C7B.02)
secondary carcinoid tumors of peritoneum (C7B.04)
Excludes2 lymph node metastases (C77.0)

● **C78.0 Secondary malignant neoplasm of lung**
- **C78.00 Secondary malignant neoplasm of unspecified lung** HCC
- **C78.01 Secondary malignant neoplasm of right lung** HCC
- **C78.02 Secondary malignant neoplasm of left lung** HCC

C78.1 Secondary malignant neoplasm of mediastinum HCC
Thoracic cavity between pleural cavities

C78.2 Secondary malignant neoplasm of pleura HCC
Serous membrane covering lungs and lining thoracic cavity

● **C78.3 Secondary malignant neoplasm of other and unspecified respiratory organs**
- **C78.30 Secondary malignant neoplasm of unspecified respiratory organ** HCC
- **C78.39 Secondary malignant neoplasm of other respiratory organs** HCC

C78.4 Secondary malignant neoplasm of small intestine HCC

C78.5 Secondary malignant neoplasm of large intestine and rectum HCC

C78.6 Secondary malignant neoplasm of retroperitoneum and peritoneum HCC
Coding Clinic: 2017, Q2, P12

C78.7 Secondary malignant neoplasm of liver and intrahepatic bile duct HCC

● **C78.8 Secondary malignant neoplasm of other and unspecified digestive organs**
- **C78.80 Secondary malignant neoplasm of unspecified digestive organ** HCC
- **C78.89 Secondary malignant neoplasm of other digestive organs** HCC
  Code also exocrine pancreatic insufficiency (K86.81)

● **C79 Secondary malignant neoplasm of other and unspecified sites**
Excludes1 secondary carcinoid tumors (C7B.-)
secondary neuroendocrine tumors (C7B.-)

● **C79.0 Secondary malignant neoplasm of kidney and renal pelvis**
- **C79.00 Secondary malignant neoplasm of unspecified kidney and renal pelvis** HCC
- **C79.01 Secondary malignant neoplasm of right kidney and renal pelvis** HCC
- **C79.02 Secondary malignant neoplasm of left kidney and renal pelvis** HCC

Item 2-6 The adrenal glands are a pair of glands situated on top of or above each kidney ("suprarenal") and chiefly responsible for regulating the stress response through the synthesis of corticosteroids and catecholamines, including cortisol and adrenaline.

● **C79.1 Secondary malignant neoplasm of bladder and other and unspecified urinary organs**

C79.10 Secondary malignant neoplasm of unspecified urinary organs

C79.11 Secondary malignant neoplasm of bladder

Excludes2 lymph node metastases (C77.Ø)

C79.19 Secondary malignant neoplasm of other urinary organs

C79.2 Secondary malignant neoplasm of skin

Excludes1 secondary Merkel cell carcinoma (C7B.1)

● **C79.3 Secondary malignant neoplasm of brain and cerebral meninges**

C79.31 Secondary malignant neoplasm of brain

C79.32 Secondary malignant neoplasm of cerebral meninges

● **C79.4 Secondary malignant neoplasm of other and unspecified parts of nervous system**

C79.40 Secondary malignant neoplasm of unspecified part of nervous system

C79.49 Secondary malignant neoplasm of other parts of nervous system

● **C79.5 Secondary malignant neoplasm of bone and bone marrow**

Excludes1 secondary carcinoid tumors of bone (C7B.Ø3)

C79.51 Secondary malignant neoplasm of bone

C79.52 Secondary malignant neoplasm of bone marrow

● **C79.6 Secondary malignant neoplasm of ovary**

C79.60 Secondary malignant neoplasm of unspecified ovary ♀

C79.61 Secondary malignant neoplasm of right ovary ♀

C79.62 Secondary malignant neoplasm of left ovary ♀

● **C79.7 Secondary malignant neoplasm of adrenal gland**

C79.70 Secondary malignant neoplasm of unspecified adrenal gland

C79.71 Secondary malignant neoplasm of right adrenal gland

C79.72 Secondary malignant neoplasm of left adrenal gland

● **C79.8 Secondary malignant neoplasm of other specified sites**

C79.81 Secondary malignant neoplasm of breast

C79.82 Secondary malignant neoplasm of genital organs

C79.89 Secondary malignant neoplasm of other specified sites

Coding Clinic: 2017, Q2, P11

C79.9 Secondary malignant neoplasm of unspecified site

Metastatic cancer NOS
Metastatic disease NOS

Excludes1 carcinomatosis NOS (C8Ø.Ø)
generalized cancer NOS (C8Ø.Ø)
malignant (primary) neoplasm of unspecified site (C8Ø.1)

OGCR Section I.C.2.j and k

Disseminated malignant neoplasm, unspecified

j. Code C8Ø.Ø, Disseminated malignant neoplasm, unspecified, is for use only in those cases where the patient has advanced metastatic disease and no known primary or secondary sites are specified. It should not be used in place of assigning codes for the primary site and all known secondary sites.

Malignant neoplasm without specification of site

k. Code C8Ø.1, Malignant (primary) neoplasm, unspecified, equates to Cancer, unspecified. This code should only be used when no determination can be made as to the primary site of a malignancy. This code should rarely be used in the inpatient setting.

● **C8Ø Malignant neoplasm without specification of site**

Excludes1 malignant carcinoid tumor of unspecified site (C7A.ØØ)
malignant neoplasm of specified multiple sites- code to each site

C8Ø.Ø Disseminated malignant neoplasm, unspecified

Carcinomatosis NOS
Generalized cancer, unspecified site (primary) (secondary)
Generalized malignancy, unspecified site (primary) (secondary)

C8Ø.1 Malignant (primary) neoplasm, unspecified

Cancer NOS
Cancer unspecified site (primary)
Carcinoma unspecified site (primary)
Malignancy unspecified site (primary)

Excludes1 secondary malignant neoplasm of unspecified site (C79.9)

C8Ø.2 Malignant neoplasm associated with transplanted organ

Code first complication of transplanted organ (T86.-)
Use additional code to identify the specific malignancy

★ **(See Plate 1 of the Anatomy Illustrations.)**

MALIGNANT NEOPLASMS OF LYMPHOID, HEMATOPOIETIC AND RELATED TISSUE (C81-C96)

Excludes2 Kaposi's sarcoma of lymph nodes (C46.3)
secondary and unspecified neoplasm of lymph nodes (C77.-)
secondary neoplasm of bone marrow (C79.52)
secondary neoplasm of spleen (C78.89)

● **C81 Hodgkin lymphoma**

Form of malignant lymphoma with four types, nodular sclerosis, mixed cellularity, lymphocyte depleted, and lymphocyte predominant

Excludes1 personal history of Hodgkin lymphoma (Z85.71)

● **C81.Ø Nodular lymphocyte predominant Hodgkin lymphoma**

Least aggressive, least common, typically no symptoms
Lymphocytic-histiocytic predominance Hodgkin's disease

C81.ØØ Nodular lymphocyte predominant Hodgkin lymphoma, unspecified site

C81.Ø1 Nodular lymphocyte predominant Hodgkin lymphoma, lymph nodes of head, face, and neck

C81.Ø2 Nodular lymphocyte predominant Hodgkin lymphoma, intrathoracic lymph nodes

C81.Ø3 Nodular lymphocyte predominant Hodgkin lymphoma, intra-abdominal lymph nodes

C81.Ø4 Nodular lymphocyte predominant Hodgkin lymphoma, lymph nodes of axilla and upper limb

C81.Ø5 Nodular lymphocyte predominant Hodgkin lymphoma, lymph nodes of inguinal region and lower limb

C81.Ø6 Nodular lymphocyte predominant Hodgkin lymphoma, intrapelvic lymph nodes

C81.Ø7 Nodular lymphocyte predominant Hodgkin lymphoma, spleen

C81.Ø8 Nodular lymphocyte predominant Hodgkin lymphoma, lymph nodes of multiple sites

C81.Ø9 Nodular lymphocyte predominant Hodgkin lymphoma, extranodal and solid organ sites

CHAPTER 2 (CØØ-D49)

C81.1 Nodular sclerosis Hodgkin lymphoma
Nodular sclerosis classical Hodgkin lymphoma
Moderately aggressive; most common in young adults

- C81.10 **Nodular sclerosis Hodgkin lymphoma, unspecified site**
- C81.11 **Nodular sclerosis Hodgkin lymphoma, lymph nodes of head, face, and neck**
- C81.12 **Nodular sclerosis Hodgkin lymphoma, intrathoracic lymph nodes**
- C81.13 **Nodular sclerosis Hodgkin lymphoma, intra-abdominal lymph nodes**
- C81.14 **Nodular sclerosis Hodgkin lymphoma, lymph nodes of axilla and upper limb**
- C81.15 **Nodular sclerosis Hodgkin lymphoma, lymph nodes of inguinal region and lower limb**
- C81.16 **Nodular sclerosis Hodgkin lymphoma, intrapelvic lymph nodes**
- C81.17 **Nodular sclerosis Hodgkin lymphoma, spleen**
- C81.18 **Nodular sclerosis Hodgkin lymphoma, lymph nodes of multiple sites**
- C81.19 **Nodular sclerosis Hodgkin lymphoma, extranodal and solid organ sites**

C81.2 Mixed cellularity Hodgkin lymphoma
Mixed cellularity classical Hodgkin lymphoma
A type of Hodgkin's that is moderately aggressive with mixed cell types

- C81.20 **Mixed cellularity Hodgkin lymphoma, unspecified site**
- C81.21 **Mixed cellularity Hodgkin lymphoma, lymph nodes of head, face, and neck**
- C81.22 **Mixed cellularity Hodgkin lymphoma, intrathoracic lymph nodes**
- C81.23 **Mixed cellularity Hodgkin lymphoma, intra-abdominal lymph nodes**
- C81.24 **Mixed cellularity Hodgkin lymphoma, lymph nodes of axilla and upper limb**
- C81.25 **Mixed cellularity Hodgkin lymphoma, lymph nodes of inguinal region and lower limb**
- C81.26 **Mixed cellularity Hodgkin lymphoma, intrapelvic lymph nodes**
- C81.27 **Mixed cellularity Hodgkin lymphoma, spleen**
- C81.28 **Mixed cellularity Hodgkin lymphoma, lymph nodes of multiple sites**
- C81.29 **Mixed cellularity Hodgkin lymphoma, extranodal and solid organ sites**

C81.3 Lymphocyte depleted Hodgkin lymphoma
Lymphocyte depleted classical Hodgkin lymphoma
Most aggressive type with poor prognosis

- C81.30 **Lymphocyte depleted Hodgkin lymphoma, unspecified site**
- C81.31 **Lymphocyte depleted Hodgkin lymphoma, lymph nodes of head, face, and neck**
- C81.32 **Lymphocyte depleted Hodgkin lymphoma, intrathoracic lymph nodes**
- C81.33 **Lymphocyte depleted Hodgkin lymphoma, intra-abdominal lymph nodes**
- C81.34 **Lymphocyte depleted Hodgkin lymphoma, lymph nodes of axilla and upper limb**
- C81.35 **Lymphocyte depleted Hodgkin lymphoma, lymph nodes of inguinal region and lower limb**
- C81.36 **Lymphocyte depleted Hodgkin lymphoma, intrapelvic lymph nodes**
- C81.37 **Lymphocyte depleted Hodgkin lymphoma, spleen**
- C81.38 **Lymphocyte depleted Hodgkin lymphoma, lymph nodes of multiple sites**
- C81.39 **Lymphocyte depleted Hodgkin lymphoma, extranodal and solid organ sites**

C81.4 Lymphocyte-rich Hodgkin lymphoma
Lymphocyte-rich classical Hodgkin lymphoma
Excludes1 nodular lymphocyte predominant Hodgkin lymphoma (C81.0-)

- C81.40 **Lymphocyte-rich Hodgkin lymphoma, unspecified site**
- C81.41 **Lymphocyte-rich Hodgkin lymphoma, lymph nodes of head, face, and neck**
- C81.42 **Lymphocyte-rich Hodgkin lymphoma, intrathoracic lymph nodes**
- C81.43 **Lymphocyte-rich Hodgkin lymphoma, intra-abdominal lymph nodes**
- C81.44 **Lymphocyte-rich Hodgkin lymphoma, lymph nodes of axilla and upper limb**
- C81.45 **Lymphocyte-rich Hodgkin lymphoma, lymph nodes of inguinal region and lower limb**
- C81.46 **Lymphocyte-rich Hodgkin lymphoma, intrapelvic lymph nodes**
- C81.47 **Lymphocyte-rich Hodgkin lymphoma, spleen**
- C81.48 **Lymphocyte-rich Hodgkin lymphoma, lymph nodes of multiple sites**
- C81.49 **Lymphocyte-rich Hodgkin lymphoma, extranodal and solid organ sites**

C81.7 Other Hodgkin lymphoma
Classical Hodgkin lymphoma NOS
Other classical Hodgkin lymphoma

- C81.70 **Other Hodgkin lymphoma, unspecified site**
- C81.71 **Other Hodgkin lymphoma, lymph nodes of head, face, and neck**
- C81.72 **Other Hodgkin lymphoma, intrathoracic lymph nodes**
- C81.73 **Other Hodgkin lymphoma, intra-abdominal lymph nodes**
- C81.74 **Other Hodgkin lymphoma, lymph nodes of axilla and upper limb**
- C81.75 **Other Hodgkin lymphoma, lymph nodes of inguinal region and lower limb**
- C81.76 **Other Hodgkin lymphoma, intrapelvic lymph nodes**
- C81.77 **Other Hodgkin lymphoma, spleen**
- C81.78 **Other Hodgkin lymphoma, lymph nodes of multiple sites**
- C81.79 **Other Hodgkin lymphoma, extranodal and solid organ sites**

C81.9 Hodgkin lymphoma, unspecified

- C81.90 **Hodgkin lymphoma, unspecified, unspecified site**
- C81.91 **Hodgkin lymphoma, unspecified, lymph nodes of head, face, and neck**
- C81.92 **Hodgkin lymphoma, unspecified, intrathoracic lymph nodes**
- C81.93 **Hodgkin lymphoma, unspecified, intra-abdominal lymph nodes**
- C81.94 **Hodgkin lymphoma, unspecified, lymph nodes of axilla and upper limb**
- C81.95 **Hodgkin lymphoma, unspecified, lymph nodes of inguinal region and lower limb**
- C81.96 **Hodgkin lymphoma, unspecified, intrapelvic lymph nodes**
- C81.97 **Hodgkin lymphoma, unspecified, spleen**
- C81.98 **Hodgkin lymphoma, unspecified, lymph nodes of multiple sites**
- C81.99 **Hodgkin lymphoma, unspecified, extranodal and solid organ sites**

C82 Follicular lymphoma
Group of malignant lymphomas
Includes follicular lymphoma with or without diffuse areas
Excludes1 mature T/NK-cell lymphomas (C84.-)
personal history of non-Hodgkin lymphoma (Z85.72)

C82.0 Follicular lymphoma grade I
- C82.00 Follicular lymphoma grade I, **unspecified site**
- C82.01 Follicular lymphoma grade I, lymph nodes of **head, face, and neck**
- C82.02 Follicular lymphoma grade I, **intrathoracic** lymph nodes
- C82.03 Follicular lymphoma grade I, **intra-abdominal** lymph nodes
- C82.04 Follicular lymphoma grade I, lymph nodes of **axilla and upper limb**
- C82.05 Follicular lymphoma grade I, lymph nodes of **inguinal region and lower limb**
- C82.06 Follicular lymphoma grade I, **intrapelvic** lymph nodes
- C82.07 Follicular lymphoma grade I, **spleen**
- C82.08 Follicular lymphoma grade I, lymph nodes of **multiple sites**
- C82.09 Follicular lymphoma grade I, **extranodal and solid organ sites**

C82.1 Follicular lymphoma grade II
- C82.10 Follicular lymphoma grade II, **unspecified site**
- C82.11 Follicular lymphoma grade II, lymph nodes of **head, face, and neck**
- C82.12 Follicular lymphoma grade II, **intrathoracic** lymph nodes
- C82.13 Follicular lymphoma grade II, **intra-abdominal** lymph nodes
- C82.14 Follicular lymphoma grade II, lymph nodes of **axilla and upper limb**
- C82.15 Follicular lymphoma grade II, lymph nodes of **inguinal region and lower limb**
- C82.16 Follicular lymphoma grade II, **intrapelvic** lymph nodes
- C82.17 Follicular lymphoma grade II, **spleen**
- C82.18 Follicular lymphoma grade II, lymph nodes of **multiple sites**
- C82.19 Follicular lymphoma grade II, **extranodal and solid organ sites**

C82.2 Follicular lymphoma grade III, unspecified
- C82.20 Follicular lymphoma grade III, unspecified, **unspecified site**
- C82.21 Follicular lymphoma grade III, unspecified, lymph nodes of **head, face, and neck**
- C82.22 Follicular lymphoma grade III, unspecified, **intrathoracic** lymph nodes
- C82.23 Follicular lymphoma grade III, unspecified, **intra-abdominal** lymph nodes
- C82.24 Follicular lymphoma grade III, unspecified, lymph nodes of **axilla and upper limb**
- C82.25 Follicular lymphoma grade III, unspecified, lymph nodes of **inguinal region and lower limb**
- C82.26 Follicular lymphoma grade III, unspecified, **intrapelvic** lymph nodes
- C82.27 Follicular lymphoma grade III, unspecified, **spleen**
- C82.28 Follicular lymphoma grade III, unspecified, lymph nodes of **multiple sites**
- C82.29 Follicular lymphoma grade III, unspecified, **extranodal and solid organ sites**

C82.3 Follicular lymphoma grade IIIa
- C82.30 Follicular lymphoma grade IIIa, **unspecified site**
- C82.31 Follicular lymphoma grade IIIa, lymph nodes of **head, face, and neck**
- C82.32 Follicular lymphoma grade IIIa, **intrathoracic** lymph nodes
- C82.33 Follicular lymphoma grade IIIa, **intra-abdominal** lymph nodes
- C82.34 Follicular lymphoma grade IIIa, lymph nodes of **axilla and upper limb**
- C82.35 Follicular lymphoma grade IIIa, lymph nodes of **inguinal region and lower limb**
- C82.36 Follicular lymphoma grade IIIa, **intrapelvic** lymph nodes
- C82.37 Follicular lymphoma grade IIIa, **spleen**
- C82.38 Follicular lymphoma grade IIIa, lymph nodes of **multiple sites**
- C82.39 Follicular lymphoma grade IIIa, **extranodal and solid organ sites**

C82.4 Follicular lymphoma grade IIIb
- C82.40 Follicular lymphoma grade IIIb, **unspecified site**
- C82.41 Follicular lymphoma grade IIIb, lymph nodes of **head, face, and neck**
- C82.42 Follicular lymphoma grade IIIb, **intrathoracic** lymph nodes
- C82.43 Follicular lymphoma grade IIIb, **intra-abdominal** lymph nodes
- C82.44 Follicular lymphoma grade IIIb, lymph nodes of **axilla and upper limb**
- C82.45 Follicular lymphoma grade IIIb, lymph nodes of **inguinal region and lower limb**
- C82.46 Follicular lymphoma grade IIIb, **intrapelvic** lymph nodes
- C82.47 Follicular lymphoma grade IIIb, **spleen**
- C82.48 Follicular lymphoma grade IIIb, lymph nodes of **multiple sites**
- C82.49 Follicular lymphoma grade IIIb, **extranodal and solid organ sites**

C82.5 Diffuse follicle center lymphoma
- C82.50 Diffuse follicle center lymphoma, **unspecified site**
- C82.51 Diffuse follicle center lymphoma, lymph nodes of **head, face, and neck**
- C82.52 Diffuse follicle center lymphoma, **intrathoracic** lymph nodes
- C82.53 Diffuse follicle center lymphoma, **intra-abdominal** lymph nodes
- C82.54 Diffuse follicle center lymphoma, lymph nodes of **axilla and upper limb**
- C82.55 Diffuse follicle center lymphoma, lymph nodes of **inguinal region and lower limb**
- C82.56 Diffuse follicle center lymphoma, **intrapelvic** lymph nodes
- C82.57 Diffuse follicle center lymphoma, **spleen**
- C82.58 Diffuse follicle center lymphoma, lymph nodes of **multiple sites**
- C82.59 Diffuse follicle center lymphoma, **extranodal and solid organ sites**

C82.6 Cutaneous follicle center lymphoma
- C82.60 Cutaneous follicle center lymphoma, **unspecified site**
- C82.61 Cutaneous follicle center lymphoma, lymph nodes of **head, face, and neck**
- C82.62 Cutaneous follicle center lymphoma, **intrathoracic** lymph nodes
- C82.63 Cutaneous follicle center lymphoma, **intra-abdominal** lymph nodes

C82.64 Cutaneous follicle center lymphoma, lymph nodes of axilla and upper limb
C82.65 Cutaneous follicle center lymphoma, lymph nodes of inguinal region and lower limb
C82.66 Cutaneous follicle center lymphoma, intrapelvic lymph nodes
C82.67 Cutaneous follicle center lymphoma, spleen
C82.68 Cutaneous follicle center lymphoma, lymph nodes of multiple sites
C82.69 Cutaneous follicle center lymphoma, extranodal and solid organ sites

● C82.8 Other types of follicular lymphoma
C82.8Ø Other types of follicular lymphoma, unspecified site
C82.81 Other types of follicular lymphoma, lymph nodes of head, face, and neck
C82.82 Other types of follicular lymphoma, intrathoracic lymph nodes
C82.83 Other types of follicular lymphoma, intra-abdominal lymph nodes
C82.84 Other types of follicular lymphoma, lymph nodes of axilla and upper limb
C82.85 Other types of follicular lymphoma, lymph nodes of inguinal region and lower limb
C82.86 Other types of follicular lymphoma, intrapelvic lymph nodes
C82.87 Other types of follicular lymphoma, spleen
C82.88 Other types of follicular lymphoma, lymph nodes of multiple sites
C82.89 Other types of follicular lymphoma, extranodal and solid organ sites

● C82.9 Follicular lymphoma, unspecified
C82.9Ø Follicular lymphoma, unspecified, unspecified site
C82.91 Follicular lymphoma, unspecified, lymph nodes of head, face, and neck
C82.92 Follicular lymphoma, unspecified, intrathoracic lymph nodes
C82.93 Follicular lymphoma, unspecified, intra-abdominal lymph nodes
C82.94 Follicular lymphoma, unspecified, lymph nodes of axilla and upper limb
C82.95 Follicular lymphoma, unspecified, lymph nodes of inguinal region and lower limb
C82.96 Follicular lymphoma, unspecified, intrapelvic lymph nodes
C82.97 Follicular lymphoma, unspecified, spleen
C82.98 Follicular lymphoma, unspecified, lymph nodes of multiple sites
C82.99 Follicular lymphoma, unspecified, extranodal and solid organ sites

● C83 Non-follicular lymphoma

Excludes1 personal history of non-Hodgkin lymphoma (Z85.72)

● C83.Ø Small cell B-cell lymphoma
Lymphoplasmacytic lymphoma
Nodal marginal zone lymphoma
Non-leukemic variant of B-CLL
Splenic marginal zone lymphoma

Excludes1 chronic lymphocytic leukemia (C91.1)
mature T/NK-cell lymphomas (C84.-)
Waldenström macroglobulinemia (C88.Ø)

C83.ØØ Small cell B-cell lymphoma, unspecified site
C83.Ø1 Small cell B-cell lymphoma, lymph nodes of head, face, and neck
C83.Ø2 Small cell B-cell lymphoma, intrathoracic lymph nodes
C83.Ø3 Small cell B-cell lymphoma, intra-abdominal lymph nodes
C83.Ø4 Small cell B-cell lymphoma, lymph nodes of axilla and upper limb
C83.Ø5 Small cell B-cell lymphoma, lymph nodes of inguinal region and lower limb
C83.Ø6 Small cell B-cell lymphoma, intrapelvic lymph nodes
C83.Ø7 Small cell B-cell lymphoma, spleen
C83.Ø8 Small cell B-cell lymphoma, lymph nodes of multiple sites
C83.Ø9 Small cell B-cell lymphoma, extranodal and solid organ sites

● C83.1 Mantle cell lymphoma
Centrocytic lymphoma
Malignant lymphomatous polyposis

C83.1Ø Mantle cell lymphoma, unspecified site
C83.11 Mantle cell lymphoma, lymph nodes of head, face, and neck
C83.12 Mantle cell lymphoma, intrathoracic lymph nodes
C83.13 Mantle cell lymphoma, intra-abdominal lymph nodes
C83.14 Mantle cell lymphoma, lymph nodes of axilla and upper limb
C83.15 Mantle cell lymphoma, lymph nodes of inguinal region and lower limb
C83.16 Mantle cell lymphoma, intrapelvic lymph nodes
C83.17 Mantle cell lymphoma, spleen
C83.18 Mantle cell lymphoma, lymph nodes of multiple sites
C83.19 Mantle cell lymphoma, extranodal and solid organ sites

● C83.3 Diffuse large B-cell lymphoma
Anaplastic diffuse large B-cell lymphoma
CD3Ø-positive diffuse large B-cell lymphoma
Centroblastic diffuse large B-cell lymphoma
Diffuse large B-cell lymphoma, subtype not specified
Immunoblastic diffuse large B-cell lymphoma
Plasmablastic diffuse large B-cell lymphoma
Diffuse large B-cell lymphoma, subtype not specified
T-cell rich diffuse large B-cell lymphoma

Excludes1 mediastinal (thymic) large B-cell lymphoma (C85.2-)
mature T/NK-cell lymphomas (C84.-)

C83.3Ø Diffuse large B-cell lymphoma, unspecified site
C83.31 Diffuse large B-cell lymphoma, lymph nodes of head, face, and neck
C83.32 Diffuse large B-cell lymphoma, intrathoracic lymph nodes
C83.33 Diffuse large B-cell lymphoma, intra-abdominal lymph nodes
C83.34 Diffuse large B-cell lymphoma, lymph nodes of axilla and upper limb
C83.35 Diffuse large B-cell lymphoma, lymph nodes of inguinal region and lower limb
C83.36 Diffuse large B-cell lymphoma, intrapelvic lymph nodes
C83.37 Diffuse large B-cell lymphoma, spleen
C83.38 Diffuse large B-cell lymphoma, lymph nodes of multiple sites
C83.39 Diffuse large B-cell lymphoma, extranodal and solid organ sites

C83.5 Lymphoblastic (diffuse) lymphoma
Highly malignant type of non-Hodgkin lymphoma with diffuse infiltration
B-precursor lymphoma
Lymphoblastic B-cell lymphoma
Lymphoblastic lymphoma NOS
Lymphoblastic T-cell lymphoma
T-precursor lymphoma

C83.50 **Lymphoblastic (diffuse) lymphoma, unspecified site**
C83.51 **Lymphoblastic (diffuse) lymphoma, lymph nodes of head, face, and neck**
C83.52 **Lymphoblastic (diffuse) lymphoma, intrathoracic lymph nodes**
C83.53 **Lymphoblastic (diffuse) lymphoma, intra-abdominal lymph nodes**
C83.54 **Lymphoblastic (diffuse) lymphoma, lymph nodes of axilla and upper limb**
C83.55 **Lymphoblastic (diffuse) lymphoma, lymph nodes of inguinal region and lower limb**
C83.56 **Lymphoblastic (diffuse) lymphoma, intrapelvic lymph nodes**
C83.57 **Lymphoblastic (diffuse) lymphoma, spleen**
C83.58 **Lymphoblastic (diffuse) lymphoma, lymph nodes of multiple sites**
C83.59 **Lymphoblastic (diffuse) lymphoma, extranodal and solid organ sites**

C83.7 Burkitt lymphoma
Form of small cell lymphoma
Atypical Burkitt lymphoma
Burkitt-like lymphoma
Excludes1 mature B-cell leukemia Burkitt type (C91.A-)

C83.70 **Burkitt lymphoma, unspecified site**
C83.71 **Burkitt lymphoma, lymph nodes of head, face, and neck**
C83.72 **Burkitt lymphoma, intrathoracic lymph nodes**
C83.73 **Burkitt lymphoma, intra-abdominal lymph nodes**
C83.74 **Burkitt lymphoma, lymph nodes of axilla and upper limb**
C83.75 **Burkitt lymphoma, lymph nodes of inguinal region and lower limb**
C83.76 **Burkitt lymphoma, intrapelvic lymph nodes**
C83.77 **Burkitt lymphoma, spleen**
C83.78 **Burkitt lymphoma, lymph nodes of multiple sites**
C83.79 **Burkitt lymphoma, extranodal and solid organ sites**

C83.8 Other non-follicular lymphoma
Intravascular large B-cell lymphoma
Lymphoid granulomatosis
Primary effusion B-cell lymphoma
Excludes1 mediastinal (thymic) large B-cell lymphoma (C85.2-)
T-cell rich B-cell lymphoma (C83.3-)

C83.80 **Other non-follicular lymphoma, unspecified site**
C83.81 **Other non-follicular lymphoma, lymph nodes of head, face, and neck**
C83.82 **Other non-follicular lymphoma, intrathoracic lymph nodes**
C83.83 **Other non-follicular lymphoma, intra-abdominal lymph nodes**
C83.84 **Other non-follicular lymphoma, lymph nodes of axilla and upper limb**
C83.85 **Other non-follicular lymphoma, lymph nodes of inguinal region and lower limb**
C83.86 **Other non-follicular lymphoma, intrapelvic lymph nodes**
C83.87 **Other non-follicular lymphoma, spleen**
C83.88 **Other non-follicular lymphoma, lymph nodes of multiple sites**
C83.89 **Other non-follicular lymphoma, extranodal and solid organ sites**

C83.9 Non-follicular (diffuse) lymphoma, unspecified

C83.90 **Non-follicular (diffuse) lymphoma, unspecified, unspecified site**
C83.91 **Non-follicular (diffuse) lymphoma, unspecified, lymph nodes of head, face, and neck**
C83.92 **Non-follicular (diffuse) lymphoma, unspecified, intrathoracic lymph nodes**
C83.93 **Non-follicular (diffuse) lymphoma, unspecified, intra-abdominal lymph nodes**
C83.94 **Non-follicular (diffuse) lymphoma, unspecified, lymph nodes of axilla and upper limb**
C83.95 **Non-follicular (diffuse) lymphoma, unspecified, lymph nodes of inguinal region and lower limb**
C83.96 **Non-follicular (diffuse) lymphoma, unspecified, intrapelvic lymph nodes**
C83.97 **Non-follicular (diffuse) lymphoma, unspecified, spleen**
C83.98 **Non-follicular (diffuse) lymphoma, unspecified, lymph nodes of multiple sites**
C83.99 **Non-follicular (diffuse) lymphoma, unspecified, extranodal and solid organ sites**

C84 Mature T/NK-cell lymphomas
Excludes1 personal history of non-Hodgkin lymphoma (Z85.72)

C84.0 Mycosis fungoides
Chronic or rapidly progressive form of cutaneous T-cell lymphoma; AKA granuloma fungoides
Excludes1 peripheral T-cell lymphoma, not classified (C84.4-)

C84.00 **Mycosis fungoides, unspecified site**
C84.01 **Mycosis fungoides, lymph nodes of head, face, and neck**
C84.02 **Mycosis fungoides, intrathoracic lymph nodes**
C84.03 **Mycosis fungoides, intra-abdominal lymph nodes**
C84.04 **Mycosis fungoides, lymph nodes of axilla and upper limb**
C84.05 **Mycosis fungoides, lymph nodes of inguinal region and lower limb**
C84.06 **Mycosis fungoides, intrapelvic lymph nodes**
C84.07 **Mycosis fungoides, spleen**
C84.08 **Mycosis fungoides, lymph nodes of multiple sites**
C84.09 **Mycosis fungoides, extranodal and solid organ sites**

C84.1 Sézary disease
Type of cutaneous lymphoma affecting T-cells

C84.10 **Sézary disease, unspecified site**
C84.11 **Sézary disease, lymph nodes of head, face, and neck**
C84.12 **Sézary disease, intrathoracic lymph nodes**
C84.13 **Sézary disease, intra-abdominal lymph nodes**
C84.14 **Sézary disease, lymph nodes of axilla and upper limb**
C84.15 **Sézary disease, lymph nodes of inguinal region and lower limb**
C84.16 **Sézary disease, intrapelvic lymph nodes**
C84.17 **Sézary disease, spleen**
C84.18 **Sézary disease, lymph nodes of multiple sites**
C84.19 **Sézary disease, extranodal and solid organ sites**

CHAPTER 2 (C00-D49)

C84.4 Peripheral T-cell lymphoma, not classified
Diverse group of blood carcinomas originating from T-cells, requiring aggressive chemotherapy
Lennert's lymphoma
Lymphoepithelioid lymphoma
Mature T-cell lymphoma, not elsewhere classified

- C84.40 **Peripheral T-cell lymphoma, not classified, unspecified site**
- C84.41 **Peripheral T-cell lymphoma, not classified, lymph nodes of head, face, and neck**
- C84.42 **Peripheral T-cell lymphoma, not classified, intrathoracic lymph nodes**
- C84.43 **Peripheral T-cell lymphoma, not classified, intra-abdominal lymph nodes**
- C84.44 **Peripheral T-cell lymphoma, not classified, lymph nodes of axilla and upper limb**
- C84.45 **Peripheral T-cell lymphoma, not classified, lymph nodes of inguinal region and lower limb**
- C84.46 **Peripheral T-cell lymphoma, not classified, intrapelvic lymph nodes**
- C84.47 **Peripheral T-cell lymphoma, not classified, spleen**
- C84.48 **Peripheral T-cell lymphoma, not classified, lymph nodes of multiple sites**
- C84.49 **Peripheral T-cell lymphoma, not classified, extranodal and solid organ sites**

C84.6 Anaplastic large cell lymphoma, ALK-positive
Anaplastic large cell lymphoma, CD30-positive

- C84.60 **Anaplastic large cell lymphoma, ALK-positive, unspecified site**
- C84.61 **Anaplastic large cell lymphoma, ALK-positive, lymph nodes of head, face, and neck**
- C84.62 **Anaplastic large cell lymphoma, ALK-positive, intrathoracic lymph nodes**
- C84.63 **Anaplastic large cell lymphoma, ALK-positive, intra-abdominal lymph nodes**
- C84.64 **Anaplastic large cell lymphoma, ALK-positive, lymph nodes of axilla and upper limb**
- C84.65 **Anaplastic large cell lymphoma, ALK-positive, lymph nodes of inguinal region and lower limb**
- C84.66 **Anaplastic large cell lymphoma, ALK-positive, intrapelvic lymph nodes**
- C84.67 **Anaplastic large cell lymphoma, ALK-positive, spleen**
- C84.68 **Anaplastic large cell lymphoma, ALK-positive, lymph nodes of multiple sites**
- C84.69 **Anaplastic large cell lymphoma, ALK-positive, extranodal and solid organ sites**

C84.7 Anaplastic large cell lymphoma, ALK-negative
Excludes1 primary cutaneous CD30-positive T-cell proliferations (C86.6-)

- C84.70 **Anaplastic large cell lymphoma, ALK-negative, unspecified site**
- C84.71 **Anaplastic large cell lymphoma, ALK-negative, lymph nodes of head, face, and neck**
- C84.72 **Anaplastic large cell lymphoma, ALK-negative, intrathoracic lymph nodes**
- C84.73 **Anaplastic large cell lymphoma, ALK-negative, intra-abdominal lymph nodes**
- C84.74 **Anaplastic large cell lymphoma, ALK-negative, lymph nodes of axilla and upper limb**
- C84.75 **Anaplastic large cell lymphoma, ALK-negative, lymph nodes of inguinal region and lower limb**
- C84.76 **Anaplastic large cell lymphoma, ALK-negative, intrapelvic lymph nodes**
- C84.77 **Anaplastic large cell lymphoma, ALK-negative, spleen**

Item 2-7 Lymphosarcoma, also known as malignant lymphoma, is a cancer of the lymph system exhibiting abnormal cells encompassing an entire lymph node creating a diffuse pattern without any definite organization. Diffuse pattern lymphoma has a more unfavorable survival outlook than those with a follicular or nodular pattern. Reticulosarcoma is the most common aggressive form of non-Hodgkin lymphoma.

- C84.78 **Anaplastic large cell lymphoma, ALK-negative, lymph nodes of multiple sites**
- C84.79 **Anaplastic large cell lymphoma, ALK-negative, extranodal and solid organ sites**

C84.A Cutaneous T-cell lymphoma, unspecified

- C84.A0 **Cutaneous T-cell lymphoma, unspecified, unspecified site**
- C84.A1 **Cutaneous T-cell lymphoma, unspecified lymph nodes of head, face, and neck**
- C84.A2 **Cutaneous T-cell lymphoma, unspecified, intrathoracic lymph nodes**
- C84.A3 **Cutaneous T-cell lymphoma, unspecified, intra-abdominal lymph nodes**
- C84.A4 **Cutaneous T-cell lymphoma, unspecified, lymph nodes of axilla and upper limb**
- C84.A5 **Cutaneous T-cell lymphoma, unspecified, lymph nodes of inguinal region and lower limb**
- C84.A6 **Cutaneous T-cell lymphoma, unspecified, intrapelvic lymph nodes**
- C84.A7 **Cutaneous T-cell lymphoma, unspecified, spleen**
- C84.A8 **Cutaneous T-cell lymphoma, unspecified, lymph nodes of multiple sites**
- C84.A9 **Cutaneous T-cell lymphoma, unspecified, extranodal and solid organ sites**

C84.Z Other mature T/NK-cell lymphomas

Note: If T-cell lineage or involvement is mentioned in conjunction with a specific lymphoma, code to the more specific description.

Excludes1 angioimmunoblastic T-cell lymphoma (C86.5)
blastic NK-cell lymphoma (C86.4)
enteropathy-type T-cell lymphoma (C86.2)
extranodal NK-cell lymphoma, nasal type (C86.0)
hepatosplenic T-cell lymphoma (C86.1)
primary cutaneous CD30-positive T-cell proliferations (C86.6)
subcutaneous panniculitis-like T-cell lymphoma (C86.3)
T-cell leukemia (C91.1-)

- C84.Z0 **Other mature T/NK-cell lymphomas, unspecified site**
- C84.Z1 **Other mature T/NK-cell lymphomas, lymph nodes of head, face, and neck**
- C84.Z2 **Other mature T/NK-cell lymphomas, intrathoracic lymph nodes**
- C84.Z3 **Other mature T/NK-cell lymphomas, intra-abdominal lymph nodes**
- C84.Z4 **Other mature T/NK-cell lymphomas, lymph nodes of axilla and upper limb**
- C84.Z5 **Other mature T/NK-cell lymphomas, lymph nodes of inguinal region and lower limb**
- C84.Z6 **Other mature T/NK-cell lymphomas, intrapelvic lymph nodes**
- C84.Z7 **Other mature T/NK-cell lymphomas, spleen**
- C84.Z8 **Other mature T/NK-cell lymphomas, lymph nodes of multiple sites**
- C84.Z9 **Other mature T/NK-cell lymphomas, extranodal and solid organ sites**

C84.9 Mature T/NK-cell lymphomas, unspecified
NK/T cell lymphoma NOS
Excludes1 mature T-cell lymphoma, not elsewhere classified (C84.4-)
C84.90 **Mature T/NK-cell lymphomas, unspecified, unspecified site**
C84.91 **Mature T/NK-cell lymphomas, unspecified, lymph nodes of head, face, and neck**
C84.92 **Mature T/NK-cell lymphomas, unspecified, intrathoracic lymph nodes**
C84.93 **Mature T/NK-cell lymphomas, unspecified, intra-abdominal lymph nodes**
C84.94 **Mature T/NK-cell lymphomas, unspecified, lymph nodes of axilla and upper limb**
C84.95 **Mature T/NK-cell lymphomas, unspecified, lymph nodes of inguinal region and lower limb**
C84.96 **Mature T/NK-cell lymphomas, unspecified, intrapelvic lymph nodes**
C84.97 **Mature T/NK-cell lymphomas, unspecified, spleen**
C84.98 **Mature T/NK-cell lymphomas, unspecified, lymph nodes of multiple sites**
C84.99 **Mature T/NK-cell lymphomas, unspecified, extranodal and solid organ sites**

C85 Other specified and unspecified types of non-Hodgkin lymphoma
Excludes1 other specified types of T/NK-cell lymphoma (C86.-)
personal history of non-Hodgkin lymphoma (Z85.72)

C85.1 Unspecified B-cell lymphoma
Note: If B-cell lineage or involvement is mentioned in conjunction with a specific lymphoma, code to the more specific description.
C85.10 **Unspecified B-cell lymphoma, unspecified site**
C85.11 **Unspecified B-cell lymphoma, lymph nodes of head, face, and neck**
C85.12 **Unspecified B-cell lymphoma, intrathoracic lymph nodes**
C85.13 **Unspecified B-cell lymphoma, intra-abdominal lymph nodes**
C85.14 **Unspecified B-cell lymphoma, lymph nodes of axilla and upper limb**
C85.15 **Unspecified B-cell lymphoma, lymph nodes of inguinal region and lower limb**
C85.16 **Unspecified B-cell lymphoma, intrapelvic lymph nodes**
C85.17 **Unspecified B-cell lymphoma, spleen**
C85.18 **Unspecified B-cell lymphoma, lymph nodes of multiple sites**
C85.19 **Unspecified B-cell lymphoma, extranodal and solid organ sites**

C85.2 Mediastinal (thymic) large B-cell lymphoma
C85.20 **Mediastinal (thymic) large B-cell lymphoma, unspecified site**
C85.21 **Mediastinal (thymic) large B-cell lymphoma, lymph nodes of head, face, and neck**
C85.22 **Mediastinal (thymic) large B-cell lymphoma, intrathoracic lymph nodes**
C85.23 **Mediastinal (thymic) large B-cell lymphoma, intra-abdominal lymph nodes**
C85.24 **Mediastinal (thymic) large B-cell lymphoma, lymph nodes of axilla and upper limb**
C85.25 **Mediastinal (thymic) large B-cell lymphoma, lymph nodes of inguinal region and lower limb**
C85.26 **Mediastinal (thymic) large B-cell lymphoma, intrapelvic lymph nodes**
C85.27 **Mediastinal (thymic) large B-cell lymphoma, spleen**
C85.28 **Mediastinal (thymic) large B-cell lymphoma, lymph nodes of multiple sites**
C85.29 **Mediastinal (thymic) large B-cell lymphoma, extranodal and solid organ sites**

C85.8 Other specified types of non-Hodgkin lymphoma
C85.80 **Other specified types of non-Hodgkin lymphoma, unspecified site**
C85.81 **Other specified types of non-Hodgkin lymphoma, lymph nodes of head, face, and neck**
C85.82 **Other specified types of non-Hodgkin lymphoma, intrathoracic lymph nodes**
C85.83 **Other specified types of non-Hodgkin lymphoma, intra-abdominal lymph nodes**
C85.84 **Other specified types of non-Hodgkin lymphoma, lymph nodes of axilla and upper limb**
C85.85 **Other specified types of non-Hodgkin lymphoma, lymph nodes of inguinal region and lower limb**
C85.86 **Other specified types of non-Hodgkin lymphoma, intrapelvic lymph nodes**
C85.87 **Other specified types of non-Hodgkin lymphoma, spleen**
C85.88 **Other specified types of non-Hodgkin lymphoma, lymph nodes of multiple sites**
C85.89 **Other specified types of non-Hodgkin lymphoma, extranodal and solid organ sites**

C85.9 Non-Hodgkin lymphoma, unspecified
Lymphoma NOS
Malignant lymphoma NOS
Non-Hodgkin lymphoma NOS
C85.90 **Non-Hodgkin lymphoma, unspecified, unspecified site**
C85.91 **Non-Hodgkin lymphoma, unspecified, lymph nodes of head, face, and neck**
C85.92 **Non-Hodgkin lymphoma, unspecified, intrathoracic lymph nodes**
C85.93 **Non-Hodgkin lymphoma, unspecified, intra-abdominal lymph nodes**
C85.94 **Non-Hodgkin lymphoma, unspecified, lymph nodes of axilla and upper limb**
C85.95 **Non-Hodgkin lymphoma, unspecified, lymph nodes of inguinal region and lower limb**
C85.96 **Non-Hodgkin lymphoma, unspecified, intrapelvic lymph nodes**
C85.97 **Non-Hodgkin lymphoma, unspecified, spleen**
C85.98 **Non-Hodgkin lymphoma, unspecified, lymph nodes of multiple sites**
C85.99 **Non-Hodgkin lymphoma, unspecified, extranodal and solid organ sites**

● **C86 Other specified types of T/NK-cell lymphoma**
Excludes1 anaplastic large cell lymphoma, ALK negative (C84.7-)
anaplastic large cell lymphoma, ALK positive (C84.6-)
mature T/NK-cell lymphomas (C84.-)
other specified types of non-Hodgkin lymphoma (C85.8-)

C86.0 Extranodal NK/T-cell lymphoma, nasal type HCC
C86.1 Hepatosplenic T-cell lymphoma HCC
Alpha-beta and gamma delta types
C86.2 Enteropathy-type (intestinal) T-cell lymphoma HCC
Enteropathy associated T-cell lymphoma
C86.3 Subcutaneous panniculitis-like T-cell lymphoma HCC
C86.4 Blastic NK-cell lymphoma HCC
Blastic plasmacytoid dendritic cell neoplasm (BPDCN)
C86.5 Angioimmunoblastic T-cell lymphoma HCC
Angioimmunoblastic lymphadenopathy with dysproteinemia (AILD)
C86.6 Primary cutaneous CD30-positive T-cell proliferations HCC
Lymphomatoid papulosis
Primary cutaneous anaplastic large cell lymphoma
Primary cutaneous CD30-positive large T-cell lymphoma

● **C88 Malignant immunoproliferative diseases and certain other B-cell lymphomas**
Diseases involving immune system
Excludes1 B-cell lymphoma, unspecified (C85.1-)
personal history of other malignant neoplasms of lymphoid, hematopoietic and related tissues (Z85.79)

C88.0 Waldenström's macroglobulinemia HCC
Lymphoplasmacytic lymphoma with IgM-production
Macroglobulinemia (idiopathic) (primary)
Excludes1 small cell B-cell lymphoma (C83.0)
C88.2 Heavy chain disease HCC
Franklin disease
Gamma heavy chain disease
Mu heavy chain disease
C88.3 Immunoproliferative small intestinal disease HCC
Alpha heavy chain disease
Mediterranean lymphoma
C88.4 Extranodal marginal zone B-cell lymphoma of mucosa-associated lymphoid tissue [MALT-lymphoma] HCC
Lymphoma of skin-associated lymphoid tissue [SALT-lymphoma]
Lymphoma of bronchial-associated lymphoid tissue [BALT-lymphoma]
Excludes1 high malignant (diffuse large B-cell) lymphoma (C83.3-)
C88.8 Other malignant immunoproliferative diseases HCC
C88.9 Malignant immunoproliferative disease, unspecified HCC
Immunoproliferative disease NOS

● **C90 Multiple myeloma and malignant plasma cell neoplasms**
Excludes1 personal history of other malignant neoplasms of lymphoid, hematopoietic and related tissues (Z85.79)

● **C90.0 Multiple myeloma**
Kahler's disease
Medullary plasmacytoma
Myelomatosis
Plasma cell myeloma
Excludes1 solitary myeloma (C90.3-)
solitary plasmacytoma (C90.3-)

C90.00 Multiple myeloma not having achieved remission HCC
Multiple myeloma with failed remission
Multiple myeloma NOS
C90.01 Multiple myeloma in remission HCC
C90.02 Multiple myeloma in relapse HCC

Item 2-8 Multiple myeloma is a cancer of a plasma cell (a type of white blood cell) and is an incurable but treatable disease. Immunoproliferative neoplasm is a term for diseases (mostly cancers) in which the immune system cells proliferate.

● **C90.1 Plasma cell leukemia**
Rare type of acute leukemia
Plasmacytic leukemia
Coding Clinic: 2019, Q2, P30

C90.10 Plasma cell leukemia not having achieved remission HCC
Plasma cell leukemia with failed remission
Plasma cell leukemia NOS
Coding Clinic: 2019, Q2, P30
C90.11 Plasma cell leukemia in remission HCC
C90.12 Plasma cell leukemia in relapse HCC

● **C90.2 Extramedullary plasmacytoma**
Malignant monoclonal plasma cell tumor growing in soft tissue; AKA plasma cell dyscrasias

C90.20 Extramedullary plasmacytoma not having achieved remission HCC
Extramedullary plasmacytoma with failed remission
Extramedullary plasmacytoma NOS
C90.21 Extramedullary plasmacytoma in remission HCC
C90.22 Extramedullary plasmacytoma in relapse HCC

● **C90.3 Solitary plasmacytoma**
Localized malignant plasma cell tumor NOS
Plasmacytoma NOS
Solitary myeloma

C90.30 Solitary plasmacytoma not having achieved remission HCC
Solitary plasmacytoma with failed remission
Solitary plasmacytoma NOS
C90.31 Solitary plasmacytoma in remission HCC
C90.32 Solitary plasmacytoma in relapse HCC

● **C91 Lymphoid leukemia**
Type of leukemia affecting circulating cells of lymphoid origin
Excludes1 personal history of leukemia (Z85.6)

● **C91.0 Acute lymphoblastic leukemia [ALL]**
Note: Codes in subcategory C91.0 should only be used for T-cell and B-cell precusor leukemia

C91.00 Acute lymphoblastic leukemia not having achieved remission HCC
Acute lymphoblastic leukemia with failed remission
Acute lymphoblastic leukemia NOS
C91.01 Acute lymphoblastic leukemia, in remission HCC
C91.02 Acute lymphoblastic leukemia, in relapse HCC

● **C91.1 Chronic lymphocytic leukemia of B-cell type**
Lymphoplasmacytic leukemia
Richter syndrome
Excludes1 lymphoplasmacytic lymphoma (C83.0-)

C91.10 Chronic lymphocytic leukemia of B-cell type not having achieved remission HCC
Chronic lymphocytic leukemia of B-cell type with failed remission
Chronic lymphocytic leukemia of B-cell type NOS
C91.11 Chronic lymphocytic leukemia of B-cell type in remission HCC
C91.12 Chronic lymphocytic leukemia of B-cell type in relapse HCC

Item 2-9 Leukemia is a cancer (acute or chronic) of the blood-forming tissues of the bone marrow. Blood cells all start out as stem cells. They mature and become red cells, white cells, or platelets. There are three main types of leukocytes (white cells that fight infection): monocytes, lymphocytes, and granulocytes. **Acute monocytic leukemia** (AML) affects monocytes. **Acute lymphoid leukemia** (ALL) affects lymphocytes, and **acute myeloid leukemia** (AML) affects cells that typically develop into white blood cells (not lymphocytes), though it may develop in other blood cells.

C91.3 Prolymphocytic leukemia of B-cell type
Chronic leukemia with symptoms of large number of circulating lymphocytes

C91.30 Prolymphocytic leukemia of B-cell type not having achieved remission
Prolymphocytic leukemia of B-cell type with failed remission
Prolymphocytic leukemia of B-cell type NOS

C91.31 Prolymphocytic leukemia of B-cell type, in remission

C91.32 Prolymphocytic leukemia of B-cell type, in relapse

C91.4 Hairy cell leukemia
Chronic leukemia with splenomegaly and excessive number of abnormal large mononuclear cells covered by hairlike villi
Leukemic reticuloendotheliosis

C91.40 Hairy cell leukemia not having achieved remission
Hairy cell leukemia with failed remission
Hairy cell leukemia NOS

C91.41 Hairy cell leukemia, in remission

C91.42 Hairy cell leukemia, in relapse

C91.5 Adult T-cell lymphoma/leukemia (HTLV-1-associated)
Acute variant of adult T-cell lymphoma/leukemia (HTLV-1-associated)
Chronic variant of adult T-cell lymphoma/leukemia (HTLV-1-associated)
Lymphomatoid variant of adult T-cell lymphoma/leukemia (HTLV-1-associated)
Smouldering variant of adult T-cell lymphoma/leukemia (HTLV-1-associated)

C91.50 Adult T-cell lymphoma/leukemia (HTLV-1-associated) not having achieved remission A
Adult T-cell lymphoma/leukemia (HTLV-1-associated) with failed remission
Adult T-cell lymphoma/leukemia (HTLV-1-associated) NOS

C91.51 Adult T-cell lymphoma/leukemia (HTLV-1-associated), in remission A

C91.52 Adult T-cell lymphoma/leukemia (HTLV-1-associated), in relapse A

C91.6 Prolymphocytic leukemia of T-cell type

C91.60 Prolymphocytic leukemia of T-cell type not having achieved remission
Prolymphocytic leukemia of T-cell type with failed remission
Prolymphocytic leukemia of T-cell type NOS

C91.61 Prolymphocytic leukemia of T-cell type, in remission

C91.62 Prolymphocytic leukemia of T-cell type, in relapse

C91.A Mature B-cell leukemia Burkitt-type
Excludes1 Burkitt lymphoma (C83.7-)

C91.A0 Mature B-cell leukemia Burkitt-type not having achieved remission
Mature B-cell leukemia Burkitt-type with failed remission
Mature B-cell leukemia Burkitt-type NOS

C91.A1 Mature B-cell leukemia Burkitt-type, in remission

C91.A2 Mature B-cell leukemia Burkitt-type, in relapse

C91.Z Other lymphoid leukemia
T-cell large granular lymphocytic leukemia (associated with rheumatoid arthritis)

C91.Z0 Other lymphoid leukemia not having achieved remission
Other lymphoid leukemia with failed remission
Other lymphoid leukemia NOS
Coding Clinic: 2019, Q2, P25

C91.Z1 Other lymphoid leukemia, in remission

C91.Z2 Other lymphoid leukemia, in relapse

C91.9 Lymphoid leukemia, unspecified

C91.90 Lymphoid leukemia, unspecified not having achieved remission
Lymphoid leukemia with failed remission
Lymphoid leukemia NOS

C91.91 Lymphoid leukemia, unspecified, in remission

C91.92 Lymphoid leukemia, unspecified, in relapse

C92 Myeloid leukemia
Includes granulocytic leukemia
myelogenous leukemia
Excludes1 personal history of leukemia (Z85.6)
Coding Clinic: 2019, Q1, P16

C92.0 Acute myeloblastic leukemia
Acute myeloblastic leukemia, minimal differentiation
Acute myeloblastic leukemia (with maturation)
Acute myeloblastic leukemia 1/ETO
Acute myeloblastic leukemia M0
Acute myeloblastic leukemia M1
Acute myeloblastic leukemia M2
Acute myeloblastic leukemia with t(8;21)
Acute myeloblastic leukemia (without a FAB classification) NOS
Refractory anemia with excess blasts in transformation [RAEB T]
Excludes1 acute exacerbation of chronic myeloid leukemia (C92.10)
refractory anemia with excess of blasts not in transformation (D46.2-)
Coding Clinic: 2018, Q4, P87

C92.00 Acute myeloblastic leukemia, not having achieved remission
Acute myeloblastic leukemia with failed remission
Acute myeloblastic leukemia NOS

C92.01 Acute myeloblastic leukemia, in remission

C92.02 Acute myeloblastic leukemia, in relapse

C92.1 Chronic myeloid leukemia, BCR/ABL-positive
Chronic myelogenous leukemia, Philadelphia chromosome (Ph1) positive
Chronic myelogenous leukemia, t(9;22) (q34;q11)
Chronic myelogenous leukemia with crisis of blast cells
Excludes1 atypical chronic myeloid leukemia BCR/ABL-negative (C92.2-)
chronic myelomonocytic leukemia (C93.1-)
chronic myeloproliferative disease (D47.1)

C92.10 Chronic myeloid leukemia, BCR/ABL-positive, not having achieved remission
Chronic myeloid leukemia, BCR/ABL-positive with failed remission
Chronic myeloid leukemia, BCR/ABL-positive NOS
Coding Clinic: 2017, Q1, P7

C92.11 Chronic myeloid leukemia, BCR/ABL-positive, in remission

C92.12 Chronic myeloid leukemia, BCR/ABL-positive, in relapse

C92.2 Atypical chronic myeloid leukemia, BCR/ABL-negative

C92.20 Atypical chronic myeloid leukemia, BCR/ABL-negative, not having achieved remission
Atypical chronic myeloid leukemia, BCR/ABL-negative with failed remission
Atypical chronic myeloid leukemia, BCR/ABL-negative NOS

C92.21 Atypical chronic myeloid leukemia, BCR/ABL-negative, in remission

C92.22 Atypical chronic myeloid leukemia, BCR/ABL-negative, in relapse

CHAPTER 2 (C00-D49)

● C92.3 **Myeloid sarcoma**
A malignant tumor of immature myeloid cells
Chloroma
Granulocytic sarcoma

C92.3Ø **Myeloid sarcoma, not having achieved remission** HCC
Myeloid sarcoma with failed remission
Myeloid sarcoma NOS

C92.31 **Myeloid sarcoma, in remission** HCC

C92.32 **Myeloid sarcoma, in relapse** HCC

● C92.4 **Acute promyelocytic leukemia**
AML M3
AML Me with t(15;17) and variants

C92.4Ø **Acute promyelocytic leukemia, not having achieved remission** HCC
Acute promyelocytic leukemia with failed remission
Acute promyelocytic leukemia NOS

C92.41 **Acute promyelocytic leukemia, in remission** HCC

C92.42 **Acute promyelocytic leukemia, in relapse** HCC

● C92.5 **Acute myelomonocytic leukemia**
AML M4
AML M4 Eo with inv(16) or t(16;16)

C92.5Ø **Acute myelomonocytic leukemia, not having achieved remission** HCC
Acute myelomonocytic leukemia with failed remission
Acute myelomonocytic leukemia NOS

C92.51 **Acute myelomonocytic leukemia, in remission** HCC

C92.52 **Acute myelomonocytic leukemia, in relapse** HCC

● C92.6 **Acute myeloid leukemia with 11q23-abnormality**
Acute myeloid leukemia with variation of MLL-gene

C92.6Ø **Acute myeloid leukemia with 11q23-abnormality not having achieved remission** HCC
Acute myeloid leukemia with 11q23-abnormality with failed remission
Acute myeloid leukemia with 11q23-abnormality NOS

C92.61 **Acute myeloid leukemia with 11q23-abnormality in remission** HCC

C92.62 **Acute myeloid leukemia with 11q23-abnormality in relapse** HCC

● C92.A **Acute myeloid leukemia with multilineage dysplasia**
Acute myeloid leukemia with dysplasia of remaining hematopoesis and/or myelodysplastic disease in its history

C92.AØ **Acute myeloid leukemia with multilineage dysplasia, not having achieved remission** HCC
Acute myeloid leukemia with multilineage dysplasia with failed remission
Acute myeloid leukemia with multilineage dysplasia NOS

C92.A1 **Acute myeloid leukemia with multilineage dysplasia, in remission** HCC

C92.A2 **Acute myeloid leukemia with multilineage dysplasia, in relapse** HCC

● C92.Z **Other myeloid leukemia**

C92.ZØ **Other myeloid leukemia not having achieved remission** HCC
Myeloid leukemia NEC with failed remission
Myeloid leukemia NEC

C92.Z1 **Other myeloid leukemia, in remission** HCC

C92.Z2 **Other myeloid leukemia, in relapse** HCC

● C92.9 **Myeloid leukemia, unspecified**

C92.9Ø **Myeloid leukemia, unspecified, not having achieved remission** HCC
Myeloid leukemia, unspecified with failed remission
Myeloid leukemia, unspecified NOS

C92.91 **Myeloid leukemia, unspecified in remission** HCC

C92.92 **Myeloid leukemia, unspecified in relapse** HCC

● C93 **Monocytic leukemia**
Includes monocytoid leukemia
Excludes1 personal history of leukemia (Z85.6)

● C93.Ø **Acute monoblastic/monocytic leukemia**
AML M5
AML M5a
AML M5b

C93.ØØ **Acute monoblastic/monocytic leukemia, not having achieved remission** HCC
Acute monoblastic/monocytic leukemia with failed remission
Acute monoblastic/monocytic leukemia NOS

C93.Ø1 **Acute monoblastic/monocytic leukemia, in remission** HCC

C93.Ø2 **Acute monoblastic/monocytic leukemia, in relapse** HCC

● C93.1 **Chronic myelomonocytic leukemia**
Chronic monocytic leukemia
CMML-1
CMML-2
CMML with eosinophilia

C93.1Ø **Chronic myelomonocytic leukemia not having achieved remission** HCC
Chronic myelomonocytic leukemia with failed remission
Chronic myelomonocytic leukemia NOS

C93.11 **Chronic myelomonocytic leukemia, in remission** HCC

C93.12 **Chronic myelomonocytic leukemia, in relapse** HCC

● C93.3 **Juvenile myelomonocytic leukemia**

C93.3Ø **Juvenile myelomonocytic leukemia, not having achieved remission** HCC P
Juvenile myelomonocytic leukemia with failed remission
Juvenile myelomonocytic leukemia NOS

C93.31 **Juvenile myelomonocytic leukemia, in remission** HCC P

C93.32 **Juvenile myelomonocytic leukemia, in relapse** HCC P

● C93.Z **Other monocytic leukemia**

C93.ZØ **Other monocytic leukemia, not having achieved remission** HCC
Other monocytic leukemia NOS

C93.Z1 **Other monocytic leukemia, in remission** HCC

C93.Z2 **Other monocytic leukemia, in relapse** HCC

● C93.9 **Monocytic leukemia, unspecified**

C93.9Ø **Monocytic leukemia, unspecified, not having achieved remission** HCC
Monocytic leukemia, unspecified with failed remission
Monocytic leukemia, unspecified NOS

C93.91 **Monocytic leukemia, unspecified in remission** HCC

C93.92 **Monocytic leukemia, unspecified in relapse** HCC

● C94 **Other leukemias of specified cell type**
Excludes1 leukemic reticuloendotheliosis (C91.4-)
myelodysplastic syndromes (D46.-)
personal history of leukemia (Z85.6)
plasma cell leukemia (C9Ø.1-)

● C94.Ø **Acute erythroid leukemia**
Acute myeloid leukemia M6(a)(b)
Erythroleukemia

C94.ØØ **Acute erythroid leukemia, not having achieved remission** HCC
Acute erythroid leukemia with failed remission
Acute erythroid leukemia NOS

C94.Ø1 **Acute erythroid leukemia, in remission** HCC

C94.Ø2 **Acute erythroid leukemia, in relapse** HCC

C94.2 Acute megakaryoblastic leukemia
Acute myeloid leukemia M7
Acute megakaryocytic leukemia

C94.20 Acute megakaryoblastic leukemia not having achieved remission
Acute megakaryoblastic leukemia with failed remission
Acute megakaryoblastic leukemia NOS

C94.21 Acute megakaryoblastic leukemia, in remission

C94.22 Acute megakaryoblastic leukemia, in relapse

C94.3 Mast cell leukemia

C94.30 Mast cell leukemia not having achieved remission
Mast cell leukemia with failed remission
Mast cell leukemia NOS

C94.31 Mast cell leukemia, in remission

C94.32 Mast cell leukemia, in relapse

C94.4 Acute panmyelosis with myelofibrosis
Acute myelofibrosis
Excludes1 myelofibrosis NOS (D75.81)
secondary myelofibrosis NOS (D75.81)

C94.40 Acute panmyelosis with myelofibrosis not having achieved remission
Acute myelofibrosis NOS
Acute panmyelosis with myelofibrosis with failed remission
Acute panmyelosis NOS

C94.41 Acute panmyelosis with myelofibrosis, in remission

C94.42 Acute panmyelosis with myelofibrosis, in relapse

C94.6 Myelodysplastic disease, not classified
Myeloproliferative disease, not classified

C94.8 Other specified leukemias
Aggressive NK-cell leukemia
Acute basophilic leukemia

C94.80 Other specified leukemias not having achieved remission
Other specified leukemia with failed remission
Other specified leukemias NOS

C94.81 Other specified leukemias, in remission

C94.82 Other specified leukemias, in relapse

C95 Leukemia of unspecified cell type
Excludes1 personal history of leukemia (Z85.6)

C95.0 Acute leukemia of unspecified cell type
Acute bilineal leukemia
Acute mixed lineage leukemia
Biphenotypic acute leukemia
Stem cell leukemia of unclear lineage
Excludes1 acute exacerbation of unspecified chronic leukemia (C95.10)

C95.00 Acute leukemia of unspecified cell type not having achieved remission
Acute leukemia of unspecified cell type with failed remission
Acute leukemia NOS

C95.01 Acute leukemia of unspecified cell type, in remission

C95.02 Acute leukemia of unspecified cell type, in relapse

C95.1 Chronic leukemia of unspecified cell type

C95.10 Chronic leukemia of unspecified cell type not having achieved remission
Chronic leukemia of unspecified cell type with failed remission
Chronic leukemia NOS

C95.11 Chronic leukemia of unspecified cell type, in remission

C95.12 Chronic leukemia of unspecified cell type, in relapse

C95.9 Leukemia, unspecified

C95.90 Leukemia, unspecified not having achieved remission
Leukemia, unspecified with failed remission
Leukemia NOS

C95.91 Leukemia, unspecified, in remission

C95.92 Leukemia, unspecified, in relapse

C96 Other and unspecified malignant neoplasms of lymphoid, hematopoietic and related tissue
Excludes1 personal history of other malignant neoplasms of lymphoid, hematopoietic and related tissues (Z85.79)

C96.0 Multifocal and multisystemic (disseminated) Langerhans-cell histiocytosis
Histiocytosis X, multisystemic
Letterer-Siwe disease
Excludes1 adult pulmonary Langerhans cell histiocytosis (J84.82)
multifocal and unisystemic Langerhans-cell histiocytosis (C96.5)
unifocal Langerhans-cell histiocytosis (C96.6)

C96.2 Malignant mast cell neoplasm
Excludes1 indolent mastocytosis (D47.02)
mast cell leukemia (C94.30)
mastocytosis (congenital) (cutaneous) (Q82.2)

C96.20 Malignant mast cell neoplasm, unspecified

C96.21 Aggressive systemic mastocytosis

C96.22 Mast cell sarcoma

C96.29 Other malignant mast cell neoplasm

C96.4 Sarcoma of dendritic cells (accessory cells)
Follicular dendritic cell sarcoma
Interdigitating dendritic cell sarcoma
Langerhans cell sarcoma

C96.5 Multifocal and unisystemic Langerhans-cell histiocytosis
Hand-Schüller-Christian disease
Histiocytosis X, multifocal
Excludes1 multifocal and multisystemic (disseminated) Langerhans-cell histiocytosis (C96.0)
unifocal Langerhans-cell histiocytosis (C96.6)

C96.6 Unifocal Langerhans-cell histiocytosis
Eosinophilic granuloma
Histiocytosis X, unifocal
Histiocytosis X NOS
Langerhans-cell histiocytosis NOS
Excludes1 multifocal and multisysemic (disseminated) Langerhans-cell histiocytosis (C96.0)
multifocal and unisystemic Langerhans-cell histiocytosis (C96.5)

C96.A Histiocytic sarcoma
Malignant histiocytosis

C96.Z Other specified malignant neoplasms of lymphoid, hematopoietic and related tissue

C96.9 Malignant neoplasm of lymphoid, hematopoietic and related tissue, unspecified

IN SITU NEOPLASMS (D00-D09)

In situ is carcinoma involving cells in localized tissues that has not spread to nearby tissues

Includes Bowen's disease
erythroplasia
grade III intraepithelial neoplasia
Queyrat's erythroplasia

● **D00 Carcinoma in situ of oral cavity, esophagus and stomach**
Excludes1 melanoma in situ (D03.-)

● **D00.0 Carcinoma in situ of lip, oral cavity and pharynx**
Use additional code to identify:
exposure to environmental tobacco smoke (Z77.22)
exposure to tobacco smoke in the perinatal period (P96.81)
history of tobacco dependence (Z87.891)
occupational exposure to environmental tobacco smoke (Z57.31)
tobacco dependence (F17.-)
tobacco use (Z72.0)
Excludes1 carcinoma in situ of aryepiglottic fold or interarytenoid fold, laryngeal aspect (D02.0)
carcinoma in situ of epiglottis NOS (D02.0)
carcinoma in situ of epiglottis suprahyoid portion (D02.0)
carcinoma in situ of skin of lip (D03.0, D04.0)

D00.00 Carcinoma in situ of oral cavity, unspecified site
D00.01 Carcinoma in situ of labial mucosa and vermilion border
D00.02 Carcinoma in situ of buccal mucosa
D00.03 Carcinoma in situ of gingiva and edentulous alveolar ridge
D00.04 Carcinoma in situ of soft palate
D00.05 Carcinoma in situ of hard palate
D00.06 Carcinoma in situ of floor of mouth
D00.07 Carcinoma in situ of tongue
D00.08 Carcinoma in situ of pharynx
Carcinoma in situ of aryepiglottic fold NOS
Carcinoma in situ of hypopharyngeal aspect of aryepiglottic fold
Carcinoma in situ of marginal zone of aryepiglottic fold

D00.1 Carcinoma in situ of esophagus
D00.2 Carcinoma in situ of stomach

● **D01 Carcinoma in situ of other and unspecified digestive organs**
Excludes1 melanoma in situ (D03.-)

D01.0 Carcinoma in situ of colon
Excludes1 carcinoma in situ of rectosigmoid junction (D01.1)

D01.1 Carcinoma in situ of rectosigmoid junction
D01.2 Carcinoma in situ of rectum
D01.3 Carcinoma in situ of anus and anal canal
Anal intraepithelial neoplasia III [AIN III]
Severe dysplasia of anus
Excludes1 anal intraepithelial neoplasia I and II [AIN I and AIN II] (K62.82)
carcinoma in situ of anal margin (D04.5)
carcinoma in situ of anal skin (D04.5)
carcinoma in situ of perianal skin (D04.5)

● **D01.4 Carcinoma in situ of other and unspecified parts of intestine**
Excludes1 carcinoma in situ of ampulla of Vater (D01.5)

D01.40 Carcinoma in situ of unspecified part of intestine
D01.49 Carcinoma in situ of other parts of intestine

D01.5 Carcinoma in situ of liver, gallbladder and bile ducts
Carcinoma in situ of ampulla of Vater
D01.7 Carcinoma in situ of other specified digestive organs
Carcinoma in situ of pancreas
D01.9 Carcinoma in situ of digestive organ, unspecified

● **D02 Carcinoma in situ of middle ear and respiratory system**
Use additional code to identify:
exposure to environmental tobacco smoke (Z77.22)
exposure to tobacco smoke in the perinatal period (P96.81)
history of tobacco dependence (Z87.891)
occupational exposure to environmental tobacco smoke (Z57.31)
tobacco dependence (F17.-)
tobacco use (Z72.0)
Excludes1 melanoma in situ (D03.-)

D02.0 Carcinoma in situ of larynx
Carcinoma in situ of aryepiglottic fold or interarytenoid fold, laryngeal aspect
Carcinoma in situ of epiglottis (suprahyoid portion)
Excludes1 carcinoma in situ of aryepiglottic fold or interarytenoid fold NOS (D00.08)
carcinoma in situ of hypopharyngeal aspect (D00.08)
carcinoma in situ of marginal zone (D00.08)

D02.1 Carcinoma in situ of trachea

● **D02.2 Carcinoma in situ of bronchus and lung**
D02.20 Carcinoma in situ of unspecified bronchus and lung
D02.21 Carcinoma in situ of right bronchus and lung
D02.22 Carcinoma in situ of left bronchus and lung

D02.3 Carcinoma in situ of other parts of respiratory system
Carcinoma in situ of accessory sinuses
Carcinoma in situ of middle ear
Carcinoma in situ of nasal cavities
Excludes1 carcinoma in situ of ear (external) (skin) (D04.2-)
carcinoma in situ of nose NOS (D09.8)
carcinoma in situ of skin of nose (D04.3)

D02.4 Carcinoma in situ of respiratory system, unspecified

● **D03 Melanoma in situ**
D03.0 Melanoma in situ of lip HCC

● **D03.1 Melanoma in situ of eyelid, including canthus**
D03.10 Melanoma in situ of unspecified eyelid, including canthus HCC
● **D03.11 Melanoma in situ of right eyelid, including canthus** HCC
D03.111 Melanoma in situ of right upper eyelid, including canthus HCC
D03.112 Melanoma in situ of right lower eyelid, including canthus HCC
● **D03.12 Melanoma in situ of left eyelid, including canthus** HCC
D03.121 Melanoma in situ of left upper eyelid, including canthus HCC
D03.122 Melanoma in situ of left lower eyelid, including canthus HCC

● **D03.2 Melanoma in situ of ear and external auricular canal**
D03.20 Melanoma in situ of unspecified ear and external auricular canal HCC
D03.21 Melanoma in situ of right ear and external auricular canal HCC
D03.22 Melanoma in situ of left ear and external auricular canal HCC

● **D03.3 Melanoma in situ of other and unspecified parts of face**
D03.30 Melanoma in situ of unspecified part of face HCC
D03.39 Melanoma in situ of other parts of face HCC

D03.4 Melanoma in situ of scalp and neck HCC

CHAPTER 2 (C00-D49)

● **D03.5 Melanoma in situ of trunk**
  D03.51 Melanoma in situ of anal skin
    Melanoma in situ of anal margin
    Melanoma in situ of perianal skin
  D03.52 Melanoma in situ of breast (skin) (soft tissue)
  D03.59 Melanoma in situ of other part of trunk
● **D03.6 Melanoma in situ of upper limb, including shoulder**
  D03.60 Melanoma in situ of unspecified upper limb, including shoulder
  D03.61 Melanoma in situ of right upper limb, including shoulder
  D03.62 Melanoma in situ of left upper limb, including shoulder
● **D03.7 Melanoma in situ of lower limb, including hip**
  D03.70 Melanoma in situ of unspecified lower limb, including hip
  D03.71 Melanoma in situ of right lower limb, including hip
  D03.72 Melanoma in situ of left lower limb, including hip
D03.8 Melanoma in situ of other sites
  Melanoma in situ of scrotum
  Excludes1 carcinoma in situ of scrotum (D07.61)
D03.9 Melanoma in situ, unspecified

● **D04 Carcinoma in situ of skin**
  Excludes1 erythroplasia of Queyrat (penis) NOS (D07.4)
  melanoma in situ (D03.-)
D04.0 Carcinoma in situ of skin of lip
  ~~**Excludes1** carcinoma in situ of vermilion border of lip (D00.01)~~
  ▶ **Excludes2** carcinoma in situ of vermilion border of lip (D00.01)
● **D04.1 Carcinoma in situ of skin of eyelid, including canthus**
  D04.10 Carcinoma in situ of skin of unspecified eyelid, including canthus
  ● **D04.11 Carcinoma in situ of skin of right eyelid, including canthus**
    D04.111 Carcinoma in situ of skin of right upper eyelid, including canthus
    D04.112 Carcinoma in situ of skin of right lower eyelid, including canthus
  ● **D04.12 Carcinoma in situ of skin of left eyelid, including canthus**
    D04.121 Carcinoma in situ of skin of left upper eyelid, including canthus
    D04.122 Carcinoma in situ of skin of left lower eyelid, including canthus
● **D04.2 Carcinoma in situ of skin of ear and external auricular canal**
  D04.20 Carcinoma in situ of skin of unspecified ear and external auricular canal
  D04.21 Carcinoma in situ of skin of right ear and external auricular canal
  D04.22 Carcinoma in situ of skin of left ear and external auricular canal
● **D04.3 Carcinoma in situ of skin of other and unspecified parts of face**
  D04.30 Carcinoma in situ of skin of unspecified part of face
  D04.39 Carcinoma in situ of skin of other parts of face
D04.4 Carcinoma in situ of skin of scalp and neck
D04.5 Carcinoma in situ of skin of trunk
  Carcinoma in situ of anal margin
  Carcinoma in situ of anal skin
  Carcinoma in situ of perianal skin
  Carcinoma in situ of skin of breast
  Excludes1 carcinoma in situ of anus NOS (D01.3)
  carcinoma in situ of scrotum (D07.61)
  carcinoma in situ of skin of genital organs (D07.-)
● **D04.6 Carcinoma in situ of skin of upper limb, including shoulder**
  D04.60 Carcinoma in situ of skin of unspecified upper limb, including shoulder
  D04.61 Carcinoma in situ of skin of right upper limb, including shoulder
  D04.62 Carcinoma in situ of skin of left upper limb, including shoulder
● **D04.7 Carcinoma in situ of skin of lower limb, including hip**
  D04.70 Carcinoma in situ of skin of unspecified lower limb, including hip
  D04.71 Carcinoma in situ of skin of right lower limb, including hip
  D04.72 Carcinoma in situ of skin of left lower limb, including hip
D04.8 Carcinoma in situ of skin of other sites
D04.9 Carcinoma in situ of skin, unspecified

● **D05 Carcinoma in situ of breast**
  Excludes1 carcinoma in situ of skin of breast (D04.5)
  melanoma in situ of breast (skin) (D03.5)
  Paget's disease of breast or nipple (C50.-)
● **D05.0 Lobular carcinoma in situ of breast**
  D05.00 Lobular carcinoma in situ of unspecified breast
  D05.01 Lobular carcinoma in situ of right breast
  D05.02 Lobular carcinoma in situ of left breast
● **D05.1 Intraductal carcinoma in situ of breast**
  D05.10 Intraductal carcinoma in situ of unspecified breast
  D05.11 Intraductal carcinoma in situ of right breast
  D05.12 Intraductal carcinoma in situ of left breast
● **D05.8 Other specified type of carcinoma in situ of breast**
  D05.80 Other specified type of carcinoma in situ of unspecified breast
  D05.81 Other specified type of carcinoma in situ of right breast
  D05.82 Other specified type of carcinoma in situ of left breast
● **D05.9 Unspecified type of carcinoma in situ of breast**
  D05.90 Unspecified type of carcinoma in situ of unspecified breast
  D05.91 Unspecified type of carcinoma in situ of right breast
  D05.92 Unspecified type of carcinoma in situ of left breast

● **D06 Carcinoma in situ of cervix uteri**
  Includes cervical adenocarcinoma in situ
  cervical intraepithelial glandular neoplasia
  cervical intraepithelial neoplasia III [CIN III]
  severe dysplasia of cervix uteri
  Excludes1 cervical intraepithelial neoplasia II [CIN II] (N87.1)
  cytologic evidence of malignancy of cervix without histologic confirmation (R87.614)
  high grade squamous intraepithelial lesion (HGSIL) of cervix (R87.613)
  melanoma in situ of cervix (D03.5)
  moderate cervical dysplasia (N87.1)
D06.0 Carcinoma in situ of endocervix ♀
D06.1 Carcinoma in situ of exocervix ♀
D06.7 Carcinoma in situ of other parts of cervix ♀
D06.9 Carcinoma in situ of cervix, unspecified ♀

CHAPTER 2 (C00-D49)

● **D07 Carcinoma in situ of other and unspecified genital organs**
Excludes1 melanoma in situ of trunk (D03.5)

D07.0 Carcinoma in situ of endometrium ♀

D07.1 Carcinoma in situ of vulva ♀
Severe dysplasia of vulva
Vulvar intraepithelial neoplasia III [VIN III]
Excludes1 moderate dysplasia of vulva (N90.1)
vulvar intraepithelial neoplasia II [VIN II] (N90.1)

D07.2 Carcinoma in situ of vagina ♀
Severe dysplasia of vagina
Vaginal intraepithelial neoplasia III [VIN III]
Excludes1 moderate dysplasia of vagina (N89.1)
vaginal intraepithelial neoplasia II [VIN II] (N89.1)

● **D07.3 Carcinoma in situ of other and unspecified female genital organs**

D07.30 Carcinoma in situ of unspecified female genital organs ♀

D07.39 Carcinoma in situ of other female genital organs ♀

D07.4 Carcinoma in situ of penis ♂
Erythroplasia of Queyrat NOS

D07.5 Carcinoma in situ of prostate ♂
Prostatic intraepithelial neoplasia III (PIN III)
Severe dysplasia of prostate
Excludes1 dysplasia (mild) (moderate) of prostate (N42.3-)
prostatic intraepithelial neoplasia II [PIN II] (N42.3-)

● **D07.6 Carcinoma in situ of other and unspecified male genital organs**

D07.60 Carcinoma in situ of unspecified male genital organs ♂

D07.61 Carcinoma in situ of scrotum ♂

D07.69 Carcinoma in situ of other male genital organs ♂

● **D09 Carcinoma in situ of other and unspecified sites**
Excludes1 melanoma in situ (D03.-)

D09.0 Carcinoma in situ of bladder

● **D09.1 Carcinoma in situ of other and unspecified urinary organs**

D09.10 Carcinoma in situ of unspecified urinary organ

D09.19 Carcinoma in situ of other urinary organs

● **D09.2 Carcinoma in situ of eye**
Excludes1 carcinoma in situ of skin of eyelid (D04.1-)

D09.20 Carcinoma in situ of unspecified eye

D09.21 Carcinoma in situ of right eye

D09.22 Carcinoma in situ of left eye

D09.3 Carcinoma in situ of thyroid and other endocrine glands
Excludes1 carcinoma in situ of endocrine pancreas (D01.7)
carcinoma in situ of ovary (D07.39)
carcinoma in situ of testis (D07.69)

D09.8 Carcinoma in situ of other specified sites

D09.9 Carcinoma in situ, unspecified

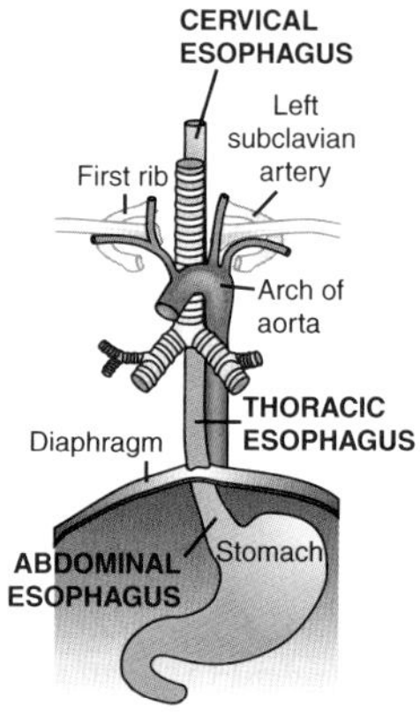

Figure 2-16 The esophagus is the muscular tube that connects the pharynx and the stomach. The 10 inch (25 cm) long esophagus is divided into three parts: **cervical, thoracic,** and **abdominal.**

BENIGN NEOPLASMS, EXCEPT BENIGN NEUROENDOCRINE TUMORS (D10-D36)

● **D10 Benign neoplasm of mouth and pharynx**

D10.0 Benign neoplasm of lip
Benign neoplasm of lip (frenulum) (inner aspect) (mucosa) (vermilion border)
Excludes1 benign neoplasm of skin of lip (D22.0, D23.0)

D10.1 Benign neoplasm of tongue
Benign neoplasm of lingual tonsil

D10.2 Benign neoplasm of floor of mouth

● **D10.3 Benign neoplasm of other and unspecified parts of mouth**

D10.30 Benign neoplasm of unspecified part of mouth

D10.39 Benign neoplasm of other parts of mouth
Benign neoplasm of minor salivary gland NOS
Excludes1 benign odontogenic neoplasms (D16.4-D16.5)
benign neoplasm of mucosa of lip (D10.0)
benign neoplasm of nasopharyngeal surface of soft palate (D10.6)

D10.4 Benign neoplasm of tonsil
Benign neoplasm of tonsil (faucial) (palatine)
Excludes1 benign neoplasm of lingual tonsil (D10.1)
benign neoplasm of pharyngeal tonsil (D10.6)
benign neoplasm of tonsillar fossa (D10.5)
benign neoplasm of tonsillar pillars (D10.5)

D10.5 Benign neoplasm of other parts of oropharynx
Division of pharynx lying between soft palate and upper edge of epiglottis
Benign neoplasm of epiglottis, anterior aspect
Benign neoplasm of tonsillar fossa
Benign neoplasm of tonsillar pillars
Benign neoplasm of vallecula
Excludes1 benign neoplasm of epiglottis NOS (D14.1)
benign neoplasm of epiglottis, suprahyoid portion (D14.1)

D10.6 Benign neoplasm of nasopharynx
Segment of pharynx that lies above soft palate
Benign neoplasm of pharyngeal tonsil
Benign neoplasm of posterior margin of septum and choanae

D10.7 Benign neoplasm of hypopharynx
Segment of pharynx that lies below upper edge of epiglottis and opens into larynx and esophagus

D10.9 Benign neoplasm of pharynx, unspecified

D11 Benign neoplasm of major salivary glands
Excludes1 benign neoplasms of specified minor salivary glands which are classified according to their anatomical location
benign neoplasms of minor salivary glands NOS (D10.39)

D11.0 Benign neoplasm of parotid gland

D11.7 Benign neoplasm of other major salivary glands
Benign neoplasm of sublingual salivary gland
Benign neoplasm of submandibular salivary gland

D11.9 Benign neoplasm of major salivary gland, unspecified

D12 Benign neoplasm of colon, rectum, anus and anal canal
Excludes1 benign carcinoid tumors of the large intestine, and rectum (D3A.02-)
polyp of colon NOS (K63.5)
Coding Clinic: 2017, Q1, P15; 2015, Q2, P14

D12.0 Benign neoplasm of cecum
Benign neoplasm of ileocecal valve

D12.1 Benign neoplasm of appendix
Excludes1 benign carcinoid tumor of the appendix (D3A.020)

D12.2 Benign neoplasm of ascending colon
Coding Clinic: 2018, Q2, P14; 2017, Q1, P15

D12.3 Benign neoplasm of transverse colon
Benign neoplasm of hepatic flexure
Benign neoplasm of splenic flexure
Flexure is a bending in a structure or organ. Note the three flexures illustrated in Figure 2–17. Hepatic = liver, sigmoid = colon, splenic = spleen.
Coding Clinic: 2017, Q1, P16

D12.4 Benign neoplasm of descending colon
Coding Clinic: 2015, Q2, P14

D12.5 Benign neoplasm of sigmoid colon

D12.6 Benign neoplasm of colon, unspecified
Adenomatosis of colon
Benign neoplasm of large intestine NOS
Polyposis (hereditary) of colon
Excludes1 inflammatory polyp of colon (K51.4-)
~~polyp of colon NOS (K63.5)~~
Coding Clinic: 2017, Q1, P8-9

D12.7 Benign neoplasm of rectosigmoid junction
Angle where sigmoid colon becomes rectum

D12.8 Benign neoplasm of rectum
Excludes1 benign carcinoid tumor of the rectum (D3A.026)
Coding Clinic: 2018, Q1, P7

D12.9 Benign neoplasm of anus and anal canal
Benign neoplasm of anus NOS
Excludes1 benign neoplasm of anal margin (D22.5, D23.5)
benign neoplasm of anal skin (D22.5, D23.5)
benign neoplasm of perianal skin (D22.5, D23.5)

D13 Benign neoplasm of other and ill-defined parts of digestive system
Excludes1 benign stromal tumors of digestive system (D21.4)

D13.0 Benign neoplasm of esophagus

D13.1 Benign neoplasm of stomach
Excludes1 benign carcinoid tumor of the stomach (D3A.092)

D13.2 Benign neoplasm of duodenum
Excludes1 benign carcinoid tumor of the duodenum (D3A.010)

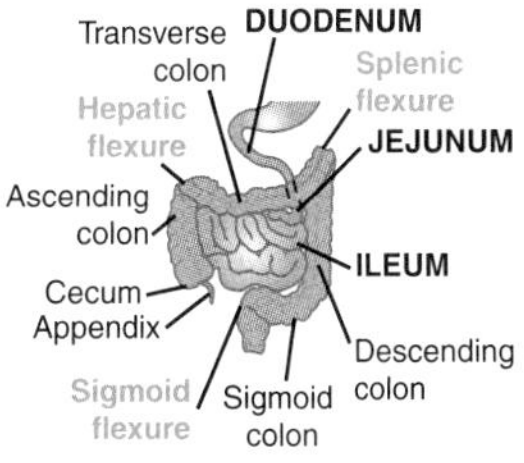

Figure 2-17 Small intestine and colon.

D13.3 Benign neoplasm of other and unspecified parts of small intestine
Excludes1 benign carcinoid tumors of the small intestine (D3A.01-)
benign neoplasm of ileocecal valve (D12.0)

D13.30 Benign neoplasm of unspecified part of small intestine

D13.39 Benign neoplasm of other parts of small intestine

D13.4 Benign neoplasm of liver
Benign neoplasm of intrahepatic bile ducts

D13.5 Benign neoplasm of extrahepatic bile ducts
Extensions of common hepatic bile duct (tube that collects bile from liver)

D13.6 Benign neoplasm of pancreas
Excludes1 benign neoplasm of endocrine pancreas (D13.7)

D13.7 Benign neoplasm of endocrine pancreas
Pancreatic islets: Cells scattered throughout pancreas
Islet cell tumor
Benign neoplasm of islets of Langerhans
Use additional code to identify any functional activity.

D13.9 Benign neoplasm of ill-defined sites within the digestive system
Benign neoplasm of digestive system NOS
Benign neoplasm of intestine NOS
Benign neoplasm of spleen

D14 Benign neoplasm of middle ear and respiratory system

D14.0 Benign neoplasm of middle ear, nasal cavity and accessory sinuses
Benign neoplasm of cartilage of nose
Excludes1 benign neoplasm of auricular canal (external) (D22.2-, D23.2-)
benign neoplasm of bone of ear (D16.4)
benign neoplasm of bone of nose (D16.4)
benign neoplasm of cartilage of ear (D21.0)
benign neoplasm of ear (external) (skin) (D22.2-, D23.2-)
benign neoplasm of nose NOS (D36.7)
benign neoplasm of skin of nose (D22.39, D23.39)
benign neoplasm of olfactory bulb (D33.3)
benign neoplasm of posterior margin of septum and choanae (D10.6)
polyp of accessory sinus (J33.8)
polyp of ear (middle) (H74.4)
polyp of nasal (cavity) (J33.-)

D14.1 Benign neoplasm of larynx
Adenomatous polyp of larynx
Benign neoplasm of epiglottis (suprahyoid portion)
Horseshoe-shaped bone in anterior midline of neck between chin and thyroid cartilage
Excludes1 benign neoplasm of epiglottis, anterior aspect (D10.5)
polyp (nonadenomatous) of vocal cord or larynx (J38.1)

D14.2 Benign neoplasm of trachea

● **D14.3 Benign neoplasm of bronchus and lung**

Excludes1 benign carcinoid tumor of the bronchus and lung (D3A.090)

D14.30 Benign neoplasm of unspecified bronchus and lung

D14.31 Benign neoplasm of right bronchus and lung

D14.32 Benign neoplasm of left bronchus and lung

D14.4 Benign neoplasm of respiratory system, unspecified

● **D15 Benign neoplasm of other and unspecified intrathoracic organs**

Excludes1 benign neoplasm of mesothelial tissue (D19.-)

D15.0 Benign neoplasm of thymus

Excludes1 benign carcinoid tumor of the thymus (D3A.091)

D15.1 Benign neoplasm of heart

Excludes1 benign neoplasm of great vessels (D21.3)

D15.2 Benign neoplasm of mediastinum

D15.7 Benign neoplasm of other specified intrathoracic organs

D15.9 Benign neoplasm of intrathoracic organ, unspecified

● **D16 Benign neoplasm of bone and articular cartilage**

Excludes1 benign neoplasm of connective tissue of ear (D21.0)
benign neoplasm of connective tissue of eyelid (D21.0)
benign neoplasm of connective tissue of larynx (D14.1)
benign neoplasm of connective tissue of nose (D14.0)
benign neoplasm of synovia (D21.-)

● **D16.0 Benign neoplasm of scapula and long bones of upper limb**

D16.00 Benign neoplasm of scapula and long bones of unspecified upper limb

D16.01 Benign neoplasm of scapula and long bones of right upper limb

D16.02 Benign neoplasm of scapula and long bones of left upper limb

● **D16.1 Benign neoplasm of short bones of upper limb**

D16.10 Benign neoplasm of short bones of unspecified upper limb

D16.11 Benign neoplasm of short bones of right upper limb

D16.12 Benign neoplasm of short bones of left upper limb

● **D16.2 Benign neoplasm of long bones of lower limb**

D16.20 Benign neoplasm of long bones of unspecified lower limb

D16.21 Benign neoplasm of long bones of right lower limb

D16.22 Benign neoplasm of long bones of left lower limb

● **D16.3 Benign neoplasm of short bones of lower limb**

D16.30 Benign neoplasm of short bones of unspecified lower limb

D16.31 Benign neoplasm of short bones of right lower limb

D16.32 Benign neoplasm of short bones of left lower limb

D16.4 Benign neoplasm of bones of skull and face
Benign neoplasm of maxilla (superior)
Benign neoplasm of orbital bone
Cavity or socket of skull in which eye and its appendages are located
Keratocyst of maxilla
Keratocystic odontogenic tumor of maxilla

Excludes2 benign neoplasm of lower jaw bone (D16.5)

D16.5 Benign neoplasm of lower jaw bone
Keratocyst of mandible
Keratocystic odontogenic tumor of mandible

D16.6 Benign neoplasm of vertebral column

Excludes1 benign neoplasm of sacrum and coccyx (D16.8)

D16.7 Benign neoplasm of ribs, sternum and clavicle

D16.8 Benign neoplasm of pelvic bones, sacrum and coccyx

D16.9 Benign neoplasm of bone and articular cartilage, unspecified

● **D17 Benign lipomatous neoplasm**
Slow-growing benign tumors (rubbery masses) of mature fat cells enclosed in a thin fibrous capsule

D17.0 Benign lipomatous neoplasm of skin and subcutaneous tissue of head, face and neck

D17.1 Benign lipomatous neoplasm of skin and subcutaneous tissue of trunk

● **D17.2 Benign lipomatous neoplasm of skin and subcutaneous tissue of limb**

D17.20 Benign lipomatous neoplasm of skin and subcutaneous tissue of unspecified limb

D17.21 Benign lipomatous neoplasm of skin and subcutaneous tissue of right arm

D17.22 Benign lipomatous neoplasm of skin and subcutaneous tissue of left arm

D17.23 Benign lipomatous neoplasm of skin and subcutaneous tissue of right leg

D17.24 Benign lipomatous neoplasm of skin and subcutaneous tissue of left leg

● **D17.3 Benign lipomatous neoplasm of skin and subcutaneous tissue of other and unspecified sites**

D17.30 Benign lipomatous neoplasm of skin and subcutaneous tissue of unspecified sites

D17.39 Benign lipomatous neoplasm of skin and subcutaneous tissue of other sites

D17.4 Benign lipomatous neoplasm of intrathoracic organs

D17.5 Benign lipomatous neoplasm of intra-abdominal organs

Excludes1 benign lipomatous neoplasm of peritoneum and retroperitoneum (D17.79)

D17.6 Benign lipomatous neoplasm of spermatic cord ♂

● **D17.7 Benign lipomatous neoplasm of other sites**

D17.71 Benign lipomatous neoplasm of kidney

D17.72 Benign lipomatous neoplasm of other genitourinary organ

D17.79 Benign lipomatous neoplasm of other sites
Benign lipomatous neoplasm of peritoneum
Benign lipomatous neoplasm of retroperitoneum

D17.9 Benign lipomatous neoplasm, unspecified
Lipoma NOS

● **D18 Hemangioma and lymphangioma, any site**

Excludes1 benign neoplasm of glomus jugulare (D35.6)
blue or pigmented nevus (D22.-)
nevus NOS (D22.-)
vascular nevus (Q82.5)

● **D18.0 Hemangioma**
Common type of vascular malformation
Angioma NOS
Cavernous nevus

D18.00 Hemangioma unspecified site

D18.01 Hemangioma of skin and subcutaneous tissue

D18.02 Hemangioma of intracranial structures (HCC)

D18.03 Hemangioma of intra-abdominal structures

D18.09 Hemangioma of other sites

D18.1 Lymphangioma, any site
Coding Clinic: 2018, Q2, P13

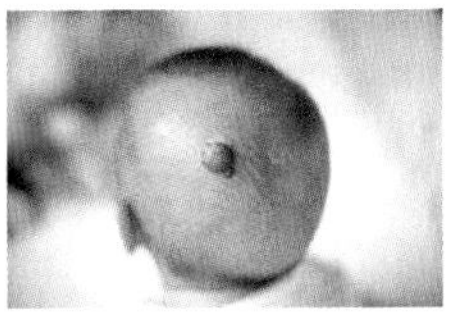

Figure 2-18 Hemangioma of skin and subcutaneous tissue. (Getty Image)

Item 2-10 Hemangiomas are abnormally dense collections of dilated capillaries that occur on the skin or in internal organs. Hemangiomas are both deep and superficial and undergo a rapid growth phase when the size increases rapidly, followed by a rest phase, in which the tumor changes very little, followed by an involutional phase in which the tumor begins to and can disappear altogether. **Lymphangiomas** or cystic hygroma are benign collections of overgrown lymph vessels and, although rare, may occur anywhere but most commonly on the head and neck of children and infants. Visceral organs, lungs, and gastrointestinal tract may also be involved.

● D19 **Benign neoplasm of mesothelial tissue**
Mesothelial tissue is the membrane lining several body cavities
D19.Ø **Benign neoplasm of mesothelial tissue of pleura**
D19.1 **Benign neoplasm of mesothelial tissue of peritoneum**
D19.7 **Benign neoplasm of mesothelial tissue of other sites**
D19.9 **Benign neoplasm of mesothelial tissue, unspecified**
Benign mesothelioma NOS

● D2Ø **Benign neoplasm of soft tissue of retroperitoneum and peritoneum**
Excludes1 benign lipomatous neoplasm of peritoneum and retroperitoneum (D17.79)
benign neoplasm of mesothelial tissue (D19.-)
D2Ø.Ø **Benign neoplasm of soft tissue of retroperitoneum**
D2Ø.1 **Benign neoplasm of soft tissue of peritoneum**

● D21 **Other benign neoplasms of connective and other soft tissue**
Includes benign neoplasm of blood vessel
benign neoplasm of bursa
benign neoplasm of cartilage
benign neoplasm of fascia
benign neoplasm of fat
benign neoplasm of ligament, except uterine
benign neoplasm of lymphatic channel
benign neoplasm of muscle
benign neoplasm of synovia
benign neoplasm of tendon (sheath)
benign stromal tumors
Excludes1 benign neoplasm of articular cartilage (D16.-)
benign neoplasm of cartilage of larynx (D14.1)
benign neoplasm of cartilage of nose (D14.Ø)
benign neoplasm of connective tissue of breast (D24.-)
benign neoplasm of peripheral nerves and autonomic nervous system (D36.1-)
benign neoplasm of peritoneum (D2Ø.1)
benign neoplasm of retroperitoneum (D2Ø.Ø)
benign neoplasm of uterine ligament, any (D28.2)
benign neoplasm of vascular tissue (D18.-)
hemangioma (D18.Ø-)
lipomatous neoplasm (D17.-)
lymphangioma (D18.1)
uterine leiomyoma (D25.-)
D21.Ø **Benign neoplasm of connective and other soft tissue of head, face and neck**
Benign neoplasm of connective tissue of ear
Benign neoplasm of connective tissue of eyelid
Excludes1 benign neoplasm of connective tissue of orbit (D31.6-)
● D21.1 **Benign neoplasm of connective and other soft tissue of upper limb, including shoulder**
D21.1Ø **Benign neoplasm of connective and other soft tissue of unspecified upper limb, including shoulder**
D21.11 **Benign neoplasm of connective and other soft tissue of right upper limb, including shoulder**
D21.12 **Benign neoplasm of connective and other soft tissue of left upper limb, including shoulder**
● D21.2 **Benign neoplasm of connective and other soft tissue of lower limb, including hip**
D21.2Ø **Benign neoplasm of connective and other soft tissue of unspecified lower limb, including hip**
D21.21 **Benign neoplasm of connective and other soft tissue of right lower limb, including hip**
D21.22 **Benign neoplasm of connective and other soft tissue of left lower limb, including hip**
D21.3 **Benign neoplasm of connective and other soft tissue of thorax**
Benign neoplasm of axilla
Benign neoplasm of diaphragm
Benign neoplasm of great vessels
Excludes1 benign neoplasm of heart (D15.1)
benign neoplasm of mediastinum (D15.2)
benign neoplasm of thymus (D15.Ø)
D21.4 **Benign neoplasm of connective and other soft tissue of abdomen**
Benign stromal tumors of abdomen
D21.5 **Benign neoplasm of connective and other soft tissue of pelvis**
Excludes1 benign neoplasm of any uterine ligament (D28.2)
uterine leiomyoma (D25.-)
D21.6 **Benign neoplasm of connective and other soft tissue of trunk, unspecified**
➡Benign neoplasm of connective and other soft tissue back NOS
D21.9 **Benign neoplasm of connective and other soft tissue, unspecified**

● D22 **Melanocytic nevi**
Includes atypical nevus
blue hairy pigmented nevus
nevus NOS
D22.Ø **Melanocytic nevi of lip**
Skin lesions composed of nests of nevus cells with macules/papules
● D22.1 **Melanocytic nevi of eyelid, including canthus**
D22.1Ø **Melanocytic nevi of unspecified eyelid, including canthus**
● D22.11 **Melanocytic nevi of right eyelid, including canthus**
D22.111 **Melanocytic nevi of right upper eyelid, including canthus**
D22.112 **Melanocytic nevi of right lower eyelid, including canthus**
● D22.12 **Melanocytic nevi of left eyelid, including canthus**
D22.121 **Melanocytic nevi of left upper eyelid, including canthus**
D22.122 **Melanocytic nevi of left lower eyelid, including canthus**
● D22.2 **Melanocytic nevi of ear and external auricular canal**
D22.2Ø **Melanocytic nevi of unspecified ear and external auricular canal**
D22.21 **Melanocytic nevi of right ear and external auricular canal**
D22.22 **Melanocytic nevi of left ear and external auricular canal**

CHAPTER 2 (CØØ-D49)

● D22.3 Melanocytic nevi of other and unspecified parts of face
D22.30 Melanocytic nevi of unspecified part of face
D22.39 Melanocytic nevi of other parts of face
D22.4 Melanocytic nevi of scalp and neck
D22.5 Melanocytic nevi of trunk
Melanocytic nevi of anal margin
Melanocytic nevi of anal skin
Melanocytic nevi of perianal skin
Melanocytic nevi of skin of breast
● D22.6 Melanocytic nevi of upper limb, including shoulder
D22.60 Melanocytic nevi of unspecified upper limb, including shoulder
D22.61 Melanocytic nevi of right upper limb, including shoulder
D22.62 Melanocytic nevi of left upper limb, including shoulder
● D22.7 Melanocytic nevi of lower limb, including hip
D22.70 Melanocytic nevi of unspecified lower limb, including hip
D22.71 Melanocytic nevi of right lower limb, including hip
D22.72 Melanocytic nevi of left lower limb, including hip
D22.9 Melanocytic nevi, unspecified

● D23 Other benign neoplasms of skin
Includes benign neoplasm of hair follicles
benign neoplasm of sebaceous glands
benign neoplasm of sweat glands
Excludes1 benign lipomatous neoplasms of skin (D17.0-D17.3)
~~melanocytic nevi (D22.-)~~
▶ **Excludes2** melanocytic nevi (D22.-)
D23.0 Other benign neoplasm of skin of lip
Excludes1 benign neoplasm of vermilion border of lip (D10.0)
● D23.1 Other benign neoplasm of skin of eyelid, including canthus
D23.10 Other benign neoplasm of skin unspecified of eyelid, including canthus
● D23.11 Other benign neoplasm of skin of right eyelid, including canthus
D23.111 Other benign neoplasm of skin of right upper eyelid, including canthus
D23.112 Other benign neoplasm of skin of right lower eyelid, including canthus
● D23.12 Other benign neoplasm of skin of left eyelid, including canthus
D23.121 Other benign neoplasm of skin of left upper eyelid, including canthus
D23.122 Other benign neoplasm of skin of left lower eyelid, including canthus
● D23.2 Other benign neoplasm of skin of ear and external auricular canal
D23.20 Other benign neoplasm of skin of unspecified ear and external auricular canal
D23.21 Other benign neoplasm of skin of right ear and external auricular canal
D23.22 Other benign neoplasm of skin of left ear and external auricular canal
● D23.3 Other benign neoplasm of skin of other and unspecified parts of face
D23.30 Other benign neoplasm of skin of unspecified part of face
D23.39 Other benign neoplasm of skin of other parts of face
D23.4 Other benign neoplasm of skin of scalp and neck
D23.5 Other benign neoplasm of skin of trunk
Other benign neoplasm of anal margin
Other benign neoplasm of anal skin
Other benign neoplasm of perianal skin
Other benign neoplasm of skin of breast
Excludes1 benign neoplasm of anus NOS (D12.9)
● D23.6 Other benign neoplasm of skin of upper limb, including shoulder
D23.60 Other benign neoplasm of skin of unspecified upper limb, including shoulder
D23.61 Other benign neoplasm of skin of right upper limb, including shoulder
D23.62 Other benign neoplasm of skin of left upper limb, including shoulder
● D23.7 Other benign neoplasm of skin of lower limb, including hip
D23.70 Other benign neoplasm of skin of unspecified lower limb, including hip
D23.71 Other benign neoplasm of skin of right lower limb, including hip
D23.72 Other benign neoplasm of skin of left lower limb, including hip
D23.9 Other benign neoplasm of skin, unspecified

● D24 Benign neoplasm of breast
Includes benign neoplasm of connective tissue of breast
benign neoplasm of soft parts of breast
fibroadenoma of breast
Excludes2 adenofibrosis of breast (N60.2)
benign cyst of breast (N60.-)
benign mammary dysplasia (N60.-)
benign neoplasm of skin of breast (D22.5, D23.5)
fibrocystic disease of breast (N60.-)
D24.1 Benign neoplasm of right breast
Coding Clinic: 2017, Q1, P5
D24.2 Benign neoplasm of left breast
D24.9 Benign neoplasm of unspecified breast

● D25 Leiomyoma of uterus
Benign tumors or nodules of the uterine wall
Includes uterine fibroid
uterine fibromyoma
uterine myoma
D25.0 Submucous leiomyoma of uterus ♀
D25.1 Intramural leiomyoma of uterus ♀
Interstitial leiomyoma of uterus
D25.2 Subserosal leiomyoma of uterus ♀
Subperitoneal leiomyoma of uterus
D25.9 Leiomyoma of uterus, unspecified ♀

● D26 Other benign neoplasms of uterus
D26.0 Other benign neoplasm of cervix uteri ♀
D26.1 Other benign neoplasm of corpus uteri ♀
D26.7 Other benign neoplasm of other parts of uterus ♀
D26.9 Other benign neoplasm of uterus, unspecified ♀

● D27 Benign neoplasm of ovary
Use additional code to identify any functional activity.
Excludes2 corpus albicans cyst (N83.2-)
corpus luteum cyst (N83.1-)
endometrial cyst (N80.1)
follicular (atretic) cyst (N83.0-)
graafian follicle cyst (N83.0-)
ovarian cyst NEC (N83.2-)
ovarian retention cyst (N83.2-)
D27.0 Benign neoplasm of right ovary ♀
D27.1 Benign neoplasm of left ovary ♀
D27.9 Benign neoplasm of unspecified ovary ♀
Ovarian teratoma

Item 2-11 Teratoma: terat = monster, oma = mass, tumor. Alternate terms: dermoid cyst of the ovary, ovarian teratoma. Teratomas are neoplasms and arise from germ cells (ovaries in female and testes in male) and can be benign or malignant. Teratomas have been known to contain hair, nails, and teeth, giving them a bizarre ("monster") appearance.

● **D28 Benign neoplasm of other and unspecified female genital organs**
Includes adenomatous polyp
benign neoplasm of skin of female genital organs
benign teratoma
Excludes1 epoophoron cyst (Q5Ø.5)
fimbrial cyst (Q5Ø.4)
Gartner's duct cyst (Q52.4)
parovarian cyst (Q5Ø.5)

D28.Ø **Benign neoplasm of vulva** ♀
D28.1 **Benign neoplasm of vagina** ♀
D28.2 **Benign neoplasm of uterine tubes and ligaments** ♀
Benign neoplasm of fallopian tube
Benign neoplasm of uterine ligament (broad) (round)
D28.7 **Benign neoplasm of other specified female genital organs** ♀
D28.9 **Benign neoplasm of female genital organ, unspecified** ♀

● **D29 Benign neoplasm of male genital organs**
Includes benign neoplasm of skin of male genital organs

D29.Ø **Benign neoplasm of penis** ♂
D29.1 **Benign neoplasm of prostate** ♂
Excludes1 enlarged prostate (N4Ø.-)
● D29.2 **Benign neoplasm of testis**
Use additional code to identify any functional activity.
D29.20 **Benign neoplasm of unspecified testis** ♂
D29.21 **Benign neoplasm of right testis** ♂
D29.22 **Benign neoplasm of left testis** ♂
● D29.3 **Benign neoplasm of epididymis**
D29.30 **Benign neoplasm of unspecified epididymis** ♂
D29.31 **Benign neoplasm of right epididymis** ♂
D29.32 **Benign neoplasm of left epididymis** ♂
D29.4 **Benign neoplasm of scrotum** ♂
Benign neoplasm of skin of scrotum
D29.8 **Benign neoplasm of other specified male genital organs** ♂
Benign neoplasm of seminal vesicle
Benign neoplasm of spermatic cord
Benign neoplasm of tunica vaginalis
D29.9 **Benign neoplasm of male genital organ, unspecified** ♂

● **D3Ø Benign neoplasm of urinary organs**
● D3Ø.Ø **Benign neoplasm of kidney**
Excludes1 benign carcinoid tumor of the kidney (D3A.Ø93)
benign neoplasm of renal calyces (D3Ø.1-)
benign neoplasm of renal pelvis (D3Ø.1-)
D3Ø.ØØ **Benign neoplasm of unspecified kidney**
D3Ø.Ø1 **Benign neoplasm of right kidney**
D3Ø.Ø2 **Benign neoplasm of left kidney**
● D3Ø.1 **Benign neoplasm of renal pelvis**
D3Ø.1Ø **Benign neoplasm of unspecified renal pelvis**
D3Ø.11 **Benign neoplasm of right renal pelvis**
D3Ø.12 **Benign neoplasm of left renal pelvis**
● D3Ø.2 **Benign neoplasm of ureter**
Excludes1 benign neoplasm of ureteric orifice of bladder (D3Ø.3)
D3Ø.2Ø **Benign neoplasm of unspecified ureter**
D3Ø.21 **Benign neoplasm of right ureter**
D3Ø.22 **Benign neoplasm of left ureter**
D3Ø.3 **Benign neoplasm of bladder**
Benign neoplasm of ureteric orifice of bladder
Benign neoplasm of urethral orifice of bladder
D3Ø.4 **Benign neoplasm of urethra**
Excludes1 benign neoplasm of urethral orifice of bladder (D3Ø.3)
D3Ø.8 **Benign neoplasm of other specified urinary organs**
Benign neoplasm of paraurethral glands
D3Ø.9 **Benign neoplasm of urinary organ, unspecified**
Benign neoplasm of urinary system NOS

● **D31 Benign neoplasm of eye and adnexa**
Excludes1 benign neoplasm of connective tissue of eyelid (D21.Ø)
benign neoplasm of optic nerve (D33.3)
benign neoplasm of skin of eyelid (D22.1-, D23.1-)

● D31.Ø **Benign neoplasm of conjunctiva**
D31.ØØ **Benign neoplasm of unspecified conjunctiva**
D31.Ø1 **Benign neoplasm of right conjunctiva**
D31.Ø2 **Benign neoplasm of left conjunctiva**
● D31.1 **Benign neoplasm of cornea**
D31.1Ø **Benign neoplasm of unspecified cornea**
D31.11 **Benign neoplasm of right cornea**
D31.12 **Benign neoplasm of left cornea**
● D31.2 **Benign neoplasm of retina**
Excludes1 dark area on retina (D49.81)
hemangioma of retina (D49.81)
neoplasm of unspecified behavior of retina and choroid (D49.81)
retinal freckle (D49.81)
D31.2Ø **Benign neoplasm of unspecified retina**
D31.21 **Benign neoplasm of right retina**
D31.22 **Benign neoplasm of left retina**
● D31.3 **Benign neoplasm of choroid**
D31.3Ø **Benign neoplasm of unspecified choroid**
D31.31 **Benign neoplasm of right choroid**
D31.32 **Benign neoplasm of left choroid**
● D31.4 **Benign neoplasm of ciliary body**
D31.4Ø **Benign neoplasm of unspecified ciliary body**
D31.41 **Benign neoplasm of right ciliary body**
D31.42 **Benign neoplasm of left ciliary body**
● D31.5 **Benign neoplasm of lacrimal gland and duct**
Benign neoplasm of lacrimal sac
Benign neoplasm of nasolacrimal duct
D31.5Ø **Benign neoplasm of unspecified lacrimal gland and duct**
D31.51 **Benign neoplasm of right lacrimal gland and duct**
D31.52 **Benign neoplasm of left lacrimal gland and duct**
● D31.6 **Benign neoplasm of unspecified site of orbit**
Benign neoplasm of connective tissue of orbit
Benign neoplasm of extraocular muscle
Benign neoplasm of peripheral nerves of orbit
Benign neoplasm of retrobulbar tissue
Benign neoplasm of retro-ocular tissue
Excludes1 benign neoplasm of orbital bone (D16.4)
D31.6Ø **Benign neoplasm of unspecified site of unspecified orbit**
D31.61 **Benign neoplasm of unspecified site of right orbit**
D31.62 **Benign neoplasm of unspecified site of left orbit**
● D31.9 **Benign neoplasm of unspecified part of eye**
Benign neoplasm of eyeball
D31.9Ø **Benign neoplasm of unspecified part of unspecified eye**
D31.91 **Benign neoplasm of unspecified part of right eye**
D31.92 **Benign neoplasm of unspecified part of left eye**

CHAPTER 2 (CØØ-D49)

D32 Benign neoplasm of meninges

D32.0 Benign neoplasm of cerebral meninges

D32.1 Benign neoplasm of spinal meninges

D32.9 Benign neoplasm of meninges, unspecified
Meningioma NOS

D33 Benign neoplasm of brain and other parts of central nervous system

Excludes1 angioma (D18.0-)
benign neoplasm of meninges (D32.-)
benign neoplasm of peripheral nerves and autonomic nervous system (D36.1-)
hemangioma (D18.0-)
neurofibromatosis (Q85.0-)
retro-ocular benign neoplasm (D31.6-)

D33.0 Benign neoplasm of brain, supratentorial
Benign neoplasm of cerebral ventricle
Benign neoplasm of cerebrum
Benign neoplasm of frontal lobe
Benign neoplasm of occipital lobe
Benign neoplasm of parietal lobe
Benign neoplasm of temporal lobe

Excludes1 benign neoplasm of fourth ventricle (D33.1)

D33.1 Benign neoplasm of brain, infratentorial
Benign neoplasm of brain stem
Benign neoplasm of cerebellum
Benign neoplasm of fourth ventricle

D33.2 Benign neoplasm of brain, unspecified

D33.3 Benign neoplasm of cranial nerves
Benign neoplasm of olfactory bulb

D33.4 Benign neoplasm of spinal cord

D33.7 Benign neoplasm of other specified parts of central nervous system

D33.9 Benign neoplasm of central nervous system, unspecified
Benign neoplasm of nervous system (central) NOS

D34 Benign neoplasm of thyroid gland
Use additional code to identify any functional activity.

D35 Benign neoplasm of other and unspecified endocrine glands
Use additional code to identify any functional activity.

Excludes1 benign neoplasm of endocrine pancreas (D13.7)
benign neoplasm of ovary (D27.-)
benign neoplasm of testis (D29.2.-)
benign neoplasm of thymus (D15.0)

D35.0 Benign neoplasm of adrenal gland

D35.00 Benign neoplasm of unspecified adrenal gland

D35.01 Benign neoplasm of right adrenal gland

D35.02 Benign neoplasm of left adrenal gland

D35.1 Benign neoplasm of parathyroid gland

D35.2 Benign neoplasm of pituitary gland

D35.3 Benign neoplasm of craniopharyngeal duct

D35.4 Benign neoplasm of pineal gland

D35.5 Benign neoplasm of carotid body

D35.6 Benign neoplasm of aortic body and other paraganglia
Benign tumor of glomus jugulare

D35.7 Benign neoplasm of other specified endocrine glands

D35.9 Benign neoplasm of endocrine gland, unspecified
Benign neoplasm of unspecified endocrine gland

D36 Benign neoplasm of other and unspecified sites

D36.0 Benign neoplasm of lymph nodes

Excludes1 lymphangioma (D18.1)

D36.1 Benign neoplasm of peripheral nerves and autonomic nervous system

Excludes1 benign neoplasm of peripheral nerves of orbit (D31.6-)
neurofibromatosis (Q85.0-)

D36.10 Benign neoplasm of peripheral nerves and autonomic nervous system, unspecified

D36.11 Benign neoplasm of peripheral nerves and autonomic nervous system of face, head, and neck

D36.12 Benign neoplasm of peripheral nerves and autonomic nervous system, upper limb, including shoulder

D36.13 Benign neoplasm of peripheral nerves and autonomic nervous system of lower limb, including hip

D36.14 Benign neoplasm of peripheral nerves and autonomic nervous system of thorax

D36.15 Benign neoplasm of peripheral nerves and autonomic nervous system of abdomen

D36.16 Benign neoplasm of peripheral nerves and autonomic nervous system of pelvis

D36.17 Benign neoplasm of peripheral nerves and autonomic nervous system of trunk, unspecified

D36.7 Benign neoplasm of other specified sites
Benign neoplasm of nose NOS
Benign neoplasm of back NOS

D36.9 Benign neoplasm, unspecified site

BENIGN NEUROENDOCRINE TUMORS (D3A)

D3A Benign neuroendocrine tumors
Code also any associated multiple endocrine neoplasia [MEN] syndromes (E31.2-)
Use additional code to identify any associated endocrine syndrome, such as:
carcinoid syndrome (E34.0)

Excludes2 benign pancreatic islet cell tumors (D13.7)

D3A.0 Benign carcinoid tumors

D3A.00 Benign carcinoid tumor of unspecified site
Carcinoid tumor NOS

D3A.01 Benign carcinoid tumors of the small intestine

D3A.010 Benign carcinoid tumor of the duodenum

D3A.011 Benign carcinoid tumor of the jejunum

D3A.012 Benign carcinoid tumor of the ileum

D3A.019 Benign carcinoid tumor of the small intestine, unspecified portion

D3A.02 Benign carcinoid tumors of the appendix, large intestine, and rectum

D3A.020 Benign carcinoid tumor of the appendix

D3A.021 Benign carcinoid tumor of the cecum

D3A.022 Benign carcinoid tumor of the ascending colon

D3A.023 Benign carcinoid tumor of the transverse colon

D3A.024 Benign carcinoid tumor of the descending colon

D3A.025 Benign carcinoid tumor of the sigmoid colon

D3A.026 Benign carcinoid tumor of the rectum

D3A.029 Benign carcinoid tumor of the large intestine, unspecified portion
Benign carcinoid tumor of the colon NOS

● D3A.09 **Benign carcinoid tumors of other sites**
D3A.090 **Benign carcinoid tumor of the bronchus and lung**
D3A.091 **Benign carcinoid tumor of the thymus**
D3A.092 **Benign carcinoid tumor of the stomach**
D3A.093 **Benign carcinoid tumor of the kidney**
D3A.094 **Benign carcinoid tumor of the foregut, unspecified**
D3A.095 **Benign carcinoid tumor of the midgut, unspecified**
D3A.096 **Benign carcinoid tumor of the hindgut, unspecified**
D3A.098 **Benign carcinoid tumors of other sites**
D3A.8 **Other benign neuroendocrine tumors**
Neuroendocrine tumor NOS

NEOPLASMS OF UNCERTAIN BEHAVIOR, POLYCYTHEMIA VERA AND MYELODYSPLASTIC SYNDROMES (D37-D48)

Note: Categories D37-D44, and D48 classify by site neoplasms of uncertain behavior, i.e., histologic confirmation whether the neoplasm is malignant or benign cannot be made.
Excludes1 neoplasms of unspecified behavior (D49.-)

● D37 **Neoplasm of uncertain behavior of oral cavity and digestive organs**
Excludes1 stromal tumors of uncertain behavior of digestive system (D48.1)

● D37.0 **Neoplasm of uncertain behavior of lip, oral cavity and pharynx**
Excludes1 neoplasm of uncertain behavior of aryepiglottic fold or interarytenoid fold, laryngeal aspect (D38.0)
neoplasm of uncertain behavior of epiglottis NOS (D38.0)
neoplasm of uncertain behavior of skin of lip (D48.5)
neoplasm of uncertain behavior of suprahyoid portion of epiglottis (D38.0)

D37.01 **Neoplasm of uncertain behavior of lip**
Neoplasm of uncertain behavior of vermilion border of lip
D37.02 **Neoplasm of uncertain behavior of tongue**
● D37.03 **Neoplasm of uncertain behavior of the major salivary glands**
D37.030 **Neoplasm of uncertain behavior of the parotid salivary glands**
D37.031 **Neoplasm of uncertain behavior of the sublingual salivary glands**
D37.032 **Neoplasm of uncertain behavior of the submandibular salivary glands**
D37.039 **Neoplasm of uncertain behavior of the major salivary glands, unspecified**

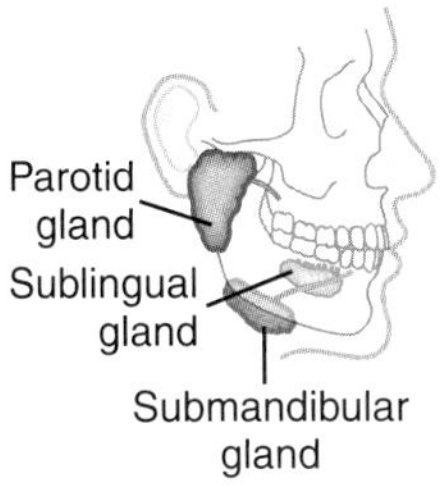

Figure 2-19 Major salivary glands.

D37.04 **Neoplasm of uncertain behavior of the minor salivary glands**
Neoplasm of uncertain behavior of submucosal salivary glands of lip
Neoplasm of uncertain behavior of submucosal salivary glands of cheek
Neoplasm of uncertain behavior of submucosal salivary glands of hard palate
Neoplasm of uncertain behavior of submucosal salivary glands of soft palate
D37.05 **Neoplasm of uncertain behavior of pharynx**
Neoplasm of uncertain behavior of aryepiglottic fold of pharynx NOS
Neoplasm of uncertain behavior of hypopharyngeal aspect of aryepiglottic fold of pharynx
Neoplasm of uncertain behavior of marginal zone of aryepiglottic fold of pharynx
D37.09 **Neoplasm of uncertain behavior of other specified sites of the oral cavity**
D37.1 **Neoplasm of uncertain behavior of stomach**
D37.2 **Neoplasm of uncertain behavior of small intestine**
D37.3 **Neoplasm of uncertain behavior of appendix**
D37.4 **Neoplasm of uncertain behavior of colon**
D37.5 **Neoplasm of uncertain behavior of rectum**
Neoplasm of uncertain behavior of rectosigmoid junction
Rectosigmoid junction: Angle where sigmoid colon becomes rectum
D37.6 **Neoplasm of uncertain behavior of liver, gallbladder and bile ducts**
Neoplasm of uncertain behavior of ampulla of Vater
Ampulla of Vater: Enlarged segment of ducts from liver and pancreas at entry point to small intestine
D37.8 **Neoplasm of uncertain behavior of other specified digestive organs**
Neoplasm of uncertain behavior of anal canal
Neoplasm of uncertain behavior of anal sphincter
Neoplasm of uncertain behavior of anus NOS
Neoplasm of uncertain behavior of esophagus
Neoplasm of uncertain behavior of intestine NOS
Neoplasm of uncertain behavior of pancreas
Excludes1 neoplasm of uncertain behavior of anal margin (D48.5)
neoplasm of uncertain behavior of anal skin (D48.5)
neoplasm of uncertain behavior of perianal skin (D48.5)
D37.9 **Neoplasm of uncertain behavior of digestive organ, unspecified**

CHAPTER 2 (C00-D49)

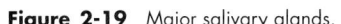

D38 Neoplasm of uncertain behavior of middle ear and respiratory and intrathoracic organs
Excludes1 neoplasm of uncertain behavior of heart (D48.7)
D38.0 Neoplasm of uncertain behavior of larynx
Neoplasm of uncertain behavior of aryepiglottic fold or interarytenoid fold, laryngeal aspect
Neoplasm of uncertain behavior of epiglottis (suprahyoid portion)
Excludes1 neoplasm of uncertain behavior of aryepiglottic fold or interarytenoid fold NOS (D37.05)
neoplasm of uncertain behavior of hypopharyngeal aspect of aryepiglottic fold (D37.05)
neoplasm of uncertain behavior of marginal zone of aryepiglottic fold (D37.05)
D38.1 Neoplasm of uncertain behavior of trachea, bronchus and lung
D38.2 Neoplasm of uncertain behavior of pleura
D38.3 Neoplasm of uncertain behavior of mediastinum
D38.4 Neoplasm of uncertain behavior of thymus
D38.5 Neoplasm of uncertain behavior of other respiratory organs
Neoplasm of uncertain behavior of accessory sinuses
Neoplasm of uncertain behavior of cartilage of nose
Neoplasm of uncertain behavior of middle ear
Neoplasm of uncertain behavior of nasal cavities
Excludes1 neoplasm of uncertain behavior of ear (external) (skin) (D48.5)
neoplasm of uncertain behavior of nose NOS (D48.7)
neoplasm of uncertain behavior of skin of nose (D48.5)
D38.6 Neoplasm of uncertain behavior of respiratory organ, unspecified

D39 Neoplasm of uncertain behavior of female genital organs
D39.0 Neoplasm of uncertain behavior of uterus ♀
D39.1 Neoplasm of uncertain behavior of ovary
Use additional code to identify any functional activity.
D39.10 Neoplasm of uncertain behavior of unspecified ovary ♀
D39.11 Neoplasm of uncertain behavior of right ovary ♀
D39.12 Neoplasm of uncertain behavior of left ovary ♀
D39.2 Neoplasm of uncertain behavior of placenta ♀M
Chorioadenoma destruens
Invasive hydatidiform mole
Malignant hydatidiform mole
Excludes1 hydatidiform mole NOS (O01.9)
D39.8 Neoplasm of uncertain behavior of other specified female genital organs ♀
Neoplasm of uncertain behavior of skin of female genital organs
D39.9 Neoplasm of uncertain behavior of female genital organ, unspecified ♀

D40 Neoplasm of uncertain behavior of male genital organs
D40.0 Neoplasm of uncertain behavior of prostate ♂
D40.1 Neoplasm of uncertain behavior of testis
D40.10 Neoplasm of uncertain behavior of unspecified testis ♂
D40.11 Neoplasm of uncertain behavior of right testis ♂
D40.12 Neoplasm of uncertain behavior of left testis ♂
D40.8 Neoplasm of uncertain behavior of other specified male genital organs ♂
Neoplasm of uncertain behavior of skin of male genital organs
D40.9 Neoplasm of uncertain behavior of male genital organ, unspecified ♂

D41 Neoplasm of uncertain behavior of urinary organs
D41.0 Neoplasm of uncertain behavior of kidney
Excludes1 neoplasm of uncertain behavior of renal pelvis (D41.1-)
D41.00 Neoplasm of uncertain behavior of unspecified kidney
D41.01 Neoplasm of uncertain behavior of right kidney
D41.02 Neoplasm of uncertain behavior of left kidney
D41.1 Neoplasm of uncertain behavior of renal pelvis
D41.10 Neoplasm of uncertain behavior of unspecified renal pelvis
D41.11 Neoplasm of uncertain behavior of right renal pelvis
D41.12 Neoplasm of uncertain behavior of left renal pelvis
D41.2 Neoplasm of uncertain behavior of ureter
D41.20 Neoplasm of uncertain behavior of unspecified ureter
D41.21 Neoplasm of uncertain behavior of right ureter
D41.22 Neoplasm of uncertain behavior of left ureter
D41.3 Neoplasm of uncertain behavior of urethra
D41.4 Neoplasm of uncertain behavior of bladder
D41.8 Neoplasm of uncertain behavior of other specified urinary organs
D41.9 Neoplasm of uncertain behavior of unspecified urinary organ

D42 Neoplasm of uncertain behavior of meninges
D42.0 Neoplasm of uncertain behavior of cerebral meninges HCC
D42.1 Neoplasm of uncertain behavior of spinal meninges HCC
D42.9 Neoplasm of uncertain behavior of meninges, unspecified HCC

D43 Neoplasm of uncertain behavior of brain and central nervous system
Excludes1 neoplasm of uncertain behavior of peripheral nerves and autonomic nervous system (D48.2)
D43.0 Neoplasm of uncertain behavior of brain, supratentorial HCC
Superior to tentorium of cerebellum
Neoplasm of uncertain behavior of cerebral ventricle
Neoplasm of uncertain behavior of cerebrum
Neoplasm of uncertain behavior of frontal lobe
Neoplasm of uncertain behavior of occipital lobe
Neoplasm of uncertain behavior of parietal lobe
Neoplasm of uncertain behavior of temporal lobe
Excludes1 neoplasm of uncertain behavior of fourth ventricle (D43.1)
D43.1 Neoplasm of uncertain behavior of brain, infratentorial HCC
Beneath the tentorium of cerebellum
Neoplasm of uncertain behavior of brain stem
Neoplasm of uncertain behavior of cerebellum
Neoplasm of uncertain behavior of fourth ventricle
D43.2 Neoplasm of uncertain behavior of brain, unspecified HCC
D43.3 Neoplasm of uncertain behavior of cranial nerves HCC
D43.4 Neoplasm of uncertain behavior of spinal cord HCC
D43.8 Neoplasm of uncertain behavior of other specified parts of central nervous system HCC
D43.9 Neoplasm of uncertain behavior of central nervous system, unspecified HCC
Neoplasm of uncertain behavior of nervous system (central) NOS

D44 Neoplasm of uncertain behavior of endocrine glands
Excludes1 multiple endocrine adenomatosis (E31.2-)
multiple endocrine neoplasia (E31.2-)
neoplasm of uncertain behavior of endocrine pancreas (D37.8)
neoplasm of uncertain behavior of ovary (D39.1-)
neoplasm of uncertain behavior of testis (D40.1-)
neoplasm of uncertain behavior of thymus (D38.4)

D44.0 Neoplasm of uncertain behavior of thyroid gland

D44.1 Neoplasm of uncertain behavior of adrenal gland
Use additional code to identify any functional activity.

D44.10 Neoplasm of uncertain behavior of unspecified adrenal gland

D44.11 Neoplasm of uncertain behavior of right adrenal gland

D44.12 Neoplasm of uncertain behavior of left adrenal gland

D44.2 Neoplasm of uncertain behavior of parathyroid gland

D44.3 Neoplasm of uncertain behavior of pituitary gland
Use additional code to identify any functional activity.

D44.4 Neoplasm of uncertain behavior of craniopharyngeal duct

D44.5 Neoplasm of uncertain behavior of pineal gland

D44.6 Neoplasm of uncertain behavior of carotid body

D44.7 Neoplasm of uncertain behavior of aortic body and other paraganglia
Coding Clinic: 2016, Q4, P26

D44.9 Neoplasm of uncertain behavior of unspecified endocrine gland

D45 Polycythemia vera
Excludes1 familial polycythemia (D75.0)
secondary polycythemia (D75.1)
Primary polycythemia. Secondary polycythemia is D75.1. Check your documentation. Polycythemia is caused by too many red blood cells, which increase the thickness of blood (viscosity). This can cause engorgement of the spleen (splenomegaly) with extra RBCs and potential clot formation.

D46 Myelodysplastic syndromes
Use additional code for adverse effect, if applicable, to identify drug (T36-T50 with fifth or sixth character 5)
Excludes2 drug-induced aplastic anemia (D61.1)

D46.0 Refractory anemia without ring sideroblasts, so stated
Refractory anemia without sideroblasts, without excess of blasts

D46.1 Refractory anemia with ring sideroblasts RARS

D46.2 Refractory anemia with excess of blasts [RAEB]
Form of myelodysplasia with increased immature white blood cells (blasts) in bone marrow

D46.20 Refractory anemia with excess of blasts, unspecified RAEB NOS

D46.21 Refractory anemia with excess of blasts 1 RAEB 1
Bone marrow disease which results in insufficient RBCs (anemia) in which level of blasts is less than 10%

D46.22 Refractory anemia with excess of blasts 2 RAEB 2
Bone marrow disease manifested by insufficient numbers of RBCs (anemia) with level of blasts 10-20%

D46.A Refractory cytopenia with multilineage dysplasia

D46.B Refractory cytopenia with multilineage dysplasia and ring sideroblasts
RCMD RS

D46.C Myelodysplastic syndrome with isolated del(5q) chromosomal abnormality
Myelodysplastic syndrome with 5q deletion
5q minus syndrome NOS

D46.4 Refractory anemia, unspecified

D46.Z Other myelodysplastic syndromes
Excludes1 chronic myelomonocytic leukemia (C93.1-)

D46.9 Myelodysplastic syndrome, unspecified
Myelodysplasia NOS

D47 Other neoplasms of uncertain behavior of lymphoid, hematopoietic and related tissue

D47.0 Mast cell neoplasms of uncertain behavior
Excludes1 congenital cutaneous mastocytosis (Q82.2)
histiocytic neoplasms of uncertain behavior (D47.Z9)
malignant mast cell neoplasm (C96.2-)

D47.01 Cutaneous mastocytosis
Diffuse cutaneous mastocytosis
Maculopapular cutaneous mastocytosis
Solitary mastocytoma
Telangiectasia macularis eruptiva perstans
Urticaria pigmentosa
Excludes1 congenital (diffuse) (maculopapular) cutaneous mastocytosis (Q82.2)
congenital urticaria pigmentosa (Q82.2)
extracutaneous mastocytoma (D47.09)

D47.02 Systemic mastocytosis
Indolent systemic mastocytosis
Isolated bone marrow mastocytosis
Smoldering systemic mastocytosis
Systemic mastocytosis, with an associated hematological non-mast cell lineage disease (SM-AHNMD)
Code also if applicable, any associated hematological non-mast cell lineage disease, such as:
acute myeloid leukemia (C92.6-, C92.A-)
chronic myelomonocytic leukemia (C93.1-)
essential thrombocytosis (D47.3)
hypereosinophilic syndrome (D72.1)
myelodysplastic syndrome (D46.9)
myeloproliferative syndrome (D47.1)
non-Hodgkin lymphoma (C82-C85)
plasma cell myeloma (C90.0-)
polycythemia vera (D45)
Excludes1 aggressive systemic mastocytosis (C96.21)
mast cell leukemia (C94.3-)

D47.09 Other mast cell neoplasms of uncertain behavior
Extracutaneous mastocytoma
Mast cell tumor NOS
Mastocytoma NOS
Mastocytosis NOS

D47.1 Chronic myeloproliferative disease
Chronic neutrophilic leukemia
Myeloproliferative disease, unspecified
Excludes1 atypical chronic myeloid leukemia BCR/ABL-negative (C92.2-)
chronic myeloid leukemia BCR/ABL-positive (C92.1-)
myelofibrosis NOS (D75.81)
myelophthisic anemia (D61.82)
myelophthisis (D61.82)
secondary myelofibrosis NOS (D75.81)

D47.2 **Monoclonal gammopathy**
Monoclonal gammopathy of undetermined significance [MGUS]

D47.3 **Essential (hemorrhagic) thrombocythemia**
Essential thrombocytosis
Idiopathic hemorrhagic thrombocythemia

D47.4 **Osteomyelofibrosis**
Chronic idiopathic myelofibrosis
Myelofibrosis (idiopathic) (with myeloid metaplasia)
Myelosclerosis (megakaryocytic) with myeloid metaplasia
Secondary myelofibrosis in myeloproliferative disease
Excludes1 acute myelofibrosis (C94.4-)

D47.Z **Other specified neoplasms of uncertain behavior of lymphoid, hematopoietic and related tissue**

D47.Z1 **Post-transplant lymphoproliferative disorder (PTLD)**
Code first complications of transplanted organs and tissue (T86.-)

D47.Z2 **Castleman disease**
Code also if applicable human herpesvirus 8 infection (B10.89)
Excludes2 Kaposi's sarcoma (C46-)
Coding Clinic: 2016, Q4, P8

D47.Z9 **Other specified neoplasms of uncertain behavior of lymphoid, hematopoietic and related tissue**
Histiocytic tumors of uncertain behavior

D47.9 **Neoplasm of uncertain behavior of lymphoid, hematopoietic and related tissue, unspecified**
Lymphoproliferative disease NOS

D48 **Neoplasm of uncertain behavior of other and unspecified sites**
Excludes1 neurofibromatosis (nonmalignant) (Q85.0-)

D48.0 **Neoplasm of uncertain behavior of bone and articular cartilage**
Excludes1 neoplasm of uncertain behavior of cartilage of ear (D48.1)
neoplasm of uncertain behavior of cartilage of larynx (D38.0)
neoplasm of uncertain behavior of cartilage of nose (D38.5)
neoplasm of uncertain behavior of connective tissue of eyelid (D48.1)
neoplasm of uncertain behavior of synovia (D48.1)

D48.1 **Neoplasm of uncertain behavior of connective and other soft tissue**
Neoplasm of uncertain behavior of connective tissue of ear
Neoplasm of uncertain behavior of connective tissue of eyelid
Stromal tumors of uncertain behavior of digestive system
Excludes1 neoplasm of uncertain behavior of articular cartilage (D48.0)
neoplasm of uncertain behavior of cartilage of larynx (D38.0)
neoplasm of uncertain behavior of cartilage of nose (D38.5)
neoplasm of uncertain behavior of connective tissue of breast (D48.6-)

D48.2 **Neoplasm of uncertain behavior of peripheral nerves and autonomic nervous system**
Excludes1 neoplasm of uncertain behavior of peripheral nerves of orbit (D48.7)

D48.3 **Neoplasm of uncertain behavior of retroperitoneum**

D48.4 **Neoplasm of uncertain behavior of peritoneum**

D48.5 **Neoplasm of uncertain behavior of skin**
Neoplasm of uncertain behavior of anal margin
Neoplasm of uncertain behavior of anal skin
Neoplasm of uncertain behavior of perianal skin
Neoplasm of uncertain behavior of skin of breast
Excludes1 neoplasm of uncertain behavior of anus NOS (D37.8)
neoplasm of uncertain behavior of skin of genital organs (D39.8, D40.8)
neoplasm of uncertain behavior of vermilion border of lip (D37.0)

D48.6 **Neoplasm of uncertain behavior of breast**
Neoplasm of uncertain behavior of connective tissue of breast
Cystosarcoma phyllodes
Excludes1 neoplasm of uncertain behavior of skin of breast (D48.5)

D48.60 **Neoplasm of uncertain behavior of unspecified breast**

D48.61 **Neoplasm of uncertain behavior of right breast**

D48.62 **Neoplasm of uncertain behavior of left breast**

D48.7 **Neoplasm of uncertain behavior of other specified sites**
Neoplasm of uncertain behavior of eye
Neoplasm of uncertain behavior of heart
Neoplasm of uncertain behavior of peripheral nerves of orbit
Excludes1 neoplasm of uncertain behavior of connective tissue (D48.1)
neoplasm of uncertain behavior of skin of eyelid (D48.5)

D48.9 **Neoplasm of uncertain behavior, unspecified**

D49 **Neoplasms of unspecified behavior**
Note: Category D49 classifies by site neoplasms of unspecified morphology and behavior. The term "mass," unless otherwise stated, is not to be regarded as a neoplastic growth.
Includes 'growth' NOS
neoplasm NOS
new growth NOS
tumor NOS
Excludes1 neoplasms of uncertain behavior (D37-D44, D48)

D49.0 **Neoplasm of unspecified behavior of digestive system**
Excludes1 neoplasm of unspecified behavior of margin of anus (D49.2)
neoplasm of unspecified behavior of perianal skin (D49.2)
neoplasm of unspecified behavior of skin of anus (D49.2)

D49.1 **Neoplasm of unspecified behavior of respiratory system**

D49.2 **Neoplasm of unspecified behavior of bone, soft tissue, and skin**
Excludes1 neoplasm of unspecified behavior of anal canal (D49.0)
neoplasm of unspecified behavior of anus NOS (D49.0)
neoplasm of unspecified behavior of bone marrow (D49.89)
neoplasm of unspecified behavior of cartilage of larynx (D49.1)
neoplasm of unspecified behavior of cartilage of nose (D49.1)
neoplasm of unspecified behavior of connective tissue of breast (D49.3)
neoplasm of unspecified behavior of skin of genital organs (D49.59)
neoplasm of unspecified behavior of vermilion border of lip (D49.0)

CHAPTER 2 (C00-D49)

D49.3 **Neoplasm of unspecified behavior of breast**
Excludes1 neoplasm of unspecified behavior of skin of breast (D49.2)

D49.4 **Neoplasm of unspecified behavior of bladder**

● D49.5 **Neoplasm of unspecified behavior of other genitourinary organs**

● D49.51 **Neoplasm of unspecified behavior of kidney**

D49.511 **Neoplasm of unspecified behavior of right kidney**
Coding Clinic: 2016, Q4, P9

D49.512 **Neoplasm of unspecified behavior of left kidney**
Coding Clinic: 2016, Q4, P9

D49.519 **Neoplasm of unspecified behavior of unspecified kidney**
Coding Clinic: 2016, Q4, P9

D49.59 **Neoplasm of unspecified behavior of other genitourinary organ**
Coding Clinic: 2016, Q4, P9

D49.6 **Neoplasm of unspecified behavior of brain**
Excludes1 neoplasm of unspecified behavior of cerebral meninges (D49.7)
neoplasm of unspecified behavior of cranial nerves (D49.7)

D49.7 **Neoplasm of unspecified behavior of endocrine glands and other parts of nervous system**
Excludes1 neoplasm of unspecified behavior of peripheral, sympathetic, and parasympathetic nerves and ganglia (D49.2)

● D49.8 **Neoplasm of unspecified behavior of other specified sites**
Excludes1 neoplasm of unspecified behavior of eyelid (skin) (D49.2)
neoplasm of unspecified behavior of eyelid cartilage (D49.2)
neoplasm of unspecified behavior of great vessels (D49.2)
neoplasm of unspecified behavior of optic nerve (D49.7)

D49.81 **Neoplasm of unspecified behavior of retina and choroid**
Dark area on retina
Retinal freckle

D49.89 **Neoplasm of unspecified behavior of other specified sites**

D49.9 **Neoplasm of unspecified behavior of unspecified site**

CHAPTER 2 (C00-D49)

OGCR Chapter-Specific Coding Guidelines

3. Chapter 3: Disease of the blood and blood-forming organs and certain disorders involving the immune mechanism (D5Ø-D89)
Reserved for future guideline expansion

CHAPTER 3

DISEASES OF THE BLOOD AND BLOOD-FORMING ORGANS AND CERTAIN DISORDERS INVOLVING THE IMMUNE MECHANISM (D5Ø-D89)

Excludes2 autoimmune disease (systemic) NOS (M35.9)
certain conditions originating in the perinatal period (PØØ-P96)
complications of pregnancy, childbirth and the puerperium (OØØ-O9A)
congenital malformations, deformations and chromosomal abnormalities (QØØ-Q99)
endocrine, nutritional and metabolic diseases (EØØ-E88)
human immunodeficiency virus [HIV] disease (B2Ø)
injury, poisoning and certain other consequences of external causes (SØØ-T88)
neoplasms (CØØ-D49)
symptoms, signs and abnormal clinical and laboratory findings, not elsewhere classified (RØØ-R94)

This chapter contains the following blocks:

D5Ø-D53	Nutritional anemias
D55-D59	Hemolytic anemias
D6Ø-D64	Aplastic and other anemias and other bone marrow failure syndromes
D65-D69	Coagulation defects, purpura and other hemorrhagic conditions
D7Ø-D77	Other disorders of blood and blood-forming organs
D78	Intraoperative and postprocedural complications of the spleen
D8Ø-D89	Certain disorders involving the immune mechanism

NUTRITIONAL ANEMIAS (D5Ø-D53)

● **D5Ø Iron deficiency anemia**
A disease characterized by a decrease in the number of red cells (hemoglobin) in the blood.
Includes asiderotic anemia
hypochromic anemia

D5Ø.Ø Iron deficiency anemia secondary to blood loss (chronic)
Posthemorrhagic anemia (chronic)
Excludes1 acute posthemorrhagic anemia (D62)
congenital anemia from fetal blood loss (P61.3)

D5Ø.1 Sideropenic dysphagia
Weblike growth of membranes in throat that makes swallowing difficult
Kelly-Paterson syndrome
Plummer-Vinson syndrome

D5Ø.8 Other iron deficiency anemias
Iron deficiency anemia due to inadequate dietary iron intake

D5Ø.9 Iron deficiency anemia, unspecified

● **D51 Vitamin B12 deficiency anemia**
Excludes1 vitamin B12 deficiency (E53.8)

D51.Ø Vitamin B12 deficiency anemia due to intrinsic factor deficiency
Addison anemia
Biermer anemia
Pernicious (congenital) anemia
Congenital intrinsic factor deficiency

D51.1 Vitamin B12 deficiency anemia due to selective vitamin B12 malabsorption with proteinuria
Imerslund (Gräsbeck) syndrome
Megaloblastic hereditary anemia

D51.2 Transcobalamin II deficiency

D51.3 Other dietary vitamin B12 deficiency anemia
Vegan anemia

D51.8 Other vitamin B12 deficiency anemias

D51.9 Vitamin B12 deficiency anemia, unspecified

● **D52 Folate deficiency anemia**
Excludes1 folate deficiency without anemia (E53.8)

D52.Ø Dietary folate deficiency anemia
Nutritional megaloblastic anemia

D52.1 Drug-induced folate deficiency anemia
Use additional code for adverse effect, if applicable, to identify drug (T36-T5Ø with fifth or sixth character 5)

D52.8 Other folate deficiency anemias

D52.9 Folate deficiency anemia, unspecified
Folic acid deficiency anemia NOS

● **D53 Other nutritional anemias**
Includes megaloblastic anemia unresponsive to vitamin B12 or folate therapy

D53.Ø Protein deficiency anemia
Amino-acid deficiency anemia
Orotaciduric anemia
Excludes1 Lesch-Nyhan syndrome (E79.1)

D53.1 Other megaloblastic anemias, not elsewhere classified
Megaloblastic anemia NOS
Excludes1 Di Guglielmo's disease (C94.Ø)

D53.2 Scorbutic anemia
Anemia resulting from deficiency of ascorbic acid (vitamin C)
Excludes1 scurvy (E54)

D53.8 Other specified nutritional anemias
Anemia associated with deficiency of copper
Anemia associated with deficiency of molybdenum
Anemia associated with deficiency of zinc
Excludes1 nutritional deficiencies without anemia, such as:
copper deficiency NOS (E61.Ø)
molybdenum deficiency NOS (E61.5)
zinc deficiency NOS (E6Ø)

D53.9 Nutritional anemia, unspecified
Simple chronic anemia
Excludes1 anemia NOS (D64.9)
Coding Clinic: 2018, Q4, P88

CHAPTER 3 (D5Ø-D89)

HEMOLYTIC ANEMIAS (D55-D59)

D55 Anemia due to enzyme disorders

Excludes1 drug-induced enzyme deficiency anemia (D59.2)

D55.0 Anemia due to glucose-6-phosphate dehydrogenase [G6PD] deficiency

Favism

G6PD deficiency anemia

Excludes1 glucose-6-phosphate dehydrogenase (G6PD) deficiency without anemia (D75.A)

D55.1 Anemia due to other disorders of glutathione metabolism

Anemia (due to) enzyme deficiencies, except G6PD, related to the hexose monophosphate [HMP] shunt pathway

Anemia (due to) hemolytic nonspherocytic (hereditary), type I

D55.2 Anemia due to disorders of glycolytic enzymes

Hemolytic nonspherocytic (hereditary) anemia, type II

Hexokinase deficiency anemia

Pyruvate kinase [PK] deficiency anemia

Triose-phosphate isomerase deficiency anemia

Excludes1 disorders of glycolysis not associated with anemia (E74.8)

D55.3 Anemia due to disorders of nucleotide metabolism

D55.8 Other anemias due to enzyme disorders

D55.9 Anemia due to enzyme disorder, unspecified

D56 Thalassemia

Hereditary disorders characterized by low production of hemoglobin or excessive destruction of red blood cells

Excludes1 sickle-cell thalassemia (D57.4-)

D56.0 Alpha thalassemia

Alpha thalassemia major

Hemoglobin H Constant Spring

Hemoglobin H disease

Hydrops fetalis due to alpha thalassemia

Severe alpha thalassemia

Triple gene defect alpha thalassemia

Use additional code, if applicable, for hydrops fetalis due to alpha thalassemia (P56.99)

Excludes1 alpha thalassemia trait or minor (D56.3)
asymptomatic alpha thalassemia (D56.3)
hydrops fetalis due to isoimmunization (P56.0)
hydrops fetalis not due to immune hemolysis (P83.2)

D56.1 Beta thalassemia

Beta thalassemia major

Cooley's anemia

Homozygous beta thalassemia

Severe beta thalassemia

Thalassemia intermedia

Thalassemia major

Excludes1 beta thalassemia minor (D56.3)
beta thalassemia trait (D56.3)
delta-beta thalassemia (D56.2)
hemoglobin E-beta thalassemia (D56.5)
sickle-cell beta thalassemia (D57.4-)

D56.2 Delta-beta thalassemia

Homozygous delta-beta thalassemia

Excludes1 delta-beta thalassemia minor (D56.3)
delta-beta thalassemia trait (D56.3)

D56.3 Thalassemia minor

Genetic disorders that have in common defective production of hemoglobin

Alpha thalassemia minor

Alpha thalassemia silent carrier

Alpha thalassemia trait

Beta thalassemia minor

Beta thalassemia trait

Delta-beta thalassemia minor

Delta-beta thalassemia trait

Thalassemia trait NOS

Excludes1 alpha thalassemia (D56.0)
beta thalassemia (D56.1)
delta-beta thalassemia (D56.2)
hemoglobin E-beta thalassemia (D56.5)
sickle-cell trait (D57.3)

D56.4 Hereditary persistence of fetal hemoglobin [HPFH]

Persistent production of hemoglobin

D56.5 Hemoglobin E-beta thalassemia

Excludes1 beta thalassemia (D56.1)
beta thalassemia minor (D56.3)
beta thalassemia trait (D56.3)
delta-beta thalassemia (D56.2)
delta-beta thalassemia trait (D56.3)
hemoglobin E disease (D58.2)
other hemoglobinopathies (D58.2)
sickle-cell beta thalassemia (D57.4-)

D56.8 Other thalassemias

Dominant thalassemia

Hemoglobin C thalassemia

Mixed thalassemia

Thalassemia with other hemoglobinopathy

Excludes1 hemoglobin C disease (D58.2)
hemoglobin E disease (D58.2)
other hemoglobinopathies (D58.2)
sickle cell anemia (D57.-)
sickle-cell thalassemia (D57.4)

D56.9 Thalassemia, unspecified

Mediterranean anemia (with other hemoglobinopathy)

D57 Sickle-cell disorders

Inherited disease in which red blood cells, normally disc-shaped, become crescent shaped

Use additional code for any associated fever (R50.81)

Excludes1 other hemoglobinopathies (D58.-)

D57.0 Hb-SS disease with crisis

Sickle-cell disease NOS with crisis

Hb-SS disease with vasoocclusive pain

D57.00 Hb-SS disease with crisis, unspecified

D57.01 Hb-SS disease with acute chest syndrome

D57.02 Hb-SS disease with splenic sequestration

D57.1 Sickle-cell disease without crisis Hb-SS disease without crisis

Sickle-cell anemia NOS

Sickle-cell disease NOS

Sickle-cell disorder NOS

D57.2 Sickle-cell/Hb-C disease

Hb-SC disease

Hb-S/Hb-C disease

D57.20 Sickle-cell/Hb-C disease without crisis

D57.21 Sickle-cell/Hb-C disease with crisis

D57.211 Sickle-cell/Hb-C disease with acute chest syndrome

D57.212 Sickle-cell/Hb-C disease with splenic sequestration

D57.219 Sickle-cell/Hb-C disease with crisis, unspecified

Sickle-cell/Hb-C disease with crisis NOS

D57.3 Sickle-cell trait
Hb-S trait
Heterozygous hemoglobin S

D57.4 Sickle-cell thalassemia
Sickle-cell beta thalassemia
Thalassemia Hb-S disease

D57.40 Sickle-cell thalassemia without crisis
Microdrepanocytosis
Sickle-cell thalassemia NOS

D57.41 Sickle-cell thalassemia with crisis
Sickle-cell "crisis" is precipitated when abnormally crescent-shaped red blood cells form clots and interrupt blood flow to major organs, causing severe pain and organ damage.
Sickle-cell thalassemia with vasoocclusive pain

D57.411 Sickle-cell thalassemia with acute chest syndrome

D57.412 Sickle-cell thalassemia with splenic sequestration

D57.419 Sickle-cell thalassemia with crisis, unspecified
Sickle-cell thalassemia with crisis NOS

D57.8 Other sickle-cell disorders
Hb-SD disease
Hb-SE disease

D57.80 Other sickle-cell disorders without crisis

D57.81 Other sickle-cell disorders with crisis

D57.811 Other sickle-cell disorders with acute chest syndrome

D57.812 Other sickle-cell disorders with splenic sequestration

D57.819 Other sickle-cell disorders with crisis, unspecified
Other sickle-cell disorders with crisis NOS

D58 Other hereditary hemolytic anemias
Genetic condition in which bone marrow is unable to compensate for premature destruction of red blood cells
Excludes1 hemolytic anemia of the newborn (P55.-)

D58.0 Hereditary spherocytosis
Presence of spherocytes (spherically shaped red blood cells)
Acholuric (familial) jaundice
Congenital (spherocytic) hemolytic icterus
Minkowski-Chauffard syndrome

D58.1 Hereditary elliptocytosis
Presence of large numbers of elliptocytes in blood
Elliptocytosis (congenital)
Ovalocytosis (congenital) (hereditary)

D58.2 Other hemoglobinopathies
Abnormal hemoglobin NOS
Congenital Heinz body anemia
Hb-C disease
Hb-D disease
Hb-E disease
Hemoglobinopathy NOS
Unstable hemoglobin hemolytic disease
Excludes1 familial polycythemia (D75.0)
Hb-M disease (D74.0)
hemoglobin E-beta thalassemia (D56.5)
hereditary persistence of fetal hemoglobin [HPFH] (D56.4)
high-altitude polycythemia (D75.1)
methemoglobinemia (D74.-)
other hemoglobinopathies with thalassemia (D56.8)

D58.8 Other specified hereditary hemolytic anemias
Stomatocytosis

D58.9 Hereditary hemolytic anemia, unspecified

D59 Acquired hemolytic anemia

D59.0 Drug-induced autoimmune hemolytic anemia
Use additional code for adverse effect, if applicable, to identify drug (T36-T50 with fifth or sixth character 5)

D59.1 Other autoimmune hemolytic anemias
Autoimmune hemolytic disease (cold type) (warm type)
Chronic cold hemagglutinin disease
Cold agglutinin disease
Cold agglutinin hemoglobinuria
Cold type (secondary) (symptomatic) hemolytic anemia
Warm type (secondary) (symptomatic) hemolytic anemia
Excludes1 Evans syndrome (D69.41)
hemolytic disease of newborn (P55.-)
paroxysmal cold hemoglobinuria (D59.6)

D59.2 Drug-induced nonautoimmune hemolytic anemia
Drug-induced enzyme deficiency anemia
Use additional code for adverse effect, if applicable, to identify drug (T36-T50 with fifth or sixth character 5)

D59.3 Hemolytic-uremic syndrome
Use additional code to identify associated:
E. coli infection (B96.2-)
Pneumococcal pneumonia (J13)
Shigella dysenteriae (A03.9)

D59.4 Other nonautoimmune hemolytic anemias
Mechanical hemolytic anemia
Microangiopathic hemolytic anemia
Toxic hemolytic anemia

D59.5 Paroxysmal nocturnal hemoglobinuria [Marchiafava-Micheli]
Excludes1 hemoglobinuria NOS (R82.3)

D59.6 Hemoglobinuria due to hemolysis from other external causes
Hemoglobinuria from exertion
March hemoglobinuria
Paroxysmal cold hemoglobinuria
Use additional code (Chapter 20) to identify external cause
Excludes1 hemoglobinuria NOS (R82.3)

D59.8 Other acquired hemolytic anemias

D59.9 Acquired hemolytic anemia, unspecified
Idiopathic hemolytic anemia, chronic

APLASTIC AND OTHER ANEMIAS AND OTHER BONE MARROW FAILURE SYNDROMES (D60-D64)

D60 Acquired pure red cell aplasia [erythroblastopenia]
Deficiency of erythroblasts
Includes red cell aplasia (acquired) (adult) (with thymoma)
Excludes1 congenital red cell aplasia (D61.01)

D60.0 Chronic acquired pure red cell aplasia
Lack of development of blood cell

D60.1 Transient acquired pure red cell aplasia

D60.8 Other acquired pure red cell aplasias

D60.9 Acquired pure red cell aplasia, unspecified

D61 Other aplastic anemias and other bone marrow failure syndromes
Excludes1 neutropenia (D70.-)

D61.0 Constitutional aplastic anemia
Condition where bone marrow is unable to produce blood cells

D61.01 Constitutional (pure) red blood cell aplasia
Blackfan-Diamond syndrome
Congenital (pure) red cell aplasia
Familial hypoplastic anemia
Primary (pure) red cell aplasia
Red cell (pure) aplasia of infants
Excludes1 acquired red cell aplasia (D60.9)

D61.09 Other constitutional aplastic anemia
Fanconi's anemia
Pancytopenia with malformations

D61.1 **Drug-induced aplastic anemia**
Use additional code for adverse effect, if applicable, to identify drug (T36-T5Ø with fifth or sixth character 5)

D61.2 **Aplastic anemia due to other external agents**
Code first, if applicable, toxic effects of substances chiefly nonmedicinal as to source (T51-T65)

D61.3 **Idiopathic aplastic anemia**

D61.8 **Other specified aplastic anemias and other bone marrow failure syndromes**

D61.81 **Pancytopenia**
Marked deficiency of all the blood elements: Red blood cells (erythrocytes), white blood cells (leukocytes), and platelets (thrombocytes). Check laboratory results.
Excludes1 pancytopenia (due to) (with) aplastic anemia (D61.9)
pancytopenia (due to) (with) bone marrow infiltration (D61.82)
pancytopenia (due to) (with) congenital (pure) red cell aplasia (D61.Ø1)
pancytopenia (due to) (with) hairy cell leukemia (C91.4-)
pancytopenia (due to) (with) human immunodeficiency virus disease (B2Ø.-)
pancytopenia (due to) (with) leukoerythroblastic anemia (D61.82)
pancytopenia (due to) (with) myeloproliferative disease (D47.1)
Excludes2 pancytopenia (due to) (with) myelodysplastic syndromes (D46.-)

D61.81Ø **Antineoplastic chemotherapy induced pancytopenia**
Excludes2 aplastic anemia due to antineoplastic chemotherapy (D61.1)

D61.811 **Other drug-induced pancytopenia**
Excludes2 aplastic anemia due to drugs (D61.1)

D61.818 **Other pancytopenia**
Coding Clinic: 2019, Q1, P16

D61.82 **Myelophthisis**
Leukoerythroblastic anemia
Myelophthisic anemia
Panmyelophthisis
Code also the underlying disorder, such as:
malignant neoplasm of breast (C5Ø.-)
tuberculosis (A15.-)
Excludes1 idiopathic myelofibrosis (D47.1)
myelofibrosis NOS (D75.81)
myelofibrosis with myeloid metaplasia (D47.4)
primary myelofibrosis (D47.1)
secondary myelofibrosis (D75.81)

D61.89 **Other specified aplastic anemias and other bone marrow failure syndromes**

D61.9 **Aplastic anemia, unspecified**
Hypoplastic anemia NOS
Medullary hypoplasia

D62 **Acute posthemorrhagic anemia**
Excludes1 anemia due to chronic blood loss (D5Ø.Ø)
blood loss anemia NOS (D5Ø.Ø)
congenital anemia from fetal blood loss (P61.3)

D63 **Anemia in chronic diseases classified elsewhere**

D63.Ø ***Anemia in neoplastic disease***
Code first neoplasm (CØØ-D49)
Excludes1 aplastic anemia due to antineoplastic chemotherapy (D61.1)
Excludes2 anemia due to antineoplastic chemotherapy (D64.81)

OGCR Section I.C.2.e.2.
2) Anemia associated with chemotherapy, immunotherapy and radiation therapy
When the admission/encounter is for management of an anemia associated with an adverse effect of the administration of chemotherapy or immunotherapy and the only treatment is for the anemia, the anemia code is sequenced first followed by the appropriate codes for the neoplasm and the adverse effect (T45.1X5, Adverse effect of antineoplastic and immunosuppressive drugs).

D63.1 ***Anemia in chronic kidney disease***
Erythropoietin resistant anemia (EPO resistant anemia)
Code first underlying chronic kidney disease (CKD) (N18.-)

D63.8 ***Anemia in other chronic diseases classified elsewhere***
Code first underlying disease, such as:
diphyllobothriasis (B7Ø.Ø)
hookworm disease (B76.Ø-B76.9)
hypothyroidism (EØØ.Ø-EØ3.9)
malaria (B5Ø.Ø-B54)
symptomatic late syphilis (A52.79)
tuberculosis (A18.89)

D64 **Other anemias**
Excludes1 refractory anemia (D46.-)
refractory anemia with excess blasts in transformation [RAEB T] (C92.Ø-)

D64.Ø **Hereditary sideroblastic anemia**
Abnormal production RBCs (erythrocytes)
Sex-linked hypochromic sideroblastic anemia

D64.1 ***Secondary sideroblastic anemia due to disease***
Code first underlying disease

D64.2 **Secondary sideroblastic anemia due to drugs and toxins**
Code first poisoning due to drug or toxin, if applicable (T36-T65 with fifth or sixth character 1-4 or 6)
Use additional code for adverse effect, if applicable, to identify drug (T36-T5Ø with fifth or sixth character 5)

D64.3 **Other sideroblastic anemias**
Sideroblastic anemia NOS
Pyridoxine-responsive sideroblastic anemia NEC

D64.4 **Congenital dyserythropoietic anemia**
Any of several rare hereditary anemias, mostly types of macrocytic anemia
Dyshematopoietic anemia (congenital)
Excludes1 Blackfan-Diamond syndrome (D61.Ø1)
Di Guglielmo's disease (C94.Ø)

D64.8 **Other specified anemias**

D64.81 **Anemia due to antineoplastic chemotherapy**
Antineoplastic chemotherapy induced anemia
Excludes1 aplastic anemia due to antineoplastic chemotherapy (D61.1)
Excludes2 anemia in neoplastic disease (D63.Ø)

D64.89 **Other specified anemias**
Infantile pseudoleukemia

D64.9 **Anemia, unspecified**
Coding Clinic: 2018, Q4, P88; 2017, Q1, P7

CHAPTER 3 (D5Ø-D89)

COAGULATION DEFECTS, PURPURA AND OTHER HEMORRHAGIC CONDITIONS (D65-D69)

D65 Disseminated intravascular coagulation [defibrination syndrome]
Blood clots form and consume all coagulation proteins and platelets and disrupt normal coagulation, resulting in abnormal bleeding
Afibrinogenemia, acquired
Consumption coagulopathy
Diffuse or disseminated intravascular coagulation [DIC]
Fibrinolytic hemorrhage, acquired
Fibrinolytic purpura
Purpura fulminans
Excludes1 disseminated intravascular coagulation (complicating):
abortion or ectopic or molar pregnancy (O00-O07, O08.1)
in newborn (P60)
pregnancy, childbirth and the puerperium (O45.0, O46.0, O67.0, O72.3)

D66 Hereditary factor VIII deficiency
Inherited coagulation disorder carried by females but most often affecting males
Classical hemophilia
Deficiency factor VIII (with functional defect)
Hemophilia NOS
Hemophilia A
Excludes1 factor VIII deficiency with vascular defect (D68.0)

D67 Hereditary factor IX deficiency
Christmas disease
Factor IX deficiency (with functional defect)
Hemophilia B
Plasma thromboplastin component [PTC] deficiency

D68 Other coagulation defects
Excludes1 abnormal coagulation profile (R79.1)
coagulation defects complicating abortion or ectopic or molar pregnancy (O00-O07, O08.1)
coagulation defects complicating pregnancy, childbirth and the puerperium (O45.0, O46.0, O67.0, O72.3)
Coding Clinic: 2016, Q1, P14

D68.0 Von Willebrand's disease
Congenital bleeding disorder
Angiohemophilia
Factor VIII deficiency with vascular defect
Vascular hemophilia
Excludes1 capillary fragility (hereditary) (D69.8)
factor VIII deficiency NOS (D66)
factor VIII deficiency with functional defect (D66)

D68.1 Hereditary factor XI deficiency
Deficiency of blood coagulation resulting in systemic blood-clotting defect
Hemophilia C
Plasma thromboplastin antecedent [PTA] deficiency
Rosenthal's disease

D68.2 Hereditary deficiency of other clotting factors
Blood clotting disorders caused by hereditary deficiencies of one or more clotting factors
AC globulin deficiency
Congenital afibrinogenemia
Deficiency of factor I [fibrinogen]
Deficiency of factor II [prothrombin]
Deficiency of factor V [labile]
Deficiency of factor VII [stable]
Deficiency of factor X [Stuart-Prower]
Deficiency of factor XII [Hageman]
Deficiency of factor XIII [fibrin stabilizing]
Dysfibrinogenemia (congenital)
Hypoproconvertinemia
Owren's disease
Proaccelerin deficiency

D68.3 Hemorrhagic disorder due to circulating anticoagulants
Blood clotting disorders caused by anticoagulants (warfarin and heparin)

D68.31 Hemorrhagic disorder due to intrinsic circulating anticoagulants, antibodies, or inhibitors

D68.311 Acquired hemophilia
Autoimmune hemophilia
Autoimmune inhibitors to clotting factors
Secondary hemophilia

D68.312 Antiphospholipid antibody with hemorrhagic disorder
Lupus anticoagulant (LAC) with hemorrhagic disorder
Systemic lupus erythematosus [SLE] inhibitor with hemorrhagic disorder
Excludes1 antiphospholipid antibody, finding without diagnosis (R76.0)
antiphospholipid antibody syndrome (D68.61)
antiphospholipid antibody with hypercoagulable state (D68.61)
lupus anticoagulant (LAC) finding without diagnosis (R76.0)
lupus anticoagulant (LAC) with hypercoagulable state (D68.62)
systemic lupus erythematosus [SLE] inhibitor finding without diagnosis (R76.0)
systemic lupus erythematosus [SLE] inhibitor with hypercoagulable state (D68.62)

D68.318 Other hemorrhagic disorder due to intrinsic circulating anticoagulants, antibodies, or inhibitors
Antithromboplastinemia
Antithromboplastinogenemia
Hemorrhagic disorder due to intrinsic increase in antithrombin
Hemorrhagic disorder due to intrinsic increase in anti-VIIIa
Hemorrhagic disorder due to intrinsic increase in anti-IXa
Hemorrhagic disorder due to intrinsic increase in anti-XIa

D68.32 Hemorrhagic disorder due to extrinsic circulating anticoagulants
Drug-induced hemorrhagic disorder
Hemorrhagic disorder due to increase in anti-IIa
Hemorrhagic disorder due to increase in anti-Xa
Hyperheparinemia
Use additional code for adverse effect, if applicable, to identify drug (T45.515, T45.525)
Coding Clinic: 2016, Q1, P14-15

CHAPTER 3 (D50-D89)

D68.4 Acquired coagulation factor deficiency
Deficiency of coagulation factor due to liver disease
Deficiency of coagulation factor due to vitamin K deficiency
Excludes1 vitamin K deficiency of newborn (P53)

D68.5 Primary thrombophilia
AKA idiopathic thrombocytopenia, may be acquired or congenital and is a common cause of coagulation disorders.
Primary hypercoagulable states
Excludes1 antiphospholipid syndrome (D68.61)
lupus anticoagulant (D68.62)
secondary activated protein C resistance (D68.69)
secondary antiphospholipid antibody syndrome (D68.69)
secondary lupus anticoagulant with hypercoagulable state (D68.69)
secondary systemic lupus erythematosus [SLE] inhibitor with hypercoagulable state (D68.69)
systemic lupus erythematosus [SLE] inhibitor finding without diagnosis (R76.0)
systemic lupus erythematosus [SLE] inhibitor with hemorrhagic disorder (D68.312)
thrombotic thrombocytopenic purpura (M31.1)

D68.51 Activated protein C resistance
Factor V Leiden mutation

D68.52 Prothrombin gene mutation

D68.59 Other primary thrombophilia
Antithrombin III deficiency
Hypercoagulable state NOS
Primary hypercoagulable state NEC
Primary thrombophilia NEC
Protein C deficiency
Protein S deficiency
Thrombophilia NOS

D68.6 Other thrombophilia
Other hypercoagulable states
Excludes1 diffuse or disseminated intravascular coagulation [DIC] (D65)
heparin induced thrombocytopenia (HIT) (D75.82)
hyperhomocysteinemia (E72.11)

D68.61 Antiphospholipid syndrome
Anticardiolipin syndrome
Antiphospholipid antibody syndrome
Excludes1 anti-phospholipid antibody, finding without diagnosis (R76.0)
anti-phospholipid antibody with hemorrhagic disorder (D68.312)
lupus anticoagulant syndrome (D68.62)

D68.62 Lupus anticoagulant syndrome
Lupus anticoagulant
Presence of systemic lupus erythematosus [SLE] inhibitor
Excludes1 anticardiolipin syndrome (D68.61)
antiphospholipid syndrome (D68.61)
lupus anticoagulant (LAC) finding without diagnosis (R76.0)
lupus anticoagulant (LAC) with hemorrhagic disorder (D68.312)

D68.69 Other thrombophilia
Hypercoagulable states NEC
Secondary hypercoagulable state NOS

D68.8 Other specified coagulation defects
Excludes1 hemorrhagic disease of newborn (P53)

D68.9 Coagulation defect, unspecified

D69 Purpura and other hemorrhagic conditions
Group of conditions characterized by small hemorrhages in skin, mucous membranes, or serosal surfaces
Excludes1 benign hypergammaglobulinemic purpura (D89.0)
cryoglobulinemic purpura (D89.1)
essential (hemorrhagic) thrombocythemia (D47.3)
hemorrhagic thrombocythemia (D47.3)
purpura fulminans (D65)
thrombotic thrombocytopenic purpura (M31.1)
Waldenström hypergammaglobulinemic purpura (D89.0)

D69.0 Allergic purpura
Allergic vasculitis
Nonthrombocytopenic hemorrhagic purpura
Nonthrombocytopenic idiopathic purpura
Purpura anaphylactoid
Purpura Henoch(-Schönlein)
Purpura rheumatica
Vascular purpura
Excludes1 thrombocytopenic hemorrhagic purpura (D69.3)

D69.1 Qualitative platelet defects
Bernard-Soulier [giant platelet] syndrome
Glanzmann's disease
Grey platelet syndrome
Thromboasthenia (hemorrhagic) (hereditary)
Thrombocytopathy
Excludes1 von Willebrand's disease (D68.0)

D69.2 Other nonthrombocytopenic purpura
Purpura NOS
Purpura simplex
Senile purpura

D69.3 Immune thrombocytopenic purpura
Hemorrhagic (thrombocytopenic) purpura
Idiopathic thrombocytopenic purpura
Tidal platelet dysgenesis

D69.4 Other primary thrombocytopenia
Excludes1 transient neonatal thrombocytopenia (P61.0)
Wiskott-Aldrich syndrome (D82.0)

D69.41 Evans syndrome
Acquired hemolytic anemia and thrombocytopenia

D69.42 Congenital and hereditary thrombocytopenia purpura
Congenital thrombocytopenia
Hereditary thrombocytopenia
Code first congential or hereditary disorder, such as:
thrombocytopenia with absent radius (TAR syndrome) (Q87.2)

D69.49 Other primary thrombocytopenia
Megakaryocytic hypoplasia
Primary thrombocytopenia NOS

D69.5 Secondary thrombocytopenia
Acquired reduction of number of platelets required for blood clotting
Excludes1 heparin induced thrombocytopenia (HIT) (D75.82)
transient thrombocytopenia of newborn (P61.0)

D69.51 Posttransfusion purpura
Posttransfusion purpura from whole blood (fresh) or blood products PTP

D69.59 Other secondary thrombocytopenia

D69.6 Thrombocytopenia, unspecified

D69.8 Other specified hemorrhagic conditions
Capillary fragility (hereditary)
Vascular pseudohemophilia

D69.9 Hemorrhagic condition, unspecified

CHAPTER 3 (D50-D89)

OTHER DISORDERS OF BLOOD AND BLOOD-FORMING ORGANS (D70-D77)

● **D70 Neutropenia**
Decrease in number of neutrophils (type of white blood cell)
Includes agranulocytosis
decreased absolute neurophile count (ANC)
Use additional code for any associated:
fever (R50.81)
mucositis (J34.81, K12.3-, K92.81, N76.81)
Excludes1 neutropenic splenomegaly (D73.81)
transient neonatal neutropenia (P61.5)

D70.0 Congenital agranulocytosis
Reduced numbers of neutrophils (type of white blood cell)
Congenital neutropenia
Infantile genetic agranulocytosis
Kostmann's disease

D70.1 Agranulocytosis secondary to cancer chemotherapy
Decreased numbers of granulocytes (type of white blood cell)
Code also *underlying neoplasm*
Use additional code for adverse effect, if applicable, to identify drug (T45.1X5)

D70.2 Other drug-induced agranulocytosis
Use additional code for adverse effect, if applicable, to identify drug (T36-T50 with fifth or sixth character 5)

D70.3 Neutropenia due to infection

D70.4 Cyclic neutropenia
Chronic neutropenia (low number of type of white blood cell)
Cyclic hematopoiesis
Periodic neutropenia

D70.8 Other neutropenia

D70.9 Neutropenia, unspecified
Coding Clinic: 2019, Q2, P25

D71 Functional disorders of polymorphonuclear neutrophils
Polymorphonuclear: varying shapes of nucleus; AKA PMNs
Cell membrane receptor complex [CR3] defect
Chronic (childhood) granulomatous disease
Congenital dysphagocytosis
Progressive septic granulomatosis

● **D72 Other disorders of white blood cells**
Excludes1 basophilia (D72.824)
immunity disorders (D80-D89)
neutropenia (D70)
preleukemia (syndrome) (D46.9)

D72.0 Genetic anomalies of leukocytes
Alder (granulation) (granulocyte) anomaly
Alder syndrome
Hereditary leukocytic hypersegmentation
Hereditary leukocytic hyposegmentation
Hereditary leukomelanopathy
May-Hegglin (granulation) (granulocyte) anomaly
May-Hegglin syndrome
Pelger-Huët (granulation) (granulocyte) anomaly
Pelger-Huët syndrome
Excludes1 Chédiak (-Steinbrinck)-Higashi syndrome (E70.330)

D72.1 Eosinophilia
Formation and accumulation of high number of white cells in blood/tissue
Allergic eosinophilia
Hereditary eosinophilia
Excludes1 Löffler's syndrome (J82)
pulmonary eosinophilia (J82)

● **D72.8 Other specified disorders of white blood cells**
Excludes1 leukemia (C91-C95)

● **D72.81 Decreased white blood cell count**
Excludes1 neutropenia (D70.-)

D72.810 Lymphocytopenia
Decreased lymphocytes
Reduction in number of lympho cytes in blood

D72.818 Other decreased white blood cell count
Basophilic leukopenia
Eosinophilic leukopenia
Monocytopenia
Other decreased leukocytes
Plasmacytopenia

D72.819 Decreased white blood cell count, unspecified
Decreased leukocytes, unspecified
Leukocytopenia, unspecified
Leukopenia
Excludes1 malignant leukopenia (D70.9)

● **D72.82 Elevated white blood cell count**
Excludes1 eosinophilia (D72.1)

D72.820 Lymphocytosis (symptomatic)
Elevated lymphocytes
Excess of normal lymphocytes

D72.821 Monocytosis (symptomatic)
Excludes1 infectious mononucleosis (B27.-)

D72.822 Plasmacytosis
Presence of excess plasma cells

D72.823 Leukemoid reaction
Basophilic leukemoid reaction
Leukemoid reaction NOS
Lymphocytic leukemoid reaction
Monocytic leukemoid reaction
Myelocytic leukemoid reaction
Neutrophilic leukemoid reaction

D72.824 Basophilia
Increase of basophils in blood

D72.825 Bandemia
Bandemia without diagnosis of specific infection
Excess number of band cells (immature white blood cells) released by bone marrow
Excludes1 confirmed infection -code to infection
leukemia (C91.-, C92.-, C93.-, C94.-, C95.-)

D72.828 Other elevated white blood cell count

D72.829 Elevated white blood cell count, unspecified
Elevated leukocytes, unspecified
Leukocytosis, unspecified

D72.89 Other specified disorders of white blood cells
Abnormality of white blood cells NEC

D72.9 Disorder of white blood cells, unspecified
Abnormal leukocyte differential NOS

CHAPTER 3 (D50-D89)

D73 Diseases of spleen

D73.Ø Hyposplenism

Diminished functioning of spleen

Atrophy of spleen

Excludes1 asplenia (congenital) (Q89.Ø1)
postsurgical absence of spleen (Z9Ø.81)

D73.1 Hypersplenism

Accelerated function of spleen

Excludes1 neutropenic splenomegaly (D73.81)
primary splenic neutropenia (D73.81)
splenitis, splenomegaly in late syphilis (A52.79)
splenitis, splenomegaly in tuberculosis (A18.85)
splenomegaly NOS (R16.1)
splenomegaly congenital (Q89.Ø)

D73.2 Chronic congestive splenomegaly

Enlargement of spleen

D73.3 Abscess of spleen

D73.4 Cyst of spleen

D73.5 Infarction of spleen

Splenic rupture, nontraumatic
Torsion of spleen

Excludes1 rupture of spleen due to Plasmodium vivax malaria (B51.Ø)
traumatic rupture of spleen (S36.Ø3-)

D73.8 Other diseases of spleen

D73.81 Neutropenic splenomegaly

Werner-Schultz disease

Enlarged spleen responding to inadequate number of neutrophils

D73.89 Other diseases of spleen

Fibrosis of spleen NOS
Perisplenitis
Splenitis NOS

D73.9 Disease of spleen, unspecified

D74 Methemoglobinemia

Excessive methemoglobin (form of hemoglobin)

D74.Ø Congenital methemoglobinemia

Congenital NADH-methemoglobin reductase deficiency
Hemoglobin-M [Hb-M] disease
Methemoglobinemia, hereditary

D74.8 Other methemoglobinemias

Acquired methemoglobinemia (with sulfhemoglobinemia)
Toxic methemoglobinemia

D74.9 Methemoglobinemia, unspecified

D75 Other and unspecified diseases of blood and blood-forming organs

Excludes2 acute lymphadenitis (LØ4.-)
chronic lymphadenitis (I88.1)
enlarged lymph nodes (R59.-)
hypergammaglobulinemia NOS (D89.2)
lymphadenitis NOS (I88.9)
mesenteric lymphadenitis (acute) (chronic) (I88.Ø)

D75.A Glucose-6-phosphate dehydrogenase (G6PD) deficiency without anemia

Excludes1 glucose-6-phosphate dehydrogenase (G6PD) deficiency with anemia (D55.Ø)

D75.Ø Familial erythrocytosis

Genetic mutation of gene that results in increased circulating RBCs

Benign polycythemia
Familial polycythemia

Excludes1 hereditary ovalocytosis (D58.1)

D75.1 Secondary polycythemia

Increase in total red cell mass

Acquired polycythemia
Emotional polycythemia
Erythrocytosis NOS
Hypoxemic polycythemia
Nephrogenous polycythemia
Polycythemia due to erythropoietin
Polycythemia due to fall in plasma volume
Polycythemia due to high altitude
Polycythemia due to stress
Polycythemia NOS
Relative polycythemia

Excludes1 polycythemia neonatorum (P61.1)
polycythemia vera (D45)

D75.8 Other specified diseases of blood and blood-forming organs

D75.81 Myelofibrosis

Replacing bone marrow by fibrous tissue

Myelofibrosis NOS
Secondary myelofibrosis NOS

Code first the underlying disorder, such as:
malignant neoplasm of breast (C5Ø.-)

Use additional code, if applicable, for associated therapy-related myelodysplastic syndrome (D46.-)

Use additional code for adverse effect, if applicable, to identify drug (T45.1X5)

Excludes1 acute myelofibrosis (C94.4-)
idiopathic myelofibrosis (D47.1)
leukoerythroblastic anemia (D61.82)
myelofibrosis with myeloid metaplasia (D47.4)
myelophthisic anemia (D61.82)
myelophthisis (D61.82)
primary myelofibrosis (D47.1)

D75.82 Heparin induced thrombocytopenia (HIT)

D75.89 Other specified diseases of blood and blood-forming organs

D75.9 Disease of blood and blood-forming organs, unspecified

D76 Other specified diseases with participation of lymphoreticular and reticulohistiocytic tissue

Excludes1 (Abt-) Letterer-Siwe disease (C96.Ø)
eosinophilic granuloma (C96.6)
Hand-Schüller-Christian disease (C96.5)
histiocytic medullary reticulosis (C96.9)
histiocytic sarcoma (C96.A)
histiocytosis X, multifocal (C96.5)
histiocytosis X, unifocal (C96.6)
Langerhans-cell histiocytosis, multifocal (C96.5)
Langerhans-cell histiocytosis NOS (C96.6)
Langerhans-cell histiocytosis, unifocal (C96.6)
leukemic reticuloendotheliosis (C91.4-)
lipomelanotic reticulosis (I89.8)
malignant histiocytosis (C96.A)
malignant reticulosis (C86.Ø)
nonlipid reticuloendotheliosis (C96.Ø)

D76.1 Hemophagocytic lymphohistiocytosis

Familial hemophagocytic reticulosis
Histiocytoses of mononuclear phagocytes

D76.2 Hemophagocytic syndrome, infection-associated

Use additional code to identify infectious agent or disease.

D76.3 Other histiocytosis syndromes

Reticulohistiocytoma (giant-cell)
Sinus histiocytosis with massive lymphadenopathy
Xanthogranuloma

CHAPTER 3 (D5Ø-D89)

D77 *Other disorders of blood and blood-forming organs in diseases classified elsewhere*

Code first underlying disease, such as:
amyloidosis (E85.-)
congenital early syphilis (A50.0)
echinococcosis (B67.0-B67.9)
malaria (B50.0-B54)
schistosomiasis [bilharziasis] (B65.0-B65.9)
vitamin C deficiency (E54)

Excludes1 rupture of spleen due to Plasmodium vivax malaria (B51.0)
splenitis, splenomegaly in late syphilis (A52.79)
splenitis, splenomegaly in tuberculosis (A18.85)

INTRAOPERATIVE AND POSTPROCEDURAL COMPLICATIONS OF THE SPLEEN (D78)

D78 Intraoperative and postprocedural complications of the spleen
Coding Clinic: 2016, Q4, P9

D78.0 **Intraoperative hemorrhage and hematoma of the spleen complicating a procedure**
Excludes1 intraoperative hemorrhage and hematoma of the spleen due to accidental puncture or laceration during a procedure (D78.1-)

D78.01 **Intraoperative hemorrhage and hematoma of the spleen complicating a procedure on the spleen**

D78.02 **Intraoperative hemorrhage and hematoma of the spleen complicating other procedure**

D78.1 **Accidental puncture and laceration of the spleen during a procedure**

D78.11 **Accidental puncture and laceration of the spleen during a procedure on the spleen**

D78.12 **Accidental puncture and laceration of the spleen during other procedure**

D78.2 **Postprocedural hemorrhage of the spleen following a procedure**

D78.21 **Postprocedural hemorrhage of the spleen following a procedure on the spleen**

D78.22 **Postprocedural hemorrhage of the spleen following other procedure**

D78.3 **Postprocedural hematoma and seroma of the spleen following a procedure**

D78.31 **Postprocedural hematoma of the spleen following a procedure on the spleen**

D78.32 **Postprocedural hematoma of the spleen following other procedure**

D78.33 **Postprocedural seroma of the spleen following a procedure on the spleen**

D78.34 **Postprocedural seroma of the spleen following other procedure**

D78.8 **Other intraoperative and postprocedural complications of the spleen**
Use additional code, if applicable, to further specify disorder

D78.81 **Other intraoperative complications of the spleen**

D78.89 **Other postprocedural complications of the spleen**

CERTAIN DISORDERS INVOLVING THE IMMUNE MECHANISM (D80-D89)

Includes defects in the complement system
immunodeficiency disorders, except human immunodeficiency virus [HIV] disease
sarcoidosis

Excludes1 autoimmune disease (systemic) NOS (M35.9)
functional disorders of polymorphonuclear neutrophils (D71)
human immunodeficiency virus [HIV] disease (B20)

D80 **Immunodeficiency with predominantly antibody defects**

D80.0 **Hereditary hypogammaglobulinemia**
Autosomal recessive agammaglobulinemia (Swiss type)
X-linked agammaglobulinemia [Bruton] (with growth hormone deficiency)

D80.1 **Nonfamilial hypogammaglobulinemia**
Abnormally low levels of all classes of immunoglobulins
Agammaglobulinemia with immunoglobulin-bearing B-lymphocytes
Common variable agammaglobulinemia [CVAgamma]
Hypogammaglobulinemia NOS

D80.2 **Selective deficiency of immunoglobulin A [IgA]**

D80.3 **Selective deficiency of immunoglobulin G [IgG] subclasses**

D80.4 **Selective deficiency of immunoglobulin M [IgM]**

D80.5 **Immunodeficiency with increased immunoglobulin M [IgM]**

D80.6 **Antibody deficiency with near-normal immunoglobulins or with hyperimmunoglobulinemia**
Abnormally high levels of immunoglobulins in serum

D80.7 **Transient hypogammaglobulinemia of infancy**

D80.8 **Other immunodeficiencies with predominantly antibody defects**
Kappa light chain deficiency

D80.9 **Immunodeficiency with predominantly antibody defects, unspecified**

D81 Combined immunodeficiencies
Excludes1 autosomal recessive agammaglobulinemia (Swiss type) (D80.0)

D81.0 **Severe combined immunodeficiency [SCID] with reticular dysgenesis**

D81.1 **Severe combined immunodeficiency [SCID] with low T- and B-cell numbers**

D81.2 **Severe combined immunodeficiency [SCID] with low or normal B-cell numbers**

D81.3 **Adenosine deaminase [ADA] deficiency**

D81.30 **Adenosine deaminase deficiency, unspecified**
ADA deficiency NOS

D81.31 **Severe combined immunodeficiency due to adenosine deaminase deficiency**
ADA deficiency with SCID
Adenosine deaminase [ADA] deficiency with severe combined immunodeficiency

D81.32 **Adenosine deaminase 2 deficiency**
ADA2 deficiency
Adenosine deaminase deficiency type 2
Code also, if applicable, any associated manifestations, such as:
polyarteritis nodosa (M30.0)
stroke (I63.-)

D81.39 **Other adenosine deaminase deficiency**
Adenosine deaminase [ADA] deficiency type 1, NOS
Adenosine deaminase [ADA] deficiency type 1, without SCID
Adenosine deaminase [ADA] deficiency type 1, without severe combined immunodeficiency
Partial ADA deficiency (type 1)
Partial adenosine deaminase deficiency (type 1)

D81.4 **Nezelof's syndrome**
D81.5 **Purine nucleoside phosphorylase [PNP] deficiency**
D81.6 **Major histocompatibility complex class I deficiency**
Bare lymphocyte syndrome
D81.7 **Major histocompatibility complex class II deficiency**
● **D81.8** **Other combined immunodeficiencies**
● **D81.81** **Biotin-dependent carboxylase deficiency**
Multiple carboxylase deficiency
Excludes1 biotin-dependent carboxylase deficiency due to dietary deficiency of biotin (E53.8)
D81.810 **Biotinidase deficiency**
D81.818 **Other biotin-dependent carboxylase deficiency**
Holocarboxylase synthetase deficiency
Other multiple carboxylase deficiency
D81.819 **Biotin-dependent carboxylase deficiency, unspecified**
Multiple carboxylase deficiency, unspecified
D81.89 **Other combined immunodeficiencies**
D81.9 **Combined immunodeficiency, unspecified**
Severe combined immunodeficiency disorder [SCID] NOS

● **D82** **Immunodeficiency associated with other major defects**
Excludes1 ataxia telangiectasia [Louis-Bar] (G11.3)
D82.0 **Wiskott-Aldrich syndrome**
X-linked immunodeficiency
Immunodeficiency with thrombocytopenia and eczema
D82.1 **Di George's syndrome**
Congenital disorder with defective development of third and fourth pharyngeal pouches
Pharyngeal pouch syndrome
Thymic alymphoplasia
Thymic aplasia or hypoplasia with immunodeficiency
D82.2 **Immunodeficiency with short-limbed stature**
D82.3 **Immunodeficiency following hereditary defective response to Epstein-Barr virus**
X-linked lymphoproliferative disease
D82.4 **Hyperimmunoglobulin E [IgE] syndrome**
Suspected genetic defect that produces high levels of antibody immunoglobulin (IgE) that causes skin and lung infections and eczema
D82.8 **Immunodeficiency associated with other specified major defects**
D82.9 **Immunodeficiency associated with major defect, unspecified**

● **D83** **Common variable immunodeficiency**
D83.0 **Common variable immunodeficiency with predominant abnormalities of B-cell numbers and function**
D83.1 **Common variable immunodeficiency with predominant immunoregulatory T-cell disorders**
D83.2 **Common variable immunodeficiency with autoantibodies to B- or T-cells**
D83.8 **Other common variable immunodeficiencies**
D83.9 **Common variable immunodeficiency, unspecified**

● **D84** **Other immunodeficiencies**
D84.0 **Lymphocyte function antigen-1 [LFA-1] defect**
D84.1 **Defects in the complement system**
C1 esterase inhibitor [C1-INH] deficiency
D84.8 **Other specified immunodeficiencies**
D84.9 **Immunodeficiency, unspecified**

Item 3-1 Sarcoidosis: A symptom of an inflammation producing tiny lumps of cells (granulomas) in various organs, most commonly the lungs and lymph nodes, that affect organ function. Cause is unknown occurring primarily in 20- to 40-year-olds, African-American, especially women, and those of Asian, German, Irish, Scandinavian, and Puerto Rican heritage.

● **D86** **Sarcoidosis**
D86.0 **Sarcoidosis of lung**
D86.1 **Sarcoidosis of lymph nodes**
D86.2 **Sarcoidosis of lung with sarcoidosis of lymph nodes**
D86.3 **Sarcoidosis of skin**
● **D86.8** **Sarcoidosis of other sites**
D86.81 **Sarcoid meningitis**
D86.82 **Multiple cranial nerve palsies in sarcoidosis**
D86.83 **Sarcoid iridocyclitis**
Rare large tumor with irregular surface of iris
D86.84 **Sarcoid pyelonephritis**
Systemic disease of unknown etiology characterized by chronic granulomatous inflammation with tissue destruction of pelvis kidney
Tubulo-interstitial nephropathy in sarcoidosis
D86.85 **Sarcoid myocarditis**
D86.86 **Sarcoid arthropathy**
Polyarthritis in sarcoidosis
D86.87 **Sarcoid myositis**
Granumloma of muscle
D86.89 **Sarcoidosis of other sites**
Hepatic granuloma
Uveoparotid fever [Heerfordt]
D86.9 **Sarcoidosis, unspecified**

● **D89** **Other disorders involving the immune mechanism, not elsewhere classified**
Excludes1 hyperglobulinemia NOS (R77.1)
monoclonal gammopathy (of undetermined significance) (D47.2)
Excludes2 transplant failure and rejection (T86.-)
D89.0 **Polyclonal hypergammaglobulinemia**
Benign hypergammaglobulinemic purpura
Polyclonal gammopathy NOS
D89.1 **Cryoglobulinemia**
Cryoglobulin (proteins) in blood that precipitate temperatures below 98.6° F; usually symptomatic of underlying disease
Cryoglobulinemic purpura
Cryoglobulinemic vasculitis
Essential cryoglobulinemia
Idiopathic cryoglobulinemia
Mixed cryoglobulinemia
Primary cryoglobulinemia
Secondary cryoglobulinemia
D89.2 **Hypergammaglobulinemia, unspecified**
D89.3 **Immune reconstitution syndrome**
Immune reconstitution inflammatory syndrome [IRIS]
Use additional code for adverse effect, if applicable, to identify drug (T36-T50 with fifth or sixth character 5)

● **D89.4   Mast cell activation syndrome and related disorders**

    Excludes1   aggressive systemic mastocytosis (C96.21)
                     congenital cutaneous mastocytosis (Q82.2)
                     (non-congenital) cutaneous mastocytosis (D47.01)
                     (indolent) systemic mastocytosis (D47.02)
                     malignant mast cell neoplasm (C96.2-)
                     malignant mastocytoma (C96.29)
                     mast cell leukemia (C94.3-)
                     mast cell sarcoma (C96.22)
                     mastocytoma NOS (D47.09)
                     other mast cell neoplasms of uncertain behavior (D47.09)
                     systemic mastocytosis associated with a clonal hematologic non-mast cell lineage disease (SM-AHNMD) (D47.02)

      Coding Clinic: 2016, Q4, P11

  D89.40   Mast cell activation, unspecified 🦠
       Mast cell activation disorder, unspecified
       Mast cell activation syndrome, NOS

  D89.41   Monoclonal mast cell activation syndrome 🦠
       Coding Clinic: 2016, Q4, P11

  D89.42   Idiopathic mast cell activation syndrome 🦠
       Coding Clinic: 2016, Q4, P11

  D89.43   Secondary mast cell activation 🦠
       Secondary mast cell activation syndrome
       Code also underlying etiology, if known
       Coding Clinic: 2016, Q4, P11

  D89.49   Other mast cell activation disorder 🦠
       Other mast cell activation syndrome
       Coding Clinic: 2016, Q4, P11

● **D89.8   Other specified disorders involving the immune mechanism, not elsewhere classified**

  ● **D89.81   Graft-versus-host disease**

      Code first underlying cause, such as:
       complications of transplanted organs and tissue (T86.-)
       complications of blood transfusion (T80.89)

      Use additional code to identify associated manifestations, such as:
       desquamative dermatitis (L30.8)
       diarrhea (R19.7)
       elevated bilirubin (R17)
       hair loss (L65.9)

    D89.810   Acute graft-versus-host disease 🦠
    D89.811   Chronic graft-versus-host disease 🦠
    D89.812   Acute on chronic graft-versus-host disease 🦠
    D89.813   Graft-versus-host disease, unspecified 🦠

  D89.82   Autoimmune lymphoproliferative syndrome [ALPS] 🦠

  D89.89   Other specified disorders involving the immune mechanism, not elsewhere classified 🦠
      Excludes1   human immunodeficiency virus disease (B20)
      Coding Clinic: 2017, Q4, P109

● **D89.9   Disorder involving the immune mechanism, unspecified** 🦠
    Immune disease NOS
    Coding Clinic: 2015, Q3, P22

CHAPTER 3 (D50-D89)

722

▶ New   ⟩ Revised   ~~deleted~~ Deleted   Excludes 1   Excludes 2   Includes   Use additional   Code first   Code also   Key words

OGCR Official Guidelines   X Assign placeholder X   ● Use Additional Character(s)   ⟩ Manifestation Code   🦠 Hierarchical Condition Category   Coding Clinic

CHAPTER 4

ENDOCRINE, NUTRITIONAL AND METABOLIC DISEASES (E00-E89)

OGCR Chapter-Specific Coding Guidelines

4. **Chapter 4: Endocrine, Nutritional, and Metabolic Diseases (E00-E89)**

a. **Diabetes mellitus**

The diabetes mellitus codes are combination codes that include the type of diabetes mellitus, the body system affected, and the complications affecting that body system. As many codes within a particular category as are necessary to describe all of the complications of the disease may be used. They should be sequenced based on the reason for a particular encounter. Assign as many codes from categories E08 – E13 as needed to identify all of the associated conditions that the patient has.

1) **Type of diabetes**

The age of a patient is not the sole determining factor, though most type 1 diabetics develop the condition before reaching puberty. For this reason type 1 diabetes mellitus is also referred to as juvenile diabetes.

2) **Type of diabetes mellitus not documented**

If the type of diabetes mellitus is not documented in the medical record the default is E11.-, Type 2 diabetes mellitus.

3) **Diabetes mellitus and the use of insulin oral hypoglycemics**

If the documentation in a medical record does not indicate the type of diabetes but does indicate that the patient uses insulin, code E11, Type 2 diabetes mellitus, should be assigned. An additional code should be assigned from category Z79 to identify the long-term (current) use of insulin or oral hypoglycemic drugs. If the patient is treated with both oral medications and insulin, only the code for long-term (current) use of insulin should be assigned. Code Z79.4 should not be assigned if insulin is given temporarily to bring a type 2 patient's blood sugar under control during an encounter.

4) **Diabetes mellitus in pregnancy and gestational diabetes**

See Section I.C.15. Diabetes mellitus in pregnancy.
See Section I.C.15. Gestational (pregnancy induced) diabetes

5) **Complications due to insulin pump malfunction**

(a) **Underdose of insulin due to insulin pump failure**

An underdose of insulin due to an insulin pump failure should be assigned to a code from subcategory T85.6, Mechanical complication of other specified internal and external prosthetic devices, implants and grafts, that specifies the type of pump malfunction, as the principal or first-listed code, followed by code T38.3X6-, Underdosing of insulin and oral hypoglycemic [antidiabetic] drugs. Additional codes for the type of diabetes mellitus and any associated complications due to the underdosing should also be assigned.

(b) **Overdose of insulin due to insulin pump failure**

The principal or first-listed code for an encounter due to an insulin pump malfunction resulting in an overdose of insulin, should also be T85.6-, Mechanical complication of other specified internal and external prosthetic devices, implants and grafts, followed by code T38.3X1-, Poisoning by insulin and oral hypoglycemic [antidiabetic] drugs, accidental (unintentional).

6) **Secondary diabetes mellitus**

Codes under categories E08, Diabetes mellitus due to underlying condition, E09, Drug or chemical induced diabetes mellitus and E13, Other specified diabetes mellitus, identify complications/manifestations associated with secondary diabetes mellitus. Secondary diabetes is always caused by another condition or event (e.g., cystic fibrosis, malignant neoplasm of pancreas, pancreatectomy, adverse effect of drug, or poisoning).

(a) **Secondary diabetes mellitus and the use of insulin or hypoglycemic drugs**

For patients with secondary diabetes mellitus who routinely use insulin or oral hypoglycemic drugs, an additional code from category Z79 should be assigned to identify the long-term (current) use of insulin or oral hypoglycemic drugs. If the patient is treated with both oral medications and insulin, only the code for long-term (current) use of insulin should be assigned. Code Z79.4 should not be assigned if insulin is given temporarily to bring a type 2 patient's blood sugar under control during an encounter.

(b) **Assigning and sequencing secondary diabetes codes and its causes**

The sequencing of the secondary diabetes codes in relationship to codes for the cause of the diabetes is based on the Tabular List instructions for categories E08, E09 and E13.

(i) **Secondary diabetes mellitus due to pancreatectomy** For postpancreatectomy diabetes mellitus (lack of insulin due to the surgical removal of all or part of the pancreas), assign code E89.1, Postprocedural hypoinsulinemia. Assign a code from category E13 and a code from subcategory Z90.41-, Acquired absence of pancreas, as additional codes.

(ii) **Secondary diabetes due to drugs** Secondary diabetes may be caused by an adverse effect of correctly administered medications, poisoning or sequela of poisoning.

See Section I.C.19.e for coding of adverse effects and poisoning, and Section I.C.20 for external cause code reporting.

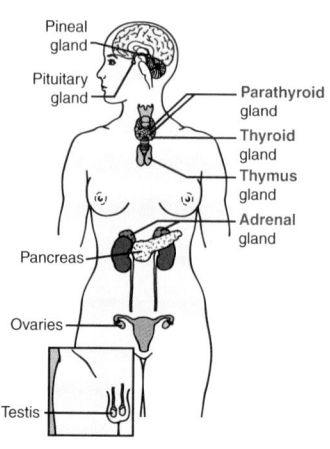

Figure 4-1   The endocrine system. (From Buck CJ: Step-by-Step Medical Coding, ed 2016, St. Louis, Elsevier, 2016)

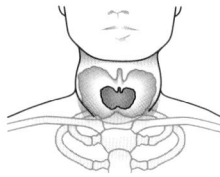

Figure 4-2   Goiter is an enlargement of the thyroid gland.

Item 4-1   Simple goiter indicates no nodules are present. The most common type of goiter is a **diffuse colloidal,** also called a **nontoxic** or **endemic** goiter.

CHAPTER 4

ENDOCRINE, NUTRITIONAL AND METABOLIC DISEASES (E00-E89)

All neoplasms, whether functionally active or not, are classified in Chapter 2. Appropriate codes in this chapter (i.e., E05.8, E07.0, E16-E31, E34.-) may be used as additional codes to indicate either functional activity by neoplasms and ectopic endocrine tissue or hyperfunction and hypofunction of endocrine glands associated with neoplasms and other conditions classified elsewhere.

> **Excludes1**   transitory endocrine and metabolic disorders specific to newborn (P70-P74)

This chapter contains the following blocks:

E00-E07	Disorders of thyroid gland
E08-E13	Diabetes mellitus
E15-E16	Other disorders of glucose regulation and pancreatic internal secretion
E20-E35	Disorders of other endocrine glands
E36	Intraoperative complications of endocrine system
E40-E46	Malnutrition
E50-E64	Other nutritional deficiencies
E65-E68	Overweight, obesity and other hyperalimentation
E70-E88	Metabolic disorders
E89	Postprocedural endocrine and metabolic complications and disorders, not elsewhere classified

DISORDERS OF THYROID GLAND (E00-E07)

● **E00   Congenital iodine-deficiency syndrome**

> Use additional code (F70-F79) to identify associated intellectual disabilities.

> **Excludes1**   subclinical iodine-deficiency hypothyroidism (E02)

E00.0   Congenital iodine-deficiency syndrome, neurological type
> Endemic cretinism, neurological type

E00.1   Congenital iodine-deficiency syndrome, myxedematous type
> *Dry, waxy type of swelling (nonpitting edema) with abnormal deposits of mucin in skin (mucinosis) and other tissues*
> Endemic hypothyroid cretinism
> Endemic cretinism, myxedematous type

E00.2   Congenital iodine-deficiency syndrome, mixed type
> Endemic cretinism, mixed type

E00.9   Congenital iodine-deficiency syndrome, unspecified
> Congenital iodine-deficiency hypothyroidism NOS
> Endemic cretinism NOS

● **E01   Iodine-deficiency related thyroid disorders and allied conditions**

> **Excludes1**   congenital iodine-deficiency syndrome (E00.-)
> subclinical iodine-deficiency hypothyroidism (E02)

E01.0   Iodine-deficiency related diffuse (endemic) goiter
> *Thyroid gland is enlarged*

E01.1   Iodine-deficiency related multinodular (endemic) goiter
> Iodine-deficiency related nodular goiter

E01.2   Iodine-deficiency related (endemic) goiter, unspecified
> Endemic goiter NOS

E01.8   Other iodine-deficiency related thyroid disorders and allied conditions
> Acquired iodine-deficiency hypothyroidism NOS

E02   Subclinical iodine-deficiency hypothyroidism

● **E03   Other hypothyroidism**

> **Excludes1**   iodine-deficiency related hypothyroidism (E00-E02)
> postprocedural hypothyroidism (E89.0)

E03.0   Congenital hypothyroidism with diffuse goiter
> Congenital parenchymatous goiter (nontoxic)
> Congenital goiter (nontoxic) NOS

> > **Excludes1**   transitory congenital goiter with normal function (P72.0)

E03.1   Congenital hypothyroidism without goiter
> Aplasia of thyroid (with myxedema)
> Congenital atrophy of thyroid
> Congenital hypothyroidism NOS

E03.2   Hypothyroidism due to medicaments and other exogenous substances
> *Code first poisoning due to drug or toxin, if applicable (T36-T65 with fifth or sixth character 1-4 or 6)*
> Use additional code for adverse effect, if applicable, to identify drug (T36-T50 with fifth or sixth character 5)

E03.3   Postinfectious hypothyroidism

E03.4   Atrophy of thyroid (acquired)
> > **Excludes1**   congenital atrophy of thyroid (E03.1)

E03.5   Myxedema coma 🖤
> *Often fatal complication of long-term hypothyroidism*

E03.8   Other specified hypothyroidism

E03.9   Hypothyroidism, unspecified
> Myxedema NOS

Item 4-2   Hypothyroidism is a condition in which there are insufficient levels of thyroxine. **Cretinism** is congenital hypothyroidism, which can result in mental and physical retardation.

▶ New   ⬛ Revised   ~~deleted~~ Deleted   Excludes 1   Excludes 2   Includes   Use additional   Code first   Code also   Key words
OGCR Official Guidelines   X Assign placeholder X   ● Use Additional Character(s)   ▶ Manifestation Code   🖤 Hierarchical Condition Category   **Coding Clinic**

E04 Other nontoxic goiter

Excludes1 congenital goiter (NOS) (diffuse) (parenchymatous) (E03.0)
iodine-deficiency related goiter (E00-E02)

E04.0 Nontoxic diffuse goiter
Thyroid gland is enlarged
Diffuse (colloid) nontoxic goiter
Simple nontoxic goiter

E04.1 Nontoxic single thyroid nodule
Colloid nodule (cystic) (thyroid)
Nontoxic uninodular goiter
Thyroid (cystic) nodule NOS

E04.2 Nontoxic multinodular goiter
Enlarged thyroid gland with multiple nodules
Cystic goiter NOS
Multinodular (cystic) goiter NOS

E04.8 Other specified nontoxic goiter

E04.9 Nontoxic goiter, unspecified
Goiter NOS
Nodular goiter (nontoxic) NOS

E05 Thyrotoxicosis [hyperthyroidism]
Enlarged thyroid gland with multiple nodules

Excludes1 chronic thyroiditis with transient thyrotoxicosis (E06.2)
neonatal thyrotoxicosis (P72.1)

E05.0 Thyrotoxicosis with diffuse goiter
Exophthalmic or toxic goiter NOS
Graves' disease
Toxic diffuse goiter

E05.00 Thyrotoxicosis with diffuse goiter without thyrotoxic crisis or storm

E05.01 Thyrotoxicosis with diffuse goiter with thyrotoxic crisis or storm

E05.1 Thyrotoxicosis with toxic single thyroid nodule
Thyrotoxicosis with toxic uninodular goiter

E05.10 Thyrotoxicosis with toxic single thyroid nodule without thyrotoxic crisis or storm

E05.11 Thyrotoxicosis with toxic single thyroid nodule with thyrotoxic crisis or storm

E05.2 Thyrotoxicosis with toxic multinodular goiter
Toxic nodular goiter NOS

E05.20 Thyrotoxicosis with toxic multinodular goiter without thyrotoxic crisis or storm

E05.21 Thyrotoxicosis with toxic multinodular goiter with thyrotoxic crisis or storm

E05.3 Thyrotoxicosis from ectopic thyroid tissue

E05.30 Thyrotoxicosis from ectopic thyroid tissue without thyrotoxic crisis or storm

E05.31 Thyrotoxicosis from ectopic thyroid tissue with thyrotoxic crisis or storm

E05.4 Thyrotoxicosis factitia

E05.40 Thyrotoxicosis factitia without thyrotoxic crisis or storm

E05.41 Thyrotoxicosis factitia with thyrotoxic crisis or storm

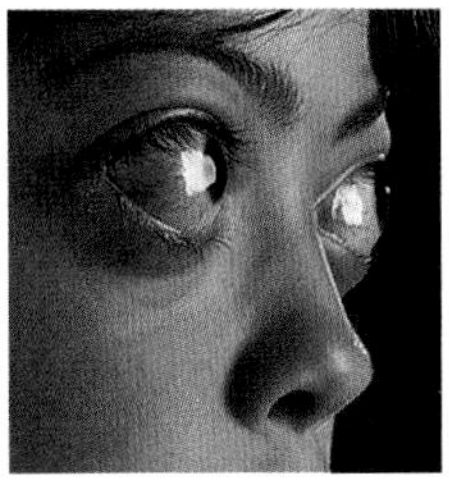

Figure 4-3 Graves' disease. In Graves' disease, exophthalmos often looks more pronounced than it actually is because of the extreme lid retraction that may occur. This patient, for instance, had minimal proptosis of the left eye but marked lid retraction. (From Lissauer T, Clayden G, and Craft A: Illustrated Textbook of Paediatrics, Edinburgh, Mosby, 2015)

Item 4–3 Thyrotoxicosis is a condition caused by excessive amounts of the thyroid hormone thyroxine production or hyperthyroidism. **Graves' disease is associated with hyperthyroidism** (known as **Basedow's disease** in Europe).

E05.8 Other thyrotoxicosis
Overproduction of thyroid-stimulating hormone

E05.80 Other thyrotoxicosis without thyrotoxic crisis or storm

E05.81 Other thyrotoxicosis with thyrotoxic crisis or storm

E05.9 Thyrotoxicosis, unspecified
Hyperthyroidism NOS

E05.90 Thyrotoxicosis, unspecified without thyrotoxic crisis or storm

E05.91 Thyrotoxicosis, unspecified with thyrotoxic crisis or storm

E06 Thyroiditis
An inflammation of the thyroid gland which results in an inability to convert iodine into thyroid hormone

Excludes1 postpartum thyroiditis (O90.5)

E06.0 Acute thyroiditis
Abscess of thyroid
Pyogenic thyroiditis
Suppurative thyroiditis
Use additional code (B95-B97) to identify infectious agent.

E06.1 Subacute thyroiditis
Inflammation of thyroid gland following viral upper respiratory infection
de Quervain thyroiditis
Giant-cell thyroiditis
Granulomatous thyroiditis
Nonsuppurative thyroiditis
Viral thyroiditis

Excludes1 autoimmune thyroiditis (E06.3)

E06.2 Chronic thyroiditis with transient thyrotoxicosis
Chronic inflammation of thyroid gland with intermittent overproduction of thyroid hormone

Excludes1 autoimmune thyroiditis (E06.3)

E06.3 Autoimmune thyroiditis
Hashimoto's thyroiditis
Hashitoxicosis (transient)
Lymphadenoid goiter
Lymphocytic thyroiditis
Struma lymphomatosa

E06.4 Drug-induced thyroiditis
Use additional code for adverse effect, if applicable, to identify drug (T36-T50 with fifth or sixth character 5)

E06.5 Other chronic thyroiditis
Chronic fibrous thyroiditis
Chronic thyroiditis NOS
Ligneous thyroiditis
Riedel thyroiditis

E06.9 Thyroiditis, unspecified

E07 Other disorders of thyroid

E07.0 Hypersecretion of calcitonin
C-cell hyperplasia of thyroid
Hypersecretion of thyrocalcitonin

E07.1 Dyshormogenetic goiter
Group of several types of goiter resulting from enzyme defects in hormone synthesis
Familial dyshormogenetic goiter
Pendred's syndrome

Excludes1 transitory congenital goiter with normal function (P72.0)

E07.8 Other specified disorders of thyroid

E07.81 Sick-euthyroid syndrome
Euthyroid sick-syndrome

E07.89 Other specified disorders of thyroid
Abnormality of thyroid-binding globulin
Hemorrhage of thyroid
Infarction of thyroid

E07.9 Disorder of thyroid, unspecified

CHAPTER 4 (E00-E90)

OGCR Section I.C.4.a.

Diabetes mellitus

The diabetes mellitus codes are combination codes that include the type of diabetes mellitus, body system affected, and the complications affecting that body system. As many codes within a particular category as are necessary to describe all of the complications of the disease may be used. They should be sequenced based on the reason for a particular visit. Assign as many codes from categories E08–E13 as needed to identify all of the associated conditions that the patient has.

DIABETES MELLITUS (E08-E13)

A metabolic disease that results in persistent hyperglycemia

Coding Clinic: 2016, Q4, P142

E08 Diabetes mellitus due to underlying condition

Code first the underlying condition, such as:
- congenital rubella (P35.0)
- Cushing's syndrome (E24.-)
- cystic fibrosis (E84.-)
- malignant neoplasm (C00-C96)
- malnutrition (E40-E46)
- pancreatitis and other diseases of the pancreas (K85-K86.-)

Use additional code to identify control using:
- insulin (Z79.4)
- oral antidiabetic drugs (Z79.84)
- oral hypoglycemic drugs (Z79.84)

Excludes1 drug or chemical induced diabetes mellitus (E09.-)
- gestational diabetes (O24.4-)
- neonatal diabetes mellitus (P70.2)
- postpancreatectomy diabetes mellitus (E13.-)
- postprocedural diabetes mellitus (E13.-)
- secondary diabetes mellitus NEC (E13.-)
- type 1 diabetes mellitus (E10.-)
- type 2 diabetes mellitus (E11.-)

E08.0 Diabetes mellitus due to underlying condition with hyperosmolarity

E08.00 Diabetes mellitus due to underlying condition with hyperosmolarity without nonketotic hyperglycemic-hyperosmolar coma (NKHHC)

E08.01 Diabetes mellitus due to underlying condition with hyperosmolarity with coma

E08.1 Diabetes mellitus due to underlying condition with ketoacidosis

E08.10 Diabetes mellitus due to underlying condition with ketoacidosis without coma

E08.11 Diabetes mellitus due to underlying condition with ketoacidosis with coma

E08.2 Diabetes mellitus due to underlying condition with kidney complications

E08.21 Diabetes mellitus due to underlying condition with diabetic nephropathy
- Diabetes mellitus due to underlying condition with intercapillary glomerulosclerosis
- Diabetes mellitus due to underlying condition with intracapillary glomerulonephrosis
- Diabetes mellitus due to underlying condition with Kimmelstiel-Wilson disease

E08.22 Diabetes mellitus due to underlying condition with diabetic chronic kidney disease

Use additional code to identify stage of chronic kidney disease (N18.1-N18.6)

E08.29 Diabetes mellitus due to underlying condition with other diabetic kidney complication
- Renal tubular degeneration in diabetes mellitus due to underlying condition

E08.3 Diabetes mellitus due to underlying condition with ophthalmic complications

Changes in blood vessels of retina in which blood vessels swell and leak fluid into retinal surface.

Coding Clinic: 2016, Q4, P11

E08.31 Diabetes mellitus due to underlying condition with unspecified diabetic retinopathy

E08.311 Diabetes mellitus due to underlying condition with unspecified diabetic retinopathy with macular edema

E08.319 Diabetes mellitus due to underlying condition with unspecified diabetic retinopathy without macular edema

E08.32 Diabetes mellitus due to underlying condition with mild nonproliferative diabetic retinopathy

Diabetes mellitus due to underlying condition with nonproliferative diabetic retinopathy NOS

One of the following 7th characters is to be assigned to codes in subcategory E08.32 to designate laterality of the disease:

1	right eye
2	left eye
3	bilateral
9	unspecified eye

E08.321 Diabetes mellitus due to underlying condition with mild nonproliferative diabetic retinopathy with macular edema

E08.329 Diabetes mellitus due to underlying condition with mild nonproliferative diabetic retinopathy without macular edema

E08.33 Diabetes mellitus due to underlying condition with moderate nonproliferative diabetic retinopathy

One of the following 7th characters is to be assigned to codes in subcategory E08.33 to designate laterality of the disease:

1	right eye
2	left eye
3	bilateral
9	unspecified eye

E08.331 Diabetes mellitus due to underlying condition with moderate nonproliferative diabetic retinopathy with macular edema

E08.339 Diabetes mellitus due to underlying condition with moderate nonproliferative diabetic retinopathy without macular edema

E08.34 Diabetes mellitus due to underlying condition with severe nonproliferative diabetic retinopathy

One of the following 7th characters is to be assigned to codes in subcategory E08.34 to designate laterality of the disease:

1	right eye
2	left eye
3	bilateral
9	unspecified eye

E08.341 Diabetes mellitus due to underlying condition with severe nonproliferative diabetic retinopathy with macular edema

E08.349 Diabetes mellitus due to underlying condition with severe nonproliferative diabetic retinopathy without macular edema

E08.35 Diabetes mellitus due to underlying condition with proliferative diabetic retinopathy

One of the following 7th characters is to be assigned to codes in subcategory E08.35 to designate laterality of the disease:

1	right eye
2	left eye
3	bilateral
9	unspecified eye

E08.351 Diabetes mellitus due to underlying condition with proliferative diabetic retinopathy with macular edema

E08.352 Diabetes mellitus due to underlying condition with proliferative diabetic retinopathy with traction retinal detachment involving the macula

E08.353 Diabetes mellitus due to underlying condition with proliferative diabetic retinopathy with traction retinal detachment not involving the macula

E08.354 Diabetes mellitus due to underlying condition with proliferative diabetic retinopathy with combined traction retinal detachment and rhegmatogenous retinal detachment

E08.355 Diabetes mellitus due to underlying condition with stable proliferative diabetic retinopathy

E08.359 Diabetes mellitus due to underlying condition with proliferative diabetic retinopathy without macular edema

E08.36 Diabetes mellitus due to underlying condition with diabetic cataract

X *E08.37 Diabetes mellitus due to underlying condition with diabetic macular edema, resolved following treatment*

One of the following 7th characters is to be assigned to code E08.37 to designate laterality of the disease:

1	right eye
2	left eye
3	bilateral
9	unspecified eye

E08.39 Diabetes mellitus due to underlying condition with other diabetic ophthalmic complication

Use additional code to identify manifestation, such as:
diabetic glaucoma (H40-H42)

E08.4 Diabetes mellitus due to underlying condition with neurological complications

E08.40 Diabetes mellitus due to underlying condition with diabetic neuropathy, unspecified

E08.41 Diabetes mellitus due to underlying condition with diabetic mononeuropathy

E08.42 Diabetes mellitus due to underlying condition with diabetic polyneuropathy

Diabetes mellitus due to underlying condition with diabetic neuralgia

E08.43 Diabetes mellitus due to underlying condition with diabetic autonomic (poly)neuropathy

Diabetes mellitus due to underlying condition with diabetic gastroparesis

E08.44 Diabetes mellitus due to underlying condition with diabetic amyotrophy

E08.49 Diabetes mellitus due to underlying condition with other diabetic neurological complication

E08.5 Diabetes mellitus due to underlying condition with circulatory complications

E08.51 Diabetes mellitus due to underlying condition with diabetic peripheral angiopathy without gangrene

E08.52 Diabetes mellitus due to underlying condition with diabetic peripheral angiopathy with gangrene

Diabetes mellitus due to underlying condition with diabetic gangrene

E08.59 Diabetes mellitus due to underlying condition with other circulatory complications

E08.6 Diabetes mellitus due to underlying condition with other specified complications

E08.61 Diabetes mellitus due to underlying condition with diabetic arthropathy

E08.610 Diabetes mellitus due to underlying condition with diabetic neuropathic arthropathy

Diabetes mellitus due to underlying condition with Charcôt's joints

E08.618 Diabetes mellitus due to underlying condition with other diabetic arthropathy

E08.62 Diabetes mellitus due to underlying condition with skin complications

E08.620 Diabetes mellitus due to underlying condition with diabetic dermatitis

Diabetes mellitus due to underlying condition with diabetic necrobiosis lipoidica

E08.621 Diabetes mellitus due to underlying condition with foot ulcer

Use additional code to identify site of ulcer (L97.4-, L97.5-)

E08.622 Diabetes mellitus due to underlying condition with other skin ulcer

Use additional code to identify site of ulcer (L97.1-L97.9, L98.41-L98.49)

E08.628 Diabetes mellitus due to underlying condition with other skin complications

E08.63 Diabetes mellitus due to underlying condition with oral complications

E08.630 Diabetes mellitus due to underlying condition with periodontal disease

E08.638 Diabetes mellitus due to underlying condition with other oral complications

E08.64 Diabetes mellitus due to underlying condition with hypoglycemia

E08.641 Diabetes mellitus due to underlying condition with hypoglycemia with coma

E08.649 Diabetes mellitus due to underlying condition with hypoglycemia without coma

E08.65 Diabetes mellitus due to underlying condition with hyperglycemia

E08.69 Diabetes mellitus due to underlying condition with other specified complication

Use additional code to identify complication

E08.8 Diabetes mellitus due to underlying condition with unspecified complications

E08.9 Diabetes mellitus due to underlying condition without complications

CHAPTER 4 (E00-E90)

● **EØ9 Drug or chemical induced diabetes mellitus**

Code first poisoning due to drug or toxin, if applicable (T36-T65 with fifth or sixth character 1-4 or 6)

Use additional code for adverse effect, if applicable, to identify drug (T36-T5Ø with fifth or sixth character 5)

Use additional code to identify control using:
- insulin (Z79.4)
- oral antidiabetic drugs (Z79.84)
- oral hypoglycemic drugs (Z79.84)

Excludes1 diabetes mellitus due to underlying condition (EØ8.-)
gestational diabetes (O24.4-)
neonatal diabetes mellitus (P7Ø.2)
postpancreatectomy diabetes mellitus (E13.-)
postprocedural diabetes mellitus (E13.-)
secondary diabetes mellitus NEC (E13.-)
type 1 diabetes mellitus (E1Ø.-)
type 2 diabetes mellitus (E11.-)

● **EØ9.Ø Drug or chemical induced diabetes mellitus with hyperosmolarity**

EØ9.ØØ Drug or chemical induced diabetes mellitus with hyperosmolarity without nonketotic hyperglycemic-hyperosmolar coma (NKHHC)

EØ9.Ø1 Drug or chemical induced diabetes mellitus with hyperosmolarity with coma

● **EØ9.1 Drug or chemical induced diabetes mellitus with ketoacidosis**

EØ9.1Ø Drug or chemical induced diabetes mellitus with ketoacidosis without coma

EØ9.11 Drug or chemical induced diabetes mellitus with ketoacidosis with coma

● **EØ9.2 Drug or chemical induced diabetes mellitus with kidney complications**

EØ9.21 Drug or chemical induced diabetes mellitus with diabetic nephropathy

Drug or chemical induced diabetes mellitus with intercapillary glomerulosclerosis
Drug or chemical induced diabetes mellitus with intracapillary glomerulonephrosis
Drug or chemical induced diabetes mellitus with Kimmelstiel-Wilson disease

EØ9.22 Drug or chemical induced diabetes mellitus with diabetic chronic kidney disease

Use additional code to identify stage of chronic kidney disease (N18.1-N18.6)

EØ9.29 Drug or chemical induced diabetes mellitus with other diabetic kidney complication

Drug or chemical induced diabetes mellitus with renal tubular degeneration

● **EØ9.3 Drug or chemical induced diabetes mellitus with ophthalmic complications**

Coding Clinic: 2016, Q4, P11

● **EØ9.31 Drug or chemical induced diabetes mellitus with unspecified diabetic retinopathy**

EØ9.311 Drug or chemical induced diabetes mellitus with unspecified diabetic retinopathy with macular edema

EØ9.319 Drug or chemical induced diabetes mellitus with unspecified diabetic retinopathy without macular edema

● **EØ9.32 Drug or chemical induced diabetes mellitus with mild nonproliferative diabetic retinopathy**

Drug or chemical induced diabetes mellitus with nonproliferative diabetic retinopathy NOS

One of the following 7th characters is to be assigned to codes in subcategory EØ9.32 to designate laterality of the disease:

1	right eye
2	left eye
3	bilateral
9	unspecified eye

● **EØ9.321 Drug or chemical induced diabetes mellitus with mild nonproliferative diabetic retinopathy with macular edema**

● **EØ9.329 Drug or chemical induced diabetes mellitus with mild nonproliferative diabetic retinopathy without macular edema**

● **EØ9.33 Drug or chemical induced diabetes mellitus with moderate nonproliferative diabetic retinopathy**

One of the following 7th characters is to be assigned to codes in subcategory EØ9.33 to designate laterality of the disease:

1	right eye
2	left eye
3	bilateral
9	unspecified eye

● **EØ9.331 Drug or chemical induced diabetes mellitus with moderate nonproliferative diabetic retinopathy with macular edema**

● **EØ9.339 Drug or chemical induced diabetes mellitus with moderate nonproliferative diabetic retinopathy without macular edema**

● **EØ9.34 Drug or chemical induced diabetes mellitus with severe nonproliferative diabetic retinopathy**

One of the following 7th characters is to be assigned to codes in subcategory EØ9.34 to designate laterality of the disease:

1	right eye
2	left eye
3	bilateral
9	unspecified eye

● **EØ9.341 Drug or chemical induced diabetes mellitus with severe nonproliferative diabetic retinopathy with macular edema**

● **EØ9.349 Drug or chemical induced diabetes mellitus with severe nonproliferative diabetic retinopathy without macular edema**

CHAPTER 4 (EØØ-E9Ø)

E09.35 Drug or chemical induced diabetes mellitus with proliferative diabetic retinopathy

One of the following 7th characters is to be assigned to codes in subcategory E09.35 to designate laterality of the disease:

1	right eye
2	left eye
3	bilateral
9	unspecified eye

E09.351 Drug or chemical induced diabetes mellitus with proliferative diabetic retinopathy with macular edema

E09.352 Drug or chemical induced diabetes mellitus with proliferative diabetic retinopathy with traction retinal detachment involving the macula

E09.353 Drug or chemical induced diabetes mellitus with proliferative diabetic retinopathy with traction retinal detachment not involving the macula

E09.354 Drug or chemical induced diabetes mellitus with proliferative diabetic retinopathy with combined traction retinal detachment and rhegmatogenous retinal detachment

E09.355 Drug or chemical induced diabetes mellitus with stable proliferative diabetic retinopathy

E09.359 Drug or chemical induced diabetes mellitus with proliferative diabetic retinopathy without macular edema

E09.36 Drug or chemical induced diabetes mellitus with diabetic cataract

X **E09.37 Drug or chemical induced diabetes mellitus with diabetic macular edema, resolved following treatment**

One of the following 7th characters is to be assigned to code E09.37 to designate laterality of the disease:

1	right eye
2	left eye
3	bilateral
9	unspecified eye

E09.39 Drug or chemical induced diabetes mellitus with other diabetic ophthalmic complication

Use additional code to identify manifestation, such as:
diabetic glaucoma (H40-H42)

E09.4 Drug or chemical induced diabetes mellitus with neurological complications

E09.40 Drug or chemical induced diabetes mellitus with neurological complications with diabetic neuropathy, unspecified

E09.41 Drug or chemical induced diabetes mellitus with neurological complications with diabetic mononeuropathy

E09.42 Drug or chemical induced diabetes mellitus with neurological complications with diabetic polyneuropathy

Drug or chemical induced diabetes mellitus with diabetic neuralgia

E09.43 Drug or chemical induced diabetes mellitus with neurological complications with diabetic autonomic (poly)neuropathy

Drug or chemical induced diabetes mellitus with diabetic gastroparesis

E09.44 Drug or chemical induced diabetes mellitus with neurological complications with diabetic amyotrophy

E09.49 Drug or chemical induced diabetes mellitus with neurological complications with other diabetic neurological complication

E09.5 Drug or chemical induced diabetes mellitus with circulatory complications

E09.51 Drug or chemical induced diabetes mellitus with diabetic peripheral angiopathy without gangrene

E09.52 Drug or chemical induced diabetes mellitus with diabetic peripheral angiopathy with gangrene

Drug or chemical induced diabetes mellitus with diabetic gangrene

E09.59 Drug or chemical induced diabetes mellitus with other circulatory complications

E09.6 Drug or chemical induced diabetes mellitus with other specified complications

E09.61 Drug or chemical induced diabetes mellitus with diabetic arthropathy

E09.610 Drug or chemical induced diabetes mellitus with diabetic neuropathic arthropathy

Drug or chemical induced diabetes mellitus with Charcôt's joints

Progressive degeneration of weight-bearing joint

E09.618 Drug or chemical induced diabetes mellitus with other diabetic arthropathy

E09.62 Drug or chemical induced diabetes mellitus with skin complications

E09.620 Drug or chemical induced diabetes mellitus with diabetic dermatitis

Drug or chemical induced diabetes mellitus with diabetic necrobiosis lipoidica

Necrotizing skin condition

E09.621 Drug or chemical induced diabetes mellitus with foot ulcer

Use additional code to identify site of ulcer (L97.4-, L97.5-)

E09.622 Drug or chemical induced diabetes mellitus with other skin ulcer

Use additional code to identify site of ulcer (L97.1-L97.9, L98.41-L98.49)

E09.628 Drug or chemical induced diabetes mellitus with other skin complications

E09.63 Drug or chemical induced diabetes mellitus with oral complications

E09.630 Drug or chemical induced diabetes mellitus with periodontal disease

E09.638 Drug or chemical induced diabetes mellitus with other oral complications

E09.64 Drug or chemical induced diabetes mellitus with hypoglycemia

E09.641 Drug or chemical induced diabetes mellitus with hypoglycemia with coma

E09.649 Drug or chemical induced diabetes mellitus with hypoglycemia without coma

E09.65 Drug or chemical induced diabetes mellitus with hyperglycemia

E09.69 Drug or chemical induced diabetes mellitus with other specified complication

Use additional code to identify complication

E09.8 Drug or chemical induced diabetes mellitus with unspecified complications

E09.9 Drug or chemical induced diabetes mellitus without complications

CHAPTER 4 (E00-E90)

E10 Type 1 diabetes mellitus

Includes brittle diabetes (mellitus)
diabetes (mellitus) due to autoimmune process
diabetes (mellitus) due to immune mediated pancreatic islet beta-cell destruction
idiopathic diabetes (mellitus)
juvenile onset diabetes (mellitus)
ketosis-prone diabetes (mellitus)

Excludes1 diabetes mellitus due to underlying condition (E08.-)
drug or chemical induced diabetes mellitus (E09.-)
gestational diabetes (O24.4-)
hyperglycemia NOS (R73.9)
neonatal diabetes mellitus (P70.2)
postpancreatectomy diabetes mellitus (E13.-)
postprocedural diabetes mellitus (E13.-)
secondary diabetes mellitus NEC (E13.-)
type 2 diabetes mellitus (E11.-)

E10.1 Type 1 diabetes mellitus with ketoacidosis

Acidosis accompanied by accumulation of ketone bodies (ketosis) in body tissues and fluids

E10.10 Type 1 diabetes mellitus with ketoacidosis without coma

Coding Clinic: 2013, Q3, P20

E10.11 Type 1 diabetes mellitus with ketoacidosis with coma

E10.2 Type 1 diabetes mellitus with kidney complications

E10.21 Type 1 diabetes mellitus with diabetic nephropathy

Type 1 diabetes mellitus with intercapillary glomerulosclerosis
Type 1 diabetes mellitus with intracapillary glomerulonephrosis
Type 1 diabetes mellitus with Kimmelstiel-Wilson disease

E10.22 Type 1 diabetes mellitus with diabetic chronic kidney disease

Use additional code to identify stage of chronic kidney disease (N18.1-N18.6)

E10.29 Type 1 diabetes mellitus with other diabetic kidney complication

Type 1 diabetes mellitus with renal tubular degeneration

Coding Clinic: 2016, Q1, P13

E10.3 Type 1 diabetes mellitus with ophthalmic complications

Coding Clinic: 2016, Q4, P11

E10.31 Type 1 diabetes mellitus with unspecified diabetic retinopathy

E10.311 Type 1 diabetes mellitus with unspecified diabetic retinopathy with macular edema

E10.319 Type 1 diabetes mellitus with unspecified diabetic retinopathy without macular edema

E10.32 Type 1 diabetes mellitus with mild nonproliferative diabetic retinopathy

Type 1 diabetes mellitus with nonproliferative diabetic retinopathy NOS

One of the following 7th characters is to be assigned to codes in subcategory E10.32 to designate laterality of the disease:

1	right eye
2	left eye
3	bilateral
9	unspecified eye

E10.321 Type 1 diabetes mellitus with mild nonproliferative diabetic retinopathy with macular edema

E10.329 Type 1 diabetes mellitus with mild nonproliferative diabetic retinopathy without macular edema

E10.33 Type 1 diabetes mellitus with moderate nonproliferative diabetic retinopathy

One of the following 7th characters is to be assigned to codes in subcategory E10.33 to designate laterality of the disease:

1	right eye
2	left eye
3	bilateral
9	unspecified eye

E10.331 Type 1 diabetes mellitus with moderate nonproliferative diabetic retinopathy with macular edema

E10.339 Type 1 diabetes mellitus with moderate nonproliferative diabetic retinopathy without macular edema

E10.34 Type 1 diabetes mellitus with severe nonproliferative diabetic retinopathy

One of the following 7th characters is to be assigned to codes in subcategory E10.34 to designate laterality of the disease:

1	right eye
2	left eye
3	bilateral
9	unspecified eye

E10.341 Type 1 diabetes mellitus with severe nonproliferative diabetic retinopathy with macular edema

E10.349 Type 1 diabetes mellitus with severe nonproliferative diabetic retinopathy without macular edema

E10.35 Type 1 diabetes mellitus with proliferative diabetic retinopathy

One of the following 7th characters is to be assigned to codes in subcategory E10.35 to designate laterality of the disease:

1	right eye
2	left eye
3	bilateral
9	unspecified eye

E10.351 Type 1 diabetes mellitus with proliferative diabetic retinopathy with macular edema

E10.352 Type 1 diabetes mellitus with proliferative diabetic retinopathy with traction retinal detachment involving the macula

E10.353 Type 1 diabetes mellitus with proliferative diabetic retinopathy with traction retinal detachment not involving the macula

E10.354 Type 1 diabetes mellitus with proliferative diabetic retinopathy with combined traction retinal detachment and rhegmatogenous retinal detachment

E10.355 Type 1 diabetes mellitus with stable proliferative diabetic retinopathy

E10.359 Type 1 diabetes mellitus with proliferative diabetic retinopathy without macular edema

E10.36 **Type 1 diabetes mellitus with diabetic cataract**

X **E10.37** **Type 1 diabetes mellitus with diabetic macular edema, resolved following treatment**

One of the following 7th characters is to be assigned to code E10.37 to designate laterality of the disease:

1	right eye
2	left eye
3	bilateral
9	unspecified eye

E10.39 **Type 1 diabetes mellitus with other diabetic ophthalmic complication**

Use additional code to identify manifestation, such as:
diabetic glaucoma (H40-H42)

E10.4 **Type 1 diabetes mellitus with neurological complications**

E10.40 **Type 1 diabetes mellitus with diabetic neuropathy, unspecified**

E10.41 **Type 1 diabetes mellitus with diabetic mononeuropathy**

E10.42 **Type 1 diabetes mellitus with diabetic polyneuropathy**

Type 1 diabetes mellitus with diabetic neuralgia

E10.43 **Type 1 diabetes mellitus with diabetic autonomic (poly)neuropathy**

Type 1 diabetes mellitus with diabetic gastroparesis

E10.44 **Type 1 diabetes mellitus with diabetic amyotrophy**

E10.49 **Type 1 diabetes mellitus with other diabetic neurological complication**

E10.5 **Type 1 diabetes mellitus with circulatory complications**

E10.51 **Type 1 diabetes mellitus with diabetic peripheral angiopathy without gangrene**

E10.52 **Type 1 diabetes mellitus with diabetic peripheral angiopathy with gangrene**

Type 1 diabetes mellitus with diabetic gangrene

E10.59 **Type 1 diabetes mellitus with other circulatory complications**

E10.6 **Type 1 diabetes mellitus with other specified complications**

E10.61 **Type 1 diabetes mellitus with diabetic arthropathy**

E10.610 **Type 1 diabetes mellitus with diabetic neuropathic arthropathy**

Type 1 diabetes mellitus with Charcôt's joints

E10.618 **Type 1 diabetes mellitus with other diabetic arthropathy**

E10.62 **Type 1 diabetes mellitus with skin complications**

E10.620 **Type 1 diabetes mellitus with diabetic dermatitis**

Type 1 diabetes mellitus with diabetic necrobiosis lipoidica

E10.621 **Type 1 diabetes mellitus with foot ulcer**

Use additional code to identify site of ulcer (L97.4-, L97.5-)

E10.622 **Type 1 diabetes mellitus with other skin ulcer**

Use additional code to identify site of ulcer (L97.1-L97.9, L98.41-L98.49)

E10.628 **Type 1 diabetes mellitus with other skin complications**

E10.63 **Type 1 diabetes mellitus with oral complications**

E10.630 **Type 1 diabetes mellitus with periodontal disease**

E10.638 **Type 1 diabetes mellitus with other oral complications**

E10.64 **Type 1 diabetes mellitus with hypoglycemia**

E10.641 **Type 1 diabetes mellitus with hypoglycemia with coma**

E10.649 **Type 1 diabetes mellitus with hypoglycemia without coma**

Coding Clinic: 2016, Q1, P13

E10.65 **Type 1 diabetes mellitus with hyperglycemia**

Coding Clinic: 2013, Q3, P20

E10.69 **Type 1 diabetes mellitus with other specified complication**

Use additional code to identify complication

E10.8 **Type 1 diabetes mellitus with unspecified complications**

E10.9 **Type 1 diabetes mellitus without complications**

E11 **Type 2 diabetes mellitus**

Includes diabetes (mellitus) due to insulin secretory defect
diabetes NOS
insulin resistant diabetes (mellitus)

Use additional code to identify control using:
insulin (Z79.4)
oral antidiabetic drugs (Z79.84)
oral hypoglycemic drugs (Z79.84)

Excludes1 diabetes mellitus due to underlying condition (E08.-)
drug or chemical induced diabetes mellitus (E09.-)
gestational diabetes (O24.4-)
neonatal diabetes mellitus (P70.2)
postpancreatectomy diabetes mellitus (E13.-)
postprocedural diabetes mellitus (E13.-)
secondary diabetes mellitus NEC (E13.-)
type 1 diabetes mellitus (E10.-)

Coding Clinic: 2016, Q4, P121, Q2, P10

E11.0 **Type 2 diabetes mellitus with hyperosmolarity**

E11.00 **Type 2 diabetes mellitus with hyperosmolarity without nonketotic hyperglycemic-hyperosmolar coma (NKHHC)**

E11.01 **Type 2 diabetes mellitus with hyperosmolarity with coma**

E11.1 **Type 2 diabetes mellitus with ketoacidosis**

E11.10 **Type 2 diabetes mellitus with ketoacidosis without coma**

Coding Clinic: 2017, Q4, P6

E11.11 **Type 2 diabetes mellitus with ketoacidosis with coma**

E11.2 **Type 2 diabetes mellitus with kidney complications**

E11.21 **Type 2 diabetes mellitus with diabetic nephropathy**

Type 2 diabetes mellitus with intercapillary glomerulosclerosis
Type 2 diabetes mellitus with intracapillary glomerulonephrosis
Type 2 diabetes mellitus with Kimmelstiel-Wilson disease

E11.22 **Type 2 diabetes mellitus with diabetic chronic kidney disease**

Use additional code to identify stage of chronic kidney disease (N18.1-N18.6)

Coding Clinic: 2018, Q4, P88; 2016, Q2, P36, Q1, P13

E11.29 **Type 2 diabetes mellitus with other diabetic kidney complication**

Type 2 diabetes mellitus with renal tubular degeneration

CHAPTER 4 (E00-E90)

● E11.3 Type 2 diabetes mellitus with ophthalmic complications
Coding Clinic: 2016, Q4, P11

● E11.31 Type 2 diabetes mellitus with unspecified diabetic retinopathy

E11.311 Type 2 diabetes mellitus with unspecified diabetic retinopathy with macular edema

E11.319 Type 2 diabetes mellitus with unspecified diabetic retinopathy without macular edema
Coding Clinic: 2013, Q3, P20

● E11.32 Type 2 diabetes mellitus with mild nonproliferative diabetic retinopathy
Type 2 diabetes mellitus with nonproliferative diabetic retinopathy NOS
One of the following 7th characters is to be assigned to codes in subcategory E11.32 to designate laterality of the disease:

1	right eye
2	left eye
3	bilateral
9	unspecified eye

● E11.321 Type 2 diabetes mellitus with mild nonproliferative diabetic retinopathy with macular edema

● E11.329 Type 2 diabetes mellitus with mild nonproliferative diabetic retinopathy without macular edema

● E11.33 Type 2 diabetes mellitus with moderate nonproliferative diabetic retinopathy
One of the following 7th characters is to be assigned to codes in subcategory E11.33 to designate laterality of the disease:

1	right eye
2	left eye
3	bilateral
9	unspecified eye

● E11.331 Type 2 diabetes mellitus with moderate nonproliferative diabetic retinopathy with macular edema

● E11.339 Type 2 diabetes mellitus with moderate nonproliferative diabetic retinopathy without macular edema

● E11.34 Type 2 diabetes mellitus with severe nonproliferative diabetic retinopathy
One of the following 7th characters is to be assigned to codes in subcategory E11.34 to designate laterality of the disease:

1	right eye
2	left eye
3	bilateral
9	unspecified eye

● E11.341 Type 2 diabetes mellitus with severe nonproliferative diabetic retinopathy with macular edema

● E11.349 Type 2 diabetes mellitus with severe nonproliferative diabetic retinopathy without macular edema

● E11.35 Type 2 diabetes mellitus with proliferative diabetic retinopathy
One of the following 7th characters is to be assigned to codes in subcategory E11.35 to designate laterality of the disease:

1	right eye
2	left eye
3	bilateral
9	unspecified eye

● E11.351 Type 2 diabetes mellitus with proliferative diabetic retinopathy with macular edema

● E11.352 Type 2 diabetes mellitus with proliferative diabetic retinopathy with traction retinal detachment involving the macula

● E11.353 Type 2 diabetes mellitus with proliferative diabetic retinopathy with traction retinal detachment not involving the macula

● E11.354 Type 2 diabetes mellitus with proliferative diabetic retinopathy with combined traction retinal detachment and rhegmatogenous retinal detachment

● E11.355 Type 2 diabetes mellitus with stable proliferative diabetic retinopathy

● E11.359 Type 2 diabetes mellitus with proliferative diabetic retinopathy without macular edema

E11.36 Type 2 diabetes mellitus with diabetic cataract
Coding Clinic: 2019, Q2, P30-31; 2016, Q2, P36

X● E11.37 Type 2 diabetes mellitus with diabetic macular edema, resolved following treatment
One of the following 7th characters is to be assigned to code E11.37 to designate laterality of the disease:

1	right eye
2	left eye
3	bilateral
9	unspecified eye

E11.39 Type 2 diabetes mellitus with other diabetic ophthalmic complication
Use additional code to identify manifestation, such as:
diabetic glaucoma (H40-H42)

● E11.4 Type 2 diabetes mellitus with neurological complications

E11.40 Type 2 diabetes mellitus with diabetic neuropathy, unspecified

E11.41 Type 2 diabetes mellitus with diabetic mononeuropathy

E11.42 Type 2 diabetes mellitus with diabetic polyneuropathy
Type 2 diabetes mellitus with diabetic neuralgia
Coding Clinic: 2016, Q1, P13

E11.43 Type 2 diabetes mellitus with diabetic autonomic (poly)neuropathy
Type 2 diabetes mellitus with diabetic gastroparesis
Coding Clinic: 2016, Q2, P36

E11.44 Type 2 diabetes mellitus with diabetic amyotrophy
Coding Clinic: 2016, Q2, P36

E11.49 Type 2 diabetes mellitus with other diabetic neurological complication

E11.5 Type 2 diabetes mellitus with circulatory complications

E11.51 **Type 2 diabetes mellitus with diabetic peripheral angiopathy without gangrene**

E11.52 **Type 2 diabetes mellitus with diabetic peripheral angiopathy with gangrene**
Type 2 diabetes mellitus with diabetic gangrene
Coding Clinic: 2017, Q4, P1Ø2

E11.59 **Type 2 diabetes mellitus with other circulatory complications**

E11.6 Type 2 diabetes mellitus with other specified complications

E11.61 Type 2 diabetes mellitus with diabetic arthropathy

E11.61Ø **Type 2 diabetes mellitus with diabetic neuropathic arthropathy**
Type 2 diabetes mellitus with Charcôt's joints
Coding Clinic: 2Ø16, Q2, P36

E11.618 **Type 2 diabetes mellitus with other diabetic arthropathy**
Coding Clinic: 2Ø18, Q2, P7; 2Ø16, Q2, P36

E11.62 Type 2 diabetes mellitus with skin complications

E11.62Ø **Type 2 diabetes mellitus with diabetic dermatitis**
Type 2 diabetes mellitus with diabetic necrobiosis lipoidica

E11.621 **Type 2 diabetes mellitus with foot ulcer**
Use additional code to identify site of ulcer (L97.4-, L97.5-)
Coding Clinic: 2Ø16, Q1, P12

E11.622 **Type 2 diabetes mellitus with other skin ulcer**
Use additional code to identify site of ulcer (L97.1-L97.9, L98.41-L98.49)
Coding Clinic: 2Ø17, Q4, P17

E11.628 **Type 2 diabetes mellitus with other skin complications**

E11.63 Type 2 diabetes mellitus with oral complications

E11.63Ø **Type 2 diabetes mellitus with periodontal disease**

E11.638 **Type 2 diabetes mellitus with other oral complications**

E11.64 Type 2 diabetes mellitus with hypoglycemia

E11.641 **Type 2 diabetes mellitus with hypoglycemia with coma**

E11.649 **Type 2 diabetes mellitus with hypoglycemia without coma**
Coding Clinic: 2Ø16, Q3, P42; 2Ø15, Q3, P21

E11.65 **Type 2 diabetes mellitus with hyperglycemia**
Coding Clinic: 2Ø13, Q3, P2Ø

E11.69 **Type 2 diabetes mellitus with other specified complication**
Use additional code to identify complication
Coding Clinic: 2Ø16, Q4, P142

E11.8 **Type 2 diabetes mellitus with unspecified complications**

E11.9 **Type 2 diabetes mellitus without complications**
Coding Clinic: 2Ø16, Q4, P142, Q2, P36

E13 Other specified diabetes mellitus

Includes diabetes mellitus due to genetic defects of beta-cell function
diabetes mellitus due to genetic defects in insulin action
postpancreatectomy diabetes mellitus
postprocedural diabetes mellitus
secondary diabetes mellitus NEC

Use additional code to identify control using:
insulin (Z79.4)
oral antidiabetic drugs (Z79.84)
oral hypoglycemic drugs (Z79.84)

Excludes1 diabetes (mellitus) due to autoimmune process (E1Ø.-)
diabetes (mellitus) due to immune mediated pancreatic islet beta-cell destruction (E1Ø.-)
diabetes mellitus due to underlying condition (EØ8.-)
drug or chemical induced diabetes mellitus (EØ9.-)
gestational diabetes (O24.4-)
neonatal diabetes mellitus (P7Ø.2)
type 1 diabetes mellitus (E1Ø.-)

E13.Ø Other specified diabetes mellitus with hyperosmolarity

E13.ØØ **Other specified diabetes mellitus with hyperosmolarity without nonketotic hyperglycemic-hyperosmolar coma (NKHHC)**
Excludes2 type 2 diabetes mellitus (E11.-)

E13.Ø1 **Other specified diabetes mellitus with hyperosmolarity with coma**

E13.1 Other specified diabetes mellitus with ketoacidosis

E13.1Ø **Other specified diabetes mellitus with ketoacidosis without coma**
Coding Clinic: 2Ø16, Q2, P1Ø; 2Ø13, Q1, P26

E13.11 **Other specified diabetes mellitus with ketoacidosis with coma**

E13.2 Other specified diabetes mellitus with kidney complications

E13.21 **Other specified diabetes mellitus with diabetic nephropathy**
Other specified diabetes mellitus with intercapillary glomerulosclerosis
Other specified diabetes mellitus with intracapillary glomerulonephrosis
Other specified diabetes mellitus with Kimmelstiel-Wilson disease

E13.22 **Other specified diabetes mellitus with diabetic chronic kidney disease**
Use additional code to identify stage of chronic kidney disease (N18.1-N18.6)

E13.29 **Other specified diabetes mellitus with other diabetic kidney complication**
Other specified diabetes mellitus with renal tubular degeneration

E13.3 Other specified diabetes mellitus with ophthalmic complications
Coding Clinic: 2Ø16, Q4, P11

E13.31 Other specified diabetes mellitus with unspecified diabetic retinopathy

E13.311 **Other specified diabetes mellitus with unspecified diabetic retinopathy with macular edema**

E13.319 **Other specified diabetes mellitus with unspecified diabetic retinopathy without macular edema**

CHAPTER 4 (EØØ-E9Ø)

● **E13.32 Other specified diabetes mellitus with mild nonproliferative diabetic retinopathy**
Other specified diabetes mellitus with nonproliferative diabetic retinopathy NOS
One of the following 7th characters is to be assigned to codes in subcategory E13.32 to designate laterality of the disease:

1	right eye
2	left eye
3	bilateral
9	unspecified eye

● **E13.321 Other specified diabetes mellitus with mild nonproliferative diabetic retinopathy with macular edema**
● **E13.329 Other specified diabetes mellitus with mild nonproliferative diabetic retinopathy without macular edema**

● **E13.33 Other specified diabetes mellitus with moderate nonproliferative diabetic retinopathy**
One of the following 7th characters is to be assigned to codes in subcategory E13.33 to designate laterality of the disease:

1	right eye
2	left eye
3	bilateral
9	unspecified eye

● **E13.331 Other specified diabetes mellitus with moderate nonproliferative diabetic retinopathy with macular edema**
● **E13.339 Other specified diabetes mellitus with moderate nonproliferative diabetic retinopathy without macular edema**

● **E13.34 Other specified diabetes mellitus with severe nonproliferative diabetic retinopathy**
One of the following 7th characters is to be assigned to codes in subcategory E13.34 to designate laterality of the disease:

1	right eye
2	left eye
3	bilateral
9	unspecified eye

● **E13.341 Other specified diabetes mellitus with severe nonproliferative diabetic retinopathy with macular edema**
● **E13.349 Other specified diabetes mellitus with severe nonproliferative diabetic retinopathy without macular edema**

● **E13.35 Other specified diabetes mellitus with proliferative diabetic retinopathy**
One of the following 7th characters is to be assigned to codes in subcategory E13.35 to designate laterality of the disease:

1	right eye
2	left eye
3	bilateral
9	unspecified eye

● **E13.351 Other specified diabetes mellitus with proliferative diabetic retinopathy with macular edema**
● **E13.352 Other specified diabetes mellitus with proliferative diabetic retinopathy with traction retinal detachment involving the macula**
● **E13.353 Other specified diabetes mellitus with proliferative diabetic retinopathy with traction retinal detachment not involving the macula**
● **E13.354 Other specified diabetes mellitus with proliferative diabetic retinopathy with combined traction retinal detachment and rhegmatogenous retinal detachment**
● **E13.355 Other specified diabetes mellitus with stable proliferative diabetic retinopathy**
● **E13.359 Other specified diabetes mellitus with proliferative diabetic retinopathy without macular edema**

E13.36 Other specified diabetes mellitus with diabetic cataract

X● **E13.37 Other specified diabetes mellitus with diabetic macular edema, resolved following treatment**
One of the following 7th characters is to be assigned to code E13.37 to designate laterality of the disease:

1	right eye
2	left eye
3	bilateral
9	unspecified eye

E13.39 Other specified diabetes mellitus with other diabetic ophthalmic complication
Use additional code to identify manifestation, such as:
diabetic glaucoma (H4Ø-H42)

● **E13.4 Other specified diabetes mellitus with neurological complications**
E13.4Ø Other specified diabetes mellitus with diabetic neuropathy, unspecified
E13.41 Other specified diabetes mellitus with diabetic mononeuropathy
E13.42 Other specified diabetes mellitus with diabetic polyneuropathy
Other specified diabetes mellitus with diabetic neuralgia
E13.43 Other specified diabetes mellitus with diabetic autonomic (poly)neuropathy
Other specified diabetes mellitus with diabetic gastroparesis
E13.44 Other specified diabetes mellitus with diabetic amyotrophy
E13.49 Other specified diabetes mellitus with other diabetic neurological complication

● **E13.5 Other specified diabetes mellitus with circulatory complications**
E13.51 Other specified diabetes mellitus with diabetic peripheral angiopathy without gangrene
E13.52 Other specified diabetes mellitus with diabetic peripheral angiopathy with gangrene
Other specified diabetes mellitus with diabetic gangrene
E13.59 Other specified diabetes mellitus with other circulatory complications

● **E13.6 Other specified diabetes mellitus with other specified complications**
● **E13.61 Other specified diabetes mellitus with diabetic arthropathy**
E13.61Ø Other specified diabetes mellitus with diabetic neuropathic arthropathy
Other specified diabetes mellitus with Charcôt's joints
E13.618 Other specified diabetes mellitus with other diabetic arthropathy

CHAPTER 4 (EØØ-E9Ø)

● E13.62 **Other specified diabetes mellitus with skin complications**

E13.620 **Other specified diabetes mellitus with diabetic dermatitis**
Other specified diabetes mellitus with diabetic necrobiosis lipoidica

E13.621 **Other specified diabetes mellitus with foot ulcer**
Use additional code to identify site of ulcer (L97.4-, L97.5-)

E13.622 **Other specified diabetes mellitus with other skin ulcer**
Use additional code to identify site of ulcer (L97.1-L97.9, L98.41-L98.49)

E13.628 **Other specified diabetes mellitus with other skin complications**

● E13.63 **Other specified diabetes mellitus with oral complications**

E13.630 **Other specified diabetes mellitus with periodontal disease**

E13.638 **Other specified diabetes mellitus with other oral complications**

● E13.64 **Other specified diabetes mellitus with hypoglycemia**

E13.641 **Other specified diabetes mellitus with hypoglycemia with coma**

E13.649 **Other specified diabetes mellitus with hypoglycemia without coma**

E13.65 **Other specified diabetes mellitus with hyperglycemia**

E13.69 **Other specified diabetes mellitus with other specified complication**
Use additional code to identify complication

E13.8 **Other specified diabetes mellitus with unspecified complications**

E13.9 **Other specified diabetes mellitus without complications**

OTHER DISORDERS OF GLUCOSE REGULATION AND PANCREATIC INTERNAL SECRETION (E15-E16)

E15 **Nondiabetic hypoglycemic coma**
Includes drug-induced insulin coma in nondiabetic
hyperinsulinism with hypoglycemic coma
hypoglycemic coma NOS

● E16 **Other disorders of pancreatic internal secretion**

E16.0 **Drug-induced hypoglycemia without coma**
Excludes1 diabetes with hypoglycemia without coma (E09.649)
Use additional code for adverse effect, if applicable, to identify drug (T36-T50 with fifth or sixth character 5)

E16.1 **Other hypoglycemia**
Functional hyperinsulinism
Functional nonhyperinsulinemic hypoglycemia
Hyperinsulinism NOS
Hyperplasia of pancreatic islet beta cells NOS
Excludes1 diabetes with hypoglycemia (E08.649, E10.649, E11.649, E13.649)
hypoglycemia in infant of diabetic mother (P70.1)
neonatal hypoglycemia (P70.4)

E16.2 **Hypoglycemia, unspecified**
Excludes1 diabetes with hypoglycemia (E08.649, E10.649, E11.649, E13.649)
Coding Clinic: 2016, Q3, P42

E16.3 **Increased secretion of glucagon**
Hyperplasia of pancreatic endocrine cells with glucagon excess

E16.4 **Increased secretion of gastrin**
Hypergastrinemia
Hyperplasia of pancreatic endocrine cells with gastrin excess
Zollinger-Ellison syndrome

E16.8 **Other specified disorders of pancreatic internal secretion**
Increased secretion from endocrine pancreas of growth hormone-releasing hormone
Increased secretion from endocrine pancreas of pancreatic polypeptide
Increased secretion from endocrine pancreas of somatostatin
Increased secretion from endocrine pancreas of vasoactive-intestinal polypeptide

E16.9 **Disorder of pancreatic internal secretion, unspecified**
Islet-cell hyperplasia NOS
Pancreatic endocrine cell hyperplasia NOS

DISORDERS OF OTHER ENDOCRINE GLANDS (E20-E35)

Excludes1 galactorrhea (N64.3)
gynecomastia (N62)

● E20 **Hypoparathyroidism**
Greatly reduced function of parathyroid glands; AKA parathyroid insufficiency
Excludes1 Di George's syndrome (D82.1)
postprocedural hypoparathyroidism (E89.2)
tetany NOS (R29.0)
transitory neonatal hypoparathyroidism (P71.4)

E20.0 **Idiopathic hypoparathyroidism**
Rare condition, unknown cause; short dwarf-like with round face

E20.1 **Pseudohypoparathyroidism**
Hereditary condition resembling hypoparathyroidism, but caused by inability to respond to parathyroid hormone

E20.8 **Other hypoparathyroidism**

E20.9 **Hypoparathyroidism, unspecified**
Parathyroid tetany

● E21 **Hyperparathyroidism and other disorders of parathyroid gland**
Excludes1 adult osteomalacia (M83.-)
ectopic hyperparathyroidism (E34.2)
familial hypocalciuric hypercalcemia (E83.52)
hungry bone syndrome (E83.81)
infantile and juvenile osteomalacia (E55.0)

E21.0 **Primary hyperparathyroidism**
Hyperplasia of parathyroid
Osteitis fibrosa cystica generalisata [von Recklinghausen's disease of bone]

E21.1 **Secondary hyperparathyroidism, not elsewhere classified**
Excludes1 secondary hyperparathyroidism of renal origin (N25.81)

E21.2 **Other hyperparathyroidism**
Tertiary hyperparathyroidism
Excludes1 familial hypocalciuric hypercalcemia (E83.52)

E21.3 **Hyperparathyroidism, unspecified**

E21.4 **Other specified disorders of parathyroid gland**

E21.5 **Disorder of parathyroid gland, unspecified**

Item 4-4 Hyperparathyroidism is an overactive parathyroid gland that secretes excessive parathormone, causing increased levels of circulating calcium. This results in a loss of calcium in the bone (osteoporosis).

Hypoparathyroidism is an underactive parathyroid gland that results in decreased levels of circulating calcium. The primary manifestation is **tetany,** a continuous muscle spasm.

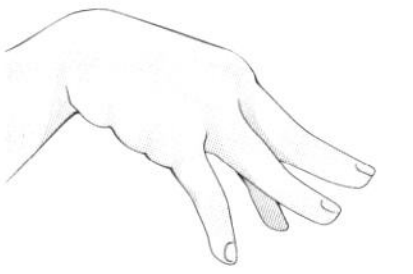

Figure 4-4 Tetany caused by hypoparathyroidism.

CHAPTER 4 (E00-E90)

Item 4–5 Hyperadrenalism is overactivity of the adrenal cortex, which secretes corticosteroid hormones. Excessive glucocorticoid hormone results in hyperglycemia **(Cushing's syndrome),** and excessive aldosterone results in **Conn's syndrome. Adrenogenital syndrome** is the result of excessive secretion of androgens, male hormones, which stimulates premature sexual development. **Hypoadrenalism, Addison's disease,** is a condition in which the adrenal glands atrophy.

● **E22 Hyperfunction of pituitary gland**

Excludes1 Cushing's syndrome (E24.-)
Nelson's syndrome (E24.1)
overproduction of ACTH not associated with Cushing's disease (E27.Ø)
overproduction of pituitary ACTH (E24.Ø)
overproduction of thyroid-stimulating hormone (EØ5.8-)

E22.Ø Acromegaly and pituitary gigantism
Chronic disease caused by hypersecretion of growth hormone
Overproduction of growth hormone
Excludes1 constitutional gigantism (E34.4)
constitutional tall stature (E34.4)
increased secretion from endocrine pancreas of growth hormone-releasing hormone (E16.8)

E22.1 Hyperprolactinemia
Increased levels of prolactin
Use additional code for adverse effect, if applicable, to identify drug (T36-T5Ø with fifth or sixth character 5)

E22.2 Syndrome of inappropriate secretion of antidiuretic hormone

E22.8 Other hyperfunction of pituitary gland
Central precocious puberty

E22.9 Hyperfunction of pituitary gland, unspecified

● **E23 Hypofunction and other disorders of the pituitary gland**

Includes the listed conditions whether the disorder is in the pituitary or the hypothalamus
Excludes1 postprocedural hypopituitarism (E89.3)

E23.Ø Hypopituitarism
Fertile eunuch syndrome
Hypogonadotropic hypogonadism
Idiopathic growth hormone deficiency
Isolated deficiency of gonadotropin
Isolated deficiency of growth hormone
Isolated deficiency of pituitary hormone
Kallmann's syndrome
Lorain-Levi short stature
Necrosis of pituitary gland (postpartum)
Panhypopituitarism
Pituitary cachexia
Pituitary insufficiency NOS
Pituitary short stature
Sheehan's syndrome
Simmonds' disease

E23.1 Drug-induced hypopituitarism
Use additional code for adverse effect, if applicable, to identify drug (T36-T5Ø with fifth or sixth character 5)

E23.2 Diabetes insipidus
Excludes1 nephrogenic diabetes insipidus (N25.1)

E23.3 Hypothalamic dysfunction, not elsewhere classified
Excludes1 Prader-Willi syndrome (Q87.11)
Russell-Silver syndrome (Q87.19)

E23.6 Other disorders of pituitary gland
Abscess of pituitary
Adiposogenital dystrophy

E23.7 Disorder of pituitary gland, unspecified

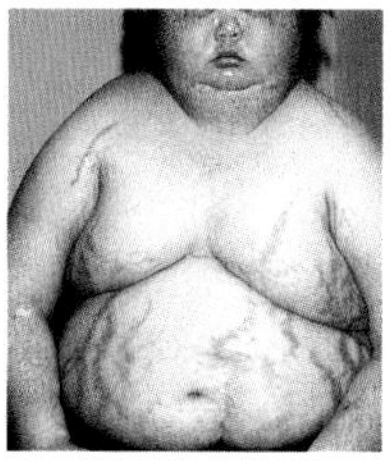

Figure 4-5 Centripetal and generalized obesity and dorsal kyphosis in a woman with Cushing's disease. (From Salvo SG: Mosby's Pathology for Massage Therapists, St. Louis, MO: Mosby/Elsevier, 2009)

● **E24 Cushing's syndrome**

Excludes1 congenital adrenal hyperplasia (E25.Ø)

E24.Ø Pituitary-dependent Cushing's disease
Overproduction of pituitary ACTH
Pituitary-dependent hypercorticalism

E24.1 Nelson's syndrome

E24.2 Drug-induced Cushing's syndrome
Use additional code for adverse effect, if applicable, to identify drug (T36-T5Ø with fifth or sixth character 5)

E24.3 Ectopic ACTH syndrome

E24.4 Alcohol-induced pseudo-Cushing's syndrome

E24.8 Other Cushing's syndrome

E24.9 Cushing's syndrome, unspecified

● **E25 Adrenogenital disorders**
Disorder of production of steroid hormone in adrenal gland

Includes adrenogenital syndromes, virilizing or feminizing, whether acquired or due to adrenal hyperplasia consequent on inborn enzyme defects in hormone synthesis
female adrenal pseudohermaphroditism
female heterosexual precocious pseudopuberty
male isosexual precocious pseudopuberty
male macrogenitosomia praecox
male sexual precocity with adrenal hyperplasia
male virilization (female)
Excludes1 indeterminate sex and pseudohermaphroditism (Q56)
chromosomal abnormalities (Q9Ø-Q99)

E25.Ø Congenital adrenogenital disorders associated with enzyme deficiency
Congenital adrenal hyperplasia
21-Hydroxylase deficiency
Salt-losing congenital adrenal hyperplasia

E25.8 Other adrenogenital disorders
Idiopathic adrenogenital disorder
Use additional code for adverse effect, if applicable, to identify drug (T36-T5Ø with fifth or sixth character 5)

E25.9 Adrenogenital disorder, unspecified
Adrenogenital syndrome NOS

● **E26 Hyperaldosteronism**
Abnormality of electrolyte metabolism caused by excessive secretion of aldosterone

● **E26.Ø Primary hyperaldosteronism**

E26.Ø1 Conn's syndrome
Code also adrenal adenoma (D35.Ø-)

E26.Ø2 Glucocorticoid-remediable aldosteronism
Familial aldosteronism type I

E26.Ø9 Other primary hyperaldosteronism
Primary aldosteronism due to adrenal hyperplasia (bilateral)

E26.1 Secondary hyperaldosteronism

● **E26.8 Other hyperaldosteronism**

E26.81 Bartter's syndrome

E26.89 Other hyperaldosteronism

E26.9 Hyperaldosteronism, unspecified
Aldosteronism NOS
Hyperaldosteronism NOS

E27 Other disorders of adrenal gland

E27.0 Other adrenocortical overactivity
Overproduction of ACTH, not associated with Cushing's disease
Premature adrenarche
Excludes1 Cushing's syndrome (E24.-)

E27.1 Primary adrenocortical insufficiency
Addison's disease
Autoimmune adrenalitis
Excludes1 Addison only phenotype adrenoleukodystrophy (E71.528)
amyloidosis (E85.-)
tuberculous Addison's disease (A18.7)
Waterhouse-Friderichsen syndrome (A39.1)

E27.2 Addisonian crisis
Acute onset of adrenocortical insufficiency
Adrenal crisis
Adrenocortical crisis

E27.3 Drug-induced adrenocortical insufficiency
Use additional code for adverse effect, if applicable, to identify drug (T36-T50 with fifth or sixth character 5)

E27.4 Other and unspecified adrenocortical insufficiency
Excludes1 adrenoleukodystrophy [Addison-Schilder] (E71.528)
Waterhouse-Friderichsen syndrome (A39.1)

E27.40 Unspecified adrenocortical insufficiency
Adrenocortical insufficiency NOS
Hypoaldosteronism

E27.49 Other adrenocortical insufficiency
Adrenal hemorrhage
Adrenal infarction

E27.5 Adrenomedullary hyperfunction
Adrenomedullary hyperplasia
Catecholamine hypersecretion

E27.8 Other specified disorders of adrenal gland
Abnormality of cortisol-binding globulin

E27.9 Disorder of adrenal gland, unspecified

E28 Ovarian dysfunction
Excludes1 isolated gonadotropin deficiency (E23.0)
postprocedural ovarian failure (E89.4-)

E28.0 Estrogen excess ♀
Use additional code for adverse effect, if applicable, to identify drug (T36-T50 with fifth or sixth character 5)

E28.1 Androgen excess ♀
Hypersecretion of ovarian androgens
Use additional code for adverse effect, if applicable, to identify drug (T36-T50 with fifth or sixth character 5)

E28.2 Polycystic ovarian syndrome ♀
Sclerocystic ovary syndrome
Stein-Leventhal syndrome

E28.3 Primary ovarian failure
Excludes1 pure gonadal dysgenesis (Q99.1)
Turner's syndrome (Q96.-)

E28.31 Premature menopause

E28.310 Symptomatic premature menopause ♀ A
Symptoms such as flushing, sleeplessness, headache, lack of concentration, associated with premature menopause

E28.319 Asymptomatic premature menopause ♀ A
Premature menopause NOS

E28.39 Other primary ovarian failure ♀
Decreased estrogen
Resistant ovary syndrome

E28.8 Other ovarian dysfunction ♀
Ovarian hyperfunction NOS
Excludes1 postprocedural ovarian failure (E89.4-)

E28.9 Ovarian dysfunction, unspecified ♀

E29 Testicular dysfunction
Excludes1 androgen insensitivity syndrome (E34.5-)
azoospermia or oligospermia NOS (N46.0-N46.1)
isolated gonadotropin deficiency (E23.0)
Klinefelter's syndrome (Q98.0-Q98.1, Q98.4)

E29.0 Testicular hyperfunction ♂
Hypersecretion of testicular hormones

E29.1 Testicular hypofunction ♂
Defective biosynthesis of testicular androgen NOS
5-delta-Reductase deficiency (with male pseudohermaphroditism)
Testicular hypogonadism NOS
Use additional code for adverse effect, if applicable, to identify drug (T36-T50 with fifth or sixth character 5)
Excludes1 postprocedural testicular hypofunction (E89.5)

E29.8 Other testicular dysfunction ♂

E29.9 Testicular dysfunction, unspecified ♂

E30 Disorders of puberty, not elsewhere classified

E30.0 Delayed puberty
Constitutional delay of puberty
Delayed sexual development

E30.1 Precocious puberty P
Sexual maturation at earlier age than normal, or before age 8 in girls and 9 in boys, usually hormonal; AKA sexual precocity or pubertas praecox
Precocious menstruation
Excludes1 Albright (-McCune) (-Sternberg) syndrome (Q78.1)
central precocious puberty (E22.8)
congenital adrenal hyperplasia (E25.0)
female heterosexual precocious pseudopuberty (E25.-)
male isosexual precocious pseudopuberty (E25.-)

E30.8 Other disorders of puberty P
Premature thelarche

E30.9 Disorder of puberty, unspecified

E31 Polyglandular dysfunction
Excludes1 ataxia telangiectasia [Louis-Bar] (G11.3)
dystrophia myotonica [Steinert] (G71.11)
pseudohypoparathyroidism (E20.1)

E31.0 Autoimmune polyglandular failure
Schmidt's syndrome

E31.1 Polyglandular hyperfunction
Excludes1 multiple endocrine adenomatosis (E31.2-)
multiple endocrine neoplasia (E31.2-)

E31.2 Multiple endocrine neoplasia [MEN] syndromes
Adenomatous hyperplasia and malignant tumors in endocrine glands
Multiple endocrine adenomatosis
Code also any associated malignancies and other conditions associated with the syndromes

E31.20 Multiple endocrine neoplasia [MEN] syndrome, unspecified
Multiple endocrine adenomatosis NOS
Multiple endocrine neoplasia [MEN] syndrome NOS

E31.21 Multiple endocrine neoplasia [MEN] type I
Wermer's syndrome

E31.22 Multiple endocrine neoplasia [MEN] type IIA
Sipple's syndrome

E31.23 Multiple endocrine neoplasia [MEN] type IIB

E31.8 Other polyglandular dysfunction

E31.9 Polyglandular dysfunction, unspecified

● **E32 Diseases of thymus**
Excludes1 aplasia or hypoplasia of thymus with immunodeficiency (D82.1)
myasthenia gravis (G70.0)
E32.0 Persistent hyperplasia of thymus
Hypertrophy of thymus
E32.1 Abscess of thymus
E32.8 Other diseases of thymus
Excludes1 aplasia or hypoplasia with immunodeficiency (D82.1)
thymoma (D15.0)
E32.9 Disease of thymus, unspecified

● **E34 Other endocrine disorders**
Excludes1 pseudohypoparathyroidism (E20.1)
E34.0 Carcinoid syndrome
Note: May be used as an additional code to identify functional activity associated with a carcinoid tumor.
E34.1 Other hypersecretion of intestinal hormones
E34.2 Ectopic hormone secretion, not elsewhere classified
Excludes1 ectopic ACTH syndrome (E24.3)
E34.3 Short stature due to endocrine disorder
Constitutional short stature
Laron-type short stature
Excludes1 achondroplastic short stature (Q77.4)
hypochondroplastic short stature (Q77.4)
nutritional short stature (E45)
pituitary short stature (E23.0)
progeria (E34.8)
renal short stature (N25.0)
Russell-Silver syndrome (Q87.19)
short-limbed stature with immunodeficiency (D82.2)
short stature in specific dysmorphic syndromes - code to syndrome - see Alphabetical Index
short stature NOS (R62.52)
E34.4 Constitutional tall stature
Constitutional gigantism
● **E34.5 Androgen insensitivity syndrome**
E34.50 Androgen insensitivity syndrome, unspecified
Androgen insensitivity NOS
E34.51 Complete androgen insensitivity syndrome
Complete androgen insensitivity
de Quervain syndrome
Goldberg-Maxwell syndrome
E34.52 Partial androgen insensitivity syndrome
Partial androgen insensitivity
Reifenstein syndrome
E34.8 Other specified endocrine disorders
Pineal gland dysfunction
Progeria
Excludes2 pseudohypoparathyroidism (E20.1)
E34.9 Endocrine disorder, unspecified
Endocrine disturbance NOS
Hormone disturbance NOS

E35 Disorders of endocrine glands in diseases classified elsewhere
Code first underlying disease, such as:
late congenital syphilis of thymus gland [Dubois disease] (A50.5)
Use additional code, if applicable, to identify:
sequelae of tuberculosis of other organs (B90.8)
Excludes1 Echinococcus granulosus infection of thyroid gland (B67.3)
meningococcal hemorrhagic adrenalitis (A39.1)
syphilis of endocrine gland (A52.79)
tuberculosis of adrenal gland, except calcification (A18.7)
tuberculosis of endocrine gland NEC (A18.82)
tuberculosis of thyroid gland (A18.81)
Waterhouse-Friderichsen syndrome (A39.1)

INTRAOPERATIVE COMPLICATIONS OF ENDOCRINE SYSTEM (E36)

● **E36 Intraoperative complications of endocrine system**
Excludes2 postprocedural endocrine and metabolic complications and disorders, not elsewhere classified (E89.-)
● **E36.0 Intraoperative hemorrhage and hematoma of an endocrine system organ or structure complicating a procedure**
Excludes1 intraoperative hemorrhage and hematoma of an endocrine system organ or structure due to accidental puncture or laceration during a procedure (E36.1-)
E36.01 Intraoperative hemorrhage and hematoma of an endocrine system organ or structure complicating an endocrine system procedure
E36.02 Intraoperative hemorrhage and hematoma of an endocrine system organ or structure complicating other procedure
● **E36.1 Accidental puncture and laceration of an endocrine system organ or structure during a procedure**
E36.11 Accidental puncture and laceration of an endocrine system organ or structure during an endocrine system procedure
E36.12 Accidental puncture and laceration of an endocrine system organ or structure during other procedure
E36.8 Other intraoperative complications of endocrine system
Use additional code, if applicable, to further specify disorder

MALNUTRITION (E40-E46)

Excludes1 intestinal malabsorption (K90.-)
sequelae of protein-calorie malnutrition (E64.0)
Excludes2 nutritional anemias (D50-D53)
starvation (T73.0)

E40 Kwashiorkor
Malnutrition produced by severe protein deficiency
Severe malnutrition with nutritional edema with dyspigmentation of skin and hair
Excludes1 marasmic kwashiorkor (E42)
Coding Clinic: 22017, Q3, P25

E41 Nutritional marasmus
Severe malnutrition with marasmus
Excludes1 marasmic kwashiorkor (E42)
Coding Clinic: 2017, Q3, P24-25

E42 Marasmic kwashiorkor
Severe protein malnutrition
Intermediate form severe protein-calorie malnutrition
Severe protein-calorie malnutrition with signs of both kwashiorkor and marasmus
Coding Clinic: 2017, Q3, P25

E43 Unspecified severe protein-calorie malnutrition
Starvation edema
Coding Clinic: 2017, Q4, P108-109; 2017, Q3, P25

● **E44 Protein-calorie malnutrition of moderate and mild degree**
E44.0 Moderate protein-calorie malnutrition
E44.1 Mild protein-calorie malnutrition

E45 Retarded development following protein-calorie malnutrition
Nutritional short stature
Nutritional stunting
Physical retardation due to malnutrition

E46 Unspecified protein-calorie malnutrition
Malnutrition NOS
Protein-calorie imbalance NOS
Excludes1 nutritional deficiency NOS (E63.9)
Coding Clinic: 2017, Q3, P25

Item 4-6 Bitot's spots are the result of a buildup of keratin debris found on the superficial surface the conjunctiva; oval, triangular, or irregular in shape; and a sign of vitamin A deficiency and associated with night blindness. The disease may progress to **keratomalacia,** which can result in eventual prolapse of the iris and loss of the lens.

Figure 4-6 Bitot's spot on the conjunctiva.

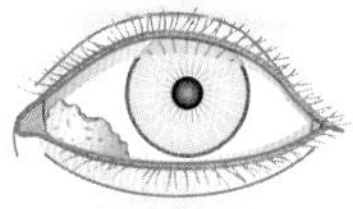

OTHER NUTRITIONAL DEFICIENCIES (E5Ø-E64)

Excludes2 nutritional anemias (D5Ø-D53)

E5Ø Vitamin A deficiency
Excludes1 sequelae of vitamin A deficiency (E64.1)
E5Ø.Ø Vitamin A deficiency with conjunctival xerosis
E5Ø.1 Vitamin A deficiency with Bitot's spot and conjunctival xerosis
Bitot's spot in the young child
E5Ø.2 Vitamin A deficiency with corneal xerosis
E5Ø.3 Vitamin A deficiency with corneal ulceration and xerosis
E5Ø.4 Vitamin A deficiency with keratomalacia
Eye disorder that results in dry cornea caused by vitamin A deficiency
E5Ø.5 Vitamin A deficiency with night blindness
E5Ø.6 Vitamin A deficiency with xerophthalmic scars of cornea
Abnormal dryness and thickening of conjunctiva and cornea due to vitamin A deficiency
E5Ø.7 Other ocular manifestations of vitamin A deficiency
Xerophthalmia NOS
E5Ø.8 Other manifestations of vitamin A deficiency
Follicular keratosis
Xeroderma
E5Ø.9 Vitamin A deficiency, unspecified
Hypovitaminosis A NOS

E51 Thiamine deficiency
Excludes1 sequelae of thiamine deficiency (E64.8)
E51.1 Beriberi
E51.11 Dry beriberi
Thiamine deficiency with nervous system manifestation most often caused by excessive alcohol consumption
Beriberi NOS
Beriberi with polyneuropathy
E51.12 Wet beriberi
Thiamine deficiency with cardiovascular manifestation most often caused by excessive alcohol consumption
Beriberi with cardiovascular manifestations
Cardiovascular beriberi
Shoshin disease
E51.2 Wernicke's encephalopathy
Acute disease of brain due to thiamine deficiency most often associated with excessive alcohol consumption
E51.8 Other manifestations of thiamine deficiency
E51.9 Thiamine deficiency, unspecified

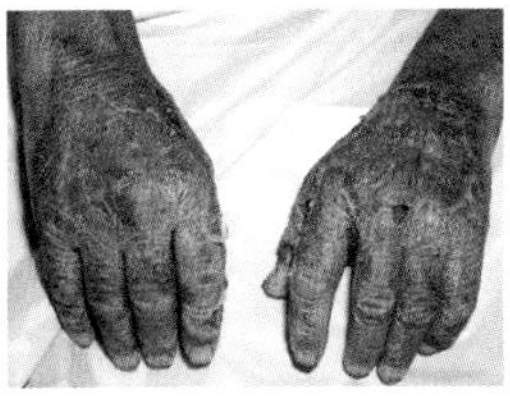

Figure 4-7 The sharply demarcated, characteristic scaling dermatitis of pellagra. (From James WD, Berger TG, Elston DM: Andrews' Diseases of the Skin: Clinical Dermatology, Philadelphia, Saunders Elsevier, 2006)

Item 4-7 Pellagra is associated with a deficiency of niacin and its precursor, **tryptophan.** Characteristics of the condition include diarrhea, dermatitis on exposed skin surfaces, dementia, and death. It is prevalent in developing countries where nutrition is inadequate. **Beriberi** is associated with thiamine deficiency.

E52 Niacin deficiency [pellagra]
Niacin (-tryptophan) deficiency
Nicotinamide deficiency
Pellagra (alcoholic)
Excludes1 sequelae of niacin deficiency (E64.8)

E53 Deficiency of other B group vitamins
Excludes1 sequelae of vitamin B deficiency (E64.8)
E53.Ø Riboflavin deficiency
Ariboflavinosis
Vitamin B2 deficiency
E53.1 Pyridoxine deficiency
Vitamin B6 deficiency
Excludes1 pyridoxine-responsive sideroblastic anemia (D64.3)
E53.8 Deficiency of other specified B group vitamins
Biotin deficiency
Cyanocobalamin deficiency
Folate deficiency
Folic acid deficiency
Pantothenic acid deficiency
Vitamin B12 deficiency
Excludes1 folate deficiency anemia (D52.-)
vitamin B12 deficiency anemia (D51.-)
E53.9 Vitamin B deficiency, unspecified

E54 Ascorbic acid deficiency
Deficiency of vitamin C
Scurvy
Excludes1 scorbutic anemia (D53.2)
sequelae of vitamin C deficiency (E64.2)

E55 Vitamin D deficiency
Excludes1 adult osteomalacia (M83.-)
osteoporosis (M8Ø.-)
sequelae of rickets (E64.3)
E55.Ø Rickets, active
Infantile osteomalacia
Juvenile osteomalacia
Softening of bone
Excludes1 celiac rickets (K9Ø.Ø)
Crohn's rickets (K5Ø.-)
hereditary vitamin D-dependent rickets (E83.32)
inactive rickets (E64.3)
renal rickets (N25.Ø)
sequelae of rickets (E64.3)
vitamin D-resistant rickets (E83.31)
E55.9 Vitamin D deficiency, unspecified
Avitaminosis D

● **E56 Other vitamin deficiencies**
Excludes1 sequelae of other vitamin deficiencies (E64.8)
E56.0 Deficiency of vitamin E
E56.1 Deficiency of vitamin K
Excludes1 deficiency of coagulation factor due to vitamin K deficiency (D68.4)
vitamin K deficiency of newborn (P53)
E56.8 Deficiency of other vitamins
E56.9 Vitamin deficiency, unspecified

E58 Dietary calcium deficiency
Excludes1 disorders of calcium metabolism (E83.5-)
sequelae of calcium deficiency (E64.8)

E59 Dietary selenium deficiency
Keshan disease
Excludes1 sequelae of selenium deficiency (E64.8)

E60 Dietary zinc deficiency

● **E61 Deficiency of other nutrient elements**
Use additional code for adverse effect, if applicable, to identify drug (T36-T50 with fifth or sixth character 5)
Excludes1 disorders of mineral metabolism (E83.-)
iodine deficiency related thyroid disorders (E00-E02)
sequelae of malnutrition and other nutritional deficiencies (E64.-)
E61.0 Copper deficiency
E61.1 Iron deficiency
Excludes1 iron deficiency anemia (D50.-)
E61.2 Magnesium deficiency
E61.3 Manganese deficiency
E61.4 Chromium deficiency
E61.5 Molybdenum deficiency
E61.6 Vanadium deficiency
E61.7 Deficiency of multiple nutrient elements
E61.8 Deficiency of other specified nutrient elements
E61.9 Deficiency of nutrient element, unspecified

● **E63 Other nutritional deficiencies**
Excludes1 dehydration (E86.0)
failure to thrive, adult (R62.7)
failure to thrive, child (R62.51)
feeding problems in newborn (P92.-)
sequelae of malnutrition and other nutritional deficiencies (E64.-)
E63.0 Essential fatty acid [EFA] deficiency
E63.1 Imbalance of constituents of food intake
E63.8 Other specified nutritional deficiencies
E63.9 Nutritional deficiency, unspecified

● **E64 Sequelae of malnutrition and other nutritional deficiencies**
Pathological condition resulting from disease, injury, or other trauma
Note: This category is to be used to indicate conditions in categories E43, E44, E46, E50-E63 as the cause of sequelae, which are themselves classified elsewhere. The "sequelae" include conditions specified as such; they also include the late effects of diseases classifiable to the above categories if the disease itself is no longer present
Code first condition resulting from (sequela) of malnutrition and other nutritional deficiencies
E64.0 Sequelae of protein-calorie malnutrition HCC
Excludes2 retarded development following protein-calorie malnutrition (E45)
E64.1 Sequelae of vitamin A deficiency
E64.2 Sequelae of vitamin C deficiency
E64.3 Sequelae of rickets
E64.8 Sequelae of other nutritional deficiencies
E64.9 Sequelae of unspecified nutritional deficiency

OVERWEIGHT, OBESITY AND OTHER HYPERALIMENTATION (E65-E68)

E65 Localized adiposity
Fat pad

● **E66 Overweight and obesity**
Code first obesity complicating pregnancy, childbirth and the puerperium, if applicable (O99.21-)
Use additional code to identify body mass index (BMI), if known (Z68.-)
Excludes1 adiposogenital dystrophy (E23.6)
lipomatosis NOS (E88.2)
lipomatosis dolorosa [Dercum] (E88.2)
➡ Prader-Willi syndrome (Q87.11)
Coding Clinic: 2018, Q4, P80
● **E66.0 Obesity due to excess calories**
E66.01 Morbid (severe) obesity due to excess calories HCC
Excludes1 morbid (severe) obesity with alveolar hypoventilation (E66.2)
Coding Clinic: 2018, Q4, P79
E66.09 Other obesity due to excess calories
E66.1 Drug-induced obesity
Use additional code for adverse effect, if applicable, to identify drug (T36-T50 with fifth or sixth character 5)
E66.2 Morbid (severe) obesity with alveolar hypoventilation HCC
Uncommon condition of unknown cause leading to inadequate ventilation in lungs, even though lungs and airways are normal
Obesity hypoventilation syndrome (OHS)
Pickwickian syndrome
E66.3 Overweight
E66.8 Other obesity
E66.9 Obesity, unspecified
Obesity NOS

● **E67 Other hyperalimentation**
Ingestion of more than optimal amount of nutrients
Excludes1 hyperalimentation NOS (R63.2)
sequelae of hyperalimentation (E68)
E67.0 Hypervitaminosis A
E67.1 Hypercarotenemia
E67.2 Megavitamin-B6 syndrome
E67.3 Hypervitaminosis D
E67.8 Other specified hyperalimentation

E68 Sequelae of hyperalimentation
Code first condition resulting from (sequela) of hyperalimentation

METABOLIC DISORDERS (E70-E88)

Excludes1 androgen insensitivity syndrome (E34.5-)
congenital adrenal hyperplasia (E25.0)
➡ Ehlers-Danlos syndrome (Q79.6-)
hemolytic anemias attributable to enzyme disorders (D55.-)
Marfan's syndrome (Q87.4)
5-alpha-reductase deficiency (E29.1)

● **E70 Disorders of aromatic amino-acid metabolism**
E70.0 Classical phenylketonuria HCC
Inherited disorder that increases to harmful levels amino acid phenylalanine
E70.1 Other hyperphenylalaninemias HCC

- **E70.2 Disorders of tyrosine metabolism**
  - **Excludes1** transitory tyrosinemia of newborn (P74.5)
  - E70.20 **Disorder of tyrosine metabolism, unspecified**
    - *Tyrosine: Nonessential amino acid occurring in most proteins*
  - E70.21 **Tyrosinemia**
    - *Congenital amino acid metabolism*
    - Hypertyrosinemia
  - E70.29 **Other disorders of tyrosine metabolism**
    - Alkaptonuria
    - Ochronosis
- **E70.3 Albinism**
  - *Congenital condition of reduced or absent pigment in eyes, skin, and hair*
  - E70.30 **Albinism, unspecified**
  - E70.31 **Ocular albinism**
    - E70.310 **X-linked ocular albinism**
    - E70.311 **Autosomal recessive ocular albinism**
    - E70.318 **Other ocular albinism**
    - E70.319 **Ocular albinism, unspecified**
  - E70.32 **Oculocutaneous albinism**
    - *Partial or total lack of melanin pigment in eyes*
    - **Excludes1** Chediak-Higashi syndrome (E70.330)
      Hermansky-Pudlak syndrome (E70.331)
    - E70.320 **Tyrosinase negative oculocutaneous albinism**
      - Albinism I
      - Oculocutaneous albinism ty-neg
    - E70.321 **Tyrosinase positive oculocutaneous albinism**
      - Albinism II
      - Oculocutaneous albinism ty-pos
    - E70.328 **Other oculocutaneous albinism**
      - Cross syndrome
    - E70.329 **Oculocutaneous albinism, unspecified**
  - E70.33 **Albinism with hematologic abnormality**
    - E70.330 **Chediak-Higashi syndrome**
    - E70.331 **Hermansky-Pudlak syndrome**
    - E70.338 **Other albinism with hematologic abnormality**
    - E70.339 **Albinism with hematologic abnormality, unspecified**
  - E70.39 **Other specified albinism**
    - Piebaldism
- **E70.4 Disorders of histidine metabolism**
  - E70.40 **Disorders of histidine metabolism, unspecified**
  - E70.41 **Histidinemia**
  - E70.49 **Other disorders of histidine metabolism**
- E70.5 **Disorders of tryptophan metabolism**
- E70.8 **Other disorders of aromatic amino-acid metabolism**
- E70.9 **Disorder of aromatic amino-acid metabolism, unspecified**

E71 Disorders of branched-chain amino-acid metabolism and fatty-acid metabolism

- E71.0 **Maple-syrup-urine disease**
  - *Due to defect in amino acid catabolism, causing severe ketoacidosis with smell of maple syrup in urine and on body*
- **E71.1 Other disorders of branched-chain amino-acid metabolism**
  - E71.11 **Branched-chain organic acidurias**
    - E71.110 **Isovaleric acidemia**
    - E71.111 **3-methylglutaconic aciduria**
    - E71.118 **Other branched-chain organic acidurias**
  - E71.12 **Disorders of propionate metabolism**
    - E71.120 **Methylmalonic acidemia**
    - E71.121 **Propionic acidemia**
    - E71.128 **Other disorders of propionate metabolism**
  - E71.19 **Other disorders of branched-chain amino-acid metabolism**
    - Hyperleucine-isoleucinemia
    - Hypervalinemia
- E71.2 **Disorder of branched-chain amino-acid metabolism, unspecified**
- **E71.3 Disorders of fatty-acid metabolism**
  - **Excludes1** peroxisomal disorders (E71.5)
    Refsum's disease (G60.1)
    Schilder's disease (G37.0)
  - **Excludes2** carnitine deficiency due to inborn error of metabolism (E71.42)
  - E71.30 **Disorder of fatty-acid metabolism, unspecified**
  - E71.31 **Disorders of fatty-acid oxidation**
    - E71.310 **Long chain/very long chain acyl CoA dehydrogenase deficiency**
      - LCAD
      - VLCAD
    - E71.311 **Medium chain acyl CoA dehydrogenase deficiency**
      - MCAD
    - E71.312 **Short chain acyl CoA dehydrogenase deficiency**
      - SCAD
    - E71.313 **Glutaric aciduria type II**
      - Glutaric aciduria type II A
      - Glutaric aciduria type II B
      - Glutaric aciduria type II C
      - **Excludes1** glutaric aciduria (type 1) NOS (E72.3)
    - E71.314 **Muscle carnitine palmitoyltransferase deficiency**
    - E71.318 **Other disorders of fatty-acid oxidation**
  - E71.32 **Disorders of ketone metabolism**
  - E71.39 **Other disorders of fatty-acid metabolism**
- **E71.4 Disorders of carnitine metabolism**
  - **Excludes1** muscle carnitine palmitoyltransferase deficiency (E71.314)
  - E71.40 **Disorder of carnitine metabolism, unspecified**
  - E71.41 **Primary carnitine deficiency**
  - E71.42 **Carnitine deficiency due to inborn errors of metabolism**
    - Code also associated inborn error or metabolism
  - E71.43 **Iatrogenic carnitine deficiency**
    - *Iatrogenic: Outcomes from activity of physicians*
    - Carnitine deficiency due to hemodialysis
    - Carnitine deficiency due to Valproic acid therapy
  - E71.44 **Other secondary carnitine deficiency**
    - E71.440 **Ruvalcaba-Myhre-Smith syndrome**
    - E71.448 **Other secondary carnitine deficiency**

CHAPTER 4 (E00-E90)

● **E71.5 Peroxisomal disorders**
Class of conditions which lead to disorders of lipid metabolism
Excludes1 Schilder's disease (G37.Ø)

E71.5Ø Peroxisomal disorder, unspecified HCC

● **E71.51 Disorders of peroxisome biogenesis**
Group 1 peroxisomal disorders
Excludes1 Refsum's disease (G6Ø.1)

E71.51Ø Zellweger syndrome HCC

E71.511 Neonatal adrenoleukodystrophy HCC
Excludes1 X-linked adrenoleukodystrophy (E71.42-)

E71.518 Other disorders of peroxisome biogenesis HCC

● **E71.52 X-linked adrenoleukodystrophy**

E71.52Ø Childhood cerebral X-linked adrenoleukodystrophy HCC

E71.521 Adolescent X-linked adrenoleukodystrophy HCC

E71.522 Adrenomyeloneuropathy HCC

E71.528 Other X-linked adrenoleukodystrophy HCC
Addison only phenotype adrenoleukodystrophy
Addison-Schilder adrenoleukodystrophy

E71.529 X-linked adrenoleukodystrophy, unspecified type HCC

E71.53 Other group 2 peroxisomal disorders HCC

● **E71.54 Other peroxisomal disorders**

E71.54Ø Rhizomelic chondrodysplasia punctata HCC
Rare, severe, inherited disorder with limb shortening, bone and cartilage abnormalities, abnormal facial appearance, severe mental retardation, psychomotor retardation, and cataracts
Excludes1 chondrodysplasia punctata NOS (Q77.3)

E71.541 Zellweger-like syndrome HCC

E71.542 Other group 3 peroxisomal disorders HCC

E71.548 Other peroxisomal disorders HCC

● **E72 Other disorders of amino-acid metabolism**
Excludes1 disorders of:
aromatic amino-acid metabolism (E7Ø.-)
branched-chain amino-acid metabolism (E71.Ø-E71.2)
fatty-acid metabolism (E71.3)
purine and pyrimidine metabolism (E79.-)
gout (M1A.-, M1Ø.-)

● **E72.Ø Disorders of amino-acid transport**
Excludes1 disorders of tryptophan metabolism (E7Ø.5)

E72.ØØ Disorders of amino-acid transport, unspecified HCC

E72.Ø1 Cystinuria HCC
Hereditary aminoaciduria due to impairment of renal transport with predominant symptom of urinary cystine calculi

E72.Ø2 Hartnup's disease HCC
Inborn error of metabolism

E72.Ø3 Lowe's syndrome HCC
X-linked disorder with rickets, hydrophthalmia, congenital glaucoma, cataracts, mental retardation, and renal tubule dysfunction
Use additional code for associated glaucoma (H42)

E72.Ø4 Cystinosis HCC
Genetic disease with excessive depostits of amino acid cystine in cells
Fanconi (-de Toni) (-Debré) syndrome with cystinosis
Excludes1 Fanconi (-de Toni) (-Debré) syndrome without cystinosis (E72.Ø9)

E72.Ø9 Other disorders of amino-acid transport HCC
Fanconi (-de Toni) (-Debré) syndrome, unspecified

● **E72.1 Disorders of sulfur-bearing amino-acid metabolism**
Excludes1 cystinosis (E72.Ø4)
cystinuria (E72.Ø1)
transcobalamin II deficiency (D51.2)

E72.1Ø Disorders of sulfur-bearing amino-acid metabolism, unspecified HCC

E72.11 Homocystinuria HCC
Cystathionine synthase deficiency

E72.12 Methylenetetrahydrofolate reductase deficiency HCC

E72.19 Other disorders of sulfur-bearing amino-acid metabolism HCC
Cystathioninuria
Methioninemia
Sulfite oxidase deficiency

● **E72.2 Disorders of urea cycle metabolism**
Excludes1 disorders of ornithine metabolism (E72.4)

E72.2Ø Disorder of urea cycle metabolism, unspecified HCC
Hyperammonemia
Elevated levels of ammonia
Excludes1 hyperammonemia-hyperornithinemia-homocitrullinemia syndrome E72.4
transient hyperammonemia of newborn (P74.6)

E72.21 Argininemia HCC
Disorder in which deficiency of enzyme arginase causes build-up of arginine and ammonia in blood

E72.22 Arginosuccinic aciduria HCC
Gene disorder of urea cycle resulting accumulation of ammonia

E72.23 Citrullinemia HCC
Urea cycle disorder that causes ammonia and other toxic substances to accumulate in blood

E72.29 Other disorders of urea cycle metabolism HCC

E72.3 Disorders of lysine and hydroxylysine metabolism HCC
Glutaric aciduria NOS
Glutaric aciduria (type I)
Hydroxylysinemia
Hyperlysinemia
Excludes1 glutaric aciduria type II (E71.313)
Refsum's disease (G6Ø.1)
Zellweger syndrome (E71.51Ø)

E72.4 Disorders of ornithine metabolism HCC
Hyperammonemia-Hyperornithinemia-Homocitrullinemia syndrome
Ornithinemia (types I, II)
Ornithine transcarbamylase deficiency
Excludes1 hereditary choroidal dystrophy (H31.2-)

CHAPTER 4 (EØØ-E9Ø)

E72.5 Disorders of glycine metabolism
- **E72.50 Disorder of glycine metabolism, unspecified**
- **E72.51 Non-ketotic hyperglycinemia**
- **E72.52 Trimethylaminuria**
- **E72.53 Primary hyperoxaluria**
  - Oxalosis
  - Oxaluria
- **E72.59 Other disorders of glycine metabolism**
  - D-glycericacidemia
  - Hyperhydroxyprolinemia
  - Hyperprolinemia (types I, II)
  - Sarcosinemia

E72.8 Other specified disorders of amino-acid metabolism
- **E72.81 Disorders of gamma aminobutyric acid metabolism**
  - 4-hydroxybutyric aciduria
  - Disorders of GABA metabolism
  - GABA metabolic defect
  - GABA transaminase deficiency
  - GABA-T deficiency
  - Gamma-hydroxybutyric aciduria
  - SSADHD
  - Succinic semialdehyde dehydrogenase deficiency
- **E72.89 Other specified disorders of amino-acid metabolism**
  - Disorders of beta-amino-acid metabolism
  - Disorders of gamma-glutamyl cycle

E72.9 Disorder of amino-acid metabolism, unspecified

E73 Lactose intolerance

Intolerance for lactose, due to inherited deficiency of lactase activity in intestinal mucosa

- **E73.0 Congenital lactase deficiency**
- **E73.1 Secondary lactase deficiency**
- **E73.8 Other lactose intolerance**
- **E73.9 Lactose intolerance, unspecified**

E74 Other disorders of carbohydrate metabolism

Excludes1 diabetes mellitus (E08-E13)
hypoglycemia NOS (E16.2)
increased secretion of glucagon (E16.3)
mucopolysaccharidosis (E76.0-E76.3)

E74.0 Glycogen storage disease
- **E74.00 Glycogen storage disease, unspecified**
- **E74.01 von Gierke's disease**
  - Type I glycogen storage disease
- **E74.02 Pompe disease**
  - Cardiac glycogenosis
  - Type II glycogen storage disease
- **E74.03 Cori disease**
  - Forbes' disease
  - Type III glycogen storage disease
- **E74.04 McArdle disease**
  - Type V glycogen storage disease
- **E74.09 Other glycogen storage disease**
  - Andersen disease
  - Hers disease
  - Tauri disease
  - Glycogen storage disease, types 0, IV, VI-XI
  - Liver phosphorylase deficiency
  - Muscle phosphofructokinase deficiency

E74.1 Disorders of fructose metabolism

Excludes1 muscle phosphofructokinase deficiency (E74.09)

- **E74.10 Disorder of fructose metabolism, unspecified**
- **E74.11 Essential fructosuria**
  - Fructokinase deficiency
- **E74.12 Hereditary fructose intolerance**
  - Fructosemia
- **E74.19 Other disorders of fructose metabolism**
  - Fructose-1, 6-diphosphatase deficiency

E74.2 Disorders of galactose metabolism
- **E74.20 Disorders of galactose metabolism, unspecified**
- **E74.21 Galactosemia**
  - *Genetic disorders resulting from defective simple sugar (galactose) metabolism*
- **E74.29 Other disorders of galactose metabolism**
  - Galactokinase deficiency

E74.3 Other disorders of intestinal carbohydrate absorption

Excludes2 lactose intolerance (E73.-)

- **E74.31 Sucrase-isomaltase deficiency**
  - *Deficiency in metabolism in intestinal mucosa results in malabsorption of sucrose and starch*
- **E74.39 Other disorders of intestinal carbohydrate absorption**
  - Disorder of intestinal carbohydrate absorption NOS
  - Glucose-galactose malabsorption
  - Sucrase deficiency

E74.4 Disorders of pyruvate metabolism and gluconeogenesis
- Deficiency of phosphoenolpyruvate carboxykinase
- Deficiency of pyruvate carboxylase
- Deficiency of pyruvate dehydrogenase

Excludes1 disorders of pyruvate metabolism and gluconeogenesis with anemia (D55.-)
Leigh's syndrome (G31.82)

E74.8 Other specified disorders of carbohydrate metabolism
- Essential pentosuria
- Renal glycosuria

E74.9 Disorder of carbohydrate metabolism, unspecified

E75 Disorders of sphingolipid metabolism and other lipid storage disorders

Excludes1 mucolipidosis, types I-III (E77.0-E77.1)
Refsum's disease (G60.1)

E75.0 GM2 gangliosidosis

Rare metabolic disorder that causes destruction of nerve cells of brain and spinal cord

- **E75.00 GM2 gangliosidosis, unspecified**
- **E75.01 Sandhoff disease**
- **E75.02 Tay-Sachs disease**
- **E75.09 Other GM2 gangliosidosis**
  - Adult GM2 gangliosidosis
  - Juvenile GM2 gangliosidosis

E75.1 Other and unspecified gangliosidosis
- **E75.10 Unspecified gangliosidosis**
  - Gangliosidosis NOS
- **E75.11 Mucolipidosis IV**
  - *Disorder with symptoms of psychomotor retardation and severe visual impairment*
- **E75.19 Other gangliosidosis**
  - GM1 gangliosidosis
  - GM3 gangliosidosis

E75.2 Other sphingolipidosis

Lysosomal (a particle in a cytoplasm cell that contains digestive enzymes) storage diseases with symptoms of abnormal storage of amino acids

Excludes1 adrenoleukodystrophy [Addison-Schilder] (E71.528)

- **E75.21 Fabry (-Anderson) disease**
- **E75.22 Gaucher disease**
- **E75.23 Krabbe disease**

Item 4-8 Leukodystrophy is characterized by degeneration and/or failure of the myelin formation of the central nervous system and sometimes of the peripheral nervous system. The disease is inherited and progressive.

CHAPTER 4 (E00-E90)

● E75.24 Niemann-Pick disease
E75.240 **Niemann-Pick disease type A** HCC
E75.241 **Niemann-Pick disease type B** HCC
E75.242 **Niemann-Pick disease type C** HCC
E75.243 **Niemann-Pick disease type D** HCC
E75.248 **Other Niemann-Pick disease** HCC
E75.249 **Niemann-Pick disease, unspecified** HCC

E75.25 **Metachromatic leukodystrophy**

E75.26 **Sulfatase deficiency**
Multiple sulfatase deficiency (MSD)

E75.29 **Other sphingolipidosis**
Farber's syndrome
Sulfatide lipidosis

E75.3 **Sphingolipidosis, unspecified** HCC

E75.4 **Neuronal ceroid lipofuscinosis**
Batten disease
Bielschowsky-Jansky disease
Kufs disease
Spielmeyer-Vogt disease

E75.5 **Other lipid storage disorders**
Cerebrotendinous cholesterosis [van Bogaert-Scherer-Epstein]
Wolman's disease

E75.6 **Lipid storage disorder, unspecified**

● E76 **Disorders of glycosaminoglycan metabolism**

● E76.0 **Mucopolysaccharidosis, type I**
Inborn metabolic disorder of enzymes that break down carbohydrates

E76.01 **Hurler's syndrome** HCC
E76.02 **Hurler-Scheie syndrome** HCC
E76.03 **Scheie's syndrome** HCC

E76.1 **Mucopolysaccharidosis, type II** HCC
Inborn metabolic disorder of enzymes that break down carbohydrates occurs in 2-4 year old males
Hunter's syndrome

● E76.2 **Other mucopolysaccharidoses**

● E76.21 **Morquio mucopolysaccharidoses**

E76.210 **Morquio A mucopolysaccharidoses** HCC
Classic Morquio syndrome
Morquio syndrome A
Mucopolysaccharidosis, type IVA

E76.211 **Morquio B mucopolysaccharidoses** HCC
Morquio-like mucopolysaccharidoses
Morquio-like syndrome
Morquio syndrome B
Mucopolysaccharidosis, type IVB

E76.219 **Morquio mucopolysaccharidoses, unspecified** HCC
Morquio syndrome
Mucopolysaccharidosis, type IV

E76.22 **Sanfilippo mucopolysaccharidoses** HCC
Mucopolysaccharidosis, type III (A) (B) (C) (D)
Sanfilippo A syndrome
Sanfilippo B syndrome
Sanfilippo C syndrome
Sanfilippo D syndrome

E76.29 **Other mucopolysaccharidoses** HCC
beta-Glucuronidase deficiency
Maroteaux-Lamy (mild) (severe) syndrome
Mucopolysaccharidosis, types VI, VII

E76.3 **Mucopolysaccharidosis, unspecified** HCC

E76.8 **Other disorders of glucosaminoglycan metabolism** HCC

E76.9 **Glucosaminoglycan metabolism disorder, unspecified** HCC

● E77 **Disorders of glycoprotein metabolism**

E77.0 **Defects in post-translational modification of lysosomal enzymes** HCC
Mucolipidosis II [I-cell disease]
Mucolipidosis III [pseudo-Hurler polydystrophy]

E77.1 **Defects in glycoprotein degradation** HCC
Aspartylglucosaminuria
Fucosidosis
Mannosidosis
Sialidosis [mucolipidosis I]

E77.8 **Other disorders of glycoprotein metabolism** HCC

E77.9 **Disorder of glycoprotein metabolism, unspecified** HCC

● E78 **Disorders of lipoprotein metabolism and other lipidemias**
Excludes1 sphingolipidosis (E75.0-E75.3)

● E78.0 **Pure hypercholesterolemia**
Coding Clinic: 2016, Q4, P13

E78.00 **Pure hypercholesterolemia, unspecified**
Fredrickson's hyperlipoproteinemia, type IIa
Hyperbetalipoproteinemia
Low-density-lipoprotein-type [LDL] hyperlipoproteinemia
(Pure) hypercholesterolemia NOS
Coding Clinic: 2016, Q4, P13

E78.01 **Familial hypercholesterolemia**
Coding Clinic: 2016, Q4, P13

E78.1 **Pure hyperglyceridemia**
Elevated fasting triglycerides
Endogenous hyperglyceridemia
Fredrickson's hyperlipoproteinemia, type IV
Hyperlipidemia, group B
Hyperprebetalipoproteinemia
Very-low-density-lipoprotein-type [VLDL] hyperlipoproteinemia

E78.2 **Mixed hyperlipidemia**
Broad- or floating-betalipoproteinemia
Combined hyperlipidemia NOS
Elevated cholesterol with elevated triglycerides NEC
Fredrickson's hyperlipoproteinemia, type IIb or III
Hyperbetalipoproteinemia with prebetalipoproteinemia
Hypercholesteremia with endogenous hyperglyceridemia
Hyperlipidemia, group C
Tubo-eruptive xanthoma
Xanthoma tuberosum
Excludes1 cerebrotendinous cholesterosis [van Bogaert-Scherer-Epstein] (E75.5)
familial combined hyperlipidemia (E78.49)

E78.3 **Hyperchylomicronemia**
Chylomicron retention disease
Fredrickson's hyperlipoproteinemia, type I or V
Hyperlipidemia, group D
Mixed hyperglyceridemia

● E78.4 **Other hyperlipidemia**

E78.41 **Elevated Lipoprotein(a)**
Elevated Lp(a)

E78.49 **Other hyperlipidemia**
Familial combined hyperlipidemia

E78.5 **Hyperlipidemia, unspecified**

E78.6 **Lipoprotein deficiency**
Abetalipoproteinemia
Depressed HDL cholesterol
High-density lipoprotein deficiency
Hypoalphalipoproteinemia
Hypobetalipoproteinemia (familial)
Lecithin cholesterol acyltransferase deficiency
Tangier disease

● E78.7 **Disorders of bile acid and cholesterol metabolism**
Excludes1 Niemann-Pick disease type C (E75.242)
E78.70 **Disorder of bile acid and cholesterol metabolism, unspecified**
E78.71 **Barth syndrome**
E78.72 **Smith-Lemli-Opitz syndrome**
E78.79 **Other disorders of bile acid and cholesterol metabolism**
● E78.8 **Other disorders of lipoprotein metabolism**
E78.81 **Lipoid dermatoarthritis**
E78.89 **Other lipoprotein metabolism disorders**
E78.9 **Disorder of lipoprotein metabolism, unspecified**

● E79 **Disorders of purine and pyrimidine metabolism**
Purines, along with pyrimidines, signal RNA and DNA production
Excludes1 Ataxia-telangiectasia (Q87.19)
Bloom's syndrome (Q82.8)
Cockayne's syndrome (Q87.19)
calculus of kidney (N20.0)
combined immunodeficiency disorders (D81.-)
Fanconi's anemia (D61.09)
gout (M1A.-, M10.-)
orotaciduric anemia (D53.0)
progeria (E34.8)
Werner's syndrome (E34.8)
xeroderma pigmentosum (Q82.1)
E79.0 **Hyperuricemia without signs of inflammatory arthritis and tophaceous disease**
Asymptomatic hyperuricemia
E79.1 **Lesch-Nyhan syndrome**
HGPRT deficiency
E79.2 **Myoadenylate deaminase deficiency**
E79.8 **Other disorders of purine and pyrimidine metabolism**
Hereditary xanthinuria
E79.9 **Disorder of purine and pyrimidine metabolism, unspecified**

● E80 **Disorders of porphyrin and bilirubin metabolism**
Group of chemical compounds in RBCs that combine with iron to form heme
Includes defects of catalase and peroxidase
E80.0 **Hereditary erythropoietic porphyria**
Congenital erythropoietic porphyria
Erythropoietic protoporphyria
E80.1 **Porphyria cutanea tarda**
● E80.2 **Other and unspecified porphyria**
E80.20 **Unspecified porphyria**
Porphyria NOS
E80.21 **Acute intermittent (hepatic) porphyria**
E80.29 **Other porphyria**
Hereditary coproporphyria
E80.3 **Defects of catalase and peroxidase**
Acatalasia [Takahara]
E80.4 **Gilbert syndrome**
E80.5 **Crigler-Najjar syndrome**
E80.6 **Other disorders of bilirubin metabolism**
Dubin-Johnson syndrome
Rotor's syndrome
E80.7 **Disorder of bilirubin metabolism, unspecified**

● E83 **Disorders of mineral metabolism**
Excludes1 dietary mineral deficiency (E58-E61)
parathyroid disorders (E20-E21)
vitamin D deficiency (E55.-)
● E83.0 **Disorders of copper metabolism**
E83.00 **Disorder of copper metabolism, unspecified**
E83.01 **Wilson's disease**
Code also associated Kayser Fleischer ring (H18.04-)
E83.09 **Other disorders of copper metabolism**
Menkes' (kinky hair) (steely hair) disease
● E83.1 **Disorders of iron metabolism**
Excludes1 iron deficiency anemia (D50.-)
sideroblastic anemia (D64.0-D64.3)
E83.10 **Disorder of iron metabolism, unspecified**
● E83.11 **Hemochromatosis**
Excludes1 GALD (P78.84)
Gestational alloimmune liver disease (P78.84)
Neonatal hemochromatosis (P78.84)
E83.110 **Hereditary hemochromatosis**
Bronzed diabetes
Pigmentary cirrhosis (of liver)
Primary (hereditary) hemochromatosis
E83.111 **Hemochromatosis due to repeated red blood cell transfusions**
Iron overload due to repeated red blood cell transfusions
Transfusion (red blood cell) associated hemochromatosis
E83.118 **Other hemochromatosis**
E83.119 **Hemochromatosis, unspecified**
E83.19 **Other disorders of iron metabolism**
Use additional code, if applicable, for idiopathic pulmonary hemosiderosis (J84.03)
E83.2 **Disorders of zinc metabolism**
Acrodermatitis enteropathica
● E83.3 **Disorders of phosphorus metabolism and phosphatases**
Excludes1 adult osteomalacia (M83.-)
osteoporosis (M80.-)
E83.30 **Disorder of phosphorus metabolism, unspecified**
E83.31 **Familial hypophosphatemia**
Vitamin D-resistant osteomalacia
Vitamin D-resistant rickets
Excludes1 vitamin D-deficiency rickets (E55.0)
E83.32 **Hereditary vitamin D-dependent rickets (type 1) (type 2)**
25-hydroxyvitamin D 1-alpha-hydroxylase deficiency
Pseudovitamin D deficiency
Vitamin D receptor defect
E83.39 **Other disorders of phosphorus metabolism**
Acid phosphatase deficiency
Hypophosphatasia
● E83.4 **Disorders of magnesium metabolism**
E83.40 **Disorders of magnesium metabolism, unspecified**
E83.41 **Hypermagnesemia**
Coding Clinic: 2016, Q4, P55
E83.42 **Hypomagnesemia**
E83.49 **Other disorders of magnesium metabolism**

CHAPTER 4 (E00-E90)

● E83.5 **Disorders of calcium metabolism**
Excludes1 chondrocalcinosis (M11.1-M11.2)
hungry bone syndrome (E83.81)
hyperparathyroidism (E21.Ø-E21.3)

E83.5Ø **Unspecified disorder of calcium metabolism**

E83.51 **Hypocalcemia**

E83.52 **Hypercalcemia**
Familial hypocalciuric hypercalcemia

E83.59 **Other disorders of calcium metabolism**
Idiopathic hypercalciuria

● E83.8 **Other disorders of mineral metabolism**

E83.81 **Hungry bone syndrome**

E83.89 **Other disorders of mineral metabolism**

E83.9 **Disorder of mineral metabolism, unspecified**

● E84 **Cystic fibrosis**
Includes mucoviscidosis
Code also exocrine pancreatic insufficiency (K86.81)

E84.Ø **Cystic fibrosis with pulmonary manifestations** HCC
Use additional code to identify any infectious organism present, such as:
Pseudomonas (B96.5)

● E84.1 **Cystic fibrosis with intestinal manifestations**

E84.11 **Meconium ileus in cystic fibrosis** HCC N
Excludes1 meconium ileus not due to cystic fibrosis (P76.Ø)

E84.19 **Cystic fibrosis with other intestinal manifestations** HCC
Distal intestinal obstruction syndrome

E84.8 **Cystic fibrosis with other manifestations** HCC

E84.9 **Cystic fibrosis, unspecified** HCC

● E85 **Amyloidosis**
A disorder resulting from the abnormal deposition of a particular protein (amyloid) into tissues of the body
Excludes2 Alzheimer's disease (G3Ø.Ø-)

E85.Ø **Non-neuropathic heredofamilial amyloidosis** HCC
Hereditary amyloid nephropathy
Code also associated disorders, such as:
autoinflammatory syndromes (M04.-)
Excludes2 Transthyretin-related (ATTR) familial amyloid cardiomyopathy (E85.4)

E85.1 **Neuropathic heredofamilial amyloidosis** HCC
Amyloid polyneuropathy (Portuguese)
Transthyretin-related (ATTR) familial amyloid polyneuropathy
Coding Clinic: 2012, Q4, P1ØØ

E85.2 **Heredofamilial amyloidosis, unspecified** HCC

E85.3 **Secondary systemic amyloidosis** HCC
Hemodialysis-associated amyloidosis

E85.4 **Organ-limited amyloidosis** HCC
Localized amyloidosis
Transthyretin-related (ATTR) familial amyloid cardiomyopathy

● E85.8 **Other amyloidosis**

E85.81 **Light chain (AL) amyloidosis** HCC

E85.82 **Wild-type transthyretin-related (ATTR) amyloidosis** HCC
Senile systemic amyloidosis (SSA)

E85.89 **Other amyloidosis** HCC

E85.9 **Amyloidosis, unspecified** HCC

Item 4-9 Circulating fluid volume is regulated by the amount of water and sodium ingested, excreted by the kidneys into the urine, and lost through the gastrointestinal tract, lungs, and skin. To maintain blood volume within a normal range, the kidneys regulate the amount of water and sodium lost into the urine. Too much **(fluid overload)** or too little fluid volume **(volume depletion)** will affect blood pressure. Severe cases of vomiting, diarrhea, bleeding, and burns (fluid loss through exposed burn surface area) can contribute to fluid loss. Internal body environment must maintain a precise balance (homeostasis) between too much fluid and too little fluid. This complex balancing mechanism is critical to good health.

● E86 **Volume depletion**
Excludes1 dehydration of newborn (P74.1)
hypovolemic shock NOS (R57.1)
postprocedural hypovolemic shock (T81.19)
traumatic hypovolemic shock (T79.4)
Use additional code(s) for any associated disorders of electrolyte and acid-base balance (E87.-)
Coding Clinic: 2019, Q2, P7

E86.Ø **Dehydration**
Excessive loss of body water
Coding Clinic: 2019, Q2, P7-8

E86.1 **Hypovolemia**
Diminished volume of circulating blood
Depletion of volume of plasma

E86.9 **Volume depletion, unspecified**
Coding Clinic: 2019, Q2, P7-8

● E87 **Other disorders of fluid, electrolyte and acid-base balance**
Excludes1 diabetes insipidus (E23.2)
electrolyte imbalance associated with hyperemesis gravidarum (O21.1)
electrolyte imbalance following ectopic or molar pregnancy (OØ8.5)
familial periodic paralysis (G72.3)

E87.Ø **Hyperosmolality and hypernatremia**
Sodium [Na] excess
Sodium [Na] overload
Coding Clinic: 2018, Q2, P6

E87.1 **Hypo-osmolality and hyponatremia**
Sodium [Na] deficiency
Excludes1 syndrome of inappropriate secretion of antidiuretic hormone (E22.2)
Coding Clinic: 2018, Q2, P6

E87.2 **Acidosis**
Acidosis NOS
Lactic acidosis
Metabolic acidosis
Respiratory acidosis
Excludes1 diabetic acidosis - see categories EØ8-E1Ø, E13 with ketoacidosis

E87.3 **Alkalosis**
Alkalosis NOS
Metabolic alkalosis
Respiratory alkalosis

E87.4 **Mixed disorder of acid-base balance**

E87.5 **Hyperkalemia**
Potassium [K] excess
Potassium [K] overload

E87.6 **Hypokalemia**
Potassium [K] deficiency

● E87.7 **Fluid overload**

Excludes1 edema NOS (R6Ø.9)
fluid retention (R6Ø.9)

E87.7Ø **Fluid overload, unspecified**

E87.71 **Transfusion associated circulatory overload**
Fluid overload due to transfusion (blood) (blood components) TACO

E87.79 **Other fluid overload**

E87.8 **Other disorders of electrolyte and fluid balance, not elsewhere classified**
Electrolyte imbalance NOS
Hyperchloremia
Hypochloremia

● E88 **Other and unspecified metabolic disorders**
Use additional codes for associated conditions

Excludes1 histiocytosis X (chronic) (C96.6)

● E88.Ø **Disorders of plasma-protein metabolism, not elsewhere classified**

Excludes1 disorder of lipoprotein metabolism (E78.-)
monoclonal gammopathy (of undetermined significance) (D47.2)
polyclonal hypergammaglobulinemia (D89.Ø)
Waldenström macroglobulinemia (C88.Ø)

E88.Ø1 **Alpha-1-antitrypsin deficiency AAT deficiency**

E88.Ø2 **Plasminogen deficiency**
Dysplasminogenemia
Hypoplasminogenemia
Type 1 plasminogen deficiency
Type 2 plasminogen deficiency

Code also, if applicable, ligneous conjunctivitis (H10.51)

Use additional code for associated findings, such as:
hydrocephalus (G91.4)
~~ligneous conjunctivitis (H10.51)~~
otitis media (H67.-)
respiratory disorder related to plasminogen deficiency (J99)

E88.Ø9 **Other disorders of plasma-protein metabolism, not elsewhere classified**
Bisalbuminemia

E88.1 **Lipodystrophy, not elsewhere classified**
Defective fat metabolism resulting in absence of subcutaneous fat
Lipodystrophy NOS

Excludes1 Whipple's disease (K9Ø.81)

E88.2 **Lipomatosis, not elsewhere classified**
Abnormal tumorlike accumulations of fat in tissue
Lipomatosis NOS
Lipomatosis (Check) dolorosa [Dercum]

E88.3 **Tumor lysis syndrome**
Tumor lysis syndrome (spontaneous)
Tumor lysis syndrome following antineoplastic drug chemotherapy

Use additional code for adverse effect, if applicable, to identify drug (T45.1X5)

Coding Clinic: 2Ø19, Q2, P25

● E88.4 **Mitochondrial metabolism disorders**
Congenital disorder of metabolism

Excludes1 disorders of pyruvate metabolism (E74.4)
Kearns-Sayre syndrome (H49.81)
Leber's disease (H47.22)
Leigh's encephalopathy (G31.82)
Mitochondrial myopathy, NEC (G71.3)
Reye's syndrome (G93.7)

E88.4Ø **Mitochondrial metabolism disorder, unspecified**

E88.41 **MELAS syndrome**
Mitochondrial myopathy, encephalopathy, lactic acidosis and stroke-like episodes

E88.42 **MERRF syndrome**
Myoclonic epilepsy associated with ragged-red fibers

Code also progressive myoclonic epilepsy (G4Ø.3-)

E88.49 **Other mitochondrial metabolism disorders**

● E88.8 **Other specified metabolic disorders**

E88.81 **Metabolic syndrome**
Dysmetabolic syndrome X

Use additional codes for associated manifestations, such as:
obesity (E66.-)

E88.89 **Other specified metabolic disorders**
Launois-Bensaude adenolipomatosis

Excludes1 adult pulmonary Langerhans cell histiocytosis (J84.82)

E88.9 **Metabolic disorder, unspecified**

POSTPROCEDURAL ENDOCRINE AND METABOLIC COMPLICATIONS AND DISORDERS, NOT ELSEWHERE CLASSIFIED (E89)

● E89 **Postprocedural endocrine and metabolic complications and disorders, not elsewhere classified**

Excludes2 intraoperative complications of endocrine system organ or structure (E36.Ø-, E36.1-, E36.8)

E89.Ø **Postprocedural hypothyroidism**
Postirradiation hypothyroidism
Postsurgical hypothyroidism

E89.1 **Postprocedural hypoinsulinemia**
Postpancreatectomy hyperglycemia
Postsurgical hypoinsulinemia

Use additional code, if applicable, to identify:
acquired absence of pancreas (Z9Ø.41-)
diabetes mellitus (postpancreatectomy) (postprocedural) (E13.-)
insulin use (Z79.4)

Excludes1 transient postprocedural hyperglycemia (R73.9)
transient postprocedural hypoglycemia (E16.2)

E89.2 **Postprocedural hypoparathyroidism**
Parathyroprival tetany

E89.3 **Postprocedural hypopituitarism**
Postirradiation hypopituitarism

● E89.4 **Postprocedural ovarian failure**

E89.4Ø **Asymptomatic postprocedural ovarian failure** ♀
Postprocedural ovarian failure NOS

E89.41 **Symptomatic postprocedural ovarian failure** ♀
Symptoms such as flushing, sleeplessness, headache, lack of concentration, associated with postprocedural menopause

CHAPTER 4 (EØØ-E9Ø)

E89.5 Postprocedural **testicular hypofunction** ♂

E89.6 Postprocedural **adrenocortical (-medullary) hypofunction** HCC

● E89.8 **Other postprocedural** endocrine and metabolic complications and disorders

Coding Clinic: 2016, Q4, P9

● E89.81 Postprocedural **hemorrhage** of an endocrine system organ or structure following a procedure

E89.810 Postprocedural hemorrhage of an endocrine system organ or structure following an **endocrine system procedure**

E89.811 Postprocedural hemorrhage of an endocrine system organ or structure following **other procedure**

● E89.82 Postprocedural **hematoma and seroma** of an endocrine system organ or structure

E89.820 Postprocedural **hematoma** of an endocrine system organ or structure following an **endocrine system procedure**

E89.821 Postprocedural **hematoma** of an endocrine system organ or structure following **other procedure**

E89.822 Postprocedural **seroma** of an endocrine system organ or structure following an **endocrine system procedure**

E89.823 Postprocedural **seroma** of an endocrine system organ or structure following **other procedure**

E89.89 **Other** postprocedural endocrine and metabolic complications and disorders

Use additional code, if applicable, to further specify disorder

CHAPTER 5

MENTAL, BEHAVIORAL AND NEURODEVELOPMENTAL DISORDERS (FØ1-F99)

OGCR Chapter-Specific Coding Guidelines

5. Chapter 5: Mental, Behavioral and Neurodevelopmental disorders (FØ1 – F99)

a. **Pain disorders related to psychological factors**

Assign code F45.41, for pain that is exclusively related to psychological disorders. As indicated by the Excludes 1 note under category G89, a code from category G89 should not be assigned with code F45.41

Code F45.42, Pain disorders with related psychological factors, should be used with a code from category G89, Pain, not elsewhere classified, if there is documentation of a psychological component for a patient with acute or chronic pain.

See Section I.C.6. Pain

b. **Mental and behavioral disorders due to psychoactive substance use**

1) **In Remission**

Selection of codes for "in remission" for categories F1Ø-F19, Mental and behavioral disorders due to psychoactive substance use (categories F1Ø-F19 with -11, -.21) requires the provider's clinical judgment. The appropriate codes for "in remission" are assigned only on the basis of provider documentation (as defined in the Official Guidelines for Coding and Reporting), unless otherwise instructed by the classification.

Mild substance use disorders in early or sustained remission are classified to the appropriate codes for substance abuse in remission, and moderate or severe substance use disorders in early or sustained remission are classified to the appropriate codes for substance dependence in remission.

2) **Psychoactive Substance Use, Abuse and Dependence**

When the provider documentation refers to use, abuse and dependence of the same substance (e.g., alcohol, opioid, cannabis, etc.), only one code should be assigned to identify the pattern of use based on the following hierarchy:

- If both use and abuse are documented, assign only the code for abuse
- If both abuse and dependence are documented, assign only the code for dependence
- If use, abuse and dependence are all documented, assign only the code for dependence
- If both use and dependence are documented, assign only the code for dependence

3) **Psychoactive Substance Use, Unspecified**

As with all other unspecified diagnoses, the codes for unspecified psychoactive substance use disorders (F1Ø.9-, F11.9-, F12.9-, F13.9-, F14.9-, F15.9-, F16.9-, F19.9-, F19.9-) should only be assigned based on provider documentation and when they meet the definition of a reportable diagnosis (see Section III, Reporting Additional Diagnoses). These codes are to be used only when the psychoactive substance use is associated with a physical, mental or behavioral disorder, and such a relationship is documented by the provider.

c. **Factitious Disorder**

Factitious disorder imposed on self or Munchausen's syndrome is a disorder in which a person falsely reports or causes his or her own physical or psychological signs or symptoms. For patients with documented factitious disorder on self or Munchausen's syndrome, assign the appropriate code from subcategory F68.1-, Factitious disorder imposed on self.

Munchausen's syndrome by proxy (MSBP) is a disorder in which a caregiver (perpetrator) falsely reports or causes an illness or injury in another person (victim) under his or her care, such as a child, an elderly adult, or a person who has a disability. The condition is also referred to as "factitious disorder imposed on another" or "factitious disorder by proxy." The perpetrator, not the victim, receives this diagnosis. Assign code F68.A, Factitious disorder imposed on another, to the perpetrator's record. For the victim of a patient suffering from MSBP, assign the appropriate code from categories T74, Adult and child abuse, neglect and other maltreatment, confirmed, or T76, Adult and child abuse, neglect and other maltreatment, suspected.

See Section I.C.19.f. Adult and child abuse, neglect and other maltreatment

CHAPTER 5

MENTAL, BEHAVIORAL AND NEURODEVELOPMENTAL DISORDERS (FØ1-F99)

Includes disorders of psychological development

Excludes2 symptoms, signs and abnormal clinical laboratory findings, not elsewhere classified (RØØ-R99)

This chapter contains the following blocks:

FØ1-FØ9	Mental disorders due to known physiological conditions
F1Ø-F19	Mental and behavioral disorders due to psychoactive substance use
F2Ø-F29	Schizophrenia, schizotypal, delusional, and other non-mood psychotic disorders
F3Ø-F39	Mood [affective] disorders
F4Ø-F48	Anxiety, dissociative, stress-related, somatoform and other nonpsychotic mental disorders
F5Ø-F59	Behavioral syndromes associated with physiological disturbances and physical factors
F6Ø-F69	Disorders of adult personality and behavior
F7Ø-F79	Intellectual disabilities
F8Ø-F89	Pervasive and specific developmental disorders
F9Ø-F98	Behavioral and emotional disorders with onset usually occurring in childhood and adolescence
F99	Unspecified mental disorder

MENTAL DISORDERS DUE TO KNOWN PHYSIOLOGICAL CONDITIONS (FØ1-FØ9)

This block comprises a range of mental disorders grouped together on the basis of their having in common a demonstrable etiology in cerebral disease, brain injury, or other insult leading to cerebral dysfunction. The dysfunction may be primary, as in diseases, injuries, and insults that affect the brain directly and selectively; or secondary, as in systemic diseases and disorders that attack the brain only as one of the multiple organs or systems of the body that are involved.

● **FØ1 Vascular dementia**

Vascular dementia as a result of infarction of the brain due to vascular disease, including hypertensive cerebrovascular disease.

Includes arteriosclerotic dementia

Code first the underlying physiological condition or sequelae of cerebrovascular disease.

● **FØ1.5 Vascular dementia**

FØ1.5Ø Vascular dementia without behavioral disturbance A

Major neurocognitive disorder without behavioral disturbance

FØ1.51 Vascular dementia with behavioral disturbance A

Major neurocognitive disorder due to vascular disease, with behavioral disturbance

Major neurocognitive disorder with aggressive behavior

Major neurocognitive disorder with combative behavior

Major neurocognitive disorder with violent behavior

Vascular dementia with aggressive behavior

Vascular dementia with combative behavior

Vascular dementia with violent behavior

Use additional code, if applicable, to identify wandering in vascular dementia (Z91.83)

F02 Dementia in other diseases classified elsewhere

Code first the underlying physiological condition, such as:
Alzheimer's (G30.-)
cerebral lipidosis (E75.4)
Creutzfeldt-Jakob disease (A81.0-)
dementia with Lewy bodies (G31.83)
dementia with Parkinsonism (G31.83)
epilepsy and recurrent seizures (G40.-)
frontotemporal dementia (G31.09)
hepatolenticular degeneration (E83.0)
human immunodeficiency virus [HIV] disease (B20)
Huntington's disease (G10)
hypercalcemia (E83.52)
hypothyroidism, acquired (E00-E03.-)
intoxications (T36-T65)
Jakob-Creutzfeldt disease (A81.0-)
multiple sclerosis (G35)
neurosyphilis (A52.17)
niacin deficiency [pellagra] (E52)
Parkinson's disease (G20)
Pick's disease (G31.01)
polyarteritis nodosa (M30.0)
prion disease (A81.9)
systemic lupus erythematosus (M32.-)
traumatic brain injury (S06.-)
trypanosomiasis (B56.-, B57.-)
vitamin B deficiency (E53.8)

Includes Major neurocognitive disorder in other diseases classified elsewhere

Excludes2 dementia in alcohol and psychoactive substance disorders (F10-F19, with .17, .27, .97)
vascular dementia (F01.5-)

Coding Clinic: 2016, Q4, P141

F02.8 Dementia in other diseases classified elsewhere

F02.80 Dementia in other diseases classified elsewhere without behavioral disturbance
Dementia in other diseases classified elsewhere NOS
Major neurocognitive disorder in other diseases classified elsewhere
Coding Clinic: 2017, Q1, P43; 2016, Q2, P6

F02.81 Dementia in other diseases classified elsewhere with behavioral disturbance
Dementia in other diseases classified elsewhere with aggressive behavior
Dementia in other diseases classified elsewhere with combative behavior
Dementia in other diseases classified elsewhere with violent behavior
Major neurocognitive disorder in other diseases classified elsewhere with aggressive behavior
Major neurocognitive disorder in other diseases classified elsewhere with combative behavior
Major neurocognitive disorder in other diseases classified elsewhere with violent behavior

Use additional code, if applicable, to identify wandering in dementia in conditions classified elsewhere (Z91.83)
Coding Clinic: 2017, Q2, P8, Q1, P43

Item 5-1 Psychosis was a term formerly applied to any mental disorder but is now restricted to disturbances of a great magnitude in which there is a personality disintegration and loss of contact with reality.

F03 Unspecified dementia
Presenile dementia NOS
Presenile psychosis NOS
Primary degenerative dementia NOS
Senile dementia NOS
Senile dementia depressed or paranoid type
Senile psychosis NOS

Excludes1 senility NOS (R41.81)

Excludes2 mild memory disturbance due to known physiological condition (F06.8)
senile dementia with delirium or acute confusional state (F05)

F03.9 Unspecified dementia

F03.90 Unspecified dementia without behavioral disturbance A
Dementia NOS
Coding Clinic: 2012, Q4, P92

F03.91 Unspecified dementia with behavioral disturbance A
Unspecified dementia with aggressive behavior
Unspecified dementia with combative behavior
Unspecified dementia with violent behavior

Use additional code, if applicable, to identify wandering in unspecified dementia (Z91.83)

F04 Amnestic disorder due to known physiological condition
Korsakov's psychosis or syndrome, nonalcoholic

Code first the underlying physiological condition

Excludes1 amnesia NOS (R41.3)
anterograde amnesia (R41.1)
dissociative amnesia (F44.0)
retrograde amnesia (R41.2)

Excludes2 alcohol-induced or unspecified Korsakov's syndrome (F10.26, F10.96)
Korsakov's syndrome induced by other psychoactive substances (F13.26, F13.96, F19.16, F19.26, F19.96)

F05 Delirium due to known physiological condition
Acute or subacute brain syndrome
Acute or subacute confusional state (nonalcoholic)
Acute or subacute infective psychosis
Acute or subacute organic reaction
Acute or subacute psycho-organic syndrome
Delirium of mixed etiology
Delirium superimposed on dementia
Sundowning

Code first the underlying physiological condition

Excludes1 delirium NOS (R41.0)

Excludes2 delirium tremens alcohol-induced or unspecified (F10.231, F10.921)

Coding Clinic: 2019, Q2, P34

F06 Other mental disorders due to known physiological condition

Includes mental disorders due to endocrine disorder
mental disorders due to exogenous hormone
mental disorders due to exogenous toxic substance
mental disorders due to primary cerebral disease
mental disorders due to somatic illness
mental disorders due to systemic disease affecting the brain

Code first the underlying physiological condition

Excludes1 unspecified dementia (F03)

Excludes2 delirium due to known physiological condition (F05)
dementia as classified in F01-F02
other mental disorders associated with alcohol and other psychoactive substances (F10-F19)

F06.0 Psychotic disorder with hallucinations due to known physiological condition
Organic hallucinatory state (nonalcoholic)
Excludes2 hallucinations and perceptual disturbance induced by alcohol and other psychoactive substances (F10-F19 with .151, .251, .951)
schizophrenia (F20.-)

F06.1 Catatonic disorder due to known physiological condition
Catatonia associated with another mental disorder
Catatonia NOS
Excludes1 catatonic stupor (R40.1)
stupor NOS (R40.1)
Excludes2 catatonic schizophrenia (F20.2)
dissociative stupor (F44.2)

F06.2 Psychotic disorder with delusions due to known physiological condition
Paranoid and paranoid-hallucinatory organic states
Schizophrenia-like psychosis in epilepsy
Excludes2 alcohol and drug-induced psychotic disorder (F10-F19 with .150, .250, .950)
brief psychotic disorder (F23)
delusional disorder (F22)
schizophrenia (F20.-)

● **F06.3 Mood disorder due to known physiological condition**
Excludes2 mood disorders due to alcohol and other psychoactive substances (F10-F19 with .14, .24, .94)
mood disorders, not due to known physiological condition or unspecified (F30-F39)

F06.30 Mood disorder due to known physiological condition, unspecified

F06.31 Mood disorder due to known physiological condition with depressive features
Depressive disorder due to known physiological condition, with depressive features

F06.32 Mood disorder due to known physiological condition with major depressive-like episode
Depressive disorder due to known physiological condition, with major depressive-like episode

F06.33 Mood disorder due to known physiological condition with manic features
Bipolar and related disorder due to a known physiological condition, with manic features
Bipolar and related disorder due to known physiological condition, with manic- or hypomanic-like episodes

F06.34 Mood disorder due to known physiological condition with mixed features
Bipolar and related disorder due to known physiological condition, with mixed features
Depressive disorder due to known physiological condition, with mixed features

F06.4 Anxiety disorder due to known physiological condition
Excludes2 anxiety disorders due to alcohol and other psychoactive substances (F10-F19 with .180, .280, .980)
anxiety disorders, not due to known physiological condition or unspecified (F40.-, F41.-)

F06.8 Other specified mental disorders due to known physiological condition
Epileptic psychosis NOS
Obsessive-compulsive and related disorder due to a known physiological condition
Organic dissociative disorder
Organic emotionally labile [asthenic] disorder

● **F07 Personality and behavioral disorders due to known physiological condition**
Code first the underlying physiological condition

F07.0 Personality change due to known physiological condition
Frontal lobe syndrome
Limbic epilepsy personality syndrome
Lobotomy syndrome
Organic personality disorder
Organic pseudopsychopathic personality
Organic pseudoretarded personality
Postleucotomy syndrome
Code first underlying physiological condition
Excludes1 mild cognitive impairment (G31.84)
postconcussional syndrome (F07.81)
postencephalitic syndrome (F07.89)
signs and symptoms involving emotional state (R45.-)
Excludes2 specific personality disorder (F60.-)

● **F07.8 Other personality and behavioral disorders due to known physiological condition**

F07.81 Postconcussional syndrome
Postcontusional syndrome (encephalopathy)
Post-traumatic brain syndrome, nonpsychotic
Use additional code to identify associated post-traumatic headache, if applicable (G44.3-)
Excludes1 current concussion (brain) (S06.0-)
postencephalitic syndrome (F07.89)

F07.89 Other personality and behavioral disorders due to known physiological condition
Postencephalitic syndrome
Damage to temporal brain lobes with memory loss and abnormal behavior
Right hemispheric organic affective disorder

F07.9 Unspecified personality and behavioral disorder due to known physiological condition
Organic psychosyndrome
Due to exposure to organic solvents

F09 Unspecified mental disorder due to known physiological condition
Mental disorder NOS due to known physiological condition
Organic brain syndrome NOS
Organic mental disorder NOS
Organic psychosis NOS
Symptomatic psychosis NOS
Code first the underlying physiological condition
Excludes1 psychosis NOS (F29)

MENTAL AND BEHAVIORAL DISORDERS DUE TO PSYCHOACTIVE SUBSTANCE USE (F10-F19)

● **F10 Alcohol related disorders**
Use additional code for blood alcohol level, if applicable (Y90.-)

● **F10.1 Alcohol abuse**
Excludes1 alcohol dependence (F10.2-)
alcohol use, unspecified (F10.9-)

F10.10 Alcohol abuse, uncomplicated
Alcohol use disorder, mild

F10.11 Alcohol abuse, in remission
Alcohol use disorder, mild, in early remission
Alcohol use disorder, mild, in sustained remission

● **F10.12 Alcohol abuse with intoxication**

F10.120 Alcohol abuse with intoxication, uncomplicated

F10.121 Alcohol abuse with intoxication, delirium

F10.129 Alcohol abuse with intoxication, unspecified

CHAPTER 5 (F01-F99)

F10.14 Alcohol abuse with alcohol-induced **mood disorder**
- Alcohol use disorder, mild, with alcohol-induced bipolar or related disorder
- Alcohol use disorder, mild, with alcohol-induced depressive disorder

F10.15 Alcohol abuse with alcohol-induced **psychotic disorder**
- **F10.150** Alcohol abuse with alcohol-induced psychotic disorder **with delusions**
- **F10.151** Alcohol abuse with alcohol-induced psychotic disorder with **hallucinations**
- **F10.159** Alcohol abuse with alcohol-induced psychotic disorder, **unspecified**

F10.18 Alcohol abuse with other alcohol-induced disorders
- **F10.180** Alcohol abuse with alcohol-induced **anxiety disorder**
- **F10.181** Alcohol abuse with alcohol-induced **sexual dysfunction**
- **F10.182** Alcohol abuse with alcohol-induced **sleep disorder**
- **F10.188** Alcohol abuse with **other** alcohol-induced disorder

F10.19 Alcohol abuse with **unspecified** alcohol-induced disorder

F10.2 Alcohol **dependence**

Excludes1 alcohol abuse (F10.1-)
alcohol use, unspecified (F10.9-)

Excludes2 toxic effect of alcohol (T51.0-)

F10.20 Alcohol dependence, **uncomplicated**
- Alcohol use disorder, moderate
- Alcohol use disorder, severe

F10.21 Alcohol dependence, **in remission**
- Alcohol use disorder, moderate, in early remission
- Alcohol use disorder, moderate, in sustained remission
- Alcohol use disorder, severe, in early remission
- Alcohol use disorder, severe, in sustained remission

F10.22 Alcohol dependence with **intoxication**
- Acute drunkenness (in alcoholism)

Excludes2 alcohol dependence with withdrawal (F10.23-)

- **F10.220** Alcohol dependence with intoxication, **uncomplicated**
- **F10.221** Alcohol dependence with intoxication **delirium**
- **F10.229** Alcohol dependence with intoxication, **unspecified**

F10.23 Alcohol dependence with **withdrawal**

Excludes2 alcohol dependence with intoxication (F10.22-)

- **F10.230** Alcohol dependence with withdrawal, **uncomplicated**
- **F10.231** Alcohol dependence with withdrawal **delirium**
- **F10.232** Alcohol dependence with withdrawal **with perceptual disturbance**
- **F10.239** Alcohol dependence with withdrawal, **unspecified**
  - Coding Clinic: 2015, Q2, P15

F10.24 Alcohol dependence with alcohol-induced **mood disorder**
- Alcohol use disorder, moderate, with alcohol-induced bipolar or related disorder
- Alcohol use disorder, moderate, with alcohol-induced depressive disorder
- Alcohol use disorder, severe, with alcohol-induced bipolar or related disorder
- Alcohol use disorder, severe, with alcohol-induced depressive disorder

F10.25 Alcohol dependence with alcohol-induced **psychotic disorder**
- **F10.250** Alcohol dependence with alcohol-induced psychotic disorder with **delusions**
- **F10.251** Alcohol dependence with alcohol-induced psychotic disorder with **hallucinations**
- **F10.259** Alcohol dependence with alcohol-induced psychotic disorder, **unspecified**

F10.26 Alcohol dependence with alcohol-induced **persisting amnestic disorder**
- Alcohol use disorder, moderate, with alcohol-induced major neurocognitive disorder, amnestic-confabulatory type
- Alcohol use disorder, severe, with alcohol-induced major neurocognitive disorder, amnestic-confabulatory type

F10.27 Alcohol dependence with alcohol-induced **persisting dementia**
- Alcohol use disorder, moderate, with alcohol-induced major neurocognitive disorder, nonamnestic-confabulatory type
- Alcohol use disorder, severe, with alcohol-induced major neurocognitive disorder, nonamnestic-confabulatory type

F10.28 Alcohol dependence with other alcohol-induced disorders
- **F10.280** Alcohol dependence with alcohol-induced **anxiety disorder**
- **F10.281** Alcohol dependence with alcohol-induced **sexual dysfunction**
- **F10.282** Alcohol dependence with alcohol-induced **sleep disorder**
- **F10.288** Alcohol dependence with **other** alcohol-induced disorder
  - Alcohol use disorder, moderate, with alcohol-induced mild neurocognitive disorder
  - Alcohol use disorder, severe, with alcohol-induced mild neurocognitive disorder

F10.29 Alcohol dependence with **unspecified** alcohol-induced disorder

F10.9 Alcohol use, **unspecified**

Excludes1 alcohol abuse (F10.1-)
alcohol dependence (F10.2-)

F10.92 Alcohol use, **unspecified with intoxication**
- **F10.920** Alcohol use, unspecified with intoxication, **uncomplicated**
- **F10.921** Alcohol use, unspecified with intoxication **delirium**
- **F10.929** Alcohol use, unspecified with intoxication, **unspecified**

F10.94 Alcohol use, **unspecified** with alcohol-induced **mood disorder**
- Alcohol-induced bipolar or related disorder, without use disorder
- Alcohol-induced depressive disorder, without use disorder

CHAPTER 5 (F01-F99)

F10.95 Alcohol use, unspecified with alcohol-induced psychotic disorder
F10.950 Alcohol use, unspecified with alcohol-induced psychotic disorder with delusions
F10.951 Alcohol use, unspecified with alcohol-induced psychotic disorder with hallucinations
F10.959 Alcohol use, unspecified with alcohol-induced psychotic disorder, unspecified
Alcohol-induced psychotic disorder without use disorder
F10.96 Alcohol use, unspecified with alcohol-induced persisting amnestic disorder
Alcohol-induced major neurocognitive disorder, amnestic-confabulatory type, without use disorder
F10.97 Alcohol use, unspecified with alcohol-induced persisting dementia
Alcohol-induced major neurocognitive disorder, nonamnestic-confabulatory type, without use disorder
F10.98 Alcohol use, unspecified with other alcohol-induced disorders
F10.980 Alcohol use, unspecified with alcohol-induced anxiety disorder
Alcohol-induced anxiety disorder, without use disorder
F10.981 Alcohol use, unspecified with alcohol-induced sexual dysfunction
Alcohol-induced sexual dysfunction, without use disorder
F10.982 Alcohol use, unspecified with alcohol-induced sleep disorder
Alcohol-induced sleep disorder, without use disorder
F10.988 Alcohol use, unspecified with other alcohol-induced disorder
Alcohol-induced mild neurocognitive disorder, without use disorder
F10.99 Alcohol use, unspecified with unspecified alcohol-induced disorder

F11 Opioid related disorders
F11.1 Opioid abuse
Excludes1 opioid dependence (F11.2-)
opioid use, unspecified (F11.9-)
F11.10 Opioid abuse, uncomplicated
Opioid use disorder, mild
F11.11 Opioid abuse, in remission
Opioid use disorder, mild, in early remission
Opioid use disorder, mild, in sustained remission
F11.12 Opioid abuse with intoxication
F11.120 Opioid abuse with intoxication, uncomplicated
F11.121 Opioid abuse with intoxication delirium
F11.122 Opioid abuse with intoxication with perceptual disturbance
F11.129 Opioid abuse with intoxication, unspecified
F11.14 Opioid abuse with opioid-induced mood disorder
Opioid use disorder, mild, with opioid-induced depressive disorder
F11.15 Opioid abuse with opioid-induced psychotic disorder
F11.150 Opioid abuse with opioid-induced psychotic disorder with delusions
F11.151 Opioid abuse with opioid-induced psychotic disorder with hallucinations
F11.159 Opioid abuse with opioid-induced psychotic disorder, unspecified
F11.18 Opioid abuse with other opioid-induced disorder
F11.181 Opioid abuse with opioid-induced sexual dysfunction
F11.182 Opioid abuse with opioid-induced sleep disorder
F11.188 Opioid abuse with other opioid-induced disorder
F11.19 Opioid abuse with unspecified opioid-induced disorder
F11.2 Opioid dependence
Excludes1 opioid abuse (F11.1-)
opioid use, unspecified (F11.9-)
Excludes2 opioid poisoning (T40.0—T40.2-)
F11.20 Opioid dependence, uncomplicated
Opioid use disorder, moderate
Opioid use disorder, severe
F11.21 Opioid dependence, in remission
Opioid use disorder, moderate, in early remission
Opioid use disorder, moderate, in sustained remission
Opioid use disorder, severe, in early remission
Opioid use disorder, severe, in sustained remission
F11.22 Opioid dependence with intoxication
Excludes1 opioid dependence with withdrawal (F11.23)
F11.220 Opioid dependence with intoxication, uncomplicated
F11.221 Opioid dependence with intoxication delirium
F11.222 Opioid dependence with intoxication with perceptual disturbance
F11.229 Opioid dependence with intoxication, unspecified
F11.23 Opioid dependence with withdrawal
Excludes1 opioid dependence with intoxication (F11.22-)
F11.24 Opioid dependence with opioid-induced mood disorder
Opioid use disorder, moderate, with opioid-induced depressive disorder
F11.25 Opioid dependence with opioid-induced psychotic disorder
F11.250 Opioid dependence with opioid-induced psychotic disorder with delusions
F11.251 Opioid dependence with opioid-induced psychotic disorder with hallucinations
F11.259 Opioid dependence with opioid-induced psychotic disorder, unspecified
F11.28 Opioid dependence with other opioid-induced disorder
F11.281 Opioid dependence with opioid-induced sexual dysfunction
F11.282 Opioid dependence with opioid-induced sleep disorder
F11.288 Opioid dependence with other opioid-induced disorder
F11.29 Opioid dependence with unspecified opioid-induced disorder

CHAPTER 5 (F01-F99)

F11.9 Opioid use, unspecified
Excludes1 opioid abuse (F11.1-)
opioid dependence (F11.2-)

F11.90 Opioid use, unspecified, uncomplicated

F11.92 Opioid use, unspecified with intoxication
Excludes1 opioid use, unspecified with withdrawal (F11.93)

F11.920 Opioid use, unspecified with intoxication, uncomplicated

F11.921 Opioid use, unspecified with intoxication delirium
Opioid-induced delirium

F11.922 Opioid use, unspecified with intoxication with perceptual disturbance

F11.929 Opioid use, unspecified with intoxication, unspecified

F11.93 Opioid use, unspecified with withdrawal
Excludes1 opioid use, unspecified with intoxication (F11.92-)

F11.94 Opioid use, unspecified with opioid-induced mood disorder
Opioid-induced depressive disorder, without use disorder

F11.95 Opioid use, unspecified with opioid-induced psychotic disorder

F11.950 Opioid use, unspecified with opioid-induced psychotic disorder with delusions

F11.951 Opioid use, unspecified with opioid-induced psychotic disorder with hallucinations

F11.959 Opioid use, unspecified with opioid-induced psychotic disorder, unspecified

F11.98 Opioid use, unspecified with other specified opioid-induced disorder

F11.981 Opioid use, unspecified with opioid-induced sexual dysfunction
Opioid-induced sexual dysfunction, without use disorder

F11.982 Opioid use, unspecified with opioid-induced sleep disorder
Opioid-induced sleep disorder, without use disorder

F11.988 Opioid use, unspecified with other opioid-induced disorder
Opioid-induced anxiety disorder, without use disorder

F11.99 Opioid use, unspecified with unspecified opioid-induced disorder

F12 Cannabis related disorders
Includes marijuana

F12.1 Cannabis abuse
Excludes1 cannabis dependence (F12.2-)
cannabis use, unspecified (F12.9-)

F12.10 Cannabis abuse, uncomplicated
Cannabis use disorder, mild

F12.11 Cannabis abuse, in remission
Cannabis use disorder, mild, in early remission
Cannabis use disorder, mild, in sustained remission

F12.12 Cannabis abuse with intoxication

F12.120 Cannabis abuse with intoxication, uncomplicated

F12.121 Cannabis abuse with intoxication delirium

F12.122 Cannabis abuse with intoxication with perceptual disturbance

F12.129 Cannabis abuse with intoxication, unspecified

F12.15 Cannabis abuse with psychotic disorder

F12.150 Cannabis abuse with psychotic disorder with delusions

F12.151 Cannabis abuse with psychotic disorder with hallucinations

F12.159 Cannabis abuse with psychotic disorder, unspecified

F12.18 Cannabis abuse with other cannabis-induced disorder

F12.180 Cannabis abuse with cannabis-induced anxiety disorder

F12.188 Cannabis abuse with other cannabis-induced disorder
Cannabis use disorder, mild, with cannabis-induced sleep disorder

F12.19 Cannabis abuse with unspecified cannabis-induced disorder

F12.2 Cannabis dependence
Excludes1 cannabis abuse (F12.1-)
cannabis use, unspecified (F12.9-)
Excludes2 cannabis poisoning (T40.7-)

F12.20 Cannabis dependence, uncomplicated
Cannabis use disorder, moderate
Cannabis use disorder, severe

F12.21 Cannabis dependence, in remission
Cannabis use disorder, moderate, in early remission
Cannabis use disorder, moderate, in sustained remission
Cannabis use disorder, severe, in early remission
Cannabis use disorder, severe, in sustained remission

F12.22 Cannabis dependence with intoxication

F12.220 Cannabis dependence with intoxication, uncomplicated

F12.221 Cannabis dependence with intoxication delirium

F12.222 Cannabis dependence with intoxication with perceptual disturbance

F12.229 Cannabis dependence with intoxication, unspecified

F12.23 Cannabis dependence with withdrawal

F12.25 Cannabis dependence with psychotic disorder

F12.250 Cannabis dependence with psychotic disorder with delusions

F12.251 Cannabis dependence with psychotic disorder with hallucinations

F12.259 Cannabis dependence with psychotic disorder, unspecified

F12.28 Cannabis dependence with other cannabis-induced disorder

F12.280 Cannabis dependence with cannabis-induced anxiety disorder

F12.288 Cannabis dependence with other cannabis-induced disorder
Cannabis use disorder, moderate, with cannabis-induced sleep disorder
Cannabis use disorder, severe, with cannabis-induced sleep disorder

F12.29 Cannabis dependence with unspecified cannabis-induced disorder

F12.9 Cannabis use, unspecified
Excludes1 cannabis abuse (F12.1-)
cannabis dependence (F12.2-)

F12.90 Cannabis use, unspecified, uncomplicated

F12.92 Cannabis use, unspecified with intoxication

F12.920 Cannabis use, unspecified with intoxication, uncomplicated

F12.921 Cannabis use, unspecified with intoxication delirium

F12.922 Cannabis use, unspecified with intoxication with perceptual disturbance

F12.929 Cannabis use, unspecified with intoxication, unspecified

F12.93 Cannabis use, unspecified with withdrawal

F12.95 Cannabis use, unspecified with psychotic disorder

F12.950 Cannabis use, unspecified with psychotic disorder with delusions

F12.951 Cannabis use, unspecified with psychotic disorder with hallucinations

F12.959 Cannabis use, unspecified with psychotic disorder, unspecified
Cannabis-induced psychotic disorder, without use disorder

F12.98 Cannabis use, unspecified with other cannabis-induced disorder

F12.980 Cannabis use, unspecified with anxiety disorder
Cannabis-induced anxiety disorder, without use disorder

F12.988 Cannabis use, unspecified with other cannabis-induced disorder
Cannabis-induced sleep disorder, without use disorder

F12.99 Cannabis use, unspecified with unspecified cannabis-induced disorder

F13 Sedative, hypnotic, or anxiolytic related disorders

F13.1 Sedative, hypnotic or anxiolytic-related abuse
Excludes1 sedative, hypnotic or anxiolytic-related dependence (F13.2-)
sedative, hypnotic, or anxiolytic use, unspecified (F13.9-)

F13.10 Sedative, hypnotic or anxiolytic abuse, uncomplicated
Sedative, hypnotic, or anxiolytic use disorder, mild

F13.11 Sedative, hypnotic or anxiolytic abuse, in remission
Sedative, hypnotic or anxiolytic use disorder, mild, in early remission
Sedative, hypnotic or anxiolytic use disorder, mild, in sustained remission

F13.12 Sedative, hypnotic or anxiolytic abuse with intoxication

F13.120 Sedative, hypnotic or anxiolytic abuse with intoxication, uncomplicated

F13.121 Sedative, hypnotic or anxiolytic abuse with intoxication delirium

F13.129 Sedative, hypnotic or anxiolytic abuse with intoxication, unspecified

F13.14 Sedative, hypnotic or anxiolytic abuse with sedative, hypnotic or anxiolytic-induced mood disorder
Sedative, hypnotic, or anxiolytic use disorder, mild, with sedative, hypnotic, or anxiolytic-induced bipolar or related disorder
Sedative, hypnotic, or anxiolytic use disorder, mild, with sedative, hypnotic, or anxiolytic-induced depressive disorder

F13.15 Sedative, hypnotic or anxiolytic abuse with sedative, hypnotic or anxiolytic-induced psychotic disorder

F13.150 Sedative, hypnotic or anxiolytic abuse with sedative, hypnotic or anxiolytic-induced psychotic disorder with delusions

F13.151 Sedative, hypnotic or anxiolytic abuse with sedative, hypnotic or anxiolytic-induced psychotic disorder with hallucinations

F13.159 Sedative, hypnotic or anxiolytic abuse with sedative, hypnotic or anxiolytic-induced psychotic disorder, unspecified

F13.18 Sedative, hypnotic or anxiolytic abuse with other sedative, hypnotic or anxiolytic-induced disorders

F13.180 Sedative, hypnotic or anxiolytic abuse with sedative, hypnotic or anxiolytic-induced anxiety disorder

F13.181 Sedative, hypnotic or anxiolytic abuse with sedative, hypnotic or anxiolytic-induced sexual dysfunction

F13.182 Sedative, hypnotic or anxiolytic abuse with sedative, hypnotic or anxiolytic-induced sleep disorder

F13.188 Sedative, hypnotic or anxiolytic abuse with other sedative, hypnotic or anxiolytic-induced disorder

F13.19 Sedative, hypnotic or anxiolytic abuse with unspecified sedative, hypnotic or anxiolytic-induced disorder

F13.2 Sedative, hypnotic or anxiolytic-related dependence
Excludes1 sedative, hypnotic or anxiolytic-related abuse (F13.1-)
sedative, hypnotic, or anxiolytic use, unspecified (F13.9-)
Excludes2 sedative, hypnotic, or anxiolytic poisoning (T42.-)

F13.20 Sedative, hypnotic or anxiolytic dependence, uncomplicated

F13.21 Sedative, hypnotic or anxiolytic dependence, in remission
Sedative, hypnotic or anxiolytic use disorder, moderate, in early remission
Sedative, hypnotic or anxiolytic use disorder, moderate, in sustained remission
Sedative, hypnotic or anxiolytic use disorder, severe, in early remission
Sedative, hypnotic or anxiolytic use disorder, severe, in sustained remission

F13.22 Sedative, hypnotic or anxiolytic dependence with intoxication
Excludes1 sedative, hypnotic or anxiolytic dependence with withdrawal (F13.23-)

F13.220 Sedative, hypnotic or anxiolytic dependence with intoxication, uncomplicated

F13.221 Sedative, hypnotic or anxiolytic dependence with intoxication delirium

F13.229 Sedative, hypnotic or anxiolytic dependence with intoxication, unspecified

● F13.23 **Sedative, hypnotic or anxiolytic dependence with withdrawal**
Sedative, hypnotic, or anxiolytic use disorder, moderate
Sedative, hypnotic, or anxiolytic use disorder, severe
Excludes1 sedative, hypnotic or anxiolytic dependence with intoxication (F13.22-)

F13.230 **Sedative, hypnotic or anxiolytic dependence with withdrawal, uncomplicated**

F13.231 **Sedative, hypnotic or anxiolytic dependence with withdrawal delirium**

F13.232 **Sedative, hypnotic or anxiolytic dependence with withdrawal with perceptual disturbance**
Sedative, hypnotic, or anxiolytic withdrawal with perceptual disturbances

F13.239 **Sedative, hypnotic or anxiolytic dependence with withdrawal, unspecified**
Sedative, hypnotic, or anxiolytic withdrawal without perceptual disturbances

F13.24 **Sedative, hypnotic or anxiolytic dependence with sedative, hypnotic or anxiolytic-induced mood disorder**
Sedative, hypnotic, or anxiolytic use disorder, moderate, with sedative, hypnotic, or anxiolytic-induced bipolar or related disorder
Sedative, hypnotic, or anxiolytic use disorder, moderate, with sedative, hypnotic, or anxiolytic-induced depressive disorder
Sedative, hypnotic, or anxiolytic use disorder, severe, with sedative, hypnotic, or anxiolytic-induced bipolar or related disorder
Sedative, hypnotic, or anxiolytic use disorder, severe, with sedative, hypnotic, or anxiolytic-induced depressive disorder

● F13.25 **Sedative, hypnotic or anxiolytic dependence with sedative, hypnotic or anxiolytic-induced psychotic disorder**

F13.250 **Sedative, hypnotic or anxiolytic dependence with sedative, hypnotic or anxiolytic-induced psychotic disorder with delusions**

F13.251 **Sedative, hypnotic or anxiolytic dependence with sedative, hypnotic or anxiolytic-induced psychotic disorder with hallucinations**

F13.259 **Sedative, hypnotic or anxiolytic dependence with sedative, hypnotic or anxiolytic-induced psychotic disorder, unspecified**

F13.26 **Sedative, hypnotic or anxiolytic dependence with sedative, hypnotic or anxiolytic-induced persisting amnestic disorder**

F13.27 **Sedative, hypnotic or anxiolytic dependence with sedative, hypnotic or anxiolytic-induced persisting dementia**
Sedative, hypnotic, or anxiolytic use disorder, moderate, with sedative, hypnotic, or anxiolytic-induced major neurocognitive disorder
Sedative, hypnotic, or anxiolytic use disorder, severe, with sedative, hypnotic, or anxiolytic-induced major neurocognitive disorder

● F13.28 **Sedative, hypnotic or anxiolytic dependence with other sedative, hypnotic or anxiolytic-induced disorders**

F13.280 **Sedative, hypnotic or anxiolytic dependence with sedative, hypnotic or anxiolytic-induced anxiety disorder**

F13.281 **Sedative, hypnotic or anxiolytic dependence with sedative, hypnotic or anxiolytic-induced sexual dysfunction**

F13.282 **Sedative, hypnotic or anxiolytic dependence with sedative, hypnotic or anxiolytic-induced sleep disorder**

F13.288 **Sedative, hypnotic or anxiolytic dependence with other sedative, hypnotic or anxiolytic-induced disorder**
Sedative, hypnotic, or anxiolytic use disorder, moderate, with sedative, hypnotic, or anxiolytic-induced mild neurocognitive disorder
Sedative, hypnotic, or anxiolytic use disorder, severe, with sedative, hypnotic, or anxiolytic-induced mild neurocognitive disorder

F13.29 **Sedative, hypnotic or anxiolytic dependence with unspecified sedative, hypnotic or anxiolytic-induced disorder**

● F13.9 **Sedative, hypnotic or anxiolytic-related use, unspecified**
Excludes1 sedative, hypnotic or anxiolytic-related abuse (F13.1-)
sedative, hypnotic or anxiolytic-related dependence (F13.2-)

F13.90 **Sedative, hypnotic, or anxiolytic use, unspecified, uncomplicated**

● F13.92 **Sedative, hypnotic or anxiolytic use, unspecified with intoxication**
Excludes1 sedative, hypnotic or anxiolytic use, unspecified with withdrawal (F13.93-)

F13.920 **Sedative, hypnotic or anxiolytic use, unspecified with intoxication, uncomplicated**

F13.921 **Sedative, hypnotic or anxiolytic use, unspecified with intoxication delirium**
Sedative, hypnotic, or anxiolytic-induced delirium

F13.929 **Sedative, hypnotic or anxiolytic use, unspecified with intoxication, unspecified**

● F13.93 **Sedative, hypnotic or anxiolytic use, unspecified with withdrawal**
Excludes1 sedative, hypnotic or anxiolytic use, unspecified with intoxication (F13.92-)

F13.930 **Sedative, hypnotic or anxiolytic use, unspecified with withdrawal, uncomplicated**

F13.931 **Sedative, hypnotic or anxiolytic use, unspecified with withdrawal delirium**

F13.932 **Sedative, hypnotic or anxiolytic use, unspecified with withdrawal with perceptual disturbances**

F13.939 **Sedative, hypnotic or anxiolytic use, unspecified with withdrawal, unspecified**

F13.94 **Sedative, hypnotic or anxiolytic use, unspecified with sedative, hypnotic or anxiolytic-induced mood disorder**
Sedative, hypnotic, or anxiolytic-induced bipolar or related disorder, without use disorder
Sedative, hypnotic, or anxiolytic-induced depressive disorder, without use disorder

F13.95 **Sedative, hypnotic or anxiolytic use, unspecified with sedative, hypnotic or anxiolytic-induced psychotic disorder**

F13.950 **Sedative, hypnotic or anxiolytic use, unspecified with sedative, hypnotic or anxiolytic-induced psychotic disorder with delusions**

F13.951 **Sedative, hypnotic or anxiolytic use, unspecified with sedative, hypnotic or anxiolytic-induced psychotic disorder with hallucinations**

F13.959 **Sedative, hypnotic or anxiolytic use, unspecified with sedative, hypnotic or anxiolytic-induced psychotic disorder, unspecified**
Sedative, hypnotic, or anxiolytic-induced psychotic disorder, without use disorder

F13.96 **Sedative, hypnotic or anxiolytic use, unspecified with sedative, hypnotic or anxiolytic-induced persisting amnestic disorder**

F13.97 **Sedative, hypnotic or anxiolytic use, unspecified with sedative, hypnotic or anxiolytic-induced persisting dementia**
Sedative, hypnotic, or anxiolytic-induced major neurocognitive disorder, without use disorder

F13.98 **Sedative, hypnotic or anxiolytic use, unspecified with other sedative, hypnotic or anxiolytic-induced disorders**

F13.980 **Sedative, hypnotic or anxiolytic use, unspecified with sedative, hypnotic or anxiolytic-induced anxiety disorder**
Sedative, hypnotic, or anxiolytic-induced anxiety disorder, without use disorder

F13.981 **Sedative, hypnotic or anxiolytic use, unspecified with sedative, hypnotic or anxiolytic-induced sexual dysfunction**
Sedative, hypnotic, or anxiolytic-induced sexual dysfunction disorder, without use disorder

F13.982 **Sedative, hypnotic or anxiolytic use, unspecified with sedative, hypnotic or anxiolytic-induced sleep disorder**
Sedative, hypnotic, or anxiolytic-induced sleep disorder, without use disorder

F13.988 **Sedative, hypnotic or anxiolytic use, unspecified with other sedative, hypnotic or anxiolytic-induced disorder**
Sedative, hypnotic, or anxiolytic-induced mild neurocognitive disorder

F13.99 **Sedative, hypnotic or anxiolytic use, unspecified with unspecified sedative, hypnotic or anxiolytic-induced disorder**

F14 **Cocaine related disorders**
Excludes2 other stimulant-related disorders (F15.-)

F14.1 **Cocaine abuse**
Excludes1 cocaine dependence (F14.2-)
cocaine use, unspecified (F14.9-)

F14.10 **Cocaine abuse, uncomplicated**
Cocaine use disorder, mild

F14.11 **Cocaine abuse, in remission**
Cocaine use disorder, mild, in early remission
Cocaine use disorder, mild, in sustained remission

F14.12 **Cocaine abuse with intoxication**

F14.120 **Cocaine abuse with intoxication, uncomplicated**

F14.121 **Cocaine abuse with intoxication with delirium**

F14.122 **Cocaine abuse with intoxication with perceptual disturbance**

F14.129 **Cocaine abuse with intoxication, unspecified**

F14.14 **Cocaine abuse with cocaine-induced mood disorder**
Cocaine use disorder, mild, with cocaine-induced bipolar or related disorder
Cocaine use disorder, mild, with cocaine-induced depressive disorder

F14.15 **Cocaine abuse with cocaine-induced psychotic disorder**

F14.150 **Cocaine abuse with cocaine-induced psychotic disorder with delusions**

F14.151 **Cocaine abuse with cocaine-induced psychotic disorder with hallucinations**

F14.159 **Cocaine abuse with cocaine-induced psychotic disorder, unspecified**

F14.18 **Cocaine abuse with other cocaine-induced disorder**

F14.180 **Cocaine abuse with cocaine-induced anxiety disorder**

F14.181 **Cocaine abuse with cocaine-induced sexual dysfunction**

F14.182 **Cocaine abuse with cocaine-induced sleep disorder**

F14.188 **Cocaine abuse with other cocaine-induced disorder**
Cocaine use disorder, mild, with cocaine-induced obsessive-compulsive or related disorder

F14.19 **Cocaine abuse with unspecified cocaine-induced disorder**

F14.2 **Cocaine dependence**
Excludes1 cocaine abuse (F14.1-)
cocaine use, unspecified (F14.9-)
Excludes2 cocaine poisoning (T40.5-)

F14.20 **Cocaine dependence, uncomplicated**
Cocaine use disorder, moderate
Cocaine use disorder, severe

F14.21 **Cocaine dependence, in remission**
Cocaine use disorder, moderate, in early remission
Cocaine use disorder, moderate, in sustained remission
Cocaine use disorder, severe, in early remission
Cocaine use disorder, severe, in sustained remission
Coding Clinic: 2017, Q2, P27

● F14.22 Cocaine dependence with intoxication
Excludes1 cocaine dependence with withdrawal (F14.23)
F14.220 Cocaine dependence with intoxication, uncomplicated
F14.221 Cocaine dependence with intoxication delirium
F14.222 Cocaine dependence with intoxication with perceptual disturbance
F14.229 Cocaine dependence with intoxication, unspecified
F14.23 Cocaine dependence with withdrawal
Excludes1 cocaine dependence with intoxication (F14.22-)
F14.24 Cocaine dependence with cocaine-induced mood disorder
Cocaine use disorder, moderate, with cocaine-induced bipolar or related disorder
Cocaine use disorder, moderate, with cocaine-induced depressive disorder
Cocaine use disorder, severe, with cocaine-induced bipolar or related disorder
Cocaine use disorder, severe, with cocaine-induced depressive disorder
● F14.25 Cocaine dependence with cocaine-induced psychotic disorder
F14.250 Cocaine dependence with cocaine-induced psychotic disorder with delusions
F14.251 Cocaine dependence with cocaine-induced psychotic disorder with hallucinations
F14.259 Cocaine dependence with cocaine-induced psychotic disorder, unspecified
● F14.28 Cocaine dependence with other cocaine-induced disorder
F14.280 Cocaine dependence with cocaine-induced anxiety disorder
F14.281 Cocaine dependence with cocaine-induced sexual dysfunction
F14.282 Cocaine dependence with cocaine-induced sleep disorder
F14.288 Cocaine dependence with other cocaine-induced disorder
Cocaine use disorder, moderate, with cocaine-induced obsessive-compulsive or related disorder
Cocaine use disorder, severe, with cocaine-induced obsessive-compulsive or related disorder
F14.29 Cocaine dependence with unspecified cocaine-induced disorder
● F14.9 Cocaine use, unspecified
Excludes1 cocaine abuse (F14.1-)
cocaine dependence (F14.2-)
F14.90 Cocaine use, unspecified, uncomplicated
Coding Clinic: 2018, Q2, P11
● F14.92 Cocaine use, unspecified with intoxication
F14.920 Cocaine use, unspecified with intoxication, uncomplicated
F14.921 Cocaine use, unspecified with intoxication delirium
F14.922 Cocaine use, unspecified with intoxication with perceptual disturbance
F14.929 Cocaine use, unspecified with intoxication, unspecified
F14.94 Cocaine use, unspecified with cocaine-induced mood disorder
Cocaine-induced bipolar or related disorder, without use disorder
Cocaine-induced depressive disorder, without use disorder
● F14.95 Cocaine use, unspecified with cocaine-induced psychotic disorder
F14.950 Cocaine use, unspecified with cocaine-induced psychotic disorder with delusions
F14.951 Cocaine use, unspecified with cocaine-induced psychotic disorder with hallucinations
F14.959 Cocaine use, unspecified with cocaine-induced psychotic disorder, unspecified
Cocaine-induced psychotic disorder, without use disorder
● F14.98 Cocaine use, unspecified with other specified cocaine-induced disorder
F14.980 Cocaine use, unspecified with cocaine-induced anxiety disorder
Cocaine-induced anxiety disorder, without use disorder
F14.981 Cocaine use, unspecified with cocaine-induced sexual dysfunction
Cocaine-induced sexual dysfunction, without use disorder
F14.982 Cocaine use, unspecified with cocaine-induced sleep disorder
Cocaine-induced sleep disorder, without use disorder
F14.988 Cocaine use, unspecified with other cocaine-induced disorder
Cocaine-induced obsessive-compulsive or related disorder
F14.99 Cocaine use, unspecified with unspecified cocaine-induced disorder

● F15 Other stimulant related disorders
Includes amphetamine-related disorders
caffeine
Excludes2 cocaine-related disorders (F14.-)
● F15.1 Other stimulant abuse
Excludes1 other stimulant dependence (F15.2-)
other stimulant use, unspecified (F15.9-)
F15.10 Other stimulant abuse, uncomplicated
Amphetamine type substance use disorder, mild
Other or unspecified stimulant use disorder, mild
F15.11 Other stimulant abuse, in remission
Amphetamine type substance use disorder, mild, in early remission
Amphetamine type substance use disorder, mild, in sustained remission
Other or unspecified stimulant use disorder, mild, in early remission
Other or unspecified stimulant use disorder, mild, in sustained remission
● F15.12 Other stimulant abuse with intoxication
F15.120 Other stimulant abuse with intoxication, uncomplicated
F15.121 Other stimulant abuse with intoxication delirium

F15.122 **Other stimulant abuse with intoxication with perceptual disturbance**
Amphetamine or other stimulant use disorder, mild, with amphetamine or other stimulant intoxication, with perceptual disturbances

F15.129 **Other stimulant abuse with intoxication, unspecified**
Amphetamine or other stimulant use disorder, mild, with amphetamine or other stimulant intoxication, without perceptual disturbances

F15.14 **Other stimulant abuse with stimulant-induced mood disorder**
Amphetamine or other stimulant use disorder, mild, with amphetamine or other stimulant-induced bipolar or related disorder
Amphetamine or other stimulant use disorder, mild, with amphetamine or other stimulant-induced depressive disorder

F15.15 **Other stimulant abuse with stimulant-induced psychotic disorder**

F15.150 **Other stimulant abuse with stimulant-induced psychotic disorder with delusions**

F15.151 **Other stimulant abuse with stimulant-induced psychotic disorder with hallucinations**

F15.159 **Other stimulant abuse with stimulant-induced psychotic disorder, unspecified**

F15.18 **Other stimulant abuse with other stimulant-induced disorder**

F15.180 **Other stimulant abuse with stimulant-induced anxiety disorder**

F15.181 **Other stimulant abuse with stimulant-induced sexual dysfunction**

F15.182 **Other stimulant abuse with stimulant-induced sleep disorder**

F15.188 **Other stimulant abuse with other stimulant-induced disorder**
Amphetamine or other stimulant use disorder, mild, with amphetamine or other stimulant-induced obsessive-compulsive or related disorder

F15.19 **Other stimulant abuse with unspecified stimulant-induced disorder**

F15.2 **Other stimulant dependence**
Excludes1 other stimulant abuse (F15.1-)
other stimulant use, unspecified (F15.9-)

F15.20 **Other stimulant dependence, uncomplicated**
Amphetamine type substance use disorder, moderate
Amphetamine type substance use disorder, severe
Other or unspecified stimulant use disorder, moderate
Other or unspecified stimulant use disorder, severe

F15.21 **Other stimulant dependence, in remission**
Amphetamine type substance use disorder, moderate, in early remission
Amphetamine type substance use disorder, moderate, in sustained remission
Amphetamine type substance use disorder, severe, in early remission
Amphetamine type substance use disorder, severe, in sustained remission
Other or unspecified stimulant use disorder, moderate, in early remission
Other or unspecified stimulant use disorder, moderate, in sustained remission
Other or unspecified stimulant use disorder, severe, in early remission
Other or unspecified stimulant use disorder, severe, in sustained remission

F15.22 **Other stimulant dependence with intoxication**
Excludes1 other stimulant dependence with withdrawal (F15.23)

F15.220 **Other stimulant dependence with intoxication, uncomplicated**

F15.221 **Other stimulant dependence with intoxication delirium**

F15.222 **Other stimulant dependence with intoxication with perceptual disturbance**
Amphetamine or other stimulant use disorder, moderate, with amphetamine or other stimulant intoxication, with perceptual disturbances
Amphetamine or other stimulant use disorder, severe, with amphetamine or other stimulant intoxication, with perceptual disturbances

F15.229 **Other stimulant dependence with intoxication, unspecified**
Amphetamine or other stimulant use disorder, moderate, with amphetamine or other stimulant intoxication, without perceptual disturbances
Amphetamine or other stimulant use disorder, severe, with amphetamine or other stimulant intoxication, without perceptual disturbances

F15.23 **Other stimulant dependence with withdrawal**
Amphetamine or other stimulant withdrawal
Excludes1 other stimulant dependence with intoxication (F15.22-)

F15.24 **Other stimulant dependence with stimulant-induced mood disorder**
Amphetamine or other stimulant use disorder, moderate, with amphetamine or other stimulant-induced bipolar or related disorder
Amphetamine or other stimulant use disorder, moderate, with amphetamine or other stimulant-induced depressive disorder
Amphetamine or other stimulant use disorder, severe, with amphetamine or other stimulant-induced bipolar or related disorder
Amphetamine or other stimulant use disorder, severe, with amphetamine or other stimulant-induced depressive disorder

F15.25 Other stimulant dependence with stimulant-induced **psychotic disorder**

- F15.250 Other stimulant dependence with stimulant-induced psychotic disorder with delusions
- F15.251 Other stimulant dependence with stimulant-induced psychotic disorder with **hallucinations**
- F15.259 Other stimulant dependence with stimulant-induced psychotic disorder, **unspecified**

F15.28 Other stimulant dependence with other stimulant-induced disorder

- F15.280 Other stimulant dependence with stimulant-induced **anxiety disorder**
- F15.281 Other stimulant dependence with stimulant-induced **sexual dysfunction**
- F15.282 Other stimulant dependence with stimulant-induced **sleep disorder**
- F15.288 Other stimulant dependence with **other** stimulant-induced disorder
  - Amphetamine or other stimulant use disorder, moderate, with amphetamine or other stimulant-induced obsessive-compulsive or related disorder
  - Amphetamine or other stimulant use disorder, severe, with amphetamine or other stimulant-induced obsessive-compulsive or related disorder

F15.29 Other stimulant dependence with **unspecified** stimulant-induced disorder

F15.9 Other stimulant use, **unspecified**

Excludes1 other stimulant abuse (F15.1-)
other stimulant dependence (F15.2-)

F15.90 Other stimulant use, **unspecified, uncomplicated**

F15.92 Other stimulant use, **unspecified with intoxication**

Excludes1 other stimulant use, unspecified with withdrawal (F15.93)

- F15.920 Other stimulant use, unspecified with intoxication, **uncomplicated**
- F15.921 Other stimulant use, unspecified with intoxication **delirium**
  - Amphetamine or other stimulant-induced delirium
- F15.922 Other stimulant use, unspecified with intoxication **with perceptual disturbance**
- F15.929 Other stimulant use, unspecified with intoxication, **unspecified**
  - Caffeine intoxication

F15.93 Other stimulant use, **unspecified with withdrawal**

Caffeine withdrawal

Excludes1 other stimulant use, unspecified with intoxication (F15.92-)

F15.94 Other stimulant use, **unspecified with** stimulant-induced **mood disorder**

- Amphetamine or other stimulant-induced bipolar or related disorder, without use disorder
- Amphetamine or other stimulant-induced depressive disorder, without use disorder

F15.95 Other stimulant use, **unspecified with** stimulant-induced **psychotic disorder**

- F15.950 Other stimulant use, unspecified with stimulant-induced psychotic disorder with delusions
- F15.951 Other stimulant use, unspecified with stimulant-induced psychotic disorder with **hallucinations**
- F15.959 Other stimulant use, unspecified with stimulant-induced psychotic disorder, **unspecified**
  - Amphetamine or other stimulant-induced psychotic disorder, without use disorder

F15.98 Other stimulant use, **unspecified** with other stimulant-induced disorder

- F15.980 Other stimulant use, unspecified with stimulant-induced **anxiety disorder**
  - Amphetamine or other stimulant-induced anxiety disorder, without use disorder
  - Caffeine-induced anxiety disorder, without use disorder
- F15.981 Other stimulant use, unspecified with stimulant-induced **sexual dysfunction**
  - Amphetamine or other stimulant-induced sexual dysfunction, without use disorder
- F15.982 Other stimulant use, unspecified with stimulant-induced **sleep disorder**
  - Amphetamine or other stimulant-induced sleep disorder, without use disorder
  - Caffeine-induced sleep disorder, without use disorder
- F15.988 Other stimulant use, unspecified with **other** stimulant-induced disorder
  - Amphetamine or other stimulant-induced obsessive-compulsive or related disorder, without use disorder

F15.99 Other stimulant use, unspecified with **unspecified** stimulant-induced disorder

F16 Hallucinogen related disorders

Includes ecstasy
PCP
phencyclidine

F16.1 Hallucinogen **abuse**

Excludes1 hallucinogen dependence (F16.2-)
hallucinogen use, unspecified (F16.9-)

F16.10 Hallucinogen abuse, **uncomplicated**

- Other hallucinogen use disorder, mild
- Phencyclidine use disorder, mild
- **Coding Clinic: 2018, Q4, P31**

F16.11 Hallucinogen abuse, **in remission**

- Other hallucinogen use disorder, mild, in early remission
- Other hallucinogen use disorder, mild, in sustained remission
- Phencyclidine use disorder, mild, in early remission
- Phencyclidine use disorder, mild, in sustained remission

F16.12 Hallucinogen abuse **with intoxication**

- F16.120 Hallucinogen abuse with intoxication, **uncomplicated**
- F16.121 Hallucinogen abuse with intoxication **with delirium**
- F16.122 Hallucinogen abuse with intoxication **with perceptual disturbance**
- F16.129 Hallucinogen abuse with intoxication, **unspecified**

F16.14 Hallucinogen abuse with hallucinogen-induced mood disorder
Other hallucinogen use disorder, mild, with other hallucinogen-induced bipolar or related disorder
Other hallucinogen use disorder, mild, with other hallucinogen-induced depressive disorder
Phencyclidine use disorder, mild, with phencyclidine-induced bipolar or related disorder
Phencyclidine use disorder, mild, with phencyclidine-induced depressive disorder

F16.15 Hallucinogen abuse with hallucinogen-induced psychotic disorder

F16.150 Hallucinogen abuse with hallucinogen-induced psychotic disorder with delusions

F16.151 Hallucinogen abuse with hallucinogen-induced psychotic disorder with hallucinations

F16.159 Hallucinogen abuse with hallucinogen-induced psychotic disorder, unspecified

F16.18 Hallucinogen abuse with other hallucinogen-induced disorder

F16.180 Hallucinogen abuse with hallucinogen-induced anxiety disorder

F16.183 Hallucinogen abuse with hallucinogen persisting perception disorder (flashbacks)

F16.188 Hallucinogen abuse with other hallucinogen-induced disorder

F16.19 Hallucinogen abuse with unspecified hallucinogen-induced disorder

F16.2 Hallucinogen dependence

Excludes1 hallucinogen abuse (F16.1-)
hallucinogen use, unspecified (F16.9-)

F16.20 Hallucinogen dependence, uncomplicated
Other hallucinogen use disorder, moderate
Other hallucinogen use disorder, severe
Phencyclidine use disorder, moderate
Phencyclidine use disorder, severe

F16.21 Hallucinogen dependence, in remission
Other hallucinogen use disorder, moderate, in early remission
Other hallucinogen use disorder, moderate, in sustained remission
Other hallucinogen use disorder, severe, in early remission
Other hallucinogen use disorder, severe, in sustained remission
Phencyclidine use disorder, moderate, in early remission
Phencyclidine use disorder, moderate, in sustained remission
Phencyclidine use disorder, severe, in early remission
Phencyclidine use disorder, severe, in sustained remission

F16.22 Hallucinogen dependence with intoxication

F16.220 Hallucinogen dependence with intoxication, uncomplicated

F16.221 Hallucinogen dependence with intoxication with delirium

F16.229 Hallucinogen dependence with intoxication, unspecified

F16.24 Hallucinogen dependence with hallucinogen-induced mood disorder
Other hallucinogen use disorder, moderate, with other hallucinogen-induced bipolar or related disorder
Other hallucinogen use disorder, moderate, with other hallucinogen-induced depressive disorder
Other hallucinogen use disorder, severe, with other hallucinogen-induced bipolar or related disorder
Other hallucinogen use disorder, severe, with other hallucinogen-induced depressive disorder
Phencyclidine use disorder, moderate, with phencyclidine-induced bipolar or related disorder
Phencyclidine use disorder, moderate, with phencyclidine-induced depressive disorder
Phencyclidine use disorder, severe, with phencyclidine-induced bipolar or related disorder
Phencyclidine use disorder, severe, with phencyclidine-induced depressive disorder

F16.25 Hallucinogen dependence with hallucinogen-induced psychotic disorder

F16.250 Hallucinogen dependence with hallucinogen-induced psychotic disorder with delusions

F16.251 Hallucinogen dependence with hallucinogen-induced psychotic disorder with hallucinations

F16.259 Hallucinogen dependence with hallucinogen-induced psychotic disorder, unspecified

F16.28 Hallucinogen dependence with other hallucinogen-induced disorder

F16.280 Hallucinogen dependence with hallucinogen-induced anxiety disorder

F16.283 Hallucinogen dependence with hallucinogen persisting perception disorder (flashbacks)

F16.288 Hallucinogen dependence with other hallucinogen-induced disorder

F16.29 Hallucinogen dependence with unspecified hallucinogen-induced disorder

F16.9 Hallucinogen use, unspecified

Excludes1 hallucinogen abuse (F16.1-)
hallucinogen dependence (F16.2-)

F16.90 Hallucinogen use, unspecified, uncomplicated

F16.92 Hallucinogen use, unspecified with intoxication

F16.920 Hallucinogen use, unspecified with intoxication, uncomplicated

F16.921 Hallucinogen use, unspecified with intoxication with delirium
Other hallucinogen intoxication delirium

F16.929 Hallucinogen use, unspecified with intoxication, unspecified

F16.94 Hallucinogen use, unspecified with hallucinogen-induced mood disorder
Other hallucinogen-induced bipolar or related disorder, without use disorder
Other hallucinogen-induced depressive disorder, without use disorder
Phencyclidine-induced bipolar or related disorder, without use disorder
Phencyclidine-induced depressive disorder, without use disorder

CHAPTER 5 (FØ1-F99)

● **F16.95** **Hallucinogen use, unspecified with hallucinogen-induced psychotic disorder**

F16.950 **Hallucinogen use, unspecified with hallucinogen-induced psychotic disorder with delusions**

F16.951 **Hallucinogen use, unspecified with hallucinogen-induced psychotic disorder with hallucinations**

F16.959 **Hallucinogen use, unspecified with hallucinogen-induced psychotic disorder, unspecified**
Other hallucinogen-induced psychotic disorder, without use disorder
Phencyclidine-induced psychotic disorder, without use disorder

● **F16.98** **Hallucinogen use, unspecified with other specified hallucinogen-induced disorder**

F16.980 **Hallucinogen use, unspecified with hallucinogen-induced anxiety disorder**
Other hallucinogen-induced anxiety disorder, without use disorder
Phencyclidine-induced anxiety disorder, without use disorder

F16.983 **Hallucinogen use, unspecified with hallucinogen persisting perception disorder (flashbacks)**

F16.988 **Hallucinogen use, unspecified with other hallucinogen-induced disorder**

F16.99 **Hallucinogen use, unspecified with unspecified hallucinogen-induced disorder**

● **F17 Nicotine dependence**

Excludes1 history of tobacco dependence (Z87.891)
tobacco use NOS (Z72.Ø)

Excludes2 tobacco use (smoking) during pregnancy, childbirth and the puerperium (O99.33-)
toxic effect of nicotine (T65.2-)

● **F17.2** **Nicotine dependence**

● **F17.2Ø** **Nicotine dependence, unspecified**

F17.2ØØ **Nicotine dependence, unspecified, uncomplicated**
Tobacco use disorder, mild
Tobacco use disorder, moderate
Tobacco use disorder, severe
Coding Clinic: 2Ø16, Q1, P37

F17.2Ø1 **Nicotine dependence, unspecified, in remission**
Tobacco use disorder, mild, in early remission
Tobacco use disorder, mild, in sustained remission
Tobacco use disorder, moderate, in early remission
Tobacco use disorder, moderate, in sustained remission
Tobacco use disorder, severe, in early remission
Tobacco use disorder, severe, in sustained remission

F17.2Ø3 **Nicotine dependence unspecified, with withdrawal**
Tobacco withdrawal

F17.2Ø8 **Nicotine dependence, unspecified, with other nicotine-induced disorders**

F17.2Ø9 **Nicotine dependence, unspecified, with unspecified nicotine-induced disorders**

● **F17.21** **Nicotine dependence, cigarettes**

F17.21Ø **Nicotine dependence, cigarettes, uncomplicated**
Coding Clinic: 2Ø17, Q2, P28-29

F17.211 **Nicotine dependence, cigarettes, in remission**
Tobacco use disorder, cigarettes, mild, in early remission
Tobacco use disorder, cigarettes, mild, in sustained remission
Tobacco use disorder, cigarettes, moderate, in early remission
Tobacco use disorder, cigarettes, moderate, in sustained remission
Tobacco use disorder, cigarettes, severe, in early remission
Tobacco use disorder, cigarettes, severe, in sustained remission

F17.213 **Nicotine dependence, cigarettes, with withdrawal**

F17.218 **Nicotine dependence, cigarettes, with other nicotine-induced disorders**

F17.219 **Nicotine dependence, cigarettes, with unspecified nicotine-induced disorders**

● **F17.22** **Nicotine dependence, chewing tobacco**

F17.22Ø **Nicotine dependence, chewing tobacco, uncomplicated**

F17.221 **Nicotine dependence, chewing tobacco, in remission**
Tobacco use disorder, chewing tobacco, mild, in early remission
Tobacco use disorder, chewing tobacco, mild, in sustained remission
Tobacco use disorder, chewing tobacco, moderate, in early remission
Tobacco use disorder, chewing tobacco, moderate, in sustained remission
Tobacco use disorder, chewing tobacco, severe, in early remission
Tobacco use disorder, chewing tobacco, severe, in sustained remission

F17.223 **Nicotine dependence, chewing tobacco, with withdrawal**

F17.228 **Nicotine dependence, chewing tobacco, with other nicotine-induced disorders**

F17.229 **Nicotine dependence, chewing tobacco, with unspecified nicotine-induced disorders**

● **F17.29** **Nicotine dependence, other tobacco product**

F17.29Ø **Nicotine dependence, other tobacco product, uncomplicated**
Coding Clinic: 2Ø17, Q2, P28-29

F17.291 **Nicotine dependence, other tobacco product, in remission**
Tobacco use disorder, other tobacco product, mild, in early remission
Tobacco use disorder, other tobacco product, mild, in sustained remission
Tobacco use disorder, other tobacco product, moderate, in early remission
Tobacco use disorder, other tobacco product, moderate, in sustained remission
Tobacco use disorder, other tobacco product, severe, in early remission
Tobacco use disorder, other tobacco product, severe, in sustained remission

F17.293 Nicotine dependence, other tobacco product, with **withdrawal**

F17.298 Nicotine dependence, other tobacco product, with **other nicotine-induced disorders**

F17.299 Nicotine dependence, other tobacco product, with **unspecified** nicotine-induced disorders

F18 Inhalant related disorders

Includes volatile solvents

F18.1 Inhalant abuse

Excludes1 inhalant dependence (F18.2-)
inhalant use, unspecified (F18.9-)

F18.10 Inhalant abuse, **uncomplicated**
Inhalant use disorder, mild

F18.11 Inhalant abuse, **in remission**
Inhalant use disorder, mild, in early remission
Inhalant use disorder, mild, in sustained remission

F18.12 Inhalant abuse with intoxication

F18.120 Inhalant abuse with intoxication, **uncomplicated**

F18.121 Inhalant abuse with intoxication **delirium**

F18.129 Inhalant abuse with intoxication, **unspecified**

F18.14 Inhalant abuse with inhalant-induced **mood disorder**
Inhalant use disorder, mild, with inhalant-induced depressive disorder

F18.15 Inhalant abuse with inhalant-induced psychotic disorder

F18.150 Inhalant abuse with inhalant-induced psychotic disorder **with delusions**

F18.151 Inhalant abuse with inhalant-induced psychotic disorder with **hallucinations**

F18.159 Inhalant abuse with inhalant-induced psychotic disorder, **unspecified**

F18.17 Inhalant abuse with inhalant-induced **dementia**
Inhalant use disorder, mild, with inhalant-induced major neurocognitive disorder

F18.18 Inhalant abuse with other inhalant-induced disorders

F18.180 Inhalant abuse with inhalant-induced **anxiety disorder**

F18.188 Inhalant abuse with **other** inhalant-induced disorder
Inhalant use disorder, mild, with inhalant-induced mild neurocognitive disorder

F18.19 Inhalant abuse with **unspecified** inhalant-induced disorder

F18.2 Inhalant dependence

Excludes1 inhalant abuse (F18.1-)
inhalant use, unspecified (F18.9-)

F18.20 Inhalant dependence, **uncomplicated**
Inhalant use disorder, moderate
Inhalant use disorder, severe

F18.21 Inhalant dependence, **in remission**
Inhalant use disorder, moderate, in early remission
Inhalant use disorder, moderate, in sustained remission
Inhalant use disorder, severe, in early remission
Inhalant use disorder, severe, in sustained remission

F18.22 Inhalant dependence with intoxication

F18.220 Inhalant dependence with intoxication, **uncomplicated**

F18.221 Inhalant dependence with intoxication **delirium**

F18.229 Inhalant dependence with intoxication, **unspecified**

F18.24 Inhalant dependence with inhalant-induced **mood disorder**
Inhalant use disorder, moderate, with inhalant-induced depressive disorder
Inhalant use disorder, severe, with inhalant-induced depressive disorder

F18.25 Inhalant dependence with inhalant-induced psychotic disorder

F18.250 Inhalant dependence with inhalant-induced psychotic disorder with **delusions**

F18.251 Inhalant dependence with inhalant-induced psychotic disorder with **hallucinations**

F18.259 Inhalant dependence with inhalant-induced psychotic disorder, **unspecified**

F18.27 Inhalant dependence with inhalant-induced **dementia**
Inhalant use disorder, moderate, with inhalant-induced major neurocognitive disorder
Inhalant use disorder, severe, with inhalant-induced major neurocognitive disorder

F18.28 Inhalant dependence with other inhalant-induced disorders

F18.280 Inhalant dependence with inhalant-induced **anxiety disorder**

F18.288 Inhalant dependence with **other** inhalant-induced disorder
Inhalant use disorder, moderate, with inhalant-induced mild neurocognitive disorder
Inhalant use disorder, severe, with inhalant-induced mild neurocognitive disorder

F18.29 Inhalant dependence with **unspecified** inhalant-induced disorder

F18.9 Inhalant use, unspecified

Excludes1 inhalant abuse (F18.1-)
inhalant dependence (F18.2-)

F18.90 Inhalant use, **unspecified, uncomplicated**

F18.92 Inhalant use, unspecified with intoxication

F18.920 Inhalant use, unspecified with intoxication, **uncomplicated**

F18.921 Inhalant use, unspecified with intoxication with **delirium**

F18.929 Inhalant use, unspecified with intoxication, **unspecified**

F18.94 Inhalant use, **unspecified** with inhalant-induced **mood disorder**
Inhalant-induced depressive disorder

F18.95 Inhalant use, unspecified with inhalant-induced psychotic disorder

F18.950 Inhalant use, unspecified with inhalant-induced psychotic disorder **with delusions**

F18.951 Inhalant use, unspecified with inhalant-induced psychotic disorder **with hallucinations**

F18.959 Inhalant use, unspecified with inhalant-induced psychotic disorder, **unspecified**

F18.97 **Inhalant use, unspecified with inhalant-induced persisting dementia**
Inhalant-induced major neurocognitive disorder

● F18.98 **Inhalant use, unspecified with other inhalant-induced disorders**

F18.980 **Inhalant use, unspecified with inhalant-induced anxiety disorder**

F18.988 **Inhalant use, unspecified with other inhalant-induced disorder**
Inhalant-induced mild neurocognitive disorder

F18.99 **Inhalant use, unspecified with unspecified inhalant-induced disorder**

● F19 **Other psychoactive substance related disorders**

Includes polysubstance drug use (indiscriminate drug use)

● F19.1 **Other psychoactive substance abuse**

Excludes1 other psychoactive substance dependence (F19.2-)
other psychoactive substance use, unspecified (F19.9-)

F19.10 **Other psychoactive substance abuse, uncomplicated**
Other (or unknown) substance use disorder, mild

F19.11 **Other psychoactive substance abuse, in remission**
Other (or unknown) substance use disorder, mild, in early remission
Other (or unknown) substance use disorder, mild, in sustained remission

● F19.12 **Other psychoactive substance abuse with intoxication**

F19.120 **Other psychoactive substance abuse with intoxication, uncomplicated**

F19.121 **Other psychoactive substance abuse with intoxication delirium**

F19.122 **Other psychoactive substance abuse with intoxication with perceptual disturbances**

F19.129 **Other psychoactive substance abuse with intoxication, unspecified**

F19.14 **Other psychoactive substance abuse with psychoactive substance-induced mood disorder**
Other (or unknown) substance use disorder, mild, with other (or unknown) substance-induced bipolar or related disorder
Other (or unknown) substance use disorder, mild, with other (or unknown) substance-induced depressive disorder

● F19.15 **Other psychoactive substance abuse with psychoactive substance-induced psychotic disorder**

F19.150 **Other psychoactive substance abuse with psychoactive substance-induced psychotic disorder with delusions**

F19.151 **Other psychoactive substance abuse with psychoactive substance-induced psychotic disorder with hallucinations**

F19.159 **Other psychoactive substance abuse with psychoactive substance-induced psychotic disorder, unspecified**

F19.16 **Other psychoactive substance abuse with psychoactive substance-induced persisting amnestic disorder**

F19.17 **Other psychoactive substance abuse with psychoactive substance-induced persisting dementia**
Other (or unknown) substance use disorder, mild, with other (or unknown) substance-induced major neurocognitive disorder

● F19.18 **Other psychoactive substance abuse with other psychoactive substance-induced disorders**

F19.180 **Other psychoactive substance abuse with psychoactive substance-induced anxiety disorder**

F19.181 **Other psychoactive substance abuse with psychoactive substance-induced sexual dysfunction**

F19.182 **Other psychoactive substance abuse with psychoactive substance-induced sleep disorder**

F19.188 **Other psychoactive substance abuse with other psychoactive substance-induced disorder**
Other (or unknown) substance use disorder, mild, with other (or unknown) substance-induced mild neurocognitive disorder
Other (or unknown) substance use disorder, mild, with other (or unknown) substance-induced obsessive-compulsive or related disorder

F19.19 **Other psychoactive substance abuse with unspecified psychoactive substance-induced disorder**

● F19.2 **Other psychoactive substance dependence**

Excludes1 other psychoactive substance abuse (F19.1-)
other psychoactive substance use, unspecified (F19.9-)

F19.20 **Other psychoactive substance dependence, uncomplicated**
Other (or unknown) substance use disorder, moderate
Other (or unknown) substance use disorder, severe

F19.21 **Other psychoactive substance dependence, in remission**
Other (or unknown) substance use disorder, moderate, in early remission
Other (or unknown) substance use disorder, moderate, in sustained remission
Other (or unknown) substance use disorder, severe, in early remission
Other (or unknown) substance use disorder, severe, in sustained remission

● F19.22 **Other psychoactive substance dependence with intoxication**

Excludes1 other psychoactive substance dependence with withdrawal (F19.23-)

F19.220 **Other psychoactive substance dependence with intoxication, uncomplicated**

F19.221 **Other psychoactive substance dependence with intoxication delirium**

F19.222 **Other psychoactive substance dependence with intoxication with perceptual disturbance**

F19.229 **Other psychoactive substance dependence with intoxication, unspecified**

CHAPTER 5 (F01-F99)

● F19.23 **Other psychoactive substance dependence with withdrawal**
Excludes1 other psychoactive substance dependence with intoxication (F19.22-)

F19.230 **Other psychoactive substance dependence with withdrawal, uncomplicated**

F19.231 **Other psychoactive substance dependence with withdrawal delirium**

F19.232 **Other psychoactive substance dependence with withdrawal with perceptual disturbance**

F19.239 **Other psychoactive substance dependence with withdrawal, unspecified**

F19.24 **Other psychoactive substance dependence with psychoactive substance-induced mood disorder**
Other (or unknown) substance use disorder, moderate, with other (or unknown) substance-induced bipolar or related disorder
Other (or unknown) substance use disorder, moderate, with other (or unknown) substance-induced depressive disorder
Other (or unknown) substance use disorder, severe, with other (or unknown) substance-induced bipolar or related disorder
Other (or unknown) substance use disorder, severe, with other (or unknown) substance-induced depressive disorder

● F19.25 **Other psychoactive substance dependence with psychoactive substance-induced psychotic disorder**

F19.250 **Other psychoactive substance dependence with psychoactive substance-induced psychotic disorder with delusions**

F19.251 **Other psychoactive substance dependence with psychoactive substance-induced psychotic disorder with hallucinations**

F19.259 **Other psychoactive substance dependence with psychoactive substance-induced psychotic disorder, unspecified**

F19.26 **Other psychoactive substance dependence with psychoactive substance-induced persisting amnestic disorder**

F19.27 **Other psychoactive substance dependence with psychoactive substance-induced persisting dementia**
Other (or unknown) substance use disorder, moderate, with other (or unknown) substance-induced major neurocognitive disorder
Other (or unknown) substance use disorder, severe, with other (or unknown) substance-induced major neurocognitive disorder

● F19.28 **Other psychoactive substance dependence with other psychoactive substance-induced disorders**

F19.280 **Other psychoactive substance dependence with psychoactive substance-induced anxiety disorder**

F19.281 **Other psychoactive substance dependence with psychoactive substance-induced sexual dysfunction**

F19.282 **Other psychoactive substance dependence with psychoactive substance-induced sleep disorder**

F19.288 **Other psychoactive substance dependence with other psychoactive substance-induced disorder**
Other (or unknown) substance use disorder, moderate, with other (or unknown) substance-induced mild neurocognitive disorder
Other (or unknown) substance use disorder, severe, with other (or unknown) substance-induced mild neurocognitive disorder
Other (or unknown) substance use disorder, moderate, with other (or unknown) substance-induced obsessive-compulsive or related disorder
Other (or unknown) substance use disorder, severe, with other (or unknown) substance-induced obsessive-compulsive or related disorder

F19.29 **Other psychoactive substance dependence with unspecified psychoactive substance-induced disorder**

● F19.9 **Other psychoactive substance use, unspecified**
Excludes1 other psychoactive substance abuse (F19.1-)
other psychoactive substance dependence (F19.2-)

F19.90 **Other psychoactive substance use, unspecified, uncomplicated**

● F19.92 **Other psychoactive substance use, unspecified with intoxication**
Excludes1 other psychoactive substance use, unspecified with withdrawal (F19.93)

F19.920 **Other psychoactive substance use, unspecified with intoxication, uncomplicated**

F19.921 **Other psychoactive substance use, unspecified with intoxication with delirium**
Other (or unknown) substance-induced delirium

F19.922 **Other psychoactive substance use, unspecified with intoxication with perceptual disturbance**

F19.929 **Other psychoactive substance use, unspecified with intoxication, unspecified**

● F19.93 **Other psychoactive substance use, unspecified with withdrawal**
Excludes1 other psychoactive substance use, unspecified with intoxication (F19.92-)

F19.930 **Other psychoactive substance use, unspecified with withdrawal, uncomplicated**

F19.931 **Other psychoactive substance use, unspecified with withdrawal delirium**

F19.932 **Other psychoactive substance use, unspecified with withdrawal with perceptual disturbance**

F19.939 **Other psychoactive substance use, unspecified with withdrawal, unspecified**

F19.94 Other psychoactive substance use, unspecified with psychoactive substance-induced mood disorder
Other (or unknown) substance-induced bipolar or related disorder, without use disorder
Other (or unknown) substance-induced depressive disorder, without use disorder

F19.95 Other psychoactive substance use, unspecified with psychoactive substance-induced psychotic disorder

F19.950 Other psychoactive substance use, unspecified with psychoactive substance-induced psychotic disorder with delusions

F19.951 Other psychoactive substance use, unspecified with psychoactive substance-induced psychotic disorder with hallucinations

F19.959 Other psychoactive substance use, unspecified with psychoactive substance-induced psychotic disorder, unspecified
Other or unknown substance-induced psychotic disorder, without use disorder

F19.96 Other psychoactive substance use, unspecified with psychoactive substance-induced persisting amnestic disorder

F19.97 Other psychoactive substance use, unspecified with psychoactive substance-induced persisting dementia
Other (or unknown) substance-induced major neurocognitive disorder, without use disorder

F19.98 Other psychoactive substance use, unspecified with other psychoactive substance-induced disorders

F19.980 Other psychoactive substance use, unspecified with psychoactive substance-induced anxiety disorder
Other (or unknown) substance-induced anxiety disorder, without use disorder

F19.981 Other psychoactive substance use, unspecified with psychoactive substance-induced sexual dysfunction
Other (or unknown) substance-induced sexual dysfunction, without use disorder

F19.982 Other psychoactive substance use, unspecified with psychoactive substance-induced sleep disorder
Other (or unknown) substance-induced sleep disorder, without use disorder

F19.988 Other psychoactive substance use, unspecified with other psychoactive substance-induced disorder
Other (or unknown) substance-induced mild neurocognitive disorder, without use disorder
Other (or unknown) substance-induced obsessive-compulsive or related disorder, without use disorder

F19.99 Other psychoactive substance use, unspecified with unspecified psychoactive substance-induced disorder

SCHIZOPHRENIA, SCHIZOTYPAL, DELUSIONAL, AND OTHER NON-MOOD PSYCHOTIC DISORDERS (F20-F29)

F20 Schizophrenia
Personality disorders characterized by multiple mental and behavioral irregularities (may exhibit disorganized thinking, delusions, and auditory hallucinations)

Excludes1 brief psychotic disorder (F23)
cyclic schizophrenia (F25.0)
mood [affective] disorders with psychotic symptoms (F30.2, F31.2, F31.5, F31.64, F32.3, F33.3)
schizoaffective disorder (F25.-)
schizophrenic reaction NOS (F23)

Excludes2 schizophrenic reaction in:
alcoholism (F10.15-, F10.25-, F10.95-)
brain disease (F06.2)
epilepsy (F06.2)
psychoactive drug use (F11-F19 with .15, .25, .95)
schizotypal disorder (F21)

Coding Clinic: 2019, Q2, P32

F20.0 Paranoid schizophrenia
Paraphrenic schizophrenia
Excludes1 involutional paranoid state (F22)
paranoia (F22)

F20.1 Disorganized schizophrenia
Hebephrenic schizophrenia
Hebephrenia

F20.2 Catatonic schizophrenia
Schizophrenic catalepsy
Schizophrenic catatonia
Schizophrenic flexibilitas cerea
Excludes1 catatonic stupor (R40.1)

F20.3 Undifferentiated schizophrenia
Atypical schizophrenia
Excludes1 acute schizophrenia-like psychotic disorder (F23)
Excludes2 post-schizophrenic depression (F32.89)

F20.5 Residual schizophrenia
Restzustand (schizophrenic)
Schizophrenic residual state

F20.8 Other schizophrenia

F20.81 Schizophreniform disorder
Schizophreniform psychosis NOS

F20.89 Other schizophrenia
Cenesthopathic schizophrenia
Simple schizophrenia

F20.9 Schizophrenia, unspecified
Coding Clinic: 2019, Q2, P32

F21 Schizotypal disorder
Personality disorder characterized by need for social isolation, odd behavior and thinking, and often unconventional beliefs
Borderline schizophrenia
Latent schizophrenia
Latent schizophrenic reaction
Prepsychotic schizophrenia
Prodromal schizophrenia
Pseudoneurotic schizophrenia
Pseudopsychopathic schizophrenia
Schizotypal personality disorder
Excludes2 Asperger's syndrome (F84.5)
schizoid personality disorder (F60.1)

F22 Delusional disorders
Delusional dysmorphophobia
Involutional paranoid state
Paranoia
Paranoia querulans
Paranoid psychosis
Paranoid state
Paraphrenia (late)
Sensitiver Beziehungswahn
Excludes1 mood [affective] disorders with psychotic symptoms (F30.2, F31.2, F31.5, F31.64, F32.3, F33.3)
paranoid schizophrenia (F20.0)
Excludes2 paranoid personality disorder (F60.0)
paranoid psychosis, psychogenic (F23)
paranoid reaction (F23)

F23 Brief psychotic disorder
Paranoid reaction
Psychogenic paranoid psychosis
Excludes2 mood [affective] disorders with psychotic symptoms (F30.2, F31.2, F31.5, F31.64, F32.3, F33.3)
Coding Clinic: 2019, Q2, P32

F24 Shared psychotic disorder
Folie à deux
Induced paranoid disorder
Induced psychotic disorder

F25 Schizoaffective disorders
Mental disorder exhibiting major depressive episode, manic episode, or mixed episode occurs with symptoms of schizophrenia, and mood disorder
Excludes1 mood [affective] disorders with psychotic symptoms (F30.2, F31.2, F31.5, F31.64, F32.3, F33.3)
schizophrenia (F20.-)

F25.0 Schizoaffective disorder, bipolar type
Cyclic schizophrenia
Schizoaffective disorder, manic type
Schizoaffective disorder, mixed type
Schizoaffective psychosis, bipolar type

F25.1 Schizoaffective disorder, depressive type
Schizoaffective psychosis, depressive type

F25.8 Other schizoaffective disorders

F25.9 Schizoaffective disorder, unspecified
Schizoaffective psychosis NOS

F28 Other psychotic disorder not due to a substance or known physiological condition
Chronic hallucinatory psychosis
Other specified schizophrenia spectrum and other psychotic disorder

F29 Unspecified psychosis not due to a substance or known physiological condition
Psychosis NOS
Unspecified schizophrenia spectrum and other psychotic disorder
Excludes1 mental disorder NOS (F99)
unspecified mental disorder due to known physiological condition (F09)

MOOD [AFFECTIVE] DISORDERS (F30-F39)

F30 Manic episode
Elevated, expansive, or irritable mood
Includes bipolar disorder, single manic episode
mixed affective episode
Excludes1 bipolar disorder (F31.-)
major depressive disorder, single episode (F32.-)
major depressive disorder, recurrent (F33.-)

F30.1 Manic episode without psychotic symptoms

F30.10 Manic episode without psychotic symptoms, unspecified

F30.11 Manic episode without psychotic symptoms, mild

F30.12 Manic episode without psychotic symptoms, moderate

F30.13 Manic episode, severe, without psychotic symptoms

F30.2 Manic episode, severe with psychotic symptoms
Manic stupor
Mania with mood-congruent psychotic symptoms
Mania with mood-incongruent psychotic symptoms

F30.3 Manic episode in partial remission

F30.4 Manic episode in full remission

F30.8 Other manic episodes
Abnormality of mood resembling mania but less intense
Hypomania

F30.9 Manic episode, unspecified
Mania NOS

F31 Bipolar disorder
Mood disorders with history of manic, mixed, or hypomanic episodes
Includes bipolar I disorder
bipolar type I disorder
manic-depressive illness
manic-depressive psychosis
manic-depressive reaction
Excludes1 bipolar disorder, single manic episode (F30.-)
major depressive disorder, single episode (F32.-)
major depressive disorder, recurrent (F33.-)
Excludes2 cyclothymia (F34.0)

F31.0 Bipolar disorder, current episode hypomanic

F31.1 Bipolar disorder, current episode manic without psychotic features

F31.10 Bipolar disorder, current episode manic without psychotic features, unspecified

F31.11 Bipolar disorder, current episode manic without psychotic features, mild

F31.12 Bipolar disorder, current episode manic without psychotic features, moderate

F31.13 Bipolar disorder, current episode manic without psychotic features, severe

F31.2 Bipolar disorder, current episode manic severe with psychotic features
Bipolar disorder, current episode manic with mood-congruent psychotic symptoms
Bipolar disorder, current episode manic with mood-incongruent psychotic symptoms
Bipolar I disorder, current or most recent episode manic with psychotic features

F31.3 Bipolar disorder, current episode depressed, mild or moderate severity

F31.30 Bipolar disorder, current episode depressed, mild or moderate severity, unspecified

F31.31 Bipolar disorder, current episode depressed, mild

F31.32 Bipolar disorder, current episode depressed, moderate

F31.4 Bipolar disorder, current episode depressed, severe, without psychotic features

F31.5 Bipolar disorder, current episode depressed, severe, with psychotic features
Bipolar disorder, current episode depressed with mood-incongruent psychotic symptoms
Bipolar disorder, current episode depressed with mood-congruent psychotic symptoms
Bipolar I disorder, current or most recent episode depressed, with psychotic features

F31.6 Bipolar disorder, current episode mixed

F31.60 Bipolar disorder, current episode mixed, unspecified

F31.61 Bipolar disorder, current episode mixed, mild

F31.62 Bipolar disorder, current episode mixed, moderate

F31.63 **Bipolar disorder, current episode mixed, severe, without psychotic features**

F31.64 **Bipolar disorder, current episode mixed, severe, with psychotic features**
Bipolar disorder, current episode mixed with mood-congruent psychotic symptoms
Bipolar disorder, current episode mixed with mood-incongruent psychotic symptoms

F31.7 **Bipolar disorder, currently in remission**

F31.70 **Bipolar disorder, currently in remission, most recent episode unspecified**

F31.71 **Bipolar disorder, in partial remission, most recent episode hypomanic**

F31.72 **Bipolar disorder, in full remission, most recent episode hypomanic**

F31.73 **Bipolar disorder, in partial remission, most recent episode manic**

F31.74 **Bipolar disorder, in full remission, most recent episode manic**

F31.75 **Bipolar disorder, in partial remission, most recent episode depressed**

F31.76 **Bipolar disorder, in full remission, most recent episode depressed**

F31.77 **Bipolar disorder, in partial remission, most recent episode mixed**

F31.78 **Bipolar disorder, in full remission, most recent episode mixed**

F31.8 **Other bipolar disorders**

F31.81 **Bipolar II disorder**
Bipolar disorder, type 2

F31.89 **Other bipolar disorder**
Recurrent manic episodes NOS

F31.9 **Bipolar disorder, unspecified**
Manic depression

F32 **Major depressive disorder, single episode**

Includes single episode of agitated depression
single episode of depressive reaction
single episode of major depression
single episode of psychogenic depression
single episode of reactive depression
single episode of vital depression

Excludes1 bipolar disorder (F31.-)
manic episode (F3Ø.-)
recurrent depressive disorder (F33.-)

Excludes2 adjustment disorder (F43.2)

F32.Ø **Major depressive disorder, single episode, mild**

F32.1 **Major depressive disorder, single episode, moderate**

F32.2 **Major depressive disorder, single episode, severe without psychotic features**

F32.3 **Major depressive disorder, single episode, severe with psychotic features**
Single episode of major depression with mood-congruent psychotic symptoms
Single episode of major depression with mood-incongruent psychotic symptoms
Single episode of major depression with psychotic symptoms
Single episode of psychogenic depressive psychosis
Single episode of psychotic depression
Single episode of reactive depressive psychosis

F32.4 **Major depressive disorder, single episode, in partial remission**

F32.5 **Major depressive disorder, single episode, in full remission**

F32.8 **Other depressive episodes**

F32.81 **Premenstrual dysphoric disorder** ♀

Excludes1 premenstrual tension syndrome (N94.3)

Coding Clinic: 2Ø16, Q4, P14

F32.89 **Other specified depressive episodes**
Atypical depression
Post-schizophrenic depression
Single episode of 'masked' depression NOS
Coding Clinic: 2Ø16, Q4, P14

F32.9 **Major depressive disorder, single episode, unspecified**
Depression NOS
Depressive disorder NOS
Major depression NOS

F33 **Major depressive disorder, recurrent**

Includes recurrent episodes of depressive reaction
recurrent episodes of endogenous depression
recurrent episodes of major depression
recurrent episodes of psychogenic depression
recurrent episodes of reactive depression
recurrent episodes of seasonal depressive disorder
recurrent episodes of vital depression

Excludes1 bipolar disorder (F31.-)
manic episode (F3Ø.-)

F33.Ø **Major depressive disorder, recurrent, mild**

F33.1 **Major depressive disorder, recurrent, moderate**

F33.2 **Major depressive disorder, recurrent severe without psychotic features**

F33.3 **Major depressive disorder, recurrent, severe with psychotic symptoms**
Endogenous depression with psychotic symptoms
Major depressive disorder, recurrent, with psychotic features
Recurrent severe episodes of major depression with mood-congruent psychotic symptoms
Recurrent severe episodes of major depression with mood-incongruent psychotic symptoms
Recurrent severe episodes of major depression with psychotic symptoms
Recurrent severe episodes of psychogenic depressive psychosis
Recurrent severe episodes of psychotic depression
Recurrent severe episodes of reactive depressive psychosis

F33.4 **Major depressive disorder, recurrent, in remission**

F33.4Ø **Major depressive disorder, recurrent, in remission, unspecified**

F33.41 **Major depressive disorder, recurrent, in partial remission**

F33.42 **Major depressive disorder, recurrent, in full remission**

F33.8 **Other recurrent depressive disorders**
Recurrent brief depressive episodes

F33.9 **Major depressive disorder, recurrent, unspecified**
Monopolar depression NOS

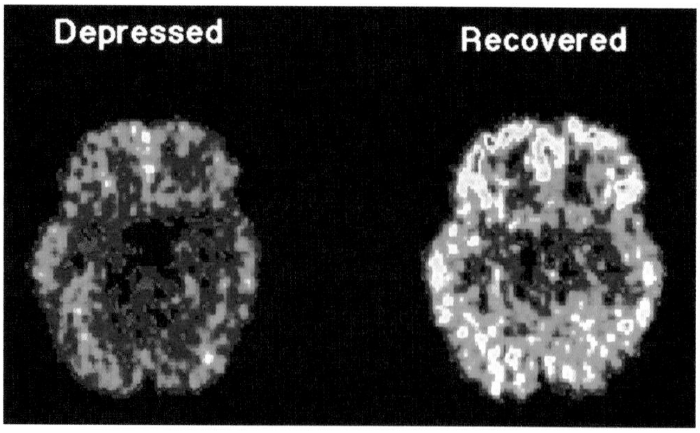

Figure 5-1 PET scan of depressed individual's brain before and after recovery. (From Fortinash KM: Psychiatric Mental Health Nursing, ed 4, St. Louis, Mosby, 2008)

F34 Persistent mood [affective] disorders

F34.0 Cyclothymic disorder
Affective personality disorder
Cycloid personality
Cyclothymia
Cyclothymic personality

F34.1 Dysthymic disorder
Depressive neurosis
Depressive personality disorder
Dysthymia
Neurotic depression
Persistent anxiety depression
Persistent depressive disorder
Excludes2 anxiety depression (mild or not persistent) (F41.8)

F34.8 Other persistent mood [affective] disorders

F34.81 Disruptive mood dysregulation disorder
Coding Clinic: 2016, Q4, P14

F34.89 Other specified persistent mood disorders
Coding Clinic: 2016, Q4, P14

F34.9 Persistent mood [affective] disorder, unspecified

F39 Unspecified mood [affective] disorder
Affective psychosis NOS

ANXIETY, DISSOCIATIVE, STRESS-RELATED, SOMATOFORM AND OTHER NONPSYCHOTIC MENTAL DISORDERS (F40-F48)

F40 Phobic anxiety disorders
Irrational fear with avoidance of the feared subject, activity, or situation even though the individual knows that the reaction is excessive

F40.0 Agoraphobia
Intense, irrational fear of open spaces

F40.00 Agoraphobia, unspecified

F40.01 Agoraphobia with panic disorder
Panic disorder with agoraphobia
Excludes1 panic disorder without agoraphobia (F41.0)

F40.02 Agoraphobia without panic disorder

F40.1 Social phobias
Anthropophobia
Social anxiety disorder
Social anxiety disorder of childhood
Social neurosis

F40.10 Social phobia, unspecified

F40.11 Social phobia, generalized

F40.2 Specific (isolated) phobias
Excludes2 dysmorphophobia (nondelusional) (F45.22)
nosophobia (F45.22)

F40.21 Animal type phobia

F40.210 Arachnophobia
Fear of spiders

F40.218 Other animal type phobia

F40.22 Natural environment type phobia

F40.220 Fear of thunderstorms

F40.228 Other natural environment type phobia

F40.23 Blood, injection, injury type phobia

F40.230 Fear of blood

F40.231 Fear of injections and transfusions

F40.232 Fear of other medical care

F40.233 Fear of injury

F40.24 Situational type phobia

F40.240 Claustrophobia
Fear of closed spaces

F40.241 Acrophobia
Fear of heights

F40.242 Fear of bridges

F40.243 Fear of flying

F40.248 Other situational type phobia

F40.29 Other specified phobia

F40.290 Androphobia
Fear of men

F40.291 Gynephobia
Fear of women

F40.298 Other specified phobia

F40.8 Other phobic anxiety disorders
Phobic anxiety disorder of childhood

F40.9 Phobic anxiety disorder, unspecified
Phobia NOS
Phobic state NOS

F41 Other anxiety disorders
Excludes2 anxiety in:
acute stress reaction (F43.0)
transient adjustment reaction (F43.2)
neurasthenia (F48.8)
psychophysiologic disorders (F45.-)
separation anxiety (F93.0)

F41.0 Panic disorder [episodic paroxysmal anxiety]
Panic attack
Panic state
Excludes1 panic disorder with agoraphobia (F40.01)

F41.1 Generalized anxiety disorder
Anxiety neurosis
Anxiety reaction
Anxiety state
Overanxious disorder
Excludes2 neurasthenia (F48.8)

F41.3 Other mixed anxiety disorders

F41.8 Other specified anxiety disorders
Anxiety depression (mild or not persistent)
Anxiety hysteria
Mixed anxiety and depressive disorder

F41.9 Anxiety disorder, unspecified
Anxiety NOS

F42 Obsessive-compulsive disorder
Anxiety disorder with recurrent obsessions or compulsions
Excludes2 obsessive-compulsive personality (disorder) (F60.5)
obsessive-compulsive symptoms occurring in depression (F32-F33)
obsessive-compulsive symptoms occurring in schizophrenia (F20.-)

F42.2 Mixed obsessional thoughts and acts
Coding Clinic: 2016, Q4, P15

F42.3 Hoarding disorder
Coding Clinic: 2016, Q4, P14-15

F42.4 Excoriation (skin-picking) disorder
Excludes1 factitial dermatitis (L98.1)
other specified behavioral and emotional disorders with onset usually occurring in early childhood and adolescence (F98.8)
Coding Clinic: 2016, Q4, P14-15

F42.8 Other obsessive-compulsive disorder
Anancastic neurosis
Obsessive-compulsive neurosis
Coding Clinic: 2016, Q4, P15

F42.9 Obsessive-compulsive disorder, unspecified
Coding Clinic: 2016, Q4, P15

F43 Reaction to severe stress and adjustment disorders

F43.0 Acute stress reaction
Acute crisis reaction
Acute reaction to stress
Combat and operational stress reaction
Combat fatigue
Crisis state
Psychic shock

CHAPTER 5 (F01-F99)

● **F43.1 Post-traumatic stress disorder (PTSD)**
Traumatic neurosis
F43.10 Post-traumatic stress disorder, unspecified
F43.11 Post-traumatic stress disorder, acute
F43.12 Post-traumatic stress disorder, chronic

● **F43.2 Adjustment disorders**
Culture shock
Grief reaction
Hospitalism in children
Excludes2 separation anxiety disorder of childhood (F93.Ø)
F43.2Ø Adjustment disorder, unspecified
F43.21 Adjustment disorder with depressed mood
F43.22 Adjustment disorder with anxiety
F43.23 Adjustment disorder with mixed anxiety and depressed mood
F43.24 Adjustment disorder with disturbance of conduct
F43.25 Adjustment disorder with mixed disturbance of emotions and conduct
F43.29 Adjustment disorder with other symptoms

F43.8 Other reactions to severe stress
Other specified trauma and stressor-related disorder

F43.9 Reaction to severe stress, unspecified
Trauma and stressor-related disorder, NOS

● **F44 Dissociative and conversion disorders**
Includes conversion hysteria
conversion reaction
hysteria
hysterical psychosis
Excludes2 malingering [conscious simulation] (Z76.5)

F44.Ø Dissociative amnesia
Sudden loss of memory for personal information
Excludes1 amnesia NOS (R41.3)
anterograde amnesia (R41.1)
dissociative amnesia with dissociative fugue (F44.1)
retrograde amnesia (R41.2)
Excludes2 alcohol or other psychoactive substance-induced amnestic disorder (F1Ø, F13, F19 with .26, .96)
amnestic disorder due to known physiological condition (FØ4)
postictal amnesia in epilepsy (G4Ø.-)

F44.1 Dissociative fugue
Characterized by episode of sudden, unexpected travel with amnesia for past and partial to total confusion about identity or assumption of new identity
Dissociative amnesia with dissociative fugue
Excludes2 postictal fugue in epilepsy (G4Ø.-)

F44.2 Dissociative stupor
Profound diminution or absence of voluntary movement and responsiveness to external stimuli
Excludes1 catatonic stupor (R4Ø.1)
stupor NOS (R4Ø.1)
Excludes2 catatonic disorder due to known physiological condition (FØ6.1)
depressive stupor (F32, F33)
manic stupor (F3Ø, F31)

F44.4 Conversion disorder with motor symptom or deficit
Conversion disorder with abnormal movement
Conversion disorder with speech symptoms
Conversion disorder with swallowing symptoms
Conversion disorder with weakness/paralysis
Dissociative motor disorders
Psychogenic aphonia
Psychogenic dysphonia

F44.5 Conversion disorder with seizures or convulsions
Conversion disorder with attacks or seizures
Dissociative convulsions
Coding Clinic: 2019, Q1, P19

F44.6 Conversion disorder with sensory symptom or deficit
Conversion disorder with anesthesia or sensory loss
Conversion disorder with special sensory symptoms
Dissociative anesthesia and sensory loss
Psychogenic deafness

F44.7 Conversion disorder with mixed symptom presentation

● **F44.8 Other dissociative and conversion disorders**
F44.81 Dissociative identity disorder
Multiple personality disorder
F44.89 Other dissociative and conversion disorders
Ganser's syndrome
Psychogenic confusion
Psychogenic twilight state
Trance and possession disorders

F44.9 Dissociative and conversion disorder, unspecified
Dissociative disorder NOS

OGCR Section I.C.5.a.

Pain disorders related to psychological factors

Assign code F45.41, for pain that is exclusively related to psychological disorders. As indicated by the Excludes 1 note under category G89, a code from category G89 should not be assigned with code F45.41

Code F45.42, Pain disorders with related psychological factors, should be used with a code from category G89, Pain, not elsewhere classified, if there is documentation of a psychological component for a patient with acute or chronic pain.

See Section I.C.6. Pain

● **F45 Somatoform disorders**
Mental disorders characterized by symptoms suggesting general medical condition
Excludes2 dissociative and conversion disorders (F44.-)
factitious disorders (F68.1-, F68.A)
hair-plucking (F63.3)
lalling (F8Ø.Ø)
lisping (F8Ø.Ø)
malingering [conscious simulation] (Z76.5)
nail-biting (F98.8)
psychological or behavioral factors associated with disorders or diseases classified elsewhere (F54)
sexual dysfunction, not due to a substance or known physiological condition (F52.-)
thumb-sucking (F98.8)
tic disorders (in childhood and adolescence) (F95.-)
Tourette's syndrome (F95.2)
trichotillomania (F63.3)

F45.Ø Somatization disorder
Briquet's disorder
Multiple psychosomatic disorder

F45.1 Undifferentiated somatoform disorder
Somatic symptom disorder
Undifferentiated psychosomatic disorder

● **F45.2 Hypochondriacal disorders**
Persistent, unrealistic preoccupation with possibility of having serious disease
Excludes2 delusional dysmorphophobia (F22)
fixed delusions about bodily functions or shape (F22)
F45.2Ø Hypochondriacal disorder, unspecified
F45.21 Hypochondriasis
Hypochondriacal neurosis
Illness anxiety disorder
F45.22 Body dysmorphic disorder
Dysmorphophobia (nondelusional)
Nosophobia
F45.29 Other hypochondriacal disorders

CHAPTER 5 (FØ1-F99)

F45.4 Pain disorders related to psychological factors
Excludes1 pain NOS (R52)
F45.41 Pain disorder exclusively related to psychological factors
Somatoform pain disorder (persistent)
F45.42 Pain disorder with related psychological factors
Code also associated acute or chronic pain (G89.-)
F45.8 Other somatoform disorders
Psychogenic dysmenorrhea
Psychogenic dysphagia, including 'globus hystericus'
Psychogenic pruritus
Psychogenic torticollis
Somatoform autonomic dysfunction
Teeth grinding
Excludes1 sleep related teeth grinding (G47.63)
Coding Clinic: 2016, Q4, P118
F45.9 Somatoform disorder, unspecified
Psychosomatic disorder NOS

F48 Other nonpsychotic mental disorders
F48.1 Depersonalization-derealization syndrome
F48.2 Pseudobulbar affect
Involuntary emotional expression disorder
Code first underlying cause, if known, such as:
amyotrophic lateral sclerosis (G12.21)
multiple sclerosis (G35)
sequelae of cerebrovascular disease (I69.-)
sequelae of traumatic intracranial injury (S06.-)
F48.8 Other specified nonpsychotic mental disorders
Dhat syndrome
Neurasthenia
Occupational neurosis, including writer's cramp
Psychasthenia
Psychasthenic neurosis
Psychogenic syncope
F48.9 Nonpsychotic mental disorder, unspecified
Neurosis NOS

BEHAVIORAL SYNDROMES ASSOCIATED WITH PHYSIOLOGICAL DISTURBANCES AND PHYSICAL FACTORS (F50-F59)

F50 Eating disorders
Excludes1 anorexia NOS (R63.0)
feeding difficulties (R63.3)
feeding problems of newborn (P92.-)
polyphagia (R63.2)
Excludes2 feeding disorder in infancy or childhood (F98.2-)
F50.0 Anorexia nervosa
Excludes1 loss of appetite (R63.0)
psychogenic loss of appetite (F50.89)
F50.00 Anorexia nervosa, unspecified
F50.01 Anorexia nervosa, restricting type
F50.02 Anorexia nervosa, binge eating/purging type
Excludes1 bulimia nervosa (F50.2)
F50.2 Bulimia nervosa
Bulimia NOS
Hyperorexia nervosa
Excludes1 anorexia nervosa, binge eating/purging type (F50.02)
F50.8 Other eating disorders
Excludes2 pica of infancy and childhood (F98.3)
F50.81 Binge eating disorder
Coding Clinic: 2016, Q4, P15
F50.82 Avoidant/restrictive food intake disorder
F50.89 Other specified eating disorder
Pica in adults
Psychogenic loss of appetite
Coding Clinic: 2016, Q4, P16
F50.9 Eating disorder, unspecified
Atypical anorexia nervosa
Atypical bulimia nervosa
Feeding or eating disorder, unspecified
Other specified feeding disorder

F51 Sleep disorders not due to a substance or known physiological condition
Excludes2 organic sleep disorders (G47.-)
F51.0 Insomnia not due to a substance or known physiological condition
Excludes2 alcohol related insomnia (F10.182, F10.282, F10.982)
drug-related insomnia (F11.182, F11.282, F11.982, F13.182, F13.282, F13.982, F14.182, F14.282, F14.982, F15.182, F15.282, F15.982, F19.182, F19.282, F19.982)
insomnia NOS (G47.0-)
insomnia due to known physiological condition (G47.0-)
organic insomnia (G47.0-)
sleep deprivation (Z72.820)
F51.01 Primary insomnia
Idiopathic insomnia
F51.02 Adjustment insomnia
F51.03 Paradoxical insomnia
F51.04 Psychophysiologic insomnia
F51.05 Insomnia due to other mental disorder
Code also associated mental disorder
F51.09 Other insomnia not due to a substance or known physiological condition
F51.1 Hypersomnia not due to a substance or known physiological condition
Hypersomnia: Excessive sleeping/sleepiness
Excludes2 alcohol related hypersomnia (F10.182, F10.282, F10.982)
drug-related hypersomnia (F11.182, F11.282, F11.982, F13.182, F13.282, F13.982, F14.182, F14.282, F14.982, F15.182, F15.282, F15.982, F19.182, F19.282, F19.982)
hypersomnia NOS (G47.10)
hypersomnia due to known physiological condition (G47.10)
idiopathic hypersomnia (G47.11, G47.12)
narcolepsy (G47.4-)
F51.11 Primary hypersomnia
F51.12 Insufficient sleep syndrome
Excludes1 sleep deprivation (Z72.820)
F51.13 Hypersomnia due to other mental disorder
Code also associated mental disorder
F51.19 Other hypersomnia not due to a substance or known physiological condition
F51.3 Sleepwalking [somnambulism]
Non-rapid eye movement sleep arousal disorders, sleepwalking type
F51.4 Sleep terrors [night terrors]
Non-rapid eye movement sleep arousal disorders, sleep terror type
F51.5 Nightmare disorder
Dream anxiety disorder
F51.8 Other sleep disorders not due to a substance or known physiological condition
F51.9 Sleep disorder not due to a substance or known physiological condition, unspecified
Emotional sleep disorder NOS

● F52 **Sexual dysfunction not due to a substance or known physiological condition**
Excludes2 Dhat syndrome (F48.8)

F52.Ø **Hypoactive sexual desire disorder**
Total loss of feeling of sexual pleasure
Lack or loss of sexual desire
Male hypoactive sexual desire disorder
Sexual anhedonia
Excludes1 decreased libido (R68.82)

F52.1 **Sexual aversion disorder**
Sexual aversion and lack of sexual enjoyment

● F52.2 **Sexual arousal disorders**
Failure of genital response

F52.21 **Male erectile disorder** ♂
Erectile disorder
Psychogenic impotence
Excludes1 impotence of organic origin (N52.-)
impotence NOS (N52.-)

F52.22 **Female sexual arousal disorder** ♀
Female sexual interest/arousal disorder

● F52.3 **Orgasmic disorder**
Inhibited orgasm
Psychogenic anorgasmy

F52.31 **Female orgasmic disorder** ♀

F52.32 **Male orgasmic disorder** ♂
Delayed ejaculation

F52.4 **Premature ejaculation** ♂

F52.5 **Vaginismus not due to a substance or known physiological condition** ♀
Psychogenic vaginismus
Excludes2 vaginismus (due to a known physiological condition) (N94.2)

F52.6 **Dyspareunia not due to a substance or known physiological condition**
Dyspareunia: Difficult or painful sexual intercourse
Genito-pelvic pain penetration disorder
Psychogenic dyspareunia
Excludes2 dyspareunia (due to a known physiological condition) (N94.1-)

F52.8 **Other sexual dysfunction not due to a substance or known physiological condition**
Excessive sexual drive
Nymphomania
Satyriasis

F52.9 **Unspecified sexual dysfunction not due to a substance or known physiological condition**
Sexual dysfunction NOS

● F53 **Mental and behavioral disorders associated with the puerperium, not elsewhere classified**
Acute mental illness with sudden onset following childbirth with symptoms of affective psychosis, disorientation, and confusion are prevalent
Excludes1 mood disorders with psychotic features (F3Ø.2, F31.2, F31.5, F31.64, F32.3, F33.3)
postpartum dysphoria (O9Ø.6)
psychosis in schizophrenia, schizotypal, delusional, and other psychotic disorders (F2Ø-F29)

F53.Ø **Postpartum depression** ♀ **M**
Postnatal depression, NOS
Postpartum depression, NOS
Coding Clinic: 2018, Q4, P8

F53.1 **Puerperal psychosis** ♀ **M**
Postpartum psychosis
Puerperal psychosis, NOS
Coding Clinic: 2018, Q4, P9

F54 ***Psychological and behavioral factors associated with disorders or diseases classified elsewhere***
Psychological factors affecting physical conditions
Code first the associated physical disorder, such as:
asthma (J45.-)
dermatitis (L23-L25)
gastric ulcer (K25.-)
mucous colitis (K58.-)
ulcerative colitis (K51.-)
urticaria (L5Ø.-)
Excludes2 tension-type headache (G44.2)

● F55 **Abuse of non-psychoactive substances**
Excludes2 abuse of psychoactive substances (F1Ø-F19)

F55.Ø **Abuse of antacids**

F55.1 **Abuse of herbal or folk remedies**

F55.2 **Abuse of laxatives**

F55.3 **Abuse of steroids or hormones**

F55.4 **Abuse of vitamins**

F55.8 **Abuse of other non-psychoactive substances**

F59 **Unspecified behavioral syndromes associated with physiological disturbances and physical factors**
Psychogenic physiological dysfunction NOS

DISORDERS OF ADULT PERSONALITY AND BEHAVIOR (F6Ø-F69)

● F6Ø **Specific personality disorders**
Long-term patterns of thoughts and behaviors causing serious problems with relationships and work

F6Ø.Ø **Paranoid personality disorder**
Hostile, devious, and combative response to disappointments
Expansive paranoid personality (disorder)
Fanatic personality (disorder)
Querulant personality (disorder)
Paranoid personality (disorder)
Sensitive paranoid personality (disorder)
Excludes2 paranoia (F22)
paranoia querulans (F22)
paranoid psychosis (F22)
paranoid schizophrenia (F2Ø.Ø)
paranoid state (F22)

F6Ø.1 **Schizoid personality disorder**
Detachment from social relationships with minimal emotional experiences and expressions
Excludes2 Asperger's syndrome (F84.5)
delusional disorder (F22)
schizoid disorder of childhood (F84.5)
schizophrenia (F2Ø.-)
schizotypal disorder (F21)

F6Ø.2 **Antisocial personality disorder**
Continuous and chronic antisocial behavior
Amoral personality (disorder)
Asocial personality (disorder)
Dissocial personality disorder
Psychopathic personality (disorder)
Sociopathic personality (disorder)
Excludes1 conduct disorders (F91.-)
Excludes2 borderline personality disorder (F6Ø.3)

F6Ø.3 **Borderline personality disorder**
Instability of mood, self-image or sense of self, and interpersonal relationships
Aggressive personality (disorder)
Emotionally unstable personality disorder
Explosive personality (disorder)
Excludes2 antisocial personality disorder (F6Ø.2)

F6Ø.4 **Histrionic personality disorder**
Personality disorder with excessive emotional and attention-seeking behavior
Hysterical personality (disorder)
Psychoinfantile personality (disorder)

F60.5 Obsessive-compulsive personality disorder
Anankastic personality (disorder)
Compulsive personality (disorder)
Obsessional personality (disorder)
Excludes2 obsessive-compulsive disorder (F42-)

F60.6 Avoidant personality disorder
Anxious personality disorder

F60.7 Dependent personality disorder
Asthenic personality (disorder)
Inadequate personality (disorder)
Passive personality (disorder)

F60.8 Other specific personality disorders

F60.81 Narcissistic personality disorder
Vanity, conceit, egotism or indifference to plight of others

F60.89 Other specific personality disorders
Eccentric personality disorder
'Haltlose' type personality disorder
Immature personality disorder
Passive-aggressive personality disorder
Psychoneurotic personality disorder
Self-defeating personality disorder

F60.9 Personality disorder, unspecified
Character disorder NOS
Character neurosis NOS
Pathological personality NOS

F63 Impulse disorders
Excludes2 habitual excessive use of alcohol or psychoactive substances (F10-F19)
impulse disorders involving sexual behavior (F65.-)

F63.0 Pathological gambling
Compulsive gambling
Gambling disorder
Excludes1 gambling and betting NOS (Z72.6)
Excludes2 excessive gambling by manic patients (F30, F31)
gambling in antisocial personality disorder (F60.2)

F63.1 Pyromania
Pathological fire-setting
Excludes2 fire-setting (by) (in):
adult with antisocial personality disorder (F60.2)
alcohol or psychoactive substance intoxication (F10-F19)
conduct disorders (F91.-)
mental disorders due to known physiological condition (F01-F09)
schizophrenia (F20.-)

F63.2 Kleptomania
Pathological stealing
Excludes1 shoplifting as the reason for observation for suspected mental disorder (Z03.8)
Excludes2 depressive disorder with stealing (F31-F33)
stealing due to underlying mental condition-code to mental condition
stealing in mental disorders due to known physiological condition (F01-F09)

F63.3 Trichotillomania
Hair plucking
Excludes2 other stereotyped movement disorder (F98.4)

F63.8 Other impulse disorders

F63.81 Intermittent explosive disorder

F63.89 Other impulse disorders

F63.9 Impulse disorder, unspecified
Impulse control disorder NOS

F64 Gender identity disorders

F64.0 Transsexualism
Gender identity disorder in adolescence and adulthood
Gender dysphoria in adolescents and adults
Coding Clinic: 2016, Q4, P16

F64.1 Dual role transvestism
Use additional code to identify sex reassignment status (Z87.890)
Excludes1 gender identity disorder in childhood (F64.2)
Excludes2 fetishistic transvestism (F65.1)
Coding Clinic: 2016, Q4, P16

F64.2 Gender identity disorder of childhood P
Gender dysphoria in children
Excludes1 gender identity disorder in adolescence and adulthood (F64.0)
Excludes2 sexual maturation disorder (F66)

F64.8 Other gender identity disorders
Other specified gender dysphoria

F64.9 Gender identity disorder, unspecified
Gender dysphoria, unspecified
Gender-role disorder NOS

F65 Paraphilias

F65.0 Fetishism
Intense sexual urges and arousing fantasies using inanimate objects
Fetishistic disorder

F65.1 Transvestic fetishism
Intense sexual urges, arousal, or orgasm associated with fantasized/actual cross-dressing
Fetishistic transvestism
Transvestic disorder

F65.2 Exhibitionism
Exhibitionistic disorder

F65.3 Voyeurism
Sexual urges or arousal involving real or fantasized observation of unsuspecting people who are naked, disrobing, or engaging in sexual activity
Voyeuristic disorder

F65.4 Pedophilia
Pedophilic disorder

F65.5 Sadomasochism

F65.50 Sadomasochism, unspecified

F65.51 Sexual masochism
Sexual masochism disorder

F65.52 Sexual sadism
Sexual sadism disorder

F65.8 Other paraphilias

F65.81 Frotteurism
Sexual arousal or orgasm is achieved by rubbing up against another person (or fantasies of), in crowded place with unsuspecting victim
Frotteuristic disorder

F65.89 Other paraphilias
Necrophilia
Other specified paraphilic disorder

F65.9 Paraphilia, unspecified
Paraphilic disorder, unspecified
Sexual deviation NOS

F66 Other sexual disorders
Sexual maturation disorder
Sexual relationship disorder

CHAPTER 5 (F01-F99)

● **F68 Other disorders of adult personality and behavior**

● **F68.1 Factitious disorder imposed on self**
Compensation neurosis
Elaboration of physical symptoms for psychological reasons
Hospital hopper syndrome
Münchhausen's syndrome
Peregrinating patient
Excludes2 factitial dermatitis (L98.1)
person feigning illness (with obvious motivation) (Z76.5)

F68.10 Factitious disorder imposed on self, unspecified

F68.11 Factitious disorder imposed on self with predominantly psychological signs and symptoms

F68.12 Factitious disorder imposed on self with predominantly physical signs and symptoms

F68.13 Factitious disorder imposed on self with combined psychological and physical signs and symptoms

F68.8 Other specified disorders of adult personality and behavior

F68.A Factitious disorder imposed on another
Factitious disorder by proxy
Münchausen's by proxy

F69 Unspecified disorder of adult personality and behavior A

INTELLECTUAL DISABILITIES (F70-F79)

Code first any associated physical or developmental disorders
Excludes1 borderline intellectual functioning, IQ above 70 to 84 (R41.83)

F70 Mild intellectual disabilities
IQ level 50-55 to approximately 70
Mild mental subnormality

F71 Moderate intellectual disabilities
IQ level 35-40 to 50-55
Moderate mental subnormality

F72 Severe intellectual disabilities
IQ 20-25 to 35-40
Severe mental subnormality

F73 Profound intellectual disabilities
IQ level below 20-25
Profound mental subnormality

F78 Other intellectual disabilities

F79 Unspecified intellectual disabilities
Mental deficiency NOS
Mental subnormality NOS

PERVASIVE AND SPECIFIC DEVELOPMENTAL DISORDERS (F80-F89)

● **F80 Specific developmental disorders of speech and language**

F80.0 Phonological disorder
Communication disorder of unknown cause, characterized by failure to use age-appropriate sounds
Dyslalia
Functional speech articulation disorder
Lalling
Lisping
Phonological developmental disorder
Speech articulation developmental disorder
Speech-sound disorder
Excludes1 speech articulation impairment due to aphasia NOS (R47.01)
speech articulation impairment due to apraxia (R48.2)
Excludes2 speech articulation impairment due to hearing loss (F80.4)
speech articulation impairment due to intellectual disabilities (F70-F79)
speech articulation impairment with expressive language developmental disorder (F80.1)
speech articulation impairment with mixed receptive expressive language developmental disorder (F80.2)

F80.1 Expressive language disorder
Developmental dysphasia or aphasia, expressive type
Excludes1 mixed receptive-expressive language disorder (F80.2)
dysphasia and aphasia NOS (R47.-)
Excludes2 acquired aphasia with epilepsy [Landau-Kleffner] (G40.80-)
intellectual disabilities (F70-F79)
pervasive developmental disorders (F84.-)
selective mutism (F94.0)

F80.2 Mixed receptive-expressive language disorder
Developmental dysphasia or aphasia, receptive type
Developmental Wernicke's aphasia
Excludes1 central auditory processing disorder (H93.25)
dysphasia or aphasia NOS (R47.-)
expressive language disorder (F80.1)
expressive type dysphasia or aphasia (F80.1)
word deafness (H93.25)
Excludes2 acquired aphasia with epilepsy [Landau-Kleffner] (G40.80-)
intellectual disabilities (F70-F79)
pervasive developmental disorders (F84.-)
selective mutism (F94.0)

F80.4 Speech and language development delay due to hearing loss
Code also type of hearing loss (H90.-, H91.-)

● **F80.8 Other developmental disorders of speech or language**

F80.81 Childhood onset fluency disorder
Cluttering NOS
Stuttering NOS
Excludes1 adult onset fluency disorder (F98.5)
fluency disorder in conditions classified elsewhere (R47.82)
fluency disorder (stuttering) following cerebrovascular disease (I69. with final characters -23)

CHAPTER 5 (F01-F99)

▶ New ➡ Revised ~~deleted~~ Deleted Excludes 1 Excludes 2 Includes Use additional Code first Code also Key words
OGCR Official Guidelines X Assign placeholder X ● Use Additional Character(s) Manifestation Code Hierarchical Condition Category Coding Clinic

F80.82 **Social pragmatic communication disorder**
Excludes1 Asperger's syndrome (F84.5)
autistic disorder (F84.0)
Coding Clinic: 2016, Q4, P16

F80.89 **Other developmental disorders of speech and language**
Coding Clinic: 2017, Q1, P27

F80.9 **Developmental disorder of speech and language, unspecified**
Communication disorder NOS
Language disorder NOS

● F81 **Specific developmental disorders of scholastic skills**

F81.0 **Specific reading disorder**
'Backward reading'
Developmental dyslexia
Specific learning disorder, with impairment in reading
Specific reading retardation
Excludes1 alexia NOS (R48.0)
dyslexia NOS (R48.0)

F81.2 **Mathematics disorder**
Developmental acalculia
Developmental arithmetical disorder
Developmental Gerstmann's syndrome
Specific learning disorder, with impairment in mathematics
Excludes1 acalculia NOS (R48.8)
Excludes2 arithmetical difficulties associated with a reading disorder (F81.0)
arithmetical difficulties associated with a spelling disorder (F81.81)
arithmetical difficulties due to inadequate teaching (Z55.8)

● F81.8 **Other developmental disorders of scholastic skills**

F81.81 **Disorder of written expression**
Specific learning disorder, with impairment in written expression
Specific spelling disorder

F81.89 **Other developmental disorders of scholastic skills**

F81.9 **Developmental disorder of scholastic skills, unspecified**
Knowledge acquisition disability NOS
Learning disability NOS
Learning disorder NOS

F82 **Specific developmental disorder of motor function**
Clumsy child syndrome
Developmental coordination disorder
Developmental dyspraxia
Excludes1 abnormalities of gait and mobility (R26.-)
lack of coordination (R27.-)
Excludes2 lack of coordination secondary to intellectual disabilities (F70-F79)

● F84 **Pervasive developmental disorders**
Use additional code to identify any associated medical condition and intellectual disabilities.

F84.0 **Autistic disorder**
Autism spectrum disorder
Infantile autism
Infantile psychosis
Kanner's syndrome
Excludes1 Asperger's syndrome (F84.5)
Coding Clinic: 2017, Q1, P27

F84.2 **Rett's syndrome**
Neurodevelopmental disorder
Excludes1 Asperger's syndrome (F84.5)
Autistic disorder (F84.0)
other childhood disintegrative disorder (F84.3)

F84.3 **Other childhood disintegrative disorder** P
Dementia infantilis
At least two years of normal development followed by significant loss of language abilities, social skills, bowel/bladder control, motor skills
Disintegrative psychosis
Heller's syndrome
At least two years of normal development followed by significant loss of language abilities, social skills, bowel/bladder control, motor skills
Symbiotic psychosis
Abnormal relationship to mothering figure, characterized by intense separation anxiety, severe regression, giving up of useful speech, and autism
Use additional code to identify any associated neurological condition.
Excludes1 Asperger's syndrome (F84.5)
Autistic disorder (F84.0)
Rett's syndrome (F84.2)

F84.5 **Asperger's syndrome**
Developmental disorder
Asperger's disorder
Autistic psychopathy
Schizoid disorder of childhood

F84.8 **Other pervasive developmental disorders**
Overactive disorder associated with intellectual disabilities and stereotyped movements

F84.9 **Pervasive developmental disorder, unspecified**
Atypical autism

F88 **Other disorders of psychological development**
Developmental agnosia
Global developmental delay
Other specified neurodevelopmental disorder

F89 **Unspecified disorder of psychological development**
Developmental disorder NOS
Neurodevelopmental disorder NOS

BEHAVIORAL AND EMOTIONAL DISORDERS WITH ONSET USUALLY OCCURRING IN CHILDHOOD AND ADOLESCENCE (F90-F98)

Note: Codes within categories F90-F98 may be used regardless of the age of a patient. These disorders generally have onset within the childhood or adolescent years, but may continue throughout life or not be diagnosed until adulthood.

● F90 **Attention-deficit hyperactivity disorders**
Attention deficit disorder with hyperactivity=ADHD
Includes attention deficit disorder with hyperactivity
attention deficit syndrome with hyperactivity
Excludes2 anxiety disorders (F40.-, F41.-)
mood [affective] disorders (F30-F39)
pervasive developmental disorders (F84.-)
schizophrenia (F20.-)

F90.0 **Attention-deficit hyperactivity disorder, predominantly inattentive type**
Attention-deficit/hyperactivity disorder, predominantly inattentive presentation

F90.1 **Attention-deficit hyperactivity disorder, predominantly hyperactive type**
Attention-deficit/hyperactivity disorder, predominantly hyperactive impulsive presentation

F90.2 **Attention-deficit hyperactivity disorder, combined type**
Attention-deficit/hyperactivity disorder, combined presentation

F90.8 **Attention-deficit hyperactivity disorder, other type**

F90.9 **Attention-deficit hyperactivity disorder, unspecified type**
Attention-deficit hyperactivity disorder of childhood or adolescence NOS
Attention-deficit hyperactivity disorder NOS

CHAPTER 5 (F01-F99)

● F91 Conduct disorders
Childhood/adolescence disruptive behavior disorder
Excludes1 antisocial behavior (Z72.81-)
antisocial personality disorder (F60.2)
Excludes2 conduct problems associated with attention-deficit hyperactivity disorder (F90.-)
mood [affective] disorders (F30-F39)
pervasive developmental disorders (F84.-)
schizophrenia (F20.-)

F91.0 Conduct disorder confined to family context

F91.1 Conduct disorder, childhood-onset type
Unsocialized conduct disorder
Conduct disorder, solitary aggressive type
Unsocialized aggressive disorder

F91.2 Conduct disorder, adolescent-onset type
Socialized conduct disorder
Conduct disorder, group type

F91.3 Oppositional defiant disorder

F91.8 Other conduct disorders
Other specified conduct disorder
Other specified disruptive disorder

F91.9 Conduct disorder, unspecified
Behavioral disorder NOS
Conduct disorder NOS
Disruptive behavior disorder NOS
Disruptive disorder NOS

● F93 Emotional disorders with onset specific to childhood

F93.0 Separation anxiety disorder of childhood
Excludes2 mood [affective] disorders (F30-F39)
nonpsychotic mental disorders (F40-F48)
phobic anxiety disorder of childhood (F40.8)
social phobia (F40.1)

F93.8 Other childhood emotional disorders
Identity disorder
Excludes2 gender identity disorder of childhood (F64.2)

F93.9 Childhood emotional disorder, unspecified

● F94 Disorders of social functioning with onset specific to childhood and adolescence

F94.0 Selective mutism
Elective mutism
Excludes2 pervasive developmental disorders (F84.-)
schizophrenia (F20.-)
specific developmental disorders of speech and language (F80.-)
transient mutism as part of separation anxiety in young children (F93.0)

F94.1 Reactive attachment disorder of childhood
Use additional code to identify any associated failure to thrive or growth retardation
Excludes1 disinhibited attachment disorder of childhood (F94.2)
normal variation in pattern of selective attachment
Excludes2 Asperger's syndrome (F84.5)
maltreatment syndromes (T74.-)
sexual or physical abuse in childhood, resulting in psychosocial problems (Z62.81-)

F94.2 Disinhibited attachment disorder of childhood
Affectionless psychopathy
Institutional syndrome
Excludes1 reactive attachment disorder of childhood (F94.1)
Excludes2 Asperger's syndrome (F84.5)
attention-deficit hyperactivity disorders (F90.-)
hospitalism in children (F43.2-)

F94.8 Other childhood disorders of social functioning

F94.9 Childhood disorder of social functioning, unspecified

● F95 Tic disorder
Involuntary twitch

F95.0 Transient tic disorder
Provisional tic disorder

F95.1 Chronic motor or vocal tic disorder

F95.2 Tourette's disorder
Combined vocal and multiple motor tic disorder [de la Tourette]
Tourette's syndrome

F95.8 Other tic disorders

F95.9 Tic disorder, unspecified
Tic NOS

● F98 Other behavioral and emotional disorders with onset usually occurring in childhood and adolescence
Excludes2 breath-holding spells (R06.89)
gender identity disorder of childhood (F64.2)
Kleine-Levin syndrome (G47.13)
obsessive-compulsive disorder (F42-)
sleep disorders not due to a substance or known physiological condition (F51.-)

F98.0 Enuresis not due to a substance or known physiological condition
Enuresis: Urinary incontinence
Enuresis (primary) (secondary) of nonorganic origin
Functional enuresis
Psychogenic enuresis
Urinary incontinence of nonorganic origin
Excludes1 enuresis NOS (R32)

F98.1 Encopresis not due to a substance or known physiological condition
Encopresis: Fecal incontinence
Functional encopresis
Incontinence of feces of nonorganic origin
Psychogenic encopresis
Use additional code to identify the cause of any coexisting constipation.
Excludes1 encopresis NOS (R15.-)

● F98.2 Other feeding disorders of infancy and childhood
Excludes1 feeding difficulties (R63.3)
Excludes2 anorexia nervosa and other eating disorders (F50.-)
feeding problems of newborn (P92.-)
pica of infancy or childhood (F98.3)

F98.21 Rumination disorder of infancy

F98.29 Other feeding disorders of infancy and early childhood

F98.3 Pica of infancy and childhood
Craving and eating substances such as paint, clay, or dirt to replace a nutritional deficit in the body.

Item 5–2 Enuresis: Bed wetting by children at night. Causes can be either psychological or medical (diabetes, urinary tract infections, or abnormalities). **Encopresis:** Overflow incontinence of bowels sometimes resulting from chronic constipation or fecal impaction. Check the documentation for additional diagnoses.

F98.4   **Stereotyped movement disorders**
       Stereotype/habit disorder

       Excludes1   abnormal involuntary movements (R25.-)

       Excludes2   compulsions in obsessive-compulsive
                 disorder (F42-)
                hair plucking (F63.3)
                movement disorders of organic origin
                 (G20-G25)
                nail-biting (F98.8)
                nose-picking (F98.8)
                stereotypies that are part of a broader
                 psychiatric condition (F01-F95)
                thumb-sucking (F98.8)
                tic disorders (F95.-)
                trichotillomania (F63.3)

F98.5   **Adult onset fluency disorder**

       Excludes1   childhood onset fluency disorder (F80.81)
                dysphasia (R47.02)
                fluency disorder in conditions classified
                 elsewhere (R47.82)
                fluency disorder (stuttering) following
                 cerebrovascular disease (I69. with
                 final characters -23)
                tic disorders (F95.-)

F98.8   **Other specified behavioral and emotional disorders with
onset usually occurring in childhood and adolescence**
       Excessive masturbation
       Nail-biting
       Nose-picking
       Thumb-sucking

F98.9   **Unspecified behavioral and emotional disorders with
onset usually occurring in childhood and adolescence**

UNSPECIFIED MENTAL DISORDER (F99)

F99   **Mental disorder, not otherwise specified**
       Mental illness NOS

       Excludes1   unspecified mental disorder due to known
                physiological condition (F09)

CHAPTER 5 (F01-F99)

CHAPTER 6

DISEASES OF THE NERVOUS SYSTEM (GØØ-G99)

OGCR Chapter-Specific Coding Guidelines

6. Chapter 6: Diseases of the Nervous System (GØØ-G99)

a. Dominant/nondominant side

Codes from category G81, Hemiplegia and hemiparesis, and subcategories, G83.1, Monoplegia of lower limb, G83.2, Monoplegia of upper limb, and G83.3, Monoplegia, unspecified, identify whether the dominant or nondominant side is affected. Should the affected side be documented, but not specified as dominant or nondominant, and the classification system does not indicate a default, code selection is as follows:

- For ambidextrous patients, the default should be dominant.
- If the left side is affected, the default is nondominant.
- If the right side is affected, the default is dominant.

b. Pain - Category G89

1) General coding information

Codes in category G89, Pain, not elsewhere classified, may be used in conjunction with codes from other categories and chapters to provide more detail about acute or chronic pain and neoplasm-related pain, unless otherwise indicated below.

If the pain is not specified as acute or chronic, post-thoracotomy, postprocedural, or neoplasm-related, do not assign codes from category G89.

A code from category G89 should not be assigned if the underlying (definitive) diagnosis is known, unless the reason for the encounter is pain control/management and not management of the underlying condition.

When an admission or encounter is for a procedure aimed at treating the underlying condition (e.g., spinal fusion, kyphoplasty), a code for the underlying condition (e.g., vertebral fracture, spinal stenosis) should be assigned as the principal diagnosis. No code from category G89 should be assigned.

(a) Category G89 Codes as Principal or First-Listed Diagnosis

Category G89 codes are acceptable as principal diagnosis or the first-listed code:

- When pain control or pain management is the reason for the admission/encounter (e.g., a patient with displaced intervertebral disc, nerve impingement and severe back pain presents for injection of steroid into the spinal canal). The underlying cause of the pain should be reported as an additional diagnosis, if known.
- When a patient is admitted for the insertion of a neurostimulator for pain control, assign the appropriate pain code as the principal or first-listed diagnosis. When an admission or encounter is for a procedure aimed at treating the underlying condition and a neurostimulator is inserted for pain control during the same admission/encounter, a code for the underlying condition should be assigned as the principal diagnosis and the appropriate pain code should be assigned as a secondary diagnosis.

(b) Use of Category G89 Codes in Conjunction with Site Specific Pain Codes

(i) Assigning Category G89 and Site-Specific Pain Codes

Codes from category G89 may be used in conjunction with codes that identify the site of pain (including codes from Chapter 18) if the category G89 code provides additional information. For example, if the code describes the site of the pain, but does not fully describe whether the pain is acute or chronic, then both codes should be assigned.

(ii) Sequencing of Category G89 Codes with Site-Specific Pain Codes

The sequencing of category G89 codes with site-specific pain codes (including Chapter 18 codes), is dependent on the circumstances of the encounter/admission as follows:

- If the encounter is for pain control or pain management, assign the code from category G89 followed by the code identifying the specific site of pain (e.g., encounter for pain management for acute neck pain from trauma is assigned code G89.11, Acute pain due to trauma, followed by code M54.2, Cervicalgia, to identify the site of pain).
- If the encounter is for any other reason except pain control or pain management, and a related definitive diagnosis has not been established (confirmed) by the provider, assign the code for the specific site of pain first, followed by the appropriate code from category G89.

2) Pain due to devices, implants and grafts

See Section I.C.19. Pain due to medical devices

3) Postoperative Pain

The provider's documentation should be used to guide the coding of postoperative pain, as well as *Section III. Reporting Additional Diagnoses* and *Section IV. Diagnostic Coding and Reporting in the Outpatient Setting.*

The default for post-thoracotomy and other postoperative pain not specified as acute or chronic is the code for the acute form.

Routine or expected postoperative pain immediately after surgery should not be coded.

(a) Postoperative pain not associated with specific postoperative complication

Postoperative pain not associated with a specific postoperative complication is assigned to the appropriate postoperative pain code in category G89.

(b) Postoperative pain associated with specific postoperative complication

Postoperative pain associated with a specific postoperative complication (such as painful wire sutures) is assigned to the appropriate code(s) found in Chapter 19, Injury, poisoning, and certain other consequences of external causes. If appropriate, use additional code(s) from category G89 to identify acute or chronic pain (G89.18 or G89.28).

4) Chronic pain

Chronic pain is classified to subcategory G89.2. There is no time frame defining when pain becomes chronic pain. The provider's documentation should be used to guide use of these codes.

5) Neoplasm Related Pain

Code G89.3 is assigned to pain documented as being related, associated or due to cancer, primary or secondary malignancy, or tumor. This code is assigned regardless of whether the pain is acute or chronic.

This code may be assigned as the principal or first-listed code when the stated reason for the admission/encounter is documented as pain control/pain management. The underlying neoplasm should be reported as an additional diagnosis.

When the reason for the admission/encounter is management of the neoplasm and the pain associated with the neoplasm is also documented, code G89.3 may be assigned as an additional diagnosis. It is not necessary to assign an additional code for the site of the pain.

See Section I.C.2 for instructions on the sequencing of neoplasms for all other stated reasons for the admission/encounter (except for pain control/pain management).

6) Chronic pain syndrome

Central pain syndrome (G89.Ø) and chronic pain syndrome (G89.4) are different than the term "chronic pain," and therefore codes should only be used when the provider has specifically documented this condition.

See Section I.C.5. Pain disorders related to psychological factors

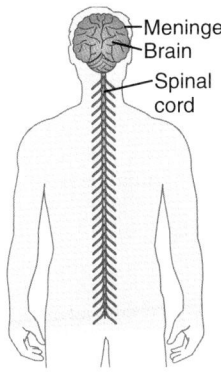

—Meninges
—Brain
—Spinal cord

Figure 6-1 The brain and spinal cord make up the central nervous system.

Item 6-1 The two major classifications of the nervous system are the peripheral nervous system and the central nervous system (CNS). The central nervous system is composed of the brain and the spinal cord. The peripheral nervous system is composed of the parasympathetic and sympathetic systems. **Encephalitis** is the swelling of the brain. **Meningitis** is swelling of the covering of the brain, the meninges. Types and causes of brain infections are:

Type	Cause
purulent	bacterial
aseptic/abacterial	viral
chronic meningitis	mycobacterial and fungal

CHAPTER 6

DISEASES OF THE NERVOUS SYSTEM (G00-G99)

Excludes2 certain conditions originating in the perinatal period (P04-P96)
certain infectious and parasitic diseases (A00-B99)
complications of pregnancy, childbirth and the puerperium (O00-O9A)
congenital malformations, deformations, and chromosomal abnormalities (Q00-Q99)
endocrine, nutritional and metabolic diseases (E00-E88)
injury, poisoning and certain other consequences of external causes (S00-T88)
neoplasms (C00-D49)
symptoms, signs and abnormal clinical and laboratory findings, not elsewhere classified (R00-R94)

This chapter contains the following blocks:

G00-G09	Inflammatory diseases of the central nervous system
G10-G14	Systemic atrophies primarily affecting the central nervous system
G20-G26	Extrapyramidal and movement disorders
G30-G32	Other degenerative diseases of the nervous system
G35-G37	Demyelinating diseases of the central nervous system
G40-G47	Episodic and paroxysmal disorders
G50-G59	Nerve, nerve root and plexus disorders
G60-G65	Polyneuropathies and other disorders of the peripheral nervous system
G70-G73	Diseases of myoneural junction and muscle
G80-G83	Cerebral palsy and other paralytic syndromes
G89-G99	Other disorders of the nervous system

INFLAMMATORY DISEASES OF THE CENTRAL NERVOUS SYSTEM (G00-G09)

● **G00 Bacterial meningitis, not elsewhere classified**
An infection of the cerebrospinal fluid surrounding the spinal cord and brain.
Includes bacterial arachnoiditis
bacterial leptomeningitis
bacterial meningitis
bacterial pachymeningitis
Excludes1 bacterial meningoencephalitis (G04.2)
bacterial meningomyelitis (G04.2)

G00.0 Hemophilus meningitis
Meningitis due to Hemophilus influenzae
G00.1 Pneumococcal meningitis
Meningitis due to Streptococcal pneumoniae
G00.2 Streptococcal meningitis
Use additional code to further identify organism (B95.0-B95.5)
G00.3 Staphylococcal meningitis
Use additional code to further identify organism (B95.61-B95.8)
G00.8 Other bacterial meningitis
Meningitis due to Escherichia coli
Meningitis due to Friedländer bacillus
Meningitis due to Klebsiella
Use additional code to further identify organism (B96.-)
G00.9 Bacterial meningitis, unspecified
Meningitis due to gram-negative bacteria, unspecified
Purulent meningitis NOS
Pyogenic meningitis NOS
Suppurative meningitis NOS

▷ **G01 *Meningitis in bacterial diseases classified elsewhere***
Code first underlying disease
Excludes1 meningitis (in):
gonococcal (A54.81)
leptospirosis (A27.81)
listeriosis (A32.11)
Lyme disease (A69.21)
meningococcal (A39.0)
neurosyphilis (A52.13)
tuberculosis (A17.0)
meningoencephalitis and meningomyelitis in bacterial diseases classified elsewhere (G05)

▷ **G02 *Meningitis in other infectious and parasitic diseases classified elsewhere***
Code first underlying disease, such as:
African trypanosomiasis (B56.-)
poliovirus infection (A80.-)
Excludes1 candidal meningitis (B37.5)
coccidioidomycosis meningitis (B38.4)
cryptococcal meningitis (B45.1)
herpesviral [herpes simplex] meningitis (B00.3)
infectious mononucleosis complicated by meningitis (B27.- with fourth character 2)
measles complicated by meningitis (B05.1)
meningoencephalitis and meningomyelitis in other infectious and parasitic diseases classified elsewhere (G05)
mumps meningitis (B26.1)
rubella meningitis (B06.02)
varicella [chickenpox] meningitis (B01.0)
zoster meningitis (B02.1)

● **G03 Meningitis due to other and unspecified causes**

Includes arachnoiditis NOS
leptomeningitis NOS
meningitis NOS
pachymeningitis NOS

Excludes1 meningoencephalitis (G04.-)
meningomyelitis (G04.-)

G03.0 Nonpyogenic meningitis
Aseptic meningitis
Nonbacterial meningitis

G03.1 Chronic meningitis

G03.2 Benign recurrent meningitis [Mollaret]

G03.8 Meningitis due to other specified causes

G03.9 Meningitis, unspecified
Arachnoiditis (spinal) NOS

● **G04 Encephalitis, myelitis and encephalomyelitis**

Includes acute ascending myelitis
meningoencephalitis
meningomyelitis

Excludes1 encephalopathy NOS (G93.40)
other noninfectious acute disseminated encephalomyelitis (noninfectious ADEM) (G04.81)

Excludes2 acute transverse myelitis (G37.3-)
alcoholic encephalopathy (G31.2)
benign myalgic encephalomyelitis (G93.3)
multiple sclerosis (G35)
subacute necrotizing myelitis (G37.4)
toxic encephalitis (G92)
toxic encephalopathy (G92)

● **G04.0 Acute disseminated encephalitis and encephalomyelitis (ADEM)**

Excludes1 acute necrotizing hemorrhagic encephalopathy (G04.3-)

G04.00 Acute disseminated encephalitis and encephalomyelitis, unspecified

G04.01 Postinfectious acute disseminated encephalitis and encephalomyelitis (postinfectious ADEM)

Excludes1 post chickenpox encephalitis (B01.1)
post measles encephalitis (B05.0)
post measles myelitis (B05.1)

G04.02 Postimmunization acute disseminated encephalitis, myelitis and encephalomyelitis
Encephalitis, post immunization
Encephalomyelitis, post immunization
Use additional code to identify the vaccine (T50.A-, T50.B-, T50.Z-)

G04.1 Tropical spastic paraplegia

G04.2 Bacterial meningoencephalitis and meningomyelitis, not elsewhere classified

● **G04.3 Acute necrotizing hemorrhagic encephalopathy**
Sudden and severe CNS disease with pathology of hemorrhages and necrosis of white matter

Excludes1 acute disseminated encephalitis and encephalomyelitis (G04.0-)

G04.30 Acute necrotizing hemorrhagic encephalopathy, unspecified

G04.31 Postinfectious acute necrotizing hemorrhagic encephalopathy

G04.32 Postimmunization acute necrotizing hemorrhagic encephalopathy
Use additional code to identify vaccine (T50.A-, T50.B-, T50.Z-)

G04.39 Other acute necrotizing hemorrhagic encephalopathy
Code also underlying etiology, if applicable

● **G04.8 Other encephalitis, myelitis and encephalomyelitis**
Code also any associated seizure (G40.-, R56.9)

G04.81 Other encephalitis and encephalomyelitis
Noninfectious acute disseminated encephalomyelitis (noninfectious ADEM)

G04.89 Other myelitis

● **G04.9 Encephalitis, myelitis and encephalomyelitis, unspecified**

G04.90 Encephalitis and encephalomyelitis, unspecified
Ventriculitis (cerebral) NOS

G04.91 Myelitis, unspecified

● **G05 Encephalitis, myelitis and encephalomyelitis in diseases classified elsewhere**

Code first underlying disease, such as:
human immunodeficiency virus [HIV] disease (B20)
poliovirus (A80.-)
suppurative otitis media (H66.01-H66.4)
trichinellosis (B75)

Excludes1 adenoviral encephalitis, myelitis and encephalomyelitis (A85.1)
congenital toxoplasmosis encephalitis, myelitis and encephalomyelitis (P37.1)
cytomegaloviral encephalitis, myelitis and encephalomyelitis (B25.8)
encephalitis, myelitis and encephalomyelitis (in) measles (B05.0)
encephalitis, myelitis and encephalomyelitis (in) systemic lupus erythematosus (M32.19)
enteroviral encephalitis, myelitis and encephalomyelitis (A85.0)
eosinophilic meningoencephalitis (B83.2)
herpesviral [herpes simplex] encephalitis, myelitis and encephalomyelitis (B00.4)
listerial encephalitis, myelitis and encephalomyelitis (A32.12)
meningococcal encephalitis, myelitis and encephalomyelitis (A39.81)
mumps encephalitis, myelitis and encephalomyelitis (B26.2)
postchickenpox encephalitis, myelitis and encephalomyelitis (B01.1-)
rubella encephalitis, myelitis and encephalomyelitis (B06.01)
toxoplasmosis encephalitis, myelitis and encephalomyelitis (B58.2)
zoster encephalitis, myelitis and encephalomyelitis (B02.0)

G05.3 Encephalitis and encephalomyelitis in diseases classified elsewhere
Meningoencephalitis in diseases classified elsewhere

G05.4 Myelitis in diseases classified elsewhere
Meningomyelitis in diseases classified elsewhere

● **G06 Intracranial and intraspinal abscess and granuloma**
An accumulation of pus in either the brain or spinal cord
Use additional code (B95-B97) to identify infectious agent.

G06.0 Intracranial abscess and granuloma
Brain [any part] abscess (embolic)
Cerebellar abscess (embolic)
Cerebral abscess (embolic)
Intracranial epidural abscess or granuloma
Intracranial extradural abscess or granuloma
Intracranial subdural abscess or granuloma
Otogenic abscess (embolic)

Excludes1 tuberculous intracranial abscess and granuloma (A17.81)

G06.1 Intraspinal abscess and granuloma
Abscess (embolic) of spinal cord [any part]
Intraspinal epidural abscess or granuloma
Intraspinal extradural abscess or granuloma
Intraspinal subdural abscess or granuloma

Excludes1 tuberculous intraspinal abscess and granuloma (A17.81)

G06.2 Extradural and subdural abscess, unspecified

G07 ***Intracranial and intraspinal abscess and granuloma in diseases classified elsewhere***

Code first underlying disease, such as:
schistosomiasis granuloma of brain (B65.-)

Excludes1 abscess of brain:
amebic (A06.6)
chromomycotic (B43.1)
gonococcal (A54.82)
tuberculous (A17.81)
tuberculoma of meninges (A17.1)

G08 Intracranial and intraspinal phlebitis and thrombophlebitis

Septic embolism of intracranial or intraspinal venous sinuses and veins
Septic endophlebitis of intracranial or intraspinal venous sinuses and veins
Septic phlebitis of intracranial or intraspinal venous sinuses and veins
Septic thrombophlebitis of intracranial or intraspinal venous sinuses and veins
Septic thrombosis of intracranial or intraspinal venous sinuses and veins

Excludes1 intracranial phlebitis and thrombophlebitis complicating:
abortion, ectopic or molar pregnancy (O00-O07, O08.7)
pregnancy, childbirth and the puerperium (O22.5, O87.3)
nonpyogenic intracranial phlebitis and thrombophlebitis (I67.6)

Excludes2 intracranial phlebitis and thrombophlebitis complicating nonpyogenic intraspinal phlebitis and thrombophlebitis (G95.1)

G09 Sequelae of inflammatory diseases of central nervous system

Note: Category G09 is to be used to indicate conditions whose primary classification is to G00-G08 as the cause of sequelae, themselves classifiable elsewhere. The 'sequelae' include conditions specified as residuals.

Code first condition resulting from (sequela) of inflammatory diseases of central nervous system

SYSTEMIC ATROPHIES PRIMARILY AFFECTING THE CENTRAL NERVOUS SYSTEM (G10-G14)

G10 Huntington's disease

Genetic disease with degeneration of cells of the nervous system, including brain
Huntington's chorea
Huntington's dementia

Code also dementia in other diseases classified elsewhere without behavioral disturbance (F02.80)

G11 Hereditary ataxia

Genetic neurological disorder affecting coordination

Excludes2 cerebral palsy (G80.-)
hereditary and idiopathic neuropathy (G60.-)
metabolic disorders (E70-E88)

G11.0 Congenital nonprogressive ataxia

G11.1 Early-onset cerebellar ataxia
Early-onset cerebellar ataxia with essential tremor
Early-onset cerebellar ataxia with myoclonus [Hunt's ataxia]
Early-onset cerebellar ataxia with retained tendon reflexes
Friedreich's ataxia (autosomal recessive)
X-linked recessive spinocerebellar ataxia

G11.2 Late-onset cerebellar ataxia A

G11.3 Cerebellar ataxia with defective DNA repair
Ataxia telangiectasia [Louis-Bar]

Excludes2 Cockayne's syndrome (Q87.19)
other disorders of purine and pyrimidine metabolism (E79.-)
xeroderma pigmentosum (Q82.1)

G11.4 Hereditary spastic paraplegia

G11.8 Other hereditary ataxias

G11.9 Hereditary ataxia, unspecified
Hereditary cerebellar ataxia NOS
Hereditary cerebellar degeneration
Hereditary cerebellar disease
Hereditary cerebellar syndrome

G12 Spinal muscular atrophy and related syndromes

G12.0 Infantile spinal muscular atrophy, type I [Werdnig-Hoffman]

G12.1 Other inherited spinal muscular atrophy
Adult form spinal muscular atrophy
Childhood form, type II spinal muscular atrophy
Distal spinal muscular atrophy
Juvenile form, type III spinal muscular atrophy [Kugelberg-Welander]
Progressive bulbar palsy of childhood [Fazio-Londe]
Scapuloperoneal form spinal muscular atrophy

G12.2 Motor neuron disease
Progressive disease of motor neurons that carry impluses to muscles to move

G12.20 Motor neuron disease, unspecified

G12.21 Amyotrophic lateral sclerosis A
Lou Gehrig's disease (ALS)

G12.22 Progressive bulbar palsy

G12.23 Primary lateral sclerosis

G12.24 Familial motor neuron disease

G12.25 Progressive spinal muscle atrophy

G12.29 Other motor neuron disease

G12.8 Other spinal muscular atrophies and related syndromes

G12.9 Spinal muscular atrophy, unspecified

G13 Systemic atrophies primarily affecting central nervous system in diseases classified elsewhere

G13.0 Paraneoplastic neuromyopathy and neuropathy
Carcinomatous neuromyopathy
Sensorial paraneoplastic neuropathy [Denny Brown]
Code first underlying neoplasm (C00-D49)

G13.1 Other systemic atrophy primarily affecting central nervous system in neoplastic disease
Paraneoplastic limbic encephalopathy
Code first underlying neoplasm (C00-D49)

G13.2 Systemic atrophy primarily affecting the central nervous system in myxedema
Code first underlying disease, such as:
hypothyroidism (E03.-)
myxedematous congenital iodine deficiency (E00.1)

G13.8 Systemic atrophy primarily affecting central nervous system in other diseases classified elsewhere
Code first underlying disease

G14 Postpolio syndrome

Includes Postpolio myelitic syndrome

Excludes1 sequelae of poliomyelitis (B91)

Item 6–2 Huntington's chorea is an inherited degenerative disorder of the central nervous system and is characterized by ceaseless, jerky movements and progressive cognitive and behavioral deterioration.

EXTRAPYRAMIDAL AND MOVEMENT DISORDERS (G20-G26)

G20 Parkinson's disease (HCC)
Progressive disease of the nervous system that affects muscle coordination
Hemiparkinsonism
Idiopathic Parkinsonism or Parkinson's disease
Paralysis agitans
Parkinsonism or Parkinson's disease NOS
Primary Parkinsonism or Parkinson's disease
Excludes1 dementia with Parkinsonism (G31.83)
Coding Clinic: 2017, Q2, P7-8; 2016, Q2, P7

● **G21 Secondary parkinsonism**
Symptoms of Parkinson's caused by medicines, illness, or other nervous system disorder
Excludes1 dementia with Parkinsonism (G31.83)
Huntington's disease (G10)
Shy-Drager syndrome (G90.3)
syphilitic Parkinsonism (A52.19)

G21.0 Malignant neuroleptic syndrome
Use additional code for adverse effect, if applicable, to identify drug (T43.3X5, T43.4X5, T43.505, T43.595)
Excludes1 neuroleptic induced parkinsonism (G21.11)

● **G21.1 Other drug-induced secondary parkinsonism**

G21.11 Neuroleptic induced parkinsonism (HCC)
Use additional code for adverse effect, if applicable, to identify drug (T43.3X5, T43.4X5, T43.505, T43.595)
Excludes1 malignant neuroleptic syndrome (G21.0)

G21.19 Other drug induced secondary parkinsonism (HCC)
Other medication-induced parkinsonism
Use additional code for adverse effect, if applicable, to identify drug (T36-T50 with fifth or sixth character 5)

G21.2 Secondary parkinsonism due to other external agents (HCC)
Code first (T51-T65) to identify external agent

G21.3 Postencephalitic parkinsonism (HCC)

G21.4 Vascular parkinsonism (HCC)

G21.8 Other secondary parkinsonism (HCC)

G21.9 Secondary parkinsonism, unspecified (HCC)

● **G23 Other degenerative diseases of basal ganglia**
Excludes2 multi-system degeneration of the autonomic nervous system (G90.3)

G23.0 Hallervorden-Spatz disease (HCC)
Pigmentary pallidal degeneration

G23.1 Progressive supranuclear ophthalmoplegia [Steele-Richardson-Olszewski] (HCC)
Progressive supranuclear palsy

G23.2 Striatonigral degeneration (HCC)

G23.8 Other specified degenerative diseases of basal ganglia (HCC)
Calcification of basal ganglia

G23.9 Degenerative disease of basal ganglia, unspecified (HCC)

● **G24 Dystonia**
Involuntary movements
Includes dyskinesia
Excludes2 athetoid cerebral palsy (G80.3)

● **G24.0 Drug induced dystonia**
Use additional code for adverse effect, if applicable, to identify drug (T36-T50 with fifth or sixth character 5)

G24.01 Drug induced subacute dyskinesia
Drug induced blepharospasm
Drug induced orofacial dyskinesia
Neuroleptic induced tardive dyskinesia
Tardive dyskinesia

G24.02 Drug induced acute dystonia
Acute dystonic reaction to drugs
Neuroleptic induced acute dystonia

G24.09 Other drug induced dystonia

G24.1 Genetic torsion dystonia
Dystonia deformans progressiva
Dystonia musculorum deformans
Familial torsion dystonia
Idiopathic familial dystonia
Idiopathic (torsion) dystonia NOS
(Schwalbe-) Ziehen-Oppenheim disease

G24.2 Idiopathic nonfamilial dystonia

G24.3 Spasmodic torticollis
Head tilts toward one side and chin is elevated and turned toward opposite side (wry neck)
Excludes1 congenital torticollis (Q68.0)
hysterical torticollis (F44.4)
ocular torticollis (R29.891)
psychogenic torticollis (F45.8)
torticollis NOS (M43.6)
traumatic recurrent torticollis (S13.4)

G24.4 Idiopathic orofacial dystonia
Orofacial dyskinesia
Excludes1 drug induced orofacial dyskinesia (G24.01)

G24.5 Blepharospasm
Tonic spasm of orbicularis oculi muscle, producing closure of eyelids
Excludes1 drug induced blepharospasm (G24.01)

G24.8 Other dystonia
Acquired torsion dystonia NOS

G24.9 Dystonia, unspecified
Dyskinesia NOS

● **G25 Other extrapyramidal and movement disorders**
Extrapyramidal: Other than pyramidal tracts
Excludes2 sleep related movement disorders (G47.6-)

G25.0 Essential tremor
Familial tremor
Excludes1 tremor NOS (R25.1)

G25.1 Drug-induced tremor
Use additional code for adverse effect, if applicable, to identify drug (T36-T50 with fifth or sixth character 5)

G25.2 Other specified forms of tremor
Intention tremor

G25.3 Myoclonus
Shocklike contractions muscle(s)
Drug-induced myoclonus
Palatal myoclonus
Use additional code for adverse effect, if applicable, to identify drug (T36-T50 with fifth or sixth character 5)
Excludes1 facial myokymia (G51.4)
myoclonic epilepsy (G40.-)

G25.4 Drug-induced chorea
Use additional code for adverse effect, if applicable, to identify drug (T36-T50 with fifth or sixth character 5)

G25.5 Other chorea
Continual, involuntary, jerky, movements
Chorea NOS
Excludes1 chorea NOS with heart involvement (I02.0)
Huntington's chorea (G10)
rheumatic chorea (I02.-)
Sydenham's chorea (I02.-)

● **G25.6 Drug induced tics and other tics of organic origin**

G25.61 Drug induced tics

Use additional code for adverse effect, if applicable, to identify drug (T36-T5Ø with fifth or sixth character 5)

G25.69 Other tics of organic origin

Excludes1 habit spasm (F95.9)
tic NOS (F95.9)
Tourette's syndrome (F95.2)

● **G25.7 Other and unspecified drug induced movement disorders**

Use additional code for adverse effect, if applicable, to identify drug (T36-T5Ø with fifth or sixth character 5)

G25.7Ø Drug induced movement disorder, unspecified

G25.71 Drug induced akathisia

Drug induced acathisia
Neuroleptic induced acute akathisia
Tardive akathisia

G25.79 Other drug induced movement disorders

● **G25.8 Other specified extrapyramidal and movement disorders**

G25.81 Restless legs syndrome

G25.82 Stiff-man syndrome

G25.83 Benign shuddering attacks

G25.89 Other specified extrapyramidal and movement disorders

G25.9 Extrapyramidal and movement disorder, unspecified

G26 Extrapyramidal and movement disorders in diseases classified elsewhere

Code first underlying disease

OTHER DEGENERATIVE DISEASES OF THE NERVOUS SYSTEM (G3Ø-G32)

● **G3Ø Alzheimer's disease**

Progressive central neurodegenerative disorder

Includes Alzheimer's dementia senile and presenile forms

Use additional code to identify:
delirium, if applicable (FØ5)
dementia with behavioral disturbance (FØ2.81)
dementia without behavioral disturbance (FØ2.8Ø)

Excludes1 senile degeneration of brain NEC (G31.1)
senile dementia NOS (FØ3)
senility NOS (R41.81)

G3Ø.Ø Alzheimer's disease with early onset

G3Ø.1 Alzheimer's disease with late onset A

G3Ø.8 Other Alzheimer's disease

G3Ø.9 Alzheimer's disease, unspecified

Coding Clinic: 2017, Q1, P43; 2016, Q2, P6; 2012, Q4, P95

● **G31 Other degenerative diseases of nervous system, not elsewhere classified**

For codes G31.Ø-G31.83, G31.85-G31.9, use additional code to identify:
dementia with behavioral disturbance (FØ2.81)
dementia without behavioral disturbance (FØ2.8Ø)

Excludes2 Reye's syndrome (G93.7)

● **G31.Ø Frontotemporal dementia**

G31.Ø1 Pick's disease

Primary progressive aphasia
Progressive isolated aphasia

G31.Ø9 Other frontotemporal dementia

Frontal dementia

G31.1 Senile degeneration of brain, not elsewhere classified

Excludes1 Alzheimer's disease (G3Ø.-)
senility NOS (R41.81)

G31.2 Degeneration of nervous system due to alcohol

Alcoholic cerebellar ataxia
Alcoholic cerebellar degeneration
Alcoholic cerebral degeneration
Alcoholic encephalopathy
Dysfunction of the autonomic nervous system due to alcohol

Code also associated alcoholism (F1Ø.-)

● **G31.8 Other specified degenerative diseases of nervous system**

G31.81 Alpers' disease

Rare neuronal degeneration of cerebral cortex disease of young children

Grey-matter degeneration

Coding Clinic: 2017, Q2, P7

G31.82 Leigh's disease

Rare neurometabolic disorder that affects central nervous system

Subacute necrotizing encephalopathy

G31.83 Dementia with Lewy bodies

Closely allied to Parkinson's Disease

Dementia with Parkinsonism
Lewy body dementia
Lewy body disease

Coding Clinic: 2017, Q2, P7; 2016, Q4, P141

G31.84 Mild cognitive impairment, so stated

Mild neurocognitive disorder

Excludes1 age related cognitive decline (R41.81)
altered mental status (R41.82)
cerebral degeneration (G31.9)
change in mental status (R41.82)
cognitive deficits following (sequelae of) cerebral hemorrhage or infarction (I69.Ø1-, I69.11-, I69.21-, I69.31-, I69.81-, I69.91-)
cognitive impairment due to intracranial or head injury (SØ6.-)
dementia (FØ1.-, FØ2.-, FØ3)
mild memory disturbance (FØ6.8)
neurologic neglect syndrome (R41.4)
personality change, nonpsychotic (F68.8)

G31.85 Corticobasal degeneration

G31.89 Other specified degenerative diseases of nervous system

G31.9 Degenerative disease of nervous system, unspecified

● **G32 Other degenerative disorders of nervous system in diseases classified elsewhere**

G32.Ø Subacute combined degeneration of spinal cord in diseases classified elsewhere

Dana-Putnam syndrome
Sclerosis of spinal cord (combined) (dorsolateral) (posterolateral)

Code first underlying disease, such as:
anemia (D51.9)
dietary (D51.3)
pernicious (D51.Ø)
vitamin B12 deficiency (E53.8)

Excludes1 syphilitic combined degeneration of spinal cord (A52.11)

● G32.8 **Other specified degenerative disorders of nervous system in diseases classified elsewhere**
Code first *underlying disease, such as:*
amyloidosis cerebral degeneration (E85.-)
cerebral degeneration (due to) hypothyroidism (E00.0-E03.9)
cerebral degeneration (due to) neoplasm (C00-D49)
cerebral degeneration (due to) vitamin B deficiency, except thiamine (E52-E53.-)
Excludes1 superior hemorrhagic polioencephalitis [Wernicke's encephalopathy] (E51.2)

G32.81 ***Cerebellar ataxia in diseases classified elsewhere***
Code first underlying disease, such as:
celiac disease (with gluten ataxia) (K90.0)
cerebellar ataxia (in) neoplastic disease (paraneoplastic cerebellar degeneration) (C00-D49)
non-celiac gluten ataxia (M35.9)
Excludes1 systemic atrophy primarily affecting the central nervous system in alcoholic cerebellar ataxia (G31.2)
systemic atrophy primarily affecting the central nervous system in myxedema (G13.2)

G32.89 ***Other specified degenerative disorders of nervous system in diseases classified elsewhere***
Degenerative encephalopathy in diseases classified elsewhere

DEMYELINATING DISEASES OF THE CENTRAL NERVOUS SYSTEM (G35-G37)

G35 **Multiple sclerosis**
Destruction of central nervous system; four types: relapsing remitting, secondary progressive, primary progressive, and progressive relapsing
Disseminated multiple sclerosis
Generalized multiple sclerosis
Multiple sclerosis NOS
Multiple sclerosis of brain stem
Multiple sclerosis of cord

● G36 **Other acute disseminated demyelination**
Excludes1 postinfectious encephalitis and encephalomyelitis NOS (G04.01)

G36.0 **Neuromyelitis optica [Devic]**
Inflammatory disorder in which immune system attacks optic nerves and spinal cord producing inflammation of optic nerve (optic neuritis) and spinal cord (myelitis)
Demyelination in optic neuritis
Excludes1 optic neuritis NOS (H46)

G36.1 **Acute and subacute hemorrhagic leukoencephalitis [Hurst]**

G36.8 **Other specified acute disseminated demyelination**

G36.9 **Acute disseminated demyelination, unspecified**

● G37 **Other demyelinating diseases of central nervous system**
Destruction of central nervous system

G37.0 **Diffuse sclerosis of central nervous system**
Periaxial encephalitis
Schilder's disease
Excludes1 X linked adrenoleukodystrophy (E71.52-)

G37.1 **Central demyelination of corpus callosum**

G37.2 **Central pontine myelinolysis**

Item 6–3 Multiple sclerosis (MS) is a nervous system disease affecting the brain and spinal cord by damaging the myelin sheath surrounding and protecting nerve cells. The damage slows down/blocks messages between the brain and body. Symptoms are visual disturbances, muscle weakness, coordination and balance issues, numbness, prickling, thinking and memory problems. The cause is unknown, though it is thought that it may be an autoimmune disease. It affects women more than men, between 20 and 40 years of age. MS can be mild, but it may cause the loss of ability to write, walk, and speak. There is no cure, but medication may slow or control symptoms.

G37.3 **Acute transverse myelitis in demyelinating disease of central nervous system**
Acute transverse myelitis NOS
Acute transverse myelopathy
Excludes1 multiple sclerosis (G35)
neuromyelitis optica [Devic] (G36.0)

G37.4 **Subacute necrotizing myelitis of central nervous system**

G37.5 **Concentric sclerosis [Baló] of central nervous system**

G37.8 **Other specified demyelinating diseases of central nervous system**

G37.9 **Demyelinating disease of central nervous system, unspecified**

EPISODIC AND PAROXYSMAL DISORDERS (G40-G47)

● G40 **Epilepsy and recurrent seizures**
Note: The following terms are to be considered equivalent to intractable: pharmacoresistant (pharmacologically resistant), treatment resistant, refractory (medically) and poorly controlled
Excludes1 conversion disorder with seizures (F44.5)
convulsions NOS (R56.9)
post traumatic seizures (R56.1)
seizure (convulsive) NOS (R56.9)
seizure of newborn (P90)
Excludes2 hippocampal sclerosis (G93.81)
mesial temporal sclerosis (G93.81)
temporal sclerosis (G93.81)
Todd's paralysis (G83.84)

● G40.0 **Localization-related (focal) (partial) idiopathic epilepsy and epileptic syndromes with seizures of localized onset**
Benign childhood epilepsy with centrotemporal EEG spikes
Childhood epilepsy with occipital EEG paroxysms
Excludes1 adult onset localization-related epilepsy (G40.1-, G40.2-)

● G40.00 **Localization-related (focal) (partial) idiopathic epilepsy and epileptic syndromes with seizures of localized onset, not intractable**
Localization-related (focal) (partial) idiopathic epilepsy and epileptic syndromes with seizures of localized onset without intractability

G40.001 **Localization-related (focal) (partial) idiopathic epilepsy and epileptic syndromes with seizures of localized onset, not intractable, with status epilepticus**

G40.009 **Localization-related (focal) (partial) idiopathic epilepsy and epileptic syndromes with seizures of localized onset, not intractable, without status epilepticus**
Localization-related (focal) (partial) idiopathic epilepsy and epileptic syndromes with seizures of localized onset NOS

● G40.01 **Localization-related (focal) (partial) idiopathic epilepsy and epileptic syndromes with seizures of localized onset, intractable**

G40.011 **Localization-related (focal) (partial) idiopathic epilepsy and epileptic syndromes with seizures of localized onset, intractable, with status epilepticus**

G40.019 **Localization-related (focal) (partial) idiopathic epilepsy and epileptic syndromes with seizures of localized onset, intractable, without status epilepticus**

- **G40.1 Localization-related (focal) (partial) symptomatic epilepsy and epileptic syndromes with simple partial seizures**
  Attacks without alteration of consciousness
  Epilepsia partialis continua [Kozhevnikof]
  Simple partial seizures developing into secondarily generalized seizures
  - **G40.10 Localization-related (focal) (partial) symptomatic epilepsy and epileptic syndromes with simple partial seizures, not intractable**
    Localization-related (focal) (partial) symptomatic epilepsy and epileptic syndromes with simple partial seizures without intractability
    - **G40.101 Localization-related (focal) (partial) symptomatic epilepsy and epileptic syndromes with simple partial seizures, not intractable, with status epilepticus**
    - **G40.109 Localization-related (focal) (partial) symptomatic epilepsy and epileptic syndromes with simple partial seizures, not intractable, without status epilepticus**
      Localization-related (focal) (partial) symptomatic epilepsy and epileptic syndromes with simple partial seizures NOS
  - **G40.11 Localization-related (focal) (partial) symptomatic epilepsy and epileptic syndromes with simple partial seizures, intractable**
    - **G40.111 Localization-related (focal) (partial) symptomatic epilepsy and epileptic syndromes with simple partial seizures, intractable, with status epilepticus**
    - **G40.119 Localization-related (focal) (partial) symptomatic epilepsy and epileptic syndromes with simple partial seizures, intractable, without status epilepticus**
- **G40.2 Localization-related (focal) (partial) symptomatic epilepsy and epileptic syndromes with complex partial seizures**
  Attacks with alteration of consciousness, often with automatisms
  Complex partial seizures developing into secondarily generalized seizures
  - **G40.20 Localization-related (focal) (partial) symptomatic epilepsy and epileptic syndromes with complex partial seizures, not intractable**
    Localization-related (focal) (partial) symptomatic epilepsy and epileptic syndromes with complex partial seizures without intractability
    - **G40.201 Localization-related (focal) (partial) symptomatic epilepsy and epileptic syndromes with complex partial seizures, not intractable, with status epilepticus**
    - **G40.209 Localization-related (focal) (partial) symptomatic epilepsy and epileptic syndromes with complex partial seizures, not intractable, without status epilepticus**
      Localization-related (focal) (partial) symptomatic epilepsy and epileptic syndromes with complex partial seizures NOS
  - **G40.21 Localization-related (focal) (partial) symptomatic epilepsy and epileptic syndromes with complex partial seizures, intractable**
    - **G40.211 Localization-related (focal) (partial) symptomatic epilepsy and epileptic syndromes with complex partial seizures, intractable, with status epilepticus**
    - **G40.219 Localization-related (focal) (partial) symptomatic epilepsy and epileptic syndromes with complex partial seizures, intractable, without status epilepticus**
- **G40.3 Generalized idiopathic epilepsy and epileptic syndromes**
  Code also MERRF syndrome, if applicable (E88.42)
  - **G40.30 Generalized idiopathic epilepsy and epileptic syndromes, not intractable**
    Generalized idiopathic epilepsy and epileptic syndromes without intractability
    - **G40.301 Generalized idiopathic epilepsy and epileptic syndromes, not intractable, with status epilepticus**
    - **G40.309 Generalized idiopathic epilepsy and epileptic syndromes, not intractable, without status epilepticus**
      Generalized idiopathic epilepsy and epileptic syndromes NOS
  - **G40.31 Generalized idiopathic epilepsy and epileptic syndromes, intractable**
    - **G40.311 Generalized idiopathic epilepsy and epileptic syndromes, intractable, with status epilepticus**
    - **G40.319 Generalized idiopathic epilepsy and epileptic syndromes, intractable, without status epilepticus**
- **G40.A Absence epileptic syndrome**
  Childhood absence epilepsy [pyknolepsy]
  Juvenile absence epilepsy
  Absence epileptic syndrome, NOS
  - **G40.A0 Absence epileptic syndrome, not intractable**
    - **G40.A01 Absence epileptic syndrome, not intractable, with status epilepticus**
    - **G40.A09 Absence epileptic syndrome, not intractable, without status epilepticus**
  - **G40.A1 Absence epileptic syndrome, intractable**
    - **G40.A11 Absence epileptic syndrome, intractable, with status epilepticus**
    - **G40.A19 Absence epileptic syndrome, intractable, without status epilepticus**
- **G40.B Juvenile myoclonic epilepsy [impulsive petit mal]**
  - **G40.B0 Juvenile myoclonic epilepsy, not intractable**
    - **G40.B01 Juvenile myoclonic epilepsy, not intractable, with status epilepticus**
    - **G40.B09 Juvenile myoclonic epilepsy, not intractable, without status epilepticus**
  - **G40.B1 Juvenile myoclonic epilepsy, intractable**
    - **G40.B11 Juvenile myoclonic epilepsy, intractable, with status epilepticus**
    - **G40.B19 Juvenile myoclonic epilepsy, intractable, without status epilepticus**

- **G40.4 Other generalized epilepsy and epileptic syndromes**
  Epilepsy with grand mal seizures on awakening
  Epilepsy with myoclonic absences
  Epilepsy with myoclonic-astatic seizures
  Grand mal seizure NOS
  Nonspecific atonic epileptic seizures
  Nonspecific clonic epileptic seizures
  Nonspecific myoclonic epileptic seizures
  Nonspecific tonic epileptic seizures
  Nonspecific tonic-clonic epileptic seizures
  Symptomatic early myoclonic encephalopathy
  - **G40.40 Other generalized epilepsy and epileptic syndromes, not intractable**
    Other generalized epilepsy and epileptic syndromes without intractability
    Other generalized epilepsy and epileptic syndromes NOS
    - **G40.401 Other generalized epilepsy and epileptic syndromes, not intractable, with status epilepticus** HCC
    - **G40.409 Other generalized epilepsy and epileptic syndromes, not intractable, without status epilepticus** HCC
  - **G40.41 Other generalized epilepsy and epileptic syndromes, intractable**
    - **G40.411 Other generalized epilepsy and epileptic syndromes, intractable, with status epilepticus** HCC
    - **G40.419 Other generalized epilepsy and epileptic syndromes, intractable, without status epilepticus** HCC
- **G40.5 Epileptic seizures related to external causes**
  Epileptic seizures related to alcohol
  Epileptic seizures related to drugs
  Epileptic seizures related to hormonal changes
  Epileptic seizures related to sleep deprivation
  Epileptic seizures related to stress
  Code also, if applicable, associated epilepsy and recurrent seizures (G40.-)
  Use additional code for adverse effect, if applicable, to identify drug (T36-T50 with fifth or sixth character 5)
  - **G40.50 Epileptic seizures related to external causes, not intractable**
    - **G40.501 Epileptic seizures related to external causes, not intractable, with status epilepticus** HCC
    - **G40.509 Epileptic seizures related to external causes, not intractable, without status epilepticus** HCC
      Epileptic seizures related to external causes, NOS
- **G40.8 Other epilepsy and recurrent seizures**
  Epilepsies and epileptic syndromes undetermined as to whether they are focal or generalized
  Landau-Kleffner syndrome
  - **G40.80 Other epilepsy**
    - **G40.801 Other epilepsy, not intractable, with status epilepticus** HCC
      Other epilepsy without intractability with status epilepticus
    - **G40.802 Other epilepsy, not intractable, without status epilepticus** HCC
      Other epilepsy NOS
      Other epilepsy without intractability without status epilepticus
    - **G40.803 Other epilepsy, intractable, with status epilepticus** HCC
    - **G40.804 Other epilepsy, intractable, without status epilepticus** HCC
  - **G40.81 Lennox-Gastaut syndrome**
    - **G40.811 Lennox-Gastaut syndrome, not intractable, with status epilepticus** HCC
    - **G40.812 Lennox-Gastaut syndrome, not intractable, without status epilepticus** HCC
    - **G40.813 Lennox-Gastaut syndrome, intractable, with status epilepticus** HCC
    - **G40.814 Lennox-Gastaut syndrome, intractable, without status epilepticus** HCC
  - **G40.82 Epileptic spasms**
    Infantile spasms
    Salaam attacks
    West's syndrome
    - **G40.821 Epileptic spasms, not intractable, with status epilepticus** HCC
    - **G40.822 Epileptic spasms, not intractable, without status epilepticus** HCC
    - **G40.823 Epileptic spasms, intractable, with status epilepticus** HCC
    - **G40.824 Epileptic spasms, intractable, without status epilepticus** HCC
  - **G40.89 Other seizures** HCC
    Excludes1 post traumatic seizures (R56.1)
    recurrent seizures NOS (G40.909)
    seizure NOS (R56.9)
- **G40.9 Epilepsy, unspecified**
  - **G40.90 Epilepsy, unspecified, not intractable**
    Epilepsy, unspecified, without intractability
    - **G40.901 Epilepsy, unspecified, not intractable, with status epilepticus** HCC
    - **G40.909 Epilepsy, unspecified, not intractable, without status epilepticus** HCC
      Epilepsy NOS
      Epileptic convulsions NOS
      Epileptic fits NOS
      Epileptic seizures NOS
      Recurrent seizures NOS
      Seizure disorder NOS
  - **G40.91 Epilepsy, unspecified, intractable**
    Intractable seizure disorder NOS
    - **G40.911 Epilepsy, unspecified, intractable, with status epilepticus** HCC
    - **G40.919 Epilepsy, unspecified, intractable, without status epilepticus** HCC

G43 Migraine

Note: The following terms are to be considered equivalent to intractable: pharmacoresistant (pharmacologically resistant), treatment resistant, refractory (medically) and poorly controlled

Use additional code for adverse effect, if applicable, to identify drug (T36-T50 with fifth or sixth character 5)

Excludes1 headache NOS (R51)
lower half migraine (G44.00)

Excludes2 headache syndromes (G44.-)

- **G43.0 Migraine without aura**
  Neurological disorder, generally recurring headaches without early symptom (aura)
  Common migraine
  Excludes1 chronic migraine without aura (G43.7-)
  - **G43.00 Migraine without aura, not intractable**
    Neurological disorder, generally recurring headaches without early symptom (aura); resistant to cure, relief, or control
    Migraine without aura without mention of refractory migraine
    - **G43.001 Migraine without aura, not intractable, with status migrainosus**
    - **G43.009 Migraine without aura, not intractable, without status migrainosus**
      Migraine without aura NOS

CHAPTER 6 (G00-G99)

Item 6–4 Migraine headache is described as an intense pulsing or throbbing pain in one area of the head. It can be accompanied by extreme sensitivity to light (photophobic) and sound and is three times more common in women than in men. Symptoms include nausea and vomiting. Research indicates migraine headaches are caused by inherited abnormalities in genes that control the activities of certain cell populations in the brain.

● **G43.01 Migraine without aura, intractable**
Intractable migraine: Not easily cured or managed; relentless pain from a migraine
Migraine without aura with refractory migraine
G43.011 Migraine without aura, intractable, with status migrainosus
G43.019 Migraine without aura, intractable, without status migrainosus

● **G43.1 Migraine with aura**
Basilar migraine
Classical migraine
Migraine equivalents
Migraine preceded or accompanied by transient focal neurological phenomena
Migraine triggered seizures
Migraine with acute-onset aura
Migraine with aura without headache (migraine equivalents)
Migraine with prolonged aura
Migraine with typical aura
Retinal migraine
Code also any associated seizure (G40.-, R56.9)
Excludes1 persistent migraine aura (G43.5-, G43.6-)

● **G43.10 Migraine with aura, not intractable**
Migraine with aura without mention of refractory migraine
G43.101 Migraine with aura, not intractable, with status migrainosus
G43.109 Migraine with aura, not intractable, without status migrainosus
Migraine with aura NOS

● **G43.11 Migraine with aura, intractable**
Migraine with aura with refractory migraine
G43.111 Migraine with aura, intractable, with status migrainosus
G43.119 Migraine with aura, intractable, without status migrainosus

● **G43.4 Hemiplegic migraine**
Inherited migraine disorder causing temporary paralysis of one side of body followed by severe headache and nausea
Familial migraine
Sporadic migraine

● **G43.40 Hemiplegic migraine, not intractable**
Hemiplegic migraine without refractory migraine
G43.401 Hemiplegic migraine, not intractable, with status migrainosus
G43.409 Hemiplegic migraine, not intractable, without status migrainosus
Hemiplegic migraine NOS

● **G43.41 Hemiplegic migraine, intractable**
Hemiplegic migraine with refractory migraine
G43.411 Hemiplegic migraine, intractable, with status migrainosus
G43.419 Hemiplegic migraine, intractable, without status migrainosus

● **G43.5 Persistent migraine aura without cerebral infarction**

● **G43.50 Persistent migraine aura without cerebral infarction, not intractable**
Persistent migraine aura without cerebral infarction, without refractory migraine
G43.501 Persistent migraine aura without cerebral infarction, not intractable, with status migrainosus
G43.509 Persistent migraine aura without cerebral infarction, not intractable, without status migrainosus
Persistent migraine aura NOS

● **G43.51 Persistent migraine aura without cerebral infarction, intractable**
Persistent migraine aura without cerebral infarction, with refractory migraine
G43.511 Persistent migraine aura without cerebral infarction, intractable, with status migrainosus
G43.519 Persistent migraine aura without cerebral infarction, intractable, without status migrainosus

● **G43.6 Persistent migraine aura with cerebral infarction**
Visual, motor, or psychic disturbances, paresthesias, and related neurologic abnormalities accompanying migraine
Code also the type of cerebral infarction (I63.-)

● **G43.60 Persistent migraine aura with cerebral infarction, not intractable**
Persistent migraine aura with cerebral infarction, without refractory migraine
G43.601 Persistent migraine aura with cerebral infarction, not intractable, with status migrainosus
G43.609 Persistent migraine aura with cerebral infarction, not intractable, without status migrainosus

● **G43.61 Persistent migraine aura with cerebral infarction, intractable**
Persistent migraine aura with cerebral infarction, with refractory migraine
G43.611 Persistent migraine aura with cerebral infarction, intractable, with status migrainosus
G43.619 Persistent migraine aura with cerebral infarction, intractable, without status migrainosus

● **G43.7 Chronic migraine without aura**
Transformed migraine
Excludes1 migraine without aura (G43.0-)

● **G43.70 Chronic migraine without aura, not intractable**
Chronic migraine without aura, without refractory migraine
G43.701 Chronic migraine without aura, not intractable, with status migrainosus
G43.709 Chronic migraine without aura, not intractable, without status migrainosus
Chronic migraine without aura NOS

● **G43.71 Chronic migraine without aura, intractable**
Chronic migraine without aura, with refractory migraine
G43.711 Chronic migraine without aura, intractable, with status migrainosus
G43.719 Chronic migraine without aura, intractable, without status migrainosus

- **G43.A Cyclical vomiting**
  - **Excludes1** cyclical vomiting syndrome unrelated to migraine (R11.15)
  - **G43.A0 Cyclical vomiting, in migraine, not intractable**
    Cyclical vomiting, without refractory migraine
  - **G43.A1 Cyclical vomiting, in migraine, intractable**
    Cyclical vomiting, with refractory migraine
- **G43.B Ophthalmoplegic migraine**
  - **G43.B0 Ophthalmoplegic migraine, not intractable**
    Ophthalmoplegic migraine, without refractory migraine
  - **G43.B1 Ophthalmoplegic migraine, intractable**
    Ophthalmoplegic migraine, with refractory migraine
- **G43.C Periodic headache syndromes in child or adult**
  - **G43.C0 Periodic headache syndromes in child or adult, not intractable**
    Periodic headache syndromes in child or adult, without refractory migraine
  - **G43.C1 Periodic headache syndromes in child or adult, intractable**
    Periodic headache syndromes in child or adult, with refractory migraine
- **G43.D Abdominal migraine**
  - **G43.D0 Abdominal migraine, not intractable**
    Abdominal migraine, without refractory migraine
  - **G43.D1 Abdominal migraine, intractable**
    Abdominal migraine, with refractory migraine
- **G43.8 Other migraine**
  - **G43.80 Other migraine, not intractable**
    Other migraine, without refractory migraine
    - **G43.801 Other migraine, not intractable, with status migrainosus**
    - **G43.809 Other migraine, not intractable, without status migrainosus**
  - **G43.81 Other migraine, intractable**
    Other migraine, with refractory migraine
    - **G43.811 Other migraine, intractable, with status migrainosus**
    - **G43.819 Other migraine, intractable, without status migrainosus**
  - **G43.82 Menstrual migraine, not intractable**
    Menstrual headache, not intractable
    Menstrual migraine, without refractory migraine
    Menstrually related migraine, not intractable
    Pre-menstrual headache, not intractable
    Pre-menstrual migraine, not intractable
    Pure menstrual migraine, not intractable
    Code also associated premenstrual tension syndrome (N94.3)
    - **G43.821 Menstrual migraine, not intractable, with status migrainosus ♀**
    - **G43.829 Menstrual migraine, not intractable, without status migrainosus ♀**
      Menstrual migraine NOS
  - **G43.83 Menstrual migraine, intractable**
    Menstrual headache, intractable
    Menstrual migraine, with refractory migraine
    Menstrually related migraine, intractable
    Pre-menstrual headache, intractable
    Pre-menstrual migraine, intractable
    Pure menstrual migraine, intractable
    Code also associated premenstrual tension syndrome (N94.3)
    - **G43.831 Menstrual migraine, intractable, with status migrainosus ♀**
    - **G43.839 Menstrual migraine, intractable, without status migrainosus ♀**
- **G43.9 Migraine, unspecified**
  - **G43.90 Migraine, unspecified, not intractable**
    Migraine, unspecified, without refractory migraine
    - **G43.901 Migraine, unspecified, not intractable, with status migrainosus**
      Status migrainosus NOS
    - **G43.909 Migraine, unspecified, not intractable, without status migrainosus**
      Migraine NOS
  - **G43.91 Migraine, unspecified, intractable**
    Migraine, unspecified, with refractory migraine
    - **G43.911 Migraine, unspecified, intractable, with status migrainosus**
    - **G43.919 Migraine, unspecified, intractable, without status migrainosus**

G44 Other headache syndromes

Excludes1 headache NOS (R51)

Excludes2 atypical facial pain (G50.1)
headache due to lumbar puncture (G97.1)
migraines (G43.-)
trigeminal neuralgia (G50.0)

- **G44.0 Cluster headaches and other trigeminal autonomic cephalgias (TAC)**
  - **G44.00 Cluster headache syndrome, unspecified**
    Ciliary neuralgia
    Cluster headache NOS
    Histamine cephalgia
    Lower half migraine
    Migrainous neuralgia
    - **G44.001 Cluster headache syndrome, unspecified, intractable**
    - **G44.009 Cluster headache syndrome, unspecified, not intractable**
      Cluster headache syndrome NOS
  - **G44.01 Episodic cluster headache**
    - **G44.011 Episodic cluster headache, intractable**
    - **G44.019 Episodic cluster headache, not intractable**
      Episodic cluster headache NOS
  - **G44.02 Chronic cluster headache**
    - **G44.021 Chronic cluster headache, intractable**
    - **G44.029 Chronic cluster headache, not intractable**
      Chronic cluster headache NOS
  - **G44.03 Episodic paroxysmal hemicrania**
    Paroxysmal hemicrania NOS
    - **G44.031 Episodic paroxysmal hemicrania, intractable**
    - **G44.039 Episodic paroxysmal hemicrania, not intractable**
      Episodic paroxysmal hemicrania NOS
  - **G44.04 Chronic paroxysmal hemicrania**
    Unilateral headache
    - **G44.041 Chronic paroxysmal hemicrania, intractable**
    - **G44.049 Chronic paroxysmal hemicrania, not intractable**
      Chronic paroxysmal hemicrania NOS

CHAPTER 6 (G00-G99)

● G44.05 **Short lasting unilateral** neuralgiform headache with conjunctival injection and tearing (SUNCT)
- G44.051 Short lasting unilateral neuralgiform headache with conjunctival injection and tearing (SUNCT), **intractable**
- G44.059 Short lasting unilateral neuralgiform headache with conjunctival injection and tearing (SUNCT), **not intractable**
  - Short lasting unilateral neuralgiform headache with conjunctival injection and tearing (SUNCT) NOS

● G44.09 **Other trigeminal autonomic cephalgias (TAC)**
Cluster headaches
- G44.091 Other trigeminal autonomic cephalgias (TAC), **intractable**
- G44.099 Other trigeminal autonomic cephalgias (TAC), **not intractable**

G44.1 **Vascular** headache, not elsewhere classified

Excludes2 cluster headache (G44.Ø)
complicated headache syndromes (G44.5-)
drug-induced headache (G44.4-)
migraine (G43.-)
other specified headache syndromes (G44.8-)
post-traumatic headache (G44.3-)
tension-type headache (G44.2-)

● G44.2 **Tension-type** headache

● G44.2Ø Tension-type headache, **unspecified**
- G44.2Ø1 Tension-type headache, unspecified, **intractable**
- G44.2Ø9 Tension-type headache, unspecified, **not intractable**
  - Tension headache NOS

● G44.21 **Episodic** tension-type headache
- G44.211 Episodic tension-type headache, **intractable**
- G44.219 Episodic tension-type headache, **not intractable**
  - Episodic tension-type headache NOS

● G44.22 **Chronic** tension-type headache
- G44.221 Chronic tension-type headache, **intractable**
- G44.229 Chronic tension-type headache, **not intractable**
  - Chronic tension-type headache NOS

● G44.3 **Post-traumatic** headache

● G44.3Ø Post-traumatic headache, **unspecified**
- G44.3Ø1 Post-traumatic headache, unspecified, **intractable**
- G44.3Ø9 Post-traumatic headache, unspecified, **not intractable**
  - Post-traumatic headache NOS

● G44.31 **Acute** post-traumatic headache
- G44.311 Acute post-traumatic headache, **intractable**
- G44.319 Acute post-traumatic headache, **not intractable**
  - Acute post-traumatic headache NOS

● G44.32 **Chronic** post-traumatic headache
- G44.321 Chronic post-traumatic headache, **intractable**
- G44.329 Chronic post-traumatic headache, **not intractable**
  - Chronic post-traumatic headache NOS

● G44.4 **Drug-induced** headache, not elsewhere classified
Medication overuse headache
Use additional code for adverse effect, if applicable, to identify drug (T36-T5Ø with fifth or sixth character 5)
- G44.4Ø Drug-induced headache, not elsewhere classified, **not intractable**
- G44.41 Drug-induced headache, not elsewhere classified, **intractable**

● G44.5 **Complicated** headache syndromes
- G44.51 **Hemicrania continua**
  - *Persistent unilateral headache*
- G44.52 **New daily persistent headache (NDPH)**
- G44.53 **Primary thunderclap headache**
- G44.59 **Other complicated headache syndrome**

● G44.8 **Other** specified headache syndromes
- G44.81 **Hypnic** headache
  - *Benign primary headaches*
- G44.82 **Headache associated with sexual activity**
  - Orgasmic headache
  - Preorgasmic headache
- G44.83 Primary **cough** headache
- G44.84 Primary **exertional** headache
- G44.85 Primary **stabbing** headache
- G44.89 **Other** headache syndrome

● G45 Transient cerebral ischemic attacks and related syndromes

Excludes1 neonatal cerebral ischemia (P91.Ø)
transient retinal artery occlusion (H34.Ø-)

Coding Clinic: 2Ø18, Q2, P9

- G45.Ø Vertebro-basilar artery syndrome
- G45.1 Carotid artery syndrome (hemispheric)
- G45.2 Multiple and bilateral precerebral artery syndromes
- G45.3 Amaurosis fugax
  - *Transient visual loss in one eye*
- G45.4 Transient global amnesia
  - *Episode of short-term memory loss, nonrecurrent, lasting few hours*
  - **Excludes1** amnesia NOS (R41.3)
- G45.8 Other transient cerebral ischemic attacks and related syndromes
- G45.9 Transient cerebral ischemic attack, **unspecified**
  - Spasm of cerebral artery
  - TIA
  - Transient cerebral ischemia NOS

● G46 Vascular syndromes of brain in cerebrovascular diseases

Code first underlying cerebrovascular disease (I6Ø-I69)

- G46.Ø **Middle** cerebral artery syndrome
- G46.1 **Anterior** cerebral artery syndrome
- G46.2 **Posterior** cerebral artery syndrome
- G46.3 **Brain stem stroke** syndrome
  - Benedikt syndrome
  - Claude syndrome
  - Foville syndrome
  - Millard-Gubler syndrome
  - Wallenberg syndrome
  - Weber syndrome
- G46.4 **Cerebellar stroke** syndrome
- G46.5 **Pure motor lacunar** syndrome
  - *Occlusion of single deep penetrating artery*
- G46.6 **Pure sensory lacunar** syndrome
- G46.7 **Other lacunar** syndromes
- G46.8 **Other** vascular syndromes of brain in cerebrovascular diseases

CHAPTER 6 (GØØ-G99)

G47 Sleep disorders

Excludes2 nightmares (F51.5)
nonorganic sleep disorders (F51.-)
sleep terrors (F51.4)
sleepwalking (F51.3)

G47.Ø Insomnia

Excludes2 alcohol related insomnia (F1Ø.182, F1Ø.282, F1Ø.982)
drug-related insomnia (F11.182, F11.282, F11.982, F13.182, F13.282, F13.982, F14.182, F14.282, F14.982, F15.182, F15.282, F15.982, F19.182, F19.282, F19.982)
idiopathic insomnia (F51.Ø1)
insomnia due to a mental disorder (F51.Ø5)
insomnia not due to a substance or known physiological condition (F51.Ø-)
nonorganic insomnia (F51.Ø-)
primary insomnia (F51.Ø1)
sleep apnea (G47.3-)

G47.ØØ Insomnia, unspecified
Insomnia NOS

G47.Ø1 Insomnia due to medical condition
Code also associated medical condition

G47.Ø9 Other insomnia

G47.1 Hypersomnia

Excludes2 alcohol-related hypersomnia (F1Ø.182, F1Ø.282, F1Ø.982)
drug-related hypersomnia (F11.182, F11.282, F11.982, F13.182, F13.282, F13.982, F14.182, F14.282, F14.982, F15.182, F15.282, F15.982, F19.182, F19.282, F19.982)
hypersomnia due to a mental disorder (F51.13)
hypersomnia not due to a substance or known physiological condition (F51.1-)
primary hypersomnia (F51.11)
sleep apnea (G47.3-)

G47.1Ø Hypersomnia, unspecified
Hypersomnia NOS

G47.11 Idiopathic hypersomnia with long sleep time
Idiopathic hypersomnia NOS

G47.12 Idiopathic hypersomnia without long sleep time

G47.13 Recurrent hypersomnia
Kleine-Levin syndrome
Menstrual related hypersomnia

G47.14 Hypersomnia due to medical condition
Code also associated medical condition

G47.19 Other hypersomnia

G47.2 Circadian rhythm sleep disorders
Disorders of the sleep wake schedule
Inversion of nyctohemeral rhythm
Inversion of sleep rhythm

G47.2Ø Circadian rhythm sleep disorder, unspecified type
Sleep wake schedule disorder NOS

G47.21 Circadian rhythm sleep disorder, delayed sleep phase type
Delayed sleep phase syndrome

G47.22 Circadian rhythm sleep disorder, advanced sleep phase type

G47.23 Circadian rhythm sleep disorder, irregular sleep wake type
Irregular sleep-wake pattern

G47.24 Circadian rhythm sleep disorder, free running type
Circadian rhythm sleep disorder, non-24-hour sleep-wake type

G47.25 Circadian rhythm sleep disorder, jet lag type

G47.26 Circadian rhythm sleep disorder, shift work type

G47.27 Circadian rhythm sleep disorder in conditions classified elsewhere
Code first underlying condition

G47.29 Other circadian rhythm sleep disorder

G47.3 Sleep apnea
Characterized by episodes in which breathing stops during sleep
Code also any associated underlying condition

Excludes1 apnea NOS (RØ6.81)
Cheyne-Stokes breathing (RØ6.3)
pickwickian syndrome (E66.2)
sleep apnea of newborn (P28.3)

G47.3Ø Sleep apnea, unspecified
Sleep apnea NOS

G47.31 Primary central sleep apnea
Idiopathic central sleep apnea

G47.32 High altitude periodic breathing

G47.33 Obstructive sleep apnea (adult) (pediatric)
Obstructive sleep apnea hypopnea

Excludes1 obstructive sleep apnea of newborn (P28.3)

G47.34 Idiopathic sleep related nonobstructive alveolar hypoventilation
Sleep related hypoxia

G47.35 Congenital central alveolar hypoventilation syndrome

G47.36 Sleep related hypoventilation in conditions classified elsewhere
Sleep related hypoxemia in conditions classified elsewhere
Code first underlying condition

G47.37 **Central** ***sleep apnea in conditions classified elsewhere***
Code first underlying condition

G47.39 Other sleep apnea

G47.4 Narcolepsy and cataplexy
***Cataplexy** is a disorder evidenced by seizures including minor slacking of the facial muscles to complete collapse and often affects people who have **narcolepsy**, a disorder in which there is great difficulty remaining awake during the daytime.*

G47.41 Narcolepsy

G47.411 Narcolepsy with cataplexy

G47.419 Narcolepsy without cataplexy
Narcolepsy NOS

G47.42 Narcolepsy in conditions classified elsewhere
Code first underlying condition

G47.421 Narcolepsy in conditions classified elsewhere with cataplexy

G47.429 Narcolepsy in conditions classified elsewhere without cataplexy

G47.5 Parasomnia

Excludes1 alcohol induced parasomnia (F1Ø.182, F1Ø.282, F1Ø.982)
drug induced parasomnia (F11.182, F11.282, F11.982, F13.182, F13.282, F13.982, F14.182, F14.282, F14.982, F15.182, F15.282, F15.982, F19.182, F19.282, F19.982)
parasomnia not due to a substance or known physiological condition (F51.8)

G47.5Ø Parasomnia, unspecified
Parasomnia NOS

G47.51 Confusional arousals

G47.52 REM sleep behavior disorder

G47.53 Recurrent isolated sleep paralysis

G47.54 Parasomnia in conditions classified elsewhere
Code first underlying condition

G47.59 Other parasomnia

● **G47.6 Sleep related movement disorders**
Excludes2 restless legs syndrome (G25.81)
G47.61 **Periodic limb movement disorder**
G47.62 **Sleep related leg cramps**
G47.63 **Sleep related bruxism**
Excludes1 psychogenic bruxism (F45.8)
Coding Clinic: 2016, Q4, P118
G47.69 **Other sleep related movement disorders**
G47.8 **Other sleep disorders**
Other specified sleep-wake disorder
G47.9 **Sleep disorder, unspecified**
Sleep disorder NOS
Unspecified sleep-wake disorder

★ **(See Plate 6 of the Anatomy Illustrations.)**

NERVE, NERVE ROOT AND PLEXUS DISORDERS (G50-G59)

Excludes1 current traumatic nerve, nerve root and plexus disorders - see Injury, nerve by body region
neuralgia NOS (M79.2)
neuritis NOS (M79.2)
peripheral neuritis in pregnancy (O26.82-)
radiculitis NOS (M54.1-)

● **G50 Disorders of trigeminal nerve**
Includes disorders of 5th cranial nerve
G50.0 **Trigeminal neuralgia**
Syndrome of paroxysmal facial pain
Tic douloureux
G50.1 **Atypical facial pain**
G50.8 **Other disorders of trigeminal nerve**
G50.9 **Disorder of trigeminal nerve, unspecified**

● **G51 Facial nerve disorders**
Includes disorders of 7th cranial nerve
G51.0 **Bell's palsy**
Facial palsy
G51.1 **Geniculate ganglionitis**
Rare disorder with symptoms of severe pain deep in ear, spreading to ear canal, outer ear, mastoid or eye regions
Excludes1 postherpetic geniculate ganglionitis (B02.21)
G51.2 **Melkersson's syndrome**
Melkersson-Rosenthal syndrome
● G51.3 **Clonic hemifacial spasm**
G51.31 **Clonic hemifacial spasm, right**
G51.32 **Clonic hemifacial spasm, left**
Coding Clinic: 2018, Q4, P10
G51.33 **Clonic hemifacial spasm, bilateral**
G51.39 **Clonic hemifacial spasm, unspecified**
G51.4 **Facial myokymia**
Involuntary facial muscle movement
G51.8 **Other disorders of facial nerve**
G51.9 **Disorder of facial nerve, unspecified**

● **G52 Disorders of other cranial nerves**
Excludes2 disorders of acoustic [8th] nerve (H93.3)
disorders of optic [2nd] nerve (H46, H47.0)
paralytic strabismus due to nerve palsy (H49.0-H49.2)
G52.0 **Disorders of olfactory nerve**
Disorders of 1st cranial nerve
G52.1 **Disorders of glossopharyngeal nerve**
Disorder of 9th cranial nerve
Glossopharyngeal neuralgia
G52.2 **Disorders of vagus nerve**
Disorders of pneumogastric [10th] nerve
G52.3 **Disorders of hypoglossal nerve**
Disorders of 12th cranial nerve
G52.7 **Disorders of multiple cranial nerves**
Polyneuritis cranialis
G52.8 **Disorders of other specified cranial nerves**
G52.9 **Cranial nerve disorder, unspecified**

G53 Cranial nerve disorders in diseases classified elsewhere
Code first underlying disease, such as:
neoplasm (C00-D49)
Excludes1 multiple cranial nerve palsy in sarcoidosis (D86.82)
multiple cranial nerve palsy in syphilis (A52.15)
postherpetic geniculate ganglionitis (B02.21)
postherpetic trigeminal neuralgia (B02.22)

● **G54 Nerve root and plexus disorders**
Raiculopathy (nerve root disorder) caused by pressure on nerve root, most common cause is herniation of intervertebral disk. Plexus disorders (plexopathies) are due to compression or injury.
Excludes1 current traumatic nerve root and plexus disorders - see nerve injury by body region
intervertebral disc disorders (M50-M51)
neuralgia or neuritis NOS (M79.2)
neuritis or radiculitis brachial NOS (M54.13)
neuritis or radiculitis lumbar NOS (M54.16)
neuritis or radiculitis lumbosacral NOS (M54.17)
neuritis or radiculitis thoracic NOS (M54.14)
radiculitis NOS (M54.10)
radiculopathy NOS (M54.10)
spondylosis (M47.-)
G54.0 **Brachial plexus disorders**
Thoracic outlet syndrome
G54.1 **Lumbosacral plexus disorders**
G54.2 **Cervical root disorders, not elsewhere classified**
G54.3 **Thoracic root disorders, not elsewhere classified**
G54.4 **Lumbosacral root disorders, not elsewhere classified**
G54.5 **Neuralgic amyotrophy**
Parsonage-Aldren-Turner syndrome
Shoulder-girdle neuritis
Excludes1 neuralgic amyotrophy in diabetes mellitus (E08-E13 with .44)
G54.6 **Phantom limb syndrome with pain**
Sensations (cramping, itching) in a limb that no longer exists
G54.7 **Phantom limb syndrome without pain**
Phantom limb syndrome NOS
G54.8 **Other nerve root and plexus disorders**
G54.9 **Nerve root and plexus disorder, unspecified**

Item 6–5 Trigeminal neuralgia, tic douloureux, is a pain syndrome diagnosed from the patient's history alone. The condition is characterized by pain and a brief facial spasm or tic. Pain is unilateral and follows the sensory distribution of cranial nerve V, typically radiating to the maxillary (V2) or mandibular (V3) area.

Item 6–6 The most common facial nerve disorder is **Bell's Palsy,** which occurs suddenly and results in facial drooping unilaterally. This disorder is the result of a reaction to a virus that causes the facial nerve in the ear to swell, resulting in pressure in the bony canal.

G55 Nerve root and plexus compressions in diseases classified elsewhere
Code first underlying disease, such as:
neoplasm (CØØ-D49)
Excludes1 nerve root compression (due to) (in) ankylosing spondylitis (M45.-)
nerve root compression (due to) (in)dorsopathies (M53.-, M54.-)
nerve root compression (due to) (in)intervertebral disc disorders (M5Ø.1.-, M51.1.-)
nerve root compression (due to) (in) spondylopathies (M46.-, M48.-)

★**(See Plates 472 and 473 on pages 56 and 57.)**

G56 Mononeuropathies of upper limb
Excludes1 current traumatic nerve disorder - see nerve injury by body region

G56.Ø Carpal tunnel syndrome
G56.ØØ Carpal tunnel syndrome, **unspecified** upper limb
G56.Ø1 Carpal tunnel syndrome, **right** upper limb
G56.Ø2 Carpal tunnel syndrome, **left** upper limb
G56.Ø3 Carpal tunnel syndrome, **bilateral** upper limbs
Coding Clinic: 2Ø16, Q4, P17

G56.1 Other lesions of median nerve
G56.1Ø Other lesions of median nerve, **unspecified** side
G56.11 Other lesions of median nerve, **right** upper limb
G56.12 Other lesions of median nerve, **left** upper limb
G56.13 Other lesions of median nerve, **bilateral** upper limbs
Coding Clinic: 2Ø16, Q4, P17

G56.2 Lesion of ulnar nerve
Tardy ulnar nerve palsy
G56.2Ø Lesion of ulnar nerve, **unspecified** upper limb
G56.21 Lesion of ulnar nerve, **right** upper limb
G56.22 Lesion of ulnar nerve, **left** upper limb
G56.23 Lesion of ulnar nerve, **bilateral** upper limbs
Coding Clinic: 2Ø16, Q4, P17

G56.3 Lesion of radial nerve
G56.3Ø Lesion of radial nerve, **unspecified** upper limb
G56.31 Lesion of radial nerve, **right** upper limb
G56.32 Lesion of radial nerve, **left** upper limb
G56.33 Lesion of radial nerve, **bilateral** upper limbs
Coding Clinic: 2Ø16, Q4, P17

G56.4 Causalgia of upper limb
Intense burning pain and sensitivity to slight touch
Complex regional pain syndrome II of upper limb
Excludes1 complex regional pain syndrome I of lower limb (G9Ø.52-)
complex regional pain syndrome I of upper limb (G9Ø.51-)
complex regional pain syndrome II of lower limb (G57.7-)
reflex sympathetic dystrophy of lower limb (G9Ø.52-)
reflex sympathetic dystrophy (G9Ø.51-)
G56.4Ø Causalgia of **unspecified** upper limb
G56.41 Causalgia of **right** upper limb
G56.42 Causalgia of **left** upper limb
G56.43 Causalgia of **bilateral** upper limbs
Coding Clinic: 2Ø16, Q4, P17

G56.8 Other specified mononeuropathies of upper limb
Disease of a single nerve
Interdigital neuroma of upper limb
G56.8Ø Other specified mononeuropathies of **unspecified** upper limb
G56.81 Other specified mononeuropathies of **right** upper limb
G56.82 Other specified mononeuropathies of **left** upper limb
G56.83 Other specified mononeuropathies of **bilateral** upper limbs
Coding Clinic: 2Ø16, Q4, P17

G56.9 Unspecified mononeuropathy of upper limb
Disease of a single nerve
G56.9Ø Unspecified mononeuropathy of **unspecified** upper limb
G56.91 Unspecified mononeuropathy of **right** upper limb
G56.92 Unspecified mononeuropathy of **left** upper limb
G56.93 Unspecified mononeuropathy of **bilateral** upper limbs
Coding Clinic: 2Ø16, Q4, P17

G57 Mononeuropathies of lower limb
Excludes1 current traumatic nerve disorder - see nerve injury by body region

★**(See Plates 544 and 545 on pages 58 and 59.)**

G57.Ø Lesion of sciatic nerve
Excludes1 sciatica NOS (M54.3-)
Excludes2 sciatica attributed to intervertebral disc disorder (M51.1.-)
G57.ØØ Lesion of sciatic nerve, **unspecified** lower limb
G57.Ø1 Lesion of sciatic nerve, **right** lower limb
G57.Ø2 Lesion of sciatic nerve, **left** lower limb
G57.Ø3 Lesion of sciatic nerve, **bilateral** lower limbs
Coding Clinic: 2Ø16, Q4, P1

G57.1 Meralgia paresthetica
Numbness or pain in outer thigh caused by injury to nerve
Lateral cutaneous nerve of thigh syndrome
G57.1Ø Meralgia paresthetica, **unspecified** lower limb
G57.11 Meralgia paresthetica, **right** lower limb
G57.12 Meralgia paresthetica, **left** lower limb
G57.13 Meralgia paresthetica, **bilateral** lower limbs
Coding Clinic: 2Ø16, Q4, P1

G57.2 Lesion of femoral nerve
G57.2Ø Lesion of femoral nerve, **unspecified** lower limb
G57.21 Lesion of femoral nerve, **right** lower limb
G57.22 Lesion of femoral nerve, **left** lower limb
G57.23 Lesion of femoral nerve, **bilateral** lower limbs
Coding Clinic: 2Ø16, Q4, P1

G57.3 Lesion of lateral popliteal nerve
Peroneal nerve palsy
G57.3Ø Lesion of lateral popliteal nerve, **unspecified** lower limb
G57.31 Lesion of lateral popliteal nerve, **right** lower limb
G57.32 Lesion of lateral popliteal nerve, **left** lower limb
G57.33 Lesion of lateral popliteal nerve, **bilateral** lower limbs
Coding Clinic: 2Ø16, Q4, P1

G57.4 Lesion of medial popliteal nerve
G57.4Ø Lesion of medial popliteal nerve, **unspecified** lower limb
G57.41 Lesion of medial popliteal nerve, **right** lower limb
G57.42 Lesion of medial popliteal nerve, **left** lower limb
G57.43 Lesion of medial popliteal nerve, **bilateral** lower limbs
Coding Clinic: 2Ø16, Q4, P1

CHAPTER 6 (GØØ-G99)

● G57.5 **Tarsal tunnel syndrome**
- G57.50 **Tarsal tunnel syndrome, unspecified lower limb**
- G57.51 **Tarsal tunnel syndrome, right lower limb**
- G57.52 **Tarsal tunnel syndrome, left lower limb**
- G57.53 **Tarsal tunnel syndrome, bilateral lower limbs**
  Coding Clinic: 2016, Q4, P1

● G57.6 **Lesion of plantar nerve**
Morton's metatarsalgia
- G57.60 **Lesion of plantar nerve, unspecified lower limb**
- G57.61 **Lesion of plantar nerve, right lower limb**
- G57.62 **Lesion of plantar nerve, left lower limb**
- G57.63 **Lesion of plantar nerve, bilateral lower limbs**
  Coding Clinic: 2016, Q4, P1

● G57.7 **Causalgia of lower limb**
Complex regional pain syndrome II of lower limb
Excludes1 complex regional pain syndrome I of lower limb (G90.52-)
complex regional pain syndrome I of upper limb (G90.51-)
complex regional pain syndrome II of upper limb (G56.4-)
reflex sympathetic dystrophy of lower limb (G90.52-)
reflex sympathetic dystrophy of upper limb (G90.51-)
- G57.70 **Causalgia of unspecified lower limb**
- G57.71 **Causalgia of right lower limb**
- G57.72 **Causalgia of left lower limb**
- G57.73 **Causalgia of bilateral lower limbs**
  Coding Clinic: 2016, Q4, P1

● G57.8 **Other specified mononeuropathies of lower limb**
Interdigital neuroma of lower limb
- G57.80 **Other specified mononeuropathies of unspecified lower limb**
- G57.81 **Other specified mononeuropathies of right lower limb**
- G57.82 **Other specified mononeuropathies of left lower limb**
- G57.83 **Other specified mononeuropathies of bilateral lower limbs**
  Coding Clinic: 2016, Q4, P17

● G57.9 **Unspecified mononeuropathy of lower limb**
- G57.90 **Unspecified mononeuropathy of unspecified lower limb**
- G57.91 **Unspecified mononeuropathy of right lower limb**
- G57.92 **Unspecified mononeuropathy of left lower limb**
- G57.93 **Unspecified mononeuropathy of bilateral lower limbs**
  Coding Clinic: 2016, Q4, P17

● G58 **Other mononeuropathies**
- G58.0 **Intercostal neuropathy**
- G58.7 **Mononeuritis multiplex**
- G58.8 **Other specified mononeuropathies**
- G58.9 **Mononeuropathy, unspecified**

G59 Mononeuropathy in diseases classified elsewhere
Code first underlying disease
Excludes1 diabetic mononeuropathy (E08-E13 with .41)
syphilitic nerve paralysis (A52.19)
syphilitic neuritis (A52.15)
tuberculous mononeuropathy (A17.83)

POLYNEUROPATHIES AND OTHER DISORDERS OF THE PERIPHERAL NERVOUS SYSTEM (G60-G65)

Excludes1 neuralgia NOS (M79.2)
neuritis NOS (M79.2)
peripheral neuritis in pregnancy (O26.82-)
radiculitis NOS (M54.10)

● G60 **Hereditary and idiopathic neuropathy**
- G60.0 **Hereditary motor and sensory neuropathy**
  Charcot-Marie-Tooth disease
  Déjerine-Sottas disease
  Hereditary motor and sensory neuropathy, types I-IV
  Hypertrophic neuropathy of infancy
  Peroneal muscular atrophy (axonal type) (hypertrophic type)
  Roussy-Lévy syndrome
- G60.1 **Refsum's disease**
  Genetic disorder affecting fatty acid metabolism
  Infantile Refsum disease
- G60.2 **Neuropathy in association with hereditary ataxia**
- G60.3 **Idiopathic progressive neuropathy**
- G60.8 **Other hereditary and idiopathic neuropathies**
  Dominantly inherited sensory neuropathy
  Morvan's disease
  Nelaton's syndrome
  Recessively inherited sensory neuropathy
- G60.9 **Hereditary and idiopathic neuropathy, unspecified**

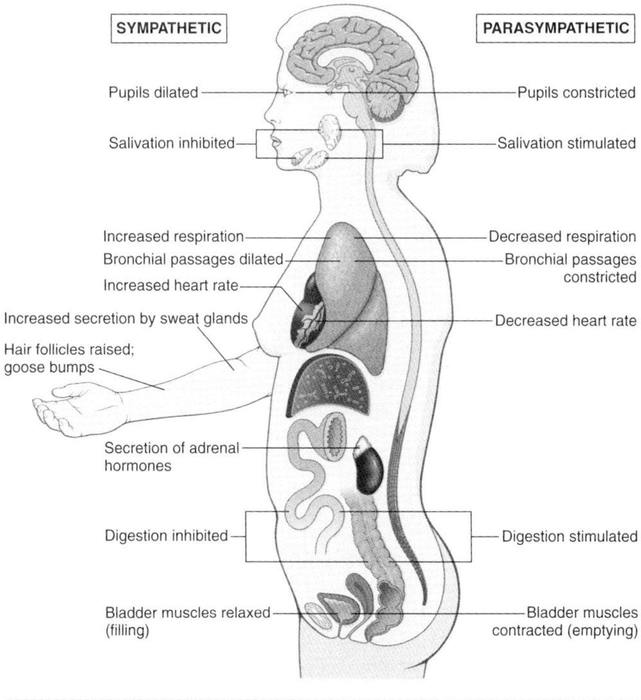

Figure 6-2 Actions of parasympathetic and sympathetic nerves. (From Chabner: The Language of Medicine, ed 9, St. Louis, Saunders, 2011)

Item 6-7 The **peripheral nervous system** consists of 31 pairs of spinal nerves, 12 pairs of cranial nerves, and the autonomic nerves, which are divided into the parasympathetic and sympathetic nerves. The cranial nerves are: olfactory (I), optic (II), oculomotor (III), trochlear (IV), trigeminal (V), abducens (VI), facial (VII), vestibulocochlear (VIII), glossopharyngeal (IX), vagus (X), accessory (XI), and hypoglossal (XII).

● G61 **Inflammatory polyneuropathy**
- G61.Ø **Guillain-Barré syndrome**
  Autoimmune disease affecting peripheral nervous system
  Acute (post-)infective polyneuritis
  Miller Fisher Syndrome
- G61.1 **Serum neuropathy**
  Use additional code for adverse effect, if applicable, to identify serum (T5Ø.-)
- ● G61.8 **Other inflammatory polyneuropathies**
  - G61.81 **Chronic inflammatory demyelinating polyneuritis**
  - G61.82 **Multifocal motor neuropathy**
    MMN
  - G61.89 **Other inflammatory polyneuropathies**
- G61.9 **Inflammatory polyneuropathy, unspecified**

● G62 **Other and unspecified polyneuropathies**
- G62.Ø **Drug-induced polyneuropathy**
  Use additional code for adverse effect, if applicable, to identify drug (T36-T5Ø with fifth or sixth character 5)
- G62.1 **Alcoholic polyneuropathy**
  Malfunction of many peripheral nerves throughout the body
- G62.2 **Polyneuropathy due to other toxic agents**
  Code first (T51-T65) to identify toxic agent
- ● G62.8 **Other specified polyneuropathies**
  - G62.81 **Critical illness polyneuropathy**
    Acute motor neuropathy
  - G62.82 **Radiation-induced polyneuropathy**
    Use additional external cause code (W88-W9Ø, X39.Ø-) to identify cause
    Coding Clinic: 2016, Q4, P18
  - G62.89 **Other specified polyneuropathies**
    Coding Clinic: 2016, Q2, P11
- G62.9 **Polyneuropathy, unspecified**
  Neuropathy NOS

G63 Polyneuropathy in diseases classified elsewhere
Code first underlying disease, such as:
amyloidosis (E85.-)
endocrine disease, except diabetes (EØØ-EØ7, E15-E16, E2Ø-E34)
metabolic diseases (E7Ø-E88)
neoplasm (CØØ-D49)
nutritional deficiency (E4Ø-E64)
Excludes1 polyneuropathy (in):
diabetes mellitus (EØ8-E13 with .42)
diphtheria (A36.83)
infectious mononucleosis (B27.Ø-B27.9 with 1)
Lyme disease (A69.22)
mumps (B26.84)
postherpetic (BØ2.23)
rheumatoid arthritis (MØ5.5-)
scleroderma (M34.83)
systemic lupus erythematosus (M32.19)
Coding Clinic: 2012, Q4, P1ØØ

G64 **Other disorders of peripheral nervous system**
Disorder of peripheral nervous system NOS

● G65 **Sequelae of inflammatory and toxic polyneuropathies**
Code first condition resulting from (sequela) of inflammatory and toxic polyneuropathies
- G65.Ø **Sequelae of Guillain-Barré syndrome**
- G65.1 **Sequelae of other inflammatory polyneuropathy**
- G65.2 **Sequelae of toxic polyneuropathy**

DISEASES OF MYONEURAL JUNCTION AND MUSCLE (G7Ø-G73)

● G7Ø **Myasthenia gravis and other myoneural disorders**
Excludes1 botulism (AØ5.1, A48.51-A48.52)
transient neonatal myasthenia gravis (P94.Ø)
- ● G7Ø.Ø **Myasthenia gravis**
  Acquired and results in fatigable muscle weakness exacerbated by activity and improved with rest
  - G7Ø.ØØ **Myasthenia gravis without (acute) exacerbation**
    Myasthenia gravis NOS
  - G7Ø.Ø1 **Myasthenia gravis with (acute) exacerbation**
    Myasthenia gravis in crisis
- G7Ø.1 **Toxic myoneural disorders**
  Dysfunction at junction of muscle and motor nerve (myoneural junction)
  Code first (T51-T65) to identify toxic agent
- G7Ø.2 **Congenital and developmental myasthenia**
- ● G7Ø.8 **Other specified myoneural disorders**
  - G7Ø.8Ø **Lambert-Eaton syndrome, unspecified**
    Lambert-Eaton syndrome NOS
  - *G7Ø.81 Lambert-Eaton syndrome in disease classified elsewhere*
    Code first underlying disease
    Excludes1 Lambert-Eaton syndrome in neoplastic disease (G73.1)
  - G7Ø.89 **Other specified myoneural disorders**
- G7Ø.9 **Myoneural disorder, unspecified**

● G71 **Primary disorders of muscles**
Excludes2 arthrogryposis multiplex congenita (Q74.3)
metabolic disorders (E7Ø-E88)
myositis (M6Ø.-)
- ● G71.Ø **Muscular dystrophy**
  - G71.ØØ **Muscular dystrophy, unspecified**
  - G71.Ø1 **Duchenne or Becker muscular dystrophy**
    Autosomal recessive, childhood type, muscular dystrophy resembling Duchenne or Becker muscular dystrophy
    Benign [Becker] muscular dystrophy
    Severe [Duchenne] muscular dystrophy
  - G71.Ø2 **Facioscapulohumeral muscular dystrophy**
    Scapulohumeral muscular dystrophy
    Coding Clinic: 2018, Q4, P12
  - G71.Ø9 **Other specified muscular dystrophies**
    Benign scapuloperoneal muscular dystrophy with early contractures [Emery-Dreifuss]
    Congenital muscular dystrophy NOS
    Congenital muscular dystrophy with specific morphological abnormalities of the muscle fiber
    Distal muscular dystrophy
    Limb-girdle muscular dystrophy
    Ocular muscular dystrophy
    Oculopharyngeal muscular dystrophy
    Scapuloperoneal muscular dystrophy

Item 6–8 Muscular dystrophies (MD) are a group of rare inherited muscle diseases. Voluntary muscles become progressively weaker. In the late stages of MD, fat and connective tissue replace muscle fibers. In some types of muscular dystrophy, heart muscles, other involuntary muscles, and other organs are affected. **Myopathies** is a general term for neuromuscular diseases in which the muscle fibers dysfunction for any one of many reasons, resulting in muscular weakness.

G71.1 Myotonic disorders
Inherited disorder that affects muscles tone

G71.11 Myotonic muscular dystrophy
Dystrophia myotonica [Steinert]
Myotonia atrophica
Myotonic dystrophy
Proximal myotonic myopathy (PROMM)
Steinert disease

G71.12 Myotonia congenita
Acetazolamide responsive myotonia congenita
Dominant myotonia congenita [Thomsen disease]
Myotonia levior
Recessive myotonia congenita [Becker disease]

G71.13 Myotonic chondrodystrophy
Chondrodystrophic myotonia
Congenital myotonic chondrodystrophy
Schwartz-Jampel disease

G71.14 Drug induced myotonia
Use additional code for adverse effect, if applicable, to identify drug (T36-T50 with fifth or sixth character 5)

G71.19 Other specified myotonic disorders
Myotonia fluctuans
Myotonia permanens
Neuromyotonia [Isaacs]
Paramyotonia congenita (of von Eulenburg)
Pseudomyotonia
Symptomatic myotonia

G71.2 Congenital myopathies
Central core disease
Fiber-type disproportion
Minicore disease
Multicore disease
Myotubular (centronuclear) myopathy
Nemaline myopathy
Excludes1 arthrogryposis multiplex congenita (Q74.3)

G71.3 Mitochondrial myopathy, not elsewhere classified
Myopathies associated with increased number of enlarged, often abnormal, mitochondria in muscle fibers
Excludes1 Kearns-Sayre syndrome (H49.81)
Leber's disease (H47.21)
Leigh's encephalopathy (G31.82)
mitochondrial metabolism disorders (E88.4.-)
Reye's syndrome (G93.7)

G71.8 Other primary disorders of muscles

G71.9 Primary disorder of muscle, unspecified
Hereditary myopathy NOS

G72 Other and unspecified myopathies
Excludes1 arthrogryposis multiplex congenita (Q74.3)
dermatopolymyositis (M33.-)
ischemic infarction of muscle (M62.2-)
myositis (M60.-)
polymyositis (M33.2.-)

G72.0 Drug-induced myopathy
Use additional code for adverse effect, if applicable, to identify drug (T36-T50 with fifth or sixth character 5)

G72.1 Alcoholic myopathy
Use additional code to identify alcoholism (F10.-)

G72.2 Myopathy due to other toxic agents
Code first (T51-T65) to identify toxic agent

G72.3 Periodic paralysis
Familial periodic paralysis
Hyperkalemic periodic paralysis (familial)
Hypokalemic periodic paralysis (familial)
Myotonic periodic paralysis (familial)
Normokalemic paralysis (familial)
Potassium sensitive periodic paralysis
Excludes1 paramyotonia congenita (of von Eulenburg) (G71.19)

G72.4 Inflammatory and immune myopathies, not elsewhere classified

G72.41 Inclusion body myositis [IBM]

G72.49 Other inflammatory and immune myopathies, not elsewhere classified
Inflammatory myopathy NOS

G72.8 Other specified myopathies

G72.81 Critical illness myopathy
Acute necrotizing myopathy
Acute quadriplegic myopathy
Intensive care (ICU) myopathy
Myopathy of critical illness

G72.89 Other specified myopathies

G72.9 Myopathy, unspecified

G73 Disorders of myoneural junction and muscle in diseases classified elsewhere

G73.1 Lambert-Eaton syndrome in neoplastic disease
Rare autoimmune disorder affecting calcium channels of nerve-muscle (neuromuscular) junction
Code first underlying neoplasm (C00-D49)
Excludes1 Lambert-Eaton syndrome not associated with neoplasm (G70.80-G70.81)

G73.3 Myasthenic syndromes in other diseases classified elsewhere
Code first underlying disease, such as:
neoplasm (C00-D49)
thyrotoxicosis (E05.-)

G73.7 Myopathy in diseases classified elsewhere
Code first underlying disease, such as:
hyperparathyroidism (E21.0, E21.3)
hypoparathyroidism (E20.-)
glycogen storage disease (E74.0)
lipid storage disorders (E75.-)
Excludes1 myopathy in:
rheumatoid arthritis (M05.32)
sarcoidosis (D86.87)
scleroderma (M34.82)
sicca syndrome [Sjögren] (M35.03)
systemic lupus erythematosus (M32.19)

CEREBRAL PALSY AND OTHER PARALYTIC SYNDROMES (G80-G83)

G80 Cerebral palsy
Excludes1 hereditary spastic paraplegia (G11.4)

G80.0 Spastic quadriplegic cerebral palsy
Congenital spastic paralysis (cerebral)

G80.1 Spastic diplegic cerebral palsy
Spastic cerebral palsy NOS

G80.2 Spastic hemiplegic cerebral palsy

G80.3 Athetoid cerebral palsy
Result of damage to cerebellum or basal ganglia responsible for processing neuromuscular signals
Double athetosis (syndrome)
Dyskinetic cerebral palsy
Dystonic cerebral palsy
Vogt disease

G80.4 Ataxic cerebral palsy
Poor muscle tone and coordination

G80.8 Other cerebral palsy
Mixed cerebral palsy syndromes

G80.9 Cerebral palsy, unspecified
Cerebral palsy NOS

CHAPTER 6 (G00-G99)

OGCR Section I.C.6.a.

Dominant/nondominant side

Codes from category G81, Hemiplegia and hemiparesis, and subcategories, G83.1, Monoplegia of lower limb, G83.2, Monoplegia of upper limb, and G83.3, Monoplegia, unspecified, identify whether the dominant and nondominant side is affected. Should the affected side be documented, but not specified as dominant or nondominant, and the classification system does not indicate a default, code selection is as follows:

- For ambidextrous patients, the default should be dominant.
- If the left side is affected, the default is nondominant.
- If the right side is affected, the default is dominant.

● G81 Hemiplegia and hemiparesis

Note: This category is to be used only when hemiplegia (complete)(incomplete) is reported without further specification, or is stated to be old or longstanding but of unspecified cause. The category is also for use in multiple coding to identify these types of hemiplegia resulting from any cause.

Excludes1 congenital cerebral palsy (G80.-)
hemiplegia and hemiparesis due to sequela of cerebrovascular disease (I69.05-, I69.15-, I69.25-, I69.35-, I69.85-, I69.95-)

Coding Clinic: 2012, Q4, P106

● G81.0 Flaccid hemiplegia
Paralysis of half of body with loss of tone of muscles of paralyzed part and absence of tendon reflexes

G81.00 **Flaccid hemiplegia affecting unspecified side**

G81.01 **Flaccid hemiplegia affecting right dominant side**

G81.02 **Flaccid hemiplegia affecting left dominant side**

G81.03 **Flaccid hemiplegia affecting right nondominant side**

G81.04 **Flaccid hemiplegia affecting left nondominant side**

● G81.1 Spastic hemiplegia
Paralysis of half of body with spasticity of muscles of paralyzed part and increased tendon reflexes

G81.10 **Spastic hemiplegia affecting unspecified side**

G81.11 **Spastic hemiplegia affecting right dominant side**

G81.12 **Spastic hemiplegia affecting left dominant side**

G81.13 **Spastic hemiplegia affecting right nondominant side**

G81.14 **Spastic hemiplegia affecting left nondominant side**

● G81.9 Hemiplegia, unspecified

G81.90 **Hemiplegia, unspecified affecting unspecified side**

G81.91 **Hemiplegia, unspecified affecting right dominant side**

G81.92 **Hemiplegia, unspecified affecting left dominant side**

G81.93 **Hemiplegia, unspecified affecting right nondominant side**

G81.94 **Hemiplegia, unspecified affecting left nondominant side**
Coding Clinic: 2015, Q1, P26

Item 6–9 Hemiplegia is complete paralysis of one side of the body—arm, leg, and trunk. **Hemiparesis** is a generalized weakness or incomplete paralysis of one side of the body. If most activities (eating, writing) are performed with the right hand, the right is the dominant side, and the left is the nondominant side. **Quadriplegia,** also called tetraplegia, is the complete paralysis of all four limbs. **Quadriparesis** is the incomplete paralysis of all four limbs. Nerve damage in C1–C4 is associated with lower limb paralysis, and C5–C7 damage is associated with upper limb paralysis. **Diplegia** is the paralysis of the upper limbs. **Monoplegia** is the complete paralysis of one limb.

● G82 Paraplegia (paraparesis) and quadriplegia (quadriparesis)

Note: This category is to be used only when the listed conditions are reported without further specification, or are stated to be old or longstanding but of unspecified cause. The category is also for use in multiple coding to identify these conditions resulting from any cause.

Excludes1 congenital cerebral palsy (G80.-)
functional quadriplegia (R53.2)
hysterical paralysis (F44.4)

● G82.2 Paraplegia
Paralysis of both lower limbs NOS
Paraparesis (lower) NOS
Paraplegia (lower) NOS

G82.20 **Paraplegia, unspecified**
Coding Clinic: 2017, Q3, P3

G82.21 **Paraplegia, complete**

G82.22 **Paraplegia, incomplete**

● G82.5 Quadriplegia
Paralysis of all limbs; AKA tetraplegia

G82.50 **Quadriplegia, unspecified**

G82.51 **Quadriplegia, C1-C4 complete**

G82.52 **Quadriplegia, C1-C4 incomplete**

G82.53 **Quadriplegia, C5-C7 complete**

G82.54 **Quadriplegia, C5-C7 incomplete**

● G83 Other paralytic syndromes

Note: This category is to be used only when the listed conditions are reported without further specification, or are stated to be old or longstanding but of unspecified cause. The category is also for use in multiple coding to identify these conditions resulting from any cause.

Includes paralysis (complete) (incomplete), except as in G80-G82

G83.0 **Diplegia of upper limbs**
Paralysis affecting limbs on both sides; AKA bilateral paralysis
Diplegia (upper)
Paralysis of both upper limbs

● G83.1 Monoplegia of lower limb
Paralysis of limb on one side
Paralysis of lower limb

Excludes1 monoplegia of lower limbs due to sequela of cerebrovascular disease (I69.04-, I69.14-, I69.24-, I69.34-, I69.84-, I69.94-)

Coding Clinic: 2012, Q4, P106

G83.10 **Monoplegia of lower limb affecting unspecified side**

G83.11 **Monoplegia of lower limb affecting right dominant side**

G83.12 **Monoplegia of lower limb affecting left dominant side**

G83.13 **Monoplegia of lower limb affecting right nondominant side**

G83.14 **Monoplegia of lower limb affecting left nondominant side**

● G83.2 Monoplegia of upper limb
Paralysis of upper limb

Excludes1 monoplegia of upper limbs due to sequela of cerebrovascular disease (I69.03-, I69.13-, I69.23-, I69.33-, I69.83-, I69.93-)

Coding Clinic: 2012, Q4, P106

G83.20 **Monoplegia of upper limb affecting unspecified side**

G83.21 **Monoplegia of upper limb affecting right dominant side**

G83.22 **Monoplegia of upper limb affecting left dominant side**

G83.23 **Monoplegia of upper limb affecting right nondominant side**

G83.24 **Monoplegia of upper limb affecting left nondominant side**

G83.3 Monoplegia, unspecified
Coding Clinic: 2012, Q4, P106

G83.30 **Monoplegia, unspecified affecting unspecified side**

G83.31 **Monoplegia, unspecified affecting right dominant side**

G83.32 **Monoplegia, unspecified affecting left dominant side**

G83.33 **Monoplegia, unspecified affecting right nondominant side**

G83.34 **Monoplegia, unspecified affecting left nondominant side**

G83.4 **Cauda equina syndrome**
Aching pain due to compression of spinal nerve roots
Neurogenic bladder due to cauda equina syndrome
Excludes1 cord bladder NOS (G95.89)
neurogenic bladder NOS (N31.9)

G83.5 **Locked-in state**

G83.8 **Other specified paralytic syndromes**
Excludes1 paralytic syndromes due to current spinal cord injury-code to spinal cord injury (S14, S24, S34)

G83.81 **Brown-Séquard syndrome**

G83.82 **Anterior cord syndrome**

G83.83 **Posterior cord syndrome**

G83.84 **Todd's paralysis (postepileptic)**

G83.89 **Other specified paralytic syndromes**

G83.9 **Paralytic syndrome, unspecified**

OTHER DISORDERS OF THE NERVOUS SYSTEM (G89-G99)

G89 Pain, not elsewhere classified
Code also related psychological factors associated with pain (F45.42)
Excludes1 generalized pain NOS (R52)
pain disorders exclusively related to psychological factors (F45.41)
pain NOS (R52)
Excludes2 atypical face pain (G50.1)
headache syndromes (G44.-)
localized pain, unspecified type - code to pain by site, such as:
abdomen pain (R10.-)
back pain (M54.9)
breast pain (N64.4)
chest pain (R07.1-R07.9)
ear pain (H92.0-)
eye pain (H57.1)
headache (R51)
joint pain (M25.5-)
limb pain (M79.6-)
lumbar region pain (M54.5)
painful urination (R30.9)
pelvic and perineal pain (R10.2)
shoulder pain (M25.51-)
spine pain (M54.-)
throat pain (R07.0)
tongue pain (K14.6)
tooth pain (K08.8)
renal colic (N23)
migraines (G43.-)
myalgia (M79.1-)
pain from prosthetic devices, implants, and grafts (T82.84, T83.84, T84.84, T85.84-)
phantom limb syndrome with pain (G54.6)
vulvar vestibulitis (N94.810)
vulvodynia (N94.81-)

G89.0 **Central pain syndrome**
Neurological condition causing intractable pain resulting from damage to CNS
Déjérine-Roussy syndrome
Myelopathic pain syndrome
Thalamic pain syndrome (hyperesthetic)

G89.1 **Acute pain, not elsewhere classified**

G89.11 **Acute pain due to trauma**

G89.12 **Acute post-thoracotomy pain**
Post-thoracotomy pain NOS

G89.18 **Other acute postprocedural pain**
Postoperative pain NOS
Postprocedural pain NOS

G89.2 **Chronic pain, not elsewhere classified**
Excludes1 causalgia, lower limb (G57.7-)
causalgia, upper limb (G56.4-)
central pain syndrome (G89.0)
chronic pain syndrome (G89.4)
complex regional pain syndrome II, lower limb (G57.7-)
complex regional pain syndrome II, upper limb (G56.4-)
neoplasm related chronic pain (G89.3)
reflex sympathetic dystrophy (G90.5-)

G89.21 **Chronic pain due to trauma**

G89.22 **Chronic post-thoracotomy pain**

G89.28 **Other chronic postprocedural pain**
Other chronic postoperative pain

G89.29 **Other chronic pain**

G89.3 **Neoplasm related pain (acute) (chronic)**
Cancer associated pain
Pain due to malignancy (primary) (secondary)
Tumor associated pain

G89.4 **Chronic pain syndrome**
Chronic pain associated with significant psychosocial dysfunction

G90 Disorders of autonomic nervous system
Excludes1 dysfunction of the autonomic nervous system due to alcohol (G31.2)

G90.0 **Idiopathic peripheral autonomic neuropathy**

G90.01 **Carotid sinus syncope**
Carotid sinus syndrome

G90.09 **Other idiopathic peripheral autonomic neuropathy**
Idiopathic peripheral autonomic neuropathy NOS

G90.1 **Familial dysautonomia [Riley-Day]**
Inherited disorder that affects nerve function

G90.2 **Horner's syndrome**
Due to damage of the sympathetic nervous system
Bernard(-Horner) syndrome
Cervical sympathetic dystrophy or paralysis

G90.3 **Multi-system degeneration of the autonomic nervous system**
Neurogenic orthostatic hypotension [Shy-Drager]
Excludes1 orthostatic hypotension NOS (I95.1)

G90.4 **Autonomic dysreflexia**
Syndrome resulting from lesions of spinal cord
Use additional code to identify the cause, such as:
fecal impaction (K56.41)
pressure ulcer (pressure area) (L89.-)
urinary tract infection (N39.0)

G90.5 **Complex regional pain syndrome I (CRPS I)**
Reflex sympathetic dystrophy
Excludes1 causalgia of lower limb (G57.7-)
causalgia of upper limb (G56.4-)
complex regional pain syndrome II of lower limb (G57.7-)
complex regional pain syndrome II of upper limb (G56.4-)

G90.50 **Complex regional pain syndrome I, unspecified**

G90.51 **Complex regional pain syndrome I of upper limb**

G90.511 **Complex regional pain syndrome I of right upper limb**

G90.512 **Complex regional pain syndrome I of left upper limb**

CHAPTER 6 (G00-G99)

G90.513 **Complex regional pain syndrome I of upper limb, bilateral**

G90.519 **Complex regional pain syndrome I of unspecified upper limb**

● G90.52 **Complex regional pain syndrome I of lower limb**

G90.521 **Complex regional pain syndrome I of right lower limb**

G90.522 **Complex regional pain syndrome I of left lower limb**

G90.523 **Complex regional pain syndrome I of lower limb, bilateral**

G90.529 **Complex regional pain syndrome I of unspecified lower limb**

G90.59 **Complex regional pain syndrome I of other specified site**

G90.8 **Other disorders of autonomic nervous system**

G90.9 **Disorder of the autonomic nervous system, unspecified**

● G91 **Hydrocephalus**

Dilatation of cerebral ventricles, accompanied by accumulation of cerebrospinal fluid

Includes acquired hydrocephalus

Excludes1 Arnold-Chiari syndrome with hydrocephalus (Q07.-)
congenital hydrocephalus (Q03.-)
spina bifida with hydrocephalus (Q05.-)

G91.0 **Communicating hydrocephalus**
Secondary normal pressure hydrocephalus

G91.1 **Obstructive hydrocephalus**

G91.2 **(Idiopathic) normal pressure hydrocephalus**
Normal pressure hydrocephalus NOS

G91.3 **Post-traumatic hydrocephalus, unspecified**

G91.4 ***Hydrocephalus in diseases classified elsewhere***

Code first underlying condition, such as:
congenital syphilis (A50.4-)
neoplasm (C00-D49)
plasminogen deficiency (E88.02)

Excludes1 hydrocephalus due to congenital toxoplasmosis (P37.1)

G91.8 **Other hydrocephalus**

G91.9 **Hydrocephalus, unspecified**

G92 **Toxic encephalopathy**

Disorder or disease of brain caused by chemicals
Toxic encephalitis
Toxic metabolic encephalopathy

Code first if applicable, drug induced (T36-T50) (T51-T65) to identify toxic agent

Coding Clinic: 2017, Q1, P39-40

● G93 **Other disorders of brain**

G93.0 **Cerebral cysts**
Arachnoid cyst
Porencephalic cyst, acquired

Excludes1 acquired periventricular cysts of newborn (P91.1)
congenital cerebral cysts (Q04.6)

G93.1 **Anoxic brain damage, not elsewhere classified** (HCC)

Permanent brain damage by lack of oxygen perfusion through brain tissues.

Excludes1 cerebral anoxia due to anesthesia during labor and delivery (O74.3)
cerebral anoxia due to anesthesia during the puerperium (O89.2)
neonatal anoxia (P84)

G93.2 **Benign intracranial hypertension**

Excludes1 hypertensive encephalopathy (I67.4)

G93.3 **Postviral fatigue syndrome**
Benign myalgic encephalomyelitis

Excludes1 chronic fatigue syndrome NOS (R53.82)

● G93.4 **Other and unspecified encephalopathy**

Excludes1 alcoholic encephalopathy (G31.2)
encephalopathy in diseases classified elsewhere (G94)
hypertensive encephalopathy (I67.4)
toxic (metabolic) encephalopathy (G92)

Coding Clinic: 2017, Q2, P9

G93.40 **Encephalopathy, unspecified**

G93.41 **Metabolic encephalopathy**
Septic encephalopathy
Coding Clinic: 2017, Q2, P8; 2016, Q3, P42; 2015, Q3, P21

G93.49 **Other encephalopathy**
Encephalopathy NEC
Coding Clinic: 2018, Q4, P16; 2018, Q2, P22; 2017, Q2, P9

G93.5 **Compression of brain** (HCC)
Arnold-Chiari type 1 compression of brain
Compression of brain (stem)
Herniation of brain (stem)

Excludes1 diffuse traumatic compression of brain (S06.2-)
focal traumatic compression of brain (S06.3-)

G93.6 **Cerebral edema** (HCC)

Excludes1 cerebral edema due to birth injury (P11.0)
traumatic cerebral edema (S06.1-)

G93.7 **Reye's syndrome** **P**

Life-threatening neurological condition, usually follows viral illness

Code first (poisoning due to salicylates, if applicable (T39.0-, with sixth character 1-4)

Use additional code for adverse effect due to salicylates, if applicable (T39.0-, with sixth character 5)

● G93.8 **Other specified disorders of brain**

G93.81 **Temporal sclerosis**
Hippocampal sclerosis
Mesial temporal sclerosis

G93.82 **Brain death**

G93.89 **Other specified disorders of brain**
Postradiation encephalopathy
Coding Clinic: 2016, Q4, P7

G93.9 **Disorder of brain, unspecified**

G94 ***Other disorders of brain in diseases classified elsewhere***

Code first underlying disease

Excludes1 encephalopathy in congenital syphilis (A50.49)
encephalopathy in influenza (J09.X9, J10.81, J11.81)
encephalopathy in syphilis (A52.19)
hydrocephalus in diseases classified elsewhere (G91.4)

Coding Clinic: 2018, Q2, P22; 2017, Q2, P8

● G95 **Other and unspecified diseases of spinal cord**

Excludes2 myelitis (G04.-)

G95.0 **Syringomyelia and syringobulbia** (HCC)

● G95.1 **Vascular myelopathies**

Excludes2 intraspinal phlebitis and thrombophlebitis, except non-pyogenic (G08)

G95.11 **Acute infarction of spinal cord (embolic) (nonembolic)** (HCC)
Anoxia of spinal cord
Arterial thrombosis of spinal cord

G95.19 **Other vascular myelopathies** (HCC)
Edema of spinal cord
Hematomyelia
Nonpyogenic intraspinal phlebitis and thrombophlebitis
Subacute necrotic myelopathy

- **G95.2** Other and unspecified cord compression
  - G95.20 Unspecified cord compression
  - G95.29 Other cord compression
- **G95.8** Other specified diseases of spinal cord
  - **Excludes1** neurogenic bladder NOS (N31.9)
    neurogenic bladder due to cauda equina syndrome (G83.4)
    neuromuscular dysfunction of bladder without spinal cord lesion (N31.-)
  - G95.81 Conus medullaris syndrome
    Damage to gray matter and/or nerve roots in lower end of spinal cord
  - G95.89 Other specified diseases of spinal cord
    Cord bladder NOS
    Drug-induced myelopathy
    Radiation-induced myelopathy
    Excludes1 myelopathy NOS (G95.9)
- G95.9 Disease of spinal cord, unspecified
  Myelopathy NOS

G96 Other disorders of central nervous system
- G96.Ø Cerebrospinal fluid leak
  Excludes1 cerebrospinal fluid leak from spinal puncture (G97.Ø)
  Coding Clinic: 2Ø18, Q2, P13
- **G96.1** Disorders of meninges, not elsewhere classified
  - G96.11 Dural tear
    Excludes1 accidental puncture or laceration of dura during a procedure (G97.41)
  - G96.12 Meningeal adhesions (cerebral) (spinal)
  - G96.19 Other disorders of meninges, not elsewhere classified
- G96.8 Other specified disorders of central nervous system
- G96.9 Disorder of central nervous system, unspecified

G97 Intraoperative and postprocedural complications and disorders of nervous system, not elsewhere classified
Excludes2 intraoperative and postprocedural cerebrovascular infarction (I97.81-, I97.82-)
Coding Clinic: 2Ø16, Q4, P9
- G97.Ø Cerebrospinal fluid leak from spinal puncture
- G97.1 Other reaction to spinal and lumbar puncture
  Headache due to lumbar puncture
- G97.2 Intracranial hypotension following ventricular shunting
- **G97.3** Intraoperative hemorrhage and hematoma of a nervous system organ or structure complicating a procedure
  Excludes1 intraoperative hemorrhage and hematoma of a nervous system organ or structure due to accidental puncture and laceration during a procedure (G97.4-)
  - G97.31 Intraoperative hemorrhage and hematoma of a nervous system organ or structure complicating a nervous system procedure
  - G97.32 Intraoperative hemorrhage and hematoma of a nervous system organ or structure complicating other procedure
- **G97.4** Accidental puncture and laceration of a nervous system organ or structure during a procedure
  - G97.41 Accidental puncture or laceration of dura during a procedure
    Incidental (inadvertent) durotomy
  - G97.48 Accidental puncture and laceration of other nervous system organ or structure during a nervous system procedure
  - G97.49 Accidental puncture and laceration of other nervous system organ or structure during other procedure
- **G97.5** Postprocedural hemorrhage of a nervous system organ or structure following a procedure
  - G97.51 Postprocedural hemorrhage of a nervous system organ or structure following a nervous system procedure
  - G97.52 Postprocedural hemorrhage of a nervous system organ or structure following other procedure
- **G97.6** Postprocedural hematoma and seroma of a nervous system organ or structure following a procedure
  - G97.61 Postprocedural hematoma of a nervous system organ or structure following a nervous system procedure
  - G97.62 Postprocedural hematoma of a nervous system organ or structure following other procedure
  - G97.63 Postprocedural seroma of a nervous system organ or structure following a nervous system procedure
  - G97.64 Postprocedural seroma of a nervous system organ or structure following other procedure
- **G97.8** Other intraoperative and postprocedural complications and disorders of nervous system
  Use additional code to further specify disorder
  - G97.81 Other intraoperative complications of nervous system
  - G97.82 Other postprocedural complications and disorders of nervous system

G98 Other disorders of nervous system not elsewhere classified
Includes nervous system disorder NOS
- G98.Ø Neurogenic arthritis, not elsewhere classified
  Nonsyphilitic neurogenic arthropathy NEC
  Nonsyphilitic neurogenic spondylopathy NEC
  Excludes1 spondylopathy (in):
  syringomyelia and syringobulbia (G95.Ø)
  tabes dorsalis (A52.11)
- G98.8 Other disorders of nervous system
  Nervous system disorder NOS

G99 Other disorders of nervous system in diseases classified elsewhere
- *G99.Ø Autonomic neuropathy in diseases classified elsewhere*
  Code first underlying disease, such as:
  amyloidosis (E85.-)
  gout (M1A.-, M1Ø.-)
  hyperthyroidism (EØ5.-)
  Excludes1 diabetic autonomic neuropathy (EØ8-E13 with .43)
- *G99.2 Myelopathy in diseases classified elsewhere*
  Code first underlying disease, such as:
  neoplasm (CØØ-D49)
  Excludes1 myelopathy in:
  intervertebral disease (M5Ø.Ø-, M51.Ø-)
  spondylosis (M47.Ø-, M47.1-)
- *G99.8 Other specified disorders of nervous system in diseases classified elsewhere*
  Code first underlying disorder, such as:
  amyloidosis (E85.-)
  avitaminosis (E56.9)
  Excludes1 nervous system involvement in:
  cysticercosis (B69.Ø)
  rubella (BØ6.Ø-)
  syphilis (A52.1-)

CHAPTER 6 (GØØ-G99)

CHAPTER 7

DISEASES OF THE EYE AND ADNEXA (HØØ-H59)

OGCR Chapter-Specific Coding Guidelines

7. Chapter 7: Diseases of the Eye and Adnexa (HØØ-H59)

a. Glaucoma

1) Assigning Glaucoma Codes

Assign as many codes from category H4Ø, Glaucoma, as needed to identify the type of glaucoma, the affected eye, and the glaucoma stage.

2) Bilateral glaucoma with same type and stage

When a patient has bilateral glaucoma and both eyes are documented as being the same type and stage, and there is a code for bilateral glaucoma, report only the code for the type of glaucoma, bilateral, with the seventh character for the stage.

When a patient has bilateral glaucoma and both eyes are documented as being the same type and stage, and the classification does not provide a code for bilateral glaucoma (i.e., subcategories H4Ø.1Ø, H4Ø.11, and H4Ø.2Ø) report only one code for the type of glaucoma with the appropriate seventh character for the stage.

3) Bilateral glaucoma stage with different types or stages

When a patient has bilateral glaucoma and each eye is documented as having a different type or stage, and the classification distinguishes laterality, assign the appropriate code for each eye rather than the code for bilateral glaucoma.

When a patient has bilateral glaucoma and each eye is documented as having a different type, and the classification does not distinguish laterality (i.e., subcategories H4Ø.1Ø, H4Ø.11 and H4Ø.2Ø), assign one code for each type of glaucoma with the appropriate seventh character for the stage.

When a patient has bilateral glaucoma and each eye is documented as having the same type, but different stage, and the classification does not distinguish laterality (i.e., subcategories H4Ø.1Ø, H4Ø.11, and H4Ø.2Ø), assign a code for the type of glaucoma for each eye with the seventh character for the specific glaucoma stage documented for each eye.

4) Patient admitted with glaucoma and stage evolves during the admission

If a patient is admitted with glaucoma and the stage progresses during the admission, assign the code for highest stage documented.

5) Indeterminate stage glaucoma

Assignment of the seventh character "4" for "indeterminate stage" should be based on the clinical documentation. The seventh character "4" is used for glaucomas whose stage cannot be clinically determined. This seventh character should not be confused with the seventh character "Ø", unspecified, which should be assigned when there is no documentation regarding the stage of the glaucoma.

b. Blindness

If "blindness" or "low vision" of both eyes is documented but the visual impairment category is not documented, assign code H54.3, Unqualified visual loss, both eyes. If "blindness" or "low vision" in one eye is documented but the visual impairment category is not documented, assign a code from H54.6-, Unqualified visual loss, one eye. If "blindness" or "visual loss" is documented without any information about whether one or both eyes are affected, assign code H54.7, Unspecified visual loss.

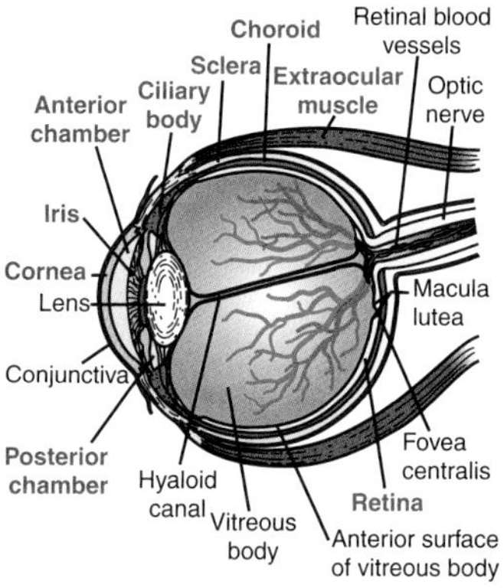

Figure 7–1 Eye and ocular adnexa. (From Buck CJ: Step-by-Step Medical Coding, ed 2016, St. Louis, Elsevier, 2016)

★ **(See Plate 15 of the Anatomy Illustrations.)**

CHAPTER 7

DISEASES OF THE EYE AND ADNEXA (HØØ-H59)

Note: Use an external cause code following the code for the eye condition, if applicable, to identify the cause of the eye condition

Excludes2 certain conditions originating in the perinatal period (PØ4-P96)
certain infectious and parasitic diseases (AØØ-B99)
complications of pregnancy, childbirth and the puerperium (OØØ-O9A)
congenital malformations, deformations, and chromosomal abnormalities (QØØ-Q99)
diabetes mellitus related eye conditions (EØ9.3-, E1Ø.3-, E11.3-, E13.3-)
endocrine, nutritional and metabolic diseases (EØØ-E88)
injury (trauma) of eye and orbit (SØ5.-)
injury, poisoning and certain other consequences of external causes (SØØ-T88)
neoplasms (CØØ-D49)
symptoms, signs and abnormal clinical and laboratory findings, not elsewhere classified (RØØ-R94)
syphilis related eye disorders (A5Ø.Ø1, A5Ø.3-, A51.43, A52.71)

This chapter contains the following blocks:

HØØ-HØ5	Disorders of eyelid, lacrimal system and orbit
H1Ø-H11	Disorders of conjunctiva
H15-H22	Disorders of sclera, cornea, iris and ciliary body
H25-H28	Disorders of lens
H3Ø-H36	Disorders of choroid and retina
H4Ø-H42	Glaucoma
H43-H44	Disorders of vitreous body and globe
H46-H47	Disorders of optic nerve and visual pathways
H49-H52	Disorders of ocular muscles, binocular movement, accommodation and refraction
H53-H54	Visual disturbances and blindness
H55-H57	Other disorders of eye and adnexa
H59	Intraoperative and postprocedural complications and disorders of eye and adnexa, not elsewhere classified

DISORDERS OF EYELID, LACRIMAL SYSTEM AND ORBIT (H00-H05)

Excludes2 open wound of eyelid (S01.1-)
superficial injury of eyelid (S00.1-, S00.2-)

● **H00** Hordeolum and chalazion
Hordeolum: inflammatory staphylococcal infection of sebaceous glands of eyelids; AKA stye. Chalazion: eyelid mass

● **H00.0** Hordeolum (externum) (internum) of eyelid
Bacterial infection (staphylococcus) of the sebaceous gland of the eyelid (stye)

● **H00.01** Hordeolum externum
Hordeolum NOS
Stye
- H00.011 Hordeolum externum **right upper** eyelid
- H00.012 Hordeolum externum **right lower** eyelid
- H00.013 Hordeolum externum **right** eye, **unspecified** eyelid
- H00.014 Hordeolum externum **left upper** eyelid
- H00.015 Hordeolum externum **left lower** eyelid
- H00.016 Hordeolum externum **left** eye, **unspecified** eyelid
- H00.019 Hordeolum externum **unspecified** eye, **unspecified** eyelid

● **H00.02** Hordeolum internum
Infection of meibomian gland
- H00.021 Hordeolum internum **right upper** eyelid
- H00.022 Hordeolum internum **right lower** eyelid
- H00.023 Hordeolum internum **right** eye, **unspecified** eyclid
- H00.024 Hordeolum internum **left upper** eyelid
- H00.025 Hordeolum internum **left lower** eyelid
- H00.026 Hordeolum internum **left** eye, **unspecified** eyelid
- H00.029 Hordeolum internum **unspecified** eye, **unspecified** eyelid

● **H00.03** Abscess of eyelid
Furuncle of eyelid
- H00.031 Abscess of **right upper** eyelid
- H00.032 Abscess of **right lower** eyelid
- H00.033 Abscess of eyelid **right** eye, **unspecified** eyelid
- H00.034 Abscess of **left upper** eyelid
- H00.035 Abscess of **left lower** eyelid
- H00.036 Abscess of eyelid **left** eye, **unspecified** eyelid
- H00.039 Abscess of eyelid **unspecified** eye, **unspecified** eyelid

● **H00.1** Chalazion
Often caused by accumulation of meibomian gland secretions resulting from a blockage of duct.
Meibomian (gland) cyst
Excludes2 infected meibomian gland (H00.02-)
- H00.11 Chalazion **right upper** eyelid
- H00.12 Chalazion **right lower** eyelid
- H00.13 Chalazion **right** eye, **unspecified** eyelid
- H00.14 Chalazion **left upper** eyelid
- H00.15 Chalazion **left lower** eyelid
- H00.16 Chalazion **left** eye, **unspecified** eyelid
- H00.19 Chalazion **unspecified** eye, **unspecified** eyelid

● **H01** Other inflammation of eyelid

● **H01.0** Blepharitis
Inflammation of eyelids
Excludes1 blepharoconjunctivitis (H10.5-)

● **H01.00** Unspecified blepharitis
- H01.001 Unspecified blepharitis **right upper** eyelid
- H01.002 Unspecified blepharitis **right lower** eyelid
- H01.003 Unspecified blepharitis **right** eye, **unspecified** eyelid
- H01.004 Unspecified blepharitis **left upper** eyelid
- H01.005 Unspecified blepharitis **left lower** eyelid
- H01.006 Unspecified blepharitis **left** eye, **unspecified** eyelid
- H01.009 Unspecified blepharitis **unspecified** eye, **unspecified** eyelid
- H01.00A Unspecified blepharitis right eye, upper and lower eyelids
- H01.00B Unspecified blepharitis left eye, upper and lower eyelids

● **H01.01** Ulcerative blepharitis
- H01.011 Ulcerative blepharitis **right upper** eyelid
- H01.012 Ulcerative blepharitis **right lower** eyelid
- H01.013 Ulcerative blepharitis **right** eye, **unspecified** eyelid
- H01.014 Ulcerative blepharitis **left upper** eyelid
- H01.015 Ulcerative blepharitis **left lower** eyelid
- H01.016 Ulcerative blepharitis **left** eye, **unspecified** eyelid
- H01.019 Ulcerative blepharitis **unspecified** eye, **unspecified** eyelid
- H01.01A Ulcerative blepharitis right eye, upper and lower eyelids
- H01.01B Ulcerative blepharitis left eye, upper and lower eyelids

● **H01.02** Squamous blepharitis
- H01.021 Squamous blepharitis **right upper** eyelid
- H01.022 Squamous blepharitis **right lower** eyelid
- H01.023 Squamous blepharitis **right** eye, **unspecified** eyelid
- H01.024 Squamous blepharitis **left upper** eyelid
- H01.025 Squamous blepharitis **left lower** eyelid
- H01.026 Squamous blepharitis **left** eye, **unspecified** eyelid
- H01.029 Squamous blepharitis **unspecified** eye, **unspecified** eyelid
- H01.02A Squamous blepharitis right eye, upper and lower eyelids
- H01.02B Squamous blepharitis left eye, upper and lower eyelids

● **H01.1** Noninfectious dermatoses of eyelid

● **H01.11** Allergic dermatitis of eyelid
Contact dermatitis of eyelid
- H01.111 Allergic dermatitis of **right upper** eyelid
- H01.112 Allergic dermatitis of **right lower** eyelid
- H01.113 Allergic dermatitis of **right** eye, **unspecified** eyelid

H01.114 Allergic dermatitis of left upper eyelid
H01.115 Allergic dermatitis of left lower eyelid
H01.116 Allergic dermatitis of left eye, unspecified eyelid
H01.119 Allergic dermatitis of unspecified eye, unspecified eyelid

● H01.12 Discoid lupus erythematosus of eyelid
H01.121 Discoid lupus erythematosus of right upper eyelid
H01.122 Discoid lupus erythematosus of right lower eyelid
H01.123 Discoid lupus erythematosus of right eye, unspecified eyelid
H01.124 Discoid lupus erythematosus of left upper eyelid
H01.125 Discoid lupus erythematosus of left lower eyelid
H01.126 Discoid lupus erythematosus of left eye, unspecified eyelid
H01.129 Discoid lupus erythematosus of unspecified eye, unspecified eyelid

● H01.13 Eczematous dermatitis of eyelid
H01.131 Eczematous dermatitis of right upper eyelid
H01.132 Eczematous dermatitis of right lower eyelid
H01.133 Eczematous dermatitis of right eye, unspecified eyelid
H01.134 Eczematous dermatitis of left upper eyelid
H01.135 Eczematous dermatitis of left lower eyelid
H01.136 Eczematous dermatitis of left eye, unspecified eyelid
H01.139 Eczematous dermatitis of unspecified eye, unspecified eyelid

● H01.14 Xeroderma of eyelid
Abnormally dry
H01.141 Xeroderma of right upper eyelid
H01.142 Xeroderma of right lower eyelid
H01.143 Xeroderma of right eye, unspecified eyelid
H01.144 Xeroderma of left upper eyelid
H01.145 Xeroderma of left lower eyelid
H01.146 Xeroderma of left eye, unspecified eyelid
H01.149 Xeroderma of unspecified eye, unspecified eyelid

H01.8 Other specified inflammations of eyelid
H01.9 Unspecified inflammation of eyelid
Inflammation of eyelid NOS

● H02 Other disorders of eyelid
Turning inward (inversion) of eyelid margin and ingrowing eyelashes
Excludes1 congenital malformations of eyelid (Q10.0-Q10.3)

● H02.0 Entropion and trichiasis of eyelid

● H02.00 Unspecified entropion of eyelid
H02.001 Unspecified entropion of right upper eyelid
H02.002 Unspecified entropion of right lower eyelid
H02.003 Unspecified entropion of right eye, unspecified eyelid
H02.004 Unspecified entropion of left upper eyelid
H02.005 Unspecified entropion of left lower eyelid

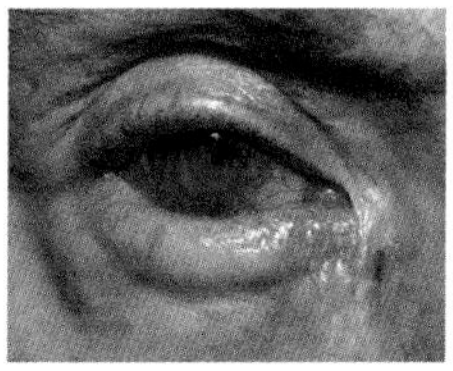

Figure 7-2 Right lower eyelid entropion. Note the inward rotation of the tarsal plate about the horizontal axis and the resultant contact between the mucocutaneous junction and ocular surface. (From Glynn M, Drake WM, Hutchison R: Hutchison's Clinical Methods: An Integrated Approach to Clinical Practice, Edinburgh, Saunders/Elsevier, 2012)

H02.006 Unspecified entropion of left eye, unspecified eyelid
H02.009 Unspecified entropion of unspecified eye, unspecified eyelid

● H02.01 Cicatricial entropion of eyelid
Scar
H02.011 Cicatricial entropion of right upper eyelid
H02.012 Cicatricial entropion of right lower eyelid
H02.013 Cicatricial entropion of right eye, unspecified eyelid
H02.014 Cicatricial entropion of left upper eyelid
H02.015 Cicatricial entropion of left lower eyelid
H02.016 Cicatricial entropion of left eye, unspecified eyelid
H02.019 Cicatricial entropion of unspecified eye, unspecified eyelid

● H02.02 Mechanical entropion of eyelid
Turning inward (inversion) of eyelid margin due to lack of support
H02.021 Mechanical entropion of right upper eyelid
H02.022 Mechanical entropion of right lower eyelid
H02.023 Mechanical entropion of right eye, unspecified eyelid
H02.024 Mechanical entropion of left upper eyelid
H02.025 Mechanical entropion of left lower eyelid
H02.026 Mechanical entropion of left eye, unspecified eyelid
H02.029 Mechanical entropion of unspecified eye, unspecified eyelid

● H02.03 Senile entropion of eyelid
Turning inward (inversion) of eyelid margin due to aging
H02.031 Senile entropion of right upper eyelid A
H02.032 Senile entropion of right lower eyelid A
H02.033 Senile entropion of right eye, unspecified eyelid A
H02.034 Senile entropion of left upper eyelid A
H02.035 Senile entropion of left lower eyelid A
H02.036 Senile entropion of left eye, unspecified eyelid A
H02.039 Senile entropion of unspecified eye, unspecified eyelid A

● H02.04 Spastic entropion of eyelid
Turning inward (inversion) of eyelid margin caused by spasm of muscle
H02.041 Spastic entropion of right upper eyelid
H02.042 Spastic entropion of right lower eyelid
H02.043 Spastic entropion of right eye, unspecified eyelid

CHAPTER 7 (H00-H59)

H02.044 Spastic entropion of left upper eyelid
H02.045 Spastic entropion of left lower eyelid
H02.046 Spastic entropion of left eye, unspecified eyelid
H02.049 Spastic entropion of unspecified eye, unspecified eyelid

● H02.05 Trichiasis without entropion
Ingrowing hairs of eyelashes
H02.051 Trichiasis without entropion right upper eyelid
H02.052 Trichiasis without entropion right lower eyelid
H02.053 Trichiasis without entropion right eye, unspecified eyelid
H02.054 Trichiasis without entropion left upper eyelid
H02.055 Trichiasis without entropion left lower eyelid
H02.056 Trichiasis without entropion left eye, unspecified eyelid
H02.059 Trichiasis without entropion unspecified eye, unspecified eyelid

● H02.1 Ectropion of eyelid
Eversion (pulling away) of eyelid

● H02.10 Unspecified ectropion of eyelid
H02.101 Unspecified ectropion of right upper eyelid
H02.102 Unspecified ectropion of right lower eyelid
H02.103 Unspecified ectropion of right eye, unspecified eyelid
H02.104 Unspecified ectropion of left upper eyelid
H02.105 Unspecified ectropion of left lower eyelid
H02.106 Unspecified ectropion of left eye, unspecified eyelid
H02.109 Unspecified ectropion of unspecified eye, unspecified eyelid

● H02.11 Cicatricial ectropion of eyelid
Pulling of eyelid down and away from eye due to scar or tightening
H02.111 Cicatricial ectropion of right upper eyelid
H02.112 Cicatricial ectropion of right lower eyelid
H02.113 Cicatricial ectropion of right eye, unspecified eyelid
H02.114 Cicatricial ectropion of left upper eyelid
H02.115 Cicatricial ectropion of left lower eyelid
H02.116 Cicatricial ectropion of left eye, unspecified eyelid
H02.119 Cicatricial ectropion of unspecified eye, unspecified eyelid

● H02.12 Mechanical ectropion of eyelid
Eversion (pulling away) of eyelid due to lack of support
H02.121 Mechanical ectropion of right upper eyelid
H02.122 Mechanical ectropion of right lower eyelid
H02.123 Mechanical ectropion of right eye, unspecified eyelid
H02.124 Mechanical ectropion of left upper eyelid
H02.125 Mechanical ectropion of left lower eyelid
H02.126 Mechanical ectropion of left eye, unspecified eyelid
H02.129 Mechanical ectropion of unspecified eye, unspecified eyelid

● H02.13 Senile ectropion of eyelid
Eversion (pulling away) of eyelid due to age
H02.131 Senile ectropion of right upper eyelid A
H02.132 Senile ectropion of right lower eyelid A
H02.133 Senile ectropion of right eye, unspecified eyelid A
H02.134 Senile ectropion of left upper eyelid A
H02.135 Senile ectropion of left lower eyelid A
H02.136 Senile ectropion of left eye, unspecified eyelid A
H02.139 Senile ectropion of unspecified eye, unspecified eyelid A

● H02.14 Spastic ectropion of eyelid
Eversion (pulling away) of eyelid due to tonic muscle spasm
H02.141 Spastic ectropion of right upper eyelid
H02.142 Spastic ectropion of right lower eyelid
H02.143 Spastic ectropion of right eye, unspecified eyelid
H02.144 Spastic ectropion of left upper eyelid
H02.145 Spastic ectropion of left lower eyelid
H02.146 Spastic ectropion of left eye, unspecified eyelid
H02.149 Spastic ectropion of unspecified eye, unspecified eyelid

● H02.15 Paralytic ectropion of eyelid
H02.151 Paralytic ectropion of right upper eyelid
H02.152 Paralytic ectropion of right lower eyelid
H02.153 Paralytic ectropion of right eye, unspecified eyelid
H02.154 Paralytic ectropion of left upper eyelid
H02.155 Paralytic ectropion of left lower eyelid
H02.156 Paralytic ectropion of left eye, unspecified eyelid
H02.159 Paralytic ectropion of unspecified eye, unspecified eyelid

● H02.2 Lagophthalmos
Condition in which eye cannot completely close

● H02.20 Unspecified lagophthalmos
H02.201 Unspecified lagophthalmos right upper eyelid
H02.202 Unspecified lagophthalmos right lower eyelid
H02.203 Unspecified lagophthalmos right eye, unspecified eyelid
H02.204 Unspecified lagophthalmos left upper eyelid
H02.205 Unspecified lagophthalmos left lower eyelid
H02.206 Unspecified lagophthalmos left eye, unspecified eyelid
H02.209 Unspecified lagophthalmos unspecified eye, unspecified eyelid
H02.20A Unspecified lagophthalmos right eye, upper and lower eyelids
H02.20B Unspecified lagophthalmos left eye, upper and lower eyelids
H02.20C Unspecified lagophthalmos, bilateral, upper and lower eyelids

● H02.21 **Cicatricial** lagophthalmos
Upper or lower eyelid does not close due to scar or tightening
H02.211 Cicatricial lagophthalmos **right upper** eyelid
H02.212 Cicatricial lagophthalmos **right lower** eyelid
H02.213 Cicatricial lagophthalmos **right** eye, **unspecified** eyelid
H02.214 Cicatricial lagophthalmos **left upper** eyelid
H02.215 Cicatricial lagophthalmos **left lower** eyelid
H02.216 Cicatricial lagophthalmos **left** eye, **unspecified** eyelid
H02.219 Cicatricial lagophthalmos **unspecified** eye, **unspecified** eyelid
H02.21A Cicatricial lagophthalmos right eye, upper and lower eyelids
H02.21B Cicatricial lagophthalmos left eye, upper and lower eyelids
H02.21C Cicatricial lagophthalmos, bilateral, upper and lower eyelids

● H02.22 **Mechanical** lagophthalmos
Inability to close lids due to structural disorder
H02.221 Mechanical lagophthalmos **right upper** eyelid
H02.222 Mechanical lagophthalmos **right lower** eyelid
H02.223 Mechanical lagophthalmos **right** eye, **unspecified** eyelid
H02.224 Mechanical lagophthalmos **left upper** eyelid
H02.225 Mechanical lagophthalmos **left lower** eyelid
H02.226 Mechanical lagophthalmos **left** eye, **unspecified** eyelid
H02.229 Mechanical lagophthalmos **unspecified** eye, **unspecified** eyelid
H02.22A Mechanical lagophthalmos right eye, upper and lower eyelids [new]
H02.22B Mechanical lagophthalmos left eye, upper and lower eyelids
H02.22C Mechanical lagophthalmos, bilateral, upper and lower eyelids

● H02.23 **Paralytic** lagophthalmos
Eyelids do not close due to paralysis
H02.231 Paralytic lagophthalmos **right upper** eyelid
H02.232 Paralytic lagophthalmos **right lower** eyelid
H02.233 Paralytic lagophthalmos **right** eye, **unspecified** eyelid
H02.234 Paralytic lagophthalmos **left upper** eyelid
H02.235 Paralytic lagophthalmos **left lower** eyelid
H02.236 Paralytic lagophthalmos **left** eye, **unspecified** eyelid
H02.239 Paralytic lagophthalmos **unspecified** eye, **unspecified** eyelid
H02.23A Paralytic lagophthalmos right eye, upper and lower eyelids
H02.23B Paralytic lagophthalmos left eye, upper and lower eyelids
H02.23C Paralytic lagophthalmos, bilateral, upper and lower eyelids

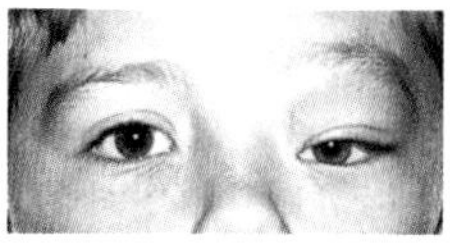

Figure 7-3 Ptosis of eyelid. (From Kanski JJ: Clinical Diagnosis in Ophthalmology, London, Elsevier Mosby, 2006)

Item 7–1 Ptosis of eyelid is drooping of the upper eyelid over the pupil when the eyes are fully opened resulting from nerve or muscle damage, which may require surgical correction.

★ **(See Plate 17 of the Anatomy Illustrations.)**

● H02.3 **Blepharochalasis**
Relaxation of skin of eyelid, due to atrophy of intercellular tissue
Pseudoptosis
H02.30 Blepharochalasis unspecified eye, **unspecified** eyelid
H02.31 Blepharochalasis **right upper** eyelid
H02.32 Blepharochalasis **right lower** eyelid
H02.33 Blepharochalasis **right** eye, **unspecified** eyelid
H02.34 Blepharochalasis **left upper** eyelid
H02.35 Blepharochalasis **left lower** eyelid
H02.36 Blepharochalasis **left** eye, **unspecified** eyelid

● H02.4 **Ptosis** of eyelid
Falling forward, drooping, sagging of eyelid

● H02.40 **Unspecified** ptosis of eyelid
H02.401 Unspecified ptosis of **right** eyelid
H02.402 Unspecified ptosis of **left** eyelid
H02.403 Unspecified ptosis of **bilateral** eyelids
H02.409 Unspecified ptosis of **unspecified** eyelid

● H02.41 **Mechanical** ptosis of eyelid
H02.411 Mechanical ptosis of **right** eyelid
H02.412 Mechanical ptosis of **left** eyelid
H02.413 Mechanical ptosis of **bilateral** eyelids
H02.419 Mechanical ptosis of **unspecified** eyelid

● H02.42 **Myogenic** ptosis of eyelid
H02.421 Myogenic ptosis of **right** eyelid
H02.422 Myogenic ptosis of **left** eyelid
H02.423 Myogenic ptosis of **bilateral** eyelids
H02.429 Myogenic ptosis of **unspecified** eyelid

● H02.43 **Paralytic** ptosis of eyelid
Neurogenic ptosis of eyelid
H02.431 Paralytic ptosis of **right** eyelid
H02.432 Paralytic ptosis of **left** eyelid
H02.433 Paralytic ptosis of **bilateral** eyelids
H02.439 Paralytic ptosis **unspecified** eyelid

● H02.5 Other disorders affecting eyelid function
Excludes2 blepharospasm (G24.5)
organic tic (G25.69)
psychogenic tic (F95.-)

● H02.51 Abnormal innervation syndrome
H02.511 Abnormal innervation syndrome **right upper** eyelid
H02.512 Abnormal innervation syndrome **right lower** eyelid
H02.513 Abnormal innervation syndrome **right** eye, **unspecified** eyelid
H02.514 Abnormal innervation syndrome **left upper** eyelid
H02.515 Abnormal innervation syndrome **left lower** eyelid
H02.516 Abnormal innervation syndrome **left** eye, **unspecified** eyelid
H02.519 Abnormal innervation syndrome **unspecified** eye, **unspecified** eyelid

CHAPTER 7 (H00-H59)

● H02.52 Blepharophimosis
Drooping of eyelid with reduced lid size
Ankyloblepharon
H02.521 Blepharophimosis **right upper** eyelid
H02.522 Blepharophimosis **right lower** eyelid
H02.523 Blepharophimosis **right** eye, **unspecified** eyelid
H02.524 Blepharophimosis **left upper** eyelid
H02.525 Blepharophimosis **left lower** eyelid
H02.526 Blepharophimosis **left** eye, **unspecified** eyelid
H02.529 Blepharophimosis **unspecified** eye, **unspecified** lid

● H02.53 Eyelid retraction
Eyelid lag
H02.531 Eyelid retraction **right upper** eyelid
H02.532 Eyelid retraction **right lower** eyelid
H02.533 Eyelid retraction **right** eye, **unspecified** eyelid
H02.534 Eyelid retraction **left upper** eyelid
H02.535 Eyelid retraction **left lower** eyelid
H02.536 Eyelid retraction **left** eye, **unspecified** eyelid
H02.539 Eyelid retraction **unspecified** eye, **unspecified** lid

H02.59 Other disorders affecting eyelid function
Deficient blink reflex
Sensory disorders

● H02.6 Xanthelasma of eyelid
Yellow-to-orange patches or pimples clustered together on eyelid
H02.60 Xanthelasma of **unspecified** eye, **unspecified** eyelid
H02.61 Xanthelasma of **right upper** eyelid
H02.62 Xanthelasma of **right lower** eyelid
H02.63 Xanthelasma of **right** eye, **unspecified** eyelid
H02.64 Xanthelasma of **left upper** eyelid
H02.65 Xanthelasma of **left lower** eyelid
H02.66 Xanthelasma of **left** eye, **unspecified** eyelid

● H02.7 Other and unspecified degenerative disorders of eyelid and periocular area
H02.70 **Unspecified** degenerative disorders of eyelid and periocular area

● H02.71 **Chloasma** of eyelid and periocular area
Dyspigmentation of eyelid
Hyperpigmentation of eyelid
H02.711 Chloasma of **right upper** eyelid and periocular area
H02.712 Chloasma of **right lower** eyelid and periocular area
H02.713 Chloasma of **right** eye, **unspecified** eyelid and periocular area
H02.714 Chloasma of **left upper** eyelid and periocular area
H02.715 Chloasma of **left lower** eyelid and periocular area
H02.716 Chloasma of **left** eye, **unspecified** eyelid and periocular area
H02.719 Chloasma of **unspecified** eye, **unspecified** eyelid and periocular area

● H02.72 **Madarosis** of eyelid and periocular area
Loss of eyelashes and/or eyebrows
Hypotrichosis of eyelid
H02.721 Madarosis of **right upper** eyelid and periocular area
H02.722 Madarosis of **right lower** eyelid and periocular area
H02.723 Madarosis of **right** eye, **unspecified** eyelid and periocular area
H02.724 Madarosis of **left upper** eyelid and periocular area
H02.725 Madarosis of **left lower** eyelid and periocular area
H02.726 Madarosis of **left** eye, **unspecified** eyelid and periocular area
H02.729 Madarosis of **unspecified** eye, **unspecified** eyelid and periocular area

● H02.73 **Vitiligo** of eyelid and periocular area
Skin pigmentation disease characterized by white patches
Hypopigmentation of eyelid
H02.731 Vitiligo of **right upper** eyelid and periocular area
H02.732 Vitiligo of **right lower** eyelid and periocular area
H02.733 Vitiligo of **right** eye, **unspecified** eyelid and periocular area
H02.734 Vitiligo of **left upper** eyelid and periocular area
H02.735 Vitiligo of **left lower** eyelid and periocular area
H02.736 Vitiligo of **left** eye, **unspecified** eyelid and periocular area
H02.739 Vitiligo of **unspecified** eye, **unspecified** eyelid and periocular area

H02.79 **Other** degenerative disorders of eyelid and periocular area

● H02.8 Other specified disorders of eyelid

● H02.81 **Retained foreign body** in eyelid
Use additional code to identify the type of retained foreign body (Z18.-)
Excludes1 laceration of eyelid with foreign body (S01.12-)
retained intraocular foreign body (H44.6-, H44.7-)
superficial foreign body of eyelid and periocular area (S00.25-)
H02.811 Retained foreign body in **right upper** eyelid
H02.812 Retained foreign body in **right lower** eyelid
H02.813 Retained foreign body in **right** eye, **unspecified** eyelid
H02.814 Retained foreign body in **left upper** eyelid
H02.815 Retained foreign body in **left lower** eyelid
H02.816 Retained foreign body in **left** eye, **unspecified** eyelid
H02.819 Retained foreign body in **unspecified** eye, **unspecified** eyelid

● H02.82 **Cysts** of eyelid
Sebaceous cyst of eyelid
H02.821 Cysts of **right upper** eyelid
H02.822 Cysts of **right lower** eyelid
H02.823 Cysts of **right** eye, **unspecified** eyelid
H02.824 Cysts of **left upper** eyelid
H02.825 Cysts of **left lower** eyelid
H02.826 Cysts of **left** eye, **unspecified** eyelid
H02.829 Cysts of **unspecified** eye, **unspecified** eyelid

● H02.83 **Dermatochalasis** of eyelid
Skin is inelastic and hangs loosely in folds
H02.831 Dermatochalasis of **right upper** eyelid
H02.832 Dermatochalasis of **right lower** eyelid
H02.833 Dermatochalasis of **right** eye, **unspecified** eyelid
H02.834 Dermatochalasis of **left upper** eyelid

H02.835 Dermatochalasis of left lower eyelid
H02.836 Dermatochalasis of left eye, unspecified eyelid
H02.839 Dermatochalasis of unspecified eye, unspecified eyelid

● H02.84 Edema of eyelid
Hyperemia of eyelid
H02.841 Edema of right upper eyelid
H02.842 Edema of right lower eyelid
H02.843 Edema of right eye, unspecified eyelid
H02.844 Edema of left upper eyelid
H02.845 Edema of left lower eyelid
H02.846 Edema of left eye, unspecified eyelid
H02.849 Edema of unspecified eye, unspecified eyelid

● H02.85 Elephantiasis of eyelid
Massive secondary lymphedema with hypertrophy of skin and subcutaneous tissues (pachyderma)
H02.851 Elephantiasis of right upper eyelid
H02.852 Elephantiasis of right lower eyelid
H02.853 Elephantiasis of right eye, unspecified eyelid
H02.854 Elephantiasis of left upper eyelid
H02.855 Elephantiasis of left lower eyelid
H02.856 Elephantiasis of left eye, unspecified eyelid
H02.859 Elephantiasis of unspecified eye, unspecified eyelid

● H02.86 Hypertrichosis of eyelid
Excessive growth of hair
H02.861 Hypertrichosis of right upper eyelid
H02.862 Hypertrichosis of right lower eyelid
H02.863 Hypertrichosis of right eye, unspecified eyelid
H02.864 Hypertrichosis of left upper eyelid
H02.865 Hypertrichosis of left lower eyelid
H02.866 Hypertrichosis of left eye, unspecified eyelid
H02.869 Hypertrichosis of unspecified eye, unspecified eyelid

● H02.87 Vascular anomalies of eyelid
H02.871 Vascular anomalies of right upper eyelid
H02.872 Vascular anomalies of right lower eyelid
H02.873 Vascular anomalies of right eye, unspecified eyelid
H02.874 Vascular anomalies of left upper eyelid
H02.875 Vascular anomalies of left lower eyelid
H02.876 Vascular anomalies of left eye, unspecified eyelid
H02.879 Vascular anomalies of unspecified eye, unspecified eyelid

● H02.88 Meibomian gland dysfunction of eyelid
H02.881 Meibomian gland dysfunction right upper eyelid
H02.882 Meibomian gland dysfunction right lower eyelid
H02.883 Meibomian gland dysfunction of right eye, unspecified eyelid
H02.884 Meibomian gland dysfunction left upper eyelid
H02.885 Meibomian gland dysfunction left lower eyelid
H02.886 Meibomian gland dysfunction of left eye, unspecified eyelid
H02.889 Meibomian gland dysfunction of unspecified eye, unspecified eyelid
H02.88A Meibomian gland dysfunction right eye, upper and lower eyelids
H02.88B Meibomian gland dysfunction left eye, upper and lower eyelids

H02.89 Other specified disorders of eyelid
Hemorrhage of eyelid

H02.9 Unspecified disorder of eyelid
Disorder of eyelid NOS

● H04 Disorders of lacrimal system
Excludes1 congenital malformations of lacrimal system (Q10.4-Q10.6)

● H04.0 Dacryoadenitis
Inflammation of lacrimal gland

● H04.00 Unspecified dacryoadenitis
H04.001 Unspecified dacryoadenitis, right lacrimal gland
H04.002 Unspecified dacryoadenitis, left lacrimal gland
H04.003 Unspecified dacryoadenitis, bilateral lacrimal glands
H04.009 Unspecified dacryoadenitis, unspecified lacrimal gland

● H04.01 Acute dacryoadenitis
H04.011 Acute dacryoadenitis, right lacrimal gland
H04.012 Acute dacryoadenitis, left lacrimal gland
H04.013 Acute dacryoadenitis, bilateral lacrimal glands
H04.019 Acute dacryoadenitis, unspecified lacrimal gland

★**(See Plate 19 of the Anatomy Illustrations.)**

● H04.02 Chronic dacryoadenitis
H04.021 Chronic dacryoadenitis, right lacrimal gland
H04.022 Chronic dacryoadenitis, left lacrimal gland
H04.023 Chronic dacryoadenitis, bilateral lacrimal gland
H04.029 Chronic dacryoadenitis, unspecified lacrimal gland

● H04.03 Chronic enlargement of lacrimal gland
H04.031 Chronic enlargement of right lacrimal gland
H04.032 Chronic enlargement of left lacrimal gland
H04.033 Chronic enlargement of bilateral lacrimal glands
H04.039 Chronic enlargement of unspecified lacrimal gland

● H04.1 Other disorders of lacrimal gland

● H04.11 Dacryops
Watery eye or distention of lacrimal duct due to fluid
H04.111 Dacryops of right lacrimal gland
H04.112 Dacryops of left lacrimal gland
H04.113 Dacryops of bilateral lacrimal glands
H04.119 Dacryops of unspecified lacrimal gland

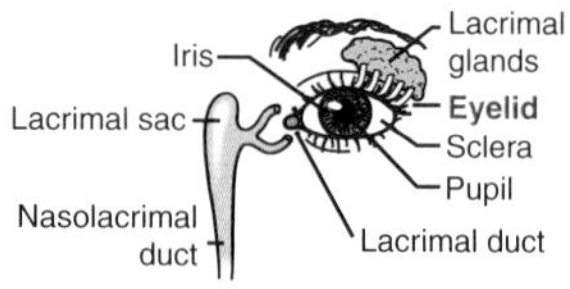

Figure 7-4 Lacrimal apparatus. (From Buck CJ: Step-by-Step Medical Coding, 2016, St. Louis, Elsevier, 2016)

CHAPTER 7 (H00-H59)

- H04.12 Dry eye syndrome
  - Tear film insufficiency, NOS
  - H04.121 Dry eye syndrome of **right** lacrimal gland
  - H04.122 Dry eye syndrome of **left** lacrimal gland
  - H04.123 Dry eye syndrome of **bilateral** lacrimal glands
  - H04.129 Dry eye syndrome of **unspecified** lacrimal gland
- H04.13 Lacrimal cyst
  - Lacrimal cystic degeneration
  - H04.131 Lacrimal cyst **right** lacrimal gland
  - H04.132 Lacrimal cyst **left** lacrimal gland
  - H04.133 Lacrimal cyst **bilateral** lacrimal glands
  - H04.139 Lacrimal cyst **unspecified** lacrimal gland
- H04.14 **Primary** lacrimal gland atrophy
  - H04.141 Primary lacrimal gland atrophy, **right** lacrimal gland
  - H04.142 Primary lacrimal gland atrophy, **left** lacrimal gland
  - H04.143 Primary lacrimal gland atrophy, **bilateral** lacrimal glands
  - H04.149 Primary lacrimal gland atrophy, **unspecified** lacrimal gland
- H04.15 **Secondary** lacrimal gland atrophy
  - H04.151 Secondary lacrimal gland atrophy, **right** lacrimal gland
  - H04.152 Secondary lacrimal gland atrophy, **left** lacrimal gland
  - H04.153 Secondary lacrimal gland atrophy, **bilateral** lacrimal glands
  - H04.159 Secondary lacrimal gland atrophy, **unspecified** lacrimal gland
- H04.16 Lacrimal gland dislocation
  - H04.161 Lacrimal gland dislocation, **right** lacrimal gland
  - H04.162 Lacrimal gland dislocation, **left** lacrimal gland
  - H04.163 Lacrimal gland dislocation, **bilateral** lacrimal glands
  - H04.169 Lacrimal gland dislocation, **unspecified** lacrimal gland
- H04.19 Other specified disorders of lacrimal gland

- H04.2 Epiphora
  - *Overflow of tears due to stricture of lacrimal passages; AKA lacrimation*
  - H04.20 **Unspecified** epiphora
    - H04.201 Unspecified epiphora, **right** side
    - H04.202 Unspecified epiphora, **left** side
    - H04.203 Unspecified epiphora, **bilateral**
    - H04.209 Unspecified epiphora, **unspecified** side
  - H04.21 Epiphora due to excess lacrimation
    - H04.211 Epiphora due to excess lacrimation, **right** lacrimal gland
    - H04.212 Epiphora due to excess lacrimation, **left** lacrimal gland
    - H04.213 Epiphora due to excess lacrimation, **bilateral** lacrimal glands
    - H04.219 Epiphora due to excess lacrimation, **unspecified** lacrimal gland
  - H04.22 Epiphora due to insufficient drainage
    - H04.221 Epiphora due to insufficient drainage, **right** side
    - H04.222 Epiphora due to insufficient drainage, **left** side
    - H04.223 Epiphora due to insufficient drainage, **bilateral**
    - H04.229 Epiphora due to insufficient drainage, **unspecified** side

- H04.3 Acute and unspecified inflammation of lacrimal passages
  - **Excludes1** neonatal dacryocystitis (P39.1)
  - H04.30 Unspecified dacryocystitis
    - H04.301 Unspecified dacryocystitis of **right** lacrimal passage
    - H04.302 Unspecified dacryocystitis of **left** lacrimal passage
    - H04.303 Unspecified dacryocystitis of **bilateral** lacrimal passages
    - H04.309 Unspecified dacryocystitis of **unspecified** lacrimal passage
  - H04.31 **Phlegmonous** dacryocystitis
    - *Cellulitis of lacrimal sac*
    - H04.311 Phlegmonous dacryocystitis of **right** lacrimal passage
    - H04.312 Phlegmonous dacryocystitis of **left** lacrimal passage
    - H04.313 Phlegmonous dacryocystitis of **bilateral** lacrimal passages
    - H04.319 Phlegmonous dacryocystitis of **unspecified** lacrimal passage
  - H04.32 **Acute** dacryocystitis
    - Acute dacryopericystitis
    - H04.321 Acute dacryocystitis of **right** lacrimal passage
    - H04.322 Acute dacryocystitis of **left** lacrimal passage
    - H04.323 Acute dacryocystitis of **bilateral** lacrimal passages
    - H04.329 Acute dacryocystitis of **unspecified** lacrimal passage
  - H04.33 Acute lacrimal **canaliculitis**
    - H04.331 Acute lacrimal canaliculitis of **right** lacrimal passage
    - H04.332 Acute lacrimal canaliculitis of **left** lacrimal passage
    - H04.333 Acute lacrimal canaliculitis of **bilateral** lacrimal passages
    - H04.339 Acute lacrimal canaliculitis of **unspecified** lacrimal passage

- H04.4 **Chronic inflammation** of lacrimal passages
  - H04.41 Chronic **dacryocystitis**
    - *Inflammation of lacrimal sac*
    - H04.411 Chronic dacryocystitis of **right** lacrimal passage
    - H04.412 Chronic dacryocystitis of **left** lacrimal passage
    - H04.413 Chronic dacryocystitis of **bilateral** lacrimal passages
    - H04.419 Chronic dacryocystitis of **unspecified** lacrimal passage
  - H04.42 Chronic lacrimal **canaliculitis**
    - *Inflammation of lacrimal ducts*
    - H04.421 Chronic lacrimal canaliculitis of **right** lacrimal passage
    - H04.422 Chronic lacrimal canaliculitis of **left** lacrimal passage
    - H04.423 Chronic lacrimal canaliculitis of **bilateral** lacrimal passages
    - H04.429 Chronic lacrimal canaliculitis of **unspecified** lacrimal passage
  - H04.43 Chronic lacrimal **mucocele**
    - *Accumulation of mucous secretion*
    - H04.431 Chronic lacrimal mucocele of **right** lacrimal passage
    - H04.432 Chronic lacrimal mucocele of **left** lacrimal passage
    - H04.433 Chronic lacrimal mucocele of **bilateral** lacrimal passages
    - H04.439 Chronic lacrimal mucocele of **unspecified** lacrimal passage

CHAPTER 7 (H00-H59)

CHAPTER 7 (H00-H59)

● H04.5 Stenosis and insufficiency of lacrimal passages

● H04.51 Dacryolith

Concretion in lacrimal sac/duct; AKA lacrimal calculus

H04.511 Dacryolith of **right** lacrimal passage

H04.512 Dacryolith of **left** lacrimal passage

H04.513 Dacryolith of **bilateral** lacrimal passages

H04.519 Dacryolith of **unspecified** lacrimal passage

● H04.52 Eversion of lacrimal punctum

Turning out of lacrimal drainage opening

H04.521 Eversion of **right** lacrimal punctum

H04.522 Eversion of **left** lacrimal punctum

H04.523 Eversion of **bilateral** lacrimal punctum

H04.529 Eversion of **unspecified** lacrimal punctum

● H04.53 Neonatal obstruction of nasolacrimal duct

Excludes1 congenital stenosis and stricture of lacrimal duct (Q10.5)

H04.531 Neonatal obstruction of **right** nasolacrimal duct N

H04.532 Neonatal obstruction of **left** nasolacrimal duct N

H04.533 Neonatal obstruction of **bilateral** nasolacrimal duct N

H04.539 Neonatal obstruction of **unspecified** nasolacrimal duct N

● H04.54 Stenosis of lacrimal canaliculi

H04.541 Stenosis of **right** lacrimal canaliculi

H04.542 Stenosis of **left** lacrimal canaliculi

H04.543 Stenosis of **bilateral** lacrimal canaliculi

H04.549 Stenosis of **unspecified** lacrimal canaliculi

● H04.55 Acquired stenosis of nasolacrimal duct

H04.551 Acquired stenosis of **right** nasolacrimal duct

H04.552 Acquired stenosis of **left** nasolacrimal duct

H04.553 Acquired stenosis of **bilateral** nasolacrimal duct

H04.559 Acquired stenosis of **unspecified** nasolacrimal duct

● H04.56 Stenosis of lacrimal punctum

H04.561 Stenosis of **right** lacrimal punctum

H04.562 Stenosis of **left** lacrimal punctum

H04.563 Stenosis of **bilateral** lacrimal punctum

H04.569 Stenosis of **unspecified** lacrimal punctum

● H04.57 Stenosis of lacrimal sac

H04.571 Stenosis of **right** lacrimal sac

H04.572 Stenosis of **left** lacrimal sac

H04.573 Stenosis of **bilateral** lacrimal sac

H04.579 Stenosis of **unspecified** lacrimal sac

● H04.6 Other changes of lacrimal passages

● H04.61 Lacrimal fistula

H04.611 Lacrimal fistula **right** lacrimal passage

H04.612 Lacrimal fistula **left** lacrimal passage

H04.613 Lacrimal fistula **bilateral** lacrimal passages

H04.619 Lacrimal fistula **unspecified** lacrimal passage

H04.69 Other changes of lacrimal passages

● H04.8 Other disorders of lacrimal system

● H04.81 Granuloma of lacrimal passages

Inflammatory response due to infectious or noninfectious agents

H04.811 Granuloma of **right** lacrimal passage

H04.812 Granuloma of **left** lacrimal passage

H04.813 Granuloma of **bilateral** lacrimal passages

H04.819 Granuloma of **unspecified** lacrimal passage

H04.89 Other disorders of lacrimal system

H04.9 Disorder of lacrimal system, **unspecified**

● H05 Disorders of orbit

Excludes1 congenital malformation of orbit (Q10.7)

● H05.0 Acute inflammation of orbit

H05.00 Unspecified acute inflammation of orbit

● H05.01 Cellulitis of orbit

Infection of soft tissue of orbit

Abscess of orbit

H05.011 Cellulitis of **right** orbit

H05.012 Cellulitis of **left** orbit

H05.013 Cellulitis of **bilateral** orbits

H05.019 Cellulitis of **unspecified** orbit

● H05.02 Osteomyelitis of orbit

Infection of boney orbit of eye

H05.021 Osteomyelitis of **right** orbit

H05.022 Osteomyelitis of **left** orbit

H05.023 Osteomyelitis of **bilateral** orbits

H05.029 Osteomyelitis of **unspecified** orbit

● H05.03 Periostitis of orbit

Inflammation of periosteum (membrane covering bone surface)

H05.031 Periostitis of **right** orbit

H05.032 Periostitis of **left** orbit

H05.033 Periostitis of **bilateral** orbits

H05.039 Periostitis of **unspecified** orbit

● H05.04 Tenonitis of orbit

Inflammation of tenon capsule (space enclosing fascia of Tenon between eyeball and fat of orbit)

H05.041 Tenonitis of **right** orbit

H05.042 Tenonitis of **left** orbit

H05.043 Tenonitis of **bilateral** orbits

H05.049 Tenonitis of **unspecified** orbit

● H05.1 Chronic inflammatory disorders of orbit

H05.10 Unspecified chronic inflammatory disorders of orbit

● H05.11 Granuloma of orbit

Pseudotumor (inflammatory) of orbit

H05.111 Granuloma of **right** orbit

H05.112 Granuloma of **left** orbit

H05.113 Granuloma of **bilateral** orbits

H05.119 Granuloma of **unspecified** orbit

● H05.12 Orbital myositis

Inflammation of extraocular muscles of orbit

H05.121 Orbital myositis, **right** orbit

H05.122 Orbital myositis, **left** orbit

H05.123 Orbital myositis, **bilateral**

H05.129 Orbital myositis, **unspecified** orbit

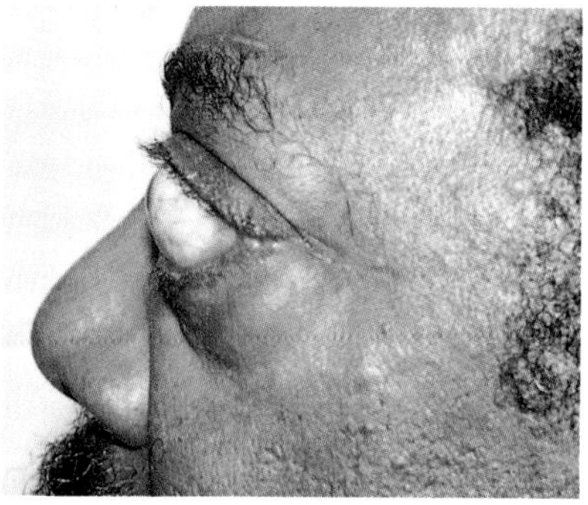

Figure 7-5 Exophthalmos. (From Black JM, Hokanson JH: Medical-Surgical Nursing: Clinical Management for Positive Outcomes, St. Louis, Saunders Elsevier, 2009)

- ● H05.2 Exophthalmic conditions
  - *Bulging eyes*
  - H05.20 Unspecified exophthalmos
  - ● H05.21 Displacement (lateral) of globe
    - H05.211 Displacement (lateral) of globe, right eye
    - H05.212 Displacement (lateral) of globe, left eye
    - H05.213 Displacement (lateral) of globe, bilateral
    - H05.219 Displacement (lateral) of globe, unspecified eye
  - ● H05.22 Edema of orbit
    - Orbital congestion
    - H05.221 Edema of right orbit
    - H05.222 Edema of left orbit
    - H05.223 Edema of bilateral orbit
    - H05.229 Edema of unspecified orbit
  - ● H05.23 Hemorrhage of orbit
    - H05.231 Hemorrhage of right orbit
    - H05.232 Hemorrhage of left orbit
    - H05.233 Hemorrhage of bilateral orbit
    - H05.239 Hemorrhage of unspecified orbit
  - ● H05.24 Constant exophthalmos
    - *Constant bulging eyes, often symptom of Graves disease*
    - H05.241 Constant exophthalmos, right eye
    - H05.242 Constant exophthalmos, left eye
    - H05.243 Constant exophthalmos, bilateral
    - H05.249 Constant exophthalmos, unspecified eye
  - ● H05.25 Intermittent exophthalmos
    - *Intermittent bulging eye occurring with bending forward or sharp turning of head*
    - H05.251 Intermittent exophthalmos, right eye
    - H05.252 Intermittent exophthalmos, left eye
    - H05.253 Intermittent exophthalmos, bilateral
    - H05.259 Intermittent exophthalmos, unspecified eye
  - ● H05.26 Pulsating exophthalmos
    - *Bulging eyes with pulsation and bruit, often due to aneurysm pushing eye forward*
    - H05.261 Pulsating exophthalmos, right eye
    - H05.262 Pulsating exophthalmos, left eye
    - H05.263 Pulsating exophthalmos, bilateral
    - H05.269 Pulsating exophthalmos, unspecified eye
- ● H05.3 Deformity of orbit
  - **Excludes1** congenital deformity of orbit (Q10.7); hypertelorism (Q75.2)
  - H05.30 Unspecified deformity of orbit
  - ● H05.31 Atrophy of orbit
    - H05.311 Atrophy of right orbit
    - H05.312 Atrophy of left orbit
    - H05.313 Atrophy of bilateral orbit
    - H05.319 Atrophy of unspecified orbit
  - ● H05.32 Deformity of orbit due to bone disease
    - Code also associated bone disease
    - H05.321 Deformity of right orbit due to bone disease
    - H05.322 Deformity of left orbit due to bone disease
    - H05.323 Deformity of bilateral orbits due to bone disease
    - H05.329 Deformity of unspecified orbit due to bone disease
  - ● H05.33 Deformity of orbit due to trauma or surgery
    - H05.331 Deformity of right orbit due to trauma or surgery
    - H05.332 Deformity of left orbit due to trauma or surgery
    - H05.333 Deformity of bilateral orbits due to trauma or surgery
    - H05.339 Deformity of unspecified orbit due to trauma or surgery
  - ● H05.34 Enlargement of orbit
    - H05.341 Enlargement of right orbit
    - H05.342 Enlargement of left orbit
    - H05.343 Enlargement of bilateral orbits
    - H05.349 Enlargement of unspecified orbit
  - ● H05.35 Exostosis of orbit
    - H05.351 Exostosis of right orbit
    - H05.352 Exostosis of left orbit
    - H05.353 Exostosis of bilateral orbits
    - H05.359 Exostosis of unspecified orbit
- ● H05.4 Enophthalmos
  - *Recessed eyeball into orbit*
  - ● H05.40 Unspecified enophthalmos
    - H05.401 Unspecified enophthalmos, right eye
    - H05.402 Unspecified enophthalmos, left eye
    - H05.403 Unspecified enophthalmos, bilateral
    - H05.409 Unspecified enophthalmos, unspecified eye
  - ● H05.41 Enophthalmos due to atrophy of orbital tissue
    - H05.411 Enophthalmos due to atrophy of orbital tissue, right eye
    - H05.412 Enophthalmos due to atrophy of orbital tissue, left eye
    - H05.413 Enophthalmos due to atrophy of orbital tissue, bilateral
    - H05.419 Enophthalmos due to atrophy of orbital tissue, unspecified eye
  - ● H05.42 Enophthalmos due to trauma or surgery
    - H05.421 Enophthalmos due to trauma or surgery, right eye
    - H05.422 Enophthalmos due to trauma or surgery, left eye
    - H05.423 Enophthalmos due to trauma or surgery, bilateral
    - H05.429 Enophthalmos due to trauma or surgery, unspecified eye

● **H05.5 Retained (old) foreign body following penetrating wound of orbit**
Retrobulbar foreign body
Use additional code to identify the type of retained foreign body (Z18.-)
Excludes1 current penetrating wound of orbit (S05.4-)
Excludes2 retained foreign body of eyelid (H02.81-)
retained intraocular foreign body (H44.6-, H44.7-)
H05.50 Retained (old) foreign body following penetrating wound of **unspecified** orbit
H05.51 Retained (old) foreign body following penetrating wound of **right** orbit
H05.52 Retained (old) foreign body following penetrating wound of **left** orbit
H05.53 Retained (old) foreign body following penetrating wound of **bilateral** orbits

● H05.8 Other disorders of orbit
● H05.81 Cyst of orbit
Encephalocele of orbit
H05.811 Cyst of **right** orbit
H05.812 Cyst of **left** orbit
H05.813 Cyst of **bilateral** orbits
H05.819 Cyst of **unspecified** orbit
● H05.82 Myopathy of extraocular muscles
Weakness of muscles of eye
H05.821 Myopathy of extraocular muscles, **right** orbit
H05.822 Myopathy of extraocular muscles, **left** orbit
H05.823 Myopathy of extraocular muscles, **bilateral**
H05.829 Myopathy of extraocular muscles, **unspecified** orbit
H05.89 Other disorders of orbit
H05.9 **Unspecified** disorder of orbit

DISORDERS OF CONJUNCTIVA (H10-H11)

★**(See Plate 18 of the Anatomy Illustrations.)**

● H10 Conjunctivitis
Inflammation of membrane of the inside of the eyelid or on surface of eye (conjunctiva)
Excludes1 keratoconjunctivitis (H16.2-)
● H10.0 **Mucopurulent** conjunctivitis
● H10.01 **Acute follicular** conjunctivitis
H10.011 Acute follicular conjunctivitis, **right** eye
H10.012 Acute follicular conjunctivitis, **left** eye
H10.013 Acute follicular conjunctivitis, **bilateral**
H10.019 Acute follicular conjunctivitis, **unspecified** eye
● H10.02 Other mucopurulent conjunctivitis
H10.021 Other mucopurulent conjunctivitis, **right** eye
H10.022 Other mucopurulent conjunctivitis, **left** eye
H10.023 Other mucopurulent conjunctivitis, **bilateral**
H10.029 Other mucopurulent conjunctivitis, **unspecified** eye
● H10.1 **Acute atopic** conjunctivitis
Acute papillary conjunctivitis
H10.10 Acute atopic conjunctivitis, **unspecified** eye
H10.11 Acute atopic conjunctivitis, **right** eye
H10.12 Acute atopic conjunctivitis, **left** eye
H10.13 Acute atopic conjunctivitis, **bilateral**

● H10.2 **Other acute** conjunctivitis
● H10.21 **Acute toxic** conjunctivitis
Acute chemical conjunctivitis
Code first (T51-T65) to identify chemical and intent
Excludes1 burn and corrosion of eye and adnexa (T26.-)
H10.211 Acute toxic conjunctivitis, **right** eye
H10.212 Acute toxic conjunctivitis, **left** eye
H10.213 Acute toxic conjunctivitis, **bilateral**
H10.219 Acute toxic conjunctivitis, **unspecified** eye
● H10.22 **Pseudomembranous** conjunctivitis
H10.221 Pseudomembranous conjunctivitis, **right** eye
H10.222 Pseudomembranous conjunctivitis, **left** eye
H10.223 Pseudomembranous conjunctivitis, **bilateral**
H10.229 Pseudomembranous conjunctivitis, **unspecified** eye
● H10.23 Serous conjunctivitis, except viral
Excludes1 viral conjunctivitis (B30.-)
H10.231 Serous conjunctivitis, except viral, **right** eye
H10.232 Serous conjunctivitis, except viral, **left** eye
H10.233 Serous conjunctivitis, except viral, **bilateral**
H10.239 Serous conjunctivitis, except viral, **unspecified** eye
● H10.3 **Unspecified acute** conjunctivitis
Excludes1 ophthalmia neonatorum NOS (P39.1)
H10.30 Unspecified acute conjunctivitis, **unspecified** eye
H10.31 Unspecified acute conjunctivitis, **right** eye
H10.32 Unspecified acute conjunctivitis, **left** eye
H10.33 Unspecified acute conjunctivitis, **bilateral**
● H10.4 **Chronic** conjunctivitis
● H10.40 **Unspecified** chronic conjunctivitis
H10.401 Unspecified chronic conjunctivitis, **right** eye
H10.402 Unspecified chronic conjunctivitis, **left** eye
H10.403 Unspecified chronic conjunctivitis, **bilateral**
H10.409 Unspecified chronic conjunctivitis, **unspecified** eye
● H10.41 Chronic **giant papillary** conjunctivitis
Inflammation of membrane of the inside of the eyelid or on surface of eye often associated with contact lens wear
H10.411 Chronic giant papillary conjunctivitis, **right** eye
H10.412 Chronic giant papillary conjunctivitis, **left** eye
H10.413 Chronic giant papillary conjunctivitis, **bilateral**
H10.419 Chronic giant papillary conjunctivitis, **unspecified** eye
● H10.42 **Simple** chronic conjunctivitis
H10.421 Simple chronic conjunctivitis, **right** eye
H10.422 Simple chronic conjunctivitis, **left** eye
H10.423 Simple chronic conjunctivitis, **bilateral**
H10.429 Simple chronic conjunctivitis, **unspecified** eye

CHAPTER 7 (H00-H59)

● H10.43 Chronic follicular conjunctivitis
Inflammation of membrane of the inside of the eyelid or on surface of eye due to topical medications or infection
H10.431 Chronic follicular conjunctivitis, right eye
H10.432 Chronic follicular conjunctivitis, left eye
H10.433 Chronic follicular conjunctivitis, bilateral
H10.439 Chronic follicular conjunctivitis, unspecified eye
H10.44 Vernal conjunctivitis
Affecting children, especially boys in which there are flattened papules with thick, gelatinous exudate on conjunctivae on inside of upper lid
Excludes1 vernal keratoconjunctivitis with limbar and corneal involvement (H16.26-)
H10.45 Other chronic allergic conjunctivitis
● H10.5 Blepharoconjunctivitis
Inflammation of eyelids and conjunctiva
● H10.50 Unspecified blepharoconjunctivitis
H10.501 Unspecified blepharoconjunctivitis, right eye
H10.502 Unspecified blepharoconjunctivitis, left eye
H10.503 Unspecified blepharoconjunctivitis, bilateral
H10.509 Unspecified blepharoconjunctivitis, unspecified eye
● H10.51 Ligneous conjunctivitis
Code also underlying condition if known, such as:
plasminogen deficiency (E88.02)
H10.511 Ligneous conjunctivitis, right eye
H10.512 Ligneous conjunctivitis, left eye
H10.513 Ligneous conjunctivitis, bilateral
H10.519 Ligneous conjunctivitis, unspecified eye
● H10.52 Angular blepharoconjunctivitis
H10.521 Angular blepharoconjunctivitis, right eye
H10.522 Angular blepharoconjunctivitis, left eye
H10.523 Angular blepharoconjunctivitis, bilateral
H10.529 Angular blepharoconjunctivitis, unspecified eye
● H10.53 Contact blepharoconjunctivitis
H10.531 Contact blepharoconjunctivitis, right eye
H10.532 Contact blepharoconjunctivitis, left eye
H10.533 Contact blepharoconjunctivitis, bilateral
H10.539 Contact blepharoconjunctivitis, unspecified eye
● H10.8 Other conjunctivitis
● H10.81 Pingueculitis
Inflammation of a yellow, raised thickening on the white of the eye associated with chronic dry eyes
Excludes1 pinguecula (H11.15-)
H10.811 Pingueculitis, right eye
H10.812 Pingueculitis, left eye
H10.813 Pingueculitis, bilateral
H10.819 Pingueculitis, unspecified eye
● H10.82 Rosacea conjunctivitis
Code first underlying rosacea dermatitis (L71.-)
H10.821 Rosacea conjunctivitis, right eye
H10.822 Rosacea conjunctivitis, left eye
H10.823 Rosacea conjunctivitis, bilateral
Coding Clinic: 2018, Q4, P15
H10.829 Rosacea conjunctivitis, unspecified eye
H10.89 Other conjunctivitis
H10.9 Unspecified conjunctivitis
● H11 Other disorders of conjunctiva
Excludes1 keratoconjunctivitis (H16.2-)
● H11.0 Pterygium of eye
Excludes1 pseudopterygium (H11.81-)
● H11.00 Unspecified pterygium of eye
H11.001 Unspecified pterygium of right eye
H11.002 Unspecified pterygium of left eye
H11.003 Unspecified pterygium of eye, bilateral
H11.009 Unspecified pterygium of unspecified eye
● H11.01 Amyloid pterygium
H11.011 Amyloid pterygium of right eye
H11.012 Amyloid pterygium of left eye
H11.013 Amyloid pterygium of eye, bilateral
H11.019 Amyloid pterygium of unspecified eye
● H11.02 Central pterygium of eye
H11.021 Central pterygium of right eye
H11.022 Central pterygium of left eye
H11.023 Central pterygium of eye, bilateral
H11.029 Central pterygium of unspecified eye
● H11.03 Double pterygium of eye
H11.031 Double pterygium of right eye
H11.032 Double pterygium of left eye
H11.033 Double pterygium of eye, bilateral
H11.039 Double pterygium of unspecified eye
● H11.04 Peripheral pterygium of eye, stationary
H11.041 Peripheral pterygium, stationary, right eye
H11.042 Peripheral pterygium, stationary, left eye
H11.043 Peripheral pterygium, stationary, bilateral
H11.049 Peripheral pterygium, stationary, unspecified eye
● H11.05 Peripheral pterygium of eye, progressive
H11.051 Peripheral pterygium, progressive, right eye
H11.052 Peripheral pterygium, progressive, left eye
H11.053 Peripheral pterygium, progressive, bilateral
H11.059 Peripheral pterygium, progressive, unspecified eye
● H11.06 Recurrent pterygium of eye
H11.061 Recurrent pterygium of right eye
H11.062 Recurrent pterygium of left eye
H11.063 Recurrent pterygium of eye, bilateral
H11.069 Recurrent pterygium of unspecified eye

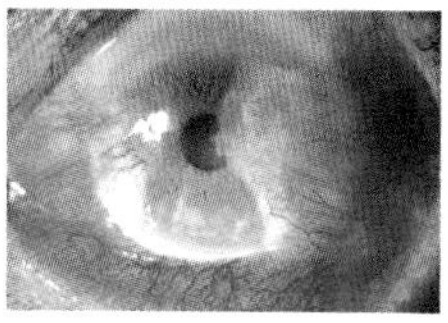

Figure 7-6 Double pterygium. Note both nasal and temporal pterygia in a 57-year-old farmer. (From Brightbill FS, McDonnell PJ: Corneal Surgery: Theory, Technique and Tissue, S.l., Mosby Elsevier, 2009)

Item 7-2 Pterygium is Greek for batlike. The condition is characterized by a membrane that extends from the limbus to the center of the cornea and resembles a wing.

● H11.1 Conjunctival degenerations and deposits
Excludes2 pseudopterygium (H11.81)
H11.10 Unspecified conjunctival degenerations
● H11.11 Conjunctival deposits
H11.111 Conjunctival deposits, right eye
H11.112 Conjunctival deposits, left eye
H11.113 Conjunctival deposits, bilateral
H11.119 Conjunctival deposits, unspecified eye
● H11.12 Conjunctival concretions
White to yellow nodules within or beneath conjunctiva
H11.121 Conjunctival concretions, right eye
H11.122 Conjunctival concretions, left eye
H11.123 Conjunctival concretions, bilateral
H11.129 Conjunctival concretions, unspecified eye
● H11.13 Conjunctival pigmentations
Conjunctival argyrosis [argyria]
H11.131 Conjunctival pigmentations, right eye
H11.132 Conjunctival pigmentations, left eye
H11.133 Conjunctival pigmentations, bilateral
H11.139 Conjunctival pigmentations, unspecified eye
● H11.14 Conjunctival xerosis, unspecified
Excludes1 xerosis of conjunctiva due to vitamin A deficiency (E50.0, E50.1)
H11.141 Conjunctival xerosis, unspecified, right eye
H11.142 Conjunctival xerosis, unspecified, left eye
H11.143 Conjunctival xerosis, unspecified, bilateral
H11.149 Conjunctival xerosis, unspecified, unspecified eye
● H11.15 Pinguecula
Yellowish spot near sclerocorneal junction, usually on nasal side; associated with aging
Excludes1 pingueculitis (H10.81-)
H11.151 Pinguecula, right eye
H11.152 Pinguecula, left eye
H11.153 Pinguecula, bilateral
H11.159 Pinguecula, unspecified eye
● H11.2 Conjunctival scars
● H11.21 Conjunctival adhesions and strands (localized)
H11.211 Conjunctival adhesions and strands (localized), right eye
H11.212 Conjunctival adhesions and strands (localized), left eye
H11.213 Conjunctival adhesions and strands (localized), bilateral
H11.219 Conjunctival adhesions and strands (localized), unspecified eye
● H11.22 Conjunctival granuloma
H11.221 Conjunctival granuloma, right eye
H11.222 Conjunctival granuloma, left eye
H11.223 Conjunctival granuloma, bilateral
H11.229 Conjunctival granuloma, unspecified
● H11.23 Symblepharon
Adhesion between tarsal conjunctiva and bulbar conjunctiva
H11.231 Symblepharon, right eye
H11.232 Symblepharon, left eye
H11.233 Symblepharon, bilateral
H11.239 Symblepharon, unspecified eye
● H11.24 Scarring of conjunctiva
H11.241 Scarring of conjunctiva, right eye
H11.242 Scarring of conjunctiva, left eye
H11.243 Scarring of conjunctiva, bilateral
H11.249 Scarring of conjunctiva, unspecified eye
● H11.3 Conjunctival hemorrhage
Subconjunctival hemorrhage
H11.30 Conjunctival hemorrhage, unspecified eye
H11.31 Conjunctival hemorrhage, right eye
H11.32 Conjunctival hemorrhage, left eye
H11.33 Conjunctival hemorrhage, bilateral
● H11.4 Other conjunctival vascular disorders and cysts
● H11.41 Vascular abnormalities of conjunctiva
Conjunctival aneurysm
H11.411 Vascular abnormalities of conjunctiva, right eye
H11.412 Vascular abnormalities of conjunctiva, left eye
H11.413 Vascular abnormalities of conjunctiva, bilateral
H11.419 Vascular abnormalities of conjunctiva, unspecified eye
● H11.42 Conjunctival edema
H11.421 Conjunctival edema, right eye
H11.422 Conjunctival edema, left eye
H11.423 Conjunctival edema, bilateral
H11.429 Conjunctival edema, unspecified eye
● H11.43 Conjunctival hyperemia
H11.431 Conjunctival hyperemia, right eye
H11.432 Conjunctival hyperemia, left eye
H11.433 Conjunctival hyperemia, bilateral
H11.439 Conjunctival hyperemia, unspecified eye
● H11.44 Conjunctival cysts
H11.441 Conjunctival cysts, right eye
H11.442 Conjunctival cysts, left eye
H11.443 Conjunctival cysts, bilateral
H11.449 Conjunctival cysts, unspecified eye
● H11.8 Other specified disorders of conjunctiva
● H11.81 Pseudopterygium of conjunctiva
Conjunctival scar attached to cornea
H11.811 Pseudopterygium of conjunctiva, right eye
H11.812 Pseudopterygium of conjunctiva, left eye
H11.813 Pseudopterygium of conjunctiva, bilateral
H11.819 Pseudopterygium of conjunctiva, unspecified eye
● H11.82 Conjunctivochalasis
Conjunctiva bulges over eyelid margin or covers lower punctum
H11.821 Conjunctivochalasis, right eye
H11.822 Conjunctivochalasis, left eye
H11.823 Conjunctivochalasis, bilateral
H11.829 Conjunctivochalasis, unspecified eye
H11.89 Other specified disorders of conjunctiva
H11.9 Unspecified disorder of conjunctiva

DISORDERS OF SCLERA, CORNEA, IRIS AND CILIARY BODY (H15-H22)

● H15 Disorders of sclera
● H15.0 Scleritis
Inflammation of the white (sclera and episclera) of the eye.
● H15.00 Unspecified scleritis
H15.001 Unspecified scleritis, **right eye**
H15.002 Unspecified scleritis, **left eye**
H15.003 Unspecified scleritis, **bilateral**
H15.009 Unspecified scleritis, **unspecified eye**
● H15.01 Anterior scleritis
H15.011 Anterior scleritis, **right eye**
H15.012 Anterior scleritis, **left eye**
H15.013 Anterior scleritis, **bilateral**
H15.019 Anterior scleritis, **unspecified eye**
● H15.02 Brawny scleritis
Swelling around the cornea that is gelantinous in appearance
H15.021 Brawny scleritis, **right eye**
H15.022 Brawny scleritis, **left eye**
H15.023 Brawny scleritis, **bilateral**
H15.029 Brawny scleritis, **unspecified eye**
● H15.03 Posterior scleritis
Sclerotenonitis
H15.031 Posterior scleritis, **right eye**
H15.032 Posterior scleritis, **left eye**
H15.033 Posterior scleritis, **bilateral**
H15.039 Posterior scleritis, **unspecified eye**
● H15.04 Scleritis with corneal involvement
H15.041 Scleritis with corneal involvement, **right eye**
H15.042 Scleritis with corneal involvement, **left eye**
H15.043 Scleritis with corneal involvement, **bilateral**
H15.049 Scleritis with corneal involvement, **unspecified eye**
● H15.05 Scleromalacia perforans
Necrotic without inflammation; usually associated with rheumatoid arthritis
H15.051 Scleromalacia perforans, **right eye**
H15.052 Scleromalacia perforans, **left eye**
H15.053 Scleromalacia perforans, **bilateral**
H15.059 Scleromalacia perforans, **unspecified eye**
● H15.09 Other scleritis
Scleral abscess
H15.091 Other scleritis, **right eye**
H15.092 Other scleritis, **left eye**
H15.093 Other scleritis, **bilateral**
H15.099 Other scleritis, **unspecified eye**
● H15.1 Episcleritis
Inflammation of the white (sclera and episclera) of the eye.
● H15.10 Unspecified episcleritis
H15.101 Unspecified episcleritis, **right eye**
H15.102 Unspecified episcleritis, **left eye**
H15.103 Unspecified episcleritis, **bilateral**
H15.109 Unspecified episcleritis, **unspecified eye**
● H15.11 Episcleritis periodica fugax
Transient, recurrent inflammation of portion of episclera (connective tissue on the surface of the sclera)
H15.111 Episcleritis periodica fugax, **right eye**
H15.112 Episcleritis periodica fugax, **left eye**
H15.113 Episcleritis periodica fugax, **bilateral**
H15.119 Episcleritis periodica fugax, **unspecified eye**
● H15.12 Nodular episcleritis
Characterized by tender, localized, moveable nodule within inflamed area
H15.121 Nodular episcleritis, **right eye**
H15.122 Nodular episcleritis, **left eye**
H15.123 Nodular episcleritis, **bilateral**
H15.129 Nodular episcleritis, **unspecified eye**
● H15.8 Other disorders of sclera
Excludes2 blue sclera (Q13.5)
degenerative myopia (H44.2-)
● H15.81 Equatorial staphyloma
H15.811 Equatorial staphyloma, **right eye**
H15.812 Equatorial staphyloma, **left eye**
H15.813 Equatorial staphyloma, **bilateral**
H15.819 Equatorial staphyloma, **unspecified eye**
● H15.82 Localized anterior staphyloma
H15.821 Localized anterior staphyloma, **right eye**
H15.822 Localized anterior staphyloma, **left eye**
H15.823 Localized anterior staphyloma, **bilateral**
H15.829 Localized anterior staphyloma, **unspecified eye**
● H15.83 Staphyloma posticum
H15.831 Staphyloma posticum, **right eye**
H15.832 Staphyloma posticum, **left eye**
H15.833 Staphyloma posticum, **bilateral**
H15.839 Staphyloma posticum, **unspecified eye**
● H15.84 Scleral ectasia
H15.841 Scleral ectasia, **right eye**
H15.842 Scleral ectasia, **left eye**
H15.843 Scleral ectasia, **bilateral**
H15.849 Scleral ectasia, **unspecified eye**
● H15.85 Ring staphyloma
H15.851 Ring staphyloma, **right eye**
H15.852 Ring staphyloma, **left eye**
H15.853 Ring staphyloma, **bilateral**
H15.859 Ring staphyloma, **unspecified eye**
H15.89 Other disorders of sclera
H15.9 Unspecified disorder of sclera

● H16 Keratitis
● H16.0 Corneal ulcer
● H16.00 Unspecified corneal ulcer
H16.001 Unspecified corneal ulcer, **right eye**
H16.002 Unspecified corneal ulcer, **left eye**
H16.003 Unspecified corneal ulcer, **bilateral**
H16.009 Unspecified corneal ulcer, **unspecified eye**
● H16.01 Central corneal ulcer
H16.011 Central corneal ulcer, **right eye**
H16.012 Central corneal ulcer, **left eye**
H16.013 Central corneal ulcer, **bilateral**
H16.019 Central corneal ulcer, **unspecified eye**
● H16.02 Ring corneal ulcer
H16.021 Ring corneal ulcer, **right eye**
H16.022 Ring corneal ulcer, **left eye**
H16.023 Ring corneal ulcer, **bilateral**
H16.029 Ring corneal ulcer, **unspecified eye**
● H16.03 Corneal ulcer with hypopyon
H16.031 Corneal ulcer with hypopyon, **right eye**
H16.032 Corneal ulcer with hypopyon, **left eye**
H16.033 Corneal ulcer with hypopyon, **bilateral**
H16.039 Corneal ulcer with hypopyon, **unspecified eye**

CHAPTER 7 (H00-H59)

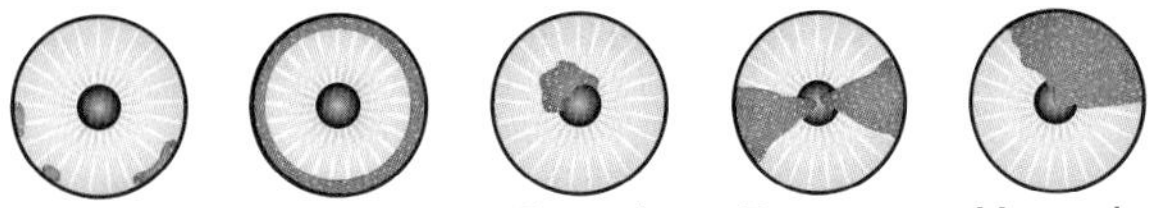

Figure 7-7 Corneal ulcers: marginal, ring, central corneal, rosacea, and Mooren's.

Item 7–3 An infected ulcer is usually called a **serpiginous** or **hypopyon** ulcer, which is a pus sac in the anterior chamber of the eye. **Marginal** ulcers are usually asymptomatic, not primary, and are often superficial and simple. More severe marginal ulcers spread to form a ring ulcer. **Ring** ulcers can extend around the entire corneal periphery. **Central corneal** ulcers develop when there is an abrasion to the epithelium and an infection develops in the eroded area. The **pyocyaneal** ulcer is the most serious corneal infection, which, if left untreated, can lead to loss of the eye.

● H16.04 **Marginal** corneal ulcer
- H16.041 Marginal corneal ulcer, **right** eye
- H16.042 Marginal corneal ulcer, **left** eye
- H16.043 Marginal corneal ulcer, **bilateral**
- H16.049 Marginal corneal ulcer, **unspecified** eye

● H16.05 **Mooren's** corneal ulcer
- H16.051 Mooren's corneal ulcer, **right** eye
- H16.052 Mooren's corneal ulcer, **left** eye
- H16.053 Mooren's corneal ulcer, **bilateral**
- H16.059 Mooren's corneal ulcer, **unspecified** eye

● H16.06 **Mycotic** corneal ulcer
- H16.061 Mycotic corneal ulcer, **right** eye
- H16.062 Mycotic corneal ulcer, **left** eye
- H16.063 Mycotic corneal ulcer, **bilateral**
- H16.069 Mycotic corneal ulcer, **unspecified** eye

● H16.07 **Perforated** corneal ulcer
- H16.071 Perforated corneal ulcer, **right** eye
- H16.072 Perforated corneal ulcer, **left** eye
- H16.073 Perforated corneal ulcer, **bilateral**
- H16.079 Perforated corneal ulcer, **unspecified** eye

● H16.1 Other and unspecified superficial keratitis without conjunctivitis

● H16.10 **Unspecified** superficial keratitis
- H16.101 Unspecified superficial keratitis, **right** eye
- H16.102 Unspecified superficial keratitis, **left** eye
- H16.103 Unspecified superficial keratitis, **bilateral**
- H16.109 Unspecified superficial keratitis, **unspecified** eye

● H16.11 **Macular** keratitis
Areolar keratitis
Nummular keratitis
Stellate keratitis
Striate keratitis
- H16.111 Macular keratitis, **right** eye
- H16.112 Macular keratitis, **left** eye
- H16.113 Macular keratitis, **bilateral**
- H16.119 Macular keratitis, **unspecified** eye

● H16.12 **Filamentary** keratitis
- H16.121 Filamentary keratitis, **right** eye
- H16.122 Filamentary keratitis, **left** eye
- H16.123 Filamentary keratitis, **bilateral**
- H16.129 Filamentary keratitis, **unspecified** eye

● H16.13 **Photokeratitis**
Snow blindness
Welders' keratitis
- H16.131 Photokeratitis, **right** eye
- H16.132 Photokeratitis, **left** eye
- H16.133 Photokeratitis, **bilateral**
- H16.139 Photokeratitis, **unspecified** eye

● H16.14 **Punctate** keratitis
- H16.141 Punctate keratitis, **right** eye
- H16.142 Punctate keratitis, **left** eye
- H16.143 Punctate keratitis, **bilateral**
- H16.149 Punctate keratitis, **unspecified** eye

● H16.2 Keratoconjunctivitis

● H16.20 **Unspecified** keratoconjunctivitis
Superficial keratitis with conjunctivitis NOS
- H16.201 Unspecified keratoconjunctivitis, **right** eye
- H16.202 Unspecified keratoconjunctivitis, **left** eye
- H16.203 Unspecified keratoconjunctivitis, **bilateral**
- H16.209 Unspecified keratoconjunctivitis, **unspecified** eye

● H16.21 **Exposure** keratoconjunctivitis
- H16.211 Exposure keratoconjunctivitis, **right** eye
- H16.212 Exposure keratoconjunctivitis, **left** eye
- H16.213 Exposure keratoconjunctivitis, **bilateral**
- H16.219 Exposure keratoconjunctivitis, **unspecified** eye

● H16.22 Keratoconjunctivitis **sicca**, not specified as Sjögren's
Excludes1 Sjogren's syndrome (M35.01)
- H16.221 Keratoconjunctivitis sicca, not specified as Sjögren's, **right** eye
- H16.222 Keratoconjunctivitis sicca, not specified as Sjögren's, **left** eye
- H16.223 Keratoconjunctivitis sicca, not specified as Sjögren's, **bilateral**
- H16.229 Keratoconjunctivitis sicca, not specified as Sjögren's, **unspecified** eye

● H16.23 **Neurotrophic** keratoconjunctivitis
- H16.231 Neurotrophic keratoconjunctivitis, **right** eye
- H16.232 Neurotrophic keratoconjunctivitis, **left** eye
- H16.233 Neurotrophic keratoconjunctivitis, **bilateral**
- H16.239 Neurotrophic keratoconjunctivitis, **unspecified** eye

● H16.24 **Ophthalmia nodosa**
- H16.241 Ophthalmia nodosa, **right** eye
- H16.242 Ophthalmia nodosa, **left** eye
- H16.243 Ophthalmia nodosa, **bilateral**
- H16.249 Ophthalmia nodosa, **unspecified** eye

● H16.25 **Phlyctenular** keratoconjunctivitis
- H16.251 Phlyctenular keratoconjunctivitis, **right** eye
- H16.252 Phlyctenular keratoconjunctivitis, **left** eye
- H16.253 Phlyctenular keratoconjunctivitis, **bilateral**
- H16.259 Phlyctenular keratoconjunctivitis, **unspecified** eye

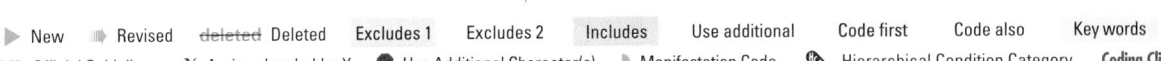

● H16.26   **Vernal keratoconjunctivitis, with limbar and corneal involvement**

> **Excludes1**   vernal conjunctivitis without limbar and corneal involvement (H10.44)

     H16.261   Vernal keratoconjunctivitis, with limbar and corneal involvement, **right eye**

     H16.262   Vernal keratoconjunctivitis, with limbar and corneal involvement, **left eye**

     H16.263   Vernal keratoconjunctivitis, with limbar and corneal involvement, **bilateral**

     H16.269   Vernal keratoconjunctivitis, with limbar and corneal involvement, **unspecified eye**

● H16.29   **Other keratoconjunctivitis**

     H16.291   Other keratoconjunctivitis, **right eye**

     H16.292   Other keratoconjunctivitis, **left eye**

     H16.293   Other keratoconjunctivitis, **bilateral**

     H16.299   Other keratoconjunctivitis, **unspecified eye**

● H16.3   **Interstitial and deep keratitis**

   ● H16.30   **Unspecified interstitial keratitis**

     H16.301   Unspecified interstitial keratitis, **right eye**

     H16.302   Unspecified interstitial keratitis, **left eye**

     H16.303   Unspecified interstitial keratitis, **bilateral**

     H16.309   Unspecified interstitial keratitis, **unspecified eye**

   ● H16.31   **Corneal abscess**

     H16.311   Corneal abscess, **right eye**

     H16.312   Corneal abscess, **left eye**

     H16.313   Corneal abscess, **bilateral**

     H16.319   Corneal abscess, **unspecified eye**

   ● H16.32   **Diffuse interstitial keratitis**
       Cogan's syndrome

     H16.321   Diffuse interstitial keratitis, **right eye**

     H16.322   Diffuse interstitial keratitis, **left eye**

     H16.323   Diffuse interstitial keratitis, **bilateral**

     H16.329   Diffuse interstitial keratitis, **unspecified eye**

   ● H16.33   **Sclerosing keratitis**

     H16.331   Sclerosing keratitis, **right eye**

     H16.332   Sclerosing keratitis, **left eye**

     H16.333   Sclerosing keratitis, **bilateral**

     H16.339   Sclerosing keratitis, **unspecified eye**

   ● H16.39   **Other interstitial and deep keratitis**

     H16.391   Other interstitial and deep keratitis, **right eye**

     H16.392   Other interstitial and deep keratitis, **left eye**

     H16.393   Other interstitial and deep keratitis, **bilateral**

     H16.399   Other interstitial and deep keratitis, **unspecified eye**

● H16.4   **Corneal neovascularization**

   ● H16.40   **Unspecified corneal neovascularization**

     H16.401   Unspecified corneal neovascularization, **right eye**

     H16.402   Unspecified corneal neovascularization, **left eye**

     H16.403   Unspecified corneal neovascularization, **bilateral**

     H16.409   Unspecified corneal neovascularization, **unspecified eye**

● H16.41   **Ghost vessels (corneal)**

     H16.411   Ghost vessels (corneal), **right eye**

     H16.412   Ghost vessels (corneal), **left eye**

     H16.413   Ghost vessels (corneal), **bilateral**

     H16.419   Ghost vessels (corneal), **unspecified eye**

● H16.42   **Pannus (corneal)**

     H16.421   Pannus (corneal), **right eye**

     H16.422   Pannus (corneal), **left eye**

     H16.423   Pannus (corneal), **bilateral**

     H16.429   Pannus (corneal), **unspecified eye**

● H16.43   **Localized vascularization of cornea**

     H16.431   Localized vascularization of cornea, **right eye**

     H16.432   Localized vascularization of cornea, **left eye**

     H16.433   Localized vascularization of cornea, **bilateral**

     H16.439   Localized vascularization of cornea, **unspecified eye**

● H16.44   **Deep vascularization of cornea**

     H16.441   Deep vascularization of cornea, **right eye**

     H16.442   Deep vascularization of cornea, **left eye**

     H16.443   Deep vascularization of cornea, **bilateral**

     H16.449   Deep vascularization of cornea, **unspecified eye**

   H16.8   **Other keratitis**

   H16.9   **Unspecified keratitis**

● H17   **Corneal scars and opacities**

   ● H17.0   **Adherent leukoma**

     H17.00   Adherent leukoma, **unspecified eye**

     H17.01   Adherent leukoma, **right eye**

     H17.02   Adherent leukoma, **left eye**

     H17.03   Adherent leukoma, **bilateral**

   ● H17.1   **Central corneal opacity**

     H17.10   Central corneal opacity, **unspecified eye**

     H17.11   Central corneal opacity, **right eye**

     H17.12   Central corneal opacity, **left eye**

     H17.13   Central corneal opacity, **bilateral**

   ● H17.8   **Other corneal scars and opacities**

    ● H17.81   **Minor opacity of cornea**
       Corneal nebula

     H17.811   Minor opacity of cornea, **right eye**

     H17.812   Minor opacity of cornea, **left eye**

     H17.813   Minor opacity of cornea, **bilateral**

     H17.819   Minor opacity of cornea, **unspecified eye**

    ● H17.82   **Peripheral opacity of cornea**

     H17.821   Peripheral opacity of cornea, **right eye**

     H17.822   Peripheral opacity of cornea, **left eye**

     H17.823   Peripheral opacity of cornea, **bilateral**

     H17.829   Peripheral opacity of cornea, **unspecified eye**

     H17.89   Other corneal scars and opacities

   H17.9   **Unspecified corneal scar and opacity**

● H18   **Other disorders of cornea**

   ● H18.0   **Corneal pigmentations and deposits**

    ● H18.00   **Unspecified corneal deposit**

     H18.001   Unspecified corneal deposit, **right eye**

     H18.002   Unspecified corneal deposit, **left eye**

     H18.003   Unspecified corneal deposit, **bilateral**

     H18.009   Unspecified corneal deposit, **unspecified eye**

CHAPTER 7 (H00–H59)

CHAPTER 7 (H00-H59)

● H18.01   **Anterior corneal pigmentations**
     Staehli's line
     H18.011   Anterior corneal pigmentations, **right eye**
     H18.012   Anterior corneal pigmentations, **left eye**
     H18.013   Anterior corneal pigmentations, **bilateral**
     H18.019   Anterior corneal pigmentations, **unspecified eye**

● H18.02   **Argentous corneal deposits**
     H18.021   Argentous corneal deposits, **right eye**
     H18.022   Argentous corneal deposits, **left eye**
     H18.023   Argentous corneal deposits, **bilateral**
     H18.029   Argentous corneal deposits, **unspecified eye**

● H18.03   **Corneal deposits in metabolic disorders**
     Code also associated metabolic disorder
     H18.031   Corneal deposits in metabolic disorders, **right eye**
     H18.032   Corneal deposits in metabolic disorders, **left eye**
     H18.033   Corneal deposits in metabolic disorders, **bilateral**
     H18.039   Corneal deposits in metabolic disorders, **unspecified eye**

● H18.04   **Kayser-Fleischer ring**
     Code also associated Wilson's disease (E83.01)
     H18.041   Kayser-Fleischer ring, **right eye**
     H18.042   Kayser-Fleischer ring, **left eye**
     H18.043   Kayser-Fleischer ring, **bilateral**
     H18.049   Kayser-Fleischer ring, **unspecified eye**

● H18.05   **Posterior corneal pigmentations**
     Krukenberg's spindle
     H18.051   Posterior corneal pigmentations, **right eye**
     H18.052   Posterior corneal pigmentations, **left eye**
     H18.053   Posterior corneal pigmentations, **bilateral**
     H18.059   Posterior corneal pigmentations, **unspecified eye**

● H18.06   **Stromal corneal pigmentations**
     Hematocornea
     H18.061   Stromal corneal pigmentations, **right eye**
     H18.062   Stromal corneal pigmentations, **left eye**
     H18.063   Stromal corneal pigmentations, **bilateral**
     H18.069   Stromal corneal pigmentations, **unspecified eye**

● H18.1   **Bullous keratopathy**
     H18.10   Bullous keratopathy, **unspecified eye**
     H18.11   Bullous keratopathy, **right eye**
     H18.12   Bullous keratopathy, **left eye**
     H18.13   Bullous keratopathy, **bilateral**

● H18.2   **Other and unspecified corneal edema**
     H18.20   Unspecified corneal edema
●   H18.21   **Corneal edema secondary to contact lens**
     Excludes2   other corneal disorders due to contact lens (H18.82-)
     H18.211   Corneal edema secondary to contact lens, **right eye**
     H18.212   Corneal edema secondary to contact lens, **left eye**
     H18.213   Corneal edema secondary to contact lens, **bilateral**
     H18.219   Corneal edema secondary to contact lens, **unspecified eye**

● H18.22   **Idiopathic corneal edema**
     H18.221   Idiopathic corneal edema, **right eye**
     H18.222   Idiopathic corneal edema, **left eye**
     H18.223   Idiopathic corneal edema, **bilateral**
     H18.229   Idiopathic corneal edema, **unspecified eye**

● H18.23   **Secondary corneal edema**
     H18.231   Secondary corneal edema, **right eye**
     H18.232   Secondary corneal edema, **left eye**
     H18.233   Secondary corneal edema, **bilateral**
     H18.239   Secondary corneal edema, **unspecified eye**

● H18.3   **Changes of corneal membranes**
     H18.30   Unspecified corneal membrane change
●   H18.31   **Folds and rupture in Bowman's membrane**
     H18.311   Folds and rupture in Bowman's membrane, **right eye**
     H18.312   Folds and rupture in Bowman's membrane, **left eye**
     H18.313   Folds and rupture in Bowman's membrane, **bilateral**
     H18.319   Folds and rupture in Bowman's membrane, **unspecified eye**

● H18.32   **Folds in Descemet's membrane**
     H18.321   Folds in Descemet's membrane, **right eye**
     H18.322   Folds in Descemet's membrane, **left eye**
     H18.323   Folds in Descemet's membrane, **bilateral**
     H18.329   Folds in Descemet's membrane, **unspecified eye**

● H18.33   **Rupture in Descemet's membrane**
     H18.331   Rupture in Descemet's membrane, **right eye**
     H18.332   Rupture in Descemet's membrane, **left eye**
     H18.333   Rupture in Descemet's membrane, **bilateral**
     H18.339   Rupture in Descemet's membrane, **unspecified eye**

● H18.4   **Corneal degeneration**
     Excludes1   Mooren's ulcer (H16.0-)
                       recurrent erosion of cornea (H18.83-)
     H18.40   Unspecified corneal degeneration
●   H18.41   **Arcus senilis**
     Senile corneal changes
     H18.411   Arcus senilis, **right eye**
     H18.412   Arcus senilis, **left eye**
     H18.413   Arcus senilis, **bilateral**
     H18.419   Arcus senilis, **unspecified eye**

● H18.42   **Band keratopathy**
     H18.421   Band keratopathy, **right eye**
     H18.422   Band keratopathy, **left eye**
     H18.423   Band keratopathy, **bilateral**
     H18.429   Band keratopathy, **unspecified eye**
     H18.43   Other calcerous corneal degeneration
●   H18.44   **Keratomalacia**
     Excludes1   keratomalacia due to vitamin A deficiency (E50.4)
     H18.441   Keratomalacia, **right eye**
     H18.442   Keratomalacia, **left eye**
     H18.443   Keratomalacia, **bilateral**
     H18.449   Keratomalacia, **unspecified eye**

▶ New   ⇒ Revised   ~~deleted~~ Deleted   Excludes 1   Excludes 2   Includes   Use additional   Code first   Code also   Key words
OGCR Official Guidelines   X Assign placeholder X   ● Use Additional Character(s)   ▶ Manifestation Code   🍁 Hierarchical Condition Category   Coding Clinic

● H18.45 Nodular corneal degeneration
H18.451 Nodular corneal degeneration, right eye
H18.452 Nodular corneal degeneration, left eye
H18.453 Nodular corneal degeneration, bilateral
H18.459 Nodular corneal degeneration, unspecified eye
● H18.46 Peripheral corneal degeneration
H18.461 Peripheral corneal degeneration, right eye
H18.462 Peripheral corneal degeneration, left eye
H18.463 Peripheral corneal degeneration, bilateral
H18.469 Peripheral corneal degeneration, unspecified eye
H18.49 Other corneal degeneration
● H18.5 Hereditary corneal dystrophies
H18.50 Unspecified hereditary corneal dystrophies
H18.51 Endothelial corneal dystrophy
Fuchs' dystrophy
H18.52 Epithelial (juvenile) corneal dystrophy
H18.53 Granular corneal dystrophy
H18.54 Lattice corneal dystrophy
H18.55 Macular corneal dystrophy
H18.59 Other hereditary corneal dystrophies
● H18.6 Keratoconus
● H18.60 Keratoconus, unspecified
H18.601 Keratoconus, unspecified, right eye
H18.602 Keratoconus, unspecified, left eye
H18.603 Keratoconus, unspecified, bilateral
H18.609 Keratoconus, unspecified, unspecified eye
● H18.61 Keratoconus, stable
H18.611 Keratoconus, stable, right eye
H18.612 Keratoconus, stable, left eye
H18.613 Keratoconus, stable, bilateral
H18.619 Keratoconus, stable, unspecified eye
● H18.62 Keratoconus, unstable
Acute hydrops
H18.621 Keratoconus, unstable, right eye
H18.622 Keratoconus, unstable, left eye
H18.623 Keratoconus, unstable, bilateral
H18.629 Keratoconus, unstable, unspecified eye

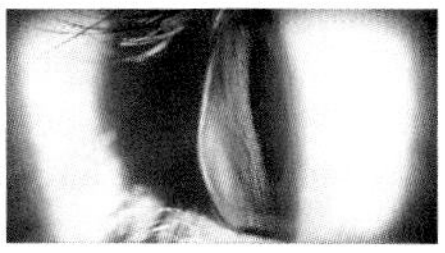

Figure 7-8 Lateral view of the displacement of the cone apex in keratoconus. (From Yanoff: Ophthalmology, ed 3, Mosby, Inc., 2008)

Item 7-4 Keratoconus results in corneal degeneration that begins in childhood, gradually changes the cornea from a round to cone shape, decreasing visual acuity. Treatment includes contact lenses. In severe cases the need for corneal transplant may be the treatment of choice; however, newer technologies may use high-frequency radio energy to shrink the edges of the cornea, pulling the central area back to a more normal shape. It can help delay or avoid the need for a corneal transplantation.

● H18.7 Other and unspecified corneal deformities
Excludes1 congenital malformations of cornea (Q13.3-Q13.4)
H18.70 Unspecified corneal deformity
● H18.71 Corneal ectasia
H18.711 Corneal ectasia, right eye
H18.712 Corneal ectasia, left eye
H18.713 Corneal ectasia, bilateral
H18.719 Corneal ectasia, unspecified eye
● H18.72 Corneal staphyloma
H18.721 Corneal staphyloma, right eye
H18.722 Corneal staphyloma, left eye
H18.723 Corneal staphyloma, bilateral
H18.729 Corneal staphyloma, unspecified eye
● H18.73 Descemetocele
H18.731 Descemetocele, right eye
H18.732 Descemetocele, left eye
H18.733 Descemetocele, bilateral
H18.739 Descemetocele, unspecified eye
● H18.79 Other corneal deformities
H18.791 Other corneal deformities, right eye
H18.792 Other corneal deformities, left eye
H18.793 Other corneal deformities, bilateral
H18.799 Other corneal deformities, unspecified eye
● H18.8 Other specified disorders of cornea
● H18.81 Anesthesia and hypoesthesia of cornea
H18.811 Anesthesia and hypoesthesia of cornea, right eye
H18.812 Anesthesia and hypoesthesia of cornea, left eye
H18.813 Anesthesia and hypoesthesia of cornea, bilateral
H18.819 Anesthesia and hypoesthesia of cornea, unspecified eye
● H18.82 Corneal disorder due to contact lens
Excludes2 corneal edema due to contact lens (H18.21-)
H18.821 Corneal disorder due to contact lens, right eye
H18.822 Corneal disorder due to contact lens, left eye
H18.823 Corneal disorder due to contact lens, bilateral
H18.829 Corneal disorder due to contact lens, unspecified eye
● H18.83 Recurrent erosion of cornea
H18.831 Recurrent erosion of cornea, right eye
H18.832 Recurrent erosion of cornea, left eye
H18.833 Recurrent erosion of cornea, bilateral
H18.839 Recurrent erosion of cornea, unspecified eye
● H18.89 Other specified disorders of cornea
H18.891 Other specified disorders of cornea, right eye
H18.892 Other specified disorders of cornea, left eye
H18.893 Other specified disorders of cornea, bilateral
H18.899 Other specified disorders of cornea, unspecified eye
H18.9 Unspecified disorder of cornea

● H20   Iridocyclitis
  ● H20.0   **Acute and subacute iridocyclitis**
      Acute anterior uveitis
      Acute cyclitis
      Acute iritis
      Subacute anterior uveitis
      Subacute cyclitis
      Subacute iritis

Excludes1   iridocyclitis, iritis, uveitis (due to) (in) diabetes mellitus (E08-E13 with .39)
iridocyclitis, iritis, uveitis (due to) (in) diphtheria (A36.89)
iridocyclitis, iritis, uveitis (due to) (in) gonococcal (A54.32)
iridocyclitis, iritis, uveitis (due to) (in) herpes (simplex) (B00.51)
iridocyclitis, iritis, uveitis (due to) (in) herpes zoster (B02.32)
iridocyclitis, iritis, uveitis (due to) (in) late congenital syphilis (A50.39)
iridocyclitis, iritis, uveitis (due to) (in) late syphilis (A52.71)
iridocyclitis, iritis, uveitis (due to) (in) sarcoidosis (D86.83)
iridocyclitis, iritis, uveitis (due to) (in) syphilis (A51.43)
iridocyclitis, iritis, uveitis (due to) (in) toxoplasmosis (B58.09)
iridocyclitis, iritis, uveitis (due to) (in) tuberculosis (A18.54)

     H20.00   Unspecified acute and subacute iridocyclitis
   ● H20.01   Primary iridocyclitis
       H20.011   Primary iridocyclitis, **right eye**
       H20.012   Primary iridocyclitis, **left eye**
       H20.013   Primary iridocyclitis, **bilateral**
       H20.019   Primary iridocyclitis, **unspecified eye**
   ● H20.02   Recurrent acute iridocyclitis
       H20.021   Recurrent acute iridocyclitis, **right eye**
       H20.022   Recurrent acute iridocyclitis, **left eye**
       H20.023   Recurrent acute iridocyclitis, **bilateral**
       H20.029   Recurrent acute iridocyclitis, **unspecified eye**
   ● H20.03   Secondary infectious iridocyclitis
       H20.031   Secondary infectious iridocyclitis, **right eye**
       H20.032   Secondary infectious iridocyclitis, **left eye**
       H20.033   Secondary infectious iridocyclitis, **bilateral**
       H20.039   Secondary infectious iridocyclitis, **unspecified eye**
   ● H20.04   Secondary noninfectious iridocyclitis
       H20.041   Secondary noninfectious iridocyclitis, **right eye**
       H20.042   Secondary noninfectious iridocyclitis, **left eye**
       H20.043   Secondary noninfectious iridocyclitis, **bilateral**
       H20.049   Secondary noninfectious iridocyclitis, **unspecified eye**
   ● H20.05   Hypopyon
       H20.051   Hypopyon, **right eye**
       H20.052   Hypopyon, **left eye**
       H20.053   Hypopyon, **bilateral**
       H20.059   Hypopyon, **unspecified eye**

● H20.1   Chronic iridocyclitis
     Use additional code for any associated cataract (H26.21-)
     Excludes2   posterior cyclitis (H30.2-)
     H20.10   Chronic iridocyclitis, **unspecified eye**
     H20.11   Chronic iridocyclitis, **right eye**
     H20.12   Chronic iridocyclitis, **left eye**
     H20.13   Chronic iridocyclitis, **bilateral**
● H20.2   Lens-induced iridocyclitis
     H20.20   Lens-induced iridocyclitis, **unspecified eye**
     H20.21   Lens-induced iridocyclitis, **right eye**
     H20.22   Lens-induced iridocyclitis, **left eye**
     H20.23   Lens-induced iridocyclitis, **bilateral**
● H20.8   Other iridocyclitis
     Excludes2   glaucomatocyclitis crises (H40.4-)
          posterior cyclitis (H30.2-)
          sympathetic uveitis (H44.13-)
   ● H20.81   Fuchs' heterochromic cyclitis
       H20.811   Fuchs' heterochromic cyclitis, **right eye**
       H20.812   Fuchs' heterochromic cyclitis, **left eye**
       H20.813   Fuchs' heterochromic cyclitis, **bilateral**
       H20.819   Fuchs' heterochromic cyclitis, **unspecified eye**
   ● H20.82   Vogt-Koyanagi syndrome
       H20.821   Vogt-Koyanagi syndrome, **right eye**
       H20.822   Vogt-Koyanagi syndrome, **left eye**
       H20.823   Vogt-Koyanagi syndrome, **bilateral**
       H20.829   Vogt-Koyanagi syndrome, **unspecified eye**
● H20.9   Unspecified iridocyclitis
     Uveitis NOS

● H21   Other disorders of iris and ciliary body
     Excludes2   sympathetic uveitis (H44.1-)
  ● H21.0   Hyphema
     Excludes1   traumatic hyphema (S05.1-)
     H21.00   Hyphema, **unspecified eye**
     H21.01   Hyphema, **right eye**
     H21.02   Hyphema, **left eye**
     H21.03   Hyphema, **bilateral**
  ● H21.1   Other vascular disorders of iris and ciliary body
     Neovascularization of iris or ciliary body
     Rubeosis iridis
     Rubeosis of iris
   ● H21.1X   Other vascular disorders of iris and ciliary body
       H21.1X1   Other vascular disorders of iris and ciliary body, **right eye**
       H21.1X2   Other vascular disorders of iris and ciliary body, **left eye**
       H21.1X3   Other vascular disorders of iris and ciliary body, **bilateral**
       H21.1X9   Other vascular disorders of iris and ciliary body, **unspecified eye**
  ● H21.2   Degeneration of iris and ciliary body
   ● H21.21   Degeneration of chamber angle
       H21.211   Degeneration of chamber angle, **right eye**
       H21.212   Degeneration of chamber angle, **left eye**
       H21.213   Degeneration of chamber angle, **bilateral**
       H21.219   Degeneration of chamber angle, **unspecified eye**

▶ New   ▶ Revised   ~~deleted~~ Deleted   Excludes 1   Excludes 2   Includes   Use additional   Code first   Code also   Key words
OGCR Official Guidelines   X Assign placeholder X   ● Use Additional Character(s)   ▶ Manifestation Code   🔾 Hierarchical Condition Category   Coding Clinic

● H21.22   Degeneration of ciliary body
     H21.221   Degeneration of ciliary body, **right eye**
     H21.222   Degeneration of ciliary body, **left eye**
     H21.223   Degeneration of ciliary body, **bilateral**
     H21.229   Degeneration of ciliary body, **unspecified eye**

● H21.23   Degeneration of **iris (pigmentary)**
     Translucency of iris
     H21.231   Degeneration of iris (pigmentary), **right eye**
     H21.232   Degeneration of iris (pigmentary), **left eye**
     H21.233   Degeneration of iris (pigmentary), **bilateral**
     H21.239   Degeneration of iris (pigmentary), **unspecified eye**

● H21.24   Degeneration of pupillary margin
     H21.241   Degeneration of pupillary margin, **right eye**
     H21.242   Degeneration of pupillary margin, **left eye**
     H21.243   Degeneration of pupillary margin, **bilateral**
     H21.249   Degeneration of pupillary margin, **unspecified eye**

● H21.25   Iridoschisis
     H21.251   Iridoschisis, **right eye**
     H21.252   Iridoschisis, **left eye**
     H21.253   Iridoschisis, **bilateral**
     H21.259   Iridoschisis, **unspecified eye**

● H21.26   Iris atrophy (essential) (progressive)
     H21.261   Iris atrophy (essential) (progressive), **right eye**
     H21.262   Iris atrophy (essential) (progressive), **left eye**
     H21.263   Iris atrophy (essential) (progressive), **bilateral**
     H21.269   Iris atrophy (essential) (progressive), **unspecified eye**

● H21.27   Miotic pupillary cyst
     H21.271   Miotic pupillary cyst, **right eye**
     H21.272   Miotic pupillary cyst, **left eye**
     H21.273   Miotic pupillary cyst, **bilateral**
     H21.279   Miotic pupillary cyst, **unspecified eye**

     H21.29   **Other iris atrophy**

● H21.3   Cyst of iris, ciliary body and anterior chamber
     Excludes2   miotic pupillary cyst (H21.27-)

● H21.30   Idiopathic cysts of iris, ciliary body or anterior chamber
     Cyst of iris, ciliary body or anterior chamber NOS
     H21.301   Idiopathic cysts of iris, ciliary body or anterior chamber, **right eye**
     H21.302   Idiopathic cysts of iris, ciliary body or anterior chamber, **left eye**
     H21.303   Idiopathic cysts of iris, ciliary body or anterior chamber, **bilateral**
     H21.309   Idiopathic cysts of iris, ciliary body or anterior chamber, **unspecified eye**

● H21.31   Exudative cysts of iris or anterior chamber
     H21.311   Exudative cysts of iris or anterior chamber, **right eye**
     H21.312   Exudative cysts of iris or anterior chamber, **left eye**
     H21.313   Exudative cysts of iris or anterior chamber, **bilateral**
     H21.319   Exudative cysts of iris or anterior chamber, **unspecified eye**

● H21.32   Implantation cysts of iris, ciliary body or anterior chamber
     H21.321   Implantation cysts of iris, ciliary body or anterior chamber, **right eye**
     H21.322   Implantation cysts of iris, ciliary body or anterior chamber, **left eye**
     H21.323   Implantation cysts of iris, ciliary body or anterior chamber, **bilateral**
     H21.329   Implantation cysts of iris, ciliary body or anterior chamber, **unspecified eye**

● H21.33   Parasitic cyst of iris, ciliary body or anterior chamber
     H21.331   Parasitic cyst of iris, ciliary body or anterior chamber, **right eye**
     H21.332   Parasitic cyst of iris, ciliary body or anterior chamber, **left eye**
     H21.333   Parasitic cyst of iris, ciliary body or anterior chamber, **bilateral**
     H21.339   Parasitic cyst of iris, ciliary body or anterior chamber, **unspecified eye**

● H21.34   Primary cyst of pars plana
     H21.341   Primary cyst of pars plana, **right eye**
     H21.342   Primary cyst of pars plana, **left eye**
     H21.343   Primary cyst of pars plana, **bilateral**
     H21.349   Primary cyst of pars plana, **unspecified eye**

● H21.35   Exudative cyst of pars plana
     H21.351   Exudative cyst of pars plana, **right eye**
     H21.352   Exudative cyst of pars plana, **left eye**
     H21.353   Exudative cyst of pars plana, **bilateral**
     H21.359   Exudative cyst of pars plana, **unspecified eye**

● H21.4   Pupillary membranes
     Iris bombé
     Pupillary occlusion
     Pupillary seclusion
     Excludes1   congenital pupillary membranes (Q13.8)
     H21.40   Pupillary membranes, **unspecified eye**
     H21.41   Pupillary membranes, **right eye**
     H21.42   Pupillary membranes, **left eye**
     H21.43   Pupillary membranes, **bilateral**

● H21.5   Other and unspecified adhesions and disruptions of iris and ciliary body
     Excludes1   corectopia (Q13.2)

● H21.50   Unspecified adhesions of iris
     Synechia (iris) NOS
     H21.501   Unspecified adhesions of iris, **right eye**
     H21.502   Unspecified adhesions of iris, **left eye**
     H21.503   Unspecified adhesions of iris, **bilateral**
     H21.509   Unspecified adhesions of iris and ciliary body, **unspecified eye**

● H21.51   Anterior synechiae (iris)
     H21.511   Anterior synechiae (iris), **right eye**
     H21.512   Anterior synechiae (iris), **left eye**
     H21.513   Anterior synechiae (iris), **bilateral**
     H21.519   Anterior synechiae (iris), **unspecified eye**

● H21.52   Goniosynechiae
     H21.521   Goniosynechiae, **right eye**
     H21.522   Goniosynechiae, **left eye**
     H21.523   Goniosynechiae, **bilateral**
     H21.529   Goniosynechiae, **unspecified eye**

CHAPTER 7 (H00–H59)

● H21.53 Iridodialysis
H21.531 Iridodialysis, **right eye**
H21.532 Iridodialysis, **left eye**
H21.533 Iridodialysis, **bilateral**
H21.539 Iridodialysis, **unspecified eye**

● H21.54 Posterior synechiae (iris)
H21.541 Posterior synechiae (iris), **right eye**
H21.542 Posterior synechiae (iris), **left eye**
H21.543 Posterior synechiae (iris), **bilateral**
H21.549 Posterior synechiae (iris), **unspecified eye**

● H21.55 Recession of chamber angle
H21.551 Recession of chamber angle, **right eye**
H21.552 Recession of chamber angle, **left eye**
H21.553 Recession of chamber angle, **bilateral**
H21.559 Recession of chamber angle, **unspecified eye**

● H21.56 Pupillary abnormalities
Deformed pupil
Ectopic pupil
Rupture of sphincter, pupil
Excludes1 congenital deformity of pupil (Q13.2-)
H21.561 Pupillary abnormality, **right eye**
H21.562 Pupillary abnormality, **left eye**
H21.563 Pupillary abnormality, **bilateral**
H21.569 Pupillary abnormality, **unspecified eye**

● H21.8 Other specified disorders of iris and ciliary body
H21.81 Floppy iris syndrome
Intraoperative floppy iris syndrome (IFIS)
Use additional code for adverse effect, if applicable, to identify drug (T36-T5Ø with fifth or sixth character 5)
H21.82 Plateau iris syndrome (post-iridectomy) (postprocedural)
H21.89 Other specified disorders of iris and ciliary body
H21.9 **Unspecified** disorder of iris and ciliary body

H22 Disorders of iris and ciliary body in diseases classified elsewhere
Code first underlying disease, such as:
gout (M1A.-, M1Ø.-)
leprosy (A3Ø.-)
parasitic disease (B89)

DISORDERS OF LENS (H25-H28)

● H25 Age-related cataract
Senile cataract
Excludes2 capsular glaucoma with pseudoexfoliation of lens (H4Ø.1-)

● H25.Ø Age-related **incipient** cataract
● H25.Ø1 Cortical age-related cataract
H25.Ø11 Cortical age-related cataract, **right eye** A
H25.Ø12 Cortical age-related cataract, **left eye** A
H25.Ø13 Cortical age-related cataract, **bilateral** A
H25.Ø19 Cortical age-related cataract, **unspecified eye** A

● H25.Ø3 **Anterior subcapsular polar** age-related cataract
H25.Ø31 Anterior subcapsular polar age-related cataract, **right eye** A
H25.Ø32 Anterior subcapsular polar age-related cataract, **left eye** A
H25.Ø33 Anterior subcapsular polar age-related cataract, **bilateral** A
H25.Ø39 Anterior subcapsular polar age-related cataract, **unspecified eye** A

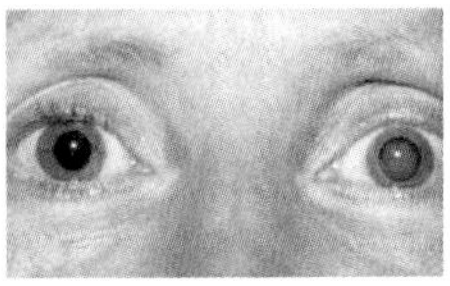

Figure 7-9 Age-related cataract. Nuclear sclerosis and cortical lens opacities are present. (From Ignatavicius DD, Workman ML: Medical-Surgical Nursing: Patient-Centered Collaborative Care, St. Louis, MO, Saunders/Elsevier, 2010)

Item 7-5 Senile cataracts are linked to the aging process. The most common area for the formation of a cataract is the cortical area of the lens. **Polar cataracts** can be either anterior or posterior. **Anterior polar cataracts** are more common and are small, white, capsular cataracts located on the anterior portion of the lens. **Total cataracts,** also called **complete** or **mature,** cause an opacity of all fibers of the lens. **Hypermature** describes a mature cataract with a swollen, milky cortex that covers the entire lens. **Immature,** also called **incipient,** cataracts have a clear cortex and are only slightly opaque. Treatment for all cataracts is the removal of the lens.

● H25.Ø4 **Posterior subcapsular polar** age-related cataract
H25.Ø41 Posterior subcapsular polar age-related cataract, **right eye** A
H25.Ø42 Posterior subcapsular polar age-related cataract, **left eye** A
H25.Ø43 Posterior subcapsular polar age-related cataract, **bilateral** A
H25.Ø49 Posterior subcapsular polar age-related cataract, **unspecified eye** A

● H25.Ø9 Other age-related incipient cataract
Coronary age-related cataract
Punctate age-related cataract
Water clefts
H25.Ø91 Other age-related incipient cataract, **right eye** A
H25.Ø92 Other age-related incipient cataract, **left eye** A
H25.Ø93 Other age-related incipient cataract, **bilateral** A
H25.Ø99 Other age-related incipient cataract, **unspecified eye** A

● H25.1 Age-related **nuclear** cataract
Cataracta brunescens
Nuclear sclerosis cataract
H25.1Ø Age-related nuclear cataract, **unspecified eye** A
H25.11 Age-related nuclear cataract, **right eye** A
Coding Clinic: 2Ø19, Q2, P3Ø
H25.12 Age-related nuclear cataract, **left eye** A
Coding Clinic: 2Ø16, Q1, P33
H25.13 Age-related nuclear cataract, **bilateral** A
Coding Clinic: 2Ø16, Q1, P32

● H25.2 Age-related cataract, **morgagnian type**
Age-related hypermature cataract
H25.2Ø Age-related cataract, morgagnian type, **unspecified eye** A
H25.21 Age-related cataract, morgagnian type, **right eye** A
H25.22 Age-related cataract, morgagnian type, **left eye** A
H25.23 Age-related cataract, morgagnian type, **bilateral** A

● H25.8 Other age-related cataract
● H25.81 **Combined forms** of age-related cataract
H25.811 Combined forms of age-related cataract, **right eye** A
H25.812 Combined forms of age-related cataract, **left eye** A
H25.813 Combined forms of age-related cataract, **bilateral** A
Coding Clinic: 2Ø19, Q2, P3Ø
H25.819 Combined forms of age-related cataract, **unspecified eye** A
H25.89 **Other** age-related cataract A
H25.9 **Unspecified** age-related cataract A

● **H26** Other cataract

Excludes1 congenital cataract (Q12.Ø)

● **H26.Ø** Infantile and juvenile cataract

● **H26.ØØ** Unspecified infantile and juvenile cataract

- H26.ØØ1 Unspecified infantile and juvenile cataract, right eye **P**
- H26.ØØ2 Unspecified infantile and juvenile cataract, left eye **P**
- H26.ØØ3 Unspecified infantile and juvenile cataract, bilateral **P**
- H26.ØØ9 Unspecified infantile and juvenile cataract, unspecified eye **P**

● **H26.Ø1** Infantile and juvenile cortical, lamellar, or zonular cataract

- H26.Ø11 Infantile and juvenile cortical, lamellar, or zonular cataract, right eye **P**
- H26.Ø12 Infantile and juvenile cortical, lamellar, or zonular cataract, left eye **P**
- H26.Ø13 Infantile and juvenile cortical, lamellar, or zonular cataract, bilateral **P**
- H26.Ø19 Infantile and juvenile cortical, lamellar, or zonular cataract, unspecified eye **P**

● **H26.Ø3** Infantile and juvenile nuclear cataract

- H26.Ø31 Infantile and juvenile nuclear cataract, right eye **P**
- H26.Ø32 Infantile and juvenile nuclear cataract, left eye **P**
- H26.Ø33 Infantile and juvenile nuclear cataract, bilateral **P**
- H26.Ø39 Infantile and juvenile nuclear cataract, unspecified eye **P**

● **H26.Ø4** Anterior subcapsular polar infantile and juvenile cataract

- H26.Ø41 Anterior subcapsular polar infantile and juvenile cataract, right eye **P**
- H26.Ø42 Anterior subcapsular polar infantile and juvenile cataract, left eye **P**
- H26.Ø43 Anterior subcapsular polar infantile and juvenile cataract, bilateral **P**
- H26.Ø49 Anterior subcapsular polar infantile and juvenile cataract, unspecified eye **P**

● **H26.Ø5** Posterior subcapsular polar infantile and juvenile cataract

- H26.Ø51 Posterior subcapsular polar infantile and juvenile cataract, right eye **P**
- H26.Ø52 Posterior subcapsular polar infantile and juvenile cataract, left eye **P**
- H26.Ø53 Posterior subcapsular polar infantile and juvenile cataract, bilateral **P**
- H26.Ø59 Posterior subcapsular polar infantile and juvenile cataract, unspecified eye **P**

● **H26.Ø6** Combined forms of infantile and juvenile cataract

- H26.Ø61 Combined forms of infantile and juvenile cataract, right eye **P**
- H26.Ø62 Combined forms of infantile and juvenile cataract, left eye **P**
- H26.Ø63 Combined forms of infantile and juvenile cataract bilateral **P**
- H26.Ø69 Combined forms of infantile and juvenile cataract, unspecified eye **P**

H26.Ø9 Other infantile and juvenile cataract **P**

● **H26.1** Traumatic cataract

Use additional code (Chapter 2Ø) to identify external cause

● **H26.1Ø** Unspecified traumatic cataract

- H26.1Ø1 Unspecified traumatic cataract, right eye
- H26.1Ø2 Unspecified traumatic cataract, left eye
- H26.1Ø3 Unspecified traumatic cataract, bilateral
- H26.1Ø9 Unspecified traumatic cataract, unspecified eye

● **H26.11** Localized traumatic opacities

- H26.111 Localized traumatic opacities, right eye
- H26.112 Localized traumatic opacities, left eye
- H26.113 Localized traumatic opacities, bilateral
- H26.119 Localized traumatic opacities, unspecified eye

● **H26.12** Partially resolved traumatic cataract

- H26.121 Partially resolved traumatic cataract, right eye
- H26.122 Partially resolved traumatic cataract, left eye
- H26.123 Partially resolved traumatic cataract, bilateral
- H26.129 Partially resolved traumatic cataract, unspecified eye

● **H26.13** Total traumatic cataract

- H26.131 Total traumatic cataract, right eye
- H26.132 Total traumatic cataract, left eye
- H26.133 Total traumatic cataract, bilateral
- H26.139 Total traumatic cataract, unspecified eye

● **H26.2** Complicated cataract

H26.2Ø Unspecified complicated cataract

Cataracta complicata NOS

● **H26.21** Cataract with neovascularization

Code also associated condition, such as:
chronic iridocyclitis (H2Ø.1-)

- H26.211 Cataract with neovascularization, right eye
- H26.212 Cataract with neovascularization, left eye
- H26.213 Cataract with neovascularization, bilateral
- H26.219 Cataract with neovascularization, unspecified eye

● **H26.22** Cataract secondary to ocular disorders (degenerative) (inflammatory)

Code also associated ocular disorder

- H26.221 Cataract secondary to ocular disorders (degenerative) (inflammatory), right eye
- H26.222 Cataract secondary to ocular disorders (degenerative) (inflammatory), left eye
- H26.223 Cataract secondary to ocular disorders (degenerative) (inflammatory), bilateral
- H26.229 Cataract secondary to ocular disorders (degenerative) (inflammatory), unspecified eye

● **H26.23** Glaucomatous flecks (subcapsular)

Code first underlying glaucoma (H4Ø-H42)

- H26.231 Glaucomatous flecks (subcapsular), right eye
- H26.232 Glaucomatous flecks (subcapsular), left eye

H26.233 Glaucomatous flecks (subcapsular), **bilateral**
H26.239 Glaucomatous flecks (subcapsular), **unspecified** eye

● H26.3 Drug-induced cataract
Toxic cataract
Use additional code for adverse effect, if applicable, to identify drug (T36-T50 with fifth or sixth character 5)
H26.30 Drug-induced cataract, **unspecified** eye
H26.31 Drug-induced cataract, **right** eye
H26.32 Drug-induced cataract, **left** eye
H26.33 Drug-induced cataract, **bilateral**

● H26.4 Secondary cataract
Coding Clinic: 2018, Q2, P14
H26.40 **Unspecified** secondary cataract
● H26.41 Soemmering's ring
H26.411 Soemmering's ring, **right** eye
H26.412 Soemmering's ring, **left** eye
H26.413 Soemmering's ring, **bilateral**
H26.419 Soemmering's ring, **unspecified** eye
● H26.49 Other secondary cataract
H26.491 Other secondary cataract, **right** eye
H26.492 Other secondary cataract, **left** eye
Coding Clinic: 2018, Q2, P13
H26.493 Other secondary cataract, **bilateral**
H26.499 Other secondary cataract, **unspecified** eye
H26.8 Other specified cataract
H26.9 Unspecified cataract

● H27 Other disorders of lens
Excludes1 congenital lens malformations (Q12.-)
mechanical complications of intraocular lens implant (T85.2)
pseudophakia (Z96.1)

● H27.0 Aphakia
Acquired absence of lens
Acquired aphakia
Aphakia due to trauma
Excludes1 cataract extraction status (Z98.4-)
congenital absence of lens (Q12.3)
congenital aphakia (Q12.3)
H27.00 Aphakia, **unspecified** eye
H27.01 Aphakia, **right** eye
H27.02 Aphakia, **left** eye
H27.03 Aphakia, **bilateral**

● H27.1 Dislocation of lens
H27.10 **Unspecified** dislocation of lens
● H27.11 **Subluxation** of lens
H27.111 Subluxation of lens, **right** eye
H27.112 Subluxation of lens, **left** eye
H27.113 Subluxation of lens, **bilateral**
H27.119 Subluxation of lens, **unspecified** eye
● H27.12 **Anterior** dislocation of lens
H27.121 Anterior dislocation of lens, **right** eye
H27.122 Anterior dislocation of lens, **left** eye
H27.123 Anterior dislocation of lens, **bilateral**
H27.129 Anterior dislocation of lens, **unspecified** eye
● H27.13 **Posterior** dislocation of lens
H27.131 Posterior dislocation of lens, **right** eye
H27.132 Posterior dislocation of lens, **left** eye
H27.133 Posterior dislocation of lens, **bilateral**
H27.139 Posterior dislocation of lens, **unspecified** eye
H27.8 Other specified disorders of lens
H27.9 Unspecified disorder of lens

H28 Cataract in diseases classified elsewhere
Code first underlying disease, such as:
hypoparathyroidism (E20.-)
myotonia (G71.1-)
myxedema (E03.-)
protein-calorie malnutrition (E40-E46)
Excludes1 cataract in diabetes mellitus (E08.36, E09.36, E10.36, E11.36, E13.36)

DISORDERS OF CHOROID AND RETINA (H30-H36)

★ **(See Plate 16 of the Anatomy Illustrations.)**

● H30 Chorioretinal inflammation

● H30.0 **Focal** chorioretinal inflammation
Focal chorioretinitis
Focal choroiditis
Focal retinitis
Focal retinochoroiditis
● H30.00 **Unspecified** focal chorioretinal inflammation
Focal chorioretinitis NOS
Focal choroiditis NOS
Focal retinitis NOS
Focal retinochoroiditis NOS
H30.001 Unspecified focal chorioretinal inflammation, **right** eye
H30.002 Unspecified focal chorioretinal inflammation, **left** eye
H30.003 Unspecified focal chorioretinal inflammation, **bilateral**
H30.009 Unspecified focal chorioretinal inflammation, **unspecified** eye
● H30.01 Focal chorioretinal inflammation, **juxtapapillary**
H30.011 Focal chorioretinal inflammation, juxtapapillary, **right** eye
H30.012 Focal chorioretinal inflammation, juxtapapillary, **left** eye
H30.013 Focal chorioretinal inflammation, juxtapapillary, **bilateral**
H30.019 Focal chorioretinal inflammation, juxtapapillary, **unspecified** eye
● H30.02 Focal chorioretinal inflammation of **posterior pole**
H30.021 Focal chorioretinal inflammation of posterior pole, **right** eye
H30.022 Focal chorioretinal inflammation of posterior pole, **left** eye
H30.023 Focal chorioretinal inflammation of posterior pole, **bilateral**
H30.029 Focal chorioretinal inflammation of posterior pole, **unspecified** eye
● H30.03 Focal chorioretinal inflammation, **peripheral**
H30.031 Focal chorioretinal inflammation, peripheral, **right** eye
H30.032 Focal chorioretinal inflammation, peripheral, **left** eye
H30.033 Focal chorioretinal inflammation, peripheral, **bilateral**
H30.039 Focal chorioretinal inflammation, peripheral, **unspecified** eye
● H30.04 Focal chorioretinal inflammation, **macular or paramacular**
H30.041 Focal chorioretinal inflammation, macular or paramacular, **right** eye
H30.042 Focal chorioretinal inflammation, macular or paramacular, **left** eye
H30.043 Focal chorioretinal inflammation, macular or paramacular, **bilateral**
H30.049 Focal chorioretinal inflammation, macular or paramacular, **unspecified** eye

H30.1 **Disseminated** chorioretinal inflammation
Disseminated chorioretinitis
Disseminated choroiditis
Disseminated retinitis
Disseminated retinochoroiditis
Excludes2 exudative retinopathy (H35.02-)

H30.10 **Unspecified** disseminated chorioretinal inflammation
Disseminated chorioretinitis NOS
Disseminated choroiditis NOS
Disseminated retinitis NOS
Disseminated retinochoroiditis NOS

H30.101 Unspecified disseminated chorioretinal inflammation, **right** eye
H30.102 Unspecified disseminated chorioretinal inflammation, **left** eye
H30.103 Unspecified disseminated chorioretinal inflammation, **bilateral**
H30.109 Unspecified disseminated chorioretinal inflammation, **unspecified** eye

H30.11 Disseminated chorioretinal inflammation of **posterior pole**
H30.111 Disseminated chorioretinal inflammation of posterior pole, **right** eye
H30.112 Disseminated chorioretinal inflammation of posterior pole, **left** eye
H30.113 Disseminated chorioretinal inflammation of posterior pole, **bilateral**
H30.119 Disseminated chorioretinal inflammation of posterior pole, **unspecified** eye

H30.12 Disseminated chorioretinal inflammation, **peripheral**
H30.121 Disseminated chorioretinal inflammation, peripheral **right** eye
H30.122 Disseminated chorioretinal inflammation, peripheral, **left** eye
H30.123 Disseminated chorioretinal inflammation, peripheral, **bilateral**
H30.129 Disseminated chorioretinal inflammation, peripheral, **unspecified** eye

H30.13 Disseminated chorioretinal inflammation, **generalized**
H30.131 Disseminated chorioretinal inflammation, generalized, **right** eye
H30.132 Disseminated chorioretinal inflammation, generalized, **left** eye
H30.133 Disseminated chorioretinal inflammation, generalized, **bilateral**
H30.139 Disseminated chorioretinal inflammation, generalized, **unspecified** eye

H30.14 **Acute posterior multifocal placoid pigment epitheliopathy**
H30.141 Acute posterior multifocal placoid pigment epitheliopathy, **right** eye
H30.142 Acute posterior multifocal placoid pigment epitheliopathy, **left** eye
H30.143 Acute posterior multifocal placoid pigment epitheliopathy, **bilateral**
H30.149 Acute posterior multifocal placoid pigment epitheliopathy, **unspecified** eye

H30.2 Posterior cyclitis
Pars planitis
H30.20 Posterior cyclitis, **unspecified** eye
H30.21 Posterior cyclitis, **right** eye
H30.22 Posterior cyclitis, **left** eye
H30.23 Posterior cyclitis, **bilateral**

H30.8 Other chorioretinal inflammations
H30.81 **Harada's** disease
H30.811 Harada's disease, **right** eye
H30.812 Harada's disease, **left** eye
H30.813 Harada's disease, **bilateral**
H30.819 Harada's disease, **unspecified** eye

H30.89 **Other** chorioretinal inflammations
H30.891 Other chorioretinal inflammations, **right** eye
H30.892 Other chorioretinal inflammations, **left** eye
H30.893 Other chorioretinal inflammations, **bilateral**
H30.899 Other chorioretinal inflammations, **unspecified** eye

H30.9 **Unspecified** chorioretinal inflammation
Chorioretinitis NOS
Choroiditis NOS
Neuroretinitis NOS
Retinitis NOS
Retinochoroiditis NOS
H30.90 Unspecified chorioretinal inflammation, **unspecified** eye
H30.91 Unspecified chorioretinal inflammation, **right** eye
H30.92 Unspecified chorioretinal inflammation, **left** eye
H30.93 Unspecified chorioretinal inflammation, **bilateral**

H31 Other disorders of choroid
H31.0 Chorioretinal **scars**
Excludes2 postsurgical chorioretinal scars (H59.81-)

H31.00 **Unspecified** chorioretinal scars
H31.001 Unspecified chorioretinal scars, **right** eye
H31.002 Unspecified chorioretinal scars, **left** eye
H31.003 Unspecified chorioretinal scars, **bilateral**
H31.009 Unspecified chorioretinal scars, **unspecified** eye

H31.01 Macula scars of posterior pole (postinflammatory) (post-traumatic)
Excludes1 postprocedural chorioretentinal scar (H59.81-)
H31.011 Macula scars of posterior pole (postinflammatory) (post-traumatic), **right** eye
H31.012 Macula scars of posterior pole (postinflammatory) (post-traumatic), **left** eye
H31.013 Macula scars of posterior pole (postinflammatory) (post-traumatic), **bilateral**
H31.019 Macula scars of posterior pole (postinflammatory) (post-traumatic), **unspecified** eye

● H31.02 Solar retinopathy
- H31.021 Solar retinopathy, right eye
- H31.022 Solar retinopathy, left eye
- H31.023 Solar retinopathy, bilateral
- H31.029 Solar retinopathy, unspecified eye

● H31.09 Other chorioretinal scars
- H31.091 Other chorioretinal scars, right eye
- H31.092 Other chorioretinal scars, left eye
- H31.093 Other chorioretinal scars, bilateral
- H31.099 Other chorioretinal scars, unspecified eye

● H31.1 Choroidal degeneration

Excludes2 angioid streaks of macula (H35.33)

● H31.10 Unspecified choroidal degeneration

Choroidal sclerosis NOS
- H31.101 Choroidal degeneration, unspecified, right eye
- H31.102 Choroidal degeneration, unspecified, left eye
- H31.103 Choroidal degeneration, unspecified, bilateral
- H31.109 Choroidal degeneration, unspecified, unspecified eye

● H31.11 Age-related choroidal atrophy
- H31.111 Age-related choroidal atrophy, right eye A
- H31.112 Age-related choroidal atrophy, left eye A
- H31.113 Age-related choroidal atrophy, bilateral A
- H31.119 Age-related choroidal atrophy, unspecified eye A

● H31.12 Diffuse secondary atrophy of choroid
- H31.121 Diffuse secondary atrophy of choroid, right eye
- H31.122 Diffuse secondary atrophy of choroid, left eye
- H31.123 Diffuse secondary atrophy of choroid, bilateral
- H31.129 Diffuse secondary atrophy of choroid, unspecified eye

● H31.2 Hereditary choroidal dystrophy

Excludes2 hyperornithinemia (E72.4)
ornithinemia (E72.4)

- H31.20 Hereditary choroidal dystrophy, unspecified
- H31.21 Choroideremia
- H31.22 Choroidal dystrophy (central areolar) (generalized) (peripapillary)
- H31.23 Gyrate atrophy, choroid
- H31.29 Other hereditary choroidal dystrophy

● H31.3 Choroidal hemorrhage and rupture

● H31.30 Unspecified choroidal hemorrhage
- H31.301 Unspecified choroidal hemorrhage, right eye
- H31.302 Unspecified choroidal hemorrhage, left eye
- H31.303 Unspecified choroidal hemorrhage, bilateral
- H31.309 Unspecified choroidal hemorrhage, unspecified eye

● H31.31 Expulsive choroidal hemorrhage
- H31.311 Expulsive choroidal hemorrhage, right eye
- H31.312 Expulsive choroidal hemorrhage, left eye
- H31.313 Expulsive choroidal hemorrhage, bilateral
- H31.319 Expulsive choroidal hemorrhage, unspecified eye

● H31.32 Choroidal rupture
- H31.321 Choroidal rupture, right eye
- H31.322 Choroidal rupture, left eye
- H31.323 Choroidal rupture, bilateral
- H31.329 Choroidal rupture, unspecified eye

● H31.4 Choroidal detachment

● H31.40 Unspecified choroidal detachment
- H31.401 Unspecified choroidal detachment, right eye
- H31.402 Unspecified choroidal detachment, left eye
- H31.403 Unspecified choroidal detachment, bilateral
- H31.409 Unspecified choroidal detachment, unspecified eye

● H31.41 Hemorrhagic choroidal detachment
- H31.411 Hemorrhagic choroidal detachment, right eye
- H31.412 Hemorrhagic choroidal detachment, left eye
- H31.413 Hemorrhagic choroidal detachment, bilateral
- H31.419 Hemorrhagic choroidal detachment, unspecified eye

● H31.42 Serous choroidal detachment
- H31.421 Serous choroidal detachment, right eye
- H31.422 Serous choroidal detachment, left eye
- H31.423 Serous choroidal detachment, bilateral
- H31.429 Serous choroidal detachment, unspecified eye

- H31.8 Other specified disorders of choroid
- H31.9 Unspecified disorder of choroid

◗ *H32 Chorioretinal disorders in diseases classified elsewhere*

Code first underlying disease, such as:
congenital toxoplasmosis (P37.1)
histoplasmosis (B39.-)
leprosy (A30.-)

Excludes1 chorioretinitis (in):
toxoplasmosis (acquired) (B58.01)
tuberculosis (A18.53)

● H33 Retinal detachments and breaks

Excludes1 detachment of retinal pigment epithelium (H35.72-, H35.73-)

● H33.0 Retinal detachment with retinal break

Rhegmatogenous retinal detachment

Excludes1 serous retinal detachment (without retinal break) (H33.2-)

● H33.00 Unspecified retinal detachment with retinal break
- H33.001 Unspecified retinal detachment with retinal break, right eye
- H33.002 Unspecified retinal detachment with retinal break, left eye

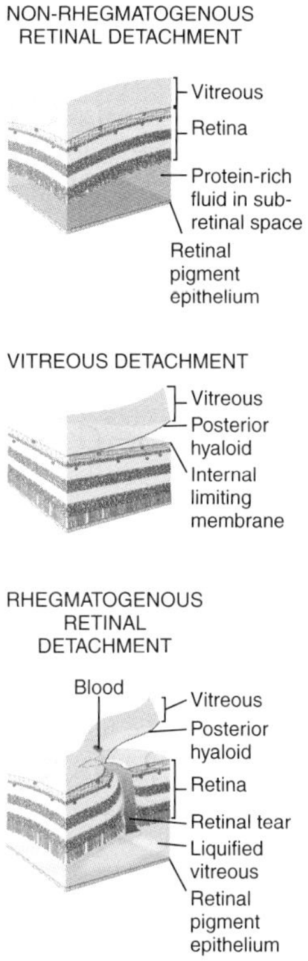

Figure 7-10 Retinal detachment. (From Kumar: Robbins and Cotran: Pathologic Basis of Disease, ed 7, Saunders, 2005)

Item 7–6 Retinal detachments and defects are conditions of the eye in which the retina separates from the underlying tissue. Initial detachment may be localized, requiring rapid treatment (medical emergency) to avoid the entire retina from detaching, which leads to vision loss and blindness.

- H33.ØØ3 Unspecified retinal detachment with retinal break, **bilateral**
- H33.ØØ9 Unspecified retinal detachment with retinal break, **unspecified eye**

● H33.Ø1 Retinal detachment with **single break**
- H33.Ø11 Retinal detachment with single break, **right eye**
- H33.Ø12 Retinal detachment with single break, **left eye**
- H33.Ø13 Retinal detachment with single break, **bilateral**
- H33.Ø19 Retinal detachment with single break, **unspecified eye**

● H33.Ø2 Retinal detachment with **multiple breaks**
- H33.Ø21 Retinal detachment with multiple breaks, **right eye**
- H33.Ø22 Retinal detachment with multiple breaks, **left eye**
- H33.Ø23 Retinal detachment with multiple breaks, **bilateral**
- H33.Ø29 Retinal detachment with multiple breaks, **unspecified eye**

● H33.Ø3 Retinal detachment with **giant retinal tear**
- H33.Ø31 Retinal detachment with giant retinal tear, **right eye**
- H33.Ø32 Retinal detachment with giant retinal tear, **left eye**
- H33.Ø33 Retinal detachment with giant retinal tear, **bilateral**
- H33.Ø39 Retinal detachment with giant retinal tear, **unspecified eye**

● H33.Ø4 Retinal detachment with **retinal dialysis**
- H33.Ø41 Retinal detachment with retinal dialysis, **right eye**
- H33.Ø42 Retinal detachment with retinal dialysis, **left eye**
- H33.Ø43 Retinal detachment with retinal dialysis, **bilateral**
- H33.Ø49 Retinal detachment with retinal dialysis, **unspecified eye**

● H33.Ø5 **Total** retinal detachment
- H33.Ø51 Total retinal detachment, **right eye**
- H33.Ø52 Total retinal detachment, **left eye**
- H33.Ø53 Total retinal detachment, **bilateral**
- H33.Ø59 Total retinal detachment, **unspecified eye**

● H33.1 Retinoschisis and retinal cysts

Excludes1 congenital retinoschisis (Q14.1)
microcystoid degeneration of retina (H35.42-)

● H33.1Ø **Unspecified** retinoschisis
- H33.1Ø1 Unspecified retinoschisis, **right eye**
- H33.1Ø2 Unspecified retinoschisis, **left eye**
- H33.1Ø3 Unspecified retinoschisis, **bilateral**
- H33.1Ø9 Unspecified retinoschisis, **unspecified eye**

● H33.11 Cyst of **ora serrata**
- H33.111 Cyst of ora serrata, **right eye**
- H33.112 Cyst of ora serrata, **left eye**
- H33.113 Cyst of ora serrata, **bilateral**
- H33.119 Cyst of ora serrata, **unspecified eye**

● H33.12 **Parasitic** cyst of retina
- H33.121 Parasitic cyst of retina, **right eye**
- H33.122 Parasitic cyst of retina, **left eye**
- H33.123 Parasitic cyst of retina, **bilateral**
- H33.129 Parasitic cyst of retina, **unspecified eye**

● H33.19 **Other** retinoschisis and retinal cysts

Pseudocyst of retina
- H33.191 Other retinoschisis and retinal cysts, **right eye**
- H33.192 Other retinoschisis and retinal cysts, **left eye**
- H33.193 Other retinoschisis and retinal cysts, **bilateral**
- H33.199 Other retinoschisis and retinal cysts, **unspecified eye**

● H33.2 Serous retinal detachment

Retinal detachment NOS
Retinal detachment without retinal break

Excludes1 central serous chorioretinopathy (H35.71-)

- H33.2Ø Serous retinal detachment, **unspecified eye**
- H33.21 Serous retinal detachment, **right eye**
- H33.22 Serous retinal detachment, **left eye**
- H33.23 Serous retinal detachment, **bilateral**

● H33.3 Retinal breaks without detachment

Excludes1 chorioretinal scars after surgery for detachment (H59.81-)
peripheral retinal degeneration without break (H35.4-)

● H33.3Ø **Unspecified** retinal break
- H33.3Ø1 Unspecified retinal break, **right eye**
- H33.3Ø2 Unspecified retinal break, **left eye**
- H33.3Ø3 Unspecified retinal break, **bilateral**
- H33.3Ø9 Unspecified retinal break, **unspecified eye**

● H33.31 **Horseshoe tear** of retina without detachment
Operculum of retina without detachment
H33.311 Horseshoe tear of retina without detachment, **right** eye
H33.312 Horseshoe tear of retina without detachment, **left** eye
H33.313 Horseshoe tear of retina without detachment, **bilateral**
H33.319 Horseshoe tear of retina without detachment, **unspecified** eye

● H33.32 **Round hole** of retina without detachment
H33.321 Round hole, **right** eye
H33.322 Round hole, **left** eye
H33.323 Round hole, **bilateral**
H33.329 Round hole, **unspecified** eye

● H33.33 **Multiple defects** of retina without detachment
H33.331 Multiple defects of retina without detachment, **right** eye
H33.332 Multiple defects of retina without detachment, **left** eye
H33.333 Multiple defects of retina without detachment, **bilateral**
H33.339 Multiple defects of retina without detachment, **unspecified** eye

● H33.4 Traction detachment of retina
Proliferative vitreo-retinopathy with retinal detachment
H33.4Ø Traction detachment of retina, **unspecified** eye
H33.41 Traction detachment of retina, **right** eye
H33.42 Traction detachment of retina, **left** eye
H33.43 Traction detachment of retina, **bilateral**

H33.8 Other retinal detachments

● H34 Retinal vascular occlusions
Blockage in vessel of the retina
Excludes1 amaurosis fugax (G45.3)

● H34.Ø **Transient** retinal artery occlusion
H34.ØØ Transient retinal artery occlusion, **unspecified** eye
H34.Ø1 Transient retinal artery occlusion, **right** eye
H34.Ø2 Transient retinal artery occlusion, **left** eye
H34.Ø3 Transient retinal artery occlusion, **bilateral**

● H34.1 **Central** retinal artery occlusion
H34.1Ø Central retinal artery occlusion, **unspecified** eye
H34.11 Central retinal artery occlusion, **right** eye
H34.12 Central retinal artery occlusion, **left** eye
H34.13 Central retinal artery occlusion, **bilateral**

● H34.2 Other retinal artery occlusions

● H34.21 **Partial** retinal artery occlusion
Hollenhorst's plaque
Retinal microembolism
H34.211 Partial retinal artery occlusion, **right** eye
H34.212 Partial retinal artery occlusion, **left** eye
H34.213 Partial retinal artery occlusion, **bilateral**
H34.219 Partial retinal artery occlusion, **unspecified** eye

● H34.23 Retinal artery **branch** occlusion
H34.231 Retinal artery branch occlusion, **right** eye
H34.232 Retinal artery branch occlusion, **left** eye
H34.233 Retinal artery branch occlusion, **bilateral**
H34.239 Retinal artery branch occlusion, **unspecified** eye

● H34.8 Other retinal vascular occlusions
Coding Clinic: 2Ø16, Q4, P19

● H34.81 **Central** retinal vein occlusion
One of the following 7th characters is to be assigned to codes in subcategory H34.81 to designate the severity of the occlusion:

Ø	with macular edema
1	with retinal neovascularization
2	stable Old central retinal vein occlusion

● H34.811 Central retinal vein occlusion, **right** eye
● H34.812 Central retinal vein occlusion, **left** eye
● H34.813 Central retinal vein occlusion, **bilateral**
● H34.819 Central retinal vein occlusion, **unspecified** eye

● H34.82 **Venous engorgement**
Incipient retinal vein occlusion
Partial retinal vein occlusion
H34.821 Venous engorgement, **right** eye
H34.822 Venous engorgement, **left** eye
H34.823 Venous engorgement, **bilateral**
H34.829 Venous engorgement, **unspecified** eye

● H34.83 **Tributary** (branch) retinal vein occlusion
One of the following 7th characters is to be assigned to codes in subcategory H34.83 to designate the severity of the occlusion:

Ø	with macular edema
1	with retinal neovascularization
2	stable Old tributary (branch) retinal vein occlusion

● H34.831 Tributary (branch) retinal vein occlusion, **right** eye
● H34.832 Tributary (branch) retinal vein occlusion, **left** eye
● H34.833 Tributary (branch) retinal vein occlusion, **bilateral**
● H34.839 Tributary (branch) retinal vein occlusion, **unspecified** eye

H34.9 **Unspecified** retinal vascular occlusion

● **H35** Other retinal disorders

Excludes2 diabetic retinal disorders (E08.311-E08.359, E09.311-E09.359, E10.311-E10.359, E11.311-E11.359, E13.311-E13.359)

● **H35.0** Background retinopathy and retinal vascular changes

Code also any associated hypertension (I10.-)

OGCR Section I. C.9.a.5.

Hypertensive Retinopathy

Subcategory H35.0, Background retinopathy and retinal vascular changes, should be used with a code from category I10–I15, Hypertensive disease to include the systemic hypertension. The sequencing is based on the reason for the encounter.

H35.00 Unspecified background retinopathy

● H35.01 Changes in retinal vascular appearance
Retinal vascular sheathing

- H35.011 Changes in retinal vascular appearance, right eye
- H35.012 Changes in retinal vascular appearance, left eye
- H35.013 Changes in retinal vascular appearance, bilateral
- H35.019 Changes in retinal vascular appearance, unspecified eye

● H35.02 Exudative retinopathy
Coats retinopathy

- H35.021 Exudative retinopathy, right eye
- H35.022 Exudative retinopathy, left eye
- H35.023 Exudative retinopathy, bilateral
- H35.029 Exudative retinopathy, unspecified eye

● H35.03 Hypertensive retinopathy

- H35.031 Hypertensive retinopathy, right eye
- H35.032 Hypertensive retinopathy, left eye
- H35.033 Hypertensive retinopathy, bilateral
- H35.039 Hypertensive retinopathy, unspecified eye

● H35.04 Retinal micro-aneurysms, unspecified

- H35.041 Retinal micro-aneurysms, unspecified, right eye
- H35.042 Retinal micro-aneurysms, unspecified, left eye
- H35.043 Retinal micro-aneurysms, unspecified, bilateral
- H35.049 Retinal micro-aneurysms, unspecified, unspecified eye

● H35.05 Retinal neovascularization, unspecified

- H35.051 Retinal neovascularization, unspecified, right eye
- H35.052 Retinal neovascularization, unspecified, left eye
- H35.053 Retinal neovascularization, unspecified, bilateral
- H35.059 Retinal neovascularization, unspecified, unspecified eye

● H35.06 Retinal vasculitis
Eales disease
Retinal perivasculitis

- H35.061 Retinal vasculitis, right eye
- H35.062 Retinal vasculitis, left eye
- H35.063 Retinal vasculitis, bilateral
- H35.069 Retinal vasculitis, unspecified eye

● H35.07 Retinal telangiectasis

- H35.071 Retinal telangiectasis, right eye
- H35.072 Retinal telangiectasis, left eye
- H35.073 Retinal telangiectasis, bilateral
- H35.079 Retinal telangiectasis, unspecified eye

H35.09 Other intraretinal microvascular abnormalities
Retinal varices

● **H35.1** Retinopathy of prematurity

● H35.10 Retinopathy of prematurity, unspecified
Retinopathy of prematurity NOS

- H35.101 Retinopathy of prematurity, unspecified, right eye
- H35.102 Retinopathy of prematurity, unspecified, left eye
- H35.103 Retinopathy of prematurity, unspecified, bilateral
- H35.109 Retinopathy of prematurity, unspecified, unspecified eye

● H35.11 Retinopathy of prematurity, stage 0

- H35.111 Retinopathy of prematurity, stage 0, right eye
- H35.112 Retinopathy of prematurity, stage 0, left eye
- H35.113 Retinopathy of prematurity, stage 0, bilateral
- H35.119 Retinopathy of prematurity, stage 0, unspecified eye

● H35.12 Retinopathy of prematurity, stage 1

- H35.121 Retinopathy of prematurity, stage 1, right eye
- H35.122 Retinopathy of prematurity, stage 1, left eye
- H35.123 Retinopathy of prematurity, stage 1, bilateral
- H35.129 Retinopathy of prematurity, stage 1, unspecified eye

● H35.13 Retinopathy of prematurity, stage 2

- H35.131 Retinopathy of prematurity, stage 2, right eye
- H35.132 Retinopathy of prematurity, stage 2, left eye
- H35.133 Retinopathy of prematurity, stage 2, bilateral
- H35.139 Retinopathy of prematurity, stage 2, unspecified eye

● H35.14 Retinopathy of prematurity, stage 3

- H35.141 Retinopathy of prematurity, stage 3, right eye
- H35.142 Retinopathy of prematurity, stage 3, left eye
- H35.143 Retinopathy of prematurity, stage 3, bilateral
- H35.149 Retinopathy of prematurity, stage 3, unspecified eye

● H35.15 Retinopathy of prematurity, stage 4

- H35.151 Retinopathy of prematurity, stage 4, right eye
- H35.152 Retinopathy of prematurity, stage 4, left eye
- H35.153 Retinopathy of prematurity, stage 4, bilateral
- H35.159 Retinopathy of prematurity, stage 4, unspecified eye

CHAPTER 7 (H00-H59)

● H35.16 Retinopathy of prematurity, **stage 5**
- H35.161 Retinopathy of prematurity, stage 5, **right eye**
- H35.162 Retinopathy of prematurity, stage 5, **left eye**
- H35.163 Retinopathy of prematurity, stage 5, **bilateral**
- H35.169 Retinopathy of prematurity, stage 5, **unspecified** eye

● H35.17 Retrolental fibroplasia
- H35.171 Retrolental fibroplasia, **right eye**
- H35.172 Retrolental fibroplasia, **left eye**
- H35.173 Retrolental fibroplasia, **bilateral**
- H35.179 Retrolental fibroplasia, **unspecified** eye

● H35.2 Other non-diabetic proliferative retinopathy
Proliferative vitreo-retinopathy
Excludes1 proliferative vitreo-retinopathy with retinal detachment (H33.4-)
- H35.20 Other non-diabetic proliferative retinopathy, unspecified eye
- H35.21 Other non-diabetic proliferative retinopathy, right eye
- H35.22 Other non-diabetic proliferative retinopathy, left eye
- H35.23 Other non-diabetic proliferative retinopathy, bilateral

● H35.3 Degeneration of macula and posterior pole
- H35.30 **Unspecified** macular degeneration A
  Age-related macular degeneration

● H35.31 **Nonexudative age-related** macular degeneration
Atrophic age-related macular degeneration
Dry age-related macular degeneration
One of the following 7th characters is to be assigned to codes in subcategory H35.31 to designate the stage of the disease:

Ø	stage unspecified
1	early dry stage
2	intermediate dry stage
3	advanced atrophic without subfoveal involvement advanced dry stage
4	advanced atrophic with subfoveal involvement

- ● H35.311 Nonexudative age-related macular degeneration, **right** eye A
  Coding Clinic: 2Ø16, Q4, P2Ø-21
- ● H35.312 Nonexudative age-related macular degeneration, **left** eye A
  Coding Clinic: 2Ø16, Q4, P2Ø-21
- ● H35.313 Nonexudative age-related macular degeneration, **bilateral** A
  Coding Clinic: 2Ø16, Q4, P2Ø
- ● H35.319 Nonexudative age-related macular degeneration, **unspecified** eye A
  Coding Clinic: 2Ø16, Q4, P2Ø

● H35.32 **Exudative age-related** macular degeneration
Wet age-related macular degeneration
One of the following 7th characters is to be assigned to codes in subcategory H35.32 to designate the stage of the disease:

Ø	stage unspecified
1	with active choroidal neovascularization
2	with inactive choroidal neovascularization with involuted or regressed neovascularization
3	with inactive scar

Coding Clinic: 2Ø16, Q4, P2Ø
- ● H35.321 Exudative age-related macular degeneration, **right** eye (HCC) A
- ● H35.322 Exudative age-related macular degeneration, **left** eye (HCC) A
- ● H35.323 Exudative age-related macular degeneration, **bilateral** (HCC) A
- ● H35.329 Exudative age-related macular degeneration, **unspecified** eye (HCC) A

H35.33 Angioid streaks of macula

● H35.34 Macular cyst, hole, or pseudohole
- H35.341 Macular cyst, hole, or pseudohole, **right** eye
- H35.342 Macular cyst, hole, or pseudohole, **left** eye
- H35.343 Macular cyst, hole, or pseudohole, **bilateral**
- H35.349 Macular cyst, hole, or pseudohole, **unspecified** eye

● H35.35 Cystoid macular degeneration
Excludes1 cystoid macular edema following cataract surgery (H59.Ø3-)
- H35.351 Cystoid macular degeneration, **right** eye
- H35.352 Cystoid macular degeneration, **left** eye
- H35.353 Cystoid macular degeneration, **bilateral**
- H35.359 Cystoid macular degeneration, **unspecified** eye

● H35.36 Drusen (degenerative) of macula
- H35.361 Drusen (degenerative) of macula, **right** eye
  Coding Clinic: 2Ø16, Q4, P21
- H35.362 Drusen (degenerative) of macula, **left** eye
  Coding Clinic: 2Ø16, Q4, P21
- H35.363 Drusen (degenerative) of macula, **bilateral**
  Coding Clinic: 2Ø17, Q1, P51
- H35.369 Drusen (degenerative) of macula, **unspecified** eye

● H35.37 Puckering of macula
- H35.371 Puckering of macula, **right** eye
- H35.372 Puckering of macula, **left** eye
- H35.373 Puckering of macula, **bilateral**
- H35.379 Puckering of macula, **unspecified** eye

Item 7–7 Macular degeneration is typically age-related, chronic, and is evidenced by deterioration of the macula (the part of the retina that provides for central field vision), resulting in blurred vision or a blind spot in the center of visual field while not affecting peripheral vision.

CHAPTER 7 (HØØ-H59)

- **H35.38 Toxic maculopathy**
  Code first poisoning due to drug or toxin, if applicable (T36-T65 with fifth or sixth character 1-4 or 6)
  Use additional code for adverse effect, if applicable, to identify drug (T36-T5Ø with fifth or sixth character 5)
  - H35.381 Toxic maculopathy, right eye
  - H35.382 Toxic maculopathy, left eye
  - H35.383 Toxic maculopathy, bilateral
  - H35.389 Toxic maculopathy, unspecified eye

H35.4 Peripheral retinal degeneration
Excludes1 hereditary retinal degeneration (dystrophy) (H35.5-)
peripheral retinal degeneration with retinal break (H33.3-)

- H35.4Ø Unspecified peripheral retinal degeneration
- **H35.41 Lattice degeneration of retina**
  Palisade degeneration of retina
  - H35.411 Lattice degeneration of retina, right eye
  - H35.412 Lattice degeneration of retina, left eye
  - H35.413 Lattice degeneration of retina, bilateral
  - H35.419 Lattice degeneration of retina, unspecified eye
- **H35.42 Microcystoid degeneration of retina**
  - H35.421 Microcystoid degeneration of retina, right eye
  - H35.422 Microcystoid degeneration of retina, left eye
  - H35.423 Microcystoid degeneration of retina, bilateral
  - H35.429 Microcystoid degeneration of retina, unspecified eye
- **H35.43 Paving stone degeneration of retina**
  - H35.431 Paving stone degeneration of retina, right eye
  - H35.432 Paving stone degeneration of retina, left eye
  - H35.433 Paving stone degeneration of retina, bilateral
  - H35.439 Paving stone degeneration of retina, unspecified eye
- **H35.44 Age-related reticular degeneration of retina**
  - H35.441 Age-related reticular degeneration of retina, right eye A
  - H35.442 Age-related reticular degeneration of retina, left eye A
  - H35.443 Age-related reticular degeneration of retina, bilateral A
  - H35.449 Age-related reticular degeneration of retina, unspecified eye A
- **H35.45 Secondary pigmentary degeneration**
  - H35.451 Secondary pigmentary degeneration, right eye
  - H35.452 Secondary pigmentary degeneration, left eye
  - H35.453 Secondary pigmentary degeneration, bilateral
  - H35.459 Secondary pigmentary degeneration, unspecified eye
- **H35.46 Secondary vitreoretinal degeneration**
  - H35.461 Secondary vitreoretinal degeneration, right eye
  - H35.462 Secondary vitreoretinal degeneration, left eye
  - H35.463 Secondary vitreoretinal degeneration, bilateral
  - H35.469 Secondary vitreoretinal degeneration, unspecified eye

H35.5 Hereditary retinal dystrophy
Excludes1 dystrophies primarily involving Bruch's membrane (H31.1-)

- H35.5Ø Unspecified hereditary retinal dystrophy
- H35.51 Vitreoretinal dystrophy
- H35.52 Pigmentary retinal dystrophy
  Albipunctate retinal dystrophy
  Retinitis pigmentosa
  Tapetoretinal dystrophy
- H35.53 Other dystrophies primarily involving the sensory retina
  Stargardt's disease
- H35.54 Dystrophies primarily involving the retinal pigment epithelium
  Vitelliform retinal dystrophy

H35.6 Retinal hemorrhage

- H35.6Ø Retinal hemorrhage, unspecified eye
- H35.61 Retinal hemorrhage, right eye
- H35.62 Retinal hemorrhage, left eye
- H35.63 Retinal hemorrhage, bilateral

H35.7 Separation of retinal layers
Excludes1 retinal detachment (serous) (H33.2-)
rhegmatogenous retinal detachment (H33.Ø-)

- H35.7Ø Unspecified separation of retinal layers
- **H35.71 Central serous chorioretinopathy**
  - H35.711 Central serous chorioretinopathy, right eye
  - H35.712 Central serous chorioretinopathy, left eye
  - H35.713 Central serous chorioretinopathy, bilateral
  - H35.719 Central serous chorioretinopathy, unspecified eye
- **H35.72 Serous detachment of retinal pigment epithelium**
  - H35.721 Serous detachment of retinal pigment epithelium, right eye
  - H35.722 Serous detachment of retinal pigment epithelium, left eye
  - H35.723 Serous detachment of retinal pigment epithelium, bilateral
  - H35.729 Serous detachment of retinal pigment epithelium, unspecified eye
- **H35.73 Hemorrhagic detachment of retinal pigment epithelium**
  - H35.731 Hemorrhagic detachment of retinal pigment epithelium, right eye
  - H35.732 Hemorrhagic detachment of retinal pigment epithelium, left eye
  - H35.733 Hemorrhagic detachment of retinal pigment epithelium, bilateral
  - H35.739 Hemorrhagic detachment of retinal pigment epithelium, unspecified eye

CHAPTER 7 (HØØ-H59)

● H35.8 Other specified retinal disorders
Excludes2 retinal hemorrhage (H35.6-)
H35.81 Retinal edema
Retinal cotton wool spots
H35.82 Retinal ischemia
H35.89 Other specified retinal disorders
H35.9 Unspecified retinal disorder

H36 Retinal disorders in diseases classified elsewhere
Code first underlying disease, such as:
lipid storage disorders (E75.-)
sickle-cell disorders (D57.-)
Excludes1 arteriosclerotic retinopathy (H35.0-)
diabetic retinopathy (E08.3-, E09.3-, E10.3-, E11.3-, E13.3-)

GLAUCOMA (H40-H42)

● H40 Glaucoma
Intraocular pressure (IOP) that is too high results from too much aqueous humor and because of excess production or inadequate drainage, optic nerve damage and vision loss may occur.
Excludes1 absolute glaucoma (H44.51-)
congenital glaucoma (Q15.0)
traumatic glaucoma due to birth injury (P15.3)

● H40.0 Glaucoma suspect
● H40.00 Preglaucoma, unspecified
H40.001 Preglaucoma, unspecified, right eye
H40.002 Preglaucoma, unspecified, left eye
H40.003 Preglaucoma, unspecified, bilateral
H40.009 Preglaucoma, unspecified, unspecified eye
● H40.01 Open angle with borderline findings, low risk
Open angle, low risk
H40.011 Open angle with borderline findings, low risk, right eye
H40.012 Open angle with borderline findings, low risk, left eye
H40.013 Open angle with borderline findings, low risk, bilateral
H40.019 Open angle with borderline findings, low risk, unspecified eye
● H40.02 Open angle with borderline findings, high risk
Open angle, high risk
H40.021 Open angle with borderline findings, high risk, right eye
H40.022 Open angle with borderline findings, high risk, left eye
H40.023 Open angle with borderline findings, high risk, bilateral
H40.029 Open angle with borderline findings, high risk, unspecified eye
● H40.03 Anatomical narrow angle
Primary angle closure suspect
H40.031 Anatomical narrow angle, right eye
H40.032 Anatomical narrow angle, left eye
H40.033 Anatomical narrow angle, bilateral
H40.039 Anatomical narrow angle, unspecified eye
● H40.04 Steroid responder
H40.041 Steroid responder, right eye
H40.042 Steroid responder, left eye
H40.043 Steroid responder, bilateral
H40.049 Steroid responder, unspecified eye
● H40.05 Ocular hypertension
H40.051 Ocular hypertension, right eye
H40.052 Ocular hypertension, left eye
H40.053 Ocular hypertension, bilateral
H40.059 Ocular hypertension, unspecified eye
● H40.06 Primary angle closure without glaucoma damage
H40.061 Primary angle closure without glaucoma damage, right eye
H40.062 Primary angle closure without glaucoma damage, left eye
H40.063 Primary angle closure without glaucoma damage, bilateral
H40.069 Primary angle closure without glaucoma damage, unspecified eye

● H40.1 Open-angle glaucoma
X● H40.10 Unspecified open-angle glaucoma
One of the following 7th characters is to be assigned to code H40.10 to designate the stage of glaucoma

0	stage unspecified
1	mild stage
2	moderate stage
3	severe stage
4	indeterminate stage

● H40.11 Primary open-angle glaucoma
Chronic simple glaucoma
One of the following 7th characters is to be assigned to each code in subcategory H40.11 to designate the stage of glaucoma

0	stage unspecified
1	mild stage
2	moderate stage
3	severe stage
4	indeterminate stage

Coding Clinic: 2016, Q4, P22
● H40.111 Primary open-angle glaucoma, right eye
Coding Clinic: 2019, Q2, P31
● H40.112 Primary open-angle glaucoma, left eye
● H40.113 Primary open-angle glaucoma, bilateral
● H40.119 Primary open-angle glaucoma, unspecified eye
● H40.12 Low-tension glaucoma
One of the following 7th characters is to be assigned to each code in subcategory H40.12 to designate the stage of glaucoma

0	stage unspecified
1	mild stage
2	moderate stage
3	severe stage
4	indeterminate stage

● H40.121 Low-tension glaucoma, right eye
● H40.122 Low-tension glaucoma, left eye
● H40.123 Low-tension glaucoma, bilateral
● H40.129 Low-tension glaucoma, unspecified eye

● **H40.13** **Pigmentary** glaucoma

One of the following 7th characters is to be assigned to each code in subcategory H40.13 to designate the stage of glaucoma

0	stage unspecified
1	mild stage
2	moderate stage
3	severe stage
4	indeterminate stage

● **H40.131** Pigmentary glaucoma, **right** eye

● **H40.132** Pigmentary glaucoma, **left** eye

● **H40.133** Pigmentary glaucoma, **bilateral**

● **H40.139** Pigmentary glaucoma, **unspecified** eye

● **H40.14** **Capsular** glaucoma **with pseudoexfoliation** of lens

One of the following 7th characters is to be assigned to each code in subcategory H40.14 to designate the stage of glaucoma

0	stage unspecified
1	mild stage
2	moderate stage
3	severe stage
4	indeterminate stage

● **H40.141** Capsular glaucoma with pseudoexfoliation of lens, **right** eye

● **H40.142** Capsular glaucoma with pseudoexfoliation of lens, **left** eye

● **H40.143** Capsular glaucoma with pseudoexfoliation of lens, **bilateral**

● **H40.149** Capsular glaucoma with pseudoexfoliation of lens, **unspecified** eye

● **H40.15** **Residual** stage of open-angle glaucoma

H40.151 Residual stage of open-angle glaucoma, **right** eye

H40.152 Residual stage of open-angle glaucoma, **left** eye

H40.153 Residual stage of open-angle glaucoma, **bilateral**

H40.159 Residual stage of open-angle glaucoma, **unspecified** eye

● **H40.2** **Primary** angle-closure glaucoma

Excludes1 aqueous misdirection (H40.83-)
malignant glaucoma (H40.83-)

X● **H40.20** **Unspecified** primary angle-closure glaucoma

One of the following 7th characters is to be assigned to code H40.20 to designate the stage of glaucoma

0	stage unspecified
1	mild stage
2	moderate stage
3	severe stage
4	indeterminate stage

● **H40.21** **Acute** angle-closure glaucoma

Acute angle-closure glaucoma attack
Acute angle-closure glaucoma crisis

H40.211 Acute angle-closure glaucoma, **right** eye

H40.212 Acute angle-closure glaucoma, **left** eye

H40.213 Acute angle-closure glaucoma, **bilateral**

H40.219 Acute angle-closure glaucoma, **unspecified** eye

● **H40.22** **Chronic** angle-closure glaucoma

Chronic primary angle closure glaucoma

One of the following 7th characters is to be assigned to each code in subcategory H40.22 to designate the stage of glaucoma

0	stage unspecified
1	mild stage
2	moderate stage
3	severe stage
4	indeterminate stage

● **H40.221** Chronic angle-closure glaucoma, **right** eye

● **H40.222** Chronic angle-closure glaucoma, **left** eye

● **H40.223** Chronic angle-closure glaucoma, **bilateral**

● **H40.229** Chronic angle-closure glaucoma, **unspecified** eye

● **H40.23** **Intermittent** angle-closure glaucoma

H40.231 Intermittent angle-closure glaucoma, **right** eye

H40.232 Intermittent angle-closure glaucoma, **left** eye

H40.233 Intermittent angle-closure glaucoma, **bilateral**

H40.239 Intermittent angle-closure glaucoma, **unspecified** eye

● **H40.24** **Residual** stage of angle-closure glaucoma

H40.241 Residual stage of angle-closure glaucoma, **right** eye

H40.242 Residual stage of angle-closure glaucoma, **left** eye

H40.243 Residual stage of angle-closure glaucoma, **bilateral**

H40.249 Residual stage of angle-closure glaucoma, **unspecified** eye

● **H40.3** Glaucoma **secondary** to eye **trauma**

Code also underlying condition

One of the following 7th characters is to be assigned to each code in subcategory H40.3 to designate the stage of glaucoma

0	stage unspecified
1	mild stage
2	moderate stage
3	severe stage
4	indeterminate stage

X● **H40.30** Glaucoma secondary to eye trauma, **unspecified** eye

X● **H40.31** Glaucoma secondary to eye trauma, **right** eye

X● **H40.32** Glaucoma secondary to eye trauma, **left** eye

X● **H40.33** Glaucoma secondary to eye trauma, **bilateral**

● **H40.4** Glaucoma secondary to eye inflammation
Code also underlying condition
One of the following 7th characters is to be assigned to each code in subcategory H40.4 to designate the stage of glaucoma

0	stage unspecified
1	mild stage
2	moderate stage
3	severe stage
4	indeterminate stage

X● **H40.40** Glaucoma secondary to eye inflammation, **unspecified eye**
X● **H40.41** Glaucoma secondary to eye inflammation, **right eye**
X● **H40.42** Glaucoma secondary to eye inflammation, **left eye**
X● **H40.43** Glaucoma secondary to eye inflammation, **bilateral**

● **H40.5** Glaucoma secondary to other eye disorders
Code also underlying eye disorder
One of the following 7th characters is to be assigned to each code in subcategory H40.5 to designate the stage of glaucoma

0	stage unspecified
1	mild stage
2	moderate stage
3	severe stage
4	indeterminate stage

X● **H40.50** Glaucoma secondary to other eye disorders, **unspecified eye**
X● **H40.51** Glaucoma secondary to other eye disorders, **right eye**
X● **H40.52** Glaucoma secondary to other eye disorders, **left eye**
X● **H40.53** Glaucoma secondary to other eye disorders, **bilateral**

● **H40.6** Glaucoma secondary to drugs
Use additional code for adverse effect, if applicable, to identify drug (T36-T50 with fifth or sixth character 5)
One of the following 7th characters is to be assigned to each code in subcategory H40.6 to designate the stage of glaucoma

0	stage unspecified
1	mild stage
2	moderate stage
3	severe stage
4	indeterminate stage

X● **H40.60** Glaucoma secondary to drugs, **unspecified eye**
X● **H40.61** Glaucoma secondary to drugs, **right eye**
X● **H40.62** Glaucoma secondary to drugs, **left eye**
X● **H40.63** Glaucoma secondary to drugs, **bilateral**

● **H40.8** Other glaucoma
● **H40.81** Glaucoma with increased episcleral venous pressure
H40.811 Glaucoma with increased episcleral venous pressure, **right eye**
H40.812 Glaucoma with increased episcleral venous pressure, **left eye**
H40.813 Glaucoma with increased episcleral venous pressure, **bilateral**
H40.819 Glaucoma with increased episcleral venous pressure, **unspecified eye**
● **H40.82** Hypersecretion glaucoma
H40.821 Hypersecretion glaucoma, **right eye**
H40.822 Hypersecretion glaucoma, **left eye**
H40.823 Hypersecretion glaucoma, **bilateral**
H40.829 Hypersecretion glaucoma, **unspecified eye**
● **H40.83** Aqueous misdirection
Malignant glaucoma
H40.831 Aqueous misdirection, **right eye**
H40.832 Aqueous misdirection, **left eye**
H40.833 Aqueous misdirection, **bilateral**
H40.839 Aqueous misdirection, **unspecified eye**
H40.89 Other specified glaucoma

H40.9 Unspecified glaucoma

H42 Glaucoma in diseases classified elsewhere
Code first underlying condition, such as:
amyloidosis (E85.-)
aniridia (Q13.1)
glaucoma (in) diabetes mellitus (E08.39, E09.39, E10.39, E11.39, E13.39)
Lowe's syndrome (E72.03)
Reiger's anomaly (Q13.81)
specified metabolic disorder (E70-E88)
Excludes1 glaucoma (in) onchocerciasis (B73.02)
glaucoma (in) syphilis (A52.71)
glaucoma (in) tuberculous (A18.59)

DISORDERS OF VITREOUS BODY AND GLOBE (H43-H44)

● **H43** Disorders of vitreous body
● **H43.0** Vitreous prolapse
Excludes1 vitreous syndrome following cataract surgery (H59.0-)
traumatic vitreous prolapse (S05.2-)
H43.00 Vitreous prolapse, **unspecified eye**
H43.01 Vitreous prolapse, **right eye**
H43.02 Vitreous prolapse, **left eye**
H43.03 Vitreous prolapse, **bilateral**
● **H43.1** Vitreous hemorrhage
H43.10 Vitreous hemorrhage, **unspecified eye** (HCC)
H43.11 Vitreous hemorrhage, **right eye** (HCC)
H43.12 Vitreous hemorrhage, **left eye** (HCC)
H43.13 Vitreous hemorrhage, **bilateral** (HCC)
● **H43.2** Crystalline deposits in vitreous body
H43.20 Crystalline deposits in vitreous body, **unspecified eye**
H43.21 Crystalline deposits in vitreous body, **right eye**
H43.22 Crystalline deposits in vitreous body, **left eye**
H43.23 Crystalline deposits in vitreous body, **bilateral**
● **H43.3** Other vitreous opacities
● **H43.31** Vitreous membranes and strands
H43.311 Vitreous membranes and strands, **right eye**
H43.312 Vitreous membranes and strands, **left eye**
H43.313 Vitreous membranes and strands, **bilateral**
H43.319 Vitreous membranes and strands, **unspecified eye**

CHAPTER 7 (H00-H59)

- H43.39 **Other vitreous opacities**
  Vitreous floaters
  Small clumps of cells that float in the vitreous of the eye, appearing as black specks or dots in the field of vision and common in the aging eye.
  - H43.391 **Other vitreous opacities, right eye**
  - H43.392 **Other vitreous opacities, left eye**
  - H43.393 **Other vitreous opacities, bilateral**
  - H43.399 **Other vitreous opacities, unspecified eye**
- H43.8 Other disorders of vitreous body
  Excludes1 proliferative vitreo-retinopathy with retinal detachment (H33.4)
  Excludes2 vitreous abscess (H44.02-)
  - H43.81 **Vitreous degeneration**
    Vitreous detachment
    - H43.811 **Vitreous degeneration, right eye**
    - H43.812 **Vitreous degeneration, left eye**
    - H43.813 **Vitreous degeneration, bilateral**
    - H43.819 **Vitreous degeneration, unspecified eye**
  - H43.82 **Vitreomacular adhesion**
    Vitreomacular traction
    - H43.821 **Vitreomacular adhesion, right eye** A
    - H43.822 **Vitreomacular adhesion, left eye** A
    - H43.823 **Vitreomacular adhesion, bilateral** A
    - H43.829 **Vitreomacular adhesion, unspecified eye** A
  - H43.89 **Other disorders of vitreous body**
- H43.9 **Unspecified disorder of vitreous body**

H44 Disorders of globe
Includes disorders affecting multiple structures of eye
- H44.0 Purulent endophthalmitis
  Use additional code to identify organism
  Excludes1 bleb associated endophthalmitis (H59.4-)
  - H44.00 Unspecified purulent endophthalmitis
    - H44.001 **Unspecified purulent endophthalmitis, right eye**
    - H44.002 **Unspecified purulent endophthalmitis, left eye**
    - H44.003 **Unspecified purulent endophthalmitis, bilateral**
    - H44.009 **Unspecified purulent endophthalmitis, unspecified eye**
  - H44.01 Panophthalmitis (acute)
    - H44.011 **Panophthalmitis (acute), right eye**
    - H44.012 **Panophthalmitis (acute), left eye**
    - H44.013 **Panophthalmitis (acute), bilateral**
    - H44.019 **Panophthalmitis (acute), unspecified eye**
  - H44.02 Vitreous abscess (chronic)
    - H44.021 **Vitreous abscess (chronic), right eye**
    - H44.022 **Vitreous abscess (chronic), left eye**
    - H44.023 **Vitreous abscess (chronic), bilateral**
    - H44.029 **Vitreous abscess (chronic), unspecified eye**
- H44.1 Other endophthalmitis
  Excludes1 bleb associated endophthalmitis (H59.4-)
  Excludes2 ophthalmia nodosa (H16.2-)
  - H44.11 Panuveitis
    - H44.111 **Panuveitis, right eye**
    - H44.112 **Panuveitis, left eye**
    - H44.113 **Panuveitis, bilateral**
    - H44.119 **Panuveitis, unspecified eye**
  - H44.12 **Parasitic endophthalmitis, unspecified**
    - H44.121 **Parasitic endophthalmitis, unspecified, right eye**
    - H44.122 **Parasitic endophthalmitis, unspecified, left eye**
    - H44.123 **Parasitic endophthalmitis, unspecified, bilateral**
    - H44.129 **Parasitic endophthalmitis, unspecified, unspecified eye**
  - H44.13 Sympathetic uveitis
    - H44.131 **Sympathetic uveitis, right eye**
    - H44.132 **Sympathetic uveitis, left eye**
    - H44.133 **Sympathetic uveitis, bilateral**
    - H44.139 **Sympathetic uveitis, unspecified eye**
  - H44.19 **Other endophthalmitis**
- H44.2 Degenerative myopia
  Malignant myopia
  - H44.20 **Degenerative myopia, unspecified eye**
  - H44.21 **Degenerative myopia, right eye**
  - H44.22 **Degenerative myopia, left eye**
  - H44.23 **Degenerative myopia, bilateral**
  - H44.2A **Degenerative myopia with choroidal neovascularization**
    Use Additional code for any associated choroid disorders (H31.-)
    - H44.2A1 **Degenerative myopia with choroidal neovascularization, right eye**
    - H44.2A2 **Degenerative myopia with choroidal neovascularization, left eye**
    - H44.2A3 **Degenerative myopia with choroidal neovascularization, bilateral eye**
    - H44.2A9 **Degenerative myopia with choroidal neovascularization, unspecified eye**
  - H44.2B **Degenerative myopia with macular hole**
    - H44.2B1 **Degenerative myopia with macular hole, right eye**
    - H44.2B2 **Degenerative myopia with macular hole, left eye**
    - H44.2B3 **Degenerative myopia with macular hole, bilateral eye**
    - H44.2B9 **Degenerative myopia with macular hole, unspecified eye**
  - H44.2C **Degenerative myopia with retinal detachment**
    Use Additional code to identify the retinal detachment (H33.-)
    - H44.2C1 **Degenerative myopia with retinal detachment, right eye**
    - H44.2C2 **Degenerative myopia with retinal detachment, left eye**
    - H44.2C3 **Degenerative myopia with retinal detachment, bilateral eye**
    - H44.2C9 **Degenerative myopia with retinal detachment, unspecified eye**
  - H44.2D **Degenerative myopia with foveoschisis**
    - H44.2D1 **Degenerative myopia with foveoschisis, right eye**
    - H44.2D2 **Degenerative myopia with foveoschisis, left eye**
    - H44.2D3 **Degenerative myopia with foveoschisis, bilateral eye**
    - H44.2D9 **Degenerative myopia with foveoschisis, unspecified eye**

- H44.2E Degenerative myopia with other maculopathy
  - H44.2E1 Degenerative myopia with other maculopathy, right eye
  - H44.2E2 Degenerative myopia with other maculopathy, left eye
  - H44.2E3 Degenerative myopia with other maculopathy, bilateral eye
  - H44.2E9 Degenerative myopia with other maculopathy, unspecified eye
- H44.3 Other and unspecified degenerative disorders of globe
  - H44.30 Unspecified degenerative disorder of globe
  - H44.31 Chalcosis
    - H44.311 Chalcosis, right eye
    - H44.312 Chalcosis, left eye
    - H44.313 Chalcosis, bilateral
    - H44.319 Chalcosis, unspecified eye
  - H44.32 Siderosis of eye
    - H44.321 Siderosis of eye, right eye
    - H44.322 Siderosis of eye, left eye
    - H44.323 Siderosis of eye, bilateral
    - H44.329 Siderosis of eye, unspecified eye
  - H44.39 Other degenerative disorders of globe
    - H44.391 Other degenerative disorders of globe, right eye
    - H44.392 Other degenerative disorders of globe, left eye
    - H44.393 Other degenerative disorders of globe, bilateral
    - H44.399 Other degenerative disorders of globe, unspecified eye
- H44.4 Hypotony of eye
  - H44.40 Unspecified hypotony of eye
  - H44.41 Flat anterior chamber hypotony of eye
    - H44.411 Flat anterior chamber hypotony of right eye
    - H44.412 Flat anterior chamber hypotony of left eye
    - H44.413 Flat anterior chamber hypotony of eye, bilateral
    - H44.419 Flat anterior chamber hypotony of unspecified eye
  - H44.42 Hypotony of eye due to ocular fistula
    - H44.421 Hypotony of right eye due to ocular fistula
    - H44.422 Hypotony of left eye due to ocular fistula
    - H44.423 Hypotony of eye due to ocular fistula, bilateral
    - H44.429 Hypotony of unspecified eye due to ocular fistula
  - H44.43 Hypotony of eye due to other ocular disorders
    - H44.431 Hypotony of eye due to other ocular disorders, right eye
    - H44.432 Hypotony of eye due to other ocular disorders, left eye
    - H44.433 Hypotony of eye due to other ocular disorders, bilateral
    - H44.439 Hypotony of eye due to other ocular disorders, unspecified eye
  - H44.44 Primary hypotony of eye
    - H44.441 Primary hypotony of right eye
    - H44.442 Primary hypotony of left eye
    - H44.443 Primary hypotony of eye, bilateral
    - H44.449 Primary hypotony of unspecified eye
- H44.5 Degenerated conditions of globe
  - H44.50 Unspecified degenerated conditions of globe
  - H44.51 Absolute glaucoma
    - H44.511 Absolute glaucoma, right eye
    - H44.512 Absolute glaucoma, left eye
    - H44.513 Absolute glaucoma, bilateral
    - H44.519 Absolute glaucoma, unspecified eye
  - H44.52 Atrophy of globe
    Phthisis bulbi
    - H44.521 Atrophy of globe, right eye
    - H44.522 Atrophy of globe, left eye
    - H44.523 Atrophy of globe, bilateral
    - H44.529 Atrophy of globe, unspecified eye
  - H44.53 Leucocoria
    - H44.531 Leucocoria, right eye
    - H44.532 Leucocoria, left eye
    - H44.533 Leucocoria, bilateral
    - H44.539 Leucocoria, unspecified eye
- H44.6 Retained (old) intraocular foreign body, magnetic
  Use additional code to identify magnetic foreign body (Z18.11)
  Excludes1 current intraocular foreign body (S05.-)
  Excludes2 retained foreign body in eyelid (H02.81-)
  retained (old) foreign body following penetrating wound of orbit (H05.5-)
  retained (old) intraocular foreign body, nonmagnetic (H44.7-)
  - H44.60 Unspecified retained (old) intraocular foreign body, magnetic
    - H44.601 Unspecified retained (old) intraocular foreign body, magnetic, right eye
    - H44.602 Unspecified retained (old) intraocular foreign body, magnetic, left eye
    - H44.603 Unspecified retained (old) intraocular foreign body, magnetic, bilateral
    - H44.609 Unspecified retained (old) intraocular foreign body, magnetic, unspecified eye
  - H44.61 Retained (old) magnetic foreign body in anterior chamber
    - H44.611 Retained (old) magnetic foreign body in anterior chamber, right eye
    - H44.612 Retained (old) magnetic foreign body in anterior chamber, left eye
    - H44.613 Retained (old) magnetic foreign body in anterior chamber, bilateral
    - H44.619 Retained (old) magnetic foreign body in anterior chamber, unspecified eye
  - H44.62 Retained (old) magnetic foreign body in iris or ciliary body
    - H44.621 Retained (old) magnetic foreign body in iris or ciliary body, right eye
    - H44.622 Retained (old) magnetic foreign body in iris or ciliary body, left eye
    - H44.623 Retained (old) magnetic foreign body in iris or ciliary body, bilateral
    - H44.629 Retained (old) magnetic foreign body in iris or ciliary body, unspecified eye
  - H44.63 Retained (old) magnetic foreign body in lens
    - H44.631 Retained (old) magnetic foreign body in lens, right eye
    - H44.632 Retained (old) magnetic foreign body in lens, left eye
    - H44.633 Retained (old) magnetic foreign body in lens, bilateral
    - H44.639 Retained (old) magnetic foreign body in lens, unspecified eye

- **H44.64** Retained (old) magnetic foreign body in **posterior wall of globe**
  - H44.641 Retained (old) magnetic foreign body in posterior wall of globe, **right eye**
  - H44.642 Retained (old) magnetic foreign body in posterior wall of globe, **left eye**
  - H44.643 Retained (old) magnetic foreign body in posterior wall of globe, **bilateral**
  - H44.649 Retained (old) magnetic foreign body in posterior wall of globe, **unspecified** eye
- **H44.65** Retained (old) magnetic foreign body in **vitreous body**
  - H44.651 Retained (old) magnetic foreign body in vitreous body, **right eye**
  - H44.652 Retained (old) magnetic foreign body in vitreous body, **left eye**
  - H44.653 Retained (old) magnetic foreign body in vitreous body, **bilateral**
  - H44.659 Retained (old) magnetic foreign body in vitreous body, **unspecified eye**
- **H44.69** Retained (old) intraocular foreign body, magnetic, in **other or multiple sites**
  - H44.691 Retained (old) intraocular foreign body, magnetic, in other or multiple sites, **right eye**
  - H44.692 Retained (old) intraocular foreign body, magnetic, in other or multiple sites, **left eye**
  - H44.693 Retained (old) intraocular foreign body, magnetic, in other or multiple sites, **bilateral**
  - H44.699 Retained (old) intraocular foreign body, magnetic, in other or multiple sites, **unspecified eye**

H44.7 Retained (old) intraocular foreign body, nonmagnetic

Use additional code to identify nonmagnetic foreign body (Z18.01-Z18.10, Z18.12, Z18.2-Z18.9)

Excludes1 current intraocular foreign body (S05.-)

Excludes2 retained foreign body in eyelid (H02.81-)
retained (old) foreign body following penetrating wound of orbit (H05.5-)
retained (old) intraocular foreign body, magnetic (H44.6-)

- **H44.70** Unspecified retained (old) intraocular foreign body, nonmagnetic
  - H44.701 Unspecified retained (old) intraocular foreign body, nonmagnetic, **right eye**
  - H44.702 Unspecified retained (old) intraocular foreign body, nonmagnetic, **left eye**
  - H44.703 Unspecified retained (old) intraocular foreign body, nonmagnetic, **bilateral**
  - H44.709 Unspecified retained (old) intraocular foreign body, nonmagnetic, **unspecified** eye
    - Retained (old) intraocular foreign body NOS
- **H44.71** Retained (nonmagnetic) (old) foreign body in **anterior chamber**
  - H44.711 Retained (nonmagnetic) (old) foreign body in anterior chamber, **right eye**
  - H44.712 Retained (nonmagnetic) (old) foreign body in anterior chamber, **left eye**
  - H44.713 Retained (nonmagnetic) (old) foreign body in anterior chamber, **bilateral**
  - H44.719 Retained (nonmagnetic) (old) foreign body in anterior chamber, **unspecified** eye
- **H44.72** Retained (nonmagnetic) (old) foreign body in **iris or ciliary body**
  - H44.721 Retained (nonmagnetic) (old) foreign body in iris or ciliary body, **right eye**
  - H44.722 Retained (nonmagnetic) (old) foreign body in iris or ciliary body, **left eye**
  - H44.723 Retained (nonmagnetic) (old) foreign body in iris or ciliary body, **bilateral**
  - H44.729 Retained (nonmagnetic) (old) foreign body in iris or ciliary body, **unspecified** eye
- **H44.73** Retained (nonmagnetic) (old) foreign body in **lens**
  - H44.731 Retained (nonmagnetic) (old) foreign body in lens, **right eye**
  - H44.732 Retained (nonmagnetic) (old) foreign body in lens, **left eye**
  - H44.733 Retained (nonmagnetic) (old) foreign body in lens, **bilateral**
  - H44.739 Retained (nonmagnetic) (old) foreign body in lens, **unspecified** eye
- **H44.74** Retained (nonmagnetic) (old) foreign body in **posterior wall of globe**
  - H44.741 Retained (nonmagnetic) (old) foreign body in posterior wall of globe, **right** eye
  - H44.742 Retained (nonmagnetic) (old) foreign body in posterior wall of globe, **left** eye
  - H44.743 Retained (nonmagnetic) (old) foreign body in posterior wall of globe, **bilateral**
  - H44.749 Retained (nonmagnetic) (old) foreign body in posterior wall of globe, **unspecified** eye
- **H44.75** Retained (nonmagnetic) (old) foreign body in **vitreous body**
  - H44.751 Retained (nonmagnetic) (old) foreign body in vitreous body, **right eye**
  - H44.752 Retained (nonmagnetic) (old) foreign body in vitreous body, **left eye**
  - H44.753 Retained (nonmagnetic) (old) foreign body in vitreous body, **bilateral**
  - H44.759 Retained (nonmagnetic) (old) foreign body in vitreous body, **unspecified** eye
- **H44.79** Retained (old) intraocular foreign body, nonmagnetic, in **other or multiple sites**
  - H44.791 Retained (old) intraocular foreign body, nonmagnetic, in other or multiple sites, **right eye**
  - H44.792 Retained (old) intraocular foreign body, nonmagnetic, in other or multiple sites, **left eye**
  - H44.793 Retained (old) intraocular foreign body, nonmagnetic, in other or multiple sites, **bilateral**
  - H44.799 Retained (old) intraocular foreign body, nonmagnetic, in other or multiple sites, **unspecified** eye

H44.8 Other disorders of globe

- **H44.81** Hemophthalmos
  - H44.811 Hemophthalmos, **right eye**
  - H44.812 Hemophthalmos, **left eye**
  - H44.813 Hemophthalmos, **bilateral**
  - H44.819 Hemophthalmos, **unspecified** eye

- H44.82 Luxation of globe
  - H44.821 Luxation of globe, **right** eye
  - H44.822 Luxation of globe, **left** eye
  - H44.823 Luxation of globe, **bilateral**
  - H44.829 Luxation of globe, **unspecified** eye
- H44.89 Other disorders of globe
- H44.9 Unspecified disorder of globe

★**(See Plate 7 of the Anatomy Illustrations.)**

DISORDERS OF OPTIC NERVE AND VISUAL PATHWAYS (H46-H47)

- H46 Optic neuritis
  - **Excludes2** ischemic optic neuropathy (H47.01-)
    neuromyelitis optica [Devic] (G36.0)
  - H46.0 Optic papillitis
    - H46.00 Optic papillitis, **unspecified** eye
    - H46.01 Optic papillitis, **right** eye
    - H46.02 Optic papillitis, **left** eye
    - H46.03 Optic papillitis, **bilateral**
  - H46.1 **Retrobulbar** neuritis
    Retrobulbar neuritis NOS
    Excludes1 syphilitic retrobulbar neuritis (A52.15)
    - H46.10 Retrobulbar neuritis, **unspecified** eye
    - H46.11 Retrobulbar neuritis, **right** eye
    - H46.12 Retrobulbar neuritis, **left** eye
    - H46.13 Retrobulbar neuritis, **bilateral**
  - H46.2 **Nutritional** optic neuropathy
  - H46.3 **Toxic** optic neuropathy
    Code first (T51-T65) to identify cause
  - H46.8 **Other** optic neuritis
  - H46.9 **Unspecified** optic neuritis
- H47 Other disorders of optic [2nd] nerve and visual pathways
  - H47.0 Disorders of optic nerve, not elsewhere classified
    - H47.01 **Ischemic** optic neuropathy
      - H47.011 Ischemic optic neuropathy, **right** eye
      - H47.012 Ischemic optic neuropathy, **left** eye
      - H47.013 Ischemic optic neuropathy, **bilateral**
      - H47.019 Ischemic optic neuropathy, **unspecified** eye
    - H47.02 **Hemorrhage** in optic nerve sheath
      - H47.021 Hemorrhage in optic nerve sheath, **right** eye
      - H47.022 Hemorrhage in optic nerve sheath, **left** eye
      - H47.023 Hemorrhage in optic nerve sheath, **bilateral**
      - H47.029 Hemorrhage in optic nerve sheath, **unspecified** eye
    - H47.03 Optic nerve **hypoplasia**
      - H47.031 Optic nerve hypoplasia, **right** eye
      - H47.032 Optic nerve hypoplasia, **left** eye
      - H47.033 Optic nerve hypoplasia, **bilateral**
      - H47.039 Optic nerve hypoplasia, **unspecified** eye
    - H47.09 **Other** disorders of optic nerve, not elsewhere classified
      Compression of optic nerve
      - H47.091 Other disorders of optic nerve, not elsewhere classified, **right** eye
      - H47.092 Other disorders of optic nerve, not elsewhere classified, **left** eye
      - H47.093 Other disorders of optic nerve, not elsewhere classified, **bilateral**
      - H47.099 Other disorders of optic nerve, not elsewhere classified, **unspecified** eye

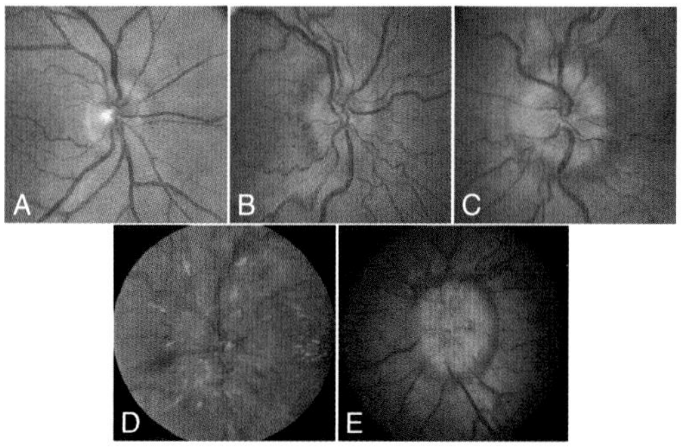

Figure 7-11 Stages of papilledema according to the Frisén grading scale. **A,** Very eary papilledema (Frisén stage 1). **B,** Early papilledema (Frisén stage 2). **C,** Moderate papilledema (Frisén stage 3). **D,** Marked papilledema (Frisén stage 4). **E,** Severe papilledema. (From Youmans JR, Winn HR: Youmans Neurological Surgery, Philadelphia, PA, Elsevier/Saunders, 2011)

Item 7-8 Papilledema is swelling of the optic disc caused by increased intracranial pressure. It is most often bilateral and occurs quickly (hours) or over weeks of time. It is a common symptom of a brain tumor. The term should not be used to describe optic disc swelling with underlying infectious, infiltrative, or inflammatory etiologies.

  - H47.1 Papilledema
    - H47.10 **Unspecified** papilledema
    - H47.11 Papilledema associated with **increased intracranial pressure**
    - H47.12 Papilledema associated with decreased **ocular pressure**
    - H47.13 Papilledema associated with **retinal disorder**
    - H47.14 Foster-Kennedy syndrome
      - H47.141 Foster-Kennedy syndrome, **right** eye
      - H47.142 Foster-Kennedy syndrome, **left** eye
      - H47.143 Foster-Kennedy syndrome, **bilateral**
      - H47.149 Foster-Kennedy syndrome, **unspecified** eye
  - H47.2 Optic atrophy
    - H47.20 **Unspecified** optic atrophy
    - H47.21 **Primary** optic atrophy
      - H47.211 Primary optic atrophy, **right** eye
      - H47.212 Primary optic atrophy, **left** eye
      - H47.213 Primary optic atrophy, **bilateral**
      - H47.219 Primary optic atrophy, **unspecified** eye
    - H47.22 **Hereditary** optic atrophy
      Leber's optic atrophy
    - H47.23 **Glaucomatous** optic atrophy
      - H47.231 Glaucomatous optic atrophy, **right** eye
      - H47.232 Glaucomatous optic atrophy, **left** eye
      - H47.233 Glaucomatous optic atrophy, **bilateral**
      - H47.239 Glaucomatous optic atrophy, **unspecified** eye
    - H47.29 **Other** optic atrophy
      Temporal pallor of optic disc
      - H47.291 Other optic atrophy, **right** eye
      - H47.292 Other optic atrophy, **left** eye
      - H47.293 Other optic atrophy, **bilateral**
      - H47.299 Other optic atrophy, **unspecified** eye
  - H47.3 Other disorders of optic disc
    - H47.31 **Coloboma** of optic disc
      - H47.311 Coloboma of optic disc, **right** eye
      - H47.312 Coloboma of optic disc, **left** eye
      - H47.313 Coloboma of optic disc, **bilateral**
      - H47.319 Coloboma of optic disc, **unspecified** eye

H47.32 Drusen of optic disc
- H47.321 Drusen of optic disc, right eye
- H47.322 Drusen of optic disc, left eye
- H47.323 Drusen of optic disc, bilateral
- H47.329 Drusen of optic disc, unspecified eye

H47.33 Pseudopapilledema of optic disc
- H47.331 Pseudopapilledema of optic disc, right eye
- H47.332 Pseudopapilledema of optic disc, left eye
- H47.333 Pseudopapilledema of optic disc, bilateral
- H47.339 Pseudopapilledema of optic disc, unspecified eye

H47.39 Other disorders of optic disc
- H47.391 Other disorders of optic disc, right eye
- H47.392 Other disorders of optic disc, left eye
- H47.393 Other disorders of optic disc, bilateral
- H47.399 Other disorders of optic disc, unspecified eye

H47.4 Disorders of optic chiasm

Code also underlying condition

- H47.41 Disorders of optic chiasm in (due to) inflammatory disorders
- H47.42 Disorders of optic chiasm in (due to) neoplasm
- H47.43 Disorders of optic chiasm in (due to) vascular disorders
- H47.49 Disorders of optic chiasm in (due to) other disorders

H47.5 Disorders of other visual pathways

Disorders of optic tracts, geniculate nuclei and optic radiations

Code also underlying condition

H47.51 Disorders of visual pathways in (due to) inflammatory disorders
- H47.511 Disorders of visual pathways in (due to) inflammatory disorders, right side
- H47.512 Disorders of visual pathways in (due to) inflammatory disorders, left side
- H47.519 Disorders of visual pathways in (due to) inflammatory disorders, unspecified side

H47.52 Disorders of visual pathways in (due to) neoplasm
- H47.521 Disorders of visual pathways in (due to) neoplasm, right side
- H47.522 Disorders of visual pathways in (due to) neoplasm, left side
- H47.529 Disorders of visual pathways in (due to) neoplasm, unspecified side

H47.53 Disorders of visual pathways in (due to) vascular disorders
- H47.531 Disorders of visual pathways in (due to) vascular disorders, right side
- H47.532 Disorders of visual pathways in (due to) vascular disorders, left side
- H47.539 Disorders of visual pathways in (due to) vascular disorders, unspecified side

H47.6 Disorders of visual cortex

Code also underlying condition

Excludes1 injury to visual cortex S04.04-

H47.61 Cortical blindness
- H47.611 Cortical blindness, right side of brain
- H47.612 Cortical blindness, left side of brain
- H47.619 Cortical blindness, unspecified side of brain

H47.62 Disorders of visual cortex in (due to) inflammatory disorders
- H47.621 Disorders of visual cortex in (due to) inflammatory disorders, right side of brain
- H47.622 Disorders of visual cortex in (due to) inflammatory disorders, left side of brain
- H47.629 Disorders of visual cortex in (due to) inflammatory disorders, unspecified side of brain

H47.63 Disorders of visual cortex in (due to) neoplasm
- H47.631 Disorders of visual cortex in (due to) neoplasm, right side of brain
- H47.632 Disorders of visual cortex in (due to) neoplasm, left side of brain
- H47.639 Disorders of visual cortex in (due to) neoplasm, unspecified side of brain

H47.64 Disorders of visual cortex in (due to) vascular disorders
- H47.641 Disorders of visual cortex in (due to) vascular disorders, right side of brain
- H47.642 Disorders of visual cortex in (due to) vascular disorders, left side of brain
- H47.649 Disorders of visual cortex in (due to) vascular disorders, unspecified side of brain

H47.9 Unspecified disorder of visual pathways

DISORDERS OF OCULAR MUSCLES, BINOCULAR MOVEMENT, ACCOMMODATION AND REFRACTION (H49-H52)

Excludes2 nystagmus and other irregular eye movements (H55)

H49 Paralytic strabismus

Excludes2 internal ophthalmoplegia (H52.51-)
internuclear ophthalmoplegia (H51.2-)
progressive supranuclear ophthalmoplegia (G23.1)

H49.0 Third [oculomotor] nerve palsy
- H49.00 Third [oculomotor] nerve palsy, unspecified eye
- H49.01 Third [oculomotor] nerve palsy, right eye
- H49.02 Third [oculomotor] nerve palsy, left eye
- H49.03 Third [oculomotor] nerve palsy, bilateral

H49.1 Fourth [trochlear] nerve palsy
- H49.10 Fourth [trochlear] nerve palsy, unspecified eye
- H49.11 Fourth [trochlear] nerve palsy, right eye
- H49.12 Fourth [trochlear] nerve palsy, left eye
- H49.13 Fourth [trochlear] nerve palsy, bilateral

H49.2 Sixth [abducent] nerve palsy
- H49.20 Sixth [abducent] nerve palsy, unspecified eye
- H49.21 Sixth [abducent] nerve palsy, right eye
- H49.22 Sixth [abducent] nerve palsy, left eye
- H49.23 Sixth [abducent] nerve palsy, bilateral

H49.3 Total (external) ophthalmoplegia
- H49.30 Total (external) ophthalmoplegia, unspecified eye
- H49.31 Total (external) ophthalmoplegia, right eye
- H49.32 Total (external) ophthalmoplegia, left eye
- H49.33 Total (external) ophthalmoplegia, bilateral

H49.4 Progressive external ophthalmoplegia

Excludes1 Kearns-Sayre syndrome (H49.81-)

- H49.40 Progressive external ophthalmoplegia, unspecified eye
- H49.41 Progressive external ophthalmoplegia, right eye
- H49.42 Progressive external ophthalmoplegia, left eye
- H49.43 Progressive external ophthalmoplegia, bilateral

Item 7-9 Strabismus or esotropia (crossed eyes) is a condition of the extraocular eye muscles, resulting in an inability of the eyes to focus and also affects depth perception.

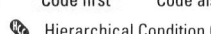

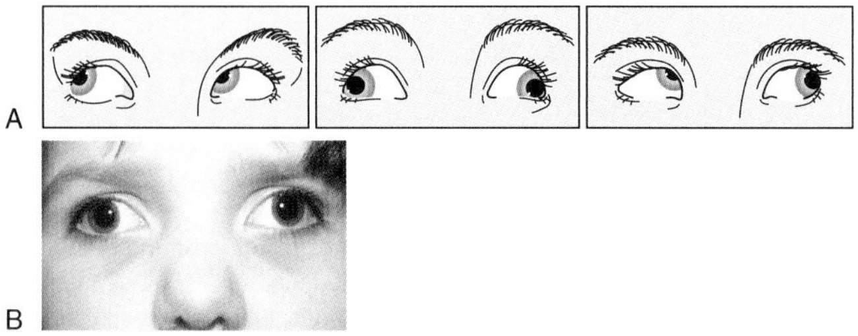

Figure 7-12 **A.** Image of strabismus. **B.** Exotropia. (**A** from Yanoff: Ophthalmology, ed 3, Mosby, Inc., 2008. **B** from Zitelli BJ, Davis HW, Pediatric Physical Diagnosis: Atlas of Pediatric Physical Diagnosis, Philadelphia, Elsevier Saunders, 2012)

● H49.8 Other paralytic strabismus
- ● H49.81 Kearns-Sayre syndrome
  - Progressive external ophthalmoplegia with pigmentary retinopathy
  - Use additional code for other manifestation, such as:
    - heart block (I45.9)
  - H49.811 Kearns-Sayre syndrome, right eye
  - H49.812 Kearns-Sayre syndrome, left eye
  - H49.813 Kearns-Sayre syndrome, bilateral
  - H49.819 Kearns-Sayre syndrome, unspecified eye
- ● H49.88 Other paralytic strabismus
  - External ophthalmoplegia NOS
  - H49.881 Other paralytic strabismus, right eye
  - H49.882 Other paralytic strabismus, left eye
  - H49.883 Other paralytic strabismus, bilateral
  - H49.889 Other paralytic strabismus, unspecified eye

H49.9 Unspecified paralytic strabismus

● H50 Other strabismus
- ● H50.0 Esotropia
  - Convergent concomitant strabismus
  - **Excludes1** intermittent esotropia (H50.31-, H50.32)
  - H50.00 Unspecified esotropia
  - ● H50.01 Monocular esotropia
    - H50.011 Monocular esotropia, right eye
    - H50.012 Monocular esotropia, left eye
  - ● H50.02 Monocular esotropia with A pattern
    - H50.021 Monocular esotropia with A pattern, right eye
    - H50.022 Monocular esotropia with A pattern, left eye
  - ● H50.03 Monocular esotropia with V pattern
    - H50.031 Monocular esotropia with V pattern, right eye
    - H50.032 Monocular esotropia with V pattern, left eye
  - ● H50.04 Monocular esotropia with other noncomitancies
    - H50.041 Monocular esotropia with other noncomitancies, right eye
    - H50.042 Monocular esotropia with other noncomitancies, left eye
  - H50.05 Alternating esotropia
  - H50.06 Alternating esotropia with A pattern
  - H50.07 Alternating esotropia with V pattern
  - H50.08 Alternating esotropia with other noncomitancies
- ● H50.1 Exotropia
  - *Misalignment in which one eye deviates outward (away from nose) while the other fixates normally*
  - Divergent concomitant strabismus
  - **Excludes1** intermittent exotropia (H50.33-, H50.34)
  - H50.10 Unspecified exotropia
  - ● H50.11 Monocular exotropia
    - H50.111 Monocular exotropia, right eye
    - H50.112 Monocular exotropia, left eye
  - ● H50.12 Monocular exotropia with A pattern
    - H50.121 Monocular exotropia with A pattern, right eye
    - H50.122 Monocular exotropia with A pattern, left eye
  - ● H50.13 Monocular exotropia with V pattern
    - H50.131 Monocular exotropia with V pattern, right eye
    - H50.132 Monocular exotropia with V pattern, left eye
  - ● H50.14 Monocular exotropia with other noncomitancies
    - H50.141 Monocular exotropia with other noncomitancies, right eye
    - H50.142 Monocular exotropia with other noncomitancies, left eye
  - H50.15 Alternating exotropia
  - H50.16 Alternating exotropia with A pattern
  - H50.17 Alternating exotropia with V pattern
  - H50.18 Alternating exotropia with other noncomitancies
- ● H50.2 Vertical strabismus
  - Hypertropia
  - H50.21 Vertical strabismus, right eye
  - H50.22 Vertical strabismus, left eye
- ● H50.3 Intermittent heterotropia
  - *Displacement of an organ or part of an organ from its normal position*
  - H50.30 Unspecified intermittent heterotropia
  - ● H50.31 Intermittent monocular esotropia
    - H50.311 Intermittent monocular esotropia, right eye
    - H50.312 Intermittent monocular esotropia, left eye
  - H50.32 Intermittent alternating esotropia
  - ● H50.33 Intermittent monocular exotropia
    - H50.331 Intermittent monocular exotropia, right eye
    - H50.332 Intermittent monocular exotropia, left eye
  - H50.34 Intermittent alternating exotropia
- ● H50.4 Other and unspecified heterotropia
  - H50.40 Unspecified heterotropia
  - ● H50.41 Cyclotropia
    - H50.411 Cyclotropia, right eye
    - H50.412 Cyclotropia, left eye
  - H50.42 Monofixation syndrome
  - H50.43 Accommodative component in esotropia
- ● H50.5 Heterophoria
  - *One or both eyes wander away from the position where both eyes are looking together in the same direction*
  - H50.50 Unspecified heterophoria
  - H50.51 Esophoria
    - *Eye deviates inward (toward the nose)*
  - H50.52 Exophoria
    - *Eye deviates outward (toward the ear)*
  - H50.53 Vertical heterophoria
  - H50.54 Cyclophoria
  - H50.55 Alternating heterophoria

● H50.6 Mechanical strabismus
H50.60 Mechanical strabismus, unspecified
● H50.61 Brown's sheath syndrome
H50.611 Brown's sheath syndrome, right eye
H50.612 Brown's sheath syndrome, left eye
H50.69 Other mechanical strabismus
Strabismus due to adhesions
Traumatic limitation of duction of eye muscle
● H50.8 Other specified strabismus
● H50.81 Duane's syndrome
H50.811 Duane's syndrome, right eye
H50.812 Duane's syndrome, left eye
H50.89 Other specified strabismus
H50.9 Unspecified strabismus

● H51 Other disorders of binocular movement
H51.0 Palsy (spasm) of conjugate gaze
● H51.1 Convergence insufficiency and excess
H51.11 Convergence insufficiency
H51.12 Convergence excess
● H51.2 Internuclear ophthalmoplegia
H51.20 Internuclear ophthalmoplegia, unspecified eye
H51.21 Internuclear ophthalmoplegia, right eye
H51.22 Internuclear ophthalmoplegia, left eye
H51.23 Internuclear ophthalmoplegia, bilateral
H51.8 Other specified disorders of binocular movement
H51.9 Unspecified disorder of binocular movement

● H52 Disorders of refraction and accommodation
● H52.0 Hypermetropia
H52.00 Hypermetropia, unspecified eye
H52.01 Hypermetropia, right eye
H52.02 Hypermetropia, left eye
H52.03 Hypermetropia, bilateral
● H52.1 Myopia
Excludes1 degenerative myopia (H44.2-)
H52.10 Myopia, unspecified eye
H52.11 Myopia, right eye
H52.12 Myopia, left eye
H52.13 Myopia, bilateral
● H52.2 Astigmatism
● H52.20 Unspecified astigmatism
H52.201 Unspecified astigmatism, right eye
H52.202 Unspecified astigmatism, left eye
H52.203 Unspecified astigmatism, bilateral
H52.209 Unspecified astigmatism, unspecified eye
● H52.21 Irregular astigmatism
H52.211 Irregular astigmatism, right eye
H52.212 Irregular astigmatism, left eye
H52.213 Irregular astigmatism, bilateral
H52.219 Irregular astigmatism, unspecified eye
● H52.22 Regular astigmatism
H52.221 Regular astigmatism, right eye
H52.222 Regular astigmatism, left eye
H52.223 Regular astigmatism, bilateral
H52.229 Regular astigmatism, unspecified eye

Item 7-10 Disorders of refraction: **Hypermetropia,** or farsightedness, means focus at a distance is adequate but not on close objects. **Myopia** is near-sightedness or short-sightedness and means the focus on nearby objects is clear but distant objects appear blurred. **Astigmatism** is warping of the curvature of the cornea so light rays entering do not meet a single focal point, resulting in a distorted image. **Anisometropia** is unequal refractive power in which one eye may be myopic (near-sighted) and the other hyperopic (far-sighted). **Presbyopia** is the loss of focus on near objects, which occurs with age because the lens loses elasticity.

● H52.3 Anisometropia and aniseikonia
H52.31 Anisometropia
H52.32 Aniseikonia
H52.4 Presbyopia
● H52.5 Disorders of accommodation
● H52.51 Internal ophthalmoplegia (complete) (total)
H52.511 Internal ophthalmoplegia (complete) (total), right eye
H52.512 Internal ophthalmoplegia (complete) (total), left eye
H52.513 Internal ophthalmoplegia (complete) (total), bilateral
H52.519 Internal ophthalmoplegia (complete) (total), unspecified eye
● H52.52 Paresis of accommodation
H52.521 Paresis of accommodation, right eye
H52.522 Paresis of accommodation, left eye
H52.523 Paresis of accommodation, bilateral
H52.529 Paresis of accommodation, unspecified eye
● H52.53 Spasm of accommodation
H52.531 Spasm of accommodation, right eye
H52.532 Spasm of accommodation, left eye
H52.533 Spasm of accommodation, bilateral
H52.539 Spasm of accommodation, unspecified eye
H52.6 Other disorders of refraction
H52.7 Unspecified disorder of refraction

VISUAL DISTURBANCES AND BLINDNESS (H53-H54)

● H53 Visual disturbances
● H53.0 Amblyopia ex anopsia
Excludes1 amblyopia due to vitamin A deficiency (E50.5)
● H53.00 Unspecified amblyopia
H53.001 Unspecified amblyopia, right eye
H53.002 Unspecified amblyopia, left eye
H53.003 Unspecified amblyopia, bilateral
H53.009 Unspecified amblyopia, unspecified eye
● H53.01 Deprivation amblyopia
H53.011 Deprivation amblyopia, right eye
H53.012 Deprivation amblyopia, left eye
H53.013 Deprivation amblyopia, bilateral
H53.019 Deprivation amblyopia, unspecified eye
● H53.02 Refractive amblyopia
H53.021 Refractive amblyopia, right eye
H53.022 Refractive amblyopia, left eye
H53.023 Refractive amblyopia, bilateral
H53.029 Refractive amblyopia, unspecified eye
● H53.03 Strabismic amblyopia
Excludes1 strabismus (H50.-)
H53.031 Strabismic amblyopia, right eye
H53.032 Strabismic amblyopia, left eye
H53.033 Strabismic amblyopia, bilateral
H53.039 Strabismic amblyopia, unspecified eye
● H53.04 Amblyopia suspect
Coding Clinic: 2016, Q4, P22
H53.041 Amblyopia suspect, right eye
H53.042 Amblyopia suspect, left eye
H53.043 Amblyopia suspect, bilateral
H53.049 Amblyopia suspect, unspecified eye

- H53.1 Subjective visual disturbances
  - **Excludes1** subjective visual disturbances due to vitamin A deficiency (E5Ø.5)
    visual hallucinations (R44.1)
  - H53.1Ø Unspecified subjective visual disturbances
  - H53.11 Day blindness
    Hemeralopia
  - H53.12 Transient visual loss
    Scintillating scotoma
    - **Excludes1** amaurosis fugax (G45.3-)
      transient retinal artery occlusion (H34.Ø-)
    - H53.121 Transient visual loss, right eye
    - H53.122 Transient visual loss, left eye
    - H53.123 Transient visual loss, bilateral
    - H53.129 Transient visual loss, unspecified eye
  - H53.13 Sudden visual loss
    - H53.131 Sudden visual loss, right eye
    - H53.132 Sudden visual loss, left eye
    - H53.133 Sudden visual loss, bilateral
    - H53.139 Sudden visual loss, unspecified eye
  - H53.14 Visual discomfort
    Asthenopia
    Photophobia
    - H53.141 Visual discomfort, right eye
    - H53.142 Visual discomfort, left eye
    - H53.143 Visual discomfort, bilateral
    - H53.149 Visual discomfort, unspecified
  - H53.15 Visual distortions of shape and size
    Metamorphopsia
  - H53.16 Psychophysical visual disturbances
  - H53.19 Other subjective visual disturbances
    Visual halos
- H53.2 Diplopia
  Double vision
- H53.3 Other and unspecified disorders of binocular vision
  - H53.3Ø Unspecified disorder of binocular vision
  - H53.31 Abnormal retinal correspondence
  - H53.32 Fusion with defective stereopsis
  - H53.33 Simultaneous visual perception without fusion
  - H53.34 Suppression of binocular vision
- H53.4 Visual field defects
  - H53.4Ø Unspecified visual field defects
  - H53.41 Scotoma involving central area
    Central scotoma
    - H53.411 Scotoma involving central area, right eye
    - H53.412 Scotoma involving central area, left eye
    - H53.413 Scotoma involving central area, bilateral
    - H53.419 Scotoma involving central area, unspecified eye
  - H53.42 Scotoma of blind spot area
    Enlarged blind spot
    - H53.421 Scotoma of blind spot area, right eye
    - H53.422 Scotoma of blind spot area, left eye
    - H53.423 Scotoma of blind spot area, bilateral
    - H53.429 Scotoma of blind spot area, unspecified eye
  - H53.43 Sector or arcuate defects
    Arcuate scotoma
    Bjerrum scotoma
    - H53.431 Sector or arcuate defects, right eye
    - H53.432 Sector or arcuate defects, left eye
    - H53.433 Sector or arcuate defects, bilateral
    - H53.439 Sector or arcuate defects, unspecified eye
  - H53.45 Other localized visual field defect
    Peripheral visual field defect
    Ring scotoma NOS
    Scotoma NOS
    - H53.451 Other localized visual field defect, right eye
    - H53.452 Other localized visual field defect, left eye
    - H53.453 Other localized visual field defect, bilateral
    - H53.459 Other localized visual field defect, unspecified eye
  - H53.46 Homonymous bilateral field defects
    Homonymous hemianopia
    Homonymous hemianopsia
    Quadrant anopia
    Quadrant anopsia
    - H53.461 Homonymous bilateral field defects, right side
    - H53.462 Homonymous bilateral field defects, left side
    - H53.469 Homonymous bilateral field defects, unspecified side
      Homonymous bilateral field defects NOS
  - H53.47 Heteronymous bilateral field defects
    Heteronymous hemianop(s)ia
  - H53.48 Generalized contraction of visual field
    - H53.481 Generalized contraction of visual field, right eye
    - H53.482 Generalized contraction of visual field, left eye
    - H53.483 Generalized contraction of visual field, bilateral
    - H53.489 Generalized contraction of visual field, unspecified eye
- H53.5 Color vision deficiencies
  Color blindness
  - **Excludes2** day blindness (H53.11)
  - H53.5Ø Unspecified color vision deficiencies
    Color blindness NOS
  - H53.51 Achromatopsia
  - H53.52 Acquired color vision deficiency
  - H53.53 Deuteranomaly
    Deuteranopia
  - H53.54 Protanomaly
    Protanopia
  - H53.55 Tritanomaly
    Tritanopia
  - H53.59 Other color vision deficiencies
- H53.6 Night blindness
  - **Excludes1** night blindness due to vitamin A deficiency (E5Ø.5)
  - H53.6Ø Unspecified night blindness
  - H53.61 Abnormal dark adaptation curve
  - H53.62 Acquired night blindness
  - H53.63 Congenital night blindness
  - H53.69 Other night blindness
- H53.7 Vision sensitivity deficiencies
  - H53.71 Glare sensitivity
  - H53.72 Impaired contrast sensitivity
- H53.8 Other visual disturbances
- H53.9 Unspecified visual disturbance

H54 Blindness and low vision

Note: For definition of visual impairment categories see table below.

Code first any associated underlying cause of the blindness

Excludes1 amaurosis fugax (G45.3)

H54.0 Blindness, both eyes

Visual impairment categories 3, 4, 5 in both eyes.

H54.0X Blindness, both eyes, different category levels

H54.0X3 Blindness right eye, category 3

H54.0X33 Blindness right eye category 3, blindness left eye category 3

H54.0X34 Blindness right eye category 3, blindness left eye category 4

H54.0X35 Blindness right eye category 3, blindness left eye category 5

H54.0X4 Blindness right eye, category 4

H54.0X43 Blindness right eye category 4, blindness left eye category 3

H54.0X44 Blindness right eye category 4, blindness left eye category 4

H54.0X45 Blindness right eye category 4, blindness left eye category 5

H54.0X5 Blindness right eye, category 5

H54.0X53 Blindness right eye category 5, blindness left eye category 3

H54.0X54 Blindness right eye category 5, blindness left eye category 4

H54.0X55 Blindness right eye category 5, blindness left eye category 5

H54.1 Blindness, one eye, low vision other eye

Visual impairment categories 3, 4, 5 in one eye, with categories 1 or 2 in the other eye.

H54.10 Blindness, one eye, low vision other eye, unspecified eyes

H54.11 Blindness, right eye, low vision left eye

H54.113 Blindness right eye category 3, low vision left eye

H54.1131 Blindness right eye category 3, low vision left eye category 1

H54.1132 Blindness right eye category 3, low vision left eye category 2

H54.114 Blindness right eye category 4, low vision left eye

H54.1141 Blindness right eye category 4, low vision left eye category 1

H54.1142 Blindness right eye category 4, low vision left eye category 2

H54.115 Blindness right eye category 5, low vision left eye

H54.1151 Blindness right eye category 5, low vision left eye category 1

H54.1152 Blindness right eye category 5, low vision left eye category 2

H54.12 Blindness, left eye, low vision right eye

H54.121 Low vision right eye category 1, blindness left eye

H54.1213 Low vision right eye category 1, blindness left eye category 3

H54.1214 Low vision right eye category 1, blindness left eye category 4

H54.1215 Low vision right eye category 1, blindness left eye category 5

H54.122 Low vision right eye category 2, blindness left eye

H54.1223 Low vision right eye category 2, blindness left eye category 3

H54.1224 Low vision right eye category 2, blindness left eye category 4

H54.1225 Low vision right eye category 2, blindness left eye category 5

H54.2 Low vision, both eyes

Visual impairment categories 1 or 2 in both eyes.

H54.2X Low vision, both eyes, different category levels

H54.2X1 Low vision, right eye, category 1

H54.2X11 Low vision right eye category 1, low vision left eye category 1

H54.2X12 Low vision right eye category 1, low vision left eye category 2

H54.2X2 Low vision, right eye, category 2

H54.2X21 Low vision right eye category 2, low vision left eye category 1

H54.2X22 Low vision right eye category 2, low vision left eye category 2

H54.3 Unqualified visual loss, both eyes

Visual impairment category 9 in both eyes.

H54.4 Blindness, one eye

Visual impairment categories 3, 4, 5 in one eye [normal vision in other eye]

H54.40 Blindness, one eye, unspecified eye

H54.41 Blindness, right eye, normal vision left eye

H54.413 Blindness, right eye, category 3

H54.413A Blindness right eye category 3, normal vision left eye

H54.414 Blindness, right eye, category 4

H54.414A Blindness right eye category 4, normal vision left eye

H54.415 Blindness, right eye, category 5

H54.415A Blindness right eye category 5, normal vision left eye

H54.42 Blindness, left eye, normal vision right eye

H54.42A Blindness, left eye, category 3-5

H54.42A3 Blindness left eye category 3, normal vision right eye

H54.42A4 Blindness left eye category 4, normal vision right eye

H54.42A5 Blindness left eye category 5, normal vision right eye

CHAPTER 7 (H00-H59)

OGCR Section I.C.7.b.

Blindness

If "blindness" or "low vision" of both eyes is documented but the visual impairment category is not documented, assign code H54.3, Unqualified visual loss, both eyes. If "blindness" or "low vision" in one eye is documented but the visual impairment category is not documented, assign a code from H54.6-, Unqualified visual loss, one eye. If "blindness" or "visual loss" is documented without any information about whether one or both eyes are affected, assign code H54.7, Unspecified visual loss.

● **H54.5 Low vision, one eye**
Visual impairment categories 1 or 2 in one eye [normal vision in other eye].
- H54.50 Low vision, one eye, **unspecified** eye
- ● H54.51 Low vision, **right** eye, normal vision left eye
  - ● H54.511 Low vision, right eye, category 1-2
    - H54.511A Low vision right eye **category 1**, normal vision left eye
    - H54.512A Low vision right eye **category 2**, normal vision left eye
- ● H54.52 Low vision, **left** eye, normal vision right eye
  - ● H54.52A Low vision, left eye, category 1-2
    - H54.52A1 Low vision left eye **category 1**, normal vision right eye
    - H54.52A2 Low vision left eye **category 2**, normal vision right eye

● **H54.6 Unqualified visual loss, one eye**
Visual impairment category 9 in one eye [normal vision in other eye].
- H54.60 Unqualified visual loss, one eye, **unspecified**
- H54.61 Unqualified visual loss, **right** eye, normal vision left eye
- H54.62 Unqualified visual loss, **left** eye, normal vision right eye

H54.7 Unspecified visual loss
Visual impairment category 9 NOS

H54.8 Legal blindness, as defined in USA
Blindness NOS according to USA definition
Excludes1 legal blindness with specification of impairment level (H54.0-H54.7)

Note: The table below gives a classification of severity of visual impairment recommended by a WHO Study Group on the Prevention of Blindness, Geneva, 6-10 November 1972.

The term "low vision" in category H54 comprises categories 1 and 2 of the table, the term "blindness" categories 3, 4, and 5, and the term "unqualified visual loss" category 9.

If the extent of the visual field is taken into account, patients with a field no greater than 10 but greater than 5 around central fixation should be placed in category 3 and patients with a field no greater than 5 around central fixation should be placed in category 4, even if the central acuity is not impaired.

(Document 508 compliance requires all cells in the following table to be filled.)

Category of visual impairment	Visual acuity with best possible correction	
	Maximum less than:	Minimum equal to or better than:
—	6/18	6/60
3/10 (0.3)	1/10 (0.1)	—
20/70	20/200	—
—	6/60	3/60
1/10 (0.1)	1/20 (0.05)	—
20/200	20/400	—
—	3/60	1/60 (finger counting at one meter)
1/20 (0.05)	1/50 (0.02)	—
20/400	5/300 (20/1200)	—
—	1/60 (finger counting at one meter)	Light perception
1/50 (0.02)	—	—
5/300	—	—
—	No light perception	—
—	Undetermined or unspecified	—

OTHER DISORDERS OF EYE AND ADNEXA (H55-H57)

● **H55 Nystagmus and other irregular eye movements**
- ● H55.0 Nystagmus
  Rapid, involuntary movements of the eyes in the horizontal or vertical direction
  - H55.00 **Unspecified** nystagmus
  - H55.01 **Congenital** nystagmus
  - H55.02 **Latent** nystagmus
  - H55.03 **Visual deprivation** nystagmus
  - H55.04 **Dissociated** nystagmus
  - H55.09 **Other forms** of nystagmus
- ● H55.8 Other irregular eye movements
  - H55.81 Saccadic eye movements
  - H55.89 Other irregular eye movements

● **H57 Other disorders of eye and adnexa**
- ● H57.0 Anomalies of pupillary function
  - H57.00 Unspecified anomaly of pupillary function
  - H57.01 Argyll Robertson pupil, atypical
    Excludes1 syphilitic Argyll Robertson pupil (A52.19)
  - H57.02 Anisocoria
  - H57.03 Miosis
  - H57.04 Mydriasis
  - ● H57.05 Tonic pupil
    - H57.051 Tonic pupil, **right** eye
    - H57.052 Tonic pupil, **left** eye
    - H57.053 Tonic pupil, **bilateral**
    - H57.059 Tonic pupil, **unspecified** eye
  - H57.09 Other anomalies of pupillary function

- H57.1 Ocular pain
  - H57.10 Ocular pain, unspecified eye
  - H57.11 Ocular pain, right eye
  - H57.12 Ocular pain, left eye
  - H57.13 Ocular pain, bilateral
- H57.8 Other specified disorders of eye and adnexa
  - H57.81 Brow ptosis
    - H57.811 Brow ptosis, right
    - H57.812 Brow ptosis, left
    - H57.813 Brow ptosis, bilateral
    - H57.819 Brow ptosis, unspecified
  - H57.89 Other specified disorders of eye and adnexa
- H57.9 Unspecified disorder of eye and adnexa

INTRAOPERATIVE AND POSTPROCEDURAL COMPLICATIONS AND DISORDERS OF EYE AND ADNEXA, NOT ELSEWHERE CLASSIFIED (H59)

H59 Intraoperative and postprocedural complications and disorders of eye and adnexa, not elsewhere classified

Excludes1 mechanical complication of intraocular lens (T85.2)
mechanical complication of other ocular prosthetic devices, implants and grafts (T85.3)
pseudophakia (Z96.1)
secondary cataracts (H26.4-)

- H59.0 Disorders of the eye following cataract surgery
  - H59.01 Keratopathy (bullous aphakic) following cataract surgery
    Vitreal corneal syndrome
    Vitreous (touch) syndrome
    - H59.011 Keratopathy (bullous aphakic) following cataract surgery, right eye
    - H59.012 Keratopathy (bullous aphakic) following cataract surgery, left eye
    - H59.013 Keratopathy (bullous aphakic) following cataract surgery, bilateral
    - H59.019 Keratopathy (bullous aphakic) following cataract surgery, unspecified eye
  - H59.02 Cataract (lens) fragments in eye following cataract surgery
    - H59.021 Cataract (lens) fragments in eye following cataract surgery, right eye
    - H59.022 Cataract (lens) fragments in eye following cataract surgery, left eye
    - H59.023 Cataract (lens) fragments in eye following cataract surgery, bilateral
    - H59.029 Cataract (lens) fragments in eye following cataract surgery, unspecified eye
  - H59.03 Cystoid macular edema following cataract surgery
    - H59.031 Cystoid macular edema following cataract surgery, right eye
    - H59.032 Cystoid macular edema following cataract surgery, left eye
    - H59.033 Cystoid macular edema following cataract surgery, bilateral
    - H59.039 Cystoid macular edema following cataract surgery, unspecified eye
  - H59.09 Other disorders of the eye following cataract surgery
    - H59.091 Other disorders of the right eye following cataract surgery
    - H59.092 Other disorders of the left eye following cataract surgery
    - H59.093 Other disorders of the eye following cataract surgery, bilateral
    - H59.099 Other disorders of unspecified eye following cataract surgery
- H59.1 Intraoperative hemorrhage and hematoma of eye and adnexa complicating a procedure

  Excludes1 intraoperative hemorrhage and hematoma of eye and adnexa due to accidental puncture or laceration during a procedure (H59.2-)
  - H59.11 Intraoperative hemorrhage and hematoma of eye and adnexa complicating an ophthalmic procedure
    - H59.111 Intraoperative hemorrhage and hematoma of right eye and adnexa complicating an ophthalmic procedure
    - H59.112 Intraoperative hemorrhage and hematoma of left eye and adnexa complicating an ophthalmic procedure
    - H59.113 Intraoperative hemorrhage and hematoma of eye and adnexa complicating an ophthalmic procedure, bilateral
    - H59.119 Intraoperative hemorrhage and hematoma of unspecified eye and adnexa complicating an ophthalmic procedure
  - H59.12 Intraoperative hemorrhage and hematoma of eye and adnexa complicating other procedure
    - H59.121 Intraoperative hemorrhage and hematoma of right eye and adnexa complicating other procedure
    - H59.122 Intraoperative hemorrhage and hematoma of left eye and adnexa complicating other procedure
    - H59.123 Intraoperative hemorrhage and hematoma of eye and adnexa complicating other procedure, bilateral
    - H59.129 Intraoperative hemorrhage and hematoma of unspecified eye and adnexa complicating other procedure
- H59.2 Accidental puncture and laceration of eye and adnexa during a procedure
  - H59.21 Accidental puncture and laceration of eye and adnexa during an ophthalmic procedure
    - H59.211 Accidental puncture and laceration of right eye and adnexa during an ophthalmic procedure
    - H59.212 Accidental puncture and laceration of left eye and adnexa during an ophthalmic procedure
    - H59.213 Accidental puncture and laceration of eye and adnexa during an ophthalmic procedure, bilateral
    - H59.219 Accidental puncture and laceration of unspecified eye and adnexa during an ophthalmic procedure
  - H59.22 Accidental puncture and laceration of eye and adnexa during other procedure
    - H59.221 Accidental puncture and laceration of right eye and adnexa during other procedure
    - H59.222 Accidental puncture and laceration of left eye and adnexa during other procedure
    - H59.223 Accidental puncture and laceration of eye and adnexa during other procedure, bilateral
    - H59.229 Accidental puncture and laceration of unspecified eye and adnexa during other procedure

- H59.3 **Postprocedural hemorrhage, hematoma, and seroma** of eye and adnexa following other procedure
  Coding Clinic: 2016, Q4, P1Ø
  - H59.31 Postprocedural **hemorrhage** of eye and adnexa following an **ophthalmic procedure**
    - H59.311 Postprocedural hemorrhage of **right** eye and adnexa following an ophthalmic procedure
    - H59.312 Postprocedural hemorrhage of **left** eye and adnexa following an ophthalmic procedure
    - H59.313 Postprocedural hemorrhage of eye and adnexa following an ophthalmic procedure, **bilateral**
    - H59.319 Postprocedural hemorrhage of **unspecified** eye and adnexa following an ophthalmic procedure
  - H59.32 Postprocedural **hemorrhage** of eye and adnexa following **other procedure**
    - H59.321 Postprocedural hemorrhage of **right** eye and adnexa following other procedure
    - H59.322 Postprocedural hemorrhage of **left** eye and adnexa following other procedure
    - H59.323 Postprocedural hemorrhage of eye and adnexa following other procedure, **bilateral**
    - H59.329 Postprocedural hemorrhage of **unspecified** eye and adnexa following other procedure
  - H59.33 Postprocedural **hematoma** of eye and adnexa following an **ophthalmic procedure**
    - H59.331 Postprocedural hematoma of **right** eye and adnexa following an ophthalmic procedure
    - H59.332 Postprocedural hematoma of **left** eye and adnexa following an ophthalmic procedure
    - H59.333 Postprocedural hematoma of eye and adnexa following an ophthalmic procedure, **bilateral**
    - H59.339 Postprocedural hematoma of **unspecified** eye and adnexa following an ophthalmic procedure
  - H59.34 Postprocedural **hematoma** of eye and adnexa following **other procedure**
    - H59.341 Postprocedural hematoma of **right** eye and adnexa following other procedure
    - H59.342 Postprocedural hematoma of **left** eye and adnexa following other procedure
    - H59.343 Postprocedural hematoma of eye and adnexa following other procedure, **bilateral**
    - H59.349 Postprocedural hematoma of **unspecified** eye and adnexa following other procedure
  - H59.35 Postprocedural **seroma** of eye and adnexa following an **ophthalmic procedure**
    - H59.351 Postprocedural seroma of **right** eye and adnexa following an ophthalmic procedure
    - H59.352 Postprocedural seroma of **left** eye and adnexa following an ophthalmic procedure
    - H59.353 Postprocedural seroma of eye and adnexa following an ophthalmic procedure, **bilateral**
    - H59.359 Postprocedural seroma of **unspecified** eye and adnexa following an ophthalmic procedure
  - H59.36 Postprocedural **seroma** of eye and adnexa following **other procedure**
    - H59.361 Postprocedural seroma of **right** eye and adnexa following other procedure
    - H59.362 Postprocedural seroma of **left** eye and adnexa following other procedure
    - H59.363 Postprocedural seroma of eye and adnexa following other procedure, **bilateral**
    - H59.369 Postprocedural seroma of **unspecified** eye and adnexa following other procedure
- H59.4 **Inflammation** (infection) of **postprocedural bleb**
  Postprocedural blebitis
  Excludes1 filtering (vitreous) bleb after glaucoma surgery status (Z98.83)
  - H59.40 Inflammation (infection) of postprocedural bleb, **unspecified**
  - H59.41 Inflammation (infection) of postprocedural bleb, **stage 1**
  - H59.42 Inflammation (infection) of postprocedural bleb, **stage 2**
  - H59.43 Inflammation (infection) of postprocedural bleb, **stage 3**
    Bleb endophthalmitis
- H59.8 **Other intraoperative and postprocedural complications** and disorders of eye and adnexa, not elsewhere classified
  - H59.81 Chorioretinal scars after surgery for detachment
    - H59.811 Chorioretinal scars after surgery for detachment, **right** eye
    - H59.812 Chorioretinal scars after surgery for detachment, **left** eye
    - H59.813 Chorioretinal **scars** after surgery for detachment, **bilateral**
    - H59.819 Chorioretinal scars after surgery for detachment, **unspecified** eye
  - H59.88 **Other intraoperative** complications of eye and adnexa, not elsewhere classified
  - H59.89 **Other postprocedural** complications and disorders of eye and adnexa, not elsewhere classified

CHAPTER 8

DISEASES OF THE EAR AND MASTOID PROCESS (H60-H95)

OGCR Chapter-Specific Coding Guidelines

8. Chapter 8: Diseases of the Ear and Mastoid Process (H60-H95)
Reserved for future guideline expansion

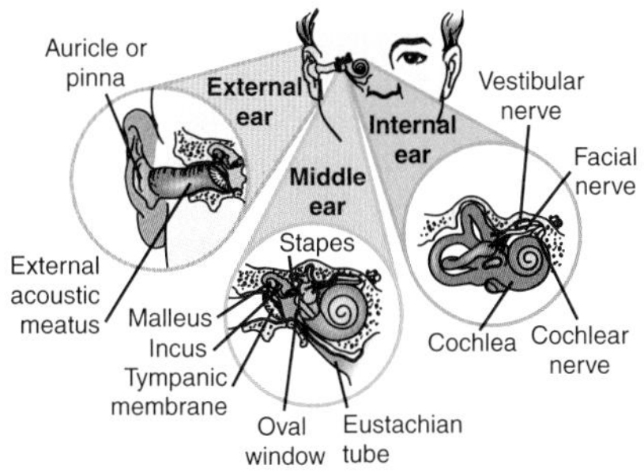

Figure 8-1 Auditory system. (From Buck CJ: Step-by-Step Medical Coding, ed 2016, St. Louis, Elsevier, 2016)

★**(See Plate 20 of the Anatomy Illustrations.)**

CHAPTER 8

DISEASES OF THE EAR AND MASTOID PROCESS (H60-H95)

Note: Use an external cause code following the code for the ear condition, if applicable, to identify the cause of the ear condition

Excludes2 certain conditions originating in the perinatal period (P04-P96)
certain infectious and parasitic diseases (A00-B99)
complications of pregnancy, childbirth and the puerperium (O00-O9A)
congenital malformations, deformations and chromosomal abnormalities (Q00-Q99)
endocrine, nutritional and metabolic diseases (E00-E88)
injury, poisoning and certain other consequences of external causes (S00-T88)
neoplasms (C00-D49)
symptoms, signs and abnormal clinical and laboratory findings, not elsewhere classified (R00-R94)

This chapter contains the following blocks:

H60-H62	Diseases of external ear
H65-H75	Diseases of middle ear and mastoid
H80-H83	Diseases of inner ear
H90-H94	Other disorders of ear
H95	Intraoperative and postprocedural complications and disorders of ear and mastoid process, not elsewhere classified

DISEASES OF EXTERNAL EAR (H60-H62)

● **H60** **Otitis externa**

● **H60.0** **Abscess of external ear**
Boil of external ear
Carbuncle of auricle or external auditory canal
Furuncle of external ear

H60.00 Abscess of external ear, **unspecified ear**
H60.01 Abscess of **right** external ear
H60.02 Abscess of **left** external ear
H60.03 Abscess of external ear, **bilateral**

● **H60.1** **Cellulitis of external ear**
Cellulitis of auricle
Cellulitis of external auditory canal

H60.10 Cellulitis of external ear, **unspecified ear**
H60.11 Cellulitis of **right** external ear
H60.12 Cellulitis of **left** external ear
H60.13 Cellulitis of external ear, **bilateral**

● **H60.2** **Malignant otitis externa**

H60.20 Malignant otitis externa, **unspecified ear**
H60.21 Malignant otitis externa, **right ear**
H60.22 Malignant otitis externa, **left ear**
H60.23 Malignant otitis externa, **bilateral**

● **H60.3** Other infective otitis externa

● **H60.31** Diffuse otitis externa

H60.311 Diffuse otitis externa, **right ear**
H60.312 Diffuse otitis externa, **left ear**
H60.313 Diffuse otitis externa, **bilateral**
H60.319 Diffuse otitis externa, **unspecified ear**

● **H60.32** Hemorrhagic otitis externa

H60.321 Hemorrhagic otitis externa, **right ear**
H60.322 Hemorrhagic otitis externa, **left ear**
H60.323 Hemorrhagic otitis externa, **bilateral**
H60.329 Hemorrhagic otitis externa, **unspecified ear**

● **H60.33** Swimmer's ear

H60.331 Swimmer's ear, **right ear**
H60.332 Swimmer's ear, **left ear**
H60.333 Swimmer's ear, **bilateral**
H60.339 Swimmer's ear, **unspecified ear**

● **H60.39** Other infective otitis externa

H60.391 Other infective otitis externa, **right ear**
H60.392 Other infective otitis externa, **left ear**
H60.393 Other infective otitis externa, **bilateral**
H60.399 Other infective otitis externa, **unspecified ear**

● **H60.4** Cholesteatoma of external ear
Keratosis obturans of external ear (canal)

Excludes2 cholesteatoma of middle ear (H71.-)
recurrent cholesteatoma of postmastoidectomy cavity (H95.0-)

H60.40 Cholesteatoma of external ear, **unspecified ear**
H60.41 Cholesteatoma of **right** external ear
H60.42 Cholesteatoma of **left** external ear
H60.43 Cholesteatoma of external ear, **bilateral**

● **H60.5** **Acute noninfective otitis externa**

● **H60.50** **Unspecified acute noninfective otitis externa**
Acute otitis externa NOS

H60.501 Unspecified acute noninfective otitis externa, **right ear**
H60.502 Unspecified acute noninfective otitis externa, **left ear**
H60.503 Unspecified acute noninfective otitis externa, **bilateral**
H60.509 Unspecified acute noninfective otitis externa, **unspecified ear**

● **H60.51** Acute **actinic** otitis externa

H60.511 Acute actinic otitis externa, **right ear**
H60.512 Acute actinic otitis externa, **left ear**
H60.513 Acute actinic otitis externa, **bilateral**
H60.519 Acute actinic otitis externa, **unspecified ear**

CHAPTER 8 (H60-H95)

- H60.52 Acute **chemical** otitis externa
  - H60.521 Acute chemical otitis externa, **right** ear
  - H60.522 Acute chemical otitis externa, **left** ear
  - H60.523 Acute chemical otitis externa, **bilateral**
  - H60.529 Acute chemical otitis externa, **unspecified** ear
- H60.53 Acute **contact** otitis externa
  - H60.531 Acute contact otitis externa, **right** ear
  - H60.532 Acute contact otitis externa, **left** ear
  - H60.533 Acute contact otitis externa, **bilateral**
  - H60.539 Acute contact otitis externa, **unspecified** ear
- H60.54 Acute eczematoid otitis externa
  - H60.541 Acute eczematoid otitis externa, right ear
  - H60.542 Acute eczematoid otitis externa, left ear
  - H60.543 Acute eczematoid otitis externa, bilateral
  - H60.549 Acute eczematoid otitis externa, **unspecified** ear
- H60.55 Acute **reactive** otitis externa
  - H60.551 Acute reactive otitis externa, **right** ear
  - H60.552 Acute reactive otitis externa, **left** ear
  - H60.553 Acute reactive otitis externa, **bilateral**
  - H60.559 Acute reactive otitis externa, **unspecified** ear
- H60.59 **Other** noninfective acute otitis externa
  - H60.591 Other noninfective acute otitis externa, **right** ear
  - H60.592 Other noninfective acute otitis externa, **left** ear
  - H60.593 Other noninfective acute otitis externa, **bilateral**
  - H60.599 Other noninfective acute otitis externa, **unspecified** ear

- H60.6 **Unspecified chronic** otitis externa
  - H60.60 Unspecified chronic otitis externa, **unspecified** ear
  - H60.61 Unspecified chronic otitis externa, **right** ear
  - H60.62 Unspecified chronic otitis externa, **left** ear
  - H60.63 Unspecified chronic otitis externa, **bilateral**
- H60.8 **Other** otitis externa
  - H60.8X Other otitis externa
    - H60.8X1 Other otitis externa, **right** ear
    - H60.8X2 Other otitis externa, **left** ear
    - H60.8X3 Other otitis externa, **bilateral**
    - H60.8X9 Other otitis externa, **unspecified** ear
- H60.9 **Unspecified** otitis externa
  - H60.90 Unspecified otitis externa, **unspecified** ear
  - H60.91 Unspecified otitis externa, **right** ear
  - H60.92 Unspecified otitis externa, **left** ear
  - H60.93 Unspecified otitis externa, **bilateral**

H61 Other disorders of external ear

- H61.0 Chondritis and perichondritis of external ear
  Chondrodermatitis nodularis chronica helicis
  Perichondritis of auricle
  Perichondritis of pinna
  - H61.00 **Unspecified perichondritis** of external ear
    - H61.001 Unspecified perichondritis of **right** external ear
    - H61.002 Unspecified perichondritis of **left** external ear
    - H61.003 Unspecified perichondritis of external ear, **bilateral**
    - H61.009 Unspecified perichondritis of external ear, **unspecified** ear
  - H61.01 **Acute perichondritis** of external ear
    - H61.011 Acute perichondritis of **right** external ear
    - H61.012 Acute perichondritis of **left** external ear
    - H61.013 Acute perichondritis of external ear, **bilateral**
    - H61.019 Acute perichondritis of external ear, **unspecified** ear
  - H61.02 **Chronic perichondritis** of external ear
    - H61.021 Chronic perichondritis of **right** external ear
    - H61.022 Chronic perichondritis of **left** external ear
    - H61.023 Chronic perichondritis of external ear, **bilateral**
    - H61.029 Chronic perichondritis of external ear, **unspecified** ear
  - H61.03 **Chondritis** of external ear
    Chondritis of auricle
    Chondritis of pinna
    - H61.031 Chondritis of **right** external ear
    - H61.032 Chondritis of **left** external ear
      Coding Clinic: 2015, Q1, P18
    - H61.033 Chondritis of external ear, **bilateral**
    - H61.039 Chondritis of external ear, **unspecified** ear
- H61.1 Noninfective disorders of pinna
  Excludes2 cauliflower ear (M95.1-)
  gouty tophi of ear (M1A.-)
  - H61.10 **Unspecified** noninfective disorders of pinna
    Disorder of pinna NOS
    - H61.101 Unspecified noninfective disorders of pinna, **right** ear
    - H61.102 Unspecified noninfective disorders of pinna, **left** ear
    - H61.103 Unspecified noninfective disorders of pinna, **bilateral**
    - H61.109 Unspecified noninfective disorders of pinna, **unspecified** ear
  - H61.11 Acquired deformity of pinna
    Acquired deformity of auricle
    Excludes2 cauliflower ear (M95.1-)
    - H61.111 Acquired deformity of pinna, **right** ear
    - H61.112 Acquired deformity of pinna, **left** ear
    - H61.113 Acquired deformity of pinna, **bilateral**
    - H61.119 Acquired deformity of pinna, **unspecified** ear
  - H61.12 Hematoma of pinna
    Hematoma of auricle
    - H61.121 Hematoma of pinna, **right** ear
    - H61.122 Hematoma of pinna, **left** ear
    - H61.123 Hematoma of pinna, **bilateral**
    - H61.129 Hematoma of pinna, **unspecified** ear
  - H61.19 Other noninfective disorders of pinna
    - H61.191 Noninfective disorders of pinna, **right** ear
    - H61.192 Noninfective disorders of pinna, **left** ear
    - H61.193 Noninfective disorders of pinna, **bilateral**
    - H61.199 Noninfective disorders of pinna, **unspecified** ear

H61.2 Impacted cerumen
Wax in ear
- H61.20 Impacted cerumen, unspecified ear
- H61.21 Impacted cerumen, right ear
- H61.22 Impacted cerumen, left ear
- H61.23 Impacted cerumen, bilateral

H61.3 Acquired stenosis of external ear canal
Collapse of external ear canal
Excludes1 postprocedural stenosis of external ear canal (H95.81-)

H61.30 Acquired stenosis of external ear canal, unspecified
- H61.301 Acquired stenosis of right external ear canal, unspecified
- H61.302 Acquired stenosis of left external ear canal, unspecified
- H61.303 Acquired stenosis of external ear canal, unspecified, bilateral
- H61.309 Acquired stenosis of external ear canal, unspecified, unspecified ear

H61.31 Acquired stenosis of external ear canal secondary to trauma
- H61.311 Acquired stenosis of right external ear canal secondary to trauma
- H61.312 Acquired stenosis of left external ear canal secondary to trauma
- H61.313 Acquired stenosis of external ear canal secondary to trauma, bilateral
- H61.319 Acquired stenosis of external ear canal secondary to trauma, unspecified ear

H61.32 Acquired stenosis of external ear canal secondary to inflammation and infection
- H61.321 Acquired stenosis of right external ear canal secondary to inflammation and infection
- H61.322 Acquired stenosis of left external ear canal secondary to inflammation and infection
- H61.323 Acquired stenosis of external ear canal secondary to inflammation and infection, bilateral
- H61.329 Acquired stenosis of external ear canal secondary to inflammation and infection, unspecified ear

H61.39 Other acquired stenosis of external ear canal
- H61.391 Other acquired stenosis of right external ear canal
- H61.392 Other acquired stenosis of left external ear canal
- H61.393 Other acquired stenosis of external ear canal, bilateral
- H61.399 Other acquired stenosis of external ear canal, unspecified ear

H61.8 Other specified disorders of external ear

H61.81 Exostosis of external canal
- H61.811 Exostosis of right external canal
- H61.812 Exostosis of left external canal
- H61.813 Exostosis of external canal, bilateral
- H61.819 Exostosis of external canal, unspecified ear

H61.89 Other specified disorders of external ear
- H61.891 Other specified disorders of right external ear
- H61.892 Other specified disorders of left external ear
- H61.893 Other specified disorders of external ear, bilateral
- H61.899 Other specified disorders of external ear, unspecified ear

H61.9 Disorder of external ear, unspecified
- H61.90 Disorder of external ear, unspecified, unspecified ear
- H61.91 Disorder of right external ear, unspecified
- H61.92 Disorder of left external ear, unspecified
- H61.93 Disorder of external ear, unspecified, bilateral

H62 Disorders of external ear in diseases classified elsewhere

H62.4 Otitis externa in other diseases classified elsewhere
Code first underlying disease, such as:
erysipelas (A46)
impetigo (L01.0)
Excludes1 otitis externa (in):
candidiasis (B37.84)
herpes viral [herpes simplex] (B00.1)
herpes zoster (B02.8)
- *H62.40 Otitis externa in other diseases classified elsewhere, unspecified ear*
- *H62.41 Otitis externa in other diseases classified elsewhere, right ear*
- *H62.42 Otitis externa in other diseases classified elsewhere, left ear*
- *H62.43 Otitis externa in other diseases classified elsewhere, bilateral*

H62.8 Other disorders of external ear in diseases classified elsewhere
Code first underlying disease, such as:
gout (M1A.-, M10.-)

H62.8X Other disorders of external ear in diseases classified elsewhere
- *H62.8X1 Other disorders of right external ear in diseases classified elsewhere*
- *H62.8X2 Other disorders of left external ear in diseases classified elsewhere*
- *H62.8X3 Other disorders of external ear in diseases classified elsewhere, bilateral*
- *H62.8X9 Other disorders of external ear in diseases classified elsewhere, unspecified ear*

DISEASES OF MIDDLE EAR AND MASTOID (H65-H75)

★**(See Plate 21 of the Anatomy Illustrations.)**

H65 Nonsuppurative otitis media
Bacterial or viral infection or inflammation of the middle ear; may result in fluid accumulation with pain and temporary hearing loss.
Includes nonsuppurative otitis media with myringitis
Use additional code for any associated perforated tympanic membrane (H72.-)
Use additional code to identify:
exposure to environmental tobacco smoke (Z77.22)
exposure to tobacco smoke in the perinatal period (P96.81)
history of tobacco dependence (Z87.891)
infectious agent (B95-B97)
occupational exposure to environmental tobacco smoke (Z57.31)
tobacco dependence (F17.-)
tobacco use (Z72.0)

H65.0 Acute serous otitis media
Acute and subacute secretory otitis
- H65.00 Acute serous otitis media, unspecified ear
- H65.01 Acute serous otitis media, right ear
- H65.02 Acute serous otitis media, left ear
- H65.03 Acute serous otitis media, bilateral
- H65.04 Acute serous otitis media, recurrent, right ear
- H65.05 Acute serous otitis media, recurrent, left ear
- H65.06 Acute serous otitis media, recurrent, bilateral
- H65.07 Acute serous otitis media, recurrent, unspecified ear

CHAPTER 8 (H60-H95)

● H65.1 Other acute nonsuppurative otitis media
Excludes1 otitic barotrauma (T70.0)
otitis media (acute) NOS (H66.9)

● H65.11 Acute and subacute allergic otitis media (mucoid) (sanguinous) (serous)
H65.111 Acute and subacute allergic otitis media (mucoid) (sanguinous) (serous), right ear
H65.112 Acute and subacute allergic otitis media (mucoid) (sanguinous) (serous), left ear
H65.113 Acute and subacute allergic otitis media (mucoid) (sanguinous) (serous), bilateral
H65.114 Acute and subacute allergic otitis media (mucoid) (sanguinous) (serous), recurrent, right ear
H65.115 Acute and subacute allergic otitis media (mucoid) (sanguinous) (serous), recurrent, left ear
H65.116 Acute and subacute allergic otitis media (mucoid) (sanguinous) (serous), recurrent, bilateral
H65.117 Acute and subacute allergic otitis media (mucoid) (sanguinous) (serous), recurrent, unspecified ear
H65.119 Acute and subacute allergic otitis media (mucoid) (sanguinous) (serous), unspecified ear

● H65.19 Other acute nonsuppurative otitis media
Acute and subacute mucoid otitis media
Acute and subacute nonsuppurative otitis media NOS
Acute and subacute sanguinous otitis media
Acute and subacute seromucinous otitis media
H65.191 Other acute nonsuppurative otitis media, right ear
H65.192 Other acute nonsuppurative otitis media, left ear
H65.193 Other acute nonsuppurative otitis media, bilateral
H65.194 Other acute nonsuppurative otitis media, recurrent, right ear
H65.195 Other acute nonsuppurative otitis media, recurrent, left ear
H65.196 Other acute nonsuppurative otitis media, recurrent, bilateral
H65.197 Other acute nonsuppurative otitis media recurrent, unspecified ear
H65.199 Other acute nonsuppurative otitis media, unspecified ear

● H65.2 Chronic serous otitis media
Chronic tubotympanal catarrh
H65.20 Chronic serous otitis media, unspecified ear
H65.21 Chronic serous otitis media, right ear
H65.22 Chronic serous otitis media, left ear
H65.23 Chronic serous otitis media, bilateral

● H65.3 Chronic mucoid otitis media
Chronic mucinous otitis media
Chronic secretory otitis media
Chronic transudative otitis media
Glue ear
Excludes1 adhesive middle ear disease (H74.1)
H65.30 Chronic mucoid otitis media, unspecified ear
H65.31 Chronic mucoid otitis media, right ear
H65.32 Chronic mucoid otitis media, left ear
H65.33 Chronic mucoid otitis media, bilateral

● H65.4 Other chronic nonsuppurative otitis media

● H65.41 Chronic allergic otitis media
H65.411 Chronic allergic otitis media, right ear
H65.412 Chronic allergic otitis media, left ear
H65.413 Chronic allergic otitis media, bilateral
H65.419 Chronic allergic otitis media, unspecified ear

● H65.49 Other chronic nonsuppurative otitis media
Chronic exudative otitis media
Chronic nonsuppurative otitis media NOS
Chronic otitis media with effusion (nonpurulent)
Chronic seromucinous otitis media
H65.491 Other chronic nonsuppurative otitis media, right ear
H65.492 Other chronic nonsuppurative otitis media, left ear
H65.493 Other chronic nonsuppurative otitis media, bilateral
H65.499 Other chronic nonsuppurative otitis media, unspecified ear

● H65.9 Unspecified nonsuppurative otitis media
Allergic otitis media NOS
Catarrhal otitis media NOS
Exudative otitis media NOS
Mucoid otitis media NOS
Otitis media with effusion (nonpurulent) NOS
Secretory otitis media NOS
Seromucinous otitis media NOS
Serous otitis media NOS
Transudative otitis media NOS
H65.90 Unspecified nonsuppurative otitis media, unspecified ear
H65.91 Unspecified nonsuppurative otitis media, right ear
H65.92 Unspecified nonsuppurative otitis media, left ear
H65.93 Unspecified nonsuppurative otitis media, bilateral

● H66 Suppurative and unspecified otitis media
Suppurative: Discharging pus
Includes suppurative and unspecified otitis media with myringitis
Use additional code to identify:
exposure to environmental tobacco smoke (Z77.22)
exposure to tobacco smoke in the perinatal period (P96.81)
history of tobacco dependence (Z87.891)
occupational exposure to environmental tobacco smoke (Z57.31)
tobacco dependence (F17.-)
tobacco use (Z72.0)

● H66.0 Acute suppurative otitis media

● H66.00 Acute suppurative otitis media without spontaneous rupture of ear drum
H66.001 Acute suppurative otitis media without spontaneous rupture of ear drum, right ear
Coding Clinic: 2016, Q1, P34
H66.002 Acute suppurative otitis media without spontaneous rupture of ear drum, left ear
H66.003 Acute suppurative otitis media without spontaneous rupture of ear drum, bilateral
H66.004 Acute suppurative otitis media without spontaneous rupture of ear drum, recurrent, right ear
H66.005 Acute suppurative otitis media without spontaneous rupture of ear drum, recurrent, left ear
H66.006 Acute suppurative otitis media without spontaneous rupture of ear drum, recurrent, bilateral
H66.007 Acute suppurative otitis media without spontaneous rupture of ear drum, recurrent, unspecified ear
H66.009 Acute suppurative otitis media without spontaneous rupture of ear drum, unspecified ear

H66.01 Acute suppurative otitis media with spontaneous rupture of ear drum
- H66.011 Acute suppurative otitis media with spontaneous rupture of ear drum, **right** ear
- H66.012 Acute suppurative otitis media with spontaneous rupture of ear drum, **left** ear
- H66.013 Acute suppurative otitis media with spontaneous rupture of ear drum, **bilateral**
- H66.014 Acute suppurative otitis media with spontaneous rupture of ear drum, **recurrent, right** ear
- H66.015 Acute suppurative otitis media with spontaneous rupture of ear drum, **recurrent, left** ear
- H66.016 Acute suppurative otitis media with spontaneous rupture of ear drum, **recurrent, bilateral**
- H66.017 Acute suppurative otitis media with spontaneous rupture of ear drum, **recurrent, unspecified** ear
- H66.019 Acute suppurative otitis media with spontaneous rupture of ear drum, **unspecified** ear

H66.1 Chronic tubotympanic suppurative otitis media
Benign chronic suppurative otitis media
Chronic tubotympanic disease
Use additional code for any associated perforated tympanic membrane (H72.-)
- H66.10 Chronic tubotympanic suppurative otitis media, **unspecified**
- H66.11 Chronic tubotympanic suppurative otitis media, **right** ear
- H66.12 Chronic tubotympanic suppurative otitis media, **left** ear
- H66.13 Chronic tubotympanic suppurative otitis media, bilateral

H66.2 Chronic atticoantral suppurative otitis media
Chronic atticoantral disease
Use additional code for any associated perforated tympanic membrane (H72.-)
- H66.20 Chronic atticoantral suppurative otitis media, **unspecified** ear
- H66.21 Chronic atticoantral suppurative otitis media, **right** ear
- H66.22 Chronic atticoantral suppurative otitis media, **left** ear
- H66.23 Chronic atticoantral suppurative otitis media, **bilateral**

H66.3 Other chronic suppurative otitis media
Chronic suppurative otitis media NOS
Use additional code for any associated perforated tympanic membrane (H72.-)
Excludes1 tuberculous otitis media (A18.6)

H66.3X Other chronic suppurative otitis media
- H66.3X1 Other chronic suppurative otitis media, **right** ear
- H66.3X2 Other chronic suppurative otitis media, **left** ear
- H66.3X3 Other chronic suppurative otitis media, **bilateral**
- H66.3X9 Other chronic suppurative otitis media, **unspecified** ear

H66.4 Suppurative otitis media, unspecified
Purulent otitis media NOS
Use additional code for any associated perforated tympanic membrane (H72.-)
- H66.40 Suppurative otitis media, unspecified, **unspecified** ear
- H66.41 Suppurative otitis media, unspecified, **right** ear
- H66.42 Suppurative otitis media, unspecified, **left** ear
- H66.43 Suppurative otitis media, unspecified, **bilateral**

H66.9 Otitis media, unspecified
Otitis media NOS
Acute otitis media NOS
Chronic otitis media NOS
Use additional code for any associated perforated tympanic membrane (H72.-)
- H66.90 Otitis media, unspecified, **unspecified** ear
- H66.91 Otitis media, unspecified, **right** ear
- H66.92 Otitis media, unspecified, **left** ear
- H66.93 Otitis media, unspecified, **bilateral**

H67 Otitis media in diseases classified elsewhere
Code first underlying disease, such as:
plasminogen deficiency (E88.02)
viral disease NEC (B00-B34)
Use additional code for any associated perforated tympanic membrane (H72.-)
Excludes1 otitis media in:
influenza (J09.X9, J10.83, J11.83)
measles (B05.3)
scarlet fever (A38.0)
tuberculosis (A18.6)
- *H67.1 Otitis media in diseases classified elsewhere, **right** ear*
- *H67.2 Otitis media in diseases classified elsewhere, **left** ear*
- *H67.3 Otitis media in diseases classified elsewhere, **bilateral***
- *H67.9 Otitis media in diseases classified elsewhere, **unspecified** ear*

H68 Eustachian salpingitis and obstruction

H68.0 Eustachian salpingitis

H68.00 Unspecified Eustachian salpingitis
- H68.001 Unspecified Eustachian salpingitis, **right** ear
- H68.002 Unspecified Eustachian salpingitis, **left** ear
- H68.003 Unspecified Eustachian salpingitis, **bilateral**
- H68.009 Unspecified Eustachian salpingitis, **unspecified** ear

H68.01 Acute Eustachian salpingitis
- H68.011 Acute Eustachian salpingitis, **right** ear
- H68.012 Acute Eustachian salpingitis, **left** ear
- H68.013 Acute Eustachian salpingitis, **bilateral**
- H68.019 Acute Eustachian salpingitis, **unspecified** ear

H68.02 Chronic Eustachian salpingitis
- H68.021 Chronic Eustachian salpingitis, **right** ear
- H68.022 Chronic Eustachian salpingitis, **left** ear
- H68.023 Chronic Eustachian salpingitis, **bilateral**
- H68.029 Chronic Eustachian salpingitis, **unspecified** ear

● H68.1 **Obstruction of Eustachian tube**
Stenosis of Eustachian tube
Stricture of Eustachian tube

● H68.10 **Unspecified obstruction of Eustachian tube**
- H68.101 Unspecified obstruction of Eustachian tube, **right** ear
- H68.102 Unspecified obstruction of Eustachian tube, **left** ear
- H68.103 Unspecified obstruction of Eustachian tube, **bilateral**
- H68.109 Unspecified obstruction of Eustachian tube, **unspecified** ear

● H68.11 **Osseous** obstruction of Eustachian tube
- H68.111 Osseous obstruction of Eustachian tube, **right** ear
- H68.112 Osseous obstruction of Eustachian tube, **left** ear
- H68.113 Osseous obstruction of Eustachian tube, **bilateral**
- H68.119 Osseous obstruction of Eustachian tube, **unspecified** ear

● H68.12 **Intrinsic cartilagenous** obstruction of Eustachian tube
- H68.121 Intrinsic cartilagenous obstruction of Eustachian tube, **right** ear
- H68.122 Intrinsic cartilagenous obstruction of Eustachian tube, **left** ear
- H68.123 Intrinsic cartilagenous obstruction of Eustachian tube, **bilateral**
- H68.129 Intrinsic cartilagenous obstruction of Eustachian tube, **unspecified** ear

● H68.13 **Extrinsic cartilagenous** obstruction of Eustachian tube
Compression of Eustachian tube
- H68.131 Extrinsic cartilagenous obstruction of Eustachian tube, **right** ear
- H68.132 Extrinsic cartilagenous obstruction of Eustachian tube, **left** ear
- H68.133 Extrinsic cartilagenous obstruction of Eustachian tube, **bilateral**
- H68.139 Extrinsic cartilagenous obstruction of Eustachian tube, **unspecified** ear

● H69 Other and unspecified disorders of Eustachian tube

● H69.0 **Patulous** Eustachian tube
- H69.00 Patulous Eustachian tube, **unspecified** ear
- H69.01 Patulous Eustachian tube, **right** ear
- H69.02 Patulous Eustachian tube, **left** ear
- H69.03 Patulous Eustachian tube, **bilateral**

● H69.8 **Other specified** disorders of Eustachian tube
- H69.80 Other specified disorders of Eustachian tube, **unspecified** ear
- H69.81 Other specified disorders of Eustachian tube, **right** ear
- H69.82 Other specified disorders of Eustachian tube, **left** ear
- H69.83 Other specified disorders of Eustachian tube, **bilateral**

● H69.9 **Unspecified** Eustachian tube disorder
- H69.90 Unspecified Eustachian tube disorder, **unspecified** ear
- H69.91 Unspecified Eustachian tube disorder, **right** ear
- H69.92 Unspecified Eustachian tube disorder, **left** ear
- H69.93 Unspecified Eustachian tube disorder, **bilateral**

● H70 Mastoiditis and related conditions

● H70.0 **Acute mastoiditis**
Abscess of mastoid
Empyema of mastoid

● H70.00 **Acute mastoiditis without complications**
- H70.001 Acute mastoiditis without complications, **right** ear
- H70.002 Acute mastoiditis without complications, **left** ear
- H70.003 Acute mastoiditis without complications, **bilateral**
- H70.009 Acute mastoiditis without complications, **unspecified** ear

● H70.01 **Subperiosteal** abscess of mastoid
- H70.011 Subperiosteal abscess of mastoid, **right** ear
- H70.012 Subperiosteal abscess of mastoid, **left** ear
- H70.013 Subperiosteal abscess of mastoid, **bilateral**
- H70.019 Subperiosteal abscess of mastoid, **unspecified** ear

● H70.09 Acute mastoiditis with other complications
- H70.091 Acute mastoiditis with other complications, **right** ear
- H70.092 Acute mastoiditis with other complications, **left** ear
- H70.093 Acute mastoiditis with other complications, **bilateral**
- H70.099 Acute mastoiditis with other complications, **unspecified** ear

● H70.1 **Chronic** mastoiditis
Caries of mastoid
Fistula of mastoid

Excludes1 tuberculous mastoiditis (A18.03)
- H70.10 Chronic mastoiditis, **unspecified** ear
- H70.11 Chronic mastoiditis, **right** ear
- H70.12 Chronic mastoiditis, **left** ear
- H70.13 Chronic mastoiditis, **bilateral**

● H70.2 Petrositis
Inflammation of petrous bone

● H70.20 **Unspecified** petrositis
- H70.201 Unspecified petrositis, **right** ear
- H70.202 Unspecified petrositis, **left** ear
- H70.203 Unspecified petrositis, **bilateral**
- H70.209 Unspecified petrositis, **unspecified** ear

● H70.21 **Acute** petrositis
- H70.211 Acute petrositis, **right** ear
- H70.212 Acute petrositis, **left** ear
- H70.213 Acute petrositis, **bilateral**
- H70.219 Acute petrositis, **unspecified** ear

● H70.22 **Chronic** petrositis
- H70.221 Chronic petrositis, **right** ear
- H70.222 Chronic petrositis, **left** ear
- H70.223 Chronic petrositis, **bilateral**
- H70.229 Chronic petrositis, **unspecified** ear

Item 8–1 **Mastoiditis** is an infection of the portion of the temporal bone of the skull that is behind the ear (mastoid process) caused by an untreated otitis media, leading to an infection of the surrounding structures which may include the brain.

H70.8 Other mastoiditis and related conditions
Excludes1 preauricular sinus and cyst (Q18.1)
sinus, fistula, and cyst of branchial cleft (Q18.0)

H70.81 Postauricular fistula
H70.811 Postauricular fistula, right ear
H70.812 Postauricular fistula, left ear
H70.813 Postauricular fistula, bilateral
H70.819 Postauricular fistula, unspecified ear

H70.89 Other mastoiditis and related conditions
H70.891 Other mastoiditis and related conditions, right ear
H70.892 Other mastoiditis and related conditions, left ear
H70.893 Other mastoiditis and related conditions, bilateral
H70.899 Other mastoiditis and related conditions, unspecified ear

H70.9 Unspecified mastoiditis
H70.90 Unspecified mastoiditis, unspecified ear
H70.91 Unspecified mastoiditis, right ear
H70.92 Unspecified mastoiditis, left ear
H70.93 Unspecified mastoiditis, bilateral

H71 Cholesteatoma of middle ear
Excludes2 cholesteatoma of external ear (H60.4-)
recurrent cholesteatoma of postmastoidectomy cavity (H95.0-)

H71.0 Cholesteatoma of attic
H71.00 Cholesteatoma of attic, unspecified ear
H71.01 Cholesteatoma of attic, right ear
H71.02 Cholesteatoma of attic, left ear
H71.03 Cholesteatoma of attic, bilateral

H71.1 Cholesteatoma of tympanum
H71.10 Cholesteatoma of tympanum, unspecified ear
H71.11 Cholesteatoma of tympanum, right ear
H71.12 Cholesteatoma of tympanum, left ear
H71.13 Cholesteatoma of tympanum, bilateral

H71.2 Cholesteatoma of mastoid
H71.20 Cholesteatoma of mastoid, unspecified ear
H71.21 Cholesteatoma of mastoid, right ear
H71.22 Cholesteatoma of mastoid, left ear
H71.23 Cholesteatoma of mastoid, bilateral

H71.3 Diffuse cholesteatosis
H71.30 Diffuse cholesteatosis, unspecified ear
H71.31 Diffuse cholesteatosis, right ear
H71.32 Diffuse cholesteatosis, left ear
H71.33 Diffuse cholesteatosis, bilateral

H71.9 Unspecified cholesteatoma
H71.90 Unspecified cholesteatoma, unspecified ear
H71.91 Unspecified cholesteatoma, right ear
H71.92 Unspecified cholesteatoma, left ear
H71.93 Unspecified cholesteatoma, bilateral

★ **(See Plate 22 of the Anatomy Illustrations.)**

H72 Perforation of tympanic membrane
Hole or rupture in ear drum
Includes persistent post-traumatic perforation of ear drum
postinflammatory perforation of ear drum
Code first any associated otitis media (H65.-, H66.1-, H66.2-, H66.3-, H66.4-, H66.9-, H67.-)
Excludes1 acute suppurative otitis media with rupture of the tympanic membrane (H66.01-)
traumatic rupture of ear drum (S09.2-)

H72.0 Central perforation of tympanic membrane
H72.00 Central perforation of tympanic membrane, unspecified ear
H72.01 Central perforation of tympanic membrane, right ear
H72.02 Central perforation of tympanic membrane, left ear
H72.03 Central perforation of tympanic membrane, bilateral

H72.1 Attic perforation of tympanic membrane
Perforation of pars flaccida
H72.10 Attic perforation of tympanic membrane, unspecified ear
H72.11 Attic perforation of tympanic membrane, right ear
H72.12 Attic perforation of tympanic membrane, left ear
H72.13 Attic perforation of tympanic membrane, bilateral

H72.2 Other marginal perforations of tympanic membrane
H72.2X Other marginal perforations of tympanic membrane
H72.2X1 Other marginal perforations of tympanic membrane, right ear
H72.2X2 Other marginal perforations of tympanic membrane, left ear
H72.2X3 Other marginal perforations of tympanic membrane, bilateral
H72.2X9 Other marginal perforations of tympanic membrane, unspecified ear

H72.8 Other perforations of tympanic membrane
H72.81 Multiple perforations of tympanic membrane
H72.811 Multiple perforations of tympanic membrane, right ear
H72.812 Multiple perforations of tympanic membrane, left ear
H72.813 Multiple perforations of tympanic membrane, bilateral
H72.819 Multiple perforations of tympanic membrane, unspecified ear

H72.82 Total perforations of tympanic membrane
H72.821 Total perforations of tympanic membrane, right ear
H72.822 Total perforations of tympanic membrane, left ear
H72.823 Total perforations of tympanic membrane, bilateral
H72.829 Total perforations of tympanic membrane, unspecified ear

H72.9 Unspecified perforation of tympanic membrane
H72.90 Unspecified perforation of tympanic membrane, unspecified ear
H72.91 Unspecified perforation of tympanic membrane, right ear
H72.92 Unspecified perforation of tympanic membrane, left ear
H72.93 Unspecified perforation of tympanic membrane, bilateral

● H73 Other disorders of tympanic membrane

● H73.0 Acute myringitis

Excludes1 acute myringitis with otitis media (H65, H66)

● H73.00 **Unspecified** acute myringitis

Acute tympanitis NOS

H73.001 Acute myringitis, **right** ear

H73.002 Acute myringitis, **left** ear

H73.003 Acute myringitis, **bilateral**

H73.009 Acute myringitis, **unspecified** ear

● H73.01 **Bullous** myringitis

H73.011 Bullous myringitis, **right** ear

H73.012 Bullous myringitis, **left** ear

H73.013 Bullous myringitis, **bilateral**

H73.019 Bullous myringitis, **unspecified** ear

● H73.09 **Other** acute myringitis

H73.091 Other acute myringitis, **right** ear

H73.092 Other acute myringitis, **left** ear

H73.093 Other acute myringitis, **bilateral**

H73.099 Other acute myringitis, **unspecified** ear

● H73.1 Chronic myringitis

Chronic tympanitis

Excludes1 chronic myringitis with otitis media (H65, H66)

H73.10 Chronic myringitis, **unspecified** ear

H73.11 Chronic myringitis, **right** ear

H73.12 Chronic myringitis, **left** ear

H73.13 Chronic myringitis, **bilateral**

● H73.2 **Unspecified** myringitis

H73.20 Unspecified myringitis, **unspecified** ear

H73.21 Unspecified myringitis, **right** ear

H73.22 Unspecified myringitis, **left** ear

H73.23 Unspecified myringitis, **bilateral**

● H73.8 Other specified disorders of tympanic membrane

● H73.81 **Atrophic flaccid** tympanic membrane

H73.811 Atrophic flaccid tympanic membrane, **right** ear

H73.812 Atrophic flaccid tympanic membrane, **left** ear

H73.813 Atrophic flaccid tympanic membrane, **bilateral**

H73.819 Atrophic flaccid tympanic membrane, **unspecified** ear

● H73.82 **Atrophic nonflaccid** tympanic membrane

H73.821 Atrophic nonflaccid tympanic membrane, **right** ear

H73.822 Atrophic nonflaccid tympanic membrane, **left** ear

H73.823 Atrophic nonflaccid tympanic membrane, **bilateral**

H73.829 Atrophic nonflaccid tympanic membrane, **unspecified** ear

● H73.89 **Other** specified disorders of tympanic membrane

H73.891 Other specified disorders of tympanic membrane, **right** ear

H73.892 Other specified disorders of tympanic membrane, **left** ear

H73.893 Other specified disorders of tympanic membrane, **bilateral**

H73.899 Other specified disorders of tympanic membrane, **unspecified** ear

● H73.9 **Unspecified** disorder of tympanic membrane

H73.90 Unspecified disorder of tympanic membrane, **unspecified** ear

H73.91 Unspecified disorder of tympanic membrane, **right** ear

H73.92 Unspecified disorder of tympanic membrane, **left** ear

H73.93 Unspecified disorder of tympanic membrane, **bilateral**

● H74 Other disorders of middle ear mastoid

Excludes2 mastoiditis (H70.-)

● H74.0 Tympanosclerosis

H74.01 Tympanosclerosis, **right** ear

H74.02 Tympanosclerosis, **left** ear

H74.03 Tympanosclerosis, **bilateral**

H74.09 Tympanosclerosis, **unspecified** ear

● H74.1 Adhesive middle ear disease

Adhesive otitis

Excludes1 glue ear (H65.3-)

H74.11 Adhesive **right** middle ear disease

H74.12 Adhesive **left** middle ear disease

H74.13 Adhesive middle ear disease, **bilateral**

H74.19 Adhesive middle ear disease, **unspecified** ear

● H74.2 Discontinuity and dislocation of ear ossicles

H74.20 Discontinuity and dislocation of ear ossicles, **unspecified** ear

H74.21 Discontinuity and dislocation of **right** ear ossicles

H74.22 Discontinuity and dislocation of **left** ear ossicles

H74.23 Discontinuity and dislocation of ear ossicles, **bilateral**

● H74.3 Other acquired abnormalities of ear ossicles

● H74.31 **Ankylosis** of ear ossicles

H74.311 Ankylosis of ear ossicles, **right** ear

H74.312 Ankylosis of ear ossicles, **left** ear

H74.313 Ankylosis of ear ossicles, **bilateral**

H74.319 Ankylosis of ear ossicles, **unspecified** ear

● H74.32 **Partial loss** of ear ossicles

H74.321 Partial loss of ear ossicles, **right** ear

H74.322 Partial loss of ear ossicles, **left** ear

H74.323 Partial loss of ear ossicles, **bilateral**

H74.329 Partial loss of ear ossicles, **unspecified** ear

● H74.39 **Other** acquired abnormalities of ear ossicles

H74.391 Other acquired abnormalities of **right** ear ossicles

H74.392 Other acquired abnormalities of **left** ear ossicles

H74.393 Other acquired abnormalities of ear ossicles, **bilateral**

H74.399 Other acquired abnormalities of ear ossicles, **unspecified** ear

● H74.4 Polyp of middle ear

H74.40 Polyp of middle ear, **unspecified** ear

H74.41 Polyp of **right** middle ear

H74.42 Polyp of **left** middle ear

H74.43 Polyp of middle ear, **bilateral**

● H74.8 Other specified disorders of middle ear and mastoid
● H74.8X Other specified disorders of middle ear and mastoid
H74.8X1 Other specified disorders of right middle ear and mastoid
H74.8X2 Other specified disorders of left middle ear and mastoid
H74.8X3 Other specified disorders of middle ear and mastoid, **bilateral**
H74.8X9 Other specified disorders of middle ear and mastoid, **unspecified** ear
● H74.9 Unspecified disorder of middle ear and mastoid
H74.90 Unspecified disorder of middle ear and mastoid, unspecified ear
H74.91 Unspecified disorder of right middle ear and mastoid
H74.92 Unspecified disorder of left middle ear and mastoid
H74.93 Unspecified disorder of middle ear and mastoid, bilateral

● H75 Other disorders of middle ear and mastoid in diseases classified elsewhere
Code first underlying disease
● H75.0 Mastoiditis in infectious and parasitic diseases classified elsewhere
Excludes1 mastoiditis (in):
syphilis (A52.77)
tuberculosis (A18.03)
*H75.00 Mastoiditis in infectious and parasitic diseases classified elsewhere, **unspecified** ear*
*H75.01 Mastoiditis in infectious and parasitic diseases classified elsewhere, **right** ear*
*H75.02 Mastoiditis in infectious and parasitic diseases classified elsewhere, **left** ear*
*H75.03 Mastoiditis in infectious and parasitic diseases classified elsewhere, **bilateral***
● H75.8 Other specified disorders of middle ear and mastoid in diseases classified elsewhere
H75.80 Other specified disorders of middle ear and mastoid in diseases classified elsewhere, unspecified ear
*H75.81 Other specified disorders of **right** middle ear and mastoid in diseases classified elsewhere*
*H75.82 Other specified disorders of **left** middle ear and mastoid in diseases classified elsewhere*
H75.83 Other specified disorders of middle ear and mastoid in diseases classified elsewhere, bilateral

DISEASES OF INNER EAR (H80-H83)

★**(See Plate 23 of the Anatomy Illustrations.)**

● H80 Otosclerosis
Inherited middle ear spongelike bone growth causing hearing loss
Includes Otospongiosis
● H80.0 Otosclerosis involving oval window, **nonobliterative**
H80.00 Otosclerosis involving oval window, nonobliterative, **unspecified** ear
H80.01 Otosclerosis involving oval window, nonobliterative, **right** ear
H80.02 Otosclerosis involving oval window, nonobliterative, **left** ear
H80.03 Otosclerosis involving oval window, nonobliterative, **bilateral**
● H80.1 Otosclerosis involving oval window, **obliterative**
H80.10 Otosclerosis involving oval window, obliterative, **unspecified** ear
H80.11 Otosclerosis involving oval window, obliterative, **right** ear
H80.12 Otosclerosis involving oval window, obliterative, **left** ear
H80.13 Otosclerosis involving oval window, obliterative, **bilateral**
● H80.2 Cochlear otosclerosis
Otosclerosis involving otic capsule
Otosclerosis involving round window
H80.20 Cochlear otosclerosis, **unspecified** ear
H80.21 Cochlear otosclerosis, **right** ear
H80.22 Cochlear otosclerosis, **left** ear
H80.23 Cochlear otosclerosis, **bilateral**
● H80.8 Other otosclerosis
H80.80 Other otosclerosis, **unspecified** ear
H80.81 Other otosclerosis, **right** ear
H80.82 Other otosclerosis, **left** ear
H80.83 Other otosclerosis, **bilateral**
● H80.9 Unspecified otosclerosis
H80.90 Unspecified otosclerosis, **unspecified** ear
H80.91 Unspecified otosclerosis, **right** ear
H80.92 Unspecified otosclerosis, **left** ear
H80.93 Unspecified otosclerosis, **bilateral**

● H81 Disorders of vestibular function
Excludes1 epidemic vertigo (A88.1)
vertigo NOS (R42)
● H81.0 Ménière's disease
Vestibular disorder that produces recurring symptoms including severe and intermittent hearing loss including the feeling of ear pressure or pain
Labyrinthine hydrops
Ménière's syndrome or vertigo
H81.01 Ménière's disease, **right** ear
H81.02 Ménière's disease, **left** ear
H81.03 Ménière's disease, **bilateral**
H81.09 Ménière's disease, **unspecified** ear
● H81.1 Benign paroxysmal vertigo
H81.10 Benign paroxysmal vertigo, **unspecified** ear
H81.11 Benign paroxysmal vertigo, **right** ear
H81.12 Benign paroxysmal vertigo, **left** ear
H81.13 Benign paroxysmal vertigo, **bilateral**
● H81.2 Vestibular neuronitis
H81.20 Vestibular neuronitis, **unspecified** ear
H81.21 Vestibular neuronitis, **right** ear
H81.22 Vestibular neuronitis, **left** ear
H81.23 Vestibular neuronitis, **bilateral**
● H81.3 Other peripheral vertigo
● H81.31 Aural vertigo
H81.311 Aural vertigo, **right** ear
H81.312 Aural vertigo, **left** ear
H81.313 Aural vertigo, **bilateral**
H81.319 Aural vertigo, **unspecified** ear
● H81.39 Other peripheral vertigo
Lermoyez' syndrome
Otogenic vertigo
Peripheral vertigo NOS
H81.391 Other peripheral vertigo, **right** ear
H81.392 Other peripheral vertigo, **left** ear
H81.393 Other peripheral vertigo, **bilateral**
H81.399 Other peripheral vertigo, **unspecified** ear
H81.4 Vertigo of central origin
Central positional nystagmus
~~H81.41 Vertigo of central origin, right ear~~
~~H81.42 Vertigo of central origin, left ear~~
~~H81.43 Vertigo of central origin, bilateral~~
~~H81.49 Vertigo of central origin, unspecified ear~~

CHAPTER 8 (H60-H95)

H81.8 Other disorders of vestibular function
H81.8X Other disorders of vestibular function
H81.8X1 Other disorders of vestibular function, right ear
H81.8X2 Other disorders of vestibular function, left ear
H81.8X3 Other disorders of vestibular function, bilateral
H81.8X9 Other disorders of vestibular function, unspecified ear
H81.9 Unspecified disorder of vestibular function
Vertiginous syndrome NOS
H81.90 Unspecified disorder of vestibular function, unspecified ear
H81.91 Unspecified disorder of vestibular function, right ear
H81.92 Unspecified disorder of vestibular function, left ear
H81.93 Unspecified disorder of vestibular function, bilateral

H82 Vertiginous syndromes in diseases classified elsewhere
Code first underlying disease
Excludes1 epidemic vertigo (A88.1)
H82.1 Vertiginous syndromes in diseases classified elsewhere, right ear
H82.2 Vertiginous syndromes in diseases classified elsewhere, left ear
H82.3 Vertiginous syndromes in diseases classified elsewhere, bilateral
H82.9 Vertiginous syndromes in diseases classified elsewhere, unspecified ear

H83 Other diseases of inner ear
H83.0 Labyrinthitis
Balance disorder that follows URI or head injury
H83.01 Labyrinthitis, right ear
H83.02 Labyrinthitis, left ear
H83.03 Labyrinthitis, bilateral
H83.09 Labyrinthitis, unspecified ear
H83.1 Labyrinthine fistula
H83.11 Labyrinthine fistula, right ear
H83.12 Labyrinthine fistula, left ear
H83.13 Labyrinthine fistula, bilateral
H83.19 Labyrinthine fistula, unspecified ear
H83.2 Labyrinthine dysfunction
Labyrinthine hypersensitivity
Labyrinthine hypofunction
Labyrinthine loss of function
H83.2X Labyrinthine dysfunction
H83.2X1 Labyrinthine dysfunction, right ear
H83.2X2 Labyrinthine dysfunction, left ear
H83.2X3 Labyrinthine dysfunction, bilateral
H83.2X9 Labyrinthine dysfunction, unspecified ear
H83.3 Noise effects on inner ear
Acoustic trauma of inner ear
Noise-induced hearing loss of inner ear
H83.3X Noise effects on inner ear
H83.3X1 Noise effects on right inner ear
H83.3X2 Noise effects on left inner ear
H83.3X3 Noise effects on inner ear, bilateral
H83.3X9 Noise effects on inner ear, unspecified ear
H83.8 Other specified diseases of inner ear
H83.8X Other specified diseases of inner ear
H83.8X1 Other specified diseases of right inner ear
H83.8X2 Other specified diseases of left inner ear
H83.8X3 Other specified diseases of inner ear, bilateral
H83.8X9 Other specified diseases of inner ear, unspecified ear
H83.9 Unspecified disease of inner ear
H83.90 Unspecified disease of inner ear, unspecified ear
H83.91 Unspecified disease of right inner ear
H83.92 Unspecified disease of left inner ear
H83.93 Unspecified disease of inner ear, bilateral

OTHER DISORDERS OF EAR (H90-H94)

H90 Conductive and sensorineural hearing loss
Excludes1 deaf nonspeaking NEC (H91.3)
deafness NOS (H91.9-)
hearing loss NOS (H91.9-)
noise-induced hearing loss (H83.3-)
ototoxic hearing loss (H91.0-)
sudden (idiopathic) hearing loss (H91.2-)
H90.0 Conductive hearing loss, bilateral
H90.1 Conductive hearing loss, unilateral with unrestricted hearing on the contralateral side
H90.11 Conductive hearing loss, unilateral, right ear, with unrestricted hearing on the contralateral side
H90.12 Conductive hearing loss, unilateral, left ear, with unrestricted hearing on the contralateral side
H90.2 Conductive hearing loss, unspecified
Conductive deafness NOS
H90.3 Sensorineural hearing loss, bilateral
H90.4 Sensorineural hearing loss, unilateral with unrestricted hearing on the contralateral side
H90.41 Sensorineural hearing loss, unilateral, right ear, with unrestricted hearing on the contralateral side
H90.42 Sensorineural hearing loss, unilateral, left ear, with unrestricted hearing on the contralateral side
H90.5 Unspecified sensorineural hearing loss
Central hearing loss NOS
Congenital deafness NOS
Neural hearing loss NOS
Perceptive hearing loss NOS
Sensorineural deafness NOS
Sensory hearing loss NOS
Excludes1 abnormal auditory perception (H93.2-)
psychogenic deafness (F44.6)
H90.6 Mixed conductive and sensorineural hearing loss, bilateral
Coding Clinic: 2015, Q2, P7
H90.7 Mixed conductive and sensorineural hearing loss, unilateral with unrestricted hearing on the contralateral side
H90.71 Mixed conductive and sensorineural hearing loss, unilateral, right ear, with unrestricted hearing on the contralateral side
H90.72 Mixed conductive and sensorineural hearing loss, unilateral, left ear, with unrestricted hearing on the contralateral side
H90.8 Mixed conductive and sensorineural hearing loss, unspecified

CHAPTER 8 (H60-H95)

H90.A Conductive and sensorineural hearing loss with **restricted hearing on the contralateral side**
Coding Clinic: 2016, Q4, P23-24
H90.A1 **Conductive** hearing loss, **unilateral**, with restricted hearing on the contralateral side
H90.A11 Conductive hearing loss, unilateral, **right** ear with restricted hearing on the contralateral side
H90.A12 Conductive hearing loss, unilateral, **left** ear with restricted hearing on the contralateral side
Coding Clinic: 2016, Q4, P25
H90.A2 **Sensorineural** hearing loss, **unilateral**, with restricted hearing on the contralateral side
H90.A21 Sensorineural hearing loss, unilateral, **right** ear, with restricted hearing on the contralateral side
H90.A22 Sensorineural hearing loss, unilateral, **left** ear, with restricted hearing on the contralateral side
H90.A3 **Mixed** conductive and sensorineural hearing loss, **unilateral** with restricted hearing on the contralateral side
H90.A31 Mixed conductive and sensorineural hearing loss, unilateral, **right** ear with restricted hearing on the contralateral side
H90.A32 Mixed conductive and sensorineural hearing loss, unilateral, **left** ear with restricted hearing on the contralateral side

H91 Other and unspecified hearing loss
Excludes1 abnormal auditory perception (H93.2-)
hearing loss as classified in H90.-
impacted cerumen (H61.2-)
noise-induced hearing loss (H83.3-)
psychogenic deafness (F44.6)
transient ischemic deafness (H93.01-)
H91.0 Ototoxic hearing loss
Code first poisoning due to drug or toxin, if applicable (T36-T65 with fifth or sixth character 1-4 or 6)
Use additional code for adverse effect, if applicable, to identify drug (T36-T50 with fifth or sixth character 5)
H91.01 Ototoxic hearing loss, **right** ear
H91.02 Ototoxic hearing loss, **left** ear
H91.03 Ototoxic hearing loss, **bilateral**
H91.09 Ototoxic hearing loss, **unspecified** ear
H91.1 Presbycusis
Presbyacusia
H91.10 Presbycusis, **unspecified** ear
H91.11 Presbycusis, **right** ear
H91.12 Presbycusis, **left** ear
H91.13 Presbycusis, **bilateral**
H91.2 Sudden idiopathic hearing loss
Sudden hearing loss NOS
H91.20 Sudden idiopathic hearing loss, **unspecified** ear
H91.21 Sudden idiopathic hearing loss, **right** ear
H91.22 Sudden idiopathic hearing loss, **left** ear
H91.23 Sudden idiopathic hearing loss, **bilateral**
H91.3 Deaf nonspeaking, not elsewhere classified
H91.8 Other specified hearing loss
H91.8X **Other** specified hearing loss
H91.8X1 Other specified hearing loss, **right** ear
H91.8X2 Other specified hearing loss, **left** ear
H91.8X3 Other specified hearing loss, **bilateral**
H91.8X9 Other specified hearing loss, **unspecified** ear
H91.9 **Unspecified** hearing loss
Deafness NOS
High frequency deafness
Low frequency deafness
H91.90 Unspecified hearing loss, **unspecified** ear
H91.91 Unspecified hearing loss, **right** ear
H91.92 Unspecified hearing loss, **left** ear
H91.93 Unspecified hearing loss, **bilateral**

H92 Otalgia and effusion of ear
H92.0 **Otalgia**
H92.01 Otalgia, **right** ear
H92.02 Otalgia, **left** ear
H92.03 Otalgia, **bilateral**
H92.09 Otalgia, **unspecified** ear
H92.1 Otorrhea
Excludes1 leakage of cerebrospinal fluid through ear (G96.0)
H92.10 Otorrhea, **unspecified** ear
H92.11 Otorrhea, **right** ear
H92.12 Otorrhea, **left** ear
H92.13 Otorrhea, **bilateral**
H92.2 Otorrhagia
Excludes1 traumatic otorrhagia - code to injury
H92.20 Otorrhagia, **unspecified** ear
H92.21 Otorrhagia, **right** ear
H92.22 Otorrhagia, **left** ear
H92.23 Otorrhagia, **bilateral**

H93 Other disorders of ear, not elsewhere classified
H93.0 Degenerative and vascular disorders of ear
Excludes1 presbycusis (H91.1)
H93.01 Transient ischemic deafness
H93.011 Transient ischemic deafness, **right** ear
H93.012 Transient ischemic deafness, **left** ear
H93.013 Transient ischemic deafness, **bilateral**
H93.019 Transient ischemic deafness, **unspecified** ear
H93.09 **Unspecified** degenerative and vascular disorders of ear
H93.091 Unspecified degenerative and vascular disorders of **right** ear
H93.092 Unspecified degenerative and vascular disorders of **left** ear
H93.093 Unspecified degenerative and vascular disorders of ear, **bilateral**
H93.099 Unspecified degenerative and vascular disorders of **unspecified** ear
H93.1 Tinnitus
Perception of sound (ringing, buzzing, humming, whistling tunes, or singing)
H93.11 Tinnitus, **right** ear
H93.12 Tinnitus, **left** ear
H93.13 Tinnitus, **bilateral**
H93.19 Tinnitus, **unspecified** ear
H93.A Pulsatile tinnitus
Coding Clinic: 2016, Q4, P25
H93.A1 Pulsatile tinnitus, **right** ear
Coding Clinic: 2016, Q4, P26
H93.A2 Pulsatile tinnitus, **left** ear
H93.A3 Pulsatile tinnitus, **bilateral**
H93.A9 Pulsatile tinnitus, **unspecified** ear

CHAPTER 8 (H60-H95)

● H93.2 Other abnormal auditory perceptions
Excludes2 auditory hallucinations (R44.Ø)
● H93.21 Auditory recruitment
H93.211 Auditory recruitment, right ear
H93.212 Auditory recruitment, left ear
H93.213 Auditory recruitment, bilateral
H93.219 Auditory recruitment, unspecified ear
● H93.22 Diplacusis
H93.221 Diplacusis, right ear
H93.222 Diplacusis, left ear
H93.223 Diplacusis, bilateral
H93.229 Diplacusis, unspecified ear
● H93.23 Hyperacusis
H93.231 Hyperacusis, right ear
H93.232 Hyperacusis, left ear
H93.233 Hyperacusis, bilateral
H93.239 Hyperacusis, unspecified ear
● H93.24 Temporary auditory threshold shift
H93.241 Temporary auditory threshold shift, right ear
H93.242 Temporary auditory threshold shift, left ear
H93.243 Temporary auditory threshold shift, bilateral
H93.249 Temporary auditory threshold shift, unspecified ear
H93.25 Central auditory processing disorder
Congenital auditory imperception
Word deafness
Excludes1 mixed receptive-expressive language disorder (F8Ø.2)
● H93.29 Other abnormal auditory perceptions
H93.291 Other abnormal auditory perceptions, right ear
H93.292 Other abnormal auditory perceptions, left ear
H93.293 Other abnormal auditory perceptions, bilateral
H93.299 Other abnormal auditory perceptions, unspecified ear
● H93.3 Disorders of acoustic nerve
Disorder of 8th cranial nerve
Excludes1 acoustic neuroma (D33.3)
syphilitic acoustic neuritis (A52.15)
● H93.3X Disorders of acoustic nerve
H93.3X1 Disorders of right acoustic nerve
H93.3X2 Disorders of left acoustic nerve
H93.3X3 Disorders of bilateral acoustic nerves
H93.3X9 Disorders of unspecified acoustic nerve
● H93.8 Other specified disorders of ear
● H93.8X Other specified disorders of ear
H93.8X1 Other specified disorders of right ear
H93.8X2 Other specified disorders of left ear
H93.8X3 Other specified disorders of ear, bilateral
H93.8X9 Other specified disorders of ear, unspecified ear
● H93.9 Unspecified disorder of ear
H93.9Ø Unspecified disorder of ear, unspecified ear
H93.91 Unspecified disorder of right ear
H93.92 Unspecified disorder of left ear
H93.93 Unspecified disorder of ear, bilateral

● H94 Other disorders of ear in diseases classified elsewhere
● H94.Ø Acoustic neuritis in infectious and parasitic diseases classified elsewhere
Code first underlying disease, such as:
parasitic disease (B65-B89)
Excludes1 acoustic neuritis (in):
herpes zoster (BØ2.29)
syphilis (A52.15)
H94.ØØ Acoustic neuritis in infectious and parasitic diseases classified elsewhere, unspecified ear
H94.Ø1 Acoustic neuritis in infectious and parasitic diseases classified elsewhere, right ear
H94.Ø2 Acoustic neuritis in infectious and parasitic diseases classified elsewhere, left ear
H94.Ø3 Acoustic neuritis in infectious and parasitic diseases classified elsewhere, bilateral
● H94.8 Other specified disorders of ear in diseases classified elsewhere
Code first underlying disease, such as:
congenital syphilis (A5Ø.Ø)
Excludes1 aural myiasis (B87.4)
syphilitic labyrinthitis (A52.79)
H94.8Ø Other specified disorders of ear in diseases classified elsewhere, unspecified ear
H94.81 Other specified disorders of right ear in diseases classified elsewhere
H94.82 Other specified disorders of left ear in diseases classified elsewhere
H94.83 Other specified disorders of ear in diseases classified elsewhere, bilateral

INTRAOPERATIVE AND POSTPROCEDURAL COMPLICATIONS AND DISORDERS OF EAR AND MASTOID PROCESS, NOT ELSEWHERE CLASSIFIED (H95)

● H95 Intraoperative and postprocedural complications and disorders of ear and mastoid process, not elsewhere classified
Coding Clinic: 2016, Q4, P1Ø
● H95.Ø Recurrent cholesteatoma of postmastoidectomy cavity
H95.ØØ Recurrent cholesteatoma of postmastoidectomy cavity, unspecified ear
H95.Ø1 Recurrent cholesteatoma of postmastoidectomy cavity, right ear
H95.Ø2 Recurrent cholesteatoma of postmastoidectomy cavity, left ear
H95.Ø3 Recurrent cholesteatoma of postmastoidectomy cavity, bilateral ears
● H95.1 Other disorders of ear and mastoid process following mastoidectomy
● H95.11 Chronic inflammation of postmastoidectomy cavity
H95.111 Chronic inflammation of postmastoidectomy cavity, right ear
H95.112 Chronic inflammation of postmastoidectomy cavity, left ear
H95.113 Chronic inflammation of postmastoidectomy cavity, bilateral ears
H95.119 Chronic inflammation of postmastoidectomy cavity, unspecified ear
● H95.12 Granulation of postmastoidectomy cavity
H95.121 Granulation of postmastoidectomy cavity, right ear
H95.122 Granulation of postmastoidectomy cavity, left ear
H95.123 Granulation of postmastoidectomy cavity, bilateral ears
H95.129 Granulation of postmastoidectomy cavity, unspecified ear

● H95.13   Mucosal cyst of postmastoidectomy cavity

    H95.131   Mucosal cyst of postmastoidectomy cavity, **right ear**

    H95.132   Mucosal cyst of postmastoidectomy cavity, **left ear**

    H95.133   Mucosal cyst of postmastoidectomy cavity, **bilateral ears**

    H95.139   Mucosal cyst of postmastoidectomy cavity, **unspecified ear**

● H95.19   Other disorders following mastoidectomy

    H95.191   Other disorders following mastoidectomy, **right ear**

    H95.192   Other disorders following mastoidectomy, **left ear**

    H95.193   Other disorders following mastoidectomy, **bilateral ears**

    H95.199   Other disorders following mastoidectomy, **unspecified ear**

● H95.2   **Intraoperative hemorrhage and hematoma of ear and mastoid process complicating a procedure**

    Excludes1   intraoperative hemorrhage and hematoma of ear and mastoid process due to accidental puncture or laceration during a procedure (H95.3-)

    H95.21   Intraoperative hemorrhage and hematoma of ear and mastoid process complicating a procedure on the ear and mastoid process

    H95.22   Intraoperative hemorrhage and hematoma of ear and mastoid process complicating **other procedure**

● H95.3   **Accidental puncture and laceration** of ear and mastoid process during a procedure

    H95.31   Accidental puncture and laceration of the ear and mastoid process during a procedure on the ear and mastoid process

    H95.32   Accidental puncture and laceration of the ear and mastoid process during **other procedure**

● H95.4   **Postprocedural hemorrhage** of ear and mastoid process following a procedure

    H95.41   Postprocedural hemorrhage of ear and mastoid process following a procedure on the **ear and mastoid process**

    H95.42   Postprocedural hemorrhage of ear and mastoid process following **other procedure**

● H95.5   **Postprocedural hematoma and seroma of ear and mastoid process following a procedure**

H95.51   Postprocedural **hematoma** of ear and mastoid process following a procedure on the **ear and mastoid process**

H95.52   Postprocedural **hematoma** of ear and mastoid process following **other procedure**

H95.53   Postprocedural **seroma** of ear and mastoid process following a procedure on the **ear and mastoid process**

H95.54   Postprocedural **seroma** of ear and mastoid process following **other procedure**

● H95.8   **Other intraoperative and postprocedural complications and disorders of the ear and mastoid process, not elsewhere classified**

    Excludes2   postprocedural complications and disorders following mastoidectomy (H95.0-, H95.1-)

● H95.81   **Postprocedural stenosis of external ear canal**

    H95.811   Postprocedural stenosis of **right** external ear canal

    H95.812   Postprocedural stenosis of **left** external ear canal

    H95.813   Postprocedural stenosis of external ear canal, **bilateral**

    H95.819   Postprocedural stenosis of **unspecified** external ear canal

H95.88   **Other intraoperative complications and disorders of the ear and mastoid process, not elsewhere classified**

    Use additional code, if applicable, to further specify disorder

H95.89   **Other postprocedural complications and disorders of the ear and mastoid process, not elsewhere classified**

    Use additional code, if applicable, to further specify disorder

CHAPTER 9

DISEASES OF THE CIRCULATORY SYSTEM (I00-I99)

OGCR Chapter-Specific Coding Guidelines

9. Chapter 9: Diseases of the Circulatory System (I00-I99)

a. **Hypertension**

The classification presumes a causal relationship between hypertension and heart involvement and between hypertension and kidney involvement, as the two conditions are linked by the term "with" in the Alphabetic Index. These conditions should be coded as related even in the absence of provider documentation explicitly linking them, unless the documentation clearly states the conditions are unrelated.

For hypertension and conditions not specifically linked by relational terms such as "with," "associated with" or "due to" in the classification, provider documentation must link the conditions in order to code them as related.

1) **Hypertension with Heart Disease**

Hypertension with heart conditions classified to I50.- or I51.4-I51.7, I51.89, I51.9, are assigned to, a code from category I11, Hypertensive heart disease. Use additional code(s) from category I50, Heart failure, to identify the type(s) of heart failure in those patients with heart failure.

The same heart conditions (I50.-, I51.4-I51.7, I51.89, I51.9) with hypertension, are coded separately if the provider has documented they are unrelated to the hypertension. Sequence according to the circumstances of the admission/encounter.

2) **Hypertensive Chronic Kidney Disease**

Assign codes from category I12, Hypertensive chronic kidney disease, when both hypertension and a condition classifiable to category N18, Chronic kidney disease (CKD), are present. CKD should not be coded as hypertensive if the provider indicates the CKD is not related to the hypertension.

The appropriate code from category N18 should be used as a secondary code with a code from category I12 to identify the stage of chronic kidney disease.

See Section I.C.14. Chronic kidney disease.

If a patient has hypertensive chronic kidney disease and acute renal failure, an additional code for the acute renal failure is required.

3) **Hypertensive Heart and Chronic Kidney Disease**

Assign codes from combination category I13, Hypertensive heart and chronic kidney disease, when there is hypertension with both heart and kidney involvement. If heart failure is present, assign an additional code from category I50 to identify the type of heart failure.

The appropriate code from category N18, Chronic kidney disease, should be used as a secondary code with a code from category I13 to identify the stage of chronic kidney disease.

See Section I.C.14. Chronic kidney disease.

The codes in category I13, Hypertensive heart and chronic kidney disease, are combination codes that include hypertension, heart disease and chronic kidney disease. The Includes note at I13 specifies that the conditions included at I11 and I12 are included together in I13. If a patient has hypertension, heart disease and chronic kidney disease then a code from I13 should be used, not individual codes for hypertension, heart disease and chronic kidney disease, or codes from I11 or I12.

For patients with both acute renal failure and chronic kidney disease an additional code for acute renal failure is required.

4) **Hypertensive Cerebrovascular Disease**

For hypertensive cerebrovascular disease, first assign the appropriate code from categories I60-I69, followed by the appropriate hypertension code.

5) **Hypertensive Retinopathy**

Subcategory H35.0, Background retinopathy and retinal vascular changes, should be used with a code from category I10 – I15, Hypertensive disease to include the systemic hypertension. The sequencing is based on the reason for the encounter.

6) **Hypertension, Secondary**

Secondary hypertension is due to an underlying condition. Two codes are required: one to identify the underlying etiology and one from category I15 to identify the hypertension. Sequencing of codes is determined by the reason for admission/encounter.

7) **Hypertension, Transient**

Assign code R03.0, Elevated blood pressure reading without diagnosis of hypertension, unless patient has an established diagnosis of hypertension. Assign code O13.-, Gestational [pregnancy-induced] hypertension without significant proteinuria, or O14.-, Pre-eclampsia, for transient hypertension of pregnancy.

8) **Hypertension, Controlled**

This diagnostic statement usually refers to an existing state of hypertension under control by therapy. Assign the appropriate code from categories I10-I15, Hypertensive diseases.

9) **Hypertension, Uncontrolled**

Uncontrolled hypertension may refer to untreated hypertension or hypertension not responding to current therapeutic regimen. In either case, assign the appropriate code from categories I10-I15, Hypertensive diseases.

10) **Hypertensive Crisis**

Assign a code from category I16, Hypertensive crisis, for documented hypertensive urgency, hypertensive emergency or unspecified hypertensive crisis. Code also any identified hypertensive disease (I10-I15). The sequencing is based on the reason for the encounter.

11) **Pulmonary Hypertension**

Pulmonary hypertension is classified to category I27, Other pulmonary heart diseases. For secondary pulmonary hypertension (I27.1, I27.2-), code also any associated conditions or adverse effects of drugs or toxins. The sequencing is based on the reason for the encounter, except for adverse effects of drugs.

*See Section I.C.19.e **Adverse Effects, Poisoning, Underdosing and Toxic Effects.***

b. **Atherosclerotic Coronary Artery Disease and Angina**

ICD-10-CM has combination codes for atherosclerotic heart disease with angina pectoris. The subcategories for these codes are I25.11, Atherosclerotic heart disease of native coronary artery with angina pectoris and I25.7, Atherosclerosis of coronary artery bypass graft(s) and coronary artery of transplanted heart with angina pectoris.

When using one of these combination codes it is not necessary to use an additional code for angina pectoris. A causal relationship can be assumed in a patient with both atherosclerosis and angina pectoris, unless the documentation indicates the angina is due to something other than the atherosclerosis.

If a patient with coronary artery disease is admitted due to an acute myocardial infarction (AMI), the AMI should be sequenced before the coronary artery disease.

See Section I.C.9. Acute myocardial infarction (AMI).

c. **Intraoperative and Postprocedural Cerebrovascular Accident**

Medical record documentation should clearly specify the cause-and-effect relationship between the medical intervention and the cerebrovascular accident in order to assign a code for intraoperative or postprocedural cerebrovascular accident.

Proper code assignment depends on whether it was an infarction or hemorrhage and whether it occurred intraoperatively or postoperatively. If it was a cerebral hemorrhage, code assignment depends on the type of procedure performed.

d. **Sequelae of Cerebrovascular Disease**

1) **Category I69, Sequelae of Cerebrovascular disease**

Category I69 is used to indicate conditions classifiable to categories I60-I67 as the causes of sequela (neurologic deficits), themselves classified elsewhere. These "late effects" include neurologic deficits that persist after initial onset of conditions classifiable to categories I60-I67. The neurologic deficits caused by cerebrovascular disease may be present from the onset or may arise at any time after the onset of the condition classifiable to categories I60-I67.

Codes from category I69, Sequelae of cerebrovascular disease, that specify hemiplegia, hemiparesis and monoplegia identify whether the dominant or nondominant side is affected. Should the affected side be documented, but not specified as dominant or nondominant, and the classification system does not indicate a default, code selection is as follows:

- For ambidextrous patients, the default should be dominant.
- If the left side is affected, the default is nondominant.
- If the right side is affected, the default is dominant.

2) **Codes from category I69 with codes from I60-I67**

Codes from category I69 may be assigned on a health care record with codes from I60-I67, if the patient has a current cerebrovascular disease and deficits from an old cerebrovascular disease.

3) Codes from category I69 and Personal history of transient ischemic attack (TIA) and cerebral infarction (Z86.73)

Codes from category I69 should not be assigned if the patient does not have neurologic deficits.

See Section I.C.21. 4. History (of) for use of personal history codes.

e. **Acute myocardial infarction (AMI)**

1) **Type 1 ST elevation myocardial infarction (STEMI) and non-ST elevation myocardial infarction (NSTEMI)**

The ICD-10-CM codes for acute type 1 myocardial infarction (AMI) identify the site, such as anterolateral wall or true posterior wall. Subcategories I21.0-I21.2 and code I21.3 are used for type 1 ST elevation myocardial infarction (STEMI). Code I21.4, non-ST elevation myocardial infarction, is used for type 1 non-ST elevation myocardial infarction (NSTEMI) and nontransmural MIs.

If a type 1 NSTEMI evolves to STEMI, assign the STEMI code. If a type 1 STEMI converts to NSTEMI due to thrombolytic therapy, it is still coded as STEMI.

For encounters occurring while the myocardial infarction is equal to, or less than, four weeks old, including transfers to another acute setting or a postacute setting, and the myocardial infarction meets the definition for "other diagnoses" (see Section III, Reporting Additional Diagnoses), codes from category I21 may continue to be reported. For encounters after the 4-week time frame and the patient is still receiving care related to the myocardial infarction, the appropriate aftercare code should be assigned, rather than a code from category I21. For old or healed myocardial infarctions not requiring further care, code I25.2, Old myocardial infarction, may be assigned.

2) **Acute myocardial infarction, unspecified**

Code I21.9, Acute myocardial infarction, unspecified, is the default for unspecified acute myocardial infarction or unspecified type. If only type 1 STEMI or transmural MI without the site is documented, assign code I21.3, ST elevation (STEMI) myocardial infarction of unspecified site.

3) **AMI documented as nontransmural or subendocardial but site provided**

If an AMI is documented as nontransmural or subendocardial, but the site is provided, it is still coded as a subendocardial AMI.

See Section I.C.21.3 for information on coding status post administration of tPA in a different facility within the last 24 hours.

4) **Subsequent acute myocardial infarction**

A code from category I22, Subsequent ST elevation (STEMI) and non-ST elevation (NSTEMI) myocardial infarction, is to be used when a patient who has suffered a type 1 or unspecified AMI has a new AMI within the 4-week time frame of the initial AMI. A code from category I22 must be used in conjunction with a code from category I21. The sequencing of the I22 and I21 codes depends on the circumstances of the encounter.

Do not assign code I22 for subsequent myocardial infarctions other than type 1 or unspecified. For subsequent type 2 AMI assign only code I21.A1. For subsequent type 4 or type 5 AMI, assign only code I21.A9.

If a subsequent myocardial infarction of one type occurs within 4 weeks of a myocardial infarction of a different type, assign the appropriate codes from category I21 to identify each type. Do not assign a code from I22. Codes from category I22 should only be assigned if both the initial and subsequent myocardial infarctions are type 1 or unspecified.

5) **Other Types of Myocardial Infarction**

The ICD-10-CM provides codes for different types of myocardial infarction. Type 1 myocardial infarctions are assigned to codes I21.0-I21.4 and I21.9.

Type 2 myocardial infarction, and myocardial infarction due to demand ischemia or secondary to ischemic balance, is assigned to code I21.A1, Myocardial infarction type 2 with a code for the underlying cause. Do not assign code I24.8, Other forms of acute ischemic heart disease for the demand ischemia. Sequencing of type 2 AMI or the underlying cause is dependent on the circumstances of admission. When a type 2 AMI code is described as NSTEMI or STEMI, only assign code I21.A1. Codes I21.01-I21.4 should only be assigned for type 1 AMIs.

Acute myocardial infarctions type 3, 4a, 4b, 4c, and 5 are assigned to code I21.A9, Other myocardial infarction type.

The "Code also" and "Code first" notes should be followed related to complications, and for coding of postprocedural myocardial infarctions during or following cardiac surgery.

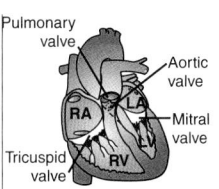

Figure 9-1 Cardiovascular valves.

Item 9–1 Rheumatic fever is the inflammation of the valve(s) of the heart, usually the mitral or aortic, which leads to valve damage. Rheumatic heart inflammations are usually **pericarditis** (sac surrounding heart), **endocarditis** (heart cavity), or **myocarditis** (heart muscle).

CHAPTER 9

DISEASES OF THE CIRCULATORY SYSTEM (I00-I99)

Excludes2   certain conditions originating in the perinatal period (P04-P96)
certain infectious and parasitic diseases (A00-B99)
complications of pregnancy, childbirth and the puerperium (O00-O9A)
congenital malformations, deformations, and chromosomal abnormalities (Q00-Q99)
endocrine, nutritional and metabolic diseases (E00-E88)
injury, poisoning and certain other consequences of external causes (S00-T88)
neoplasms (C00-D49)
symptoms, signs and abnormal clinical and laboratory findings, not elsewhere classified (R00-R94)
systemic connective tissue disorders (M30-M36)
transient cerebral ischemic attacks and related syndromes (G45.-)

This chapter contains the following blocks:

I00-I02	Acute rheumatic fever
I05-I09	Chronic rheumatic heart diseases
I10-I16	Hypertensive diseases
I20-I25	Ischemic heart diseases
I26-I28	Pulmonary heart disease and diseases of pulmonary circulation
I30-I52	Other forms of heart disease
I60-I69	Cerebrovascular diseases
I70-I79	Diseases of arteries, arterioles and capillaries
I80-I89	Diseases of veins, lymphatic vessels and lymph nodes, not elsewhere classified
I95-I99	Other and unspecified disorders of the circulatory system

ACUTE RHEUMATIC FEVER (I00-I02)

I00   **Rheumatic fever without heart involvement**

     Includes   arthritis, rheumatic, acute or subacute

     Excludes1   rheumatic fever with heart involvement (I01.0-I01.9)

● **I01**   **Rheumatic fever with heart involvement**

     Excludes1   chronic diseases of rheumatic origin (I05-I09) unless rheumatic fever is also present or there is evidence of reactivation or activity of the rheumatic process.

     I01.0   **Acute rheumatic pericarditis**
         Any condition in I00 with pericarditis
         Rheumatic pericarditis (acute)

         Excludes1   acute pericarditis not specified as rheumatic (I30.-)

     I01.1   **Acute rheumatic endocarditis**
         Any condition in I00 with endocarditis or valvulitis
         Acute rheumatic valvulitis

Item 9–2 Rheumatic chorea, also called Sydenham's, juvenile, minor, simple, or St. Vitus' dance, is a major symptom of rheumatic fever and is characterized by ceaseless, involuntary, jerky, purposeless movements.

I01.2 **Acute rheumatic myocarditis**
Any condition in I00 with myocarditis

I01.8 **Other acute rheumatic heart disease**
Any condition in I00 with other or multiple types of heart involvement
Acute rheumatic pancarditis

I01.9 **Acute rheumatic heart disease, unspecified**
Any condition in I00 with unspecified type of heart involvement
Rheumatic carditis, acute
Rheumatic heart disease, active or acute

● I02 **Rheumatic chorea**
Includes Sydenham's chorea
Excludes1 chorea NOS (G25.5)
Huntington's chorea (G10)

I02.0 **Rheumatic chorea with heart involvement**
Chorea NOS with heart involvement
Rheumatic chorea with heart involvement of any type classifiable under I01.-

I02.9 **Rheumatic chorea without heart involvement**
Rheumatic chorea NOS

CHRONIC RHEUMATIC HEART DISEASES (I05-I09)

● I05 **Rheumatic mitral valve diseases**
Includes conditions classifiable to both I05.0 and I05.2-I05.9, whether specified as rheumatic or not
Excludes1 mitral valve disease specified as nonrheumatic (I34.-)
mitral valve disease with aortic and/or tricuspid valve involvement (I08.-)

I05.0 **Rheumatic mitral stenosis**
Mitral (valve) obstruction (rheumatic)

I05.1 **Rheumatic mitral insufficiency**
Rheumatic mitral incompetence
Rheumatic mitral regurgitation
Excludes1 mitral insufficiency not specified as rheumatic (I34.0)

I05.2 **Rheumatic mitral stenosis with insufficiency**
Rheumatic mitral stenosis with incompetence or regurgitation

I05.8 **Other rheumatic mitral valve diseases**
Rheumatic mitral (valve) failure

I05.9 **Rheumatic mitral valve disease, unspecified**
Rheumatic mitral (valve) disorder (chronic) NOS

● I06 **Rheumatic aortic valve diseases**
Excludes1 aortic valve disease not specified as rheumatic (I35.-)
aortic valve disease with mitral and/or tricuspid valve involvement (I08.-)

I06.0 **Rheumatic aortic stenosis**
Rheumatic aortic (valve) obstruction

I06.1 **Rheumatic aortic insufficiency**
Rheumatic aortic incompetence
Rheumatic aortic regurgitation

I06.2 **Rheumatic aortic stenosis with insufficiency**
Rheumatic aortic stenosis with incompetence or regurgitation

★ **(See Plate 33 of the Anatomy Illustrations.)**

Item 9–3 Mitral stenosis is the narrowing of the mitral valve separating the left atrium from the left ventricle. **Mitral insufficiency** is the improper closure of the mitral valve, which may lead to enlargement (hypertrophy) of the left atrium.

Item 9–4 Aortic stenosis is the narrowing of the aortic valve located between the left ventricle and the aorta. **Aortic insufficiency** is the improper closure of the aortic valve, which may lead to enlargement (hypertrophy) of the left ventricle.

I06.8 **Other rheumatic aortic valve diseases**

I06.9 **Rheumatic aortic valve disease, unspecified**
Rheumatic aortic (valve) disease NOS

● I07 **Rheumatic tricuspid valve diseases**
Includes rheumatic tricuspid valve diseases specified as rheumatic or unspecified
Excludes1 tricuspid valve disease specified as nonrheumatic (I36.-)
tricuspid valve disease with aortic and/or mitral valve involvement (I08.-)

I07.0 **Rheumatic tricuspid stenosis**
Tricuspid (valve) stenosis (rheumatic)

I07.1 **Rheumatic tricuspid insufficiency**
Tricuspid (valve) insufficiency (rheumatic)

I07.2 **Rheumatic tricuspid stenosis and insufficiency**

I07.8 **Other rheumatic tricuspid valve diseases**

I07.9 **Rheumatic tricuspid valve disease, unspecified**
Rheumatic tricuspid valve disorder NOS

● I08 **Multiple valve diseases**
Includes multiple valve diseases specified as rheumatic or unspecified
Excludes1 endocarditis, valve unspecified (I38)
multiple valve disease specified a nonrheumatic (I34.-, I35.-, I36.-, I37.-, I38.-, Q22.-, Q23.-, Q24.8-)
rheumatic valve disease NOS (I09.1)
Coding Clinic: 2019, Q2, P5

I08.0 **Rheumatic disorders of both mitral and aortic valves**
Involvement of both mitral and aortic valves specified as rheumatic or unspecified
Coding Clinic: 2019, Q2, P5

I08.1 **Rheumatic disorders of both mitral and tricuspid valves**

I08.2 **Rheumatic disorders of both aortic and tricuspid valves**

I08.3 **Combined rheumatic disorders of mitral, aortic and tricuspid valves**

I08.8 **Other rheumatic multiple valve diseases**

I08.9 **Rheumatic multiple valve disease, unspecified**

● I09 **Other rheumatic heart diseases**

I09.0 **Rheumatic myocarditis**
Excludes1 myocarditis not specified as rheumatic (I51.4)

I09.1 **Rheumatic diseases of endocardium, valve unspecified**
Rheumatic endocarditis (chronic)
Rheumatic valvulitis (chronic)
Excludes1 endocarditis, valve unspecified (I38)

I09.2 **Chronic rheumatic pericarditis**
Adherent pericardium, rheumatic
Chronic rheumatic mediastinopericarditis
Chronic rheumatic myopericarditis
Excludes1 chronic pericarditis not specified as rheumatic (I31.-)

● I09.8 **Other specified rheumatic heart diseases**

I09.81 **Rheumatic heart failure** (HCC)
Use additional code to identify type of heart failure (I50.-)

I09.89 **Other specified rheumatic heart diseases**
Rheumatic disease of pulmonary valve

I09.9 **Rheumatic heart disease, unspecified**
Rheumatic carditis
Excludes1 rheumatoid carditis (M05.31)

Item 9–5 Hypertension is caused by high arterial blood pressure in the arteries. **Essential, primary,** or **idiopathic** hypertension occurs without identifiable organic cause. **Secondary** hypertension is that which has an organic cause. **Malignant** hypertension is severely elevated blood pressure. **Benign** hypertension is mildly elevated blood pressure.

HYPERTENSIVE DISEASES (I10-I16)

Use additional code to identify:
exposure to environmental tobacco smoke (Z77.22)
history of tobacco dependence (Z87.891)
occupational exposure to environmental tobacco smoke (Z57.31)
tobacco dependence (F17.-)
tobacco use (Z72.0)

Excludes1 neonatal hypertension (P29.2)
primary pulmonary hypertension (I27.0)

Excludes2 hypertensive disease complicating pregnancy, childbirth and the puerperium (O10-O11, O13-O16)

I10 Essential (primary) hypertension

Includes high blood pressure
hypertension (arterial) (benign) (essential) (malignant) (primary) (systemic)

Excludes1 hypertensive disease complicating pregnancy, childbirth and the puerperium (O10-O11, O13-O16)

Excludes2 essential (primary) hypertension involving vessels of brain (I60-I69)
essential (primary) hypertension involving vessels of eye (H35.0-)

● **I11 Hypertensive heart disease**

Includes any condition in I50.-, I51.4-I51.9 due to hypertension

I11.0 Hypertensive heart disease with heart failure
Hypertensive heart failure
Use additional code to identify type of heart failure (I50.-)
Coding Clinic: 2017, Q1, P47

I11.9 Hypertensive heart disease without heart failure
Hypertensive heart disease NOS

OGCR Section I.C.9.a.2.

Hypertensive Chronic Kidney Disease

Assign codes from category I12, Hypertensive chronic kidney disease, when both hypertension and a condition classifiable to category N18, Chronic kidney disease (CKD), are present. **CKD should not be coded as hypertensive if the physician has specifically documented a different cause.**

The appropriate code from category N18 should be used as a secondary code with a code from category I12 to identify the stage of chronic kidney disease.

See Section I.C.14. Chronic kidney disease.

If a patient has hypertensive chronic kidney disease and acute renal failure, an additional code for the acute renal failure is required.

● **I12 Hypertensive chronic kidney disease**

Includes any condition in N18 and N26 - due to hypertension
arteriosclerosis of kidney
arteriosclerotic nephritis (chronic) (interstitial)
hypertensive nephropathy
nephrosclerosis

Excludes1 hypertension due to kidney disease (I15.0, I15.1)
renovascular hypertension (I15.0)
secondary hypertension (I15.-)

Excludes2 acute kidney failure (N17.-)

Coding Clinic: 2018, Q4, P89; 2016, Q4, P123

I12.0 Hypertensive chronic kidney disease with stage 5 chronic kidney disease or end stage renal disease
Use additional code to identify the stage of chronic kidney disease (N18.5, N18.6)
Coding Clinic: 2016, Q3, P23

I12.9 Hypertensive chronic kidney disease with stage 1 through stage 4 chronic kidney disease, or unspecified chronic kidney disease
Hypertensive chronic kidney disease NOS
Hypertensive renal disease NOS
Use additional code to identify the stage of chronic kidney disease (N18.1-N18.4, N18.9)
Coding Clinic: 2018, Q4, P88

OGCR Section I.c.9.a.3.

Hypertensive Heart and Chronic Kidney Disease

Assign codes from combination category I13, Hypertensive heart and chronic kidney disease, when **there is hypertension with both heart and kidney involvement.** If heart failure is present, assign an additional code from category I50 to identify the type of heart failure.

The appropriate code from category N18, Chronic kidney disease, should be used as a secondary code with a code from category I13 to identify the stage of chronic kidney disease.

See Section I.C.14. Chronic kidney disease.

The codes in category I13, Hypertensive heart and chronic kidney disease, are combination codes that include hypertension, heart disease and chronic kidney disease. The Includes note at I13 specifies that the conditions included at I11 and I12 are included together in I13. If a patient has hypertension, heart disease and chronic kidney disease then a code from I13 should be used, not individual codes for hypertension, heart disease and chronic kidney disease, or codes from I11 or I12.

For patients with both acute renal failure and chronic kidney disease an additional code for acute renal failure is required.

● **I13 Hypertensive heart and chronic kidney disease**

Includes any condition in I11.- with any condition in I12.-
cardiorenal disease
cardiovascular renal disease

Coding Clinic: 2016, Q4, P123

I13.0 Hypertensive heart and chronic kidney disease with heart failure and stage 1 through stage 4 chronic kidney disease, or unspecified chronic kidney disease
Use additional code to identify type of heart failure (I50.-)
Use additional code to identify stage of chronic kidney disease (N18.1-N18.4, N18.9)

● **I13.1 Hypertensive heart and chronic kidney disease without heart failure**

I13.10 Hypertensive heart and chronic kidney disease without heart failure, with stage 1 through stage 4 chronic kidney disease, or unspecified chronic kidney disease
Hypertensive heart disease and hypertensive chronic kidney disease NOS
Use additional code to identify the stage of chronic kidney disease (N18.1-N18.4, N18.9)

I13.11 Hypertensive heart and chronic kidney disease without heart failure, with stage 5 chronic kidney disease, or end stage renal disease
Use additional code to identify the stage of chronic kidney disease (N18.5, N18.6)

I13.2 Hypertensive heart and chronic kidney disease with heart failure and with stage 5 chronic kidney disease, or end stage renal disease
Use additional code to identify type of heart failure (I50.-)
Use additional code to identify the stage of chronic kidney disease (N18.5, N18.6)

OGCR Section I.9.a.6.

Hypertension, Secondary

Secondary hypertension is due to an underlying condition. Two codes are required: one to identify the underlying etiology and one from category I15 to identify the hypertension. Sequencing of codes is determined by the reason for admission/encounter.

● **I15 Secondary hypertension**

Code also underlying condition

Excludes1 postprocedural hypertension (I97.3)

Excludes2 secondary hypertension involving vessels of brain (I60-I69)
secondary hypertension involving vessels of eye (H35.0-)

I15.0 Renovascular hypertension

I15.1 Hypertension secondary to other renal disorders
Coding Clinic: 2016, Q3, P23

I15.2 Hypertension secondary to endocrine disorders

I15.8 Other secondary hypertension

I15.9 Secondary hypertension, unspecified

● **I16 Hypertensive crisis**

Code also any identified hypertensive disease (I10-I15)
Coding Clinic: 2016, Q4, P26-27, 123

I16.0 Hypertensive urgency

I16.1 Hypertensive emergency

I16.9 Hypertensive crisis, unspecified

ISCHEMIC HEART DISEASES (I20-I25)

Use additional code to identify presence of hypertension (I10-I16)

● **I20 Angina pectoris**

Chest pain/discomfort due to lack of oxygen to the heart muscle. Principal symptom of myocardial infarction.

Use additional code to identify:
exposure to environmental tobacco smoke (Z77.22)
history of tobacco dependence (Z87.891)
occupational exposure to environmental tobacco smoke (Z57.31)
tobacco dependence (F17.-)
tobacco use (Z72.0)

Excludes1 angina pectoris with atherosclerotic heart disease of native coronary arteries (I25.1-)
atherosclerosis of coronary artery bypass graft(s) and coronary artery of transplanted heart with angina pectoris (I25.7-)
postinfarction angina (I23.7)

I20.0 Unstable angina HCC
Accelerated angina
Crescendo angina
De novo effort angina
Intermediate coronary syndrome
Preinfarction syndrome
Worsening effort angina

I20.1 Angina pectoris with documented spasm HCC
Angiospastic angina
Prinzmetal angina
Spasm-induced angina
Variant angina

I20.8 Other forms of angina pectoris HCC
Angina equivalent
Angina of effort
Coronary slow flow syndrome
Stable angina
Stenocardia

Use additional code(s) for symptoms associated with angina equivalent

I20.9 Angina pectoris, unspecified HCC
Angina NOS
Anginal syndrome
Cardiac angina
Ischemic chest pain

● **I21 Acute myocardial infarction**

Includes cardiac infarction
coronary (artery) embolism
coronary (artery) occlusion
coronary (artery) rupture
coronary (artery) thrombosis
infarction of heart, myocardium, or ventricle
myocardial infarction specified as acute or with a stated duration of 4 weeks (28 days) or less from onset

Use additional code, if applicable, to identify:
exposure to environmental tobacco smoke (Z77.22)
history of tobacco dependence (Z87.891)
occupational exposure to environmental tobacco smoke (Z57.31)
status post administration of tPA (rtPA) in a different facility within the last 24 hours prior to admission to current facility (Z92.82)
tobacco dependence (F17.-)
tobacco use (Z72.0)

Excludes2 old myocardial infarction (I25.2)
postmyocardial infarction syndrome (I24.1)
subsequent type 1 myocardial infarction (I22.-)

Coding Clinic: 2016, Q4, P140; 2013, Q1, P25-26; 2012, Q4, P103

● **I21.0 ST elevation (STEMI) myocardial infarction of anterior wall**
Type 1 ST elevation myocardial infarction of anterior wall
Coding Clinic: 2013, Q1, P26

I21.01 ST elevation (STEMI) myocardial infarction involving left main coronary artery HCC

I21.02 ST elevation (STEMI) myocardial infarction involving left anterior descending coronary artery HCC
ST elevation (STEMI) myocardial infarction involving diagonal coronary artery
Coding Clinic: 2013, Q1, P26

I21.09 ST elevation (STEMI) myocardial infarction involving other coronary artery of anterior wall HCC
Acute transmural myocardial infarction of anterior wall
Anteroapical transmural (Q wave) infarction (acute)
Anterolateral transmural (Q wave) infarction (acute)
Anteroseptal transmural (Q wave) infarction (acute)
Transmural (Q wave) infarction (acute) (of) anterior (wall) NOS
Coding Clinic: 2012, Q4, P102, 104

● **I21.1 ST elevation (STEMI) myocardial infarction of inferior wall**
Type 1 ST elevation myocardial infarction of inferior wall
Coding Clinic: 2013, Q1, P26

I21.11 ST elevation (STEMI) myocardial infarction involving right coronary artery HCC
Inferoposterior transmural (Q wave) infarction (acute)

I21.19 ST elevation (STEMI) myocardial infarction involving other coronary artery of inferior wall HCC
Acute transmural myocardial infarction of inferior wall
Inferolateral transmural (Q wave) infarction (acute)
Transmural (Q wave) infarction (acute) (of) diaphragmatic wall
Transmural (Q wave) infarction (acute) (of) inferior (wall) NOS

Excludes2 ST elevation (STEMI) myocardial infarction involving left circumflex coronary artery (I21.21)

Coding Clinic: 2012, Q4, P97

I21.2 ST elevation (STEMI) myocardial infarction of other sites
Type 1 ST elevation myocardial infarction of other sites
Coding Clinic: 2013, Q1, P26

I21.21 ST elevation (STEMI) myocardial infarction involving left circumflex coronary artery
ST elevation (STEMI) myocardial infarction involving oblique marginal coronary artery

I21.29 ST elevation (STEMI) myocardial infarction involving other sites
Acute transmural myocardial infarction of other sites
Apical-lateral transmural (Q wave) infarction (acute)
Basal-lateral transmural (Q wave) infarction (acute)
High lateral transmural (Q wave) infarction (acute)
Lateral (wall) NOS transmural (Q wave) infarction (acute)
Posterior (true) transmural (Q wave) infarction (acute)
Posterobasal transmural (Q wave) infarction (acute)
Posterolateral transmural (Q wave) infarction (acute)
Posteroseptal transmural (Q wave) infarction (acute)
Septal transmural (Q wave) infarction (acute) NOS

OGCR Section I.c.9.e.2.

Acute myocardial infarction, unspecified

Code I21.9, Acute myocardial infarction, unspecified, is the default for unspecified acute myocardial infarction or unspecified type. If only type 1 STEMI or transmural MI without the site is documented, assign I21.3, ST elevation (STEMI) myocardial infarction of unspecified site.

I21.3 ST elevation (STEMI) myocardial infarction of unspecified site
Acute transmural myocardial infarction of unspecified site
Transmural (Q wave) myocardial infarction NOS
Type 1 ST elevation myocardial infarction of unspecified site
Coding Clinic: 2013, Q1, P26

I21.4 Non-ST elevation (NSTEMI) myocardial infarction
Acute subendocardial myocardial infarction
Non-Q wave myocardial infarction NOS
Nontransmural myocardial infarction NOS
Type 1 non-ST elevation myocardial infarction
Coding Clinic: 2017, Q1, P44; 2015, Q2, P16; 2013, Q1, P26

I21.9 Acute myocardial infarction, unspecified
Myocardial infarction (acute) NOS

I21.A Other type of myocardial infarction

I21.A1 Myocardial infarction type 2
Myocardial infarction due to demand ischemia
Myocardial infarction secondary to ischemic imbalance
~~Code also the underlying cause, if known and applicable, such as:~~
~~anemia (D50.0-D64.9)~~
~~chronic obstructive pulmonary disease (J44.-)~~
~~heart failure (I50.-)~~
~~paroxysmal tachycardia (I47.0-I47.9)~~
~~renal failure (N17.0-N19)~~
~~shock (R57.0-R57.9)~~
Code first the underlying cause, such as:
anemia (D50.0-D64.9)
chronic obstructive pulmonary disease (J44.-)
paroxysmal tachycardia (I47.0-I47.9)
shock (R57.0-R57.9)
Coding Clinic: 2017, Q4, P13-14

I21.A9 Other myocardial infarction type
Myocardial infarction associated with revascularization procedure
Myocardial infarction type 3
Myocardial infarction type 4a
Myocardial infarction type 4b
Myocardial infarction type 4c
Myocardial infarction type 5
Code first, if applicable, postprocedural myocardial infarction following cardiac surgery (I97.190), or postprocedural myocardial infarction during cardiac surgery (I97.790)
Code also complication, if known and applicable, such as:
(acute) stent occlusion (T82.897-)
(acute) stent stenosis (T82.857-)
(acute) stent thrombosis (T82.865-)
cardiac arrest due to underlying cardiac condition (I46.2)
complication of percutaneous coronary intervention (PCI) (I97.89)
occlusion of coronary artery bypass graft (T82.218-)
Coding Clinic: 2019, Q2, P32-33

I22 Subsequent ST elevation (STEMI) and non-ST elevation (NSTEMI) myocardial infarction

Includes acute myocardial infarction occurring within four weeks (28 days) of a previous acute myocardial infarction, regardless of site
cardiac infarction
coronary (artery) embolism
coronary (artery) occlusion
coronary (artery) rupture
coronary (artery) thrombosis
infarction of heart, myocardium, or ventricle
recurrent myocardial infarction
reinfarction of myocardium
rupture of heart, myocardium, or ventricle
subsequent type 1 myocardial infarction

Excludes1 subsequent myocardial infarction, type 2 (I21.A1)
subsequent myocardial infarction of other type (type 3) (type 4) (type 5) (I21.A9)

Use additional code, if applicable, to identify:
exposure to environmental tobacco smoke (Z77.22)
history of tobacco dependence (Z87.891)
occupational exposure to environmental tobacco smoke (Z57.31)
status post administration of tPA (rtPA) in a different facility within the last 24 hours prior to admission to current facility (Z92.82)
tobacco dependence (F17.-)
tobacco use (Z72.0)
Coding Clinic: 2017, Q4, P14; 2013, Q1, P25; 2012, Q4, P103

I22.0 Subsequent ST elevation (STEMI) myocardial infarction of anterior wall
Subsequent acute transmural myocardial infarction of anterior wall
Subsequent transmural (Q wave) infarction (acute)(of) anterior (wall) NOS
Subsequent anteroapical transmural (Q wave) infarction (acute)
Subsequent anterolateral transmural (Q wave) infarction (acute)
Subsequent anteroseptal transmural (Q wave) infarction (acute)

I22.1 Subsequent ST elevation (STEMI) myocardial infarction of inferior wall
Subsequent acute transmural myocardial infarction of inferior wall
Subsequent transmural (Q wave) infarction (acute)(of) diaphragmatic wall
Subsequent transmural (Q wave) infarction (acute)(of) inferior (wall) NOS
Subsequent inferolateral transmural (Q wave) infarction (acute)
Subsequent inferoposterior transmural (Q wave) infarction (acute)
Coding Clinic: 2012, Q4, P97, 102, 104

CHAPTER 9 (I00-I99)

I22.2   **Subsequent non-ST elevation (NSTEMI) myocardial infarction** 🝕
  Subsequent acute subendocardial myocardial infarction
  Subsequent non-Q wave myocardial infarction NOS
  Subsequent nontransmural myocardial infarction NOS

I22.8   **Subsequent ST elevation (STEMI) myocardial infarction of other sites** 🝕
  Subsequent acute transmural myocardial infarction of other sites
  Subsequent apical-lateral transmural (Q wave) myocardial infarction (acute)
  Subsequent basal-lateral transmural (Q wave) myocardial infarction (acute)
  Subsequent high lateral transmural (Q wave) myocardial infarction (acute)
  Subsequent transmural (Q wave) myocardial infarction (acute)(of) lateral (wall) NOS
  Subsequent posterior (true) transmural (Q wave) myocardial infarction (acute)
  Subsequent posterobasal transmural (Q wave) myocardial infarction (acute)
  Subsequent posterolateral transmural (Q wave) myocardial infarction (acute)
  Subsequent posteroseptal transmural (Q wave) myocardial infarction (acute)
  Subsequent septal NOS transmural (Q wave) myocardial infarction (acute)

I22.9   **Subsequent ST elevation (STEMI) myocardial infarction of unspecified site** 🝕
  Subsequent acute myocardial infarction of unspecified site
  Subsequent myocardial infarction (acute) NOS

● **I23**   **Certain current complications following ST elevation (STEMI) and non-ST elevation (NSTEMI) myocardial infarction (within the 28 day period)**
  Coding Clinic: 2017, Q2, P11

I23.0   **Hemopericardium as current complication following acute myocardial infarction** 🝕   A
  Excludes1   hemopericardium not specified as current complication following acute myocardial infarction (I31.2)

I23.1   **Atrial septal defect as current complication following acute myocardial infarction** 🝕   A
  Excludes1   acquired atrial septal defect not specified as current complication following acute myocardial infarction (I51.0)

I23.2   **Ventricular septal defect as current complication following acute myocardial infarction** 🝕   A
  Excludes1   acquired ventricular septal defect not specified as current complication following acute myocardial infarction (I51.0)

I23.3   **Rupture of cardiac wall without hemopericardium as current complication following acute myocardial infarction** 🝕   A
  Coding Clinic: 2017, Q2, P11

I23.4   **Rupture of chordae tendineae as current complication following acute myocardial infarction** 🝕
  Excludes1   rupture of chordae tendineae not specified as current complication following acute myocardial infarction (I51.1)

I23.5   **Rupture of papillary muscle as current complication following acute myocardial infarction** 🝕
  Excludes1   rupture of papillary muscle not specified as current complication following acute myocardial infarction (I51.2)

I23.6   **Thrombosis of atrium, auricular appendage, and ventricle as current complications following acute myocardial infarction** 🝕   A
  Excludes1   thrombosis of atrium, auricular appendage, and ventricle not specified as current complication following acute myocardial infarction (I51.3)

I23.7   **Postinfarction angina** 🝕   A
  Coding Clinic: 2015, Q2, P16-17

I23.8   **Other current complications following acute myocardial infarction** 🝕   A

● **I24**   **Other acute ischemic heart diseases**
  Excludes1   angina pectoris (I20.-)
    transient myocardial ischemia in newborn (P29.4)

I24.0   **Acute coronary thrombosis not resulting in myocardial infarction** 🝕
  Acute coronary (artery) (vein) embolism not resulting in myocardial infarction
  Acute coronary (artery) (vein) occlusion not resulting in myocardial infarction
  Acute coronary (artery) (vein) thromboembolism not resulting in myocardial infarction
  Excludes1   atherosclerotic heart disease (I25.1-)
  Coding Clinic: 2013, Q1, P24

I24.1   **Dressler's syndrome** 🝕
  Postmyocardial infarction syndrome
  Excludes1   postinfarction angina (I23.7)

I24.8   **Other forms of acute ischemic heart disease** 🝕
  Excludes1   myocardial infarction due to demand ischemia (I21.A1)
  Coding Clinic: 2017, Q4, P13

I24.9   **Acute ischemic heart disease, unspecified** 🝕
  Excludes1   ischemic heart disease (chronic) NOS (I25.9)

● **I25**   **Chronic ischemic heart disease**
  Use additional code to identify:
    chronic total occlusion of coronary artery (I25.82)
    exposure to environmental tobacco smoke (Z77.22)
    history of tobacco dependence (Z87.891)
    occupational exposure to environmental tobacco smoke (Z57.31)
    tobacco dependence (F17.-)
    tobacco use (Z72.0)

★ **(See Plates 218 and 219 on pages 74 and 75.)**

● **I25.1**   **Atherosclerotic heart disease of native coronary artery**
  Disease in which fatty deposits form on the walls of arteries
  Atherosclerotic cardiovascular disease
  Coronary (artery) atheroma
  Coronary (artery) atherosclerosis
  Coronary (artery) disease
  Coronary (artery) sclerosis
  Use additional code, if applicable, to identify:
    coronary atherosclerosis due to calcified coronary lesion (I25.84)
    coronary atherosclerosis due to lipid rich plaque (I25.83)
  Excludes2   atheroembolism (I75.-)
    atherosclerosis of coronary artery bypass graft(s) and transplanted heart (I25.7-)

I25.10   **Atherosclerotic heart disease of native coronary artery without angina pectoris**   A
  Atherosclerotic heart disease NOS
  Coding Clinic: 2015, Q2, P17; 2012, Q4, P92

Item 9-6 Classification is based on the location of the atherosclerosis. **"Of native coronary artery"** indicates the atherosclerosis is within an original heart artery. **"Of autologous vein bypass graft"** indicates that the atherosclerosis is within a vein graft that was taken from within the patient. **"Of nonautologous biological bypass graft"** indicates the atherosclerosis is within a vessel grafted from other than the patient. **"Of artery bypass graft"** indicates the atherosclerosis is within an artery that was grafted from within the patient.

▶ New   ⇒ Revised   ~~deleted~~ Deleted   Excludes 1   Excludes 2   Includes   Use additional   Code first   Code also   Key words
OGCR Official Guidelines   X Assign placeholder X   ● Use Additional Character(s)   ▷ Manifestation Code   🝕 Hierarchical Condition Category   Coding Clinic

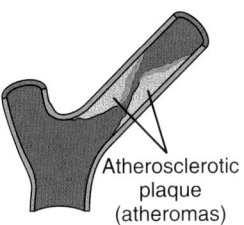

Figure 9-2   Atherosclerotic plaque.

Atherosclerotic plaque (atheromas)

OGCR   See Section I.9.b.

Atherosclerotic Coronary Artery Disease and Angina

ICD-10-CM has combination codes for atherosclerotic heart disease with angina pectoris. The subcategories for these codes are I25.11, Atherosclerotic heart disease of native coronary artery with angina pectoris and I25.7, Atherosclerosis of coronary artery bypass graft(s) and coronary artery of transplanted heart with angina pectoris.

When using one of these combination codes it is not necessary to use an additional code for angina pectoris. A causal relationship can be assumed in a patient with both atherosclerosis and angina pectoris, unless the documentation indicates the angina is due to something other than the atherosclerosis.

If a patient with coronary artery disease is admitted due to an acute myocardial infarction (AMI), the AMI should be sequenced before the coronary artery disease.

See Section I.C.9. Acute myocardial infarction (AMI).

● **I25.11**   **Atherosclerotic heart disease of native coronary artery with angina pectoris**

     I25.110   **Atherosclerotic heart disease of native coronary artery with unstable angina pectoris** 🔖   **A**

         Excludes1   unstable angina without atherosclerotic heart disease (I20.0)

     I25.111   **Atherosclerotic heart disease of native coronary artery with angina pectoris with documented spasm** 🔖   **A**

         Excludes1   angina pectoris with documented spasm without atherosclerotic heart disease (I20.1)

     I25.118   **Atherosclerotic heart disease of native coronary artery with other forms of angina pectoris** 🔖   **A**

         Excludes1   other forms of angina pectoris without atherosclerotic heart disease (I20.8)

         Coding Clinic: 2015, Q2, P16-17

     I25.119   **Atherosclerotic heart disease of native coronary artery with unspecified angina pectoris** 🔖   **A**

         Atherosclerotic heart disease with angina NOS

         Atherosclerotic heart disease with ischemic chest pain

         Excludes1   unspecified angina pectoris without atherosclerotic heart disease (I20.9)

I25.2   **Old myocardial infarction**

     Healed myocardial infarction

     Past myocardial infarction diagnosed by ECG or other investigation, but currently presenting no symptoms

I25.3   **Aneurysm of heart**

     Mural aneurysm

     Ventricular aneurysm

● **I25.4**   **Coronary artery aneurysm and dissection**

     I25.41   **Coronary artery aneurysm**

         Coronary arteriovenous fistula, acquired

         Excludes1   congenital coronary (artery) aneurysm (Q24.5)

     I25.42   **Coronary artery dissection**

I25.5   **Ischemic cardiomyopathy**

     Excludes2   coronary atherosclerosis (I25.1-, I25.7-)

I25.6   **Silent myocardial ischemia**

● **I25.7**   **Atherosclerosis of coronary artery bypass graft(s) and coronary artery of transplanted heart with angina pectoris**

     Use additional code, if applicable, to identify:

         coronary atherosclerosis due to calcified coronary lesion (I25.84)

         coronary atherosclerosis due to lipid rich plaque (I25.83)

     Excludes1   atherosclerosis of bypass graft(s) of transplanted heart without angina pectoris (I25.812)

               atherosclerosis of coronary artery bypass graft(s) without angina pectoris (I25.810)

               atherosclerosis of native coronary artery of transplanted heart without angina pectoris (I25.811)

● **I25.70**   **Atherosclerosis of coronary artery bypass graft(s), unspecified, with angina pectoris**

     I25.700   **Atherosclerosis of coronary artery bypass graft(s), unspecified, with unstable angina pectoris** 🔖   **A**

         Excludes1   unstable angina pectoris without atherosclerosis of coronary artery bypass graft (I20.0)

     I25.701   **Atherosclerosis of coronary artery bypass graft(s), unspecified, with angina pectoris with documented spasm** 🔖   **A**

         Excludes1   angina pectoris with documented spasm without atherosclerosis of coronary artery bypass graft (I20.1)

     I25.708   **Atherosclerosis of coronary artery bypass graft(s), unspecified, with other forms of angina pectoris** 🔖   **A**

         Excludes1   other forms of angina pectoris without atherosclerosis of coronary artery bypass graft (I20.8)

     I25.709   **Atherosclerosis of coronary artery bypass graft(s), unspecified, with unspecified angina pectoris** 🔖   **A**

         Excludes1   unspecified angina pectoris without atherosclerosis of coronary artery bypass graft (I20.9)

CHAPTER 9 (I00-I99)

● **I25.71** Atherosclerosis of **autologous vein** coronary artery bypass graft(s) with angina pectoris

    I25.710 Atherosclerosis of autologous vein coronary artery bypass graft(s) with **unstable** angina pectoris 🍥   A

        Excludes1 unstable angina without atherosclerosis of autologous vein coronary artery bypass graft(s) (I20.0)

        Excludes2 embolism or thrombus of coronary artery bypass graft(s) (T82.8-)

    I25.711 Atherosclerosis of autologous vein coronary artery bypass graft(s) with angina pectoris with **documented spasm** 🍥   A

        Excludes1 angina pectoris with documented spasm without atherosclerosis of autologous vein coronary artery bypass graft(s) (I20.1)

    I25.718 Atherosclerosis of autologous vein coronary artery bypass graft(s) with **other forms of angina pectoris** 🍥   A

        Excludes1 other forms of angina pectoris without atherosclerosis of autologous vein coronary artery bypass graft(s) (I20.8)

    I25.719 Atherosclerosis of autologous vein coronary artery bypass graft(s) with **unspecified angina pectoris** 🍥   A

        Excludes1 unspecified angina pectoris without atherosclerosis of autologous vein coronary artery bypass graft(s) (I20.9)

● **I25.72** Atherosclerosis of **autologous artery** coronary artery bypass graft(s) with angina pectoris

    Atherosclerosis of internal mammary artery graft with angina pectoris

    I25.720 Atherosclerosis of autologous artery coronary artery bypass graft(s) with **unstable** angina pectoris 🍥   A

        Excludes1 unstable angina without atherosclerosis of autologous artery coronary artery bypass graft(s) (I20.0)

    I25.721 Atherosclerosis of autologous artery coronary artery bypass graft(s) with angina pectoris with **documented spasm** 🍥   A

        Excludes1 angina pectoris with documented spasm without atherosclerosis of autologous artery coronary artery bypass graft(s) (I20.1)

    I25.728 Atherosclerosis of autologous artery coronary artery bypass graft(s) with **other forms of angina pectoris** 🍥   A

        Excludes1 other forms of angina pectoris without atherosclerosis of autologous artery coronary artery bypass graft(s) (I20.8)

    I25.729 Atherosclerosis of autologous artery coronary artery bypass graft(s) with **unspecified angina pectoris** 🍥   A

        Excludes1 unspecified angina pectoris without atherosclerosis of autologous artery coronary artery bypass graft(s) (I20.9)

● **I25.73** Atherosclerosis of **nonautologous biological** coronary artery bypass graft(s) with angina pectoris

    I25.730 Atherosclerosis of nonautologous biological coronary artery bypass graft(s) with **unstable angina pectoris** 🍥   A

        Excludes1 unstable angina without atherosclerosis of nonautologous biological coronary artery bypass graft(s) (I20.0)

    I25.731 Atherosclerosis of nonautologous biological coronary artery bypass graft(s) with angina pectoris with **documented spasm** 🍥   A

        Excludes1 angina pectoris with documented spasm without atherosclerosis of nonautologous biological coronary artery bypass graft(s) (I20.1)

    I25.738 Atherosclerosis of nonautologous biological coronary artery bypass graft(s) with **other forms of angina pectoris** 🍥   A

        Excludes1 other forms of angina pectoris without atherosclerosis of nonautologous biological coronary artery bypass graft(s) (I20.8)

    I25.739 Atherosclerosis of nonautologous biological coronary artery bypass graft(s) with **unspecified angina pectoris** 🍥   A

        Excludes1 unspecified angina pectoris without atherosclerosis of nonautologous biological coronary artery bypass graft(s) (I20.9)

▶ New   ⇒ Revised   ~~deleted~~ Deleted   Excludes 1   Excludes 2   Includes   Use additional   Code first   Code also   Key words

OGCR Official Guidelines   X Assign placeholder X   ● Use Additional Character(s)   ▷ Manifestation Code   🍥 Hierarchical Condition Category   **Coding Clinic**

● **I25.75**   Atherosclerosis of native coronary artery of transplanted heart with angina pectoris

     Excludes1   atherosclerosis of native coronary artery of transplanted heart without angina pectoris (I25.811)

   I25.750   Atherosclerosis of native coronary artery of transplanted heart with unstable angina 🔒

   I25.751   Atherosclerosis of native coronary artery of transplanted heart with angina pectoris with documented spasm 🔒

   I25.758   Atherosclerosis of native coronary artery of transplanted heart with other forms of angina pectoris 🔒

   I25.759   Atherosclerosis of native coronary artery of transplanted heart with unspecified angina pectoris 🔒

● **I25.76**   Atherosclerosis of bypass graft of coronary artery of transplanted heart with angina pectoris

     Excludes1   atherosclerosis of bypass graft of coronary artery of transplanted heart without angina pectoris (I25.812)

   I25.760   Atherosclerosis of bypass graft of coronary artery of transplanted heart with unstable angina 🔒   A

   I25.761   Atherosclerosis of bypass graft of coronary artery of transplanted heart with angina pectoris with documented spasm 🔒   A

   I25.768   Atherosclerosis of bypass graft of coronary artery of transplanted heart with other forms of angina pectoris 🔒   A

   I25.769   Atherosclerosis of bypass graft of coronary artery of transplanted heart with unspecified angina pectoris 🔒   A

● **I25.79**   Atherosclerosis of other coronary artery bypass graft(s) with angina pectoris   A

   I25.790   Atherosclerosis of other coronary artery bypass graft(s) with unstable angina pectoris 🔒

     Excludes1   unstable angina without atherosclerosis of other coronary artery bypass graft(s) (I20.0)

   I25.791   Atherosclerosis of other coronary artery bypass graft(s) with angina pectoris with documented spasm 🔒   A

     Excludes1   angina pectoris with documented spasm without atherosclerosis of other coronary artery bypass graft(s) (I20.1)

   I25.798   Atherosclerosis of other coronary artery bypass graft(s) with other forms of angina pectoris 🔒   A

     Excludes1   other forms of angina pectoris without atherosclerosis of other coronary artery bypass graft(s) (I20.8)

   I25.799   Atherosclerosis of other coronary artery bypass graft(s) with unspecified angina pectoris 🔒   A

     Excludes1   unspecified angina pectoris without atherosclerosis of other coronary artery bypass graft(s) (I20.9)

● **I25.8**   Other forms of chronic ischemic heart disease

● **I25.81**   Atherosclerosis of other coronary vessels without angina pectoris

     Use additional code, if applicable, to identify:
coronary atherosclerosis due to calcified coronary lesion (I25.84)
coronary atherosclerosis due to lipid rich plaque (I25.83)

     ~~**Excludes1** atherosclerotic heart disease of native coronary artery without angina pectoris (I25.10)~~

     ▶ **Excludes2**   atherosclerotic heart disease of native coronary artery without angina pectoris (I25.10)

   I25.810   Atherosclerosis of coronary artery bypass graft(s) without angina pectoris   A

     Atherosclerosis of coronary artery bypass graft NOS

     Excludes1   atherosclerosis of coronary bypass graft(s) with angina pectoris (I25.70- -I25.73-, I25.79-)

     Coding Clinic: 2016, Q4, P86

   I25.811   Atherosclerosis of native coronary artery of transplanted heart without angina pectoris

     Atherosclerosis of native coronary artery of transplanted heart NOS

     Excludes1   atherosclerosis of native coronary artery of transplanted heart with angina pectoris (I25.75-)

   I25.812   Atherosclerosis of bypass graft of coronary artery of transplanted heart without angina pectoris   A

     Atherosclerosis of bypass graft of transplanted heart NOS

     Excludes1   atherosclerosis of bypass graft of transplanted heart with angina pectoris (I25.76)

I25.82   **Chronic total occlusion of coronary artery**
Complete occlusion of coronary artery
Total occlusion of coronary artery
Code first coronary atherosclerosis (I25.1-, I25.7-, I25.81-)

> **Excludes1**   acute coronary occlusion with myocardial infarction (I21.0-I21.9, I22.-)
> acute coronary occlusion without myocardial infarction (I24.0)

I25.83   **Coronary atherosclerosis due to lipid rich plaque**   A
Code first coronary atherosclerosis (I25.1-, I25.7-, I25.81-)

I25.84   **Coronary atherosclerosis due to calcified coronary lesion**
Coronary atherosclerosis due to severely calcified coronary lesion
Code first coronary atherosclerosis (I25.1-, I25.7-, I25.81-)

I25.89   **Other forms of chronic ischemic heart disease**

I25.9   **Chronic ischemic heart disease, unspecified**
Ischemic heart disease (chronic) NOS

PULMONARY HEART DISEASE AND DISEASES OF PULMONARY CIRCULATION (I26-I28)

● **I26**   **Pulmonary embolism**
> **Includes**   pulmonary (acute)(artery)(vein) infarction
> pulmonary (acute)(artery)(vein) thromboembolism
> pulmonary (acute)(artery)(vein) thrombosis

> **Excludes2**   chronic pulmonary embolism (I27.82)
> personal history of pulmonary embolism (Z86.711)
> pulmonary embolism due to trauma (T79.0, T79.1)
> pulmonary embolism due to complications of surgical and medical care (T80.0, T81.7-, T82.8-)
> pulmonary embolism complicating abortion, ectopic or molar pregnancy (O00-O07, O08.2)
> pulmonary embolism complicating pregnancy, childbirth and the puerperium (O88.-)
> septic (non-pulmonary) arterial embolism (I76)

● **I26.0**   **Pulmonary embolism with acute cor pulmonale**

     I26.01   **Septic pulmonary embolism with acute cor pulmonale** 🔹
Code first underlying infection

     I26.02   **Saddle embolus of pulmonary artery with acute cor pulmonale** 🔹

     I26.09   **Other pulmonary embolism with acute cor pulmonale** 🔹
Acute cor pulmonale NOS

● **I26.9**   **Pulmonary embolism without acute cor pulmonale**

     I26.90   **Septic pulmonary embolism without acute cor pulmonale** 🔹
Code first underlying infection

     I26.92   **Saddle embolus of pulmonary artery without acute cor pulmonale** 🔹

     ▶**I26.93**   **Single subsegmental pulmonary embolism without acute cor pulmonale**
▶Subsegmental pulmonary embolism NOS

     ▶**I26.94**   **Multiple subsegmental pulmonary emboli without acute cor pulmonale**

     I26.99   **Other pulmonary embolism without acute cor pulmonale** 🔹
Acute pulmonary embolism NOS
Pulmonary embolism NOS
Coding Clinic: 2019, Q2, P22-23

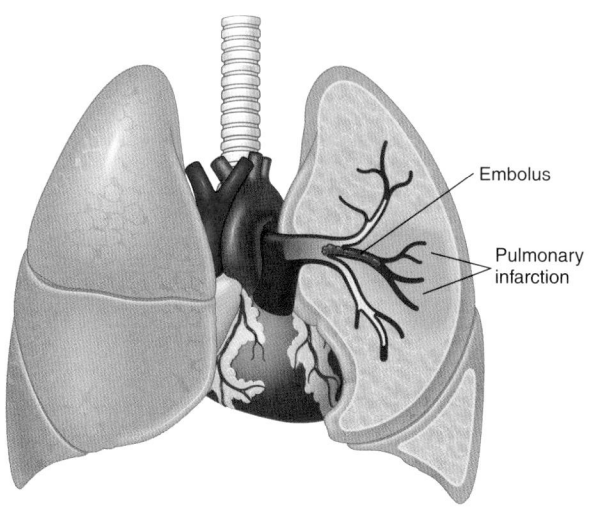

Figure 9-3   Pulmonary embolism. (From Chabner: The Language of Medicine, ed 8, St. Louis, Saunders, 2007)

Item 9–7   Pulmonary heart disease or **cor pulmonale** is right ventricle hypertrophy or RVH as a result of a respiratory disorder increasing back flow pressure to the right ventricle. Left untreated, cor pulmonale leads to right-heart failure and death.

● **I27**   **Other pulmonary heart diseases**

     I27.0   **Primary pulmonary hypertension** 🔹
Heritable pulmonary arterial hypertension
Idiopathic pulmonary arterial hypertension
Primary group 1 pulmonary hypertension
Primary pulmonary arterial hypertension

> **Excludes1**   persistent pulmonary hypertension of newborn (P29.30)
> pulmonary hypertension NOS (I27.20)
> secondary pulmonary arterial hypertension (I27.21)
> secondary pulmonary hypertension (I27.29)

     I27.1   **Kyphoscoliotic heart disease** 🔹

● **I27.2**   **Other secondary pulmonary hypertension**
Code also associated underlying condition
> **Excludes1**   Eisenmenger's syndrome (I27.83)
Coding Clinic: 2016, Q2, P8

     I27.20   **Pulmonary hypertension, unspecified** 🔹
Pulmonary hypertension NOS

     I27.21   **Secondary pulmonary arterial hypertension** 🔹
(Associated) (drug-induced) (toxin-induced) pulmonary arterial hypertension NOS
(Associated) (drug-induced) (toxin-induced) (secondary) group 1 pulmonary hypertension
Code also associated conditions if applicable, or adverse effects of drugs or toxins, such as:
adverse effect of appetite depressants (T50.5X5)
congenital heart disease (Q20-Q28)
human immunodeficiency virus [HIV] disease (B20)
polymyositis (M33.2-)
portal hypertension (K76.6)
rheumatoid arthritis (M05.-)
schistosomiasis (B65.-)
Sjögren syndrome (M35.0-)
systemic sclerosis (M34.-)

▶ New   ⇒ Revised   ~~deleted~~ Deleted   Excludes 1   Excludes 2   Includes   Use additional   Code first   Code also   Key words

868   OGCR Official Guidelines   X Assign placeholder X   ● Use Additional Character(s)   ▶ Manifestation Code   🔹 Hierarchical Condition Category   Coding Clinic

I27.22 **Pulmonary hypertension due to left heart disease**
Group 2 pulmonary hypertension
Code also associated left heart disease, if known, such as:
multiple valve disease (I08.-)
rheumatic mitral valve diseases (I05.-)
rheumatic aortic valve diseases (I06.-)

I27.23 **Pulmonary hypertension due to lung diseases and hypoxia**
Group 3 pulmonary hypertension
Code also associated lung disease, if known, such as:
bronchiectasis (J47.-)
cystic fibrosis with pulmonary manifestations (E84.0)
interstitial lung disease (J84.-)
pleural effusion (J90)
sleep apnea (G47.3-)

I27.24 **Chronic thromboembolic pulmonary hypertension**
Group 4 pulmonary hypertension
Code also associated pulmonary embolism, if applicable (I26.-, I27.82)

I27.29 **Other secondary pulmonary hypertension**
Group 5 pulmonary hypertension
Pulmonary hypertension with unclear multifactorial mechanisms
Pulmonary hypertension due to hematologic disorders
Pulmonary hypertension due to metabolic disorders
Pulmonary hypertension due to other systemic disorders
Code also other associated disorders, if known, such as:
chronic myeloid leukemia (C92.10- C92.22)
essential thrombocythemia (D47.3)
Gaucher disease (E75.22)
hypertensive chronic kidney disease with end stage renal disease (I12.0, I13.11,I13.2)
hyperthyroidism (E05.-)
hypothyroidism (E00-E03)
polycythemia vera (D45)
sarcoidosis (D86.-)

● I27.8 **Other specified pulmonary heart diseases**

I27.81 **Cor pulmonale (chronic)**
Cor pulmonale NOS
Excludes1 acute cor pulmonale (I26.0-)

I27.82 **Chronic pulmonary embolism**
Use additional code, if applicable, for associated long-term (current) use of anticoagulants (Z79.01)
Excludes1 personal history of pulmonary embolism (Z86.711)

I27.83 **Eisenmenger's syndrome**
Eisenmenger's complex
(Irreversible) Eisenmenger's disease
Pulmonary hypertension with right to left shunt related to congenital heart disease
Code also underlying heart defect, if known, such as:
atrial septal defect (Q21.1)
Eisenmenger's defect (Q21.8)
patent ductus arteriosus (Q25.0)
ventricular septal defect (Q21.0)

I27.89 **Other specified pulmonary heart diseases**

I27.9 **Pulmonary heart disease, unspecified**
Chronic cardiopulmonary disease

● I28 **Other diseases of pulmonary vessels**

I28.0 **Arteriovenous fistula of pulmonary vessels**
Excludes1 congenital arteriovenous fistula (Q25.72)

I28.1 **Aneurysm of pulmonary artery**
Excludes1 congenital aneurysm (Q25.79)
congenital arteriovenous aneurysm (Q25.72)

I28.8 **Other diseases of pulmonary vessels**
Pulmonary arteritis
Pulmonary endarteritis
Rupture of pulmonary vessels
Stenosis of pulmonary vessels
Stricture of pulmonary vessels

I28.9 **Disease of pulmonary vessels, unspecified**

OTHER FORMS OF HEART DISEASE (I30-I52)

● I30 **Acute pericarditis**
Inflammation of pericardium (sac surrounding the heart) caused by an infection
Includes acute mediastinopericarditis
acute myopericarditis
acute pericardial effusion
acute pleuropericarditis
acute pneumopericarditis
Excludes1 Dressler's syndrome (I24.1)
rheumatic pericarditis (acute) (I01.0)
viral pericarditis due to Coxsakie virus (B33.23)

I30.0 **Acute nonspecific idiopathic pericarditis**

I30.1 **Infective pericarditis**
Pneumococcal pericarditis
Pneumopyopericardium
Purulent pericarditis
Pyopericarditis
Pyopericardium
Pyopneumopericardium
Staphylococcal pericarditis
Streptococcal pericarditis
Suppurative pericarditis
Viral pericarditis
Use additional code (B95-B97) to identify infectious agent

I30.8 **Other forms of acute pericarditis**

I30.9 **Acute pericarditis, unspecified**

● I31 **Other diseases of pericardium**
Excludes1 diseases of pericardium specified as rheumatic (I09.2)
postcardiotomy syndrome (I97.0)
traumatic injury to pericardium (S26.-)

I31.0 **Chronic adhesive pericarditis**
Accretio cordis
Adherent pericardium
Adhesive mediastinopericarditis

I31.1 **Chronic constrictive pericarditis**
Concretio cordis
Pericardial calcification

I31.2 **Hemopericardium, not elsewhere classified**
Excludes1 hemopericardium as current complication following acute myocardial infarction (I23.0)

I31.3 **Pericardial effusion (noninflammatory)**
Chylopericardium
Excludes1 acute pericardial effusion (I30.9)
Coding Clinic: 2019, Q1, P16

I31.4 **Cardiac tamponade**
Code first underlying cause

I31.8 **Other specified diseases of pericardium**
Epicardial plaques
Focal pericardial adhesions

I31.9 **Disease of pericardium, unspecified**
Pericarditis (chronic) NOS

CHAPTER 9 (I00-I99)

I32 *Pericarditis in diseases classified elsewhere*
Code first underlying disease
Excludes1 pericarditis (in):
coxsackie (virus) (B33.23)
gonococcal (A54.83)
meningococcal (A39.53)
rheumatoid (arthritis) (M05.31)
syphilitic (A52.06)
systemic lupus erythematosus (M32.12)
tuberculosis (A18.84)

I33 **Acute and subacute endocarditis**
Inflammation/infection of lining of heart, affecting heart valves including replacement valves and is usually caused by a bacterial infection
Excludes1 acute rheumatic endocarditis (I01.1)
endocarditis NOS (I38)

I33.0 **Acute and subacute infective endocarditis**
Bacterial endocarditis (acute) (subacute)
Infective endocarditis (acute) (subacute) NOS
Endocarditis lenta (acute) (subacute)
Malignant endocarditis (acute) (subacute)
Purulent endocarditis (acute) (subacute)
Septic endocarditis (acute) (subacute)
Ulcerative endocarditis (acute) (subacute)
Vegetative endocarditis (acute) (subacute)
Use additional code (B95-B97) to identify infectious agent

I33.9 **Acute and subacute endocarditis, unspecified**
Acute endocarditis NOS
Acute myoendocarditis NOS
Acute periendocarditis NOS
Subacute endocarditis NOS
Subacute myoendocarditis NOS
Subacute periendocarditis NOS

I34 **Nonrheumatic mitral valve disorders**
Excludes1 mitral valve disease (I05.9)
mitral valve failure (I05.8)
mitral valve stenosis (I05.0)
mitral valve disorder of unspecified cause with diseases of aortic and/or tricuspid valve(s) (I08.-)
mitral valve disorder of unspecified cause with mitral stenosis or obstruction (I05.0)
mitral valve disorder specified as congenital (Q23.2, Q23.9)
mitral valve disorder specified as rheumatic (I05.-)

I34.0 **Nonrheumatic mitral (valve) insufficiency**
Nonrheumatic mitral (valve) incompetence NOS
Nonrheumatic mitral (valve) regurgitation NOS

I34.1 **Nonrheumatic mitral (valve) prolapse**
Floppy nonrheumatic mitral valve syndrome
Excludes1 Marfan's syndrome (Q87.4-)

I34.2 **Nonrheumatic mitral (valve) stenosis**

I34.8 **Other nonrheumatic mitral valve disorders**

I34.9 **Nonrheumatic mitral valve disorder, unspecified**

I35 **Nonrheumatic aortic valve disorders**
Excludes1 aortic valve disorder of unspecified cause but with diseases of mitral and/or tricuspid valve(s) (I08.-)
aortic valve disorder specified as congenital (Q23.0, Q23.1)
aortic valve disorder specified as rheumatic (I06.-)
hypertrophic subaortic stenosis (I42.1)

I35.0 **Nonrheumatic aortic (valve) stenosis**

I35.1 **Nonrheumatic aortic (valve) insufficiency**
Nonrheumatic aortic (valve) incompetence NOS
Nonrheumatic aortic (valve) regurgitation NOS

I35.2 **Nonrheumatic aortic (valve) stenosis with insufficiency**

I35.8 **Other nonrheumatic aortic valve disorders**

I35.9 **Nonrheumatic aortic valve disorder, unspecified**

I36 **Nonrheumatic tricuspid valve disorders**
Excludes1 tricuspid valve disorders of unspecified cause (I07.-)
tricuspid valve disorders specified as congenital (Q22.4, Q22.8, Q22.9)
tricuspid valve disorders specified as rheumatic (I07.-)
tricuspid valve disorders with aortic and/or mitral valve involvement (I08.-)

I36.0 **Nonrheumatic tricuspid (valve) stenosis**

I36.1 **Nonrheumatic tricuspid (valve) insufficiency**
Nonrheumatic tricuspid (valve) incompetence
Nonrheumatic tricuspid (valve) regurgitation

I36.2 **Nonrheumatic tricuspid (valve) stenosis with insufficiency**

I36.8 **Other nonrheumatic tricuspid valve disorders**

I36.9 **Nonrheumatic tricuspid valve disorder, unspecified**

I37 **Nonrheumatic pulmonary valve disorders**
Excludes1 pulmonary valve disorder specified as congenital (Q22.1, Q22.2, Q22.3)
pulmonary valve disorder specified as rheumatic (I09.89)

I37.0 **Nonrheumatic pulmonary valve stenosis**

I37.1 **Nonrheumatic pulmonary valve insufficiency**
Nonrheumatic pulmonary valve incompetence
Nonrheumatic pulmonary valve regurgitation

I37.2 **Nonrheumatic pulmonary valve stenosis with insufficiency**

I37.8 **Other nonrheumatic pulmonary valve disorders**

I37.9 **Nonrheumatic pulmonary valve disorder, unspecified**

I38 **Endocarditis, valve unspecified**
Includes endocarditis (chronic) NOS
valvular incompetence NOS
valvular insufficiency NOS
valvular regurgitation NOS
valvular stenosis NOS
valvulitis (chronic) NOS
Excludes1 congenital insufficiency of cardiac valve NOS (Q24.8)
congenital stenosis of cardiac valve NOS (Q24.8)
endocardial fibroelastosis (I42.4)
endocarditis specified as rheumatic (I09.1)

I39 *Endocarditis and heart valve disorders in diseases classified elsewhere*
Code first underlying disease, such as:
Q fever (A78)
Excludes1 endocardial involvement in:
candidiasis (B37.6)
gonococcal infection (A54.83)
Libman-Sacks disease (M32.11)
listerosis (A32.82)
meningococcal infection (A39.51)
rheumatoid arthritis (M05.31)
syphilis (A52.03)
tuberculosis (A18.84)
typhoid fever (A01.02)

I40 **Acute myocarditis**
Inflammation of heart muscle due to infection (viral/bacterial)
Includes subacute myocarditis
Excludes1 acute rheumatic myocarditis (I01.2)

I40.0 **Infective myocarditis**
Septic myocarditis
Use additional code (B95-B97) to identify infectious agent

I40.1 **Isolated myocarditis**
Fiedler's myocarditis
Giant cell myocarditis
Idiopathic myocarditis

I40.8 **Other acute myocarditis**

I40.9 **Acute myocarditis, unspecified**

I41 *Myocarditis in diseases classified elsewhere*

Code first underlying disease, such as:
typhus (A75.Ø-A75.9)

Excludes1 myocarditis (in):
Chagas' disease (chronic) (B57.2)
acute (B57.Ø)
coxsackie (virus) infection (B33.22)
diphtheritic (A36.81)
gonococcal (A54.83)
influenzal (JØ9.X9, J1Ø.82, J11.82)
meningococcal (A39.52)
mumps (B26.82)
rheumatoid arthritis (MØ5.31)
sarcoid (D86.85)
syphilis (A52.Ø6)
toxoplasmosis (B58.81)
tuberculous (A18.84)

I42 Cardiomyopathy

Disease of the heart muscle resulting in an abnormally enlarged, weakened, thickened, and/or stiffened muscles

Includes myocardiopathy

Code first pre-existing cardiomyopathy complicating pregnancy and puerperium (O99.4)

Excludes2 ischemic cardiomyopathy (I25.5)
peripartum cardiomyopathy (O9Ø.3)
ventricular hypertrophy (I51.7)

I42.Ø Dilated cardiomyopathy
Congestive cardiomyopathy

I42.1 Obstructive hypertrophic cardiomyopathy
Hypertrophic subaortic stenosis (idiopathic)

I42.2 Other hypertrophic cardiomyopathy
Nonobstructive hypertrophic cardiomyopathy

I42.3 Endomyocardial (eosinophilic) disease
Endomyocardial (tropical) fibrosis
Löffler's endocarditis

I42.4 Endocardial fibroelastosis
Congenital cardiomyopathy
Elastomyofibrosis

I42.5 Other restrictive cardiomyopathy
Constrictive cardiomyopathy NOS

I42.6 Alcoholic cardiomyopathy
Code also presence of alcoholism (F1Ø.-)

I42.7 Cardiomyopathy due to drug and external agent
Code first poisoning due to drug or toxin, if applicable (T36-T65 with fifth or sixth character 1-4 or 6)
Use additional code for adverse effect, if applicable, to identify drug (T36-T5Ø with fifth or sixth character 5)

I42.8 Other cardiomyopathies

I42.9 Cardiomyopathy, unspecified
Cardiomyopathy (primary) (secondary) NOS

I43 *Cardiomyopathy in diseases classified elsewhere*

Code first underlying disease, such as:
amyloidosis (E85.-)
glycogen storage disease (E74.Ø)
gout (M1Ø.Ø-)
thyrotoxicosis (EØ5.Ø-EØ5.9-)

Excludes1 cardiomyopathy (in):
coxsackie (virus) (B33.24)
diphtheria (A36.81)
sarcoidosis (D86.85)
tuberculosis (A18.84)

I44 Atrioventricular and left bundle-branch block

Conduction problem resulting in arrhythmias/dysrhythmias due to a lack of electrical impulses being transmitted normally through the heart

I44.Ø Atrioventricular block, first degree

I44.1 Atrioventricular block, second degree
Atrioventricular block, type I and II
Möbitz block, type I and II
Second degree block, type I and II
Wenckebach's block

I44.2 Atrioventricular block, complete
Complete heart block NOS
Third degree block
Coding Clinic: 2019, Q2, P4

I44.3 Other and unspecified atrioventricular block
Atrioventricular block NOS

I44.30 Unspecified atrioventricular block

I44.39 Other atrioventricular block

I44.4 Left anterior fascicular block

I44.5 Left posterior fascicular block

I44.6 Other and unspecified fascicular block

I44.6Ø Unspecified fascicular block
Left bundle-branch hemiblock NOS

I44.69 Other fascicular block

I44.7 Left bundle-branch block, unspecified

I45 Other conduction disorders

I45.Ø Right fascicular block

I45.1 Other and unspecified right bundle-branch block

I45.1Ø Unspecified right bundle-branch block
Right bundle-branch block NOS

I45.19 Other right bundle-branch block

I45.2 Bifascicular block

I45.3 Trifascicular block

I45.4 Nonspecific intraventricular block
Bundle-branch block NOS

I45.5 Other specified heart block
Sinoatrial block
Sinoauricular block

Excludes1 heart block NOS (I45.9)

I45.6 Pre-excitation syndrome
Accelerated atrioventricular conduction
Accessory atrioventricular conduction
Anomalous atrioventricular excitation
Lown-Ganong-Levine syndrome
Pre-excitation atrioventricular conduction
Wolff-Parkinson-White syndrome

I45.8 Other specified conduction disorders

I45.81 Long QT syndrome

I45.89 Other specified conduction disorders
Atrioventricular [AV] dissociation
Interference dissociation
Isorhythmic dissociation
Nonparoxysmal AV nodal tachycardia
Coding Clinic: 2013, Q2, P32

I45.9 Conduction disorder, unspecified
Heart block NOS
Stokes-Adams syndrome

I46 Cardiac arrest

Excludes1 cardiogenic shock (R57.Ø)

I46.2 Cardiac arrest due to underlying cardiac condition
Code first underlying cardiac condition

I46.8 Cardiac arrest due to other underlying condition
Code first underlying condition

I46.9 Cardiac arrest, cause unspecified

CHAPTER 9 (IØØ-I99)

I47 Paroxysmal tachycardia

Code first tachycardia complicating:
abortion or ectopic or molar pregnancy (O00-O07, O08.8)
obstetric surgery and procedures (O75.4)

Excludes1 tachycardia NOS (R00.0)
sinoauricular tachycardia NOS (R00.0)
sinus [sinusal] tachycardia NOS (R00.0)

I47.0 **Re-entry ventricular arrhythmia**

I47.1 **Supraventricular tachycardia**
Atrial (paroxysmal) tachycardia
Atrioventricular [AV] (paroxysmal) tachycardia
Atrioventricular re-entrant (nodal) tachycardia [AVNRT] [AVRT]
Junctional (paroxysmal) tachycardia
Nodal (paroxysmal) tachycardia

I47.2 **Ventricular tachycardia**
Coding Clinic: 2013, Q3, P23

I47.9 **Paroxysmal tachycardia, unspecified**
Bouveret (-Hoffman) syndrome

I48 Atrial fibrillation and flutter

Most common abnormal heart rhythm (arrhythmia) presenting as irregular, rapid beating (tachycardia) of the heart's upper chamber.

I48.0 **Paroxysmal atrial fibrillation**

I48.1 **Persistent atrial fibrillation**
Rapid contractions of the upper heart chamber

Excludes1 Permanent atrial fibrillation (I48.21)

Coding Clinic: 2019, Q2, P3-4

I48.11 **Longstanding persistent atrial fibrillation**

I48.19 **Other persistent atrial fibrillation**
Chronic persistent atrial fibrillation
Persistent atrial fibrillation, NOS

I48.2 **Chronic atrial fibrillation**
~~Permanent atrial fibrillation~~
Coding Clinic: 2019, Q2, P3

I48.20 **Chronic atrial fibrillation, unspecified**

Excludes1 Chronic persistent atrial fibrillation (I48.19)

I48.21 **Permanent atrial fibrillation**

I48.3 **Typical atrial flutter**
Type I atrial flutter

I48.4 **Atypical atrial flutter**
Type II atrial flutter

I48.9 **Unspecified atrial fibrillation and atrial flutter**

I48.91 **Unspecified atrial fibrillation**

I48.92 **Unspecified atrial flutter**

I49 Other cardiac arrhythmias

Code first cardiac arrhythmia complicating:
abortion or ectopic or molar pregnancy (O00-O07, O08.8)
obstetric surgery and procedures (O75.4)

Excludes1 neonatal dysrhythmia (P29.1-)
sinoatrial bradycardia (R00.1)
sinus bradycardia (R00.1)
vagal bradycardia (R00.1)

Excludes2 bradycardia NOS (R00.1)

I49.0 **Ventricular fibrillation and flutter**

I49.01 **Ventricular fibrillation**

I49.02 **Ventricular flutter**

I49.1 **Atrial premature depolarization**
Atrial premature beats

I49.2 **Junctional premature depolarization**

I49.3 **Ventricular premature depolarization**

I49.4 **Other and unspecified premature depolarization**

I49.40 **Unspecified premature depolarization**
Premature beats NOS

I49.49 **Other premature depolarization**
Ectopic beats
Extrasystoles
Extrasystolic arrhythmias
Premature contractions

I49.5 **Sick sinus syndrome**
Tachycardia-bradycardia syndrome
Coding Clinic: 2019, Q1, P33

I49.8 **Other specified cardiac arrhythmias**
Brugada syndrome
Coronary sinus rhythm disorder
Ectopic rhythm disorder
Nodal rhythm disorder

I49.9 **Cardiac arrhythmia, unspecified**
Arrhythmia (cardiac) NOS

I50 Heart failure

Code first heart failure complicating abortion or ectopic or molar pregnancy (O00-O07, O08.8)
heart failure due to hypertension (I11.0)
heart failure due to hypertension with chronic kidney disease (I13.-)
heart failure following surgery (I97.13-)
obstetric surgery and procedures (O75.4)
rheumatic heart failure (I09.81)

Excludes1 neonatal cardiac failure (P29.0)

Excludes2 cardiac arrest (I46.-)

Coding Clinic: 2017, Q1, P47; 2016, Q4, P122-123, Q1, P38; 2015, Q2, P15

I50.1 **Left ventricular failure, unspecified**
Cardiac asthma
Edema of lung with heart disease NOS
Edema of lung with heart failure
Left heart failure
Pulmonary edema with heart disease NOS
Pulmonary edema with heart failure

Excludes1 edema of lung without heart disease or heart failure (J81.-)
pulmonary edema without heart disease or failure (J81.-)

I50.2 **Systolic (congestive) heart failure**
Heart failure with reduced ejection fraction [HFrEF]
Systolic left ventricular heart failure

Code also end stage heart failure, if applicable (I50.84)

Excludes1 combined systolic (congestive) and diastolic (congestive) heart failure (I50.4-)

I50.20 **Unspecified systolic (congestive) heart failure**

I50.21 **Acute systolic (congestive) heart failure**
Presenting a short and relatively severe episode

I50.22 **Chronic systolic (congestive) heart failure**
Long-lasting, presenting over time

I50.23 **Acute on chronic systolic (congestive) heart failure**
Combination code. What was a chronic condition now has an acute exacerbation (to make more severe).
Coding Clinic: 2013, Q2, P33

I50.3 **Diastolic (congestive) heart failure**
Diastolic left ventricular heart failure
Heart failure with normal ejection fraction
Heart failure with preserved ejection fraction [HFpEF]

Code also end stage heart failure, if applicable (I50.84)

Excludes1 combined systolic (congestive) and diastolic (congestive) heart failure (I50.4-)

I50.30 **Unspecified diastolic (congestive) heart failure**

I50.31 **Acute diastolic (congestive) heart failure**
Coding Clinic: 2017, Q1, P46

I50.32 **Chronic diastolic (congestive) heart failure**

I50.33 **Acute on chronic diastolic (congestive) heart failure**

Item 9–8 Congestive heart failure (CHF) is a condition in which the left ventricle of the heart cannot pump enough blood to the body. The blood flow from the heart slows or returns to the heart from the venous system (back flow) resulting in congestion (fluid accumulation) particularly in the abdomen. Most commonly, fluid collects in the lungs and results in shortness of breath, especially when in a reclining position.

I50.4 Combined systolic (congestive) and diastolic (congestive) heart failure
Combined systolic and diastolic left ventricular heart failure
Heart failure with reduced ejection fraction and diastolic dysfunction
Code also end stage heart failure, if applicable (I50.84)

I50.40 Unspecified combined systolic (congestive) and diastolic (congestive) heart failure

I50.41 Acute combined systolic (congestive) and diastolic (congestive) heart failure

I50.42 Chronic combined systolic (congestive) and diastolic (congestive) heart failure

I50.43 Acute on chronic combined systolic (congestive) and diastolic (congestive) heart failure

I50.8 Other heart failure

I50.81 Right heart failure
Right ventricular failure

I50.810 Right heart failure, unspecified
Right heart failure without mention of left heart failure
Right ventricular failure NOS

I50.811 Acute right heart failure
Acute isolated right heart failure
Acute (isolated) right ventricular failure

I50.812 Chronic right heart failure
Chronic isolated right heart failure
Chronic (isolated) right ventricular failure

I50.813 Acute on chronic right heart failure
Acute on chronic isolated right heart failure
Acute on chronic (isolated) right ventricular failure
Acute decompensation of chronic (isolated) right ventricular failure
Acute exacerbation of chronic (isolated) right ventricular failure

I50.814 Right heart failure due to left heart failure
Right ventricular failure secondary to left ventricular failure
Code also the type of left ventricular failure, if known (I50.2-I50.43)
Excludes1 Right heart failure with but not due to left heart failure (I50.82)

I50.82 Biventricular heart failure
Code also the type of left ventricular failure as systolic, diastolic, or combined, if known **(I50.2-I50.43)**

I50.83 High output heart failure

I50.84 End stage heart failure
Stage D heart failure
Code also the type of heart failure as systolic, diastolic, or combined, if known (I50.2-I50.43)

I50.89 Other heart failure

I50.9 Heart failure, unspecified
Cardiac, heart or myocardial failure NOS
Congestive heart disease
Congestive heart failure NOS
Excludes2 fluid overload unrelated to congestive heart failure (E87.70)
Coding Clinic: 2017, Q1, P45-46; 2015, Q2, P15; 2012, Q4, P92

I51 Complications and ill-defined descriptions of heart disease
Excludes1 any condition in I51.4-I51.9 due to hypertension (I11.-)
any condition in I51.4-I51.9 due to hypertension and chronic kidney disease (I13.-)
heart disease specified as rheumatic (I00-I09)

I51.0 Cardiac septal defect, acquired A
Acquired septal atrial defect (old)
Acquired septal auricular defect (old)
Acquired septal ventricular defect (old)
Excludes1 cardiac septal defect as current complication following acute myocardial infarction (I23.1, I23.2)

I51.1 Rupture of chordae tendineae, not elsewhere classified
Excludes1 rupture of chordae tendineae as current complication following acute myocardial infarction (I23.4)

I51.2 Rupture of papillary muscle, not elsewhere classified
Excludes1 rupture of papillary muscle as current complication following acute myocardial infarction (I23.5)

I51.3 Intracardiac thrombosis, not elsewhere classified
Apical thrombosis (old)
Atrial thrombosis (old)
Auricular thrombosis (old)
Mural thrombosis (old)
Ventricular thrombosis (old)
Excludes1 intracardiac thrombosis as current complication following acute myocardial infarction (I23.6)
Coding Clinic: 2013, Q1, P24

I51.4 Myocarditis, unspecified
Chronic (interstitial) myocarditis
Myocardial fibrosis
Myocarditis NOS
Excludes1 acute or subacute myocarditis (I40.-)
Coding Clinic: 2016, Q4, P122

I51.5 Myocardial degeneration
Fatty degeneration of heart or myocardium
Myocardial disease
Senile degeneration of heart or myocardium
Coding Clinic: 2016, Q4, P122

I51.7 Cardiomegaly
Cardiac dilatation
Cardiac hypertrophy
Ventricular dilatation
Coding Clinic: 2016, Q4, P122

I51.8 Other ill-defined heart diseases
Coding Clinic: 2016, Q4, P122

I51.81 Takotsubo syndrome
Reversible left ventricular dysfunction following sudden emotional stress
Stress induced cardiomyopathy
Takotsubo cardiomyopathy
Transient left ventricular apical ballooning syndrome

I51.89 Other ill-defined heart diseases
Carditis (acute)(chronic)
Pancarditis (acute)(chronic)
Coding Clinic: 2019, Q2, P6

I51.9 Heart disease, unspecified
Coding Clinic: 2016, Q4, P122

I52 *Other heart disorders in diseases classified elsewhere*
Code first underlying disease, such as:
congenital syphilis (A50.5)
mucopolysaccharidosis (E76.3)
schistosomiasis (B65.0-B65.9)
Excludes1 heart disease (in):
gonococcal infection (A54.83)
meningococcal infection (A39.50)
rheumatoid arthritis (M05.31)
syphilis (A52.06)

CEREBROVASCULAR DISEASES (I60-I69)

Use additional code to identify presence of:
alcohol abuse and dependence (F10.-)
exposure to environmental tobacco smoke (Z77.22)
history of tobacco dependence (Z87.891)
hypertension (I10-I16)
occupational exposure to environmental tobacco smoke (Z57.31)
tobacco dependence (F17.-)
tobacco use (Z72.0)
Excludes1 traumatic intracranial hemorrhage (S06.-)
Coding Clinic: 2015, Q4, P40

I60 Nontraumatic subarachnoid hemorrhage
Excludes1 syphilitic ruptured cerebral aneurysm (A52.05)
Excludes2 sequelae of subarachnoid hemorrhage (I69.0-)

I60.0 Nontraumatic subarachnoid hemorrhage from carotid siphon and bifurcation
I60.00 Nontraumatic subarachnoid hemorrhage from unspecified carotid siphon and bifurcation
I60.01 Nontraumatic subarachnoid hemorrhage from right carotid siphon and bifurcation
I60.02 Nontraumatic subarachnoid hemorrhage from left carotid siphon and bifurcation

I60.1 Nontraumatic subarachnoid hemorrhage from middle cerebral artery
I60.10 Nontraumatic subarachnoid hemorrhage from unspecified middle cerebral artery
I60.11 Nontraumatic subarachnoid hemorrhage from right middle cerebral artery
I60.12 Nontraumatic subarachnoid hemorrhage from left middle cerebral artery

I60.2 Nontraumatic subarachnoid hemorrhage from anterior communicating artery

I60.3 Nontraumatic subarachnoid hemorrhage from posterior communicating artery
I60.30 Nontraumatic subarachnoid hemorrhage from unspecified posterior communicating artery
I60.31 Nontraumatic subarachnoid hemorrhage from right posterior communicating artery
I60.32 Nontraumatic subarachnoid hemorrhage from left posterior communicating artery

I60.4 Nontraumatic subarachnoid hemorrhage from basilar artery

I60.5 Nontraumatic subarachnoid hemorrhage from vertebral artery
I60.50 Nontraumatic subarachnoid hemorrhage from unspecified vertebral artery
I60.51 Nontraumatic subarachnoid hemorrhage from right vertebral artery
I60.52 Nontraumatic subarachnoid hemorrhage from left vertebral artery

I60.6 Nontraumatic subarachnoid hemorrhage from other intracranial arteries

I60.7 Nontraumatic subarachnoid hemorrhage from unspecified intracranial artery
Ruptured (congenital) berry aneurysm
Ruptured (congenital) cerebral aneurysm
Subarachnoid hemorrhage (nontraumatic) from cerebral artery NOS
Subarachnoid hemorrhage (nontraumatic) from communicating artery NOS
Excludes1 berry aneurysm, nonruptured (I67.1)

I60.8 Other nontraumatic subarachnoid hemorrhage
Meningeal hemorrhage
Rupture of cerebral arteriovenous malformation

I60.9 Nontraumatic subarachnoid hemorrhage, unspecified

I61 Nontraumatic intracerebral hemorrhage
Excludes2 sequelae of intracerebral hemorrhage (I69.1-)
Coding Clinic: 2017, Q2, P10

I61.0 Nontraumatic intracerebral hemorrhage in hemisphere, subcortical
Deep intracerebral hemorrhage (nontraumatic)
Coding Clinic: 2016, Q4, P27

I61.1 Nontraumatic intracerebral hemorrhage in hemisphere, cortical
Cerebral lobe hemorrhage (nontraumatic)
Superficial intracerebral hemorrhage (nontraumatic)
Coding Clinic: 2016, Q4, P28

I61.2 Nontraumatic intracerebral hemorrhage in hemisphere, unspecified
I61.3 Nontraumatic intracerebral hemorrhage in brain stem
I61.4 Nontraumatic intracerebral hemorrhage in cerebellum
I61.5 Nontraumatic intracerebral hemorrhage, intraventricular
I61.6 Nontraumatic intracerebral hemorrhage, multiple localized
I61.8 Other nontraumatic intracerebral hemorrhage
I61.9 Nontraumatic intracerebral hemorrhage, unspecified

I62 Other and unspecified nontraumatic intracranial hemorrhage
Excludes2 sequelae of intracranial hemorrhage (I69.2)

I62.0 Nontraumatic subdural hemorrhage
I62.00 Nontraumatic subdural hemorrhage, unspecified
I62.01 Nontraumatic acute subdural hemorrhage
I62.02 Nontraumatic subacute subdural hemorrhage
I62.03 Nontraumatic chronic subdural hemorrhage

I62.1 Nontraumatic extradural hemorrhage
Nontraumatic epidural hemorrhage

I62.9 Nontraumatic intracranial hemorrhage, unspecified

★(See Plate 31 of the Anatomy Illustrations.)

I63 Cerebral infarction
Includes occlusion and stenosis of cerebral and precerebral arteries, resulting in cerebral infarction
Use additional code, if applicable, to identify status post administration of tPA (rtPA) in a different facility within the last 24 hours prior to admission to current facility (Z92.82)
Use additional code, if known, to indicate National Institutes of Health Stroke Scale (NIHSS) score (R29.7-)
Excludes2 sequelae of cerebral infarction (I69.3-)
Coding Clinic: 2016, Q4, P28, 61, 127

I63.0 Cerebral infarction due to thrombosis of precerebral arteries
I63.00 Cerebral infarction due to thrombosis of unspecified precerebral artery

CHAPTER 9 (I00-I99)

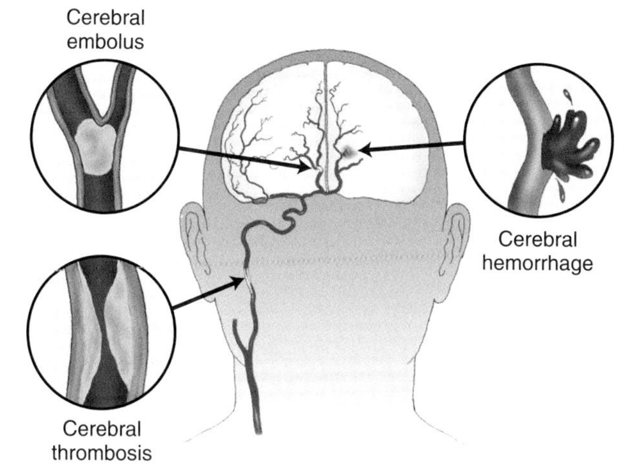

Figure 9-4 Events causing a stroke. (From Shiland: Mastering Healthcare Terminology, ed 1, St. Louis, Mosby, 2003)

- **I63.Ø1** Cerebral infarction due to thrombosis of vertebral artery
  - I63.Ø11 Cerebral infarction due to thrombosis of right vertebral artery
  - I63.Ø12 Cerebral infarction due to thrombosis of left vertebral artery
  - I63.Ø13 Cerebral infarction due to thrombosis of bilateral vertebral arteries
  - I63.Ø19 Cerebral infarction due to thrombosis of unspecified vertebral artery
- I63.Ø2 Cerebral infarction due to thrombosis of basilar artery
- **I63.Ø3** Cerebral infarction due to thrombosis of carotid artery
  - I63.Ø31 Cerebral infarction due to thrombosis of right carotid artery
  - I63.Ø32 Cerebral infarction due to thrombosis of left carotid artery
  - I63.Ø33 Cerebral infarction due to thrombosis of bilateral carotid arteries
  - I63.Ø39 Cerebral infarction due to thrombosis of unspecified carotid artery
- I63.Ø9 Cerebral infarction due to thrombosis of other precerebral artery

I63.1 Cerebral infarction due to embolism of precerebral arteries
- I63.1Ø Cerebral infarction due to embolism of unspecified precerebral artery
- **I63.11** Cerebral infarction due to embolism of vertebral artery
  - I63.111 Cerebral infarction due to embolism of right vertebral artery
  - I63.112 Cerebral infarction due to embolism of left vertebral artery
  - I63.113 Cerebral infarction due to embolism of bilateral vertebral arteries
  - I63.119 Cerebral infarction due to embolism of unspecified vertebral artery
- I63.12 Cerebral infarction due to embolism of basilar artery
- **I63.13** Cerebral infarction due to embolism of carotid artery
  - I63.131 Cerebral infarction due to embolism of right carotid artery
  - I63.132 Cerebral infarction due to embolism of left carotid artery
  - I63.133 Cerebral infarction due to embolism of bilateral carotid arteries
  - I63.139 Cerebral infarction due to embolism of unspecified carotid artery
- I63.19 Cerebral infarction due to embolism of other precerebral artery

I63.2 Cerebral infarction due to unspecified occlusion or stenosis of precerebral arteries
- I63.2Ø Cerebral infarction due to unspecified occlusion or stenosis of unspecified precerebral arteries
- **I63.21** Cerebral infarction due to unspecified occlusion or stenosis of vertebral arteries
  - I63.211 Cerebral infarction due to unspecified occlusion or stenosis of right vertebral artery
  - I63.212 Cerebral infarction due to unspecified occlusion or stenosis of left vertebral artery
  - I63.213 Cerebral infarction due to unspecified occlusion or stenosis of bilateral vertebral arteries
  - I63.219 Cerebral infarction due to unspecified occlusion or stenosis of unspecified vertebral artery
- I63.22 Cerebral infarction due to unspecified occlusion or stenosis of basilar artery
- **I63.23** Cerebral infarction due to unspecified occlusion or stenosis of carotid arteries
  - I63.231 Cerebral infarction due to unspecified occlusion or stenosis of right carotid arteries
  - I63.232 Cerebral infarction due to unspecified occlusion or stenosis of left carotid arteries
  - I63.233 Cerebral infarction due to unspecified occlusion or stenosis of bilateral carotid arteries
  - I63.239 Cerebral infarction due to unspecified occlusion or stenosis of unspecified carotid artery
- I63.29 Cerebral infarction due to unspecified occlusion or stenosis of other precerebral arteries

I63.3 Cerebral infarction due to thrombosis of cerebral arteries
- I63.3Ø Cerebral infarction due to thrombosis of unspecified cerebral artery
- **I63.31** Cerebral infarction due to thrombosis of middle cerebral artery
  - I63.311 Cerebral infarction due to thrombosis of right middle cerebral artery
  - I63.312 Cerebral infarction due to thrombosis of left middle cerebral artery
  - I63.313 Cerebral infarction due to thrombosis of bilateral middle cerebral arteries
  - I63.319 Cerebral infarction due to thrombosis of unspecified middle cerebral artery
- **I63.32** Cerebral infarction due to thrombosis of anterior cerebral artery
  - I63.321 Cerebral infarction due to thrombosis of right anterior cerebral artery
  - I63.322 Cerebral infarction due to thrombosis of left anterior cerebral artery
  - I63.323 Cerebral infarction due to thrombosis of bilateral anterior cerebral arteries
  - I63.329 Cerebral infarction due to thrombosis of unspecified anterior cerebral artery

- I63.33 Cerebral infarction due to thrombosis of posterior cerebral artery
  - I63.331 Cerebral infarction due to thrombosis of right posterior cerebral artery
  - I63.332 Cerebral infarction due to thrombosis of left posterior cerebral artery
  - I63.333 Cerebral infarction due to thrombosis of bilateral posterior cerebral arteries
  - I63.339 Cerebral infarction due to thrombosis of unspecified posterior cerebral artery
- I63.34 Cerebral infarction due to thrombosis of cerebellar artery
  - I63.341 Cerebral infarction due to thrombosis of right cerebellar artery
  - I63.342 Cerebral infarction due to thrombosis of left cerebellar artery
  - I63.343 Cerebral infarction due to thrombosis of bilateral cerebellar arteries
  - I63.349 Cerebral infarction due to thrombosis of unspecified cerebellar artery
- I63.39 Cerebral infarction due to thrombosis of other cerebral artery

I63.4 Cerebral infarction due to embolism of cerebral arteries

- I63.40 Cerebral infarction due to embolism of unspecified cerebral artery
- I63.41 Cerebral infarction due to embolism of middle cerebral artery
  - I63.411 Cerebral infarction due to embolism of right middle cerebral artery
  - I63.412 Cerebral infarction due to embolism of left middle cerebral artery
  - I63.413 Cerebral infarction due to embolism of bilateral middle cerebral arteries
  - I63.419 Cerebral infarction due to embolism of unspecified middle cerebral artery
- I63.42 Cerebral infarction due to embolism of anterior cerebral artery
  - I63.421 Cerebral infarction due to embolism of right anterior cerebral artery
  - I63.422 Cerebral infarction due to embolism of left anterior cerebral artery
  - I63.423 Cerebral infarction due to embolism of bilateral anterior cerebral arteries
  - I63.429 Cerebral infarction due to embolism of unspecified anterior cerebral artery
- I63.43 Cerebral infarction due to embolism of posterior cerebral artery
  - I63.431 Cerebral infarction due to embolism of right posterior cerebral artery
  - I63.432 Cerebral infarction due to embolism of left posterior cerebral artery
  - I63.433 Cerebral infarction due to embolism of bilateral posterior cerebral arteries
  - I63.439 Cerebral infarction due to embolism of unspecified posterior cerebral artery
- I63.44 Cerebral infarction due to embolism of cerebellar artery
  - I63.441 Cerebral infarction due to embolism of right cerebellar artery
  - I63.442 Cerebral infarction due to embolism of left cerebellar artery
  - I63.443 Cerebral infarction due to embolism of bilateral cerebellar arteries
  - I63.449 Cerebral infarction due to embolism of unspecified cerebellar artery
- I63.49 Cerebral infarction due to embolism of other cerebral artery

I63.5 Cerebral infarction due to unspecified occlusion or stenosis of cerebral arteries

- I63.5Ø Cerebral infarction due to unspecified occlusion or stenosis of unspecified cerebral artery
- I63.51 Cerebral infarction due to unspecified occlusion or stenosis of middle cerebral artery
  - I63.511 Cerebral infarction due to unspecified occlusion or stenosis of right middle cerebral artery
  - I63.512 Cerebral infarction due to unspecified occlusion or stenosis of left middle cerebral artery
  - I63.513 Cerebral infarction due to unspecified occlusion or stenosis of bilateral middle cerebral arteries
  - I63.519 Cerebral infarction due to unspecified occlusion or stenosis of unspecified middle cerebral artery
- I63.52 Cerebral infarction due to unspecified occlusion or stenosis of anterior cerebral artery
  - I63.521 Cerebral infarction due to unspecified occlusion or stenosis of right anterior cerebral artery
  - I63.522 Cerebral infarction due to unspecified occlusion or stenosis of left anterior cerebral artery
  - I63.523 Cerebral infarction due to unspecified occlusion or stenosis of bilateral anterior cerebral arteries
  - I63.529 Cerebral infarction due to unspecified occlusion or stenosis of unspecified anterior cerebral artery
- I63.53 Cerebral infarction due to unspecified occlusion or stenosis of posterior cerebral artery
  - I63.531 Cerebral infarction due to unspecified occlusion or stenosis of right posterior cerebral artery
  - I63.532 Cerebral infarction due to unspecified occlusion or stenosis of left posterior cerebral artery
    Coding Clinic: 2Ø17, Q2, P1Ø
  - I63.533 Cerebral infarction due to unspecified occlusion or stenosis of bilateral posterior cerebral arteries
  - I63.539 Cerebral infarction due to unspecified occlusion or stenosis of unspecified posterior cerebral artery

● I63.54   Cerebral infarction due to unspecified occlusion or stenosis of cerebellar artery

    I63.541   Cerebral infarction due to unspecified occlusion or stenosis of **right cerebellar artery** 🔖

    I63.542   Cerebral infarction due to unspecified occlusion or stenosis of **left cerebellar artery** 🔖

    I63.543   Cerebral infarction due to unspecified occlusion or stenosis of **bilateral cerebellar arteries** 🔖

    I63.549   Cerebral infarction due to unspecified occlusion or stenosis of **unspecified cerebellar artery** 🔖

   I63.59   Cerebral infarction due to unspecified occlusion or stenosis of **other cerebral artery** 🔖

I63.6   Cerebral infarction due to cerebral venous thrombosis, **nonpyogenic** 🔖

● I63.8   Other cerebral infarction 🔖

   I63.81   Other cerebral infarction due to occlusion or stenosis of **small artery** 🔖
      Lacunar infarction
      Coding Clinic: 2018, Q4, P16

   I63.89   Other cerebral infarction 🔖
      Coding Clinic: 2017, Q2, P9

I63.9   Cerebral infarction, **unspecified** 🔖
     Stroke NOS

     Excludes2   transient cerebral ischemic attacks and related syndromes (G45.-)
     Coding Clinic: 2016, Q4, P62; 2015, Q1, P26

● I65   Occlusion and stenosis of **precerebral arteries, not resulting in cerebral infarction**

   Includes   embolism of precerebral artery
     narrowing of precerebral artery
     obstruction (complete) (partial) of precerebral artery
     thrombosis of precerebral artery

   Excludes1   insufficiency, NOS, of precerebral artery (G45.-)
     insufficiency of precerebral arteries causing cerebral infarction (I63.0-I63.2)

● I65.0   Occlusion and stenosis of **vertebral artery**

   I65.01   Occlusion and stenosis of **right vertebral artery**
   I65.02   Occlusion and stenosis of **left vertebral artery**
   I65.03   Occlusion and stenosis of **bilateral vertebral arteries**
   I65.09   Occlusion and stenosis of **unspecified vertebral artery**

I65.1   Occlusion and stenosis of **basilar artery**

● I65.2   Occlusion and stenosis of **carotid artery**

   I65.21   Occlusion and stenosis of **right carotid artery**
   I65.22   Occlusion and stenosis of **left carotid artery**
   I65.23   Occlusion and stenosis of **bilateral carotid arteries**
   I65.29   Occlusion and stenosis of **unspecified carotid artery**

I65.8   Occlusion and stenosis of **other precerebral arteries**

I65.9   Occlusion and stenosis of **unspecified precerebral artery**
     Occlusion and stenosis of precerebral artery NOS

● I66   Occlusion and stenosis of **cerebral arteries, not resulting in cerebral infarction**

   Includes   embolism of cerebral artery
     narrowing of cerebral artery
     obstruction (complete) (partial) of cerebral artery
     thrombosis of cerebral artery

   Excludes1   occlusion and stenosis of cerebral artery causing cerebral infarction (I63.3-I63.5)

● I66.0   Occlusion and stenosis of **middle cerebral artery**

   I66.01   Occlusion and stenosis of **right middle cerebral artery**
   I66.02   Occlusion and stenosis of **left middle cerebral artery**
   I66.03   Occlusion and stenosis of **bilateral middle cerebral arteries**
   I66.09   Occlusion and stenosis of **unspecified middle cerebral artery**

● I66.1   Occlusion and stenosis of **anterior cerebral artery**

   I66.11   Occlusion and stenosis of **right anterior cerebral artery**
   I66.12   Occlusion and stenosis of **left anterior cerebral artery**
   I66.13   Occlusion and stenosis of **bilateral anterior cerebral arteries**
   I66.19   Occlusion and stenosis of **unspecified anterior cerebral artery**

● I66.2   Occlusion and stenosis of **posterior cerebral artery**

   I66.21   Occlusion and stenosis of **right posterior cerebral artery**
   I66.22   Occlusion and stenosis of **left posterior cerebral artery**
   I66.23   Occlusion and stenosis of **bilateral posterior cerebral arteries**
   I66.29   Occlusion and stenosis of **unspecified posterior cerebral artery**

I66.3   Occlusion and stenosis of **cerebellar arteries**

I66.8   Occlusion and stenosis of **other cerebral arteries**
     Occlusion and stenosis of perforating arteries

I66.9   Occlusion and stenosis of **unspecified cerebral artery**

● I67   Other cerebrovascular diseases

   Excludes2   sequelae of the listed conditions (I69.8)

   I67.0   Dissection of cerebral arteries, **nonruptured** 🔖

     Excludes1   ruptured cerebral arteries (I60.7)

   I67.1   Cerebral aneurysm, **nonruptured**
     Cerebral aneurysm NOS
     Cerebral arteriovenous fistula, acquired
     Internal carotid artery aneurysm, intracranial portion
     Internal carotid artery aneurysm, NOS

     Excludes1   congenital cerebral aneurysm, nonruptured (Q28.-)
       ruptured cerebral aneurysm (I60.7)

   I67.2   Cerebral atherosclerosis   A
     Atheroma of cerebral and precerebral arteries

   I67.3   Progressive vascular leukoencephalopathy
     Binswanger's disease

   I67.4   Hypertensive encephalopathy

     Excludes2   insufficiency, NOS, of precerebral arteries (G45.2)

   I67.5   Moyamoya disease

   I67.6   Nonpyogenic thrombosis of **intracranial venous system**
     Nonpyogenic thrombosis of cerebral vein
     Nonpyogenic thrombosis of intracranial venous sinus

     Excludes1   nonpyogenic thrombosis of intracranial venous system causing infarction (I63.6)

   I67.7   Cerebral arteritis, not elsewhere classified
     Granulomatous angiitis of the nervous system

     Excludes1   allergic granulomatous angiitis (M30.1)

● **I67.8**   **Other specified cerebrovascular diseases**

  I67.81   **Acute cerebrovascular insufficiency**
             Acute cerebrovascular insufficiency
                 unspecified as to location or reversibility

  I67.82   **Cerebral ischemia**
             Chronic cerebral ischemia

  I67.83   **Posterior reversible encephalopathy syndrome**
             PRES

● **I67.84**   **Cerebral vasospasm and vasoconstriction**

  I67.841   **Reversible cerebrovascular vasoconstriction syndrome**
             Call-Fleming syndrome

             Code first underlying condition, if applicable, such as eclampsia (O15.00-O15.9)

  I67.848   **Other cerebrovascular vasospasm and vasoconstriction**

● **I67.85**   **Hereditary cerebrovascular diseases**

  I67.850   **Cerebral autosomal dominant arteriopathy with subcortical infarcts and leukoencephalopathy**
             CADASIL

             Code also any associated diagnoses, such as:
                 epilepsy (G40.-), stroke (I63.-)
                 vascular dementia (F01.-)

  I67.858   **Other hereditary cerebrovascular disease**

  I67.89   **Other cerebrovascular disease**

  I67.9   **Cerebrovascular disease, unspecified**

● **I68**   **Cerebrovascular disorders in diseases classified elsewhere**

▶ *I68.0*   *Cerebral amyloid angiopathy*
             Code first underlying amyloidosis (E85.-)

▶ *I68.2*   *Cerebral arteritis in other diseases classified elsewhere*
             Code first underlying disease

             Excludes1   cerebral arteritis (in):
                 listerosis (A32.89)
                 systemic lupus erythematosus (M32.19)
                 syphilis (A52.04)
                 tuberculosis (A18.89)

▶ *I68.8*   *Other cerebrovascular disorders in diseases classified elsewhere*
             Code first underlying disease

             Excludes1   syphilitic cerebral aneurysm (A52.05)

OGCR Section I.c.9.d.

Sequelae of Cerebrovascular Disease

1) Category I69, Sequelae of Cerebrovascular disease

Category I69 is used to indicate conditions classifiable to categories I60-I67 as the causes of sequela (neurologic deficits), themselves classified elsewhere. These "late effects" include neurologic deficits that persist after initial onset of conditions classifiable to categories I60-I67. The neurologic deficits caused by cerebrovascular disease may be present from the onset of may arise at any time after the onset of the condition classifiable to categories I60-I67.

Codes from category I69, Sequelae of cerebrovascular disease, that specify hemiplegia, hemiparesis and monoplegia identify whether the dominant or nondominant side is affected. Should the affected side be documented, but not specified as dominant or nondominant, and the classification system does not indicate a default, code selection is as follows:

For ambidextrous patients, the default should be dominant.

If the left side is affected, the default is nondominant.

If the right side is affected, the default is dominant.

2) Codes from category I69 with codes from I60-I67

Codes from category I69 may be assigned on a health care record with codes from I60-I67, if the patient has a current cerebrovascular disease and deficits from an old cerebrovascular disease.

● **I69**   **Sequelae of cerebrovascular disease**

  Note: Category I69 is to be used to indicate conditions in I60-I67 as the cause of sequelae. The 'sequelae' include conditions specified as such or as residuals which may occur at any time after the onset of the causal condition.

  Excludes1   personal history of cerebral infarction without residual deficit (Z86.73)
             personal history of prolonged reversible ischemic neurologic deficit (PRIND) (Z86.73)
             personal history of reversible ischemic neurologcal deficit (RIND) (Z86.73)
             sequelae of traumatic intracranial injury (S06.-)

  Coding Clinic: 2016, Q4, P28; 2015, Q4, P40; 2012, Q4, P107

● **I69.0**   **Sequelae of nontraumatic subarachnoid hemorrhage**

  I69.00   **Unspecified sequelae of nontraumatic subarachnoid hemorrhage**

● **I69.01**   **Cognitive deficits following nontraumatic subarachnoid hemorrhage**

  I69.010   **Attention and concentration deficit following nontraumatic subarachnoid hemorrhage**

  I69.011   **Memory deficit following nontraumatic subarachnoid hemorrhage**

  I69.012   **Visuospatial deficit and spatial neglect following nontraumatic subarachnoid hemorrhage**

  I69.013   **Psychomotor deficit following nontraumatic subarachnoid hemorrhage**

  I69.014   **Frontal lobe and executive function deficit following nontraumatic subarachnoid hemorrhage**

  I69.015   **Cognitive social or emotional deficit following nontraumatic subarachnoid hemorrhage**

  I69.018   **Other symptoms and signs involving cognitive functions following nontraumatic subarachnoid hemorrhage**

  I69.019   **Unspecified symptoms and signs involving cognitive functions following nontraumatic subarachnoid hemorrhage**

● **I69.02**   **Speech and language deficits following nontraumatic subarachnoid hemorrhage**

  I69.020   **Aphasia following nontraumatic subarachnoid hemorrhage**

  I69.021   **Dysphasia following nontraumatic subarachnoid hemorrhage**

  I69.022   **Dysarthria following nontraumatic subarachnoid hemorrhage**

  I69.023   **Fluency disorder following nontraumatic subarachnoid hemorrhage**
             Stuttering following nontraumatic subarachnoid hemorrhage

  I69.028   **Other speech and language deficits following nontraumatic subarachnoid hemorrhage**

▶ New   ⏩ Revised   ~~deleted~~ Deleted   Excludes 1   Excludes 2   Includes   Use additional   Code first   Code also   Key words

OGCR Official Guidelines   X Assign placeholder X   ● Use Additional Character(s)   ▶ Manifestation Code   🞈 Hierarchical Condition Category   Coding Clinic

● **I69.03 Monoplegia of upper limb following nontraumatic subarachnoid hemorrhage**

    I69.031 Monoplegia of upper limb following nontraumatic subarachnoid hemorrhage affecting **right dominant side** 🦠

    I69.032 Monoplegia of upper limb following nontraumatic subarachnoid hemorrhage affecting **left dominant side** 🦠

    I69.033 Monoplegia of upper limb following nontraumatic subarachnoid hemorrhage affecting **right non-dominant side** 🦠

    I69.034 Monoplegia of upper limb following nontraumatic subarachnoid hemorrhage affecting **left non-dominant side** 🦠

    I69.039 Monoplegia of upper limb following nontraumatic subarachnoid hemorrhage affecting **unspecified side** 🦠

● **I69.04 Monoplegia of lower limb following nontraumatic subarachnoid hemorrhage**

    I69.041 Monoplegia of lower limb following nontraumatic subarachnoid hemorrhage affecting **right dominant side** 🦠

    I69.042 Monoplegia of lower limb following nontraumatic subarachnoid hemorrhage affecting **left dominant side** 🦠

    I69.043 Monoplegia of lower limb following nontraumatic subarachnoid hemorrhage affecting **right non-dominant side** 🦠

    I69.044 Monoplegia of lower limb following nontraumatic subarachnoid hemorrhage affecting **left non-dominant side** 🦠

    I69.049 Monoplegia of lower limb following nontraumatic subarachnoid hemorrhage affecting **unspecified side** 🦠

● **I69.05 Hemiplegia and hemiparesis following nontraumatic subarachnoid hemorrhage**

    I69.051 Hemiplegia and hemiparesis following nontraumatic subarachnoid hemorrhage affecting **right dominant side** 🦠

    I69.052 Hemiplegia and hemiparesis following nontraumatic subarachnoid hemorrhage affecting **left dominant side** 🦠

    I69.053 Hemiplegia and hemiparesis following nontraumatic subarachnoid hemorrhage affecting **right non-dominant side** 🦠

    I69.054 Hemiplegia and hemiparesis following nontraumatic subarachnoid hemorrhage affecting **left non-dominant side** 🦠

    I69.059 Hemiplegia and hemiparesis following nontraumatic subarachnoid hemorrhage affecting **unspecified side** 🦠

● **I69.06 Other paralytic syndrome following nontraumatic subarachnoid hemorrhage**

    Use additional code to identify type of paralytic syndrome, such as:
    locked-in state (G83.5)
    quadriplegia (G82.5-)

    Excludes1 hemiplegia/hemiparesis following nontraumatic subarachnoid hemorrhage (I69.05-)
                monoplegia of lower limb following nontraumatic subarachnoid hemorrhage (I69.04-)
                monoplegia of upper limb following nontraumatic subarachnoid hemorrhage (I69.03-)

    I69.061 Other paralytic syndrome following nontraumatic subarachnoid hemorrhage affecting **right dominant side** 🦠

    I69.062 Other paralytic syndrome following nontraumatic subarachnoid hemorrhage affecting **left dominant side** 🦠

    I69.063 Other paralytic syndrome following nontraumatic subarachnoid hemorrhage affecting **right non-dominant side** 🦠

    I69.064 Other paralytic syndrome following nontraumatic subarachnoid hemorrhage affecting **left non-dominant side** 🦠

    I69.065 Other paralytic syndrome following nontraumatic subarachnoid hemorrhage, **bilateral** 🦠

    I69.069 Other paralytic syndrome following nontraumatic subarachnoid hemorrhage affecting **unspecified side** 🦠

● **I69.09 Other sequelae of nontraumatic subarachnoid hemorrhage**

    I69.090 **Apraxia following nontraumatic subarachnoid hemorrhage**

    I69.091 **Dysphagia following nontraumatic subarachnoid hemorrhage**

        Use additional code to identify the type of dysphagia, if known (R13.1-)

    I69.092 **Facial weakness following nontraumatic subarachnoid hemorrhage**
        Facial droop following nontraumatic subarachnoid hemorrhage

    I69.093 **Ataxia following nontraumatic subarachnoid hemorrhage**

    I69.098 **Other sequelae following nontraumatic subarachnoid hemorrhage**
        Alterations of sensation following nontraumatic subarachnoid hemorrhage
        Disturbance of vision following nontraumatic subarachnoid hemorrhage
        Use additional code to identify the sequelae

CHAPTER 9 (I00-I99)

- I69.1 Sequelae of nontraumatic **intracerebral** hemorrhage
  - I69.10 **Unspecified** sequelae of nontraumatic intracerebral hemorrhage
  - I69.11 **Cognitive deficits** following nontraumatic intracerebral hemorrhage
    - I69.110 **Attention and concentration** deficit following nontraumatic intracerebral hemorrhage
    - I69.111 **Memory** deficit following nontraumatic intracerebral hemorrhage
    - I69.112 **Visuospatial** deficit and spatial neglect following nontraumatic intracerebral hemorrhage
    - I69.113 **Psychomotor** deficit following nontraumatic intracerebral hemorrhage
    - I69.114 **Frontal lobe and executive function** deficit following nontraumatic intracerebral hemorrhage
    - I69.115 **Cognitive social or emotional deficit** following nontraumatic intracerebral hemorrhage
    - I69.118 **Other symptoms and signs** involving cognitive functions following nontraumatic intracerebral hemorrhage
    - I69.119 **Unspecified** symptoms and signs involving cognitive functions following nontraumatic intracerebral hemorrhage
  - I69.12 **Speech and language deficits** following nontraumatic intracerebral hemorrhage
    - I69.120 **Aphasia** following nontraumatic intracerebral hemorrhage
    - I69.121 **Dysphasia** following nontraumatic intracerebral hemorrhage
    - I69.122 **Dysarthria** following nontraumatic intracerebral hemorrhage
    - I69.123 **Fluency disorder** following nontraumatic intracerebral hemorrhage
      Stuttering following nontraumatic intracerebral hemorrhage
    - I69.128 **Other** speech and language deficits following nontraumatic intracerebral hemorrhage
  - I69.13 **Monoplegia of upper limb** following nontraumatic intracerebral hemorrhage
    - I69.131 Monoplegia of upper limb following nontraumatic intracerebral hemorrhage affecting **right dominant** side HCC
    - I69.132 Monoplegia of upper limb following nontraumatic intracerebral hemorrhage affecting **left dominant** side HCC
    - I69.133 Monoplegia of upper limb following nontraumatic intracerebral hemorrhage affecting **right non-dominant side** HCC
    - I69.134 Monoplegia of upper limb following nontraumatic intracerebral hemorrhage affecting left non-dominant side HCC
    - I69.139 Monoplegia of upper limb following nontraumatic intracerebral hemorrhage affecting **unspecified** side HCC
  - I69.14 **Monoplegia of lower limb** following nontraumatic intracerebral hemorrhage
    - I69.141 Monoplegia of lower limb following nontraumatic intracerebral hemorrhage affecting **right dominant** side HCC
    - I69.142 Monoplegia of lower limb following nontraumatic intracerebral hemorrhage affecting **left dominant** side HCC
    - I69.143 Monoplegia of lower limb following nontraumatic intracerebral hemorrhage affecting **right non-dominant side** HCC
    - I69.144 Monoplegia of lower limb following nontraumatic intracerebral hemorrhage affecting **left non-dominant side** HCC
    - I69.149 Monoplegia of lower limb following nontraumatic intracerebral hemorrhage affecting **unspecified** side HCC
  - I69.15 **Hemiplegia and hemiparesis** following nontraumatic intracerebral hemorrhage
    - I69.151 Hemiplegia and hemiparesis following nontraumatic intracerebral hemorrhage affecting **right dominant** side HCC
    - I69.152 Hemiplegia and hemiparesis following nontraumatic intracerebral hemorrhage affecting **left dominant** side HCC
    - I69.153 Hemiplegia and hemiparesis following nontraumatic intracerebral hemorrhage affecting **right non-dominant side** HCC
    - I69.154 Hemiplegia and hemiparesis following nontraumatic intracerebral hemorrhage affecting **left non-dominant side** HCC
    - I69.159 Hemiplegia and hemiparesis following nontraumatic intracerebral hemorrhage affecting **unspecified** side HCC
  - I69.16 **Other paralytic syndrome** following nontraumatic intracerebral hemorrhage

    Use additional code to identify type of paralytic syndrome, such as:
    locked-in state (G83.5)
    quadriplegia (G82.5-)

    Excludes1 hemiplegia/hemiparesis following nontraumatic intracerebral hemorrhage (I69.15-)
    monoplegia of lower limb following nontraumatic intracerebral hemorrhage (I69.14-)
    monoplegia of upper limb following nontraumatic intracerebral hemorrhage (I69.13-)
    - I69.161 Other paralytic syndrome following nontraumatic intracerebral hemorrhage affecting **right dominant** side HCC
    - I69.162 Other paralytic syndrome following nontraumatic intracerebral hemorrhage affecting **left dominant** side HCC
    - I69.163 Other paralytic syndrome following nontraumatic intracerebral hemorrhage affecting **right non-dominant side** HCC

CHAPTER 9 (I00-I99)

New | Revised | ~~deleted~~ Deleted | Excludes 1 | Excludes 2 | Includes | Use additional | Code first | Code also | Key words
OGCR Official Guidelines | X Assign placeholder X | Use Additional Character(s) | Manifestation Code | Hierarchical Condition Category | Coding Clinic

I69.164   Other paralytic syndrome following nontraumatic intracerebral hemorrhage affecting **left non-dominant side** 🔖

I69.165   Other paralytic syndrome following nontraumatic intracerebral hemorrhage, **bilateral** 🔖

I69.169   Other paralytic syndrome following nontraumatic intracerebral hemorrhage affecting **unspecified side** 🔖

● I69.19   **Other sequelae** of nontraumatic intracerebral hemorrhage

I69.190   **Apraxia** following nontraumatic intracerebral hemorrhage

I69.191   **Dysphagia** following nontraumatic intracerebral hemorrhage

Use additional code to identify the type of dysphagia, if known (R13.1-)

I69.192   **Facial weakness** following nontraumatic intracerebral hemorrhage

Facial droop following nontraumatic intracerebral hemorrhage

I69.193   **Ataxia** following nontraumatic intracerebral hemorrhage

I69.198   **Other sequelae** of nontraumatic intracerebral hemorrhage

Alteration of sensations following nontraumatic intracerebral hemorrhage

Disturbance of vision following nontraumatic intracerebral hemorrhage

Use additional code to identify the sequelae

● I69.2   **Sequelae of other nontraumatic intracranial hemorrhage**

I69.20   **Unspecified sequelae** of other nontraumatic intracranial hemorrhage

● I69.21   **Cognitive deficits** following other nontraumatic intracranial hemorrhage

I69.210   **Attention and concentration deficit** following other nontraumatic intracranial hemorrhage

I69.211   **Memory** deficit following other nontraumatic intracranial hemorrhage

I69.212   **Visuospatial** deficit and spatial neglect following other nontraumatic intracranial hemorrhage

I69.213   **Psychomotor** deficit following other nontraumatic intracranial hemorrhage

I69.214   **Frontal lobe and executive function** deficit following other nontraumatic intracranial hemorrhage

I69.215   **Cognitive social or emotional** deficit following other nontraumatic intracranial hemorrhage

I69.218   **Other** symptoms and signs involving cognitive functions following other nontraumatic intracranial hemorrhage

I69.219   **Unspecified** symptoms and signs involving cognitive functions following other nontraumatic intracranial hemorrhage

● I69.22   **Speech and language deficits** following other nontraumatic intracranial hemorrhage

I69.220   **Aphasia** following other nontraumatic intracranial hemorrhage

I69.221   **Dysphasia** following other nontraumatic intracranial hemorrhage

I69.222   **Dysarthria** following other nontraumatic intracranial hemorrhage

I69.223   **Fluency disorder** following other nontraumatic intracranial hemorrhage

Stuttering following other nontraumatic intracranial hemorrhage

I69.228   **Other speech and language deficits** following other nontraumatic intracranial hemorrhage

● I69.23   **Monoplegia of upper limb** following other nontraumatic intracranial hemorrhage

I69.231   Monoplegia of upper limb following other nontraumatic intracranial hemorrhage affecting **right dominant side** 🔖

I69.232   Monoplegia of upper limb following other nontraumatic intracranial hemorrhage affecting **left dominant side** 🔖

I69.233   Monoplegia of upper limb following other nontraumatic intracranial hemorrhage affecting **right non-dominant side** 🔖

I69.234   Monoplegia of upper limb following other nontraumatic intracranial hemorrhage affecting **left non-dominant side** 🔖

I69.239   Monoplegia of upper limb following other nontraumatic intracranial hemorrhage affecting **unspecified side** 🔖

● I69.24   **Monoplegia of lower limb** following other nontraumatic intracranial hemorrhage

I69.241   Monoplegia of lower limb following other nontraumatic intracranial hemorrhage affecting **right dominant side** 🔖

I69.242   Monoplegia of lower limb following other nontraumatic intracranial hemorrhage affecting **left dominant side** 🔖

I69.243   Monoplegia of lower limb following other nontraumatic intracranial hemorrhage affecting **right non-dominant side** 🔖

I69.244   Monoplegia of lower limb following other nontraumatic intracranial hemorrhage affecting **left non-dominant side** 🔖

I69.249   Monoplegia of lower limb following other nontraumatic intracranial hemorrhage affecting **unspecified side** 🔖

● I69.25   **Hemiplegia and hemiparesis** following other nontraumatic intracranial hemorrhage

I69.251   Hemiplegia and hemiparesis following other nontraumatic intracranial hemorrhage affecting **right dominant side** 🔖

I69.252   Hemiplegia and hemiparesis following other nontraumatic intracranial hemorrhage affecting **left dominant side** 🔖

I69.253   Hemiplegia and hemiparesis following other nontraumatic intracranial hemorrhage affecting **right non-dominant side** 🔖

I69.254   Hemiplegia and hemiparesis following other nontraumatic intracranial hemorrhage affecting **left non-dominant side** 🔖

I69.259   Hemiplegia and hemiparesis following other nontraumatic intracranial hemorrhage affecting **unspecified side** 🔖

CHAPTER 9 (I00–I99)

● **I69.26**   **Other paralytic syndrome following other nontraumatic intracranial hemorrhage**

Use additional code to identify type of paralytic syndrome, such as:
locked-in state (G83.5)
quadriplegia (G82.5-)

Excludes1   hemiplegia/hemiparesis following other nontraumatic intracranial hemorrhage (I69.25-)
monoplegia of lower limb following other nontraumatic intracranial hemorrhage (I69.24-)
monoplegia of upper limb following other nontraumatic intracranial hemorrhage (I69.23-)

I69.261   Other paralytic syndrome following other nontraumatic intracranial hemorrhage affecting **right dominant side** 🐾

I69.262   Other paralytic syndrome following other nontraumatic intracranial hemorrhage affecting **left dominant side** 🐾

I69.263   Other paralytic syndrome following other nontraumatic intracranial hemorrhage affecting **right non-dominant side** 🐾

I69.264   Other paralytic syndrome following other nontraumatic intracranial hemorrhage affecting **left non-dominant side** 🐾

I69.265   Other paralytic syndrome following other nontraumatic intracranial hemorrhage, **bilateral** 🐾

I69.269   Other paralytic syndrome following other nontraumatic intracranial hemorrhage affecting **unspecified side** 🐾

● **I69.29**   **Other sequelae of other nontraumatic intracranial hemorrhage**

I69.290   **Apraxia** following other nontraumatic intracranial hemorrhage

I69.291   **Dysphagia** following other nontraumatic intracranial hemorrhage

Use additional code to identify the type of dysphagia, if known (R13.1-)

I69.292   **Facial weakness** following other nontraumatic intracranial hemorrhage
Facial droop following other nontraumatic intracranial hemorrhage

I69.293   **Ataxia** following other nontraumatic intracranial hemorrhage

I69.298   **Other sequelae** of other nontraumatic intracranial hemorrhage
Alteration of sensation following other nontraumatic intracranial hemorrhage
Disturbance of vision following other nontraumatic intracranial hemorrhage
Use additional code to identify the sequelae

● **I69.3**   **Sequelae of cerebral infarction**
Sequelae of stroke NOS
Coding Clinic: 2012, Q4, P92, 95

I69.30   **Unspecified sequelae** of cerebral infarction

● **I69.31**   **Cognitive deficits following cerebral infarction**

I69.310   **Attention and concentration deficit** following cerebral infarction

I69.311   **Memory deficit** following cerebral infarction

I69.312   **Visuospatial deficit and spatial neglect** following cerebral infarction

I69.313   **Psychomotor deficit** following cerebral infarction

I69.314   **Frontal lobe and executive function deficit** following cerebral infarction

I69.315   **Cognitive social or emotional deficit** following cerebral infarction

I69.318   **Other symptoms and signs involving cognitive functions** following cerebral infarction

I69.319   **Unspecified symptoms and signs involving cognitive functions** following cerebral infarction

● **I69.32**   **Speech and language deficits following cerebral infarction**

I69.320   **Aphasia** following cerebral infarction

I69.321   **Dysphasia** following cerebral infarction
Coding Clinic: 2012, Q4, P91

I69.322   **Dysarthria** following cerebral infarction

Excludes2   transient ischemic attack (TIA) (G45.9)

I69.323   **Fluency disorder** following cerebral infarction
Stuttering following cerebral infarction

I69.328   **Other speech and language deficits** following cerebral infarction

● **I69.33**   **Monoplegia of upper limb following cerebral infarction**
Coding Clinic: 2017, Q1, P47

I69.331   Monoplegia of upper limb following cerebral infarction affecting **right dominant side** 🐾

I69.332   Monoplegia of upper limb following cerebral infarction affecting **left dominant side** 🐾

I69.333   Monoplegia of upper limb following cerebral infarction affecting **right non-dominant side** 🐾

I69.334   Monoplegia of upper limb following cerebral infarction affecting **left non-dominant side** 🐾

I69.339   Monoplegia of upper limb following cerebral infarction affecting **unspecified side** 🐾

● **I69.34**   **Monoplegia of lower limb following cerebral infarction**
Coding Clinic: 2017, Q1, P47

I69.341   Monoplegia of lower limb following cerebral infarction affecting **right dominant side** 🐾

I69.342   Monoplegia of lower limb following cerebral infarction affecting **left dominant side** 🐾

I69.343   Monoplegia of lower limb following cerebral infarction affecting **right non-dominant side** 🐾

CHAPTER 9 (I00-I99)

▶ New   ⇒ Revised   ~~deleted~~ Deleted   Excludes 1   Excludes 2   Includes   Use additional   Code first   Code also   Key words

OGCR Official Guidelines   X Assign placeholder X   ● Use Additional Character(s)   ▌ Manifestation Code   🐾 Hierarchical Condition Category   Coding Clinic

I69.344   Monoplegia of lower limb following cerebral infarction affecting left non-dominant side 🔓

I69.349   Monoplegia of lower limb following cerebral infarction affecting unspecified side 🔓

● I69.35   **Hemiplegia and hemiparesis following cerebral infarction**

     I69.351   **Hemiplegia and hemiparesis following cerebral infarction affecting right dominant side** 🔓

         Excludes2   transient ischemic attack (TIA) (G45.9)

         Coding Clinic: 2015, Q1, P25

     I69.352   **Hemiplegia and hemiparesis following cerebral infarction affecting left dominant side** 🔓

     I69.353   **Hemiplegia and hemiparesis following cerebral infarction affecting right non-dominant side** 🔓

     I69.354   **Hemiplegia and hemiparesis following cerebral infarction affecting left non-dominant side** 🔓

         Coding Clinic: 2012, Q4, P91

     I69.359   **Hemiplegia and hemiparesis following cerebral infarction affecting unspecified side** 🔓

● I69.36   **Other paralytic syndrome following cerebral infarction**

     Use additional code to identify type of paralytic syndrome, such as:
     locked-in state (G83.5)
     quadriplegia (G82.5-)

     Excludes1   hemiplegia/hemiparesis following cerebral infarction (I69.35-)
         monoplegia of lower limb following cerebral infarction (I69.34-)
         monoplegia of upper limb following cerebral infarction (I69.33-)

     I69.361   **Other paralytic syndrome following cerebral infarction affecting right dominant side** 🔓

     I69.362   **Other paralytic syndrome following cerebral infarction affecting left dominant side** 🔓

     I69.363   **Other paralytic syndrome following cerebral infarction affecting right non-dominant side** 🔓

     I69.364   **Other paralytic syndrome following cerebral infarction affecting left non-dominant side** 🔓

     I69.365   **Other paralytic syndrome following cerebral infarction, bilateral** 🔓

     I69.369   **Other paralytic syndrome following cerebral infarction affecting unspecified side** 🔓

● I69.39   **Other sequelae of cerebral infarction**

     I69.390   **Apraxia following cerebral infarction**

     I69.391   **Dysphagia following cerebral infarction**

         Use additional code to identify the type of dysphagia, if known (R13.1-)

     I69.392   **Facial weakness following cerebral infarction**

         Facial droop following cerebral infarction

     I69.393   **Ataxia following cerebral infarction**

     I69.398   **Other sequelae of cerebral infarction**

         Alteration of sensation following cerebral infarction
         Disturbance of vision following cerebral infarction

         Use additional code to identify the sequelae

● I69.8   **Sequelae of other cerebrovascular diseases**

     Excludes1   sequelae of traumatic intracranial injury (S06.-)

   I69.80   **Unspecified sequelae of other cerebrovascular disease**

● I69.81   **Cognitive deficits following other cerebrovascular disease**

     I69.810   **Attention and concentration deficit following other cerebrovascular disease**

     I69.811   **Memory deficit following other cerebrovascular disease**

     I69.812   **Visuospatial deficit and spatial neglect following other cerebrovascular disease**

     I69.813   **Psychomotor deficit following other cerebrovascular disease**

     I69.814   **Frontal lobe and executive function deficit following other cerebrovascular disease**

     I69.815   **Cognitive social or emotional deficit following other cerebrovascular disease**

     I69.818   **Other symptoms and signs involving cognitive functions following other cerebrovascular disease**

     I69.819   **Unspecified symptoms and signs involving cognitive functions following other cerebrovascular disease**

● I69.82   **Speech and language deficits following other cerebrovascular disease**

     I69.820   **Aphasia following other cerebrovascular disease**

     I69.821   **Dysphasia following other cerebrovascular disease**

     I69.822   **Dysarthria following other cerebrovascular disease**

     I69.823   **Fluency disorder following other cerebrovascular disease**

         Stuttering following other cerebrovascular disease

     I69.828   **Other speech and language deficits following other cerebrovascular disease**

● I69.83   **Monoplegia of upper limb following other cerebrovascular disease**

     I69.831   **Monoplegia of upper limb following other cerebrovascular disease affecting right dominant side** 🔓

     I69.832   **Monoplegia of upper limb following other cerebrovascular disease affecting left dominant side** 🔓

     I69.833   **Monoplegia of upper limb following other cerebrovascular disease affecting right non-dominant side** 🔓

     I69.834   **Monoplegia of upper limb following other cerebrovascular disease affecting left non-dominant side** 🔓

     I69.839   **Monoplegia of upper limb following other cerebrovascular disease affecting unspecified side** 🔓

CHAPTER 9 (I00-I99)

● **I69.84**   **Monoplegia of lower limb following other cerebrovascular disease**

     I69.841   Monoplegia of lower limb following other cerebrovascular disease affecting **right dominant side** 🦠

     I69.842   Monoplegia of lower limb following other cerebrovascular disease affecting **left dominant side** 🦠

     I69.843   Monoplegia of lower limb following other cerebrovascular disease affecting **right non-dominant side** 🦠

     I69.844   Monoplegia of lower limb following other cerebrovascular disease affecting **left non-dominant side** 🦠

     I69.849   Monoplegia of lower limb following other cerebrovascular disease affecting **unspecified side** 🦠

● **I69.85**   **Hemiplegia and hemiparesis following other cerebrovascular disease**

     I69.851   Hemiplegia and hemiparesis following other cerebrovascular disease affecting **right dominant side** 🦠

     I69.852   Hemiplegia and hemiparesis following other cerebrovascular disease affecting **left dominant side** 🦠

     I69.853   Hemiplegia and hemiparesis following other cerebrovascular disease affecting **right non-dominant side** 🦠

     I69.854   Hemiplegia and hemiparesis following other cerebrovascular disease affecting **left non-dominant side** 🦠

     I69.859   Hemiplegia and hemiparesis following other cerebrovascular disease affecting **unspecified side** 🦠

● **I69.86**   **Other paralytic syndrome following other cerebrovascular disease**

     Use additional code to identify type of paralytic syndrome, such as:
     locked-in state (G83.5)
     quadriplegia (G82.5-)

     Excludes1   hemiplegia/hemiparesis following other cerebrovascular disease (I69.85-)
                 monoplegia of lower limb following other cerebrovascular disease (I69.84-)
                 monoplegia of upper limb following other cerebrovascular disease (I69.83-)

     I69.861   Other paralytic syndrome following other cerebrovascular disease affecting **right dominant side** 🦠

     I69.862   Other paralytic syndrome following other cerebrovascular disease affecting **left dominant side** 🦠

     I69.863   Other paralytic syndrome following other cerebrovascular disease affecting **right non-dominant side** 🦠

     I69.864   Other paralytic syndrome following other cerebrovascular disease affecting **left non-dominant side** 🦠

     I69.865   Other paralytic syndrome following other cerebrovascular disease, **bilateral** 🦠

     I69.869   Other paralytic syndrome following other cerebrovascular disease affecting **unspecified side** 🦠

● **I69.89**   **Other sequelae of other cerebrovascular disease**

     I69.890   **Apraxia** following other cerebrovascular disease

     I69.891   **Dysphagia** following other cerebrovascular disease
           Use additional code to identify the type of dysphagia, if known (R13.1-)

     I69.892   **Facial weakness** following other cerebrovascular disease
           Facial droop following other cerebrovascular disease

     I69.893   **Ataxia** following other cerebrovascular disease

     I69.898   **Other sequelae of other cerebrovascular disease**
           Alteration of sensation following other cerebrovascular disease
           Disturbance of vision following other cerebrovascular disease
           Use additional code to identify the sequelae

● **I69.9**   **Sequelae of unspecified cerebrovascular diseases**

     Excludes1   sequelae of stroke (I69.3)
                 sequelae of traumatic intracranial injury (S06.-)

     I69.90   **Unspecified sequelae of unspecified cerebrovascular disease**

● **I69.91**   **Cognitive deficits following unspecified cerebrovascular disease**

     I69.910   **Attention and concentration deficit** following unspecified cerebrovascular disease

     I69.911   **Memory deficit** following unspecified cerebrovascular disease

     I69.912   **Visuospatial deficit and spatial neglect** following unspecified cerebrovascular disease

     I69.913   **Psychomotor deficit** following unspecified cerebrovascular disease

     I69.914   **Frontal lobe and executive function deficit** following unspecified cerebrovascular disease

     I69.915   **Cognitive social or emotional deficit** following unspecified cerebrovascular disease

     I69.918   **Other symptoms and signs involving cognitive functions** following unspecified cerebrovascular disease

     I69.919   **Unspecified symptoms and signs involving cognitive functions** following unspecified cerebrovascular disease

▶ New   ⇒ Revised   ~~deleted~~ Deleted   Excludes 1   Excludes 2   Includes   Use additional   Code first   Code also   Key words

OGCR Official Guidelines   X Assign placeholder X   ● Use Additional Character(s)   ▶ Manifestation Code   🦠 Hierarchical Condition Category   **Coding Clinic**

● **I69.92** **Speech and language deficits following unspecified cerebrovascular disease**

 I69.920 **Aphasia following unspecified cerebrovascular disease**

 I69.921 **Dysphasia following unspecified cerebrovascular disease**

 I69.922 **Dysarthria following unspecified cerebrovascular disease**

 I69.923 **Fluency disorder following unspecified cerebrovascular disease**
 Stuttering following unspecified cerebrovascular disease

 I69.928 **Other speech and language deficits following unspecified cerebrovascular disease**

● **I69.93** **Monoplegia of upper limb following unspecified cerebrovascular disease**

 I69.931 **Monoplegia of upper limb following unspecified cerebrovascular disease affecting right dominant side** 🔒

 I69.932 **Monoplegia of upper limb following unspecified cerebrovascular disease affecting left dominant side** 🔒

 I69.933 **Monoplegia of upper limb following unspecified cerebrovascular disease affecting right non-dominant side** 🔒

 I69.934 **Monoplegia of upper limb following unspecified cerebrovascular disease affecting left non-dominant side** 🔒

 I69.939 **Monoplegia of upper limb following unspecified cerebrovascular disease affecting unspecified side** 🔒

● **I69.94** **Monoplegia of lower limb following unspecified cerebrovascular disease**

 I69.941 **Monoplegia of lower limb following unspecified cerebrovascular disease affecting right dominant side** 🔒

 I69.942 **Monoplegia of lower limb following unspecified cerebrovascular disease affecting left dominant side** 🔒

 I69.943 **Monoplegia of lower limb following unspecified cerebrovascular disease affecting right non-dominant side** 🔒

 I69.944 **Monoplegia of lower limb following unspecified cerebrovascular disease affecting left non-dominant side** 🔒

 I69.949 **Monoplegia of lower limb following unspecified cerebrovascular disease affecting unspecified side** 🔒

● **I69.95** **Hemiplegia and hemiparesis following unspecified cerebrovascular disease**

 I69.951 **Hemiplegia and hemiparesis following unspecified cerebrovascular disease affecting right dominant side** 🔒

 I69.952 **Hemiplegia and hemiparesis following unspecified cerebrovascular disease affecting left dominant side** 🔒

 I69.953 **Hemiplegia and hemiparesis following unspecified cerebrovascular disease affecting right non-dominant side** 🔒

 I69.954 **Hemiplegia and hemiparesis following unspecified cerebrovascular disease affecting left non-dominant side** 🔒

 I69.959 **Hemiplegia and hemiparesis following unspecified cerebrovascular disease affecting unspecified side** 🔒

● **I69.96** **Other paralytic syndrome following unspecified cerebrovascular disease**
 Use additional code to identify type of paralytic syndrome, such as:
 locked-in state (G83.5)
 quadriplegia (G82.5-)

 Excludes1 hemiplegia/hemiparesis following unspecified cerebrovascular disease (I69.95-)
 monoplegia of lower limb following unspecified cerebrovascular disease (I69.94-)
 monoplegia of upper limb following unspecified cerebrovascular disease (I69.93-)

 I69.961 **Other paralytic syndrome following unspecified cerebrovascular disease affecting right dominant side** 🔒

 I69.962 **Other paralytic syndrome following unspecified cerebrovascular disease affecting left dominant side** 🔒

 I69.963 **Other paralytic syndrome following unspecified cerebrovascular disease affecting right non-dominant side** 🔒

 I69.964 **Other paralytic syndrome following unspecified cerebrovascular disease affecting left non-dominant side** 🔒

 I69.965 **Other paralytic syndrome following unspecified cerebrovascular disease, bilateral** 🔒

 I69.969 **Other paralytic syndrome following unspecified cerebrovascular disease affecting unspecified side** 🔒

● **I69.99** **Other sequelae of unspecified cerebrovascular disease**

 I69.990 **Apraxia following unspecified cerebrovascular disease**

 I69.991 **Dysphagia following unspecified cerebrovascular disease**
 Use additional code to identify the type of dysphagia, if known (R13.1-)

 I69.992 **Facial weakness following unspecified cerebrovascular disease**
 Facial droop following unspecified cerebrovascular disease

 I69.993 **Ataxia following unspecified cerebrovascular disease**

 I69.998 **Other sequelae following unspecified cerebrovascular disease**
 Alteration in sensation following unspecified cerebrovascular disease
 Disturbance of vision following unspecified cerebrovascular disease
 Use additional code to identify the sequelae

CHAPTER 9 (I00-I99)

DISEASES OF ARTERIES, ARTERIOLES AND CAPILLARIES (I70-I79)

● **I70**   **Atherosclerosis**

   Includes   arteriolosclerosis
   arterial degeneration
   arteriosclerosis
   arteriosclerotic vascular disease
   arteriovascular degeneration
   atheroma
   endarteritis deformans or obliterans
   senile arteritis
   senile endarteritis
   vascular degeneration

   Use additional code to identify:
   exposure to environmental tobacco smoke (Z77.22)
   history of tobacco dependence (Z87.891)
   occupational exposure to environmental tobacco smoke
   (Z57.31)
   tobacco dependence (F17.-)
   tobacco use (Z72.0)

   Excludes2   arteriosclerotic cardiovascular disease (I25.1-)
   arteriosclerotic heart disease (I25.1-)
   atheroembolism (I75.-)
   cerebral atherosclerosis (I67.2)
   coronary atherosclerosis (I25.1-)
   mesenteric atherosclerosis (K55.1)
   precerebral atherosclerosis (I67.2)
   primary pulmonary atherosclerosis (I27.0)

   I70.0   **Atherosclerosis of aorta** 🐾   A

   I70.1   **Atherosclerosis of renal artery** 🐾   A
   Goldblatt's kidney
      Excludes2   atherosclerosis of renal arterioles (I12.-)

★ **(See Plates 500, 501, and 502 on pages 60 – 62.)**

   ● I70.2   **Atherosclerosis of native arteries of the extremities**
   Mönckeberg's (medial) sclerosis
      Use additional code, if applicable, to identify chronic
      total occlusion of artery of extremity (I70.92)
      Excludes2   atherosclerosis of bypass graft of
      extremities (I70.30-I70.79)

      ● I70.20   **Unspecified atherosclerosis of native arteries of
      extremities**
         I70.201   **Unspecified atherosclerosis of native
         arteries of extremities, right leg** 🐾   A
         I70.202   **Unspecified atherosclerosis of native
         arteries of extremities, left leg** 🐾   A
         I70.203   **Unspecified atherosclerosis of native
         arteries of extremities, bilateral
         legs** 🐾   A
         I70.208   **Unspecified atherosclerosis of native
         arteries of extremities, other
         extremity** 🐾   A
         I70.209   **Unspecified atherosclerosis of native
         arteries of extremities, unspecified
         extremity** 🐾   A

      ● I70.21   **Atherosclerosis of native arteries of extremities
      with intermittent claudication**
         I70.211   **Atherosclerosis of native arteries
         of extremities with intermittent
         claudication, right leg** 🐾   A
         I70.212   **Atherosclerosis of native arteries
         of extremities with intermittent
         claudication, left leg** 🐾   A
         I70.213   **Atherosclerosis of native arteries
         of extremities with intermittent
         claudication, bilateral legs** 🐾   A
         I70.218   **Atherosclerosis of native arteries
         of extremities with intermittent
         claudication, other extremity** 🐾   A
         I70.219   **Atherosclerosis of native arteries
         of extremities with intermittent
         claudication, unspecified
         extremity** 🐾   A

   ● I70.22   **Atherosclerosis of native arteries of extremities
   with rest pain**
      Includes   any condition classifiable to
      I70.21-
      I70.221   **Atherosclerosis of native arteries of
      extremities with rest pain, right leg** 🐾
      A
      I70.222   **Atherosclerosis of native arteries of
      extremities with rest pain, left leg** 🐾   A
      I70.223   **Atherosclerosis of native arteries of
      extremities with rest pain, bilateral
      legs** 🐾   A
      I70.228   **Atherosclerosis of native arteries of
      extremities with rest pain, other
      extremity** 🐾   A
      I70.229   **Atherosclerosis of native arteries of
      extremities with rest pain, unspecified
      extremity** 🐾   A

   ● I70.23   **Atherosclerosis of native arteries of right leg
   with ulceration**
      Includes   any condition classifiable to
      I70.211 and I70.221
      Use additional code to identify severity of
      ulcer (L97.-)
      I70.231   **Atherosclerosis of native arteries of
      right leg with ulceration of thigh** 🐾   A
      I70.232   **Atherosclerosis of native arteries of
      right leg with ulceration of calf** 🐾   A
      I70.233   **Atherosclerosis of native arteries of
      right leg with ulceration of ankle** 🐾   A
      I70.234   **Atherosclerosis of native arteries of
      right leg with ulceration of heel and
      midfoot** 🐾   A
         Atherosclerosis of native arteries
         of right leg with ulceration of
         plantar surface of midfoot
      I70.235   **Atherosclerosis of native arteries of
      right leg with ulceration of other part
      of foot** 🐾   A
         Atherosclerosis of native arteries
         of right leg extremities with
         ulceration of toe
      ➠ I70.238   **Atherosclerosis of native arteries of
      right leg with ulceration of other part
      of lower leg** 🐾   A
      I70.239   **Atherosclerosis of native arteries of
      right leg with ulceration of
      unspecified site** 🐾   A

   ● I70.24   **Atherosclerosis of native arteries of left leg
   with ulceration**
      Includes   any condition classifiable to
      I70.212 and I70.222
      Use additional code to identify severity of
      ulcer (L97.-)
      I70.241   **Atherosclerosis of native arteries of
      left leg with ulceration of thigh** 🐾   A
      I70.242   **Atherosclerosis of native arteries of
      left leg with ulceration of calf** 🐾   A
      I70.243   **Atherosclerosis of native arteries of
      left leg with ulceration of ankle** 🐾   A
      I70.244   **Atherosclerosis of native arteries of
      left leg with ulceration of heel and
      midfoot** 🐾   A
         Atherosclerosis of native arteries
         of left leg with ulceration of
         plantar surface of midfoot
      I70.245   **Atherosclerosis of native arteries of
      left leg with ulceration of other part
      of foot** 🐾   A
         Atherosclerosis of native arteries
         of left leg extremities with
         ulceration of toe

▶ New   ➠ Revised   ~~deleted~~ Deleted   Excludes 1   Excludes 2   Includes   Use additional   Code first   Code also   Key words

OGCR Official Guidelines   X Assign placeholder X   ● Use Additional Character(s)   ▷ Manifestation Code   🐾 Hierarchical Condition Category   **Coding Clinic**

▪I70.248   Atherosclerosis of native arteries of left leg with ulceration of **other part of lower leg** ✇   A

I70.249   Atherosclerosis of native arteries of left leg with ulceration of **unspecified site** ✇   A

I70.25   Atherosclerosis of native arteries of other extremities with ulceration ✇   A

Includes   any condition classifiable to I70.218 and I70.228

Use additional code to identify the severity of the ulcer (L98.49-)

●I70.26   Atherosclerosis of native arteries of extremities with gangrene

Includes   any condition classifiable to I70.21-, I70.22-, I70.23-, I70.24-, and I70.25-

Use additional code to identify the severity of any ulcer (L97.-, L98.49-), if applicable

I70.261   Atherosclerosis of native arteries of extremities with gangrene, **right leg**   A

I70.262   Atherosclerosis of native arteries of extremities with gangrene, **left leg** ✇A

I70.263   Atherosclerosis of native arteries of extremities with gangrene, **bilateral legs** ✇   A

I70.268   Atherosclerosis of native arteries of extremities with gangrene, **other extremity** ✇   A

I70.269   Atherosclerosis of native arteries of extremities with gangrene, **unspecified extremity** ✇   A

●I70.29   Other atherosclerosis of native arteries of extremities

I70.291   Other atherosclerosis of native arteries of extremities, **right leg** ✇   A

I70.292   Other atherosclerosis of native arteries of extremities, **left leg** ✇   A

I70.293   Other atherosclerosis of native arteries of extremities, **bilateral legs** ✇   A

I70.298   Other atherosclerosis of native arteries of extremities, **other extremity** ✇   A

I70.299   Other atherosclerosis of native arteries of extremities, **unspecified extremity** ✇   A

●I70.3   Atherosclerosis of **unspecified type of bypass graft(s) of the extremities**

Use additional code, if applicable, to identify chronic total occlusion of artery of extremity (I70.92)

Excludes1   embolism or thrombus of bypass graft(s) of extremities (T82.8-)

●I70.30   Unspecified atherosclerosis of **unspecified** type of bypass graft(s) of the extremities

I70.301   Unspecified atherosclerosis of unspecified type of bypass graft(s) of the extremities, **right leg** ✇   A

I70.302   Unspecified atherosclerosis of unspecified type of bypass graft(s) of the extremities, **left leg** ✇   A

I70.303   Unspecified atherosclerosis of unspecified type of bypass graft(s) of the extremities, **bilateral legs** ✇   A

I70.308   Unspecified atherosclerosis of unspecified type of bypass graft(s) of the extremities, **other extremity** ✇   A

I70.309   Unspecified atherosclerosis of unspecified type of bypass graft(s) of the extremities, **unspecified extremity** ✇   A

●I70.31   Atherosclerosis of **unspecified type of bypass graft(s) of the extremities with intermittent claudication**

I70.311   Atherosclerosis of unspecified type of bypass graft(s) of the extremities with intermittent claudication, **right leg** ✇ A

I70.312   Atherosclerosis of unspecified type of bypass graft(s) of the extremities with intermittent claudication, **left leg** ✇   A

I70.313   Atherosclerosis of unspecified type of bypass graft(s) of the extremities with intermittent claudication, **bilateral legs** ✇   A

I70.318   Atherosclerosis of unspecified type of bypass graft(s) of the extremities with intermittent claudication, **other extremity** ✇   A

I70.319   Atherosclerosis of unspecified type of bypass graft(s) of the extremities with intermittent claudication, **unspecified extremity** ✇   A

●I70.32   Atherosclerosis of **unspecified type of bypass graft(s) of the extremities with rest pain**

Includes   any condition classifiable to I70.31-

I70.321   Atherosclerosis of unspecified type of bypass graft(s) of the extremities with rest pain, **right leg** ✇   A

I70.322   Atherosclerosis of unspecified type of bypass graft(s) of the extremities with rest pain, **left leg** ✇   A

I70.323   Atherosclerosis of unspecified type of bypass graft(s) of the extremities with rest pain, **bilateral legs** ✇   A

I70.328   Atherosclerosis of unspecified type of bypass graft(s) of the extremities with rest pain, **other extremity** ✇   A

I70.329   Atherosclerosis of unspecified type of bypass graft(s) of the extremities with rest pain, **unspecified extremity** ✇   A

●I70.33   Atherosclerosis of **unspecified type of bypass graft(s) of the right leg with ulceration**

Includes   any condition classifiable to I70.311 and I70.321

Use additional code to identify severity of ulcer (L97.-)

I70.331   Atherosclerosis of unspecified type of bypass graft(s) of the right leg with ulceration of **thigh** ✇   A

I70.332   Atherosclerosis of unspecified type of bypass graft(s) of the right leg with ulceration of **calf** ✇   A

I70.333   Atherosclerosis of unspecified type of bypass graft(s) of the right leg with ulceration of **ankle** ✇   A

I70.334   Atherosclerosis of unspecified type of bypass graft(s) of the right leg with ulceration of **heel and midfoot** ✇   A

Atherosclerosis of unspecified type of bypass graft(s) of right leg with ulceration of plantar surface of midfoot

I70.335   Atherosclerosis of unspecified type of bypass graft(s) of the right leg with ulceration of **other part of foot** ✇   A

Atherosclerosis of unspecified type of bypass graft(s) of the right leg with ulceration of toe

I70.338   Atherosclerosis of unspecified type of bypass graft(s) of the right leg with ulceration of **other part of lower leg** ✇A

I70.339   Atherosclerosis of unspecified type of bypass graft(s) of the right leg with ulceration of **unspecified site** ✇   A

CHAPTER 9 (I00-I99)

● **I70.34** **Atherosclerosis of unspecified type of bypass graft(s) of the left leg with ulceration**

> **Includes** any condition classifiable to I70.312 and I70.322

Use additional code to identify severity of ulcer (L97.-)

 I70.341 Atherosclerosis of unspecified type of bypass graft(s) of the left leg with ulceration of **thigh** 🐾 A

 I70.342 Atherosclerosis of unspecified type of bypass graft(s) of the left leg with ulceration of **calf** 🐾 A

 I70.343 Atherosclerosis of unspecified type of bypass graft(s) of the left leg with ulceration of **ankle** 🐾 A

 I70.344 Atherosclerosis of unspecified type of bypass graft(s) of the left leg with ulceration of **heel and midfoot** 🐾 A
> Atherosclerosis of unspecified type of bypass graft(s) of left leg with ulceration of plantar surface of midfoot

 I70.345 Atherosclerosis of unspecified type of bypass graft(s) of the left leg with ulceration of **other part of foot** 🐾 A
> Atherosclerosis of unspecified type of bypass graft(s) of the left leg with ulceration of toe

 I70.348 Atherosclerosis of unspecified type of bypass graft(s) of the left leg with ulceration of **other part of lower leg** 🐾 A

 I70.349 Atherosclerosis of unspecified type of bypass graft(s) of the left leg with ulceration of **unspecified site** 🐾 A

 I70.35 **Atherosclerosis of unspecified type of bypass graft(s) of other extremity with ulceration** 🐾 A

> **Includes** any condition classifiable to I70.318 and I70.328

Use additional code to identify severity of ulcer (L98.49-)

● **I70.36** **Atherosclerosis of unspecified type of bypass graft(s) of the extremities with gangrene**

> **Includes** any condition classifiable to I70.31-, I70.32-, I70.33-, I70.34-, I70.35

Use additional code to identify the severity of any ulcer (L97.-, L98.49-), if applicable

 I70.361 Atherosclerosis of unspecified type of bypass graft(s) of the extremities with gangrene, **right leg** 🐾 A

 I70.362 Atherosclerosis of unspecified type of bypass graft(s) of the extremities with gangrene, **left leg** 🐾 A

 I70.363 Atherosclerosis of unspecified type of bypass graft(s) of the extremities with gangrene, **bilateral legs** 🐾 A

 I70.368 Atherosclerosis of unspecified type of bypass graft(s) of the extremities with gangrene, **other extremity** 🐾 A

 I70.369 Atherosclerosis of unspecified type of bypass graft(s) of the extremities with gangrene, **unspecified extremity** 🐾 A

● **I70.39** **Other atherosclerosis of unspecified type of bypass graft(s) of the extremities**

 I70.391 Other atherosclerosis of unspecified type of bypass graft(s) of the extremities, **right leg** 🐾 A

 I70.392 Other atherosclerosis of unspecified type of bypass graft(s) of the extremities, **left leg** 🐾 A

 I70.393 Other atherosclerosis of unspecified type of bypass graft(s) of the extremities, **bilateral legs** 🐾 A

 I70.398 Other atherosclerosis of unspecified type of bypass graft(s) of the extremities, **other extremity** 🐾 A

 I70.399 Other atherosclerosis of unspecified type of bypass graft(s) of the extremities, **unspecified extremity** 🐾 A

● **I70.4** **Atherosclerosis of autologous vein bypass graft(s) of the extremities**

> Use additional code, if applicable, to identify chronic total occlusion of artery of extremity (I70.92)

● **I70.40** **Unspecified atherosclerosis of autologous vein bypass graft(s) of the extremities**

 I70.401 Unspecified atherosclerosis of autologous vein bypass graft(s) of the extremities, **right leg** 🐾 A

 I70.402 Unspecified atherosclerosis of autologous vein bypass graft(s) of the extremities, **left leg** 🐾 A

 I70.403 Unspecified atherosclerosis of autologous vein bypass graft(s) of the extremities, **bilateral legs** 🐾 A

 I70.408 Unspecified atherosclerosis of autologous vein bypass graft(s) of the extremities, **other extremity** 🐾 A

 I70.409 Unspecified atherosclerosis of autologous vein bypass graft(s) of the extremities, **unspecified extremity** 🐾 A

● **I70.41** **Atherosclerosis of autologous vein bypass graft(s) of the extremities with intermittent claudication**

 I70.411 Atherosclerosis of autologous vein bypass graft(s) of the extremities with intermittent claudication, **right leg** 🐾 A

 I70.412 Atherosclerosis of autologous vein bypass graft(s) of the extremities with intermittent claudication, **left leg** 🐾 A

 I70.413 Atherosclerosis of autologous vein bypass graft(s) of the extremities with intermittent claudication, **bilateral legs** 🐾 A

 I70.418 Atherosclerosis of autologous vein bypass graft(s) of the extremities with intermittent claudication, **other extremity** 🐾 A

 I70.419 Atherosclerosis of autologous vein bypass graft(s) of the extremities with intermittent claudication, **unspecified extremity** 🐾 A

● **I70.42** **Atherosclerosis of autologous vein bypass graft(s) of the extremities with rest pain**

> **Includes** any condition classifiable to I70.41-

 I70.421 Atherosclerosis of autologous vein bypass graft(s) of the extremities with rest pain, **right leg** 🐾 A

 I70.422 Atherosclerosis of autologous vein bypass graft(s) of the extremities with rest pain, **left leg** 🐾 A

 I70.423 Atherosclerosis of autologous vein bypass graft(s) of the extremities with rest pain, **bilateral legs** 🐾 A

 I70.428 Atherosclerosis of autologous vein bypass graft(s) of the extremities with rest pain, **other extremity** 🐾 A

 I70.429 Atherosclerosis of autologous vein bypass graft(s) of the extremities with rest pain, **unspecified extremity** 🐾 A

▶ New ⟹ Revised ~~deleted~~ Deleted Excludes 1 Excludes 2 Includes Use additional Code first Code also Key words
OGCR Official Guidelines X Assign placeholder X ● Use Additional Character(s) ▶ Manifestation Code 🐾 Hierarchical Condition Category **Coding Clinic**

● I70.43   Atherosclerosis of autologous vein bypass graft(s) of the right leg with ulceration

    Includes   any condition classifiable to I70.411 and I70.421

    Use additional code to identify severity of ulcer (L97.-)

    I70.431   Atherosclerosis of autologous vein bypass graft(s) of the right leg with ulceration of **thigh** 🦠   A

    I70.432   Atherosclerosis of autologous vein bypass graft(s) of the right leg with ulceration of **calf** 🦠   A

    I70.433   Atherosclerosis of autologous vein bypass graft(s) of the right leg with ulceration of **ankle** 🦠   A

    I70.434   Atherosclerosis of autologous vein bypass graft(s) of the right leg with ulceration of **heel and midfoot** 🦠   A

        Atherosclerosis of autologous vein bypass graft(s) of right leg with ulceration of plantar surface of midfoot

    I70.435   Atherosclerosis of autologous vein bypass graft(s) of the right leg with ulceration of **other part of foot** 🦠   A

        Atherosclerosis of autologous vein bypass graft(s) of right leg with ulceration of toe

    I70.438   Atherosclerosis of autologous vein bypass graft(s) of the right leg with ulceration of **other part of lower leg** 🦠   A

    I70.439   Atherosclerosis of autologous vein bypass graft(s) of the right leg with ulceration of **unspecified site** 🦠   A

● I70.44   Atherosclerosis of autologous vein bypass graft(s) of the left leg with ulceration

    Includes   any condition classifiable to I70.412 and I70.422

    Use additional code to identify severity of ulcer (L97.-)

    I70.441   Atherosclerosis of autologous vein bypass graft(s) of the left leg with ulceration of **thigh** 🦠   A

    I70.442   Atherosclerosis of autologous vein bypass graft(s) of the left leg with ulceration of **calf** 🦠   A

    I70.443   Atherosclerosis of autologous vein bypass graft(s) of the left leg with ulceration of **ankle** 🦠   A

    I70.444   Atherosclerosis of autologous vein bypass graft(s) of the left leg with ulceration of **heel and midfoot** 🦠   A

        Atherosclerosis of autologous vein bypass graft(s) of left leg with ulceration of plantar surface of midfoot

    I70.445   Atherosclerosis of autologous vein bypass graft(s) of the left leg with ulceration of **other part of foot** 🦠   A

        Atherosclerosis of autologous vein bypass graft(s) of left leg with ulceration of toe

    I70.448   Atherosclerosis of autologous vein bypass graft(s) of the left leg with ulceration of **other part of lower leg** 🦠   A

    I70.449   Atherosclerosis of autologous vein bypass graft(s) of the left leg with ulceration of **unspecified site** 🦠   A

I70.45   Atherosclerosis of autologous vein bypass graft(s) of **other extremity** with ulceration 🦠   A

    Includes   any condition classifiable to I70.418, I70.428, and I70.438

    Use additional code to identify severity of ulcer (L98.49-)

● I70.46   Atherosclerosis of autologous vein bypass graft(s) of the extremities **with gangrene**

    Includes   any condition classifiable to I70.41-, I70.42-, and I70.43-, I70.44-, I70.45

    Use additional code to identify the severity of any ulcer (L97.-, L98.49-), if applicable

    I70.461   Atherosclerosis of autologous vein bypass graft(s) of the extremities with gangrene, **right leg**   A

    I70.462   Atherosclerosis of autologous vein bypass graft(s) of the extremities with gangrene, **left leg** 🦠   A

    I70.463   Atherosclerosis of autologous vein bypass graft(s) of the extremities with gangrene, **bilateral legs** 🦠   A

    I70.468   Atherosclerosis of autologous vein bypass graft(s) of the extremities with gangrene, **other extremity** 🦠   A

    I70.469   Atherosclerosis of autologous vein bypass graft(s) of the extremities with gangrene, **unspecified extremity** 🦠   A

● I70.49   Other atherosclerosis of autologous vein bypass graft(s) of the extremities

    I70.491   Other atherosclerosis of autologous vein bypass graft(s) of the extremities, **right leg** 🦠   A

    I70.492   Other atherosclerosis of autologous vein bypass graft(s) of the extremities, **left leg** 🦠   A

    I70.493   Other atherosclerosis of autologous vein bypass graft(s) of the extremities, **bilateral legs** 🦠   A

    I70.498   Other atherosclerosis of autologous vein bypass graft(s) of the extremities, **other extremity** 🦠   A

    I70.499   Other atherosclerosis of autologous vein bypass graft(s) of the extremities, **unspecified extremity** 🦠   A

● I70.5   Atherosclerosis of **nonautologous biological** bypass graft(s) of the extremities

    Use additional code, if applicable, to identify chronic total occlusion of artery of extremity (I70.92)

● I70.50   **Unspecified** atherosclerosis of nonautologous biological bypass graft(s) of the extremities

    I70.501   Unspecified atherosclerosis of nonautologous biological bypass graft(s) of the extremities, **right leg** 🦠   A

    I70.502   Unspecified atherosclerosis of nonautologous biological bypass graft(s) of the extremities, **left leg** 🦠 A

    I70.503   Unspecified atherosclerosis of nonautologous biological bypass graft(s) of the extremities, **bilateral legs** 🦠   A

    I70.508   Unspecified atherosclerosis of nonautologous biological bypass graft(s) of the extremities, **other extremity** 🦠   A

    I70.509   Unspecified atherosclerosis of nonautologous biological bypass graft(s) of the extremities, **unspecified extremity** 🦠   A

CHAPTER 9 (I00-I99)

● **I70.51** Atherosclerosis of nonautologous biological bypass graft(s) of the extremities **intermittent claudication**

 I70.511 Atherosclerosis of nonautologous biological bypass graft(s) of the extremities with intermittent claudication, **right leg** 🖉 A

 I70.512 Atherosclerosis of nonautologous biological bypass graft(s) of the extremities with intermittent claudication, **left leg** 🖉 A

 I70.513 Atherosclerosis of nonautologous biological bypass graft(s) of the extremities with intermittent claudication, **bilateral legs** 🖉 A

 I70.518 Atherosclerosis of nonautologous biological bypass graft(s) of the extremities with intermittent claudication, **other extremity** 🖉 A

 I70.519 Atherosclerosis of nonautologous biological bypass graft(s) of the extremities with intermittent claudication, **unspecified extremity** 🖉 A

● **I70.52** Atherosclerosis of nonautologous biological bypass graft(s) of the extremities **with rest pain**

 Includes any condition classifiable to I70.51-

 I70.521 Atherosclerosis of nonautologous biological bypass graft(s) of the extremities with rest pain, **right leg** 🖉 A

 I70.522 Atherosclerosis of nonautologous biological bypass graft(s) of the extremities with rest pain, **left leg** 🖉 A

 I70.523 Atherosclerosis of nonautologous biological bypass graft(s) of the extremities with rest pain, **bilateral legs** 🖉 A

 I70.528 Atherosclerosis of nonautologous biological bypass graft(s) of the extremities with rest pain, **other extremity** 🖉 A

 I70.529 Atherosclerosis of nonautologous biological bypass graft(s) of the extremities with rest pain, **unspecified extremity** 🖉 A

● **I70.53** Atherosclerosis of nonautologous biological bypass graft(s) of the **right leg with ulceration**

 Includes any condition classifiable to I70.511 and I70.521

 Use additional code to identify severity of ulcer (L97.-)

 I70.531 Atherosclerosis of nonautologous biological bypass graft(s) of the right leg with ulceration of **thigh** 🖉 A

 I70.532 Atherosclerosis of nonautologous biological bypass graft(s) of the right leg with ulceration of **calf** 🖉 A

 I70.533 Atherosclerosis of nonautologous biological bypass graft(s) of the right leg with ulceration of **ankle** 🖉 A

 I70.534 Atherosclerosis of nonautologous biological bypass graft(s) of the right leg with ulceration of **heel and midfoot** 🖉 A

 Atherosclerosis of nonautologous biological bypass graft(s) of right leg with ulceration of plantar surface of midfoot

 I70.535 Atherosclerosis of nonautologous biological bypass graft(s) of the right leg with ulceration of **other part of foot** 🖉 A

 Atherosclerosis of nonautologous biological bypass graft(s) of the right leg with ulceration of toe

 I70.538 Atherosclerosis of nonautologous biological bypass graft(s) of the right leg with ulceration of **other part of lower leg** 🖉 A

 I70.539 Atherosclerosis of nonautologous biological bypass graft(s) of the right leg with ulceration of **unspecified site** 🖉 A

● **I70.54** Atherosclerosis of nonautologous biological bypass graft(s) of the **left leg with ulceration**

 Includes any condition classifiable to I70.512 and I70.522

 Use additional code to identify severity of ulcer (L97.-)

 I70.541 Atherosclerosis of nonautologous biological bypass graft(s) of the left leg with ulceration of **thigh** 🖉 A

 I70.542 Atherosclerosis of nonautologous biological bypass graft(s) of the left leg with ulceration of **calf** 🖉 A

 I70.543 Atherosclerosis of nonautologous biological bypass graft(s) of the left leg with ulceration of **ankle** 🖉 A

 I70.544 Atherosclerosis of nonautologous biological bypass graft(s) of the left leg with ulceration of **heel and midfoot** 🖉 A

 Atherosclerosis of nonautologous biological bypass graft(s) of left leg with ulceration of plantar surface of midfoot

 I70.545 Atherosclerosis of nonautologous biological bypass graft(s) of the left leg with ulceration of **other part of foot** 🖉 A

 Atherosclerosis of nonautologous biological bypass graft(s) of the left leg with ulceration of toe

 I70.548 Atherosclerosis of nonautologous biological bypass graft(s) of the left leg with ulceration of **other part of lower leg** 🖉 A

 I70.549 Atherosclerosis of nonautologous biological bypass graft(s) of the left leg with ulceration of **unspecified site** 🖉 A

I70.55 Atherosclerosis of nonautologous biological bypass graft(s) of **other extremity with ulceration** 🖉 A

 Includes any condition classifiable to I70.518, I70.528, and I70.538

 Use additional code to identify severity of ulcer (L98.49)

▶ New ⇒ Revised ~~deleted~~ Deleted Excludes 1 Excludes 2 Includes Use additional Code first Code also Key words

OGCR Official Guidelines X Assign placeholder X ● Use Additional Character(s) ❭ Manifestation Code 🖉 Hierarchical Condition Category **Coding Clinic**

● **I70.56** **Atherosclerosis of nonautologous biological bypass graft(s) of the extremities with gangrene**

Includes   any condition classifiable to I70.51-, I70.52-, and I70.53-, I70.54-, I70.55

Use additional code to identify the severity of any ulcer (L97.-, L98.49-), if applicable

I70.561 Atherosclerosis of nonautologous biological bypass graft(s) of the extremities with gangrene, right leg 🐾   A

I70.562 Atherosclerosis of nonautologous biological bypass graft(s) of the extremities with gangrene, left leg 🐾A

I70.563 Atherosclerosis of nonautologous biological bypass graft(s) of the extremities with gangrene, bilateral legs 🐾   A

I70.568 Atherosclerosis of nonautologous biological bypass graft(s) of the extremities with gangrene, other extremity 🐾   A

I70.569 Atherosclerosis of nonautologous biological bypass graft(s) of the extremities with gangrene, unspecified extremity 🐾   A

● **I70.59** **Other atherosclerosis of nonautologous biological bypass graft(s) of the extremities**

I70.591 Other atherosclerosis of nonautologous biological bypass graft(s) of the extremities, right leg 🐾   A

I70.592 Other atherosclerosis of nonautologous biological bypass graft(s) of the extremities, left leg 🐾   A

I70.593 Other atherosclerosis of nonautologous biological bypass graft(s) of the extremities, bilateral legs 🐾   A

I70.598 Other atherosclerosis of nonautologous biological bypass graft(s) of the extremities, other extremity 🐾   A

I70.599 Other atherosclerosis of nonautologous biological bypass graft(s) of the extremities, unspecified extremity 🐾   A

● **I70.6** **Atherosclerosis of nonbiological bypass graft(s) of the extremities**

Use additional code, if applicable, to identify chronic total occlusion of artery of extremity (I70.92)

● **I70.60** **Unspecified atherosclerosis of nonbiological bypass graft(s) of the extremities**

I70.601 Unspecified atherosclerosis of nonbiological bypass graft(s) of the extremities, right leg 🐾   A

I70.602 Unspecified atherosclerosis of nonbiological bypass graft(s) of the extremities, left leg 🐾   A

I70.603 Unspecified atherosclerosis of nonbiological bypass graft(s) of the extremities, bilateral legs 🐾   A

I70.608 Unspecified atherosclerosis of nonbiological bypass graft(s) of the extremities, other extremity 🐾   A

I70.609 Unspecified atherosclerosis of nonbiological bypass graft(s) of the extremities, unspecified extremity 🐾A

● **I70.61** **Atherosclerosis of nonbiological bypass graft(s) of the extremities with intermittent claudication**

I70.611 Atherosclerosis of nonbiological bypass graft(s) of the extremities with intermittent claudication, right leg 🐾   A

I70.612 Atherosclerosis of nonbiological bypass graft(s) of the extremities with intermittent claudication, left leg 🐾 A

I70.613 Atherosclerosis of nonbiological bypass graft(s) of the extremities with intermittent claudication, bilateral legs 🐾   A

I70.618 Atherosclerosis of nonbiological bypass graft(s) of the extremities with intermittent claudication, other extremity 🐾   A

I70.619 Atherosclerosis of nonbiological bypass graft(s) of the extremities with intermittent claudication, unspecified extremity 🐾   A

● **I70.62** **Atherosclerosis of nonbiological bypass graft(s) of the extremities with rest pain**

Includes   any condition classifiable to I70.61-

I70.621 Atherosclerosis of nonbiological bypass graft(s) of the extremities with rest pain, right leg 🐾   A

I70.622 Atherosclerosis of nonbiological bypass graft(s) of the extremities with rest pain, left leg 🐾   A

I70.623 Atherosclerosis of nonbiological bypass graft(s) of the extremities with rest pain, bilateral legs 🐾   A

I70.628 Atherosclerosis of nonbiological bypass graft(s) of the extremities with rest pain, other extremity 🐾   A

I70.629 Atherosclerosis of nonbiological bypass graft(s) of the extremities with rest pain, unspecified extremity 🐾   A

● **I70.63** **Atherosclerosis of nonbiological bypass graft(s) of the right leg with ulceration**

Includes   any condition classifiable to I70.611 and I70.621

Use additional code to identify severity of ulcer (L97.-)

I70.631 Atherosclerosis of nonbiological bypass graft(s) of the right leg with ulceration of thigh 🐾   A

I70.632 Atherosclerosis of nonbiological bypass graft(s) of the right leg with ulceration of calf 🐾   A

I70.633 Atherosclerosis of nonbiological bypass graft(s) of the right leg with ulceration of ankle 🐾   A

I70.634 Atherosclerosis of nonbiological bypass graft(s) of the right leg with ulceration of heel and midfoot 🐾   A

Atherosclerosis of nonbiological bypass graft(s) of right leg with ulceration of plantar surface of midfoot

I70.635 Atherosclerosis of nonbiological bypass graft(s) of the right leg with ulceration of other part of foot 🐾   A

Atherosclerosis of nonbiological bypass graft(s) of the right leg with ulceration of toe

I70.638 Atherosclerosis of nonbiological bypass graft(s) of the right leg with ulceration of other part of lower leg 🐾   A

I70.639 Atherosclerosis of nonbiological bypass graft(s) of the right leg with ulceration of unspecified site 🐾   A

CHAPTER 9 (I00-I99)

CHAPTER 9 (I00-I99)

● **I70.64**   **Atherosclerosis of nonbiological bypass graft(s) of the left leg with ulceration**

> **Includes**   any condition classifiable to I70.612 and I70.622

> Use additional code to identify severity of ulcer (L97.-)

    I70.641   Atherosclerosis of nonbiological bypass graft(s) of the left leg with ulceration of **thigh** 🐾   A

    I70.642   Atherosclerosis of nonbiological bypass graft(s) of the left leg with ulceration of **calf** 🐾   A

    I70.643   Atherosclerosis of nonbiological bypass graft(s) of the left leg with ulceration of **ankle** 🐾   A

    I70.644   Atherosclerosis of nonbiological bypass graft(s) of the left leg with ulceration of **heel and midfoot** 🐾   A
> Atherosclerosis of nonbiological bypass graft(s) of left leg with ulceration of plantar surface of midfoot

    I70.645   Atherosclerosis of nonbiological bypass graft(s) of the left leg with ulceration of **other part of foot** 🐾   A
> Atherosclerosis of nonbiological bypass graft(s) of the left leg with ulceration of toe

    I70.648   Atherosclerosis of nonbiological bypass graft(s) of the left leg with ulceration of **other part of lower leg** 🐾   A

    I70.649   Atherosclerosis of nonbiological bypass graft(s) of the left leg with ulceration of **unspecified site** 🐾   A

  I70.65   Atherosclerosis of nonbiological bypass graft(s) of other extremity with ulceration 🐾   A

> **Includes**   any condition classifiable to I70.618 and I70.628

> Use additional code to identify severity of ulcer (L98.49-)

● **I70.66**   **Atherosclerosis of nonbiological bypass graft(s) of the extremities with gangrene**

> **Includes**   any condition classifiable to I70.61-, I70.62-, I70.63-, I70.64-, I70.65

> Use additional code to identify the severity of any ulcer (L97.-, L98.49-), if applicable

    I70.661   Atherosclerosis of nonbiological bypass graft(s) of the extremities with gangrene, **right leg** 🐾   A

    I70.662   Atherosclerosis of nonbiological bypass graft(s) of the extremities with gangrene, **left leg** 🐾   A

    I70.663   Atherosclerosis of nonbiological bypass graft(s) of the extremities with gangrene, **bilateral legs** 🐾   A

    I70.668   Atherosclerosis of nonbiological bypass graft(s) of the extremities with gangrene, **other extremity** 🐾   A

    I70.669   Atherosclerosis of nonbiological bypass graft(s) of the extremities with gangrene, **unspecified extremity** 🐾   A

● **I70.69**   **Other atherosclerosis of nonbiological bypass graft(s) of the extremities**

    I70.691   Other atherosclerosis of nonbiological bypass graft(s) of the extremities, **right leg** 🐾   A

    I70.692   Other atherosclerosis of nonbiological bypass graft(s) of the extremities, **left leg** 🐾   A

    I70.693   Other atherosclerosis of nonbiological bypass graft(s) of the extremities, **bilateral legs** 🐾   A

    I70.698   Other atherosclerosis of nonbiological bypass graft(s) of the extremities, **other extremity** 🐾   A

    I70.699   Other atherosclerosis of nonbiological bypass graft(s) of the extremities, **unspecified extremity** 🐾   A

● **I70.7**   **Atherosclerosis of other type of bypass graft(s) of the extremities**

> Use additional code, if applicable, to identify chronic total occlusion of artery of extremity (I70.92)

● **I70.70**   **Unspecified atherosclerosis of other type of bypass graft(s) of the extremities**

    I70.701   Unspecified atherosclerosis of other type of bypass graft(s) of the extremities, **right leg** 🐾   A

    I70.702   Unspecified atherosclerosis of other type of bypass graft(s) of the extremities, **left leg** 🐾   A

    I70.703   Unspecified atherosclerosis of other type of bypass graft(s) of the extremities, **bilateral legs** 🐾   A

    I70.708   Unspecified atherosclerosis of other type of bypass graft(s) of the extremities, **other extremity** 🐾   A

    I70.709   Unspecified atherosclerosis of other type of bypass graft(s) of the extremities, **unspecified extremity** 🐾 A

● **I70.71**   **Atherosclerosis of other type of bypass graft(s) of the extremities with intermittent claudication**

    I70.711   Atherosclerosis of other type of bypass graft(s) of the extremities with intermittent claudication, **right leg** 🐾 A

    I70.712   Atherosclerosis of other type of bypass graft(s) of the extremities with intermittent claudication, **left leg** 🐾   A

    I70.713   Atherosclerosis of other type of bypass graft(s) of the extremities with intermittent claudication, **bilateral legs** 🐾   A

    I70.718   Atherosclerosis of other type of bypass graft(s) of the extremities with intermittent claudication, **other extremity** 🐾   A

    I70.719   Atherosclerosis of other type of bypass graft(s) of the extremities with intermittent claudication, **unspecified extremity** 🐾   A

● **I70.72**   **Atherosclerosis of other type of bypass graft(s) of the extremities with rest pain**

> **Includes**   any condition classifiable to I70.71-

    I70.721   Atherosclerosis of other type of bypass graft(s) of the extremities with rest pain, **right leg** 🐾   A

    I70.722   Atherosclerosis of other type of bypass graft(s) of the extremities with rest pain, **left leg** 🐾   A

    I70.723   Atherosclerosis of other type of bypass graft(s) of the extremities with rest pain, **bilateral legs** 🐾   A

    I70.728   Atherosclerosis of other type of bypass graft(s) of the extremities with rest pain, **other extremity** 🐾   A

    I70.729   Atherosclerosis of other type of bypass graft(s) of the extremities with rest pain, **unspecified extremity** 🐾   A

▶ New   ⇒ Revised   ~~deleted~~ Deleted   Excludes 1   Excludes 2   Includes   Use additional   Code first   Code also   Key words

OGCR Official Guidelines   X Assign placeholder X   ● Use Additional Character(s)   ▶ Manifestation Code   🐾 Hierarchical Condition Category   **Coding Clinic**

● **I70.73** **Atherosclerosis of other type of bypass graft(s) of the right leg with ulceration**

> **Includes** any condition classifiable to I70.711 and I70.721

> Use additional code to identify severity of ulcer (L97.-)

 I70.731 Atherosclerosis of other type of bypass graft(s) of the right leg with ulceration of **thigh** 🔁 A

 I70.732 Atherosclerosis of other type of bypass graft(s) of the right leg with ulceration of **calf** 🔁 A

 I70.733 Atherosclerosis of other type of bypass graft(s) of the right leg with ulceration of **ankle** 🔁 A

 I70.734 Atherosclerosis of other type of bypass graft(s) of the right leg with ulceration of **heel and midfoot** 🔁 A

> Atherosclerosis of other type of bypass graft(s) of right leg with ulceration of plantar surface of midfoot

 I70.735 Atherosclerosis of other type of bypass graft(s) of the right leg with ulceration of **other part of foot** 🔁 A

> Atherosclerosis of other type of bypass graft(s) of right leg with ulceration of toe

 I70.738 Atherosclerosis of other type of bypass graft(s) of the right leg with ulceration of **other part of lower leg** 🔁 A

 I70.739 Atherosclerosis of other type of bypass graft(s) of the right leg with ulceration of **unspecified site** 🔁 A

● **I70.74** **Atherosclerosis of other type of bypass graft(s) of the left leg with ulceration**

> **Includes** any condition classifiable to I70.712 and I70.722

> Use additional code to identify severity of ulcer (L97.-)

 I70.741 Atherosclerosis of other type of bypass graft(s) of the left leg with ulceration of **thigh** 🔁 A

 I70.742 Atherosclerosis of other type of bypass graft(s) of the left leg with ulceration of **calf** 🔁 A

 I70.743 Atherosclerosis of other type of bypass graft(s) of the left leg with ulceration of **ankle** 🔁 A

 I70.744 Atherosclerosis of other type of bypass graft(s) of the left leg with ulceration of **heel and midfoot** 🔁 A

> Atherosclerosis of other type of bypass graft(s) of left leg with ulceration of plantar surface of midfoot

 I70.745 Atherosclerosis of other type of bypass graft(s) of the left leg with ulceration of **other part of foot** 🔁 A

> Atherosclerosis of other type of bypass graft(s) of left leg with ulceration of toe

 I70.748 Atherosclerosis of other type of bypass graft(s) of the left leg with ulceration of **other part of lower leg** 🔁 A

 I70.749 Atherosclerosis of other type of bypass graft(s) of the left leg with ulceration of **unspecified site** 🔁 A

 I70.75 **Atherosclerosis of other type of bypass graft(s) of other extremity with ulceration** 🔁 A

> **Includes** any condition classifiable to I70.718 and I70.728

> Use additional code to identify severity of ulcer (L98.49)

● **I70.76** **Atherosclerosis of other type of bypass graft(s) of the extremities with gangrene**

> **Includes** any condition classifiable to I70.71-, I70.72-, I70.73-, I70.74-, I70.75

> Use additional code to identify the severity of any ulcer (L97.-, L98.49-), if applicable

 I70.761 Atherosclerosis of other type of bypass graft(s) of the extremities with gangrene, **right leg** 🔁 A

 I70.762 Atherosclerosis of other type of bypass graft(s) of the extremities with gangrene, **left leg** 🔁 A

 I70.763 Atherosclerosis of other type of bypass graft(s) of the extremities with gangrene, **bilateral legs** 🔁 A

 I70.768 Atherosclerosis of other type of bypass graft(s) of the extremities with gangrene, **other extremity** 🔁 A

 I70.769 Atherosclerosis of other type of bypass graft(s) of the extremities with gangrene, **unspecified extremity** 🔁 A

● **I70.79** **Other atherosclerosis of other type of bypass graft(s) of the extremities**

 I70.791 Other atherosclerosis of other type of bypass graft(s) of the extremities, **right leg** 🔁 A

 I70.792 Other atherosclerosis of other type of bypass graft(s) of the extremities, **left leg** 🔁 A

 I70.793 Other atherosclerosis of other type of bypass graft(s) of the extremities, **bilateral legs** 🔁 A

 I70.798 Other atherosclerosis of other type of bypass graft(s) of the extremities, **other extremity** 🔁 A

 I70.799 Other atherosclerosis of other type of bypass graft(s) of the extremities, **unspecified extremity** 🔁 A

 I70.8 Atherosclerosis of other arteries A

● **I70.9** Other and unspecified atherosclerosis

 I70.90 **Unspecified atherosclerosis** A

 I70.91 **Generalized atherosclerosis** A

 I70.92 **Chronic total occlusion of artery of the extremities** 🔁 A

> Complete occlusion of artery of the extremities
> Total occlusion of artery of the extremities
> *Code first atherosclerosis of arteries of the extremities (I70.2-, I70.3-, I70.4-, I70.5-, I70.6-, I70.7-)*

CHAPTER 9 (I00-I99)

CHAPTER 9 (I00-I99)

● **I71**   **Aortic aneurysm and dissection**
      Excludes1   aortic ectasia (I77.81-)
                        syphilitic aortic aneurysm (A52.01)
                        traumatic aortic aneurysm (S25.09, S35.09)

  ● **I71.0**   **Dissection of aorta**
      I71.00   **Dissection of unspecified site of aorta** 🗖
      I71.01   **Dissection of thoracic aorta** 🗖
      I71.02   **Dissection of abdominal aorta** 🗖
      I71.03   **Dissection of thoracoabdominal aorta** 🗖

  I71.1   **Thoracic aortic aneurysm, ruptured** 🗖
  I71.2   **Thoracic aortic aneurysm, without rupture** 🗖
  I71.3   **Abdominal aortic aneurysm, ruptured** 🗖
  I71.4   **Abdominal aortic aneurysm, without rupture** 🗖
  I71.5   **Thoracoabdominal aortic aneurysm, ruptured** 🗖
  I71.6   **Thoracoabdominal aortic aneurysm, without rupture** 🗖
  I71.8   **Aortic aneurysm of unspecified site, ruptured** 🗖
      Rupture of aorta NOS
  I71.9   **Aortic aneurysm of unspecified site, without rupture** 🗖
      Aneurysm of aorta
      Dilatation of aorta
      Hyaline necrosis of aorta

● **I72**   **Other aneurysm**
      Includes   aneurysm (cirsoid) (false) (ruptured)
      Excludes2   acquired aneurysm (I77.0)
                     aneurysm (of) aorta (I71.-)
                     aneurysm (of) arteriovenous NOS (Q27.3-)
                     carotid artery dissection (I77.71)
                     cerebral (nonruptured) aneurysm (I67.1)
                     coronary aneurysm (I25.4)
                     coronary artery dissection (I25.42)
                     dissection of artery NEC (I77.79)
                     dissection of precerebral artery, congenital
                       (nonruptured) (Q28.1)
                     heart aneurysm (I25.3)
                     iliac artery dissection (I77.72)
                     precerebral artery, congenital (nonruptured) (Q28.1)
                     pulmonary artery aneurysm (I28.1)
                     renal artery dissection (I77.73)
                     retinal aneurysm (H35.0)
                     ruptured cerebral aneurysm (I60.7)
                     varicose aneurysm (I77.0)
                     vertebral artery dissection (I77.74)

  I72.0   **Aneurysm of carotid artery** 🗖
      Aneurysm of common carotid artery
      Aneurysm of external carotid artery
      Aneurysm of internal carotid artery, extracranial
        portion
      Excludes1   aneurysm of internal carotid artery,
                    intracranial portion (I67.1)
                    aneurysm of internal carotid artery NOS
                    (I67.1)

  I72.1   **Aneurysm of artery of upper extremity** 🗖
  I72.2   **Aneurysm of renal artery** 🗖
  I72.3   **Aneurysm of iliac artery** 🗖
  I72.4   **Aneurysm of artery of lower extremity** 🗖
      Coding Clinic: 2019, Q2, P22
  I72.5   **Aneurysm of other precerebral arteries** 🗖
      Aneurysm of basilar artery (trunk)
      Excludes2   aneurysm of carotid artery (I72.0)
                    aneurysm of vertebral artery (I72.6)
                    dissection of carotid artery (I77.71)
                    dissection of other precerebral arteries
                     (I77.75)
                    dissection of vertebral artery (I77.74)
      Coding Clinic 2016, Q4, P28
  I72.6   **Aneurysm of vertebral artery** 🗖
      Excludes2   dissection of vertebral artery (I77.74)
      Coding Clinic 2016, Q4, P28
  I72.8   **Aneurysm of other specified arteries** 🗖
  I72.9   **Aneurysm of unspecified site** 🗖

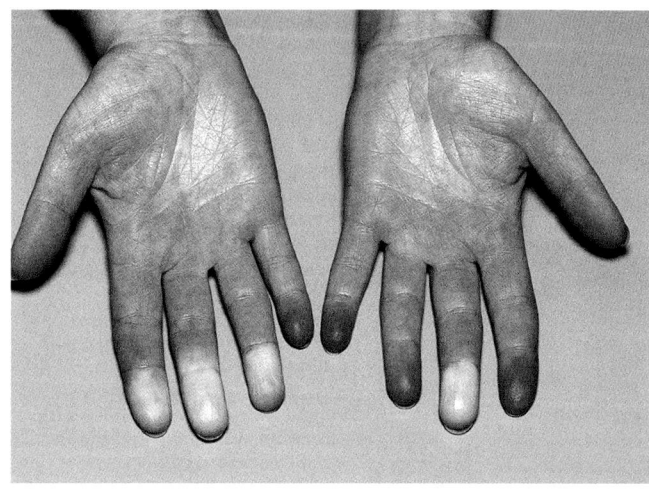

Figure 9-5   Raynaud's syndrome. (From Hallett: Comprehensive Vascular and Endovascular Surgery, ed 2, Philadelphia, Mosby Ltd., 2010)

● **I73**   **Other peripheral vascular diseases**
      Excludes2   chilblains (T69.1)
                    frostbite (T33-T34)
                    immersion hand or foot (T69.0-)
                    spasm of cerebral artery (G45.9)
    Coding Clinic: 2018, Q4, P87-88

  ● **I73.0**   **Raynaud's syndrome**
      Diminishing oxygen supply to fingers, toes, nose, and ears when exposed to temperature changes or stress
      Raynaud's disease
      Raynaud's phenomenon (secondary)
      I73.00   **Raynaud's syndrome without gangrene**
      I73.01   **Raynaud's syndrome with gangrene** 🗖

  I73.1   **Thromboangiitis obliterans [Buerger's disease]** 🗖
      Inflammatory occlusive disease resulting in poor circulation to the legs, feet, and sometimes the hands due to progressive inflammatory narrowing and eventually obliteration of the small arteries

  ● **I73.8**   **Other specified peripheral vascular diseases**
      Excludes1   diabetic (peripheral) angiopathy
                    (E08-E13 with .51-.52)
      I73.81   **Erythromelalgia** 🗖
      I73.89   **Other specified peripheral vascular diseases** 🗖
          Acrocyanosis
          Erythrocyanosis
          Simple acroparesthesia [Schultze's type]
          Vasomotor acroparesthesia [Nothnagel's type]

  I73.9   **Peripheral vascular disease, unspecified** 🗖
      Intermittent claudication
      Peripheral angiopathy NOS
      Spasm of artery
      Excludes1   atherosclerosis of the extremities
                    (I70.2—I70.7-)
    Coding Clinic: 2018, Q4, P87

▶ New   ⇒ Revised   ~~deleted~~ Deleted   Excludes 1   Excludes 2   Includes   Use additional   Code first   Code also   Key words

894   OGCR Official Guidelines   X Assign placeholder X   ● Use Additional Character(s)   ▶ Manifestation Code   🗖 Hierarchical Condition Category   **Coding Clinic**

Item 9–9   An **embolus** is a mass of undissolved matter present in the blood that is transported by the blood current. A **thrombus** is a blood clot that occludes or shuts off a vessel. When a thrombus is dislodged, it becomes an embolus.

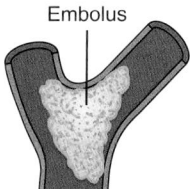
Embolus

Figure 9-6   An arterial embolus.

● I74   **Arterial embolism and thrombosis**

    Includes   embolic infarction
                embolic occlusion
                thrombotic infarction
                thrombotic occlusion

    Code first embolism and thrombosis complicating abortion or ectopic or molar pregnancy (O00-O07, O08.2)
       embolism and thrombosis complicating pregnancy, childbirth and the puerperium (O88.-)

    Excludes2   atheroembolism (I75.-)
               basilar embolism and thrombosis (I63.0-I63.2, I65.1)
               carotid embolism and thrombosis (I63.0-I63.2, I65.2)
               cerebral embolism and thrombosis (I63.3-I63.5, I66.-)
               coronary embolism and thrombosis (I21-I25)
               mesenteric embolism and thrombosis (K55.0-)
               ophthalmic embolism and thrombosis (H34.-)
               precerebral embolism and thrombosis NOS (I63.0-I63.2, I65.9)
               pulmonary embolism and thrombosis (I26.-)
               renal embolism and thrombosis (N28.0)
               retinal embolism and thrombosis (H34.-)
               septic embolism and thrombosis (I76)
               vertebral embolism and thrombosis (I63.0-I63.2, I65.0)

● **I74.0**   **Embolism and thrombosis of abdominal aorta**

    I74.01   **Saddle embolus of abdominal aorta** 🔖

    I74.09   **Other arterial embolism and thrombosis of abdominal aorta** 🔖
           Aortic bifurcation syndrome
           Aortoiliac obstruction
           Leriche's syndrome

● **I74.1**   **Embolism and thrombosis of other and unspecified parts of aorta**

    I74.10   **Embolism and thrombosis of unspecified parts of aorta** 🔖

    I74.11   **Embolism and thrombosis of thoracic aorta** 🔖

    I74.19   **Embolism and thrombosis of other parts of aorta** 🔖

   I74.2   **Embolism and thrombosis of arteries of the upper extremities** 🔖

   I74.3   **Embolism and thrombosis of arteries of the lower extremities** 🔖

   I74.4   **Embolism and thrombosis of arteries of extremities, unspecified** 🔖
       Peripheral arterial embolism NOS

   I74.5   **Embolism and thrombosis of iliac artery** 🔖

   I74.8   **Embolism and thrombosis of other arteries** 🔖

   I74.9   **Embolism and thrombosis of unspecified artery** 🔖

● I75   **Atheroembolism**

    Includes   atherothrombotic microembolism
                cholesterol embolism

● **I75.0**   **Atheroembolism of extremities**

   ● **I75.01**   **Atheroembolism of upper extremity**

       I75.011   **Atheroembolism of right upper extremity** 🔖

       I75.012   **Atheroembolism of left upper extremity** 🔖

       I75.013   **Atheroembolism of bilateral upper extremities** 🔖

       I75.019   **Atheroembolism of unspecified upper extremity** 🔖

   ● **I75.02**   **Atheroembolism of lower extremity**

       I75.021   **Atheroembolism of right lower extremity** 🔖

       I75.022   **Atheroembolism of left lower extremity** 🔖

       I75.023   **Atheroembolism of bilateral lower extremities** 🔖

       I75.029   **Atheroembolism of unspecified lower extremity** 🔖

● **I75.8**   **Atheroembolism of other sites**

    I75.81   **Atheroembolism of kidney** 🔖
         Use additional code for any associated acute kidney failure and chronic kidney disease (N17.-, N18.-)

    I75.89   **Atheroembolism of other site** 🔖

I76   **Septic arterial embolism** 🔖

    Code first underlying infection, such as:
      infective endocarditis (I33.0)
      lung abscess (J85.-)
    Use additional code to identify the site of the embolism (I74.-)

    Excludes2   septic pulmonary embolism (I26.01, I26.90)

● I77   **Other disorders of arteries and arterioles**

    Excludes2   collagen (vascular) diseases (M30-M36)
               hypersensitivity angiitis (M31.0)
               pulmonary artery (I28.-)

   I77.0   **Arteriovenous fistula, acquired** 🔖
      Aneurysmal varix
      Arteriovenous aneurysm, acquired

    Excludes1   arteriovenous aneurysm NOS (Q27.3-)
               presence of arteriovenous shunt (fistula) for dialysis (Z99.2)
               traumatic - see injury of blood vessel by body region

    Excludes2   cerebral (I67.1)
               coronary (I25.4)

   I77.1   **Stricture of artery** 🔖
      Narrowing of artery

   I77.2   **Rupture of artery** 🔖
      Erosion of artery
      Fistula of artery
      Ulcer of artery

    Excludes1   traumatic rupture of artery - see injury of blood vessel by body region

   I77.3   **Arterial fibromuscular dysplasia** 🔖
      Fibromuscular hyperplasia (of) carotid artery
      Fibromuscular hyperplasia (of) renal artery

   I77.4   **Celiac artery compression syndrome** 🔖

   I77.5   **Necrosis of artery** 🔖

CHAPTER 9 (I00-I99)

I77.6 **Arteritis, unspecified**
Aortitis NOS
Endarteritis NOS
Excludes1 arteritis or endarteritis:
aortic arch (M31.4)
cerebral NEC (I67.7)
coronary (I25.89)
deformans (I70.-)
giant cell (M31.5, M31.6)
obliterans (I70.-)
senile (I70.-)

I77.7 **Other arterial dissection**
Excludes2 dissection of aorta (I71.0-)
dissection of coronary artery (I25.42)

I77.70 **Dissection of unspecified artery**
Coding Clinic 2016, Q4, P28

I77.71 **Dissection of carotid artery**

I77.72 **Dissection of iliac artery**

I77.73 **Dissection of renal artery**

I77.74 **Dissection of vertebral artery**
Excludes2 aneurysm of vertebral artery (I72.6)

I77.75 **Dissection of other precerebral arteries**
Dissection of basilar artery (trunk)
Excludes2 aneurysm of carotid artery (I72.0)
aneurysm of other precerebral arteries (I72.5)
aneurysm of vertebral artery (I72.6)
dissection of carotid artery (I77.71)
dissection of vertebral artery (I77.74)
Coding Clinic 2016, Q4, P28

I77.76 **Dissection of artery of upper extremity**
Coding Clinic 2016, Q4, P28

I77.77 **Dissection of artery of lower extremity**
Coding Clinic 2016, Q4, P28

I77.79 **Dissection of other specified artery**
Coding Clinic 2016, Q4, P28

I77.8 **Other specified disorders of arteries and arterioles**

I77.81 **Aortic ectasia**
Ectasis aorta
Excludes1 aortic aneurysm and dissection (I71.0-)

I77.810 **Thoracic aortic ectasia**

I77.811 **Abdominal aortic ectasia**

I77.812 **Thoracoabdominal aortic ectasia**

I77.819 **Aortic ectasia, unspecified site**

I77.89 **Other specified disorders of arteries and arterioles**

I77.9 **Disorder of arteries and arterioles, unspecified**

I78 **Diseases of capillaries**

I78.0 **Hereditary hemorrhagic telangiectasia**
Rendu-Osler-Weber disease

I78.1 **Nevus, non-neoplastic**
Araneus nevus
Senile nevus
Spider nevus
Stellar nevus
Excludes1 nevus NOS (D22.-)
vascular NOS (Q82.5)
Excludes2 blue nevus (D22.-)
flammeus nevus (Q82.5)
hairy nevus (D22.-)
melanocytic nevus (D22.-)
pigmented nevus (D22.-)
portwine nevus (Q82.5)
sanguineous nevus (Q82.5)
strawberry nevus (Q82.5)
verrucous nevus (Q82.5)
Coding Clinic: 2019, Q1, P21

I78.8 **Other diseases of capillaries**

I78.9 **Disease of capillaries, unspecified**

I79 **Disorders of arteries, arterioles and capillaries in diseases classified elsewhere**

I79.0 ***Aneurysm of aorta in diseases classified elsewhere***
Code first underlying disease
Excludes1 syphilitic aneurysm (A52.01)

I79.1 ***Aortitis in diseases classified elsewhere***
Code first underlying disease
Excludes1 syphilitic aortitis (A52.02)

I79.8 ***Other disorders of arteries, arterioles and capillaries in diseases classified elsewhere***
Code first underlying disease, such as:
amyloidosis (E85.-)
Excludes1 diabetic (peripheral) angiopathy (E08-E13 with .51-.52)
syphilitic endarteritis (A52.09)
tuberculous endarteritis (A18.89)

DISEASES OF VEINS, LYMPHATIC VESSELS AND LYMPH NODES, NOT ELSEWHERE CLASSIFIED (I80-I89)

I80 **Phlebitis and thrombophlebitis**
Inflammation of a vein with infiltration of walls (phlebitis)
Includes endophlebitis
inflammation, vein
periphlebitis
suppurative phlebitis
Code first phlebitis and thrombophlebitis complicating abortion, ectopic or molar pregnancy (O00-O07, O08.7)
phlebitis and thrombophlebitis complicating pregnancy, childbirth and the puerperium (O22.-, O87.-)
Excludes1 venous embolism and thrombosis of lower extremities (I82.4-, I82.5-, I82.81-)

I80.0 **Phlebitis and thrombophlebitis of superficial vessels of lower extremities**
Phlebitis and thrombophlebitis of femoropopliteal vein

I80.00 **Phlebitis and thrombophlebitis of superficial vessels of unspecified lower extremity**

I80.01 **Phlebitis and thrombophlebitis of superficial vessels of right lower extremity**

I80.02 **Phlebitis and thrombophlebitis of superficial vessels of left lower extremity**

I80.03 **Phlebitis and thrombophlebitis of superficial vessels of lower extremities, bilateral**

I80.1 **Phlebitis and thrombophlebitis of femoral vein**
▶Phlebitis and thrombophlebitis of common femoral vein
▶Phlebitis and thrombophlebitis of deep femoral vein

I80.10 **Phlebitis and thrombophlebitis of unspecified femoral vein**

I80.11 **Phlebitis and thrombophlebitis of right femoral vein**

I80.12 **Phlebitis and thrombophlebitis of left femoral vein**

I80.13 **Phlebitis and thrombophlebitis of femoral vein, bilateral**

I80.2 **Phlebitis and thrombophlebitis of other and unspecified deep vessels of lower extremities**

I80.20 **Phlebitis and thrombophlebitis of unspecified deep vessels of lower extremities**

I80.201 **Phlebitis and thrombophlebitis of unspecified deep vessels of right lower extremity**

I80.202 **Phlebitis and thrombophlebitis of unspecified deep vessels of left lower extremity**

I80.203 **Phlebitis and thrombophlebitis of unspecified deep vessels of lower extremities, bilateral**

I80.209 **Phlebitis and thrombophlebitis of unspecified deep vessels of unspecified lower extremity**

● I80.21 **Phlebitis and thrombophlebitis of iliac vein**
▶Phlebitis and thrombophlebitis of common iliac vein
▶Phlebitis and thrombophlebitis of external iliac vein
▶Phlebitis and thrombophlebitis of internal iliac vein

I80.211 **Phlebitis and thrombophlebitis of right iliac vein**

I80.212 **Phlebitis and thrombophlebitis of left iliac vein**

I80.213 **Phlebitis and thrombophlebitis of iliac vein, bilateral**

I80.219 **Phlebitis and thrombophlebitis of unspecified iliac vein**

● I80.22 **Phlebitis and thrombophlebitis of popliteal vein**

I80.221 **Phlebitis and thrombophlebitis of right popliteal vein**

I80.222 **Phlebitis and thrombophlebitis of left popliteal vein**

I80.223 **Phlebitis and thrombophlebitis of popliteal vein, bilateral**

I80.229 **Phlebitis and thrombophlebitis of unspecified popliteal vein**

● I80.23 **Phlebitis and thrombophlebitis of tibial vein**
▶Phlebitis and thrombophlebitis of anterior tibial vein
▶Phlebitis and thrombophlebitis of posterior tibial vein

I80.231 **Phlebitis and thrombophlebitis of right tibial vein**

I80.232 **Phlebitis and thrombophlebitis of left tibial vein**

I80.233 **Phlebitis and thrombophlebitis of tibial vein, bilateral**

I80.239 **Phlebitis and thrombophlebitis of unspecified tibial vein**

▶● I80.24 **Phlebitis and thrombophlebitis of peroneal vein**

▶I80.241 **Phlebitis and thrombophlebitis of right peroneal vein**

▶I80.242 **Phlebitis and thrombophlebitis of left peroneal vein**

▶I80.243 **Phlebitis and thrombophlebitis of peroneal vein, bilateral**

▶I80.249 **Phlebitis and thrombophlebitis of unspecified peroneal vein**

▶● I80.25 **Phlebitis and thrombophlebitis of calf muscular vein**
▶Phlebitis and thrombophlebitis of calf muscular vein, NOS
▶Phlebitis and thrombophlebitis of gastrocnemial vein
▶Phlebitis and thrombophlebitis of soleal vein

▶ I80.251 **Phlebitis and thrombophlebitis of right calf muscular vein**

▶ I80.252 **Phlebitis and thrombophlebitis of left calf muscular vein**

▶ I80.253 **Phlebitis and thrombophlebitis of calf muscular vein, bilateral**

▶ I80.259 **Phlebitis and thrombophlebitis of unspecified calf muscular vein**

● I80.29 **Phlebitis and thrombophlebitis of other deep vessels of lower extremities**

I80.291 **Phlebitis and thrombophlebitis of other deep vessels of right lower extremity**

I80.292 **Phlebitis and thrombophlebitis of other deep vessels of left lower extremity**

I80.293 **Phlebitis and thrombophlebitis of other deep vessels of lower extremity, bilateral**

I80.299 **Phlebitis and thrombophlebitis of other deep vessels of unspecified lower extremity**

I80.3 **Phlebitis and thrombophlebitis of lower extremities, unspecified**

I80.8 **Phlebitis and thrombophlebitis of other sites**

I80.9 **Phlebitis and thrombophlebitis of unspecified site**

I81 **Portal vein thrombosis**
Portal (vein) obstruction
Excludes2 hepatic vein thrombosis (I82.0)
phlebitis of portal vein (K75.1)

● I82 **Other venous embolism and thrombosis**
Code first venous embolism and thrombosis complicating:
abortion, ectopic or molar pregnancy (O00-O07, O08.7)
pregnancy, childbirth and the puerperium (O22.-, O87.-)
Excludes2 venous embolism and thrombosis (of):
cerebral (I63.6, I67.6)
coronary (I21-I25)
intracranial and intraspinal, septic or NOS (G08)
intracranial, nonpyogenic (I67.6)
intraspinal, nonpyogenic (G95.1)
mesenteric (K55.0-)
portal (I81)
pulmonary (I26.-)

I82.0 **Budd-Chiari syndrome**
Hepatic vein thrombosis

I82.1 **Thrombophlebitis migrans**
"White leg" is the other term to describe a migrating thrombus.

● I82.2 **Embolism and thrombosis of vena cava and other thoracic veins**

● I82.21 **Embolism and thrombosis of superior vena cava**

I82.210 **Acute embolism and thrombosis of superior vena cava**
Embolism and thrombosis of superior vena cava NOS

I82.211 **Chronic embolism and thrombosis of superior vena cava**

● I82.22 **Embolism and thrombosis of inferior vena cava**

I82.220 **Acute embolism and thrombosis of inferior vena cava**
Embolism and thrombosis of inferior vena cava NOS

I82.221 **Chronic embolism and thrombosis of inferior vena cava**

● I82.29 **Embolism and thrombosis of other thoracic veins**
Embolism and thrombosis of brachiocephalic (innominate) vein

I82.290 **Acute embolism and thrombosis of other thoracic veins**

I82.291 **Chronic embolism and thrombosis of other thoracic veins**

I82.3 **Embolism and thrombosis of renal vein**

I82.4 Acute embolism and thrombosis of deep veins of lower extremity

I82.40 Acute embolism and thrombosis of unspecified deep veins of lower extremity

Deep vein thrombosis NOS
DVT NOS

Excludes1 acute embolism and thrombosis of unspecified deep veins of distal lower extremity (I82.4Z-)
acute embolism and thrombosis of unspecified deep veins of proximal lower extremity (I82.4Y-)

I82.401 Acute embolism and thrombosis of unspecified deep veins of right lower extremity

I82.402 Acute embolism and thrombosis of unspecified deep veins of left lower extremity

I82.403 Acute embolism and thrombosis of unspecified deep veins of lower extremity, bilateral

I82.409 Acute embolism and thrombosis of unspecified deep veins of unspecified lower extremity

I82.41 Acute embolism and thrombosis of femoral vein

Acute embolism and thrombosis of common femoral vein
Acute embolism and thrombosis of deep femoral vein

I82.411 Acute embolism and thrombosis of right femoral vein

I82.412 Acute embolism and thrombosis of left femoral vein

I82.413 Acute embolism and thrombosis of femoral vein, bilateral

I82.419 Acute embolism and thrombosis of unspecified femoral vein

I82.42 Acute embolism and thrombosis of iliac vein

Acute embolism and thrombosis of common iliac vein
Acute embolism and thrombosis of external iliac vein
Acute embolism and thrombosis of internal iliac vein

I82.421 Acute embolism and thrombosis of right iliac vein

I82.422 Acute embolism and thrombosis of left iliac vein

I82.423 Acute embolism and thrombosis of iliac vein, bilateral

I82.429 Acute embolism and thrombosis of unspecified iliac vein

I82.43 Acute embolism and thrombosis of popliteal vein

I82.431 Acute embolism and thrombosis of right popliteal vein

I82.432 Acute embolism and thrombosis of left popliteal vein

I82.433 Acute embolism and thrombosis of popliteal vein, bilateral

I82.439 Acute embolism and thrombosis of unspecified popliteal vein

I82.44 Acute embolism and thrombosis of tibial vein

Acute embolism and thrombosis of anterior tibial vein
Acute embolism and thrombosis of posterior tibial vein

I82.441 Acute embolism and thrombosis of right tibial vein

I82.442 Acute embolism and thrombosis of left tibial vein

I82.443 Acute embolism and thrombosis of tibial vein, bilateral

I82.449 Acute embolism and thrombosis of unspecified tibial vein

I82.45 Acute embolism and thrombosis of peroneal vein

I82.451 Acute embolism and thrombosis of right peroneal vein

I82.452 Acute embolism and thrombosis of left peroneal vein

I82.453 Acute embolism and thrombosis of peroneal vein, bilateral

I82.459 Acute embolism and thrombosis of unspecified peroneal vein

I82.46 Acute embolism and thrombosis of calf muscular vein

Acute embolism and thrombosis of calf muscular vein, NOS
Acute embolism and thrombosis of gastrocnemial vein
Acute embolism and thrombosis of soleal vein

I82.461 Acute embolism and thrombosis of right calf muscular vein

I82.462 Acute embolism and thrombosis of left calf muscular vein

I82.463 Acute embolism and thrombosis of calf muscular vein, bilateral

I82.469 Acute embolism and thrombosis of unspecified calf muscular vein

I82.49 Acute embolism and thrombosis of other specified deep vein of lower extremity

I82.491 Acute embolism and thrombosis of other specified deep vein of right lower extremity

I82.492 Acute embolism and thrombosis of other specified deep vein of left lower extremity

I82.493 Acute embolism and thrombosis of other specified deep vein of lower extremity, bilateral

I82.499 Acute embolism and thrombosis of other specified deep vein of unspecified lower extremity

I82.4Y Acute embolism and thrombosis of unspecified deep veins of proximal lower extremity

Acute embolism and thrombosis of deep vein of thigh NOS
Acute embolism and thrombosis of deep vein of upper leg NOS

I82.4Y1 Acute embolism and thrombosis of unspecified deep veins of right proximal lower extremity

I82.4Y2 Acute embolism and thrombosis of unspecified deep veins of left proximal lower extremity

I82.4Y3 Acute embolism and thrombosis of unspecified deep veins of proximal lower extremity, bilateral

I82.4Y9 Acute embolism and thrombosis of unspecified deep veins of unspecified proximal lower extremity

● I82.4Z **Acute embolism and thrombosis of unspecified deep veins of distal lower extremity**
Acute embolism and thrombosis of deep vein of calf NOS
Acute embolism and thrombosis of deep vein of lower leg NOS
I82.4Z1 **Acute embolism and thrombosis of unspecified deep veins of right distal lower extremity**
I82.4Z2 **Acute embolism and thrombosis of unspecified deep veins of left distal lower extremity**
I82.4Z3 **Acute embolism and thrombosis of unspecified deep veins of distal lower extremity, bilateral**
I82.4Z9 **Acute embolism and thrombosis of unspecified deep veins of unspecified distal lower extremity**

● I82.5 **Chronic embolism and thrombosis of deep veins of lower extremity**
Use additional code, if applicable, for associated long-term (current) use of anticoagulants (Z79.01)
Excludes1 personal history of venous embolism and thrombosis (Z86.718)

● I82.50 **Chronic embolism and thrombosis of unspecified deep veins of lower extremity**
Excludes1 chronic embolism and thrombosis of unspecified deep veins of distal lower extremity (I82.5Z-)
chronic embolism and thrombosis of unspecified deep veins of proximal lower extremity (I82.5Y-)
I82.501 **Chronic embolism and thrombosis of unspecified deep veins of right lower extremity**
I82.502 **Chronic embolism and thrombosis of unspecified deep veins of left lower extremity**
I82.503 **Chronic embolism and thrombosis of unspecified deep veins of lower extremity, bilateral**
I82.509 **Chronic embolism and thrombosis of unspecified deep veins of unspecified lower extremity**

● I82.51 **Chronic embolism and thrombosis of femoral vein**
▶Chronic embolism and thrombosis of common femoral vein
▶Chronic embolism and thrombosis of deep femoral vein
I82.511 **Chronic embolism and thrombosis of right femoral vein**
I82.512 **Chronic embolism and thrombosis of left femoral vein**
I82.513 **Chronic embolism and thrombosis of femoral vein, bilateral**
I82.519 **Chronic embolism and thrombosis of unspecified femoral vein**

● I82.52 **Chronic embolism and thrombosis of iliac vein**
▶Chronic embolism and thrombosis of common iliac vein
▶Chronic embolism and thrombosis of external iliac vein
▶Chronic embolism and thrombosis of internal iliac vein
I82.521 **Chronic embolism and thrombosis of right iliac vein**
I82.522 **Chronic embolism and thrombosis of left iliac vein**

Item 9–10 Varicose/Varicosities (varix = singular, varices = plural): Enlarged, engorged, tortuous, twisted vascular vessels (veins, arteries, lymphatics). As such, the condition can present in various parts of the body, although the most familiar locations are the lower extremities. A common complication of varices is thrombophlebitis. Varicosities of the anus and rectum are called hemorrhoids.

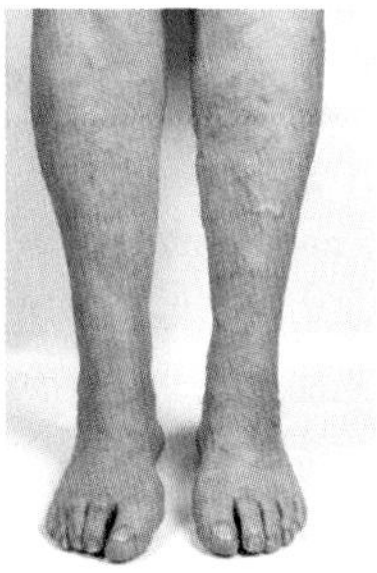

Figure 9-7 Varicose veins of the legs. (Getty Image)

I82.523 **Chronic embolism and thrombosis of iliac vein, bilateral**
I82.529 **Chronic embolism and thrombosis of unspecified iliac vein**

● I82.53 **Chronic embolism and thrombosis of popliteal vein**
I82.531 **Chronic embolism and thrombosis of right popliteal vein**
I82.532 **Chronic embolism and thrombosis of left popliteal vein**
I82.533 **Chronic embolism and thrombosis of popliteal vein, bilateral**
I82.539 **Chronic embolism and thrombosis of unspecified popliteal vein**

● I82.54 **Chronic embolism and thrombosis of tibial vein**
▶Chronic embolism and thrombosis of anterior tibial vein
▶Chronic embolism and thrombosis of posterior tibial vein
I82.541 **Chronic embolism and thrombosis of right tibial vein**
I82.542 **Chronic embolism and thrombosis of left tibial vein**
I82.543 **Chronic embolism and thrombosis of tibial vein, bilateral**
I82.549 **Chronic embolism and thrombosis of unspecified tibial vein**

▶● I82.55 **Chronic embolism and thrombosis of peroneal vein**
▶I82.551 **Chronic embolism and thrombosis of right peroneal vein**
▶I82.552 **Chronic embolism and thrombosis of left peroneal vein**
▶I82.553 **Chronic embolism and thrombosis of peroneal vein, bilateral**
▶I82.559 **Chronic embolism and thrombosis of unspecified peroneal vein**

▶● I82.56 **Chronic embolism and thrombosis of calf muscular vein**
▶Chronic embolism and thrombosis of calf muscular vein NOS
▶Chronic embolism and thrombosis of gastrocnemial vein
▶Chronic embolism and thrombosis of soleal vein
▶I82.561 **Chronic embolism and thrombosis of right calf muscular vein**
▶I82.562 **Chronic embolism and thrombosis of left calf muscular vein**
▶I82.563 **Chronic embolism and thrombosis of calf muscular vein, bilateral**
▶I82.569 **Chronic embolism and thrombosis of unspecified calf muscular vein**

CHAPTER 9 (I00-I99)

- I82.59 **Chronic embolism and thrombosis of other specified deep vein of lower extremity**
  - I82.591 **Chronic embolism and thrombosis of other specified deep vein of right lower extremity**
  - I82.592 **Chronic embolism and thrombosis of other specified deep vein of left lower extremity**
  - I82.593 **Chronic embolism and thrombosis of other specified deep vein of lower extremity, bilateral**
  - I82.599 **Chronic embolism and thrombosis of other specified deep vein of unspecified lower extremity**
- I82.5Y **Chronic embolism and thrombosis of unspecified deep veins of proximal lower extremity**
  Chronic embolism and thrombosis of deep veins of thigh NOS
  Chronic embolism and thrombosis of deep veins of upper leg NOS
  - I82.5Y1 **Chronic embolism and thrombosis of unspecified deep veins of right proximal lower extremity**
  - I82.5Y2 **Chronic embolism and thrombosis of unspecified deep veins of left proximal lower extremity**
  - I82.5Y3 **Chronic embolism and thrombosis of unspecified deep veins of proximal lower extremity, bilateral**
  - I82.5Y9 **Chronic embolism and thrombosis of unspecified deep veins of unspecified proximal lower extremity**
- I82.5Z **Chronic embolism and thrombosis of unspecified deep veins of distal lower extremity**
  Chronic embolism and thrombosis of deep veins of calf NOS
  Chronic embolism and thrombosis of deep veins of lower leg NOS
  - I82.5Z1 **Chronic embolism and thrombosis of unspecified deep veins of right distal lower extremity**
  - I82.5Z2 **Chronic embolism and thrombosis of unspecified deep veins of left distal lower extremity**
  - I82.5Z3 **Chronic embolism and thrombosis of unspecified deep veins of distal lower extremity, bilateral**
  - I82.5Z9 **Chronic embolism and thrombosis of unspecified deep veins of unspecified distal lower extremity**

I82.6 **Acute embolism and thrombosis of veins of upper extremity**
- I82.60 **Acute embolism and thrombosis of unspecified veins of upper extremity**
  - I82.601 **Acute embolism and thrombosis of unspecified veins of right upper extremity**
  - I82.602 **Acute embolism and thrombosis of unspecified veins of left upper extremity**
  - I82.603 **Acute embolism and thrombosis of unspecified veins of upper extremity, bilateral**
  - I82.609 **Acute embolism and thrombosis of unspecified veins of unspecified upper extremity**
- I82.61 **Acute embolism and thrombosis of superficial veins of upper extremity**
  Acute embolism and thrombosis of antecubital vein
  Acute embolism and thrombosis of basilic vein
  Acute embolism and thrombosis of cephalic vein
  - I82.611 **Acute embolism and thrombosis of superficial veins of right upper extremity**
  - I82.612 **Acute embolism and thrombosis of superficial veins of left upper extremity**
  - I82.613 **Acute embolism and thrombosis of superficial veins of upper extremity, bilateral**
  - I82.619 **Acute embolism and thrombosis of superficial veins of unspecified upper extremity**
- I82.62 **Acute embolism and thrombosis of deep veins of upper extremity**
  Acute embolism and thrombosis of brachial vein
  Acute embolism and thrombosis of radial vein
  Acute embolism and thrombosis of ulnar vein
  - I82.621 **Acute embolism and thrombosis of deep veins of right upper extremity**
  - I82.622 **Acute embolism and thrombosis of deep veins of left upper extremity**
  - I82.623 **Acute embolism and thrombosis of deep veins of upper extremity, bilateral**
  - I82.629 **Acute embolism and thrombosis of deep veins of unspecified upper extremity**

I82.7 **Chronic embolism and thrombosis of veins of upper extremity**
Use additional code, if applicable, for associated long-term (current) use of anticoagulants (Z79.01)
Excludes1 personal history of venous embolism and thrombosis (Z86.718)
- I82.70 **Chronic embolism and thrombosis of unspecified veins of upper extremity**
  - I82.701 **Chronic embolism and thrombosis of unspecified veins of right upper extremity**
  - I82.702 **Chronic embolism and thrombosis of unspecified veins of left upper extremity**
  - I82.703 **Chronic embolism and thrombosis of unspecified veins of upper extremity, bilateral**
  - I82.709 **Chronic embolism and thrombosis of unspecified veins of unspecified upper extremity**
- I82.71 **Chronic embolism and thrombosis of superficial veins of upper extremity**
  Chronic embolism and thrombosis of antecubital vein
  Chronic embolism and thrombosis of basilic vein
  Chronic embolism and thrombosis of cephalic vein
  - I82.711 **Chronic embolism and thrombosis of superficial veins of right upper extremity**
  - I82.712 **Chronic embolism and thrombosis of superficial veins of left upper extremity**
  - I82.713 **Chronic embolism and thrombosis of superficial veins of upper extremity, bilateral**
  - I82.719 **Chronic embolism and thrombosis of superficial veins of unspecified upper extremity**

- I82.72 Chronic embolism and thrombosis of deep veins of upper extremity
  - Chronic embolism and thrombosis of brachial vein
  - Chronic embolism and thrombosis of radial vein
  - Chronic embolism and thrombosis of ulnar vein
  - I82.721 Chronic embolism and thrombosis of deep veins of **right** upper extremity
  - I82.722 Chronic embolism and thrombosis of deep veins of **left** upper extremity
  - I82.723 Chronic embolism and thrombosis of deep veins of upper extremity, **bilateral**
  - I82.729 Chronic embolism and thrombosis of deep veins of **unspecified** upper extremity

- I82.A Embolism and thrombosis of **axillary vein**
  - I82.A1 **Acute** embolism and thrombosis of axillary vein
    - I82.A11 Acute embolism and thrombosis of **right** axillary vein
    - I82.A12 Acute embolism and thrombosis of **left** axillary vein
    - I82.A13 Acute embolism and thrombosis of axillary vein, **bilateral**
    - I82.A19 Acute embolism and thrombosis of **unspecified** axillary vein
  - I82.A2 **Chronic** embolism and thrombosis of axillary vein
    - I82.A21 Chronic embolism and thrombosis of **right** axillary vein
    - I82.A22 Chronic embolism and thrombosis of **left** axillary vein
    - I82.A23 Chronic embolism and thrombosis of axillary vein, **bilateral**
    - I82.A29 Chronic embolism and thrombosis of **unspecified** axillary vein

- I82.B Embolism and thrombosis of **subclavian vein**
  - I82.B1 **Acute** embolism and thrombosis of subclavian vein
    - I82.B11 Acute embolism and thrombosis of **right** subclavian vein
    - I82.B12 Acute embolism and thrombosis of **left** subclavian vein
    - I82.B13 Acute embolism and thrombosis of subclavian vein, **bilateral**
    - I82.B19 Acute embolism and thrombosis of **unspecified** subclavian vein
  - I82.B2 **Chronic** embolism and thrombosis of subclavian vein
    - I82.B21 Chronic embolism and thrombosis of **right** subclavian vein
    - I82.B22 Chronic embolism and thrombosis of **left** subclavian vein
    - I82.B23 Chronic embolism and thrombosis of subclavian vein, **bilateral**
    - I82.B29 Chronic embolism and thrombosis of **unspecified** subclavian vein

- I82.C Embolism and thrombosis of **internal jugular vein**
  - I82.C1 **Acute** embolism and thrombosis of internal jugular vein
    - I82.C11 Acute embolism and thrombosis of **right** internal jugular vein
    - I82.C12 Acute embolism and thrombosis of **left** internal jugular vein
    - I82.C13 Acute embolism and thrombosis of internal jugular vein, **bilateral**
    - I82.C19 Acute embolism and thrombosis of **unspecified** internal jugular vein
  - I82.C2 **Chronic** embolism and thrombosis of internal jugular vein
    - I82.C21 Chronic embolism and thrombosis of **right** internal jugular vein
    - I82.C22 Chronic embolism and thrombosis of **left** internal jugular vein
    - I82.C23 Chronic embolism and thrombosis of internal jugular vein, **bilateral**
    - I82.C29 Chronic embolism and thrombosis of **unspecified** internal jugular vein

- I82.8 Embolism and thrombosis of **other specified veins**
  - Use additional code, if applicable, for associated long-term (current) use of anticoagulants (Z79.01)
  - I82.81 Embolism and thrombosis of **superficial veins of lower extremities**
    - Embolism and thrombosis of saphenous vein (greater) (lesser)
    - I82.811 Embolism and thrombosis of superficial veins of **right** lower extremity
    - I82.812 Embolism and thrombosis of superficial veins of **left** lower extremity
    - I82.813 Embolism and thrombosis of superficial veins of lower extremities, **bilateral**
    - I82.819 Embolism and thrombosis of superficial veins of **unspecified** lower extremity
  - I82.89 Embolism and thrombosis of **other specified** veins
    - I82.890 **Acute** embolism and thrombosis of other specified veins
    - I82.891 **Chronic** embolism and thrombosis of other specified veins

- I82.9 Embolism and thrombosis of **unspecified vein**
  - I82.90 **Acute** embolism and thrombosis of unspecified vein
    - Embolism of vein NOS
    - Thrombosis (vein) NOS
  - I82.91 **Chronic** embolism and thrombosis of unspecified vein

I83 Varicose veins of lower extremities

Excludes1 varicose veins complicating pregnancy (O22.0-)
varicose veins complicating the puerperium (O87.4)

- I83.0 Varicose veins of lower extremities **with ulcer**
  - Use additional code to identify severity of ulcer (L97.-)
  - I83.00 Varicose veins of **unspecified** lower extremity with ulcer
    - I83.001 Varicose veins of unspecified lower extremity with ulcer of **thigh** A
    - I83.002 Varicose veins of unspecified lower extremity with ulcer of **calf** A
    - I83.003 Varicose veins of unspecified lower extremity with ulcer of **ankle** A
    - I83.004 Varicose veins of unspecified lower extremity with ulcer of **heel and midfoot** A
      - Varicose veins of unspecified lower extremity with ulcer of plantar surface of midfoot
    - I83.005 Varicose veins of unspecified lower extremity with ulcer **other part of foot** A
      - Varicose veins of unspecified lower extremity with ulcer of toe
    - I83.008 Varicose veins of unspecified lower extremity with ulcer **other part of lower leg** A
    - I83.009 Varicose veins of unspecified lower extremity with ulcer of **unspecified site** A

CHAPTER 9 (I00-I99)

● I83.01 Varicose veins of **right** lower extremity with ulcer

I83.011 Varicose veins of right lower extremity with ulcer of **thigh** A

I83.012 Varicose veins of right lower extremity with ulcer of **calf** A

I83.013 Varicose veins of right lower extremity with ulcer of **ankle** A

I83.014 Varicose veins of right lower extremity with ulcer of **heel and midfoot** A

Varicose veins of right lower extremity with ulcer of plantar surface of midfoot

I83.015 Varicose veins of right lower extremity with ulcer **other part of foot** A

Varicose veins of right lower extremity with ulcer of toe

I83.018 Varicose veins of right lower extremity with ulcer **other part of lower leg** A

I83.019 Varicose veins of right lower extremity with ulcer of **unspecified** site A

● I83.02 Varicose veins of **left** lower extremity with ulcer

I83.021 Varicose veins of left lower extremity with ulcer of **thigh** A

I83.022 Varicose veins of left lower extremity with ulcer of **calf** A

I83.023 Varicose veins of left lower extremity with ulcer of **ankle** A

I83.024 Varicose veins of left lower extremity with ulcer of **heel and midfoot** A

Varicose veins of left lower extremity with ulcer of plantar surface of midfoot

I83.025 Varicose veins of left lower extremity with ulcer **other part of foot** A

Varicose veins of left lower extremity with ulcer of toe

I83.028 Varicose veins of left lower extremity with ulcer **other part of lower leg** A

I83.029 Varicose veins of left lower extremity with ulcer of **unspecified** site A

● I83.1 Varicose veins of lower extremities with **inflammation**

I83.10 Varicose veins of **unspecified** lower extremity with inflammation A

I83.11 Varicose veins of **right** lower extremity with inflammation A

I83.12 Varicose veins of **left** lower extremity with inflammation A

● I83.2 Varicose veins of lower extremities with both **ulcer and inflammation**

Use additional code to identify severity of ulcer (L97.-)

● I83.20 Varicose veins of **unspecified** lower extremity with both ulcer and inflammation

I83.201 Varicose veins of unspecified lower extremity with both ulcer of **thigh** and inflammation A

I83.202 Varicose veins of unspecified lower extremity with both ulcer of **calf** and inflammation A

I83.203 Varicose veins of unspecified lower extremity with both ulcer of **ankle** and inflammation A

I83.204 Varicose veins of unspecified lower extremity with both ulcer of **heel and midfoot** and inflammation A

Varicose veins of unspecified lower extremity with both ulcer of plantar surface of midfoot and inflammation

I83.205 Varicose veins of unspecified lower extremity with both ulcer **other part of foot** and inflammation A

Varicose veins of unspecified lower extremity with both ulcer of toe and inflammation

I83.208 Varicose veins of unspecified lower extremity with both ulcer of **other part of lower extremity** and inflammation A

I83.209 Varicose veins of unspecified lower extremity with both ulcer of **unspecified** site and inflammation A

● I83.21 Varicose veins of **right** lower extremity with both ulcer and inflammation

I83.211 Varicose veins of right lower extremity with both ulcer of **thigh** and inflammation A

I83.212 Varicose veins of right lower extremity with both ulcer of **calf** and inflammation A

I83.213 Varicose veins of right lower extremity with both ulcer of **ankle** and inflammation A

I83.214 Varicose veins of right lower extremity with both ulcer of **heel and midfoot** and inflammation A

Varicose veins of right lower extremity with both ulcer of plantar surface of midfoot and inflammation

I83.215 Varicose veins of right lower extremity with both ulcer **other part of foot** and inflammation A

Varicose veins of right lower extremity with both ulcer of toe and inflammation

I83.218 Varicose veins of right lower extremity with both ulcer of **other part of lower extremity** and inflammation A

I83.219 Varicose veins of right lower extremity with both ulcer of **unspecified** site and inflammation A

● I83.22 Varicose veins of **left** lower extremity with both ulcer and inflammation

I83.221 Varicose veins of left lower extremity with both ulcer of **thigh** and inflammation A

I83.222 Varicose veins of left lower extremity with both ulcer of **calf** and inflammation A

I83.223 Varicose veins of left lower extremity with both ulcer of **ankle** and inflammation A

I83.224 Varicose veins of left lower extremity with both ulcer of **heel and midfoot** and inflammation A

Varicose veins of left lower extremity with both ulcer of plantar surface of midfoot and inflammation

I83.225 Varicose veins of left lower extremity with both ulcer **other part of foot** and inflammation A

Varicose veins of left lower extremity with both ulcer of toe and inflammation

I83.228 Varicose veins of left lower extremity with both ulcer of **other part of lower extremity** and inflammation A

I83.229 Varicose veins of left lower extremity with both ulcer of **unspecified** site and inflammation A

I83.8 Varicose veins of lower extremities with other complications

I83.81 Varicose veins of lower extremities with pain

- **I83.811 Varicose veins of right lower extremity with pain** A
- **I83.812 Varicose veins of left lower extremity with pain** A
- **I83.813 Varicose veins of bilateral lower extremities with pain** A
- **I83.819 Varicose veins of unspecified lower extremity with pain** A

I83.89 Varicose veins of lower extremities with other complications

Varicose veins of lower extremities with edema
Varicose veins of lower extremities with swelling

- **I83.891 Varicose veins of right lower extremity with other complications** A
- **I83.892 Varicose veins of left lower extremity with other complications** A
- **I83.893 Varicose veins of bilateral lower extremities with other complications** A
- **I83.899 Varicose veins of unspecified lower extremity with other complications** A

I83.9 Asymptomatic varicose veins of lower extremities

Phlebectasia of lower extremities
Varicose veins of lower extremities
Varix of lower extremities

- **I83.9Ø Asymptomatic varicose veins of unspecified lower extremity** A
  Varicose veins NOS
- **I83.91 Asymptomatic varicose veins of right lower extremity** A
- **I83.92 Asymptomatic varicose veins of left lower extremity** A
- **I83.93 Asymptomatic varicose veins of bilateral lower extremities** A

I85 Esophageal varices

Use additional code to identify:
alcohol abuse and dependence (F1Ø.-)

I85.Ø Esophageal varices

Idiopathic esophageal varices
Primary esophageal varices

- **I85.ØØ Esophageal varices without bleeding**
  Esophageal varices NOS
- **I85.Ø1 Esophageal varices with bleeding**

I85.1 Secondary esophageal varices

Esophageal varices secondary to alcoholic liver disease
Esophageal varices secondary to cirrhosis of liver
Esophageal varices secondary to schistosomiasis
Esophageal varices secondary to toxic liver disease

Code first underlying disease

- **I85.1Ø Secondary esophageal varices without bleeding**
- **I85.11 Secondary esophageal varices with bleeding**

I86 Varicose veins of other sites

Excludes1 varicose veins of unspecified site (I83.9-)
Excludes2 retinal varices (H35.Ø-)

- **I86.Ø Sublingual varices**
- **I86.1 Scrotal varices** ♂
  Varicocele
- **I86.2 Pelvic varices**
- **I86.3 Vulval varices** ♀
  Excludes1 vulval varices complicating childbirth and the puerperium (O87.8)
  vulval varices complicating pregnancy (O22.1-)
- **I86.4 Gastric varices**
- **I86.8 Varicose veins of other specified sites** A
  Varicose ulcer of nasal septum

I87 Other disorders of veins

I87.Ø Postthrombotic syndrome

Chronic venous hypertension due to deep vein thrombosis
Postphlebitic syndrome

Excludes1 chronic venous hypertension without deep vein thrombosis (I87.3-)

I87.ØØ Postthrombotic syndrome without complications

Asymptomatic Postthrombotic syndrome

- **I87.ØØ1 Postthrombotic syndrome without complications of right lower extremity**
- **I87.ØØ2 Postthrombotic syndrome without complications of left lower extremity**
- **I87.ØØ3 Postthrombotic syndrome without complications of bilateral lower extremity**
- **I87.ØØ9 Postthrombotic syndrome without complications of unspecified extremity**
  Postthrombotic syndrome NOS

I87.Ø1 Postthrombotic syndrome with ulcer

Use additional code to specify site and severity of ulcer (L97.-)

- **I87.Ø11 Postthrombotic syndrome with ulcer of right lower extremity**
- **I87.Ø12 Postthrombotic syndrome with ulcer of left lower extremity**
- **I87.Ø13 Postthrombotic syndrome with ulcer of bilateral lower extremity**
- **I87.Ø19 Postthrombotic syndrome with ulcer of unspecified lower extremity**

I87.Ø2 Postthrombotic syndrome with inflammation

- **I87.Ø21 Postthrombotic syndrome with inflammation of right lower extremity**
- **I87.Ø22 Postthrombotic syndrome with inflammation of left lower extremity**
- **I87.Ø23 Postthrombotic syndrome with inflammation of bilateral lower extremity**
- **I87.Ø29 Postthrombotic syndrome with inflammation of unspecified lower extremity**

I87.Ø3 Postthrombotic syndrome with ulcer and inflammation

Use additional code to specify site and severity of ulcer (L97.-)

- **I87.Ø31 Postthrombotic syndrome with ulcer and inflammation of right lower extremity**
- **I87.Ø32 Postthrombotic syndrome with ulcer and inflammation of left lower extremity**
- **I87.Ø33 Postthrombotic syndrome with ulcer and inflammation of bilateral lower extremity**
- **I87.Ø39 Postthrombotic syndrome with ulcer and inflammation of unspecified lower extremity**

I87.Ø9 Postthrombotic syndrome with other complications

- **I87.Ø91 Postthrombotic syndrome with other complications of right lower extremity**
- **I87.Ø92 Postthrombotic syndrome with other complications of left lower extremity**
- **I87.Ø93 Postthrombotic syndrome with other complications of bilateral lower extremity**
- **I87.Ø99 Postthrombotic syndrome with other complications of unspecified lower extremity**

I87.1 **Compression of vein**
Stricture of vein
Vena cava syndrome (inferior) (superior)
Excludes2 compression of pulmonary vein (I28.8)

I87.2 **Venous insufficiency (chronic) (peripheral)**
Stasis dermatitis
Excludes1 stasis dermatitis with varicose veins of lower extremities (I83.1-, I83.2-)

● I87.3 **Chronic venous hypertension (idiopathic)**
Stasis edema
Excludes1 chronic venous hypertension due to deep vein thrombosis (I87.Ø-)
varicose veins of lower extremities (I83.-)

● I87.3Ø **Chronic venous hypertension (idiopathic) without complications**
Asymptomatic chronic venous hypertension (idiopathic)

I87.3Ø1 **Chronic venous hypertension (idiopathic) without complications of right lower extremity**

I87.3Ø2 **Chronic venous hypertension (idiopathic) without complications of left lower extremity**

I87.3Ø3 **Chronic venous hypertension (idiopathic) without complications of bilateral lower extremity**

I87.3Ø9 **Chronic venous hypertension (idiopathic) without complications of unspecified lower extremity**
Chronic venous hypertension NOS

● I87.31 **Chronic venous hypertension (idiopathic) with ulcer**
Use additional code to specify site and severity of ulcer (L97.-)

I87.311 **Chronic venous hypertension (idiopathic) with ulcer of right lower extremity** HCC

I87.312 **Chronic venous hypertension (idiopathic) with ulcer of left lower extremity** HCC

I87.313 **Chronic venous hypertension (idiopathic) with ulcer of bilateral lower extremity** HCC

I87.319 **Chronic venous hypertension (idiopathic) with ulcer of unspecified lower extremity** HCC

● I87.32 **Chronic venous hypertension (idiopathic) with inflammation**

I87.321 **Chronic venous hypertension (idiopathic) with inflammation of right lower extremity**

I87.322 **Chronic venous hypertension (idiopathic) with inflammation of left lower extremity**

I87.323 **Chronic venous hypertension (idiopathic) with inflammation of bilateral lower extremity**

I87.329 **Chronic venous hypertension (idiopathic) with inflammation of unspecified lower extremity**

● I87.33 **Chronic venous hypertension (idiopathic) with ulcer and inflammation**
Use additional code to specify site and severity of ulcer (L97.-)

I87.331 **Chronic venous hypertension (idiopathic) with ulcer and inflammation of right lower extremity** HCC

I87.332 **Chronic venous hypertension (idiopathic) with ulcer and inflammation of left lower extremity** HCC

I87.333 **Chronic venous hypertension (idiopathic) with ulcer and inflammation of bilateral lower extremity** HCC

I87.339 **Chronic venous hypertension (idiopathic) with ulcer and inflammation of unspecified lower extremity** HCC

● I87.39 **Chronic venous hypertension (idiopathic) with other complications**

I87.391 **Chronic venous hypertension (idiopathic) with other complications of right lower extremity**

I87.392 **Chronic venous hypertension (idiopathic) with other complications of left lower extremity**

I87.393 **Chronic venous hypertension (idiopathic) with other complications of bilateral lower extremity**

I87.399 **Chronic venous hypertension (idiopathic) with other complications of unspecified lower extremity**

I87.8 **Other specified disorders of veins**
Phlebosclerosis
Venofibrosis

I87.9 **Disorder of vein, unspecified**

● I88 **Nonspecific lymphadenitis**
Excludes1 acute lymphadenitis, except mesenteric (LØ4.-)
enlarged lymph nodes NOS (R59.-)
human immunodeficiency virus [HIV] disease resulting in generalized lymphadenopathy (B2Ø)

I88.Ø **Nonspecific mesenteric lymphadenitis**
Mesenteric lymphadenitis (acute)(chronic)

I88.1 **Chronic lymphadenitis, except mesenteric**
Adenitis
Lymphadenitis

I88.8 **Other nonspecific lymphadenitis**

I88.9 **Nonspecific lymphadenitis, unspecified**
Lymphadenitis NOS

● I89 **Other noninfective disorders of lymphatic vessels and lymph nodes**
Excludes1 chylocele, tunica vaginalis (nonfilarial) NOS (N5Ø.89)
enlarged lymph nodes NOS (R59.-)
filarial chylocele (B74.-)
hereditary lymphedema (Q82.Ø)

I89.Ø **Lymphedema, not elsewhere classified**
Elephantiasis (nonfilarial) NOS
Lymphangiectasis
Obliteration, lymphatic vessel
Praecox lymphedema
Secondary lymphedema
Excludes1 postmastectomy lymphedema (I97.2)

I89.1 **Lymphangitis**
Chronic lymphangitis
Lymphangitis NOS
Subacute lymphangitis
Excludes1 acute lymphangitis (LØ3.-)

I89.8 **Other specified noninfective disorders of lymphatic vessels and lymph nodes**
Chylocele (nonfilarial)
Chylous ascites
Chylous cyst
Lipomelanotic reticulosis
Lymph node or vessel fistula
Lymph node or vessel infarction
Lymph node or vessel rupture

I89.9 **Noninfective disorder of lymphatic vessels and lymph nodes, unspecified**
Disease of lymphatic vessels NOS

OTHER AND UNSPECIFIED DISORDERS OF THE CIRCULATORY SYSTEM (I95-I99)

● **I95 Hypotension**
Subnormal arterial blood pressure
Excludes1 cardiovascular collapse (R57.9)
maternal hypotension syndrome (O26.5-)
nonspecific low blood pressure reading NOS (RØ3.1)

I95.Ø Idiopathic hypotension

I95.1 Orthostatic hypotension
Hypotension, postural
Moving from a sitting or reclining position to a standing position precipitates a sudden drop in blood pressure (hypotension).
Excludes1 neurogenic orthostatic hypotension [Shy-Drager] (G9Ø.3)
orthostatic hypotension due to drugs (I95.2)

I95.2 Hypotension due to drugs
Orthostatic hypotension due to drugs
Use additional code for adverse effect, if applicable, to identify drug (T36-T5Ø with fifth or sixth character 5)

I95.3 Hypotension of hemodialysis
Intra-dialytic hypotension

● **I95.8 Other hypotension**

I95.81 Postprocedural hypotension

I95.89 Other hypotension
Chronic hypotension

I95.9 Hypotension, unspecified

I96 Gangrene, not elsewhere classified
Gangrenous cellulitis
Excludes1 gangrene in atherosclerosis of native arteries of the extremities (I7Ø.26)
gangrene of certain specified sites - *see* Alphabetical Index
gangrene in hernia (K4Ø.1, K4Ø.4, K41.1, K41.4, K42.1, K43.1-, K44.1, K45.1, K46.1)
gangrene in other peripheral vascular diseases (I73.-)
gas gangrene (A48.Ø)
pyoderma gangrenosum (L88)
Excludes2 gangrene in diabetes mellitus (EØ8-E13 with .52)
Coding Clinic: 2Ø18, Q4, P87; 2Ø17, Q3, P6; 2Ø13, Q2, P35

● **I97 Intraoperative and postprocedural complications and disorders of circulatory system, not elsewhere classified**
Excludes2 postprocedural shock (T81.1-)
Coding Clinic: 2Ø19, Q2, P22

I97.Ø Postcardiotomy syndrome

● **I97.1 Other postprocedural cardiac functional disturbances**
Excludes2 acute pulmonary insufficiency following thoracic surgery (J95.1)
intraoperative cardiac functional disturbances (I97.7-)

● **I97.11 Postprocedural cardiac insufficiency**

I97.11Ø Postprocedural cardiac insufficiency following cardiac surgery

I97.111 Postprocedural cardiac insufficiency following other surgery

● **I97.12 Postprocedural cardiac arrest**

I97.12Ø Postprocedural cardiac arrest following cardiac surgery

I97.121 Postprocedural cardiac arrest following other surgery

● **I97.13 Postprocedural heart failure**
Use additional code to identify the heart failure (I5Ø.-)

I97.13Ø Postprocedural heart failure following cardiac surgery

I97.131 Postprocedural heart failure following other surgery

● **I97.19 Other postprocedural cardiac functional disturbances**
Use additional code, if applicable, to further specify disorder

I97.19Ø Other postprocedural cardiac functional disturbances following cardiac surgery
Use Additional code, if applicable, for type 4 or type 5 myocardial infarction, to further specify disorder
Coding Clinic: 2Ø19, Q2, P32-33

I97.191 Other postprocedural cardiac functional disturbances following other surgery

I97.2 Postmastectomy lymphedema syndrome A
Elephantiasis due to mastectomy
Obliteration of lymphatic vessels

I97.3 Postprocedural hypertension

● **I97.4 Intraoperative hemorrhage and hematoma of a circulatory system organ or structure complicating a procedure**
Excludes1 intraoperative hemorrhage and hematoma of a circulatory system organ or structure due to accidental puncture and laceration during a procedure (I97.5-)
Excludes2 intraoperative cerebrovascular hemorrhage complicating a procedure (G97.3-)

● **I97.41 Intraoperative hemorrhage and hematoma of a circulatory system organ or structure complicating a circulatory system procedure**

I97.41Ø Intraoperative hemorrhage and hematoma of a circulatory system organ or structure complicating a cardiac catheterization

I97.411 Intraoperative hemorrhage and hematoma of a circulatory system organ or structure complicating a cardiac bypass

I97.418 Intraoperative hemorrhage and hematoma of a circulatory system organ or structure complicating other circulatory system procedure

I97.42 Intraoperative hemorrhage and hematoma of a circulatory system organ or structure complicating other procedure
Coding Clinic: 2Ø16, Q4, P1ØØ

● **I97.5 Accidental puncture and laceration of a circulatory system organ or structure during a procedure**
Excludes2 accidental puncture and laceration of brain during a procedure (G97.4-)

I97.51 Accidental puncture and laceration of a circulatory system organ or structure during a circulatory system procedure
Coding Clinic: 2Ø19, Q2, P24

I97.52 Accidental puncture and laceration of a circulatory system organ or structure during other procedure

● **I97.6** **Postprocedural hemorrhage, hematoma and seroma of a circulatory system organ or structure following a procedure**
 Excludes2 postprocedural cerebrovascular hemorrhage complicating a procedure (G97.5-)
 Coding Clinic: 2016, Q4, P10

● **I97.61** Postprocedural **hemorrhage** of a circulatory system organ or structure following a **circulatory system procedure**
 I97.610 Postprocedural hemorrhage of a circulatory system organ or structure following a **cardiac catheterization**
 I97.611 Postprocedural hemorrhage of a circulatory system organ or structure following **cardiac bypass**
 I97.618 Postprocedural hemorrhage of a circulatory system organ or structure following **other circulatory system procedure**

● **I97.62** Postprocedural **hemorrhage, hematoma and seroma** of a circulatory system organ or structure following **other procedure**
 I97.620 Postprocedural **hemorrhage** of a circulatory system organ or structure following other procedure
 I97.621 Postprocedural **hematoma** of a circulatory system organ or structure following other procedure
 I97.622 Postprocedural **seroma** of a circulatory system organ or structure following other procedure

● **I97.63** Postprocedural **hematoma** of a circulatory system organ or structure following a **circulatory system procedure**
 I97.630 Postprocedural hematoma of a circulatory system organ or structure following a **cardiac catheterization**
 I97.631 Postprocedural hematoma of a circulatory system organ or structure following **cardiac bypass**
 I97.638 Postprocedural hematoma of a circulatory system organ or structure following **other circulatory system procedure**

● **I97.64** Postprocedural **seroma** of a circulatory system organ or structure following a **circulatory system procedure**
 I97.640 Postprocedural seroma of a circulatory system organ or structure following a **cardiac catheterization**
 I97.641 Postprocedural seroma of a circulatory system organ or structure following **cardiac bypass**
 I97.648 Postprocedural seroma of a circulatory system organ or structure following **other circulatory system procedure**

● **I97.7** **Intraoperative cardiac functional disturbances**
 Excludes2 acute pulmonary insufficiency following thoracic surgery (J95.1)
 postprocedural cardiac functional disturbances (I97.1-)

● **I97.71** Intraoperative cardiac arrest
 I97.710 Intraoperative cardiac arrest during **cardiac surgery**
 I97.711 Intraoperative cardiac arrest during **other surgery**

● **I97.79** Other intraoperative cardiac functional disturbances
 Use additional code, if applicable, to further specify disorder
 I97.790 Other intraoperative cardiac functional disturbances during **cardiac surgery**
 I97.791 Other intraoperative cardiac functional disturbances during **other surgery**

● **I97.8** Other intraoperative and postprocedural complications and disorders of the circulatory system, not elsewhere classified
 Use additional code, if applicable, to further specify disorder

● **I97.81** Intraoperative cerebrovascular infarction
 I97.810 Intraoperative cerebrovascular infarction during **cardiac surgery** 🐾
 I97.811 Intraoperative cerebrovascular infarction during **other surgery** 🐾

● **I97.82** Postprocedural cerebrovascular infarction
 I97.820 Postprocedural cerebrovascular infarction following **cardiac surgery** 🐾
 I97.821 Postprocedural cerebrovascular infarction following **other surgery** 🐾

 I97.88 Other intraoperative complications of the circulatory system, not elsewhere classified
 I97.89 Other **postprocedural** complications and disorders of the circulatory system, not elsewhere classified
 Coding Clinic: 2019, Q2, P32-33

● **I99** Other and unspecified disorders of circulatory system
 I99.8 Other disorder of circulatory system
 I99.9 **Unspecified** disorder of circulatory system

▶ New ➟ Revised ~~deleted~~ Deleted Excludes 1 Excludes 2 Includes Use additional Code first Code also Key words
OGCR Official Guidelines X Assign placeholder X ● Use Additional Character(s) ⫿ Manifestation Code 🐾 Hierarchical Condition Category Coding Clinic

CHAPTER 10

DISEASES OF THE RESPIRATORY SYSTEM
(J00-J99)

OGCR Chapter-Specific Coding Guidelines

10. Chapter 10: Diseases of the Respiratory System (J00-J99)

a. Chronic Obstructive Pulmonary Disease [COPD] and Asthma

1) Acute exacerbation of chronic obstructive bronchitis and asthma

The codes in categories J44 and J45 distinguish between uncomplicated cases and those in acute exacerbation. An acute exacerbation is a worsening or a decompensation of a chronic condition. An acute exacerbation is not equivalent to an infection superimposed on a chronic condition, though an exacerbation may be triggered by an infection.

b. Acute Respiratory Failure

1) Acute respiratory failure as principal diagnosis

A code from subcategory J96.0, Acute respiratory failure, or subcategory J96.2, Acute and chronic respiratory failure, may be assigned as a principal diagnosis when it is the condition established after study to be chiefly responsible for occasioning the admission to the hospital, and the selection is supported by the Alphabetic Index and Tabular List. However, chapter-specific coding guidelines (such as obstetrics, poisoning, HIV, newborn) that provide sequencing direction take precedence.

2) Acute respiratory failure as secondary diagnosis

Respiratory failure may be listed as a secondary diagnosis if it occurs after admission, or if it is present on admission, but does not meet the definition of principal diagnosis.

3) Sequencing of acute respiratory failure and another acute condition

When a patient is admitted with respiratory failure and another acute condition (e.g., myocardial infarction, cerebrovascular accident, aspiration pneumonia), the principal diagnosis will not be the same in every situation. This applies whether the other acute condition is a respiratory or nonrespiratory condition. Selection of the principal diagnosis will be dependent on the circumstances of admission. If both the respiratory failure and the other acute condition are equally responsible for occasioning the admission to the hospital, and there are no chapter-specific sequencing rules, the guideline regarding two or more diagnoses that equally meet the definition for principal diagnosis (*Section II, C.*) may be applied in these situations.

If the documentation is not clear as to whether acute respiratory failure and another condition are equally responsible for occasioning the admission, query the provider for clarification.

c. Influenza due to certain identified influenza viruses

Code only confirmed cases of influenza due to certain identified influenza viruses (category J09), and due to other identified influenza virus (category J10). This is an exception to the hospital inpatient guideline Section II, H. (Uncertain Diagnosis).

In this context, "confirmation" does not require documentation of positive laboratory testing specific for avian or other novel influenza A or other identified influenza virus. However, coding should be based on the provider's diagnostic statement that the patient has avian influenza, or other novel influenza A, for category J09, or has another particular identified strain of influenza, such as H1N1 or H3N2, but not identified as novel or variant, for category J10.

If the provider records "suspected" or "possible" or "probable" avian influenza, or novel influenza, or other identified influenza, then the appropriate influenza code from category J11, Influenza due to unidentified influenza virus, should be assigned. A code from category J09, Influenza due to certain identified influenza viruses, should not be assigned nor should a code from category J10, Influenza due to other identified influenza virus.

d. Ventilator associated Pneumonia

1) Documentation of Ventilator associated Pneumonia

As with all procedural or postprocedural complications, code assignment is based on the provider's documentation of the relationship between the condition and the procedure.

Code J95.851, Ventilator associated pneumonia, should be assigned only when the provider has documented ventilator associated pneumonia (VAP). An additional code to identify the organism (e.g., Pseudomonas aeruginosa, code B96.5) should also be assigned. Do not assign an additional code from categories J12-J18 to identify the type of pneumonia.

Code J95.851 should not be assigned for cases where the patient has pneumonia and is on a mechanical ventilator and the provider has not specifically stated that the pneumonia is ventilator associated pneumonia. If the documentation is unclear as to whether the patient has a pneumonia that is a complication attributable to the mechanical ventilator, query the provider.

2) Ventilator associated Pneumonia Develops after Admission

A patient may be admitted with one type of pneumonia (e.g., code J13, Pneumonia due to Streptococcus pneumonia) and subsequently develop VAP. In this instance, the principal diagnosis would be the appropriate code from categories J12-J18 for the pneumonia diagnosed at the time of admission. Code J95.851, Ventilator associated pneumonia, would be assigned as an additional diagnosis when the provider has also documented the presence of ventilator associated pneumonia.

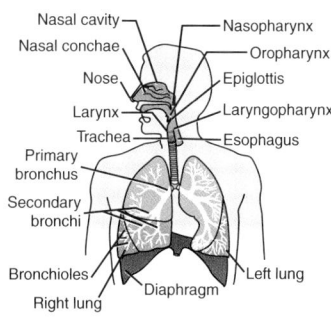

Figure 10-1 Respiratory system. (From Buck CJ: Step-by-Step Medical Coding, ed 2016, St. Louis, Elsevier, 2016)

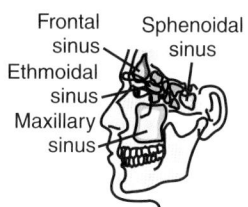

Figure 10-2 Paranasal sinuses. (From Buck CJ: Step-by-Step Medical Coding, ed 2016, St. Louis, Elsevier, 2016)

Item 10-1 Pharyngitis is painful inflammation of the pharynx (sore throat). Ninety percent of the infections are caused by a virus with the remaining being bacterial and rarely a fungus (candidiasis). Other irritants such as pollutants, chemicals, or smoke may cause similar symptoms.

CHAPTER 10

DISEASES OF THE RESPIRATORY SYSTEM (J00-J99)

Note: When a respiratory condition is described as occurring in more than one site and is not specifically indexed, it should be classified to the lower anatomic site (e.g., tracheobronchitis to bronchitis in J40).

Use additional code, where applicable, to identify:
exposure to environmental tobacco smoke (Z77.22)
exposure to tobacco smoke in the perinatal period (P96.81)
history of tobacco dependence (Z87.891)
occupational exposure to environmental tobacco smoke (Z57.31)
tobacco dependence (F17.-)
tobacco use (Z72.0)

Excludes2   certain conditions originating in the perinatal period (P04-P96)
certain infectious and parasitic diseases (A00-B99)
complications of pregnancy, childbirth and the puerperium (O00-O99A)
congenital malformations, deformations and chromosomal abnormalities (Q00-Q99)
endocrine, nutritional and metabolic diseases (E00-E88)
injury, poisoning and certain other consequences of external causes (S00-T88)
neoplasms (C00-D49)
smoke inhalation (T59.81-)
symptoms, signs and abnormal clinical and laboratory findings, not elsewhere classified (R00-R94)

This chapter contains the following blocks:

J00-J06	Acute upper respiratory infections
J09-J18	Influenza and pneumonia
J20-J22	Other acute lower respiratory infections
J30-J39	Other diseases of upper respiratory tract
J40-J47	Chronic lower respiratory diseases
J60-J70	Lung diseases due to external agents
J80-J84	Other respiratory diseases principally affecting the interstitium
J85-J86	Suppurative and necrotic conditions of the lower respiratory tract
J90-J94	Other diseases of the pleura
J95	Intraoperative and postprocedural complications and disorders of respiratory system, not elsewhere classified
J96-J99	Other diseases of the respiratory system

ACUTE UPPER RESPIRATORY INFECTIONS (J00-J06)

Excludes1   chronic obstructive pulmonary disease with acute lower respiratory infection (J44.0)
influenza virus with other respiratory manifestations (J09.X2, J10.1, J11.1)

J00   **Acute nasopharyngitis [common cold]**
Acute rhinitis
Coryza (acute)
Infective nasopharyngitis NOS
Infective rhinitis
Nasal catarrh, acute
Nasopharyngitis NOS

Excludes1   acute pharyngitis (J02.-)
acute sore throat NOS (J02.9)
pharyngitis NOS (J02.9)
rhinitis NOS (J31.0)
sore throat NOS (J02.9)

Excludes2   allergic rhinitis (J30.1-J30.9)
chronic pharyngitis (J31.2)
chronic rhinitis (J31.0)
chronic sore throat (J31.2)
nasopharyngitis, chronic (J31.1)
vasomotor rhinitis (J30.0)

★ **(See Plate 27 of the Anatomy Illustrations.)**

● **J01**   **Acute sinusitis**

     Includes   acute abscess of sinus
acute empyema of sinus
acute infection of sinus
acute inflammation of sinus
acute suppuration of sinus

Use additional code (B95-B97) to identify infectious agent.

     Excludes1   sinusitis NOS (J32.9)

     Excludes2   chronic sinusitis (J32.0-J32.8)

● **J01.0**   **Acute maxillary sinusitis**
     Acute antritis

     J01.00   Acute maxillary sinusitis, **unspecified**

     J01.01   Acute **recurrent** maxillary sinusitis

● **J01.1**   **Acute frontal sinusitis**

     J01.10   Acute frontal sinusitis, **unspecified**

     J01.11   Acute **recurrent** frontal sinusitis

● **J01.2**   **Acute ethmoidal sinusitis**

     J01.20   Acute ethmoidal sinusitis, **unspecified**

     J01.21   Acute **recurrent** ethmoidal sinusitis

● **J01.3**   **Acute sphenoidal sinusitis**

     J01.30   Acute sphenoidal sinusitis, **unspecified**

     J01.31   Acute **recurrent** sphenoidal sinusitis

● **J01.4**   **Acute pansinusitis**

     J01.40   Acute pansinusitis, **unspecified**

     J01.41   Acute **recurrent** pansinusitis

● **J01.8 Other acute sinusitis**

J01.80 Other acute sinusitis
Acute sinusitis involving more than one sinus but not pansinusitis

J01.81 Other acute recurrent sinusitis
Acute recurrent sinusitis involving more than one sinus but not pansinusitis

● **J01.9 Acute sinusitis, unspecified**

J01.90 Acute sinusitis, unspecified

J01.91 Acute recurrent sinusitis, unspecified

● **J02 Acute pharyngitis**

Includes acute sore throat

Excludes1 acute laryngopharyngitis (J06.0)
peritonsillar abscess (J36)
pharyngeal abscess (J39.1)
retropharyngeal abscess (J39.0)

Excludes2 chronic pharyngitis (J31.2)

J02.0 Streptococcal pharyngitis
Septic pharyngitis
Streptococcal sore throat

Excludes2 scarlet fever (A38.-)

J02.8 Acute pharyngitis due to other specified organisms
Use additional code (B95-B97) to identify infectious agent

Excludes1 pharyngitis due to coxsackie virus (B08.5)
pharyngitis due to gonococcus (A54.5)
acute pharyngitis due to herpes [simplex] virus (B00.2)
acute pharyngitis due to infectious mononucleosis (B27.-)
enteroviral vesicular pharyngitis (B08.5)

J02.9 Acute pharyngitis, unspecified
Gangrenous pharyngitis (acute)
Infective pharyngitis (acute) NOS
Pharyngitis (acute) NOS
Sore throat (acute) NOS
Suppurative pharyngitis (acute)
Ulcerative pharyngitis (acute)

● **J03 Acute tonsillitis**
Inflammation of pharyngeal tonsils caused by virus or bacteria

Excludes1 acute sore throat (J02.-)
hypertrophy of tonsils (J35.1)
peritonsillar abscess (J36)
sore throat NOS (J02.9)
streptococcal sore throat (J02.0)

Excludes2 chronic tonsillitis (J35.0)

● **J03.0 Streptococcal tonsillitis**

J03.00 Acute streptococcal tonsillitis, unspecified

J03.01 Acute recurrent streptococcal tonsillitis

● **J03.8 Acute tonsillitis due to other specified organisms**
Use additional code (B95-B97) to identify infectious agent.

Excludes1 diphtheritic tonsillitis (A36.0)
herpesviral pharyngotonsillitis (B00.2)
streptococcal tonsillitis (J03.0)
tuberculous tonsillitis (A15.8)
Vincent's tonsillitis (A69.1)

J03.80 Acute tonsillitis due to other specified organisms

J03.81 Acute recurrent tonsillitis due to other specified organisms

● **J03.9 Acute tonsillitis, unspecified**
Follicular tonsillitis (acute)
Gangrenous tonsillitis (acute)
Infective tonsillitis (acute)
Tonsillitis (acute) NOS
Ulcerative tonsillitis (acute)

J03.90 Acute tonsillitis, unspecified

J03.91 Acute recurrent tonsillitis, unspecified

Item 10–2 Laryngitis is an inflammation of the larynx (voice box) resulting in hoarse voice or the complete loss of the voice. **Tracheitis** is an inflammation of the trachea (often following a URI) commonly caused by *staphylococcus aureus* resulting in inspiratory stridor (crowing sound on inspiration) and a crouplike cough.

● **J04 Acute laryngitis and tracheitis**
Use additional code (B95-B97) to identify infectious agent.

Excludes1 acute obstructive laryngitis [croup] and epiglottitis (J05.-)

Excludes2 laryngismus (stridulus) (J38.5)

J04.0 Acute laryngitis
Edematous laryngitis (acute)
Laryngitis (acute) NOS
Subglottic laryngitis (acute)
Suppurative laryngitis (acute)
Ulcerative laryngitis (acute)

Excludes1 acute obstructive laryngitis (J05.0)

Excludes2 chronic laryngitis (J37.0)

● **J04.1 Acute tracheitis**
Acute viral tracheitis
Catarrhal tracheitis (acute)
Tracheitis (acute) NOS

Excludes2 chronic tracheitis (J42)

J04.10 Acute tracheitis without obstruction

J04.11 Acute tracheitis with obstruction

J04.2 Acute laryngotracheitis
Laryngotracheitis NOS
Tracheitis (acute) with laryngitis (acute)

Excludes1 acute obstructive laryngotracheitis (J05.0)

Excludes2 chronic laryngotracheitis (J37.1)

● **J04.3 Supraglottitis, unspecified**

J04.30 Supraglottitis, unspecified, without obstruction

J04.31 Supraglottitis, unspecified, with obstruction

● **J05 Acute obstructive laryngitis [croup] and epiglottitis**
Use additional code (B95-B97) to identify infectious agent.

J05.0 Acute obstructive laryngitis [croup]
Obstructive laryngitis (acute) NOS
Obstructive laryngotracheitis NOS

● **J05.1 Acute epiglottitis**

Excludes2 epiglottitis, chronic (J37.0)

J05.10 Acute epiglottitis without obstruction
Epiglottitis NOS

J05.11 Acute epiglottitis with obstruction

● **J06 Acute upper respiratory infections of multiple and unspecified sites**

Excludes1 acute respiratory infection NOS (J22)
streptococcal pharyngitis (J02.0)

J06.0 Acute laryngopharyngitis

J06.9 Acute upper respiratory infection, unspecified
Upper respiratory disease, acute
Upper respiratory infection NOS
▶ Use additional code (B95-B97) to identify infectious agent, if known, such as:
▶ respiratory syncytial virus (RSV) (B97.4)

CHAPTER 10 (J00-J99)

INFLUENZA AND PNEUMONIA (J09-J18)

Excludes2 allergic or eosinophilic pneumonia (J82)
aspiration pneumonia NOS (J69.0)
meconium pneumonia (P24.01)
neonatal aspiration pneumonia (P24.-)
pneumonia due to solids and liquids (J69.-)
congenital pneumonia (P23.9)
lipid pneumonia (J69.1)
rheumatic pneumonia (I00)
ventilator associated pneumonia (J95.851)

● **J09 Influenza due to certain identified influenza viruses**

Excludes1 influenza A/H1N1 (J10.-)
influenza due to other influenza viruses (J10.-)
influenza due to unidentified influenza virus (J11.-)
seasonal influenza due to other identified influenza virus (J10.-)
seasonal influenza due to unidentified influenza virus (J11.-)

● **J09.X Influenza due to identified novel influenza A virus**

Avian influenza
Bird influenza
Influenza A/H5N1
Influenza of other animal origin, not bird or swine
Swine influenza virus (viruses that normally cause infections in pigs)
Coding Clinic: 2016, Q3, P11

J09.X1 Influenza due to identified novel influenza A virus with pneumonia

Code also , if applicable, associated:
lung abscess (J85.1)
other specified type of pneumonia

J09.X2 Influenza due to identified novel influenza A virus with other respiratory manifestations

Influenza due to identified novel influenza A virus NOS
Influenza due to identified novel influenza A virus with laryngitis
Influenza due to identified novel influenza A virus with pharyngitis
Influenza due to identified novel influenza A virus with upper respiratory symptoms

Use additional code, if applicable, for associated:
pleural effusion (J91.8)
sinusitis (J01.-)

J09.X3 Influenza due to identified novel influenza A virus with gastrointestinal manifestations

Influenza due to identified novel influenza A virus gastroenteritis

Excludes1 'intestinal flu' [viral gastroenteritis] (A08.-)

J09.X9 Influenza due to identified novel influenza A virus with other manifestations

Influenza due to identified novel influenza A virus with encephalopathy
Influenza due to identified novel influenza A virus with myocarditis
Influenza due to identified novel influenza A virus with otitis media

Use additional code to identify manifestation

● **J10 Influenza due to other identified influenza virus**

Excludes1 influenza due to avian influenza virus (J09.X-)
influenza due to swine flu (J09.X-)
influenza due to unidentified influenza virus (J11.-)

● **J10.0 Influenza due to other identified influenza virus with pneumonia**

Code also associated lung abscess, if applicable (J85.1)

J10.00 Influenza due to other identified influenza virus with unspecified type of pneumonia

J10.01 Influenza due to other identified influenza virus with the same other identified influenza virus pneumonia

J10.08 Influenza due to other identified influenza virus with other specified pneumonia

Code also other specified type of pneumonia
Coding Clinic: 2017, Q4, P96

J10.1 Influenza due to other identified influenza virus with other respiratory manifestations

Influenza due to other identified influenza virus NOS
Influenza due to other identified influenza virus with laryngitis
Influenza due to other identified influenza virus with pharyngitis
Influenza due to other identified influenza virus with upper respiratory symptoms

Use additional code for associated pleural effusion, if applicable (J91.8)

Use additional code for associated sinusitis, if applicable (J01.-)
Coding Clinic: 2016, Q3, P11

J10.2 Influenza due to other identified influenza virus with gastrointestinal manifestations

Influenza due to other identified influenza virus gastroenteritis

Excludes1 'intestinal flu' [viral gastroenteritis] (A08.-)

● **J10.8 Influenza due to other identified influenza virus with other manifestations**

J10.81 Influenza due to other identified influenza virus with encephalopathy

J10.82 Influenza due to other identified influenza virus with myocarditis

J10.83 Influenza due to other identified influenza virus with otitis media

Use additional code for any associated perforated tympanic membrane (H72.-)

J10.89 Influenza due to other identified influenza virus with other manifestations

Use additional codes to identify the manifestations

● **J11 Influenza due to unidentified influenza virus**

● **J11.0 Influenza due to unidentified influenza virus with pneumonia**

Code also associated lung abscess, if applicable (J85.1)

J11.00 Influenza due to unidentified influenza virus with unspecified type of pneumonia

Influenza with pneumonia NOS
Coding Clinic: 2016, Q3, P12

J11.08 Influenza due to unidentified influenza virus with specified pneumonia

Code also other specified type of pneumonia

CHAPTER 10 (J00-J99)

▶ New ➡ Revised ~~deleted~~ Deleted Excludes 1 Excludes 2 Includes Use additional Code first Code also Key words
OGCR Official Guidelines X Assign placeholder X ● Use Additional Character(s) ◗ Manifestation Code Hierarchical Condition Category Coding Clinic

J11.1 Influenza due to unidentified influenza virus with other respiratory manifestations
Influenza NOS
Influenzal laryngitis NOS
Influenzal pharyngitis NOS
Influenza with upper respiratory symptoms NOS
Use additional code for associated pleural effusion, if applicable (J91.8)
Use additional code for associated sinusitis, if applicable (J01.-)

J11.2 Influenza due to unidentified influenza virus with gastrointestinal manifestations
Influenza gastroenteritis NOS
Excludes1 'intestinal flu' [viral gastroenteritis] (A08.-)

● **J11.8 Influenza due to unidentified influenza virus with other manifestations**

J11.81 Influenza due to unidentified influenza virus with encephalopathy
Influenzal encephalopathy NOS

J11.82 Influenza due to unidentified influenza virus with myocarditis
Influenzal myocarditis NOS

J11.83 Influenza due to unidentified influenza virus with otitis media
Influenzal otitis media NOS
Use additional code for any associated perforated tympanic membrane (H72.-)

J11.89 Influenza due to unidentified influenza virus with other manifestations
Use additional codes to identify the manifestations

● **J12 Viral pneumonia, not elsewhere classified**
Includes bronchopneumonia due to viruses other than influenza viruses
Code first associated influenza, if applicable (J09.X1, J10.0-, J11.0-)
Code also associated abscess, if applicable (J85.1)
Excludes1 aspiration pneumonia due to anesthesia during labor and delivery (O74.0)
aspiration pneumonia due to anesthesia during pregnancy (O29)
aspiration pneumonia due to anesthesia during puerperium (O89.0)
aspiration pneumonia due to solids and liquids (J69.-)
aspiration pneumonia NOS (J69.0)
congenital pneumonia (P23.0)
congenital rubella pneumonitis (P35.0)
interstitial pneumonia NOS (J84.9)
lipid pneumonia (J69.1)
neonatal aspiration pneumonia (P24.-)

J12.0 Adenoviral pneumonia

J12.1 Respiratory syncytial virus pneumonia
▶RSV pneumonia

J12.2 Parainfluenza virus pneumonia

J12.3 Human metapneumovirus pneumonia

● **J12.8 Other viral pneumonia**

J12.81 Pneumonia due to SARS-associated coronavirus
Severe acute respiratory syndrome NOS

J12.89 Other viral pneumonia

J12.9 Viral pneumonia, unspecified

Item 10–3 Pneumonia is an infection of the lungs, caused by a variety of microorganisms, including viruses, most commonly the Streptococcus pneumoniae (pneumococcus) bacteria, fungi, and parasites. Pneumonia occurs when the immune system is weakened, often by a URI or influenza.

J13 Pneumonia due to Streptococcus pneumoniae ℞
Bronchopneumonia due to S. pneumoniae
Code first associated influenza, if applicable (J09.X1, J10.0-, J11.0-)
Code also associated abscess, if applicable (J85.1)
Excludes1 congenital pneumonia due to S. pneumoniae (P23.6)
lobar pneumonia, unspecified organism (J18.1)
pneumonia due to other streptococci (J15.3-J15.4)

J14 Pneumonia due to Hemophilus influenzae ℞
Bronchopneumonia due to H. influenzae
Code first associated influenza, if applicable (J09.X1, J10.0-, J11.0-)
Code also associated abscess, if applicable (J85.1)
Excludes1 congenital pneumonia due to H. influenzae (P23.6)

● **J15 Bacterial pneumonia, not elsewhere classified**
Includes bronchopneumonia due to bacteria other than S. pneumoniae and H. influenzae
Code first associated influenza, if applicable (J09.X1, J10.0-, J11.0-)
Code also associated abscess, if applicable (J85.1)
Excludes1 chlamydial pneumonia (J16.0)
congenital pneumonia (P23.-)
Legionnaires' disease (A48.1)
spirochetal pneumonia (A69.8)

J15.0 Pneumonia due to Klebsiella pneumoniae ℞

J15.1 Pneumonia due to Pseudomonas ℞

● **J15.2 Pneumonia due to staphylococcus**

J15.20 Pneumonia due to staphylococcus, unspecified ℞

● **J15.21 Pneumonia due to staphylococcus aureus**

J15.211 Pneumonia due to Methicillin susceptible Staphylococcus aureus ℞
MSSA pneumonia
Pneumonia due to Staphylococcus aureus NOS

J15.212 Pneumonia due to Methicillin resistant Staphylococcus aureus ℞

J15.29 Pneumonia due to other staphylococcus ℞

J15.3 Pneumonia due to streptococcus, group B ℞

J15.4 Pneumonia due to other streptococci ℞
Excludes1 pneumonia due to streptococcus, group B (J15.3)
pneumonia due to Streptococcus pneumoniae (J13)

J15.5 Pneumonia due to Escherichia coli ℞

J15.6 Pneumonia due to other Gram-negative bacteria ℞
Pneumonia due to other aerobic Gram-negative bacteria
Pneumonia due to Serratia marcescens

J15.7 Pneumonia due to Mycoplasma pneumoniae

J15.8 Pneumonia due to other specified bacteria ℞

J15.9 Unspecified bacterial pneumonia
Pneumonia due to gram-positive bacteria
Coding Clinic: 2017, Q4, P96

J16 Pneumonia due to other infectious organisms, not elsewhere classified

Code first associated influenza, if applicable (J09.X1, J10.0-, J11.0-)

Code also associated abscess, if applicable (J85.1)

Excludes1 congenital pneumonia (P23.-)
ornithosis (A70)
pneumocystosis (B59)
pneumonia NOS (J18.9)

J16.0 Chlamydial pneumonia

J16.8 Pneumonia due to other specified infectious organisms

J17 Pneumonia in diseases classified elsewhere

Code first underlying disease, such as:
Q fever (A78)
rheumatic fever (I00)
schistosomiasis (B65.0-B65.9)

Excludes1 candidial pneumonia (B37.1)
chlamydial pneumonia (J16.0)
gonorrheal pneumonia (A54.84)
histoplasmosis pneumonia (B39.0-B39.2)
measles pneumonia (B05.2)
nocardiosis pneumonia (A43.0)
pneumocystosis (B59)
pneumonia due to Pneumocystis carinii (B59)
pneumonia due to Pneumocystis jiroveci (B59)
pneumonia in actinomycosis (A42.0)
pneumonia in anthrax (A22.1)
pneumonia in ascariasis (B77.81)
pneumonia in aspergillosis (B44.0-B44.1)
pneumonia in coccidioidomycosis (B38.0-B38.2)
pneumonia in cytomegalovirus disease (B25.0)
pneumonia in toxoplasmosis (B58.3)
rubella pneumonia (B06.81)
salmonella pneumonia (A02.22)
spirochetal infection NEC with pneumonia (A69.8)
tularemia pneumonia (A21.2)
typhoid fever with pneumonia (A01.03)
varicella pneumonia (B01.2)
whooping cough with pneumonia (A37 with fifth-character 1)

J18 Pneumonia, unspecified organism

Code first associated influenza, if applicable (J09.X1, J10.0-, J11.0-)

Excludes1 abscess of lung with pneumonia (J85.1)
aspiration pneumonia due to anesthesia during labor and delivery (O74.0)
aspiration pneumonia due to anesthesia during pregnancy (O29)
aspiration pneumonia due to anesthesia during puerperium (O89.0)
aspiration pneumonia due to solids and liquids (J69.-)
aspiration pneumonia NOS (J69.0)
congenital pneumonia (P23.0)
drug-induced interstitial lung disorder (J70.2-J70.4)
interstitial pneumonia NOS (J84.9)
lipid pneumonia (J69.1)
neonatal aspiration pneumonia (P24.-)
pneumonitis due to external agents (J67-J70)
pneumonitis due to fumes and vapors (J68.0)
usual interstitial pneumonia (J84.17)

J18.0 Bronchopneumonia, unspecified organism

Excludes1 hypostatic bronchopneumonia (J18.2)
lipid pneumonia (J69.1)

Excludes2 acute bronchiolitis (J21.-)
chronic bronchiolitis (J44.9)

J18.1 Lobar pneumonia, unspecified organism
Coding Clinic: 2016, Q3, P15

J18.2 Hypostatic pneumonia, unspecified organism
Hypostatic bronchopneumonia
Passive pneumonia

J18.8 Other pneumonia, unspecified organism

J18.9 Pneumonia, unspecified organism
Coding Clinic: 2019, Q2, P28; Q1, P36; 2016, Q3, P15; 2012, Q4, P94

OTHER ACUTE LOWER RESPIRATORY INFECTIONS (J20-J22)

Excludes2 chronic obstructive pulmonary disease with acute lower respiratory infection (J44.0)

J20 Acute bronchitis

Inflammation/irritation of the bronchial tubes lasting 2-3 weeks, most commonly caused by a virus

Includes acute and subacute bronchitis (with) bronchospasm
acute and subacute bronchitis (with) tracheitis
acute and subacute bronchitis (with) tracheobronchitis, acute
acute and subacute fibrinous bronchitis
acute and subacute membranous bronchitis
acute and subacute purulent bronchitis
acute and subacute septic bronchitis

Excludes1 bronchitis NOS (J40)
tracheobronchitis NOS (J40)

Excludes2 acute bronchitis with bronchiectasis (J47.0)
acute bronchitis with chronic obstructive asthma (J44.0)
acute bronchitis with chronic obstructive pulmonary disease (J44.0)
allergic bronchitis NOS (J45.909-)
bronchitis due to chemicals, fumes and vapors (J68.0)
chronic bronchitis NOS (J42)
chronic mucopurulent bronchitis (J41.1)
chronic obstructive bronchitis (J44.-)
chronic obstructive tracheobronchitis (J44.-)
chronic simple bronchitis (J41.0)
chronic tracheobronchitis (J42)

J20.0 Acute bronchitis due to Mycoplasma pneumoniae

J20.1 Acute bronchitis due to Hemophilus influenzae

J20.2 Acute bronchitis due to streptococcus

J20.3 Acute bronchitis due to coxsackievirus

J20.4 Acute bronchitis due to parainfluenza virus

J20.5 Acute bronchitis due to respiratory syncytial virus
▶Acute bronchitis due to RSV

J20.6 Acute bronchitis due to rhinovirus
Coding Clinic: 2016, Q3, P10

J20.7 Acute bronchitis due to echovirus

J20.8 Acute bronchitis due to other specified organisms
Coding Clinic: 2016, Q3, P11

J20.9 Acute bronchitis, unspecified
Coding Clinic: 2019, Q1, P35; 2016, Q3, P16

J21 Acute bronchiolitis

Bronchiolitis obliterans with organizing pneumonia (BOOP) inflammation of bronchioles and surrounding tissue in lung

Includes acute bronchiolitis with bronchospasm

Excludes2 respiratory bronchiolitis interstitial lung disease (J84.115)

J21.0 Acute bronchiolitis due to respiratory syncytial virus
▶Acute bronchitis due to RSV

J21.1 Acute bronchiolitis due to human metapneumovirus

J21.8 Acute bronchiolitis due to other specified organisms

J21.9 Acute bronchiolitis, unspecified
Bronchiolitis (acute)

Excludes1 chronic bronchiolitis (J44.-)

J22 Unspecified acute lower respiratory infection
Acute (lower) respiratory (tract) infection NOS

Excludes1 upper respiratory infection (acute) (J06.9)

OTHER DISEASES OF UPPER RESPIRATORY TRACT (J3Ø-J39)

J3Ø Vasomotor and allergic rhinitis
- **Includes** spasmodic rhinorrhea
- **Excludes1** allergic rhinitis with asthma (bronchial) (J45.9Ø9); rhinitis NOS (J31.Ø)

J3Ø.Ø **Vasomotor rhinitis**

J3Ø.1 **Allergic rhinitis due to pollen**
Allergy NOS due to pollen
Hay fever
Pollinosis

J3Ø.2 **Other seasonal allergic rhinitis**

J3Ø.5 **Allergic rhinitis due to food**

J3Ø.8 **Other allergic rhinitis**

J3Ø.81 **Allergic rhinitis due to animal (cat) (dog) hair and dander**

J3Ø.89 **Other allergic rhinitis**
Perennial allergic rhinitis

J3Ø.9 **Allergic rhinitis, unspecified**

J31 **Chronic rhinitis, nasopharyngitis and pharyngitis**
Use additional code to identify:
exposure to environmental tobacco smoke (Z77.22)
exposure to tobacco smoke in the perinatal period (P96.81)
history of tobacco dependence (Z87.891)
occupational exposure to environmental tobacco smoke (Z57.31)
tobacco dependence (F17.-)
tobacco use (Z72.Ø)

J31.Ø **Chronic rhinitis**
Atrophic rhinitis (chronic)
Granulomatous rhinitis (chronic)
Hypertrophic rhinitis (chronic)
Obstructive rhinitis (chronic)
Ozena
Purulent rhinitis (chronic)
Rhinitis (chronic) NOS
Ulcerative rhinitis (chronic)
- **Excludes1** allergic rhinitis (J3Ø.1-J3Ø.9); vasomotor rhinitis (J3Ø.Ø)

J31.1 **Chronic nasopharyngitis**
- **Excludes2** acute nasopharyngitis (JØØ)

J31.2 **Chronic pharyngitis**
Chronic sore throat
Atrophic pharyngitis (chronic)
Granular pharyngitis (chronic)
Hypertrophic pharyngitis (chronic)
- **Excludes2** acute pharyngitis (JØ2.9)

J32 Chronic sinusitis
- **Includes** sinus abscess; sinus empyema; sinus infection; sinus suppuration

Use additional code to identify:
exposure to environmental tobacco smoke (Z77.22)
exposure to tobacco smoke in the perinatal period (P96.81)
history of tobacco dependence (Z87.891)
infectious agent (B95-B97)
occupational exposure to environmental tobacco smoke (Z57.31)
tobacco dependence (F17.-)
tobacco use (Z72.Ø)
- **Excludes2** acute sinusitis (JØ1.-)

J32.Ø **Chronic maxillary sinusitis**
Antritis (chronic)
Maxillary sinusitis NOS

J32.1 **Chronic frontal sinusitis**
Frontal sinusitis NOS

Item 10–4 **Nasal polyps** are an abnormal growth of tissue (tumor) projecting from a mucous membrane and attached to the surface by a narrow elongated stalk (pedunculated). Nasal polyps usually originate in the ethmoid sinus but also may occur in the maxillary sinus. Symptoms are nasal block, sinusitis, anosmia, and secondary infections.

J32.2 **Chronic ethmoidal sinusitis**
Ethmoidal sinusitis NOS
- **Excludes1** Woakes' ethmoiditis (J33.1)

J32.3 **Chronic sphenoidal sinusitis**
Sphenoidal sinusitis NOS

J32.4 **Chronic pansinusitis**
Pansinusitis NOS

J32.8 **Other chronic sinusitis**
Sinusitis (chronic) involving more than one sinus but not pansinusitis

J32.9 **Chronic sinusitis, unspecified**
Sinusitis (chronic) NOS

J33 Nasal polyp
Use additional code to identify:
exposure to environmental tobacco smoke (Z77.22)
exposure to tobacco smoke in the perinatal period (P96.81)
history of tobacco dependence (Z87.891)
occupational exposure to environmental tobacco smoke (Z57.31)
tobacco dependence (F17.-)
tobacco use (Z72.Ø)
- **Excludes1** adenomatous polyps (D14.Ø)

J33.Ø **Polyp of nasal cavity**
Choanal polyp
Nasopharyngeal polyp

J33.1 **Polypoid sinus degeneration**
Woakes' syndrome or ethmoiditis

J33.8 **Other polyp of sinus**
Accessory polyp of sinus
Ethmoidal polyp of sinus
Maxillary polyp of sinus
Sphenoidal polyp of sinus

J33.9 **Nasal polyp, unspecified**

J34 Other and unspecified disorders of nose and nasal sinuses
- **Excludes2** varicose ulcer of nasal septum (I86.8)

J34.Ø **Abscess, furuncle and carbuncle of nose**
Cellulitis of nose
Necrosis of nose
Ulceration of nose

J34.1 **Cyst and mucocele of nose and nasal sinus**

J34.2 **Deviated nasal septum**
Deflection or deviation of septum (nasal) (acquired)
- **Excludes1** congenital deviated nasal septum (Q67.4)

J34.3 **Hypertrophy of nasal turbinates**

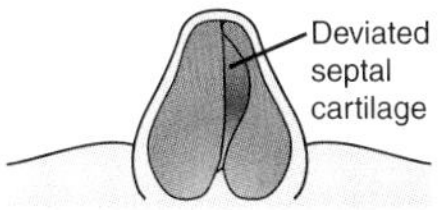

Figure 10-3 Deviated nasal septum.

Item 10–5 A **deviated nasal septum** is the displacement of the septal cartilage that separates the nares. This displacement causes obstructed air flow through the nasal passages. A child can be born with this displacement (congenital), or the condition may be acquired through trauma, such as a sports injury. Symptoms include nasal block, sinusitis, and related secondary infections. Septoplasty is surgical repair of this condition.

J34.8 Other specified disorders of nose and nasal sinuses

J34.81 Nasal mucositis (ulcerative)

Code also type of associated therapy, such as:
antineoplastic and immunosuppressive drugs (T45.1X-)
radiological procedure and radiotherapy (Y84.2)

Excludes2 gastrointestinal mucositis (ulcerative) (K92.81)
mucositis (ulcerative) of vagina and vulva (N76.81)
oral mucositis (ulcerative) (K12.3-)

J34.89 Other specified disorders of nose and nasal sinuses
Perforation of nasal septum NOS
Rhinolith

J34.9 Unspecified disorder of nose and nasal sinuses

J35 Chronic diseases of tonsils and adenoids

Use additional code to identify:
exposure to environmental tobacco smoke (Z77.22)
exposure to tobacco smoke in the perinatal period (P96.81)
history of tobacco dependence (Z87.891)
occupational exposure to environmental tobacco smoke (Z57.31)
tobacco dependence (F17.-)
tobacco use (Z72.Ø)

J35.Ø Chronic tonsillitis and adenoiditis

Excludes2 acute tonsillitis (JØ3.-)

J35.Ø1 Chronic tonsillitis

J35.Ø2 Chronic adenoiditis

J35.Ø3 Chronic tonsillitis and adenoiditis

J35.1 Hypertrophy of tonsils
Enlargement of tonsils

Excludes1 hypertrophy of tonsils with tonsillitis (J35.Ø-)

J35.2 Hypertrophy of adenoids
Enlargement of adenoids

Excludes1 hypertrophy of adenoids with adenoiditis (J35.Ø-)

J35.3 Hypertrophy of tonsils with hypertrophy of adenoids

Excludes1 hypertrophy of tonsils and adenoids with tonsillitis and adenoiditis (J35.Ø3)

J35.8 Other chronic diseases of tonsils and adenoids
Adenoid vegetations
Amygdalolith
Calculus, tonsil
Cicatrix of tonsil (and adenoid)
Tonsillar tag
Ulcer of tonsil

J35.9 Chronic disease of tonsils and adenoids, unspecified
Disease (chronic) of tonsils and adenoids NOS

J36 Peritonsillar abscess

Includes abscess of tonsil
peritonsillar cellulitis
quinsy

Use additional code (B95-B97) to identify infectious agent.

Excludes1 acute tonsillitis (JØ3.-)
chronic tonsillitis (J35.Ø)
retropharyngeal abscess (J39.Ø)
tonsillitis NOS (JØ3.9-)

J37 Chronic laryngitis and laryngotracheitis

Use additional code to identify:
exposure to environmental tobacco smoke (Z77.22)
exposure to tobacco smoke in the perinatal period (P96.81)
history of tobacco dependence (Z87.891)
infectious agent (B95-B97)
occupational exposure to environmental tobacco smoke (Z57.31)
tobacco dependence (F17.-)
tobacco use (Z72.Ø)

J37.Ø Chronic laryngitis
Catarrhal laryngitis
Hypertrophic laryngitis
Sicca laryngitis

Excludes2 acute laryngitis (JØ4.Ø)
obstructive (acute) laryngitis (JØ5.Ø)

J37.1 Chronic laryngotracheitis
Laryngitis, chronic, with tracheitis (chronic)
Tracheitis, chronic, with laryngitis

Excludes1 chronic tracheitis (J42)

Excludes2 acute laryngotracheitis (JØ4.2)
acute tracheitis (JØ4.1)

J38 Diseases of vocal cords and larynx, not elsewhere classified

Use additional code to identify:
exposure to environmental tobacco smoke (Z77.22)
exposure to tobacco smoke in the perinatal period (P96.81)
history of tobacco dependence (Z87.891)
occupational exposure to environmental tobacco smoke (Z57.31)
tobacco dependence (F17.-)
tobacco use (Z72.Ø)

Excludes1 congenital laryngeal stridor (P28.89)
obstructive laryngitis (acute) (JØ5.Ø)
postprocedural subglottic stenosis (J95.5)
stridor (RØ6.1)
ulcerative laryngitis (JØ4.Ø)

J38.Ø Paralysis of vocal cords and larynx
Laryngoplegia
Paralysis of glottis

J38.ØØ Paralysis of vocal cords and larynx, unspecified

J38.Ø1 Paralysis of vocal cords and larynx, unilateral

J38.Ø2 Paralysis of vocal cords and larynx, bilateral

J38.1 Polyp of vocal cord and larynx

Excludes1 adenomatous polyps (D14.1)

J38.2 Nodules of vocal cords
Chorditis (fibrinous)(nodosa)(tuberosa)
Singer's nodes
Teacher's nodes

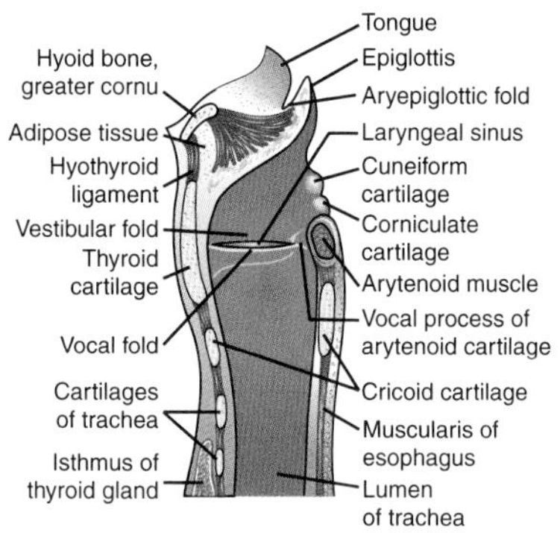

Figure 10-4 Coronal section of the larynx.

Item 10–6 The **larynx** extends from the tongue to the trachea and is divided into an upper and lower portion separated by folds. The framework of the larynx is cartilage composed of the single cricoid, thyroid, and epiglottic cartilages, and the paired arytenoid, cuneiform, and corniculate cartilages.

J38.3 Other diseases of vocal cords
Abscess of vocal cords
Cellulitis of vocal cords
Granuloma of vocal cords
Leukokeratosis of vocal cords
Leukoplakia of vocal cords

J38.4 Edema of larynx
Edema (of) glottis
Subglottic edema
Supraglottic edema
Excludes1 acute obstructive laryngitis [croup] (J05.0)
edematous laryngitis (J04.0)

J38.5 Laryngeal spasm
Laryngismus (stridulus)

J38.6 Stenosis of larynx

J38.7 Other diseases of larynx
Abscess of larynx
Cellulitis of larynx
Disease of larynx NOS
Necrosis of larynx
Pachyderma of larynx
Perichondritis of larynx
Ulcer of larynx

● **J39 Other diseases of upper respiratory tract**
Excludes1 acute respiratory infection NOS (J22)
acute upper respiratory infection (J06.9)
upper respiratory inflammation due to chemicals, gases, fumes or vapors (J68.2)

J39.0 Retropharyngeal and parapharyngeal abscess
Peripharyngeal abscess
Excludes1 peritonsillar abscess (J36)

J39.1 Other abscess of pharynx
Cellulitis of pharynx
Nasopharyngeal abscess

J39.2 Other diseases of pharynx
Cyst of pharynx
Edema of pharynx
Excludes2 chronic pharyngitis (J31.2)
ulcerative pharyngitis (J02.9)

J39.3 Upper respiratory tract hypersensitivity reaction, site unspecified
Excludes1 hypersensitivity reaction of upper respiratory tract, such as:
extrinsic allergic alveolitis (J67.9)
pneumoconiosis (J60-J67.9)

J39.8 Other specified diseases of upper respiratory tract

J39.9 Disease of upper respiratory tract, unspecified

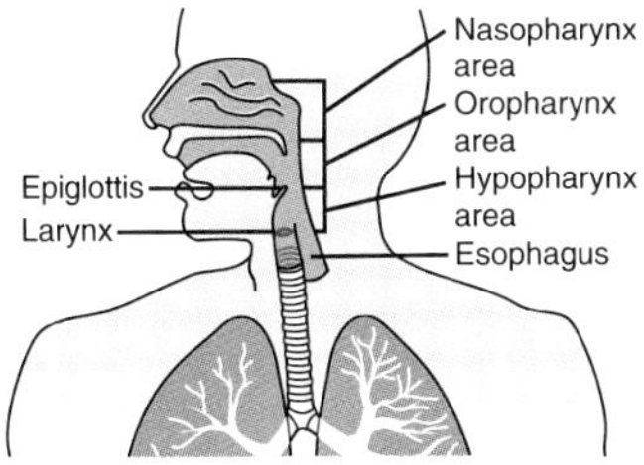

Figure 10-5 The pharynx.

Item 10–7 The **pharynx** is the passage for both food and air between the mouth and the esophagus and is divided into three areas: nasopharynx, oropharynx, and hypopharynx. The hypopharynx branches into the esophagus and the voice box.

Item 10–8 Chronic bronchitis is usually defined as being present in any patient who has persistent cough with sputum production for at least three months in at least two consecutive years. **Simple chronic bronchitis** is marked by a productive cough but no pathological airflow obstruction. **Chronic obstructive pulmonary disease (COPD)** is a group of conditions—bronchitis, emphysema, asthma, bronchiectasis, allergic alveolitis—marked by dyspnea. **Catarrhal** bronchitis is an acute form of bronchitis marked by profuse mucus and pus production (**mucopurulent** discharge). **Croupous** bronchitis, also known as pseudomembranous, fibrinous, plastic, exudative, or membranous, is marked by a violent cough and dyspnea.

CHRONIC LOWER RESPIRATORY DISEASES (J40-J47)

Excludes1 bronchitis due to chemicals, gases, fumes and vapors (J68.0)
Excludes2 cystic fibrosis (E84.-)

J40 Bronchitis, not specified as acute or chronic
Bronchitis NOS
Catarrhal bronchitis
Bronchitis with tracheitis NOS
Tracheobronchitis NOS
Use additional code to identify:
exposure to environmental tobacco smoke (Z77.22)
exposure to tobacco smoke in the perinatal period (P96.81)
history of tobacco dependence (Z87.891)
occupational exposure to environmental tobacco smoke (Z57.31)
tobacco dependence (F17.-)
tobacco use (Z72.0)
Excludes1 acute bronchitis (J20.-)
allergic bronchitis NOS (J45.909-)
asthmatic bronchitis NOS (J45.9-)
bronchitis due to chemicals, gases, fumes and vapors (J68.0)

● **J41 Simple and mucopurulent chronic bronchitis**
Use additional code to identify:
exposure to environmental tobacco smoke (Z77.22)
exposure to tobacco smoke in the perinatal period (P96.81)
history of tobacco dependence (Z87.891)
occupational exposure to environmental tobacco smoke (Z57.31)
tobacco dependence (F17.-)
tobacco use (Z72.0)
Excludes1 chronic bronchitis NOS (J42)
chronic obstructive bronchitis (J44.-)

J41.0 Simple chronic bronchitis

J41.1 Mucopurulent chronic bronchitis

J41.8 Mixed simple and mucopurulent chronic bronchitis

J42 Unspecified chronic bronchitis
Chronic bronchitis NOS
Chronic tracheitis
Chronic tracheobronchitis
Use additional code to identify:
exposure to environmental tobacco smoke (Z77.22)
exposure to tobacco smoke in the perinatal period (P96.81)
history of tobacco dependence (Z87.891)
occupational exposure to environmental tobacco smoke (Z57.31)
tobacco dependence (F17.-)
tobacco use (Z72.0)
Excludes1 chronic asthmatic bronchitis (J44.-)
chronic bronchitis with airways obstruction (J44.-)
chronic emphysematous bronchitis (J44.-)
chronic obstructive pulmonary disease NOS (J44.9)
simple and mucopurulent chronic bronchitis (J41.-)

J43 Emphysema

Use additional code to identify:
exposure to environmental tobacco smoke (Z77.22)
history of tobacco dependence (Z87.891)
occupational exposure to environmental tobacco smoke (Z57.31)
tobacco dependence (F17.-)
tobacco use (Z72.Ø)

Excludes1 compensatory emphysema (J98.3)
emphysema due to inhalation of chemicals, gases, fumes or vapors (J68.4)
emphysema with chronic (obstructive) bronchitis (J44.-)
emphysematous (obstructive) bronchitis (J44.-)
interstitial emphysema (J98.2)
mediastinal emphysema (J98.2)
neonatal interstitial emphysema (P25.Ø)
surgical (subcutaneous) emphysema (T81.82)
traumatic subcutaneous emphysema (T79.7)

J43.Ø Unilateral pulmonary emphysema [MacLeod's syndrome]
Swyer-James syndrome
Unilateral emphysema
Unilateral hyperlucent lung
Unilateral pulmonary artery functional hypoplasia
Unilateral transparency of lung

J43.1 Panlobular emphysema
Panacinar emphysema

J43.2 Centrilobular emphysema

J43.8 Other emphysema

J43.9 Emphysema, unspecified
Bullous emphysema (lung)(pulmonary)
Emphysema (lung)(pulmonary) NOS
Emphysematous bleb
Vesicular emphysema (lung)(pulmonary)
Coding Clinic: 2Ø19, Q1, P35-37; 2Ø17, Q4, P97-98

J44 Other chronic obstructive pulmonary disease

Includes asthma with chronic obstructive pulmonary disease
chronic asthmatic (obstructive) bronchitis
chronic bronchitis with airways obstruction
chronic bronchitis with emphysema
chronic emphysematous bronchitis
chronic obstructive asthma
chronic obstructive bronchitis
chronic obstructive tracheobronchitis

Code also type of asthma, if applicable (J45.-)

Use additional code to identify:
exposure to environmental tobacco smoke (Z77.22)
history of tobacco dependence (Z87.891)
occupational exposure to environmental tobacco smoke (Z57.31)
tobacco dependence (F17.-)
tobacco use (Z72.Ø)

Excludes1 bronchiectasis (J47.-)
chronic bronchitis NOS (J42)
chronic simple and mucopurulent bronchitis (J41.-)
chronic tracheitis (J42)
chronic tracheobronchitis (J42)
emphysema without chronic bronchitis (J43.-)

Coding Clinic: 2Ø19, Q1, P34-36; 2Ø17, Q4, P97; 2Ø17, Q1, P25; 2Ø16, Q3, P16

J44.Ø Chronic obstructive pulmonary disease with (acute) lower respiratory infection
Code also to identify the infection
Coding Clinic: 2Ø19, Q1, P35-36; 2Ø17, Q4, P96; 2Ø17, Q2, P3Ø, Q1, P24-25; 2Ø16, Q3, P15-16

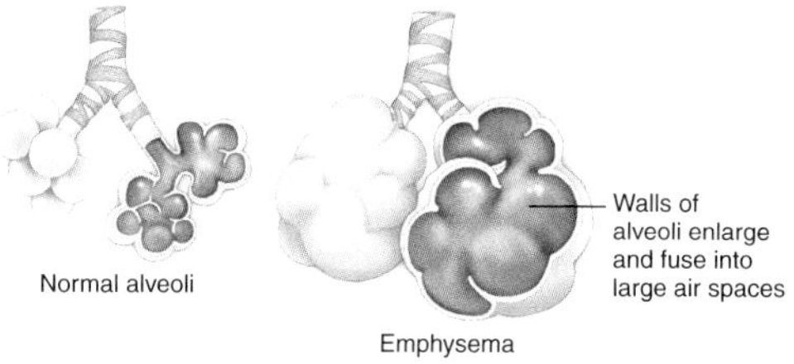

Figure 10-6 Emphysema. (From Shiland, BJ: Medical Terminology & Anatomy for ICD-10 Coding, ed 2, Mosby, 2015)

J44.1 Chronic obstructive pulmonary disease with (acute) exacerbation
Decompensated COPD
Decompensated COPD with (acute) exacerbation

Excludes2 chronic obstructive pulmonary disease [COPD] with acute bronchitis (J44.Ø)
lung diseases due to external agents (J6Ø-J7Ø)

Coding Clinic: 2Ø19, Q1, P34-35; 2Ø17, Q4, P96; 2Ø17, Q1, P26; 2Ø16, Q3, P15-16, Q1, P36

J44.9 Chronic obstructive pulmonary disease, unspecified
Chronic obstructive airway disease NOS
Chronic obstructive lung disease NOS

Excludes2 lung diseases due to external agents (J6Ø-J7Ø)

Coding Clinic: 2Ø19, Q1, P36; 2Ø17, Q4, P96-97; 2Ø17, Q1, P24-25; 2Ø16, Q1, P37

J45 Asthma
Allergic (predominantly) asthma
Allergic bronchitis NOS
Allergic rhinitis with asthma
Atopic asthma
Extrinsic allergic asthma
Hay fever with asthma
Idiosyncratic asthma
Intrinsic nonallergic asthma
Nonallergic asthma

Use additional code to identify:
exposure to environmental tobacco smoke (Z77.22)
exposure to tobacco smoke in the perinatal period (P96.81)
history of tobacco dependence (Z87.891)
occupational exposure to environmental tobacco smoke (Z57.31)
tobacco dependence (F17.-)
tobacco use (Z72.Ø)

Excludes1 detergent asthma (J69.8)
eosinophilic asthma (J82)
miner's asthma (J6Ø)
wheezing NOS (RØ6.2)
wood asthma (J67.8)

Excludes2 asthma with chronic obstructive pulmonary disease (J44.9)
chronic asthmatic (obstructive) bronchitis (J44.9)
chronic obstructive asthma (J44.9)

Coding Clinic: 2Ø19, Q1, P37; 2Ø17, Q1, P25

J45.2 Mild intermittent asthma

J45.2Ø Mild intermittent asthma, uncomplicated
Mild intermittent asthma NOS

J45.21 Mild intermittent asthma with (acute) exacerbation

J45.22 Mild intermittent asthma with status asthmaticus

Item 10–9 Asthma is a bronchial condition marked by airway obstruction, hyper-responsiveness, and inflammation. **Extrinsic** asthma, also known as allergic asthma, is characterized by the same symptoms that occur with exposure to allergens and is divided into the following types: **atopic, occupational,** and **allergic bronchopulmonary aspergillosis. Intrinsic** asthma occurs in patients who have no history of allergy or sensitivities to allergens and is divided into the following types: **nonreaginic** and **pharmacologic. Status asthmaticus** is the most severe form of asthma attack and can last for days or weeks.

New Revised ~~deleted~~ Deleted Excludes 1 Excludes 2 Includes Use additional Code first Code also Key words
OGCR Official Guidelines X Assign placeholder X Use Additional Character(s) Manifestation Code Hierarchical Condition Category Coding Clinic

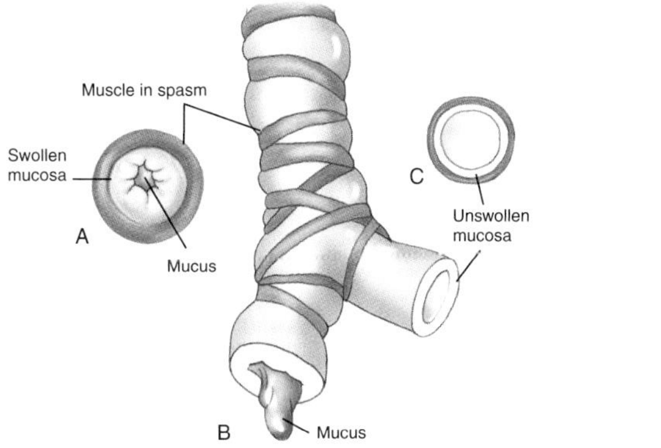

Figure 10-7 Factors causing expiratory obstruction in asthma. **A.** Cross section of a bronchiole occluded by muscle spasm, swollen mucosa, and mucus. **B.** Longitudinal section of an obstructed bronchiole. **C.** Cross section of a clear bronchiole. (From Shiland: Mastering Healthcare Terminology, ed 1, St. Louis, Mosby, 2003)

● J45.3 **Mild persistent asthma**

J45.3Ø **Mild persistent asthma, uncomplicated**
Mild persistent asthma NOS

J45.31 **Mild persistent asthma with (acute) exacerbation**
Coding Clinic: 2016, Q1, P35

J45.32 **Mild persistent asthma with status asthmaticus**

● J45.4 **Moderate persistent asthma**

J45.4Ø **Moderate persistent asthma, uncomplicated**
Moderate persistent asthma NOS

J45.41 **Moderate persistent asthma with (acute) exacerbation**
Coding Clinic: 2017, Q1, P26

J45.42 **Moderate persistent asthma with status asthmaticus**

● J45.5 **Severe persistent asthma**

J45.5Ø **Severe persistent asthma, uncomplicated**
Severe persistent asthma NOS

J45.51 **Severe persistent asthma with (acute) exacerbation**

J45.52 **Severe persistent asthma with status asthmaticus**

● J45.9 **Other and unspecified asthma**

● J45.9Ø **Unspecified asthma**
Asthmatic bronchitis NOS
Childhood asthma NOS
Late onset asthma

J45.9Ø1 **Unspecified asthma with (acute) exacerbation**
Coding Clinic: 2017, Q4, P96

J45.9Ø2 **Unspecified asthma with status asthmaticus**

J45.9Ø9 **Unspecified asthma, uncomplicated**
Asthma NOS
Excludes2 lung diseases due to external agents (J6Ø-J7Ø)
Coding Clinic: 2017, Q4, P96; 2017, Q1, P25

● J45.99 Other asthma

J45.99Ø **Exercise induced bronchospasm**

J45.991 **Cough variant asthma**

J45.998 **Other asthma**

● J47 **Bronchiectasis**
Includes bronchiolectasis
Use additional code to identify:
exposure to environmental tobacco smoke (Z77.22)
exposure to tobacco smoke in the perinatal period (P96.81)
history of tobacco dependence (Z87.891)
occupational exposure to environmental tobacco smoke (Z57.31)
tobacco dependence (F17.-)
tobacco use (Z72.Ø)
Excludes1 congenital bronchiectasis (Q33.4)
tuberculous bronchiectasis (current disease) (A15.Ø)

J47.Ø **Bronchiectasis with acute lower respiratory infection**
Bronchiectasis with acute bronchitis
Use additional code to identify the infection

J47.1 **Bronchiectasis with (acute) exacerbation**

J47.9 **Bronchiectasis, uncomplicated**
Bronchiectasis NOS

LUNG DISEASES DUE TO EXTERNAL AGENTS (J6Ø-J7Ø)

Excludes2 asthma (J45.-)
malignant neoplasm of bronchus and lung (C34.-)

J6Ø **Coalworker's pneumoconiosis** A
Anthracosilicosis
Anthracosis
Black lung disease
Coalworker's lung
Excludes1 coalworker pneumoconiosis with tuberculosis, any type in A15 (J65)

J61 **Pneumoconiosis due to asbestos and other mineral fibers** A
Asbestosis
Excludes1 pleural plaque with asbestosis (J92.Ø)
pneumoconiosis with tuberculosis, any type in A15 (J65)

● J62 **Pneumoconiosis due to dust containing silica**
Includes silicotic fibrosis (massive) of lung
Excludes1 pneumoconiosis with tuberculosis, any type in A15 (J65)

J62.Ø **Pneumoconiosis due to talc dust**

J62.8 **Pneumoconiosis due to other dust containing silica**
Silicosis NOS

● J63 **Pneumoconiosis due to other inorganic dusts**
Excludes1 pneumoconiosis with tuberculosis, any type in A15 (J65)

J63.Ø **Aluminosis (of lung)**

J63.1 **Bauxite fibrosis (of lung)**

J63.2 **Berylliosis**

J63.3 **Graphite fibrosis (of lung)**

J63.4 **Siderosis**

J63.5 **Stannosis**

J63.6 **Pneumoconiosis due to other specified inorganic dusts**

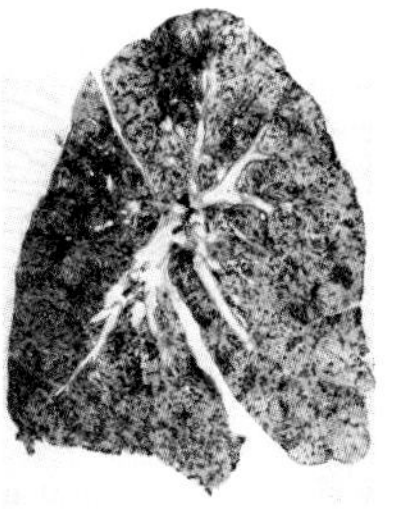

Figure 10-8 Progressive massive fibrosis superimposed on coal workers' pneumoconiosis. The large, blackened scars are located principally in the upper lobe. (From Frazier MS, Drzymkowski JW: Essentials of Human Diseases and Conditions, St. Louis, MO, Saunders, 2004)

Item 10-10 Pneumoconiosis refers to a lung condition resulting from exposure to inorganic or organic airborne particles, such as coal dust or moldy hay, as well as chemical fumes and vapors, such as insecticides. In this condition, the lungs retain the airborne particles.

J64 Unspecified pneumoconiosis
Excludes1 pneumonoconiosis with tuberculosis, any type in A15 (J65)

J65 Pneumoconiosis associated with tuberculosis
Any condition in J60-J64 with tuberculosis, any type in A15
Silicotuberculosis

J66 Airway disease due to specific organic dust
Excludes2 allergic alveolitis (J67.-)
asbestosis (J61)
bagassosis (J67.1)
farmer's lung (J67.0)
hypersensitivity pneumonitis due to organic dust (J67.-)
reactive airways dysfunction syndrome (J68.3)

J66.0 **Byssinosis**
Airway disease due to cotton dust

J66.1 **Flax-dressers' disease**

J66.2 **Cannabinosis**

J66.8 **Airway disease due to other specific organic dusts**

J67 Hypersensitivity pneumonitis due to organic dust
Includes allergic alveolitis and pneumonitis due to inhaled organic dust and particles of fungal, actinomycetic or other origin
Excludes1 pneumonitis due to inhalation of chemicals, gases, fumes or vapors (J68.0)

J67.0 **Farmer's lung**
Harvester's lung
Haymaker's lung
Moldy hay disease

J67.1 **Bagassosis**
Bagasse disease
Bagasse pneumonitis

J67.2 **Bird fancier's lung**
Budgerigar fancier's disease or lung
Pigeon fancier's disease or lung

J67.3 **Suberosis**
Corkhandler's disease or lung
Corkworker's disease or lung

J67.4 **Maltworker's lung**
Alveolitis due to Aspergillus clavatus

J67.5 **Mushroom-worker's lung**

J67.6 **Maple-bark-stripper's lung**
Alveolitis due to Cryptostroma corticale
Cryptostromosis

J67.7 **Air conditioner and humidifier lung**
Allergic alveolitis due to fungal, thermophilic actinomycetes and other organisms growing in ventilation [air conditioning] systems

J67.8 **Hypersensitivity pneumonitis due to other organic dusts**
Cheese-washer's lung
Coffee-worker's lung
Fish-meal worker's lung
Furrier's lung
Sequoiosis

J67.9 **Hypersensitivity pneumonitis due to unspecified organic dust**
Allergic alveolitis (extrinsic) NOS
Hypersensitivity pneumonitis NOS

J68 Respiratory conditions due to inhalation of chemicals, gases, fumes and vapors
Code first (T51-T65) to identify cause
Use additional code to identify associated respiratory conditions, such as:
acute respiratory failure (J96.0-)

J68.0 **Bronchitis and pneumonitis due to chemicals, gases, fumes and vapors**
Chemical bronchitis (acute)
Coding Clinic: 2019, Q2, P31-32

J68.1 **Pulmonary edema due to chemicals, gases, fumes and vapors**
Chemical pulmonary edema (acute) (chronic)
Excludes1 pulmonary edema (acute) (chronic) NOS (J81.-)

J68.2 **Upper respiratory inflammation due to chemicals, gases, fumes and vapors, not elsewhere classified**

J68.3 **Other acute and subacute respiratory conditions due to chemicals, gases, fumes and vapors**
Reactive airways dysfunction syndrome

J68.4 **Chronic respiratory conditions due to chemicals, gases, fumes and vapors**
Emphysema (diffuse) (chronic) due to inhalation of chemicals, gases, fumes and vapors
Obliterative bronchiolitis (chronic) (subacute) due to inhalation of chemicals, gases, fumes and vapors
Pulmonary fibrosis (chronic) due to inhalation of chemicals, gases, fumes and vapors
Excludes1 chronic pulmonary edema due to chemicals, gases, fumes and vapors (J68.1)

J68.8 **Other respiratory conditions due to chemicals, gases, fumes and vapors**

J68.9 **Unspecified respiratory condition due to chemicals, gases, fumes and vapors**

J69 Pneumonitis due to solids and liquids
Excludes1 neonatal aspiration syndromes (P24.-)
postprocedural pneumonitis (J95.4)

J69.0 **Pneumonitis due to inhalation of food and vomit**
Aspiration pneumonia NOS
Aspiration pneumonia (due to) food (regurgitated)
Aspiration pneumonia (due to) gastric secretions
Aspiration pneumonia (due to) milk
Aspiration pneumonia (due to) vomit
Code also any associated foreign body in respiratory tract (T17.-)
Excludes1 chemical pneumonitis due to anesthesia (J95.4)
obstetric aspiration pneumonitis (O74.0)
Coding Clinic: 2019, Q2, P7, 31-32; 2017, Q1, P24

J69.1 **Pneumonitis due to inhalation of oils and essences**
Exogenous lipoid pneumonia
Lipid pneumonia NOS
Code first (T51-T65) to identify substance
Excludes1 endogenous lipoid pneumonia (J84.89)

J69.8 **Pneumonitis due to inhalation of other solids and liquids**
Pneumonitis due to aspiration of blood
Pneumonitis due to aspiration of detergent
Code first (T51-T65) to identify substance

J70 Respiratory conditions due to other external agents

J70.0 Acute pulmonary manifestations due to radiation
Radiation pneumonitis
Use additional code (W88-W90, X39.0-) to identify the external cause

J70.1 Chronic and other pulmonary manifestations due to radiation
Fibrosis of lung following radiation
Use additional code (W88-W90, X39.0-) to identify the external cause

J70.2 Acute drug-induced interstitial lung disorders
Use additional code for adverse effect, if applicable, to identify drug (T36-T50 with fifth or sixth character 5)
Excludes1 interstitial pneumonia NOS (J84.9)
lymphoid interstitial pneumonia (J84.2)
Coding Clinic: 2019, Q2, P28

J70.3 Chronic drug-induced interstitial lung disorders
Use additional code for adverse effect, if applicable, to identify drug (T36-T50 with fifth or sixth character 5)
Excludes1 interstitial pneumonia NOS (J84.9)
lymphoid interstitial pneumonia (J84.2)

J70.4 Drug-induced interstitial lung disorders, unspecified
Use additional code for adverse effect, if applicable, to identify drug (T36-T50 with fifth or sixth character 5)
Excludes1 interstitial pneumonia NOS (J84.9)
lymphoid interstitial pneumonia (J84.2)
Coding Clinic: 2019, Q2, P28

J70.5 Respiratory conditions due to smoke inhalation
Smoke inhalation NOS
Excludes1 smoke inhalation due to chemicals, gases, fumes and vapors (J68.9)

J70.8 Respiratory conditions due to other specified external agents
Code first (T51-T65) to identify the external agent

J70.9 Respiratory conditions due to unspecified external agent
Code first (T51-T65) to identify the external agent

OTHER RESPIRATORY DISEASES PRINCIPALLY AFFECTING THE INTERSTITIUM (J80-J84)

J80 Acute respiratory distress syndrome
Acute respiratory distress syndrome in adult or child
Adult hyaline membrane disease
Excludes1 respiratory distress syndrome in newborn (perinatal) (P22.0)
Coding Clinic: 2017, Q1, P26-27

J81 Pulmonary edema
Use additional code to identify:
exposure to environmental tobacco smoke (Z77.22)
history of tobacco dependence (Z87.891)
occupational exposure to environmental tobacco smoke (Z57.31)
tobacco dependence (F17.-)
tobacco use (Z72.0)
Excludes1 chemical (acute) pulmonary edema (J68.1)
hypostatic pneumonia (J18.2)
passive pneumonia (J18.2)
pulmonary edema due to external agents (J60-J70)
pulmonary edema with heart disease NOS (I50.1)
pulmonary edema with heart failure (I50.1)

J81.0 Acute pulmonary edema
Acute edema of lung
Coding Clinic: 2017, Q1, P26

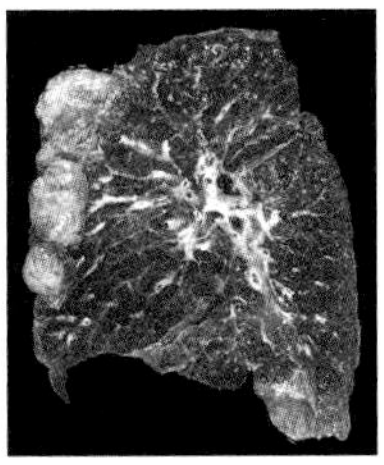

Figure 10-9 Bullous emphysema with large subpleural bullae *(upper left)*. (From Kumar: Robbins and Cotran: Pathologic Basis of Disease, ed 8, Saunders, An Imprint of Elsevier, 2009)

J81.1 Chronic pulmonary edema
Pulmonary congestion (chronic) (passive)
Pulmonary edema NOS

J82 Pulmonary eosinophilia, not elsewhere classified
Allergic pneumonia
Eosinophilic asthma
Eosinophilic pneumonia
Löffler's pneumonia
Tropical (pulmonary) eosinophilia NOS
Excludes1 pulmonary eosinophilia due to aspergillosis (B44.-)
pulmonary eosinophilia due to drugs (J70.2-J70.4)
pulmonary eosinophilia due to specified parasitic infection (B50-B83)
pulmonary eosinophilia due to systemic connective tissue disorders (M30-M36)
pulmonary infiltrate NOS (R91.8)

J84 Other interstitial pulmonary diseases
Excludes1 drug-induced interstitial lung disorders (J70.2-J70.4)
interstitial emphysema (J98.2)
Excludes2 lung diseases due to external agents (J60-J70)
Coding Clinic: 2019, Q2, P28

J84.0 Alveolar and parieto-alveolar conditions

J84.01 Alveolar proteinosis

J84.02 Pulmonary alveolar microlithiasis

J84.03 Idiopathic pulmonary hemosiderosis
Essential brown induration of lung
Code first underlying disease, such as:
disorders of iron metabolism (E83.1-)
Excludes1 acute idiopathic pulmonary hemorrhage in infants [AIPHI] (R04.81)

J84.09 Other alveolar and parieto-alveolar conditions

J84.1 Other interstitial pulmonary diseases with fibrosis
Excludes1 pulmonary fibrosis (chronic) due to inhalation of chemicals, gases, fumes or vapors (J68.4)
pulmonary fibrosis (chronic) following radiation (J70.1)

J84.10 Pulmonary fibrosis, unspecified
Capillary fibrosis of lung
Cirrhosis of lung (chronic) NOS
Fibrosis of lung (atrophic) (chronic) (confluent) (massive) (perialveolar) (peribronchial) NOS
Induration of lung (chronic) NOS
Postinflammatory pulmonary fibrosis

CHAPTER 10 (J00-J99)

J84.11 Idiopathic interstitial pneumonia

Excludes1 lymphoid interstitial pneumonia (J84.2)
pneumocystis pneumonia (B59)

J84.111 **Idiopathic interstitial pneumonia, not otherwise specified** HCC

J84.112 **Idiopathic pulmonary fibrosis** HCC
Cryptogenic fibrosing alveolitis
Idiopathic fibrosing alveolitis

J84.113 **Idiopathic non-specific interstitial pneumonitis** HCC
Excludes1 non-specific interstitial pneumonia NOS, or due to known underlying cause (J84.89)

J84.114 **Acute interstitial pneumonitis** HCC
Hamman-Rich syndrome
Excludes1 pneumocystis pneumonia (B59)

J84.115 **Respiratory bronchiolitis interstitial lung disease** HCC

J84.116 **Cryptogenic organizing pneumonia** HCC
Excludes1 organizing pneumonia NOS, or due to known underlying cause (J84.89)

J84.117 **Desquamative interstitial pneumonia** HCC

J84.17 Other interstitial pulmonary diseases with fibrosis in diseases classified elsewhere HCC
Interstitial pneumonia (nonspecific) (usual) due to collagen vascular disease
Interstitial pneumonia (nonspecific) (usual) in diseases classified elsewhere
Organizing pneumonia due to collagen vascular disease
Organizing pneumonia in diseases classified elsewhere
Code first underlying disease, such as:
progressive systemic sclerosis (M34.Ø)
rheumatoid arthritis (MØ5.ØØ-MØ6.9)
systemic lupus erythematosis (M32.Ø-M32.9)

J84.2 **Lymphoid interstitial pneumonia** HCC
Lymphoid interstitial pneumonitis

J84.8 **Other specified interstitial pulmonary diseases**
Excludes1 exogenous lipoid pneumonia (J69.1)
unspecified lipoid pneumonia (J69.1)

J84.81 **Lymphangioleiomyomatosis** HCC
Lymphangiomyomatosis

J84.82 **Adult pulmonary Langerhans cell histiocytosis** HCC A
Adult PLCH

J84.83 **Surfactant mutations of the lung** HCC

J84.84 **Other interstitial lung diseases of childhood**

J84.841 **Neuroendocrine cell hyperplasia of infancy** HCC

J84.842 **Pulmonary interstitial glycogenosis** HCC

J84.843 **Alveolar capillary dysplasia with vein misalignment** HCC

J84.848 **Other interstitial lung diseases of childhood** HCC

J84.89 **Other specified interstitial pulmonary diseases** HCC
Endogenous lipoid pneumonia
Interstitial pneumonitis
Non-specific interstitial pneumonitis NOS
Organizing pneumonia NOS
Code first, if applicable:
poisoning due to drug or toxin (T51-T65 with fifth or sixth character to indicate intent), for toxic pneumonopathy
underlying cause of pneumonopathy, if known
Use additional code, for adverse effect, to identify drug (T36-T5Ø with fifth or sixth character 5), if drug-induced
Excludes1 cryptogenic organizing pneumonia (J84.116)
idiopathic non-specific interstitial pneumonitis (J84.113)
lipoid pneumonia, exogenous or unspecified (J69.1)
lymphoid interstitial pneumonia (J84.2)

Coding Clinic: 2019, Q2, P28

J84.9 **Interstitial pulmonary disease, unspecified** HCC
Interstitial pneumonia NOS

SUPPURATIVE AND NECROTIC CONDITIONS OF THE LOWER RESPIRATORY TRACT (J85-J86)

J85 Abscess of lung and mediastinum
Use additional code (B95-B97) to identify infectious agent.

J85.Ø **Gangrene and necrosis of lung** HCC

J85.1 **Abscess of lung with pneumonia** HCC
Code also the type of pneumonia

J85.2 **Abscess of lung without pneumonia** HCC
Abscess of lung NOS

J85.3 **Abscess of mediastinum** HCC

J86 Pyothorax
Use additional code (B95-B97) to identify infectious agent.
Excludes1 abscess of lung (J85.-)
pyothorax due to tuberculosis (A15.6)

J86.Ø **Pyothorax with fistula** HCC
Bronchocutaneous fistula
Bronchopleural fistula
Hepatopleural fistula
Mediastinal fistula
Pleural fistula
Thoracic fistula
Any condition classifiable to J86.9 with fistula

J86.9 **Pyothorax without fistula** HCC
Abscess of pleura
Abscess of thorax
Empyema (chest) (lung) (pleura)
Fibrinopurulent pleurisy
Purulent pleurisy
Pyopneumothorax
Septic pleurisy
Seropurulent pleurisy
Suppurative pleurisy

Item 10-11 Empyema is a condition in which pus accumulates in a body cavity. Empyema **with fistula** occurs when the pus passes from one cavity to another organ or structure.

OTHER DISEASES OF THE PLEURA (J90-J94)

J90 Pleural effusion, not elsewhere classified
Encysted pleurisy
Pleural effusion NOS
Pleurisy with effusion (exudative) (serous)
Excludes1 chylous (pleural) effusion (J94.0)
malignant pleural effusion (J91.0))
pleurisy NOS (R09.1)
tuberculous pleural effusion (A15.6)
Coding Clinic: 2015, Q2, P16

J91 Pleural effusion in conditions classified elsewhere
Excludes2 pleural effusion in heart failure (I50.-)
pleural effusion in systemic lupus erythematosus (M32.13)

J91.0 Malignant pleural effusion
Code first underlying neoplasm

J91.8 Pleural effusion in other conditions classified elsewhere
Code first underlying disease, such as:
filariasis (B74.0-B74.9)
influenza (J09.X2, J10.1, J11.1)
Coding Clinic: 2015, Q2, P16

J92 Pleural plaque
Includes pleural thickening
J92.0 Pleural plaque with presence of asbestos
J92.9 Pleural plaque without asbestos
Pleural plaque NOS

J93 Pneumothorax and air leak
Collapsed lung
Excludes1 congenital or perinatal pneumothorax (P25.1)
postprocedural air leak (J95.812)
postprocedural pneumothorax (J95.811)
traumatic pneumothorax (S27.0)
tuberculous (current disease) pneumothorax (A15.-)
pyopneumothorax (J86.-)

J93.0 Spontaneous tension pneumothorax
Tension pneumothorax (most serious type) occurs when air (positive pressure) collects in the pleural space

J93.1 Other spontaneous pneumothorax
J93.11 Primary spontaneous pneumothorax
J93.12 Secondary spontaneous pneumothorax
Code first underlying condition, such as:
catamenial pneumothorax due to endometriosis (N80.8)
cystic fibrosis (E84.-)
eosinophilic pneumonia (J82)
lymphangioleiomyomatosis (J84.81)
malignant neoplasm of bronchus and lung (C34.-)
Marfan's syndrome (Q87.4)
pneumonia due to Pneumocystis carinii (B59)
secondary malignant neoplasm of lung (C78.0-)
spontaneous rupture of the esophagus (K22.3)

J93.8 Other pneumothorax and air leak
J93.81 Chronic pneumothorax
J93.82 Other air leak
Persistent air leak
J93.83 Other pneumothorax
Acute pneumothorax
Spontaneous pneumothorax NOS

J93.9 Pneumothorax, unspecified
Pneumothorax NOS

J94 Other pleural conditions
Excludes1 pleurisy NOS (R09.1)
traumatic hemopneumothorax (S27.2)
traumatic hemothorax (S27.1)
tuberculous pleural conditions (current disease) (A15.-)

J94.0 Chylous effusion
Chyliform effusion
J94.1 Fibrothorax
J94.2 Hemothorax
Hemopneumothorax
J94.8 Other specified pleural conditions
Hydropneumothorax
Hydrothorax
J94.9 Pleural condition, unspecified

INTRAOPERATIVE AND POSTPROCEDURAL COMPLICATIONS AND DISORDERS OF RESPIRATORY SYSTEM, NOT ELSEWHERE CLASSIFIED (J95)

J95 Intraoperative and postprocedural complications and disorders of respiratory system, not elsewhere classified
Excludes2 aspiration pneumonia (J69.-)
emphysema (subcutaneous) resulting from a procedure (T81.82)
hypostatic pneumonia (J18.2)
pulmonary manifestations due to radiation (J70.0- J70.1)

J95.0 Tracheostomy complications
J95.00 Unspecified tracheostomy complication
J95.01 Hemorrhage from tracheostomy stoma
J95.02 Infection of tracheostomy stoma
Use additional code to identify type of infection, such as:
cellulitis of neck (L03.221)
sepsis (A40, A41.-)
J95.03 Malfunction of tracheostomy stoma
Mechanical complication of tracheostomy stoma
Obstruction of tracheostomy airway
Tracheal stenosis due to tracheostomy
J95.04 Tracheo-esophageal fistula following tracheostomy
J95.09 Other tracheostomy complication

J95.1 Acute pulmonary insufficiency following thoracic surgery
Excludes2 functional disturbances following cardiac surgery (I97.0, I97.1-)

J95.2 Acute pulmonary insufficiency following nonthoracic surgery
Excludes2 functional disturbances following cardiac surgery (I97.0, I97.1-)

J95.3 Chronic pulmonary insufficiency following surgery
Excludes2 functional disturbances following cardiac surgery (I97.0, I97.1-)

J95.4 Chemical pneumonitis due to anesthesia
Mendelson's syndrome
Postprocedural aspiration pneumonia
Use additional code for adverse effect, if applicable, to identify drug (T41.- with fifth or sixth character 5)
Excludes1 aspiration pneumonitis due to anesthesia complicating labor and delivery (O74.0)
aspiration pneumonitis due to anesthesia complicating pregnancy (O29)
aspiration pneumonitis due to anesthesia complicating the puerperium (O89.01)

J95.5 Postprocedural subglottic stenosis

CHAPTER 10 (J00-J99)

J95.6 **Intraoperative hemorrhage and hematoma of a respiratory system organ or structure complicating a procedure**

Excludes1 intraoperative hemorrhage and hematoma of a respiratory system organ or structure due to accidental puncture and laceration during procedure (J95.7-)

J95.61 **Intraoperative hemorrhage and hematoma of a respiratory system organ or structure complicating a respiratory system procedure**

J95.62 **Intraoperative hemorrhage and hematoma of a respiratory system organ or structure complicating other procedure**

J95.7 **Accidental puncture and laceration of a respiratory system organ or structure during a procedure**

Excludes2 postprocedural pneumothorax (J95.811)

J95.71 **Accidental puncture and laceration of a respiratory system organ or structure during a respiratory system procedure**

J95.72 **Accidental puncture and laceration of a respiratory system organ or structure during other procedure**

J95.8 **Other intraoperative and postprocedural complications and disorders of respiratory system, not elsewhere classified**

Coding Clinic: 2016, Q4, P10

J95.81 **Postprocedural pneumothorax and air leak**

J95.811 **Postprocedural pneumothorax**

J95.812 **Postprocedural air leak**

J95.82 **Postprocedural respiratory failure**

Excludes1 Respiratory failure in other conditions (J96.-)

J95.821 **Acute postprocedural respiratory failure**

Postprocedural respiratory failure NOS

J95.822 **Acute and chronic postprocedural respiratory failure**

J95.83 **Postprocedural hemorrhage of a respiratory system organ or structure following a procedure**

J95.830 **Postprocedural hemorrhage of a respiratory system organ or structure following a respiratory system procedure**

J95.831 **Postprocedural hemorrhage of a respiratory system organ or structure following other procedure**

J95.84 **Transfusion-related acute lung injury (TRALI)**

J95.85 **Complication of respirator [ventilator]**

J95.850 **Mechanical complication of respirator**

Excludes1 encounter for respirator [ventilator] dependence during power failure (Z99.12)

J95.851 **Ventilator associated pneumonia**

Ventilator associated pneumonitis

Use additional code to identify the organism, if known (B95.-, B96.-, B97.-)

Excludes1 ventilator lung in newborn (P27.8)

Coding Clinic: 2017, Q1, P25

J95.859 **Other complication of respirator [ventilator]**

J95.86 **Postprocedural hematoma and seroma of a respiratory system organ or structure following a procedure**

J95.860 **Postprocedural hematoma of a respiratory system organ or structure following a respiratory system procedure**

J95.861 **Postprocedural hematoma of a respiratory system organ or structure following other procedure**

J95.862 **Postprocedural seroma of a respiratory system organ or structure following a respiratory system procedure**

J95.863 **Postprocedural seroma of a respiratory system organ or structure following other procedure**

J95.88 **Other intraoperative complications of respiratory system, not elsewhere classified**

J95.89 **Other postprocedural complications and disorders of respiratory system, not elsewhere classified**

Use additional code to identify disorder, such as:
aspiration pneumonia (J69.-)
bacterial or viral pneumonia (J12-J18)

Excludes2 acute pulmonary insufficiency following thoracic surgery (J95.1)
postprocedural subglottic stenosis (J95.5)

OTHER DISEASES OF THE RESPIRATORY SYSTEM (J96-J99)

J96 **Respiratory failure, not elsewhere classified**

Excludes1 acute respiratory distress syndrome (J80)
cardiorespiratory failure (R09.2)
newborn respiratory distress syndrome (P22.0)
postprocedural respiratory failure (J95.82-)
respiratory arrest (R09.2)
respiratory arrest of newborn (P28.81)
respiratory failure of newborn (P28.5)

J96.0 **Acute respiratory failure**

J96.00 **Acute respiratory failure, unspecified whether with hypoxia or hypercapnia**

Coding Clinic: 2016, Q3, P14

J96.01 **Acute respiratory failure with hypoxia**

J96.02 **Acute respiratory failure with hypercapnia**

J96.1 **Chronic respiratory failure**

J96.10 **Chronic respiratory failure, unspecified whether with hypoxia or hypercapnia**

Coding Clinic: 2016, Q1, P38; 2015, Q1, P21

J96.11 **Chronic respiratory failure with hypoxia**

J96.12 **Chronic respiratory failure with hypercapnia**

J96.2 **Acute and chronic respiratory failure**

Acute on chronic respiratory failure

J96.20 **Acute and chronic respiratory failure, unspecified whether with hypoxia or hypercapnia**

J96.21 **Acute and chronic respiratory failure with hypoxia**

J96.22 **Acute and chronic respiratory failure with hypercapnia**

J96.9 **Respiratory failure, unspecified**

J96.90 **Respiratory failure, unspecified, unspecified whether with hypoxia or hypercapnia**

J96.91 **Respiratory failure, unspecified with hypoxia**

J96.92 **Respiratory failure, unspecified with hypercapnia**

J98 Other respiratory disorders
Use additional code to identify:
exposure to environmental tobacco smoke (Z77.22)
exposure to tobacco smoke in the perinatal period (P96.81)
history of tobacco dependence (Z87.891)
occupational exposure to environmental tobacco smoke (Z57.31)
tobacco dependence (F17.-)
tobacco use (Z72.Ø)
Excludes1 newborn apnea (P28.4)
newborn sleep apnea (P28.3)
Excludes2 apnea NOS (RØ6.81)
sleep apnea (G47.3-)

J98.Ø Diseases of bronchus, not elsewhere classified

J98.Ø1 Acute bronchospasm
Excludes1 acute bronchiolitis with bronchospasm (J21.-)
acute bronchitis with bronchospasm (J2Ø.-)
asthma (J45.-)
exercise induced bronchospasm (J45.99Ø)

J98.Ø9 Other diseases of bronchus, not elsewhere classified
Broncholithiasis
Calcification of bronchus
Stenosis of bronchus
Tracheobronchial collapse
Tracheobronchial dyskinesia
Ulcer of bronchus

J98.1 Pulmonary collapse
Excludes1 therapeutic collapse of lung status (Z98.3)

J98.11 Atelectasis
Excludes1 newborn atelectasis
tuberculous atelectasis (current disease) (A15)

J98.19 Other pulmonary collapse

J98.2 Interstitial emphysema
Mediastinal emphysema
Excludes1 emphysema NOS (J43.9)
emphysema in newborn (P25.Ø)
surgical emphysema (subcutaneous) (T81.82)
traumatic subcutaneous emphysema (T79.7)

J98.3 Compensatory emphysema

J98.4 Other disorders of lung
Calcification of lung
Cystic lung disease (acquired)
Lung disease NOS
Pulmolithiasis
Excludes1 acute interstitial pneumonitis (J84.114)
pulmonary insufficiency following surgery (J95.1-J95.2)

J98.5 Diseases of mediastinum, not elsewhere classified
Excludes2 abscess of mediastinum (J85.3)
Coding Clinic: 2Ø16, Q4, P29

J98.51 Mediastinitis
Code first underlying condition, if applicable, such as postoperative mediastinitis (T81.-)

J98.59 Other diseases of mediastinum, not elsewhere classified
Fibrosis of mediastinum
Hernia of mediastinum
Retraction of mediastinum

J98.6 Disorders of diaphragm
Diaphragmatitis
Paralysis of diaphragm
Relaxation of diaphragm
Excludes1 congenital malformation of diaphragm NEC (Q79.1)
congenital diaphragmatic hernia (Q79.Ø)
Excludes2 diaphragmatic hernia (K44.-)

J98.8 Other specified respiratory disorders

J98.9 Respiratory disorder, unspecified
Respiratory disease (chronic) NOS

J99 Respiratory disorders in diseases classified elsewhere
Code first underlying disease, such as:
amyloidosis (E85.-)
ankylosing spondylitis (M45)
congenital syphilis (A5Ø.5)
cryoglobulinemia (D89.1)
early congenital syphilis (A5Ø.Ø)
plasminogen deficiency (E88.Ø2)
schistosomiasis (B65.Ø-B65.9)
Excludes1 respiratory disorders in:
amebiasis (AØ6.5)
blastomycosis (B4Ø.Ø-B4Ø.2)
candidiasis (B37.1)
coccidioidomycosis (B38.Ø-B38.2)
cystic fibrosis with pulmonary manifestations (E84.Ø)
dermatomyositis (M33.Ø1, M33.11)
histoplasmosis (B39.Ø-B39.2)
late syphilis (A52.72, A52.73)
polymyositis (M33.21)
sicca syndrome (M35.Ø2)
systemic lupus erythematosus (M32.13)
systemic sclerosis (M34.81)
Wegener's granulomatosis (M31.3Ø-M31.31)

CHAPTER 11

DISEASES OF THE DIGESTIVE SYSTEM (KØØ-K95)

OGCR Chapter-Specific Coding Guidelines

11. Chapter 11: Diseases of the Digestive System (KØØ-K95)
Reserved for future guideline expansion

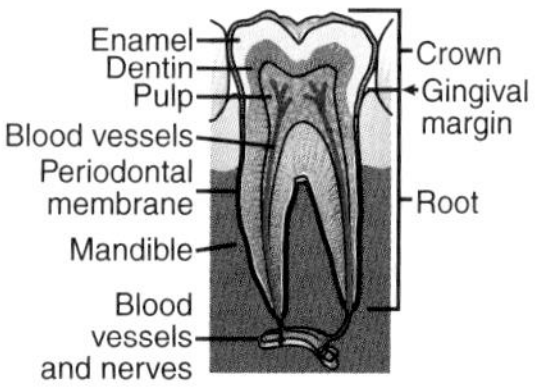

Figure 11-1 Anatomy of a tooth.

Item 11-1 **Anodontia** is the congenital absence of teeth. **Hypodontia** is partial anodontia. **Oligodontia** is the congenital absence of some teeth, whereas **supernumerary** is having more teeth than the normal number. **Mesiodens** are small extra teeth that often appear in pairs, although single small teeth are not uncommon.

CHAPTER 11

DISEASES OF THE DIGESTIVE SYSTEM (KØØ-K95)

Excludes2 certain conditions originating in the perinatal period (PØ4-P96)
certain infectious and parasitic diseases (AØØ-B99)
complications of pregnancy, childbirth and the puerperium (OØØ-O9A)
congenital malformations, deformations and chromosomal abnormalities (QØØ-Q99)
endocrine, nutritional and metabolic diseases (EØØ-E88)
injury, poisoning and certain other consequences of external causes (SØØ-T88)
neoplasms (CØØ-D49)
symptoms, signs and abnormal clinical and laboratory findings, not elsewhere classified (RØØ-R94)

This chapter contains the following blocks:

KØØ-K14	Diseases of oral cavity and salivary glands
K2Ø-K31	Diseases of esophagus, stomach and duodenum
K35-K38	Diseases of appendix
K4Ø-K46	Hernia
K5Ø-K52	Noninfective enteritis and colitis
K55-K64	Other diseases of intestines
K65-K68	Diseases of peritoneum and retroperitoneum
K7Ø-K77	Diseases of liver
K8Ø-K87	Disorders of gallbladder, biliary tract and pancreas
K9Ø-K95	Other diseases of the digestive system

DISEASES OF ORAL CAVITY AND SALIVARY GLANDS (KØØ-K14)

● **KØØ Disorders of tooth development and eruption**
Excludes2 embedded and impacted teeth (KØ1.-)

KØØ.Ø Anodontia
Hypodontia
Oligodontia
Excludes1 acquired absence of teeth (KØ8.1-)

KØØ.1 Supernumerary teeth
Distomolar
Fourth molar
Mesiodens
Paramolar
Supplementary teeth
Excludes2 supernumerary roots (KØØ.2)

KØØ.2 Abnormalities of size and form of teeth
Concrescence of teeth
Fusion of teeth
Gemination of teeth
Dens evaginatus
Dens in dente
Dens invaginatus
Enamel pearls
Macrodontia
Microdontia
Peg-shaped [conical] teeth
Supernumerary roots
Taurodontism
Tuberculum paramolare
Excludes1 abnormalities of teeth due to congenital syphilis (A5Ø.5)
tuberculum Carabelli, which is regarded as a normal variation and should not be coded

KØØ.3 Mottled teeth
Dental fluorosis
Mottling of enamel
Nonfluoride enamel opacities
Excludes2 deposits [accretions] on teeth (KØ3.6)

KØØ.4 Disturbances in tooth formation
Aplasia and hypoplasia of cementum
Dilaceration of tooth
Enamel hypoplasia (neonatal) (postnatal) (prenatal)
Regional odontodysplasia
Turner's tooth
Excludes1 Hutchinson's teeth and mulberry molars in congenital syphilis (A5Ø.5)
Excludes2 mottled teeth (KØØ.3)

KØØ.5 Hereditary disturbances in tooth structure, not elsewhere classified
Amelogenesis imperfecta
Dentinogenesis imperfecta
Odontogenesis imperfecta
Dentinal dysplasia
Shell teeth

KØØ.6 Disturbances in tooth eruption
Dentia praecox
Natal tooth
Neonatal tooth
Premature eruption of tooth
Premature shedding of primary [deciduous] tooth
Prenatal teeth
Retained [persistent] primary tooth
Excludes2 embedded and impacted teeth (KØ1.-)

KØØ.7 Teething syndrome

KØØ.8 Other disorders of tooth development
Color changes during tooth formation
Intrinsic staining of teeth NOS
Excludes2 posteruptive color changes (KØ3.7)

KØØ.9 Disorder of tooth development, unspecified
Disorder of odontogenesis NOS

● **KØ1 Embedded and impacted teeth**
Excludes1 abnormal position of fully erupted teeth (M26.3-)

KØ1.Ø Embedded teeth

KØ1.1 Impacted teeth

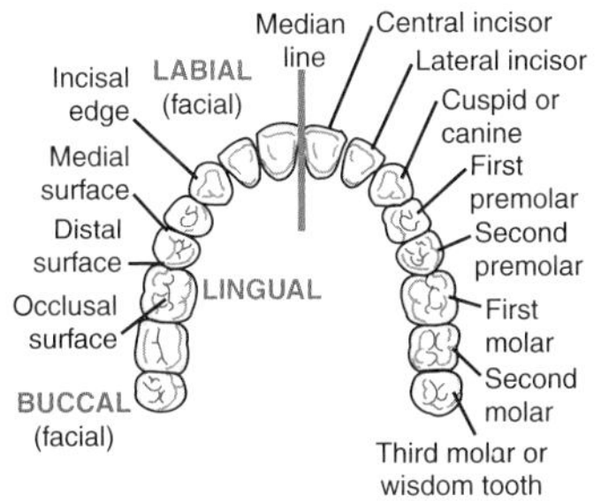

Figure 11-2 The permanent teeth within the dental arch.

Item 11-2 Each dental arch (jaw) normally contains 16 teeth. Tooth decay or **dental caries** is a disease of the enamel, dentin, and cementum of the tooth and can result in a cavity.

KØ2 Dental caries
Includes caries of dentine
dental cavities
early childhood caries
pre-eruptive caries
recurrent caries (dentino enamel junction) (enamel) (to the pulp)
tooth decay

KØ2.3 Arrested dental caries
Arrested coronal and root caries

KØ2.5 Dental caries on pit and fissure surface
Dental caries on chewing surface of tooth

KØ2.51 Dental caries on pit and fissure surface limited to enamel
White spot lesions [initial caries] on pit and fissure surface of tooth

KØ2.52 Dental caries on pit and fissure surface penetrating into dentin
Primary dental caries, cervical origin

KØ2.53 Dental caries on pit and fissure surface penetrating into pulp

KØ2.6 Dental caries on smooth surface

KØ2.61 Dental caries on smooth surface limited to enamel
White spot lesions [initial caries] on smooth surface of tooth

KØ2.62 Dental caries on smooth surface penetrating into dentin

KØ2.63 Dental caries on smooth surface penetrating into pulp

KØ2.7 Dental root caries

KØ2.9 Dental caries, unspecified

KØ3 Other diseases of hard tissues of teeth
Excludes2 bruxism (F45.8)
dental caries (KØ2.-)
teeth-grinding NOS (F45.8)

KØ3.Ø Excessive attrition of teeth
Approximal wear of teeth
Occlusal wear of teeth

KØ3.1 Abrasion of teeth
Dentifrice abrasion of teeth
Habitual abrasion of teeth
Occupational abrasion of teeth
Ritual abrasion of teeth
Traditional abrasion of teeth
Wedge defect NOS

KØ3.2 Erosion of teeth
Erosion of teeth due to diet
Erosion of teeth due to drugs and medicaments
Erosion of teeth due to persistent vomiting
Erosion of teeth NOS
Idiopathic erosion of teeth
Occupational erosion of teeth

KØ3.3 Pathological resorption of teeth
Internal granuloma of pulp
Resorption of teeth (external)

KØ3.4 Hypercementosis
Cementation hyperplasia

KØ3.5 Ankylosis of teeth

KØ3.6 Deposits [accretions] on teeth
Betel deposits [accretions] on teeth
Black deposits [accretions] on teeth
Extrinsic staining of teeth NOS
Green deposits [accretions] on teeth
Materia alba deposits [accretions] on teeth
Orange deposits [accretions] on teeth
Staining of teeth NOS
Subgingival dental calculus
Supragingival dental calculus
Tobacco deposits [accretions] on teeth

KØ3.7 Posteruptive color changes of dental hard tissues
Excludes2 deposits [accretions] on teeth (KØ3.6)

KØ3.8 Other specified diseases of hard tissues of teeth

KØ3.81 Cracked tooth
Excludes1 asymptomatic craze lines in enamel - omit code
broken or fractured tooth due to trauma (SØ2.5)

KØ3.89 Other specified diseases of hard tissues of teeth

KØ3.9 Disease of hard tissues of teeth, unspecified

KØ4 Diseases of pulp and periapical tissues
Coding Clinic: 2016, Q4, P29

KØ4.Ø Pulpitis
Acute pulpitis
Chronic (hyperplastic) (ulcerative) pulpitis

KØ4.Ø1 Reversible pulpitis

KØ4.Ø2 Irreversible pulpitis

KØ4.1 Necrosis of pulp
Pulpal gangrene

KØ4.2 Pulp degeneration
Denticles
Pulpal calcifications
Pulpal stones

KØ4.3 Abnormal hard tissue formation in pulp
Secondary or irregular dentine

KØ4.4 Acute apical periodontitis of pulpal origin
Acute apical periodontitis NOS
Excludes1 acute periodontitis (KØ5.2-)

KØ4.5 Chronic apical periodontitis
Apical or periapical granuloma
Apical periodontitis NOS
Excludes1 chronic periodontitis (KØ5.3-)

KØ4.6 Periapical abscess with sinus
Dental abscess with sinus
Dentoalveolar abscess with sinus

KØ4.7 Periapical abscess without sinus
Dental abscess without sinus
Dentoalveolar abscess without sinus

KØ4.8 Radicular cyst
Apical (periodontal) cyst
Periapical cyst
Residual radicular cyst
Excludes2 lateral periodontal cyst (KØ9.Ø)

KØ4.9 Other and unspecified diseases of pulp and periapical tissues

KØ4.90 Unspecified diseases of pulp and periapical tissues

KØ4.99 Other diseases of pulp and periapical tissues

Item 11–3 **Acute gingivitis,** also known as orilitis or ulitis, is the short-term, severe inflammation of the gums (gingiva) caused by bacteria. **Chronic gingivitis** is persistent inflammation of the gums. When the gingivitis moves into the periodontium it is called periodontitis, also known as paradentitis.

● **KØ5 Gingivitis and periodontal diseases**
Use additional code to identify:
alcohol abuse and dependence (F1Ø.-)
exposure to environmental tobacco smoke (Z77.22)
exposure to tobacco smoke in the perinatal period (P96.81)
history of tobacco dependence (Z87.891)
occupational exposure to environmental tobacco smoke (Z57.31)
tobacco dependence (F17.-)
tobacco use (Z72.Ø)
Coding Clinic: 2016, Q4, P29

● **KØ5.Ø Acute gingivitis**
Excludes1 acute necrotizing ulcerative gingivitis (A69.1)
herpesviral [herpes simplex] gingivostomatitis (BØØ.2)

KØ5.ØØ Acute gingivitis, plaque induced
Acute gingivitis NOS
Plaque induced gingival disease

KØ5.Ø1 Acute gingivitis, non-plaque induced

● **KØ5.1 Chronic gingivitis**
Desquamative gingivitis (chronic)
Gingivitis (chronic) NOS
Hyperplastic gingivitis (chronic)
Pregnancy associated gingivitis
Simple marginal gingivitis (chronic)
Ulcerative gingivitis (chronic)
Code first, if applicable, diseases of the digestive system complicating pregnancy (O99.61-)

KØ5.1Ø Chronic gingivitis, plaque induced
Chronic gingivitis NOS
Gingivitis NOS

KØ5.11 Chronic gingivitis, non-plaque induced

● **KØ5.2 Aggressive periodontitis**
Acute pericoronitis
Excludes1 acute apical periodontitis (KØ4.4)
periapical abscess (KØ4.7)
periapical abscess with sinus (KØ4.6)

KØ5.2Ø Aggressive periodontitis, unspecified

● **KØ5.21 Aggressive periodontitis, localized**
Periodontal abscess

KØ5.211 Aggressive periodontitis, localized, slight

KØ5.212 Aggressive periodontitis, localized, moderate

KØ5.213 Aggressive periodontitis, localized, severe

KØ5.219 Aggressive periodontitis, localized, unspecified severity

● **KØ5.22 Aggressive periodontitis, generalized**

KØ5.221 Aggressive periodontitis, generalized, slight

KØ5.222 Aggressive periodontitis, generalized, moderate

KØ5.223 Aggressive periodontitis, generalized, severe

KØ5.229 Aggressive periodontitis, generalized, unspecified severity

● **KØ5.3 Chronic periodontitis**
Chronic pericoronitis
Complex periodontitis
Periodontitis NOS
Simplex periodontitis
Excludes1 chronic apical periodontitis (KØ4.5)

KØ5.3Ø Chronic periodontitis, unspecified

● **KØ5.31 Chronic periodontitis, localized**

KØ5.311 Chronic periodontitis, localized, slight

KØ5.312 Chronic periodontitis, localized, moderate

KØ5.313 Chronic periodontitis, localized, severe

KØ5.319 Chronic periodontitis, localized, unspecified severity

● **KØ5.32 Chronic periodontitis, generalized**

KØ5.321 Chronic periodontitis, generalized, slight

KØ5.322 Chronic periodontitis, generalized, moderate

KØ5.323 Chronic periodontitis, generalized, severe

KØ5.329 Chronic periodontitis, generalized, unspecified severity

KØ5.4 Periodontosis
Juvenile periodontosis

KØ5.5 Other periodontal diseases
Combined periodontic-endodontic lesion
Narrow gingival width (of periodontal soft tissue)
Excludes2 leukoplakia of gingiva (K13.21)

KØ5.6 Periodontal disease, unspecified

● **KØ6 Other disorders of gingiva and edentulous alveolar ridge**
Excludes2 acute gingivitis (KØ5.Ø)
atrophy of edentulous alveolar ridge (KØ8.2)
chronic gingivitis (KØ5.1)
gingivitis NOS (KØ5.1)
Coding Clinic: 2016, Q4, P29

● **KØ6.Ø Gingival recession**
Gingival recession (postinfective) (postprocedural)

● **KØ6.Ø1 Gingival recession, localized**

KØ6.Ø1Ø Localized gingival recession, unspecified
Localized gingival recession, NOS

KØ6.Ø11 Localized gingival recession, minimal

KØ6.Ø12 Localized gingival recession, moderate

KØ6.Ø13 Localized gingival recession, severe

● **KØ6.Ø2 Gingival recession, generalized**

KØ6.Ø2Ø Generalized gingival recession, unspecified
Generalized gingival recession, NOS

KØ6.Ø21 Generalized gingival recession, minimal

KØ6.Ø22 Generalized gingival recession, moderate

KØ6.Ø23 Generalized gingival recession, severe

KØ6.1 Gingival enlargement
Gingival fibromatosis

KØ6.2 Gingival and edentulous alveolar ridge lesions associated with trauma
Irritative hyperplasia of edentulous ridge [denture hyperplasia]
Use additional code (Chapter 2Ø) to identify external cause or denture status (Z97.2)

KØ6.3 Horizontal alveolar bone loss

CHAPTER 11 (KØØ-K95)

KØ6.8 **Other specified disorders of gingiva and edentulous alveolar ridge**
Fibrous epulis
Flabby alveolar ridge
Giant cell epulis
Peripheral giant cell granuloma of gingiva
Pyogenic granuloma of gingiva
Vertical ridge deficiency
Excludes2 gingival cyst (KØ9.Ø)

KØ6.9 **Disorder of gingiva and edentulous alveolar ridge, unspecified**

KØ8 **Other disorders of teeth and supporting structures**
Excludes2 dentofacial anomalies [including malocclusion] (M26.-)
disorders of jaw (M27.-)
Coding Clinic: 2016, Q4, P29

KØ8.Ø **Exfoliation of teeth due to systemic causes**
Code also underlying systemic condition

KØ8.1 **Complete loss of teeth**
Acquired loss of teeth, complete
Excludes1 congenital absence of teeth (KØØ.Ø)
exfoliation of teeth due to systemic causes (KØ8.Ø)
partial loss of teeth (KØ8.4-)

KØ8.1Ø **Complete loss of teeth, unspecified cause**
KØ8.1Ø1 **Complete loss of teeth, unspecified cause, class I**
KØ8.1Ø2 **Complete loss of teeth, unspecified cause, class II**
KØ8.1Ø3 **Complete loss of teeth, unspecified cause, class III**
KØ8.1Ø4 **Complete loss of teeth, unspecified cause, class IV**
KØ8.1Ø9 **Complete loss of teeth, unspecified cause, unspecified class**
Edentulism NOS

KØ8.11 **Complete loss of teeth due to trauma**
KØ8.111 **Complete loss of teeth due to trauma, class I**
KØ8.112 **Complete loss of teeth due to trauma, class II**
KØ8.113 **Complete loss of teeth due to trauma, class III**
KØ8.114 **Complete loss of teeth due to trauma, class IV**
KØ8.119 **Complete loss of teeth due to trauma, unspecified class**

KØ8.12 **Complete loss of teeth due to periodontal diseases**
KØ8.121 **Complete loss of teeth due to periodontal diseases, class I**
KØ8.122 **Complete loss of teeth due to periodontal diseases, class II**
KØ8.123 **Complete loss of teeth due to periodontal diseases, class III**
KØ8.124 **Complete loss of teeth due to periodontal diseases, class IV**
KØ8.129 **Complete loss of teeth due to periodontal diseases, unspecified class**

KØ8.13 **Complete loss of teeth due to caries**
KØ8.131 **Complete loss of teeth due to caries, class I**
KØ8.132 **Complete loss of teeth due to caries, class II**
KØ8.133 **Complete loss of teeth due to caries, class III**
KØ8.134 **Complete loss of teeth due to caries, class IV**
KØ8.139 **Complete loss of teeth due to caries, unspecified class**

KØ8.19 **Complete loss of teeth due to other specified cause**
KØ8.191 **Complete loss of teeth due to other specified cause, class I**
KØ8.192 **Complete loss of teeth due to other specified cause, class II**
KØ8.193 **Complete loss of teeth due to other specified cause, class III**
KØ8.194 **Complete loss of teeth due to other specified cause, class IV**
KØ8.199 **Complete loss of teeth due to other specified cause, unspecified class**

KØ8.2 **Atrophy of edentulous alveolar ridge**
KØ8.2Ø **Unspecified atrophy of edentulous alveolar ridge**
Atrophy of the mandible NOS
Atrophy of the maxilla NOS
KØ8.21 **Minimal atrophy of the mandible**
Minimal atrophy of the edentulous mandible
KØ8.22 **Moderate atrophy of the mandible**
Moderate atrophy of the edentulous mandible
KØ8.23 **Severe atrophy of the mandible**
Severe atrophy of the edentulous mandible
KØ8.24 **Minimal atrophy of maxilla**
Minimal atrophy of the edentulous maxilla
KØ8.25 **Moderate atrophy of the maxilla**
Moderate atrophy of the edentulous maxilla
KØ8.26 **Severe atrophy of the maxilla**
Severe atrophy of the edentulous maxilla

KØ8.3 **Retained dental root**

KØ8.4 **Partial loss of teeth**
Acquired loss of teeth, partial
Excludes1 complete loss of teeth (KØ8.1-)
congenital absence of teeth (KØØ.Ø)
Excludes2 exfoliation of teeth due to systemic causes (KØ8.Ø)

KØ8.4Ø **Partial loss of teeth, unspecified cause**
KØ8.4Ø1 **Partial loss of teeth, unspecified cause, class I**
KØ8.4Ø2 **Partial loss of teeth, unspecified cause, class II**
KØ8.4Ø3 **Partial loss of teeth, unspecified cause, class III**
KØ8.4Ø4 **Partial loss of teeth, unspecified cause, class IV**
KØ8.4Ø9 **Partial loss of teeth, unspecified cause, unspecified class**
Tooth extraction status NOS

KØ8.41 **Partial loss of teeth due to trauma**
KØ8.411 **Partial loss of teeth due to trauma, class I**
KØ8.412 **Partial loss of teeth due to trauma, class II**
KØ8.413 **Partial loss of teeth due to trauma, class III**
KØ8.414 **Partial loss of teeth due to trauma, class IV**
KØ8.419 **Partial loss of teeth due to trauma, unspecified class**

KØ8.42 **Partial loss of teeth due to periodontal diseases**
KØ8.421 **Partial loss of teeth due to periodontal diseases, class I**
KØ8.422 **Partial loss of teeth due to periodontal diseases, class II**
KØ8.423 **Partial loss of teeth due to periodontal diseases, class III**
KØ8.424 **Partial loss of teeth due to periodontal diseases, class IV**
KØ8.429 **Partial loss of teeth due to periodontal diseases, unspecified class**

● KØ8.43 Partial loss of teeth due to caries
- KØ8.431 Partial loss of teeth due to caries, class I
- KØ8.432 Partial loss of teeth due to caries, class II
- KØ8.433 Partial loss of teeth due to caries, class III
- KØ8.434 Partial loss of teeth due to caries, class IV
- KØ8.439 Partial loss of teeth due to caries, unspecified class

● KØ8.49 Partial loss of teeth due to other specified cause
- KØ8.491 Partial loss of teeth due to other specified cause, class I
- KØ8.492 Partial loss of teeth due to other specified cause, class II
- KØ8.493 Partial loss of teeth due to other specified cause, class III
- KØ8.494 Partial loss of teeth due to other specified cause, class IV
- KØ8.499 Partial loss of teeth due to other specified cause, unspecified class

● KØ8.5 Unsatisfactory restoration of tooth
Defective bridge, crown, filling
Defective dental restoration

Excludes1 dental restoration status (Z98.811)

Excludes2 endosseous dental implant failure (M27.6-)
unsatisfactory endodontic treatment (M27.5-)

KØ8.5Ø Unsatisfactory restoration of tooth, unspecified
Defective dental restoration NOS

KØ8.51 Open restoration margins of tooth
Dental restoration failure of marginal integrity
Open margin on tooth restoration
Poor gingival margin to tooth restoration

KØ8.52 Unrepairable overhanging of dental restorative materials
Overhanging of tooth restoration

● KØ8.53 Fractured dental restorative material

Excludes1 cracked tooth (KØ3.81)
traumatic fracture of tooth (SØ2.5)

- KØ8.53Ø Fractured dental restorative material without loss of material
- KØ8.531 Fractured dental restorative material with loss of material
- KØ8.539 Fractured dental restorative material, unspecified

KØ8.54 Contour of existing restoration of tooth biologically incompatible with oral health
Dental restoration failure of periodontal anatomical integrity
Unacceptable contours of existing restoration of tooth
Unacceptable morphology of existing restoration of tooth

KØ8.55 Allergy to existing dental restorative material
Use additional code to identify the specific type of allergy

KØ8.56 Poor aesthetic of existing restoration of tooth
Dental restoration aesthetically inadequate or displeasing

KØ8.59 Other unsatisfactory restoration of tooth
Other defective dental restoration

● KØ8.8 Other specified disorders of teeth and supporting structures
- KØ8.81 Primary occlusal trauma
- KØ8.82 Secondary occlusal trauma
- KØ8.89 Other specified disorders of teeth and supporting structures
  Enlargement of alveolar ridge NOS
  Insufficient anatomic crown height
  Insufficient clinical crown length
  Irregular alveolar process
  Toothache NOS

KØ8.9 Disorder of teeth and supporting structures, unspecified

● KØ9 Cysts of oral region, not elsewhere classified

Includes lesions showing histological features both of aneurysmal cyst and of another fibro-osseous lesion

Excludes2 cysts of jaw (M27.Ø-, M27.4-)
radicular cyst (KØ4.8)

KØ9.Ø Developmental odontogenic cysts
Dentigerous cyst
Eruption cyst
Follicular cyst
Gingival cyst
Lateral periodontal cyst
Primordial cyst

Excludes2 keratocysts (D16.4, D16.5)
odontogenic keratocystic tumors (D16.4, D16.5)

KØ9.1 Developmental (nonodontogenic) cysts of oral region
Cyst (of) incisive canal
Cyst (of) palatine of papilla
Globulomaxillary cyst
Median palatal cyst
Nasoalveolar cyst
Nasolabial cyst
Nasopalatine duct cyst

KØ9.8 Other cysts of oral region, not elsewhere classified
Dermoid cyst
Epidermoid cyst
Lymphoepithelial cyst
Epstein's pearl

KØ9.9 Cyst of oral region, unspecified

★ **(See Plate 28 of the Anatomy Illustrations.)**

● K11 Diseases of salivary glands
Use additional code to identify:
alcohol abuse and dependence (F1Ø.-)
exposure to environmental tobacco smoke (Z77.22)
exposure to tobacco smoke in the perinatal period (P96.81)
history of tobacco dependence (Z87.891)
occupational exposure to environmental tobacco smoke (Z57.31)
tobacco dependence (F17.-)
tobacco use (Z72.Ø)

K11.Ø Atrophy of salivary gland

K11.1 Hypertrophy of salivary gland

Item 11–4 Atrophy is wasting away of a tissue or organ, whereas **hypertrophy** is overdevelopment or enlargement of a tissue or organ. **Sialoadenitis** is salivary gland inflammation. **Parotitis** is the inflammation of the parotid gland. In the epidemic form, parotitis is also known as mumps. **Sialolithiasis** is the formation of calculus within a salivary gland. **Mucocele** is a polyp composed of mucus.

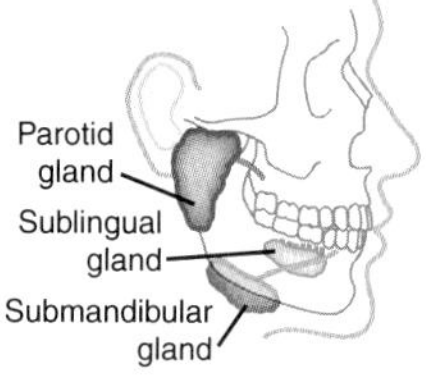

Figure 11-3 Major salivary glands.

● **K11.2 Sialoadenitis**
Parotitis
Excludes1 epidemic parotitis (B26.-)
mumps (B26.-)
uveoparotid fever [Heerfordt] (D86.89)

K11.20 Sialoadenitis, unspecified

K11.21 Acute sialoadenitis
Excludes1 acute recurrent sialoadenitis (K11.22)

K11.22 Acute recurrent sialoadenitis

K11.23 Chronic sialoadenitis

K11.3 Abscess of salivary gland

K11.4 Fistula of salivary gland
Excludes1 congenital fistula of salivary gland (Q38.4)

K11.5 Sialolithiasis
Calculus of salivary gland or duct
Stone of salivary gland or duct

K11.6 Mucocele of salivary gland
Mucous extravasation cyst of salivary gland
Mucous retention cyst of salivary gland
Ranula

K11.7 Disturbances of salivary secretion
Hypoptyalism
Ptyalism
Xerostomia
Excludes2 dry mouth NOS (R68.2)

K11.8 Other diseases of salivary glands
Benign lymphoepithelial lesion of salivary gland
Mikulicz' disease
Necrotizing sialometaplasia
Sialectasia
Stenosis of salivary duct
Stricture of salivary duct
Excludes1 sicca syndrome [Sjögren] (M35.Ø-)

K11.9 Disease of salivary gland, unspecified
Sialoadenopathy NOS

● **K12 Stomatitis and related lesions**
Use additional code to identify:
alcohol abuse and dependence (F1Ø.-)
exposure to environmental tobacco smoke (Z77.22)
exposure to tobacco smoke in the perinatal period (P96.81)
history of tobacco dependence (Z87.891)
occupational exposure to environmental tobacco smoke (Z57.31)
tobacco dependence (F17.-)
tobacco use (Z72.Ø)
Excludes1 cancrum oris (A69.Ø)
cheilitis (K13.Ø)
gangrenous stomatitis (A69.Ø)
herpesviral [herpes simplex] gingivostomatitis (BØØ.2)
noma (A69.Ø)

K12.Ø Recurrent oral aphthae
Aphthous stomatitis (major) (minor)
Bednar's aphthae
Periadenitis mucosa necrotica recurrens
Recurrent aphthous ulcer
Stomatitis herpetiformis

K12.1 Other forms of stomatitis
Stomatitis NOS
Denture stomatitis
Ulcerative stomatitis
Vesicular stomatitis
Excludes1 acute necrotizing ulcerative stomatitis (A69.1)
Vincent's stomatitis (A69.1)

Item 11-5 Stomatitis is the inflammation of the oral mucosa. **Mucositis** is the inflammation of the mucous membranes lining the digestive tract from the mouth to the anus. It is a common side effect of chemotherapy and of radiotherapy that involves any part of the digestive tract.

K12.2 Cellulitis and abscess of mouth
Cellulitis of mouth (floor)
Submandibular abscess
Excludes2 abscess of salivary gland (K11.3)
abscess of tongue (K14.Ø)
periapical abscess (KØ4.6-KØ4.7)
periodontal abscess (KØ5.21)
peritonsillar abscess (J36)

● **K12.3 Oral mucositis (ulcerative)**
Mucositis (oral) (oropharyneal)
Excludes2 gastrointestinal mucositis (ulcerative) (K92.81)
mucositis (ulcerative) of vagina and vulva (N76.81)
nasal mucositis (ulcerative) (J34.81)

K12.3Ø Oral mucositis (ulcerative), unspecified

K12.31 Oral mucositis (ulcerative) due to antineoplastic therapy
Use additional code for adverse effect, if applicable, to identify antineoplastic and immunosuppressive drugs (T45.1X5)
Use additional code for other antineoplastic therapy, such as:
radiological procedure and radiotherapy (Y84.2)

K12.32 Oral mucositis (ulcerative) due to other drugs
Use additional code for adverse effect, if applicable, to identify drug (T36-T5Ø with fifth or sixth character 5)

K12.33 Oral mucositis (ulcerative) due to radiation
Use additional external cause code (W88-W9Ø, X39.Ø-) to identify cause

K12.39 Other oral mucositis (ulcerative)
Viral oral mucositis (ulcerative)

● **K13 Other diseases of lip and oral mucosa**
Includes epithelial disturbances of tongue
Use additional code to identify:
alcohol abuse and dependence (F1Ø.-)
exposure to environmental tobacco smoke (Z77.22)
exposure to tobacco smoke in the perinatal period (P96.81)
history of tobacco dependence (Z87.891)
occupational exposure to environmental tobacco smoke (Z57.31)
tobacco dependence (F17.-)
tobacco use (Z72.Ø)
Excludes2 certain disorders of gingiva and edentulous alveolar ridge (KØ5-KØ6)
cysts of oral region (KØ9.-)
diseases of tongue (K14.-)
stomatitis and related lesions (K12.-)

K13.Ø Diseases of lips
Abscess of lips
Angular cheilitis
Cellulitis of lips
Cheilitis NOS
Cheilodynia
Cheilosis
Exfoliative cheilitis
Fistula of lips
Glandular cheilitis
Hypertrophy of lips
Perlèche NEC
Excludes1 ariboflavinosis (E53.Ø)
cheilitis due to radiation-related disorders (L55-L59)
congenital fistula of lips (Q38.Ø)
congenital hypertrophy of lips (Q18.6)
Perlèche due to candidiasis (B37.83)
Perlèche due to riboflavin deficiency (E53.Ø)

K13.1 Cheek and lip biting

CHAPTER 11 (KØØ-K95)

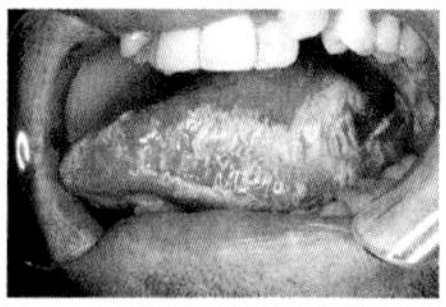

Figure 11-4 Oral leukoplakia and associated. (From Swartz MH: Textbook of Physical Diagnosis: History and Examination, Philadelphia, PA, Saunders/Elsevier, 2010)

● **K13.2 Leukoplakia and other disturbances of oral epithelium, including tongue**
Excludes1 carcinoma in situ of oral epithelium (DØØ.Ø-)
hairy leukoplakia (K13.3)

K13.21 Leukoplakia of oral mucosa, including tongue
Considered precancerous and evidenced by thickened white patches of epithelium on mucous membranes
Leukokeratosis of oral mucosa
Leukoplakia of gingiva, lips, tongue
Excludes1 hairy leukoplakia (K13.3)
leukokeratosis nicotina palati (K13.24)

K13.22 Minimal keratinized residual ridge mucosa
Minimal keratinization of alveolar ridge mucosa

K13.23 Excessive keratinized residual ridge mucosa
Excessive keratinization of alveolar ridge mucosa

K13.24 Leukokeratosis nicotina palati
Smoker's palate

K13.29 Other disturbances of oral epithelium, including tongue
Erythroplakia of mouth or tongue
Focal epithelial hyperplasia of mouth or tongue
Leukoedema of mouth or tongue
Other oral epithelium disturbances

K13.3 Hairy leukoplakia

K13.4 Granuloma and granuloma-like lesions of oral mucosa
Eosinophilic granuloma
Granuloma pyogenicum
Verrucous xanthoma

K13.5 Oral submucous fibrosis
Submucous fibrosis of tongue

K13.6 Irritative hyperplasia of oral mucosa
Excludes2 irritative hyperplasia of edentulous ridge [denture hyperplasia] (KØ6.2)

● **K13.7 Other and unspecified lesions of oral mucosa**

K13.7Ø Unspecified lesions of oral mucosa

K13.79 Other lesions of oral mucosa
Focal oral mucinosis

★**(See Plate 26 of the Anatomy Illustrations.)**

● **K14 Diseases of tongue**
Use additional code to identify:
alcohol abuse and dependence (F1Ø.-)
exposure to environmental tobacco smoke (Z77.22)
history of tobacco dependence (Z87.891)
occupational exposure to environmental tobacco smoke (Z57.31)
tobacco dependence (F17.-)
tobacco use (Z72.Ø)
Excludes2 erythroplakia (K13.29)
focal epithelial hyperplasia (K13.29)
leukedema of tongue (K13.29)
leukoplakia of tongue (K13.21)
hairy leukoplakia (K13.3)
macroglossia (congenital) (Q38.2)
submucous fibrosis of tongue (K13.5)

K14.Ø Glossitis
Abscess of tongue
Ulceration (traumatic) of tongue
Excludes1 atrophic glossitis (K14.4)

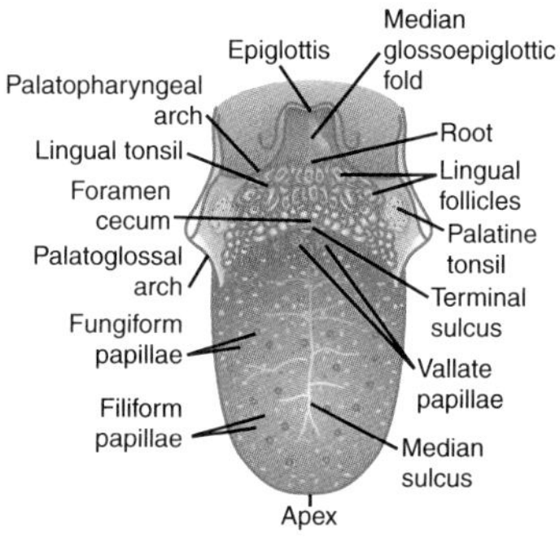

Figure 11-5 Structure of the tongue.

K14.1 Geographic tongue
Benign migratory glossitis
Glossitis areata exfoliativa

K14.2 Median rhomboid glossitis

K14.3 Hypertrophy of tongue papillae
Black hairy tongue
Coated tongue
Hypertrophy of foliate papillae
Lingua villosa nigra

K14.4 Atrophy of tongue papillae
Atrophic glossitis

K14.5 Plicated tongue
Fissured tongue
Furrowed tongue
Scrotal tongue
Excludes1 fissured tongue, congenital (Q38.3)

K14.6 Glossodynia
Glossopyrosis
Painful tongue

K14.8 Other diseases of tongue
Atrophy of tongue
Crenated tongue
Enlargement of tongue
Glossocele
Glossoptosis
Hypertrophy of tongue

K14.9 Disease of tongue, unspecified
Glossopathy NOS

DISEASES OF ESOPHAGUS, STOMACH AND DUODENUM (K2Ø-K31)

Excludes2 hiatus hernia (K44.-)

● **K2Ø Esophagitis**
Use additional code to identify:
alcohol abuse and dependence (F1Ø.-)
Excludes1 erosion of esophagus (K22.1-)
esophagitis with gastro-esophageal reflux disease (K21.Ø)
reflux esophagitis (K21.Ø)
ulcerative esophagitis (K22.1-)
Excludes2 eosinophilic gastritis or gastroenteritis (K52.81)

K2Ø.Ø Eosinophilic esophagitis

K2Ø.8 Other esophagitis
Abscess of esophagus

K2Ø.9 Esophagitis, unspecified
Esophagitis NOS

● **K21 Gastro-esophageal reflux disease**
Excludes1 newborn esophageal reflux (P78.83)

K21.Ø Gastro-esophageal reflux disease with esophagitis
Reflux esophagitis

K21.9 Gastro-esophageal reflux disease without esophagitis
Esophageal reflux NOS
Coding Clinic: 2Ø16, Q1, P18

Item 11-6 **Esophageal reflux** is the return flow of the contents of the stomach to the esophagus and is referred to as GERD and/or "heartburn." **Gastroesophageal reflux** is the return flow of the contents of the stomach and duodenum to the esophagus. **Esophageal leukoplakia** are white areas on the mucous membrane of the esophagus for which no specific cause can be identified.

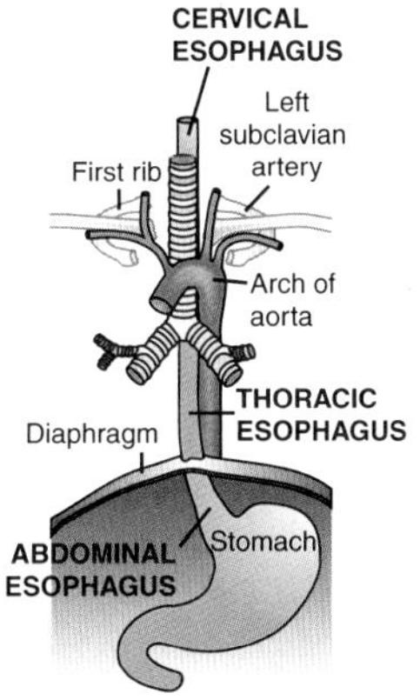

Figure 11-6 The esophagus is the muscular tube that connects the pharynx and the stomach. The 1Ø-inch (25 cm) long esophagus is divided into three parts: **cervical, thoracic,** and **abdominal.**

K22 Other diseases of esophagus
Excludes2 esophageal varices (I85.-)

K22.Ø **Achalasia of cardia**
Achalasia NOS
Cardiospasm
Excludes1 congenital cardiospasm (Q39.5)

K22.1 **Ulcer of esophagus**
Barrett's ulcer
Erosion of esophagus
Fungal ulcer of esophagus
Peptic ulcer of esophagus
Ulcer of esophagus due to ingestion of chemicals
Ulcer of esophagus due to ingestion of drugs and medicaments
Ulcerative esophagitis
Code first poisoning due to drug or toxin, if applicable (T36-T65 with fifth or sixth character 1-4 or 6)
Use additional code for adverse effect, if applicable, to identify drug (T36-T5Ø with fifth or sixth character 5)
Excludes1 Barrett's esophagus (K22.87-)

K22.1Ø **Ulcer of esophagus without bleeding**
Ulcer of esophagus NOS

K22.11 **Ulcer of esophagus with bleeding**
Excludes2 bleeding esophageal varices (I85.Ø1, I85.11)

K22.2 **Esophageal obstruction**
Compression of esophagus
Constriction of esophagus
Stenosis of esophagus
Stricture of esophagus
Excludes1 congenital stenosis or stricture of esophagus (Q39.3)

K22.3 **Perforation of esophagus**
Rupture of esophagus
Excludes1 traumatic perforation of (thoracic) esophagus (S27.8-)

K22.4 **Dyskinesia of esophagus**
Difficulty in moving
Corkscrew esophagus
Diffuse esophageal spasm
Spasm of esophagus
Excludes1 cardiospasm (K22.Ø)

K22.5 **Diverticulum of esophagus, acquired**
Esophageal pouch, acquired
Excludes1 diverticulum of esophagus (congenital) (Q39.6)

K22.6 **Gastro-esophageal laceration-hemorrhage syndrome**
Mallory-Weiss syndrome

Item 11-7 **Achalasia** is a condition in which the smooth muscle fibers of the esophagus do not relax. Most frequently, this condition occurs at the esophagogastric sphincter. **Cardiospasm,** also known as **megaesophagus,** is achalasia of the thoracic esophagus.

K22.7 **Barrett's esophagus**
Barrett's disease
Barrett's syndrome
Excludes1 Barrett's ulcer (K22.1)
malignant neoplasm of esophagus (C15.-)

K22.7Ø **Barrett's esophagus without dysplasia**
Barrett's esophagus NOS

K22.71 **Barrett's esophagus with dysplasia**

K22.71Ø **Barrett's esophagus with low grade dysplasia**

K22.711 **Barrett's esophagus with high grade dysplasia**

K22.719 **Barrett's esophagus with dysplasia, unspecified**

K22.8 **Other specified diseases of esophagus**
Hemorrhage of esophagus NOS
Excludes2 esophageal varices (I85.-)
Paterson-Kelly syndrome (D5Ø.1)

K22.9 **Disease of esophagus, unspecified**

K23 Disorders of esophagus in diseases classified elsewhere
Code first underlying disease, such as:
congenital syphilis (A5Ø.5)
Excludes1 late syphilis (A52.79)
megaesophagus due to Chagas' disease (B57.31)
tuberculosis (A18.83)

K25 Gastric ulcer
Includes erosion (acute) of stomach
pylorus ulcer (peptic)
stomach ulcer (peptic)
Use additional code to identify:
alcohol abuse and dependence (F1Ø.-)
Excludes1 acute gastritis (K29.Ø-)
peptic ulcer NOS (K27.-)

K25.Ø **Acute gastric ulcer with hemorrhage**

K25.1 **Acute gastric ulcer with perforation**

K25.2 **Acute gastric ulcer with both hemorrhage and perforation**

K25.3 **Acute gastric ulcer without hemorrhage or perforation**

K25.4 **Chronic or unspecified gastric ulcer with hemorrhage**
Coding Clinic: 2017, Q3, P27

K25.5 **Chronic or unspecified gastric ulcer with perforation**

K25.6 **Chronic or unspecified gastric ulcer with both hemorrhage and perforation**

K25.7 **Chronic gastric ulcer without hemorrhage or perforation**

K25.9 **Gastric ulcer, unspecified as acute or chronic, without hemorrhage or perforation**

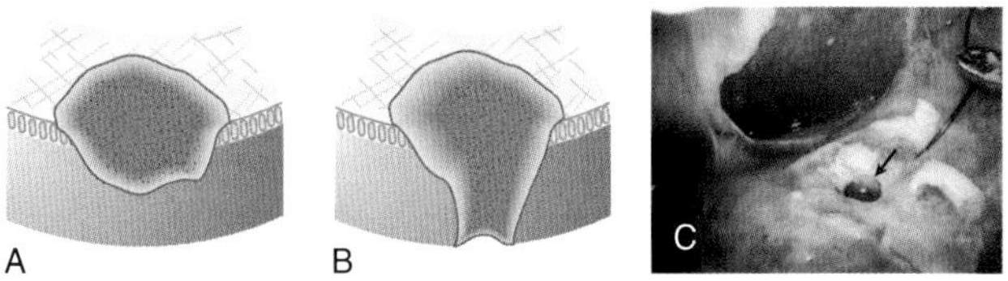

Figure 11-7 **A.** Ulcer. **B.** Perforated ulcer. **C.** Laparoscopic view of a perforated duodenal ulcer *(arrow)* with fibrinous exudate on the adjacent peritoneum. (**C** from Feldman: Sleisenger & Fordtran's Gastrointestinal and Liver Disease, ed 8, Saunders, An Imprint of Elsevier, 2006)

Item 11-8 **Gastric ulcers** are lesions of the stomach that result in the death of the tissue and a defect of the surface. **Perforated ulcers** are those in which the lesion penetrates the gastric wall, leaving a hole. **Peptic ulcers** are lesions of the stomach or the duodenum. **Peptic** refers to the gastric juice, pepsin.

K26 Duodenal ulcer

Includes erosion (acute) of duodenum
duodenum ulcer (peptic)
postpyloric ulcer (peptic)

Use additional code to identify:
alcohol abuse and dependence (F10.-)

Excludes1 peptic ulcer NOS (K27.-)

K26.0 Acute duodenal ulcer with hemorrhage
K26.1 Acute duodenal ulcer with perforation
K26.2 Acute duodenal ulcer with both hemorrhage and perforation
K26.3 Acute duodenal ulcer without hemorrhage or perforation
K26.4 Chronic or unspecified duodenal ulcer with hemorrhage
Coding Clinic: 2016, Q1, P14
K26.5 Chronic or unspecified duodenal ulcer with perforation
K26.6 Chronic or unspecified duodenal ulcer with both hemorrhage and perforation
K26.7 Chronic duodenal ulcer without hemorrhage or perforation
K26.9 Duodenal ulcer, unspecified as acute or chronic, without hemorrhage or perforation

K27 Peptic ulcer, site unspecified

Includes gastroduodenal ulcer NOS
peptic ulcer NOS

Use additional code to identify:
alcohol abuse and dependence (F10.-)

Excludes1 peptic ulcer of newborn (P78.82)

K27.0 Acute peptic ulcer, site unspecified, with hemorrhage
K27.1 Acute peptic ulcer, site unspecified, with perforation
K27.2 Acute peptic ulcer, site unspecified, with both hemorrhage and perforation
K27.3 Acute peptic ulcer, site unspecified, without hemorrhage or perforation
K27.4 Chronic or unspecified peptic ulcer, site unspecified, with hemorrhage
K27.5 Chronic or unspecified peptic ulcer, site unspecified, with perforation
K27.6 Chronic or unspecified peptic ulcer, site unspecified, with both hemorrhage and perforation
K27.7 Chronic peptic ulcer, site unspecified, without hemorrhage or perforation
K27.9 Peptic ulcer, site unspecified, unspecified as acute or chronic, without hemorrhage or perforation

K28 Gastrojejunal ulcer

Includes anastomotic ulcer (peptic) or erosion
gastrocolic ulcer (peptic) or erosion
gastrointestinal ulcer (peptic) or erosion
gastrojejunal ulcer (peptic) or erosion
jejunal ulcer (peptic) or erosion
marginal ulcer (peptic) or erosion
stomal ulcer (peptic) or erosion

Use additional code to identify:
alcohol abuse and dependence (F10.-)

Excludes1 primary ulcer of small intestine (K63.3)

K28.0 Acute gastrojejunal ulcer with hemorrhage
K28.1 Acute gastrojejunal ulcer with perforation
K28.2 Acute gastrojejunal ulcer with both hemorrhage and perforation
K28.3 Acute gastrojejunal ulcer without hemorrhage or perforation
K28.4 Chronic or unspecified gastrojejunal ulcer with hemorrhage
K28.5 Chronic or unspecified gastrojejunal ulcer with perforation
K28.6 Chronic or unspecified gastrojejunal ulcer with both hemorrhage and perforation
K28.7 Chronic gastrojejunal ulcer without hemorrhage or perforation
K28.9 Gastrojejunal ulcer, unspecified as acute or chronic, without hemorrhage or perforation

K29 Gastritis and duodenitis

Excludes1 eosinophilic gastritis or gastroenteritis (K52.81)
Zollinger-Ellison syndrome (E16.4)

K29.0 Acute gastritis
Use additional code to identify:
alcohol abuse and dependence (F10.-)
Excludes1 erosion (acute) of stomach (K25.-)
K29.00 Acute gastritis without bleeding
K29.01 Acute gastritis with bleeding

K29.2 Alcoholic gastritis
Use additional code to identify:
alcohol abuse and dependence (F10.-)
K29.20 Alcoholic gastritis without bleeding
K29.21 Alcoholic gastritis with bleeding

K29.3 Chronic superficial gastritis
K29.30 Chronic superficial gastritis without bleeding
K29.31 Chronic superficial gastritis with bleeding

K29.4 Chronic atrophic gastritis
Gastric atrophy
K29.40 Chronic atrophic gastritis without bleeding
K29.41 Chronic atrophic gastritis with bleeding

K29.5 Unspecified chronic gastritis
Chronic antral gastritis
Chronic fundal gastritis
K29.50 Unspecified chronic gastritis without bleeding
K29.51 Unspecified chronic gastritis with bleeding

K29.6 Other gastritis
Giant hypertrophic gastritis
Granulomatous gastritis
Ménétrier's disease
K29.60 Other gastritis without bleeding
K29.61 Other gastritis with bleeding

K29.7 Gastritis, unspecified
K29.70 Gastritis, unspecified, without bleeding
K29.71 Gastritis, unspecified, with bleeding

K29.8 Duodenitis
K29.80 Duodenitis without bleeding
K29.81 Duodenitis with bleeding

K29.9 Gastroduodenitis, unspecified
K29.90 Gastroduodenitis, unspecified, without bleeding
K29.91 Gastroduodenitis, unspecified, with bleeding

K30 Functional dyspepsia
Indigestion

Excludes1 dyspepsia NOS (R10.13)
heartburn (R12)
nervous dyspepsia (F45.8)
neurotic dyspepsia (F45.8)
psychogenic dyspepsia (F45.8)

Item 11-9 Gastritis is a severe inflammation of the stomach. **Atrophic gastritis** is a chronic inflammation of the stomach that results in destruction of the cells of the mucosa of the stomach. Duodenitis is an inflammation of the duodenum, the first section of the small intestine.

CHAPTER 11 (K00-K95)

Item 11-10 Achlorhydria, also known as gastric anacidity, is the absence of gastric acid.

● K31 **Other diseases of stomach and duodenum**
Includes functional disorders of stomach
Excludes2 diabetic gastroparesis (E08.43, E09.43, E10.43, E11.43, E13.43)
diverticulum of duodenum (K57.00-K57.13)

K31.0 **Acute dilatation of stomach**
Acute distention of stomach

K31.1 **Adult hypertrophic pyloric stenosis** A
Pyloric stenosis NOS
Excludes1 congenital or infantile pyloric stenosis (Q40.0)

K31.2 **Hourglass stricture and stenosis of stomach**
Excludes1 congenital hourglass stomach (Q40.2)
hourglass contraction of stomach (K31.89)

K31.3 **Pylorospasm, not elsewhere classified**
Excludes1 congenital or infantile pylorospasm (Q40.0)
neurotic pylorospasm (F45.8)
psychogenic pylorospasm (F45.8)

K31.4 **Gastric diverticulum**
Excludes1 congenital diverticulum of stomach (Q40.2)

K31.5 **Obstruction of duodenum**
Constriction of duodenum
Duodenal ileus (chronic)
Stenosis of duodenum
Narrowing
Stricture of duodenum
Narrowing
Volvulus of duodenum
Twisting/knotting
Excludes1 congenital stenosis of duodenum (Q41.0)

K31.6 **Fistula of stomach and duodenum**
Gastrocolic fistula
Gastrojejunocolic fistula

K31.7 **Polyp of stomach and duodenum**
Excludes1 adenomatous polyp of stomach (D13.1)

● K31.8 **Other specified diseases of stomach and duodenum**

● K31.81 **Angiodysplasia of stomach and duodenum**

K31.811 **Angiodysplasia of stomach and duodenum with bleeding**

K31.819 **Angiodysplasia of stomach and duodenum without bleeding**
Angiodysplasia of stomach and duodenum NOS

K31.82 **Dieulafoy lesion (hemorrhagic) of stomach and duodenum**
Excludes2 Dieulafoy lesion of intestine (K63.81)

K31.83 **Achlorhydria**

K31.84 **Gastroparesis**
Gastroparalysis
Code first underlying disease, if known, such as:
anorexia nervosa (F50.0-)
diabetes mellitus (E08.43, E09.43, E10.43, E11.43, E13.43)
scleroderma (M34.-)

K31.89 **Other diseases of stomach and duodenum**
Coding Clinic: 2017, Q1, P28

K31.9 **Disease of stomach and duodenum, unspecified**

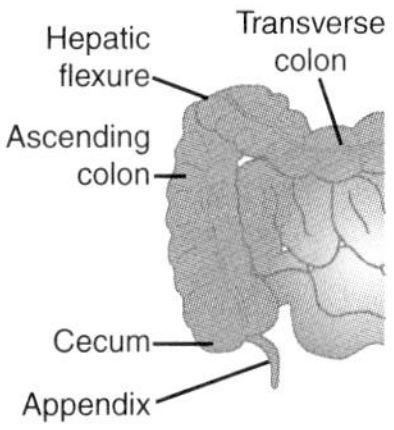

Figure 11-8 Acute appendicitis is the inflammation of the appendix, usually associated with obstruction. Most often this is a disease of adolescents and young adults.

DISEASES OF APPENDIX (K35-K38)

● K35 **Acute appendicitis**

● K35.2 **Acute appendicitis with generalized peritonitis**
Appendicitis (acute) with generalized (diffuse) peritonitis following rupture or perforation of appendix

K35.20 **Acute appendicitis with generalized peritonitis, without abscess (Acute) appendicitis with generalized peritonitis NOS**
Coding Clinic: 2018, Q4, P18

K35.21 **Acute appendicitis with generalized peritonitis, with abscess**

● K35.3 **Acute appendicitis with localized peritonitis**

K35.30 **Acute appendicitis with localized peritonitis, without perforation or gangrene**
Acute appendicitis with localized peritonitis NOS

K35.31 **Acute appendicitis with localized peritonitis and gangrene, without perforation**

K35.32 **Acute appendicitis with perforation and localized peritonitis, without abscess**
(Acute) appendicitis with perforation NOS
Perforated appendix NOS
Ruptured appendix (with localized peritonitis) NOS
Coding Clinic: 2018, Q4, P18

K35.33 **Acute appendicitis with perforation and localized peritonitis, with abscess**
(Acute) appendicitis with (peritoneal) abscess NOS
Ruptured appendix with localized peritonitis and abscess

● K35.8 **Other and unspecified acute appendicitis**

K35.80 **Unspecified acute appendicitis**
Acute appendicitis NOS
Acute appendicitis without (localized) (generalized) peritonitis

● K35.89 **Other acute appendicitis**

K35.890 **Other acute appendicitis without perforation or gangrene**

K35.891 **Other acute appendicitis without perforation, with gangrene**
(Acute) appendicitis with gangrene NOS

K36 **Other appendicitis**
Chronic appendicitis
Recurrent appendicitis

K37 **Unspecified appendicitis**
Excludes1 -unspecified appendicitis with peritonitis (K35.2-, K35.3)

● K38 **Other diseases of appendix**

K38.0 **Hyperplasia of appendix**

K38.1 **Appendicular concretions**
Fecalith of appendix
Stercolith of appendix

K38.2 **Diverticulum of appendix**

K38.3 **Fistula of appendix**

K38.8 **Other specified diseases of appendix**
Intussusception of appendix

K38.9 **Disease of appendix, unspecified**

Item 11–11 **Hernias** of the groin are the most common type, accounting for 80 percent of all hernias. There are two major types of inguinal hernias: indirect (oblique) affecting men only and direct. **Indirect inguinal hernias** result when the intestines emerge through the abdominal wall in an indirect fashion through the inguinal canal. **Direct inguinal hernias** penetrate through the abdominal wall in a direct fashion. **Femoral hernias** occur at the femoral ring where the femoral vessels enter the thigh and is most common in women. An abdominal wall hernia is also called a ventral or epigastric hernia and occurs in both sexes. Classification is based on location of the hernia and whether there is obstruction or gangrene.

Ventral, epigastric, or incisional hernia occurs on the abdominal surface caused by musculature weakness or a tear at a previous surgical site and is evidenced by a bulge that changes in size, becoming larger with exertion. An **incarcerated** hernia is one in which the intestines become trapped in the hernia. A **strangulated** hernia is one in which the blood supply to the intestines is lost. **Hiatal hernia** occurs when a loop of the stomach protrudes upward through the small opening in the diaphragm through which the esophagus passes, leaving the abdominal cavity and entering the chest. It occurs in both sexes.

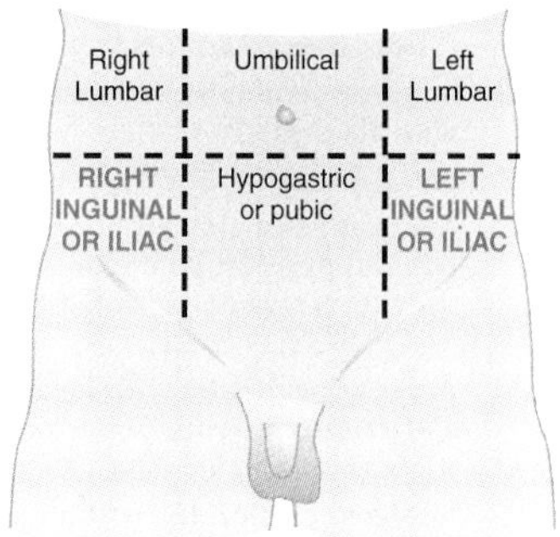

Figure 11-9 Inguinal hernias are those that are located in the inguinal or iliac areas of the abdomen.

HERNIA (K40-K46)

Note: Hernia with both gangrene and obstruction is classified to hernia with gangrene.

Includes acquired hernia
congenital [except diaphragmatic or hiatus] hernia
recurrent hernia

K40 Inguinal hernia

Includes bubonocele
direct inguinal hernia
double inguinal hernia
indirect inguinal hernia
inguinal hernia NOS
oblique inguinal hernia
scrotal hernia

K40.0 Bilateral inguinal hernia, with obstruction, without gangrene
Inguinal hernia (bilateral) causing obstruction without gangrene
Incarcerated inguinal hernia (bilateral) without gangrene
Irreducible inguinal hernia (bilateral) without gangrene
Strangulated inguinal hernia (bilateral) without gangrene

K40.00 Bilateral inguinal hernia, with obstruction, without gangrene, not specified as recurrent
Bilateral inguinal hernia, with obstruction, without gangrene NOS

K40.01 Bilateral inguinal hernia, with obstruction, without gangrene, recurrent

K40.1 Bilateral inguinal hernia, with gangrene

K40.10 Bilateral inguinal hernia, with gangrene, not specified as recurrent
Bilateral inguinal hernia, with gangrene NOS

K40.11 Bilateral inguinal hernia, with gangrene, recurrent

K40.2 Bilateral inguinal hernia, without obstruction or gangrene

K40.20 Bilateral inguinal hernia, without obstruction or gangrene, not specified as recurrent
Bilateral inguinal hernia NOS

K40.21 Bilateral inguinal hernia, without obstruction or gangrene, recurrent

K40.3 Unilateral inguinal hernia, with obstruction, without gangrene
Inguinal hernia (unilateral) causing obstruction without gangrene
Incarcerated inguinal hernia (unilateral) without gangrene
Irreducible inguinal hernia (unilateral) without gangrene
Strangulated inguinal hernia (unilateral) without gangrene

K40.30 Unilateral inguinal hernia, with obstruction, without gangrene, not specified as recurrent
Inguinal hernia, with obstruction NOS
Unilateral inguinal hernia, with obstruction, without gangrene NOS

K40.31 Unilateral inguinal hernia, with obstruction, without gangrene, recurrent

K40.4 Unilateral inguinal hernia, with gangrene

K40.40 Unilateral inguinal hernia, with gangrene, not specified as recurrent
Inguinal hernia with gangrene NOS
Unilateral inguinal hernia with gangrene NOS

K40.41 Unilateral inguinal hernia, with gangrene, recurrent

K40.9 Unilateral inguinal hernia, without obstruction or gangrene

K40.90 Unilateral inguinal hernia, without obstruction or gangrene, not specified as recurrent
Inguinal hernia NOS
Unilateral inguinal hernia NOS

K40.91 Unilateral inguinal hernia, without obstruction or gangrene, recurrent

K41 Femoral hernia

K41.0 Bilateral femoral hernia, with obstruction, without gangrene
Femoral hernia (bilateral) causing obstruction, without gangrene
Incarcerated femoral hernia (bilateral), without gangrene
Irreducible femoral hernia (bilateral), without gangrene
Strangulated femoral hernia (bilateral), without gangrene

K41.00 Bilateral femoral hernia, with obstruction, without gangrene, not specified as recurrent
Bilateral femoral hernia, with obstruction, without gangrene NOS

K41.01 Bilateral femoral hernia, with obstruction, without gangrene, recurrent

K41.1 Bilateral femoral hernia, with gangrene

K41.10 Bilateral femoral hernia, with gangrene, not specified as recurrent
Bilateral femoral hernia, with gangrene NOS

K41.11 Bilateral femoral hernia, with gangrene, recurrent

● K41.2 **Bilateral femoral hernia, without obstruction or gangrene**
  K41.20 **Bilateral femoral hernia, without obstruction or gangrene, not specified as recurrent**
    Bilateral femoral hernia NOS
  K41.21 **Bilateral femoral hernia, without obstruction or gangrene, recurrent**
● K41.3 **Unilateral femoral hernia, with obstruction, without gangrene**
  Femoral hernia (unilateral) causing obstruction, without gangrene
  Incarcerated femoral hernia (unilateral), without gangrene
  Irreducible femoral hernia (unilateral), without gangrene
  Strangulated femoral hernia (unilateral), without gangrene
  K41.30 **Unilateral femoral hernia, with obstruction, without gangrene, not specified as recurrent**
    Femoral hernia, with obstruction NOS
    Unilateral femoral hernia, with obstruction NOS
  K41.31 **Unilateral femoral hernia, with obstruction, without gangrene, recurrent**
● K41.4 **Unilateral femoral hernia, with gangrene**
  K41.40 **Unilateral femoral hernia, with gangrene, not specified as recurrent**
    Femoral hernia, with gangrene NOS
    Unilateral femoral hernia, with gangrene NOS
  K41.41 **Unilateral femoral hernia, with gangrene, recurrent**
● K41.9 **Unilateral femoral hernia, without obstruction or gangrene**
  K41.90 **Unilateral femoral hernia, without obstruction or gangrene, not specified as recurrent**
    Femoral hernia NOS
    Unilateral femoral hernia NOS
  K41.91 **Unilateral femoral hernia, without obstruction or gangrene, recurrent**

● K42 **Umbilical hernia**
  Includes paraumbilical hernia
  Excludes1 omphalocele (Q79.2)
K42.0 **Umbilical hernia with obstruction, without gangrene**
  Umbilical hernia causing obstruction, without gangrene
  Incarcerated umbilical hernia, without gangrene
  Irreducible umbilical hernia, without gangrene
  Strangulated umbilical hernia, without gangrene
K42.1 **Umbilical hernia with gangrene**
  Gangrenous umbilical hernia
K42.9 **Umbilical hernia without obstruction or gangrene**
  Umbilical hernia NOS

● K43 **Ventral hernia**
K43.0 **Incisional hernia with obstruction, without gangrene**
  Incisional hernia causing obstruction, without gangrene
  Incarcerated incisional hernia, without gangrene
  Irreducible incisional hernia, without gangrene
  Strangulated incisional hernia, without gangrene
K43.1 **Incisional hernia with gangrene**
  Gangrenous incisional hernia
K43.2 **Incisional hernia without obstruction or gangrene**
  Incisional hernia NOS
K43.3 **Parastomal hernia with obstruction, without gangrene**
  Incarcerated parastomal hernia, without gangrene
  Irreducible parastomal hernia, without gangrene
  Parastomal hernia causing obstruction, without gangrene
  Strangulated parastomal hernia, without gangrene
K43.4 **Parastomal hernia with gangrene**
  Gangrenous parastomal hernia
K43.5 **Parastomal hernia without obstruction or gangrene**
  Parastomal hernia NOS
K43.6 **Other and unspecified ventral hernia with obstruction, without gangrene**
  Epigastric hernia causing obstruction, without gangrene
  Hypogastric hernia causing obstruction, without gangrene
  Incarcerated epigastric hernia without gangrene
  Incarcerated hypogastric hernia without gangrene
  Incarcerated midline hernia without gangrene
  Incarcerated spigelian hernia without gangrene
  Incarcerated subxiphoid hernia without gangrene
  Irreducible epigastric hernia without gangrene
  Irreducible hypogastric hernia without gangrene
  Irreducible midline hernia without gangrene
  Irreducible spigelian hernia without gangrene
  Irreducible subxiphoid hernia without gangrene
  Midline hernia causing obstruction, without gangrene
  Spigelian hernia causing obstruction, without gangrene
  Strangulated epigastric hernia without gangrene
  Strangulated hypogastric hernia without gangrene
  Strangulated midline hernia without gangrene
  Strangulated spigelian hernia without gangrene
  Strangulated subxiphoid hernia without gangrene
  Subxiphoid hernia causing obstruction, without gangrene
K43.7 **Other and unspecified ventral hernia with gangrene**
  Any condition listed under K43.6 specified as gangrenous
K43.9 **Ventral hernia without obstruction or gangrene**
  Epigastric hernia
  Ventral hernia NOS

● K44 **Diaphragmatic hernia**
  Includes hiatus hernia (esophageal) (sliding)
  paraesophageal hernia
  Excludes1 congenital diaphragmatic hernia (Q79.0)
  congenital hiatus hernia (Q40.1)
K44.0 **Diaphragmatic hernia with obstruction, without gangrene**
  Diaphragmatic hernia causing obstruction
  Incarcerated diaphragmatic hernia
  Irreducible diaphragmatic hernia
  Strangulated diaphragmatic hernia
K44.1 **Diaphragmatic hernia with gangrene**
  Gangrenous diaphragmatic hernia
K44.9 **Diaphragmatic hernia without obstruction or gangrene**
  Diaphragmatic hernia NOS
  Coding Clinic: 2017, Q1, P7

● K45 **Other abdominal hernia**
  Includes abdominal hernia, specified site NEC
  lumbar hernia
  obturator hernia
  pudendal hernia
  retroperitoneal hernia
  sciatic hernia
K45.0 **Other specified abdominal hernia with obstruction, without gangrene**
  Other specified abdominal hernia causing obstruction
  Other specified incarcerated abdominal hernia
  Other specified irreducible abdominal hernia
  Other specified strangulated abdominal hernia
K45.1 **Other specified abdominal hernia with gangrene**
  Any condition listed under K45 specified as gangrenous
K45.8 **Other specified abdominal hernia without obstruction or gangrene**

K46 Unspecified abdominal hernia

Includes enterocele
epiplocele
hernia NOS
interstitial hernia
intestinal hernia
intra-abdominal hernia

Excludes1 vaginal enterocele (N81.5)

K46.Ø Unspecified abdominal hernia with obstruction, without gangrene
Unspecified abdominal hernia causing obstruction
Unspecified incarcerated abdominal hernia
Unspecified irreducible abdominal hernia
Unspecified strangulated abdominal hernia

K46.1 Unspecified abdominal hernia with gangrene
Any condition listed under K46 specified as gangrenous

K46.9 Unspecified abdominal hernia without obstruction or gangrene
Abdominal hernia NOS

★ **(See Plate 32 of the Anatomy Illustrations.)**

NONINFECTIVE ENTERITIS AND COLITIS (K5Ø-K52)

Includes noninfective inflammatory bowel disease

Excludes1 irritable bowel syndrome (K58.-)
megacolon (K59.3-)

K5Ø Crohn's disease [regional enteritis]

Includes granulomatous enteritis

Use additional code to identify manifestations, such as:
pyoderma gangrenosum (L88)

Excludes1 ulcerative colitis (K51.-)

K5Ø.Ø Crohn's disease of small intestine
Crohn's disease [regional enteritis] of duodenum
Crohn's disease [regional enteritis] of ileum
Crohn's disease [regional enteritis] of jejunum
Regional ileitis
Terminal ileitis

Excludes1 Crohn's disease of both small and large intestine (K5Ø.8-)

K5Ø.ØØ Crohn's disease of small intestine without complications

K5Ø.Ø1 Crohn's disease of small intestine with complications

K5Ø.Ø11 Crohn's disease of small intestine with rectal bleeding

K5Ø.Ø12 Crohn's disease of small intestine with intestinal obstruction

K5Ø.Ø13 Crohn's disease of small intestine with fistula

K5Ø.Ø14 Crohn's disease of small intestine with abscess
Coding Clinic: 2Ø12, Q4, P1Ø4

K5Ø.Ø18 Crohn's disease of small intestine with other complication

K5Ø.Ø19 Crohn's disease of small intestine with unspecified complications

Item 11-12 Crohn's disease, also known as **regional enteritis,** is a chronic inflammatory disease of the intestines. Classification is based on location in the small (duodenum, ileum, jejunum) or large (cecum, colon, rectum, anal canal) intestine.

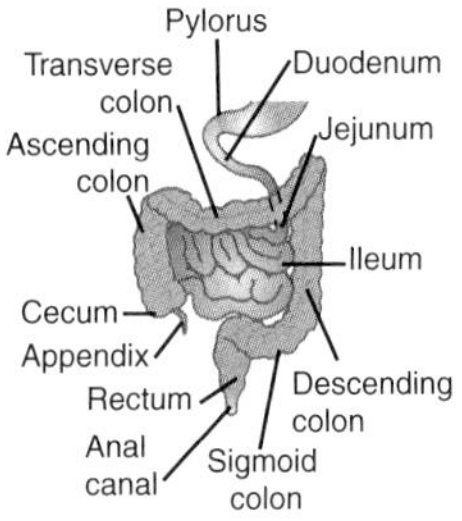

Figure 11-10 Small and large intestines.

K5Ø.1 Crohn's disease of large intestine
Crohn's disease [regional enteritis] of colon
Crohn's disease [regional enteritis] of large bowel
Crohn's disease [regional enteritis] of rectum
Granulomatous colitis
Regional colitis

Excludes1 Crohn's disease of both small and large intestine (K5Ø.8)

K5Ø.1Ø Crohn's disease of large intestine without complications

K5Ø.11 Crohn's disease of large intestine with complications

K5Ø.111 Crohn's disease of large intestine with rectal bleeding

K5Ø.112 Crohn's disease of large intestine with intestinal obstruction

K5Ø.113 Crohn's disease of large intestine with fistula

K5Ø.114 Crohn's disease of large intestine with abscess
Coding Clinic: 2Ø12, Q4, P1Ø4

K5Ø.118 Crohn's disease of large intestine with other complication

K5Ø.119 Crohn's disease of large intestine with unspecified complications

K5Ø.8 Crohn's disease of both small and large intestine

K5Ø.8Ø Crohn's disease of both small and large intestine without complications

K5Ø.81 Crohn's disease of both small and large intestine with complications

K5Ø.811 Crohn's disease of both small and large intestine with rectal bleeding

K5Ø.812 Crohn's disease of both small and large intestine with intestinal obstruction

K5Ø.813 Crohn's disease of both small and large intestine with fistula

K5Ø.814 Crohn's disease of both small and large intestine with abscess
Coding Clinic: 2Ø12, Q4, P1Ø4

K5Ø.818 Crohn's disease of both small and large intestine with other complication

K5Ø.819 Crohn's disease of both small and large intestine with unspecified complications

K5Ø.9 Crohn's disease, unspecified

K5Ø.9Ø Crohn's disease, unspecified, without complications
Crohn's disease NOS
Regional enteritis NOS

K5Ø.91 Crohn's disease, unspecified, with complications

K5Ø.911 Crohn's disease, unspecified, with rectal bleeding

K5Ø.912 Crohn's disease, unspecified, with intestinal obstruction

K5Ø.913 Crohn's disease, unspecified, with fistula

K5Ø.914 Crohn's disease, unspecified, with abscess
Coding Clinic: 2Ø12, Q4, P1Ø4

K5Ø.918 Crohn's disease, unspecified, with other complication

K5Ø.919 Crohn's disease, unspecified, with unspecified complications

Item 11–13 Ulcerative colitis attacks the colonic mucosa and forms abscesses. The disease involves the intestines. Classification is based on the location:
- Enterocolitis: large and small intestine
- Ileocolitis: ileum and colon
- Proctitis: rectum
- Proctosigmoiditis: sigmoid colon and rectum

● **K51 Ulcerative colitis**

Use additional code to identify manifestations, such as: pyoderma gangrenosum (L88)

Excludes1 Crohn's disease [regional enteritis] (K50.-)

● **K51.0 Ulcerative (chronic) pancolitis**
Backwash ileitis

K51.00 Ulcerative (chronic) pancolitis without complications 🐾
Ulcerative (chronic) pancolitis NOS

● **K51.01 Ulcerative (chronic) pancolitis with complications**

K51.011 Ulcerative (chronic) pancolitis with rectal bleeding 🐾

K51.012 Ulcerative (chronic) pancolitis with intestinal obstruction 🐾

K51.013 Ulcerative (chronic) pancolitis with fistula 🐾

K51.014 Ulcerative (chronic) pancolitis with abscess 🐾

K51.018 Ulcerative (chronic) pancolitis with other complication 🐾

K51.019 Ulcerative (chronic) pancolitis with unspecified complications 🐾

● **K51.2 Ulcerative (chronic) proctitis**

K51.20 Ulcerative (chronic) proctitis without complications 🐾
Ulcerative (chronic) proctitis NOS

● **K51.21 Ulcerative (chronic) proctitis with complications**

K51.211 Ulcerative (chronic) proctitis with rectal bleeding 🐾

K51.212 Ulcerative (chronic) proctitis with intestinal obstruction 🐾

K51.213 Ulcerative (chronic) proctitis with fistula 🐾

K51.214 Ulcerative (chronic) proctitis with abscess 🐾

K51.218 Ulcerative (chronic) proctitis with other complication 🐾

K51.219 Ulcerative (chronic) proctitis with unspecified complications 🐾

● **K51.3 Ulcerative (chronic) rectosigmoiditis**

K51.30 Ulcerative (chronic) rectosigmoiditis without complications 🐾
Ulcerative (chronic) rectosigmoiditis NOS

● **K51.31 Ulcerative (chronic) rectosigmoiditis with complications**

K51.311 Ulcerative (chronic) rectosigmoiditis with rectal bleeding 🐾

K51.312 Ulcerative (chronic) rectosigmoiditis with intestinal obstruction 🐾

K51.313 Ulcerative (chronic) rectosigmoiditis with fistula 🐾

K51.314 Ulcerative (chronic) rectosigmoiditis with abscess 🐾

K51.318 Ulcerative (chronic) rectosigmoiditis with other complication 🐾

K51.319 Ulcerative (chronic) rectosigmoiditis with unspecified complications 🐾

● **K51.4 Inflammatory polyps of colon**

Excludes1 adenomatous polyp of colon (D12.6)
polyposis of colon (D12.6)
polyps of colon NOS (K63.5)

K51.40 Inflammatory polyps of colon without complications 🐾
Inflammatory polyps of colon NOS

● **K51.41 Inflammatory polyps of colon with complications**

K51.411 Inflammatory polyps of colon with rectal bleeding 🐾

K51.412 Inflammatory polyps of colon with intestinal obstruction 🐾

K51.413 Inflammatory polyps of colon with fistula 🐾

K51.414 Inflammatory polyps of colon with abscess 🐾

K51.418 Inflammatory polyps of colon with other complication 🐾

K51.419 Inflammatory polyps of colon with unspecified complications 🐾

● **K51.5 Left sided colitis**
Left hemicolitis

K51.50 Left sided colitis without complications 🐾
Left sided colitis NOS

● **K51.51 Left sided colitis with complications**

K51.511 Left sided colitis with rectal bleeding 🐾

K51.512 Left sided colitis with intestinal obstruction 🐾

K51.513 Left sided colitis with fistula 🐾

K51.514 Left sided colitis with abscess 🐾

K51.518 Left sided colitis with other complication 🐾

K51.519 Left sided colitis with unspecified complications 🐾

● **K51.8 Other ulcerative colitis**

K51.80 Other ulcerative colitis without complications 🐾

● **K51.81 Other ulcerative colitis with complications**

K51.811 Other ulcerative colitis with rectal bleeding 🐾

K51.812 Other ulcerative colitis with intestinal obstruction 🐾

K51.813 Other ulcerative colitis with fistula 🐾

K51.814 Other ulcerative colitis with abscess 🐾

K51.818 Other ulcerative colitis with other complication 🐾

K51.819 Other ulcerative colitis with unspecified complications 🐾

● **K51.9 Ulcerative colitis, unspecified**

K51.90 Ulcerative colitis, unspecified, without complications 🐾

● **K51.91 Ulcerative colitis, unspecified, with complications**

K51.911 Ulcerative colitis, unspecified with rectal bleeding 🐾

K51.912 Ulcerative colitis, unspecified with intestinal obstruction 🐾

K51.913 Ulcerative colitis, unspecified with fistula 🐾

K51.914 Ulcerative colitis, unspecified with abscess 🐾

K51.918 Ulcerative colitis, unspecified with other complication 🐾

K51.919 Ulcerative colitis, unspecified with unspecified complications 🐾

CHAPTER 11 (K00-K95)

● **K52**   **Other and unspecified noninfective gastroenteritis and colitis**

    K52.0   **Gastroenteritis and colitis due to radiation**

    K52.1   **Toxic gastroenteritis and colitis**

          Drug-induced gastroenteritis and colitis

          Code first (T51-T65) to identify toxic agent

          Use additional code for adverse effect, if applicable, to identify drug (T36-T50 with fifth or sixth character 5)

          Coding Clinic: 2019, Q1, P17

●   **K52.2**   **Allergic and dietetic gastroenteritis and colitis**

          Food hypersensitivity gastroenteritis or colitis

          Use additional code to identify type of food allergy (Z91.01-, Z91.02-)

          Excludes2   allergic eosinophilic colitis (K52.82)
                           allergic eosinophilic esophagitis (K20.0)
                           allergic eosinophilic gastritis (K52.81)
                           allergic eosinophilic gastroenteritis (K52.81)
                           food protein-induced proctocolitis (K52.82)

          Coding Clinic: 2016, Q4, P30-31

       K52.21   **Food protein-induced enterocolitis syndrome**

             FPIES

             Use additional code for hypovolemic shock, if present (R57.1)

       K52.22   **Food protein-induced enteropathy**

       K52.29   **Other allergic and dietetic gastroenteritis and colitis**

             Food hypersensitivity gastroenteritis or colitis

             Immediate gastrointestinal hypersensitivity

    K52.3   **Indeterminate colitis**

          Colonic inflammatory bowel disease unclassified (IBDU)

          Excludes1   unspecified colitis (K52.9)

●   **K52.8**   **Other specified noninfective gastroenteritis and colitis**

       K52.81   **Eosinophilic gastritis or gastroenteritis**

             Eosinophilic enteritis

             Excludes2   eosinophilic esophagitis (K20.0)

       K52.82   **Eosinophilic colitis**

             Allergic proctocolitis

             Food-induced eosinophilic proctocolitis

             Food protein-induced proctocolitis

             Milk protein-induced proctocolitis

●   **K52.83**   **Microscopic colitis**

             Coding Clinic: 2016, Q4, P30-31

          K52.831   **Collagenous colitis**

          K52.832   **Lymphocytic colitis**

          K52.838   **Other microscopic colitis**

          K52.839   **Microscopic colitis, unspecified**

       K52.89   **Other specified noninfective gastroenteritis and colitis**

             Coding Clinic: 2019, Q1, P21

    K52.9   **Noninfective gastroenteritis and colitis, unspecified**

          Colitis NOS   Ileitis NOS

          Enteritis NOS   Jejunitis NOS

          Gastroenteritis NOS   Sigmoiditis NOS

          Excludes1   diarrhea NOS (R19.7)
                          functional diarrhea (K59.1)
                          infectious gastroenteritis and colitis NOS (A09)
                          neonatal diarrhea (noninfective) (P78.3)
                          psychogenic diarrhea (F45.8)

OTHER DISEASES OF INTESTINES (K55-K64)

● **K55**   **Vascular disorders of intestine**

    Excludes1   necrotizing enterocolitis of newborn (P77.-)

●   **K55.0**   **Acute vascular disorders of intestine**

          Infarction of appendices epiploicae

          Mesenteric (artery) (vein) embolism

          Mesenteric (artery) (vein) infarction

          Mesenteric (artery) (vein) thrombosis

●   **K55.01**   **Acute (reversible) ischemia of small intestine**

             Coding Clinic: 2016, Q4, P32

          K55.011   **Focal (segmental) acute (reversible) ischemia of small intestine** 🍗

          K55.012   **Diffuse acute (reversible) ischemia of small intestine** 🍗

          K55.019   **Acute (reversible) ischemia of small intestine, extent unspecified** 🍗

●   **K55.02**   **Acute infarction of small intestine**

          Gangrene of small intestine

          Necrosis of small intestine

          Coding Clinic: 2016, Q4, P32

          K55.021   **Focal (segmental) acute infarction of small intestine** 🍗

          K55.022   **Diffuse acute infarction of small intestine** 🍗

          K55.029   **Acute infarction of small intestine, extent unspecified** 🍗

●   **K55.03**   **Acute (reversible) ischemia of large intestine**

          Acute fulminant ischemic colitis

          Subacute ischemic colitis

          Coding Clinic: 2016, Q4, P32

          K55.031   **Focal (segmental) acute (reversible) ischemia of large intestine** 🍗

          K55.032   **Diffuse acute (reversible) ischemia of large intestine** 🍗

          K55.039   **Acute (reversible) ischemia of large intestine, extent unspecified** 🍗

●   **K55.04**   **Acute infarction of large intestine**

          Gangrene of large intestine

          Necrosis of large intestine

          Coding Clinic: 2016, Q4, P32

          K55.041   **Focal (segmental) acute infarction of large intestine** 🍗

          K55.042   **Diffuse acute infarction of large intestine** 🍗

          K55.049   **Acute infarction of large intestine, extent unspecified** 🍗

●   **K55.05**   **Acute (reversible) ischemia of intestine, part unspecified**

          K55.051   **Focal (segmental) acute (reversible) ischemia of intestine, part unspecified** 🍗

          K55.052   **Diffuse acute (reversible) ischemia of intestine, part unspecified** 🍗

          K55.059   **Acute (reversible) ischemia of intestine, part and extent unspecified** 🍗

▶ New   ⬛ Revised   ~~deleted~~ Deleted   Excludes 1   Excludes 2   Includes   Use additional   Code first   Code also   Key words

OGCR Official Guidelines   X Assign placeholder X   ● Use Additional Character(s)   ▶ Manifestation Code   🍗 Hierarchical Condition Category   Coding Clinic

● **K55.06** **Acute infarction of intestine, part unspecified**
Acute intestinal infarction
Gangrene of intestine
Necrosis of intestine

 K55.061 **Focal (segmental) acute infarction of intestine, part unspecified** 🔖

 K55.062 **Diffuse acute infarction of intestine, part unspecified** 🔖

 K55.069 **Acute infarction of intestine, part and extent unspecified** 🔖

K55.1 **Chronic vascular disorders of intestine** 🔖
Chronic ischemic colitis
Chronic ischemic enteritis
Chronic ischemic enterocolitis
Ischemic stricture of intestine
Mesenteric atherosclerosis
Mesenteric vascular insufficiency

● **K55.2** **Angiodysplasia of colon**

 K55.20 **Angiodysplasia of colon without hemorrhage**

 K55.21 **Angiodysplasia of colon with hemorrhage**

● **K55.3** **Necrotizing enterocolitis**

 Excludes1 necrotizing enterocolitis of newborn (P77.-)

 Excludes2 necrotizing enterocolitis due to Clostridium difficile (A04.7-)

 K55.30 **Necrotizing enterocolitis, unspecified** 🔖
Necrotizing enterocolitis, NOS

 K55.31 **Stage 1 necrotizing enterocolitis** 🔖
Necrotizing enterocolitis without pneumatosis, without perforation
Coding Clinic: 2016, Q4, P32

 K55.32 **Stage 2 necrotizing enterocolitis** 🔖
Necrotizing enterocolitis with pneumatosis, without perforation
Coding Clinic: 2016, Q4, P32

 K55.33 **Stage 3 necrotizing enterocolitis** 🔖
Necrotizing enterocolitis with perforation
Necrotizing enterocolitis with pneumatosis and perforation
Coding Clinic: 2016, Q4, P32

K55.8 **Other vascular disorders of intestine** 🔖

K55.9 **Vascular disorder of intestine, unspecified** 🔖
Ischemic colitis
Ischemic enteritis
Ischemic enterocolitis

● **K56** **Paralytic ileus and intestinal obstruction without hernia**

 Excludes1 congenital stricture or stenosis of intestine (Q41-Q42)
cystic fibrosis with meconium ileus (E84.11)
ischemic stricture of intestine (K55.1)
meconium ileus NOS (P76.0)
neonatal intestinal obstructions classifiable to P76.-
obstruction of duodenum (K31.5)
postprocedural intestinal obstruction (K91.3-)
stenosis of anus or rectum (K62.4)

K56.0 **Paralytic ileus** 🔖
Paralysis of bowel
Paralysis of colon
Paralysis of intestine

 Excludes1 gallstone ileus (K56.3)
ileus NOS (K56.7)
obstructive ileus NOS (K56.69-)

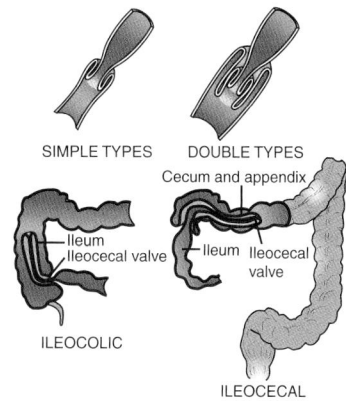

SIMPLE TYPES DOUBLE TYPES

Cecum and appendix

Ileum — Ileocecal valve Ileum — Ileocecal valve

ILEOCOLIC ILEOCECAL

Figure 11-11 Types of intussusception.

Item 11–14 Intussusception is the prolapse (telescoping) of a part of the intestine into another adjacent part of the intestine. Intussusception may be enteric (ileoileal, jejunoileal, jejunojejunal), colic (colocolic), or intracolic (ileocecal, ileocolic).

Item 11–15 Volvulus is the twisting of a segment of the intestine, resulting in obstruction. Paralytic ileus is paralysis of the intestine. It need not be a complete paralysis, but it must prohibit the passage of food through the intestine and lead to intestinal blockage. It is a common aftermath of some types of surgery.

K56.1 **Intussusception** 🔖
Intussusception or invagination of bowel
Intussusception or invagination of colon
Intussusception or invagination of intestine
Intussusception or invagination of rectum

 Excludes2 intussusception of appendix (K38.8)

K56.2 **Volvulus** 🔖
Strangulation of colon or intestine
Torsion of colon or intestine
Twist of colon or intestine

 Excludes2 volvulus of duodenum (K31.5)

K56.3 **Gallstone ileus** 🔖
Obstruction of intestine by gallstone

● **K56.4** **Other impaction of intestine**

 K56.41 **Fecal impaction** 🔖

  Excludes1 constipation (K59.0-)
incomplete defecation (R15.0)

 K56.49 **Other impaction of intestine** 🔖

● **K56.5** **Intestinal adhesions [bands] with obstruction (postinfection)**
Abdominal hernia due to adhesions with obstruction
Peritoneal adhesions [bands] with intestinal obstruction (postinfection)

 K56.50 **Intestinal adhesions [bands], unspecified as to partial versus complete obstruction** 🔖
Intestinal adhesions with obstruction NOS

 K56.51 **Intestinal adhesions [bands], with partial obstruction** 🔖
Intestinal adhesions with incomplete obstruction

 K56.52 **Intestinal adhesions [bands] with complete obstruction** 🔖

CHAPTER 11 (K00-K95)

●K56.6   **Other and unspecified intestinal obstruction**
   ●K56.60   **Unspecified intestinal obstruction**
       Excludes1   intestinal obstruction due to specified condition-code to condition
       Coding Clinic: 2017, Q2, P12

      K56.600   **Partial intestinal obstruction, unspecified as to cause** 🅱
         Incomplete intestinal obstruction, NOS

      K56.601   **Complete intestinal obstruction, unspecified as to cause** 🅱

      K56.609   **Unspecified intestinal obstruction, unspecified as to partial versus complete obstruction** 🅱
         Intestinal obstruction NOS

   ●K56.69   **Other intestinal obstruction**
       Enterostenosis NOS
       Obstructive ileus NOS
       Occlusion of colon or intestine NOS
       Stenosis of colon or intestine NOS
       Stricture of colon or intestine NOS
       Excludes1   intestinal obstruction due to specified condition-code to condition
       Coding Clinic: 2017, Q2, P12

      K56.690   **Other partial intestinal obstruction** 🅱
         Other incomplete intestinal obstruction

      K56.691   **Other complete intestinal obstruction** 🅱

      K56.699   **Other intestinal obstruction unspecified as to partial versus complete obstruction** 🅱
         Other intestinal obstruction, NEC

    K56.7   **Ileus, unspecified** 🅱
       Excludes1   obstructive ileus (K56.69-)
       Excludes2   intestinal obstruction with hernia (K40-K46)
       Coding Clinic: 2017, Q1, P41

●K57   **Diverticular disease of intestine**
      Code also if applicable peritonitis K65.-
      Excludes1   congenital diverticulum of intestine (Q43.8)
           Meckel's diverticulum (Q43.0)
      Excludes2   diverticulum of appendix (K38.2)

●K57.0   **Diverticulitis of small intestine with perforation and abscess**
      Diverticulitis of small intestine with peritonitis
      Excludes1   diverticulitis of both small and large intestine with perforation and abscess (K57.4-)

    K57.00   **Diverticulitis of small intestine with perforation and abscess without bleeding**

    K57.01   **Diverticulitis of small intestine with perforation and abscess with bleeding**

●K57.1   **Diverticular disease of small intestine without perforation or abscess**
      Excludes1   diverticular disease of both small and large intestine without perforation or abscess (K57.5-)

    K57.10   **Diverticulosis of small intestine without perforation or abscess without bleeding**
       Diverticular disease of small intestine NOS

    K57.11   **Diverticulosis of small intestine without perforation or abscess with bleeding**

    K57.12   **Diverticulitis of small intestine without perforation or abscess without bleeding**

    K57.13   **Diverticulitis of small intestine without perforation or abscess with bleeding**

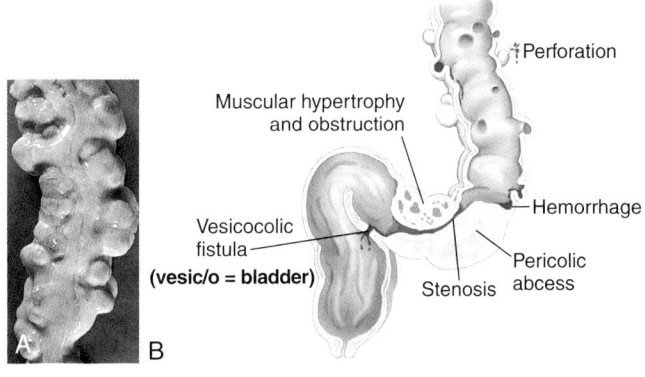

Figure 11-12   Diverticulosis. (From Shiland: Mastering Healthcare Terminology, ed 4, St. Louis, Mosby, 2012)

Item 11–16 Diverticula of the intestines are acquired herniations of the mucosa. Diverticulum (singular): Pocket or pouch that bulges outward through a weak spot (herniation) in the colon. Diverticula (plural). **Diverticulosis** is the condition of having diverticula. **Diverticulitis** is inflammation of these pouches or herniations. Classification is based on location (small intestine or colon) and whether it occurs with or without hemorrhage.

●K57.2   **Diverticulitis of large intestine with perforation and abscess**
      Diverticulitis of colon with peritonitis
      Excludes1   diverticulitis of both small and large intestine with perforation and abscess (K57.4-)

    K57.20   **Diverticulitis of large intestine with perforation and abscess without bleeding**

    K57.21   **Diverticulitis of large intestine with perforation and abscess with bleeding**

●K57.3   **Diverticular disease of large intestine without perforation or abscess**
      Excludes1   diverticular disease of both small and large intestine without perforation or abscess (K57.5-)

    K57.30   **Diverticulosis of large intestine without perforation or abscess without bleeding**
       Diverticular disease of colon NOS

    K57.31   **Diverticulosis of large intestine without perforation or abscess with bleeding**

    K57.32   **Diverticulitis of large intestine without perforation or abscess without bleeding**

    K57.33   **Diverticulitis of large intestine without perforation or abscess with bleeding**

●K57.4   **Diverticulitis of both small and large intestine with perforation and abscess**
      Diverticulitis of both small and large intestine with peritonitis

    K57.40   **Diverticulitis of both small and large intestine with perforation and abscess without bleeding**

    K57.41   **Diverticulitis of both small and large intestine with perforation and abscess with bleeding**

●K57.5   **Diverticular disease of both small and large intestine without perforation or abscess**

    K57.50   **Diverticulosis of both small and large intestine without perforation or abscess without bleeding**
       Diverticular disease of both small and large intestine NOS

    K57.51   **Diverticulosis of both small and large intestine without perforation or abscess with bleeding**

    K57.52   **Diverticulitis of both small and large intestine without perforation or abscess without bleeding**

    K57.53   **Diverticulitis of both small and large intestine without perforation or abscess with bleeding**

▶ New   ▶ Revised   ~~deleted~~ Deleted   Excludes 1   Excludes 2   Includes   Use additional   Code first   Code also   Key words

OGCR Official Guidelines   X Assign placeholder X   ● Use Additional Character(s)   ▶ Manifestation Code   🅱 Hierarchical Condition Category   **Coding Clinic**

● **K57.8 Diverticulitis of intestine, part unspecified, with perforation and abscess**
     Diverticulitis of intestine NOS with peritonitis

     K57.80 Diverticulitis of intestine, part unspecified, with perforation and abscess without bleeding

     K57.81 Diverticulitis of intestine, part unspecified, with perforation and abscess with bleeding

● **K57.9 Diverticular disease of intestine, part unspecified, without perforation or abscess**

     K57.90 Diverticulosis of intestine, part unspecified, without perforation or abscess without bleeding
         Diverticular disease of intestine NOS

     K57.91 Diverticulosis of intestine, part unspecified, without perforation or abscess with bleeding

     K57.92 Diverticulitis of intestine, part unspecified, without perforation or abscess without bleeding

     K57.93 Diverticulitis of intestine, part unspecified, without perforation or abscess with bleeding

● **K58 Irritable bowel syndrome**

     Includes   irritable colon
                   spastic colon

     K58.0 Irritable bowel syndrome with diarrhea

     K58.1 Irritable bowel syndrome with constipation
         Coding Clinic: 2016, Q4, P32

     K58.2 Mixed irritable bowel syndrome
         Coding Clinic: 2016, Q4, P32

     K58.8 Other irritable bowel syndrome
         Coding Clinic: 2016, Q4, P32

     K58.9 Irritable bowel syndrome without diarrhea
         Irritable bowel syndrome NOS

● **K59 Other functional intestinal disorders**

     Excludes1   change in bowel habit NOS (R19.4)
                 intestinal malabsorption (K90.-)
                 psychogenic intestinal disorders (F45.8)

     Excludes2   functional disorders of stomach (K31.-)

● **K59.0 Constipation**

         ~~Use additional code for adverse effect, if applicable, to identify drug (T36-T50 with fifth or sixth character 5)~~

     Excludes1   fecal impaction (K56.41)
                 incomplete defecation (R15.0)

     K59.00 Constipation, unspecified

     K59.01 Slow transit constipation

     K59.02 Outlet dysfunction constipation

     K59.03 Drug induced constipation
         Use additional code for adverse effect, if applicable, to identify drug (T36-T50 with fifth or sixth character 5)
         Coding Clinic: 2016, Q4, P33

     K59.04 Chronic idiopathic constipation
         Functional constipation
         Coding Clinic: 2016, Q4, P33

     K59.09 Other constipation
         Chronic constipation

     K59.1 Functional diarrhea

     Excludes1   diarrhea NOS (R19.7)
                 irritable bowel syndrome with diarrhea (K58.0)

     K59.2 Neurogenic bowel, not elsewhere classified

Item 11–17   A **fissure** is a groove in the surface, whereas a **fistula** is an abnormal passage. An **abscess** is an accumulation of pus in a tissue cavity resulting from a bacterial or parasitic infection.

● **K59.3 Megacolon, not elsewhere classified**
     Dilatation of colon
     Code first, if applicable (T51-T65) to identify toxic agent

     Excludes1   congenital megacolon (aganglionic) (Q43.1)
                 megacolon (due to) (in) Chagas' disease (B57.32)
                 megacolon (due to) (in) Clostridium difficile (A04.7-)
                 megacolon (due to) (in) Hirschsprung's disease (Q43.1)
     Coding Clinic: 2016, Q4, P33

     K59.31 Toxic megacolon 🔁

     K59.39 Other megacolon
         Megacolon NOS

     K59.4 Anal spasm
         Proctalgia fugax

     K59.8 Other specified functional intestinal disorders
         Atony of colon Pseudo-obstruction (acute) (chronic) of intestine

     K59.9 Functional intestinal disorder, unspecified

● **K60 Fissure and fistula of anal and rectal regions**

     Excludes1   fissure and fistula of anal and rectal regions with abscess or cellulitis (K61.-)

     Excludes2   anal sphincter tear (healed) (nontraumatic) (old) (K62.81)

     K60.0 Acute anal fissure

     K60.1 Chronic anal fissure

     K60.2 Anal fissure, unspecified

     K60.3 Anal fistula

     K60.4 Rectal fistula
         Fistula of rectum to skin

         Excludes1   rectovaginal fistula (N82.3)
                     vesicorectal fistula (N32.1)

     K60.5 Anorectal fistula

● **K61 Abscess of anal and rectal regions**

     Includes   abscess of anal and rectal regions
                 cellulitis of anal and rectal regions

     K61.0 Anal abscess
         Perianal abscess

         Excludes2   intrasphincteric abscess (K61.4)

     K61.1 Rectal abscess
         Perirectal abscess

         Excludes1   ischiorectal abscess (K61.39)
         Coding Clinic: 2012, Q4, P104

     K61.2 Anorectal abscess

     K61.3 Ischiorectal abscess

     K61.31 Horseshoe abscess

     K61.39 Other ischiorectal abscess
         Abscess of ischiorectal fossa
         Ischiorectal abscess, NOS

     K61.4 Intrasphincteric abscess
         Intersphincteric abscess

     K61.5 Supralevator abscess

● **K62 Other diseases of anus and rectum**

Includes anal canal

Excludes2 colostomy and enterostomy malfunction (K94.Ø-, K91.4-)
fecal incontinence (R15.-)
hemorrhoids (K64.-)

K62.Ø Anal polyp
Coding Clinic: 2018, Q1, P7

K62.1 Rectal polyp
Excludes1 adenomatous polyp (D12.8)
Coding Clinic: 2018, Q1, P7

K62.2 Anal prolapse
Prolapse of anal canal

K62.3 Rectal prolapse
Prolapse of rectal mucosa

K62.4 Stenosis of anus and rectum
Stricture of anus (sphincter)
Coding Clinic: 2019, Q2, P13

K62.5 Hemorrhage of anus and rectum
Excludes1 gastrointestinal bleeding NOS (K92.2)
melena (K92.1)
neonatal rectal hemorrhage (P54.2)

K62.6 Ulcer of anus and rectum
Solitary ulcer of anus and rectum
Stercoral ulcer of anus and rectum
Excludes1 fissure and fistula of anus and rectum (K6Ø.-)
ulcerative colitis (K51.-)

K62.7 Radiation proctitis
Use additional code to identify the type of radiation (W9Ø.-)
Coding Clinic: 2019, Q1, P21

● **K62.8 Other specified diseases of anus and rectum**
Excludes2 ulcerative proctitis (K51.2)

K62.81 Anal sphincter tear (healed) (nontraumatic) (old)
Tear of anus, nontraumatic
Use additional code for any associated fecal incontinence (R15.-)
Excludes2 anal fissure (K6Ø.-)
anal sphincter tear (healed) (old) complicating delivery (O34.7-)
traumatic tear of anal sphincter (S31.831)

K62.82 Dysplasia of anus
Anal intraepithelial neoplasia I and II (AIN I and II) (histologically confirmed)
Dysplasia of anus NOS
Mild and moderate dysplasia of anus (histologically confirmed)
Excludes1 abnormal results from anal cytologic examination without histologic confirmation (R85.61-)
anal intraepithelial neoplasia III (DØ1.3)
carcinoma in situ of anus (DØ1.3)
HGSIL of anus (R85.613)
severe dysplasia of anus (DØ1.3)

K62.89 Other specified diseases of anus and rectum
Proctitis NOS
Use additional code for any associated fecal incontinence (R15.-)

K62.9 Disease of anus and rectum, unspecified

● **K63 Other diseases of intestine**

K63.Ø Abscess of intestine
Excludes1 abscess of intestine with Crohn's disease (K5Ø.Ø14, K5Ø.114, K5Ø.814, K5Ø.914)
abscess of intestine with diverticular disease (K57.Ø, K57.2, K57.4, K57.8)
abscess of intestine with ulcerative colitis (K51.Ø14, K51.214, K51.314, K51.414, K51.514, K51.814, K51.914)
Excludes2 abscess of anal and rectal regions (K61.-)
abscess of appendix (K35.3-)

K63.1 Perforation of intestine (nontraumatic) HCC
Perforation (nontraumatic) of rectum
Excludes1 perforation (nontraumatic) of duodenum (K26.-)
perforation (nontraumatic) of intestine with diverticular disease (K57.Ø, K57.2, K57.4, K57.8)
Excludes2 perforation (nontraumatic) of appendix (K35.2-, K35.3)

K63.2 Fistula of intestine
Excludes1 fistula of duodenum (K31.6)
fistula of intestine with Crohn's disease (K5Ø.Ø13, K5Ø.113, K5Ø.813, K5Ø.913)
fistula of intestine with ulcerative colitis (K51.Ø13, K51.213, K51.313, K51.413, K51.513, K51.813, K51.913)
Excludes2 fistula of anal and rectal regions (K6Ø.-)
fistula of appendix (K38.3)
intestinal-genital fistula, female (N82.2-N82.4)
vesicointestinal fistula (N32.1)
Coding Clinic: 2017, Q3, P4

K63.3 Ulcer of intestine
Primary ulcer of small intestine
Excludes1 duodenal ulcer (K26.-)
gastrointestinal ulcer (K28.-)
gastrojejunal ulcer (K28.-)
jejunal ulcer (K28.-)
peptic ulcer, site unspecified (K27.-)
ulcer of intestine with perforation (K63.1)
ulcer of anus or rectum (K62.6)
ulcerative colitis (K51.-)

K63.4 Enteroptosis

K63.5 Polyp of colon
Excludes1 adenomatous polyp of colon (D12.-)
inflammatory polyp of colon (K51.4-)
polyposis of colon (D12.6)
Coding Clinic: 2019, Q1, P33; 2017, Q1, P15-16; 2015, Q2, P14

● **K63.8 Other specified diseases of intestine**

K63.81 Dieulafoy lesion of intestine
Excludes2 Dieulafoy lesion of stomach and duodenum (K31.82)

K63.89 Other specified diseases of intestine
Coding Clinic: 2013, Q2, P31

K63.9 Disease of intestine, unspecified

● **K64 Hemorrhoids and perianal venous thrombosis**

Includes piles

Excludes1 hemorrhoids complicating childbirth and the puerperium (O87.2)
hemorrhoids complicating pregnancy (O22.4)

K64.Ø First degree hemorrhoids
Grade/stage I hemorrhoids
Hemorrhoids (bleeding) without prolapse outside of anal canal

K64.1 Second degree hemorrhoids
Grade/stage II hemorrhoids
Hemorrhoids (bleeding) that prolapse with straining, but retract spontaneously

CHAPTER 11 (KØØ-K95)

K64.2 **Third degree hemorrhoids**
Grade/stage III hemorrhoids
Hemorrhoids (bleeding) that prolapse with straining and require manual replacement back inside anal canal

K64.3 **Fourth degree hemorrhoids**
Grade/stage IV hemorrhoids
Hemorrhoids (bleeding) with prolapsed tissue that cannot be manually replaced

K64.4 **Residual hemorrhoidal skin tags**
External hemorrhoids, NOS
Skin tags of anus

K64.5 **Perianal venous thrombosis**
External hemorrhoids with thrombosis
Perianal hematoma
Thrombosed hemorrhoids NOS

K64.8 **Other hemorrhoids**
Internal hemorrhoids, without mention of degree
Prolapsed hemorrhoids, degree not specified

K64.9 **Unspecified hemorrhoids**
Hemorrhoids (bleeding) NOS
Hemorrhoids (bleeding) without mention of degree

DISEASES OF PERITONEUM AND RETROPERITONEUM (K65-K68)

● K65 Peritonitis
Use additional code (B95-B97), to identify infectious agent, if known
Code also if applicable diverticular disease of intestine (K57.-)
Excludes1 acute appendicitis with generalized peritonitis (K35.2-)
aseptic peritonitis (T81.6)
benign paroxysmal peritonitis (E85.Ø)
chemical peritonitis (T81.6)
gonococcal peritonitis (A54.85)
neonatal peritonitis (P78.Ø-P78.1)
pelvic peritonitis, female (N73.3-N73.5)
periodic familial peritonitis (E85.Ø)
peritonitis due to talc or other foreign substance (T81.6)
peritonitis in chlamydia (A74.81)
peritonitis in diphtheria (A36.89)
peritonitis in syphilis (late) (A52.74)
peritonitis in tuberculosis (A18.31)
peritonitis with or following abortion or ectopic or molar pregnancy (OØØ-OØ7, OØ8.Ø)
peritonitis with or following appendicitis (K35.-)
puerperal peritonitis (O85)
retroperitoneal infections (K68.-)

K65.Ø **Generalized (acute) peritonitis**
Pelvic peritonitis (acute), male
Subphrenic peritonitis (acute)
Suppurative peritonitis (acute)

K65.1 **Peritoneal abscess**
Abdominopelvic abscess
Abscess (of) omentum
Abscess (of) peritoneum
Mesenteric abscess
Retrocecal abscess
Subdiaphragmatic abscess
Subhepatic abscess
Subphrenic abscess
Coding Clinic: 2Ø19, Q1, P15

K65.2 **Spontaneous bacterial peritonitis**
Excludes1 bacterial peritonitis NOS (K65.9)

K65.3 **Choleperitonitis**
Peritonitis due to bile

K65.4 **Sclerosing mesenteritis**
Fat necrosis of peritoneum
(Idiopathic) sclerosing mesenteric fibrosis
Mesenteric lipodystrophy
Mesenteric panniculitis
Retractile mesenteritis

Item 11-18 Peritonitis is an inflammation of the lining (peritoneum) of the abdominal cavity and surface of the intestines.

Item 11-19 Retroperitoneal infections occur between the posterior parietal peritoneum and posterior abdominal wall where the kidneys, adrenal glands, ureters, duodenum, ascending colon, descending colon, pancreas, and the large vessels and nerves are located.

K65.8 **Other peritonitis**
Chronic proliferative peritonitis
Peritonitis due to urine

K65.9 **Peritonitis, unspecified**
Bacterial peritonitis NOS
Coding Clinic: 2Ø13, Q2, P31

● K66 Other disorders of peritoneum
Excludes2 ascites (R18.-)
peritoneal effusion (chronic) (R18.8)

K66.Ø **Peritoneal adhesions (postprocedural) (postinfection)**
Adhesions (of) abdominal (wall)
Adhesions (of) diaphragm
Adhesions (of) intestine
Adhesions (of) male pelvis
Adhesions (of) omentum
Adhesions (of) stomach
Adhesive bands
Mesenteric adhesions
Excludes1 female pelvic adhesions [bands] (N73.6)
peritoneal adhesions with intestinal obstruction (K56.5-)

K66.1 **Hemoperitoneum**
Excludes1 traumatic hemoperitoneum (S36.8-)

K66.8 **Other specified disorders of peritoneum**

K66.9 **Disorder of peritoneum, unspecified**

K67 *Disorders of peritoneum in infectious diseases classified elsewhere*
Code first underlying disease, such as:
congenital syphilis (A5Ø.Ø)
helminthiasis (B65.Ø-B83.9)
Excludes1 peritonitis in chlamydia (A74.81)
peritonitis in diphtheria (A36.89)
peritonitis in gonococcal (A54.85)
peritonitis in syphilis (late) (A52.74)
peritonitis in tuberculosis (A18.31)

● K68 Disorders of retroperitoneum

● K68.1 **Retroperitoneal abscess**

K68.11 **Postprocedural retroperitoneal abscess**
Excludes2 infection following procedure (T81.44)

K68.12 **Psoas muscle abscess**

K68.19 **Other retroperitoneal abscess**
Coding Clinic: 2Ø19, Q1, P15

K68.9 **Other disorders of retroperitoneum**

DISEASES OF LIVER (K7Ø-K77)

Excludes1 jaundice NOS (R17)
Excludes2 hemochromatosis (E83.11-)
Reye's syndrome (G93.7)
viral hepatitis (B15-B19)
Wilson's disease (E83.Ø)

● K7Ø Alcoholic liver disease
Use additional code to identify:
alcohol abuse and dependence (F1Ø.-)

K7Ø.Ø **Alcoholic fatty liver** A

● K7Ø.1 **Alcoholic hepatitis**

K7Ø.1Ø **Alcoholic hepatitis without ascites** A

K7Ø.11 **Alcoholic hepatitis with ascites** A

K7Ø.2 **Alcoholic fibrosis and sclerosis of liver** A

CHAPTER 11 (KØØ-K95)

Item 11-20 **Cirrhosis** is the progressive fibrosis of the liver resulting in loss of liver function. The main causes of cirrhosis of the liver are alcohol abuse, chronic hepatitis (inflammation of the liver), biliary disease, and excessive amounts of iron. **Alcoholic cirrhosis of the liver** is also called portal, Laënnec's, or fatty nutritional cirrhosis.

● K70.3 **Alcoholic cirrhosis of liver**
Alcoholic cirrhosis NOS
K70.30 **Alcoholic cirrhosis of liver without ascites** HCC A
K70.31 **Alcoholic cirrhosis of liver with ascites** HCC A
Coding Clinic: 2018, Q1, P5

● K70.4 **Alcoholic hepatic failure**
Acute alcoholic hepatic failure
Alcoholic hepatic failure NOS
Chronic alcoholic hepatic failure
Subacute alcoholic hepatic failure
K70.40 **Alcoholic hepatic failure without coma** HCC A
K70.41 **Alcoholic hepatic failure with coma** HCC A

K70.9 **Alcoholic liver disease, unspecified** HCC A

● K71 **Toxic liver disease**
Includes drug-induced idiosyncratic (unpredictable) liver disease
drug-induced toxic (predictable) liver disease
Code first poisoning due to drug or toxin, if applicable (T36-T65 with fifth or sixth character 1-4 or 6)
Use additional code for adverse effect, if applicable, to identify drug (T36-T50 with fifth or sixth character 5)
Excludes2 alcoholic liver disease (K70.-)
Budd-Chiari syndrome (I82.0)

K71.0 **Toxic liver disease with cholestasis**
Cholestasis with hepatocyte injury
'Pure' cholestasis

● K71.1 **Toxic liver disease with hepatic necrosis**
Hepatic failure (acute) (chronic) due to drugs
K71.10 **Toxic liver disease with hepatic necrosis, without coma**
K71.11 **Toxic liver disease with hepatic necrosis, with coma** HCC

K71.2 **Toxic liver disease with acute hepatitis**
K71.3 **Toxic liver disease with chronic persistent hepatitis**
K71.4 **Toxic liver disease with chronic lobular hepatitis**

● K71.5 **Toxic liver disease with chronic active hepatitis**
Toxic liver disease with lupoid hepatitis
K71.50 **Toxic liver disease with chronic active hepatitis without ascites**
K71.51 **Toxic liver disease with chronic active hepatitis with ascites**
Coding Clinic: 2018, Q1, P4

K71.6 **Toxic liver disease with hepatitis, not elsewhere classified**
K71.7 **Toxic liver disease with fibrosis and cirrhosis of liver**
K71.8 **Toxic liver disease with other disorders of liver**
Toxic liver disease with focal nodular hyperplasia
Toxic liver disease with hepatic granulomas
Toxic liver disease with peliosis hepatis
Toxic liver disease with veno-occlusive disease of liver
K71.9 **Toxic liver disease, unspecified**

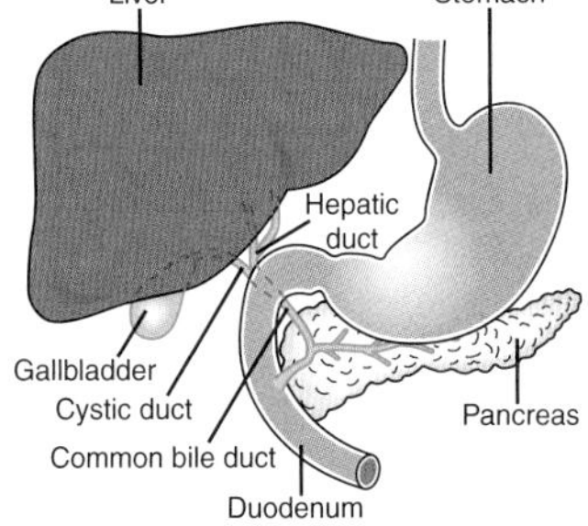

Figure 11-13 Liver and bile ducts.

● K72 **Hepatic failure, not elsewhere classified**
Includes fulminant hepatitis NEC, with hepatic failure
hepatic encephalopathy NOS
liver (cell) necrosis with hepatic failure
malignant hepatitis NEC, with hepatic failure
yellow liver atrophy or dystrophy
Excludes1 alcoholic hepatic failure (K70.4)
hepatic failure with toxic liver disease (K71.1-)
icterus of newborn (P55-P59)
postprocedural hepatic failure (K91.82)
Excludes2 hepatic failure complicating abortion or ectopic or molar pregnancy (O00-O07, O08.8)
hepatic failure complicating pregnancy, childbirth and the puerperium (O26.6-)
viral hepatitis with hepatic coma (B15-B19)

● K72.0 **Acute and subacute hepatic failure**
Acute non-viral hepatitis NOS
Coding Clinic: 2015, Q2, P17
K72.00 **Acute and subacute hepatic failure without coma**
Coding Clinic: 2015, Q2, P17
K72.01 **Acute and subacute hepatic failure with coma** HCC

● K72.1 **Chronic hepatic failure**
K72.10 **Chronic hepatic failure without coma** HCC
Coding Clinic: 2017, Q1, P41
K72.11 **Chronic hepatic failure with coma** HCC

● K72.9 **Hepatic failure, unspecified**
K72.90 **Hepatic failure, unspecified without coma** HCC
Coding Clinic: 2018, Q4, P21
K72.91 **Hepatic failure, unspecified with coma** HCC
Hepatic coma NOS
Coding Clinic: 2016, Q2, P35

● K73 **Chronic hepatitis, not elsewhere classified**
Excludes1 alcoholic hepatitis (chronic) (K70.1-)
drug-induced hepatitis (chronic) (K71.-)
granulomatous hepatitis (chronic) NEC (K75.3)
reactive, nonspecific hepatitis (chronic) (K75.2)
viral hepatitis (chronic) (B15-B19)

K73.0 **Chronic persistent hepatitis, not elsewhere classified** HCC
K73.1 **Chronic lobular hepatitis, not elsewhere classified** HCC
K73.2 **Chronic active hepatitis, not elsewhere classified** HCC
K73.8 **Other chronic hepatitis, not elsewhere classified** HCC
K73.9 **Chronic hepatitis, unspecified** HCC

● K74 **Fibrosis and cirrhosis of liver**
Code also, if applicable, viral hepatitis (acute) (chronic) (B15-B19)
Excludes1 alcoholic cirrhosis (of liver) (K70.3)
alcoholic fibrosis of liver (K70.2)
cardiac sclerosis of liver (K76.1)
cirrhosis (of liver) with toxic liver disease (K71.7)
congenital cirrhosis (of liver) (P78.81)
pigmentary cirrhosis (of liver) (E83.110)

K74.0 **Hepatic fibrosis**
K74.1 **Hepatic sclerosis**
K74.2 **Hepatic fibrosis with hepatic sclerosis**
K74.3 **Primary biliary cirrhosis** HCC
Chronic nonsuppurative destructive cholangitis
Primary biliary cholangitis
➡ **Excludes2** primary sclerosing cholangitis (K83.01)
K74.4 **Secondary biliary cirrhosis** HCC
K74.5 **Biliary cirrhosis, unspecified** HCC

K74.6 Other and unspecified cirrhosis of liver

K74.60 Unspecified cirrhosis of liver
Cirrhosis (of liver) NOS
Coding Clinic: 2018, Q1, P4

K74.69 Other cirrhosis of liver
Cryptogenic cirrhosis (of liver)
Macronodular cirrhosis (of liver)
Micronodular cirrhosis (of liver)
Mixed type cirrhosis (of liver)
Portal cirrhosis (of liver)
Postnecrotic cirrhosis (of liver)

K75 Other inflammatory liver diseases
Excludes2 toxic liver disease (K71.-)

K75.0 Abscess of liver
Cholangitic hepatic abscess
Hematogenic hepatic abscess
Hepatic abscess NOS
Lymphogenic hepatic abscess
Pylephlebitic hepatic abscess
Excludes1 amebic liver abscess (A06.4)
cholangitis without liver abscess (K83.09)
pylephlebitis without liver abscess (K75.1)
Excludes2 acute or subacute hepatitis NOS (B17.9)
acute or subacute non-viral hepatitis (K72.0)
chronic hepatitis NEC (K73.8)

K75.1 Phlebitis of portal vein
Pylephlebitis
Excludes1 pylephlebitic liver abscess (K75.0)

K75.2 Nonspecific reactive hepatitis
Excludes1 acute or subacute hepatitis (K72.0-)
chronic hepatitis NEC (K73.-)
viral hepatitis (B15-B19)

K75.3 Granulomatous hepatitis, not elsewhere classified
Excludes1 acute or subacute hepatitis (K72.0-)
chronic hepatitis NEC (K73.-)
viral hepatitis (B15-B19)

K75.4 Autoimmune hepatitis
Lupoid hepatitis NEC

K75.8 Other specified inflammatory liver diseases

K75.81 Nonalcoholic steatohepatitis (NASH)

K75.89 Other specified inflammatory liver diseases

K75.9 Inflammatory liver disease, unspecified
Hepatitis NOS
Excludes1 acute or subacute hepatitis (K72.0-)
chronic hepatitis NEC (K73.-)
viral hepatitis (B15-B19)
Coding Clinic: 2015, Q2, P17

K76 Other diseases of liver
Excludes2 alcoholic liver disease (K70.-)
amyloid degeneration of liver (E85.-)
cystic disease of liver (congenital) (Q44.6)
hepatic vein thrombosis (I82.0)
hepatomegaly NOS (R16.0)
pigmentary cirrhosis (of liver) (E83.110)
portal vein thrombosis (I81)
toxic liver disease (K71.-)

K76.0 Fatty (change of) liver, not elsewhere classified
Nonalcoholic fatty liver disease (NAFLD)
Excludes1 nonalcoholic steatohepatitis (NASH) (K75.81)

K76.1 Chronic passive congestion of liver
Cardiac cirrhosis
Cardiac sclerosis

K76.2 Central hemorrhagic necrosis of liver
Excludes1 liver necrosis with hepatic failure (K72.-)

K76.3 Infarction of liver

K76.4 Peliosis hepatis
Hepatic angiomatosis

K76.5 Hepatic veno-occlusive disease
Excludes1 Budd-Chiari syndrome (I82.0)

K76.6 Portal hypertension
Use additional code for any associated complications, such as:
portal hypertensive gastropathy (K31.89)

K76.7 Hepatorenal syndrome
Excludes1 hepatorenal syndrome following labor and delivery (O90.4)
postprocedural hepatorenal syndrome (K91.83)

K76.8 Other specified diseases of liver

K76.81 Hepatopulmonary syndrome
Code first underlying liver disease, such as:
alcoholic cirrhosis of liver (K70.3-)
cirrhosis of liver without mention of alcohol (K74.6-)

K76.89 Other specified diseases of liver
Cyst (simple) of liver
Focal nodular hyperplasia of liver
Hepatoptosis

K76.9 Liver disease, unspecified

K77 Liver disorders in diseases classified elsewhere
Code first underlying disease, such as:
amyloidosis (E85.-)
congenital syphilis (A50.0, A50.5)
congenital toxoplasmosis (P37.1)
schistosomiasis (B65.0-B65.9)
Excludes1 alcoholic hepatitis (K70.1-)
alcoholic liver disease (K70.-)
cytomegaloviral hepatitis (B25.1)
herpesviral [herpes simplex] hepatitis (B00.81)
infectious mononucleosis with liver disease (B27.0-B27.9 with .9)
mumps hepatitis (B26.81)
sarcoidosis with liver disease (D86.89)
secondary syphilis with liver disease (A51.45)
syphilis (late) with liver disease (A52.74)
toxoplasmosis (acquired) hepatitis (B58.1)
tuberculosis with liver disease (A18.83)

DISORDERS OF GALLBLADDER, BILIARY TRACT AND PANCREAS (K80–K87)

K80 Cholelithiasis
Presence or formation of gallstones
Excludes1 retained cholelithiasis following cholecystectomy (K91.86)

K80.0 Calculus of gallbladder with acute cholecystitis
Any condition listed in K80.2 with acute cholecystitis
Use additional code if applicable for associated gangrene of gallbladder (K82.A1), or perforation of gallbladder (K82.A2)
Check documentation for acute/chronic gallbladder/common bile duct either with or without obstruction.

K80.00 Calculus of gallbladder with acute cholecystitis without obstruction
Coding Clinic: 2018, Q4, P20

K80.01 Calculus of gallbladder with acute cholecystitis with obstruction

K80.1 Calculus of gallbladder with other cholecystitis
Use additional code if applicable for associated gangrene of gallbladder (K82.A1), or perforation of gallbladder (K82.A2)

K80.10 Calculus of gallbladder with chronic cholecystitis without obstruction
Cholelithiasis with cholecystitis NOS

K80.11 Calculus of gallbladder with chronic cholecystitis with obstruction

K80.12 Calculus of gallbladder with acute and chronic cholecystitis without obstruction

K80.13 Calculus of gallbladder with acute and chronic cholecystitis with obstruction

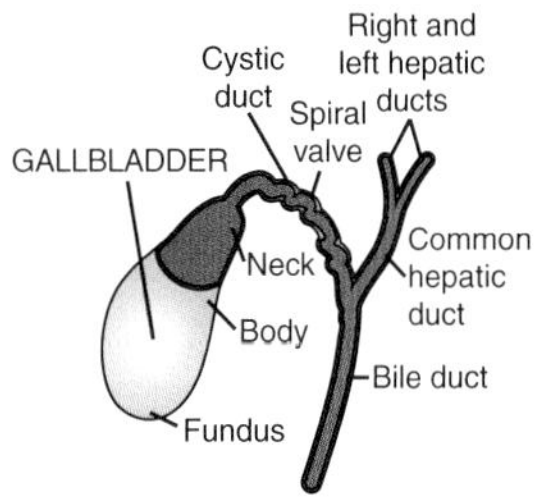

Figure 11-14 Gallbladder and bile ducts.

K80.18 **Calculus of gallbladder with other cholecystitis without obstruction**

K80.19 **Calculus of gallbladder with other cholecystitis with obstruction**

● K80.2 **Calculus of gallbladder without cholecystitis**
Cholecystolithiasis without cholecystitis
Cholelithiasis (without cholecystitis)
Colic (recurrent) of gallbladder (without cholecystitis)
Gallstone (impacted) of cystic duct (without cholecystitis)
Gallstone (impacted) of gallbladder (without cholecystitis)

K80.20 **Calculus of gallbladder without cholecystitis without obstruction**

K80.21 **Calculus of gallbladder without cholecystitis with obstruction**

● K80.3 **Calculus of bile duct with cholangitis**
Any condition listed in K80.5 with cholangitis

K80.30 **Calculus of bile duct with cholangitis, unspecified, without obstruction**

K80.31 **Calculus of bile duct with cholangitis, unspecified, with obstruction**

K80.32 **Calculus of bile duct with acute cholangitis without obstruction**

K80.33 **Calculus of bile duct with acute cholangitis with obstruction**

K80.34 **Calculus of bile duct with chronic cholangitis without obstruction**

K80.35 **Calculus of bile duct with chronic cholangitis with obstruction**

K80.36 **Calculus of bile duct with acute and chronic cholangitis without obstruction**

K80.37 **Calculus of bile duct with acute and chronic cholangitis with obstruction**

● K80.4 **Calculus of bile duct with cholecystitis**
Any condition listed in K80.5 with cholecystitis (with cholangitis)
Use additional code if applicable for associated gangrene of gallbladder (K82.A1), or perforation of gallbladder (K82.A2)

K80.40 **Calculus of bile duct with cholecystitis, unspecified, without obstruction**

K80.41 **Calculus of bile duct with cholecystitis, unspecified, with obstruction**
Coding Clinic: 2019, Q1, P18

K80.42 **Calculus of bile duct with acute cholecystitis without obstruction**

K80.43 **Calculus of bile duct with acute cholecystitis with obstruction**

K80.44 **Calculus of bile duct with chronic cholecystitis without obstruction**

K80.45 **Calculus of bile duct with chronic cholecystitis with obstruction**

K80.46 **Calculus of bile duct with acute and chronic cholecystitis without obstruction**

K80.47 **Calculus of bile duct with acute and chronic cholecystitis with obstruction**

● K80.5 **Calculus of bile duct without cholangitis or cholecystitis**
Choledocholithiasis (without cholangitis or cholecystitis)
Gallstone (impacted) of bile duct NOS (without cholangitis or cholecystitis)
Gallstone (impacted) of common duct (without cholangitis or cholecystitis)
Gallstone (impacted) of hepatic duct (without cholangitis or cholecystitis)
Hepatic cholelithiasis (without cholangitis or cholecystitis)
Hepatic colic (recurrent) (without cholangitis or cholecystitis)

K80.50 **Calculus of bile duct without cholangitis or cholecystitis without obstruction**

K80.51 **Calculus of bile duct without cholangitis or cholecystitis with obstruction**

● K80.6 **Calculus of gallbladder and bile duct with cholecystitis**
Use additional code if applicable for associated gangrene of gallbladder (K82.A1), or perforation of gallbladder (K82.A2)

K80.60 **Calculus of gallbladder and bile duct with cholecystitis, unspecified, without obstruction**

K80.61 **Calculus of gallbladder and bile duct with cholecystitis, unspecified, with obstruction**

K80.62 **Calculus of gallbladder and bile duct with acute cholecystitis without obstruction**

K80.63 **Calculus of gallbladder and bile duct with acute cholecystitis with obstruction**

K80.64 **Calculus of gallbladder and bile duct with chronic cholecystitis without obstruction**

K80.65 **Calculus of gallbladder and bile duct with chronic cholecystitis with obstruction**

K80.66 **Calculus of gallbladder and bile duct with acute and chronic cholecystitis without obstruction**

K80.67 **Calculus of gallbladder and bile duct with acute and chronic cholecystitis with obstruction**

● K80.7 **Calculus of gallbladder and bile duct without cholecystitis**

K80.70 **Calculus of gallbladder and bile duct without cholecystitis without obstruction**

K80.71 **Calculus of gallbladder and bile duct without cholecystitis with obstruction**

● K80.8 **Other cholelithiasis**

K80.80 **Other cholelithiasis without obstruction**

K80.81 **Other cholelithiasis with obstruction**

● K81 **Cholecystitis**
Chronic or acute inflammation of the gallbladder
Use additional code if applicable for associated gangrene of gallbladder (K82.A1), or perforation of gallbladder (K82.A2)
Excludes1 cholecystitis with cholelithiasis (K80.-)

K81.0 **Acute cholecystitis**
Abscess of gallbladder
Angiocholecystitis
Emphysematous (acute) cholecystitis
Empyema of gallbladder
Gangrene of gallbladder
Gangrenous cholecystitis
Suppurative cholecystitis

K81.1 **Chronic cholecystitis**

K81.2 **Acute cholecystitis with chronic cholecystitis**

K81.9 **Cholecystitis, unspecified**

CHAPTER 11 (K00-K95)

K82 Other diseases of gallbladder
Excludes1 nonvisualization of gallbladder (R93.2)
postcholecystectomy syndrome (K91.5)

K82.0 Obstruction of gallbladder
Occlusion of cystic duct or gallbladder without cholelithiasis
Stenosis of cystic duct or gallbladder without cholelithiasis
Stricture of cystic duct or gallbladder without cholelithiasis
Excludes1 obstruction of gallbladder with cholelithiasis (K80.-)

K82.1 Hydrops of gallbladder
Mucocele of gallbladder

K82.2 Perforation of gallbladder
Rupture of cystic duct or gallbladder
Excludes1 Perforation of gallbladder in cholecystitis (K82.A2)

K82.3 Fistula of gallbladder
Cholecystocolic fistula
Cholecystoduodenal fistula
Coding Clinic: 2019, Q1, P18

K82.4 Cholesterolosis of gallbladder
Strawberry gallbladder
Excludes1 cholesterolosis of gallbladder with cholecystitis (K81.-)
cholesterolosis of gallbladder with cholelithiasis (K80.-)

K82.8 Other specified diseases of gallbladder
Adhesions of cystic duct or gallbladder
Atrophy of cystic duct or gallbladder
Cyst of cystic duct or gallbladder
Dyskinesia of cystic duct or gallbladder
Hypertrophy of cystic duct or gallbladder
Nonfunctioning of cystic duct or gallbladder
Ulcer of cystic duct or gallbladder

K82.9 Disease of gallbladder, unspecified

K82.A Disorders of gallbladder in diseases classified elsewhere
Code first the type of cholecystitis (K81.-), or cholelithiasis with cholecystitis (K80.00-K80.19, K80.40-K80.47, K80.60-K80.67)

K82.A1 Gangrene of gallbladder in cholecystitis
Coding Clinic: 2018, Q4, P20

K82.A2 Perforation of gallbladder in cholecystitis
Coding Clinic: 2018, Q4, P20

K83 Other diseases of biliary tract
Excludes1 postcholecystectomy syndrome (K91.5)
Excludes2 conditions involving the gallbladder (K81-K82)
conditions involving the cystic duct (K81-K82)

K83.0 Cholangitis
Excludes1 cholangitic liver abscess (K75.0)
cholangitis with choledocholithiasis (K80.3-, K80.4-)
Excludes2 chronic nonsuppurative destructive cholangitis (K74.3)
primary biliary cholangitis (K74.3)
primary biliary cirrhosis (K74.3)

K83.01 Primary sclerosing cholangitis
Coding Clinic: 2018, Q4, P21

K83.09 Other cholangitis
Ascending cholangitis
Cholangitis NOS
Primary cholangitis
Recurrent cholangitis
Sclerosing cholangitis
Secondary cholangitis
Stenosing cholangitis
Suppurative cholangitis

K83.1 Obstruction of bile duct
Occlusion of bile duct without cholelithiasis
Stenosis of bile duct without cholelithiasis
Stricture of bile duct without cholelithiasis
Excludes1 congenital obstruction of bile duct (Q44.3)
obstruction of bile duct with cholelithiasis (K80.-)
Coding Clinic: 2016, Q1, P18

K83.2 Perforation of bile duct
Rupture of bile duct

K83.3 Fistula of bile duct
Choledochoduodenal fistula

K83.4 Spasm of sphincter of Oddi

K83.5 Biliary cyst

K83.8 Other specified diseases of biliary tract
Adhesions of biliary tract
Atrophy of biliary tract
Hypertrophy of biliary tract
Ulcer of biliary tract

K83.9 Disease of biliary tract, unspecified

K85 Acute pancreatitis
Inflammatory process in which pancreatic enzymes autodigest the gland
Includes acute (recurrent) pancreatitis
subacute pancreatitis
Coding Clinic: 2016, Q4, P34

K85.0 Idiopathic acute pancreatitis
K85.00 Idiopathic acute pancreatitis without necrosis or infection
K85.01 Idiopathic acute pancreatitis with uninfected necrosis
K85.02 Idiopathic acute pancreatitis with infected necrosis

K85.1 Biliary acute pancreatitis
Gallstone pancreatitis
K85.10 Biliary acute pancreatitis without necrosis or infection
K85.11 Biliary acute pancreatitis with uninfected necrosis
K85.12 Biliary acute pancreatitis with infected necrosis

K85.2 Alcohol induced acute pancreatitis
Excludes2 alcohol induced chronic pancreatitis (K86.0)
K85.20 Alcohol induced acute pancreatitis without necrosis or infection
K85.21 Alcohol induced acute pancreatitis with uninfected necrosis
K85.22 Alcohol induced acute pancreatitis with infected necrosis

K85.3 Drug induced acute pancreatitis
Use additional code for adverse effect, if applicable, to identify drug (T36-T50 with fifth or sixth character 5)
Use additional code to identify drug abuse and dependence (F11.-F17.-)
K85.30 Drug induced acute pancreatitis without necrosis or infection
K85.31 Drug induced acute pancreatitis with uninfected necrosis
K85.32 Drug induced acute pancreatitis with infected necrosis

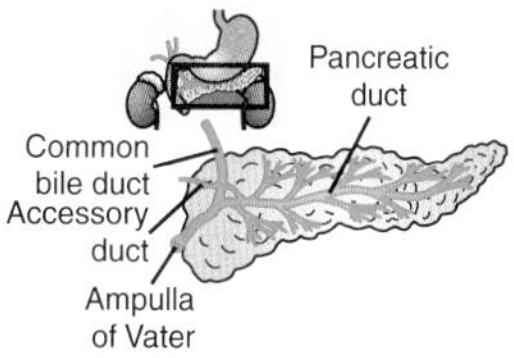

Figure 11-15 Pancreatic ductal system.

K85.8 Other acute pancreatitis
K85.80 Other acute pancreatitis without necrosis or infection
K85.81 Other acute pancreatitis with uninfected necrosis
K85.82 Other acute pancreatitis with infected necrosis
K85.9 Acute pancreatitis, unspecified
Pancreatitis NOS
K85.90 Acute pancreatitis without necrosis or infection, unspecified
K85.91 Acute pancreatitis with uninfected necrosis, unspecified
K85.92 Acute pancreatitis with infected necrosis, unspecified

K86 Other diseases of pancreas
Excludes2 fibrocystic disease of pancreas (E84.-)
islet cell tumor (of pancreas) (D13.7)
pancreatic steatorrhea (K90.3)
K86.0 Alcohol-induced chronic pancreatitis
Use additional code to identify:
alcohol abuse and dependence (F10.-)
Code also exocrine pancreatic insufficiency (K86.81)
Excludes2 alcohol induced acute pancreatitis (K85.2-)
K86.1 Other chronic pancreatitis
Chronic pancreatitis NOS
Infectious chronic pancreatitis
Recurrent chronic pancreatitis
Relapsing chronic pancreatitis
Code also exocrine pancreatic insufficiency (K86.81)
K86.2 Cyst of pancreas
K86.3 Pseudocyst of pancreas
K86.8 Other specified diseases of pancreas
Coding Clinic: 2016, Q4, P34
K86.81 Exocrine pancreatic insufficiency
K86.89 Other specified diseases of pancreas
Aseptic pancreatic necrosis, unrelated to acute pancreatitis
Atrophy of pancreas
Calculus of pancreas
Cirrhosis of pancreas
Fibrosis of pancreas
Pancreatic fat necrosis, unrelated to acute pancreatitis
Pancreatic infantilism
Pancreatic necrosis NOS, unrelated to acute pancreatitis
K86.9 Disease of pancreas, unspecified

K87 *Disorders of gallbladder, biliary tract and pancreas in diseases classified elsewhere*
Code first underlying disease
Excludes1 cytomegaloviral pancreatitis (B25.2)
mumps pancreatitis (B26.3)
syphilitic gallbladder (A52.74)
syphilitic pancreas (A52.74)
tuberculosis of gallbladder (A18.83)
tuberculosis of pancreas (A18.83)

OTHER DISEASES OF THE DIGESTIVE SYSTEM (K90-K95)

K90 Intestinal malabsorption
Excludes1 intestinal malabsorption following gastrointestinal surgery (K91.2)
K90.0 Celiac disease
Celiac disease with steatorrhea
Celiac gluten-sensitive enteropathy
Nontropical sprue
Use additional code for associated disorders including:
dermatitis herpetiformis (L13.0)
gluten ataxia (G32.81)
Code also exocrine pancreatic insufficiency (K86.81)
K90.1 Tropical sprue
Sprue NOS
Tropical steatorrhea
K90.2 Blind loop syndrome, not elsewhere classified
Blind loop syndrome NOS
Excludes1 congenital blind loop syndrome (Q43.8)
postsurgical blind loop syndrome (K91.2)
K90.3 Pancreatic steatorrhea
K90.4 Other malabsorption due to intolerance
Excludes2 celiac gluten-sensitive enteropathy (K90.0)
lactose intolerance (E73.-)
Coding Clinic: 2016, Q4, P35-36
K90.41 Non-celiac gluten sensitivity
Gluten sensitivity NOS
Non-celiac gluten sensitive enteropathy
K90.49 Malabsorption due to intolerance, not elsewhere classified
Malabsorption due to intolerance to carbohydrate
Malabsorption due to intolerance to fat
Malabsorption due to intolerance to protein
Malabsorption due to intolerance to starch
K90.8 Other intestinal malabsorption
K90.81 Whipple's disease
K90.89 Other intestinal malabsorption
K90.9 Intestinal malabsorption, unspecified
Coding Clinic: 2017, Q4, P108-109

K91 Intraoperative and postprocedural complications and disorders of digestive system, not elsewhere classified
Excludes2 complications of artificial opening of digestive system (K94.-)
complications of bariatric procedures (K95.-)
gastrojejunal ulcer (K28.-)
postprocedural (radiation) retroperitoneal abscess (K68.11)
radiation colitis (K52.0)
radiation gastroenteritis (K52.0)
radiation proctitis (K62.7)
Coding Clinic: 2016, Q4, P10
K91.0 Vomiting following gastrointestinal surgery
K91.1 Postgastric surgery syndromes
Dumping syndrome
Postgastrectomy syndrome
Postvagotomy syndrome
K91.2 Postsurgical malabsorption, not elsewhere classified
Postsurgical blind loop syndrome
Excludes1 malabsorption osteomalacia in adults (M83.2)
malabsorption osteoporosis, postsurgical (M80.8-, M81.8)
K91.3 Postprocedural intestinal obstruction
Coding Clinic: 2017, Q1, P40-41
K91.30 Postprocedural intestinal obstruction, unspecified as to partial versus complete
Postprocedural intestinal obstruction NOS
K91.31 Postprocedural partial intestinal obstruction
Postprocedural incomplete intestinal obstruction
K91.32 Postprocedural complete intestinal obstruction

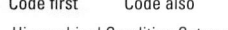

K91.5 **Postcholecystectomy syndrome**

● K91.6 **Intraoperative hemorrhage and hematoma of a digestive system organ or structure complicating a procedure**

Excludes1 intraoperative hemorrhage and hematoma of a digestive system organ or structure due to accidental puncture and laceration during a procedure (K91.7-)

K91.61 **Intraoperative hemorrhage and hematoma of a digestive system organ or structure complicating a digestive system procedure**

K91.62 **Intraoperative hemorrhage and hematoma of a digestive system organ or structure complicating other procedure**

● K91.7 **Accidental puncture and laceration of a digestive system organ or structure during a procedure**

K91.71 **Accidental puncture and laceration of a digestive system organ or structure during a digestive system procedure**

K91.72 **Accidental puncture and laceration of a digestive system organ or structure during other procedure**

Coding Clinic: 2019, Q2, P24

● K91.8 **Other intraoperative and postprocedural complications and disorders of digestive system**

K91.81 **Other intraoperative complications of digestive system**

K91.82 **Postprocedural hepatic failure**

K91.83 **Postprocedural hepatorenal syndrome**

● K91.84 **Postprocedural hemorrhage of a digestive system organ or structure following a procedure**

K91.840 **Postprocedural hemorrhage of a digestive system organ or structure following a digestive system procedure**

Coding Clinic: 2016, Q1, P15

K91.841 **Postprocedural hemorrhage of a digestive system organ or structure following other procedure**

● K91.85 **Complications of intestinal pouch**

K91.850 **Pouchitis**

Inflammation of internal ileoanal pouch

K91.858 **Other complications of intestinal pouch**

Coding Clinic: 2019, Q2, P13

K91.86 **Retained cholelithiasis following cholecystectomy**

● K91.87 **Postprocedural hematoma and seroma of a digestive system organ or structure following a procedure**

K91.870 **Postprocedural hematoma of a digestive system organ or structure following a digestive system procedure**

K91.871 **Postprocedural hematoma of a digestive system organ or structure following other procedure**

K91.872 **Postprocedural seroma of a digestive system organ or structure following a digestive system procedure**

K91.873 **Postprocedural seroma of a digestive system organ or structure following other procedure**

K91.89 **Other postprocedural complications and disorders of digestive system**

Use additional code, if applicable, to further specify disorder

Excludes2 postprocedural retroperitoneal abscess (K68.11)

Coding Clinic: 2017, Q1, P41

● K92 **Other diseases of digestive system**

Excludes1 neonatal gastrointestinal hemorrhage (P54.0-P54.3)

K92.0 **Hematemesis**

K92.1 **Melena**

Excludes1 occult blood in feces (R19.5)

K92.2 **Gastrointestinal hemorrhage, unspecified**

Gastric hemorrhage NOS
Intestinal hemorrhage NOS

Excludes1 acute hemorrhagic gastritis (K29.01)
hemorrhage of anus and rectum (K62.5)
angiodysplasia of stomach with hemorrhage (K31.811)
diverticular disease with hemorrhage (K57.-)
gastritis and duodenitis with hemorrhage (K29.-)
peptic ulcer with hemorrhage (K25-K28)

● K92.8 **Other specified diseases of the digestive system**

K92.81 **Gastrointestinal mucositis (ulcerative)**

Code also type of associated therapy, such as:
antineoplastic and immunosuppressive drugs (T45.1X-)
radiological procedure and radiotherapy (Y84.2)

Excludes2 mucositis (ulcerative) of vagina and vulva (N76.81)
nasal mucositis (ulcerative) (J34.81)
oral mucositis (ulcerative) (K12.3-)

K92.89 **Other specified diseases of the digestive system**

K92.9 **Disease of digestive system, unspecified**

● K94 **Complications of artificial openings of the digestive system**

● K94.0 **Colostomy complications**

K94.00 **Colostomy complication, unspecified**

K94.01 **Colostomy hemorrhage**

K94.02 **Colostomy infection**

Use additional code to specify type of infection, such as:
cellulitis of abdominal wall (L03.311)
sepsis (A40.-, A41.-)

K94.03 **Colostomy malfunction**

Mechanical complication of colostomy

K94.09 **Other complications of colostomy**

● K94.1 **Enterostomy complications**

K94.10 **Enterostomy complication, unspecified**

K94.11 **Enterostomy hemorrhage**

K94.12 **Enterostomy infection**

Use additional code to specify type of infection, such as:
cellulitis of abdominal wall (L03.311)
sepsis (A40.-, A41.-)

K94.13 **Enterostomy malfunction**

Mechanical complication of enterostomy

K94.19 **Other complications of enterostomy**

● K94.2 **Gastrostomy complications**

K94.20 **Gastrostomy complication, unspecified**

K94.21 **Gastrostomy hemorrhage**

K94.22 **Gastrostomy infection**

Use additional code to specify type of infection, such as:
cellulitis of abdominal wall (L03.311)
sepsis (A40.-, A41.-)

K94.23 **Gastrostomy malfunction**

Mechanical complication of gastrostomy

K94.29 **Other complications of gastrostomy**

- K94.3 Esophagostomy complications
  - K94.30 Esophagostomy complications, unspecified
  - K94.31 Esophagostomy hemorrhage
  - K94.32 Esophagostomy infection
    - Use additional code to identify the infection
  - K94.33 Esophagostomy malfunction
    - Mechanical complication of esophagostomy
  - K94.39 Other complications of esophagostomy

- K95 Complications of bariatric procedures
  - K95.Ø Complications of gastric band procedure
    - K95.Ø1 Infection due to gastric band procedure
      - Use additional code to specify type of infection or organism, such as:
        - bacterial and viral infectious agents (B95.-, B96.-)
        - cellulitis of abdominal wall (LØ3.311)
        - sepsis (A4Ø.-, A41.-)
    - K95.Ø9 Other complications of gastric band procedure
      - Use additional code, if applicable, to further specify complication
  - K95.8 Complications of other bariatric procedure
    - **Excludes1** complications of gastric band surgery (K95.Ø-)
    - K95.81 Infection due to other bariatric procedure
      - Use additional code to specify type of infection or organism, such as:
        - bacterial and viral infectious agents (B95.-, B96.-)
        - cellulitis of abdominal wall (LØ3.311)
        - sepsis (A4Ø.-, A41.-)
    - K95.89 Other complications of other bariatric procedure
      - Use additional code, if applicable, to further specify complication

CHAPTER 12

DISEASES OF THE SKIN AND SUBCUTANEOUS TISSUE (LØØ-L99)

OGCR Chapter-Specific Coding Guidelines

12. Chapter 12: Diseases of the Skin and Subcutaneous Tissue (LØØ-L99)

a. Pressure ulcer stage codes

1) Pressure ulcer stages

Codes from category L89, Pressure ulcer, identify the site of the pressure ulcer as well as the stage of the ulcer.

The ICD-10-CM classifies pressure ulcer stages based on severity, which is designated by stages 1-4, unspecified stage and unstageable.

Assign as many codes from category L89 as needed to identify all the pressure ulcers the patient has, if applicable.

See Section I.B.14 for pressure ulcer stage documentation by clinicians other than patient's provider.

2) Unstageable pressure ulcers

Assignment of the code for unstageable pressure ulcer (L89.--Ø) should be based on the clinical documentation. These codes are used for pressure ulcers whose stage cannot be clinically determined (e.g., the ulcer is covered by eschar or has been treated with a skin or muscle graft) and pressure ulcers that are documented as deep tissue injury but not documented as due to trauma. This code should not be confused with the codes for unspecified stage (L89.--9). When there is no documentation regarding the stage of the pressure ulcer, assign the appropriate code for unspecified stage (L89.--9).

3) Documented pressure ulcer stage

Assignment of the pressure ulcer stage code should be guided by clinical documentation of the stage or documentation of the terms found in the Alphabetic Index. For clinical terms describing the stage that are not found in the Alphabetic Index, and there is no documentation of the stage, the provider should be queried.

4) Patients admitted with pressure ulcers documented as healed

No code is assigned if the documentation states that the pressure ulcer is completely healed.

5) Patients admitted with pressure ulcers documented as healing

Pressure ulcers described as healing should be assigned the appropriate pressure ulcer stage code based on the documentation in the medical record. If the documentation does not provide information about the stage of the healing pressure ulcer, assign the appropriate code for unspecified stage.

If the documentation is unclear as to whether the patient has a current (new) pressure ulcer or if the patient is being treated for a healing pressure ulcer, query the provider.

For ulcers that were present on admission but healed at the time of discharge, assign the code for the site and stage of the pressure ulcer at the time of admission.

6) Patient admitted with pressure ulcer evolving into another stage during the admission

If a patient is admitted to an inpatient hospital with a pressure ulcer at one stage and it progresses to a higher stage, two separate codes should be assigned: one code for the site and stage of the ulcer on admission and a second code for the same ulcer site and the highest stage reported during the stay.

b. Non-Pressure Chronic Ulcers

1) Patients admitted with non-pressure ulcers documented as healed

No code is assigned if the documentation states that the non-pressure ulcer is completely healed.

2) Patients admitted with non-pressure ulcers documented as healing

Non-pressure ulcers described as healing should be assigned the appropriate non-pressure ulcer code based on the documentation in the medical record. If the documentation does not provide information about the severity of the healing non-pressure ulcer, assign the appropriate code for unspecified severity.

If the documentation is unclear as to whether the patient has a current (new) non-pressure ulcer or if the patient is being treated for a healing non-pressure ulcer, query the provider.

For ulcers that were present on admission but healed at the time of discharge, assign the code for the site and severity of the non-pressure ulcer at the time of admission.

3) Patient admitted with non-pressure ulcer that progresses to another severity level during the admission

If a patient is admitted to an inpatient hospital with a non-pressure ulcer at one severity level and it progresses to a higher severity level, two separate codes should be assigned: one code for the site and severity level of the ulcer on admission and a second code for the same ulcer site and the highest severity level reported during the stay.

See Section I.B.14 for pressure ulcer stage documentation by clinicians other than patient's provider.

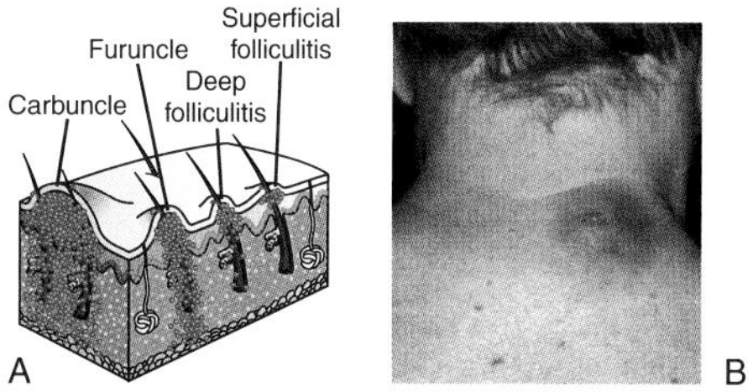

Figure 12-1 Furuncle, also known as a boil, is a staphylococcal infection. The organism enters the body through a hair follicle and so furuncles usually appear in hairy areas of the body. A cluster of furuncles is known as a carbuncle and involves infection into the deep subcutaneous fascia. These usually appear on the back and neck. (**B** from Habif TP, Binnick AN, Meyerson LB: Clinical Dermatology: A Color Guide to Diagnosis and Therapy, S.l., Mosby Elsevier, 2010)

CHAPTER 12

DISEASES OF THE SKIN AND SUBCUTANEOUS TISSUE (LØØ-L99)

Excludes2 certain conditions originating in the perinatal period (PØ4-P96)
certain infectious and parasitic diseases (AØØ-B99)
complications of pregnancy, childbirth and the puerperium (OØØ-O9A)
congenital malformations, deformations, and chromosomal abnormalities (QØØ-Q99)
endocrine, nutritional and metabolic diseases (EØØ-E88)
lipomelanotic reticulosis (I89.8)
neoplasms (CØØ-D49)
symptoms, signs and abnormal clinical and laboratory findings, not elsewhere classified (RØØ-R94)
systemic connective tissue disorders (M3Ø-M36)
viral warts (BØ7.-)

This chapter contains the following blocks:

LØØ-LØ8	Infections of the skin and subcutaneous tissue
L1Ø-L14	Bullous disorders
L2Ø-L3Ø	Dermatitis and eczema
L4Ø-L45	Papulosquamous disorders
L49-L54	Urticaria and erythema
L55-L59	Radiation-related disorders of the skin and subcutaneous tissue
L6Ø-L75	Disorders of skin appendages
L76	Intraoperative and postprocedural complications of skin and subcutaneous tissue
L8Ø-L99	Other disorders of the skin and subcutaneous tissue

INFECTIONS OF THE SKIN AND SUBCUTANEOUS TISSUE (LØØ-LØ8)

Use additional code (B95-B97) to identify infectious agent.

Excludes2 hordeolum (HØØ.Ø)
infective dermatitis (L3Ø.3)
local infections of skin classified in Chapter 1
lupus panniculitis (L93.2)
panniculitis NOS (M79.3)
panniculitis of neck and back (M54.Ø-)
Perlèche NOS (K13.Ø)
Perlèche due to candidiasis (B37.Ø)
Perlèche due to riboflavin deficiency (E53.Ø)
pyogenic granuloma (L98.Ø)
relapsing panniculitis [Weber-Christian] (M35.6)
viral warts (BØ7.-)
zoster (BØ2.-)

LØØ Staphylococcal scalded skin syndrome
Ritter's disease
Use additional code to identify percentage of skin exfoliation (L49.-)
Excludes1 bullous impetigo (LØ1.Ø3)
pemphigus neonatorum (LØ1.Ø3)
toxic epidermal necrolysis [Lyell] (L51.2)

● **LØ1 Impetigo**
Contagious skin infection caused by a streptococcus or staphylococcus aureus, common skin infections among children
Excludes1 impetigo herpetiformis (L4Ø.1)

● **LØ1.Ø Impetigo**
Impetigo contagiosa
Impetigo vulgaris

LØ1.ØØ Impetigo, unspecified
Impetigo NOS

LØ1.Ø1 Non-bullous impetigo

LØ1.Ø2 Bockhart's impetigo
Impetigo follicularis
Perifolliculitis NOS
Superficial pustular perifolliculitis

LØ1.Ø3 Bullous impetigo
Impetigo neonatorum
Pemphigus neonatorum
Neonate = newborn

LØ1.Ø9 Other impetigo
Ulcerative impetigo

LØ1.1 Impetiginization of other dermatoses

● **LØ2 Cutaneous abscess, furuncle and carbuncle**
Use additional code to identify organism (B95-B96)
Excludes2 abscess of anus and rectal regions (K61.-)
abscess of female genital organs (external) (N76.4)
abscess of male genital organs (external) (N48.2, N49.-)

● **LØ2.Ø Cutaneous abscess, furuncle and carbuncle of face**
Excludes2 abscess of ear, external (H6Ø.Ø)
abscess of eyelid (HØØ.Ø)
abscess of head [any part, except face] (LØ2.8)
abscess of lacrimal gland (HØ4.Ø)
abscess of lacrimal passages (HØ4.3)
abscess of mouth (K12.2)
abscess of nose (J34.Ø)
abscess of orbit (HØ5.Ø)
submandibular abscess (K12.2)

LØ2.Ø1 Cutaneous abscess of face

LØ2.Ø2 Furuncle of face
Boil of face
Folliculitis of face

LØ2.Ø3 Carbuncle of face

● **LØ2.1 Cutaneous abscess, furuncle and carbuncle of neck**

LØ2.11 Cutaneous abscess of neck

LØ2.12 Furuncle of neck
Boil of neck
Folliculitis of neck

LØ2.13 Carbuncle of neck

● **LØ2.2 Cutaneous abscess, furuncle and carbuncle of trunk**
Excludes1 non-newborn omphalitis (LØ8.82)
omphalitis of newborn (P38.-)
Excludes2 abscess of breast (N61.1)
abscess of buttocks (LØ2.3)
abscess of female external genital organs (N76.4)
abscess of male external genital organs (N48.2, N49.-)
abscess of hip (LØ2.4)

● **LØ2.21 Cutaneous abscess of trunk**
LØ2.211 Cutaneous abscess of abdominal wall
LØ2.212 Cutaneous abscess of back [any part, except buttock]
LØ2.213 Cutaneous abscess of chest wall
LØ2.214 Cutaneous abscess of groin
LØ2.215 Cutaneous abscess of perineum
LØ2.216 Cutaneous abscess of umbilicus
LØ2.219 Cutaneous abscess of trunk, unspecified

● **LØ2.22 Furuncle of trunk**
Boil of trunk
Folliculitis of trunk
LØ2.221 Furuncle of abdominal wall
LØ2.222 Furuncle of back [any part, except buttock]
LØ2.223 Furuncle of chest wall
LØ2.224 Furuncle of groin
LØ2.225 Furuncle of perineum
LØ2.226 Furuncle of umbilicus
LØ2.229 Furuncle of trunk, unspecified

● **LØ2.23 Carbuncle of trunk**
LØ2.231 Carbuncle of abdominal wall
LØ2.232 Carbuncle of back [any part, except buttock]
LØ2.233 Carbuncle of chest wall
LØ2.234 Carbuncle of groin
LØ2.235 Carbuncle of perineum
LØ2.236 Carbuncle of umbilicus
LØ2.239 Carbuncle of trunk, unspecified

● **LØ2.3 Cutaneous abscess, furuncle and carbuncle of buttock**
Excludes1 pilonidal cyst with abscess (LØ5.Ø1)

LØ2.31 Cutaneous abscess of buttock
Cutaneous abscess of gluteal region

LØ2.32 Furuncle of buttock
Boil of buttock
Folliculitis of buttock
Furuncle of gluteal region

LØ2.33 Carbuncle of buttock
Carbuncle of gluteal region

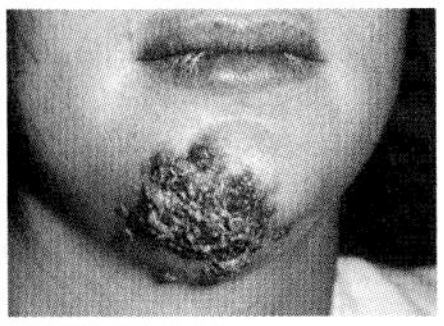

Figure 12-2 Impetigo. A thick, honey-yellow adherent crust covers the entire eroded surface. (From James WD, Elston DM, Berger TG, Andrews GC: Andrews' Diseases of the Skin: Clinical Dermatology, London, Saunders/Elsevier, 2011)

CHAPTER 12 (LØØ-L99)

● LØ2.4 Cutaneous abscess, furuncle and carbuncle of limb
Excludes2 Cutaneous abscess, furuncle and carbuncle of groin (LØ2.214, LØ2.224, LØ2.234)
Cutaneous abscess, furuncle and carbuncle of hand (LØ2.5-)
Cutaneous abscess, furuncle and carbuncle of foot (LØ2.6-)
● LØ2.41 Cutaneous abscess of limb
LØ2.411 Cutaneous abscess of right axilla
LØ2.412 Cutaneous abscess of left axilla
LØ2.413 Cutaneous abscess of right upper limb
LØ2.414 Cutaneous abscess of left upper limb
LØ2.415 Cutaneous abscess of right lower limb
LØ2.416 Cutaneous abscess of left lower limb
LØ2.419 Cutaneous abscess of limb, unspecified
● LØ2.42 Furuncle of limb
Boil of limb
Folliculitis of limb
LØ2.421 Furuncle of right axilla
LØ2.422 Furuncle of left axilla
LØ2.423 Furuncle of right upper limb
LØ2.424 Furuncle of left upper limb
LØ2.425 Furuncle of right lower limb
LØ2.426 Furuncle of left lower limb
LØ2.429 Furuncle of limb, unspecified
● LØ2.43 Carbuncle of limb
LØ2.431 Carbuncle of right axilla
LØ2.432 Carbuncle of left axilla
LØ2.433 Carbuncle of right upper limb
LØ2.434 Carbuncle of left upper limb
LØ2.435 Carbuncle of right lower limb
LØ2.436 Carbuncle of left lower limb
LØ2.439 Carbuncle of limb, unspecified
● LØ2.5 Cutaneous abscess, furuncle and carbuncle of hand
● LØ2.51 Cutaneous abscess of hand
LØ2.511 Cutaneous abscess of right hand
LØ2.512 Cutaneous abscess of left hand
LØ2.519 Cutaneous abscess of unspecified hand
● LØ2.52 Furuncle hand
Boil of hand
Folliculitis of hand
LØ2.521 Furuncle right hand
LØ2.522 Furuncle left hand
LØ2.529 Furuncle unspecified hand
● LØ2.53 Carbuncle of hand
LØ2.531 Carbuncle of right hand
LØ2.532 Carbuncle of left hand
LØ2.539 Carbuncle of unspecified hand
● LØ2.6 Cutaneous abscess, furuncle and carbuncle of foot
● LØ2.61 Cutaneous abscess of foot
LØ2.611 Cutaneous abscess of right foot
LØ2.612 Cutaneous abscess of left foot
LØ2.619 Cutaneous abscess of unspecified foot
● LØ2.62 Furuncle of foot
Boil of foot
Folliculitis of foot
LØ2.621 Furuncle of right foot
LØ2.622 Furuncle of left foot
LØ2.629 Furuncle of unspecified foot
● LØ2.63 Carbuncle of foot
LØ2.631 Carbuncle of right foot
LØ2.632 Carbuncle of left foot
LØ2.639 Carbuncle of unspecified foot

● LØ2.8 Cutaneous abscess, furuncle and carbuncle of other sites
● LØ2.81 Cutaneous abscess of other sites
LØ2.811 Cutaneous abscess of head [any part, except face]
LØ2.818 Cutaneous abscess of other sites
● LØ2.82 Furuncle of other sites
Boil of other sites
Folliculitis of other sites
LØ2.821 Furuncle of head [any part, except face]
LØ2.828 Furuncle of other sites
● LØ2.83 Carbuncle of other sites
LØ2.831 Carbuncle of head [any part, except face]
LØ2.838 Carbuncle of other sites
● LØ2.9 Cutaneous abscess, furuncle and carbuncle, unspecified
LØ2.91 Cutaneous abscess, unspecified
LØ2.92 Furuncle, unspecified
Boil NOS
Furunculosis NOS
LØ2.93 Carbuncle, unspecified

● LØ3 Cellulitis and acute lymphangitis
Excludes2 cellulitis of anal and rectal region (K61.-)
cellulitis of external auditory canal (H6Ø.1)
cellulitis of eyelid (HØØ.Ø)
cellulitis of female external genital organs (N76.4)
cellulitis of lacrimal apparatus (HØ4.3)
cellulitis of male external genital organs (N48.2, N49.-)
cellulitis of mouth (K12.2)
cellulitis of nose (J34.Ø)
eosinophilic cellulitis [Wells] (L98.3)
febrile neutrophilic dermatosis [Sweet] (L98.2)
lymphangitis (chronic) (subacute) (I89.1)
● LØ3.Ø Cellulitis and acute lymphangitis of finger and toe
Infection of nail
Onychia
Paronychia
Perionychia
● LØ3.Ø1 Cellulitis of finger
Felon
Whitlow
Excludes1 herpetic whitlow (BØØ.89)
LØ3.Ø11 Cellulitis of right finger
LØ3.Ø12 Cellulitis of left finger
LØ3.Ø19 Cellulitis of unspecified finger
● LØ3.Ø2 Acute lymphangitis of finger
Hangnail with lymphangitis of finger
LØ3.Ø21 Acute lymphangitis of right finger
LØ3.Ø22 Acute lymphangitis of left finger
LØ3.Ø29 Acute lymphangitis of unspecified finger
● LØ3.Ø3 Cellulitis of toe
LØ3.Ø31 Cellulitis of right toe
LØ3.Ø32 Cellulitis of left toe
LØ3.Ø39 Cellulitis of unspecified toe
● LØ3.Ø4 Acute lymphangitis of toe
Hangnail with lymphangitis of toe
LØ3.Ø41 Acute lymphangitis of right toe
LØ3.Ø42 Acute lymphangitis of left toe
LØ3.Ø49 Acute lymphangitis of unspecified toe

Item 12-1 **Onychia** is an inflammation of the tissue surrounding the nail with pus accumulation and loss of the nail, resulting from microscopic pathogens entering through small wounds. **Paronychia** is a nail disease also known as felon or whitlow and is a bacterial or fungal infection.

Item 12–2 Cellulitis is an acute spreading bacterial infection below the surface of the skin characterized by redness (erythema), warmth, swelling, pain, fever, chills, and enlarged lymph nodes ("swollen glands").

● LØ3.1 Cellulitis and acute lymphangitis of other parts of limb
● LØ3.11 Cellulitis of other parts of limb
Excludes2 cellulitis of fingers (LØ3.Ø1-)
cellulitis of toes (LØ3.Ø3-)
groin (LØ3.314)
LØ3.111 Cellulitis of right axilla
LØ3.112 Cellulitis of left axilla
LØ3.113 Cellulitis of right upper limb
LØ3.114 Cellulitis of left upper limb
Coding Clinic: 2019, Q1, P13
LØ3.115 Cellulitis of right lower limb
LØ3.116 Cellulitis of left lower limb
LØ3.119 Cellulitis of unspecified part of limb
● LØ3.12 Acute lymphangitis of other parts of limb
Excludes2 acute lymphangitis of fingers (LØ3.2-)
acute lymphangitis of toes (LØ3.Ø4-)
acute lymphangitis of groin (LØ3.324)
LØ3.121 Acute lymphangitis of right axilla
LØ3.122 Acute lymphangitis of left axilla
LØ3.123 Acute lymphangitis of right upper limb
LØ3.124 Acute lymphangitis of left upper limb
LØ3.125 Acute lymphangitis of right lower limb
LØ3.126 Acute lymphangitis of left lower limb
LØ3.129 Acute lymphangitis of unspecified part of limb
● LØ3.2 Cellulitis and acute lymphangitis of face and neck
● LØ3.21 Cellulitis and acute lymphangitis of face
LØ3.211 Cellulitis of face
Excludes2 abscess of orbit (HØ5.Ø1-)
cellulitis of ear (H6Ø.1-)
cellulitis of eyelid (HØØ.Ø-)
cellulitis of head (LØ3.81)
cellulitis of lacrimal apparatus (HØ4.3)
cellulitis of lip (K13.Ø)
cellulitis of mouth (K12.2)
cellulitis of nose (internal) (J34.Ø)
cellulitis of orbit (HØ5.Ø1-)
cellulitis of scalp (LØ3.81)
LØ3.212 Acute lymphangitis of face
LØ3.213 Periorbital cellulitis
Preseptal cellulitis
Coding Clinic: 2016, Q4, P36
● LØ3.22 Cellulitis and acute lymphangitis of neck
LØ3.221 Cellulitis of neck
LØ3.222 Acute lymphangitis of neck

● LØ3.3 Cellulitis and acute lymphangitis of trunk
● LØ3.31 Cellulitis of trunk
Excludes2 cellulitis of anal and rectal regions (K61.-)
cellulitis of breast NOS (N61.Ø)
cellulitis of female external genital organs (N76.4)
cellulitis of male external genital organs (N48.2, N49.-)
omphalitis of newborn (P38.-)
puerperal cellulitis of breast (O91.2)
LØ3.311 Cellulitis of abdominal wall
Excludes2 cellulitis of umbilicus (LØ3.316)
cellulitis of groin (LØ3.314)
LØ3.312 Cellulitis of back [any part except buttock]
LØ3.313 Cellulitis of chest wall
LØ3.314 Cellulitis of groin
LØ3.315 Cellulitis of perineum
LØ3.316 Cellulitis of umbilicus
LØ3.317 Cellulitis of buttock
LØ3.319 Cellulitis of trunk, unspecified
● LØ3.32 Acute lymphangitis of trunk
LØ3.321 Acute lymphangitis of abdominal wall
LØ3.322 Acute lymphangitis of back [any part except buttock]
LØ3.323 Acute lymphangitis of chest wall
LØ3.324 Acute lymphangitis of groin
LØ3.325 Acute lymphangitis of perineum
LØ3.326 Acute lymphangitis of umbilicus
LØ3.327 Acute lymphangitis of buttock
LØ3.329 Acute lymphangitis of trunk, unspecified
● LØ3.8 Cellulitis and acute lymphangitis of other sites
● LØ3.81 Cellulitis of other sites
LØ3.811 Cellulitis of head [any part, except face]
Cellulitis of scalp
Excludes2 cellulitis of face (LØ3.211)
LØ3.818 Cellulitis of other sites
● LØ3.89 Acute lymphangitis of other sites
LØ3.891 Acute lymphangitis of head [any part, except face]
LØ3.898 Acute lymphangitis of other sites
● LØ3.9 Cellulitis and acute lymphangitis, unspecified
LØ3.90 Cellulitis, unspecified
LØ3.91 Acute lymphangitis, unspecified
Excludes1 lymphangitis NOS (I89.1)

Item 12–3 **Abscess** is a localized collection of pus in tissues or organs and is a sign of infection, resulting in swelling and inflammation.

Item 12–4 **Pilonidal cyst,** also called a coccygeal cyst, is the result of a disorder called pilonidal disease. The cyst usually contains hair and pus.

● L04 Acute lymphadenitis
Short-term inflammation of lymph nodes which can be regionalized to involve a given area of the lymph system or systemic involving much of the body
Includes abscess (acute) of lymph nodes, except mesenteric
acute lymphadenitis, except mesenteric
Excludes1 chronic or subacute lymphadenitis, except mesenteric (I88.1)
enlarged lymph nodes (R59.-)
human immunodeficiency virus [HIV] disease resulting in generalized lymphadenopathy (B20)
lymphadenitis NOS (I88.9)
nonspecific mesenteric lymphadenitis (I88.0)

L04.0 Acute lymphadenitis of face, head and neck
L04.1 Acute lymphadenitis of trunk
L04.2 Acute lymphadenitis of upper limb
Acute lymphadenitis of axilla
Acute lymphadenitis of shoulder
L04.3 Acute lymphadenitis of lower limb
Acute lymphadenitis of hip
Excludes2 acute lymphadenitis of groin (L04.1)
L04.8 Acute lymphadenitis of other sites
L04.9 Acute lymphadenitis, unspecified

● L05 Pilonidal cyst and sinus
● **L05.0 Pilonidal cyst and sinus with abscess**
L05.01 Pilonidal cyst with abscess
Pilonidal abscess
Pilonidal dimple with abscess
Postanal dimple with abscess
Excludes2 congenital sacral dimple (Q82.6)
parasacral dimple (Q82.6)
L05.02 Pilonidal sinus with abscess
Coccygeal fistula with abscess
Coccygeal sinus with abscess
Pilonidal fistula with abscess
● **L05.9 Pilonidal cyst and sinus without abscess**
L05.91 Pilonidal cyst without abscess
Pilonidal dimple
Postanal dimple
Pilonidal cyst NOS
Excludes2 congenital sacral dimple (Q82.6)
parasacral dimple (Q82.6)
L05.92 Pilonidal sinus without abscess
Coccygeal fistula
Coccygeal sinus without abscess
Pilonidal fistula

● L08 Other local infections of skin and subcutaneous tissue
L08.0 Pyoderma
Dermatitis gangrenosa
Purulent dermatitis
Septic dermatitis
Suppurative dermatitis
Excludes1 pyoderma gangrenosum (L88)
pyoderma vegetans (L08.81)
L08.1 Erythrasma
● **L08.8 Other specified local infections of the skin and subcutaneous tissue**
L08.81 Pyoderma vegetans
Excludes1 pyoderma gangrenosum (L88)
pyoderma NOS (L08.0)
L08.82 Omphalitis not of newborn
Excludes1 omphalitis of newborn (P38.-)
L08.89 Other specified local infections of the skin and subcutaneous tissue
L08.9 Local infection of the skin and subcutaneous tissue, unspecified

BULLOUS DISORDERS (L10-L14)

Excludes1 benign familial pemphigus [Hailey-Hailey] (Q82.8)
staphylococcal scalded skin syndrome (L00)
toxic epidermal necrolysis [Lyell] (L51.2)

● L10 Pemphigus
Excludes1 pemphigus neonatorum (L01.03)
L10.0 Pemphigus vulgaris
L10.1 Pemphigus vegetans
L10.2 Pemphigus foliaceous
L10.3 Brazilian pemphigus [fogo selvagem]
L10.4 Pemphigus erythematosus
Senear-Usher syndrome
L10.5 Drug-induced pemphigus
Use additional code for adverse effect, if applicable, to identify drug (T36-T50 with fifth or sixth character 5)
● **L10.8 Other pemphigus**
L10.81 Paraneoplastic pemphigus
L10.89 Other pemphigus
L10.9 Pemphigus, unspecified

● L11 Other acantholytic disorders
L11.0 Acquired keratosis follicularis
Excludes1 keratosis follicularis (congenital) [Darier-White] (Q82.8)
L11.1 Transient acantholytic dermatosis [Grover]
L11.8 Other specified acantholytic disorders
L11.9 Acantholytic disorder, unspecified

● L12 Pemphigoid
Excludes1 herpes gestationis (O26.4-)
impetigo herpetiformis (L40.1)
L12.0 Bullous pemphigoid
L12.1 Cicatricial pemphigoid
Benign mucous membrane pemphigoid
L12.2 Chronic bullous disease of childhood P
Juvenile dermatitis herpetiformis
● **L12.3 Acquired epidermolysis bullosa**
Excludes1 epidermolysis bullosa (congenital) (Q81.-)
L12.30 Acquired epidermolysis bullosa, unspecified
L12.31 Epidermolysis bullosa due to drug
Use additional code for adverse effect, if applicable, to identify drug (T36-T50 with fifth or sixth character 5)
L12.35 Other acquired epidermolysis bullosa
L12.8 Other pemphigoid
L12.9 Pemphigoid, unspecified

CHAPTER 12 (L00-L99)

Item 12-5 Dermatitis herpetiformis, also known as Duhring's disease, is a systemic disease characterized by small blisters (3 to 5 mm) and occasionally large bullae (> 5 mm).

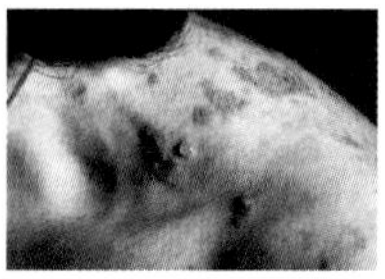

Figure 12-3 Dermatitis herpetiformis. (From Terhorst D: BASICS Dermatologie, München, Elsevier, Urban & Fischer, 2011)

● L13 **Other bullous disorders**

L13.Ø **Dermatitis herpetiformis**
Duhring's disease
Hydroa herpetiformis
Excludes1 juvenile dermatitis herpetiformis (L12.2)
senile dermatitis herpetiformis (L12.Ø)

L13.1 **Subcorneal pustular dermatitis**
Sneddon-Wilkinson disease

L13.8 **Other specified bullous disorders**

L13.9 **Bullous disorder, unspecified**

L14 Bullous disorders in diseases classified elsewhere
Code first underlying disease

DERMATITIS AND ECZEMA (L2Ø-L3Ø)

Note: In this block the terms dermatitis and eczema are used synonymously and interchangeably.

Excludes2 chronic (childhood) granulomatous disease (D71)
dermatitis gangrenosa (LØ8.Ø)
dermatitis herpetiformis (L13.Ø)
dry skin dermatitis (L85.3)
factitial dermatitis (L98.1)
perioral dermatitis (L71.Ø)
radiation-related disorders of the skin and subcutaneous tissue (L55-L59)
stasis dermatitis (I87.2)

● L2Ø **Atopic dermatitis**

L2Ø.Ø **Besnier's prurigo**

● L2Ø.8 **Other atopic dermatitis**
Excludes2 circumscribed neurodermatitis (L28.Ø)

L2Ø.81 **Atopic neurodermatitis**
Diffuse neurodermatitis

L2Ø.82 **Flexural eczema**

L2Ø.83 **Infantile (acute) (chronic) eczema** P

L2Ø.84 **Intrinsic (allergic) eczema**

L2Ø.89 **Other atopic dermatitis**

L2Ø.9 **Atopic dermatitis, unspecified**

● L21 **Seborrheic dermatitis**
Excludes2 infective dermatitis (L3Ø.3)
seborrheic keratosis (L82.-)

L21.Ø **Seborrhea capitis**
Cradle cap
Coding Clinic: 2018, Q1, P6

L21.1 **Seborrheic infantile dermatitis** P

L21.8 **Other seborrheic dermatitis**

L21.9 **Seborrheic dermatitis, unspecified**
Seborrhea NOS

Item 12-6 Seborrheic dermatitis is characterized by greasy, scaly, red patches and is associated with oily skin and scalp.

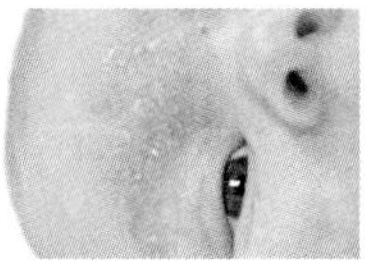

Figure 12-4 Seborrheic dermatitis. (Getty Image)

Item 12-7 Atopic dermatitis, also known as atopic eczema, infantile eczema, disseminated neuro dermatitis, flexural eczema, and *prurigo diathesique* (Besnier), is characterized by intense itching and is often hereditary.

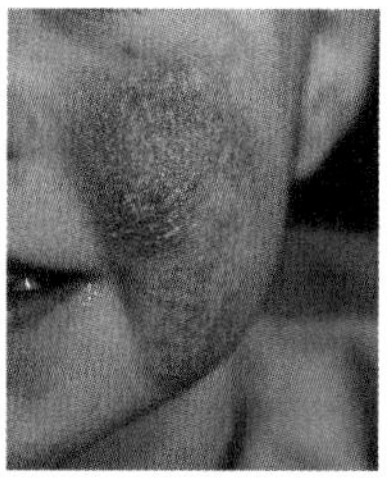

Figure 12-5 Atopic dermatitis. (From Chabner D-E: The Language of Medicine, St. Louis, MO, Saunders/Elsevier, 2007)

L22 **Diaper dermatitis**
Diaper erythema
Diaper rash
Psoriasiform diaper rash

● L23 **Allergic contact dermatitis**
Excludes1 allergy NOS (T78.4Ø)
contact dermatitis NOS (L25.9)
dermatitis NOS (L3Ø.9)
Excludes2 dermatitis due to substances taken internally (L27.-)
dermatitis of eyelid (HØ1.1-)
diaper dermatitis (L22)
eczema of external ear (H6Ø.5-)
irritant contact dermatitis (L24.-)
perioral dermatitis (L71.Ø)
radiation-related disorders of the skin and subcutaneous tissue (L55-L59)

L23.Ø **Allergic contact dermatitis due to metals**
Allergic contact dermatitis due to chromium
Allergic contact dermatitis due to nickel

L23.1 **Allergic contact dermatitis due to adhesives**

L23.2 **Allergic contact dermatitis due to cosmetics**

L23.3 **Allergic contact dermatitis due to drugs in contact with skin**
Use additional code for adverse effect, if applicable, to identify drug (T36-T5Ø with fifth or sixth character 5)
Excludes2 dermatitis due to ingested drugs and medicaments (L27.Ø-L27.1)

L23.4 **Allergic contact dermatitis due to dyes**

L23.5 **Allergic contact dermatitis due to other chemical products**
Allergic contact dermatitis due to cement
Allergic contact dermatitis due to insecticide
Allergic contact dermatitis due to plastic
Allergic contact dermatitis due to rubber

L23.6 **Allergic contact dermatitis due to food in contact with the skin**
Excludes2 dermatitis due to ingested food (L27.2)

L23.7 **Allergic contact dermatitis due to plants, except food**
Excludes2 allergy NOS due to pollen (J3Ø.1)

● L23.8 **Allergic contact dermatitis due to other agents**

L23.81 **Allergic contact dermatitis due to animal (cat) (dog) dander**
Allergic contact dermatitis due to animal (cat) (dog) hair

L23.89 **Allergic contact dermatitis due to other agents**

L23.9 **Allergic contact dermatitis, unspecified cause**
Allergic contact eczema NOS

● **L24 Irritant contact dermatitis**

Excludes1 allergy NOS (T78.40)
contact dermatitis NOS (L25.9)
dermatitis NOS (L30.9)

Excludes2 allergic contact dermatitis (L23.-)
dermatitis due to substances taken internally (L27.-)
dermatitis of eyelid (H01.1-)
diaper dermatitis (L22)
eczema of external ear (H60.5-)
perioral dermatitis (L71.0)
radiation-related disorders of the skin and subcutaneous tissue (L55-L59)

L24.0 Irritant contact dermatitis due to detergents

L24.1 Irritant contact dermatitis due to oils and greases

L24.2 Irritant contact dermatitis due to solvents
Irritant contact dermatitis due to chlorocompound
Irritant contact dermatitis due to cyclohexane
Irritant contact dermatitis due to ester
Irritant contact dermatitis due to glycol
Irritant contact dermatitis due to hydrocarbon
Irritant contact dermatitis due to ketone

L24.3 Irritant contact dermatitis due to cosmetics

L24.4 Irritant contact dermatitis due to drugs in contact with skin
Use additional code for adverse effect, if applicable, to identify drug (T36-T50 with fifth or sixth character 5)

L24.5 Irritant contact dermatitis due to other chemical products
Irritant contact dermatitis due to cement
Irritant contact dermatitis due to insecticide
Irritant contact dermatitis due to plastic
Irritant contact dermatitis due to rubber

L24.6 Irritant contact dermatitis due to food in contact with skin
Excludes2 dermatitis due to ingested food (L27.2)

L24.7 Irritant contact dermatitis due to plants, except food
Excludes2 allergy NOS to pollen (J30.1)

● **L24.8 Irritant contact dermatitis due to other agents**

L24.81 Irritant contact dermatitis due to metals
Irritant contact dermatitis due to chromium
Irritant contact dermatitis due to nickel

L24.89 Irritant contact dermatitis due to other agents
Irritant contact dermatitis due to dyes

L24.9 Irritant contact dermatitis, unspecified cause
Irritant contact eczema NOS

● **L25 Unspecified contact dermatitis**

Excludes1 allergic contact dermatitis (L23.-)
allergy NOS (T78.40)
dermatitis NOS (L30.9)
irritant contact dermatitis (L24.-)

Excludes2 dermatitis due to ingested substances (L27.-)
dermatitis of eyelid (H01.1-)
eczema of external ear (H60.5-)
perioral dermatitis (L71.0)
radiation-related disorders of the skin and subcutaneous tissue (L55-L59)

L25.0 Unspecified contact dermatitis due to cosmetics

L25.1 Unspecified contact dermatitis due to drugs in contact with skin
Use additional code for adverse effect, if applicable, to identify drug (T36-T50 with fifth or sixth character 5)
Excludes2 dermatitis due to ingested drugs and medicaments (L27.0-L27.1)

L25.2 Unspecified contact dermatitis due to dyes

L25.3 Unspecified contact dermatitis due to other chemical products
Unspecified contact dermatitis due to cement
Unspecified contact dermatitis due to insecticide

L25.4 Unspecified contact dermatitis due to food in contact with skin
Excludes2 dermatitis due to ingested food (L27.2)

L25.5 Unspecified contact dermatitis due to plants, except food
Excludes1 nettle rash (L50.9)
Excludes2 allergy NOS due to pollen (J30.1)

L25.8 Unspecified contact dermatitis due to other agents

L25.9 Unspecified contact dermatitis, unspecified cause
Contact dermatitis (occupational) NOS
Contact eczema (occupational) NOS

L26 Exfoliative dermatitis
Hebra's pityriasis
Excludes1 Ritter's disease (L00)

● **L27 Dermatitis due to substances taken internally**

Excludes1 allergy NOS (T78.40)

Excludes2 adverse food reaction, except dermatitis (T78.0-T78.1)
contact dermatitis (L23-L25)
drug photoallergic response (L56.1)
drug phototoxic response (L56.0)
urticaria (L50.-)

L27.0 Generalized skin eruption due to drugs and medicaments taken internally
Use additional code for adverse effect, if applicable, to identify drug (T36-T50 with fifth or sixth character 5)

L27.1 Localized skin eruption due to drugs and medicaments taken internally
Use additional code for adverse effect, if applicable, to identify drug (T36-T50 with fifth or sixth character 5)

L27.2 Dermatitis due to ingested food
Excludes2 dermatitis due to food in contact with skin (L23.6, L24.6, L25.4)

L27.8 Dermatitis due to other substances taken internally

L27.9 Dermatitis due to unspecified substance taken internally

● **L28 Lichen simplex chronicus and prurigo**

L28.0 Lichen simplex chronicus
Circumscribed neurodermatitis
Lichen NOS

L28.1 Prurigo nodularis

L28.2 Other prurigo
Prurigo NOS
Prurigo Hebra
Prurigo mitis
Urticaria papulosa

● **L29 Pruritus**

Excludes1 neurotic excoriation (L98.1)
psychogenic pruritus (F45.8)

L29.0 Pruritus ani

L29.1 Pruritus scroti ♂

L29.2 Pruritus vulvae ♀

L29.3 Anogenital pruritus, unspecified

L29.8 Other pruritus

L29.9 Pruritus, unspecified
Itch NOS

● L30 Other and unspecified dermatitis
Excludes2 contact dermatitis (L23-L25)
dry skin dermatitis (L85.3)
small plaque parapsoriasis (L41.3)
stasis dermatitis (I87.2)

L30.0 **Nummular dermatitis**

L30.1 **Dyshidrosis [pompholyx]**

L30.2 **Cutaneous autosensitization**
Candidid [levurid] Eczematid
Dermatophytid

L30.3 **Infective dermatitis**
Infectious eczematoid dermatitis

L30.4 **Erythema intertrigo**

L30.5 **Pityriasis alba**
Coding Clinic: 2018, Q1, P6

L30.8 **Other specified dermatitis**

L30.9 **Dermatitis, unspecified**
Eczema NOS

PAPULOSQUAMOUS DISORDERS (L40-L45)

● L40 Psoriasis

L40.0 **Psoriasis vulgaris**
Nummular psoriasis Plaque psoriasis

L40.1 **Generalized pustular psoriasis**
Impetigo herpetiformis Von Zumbusch's disease

L40.2 **Acrodermatitis continua**

L40.3 **Pustulosis palmaris et plantaris**

L40.4 **Guttate psoriasis**

● L40.5 **Arthropathic psoriasis**

L40.50 **Arthropathic psoriasis, unspecified** HCC

L40.51 **Distal interphalangeal psoriatic arthropathy** HCC

L40.52 **Psoriatic arthritis mutilans** HCC

L40.53 **Psoriatic spondylitis** HCC

L40.54 **Psoriatic juvenile arthropathy** HCC

L40.59 **Other psoriatic arthropathy** HCC

L40.8 **Other psoriasis**
Flexural psoriasis

L40.9 **Psoriasis, unspecified**

● L41 Parapsoriasis
Excludes1 poikiloderma vasculare atrophicans (L94.5)

L41.0 **Pityriasis lichenoides et varioliformis acuta**
Mucha-Habermann disease

L41.1 **Pityriasis lichenoides chronica**

L41.3 **Small plaque parapsoriasis**

L41.4 **Large plaque parapsoriasis**

L41.5 **Retiform parapsoriasis**

L41.8 **Other parapsoriasis**

L41.9 **Parapsoriasis, unspecified**

L42 Pityriasis rosea

● L43 Lichen planus
Excludes1 lichen planopilaris (L66.1)

L43.0 **Hypertrophic lichen planus**

L43.1 **Bullous lichen planus**

L43.2 **Lichenoid drug reaction**
Use additional code for adverse effect, if applicable, to identify drug (T36-T50 with fifth or sixth character 5)

L43.3 **Subacute (active) lichen planus**
Lichen planus tropicus

L43.8 **Other lichen planus**

L43.9 **Lichen planus, unspecified**

Item 12-8 Psoriasis is a chronic, recurrent inflammatory skin disease characterized by small patches covered with thick, silvery scales. **Parapsoriasis** is a treatment-resistant erythroderma. **Pityriasis rosea** is characterized by a herald patch that is a single large lesion and that usually appears on the trunk and is followed by scattered, smaller lesions.

● L44 Other papulosquamous disorders

L44.0 **Pityriasis rubra pilaris**

L44.1 **Lichen nitidus**

L44.2 **Lichen striatus**

L44.3 **Lichen ruber moniliformis**

L44.4 **Infantile papular acrodermatitis [Gianotti-Crosti]** P

L44.8 **Other specified papulosquamous disorders**

L44.9 **Papulosquamous disorder, unspecified**

L45 *Papulosquamous disorders in diseases classified elsewhere*
Code first underlying disease

URTICARIA AND ERYTHEMA (L49-L54)

Excludes1 Lyme disease (A69.2-)
rosacea (L71.-)

● L49 Exfoliation due to erythematous conditions according to extent of body surface involved
Code first erythematous condition causing exfoliation, such as:
Ritter's disease (L00)
(Staphylococcal) scalded skin syndrome (L00)
Stevens-Johnson syndrome (L51.1)
Stevens-Johnson syndrome-toxic epidermal necrolysis overlap syndrome (L51.3)
Toxic epidermal necrolysis (L51.2)

L49.0 **Exfoliation due to erythematous condition involving less than 10 percent of body surface**
Exfoliation due to erythematous condition NOS

L49.1 **Exfoliation due to erythematous condition involving 10-19 percent of body surface**

L49.2 **Exfoliation due to erythematous condition involving 20-29 percent of body surface**

L49.3 **Exfoliation due to erythematous condition involving 30-39 percent of body surface**

L49.4 **Exfoliation due to erythematous condition involving 40-49 percent of body surface**

L49.5 **Exfoliation due to erythematous condition involving 50-59 percent of body surface**

L49.6 **Exfoliation due to erythematous condition involving 60-69 percent of body surface**

L49.7 **Exfoliation due to erythematous condition involving 70-79 percent of body surface**

L49.8 **Exfoliation due to erythematous condition involving 80-89 percent of body surface**

L49.9 **Exfoliation due to erythematous condition involving 90 or more percent of body surface**

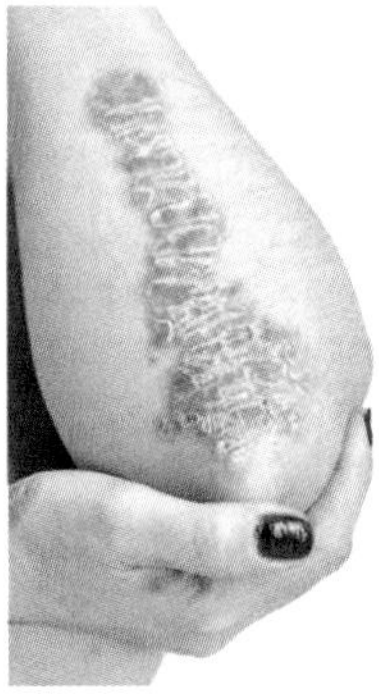

Figure 12-6 Erythematous plaques with silvery scales in a patient with psoriasis. (Getty Image)

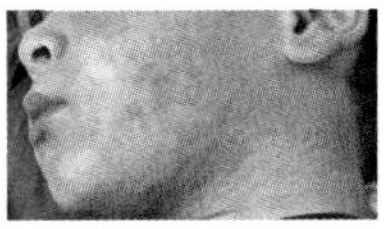

Figure 12-7 Urticaria (hives). *(Courtesy of David Effron, MD.)* (Getty Image)

Item 12-9 Urticaria is a vascular reaction in which wheals surrounded by a red halo appear and cause severe itching. The causes of urticaria or hives are extensive and varied (e.g., food, heat, cold, drugs, stress, infections).

L5Ø Urticaria

Excludes1 allergic contact dermatitis (L23.-)
angioneurotic edema (T78.3)
giant urticaria (T78.3)
hereditary angio-edema (D84.1)
Quincke's edema (T78.3)
serum urticaria (T8Ø.6-)
solar urticaria (L56.3)
urticaria neonatorum (P83.8)
urticaria papulosa (L28.2)
urticaria pigmentosa (D47.Ø1)

L5Ø.Ø Allergic urticaria

L5Ø.1 Idiopathic urticaria

L5Ø.2 Urticaria due to cold and heat
Excludes2 familial cold urticaria (MØ4.2)

L5Ø.3 Dermatographic urticaria

L5Ø.4 Vibratory urticaria

L5Ø.5 Cholinergic urticaria

L5Ø.6 Contact urticaria

L5Ø.8 Other urticaria
Chronic urticaria
Recurrent periodic urticaria

L5Ø.9 Urticaria, unspecified

L51 Erythema multiforme

Use additional code for adverse effect, if applicable, to identify drug (T36-T5Ø with fifth or sixth character 5)

Use additional code to identify associated manifestations, such as:
arthropathy associated with dermatological disorders (M14.8-)
conjunctival edema (H11.42)
conjunctivitis (H1Ø.22-)
corneal scars and opacities (H17.-)
corneal ulcer (H16.Ø-)
edema of eyelid (HØ2.84-)
inflammation of eyelid (HØ1.8)
keratoconjunctivitis sicca (H16.22-)
mechanical lagophthalmos (HØ2.22-)
stomatitis (K12.-)
symblepharon (H11.23-)

Use additional code to identify percentage of skin exfoliation (L49.-)

Excludes1 staphylococcal scalded skin syndrome (LØØ)
Ritter's disease (LØØ)

L51.Ø Nonbullous erythema multiforme

L51.1 Stevens-Johnson syndrome

L51.2 Toxic epidermal necrolysis [Lyell]

L51.3 Stevens-Johnson syndrome-toxic epidermal necrolysis overlap syndrome
SJS-TEN overlap syndrome

L51.8 Other erythema multiforme

L51.9 Erythema multiforme, unspecified
Erythema iris
Erythema multiforme major NOS
Erythema multiforme minor NOS
Herpes iris

L52 Erythema nodosum

Excludes1 tuberculous erythema nodosum (A18.4)

L53 Other erythematous conditions

Excludes1 erythema ab igne (L59.Ø)
erythema due to external agents in contact with skin (L23-L25)
erythema intertrigo (L3Ø.4)

L53.Ø Toxic erythema
Code first poisoning due to drug or toxin, if applicable (T36-T65 with fifth or sixth character 1-4 or 6)
Use additional code for adverse effect, if applicable, to identify drug (T36-T5Ø with fifth or sixth character 5)
Excludes1 neonatal erythema toxicum (P83.1)

L53.1 Erythema annulare centrifugum

L53.2 Erythema marginatum

L53.3 Other chronic figurate erythema

L53.8 Other specified erythematous conditions

L53.9 Erythematous condition, unspecified
Erythema NOS
Erythroderma NOS

L54 Erythema in diseases classified elsewhere
Code first underlying disease

RADIATION-RELATED DISORDERS OF THE SKIN AND SUBCUTANEOUS TISSUE (L55-L59)

L55 Sunburn

L55.Ø Sunburn of first degree

L55.1 Sunburn of second degree

L55.2 Sunburn of third degree

L55.9 Sunburn, unspecified

L56 Other acute skin changes due to ultraviolet radiation

Use additional code to identify the source of the ultraviolet radiation (W89, X32)

L56.Ø Drug phototoxic response
Use additional code for adverse effect, if applicable, to identify drug (T36-T5Ø with fifth or sixth character 5)

L56.1 Drug photoallergic response
Use additional code for adverse effect, if applicable, to identify drug (T36-T5Ø with fifth or sixth character 5)

L56.2 Photocontact dermatitis [berloque dermatitis]

L56.3 Solar urticaria

L56.4 Polymorphous light eruption

L56.5 Disseminated superficial actinic porokeratosis (DSAP)

L56.8 Other specified acute skin changes due to ultraviolet radiation

L56.9 Acute skin change due to ultraviolet radiation, unspecified

L57 Skin changes due to chronic exposure to nonionizing radiation

Use additional code to identify the source of the ultraviolet radiation (W89)

L57.Ø Actinic keratosis
Keratosis NOS
Senile keratosis
Solar keratosis

L57.1 Actinic reticuloid

L57.2 Cutis rhomboidalis nuchae

L57.3 Poikiloderma of Civatte

L57.4 Cutis laxa senilis
Elastosis senilis

L57.5 Actinic granuloma

L57.8 Other skin changes due to chronic exposure to nonionizing radiation
Farmer's skin
Sailor's skin
Solar dermatitis

L57.9 Skin changes due to chronic exposure to nonionizing radiation, unspecified

L58 Radiodermatitis
Use additional code to identify the source of the radiation (W88, W90)
- L58.0 **Acute radiodermatitis**
- L58.1 **Chronic radiodermatitis**
- L58.9 **Radiodermatitis, unspecified**

L59 Other disorders of skin and subcutaneous tissue related to radiation
- L59.0 **Erythema ab igne [dermatitis ab igne]**
- L59.8 **Other specified disorders of the skin and subcutaneous tissue related to radiation**
  Coding Clinic: 2017, Q1, P34
- L59.9 **Disorder of the skin and subcutaneous tissue related to radiation, unspecified**

DISORDERS OF SKIN APPENDAGES (L60-L75)

Excludes1 congenital malformations of integument (Q84.-)

L60 Nail disorders
Excludes2 clubbing of nails (R68.3)
onychia and paronychia (L03.0-)
- L60.0 **Ingrowing nail**
- L60.1 **Onycholysis**
- L60.2 **Onychogryphosis**
- L60.3 **Nail dystrophy**
- L60.4 **Beau's lines**
- L60.5 **Yellow nail syndrome**
- L60.8 **Other nail disorders**
- L60.9 **Nail disorder, unspecified**

L62 Nail disorders in diseases classified elsewhere
Code first underlying disease, such as:
pachydermoperiostosis (M89.4-)

L63 Alopecia areata
- L63.0 **Alopecia (capitis) totalis**
- L63.1 **Alopecia universalis**
- L63.2 **Ophiasis**
- L63.8 **Other alopecia areata**
- L63.9 **Alopecia areata, unspecified**

Item 12-10 Alopecia is lack of hair and takes many forms. The most common is male pattern alopecia, also known as **androgenetic alopecia. Telogen effluvium** is early and excessive loss of hair resulting from a trauma to the hair follicle (fever, drugs, surgery, etc.).

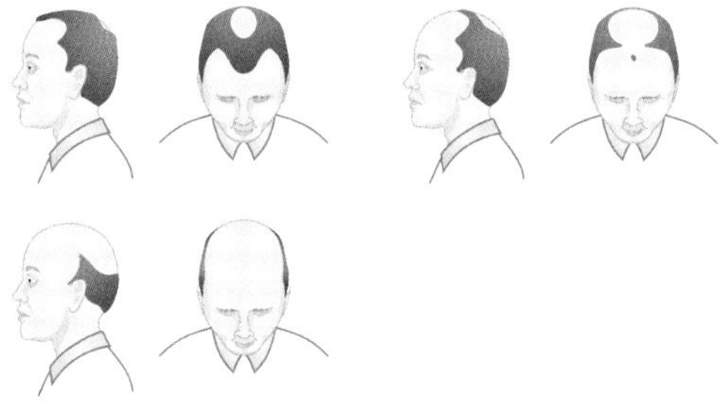

Figure 12-8 Male pattern alopecia.

L64 Androgenic alopecia
Includes male-pattern baldness
- L64.0 **Drug-induced androgenic alopecia**
  Use additional code for adverse effect, if applicable, to identify drug (T36-T50 with fifth or sixth character 5)
- L64.8 **Other androgenic alopecia**
- L64.9 **Androgenic alopecia, unspecified**

L65 Other nonscarring hair loss
Use additional code for adverse effect, if applicable, to identify drug (T36-T50 with fifth or sixth character 5)
Excludes1 trichotillomania (F63.3)
- L65.0 **Telogen effluvium**
- L65.1 **Anagen effluvium**
- L65.2 **Alopecia mucinosa**
- L65.8 **Other specified nonscarring hair loss**
- L65.9 **Nonscarring hair loss, unspecified**
  Alopecia NOS

L66 Cicatricial alopecia [scarring hair loss]
- L66.0 **Pseudopelade**
- L66.1 **Lichen planopilaris**
  Follicular lichen planus
- L66.2 **Folliculitis decalvans**
- L66.3 **Perifolliculitis capitis abscedens**
- L66.4 **Folliculitis ulerythematosa reticulata**
- L66.8 **Other cicatricial alopecia**
  Coding Clinic: 2015, Q1, P19
- L66.9 **Cicatricial alopecia, unspecified**

L67 Hair color and hair shaft abnormalities
Excludes1 monilethrix (Q84.1)
pili annulati (Q84.1)
telogen effluvium (L65.0)
- L67.0 **Trichorrhexis nodosa**
- L67.1 **Variations in hair color**
  Canities
  Greyness, hair (premature)
  Heterochromia of hair
  Poliosis circumscripta, acquired
  Poliosis NOS
- L67.8 **Other hair color and hair shaft abnormalities**
  Fragilitas crinium
- L67.9 **Hair color and hair shaft abnormality, unspecified**

L68 Hypertrichosis
Includes excess hair
Excludes1 congenital hypertrichosis (Q84.2)
persistent lanugo (Q84.2)
- L68.0 **Hirsutism**
  Excessive growth of hair
- L68.1 **Acquired hypertrichosis lanuginosa**
- L68.2 **Localized hypertrichosis**
- L68.3 **Polytrichia**
- L68.8 **Other hypertrichosis**
- L68.9 **Hypertrichosis, unspecified**

L70 Acne
Excludes2 acne keloid (L73.0)
- L70.0 Acne vulgaris
- L70.1 Acne conglobata
- L70.2 Acne varioliformis
  Acne necrotica miliaris
- L70.3 Acne tropica
- L70.4 Infantile acne P
- L70.5 Acné excoriée
  Acné excoriée des jeunes filles
  Picker's acne
- L70.8 Other acne
- L70.9 Acne, unspecified

L71 Rosacea
Use additional code for adverse effect, if applicable, to identify drug (T36-T50 with fifth or sixth character 5)
- L71.0 Perioral dermatitis
- L71.1 Rhinophyma
- L71.8 Other rosacea
  Coding Clinic: 2018, Q4, P15
- L71.9 Rosacea, unspecified

L72 Follicular cysts of skin and subcutaneous tissue
- L72.0 Epidermal cyst
- L72.1 Pilar and trichodermal cyst
  - L72.11 Pilar cyst
  - L72.12 Trichodermal cyst
    Trichilemmal (proliferating) cyst
- L72.3 Sebaceous cyst
  Excludes2 pilar cyst (L72.11)
  trichilemmal (proliferating) cyst (L72.12)
- L72.2 Steatocystoma multiplex
- L72.8 Other follicular cysts of the skin and subcutaneous tissue
- L72.9 Follicular cyst of the skin and subcutaneous tissue, unspecified

L73 Other follicular disorders
- L73.0 Acne keloid
- L73.1 Pseudofolliculitis barbae
- L73.2 Hidradenitis suppurativa
- L73.8 Other specified follicular disorders
  Sycosis barbae
- L73.9 Follicular disorder, unspecified

L74 Eccrine sweat disorders
Excludes2 generalized hyperhidrosis (R61)
- L74.0 Miliaria rubra
- L74.1 Miliaria crystallina
- L74.2 Miliaria profunda
  Miliaria tropicalis
- L74.3 Miliaria, unspecified
- L74.4 Anhidrosis
  Hypohidrosis
- L74.5 Focal hyperhidrosis
  - L74.51 Primary focal hyperhidrosis
    - L74.510 Primary focal hyperhidrosis, axilla
    - L74.511 Primary focal hyperhidrosis, face
    - L74.512 Primary focal hyperhidrosis, palms
    - L74.513 Primary focal hyperhidrosis, soles
    - L74.519 Primary focal hyperhidrosis, unspecified
  - L74.52 Secondary focal hyperhidrosis
    Frey's syndrome
- L74.8 Other eccrine sweat disorders
- L74.9 Eccrine sweat disorder, unspecified
  Sweat gland disorder NOS

L75 Apocrine sweat disorders
Excludes1 dyshidrosis (L30.1)
hidradenitis suppurativa (L73.2)
- L75.0 Bromhidrosis
- L75.1 Chromhidrosis
- L75.2 Apocrine miliaria
  Fox-Fordyce disease
- L75.8 Other apocrine sweat disorders
- L75.9 Apocrine sweat disorder, unspecified
  Intraoperative and postprocedural complications of skin and subcutaneous tissue (L76)

INTRAOPERATIVE AND POSTPROCEDURAL COMPLICATIONS OF SKIN AND SUBCUTANEOUS TISSUE (L76)

L76 Intraoperative and postprocedural complications of skin and subcutaneous tissue
Coding Clinic: 2016, Q4, P10
- L76.0 Intraoperative hemorrhage and hematoma of skin and subcutaneous tissue complicating a procedure
  Excludes1 intraoperative hemorrhage and hematoma of skin and subcutaneous tissue due to accidental puncture and laceration during a procedure (L76.1-)
  - L76.01 Intraoperative hemorrhage and hematoma of skin and subcutaneous tissue complicating a dermatologic procedure
  - L76.02 Intraoperative hemorrhage and hematoma of skin and subcutaneous tissue complicating other procedure
- L76.1 Accidental puncture and laceration of skin and subcutaneous tissue during a procedure
  - L76.11 Accidental puncture and laceration of skin and subcutaneous tissue during a dermatologic procedure
  - L76.12 Accidental puncture and laceration of skin and subcutaneous tissue during other procedure
- L76.2 Postprocedural hemorrhage of skin and subcutaneous tissue following a procedure
  - L76.21 Postprocedural hemorrhage of skin and subcutaneous tissue following a dermatologic procedure
  - L76.22 Postprocedural hemorrhage of skin and subcutaneous tissue following other procedure
- L76.3 Postprocedural hematoma and seroma of skin and subcutaneous tissue following a procedure
  - L76.31 Postprocedural hematoma of skin and subcutaneous tissue following a dermatologic procedure
  - L76.32 Postprocedural hematoma of skin and subcutaneous tissue following other procedure
  - L76.33 Postprocedural seroma of skin and subcutaneous tissue following a dermatologic procedure
  - L76.34 Postprocedural seroma of skin and subcutaneous tissue following other procedure
- L76.8 Other intraoperative and postprocedural complications of skin and subcutaneous tissue
  Use additional code, if applicable, to further specify disorder
  - L76.81 Other intraoperative complications of skin and subcutaneous tissue
  - L76.82 Other postprocedural complications of skin and subcutaneous tissue
    Coding Clinic: 2017, Q3, P6

CHAPTER 12 (L00-L99)

OTHER DISORDERS OF THE SKIN AND SUBCUTANEOUS TISSUE (L80-L99)

L80 Vitiligo
Excludes2 vitiligo of eyelids (H02.73-)
vitiligo of vulva (N90.89)

L81 Other disorders of pigmentation
Excludes1 birthmark NOS (Q82.5)
Peutz-Jeghers syndrome (Q85.8)
Excludes2 nevus - see Alphabetical Index
L81.0 Postinflammatory hyperpigmentation
L81.1 Chloasma
L81.2 Freckles
L81.3 Café au lait spots
L81.4 Other melanin hyperpigmentation
Lentigo
L81.5 Leukoderma, not elsewhere classified
L81.6 Other disorders of diminished melanin formation
L81.7 Pigmented purpuric dermatosis
Angioma serpiginosum
L81.8 Other specified disorders of pigmentation
Iron pigmentation
Tattoo pigmentation
L81.9 Disorder of pigmentation, unspecified

L82 Seborrheic keratosis
Includes basal cell papilloma
dermatosis papulosa nigra
Leser-Trélat disease
Excludes2 seborrheic dermatitis (L21.-)
L82.0 Inflamed seborrheic keratosis
L82.1 Other seborrheic keratosis
Seborrheic keratosis NOS

L83 Acanthosis nigricans
Confluent and reticulated papillomatosis

L84 Corns and callosities
Callus
Clavus

L85 Other epidermal thickening
Excludes2 hypertrophic disorders of the skin (L91.-)
L85.0 Acquired ichthyosis
Excludes1 congenital ichthyosis (Q80.-)
L85.1 Acquired keratosis [keratoderma] palmaris et plantaris
Excludes1 inherited keratosis palmaris et plantaris (Q82.8)
L85.2 Keratosis punctata (palmaris et plantaris)
L85.3 Xerosis cutis
Dry skin dermatitis
L85.8 Other specified epidermal thickening
Cutaneous horn
L85.9 Epidermal thickening, unspecified

L86 Keratoderma in diseases classified elsewhere
Firm horny papules that have a cobblestone appearance
Code first underlying disease, such as:
Reiter's disease (M02.3-)
Excludes1 gonococcal keratoderma (A54.89)
gonococcal keratosis (A54.89)
keratoderma due to vitamin A deficiency (E50.8)
keratosis due to vitamin A deficiency (E50.8)
xeroderma due to vitamin A deficiency (E50.8)

L87 Transepidermal elimination disorders
Excludes1 granuloma annulare (perforating) (L92.0)
L87.0 Keratosis follicularis et parafollicularis in cutem penetrans
Kyrle disease
Hyperkeratosis follicularis penetrans
L87.1 Reactive perforating collagenosis
L87.2 Elastosis perforans serpiginosa
L87.8 Other transepidermal elimination disorders
L87.9 Transepidermal elimination disorder, unspecified

L88 Pyoderma gangrenosum
Phagedenic pyoderma
Excludes1 dermatitis gangrenosa (L08.0)

OGCR Section I.B.14.

General Coding Guidelines

Documentation for BMI, *Depth of* Non-pressure ulcers, Pressure Ulcer Stages, **Coma Scale, and *NIH Stroke Scale***

For the Body Mass Index (BMI), depth of non-pressure chronic ulcers, pressure ulcer stage**, coma scale, and NIH stroke scale (NIHSS) codes,** code assignment may be based on medical record documentation from clinicians who are not the patient's provider (i.e., physician or other qualified healthcare practitioner legally accountable for establishing the patient's diagnosis), since this information is typically documented by other clinicians involved in the care of the patient (e.g., a dietitian often documents the BMI, a nurse often documents the pressure ulcer stages**, and an emergency medical technician often documents the coma scale**). However, the associated diagnosis (such as overweight, obesity, **acute stroke,** or pressure ulcer) must be documented by the patient's provider. If there is conflicting medical record documentation, either from the same clinician or different clinicians, the patient's attending provider should be queried for clarification.

The BMI, **coma scale, and NIHSS** codes should only be reported as secondary diagnoses.

L89 Pressure ulcer
Includes bed sore, decubitus ulcer, plaster ulcer, pressure area, pressure sore
Code first any associated gangrene (I96)
Excludes2 decubitus (trophic) ulcer of cervix (uteri) (N86)
diabetic ulcers (E08.621, E08.622, E09.621, E09.622, E10.621, E10.622, E11.621, E11.622, E13.621, E13.622)
non-pressure chronic ulcer of skin (L97.-)
skin infections (L00-L08)
varicose ulcer (I83.0, I83.2)
Coding Clinic: 2018, Q2, P22; 2016, Q4, P124
L89.0 Pressure ulcer of elbow
L89.00 Pressure ulcer of unspecified elbow
L89.000 Pressure ulcer of unspecified elbow, unstageable
L89.001 Pressure ulcer of unspecified elbow, stage 1
Healing pressure ulcer of unspecified elbow, stage 1
Pressure pre-ulcer skin changes limited to persistent focal edema, unspecified elbow
L89.002 Pressure ulcer of unspecified elbow, stage 2
Healing pressure ulcer of unspecified elbow, stage 2
Pressure ulcer with abrasion, blister, partial thickness skin loss involving epidermis and/or dermis, unspecified elbow

CHAPTER 12 (L00-L99)

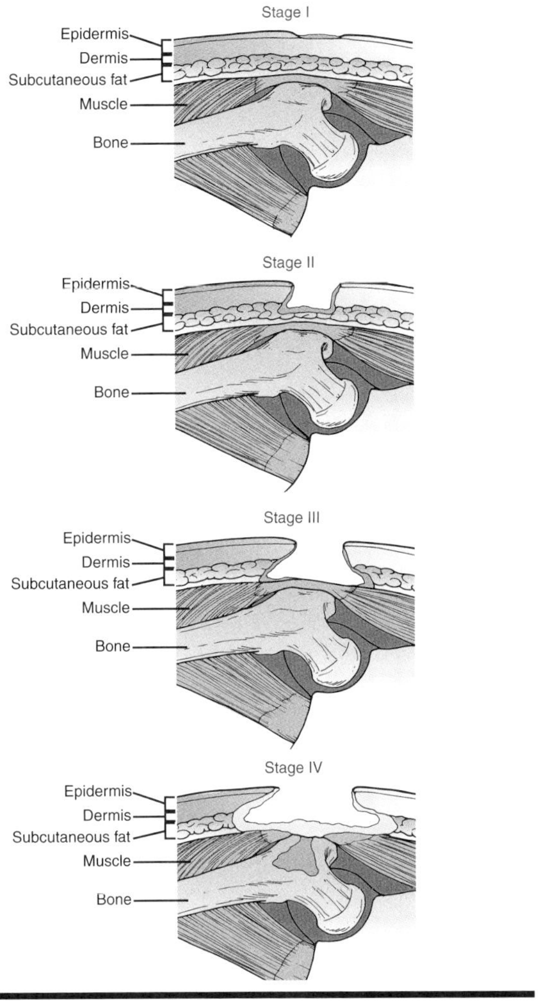

Figure 12-9 Stage I, II, III, and IV of pressure ulcers.

L89.ØØ3 Pressure ulcer of unspecified elbow, stage 3
- Healing pressure ulcer of unspecified elbow, stage 3
- Pressure ulcer with full thickness skin loss involving damage or necrosis of subcutaneous tissue, unspecified elbow

L89.ØØ4 Pressure ulcer of unspecified elbow, stage 4
- Healing pressure ulcer of unspecified elbow, stage 4
- Pressure ulcer with necrosis of soft tissues through to underlying muscle, tendon, or bone, unspecified elbow

▶ **L89.ØØ6 Pressure-induced deep tissue damage of unspecified elbow**

L89.ØØ9 Pressure ulcer of unspecified elbow, unspecified stage
- Healing pressure ulcer of elbow NOS
- Healing pressure ulcer of unspecified elbow, unspecified stage

● **L89.Ø1 Pressure ulcer of right elbow**

L89.Ø1Ø Pressure ulcer of right elbow, unstageable

L89.Ø11 Pressure ulcer of right elbow, stage 1
- Healing pressure ulcer of right elbow, stage 1
- Pressure pre-ulcer skin changes limited to persistent focal edema, right elbow

L89.Ø12 Pressure ulcer of right elbow, stage 2
- Healing pressure ulcer of right elbow, stage 2
- Pressure ulcer with abrasion, blister, partial thickness skin loss involving epidermis and/or dermis, right elbow

L89.Ø13 Pressure ulcer of right elbow, stage 3
- Healing pressure ulcer of right elbow, stage 3
- Pressure ulcer with full thickness skin loss involving damage or necrosis of subcutaneous tissue, right elbow

L89.Ø14 Pressure ulcer of right elbow, stage 4
- Healing pressure ulcer of right elbow, stage 4
- Pressure ulcer with necrosis of soft tissues through to underlying muscle, tendon, or bone, right elbow

▶ **L89.Ø16 Pressure-induced deep tissue damage of right elbow**

L89.Ø19 Pressure ulcer of right elbow, unspecified stage
- Healing pressure right of elbow NOS
- Healing pressure ulcer of right elbow, unspecified stage

● **L89.Ø2 Pressure ulcer of left elbow**

L89.Ø2Ø Pressure ulcer of left elbow, unstageable

L89.Ø21 Pressure ulcer of left elbow, stage 1
- Healing pressure ulcer of left elbow, stage 1
- Pressure pre-ulcer skin changes limited to persistent focal edema, left elbow

L89.Ø22 Pressure ulcer of left elbow, stage 2
- Healing pressure ulcer of left elbow, stage 2
- Pressure ulcer with abrasion, blister, partial thickness skin loss involving epidermis and/or dermis, left elbow

L89.Ø23 Pressure ulcer of left elbow, stage 3
- Healing pressure ulcer of left elbow, stage 3
- Pressure ulcer with full thickness skin loss involving damage or necrosis of subcutaneous tissue, left elbow

L89.Ø24 Pressure ulcer of left elbow, stage 4
- Healing pressure ulcer of left elbow, stage 4
- Pressure ulcer with necrosis of soft tissues through to underlying muscle, tendon, or bone, left elbow

▶L89.026 **Pressure-induced deep tissue damage of left elbow**

L89.029 **Pressure ulcer of left elbow, unspecified stage**
Healing pressure ulcer of left of elbow NOS
Healing pressure ulcer of left elbow, unspecified stage

● L89.1 **Pressure ulcer of back**

● L89.10 **Pressure ulcer of unspecified part of back**

L89.100 **Pressure ulcer of unspecified part of back, unstageable** HCC

L89.101 **Pressure ulcer of unspecified part of back, stage 1**
Healing pressure ulcer of unspecified part of back, stage 1
Pressure pre-ulcer skin changes limited to persistent focal edema, unspecified part of back

L89.102 **Pressure ulcer of unspecified part of back, stage 2**
Healing pressure ulcer of unspecified part of back, stage 2
Pressure ulcer with abrasion, blister, partial thickness skin loss involving epidermis and/or dermis, unspecified part of back

L89.103 **Pressure ulcer of unspecified part of back, stage 3** HCC
Healing pressure ulcer of unspecified part of back, stage 3
Pressure ulcer with full thickness skin loss involving damage or necrosis of subcutaneous tissue, unspecified part of back

L89.104 **Pressure ulcer of unspecified part of back, stage 4** HCC
Healing pressure ulcer of unspecified part of back, stage 4
Pressure ulcer with necrosis of soft tissues through to underlying muscle, tendon, or bone, unspecified part of back

▶L89.106 **Pressure-induced deep tissue damage of unspecified part of back**

L89.109 **Pressure ulcer of unspecified part of back, unspecified stage**
Healing pressure ulcer of unspecified part of back NOS
Healing pressure ulcer of unspecified part of back, unspecified stage

● L89.11 **Pressure ulcer of right upper back**
Pressure ulcer of right shoulder blade

L89.110 **Pressure ulcer of right upper back, unstageable** HCC

L89.111 **Pressure ulcer of right upper back, stage 1**
Healing pressure ulcer of right upper back, stage 1
Pressure pre-ulcer skin changes limited to persistent focal edema, right upper back

L89.112 **Pressure ulcer of right upper back, stage 2**
Healing pressure ulcer of right upper back, stage 2
Pressure ulcer with abrasion, blister, partial thickness skin loss involving epidermis and/or dermis, right upper back

L89.113 **Pressure ulcer of right upper back, stage 3** HCC
Healing pressure ulcer of right upper back, stage 3
Pressure ulcer with full thickness skin loss involving damage or necrosis of subcutaneous tissue, right upper back

L89.114 **Pressure ulcer of right upper back, stage 4** HCC
Healing pressure ulcer of right upper back, stage 4
Pressure ulcer with necrosis of soft tissues through to underlying muscle, tendon, or bone, right upper back

▶L89.116 **Pressure-induced deep tissue damage of right upper back**

L89.119 **Pressure ulcer of right upper back, unspecified stage**
Healing pressure ulcer of right upper back NOS
Healing pressure ulcer of right upper back, unspecified stage

● L89.12 **Pressure ulcer of left upper back**
Pressure ulcer of left shoulder blade

L89.120 **Pressure ulcer of left upper back, unstageable** HCC

L89.121 **Pressure ulcer of left upper back, stage 1**
Healing pressure ulcer of left upper back, stage 1
Pressure pre-ulcer skin changes limited to persistent focal edema, left upper back

L89.122 **Pressure ulcer of left upper back, stage 2**
Healing pressure ulcer of left upper back, stage 2
Pressure ulcer with abrasion, blister, partial thickness skin loss involving epidermis and/or dermis, left upper back

L89.123 **Pressure ulcer of left upper back, stage 3** HCC
Healing pressure ulcer of left upper back, stage 3
Pressure ulcer with full thickness skin loss involving damage or necrosis of subcutaneous tissue, left upper back

L89.124 **Pressure ulcer of left upper back, stage 4** HCC
Healing pressure ulcer of left upper back, stage 4
Pressure ulcer with necrosis of soft tissues through to underlying muscle, tendon, or bone, left upper back

▶L89.126 **Pressure-induced deep tissue damage of left upper back**

L89.129 **Pressure ulcer of left upper back, unspecified stage**
Healing pressure ulcer of left upper back NOS
Healing pressure ulcer of left upper back, unspecified stage

- **L89.13 Pressure ulcer of right lower back**
  - **L89.130 Pressure ulcer of right lower back, unstageable**
  - **L89.131 Pressure ulcer of right lower back, stage 1**
    - Healing pressure ulcer of right lower back, stage 1
    - Pressure pre-ulcer skin changes limited to persistent focal edema, right lower back
  - **L89.132 Pressure ulcer of right lower back, stage 2**
    - Healing pressure ulcer of right lower back, stage 2
    - Pressure ulcer with abrasion, blister, partial thickness skin loss involving epidermis and/or dermis, right lower back
  - **L89.133 Pressure ulcer of right lower back, stage 3**
    - Healing pressure ulcer of right lower back, stage 3
    - Pressure ulcer with full thickness skin loss involving damage or necrosis of subcutaneous tissue, right lower back
  - **L89.134 Pressure ulcer of right lower back, stage 4**
    - Healing pressure ulcer of right lower back, stage 4
    - Pressure ulcer with necrosis of soft tissues through to underlying muscle, tendon, or bone, right lower back
  - **L89.136 Pressure-induced deep tissue damage of right lower back**
  - **L89.139 Pressure ulcer of right lower back, unspecified stage**
    - Healing pressure ulcer of right lower back NOS
    - Healing pressure ulcer of right lower back, unspecified stage
- **L89.14 Pressure ulcer of left lower back**
  - **L89.140 Pressure ulcer of left lower back, unstageable**
  - **L89.141 Pressure ulcer of left lower back, stage 1**
    - Healing pressure ulcer of left lower back, stage 1
    - Pressure pre-ulcer skin changes limited to persistent focal edema, left lower back
  - **L89.142 Pressure ulcer of left lower back, stage 2**
    - Healing pressure ulcer of left lower back, stage 2
    - Pressure ulcer with abrasion, blister, partial thickness skin loss involving epidermis and/or dermis, left lower back
  - **L89.143 Pressure ulcer of left lower back, stage 3**
    - Healing pressure ulcer of left lower back, stage 3
    - Pressure ulcer with full thickness skin loss involving damage or necrosis of subcutaneous tissue, left lower back
  - **L89.144 Pressure ulcer of left lower back, stage 4**
    - Healing pressure ulcer of left lower back, stage 4
    - Pressure ulcer with necrosis of soft tissues through to underlying muscle, tendon, or bone, left lower back
  - **L89.146 Pressure-induced deep tissue damage of left lower back**
  - **L89.149 Pressure ulcer of left lower back, unspecified stage**
    - Healing pressure ulcer of left lower back NOS
    - Healing pressure ulcer of left lower back, unspecified stage
- **L89.15 Pressure ulcer of sacral region**
  - Pressure ulcer of coccyx
  - Pressure ulcer of tailbone
  - **L89.150 Pressure ulcer of sacral region, unstageable**
  - **L89.151 Pressure ulcer of sacral region, stage 1**
    - Healing pressure ulcer of sacral region, stage 1
    - Pressure pre-ulcer skin changes limited to persistent focal edema, sacral region
  - **L89.152 Pressure ulcer of sacral region, stage 2**
    - Healing pressure ulcer of sacral region, stage 2
    - Pressure ulcer with abrasion, blister, partial thickness skin loss involving epidermis and/or dermis, sacral region
  - **L89.153 Pressure ulcer of sacral region, stage 3**
    - Healing pressure ulcer of sacral region, stage 3
    - Pressure ulcer with full thickness skin loss involving damage or necrosis of subcutaneous tissue, sacral region
  - **L89.154 Pressure ulcer of sacral region, stage 4**
    - Healing pressure ulcer of sacral region, stage 4
    - Pressure ulcer with necrosis of soft tissues through to underlying muscle, tendon, or bone, sacral region
  - **L89.156 Pressure-induced deep tissue damage of sacral region**
  - **L89.159 Pressure ulcer of sacral region, unspecified stage**
    - Healing pressure ulcer of sacral region NOS
    - Healing pressure ulcer of sacral region, unspecified stage
- **L89.2 Pressure ulcer of hip**
  - **L89.20 Pressure ulcer of unspecified hip**
    - **L89.200 Pressure ulcer of unspecified hip, unstageable**
    - **L89.201 Pressure ulcer of unspecified hip, stage 1**
      - Healing pressure ulcer of unspecified hip back, stage 1
      - Pressure pre-ulcer skin changes limited to persistent focal edema, unspecified hip

L89.202 Pressure ulcer of unspecified hip, stage 2
Healing pressure ulcer of unspecified hip, stage 2
Pressure ulcer with abrasion, blister, partial thickness skin loss involving epidermis and/or dermis, unspecified hip

L89.203 Pressure ulcer of unspecified hip, stage 3
Healing pressure ulcer of unspecified hip, stage 3
Pressure ulcer with full thickness skin loss involving damage or necrosis of subcutaneous tissue, unspecified hip

L89.204 Pressure ulcer of unspecified hip, stage 4
Healing pressure ulcer of unspecified hip, stage 4
Pressure ulcer with necrosis of soft tissues through to underlying muscle, tendon, or bone, unspecified hip

L89.206 Pressure-induced deep tissue damage of unspecified hip

L89.209 Pressure ulcer of unspecified hip, unspecified stage
Healing pressure ulcer of unspecified hip NOS
Healing pressure ulcer of unspecified hip, unspecified stage

L89.21 Pressure ulcer of right hip

L89.210 Pressure ulcer of right hip, unstageable

L89.211 Pressure ulcer of right hip, stage 1
Healing pressure ulcer of right hip back, stage 1
Pressure pre-ulcer skin changes limited to persistent focal edema, right hip

L89.212 Pressure ulcer of right hip, stage 2
Healing pressure ulcer of right hip, stage 2
Pressure ulcer with abrasion, blister, partial thickness skin loss involving epidermis and/or dermis, right hip

L89.213 Pressure ulcer of right hip, stage 3
Healing pressure ulcer of right hip, stage 3
Pressure ulcer with full thickness skin loss involving damage or necrosis of subcutaneous tissue, right hip

L89.214 Pressure ulcer of right hip, stage 4
Healing pressure ulcer of right hip, stage 4
Pressure ulcer with necrosis of soft tissues through to underlying muscle, tendon, or bone, right hip

L89.216 Pressure-induced deep tissue damage of right hip

L89.219 Pressure ulcer of right hip, unspecified stage
Healing pressure ulcer of right hip NOS
Healing pressure ulcer of right hip, unspecified stage

L89.22 Pressure ulcer of left hip

L89.220 Pressure ulcer of left hip, unstageable

L89.221 Pressure ulcer of left hip, stage 1
Healing pressure ulcer of left hip back, stage 1
Pressure pre-ulcer skin changes limited to persistent focal edema, left hip

L89.222 Pressure ulcer of left hip, stage 2
Healing pressure ulcer of left hip, stage 2
Pressure ulcer with abrasion, blister, partial thickness skin loss involving epidermis and/or dermis, left hip

L89.223 Pressure ulcer of left hip, stage 3
Healing pressure ulcer of left hip, stage 3
Pressure ulcer with full thickness skin loss involving damage or necrosis of subcutaneous tissue, left hip

L89.224 Pressure ulcer of left hip, stage 4
Healing pressure ulcer of left hip, stage 4
Pressure ulcer with necrosis of soft tissues through to underlying muscle, tendon, or bone, left hip

L89.226 Pressure-induced deep tissue damage of left hip

L89.229 Pressure ulcer of left hip, unspecified stage
Healing pressure ulcer of left hip NOS
Healing pressure ulcer of left hip, unspecified stage

L89.3 Pressure ulcer of buttock

L89.30 Pressure ulcer of unspecified buttock

L89.300 Pressure ulcer of unspecified buttock, unstageable

L89.301 Pressure ulcer of unspecified buttock, stage 1
Healing pressure ulcer of unspecified buttock, stage 1
Pressure pre-ulcer skin changes limited to persistent focal edema, unspecified buttock

L89.302 Pressure ulcer of unspecified buttock, stage 2
Healing pressure ulcer of unspecified buttock, stage 2
Pressure ulcer with abrasion, blister, partial thickness skin loss involving epidermis and/or dermis, unspecified buttock

L89.303 Pressure ulcer of unspecified buttock, stage 3
Healing pressure ulcer of unspecified buttock, stage 3
Pressure ulcer with full thickness skin loss involving damage or necrosis of subcutaneous tissue, unspecified buttock

L89.304 Pressure ulcer of unspecified buttock, stage 4
Healing pressure ulcer of unspecified buttock, stage 4
Pressure ulcer with necrosis of soft tissues through to underlying muscle, tendon, or bone, unspecified buttock

▶L89.306 **Pressure-induced deep tissue damage of unspecified buttock**

L89.309 **Pressure ulcer of unspecified buttock, unspecified stage**
Healing pressure ulcer of unspecified buttock NOS
Healing pressure ulcer of unspecified buttock, unspecified stage

● L89.31 **Pressure ulcer of right buttock**

L89.310 **Pressure ulcer of right buttock, unstageable**

L89.311 **Pressure ulcer of right buttock, stage 1**
Healing pressure ulcer of right buttock, stage 1
Pressure pre-ulcer skin changes limited to persistent focal edema, right buttock

L89.312 **Pressure ulcer of right buttock, stage 2**
Healing pressure ulcer of right buttock, stage 2
Pressure ulcer with abrasion, blister, partial thickness skin loss involving epidermis and/or dermis, right buttock

L89.313 **Pressure ulcer of right buttock, stage 3**
Healing pressure ulcer of right buttock, stage 3
Pressure ulcer with full thickness skin loss involving damage or necrosis of subcutaneous tissue, right buttock

L89.314 **Pressure ulcer of right buttock, stage 4**
Healing pressure ulcer of right buttock, stage 4
Pressure ulcer with necrosis of soft tissues through to underlying muscle, tendon, or bone, right buttock

▶L89.316 **Pressure-induced deep tissue damage of right buttock**

L89.319 **Pressure ulcer of right buttock, unspecified stage**
Healing pressure ulcer of right buttock NOS
Healing pressure ulcer of right buttock, unspecified stage

● L89.32 **Pressure ulcer of left buttock**

L89.320 **Pressure ulcer of left buttock, unstageable**

L89.321 **Pressure ulcer of left buttock, stage 1**
Healing pressure ulcer of left buttock, stage 1
Pressure pre-ulcer skin changes limited to persistent focal edema, left buttock

L89.322 **Pressure ulcer of left buttock, stage 2**
Healing pressure ulcer of left buttock, stage 2
Pressure ulcer with abrasion, blister, partial thickness skin loss involving epidermis and/or dermis, left buttock

L89.323 **Pressure ulcer of left buttock, stage 3**
Healing pressure ulcer of left buttock, stage 3
Pressure ulcer with full thickness skin loss involving damage or necrosis of subcutaneous tissue, left buttock

L89.324 **Pressure ulcer of left buttock, stage 4**
Healing pressure ulcer of left buttock, stage 4
Pressure ulcer with necrosis of soft tissues through to underlying muscle, tendon, or bone, left buttock

▶L89.326 **Pressure-induced deep tissue damage of left buttock**

L89.329 **Pressure ulcer of left buttock, unspecified stage**
Healing pressure ulcer of left buttock NOS
Healing pressure ulcer of left buttock, unspecified stage

● L89.4 **Pressure ulcer of contiguous site of back, buttock and hip**

L89.40 **Pressure ulcer of contiguous site of back, buttock and hip, unspecified stage**
Healing pressure ulcer of contiguous site of back, buttock and hip NOS
Healing pressure ulcer of contiguous site of back, buttock and hip, unspecified stage

L89.41 **Pressure ulcer of contiguous site of back, buttock and hip, stage 1**
Healing pressure ulcer of contiguous site of back, buttock and hip, stage 1
Pressure pre-ulcer skin changes limited to persistent focal edema, contiguous site of back, buttock and hip

L89.42 **Pressure ulcer of contiguous site of back, buttock and hip, stage 2**
Healing pressure ulcer of contiguous site of back, buttock and hip, stage 2
Pressure ulcer with abrasion, blister, partial thickness skin loss involving epidermis and/or dermis, contiguous site of back, buttock and hip

L89.43 **Pressure ulcer of contiguous site of back, buttock and hip, stage 3**
Healing pressure ulcer of contiguous site of back, buttock and hip, stage 3
Pressure ulcer with full thickness skin loss involving damage or necrosis of subcutaneous tissue, contiguous site of back, buttock and hip

L89.44 **Pressure ulcer of contiguous site of back, buttock and hip, stage 4**
Healing pressure ulcer of contiguous site of back, buttock and hip, stage 4
Pressure ulcer with necrosis of soft tissues through to underlying muscle, tendon, or bone, contiguous site of back, buttock and hip

L89.45 **Pressure ulcer of contiguous site of back, buttock and hip, unstageable**

▶L89.46 **Pressure-induced deep tissue damage of contiguous site of back, buttock and hip**

- L89.5 **Pressure ulcer of ankle**
  - L89.50 **Pressure ulcer of unspecified ankle**
    - L89.500 **Pressure ulcer of unspecified ankle, unstageable**
    - L89.501 **Pressure ulcer of unspecified ankle, stage 1**
      Healing pressure ulcer of unspecified ankle, stage 1
      Pressure pre-ulcer skin changes limited to persistent focal edema, unspecified ankle
    - L89.502 **Pressure ulcer of unspecified ankle, stage 2**
      Healing pressure ulcer of unspecified ankle, stage 2
      Pressure ulcer with abrasion, blister, partial thickness skin loss involving epidermis and/or dermis, unspecified ankle
    - L89.503 **Pressure ulcer of unspecified ankle, stage 3**
      Healing pressure ulcer of unspecified ankle, stage 3
      Pressure ulcer with full thickness skin loss involving damage or necrosis of subcutaneous tissue, unspecified ankle
    - L89.504 **Pressure ulcer of unspecified ankle, stage 4**
      Healing pressure ulcer of unspecified ankle, stage 4
      Pressure ulcer with necrosis of soft tissues through to underlying muscle, tendon, or bone, unspecified ankle
    - L89.506 **Pressure-induced deep tissue damage of unspecified ankle**
    - L89.509 **Pressure ulcer of unspecified ankle, unspecified stage**
      Healing pressure ulcer of unspecified ankle NOS
      Healing pressure ulcer of unspecified ankle, unspecified stage
  - L89.51 **Pressure ulcer of right ankle**
    - L89.510 **Pressure ulcer of right ankle, unstageable**
    - L89.511 **Pressure ulcer of right ankle, stage 1**
      Healing pressure ulcer of right ankle, stage 1
      Pressure pre-ulcer skin changes limited to persistent focal edema, right ankle
    - L89.512 **Pressure ulcer of right ankle, stage 2**
      Healing pressure ulcer of right ankle, stage 2
      Pressure ulcer with abrasion, blister, partial thickness skin loss involving epidermis and/or dermis, right ankle
    - L89.513 **Pressure ulcer of right ankle, stage 3**
      Healing pressure ulcer of right ankle, stage 3
      Pressure ulcer with full thickness skin loss involving damage or necrosis of subcutaneous tissue, right ankle
    - L89.514 **Pressure ulcer of right ankle, stage 4**
      Healing pressure ulcer of right ankle, stage 4
      Pressure ulcer with necrosis of soft tissues through to underlying muscle, tendon, or bone, right ankle
    - L89.516 **Pressure-induced deep tissue damage of right ankle**
    - L89.519 **Pressure ulcer of right ankle, unspecified stage**
      Healing pressure ulcer of right ankle NOS
      Healing pressure ulcer of right ankle, unspecified stage
  - L89.52 **Pressure ulcer of left ankle**
    - L89.520 **Pressure ulcer of left ankle, unstageable**
    - L89.521 **Pressure ulcer of left ankle, stage 1**
      Healing pressure ulcer of left ankle, stage 1
      Pressure pre-ulcer skin changes limited to persistent focal edema, left ankle
    - L89.522 **Pressure ulcer of left ankle, stage 2**
      Healing pressure ulcer of left ankle, stage 2
      Pressure ulcer with abrasion, blister, partial thickness skin loss involving epidermis and/or dermis, left ankle
    - L89.523 **Pressure ulcer of left ankle, stage 3**
      Healing pressure ulcer of left ankle, stage 3
      Pressure ulcer with full thickness skin loss involving damage or necrosis of subcutaneous tissue, left ankle
    - L89.524 **Pressure ulcer of left ankle, stage 4**
      Healing pressure ulcer of left ankle, stage 4
      Pressure ulcer with necrosis of soft tissues through to underlying muscle, tendon, or bone, left ankle
    - L89.526 **Pressure-induced deep tissue damage of left ankle**
    - L89.529 **Pressure ulcer of left ankle, unspecified stage**
      Healing pressure ulcer of left ankle NOS
      Healing pressure ulcer of left ankle, unspecified stage
- L89.6 **Pressure ulcer of heel**
  - L89.60 **Pressure ulcer of unspecified heel**
    - L89.600 **Pressure ulcer of unspecified heel, unstageable**
    - L89.601 **Pressure ulcer of unspecified heel, stage 1**
      Healing pressure ulcer of unspecified heel, stage 1
      Pressure pre-ulcer skin changes limited to persistent focal edema, unspecified heel
    - L89.602 **Pressure ulcer of unspecified heel, stage 2**
      Healing pressure ulcer of unspecified heel, stage 2
      Pressure ulcer with abrasion, blister, partial thickness skin loss involving epidermis and/or dermis, unspecified heel
    - L89.603 **Pressure ulcer of unspecified heel, stage 3**
      Healing pressure ulcer of unspecified heel, stage 3
      Pressure ulcer with full thickness skin loss involving damage or necrosis of subcutaneous tissue, unspecified heel

L89.604 **Pressure ulcer of unspecified heel, stage 4**
Healing pressure ulcer of unspecified heel, stage 4
Pressure ulcer with necrosis of soft tissues through to underlying muscle, tendon, or bone, unspecified heel

L89.606 **Pressure-induced deep tissue damage of unspecified heel**

L89.609 **Pressure ulcer of unspecified heel, unspecified stage**
Healing pressure ulcer of unspecified heel NOS
Healing pressure ulcer of unspecified heel, unspecified stage

L89.61 Pressure ulcer of **right heel**

L89.610 **Pressure ulcer of right heel, unstageable**

L89.611 **Pressure ulcer of right heel, stage 1**
Healing pressure ulcer of right heel, stage 1
Pressure pre-ulcer skin changes limited to persistent focal edema, right heel

L89.612 **Pressure ulcer of right heel, stage 2**
Healing pressure ulcer of right heel, stage 2
Pressure ulcer with abrasion, blister, partial thickness skin loss involving epidermis and/or dermis, right heel

L89.613 **Pressure ulcer of right heel, stage 3**
Healing pressure ulcer of right heel, stage 3
Pressure ulcer with full thickness skin loss involving damage or necrosis of subcutaneous tissue, right heel

L89.614 **Pressure ulcer of right heel, stage 4**
Healing pressure ulcer of right heel, stage 4
Pressure ulcer with necrosis of soft tissues through to underlying muscle, tendon, or bone, right heel

L89.616 **Pressure-induced deep tissue damage of right heel**

L89.619 **Pressure ulcer of right heel, unspecified stage**
Healing pressure ulcer of right heel NOS
Healing pressure ulcer of right heel, unspecified stage

L89.62 Pressure ulcer of **left heel**

L89.620 **Pressure ulcer of left heel, unstageable**

L89.621 **Pressure ulcer of left heel, stage 1**
Healing pressure ulcer of left heel, stage 1
Pressure pre-ulcer skin changes limited to persistent focal edema, left heel

L89.622 **Pressure ulcer of left heel, stage 2**
Healing pressure ulcer of left heel, stage 2
Pressure ulcer with abrasion, blister, partial thickness skin loss involving epidermis and/or dermis, left heel
Coding Clinic: 2016, Q4, P142

L89.623 **Pressure ulcer of left heel, stage 3**
Healing pressure ulcer of left heel, stage 3
Pressure ulcer with full thickness skin loss involving damage or necrosis of subcutaneous tissue, left heel
Coding Clinic: 2016, Q4, P142

L89.624 **Pressure ulcer of left heel, stage 4**
Healing pressure ulcer of left heel, stage 4
Pressure ulcer with necrosis of soft tissues through to underlying muscle, tendon, or bone, left heel

L89.626 **Pressure-induced deep tissue damage of left heel**

L89.629 **Pressure ulcer of left heel, unspecified stage**
Healing pressure ulcer of left heel NOS
Healing pressure ulcer of left heel, unspecified stage

L89.8 Pressure ulcer of **other site**

L89.81 Pressure ulcer of **head**
Pressure ulcer of face

L89.810 **Pressure ulcer of head, unstageable**

L89.811 **Pressure ulcer of head, stage 1**
Healing pressure ulcer of head, stage 1
Pressure pre-ulcer skin changes limited to persistent focal edema, head

L89.812 **Pressure ulcer of head, stage 2**
Healing pressure ulcer of head, stage 2
Pressure ulcer with abrasion, blister, partial thickness skin loss involving epidermis and/or dermis, head

L89.813 **Pressure ulcer of head, stage 3**
Healing pressure ulcer of head, stage 3
Pressure ulcer with full thickness skin loss involving damage or necrosis of subcutaneous tissue, head

L89.814 **Pressure ulcer of head, stage 4**
Healing pressure ulcer of head, stage 4
Pressure ulcer with necrosis of soft tissues through to underlying muscle, tendon, or bone, head

L89.816 **Pressure-induced deep tissue damage of head**

L89.819 **Pressure ulcer of head, unspecified stage**
Healing pressure ulcer of head NOS
Healing pressure ulcer of head, unspecified stage

L89.89 Pressure ulcer of **other site**

L89.890 **Pressure ulcer of other site, unstageable**

L89.891 **Pressure ulcer of other site, stage 1**
Healing pressure ulcer of other site, stage 1
Pressure pre-ulcer skin changes limited to persistent focal edema, other site

L89.892 **Pressure ulcer of other site, stage 2**
Healing pressure ulcer of other site, stage 2
Pressure ulcer with abrasion, blister, partial thickness skin loss involving epidermis and/or dermis, other site

L89.893 **Pressure ulcer of other site, stage 3**
Healing pressure ulcer of other site, stage 3
Pressure ulcer with full thickness skin loss involving damage or necrosis of subcutaneous tissue, other site

L89.894 **Pressure ulcer of other site, stage 4**
Healing pressure ulcer of other site, stage 4
Pressure ulcer with necrosis of soft tissues through to underlying muscle, tendon, or bone, other site

L89.899 **Pressure ulcer of other site, unspecified stage**
Healing pressure ulcer of other site NOS
Healing pressure ulcer of other site, unspecified stage

● L89.9 **Pressure ulcer of unspecified site**

L89.90 **Pressure ulcer of unspecified site, unspecified stage**
Healing pressure ulcer of unspecified site NOS
Healing pressure ulcer of unspecified site, unspecified stage

L89.91 **Pressure ulcer of unspecified site, stage 1**
Healing pressure ulcer of unspecified site, stage 1
Pressure pre-ulcer skin changes limited to persistent focal edema, unspecified site

L89.92 **Pressure ulcer of unspecified site, stage 2**
Healing pressure ulcer of unspecified site, stage 2
Pressure ulcer with abrasion, blister, partial thickness skin loss involving epidermis and/or dermis, unspecified site

L89.93 **Pressure ulcer of unspecified site, stage 3**
Healing pressure ulcer of unspecified site, stage 3
Pressure ulcer with full thickness skin loss involving damage or necrosis of subcutaneous tissue, unspecified site

L89.94 **Pressure ulcer of unspecified site, stage 4**
Healing pressure ulcer of unspecified site, stage 4
Pressure ulcer with necrosis of soft tissues through to underlying muscle, tendon, or bone, unspecified site

L89.95 **Pressure ulcer of unspecified site, unstageable**

▶ L89.96 **Pressure-induced deep tissue damage of unspecified site**

● L90 **Atrophic disorders of skin**

L90.0 **Lichen sclerosus et atrophicus**
Excludes2 lichen sclerosus of external female genital organs (N90.4)
lichen sclerosus of external male genital organs (N48.0)

L90.1 **Anetoderma of Schweninger-Buzzi**

L90.2 **Anetoderma of Jadassohn-Pellizzari**

L90.3 **Atrophoderma of Pasini and Pierini**

L90.4 **Acrodermatitis chronica atrophicans**

L90.5 **Scar conditions and fibrosis of skin**
Adherent scar (skin)
Cicatrix
Disfigurement of skin due to scar
Fibrosis of skin NOS
Scar NOS
Excludes2 hypertrophic scar (L91.0)
keloid scar (L91.0)
Coding Clinic: 2016, Q2, P5; 2015, Q1, P19

Item 12-11 Scleroderma means hard skin. It is a group of diseases that causes abnormal growth of connective tissues that support the skin and organs. There are two types: localized scleroderma affecting the skin and systemic scleroderma affecting blood vessels and internal organs and the skin.

L90.6 **Striae atrophicae**

L90.8 **Other atrophic disorders of skin**

L90.9 **Atrophic disorder of skin, unspecified**

● L91 **Hypertrophic disorders of skin**

L91.0 **Keloid scar**
Hypertrophic scar
Keloid
Excludes2 acne keloid (L73.0)
scar NOS (L90.5)

L91.8 **Other hypertrophic disorders of the skin**

L91.9 **Hypertrophic disorder of the skin, unspecified**

● L92 **Granulomatous disorders of skin and subcutaneous tissue**
Excludes2 actinic granuloma (L57.5)

L92.0 **Granuloma annulare**
Perforating granuloma annulare

L92.1 **Necrobiosis lipoidica, not elsewhere classified**
Excludes1 necrobiosis lipoidica associated with diabetes mellitus (E08-E13 with .620)

L92.2 **Granuloma faciale [eosinophilic granuloma of skin]**

L92.3 **Foreign body granuloma of the skin and subcutaneous tissue**
Use additional code to identify the type of retained foreign body (Z18.-)

L92.8 **Other granulomatous disorders of the skin and subcutaneous tissue**

L92.9 **Granulomatous disorder of the skin and subcutaneous tissue, unspecified**
Excludes2 umbilical granuloma (P83.81)

● L93 **Lupus erythematosus**
Use additional code for adverse effect, if applicable, to identify drug (T36-T50 with fifth or sixth character 5)
Excludes1 lupus exedens (A18.4)
lupus vulgaris (A18.4)
scleroderma (M34.-)
systemic lupus erythematosus (M32.-)

L93.0 **Discoid lupus erythematosus**
Lupus erythematosus NOS

L93.1 **Subacute cutaneous lupus erythematosus**

L93.2 **Other local lupus erythematosus**
Lupus erythematosus profundus
Lupus panniculitis

● L94 **Other localized connective tissue disorders**
Excludes1 systemic connective tissue disorders (M30-M36)

L94.0 **Localized scleroderma [morphea]**
Circumscribed scleroderma

L94.1 **Linear scleroderma**
En coup de sabre lesion

L94.2 **Calcinosis cutis**

L94.3 **Sclerodactyly**

L94.4 **Gottron's papules**

L94.5 **Poikiloderma vasculare atrophicans**

L94.6 **Ainhum**

L94.8 **Other specified localized connective tissue disorders**

L94.9 **Localized connective tissue disorder, unspecified**

L95 Vasculitis limited to skin, not elsewhere classified

Excludes1 angioma serpiginosum (L81.7)
Henoch(-Schönlein) purpura (D69.0)
hypersensitivity angiitis (M31.0)
lupus panniculitis (L93.2)
panniculitis NOS (M79.3)
panniculitis of neck and back (M54.0-)
polyarteritis nodosa (M30.0)
relapsing panniculitis (M35.6)
rheumatoid vasculitis (M05.2)
serum sickness (T80.6-)
urticaria (L50.-)
Wegener's granulomatosis (M31.3-)

L95.0 Livedoid vasculitis
Atrophie blanche (en plaque)

L95.1 Erythema elevatum diutinum

L95.8 Other vasculitis limited to the skin

L95.9 Vasculitis limited to the skin, unspecified

L97 Non-pressure chronic ulcer of lower limb, not elsewhere classified

Includes chronic ulcer of skin of lower limb NOS
non-healing ulcer of skin
non-infected sinus of skin
trophic ulcer NOS
tropical ulcer NOS
ulcer of skin of lower limb NOS

Code first any associated underlying condition, such as:
any associated gangrene (I96)
atherosclerosis of the lower extremities (I70.23-, I70.24-, I70.33-, I70.34-, I70.43-, I70.44-, I70.53-, I70.54-, I70.63-, I70.64-, I70.73-, I70.74-)
chronic venous hypertension (I87.31-, I87.33-)
diabetic ulcers (E08.621, E08.622, E09.621, E09.622, E10.621, E10.622, E11.621, E11.622, E13.621, E13.622)
postphlebitic syndrome (I87.01-, I87.03-)
postthrombotic syndrome (I87.01-, I87.03-)
varicose ulcer (I83.0 , I83.2-)

Excludes2 pressure ulcer (pressure area) (L89.-)
skin infections (L00-L08)
specific infections classified to A00-B99

L97.1 Non-pressure chronic ulcer of thigh

L97.10 Non-pressure chronic ulcer of unspecified thigh

L97.101 Non-pressure chronic ulcer of unspecified thigh limited to breakdown of skin

L97.102 Non-pressure chronic ulcer of unspecified thigh with fat layer exposed

L97.103 Non-pressure chronic ulcer of unspecified thigh with necrosis of muscle

L97.104 Non-pressure chronic ulcer of unspecified thigh with necrosis of bone

L97.105 Non-pressure chronic ulcer of unspecified thigh with muscle involvement without evidence of necrosis

L97.106 Non-pressure chronic ulcer of unspecified thigh with bone involvement without evidence of necrosis

L97.108 Non-pressure chronic ulcer of unspecified thigh with other specified severity

L97.109 Non-pressure chronic ulcer of unspecified thigh with unspecified severity

L97.11 Non-pressure chronic ulcer of right thigh

L97.111 Non-pressure chronic ulcer of right thigh limited to breakdown of skin

L97.112 Non-pressure chronic ulcer of right thigh with fat layer exposed

L97.113 Non-pressure chronic ulcer of right thigh with necrosis of muscle

L97.114 Non-pressure chronic ulcer of right thigh with necrosis of bone

L97.115 Non-pressure chronic ulcer of right thigh with muscle involvement without evidence of necrosis

L97.116 Non-pressure chronic ulcer of right thigh with bone involvement without evidence of necrosis

L97.118 Non-pressure chronic ulcer of right thigh with other specified severity

L97.119 Non-pressure chronic ulcer of right thigh with unspecified severity

L97.12 Non-pressure chronic ulcer of left thigh

L97.121 Non-pressure chronic ulcer of left thigh limited to breakdown of skin

L97.122 Non-pressure chronic ulcer of left thigh with fat layer exposed

L97.123 Non-pressure chronic ulcer of left thigh with necrosis of muscle

L97.124 Non-pressure chronic ulcer of left thigh with necrosis of bone

L97.125 Non-pressure chronic ulcer of left thigh with muscle involvement without evidence of necrosis

L97.126 Non-pressure chronic ulcer of left thigh with bone involvement without evidence of necrosis

L97.128 Non-pressure chronic ulcer of left thigh with other specified severity

L97.129 Non-pressure chronic ulcer of left thigh with unspecified severity

L97.2 Non-pressure chronic ulcer of calf

L97.20 Non-pressure chronic ulcer of unspecified calf

L97.201 Non-pressure chronic ulcer of unspecified calf limited to breakdown of skin

L97.202 Non-pressure chronic ulcer of unspecified calf with fat layer exposed

L97.203 Non-pressure chronic ulcer of unspecified calf with necrosis of muscle

L97.204 Non-pressure chronic ulcer of unspecified calf with necrosis of bone

L97.205 Non-pressure chronic ulcer of unspecified calf with muscle involvement without evidence of necrosis

L97.206 Non-pressure chronic ulcer of unspecified calf with bone involvement without evidence of necrosis

L97.208 Non-pressure chronic ulcer of unspecified calf with other specified severity

L97.209 Non-pressure chronic ulcer of unspecified calf with unspecified severity

L97.21 Non-pressure chronic ulcer of right calf

L97.211 Non-pressure chronic ulcer of right calf limited to breakdown of skin

L97.212 Non-pressure chronic ulcer of right calf with fat layer exposed

L97.213 Non-pressure chronic ulcer of right calf with necrosis of muscle

CHAPTER 12 (L00-L99)

L97.214 Non-pressure chronic ulcer of right calf with **necrosis of bone** HCC

L97.215 Non-pressure chronic ulcer of right calf with **muscle involvement** without evidence of necrosis HCC

L97.216 Non-pressure chronic ulcer of right calf with **bone involvement** without evidence of necrosis HCC

L97.218 Non-pressure chronic ulcer of right calf with **other specified severity** HCC

L97.219 Non-pressure chronic ulcer of right calf with **unspecified severity** HCC

● L97.22 Non-pressure chronic ulcer of **left calf**

L97.221 Non-pressure chronic ulcer of left calf limited to **breakdown of skin** HCC

L97.222 Non-pressure chronic ulcer of left calf with **fat layer exposed** HCC

L97.223 Non-pressure chronic ulcer of left calf with **necrosis of muscle** HCC

L97.224 Non-pressure chronic ulcer of left calf with **necrosis of bone** HCC

L97.225 Non-pressure chronic ulcer of left calf with **muscle involvement** without evidence of necrosis HCC

L97.226 Non-pressure chronic ulcer of left calf with **bone involvement** without evidence of necrosis HCC

L97.228 Non-pressure chronic ulcer of left calf with **other specified severity** HCC

L97.229 Non-pressure chronic ulcer of left calf with **unspecified severity** HCC

● L97.3 Non-pressure chronic ulcer of **ankle**

● L97.30 Non-pressure chronic ulcer of **unspecified** ankle

L97.301 Non-pressure chronic ulcer of unspecified ankle limited to **breakdown of skin** HCC

L97.302 Non-pressure chronic ulcer of unspecified ankle with **fat layer exposed** HCC

L97.303 Non-pressure chronic ulcer of unspecified ankle with **necrosis of muscle** HCC

L97.304 Non-pressure chronic ulcer of unspecified ankle with **necrosis of bone** HCC

L97.305 Non-pressure chronic ulcer of unspecified ankle with **muscle involvement** without evidence of necrosis HCC

L97.306 Non-pressure chronic ulcer of unspecified ankle with **bone involvement** without evidence of necrosis HCC

L97.308 Non-pressure chronic ulcer of unspecified ankle with **other specified severity** HCC

L97.309 Non-pressure chronic ulcer of unspecified ankle with **unspecified severity** HCC

● L97.31 Non-pressure chronic ulcer of **right ankle**

L97.311 Non-pressure chronic ulcer of right ankle limited to **breakdown of skin** HCC

L97.312 Non-pressure chronic ulcer of right ankle with **fat layer exposed** HCC

L97.313 Non-pressure chronic ulcer of right ankle with **necrosis of muscle** HCC

L97.314 Non-pressure chronic ulcer of right ankle with **necrosis of bone** HCC

L97.315 Non-pressure chronic ulcer of right ankle with **muscle involvement** without evidence of necrosis HCC
Coding Clinic: 2017, Q4, P17

L97.316 Non-pressure chronic ulcer of right ankle with **bone involvement** without evidence of necrosis HCC

L97.318 Non-pressure chronic ulcer of right ankle with **other specified severity** HCC

L97.319 Non-pressure chronic ulcer of right ankle with **unspecified severity** HCC

● L97.32 Non-pressure chronic ulcer of **left ankle**

L97.321 Non-pressure chronic ulcer of left ankle limited to **breakdown of skin** HCC

L97.322 Non-pressure chronic ulcer of left ankle with **fat layer exposed** HCC

L97.323 Non-pressure chronic ulcer of left ankle with **necrosis of muscle** HCC

L97.324 Non-pressure chronic ulcer of left ankle with **necrosis of bone** HCC

L97.325 Non-pressure chronic ulcer of left ankle with **muscle involvement** without evidence of necrosis HCC

L97.326 Non-pressure chronic ulcer of left ankle with **bone involvement** without evidence of necrosis HCC

L97.328 Non-pressure chronic ulcer of left ankle with **other specified severity** HCC

L97.329 Non-pressure chronic ulcer of left ankle with **unspecified severity** HCC

● L97.4 Non-pressure chronic ulcer of **heel and midfoot**
Non-pressure chronic ulcer of plantar surface of midfoot

● L97.40 Non-pressure chronic ulcer of **unspecified** heel and midfoot

L97.401 Non-pressure chronic ulcer of unspecified heel and midfoot limited to **breakdown of skin** HCC

L97.402 Non-pressure chronic ulcer of unspecified heel and midfoot with **fat layer exposed** HCC

L97.403 Non-pressure chronic ulcer of unspecified heel and midfoot with **necrosis of muscle** HCC

L97.404 Non-pressure chronic ulcer of unspecified heel and midfoot with **necrosis of bone** HCC

L97.405 Non-pressure chronic ulcer of unspecified heel and midfoot with **muscle involvement** without evidence of necrosis HCC

L97.406 Non-pressure chronic ulcer of unspecified heel and midfoot with **bone involvement** without evidence of necrosis HCC

L97.408 Non-pressure chronic ulcer of unspecified heel and midfoot with **other specified severity** HCC

L97.409 Non-pressure chronic ulcer of unspecified heel and midfoot with **unspecified severity** HCC

● L97.41 Non-pressure chronic ulcer of **right heel and midfoot**

L97.411 Non-pressure chronic ulcer of right heel and midfoot limited to **breakdown of skin** HCC

L97.412 Non-pressure chronic ulcer of right heel and midfoot with **fat layer exposed** HCC

L97.413 Non-pressure chronic ulcer of right heel and midfoot with **necrosis of muscle** HCC

L97.414 Non-pressure chronic ulcer of right heel and midfoot with necrosis of bone
L97.415 Non-pressure chronic ulcer of right heel and midfoot with muscle involvement without evidence of necrosis
L97.416 Non-pressure chronic ulcer of right heel and midfoot with bone involvement without evidence of necrosis
L97.418 Non-pressure chronic ulcer of right heel and midfoot with other specified severity
L97.419 Non-pressure chronic ulcer of right heel and midfoot with unspecified severity

● L97.42 Non-pressure chronic ulcer of left heel and midfoot
L97.421 Non-pressure chronic ulcer of left heel and midfoot limited to breakdown of skin
Coding Clinic: 2016, Q1, P13
L97.422 Non-pressure chronic ulcer of left heel and midfoot with fat layer exposed
L97.423 Non-pressure chronic ulcer of left heel and midfoot with necrosis of muscle
L97.424 Non-pressure chronic ulcer of left heel and midfoot with necrosis of bone
L97.425 Non-pressure chronic ulcer of left heel and midfoot with muscle involvement without evidence of necrosis
L97.426 Non-pressure chronic ulcer of left heel and midfoot with bone involvement without evidence of necrosis
L97.428 Non-pressure chronic ulcer of left heel and midfoot with other specified severity
L97.429 Non-pressure chronic ulcer of left heel and midfoot with unspecified severity

● L97.5 Non-pressure chronic ulcer of other part of foot
Non-pressure chronic ulcer of toe

● L97.50 Non-pressure chronic ulcer of other part of unspecified foot
L97.501 Non-pressure chronic ulcer of other part of unspecified foot limited to breakdown of skin
L97.502 Non-pressure chronic ulcer of other part of unspecified foot with fat layer exposed
L97.503 Non-pressure chronic ulcer of other part of unspecified foot with necrosis of muscle
L97.504 Non-pressure chronic ulcer of other part of unspecified foot with necrosis of bone
L97.505 Non-pressure chronic ulcer of other part of unspecified foot with muscle involvement without evidence of necrosis
L97.506 Non-pressure chronic ulcer of other part of unspecified foot with bone involvement without evidence of necrosis
L97.508 Non-pressure chronic ulcer of other part of unspecified foot with other specified severity
L97.509 Non-pressure chronic ulcer of other part of unspecified foot with unspecified severity

● L97.51 Non-pressure chronic ulcer of other part of right foot
L97.511 Non-pressure chronic ulcer of other part of right foot limited to breakdown of skin
L97.512 Non-pressure chronic ulcer of other part of right foot with fat layer exposed
L97.513 Non-pressure chronic ulcer of other part of right foot with necrosis of muscle
L97.514 Non-pressure chronic ulcer of other part of right foot with necrosis of bone
L97.515 Non-pressure chronic ulcer of other part of right foot with muscle involvement without evidence of necrosis
L97.516 Non-pressure chronic ulcer of other part of right foot with bone involvement without evidence of necrosis
L97.518 Non-pressure chronic ulcer of other part of right foot with other specified severity
L97.519 Non-pressure chronic ulcer of other part of right foot with unspecified severity

● L97.52 Non-pressure chronic ulcer of other part of left foot
L97.521 Non-pressure chronic ulcer of other part of left foot limited to breakdown of skin
L97.522 Non-pressure chronic ulcer of other part of left foot with fat layer exposed
L97.523 Non-pressure chronic ulcer of other part of left foot with necrosis of muscle
L97.524 Non-pressure chronic ulcer of other part of left foot with necrosis of bone
L97.525 Non-pressure chronic ulcer of other part of left foot with muscle involvement without evidence of necrosis
L97.526 Non-pressure chronic ulcer of other part of left foot with bone involvement without evidence of necrosis
L97.528 Non-pressure chronic ulcer of other part of left foot with other specified severity
L97.529 Non-pressure chronic ulcer of other part of left foot with unspecified severity

● L97.8 Non-pressure chronic ulcer of other part of lower leg

● L97.80 Non-pressure chronic ulcer of other part of unspecified lower leg
L97.801 Non-pressure chronic ulcer of other part of unspecified lower leg limited to breakdown of skin
L97.802 Non-pressure chronic ulcer of other part of unspecified lower leg with fat layer exposed

L97.803 Non-pressure chronic ulcer of other part of unspecified lower leg with **necrosis of muscle**

L97.804 Non-pressure chronic ulcer of other part of unspecified lower leg with **necrosis of bone**

L97.805 Non-pressure chronic ulcer of other part of unspecified lower leg with **muscle involvement** without evidence of necrosis

L97.806 Non-pressure chronic ulcer of other part of unspecified lower leg with **bone involvement** without evidence of necrosis

L97.808 Non-pressure chronic ulcer of other part of unspecified lower leg with **other specified severity**

L97.809 Non-pressure chronic ulcer of other part of unspecified lower leg with **unspecified severity**

● L97.81 Non-pressure chronic ulcer of other part of **right lower leg**

L97.811 Non-pressure chronic ulcer of other part of right lower leg limited to **breakdown of skin**

L97.812 Non-pressure chronic ulcer of other part of right lower leg with **fat layer exposed**

L97.813 Non-pressure chronic ulcer of other part of right lower leg with **necrosis of muscle**

L97.814 Non-pressure chronic ulcer of other part of right lower leg with **necrosis of bone**

L97.815 Non-pressure chronic ulcer of other part of right lower leg with **muscle involvement** without evidence of necrosis

L97.816 Non-pressure chronic ulcer of other part of right lower leg with **bone involvement** without evidence of necrosis

L97.818 Non-pressure chronic ulcer of other part of right lower leg with **other specified severity**

L97.819 Non-pressure chronic ulcer of other part of right lower leg with **unspecified severity**

● L97.82 Non-pressure chronic ulcer of other part of **left lower leg**

L97.821 Non-pressure chronic ulcer of other part of left lower leg limited to **breakdown of skin**

L97.822 Non-pressure chronic ulcer of other part of left lower leg with **fat layer exposed**

L97.823 Non-pressure chronic ulcer of other part of left lower leg with **necrosis of muscle**

L97.824 Non-pressure chronic ulcer of other part of left lower leg with **necrosis of bone**

L97.825 Non-pressure chronic ulcer of other part of left lower leg with **muscle involvement** without evidence of necrosis

L97.826 Non-pressure chronic ulcer of other part of left lower leg with **bone involvement** without evidence of necrosis

L97.828 Non-pressure chronic ulcer of other part of left lower leg with **other specified severity**

L97.829 Non-pressure chronic ulcer of other part of left lower leg with **unspecified severity**

● L97.9 Non-pressure chronic ulcer of **unspecified part of lower leg**

● L97.90 Non-pressure chronic ulcer of unspecified part of **unspecified lower leg**

L97.901 Non-pressure chronic ulcer of unspecified part of unspecified lower leg limited to **breakdown of skin**

L97.902 Non-pressure chronic ulcer of unspecified part of unspecified lower leg with **fat layer exposed**

L97.903 Non-pressure chronic ulcer of unspecified part of unspecified lower leg with **necrosis of muscle**

L97.904 Non-pressure chronic ulcer of unspecified part of unspecified lower leg with **necrosis of bone**

L97.905 Non-pressure chronic ulcer of unspecified part of unspecified lower leg with **muscle involvement** without evidence of necrosis

L97.906 Non-pressure chronic ulcer of unspecified part of unspecified lower leg with **bone involvement** without evidence of necrosis

L97.908 Non-pressure chronic ulcer of unspecified part of unspecified lower leg with **other specified severity**

L97.909 Non-pressure chronic ulcer of unspecified part of unspecified lower leg with **unspecified severity**

● L97.91 Non-pressure chronic ulcer of **unspecified part of right lower leg**

L97.911 Non-pressure chronic ulcer of unspecified part of right lower leg limited to **breakdown of skin**

L97.912 Non-pressure chronic ulcer of unspecified part of right lower leg with **fat layer exposed**

L97.913 Non-pressure chronic ulcer of unspecified part of right lower leg with **necrosis of muscle**

L97.914 Non-pressure chronic ulcer of unspecified part of right lower leg with **necrosis of bone**

L97.915 Non-pressure chronic ulcer of unspecified part of right lower leg with **muscle involvement** without evidence of necrosis

L97.916 Non-pressure chronic ulcer of unspecified part of right lower leg with **bone involvement** without evidence of necrosis

L97.918 Non-pressure chronic ulcer of unspecified part of right lower leg with **other specified severity**

L97.919 Non-pressure chronic ulcer of unspecified part of right lower leg with **unspecified severity**

● L97.92 Non-pressure chronic ulcer of **unspecified part of left lower leg**

L97.921 Non-pressure chronic ulcer of unspecified part of left lower leg limited to **breakdown of skin**

L97.922 Non-pressure chronic ulcer of unspecified part of left lower leg with **fat layer exposed**

L97.923 Non-pressure chronic ulcer of unspecified part of left lower leg with **necrosis of muscle**

L97.924 Non-pressure chronic ulcer of unspecified part of left lower leg with **necrosis of bone**

L97.925 Non-pressure chronic ulcer of unspecified part of left lower leg with **muscle involvement** without evidence of necrosis

L97.926 Non-pressure chronic ulcer of unspecified part of left lower leg with **bone involvement** without evidence of necrosis

L97.928 Non-pressure chronic ulcer of unspecified part of left lower leg with **other specified severity**

L97.929 Non-pressure chronic ulcer of unspecified part of left lower leg with **unspecified severity**

● L98 Other disorders of skin and subcutaneous tissue, not elsewhere classified

L98.Ø Pyogenic granuloma

Excludes2 pyogenic granuloma of gingiva (KØ6.8)
pyogenic granuloma of maxillary alveolar ridge (KØ4.5)
pyogenic granuloma of oral mucosa (K13.4)

L98.1 Factitial dermatitis
Neurotic excoriation

Excludes1 Excoriation (skin-picking) disorder (F42.4)
Coding Clinic: 2Ø16, Q4, P15

L98.2 Febrile neutrophilic dermatosis [Sweet]

L98.3 Eosinophilic cellulitis [Wells]

● L98.4 Non-pressure chronic ulcer of skin, not elsewhere classified
Chronic ulcer of skin NOS
Tropical ulcer NOS
Ulcer of skin NOS

Excludes2 pressure ulcer (pressure area) (L89.-)
gangrene (I96)
skin infections (LØØ-LØ8)
specific infections classified to AØØ-B99
ulcer of lower limb NEC (L97.-)
varicose ulcer (I83.Ø-I82.2)

● L98.41 Non-pressure chronic ulcer of **buttock**

L98.411 Non-pressure chronic ulcer of buttock limited to **breakdown of skin**

L98.412 Non-pressure chronic ulcer of buttock with **fat layer exposed**

L98.413 Non-pressure chronic ulcer of buttock with **necrosis of muscle**

L98.414 Non-pressure chronic ulcer of buttock with **necrosis of bone**

L98.415 Non-pressure chronic ulcer of buttock with **muscle involvement** without evidence of necrosis

L98.416 Non-pressure chronic ulcer of buttock with **bone involvement** without evidence of necrosis

L98.418 Non-pressure chronic ulcer of buttock with **other specified severity**

L98.419 Non-pressure chronic ulcer of buttock with **unspecified severity**

● L98.42 Non-pressure chronic ulcer of **back**

L98.421 Non-pressure chronic ulcer of back limited to **breakdown of skin**

L98.422 Non-pressure chronic ulcer of back with **fat layer exposed**

L98.423 Non-pressure chronic ulcer of back with **necrosis of muscle**

L98.424 Non-pressure chronic ulcer of back with **necrosis of bone**

L98.425 Non-pressure chronic ulcer of back with **muscle involvement** without evidence of necrosis

L98.426 Non-pressure chronic ulcer of back with **bone involvement** without evidence of necrosis

L98.428 Non-pressure chronic ulcer of back with **other specified severity**

L98.429 Non-pressure chronic ulcer of back with **unspecified severity**

● L98.49 Non-pressure chronic ulcer of skin of **other sites**
Non-pressure chronic ulcer of skin NOS

L98.491 Non-pressure chronic ulcer of skin of other sites limited to **breakdown of skin**

L98.492 Non-pressure chronic ulcer of skin of other sites with **fat layer exposed**

L98.493 Non-pressure chronic ulcer of skin of other sites with **necrosis of muscle**

L98.494 Non-pressure chronic ulcer of skin of other sites with **necrosis of bone**

L98.495 Non-pressure chronic ulcer of skin of other sites with **muscle involvement** without evidence of necrosis

L98.496 Non-pressure chronic ulcer of skin of other sites with **bone involvement** without evidence of necrosis

L98.498 Non-pressure chronic ulcer of skin of other sites with **other specified severity**

L98.499 Non-pressure chronic ulcer of skin of other sites with **unspecified severity**

L98.5 Mucinosis of the skin
Focal mucinosis
Lichen myxedematosus
Reticular erythematous mucinosis

Excludes1 focal oral mucinosis (K13.79)
myxedema (EØ3.9)

L98.6 Other infiltrative disorders of the skin and subcutaneous tissue

Excludes1 hyalinosis cutis et mucosae (E78.89)

L98.7 Excessive and redundant skin and subcutaneous tissue
Loose or sagging skin following bariatric surgery weight loss
Loose or sagging skin following dietary weight loss
Loose or sagging skin, NOS

Excludes2 acquired excess or redundant skin of eyelid (HØ2.3-)
congenital excess or redundant skin of eyelid (Q1Ø.3)
skin changes due to chronic exposure to nonionizing radiation (L57.-)
Coding Clinic: 2Ø16, Q4, P36

L98.8 Other specified disorders of the skin and subcutaneous tissue
Coding Clinic: 2Ø13, Q2, P32

L98.9 Disorder of the skin and subcutaneous tissue, unspecified

L99 Other disorders of skin and subcutaneous tissue in diseases classified elsewhere

Code first underlying disease, such as:
amyloidosis (E85.-)

Excludes1 skin disorders in diabetes (EØ8-E13 with .62)
skin disorders in gonorrhea (A54.89)
skin disorders in syphilis (A51.31, A52.79)

CHAPTER 12 (LØØ-L99)

CHAPTER 13

DISEASES OF THE MUSCULOSKELETAL SYSTEM AND CONNECTIVE TISSUE (MØØ-M99)

OGCR Chapter-Specific Coding Guidelines

13. Chapter 13: Diseases of the Musculoskeletal System and Connective Tissue (MØØ-M99)

a. Site and laterality

Most of the codes within Chapter 13 have site and laterality designations. The site represents the bone, joint or the muscle involved. For some conditions where more than one bone, joint or muscle is usually involved, such as osteoarthritis, there is a "multiple sites" code available. For categories where no multiple site code is provided and more than one bone, joint or muscle is involved, multiple codes should be used to indicate the different sites involved.

1) Bone versus joint

For certain conditions, the bone may be affected at the upper or lower end (e.g., avascular necrosis of bone, M87, Osteoporosis, M8Ø, M81). Though the portion of the bone affected may be at the joint, the site designation will be the bone, not the joint.

b. Acute traumatic versus chronic or recurrent musculoskeletal conditions

Many musculoskeletal conditions are a result of previous injury or trauma to a site, or are recurrent conditions. Bone, joint or muscle conditions that are the result of a healed injury are usually found in Chapter 13. Recurrent bone, joint or muscle conditions are also usually found in Chapter 13. Any current, acute injury should be coded to the appropriate injury code from Chapter 19. Chronic or recurrent conditions should generally be coded with a code from Chapter 13. If it is difficult to determine from the documentation in the record which code is best to describe a condition, query the provider.

c. Coding of Pathologic Fractures

7th character A is for use as long as the patient is receiving active treatment for the fracture. While the patient may be seen by a new or different provider over the course of treatment for a pathological fracture, assignment of the 7th character is based on whether the patient is undergoing active treatment and not whether the provider is seeing the patient for the first time.

7th character, D is to be used for encounters after the patient has completed active treatment for the fracture and is receiving routine care for the fracture during the healing or recovery phase. The other 7th characters, listed under each subcategory in the Tabular List, are to be used for subsequent encounters for treatment of problems associated with the healing, such as malunions, nonunions, and sequelae.

Care for complications of surgical treatment for fracture repairs during the healing or recovery phase should be coded with the appropriate complication codes.

See Section I.C.19. Coding of traumatic fractures.

d. Osteoporosis

Osteoporosis is a systemic condition, meaning that all bones of the musculoskeletal system are affected. Therefore, site is not a component of the codes under category M81, Osteoporosis without current pathological fracture. The site codes under category M8Ø, Osteoporosis with current pathological fracture, identify the site of the fracture, not the osteoporosis.

1) Osteoporosis without pathological fracture

Category M81, Osteoporosis without current pathological fracture, is for use for patients with osteoporosis who do not currently have a pathologic fracture due to the osteoporosis, even if they have had a fracture in the past. For patients with a history of osteoporosis fractures, status code Z87.31Ø, Personal history of (healed) osteoporosis fracture, should follow the code from M81.

2) Osteoporosis with current pathological fracture

Category M8Ø, Osteoporosis with current pathological fracture, is for patients who have a current pathologic fracture at the time of an encounter. The codes under M8Ø identify the site of the fracture. A code from category M8Ø, not a traumatic fracture code, should be used for any patient with known osteoporosis who suffers a fracture, even if the patient had a minor fall or trauma, if that fall or trauma would not usually break a normal, healthy bone.

CHAPTER 13

DISEASES OF THE MUSCULOSKELETAL SYSTEM AND CONNECTIVE TISSUE (MØØ-M99)

Note: Use an external cause code following the code for the musculoskeletal condition, if applicable, to identify the cause of the musculoskeletal condition

Excludes2 arthropathic psoriasis (L4Ø.5-)
certain conditions originating in the perinatal period (PØ4-P96)
certain infectious and parasitic diseases (AØØ-B99)
compartment syndrome (traumatic) (T79.A-)
complications of pregnancy, childbirth and the puerperium (OØØ-O9A)
congenital malformations, deformations, and chromosomal abnormalities (QØØ-Q99)
endocrine, nutritional and metabolic diseases (EØØ-E88)
injury, poisoning and certain other consequences of external causes (SØØ-T88)
neoplasms (CØØ-D49)
symptoms, signs and abnormal clinical and laboratory findings, not elsewhere classified (RØØ-R94)

This chapter contains the following blocks:

MØØ-MØ2	Infectious arthropathies
MØ4	Autoinflammatory syndromes
MØ5-M14	Inflammatory polyarthropathies
M15-M19	Osteoarthritis
M2Ø-M25	Other joint disorders
M26-M27	Dentofacial anomalies [including malocclusion] and other disorders of jaw
M3Ø-M36	Systemic connective tissue disorders
M4Ø-M43	Deforming dorsopathies
M45-M49	Spondylopathies
M5Ø-M54	Other dorsopathies
M6Ø-M63	Disorders of muscles
M65-M67	Disorders of synovium and tendon
M7Ø-M79	Other soft tissue disorders
M8Ø-M85	Disorders of bone density and structure
M86-M9Ø	Other osteopathies
M91-M94	Chondropathies
M95	Other disorders of the musculoskeletal system and connective tissue
M96	Intraoperative and postprocedural complications and disorders of musculoskeletal system, not elsewhere classified
M97	Periprosthetic fracture around internal prosthetic joint
M99	Biomechanical lesions, not elsewhere classified

Coding Clinic: 2Ø16, Q4, P124

ARTHROPATHIES (MØØ-M25)

Includes Disorders affecting predominantly peripheral (limb) joints

INFECTIOUS ARTHROPATHIES (MØØ-MØ2)

Note: This block comprises arthropathies due to microbiological agents.

Distinction is made between the following types of etiological relationship:

a) direct infection of joint, where organisms invade synovial tissue and microbial antigen is present in the joint;

b) indirect infection, which may be of two types: a reactive arthropathy, where microbial infection of the body is established but neither organisms nor antigens can be identified in the joint, and a postinfective arthropathy, where microbial antigen is present but recovery of an organism is inconstant and evidence of local multiplication is lacking.

M00 Pyogenic arthritis

M00.0 Staphylococcal arthritis and polyarthritis

Use additional code (B95.61-B95.8) to identify bacterial agent

Excludes2 infection and inflammatory reaction due to internal joint prosthesis (T84.5-)

M00.00 Staphylococcal arthritis, unspecified joint

M00.01 Staphylococcal arthritis, shoulder

- M00.011 Staphylococcal arthritis, right shoulder
- M00.012 Staphylococcal arthritis, left shoulder
- M00.019 Staphylococcal arthritis, unspecified shoulder

M00.02 Staphylococcal arthritis, elbow

- M00.021 Staphylococcal arthritis, right elbow
- M00.022 Staphylococcal arthritis, left elbow
- M00.029 Staphylococcal arthritis, unspecified elbow

M00.03 Staphylococcal arthritis, wrist

Staphylococcal arthritis of carpal bones

- M00.031 Staphylococcal arthritis, right wrist
- M00.032 Staphylococcal arthritis, left wrist
- M00.039 Staphylococcal arthritis, unspecified wrist

M00.04 Staphylococcal arthritis, hand

Staphylococcal arthritis of metacarpus and phalanges

- M00.041 Staphylococcal arthritis, right hand
- M00.042 Staphylococcal arthritis, left hand
- M00.049 Staphylococcal arthritis, unspecified hand

M00.05 Staphylococcal arthritis, hip

- M00.051 Staphylococcal arthritis, right hip
- M00.052 Staphylococcal arthritis, left hip
- M00.059 Staphylococcal arthritis, unspecified hip

M00.06 Staphylococcal arthritis, knee

- M00.061 Staphylococcal arthritis, right knee
- M00.062 Staphylococcal arthritis, left knee
- M00.069 Staphylococcal arthritis, unspecified knee

M00.07 Staphylococcal arthritis, ankle and foot

Staphylococcal arthritis, tarsus, metatarsus and phalanges

- M00.071 Staphylococcal arthritis, right ankle and foot
- M00.072 Staphylococcal arthritis, left ankle and foot
- M00.079 Staphylococcal arthritis, unspecified ankle and foot

M00.08 Staphylococcal arthritis, vertebrae

M00.09 Staphylococcal polyarthritis

M00.1 Pneumococcal arthritis and polyarthritis

M00.10 Pneumococcal arthritis, unspecified joint

M00.11 Pneumococcal arthritis, shoulder

- M00.111 Pneumococcal arthritis, right shoulder
- M00.112 Pneumococcal arthritis, left shoulder
- M00.119 Pneumococcal arthritis, unspecified shoulder

M00.12 Pneumococcal arthritis, elbow

- M00.121 Pneumococcal arthritis, right elbow
- M00.122 Pneumococcal arthritis, left elbow
- M00.129 Pneumococcal arthritis, unspecified elbow

M00.13 Pneumococcal arthritis, wrist

Pneumococcal arthritis of carpal bones

- M00.131 Pneumococcal arthritis, right wrist
- M00.132 Pneumococcal arthritis, left wrist
- M00.139 Pneumococcal arthritis, unspecified wrist

M00.14 Pneumococcal arthritis, hand

Pneumococcal arthritis of metacarpus and phalanges

- M00.141 Pneumococcal arthritis, right hand
- M00.142 Pneumococcal arthritis, left hand
- M00.149 Pneumococcal arthritis, unspecified hand

M00.15 Pneumococcal arthritis, hip

- M00.151 Pneumococcal arthritis, right hip
- M00.152 Pneumococcal arthritis, left hip
- M00.159 Pneumococcal arthritis, unspecified hip

M00.16 Pneumococcal arthritis, knee

- M00.161 Pneumococcal arthritis, right knee
- M00.162 Pneumococcal arthritis, left knee
- M00.169 Pneumococcal arthritis, unspecified knee

M00.17 Pneumococcal arthritis, ankle and foot

Pneumococcal arthritis, tarsus, metatarsus and phalanges

- M00.171 Pneumococcal arthritis, right ankle and foot
- M00.172 Pneumococcal arthritis, left ankle and foot
- M00.179 Pneumococcal arthritis, unspecified ankle and foot

M00.18 Pneumococcal arthritis, vertebrae

M00.19 Pneumococcal polyarthritis

M00.2 Other streptococcal arthritis and polyarthritis

Use additional code (B95.0-B95.2, B95.4-B95.5) to identify bacterial agent

M00.20 Other streptococcal arthritis, unspecified joint

M00.21 Other streptococcal arthritis, shoulder

- M00.211 Other streptococcal arthritis, right shoulder
- M00.212 Other streptococcal arthritis, left shoulder
- M00.219 Other streptococcal arthritis, unspecified shoulder

M00.22 Other streptococcal arthritis, elbow

- M00.221 Other streptococcal arthritis, right elbow
- M00.222 Other streptococcal arthritis, left elbow
- M00.229 Other streptococcal arthritis, unspecified elbow

M00.23 Other streptococcal arthritis, wrist

Other streptococcal arthritis of carpal bones

- M00.231 Other streptococcal arthritis, right wrist
- M00.232 Other streptococcal arthritis, left wrist
- M00.239 Other streptococcal arthritis, unspecified wrist

M00.24 Other streptococcal arthritis, hand

Other streptococcal arthritis metacarpus and phalanges

- M00.241 Other streptococcal arthritis, right hand
- M00.242 Other streptococcal arthritis, left hand
- M00.249 Other streptococcal arthritis, unspecified hand

- MØØ.25 Other streptococcal arthritis, hip
  - MØØ.251 Other streptococcal arthritis, right hip
  - MØØ.252 Other streptococcal arthritis, left hip
  - MØØ.259 Other streptococcal arthritis, unspecified hip
- MØØ.26 Other streptococcal arthritis, knee
  - MØØ.261 Other streptococcal arthritis, right knee
  - MØØ.262 Other streptococcal arthritis, left knee
  - MØØ.269 Other streptococcal arthritis, unspecified knee
- MØØ.27 Other streptococcal arthritis, ankle and foot
  Other streptococcal arthritis, tarsus, metatarsus and phalanges
  - MØØ.271 Other streptococcal arthritis, right ankle and foot
  - MØØ.272 Other streptococcal arthritis, left ankle and foot
  - MØØ.279 Other streptococcal arthritis, unspecified ankle and foot
- MØØ.28 Other streptococcal arthritis, vertebrae
- MØØ.29 Other streptococcal polyarthritis

MØØ.8 Arthritis and polyarthritis due to other bacteria
Use additional code (B96) to identify bacteria

- MØØ.8Ø Arthritis due to other bacteria, unspecified joint
- MØØ.81 Arthritis due to other bacteria, shoulder
  - MØØ.811 Arthritis due to other bacteria, right shoulder
  - MØØ.812 Arthritis due to other bacteria, left shoulder
  - MØØ.819 Arthritis due to other bacteria, unspecified shoulder
- MØØ.82 Arthritis due to other bacteria, elbow
  - MØØ.821 Arthritis due to other bacteria, right elbow
  - MØØ.822 Arthritis due to other bacteria, left elbow
  - MØØ.829 Arthritis due to other bacteria, unspecified elbow
- MØØ.83 Arthritis due to other bacteria, wrist
  Arthritis due to other bacteria, carpal bones
  - MØØ.831 Arthritis due to other bacteria, right wrist
  - MØØ.832 Arthritis due to other bacteria, left wrist
  - MØØ.839 Arthritis due to other bacteria, unspecified wrist
- MØØ.84 Arthritis due to other bacteria, hand
  Arthritis due to other bacteria, metacarpus and phalanges
  - MØØ.841 Arthritis due to other bacteria, right hand
  - MØØ.842 Arthritis due to other bacteria, left hand
  - MØØ.849 Arthritis due to other bacteria, unspecified hand
- MØØ.85 Arthritis due to other bacteria, hip
  - MØØ.851 Arthritis due to other bacteria, right hip
  - MØØ.852 Arthritis due to other bacteria, left hip
  - MØØ.859 Arthritis due to other bacteria, unspecified hip
- MØØ.86 Arthritis due to other bacteria, knee
  - MØØ.861 Arthritis due to other bacteria, right knee
  - MØØ.862 Arthritis due to other bacteria, left knee
  - MØØ.869 Arthritis due to other bacteria, unspecified knee
- MØØ.87 Arthritis due to other bacteria, ankle and foot
  Arthritis due to other bacteria, tarsus, metatarsus, and phalanges
  - MØØ.871 Arthritis due to other bacteria, right ankle and foot
  - MØØ.872 Arthritis due to other bacteria, left ankle and foot
  - MØØ.879 Arthritis due to other bacteria, unspecified ankle and foot
- MØØ.88 Arthritis due to other bacteria, vertebrae
- MØØ.89 Polyarthritis due to other bacteria

MØØ.9 Pyogenic arthritis, unspecified
Infective arthritis NOS

MØ1 Direct infections of joint in infectious and parasitic diseases classified elsewhere

Code first underlying disease, such as:
leprosy [Hansen's disease] (A3Ø.-)
mycoses (B35-B49)
O'nyong-nyong fever (A92.1)
paratyphoid fever (AØ1.1-AØ1.4)

Excludes1 arthropathy in Lyme disease (A69.23)
gonococcal arthritis (A54.42)
meningococcal arthritis (A39.83)
mumps arthritis (B26.85)
postinfective arthropathy (MØ2.-)
postmeningococcal arthritis (A39.84)
reactive arthritis (MØ2.3)
rubella arthritis (BØ6.82)
sarcoidosis arthritis (D86.86)
typhoid fever arthritis (AØ1.Ø4)
tuberculosis arthritis (A18.Ø1-A18.Ø2)

MØ1.X Direct infection of joint in infectious and parasitic diseases classified elsewhere

- *MØ1.XØ Direct infection of unspecified joint in infectious and parasitic diseases classified elsewhere*
- MØ1.X1 Direct infection of shoulder joint in infectious and parasitic diseases classified elsewhere
  - *MØ1.X11 Direct infection of right shoulder in infectious and parasitic diseases classified elsewhere*
  - *MØ1.X12 Direct infection of left shoulder in infectious and parasitic diseases classified elsewhere*
  - *MØ1.X19 Direct infection of unspecified shoulder in infectious and parasitic diseases classified elsewhere*
- MØ1.X2 Direct infection of elbow in infectious and parasitic diseases classified elsewhere
  - *MØ1.X21 Direct infection of right elbow in infectious and parasitic diseases classified elsewhere*
  - *MØ1.X22 Direct infection of left elbow in infectious and parasitic diseases classified elsewhere*
  - *MØ1.X29 Direct infection of unspecified elbow in infectious and parasitic diseases classified elsewhere*

MØ1.X3 Direct infection of wrist in infectious and parasitic diseases classified elsewhere
Direct infection of carpal bones in infectious and parasitic diseases classified elsewhere

MØ1.X31 Direct infection of right wrist in infectious and parasitic diseases classified elsewhere

MØ1.X32 Direct infection of left wrist in infectious and parasitic diseases classified elsewhere

MØ1.X39 Direct infection of unspecified wrist in infectious and parasitic diseases classified elsewhere

MØ1.X4 Direct infection of hand in infectious and parasitic diseases classified elsewhere
Direct infection of metacarpus and phalanges in infectious and parasitic diseases classified elsewhere

MØ1.X41 Direct infection of right hand in infectious and parasitic diseases classified elsewhere

MØ1.X42 Direct infection of left hand in infectious and parasitic diseases classified elsewhere

MØ1.X49 Direct infection of unspecified hand in infectious and parasitic diseases classified elsewhere

MØ1.X5 Direct infection of hip in infectious and parasitic diseases classified elsewhere

MØ1.X51 Direct infection of right hip in infectious and parasitic diseases classified elsewhere

MØ1.X52 Direct infection of left hip in infectious and parasitic diseases classified elsewhere

MØ1.X59 Direct infection of unspecified hip in infectious and parasitic diseases classified elsewhere

MØ1.X6 Direct infection of knee in infectious and parasitic diseases classified elsewhere

MØ1.X61 Direct infection of right knee in infectious and parasitic diseases classified elsewhere

MØ1.X62 Direct infection of left knee in infectious and parasitic diseases classified elsewhere

MØ1.X69 Direct infection of unspecified knee in infectious and parasitic diseases classified elsewhere

MØ1.X7 Direct infection of ankle and foot in infectious and parasitic diseases classified elsewhere
Direct infection of tarsus, metatarsus and phalanges in infectious and parasitic diseases classified elsewhere

MØ1.X71 Direct infection of right ankle and foot in infectious and parasitic diseases classified elsewhere

MØ1.X72 Direct infection of left ankle and foot in infectious and parasitic diseases classified elsewhere

MØ1.X79 Direct infection of unspecified ankle and foot in infectious and parasitic diseases classified elsewhere

MØ1.X8 Direct infection of vertebrae in infectious and parasitic diseases classified elsewhere

MØ1.X9 Direct infection of multiple joints in infectious and parasitic diseases classified elsewhere

MØ2 Postinfective and reactive arthropathies
Code first underlying disease, such as:
congenital syphilis [Clutton's joints] (A5Ø.5)
enteritis due to Yersinia enterocolitica (AØ4.6)
infective endocarditis (I33.Ø)
viral hepatitis (B15-B19)

Excludes1 Behçet's disease (M35.2)
direct infections of joint in infectious and parasitic diseases classified elsewhere (MØ1.-)
postmeningococcal arthritis (A39.84)
mumps arthritis (B26.85)
rubella arthritis (BØ6.82)
syphilis arthritis (late) (A52.77)
rheumatic fever (IØØ)
tabetic arthropathy [Charcôt's] (A52.16)

MØ2.Ø Arthropathy following intestinal bypass

MØ2.ØØ Arthropathy following intestinal bypass, unspecified site

MØ2.Ø1 Arthropathy following intestinal bypass, shoulder

MØ2.Ø11 Arthropathy following intestinal bypass, right shoulder

MØ2.Ø12 Arthropathy following intestinal bypass, left shoulder

MØ2.Ø19 Arthropathy following intestinal bypass, unspecified shoulder

MØ2.Ø2 Arthropathy following intestinal bypass, elbow

MØ2.Ø21 Arthropathy following intestinal bypass, right elbow

MØ2.Ø22 Arthropathy following intestinal bypass, left elbow

MØ2.Ø29 Arthropathy following intestinal bypass, unspecified elbow

MØ2.Ø3 Arthropathy following intestinal bypass, wrist
Arthropathy following intestinal bypass, carpal bones

MØ2.Ø31 Arthropathy following intestinal bypass, right wrist

MØ2.Ø32 Arthropathy following intestinal bypass, left wrist

MØ2.Ø39 Arthropathy following intestinal bypass, unspecified wrist

MØ2.Ø4 Arthropathy following intestinal bypass, hand
Arthropathy following intestinal bypass, metacarpals and phalanges

MØ2.Ø41 Arthropathy following intestinal bypass, right hand

MØ2.Ø42 Arthropathy following intestinal bypass, left hand

MØ2.Ø49 Arthropathy following intestinal bypass, unspecified hand

MØ2.Ø5 Arthropathy following intestinal bypass, hip

MØ2.Ø51 Arthropathy following intestinal bypass, right hip

MØ2.Ø52 Arthropathy following intestinal bypass, left hip

MØ2.Ø59 Arthropathy following intestinal bypass, unspecified hip

MØ2.Ø6 Arthropathy following intestinal bypass, knee

MØ2.Ø61 Arthropathy following intestinal bypass, right knee

MØ2.Ø62 Arthropathy following intestinal bypass, left knee

MØ2.Ø69 Arthropathy following intestinal bypass, unspecified knee

M02.07 Arthropathy following intestinal bypass, ankle and foot
Arthropathy following intestinal bypass, tarsus, metatarsus and phalanges
M02.071 Arthropathy following intestinal bypass, right ankle and foot
M02.072 Arthropathy following intestinal bypass, left ankle and foot
M02.079 Arthropathy following intestinal bypass, unspecified ankle and foot
M02.08 Arthropathy following intestinal bypass, vertebrae
M02.09 Arthropathy following intestinal bypass, multiple sites
M02.1 Postdysenteric arthropathy
M02.10 Postdysenteric arthropathy, unspecified site
M02.11 Postdysenteric arthropathy, shoulder
M02.111 Postdysenteric arthropathy, right shoulder
M02.112 Postdysenteric arthropathy, left shoulder
M02.119 Postdysenteric arthropathy, unspecified shoulder
M02.12 Postdysenteric arthropathy, elbow
M02.121 Postdysenteric arthropathy, right elbow
M02.122 Postdysenteric arthropathy, left elbow
M02.129 Postdysenteric arthropathy, unspecified elbow
M02.13 Postdysenteric arthropathy, wrist
Postdysenteric arthropathy, carpal bones
M02.131 Postdysenteric arthropathy, right wrist
M02.132 Postdysenteric arthropathy, left wrist
M02.139 Postdysenteric arthropathy, unspecified wrist
M02.14 Postdysenteric arthropathy, hand
Postdysenteric arthropathy, metacarpus and phalanges
M02.141 Postdysenteric arthropathy, right hand
M02.142 Postdysenteric arthropathy, left hand
M02.149 Postdysenteric arthropathy, unspecified hand
M02.15 Postdysenteric arthropathy, hip
M02.151 Postdysenteric arthropathy, right hip
M02.152 Postdysenteric arthropathy, left hip
M02.159 Postdysenteric arthropathy, unspecified hip
M02.16 Postdysenteric arthropathy, knee
M02.161 Postdysenteric arthropathy, right knee
M02.162 Postdysenteric arthropathy, left knee
M02.169 Postdysenteric arthropathy, unspecified knee
M02.17 Postdysenteric arthropathy, ankle and foot
Postdysenteric arthropathy, tarsus, metatarsus and phalanges
M02.171 Postdysenteric arthropathy, right ankle and foot
M02.172 Postdysenteric arthropathy, left ankle and foot
M02.179 Postdysenteric arthropathy, unspecified ankle and foot
M02.18 Postdysenteric arthropathy, vertebrae
M02.19 Postdysenteric arthropathy, multiple sites

M02.2 Postimmunization arthropathy
M02.20 Postimmunization arthropathy, unspecified site
M02.21 Postimmunization arthropathy, shoulder
M02.211 Postimmunization arthropathy, right shoulder
M02.212 Postimmunization arthropathy, left shoulder
M02.219 Postimmunization arthropathy, unspecified shoulder
M02.22 Postimmunization arthropathy, elbow
M02.221 Postimmunization arthropathy, right elbow
M02.222 Postimmunization arthropathy, left elbow
M02.229 Postimmunization arthropathy, unspecified elbow
M02.23 Postimmunization arthropathy, wrist
Postimmunization arthropathy, carpal bones
M02.231 Postimmunization arthropathy, right wrist
M02.232 Postimmunization arthropathy, left wrist
M02.239 Postimmunization arthropathy, unspecified wrist
M02.24 Postimmunization arthropathy, hand
Postimmunization arthropathy, metacarpus and phalanges
M02.241 Postimmunization arthropathy, right hand
M02.242 Postimmunization arthropathy, left hand
M02.249 Postimmunization arthropathy, unspecified hand
M02.25 Postimmunization arthropathy, hip
M02.251 Postimmunization arthropathy, right hip
M02.252 Postimmunization arthropathy, left hip
M02.259 Postimmunization arthropathy, unspecified hip
M02.26 Postimmunization arthropathy, knee
M02.261 Postimmunization arthropathy, right knee
M02.262 Postimmunization arthropathy, left knee
M02.269 Postimmunization arthropathy, unspecified knee
M02.27 Postimmunization arthropathy, ankle and foot
Postimmunization arthropathy, tarsus, metatarsus and phalanges
M02.271 Postimmunization arthropathy, right ankle and foot
M02.272 Postimmunization arthropathy, left ankle and foot
M02.279 Postimmunization arthropathy, unspecified ankle and foot
M02.28 Postimmunization arthropathy, vertebrae
M02.29 Postimmunization arthropathy, multiple sites
M02.3 Reiter's disease
Reactive arthritis
M02.30 Reiter's disease, unspecified site
M02.31 Reiter's disease, shoulder
M02.311 Reiter's disease, right shoulder
M02.312 Reiter's disease, left shoulder
M02.319 Reiter's disease, unspecified shoulder

M02.32 Reiter's disease, elbow
M02.321 Reiter's disease, right elbow
M02.322 Reiter's disease, left elbow
M02.329 Reiter's disease, unspecified elbow
M02.33 Reiter's disease, wrist
Reiter's disease, carpal bones
M02.331 Reiter's disease, right wrist
M02.332 Reiter's disease, left wrist
M02.339 Reiter's disease, unspecified wrist
M02.34 Reiter's disease, hand
Reiter's disease, metacarpus and phalanges
M02.341 Reiter's disease, right hand
M02.342 Reiter's disease, left hand
M02.349 Reiter's disease, unspecified hand
M02.35 Reiter's disease, hip
M02.351 Reiter's disease, right hip
M02.352 Reiter's disease, left hip
M02.359 Reiter's disease, unspecified hip
M02.36 Reiter's disease, knee
M02.361 Reiter's disease, right knee
M02.362 Reiter's disease, left knee
M02.369 Reiter's disease, unspecified knee
M02.37 Reiter's disease, ankle and foot
Reiter's disease, tarsus, metatarsus and phalanges
M02.371 Reiter's disease, right ankle and foot
M02.372 Reiter's disease, left ankle and foot
M02.379 Reiter's disease, unspecified ankle and foot
M02.38 Reiter's disease, vertebrae
M02.39 Reiter's disease, multiple sites
M02.8 Other reactive arthropathies
M02.80 Other reactive arthropathies, unspecified site
M02.81 Other reactive arthropathies, shoulder
M02.811 Other reactive arthropathies, right shoulder
M02.812 Other reactive arthropathies, left shoulder
M02.819 Other reactive arthropathies, unspecified shoulder
M02.82 Other reactive arthropathies, elbow
M02.821 Other reactive arthropathies, right elbow
M02.822 Other reactive arthropathies, left elbow
M02.829 Other reactive arthropathies, unspecified elbow
M02.83 Other reactive arthropathies, wrist
Other reactive arthropathies, carpal bones
M02.831 Other reactive arthropathies, right wrist
M02.832 Other reactive arthropathies, left wrist
M02.839 Other reactive arthropathies, unspecified wrist
M02.84 Other reactive arthropathies, hand
Other reactive arthropathies, metacarpus and phalanges
M02.841 Other reactive arthropathies, right hand
M02.842 Other reactive arthropathies, left hand
M02.849 Other reactive arthropathies, unspecified hand
M02.85 Other reactive arthropathies, hip
M02.851 Other reactive arthropathies, right hip
M02.852 Other reactive arthropathies, left hip
M02.859 Other reactive arthropathies, unspecified hip
M02.86 Other reactive arthropathies, knee
M02.861 Other reactive arthropathies, right knee
M02.862 Other reactive arthropathies, left knee
M02.869 Other reactive arthropathies, unspecified knee
M02.87 Other reactive arthropathies, ankle and foot
Other reactive arthropathies, tarsus, metatarsus and phalanges
M02.871 Other reactive arthropathies, right ankle and foot
M02.872 Other reactive arthropathies, left ankle and foot
M02.879 Other reactive arthropathies, unspecified ankle and foot
M02.88 Other reactive arthropathies, vertebrae
M02.89 Other reactive arthropathies, multiple sites
M02.9 Reactive arthropathy, unspecified

AUTOINFLAMMATORY SYNDROMES (M04)

M04 Autoinflammatory syndromes
Excludes2 Crohn's disease (K50.-)
Coding Clinic: 2016, Q4, P37
M04.1 Periodic fever syndromes
Familial Mediterranean fever
Hyperimmunoglobin D syndrome
Mevalonate kinase deficiency
Tumor necrosis factor receptor associated periodic syndrome [TRAPS]
M04.2 Cryopyrin-associated periodic syndromes
Chronic infantile neurological, cutaneous and articular syndrome [CINCA]
Familial cold autoinflammatory syndrome
Familial cold urticaria
Muckle-Wells syndrome
Neonatal onset multisystemic inflammatory disorder [NOMID]
M04.8 Other autoinflammatory syndromes
Blau syndrome
Deficiency of interleukin 1 receptor antagonist [DIRA]
Majeed syndrome
Periodic fever, aphthous stomatitis, pharyngitis, and adenopathy syndrome [PFAPA]
Pyogenic arthritis, pyoderma gangrenosum, and acne syndrome [PAPA]
M04.9 Autoinflammatory syndrome, unspecified

INFLAMMATORY POLYARTHROPATHIES (M05-M14)

M05 Rheumatoid arthritis with rheumatoid factor
Excludes1 rheumatic fever (I00)
juvenile rheumatoid arthritis (M08.-)
rheumatoid arthritis of spine (M45.-)
M05.0 Felty's syndrome
Rheumatoid arthritis with splenoadenomegaly and leukopenia
M05.00 Felty's syndrome, unspecified site
M05.01 Felty's syndrome, shoulder
M05.011 Felty's syndrome, right shoulder
M05.012 Felty's syndrome, left shoulder
M05.019 Felty's syndrome, unspecified shoulder

CHAPTER 13 (M00-M99)

- M05.02 Felty's syndrome, **elbow**
  - M05.021 Felty's syndrome, **right** elbow
  - M05.022 Felty's syndrome, **left** elbow
  - M05.029 Felty's syndrome, **unspecified** elbow
- M05.03 Felty's syndrome, **wrist**
  - Felty's syndrome, carpal bones
  - M05.031 Felty's syndrome, **right** wrist
  - M05.032 Felty's syndrome, **left** wrist
  - M05.039 Felty's syndrome, **unspecified** wrist
- M05.04 Felty's syndrome, **hand**
  - Felty's syndrome, metacarpus and phalanges
  - M05.041 Felty's syndrome, **right** hand
  - M05.042 Felty's syndrome, **left** hand
  - M05.049 Felty's syndrome, **unspecified** hand
- M05.05 Felty's syndrome, **hip**
  - M05.051 Felty's syndrome, **right** hip
  - M05.052 Felty's syndrome, **left** hip
  - M05.059 Felty's syndrome, **unspecified** hip
- M05.06 Felty's syndrome, **knee**
  - M05.061 Felty's syndrome, **right** knee
  - M05.062 Felty's syndrome, **left** knee
  - M05.069 Felty's syndrome, **unspecified** knee
- M05.07 Felty's syndrome, **ankle and foot**
  - Felty's syndrome, tarsus, metatarsus and phalanges
  - M05.071 Felty's syndrome, **right** ankle and foot
  - M05.072 Felty's syndrome, **left** ankle and foot
  - M05.079 Felty's syndrome, **unspecified** ankle and foot
- M05.09 Felty's syndrome, **multiple sites**

- M05.1 Rheumatoid **lung disease with rheumatoid arthritis**
  - M05.10 Rheumatoid lung disease with rheumatoid arthritis of **unspecified** site
  - M05.11 Rheumatoid lung disease with rheumatoid arthritis of **shoulder**
    - M05.111 Rheumatoid lung disease with rheumatoid arthritis of **right** shoulder
    - M05.112 Rheumatoid lung disease with rheumatoid arthritis of **left** shoulder
    - M05.119 Rheumatoid lung disease with rheumatoid arthritis of **unspecified** shoulder
  - M05.12 Rheumatoid lung disease with rheumatoid arthritis of **elbow**
    - M05.121 Rheumatoid lung disease with rheumatoid arthritis of **right** elbow
    - M05.122 Rheumatoid lung disease with rheumatoid arthritis of **left** elbow
    - M05.129 Rheumatoid lung disease with rheumatoid arthritis of **unspecified** elbow
  - M05.13 Rheumatoid lung disease with rheumatoid arthritis of **wrist**
    - Rheumatoid lung disease with rheumatoid arthritis, carpal bones
    - M05.131 Rheumatoid lung disease with rheumatoid arthritis of **right** wrist
    - M05.132 Rheumatoid lung disease with rheumatoid arthritis of **left** wrist
    - M05.139 Rheumatoid lung disease with rheumatoid arthritis of **unspecified** wrist
  - M05.14 Rheumatoid lung disease with rheumatoid arthritis of **hand**
    - Rheumatoid lung disease with rheumatoid arthritis, metacarpus and phalanges
    - M05.141 Rheumatoid lung disease with rheumatoid arthritis of **right** hand
    - M05.142 Rheumatoid lung disease with rheumatoid arthritis of **left** hand
    - M05.149 Rheumatoid lung disease with rheumatoid arthritis of **unspecified** hand
  - M05.15 Rheumatoid lung disease with rheumatoid arthritis of **hip**
    - M05.151 Rheumatoid lung disease with rheumatoid arthritis of **right** hip
    - M05.152 Rheumatoid lung disease with rheumatoid arthritis of **left** hip
    - M05.159 Rheumatoid lung disease with rheumatoid arthritis of **unspecified** hip
  - M05.16 Rheumatoid lung disease with rheumatoid arthritis of **knee**
    - M05.161 Rheumatoid lung disease with rheumatoid arthritis of **right** knee
    - M05.162 Rheumatoid lung disease with rheumatoid arthritis of **left** knee
    - M05.169 Rheumatoid lung disease with rheumatoid arthritis of **unspecified** knee
  - M05.17 Rheumatoid lung disease with rheumatoid arthritis of **ankle and foot**
    - Rheumatoid lung disease with rheumatoid arthritis, tarsus, metatarsus and phalanges
    - M05.171 Rheumatoid lung disease with rheumatoid arthritis of **right** ankle and foot
    - M05.172 Rheumatoid lung disease with rheumatoid arthritis of **left** ankle and foot
    - M05.179 Rheumatoid lung disease with rheumatoid arthritis of **unspecified** ankle and foot
  - M05.19 Rheumatoid lung disease with rheumatoid arthritis of **multiple sites**

- M05.2 Rheumatoid **vasculitis with rheumatoid arthritis**
  - M05.20 Rheumatoid vasculitis with rheumatoid arthritis of **unspecified** site
  - M05.21 Rheumatoid vasculitis with rheumatoid arthritis of **shoulder**
    - M05.211 Rheumatoid vasculitis with rheumatoid arthritis of **right** shoulder
    - M05.212 Rheumatoid vasculitis with rheumatoid arthritis of **left** shoulder
    - M05.219 Rheumatoid vasculitis with rheumatoid arthritis of **unspecified** shoulder

Item 13–1 Rheumatoid arthritis (RA) is a chronic systemic inflammatory autoimmune disease of undetermined etiology involving primarily the synovial membranes and articular structures of multiple joints. It can also affect other organs, including the eyes, blood vessels, heart, and lungs. The disease is often progressive. In late stages, deformity, ankylosis, and other **inflammatory polyarthropathies** develop.

● M05.22 Rheumatoid vasculitis with rheumatoid arthritis of **elbow**
- M05.221 Rheumatoid vasculitis with rheumatoid arthritis of **right** elbow
- M05.222 Rheumatoid vasculitis with rheumatoid arthritis of **left** elbow
- M05.229 Rheumatoid vasculitis with rheumatoid arthritis of **unspecified** elbow

● M05.23 Rheumatoid vasculitis with rheumatoid arthritis of **wrist**

Rheumatoid vasculitis with rheumatoid arthritis, carpal bones
- M05.231 Rheumatoid vasculitis with rheumatoid arthritis of **right** wrist
- M05.232 Rheumatoid vasculitis with rheumatoid arthritis of **left** wrist
- M05.239 Rheumatoid vasculitis with rheumatoid arthritis of **unspecified** wrist

● M05.24 Rheumatoid vasculitis with rheumatoid arthritis of **hand**

Rheumatoid vasculitis with rheumatoid arthritis, metacarpus and phalanges
- M05.241 Rheumatoid vasculitis with rheumatoid arthritis of **right** hand
- M05.242 Rheumatoid vasculitis with rheumatoid arthritis of **left** hand
- M05.249 Rheumatoid vasculitis with rheumatoid arthritis of **unspecified** hand

● M05.25 Rheumatoid vasculitis with rheumatoid arthritis of **hip**
- M05.251 Rheumatoid vasculitis with rheumatoid arthritis of **right** hip
- M05.252 Rheumatoid vasculitis with rheumatoid arthritis of **left** hip
- M05.259 Rheumatoid vasculitis with rheumatoid arthritis of **unspecified** hip

● M05.26 Rheumatoid vasculitis with rheumatoid arthritis of **knee**
- M05.261 Rheumatoid vasculitis with rheumatoid arthritis of **right** knee
- M05.262 Rheumatoid vasculitis with rheumatoid arthritis of **left** knee
- M05.269 Rheumatoid vasculitis with rheumatoid arthritis of **unspecified** knee

● M05.27 Rheumatoid vasculitis with rheumatoid arthritis of **ankle and foot**

Rheumatoid vasculitis with rheumatoid arthritis, tarsus, metatarsus and phalanges
- M05.271 Rheumatoid vasculitis with rheumatoid arthritis of **right** ankle and foot
- M05.272 Rheumatoid vasculitis with rheumatoid arthritis of **left** ankle and foot
- M05.279 Rheumatoid vasculitis with rheumatoid arthritis of **unspecified** ankle and foot

M05.29 Rheumatoid vasculitis with rheumatoid arthritis of **multiple sites**

● M05.3 Rheumatoid **heart disease with rheumatoid arthritis**

Rheumatoid carditis
Rheumatoid endocarditis
Rheumatoid myocarditis
Rheumatoid pericarditis

M05.30 Rheumatoid heart disease with rheumatoid arthritis of **unspecified** site

● M05.31 Rheumatoid heart disease with rheumatoid arthritis of **shoulder**
- M05.311 Rheumatoid heart disease with rheumatoid arthritis of **right** shoulder
- M05.312 Rheumatoid heart disease with rheumatoid arthritis of **left** shoulder
- M05.319 Rheumatoid heart disease with rheumatoid arthritis of **unspecified** shoulder

● M05.32 Rheumatoid heart disease with rheumatoid arthritis of **elbow**
- M05.321 Rheumatoid heart disease with rheumatoid arthritis of **right** elbow
- M05.322 Rheumatoid heart disease with rheumatoid arthritis of **left** elbow
- M05.329 Rheumatoid heart disease with rheumatoid arthritis of **unspecified** elbow

● M05.33 Rheumatoid heart disease with rheumatoid arthritis of **wrist**

Rheumatoid heart disease with rheumatoid arthritis, carpal bones
- M05.331 Rheumatoid heart disease with rheumatoid arthritis of **right** wrist
- M05.332 Rheumatoid heart disease with rheumatoid arthritis of **left** wrist
- M05.339 Rheumatoid heart disease with rheumatoid arthritis of **unspecified** wrist

● M05.34 Rheumatoid heart disease with rheumatoid arthritis of **hand**

Rheumatoid heart disease with rheumatoid arthritis, metacarpus and phalanges
- M05.341 Rheumatoid heart disease with rheumatoid arthritis of **right** hand
- M05.342 Rheumatoid heart disease with rheumatoid arthritis of **left** hand
- M05.349 Rheumatoid heart disease with rheumatoid arthritis of **unspecified** hand

● M05.35 Rheumatoid heart disease with rheumatoid arthritis of **hip**
- M05.351 Rheumatoid heart disease with rheumatoid arthritis of **right** hip
- M05.352 Rheumatoid heart disease with rheumatoid arthritis of **left** hip
- M05.359 Rheumatoid heart disease with rheumatoid arthritis of **unspecified** hip

● M05.36 Rheumatoid heart disease with rheumatoid arthritis of **knee**
- M05.361 Rheumatoid heart disease with rheumatoid arthritis of **right** knee
- M05.362 Rheumatoid heart disease with rheumatoid arthritis of **left** knee
- M05.369 Rheumatoid heart disease with rheumatoid arthritis of **unspecified** knee

MØ5.37 Rheumatoid heart disease with rheumatoid arthritis of ankle and foot
Rheumatoid heart disease with rheumatoid arthritis, tarsus, metatarsus and phalanges
MØ5.371 Rheumatoid heart disease with rheumatoid arthritis of right ankle and foot
MØ5.372 Rheumatoid heart disease with rheumatoid arthritis of left ankle and foot
MØ5.379 Rheumatoid heart disease with rheumatoid arthritis of unspecified ankle and foot
MØ5.39 Rheumatoid heart disease with rheumatoid arthritis of multiple sites

MØ5.4 Rheumatoid myopathy with rheumatoid arthritis
MØ5.4Ø Rheumatoid myopathy with rheumatoid arthritis of unspecified site
MØ5.41 Rheumatoid myopathy with rheumatoid arthritis of shoulder
MØ5.411 Rheumatoid myopathy with rheumatoid arthritis of right shoulder
MØ5.412 Rheumatoid myopathy with rheumatoid arthritis of left shoulder
MØ5.419 Rheumatoid myopathy with rheumatoid arthritis of unspecified shoulder
MØ5.42 Rheumatoid myopathy with rheumatoid arthritis of elbow
MØ5.421 Rheumatoid myopathy with rheumatoid arthritis of right elbow
MØ5.422 Rheumatoid myopathy with rheumatoid arthritis of left elbow
MØ5.429 Rheumatoid myopathy with rheumatoid arthritis of unspecified elbow
MØ5.43 Rheumatoid myopathy with rheumatoid arthritis of wrist
Rheumatoid myopathy with rheumatoid arthritis, carpal bones
MØ5.431 Rheumatoid myopathy with rheumatoid arthritis of right wrist
MØ5.432 Rheumatoid myopathy with rheumatoid arthritis of left wrist
MØ5.439 Rheumatoid myopathy with rheumatoid arthritis of unspecified wrist
MØ5.44 Rheumatoid myopathy with rheumatoid arthritis of hand
Rheumatoid myopathy with rheumatoid arthritis, metacarpus and phalanges
MØ5.441 Rheumatoid myopathy with rheumatoid arthritis of right hand
MØ5.442 Rheumatoid myopathy with rheumatoid arthritis of left hand
MØ5.449 Rheumatoid myopathy with rheumatoid arthritis of unspecified hand
MØ5.45 Rheumatoid myopathy with rheumatoid arthritis of hip
MØ5.451 Rheumatoid myopathy with rheumatoid arthritis of right hip
MØ5.452 Rheumatoid myopathy with rheumatoid arthritis of left hip
MØ5.459 Rheumatoid myopathy with rheumatoid arthritis of unspecified hip
MØ5.46 Rheumatoid myopathy with rheumatoid arthritis of knee
MØ5.461 Rheumatoid myopathy with rheumatoid arthritis of right knee
MØ5.462 Rheumatoid myopathy with rheumatoid arthritis of left knee
MØ5.469 Rheumatoid myopathy with rheumatoid arthritis of unspecified knee
MØ5.47 Rheumatoid myopathy with rheumatoid arthritis of ankle and foot
Rheumatoid myopathy with rheumatoid arthritis, tarsus, metatarsus and phalanges
MØ5.471 Rheumatoid myopathy with rheumatoid arthritis of right ankle and foot
MØ5.472 Rheumatoid myopathy with rheumatoid arthritis of left ankle and foot
MØ5.479 Rheumatoid myopathy with rheumatoid arthritis of unspecified ankle and foot
MØ5.49 Rheumatoid myopathy with rheumatoid arthritis of multiple sites

MØ5.5 Rheumatoid polyneuropathy with rheumatoid arthritis
MØ5.5Ø Rheumatoid polyneuropathy with rheumatoid arthritis of unspecified site
MØ5.51 Rheumatoid polyneuropathy with rheumatoid arthritis of shoulder
MØ5.511 Rheumatoid polyneuropathy with rheumatoid arthritis of right shoulder
MØ5.512 Rheumatoid polyneuropathy with rheumatoid arthritis of left shoulder
MØ5.519 Rheumatoid polyneuropathy with rheumatoid arthritis of unspecified shoulder
MØ5.52 Rheumatoid polyneuropathy with rheumatoid arthritis of elbow
MØ5.521 Rheumatoid polyneuropathy with rheumatoid arthritis of right elbow
MØ5.522 Rheumatoid polyneuropathy with rheumatoid arthritis of left elbow
MØ5.529 Rheumatoid polyneuropathy with rheumatoid arthritis of unspecified elbow
MØ5.53 Rheumatoid polyneuropathy with rheumatoid arthritis of wrist
Rheumatoid polyneuropathy with rheumatoid arthritis, carpal bones
MØ5.531 Rheumatoid polyneuropathy with rheumatoid arthritis of right wrist
MØ5.532 Rheumatoid polyneuropathy with rheumatoid arthritis of left wrist
MØ5.539 Rheumatoid polyneuropathy with rheumatoid arthritis of unspecified wrist
MØ5.54 Rheumatoid polyneuropathy with rheumatoid arthritis of hand
Rheumatoid polyneuropathy with rheumatoid arthritis, metacarpus and phalanges
MØ5.541 Rheumatoid polyneuropathy with rheumatoid arthritis of right hand
MØ5.542 Rheumatoid polyneuropathy with rheumatoid arthritis of left hand
MØ5.549 Rheumatoid polyneuropathy with rheumatoid arthritis of unspecified hand

● **M05.55** Rheumatoid polyneuropathy with rheumatoid arthritis of **hip**
- **M05.551** Rheumatoid polyneuropathy with rheumatoid arthritis of **right** hip
- **M05.552** Rheumatoid polyneuropathy with rheumatoid arthritis of **left** hip
- **M05.559** Rheumatoid polyneuropathy with rheumatoid arthritis of **unspecified** hip

● **M05.56** Rheumatoid polyneuropathy with rheumatoid arthritis of **knee**
- **M05.561** Rheumatoid polyneuropathy with rheumatoid arthritis of **right** knee
- **M05.562** Rheumatoid polyneuropathy with rheumatoid arthritis of **left** knee
- **M05.569** Rheumatoid polyneuropathy with rheumatoid arthritis of **unspecified** knee

● **M05.57** Rheumatoid polyneuropathy with rheumatoid arthritis of **ankle and foot**
Rheumatoid polyneuropathy with rheumatoid arthritis, tarsus, metatarsus and phalanges
- **M05.571** Rheumatoid polyneuropathy with rheumatoid arthritis of **right** ankle and foot
- **M05.572** Rheumatoid polyneuropathy with rheumatoid arthritis of **left** ankle and foot
- **M05.579** Rheumatoid polyneuropathy with rheumatoid arthritis of **unspecified** ankle and foot

M05.59 Rheumatoid polyneuropathy with rheumatoid arthritis of **multiple sites**

● **M05.6** Rheumatoid arthritis with involvement of other organs and systems

M05.60 Rheumatoid arthritis of **unspecified** site with involvement of other organs and systems

● **M05.61** Rheumatoid arthritis of **shoulder** with involvement of other organs and systems
- **M05.611** Rheumatoid arthritis of **right** shoulder with involvement of other organs and systems
- **M05.612** Rheumatoid arthritis of **left** shoulder with involvement of other organs and systems
- **M05.619** Rheumatoid arthritis of **unspecified** shoulder with involvement of other organs and systems

● **M05.62** Rheumatoid arthritis of **elbow** with involvement of other organs and systems
- **M05.621** Rheumatoid arthritis of **right** elbow with involvement of other organs and systems
- **M05.622** Rheumatoid arthritis of **left** elbow with involvement of other organs and systems
- **M05.629** Rheumatoid arthritis of **unspecified** elbow with involvement of other organs and systems

● **M05.63** Rheumatoid arthritis of **wrist** with involvement of other organs and systems
Rheumatoid arthritis of carpal bones with involvement of other organs and systems
- **M05.631** Rheumatoid arthritis of **right** wrist with involvement of other organs and systems
- **M05.632** Rheumatoid arthritis of **left** wrist with involvement of other organs and systems
- **M05.639** Rheumatoid arthritis of **unspecified** wrist with involvement of other organs and systems

● **M05.64** Rheumatoid arthritis of **hand** with involvement of other organs and systems
Rheumatoid arthritis of metacarpus and phalanges with involvement of other organs and systems
- **M05.641** Rheumatoid arthritis of **right** hand with involvement of other organs and systems
- **M05.642** Rheumatoid arthritis of **left** hand with involvement of other organs and systems
- **M05.649** Rheumatoid arthritis of **unspecified** hand with involvement of other organs and systems

● **M05.65** Rheumatoid arthritis of **hip** with involvement of other organs and systems
- **M05.651** Rheumatoid arthritis of **right** hip with involvement of other organs and systems
- **M05.652** Rheumatoid arthritis of **left** hip with involvement of other organs and systems
- **M05.659** Rheumatoid arthritis of **unspecified** hip with involvement of other organs and systems

● **M05.66** Rheumatoid arthritis of **knee** with involvement of other organs and systems
- **M05.661** Rheumatoid arthritis of **right** knee with involvement of other organs and systems
- **M05.662** Rheumatoid arthritis of **left** knee with involvement of other organs and systems
- **M05.669** Rheumatoid arthritis of **unspecified** knee with involvement of other organs and systems

● **M05.67** Rheumatoid arthritis of **ankle and foot** with involvement of other organs and systems
Rheumatoid arthritis of tarsus, metatarsus and phalanges with involvement of other organs and systems
- **M05.671** Rheumatoid arthritis of **right** ankle and foot with involvement of other organs and systems
- **M05.672** Rheumatoid arthritis of **left** ankle and foot with involvement of other organs and systems
- **M05.679** Rheumatoid arthritis of **unspecified** ankle and foot with involvement of other organs and systems

M05.69 Rheumatoid arthritis of **multiple sites** with involvement of other organs and systems

● **M05.7** Rheumatoid arthritis with rheumatoid factor without organ or systems involvement

M05.70 Rheumatoid arthritis with rheumatoid factor of **unspecified** site without organ or systems involvement

● **M05.71** Rheumatoid arthritis with rheumatoid factor of **shoulder** without organ or systems involvement
- **M05.711** Rheumatoid arthritis with rheumatoid factor of **right** shoulder without organ or systems involvement
- **M05.712** Rheumatoid arthritis with rheumatoid factor of **left** shoulder without organ or systems involvement
- **M05.719** Rheumatoid arthritis with rheumatoid factor of **unspecified** shoulder without organ or systems involvement

M05.72 Rheumatoid arthritis with rheumatoid factor of **elbow** without organ or systems involvement
- M05.721 Rheumatoid arthritis with rheumatoid factor of **right** elbow without organ or systems involvement
- M05.722 Rheumatoid arthritis with rheumatoid factor of **left** elbow without organ or systems involvement
- M05.729 Rheumatoid arthritis with rheumatoid factor of **unspecified** elbow without organ or systems involvement

M05.73 Rheumatoid arthritis with rheumatoid factor of **wrist** without organ or systems involvement
- M05.731 Rheumatoid arthritis with rheumatoid factor of **right** wrist without organ or systems involvement
- M05.732 Rheumatoid arthritis with rheumatoid factor of **left** wrist without organ or systems involvement
- M05.739 Rheumatoid arthritis with rheumatoid factor of **unspecified** wrist without organ or systems involvement

M05.74 Rheumatoid arthritis with rheumatoid factor of **hand** without organ or systems involvement
- M05.741 Rheumatoid arthritis with rheumatoid factor of **right** hand without organ or systems involvement
- M05.742 Rheumatoid arthritis with rheumatoid factor of **left** hand without organ or systems involvement
- M05.749 Rheumatoid arthritis with rheumatoid factor of **unspecified** hand without organ or systems involvement

M05.75 Rheumatoid arthritis with rheumatoid factor of **hip** without organ or systems involvement
- M05.751 Rheumatoid arthritis with rheumatoid factor of **right** hip without organ or systems involvement
- M05.752 Rheumatoid arthritis with rheumatoid factor of **left** hip without organ or systems involvement
- M05.759 Rheumatoid arthritis with rheumatoid factor of **unspecified** hip without organ or systems involvement

M05.76 Rheumatoid arthritis with rheumatoid factor of **knee** without organ or systems involvement
- M05.761 Rheumatoid arthritis with rheumatoid factor of **right** knee without organ or systems involvement
- M05.762 Rheumatoid arthritis with rheumatoid factor of **left** knee without organ or systems involvement
- M05.769 Rheumatoid arthritis with rheumatoid factor of **unspecified** knee without organ or systems involvement

M05.77 Rheumatoid arthritis with rheumatoid factor of **ankle and foot** without organ or systems involvement
- M05.771 Rheumatoid arthritis with rheumatoid factor of **right** ankle and foot without organ or systems involvement
- M05.772 Rheumatoid arthritis with rheumatoid factor of **left** ankle and foot without organ or systems involvement
- M05.779 Rheumatoid arthritis with rheumatoid factor of **unspecified** ankle and foot without organ or systems involvement

M05.79 Rheumatoid arthritis with rheumatoid factor of **multiple sites** without organ or systems involvement

M05.8 **Other** rheumatoid arthritis with **rheumatoid factor**

M05.80 Other rheumatoid arthritis with rheumatoid factor of **unspecified** site

M05.81 Other rheumatoid arthritis with rheumatoid factor of **shoulder**
- M05.811 Other rheumatoid arthritis with rheumatoid factor of **right** shoulder
- M05.812 Other rheumatoid arthritis with rheumatoid factor of **left** shoulder
- M05.819 Other rheumatoid arthritis with rheumatoid factor of **unspecified** shoulder

M05.82 Other rheumatoid arthritis with rheumatoid factor of **elbow**
- M05.821 Other rheumatoid arthritis with rheumatoid factor of **right** elbow
- M05.822 Other rheumatoid arthritis with rheumatoid factor of **left** elbow
- M05.829 Other rheumatoid arthritis with rheumatoid factor of **unspecified** elbow

M05.83 Other rheumatoid arthritis with rheumatoid factor of **wrist**
- M05.831 **Other** rheumatoid arthritis with rheumatoid factor of **right** wrist
- M05.832 Other rheumatoid arthritis with rheumatoid factor of **left** wrist
- M05.839 Other rheumatoid arthritis with rheumatoid factor of **unspecified** wrist

M05.84 Other rheumatoid arthritis with rheumatoid factor of **hand**
- M05.841 Other rheumatoid arthritis with rheumatoid factor of **right** hand
- M05.842 Other rheumatoid arthritis with rheumatoid factor of **left** hand
- M05.849 Other rheumatoid arthritis with rheumatoid factor of **unspecified** hand

M05.85 Other rheumatoid arthritis with rheumatoid factor of **hip**
- M05.851 Other rheumatoid arthritis with rheumatoid factor of **right** hip
- M05.852 Other rheumatoid arthritis with rheumatoid factor of **left** hip
- M05.859 Other rheumatoid arthritis with rheumatoid factor of **unspecified** hip

MØ5.86 Other rheumatoid arthritis with rheumatoid factor of knee
- MØ5.861 Other rheumatoid arthritis with rheumatoid factor of right knee
- MØ5.862 Other rheumatoid arthritis with rheumatoid factor of left knee
- MØ5.869 Other rheumatoid arthritis with rheumatoid factor of unspecified knee

MØ5.87 Other rheumatoid arthritis with rheumatoid factor of ankle and foot
- MØ5.871 Other rheumatoid arthritis with rheumatoid factor of right ankle and foot
- MØ5.872 Other rheumatoid arthritis with rheumatoid factor of left ankle and foot
- MØ5.879 Other rheumatoid arthritis with rheumatoid factor of unspecified ankle and foot

MØ5.89 Other rheumatoid arthritis with rheumatoid factor of multiple sites

MØ5.9 Rheumatoid arthritis with rheumatoid factor, unspecified

MØ6 Other rheumatoid arthritis

MØ6.Ø Rheumatoid arthritis without rheumatoid factor

MØ6.ØØ Rheumatoid arthritis without rheumatoid factor, unspecified site

MØ6.Ø1 Rheumatoid arthritis without rheumatoid factor, shoulder
- MØ6.Ø11 Rheumatoid arthritis without rheumatoid factor, right shoulder
- MØ6.Ø12 Rheumatoid arthritis without rheumatoid factor, left shoulder
- MØ6.Ø19 Rheumatoid arthritis without rheumatoid factor, unspecified shoulder

MØ6.Ø2 Rheumatoid arthritis without rheumatoid factor, elbow
- MØ6.Ø21 Rheumatoid arthritis without rheumatoid factor, right elbow
- MØ6.Ø22 Rheumatoid arthritis without rheumatoid factor, left elbow
- MØ6.Ø29 Rheumatoid arthritis without rheumatoid factor, unspecified elbow

MØ6.Ø3 Rheumatoid arthritis without rheumatoid factor, wrist
- MØ6.Ø31 Rheumatoid arthritis without rheumatoid factor, right wrist
- MØ6.Ø32 Rheumatoid arthritis without rheumatoid factor, left wrist
- MØ6.Ø39 Rheumatoid arthritis without rheumatoid factor, unspecified wrist

MØ6.Ø4 Rheumatoid arthritis without rheumatoid factor, hand
- MØ6.Ø41 Rheumatoid arthritis without rheumatoid factor, right hand
- MØ6.Ø42 Rheumatoid arthritis without rheumatoid factor, left hand
- MØ6.Ø49 Rheumatoid arthritis without rheumatoid factor, unspecified hand

MØ6.Ø5 Rheumatoid arthritis without rheumatoid factor, hip
- MØ6.Ø51 Rheumatoid arthritis without rheumatoid factor, right hip
- MØ6.Ø52 Rheumatoid arthritis without rheumatoid factor, left hip
- MØ6.Ø59 Rheumatoid arthritis without rheumatoid factor, unspecified hip

MØ6.Ø6 Rheumatoid arthritis without rheumatoid factor, knee
- MØ6.Ø61 Rheumatoid arthritis without rheumatoid factor, right knee
- MØ6.Ø62 Rheumatoid arthritis without rheumatoid factor, left knee
- MØ6.Ø69 Rheumatoid arthritis without rheumatoid factor, unspecified knee

MØ6.Ø7 Rheumatoid arthritis without rheumatoid factor, ankle and foot
- MØ6.Ø71 Rheumatoid arthritis without rheumatoid factor, right ankle and foot
- MØ6.Ø72 Rheumatoid arthritis without rheumatoid factor, left ankle and foot
- MØ6.Ø79 Rheumatoid arthritis without rheumatoid factor, unspecified ankle and foot

MØ6.Ø8 Rheumatoid arthritis without rheumatoid factor, vertebrae

MØ6.Ø9 Rheumatoid arthritis without rheumatoid factor, multiple sites

MØ6.1 Adult-onset Still's disease A

Excludes1 Still's disease NOS (MØ8.2-)

MØ6.2 Rheumatoid bursitis

MØ6.2Ø Rheumatoid bursitis, unspecified site

MØ6.21 Rheumatoid bursitis, shoulder
- MØ6.211 Rheumatoid bursitis, right shoulder
- MØ6.212 Rheumatoid bursitis, left shoulder
- MØ6.219 Rheumatoid bursitis, unspecified shoulder

MØ6.22 Rheumatoid bursitis, elbow
- MØ6.221 Rheumatoid bursitis, right elbow
- MØ6.222 Rheumatoid bursitis, left elbow
- MØ6.229 Rheumatoid bursitis, unspecified elbow

MØ6.23 Rheumatoid bursitis, wrist
- MØ6.231 Rheumatoid bursitis, right wrist
- MØ6.232 Rheumatoid bursitis, left wrist
- MØ6.239 Rheumatoid bursitis, unspecified wrist

MØ6.24 Rheumatoid bursitis, hand
- MØ6.241 Rheumatoid bursitis, right hand
- MØ6.242 Rheumatoid bursitis, left hand
- MØ6.249 Rheumatoid bursitis, unspecified hand

MØ6.25 Rheumatoid bursitis, hip
- MØ6.251 Rheumatoid bursitis, right hip
- MØ6.252 Rheumatoid bursitis, left hip
- MØ6.259 Rheumatoid bursitis, unspecified hip

MØ6.26 Rheumatoid bursitis, knee
- MØ6.261 Rheumatoid bursitis, right knee
- MØ6.262 Rheumatoid bursitis, left knee
- MØ6.269 Rheumatoid bursitis, unspecified knee

CHAPTER 13 (MØØ-M99)

● MØ6.27 Rheumatoid bursitis, **ankle and foot**
- MØ6.271 Rheumatoid bursitis, **right** ankle and foot
- MØ6.272 Rheumatoid bursitis, **left** ankle and foot
- MØ6.279 Rheumatoid bursitis, **unspecified** ankle and foot

MØ6.28 Rheumatoid bursitis, **vertebrae**

MØ6.29 Rheumatoid bursitis, **multiple sites**

● MØ6.3 **Rheumatoid nodule**

MØ6.3Ø Rheumatoid nodule, **unspecified** site

● MØ6.31 Rheumatoid nodule, **shoulder**
- MØ6.311 Rheumatoid nodule, **right** shoulder
- MØ6.312 Rheumatoid nodule, **left** shoulder
- MØ6.319 Rheumatoid nodule, **unspecified** shoulder

● MØ6.32 Rheumatoid nodule, **elbow**
- MØ6.321 Rheumatoid nodule, **right** elbow
- MØ6.322 Rheumatoid nodule, **left** elbow
- MØ6.329 Rheumatoid nodule, **unspecified** elbow

● MØ6.33 Rheumatoid nodule, **wrist**
- MØ6.331 Rheumatoid nodule, **right** wrist
- MØ6.332 Rheumatoid nodule, **left** wrist
- MØ6.339 Rheumatoid nodule, **unspecified** wrist

● MØ6.34 Rheumatoid nodule, **hand**
- MØ6.341 Rheumatoid nodule, **right** hand
- MØ6.342 Rheumatoid nodule, **left** hand
- MØ6.349 Rheumatoid nodule, **unspecified** hand

● MØ6.35 Rheumatoid nodule, **hip**
- MØ6.351 Rheumatoid nodule, **right** hip
- MØ6.352 Rheumatoid nodule, **left** hip
- MØ6.359 Rheumatoid nodule, **unspecified** hip

● MØ6.36 Rheumatoid nodule, **knee**
- MØ6.361 Rheumatoid nodule, **right** knee
- MØ6.362 Rheumatoid nodule, **left** knee
- MØ6.369 Rheumatoid nodule, **unspecified** knee

● MØ6.37 Rheumatoid nodule, **ankle and foot**
- MØ6.371 Rheumatoid nodule, **right** ankle and foot
- MØ6.372 Rheumatoid nodule, **left** ankle and foot
- MØ6.379 Rheumatoid nodule, **unspecified** ankle and foot

MØ6.38 Rheumatoid nodule, **vertebrae**

MØ6.39 Rheumatoid nodule, **multiple sites**

MØ6.4 Inflammatory polyarthropathy

Excludes1 polyarthritis NOS (M13.Ø)

● MØ6.8 **Other specified** rheumatoid arthritis

MØ6.8Ø Other specified rheumatoid arthritis, **unspecified** site

● MØ6.81 Other specified rheumatoid arthritis, **shoulder**
- MØ6.811 Other specified rheumatoid arthritis, **right** shoulder
- MØ6.812 Other specified rheumatoid arthritis, **left** shoulder
- MØ6.819 Other specified rheumatoid arthritis, **unspecified** shoulder

● MØ6.82 Other specified rheumatoid arthritis, **elbow**
- MØ6.821 Other specified rheumatoid arthritis, **right** elbow
- MØ6.822 Other specified rheumatoid arthritis, **left** elbow
- MØ6.829 Other specified rheumatoid arthritis, **unspecified** elbow

● MØ6.83 Other specified rheumatoid arthritis, **wrist**
- MØ6.831 Other specified rheumatoid arthritis, **right** wrist
- MØ6.832 Other specified rheumatoid arthritis, **left** wrist
- MØ6.839 Other specified rheumatoid arthritis, **unspecified** wrist

● MØ6.84 Other specified rheumatoid arthritis, **hand**
- MØ6.841 Other specified rheumatoid arthritis, **right** hand
- MØ6.842 Other specified rheumatoid arthritis, **left** hand
- MØ6.849 Other specified rheumatoid arthritis, **unspecified** hand

● MØ6.85 Other specified rheumatoid arthritis, **hip**
- MØ6.851 Other specified rheumatoid arthritis, **right** hip
- MØ6.852 Other specified rheumatoid arthritis, **left** hip
- MØ6.859 Other specified rheumatoid arthritis, **unspecified** hip

● MØ6.86 Other specified rheumatoid arthritis, **knee**
- MØ6.861 Other specified rheumatoid arthritis, **right** knee
- MØ6.862 Other specified rheumatoid arthritis, **left** knee
- MØ6.869 Other specified rheumatoid arthritis, **unspecified** knee

● MØ6.87 Other specified rheumatoid arthritis, **ankle and foot**
- MØ6.871 Other specified rheumatoid arthritis, **right** ankle and foot
- MØ6.872 Other specified rheumatoid arthritis, **left** ankle and foot
- MØ6.879 Other specified rheumatoid arthritis, **unspecified** ankle and foot

MØ6.88 Other specified rheumatoid arthritis, **vertebrae**

MØ6.89 Other specified rheumatoid arthritis, **multiple sites**

MØ6.9 Rheumatoid arthritis, **unspecified**

● MØ7 Enteropathic arthropathies

Code also associated enteropathy, such as:
- regional enteritis [Crohn's disease] (K5Ø.-)
- ulcerative colitis (K51.-)

Excludes1 psoriatic arthropathies (L4Ø.5-)

● MØ7.6 Enteropathic arthropathies

MØ7.6Ø Enteropathic arthropathies, **unspecified** site

● MØ7.61 Enteropathic arthropathies, **shoulder**
- MØ7.611 Enteropathic arthropathies, **right** shoulder
- MØ7.612 Enteropathic arthropathies, **left** shoulder
- MØ7.619 Enteropathic arthropathies, **unspecified** shoulder

● MØ7.62 Enteropathic arthropathies, **elbow**
- MØ7.621 Enteropathic arthropathies, **right** elbow
- MØ7.622 Enteropathic arthropathies, **left** elbow
- MØ7.629 Enteropathic arthropathies, **unspecified** elbow

M07.63 Enteropathic arthropathies, wrist
- M07.631 Enteropathic arthropathies, right wrist
- M07.632 Enteropathic arthropathies, left wrist
- M07.639 Enteropathic arthropathies, unspecified wrist

M07.64 Enteropathic arthropathies, hand
- M07.641 Enteropathic arthropathies, right hand
- M07.642 Enteropathic arthropathies, left hand
- M07.649 Enteropathic arthropathies, unspecified hand

M07.65 Enteropathic arthropathies, hip
- M07.651 Enteropathic arthropathies, right hip
- M07.652 Enteropathic arthropathies, left hip
- M07.659 Enteropathic arthropathies, unspecified hip

M07.66 Enteropathic arthropathies, knee
- M07.661 Enteropathic arthropathies, right knee
- M07.662 Enteropathic arthropathies, left knee
- M07.669 Enteropathic arthropathies, unspecified knee

M07.67 Enteropathic arthropathies, ankle and foot
- M07.671 Enteropathic arthropathies, right ankle and foot
- M07.672 Enteropathic arthropathies, left ankle and foot
- M07.679 Enteropathic arthropathies, unspecified ankle and foot

M07.68 Enteropathic arthropathies, vertebrae

M07.69 Enteropathic arthropathies, multiple sites

M08 Juvenile arthritis

Code also any associated underlying condition, such as:
regional enteritis [Crohn's disease] (K50.-)
ulcerative colitis (K51.-)

Excludes1 arthropathy in Whipple's disease (M14.8)
Felty's syndrome (M05.0)
juvenile dermatomyositis (M33.0-)
psoriatic juvenile arthropathy (L40.54)

M08.0 Unspecified juvenile rheumatoid arthritis
Juvenile rheumatoid arthritis with or without rheumatoid factor

M08.00 Unspecified juvenile rheumatoid arthritis of unspecified site

M08.01 Unspecified juvenile rheumatoid arthritis, shoulder
- M08.011 Unspecified juvenile rheumatoid arthritis, right shoulder
- M08.012 Unspecified juvenile rheumatoid arthritis, left shoulder
- M08.019 Unspecified juvenile rheumatoid arthritis, unspecified shoulder

M08.02 Unspecified juvenile rheumatoid arthritis of elbow
- M08.021 Unspecified juvenile rheumatoid arthritis, right elbow
- M08.022 Unspecified juvenile rheumatoid arthritis, left elbow
- M08.029 Unspecified juvenile rheumatoid arthritis, unspecified elbow

M08.03 Unspecified juvenile rheumatoid arthritis, wrist
- M08.031 Unspecified juvenile rheumatoid arthritis, right wrist
- M08.032 Unspecified juvenile rheumatoid arthritis, left wrist
- M08.039 Unspecified juvenile rheumatoid arthritis, unspecified wrist

M08.04 Unspecified juvenile rheumatoid arthritis, hand
- M08.041 Unspecified juvenile rheumatoid arthritis, right hand
- M08.042 Unspecified juvenile rheumatoid arthritis, left hand
- M08.049 Unspecified juvenile rheumatoid arthritis, unspecified hand

M08.05 Unspecified juvenile rheumatoid arthritis, hip
- M08.051 Unspecified juvenile rheumatoid arthritis, right hip
- M08.052 Unspecified juvenile rheumatoid arthritis, left hip
- M08.059 Unspecified juvenile rheumatoid arthritis, unspecified hip

M08.06 Unspecified juvenile rheumatoid arthritis, knee
- M08.061 Unspecified juvenile rheumatoid arthritis, right knee
- M08.062 Unspecified juvenile rheumatoid arthritis, left knee
- M08.069 Unspecified juvenile rheumatoid arthritis, unspecified knee

M08.07 Unspecified juvenile rheumatoid arthritis, ankle and foot
- M08.071 Unspecified juvenile rheumatoid arthritis, right ankle and foot
- M08.072 Unspecified juvenile rheumatoid arthritis, left ankle and foot
- M08.079 Unspecified juvenile rheumatoid arthritis, unspecified ankle and foot

M08.08 Unspecified juvenile rheumatoid arthritis, vertebrae

M08.09 Unspecified juvenile rheumatoid arthritis, multiple sites

M08.1 Juvenile ankylosing spondylitis

Excludes1 ankylosing spondylitis in adults (M45.0-)

M08.2 Juvenile rheumatoid arthritis with systemic onset
Still's disease NOS

Excludes1 adult-onset Still's disease (M06.1-)

M08.20 Juvenile rheumatoid arthritis with systemic onset, unspecified site

M08.21 Juvenile rheumatoid arthritis with systemic onset, shoulder
- M08.211 Juvenile rheumatoid arthritis with systemic onset, right shoulder
- M08.212 Juvenile rheumatoid arthritis with systemic onset, left shoulder
- M08.219 Juvenile rheumatoid arthritis with systemic onset, unspecified shoulder

M08.22 Juvenile rheumatoid arthritis with systemic onset, elbow
- M08.221 Juvenile rheumatoid arthritis with systemic onset, right elbow
- M08.222 Juvenile rheumatoid arthritis with systemic onset, left elbow
- M08.229 Juvenile rheumatoid arthritis with systemic onset, unspecified elbow

M08.23 Juvenile rheumatoid arthritis with systemic onset, wrist
- M08.231 Juvenile rheumatoid arthritis with systemic onset, right wrist
- M08.232 Juvenile rheumatoid arthritis with systemic onset, left wrist
- M08.239 Juvenile rheumatoid arthritis with systemic onset, unspecified wrist

M08.24 Juvenile rheumatoid arthritis with systemic onset, **hand**
- M08.241 Juvenile rheumatoid arthritis with systemic onset, **right** hand
- M08.242 Juvenile rheumatoid arthritis with systemic onset, **left** hand
- M08.249 Juvenile rheumatoid arthritis with systemic onset, **unspecified** hand

M08.25 Juvenile rheumatoid arthritis with systemic onset, **hip**
- M08.251 Juvenile rheumatoid arthritis with systemic onset, **right** hip
- M08.252 Juvenile rheumatoid arthritis with systemic onset, **left** hip
- M08.259 Juvenile rheumatoid arthritis with systemic onset, **unspecified** hip

M08.26 Juvenile rheumatoid arthritis with systemic onset, **knee**
- M08.261 Juvenile rheumatoid arthritis with systemic onset, **right** knee
- M08.262 Juvenile rheumatoid arthritis with systemic onset, **left** knee
- M08.269 Juvenile rheumatoid arthritis with systemic onset, **unspecified** knee

M08.27 Juvenile rheumatoid arthritis with systemic onset, **ankle and foot**
- M08.271 Juvenile rheumatoid arthritis with systemic onset, **right** ankle and foot
- M08.272 Juvenile rheumatoid arthritis with systemic onset, **left** ankle and foot
- M08.279 Juvenile rheumatoid arthritis with systemic onset, **unspecified** ankle and foot

M08.28 Juvenile rheumatoid arthritis with systemic onset, **vertebrae**

M08.29 Juvenile rheumatoid arthritis with systemic onset, **multiple sites**

M08.3 Juvenile rheumatoid **polyarthritis** (seronegative)

M08.4 **Pauciarticular** juvenile rheumatoid arthritis

M08.40 Pauciarticular juvenile rheumatoid arthritis, **unspecified** site

M08.41 Pauciarticular juvenile rheumatoid arthritis, **shoulder**
- M08.411 Pauciarticular juvenile rheumatoid arthritis, **right** shoulder
- M08.412 Pauciarticular juvenile rheumatoid arthritis, **left** shoulder
- M08.419 Pauciarticular juvenile rheumatoid arthritis, **unspecified** shoulder

M08.42 Pauciarticular juvenile rheumatoid arthritis, **elbow**
- M08.421 Pauciarticular juvenile rheumatoid arthritis, **right** elbow
- M08.422 Pauciarticular juvenile rheumatoid arthritis, **left** elbow
- M08.429 Pauciarticular juvenile rheumatoid arthritis, **unspecified** elbow

M08.43 Pauciarticular juvenile rheumatoid arthritis, **wrist**
- M08.431 Pauciarticular juvenile rheumatoid arthritis, **right** wrist
- M08.432 Pauciarticular juvenile rheumatoid arthritis, **left** wrist
- M08.439 Pauciarticular juvenile rheumatoid arthritis, **unspecified** wrist

M08.44 Pauciarticular juvenile rheumatoid arthritis, **hand**
- M08.441 Pauciarticular juvenile rheumatoid arthritis, **right** hand
- M08.442 Pauciarticular juvenile rheumatoid arthritis, **left** hand
- M08.449 Pauciarticular juvenile rheumatoid arthritis, **unspecified** hand

M08.45 Pauciarticular juvenile rheumatoid arthritis, **hip**
- M08.451 Pauciarticular juvenile rheumatoid arthritis, **right** hip
- M08.452 Pauciarticular juvenile rheumatoid arthritis, **left** hip
- M08.459 Pauciarticular juvenile rheumatoid arthritis, **unspecified** hip

M08.46 Pauciarticular juvenile rheumatoid arthritis, **knee**
- M08.461 Pauciarticular juvenile rheumatoid arthritis, **right** knee
- M08.462 Pauciarticular juvenile rheumatoid arthritis, **left** knee
- M08.469 Pauciarticular juvenile rheumatoid arthritis, **unspecified** knee

M08.47 Pauciarticular juvenile rheumatoid arthritis, **ankle and foot**
- M08.471 Pauciarticular juvenile rheumatoid arthritis, **right** ankle and foot
- M08.472 Pauciarticular juvenile rheumatoid arthritis, **left** ankle and foot
- M08.479 Pauciarticular juvenile rheumatoid arthritis, **unspecified** ankle and foot

M08.48 Pauciarticular juvenile rheumatoid arthritis, **vertebrae**

M08.8 **Other** juvenile arthritis

M08.80 Other juvenile arthritis, **unspecified** site

M08.81 Other juvenile arthritis, **shoulder**
- M08.811 Other juvenile arthritis, **right** shoulder
- M08.812 Other juvenile arthritis, **left** shoulder
- M08.819 Other juvenile arthritis, **unspecified** shoulder

M08.82 Other juvenile arthritis, **elbow**
- M08.821 Other juvenile arthritis, **right** elbow
- M08.822 Other juvenile arthritis, **left** elbow
- M08.829 Other juvenile arthritis, **unspecified** elbow

M08.83 Other juvenile arthritis, **wrist**
- M08.831 Other juvenile arthritis, **right** wrist
- M08.832 Other juvenile arthritis, **left** wrist
- M08.839 Other juvenile arthritis, **unspecified** wrist

M08.84 Other juvenile arthritis, **hand**
- M08.841 Other juvenile arthritis, **right** hand
- M08.842 Other juvenile arthritis, **left** hand
- M08.849 Other juvenile arthritis, **unspecified** hand

M08.85 Other juvenile arthritis, **hip**
- M08.851 Other juvenile arthritis, **right** hip
- M08.852 Other juvenile arthritis, **left** hip
- M08.859 Other juvenile arthritis, **unspecified** hip

● MØ8.86 Other juvenile arthritis, knee
MØ8.861 Other juvenile arthritis, right knee
MØ8.862 Other juvenile arthritis, left knee
MØ8.869 Other juvenile arthritis, unspecified knee
● MØ8.87 Other juvenile arthritis, ankle and foot
MØ8.871 Other juvenile arthritis, right ankle and foot
MØ8.872 Other juvenile arthritis, left ankle and foot
MØ8.879 Other juvenile arthritis, unspecified ankle and foot
MØ8.88 Other juvenile arthritis, other specified site
Other juvenile arthritis, vertebrae
MØ8.89 Other juvenile arthritis, multiple sites
● MØ8.9 Juvenile arthritis, unspecified
Excludes1 juvenile rheumatoid arthritis, unspecified (MØ8.Ø-)
MØ8.9Ø Juvenile arthritis, unspecified, unspecified site
● MØ8.91 Juvenile arthritis, unspecified, shoulder
MØ8.911 Juvenile arthritis, unspecified, right shoulder
MØ8.912 Juvenile arthritis, unspecified, left shoulder
MØ8.919 Juvenile arthritis, unspecified, unspecified shoulder
● MØ8.92 Juvenile arthritis, unspecified, elbow
MØ8.921 Juvenile arthritis, unspecified, right elbow
MØ8.922 Juvenile arthritis, unspecified, left elbow
MØ8.929 Juvenile arthritis, unspecified, unspecified elbow
● MØ8.93 Juvenile arthritis, unspecified, wrist
MØ8.931 Juvenile arthritis, unspecified, right wrist
MØ8.932 Juvenile arthritis, unspecified, left wrist
MØ8.939 Juvenile arthritis, unspecified, unspecified wrist
● MØ8.94 Juvenile arthritis, unspecified, hand
MØ8.941 Juvenile arthritis, unspecified, right hand
MØ8.942 Juvenile arthritis, unspecified, left hand
MØ8.949 Juvenile arthritis, unspecified, unspecified hand
● MØ8.95 Juvenile arthritis, unspecified, hip
MØ8.951 Juvenile arthritis, unspecified, right hip
MØ8.952 Juvenile arthritis, unspecified, left hip
MØ8.959 Juvenile arthritis, unspecified, unspecified hip
● MØ8.96 Juvenile arthritis, unspecified, knee
MØ8.961 Juvenile arthritis, unspecified, right knee
MØ8.962 Juvenile arthritis, unspecified, left knee
MØ8.969 Juvenile arthritis, unspecified, unspecified knee
● MØ8.97 Juvenile arthritis, unspecified, ankle and foot
MØ8.971 Juvenile arthritis, unspecified, right ankle and foot
MØ8.972 Juvenile arthritis, unspecified, left ankle and foot
MØ8.979 Juvenile arthritis, unspecified, unspecified ankle and foot
MØ8.98 Juvenile arthritis, unspecified, vertebrae
MØ8.99 Juvenile arthritis, unspecified, multiple sites

● M1A Chronic gout
Use additional code to identify:
Autonomic neuropathy in diseases classified elsewhere (G99.Ø)
Calculus of urinary tract in diseases classified elsewhere (N22)
Cardiomyopathy in diseases classified elsewhere (I43)
Disorders of external ear in diseases classified elsewhere (H61.1-, H62.8-)
Disorders of iris and ciliary body in diseases classified elsewhere (H22)
Glomerular disorders in diseases classified elsewhere (NØ8)
Excludes1 gout NOS (M10.-)
Excludes2 acute gout (M1Ø.-)
The appropriate 7th character is to be added to each code from category M1A

Ø	without tophus (tophi)
1	with tophus (tophi)

● M1A.Ø Idiopathic chronic gout
Chronic gouty bursitis
Primary chronic gout
X● M1A.ØØ Idiopathic chronic gout, unspecified site
● M1A.Ø1 Idiopathic chronic gout, shoulder
● M1A.Ø11 Idiopathic chronic gout, right shoulder
● M1A.Ø12 Idiopathic chronic gout, left shoulder
● M1A.Ø19 Idiopathic chronic gout, unspecified shoulder
● M1A.Ø2 Idiopathic chronic gout, elbow
● M1A.Ø21 Idiopathic chronic gout, right elbow
● M1A.Ø22 Idiopathic chronic gout, left elbow
● M1A.Ø29 Idiopathic chronic gout, unspecified elbow
● M1A.Ø3 Idiopathic chronic gout, wrist
● M1A.Ø31 Idiopathic chronic gout, right wrist
● M1A.Ø32 Idiopathic chronic gout, left wrist
● M1A.Ø39 Idiopathic chronic gout, unspecified wrist
● M1A.Ø4 Idiopathic chronic gout, hand
● M1A.Ø41 Idiopathic chronic gout, right hand
● M1A.Ø42 Idiopathic chronic gout, left hand
● M1A.Ø49 Idiopathic chronic gout, unspecified hand
● M1A.Ø5 Idiopathic chronic gout, hip
● M1A.Ø51 Idiopathic chronic gout, right hip
● M1A.Ø52 Idiopathic chronic gout, left hip
● M1A.Ø59 Idiopathic chronic gout, unspecified hip
● M1A.Ø6 Idiopathic chronic gout, knee
● M1A.Ø61 Idiopathic chronic gout, right knee
● M1A.Ø62 Idiopathic chronic gout, left knee
● M1A.Ø69 Idiopathic chronic gout, unspecified knee
● M1A.Ø7 Idiopathic chronic gout, ankle and foot
● M1A.Ø71 Idiopathic chronic gout, right ankle and foot
● M1A.Ø72 Idiopathic chronic gout, left ankle and foot
● M1A.Ø79 Idiopathic chronic gout, unspecified ankle and foot
X● M1A.Ø8 Idiopathic chronic gout, vertebrae
X● M1A.Ø9 Idiopathic chronic gout, multiple sites

● M1A.1 Lead-induced chronic gout
Code first toxic effects of lead and its compounds (T56.Ø-)
X● M1A.1Ø Lead-induced chronic gout, **unspecified** site
● M1A.11 Lead-induced chronic gout, **shoulder**
● M1A.111 Lead-induced chronic gout, **right** shoulder
● M1A.112 Lead-induced chronic gout, **left** shoulder
● M1A.119 Lead-induced chronic gout, **unspecified** shoulder
● M1A.12 Lead-induced chronic gout, **elbow**
● M1A.121 Lead-induced chronic gout, **right** elbow
● M1A.122 Lead-induced chronic gout, **left** elbow
● M1A.129 Lead-induced chronic gout, **unspecified** elbow
● M1A.13 Lead-induced chronic gout, **wrist**
● M1A.131 Lead-induced chronic gout, **right** wrist
● M1A.132 Lead-induced chronic gout, **left** wrist
● M1A.139 Lead-induced chronic gout, **unspecified** wrist
● M1A.14 Lead-induced chronic gout, **hand**
● M1A.141 Lead-induced chronic gout, **right** hand
● M1A.142 Lead-induced chronic gout, **left** hand
● M1A.149 Lead-induced chronic gout, **unspecified** hand
● M1A.15 Lead-induced chronic gout, **hip**
● M1A.151 Lead-induced chronic gout, **right** hip
● M1A.152 Lead-induced chronic gout, **left** hip
● M1A.159 Lead-induced chronic gout, **unspecified** hip
● M1A.16 Lead-induced chronic gout, **knee**
● M1A.161 Lead-induced chronic gout, **right** knee
● M1A.162 Lead-induced chronic gout, **left** knee
● M1A.169 Lead-induced chronic gout, **unspecified** knee
● M1A.17 Lead-induced chronic gout, **ankle and foot**
● M1A.171 Lead-induced chronic gout, **right** ankle and foot
● M1A.172 Lead-induced chronic gout, **left** ankle and foot
● M1A.179 Lead-induced chronic gout, **unspecified** ankle and foot
X● M1A.18 Lead-induced chronic gout, **vertebrae**
X● M1A.19 Lead-induced chronic gout, **multiple sites**
● M1A.2 Drug-induced chronic gout
Use additional code for adverse effect, if applicable, to identify drug (T36-T5Ø with fifth or sixth character 5)
X● M1A.2Ø Drug-induced chronic gout, **unspecified** site
● M1A.21 Drug-induced chronic gout, **shoulder**
● M1A.211 Drug-induced chronic gout, **right** shoulder
● M1A.212 Drug-induced chronic gout, **left** shoulder
● M1A.219 Drug-induced chronic gout, **unspecified** shoulder
● M1A.22 Drug-induced chronic gout, **elbow**
● M1A.221 Drug-induced chronic gout, **right** elbow
● M1A.222 Drug-induced chronic gout, **left** elbow
● M1A.229 Drug-induced chronic gout, **unspecified** elbow
● M1A.23 Drug-induced chronic gout, **wrist**
● M1A.231 Drug-induced chronic gout, **right** wrist
● M1A.232 Drug-induced chronic gout, **left** wrist
● M1A.239 Drug-induced chronic gout, **unspecified** wrist
● M1A.24 Drug-induced chronic gout, **hand**
● M1A.241 Drug-induced chronic gout, **right** hand
● M1A.242 Drug-induced chronic gout, **left** hand
● M1A.249 Drug-induced chronic gout, **unspecified** hand
● M1A.25 Drug-induced chronic gout, **hip**
● M1A.251 Drug-induced chronic gout, **right** hip
● M1A.252 Drug-induced chronic gout, **left** hip
● M1A.259 Drug-induced chronic gout, **unspecified** hip
● M1A.26 Drug-induced chronic gout, **knee**
● M1A.261 Drug-induced chronic gout, **right** knee
● M1A.262 Drug-induced chronic gout, **left** knee
● M1A.269 Drug-induced chronic gout, **unspecified** knee
● M1A.27 Drug-induced chronic gout, **ankle and foot**
● M1A.271 Drug-induced chronic gout, **right** ankle and foot
● M1A.272 Drug-induced chronic gout, **left** ankle and foot
● M1A.279 Drug-induced chronic gout, **unspecified** ankle and foot
X● M1A.28 Drug-induced chronic gout, **vertebrae**
X● M1A.29 Drug-induced chronic gout, **multiple sites**
● M1A.3 Chronic gout due to renal impairment
Code first associated renal disease
X● M1A.3Ø Chronic gout due to renal impairment, **unspecified** site
● M1A.31 Chronic gout due to renal impairment, **shoulder**
● M1A.311 Chronic gout due to renal impairment, **right** shoulder
● M1A.312 Chronic gout due to renal impairment, **left** shoulder
● M1A.319 Chronic gout due to renal impairment, **unspecified** shoulder
● M1A.32 Chronic gout due to renal impairment, **elbow**
● M1A.321 Chronic gout due to renal impairment, **right** elbow
● M1A.322 Chronic gout due to renal impairment, **left** elbow
● M1A.329 Chronic gout due to renal impairment, **unspecified** elbow
● M1A.33 Chronic gout due to renal impairment, **wrist**
● M1A.331 Chronic gout due to renal impairment, **right** wrist
● M1A.332 Chronic gout due to renal impairment, **left** wrist
● M1A.339 Chronic gout due to renal impairment, **unspecified** wrist
● M1A.34 Chronic gout due to renal impairment, **hand**
● M1A.341 Chronic gout due to renal impairment, **right** hand
● M1A.342 Chronic gout due to renal impairment, **left** hand
● M1A.349 Chronic gout due to renal impairment, **unspecified** hand

CHAPTER 13 (MØØ-M99)

● **M1A.35** Chronic gout due to renal impairment, **hip**
- ● **M1A.351** Chronic gout due to renal impairment, **right** hip
- ● **M1A.352** Chronic gout due to renal impairment, **left** hip
- ● **M1A.359** Chronic gout due to renal impairment, **unspecified** hip

● **M1A.36** Chronic gout due to renal impairment, **knee**
- ● **M1A.361** Chronic gout due to renal impairment, **right** knee
- ● **M1A.362** Chronic gout due to renal impairment, **left** knee
- ● **M1A.369** Chronic gout due to renal impairment, **unspecified** knee

● **M1A.37** Chronic gout due to renal impairment, **ankle and foot**
- ● **M1A.371** Chronic gout due to renal impairment, **right** ankle and foot
- ● **M1A.372** Chronic gout due to renal impairment, **left** ankle and foot
- ● **M1A.379** Chronic gout due to renal impairment, **unspecified** ankle and foot

X● **M1A.38** Chronic gout due to renal impairment, **vertebrae**

X● **M1A.39** Chronic gout due to renal impairment, **multiple sites**

● **M1A.4** **Other secondary** chronic gout

Code first associated condition

X● **M1A.40** Other secondary chronic gout, **unspecified site**

● **M1A.41** Other secondary chronic gout, **shoulder**
- ● **M1A.411** Other secondary chronic gout, **right** shoulder
- ● **M1A.412** Other secondary chronic gout, **left** shoulder
- ● **M1A.419** Other secondary chronic gout, **unspecified** shoulder

● **M1A.42** Other secondary chronic gout, **elbow**
- ● **M1A.421** Other secondary chronic gout, **right** elbow
- ● **M1A.422** Other secondary chronic gout, **left** elbow
- ● **M1A.429** Other secondary chronic gout, **unspecified** elbow

● **M1A.43** Other secondary chronic gout, **wrist**
- ● **M1A.431** Other secondary chronic gout, **right** wrist
- ● **M1A.432** Other secondary chronic gout, **left** wrist
- ● **M1A.439** Other secondary chronic gout, **unspecified** wrist

● **M1A.44** Other secondary chronic gout, **hand**
- ● **M1A.441** Other secondary chronic gout, **right** hand
- ● **M1A.442** Other secondary chronic gout, **left** hand
- ● **M1A.449** Other secondary chronic gout, **unspecified** hand

● **M1A.45** Other secondary chronic gout, **hip**
- ● **M1A.451** Other secondary chronic gout, **right** hip
- ● **M1A.452** Other secondary chronic gout, **left** hip
- ● **M1A.459** Other secondary chronic gout, **unspecified** hip

● **M1A.46** Other secondary chronic gout, **knee**
- ● **M1A.461** Other secondary chronic gout, **right** knee
- ● **M1A.462** Other secondary chronic gout, **left** knee
- ● **M1A.469** Other secondary chronic gout, **unspecified** knee

● **M1A.47** Other secondary chronic gout, **ankle and foot**
- ● **M1A.471** Other secondary chronic gout, **right** ankle and foot
- ● **M1A.472** Other secondary chronic gout, **left** ankle and foot
- ● **M1A.479** Other secondary chronic gout, **unspecified** ankle and foot

X● **M1A.48** Other secondary chronic gout, **vertebrae**

X● **M1A.49** Other secondary chronic gout, **multiple sites**

X● **M1A.9** Chronic gout, **unspecified**

● **M10** Gout

Accumulation of uric acid that results in swollen, red, hot, painful, stiff joints

Acute gout
Gout attack
Gout flare
Podagra

Use additional code to identify:
- Autonomic neuropathy in diseases classified elsewhere (G99.0)
- Calculus of urinary tract in diseases classified elsewhere (N22)
- Cardiomyopathy in diseases classified elsewhere (I43)
- Disorders of external ear in diseases classified elsewhere (H61.1-, H62.8-)
- Disorders of iris and ciliary body in diseases classified elsewhere (H22)
- Glomerular disorders in diseases classified elsewhere (N08)

Excludes2 chronic gout (M1A.-)

● **M10.0** **Idiopathic gout**

Gouty bursitis
Primary gout

M10.00 Idiopathic gout, **unspecified site**

● **M10.01** Idiopathic gout, **shoulder**
- **M10.011** Idiopathic gout, **right** shoulder
- **M10.012** Idiopathic gout, **left** shoulder
- **M10.019** Idiopathic gout, **unspecified** shoulder

● **M10.02** Idiopathic gout, **elbow**
- **M10.021** Idiopathic gout, **right** elbow
- **M10.022** Idiopathic gout, **left** elbow
- **M10.029** Idiopathic gout, **unspecified** elbow

● **M10.03** Idiopathic gout, **wrist**
- **M10.031** Idiopathic gout, **right** wrist
- **M10.032** Idiopathic gout, **left** wrist
- **M10.039** Idiopathic gout, **unspecified** wrist

● **M10.04** Idiopathic gout, **hand**
- **M10.041** Idiopathic gout, **right** hand
- **M10.042** Idiopathic gout, **left** hand
- **M10.049** Idiopathic gout, **unspecified** hand

● **M10.05** Idiopathic gout, **hip**
- **M10.051** Idiopathic gout, **right** hip
- **M10.052** Idiopathic gout, **left** hip
- **M10.059** Idiopathic gout, **unspecified** hip

● **M10.06** Idiopathic gout, **knee**
- **M10.061** Idiopathic gout, **right** knee
- **M10.062** Idiopathic gout, **left** knee
- **M10.069** Idiopathic gout, **unspecified** knee

- M10.07 Idiopathic gout, **ankle and foot**
  - M10.071 Idiopathic gout, **right** ankle and foot
  - M10.072 Idiopathic gout, **left** ankle and foot
  - M10.079 Idiopathic gout, **unspecified** ankle and foot
- M10.08 Idiopathic gout, **vertebrae**
- M10.09 Idiopathic gout, **multiple sites**

M10.1 Lead-induced gout

Code first toxic effects of lead and its compounds (T56.0-)

- M10.10 Lead-induced gout, **unspecified** site
- M10.11 Lead-induced gout, **shoulder**
  - M10.111 Lead-induced gout, **right** shoulder
  - M10.112 Lead-induced gout, **left** shoulder
  - M10.119 Lead-induced gout, **unspecified** shoulder
- M10.12 Lead-induced gout, **elbow**
  - M10.121 Lead-induced gout, **right** elbow
  - M10.122 Lead-induced gout, **left** elbow
  - M10.129 Lead-induced gout, **unspecified** elbow
- M10.13 Lead-induced gout, **wrist**
  - M10.131 Lead-induced gout, **right** wrist
  - M10.132 Lead-induced gout, **left** wrist
  - M10.139 Lead-induced gout, **unspecified** wrist
- M10.14 Lead-induced gout, **hand**
  - M10.141 Lead-induced gout, **right** hand
  - M10.142 Lead-induced gout, **left** hand
  - M10.149 Lead-induced gout, **unspecified** hand
- M10.15 Lead-induced gout, **hip**
  - M10.151 Lead-induced gout, **right** hip
  - M10.152 Lead-induced gout, **left** hip
  - M10.159 Lead-induced gout, **unspecified** hip
- M10.16 Lead-induced gout, **knee**
  - M10.161 Lead-induced gout, **right** knee
  - M10.162 Lead-induced gout, **left** knee
  - M10.169 Lead-induced gout, **unspecified** knee
- M10.17 Lead-induced gout, **ankle and foot**
  - M10.171 Lead-induced gout, **right** ankle and foot
  - M10.172 Lead-induced gout, **left** ankle and foot
  - M10.179 Lead-induced gout, **unspecified** ankle and foot
- M10.18 Lead-induced gout, **vertebrae**
- M10.19 Lead-induced gout, **multiple sites**

M10.2 Drug-induced gout

Use additional code for adverse effect, if applicable, to identify drug (T36-T50 with fifth or sixth character 5)

- M10.20 Drug-induced gout, **unspecified** site
- M10.21 Drug-induced gout, **shoulder**
  - M10.211 Drug-induced gout, **right** shoulder
  - M10.212 Drug-induced gout, **left** shoulder
  - M10.219 Drug-induced gout, **unspecified** shoulder
- M10.22 Drug-induced gout, **elbow**
  - M10.221 Drug-induced gout, **right** elbow
  - M10.222 Drug-induced gout, **left** elbow
  - M10.229 Drug-induced gout, **unspecified** elbow
- M10.23 Drug-induced gout, **wrist**
  - M10.231 Drug-induced gout, **right** wrist
  - M10.232 Drug-induced gout, **left** wrist
  - M10.239 Drug-induced gout, **unspecified** wrist
- M10.24 Drug-induced gout, **hand**
  - M10.241 Drug-induced gout, **right** hand
  - M10.242 Drug-induced gout, **left** hand
  - M10.249 Drug-induced gout, **unspecified** hand
- M10.25 Drug-induced gout, **hip**
  - M10.251 Drug-induced gout, **right** hip
  - M10.252 Drug-induced gout, **left** hip
  - M10.259 Drug-induced gout, **unspecified** hip
- M10.26 Drug-induced gout, **knee**
  - M10.261 Drug-induced gout, **right** knee
  - M10.262 Drug-induced gout, **left** knee
  - M10.269 Drug-induced gout, **unspecified** knee
- M10.27 Drug-induced gout, **ankle and foot**
  - M10.271 Drug-induced gout, **right** ankle and foot
  - M10.272 Drug-induced gout, **left** ankle and foot
  - M10.279 Drug-induced gout, **unspecified** ankle and foot
- M10.28 Drug-induced gout, **vertebrae**
- M10.29 Drug-induced gout, **multiple sites**

M10.3 Gout due to renal impairment

Code also associated renal disease

- M10.30 Gout due to renal impairment, **unspecified** site
- M10.31 Gout due to renal impairment, **shoulder**
  - M10.311 Gout due to renal impairment, **right** shoulder
  - M10.312 Gout due to renal impairment, **left** shoulder
  - M10.319 Gout due to renal impairment, **unspecified** shoulder
- M10.32 Gout due to renal impairment, **elbow**
  - M10.321 Gout due to renal impairment, **right** elbow
  - M10.322 Gout due to renal impairment, **left** elbow
  - M10.329 Gout due to renal impairment, **unspecified** elbow
- M10.33 Gout due to renal impairment, **wrist**
  - M10.331 Gout due to renal impairment, **right** wrist
  - M10.332 Gout due to renal impairment, **left** wrist
  - M10.339 Gout due to renal impairment, **unspecified** wrist
- M10.34 Gout due to renal impairment, **hand**
  - M10.341 Gout due to renal impairment, **right** hand
  - M10.342 Gout due to renal impairment, **left** hand
  - M10.349 Gout due to renal impairment, **unspecified** hand
- M10.35 Gout due to renal impairment, **hip**
  - M10.351 Gout due to renal impairment, **right** hip
  - M10.352 Gout due to renal impairment, **left** hip
  - M10.359 Gout due to renal impairment, **unspecified** hip
- M10.36 Gout due to renal impairment, **knee**
  - M10.361 Gout due to renal impairment, **right** knee
  - M10.362 Gout due to renal impairment, **left** knee
  - M10.369 Gout due to renal impairment, **unspecified** knee

M10.37 Gout due to renal impairment, ankle and foot
M10.371 Gout due to renal impairment, right ankle and foot
M10.372 Gout due to renal impairment, left ankle and foot
M10.379 Gout due to renal impairment, unspecified ankle and foot
M10.38 Gout due to renal impairment, vertebrae
M10.39 Gout due to renal impairment, multiple sites
M10.4 Other secondary gout
Code first associated condition
M10.40 Other secondary gout, unspecified site
M10.41 Other secondary gout, shoulder
M10.411 Other secondary gout, right shoulder
M10.412 Other secondary gout, left shoulder
M10.419 Other secondary gout, unspecified shoulder
M10.42 Other secondary gout, elbow
M10.421 Other secondary gout, right elbow
M10.422 Other secondary gout, left elbow
M10.429 Other secondary gout, unspecified elbow
M10.43 Other secondary gout, wrist
M10.431 Other secondary gout, right wrist
M10.432 Other secondary gout, left wrist
M10.439 Other secondary gout, unspecified wrist
M10.44 Other secondary gout, hand
M10.441 Other secondary gout, right hand
M10.442 Other secondary gout, left hand
M10.449 Other secondary gout, unspecified hand
M10.45 Other secondary gout, hip
M10.451 Other secondary gout, right hip
M10.452 Other secondary gout, left hip
M10.459 Other secondary gout, unspecified hip
M10.46 Other secondary gout, knee
M10.461 Other secondary gout, right knee
M10.462 Other secondary gout, left knee
M10.469 Other secondary gout, unspecified knee
M10.47 Other secondary gout, ankle and foot
M10.471 Other secondary gout, right ankle and foot
M10.472 Other secondary gout, left ankle and foot
M10.479 Other secondary gout, unspecified ankle and foot
M10.48 Other secondary gout, vertebrae
M10.49 Other secondary gout, multiple sites
M10.9 Gout, unspecified
Gout NOS

M11 Other crystal arthropathies
M11.0 Hydroxyapatite deposition disease
M11.00 Hydroxyapatite deposition disease, unspecified site
M11.01 Hydroxyapatite deposition disease, shoulder
M11.011 Hydroxyapatite deposition disease, right shoulder
M11.012 Hydroxyapatite deposition disease, left shoulder
M11.019 Hydroxyapatite deposition disease, unspecified shoulder
M11.02 Hydroxyapatite deposition disease, elbow
M11.021 Hydroxyapatite deposition disease, right elbow
M11.022 Hydroxyapatite deposition disease, left elbow
M11.029 Hydroxyapatite deposition disease, unspecified elbow
M11.03 Hydroxyapatite deposition disease, wrist
M11.031 Hydroxyapatite deposition disease, right wrist
M11.032 Hydroxyapatite deposition disease, left wrist
M11.039 Hydroxyapatite deposition disease, unspecified wrist
M11.04 Hydroxyapatite deposition disease, hand
M11.041 Hydroxyapatite deposition disease, right hand
M11.042 Hydroxyapatite deposition disease, left hand
M11.049 Hydroxyapatite deposition disease, unspecified hand
M11.05 Hydroxyapatite deposition disease, hip
M11.051 Hydroxyapatite deposition disease, right hip
M11.052 Hydroxyapatite deposition disease, left hip
M11.059 Hydroxyapatite deposition disease, unspecified hip
M11.06 Hydroxyapatite deposition disease, knee
M11.061 Hydroxyapatite deposition disease, right knee
M11.062 Hydroxyapatite deposition disease, left knee
M11.069 Hydroxyapatite deposition disease, unspecified knee
M11.07 Hydroxyapatite deposition disease, ankle and foot
M11.071 Hydroxyapatite deposition disease, right ankle and foot
M11.072 Hydroxyapatite deposition disease, left ankle and foot
M11.079 Hydroxyapatite deposition disease, unspecified ankle and foot
M11.08 Hydroxyapatite deposition disease, vertebrae
M11.09 Hydroxyapatite deposition disease, multiple sites
M11.1 Familial chondrocalcinosis
M11.10 Familial chondrocalcinosis, unspecified site
M11.11 Familial chondrocalcinosis, shoulder
M11.111 Familial chondrocalcinosis, right shoulder
M11.112 Familial chondrocalcinosis, left shoulder
M11.119 Familial chondrocalcinosis, unspecified shoulder
M11.12 Familial chondrocalcinosis, elbow
M11.121 Familial chondrocalcinosis, right elbow
M11.122 Familial chondrocalcinosis, left elbow
M11.129 Familial chondrocalcinosis, unspecified elbow
M11.13 Familial chondrocalcinosis, wrist
M11.131 Familial chondrocalcinosis, right wrist
M11.132 Familial chondrocalcinosis, left wrist
M11.139 Familial chondrocalcinosis, unspecified wrist

● M11.14 Familial chondrocalcinosis, **hand**
M11.141 Familial chondrocalcinosis, **right** hand
M11.142 Familial chondrocalcinosis, **left** hand
M11.149 Familial chondrocalcinosis, **unspecified** hand
● M11.15 Familial chondrocalcinosis, **hip**
M11.151 Familial chondrocalcinosis, **right** hip
M11.152 Familial chondrocalcinosis, **left** hip
M11.159 Familial chondrocalcinosis, **unspecified** hip
● M11.16 Familial chondrocalcinosis, **knee**
M11.161 Familial chondrocalcinosis, **right** knee
M11.162 Familial chondrocalcinosis, **left** knee
M11.169 Familial chondrocalcinosis, **unspecified** knee
● M11.17 Familial chondrocalcinosis, **ankle and foot**
M11.171 Familial chondrocalcinosis, **right** ankle and foot
M11.172 Familial chondrocalcinosis, **left** ankle and foot
M11.179 Familial chondrocalcinosis, **unspecified** ankle and foot
M11.18 Familial chondrocalcinosis, **vertebrae**
M11.19 Familial chondrocalcinosis, **multiple sites**
● M11.2 **Other** chondrocalcinosis
Chondrocalcinosis NOS
M11.20 Other chondrocalcinosis, **unspecified** site
● M11.21 Other chondrocalcinosis, **shoulder**
M11.211 Other chondrocalcinosis, **right** shoulder
M11.212 Other chondrocalcinosis, **left** shoulder
M11.219 Other chondrocalcinosis, **unspecified** shoulder
● M11.22 Other chondrocalcinosis, **elbow**
M11.221 Other chondrocalcinosis, **right** elbow
M11.222 Other chondrocalcinosis, **left** elbow
M11.229 Other chondrocalcinosis, **unspecified** elbow
● M11.23 Other chondrocalcinosis, **wrist**
M11.231 Other chondrocalcinosis, **right** wrist
M11.232 Other chondrocalcinosis, **left** wrist
M11.239 Other chondrocalcinosis, **unspecified** wrist
● M11.24 Other chondrocalcinosis, **hand**
M11.241 Other chondrocalcinosis, **right** hand
M11.242 Other chondrocalcinosis, **left** hand
M11.249 Other chondrocalcinosis, **unspecified** hand
● M11.25 Other chondrocalcinosis, **hip**
M11.251 Other chondrocalcinosis, **right** hip
M11.252 Other chondrocalcinosis, **left** hip
M11.259 Other chondrocalcinosis, **unspecified** hip
● M11.26 Other chondrocalcinosis, **knee**
M11.261 Other chondrocalcinosis, **right** knee
M11.262 Other chondrocalcinosis, **left** knee
M11.269 Other chondrocalcinosis, **unspecified** knee
● M11.27 Other chondrocalcinosis, **ankle and foot**
M11.271 Other chondrocalcinosis, **right** ankle and foot
M11.272 Other chondrocalcinosis, **left** ankle and foot
M11.279 Other chondrocalcinosis, **unspecified** ankle and foot
M11.28 Other chondrocalcinosis, **vertebrae**
M11.29 Other chondrocalcinosis, **multiple sites**
● M11.8 **Other specified** crystal arthropathies
M11.80 Other specified crystal arthropathies, **unspecified** site
● M11.81 Other specified crystal arthropathies, **shoulder**
M11.811 Other specified crystal arthropathies, **right** shoulder
M11.812 Other specified crystal arthropathies, **left** shoulder
M11.819 Other specified crystal arthropathies, **unspecified** shoulder
● M11.82 Other specified crystal arthropathies, **elbow**
M11.821 Other specified crystal arthropathies, **right** elbow
M11.822 Other specified crystal arthropathies, **left** elbow
M11.829 Other specified crystal arthropathies, **unspecified** elbow
● M11.83 Other specified crystal arthropathies, **wrist**
M11.831 Other specified crystal arthropathies, **right** wrist
M11.832 Other specified crystal arthropathies, **left** wrist
M11.839 Other specified crystal arthropathies, **unspecified** wrist
● M11.84 Other specified crystal arthropathies, **hand**
M11.841 Other specified crystal arthropathies, **right** hand
M11.842 Other specified crystal arthropathies, **left** hand
M11.849 Other specified crystal arthropathies, **unspecified** hand
● M11.85 Other specified crystal arthropathies, **hip**
M11.851 Other specified crystal arthropathies, **right** hip
M11.852 Other specified crystal arthropathies, **left** hip
M11.859 Other specified crystal arthropathies, **unspecified** hip
● M11.86 Other specified crystal arthropathies, **knee**
M11.861 Other specified crystal arthropathies, **right** knee
M11.862 Other specified crystal arthropathies, **left** knee
M11.869 Other specified crystal arthropathies, **unspecified** knee
● M11.87 Other specified crystal arthropathies, **ankle and foot**
M11.871 Other specified crystal arthropathies, **right** ankle and foot
M11.872 Other specified crystal arthropathies, **left** ankle and foot
M11.879 Other specified crystal arthropathies, **unspecified** ankle and foot
M11.88 Other specified crystal arthropathies, **vertebrae**
M11.89 Other specified crystal arthropathies, **multiple sites**
M11.9 Crystal arthropathy, **unspecified**

- **M12 Other and unspecified arthropathy**
  - **Excludes1** arthrosis (M15-M19)
    cricoarytenoid arthropathy (J38.7)
  - **M12.0 Chronic postrheumatic arthropathy [Jaccoud]**
    - M12.00 Chronic postrheumatic arthropathy [Jaccoud], **unspecified site**
    - M12.01 Chronic postrheumatic arthropathy [Jaccoud], **shoulder**
      - M12.011 Chronic postrheumatic arthropathy [Jaccoud], **right shoulder**
      - M12.012 Chronic postrheumatic arthropathy [Jaccoud], **left shoulder**
      - M12.019 Chronic postrheumatic arthropathy [Jaccoud], **unspecified shoulder**
    - M12.02 Chronic postrheumatic arthropathy [Jaccoud], **elbow**
      - M12.021 Chronic postrheumatic arthropathy [Jaccoud], **right elbow**
      - M12.022 Chronic postrheumatic arthropathy [Jaccoud], **left elbow**
      - M12.029 Chronic postrheumatic arthropathy [Jaccoud], **unspecified elbow**
    - M12.03 Chronic postrheumatic arthropathy [Jaccoud], **wrist**
      - M12.031 Chronic postrheumatic arthropathy [Jaccoud], **right wrist**
      - M12.032 Chronic postrheumatic arthropathy [Jaccoud], **left wrist**
      - M12.039 Chronic postrheumatic arthropathy [Jaccoud], **unspecified wrist**
    - M12.04 Chronic postrheumatic arthropathy [Jaccoud], **hand**
      - M12.041 Chronic postrheumatic arthropathy [Jaccoud], **right hand**
      - M12.042 Chronic postrheumatic arthropathy [Jaccoud], **left hand**
      - M12.049 Chronic postrheumatic arthropathy [Jaccoud], **unspecified hand**
    - M12.05 Chronic postrheumatic arthropathy [Jaccoud], **hip**
      - M12.051 Chronic postrheumatic arthropathy [Jaccoud], **right hip**
      - M12.052 Chronic postrheumatic arthropathy [Jaccoud], **left hip**
      - M12.059 Chronic postrheumatic arthropathy [Jaccoud], **unspecified hip**
    - M12.06 Chronic postrheumatic arthropathy [Jaccoud], **knee**
      - M12.061 Chronic postrheumatic arthropathy [Jaccoud], **right knee**
      - M12.062 Chronic postrheumatic arthropathy [Jaccoud], **left knee**
      - M12.069 Chronic postrheumatic arthropathy [Jaccoud], **unspecified knee**
    - M12.07 Chronic postrheumatic arthropathy [Jaccoud], **ankle and foot**
      - M12.071 Chronic postrheumatic arthropathy [Jaccoud], **right ankle and foot**
      - M12.072 Chronic postrheumatic arthropathy [Jaccoud], **left ankle and foot**
      - M12.079 Chronic postrheumatic arthropathy [Jaccoud], **unspecified ankle and foot**
    - M12.08 Chronic postrheumatic arthropathy [Jaccoud], **other specified site**
      Chronic postrheumatic arthropathy [Jaccoud], vertebrae
    - M12.09 Chronic postrheumatic arthropathy [Jaccoud], **multiple sites**
  - **M12.1 Kaschin-Beck disease**
    Osteochondroarthrosis deformans endemica
    - M12.10 Kaschin-Beck disease, **unspecified site**
    - M12.11 Kaschin-Beck disease, **shoulder**
      - M12.111 Kaschin-Beck disease, **right shoulder**
      - M12.112 Kaschin-Beck disease, **left shoulder**
      - M12.119 Kaschin-Beck disease, **unspecified shoulder**
    - M12.12 Kaschin-Beck disease, **elbow**
      - M12.121 Kaschin-Beck disease, **right elbow**
      - M12.122 Kaschin-Beck disease, **left elbow**
      - M12.129 Kaschin-Beck disease, **unspecified elbow**
    - M12.13 Kaschin-Beck disease, **wrist**
      - M12.131 Kaschin-Beck disease, **right wrist**
      - M12.132 Kaschin-Beck disease, **left wrist**
      - M12.139 Kaschin-Beck disease, **unspecified wrist**
    - M12.14 Kaschin-Beck disease, **hand**
      - M12.141 Kaschin-Beck disease, **right hand**
      - M12.142 Kaschin-Beck disease, **left hand**
      - M12.149 Kaschin-Beck disease, **unspecified hand**
    - M12.15 Kaschin-Beck disease, **hip**
      - M12.151 Kaschin-Beck disease, **right hip**
      - M12.152 Kaschin-Beck disease, **left hip**
      - M12.159 Kaschin-Beck disease, **unspecified hip**
    - M12.16 Kaschin-Beck disease, **knee**
      - M12.161 Kaschin-Beck disease, **right knee**
      - M12.162 Kaschin-Beck disease, **left knee**
      - M12.169 Kaschin-Beck disease, **unspecified knee**
    - M12.17 Kaschin-Beck disease, **ankle and foot**
      - M12.171 Kaschin-Beck disease, **right ankle and foot**
      - M12.172 Kaschin-Beck disease, **left ankle and foot**
      - M12.179 Kaschin-Beck disease, **unspecified ankle and foot**
    - M12.18 Kaschin-Beck disease, **vertebrae**
    - M12.19 Kaschin-Beck disease, **multiple sites**
  - **M12.2 Villonodular synovitis (pigmented)**
    - M12.20 Villonodular synovitis (pigmented), **unspecified site**
    - M12.21 Villonodular synovitis (pigmented), **shoulder**
      - M12.211 Villonodular synovitis (pigmented), **right shoulder**
      - M12.212 Villonodular synovitis (pigmented), **left shoulder**
      - M12.219 Villonodular synovitis (pigmented), **unspecified shoulder**
    - M12.22 Villonodular synovitis (pigmented), **elbow**
      - M12.221 Villonodular synovitis (pigmented), **right elbow**
      - M12.222 Villonodular synovitis (pigmented), **left elbow**
      - M12.229 Villonodular synovitis (pigmented), **unspecified elbow**
    - M12.23 Villonodular synovitis (pigmented), **wrist**
      - M12.231 Villonodular synovitis (pigmented), **right wrist**
      - M12.232 Villonodular synovitis (pigmented), **left wrist**
      - M12.239 Villonodular synovitis (pigmented), **unspecified wrist**

CHAPTER 13 (M00-M99)

- ● M12.24 Villonodular synovitis (pigmented), **hand**
  - M12.241 Villonodular synovitis (pigmented), **right hand**
  - M12.242 Villonodular synovitis (pigmented), **left hand**
  - M12.249 Villonodular synovitis (pigmented), **unspecified hand**
- ● M12.25 Villonodular synovitis (pigmented), **hip**
  - M12.251 Villonodular synovitis (pigmented), **right hip**
  - M12.252 Villonodular synovitis (pigmented), **left hip**
  - M12.259 Villonodular synovitis (pigmented), **unspecified hip**
- ● M12.26 Villonodular synovitis (pigmented), **knee**
  - M12.261 Villonodular synovitis (pigmented), **right knee**
  - M12.262 Villonodular synovitis (pigmented), **left knee**
  - M12.269 Villonodular synovitis (pigmented), **unspecified knee**
- ● M12.27 Villonodular synovitis (pigmented), **ankle and foot**
  - M12.271 Villonodular synovitis (pigmented), **right ankle and foot**
  - M12.272 Villonodular synovitis (pigmented), **left ankle and foot**
  - M12.279 Villonodular synovitis (pigmented), **unspecified ankle and foot**
- M12.28 Villonodular synovitis (pigmented), **other specified site**
  - Villonodular synovitis (pigmented), vertebrae
- M12.29 Villonodular synovitis (pigmented), **multiple sites**

● M12.3 **Palindromic rheumatism**

- M12.3Ø Palindromic rheumatism, **unspecified site**
- ● M12.31 Palindromic rheumatism, **shoulder**
  - M12.311 Palindromic rheumatism, **right shoulder**
  - M12.312 Palindromic rheumatism, **left shoulder**
  - M12.319 Palindromic rheumatism, **unspecified shoulder**
- ● M12.32 Palindromic rheumatism, **elbow**
  - M12.321 Palindromic rheumatism, **right elbow**
  - M12.322 Palindromic rheumatism, **left elbow**
  - M12.329 Palindromic rheumatism, **unspecified elbow**
- ● M12.33 Palindromic rheumatism, **wrist**
  - M12.331 Palindromic rheumatism, **right wrist**
  - M12.332 Palindromic rheumatism, **left wrist**
  - M12.339 Palindromic rheumatism, **unspecified wrist**
- ● M12.34 Palindromic rheumatism, **hand**
  - M12.341 Palindromic rheumatism, **right hand**
  - M12.342 Palindromic rheumatism, **left hand**
  - M12.349 Palindromic rheumatism, **unspecified hand**
- ● M12.35 Palindromic rheumatism, **hip**
  - M12.351 Palindromic rheumatism, **right hip**
  - M12.352 Palindromic rheumatism, **left hip**
  - M12.359 Palindromic rheumatism, **unspecified hip**
- ● M12.36 Palindromic rheumatism, **knee**
  - M12.361 Palindromic rheumatism, **right knee**
  - M12.362 Palindromic rheumatism, **left knee**
  - M12.369 Palindromic rheumatism, **unspecified knee**
- ● M12.37 Palindromic rheumatism, **ankle and foot**
  - M12.371 Palindromic rheumatism, **right ankle and foot**
  - M12.372 Palindromic rheumatism, **left ankle and foot**
  - M12.379 Palindromic rheumatism, **unspecified ankle and foot**
- M12.38 Palindromic rheumatism, **other specified site**
  - Palindromic rheumatism, vertebrae
- M12.39 Palindromic rheumatism, **multiple sites**

● M12.4 **Intermittent hydrarthrosis**

- M12.4Ø Intermittent hydrarthrosis, **unspecified site**
- ● M12.41 Intermittent hydrarthrosis, **shoulder**
  - M12.411 Intermittent hydrarthrosis, **right shoulder**
  - M12.412 Intermittent hydrarthrosis, **left shoulder**
  - M12.419 Intermittent hydrarthrosis, **unspecified shoulder**
- ● M12.42 Intermittent hydrarthrosis, **elbow**
  - M12.421 Intermittent hydrarthrosis, **right elbow**
  - M12.422 Intermittent hydrarthrosis, **left elbow**
  - M12.429 Intermittent hydrarthrosis, **unspecified elbow**
- ● M12.43 Intermittent hydrarthrosis, **wrist**
  - M12.431 Intermittent hydrarthrosis, **right wrist**
  - M12.432 Intermittent hydrarthrosis, **left wrist**
  - M12.439 Intermittent hydrarthrosis, **unspecified wrist**
- ● M12.44 Intermittent hydrarthrosis, **hand**
  - M12.441 Intermittent hydrarthrosis, **right hand**
  - M12.442 Intermittent hydrarthrosis, **left hand**
  - M12.449 Intermittent hydrarthrosis, **unspecified hand**
- ● M12.45 Intermittent hydrarthrosis, **hip**
  - M12.451 Intermittent hydrarthrosis, **right hip**
  - M12.452 Intermittent hydrarthrosis, **left hip**
  - M12.459 Intermittent hydrarthrosis, **unspecified hip**
- ● M12.46 Intermittent hydrarthrosis, **knee**
  - M12.461 Intermittent hydrarthrosis, **right knee**
  - M12.462 Intermittent hydrarthrosis, **left knee**
  - M12.469 Intermittent hydrarthrosis, **unspecified knee**
- ● M12.47 Intermittent hydrarthrosis, **ankle and foot**
  - M12.471 Intermittent hydrarthrosis, **right ankle and foot**
  - M12.472 Intermittent hydrarthrosis, **left ankle and foot**
  - M12.479 Intermittent hydrarthrosis, **unspecified ankle and foot**
- M12.48 Intermittent hydrarthrosis, **other site**
- M12.49 Intermittent hydrarthrosis, **multiple sites**

● M12.5 **Traumatic arthropathy**

Excludes1 current injury-see Alphabetic Index
post-traumatic osteoarthritis of first carpometacarpal joint (M18.2-M18.3)
post-traumatic osteoarthritis of hip (M16.4-M16.5)
post-traumatic osteoarthritis of knee (M17.2-M17.3)
post-traumatic osteoarthritis NOS (M19.1-)
post-traumatic osteoarthritis of other single joints (M19.1-)

M12.50 **Traumatic arthropathy, unspecified site**

● M12.51 **Traumatic arthropathy, shoulder**

M12.511 **Traumatic arthropathy, right shoulder**

M12.512 **Traumatic arthropathy, left shoulder**

M12.519 **Traumatic arthropathy, unspecified shoulder**

● M12.52 **Traumatic arthropathy, elbow**

M12.521 **Traumatic arthropathy, right elbow**

M12.522 **Traumatic arthropathy, left elbow**

M12.529 **Traumatic arthropathy, unspecified elbow**

● M12.53 **Traumatic arthropathy, wrist**

M12.531 **Traumatic arthropathy, right wrist**

M12.532 **Traumatic arthropathy, left wrist**

M12.539 **Traumatic arthropathy, unspecified wrist**

● M12.54 **Traumatic arthropathy, hand**

M12.541 **Traumatic arthropathy, right hand**

M12.542 **Traumatic arthropathy, left hand**

M12.549 **Traumatic arthropathy, unspecified hand**

● M12.55 **Traumatic arthropathy, hip**

M12.551 **Traumatic arthropathy, right hip**

M12.552 **Traumatic arthropathy, left hip**
Coding Clinic: 2015, Q1, P17

M12.559 **Traumatic arthropathy, unspecified hip**

● M12.56 **Traumatic arthropathy, knee**

M12.561 **Traumatic arthropathy, right knee**

M12.562 **Traumatic arthropathy, left knee**

M12.569 **Traumatic arthropathy, unspecified knee**

● M12.57 **Traumatic arthropathy, ankle and foot**

M12.571 **Traumatic arthropathy, right ankle and foot**

M12.572 **Traumatic arthropathy, left ankle and foot**

M12.579 **Traumatic arthropathy, unspecified ankle and foot**

M12.58 **Traumatic arthropathy, other specified site**
Traumatic arthropathy, vertebrae

M12.59 **Traumatic arthropathy, multiple sites**

● M12.8 **Other specific arthropathies, not elsewhere classified**
Transient arthropathy

M12.80 **Other specific arthropathies, not elsewhere classified, unspecified site**

● M12.81 **Other specific arthropathies, not elsewhere classified, shoulder**

M12.811 **Other specific arthropathies, not elsewhere classified, right shoulder**

M12.812 **Other specific arthropathies, not elsewhere classified, left shoulder**

M12.819 **Other specific arthropathies, not elsewhere classified, unspecified shoulder**

● M12.82 **Other specific arthropathies, not elsewhere classified, elbow**

M12.821 **Other specific arthropathies, not elsewhere classified, right elbow**

M12.822 **Other specific arthropathies, not elsewhere classified, left elbow**

M12.829 **Other specific arthropathies, not elsewhere classified, unspecified elbow**

● M12.83 **Other specific arthropathies, not elsewhere classified, wrist**

M12.831 **Other specific arthropathies, not elsewhere classified, right wrist**

M12.832 **Other specific arthropathies, not elsewhere classified, left wrist**

M12.839 **Other specific arthropathies, not elsewhere classified, unspecified wrist**

● M12.84 **Other specific arthropathies, not elsewhere classified, hand**

M12.841 **Other specific arthropathies, not elsewhere classified, right hand**

M12.842 **Other specific arthropathies, not elsewhere classified, left hand**

M12.849 **Other specific arthropathies, not elsewhere classified, unspecified hand**

● M12.85 **Other specific arthropathies, not elsewhere classified, hip**

M12.851 **Other specific arthropathies, not elsewhere classified, right hip**

M12.852 **Other specific arthropathies, not elsewhere classified, left hip**

M12.859 **Other specific arthropathies, not elsewhere classified, unspecified hip**

● M12.86 **Other specific arthropathies, not elsewhere classified, knee**

M12.861 **Other specific arthropathies, not elsewhere classified, right knee**

M12.862 **Other specific arthropathies, not elsewhere classified, left knee**

M12.869 **Other specific arthropathies, not elsewhere classified, unspecified knee**

● M12.87 **Other specific arthropathies, not elsewhere classified, ankle and foot**

M12.871 **Other specific arthropathies, not elsewhere classified, right ankle and foot**

M12.872 **Other specific arthropathies, not elsewhere classified, left ankle and foot**

M12.879 **Other specific arthropathies, not elsewhere classified, unspecified ankle and foot**

M12.88 **Other specific arthropathies, not elsewhere classified, other specified site**
Other specific arthropathies, not elsewhere classified, vertebrae

M12.89 **Other specific arthropathies, not elsewhere classified, multiple sites**

M12.9 **Arthropathy, unspecified**

- **M13 Other arthritis**
  - **Excludes1** arthrosis (M15-M19)
    osteoarthritis (M15-M19)
  - **M13.Ø Polyarthritis, unspecified**
  - **M13.1 Monoarthritis, not elsewhere classified**
    - M13.1Ø Monoarthritis, not elsewhere classified, **unspecified** site
    - M13.11 Monoarthritis, not elsewhere classified, **shoulder**
      - M13.111 Monoarthritis, not elsewhere classified, **right** shoulder
      - M13.112 Monoarthritis, not elsewhere classified, **left** shoulder
      - M13.119 Monoarthritis, not elsewhere classified, **unspecified** shoulder
    - M13.12 Monoarthritis, not elsewhere classified, **elbow**
      - M13.121 Monoarthritis, not elsewhere classified, **right** elbow
      - M13.122 Monoarthritis, not elsewhere classified, **left** elbow
      - M13.129 Monoarthritis, not elsewhere classified, **unspecified** elbow
    - M13.13 Monoarthritis, not elsewhere classified, **wrist**
      - M13.131 Monoarthritis, not elsewhere classified, **right** wrist
      - M13.132 Monoarthritis, not elsewhere classified, **left** wrist
      - M13.139 Monoarthritis, not elsewhere classified, **unspecified** wrist
    - M13.14 Monoarthritis, not elsewhere classified, **hand**
      - M13.141 Monoarthritis, not elsewhere classified, **right** hand
      - M13.142 Monoarthritis, not elsewhere classified, **left** hand
      - M13.149 Monoarthritis, not elsewhere classified, **unspecified** hand
    - M13.15 Monoarthritis, not elsewhere classified, **hip**
      - M13.151 Monoarthritis, not elsewhere classified, **right** hip
      - M13.152 Monoarthritis, not elsewhere classified, **left** hip
      - M13.159 Monoarthritis, not elsewhere classified, **unspecified** hip
    - M13.16 Monoarthritis, not elsewhere classified, **knee**
      - M13.161 Monoarthritis, not elsewhere classified, **right** knee
      - M13.162 Monoarthritis, not elsewhere classified, **left** knee
      - M13.169 Monoarthritis, not elsewhere classified, **unspecified** knee
    - M13.17 Monoarthritis, not elsewhere classified, **ankle and foot**
      - M13.171 Monoarthritis, not elsewhere classified, **right** ankle and foot
      - M13.172 Monoarthritis, not elsewhere classified, **left** ankle and foot
      - M13.179 Monoarthritis, not elsewhere classified, **unspecified** ankle and foot
  - **M13.8 Other specified arthritis**
    Allergic arthritis
    - **Excludes1** osteoarthritis (M15-M19)
    - M13.8Ø Other specified arthritis, **unspecified** site
    - M13.81 Other specified arthritis, **shoulder**
      - M13.811 Other specified arthritis, **right** shoulder
      - M13.812 Other specified arthritis, **left** shoulder
      - M13.819 Other specified arthritis, **unspecified** shoulder
    - M13.82 Other specified arthritis, **elbow**
      - M13.821 Other specified arthritis, **right** elbow
      - M13.822 Other specified arthritis, **left** elbow
      - M13.829 Other specified arthritis, **unspecified** elbow
    - M13.83 Other specified arthritis, **wrist**
      - M13.831 Other specified arthritis, **right** wrist
      - M13.832 Other specified arthritis, **left** wrist
      - M13.839 Other specified arthritis, **unspecified** wrist
    - M13.84 Other specified arthritis, **hand**
      - M13.841 Other specified arthritis, **right** hand
      - M13.842 Other specified arthritis, **left** hand
      - M13.849 Other specified arthritis, **unspecified** hand
    - M13.85 Other specified arthritis, **hip**
      - M13.851 Other specified arthritis, **right** hip
      - M13.852 Other specified arthritis, **left** hip
      - M13.859 Other specified arthritis, **unspecified** hip
    - M13.86 Other specified arthritis, **knee**
      - M13.861 Other specified arthritis, **right** knee
      - M13.862 Other specified arthritis, **left** knee
      - M13.869 Other specified arthritis, **unspecified** knee
    - M13.87 Other specified arthritis, **ankle and foot**
      - M13.871 Other specified arthritis, **right** ankle and foot
      - M13.872 Other specified arthritis, **left** ankle and foot
      - M13.879 Other specified arthritis, **unspecified** ankle and foot
    - M13.88 Other specified arthritis, **other site**
    - M13.89 Other specified arthritis, **multiple sites**

- **M14 Arthropathies in other diseases classified elsewhere**
  - **Excludes1** arthropathy in:
    - diabetes mellitus (EØ8-E13 with .61-)
    - hematological disorders (M36.2-M36.3)
    - hypersensitivity reactions (M36.4)
    - neoplastic disease (M36.1)
    - neurosyphillis (A52.16)
    - sarcoidosis (D86.86)

    enteropathic arthropathies (MØ7.Ø-)
    juvenile psoriatic arthropathy (L4Ø.54)
    lipoid dermatoarthritis (E78.81)
  - **M14.6 Charcôt's joint**
    Neuropathic arthropathy
    - **Excludes1** Charcôt's joint in diabetes mellitus (EØ8-E13 with .61Ø)
      Charcôt's joint in tabes dorsalis (A52.16)
    - M14.6Ø Charcôt's joint, **unspecified** site
    - M14.61 Charcôt's joint, **shoulder**
      - M14.611 Charcôt's joint, **right** shoulder
      - M14.612 Charcôt's joint, **left** shoulder
      - M14.619 Charcôt's joint, **unspecified** shoulder
    - M14.62 Charcôt's joint, **elbow**
      - M14.621 Charcôt's joint, **right** elbow
      - M14.622 Charcôt's joint, **left** elbow
      - M14.629 Charcôt's joint, **unspecified** elbow
    - M14.63 Charcôt's joint, **wrist**
      - M14.631 Charcôt's joint, **right** wrist
      - M14.632 Charcôt's joint, **left** wrist
      - M14.639 Charcôt's joint, **unspecified** wrist

M14.64 Charcôt's joint, hand
M14.641 Charcôt's joint, right hand
M14.642 Charcôt's joint, left hand
M14.649 Charcôt's joint, unspecified hand
M14.65 Charcôt's joint, hip
M14.651 Charcôt's joint, right hip
M14.652 Charcôt's joint, left hip
M14.659 Charcôt's joint, unspecified hip
M14.66 Charcôt's joint, knee
M14.661 Charcôt's joint, right knee
M14.662 Charcôt's joint, left knee
M14.669 Charcôt's joint, unspecified knee
M14.67 Charcôt's joint, ankle and foot
M14.671 Charcôt's joint, right ankle and foot
M14.672 Charcôt's joint, left ankle and foot
M14.679 Charcôt's joint, unspecified ankle and foot
M14.68 Charcôt's joint, vertebrae
M14.69 Charcôt's joint, multiple sites

M14.8 Arthropathies in other specified diseases classified elsewhere

Code first underlying disease, such as:
amyloidosis (E85.-)
erythema multiforme (L51.-)
erythema nodosum (L52)
hemochromatosis (E83.11-)
hyperparathyroidism (E21.-)
hypothyroidism (E00-E03)
sickle-cell disorders (D57.-)
thyrotoxicosis [hyperthyroidism] (E05.-)
Whipple's disease (K90.81)

M14.80 Arthropathies in other specified diseases classified elsewhere, unspecified site
M14.81 Arthropathies in other specified diseases classified elsewhere, shoulder
M14.811 Arthropathies in other specified diseases classified elsewhere, right shoulder
M14.812 Arthropathies in other specified diseases classified elsewhere, left shoulder
M14.819 Arthropathies in other specified diseases classified elsewhere, unspecified shoulder
M14.82 Arthropathies in other specified diseases classified elsewhere, elbow
M14.821 Arthropathies in other specified diseases classified elsewhere, right elbow
M14.822 Arthropathies in other specified diseases classified elsewhere, left elbow
M14.829 Arthropathies in other specified diseases classified elsewhere, unspecified elbow
M14.83 Arthropathies in other specified diseases classified elsewhere, wrist
M14.831 Arthropathies in other specified diseases classified elsewhere, right wrist
M14.832 Arthropathies in other specified diseases classified elsewhere, left wrist
M14.839 Arthropathies in other specified diseases classified elsewhere, unspecified wrist
M14.84 Arthropathies in other specified diseases classified elsewhere, hand
M14.841 Arthropathies in other specified diseases classified elsewhere, right hand
M14.842 Arthropathies in other specified diseases classified elsewhere, left hand
M14.849 Arthropathies in other specified diseases classified elsewhere, unspecified hand
M14.85 Arthropathies in other specified diseases classified elsewhere, hip
M14.851 Arthropathies in other specified diseases classified elsewhere, right hip
M14.852 Arthropathies in other specified diseases classified elsewhere, left hip
M14.859 Arthropathies in other specified diseases classified elsewhere, unspecified hip
M14.86 Arthropathies in other specified diseases classified elsewhere, knee
M14.861 Arthropathies in other specified diseases classified elsewhere, right knee
M14.862 Arthropathies in other specified diseases classified elsewhere, left knee
M14.869 Arthropathies in other specified diseases classified elsewhere, unspecified knee
M14.87 Arthropathies in other specified diseases classified elsewhere, ankle and foot
M14.871 Arthropathies in other specified diseases classified elsewhere, right ankle and foot
M14.872 Arthropathies in other specified diseases classified elsewhere, left ankle and foot
M14.879 Arthropathies in other specified diseases classified elsewhere, unspecified ankle and foot
M14.88 Arthropathies in other specified diseases classified elsewhere, vertebrae
M14.89 Arthropathies in other specified diseases classified elsewhere, multiple sites

OSTEOARTHRITIS (M15-M19)

Osteoarthritis is the most common degenerative joint disease and form of arthritis that breaks down the cartilage causing pain, swelling, and reduced motion in the joints.

Excludes2 osteoarthritis of spine (M47.-)

M15 Polyosteoarthritis
Includes arthritis of multiple sites
Excludes1 bilateral involvement of single joint (M16-M19)
M15.0 Primary generalized (osteo)arthritis
M15.1 Heberden's nodes (with arthropathy)
Interphalangeal distal osteoarthritis
M15.2 Bouchard's nodes (with arthropathy)
Juxtaphalangeal distal osteoarthritis
M15.3 Secondary multiple arthritis
Post-traumatic polyosteoarthritis
M15.4 Erosive (osteo)arthritis
M15.8 Other polyosteoarthritis
M15.9 Polyosteoarthritis, unspecified
Generalized osteoarthritis NOS

CHAPTER 13 (M00-M99)

● **M16 Osteoarthritis of hip**
M16.0 **Bilateral primary** osteoarthritis of hip
Coding Clinic: 2018, Q2, P15; 2016, Q4, P146
● M16.1 **Unilateral primary** osteoarthritis of hip
Primary osteoarthritis of hip NOS
M16.10 Unilateral primary osteoarthritis, **unspecified** hip
M16.11 Unilateral primary osteoarthritis, **right** hip
M16.12 Unilateral primary osteoarthritis, **left** hip
M16.2 **Bilateral** osteoarthritis resulting from **hip dysplasia**
● M16.3 **Unilateral** osteoarthritis resulting from **hip dysplasia**
Dysplastic osteoarthritis of hip NOS
M16.30 Unilateral osteoarthritis resulting from hip dysplasia, **unspecified** hip
M16.31 Unilateral osteoarthritis resulting from hip dysplasia, **right** hip
M16.32 Unilateral osteoarthritis resulting from hip dysplasia, **left** hip
M16.4 **Bilateral post-traumatic** osteoarthritis of hip
● M16.5 **Unilateral post-traumatic** osteoarthritis of hip
Post-traumatic osteoarthritis of hip NOS
M16.50 Unilateral post-traumatic osteoarthritis, **unspecified** hip
M16.51 Unilateral post-traumatic osteoarthritis, **right** hip
M16.52 Unilateral post-traumatic osteoarthritis, **left** hip
M16.6 **Other bilateral secondary** osteoarthritis of hip
M16.7 **Other unilateral secondary** osteoarthritis of hip
Secondary osteoarthritis of hip NOS
M16.9 Osteoarthritis of hip, **unspecified**

● **M17 Osteoarthritis of knee**
M17.0 **Bilateral primary** osteoarthritis of knee
● M17.1 **Unilateral primary** osteoarthritis of knee
Primary osteoarthritis of knee NOS
M17.10 Unilateral primary osteoarthritis, **unspecified** knee
Coding Clinic: 2016, Q4, P147
M17.11 Unilateral primary osteoarthritis, **right** knee
M17.12 Unilateral primary osteoarthritis, **left** knee
Coding Clinic: 2016, Q4, P146
M17.2 **Bilateral post-traumatic** osteoarthritis of knee
● M17.3 **Unilateral post-traumatic** osteoarthritis of knee
Post-traumatic osteoarthritis of knee NOS
M17.30 Unilateral post-traumatic osteoarthritis, **unspecified** knee
M17.31 Unilateral post-traumatic osteoarthritis, **right** knee
M17.32 Unilateral post-traumatic osteoarthritis, **left** knee
M17.4 **Other bilateral secondary** osteoarthritis of knee
M17.5 **Other unilateral secondary** osteoarthritis of knee
Secondary osteoarthritis of knee NOS
M17.9 Osteoarthritis of knee, **unspecified**
Coding Clinic: 2016, Q4, P146

● **M18 Osteoarthritis of first carpometacarpal joint**
M18.0 **Bilateral primary** osteoarthritis of first carpometacarpal joints
● M18.1 **Unilateral primary** osteoarthritis of first carpometacarpal joint
Primary osteoarthritis of first carpometacarpal joint NOS
M18.10 Unilateral primary osteoarthritis of first carpometacarpal joint, **unspecified** hand
M18.11 Unilateral primary osteoarthritis of first carpometacarpal joint, **right** hand
M18.12 Unilateral primary osteoarthritis of first carpometacarpal joint, **left** hand
M18.2 **Bilateral post-traumatic** osteoarthritis of first carpometacarpal joints
● M18.3 **Unilateral post-traumatic** osteoarthritis of first carpometacarpal joint
Post-traumatic osteoarthritis of first carpometacarpal joint NOS
M18.30 Unilateral post-traumatic osteoarthritis of first carpometacarpal joint, **unspecified** hand
M18.31 Unilateral post-traumatic osteoarthritis of first carpometacarpal joint, **right** hand
M18.32 Unilateral post-traumatic osteoarthritis of first carpometacarpal joint, **left** hand
M18.4 **Other bilateral secondary** osteoarthritis of first carpometacarpal joints
● M18.5 **Other unilateral secondary** osteoarthritis of first carpometacarpal joint
Secondary osteoarthritis of first carpometacarpal joint NOS
M18.50 Other unilateral secondary osteoarthritis of first carpometacarpal joint, **unspecified** hand
M18.51 Other unilateral secondary osteoarthritis of first carpometacarpal joint, **right** hand
M18.52 Other unilateral secondary osteoarthritis of first carpometacarpal joint, **left** hand
M18.9 Osteoarthritis of first carpometacarpal joint, **unspecified**

● **M19 Other and unspecified osteoarthritis**
Excludes1 polyarthritis (M15.-)
Excludes2 arthrosis of spine (M47.-)
hallux rigidus (M20.2)
osteoarthritis of spine (M47.-)
● M19.0 **Primary** osteoarthritis of other joints
● M19.01 Primary osteoarthritis, **shoulder**
M19.011 Primary osteoarthritis, **right** shoulder
Coding Clinic: 2016, Q4, P145
M19.012 Primary osteoarthritis, **left** shoulder
M19.019 Primary osteoarthritis, **unspecified** shoulder
● M19.02 Primary osteoarthritis, **elbow**
M19.021 Primary osteoarthritis, **right** elbow
M19.022 Primary osteoarthritis, **left** elbow
M19.029 Primary osteoarthritis, **unspecified** elbow
● M19.03 Primary osteoarthritis, **wrist**
M19.031 Primary osteoarthritis, **right** wrist
M19.032 Primary osteoarthritis, **left** wrist
M19.039 Primary osteoarthritis, **unspecified** wrist
● M19.04 Primary osteoarthritis, **hand**
Excludes2 primary osteoarthritis of first carpometacarpal joint (M18.0-, M18.1-)
M19.041 Primary osteoarthritis, **right** hand
M19.042 Primary osteoarthritis, **left** hand
M19.049 Primary osteoarthritis, **unspecified** hand
● M19.07 Primary osteoarthritis **ankle and foot**
M19.071 Primary osteoarthritis, **right** ankle and foot
M19.072 Primary osteoarthritis, **left** ankle and foot
M19.079 Primary osteoarthritis, **unspecified** ankle and foot

M19.1 Post-traumatic osteoarthritis of other joints
M19.11 Post-traumatic osteoarthritis, shoulder
M19.111 Post-traumatic osteoarthritis, right shoulder
M19.112 Post-traumatic osteoarthritis, left shoulder
M19.119 Post-traumatic osteoarthritis, unspecified shoulder
M19.12 Post-traumatic osteoarthritis, elbow
M19.121 Post-traumatic osteoarthritis, right elbow
M19.122 Post-traumatic osteoarthritis, left elbow
M19.129 Post-traumatic osteoarthritis, unspecified elbow
M19.13 Post-traumatic osteoarthritis, wrist
M19.131 Post-traumatic osteoarthritis, right wrist
M19.132 Post-traumatic osteoarthritis, left wrist
M19.139 Post-traumatic osteoarthritis, unspecified wrist
M19.14 Post-traumatic osteoarthritis, hand
Excludes2 post-traumatic osteoarthritis of first carpometacarpal joint (M18.2-, M18.3-)
M19.141 Post-traumatic osteoarthritis, right hand
M19.142 Post-traumatic osteoarthritis, left hand
M19.149 Post-traumatic osteoarthritis, unspecified hand
M19.17 Post-traumatic osteoarthritis, ankle and foot
M19.171 Post-traumatic osteoarthritis, right ankle and foot
M19.172 Post-traumatic osteoarthritis, left ankle and foot
M19.179 Post-traumatic osteoarthritis, unspecified ankle and foot
M19.2 Secondary osteoarthritis of other joints
M19.21 Secondary osteoarthritis, shoulder
M19.211 Secondary osteoarthritis, right shoulder
M19.212 Secondary osteoarthritis, left shoulder
M19.219 Secondary osteoarthritis, unspecified shoulder
M19.22 Secondary osteoarthritis, elbow
M19.221 Secondary osteoarthritis, right elbow
M19.222 Secondary osteoarthritis, left elbow
M19.229 Secondary osteoarthritis, unspecified elbow
M19.23 Secondary osteoarthritis, wrist
M19.231 Secondary osteoarthritis, right wrist
M19.232 Secondary osteoarthritis, left wrist
M19.239 Secondary osteoarthritis, unspecified wrist
M19.24 Secondary osteoarthritis, hand
M19.241 Secondary osteoarthritis, right hand
M19.242 Secondary osteoarthritis, left hand
M19.249 Secondary osteoarthritis, unspecified hand
M19.27 Secondary osteoarthritis, ankle and foot
M19.271 Secondary osteoarthritis, right ankle and foot
M19.272 Secondary osteoarthritis, left ankle and foot
M19.279 Secondary osteoarthritis, unspecified ankle and foot

M19.9 Osteoarthritis, unspecified site
M19.90 Unspecified osteoarthritis, unspecified site
Arthrosis NOS
Arthritis NOS
Osteoarthritis NOS
Coding Clinic: 2016, Q4, P147
M19.91 Primary osteoarthritis, unspecified site
Primary osteoarthritis NOS
M19.92 Post-traumatic osteoarthritis, unspecified site
Post-traumatic osteoarthritis NOS
M19.93 Secondary osteoarthritis, unspecified site
Secondary osteoarthritis NOS

OTHER JOINT DISORDERS (M20-M25)

Excludes2 joints of the spine (M40-M54)

M20 Acquired deformities of fingers and toes
Excludes1 acquired absence of fingers and toes (Z89.-)
congenital absence of fingers and toes (Q71.3-, Q72.3-)
congenital deformities and malformations of fingers and toes (Q66.-, Q68-Q70, Q74.-)
M20.0 Deformity of finger(s)
Excludes1 clubbing of fingers (R68.3)
palmar fascial fibromatosis [Dupuytren] (M72.0)
trigger finger (M65.3)
M20.00 Unspecified deformity of finger(s)
M20.001 Unspecified deformity of right finger(s)
M20.002 Unspecified deformity of left finger(s)
M20.009 Unspecified deformity of unspecified finger(s)
M20.01 Mallet finger
M20.011 Mallet finger of right finger(s)
M20.012 Mallet finger of left finger(s)
M20.019 Mallet finger of unspecified finger(s)
M20.02 Boutonnière deformity
M20.021 Boutonnière deformity of right finger(s)
M20.022 Boutonnière deformity of left finger(s)
M20.029 Boutonnière deformity of unspecified finger(s)
M20.03 Swan-neck deformity
M20.031 Swan-neck deformity of right finger(s)
M20.032 Swan-neck deformity of left finger(s)
M20.039 Swan-neck deformity of unspecified finger(s)
M20.09 Other deformity of finger(s)
M20.091 Other deformity of right finger(s)
M20.092 Other deformity of left finger(s)
M20.099 Other deformity of finger(s), unspecified finger(s)
M20.1 Hallux valgus (acquired)
Excludes2 bunion (M21.6-)
Coding Clinic: 2016, Q4, P38
M20.10 Hallux valgus (acquired), unspecified foot
M20.11 Hallux valgus (acquired), right foot
M20.12 Hallux valgus (acquired), left foot
M20.2 Hallux rigidus
M20.20 Hallux rigidus, unspecified foot
M20.21 Hallux rigidus, right foot
M20.22 Hallux rigidus, left foot

CHAPTER 13 (M00-M99)

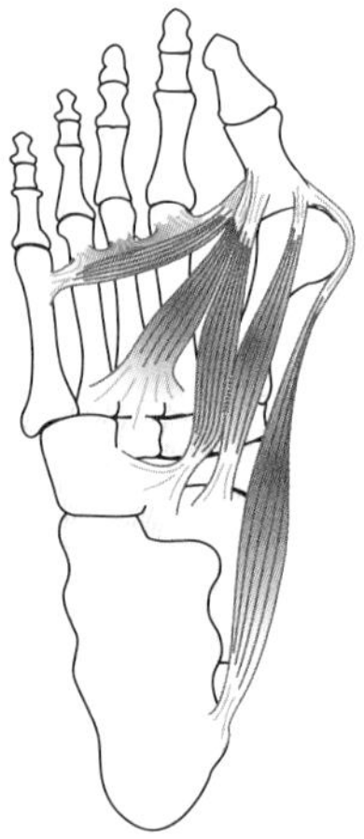

Figure 13-1 Hallux valgus.

Item 13–2 Hallux valgus is a sometimes painful structural deformity caused by an inflammation of the bursal sac at the base of the metatarsophalangeal joint (big toe). **Hallus varus** is a deviation of the great toe to the inner side of the foot or away from the next toe.

● **M20.3** **Hallux varus (acquired)**
- **M20.30** **Hallux varus (acquired), unspecified foot**
- **M20.31** **Hallux varus (acquired), right foot**
- **M20.32** **Hallux varus (acquired), left foot**

● **M20.4** **Other hammer toe(s) (acquired)**
- **M20.40** **Other hammer toe(s) (acquired), unspecified foot**
- **M20.41** **Other hammer toe(s) (acquired), right foot**
- **M20.42** **Other hammer toe(s) (acquired), left foot**

● **M20.5** **Other deformities of toe(s) (acquired)**
- ● **M20.5X** **Other deformities of toe(s) (acquired)**
  - **M20.5X1** **Other deformities of toe(s) (acquired), right foot**
  - **M20.5X2** **Other deformities of toe(s) (acquired), left foot**
  - **M20.5X9** **Other deformities of toe(s) (acquired), unspecified foot**

● **M20.6** **Acquired deformities of toe(s), unspecified**
- **M20.60** **Acquired deformities of toe(s), unspecified, unspecified foot**
- **M20.61** **Acquired deformities of toe(s), unspecified, right foot**
- **M20.62** **Acquired deformities of toe(s), unspecified, left foot**

● **M21** **Other acquired deformities of limbs**

Excludes1 acquired absence of limb (Z89.-)
congenital absence of limbs (Q71-Q73)
congenital deformities and malformations of limbs (Q65-Q66, Q68-Q74)

Excludes2 acquired deformities of fingers or toes (M20.-)
coxa plana (M91.2)

● **M21.0** **Valgus deformity, not elsewhere classified**

Excludes1 metatarsus valgus (Q66.6)
talipes calcaneovalgus (Q66.4-)

- **M21.00** **Valgus deformity, not elsewhere classified, unspecified site**
- ● **M21.02** **Valgus deformity, not elsewhere classified, elbow**
  Cubitus valgus
  - **M21.021** **Valgus deformity, not elsewhere classified, right elbow**
  - **M21.022** **Valgus deformity, not elsewhere classified, left elbow**
  - **M21.029** **Valgus deformity, not elsewhere classified, unspecified elbow**

Item 13–3 Cubitus valgus is a deformity of the elbow resulting in an increased carrying angle in which the arm extends at the side and the palm faces forward, which results in the forearm and hand extended at greater than 15 degrees.

Item 13–4 Cubitus varus is a deformity of the elbow resulting in the arm extended at the side and the palm facing forward so that the forearm and hand are held at less than 5 degrees, decreasing the carrying angle.

- ● **M21.05** **Valgus deformity, not elsewhere classified, hip**
  - **M21.051** **Valgus deformity, not elsewhere classified, right hip**
  - **M21.052** **Valgus deformity, not elsewhere classified, left hip**
  - **M21.059** **Valgus deformity, not elsewhere classified, unspecified hip**
- ● **M21.06** **Valgus deformity, not elsewhere classified, knee**
  Genu valgum
  Knock knee
  - **M21.061** **Valgus deformity, not elsewhere classified, right knee**
  - **M21.062** **Valgus deformity, not elsewhere classified, left knee**
  - **M21.069** **Valgus deformity, not elsewhere classified, unspecified knee**
- ● **M21.07** **Valgus deformity, not elsewhere classified, ankle**
  - **M21.071** **Valgus deformity, not elsewhere classified, right ankle**
  - **M21.072** **Valgus deformity, not elsewhere classified, left ankle**
  - **M21.079** **Valgus deformity, not elsewhere classified, unspecified ankle**

● **M21.1** **Varus deformity, not elsewhere classified**

Excludes1 metatarsus varus (Q66.22-)
tibia vara (M92.5)

- **M21.10** **Varus deformity, not elsewhere classified, unspecified site**
- ● **M21.12** **Varus deformity, not elsewhere classified, elbow**
  Cubitus varus, elbow
  - **M21.121** **Varus deformity, not elsewhere classified, right elbow**
  - **M21.122** **Varus deformity, not elsewhere classified, left elbow**
  - **M21.129** **Varus deformity, not elsewhere classified, unspecified elbow**
- ● **M21.15** **Varus deformity, not elsewhere classified, hip**
  - **M21.151** **Varus deformity, not elsewhere classified, right hip**
  - **M21.152** **Varus deformity, not elsewhere classified, left hip**
  - **M21.159** **Varus deformity, not elsewhere classified, unspecified**
- ● **M21.16** **Varus deformity, not elsewhere classified, knee**
  Bow leg
  Genu varum
  - **M21.161** **Varus deformity, not elsewhere classified, right knee**
  - **M21.162** **Varus deformity, not elsewhere classified, left knee**
  - **M21.169** **Varus deformity, not elsewhere classified, unspecified knee**
- ● **M21.17** **Varus deformity, not elsewhere classified, ankle**
  - **M21.171** **Varus deformity, not elsewhere classified, right ankle**
  - **M21.172** **Varus deformity, not elsewhere classified, left ankle**
  - **M21.179** **Varus deformity, not elsewhere classified, unspecified ankle**

● M21.2 Flexion deformity
- M21.20 Flexion deformity, unspecified site
- ● M21.21 Flexion deformity, shoulder
  - M21.211 Flexion deformity, right shoulder
  - M21.212 Flexion deformity, left shoulder
  - M21.219 Flexion deformity, unspecified shoulder
- ● M21.22 Flexion deformity, elbow
  - M21.221 Flexion deformity, right elbow
  - M21.222 Flexion deformity, left elbow
  - M21.229 Flexion deformity, unspecified elbow
- ● M21.23 Flexion deformity, wrist
  - M21.231 Flexion deformity, right wrist
  - M21.232 Flexion deformity, left wrist
  - M21.239 Flexion deformity, unspecified wrist
- ● M21.24 Flexion deformity, finger joints
  - M21.241 Flexion deformity, right finger joints
  - M21.242 Flexion deformity, left finger joints
  - M21.249 Flexion deformity, unspecified finger joints
- ● M21.25 Flexion deformity, hip
  - M21.251 Flexion deformity, right hip
  - M21.252 Flexion deformity, left hip
  - M21.259 Flexion deformity, unspecified hip
- ● M21.26 Flexion deformity, knee
  - M21.261 Flexion deformity, right knee
  - M21.262 Flexion deformity, left knee
  - M21.269 Flexion deformity, unspecified knee
- ● M21.27 Flexion deformity, ankle and toes
  - M21.271 Flexion deformity, right ankle and toes
  - M21.272 Flexion deformity, left ankle and toes
  - M21.279 Flexion deformity, unspecified ankle and toes

● M21.3 Wrist or foot drop (acquired)
- ● M21.33 Wrist drop (acquired)
  - M21.331 Wrist drop, right wrist
  - M21.332 Wrist drop, left wrist
  - M21.339 Wrist drop, unspecified wrist
- ● M21.37 Foot drop (acquired)
  - M21.371 Foot drop, right foot
  - M21.372 Foot drop, left foot
  - M21.379 Foot drop, unspecified foot

● M21.4 Flat foot [pes planus] (acquired)

Excludes1 congenital pes planus (Q66.5-)

- M21.40 Flat foot [pes planus] (acquired), unspecified foot
- M21.41 Flat foot [pes planus] (acquired), right foot
- M21.42 Flat foot [pes planus] (acquired), left foot

● M21.5 Acquired clawhand, clubhand, clawfoot and clubfoot

Excludes1 clubfoot, not specified as acquired (Q66.89)

- ● M21.51 Acquired clawhand
  - M21.511 Acquired clawhand, right hand
  - M21.512 Acquired clawhand, left hand
  - M21.519 Acquired clawhand, unspecified hand
- ● M21.52 Acquired clubhand
  - M21.521 Acquired clubhand, right hand
  - M21.522 Acquired clubhand, left hand
  - M21.529 Acquired clubhand, unspecified hand
- ● M21.53 Acquired clawfoot
  - M21.531 Acquired clawfoot, right foot
  - M21.532 Acquired clawfoot, left foot
  - M21.539 Acquired clawfoot, unspecified foot
- ● M21.54 Acquired clubfoot
  - M21.541 Acquired clubfoot, right foot
  - M21.542 Acquired clubfoot, left foot
  - M21.549 Acquired clubfoot, unspecified foot

● M21.6 Other acquired deformities of foot

Excludes2 deformities of toe (acquired) (M20.1-M20.6-)

- ● M21.61 Bunion
  - Coding Clinic: 2016, Q4, P38
  - M21.611 Bunion of right foot
  - M21.612 Bunion of left foot
  - M21.619 Bunion of unspecified foot
- ● M21.62 Bunionette
  - Coding Clinic: 2016, Q4, P38
  - M21.621 Bunionette of right foot
  - M21.622 Bunionette of left foot
  - M21.629 Bunionette of unspecified foot
- ● M21.6X Other acquired deformities of foot
  - M21.6X1 Other acquired deformities of right foot
  - M21.6X2 Other acquired deformities of left foot
  - M21.6X9 Other acquired deformities of unspecified foot

● M21.7 Unequal limb length (acquired)

Note: The site used should correspond to the shorter limb.

- M21.70 Unequal limb length (acquired), unspecified site
- ● M21.72 Unequal limb length (acquired), humerus
  - M21.721 Unequal limb length (acquired), right humerus
  - M21.722 Unequal limb length (acquired), left humerus
  - M21.729 Unequal limb length (acquired), unspecified humerus
- ● M21.73 Unequal limb length (acquired), ulna and radius
  - M21.731 Unequal limb length (acquired), right ulna
  - M21.732 Unequal limb length (acquired), left ulna
  - M21.733 Unequal limb length (acquired), right radius
  - M21.734 Unequal limb length (acquired), left radius
  - M21.739 Unequal limb length (acquired), unspecified ulna and radius
- ● M21.75 Unequal limb length (acquired), femur
  - M21.751 Unequal limb length (acquired), right femur
  - M21.752 Unequal limb length (acquired), left femur
  - M21.759 Unequal limb length (acquired), unspecified femur
- ● M21.76 Unequal limb length (acquired), tibia and fibula
  - M21.761 Unequal limb length (acquired), right tibia
  - M21.762 Unequal limb length (acquired), left tibia
  - M21.763 Unequal limb length (acquired), right fibula
  - M21.764 Unequal limb length (acquired), left fibula
  - M21.769 Unequal limb length (acquired), unspecified tibia and fibula

- M21.8 Other specified acquired deformities of limbs
  - **Excludes2** coxa plana (M91.2)
  - M21.80 Other specified acquired deformities of unspecified limb
  - M21.82 Other specified acquired deformities of upper arm
    - M21.821 Other specified acquired deformities of right upper arm
    - M21.822 Other specified acquired deformities of left upper arm
    - M21.829 Other specified acquired deformities of unspecified upper arm
  - M21.83 Other specified acquired deformities of forearm
    - M21.831 Other specified acquired deformities of right forearm
    - M21.832 Other specified acquired deformities of left forearm
    - M21.839 Other specified acquired deformities of unspecified forearm
  - M21.85 Other specified acquired deformities of thigh
    - M21.851 Other specified acquired deformities of right thigh
    - M21.852 Other specified acquired deformities of left thigh
    - M21.859 Other specified acquired deformities of unspecified thigh
  - M21.86 Other specified acquired deformities of lower leg
    - M21.861 Other specified acquired deformities of right lower leg
    - M21.862 Other specified acquired deformities of left lower leg
    - M21.869 Other specified acquired deformities of unspecified lower leg
- M21.9 Unspecified acquired deformity of limb and hand
  - M21.90 Unspecified acquired deformity of unspecified limb
  - M21.92 Unspecified acquired deformity of upper arm
    - M21.921 Unspecified acquired deformity of right upper arm
    - M21.922 Unspecified acquired deformity of left upper arm
    - M21.929 Unspecified acquired deformity of unspecified upper arm
  - M21.93 Unspecified acquired deformity of forearm
    - M21.931 Unspecified acquired deformity of right forearm
    - M21.932 Unspecified acquired deformity of left forearm
    - M21.939 Unspecified acquired deformity of unspecified forearm
  - M21.94 Unspecified acquired deformity of hand
    - M21.941 Unspecified acquired deformity of hand, right hand
    - M21.942 Unspecified acquired deformity of hand, left hand
    - M21.949 Unspecified acquired deformity of hand, unspecified hand
  - M21.95 Unspecified acquired deformity of thigh
    - M21.951 Unspecified acquired deformity of right thigh
    - M21.952 Unspecified acquired deformity of left thigh
    - M21.959 Unspecified acquired deformity of unspecified thigh
  - M21.96 Unspecified acquired deformity of lower leg
    - M21.961 Unspecified acquired deformity of right lower leg
    - M21.962 Unspecified acquired deformity of left lower leg
    - M21.969 Unspecified acquired deformity of unspecified lower leg

- M22 Disorder of patella
  - **Excludes1** traumatic dislocation of patella (S83.0-)
  - M22.0 Recurrent dislocation of patella
    - M22.00 Recurrent dislocation of patella, unspecified knee
    - M22.01 Recurrent dislocation of patella, right knee
    - M22.02 Recurrent dislocation of patella, left knee
  - M22.1 Recurrent subluxation of patella
    - Incomplete dislocation of patella
    - M22.10 Recurrent subluxation of patella, unspecified knee
    - M22.11 Recurrent subluxation of patella, right knee
    - M22.12 Recurrent subluxation of patella, left knee
  - M22.2 Patellofemoral disorders
    - M22.2X Patellofemoral disorders
      - M22.2X1 Patellofemoral disorders, right knee
      - M22.2X2 Patellofemoral disorders, left knee
      - M22.2X9 Patellofemoral disorders, unspecified knee
  - M22.3 Other derangements of patella
    - M22.3X Other derangements of patella
      - M22.3X1 Other derangements of patella, right knee
      - M22.3X2 Other derangements of patella, left knee
      - M22.3X9 Other derangements of patella, unspecified knee
  - M22.4 Chondromalacia patellae
    - M22.40 Chondromalacia patellae, unspecified knee
    - M22.41 Chondromalacia patellae, right knee
    - M22.42 Chondromalacia patellae, left knee
  - M22.8 Other disorders of patella
    - M22.8X Other disorders of patella
      - M22.8X1 Other disorders of patella, right knee
      - M22.8X2 Other disorders of patella, left knee
      - M22.8X9 Other disorders of patella, unspecified knee
  - M22.9 Unspecified disorder of patella
    - M22.90 Unspecified disorder of patella, unspecified knee
    - M22.91 Unspecified disorder of patella, right knee
    - M22.92 Unspecified disorder of patella, left knee

M23 Internal derangement of knee

Excludes1 ankylosis (M24.66)
current injury - see injury of knee and lower leg (S80-S89)
deformity of knee (M21.-)
osteochondritis dissecans (M93.2)
recurrent dislocation or subluxation of joints (M24.4)
recurrent dislocation or subluxation of patella (M22.0-M22.1)

Coding Clinic: 2019, Q2, P26

M23.0 Cystic meniscus

M23.00 Cystic meniscus, unspecified meniscus
Cystic meniscus, unspecified lateral meniscus
Cystic meniscus, unspecified medial meniscus

M23.000 Cystic meniscus, unspecified lateral meniscus, right knee
M23.001 Cystic meniscus, unspecified lateral meniscus, left knee
M23.002 Cystic meniscus, unspecified lateral meniscus, unspecified knee
M23.003 Cystic meniscus, unspecified medial meniscus, right knee
M23.004 Cystic meniscus, unspecified medial meniscus, left knee
M23.005 Cystic meniscus, unspecified medial meniscus, unspecified knee
M23.006 Cystic meniscus, unspecified meniscus, right knee
M23.007 Cystic meniscus, unspecified meniscus, left knee
M23.009 Cystic meniscus, unspecified meniscus, unspecified knee

M23.01 Cystic meniscus, anterior horn of medial meniscus

M23.011 Cystic meniscus, anterior horn of medial meniscus, right knee
M23.012 Cystic meniscus, anterior horn of medial meniscus, left knee
M23.019 Cystic meniscus, anterior horn of medial meniscus, unspecified knee

M23.02 Cystic meniscus, posterior horn of medial meniscus

M23.021 Cystic meniscus, posterior horn of medial meniscus, right knee
M23.022 Cystic meniscus, posterior horn of medial meniscus, left knee
M23.029 Cystic meniscus, posterior horn of medial meniscus, unspecified knee

M23.03 Cystic meniscus, other medial meniscus

M23.031 Cystic meniscus, other medial meniscus, right knee
M23.032 Cystic meniscus, other medial meniscus, left knee
M23.039 Cystic meniscus, other medial meniscus, unspecified knee

M23.04 Cystic meniscus, anterior horn of lateral meniscus

M23.041 Cystic meniscus, anterior horn of lateral meniscus, right knee
M23.042 Cystic meniscus, anterior horn of lateral meniscus, left knee
M23.049 Cystic meniscus, anterior horn of lateral meniscus, unspecified knee

M23.05 Cystic meniscus, posterior horn of lateral meniscus

M23.051 Cystic meniscus, posterior horn of lateral meniscus, right knee
M23.052 Cystic meniscus, posterior horn of lateral meniscus, left knee
M23.059 Cystic meniscus, posterior horn of lateral meniscus, unspecified knee

M23.06 Cystic meniscus, other lateral meniscus

M23.061 Cystic meniscus, other lateral meniscus, right knee
M23.062 Cystic meniscus, other lateral meniscus, left knee
M23.069 Cystic meniscus, other lateral meniscus, unspecified knee

★**(See Plate 34 of the Anatomy Illustrations.)**

M23.2 Derangement of meniscus due to old tear or injury
Old bucket-handle tear

M23.20 Derangement of unspecified meniscus due to old tear or injury
Derangement of unspecified lateral meniscus due to old tear or injury
Derangement of unspecified medial meniscus due to old tear or injury

M23.200 Derangement of unspecified lateral meniscus due to old tear or injury, right knee
M23.201 Derangement of unspecified lateral meniscus due to old tear or injury, left knee
M23.202 Derangement of unspecified lateral meniscus due to old tear or injury, unspecified knee
M23.203 Derangement of unspecified medial meniscus due to old tear or injury, right knee
M23.204 Derangement of unspecified medial meniscus due to old tear or injury, left knee
M23.205 Derangement of unspecified medial meniscus due to old tear or injury, unspecified knee
M23.206 Derangement of unspecified meniscus due to old tear or injury, right knee
M23.207 Derangement of unspecified meniscus due to old tear or injury, left knee
M23.209 Derangement of unspecified meniscus due to old tear or injury, unspecified knee

M23.21 Derangement of anterior horn of medial meniscus due to old tear or injury

M23.211 Derangement of anterior horn of medial meniscus due to old tear or injury, right knee
M23.212 Derangement of anterior horn of medial meniscus due to old tear or injury, left knee
M23.219 Derangement of anterior horn of medial meniscus due to old tear or injury, unspecified knee

M23.22 Derangement of posterior horn of medial meniscus due to old tear or injury

M23.221 Derangement of posterior horn of medial meniscus due to old tear or injury, right knee
M23.222 Derangement of posterior horn of medial meniscus due to old tear or injury, left knee
M23.229 Derangement of posterior horn of medial meniscus due to old tear or injury, unspecified knee

● M23.23 Derangement of **other medial** meniscus due to old tear or injury
- M23.231 Derangement of other medial meniscus due to old tear or injury, **right** knee
- M23.232 Derangement of other medial meniscus due to old tear or injury, **left** knee
- M23.239 Derangement of other medial meniscus due to old tear or injury, **unspecified** knee

● M23.24 Derangement of **anterior horn** of lateral meniscus due to old tear or injury
- M23.241 Derangement of anterior horn of lateral meniscus due to old tear or injury, **right** knee
- M23.242 Derangement of anterior horn of lateral meniscus due to old tear or injury, **left** knee
- M23.249 Derangement of anterior horn of lateral meniscus due to old tear or injury, **unspecified** knee

● M23.25 Derangement of **posterior horn** of lateral meniscus due to old tear or injury
- M23.251 Derangement of posterior horn of lateral meniscus due to old tear or injury, **right** knee
- M23.252 Derangement of posterior horn of lateral meniscus due to old tear or injury, **left** knee
- M23.259 Derangement of posterior horn of lateral meniscus due to old tear or injury, **unspecified** knee

● M23.26 Derangement of **other lateral** meniscus due to old tear or injury
- M23.261 Derangement of other lateral meniscus due to old tear or injury, **right** knee
- M23.262 Derangement of other lateral meniscus due to old tear or injury, **left** knee
- M23.269 Derangement of other lateral meniscus due to old tear or injury, **unspecified** knee

● M23.3 Other meniscus derangements

Degenerate meniscus
Detached meniscus
Retained meniscus

● M23.30 Other meniscus derangements, **unspecified meniscus**

Other meniscus derangements, unspecified lateral meniscus
Other meniscus derangements, unspecified medial meniscus

- M23.300 Other meniscus derangements, unspecified **lateral** meniscus, **right** knee
- M23.301 Other meniscus derangements, unspecified **lateral** meniscus, **left** knee
- M23.302 Other meniscus derangements, unspecified **lateral** meniscus, **unspecified** knee
- M23.303 Other meniscus derangements, unspecified **medial** meniscus, **right** knee
- M23.304 Other meniscus derangements, unspecified **medial** meniscus, **left** knee
- M23.305 Other meniscus derangements, unspecified **medial** meniscus, **unspecified** knee
- M23.306 Other meniscus derangements, unspecified meniscus, **right** knee
- M23.307 Other meniscus derangements, unspecified meniscus, **left** knee
- M23.309 Other meniscus derangements, unspecified meniscus, **unspecified** knee

● M23.31 Other meniscus derangements, **anterior horn of medial** meniscus
- M23.311 Other meniscus derangements, anterior horn of medial meniscus, **right** knee
- M23.312 Other meniscus derangements, anterior horn of medial meniscus, **left** knee
- M23.319 Other meniscus derangements, anterior horn of medial meniscus, **unspecified** knee

● M23.32 Other meniscus derangements, **posterior horn of medial** meniscus
- M23.321 Other meniscus derangements, posterior horn of medial meniscus, **right** knee
- M23.322 Other meniscus derangements, posterior horn of medial meniscus, **left** knee
- M23.329 Other meniscus derangements, posterior horn of medial meniscus, **unspecified** knee

● M23.33 Other meniscus derangements, **other medial** meniscus
- M23.331 Other meniscus derangements, other medial meniscus, **right** knee
- M23.332 Other meniscus derangements, other medial meniscus, **left** knee
- M23.339 Other meniscus derangements, other medial meniscus, **unspecified** knee

● M23.34 Other meniscus derangements, **anterior horn of lateral** meniscus
- M23.341 Other meniscus derangements, anterior horn of lateral meniscus, **right** knee
- M23.342 Other meniscus derangements, anterior horn of lateral meniscus, **left** knee
- M23.349 Other meniscus derangements, anterior horn of lateral meniscus, **unspecified** knee

● M23.35 Other meniscus derangements, **posterior horn of lateral** meniscus
- M23.351 Other meniscus derangements, posterior horn of lateral meniscus, **right** knee
- M23.352 Other meniscus derangements, posterior horn of lateral meniscus, **left** knee
- M23.359 Other meniscus derangements, posterior horn of lateral meniscus, **unspecified** knee

● M23.36 Other meniscus derangements, **other lateral** meniscus
- M23.361 Other meniscus derangements, other lateral meniscus, **right** knee
- M23.362 Other meniscus derangements, other lateral meniscus, **left** knee
- M23.369 Other meniscus derangements, other lateral meniscus, **unspecified** knee

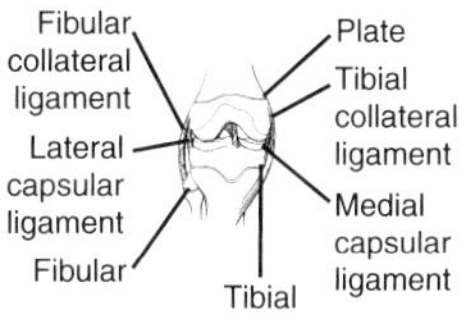

Figure 13-2 Collateral and cruciate ligament of knee. (From DeLee: DeLee and Drez's Orthopaedic Sports Medicine, ed 3, Saunders, 2009)

- ● M23.4 Loose body in knee
  - M23.40 Loose body in knee, unspecified knee
  - M23.41 Loose body in knee, right knee
  - M23.42 Loose body in knee, left knee
- ● M23.5 Chronic instability of knee
  - M23.50 Chronic instability of knee, unspecified knee
  - M23.51 Chronic instability of knee, right knee
  - M23.52 Chronic instability of knee, left knee
- ● M23.6 Other spontaneous disruption of ligament(s) of knee
  - ● M23.60 Other spontaneous disruption of unspecified ligament of knee
    - M23.601 Other spontaneous disruption of unspecified ligament of right knee
    - M23.602 Other spontaneous disruption of unspecified ligament of left knee
    - M23.609 Other spontaneous disruption of unspecified ligament of unspecified knee
  - ● M23.61 Other spontaneous disruption of anterior cruciate ligament of knee
    - M23.611 Other spontaneous disruption of anterior cruciate ligament of right knee
    - M23.612 Other spontaneous disruption of anterior cruciate ligament of left knee
    - M23.619 Other spontaneous disruption of anterior cruciate ligament of unspecified knee
  - ● M23.62 Other spontaneous disruption of posterior cruciate ligament of knee
    - M23.621 Other spontaneous disruption of posterior cruciate ligament of right knee
    - M23.622 Other spontaneous disruption of posterior cruciate ligament of left knee
    - M23.629 Other spontaneous disruption of posterior cruciate ligament of unspecified knee
  - ● M23.63 Other spontaneous disruption of medial collateral ligament of knee
    - M23.631 Other spontaneous disruption of medial collateral ligament of right knee
    - M23.632 Other spontaneous disruption of medial collateral ligament of left knee
    - M23.639 Other spontaneous disruption of medial collateral ligament of unspecified knee
  - ● M23.64 Other spontaneous disruption of lateral collateral ligament of knee
    - M23.641 Other spontaneous disruption of lateral collateral ligament of right knee
    - M23.642 Other spontaneous disruption of lateral collateral ligament of left knee
    - M23.649 Other spontaneous disruption of lateral collateral ligament of unspecified knee
  - ● M23.67 Other spontaneous disruption of capsular ligament of knee
    - M23.671 Other spontaneous disruption of capsular ligament of right knee
    - M23.672 Other spontaneous disruption of capsular ligament of left knee
    - M23.679 Other spontaneous disruption of capsular ligament of unspecified knee
- ● M23.8 Other internal derangements of knee
  - Laxity of ligament of knee
  - Snapping knee
  - ● M23.8X Other internal derangements of knee
    - M23.8X1 Other internal derangements of right knee
    - M23.8X2 Other internal derangements of left knee
    - M23.8X9 Other internal derangements of unspecified knee
- ● M23.9 Unspecified internal derangement of knee
  - M23.90 Unspecified internal derangement of unspecified knee
  - M23.91 Unspecified internal derangement of right knee
  - M23.92 Unspecified internal derangement of left knee

● M24 Other specific joint derangements

Excludes1 current injury - see injury of joint by body region

Excludes2 ganglion (M67.4)
snapping knee (M23.8-)
temporomandibular joint disorders (M26.6-)

- ● M24.0 Loose body in joint
  - **Excludes2** loose body in knee (M23.4)
  - M24.00 Loose body in unspecified joint
  - ● M24.01 Loose body in shoulder
    - M24.011 Loose body in right shoulder
    - M24.012 Loose body in left shoulder
    - M24.019 Loose body in unspecified shoulder
  - ● M24.02 Loose body in elbow
    - M24.021 Loose body in right elbow
    - M24.022 Loose body in left elbow
    - M24.029 Loose body in unspecified elbow
  - ● M24.03 Loose body in wrist
    - M24.031 Loose body in right wrist
    - M24.032 Loose body in left wrist
    - M24.039 Loose body in unspecified wrist
  - ● M24.04 Loose body in finger joints
    - M24.041 Loose body in right finger joint(s)
    - M24.042 Loose body in left finger joint(s)
    - M24.049 Loose body in unspecified finger joint(s)
  - ● M24.05 Loose body in hip
    - M24.051 Loose body in right hip
    - M24.052 Loose body in left hip
    - M24.059 Loose body in unspecified hip
  - ● M24.07 Loose body in ankle and toe joints
    - M24.071 Loose body in right ankle
    - M24.072 Loose body in left ankle
    - M24.073 Loose body in unspecified ankle
    - M24.074 Loose body in right toe joint(s)
    - M24.075 Loose body in left toe joint(s)
    - M24.076 Loose body in unspecified toe joints
  - M24.08 Loose body, other site

● M24.1 Other articular cartilage disorders

Excludes2 chondrocalcinosis (M11.1, M11.2-)
internal derangement of knee (M23.-)
metastatic calcification (E83.5)
ochronosis (E70.2)

M24.10 Other articular cartilage disorders, unspecified site

● M24.11 Other articular cartilage disorders, shoulder

M24.111 Other articular cartilage disorders, right shoulder

M24.112 Other articular cartilage disorders, left shoulder

M24.119 Other articular cartilage disorders, unspecified shoulder

● M24.12 Other articular cartilage disorders, elbow

M24.121 Other articular cartilage disorders, right elbow

M24.122 Other articular cartilage disorders, left elbow

M24.129 Other articular cartilage disorders, unspecified elbow

● M24.13 Other articular cartilage disorders, wrist

M24.131 Other articular cartilage disorders, right wrist

M24.132 Other articular cartilage disorders, left wrist

M24.139 Other articular cartilage disorders, unspecified wrist

● M24.14 Other articular cartilage disorders, hand

M24.141 Other articular cartilage disorders, right hand

M24.142 Other articular cartilage disorders, left hand

M24.149 Other articular cartilage disorders, unspecified hand

● M24.15 Other articular cartilage disorders, hip

M24.151 Other articular cartilage disorders, right hip

M24.152 Other articular cartilage disorders, left hip

M24.159 Other articular cartilage disorders, unspecified hip

● M24.17 Other articular cartilage disorders, ankle and foot

M24.171 Other articular cartilage disorders, right ankle

M24.172 Other articular cartilage disorders, left ankle

M24.173 Other articular cartilage disorders, unspecified ankle

M24.174 Other articular cartilage disorders, right foot

M24.175 Other articular cartilage disorders, left foot

M24.176 Other articular cartilage disorders, unspecified foot

● M24.2 Disorder of ligament

Instability secondary to old ligament injury
Ligamentous laxity NOS

Excludes1 familial ligamentous laxity (M35.7)

Excludes2 internal derangement of knee (M23.5-M23.8X9)

M24.20 Disorder of ligament, unspecified site

● M24.21 Disorder of ligament, shoulder

M24.211 Disorder of ligament, right shoulder

M24.212 Disorder of ligament, left shoulder

M24.219 Disorder of ligament, unspecified shoulder

● M24.22 Disorder of ligament, elbow

M24.221 Disorder of ligament, right elbow

M24.222 Disorder of ligament, left elbow

M24.229 Disorder of ligament, unspecified elbow

● M24.23 Disorder of ligament, wrist

M24.231 Disorder of ligament, right wrist

M24.232 Disorder of ligament, left wrist

M24.239 Disorder of ligament, unspecified wrist

● M24.24 Disorder of ligament, hand

M24.241 Disorder of ligament, right hand

M24.242 Disorder of ligament, left hand

M24.249 Disorder of ligament, unspecified hand

● M24.25 Disorder of ligament, hip

M24.251 Disorder of ligament, right hip

M24.252 Disorder of ligament, left hip

M24.259 Disorder of ligament, unspecified hip

● M24.27 Disorder of ligament, ankle and foot

M24.271 Disorder of ligament, right ankle

M24.272 Disorder of ligament, left ankle

M24.273 Disorder of ligament, unspecified ankle

M24.274 Disorder of ligament, right foot

M24.275 Disorder of ligament, left foot

M24.276 Disorder of ligament, unspecified foot

M24.28 Disorder of ligament, vertebrae

● M24.3 Pathological dislocation of joint, not elsewhere classified

Excludes1 congenital dislocation or displacement of joint - see congenital malformations and deformations of the musculoskeletal system (Q65-Q79)
current injury - see injury of joints and ligaments by body region
recurrent dislocation of joint (M24.4-)

M24.30 Pathological dislocation of unspecified joint, not elsewhere classified

● M24.31 Pathological dislocation of shoulder, not elsewhere classified

M24.311 Pathological dislocation of right shoulder, not elsewhere classified

M24.312 Pathological dislocation of left shoulder, not elsewhere classified

M24.319 Pathological dislocation of unspecified shoulder, not elsewhere classified

● M24.32 Pathological dislocation of elbow, not elsewhere classified

M24.321 Pathological dislocation of right elbow, not elsewhere classified

M24.322 Pathological dislocation of left elbow, not elsewhere classified

M24.329 Pathological dislocation of unspecified elbow, not elsewhere classified

● M24.33 Pathological dislocation of wrist, not elsewhere classified

M24.331 Pathological dislocation of right wrist, not elsewhere classified

M24.332 Pathological dislocation of left wrist, not elsewhere classified

M24.339 Pathological dislocation of unspecified wrist, not elsewhere classified

● M24.34 Pathological dislocation of hand, not elsewhere classified
- M24.341 Pathological dislocation of right hand, not elsewhere classified
- M24.342 Pathological dislocation of left hand, not elsewhere classified
- M24.349 Pathological dislocation of unspecified hand, not elsewhere classified

● M24.35 Pathological dislocation of hip, not elsewhere classified
- M24.351 Pathological dislocation of right hip, not elsewhere classified
- M24.352 Pathological dislocation of left hip, not elsewhere classified
- M24.359 Pathological dislocation of unspecified hip, not elsewhere classified

● M24.36 Pathological dislocation of knee, not elsewhere classified
- M24.361 Pathological dislocation of right knee, not elsewhere classified
- M24.362 Pathological dislocation of left knee, not elsewhere classified
- M24.369 Pathological dislocation of unspecified knee, not elsewhere classified

● M24.37 Pathological dislocation of ankle and foot, not elsewhere classified
- M24.371 Pathological dislocation of right ankle, not elsewhere classified
- M24.372 Pathological dislocation of left ankle, not elsewhere classified
- M24.373 Pathological dislocation of unspecified ankle, not elsewhere classified
- M24.374 Pathological dislocation of right foot, not elsewhere classified
- M24.375 Pathological dislocation of left foot, not elsewhere classified
- M24.376 Pathological dislocation of unspecified foot, not elsewhere classified

● M24.4 Recurrent dislocation of joint

Recurrent subluxation of joint

Excludes2 recurrent dislocation of patella (M22.Ø-M22.1)
recurrent vertebral dislocation (M43.3-, M43.4, M43.5-)

M24.4Ø Recurrent dislocation, unspecified joint

● M24.41 Recurrent dislocation, shoulder
- M24.411 Recurrent dislocation, right shoulder
- M24.412 Recurrent dislocation, left shoulder
- M24.419 Recurrent dislocation, unspecified shoulder

● M24.42 Recurrent dislocation, elbow
- M24.421 Recurrent dislocation, right elbow
- M24.422 Recurrent dislocation, left elbow
- M24.429 Recurrent dislocation, unspecified elbow

● M24.43 Recurrent dislocation, wrist
- M24.431 Recurrent dislocation, right wrist
- M24.432 Recurrent dislocation, left wrist
- M24.439 Recurrent dislocation, unspecified wrist

● M24.44 Recurrent dislocation, hand and finger(s)
- M24.441 Recurrent dislocation, right hand
- M24.442 Recurrent dislocation, left hand
- M24.443 Recurrent dislocation, unspecified hand
- M24.444 Recurrent dislocation, right finger
- M24.445 Recurrent dislocation, left finger
- M24.446 Recurrent dislocation, unspecified finger

● M24.45 Recurrent dislocation, hip
- M24.451 Recurrent dislocation, right hip
- M24.452 Recurrent dislocation, left hip
- M24.459 Recurrent dislocation, unspecified hip

● M24.46 Recurrent dislocation, knee
- M24.461 Recurrent dislocation, right knee
- M24.462 Recurrent dislocation, left knee
- M24.469 Recurrent dislocation, unspecified knee

● M24.47 Recurrent dislocation, ankle, foot and toes
- M24.471 Recurrent dislocation, right ankle
- M24.472 Recurrent dislocation, left ankle
- M24.473 Recurrent dislocation, unspecified ankle
- M24.474 Recurrent dislocation, right foot
- M24.475 Recurrent dislocation, left foot
- M24.476 Recurrent dislocation, unspecified foot
- M24.477 Recurrent dislocation, right toe(s)
- M24.478 Recurrent dislocation, left toe(s)
- M24.479 Recurrent dislocation, unspecified toe(s)

● M24.5 Contracture of joint

Excludes1 contracture of muscle without contracture of joint (M62.4-)
contracture of tendon (sheath) without contracture of joint (M62.4-)
Dupuytren's contracture (M72.Ø)

Excludes2 acquired deformities of limbs (M2Ø-M21)

M24.5Ø Contracture, unspecified joint

● M24.51 Contracture, shoulder
- M24.511 Contracture, right shoulder
- M24.512 Contracture, left shoulder
- M24.519 Contracture, unspecified shoulder

● M24.52 Contracture, elbow
- M24.521 Contracture, right elbow
- M24.522 Contracture, left elbow
- M24.529 Contracture, unspecified elbow

● M24.53 Contracture, wrist
- M24.531 Contracture, right wrist
- M24.532 Contracture, left wrist
- M24.539 Contracture, unspecified wrist

● M24.54 Contracture, hand
- M24.541 Contracture, right hand
- M24.542 Contracture, left hand
- M24.549 Contracture, unspecified hand

● M24.55 Contracture, hip
- M24.551 Contracture, right hip
  Coding Clinic: 2Ø16, Q2, P6
- M24.552 Contracture, left hip
  Coding Clinic: 2Ø16, Q2, P6
- M24.559 Contracture, unspecified hip

Item 13–5 **Ankylosis** or arthrokleisis is a consolidation of a joint due to disease, injury, or surgical procedure. Spondylosis is the degeneration of the vertebral processes and formation of osteophytes and commonly occurs with age. **Spondylitis** or ankylosing spondylitis is a type of arthritis that affects the spine or backbone, causing back pain and stiffness.

● M24.56 Contracture, knee
- M24.561 Contracture, right knee
  Coding Clinic: 2016, Q2, P6
- M24.562 Contracture, left knee
  Coding Clinic: 2016, Q2, P6
- M24.569 Contracture, unspecified knee

● M24.57 Contracture, ankle and foot
- M24.571 Contracture, right ankle
- M24.572 Contracture, left ankle
- M24.573 Contracture, unspecified ankle
- M24.574 Contracture, right foot
- M24.575 Contracture, left foot
- M24.576 Contracture, unspecified foot

● M24.6 Ankylosis of joint

Excludes1 stiffness of joint without ankylosis (M25.6-)

Excludes2 spine (M43.2-)

M24.60 Ankylosis, unspecified joint

● M24.61 Ankylosis, shoulder
- M24.611 Ankylosis, right shoulder
- M24.612 Ankylosis, left shoulder
- M24.619 Ankylosis, unspecified shoulder

● M24.62 Ankylosis, elbow
- M24.621 Ankylosis, right elbow
- M24.622 Ankylosis, left elbow
- M24.629 Ankylosis, unspecified elbow

● M24.63 Ankylosis, wrist
- M24.631 Ankylosis, right wrist
- M24.632 Ankylosis, left wrist
- M24.639 Ankylosis, unspecified wrist

● M24.64 Ankylosis, hand
- M24.641 Ankylosis, right hand
- M24.642 Ankylosis, left hand
- M24.649 Ankylosis, unspecified hand

● M24.65 Ankylosis, hip
- M24.651 Ankylosis, right hip
- M24.652 Ankylosis, left hip
- M24.659 Ankylosis, unspecified hip

● M24.66 Ankylosis, knee
- M24.661 Ankylosis, right knee
- M24.662 Ankylosis, left knee
- M24.669 Ankylosis, unspecified knee

● M24.67 Ankylosis, ankle and foot
- M24.671 Ankylosis, right ankle
- M24.672 Ankylosis, left ankle
- M24.673 Ankylosis, unspecified ankle
- M24.674 Ankylosis, right foot
- M24.675 Ankylosis, left foot
- M24.676 Ankylosis, unspecified foot

M24.7 Protrusio acetabuli

● M24.8 Other specific joint derangements, not elsewhere classified

Excludes2 iliotibial band syndrome (M76.3)

M24.80 Other specific joint derangements of unspecified joint, not elsewhere classified

● M24.81 Other specific joint derangements of shoulder, not elsewhere classified
- M24.811 Other specific joint derangements of right shoulder, not elsewhere classified
- M24.812 Other specific joint derangements of left shoulder, not elsewhere classified
- M24.819 Other specific joint derangements of unspecified shoulder, not elsewhere classified

● M24.82 Other specific joint derangements of elbow, not elsewhere classified
- M24.821 Other specific joint derangements of right elbow, not elsewhere classified
- M24.822 Other specific joint derangements of left elbow, not elsewhere classified
- M24.829 Other specific joint derangements of unspecified elbow, not elsewhere classified

● M24.83 Other specific joint derangements of wrist, not elsewhere classified
- M24.831 Other specific joint derangements of right wrist, not elsewhere classified
- M24.832 Other specific joint derangements of left wrist, not elsewhere classified
- M24.839 Other specific joint derangements of unspecified wrist, not elsewhere classified

● M24.84 Other specific joint derangements of hand, not elsewhere classified
- M24.841 Other specific joint derangements of right hand, not elsewhere classified
- M24.842 Other specific joint derangements of left hand, not elsewhere classified
- M24.849 Other specific joint derangements of unspecified hand, not elsewhere classified

● M24.85 Other specific joint derangements of hip, not elsewhere classified

Irritable hip
- M24.851 Other specific joint derangements of right hip, not elsewhere classified
- M24.852 Other specific joint derangements of left hip, not elsewhere classified
- M24.859 Other specific joint derangements of unspecified hip, not elsewhere classified

● M24.87 Other specific joint derangements of ankle and foot, not elsewhere classified
- M24.871 Other specific joint derangements of right ankle, not elsewhere classified
- M24.872 Other specific joint derangements of left ankle, not elsewhere classified
- M24.873 Other specific joint derangements of unspecified ankle, not elsewhere classified
- M24.874 Other specific joint derangements of right foot, not elsewhere classified
- M24.875 Other specific joint derangements left foot, not elsewhere classified
- M24.876 Other specific joint derangements of unspecified foot, not elsewhere classified

M24.9 Joint derangement, unspecified

M25 Other joint disorder, not elsewhere classified

Excludes2 abnormality of gait and mobility (R26.-)
acquired deformities of limb (M2Ø-M21)
calcification of bursa (M71.4-)
calcification of shoulder (joint) (M75.3)
calcification of tendon (M65.2-)
difficulty in walking (R26.2)
temporomandibular joint disorder (M26.6-)

M25.Ø Hemarthrosis

Excludes1 current injury - see injury of joint by body region
hemophilic arthropathy (M36.2)

M25.ØØ Hemarthrosis, unspecified joint

M25.Ø1 Hemarthrosis, shoulder

M25.Ø11 Hemarthrosis, right shoulder
M25.Ø12 Hemarthrosis, left shoulder
M25.Ø19 Hemarthrosis, unspecified shoulder

M25.Ø2 Hemarthrosis, elbow

M25.Ø21 Hemarthrosis, right elbow
M25.Ø22 Hemarthrosis, left elbow
M25.Ø29 Hemarthrosis, unspecified elbow

M25.Ø3 Hemarthrosis, wrist

M25.Ø31 Hemarthrosis, right wrist
M25.Ø32 Hemarthrosis, left wrist
M25.Ø39 Hemarthrosis, unspecified wrist

M25.Ø4 Hemarthrosis, hand

M25.Ø41 Hemarthrosis, right hand
M25.Ø42 Hemarthrosis, left hand
M25.Ø49 Hemarthrosis, unspecified hand

M25.Ø5 Hemarthrosis, hip

M25.Ø51 Hemarthrosis, right hip
M25.Ø52 Hemarthrosis, left hip
M25.Ø59 Hemarthrosis, unspecified hip

M25.Ø6 Hemarthrosis, knee

M25.Ø61 Hemarthrosis, right knee
M25.Ø62 Hemarthrosis, left knee
M25.Ø69 Hemarthrosis, unspecified knee

M25.Ø7 Hemarthrosis, ankle and foot

M25.Ø71 Hemarthrosis, right ankle
M25.Ø72 Hemarthrosis, left ankle
M25.Ø73 Hemarthrosis, unspecified ankle
M25.Ø74 Hemarthrosis, right foot
M25.Ø75 Hemarthrosis, left foot
M25.Ø76 Hemarthrosis, unspecified foot

M25.Ø8 Hemarthrosis, other specified site
Hemarthrosis, vertebrae

M25.1 Fistula of joint

M25.1Ø Fistula, unspecified joint

M25.11 Fistula, shoulder

M25.111 Fistula, right shoulder
M25.112 Fistula, left shoulder
M25.119 Fistula, unspecified shoulder

M25.12 Fistula, elbow

M25.121 Fistula, right elbow
M25.122 Fistula, left elbow
M25.129 Fistula, unspecified elbow

M25.13 Fistula, wrist

M25.131 Fistula, right wrist
M25.132 Fistula, left wrist
M25.139 Fistula, unspecified wrist

M25.14 Fistula, hand

M25.141 Fistula, right hand
M25.142 Fistula, left hand
M25.149 Fistula, unspecified hand

M25.15 Fistula, hip

M25.151 Fistula, right hip
M25.152 Fistula, left hip
M25.159 Fistula, unspecified hip

M25.16 Fistula, knee

M25.161 Fistula, right knee
M25.162 Fistula, left knee
M25.169 Fistula, unspecified knee

M25.17 Fistula, ankle and foot

M25.171 Fistula, right ankle
M25.172 Fistula, left ankle
M25.173 Fistula, unspecified ankle
M25.174 Fistula, right foot
M25.175 Fistula, left foot
M25.176 Fistula, unspecified foot

M25.18 Fistula, other specified site
Fistula, vertebrae

M25.2 Flail joint

M25.2Ø Flail joint, unspecified joint

M25.21 Flail joint, shoulder

M25.211 Flail joint, right shoulder
M25.212 Flail joint, left shoulder
M25.219 Flail joint, unspecified shoulder

M25.22 Flail joint, elbow

M25.221 Flail joint, right elbow
M25.222 Flail joint, left elbow
M25.229 Flail joint, unspecified elbow

M25.23 Flail joint, wrist

M25.231 Flail joint, right wrist
M25.232 Flail joint, left wrist
M25.239 Flail joint, unspecified wrist

M25.24 Flail joint, hand

M25.241 Flail joint, right hand
M25.242 Flail joint, left hand
M25.249 Flail joint, unspecified hand

M25.25 Flail joint, hip

M25.251 Flail joint, right hip
M25.252 Flail joint, left hip
M25.259 Flail joint, unspecified hip

M25.26 Flail joint, knee

M25.261 Flail joint, right knee
M25.262 Flail joint, left knee
M25.269 Flail joint, unspecified knee

M25.27 Flail joint, ankle and foot

M25.271 Flail joint, right ankle and foot
M25.272 Flail joint, left ankle and foot
M25.279 Flail joint, unspecified ankle and foot

M25.28 Flail joint, other site

M25.3 Other instability of joint

Excludes1 instability of joint secondary to old ligament injury (M24.2-)
instability of joint secondary to removal of joint prosthesis (M96.8-)

Excludes2 spinal instabilities (M53.2-)

M25.3Ø Other instability, unspecified joint

M25.31 Other instability, shoulder

M25.311 Other instability, right shoulder
M25.312 Other instability, left shoulder
M25.319 Other instability, unspecified shoulder

M25.32 Other instability, elbow

M25.321 Other instability, right elbow
M25.322 Other instability, left elbow
M25.329 Other instability, unspecified elbow

● M25.33 Other instability, wrist
M25.331 Other instability, right wrist
M25.332 Other instability, left wrist
M25.339 Other instability, unspecified wrist
● M25.34 Other instability, hand
M25.341 Other instability, right hand
M25.342 Other instability, left hand
M25.349 Other instability, unspecified hand
● M25.35 Other instability, hip
M25.351 Other instability, right hip
M25.352 Other instability, left hip
M25.359 Other instability, unspecified hip
● M25.36 Other instability, knee
M25.361 Other instability, right knee
M25.362 Other instability, left knee
M25.369 Other instability, unspecified knee
● M25.37 Other instability, ankle and foot
M25.371 Other instability, right ankle
M25.372 Other instability, left ankle
M25.373 Other instability, unspecified ankle
M25.374 Other instability, right foot
M25.375 Other instability, left foot
M25.376 Other instability, unspecified foot
● M25.4 Effusion of joint
Excludes1 hydrarthrosis in yaws (A66.6)
intermittent hydrarthrosis (M12.4-)
other infective (teno)synovitis (M65.1-)
M25.40 Effusion, unspecified joint
● M25.41 Effusion, shoulder
M25.411 Effusion, right shoulder
M25.412 Effusion, left shoulder
M25.419 Effusion, unspecified shoulder
● M25.42 Effusion, elbow
M25.421 Effusion, right elbow
M25.422 Effusion, left elbow
M25.429 Effusion, unspecified elbow
● M25.43 Effusion, wrist
M25.431 Effusion, right wrist
M25.432 Effusion, left wrist
M25.439 Effusion, unspecified wrist
● M25.44 Effusion, hand
M25.441 Effusion, right hand
M25.442 Effusion, left hand
M25.449 Effusion, unspecified hand
● M25.45 Effusion, hip
M25.451 Effusion, right hip
M25.452 Effusion, left hip
M25.459 Effusion, unspecified hip
● M25.46 Effusion, knee
M25.461 Effusion, right knee
M25.462 Effusion, left knee
M25.469 Effusion, unspecified knee
● M25.47 Effusion, ankle and foot
M25.471 Effusion, right ankle
M25.472 Effusion, left ankle
M25.473 Effusion, unspecified ankle
M25.474 Effusion, right foot
M25.475 Effusion, left foot
M25.476 Effusion, unspecified foot
M25.48 Effusion, other site

● M25.5 Pain in joint
Excludes2 pain in hand (M79.64-)
pain in fingers (M79.64-)
pain in foot (M79.67-)
pain in limb (M79.6-)
pain in toes (M79.67-)
M25.50 Pain in unspecified joint
● M25.51 Pain in shoulder
M25.511 Pain in right shoulder
M25.512 Pain in left shoulder
M25.519 Pain in unspecified shoulder
● M25.52 Pain in elbow
M25.521 Pain in right elbow
M25.522 Pain in left elbow
M25.529 Pain in unspecified elbow
● M25.53 Pain in wrist
M25.531 Pain in right wrist
M25.532 Pain in left wrist
M25.539 Pain in unspecified wrist
● M25.54 Pain in joints of hand
Coding Clinic: 2016, Q4, P38
M25.541 Pain in joints of right hand
M25.542 Pain in joints of left hand
M25.549 Pain in joints of unspecified hand
Pain in joints of hand NOS
● M25.55 Pain in hip
M25.551 Pain in right hip
M25.552 Pain in left hip
M25.559 Pain in unspecified hip
● M25.56 Pain in knee
M25.561 Pain in right knee
M25.562 Pain in left knee
M25.569 Pain in unspecified knee
● M25.57 Pain in ankle and joints of foot
M25.571 Pain in right ankle and joints of right foot
M25.572 Pain in left ankle and joints of left foot
M25.579 Pain in unspecified ankle and joints of unspecified foot
● M25.6 Stiffness of joint, not elsewhere classified
Excludes1 ankylosis of joint (M24.6-)
contracture of joint (M24.5-)
M25.60 Stiffness of unspecified joint, not elsewhere classified
● M25.61 Stiffness of shoulder, not elsewhere classified
M25.611 Stiffness of right shoulder, not elsewhere classified
M25.612 Stiffness of left shoulder, not elsewhere classified
M25.619 Stiffness of unspecified shoulder, not elsewhere classified
● M25.62 Stiffness of elbow, not elsewhere classified
M25.621 Stiffness of right elbow, not elsewhere classified
M25.622 Stiffness of left elbow, not elsewhere classified
M25.629 Stiffness of unspecified elbow, not elsewhere classified
● M25.63 Stiffness of wrist, not elsewhere classified
M25.631 Stiffness of right wrist, not elsewhere classified
M25.632 Stiffness of left wrist, not elsewhere classified
M25.639 Stiffness of unspecified wrist, not elsewhere classified

● M25.64 Stiffness of **hand**, not elsewhere classified
- M25.641 Stiffness of **right** hand, not elsewhere classified
- M25.642 Stiffness of **left** hand, not elsewhere classified
- M25.649 Stiffness of **unspecified** hand, not elsewhere classified

● M25.65 Stiffness of **hip**, not elsewhere classified
- M25.651 Stiffness of **right** hip, not elsewhere classified
- M25.652 Stiffness of **left** hip, not elsewhere classified
- M25.659 Stiffness of **unspecified** hip, not elsewhere classified

● M25.66 Stiffness of **knee**, not elsewhere classified
- M25.661 Stiffness of **right** knee, not elsewhere classified
- M25.662 Stiffness of **left** knee, not elsewhere classified
- M25.669 Stiffness of **unspecified** knee, not elsewhere classified

● M25.67 Stiffness of **ankle and foot**, not elsewhere classified
- M25.671 Stiffness of **right ankle**, not elsewhere classified
- M25.672 Stiffness of **left ankle**, not elsewhere classified
- M25.673 Stiffness of **unspecified ankle**, not elsewhere classified
- M25.674 Stiffness of **right foot**, not elsewhere classified
- M25.675 Stiffness of **left foot**, not elsewhere classified
- M25.676 Stiffness of **unspecified foot**, not elsewhere classified

● M25.7 Osteophyte

M25.70 Osteophyte, **unspecified** joint

● M25.71 Osteophyte, **shoulder**
- M25.711 Osteophyte, **right** shoulder
- M25.712 Osteophyte, **left** shoulder
- M25.719 Osteophyte, **unspecified** shoulder

● M25.72 Osteophyte, **elbow**
- M25.721 Osteophyte, **right** elbow
- M25.722 Osteophyte, **left** elbow
- M25.729 Osteophyte, **unspecified** elbow

● M25.73 Osteophyte, **wrist**
- M25.731 Osteophyte, **right** wrist
- M25.732 Osteophyte, **left** wrist
- M25.739 Osteophyte, **unspecified** wrist

● M25.74 Osteophyte, **hand**
- M25.741 Osteophyte, **right** hand
- M25.742 Osteophyte, **left** hand
- M25.749 Osteophyte, **unspecified** hand

● M25.75 Osteophyte, **hip**
- M25.751 Osteophyte, **right** hip
- M25.752 Osteophyte, **left** hip
- M25.759 Osteophyte, **unspecified** hip

● M25.76 Osteophyte, **knee**
- M25.761 Osteophyte, **right** knee
- M25.762 Osteophyte, **left** knee
- M25.769 Osteophyte, **unspecified** knee

● M25.77 Osteophyte, **ankle and foot**
- M25.771 Osteophyte, **right ankle**
- M25.772 Osteophyte, **left ankle**
- M25.773 Osteophyte, **unspecified ankle**
- M25.774 Osteophyte, **right foot**
- M25.775 Osteophyte, **left foot**
- M25.776 Osteophyte, **unspecified foot**

M25.78 Osteophyte, **vertebrae**

● M25.8 Other specified joint disorders

M25.80 Other specified joint disorders, **unspecified** joint

● M25.81 Other specified joint disorders, **shoulder**
- M25.811 Other specified joint disorders, **right** shoulder
- M25.812 Other specified joint disorders, **left** shoulder
- M25.819 Other specified joint disorders, **unspecified** shoulder

● M25.82 Other specified joint disorders, **elbow**
- M25.821 Other specified joint disorders, **right** elbow
- M25.822 Other specified joint disorders, **left** elbow
- M25.829 Other specified joint disorders, **unspecified** elbow

● M25.83 Other specified joint disorders, **wrist**
- M25.831 Other specified joint disorders, **right** wrist
- M25.832 Other specified joint disorders, **left** wrist
- M25.839 Other specified joint disorders, **unspecified** wrist

● M25.84 Other specified joint disorders, **hand**
- M25.841 Other specified joint disorders, **right** hand
- M25.842 Other specified joint disorders, **left** hand
- M25.849 Other specified joint disorders, **unspecified** hand

● M25.85 Other specified joint disorders, **hip**
- M25.851 Other specified joint disorders, **right** hip
- M25.852 Other specified joint disorders, **left** hip
- M25.859 Other specified joint disorders, **unspecified** hip

● M25.86 Other specified joint disorders, **knee**
- M25.861 Other specified joint disorders, **right** knee
- M25.862 Other specified joint disorders, **left** knee
- M25.869 Other specified joint disorders, **unspecified** knee

● M25.87 Other specified joint disorders, **ankle and foot**
- M25.871 Other specified joint disorders, **right** ankle and foot
- M25.872 Other specified joint disorders, **left** ankle and foot
- M25.879 Other specified joint disorders, **unspecified** ankle and foot

M25.9 Joint disorder, unspecified

CHAPTER 13 (MØØ-M99)

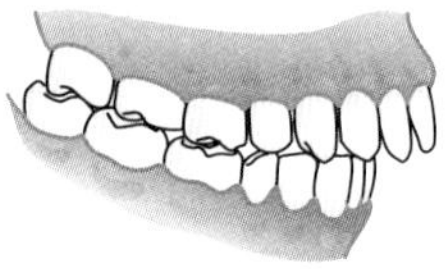

Figure 13-3 Dentofacial malocclusion.

Item 13–6 **Hyperplasia** is a condition of overdevelopment, whereas **hypoplasia** is a condition of underdevelopment. **Macrogenia** is overdevelopment of the chin, whereas **microgenia** is underdevelopment of the chin.

DENTOFACIAL ANOMALIES [INCLUDING MALOCCLUSION] AND OTHER DISORDERS OF JAW (M26-M27)

Excludes1 hemifacial atrophy or hypertrophy (Q67.4)
unilateral condylar hyperplasia or hypoplasia (M27.8)

● **M26 Dentofacial anomalies [including malocclusion]**

● **M26.Ø Major anomalies of jaw size**

Excludes1 acromegaly (E22.Ø)
Robin's syndrome (Q87.Ø)

M26.ØØ Unspecified anomaly of jaw size

M26.Ø1 Maxillary hyperplasia

M26.Ø2 Maxillary hypoplasia

M26.Ø3 Mandibular hyperplasia

M26.Ø4 Mandibular hypoplasia

M26.Ø5 Macrogenia

M26.Ø6 Microgenia

M26.Ø7 Excessive tuberosity of jaw
Entire maxillary tuberosity

M26.Ø9 Other specified anomalies of jaw size

● **M26.1 Anomalies of jaw-cranial base relationship**

M26.1Ø Unspecified anomaly of jaw-cranial base relationship

M26.11 Maxillary asymmetry

M26.12 Other jaw asymmetry

M26.19 Other specified anomalies of jaw-cranial base relationship

● **M26.2 Anomalies of dental arch relationship**

M26.2Ø Unspecified anomaly of dental arch relationship

● **M26.21 Malocclusion, Angle's class**

M26.211 Malocclusion, Angle's class I
Neutro-occlusion

M26.212 Malocclusion, Angle's class II
Disto-occlusion Division I
Disto-occlusion Division II

M26.213 Malocclusion, Angle's class III
Mesio-occlusion

M26.219 Malocclusion, Angle's class, unspecified

● **M26.22 Open occlusal relationship**

M26.22Ø Open anterior occlusal relationship
Anterior open bite

M26.221 Open posterior occlusal relationship
Posterior open bite

M26.23 Excessive horizontal overlap
Excessive horizontal overjet

M26.24 Reverse articulation
Crossbite (anterior) (posterior)

M26.25 Anomalies of interarch distance

M26.29 Other anomalies of dental arch relationship
Midline deviation of dental arch
Overbite (excessive) deep
Overbite (excessive) horizontal
Overbite (excessive) vertical
Posterior lingual occlusion of mandibular teeth

● **M26.3 Anomalies of tooth position of fully erupted tooth or teeth**

Excludes2 embedded and impacted teeth (KØ1.-)

M26.3Ø Unspecified anomaly of tooth position of fully erupted tooth or teeth
Abnormal spacing of fully erupted tooth or teeth NOS
Displacement of fully erupted tooth or teeth NOS
Transposition of fully erupted tooth or teeth NOS

M26.31 Crowding of fully erupted teeth

M26.32 Excessive spacing of fully erupted teeth
Diastema of fully erupted tooth or teeth NOS

M26.33 Horizontal displacement of fully erupted tooth or teeth
Tipped tooth or teeth
Tipping of fully erupted tooth

M26.34 Vertical displacement of fully erupted tooth or teeth
Extruded tooth
Infraeruption of tooth or teeth
Supraeruption of tooth or teeth

M26.35 Rotation of fully erupted tooth or teeth

M26.36 Insufficient interocclusal distance of fully erupted teeth (ridge)
Lack of adequate intermaxillary vertical dimension of fully erupted teeth

M26.37 Excessive interocclusal distance of fully erupted teeth
Excessive intermaxillary vertical dimension of fully erupted teeth
Loss of occlusal vertical dimension of fully erupted teeth

M26.39 Other anomalies of tooth position of fully erupted tooth or teeth

M26.4 Malocclusion, unspecified

● **M26.5 Dentofacial functional abnormalities**

Excludes1 bruxism (F45.8)
teeth-grinding NOS (F45.8)

M26.5Ø Dentofacial functional abnormalities, unspecified

M26.51 Abnormal jaw closure

M26.52 Limited mandibular range of motion

M26.53 Deviation in opening and closing of the mandible

M26.54 Insufficient anterior guidance
Insufficient anterior occlusal guidance

M26.55 Centric occlusion maximum intercuspation discrepancy

Excludes1 centric occlusion NOS (M26.59)

M26.56 Non-working side interference
Balancing side interference

M26.57 Lack of posterior occlusal support

M26.59 Other dentofacial functional abnormalities
Centric occlusion (of teeth) NOS
Malocclusion due to abnormal swallowing
Malocclusion due to mouth breathing
Malocclusion due to tongue, lip or finger habits

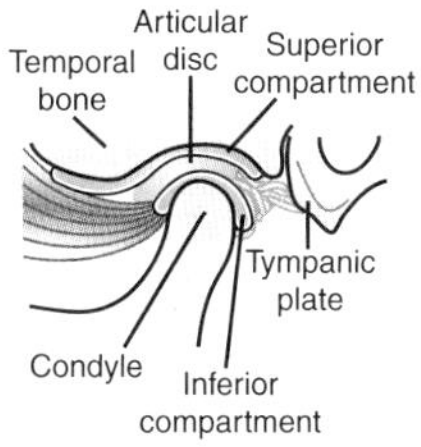

Figure 13-4 Temporomandibular joint.

Item 13–7 Dysfunction of the temporomandibular joint is termed **temporomandibular joint (TMJ) syndrome** and is characterized by pain and tenderness/spasm of the muscles of mastication, joint noise, and in the later stages, limited mandibular movement.

● M26.6 **Temporomandibular joint disorders**
Excludes2 current temporomandibular joint dislocation (SØ3.Ø)
current temporomandibular joint sprain (SØ3.4)
Coding Clinic: 2016, Q4, P38-39
● M26.6Ø **Temporomandibular joint disorder, unspecified**
M26.6Ø1 **Right temporomandibular joint disorder, unspecified**
M26.6Ø2 **Left temporomandibular joint disorder, unspecified**
M26.6Ø3 **Bilateral temporomandibular joint disorder, unspecified**
M26.6Ø9 **Unspecified temporomandibular joint disorder, unspecified side**
Temporomandibular joint disorder NOS
● M26.61 **Adhesions and ankylosis of temporomandibular joint**
M26.611 **Adhesions and ankylosis of right temporomandibular joint**
M26.612 **Adhesions and ankylosis of left temporomandibular joint**
M26.613 **Adhesions and ankylosis of bilateral temporomandibular joint**
M26.619 **Adhesions and ankylosis of temporomandibular joint, unspecified side**
● M26.62 **Arthralgia of temporomandibular joint**
M26.621 **Arthralgia of right temporomandibular joint**
M26.622 **Arthralgia of left temporomandibular joint**
M26.623 **Arthralgia of bilateral temporomandibular joint**
M26.629 **Arthralgia of temporomandibular joint, unspecified side**
● M26.63 **Articular disc disorder of temporomandibular joint**
M26.631 **Articular disc disorder of right temporomandibular joint**
M26.632 **Articular disc disorder of left temporomandibular joint**
M26.633 **Articular disc disorder of bilateral temporomandibular joint**
M26.639 **Articular disc disorder of temporomandibular joint, unspecified side**
M26.69 **Other specified disorders of temporomandibular joint**

● M26.7 **Dental alveolar anomalies**
M26.7Ø **Unspecified alveolar anomaly**
M26.71 **Alveolar maxillary hyperplasia**
M26.72 **Alveolar mandibular hyperplasia**
M26.73 **Alveolar maxillary hypoplasia**
M26.74 **Alveolar mandibular hypoplasia**
M26.79 **Other specified alveolar anomalies**
● M26.8 **Other dentofacial anomalies**
M26.81 **Anterior soft tissue impingement**
Anterior soft tissue impingement on teeth
M26.82 **Posterior soft tissue impingement**
Posterior soft tissue impingement on teeth
M26.89 **Other dentofacial anomalies**
M26.9 **Dentofacial anomaly, unspecified**

● M27 **Other diseases of jaws**
M27.Ø **Developmental disorders of jaws**
Latent bone cyst of jaw
Stafne's cyst
Torus mandibularis
Torus palatinus
M27.1 **Giant cell granuloma, central**
Giant cell granuloma NOS
Excludes1 peripheral giant cell granuloma (KØ6.8)
M27.2 **Inflammatory conditions of jaws**
Osteitis of jaw(s)
Osteomyelitis (neonatal) jaw(s)
Osteoradionecrosis jaw(s)
Periostitis jaw(s)
Sequestrum of jaw bone
Use additional code (W88-W9Ø, X39.Ø) to identify radiation, if radiation-induced
Excludes2 osteonecrosis of jaw due to drug (M87.18Ø)
M27.3 **Alveolitis of jaws**
Alveolar osteitis
Dry socket
● M27.4 **Other and unspecified cysts of jaw**
Excludes1 cysts of oral region (KØ9.-)
latent bone cyst of jaw (M27.Ø)
Stafne's cyst (M27.Ø)
M27.4Ø **Unspecified cyst of jaw**
Cyst of jaw NOS
M27.49 **Other cysts of jaw**
Aneurysmal cyst of jaw
Hemorrhagic cyst of jaw
Traumatic cyst of jaw
● M27.5 **Periradicular pathology associated with previous endodontic treatment**
M27.51 **Perforation of root canal space due to endodontic treatment**
M27.52 **Endodontic overfill**
M27.53 **Endodontic underfill**
M27.59 **Other periradicular pathology associated with previous endodontic treatment**
● M27.6 **Endosseous dental implant failure**
M27.61 **Osseointegration failure of dental implant**
Hemorrhagic complications of dental implant placement
Iatrogenic osseointegration failure of dental implant
Osseointegration failure of dental implant due to complications of systemic disease
Osseointegration failure of dental implant due to poor bone quality
Pre-integration failure of dental implant NOS
Pre-osseointegration failure of dental implant

CHAPTER 13 (MØØ-M99)

M27.62 **Post-osseointegration biological failure of dental implant**
Failure of dental implant due to lack of attached gingiva
Failure of dental implant due to occlusal trauma (caused by poor prosthetic design)
Failure of dental implant due to parafunctional habits
Failure of dental implant due to periodontal infection (peri mplantitis)
Failure of dental implant due to poor oral hygiene
Iatrogenic post-osseointegration failure of dental implant
Post-osseointegration failure of dental implant due to complications of systemic disease

M27.63 **Post-osseointegration mechanical failure of dental implant**
Failure of dental prosthesis causing loss of dental implant
Fracture of dental implant
Excludes2 cracked tooth (KØ3.81)
fractured dental restorative material with loss of material (KØ8.531)
fractured dental restorative material without loss of material (KØ8.53Ø)
fractured tooth (SØ2.5)

M27.69 **Other endosseous dental implant failure**
Dental implant failure NOS

M27.8 **Other specified diseases of jaws**
Cherubism
Exostosis
Fibrous dysplasia
Unilateral condylar hyperplasia
Unilateral condylar hypoplasia
Excludes1 jaw pain (R68.84)

M27.9 **Disease of jaws, unspecified**

SYSTEMIC CONNECTIVE TISSUE DISORDERS (M3Ø-M36)

Includes autoimmune disease NOS
collagen (vascular) disease NOS
systemic autoimmune disease
systemic collagen (vascular) disease

Excludes1 autoimmune disease, single organ or single cell-type - code to relevant condition category

● M3Ø **Polyarteritis nodosa and related conditions**
Excludes1 microscopic polyarteritis (M31.7)

M3Ø.Ø **Polyarteritis nodosa** HCC
M3Ø.1 **Polyarteritis with lung involvement [Churg-Strauss]** HCC
Allergic granulomatous angiitis
M3Ø.2 **Juvenile polyarteritis** HCC
M3Ø.3 **Mucocutaneous lymph node syndrome [Kawasaki]** HCC
M3Ø.8 **Other conditions related to polyarteritis nodosa** HCC
Polyangiitis overlap syndrome

● M31 **Other necrotizing vasculopathies**

M31.Ø **Hypersensitivity angiitis** HCC
Goodpasture's syndrome
M31.1 **Thrombotic microangiopathy** HCC
Thrombotic thrombocytopenic purpura
M31.2 **Lethal midline granuloma** HCC
● M31.3 **Wegener's granulomatosis**
Necrotizing respiratory granulomatosis
M31.3Ø **Wegener's granulomatosis without renal involvement** HCC
Wegener's granulomatosis NOS
M31.31 **Wegener's granulomatosis with renal involvement** HCC
M31.4 **Aortic arch syndrome [Takayasu]** HCC
M31.5 **Giant cell arteritis with polymyalgia rheumatica** HCC
M31.6 **Other giant cell arteritis** HCC
M31.7 **Microscopic polyangiitis** HCC
Microscopic polyarteritis
Excludes1 polyarteritis nodosa (M3Ø.Ø)
M31.8 **Other specified necrotizing vasculopathies** HCC
Hypocomplementemic vasculitis
Septic vasculitis
M31.9 **Necrotizing vasculopathy, unspecified** HCC

● M32 **Systemic lupus erythematosus (SLE)**
Autoimmune inflammatory connective tissue disease of unknown cause that occurs most often in women
Excludes1 lupus erythematosus (discoid) (NOS) (L93.Ø)

M32.Ø **Drug-induced systemic lupus erythematosus** HCC
Use additional code for adverse effect, if applicable, to identify drug (T36-T5Ø with fifth or sixth character 5)
● M32.1 **Systemic lupus erythematosus with organ or system involvement**
M32.1Ø **Systemic lupus erythematosus, organ or system involvement unspecified** HCC
M32.11 **Endocarditis in systemic lupus erythematosus** HCC
Libman-Sacks disease
M32.12 **Pericarditis in systemic lupus erythematosus** HCC
Lupus pericarditis
M32.13 **Lung involvement in systemic lupus erythematosus** HCC
Pleural effusion due to systemic lupus erythematosus
M32.14 **Glomerular disease in systemic lupus erythematosus** HCC
Lupus renal disease NOS
M32.15 **Tubulo-interstitial nephropathy in systemic lupus erythematosus** HCC
M32.19 **Other organ or system involvement in systemic lupus erythematosus** HCC
M32.8 **Other forms of systemic lupus erythematosus** HCC
M32.9 **Systemic lupus erythematosus, unspecified** HCC
SLE NOS
Systemic lupus erythematosus NOS
Systemic lupus erythematosus without organ involvement

● M33 **Dermatopolymyositis**
● M33.Ø **Juvenile dermatomyositis**
M33.ØØ **Juvenile dermatomyositis, organ involvement unspecified** HCC
M33.Ø1 **Juvenile dermatomyositis with respiratory involvement** HCC
M33.Ø2 **Juvenile dermatomyositis with myopathy** HCC
M33.Ø3 **Juvenile dermatomyositis without myopathy** HCC
M33.Ø9 **Juvenile dermatomyositis with other organ involvement** HCC
● M33.1 **Other dermatomyositis**
Adult dermatomyositis
M33.1Ø **Other dermatomyositis, organ involvement unspecified** HCC
M33.11 **Other dermatomyositis with respiratory involvement** HCC
M33.12 **Other dermatomyositis with myopathy** HCC
M33.13 **Other dermatomyositis without myopathy** HCC
Dermatomyositis NOS
M33.19 **Other dermatomyositis with other organ involvement** HCC

Item 13-8 Polymyalgia rheumatica is a syndrome characterized by aching and morning stiffness and is related to aging and hereditary predisposition.

M33.2 Polymyositis
- **M33.20 Polymyositis, organ involvement unspecified**
- **M33.21 Polymyositis with respiratory involvement**
- **M33.22 Polymyositis with myopathy**
- **M33.29 Polymyositis with other organ involvement**

M33.9 Dermatopolymyositis, unspecified
- **M33.90 Dermatopolymyositis, unspecified, organ involvement unspecified**
- **M33.91 Dermatopolymyositis, unspecified with respiratory involvement**
- **M33.92 Dermatopolymyositis, unspecified with myopathy**
- **M33.93 Dermatopolymyositis, unspecified without myopathy**
- **M33.99 Dermatopolymyositis, unspecified with other organ involvement**

M34 Systemic sclerosis [scleroderma]

Excludes1 circumscribed scleroderma (L94.0)
neonatal scleroderma (P83.88)

M34.0 Progressive systemic sclerosis

M34.1 CR(E)ST syndrome
Combination of calcinosis, Raynaud's phenomenon, esophageal dysfunction, sclerodactyly, telangiectasia

M34.2 Systemic sclerosis induced by drug and chemical
Code first poisoning due to drug or toxin, if applicable (T36-T65 with fifth or sixth character 1-4 or 6)
Use additional code for adverse effect, if applicable, to identify drug (T36-T50 with fifth or sixth character 5)

M34.8 Other forms of systemic sclerosis
- **M34.81 Systemic sclerosis with lung involvement**
- **M34.82 Systemic sclerosis with myopathy**
- **M34.83 Systemic sclerosis with polyneuropathy**
- **M34.89 Other systemic sclerosis**

M34.9 Systemic sclerosis, unspecified

M35 Other systemic involvement of connective tissue

Excludes1 reactive perforating collagenosis (L87.1)

M35.0 Sicca syndrome [Sjögren]
- **M35.00 Sicca syndrome, unspecified**
- **M35.01 Sicca syndrome with keratoconjunctivitis**
- **M35.02 Sicca syndrome with lung involvement**
- **M35.03 Sicca syndrome with myopathy**
- **M35.04 Sicca syndrome with tubulo-interstitial nephropathy**
  Renal tubular acidosis in sicca syndrome
- **M35.09 Sicca syndrome with other organ involvement**

M35.1 Other overlap syndromes
Mixed connective tissue disease
Excludes1 polyangiitis overlap syndrome (M30.8)

M35.2 Behçet's disease

M35.3 Polymyalgia rheumatica
Excludes1 polymyalgia rheumatica with giant cell arteritis (M31.5)

M35.4 Diffuse (eosinophilic) fasciitis

M35.5 Multifocal fibrosclerosis

M35.6 Relapsing panniculitis [Weber-Christian]
Excludes1 lupus panniculitis (L93.2)
panniculitis NOS (M79.3-)

M35.7 Hypermobility syndrome
Familial ligamentous laxity
Excludes1 Ehlers-Danlos syndrome (Q79.6-)
ligamentous laxity, NOS (M24.2-)

M35.8 Other specified systemic involvement of connective tissue

M35.9 Systemic involvement of connective tissue, unspecified
Autoimmune disease (systemic) NOS
Collagen (vascular) disease NOS

M36 Systemic disorders of connective tissue in diseases classified elsewhere

Excludes2 arthropathies in diseases classified elsewhere (M14.-)

M36.0 Dermato(poly)myositis in neoplastic disease
Code first underlying neoplasm (C00-D49)

M36.1 Arthropathy in neoplastic disease
Code first underlying neoplasm, such as:
leukemia (C91-C95)
malignant histiocytosis (C96.A)
multiple myeloma (C90.0)

M36.2 Hemophilic arthropathy
Hemarthrosis in hemophilic arthropathy
Code first underlying disease, such as:
factor VIII deficiency (D66)
with vascular defect (D68.0)
factor IX deficiency (D67)
hemophilia (classical) (D66)
hemophilia B (D67)
hemophilia C (D68.1)

M36.3 Arthropathy in other blood disorders

M36.4 Arthropathy in hypersensitivity reactions classified elsewhere
Code first underlying disease, such as:
Henoch (-Schönlein) purpura (D69.0)
serum sickness (T80.6-)

M36.8 Systemic disorders of connective tissue in other diseases classified elsewhere
Code first underlying disease, such as:
alkaptonuria (E70.2)
hypogammaglobulinemia (D80.-)
ochronosis (E70.2)

DORSOPATHIES (M40-M54)

DEFORMING DORSOPATHIES (M40-M43)

M40 Kyphosis and lordosis

Excludes1 congenital kyphosis and lordosis (Q76.4)
kyphoscoliosis (M41.-)
postprocedural kyphosis and lordosis (M96.-)

M40.0 Postural kyphosis
Excludes1 osteochondrosis of spine (M42.-)
- **M40.00 Postural kyphosis, site unspecified**
- **M40.03 Postural kyphosis, cervicothoracic region**
- **M40.04 Postural kyphosis, thoracic region**
- **M40.05 Postural kyphosis, thoracolumbar region**

CHAPTER 13 (M00-M99)

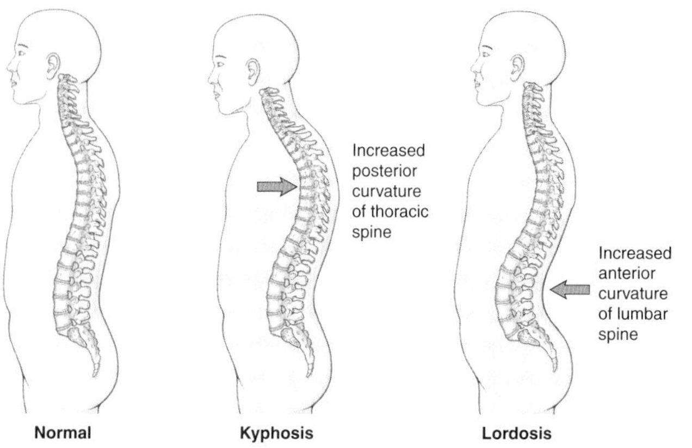

Figure 13-5 Kyphosis, Lordosis, Scoliosis. (From Chabner: The Language of Medicine, ed 8, St. Louis, Saunders, 2007)

Item 13–9 Kyphosis is an abnormal curvature of the spine. **Senile kyphosis** is a result of disc degeneration causing ossification (turning to bone). **Adolescent** or **juvenile** kyphosis is also known as **Scheuermann's disease,** a condition in which the discs of the lower thoracic spine herniate, causing the disc space to narrow and the spine to tilt forward. This condition is attributed to poor posture. **Lordosis or swayback** is an abnormal curvature of the spine resulting in an inward curve of the lumbar spine just above the buttocks. **Scoliosis** causes a sideways curve to the spine. The curves are S- or C-shaped, and it is most commonly acquired in late childhood and early teen years, when growth is fast.

● M40.1 Other secondary kyphosis
- M40.10 Other secondary kyphosis, site **unspecified**
- M40.12 Other secondary kyphosis, **cervical** region
- M40.13 Other secondary kyphosis, **cervicothoracic** region
- M40.14 Other secondary kyphosis, **thoracic** region
- M40.15 Other secondary kyphosis, **thoracolumbar** region

● M40.2 Other and unspecified kyphosis
- ● M40.20 Unspecified kyphosis
  - M40.202 Unspecified kyphosis, **cervical** region
  - M40.203 Unspecified kyphosis, **cervicothoracic** region
  - M40.204 Unspecified kyphosis, **thoracic** region
  - M40.205 Unspecified kyphosis, **thoracolumbar** region
  - M40.209 Unspecified kyphosis, site **unspecified**
- ● M40.29 Other kyphosis
  - M40.292 Other kyphosis, **cervical** region
  - M40.293 Other kyphosis, **cervicothoracic** region
  - M40.294 Other kyphosis, **thoracic** region
  - M40.295 Other kyphosis, **thoracolumbar** region
  - M40.299 Other kyphosis, site **unspecified**

● M40.3 Flatback syndrome
- M40.30 Flatback syndrome, site **unspecified**
- M40.35 Flatback syndrome, **thoracolumbar** region
- M40.36 Flatback syndrome, **lumbar** region
- M40.37 Flatback syndrome, **lumbosacral** region

● M40.4 Postural lordosis

Abnormal increase in the normal curvature of the lumbar spine (sway back)

Acquired lordosis
- M40.40 Postural lordosis, site **unspecified**
- M40.45 Postural lordosis, **thoracolumbar** region
- M40.46 Postural lordosis, **lumbar** region
- M40.47 Postural lordosis, **lumbosacral** region

● M40.5 Lordosis, unspecified
- M40.50 Lordosis, unspecified, site **unspecified**
- M40.55 Lordosis, unspecified, **thoracolumbar** region
- M40.56 Lordosis, unspecified, **lumbar** region
- M40.57 Lordosis, unspecified, **lumbosacral** region

● M41 Scoliosis

Includes kyphoscoliosis

Excludes1 congenital scoliosis NOS (Q67.5)
congenital scoliosis due to bony malformation (Q76.3)
postural congenital scoliosis (Q67.5)
kyphoscoliotic heart disease (I27.1)
postprocedural scoliosis (M96.-)

● M41.0 Infantile idiopathic scoliosis
- M41.00 Infantile idiopathic scoliosis, site **unspecified**
- M41.02 Infantile idiopathic scoliosis, **cervical** region
- M41.03 Infantile idiopathic scoliosis, **cervicothoracic** region
- M41.04 Infantile idiopathic scoliosis, **thoracic** region
- M41.05 Infantile idiopathic scoliosis, **thoracolumbar** region
- M41.06 Infantile idiopathic scoliosis, **lumbar** region
- M41.07 Infantile idiopathic scoliosis, **lumbosacral** region
- M41.08 Infantile idiopathic scoliosis, **sacral and sacrococcygeal** region

● M41.1 Juvenile and adolescent idiopathic scoliosis
- ● M41.11 **Juvenile idiopathic** scoliosis
  - M41.112 Juvenile idiopathic scoliosis, **cervical** region
  - M41.113 Juvenile idiopathic scoliosis, **cervicothoracic** region
  - M41.114 Juvenile idiopathic scoliosis, **thoracic** region
  - M41.115 Juvenile idiopathic scoliosis, **thoracolumbar** region
  - M41.116 Juvenile idiopathic scoliosis, **lumbar** region
  - M41.117 Juvenile idiopathic scoliosis, **lumbosacral** region
  - M41.119 Juvenile idiopathic scoliosis, site **unspecified**
- ● M41.12 Adolescent scoliosis
  - M41.122 Adolescent idiopathic scoliosis, **cervical** region
  - M41.123 Adolescent idiopathic scoliosis, **cervicothoracic** region
  - M41.124 Adolescent idiopathic scoliosis, **thoracic** region
  - M41.125 Adolescent idiopathic scoliosis, **thoracolumbar** region
  - M41.126 Adolescent idiopathic scoliosis, **lumbar** region
  - M41.127 Adolescent idiopathic scoliosis, **lumbosacral** region
  - M41.129 Adolescent idiopathic scoliosis, site **unspecified**

● M41.2 Other idiopathic scoliosis
- M41.20 Other idiopathic scoliosis, site unspecified
- M41.22 Other idiopathic scoliosis, cervical region
- M41.23 Other idiopathic scoliosis, cervicothoracic region
- M41.24 Other idiopathic scoliosis, thoracic region
- M41.25 Other idiopathic scoliosis, thoracolumbar region
- M41.26 Other idiopathic scoliosis, lumbar region
- M41.27 Other idiopathic scoliosis, lumbosacral region

● M41.3 Thoracogenic scoliosis
- M41.30 Thoracogenic scoliosis, site unspecified
- M41.34 Thoracogenic scoliosis, thoracic region
- M41.35 Thoracogenic scoliosis, thoracolumbar region

● M41.4 Neuromuscular scoliosis

Scoliosis secondary to cerebral palsy, Friedreich's ataxia, poliomyelitis and other neuromuscular disorders

Code also underlying condition
- M41.40 Neuromuscular scoliosis, site unspecified
- M41.41 Neuromuscular scoliosis, occipito-atlanto-axial region
- M41.42 Neuromuscular scoliosis, cervical region
- M41.43 Neuromuscular scoliosis, cervicothoracic region
- M41.44 Neuromuscular scoliosis, thoracic region
- M41.45 Neuromuscular scoliosis, thoracolumbar region
- M41.46 Neuromuscular scoliosis, lumbar region
- M41.47 Neuromuscular scoliosis, lumbosacral region

● M41.5 Other secondary scoliosis

Coding Clinic: 2019, Q1, P19
- M41.50 Other secondary scoliosis, site unspecified
- M41.52 Other secondary scoliosis, cervical region
- M41.53 Other secondary scoliosis, cervicothoracic region
- M41.54 Other secondary scoliosis, thoracic region
- M41.55 Other secondary scoliosis, thoracolumbar region
- M41.56 Other secondary scoliosis, lumbar region
- M41.57 Other secondary scoliosis, lumbosacral region

● M41.8 Other forms of scoliosis
- M41.80 Other forms of scoliosis, site unspecified
- M41.82 Other forms of scoliosis, cervical region
- M41.83 Other forms of scoliosis, cervicothoracic region
- M41.84 Other forms of scoliosis, thoracic region
- M41.85 Other forms of scoliosis, thoracolumbar region
- M41.86 Other forms of scoliosis, lumbar region
- M41.87 Other forms of scoliosis, lumbosacral region

M41.9 Scoliosis, unspecified

● M42 Spinal osteochondrosis

● M42.0 Juvenile osteochondrosis of spine

Calvé's disease

Scheuermann's disease

Excludes1 postural kyphosis (M40.0)
- M42.00 Juvenile osteochondrosis of spine, site unspecified
- M42.01 Juvenile osteochondrosis of spine, occipito-atlanto-axial region
- M42.02 Juvenile osteochondrosis of spine, cervical region
- M42.03 Juvenile osteochondrosis of spine, cervicothoracic region
- M42.04 Juvenile osteochondrosis of spine, thoracic region
- M42.05 Juvenile osteochondrosis of spine, thoracolumbar region
- M42.06 Juvenile osteochondrosis of spine, lumbar region
- M42.07 Juvenile osteochondrosis of spine, lumbosacral region
- M42.08 Juvenile osteochondrosis of spine, sacral and sacrococcygeal region
- M42.09 Juvenile osteochondrosis of spine, multiple sites in spine

● M42.1 Adult osteochondrosis of spine
- M42.10 Adult osteochondrosis of spine, site unspecified A
- M42.11 Adult osteochondrosis of spine, occipitoatlanto-axial region A
- M42.12 Adult osteochondrosis of spine, cervical region A
- M42.13 Adult osteochondrosis of spine, cervicothoracic region A
- M42.14 Adult osteochondrosis of spine, thoracic region A
- M42.15 Adult osteochondrosis of spine, thoracolumbar region A
- M42.16 Adult osteochondrosis of spine, lumbar region A
- M42.17 Adult osteochondrosis of spine, lumbosacral region A
- M42.18 Adult osteochondrosis of spine, sacral and sacrococcygeal region A
- M42.19 Adult osteochondrosis of spine, multiple sites in spine A

M42.9 Spinal osteochondrosis, unspecified

● M43 Other deforming dorsopathies

Excludes1 congenital spondylolysis and spondylolisthesis (Q76.2)
hemivertebra (Q76.3-Q76.4)
Klippel-Feil syndrome (Q76.1)
lumbarization and sacralization (Q76.4)
platyspondylisis (Q76.4)
spina bifida occulta (Q76.0)
spinal curvature in osteoporosis (M80.-)
spinal curvature in Paget's disease of bone [osteitis deformans] (M88.-)

● M43.0 Spondylolysis

Excludes1 congenital spondylolysis (Q76.2)
spondylolisthesis (M43.1)
- M43.00 Spondylolysis, site unspecified
- M43.01 Spondylolysis, occipito-atlanto-axial region
- M43.02 Spondylolysis, cervical region
- M43.03 Spondylolysis, cervicothoracic region
- M43.04 Spondylolysis, thoracic region
- M43.05 Spondylolysis, thoracolumbar region
- M43.06 Spondylolysis, lumbar region
- M43.07 Spondylolysis, lumbosacral region
- M43.08 Spondylolysis, sacral and sacrococcygeal region
- M43.09 Spondylolysis, multiple sites in spine

● M43.1 Spondylolisthesis

Excludes1 acute traumatic of lumbosacral region (S33.1)
acute traumatic of sites other than lumbosacral - code to Fracture, vertebra, by region
congenital spondylolisthesis (Q76.2)
- M43.10 Spondylolisthesis, site unspecified
- M43.11 Spondylolisthesis, occipito-atlanto-axial region
- M43.12 Spondylolisthesis, cervical region
- M43.13 Spondylolisthesis, cervicothoracic region
- M43.14 Spondylolisthesis, thoracic region
- M43.15 Spondylolisthesis, thoracolumbar region
- M43.16 Spondylolisthesis, lumbar region
- M43.17 Spondylolisthesis, lumbosacral region
- M43.18 Spondylolisthesis, sacral and sacrococcygeal region
- M43.19 Spondylolisthesis, multiple sites in spine

Item 13–10 Spondylolisthesis is a condition caused by the slipping forward of one disc over another.

● **M43.2 Fusion of spine**
Ankylosis of spinal joint
Excludes1 ankylosing spondylitis (M45.Ø-)
congenital fusion of spine (Q76.4)
Excludes2 arthrodesis status (Z98.1)
pseudoarthrosis after fusion or arthrodesis (M96.Ø)

M43.2Ø Fusion of spine, site unspecified
M43.21 Fusion of spine, occipito-atlanto-axial region
M43.22 Fusion of spine, cervical region
M43.23 Fusion of spine, cervicothoracic region
M43.24 Fusion of spine, thoracic region
M43.25 Fusion of spine, thoracolumbar region
M43.26 Fusion of spine, lumbar region
M43.27 Fusion of spine, lumbosacral region
M43.28 Fusion of spine, sacral and sacrococcygeal region

M43.3 Recurrent atlantoaxial dislocation with myelopathy
M43.4 Other recurrent atlantoaxial dislocation
● **M43.5 Other recurrent vertebral dislocation**
Excludes1 biomechanical lesions NEC (M99.-)

● **M43.5X Other recurrent vertebral dislocation**
M43.5X2 Other recurrent vertebral dislocation, cervical region
M43.5X3 Other recurrent vertebral dislocation, cervicothoracic region
M43.5X4 Other recurrent vertebral dislocation, thoracic region
M43.5X5 Other recurrent vertebral dislocation, thoracolumbar region
M43.5X6 Other recurrent vertebral dislocation, lumbar region
M43.5X7 Other recurrent vertebral dislocation, lumbosacral region
M43.5X8 Other recurrent vertebral dislocation, sacral and sacrococcygeal region
M43.5X9 Other recurrent vertebral dislocation, site unspecified

M43.6 Torticollis
Excludes1 congenital (sternomastoid) torticollis (Q68.Ø)
current injury - see Injury, of spine, by body region ocular torticollis (R29.891)
psychogenic torticollis (F45.8)
spasmodic torticollis (G24.3)
torticollis due to birth injury (P15.2)

● **M43.8 Other specified deforming dorsopathies**
Excludes2 kyphosis and lordosis (M4Ø.-)
scoliosis (M41.-)

● **M43.8X Other specified deforming dorsopathies**
M43.8X1 Other specified deforming dorsopathies, occipito-atlanto-axial region
M43.8X2 Other specified deforming dorsopathies, cervical region
M43.8X3 Other specified deforming dorsopathies, cervicothoracic region
M43.8X4 Other specified deforming dorsopathies, thoracic region
M43.8X5 Other specified deforming dorsopathies, thoracolumbar region
M43.8X6 Other specified deforming dorsopathies, lumbar region
M43.8X7 Other specified deforming dorsopathies, lumbosacral region
M43.8X8 Other specified deforming dorsopathies, sacral and sacrococcygeal region
M43.8X9 Other specified deforming dorsopathies, site unspecified

M43.9 Deforming dorsopathy, unspecified
Curvature of spine NOS

SPONDYLOPATHIES (M45-M49)

● **M45 Ankylosing spondylitis**
Rheumatoid arthritis of spine
Excludes1 arthropathy in Reiter's disease (MØ2.3-)
juvenile (ankylosing) spondylitis (MØ8.1)
Excludes2 Behçet's disease (M35.2)

M45.Ø Ankylosing spondylitis of multiple sites in spine HCC
M45.1 Ankylosing spondylitis of occipito-atlanto-axial region HCC
M45.2 Ankylosing spondylitis of cervical region HCC
M45.3 Ankylosing spondylitis of cervicothoracic region HCC
M45.4 Ankylosing spondylitis of thoracic region HCC
M45.5 Ankylosing spondylitis of thoracolumbar region HCC
M45.6 Ankylosing spondylitis lumbar region HCC
M45.7 Ankylosing spondylitis of lumbosacral region HCC
M45.8 Ankylosing spondylitis sacral and sacrococcygeal region HCC
M45.9 Ankylosing spondylitis of unspecified sites in spine HCC

● **M46 Other inflammatory spondylopathies**
● **M46.Ø Spinal enthesopathy**
Disorder of ligamentous or muscular attachments of spine

M46.ØØ Spinal enthesopathy, site unspecified HCC
M46.Ø1 Spinal enthesopathy, occipito-atlanto-axial region HCC
M46.Ø2 Spinal enthesopathy, cervical region HCC
M46.Ø3 Spinal enthesopathy, cervicothoracic region HCC
M46.Ø4 Spinal enthesopathy, thoracic region HCC
M46.Ø5 Spinal enthesopathy, thoracolumbar region HCC
M46.Ø6 Spinal enthesopathy, lumbar region HCC
M46.Ø7 Spinal enthesopathy, lumbosacral region HCC
M46.Ø8 Spinal enthesopathy, sacral and sacrococcygeal region HCC
M46.Ø9 Spinal enthesopathy, multiple sites in spine HCC

M46.1 Sacroiliitis, not elsewhere classified HCC
● **M46.2 Osteomyelitis of vertebra**
M46.2Ø Osteomyelitis of vertebra, site unspecified HCC
M46.21 Osteomyelitis of vertebra, occipito-atlanto-axial region HCC
M46.22 Osteomyelitis of vertebra, cervical region HCC
M46.23 Osteomyelitis of vertebra, cervicothoracic region HCC
M46.24 Osteomyelitis of vertebra, thoracic region HCC
M46.25 Osteomyelitis of vertebra, thoracolumbar region HCC
M46.26 Osteomyelitis of vertebra, lumbar region HCC
M46.27 Osteomyelitis of vertebra, lumbosacral region HCC
M46.28 Osteomyelitis of vertebra, sacral and sacrococcygeal region HCC

- **M46.3** Infection of intervertebral disc (pyogenic)
  Use additional code (B95-B97) to identify infectious agent
  - M46.30 Infection of intervertebral disc (pyogenic), site unspecified
  - M46.31 Infection of intervertebral disc (pyogenic), occipito-atlanto-axial region
  - M46.32 Infection of intervertebral disc (pyogenic), cervical region
  - M46.33 Infection of intervertebral disc (pyogenic), cervicothoracic region
  - M46.34 Infection of intervertebral disc (pyogenic), thoracic region
  - M46.35 Infection of intervertebral disc (pyogenic), thoracolumbar region
  - M46.36 Infection of intervertebral disc (pyogenic), lumbar region
  - M46.37 Infection of intervertebral disc (pyogenic), lumbosacral region
  - M46.38 Infection of intervertebral disc (pyogenic), sacral and sacrococcygeal region
  - M46.39 Infection of intervertebral disc (pyogenic), multiple sites in spine
- **M46.4** Discitis, unspecified
  - M46.40 Discitis, unspecified, site unspecified
  - M46.41 Discitis, unspecified, occipito-atlanto-axial region
  - M46.42 Discitis, unspecified, cervical region
  - M46.43 Discitis, unspecified, cervicothoracic region
  - M46.44 Discitis, unspecified, thoracic region
  - M46.45 Discitis, unspecified, thoracolumbar region
  - M46.46 Discitis, unspecified, lumbar region
  - M46.47 Discitis, unspecified, lumbosacral region
  - M46.48 Discitis, unspecified, sacral and sacrococcygeal region
  - M46.49 Discitis, unspecified, multiple sites in spine
- **M46.5** Other infective spondylopathies
  - M46.50 Other infective spondylopathies, site unspecified
  - M46.51 Other infective spondylopathies, occipitoatlanto-axial region
  - M46.52 Other infective spondylopathies, cervical region
  - M46.53 Other infective spondylopathies, cervicothoracic region
  - M46.54 Other infective spondylopathies, thoracic region
  - M46.55 Other infective spondylopathies, thoracolumbar region
  - M46.56 Other infective spondylopathies, lumbar region
  - M46.57 Other infective spondylopathies, lumbosacral region
  - M46.58 Other infective spondylopathies, sacral and sacrococcygeal region
  - M46.59 Other infective spondylopathies, multiple sites in spine
- **M46.8** Other specified inflammatory spondylopathies
  - M46.80 Other specified inflammatory spondylopathies, site unspecified
  - M46.81 Other specified inflammatory spondylopathies, occipito-atlanto-axial region
  - M46.82 Other specified inflammatory spondylopathies, cervical region
  - M46.83 Other specified inflammatory spondylopathies, cervicothoracic region
  - M46.84 Other specified inflammatory spondylopathies, thoracic region
  - M46.85 Other specified inflammatory spondylopathies, thoracolumbar region
  - M46.86 Other specified inflammatory spondylopathies, lumbar region
  - M46.87 Other specified inflammatory spondylopathies, lumbosacral region
  - M46.88 Other specified inflammatory spondylopathies, sacral and sacrococcygeal region
  - M46.89 Other specified inflammatory spondylopathies, multiple sites in spine
- **M46.9** Unspecified inflammatory spondylopathy
  - M46.90 Unspecified inflammatory spondylopathy, site unspecified
  - M46.91 Unspecified inflammatory spondylopathy, occipito-atlanto-axial region
  - M46.92 Unspecified inflammatory spondylopathy, cervical region
  - M46.93 Unspecified inflammatory spondylopathy, cervicothoracic region
  - M46.94 Unspecified inflammatory spondylopathy, thoracic region
  - M46.95 Unspecified inflammatory spondylopathy, thoracolumbar region
  - M46.96 Unspecified inflammatory spondylopathy, lumbar region
  - M46.97 Unspecified inflammatory spondylopathy, lumbosacral region
  - M46.98 Unspecified inflammatory spondylopathy, sacral and sacrococcygeal region
  - M46.99 Unspecified inflammatory spondylopathy, multiple sites in spine

M47 Spondylosis

Includes arthrosis or osteoarthritis of spine
degeneration of facet joints

- **M47.0** Anterior spinal and vertebral artery compression syndromes
  - **M47.01** Anterior spinal artery compression syndromes
    - M47.011 Anterior spinal artery compression syndromes, occipito-atlanto-axial region
    - M47.012 Anterior spinal artery compression syndromes, cervical region
    - M47.013 Anterior spinal artery compression syndromes, cervicothoracic region
    - M47.014 Anterior spinal artery compression syndromes, thoracic region
    - M47.015 Anterior spinal artery compression syndromes, thoracolumbar region
    - M47.016 Anterior spinal artery compression syndromes, lumbar region
    - M47.019 Anterior spinal artery compression syndromes, site unspecified
  - **M47.02** Vertebral artery compression syndromes
    - M47.021 Vertebral artery compression syndromes, occipito-atlanto-axial region
    - M47.022 Vertebral artery compression syndromes, cervical region
    - M47.029 Vertebral artery compression syndromes, site unspecified

● M47.1 Other spondylosis with myelopathy
Spondylogenic compression of spinal cord
Excludes1 vertebral subluxation (M43.3-M43.5X9)
M47.10 Other spondylosis with myelopathy, site unspecified
M47.11 Other spondylosis with myelopathy, occipito-atlanto-axial region
M47.12 Other spondylosis with myelopathy, cervical region
M47.13 Other spondylosis with myelopathy, cervicothoracic region
M47.14 Other spondylosis with myelopathy, thoracic region
M47.15 Other spondylosis with myelopathy, thoracolumbar region
M47.16 Other spondylosis with myelopathy, lumbar region

● M47.2 Other spondylosis with radiculopathy
M47.20 Other spondylosis with radiculopathy, site unspecified
M47.21 Other spondylosis with radiculopathy, occipito-atlanto-axial region
M47.22 Other spondylosis with radiculopathy, cervical region
M47.23 Other spondylosis with radiculopathy, cervicothoracic region
M47.24 Other spondylosis with radiculopathy, thoracic region
M47.25 Other spondylosis with radiculopathy, thoracolumbar region
M47.26 Other spondylosis with radiculopathy, lumbar region
M47.27 Other spondylosis with radiculopathy, lumbosacral region
M47.28 Other spondylosis with radiculopathy, sacral and sacrococcygeal region

● M47.8 Other spondylosis
● M47.81 Spondylosis without myelopathy or radiculopathy
M47.811 Spondylosis without myelopathy or radiculopathy, occipito-atlanto-axial region
M47.812 Spondylosis without myelopathy or radiculopathy, cervical region
Coding Clinic: 2018, Q2, P15
M47.813 Spondylosis without myelopathy or radiculopathy, cervicothoracic region
M47.814 Spondylosis without myelopathy or radiculopathy, thoracic region
M47.815 Spondylosis without myelopathy or radiculopathy, thoracolumbar region
M47.816 Spondylosis without myelopathy or radiculopathy, lumbar region
M47.817 Spondylosis without myelopathy or radiculopathy, lumbosacral region
M47.818 Spondylosis without myelopathy or radiculopathy, sacral and sacrococcygeal region
M47.819 Spondylosis without myelopathy or radiculopathy, site unspecified

● M47.89 Other spondylosis
M47.891 Other spondylosis, occipito-atlanto-axial region
M47.892 Other spondylosis, cervical region
M47.893 Other spondylosis, cervicothoracic region
M47.894 Other spondylosis, thoracic region
M47.895 Other spondylosis, thoracolumbar region
M47.896 Other spondylosis, lumbar region
M47.897 Other spondylosis, lumbosacral region
M47.898 Other spondylosis, sacral and sacrococcygeal region
M47.899 Other spondylosis, site unspecified

M47.9 Spondylosis, unspecified

● M48 Other spondylopathies
● M48.0 Spinal stenosis
Caudal stenosis
M48.00 Spinal stenosis, site unspecified
M48.01 Spinal stenosis, occipito-atlanto-axial region
M48.02 Spinal stenosis, cervical region
M48.03 Spinal stenosis, cervicothoracic region
M48.04 Spinal stenosis, thoracic region
M48.05 Spinal stenosis, thoracolumbar region
● M48.06 Spinal stenosis, lumbar region
Coding Clinic: 2017, Q3, P24
M48.061 Spinal stenosis, lumbar region without neurogenic claudication
Spinal stenosis, lumbar region NOS
M48.062 Spinal stenosis, lumbar region with neurogenic claudication
Coding Clinic: 2017, Q4, P19
M48.07 Spinal stenosis, lumbosacral region
M48.08 Spinal stenosis, sacral and sacrococcygeal region

● M48.1 Ankylosing hyperostosis [Forestier]
Diffuse idiopathic skeletal hyperostosis [DISH]
M48.10 Ankylosing hyperostosis [Forestier], site unspecified
M48.11 Ankylosing hyperostosis [Forestier], occipito-atlanto-axial region
M48.12 Ankylosing hyperostosis [Forestier], cervical region
M48.13 Ankylosing hyperostosis [Forestier], cervicothoracic region
M48.14 Ankylosing hyperostosis [Forestier], thoracic region
M48.15 Ankylosing hyperostosis [Forestier], thoracolumbar region
M48.16 Ankylosing hyperostosis [Forestier], lumbar region
M48.17 Ankylosing hyperostosis [Forestier], lumbosacral region
M48.18 Ankylosing hyperostosis [Forestier], sacral and sacrococcygeal region
M48.19 Ankylosing hyperostosis [Forestier], multiple sites in spine

● M48.2 Kissing spine

M48.20 Kissing spine, site unspecified

M48.21 Kissing spine, occipito-atlanto-axial region

M48.22 Kissing spine, cervical region

M48.23 Kissing spine, cervicothoracic region

M48.24 Kissing spine, thoracic region

M48.25 Kissing spine, thoracolumbar region

M48.26 Kissing spine, lumbar region

M48.27 Kissing spine, lumbosacral region

● M48.3 Traumatic spondylopathy

M48.30 Traumatic spondylopathy, site unspecified

M48.31 Traumatic spondylopathy, occipito-atlanto-axial region

M48.32 Traumatic spondylopathy, cervical region

M48.33 Traumatic spondylopathy, cervicothoracic region

M48.34 Traumatic spondylopathy, thoracic region

M48.35 Traumatic spondylopathy, thoracolumbar region

M48.36 Traumatic spondylopathy, lumbar region

M48.37 Traumatic spondylopathy, lumbosacral region

M48.38 Traumatic spondylopathy, sacral and sacrococcygeal region

● M48.4 Fatigue fracture of vertebra

Stress fracture of vertebra

Excludes1 pathological fracture NOS (M84.4-)
pathological fracture of vertebra due to neoplasm (M84.58)
pathological fracture of vertebra due to other diagnosis (M84.68)
pathological fracture of vertebra due to osteoporosis (M8Ø.-)
traumatic fracture of vertebrae (S12.Ø-S12.3-, S22.Ø-, S32.Ø-)

The appropriate 7th character is to be added to each code from subcategory M48.4:

A	initial encounter for fracture
D	subsequent encounter for fracture with routine healing
G	subsequent encounter for fracture with delayed healing
S	sequela of fracture

X● M48.4Ø Fatigue fracture of vertebra, site unspecified

X● M48.41 Fatigue fracture of vertebra, occipitoatlanto-axial region

X● M48.42 Fatigue fracture of vertebra, cervical region

X● M48.43 Fatigue fracture of vertebra, cervicothoracic region

X● M48.44 Fatigue fracture of vertebra, thoracic region

X● M48.45 Fatigue fracture of vertebra, thoracolumbar region

X● M48.46 Fatigue fracture of vertebra, lumbar region

X● M48.47 Fatigue fracture of vertebra, lumbosacral region

X● M48.48 Fatigue fracture of vertebra, sacral and sacrococcygeal region

● M48.5 Collapsed vertebra, not elsewhere classified

Collapsed vertebra NOS
Compression fracture of vertebra NOS
Wedging of vertebra NOS

Excludes1 current injury - see Injury of spine, by body region
fatigue fracture of vertebra (M48.4)
pathological fracture of vertebra due to neoplasm (M84.58)
pathological fracture of vertebra due to other diagnosis (M84.68)
pathological fracture of vertebra due to osteoporosis (M8Ø.-)
pathological fracture NOS (M84.4-)
stress fracture of vertebra (M48.4-)
traumatic fracture of vertebra (S12.-, S22.-, S32.-)

The appropriate 7th character is to be added to each code from subcategory M48.5:

A	initial encounter for fracture
D	subsequent encounter for fracture with routine healing
G	subsequent encounter for fracture with delayed healing
S	sequela of fracture

X● M48.5Ø Collapsed vertebra, not elsewhere classified, site unspecified A

X● M48.51 Collapsed vertebra, not elsewhere classified, occipito-atlanto-axial region A

X● M48.52 Collapsed vertebra, not elsewhere classified, cervical region A

X● M48.53 Collapsed vertebra, not elsewhere classified, cervicothoracic region A

X● M48.54 Collapsed vertebra, not elsewhere classified, thoracic region A

X● M48.55 Collapsed vertebra, not elsewhere classified, thoracolumbar region A

X● M48.56 Collapsed vertebra, not elsewhere classified, lumbar region A

X● M48.57 Collapsed vertebra, not elsewhere classified, lumbosacral region A

X● M48.58 Collapsed vertebra, not elsewhere classified, sacral and sacrococcygeal region A

● M48.8 Other specified spondylopathies

Ossification of posterior longitudinal ligament

● M48.8X Other specified spondylopathies

M48.8X1 Other specified spondylopathies, occipito-atlanto-axial region

M48.8X2 Other specified spondylopathies, cervical region

M48.8X3 Other specified spondylopathies, cervicothoracic region

M48.8X4 Other specified spondylopathies, thoracic region

M48.8X5 Other specified spondylopathies, thoracolumbar region

M48.8X6 Other specified spondylopathies, lumbar region

M48.8X7 Other specified spondylopathies, lumbosacral region

M48.8X8 Other specified spondylopathies, sacral and sacrococcygeal region

M48.8X9 Other specified spondylopathies, site unspecified

M48.9 Spondylopathy, unspecified

M49 Spondylopathies in diseases classified elsewhere

Includes curvature of spine in diseases classified elsewhere
deformity of spine in diseases classified elsewhere
kyphosis in diseases classified elsewhere
scoliosis in diseases classified elsewhere
spondylopathy in diseases classified elsewhere

Code first underlying disease, such as:
brucellosis (A23.-)
Charcot-Marie-Tooth disease (G60.0)
enterobacterial infections (A01-A04)
osteitis fibrosa cystica (E21.0)

Excludes1 curvature of spine in tuberculosis [Pott's] (A18.01)
enteropathic arthropathies (M07.-)
gonococcal spondylitis (A54.41)
neuropathic [tabes dorsalis] spondylitis (A52.11)
neuropathic spondylopathy in syringomyelia (G95.0)
neuropathic spondylopathy in tabes dorsalis (A52.11)
nonsyphilitic neuropathic spondylopathy NEC (G98.0)
spondylitis in syphilis (acquired) (A52.77)
tuberculous spondylitis (A18.01)
typhoid fever spondylitis (A01.05)

M49.8 Spondylopathy in diseases classified elsewhere

M49.80 Spondylopathy in diseases classified elsewhere, site unspecified

M49.81 Spondylopathy in diseases classified elsewhere, occipito-atlanto-axial region

M49.82 Spondylopathy in diseases classified elsewhere, cervical region

M49.83 Spondylopathy in diseases classified elsewhere, cervicothoracic region

M49.84 Spondylopathy in diseases classified elsewhere, thoracic region

M49.85 Spondylopathy in diseases classified elsewhere, thoracolumbar region

M49.86 Spondylopathy in diseases classified elsewhere, lumbar region

M49.87 Spondylopathy in diseases classified elsewhere, lumbosacral region

M49.88 Spondylopathy in diseases classified elsewhere, sacral and sacrococcygeal region

M49.89 Spondylopathy in diseases classified elsewhere, multiple sites in spine

OTHER DORSOPATHIES (M50-M54)

Excludes1 current injury - see injury of spine by body region
discitis NOS (M46.4-)

M50 Cervical disc disorders

Note: Code to the most superior level of disorder.

Includes cervicothoracic disc disorders with cervicalgia
cervicothoracic disc disorders

Coding Clinic: 2016, Q1, P17

M50.0 Cervical disc disorder with myelopathy

M50.00 Cervical disc disorder with myelopathy, unspecified cervical region

M50.01 Cervical disc disorder with myelopathy, high cervical region
C2-C3 disc disorder with myelopathy
C3-C4 disc disorder with myelopathy
Coding Clinic: 2016, Q1, P17

M50.02 Cervical disc disorder with myelopathy, mid-cervical region
Coding Clinic: 2016, Q4, P39-40

M50.020 Cervical disc disorder with myelopathy, mid-cervical region, unspecified level

M50.021 Cervical disc disorder at C4-C5 level with myelopathy
C4-C5 disc disorder with myelopathy

M50.022 Cervical disc disorder at C5-C6 level with myelopathy
C5-C6 disc disorder with myelopathy

M50.023 Cervical disc disorder at C6-C7 level with myelopathy
C6-C7 disc disorder with myelopathy

M50.03 Cervical disc disorder with myelopathy, cervicothoracic region
C7-T1 disc disorder with myelopathy

M50.1 Cervical disc disorder with radiculopathy

Excludes2 brachial radiculitis NOS (M54.13)

M50.10 Cervical disc disorder with radiculopathy, unspecified cervical region

M50.11 Cervical disc disorder with radiculopathy, high cervical region
C2-C3 disc disorder with radiculopathy
C3 radiculopathy due to disc disorder
C3-C4 disc disorder with radiculopathy
C4 radiculopathy due to disc disorder

M50.12 Cervical disc disorder with radiculopathy, mid-cervical region
Coding Clinic: 2016, Q4, P39-40

M50.120 Mid-cervical disc disorder, unspecified level

M50.121 Cervical disc disorder at C4-C5 level with radiculopathy
C4-C5 disc disorder with radiculopathy
C5 radiculopathy due to disc disorder

M50.122 Cervical disc disorder at C5-C6 level with radiculopathy
C5-C6 disc disorder with radiculopathy
C6 radiculopathy due to disc disorder

M50.123 Cervical disc disorder at C6-C7 level with radiculopathy
C6-C7 disc disorder with radiculopathy
C7 radiculopathy due to disc disorder

M50.13 Cervical disc disorder with radiculopathy, cervicothoracic region
C7-T1 disc disorder with radiculopathy
C8 radiculopathy due to disc disorder

M50.2 Other cervical disc displacement
Coding Clinic: 2016, Q4, P40

M50.20 Other cervical disc displacement, unspecified cervical region

M50.21 Other cervical disc displacement, high cervical region
Other C2-C3 cervical disc displacement
Other C3-C4 cervical disc displacement

● M50.22 Other cervical disc displacement, **mid-cervical region**

M50.220 Other cervical disc displacement, mid-cervical region, **unspecified level**

M50.221 Other cervical disc displacement at **C4-C5 level**
Other C4-C5 cervical disc displacement

M50.222 Other cervical disc displacement at **C5-C6 level**
Other C5-C6 cervical disc displacement

M50.223 Other cervical disc displacement at **C6-C7 level**
Other C6-C7 cervical disc displacement

M50.23 Other cervical disc displacement, **cervicothoracic region**
Other C7-T1 cervical disc displacement

● M50.3 Other cervical disc degeneration
Coding Clinic: 2016, Q4, P40

M50.30 Other cervical disc degeneration, **unspecified cervical region**

M50.31 Other cervical disc degeneration, **high cervical region**
Other C2-C3 cervical disc degeneration
Other C3-C4 cervical disc degeneration

● M50.32 Other cervical disc degeneration, **mid-cervical region**

M50.320 Other cervical disc degeneration, mid-cervical region, **unspecified level**

M50.321 Other cervical disc degeneration at **C4-C5 level**
Other C4-C5 cervical disc degeneration

M50.322 Other cervical disc degeneration at **C5-C6 level**
Other C5-C6 cervical disc degeneration

M50.323 Other cervical disc degeneration at **C6-C7 level**
Other C6-C7 cervical disc degeneration

M50.33 Other cervical disc degeneration, **cervicothoracic region**
Other C7-T1 cervical disc degeneration

● M50.8 Other cervical disc disorders
Coding Clinic: 2016, Q4, P40

M50.80 Other cervical disc disorders, **unspecified cervical region**

M50.81 Other cervical disc disorders, **high cervical region**
Other C2-C3 cervical disc disorders
Other C3-C4 cervical disc disorders

● M50.82 Other cervical disc disorders, **mid-cervical region**

M50.820 Other cervical disc disorders, mid-cervical region, **unspecified level**

M50.821 Other cervical disc disorders at **C4-C5 level**
Other C4-C5 cervical disc disorders

M50.822 Other cervical disc disorders at **C5-C6 level**
Other C5-C6 cervical disc disorders

M50.823 Other cervical disc disorders at **C6-C7 level**
Other C6-C7 cervical disc disorders

M50.83 Other cervical disc disorders, **cervicothoracic region**
Other C7-T1 cervical disc disorders

● M50.9 Cervical disc disorder, **unspecified**
Coding Clinic: 2016, Q4, P40

M50.90 Cervical disc disorder, unspecified, **unspecified cervical region**

M50.91 Cervical disc disorder, unspecified, **high cervical region**
C2-C3 cervical disc disorder, unspecified
C3-C4 cervical disc disorder, unspecified

● M50.92 Cervical disc disorder, unspecified, **mid-cervical region**

M50.920 Unspecified cervical disc disorder, mid-cervical region, **unspecified level**

M50.921 Unspecified cervical disc disorder at **C4-C5 level**
Unspecified C4-C5 cervical disc disorder

M50.922 Unspecified cervical disc disorder at **C5-C6 level**
Unspecified C5-C6 cervical disc disorder

M50.923 Unspecified cervical disc disorder at **C6-C7 level**
Unspecified C6-C7 cervical disc disorder

M50.93 Cervical disc disorder, unspecified, **cervicothoracic region**
C7-T1 cervical disc disorder, unspecified

● M51 Thoracic, thoracolumbar, and lumbosacral intervertebral disc disorders

Excludes2 cervical and cervicothoracic disc disorders (M50.-)
sacral and sacrococcygeal disorders (M53.3)

● M51.0 Thoracic, thoracolumbar and lumbosacral intervertebral disc disorders **with myelopathy**

M51.04 Intervertebral disc disorders with myelopathy, **thoracic region**

M51.05 Intervertebral disc disorders with myelopathy, **thoracolumbar region**

M51.06 Intervertebral disc disorders with myelopathy, **lumbar region**

● M51.1 Thoracic, thoracolumbar and lumbosacral intervertebral disc disorders **with radiculopathy**
Sciatica due to intervertebral disc disorder

Excludes1 lumbar radiculitis NOS (M54.16)
sciatica NOS (M54.3)

M51.14 Intervertebral disc disorders with radiculopathy, **thoracic region**

M51.15 Intervertebral disc disorders with radiculopathy, **thoracolumbar region**

M51.16 Intervertebral disc disorders with radiculopathy, **lumbar region**

M51.17 Intervertebral disc disorders with radiculopathy, **lumbosacral region**

CHAPTER 13 (M00-M99)

- M51.2 Other thoracic, thoracolumbar and lumbosacral intervertebral disc **displacement**
  Lumbago due to displacement of intervertebral disc
  - M51.24 Other intervertebral disc displacement, **thoracic** region
  - M51.25 Other intervertebral disc displacement, **thoracolumbar** region
  - M51.26 Other intervertebral disc displacement, **lumbar** region
  - M51.27 Other intervertebral disc displacement, **lumbosacral** region
- M51.3 Other thoracic, thoracolumbar and lumbosacral intervertebral disc **degeneration**
  Coding Clinic: 2013, Q3, P22
  - M51.34 Other intervertebral disc degeneration, **thoracic** region
  - M51.35 Other intervertebral disc degeneration, **thoracolumbar** region
  - M51.36 Other intervertebral disc degeneration, **lumbar** region
    Coding Clinic: 2018, Q2, P15
  - M51.37 Other intervertebral disc degeneration, **lumbosacral** region
- M51.4 Schmorl's nodes
  - M51.44 Schmorl's nodes, **thoracic** region
  - M51.45 Schmorl's nodes, **thoracolumbar** region
  - M51.46 Schmorl's nodes, **lumbar** region
  - M51.47 Schmorl's nodes, **lumbosacral** region
- M51.8 Other thoracic, thoracolumbar and lumbosacral intervertebral disc **disorders**
  - M51.84 Other intervertebral disc disorders, **thoracic** region
  - M51.85 Other intervertebral disc disorders, **thoracolumbar** region
  - M51.86 Other intervertebral disc disorders, **lumbar** region
  - M51.87 Other intervertebral disc disorders, **lumbosacral** region
- M51.9 **Unspecified** thoracic, thoracolumbar and lumbosacral intervertebral disc disorder

M53 Other and unspecified dorsopathies, not elsewhere classified

- M53.0 Cervicocranial syndrome
  Posterior cervical sympathetic syndrome
- M53.1 Cervicobrachial syndrome
  Excludes2 cervical disc disorder (M50.-)
  thoracic outlet syndrome (G54.0)
- M53.2 Spinal instabilities
  - M53.2X Spinal **instabilities**
    - M53.2X1 Spinal instabilities, **occipito-atlanto-axial** region
    - M53.2X2 Spinal instabilities, **cervical** region
    - M53.2X3 Spinal instabilities, **cervicothoracic** region
    - M53.2X4 Spinal instabilities, **thoracic** region
    - M53.2X5 Spinal instabilities, **thoracolumbar** region
    - M53.2X6 Spinal instabilities, **lumbar** region
    - M53.2X7 Spinal instabilities, **lumbosacral** region
    - M53.2X8 Spinal instabilities, **sacral and sacrococcygeal** region
    - M53.2X9 Spinal instabilities, site **unspecified**
- M53.3 Sacrococcygeal disorders, not elsewhere classified
  Coccygodynia
- M53.8 Other specified dorsopathies
  - M53.80 Other specified dorsopathies, site **unspecified**
  - M53.81 Other specified dorsopathies, **occipito-atlanto-axial** region
  - M53.82 Other specified dorsopathies, **cervical** region
  - M53.83 Other specified dorsopathies, **cervicothoracic** region
  - M53.84 Other specified dorsopathies, **thoracic** region
  - M53.85 Other specified dorsopathies, **thoracolumbar** region
  - M53.86 Other specified dorsopathies, **lumbar** region
  - M53.87 Other specified dorsopathies, **lumbosacral** region
  - M53.88 Other specified dorsopathies, **sacral and sacrococcygeal** region
- M53.9 Dorsopathy, **unspecified**

M54 Dorsalgia

Excludes1 psychogenic dorsalgia (F45.41)

- M54.0 Panniculitis affecting regions of neck and back
  Excludes1 lupus panniculitis (L93.2)
  panniculitis NOS (M79.3)
  relapsing [Weber-Christian] panniculitis (M35.6)
  - M54.00 Panniculitis affecting regions of neck and back, site **unspecified**
  - M54.01 Panniculitis affecting regions of neck and back, **occipito-atlanto-axial** region
  - M54.02 Panniculitis affecting regions of neck and back, **cervical** region
  - M54.03 Panniculitis affecting regions of neck and back, **cervicothoracic** region
  - M54.04 Panniculitis affecting regions of neck and back, **thoracic** region
  - M54.05 Panniculitis affecting regions of neck and back, **thoracolumbar** region
  - M54.06 Panniculitis affecting regions of neck and back, **lumbar** region
  - M54.07 Panniculitis affecting regions of neck and back, **lumbosacral** region
  - M54.08 Panniculitis affecting regions of neck and back, **sacral and sacrococcygeal** region
  - M54.09 Panniculitis affecting regions, neck and back, **multiple sites in spine**
- M54.1 Radiculopathy
  Brachial neuritis or radiculitis NOS
  Lumbar neuritis or radiculitis NOS
  Lumbosacral neuritis or radiculitis NOS
  Thoracic neuritis or radiculitis NOS
  Radiculitis NOS
  Excludes1 neuralgia and neuritis NOS (M79.2)
  radiculopathy with cervical disc disorder (M50.1)
  radiculopathy with lumbar and other intervertebral disc disorder (M51.1-)
  radiculopathy with spondylosis (M47.2-)
  - M54.10 Radiculopathy, site **unspecified**
  - M54.11 Radiculopathy, **occipito-atlanto-axial** region
  - M54.12 Radiculopathy, **cervical** region
  - M54.13 Radiculopathy, **cervicothoracic** region
  - M54.14 Radiculopathy, **thoracic** region
  - M54.15 Radiculopathy, **thoracolumbar** region
  - M54.16 Radiculopathy, **lumbar** region
  - M54.17 Radiculopathy, **lumbosacral** region
  - M54.18 Radiculopathy, **sacral and sacrococcygeal** region

CHAPTER 13 (M00-M99)

M54.2 Cervicalgia
Excludes1 cervicalgia due to intervertebral cervical disc disorder (M50.-)

M54.3 Sciatica
Excludes1 lesion of sciatic nerve (G57.0)
sciatica due to intervertebral disc disorder (M51.1-)
sciatica with lumbago (M54.4-)

M54.30 **Sciatica, unspecified side**
M54.31 **Sciatica, right side**
M54.32 **Sciatica, left side**

M54.4 Lumbago with sciatica
Excludes1 lumbago with sciatica due to intervertebral disc disorder (M51.1-)

M54.40 **Lumbago with sciatica, unspecified side**
M54.41 **Lumbago with sciatica, right side**
M54.42 **Lumbago with sciatica, left side**
Coding Clinic: 2016, Q2, P7

M54.5 **Low back pain**
Loin pain
Lumbago NOS
Excludes1 low back strain (S39.012)
lumbago due to intervertebral disc displacement (M51.2-)
lumbago with sciatica (M54.4-)

M54.6 **Pain in thoracic spine**
Excludes1 pain in thoracic spine due to intervertebral disc disorder (M51.)

M54.8 Other dorsalgia
Excludes1 dorsalgia in thoracic region (M54.6)
low back pain (M54.5)

M54.81 **Occipital neuralgia**
M54.89 **Other dorsalgia**

M54.9 **Dorsalgia, unspecified**
Backache NOS
Back pain NOS

SOFT TISSUE DISORDERS (M60-M79)

DISORDERS OF MUSCLES (M60-M63)

Excludes1 dermatopolymyositis (M33.-)
muscular dystrophies and myopathies (G71-G72)
myopathy in amyloidosis (E85.-)
myopathy in polyarteritis nodosa (M30.0)
myopathy in rheumatoid arthritis (M05.32)
myopathy in scleroderma (M34.-)
myopathy in Sjögren's syndrome (M35.03)
myopathy in systemic lupus erythematosus (M32.-)

M60 Myositis
Excludes2 inclusion body myositis [IBM] (G72.41)

M60.0 Infective myositis
Tropical pyomyositis
Use additional code (B95-B97) to identify infectious agent

M60.00 **Infective myositis, unspecified site**
M60.000 **Infective myositis, unspecified right arm**
Infective myositis, right upper limb NOS
M60.001 **Infective myositis, unspecified left arm**
Infective myositis, left upper limb NOS
M60.002 **Infective myositis, unspecified arm**
Infective myositis, upper limb NOS
M60.003 **Infective myositis, unspecified right leg**
Infective myositis, right lower limb NOS
M60.004 **Infective myositis, unspecified left leg**
Infective myositis, left lower limb NOS
M60.005 **Infective myositis, unspecified leg**
Infective myositis, lower limb NOS
M60.009 **Infective myositis, unspecified site**

M60.01 Infective myositis, shoulder
M60.011 **Infective myositis, right shoulder**
M60.012 **Infective myositis, left shoulder**
M60.019 **Infective myositis, unspecified shoulder**

M60.02 Infective myositis, upper arm
M60.021 **Infective myositis, right upper arm**
M60.022 **Infective myositis, left upper arm**
M60.029 **Infective myositis, unspecified upper arm**

M60.03 Infective myositis, forearm
M60.031 **Infective myositis, right forearm**
M60.032 **Infective myositis, left forearm**
M60.039 **Infective myositis, unspecified forearm**

M60.04 Infective myositis, hand and fingers
M60.041 **Infective myositis, right hand**
M60.042 **Infective myositis, left hand**
M60.043 **Infective myositis, unspecified hand**
M60.044 **Infective myositis, right finger(s)**
M60.045 **Infective myositis, left finger(s)**
M60.046 **Infective myositis, unspecified finger(s)**

M60.05 Infective myositis, thigh
M60.051 **Infective myositis, right thigh**
M60.052 **Infective myositis, left thigh**
M60.059 **Infective myositis, unspecified thigh**

M60.06 Infective myositis, lower leg
M60.061 **Infective myositis, right lower leg**
M60.062 **Infective myositis, left lower leg**
M60.069 **Infective myositis, unspecified lower leg**

M60.07 Infective myositis, ankle, foot and toes
M60.070 **Infective myositis, right ankle**
M60.071 **Infective myositis, left ankle**
M60.072 **Infective myositis, unspecified ankle**
M60.073 **Infective myositis, right foot**
M60.074 **Infective myositis, left foot**
M60.075 **Infective myositis, unspecified foot**
M60.076 **Infective myositis, right toe(s)**
M60.077 **Infective myositis, left toe(s)**
M60.078 **Infective myositis, unspecified toe(s)**

M60.08 **Infective myositis, other site**
M60.09 **Infective myositis, multiple sites**

M60.1 Interstitial myositis
M60.10 **Interstitial myositis of unspecified site**

M60.11 Interstitial myositis, shoulder
M60.111 **Interstitial myositis, right shoulder**
M60.112 **Interstitial myositis, left shoulder**
M60.119 **Interstitial myositis, unspecified shoulder**

M60.12 Interstitial myositis, upper arm
M60.121 **Interstitial myositis, right upper arm**
M60.122 **Interstitial myositis, left upper arm**
M60.129 **Interstitial myositis, unspecified upper arm**

● M60.13 Interstitial myositis, **forearm**
- M60.131 Interstitial myositis, **right** forearm
- M60.132 Interstitial myositis, **left** forearm
- M60.139 Interstitial myositis, **unspecified** forearm

● M60.14 Interstitial myositis, **hand**
- M60.141 Interstitial myositis, **right** hand
- M60.142 Interstitial myositis, **left** hand
- M60.149 Interstitial myositis, **unspecified** hand

● M60.15 Interstitial myositis, **thigh**
- M60.151 Interstitial myositis, **right** thigh
- M60.152 Interstitial myositis, **left** thigh
- M60.159 Interstitial myositis, **unspecified** thigh

● M60.16 Interstitial myositis, **lower leg**
- M60.161 Interstitial myositis, **right** lower leg
- M60.162 Interstitial myositis, **left** lower leg
- M60.169 Interstitial myositis, **unspecified** lower leg

● M60.17 Interstitial myositis, **ankle and foot**
- M60.171 Interstitial myositis, **right** ankle and foot
- M60.172 Interstitial myositis, **left** ankle and foot
- M60.179 Interstitial myositis, **unspecified** ankle and foot

M60.18 Interstitial myositis, **other site**

M60.19 Interstitial myositis, **multiple sites**

● M60.2 Foreign body granuloma of soft tissue, not elsewhere classified

Use additional code to identify the type of retained foreign body (Z18.-)

Excludes1 foreign body granuloma of skin and subcutaneous tissue (L92.3)

M60.20 Foreign body granuloma of soft tissue, not elsewhere classified, **unspecified site**

● M60.21 Foreign body granuloma of soft tissue, not elsewhere classified, **shoulder**
- M60.211 Foreign body granuloma of soft tissue, not elsewhere classified, **right** shoulder
- M60.212 Foreign body granuloma of soft tissue, not elsewhere classified, **left** shoulder
- M60.219 Foreign body granuloma of soft tissue, not elsewhere classified, **unspecified** shoulder

● M60.22 Foreign body granuloma of soft tissue, not elsewhere classified, **upper arm**
- M60.221 Foreign body granuloma of soft tissue, not elsewhere classified, **right** upper arm
- M60.222 Foreign body granuloma of soft tissue, not elsewhere classified, **left** upper arm
- M60.229 Foreign body granuloma of soft tissue, not elsewhere classified, **unspecified** upper arm

● M60.23 Foreign body granuloma of soft tissue, not elsewhere classified, **forearm**
- M60.231 Foreign body granuloma of soft tissue, not elsewhere classified, **right** forearm
- M60.232 Foreign body granuloma of soft tissue, not elsewhere classified, **left** forearm
- M60.239 Foreign body granuloma of soft tissue, not elsewhere classified, **unspecified** forearm

● M60.24 Foreign body granuloma of soft tissue, not elsewhere classified, **hand**
- M60.241 Foreign body granuloma of soft tissue, not elsewhere classified, **right** hand
- M60.242 Foreign body granuloma of soft tissue, not elsewhere classified, **left** hand
- M60.249 Foreign body granuloma of soft tissue, not elsewhere classified, **unspecified** hand

● M60.25 Foreign body granuloma of soft tissue, not elsewhere classified, **thigh**
- M60.251 Foreign body granuloma of soft tissue, not elsewhere classified, **right** thigh
- M60.252 Foreign body granuloma of soft tissue, not elsewhere classified, **left** thigh
- M60.259 Foreign body granuloma of soft tissue, not elsewhere classified, **unspecified** thigh

● M60.26 Foreign body granuloma of soft tissue, not elsewhere classified, **lower leg**
- M60.261 Foreign body granuloma of soft tissue, not elsewhere classified, **right** lower leg
- M60.262 Foreign body granuloma of soft tissue, not elsewhere classified, **left** lower leg
- M60.269 Foreign body granuloma of soft tissue, not elsewhere classified, **unspecified** lower leg

● M60.27 Foreign body granuloma of soft tissue, not elsewhere classified, **ankle and foot**
- M60.271 Foreign body granuloma of soft tissue, not elsewhere classified, **right** ankle and foot
- M60.272 Foreign body granuloma of soft tissue, not elsewhere classified, **left** ankle and foot
- M60.279 Foreign body granuloma of soft tissue, not elsewhere classified, **unspecified** ankle and foot

M60.28 Foreign body granuloma of soft tissue, not elsewhere classified, **other site**

● M60.8 Other myositis

M60.80 Other myositis, **unspecified** site

● M60.81 Other myositis shoulder
- M60.811 Other myositis, **right** shoulder
- M60.812 Other myositis, **left** shoulder
- M60.819 Other myositis, **unspecified** shoulder

● M60.82 Other myositis, **upper arm**
- M60.821 Other myositis, **right** upper arm
- M60.822 Other myositis, **left** upper arm
- M60.829 Other myositis, **unspecified** upper arm

● M60.83 Other myositis, **forearm**
- M60.831 Other myositis, **right** forearm
- M60.832 Other myositis, **left** forearm
- M60.839 Other myositis, **unspecified** forearm

● M60.84 Other myositis, **hand**
- M60.841 Other myositis, **right** hand
- M60.842 Other myositis, **left** hand
- M60.849 Other myositis, **unspecified** hand

● M60.85 Other myositis, **thigh**
- M60.851 Other myositis, **right** thigh
- M60.852 Other myositis, **left** thigh
- M60.859 Other myositis, **unspecified** thigh

- M60.86 Other myositis, lower leg
  - M60.861 Other myositis, right lower leg
  - M60.862 Other myositis, left lower leg
  - M60.869 Other myositis, unspecified lower leg
- M60.87 Other myositis, ankle and foot
  - M60.871 Other myositis, right ankle and foot
  - M60.872 Other myositis, left ankle and foot
  - M60.879 Other myositis, unspecified ankle and foot
- M60.88 Other myositis, other site
- M60.89 Other myositis, multiple sites

M60.9 Myositis, unspecified

M61 Calcification and ossification of muscle

- M61.0 Myositis ossificans traumatica
  - M61.00 Myositis ossificans traumatica, unspecified site
  - M61.01 Myositis ossificans traumatica, shoulder
    - M61.011 Myositis ossificans traumatica, right shoulder
    - M61.012 Myositis ossificans traumatica, left shoulder
    - M61.019 Myositis ossificans traumatica, unspecified shoulder
  - M61.02 Myositis ossificans traumatica, upper arm
    - M61.021 Myositis ossificans traumatica, right upper arm
    - M61.022 Myositis ossificans traumatica, left upper arm
    - M61.029 Myositis ossificans traumatica, unspecified upper arm
  - M61.03 Myositis ossificans traumatica, forearm
    - M61.031 Myositis ossificans traumatica, right forearm
    - M61.032 Myositis ossificans traumatica, left forearm
    - M61.039 Myositis ossificans traumatica, unspecified forearm
  - M61.04 Myositis ossificans traumatica, hand
    - M61.041 Myositis ossificans traumatica, right hand
    - M61.042 Myositis ossificans traumatica, left hand
    - M61.049 Myositis ossificans traumatica, unspecified hand
  - M61.05 Myositis ossificans traumatica, thigh
    - M61.051 Myositis ossificans traumatica, right thigh
    - M61.052 Myositis ossificans traumatica, left thigh
    - M61.059 Myositis ossificans traumatica, unspecified thigh
  - M61.06 Myositis ossificans traumatica, lower leg
    - M61.061 Myositis ossificans traumatica, right lower leg
    - M61.062 Myositis ossificans traumatica, left lower leg
    - M61.069 Myositis ossificans traumatica, unspecified lower leg
  - M61.07 Myositis ossificans traumatica, ankle and foot
    - M61.071 Myositis ossificans traumatica, right ankle and foot
    - M61.072 Myositis ossificans traumatica, left ankle and foot
    - M61.079 Myositis ossificans traumatica, unspecified ankle and foot
  - M61.08 Myositis ossificans traumatica, other site
  - M61.09 Myositis ossificans traumatica, multiple sites
- M61.1 Myositis ossificans progressiva
  Fibrodysplasia ossificans progressiva
  - M61.10 Myositis ossificans progressiva, unspecified site
  - M61.11 Myositis ossificans progressiva, shoulder
    - M61.111 Myositis ossificans progressiva, right shoulder
    - M61.112 Myositis ossificans progressiva, left shoulder
    - M61.119 Myositis ossificans progressiva, unspecified shoulder
  - M61.12 Myositis ossificans progressiva, upper arm
    - M61.121 Myositis ossificans progressiva, right upper arm
    - M61.122 Myositis ossificans progressiva, left upper arm
    - M61.129 Myositis ossificans progressiva, unspecified arm
  - M61.13 Myositis ossificans progressiva, forearm
    - M61.131 Myositis ossificans progressiva, right forearm
    - M61.132 Myositis ossificans progressiva, left forearm
    - M61.139 Myositis ossificans progressiva, unspecified forearm
  - M61.14 Myositis ossificans progressiva, hand and finger(s)
    - M61.141 Myositis ossificans progressiva, right hand
    - M61.142 Myositis ossificans progressiva, left hand
    - M61.143 Myositis ossificans progressiva, unspecified hand
    - M61.144 Myositis ossificans progressiva, right finger(s)
    - M61.145 Myositis ossificans progressiva, left finger(s)
    - M61.146 Myositis ossificans progressiva, unspecified finger(s)
  - M61.15 Myositis ossificans progressiva, thigh
    - M61.151 Myositis ossificans progressiva, right thigh
    - M61.152 Myositis ossificans progressiva, left thigh
    - M61.159 Myositis ossificans progressiva, unspecified thigh
  - M61.16 Myositis ossificans progressiva, lower leg
    - M61.161 Myositis ossificans progressiva, right lower leg
    - M61.162 Myositis ossificans progressiva, left lower leg
    - M61.169 Myositis ossificans progressiva, unspecified lower leg
  - M61.17 Myositis ossificans progressiva, ankle, foot and toe(s)
    - M61.171 Myositis ossificans progressiva, right ankle
    - M61.172 Myositis ossificans progressiva, left ankle
    - M61.173 Myositis ossificans progressiva, unspecified ankle
    - M61.174 Myositis ossificans progressiva, right foot
    - M61.175 Myositis ossificans progressiva, left foot
    - M61.176 Myositis ossificans progressiva, unspecified foot
    - M61.177 Myositis ossificans progressiva, right toe(s)
    - M61.178 Myositis ossificans progressiva, left toe(s)
    - M61.179 Myositis ossificans progressiva, unspecified toe(s)

M61.18 Myositis ossificans progressiva, **other site**

M61.19 Myositis ossificans progressiva, **multiple sites**

● **M61.2 Paralytic calcification and ossification of muscle**

Myositis ossificans associated with quadriplegia or paraplegia

M61.20 Paralytic calcification and ossification of muscle, **unspecified** site

● M61.21 Paralytic calcification and ossification of muscle, **shoulder**

M61.211 Paralytic calcification and ossification of muscle, **right** shoulder

M61.212 Paralytic calcification and ossification of muscle, **left** shoulder

M61.219 Paralytic calcification and ossification of muscle, **unspecified** shoulder

● M61.22 Paralytic calcification and ossification of muscle, **upper arm**

M61.221 Paralytic calcification and ossification of muscle, **right** upper arm

M61.222 Paralytic calcification and ossification of muscle, **left** upper arm

M61.229 Paralytic calcification and ossification of muscle, **unspecified** upper arm

● M61.23 Paralytic calcification and ossification of muscle, **forearm**

M61.231 Paralytic calcification and ossification of muscle, **right** forearm

M61.232 Paralytic calcification and ossification of muscle, **left** forearm

M61.239 Paralytic calcification and ossification of muscle, **unspecified** forearm

● M61.24 Paralytic calcification and ossification of muscle, **hand**

M61.241 Paralytic calcification and ossification of muscle, **right** hand

M61.242 Paralytic calcification and ossification of muscle, **left** hand

M61.249 Paralytic calcification and ossification of muscle, **unspecified** hand

● M61.25 Paralytic calcification and ossification of muscle, **thigh**

M61.251 Paralytic calcification and ossification of muscle, **right** thigh

M61.252 Paralytic calcification and ossification of muscle, **left** thigh

M61.259 Paralytic calcification and ossification of muscle, **unspecified** thigh

● M61.26 Paralytic calcification and ossification of muscle, **lower leg**

M61.261 Paralytic calcification and ossification of muscle, **right** lower leg

M61.262 Paralytic calcification and ossification of muscle, **left** lower leg

M61.269 Paralytic calcification and ossification of muscle, **unspecified** lower leg

● M61.27 Paralytic calcification and ossification of muscle, **ankle and foot**

M61.271 Paralytic calcification and ossification of muscle, **right** ankle and foot

M61.272 Paralytic calcification and ossification of muscle, **left** ankle and foot

M61.279 Paralytic calcification and ossification of muscle, **unspecified** ankle and foot

M61.28 Paralytic calcification and ossification of muscle, **other site**

M61.29 Paralytic calcification and ossification of muscle, **multiple sites**

● **M61.3 Calcification and ossification of muscles associated with burns**

Myositis ossificans associated with burns

M61.30 Calcification and ossification of muscles associated with burns, **unspecified** site

● M61.31 Calcification and ossification of muscles associated with burns, **shoulder**

M61.311 Calcification and ossification of muscles associated with burns, **right** shoulder

M61.312 Calcification and ossification of muscles associated with burns, **left** shoulder

M61.319 Calcification and ossification of muscles associated with burns, **unspecified** shoulder

● M61.32 Calcification and ossification of muscles associated with burns, **upper arm**

M61.321 Calcification and ossification of muscles associated with burns, **right** upper arm

M61.322 Calcification and ossification of muscles associated with burns, **left** upper arm

M61.329 Calcification and ossification of muscles associated with burns, **unspecified** upper arm

● M61.33 Calcification and ossification of muscles associated with burns, **forearm**

M61.331 Calcification and ossification of muscles associated with burns, **right** forearm

M61.332 Calcification and ossification of muscles associated with burns, **left** forearm

M61.339 Calcification and ossification of muscles associated with burns, **unspecified** forearm

● M61.34 Calcification and ossification of muscles associated with burns, **hand**

M61.341 Calcification and ossification of muscles associated with burns, **right** hand

M61.342 Calcification and ossification of muscles associated with burns, **left** hand

M61.349 Calcification and ossification of muscles associated with burns, **unspecified** hand

● M61.35 Calcification and ossification of muscles associated with burns, **thigh**

M61.351 Calcification and ossification of muscles associated with burns, **right** thigh

M61.352 Calcification and ossification of muscles associated with burns, **left** thigh

M61.359 Calcification and ossification of muscles associated with burns, **unspecified** thigh

● M61.36 Calcification and ossification of muscles associated with burns, **lower leg**

M61.361 Calcification and ossification of muscles associated with burns, **right** lower leg

M61.362 Calcification and ossification of muscles associated with burns, **left** lower leg

M61.369 Calcification and ossification of muscles associated with burns, **unspecified** lower leg

- ● M61.37 Calcification and ossification of muscles associated with burns, **ankle and foot**
  - M61.371 Calcification and ossification of muscles associated with burns, **right** ankle and foot
  - M61.372 Calcification and ossification of muscles associated with burns, **left** ankle and foot
  - M61.379 Calcification and ossification of muscles associated with burns, **unspecified** ankle and foot
- M61.38 Calcification and ossification of muscles associated with burns, **other site**
- M61.39 Calcification and ossification of muscles associated with burns, **multiple sites**

● M61.4 Other calcification of muscle

Excludes1 calcific tendinitis NOS (M65.2-)
calcific tendinitis of shoulder (M75.3)

- M61.40 Other calcification of muscle, **unspecified** site
- ● M61.41 Other calcification of muscle, **shoulder**
  - M61.411 Other calcification of muscle, **right** shoulder
  - M61.412 Other calcification of muscle, **left** shoulder
  - M61.419 Other calcification of muscle, **unspecified** shoulder
- ● M61.42 Other calcification of muscle, **upper arm**
  - M61.421 Other calcification of muscle, **right** upper arm
  - M61.422 Other calcification of muscle, **left** upper arm
  - M61.429 Other calcification of muscle, **unspecified** upper arm
- ● M61.43 Other calcification of muscle, **forearm**
  - M61.431 Other calcification of muscle, **right** forearm
  - M61.432 Other calcification of muscle, **left** forearm
  - M61.439 Other calcification of muscle, **unspecified** forearm
- ● M61.44 Other calcification of muscle, **hand**
  - M61.441 Other calcification of muscle, **right** hand
  - M61.442 Other calcification of muscle, **left** hand
  - M61.449 Other calcification of muscle, **unspecified** hand
- ● M61.45 Other calcification of muscle, **thigh**
  - M61.451 Other calcification of muscle, **right** thigh
  - M61.452 Other calcification of muscle, **left** thigh
  - M61.459 Other calcification of muscle, **unspecified** thigh
- ● M61.46 Other calcification of muscle, **lower leg**
  - M61.461 Other calcification of muscle, **right** lower leg
  - M61.462 Other calcification of muscle, **left** lower leg
  - M61.469 Other calcification of muscle, **unspecified** lower leg
- ● M61.47 Other calcification of muscle, **ankle and foot**
  - M61.471 Other calcification of muscle, **right** ankle and foot
  - M61.472 Other calcification of muscle, **left** ankle and foot
  - M61.479 Other calcification of muscle, **unspecified** ankle and foot
- M61.48 Other calcification of muscle, **other site**
- M61.49 Other calcification of muscle, **multiple sites**

● M61.5 Other ossification of muscle

- M61.50 Other ossification of muscle, **unspecified** site
- ● M61.51 Other ossification of muscle, **shoulder**
  - M61.511 Other ossification of muscle, **right** shoulder
  - M61.512 Other ossification of muscle, **left** shoulder
  - M61.519 Other ossification of muscle, **unspecified** shoulder
- ● M61.52 Other ossification of muscle, **upper arm**
  - M61.521 Other ossification of muscle, **right** upper arm
  - M61.522 Other ossification of muscle, **left** upper arm
  - M61.529 Other ossification of muscle, **unspecified** upper arm
- ● M61.53 Other ossification of muscle, **forearm**
  - M61.531 Other ossification of muscle, **right** forearm
  - M61.532 Other ossification of muscle, **left** forearm
  - M61.539 Other ossification of muscle, **unspecified** forearm
- ● M61.54 Other ossification of muscle, **hand**
  - M61.541 Other ossification of muscle, **right** hand
  - M61.542 Other ossification of muscle, **left** hand
  - M61.549 Other ossification of muscle, **unspecified** hand
- ● M61.55 Other ossification of muscle, **thigh**
  - M61.551 Other ossification of muscle, **right** thigh
  - M61.552 Other ossification of muscle, **left** thigh
  - M61.559 Other ossification of muscle, **unspecified** thigh
- ● M61.56 Other ossification of muscle, **lower leg**
  - M61.561 Other ossification of muscle, **right** lower leg
  - M61.562 Other ossification of muscle, **left** lower leg
  - M61.569 Other ossification of muscle, **unspecified** lower leg
- ● M61.57 Other ossification of muscle, **ankle and foot**
  - M61.571 Other ossification of muscle, **right** ankle and foot
  - M61.572 Other ossification of muscle, **left** ankle and foot
  - M61.579 Other ossification of muscle, **unspecified** ankle and foot
- M61.58 Other ossification of muscle, **other site**
- M61.59 Other ossification of muscle, **multiple sites**

M61.9 Calcification and ossification of muscle, **unspecified**

M62 Other disorders of muscle

Excludes1 alcoholic myopathy (G72.1)
cramp and spasm (R25.2)
drug-induced myopathy (G72.0)
myalgia (M79.1-)
stiff-man syndrome (G25.82)

Excludes2 nontraumatic hematoma of muscle (M79.81)

M62.0 Separation of muscle (nontraumatic)
Diastasis of muscle

Excludes1 diastasis recti complicating pregnancy, labor and delivery (O71.8)
traumatic separation of muscle - see strain of muscle by body region

M62.00 Separation of muscle (nontraumatic), unspecified site

M62.01 Separation of muscle (nontraumatic), shoulder
M62.011 Separation of muscle (nontraumatic), right shoulder
M62.012 Separation of muscle (nontraumatic), left shoulder
M62.019 Separation of muscle (nontraumatic), unspecified shoulder

M62.02 Separation of muscle (nontraumatic), upper arm
M62.021 Separation of muscle (nontraumatic), right upper arm
M62.022 Separation of muscle (nontraumatic), left upper arm
M62.029 Separation of muscle (nontraumatic), unspecified upper arm

M62.03 Separation of muscle (nontraumatic), forearm
M62.031 Separation of muscle (nontraumatic), right forearm
M62.032 Separation of muscle (nontraumatic), left forearm
M62.039 Separation of muscle (nontraumatic), unspecified forearm

M62.04 Separation of muscle (nontraumatic), hand
M62.041 Separation of muscle (nontraumatic), right hand
M62.042 Separation of muscle (nontraumatic), left hand
M62.049 Separation of muscle (nontraumatic), unspecified hand

M62.05 Separation of muscle (nontraumatic), thigh
M62.051 Separation of muscle (nontraumatic), right thigh
M62.052 Separation of muscle (nontraumatic), left thigh
M62.059 Separation of muscle (nontraumatic), unspecified thigh

M62.06 Separation of muscle (nontraumatic), lower leg
M62.061 Separation of muscle (nontraumatic), right lower leg
M62.062 Separation of muscle (nontraumatic), left lower leg
M62.069 Separation of muscle (nontraumatic), unspecified lower leg

M62.07 Separation of muscle (nontraumatic), ankle and foot
M62.071 Separation of muscle (nontraumatic), right ankle and foot
M62.072 Separation of muscle (nontraumatic), left ankle and foot
M62.079 Separation of muscle (nontraumatic), unspecified ankle and foot

M62.08 Separation of muscle (nontraumatic), other site

M62.1 Other rupture of muscle (nontraumatic)

Excludes1 traumatic rupture of muscle - see strain of muscle by body region

Excludes2 rupture of tendon (M66.-)

M62.10 Other rupture of muscle (nontraumatic), unspecified site

M62.11 Other rupture of muscle (nontraumatic), shoulder
M62.111 Other rupture of muscle (nontraumatic), right shoulder
M62.112 Other rupture of muscle (nontraumatic), left shoulder
M62.119 Other rupture of muscle (nontraumatic), unspecified shoulder

M62.12 Other rupture of muscle (nontraumatic), upper arm
M62.121 Other rupture of muscle (nontraumatic), right upper arm
M62.122 Other rupture of muscle (nontraumatic), left upper arm
M62.129 Other rupture of muscle (nontraumatic), unspecified upper arm

M62.13 Other rupture of muscle (nontraumatic), forearm
M62.131 Other rupture of muscle (nontraumatic), right forearm
M62.132 Other rupture of muscle (nontraumatic), left forearm
M62.139 Other rupture of muscle (nontraumatic), unspecified forearm

M62.14 Other rupture of muscle (nontraumatic), hand
M62.141 Other rupture of muscle (nontraumatic), right hand
M62.142 Other rupture of muscle (nontraumatic), left hand
M62.149 Other rupture of muscle (nontraumatic), unspecified hand

M62.15 Other rupture of muscle (nontraumatic), thigh
M62.151 Other rupture of muscle (nontraumatic), right thigh
M62.152 Other rupture of muscle (nontraumatic), left thigh
M62.159 Other rupture of muscle (nontraumatic), unspecified thigh

M62.16 Other rupture of muscle (nontraumatic), lower leg
M62.161 Other rupture of muscle (nontraumatic), right lower leg
M62.162 Other rupture of muscle (nontraumatic), left lower leg
M62.169 Other rupture of muscle (nontraumatic), unspecified lower leg

M62.17 Other rupture of muscle (nontraumatic), ankle and foot
M62.171 Other rupture of muscle (nontraumatic), right ankle and foot
M62.172 Other rupture of muscle (nontraumatic), left ankle and foot
M62.179 Other rupture of muscle (nontraumatic), unspecified ankle and foot

M62.18 Other rupture of muscle (nontraumatic), other site

● **M62.2 Nontraumatic ischemic infarction of muscle**

Excludes1 compartment syndrome (traumatic) (T79.A-)
nontraumatic compartment syndrome (M79.A-)
traumatic ischemia of muscle (T79.6)
rhabdomyolysis (M62.82)
Volkmann's ischemic contracture (T79.6)

M62.20 Nontraumatic ischemic infarction of muscle, unspecified site

● **M62.21 Nontraumatic ischemic infarction of muscle, shoulder**

M62.211 Nontraumatic ischemic infarction of muscle, **right shoulder**

M62.212 Nontraumatic ischemic infarction of muscle, **left shoulder**

M62.219 Nontraumatic ischemic infarction of muscle, **unspecified shoulder**

● **M62.22 Nontraumatic ischemic infarction of muscle, upper arm**

M62.221 Nontraumatic ischemic infarction of muscle, **right upper arm**

M62.222 Nontraumatic ischemic infarction of muscle, **left upper arm**

M62.229 Nontraumatic ischemic infarction of muscle, **unspecified upper arm**

● **M62.23 Nontraumatic ischemic infarction of muscle, forearm**

M62.231 Nontraumatic ischemic infarction of muscle, **right forearm**

M62.232 Nontraumatic ischemic infarction of muscle, **left forearm**

M62.239 Nontraumatic ischemic infarction of muscle, **unspecified forearm**

● **M62.24 Nontraumatic ischemic infarction of muscle, hand**

M62.241 Nontraumatic ischemic infarction of muscle, **right hand**

M62.242 Nontraumatic ischemic infarction of muscle, **left hand**

M62.249 Nontraumatic ischemic infarction of muscle, **unspecified hand**

● **M62.25 Nontraumatic ischemic infarction of muscle, thigh**

M62.251 Nontraumatic ischemic infarction of muscle, **right thigh**

M62.252 Nontraumatic ischemic infarction of muscle, **left thigh**

M62.259 Nontraumatic ischemic infarction of muscle, **unspecified thigh**

● **M62.26 Nontraumatic ischemic infarction of muscle, lower leg**

M62.261 Nontraumatic ischemic infarction of muscle, **right lower leg**

M62.262 Nontraumatic ischemic infarction of muscle, **left lower leg**

M62.269 Nontraumatic ischemic infarction of muscle, **unspecified lower leg**

● **M62.27 Nontraumatic ischemic infarction of muscle, ankle and foot**

M62.271 Nontraumatic ischemic infarction of muscle, **right ankle and foot**

M62.272 Nontraumatic ischemic infarction of muscle, **left ankle and foot**

M62.279 Nontraumatic ischemic infarction of muscle, **unspecified ankle and foot**

M62.28 Nontraumatic ischemic infarction of muscle, other site

M62.3 Immobility syndrome (paraplegic)

M62.4 Contracture of muscle

Contracture of tendon (sheath)

Excludes1 contracture of joint (M24.5-)

M62.40 Contracture of muscle, unspecified site

● **M62.41 Contracture of muscle, shoulder**

M62.411 Contracture of muscle, **right shoulder**

M62.412 Contracture of muscle, **left shoulder**

M62.419 Contracture of muscle, **unspecified shoulder**

● **M62.42 Contracture of muscle, upper arm**

M62.421 Contracture of muscle, **right upper arm**

M62.422 Contracture of muscle, **left upper arm**

M62.429 Contracture of muscle, **unspecified upper arm**

● **M62.43 Contracture of muscle, forearm**

M62.431 Contracture of muscle, **right forearm**

M62.432 Contracture of muscle, **left forearm**

M62.439 Contracture of muscle, **unspecified forearm**

● **M62.44 Contracture of muscle, hand**

M62.441 Contracture of muscle, **right hand**

M62.442 Contracture of muscle, **left hand**

M62.449 Contracture of muscle, **unspecified hand**

● **M62.45 Contracture of muscle, thigh**

M62.451 Contracture of muscle, **right thigh**

M62.452 Contracture of muscle, **left thigh**

M62.459 Contracture of muscle, **unspecified thigh**

● **M62.46 Contracture of muscle, lower leg**

M62.461 Contracture of muscle, **right lower leg**

M62.462 Contracture of muscle, **left lower leg**

M62.469 Contracture of muscle, **unspecified lower leg**

● **M62.47 Contracture of muscle, ankle and foot**

M62.471 Contracture of muscle, **right ankle and foot**

M62.472 Contracture of muscle, **left ankle and foot**

M62.479 Contracture of muscle, **unspecified ankle and foot**

M62.48 Contracture of muscle, other site

M62.49 Contracture of muscle, multiple sites

● **M62.5 Muscle wasting and atrophy, not elsewhere classified**

Disuse atrophy NEC

Excludes1 neuralgic amyotrophy (G54.5)
progressive muscular atrophy (G12.21)
sarcopenia (M62.84)

Excludes2 pelvic muscle wasting (N81.84)

M62.50 Muscle wasting and atrophy, not elsewhere classified, unspecified site

● **M62.51 Muscle wasting and atrophy, not elsewhere classified, shoulder**

M62.511 Muscle wasting and atrophy, not elsewhere classified, **right shoulder**

M62.512 Muscle wasting and atrophy, not elsewhere classified, **left shoulder**

M62.519 Muscle wasting and atrophy, not elsewhere classified, **unspecified shoulder**

CHAPTER 13 (MØØ-M99)

- M62.52 Muscle wasting and atrophy, not elsewhere classified, **upper arm**
  - M62.521 Muscle wasting and atrophy, not elsewhere classified, **right upper arm**
  - M62.522 Muscle wasting and atrophy, not elsewhere classified, **left upper arm**
  - M62.529 Muscle wasting and atrophy, not elsewhere classified, **unspecified** upper arm
- M62.53 Muscle wasting and atrophy, not elsewhere classified, **forearm**
  - M62.531 Muscle wasting and atrophy, not elsewhere classified, **right forearm**
  - M62.532 Muscle wasting and atrophy, not elsewhere classified, **left forearm**
  - M62.539 Muscle wasting and atrophy, not elsewhere classified, **unspecified** forearm
- M62.54 Muscle wasting and atrophy, not elsewhere classified, **hand**
  - M62.541 Muscle wasting and atrophy, not elsewhere classified, **right hand**
  - M62.542 Muscle wasting and atrophy, not elsewhere classified, **left hand**
  - M62.549 Muscle wasting and atrophy, not elsewhere classified, **unspecified hand**
- M62.55 Muscle wasting and atrophy, not elsewhere classified, **thigh**
  - M62.551 Muscle wasting and atrophy, not elsewhere classified, **right thigh**
  - M62.552 Muscle wasting and atrophy, not elsewhere classified, **left thigh**
  - M62.559 Muscle wasting and atrophy, not elsewhere classified, **unspecified** thigh
- M62.56 Muscle wasting and atrophy, not elsewhere classified, **lower leg**
  - M62.561 Muscle wasting and atrophy, not elsewhere classified, **right lower leg**
  - M62.562 Muscle wasting and atrophy, not elsewhere classified, **left lower leg**
  - M62.569 Muscle wasting and atrophy, not elsewhere classified, **unspecified** lower leg
- M62.57 Muscle wasting and atrophy, not elsewhere classified, **ankle and foot**
  - M62.571 Muscle wasting and atrophy, not elsewhere classified, **right ankle and foot**
  - M62.572 Muscle wasting and atrophy, not elsewhere classified, **left ankle and foot**
  - M62.579 Muscle wasting and atrophy, not elsewhere classified, **unspecified** ankle and foot
- M62.58 Muscle wasting and atrophy, not elsewhere classified, **other site**
- M62.59 Muscle wasting and atrophy, not elsewhere classified, **multiple sites**

M62.8 Other specified disorders of muscle

Excludes2 nontraumatic hematoma of muscle (M79.81)

- M62.81 Muscle weakness (generalized)
  - **Excludes1** muscle weakness in sarcopenia (M62.84)
- M62.82 Rhabdomyolysis
  - **Excludes1** traumatic rhabdomyolysis (T79.6)
  - **Coding Clinic: 2019, Q2, P12**
- M62.83 Muscle spasm
  - M62.830 Muscle spasm of back
  - M62.831 Muscle spasm of calf
    - Charley-horse
  - M62.838 Other muscle spasm
- M62.84 Sarcopenia
  - Age-related sarcopenia
  - *Code first underlying disease, if applicable, such as:*
    - disorders of myoneural junction and muscle disease in diseases classified elsewhere (G73.-)
    - other and unspecified myopathies (G72.-)
    - primary disorders of muscles (G71.-)
  - **Coding Clinic: 2016, Q4, P41**
- M62.89 Other specified disorders of muscle
  - Muscle (sheath) hernia

M62.9 Disorder of muscle, **unspecified**

M63 Disorders of muscle in diseases classified elsewhere

Code first underlying disease, such as:
- leprosy (A3Ø.-)
- neoplasm (C49.-, C79.89, D21.-, D48.1)
- schistosomiasis (B65.-)
- trichinellosis (B75)

Excludes1
- myopathy in cysticercosis (B69.81)
- myopathy in endocrine diseases (G73.7)
- myopathy in metabolic diseases (G73.7)
- myopathy in sarcoidosis (D86.87)
- myopathy in secondary syphilis (A51.49)
- myopathy in syphilis (late) (A52.78)
- myopathy in toxoplasmosis (B58.82)
- myopathy in tuberculosis (A18.Ø9)

M63.8 Disorders of muscle in diseases classified elsewhere

- *M63.8Ø Disorders of muscle in diseases classified elsewhere, **unspecified site***
- M63.81 Disorders of muscle in diseases classified elsewhere, **shoulder**
  - *M63.811 Disorders of muscle in diseases classified elsewhere, **right shoulder***
  - *M63.812 Disorders of muscle in diseases classified elsewhere, **left shoulder***
  - *M63.819 Disorders of muscle in diseases classified elsewhere, **unspecified** shoulder*
- M63.82 Disorders of muscle in diseases classified elsewhere, **upper arm**
  - *M63.821 Disorders of muscle in diseases classified elsewhere, **right upper arm***
  - *M63.822 Disorders of muscle in diseases classified elsewhere, **left upper arm***
  - *M63.829 Disorders of muscle in diseases classified elsewhere, **unspecified** upper arm*
- M63.83 Disorders of muscle in diseases classified elsewhere, **forearm**
  - *M63.831 Disorders of muscle in diseases classified elsewhere, **right forearm***
  - *M63.832 Disorders of muscle in diseases classified elsewhere, **left forearm***
  - *M63.839 Disorders of muscle in diseases classified elsewhere, **unspecified** forearm*
- M63.84 Disorders of muscle in diseases classified elsewhere, **hand**
  - *M63.841 Disorders of muscle in diseases classified elsewhere, **right hand***
  - *M63.842 Disorders of muscle in diseases classified elsewhere, **left hand***
  - *M63.849 Disorders of muscle in diseases classified elsewhere, **unspecified hand***

M63.85 Disorders of muscle in diseases classified elsewhere, thigh
- *M63.851 Disorders of muscle in diseases classified elsewhere, right thigh*
- *M63.852 Disorders of muscle in diseases classified elsewhere, left thigh*
- *M63.859 Disorders of muscle in diseases classified elsewhere, unspecified thigh*

M63.86 Disorders of muscle in diseases classified elsewhere, lower leg
- *M63.861 Disorders of muscle in diseases classified elsewhere, right lower leg*
- *M63.862 Disorders of muscle in diseases classified elsewhere, left lower leg*
- *M63.869 Disorders of muscle in diseases classified elsewhere, unspecified lower leg*

M63.87 Disorders of muscle in diseases classified elsewhere, ankle and foot
- *M63.871 Disorders of muscle in diseases classified elsewhere, right ankle and foot*
- *M63.872 Disorders of muscle in diseases classified elsewhere, left ankle and foot*
- *M63.879 Disorders of muscle in diseases classified elsewhere, unspecified ankle and foot*

M63.88 Disorders of muscle in diseases classified elsewhere, other site

M63.89 Disorders of muscle in diseases classified elsewhere, multiple sites

DISORDERS OF SYNOVIUM AND TENDON (M65-M67)

M65 Synovitis and tenosynovitis

Excludes1 chronic crepitant synovitis of hand and wrist (M70.0-)
current injury - see injury of ligament or tendon by body region
soft tissue disorders related to use, overuse and pressure (M70.-)

M65.0 Abscess of tendon sheath

Use additional code (B95-B96) to identify bacterial agent

M65.00 Abscess of tendon sheath, unspecified site

M65.01 Abscess of tendon sheath, shoulder
- M65.011 Abscess of tendon sheath, right shoulder
- M65.012 Abscess of tendon sheath, left shoulder
- M65.019 Abscess of tendon sheath, unspecified shoulder

M65.02 Abscess of tendon sheath, upper arm
- M65.021 Abscess of tendon sheath, right upper arm
- M65.022 Abscess of tendon sheath, left upper arm
- M65.029 Abscess of tendon sheath, unspecified upper arm

Item 13-11 Synovitis is an inflammation of a synovial membrane resulting in pain on motion and is characterized by fluctuating swelling due to effusion in a synovial sac. **Tenosynovitis** is an inflammation of a tendon sheath and occurs most commonly in the wrists, hands, and feet. Bursitis is inflammation of a bursa (fluid-filled sac) caused by repetitive use, trauma, infection, or systemic inflammatory disease. Bursae act as protectors and facilitate movement between bones and overlapping muscles (deep bursae) or between bones and tendons/skin (superficial bursae).

M65.03 Abscess of tendon sheath, forearm
- M65.031 Abscess of tendon sheath, right forearm
- M65.032 Abscess of tendon sheath, left forearm
- M65.039 Abscess of tendon sheath, unspecified forearm

M65.04 Abscess of tendon sheath, hand
- M65.041 Abscess of tendon sheath, right hand
- M65.042 Abscess of tendon sheath, left hand
- M65.049 Abscess of tendon sheath, unspecified hand

M65.05 Abscess of tendon sheath, thigh
- M65.051 Abscess of tendon sheath, right thigh
- M65.052 Abscess of tendon sheath, left thigh
- M65.059 Abscess of tendon sheath, unspecified thigh

M65.06 Abscess of tendon sheath, lower leg
- M65.061 Abscess of tendon sheath, right lower leg
- M65.062 Abscess of tendon sheath, left lower leg
- M65.069 Abscess of tendon sheath, unspecified lower leg

M65.07 Abscess of tendon sheath, ankle and foot
- M65.071 Abscess of tendon sheath, right ankle and foot
- M65.072 Abscess of tendon sheath, left ankle and foot
- M65.079 Abscess of tendon sheath, unspecified ankle and foot

M65.08 Abscess of tendon sheath, other site

M65.1 Other infective (teno)synovitis

M65.10 Other infective (teno)synovitis, unspecified site

M65.11 Other infective (teno)synovitis, shoulder
- M65.111 Other infective (teno)synovitis, right shoulder
- M65.112 Other infective (teno)synovitis, left shoulder
- M65.119 Other infective (teno)synovitis, unspecified shoulder

M65.12 Other infective (teno)synovitis, elbow
- M65.121 Other infective (teno)synovitis, right elbow
- M65.122 Other infective (teno)synovitis, left elbow
- M65.129 Other infective (teno)synovitis, unspecified elbow

M65.13 Other infective (teno)synovitis, wrist
- M65.131 Other infective (teno)synovitis, right wrist
- M65.132 Other infective (teno)synovitis, left wrist
- M65.139 Other infective (teno)synovitis, unspecified wrist

M65.14 Other infective (teno)synovitis, hand
- M65.141 Other infective (teno)synovitis, right hand
- M65.142 Other infective (teno)synovitis, left hand
- M65.149 Other infective (teno)synovitis, unspecified hand

M65.15 Other infective (teno)synovitis, hip
- M65.151 Other infective (teno)synovitis, right hip
- M65.152 Other infective (teno)synovitis, left hip
- M65.159 Other infective (teno)synovitis, unspecified hip

CHAPTER 13 (M00-M99)

- ● M65.16 Other infective (teno)synovitis, **knee**
  - M65.161 Other infective (teno)synovitis, **right** knee
  - M65.162 Other infective (teno)synovitis, **left** knee
  - M65.169 Other infective (teno)synovitis, **unspecified** knee
- ● M65.17 Other infective (teno)synovitis, **ankle and foot**
  - M65.171 Other infective (teno)synovitis, **right** ankle and foot
  - M65.172 Other infective (teno)synovitis, **left** ankle and foot
  - M65.179 Other infective (teno)synovitis, **unspecified** ankle and foot
- M65.18 Other infective (teno)synovitis, **other site**
- M65.19 Other infective (teno)synovitis, **multiple sites**

● M65.2 Calcific tendinitis

Excludes1 tendinitis as classified in M75-M77
calcified tendinitis of shoulder (M75.3)

- M65.20 Calcific tendinitis, **unspecified** site
- ● M65.22 Calcific tendinitis, **upper arm**
  - M65.221 Calcific tendinitis, **right** upper arm
  - M65.222 Calcific tendinitis, **left** upper arm
  - M65.229 Calcific tendinitis, **unspecified** upper arm
- ● M65.23 Calcific tendinitis, **forearm**
  - M65.231 Calcific tendinitis, **right** forearm
  - M65.232 Calcific tendinitis, **left** forearm
  - M65.239 Calcific tendinitis, **unspecified** forearm
- ● M65.24 Calcific tendinitis, **hand**
  - M65.241 Calcific tendinitis, **right** hand
  - M65.242 Calcific tendinitis, **left** hand
  - M65.249 Calcific tendinitis, **unspecified** hand
- ● M65.25 Calcific tendinitis, **thigh**
  - M65.251 Calcific tendinitis, **right** thigh
  - M65.252 Calcific tendinitis, **left** thigh
  - M65.259 Calcific tendinitis, **unspecified** thigh
- ● M65.26 Calcific tendinitis, **lower leg**
  - M65.261 Calcific tendinitis, **right** lower leg
  - M65.262 Calcific tendinitis, **left** lower leg
  - M65.269 Calcific tendinitis, **unspecified** lower leg
- ● M65.27 Calcific tendinitis, **ankle and foot**
  - M65.271 Calcific tendinitis, **right** ankle and foot
  - M65.272 Calcific tendinitis, **left** ankle and foot
  - M65.279 Calcific tendinitis, **unspecified** ankle and foot
- M65.28 Calcific tendinitis, **other site**
- M65.29 Calcific tendinitis, **multiple sites**

● M65.3 Trigger finger

Nodular tendinous disease

- M65.30 Trigger finger, **unspecified** finger
- ● M65.31 Trigger **thumb**
  - M65.311 Trigger thumb, **right** thumb
  - M65.312 Trigger thumb, **left** thumb
  - M65.319 Trigger thumb, **unspecified** thumb
- ● M65.32 Trigger finger, **index** finger
  - M65.321 Trigger finger, **right** index finger
  - M65.322 Trigger finger, **left** index finger
  - M65.329 Trigger finger, **unspecified** index finger
- ● M65.33 Trigger finger, **middle** finger
  - M65.331 Trigger finger, **right** middle finger
  - M65.332 Trigger finger, **left** middle finger
  - M65.339 Trigger finger, **unspecified** middle finger
- ● M65.34 Trigger finger, **ring** finger
  - M65.341 Trigger finger, **right** ring finger
  - M65.342 Trigger finger, **left** ring finger
  - M65.349 Trigger finger, **unspecified** ring finger
- ● M65.35 Trigger finger, **little** finger
  - M65.351 Trigger finger, **right** little finger
  - M65.352 Trigger finger, **left** little finger
  - M65.359 Trigger finger, **unspecified** little finger

M65.4 Radial styloid tenosynovitis [de Quervain]

● M65.8 Other synovitis and tenosynovitis

- M65.80 Other synovitis and tenosynovitis, **unspecified** site
- ● M65.81 Other synovitis and tenosynovitis, **shoulder**
  - M65.811 Other synovitis and tenosynovitis, **right** shoulder
  - M65.812 Other synovitis and tenosynovitis, **left** shoulder
  - M65.819 Other synovitis and tenosynovitis, **unspecified** shoulder
- ● M65.82 Other synovitis and tenosynovitis, **upper arm**
  - M65.821 Other synovitis and tenosynovitis, **right** upper arm
  - M65.822 Other synovitis and tenosynovitis, **left** upper arm
  - M65.829 Other synovitis and tenosynovitis, **unspecified** upper arm
- ● M65.83 Other synovitis and tenosynovitis, **forearm**
  - M65.831 Other synovitis and tenosynovitis, **right** forearm
  - M65.832 Other synovitis and tenosynovitis, **left** forearm
  - M65.839 Other synovitis and tenosynovitis, **unspecified** forearm
- ● M65.84 Other synovitis and tenosynovitis, **hand**
  - M65.841 Other synovitis and tenosynovitis, **right** hand
  - M65.842 Other synovitis and tenosynovitis, **left** hand
  - M65.849 Other synovitis and tenosynovitis, **unspecified** hand
- ● M65.85 Other synovitis and tenosynovitis, **thigh**
  - M65.851 Other synovitis and tenosynovitis, **right** thigh
  - M65.852 Other synovitis and tenosynovitis, **left** thigh
  - M65.859 Other synovitis and tenosynovitis, **unspecified** thigh
- ● M65.86 Other synovitis and tenosynovitis, **lower leg**
  - M65.861 Other synovitis and tenosynovitis, **right** lower leg
  - M65.862 Other synovitis and tenosynovitis, **left** lower leg
  - M65.869 Other synovitis and tenosynovitis, **unspecified** lower leg
- ● M65.87 Other synovitis and tenosynovitis, **ankle and foot**
  - M65.871 Other synovitis and tenosynovitis, **right** ankle and foot
  - M65.872 Other synovitis and tenosynovitis, **left** ankle and foot
  - M65.879 Other synovitis and tenosynovitis, **unspecified** ankle and foot
- M65.88 Other synovitis and tenosynovitis, **other site**
- M65.89 Other synovitis and tenosynovitis, **multiple sites**

M65.9 Synovitis and tenosynovitis, **unspecified**

● M66 Spontaneous rupture of synovium and tendon

Includes rupture that occurs when a normal force is applied to tissues that are inferred to have less than normal strength

Excludes2 rotator cuff syndrome (M75.1-)
rupture where an abnormal force is applied to normal tissue - see injury of tendon by body region

M66.Ø Rupture of popliteal cyst

● M66.1 Rupture of synovium
Rupture of synovial cyst
Excludes2 rupture of popliteal cyst (M66.Ø)

M66.1Ø Rupture of synovium, unspecified joint

● M66.11 Rupture of synovium, shoulder
M66.111 Rupture of synovium, right shoulder
M66.112 Rupture of synovium, left shoulder
M66.119 Rupture of synovium, unspecified shoulder

● M66.12 Rupture of synovium, elbow
M66.121 Rupture of synovium, right elbow
M66.122 Rupture of synovium, left elbow
M66.129 Rupture of synovium, unspecified elbow

● M66.13 Rupture of synovium, wrist
M66.131 Rupture of synovium, right wrist
M66.132 Rupture of synovium, left wrist
M66.139 Rupture of synovium, unspecified wrist

● M66.14 Rupture of synovium, hand and fingers
M66.141 Rupture of synovium, right hand
M66.142 Rupture of synovium, left hand
M66.143 Rupture of synovium, unspecified hand
M66.144 Rupture of synovium, right finger(s)
M66.145 Rupture of synovium, left finger(s)
M66.146 Rupture of synovium, unspecified finger(s)

● M66.15 Rupture of synovium, hip
M66.151 Rupture of synovium, right hip
M66.152 Rupture of synovium, left hip
M66.159 Rupture of synovium, unspecified hip

● M66.17 Rupture of synovium, ankle, foot and toes
M66.171 Rupture of synovium, right ankle
M66.172 Rupture of synovium, left ankle
M66.173 Rupture of synovium, unspecified ankle
M66.174 Rupture of synovium, right foot
M66.175 Rupture of synovium, left foot
M66.176 Rupture of synovium, unspecified foot
M66.177 Rupture of synovium, right toe(s)
M66.178 Rupture of synovium, left toe(s)
M66.179 Rupture of synovium, unspecified toe(s)

M66.18 Rupture of synovium, other site

● M66.2 Spontaneous rupture of extensor tendons

M66.2Ø Spontaneous rupture of extensor tendons, unspecified site

● M66.21 Spontaneous rupture of extensor tendons, shoulder
M66.211 Spontaneous rupture of extensor tendons, right shoulder
M66.212 Spontaneous rupture of extensor tendons, left shoulder
M66.219 Spontaneous rupture of extensor tendons, unspecified shoulder

● M66.22 Spontaneous rupture of extensor tendons, upper arm
M66.221 Spontaneous rupture of extensor tendons, right upper arm
M66.222 Spontaneous rupture of extensor tendons, left upper arm
M66.229 Spontaneous rupture of extensor tendons, unspecified upper arm

● M66.23 Spontaneous rupture of extensor tendons, forearm
M66.231 Spontaneous rupture of extensor tendons, right forearm
M66.232 Spontaneous rupture of extensor tendons, left forearm
M66.239 Spontaneous rupture of extensor tendons, unspecified forearm

● M66.24 Spontaneous rupture of extensor tendons, hand
M66.241 Spontaneous rupture of extensor tendons, right hand
M66.242 Spontaneous rupture of extensor tendons, left hand
M66.249 Spontaneous rupture of extensor tendons, unspecified hand

● M66.25 Spontaneous rupture of extensor tendons, thigh
M66.251 Spontaneous rupture of extensor tendons, right thigh
M66.252 Spontaneous rupture of extensor tendons, left thigh
M66.259 Spontaneous rupture of extensor tendons, unspecified thigh

● M66.26 Spontaneous rupture of extensor tendons, lower leg
M66.261 Spontaneous rupture of extensor tendons, right lower leg
M66.262 Spontaneous rupture of extensor tendons, left lower leg
M66.269 Spontaneous rupture of extensor tendons, unspecified lower leg

● M66.27 Spontaneous rupture of extensor tendons, ankle and foot
M66.271 Spontaneous rupture of extensor tendons, right ankle and foot
M66.272 Spontaneous rupture of extensor tendons, left ankle and foot
M66.279 Spontaneous rupture of extensor tendons, unspecified ankle and foot

M66.28 Spontaneous rupture of extensor tendons, other site

M66.29 Spontaneous rupture of extensor tendons, multiple sites

● M66.3 Spontaneous rupture of flexor tendons

M66.3Ø Spontaneous rupture of flexor tendons, unspecified site

● M66.31 Spontaneous rupture of flexor tendons, shoulder
M66.311 Spontaneous rupture of flexor tendons, right shoulder
M66.312 Spontaneous rupture of flexor tendons, left shoulder
M66.319 Spontaneous rupture of flexor tendons, unspecified shoulder

● M66.32 Spontaneous rupture of flexor tendons, upper arm
M66.321 Spontaneous rupture of flexor tendons, right upper arm
M66.322 Spontaneous rupture of flexor tendons, left upper arm
M66.329 Spontaneous rupture of flexor tendons, unspecified upper arm

● M66.33 Spontaneous rupture of flexor tendons, **forearm**
- M66.331 Spontaneous rupture of flexor tendons, **right forearm**
- M66.332 Spontaneous rupture of flexor tendons, **left forearm**
- M66.339 Spontaneous rupture of flexor tendons, **unspecified forearm**

● M66.34 Spontaneous rupture of flexor tendons, **hand**
- M66.341 Spontaneous rupture of flexor tendons, **right hand**
- M66.342 Spontaneous rupture of flexor tendons, **left hand**
- M66.349 Spontaneous rupture of flexor tendons, **unspecified hand**

● M66.35 Spontaneous rupture of flexor tendons, **thigh**
- M66.351 Spontaneous rupture of flexor tendons, **right thigh**
- M66.352 Spontaneous rupture of flexor tendons, **left thigh**
- M66.359 Spontaneous rupture of flexor tendons, **unspecified thigh**

● M66.36 Spontaneous rupture of flexor tendons, **lower leg**
- M66.361 Spontaneous rupture of flexor tendons, **right lower leg**
- M66.362 Spontaneous rupture of flexor tendons, **left lower leg**
- M66.369 Spontaneous rupture of flexor tendons, **unspecified lower leg**

● M66.37 Spontaneous rupture of flexor tendons, **ankle and foot**
- M66.371 Spontaneous rupture of flexor tendons, **right ankle and foot**
- M66.372 Spontaneous rupture of flexor tendons, **left ankle and foot**
- M66.379 Spontaneous rupture of flexor tendons, **unspecified ankle and foot**

M66.38 Spontaneous rupture of flexor tendons, **other site**

M66.39 Spontaneous rupture of flexor tendons, **multiple sites**

● M66.8 Spontaneous rupture of other tendons

M66.8Ø Spontaneous rupture of other tendons, **unspecified site**

● M66.81 Spontaneous rupture of other tendons, **shoulder**
- M66.811 Spontaneous rupture of other tendons, **right shoulder**
- M66.812 Spontaneous rupture of other tendons, **left shoulder**
- M66.819 Spontaneous rupture of other tendons, **unspecified shoulder**

● M66.82 Spontaneous rupture of other tendons, **upper arm**
- M66.821 Spontaneous rupture of other tendons, **right upper arm**
- M66.822 Spontaneous rupture of other tendons, **left upper arm**
- M66.829 Spontaneous rupture of other tendons, **unspecified upper arm**

● M66.83 Spontaneous rupture of other tendons, **forearm**
- M66.831 Spontaneous rupture of other tendons, **right forearm**
- M66.832 Spontaneous rupture of other tendons, **left forearm**
- M66.839 Spontaneous rupture of other tendons, **unspecified forearm**

● M66.84 Spontaneous rupture of other tendons, **hand**
- M66.841 Spontaneous rupture of other tendons, **right hand**
- M66.842 Spontaneous rupture of other tendons, **left hand**
- M66.849 Spontaneous rupture of other tendons, **unspecified hand**

● M66.85 Spontaneous rupture of other tendons, **thigh**
- M66.851 Spontaneous rupture of other tendons, **right thigh**
- M66.852 Spontaneous rupture of other tendons, **left thigh**
- M66.859 Spontaneous rupture of other tendons, **unspecified thigh**

● M66.86 Spontaneous rupture of other tendons, **lower leg**
- M66.861 Spontaneous rupture of other tendons, **right lower leg**
- M66.862 Spontaneous rupture of other tendons, **left lower leg**
- M66.869 Spontaneous rupture of other tendons, **unspecified lower leg**

● M66.87 Spontaneous rupture of other tendons, **ankle and foot**
- M66.871 Spontaneous rupture of other tendons, **right ankle and foot**
- M66.872 Spontaneous rupture of other tendons, **left ankle and foot**
- M66.879 Spontaneous rupture of other tendons, **unspecified ankle and foot**

M66.88 Spontaneous rupture of other tendons, **other sites**

M66.89 Spontaneous rupture of other tendons, **multiple sites**

M66.9 Spontaneous rupture of **unspecified** tendon
Rupture at musculotendinous junction, nontraumatic

● M67 Other disorders of synovium and tendon

Excludes1 palmar fascial fibromatosis [Dupuytren] (M72.Ø)
tendinitis NOS (M77.9-)
xanthomatosis localized to tendons (E78.2)

● M67.Ø Short Achilles tendon (acquired)
- M67.ØØ Short Achilles tendon (acquired), **unspecified ankle**
- M67.Ø1 Short Achilles tendon (acquired), **right ankle**
- M67.Ø2 Short Achilles tendon (acquired), **left ankle**

● M67.2 Synovial hypertrophy, not elsewhere classified

Excludes1 villonodular synovitis (pigmented) (M12.2-)

M67.2Ø Synovial hypertrophy, not elsewhere classified, **unspecified site**

● M67.21 Synovial hypertrophy, not elsewhere classified, **shoulder**
- M67.211 Synovial hypertrophy, not elsewhere classified, **right shoulder**
- M67.212 Synovial hypertrophy, not elsewhere classified, **left shoulder**
- M67.219 Synovial hypertrophy, not elsewhere classified, **unspecified shoulder**

● M67.22 Synovial hypertrophy, not elsewhere classified, **upper arm**
- M67.221 Synovial hypertrophy, not elsewhere classified, **right upper arm**
- M67.222 Synovial hypertrophy, not elsewhere classified, **left upper arm**
- M67.229 Synovial hypertrophy, not elsewhere classified, **unspecified upper arm**

● M67.23 Synovial hypertrophy, not elsewhere classified, **forearm**
M67.231 Synovial hypertrophy, not elsewhere classified, **right forearm**
M67.232 Synovial hypertrophy, not elsewhere classified, **left forearm**
M67.239 Synovial hypertrophy, not elsewhere classified, **unspecified forearm**
● M67.24 Synovial hypertrophy, not elsewhere classified, **hand**
M67.241 Synovial hypertrophy, not elsewhere classified, **right hand**
M67.242 Synovial hypertrophy, not elsewhere classified, **left hand**
M67.249 Synovial hypertrophy, not elsewhere classified, **unspecified hand**
● M67.25 Synovial hypertrophy, not elsewhere classified, **thigh**
M67.251 Synovial hypertrophy, not elsewhere classified, **right thigh**
M67.252 Synovial hypertrophy, not elsewhere classified, **left thigh**
M67.259 Synovial hypertrophy, not elsewhere classified, **unspecified thigh**
● M67.26 Synovial hypertrophy, not elsewhere classified, **lower leg**
M67.261 Synovial hypertrophy, not elsewhere classified, **right lower leg**
M67.262 Synovial hypertrophy, not elsewhere classified, **left lower leg**
M67.269 Synovial hypertrophy, not elsewhere classified, **unspecified lower leg**
● M67.27 Synovial hypertrophy, not elsewhere classified, **ankle and foot**
M67.271 Synovial hypertrophy, not elsewhere classified, **right ankle and foot**
M67.272 Synovial hypertrophy, not elsewhere classified, **left ankle and foot**
M67.279 Synovial hypertrophy, not elsewhere classified, **unspecified ankle and foot**
M67.28 Synovial hypertrophy, not elsewhere classified, **other site**
M67.29 Synovial hypertrophy, not elsewhere classified, **multiple sites**

● M67.3 Transient synovitis
Toxic synovitis
Excludes1 palindromic rheumatism (M12.3-)
M67.30 Transient synovitis, **unspecified site**
● M67.31 Transient synovitis, **shoulder**
M67.311 Transient synovitis, **right shoulder**
M67.312 Transient synovitis, **left shoulder**
M67.319 Transient synovitis, **unspecified shoulder**
● M67.32 Transient synovitis, **elbow**
M67.321 Transient synovitis, **right elbow**
M67.322 Transient synovitis, **left elbow**
M67.329 Transient synovitis, **unspecified elbow**
● M67.33 Transient synovitis, **wrist**
M67.331 Transient synovitis, **right wrist**
M67.332 Transient synovitis, **left wrist**
M67.339 Transient synovitis, **unspecified wrist**
● M67.34 Transient synovitis, **hand**
M67.341 Transient synovitis, **right hand**
M67.342 Transient synovitis, **left hand**
M67.349 Transient synovitis, **unspecified hand**
● M67.35 Transient synovitis, **hip**
M67.351 Transient synovitis, **right hip**
M67.352 Transient synovitis, **left hip**
M67.359 Transient synovitis, **unspecified hip**
● M67.36 Transient synovitis, **knee**
M67.361 Transient synovitis, **right knee**
M67.362 Transient synovitis, **left knee**
M67.369 Transient synovitis, **unspecified knee**
● M67.37 Transient synovitis, **ankle and foot**
M67.371 Transient synovitis, **right ankle and foot**
M67.372 Transient synovitis, **left ankle and foot**
M67.379 Transient synovitis, **unspecified ankle and foot**
M67.38 Transient synovitis, **other site**
M67.39 Transient synovitis, **multiple sites**

● M67.4 Ganglion
Ganglion of joint or tendon (sheath)
Excludes1 ganglion in yaws (A66.6)
Excludes2 cyst of bursa (M71.2-M71.3)
cyst of synovium (M71.2-M71.3)
M67.40 Ganglion, **unspecified site**
● M67.41 Ganglion, **shoulder**
M67.411 Ganglion, **right shoulder**
M67.412 Ganglion, **left shoulder**
M67.419 Ganglion, **unspecified shoulder**
● M67.42 Ganglion, **elbow**
M67.421 Ganglion, **right elbow**
M67.422 Ganglion, **left elbow**
M67.429 Ganglion, **unspecified elbow**
● M67.43 Ganglion, **wrist**
M67.431 Ganglion, **right wrist**
M67.432 Ganglion, **left wrist**
M67.439 Ganglion, **unspecified wrist**
● M67.44 Ganglion, **hand**
M67.441 Ganglion, **right hand**
M67.442 Ganglion, **left hand**
M67.449 Ganglion, **unspecified hand**
● M67.45 Ganglion, **hip**
M67.451 Ganglion, **right hip**
M67.452 Ganglion, **left hip**
M67.459 Ganglion, **unspecified hip**
● M67.46 Ganglion, **knee**
M67.461 Ganglion, **right knee**
M67.462 Ganglion, **left knee**
M67.469 Ganglion, **unspecified knee**
● M67.47 Ganglion, **ankle and foot**
M67.471 Ganglion, **right ankle and foot**
M67.472 Ganglion, **left ankle and foot**
M67.479 Ganglion, **unspecified ankle and foot**
M67.48 Ganglion, **other site**
M67.49 Ganglion, **multiple sites**

● M67.5 Plica syndrome
Plica knee
M67.50 Plica syndrome, **unspecified knee**
M67.51 Plica syndrome, **right knee**
M67.52 Plica syndrome, **left knee**

● M67.8 Other specified disorders of synovium and tendon
M67.80 Other specified disorders of synovium and tendon, **unspecified** site
● M67.81 Other specified disorders of synovium and tendon, **shoulder**
M67.811 Other specified disorders of **synovium, right** shoulder
M67.812 Other specified disorders of **synovium, left** shoulder
M67.813 Other specified disorders of **tendon, right** shoulder
M67.814 Other specified disorders of **tendon, left** shoulder
M67.819 Other specified disorders of synovium and tendon, **unspecified** shoulder
● M67.82 Other specified disorders of synovium and tendon, **elbow**
M67.821 Other specified disorders of **synovium, right** elbow
M67.822 Other specified disorders of **synovium, left** elbow
M67.823 Other specified disorders of **tendon, right** elbow
M67.824 Other specified disorders of **tendon, left** elbow
M67.829 Other specified disorders of synovium and tendon, **unspecified** elbow
● M67.83 Other specified disorders of synovium and tendon, **wrist**
M67.831 Other specified disorders of **synovium, right** wrist
M67.832 Other specified disorders of **synovium, left** wrist
M67.833 Other specified disorders of **tendon, right** wrist
M67.834 Other specified disorders of **tendon, left** wrist
M67.839 Other specified disorders of synovium and tendon, **unspecified** wrist
● M67.84 Other specified disorders of synovium and tendon, **hand**
M67.841 Other specified disorders of **synovium, right** hand
M67.842 Other specified disorders of **synovium, left** hand
M67.843 Other specified disorders of **tendon, right** hand
M67.844 Other specified disorders of **tendon, left** hand
M67.849 Other specified disorders of synovium and tendon, **unspecified** hand
● M67.85 Other specified disorders of synovium and tendon, **hip**
M67.851 Other specified disorders of **synovium, right** hip
M67.852 Other specified disorders of **synovium, left** hip
M67.853 Other specified disorders of **tendon, right** hip
M67.854 Other specified disorders of **tendon, left** hip
M67.859 Other specified disorders of synovium and tendon, **unspecified** hip
● M67.86 Other specified disorders of synovium and tendon, **knee**
M67.861 Other specified disorders of **synovium, right** knee
M67.862 Other specified disorders of **synovium, left** knee
M67.863 Other specified disorders of **tendon, right** knee
M67.864 Other specified disorders of **tendon, left** knee
M67.869 Other specified disorders of synovium and tendon, **unspecified** knee
● M67.87 Other specified disorders of synovium and tendon, **ankle and foot**
M67.871 Other specified disorders of **synovium, right** ankle and foot
M67.872 Other specified disorders of **synovium, left** ankle and foot
M67.873 Other specified disorders of **tendon, right** ankle and foot
M67.874 Other specified disorders of **tendon, left** ankle and foot
M67.879 Other specified disorders of synovium and tendon, **unspecified** ankle and foot
M67.88 Other specified disorders of synovium and tendon, **other site**
M67.89 Other specified disorders of synovium and tendon, **multiple sites**
● M67.9 **Unspecified** disorder of synovium and tendon
M67.90 Unspecified disorder of synovium and tendon, **unspecified** site
● M67.91 Unspecified disorder of synovium and tendon, **shoulder**
M67.911 Unspecified disorder of synovium and tendon, **right** shoulder
M67.912 Unspecified disorder of synovium and tendon, **left** shoulder
M67.919 Unspecified disorder of synovium and tendon, **unspecified** shoulder
● M67.92 Unspecified disorder of synovium and tendon, **upper arm**
M67.921 Unspecified disorder of synovium and tendon, **right** upper arm
M67.922 Unspecified disorder of synovium and tendon, **left** upper arm
M67.929 Unspecified disorder of synovium and tendon, **unspecified** upper arm
● M67.93 Unspecified disorder of synovium and tendon, **forearm**
M67.931 Unspecified disorder of synovium and tendon, **right** forearm
M67.932 Unspecified disorder of synovium and tendon, **left** forearm
M67.939 Unspecified disorder of synovium and tendon, **unspecified** forearm
● M67.94 Unspecified disorder of synovium and tendon, **hand**
M67.941 Unspecified disorder of synovium and tendon, **right** hand
M67.942 Unspecified disorder of synovium and tendon, **left** hand
M67.949 Unspecified disorder of synovium and tendon, **unspecified** hand

- ● M67.95 Unspecified disorder of synovium and tendon, thigh
  - M67.951 Unspecified disorder of synovium and tendon, right thigh
  - M67.952 Unspecified disorder of synovium and tendon, left thigh
  - M67.959 Unspecified disorder of synovium and tendon, unspecified thigh
- ● M67.96 Unspecified disorder of synovium and tendon, lower leg
  - M67.961 Unspecified disorder of synovium and tendon, right lower leg
  - M67.962 Unspecified disorder of synovium and tendon, left lower leg
  - M67.969 Unspecified disorder of synovium and tendon, unspecified lower leg
- ● M67.97 Unspecified disorder of synovium and tendon, ankle and foot
  - M67.971 Unspecified disorder of synovium and tendon, right ankle and foot
  - M67.972 Unspecified disorder of synovium and tendon, left ankle and foot
  - M67.979 Unspecified disorder of synovium and tendon, unspecified ankle and foot
- M67.98 Unspecified disorder of synovium and tendon, other site
- M67.99 Unspecified disorder of synovium and tendon, multiple sites

OTHER SOFT TISSUE DISORDERS (M70-M79)

● M70 Soft tissue disorders related to use, overuse and pressure

Includes soft tissue disorders of occupational origin

Use additional external cause code to identify activity causing disorder (Y93.-)

Excludes1 bursitis NOS (M71.9-)

Excludes2 bursitis of shoulder (M75.5)
enthesopathies (M76-M77)
pressure ulcer (pressure area) (L89.-)

- ● M70.0 Crepitant synovitis (acute) (chronic) of hand and wrist
  - ● M70.03 Crepitant synovitis (acute) (chronic), wrist
    - M70.031 Crepitant synovitis (acute) (chronic), right wrist
    - M70.032 Crepitant synovitis (acute) (chronic), left wrist
    - M70.039 Crepitant synovitis (acute) (chronic), unspecified wrist
  - ● M70.04 Crepitant synovitis (acute) (chronic), hand
    - M70.041 Crepitant synovitis (acute) (chronic), right hand
    - M70.042 Crepitant synovitis (acute) (chronic), left hand
    - M70.049 Crepitant synovitis (acute) (chronic), unspecified hand
- ● M70.1 Bursitis of hand
  - M70.10 Bursitis, unspecified hand
  - M70.11 Bursitis, right hand
  - M70.12 Bursitis, left hand
- ● M70.2 Olecranon bursitis
  - M70.20 Olecranon bursitis, unspecified elbow
  - M70.21 Olecranon bursitis, right elbow
  - M70.22 Olecranon bursitis, left elbow
- ● M70.3 Other bursitis of elbow
  - M70.30 Other bursitis of elbow, unspecified elbow
  - M70.31 Other bursitis of elbow, right elbow
  - M70.32 Other bursitis of elbow, left elbow
- ● M70.4 Prepatellar bursitis
  - M70.40 Prepatellar bursitis, unspecified knee
  - M70.41 Prepatellar bursitis, right knee
  - M70.42 Prepatellar bursitis, left knee
- ● M70.5 Other bursitis of knee
  - M70.50 Other bursitis of knee, unspecified knee
  - M70.51 Other bursitis of knee, right knee
  - M70.52 Other bursitis of knee, left knee
- ● M70.6 Trochanteric bursitis
  Trochanteric tendinitis
  - M70.60 Trochanteric bursitis, unspecified hip
  - M70.61 Trochanteric bursitis, right hip
  - M70.62 Trochanteric bursitis, left hip
- ● M70.7 Other bursitis of hip
  Ischial bursitis
  - M70.70 Other bursitis of hip, unspecified hip
  - M70.71 Other bursitis of hip, right hip
  - M70.72 Other bursitis of hip, left hip
- ● M70.8 Other soft tissue disorders related to use, overuse and pressure
  - M70.80 Other soft tissue disorders related to use, overuse and pressure of unspecified site
  - ● M70.81 Other soft tissue disorders related to use, overuse and pressure of shoulder
    - M70.811 Other soft tissue disorders related to use, overuse and pressure, right shoulder
    - M70.812 Other soft tissue disorders related to use, overuse and pressure, left shoulder
    - M70.819 Other soft tissue disorders related to use, overuse and pressure, unspecified shoulder
  - ● M70.82 Other soft tissue disorders related to use, overuse and pressure of upper arm
    - M70.821 Other soft tissue disorders related to use, overuse and pressure, right upper arm
    - M70.822 Other soft tissue disorders related to use, overuse and pressure, left upper arm
    - M70.829 Other soft tissue disorders related to use, overuse and pressure, unspecified upper arms
  - ● M70.83 Other soft tissue disorders related to use, overuse and pressure of forearm
    - M70.831 Other soft tissue disorders related to use, overuse and pressure, right forearm
    - M70.832 Other soft tissue disorders related to use, overuse and pressure, left forearm
    - M70.839 Other soft tissue disorders related to use, overuse and pressure, unspecified forearm
  - ● M70.84 Other soft tissue disorders related to use, overuse and pressure of hand
    - M70.841 Other soft tissue disorders related to use, overuse and pressure, right hand
    - M70.842 Other soft tissue disorders related to use, overuse and pressure, left hand
    - M70.849 Other soft tissue disorders related to use, overuse and pressure, unspecified hand

- M70.85 Other soft tissue disorders related to use, overuse and pressure of **thigh**
  - M70.851 Other soft tissue disorders related to use, overuse and pressure, **right** thigh
  - M70.852 Other soft tissue disorders related to use, overuse and pressure, **left** thigh
  - M70.859 Other soft tissue disorders related to use, overuse and pressure, **unspecified** thigh
- M70.86 Other soft tissue disorders related to use, overuse and pressure **lower leg**
  - M70.861 Other soft tissue disorders related to use, overuse and pressure, **right** lower leg
  - M70.862 Other soft tissue disorders related to use, overuse and pressure, **left** lower leg
  - M70.869 Other soft tissue disorders related to use, overuse and pressure, **unspecified** leg
- M70.87 Other soft tissue disorders related to use, overuse and pressure of **ankle and foot**
  - M70.871 Other soft tissue disorders related to use, overuse and pressure, **right** ankle and foot
  - M70.872 Other soft tissue disorders related to use, overuse and pressure, **left** ankle and foot
  - M70.879 Other soft tissue disorders related to use, overuse and pressure, **unspecified** ankle and foot
- M70.88 Other soft tissue disorders related to use, overuse and pressure **other site**
- M70.89 Other soft tissue disorders related to use, overuse and pressure **multiple sites**

M70.9 **Unspecified** soft tissue disorder related to use, overuse and pressure

- M70.90 Unspecified soft tissue disorder related to use, overuse and pressure of **unspecified site**
- M70.91 Unspecified soft tissue disorder related to use, overuse and pressure of **shoulder**
  - M70.911 Unspecified soft tissue disorder related to use, overuse and pressure, **right** shoulder
  - M70.912 Unspecified soft tissue disorder related to use, overuse and pressure, **left** shoulder
  - M70.919 Unspecified soft tissue disorder related to use, overuse and pressure, **unspecified** shoulder
- M70.92 Unspecified soft tissue disorder related to use, overuse and pressure of **upper arm**
  - M70.921 Unspecified soft tissue disorder related to use, overuse and pressure, **right** upper arm
  - M70.922 Unspecified soft tissue disorder related to use, overuse and pressure, **left** upper arm
  - M70.929 Unspecified soft tissue disorder related to use, overuse and pressure, **unspecified** upper arm
- M70.93 Unspecified soft tissue disorder related to use, overuse and pressure of **forearm**
  - M70.931 Unspecified soft tissue disorder related to use, overuse and pressure, **right** forearm
  - M70.932 Unspecified soft tissue disorder related to use, overuse and pressure, **left** forearm
  - M70.939 Unspecified soft tissue disorder related to use, overuse and pressure, **unspecified** forearm
- M70.94 Unspecified soft tissue disorder related to use, overuse and pressure of **hand**
  - M70.941 Unspecified soft tissue disorder related to use, overuse and pressure, **right** hand
  - M70.942 Unspecified soft tissue disorder related to use, overuse and pressure, **left** hand
  - M70.949 Unspecified soft tissue disorder related to use, overuse and pressure, **unspecified** hand
- M70.95 Unspecified soft tissue disorder related to use, overuse and pressure of **thigh**
  - M70.951 Unspecified soft tissue disorder related to use, overuse and pressure, **right** thigh
  - M70.952 Unspecified soft tissue disorder related to use, overuse and pressure, **left** thigh
  - M70.959 Unspecified soft tissue disorder related to use, overuse and pressure, **unspecified** thigh
- M70.96 Unspecified soft tissue disorder related to use, overuse and pressure **lower leg**
  - M70.961 Unspecified soft tissue disorder related to use, overuse and pressure, **right** lower leg
  - M70.962 Unspecified soft tissue disorder related to use, overuse and pressure, **left** lower leg
  - M70.969 Unspecified soft tissue disorder related to use, overuse and pressure, **unspecified** lower leg
- M70.97 Unspecified soft tissue disorder related to use, overuse and pressure of **ankle and foot**
  - M70.971 Unspecified soft tissue disorder related to use, overuse and pressure, **right** ankle and foot
  - M70.972 Unspecified soft tissue disorder related to use, overuse and pressure, **left** ankle and foot
  - M70.979 Unspecified soft tissue disorder related to use, overuse and pressure, **unspecified** ankle and foot
- M70.98 Unspecified soft tissue disorder related to use, overuse and pressure **other**
- M70.99 Unspecified soft tissue disorder related to use, overuse and pressure **multiple sites**

M71 Other bursopathies

Excludes1 bunion (M20.1)
bursitis related to use, overuse or pressure (M70.-)
enthesopathies (M76-M77)

M71.0 Abscess of bursa

Use additional code (B95.-, B96.-) to identify causative organism

- M71.00 Abscess of bursa, **unspecified** site
- M71.01 Abscess of bursa, **shoulder**
  - M71.011 Abscess of bursa, **right** shoulder
  - M71.012 Abscess of bursa, **left** shoulder
  - M71.019 Abscess of bursa, **unspecified** shoulder
- M71.02 Abscess of bursa, **elbow**
  - M71.021 Abscess of bursa, **right** elbow
  - M71.022 Abscess of bursa, **left** elbow
  - M71.029 Abscess of bursa, **unspecified** elbow
- M71.03 Abscess of bursa, **wrist**
  - M71.031 Abscess of bursa, **right** wrist
  - M71.032 Abscess of bursa, **left** wrist
  - M71.039 Abscess of bursa, **unspecified** wrist

- M71.04 Abscess of bursa, hand
  - M71.041 Abscess of bursa, right hand
  - M71.042 Abscess of bursa, left hand
  - M71.049 Abscess of bursa, unspecified hand
- M71.05 Abscess of bursa, hip
  - M71.051 Abscess of bursa, right hip
  - M71.052 Abscess of bursa, left hip
  - M71.059 Abscess of bursa, unspecified hip
- M71.06 Abscess of bursa, knee
  - M71.061 Abscess of bursa, right knee
  - M71.062 Abscess of bursa, left knee
  - M71.069 Abscess of bursa, unspecified knee
- M71.07 Abscess of bursa, ankle and foot
  - M71.071 Abscess of bursa, right ankle and foot
  - M71.072 Abscess of bursa, left ankle and foot
  - M71.079 Abscess of bursa, unspecified ankle and foot
- M71.08 Abscess of bursa, other site
- M71.09 Abscess of bursa, multiple sites

M71.1 Other infective bursitis

Use additional code (B95.-, B96.-) to identify causative organism

- M71.10 Other infective bursitis, unspecified site
- M71.11 Other infective bursitis, shoulder
  - M71.111 Other infective bursitis, right shoulder
  - M71.112 Other infective bursitis, left shoulder
  - M71.119 Other infective bursitis, unspecified shoulder
- M71.12 Other infective bursitis, elbow
  - M71.121 Other infective bursitis, right elbow
  - M71.122 Other infective bursitis, left elbow
  - M71.129 Other infective bursitis, unspecified elbow
- M71.13 Other infective bursitis, wrist
  - M71.131 Other infective bursitis, right wrist
  - M71.132 Other infective bursitis, left wrist
  - M71.139 Other infective bursitis, unspecified wrist
- M71.14 Other infective bursitis, hand
  - M71.141 Other infective bursitis, right hand
  - M71.142 Other infective bursitis, left hand
  - M71.149 Other infective bursitis, unspecified hand
- M71.15 Other infective bursitis, hip
  - M71.151 Other infective bursitis, right hip
  - M71.152 Other infective bursitis, left hip
  - M71.159 Other infective bursitis, unspecified hip
- M71.16 Other infective bursitis, knee
  - M71.161 Other infective bursitis, right knee
  - M71.162 Other infective bursitis, left knee
  - M71.169 Other infective bursitis, unspecified knee
- M71.17 Other infective bursitis, ankle and foot
  - M71.171 Other infective bursitis, right ankle and foot
  - M71.172 Other infective bursitis, left ankle and foot
  - M71.179 Other infective bursitis, unspecified ankle and foot
- M71.18 Other infective bursitis, other site
- M71.19 Other infective bursitis, multiple sites

M71.2 Synovial cyst of popliteal space [Baker]

Popliteal space = popliteal cavity, popliteal fossa. Depression in the posterior aspect of the knee (behind the knee).

Excludes1 synovial cyst of popliteal space with rupture (M66.0)

- M71.20 Synovial cyst of popliteal space [Baker], unspecified knee
- M71.21 Synovial cyst of popliteal space [Baker], right knee
- M71.22 Synovial cyst of popliteal space [Baker], left knee

M71.3 Other bursal cyst

Synovial cyst NOS

Excludes1 synovial cyst with rupture (M66.1-)

- M71.30 Other bursal cyst, unspecified site
- M71.31 Other bursal cyst, shoulder
  - M71.311 Other bursal cyst, right shoulder
  - M71.312 Other bursal cyst, left shoulder
  - M71.319 Other bursal cyst, unspecified shoulder
- M71.32 Other bursal cyst, elbow
  - M71.321 Other bursal cyst, right elbow
  - M71.322 Other bursal cyst, left elbow
  - M71.329 Other bursal cyst, unspecified elbow
- M71.33 Other bursal cyst, wrist
  - M71.331 Other bursal cyst, right wrist
  - M71.332 Other bursal cyst, left wrist
  - M71.339 Other bursal cyst, unspecified wrist
- M71.34 Other bursal cyst, hand
  - M71.341 Other bursal cyst, right hand
  - M71.342 Other bursal cyst, left hand
  - M71.349 Other bursal cyst, unspecified hand
- M71.35 Other bursal cyst, hip
  - M71.351 Other bursal cyst, right hip
  - M71.352 Other bursal cyst, left hip
  - M71.359 Other bursal cyst, unspecified hip
- M71.37 Other bursal cyst, ankle and foot
  - M71.371 Other bursal cyst, right ankle and foot
  - M71.372 Other bursal cyst, left ankle and foot
  - M71.379 Other bursal cyst, unspecified ankle and foot
- M71.38 Other bursal cyst, other site
- M71.39 Other bursal cyst, multiple sites

M71.4 Calcium deposit in bursa

Excludes2 calcium deposit in bursa of shoulder (M75.3)

- M71.40 Calcium deposit in bursa, unspecified site
- M71.42 Calcium deposit in bursa, elbow
  - M71.421 Calcium deposit in bursa, right elbow
  - M71.422 Calcium deposit in bursa, left elbow
  - M71.429 Calcium deposit in bursa, unspecified elbow
- M71.43 Calcium deposit in bursa, wrist
  - M71.431 Calcium deposit in bursa, right wrist
  - M71.432 Calcium deposit in bursa, left wrist
  - M71.439 Calcium deposit in bursa, unspecified wrist
- M71.44 Calcium deposit in bursa, hand
  - M71.441 Calcium deposit in bursa, right hand
  - M71.442 Calcium deposit in bursa, left hand
  - M71.449 Calcium deposit in bursa, unspecified hand

CHAPTER 13 (M00-M99)

- ● M71.45 Calcium deposit in bursa, **hip**
  - M71.451 Calcium deposit in bursa, **right** hip
  - M71.452 Calcium deposit in bursa, **left** hip
  - M71.459 Calcium deposit in bursa, **unspecified** hip
- ● M71.46 Calcium deposit in bursa, **knee**
  - M71.461 Calcium deposit in bursa, **right** knee
  - M71.462 Calcium deposit in bursa, **left** knee
  - M71.469 Calcium deposit in bursa, **unspecified** knee
- ● M71.47 Calcium deposit in bursa, **ankle and foot**
  - M71.471 Calcium deposit in bursa, **right** ankle and foot
  - M71.472 Calcium deposit in bursa, **left** ankle and foot
  - M71.479 Calcium deposit in bursa, **unspecified** ankle and foot
- M71.48 Calcium deposit in bursa, **other site**
- M71.49 Calcium deposit in bursa, **multiple sites**

● M71.5 Other bursitis, not elsewhere classified

Excludes1 bursitis NOS (M71.9-)

Excludes2 bursitis of shoulder (M75.5)
bursitis of tibial collateral [Pellegrini-Stieda] (M76.4-)

- M71.50 Other bursitis, not elsewhere classified, **unspecified** site
- ● M71.52 Other bursitis, not elsewhere classified, **elbow**
  - M71.521 Other bursitis, not elsewhere classified, **right** elbow
  - M71.522 Other bursitis, not elsewhere classified, **left** elbow
  - M71.529 Other bursitis, not elsewhere classified, **unspecified** elbow
- ● M71.53 Other bursitis, not elsewhere classified, **wrist**
  - M71.531 Other bursitis, not elsewhere classified, **right** wrist
  - M71.532 Other bursitis, not elsewhere classified, **left** wrist
  - M71.539 Other bursitis, not elsewhere classified, **unspecified** wrist
- ● M71.54 Other bursitis, not elsewhere classified, **hand**
  - M71.541 Other bursitis, not elsewhere classified, **right** hand
  - M71.542 Other bursitis, not elsewhere classified, **left** hand
  - M71.549 Other bursitis, not elsewhere classified, **unspecified** hand
- ● M71.55 Other bursitis, not elsewhere classified, **hip**
  - M71.551 Other bursitis, not elsewhere classified, **right** hip
  - M71.552 Other bursitis, not elsewhere classified, **left** hip
  - M71.559 Other bursitis, not elsewhere classified, **unspecified** hip
- ● M71.56 Other bursitis, not elsewhere classified, **knee**
  - M71.561 Other bursitis, not elsewhere classified, **right** knee
  - M71.562 Other bursitis, not elsewhere classified, **left** knee
  - M71.569 Other bursitis, not elsewhere classified, **unspecified** knee
- ● M71.57 Other bursitis, not elsewhere classified, **ankle and foot**
  - M71.571 Other bursitis, not elsewhere classified, **right** ankle and foot
  - M71.572 Other bursitis, not elsewhere classified, **left** ankle and foot
  - M71.579 Other bursitis, not elsewhere classified, **unspecified** ankle and foot
- M71.58 Other bursitis, not elsewhere classified, **other site**

● M71.8 Other specified bursopathies

- M71.80 Other specified bursopathies, **unspecified** site
- ● M71.81 Other specified bursopathies, **shoulder**
  - M71.811 Other specified bursopathies, **right** shoulder
  - M71.812 Other specified bursopathies, **left** shoulder
  - M71.819 Other specified bursopathies, **unspecified** shoulder
- ● M71.82 Other specified bursopathies, **elbow**
  - M71.821 Other specified bursopathies, **right** elbow
  - M71.822 Other specified bursopathies, **left** elbow
  - M71.829 Other specified bursopathies, **unspecified** elbow
- ● M71.83 Other specified bursopathies, **wrist**
  - M71.831 Other specified bursopathies, **right** wrist
  - M71.832 Other specified bursopathies, **left** wrist
  - M71.839 Other specified bursopathies, **unspecified** wrist
- ● M71.84 Other specified bursopathies, **hand**
  - M71.841 Other specified bursopathies, **right** hand
  - M71.842 Other specified bursopathies, **left** hand
  - M71.849 Other specified bursopathies, **unspecified** hand
- ● M71.85 Other specified bursopathies, **hip**
  - M71.851 Other specified bursopathies, **right** hip
  - M71.852 Other specified bursopathies, **left** hip
  - M71.859 Other specified bursopathies, **unspecified** hip
- ● M71.86 Other specified bursopathies, **knee**
  - M71.861 Other specified bursopathies, **right** knee
  - M71.862 Other specified bursopathies, **left** knee
  - M71.869 Other specified bursopathies, **unspecified** knee
- ● M71.87 Other specified bursopathies, **ankle and foot**
  - M71.871 Other specified bursopathies, **right** ankle and foot
  - M71.872 Other specified bursopathies, **left** ankle and foot
  - M71.879 Other specified bursopathies, **unspecified** ankle and foot
- M71.88 Other specified bursopathies, **other site**
- M71.89 Other specified bursopathies, **multiple sites**

M71.9 Bursopathy, **unspecified**
Bursitis NOS

M72 Fibroblastic disorders

Excludes2 retroperitoneal fibromatosis (D48.3)

M72.0 Palmar fascial fibromatosis [Dupuytren] A

M72.1 Knuckle pads

M72.2 Plantar fascial fibromatosis
Plantar fasciitis

M72.4 Pseudosarcomatous fibromatosis
Nodular fasciitis

M72.6 Necrotizing fasciitis

Use additional code (B95.-, B96.-) to identify causative organism

M72.8 Other fibroblastic disorders
Abscess of fascia
Fasciitis NEC
Other infective fasciitis

Use additional code to (B95.-, B96.-) identify causative organism

Excludes1 diffuse (eosinophilic) fasciitis (M35.4)
necrotizing fasciitis (M72.6)
nodular fasciitis (M72.4)
perirenal fasciitis NOS (N13.5)
perirenal fasciitis with infection (N13.6)
plantar fasciitis (M72.2)

M72.9 Fibroblastic disorder, unspecified
Fasciitis NOS
Fibromatosis NOS

M75 Shoulder lesions

Excludes2 shoulder-hand syndrome (M89.0-)

M75.0 Adhesive capsulitis of shoulder
Frozen shoulder
Periarthritis of shoulder

M75.00 Adhesive capsulitis of unspecified shoulder

M75.01 Adhesive capsulitis of right shoulder

M75.02 Adhesive capsulitis of left shoulder
Coding Clinic: 2015, Q2, P23

M75.1 Rotator cuff tear or rupture, not specified as traumatic
Rotator cuff syndrome
Supraspinatus syndrome
Supraspinatus tear or rupture, not specified as traumatic

Excludes1 tear of rotator cuff, traumatic (S46.01-)

Gradual onset due to repetitive stress to rotator cuff

M75.10 Unspecified rotator cuff tear or rupture, not specified as traumatic

M75.100 Unspecified rotator cuff tear or rupture of unspecified shoulder, not specified as traumatic

M75.101 Unspecified rotator cuff tear or rupture of right shoulder, not specified as traumatic

M75.102 Unspecified rotator cuff tear or rupture of left shoulder, not specified as traumatic

M75.11 Incomplete rotator cuff tear or rupture not specified as traumatic

M75.110 Incomplete rotator cuff tear or rupture of unspecified shoulder, not specified as traumatic

M75.111 Incomplete rotator cuff tear or rupture of right shoulder, not specified as traumatic

M75.112 Incomplete rotator cuff tear or rupture of left shoulder, not specified as traumatic

M75.12 Complete rotator cuff tear or rupture not specified as traumatic

M75.120 Complete rotator cuff tear or rupture of unspecified shoulder, not specified as traumatic

M75.121 Complete rotator cuff tear or rupture of right shoulder, not specified as traumatic

M75.122 Complete rotator cuff tear or rupture of left shoulder, not specified as traumatic

M75.2 Bicipital tendinitis

M75.20 Bicipital tendinitis, unspecified shoulder

M75.21 Bicipital tendinitis, right shoulder

M75.22 Bicipital tendinitis, left shoulder

M75.3 Calcific tendinitis of shoulder
Calcified bursa of shoulder

M75.30 Calcific tendinitis of unspecified shoulder

M75.31 Calcific tendinitis of right shoulder

M75.32 Calcific tendinitis of left shoulder

M75.4 Impingement syndrome of shoulder

M75.40 Impingement syndrome of unspecified shoulder

M75.41 Impingement syndrome of right shoulder

M75.42 Impingement syndrome of left shoulder

M75.5 Bursitis of shoulder

M75.50 Bursitis of unspecified shoulder

M75.51 Bursitis of right shoulder

M75.52 Bursitis of left shoulder

M75.8 Other shoulder lesions

M75.80 Other shoulder lesions, unspecified shoulder

M75.81 Other shoulder lesions, right shoulder

M75.82 Other shoulder lesions, left shoulder

M75.9 Shoulder lesion, unspecified

M75.90 Shoulder lesion, unspecified, unspecified shoulder

M75.91 Shoulder lesion, unspecified, right shoulder

M75.92 Shoulder lesion, unspecified, left shoulder

M76 Enthesopathies, lower limb, excluding foot

Excludes2 bursitis due to use, overuse and pressure (M70.-)
enthesopathies of ankle and foot (M77.5-)

M76.0 Gluteal tendinitis

M76.00 Gluteal tendinitis, unspecified hip

M76.01 Gluteal tendinitis, right hip

M76.02 Gluteal tendinitis, left hip

M76.1 Psoas tendinitis

M76.10 Psoas tendinitis, unspecified hip

M76.11 Psoas tendinitis, right hip

M76.12 Psoas tendinitis, left hip

M76.2 Iliac crest spur

M76.20 Iliac crest spur, unspecified hip

M76.21 Iliac crest spur, right hip

M76.22 Iliac crest spur, left hip

M76.3 Iliotibial band syndrome

M76.30 Iliotibial band syndrome, unspecified leg

M76.31 Iliotibial band syndrome, right leg

M76.32 Iliotibial band syndrome, left leg

M76.4 Tibial collateral bursitis [Pellegrini-Stieda]

M76.40 Tibial collateral bursitis [Pellegrini-Stieda], unspecified leg

M76.41 Tibial collateral bursitis [Pellegrini-Stieda], right leg

M76.42 Tibial collateral bursitis [Pellegrini-Stieda], left leg

- M76.5 **Patellar tendinitis**
  - M76.50 **Patellar tendinitis, unspecified knee**
  - M76.51 **Patellar tendinitis, right knee**
  - M76.52 **Patellar tendinitis, left knee**
- M76.6 **Achilles tendinitis**
  - Achilles bursitis
  - M76.60 **Achilles tendinitis, unspecified leg**
  - M76.61 **Achilles tendinitis, right leg**
  - M76.62 **Achilles tendinitis, left leg**
- M76.7 **Peroneal tendinitis**
  - M76.70 **Peroneal tendinitis, unspecified leg**
  - M76.71 **Peroneal tendinitis, right leg**
  - M76.72 **Peroneal tendinitis, left leg**
- M76.8 **Other specified enthesopathies of lower limb, excluding foot**
  - M76.81 **Anterior tibial syndrome**
    - M76.811 **Anterior tibial syndrome, right leg**
    - M76.812 **Anterior tibial syndrome, left leg**
    - M76.819 **Anterior tibial syndrome, unspecified leg**
  - M76.82 **Posterior tibial tendinitis**
    - M76.821 **Posterior tibial tendinitis, right leg**
    - M76.822 **Posterior tibial tendinitis, left leg**
    - M76.829 **Posterior tibial tendinitis, unspecified leg**
  - M76.89 **Other specified enthesopathies of lower limb, excluding foot**
    - M76.891 **Other specified enthesopathies of right lower limb, excluding foot**
    - M76.892 **Other specified enthesopathies of left lower limb, excluding foot**
    - M76.899 **Other specified enthesopathies of unspecified lower limb, excluding foot**
- M76.9 **Unspecified enthesopathy, lower limb, excluding foot**

M77 Other enthesopathies

Excludes1 bursitis NOS (M71.9-)

Excludes2 bursitis due to use, overuse and pressure (M7Ø.-)
osteophyte (M25.7)
spinal enthesopathy (M46.Ø-)

- M77.Ø **Medial epicondylitis**
  - M77.ØØ **Medial epicondylitis, unspecified elbow**
  - M77.Ø1 **Medial epicondylitis, right elbow**
  - M77.Ø2 **Medial epicondylitis, left elbow**
- M77.1 **Lateral epicondylitis**
  - Tennis elbow
  - M77.1Ø **Lateral epicondylitis, unspecified elbow**
  - M77.11 **Lateral epicondylitis, right elbow**
  - M77.12 **Lateral epicondylitis, left elbow**
- M77.2 **Periarthritis of wrist**
  - M77.2Ø **Periarthritis, unspecified wrist**
  - M77.21 **Periarthritis, right wrist**
  - M77.22 **Periarthritis, left wrist**
- M77.3 **Calcaneal spur**
  - M77.3Ø **Calcaneal spur, unspecified foot**
  - M77.31 **Calcaneal spur, right foot**
  - M77.32 **Calcaneal spur, left foot**
- M77.4 **Metatarsalgia**
  - **Excludes1** Morton's metatarsalgia (G57.6)
  - M77.4Ø **Metatarsalgia, unspecified foot**
  - M77.41 **Metatarsalgia, right foot**
  - M77.42 **Metatarsalgia, left foot**
- M77.5 **Other enthesopathy of foot and ankle**
  - M77.5Ø **Other enthesopathy of unspecified foot and ankle**
  - M77.51 **Other enthesopathy of right foot and ankle**
  - M77.52 **Other enthesopathy of left foot and ankle**
- M77.8 **Other enthesopathies, not elsewhere classified**
- M77.9 **Enthesopathy, unspecified**
  - Bone spur NOS
  - Capsulitis NOS
  - Periarthritis NOS
  - Tendinitis NOS

M79 Other and unspecified soft tissue disorders, not elsewhere classified

Excludes1 psychogenic rheumatism (F45.8)
soft tissue pain, psychogenic (F45.41)

- M79.Ø **Rheumatism, unspecified**
  - **Excludes1** fibromyalgia (M79.7)
    palindromic rheumatism (M12.3-)
- M79.1 **Myalgia**
  - Myofascial pain syndrome
  - M79.1Ø **Myalgia, unspecified site**
  - M79.11 **Myalgia of mastication muscle**
  - M79.12 **Myalgia of auxiliary muscles, head and neck**
  - M79.18 **Myalgia, other site**
    - **Excludes1** fibromyalgia (M79.7)
      myositis (M6Ø.-)
- M79.2 **Neuralgia and neuritis, unspecified**
  - **Excludes1** brachial radiculitis NOS (M54.1)
    lumbosacral radiculitis NOS (M54.1)
    mononeuropathies (G56-G58)
    radiculitis NOS (M54.1)
    sciatica (M54.3-M54.4)
- M79.3 **Panniculitis, unspecified**
  - **Excludes1** lupus panniculitis (L93.2)
    neck and back panniculitis (M54.Ø-)
    relapsing [Weber-Christian] panniculitis (M35.6)
- M79.4 **Hypertrophy of (infrapatellar) fat pad**
- M79.5 **Residual foreign body in soft tissue**
  - **Excludes1** foreign body granuloma of skin and subcutaneous tissue (L92.3)
    foreign body granuloma of soft tissue (M6Ø.2-)
- M79.6 **Pain in limb, hand, foot, fingers and toes**
  - **Excludes2** pain in joint (M25.5-)
  - M79.6Ø **Pain in limb, unspecified**
    - M79.6Ø1 **Pain in right arm**
      - Pain in right upper limb NOS
    - M79.6Ø2 **Pain in left arm**
      - Pain in left upper limb NOS
    - M79.6Ø3 **Pain in arm, unspecified**
      - Pain in upper limb NOS
    - M79.6Ø4 **Pain in right leg**
      - Pain in right lower limb NOS
    - M79.6Ø5 **Pain in left leg**
      - Pain in left lower limb NOS
    - M79.6Ø6 **Pain in leg, unspecified**
      - Pain in lower limb NOS
    - M79.6Ø9 **Pain in unspecified limb**
      - Pain in limb NOS
  - M79.62 **Pain in upper arm**
    - Pain in axillary region
    - M79.621 **Pain in right upper arm**
    - M79.622 **Pain in left upper arm**
    - M79.629 **Pain in unspecified upper arm**
  - M79.63 **Pain in forearm**
    - M79.631 **Pain in right forearm**
    - M79.632 **Pain in left forearm**
    - M79.639 **Pain in unspecified forearm**

CHAPTER 13 (MØØ-M99)

M79.64 Pain in hand and fingers
- M79.641 Pain in right hand
- M79.642 Pain in left hand
- M79.643 Pain in unspecified hand
- M79.644 Pain in right finger(s)
- M79.645 Pain in left finger(s)
- M79.646 Pain in unspecified finger(s)

M79.65 Pain in thigh
- M79.651 Pain in right thigh
- M79.652 Pain in left thigh
- M79.659 Pain in unspecified thigh

M79.66 Pain in lower leg
- M79.661 Pain in right lower leg
- M79.662 Pain in left lower leg
- M79.669 Pain in unspecified lower leg

M79.67 Pain in foot and toes
- M79.671 Pain in right foot
- M79.672 Pain in left foot
- M79.673 Pain in unspecified foot
- M79.674 Pain in right toe(s)
- M79.675 Pain in left toe(s)
- M79.676 Pain in unspecified toe(s)

M79.7 Fibromyalgia
Fibromyositis
Fibrositis
Myofibrositis

M79.A Nontraumatic compartment syndrome
Code first, if applicable, associated postprocedural complication
Excludes1 compartment syndrome NOS (T79.A-)
fibromyalgia (M79.7) nontraumatic ischemic infarction of muscle (M62.2-)
traumatic compartment syndrome (T79.A-)

M79.A1 Nontraumatic compartment syndrome of upper extremity
Nontraumatic compartment syndrome of shoulder, arm, forearm, wrist, hand, and fingers
- M79.A11 Nontraumatic compartment syndrome of right upper extremity
- M79.A12 Nontraumatic compartment syndrome of left upper extremity
- M79.A19 Nontraumatic compartment syndrome of unspecified upper extremity

M79.A2 Nontraumatic compartment syndrome of lower extremity
Nontraumatic compartment syndrome of hip, buttock, thigh, leg, foot, and toes
- M79.A21 Nontraumatic compartment syndrome of right lower extremity
- M79.A22 Nontraumatic compartment syndrome of left lower extremity
- M79.A29 Nontraumatic compartment syndrome of unspecified lower extremity

M79.A3 Nontraumatic compartment syndrome of abdomen

M79.A9 Nontraumatic compartment syndrome of other sites

M79.8 Other specified soft tissue disorders
- M79.81 Nontraumatic hematoma of soft tissue
  Nontraumatic hematoma of muscle
  Nontraumatic seroma of muscle and soft tissue
- M79.89 Other specified soft tissue disorders
  Polyalgia

M79.9 Soft tissue disorder, unspecified

OGCR See Section I.C., Chapter 13.d.

Osteoporosis

Osteoporosis is a systemic condition, meaning that all bones of the musculoskeletal system are affected. Therefore, site is not a component of the codes under category M81, Osteoporosis without current pathological fracture. The site codes under category M80, Osteoporosis with current pathological fracture, identify the site of the fracture, not the osteoporosis.

1) Osteoporosis without pathological fracture

Category M81, Osteoporosis without current pathological fracture, is for use for patients with osteoporosis who do not currently have a pathologic fracture due to the osteoporosis, even if they have had a fracture in the past. For patients with a history of osteoporosis fractures, status code Z87.310, Personal history of (healed) osteoporosis fracture, should follow the code from M81.

2) Osteoporosis with current pathological fracture

Category M80, Osteoporosis with current pathological fracture, is for patients who have a current pathologic fracture at the time of an encounter. The codes under M80 identify the site of the fracture. A code from category M80, not a traumatic fracture code, should be used for any patient with known osteoporosis who suffers a fracture, even if the patient had a minor fall or trauma, if that fall or trauma would not usually break a normal, healthy bone.

OSTEOPATHIES AND CHONDROPATHIES (M80-M94)

DISORDERS OF BONE DENSITY AND STRUCTURE (M80-M85)

M80 Osteoporosis with current pathological fracture
Excessive skeletal fragility (porous bone) resulting in bone fractures
Includes osteoporosis with current fragility fracture
Use additional code to identify major osseous defect, if applicable (M89.7-)
Excludes1 collapsed vertebra NOS (M48.5)
pathological fracture NOS (M84.4)
wedging of vertebra NOS (M48.5)
Excludes2 personal history of (healed) osteoporosis fracture (Z87.310)
Coding Clinic: 2018, Q2, P12
The appropriate 7th character is to be added to each code from category M80:

A	initial encounter for fracture *All encounters involving diagnosis and treatment*
D	subsequent encounter for fracture with routine healing
G	subsequent encounter for fracture with delayed healing *Encounters for attention to casting or fixation devices, medication, and follow-up visits during the healing phase*
K	subsequent encounter for fracture with nonunion *Total failure of fracture healing*
P	subsequent encounter for fracture with malunion *Fracture ends do not heal together correctly.*
S	sequela

M80.0 Age-related osteoporosis with current pathological fracture
Involutional osteoporosis with current pathological fracture
Osteoporosis NOS with current pathological fracture
Postmenopausal osteoporosis with current pathological fracture
Senile osteoporosis with current pathological fracture
- X M80.00 Age-related osteoporosis with current pathological fracture, unspecified site A
- M80.01 Age-related osteoporosis with current pathological fracture, shoulder
  - M80.011 Age-related osteoporosis with current pathological fracture, right shoulder A
  - M80.012 Age-related osteoporosis with current pathological fracture, left shoulder A
  - M80.019 Age-related osteoporosis with current pathological fracture, unspecified shoulder A

CHAPTER 13 (M00-M99)

M80.02 Age-related osteoporosis with current pathological fracture, **humerus**

M80.021 Age-related osteoporosis with current pathological fracture, **right humerus** A

M80.022 Age-related osteoporosis with current pathological fracture, **left humerus** A

M80.029 Age-related osteoporosis with current pathological fracture, **unspecified** humerus A

M80.03 Age-related osteoporosis with current pathological fracture, **forearm**

Age-related osteoporosis with current pathological fracture of wrist

M80.031 Age-related osteoporosis with current pathological fracture, **right forearm** A

M80.032 Age-related osteoporosis with current pathological fracture, **left forearm** A

M80.039 Age-related osteoporosis with current pathological fracture, **unspecified** forearm A

M80.04 Age-related osteoporosis with current pathological fracture, **hand**

M80.041 Age-related osteoporosis with current pathological fracture, **right hand** A

M80.042 Age-related osteoporosis with current pathological fracture, **left hand** A

M80.049 Age-related osteoporosis with current pathological fracture, **unspecified** hand A

M80.05 Age-related osteoporosis with current pathological fracture, **femur**

Age-related osteoporosis with current pathological fracture of hip

M80.051 Age-related osteoporosis with current pathological fracture, **right** femur A A

M80.052 Age-related osteoporosis with current pathological fracture, **left femur** A A

Coding Clinic: 2018, Q2, P12

M80.059 Age-related osteoporosis with current pathological fracture, **unspecified** femur A A

M80.06 Age-related osteoporosis with current pathological fracture, **lower leg**

M80.061 Age-related osteoporosis with current pathological fracture, **right** lower leg A

M80.062 Age-related osteoporosis with current pathological fracture, **left** lower leg A

M80.069 Age-related osteoporosis with current pathological fracture, **unspecified** lower leg A

M80.07 Age-related osteoporosis with current pathological fracture, **ankle and foot**

M80.071 Age-related osteoporosis with current pathological fracture, **right** ankle and foot A

M80.072 Age-related osteoporosis with current pathological fracture, **left** ankle and foot A

M80.079 Age-related osteoporosis with current pathological fracture, **unspecified** ankle and foot A

X M80.08 Age-related osteoporosis with current pathological fracture, **vertebra(e)** A A

M80.8 Other osteoporosis with current pathological fracture

Drug-induced osteoporosis with current pathological fracture

Idiopathic osteoporosis with current pathological fracture

Osteoporosis of disuse with current pathological fracture

Postoophorectomy osteoporosis with current pathological fracture

Postsurgical malabsorption osteoporosis with current pathological fracture

Post-traumatic osteoporosis with current pathological fracture

Use additional code for adverse effect, if applicable, to identify drug (T36-T50 with fifth or sixth character 5)

X M80.80 Other osteoporosis with current pathological fracture, **unspecified site** A

M80.81 Other osteoporosis with pathological fracture, **shoulder**

M80.811 Other osteoporosis with current pathological fracture, **right shoulder**

M80.812 Other osteoporosis with current pathological fracture, **left shoulder**

M80.819 Other osteoporosis with current pathological fracture, **unspecified** shoulder

M80.82 Other osteoporosis with current pathological fracture, **humerus**

M80.821 Other osteoporosis with current pathological fracture, **right humerus**

M80.822 Other osteoporosis with current pathological fracture, **left humerus**

M80.829 Other osteoporosis with current pathological fracture, **unspecified** humerus

M80.83 Other osteoporosis with current pathological fracture, **forearm**

Other osteoporosis with current pathological fracture of wrist

M80.831 Other osteoporosis with current pathological fracture, **right forearm**

M80.832 Other osteoporosis with current pathological fracture, **left forearm**

M80.839 Other osteoporosis with current pathological fracture, **unspecified** forearm

M80.84 Other osteoporosis with current pathological fracture, **hand**

M80.841 Other osteoporosis with current pathological fracture, **right hand**

M80.842 Other osteoporosis with current pathological fracture, **left hand**

M80.849 Other osteoporosis with current pathological fracture, **unspecified** hand

M80.85 Other osteoporosis with current pathological fracture, **femur**

Other osteoporosis with current pathological fracture of hip

M80.851 Other osteoporosis with current pathological fracture, **right** femur A

M80.852 Other osteoporosis with current pathological fracture, **left femur** A

M80.859 Other osteoporosis with current pathological fracture, **unspecified** femur A

M80.86 Other osteoporosis with current pathological fracture, lower leg
M80.861 Other osteoporosis with current pathological fracture, right lower leg
M80.862 Other osteoporosis with current pathological fracture, left lower leg
M80.869 Other osteoporosis with current pathological fracture, unspecified lower leg
M80.87 Other osteoporosis with current pathological fracture, ankle and foot
M80.871 Other osteoporosis with current pathological fracture, right ankle and foot
M80.872 Other osteoporosis with current pathological fracture, left ankle and foot
M80.879 Other osteoporosis with current pathological fracture, unspecified ankle and foot
X M80.88 Other osteoporosis with current pathological fracture, vertebra(e) A

M81 Osteoporosis without current pathological fracture
Use additional code to identify:
major osseous defect, if applicable (M89.7-)
personal history of (healed) osteoporosis fracture, if applicable (Z87.310)
Excludes1 osteoporosis with current pathological fracture (M80.-)
Sudeck's atrophy (M89.0)

M81.0 Age-related osteoporosis without current pathological fracture A
Involutional osteoporosis without current pathological fracture
Osteoporosis NOS
Postmenopausal osteoporosis without current pathological fracture
Senile osteoporosis without current pathological fracture

M81.6 Localized osteoporosis [Lequesne]
Excludes1 Sudeck's atrophy (M89.0)

M81.8 Other osteoporosis without current pathological fracture
Drug-induced osteoporosis without current pathological fracture
Idiopathic osteoporosis without current pathological fracture
Osteoporosis of disuse without current pathological fracture
Postoophorectomy osteoporosis without current pathological fracture
Postsurgical malabsorption osteoporosis without current pathological fracture
Post-traumatic osteoporosis without current pathological fracture
Use additional code for adverse effect, if applicable, to identify drug (T36-T50 with fifth or sixth character 5)

M83 Adult osteomalacia
Excludes1 infantile and juvenile osteomalacia (E55.0)
renal osteodystrophy (N25.0)
rickets (active) (E55.0)
rickets (active) sequelae (E64.3)
vitamin D-resistant osteomalacia (E83.3)
vitamin D-resistant rickets (active) (E83.3)

M83.0 Puerperal osteomalacia ♀ M
M83.1 Senile osteomalacia A
M83.2 Adult osteomalacia due to malabsorption A
Postsurgical malabsorption osteomalacia in adults
M83.3 Adult osteomalacia due to malnutrition A
M83.4 Aluminum bone disease
M83.5 Other drug-induced osteomalacia in adults A
Use additional code for adverse effect, if applicable, to identify drug (T36-T50 with fifth or sixth character 5)
M83.8 Other adult osteomalacia A
M83.9 Adult osteomalacia, unspecified A

M84 Disorder of continuity of bone
Excludes2 traumatic fracture of bone-see fracture, by site

M84.3 Stress fracture
Fatigue fracture
March fracture
Stress fracture NOS
Stress reaction
Use additional external cause code(s) to identify the cause of the stress fracture
Excludes1 pathological fracture NOS (M84.4.-)
pathological fracture due to osteoporosis (M80.-)
traumatic fracture (S12.-, S22.-, S32.-, S42.-, S52.-, S62.-, S72.-, S82.-, S92.-)
Excludes2 personal history of (healed) stress (fatigue) fracture (Z87.312)
stress fracture of vertebra (M48.4-)
The appropriate 7th character is to be added to each code from subcategory M84.3:

A	initial encounter for fracture
D	subsequent encounter for fracture with routine healing
G	subsequent encounter for fracture with delayed healing
K	subsequent encounter for fracture with nonunion
P	subsequent encounter for fracture with malunion
S	sequela

X M84.30 Stress fracture, unspecified site
M84.31 Stress fracture, shoulder
M84.311 Stress fracture, right shoulder
M84.312 Stress fracture, left shoulder
M84.319 Stress fracture, unspecified shoulder
M84.32 Stress fracture, humerus
M84.321 Stress fracture, right humerus
M84.322 Stress fracture, left humerus
M84.329 Stress fracture, unspecified humerus
M84.33 Stress fracture, ulna and radius
M84.331 Stress fracture, right ulna
M84.332 Stress fracture, left ulna
M84.333 Stress fracture, right radius
M84.334 Stress fracture, left radius
M84.339 Stress fracture, unspecified ulna and radius
M84.34 Stress fracture, hand and fingers
M84.341 Stress fracture, right hand
M84.342 Stress fracture, left hand
M84.343 Stress fracture, unspecified hand
M84.344 Stress fracture, right finger(s)
M84.345 Stress fracture, left finger(s)
M84.346 Stress fracture, unspecified finger(s)
M84.35 Stress fracture, pelvis and femur
Stress fracture, hip
M84.350 Stress fracture, pelvis
M84.351 Stress fracture, right femur
M84.352 Stress fracture, left femur
M84.353 Stress fracture, unspecified femur
M84.359 Stress fracture, hip, unspecified
M84.36 Stress fracture, tibia and fibula
M84.361 Stress fracture, right tibia
M84.362 Stress fracture, left tibia
M84.363 Stress fracture, right fibula
M84.364 Stress fracture, left fibula
M84.369 Stress fracture, unspecified tibia and fibula

CHAPTER 13 (M00-M99)

● M84.37 Stress fracture, **ankle, foot and toes**

- ● M84.371 Stress fracture, **right ankle**
- ● M84.372 Stress fracture, **left ankle**
- ● M84.373 Stress fracture, **unspecified ankle**
- ● M84.374 Stress fracture, **right foot**
- ● M84.375 Stress fracture, **left foot**
- ● M84.376 Stress fracture, **unspecified foot**
- ● M84.377 Stress fracture, **right toe(s)**
- ● M84.378 Stress fracture, **left toe(s)**
- ● M84.379 Stress fracture, **unspecified toe(s)**

X● M84.38 Stress fracture, **other site**

Excludes2 stress fracture of vertebra (M48.4-)

● **M84.4 Pathological fracture, not elsewhere classified**

Chronic fracture
Pathological fracture NOS

Excludes1 collapsed vertebra NEC (M48.5)
pathological fracture in neoplastic disease (M84.5-)
pathological fracture in osteoporosis (M8Ø.-)
pathological fracture in other disease (M84.6-)
stress fracture (M84.3-)
traumatic fracture (S12.-, S22.-, S32.-, S42.-, S52.-, S62.-, S72.-, S82.-, S92.-)

Excludes2 personal history of (healed) pathological fracture (Z87.311)

The appropriate 7th character is to be added to each code from subcategory M84.4:

A	initial encounter for fracture
D	subsequent encounter for fracture with routine healing
G	subsequent encounter for fracture with delayed healing
K	subsequent encounter for fracture with nonunion
P	subsequent encounter for fracture with malunion
S	sequela

X● M84.4Ø Pathological fracture, **unspecified site**

● M84.41 Pathological fracture, **shoulder**

- ● M84.411 Pathological fracture, **right shoulder**
- ● M84.412 Pathological fracture, **left shoulder**
- ● M84.419 Pathological fracture, **unspecified shoulder**

● M84.42 Pathological fracture, **humerus**

- ● M84.421 Pathological fracture, **right humerus**
- ● M84.422 Pathological fracture, **left humerus**
- ● M84.429 Pathological fracture, **unspecified humerus**

● M84.43 Pathological fracture, **ulna and radius**

- ● M84.431 Pathological fracture, **right ulna**
- ● M84.432 Pathological fracture, **left ulna**
- ● M84.433 Pathological fracture, **right radius**
- ● M84.434 Pathological fracture, **left radius**
- ● M84.439 Pathological fracture, **unspecified ulna and radius**

● M84.44 Pathological fracture, **hand and fingers**

- ● M84.441 Pathological fracture, **right hand**
- ● M84.442 Pathological fracture, **left hand**
- ● M84.443 Pathological fracture, **unspecified hand**
- ● M84.444 Pathological fracture, **right finger(s)**
- ● M84.445 Pathological fracture, **left finger(s)**
- ● M84.446 Pathological fracture, **unspecified finger(s)**

● M84.45 Pathological fracture, **femur and pelvis**

- ● M84.451 Pathological fracture, **right femur** A
- ● M84.452 Pathological fracture, **left femur** A
- ● M84.453 Pathological fracture, **unspecified femur** A
- ● M84.454 Pathological fracture, **pelvis** A
  Coding Clinic: 2Ø16, Q4, P43
- ● M84.459 Pathological fracture, **hip, unspecified** A

● M84.46 Pathological fracture, **tibia and fibula**

- ● M84.461 Pathological fracture, **right tibia**
- ● M84.462 Pathological fracture, **left tibia**
- ● M84.463 Pathological fracture, **right fibula**
- ● M84.464 Pathological fracture, **left fibula**
- ● M84.469 Pathological fracture, **unspecified tibia and fibula**

● M84.47 Pathological fracture, **ankle, foot and toes**

- ● M84.471 Pathological fracture, **right ankle**
- ● M84.472 Pathological fracture, **left ankle**
- ● M84.473 Pathological fracture, **unspecified ankle**
- ● M84.474 Pathological fracture, **right foot**
- ● M84.475 Pathological fracture, **left foot**
- ● M84.476 Pathological fracture, **unspecified foot**
- ● M84.477 Pathological fracture, **right toe(s)**
- ● M84.478 Pathological fracture, **left toe(s)**
- ● M84.479 Pathological fracture, **unspecified toe(s)**

X● M84.48 Pathological fracture, **other site**

OGCR Section I.C. 13.C.

Coding of Pathologic Fractures

7th character A is for use as long as the patient is receiving active treatment for the fracture. While the patient may be seen by a new or different provider over the course of treatment for a pathological fracture, assignment of the 7th character is based on whether the patient is undergoing active treatment and not whether the provider is seeing the patient for the first time.

7th character, D is to be used for encounters after the patient has completed active treatment for the fracture and is receiving routine care for the fracture during the healing or recovery phase. The other 7th characters, listed under each subcategory in the Tabular List, are to be used for subsequent encounters for treatment of problems associated with the healing, such as malunions, nonunions, and sequelae.

Care for complications of surgical treatment for fracture repairs during the healing or recovery phase should be coded with the appropriate complication codes.

See Section I.C.19. Coding of traumatic fractures.

● **M84.5 Pathological fracture in neoplastic disease**

Code also underlying neoplasm

The appropriate 7th character is to be added to each code from subcategory M84.5:

A	initial encounter for fracture
D	subsequent encounter for fracture with routine healing
G	subsequent encounter for fracture with delayed healing
K	subsequent encounter for fracture with nonunion
P	subsequent encounter for fracture with malunion
S	sequela

X● M84.5Ø Pathological fracture in neoplastic disease, **unspecified site**

● M84.51 Pathological fracture in neoplastic disease, **shoulder**

- ● M84.511 Pathological fracture in neoplastic disease, **right shoulder**
- ● M84.512 Pathological fracture in neoplastic disease, **left shoulder**
- ● M84.519 Pathological fracture in neoplastic disease, **unspecified shoulder**

New Revised ~~deleted~~ Deleted Excludes 1 Excludes 2 Includes Use additional Code first Code also Key words
OGCR Official Guidelines X Assign placeholder X ● Use Additional Character(s) Manifestation Code Hierarchical Condition Category Coding Clinic

M84.52 Pathological fracture in neoplastic disease, humerus
- M84.521 Pathological fracture in neoplastic disease, right humerus
- M84.522 Pathological fracture in neoplastic disease, left humerus
- M84.529 Pathological fracture in neoplastic disease, unspecified humerus

M84.53 Pathological fracture in neoplastic disease, ulna and radius
- M84.531 Pathological fracture in neoplastic disease, right ulna
- M84.532 Pathological fracture in neoplastic disease, left ulna
- M84.533 Pathological fracture in neoplastic disease, right radius
- M84.534 Pathological fracture in neoplastic disease, left radius
- M84.539 Pathological fracture in neoplastic disease, unspecified ulna and radius

M84.54 Pathological fracture in neoplastic disease, hand
- M84.541 Pathological fracture in neoplastic disease, right hand
- M84.542 Pathological fracture in neoplastic disease, left hand
- M84.549 Pathological fracture in neoplastic disease, unspecified hand

M84.55 Pathological fracture in neoplastic disease, pelvis and femur
- M84.550 Pathological fracture in neoplastic disease, pelvis
- M84.551 Pathological fracture in neoplastic disease, right femur A
- M84.552 Pathological fracture in neoplastic disease, left femur A
- M84.553 Pathological fracture in neoplastic disease, unspecified femur A
- M84.559 Pathological fracture in neoplastic disease, hip, unspecified A

M84.56 Pathological fracture in neoplastic disease, tibia and fibula
- M84.561 Pathological fracture in neoplastic disease, right tibia
- M84.562 Pathological fracture in neoplastic disease, left tibia
- M84.563 Pathological fracture in neoplastic disease, right fibula
- M84.564 Pathological fracture in neoplastic disease, left fibula
- M84.569 Pathological fracture in neoplastic disease, unspecified tibia and fibula

M84.57 Pathological fracture in neoplastic disease, ankle and foot
- M84.571 Pathological fracture in neoplastic disease, right ankle
- M84.572 Pathological fracture in neoplastic disease, left ankle
- M84.573 Pathological fracture in neoplastic disease, unspecified ankle
- M84.574 Pathological fracture in neoplastic disease, right foot
- M84.575 Pathological fracture in neoplastic disease, left foot
- M84.576 Pathological fracture in neoplastic disease, unspecified foot

X M84.58 Pathological fracture in neoplastic disease, other specified site

Pathological fracture in neoplastic disease, vertebrae

M84.6 Pathological fracture in other disease

Code also underlying condition

Excludes1 pathological fracture in osteoporosis (M8Ø.-)

The appropriate 7th character is to be added to each code from subcategory M84.6:

A	initial encounter for fracture
D	subsequent encounter for fracture with routine healing
G	subsequent encounter for fracture with delayed healing
K	subsequent encounter for fracture with nonunion
P	subsequent encounter for fracture with malunion
S	sequela

X M84.6Ø Pathological fracture in other disease, unspecified site

M84.61 Pathological fracture in other disease, shoulder
- M84.611 Pathological fracture in other disease, right shoulder
- M84.612 Pathological fracture in other disease, left shoulder
- M84.619 Pathological fracture in other disease, unspecified shoulder

M84.62 Pathological fracture in other disease, humerus
- M84.621 Pathological fracture in other disease, right humerus
- M84.622 Pathological fracture in other disease, left humerus
- M84.629 Pathological fracture in other disease, unspecified humerus

M84.63 Pathological fracture in other disease, ulna and radius
- M84.631 Pathological fracture in other disease, right ulna
- M84.632 Pathological fracture in other disease, left ulna
- M84.633 Pathological fracture in other disease, right radius
- M84.634 Pathological fracture in other disease, left radius
- M84.639 Pathological fracture in other disease, unspecified ulna and radius

M84.64 Pathological fracture in other disease, hand
- M84.641 Pathological fracture in other disease, right hand
- M84.642 Pathological fracture in other disease, left hand
- M84.649 Pathological fracture in other disease, unspecified hand

M84.65 Pathological fracture in other disease, pelvis and femur
- M84.65Ø Pathological fracture in other disease, pelvis
- M84.651 Pathological fracture in other disease, right femur A
- M84.652 Pathological fracture in other disease, left femur A
- M84.653 Pathological fracture in other disease, unspecified femur A
- M84.659 Pathological fracture in other disease, hip, unspecified A

CHAPTER 13 (MØØ-M99)

● M84.66 Pathological fracture in other disease, **tibia and fibula**
● M84.661 Pathological fracture in other disease, **right tibia**
● M84.662 Pathological fracture in other disease, **left tibia**
● M84.663 Pathological fracture in other disease, **right fibula**
● M84.664 Pathological fracture in other disease, **left fibula**
● M84.669 Pathological fracture in other disease, **unspecified tibia and fibula**
● M84.67 Pathological fracture in other disease, **ankle and foot**
● M84.671 Pathological fracture in other disease, **right ankle**
● M84.672 Pathological fracture in other disease, **left ankle**
● M84.673 Pathological fracture in other disease, **unspecified ankle**
● M84.674 Pathological fracture in other disease, **right foot**
● M84.675 Pathological fracture in other disease, **left foot**
● M84.676 Pathological fracture in other disease, **unspecified foot**
X● M84.68 Pathological fracture in other disease, **other site**
● M84.7 Nontraumatic fracture, not elsewhere classified
● M84.75 Atypical femoral fracture

The appropriate 7th character is to be added to each code from M84.75:

A	initial encounter for fracture
D	subsequent encounter for fracture with routine healing
G	subsequent encounter for fracture with delayed healing
K	subsequent encounter for fracture with nonunion
P	subsequent encounter for fracture with malunion
S	sequela

Coding Clinic: 2016, Q4, P41

● M84.750 Atypical femoral fracture, **unspecified**
● M84.751 **Incomplete** atypical femoral fracture, **right leg**
● M84.752 **Incomplete** atypical femoral fracture, **left leg**
● M84.753 **Incomplete** atypical femoral fracture, **unspecified leg**
● M84.754 **Complete transverse** atypical femoral fracture, **right leg** A HCC
● M84.755 **Complete transverse** atypical femoral fracture, **left leg** A HCC
● M84.756 **Complete transverse** atypical femoral fracture, **unspecified leg** A HCC
● M84.757 **Complete oblique** atypical femoral fracture, **right leg** A HCC
● M84.758 **Complete oblique** atypical femoral fracture, **left leg** A HCC
● M84.759 **Complete oblique** atypical femoral fracture, **unspecified leg** , A HCC

● M84.8 Other disorders of continuity of bone
M84.80 Other disorders of continuity of bone, **unspecified site**
● M84.81 Other disorders of continuity of bone, **shoulder**
M84.811 Other disorders of continuity of bone, **right shoulder**
M84.812 Other disorders of continuity of bone, **left shoulder**
M84.819 Other disorders of continuity of bone, **unspecified shoulder**
● M84.82 Other disorders of continuity of bone, **humerus**
M84.821 Other disorders of continuity of bone, **right humerus**
M84.822 Other disorders of continuity of bone, **left humerus**
M84.829 Other disorders of continuity of bone, **unspecified humerus**
● M84.83 Other disorders of continuity of bone, **ulna and radius**
M84.831 Other disorders of continuity of bone, **right ulna**
M84.832 Other disorders of continuity of bone, **left ulna**
M84.833 Other disorders of continuity of bone, **right radius**
M84.834 Other disorders of continuity of bone, **left radius**
M84.839 Other disorders of continuity of bone, **unspecified ulna and radius**
● M84.84 Other disorders of continuity of bone, **hand**
M84.841 Other disorders of continuity of bone, **right hand**
M84.842 Other disorders of continuity of bone, **left hand**
M84.849 Other disorders of continuity of bone, **unspecified hand**
● M84.85 Other disorders of continuity of bone, **pelvic region and thigh**
M84.851 Other disorders of continuity of bone, **right pelvic region and thigh**
M84.852 Other disorders of continuity of bone, **left pelvic region and thigh**
M84.859 Other disorders of continuity of bone, **unspecified pelvic region and thigh**
● M84.86 Other disorders of continuity of bone, **tibia and fibula**
M84.861 Other disorders of continuity of bone, **right tibia**
M84.862 Other disorders of continuity of bone, **left tibia**
M84.863 Other disorders of continuity of bone, **right fibula**
M84.864 Other disorders of continuity of bone, **left fibula**
M84.869 Other disorders of continuity of bone, **unspecified tibia and fibula**
● M84.87 Other disorders of continuity of bone, **ankle and foot**
M84.871 Other disorders of continuity of bone, **right ankle and foot**
M84.872 Other disorders of continuity of bone, **left ankle and foot**
M84.879 Other disorders of continuity of bone, **unspecified ankle and foot**
M84.88 Other disorders of continuity of bone, **other site**
M84.9 Disorder of continuity of bone, **unspecified**

M85 Other disorders of bone density and structure

Excludes1 osteogenesis imperfecta (Q78.Ø)
osteopetrosis (Q78.2)
osteopoikilosis (Q78.8)
polyostotic fibrous dysplasia (Q78.1)

M85.Ø Fibrous dysplasia (monostotic)

Excludes2 fibrous dysplasia of jaw (M27.8)

M85.ØØ Fibrous dysplasia (monostotic), unspecified site
M85.Ø1 Fibrous dysplasia (monostotic), shoulder
M85.Ø11 Fibrous dysplasia (monostotic), right shoulder
M85.Ø12 Fibrous dysplasia (monostotic), left shoulder
M85.Ø19 Fibrous dysplasia (monostotic), unspecified shoulder
M85.Ø2 Fibrous dysplasia (monostotic), upper arm
M85.Ø21 Fibrous dysplasia (monostotic), right upper arm
M85.Ø22 Fibrous dysplasia (monostotic), left upper arm
M85.Ø29 Fibrous dysplasia (monostotic), unspecified upper arm
M85.Ø3 Fibrous dysplasia (monostotic), forearm
M85.Ø31 Fibrous dysplasia (monostotic), right forearm
M85.Ø32 Fibrous dysplasia (monostotic), left forearm
M85.Ø39 Fibrous dysplasia (monostotic), unspecified forearm
M85.Ø4 Fibrous dysplasia (monostotic), hand
M85.Ø41 Fibrous dysplasia (monostotic), right hand
M85.Ø42 Fibrous dysplasia (monostotic), left hand
M85.Ø49 Fibrous dysplasia (monostotic), unspecified hand
M85.Ø5 Fibrous dysplasia (monostotic), thigh
M85.Ø51 Fibrous dysplasia (monostotic), right thigh
M85.Ø52 Fibrous dysplasia (monostotic), left thigh
M85.Ø59 Fibrous dysplasia (monostotic), unspecified thigh
M85.Ø6 Fibrous dysplasia (monostotic), lower leg
M85.Ø61 Fibrous dysplasia (monostotic), right lower leg
M85.Ø62 Fibrous dysplasia (monostotic), left lower leg
M85.Ø69 Fibrous dysplasia (monostotic), unspecified lower leg
M85.Ø7 Fibrous dysplasia (monostotic), ankle and foot
M85.Ø71 Fibrous dysplasia (monostotic), right ankle and foot
M85.Ø72 Fibrous dysplasia (monostotic), left ankle and foot
M85.Ø79 Fibrous dysplasia (monostotic), unspecified ankle and foot
M85.Ø8 Fibrous dysplasia (monostotic), other site
M85.Ø9 Fibrous dysplasia (monostotic), multiple sites

M85.1 Skeletal fluorosis

M85.1Ø Skeletal fluorosis, unspecified site
M85.11 Skeletal fluorosis, shoulder
M85.111 Skeletal fluorosis, right shoulder
M85.112 Skeletal fluorosis, left shoulder
M85.119 Skeletal fluorosis, unspecified shoulder
M85.12 Skeletal fluorosis, upper arm
M85.121 Skeletal fluorosis, right upper arm
M85.122 Skeletal fluorosis, left upper arm
M85.129 Skeletal fluorosis, unspecified upper arm
M85.13 Skeletal fluorosis, forearm
M85.131 Skeletal fluorosis, right forearm
M85.132 Skeletal fluorosis, left forearm
M85.139 Skeletal fluorosis, unspecified forearm
M85.14 Skeletal fluorosis, hand
M85.141 Skeletal fluorosis, right hand
M85.142 Skeletal fluorosis, left hand
M85.149 Skeletal fluorosis, unspecified hand
M85.15 Skeletal fluorosis, thigh
M85.151 Skeletal fluorosis, right thigh
M85.152 Skeletal fluorosis, left thigh
M85.159 Skeletal fluorosis, unspecified thigh
M85.16 Skeletal fluorosis, lower leg
M85.161 Skeletal fluorosis, right lower leg
M85.162 Skeletal fluorosis, left lower leg
M85.169 Skeletal fluorosis, unspecified lower leg
M85.17 Skeletal fluorosis, ankle and foot
M85.171 Skeletal fluorosis, right ankle and foot
M85.172 Skeletal fluorosis, left ankle and foot
M85.179 Skeletal fluorosis, unspecified ankle and foot
M85.18 Skeletal fluorosis, other site
M85.19 Skeletal fluorosis, multiple sites

M85.2 Hyperostosis of skull

M85.3 Osteitis condensans

M85.3Ø Osteitis condensans, unspecified site
M85.31 Osteitis condensans, shoulder
M85.311 Osteitis condensans, right shoulder
M85.312 Osteitis condensans, left shoulder
M85.319 Osteitis condensans, unspecified shoulder
M85.32 Osteitis condensans, upper arm
M85.321 Osteitis condensans, right upper arm
M85.322 Osteitis condensans, left upper arm
M85.329 Osteitis condensans, unspecified upper arm
M85.33 Osteitis condensans, forearm
M85.331 Osteitis condensans, right forearm
M85.332 Osteitis condensans, left forearm
M85.339 Osteitis condensans, unspecified forearm
M85.34 Osteitis condensans, hand
M85.341 Osteitis condensans, right hand
M85.342 Osteitis condensans, left hand
M85.349 Osteitis condensans, unspecified hand
M85.35 Osteitis condensans, thigh
M85.351 Osteitis condensans, right thigh
M85.352 Osteitis condensans, left thigh
M85.359 Osteitis condensans, unspecified thigh
M85.36 Osteitis condensans, lower leg
M85.361 Osteitis condensans, right lower leg
M85.362 Osteitis condensans, left lower leg
M85.369 Osteitis condensans, unspecified lower leg

- M85.37 Osteitis condensans, **ankle and foot**
  - M85.371 Osteitis condensans, **right ankle and foot**
  - M85.372 Osteitis condensans, **left ankle and foot**
  - M85.379 Osteitis condensans, **unspecified ankle and foot**
- M85.38 Osteitis condensans, **other site**
- M85.39 Osteitis condensans, **multiple sites**

M85.4 Solitary bone cyst

Excludes2 solitary cyst of jaw (M27.4)

- M85.40 Solitary bone cyst, **unspecified site**
- M85.41 Solitary bone cyst, **shoulder**
  - M85.411 Solitary bone cyst, **right shoulder**
  - M85.412 Solitary bone cyst, **left shoulder**
  - M85.419 Solitary bone cyst, **unspecified shoulder**
- M85.42 Solitary bone cyst, **humerus**
  - M85.421 Solitary bone cyst, **right humerus**
  - M85.422 Solitary bone cyst, **left humerus**
  - M85.429 Solitary bone cyst, **unspecified humerus**
- M85.43 Solitary bone cyst, **ulna and radius**
  - M85.431 Solitary bone cyst, **right ulna and radius**
  - M85.432 Solitary bone cyst, **left ulna and radius**
  - M85.439 Solitary bone cyst, **unspecified ulna and radius**
- M85.44 Solitary bone cyst, **hand**
  - M85.441 Solitary bone cyst, **right hand**
  - M85.442 Solitary bone cyst, **left hand**
  - M85.449 Solitary bone cyst, **unspecified hand**
- M85.45 Solitary bone cyst, **pelvis**
  - M85.451 Solitary bone cyst, **right pelvis**
  - M85.452 Solitary bone cyst, **left pelvis**
  - M85.459 Solitary bone cyst, **unspecified pelvis**
- M85.46 Solitary bone cyst, **tibia and fibula**
  - M85.461 Solitary bone cyst, **right tibia and fibula**
  - M85.462 Solitary bone cyst, **left tibia and fibula**
  - M85.469 Solitary bone cyst, **unspecified tibia and fibula**
- M85.47 Solitary bone cyst, **ankle and foot**
  - M85.471 Solitary bone cyst, **right ankle and foot**
  - M85.472 Solitary bone cyst, **left ankle and foot**
  - M85.479 Solitary bone cyst, **unspecified ankle and foot**
- M85.48 Solitary bone cyst, **other site**

M85.5 Aneurysmal bone cyst

Excludes2 aneurysmal cyst of jaw (M27.4)

- M85.50 Aneurysmal bone cyst, **unspecified site**
- M85.51 Aneurysmal bone cyst, **shoulder**
  - M85.511 Aneurysmal bone cyst, **right shoulder**
  - M85.512 Aneurysmal bone cyst, **left shoulder**
  - M85.519 Aneurysmal bone cyst, **unspecified shoulder**
- M85.52 Aneurysmal bone cyst, **upper arm**
  - M85.521 Aneurysmal bone cyst, **right upper arm**
  - M85.522 Aneurysmal bone cyst, **left upper arm**
  - M85.529 Aneurysmal bone cyst, **unspecified upper arm**
- M85.53 Aneurysmal bone cyst, **forearm**
  - M85.531 Aneurysmal bone cyst, **right forearm**
  - M85.532 Aneurysmal bone cyst, **left forearm**
  - M85.539 Aneurysmal bone cyst, **unspecified forearm**
- M85.54 Aneurysmal bone cyst, **hand**
  - M85.541 Aneurysmal bone cyst, **right hand**
  - M85.542 Aneurysmal bone cyst, **left hand**
  - M85.549 Aneurysmal bone cyst, **unspecified hand**
- M85.55 Aneurysmal bone cyst, **thigh**
  - M85.551 Aneurysmal bone cyst, **right thigh**
  - M85.552 Aneurysmal bone cyst, **left thigh**
  - M85.559 Aneurysmal bone cyst, **unspecified thigh**
- M85.56 Aneurysmal bone cyst, **lower leg**
  - M85.561 Aneurysmal bone cyst, **right lower leg**
  - M85.562 Aneurysmal bone cyst, **left lower leg**
  - M85.569 Aneurysmal bone cyst, **unspecified lower leg**
- M85.57 Aneurysmal bone cyst, **ankle and foot**
  - M85.571 Aneurysmal bone cyst, **right ankle and foot**
  - M85.572 Aneurysmal bone cyst, **left ankle and foot**
  - M85.579 Aneurysmal bone cyst, **unspecified ankle and foot**
- M85.58 Aneurysmal bone cyst, **other site**
- M85.59 Aneurysmal bone cyst, **multiple sites**

M85.6 Other cyst of bone

Excludes1 cyst of jaw NEC (M27.4)
osteitis fibrosa cystica generalisata [von Recklinghausen's disease of bone] (E21.0)

- M85.60 Other cyst of bone, **unspecified site**
- M85.61 Other cyst of bone, **shoulder**
  - M85.611 Other cyst of bone, **right shoulder**
  - M85.612 Other cyst of bone, **left shoulder**
  - M85.619 Other cyst of bone, **unspecified shoulder**
- M85.62 Other cyst of bone, **upper arm**
  - M85.621 Other cyst of bone, **right upper arm**
  - M85.622 Other cyst of bone, **left upper arm**
  - M85.629 Other cyst of bone, **unspecified upper arm**
- M85.63 Other cyst of bone, **forearm**
  - M85.631 Other cyst of bone, **right forearm**
  - M85.632 Other cyst of bone, **left forearm**
  - M85.639 Other cyst of bone, **unspecified forearm**
- M85.64 Other cyst of bone, **hand**
  - M85.641 Other cyst of bone, **right hand**
  - M85.642 Other cyst of bone, **left hand**
  - M85.649 Other cyst of bone, **unspecified hand**
- M85.65 Other cyst of bone, **thigh**
  - M85.651 Other cyst of bone, **right thigh**
  - M85.652 Other cyst of bone, **left thigh**
  - M85.659 Other cyst of bone, **unspecified thigh**
- M85.66 Other cyst of bone, **lower leg**
  - M85.661 Other cyst of bone, **right lower leg**
  - M85.662 Other cyst of bone, **left lower leg**
  - M85.669 Other cyst of bone, **unspecified lower leg**

● M85.67 Other cyst of bone, **ankle and foot**
- M85.671 Other cyst of bone, **right** ankle and foot
- M85.672 Other cyst of bone, **left** ankle and foot
- M85.679 Other cyst of bone, **unspecified** ankle and foot

M85.68 Other cyst of bone, **other site**

M85.69 Other cyst of bone, **multiple sites**

● M85.8 Other specified disorders of bone density and structure
Hyperostosis of bones, except skull
Osteosclerosis, acquired

Excludes1 diffuse idiopathic skeletal hyperostosis [DISH] (M48.1)
osteosclerosis congenita (Q77.4)
osteosclerosis fragilitas (generalista) (Q78.2)
osteosclerosis myelofibrosis (D75.81)

M85.8Ø Other specified disorders of bone density and structure, **unspecified** site

● M85.81 Other specified disorders of bone density and structure, **shoulder**
- M85.811 Other specified disorders of bone density and structure, **right** shoulder
- M85.812 Other specified disorders of bone density and structure, **left** shoulder
- M85.819 Other specified disorders of bone density and structure, **unspecified** shoulder

● M85.82 Other specified disorders of bone density and structure, **upper arm**
- M85.821 Other specified disorders of bone density and structure, **right** upper arm
- M85.822 Other specified disorders of bone density and structure, **left** upper arm
- M85.829 Other specified disorders of bone density and structure, **unspecified** upper arm

● M85.83 Other specified disorders of bone density and structure, **forearm**
- M85.831 Other specified disorders of bone density and structure, **right** forearm
- M85.832 Other specified disorders of bone density and structure, **left** forearm
- M85.839 Other specified disorders of bone density and structure, **unspecified** forearm

● M85.84 Other specified disorders of bone density and structure, **hand**
- M85.841 Other specified disorders of bone density and structure, **right** hand
- M85.842 Other specified disorders of bone density and structure, **left** hand
- M85.849 Other specified disorders of bone density and structure, **unspecified** hand

● M85.85 Other specified disorders of bone density and structure, **thigh**
- M85.851 Other specified disorders of bone density and structure, **right** thigh
- M85.852 Other specified disorders of bone density and structure, **left** thigh
- M85.859 Other specified disorders of bone density and structure, **unspecified** thigh

● M85.86 Other specified disorders of bone density and structure, **lower leg**
- M85.861 Other specified disorders of bone density and structure, **right** lower leg
- M85.862 Other specified disorders of bone density and structure, **left** lower leg
- M85.869 Other specified disorders of bone density and structure, **unspecified** lower leg

● M85.87 Other specified disorders of bone density and structure, **ankle and foot**
- M85.871 Other specified disorders of bone density and structure, **right** ankle and foot
- M85.872 Other specified disorders of bone density and structure, **left** ankle and foot
- M85.879 Other specified disorders of bone density and structure, **unspecified** ankle and foot

M85.88 Other specified disorders of bone density and structure, **other site**

M85.89 Other specified disorders of bone density and structure, **multiple sites**

M85.9 Disorder of bone density and structure, **unspecified**

OTHER OSTEOPATHIES (M86-M9Ø)

Excludes1 postprocedural osteopathies (M96.-)

● M86 **Osteomyelitis**
Use additional code (B95-B97) to identify infectious agent
Use additional code to identify major osseous defect, if applicable (M89.7-)

Excludes1 osteomyelitis due to:
echinococcus (B67.2)
gonococcus (A54.43)
salmonella (AØ2.24)

Excludes2 ostemyelitis of:
orbit (HØ5.Ø-)
petrous bone (H7Ø.2-)
vertebra (M46.2-)

● M86.Ø Acute hematogenous osteomyelitis

M86.ØØ Acute hematogenous osteomyelitis, **unspecified** site

● M86.Ø1 Acute hematogenous osteomyelitis, **shoulder**
- M86.Ø11 Acute hematogenous osteomyelitis, **right** shoulder
- M86.Ø12 Acute hematogenous osteomyelitis, **left** shoulder
- M86.Ø19 Acute hematogenous osteomyelitis, **unspecified** shoulder

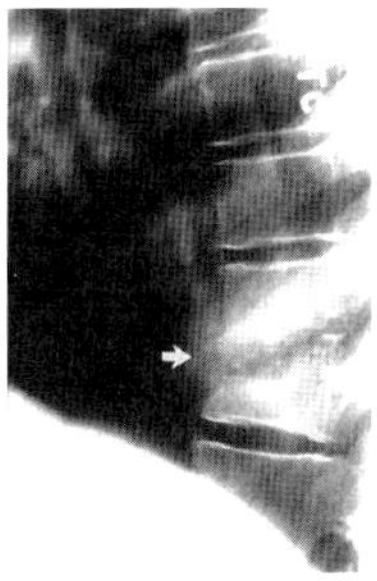

Figure 13-6 Osteomyelitis of the spine. A lateral view of the lower thoracic spine demonstrates destruction of the disk space *(arrow)* as well as destruction of the adjoining vertebral bodies. (From Mettler: Essentials of Radiology, ed 2, Saunders, An Imprint of Elsevier, 2005)

Item 13–12 Osteomyelitis is an inflammation of the bone. **Acute osteomyelitis** is a rapidly destructive, pus-producing infection capable of causing severe bone destruction. **Chronic osteomyelitis** can remain long after the initial acute episode has passed and may lead to a recurrence of the acute phase. **Brodie's abscess** is an encapsulated focal abscess that must be surgically drained. **Periostitis** is an inflammation of the periosteum, a dense membrane composed of fibrous connective tissue that closely wraps all bone, except those with articulating surfaces in joints, which are covered by synovial membranes.

M86.02 Acute hematogenous osteomyelitis, **humerus**
- M86.021 Acute hematogenous osteomyelitis, **right humerus**
- M86.022 Acute hematogenous osteomyelitis, **left humerus**
- M86.029 Acute hematogenous osteomyelitis, **unspecified humerus**

M86.03 Acute hematogenous osteomyelitis, **radius and ulna**
- M86.031 Acute hematogenous osteomyelitis, **right radius and ulna**
- M86.032 Acute hematogenous osteomyelitis, **left radius and ulna**
- M86.039 Acute hematogenous osteomyelitis, **unspecified radius and ulna**

M86.04 Acute hematogenous osteomyelitis, **hand**
- M86.041 Acute hematogenous osteomyelitis, **right hand**
- M86.042 Acute hematogenous osteomyelitis, **left hand**
- M86.049 Acute hematogenous osteomyelitis, **unspecified hand**

M86.05 Acute hematogenous osteomyelitis, **femur**
- M86.051 Acute hematogenous osteomyelitis, **right femur**
- M86.052 Acute hematogenous osteomyelitis, **left femur**
- M86.059 Acute hematogenous osteomyelitis, **unspecified femur**

M86.06 Acute hematogenous osteomyelitis, **tibia and fibula**
- M86.061 Acute hematogenous osteomyelitis, **right tibia and fibula**
- M86.062 Acute hematogenous osteomyelitis, **left tibia and fibula**
- M86.069 Acute hematogenous osteomyelitis, **unspecified tibia and fibula**

M86.07 Acute hematogenous osteomyelitis, **ankle and foot**
- M86.071 Acute hematogenous osteomyelitis, **right ankle and foot**
- M86.072 Acute hematogenous osteomyelitis, **left ankle and foot**
- M86.079 Acute hematogenous osteomyelitis, **unspecified ankle and foot**

M86.08 Acute hematogenous osteomyelitis, **other sites**

M86.09 Acute hematogenous osteomyelitis, **multiple sites**

M86.1 Other acute osteomyelitis

M86.10 Other acute osteomyelitis, **unspecified site**

M86.11 Other acute osteomyelitis, **shoulder**
- M86.111 Other acute osteomyelitis, **right shoulder**
- M86.112 Other acute osteomyelitis, **left shoulder**
- M86.119 Other acute osteomyelitis, **unspecified shoulder**

M86.12 Other acute osteomyelitis, **humerus**
- M86.121 Other acute osteomyelitis, **right humerus**
- M86.122 Other acute osteomyelitis, **left humerus**
- M86.129 Other acute osteomyelitis, **unspecified humerus**

M86.13 Other acute osteomyelitis, **radius and ulna**
- M86.131 Other acute osteomyelitis, **right radius and ulna**
- M86.132 Other acute osteomyelitis, **left radius and ulna**
- M86.139 Other acute osteomyelitis, **unspecified radius and ulna**

M86.14 Other acute osteomyelitis, **hand**
- M86.141 Other acute osteomyelitis, **right hand**
- M86.142 Other acute osteomyelitis, **left hand**
- M86.149 Other acute osteomyelitis, **unspecified hand**

M86.15 Other acute osteomyelitis, **femur**
- M86.151 Other acute osteomyelitis, **right femur**
- M86.152 Other acute osteomyelitis, **left femur**
- M86.159 Other acute osteomyelitis, **unspecified femur**

M86.16 Other acute osteomyelitis, **tibia and fibula**
- M86.161 Other acute osteomyelitis, **right tibia and fibula**
- M86.162 Other acute osteomyelitis, **left tibia and fibula**
- M86.169 Other acute osteomyelitis, **unspecified tibia and fibula**

M86.17 Other acute osteomyelitis, **ankle and foot**
- M86.171 Other acute osteomyelitis, **right ankle and foot**
- M86.172 Other acute osteomyelitis, **left ankle and foot**
- M86.179 Other acute osteomyelitis, **unspecified ankle and foot**

M86.18 Other acute osteomyelitis, **other site**

M86.19 Other acute osteomyelitis, **multiple sites**

M86.2 Subacute osteomyelitis

M86.20 Subacute osteomyelitis, **unspecified site**

M86.21 Subacute osteomyelitis, **shoulder**
- M86.211 Subacute osteomyelitis, **right shoulder**
- M86.212 Subacute osteomyelitis, **left shoulder**
- M86.219 Subacute osteomyelitis, **unspecified shoulder**

M86.22 Subacute osteomyelitis, **humerus**
- M86.221 Subacute osteomyelitis, **right humerus**
- M86.222 Subacute osteomyelitis, **left humerus**
- M86.229 Subacute osteomyelitis, **unspecified humerus**

M86.23 Subacute osteomyelitis, **radius and ulna**
- M86.231 Subacute osteomyelitis, **right radius and ulna**
- M86.232 Subacute osteomyelitis, **left radius and ulna**
- M86.239 Subacute osteomyelitis, **unspecified radius and ulna**

M86.24 Subacute osteomyelitis, **hand**
- M86.241 Subacute osteomyelitis, **right hand**
- M86.242 Subacute osteomyelitis, **left hand**
- M86.249 Subacute osteomyelitis, **unspecified hand**

● M86.25 Subacute osteomyelitis, femur
M86.251 Subacute osteomyelitis, right femur
M86.252 Subacute osteomyelitis, left femur
M86.259 Subacute osteomyelitis, unspecified femur
● M86.26 Subacute osteomyelitis, tibia and fibula
M86.261 Subacute osteomyelitis, right tibia and fibula
M86.262 Subacute osteomyelitis, left tibia and fibula
M86.269 Subacute osteomyelitis, unspecified tibia and fibula
● M86.27 Subacute osteomyelitis, ankle and foot
M86.271 Subacute osteomyelitis, right ankle and foot
M86.272 Subacute osteomyelitis, left ankle and foot
M86.279 Subacute osteomyelitis, unspecified ankle and foot
M86.28 Subacute osteomyelitis, other site
M86.29 Subacute osteomyelitis, multiple sites
● M86.3 Chronic multifocal osteomyelitis
M86.3Ø Chronic multifocal osteomyelitis, unspecified site
● M86.31 Chronic multifocal osteomyelitis, shoulder
M86.311 Chronic multifocal osteomyelitis, right shoulder
M86.312 Chronic multifocal osteomyelitis, left shoulder
M86.319 Chronic multifocal osteomyelitis, unspecified shoulder
● M86.32 Chronic multifocal osteomyelitis, humerus
M86.321 Chronic multifocal osteomyelitis, right humerus
M86.322 Chronic multifocal osteomyelitis, left humerus
M86.329 Chronic multifocal osteomyelitis, unspecified humerus
● M86.33 Chronic multifocal osteomyelitis, radius and ulna
M86.331 Chronic multifocal osteomyelitis, right radius and ulna
M86.332 Chronic multifocal osteomyelitis, left radius and ulna
M86.339 Chronic multifocal osteomyelitis, unspecified radius and ulna
● M86.34 Chronic multifocal osteomyelitis, hand
M86.341 Chronic multifocal osteomyelitis, right hand
M86.342 Chronic multifocal osteomyelitis, left hand
M86.349 Chronic multifocal osteomyelitis, unspecified hand
● M86.35 Chronic multifocal osteomyelitis, femur
M86.351 Chronic multifocal osteomyelitis, right femur
M86.352 Chronic multifocal osteomyelitis, left femur
M86.359 Chronic multifocal osteomyelitis, unspecified femur
● M86.36 Chronic multifocal osteomyelitis, tibia and fibula
M86.361 Chronic multifocal osteomyelitis, right tibia and fibula
M86.362 Chronic multifocal osteomyelitis, left tibia and fibula
M86.369 Chronic multifocal osteomyelitis, unspecified tibia and fibula
● M86.37 Chronic multifocal osteomyelitis, ankle and foot
M86.371 Chronic multifocal osteomyelitis, right ankle and foot
M86.372 Chronic multifocal osteomyelitis, left ankle and foot
M86.379 Chronic multifocal osteomyelitis, unspecified ankle and foot
M86.38 Chronic multifocal osteomyelitis, other site
M86.39 Chronic multifocal osteomyelitis, multiple sites
● M86.4 Chronic osteomyelitis with draining sinus
M86.4Ø Chronic osteomyelitis with draining sinus, unspecified site
● M86.41 Chronic osteomyelitis with draining sinus, shoulder
M86.411 Chronic osteomyelitis with draining sinus, right shoulder
M86.412 Chronic osteomyelitis with draining sinus, left shoulder
M86.419 Chronic osteomyelitis with draining sinus, unspecified shoulder
● M86.42 Chronic osteomyelitis with draining sinus, humerus
M86.421 Chronic osteomyelitis with draining sinus, right humerus
M86.422 Chronic osteomyelitis with draining sinus, left humerus
M86.429 Chronic osteomyelitis with draining sinus, unspecified humerus
● M86.43 Chronic osteomyelitis with draining sinus, radius and ulna
M86.431 Chronic osteomyelitis with draining sinus, right radius and ulna
M86.432 Chronic osteomyelitis with draining sinus, left radius and ulna
M86.439 Chronic osteomyelitis with draining sinus, unspecified radius and ulna
● M86.44 Chronic osteomyelitis with draining sinus, hand
M86.441 Chronic osteomyelitis with draining sinus, right hand
M86.442 Chronic osteomyelitis with draining sinus, left hand
M86.449 Chronic osteomyelitis with draining sinus, unspecified hand
● M86.45 Chronic osteomyelitis with draining sinus, femur
M86.451 Chronic osteomyelitis with draining sinus, right femur
M86.452 Chronic osteomyelitis with draining sinus, left femur
M86.459 Chronic osteomyelitis with draining sinus, unspecified femur
● M86.46 Chronic osteomyelitis with draining sinus, tibia and fibula
M86.461 Chronic osteomyelitis with draining sinus, right tibia and fibula
M86.462 Chronic osteomyelitis with draining sinus, left tibia and fibula
M86.469 Chronic osteomyelitis with draining sinus, unspecified tibia and fibula

M86.47 Chronic osteomyelitis with draining sinus, **ankle and foot**
- M86.471 Chronic osteomyelitis with draining sinus, **right** ankle and foot
- M86.472 Chronic osteomyelitis with draining sinus, **left** ankle and foot
- M86.479 Chronic osteomyelitis with draining sinus, **unspecified** ankle and foot

M86.48 Chronic osteomyelitis with draining sinus, **other site**

M86.49 Chronic osteomyelitis with draining sinus, **multiple sites**

M86.5 **Other chronic hematogenous** osteomyelitis

M86.50 Other chronic hematogenous osteomyelitis, **unspecified** site

M86.51 Other chronic hematogenous osteomyelitis, **shoulder**
- M86.511 Other chronic hematogenous osteomyelitis, **right** shoulder
- M86.512 Other chronic hematogenous osteomyelitis, **left** shoulder
- M86.519 Other chronic hematogenous osteomyelitis, **unspecified** shoulder

M86.52 Other chronic hematogenous osteomyelitis, **humerus**
- M86.521 Other chronic hematogenous osteomyelitis, **right** humerus
- M86.522 Other chronic hematogenous osteomyelitis, **left** humerus
- M86.529 Other chronic hematogenous osteomyelitis, **unspecified** humerus

M86.53 Other chronic hematogenous osteomyelitis, **radius and ulna**
- M86.531 Other chronic hematogenous osteomyelitis, **right** radius and ulna
- M86.532 Other chronic hematogenous osteomyelitis, **left** radius and ulna
- M86.539 Other chronic hematogenous osteomyelitis, **unspecified** radius and ulna

M86.54 Other chronic hematogenous osteomyelitis, **hand**
- M86.541 Other chronic hematogenous osteomyelitis, **right** hand
- M86.542 Other chronic hematogenous osteomyelitis, **left** hand
- M86.549 Other chronic hematogenous osteomyelitis, **unspecified** hand

M86.55 Other chronic hematogenous osteomyelitis, **femur**
- M86.551 Other chronic hematogenous osteomyelitis, **right** femur
- M86.552 Other chronic hematogenous osteomyelitis, **left** femur
- M86.559 Other chronic hematogenous osteomyelitis, **unspecified** femur

M86.56 Other chronic hematogenous osteomyelitis, **tibia and fibula**
- M86.561 Other chronic hematogenous osteomyelitis, **right** tibia and fibula
- M86.562 Other chronic hematogenous osteomyelitis, **left** tibia and fibula
- M86.569 Other chronic hematogenous osteomyelitis, **unspecified** tibia and fibula

M86.57 Other chronic hematogenous osteomyelitis, **ankle and foot**
- M86.571 Other chronic hematogenous osteomyelitis, **right** ankle and foot
- M86.572 Other chronic hematogenous osteomyelitis, **left** ankle and foot
- M86.579 Other chronic hematogenous osteomyelitis, **unspecified** ankle and foot

M86.58 Other chronic hematogenous osteomyelitis, **other site**

M86.59 Other chronic hematogenous osteomyelitis, **multiple sites**

M86.6 **Other chronic** osteomyelitis

M86.60 Other chronic osteomyelitis, **unspecified** site

M86.61 Other chronic osteomyelitis, **shoulder**
- M86.611 Other chronic osteomyelitis, **right** shoulder
- M86.612 Other chronic osteomyelitis, **left** shoulder
- M86.619 Other chronic osteomyelitis, **unspecified** shoulder

M86.62 Other chronic osteomyelitis, **humerus**
- M86.621 Other chronic osteomyelitis, **right** humerus
- M86.622 Other chronic osteomyelitis, **left** humerus
- M86.629 Other chronic osteomyelitis, **unspecified** humerus

M86.63 Other chronic osteomyelitis, **radius and ulna**
- M86.631 Other chronic osteomyelitis, **right** radius and ulna
- M86.632 Other chronic osteomyelitis, **left** radius and ulna
- M86.639 Other chronic osteomyelitis, **unspecified** radius and ulna

M86.64 Other chronic osteomyelitis, **hand**
- M86.641 Other chronic osteomyelitis, **right** hand
- M86.642 Other chronic osteomyelitis, **left** hand
- M86.649 Other chronic osteomyelitis, **unspecified** hand

M86.65 Other chronic osteomyelitis, **thigh**
- M86.651 Other chronic osteomyelitis, **right** thigh
- M86.652 Other chronic osteomyelitis, **left** thigh
- M86.659 Other chronic osteomyelitis, **unspecified** thigh

M86.66 Other chronic osteomyelitis, **tibia and fibula**
- M86.661 Other chronic osteomyelitis, **right** tibia and fibula
- M86.662 Other chronic osteomyelitis, **left** tibia and fibula
- M86.669 Other chronic osteomyelitis, **unspecified** tibia and fibula

M86.67 Other chronic osteomyelitis, **ankle and foot**
- M86.671 Other chronic osteomyelitis, **right** ankle and foot
  Coding Clinic: 2016, Q1, P13
- M86.672 Other chronic osteomyelitis, **left** ankle and foot
- M86.679 Other chronic osteomyelitis, **unspecified** ankle and foot

M86.68 Other chronic osteomyelitis, **other site**

M86.69 Other chronic osteomyelitis, **multiple sites**

CHAPTER 13 (MØØ-M99)

New Revised ~~deleted~~ Deleted Excludes 1 Excludes 2 Includes Use additional Code first Code also Key words
OGCR Official Guidelines X Assign placeholder X Use Additional Character(s) Manifestation Code Hierarchical Condition Category Coding Clinic

M86.8 Other osteomyelitis
Brodie's abscess

M86.8X Other osteomyelitis

- M86.8X0 Other osteomyelitis, **multiple sites**
- M86.8X1 Other osteomyelitis, **shoulder**
- M86.8X2 Other osteomyelitis, **upper arm**
- M86.8X3 Other osteomyelitis, **forearm**
- M86.8X4 Other osteomyelitis, **hand**
- M86.8X5 Other osteomyelitis, **thigh**
- M86.8X6 Other osteomyelitis, **lower leg**
- M86.8X7 Other osteomyelitis, **ankle and foot**
- M86.8X8 Other osteomyelitis, **other site**
- M86.8X9 Other osteomyelitis, **unspecified sites**

M86.9 Osteomyelitis, unspecified
Infection of bone NOS
Periostitis without osteomyelitis

M87 Osteonecrosis

Includes avascular necrosis of bone

Use additional code to identify major osseous defect, if applicable (M89.7-)

Excludes1 juvenile osteonecrosis (M91-M92)
osteochondropathies (M90-M93)

M87.0 Idiopathic aseptic necrosis of bone

- M87.00 Idiopathic aseptic necrosis of **unspecified bone**

M87.01 Idiopathic aseptic necrosis of shoulder
Idiopathic aseptic necrosis of clavicle and scapula

- M87.011 Idiopathic aseptic necrosis of **right shoulder**
- M87.012 Idiopathic aseptic necrosis of **left shoulder**
- M87.019 Idiopathic aseptic necrosis of **unspecified shoulder**

M87.02 Idiopathic aseptic necrosis of humerus

- M87.021 Idiopathic aseptic necrosis of **right humerus**
- M87.022 Idiopathic aseptic necrosis of **left humerus**
- M87.029 Idiopathic aseptic necrosis of **unspecified humerus**

M87.03 Idiopathic aseptic necrosis of radius, ulna and carpus

- M87.031 Idiopathic aseptic necrosis of **right radius**
- M87.032 Idiopathic aseptic necrosis of **left radius**
- M87.033 Idiopathic aseptic necrosis of **unspecified radius**
- M87.034 Idiopathic aseptic necrosis of **right ulna**
- M87.035 Idiopathic aseptic necrosis of **left ulna**
- M87.036 Idiopathic aseptic necrosis of **unspecified ulna**
- M87.037 Idiopathic aseptic necrosis of **right carpus**
- M87.038 Idiopathic aseptic necrosis of **left carpus**
- M87.039 Idiopathic aseptic necrosis of **unspecified carpus**

M87.04 Idiopathic aseptic necrosis of hand and fingers
Idiopathic aseptic necrosis of metacarpals and phalanges of hands

- M87.041 Idiopathic aseptic necrosis of **right hand**
- M87.042 Idiopathic aseptic necrosis of **left hand**
- M87.043 Idiopathic aseptic necrosis of **unspecified hand**
- M87.044 Idiopathic aseptic necrosis of **right finger(s)**
- M87.045 Idiopathic aseptic necrosis of **left finger(s)**
- M87.046 Idiopathic aseptic necrosis of **unspecified finger(s)**

M87.05 Idiopathic aseptic necrosis of pelvis and femur

- M87.050 Idiopathic aseptic necrosis of **pelvis**
- M87.051 Idiopathic aseptic necrosis of **right femur**
- M87.052 Idiopathic aseptic necrosis of **left femur**
- M87.059 Idiopathic aseptic necrosis of **unspecified femur**
  Idiopathic aseptic necrosis of hip NOS

M87.06 Idiopathic aseptic necrosis of tibia and fibula

- M87.061 Idiopathic aseptic necrosis of **right tibia**
- M87.062 Idiopathic aseptic necrosis of **left tibia**
- M87.063 Idiopathic aseptic necrosis of **unspecified tibia**
- M87.064 Idiopathic aseptic necrosis of **right fibula**
- M87.065 Idiopathic aseptic necrosis of **left fibula**
- M87.066 Idiopathic aseptic necrosis of **unspecified fibula**

M87.07 Idiopathic aseptic necrosis of ankle, foot and toes
Idiopathic aseptic necrosis of metatarsus, tarsus, and phalanges of toes

- M87.071 Idiopathic aseptic necrosis of **right ankle**
- M87.072 Idiopathic aseptic necrosis of **left ankle**
- M87.073 Idiopathic aseptic necrosis of **unspecified ankle**
- M87.074 Idiopathic aseptic necrosis of **right foot**
- M87.075 Idiopathic aseptic necrosis of **left foot**
- M87.076 Idiopathic aseptic necrosis of **unspecified foot**
- M87.077 Idiopathic aseptic necrosis of **right toe(s)**
- M87.078 Idiopathic aseptic necrosis of **left toe(s)**
- M87.079 Idiopathic aseptic necrosis of **unspecified toe(s)**

M87.08 Idiopathic aseptic necrosis of bone, **other site**

M87.09 Idiopathic aseptic necrosis of bone, **multiple sites**

CHAPTER 13 (M00-M99)

● M87.1 Osteonecrosis due to drugs
Use additional code for adverse effect, if applicable, to identify drug (T36-T5Ø with fifth or sixth character 5)

M87.1Ø Osteonecrosis due to drugs, unspecified bone

● M87.11 Osteonecrosis due to drugs, shoulder
- M87.111 Osteonecrosis due to drugs, right shoulder
- M87.112 Osteonecrosis due to drugs, left shoulder
- M87.119 Osteonecrosis due to drugs, unspecified shoulder

● M87.12 Osteonecrosis due to drugs, humerus
- M87.121 Osteonecrosis due to drugs, right humerus
- M87.122 Osteonecrosis due to drugs, left humerus
- M87.129 Osteonecrosis due to drugs, unspecified humerus

● M87.13 Osteonecrosis due to drugs of radius, ulna and carpus
- M87.131 Osteonecrosis due to drugs of right radius
- M87.132 Osteonecrosis due to drugs of left radius
- M87.133 Osteonecrosis due to drugs of unspecified radius
- M87.134 Osteonecrosis due to drugs of right ulna
- M87.135 Osteonecrosis due to drugs of left ulna
- M87.136 Osteonecrosis due to drugs of unspecified ulna
- M87.137 Osteonecrosis due to drugs of right carpus
- M87.138 Osteonecrosis due to drugs of left carpus
- M87.139 Osteonecrosis due to drugs of unspecified carpus

● M87.14 Osteonecrosis due to drugs, hand and fingers
- M87.141 Osteonecrosis due to drugs, right hand
- M87.142 Osteonecrosis due to drugs, left hand
- M87.143 Osteonecrosis due to drugs, unspecified hand
- M87.144 Osteonecrosis due to drugs, right finger(s)
- M87.145 Osteonecrosis due to drugs, left finger(s)
- M87.146 Osteonecrosis due to drugs, unspecified finger(s)

● M87.15 Osteonecrosis due to drugs, pelvis and femur
- M87.15Ø Osteonecrosis due to drugs, pelvis
- M87.151 Osteonecrosis due to drugs, right femur
- M87.152 Osteonecrosis due to drugs, left femur
- M87.159 Osteonecrosis due to drugs, unspecified femur

● M87.16 Osteonecrosis due to drugs, tibia and fibula
- M87.161 Osteonecrosis due to drugs, right tibia
- M87.162 Osteonecrosis due to drugs, left tibia
- M87.163 Osteonecrosis due to drugs, unspecified tibia
- M87.164 Osteonecrosis due to drugs, right fibula
- M87.165 Osteonecrosis due to drugs, left fibula
- M87.166 Osteonecrosis due to drugs, unspecified fibula

● M87.17 Osteonecrosis due to drugs, ankle, foot and toes
- M87.171 Osteonecrosis due to drugs, right ankle
- M87.172 Osteonecrosis due to drugs, left ankle
- M87.173 Osteonecrosis due to drugs, unspecified ankle
- M87.174 Osteonecrosis due to drugs, right foot
- M87.175 Osteonecrosis due to drugs, left foot
- M87.176 Osteonecrosis due to drugs, unspecified foot
- M87.177 Osteonecrosis due to drugs, right toe(s)
- M87.178 Osteonecrosis due to drugs, left toe(s)
- M87.179 Osteonecrosis due to drugs, unspecified toe(s)

● M87.18 Osteonecrosis due to drugs, other site
- M87.18Ø Osteonecrosis due to drugs, jaw
- M87.188 Osteonecrosis due to drugs, other site

M87.19 Osteonecrosis due to drugs, multiple sites

● M87.2 Osteonecrosis due to previous trauma

M87.2Ø Osteonecrosis due to previous trauma, unspecified bone

● M87.21 Osteonecrosis due to previous trauma, shoulder
- M87.211 Osteonecrosis due to previous trauma, right shoulder
- M87.212 Osteonecrosis due to previous trauma, left shoulder
- M87.219 Osteonecrosis due to previous trauma, unspecified shoulder

● M87.22 Osteonecrosis due to previous trauma, humerus
- M87.221 Osteonecrosis due to previous trauma, right humerus
- M87.222 Osteonecrosis due to previous trauma, left humerus
- M87.229 Osteonecrosis due to previous trauma, unspecified humerus

● M87.23 Osteonecrosis due to previous trauma of radius, ulna and carpus
- M87.231 Osteonecrosis due to previous trauma of right radius
- M87.232 Osteonecrosis due to previous trauma of left radius
- M87.233 Osteonecrosis due to previous trauma of unspecified radius
- M87.234 Osteonecrosis due to previous trauma of right ulna
- M87.235 Osteonecrosis due to previous trauma of left ulna
- M87.236 Osteonecrosis due to previous trauma of unspecified ulna
- M87.237 Osteonecrosis due to previous trauma of right carpus
- M87.238 Osteonecrosis due to previous trauma of left carpus
- M87.239 Osteonecrosis due to previous trauma of unspecified carpus

M87.24 Osteonecrosis due to previous trauma, hand and fingers
M87.241 Osteonecrosis due to previous trauma, right hand
M87.242 Osteonecrosis due to previous trauma, left hand
M87.243 Osteonecrosis due to previous trauma, unspecified hand
M87.244 Osteonecrosis due to previous trauma, right finger(s)
M87.245 Osteonecrosis due to previous trauma, left finger(s)
M87.246 Osteonecrosis due to previous trauma, unspecified finger(s)
M87.25 Osteonecrosis due to previous trauma, pelvis and femur
M87.250 Osteonecrosis due to previous trauma, pelvis
M87.251 Osteonecrosis due to previous trauma, right femur
M87.252 Osteonecrosis due to previous trauma, left femur
M87.256 Osteonecrosis due to previous trauma, unspecified femur
M87.26 Osteonecrosis due to previous trauma, tibia and fibula
M87.261 Osteonecrosis due to previous trauma, right tibia
M87.262 Osteonecrosis due to previous trauma, left tibia
M87.263 Osteonecrosis due to previous trauma, unspecified tibia
M87.264 Osteonecrosis due to previous trauma, right fibula
M87.265 Osteonecrosis due to previous trauma, left fibula
M87.266 Osteonecrosis due to previous trauma, unspecified fibula
M87.27 Osteonecrosis due to previous trauma, ankle, foot and toes
M87.271 Osteonecrosis due to previous trauma, right ankle
M87.272 Osteonecrosis due to previous trauma, left ankle
M87.273 Osteonecrosis due to previous trauma, unspecified ankle
M87.274 Osteonecrosis due to previous trauma, right foot
M87.275 Osteonecrosis due to previous trauma, left foot
M87.276 Osteonecrosis due to previous trauma, unspecified foot
M87.277 Osteonecrosis due to previous trauma, right toe(s)
M87.278 Osteonecrosis due to previous trauma, left toe(s)
M87.279 Osteonecrosis due to previous trauma, unspecified toe(s)
M87.28 Osteonecrosis due to previous trauma, other site
M87.29 Osteonecrosis due to previous trauma, multiple sites

M87.3 Other secondary osteonecrosis
M87.30 Other secondary osteonecrosis, unspecified bone
M87.31 Other secondary osteonecrosis, shoulder
M87.311 Other secondary osteonecrosis, right shoulder
M87.312 Other secondary osteonecrosis, left shoulder
M87.319 Other secondary osteonecrosis, unspecified shoulder
M87.32 Other secondary osteonecrosis, humerus
M87.321 Other secondary osteonecrosis, right humerus
M87.322 Other secondary osteonecrosis, left humerus
M87.329 Other secondary osteonecrosis, unspecified humerus
M87.33 Other secondary osteonecrosis of radius, ulna and carpus
M87.331 Other secondary osteonecrosis of right radius
M87.332 Other secondary osteonecrosis of left radius
M87.333 Other secondary osteonecrosis of unspecified radius
M87.334 Other secondary osteonecrosis of right ulna
M87.335 Other secondary osteonecrosis of left ulna
M87.336 Other secondary osteonecrosis of unspecified ulna
M87.337 Other secondary osteonecrosis of right carpus
M87.338 Other secondary osteonecrosis of left carpus
M87.339 Other secondary osteonecrosis of unspecified carpus
M87.34 Other secondary osteonecrosis, hand and fingers
M87.341 Other secondary osteonecrosis, right hand
M87.342 Other secondary osteonecrosis, left hand
M87.343 Other secondary osteonecrosis, unspecified hand
M87.344 Other secondary osteonecrosis, right finger(s)
M87.345 Other secondary osteonecrosis, left finger(s)
M87.346 Other secondary osteonecrosis, unspecified finger(s)
M87.35 Other secondary osteonecrosis, pelvis and femur
M87.350 Other secondary osteonecrosis, pelvis
M87.351 Other secondary osteonecrosis, right femur
M87.352 Other secondary osteonecrosis, left femur
M87.353 Other secondary osteonecrosis, unspecified femur

CHAPTER 13 (M00-M99)

● M87.36 Other secondary osteonecrosis, tibia and fibula
- M87.361 Other secondary osteonecrosis, right tibia
- M87.362 Other secondary osteonecrosis, left tibia
- M87.363 Other secondary osteonecrosis, unspecified tibia
- M87.364 Other secondary osteonecrosis, right fibula
- M87.365 Other secondary osteonecrosis, left fibula
- M87.366 Other secondary osteonecrosis, unspecified fibula

● M87.37 Other secondary osteonecrosis, ankle and foot
- M87.371 Other secondary osteonecrosis, right ankle
- M87.372 Other secondary osteonecrosis, left ankle
- M87.373 Other secondary osteonecrosis, unspecified ankle
- M87.374 Other secondary osteonecrosis, right foot
- M87.375 Other secondary osteonecrosis, left foot
- M87.376 Other secondary osteonecrosis, unspecified foot
- M87.377 Other secondary osteonecrosis, right toe(s)
- M87.378 Other secondary osteonecrosis, left toe(s)
- M87.379 Other secondary osteonecrosis, unspecified toe(s)

M87.38 Other secondary osteonecrosis, other site

M87.39 Other secondary osteonecrosis, multiple sites

● M87.8 Other osteonecrosis

M87.80 Other osteonecrosis, unspecified bone

● M87.81 Other osteonecrosis, shoulder
- M87.811 Other osteonecrosis, right shoulder
- M87.812 Other osteonecrosis, left shoulder
- M87.819 Other osteonecrosis, unspecified shoulder

● M87.82 Other osteonecrosis, humerus
- M87.821 Other osteonecrosis, right humerus
- M87.822 Other osteonecrosis, left humerus
- M87.829 Other osteonecrosis, unspecified humerus

● M87.83 Other osteonecrosis of radius, ulna and carpus
- M87.831 Other osteonecrosis of right radius
- M87.832 Other osteonecrosis of left radius
- M87.833 Other osteonecrosis of unspecified radius
- M87.834 Other osteonecrosis of right ulna
- M87.835 Other osteonecrosis of left ulna
- M87.836 Other osteonecrosis of unspecified ulna
- M87.837 Other osteonecrosis of right carpus
- M87.838 Other osteonecrosis of left carpus
- M87.839 Other osteonecrosis of unspecified carpus

● M87.84 Other osteonecrosis, hand and fingers
- M87.841 Other osteonecrosis, right hand
- M87.842 Other osteonecrosis, left hand
- M87.843 Other osteonecrosis, unspecified hand
- M87.844 Other osteonecrosis, right finger(s)
- M87.845 Other osteonecrosis, left finger(s)
- M87.849 Other osteonecrosis, unspecified finger(s)

● M87.85 Other osteonecrosis, pelvis and femur
- M87.850 Other osteonecrosis, pelvis
- M87.851 Other osteonecrosis, right femur
- M87.852 Other osteonecrosis, left femur
- M87.859 Other osteonecrosis, unspecified femur

● M87.86 Other osteonecrosis, tibia and fibula
- M87.861 Other osteonecrosis, right tibia
- M87.862 Other osteonecrosis, left tibia
- M87.863 Other osteonecrosis, unspecified tibia
- M87.864 Other osteonecrosis, right fibula
- M87.865 Other osteonecrosis, left fibula
- M87.869 Other osteonecrosis, unspecified fibula

● M87.87 Other osteonecrosis, ankle, foot and toes
- M87.871 Other osteonecrosis, right ankle
- M87.872 Other osteonecrosis, left ankle
- M87.873 Other osteonecrosis, unspecified ankle
- M87.874 Other osteonecrosis, right foot
- M87.875 Other osteonecrosis, left foot
- M87.876 Other osteonecrosis, unspecified foot
- M87.877 Other osteonecrosis, right toe(s)
- M87.878 Other osteonecrosis, left toe(s)
- M87.879 Other osteonecrosis, unspecified toe(s)

M87.88 Other osteonecrosis, other site

M87.89 Other osteonecrosis, multiple sites

M87.9 Osteonecrosis, unspecified

Necrosis of bone NOS

● M88 Osteitis deformans [Paget's disease of bone]

Chronic disorder that results in enlarged and deformed bones. The excessive breakdown and formation of bone tissue causes bones to weaken and results in bone pain, arthritis, deformities, and fractures.

Excludes1 osteitis deformans in neoplastic disease (M90.6)

M88.0 Osteitis deformans of skull

M88.1 Osteitis deformans of vertebrae

● M88.8 Osteitis deformans of other bones

● M88.81 Osteitis deformans of shoulder
- M88.811 Osteitis deformans of right shoulder
- M88.812 Osteitis deformans of left shoulder
- M88.819 Osteitis deformans of unspecified shoulder

● M88.82 Osteitis deformans of upper arm
- M88.821 Osteitis deformans of right upper arm
- M88.822 Osteitis deformans of left upper arm
- M88.829 Osteitis deformans of unspecified upper arm

● M88.83 Osteitis deformans of forearm
- M88.831 Osteitis deformans of right forearm
- M88.832 Osteitis deformans of left forearm
- M88.839 Osteitis deformans of unspecified forearm

● M88.84 Osteitis deformans of hand
- M88.841 Osteitis deformans of right hand
- M88.842 Osteitis deformans of left hand
- M88.849 Osteitis deformans of unspecified hand

● M88.85 Osteitis deformans of thigh
- M88.851 Osteitis deformans of right thigh
- M88.852 Osteitis deformans of left thigh
- M88.859 Osteitis deformans of unspecified thigh

M88.86 Osteitis deformans of lower leg
M88.861 Osteitis deformans of right lower leg
M88.862 Osteitis deformans of left lower leg
M88.869 Osteitis deformans of unspecified lower leg
M88.87 Osteitis deformans of ankle and foot
M88.871 Osteitis deformans of right ankle and foot
M88.872 Osteitis deformans of left ankle and foot
M88.879 Osteitis deformans of unspecified ankle and foot
M88.88 Osteitis deformans of other bones
Excludes2 osteitis deformans of skull (M88.Ø)
osteitis deformans of vertebrae (M88.1)
M88.89 Osteitis deformans of multiple sites
M88.9 Osteitis deformans of unspecified bone

M89 Other disorders of bone
M89.Ø Algoneurodystrophy
Shoulder-hand syndrome
Sudeck's atrophy
Excludes1 causalgia, lower limb (G57.7-)
causalgia, upper limb (G56.4-)
complex regional pain syndrome II, lower limb (G57.7-)
complex regional pain syndrome II, upper limb (G56.4-)
reflex sympathetic dystrophy (G9Ø.5-)
M89.ØØ Algoneurodystrophy, unspecified site
M89.Ø1 Algoneurodystrophy, shoulder
M89.Ø11 Algoneurodystrophy, right shoulder
M89.Ø12 Algoneurodystrophy, left shoulder
M89.Ø19 Algoneurodystrophy, unspecified shoulder
M89.Ø2 Algoneurodystrophy, upper arm
M89.Ø21 Algoneurodystrophy, right upper arm
M89.Ø22 Algoneurodystrophy, left upper arm
M89.Ø29 Algoneurodystrophy, unspecified upper arm
M89.Ø3 Algoneurodystrophy, forearm
M89.Ø31 Algoneurodystrophy, right forearm
M89.Ø32 Algoneurodystrophy, left forearm
M89.Ø39 Algoneurodystrophy, unspecified forearm
M89.Ø4 Algoneurodystrophy, hand
M89.Ø41 Algoneurodystrophy, right hand
M89.Ø42 Algoneurodystrophy, left hand
M89.Ø49 Algoneurodystrophy, unspecified hand
M89.Ø5 Algoneurodystrophy, thigh
M89.Ø51 Algoneurodystrophy, right thigh
M89.Ø52 Algoneurodystrophy, left thigh
M89.Ø59 Algoneurodystrophy, unspecified thigh
M89.Ø6 Algoneurodystrophy, lower leg
M89.Ø61 Algoneurodystrophy, right lower leg
M89.Ø62 Algoneurodystrophy, left lower leg
M89.Ø69 Algoneurodystrophy, unspecified lower leg
M89.Ø7 Algoneurodystrophy, ankle and foot
M89.Ø71 Algoneurodystrophy, right ankle and foot
M89.Ø72 Algoneurodystrophy, left ankle and foot
M89.Ø79 Algoneurodystrophy, unspecified ankle and foot
M89.Ø8 Algoneurodystrophy, other site
M89.Ø9 Algoneurodystrophy, multiple sites
M89.1 Physeal arrest
Arrest of growth plate
Epiphyseal arrest
Growth plate arrest
M89.12 Physeal arrest, humerus
M89.121 Complete physeal arrest, right proximal humerus
M89.122 Complete physeal arrest, left proximal humerus
M89.123 Partial physeal arrest, right proximal humerus
M89.124 Partial physeal arrest, left proximal humerus
M89.125 Complete physeal arrest, right distal humerus
M89.126 Complete physeal arrest, left distal humerus
M89.127 Partial physeal arrest, right distal humerus
M89.128 Partial physeal arrest, left distal humerus
M89.129 Physeal arrest, humerus, unspecified
M89.13 Physeal arrest, forearm
M89.131 Complete physeal arrest, right distal radius
M89.132 Complete physeal arrest, left distal radius
M89.133 Partial physeal arrest, right distal radius
M89.134 Partial physeal arrest, left distal radius
M89.138 Other physeal arrest of forearm
M89.139 Physeal arrest, forearm, unspecified
M89.15 Physeal arrest, femur
M89.151 Complete physeal arrest, right proximal femur
M89.152 Complete physeal arrest, left proximal femur
M89.153 Partial physeal arrest, right proximal femur
M89.154 Partial physeal arrest, left proximal femur
M89.155 Complete physeal arrest, right distal femur
M89.156 Complete physeal arrest, left distal femur
M89.157 Partial physeal arrest, right distal femur
M89.158 Partial physeal arrest, left distal femur
M89.159 Physeal arrest, femur, unspecified

● M89.16 Physeal arrest, lower leg
M89.160 Complete physeal arrest, right proximal tibia
M89.161 Complete physeal arrest, left proximal tibia
M89.162 Partial physeal arrest, right proximal tibia
M89.163 Partial physeal arrest, left proximal tibia
M89.164 Complete physeal arrest, right distal tibia
M89.165 Complete physeal arrest, left distal tibia
M89.166 Partial physeal arrest, right distal tibia
M89.167 Partial physeal arrest, left distal tibia
M89.168 Other physeal arrest of lower leg
M89.169 Physeal arrest, lower leg, unspecified
M89.18 Physeal arrest, other site
● M89.2 Other disorders of bone development and growth
M89.20 Other disorders of bone development and growth, unspecified site
● M89.21 Other disorders of bone development and growth, shoulder
M89.211 Other disorders of bone development and growth, right shoulder
M89.212 Other disorders of bone development and growth, left shoulder
M89.219 Other disorders of bone development and growth, unspecified shoulder
● M89.22 Other disorders of bone development and growth, humerus
M89.221 Other disorders of bone development and growth, right humerus
M89.222 Other disorders of bone development and growth, left humerus
M89.229 Other disorders of bone development and growth, unspecified humerus
● M89.23 Other disorders of bone development and growth, ulna and radius
M89.231 Other disorders of bone development and growth, right ulna
M89.232 Other disorders of bone development and growth, left ulna
M89.233 Other disorders of bone development and growth, right radius
M89.234 Other disorders of bone development and growth, left radius
M89.239 Other disorders of bone development and growth, unspecified ulna and radius
● M89.24 Other disorders of bone development and growth, hand
M89.241 Other disorders of bone development and growth, right hand
M89.242 Other disorders of bone development and growth, left hand
M89.249 Other disorders of bone development and growth, unspecified hand
● M89.25 Other disorders of bone development and growth, femur
M89.251 Other disorders of bone development and growth, right femur
M89.252 Other disorders of bone development and growth, left femur
M89.259 Other disorders of bone development and growth, unspecified femur
● M89.26 Other disorders of bone development and growth, tibia and fibula
M89.261 Other disorders of bone development and growth, right tibia
M89.262 Other disorders of bone development and growth, left tibia
M89.263 Other disorders of bone development and growth, right fibula
M89.264 Other disorders of bone development and growth, left fibula
M89.269 Other disorders of bone development and growth, unspecified lower leg
● M89.27 Other disorders of bone development and growth, ankle and foot
M89.271 Other disorders of bone development and growth, right ankle and foot
M89.272 Other disorders of bone development and growth, left ankle and foot
M89.279 Other disorders of bone development and growth, unspecified ankle and foot
M89.28 Other disorders of bone development and growth, other site
M89.29 Other disorders of bone development and growth, multiple sites
● M89.3 Hypertrophy of bone
M89.30 Hypertrophy of bone, unspecified site
● M89.31 Hypertrophy of bone, shoulder
M89.311 Hypertrophy of bone, right shoulder
M89.312 Hypertrophy of bone, left shoulder
M89.319 Hypertrophy of bone, unspecified shoulder
● M89.32 Hypertrophy of bone, humerus
M89.321 Hypertrophy of bone, right humerus
M89.322 Hypertrophy of bone, left humerus
M89.329 Hypertrophy of bone, unspecified humerus
● M89.33 Hypertrophy of bone, ulna and radius
M89.331 Hypertrophy of bone, right ulna
M89.332 Hypertrophy of bone, left ulna
M89.333 Hypertrophy of bone, right radius
M89.334 Hypertrophy of bone, left radius
M89.339 Hypertrophy of bone, unspecified ulna and radius
● M89.34 Hypertrophy of bone, hand
M89.341 Hypertrophy of bone, right hand
M89.342 Hypertrophy of bone, left hand
M89.349 Hypertrophy of bone, unspecified hand
● M89.35 Hypertrophy of bone, femur
M89.351 Hypertrophy of bone, right femur
M89.352 Hypertrophy of bone, left femur
M89.359 Hypertrophy of bone, unspecified femur
● M89.36 Hypertrophy of bone, tibia and fibula
M89.361 Hypertrophy of bone, right tibia
M89.362 Hypertrophy of bone, left tibia
M89.363 Hypertrophy of bone, right fibula
M89.364 Hypertrophy of bone, left fibula
M89.369 Hypertrophy of bone, unspecified tibia and fibula

● M89.37 Hypertrophy of bone, ankle and foot
M89.371 Hypertrophy of bone, right ankle and foot
M89.372 Hypertrophy of bone, left ankle and foot
M89.379 Hypertrophy of bone, unspecified ankle and foot
M89.38 Hypertrophy of bone, other site
M89.39 Hypertrophy of bone, multiple sites

● M89.4 Other hypertrophic osteoarthropathy
Marie-Bamberger disease
Pachydermoperiostosis
M89.40 Other hypertrophic osteoarthropathy, unspecified site
● M89.41 Other hypertrophic osteoarthropathy, shoulder
M89.411 Other hypertrophic osteoarthropathy, right shoulder
M89.412 Other hypertrophic osteoarthropathy, left shoulder
M89.419 Other hypertrophic osteoarthropathy, unspecified shoulder
● M89.42 Other hypertrophic osteoarthropathy, upper arm
M89.421 Other hypertrophic osteoarthropathy, right upper arm
M89.422 Other hypertrophic osteoarthropathy, left upper arm
M89.429 Other hypertrophic osteoarthropathy, unspecified upper arm
● M89.43 Other hypertrophic osteoarthropathy, forearm
M89.431 Other hypertrophic osteoarthropathy, right forearm
M89.432 Other hypertrophic osteoarthropathy, left forearm
M89.439 Other hypertrophic osteoarthropathy, unspecified forearm
● M89.44 Other hypertrophic osteoarthropathy, hand
M89.441 Other hypertrophic osteoarthropathy, right hand
M89.442 Other hypertrophic osteoarthropathy, left hand
M89.449 Other hypertrophic osteoarthropathy, unspecified hand
● M89.45 Other hypertrophic osteoarthropathy, thigh
M89.451 Other hypertrophic osteoarthropathy, right thigh
M89.452 Other hypertrophic osteoarthropathy, left thigh
M89.459 Other hypertrophic osteoarthropathy, unspecified thigh
● M89.46 Other hypertrophic osteoarthropathy, lower leg
M89.461 Other hypertrophic osteoarthropathy, right lower leg
M89.462 Other hypertrophic osteoarthropathy, left lower leg
M89.469 Other hypertrophic osteoarthropathy, unspecified lower leg
● M89.47 Other hypertrophic osteoarthropathy, ankle and foot
M89.471 Other hypertrophic osteoarthropathy, right ankle and foot
M89.472 Other hypertrophic osteoarthropathy, left ankle and foot
M89.479 Other hypertrophic osteoarthropathy, unspecified ankle and foot
M89.48 Other hypertrophic osteoarthropathy, other site
M89.49 Other hypertrophic osteoarthropathy, multiple sites

● M89.5 Osteolysis
Use additional code to identify major osseous defect, if applicable (M89.7-)
Excludes2 periprosthetic osteolysis of internal prosthetic joint (T84.05-)
M89.50 Osteolysis, unspecified site
● M89.51 Osteolysis, shoulder
M89.511 Osteolysis, right shoulder
M89.512 Osteolysis, left shoulder
M89.519 Osteolysis, unspecified shoulder
● M89.52 Osteolysis, upper arm
M89.521 Osteolysis, right upper arm
M89.522 Osteolysis, left upper arm
M89.529 Osteolysis, unspecified upper arm
● M89.53 Osteolysis, forearm
M89.531 Osteolysis, right forearm
M89.532 Osteolysis, left forearm
M89.539 Osteolysis, unspecified forearm
● M89.54 Osteolysis, hand
M89.541 Osteolysis, right hand
M89.542 Osteolysis, left hand
M89.549 Osteolysis, unspecified hand
● M89.55 Osteolysis, thigh
M89.551 Osteolysis, right thigh
M89.552 Osteolysis, left thigh
M89.559 Osteolysis, unspecified thigh
● M89.56 Osteolysis, lower leg
M89.561 Osteolysis, right lower leg
M89.562 Osteolysis, left lower leg
M89.569 Osteolysis, unspecified lower leg
● M89.57 Osteolysis, ankle and foot
M89.571 Osteolysis, right ankle and foot
M89.572 Osteolysis, left ankle and foot
M89.579 Osteolysis, unspecified ankle and foot
M89.58 Osteolysis, other site
M89.59 Osteolysis, multiple sites

● M89.6 Osteopathy after poliomyelitis
Use additional code (B91) to identify previous poliomyelitis
Excludes1 postpolio syndrome (G14)
M89.60 Osteopathy after poliomyelitis, unspecified site
● M89.61 Osteopathy after poliomyelitis, shoulder
M89.611 Osteopathy after poliomyelitis, right shoulder
M89.612 Osteopathy after poliomyelitis, left shoulder
M89.619 Osteopathy after poliomyelitis, unspecified shoulder
● M89.62 Osteopathy after poliomyelitis, upper arm
M89.621 Osteopathy after poliomyelitis, right upper arm
M89.622 Osteopathy after poliomyelitis, left upper arm
M89.629 Osteopathy after poliomyelitis, unspecified upper arm
● M89.63 Osteopathy after poliomyelitis, forearm
M89.631 Osteopathy after poliomyelitis, right forearm
M89.632 Osteopathy after poliomyelitis, left forearm
M89.639 Osteopathy after poliomyelitis, unspecified forearm

● M89.64 Osteopathy after poliomyelitis, hand
M89.641 Osteopathy after poliomyelitis, right hand
M89.642 Osteopathy after poliomyelitis, left hand
M89.649 Osteopathy after poliomyelitis, unspecified hand
● M89.65 Osteopathy after poliomyelitis, thigh
M89.651 Osteopathy after poliomyelitis, right thigh
M89.652 Osteopathy after poliomyelitis, left thigh
M89.659 Osteopathy after poliomyelitis, unspecified thigh
● M89.66 Osteopathy after poliomyelitis, lower leg
M89.661 Osteopathy after poliomyelitis, right lower leg
M89.662 Osteopathy after poliomyelitis, left lower leg
M89.669 Osteopathy after poliomyelitis, unspecified lower leg
● M89.67 Osteopathy after poliomyelitis, ankle and foot
M89.671 Osteopathy after poliomyelitis, right ankle and foot
M89.672 Osteopathy after poliomyelitis, left ankle and foot
M89.679 Osteopathy after poliomyelitis, unspecified ankle and foot
M89.68 Osteopathy after poliomyelitis, other site
M89.69 Osteopathy after poliomyelitis, multiple sites

● M89.7 **Major osseous defect**

Code first underlying disease, if known, such as:
aseptic necrosis of bone (M87.-)
malignant neoplasm of bone (C4Ø.-)
osteolysis (M89.5)
osteomyelitis (M86.-)
osteonecrosis (M87.-)
osteoporosis (M8Ø.-, M81.-)
periprosthetic osteolysis (T84.Ø5-)

M89.7Ø Major osseous defect, unspecified site
● M89.71 Major osseous defect, shoulder region
Major osseous defect clavicle or scapula
M89.711 Major osseous defect, right shoulder region
M89.712 Major osseous defect, left shoulder region
M89.719 Major osseous defect, unspecified shoulder region
● M89.72 Major osseous defect, humerus
M89.721 Major osseous defect, right humerus
M89.722 Major osseous defect, left humerus
M89.729 Major osseous defect, unspecified humerus
● M89.73 Major osseous defect, forearm
Major osseous defect of radius and ulna
M89.731 Major osseous defect, right forearm
M89.732 Major osseous defect, left forearm
M89.739 Major osseous defect, unspecified forearm
● M89.74 Major osseous defect, hand
Major osseous defect of carpus, fingers, metacarpus
M89.741 Major osseous defect, right hand
M89.742 Major osseous defect, left hand
M89.749 Major osseous defect, unspecified hand
● M89.75 Major osseous defect, pelvic region and thigh
Major osseous defect of femur and pelvis
M89.751 Major osseous defect, right pelvic region and thigh
M89.752 Major osseous defect, left pelvic region and thigh
M89.759 Major osseous defect, unspecified pelvic region and thigh
● M89.76 Major osseous defect, lower leg
Major osseous defect of fibula and tibia
M89.761 Major osseous defect, right lower leg
M89.762 Major osseous defect, left lower leg
M89.769 Major osseous defect, unspecified lower leg
● M89.77 Major osseous defect, ankle and foot
Major osseous defect of metatarsus, tarsus, toes
M89.771 Major osseous defect, right ankle and foot
M89.772 Major osseous defect, left ankle and foot
M89.779 Major osseous defect, unspecified ankle and foot
M89.78 Major osseous defect, other site
M89.79 Major osseous defect, multiple sites

● M89.8 **Other specified disorders of bone**
Infantile cortical hyperostoses
Post-traumatic subperiosteal ossification
● M89.8X Other specified disorders of bone
M89.8XØ Other specified disorders of bone, multiple sites
M89.8X1 Other specified disorders of bone, shoulder
M89.8X2 Other specified disorders of bone, upper arm
M89.8X3 Other specified disorders of bone, forearm
M89.8X4 Other specified disorders of bone, hand
M89.8X5 Other specified disorders of bone, thigh
M89.8X6 Other specified disorders of bone, lower leg
M89.8X7 Other specified disorders of bone, ankle and foot
M89.8X8 Other specified disorders of bone, other site
M89.8X9 Other specified disorders of bone, unspecified site

M89.9 **Disorder of bone, unspecified**

M90 Osteopathies in diseases classified elsewhere

Excludes1 osteochondritis, osteomyelitis, and osteopathy (in):
cryptococcosis (B45.3)
diabetes mellitus (E08-E13 with .69-)
gonococcal (A54.43)
neurogenic syphilis (A52.11)
renal osteodystrophy (N25.0)
salmonellosis (A02.24)
secondary syphilis (A51.46)
syphilis (late) (A52.77)

M90.5 Osteonecrosis in diseases classified elsewhere

Code first underlying disease, such as:
caisson disease (T70.3)
hemoglobinopathy (D50-D64)

M90.50 Osteonecrosis in diseases classified elsewhere, unspecified site

M90.51 Osteonecrosis in diseases classified elsewhere, shoulder

M90.511 Osteonecrosis in diseases classified elsewhere, right shoulder
M90.512 Osteonecrosis in diseases classified elsewhere, left shoulder
M90.519 Osteonecrosis in diseases classified elsewhere, unspecified shoulder

M90.52 Osteonecrosis in diseases classified elsewhere, upper arm

M90.521 Osteonecrosis in diseases classified elsewhere, right upper arm
M90.522 Osteonecrosis in diseases classified elsewhere, left upper arm
M90.529 Osteonecrosis in diseases classified elsewhere, unspecified upper arm

M90.53 Osteonecrosis in diseases classified elsewhere, forearm

M90.531 Osteonecrosis in diseases classified elsewhere, right forearm
M90.532 Osteonecrosis in diseases classified elsewhere, left forearm
M90.539 Osteonecrosis in diseases classified elsewhere, unspecified forearm

M90.54 Osteonecrosis in diseases classified elsewhere, hand

M90.541 Osteonecrosis in diseases classified elsewhere, right hand
M90.542 Osteonecrosis in diseases classified elsewhere, left hand
M90.549 Osteonecrosis in diseases classified elsewhere, unspecified hand

M90.55 Osteonecrosis in diseases classified elsewhere, thigh

M90.551 Osteonecrosis in diseases classified elsewhere, right thigh
M90.552 Osteonecrosis in diseases classified elsewhere, left thigh
M90.559 Osteonecrosis in diseases classified elsewhere, unspecified thigh

M90.56 Osteonecrosis in diseases classified elsewhere, lower leg

M90.561 Osteonecrosis in diseases classified elsewhere, right lower leg
M90.562 Osteonecrosis in diseases classified elsewhere, left lower leg
M90.569 Osteonecrosis in diseases classified elsewhere, unspecified lower leg

M90.57 Osteonecrosis in diseases classified elsewhere, ankle and foot

M90.571 Osteonecrosis in diseases classified elsewhere, right ankle and foot
M90.572 Osteonecrosis in diseases classified elsewhere, left ankle and foot
M90.579 Osteonecrosis in diseases classified elsewhere, unspecified ankle and foot

M90.58 Osteonecrosis in diseases classified elsewhere, other site
M90.59 Osteonecrosis in diseases classified elsewhere, multiple sites

M90.6 Osteitis deformans in neoplastic diseases

Osteitis deformans in malignant neoplasm of bone
Code first the neoplasm (C40.-, C41.-)

Excludes1 osteitis deformans [Paget's disease of bone] (M88.-)

M90.60 Osteitis deformans in neoplastic diseases, unspecified site

M90.61 Osteitis deformans in neoplastic diseases, shoulder

M90.611 Osteitis deformans in neoplastic diseases, right shoulder
M90.612 Osteitis deformans in neoplastic diseases, left shoulder
M90.619 Osteitis deformans in neoplastic diseases, unspecified shoulder

M90.62 Osteitis deformans in neoplastic diseases, upper arm

M90.621 Osteitis deformans in neoplastic diseases, right upper arm
M90.622 Osteitis deformans in neoplastic diseases, left upper arm
M90.629 Osteitis deformans in neoplastic diseases, unspecified upper arm

M90.63 Osteitis deformans in neoplastic diseases, forearm

M90.631 Osteitis deformans in neoplastic diseases, right forearm
M90.632 Osteitis deformans in neoplastic diseases, left forearm
M90.639 Osteitis deformans in neoplastic diseases, unspecified forearm

M90.64 Osteitis deformans in neoplastic diseases, hand

M90.641 Osteitis deformans in neoplastic diseases, right hand
M90.642 Osteitis deformans in neoplastic diseases, left hand
M90.649 Osteitis deformans in neoplastic diseases, unspecified hand

M90.65 Osteitis deformans in neoplastic diseases, thigh

M90.651 Osteitis deformans in neoplastic diseases, right thigh
M90.652 Osteitis deformans in neoplastic diseases, left thigh
M90.659 Osteitis deformans in neoplastic diseases, unspecified thigh

M90.66 Osteitis deformans in neoplastic diseases, lower leg

M90.661 Osteitis deformans in neoplastic diseases, right lower leg
M90.662 Osteitis deformans in neoplastic diseases, left lower leg
M90.669 Osteitis deformans in neoplastic diseases, unspecified lower leg

M90.67 Osteitis deformans in neoplastic diseases, ankle and foot

M90.671 Osteitis deformans in neoplastic diseases, right ankle and foot

M90.672 Osteitis deformans in neoplastic diseases, left ankle and foot

M90.679 Osteitis deformans in neoplastic diseases, unspecified ankle and foot

M90.68 Osteitis deformans in neoplastic diseases, other site

M90.69 Osteitis deformans in neoplastic diseases, multiple sites

M90.8 Osteopathy in diseases classified elsewhere

Code first underlying disease, such as:
rickets (E55.0)
vitamin-D-resistant rickets (E83.3)

M90.80 Osteopathy in diseases classified elsewhere, unspecified site

M90.81 Osteopathy in diseases classified elsewhere, shoulder

M90.811 Osteopathy in diseases classified elsewhere, right shoulder

M90.812 Osteopathy in diseases classified elsewhere, left shoulder

M90.819 Osteopathy in diseases classified elsewhere, unspecified shoulder

M90.82 Osteopathy in diseases classified elsewhere, upper arm

M90.821 Osteopathy in diseases classified elsewhere, right upper arm

M90.822 Osteopathy in diseases classified elsewhere, left upper arm

M90.829 Osteopathy in diseases classified elsewhere, unspecified upper arm

M90.83 Osteopathy in diseases classified elsewhere, forearm

M90.831 Osteopathy in diseases classified elsewhere, right forearm

M90.832 Osteopathy in diseases classified elsewhere, left forearm

M90.839 Osteopathy in diseases classified elsewhere, unspecified forearm

M90.84 Osteopathy in diseases classified elsewhere, hand

M90.841 Osteopathy in diseases classified elsewhere, right hand

M90.842 Osteopathy in diseases classified elsewhere, left hand

M90.849 Osteopathy in diseases classified elsewhere, unspecified hand

M90.85 Osteopathy in diseases classified elsewhere, thigh

M90.851 Osteopathy in diseases classified elsewhere, right thigh

M90.852 Osteopathy in diseases classified elsewhere, left thigh

M90.859 Osteopathy in diseases classified elsewhere, unspecified thigh

M90.86 Osteopathy in diseases classified elsewhere, lower leg

M90.861 Osteopathy in diseases classified elsewhere, right lower leg

M90.862 Osteopathy in diseases classified elsewhere, left lower leg

M90.869 Osteopathy in diseases classified elsewhere, unspecified lower leg

M90.87 Osteopathy in diseases classified elsewhere, ankle and foot

M90.871 Osteopathy in diseases classified elsewhere, right ankle and foot

M90.872 Osteopathy in diseases classified elsewhere, left ankle and foot

M90.879 Osteopathy in diseases classified elsewhere, unspecified ankle and foot

M90.88 Osteopathy in diseases classified elsewhere, other site

M90.89 Osteopathy in diseases classified elsewhere, multiple sites

CHONDROPATHIES (M91-M94)

Excludes1 postprocedural chondropathies (M96.-)

M91 Juvenile osteochondrosis of hip and pelvis

Excludes1 slipped upper femoral epiphysis (nontraumatic) (M93.0)

M91.0 Juvenile osteochondrosis of pelvis

Osteochondrosis (juvenile) of acetabulum
Osteochondrosis (juvenile) of iliac crest [Buchanan]
Osteochondrosis (juvenile) of ischiopubic synchondrosis [van Neck]
Osteochondrosis (juvenile) of symphysis pubis [Pierson]

M91.1 Juvenile osteochondrosis of head of femur [Legg-Calvé-Perthes]

M91.10 Juvenile osteochondrosis of head of femur [Legg-Calvé-Perthes], unspecified leg

M91.11 Juvenile osteochondrosis of head of femur [Legg-Calvé-Perthes], right leg

M91.12 Juvenile osteochondrosis of head of femur [Legg-Calvé-Perthes], left leg

M91.2 Coxa plana

Hip deformity due to previous juvenile osteochondrosis

M91.20 Coxa plana, unspecified hip

M91.21 Coxa plana, right hip

M91.22 Coxa plana, left hip

M91.3 Pseudocoxalgia

M91.30 Pseudocoxalgia, unspecified hip

M91.31 Pseudocoxalgia, right hip

M91.32 Pseudocoxalgia, left hip

M91.4 Coxa magna

M91.40 Coxa magna, unspecified hip

M91.41 Coxa magna, right hip

M91.42 Coxa magna, left hip

M91.8 Other juvenile osteochondrosis of hip and pelvis

Juvenile osteochondrosis after reduction of congenital dislocation of hip

M91.80 Other juvenile osteochondrosis of hip and pelvis, unspecified leg

M91.81 Other juvenile osteochondrosis of hip and pelvis, right leg

M91.82 Other juvenile osteochondrosis of hip and pelvis, left leg

M91.9 Juvenile osteochondrosis of hip and pelvis, unspecified

M91.90 Juvenile osteochondrosis of hip and pelvis, unspecified, unspecified leg

M91.91 Juvenile osteochondrosis of hip and pelvis, unspecified, right leg

M91.92 Juvenile osteochondrosis of hip and pelvis, unspecified, left leg

M92 Other juvenile osteochondrosis

M92.0 Juvenile osteochondrosis of humerus
Osteochondrosis (juvenile) of capitulum of humerus [Panner]
Osteochondrosis (juvenile) of head of humerus [Haas]

M92.00 Juvenile osteochondrosis of humerus, unspecified arm
M92.01 Juvenile osteochondrosis of humerus, right arm
M92.02 Juvenile osteochondrosis of humerus, left arm

M92.1 Juvenile osteochondrosis of radius and ulna
Osteochondrosis (juvenile) of lower ulna [Burns]
Osteochondrosis (juvenile) of radial head [Brailsford]

M92.10 Juvenile osteochondrosis of radius and ulna, unspecified arm
M92.11 Juvenile osteochondrosis of radius and ulna, right arm
M92.12 Juvenile osteochondrosis of radius and ulna, left arm

M92.2 Juvenile osteochondrosis, hand

M92.20 Unspecified juvenile osteochondrosis, hand
M92.201 Unspecified juvenile osteochondrosis, right hand
M92.202 Unspecified juvenile osteochondrosis, left hand
M92.209 Unspecified juvenile osteochondrosis, unspecified hand

M92.21 Osteochondrosis (juvenile) of carpal lunate [Kienböck]
M92.211 Osteochondrosis (juvenile) of carpal lunate [Kienböck], right hand
M92.212 Osteochondrosis (juvenile) of carpal lunate [Kienböck], left hand
M92.219 Osteochondrosis (juvenile) of carpal lunate [Kienböck], unspecified hand

M92.22 Osteochondrosis (juvenile) of metacarpal heads [Mauclaire]
M92.221 Osteochondrosis (juvenile) of metacarpal heads [Mauclaire], right hand
M92.222 Osteochondrosis (juvenile) of metacarpal heads [Mauclaire], left hand
M92.229 Osteochondrosis (juvenile) of metacarpal heads [Mauclaire], unspecified hand

M92.29 Other juvenile osteochondrosis, hand
M92.291 Other juvenile osteochondrosis, right hand
M92.292 Other juvenile osteochondrosis, left hand
M92.299 Other juvenile osteochondrosis, unspecified hand

M92.3 Other juvenile osteochondrosis, upper limb
M92.30 Other juvenile osteochondrosis, unspecified upper limb
M92.31 Other juvenile osteochondrosis, right upper limb
M92.32 Other juvenile osteochondrosis, left upper limb

M92.4 Juvenile osteochondrosis of patella
Osteochondrosis (juvenile) of primary patellar center [Köhler]
Osteochondrosis (juvenile) of secondary patellar center [Sinding Larsen]

M92.40 Juvenile osteochondrosis of patella, unspecified knee
M92.41 Juvenile osteochondrosis of patella, right knee
M92.42 Juvenile osteochondrosis of patella, left knee

M92.5 Juvenile osteochondrosis of tibia and fibula
Osteochondrosis (juvenile) of proximal tibia [Blount]
Osteochondrosis (juvenile) of tibial tubercle [Osgood-Schlatter]
Tibia vara

M92.50 Juvenile osteochondrosis of tibia and fibula, unspecified leg
M92.51 Juvenile osteochondrosis of tibia and fibula, right leg
M92.52 Juvenile osteochondrosis of tibia and fibula, left leg

M92.6 Juvenile osteochondrosis of tarsus
Osteochondrosis (juvenile) of calcaneum [Sever]
Osteochondrosis (juvenile) of os tibiale externum [Haglund]
Osteochondrosis (juvenile) of talus [Diaz]
Osteochondrosis (juvenile) of tarsal navicular [Köhler]

M92.60 Juvenile osteochondrosis of tarsus, unspecified ankle
M92.61 Juvenile osteochondrosis of tarsus, right ankle
M92.62 Juvenile osteochondrosis of tarsus, left ankle

M92.7 Juvenile osteochondrosis of metatarsus
Osteochondrosis (juvenile) of fifth metatarsus [Iselin]
Osteochondrosis (juvenile) of second metatarsus [Freiberg]

M92.70 Juvenile osteochondrosis of metatarsus, unspecified foot
M92.71 Juvenile osteochondrosis of metatarsus, right foot
M92.72 Juvenile osteochondrosis of metatarsus, left foot

M92.8 Other specified juvenile osteochondrosis
Calcaneal apophysitis

M92.9 Juvenile osteochondrosis, unspecified
Juvenile apophysitis NOS
Juvenile epiphysitis NOS
Juvenile osteochondritis NOS
Juvenile osteochondrosis NOS

M93 Other osteochondropathies
Excludes2 osteochondrosis of spine (M42.-)

M93.0 Slipped upper femoral epiphysis (nontraumatic)
Use additional code for associated chondrolysis (M94.3)

M93.00 Unspecified slipped upper femoral epiphysis (nontraumatic)
M93.001 Unspecified slipped upper femoral epiphysis (nontraumatic), right hip
M93.002 Unspecified slipped upper femoral epiphysis (nontraumatic), left hip
M93.003 Unspecified slipped upper femoral epiphysis (nontraumatic), unspecified hip

M93.01 Acute slipped upper femoral epiphysis (nontraumatic)
M93.011 Acute slipped upper femoral epiphysis (nontraumatic), right hip
M93.012 Acute slipped upper femoral epiphysis (nontraumatic), left hip
M93.013 Acute slipped upper femoral epiphysis (nontraumatic), unspecified hip

M93.02 Chronic slipped upper femoral epiphysis (nontraumatic)
M93.021 Chronic slipped upper femoral epiphysis (nontraumatic), right hip
M93.022 Chronic slipped upper femoral epiphysis (nontraumatic), left hip
M93.023 Chronic slipped upper femoral epiphysis (nontraumatic), unspecified hip

● M93.03 Acute on chronic slipped upper femoral epiphysis (nontraumatic)
- M93.031 Acute on chronic slipped upper femoral epiphysis (nontraumatic), right hip
- M93.032 Acute on chronic slipped upper femoral epiphysis (nontraumatic), left hip
- M93.033 Acute on chronic slipped upper femoral epiphysis (nontraumatic), unspecified hip

M93.1 Kienböck's disease of adults A
Adult osteochondrosis of carpal lunates

● M93.2 Osteochondritis dissecans
- M93.20 Osteochondritis dissecans of unspecified site

● M93.21 Osteochondritis dissecans of shoulder
- M93.211 Osteochondritis dissecans, right shoulder
- M93.212 Osteochondritis dissecans, left shoulder
- M93.219 Osteochondritis dissecans, unspecified shoulder

● M93.22 Osteochondritis dissecans of elbow
- M93.221 Osteochondritis dissecans, right elbow
- M93.222 Osteochondritis dissecans, left elbow
- M93.229 Osteochondritis dissecans, unspecified elbow

● M93.23 Osteochondritis dissecans of wrist
- M93.231 Osteochondritis dissecans, right wrist
- M93.232 Osteochondritis dissecans, left wrist
- M93.239 Osteochondritis dissecans, unspecified wrist

● M93.24 Osteochondritis dissecans of joints of hand
- M93.241 Osteochondritis dissecans, joints of right hand
- M93.242 Osteochondritis dissecans, joints of left hand
- M93.249 Osteochondritis dissecans, joints of unspecified hand

● M93.25 Osteochondritis dissecans of hip
- M93.251 Osteochondritis dissecans, right hip
- M93.252 Osteochondritis dissecans, left hip
- M93.259 Osteochondritis dissecans, unspecified hip

● M93.26 Osteochondritis dissecans knee
- M93.261 Osteochondritis dissecans, right knee
- M93.262 Osteochondritis dissecans, left knee
- M93.269 Osteochondritis dissecans, unspecified knee

● M93.27 Osteochondritis dissecans of ankle and joints of foot
- M93.271 Osteochondritis dissecans, right ankle and joints of right foot
- M93.272 Osteochondritis dissecans, left ankle and joints of left foot
- M93.279 Osteochondritis dissecans, unspecified ankle and joints of foot

M93.28 Osteochondritis dissecans other site

M93.29 Osteochondritis dissecans multiple sites

● M93.8 Other specified osteochondropathies
- M93.80 Other specified osteochondropathies of unspecified site

● M93.81 Other specified osteochondropathies of shoulder
- M93.811 Other specified osteochondropathies, right shoulder
- M93.812 Other specified osteochondropathies, left shoulder
- M93.819 Other specified osteochondropathies, unspecified shoulder

● M93.82 Other specified osteochondropathies of upper arm
- M93.821 Other specified osteochondropathies, right upper arm
- M93.822 Other specified osteochondropathies, left upper arm
- M93.829 Other specified osteochondropathies, unspecified upper arm

● M93.83 Other specified osteochondropathies of forearm
- M93.831 Other specified osteochondropathies, right forearm
- M93.832 Other specified osteochondropathies, left forearm
- M93.839 Other specified osteochondropathies, unspecified forearm

● M93.84 Other specified osteochondropathies of hand
- M93.841 Other specified osteochondropathies, right hand
- M93.842 Other specified osteochondropathies, left hand
- M93.849 Other specified osteochondropathies, unspecified hand

● M93.85 Other specified osteochondropathies of thigh
- M93.851 Other specified osteochondropathies, right thigh
- M93.852 Other specified osteochondropathies, left thigh
- M93.859 Other specified osteochondropathies, unspecified thigh

● M93.86 Other specified osteochondropathies lower leg
- M93.861 Other specified osteochondropathies, right lower leg
- M93.862 Other specified osteochondropathies, left lower leg
- M93.869 Other specified osteochondropathies, unspecified lower leg

● M93.87 Other specified osteochondropathies of ankle and foot
- M93.871 Other specified osteochondropathies, right ankle and foot
- M93.872 Other specified osteochondropathies, left ankle and foot
- M93.879 Other specified osteochondropathies, unspecified ankle and foot

M93.88 Other specified osteochondropathies other

M93.89 Other specified osteochondropathies multiple sites

M93.9 Osteochondropathy, unspecified
Apophysitis NOS
Epiphysitis NOS
Osteochondritis NOS
Osteochondrosis NOS

M93.90 Osteochondropathy, unspecified of unspecified site

● M93.91 Osteochondropathy, unspecified of shoulder
- M93.911 Osteochondropathy, unspecified, right shoulder
- M93.912 Osteochondropathy, unspecified, left shoulder
- M93.919 Osteochondropathy, unspecified, unspecified shoulder

● M93.92 Osteochondropathy, unspecified of upper arm
- M93.921 Osteochondropathy, unspecified, right upper arm
- M93.922 Osteochondropathy, unspecified, left upper arm
- M93.929 Osteochondropathy, unspecified, unspecified upper arm

- M93.93 Osteochondropathy, unspecified of **forearm**
  - M93.931 Osteochondropathy, unspecified, **right** forearm
  - M93.932 Osteochondropathy, unspecified, **left** forearm
  - M93.939 Osteochondropathy, unspecified, **unspecified** forearm
- M93.94 Osteochondropathy, unspecified of **hand**
  - M93.941 Osteochondropathy, unspecified, **right** hand
  - M93.942 Osteochondropathy, unspecified, **left** hand
  - M93.949 Osteochondropathy, unspecified, **unspecified** hand
- M93.95 Osteochondropathy, unspecified of **thigh**
  - M93.951 Osteochondropathy, unspecified, **right** thigh
  - M93.952 Osteochondropathy, unspecified, **left** thigh
  - M93.959 Osteochondropathy, unspecified, **unspecified** thigh
- M93.96 Osteochondropathy, unspecified **lower leg**
  - M93.961 Osteochondropathy, unspecified, **right** lower leg
  - M93.962 Osteochondropathy, unspecified, **left** lower leg
  - M93.969 Osteochondropathy, unspecified, **unspecified** lower leg
- M93.97 Osteochondropathy, unspecified of **ankle and foot**
  - M93.971 Osteochondropathy, unspecified, **right** ankle and foot
  - M93.972 Osteochondropathy, unspecified, **left** ankle and foot
  - M93.979 Osteochondropathy, unspecified, **unspecified** ankle and foot
- M93.98 Osteochondropathy, **unspecified other**
- M93.99 Osteochondropathy, **unspecified multiple sites**

M94 Other disorders of cartilage

- M94.0 Chondrocostal junction syndrome [Tietze]
  Costochondritis
- M94.1 Relapsing polychondritis
- M94.2 **Chondromalacia**
  Excludes1 chondromalacia patellae (M22.4)
  - M94.20 Chondromalacia, **unspecified** site
  - M94.21 Chondromalacia, **shoulder**
    - M94.211 Chondromalacia, **right** shoulder
    - M94.212 Chondromalacia, **left** shoulder
    - M94.219 Chondromalacia, **unspecified** shoulder
  - M94.22 Chondromalacia, **elbow**
    - M94.221 Chondromalacia, **right** elbow
    - M94.222 Chondromalacia, **left** elbow
    - M94.229 Chondromalacia, **unspecified** elbow
  - M94.23 Chondromalacia, **wrist**
    - M94.231 Chondromalacia, **right** wrist
    - M94.232 Chondromalacia, **left** wrist
    - M94.239 Chondromalacia, **unspecified** wrist
  - M94.24 Chondromalacia, joints of **hand**
    - M94.241 Chondromalacia, joints of **right** hand
    - M94.242 Chondromalacia, joints of **left** hand
    - M94.249 Chondromalacia, joints of **unspecified** hand
  - M94.25 Chondromalacia, **hip**
    - M94.251 Chondromalacia, **right** hip
    - M94.252 Chondromalacia, **left** hip
    - M94.259 Chondromalacia, **unspecified** hip
  - M94.26 Chondromalacia, **knee**
    - M94.261 Chondromalacia, **right** knee
    - M94.262 Chondromalacia, **left** knee
    - M94.269 Chondromalacia, **unspecified** knee
  - M94.27 Chondromalacia, **ankle and joints of foot**
    - M94.271 Chondromalacia, **right** ankle and joints of right foot
    - M94.272 Chondromalacia, **left** ankle and joints of left foot
    - M94.279 Chondromalacia, **unspecified** ankle and joints of foot
  - M94.28 Chondromalacia, **other site**
  - M94.29 Chondromalacia, **multiple sites**
- M94.3 **Chondrolysis**
  Code first any associated slipped upper femoral epiphysis (nontraumatic) (M93.0-)
  - M94.35 Chondrolysis, **hip**
    - M94.351 Chondrolysis, **right** hip
    - M94.352 Chondrolysis, **left** hip
    - M94.359 Chondrolysis, **unspecified** hip
- M94.8 Other specified disorders of cartilage
  - M94.8X Other specified disorders of **cartilage**
    - M94.8X0 Other specified disorders of cartilage, **multiple sites**
    - M94.8X1 Other specified disorders of cartilage, **shoulder**
    - M94.8X2 Other specified disorders of cartilage, **upper arm**
    - M94.8X3 Other specified disorders of cartilage, **forearm**
    - M94.8X4 Other specified disorders of cartilage, **hand**
    - M94.8X5 Other specified disorders of cartilage, **thigh**
    - M94.8X6 Other specified disorders of cartilage, **lower leg**
    - M94.8X7 Other specified disorders of cartilage, **ankle and foot**
    - M94.8X8 Other specified disorders of cartilage, **other site**
    - M94.8X9 Other specified disorders of cartilage, **unspecified sites**
- M94.9 Disorder of cartilage, **unspecified**

OTHER DISORDERS OF THE MUSCULOSKELETAL SYSTEM AND CONNECTIVE TISSUE (M95)

M95 Other acquired deformities of musculoskeletal system and connective tissue

Excludes2 acquired absence of limbs and organs (Z89-Z90)
acquired deformities of limbs (M20-M21)
congenital malformations and deformations of the musculoskeletal system (Q65-Q79)
deforming dorsopathies (M40-M43)
dentofacial anomalies [including malocclusion] (M26.-)
postprocedural musculoskeletal disorders (M96.-)

- M95.0 Acquired deformity of nose
  Excludes2 deviated nasal septum (J34.2)
- M95.1 Cauliflower ear
  Excludes2 other acquired deformities of ear (H61.1)
  - M95.10 Cauliflower ear, **unspecified** ear
  - M95.11 Cauliflower ear, **right** ear
  - M95.12 Cauliflower ear, **left** ear
- M95.2 Other acquired deformity of head
- M95.3 Acquired deformity of neck
- M95.4 Acquired deformity of chest and rib
- M95.5 Acquired deformity of pelvis
  Excludes1 maternal care for known or suspected disproportion (O33.-)

M95.8 Other specified acquired deformities of musculoskeletal system

M95.9 Acquired deformity of musculoskeletal system, unspecified

INTRAOPERATIVE AND POSTPROCEDURAL COMPLICATIONS AND DISORDERS OF MUSCULOSKELETAL SYSTEM, NOT ELSEWHERE CLASSIFIED (M96)

● M96 Intraoperative and postprocedural complications and disorders of musculoskeletal system, not elsewhere classified

Excludes2 arthropathy following intestinal bypass (MØ2.Ø-)
complications of internal orthopedic prosthetic devices, implants and grafts (T84.-)
disorders associated with osteoporosis (M8Ø)
periprosthetic fracture around internal prosthetic joint (M97.-)
presence of functional implants and other devices (Z96-Z97)

M96.Ø Pseudarthrosis after fusion or arthrodesis

M96.1 Postlaminectomy syndrome, not elsewhere classified

M96.2 Postradiation kyphosis

M96.3 Postlaminectomy kyphosis

M96.4 Postsurgical lordosis

M96.5 Postradiation scoliosis

● M96.6 Fracture of bone following insertion of orthopedic implant, joint prosthesis, or bone plate
Intraoperative fracture of bone during insertion of orthopedic implant, joint prosthesis, or bone plate

Excludes2 complication of internal orthopedic devices, implants or grafts (T84.-)

● M96.62 Fracture of humerus following insertion of orthopedic implant, joint prosthesis, or bone plate

M96.621 Fracture of humerus following insertion of orthopedic implant, joint prosthesis, or bone plate, right arm HCC

M96.622 Fracture of humerus following insertion of orthopedic implant, joint prosthesis, or bone plate, left arm HCC

M96.629 Fracture of humerus following insertion of orthopedic implant, joint prosthesis, or bone plate, unspecified arm HCC

● M96.63 Fracture of radius or ulna following insertion of orthopedic implant, joint prosthesis, or bone plate

M96.631 Fracture of radius or ulna following insertion of orthopedic implant, joint prosthesis, or bone plate, right arm HCC

M96.632 Fracture of radius or ulna following insertion of orthopedic implant, joint prosthesis, or bone plate, left arm HCC

M96.639 Fracture of radius or ulna following insertion of orthopedic implant, joint prosthesis, or bone plate, unspecified arm HCC

M96.65 Fracture of pelvis following insertion of orthopedic implant, joint prosthesis, or bone plate HCC

● M96.66 Fracture of femur following insertion of orthopedic implant, joint prosthesis, or bone plate

M96.661 Fracture of femur following insertion of orthopedic implant, joint prosthesis, or bone plate, right leg HCC

M96.662 Fracture of femur following insertion of orthopedic implant, joint prosthesis, or bone plate, left leg HCC

M96.669 Fracture of femur following insertion of orthopedic implant, joint prosthesis, or bone plate, unspecified leg HCC

● M96.67 Fracture of tibia or fibula following insertion of orthopedic implant, joint prosthesis, or bone plate

M96.671 Fracture of tibia or fibula following insertion of orthopedic implant, joint prosthesis, or bone plate, right leg HCC

M96.672 Fracture of tibia or fibula following insertion of orthopedic implant, joint prosthesis, or bone plate, left leg HCC

M96.679 Fracture of tibia or fibula following insertion of orthopedic implant, joint prosthesis, or bone plate, unspecified leg HCC

M96.69 Fracture of other bone following insertion of orthopedic implant, joint prosthesis, or bone plate HCC

● M96.8 Other intraoperative and postprocedural complications and disorders of musculoskeletal system, not elsewhere classified
Coding Clinic: 2Ø16, Q4, P1Ø

● M96.81 Intraoperative hemorrhage and hematoma of a musculoskeletal structure complicating a procedure

Excludes1 intraoperative hemorrhage and hematoma of a musculoskeletal structure due to accidental puncture and laceration during a procedure (M96.82-)

M96.81Ø Intraoperative hemorrhage and hematoma of a musculoskeletal structure complicating a musculoskeletal system procedure

M96.811 Intraoperative hemorrhage and hematoma of a musculoskeletal structure complicating other procedure

● M96.82 Accidental puncture and laceration of a musculoskeletal structure during a procedure

M96.82Ø Accidental puncture and laceration of a musculoskeletal structure during a musculoskeletal system procedure

M96.821 Accidental puncture and laceration of a musculoskeletal structure during other procedure

● M96.83 Postprocedural hemorrhage of a musculoskeletal structure following a procedure

M96.83Ø Postprocedural hemorrhage of a musculoskeletal structure following a musculoskeletal system procedure

M96.831 Postprocedural hemorrhage of a musculoskeletal structure following other procedure

● M96.84 Postprocedural hematoma and seroma of a musculoskeletal structure following a procedure

M96.84Ø Postprocedural hematoma of a musculoskeletal structure following a musculoskeletal system procedure

M96.841 Postprocedural hematoma of a musculoskeletal structure following other procedure
Coding Clinic: 2Ø16, Q4, P1Ø

M96.842 Postprocedural seroma of a musculoskeletal structure following a musculoskeletal system procedure

M96.843 Postprocedural seroma of a musculoskeletal structure following other procedure

CHAPTER 13 (MØØ-M99)

M96.89 **Other intraoperative and postprocedural complications and disorders of the musculoskeletal system**
Instability of joint secondary to removal of joint prosthesis
Use additional code, if applicable, to further specify disorder

PERIPROSTHETIC FRACTURE AROUND INTERNAL PROSTHETIC JOINT (M97)

M97 Periprosthetic fracture around internal prosthetic joint
Excludes2 fracture of bone following insertion of orthopedic implant, joint prosthesis or bone plate (M96.6-)
breakage (fracture) of prosthetic joint (T84.01-)
Coding Clinic: 2016, Q4, P42
The appropriate 7th character is to be added to each code from category M97:

A	initial encounter
D	subsequent encounter
S	sequela

M97.0 Periprosthetic fracture around internal prosthetic hip joint
X M97.01 **Periprosthetic fracture around internal prosthetic right hip joint**
Coding Clinic: 2016, Q4, P43
X M97.02 **Periprosthetic fracture around internal prosthetic left hip joint**
M97.1 Periprosthetic fracture around internal prosthetic knee joint
X M97.11 **Periprosthetic fracture around internal prosthetic right knee joint**
X M97.12 **Periprosthetic fracture around internal prosthetic left knee joint**
M97.2 Periprosthetic fracture around internal prosthetic ankle joint
X M97.21 **Periprosthetic fracture around internal prosthetic right ankle joint**
X M97.22 **Periprosthetic fracture around internal prosthetic left ankle joint**
M97.3 Periprosthetic fracture around internal prosthetic shoulder joint
X M97.31 **Periprosthetic fracture around internal prosthetic right shoulder joint**
X M97.32 **Periprosthetic fracture around internal prosthetic left shoulder joint**
M97.4 Periprosthetic fracture around internal prosthetic elbow joint
X M97.41 **Periprosthetic fracture around internal prosthetic right elbow joint**
X M97.42 **Periprosthetic fracture around internal prosthetic left elbow joint**
X **M97.8 Periprosthetic fracture around other internal prosthetic joint**
Periprosthetic fracture around internal prosthetic finger joint
Periprosthetic fracture around internal prosthetic spinal joint
Periprosthetic fracture around internal prosthetic toe joint
Periprosthetic fracture around internal prosthetic wrist joint
Use additional code to identify the joint (Z96.6-)
X **M97.9 Periprosthetic fracture around unspecified internal prosthetic joint**

BIOMECHANICAL LESIONS, NOT ELSEWHERE CLASSIFIED (M99)

M99 Biomechanical lesions, not elsewhere classified
Note: This category should not be used if the condition can be classified elsewhere.
M99.0 Segmental and somatic dysfunction
M99.00 **Segmental and somatic dysfunction of head region**
M99.01 **Segmental and somatic dysfunction of cervical region**
M99.02 **Segmental and somatic dysfunction of thoracic region**
M99.03 **Segmental and somatic dysfunction of lumbar region**
M99.04 **Segmental and somatic dysfunction of sacral region**
M99.05 **Segmental and somatic dysfunction of pelvic region**
M99.06 **Segmental and somatic dysfunction of lower extremity**
M99.07 **Segmental and somatic dysfunction of upper extremity**
M99.08 **Segmental and somatic dysfunction of rib cage**
M99.09 **Segmental and somatic dysfunction of abdomen and other regions**
M99.1 Subluxation complex (vertebral)
M99.10 **Subluxation complex (vertebral) of head region**
M99.11 **Subluxation complex (vertebral) of cervical region**
M99.12 **Subluxation complex (vertebral) of thoracic region**
M99.13 **Subluxation complex (vertebral) of lumbar region**
M99.14 **Subluxation complex (vertebral) of sacral region**
M99.15 **Subluxation complex (vertebral) of pelvic region**
M99.16 **Subluxation complex (vertebral) of lower extremity**
M99.17 **Subluxation complex (vertebral) of upper extremity**
M99.18 **Subluxation complex (vertebral) of rib cage**
M99.19 **Subluxation complex (vertebral) of abdomen and other regions**
M99.2 Subluxation stenosis of neural canal
M99.20 **Subluxation stenosis of neural canal of head region**
M99.21 **Subluxation stenosis of neural canal of cervical region**
M99.22 **Subluxation stenosis of neural canal of thoracic region**
M99.23 **Subluxation stenosis of neural canal of lumbar region**
M99.24 **Subluxation stenosis of neural canal of sacral region**
M99.25 **Subluxation stenosis of neural canal of pelvic region**
M99.26 **Subluxation stenosis of neural canal of lower extremity**
M99.27 **Subluxation stenosis of neural canal of upper extremity**
M99.28 **Subluxation stenosis of neural canal of rib cage**
M99.29 **Subluxation stenosis of neural canal of abdomen and other regions**

- M99.3 Osseous stenosis of neural canal
  - M99.30 Osseous stenosis of neural canal of head region
  - M99.31 Osseous stenosis of neural canal of cervical region
  - M99.32 Osseous stenosis of neural canal of thoracic region
  - M99.33 Osseous stenosis of neural canal of lumbar region
  - M99.34 Osseous stenosis of neural canal of sacral region
  - M99.35 Osseous stenosis of neural canal of pelvic region
  - M99.36 Osseous stenosis of neural canal of lower extremity
  - M99.37 Osseous stenosis of neural canal of upper extremity
  - M99.38 Osseous stenosis of neural canal of rib cage
  - M99.39 Osseous stenosis of neural canal of abdomen and other regions
- M99.4 Connective tissue stenosis of neural canal
  - M99.40 Connective tissue stenosis of neural canal of head region
  - M99.41 Connective tissue stenosis of neural canal of cervical region
  - M99.42 Connective tissue stenosis of neural canal of thoracic region
  - M99.43 Connective tissue stenosis of neural canal of lumbar region
  - M99.44 Connective tissue stenosis of neural canal of sacral region
  - M99.45 Connective tissue stenosis of neural canal of pelvic region
  - M99.46 Connective tissue stenosis of neural canal of lower extremity
  - M99.47 Connective tissue stenosis of neural canal of upper extremity
  - M99.48 Connective tissue stenosis of neural canal of rib cage
  - M99.49 Connective tissue stenosis of neural canal of abdomen and other regions
- M99.5 Intervertebral disc stenosis of neural canal
  - M99.50 Intervertebral disc stenosis of neural canal of head region
  - M99.51 Intervertebral disc stenosis of neural canal of cervical region
  - M99.52 Intervertebral disc stenosis of neural canal of thoracic region
  - M99.53 Intervertebral disc stenosis of neural canal of lumbar region
  - M99.54 Intervertebral disc stenosis of neural canal of sacral region
  - M99.55 Intervertebral disc stenosis of neural canal of pelvic region
  - M99.56 Intervertebral disc stenosis of neural canal of lower extremity
  - M99.57 Intervertebral disc stenosis of neural canal of upper extremity
  - M99.58 Intervertebral disc stenosis of neural canal of rib cage
  - M99.59 Intervertebral disc stenosis of neural canal of abdomen and other regions
- M99.6 Osseous and subluxation stenosis of intervertebral foramina
  - M99.60 Osseous and subluxation stenosis of intervertebral foramina of head region
  - M99.61 Osseous and subluxation stenosis of intervertebral foramina of cervical region
  - M99.62 Osseous and subluxation stenosis of intervertebral foramina of thoracic region
  - M99.63 Osseous and subluxation stenosis of intervertebral foramina of lumbar region
  - M99.64 Osseous and subluxation stenosis of intervertebral foramina of sacral region
  - M99.65 Osseous and subluxation stenosis of intervertebral foramina of pelvic region
  - M99.66 Osseous and subluxation stenosis of intervertebral foramina of lower extremity
  - M99.67 Osseous and subluxation stenosis of intervertebral foramina of upper extremity
  - M99.68 Osseous and subluxation stenosis of intervertebral foramina of rib cage
  - M99.69 Osseous and subluxation stenosis of intervertebral foramina of abdomen and other regions
- M99.7 Connective tissue and disc stenosis of intervertebral foramina
  - M99.70 Connective tissue and disc stenosis of intervertebral foramina of head region
  - M99.71 Connective tissue and disc stenosis of intervertebral foramina of cervical region
  - M99.72 Connective tissue and disc stenosis of intervertebral foramina of thoracic region
  - M99.73 Connective tissue and disc stenosis of intervertebral foramina of lumbar region
  - M99.74 Connective tissue and disc stenosis of intervertebral foramina of sacral region
  - M99.75 Connective tissue and disc stenosis of intervertebral foramina of pelvic region
  - M99.76 Connective tissue and disc stenosis of intervertebral foramina of lower extremity
  - M99.77 Connective tissue and disc stenosis of intervertebral foramina of upper extremity
  - M99.78 Connective tissue and disc stenosis of intervertebral foramina of rib cage
  - M99.79 Connective tissue and disc stenosis of intervertebral foramina of abdomen and other regions
- M99.8 Other biomechanical lesions
  - M99.80 Other biomechanical lesions of head region
  - M99.81 Other biomechanical lesions of cervical region
  - M99.82 Other biomechanical lesions of thoracic region
  - M99.83 Other biomechanical lesions of lumbar region
  - M99.84 Other biomechanical lesions of sacral region
  - M99.85 Other biomechanical lesions of pelvic region
  - M99.86 Other biomechanical lesions of lower extremity
  - M99.87 Other biomechanical lesions of upper extremity
  - M99.88 Other biomechanical lesions of rib cage
  - M99.89 Other biomechanical lesions of abdomen and other regions
- M99.9 Biomechanical lesion, unspecified

CHAPTER 14

DISEASES OF THE GENITOURINARY SYSTEM (NØØ-N99)

OGCR Chapter-Specific Coding Guidelines

14. Chapter 14: Diseases of Genitourinary System (NØØ-N99)

a. Chronic kidney disease

1) Stages of chronic kidney disease (CKD)

The ICD-10-CM classifies CKD based on severity. The severity of CKD is designated by stages 1-5. Stage 2, code N18.2, equates to mild CKD; stage 3, code N18.3, equates to moderate CKD; and stage 4, code N18.4, equates to severe CKD. Code N18.6, End stage renal disease (ESRD), is assigned when the provider has documented end-stage-renal disease (ESRD).

If both a stage of CKD and ESRD are documented, assign code N18.6 only.

2) Chronic kidney disease and kidney transplant status

Patients who have undergone kidney transplant may still have some form of chronic kidney disease CKD because the kidney transplant may not fully restore kidney function. Therefore, the presence of CKD alone does not constitute a transplant complication. Assign the appropriate N18 code for the patient's stage of CKD and code Z94.Ø, Kidney transplant status. If a transplant complication such as failure or rejection or other transplant complication is documented, see Section I.C.19.g for information on coding complications of a kidney transplant. If the documentation is unclear as to whether the patient has a complication of the transplant, query the provider.

3) Chronic kidney disease with other conditions

Patients with CKD may also suffer from other serious conditions, most commonly diabetes mellitus and hypertension. The sequencing of the CKD code in relationship to codes for other contributing conditions is based on the conventions in the Tabular List.

See I.C.9. Hypertensive chronic kidney disease.

See I.C.19. Chronic kidney disease and kidney transplant complications.

Item 14–1 Nephritis (inflammation) or **nephropathy** (disease) **with lesion of proliferative glomerulonephritis** results from a streptococcal infection.

Nephritis (inflammation) or **nephropathy** (disease) **with lesion of membranous glomerulonephritis** is characterized by deposits along the epithelial side of the basement membrane.

Nephritis (inflammation) or **nephropathy** (disease) **with lesion of membranoproliferative glomerulonephritis** is characterized by alterations in the basement membranes of the kidney and the glomerular cells.

Nephritis (inflammation) or **nephropathy** (disease) **with lesion of rapidly progressive glomerulonephritis** is characterized by rapid and progressive decline in renal function.

Nephritis (inflammation) or **nephropathy** (disease) **with lesion of renal cortical necrosis** is characterized by death of the cortical tissues.

Nephritis (inflammation) or **nephropathy** (disease) **with lesion of renal medullary necrosis** is characterized by death of the tissues that collect urine.

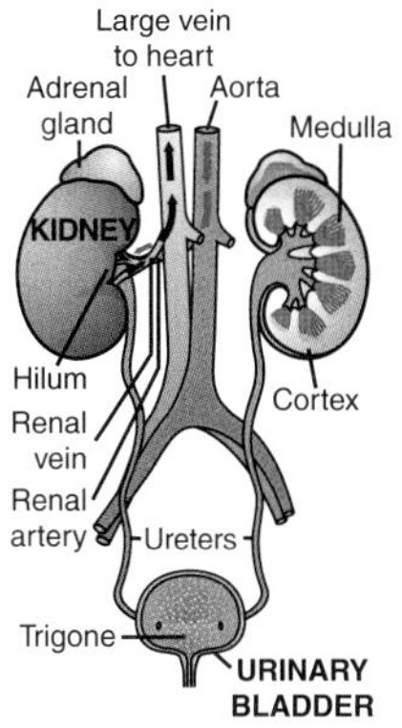

Figure 14-1 Kidneys within the urinary system.

Item 14–2 Glomerulonephritis is nephritis accompanied by inflammation of the glomeruli of the kidney, resulting in the degeneration of the glomeruli and the nephrons.

Acute glomerulonephritis primarily affects children and young adults and is usually a result of a streptococcal infection.

Proliferative glomerulonephritis is the acute form of the disease resulting from a streptococcal infection.

Rapidly progressive glomerulonephritis, also known as **crescentic** or **malignant glomerulonephritis**, is the acute form of the disease, which leads quickly to rapid and progressive decline in renal function.

CHAPTER 14

DISEASES OF THE GENITOURINARY SYSTEM (NØØ-N99)

Excludes2 certain conditions originating in the perinatal period (PØ4-P96)
certain infectious and parasitic diseases (AØØ-B99)
complications of pregnancy, childbirth and the puerperium (OØØ-O9A)
congenital malformations, deformations and chromosomal abnormalities (QØØ-Q99)
endocrine, nutritional and metabolic diseases (EØØ-E88)
injury, poisoning and certain other consequences of external causes (SØØ-T88)
neoplasms (CØØ-D49)
symptoms, signs and abnormal clinical and laboratory findings, not elsewhere classified (RØØ-R94)

This chapter contains the following blocks:

NØØ-NØ8	Glomerular diseases
N1Ø-N16	Renal tubulo-interstitial diseases
N17-N19	Acute kidney failure and chronic kidney disease
N2Ø-N23	Urolithiasis
N25-N29	Other disorders of kidney and ureter
N3Ø-N39	Other diseases of the urinary system
N4Ø-N53	Diseases of male genital organs
N6Ø-N65	Disorders of breast
N7Ø-N77	Inflammatory diseases of female pelvic organs
N8Ø-N98	Noninflammatory disorders of female genital tract
N99	Intraoperative and postprocedural complications and disorders of genitourinary system, not elsewhere classified

GLOMERULAR DISEASES (NØØ-NØ8)

Code also any associated kidney failure (N17-N19)

Excludes1 hypertensive chronic kidney disease (I12.-)

● **NØØ Acute nephritic syndrome**

Includes acute glomerular disease
acute glomerulonephritis
acute nephritis

Excludes1 acute tubulo-interstitial nephritis (N1Ø)
nephritic syndrome NOS (NØ5.-)

NØØ.Ø Acute nephritic syndrome with minor glomerular abnormality
Acute nephritic syndrome with minimal change lesion

NØØ.1 Acute nephritic syndrome with focal and segmental glomerular lesions
Acute nephritic syndrome with focal and segmental hyalinosis
Acute nephritic syndrome with focal and segmental sclerosis
Acute nephritic syndrome with focal glomerulonephritis

NØØ.2 Acute nephritic syndrome with diffuse membranous glomerulonephritis

NØØ.3 Acute nephritic syndrome with diffuse mesangial proliferative glomerulonephritis

NØØ.4 Acute nephritic syndrome with diffuse endocapillary proliferative glomerulonephritis

NØØ.5 Acute nephritic syndrome with diffuse mesangiocapillary glomerulonephritis
Acute nephritic syndrome with membranoproliferative glomerulonephritis, types 1 and 3, or NOS

NØØ.6 Acute nephritic syndrome with dense deposit disease
Acute nephritic syndrome with membranoproliferative glomerulonephritis, type 2

NØØ.7 Acute nephritic syndrome with diffuse crescentic glomerulonephritis
Acute nephritic syndrome with extracapillary glomerulonephritis

NØØ.8 Acute nephritic syndrome with other morphologic changes
Acute nephritic syndrome with proliferative glomerulonephritis NOS

NØØ.9 Acute nephritic syndrome with unspecified morphologic changes

● **NØ1 Rapidly progressive nephritic syndrome**

Includes rapidly progressive glomerular disease
rapidly progressive glomerulonephritis
rapidly progressive nephritis

Excludes1 nephritic syndrome NOS (NØ5.-)

NØ1.Ø Rapidly progressive nephritic syndrome with minor glomerular abnormality
Rapidly progressive nephritic syndrome with minimal change lesion

NØ1.1 Rapidly progressive nephritic syndrome with focal and segmental glomerular lesions
Rapidly progressive nephritic syndrome with focal and segmental hyalinosis
Rapidly progressive nephritic syndrome with focal and segmental sclerosis
Rapidly progressive nephritic syndrome with focal glomerulonephritis

NØ1.2 Rapidly progressive nephritic syndrome with diffuse membranous glomerulonephritis

NØ1.3 Rapidly progressive nephritic syndrome with diffuse mesangial proliferative glomerulonephritis

NØ1.4 Rapidly progressive nephritic syndrome with diffuse endocapillary proliferative glomerulonephritis

NØ1.5 Rapidly progressive nephritic syndrome with diffuse mesangiocapillary glomerulonephritis
Rapidly progressive nephritic syndrome with membranoproliferative glomerulonephritis, types 1 and 3, or NOS

NØ1.6 Rapidly progressive nephritic syndrome with dense deposit disease
Rapidly progressive nephritic syndrome with membranoproliferative glomerulonephritis, type 2

NØ1.7 Rapidly progressive nephritic syndrome with diffuse crescentic glomerulonephritis
Rapidly progressive nephritic syndrome with extracapillary glomerulonephritis

NØ1.8 Rapidly progressive nephritic syndrome with other morphologic changes
Rapidly progressive nephritic syndrome with proliferative glomerulonephritis NOS

NØ1.9 Rapidly progressive nephritic syndrome with unspecified morphologic changes

● **NØ2 Recurrent and persistent hematuria**

Excludes1 acute cystitis with hematuria (N3Ø.Ø1)
hematuria NOS (R31.9)
hematuria not associated with specified morphologic lesions (R31.-)

NØ2.Ø Recurrent and persistent hematuria with minor glomerular abnormality
Recurrent and persistent hematuria with minimal change lesion

NØ2.1 Recurrent and persistent hematuria with focal and segmental glomerular lesions
Recurrent and persistent hematuria with focal and segmental hyalinosis
Recurrent and persistent hematuria with focal and segmental sclerosis
Recurrent and persistent hematuria with focal glomerulonephritis

NØ2.2 Recurrent and persistent hematuria with diffuse membranous glomerulonephritis

NØ2.3 Recurrent and persistent hematuria with diffuse mesangial proliferative glomerulonephritis

NØ2.4 Recurrent and persistent hematuria with diffuse endocapillary proliferative glomerulonephritis

NØ2.5 Recurrent and persistent hematuria with diffuse mesangiocapillary glomerulonephritis
Recurrent and persistent hematuria with membranoproliferative glomerulonephritis, types 1 and 3, or NOS

NØ2.6 Recurrent and persistent hematuria with dense deposit disease
Recurrent and persistent hematuria with membranoproliferative glomerulonephritis, type 2

NØ2.7 Recurrent and persistent hematuria with diffuse crescentic glomerulonephritis
Recurrent and persistent hematuria with extracapillary glomerulonephritis

NØ2.8 Recurrent and persistent hematuria with other morphologic changes
Recurrent and persistent hematuria with proliferative glomerulonephritis NOS

NØ2.9 Recurrent and persistent hematuria with unspecified morphologic changes
Coding Clinic: 2017, Q2, P5

● **NØ3 Chronic nephritic syndrome**

Includes chronic glomerular disease
chronic glomerulonephritis
chronic nephritis

Excludes1 chronic tubulo-interstitial nephritis (N11.-)
diffuse sclerosing glomerulonephritis (NØ5.8-)
nephritic syndrome NOS (NØ5.-)

NØ3.Ø Chronic nephritic syndrome with minor glomerular abnormality
Chronic nephritic syndrome with minimal change lesion

NØ3.1 Chronic nephritic syndrome with focal and segmental glomerular lesions
Chronic nephritic syndrome with focal and segmental hyalinosis
Chronic nephritic syndrome with focal and segmental sclerosis
Chronic nephritic syndrome with focal glomerulonephritis

NØ3.2 Chronic nephritic syndrome with diffuse membranous glomerulonephritis

NØ3.3 Chronic nephritic syndrome with diffuse mesangial proliferative glomerulonephritis

NØ3.4 Chronic nephritic syndrome with diffuse endocapillary proliferative glomerulonephritis

Item 14–3 Chronic glomerulonephritis (GN) persists over a period of years, with remissions and exacerbation.

Chronic GN with lesion of proliferative glomerulonephritis results from a streptococcal infection.

Chronic GN with lesion of membranous glomerulonephritis, also known as membranous nephropathy, is characterized by deposits along the epithelial side of the basement membrane.

Chronic GN with lesion of membrano-proliferative glomerulonephritis (MPGN) is a group of disorders characterized by alterations in the basement membranes of the kidney and the glomerular cells.

Chronic GN with lesion of rapidly progressive glomerulonephritis is characterized by necrosis, endothelial proliferation, and mesangial proliferation. The condition is marked by rapid and progressive decline in renal function.

N03.5 Chronic nephritic syndrome with diffuse mesangiocapillary glomerulonephritis
Chronic nephritic syndrome with membranoproliferative glomerulonephritis, types 1 and 3, or NOS

N03.6 Chronic nephritic syndrome with dense deposit disease
Chronic nephritic syndrome with membranoproliferative glomerulonephritis, type 2

N03.7 Chronic nephritic syndrome with diffuse crescentic glomerulonephritis
Chronic nephritic syndrome with extracapillary glomerulonephritis

N03.8 Chronic nephritic syndrome with other morphologic changes
Chronic nephritic syndrome with proliferative glomerulonephritis NOS

N03.9 Chronic nephritic syndrome with unspecified morphologic changes

● **N04 Nephrotic syndrome**

Includes congenital nephrotic syndrome
lipoid nephrosis

N04.0 Nephrotic syndrome with minor glomerular abnormality
Nephrotic syndrome with minimal change lesion

N04.1 Nephrotic syndrome with focal and segmental glomerular lesions
Nephrotic syndrome with focal and segmental hyalinosis
Nephrotic syndrome with focal and segmental sclerosis
Nephrotic syndrome with focal glomerulonephritis

N04.2 Nephrotic syndrome with diffuse membranous glomerulonephritis

N04.3 Nephrotic syndrome with diffuse mesangial proliferative glomerulonephritis

N04.4 Nephrotic syndrome with diffuse endocapillary proliferative glomerulonephritis

N04.5 Nephrotic syndrome with diffuse mesangiocapillary glomerulonephritis
Nephrotic syndrome with membranoproliferative glomerulonephritis, types 1 and 3, or NOS

N04.6 Nephrotic syndrome with dense deposit disease
Nephrotic syndrome with membranoproliferative glomerulonephritis, type 2

N04.7 Nephrotic syndrome with diffuse crescentic glomerulonephritis
Nephrotic syndrome with extracapillary glomerulonephritis

N04.8 Nephrotic syndrome with other morphologic changes
Nephrotic syndrome with proliferative glomerulonephritis NOS

N04.9 Nephrotic syndrome with unspecified morphologic changes

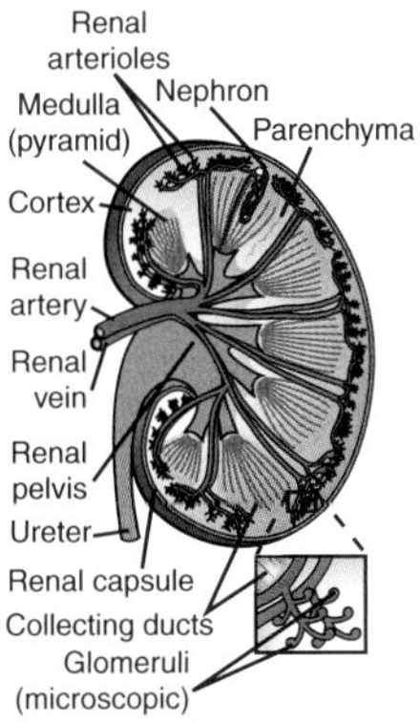

Figure 14-2 Kidney cross section.

Item 14–4 Nephrotic syndrome (NS) is marked by massive proteinuria (protein in the urine) and water retention. Patients with NS are particularly vulnerable to staphylococcal and pneumococcal infections. NS with lesion of proliferative glomerulonephritis results from a streptococcal infection. NS with lesion of membranous glomerulonephritis results in thickening of the capillary walls. NS with lesion of minimal change glomerulonephritis is usually a benign disorder that occurs mostly in children and requires electron microscopy (biopsy) to verify changes in the glomeruli.

● **N05 Unspecified nephritic syndrome**

Includes glomerular disease NOS
glomerulonephritis NOS
nephritis NOS
nephropathy NOS and renal disease NOS with morphological lesion specified in .0-.8

Excludes1 nephropathy NOS with no stated morphological lesion (N28.9)
renal disease NOS with no stated morphological lesion (N28.9)
tubulo-interstitial nephritis NOS (N12)

N05.0 Unspecified nephritic syndrome with minor glomerular abnormality
Unspecified nephritic syndrome with minimal change lesion

N05.1 Unspecified nephritic syndrome with focal and segmental glomerular lesions
Unspecified nephritic syndrome with focal and segmental hyalinosis
Unspecified nephritic syndrome with focal and segmental sclerosis
Unspecified nephritic syndrome with focal glomerulonephritis

N05.2 Unspecified nephritic syndrome with diffuse membranous glomerulonephritis

N05.3 Unspecified nephritic syndrome with diffuse mesangial proliferative glomerulonephritis

N05.4 Unspecified nephritic syndrome with diffuse endocapillary proliferative glomerulonephritis

N05.5 Unspecified nephritic syndrome with diffuse mesangiocapillary glomerulonephritis
Unspecified nephritic syndrome with membranoproliferative glomerulonephritis, types 1 and 3, or NOS

N05.6 Unspecified nephritic syndrome with dense deposit disease
Unspecified nephritic syndrome with membranoproliferative glomerulonephritis, type 2

N05.7 Unspecified nephritic syndrome with diffuse crescentic glomerulonephritis
Unspecified nephritic syndrome with extracapillary glomerulonephritis

N05.8 Unspecified nephritic syndrome with other morphologic changes
Unspecified nephritic syndrome with proliferative glomerulonephritis NOS

N05.9 Unspecified nephritic syndrome with unspecified morphologic changes

CHAPTER 14 (N00-N99)

● N06 Isolated proteinuria with specified morphological lesion

Excludes1 proteinuria not associated with specific morphologic lesions (R80.0)

N06.0 Isolated proteinuria with minor glomerular abnormality
Isolated proteinuria with minimal change lesion

N06.1 Isolated proteinuria with focal and segmental glomerular lesions
Isolated proteinuria with focal and segmental hyalinosis
Isolated proteinuria with focal and segmental sclerosis
Isolated proteinuria with focal glomerulonephritis

N06.2 Isolated proteinuria with diffuse membranous glomerulonephritis

N06.3 Isolated proteinuria with diffuse mesangial proliferative glomerulonephritis

N06.4 Isolated proteinuria with diffuse endocapillary proliferative glomerulonephritis

N06.5 Isolated proteinuria with diffuse mesangiocapillary glomerulonephritis
Isolated proteinuria with membranoproliferative glomerulonephritis, types 1 and 3, or NOS

N06.6 Isolated proteinuria with dense deposit disease
Isolated proteinuria with membranoproliferative glomerulonephritis, type 2

N06.7 Isolated proteinuria with diffuse crescentic glomerulonephritis
Isolated proteinuria with extracapillary glomerulonephritis

N06.8 Isolated proteinuria with other morphologic lesion
Isolated proteinuria with proliferative glomerulonephritis NOS

N06.9 Isolated proteinuria with unspecified morphologic lesion

● N07 Hereditary nephropathy, not elsewhere classified

Excludes2 Alport's syndrome (Q87.81-)
hereditary amyloid nephropathy (E85.-)
nail patella syndrome (Q87.2)
non-neuropathic heredofamilial amyloidosis (E85.-)

N07.0 Hereditary nephropathy, not elsewhere classified with minor glomerular abnormality
Hereditary nephropathy, not elsewhere classified with minimal change lesion

N07.1 Hereditary nephropathy, not elsewhere classified with focal and segmental glomerular lesions
Hereditary nephropathy, not elsewhere classified with focal and segmental hyalinosis
Hereditary nephropathy, not elsewhere classified with focal and segmental sclerosis
Hereditary nephropathy, not elsewhere classified with focal glomerulonephritis

N07.2 Hereditary nephropathy, not elsewhere classified with diffuse membranous glomerulonephritis

N07.3 Hereditary nephropathy, not elsewhere classified with diffuse mesangial proliferative glomerulonephritis

N07.4 Hereditary nephropathy, not elsewhere classified with diffuse endocapillary proliferative glomerulonephritis

N07.5 Hereditary nephropathy, not elsewhere classified with diffuse mesangiocapillary glomerulonephritis
Hereditary nephropathy, not elsewhere classified with membranoproliferative glomerulonephritis, types 1 and 3, or NOS

N07.6 Hereditary nephropathy, not elsewhere classified with dense deposit disease
Hereditary nephropathy, not elsewhere classified with membranoproliferative glomerulonephritis, type 2

N07.7 Hereditary nephropathy, not elsewhere classified with diffuse crescentic glomerulonephritis
Hereditary nephropathy, not elsewhere classified with extracapillary glomerulonephritis

N07.8 Hereditary nephropathy, not elsewhere classified with other morphologic lesions
Hereditary nephropathy, not elsewhere classified with proliferative glomerulonephritis NOS

N07.9 Hereditary nephropathy, not elsewhere classified with unspecified morphologic lesions

N08 Glomerular disorders in diseases classified elsewhere
Glomerulonephritis
Nephritis
Nephropathy

Code first underlying disease, such as:
amyloidosis (E85.-)
congenital syphilis (A50.5)
cryoglobulinemia (D89.1)
disseminated intravascular coagulation (D65)
gout (M1A.-, M10.-)
microscopic polyangiitis (M31.7)
multiple myeloma (C90.0-)
sepsis (A40.0-A41.9)
sickle-cell disease (D57.0-D57.8)

Excludes1 glomerulonephritis, nephritis and nephropathy (in):
antiglomerular basement membrane disease (M31.0)
diabetes (E08-E13 with .21)
gonococcal (A54.21)
Goodpasture's syndrome (M31.0)
hemolytic-uremic syndrome (D59.3)
lupus (M32.14)
mumps (B26.83)
syphilis (A52.75)
systemic lupus erythematosus (M32.14)
Wegener's granulomatosis (M31.31)
pyelonephritis in diseases classified elsewhere (N16)
renal tubulo-interstitial disorders classified elsewhere (N16)

RENAL TUBULO-INTERSTITIAL DISEASES (N10-N16)

Includes pyelonephritis

Excludes1 pyeloureteritis cystica (N28.85)

N10 Acute pyelonephritis
Acute infectious interstitial nephritis
Acute pyelitis
Acute tubulo-interstitial nephritis
Hemoglobin nephrosis
Myoglobin nephrosis
Use additional code (B95-B97), to identify infectious agent

● N11 Chronic tubulo-interstitial nephritis

Includes chronic infectious interstitial nephritis
chronic pyelitis
chronic pyelonephritis

Use additional code (B95-B97), to identify infectious agent

N11.0 Nonobstructive reflux-associated chronic pyelonephritis
Pyelonephritis (chronic) associated with (vesicoureteral) reflux

Excludes1 vesicoureteral reflux NOS (N13.70)

N11.1 Chronic obstructive pyelonephritis
Pyelonephritis (chronic) associated with anomaly of pelviureteric junction
Pyelonephritis (chronic) associated with anomaly of pyeloureteric junction
Pyelonephritis (chronic) associated with crossing of vessel
Pyelonephritis (chronic) associated with kinking of ureter
Pyelonephritis (chronic) associated with obstruction of ureter
Pyelonephritis (chronic) associated with stricture of pelviureteric junction
Pyelonephritis (chronic) associated with stricture of ureter

Excludes1 calculous pyelonephritis (N20.9)
obstructive uropathy (N13.-)

N11.8 Other chronic tubulo-interstitial nephritis
Nonobstructive chronic pyelonephritis NOS

N11.9 Chronic tubulo-interstitial nephritis, unspecified
Chronic interstitial nephritis NOS
Chronic pyelitis NOS
Chronic pyelonephritis NOS

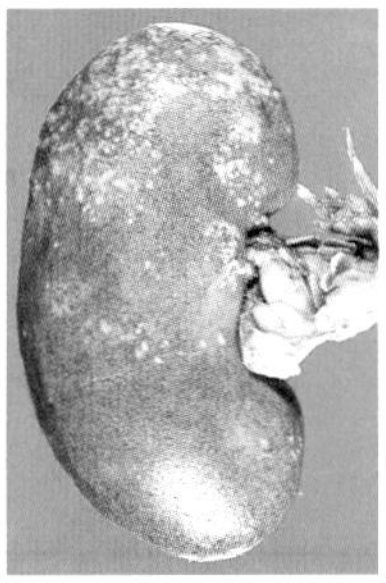

Figure 14-3 Acute pyelonephritis. Cortical surface exhibits grayish white areas of inflammation and abscess formation. (From Frazier MS, Drzymkowski JW: Essentials of Human Diseases and Conditions, St. Louis, Saunders/Elsevier, 2009)

Item 14–5 Pyelonephritis is an infection of the kidneys and ureters and may be chronic or acute in one or both kidneys.

N12 Tubulo-interstitial nephritis, not specified as acute or chronic
Interstitial nephritis NOS
Pyelitis NOS
Pyelonephritis NOS
Excludes1 calculous pyelonephritis (N2Ø.9)

● **N13 Obstructive and reflux uropathy**
Excludes2 calculus of kidney and ureter without hydronephrosis (N2Ø.-)
congenital obstructive defects of renal pelvis and ureter (Q62.Ø-Q62.3)
hydronephrosis with ureteropelvic junction obstruction (Q62.11)
obstructive pyelonephritis (N11.1)

N13.Ø Hydronephrosis with ureteropelvic junction obstruction
Hydronephrosis due to acquired occlusion of ureteropelvic junction
Excludes2 Hydronephrosis with ureteropelvic junction obstruction due to calculus (N13.2)
Coding Clinic: 2Ø16, Q4, P43

N13.1 Hydronephrosis with ureteral stricture, not elsewhere classified
Excludes1 hydronephrosis with ureteral stricture with infection (N13.6)

N13.2 Hydronephrosis with renal and ureteral calculous obstruction
Excludes1 hydronephrosis with renal and ureteral calculous obstruction with infection (N13.6)

● **N13.3 Other and unspecified hydronephrosis**
Excludes1 hydronephrosis with infection (N13.6)
N13.3Ø Unspecified hydronephrosis
N13.39 Other hydronephrosis

N13.4 Hydroureter
Excludes1 congenital hydroureter (Q62.3-)
hydroureter with infection (N13.6)
vesicoureteral-reflux with hydroureter (N13.73-)

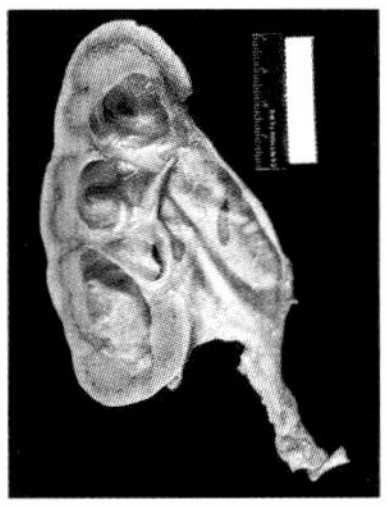

Figure 14-4 Hydronephrosis of the kidney, with marked dilatation of pelvis and calyces and thinning of renal parenchyma. (From Kumar: Robbins and Cotran: Pathologic Basis of Disease, ed 8, Saunders, An Imprint of Elsevier, 2009)

N13.5 Crossing vessel and stricture of ureter without hydronephrosis
Kinking and stricture of ureter without hydronephrosis
Excludes1 crossing vessel and stricture of ureter without hydronephrosis with infection (N13.6)
Coding Clinic: 2Ø16, Q4, P43

N13.6 Pyonephrosis
Conditions in N13.Ø-N13.5 with infection
Obstructive uropathy with infection
Use additional code (B95-B97), to identify infectious agent
Coding Clinic: 2Ø18, Q2, P21

● **N13.7 Vesicoureteral-reflux**
Excludes1 reflux-associated pyelonephritis (N11.Ø)
N13.7Ø Vesicoureteral-reflux, unspecified
Occurs when urine flows from bladder back into ureters
Vesicoureteral-reflux NOS
N13.71 Vesicoureteral-reflux without reflux nephropathy
● **N13.72 Vesicoureteral-reflux with reflux nephropathy without hydroureter**
N13.721 Vesicoureteral-reflux with reflux nephropathy without hydroureter, unilateral
N13.722 Vesicoureteral-reflux with reflux nephropathy without hydroureter, bilateral
N13.729 Vesicoureteral-reflux with reflux nephropathy without hydroureter, unspecified
● **N13.73 Vesicoureteral-reflux with reflux nephropathy with hydroureter**
N13.731 Vesicoureteral-reflux with reflux nephropathy with hydroureter, unilateral
N13.732 Vesicoureteral-reflux with reflux nephropathy with hydroureter, bilateral
N13.739 Vesicoureteral-reflux with reflux nephropathy with hydroureter, unspecified

N13.8 Other obstructive and reflux uropathy
Urinary tract obstruction due to specified cause
Code first, if applicable, any causal condition first, such as:
enlarged prostate (N4Ø.1)

N13.9 Obstructive and reflux uropathy, unspecified
Urinary tract obstruction NOS

● **N14 Drug- and heavy-metal-induced tubulo-interstitial and tubular conditions**
Code first poisoning due to drug or toxin, if applicable (T36-T65 with fifth or sixth character 1-4 or 6)
Use additional code for adverse effect, if applicable, to identify drug (T36-T5Ø with fifth or sixth character 5)
N14.Ø Analgesic nephropathy
N14.1 Nephropathy induced by other drugs, medicaments and biological substances
N14.2 Nephropathy induced by unspecified drug, medicament or biological substance
N14.3 Nephropathy induced by heavy metals
N14.4 Toxic nephropathy, not elsewhere classified

● **N15 Other renal tubulo-interstitial diseases**
N15.Ø Balkan nephropathy
Balkan endemic nephropathy
N15.1 Renal and perinephric abscess
N15.8 Other specified renal tubulo-interstitial diseases
N15.9 Renal tubulo-interstitial disease, unspecified
Infection of kidney NOS
Excludes1 urinary tract infection NOS (N39.Ø)

CHAPTER 14 (NØØ-N99)

N16 ***Renal tubulo-interstitial disorders in diseases classified elsewhere***
Pyelonephritis
Tubulo-interstitial nephritis
Code first underlying disease, such as:
brucellosis (A23.Ø-A23.9)
cryoglobulinemia (D89.1)
glycogen storage disease (E74.Ø)
leukemia (C91-C95)
lymphoma (C81.Ø-C85.9, C96.Ø-C96.9)
multiple myeloma (C9Ø.Ø-)
sepsis (A4Ø.Ø-A41.9)
Wilson's disease (E83.Ø)
Excludes1 diphtheritic pyelonephritis and tubulo-interstitial nephritis (A36.84)
pyelonephritis and tubulo-interstitial nephritis in candidiasis (B37.49)
pyelonephritis and tubulo-interstitial nephritis in cystinosis (E72.Ø4)
pyelonephritis and tubulo-interstitial nephritis in salmonella infection (AØ2.25)
pyelonephritis and tubulo-interstitial nephritis in sarcoidosis (D86.84)
pyelonephritis and tubulo-interstitial nephritis in sicca syndrome [Sjogren's] (M35.Ø4)
pyelonephritis and tubulo-interstitial nephritis in systemic lupus erythematosus (M32.15)
pyelonephritis and tubulo-interstitial nephritis in toxoplasmosis (B58.83)
renal tubular degeneration in diabetes (EØ8-E13 with .29)
syphilitic pyelonephritis and tubulo-interstitial nephritis (A52.75)

ACUTE KIDNEY FAILURE AND CHRONIC KIDNEY DISEASE (N17-N19)

Excludes2 congenital renal failure (P96.Ø)
drug- and heavy-metal-induced tubulo-interstitial and tubular conditions (N14.-)
extrarenal uremia (R39.2)
hemolytic-uremic syndrome (D59.3)
hepatorenal syndrome (K76.7)
postpartum hepatorenal syndrome (O9Ø.4)
posttraumatic renal failure (T79.5)
prerenal uremia (R39.2)
renal failure complicating abortion or ectopic or molar pregnancy (OØØ-OØ7, OØ8.4)
renal failure following labor and delivery (O9Ø.4)
renal failure postprocedural (N99.Ø)

N17 Acute kidney failure
Code also associated underlying condition
Excludes1 posttraumatic renal failure (T79.5)

N17.Ø Acute kidney failure with tubular necrosis
Acute tubular necrosis
Renal tubular necrosis
Tubular necrosis NOS

N17.1 Acute kidney failure with acute cortical necrosis
Acute cortical necrosis
Cortical necrosis NOS
Renal cortical necrosis

N17.2 Acute kidney failure with medullary necrosis
Medullary [papillary] necrosis NOS
Acute medullary [papillary] necrosis
Renal medullary [papillary] necrosis

N17.8 Other acute kidney failure

N17.9 Acute kidney failure, unspecified
Acute kidney injury (nontraumatic)
Excludes2 traumatic kidney injury (S37.Ø-)
Coding Clinic: 2Ø19, Q2, P7,25

Item 14-6 Decreased blood flow is the usual cause of **acute renal failure** that offers a good prognosis for recovery.

Chronic renal failure is usually the result of long-standing kidney disease and is a very serious condition that generally results in death.

N18 Chronic kidney disease (CKD)
Code first any associated:
diabetic chronic kidney disease (EØ8.22, EØ9.22, E1Ø.22, E11.22, E13.22)
hypertensive chronic kidney disease (I12.-, I13.-)
Use additional code to identify kidney transplant status, if applicable, (Z94.Ø)
Coding Clinic: 2018, Q4, P89; 2016, Q4, P123

N18.1 Chronic kidney disease, stage 1

N18.2 Chronic kidney disease, stage 2 (mild)

N18.3 Chronic kidney disease, stage 3 (moderate)

N18.4 Chronic kidney disease, stage 4 (severe)
Coding Clinic: 2Ø13, Q1, P24

N18.5 Chronic kidney disease, stage 5
Excludes1 chronic kidney disease, stage 5 requiring chronic dialysis (N18.6)

N18.6 End stage renal disease
Chronic kidney disease requiring chronic dialysis
Use additional code to identify dialysis status (Z99.2)
Coding Clinic: 2Ø16, Q3, P23, Q1, P13

N18.9 Chronic kidney disease, unspecified
Chronic renal disease
Chronic renal failure NOS
Chronic renal insufficiency
Chronic uremia NOS
Diffuse sclerosing glomerulonephritis NOS
Coding Clinic: 2Ø18, Q4, P88

N19 Unspecified kidney failure
Uremia NOS
Excludes1 acute kidney failure (N17.-)
chronic kidney disease (N18.-)
chronic uremia (N18.9)
extrarenal uremia (R39.2)
prerenal uremia (R39.2)
renal insufficiency (acute) (N28.9)
uremia of newborn (P96.Ø)

UROLITHIASIS (N2Ø-N23)

N2Ø Calculus of kidney and ureter
Calculous pyelonephritis
Excludes1 nephrocalcinosis (E83.5)
that with hydronephrosis (N13.2)

N2Ø.Ø Calculus of kidney
Nephrolithiasis NOS
Renal calculus
Renal stone
Staghorn calculus
Stone in kidney
Coding Clinic: 2Ø17, Q1, P5

N2Ø.1 Calculus of ureter
Ureteric stone
Coding Clinic: 2Ø16, Q3, P24

N2Ø.2 Calculus of kidney with calculus of ureter

N2Ø.9 Urinary calculus, unspecified

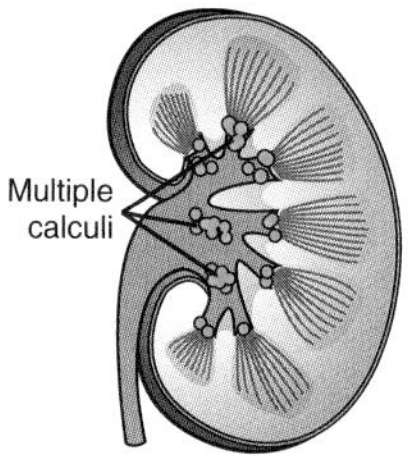

Figure 14-5 Multiple urinary calculi.

N21 Calculus of lower urinary tract
Includes calculus of lower urinary tract with cystitis and urethritis

N21.0 Calculus in bladder
Calculus in diverticulum of bladder
Urinary bladder stone
Excludes2 staghorn calculus (N20.0)
Coding Clinic: 2015, Q2, P9

N21.1 Calculus in urethra
Excludes2 calculus of prostate (N42.0)

N21.8 Other lower urinary tract calculus

N21.9 Calculus of lower urinary tract, unspecified
Excludes1 calculus of urinary tract NOS (N20.9)

N22 Calculus of urinary tract in diseases classified elsewhere
Code first underlying disease, such as:
gout (M1A.-, M10.-)
schistosomiasis (B65.0-B65.9)

N23 Unspecified renal colic

OTHER DISORDERS OF KIDNEY AND URETER (N25-N29)

Excludes2 disorders of kidney and ureter with urolithiasis (N20-N23)

N25 Disorders resulting from impaired renal tubular function

N25.0 Renal osteodystrophy
Azotemic osteodystrophy
Phosphate-losing tubular disorders
Renal rickets
Renal short stature
Excludes2 metabolic disorders classifiable to E70-E88

N25.1 Nephrogenic diabetes insipidus
Excludes1 diabetes insipidus NOS (E23.2)

N25.8 Other disorders resulting from impaired renal tubular function

N25.81 Secondary hyperparathyroidism of renal origin
Excludes1 secondary hyperparathyroidism, non-renal (E21.1)
Excludes2 metabolic disorders classifiable to E70-E88

N25.89 Other disorders resulting from impaired renal tubular function
Hypokalemic nephropathy
Lightwood-Albright syndrome
Renal tubular acidosis NOS

N25.9 Disorder resulting from impaired renal tubular function, unspecified

N26 Unspecified contracted kidney
Excludes1 contracted kidney due to hypertension (I12.-)
diffuse sclerosing glomerulonephritis (N05.8.-)
hypertensive nephrosclerosis (arteriolar) (arteriosclerotic) (I12.-)
small kidney of unknown cause (N27.-)

N26.1 Atrophy of kidney (terminal)

N26.2 Page kidney

N26.9 Renal sclerosis, unspecified

N27 Small kidney of unknown cause
Includes oligonephronia

N27.0 Small kidney, unilateral

N27.1 Small kidney, bilateral

N27.9 Small kidney, unspecified

N28 Other disorders of kidney and ureter, not elsewhere classified

N28.0 Ischemia and infarction of kidney
Renal artery embolism
Renal artery obstruction
Renal artery occlusion
Renal artery thrombosis
Renal infarct
Excludes1 atherosclerosis of renal artery (extrarenal part) (I70.1)
congenital stenosis of renal artery (Q27.1)
Goldblatt's kidney (I70.1)

N28.1 Cyst of kidney, acquired
Cyst (multiple) (solitary) of kidney, (acquired)
Excludes1 cystic kidney disease (congenital) (Q61.-)

N28.8 Other specified disorders of kidney and ureter
Excludes1 hydroureter (N13.4)
ureteric stricture with hydronephrosis (N13.1)
ureteric stricture without hydronephrosis (N13.5)

N28.81 Hypertrophy of kidney

N28.82 Megaloureter

N28.83 Nephroptosis

N28.84 Pyelitis cystica

N28.85 Pyeloureteritis cystica

N28.86 Ureteritis cystica

N28.89 Other specified disorders of kidney and ureter

N28.9 Disorder of kidney and ureter, unspecified
Nephropathy NOS
Renal disease (acute) NOS
Renal insufficiency (acute)
Excludes1 chronic renal insufficiency (N18.9)
unspecified nephritic syndrome (N05.-)
Coding Clinic: 2016, Q1, P13

N29 Other disorders of kidney and ureter in diseases classified elsewhere
Code first underlying disease, such as:
amyloidosis (E85.-)
nephrocalcinosis (E83.5)
schistosomiasis (B65.0-B65.9)
Excludes1 disorders of kidney and ureter in:
cystinosis (E72.0)
gonorrhea (A54.21)
syphilis (A52.75)
tuberculosis (A18.11)

OTHER DISEASES OF THE URINARY SYSTEM (N30-N39)

Excludes1 urinary infection (complicating):
abortion or ectopic or molar pregnancy (O00-O07, O08.8)
pregnancy, childbirth and the puerperium (O23.-, O75.3, O86.2-)

N30 Cystitis
Infection of bladder and irritation in lower urinary tract
Use additional code to identify infectious agent (B95-B97)
Excludes1 prostatocystitis (N41.3)

N30.0 Acute cystitis
Excludes1 irradiation cystitis (N30.4-)
trigonitis (N30.3-)

N30.00 Acute cystitis without hematuria

N30.01 Acute cystitis with hematuria

N30.1 Interstitial cystitis (chronic)
Ongoing infection of kidney glomeruli and tubules

N30.10 Interstitial cystitis (chronic) without hematuria

N30.11 Interstitial cystitis (chronic) with hematuria

N30.2 Other chronic cystitis

N30.20 Other chronic cystitis without hematuria

N30.21 Other chronic cystitis with hematuria

● **N30.3 Trigonitis**
Inflammation of triangular area of bladder (where the ureters and urethra come together)
Urethrotrigonitis
N30.30 Trigonitis without hematuria
N30.31 Trigonitis with hematuria

● **N30.4 Irradiation cystitis**
N30.40 Irradiation cystitis without hematuria
N30.41 Irradiation cystitis with hematuria

● **N30.8 Other cystitis**
Abscess of bladder
N30.80 Other cystitis without hematuria
N30.81 Other cystitis with hematuria

● **N30.9 Cystitis, unspecified**
N30.90 Cystitis, unspecified without hematuria
N30.91 Cystitis, unspecified with hematuria

● **N31 Neuromuscular dysfunction of bladder, not elsewhere classified**
Use additional code to identify any associated urinary incontinence (N39.3-N39.4-)
Excludes1 cord bladder NOS (G95.89)
neurogenic bladder due to cauda equina syndrome (G83.4)
neuromuscular dysfunction due to spinal cord lesion (G95.89)

N31.0 Uninhibited neuropathic bladder, not elsewhere classified
N31.1 Reflex neuropathic bladder, not elsewhere classified
N31.2 Flaccid neuropathic bladder, not elsewhere classified
Atonic (motor) (sensory) neuropathic bladder
Diminished tone of bladder muscle
Autonomous neuropathic bladder
Nonreflex neuropathic bladder
N31.8 Other neuromuscular dysfunction of bladder
N31.9 Neuromuscular dysfunction of bladder, unspecified
Neurogenic bladder dysfunction NOS

● **N32 Other disorders of bladder**
Excludes2 calculus of bladder (N21.0)
cystocele (N81.1-)
hernia or prolapse of bladder, female (N81.1-)

N32.0 Bladder-neck obstruction
Bladder-neck stenosis (acquired)
Excludes1 congenital bladder-neck obstruction (Q64.3-)
N32.1 Vesicointestinal fistula
Vesicorectal fistula
N32.2 Vesical fistula, not elsewhere classified
Excludes1 fistula between bladder and female genital tract (N82.0-N82.1)
N32.3 Diverticulum of bladder
Formation of sac from a herniation of wall of bladder
Excludes1 congenital diverticulum of bladder (Q64.6)
diverticulitis of bladder (N30.8-)

● **N32.8 Other specified disorders of bladder**
N32.81 Overactive bladder
Detrusor muscle hyperactivity
Excludes1 frequent urination due to specified bladder condition- code to condition
N32.89 Other specified disorders of bladder
Bladder hemorrhage
Bladder hypertrophy
Calcified bladder
Contracted bladder

N32.9 Bladder disorder, unspecified

N33 Bladder disorders in diseases classified elsewhere
Code first underlying disease, such as:
schistosomiasis (B65.0-B65.9)
Excludes1 bladder disorder in syphilis (A52.76)
bladder disorder in tuberculosis (A18.12)
candidal cystitis (B37.41)
chlamydial cystitis(A56.01)
cystitis in gonorrhea (A54.01)
cystitis in neurogenic bladder (N31.-)
diphtheritic cystitis (A36.85)
syphilitic cystitis (A52.76)
trichomonal cystitis (A59.03)

● **N34 Urethritis and urethral syndrome**
Use additional code (B95-B97), to identify infectious agent
Excludes2 Reiter's disease (M02.3-)
urethritis in diseases with a predominantly sexual mode of transmission (A50-A64)
urethrotrigonitis (N30.3-)

N34.0 Urethral abscess
Abscess (of) Cowper's gland
Abscess (of) Littré's gland
Abscess (of) urethral (gland)
Periurethral abscess
Excludes1 urethral caruncle (N36.2)
N34.1 Nonspecific urethritis
Nongonococcal urethritis
Nonvenereal urethritis
N34.2 Other urethritis
Inflammation of urethra
Meatitis, urethral
Postmenopausal urethritis
Ulcer of urethra (meatus)
Urethritis NOS
N34.3 Urethral syndrome, unspecified

● **N35 Urethral stricture**
Narrowing of lumen of urethra caused by scarring due to infection or injury
Excludes1 congenital urethral stricture (Q64.3-)
postprocedural urethral stricture (N99.1-)

● **N35.0 Post-traumatic urethral stricture**
Urethral stricture due to injury
Excludes1 postprocedural urethral stricture (N99.1-)
● **N35.01 Post-traumatic urethral stricture, male**
N35.010 Post-traumatic urethral stricture, male, meatal ♂
N35.011 Post-traumatic bulbous urethral stricture ♂
N35.012 Post-traumatic membranous urethral stricture ♂
N35.013 Post-traumatic anterior urethral stricture ♂
N35.014 Post-traumatic urethral stricture, male, unspecified ♂
N35.016 Post-traumatic urethral stricture, male, overlapping sites ♂
● **N35.02 Post-traumatic urethral stricture, female**
N35.021 Urethral stricture due to childbirth ♀
N35.028 Other post-traumatic urethral stricture, female ♀

● **N35.1 Postinfective urethral stricture, not elsewhere classified**
Excludes1 urethral stricture associated with schistosomiasis (B65.-, N29)
gonococcal urethral stricture (A54.01)
syphilitic urethral stricture (A52.76)
● **N35.11 Postinfective urethral stricture, not elsewhere classified, male**
N35.111 Postinfective urethral stricture, not elsewhere classified, male, meatal ♂
N35.112 Postinfective bulbous urethral stricture, not elsewhere classified, male ♂

N35.113 Postinfective membranous urethral stricture, not elsewhere classified, male ♂

N35.114 Postinfective anterior urethral stricture, not elsewhere classified, male ♂

N35.116 Postinfective urethral stricture, not elsewhere classified, male, overlapping sites ♂

N35.119 Postinfective urethral stricture, not elsewhere classified, male, unspecified ♂

N35.12 Postinfective urethral stricture, not elsewhere classified, female ♀

N35.8 Other urethral stricture

Excludes1 postprocedural urethral stricture (N99.1-)

N35.81 Other urethral stricture, male

N35.811 Other urethral stricture, male, meatal ♂

N35.812 Other urethral bulbous stricture, male ♂

N35.813 Other membranous urethral stricture, male ♂

N35.814 Other anterior urethral stricture, male ♂

N35.816 Other urethral stricture, male, overlapping sites ♂

N35.819 Other urethral stricture, male, unspecified site ♂

N35.82 Other urethral stricture, female ♀

N35.9 Urethral stricture, unspecified

N35.91 Urethral stricture, unspecified, male

N35.911 Unspecified urethral stricture, male, meatal ♂

N35.912 Unspecified bulbous urethral stricture, male ♂

N35.913 Unspecified membranous urethral stricture, male ♂

N35.914 Unspecified anterior urethral stricture, male ♂

N35.916 Unspecified urethral stricture, male, overlapping sites ♂

N35.919 Unspecified urethral stricture, male, unspecified site ♂
Pinhole meatus NOS
Urethral stricture NOS

N35.92 Unspecified urethral stricture, female ♀

N36 Other disorders of urethra

N36.0 Urethral fistula
Urethroperineal fistula
Urethrorectal fistula
Urinary fistula NOS

Excludes1 urethroscrotal fistula (N50.89)
urethrovaginal fistula (N82.1)
urethrovesicovaginal fistula (N82.1)

N36.1 Urethral diverticulum

N36.2 Urethral caruncle

N36.4 Urethral functional and muscular disorders
Use additional code to identify associated urinary stress incontinence (N39.3)

N36.41 Hypermobility of urethra

N36.42 Intrinsic sphincter deficiency (ISD)

N36.43 Combined hypermobility of urethra and intrinsic sphincter deficiency

N36.44 Muscular disorders of urethra
Bladder sphincter dyssynergy

N36.5 Urethral false passage

N36.8 Other specified disorders of urethra

Excludes1 congenital urethrocele (Q64.7)
female urethrocele (N81.0)

N36.9 Urethral disorder, unspecified

N37 Urethral disorders in diseases classified elsewhere
Code first underlying disease

Excludes1 urethritis (in):
candidal infection (B37.41)
chlamydial (A56.01)
gonorrhea (A54.01)
syphilis (A52.76)
trichomonal infection (A59.03)
tuberculosis (A18.13)

N39 Other disorders of urinary system

Excludes2 hematuria NOS (R31.-)
recurrent or persistent hematuria (N02.-)
recurrent or persistent hematuria with specified morphological lesion (N02.-)
proteinuria NOS (R80.-)

N39.0 Urinary tract infection, site not specified
Use additional code (B95-B97), to identify infectious agent

Excludes1 candidiasis of urinary tract (B37.4-)
neonatal urinary tract infection (P39.3)
pyuria (R82.81)
urinary tract infection of specified site, such as:
cystitis (N30.-)
urethritis (N34.-)

Coding Clinic: 2018, Q2, P22; Q1, P16; 2012, Q4, P94

N39.3 Stress incontinence (female) (male)
Code also any associated overactive bladder (N32.81)

Excludes1 mixed incontinence (N39.46)

N39.4 Other specified urinary incontinence
Code also any associated overactive bladder (N32.81)

Excludes1 enuresis NOS (R32)
functional urinary incontinence (R39.81)
urinary incontinence associated with cognitive impairment (R39.81)
urinary incontinence NOS (R32)
urinary incontinence of nonorganic origin (F98.0)

N39.41 Urge incontinence

Excludes1 mixed incontinence (N39.46)

N39.42 Incontinence without sensory awareness
Insensible (urinary) incontinence

N39.43 Post-void dribbling

N39.44 Nocturnal enuresis

N39.45 Continuous leakage

N39.46 Mixed incontinence
Urge and stress incontinence

N39.49 Other specified urinary incontinence

N39.490 Overflow incontinence

N39.491 Coital incontinence
Coding Clinic: 2016, Q4, P44

N39.492 Postural (urinary) incontinence
Coding Clinic: 2016, Q4, P44

N39.498 Other specified urinary incontinence
Reflex incontinence
Total incontinence

N39.8 Other specified disorders of urinary system

N39.9 Disorder of urinary system, unspecified

CHAPTER 14 (N00-N99)

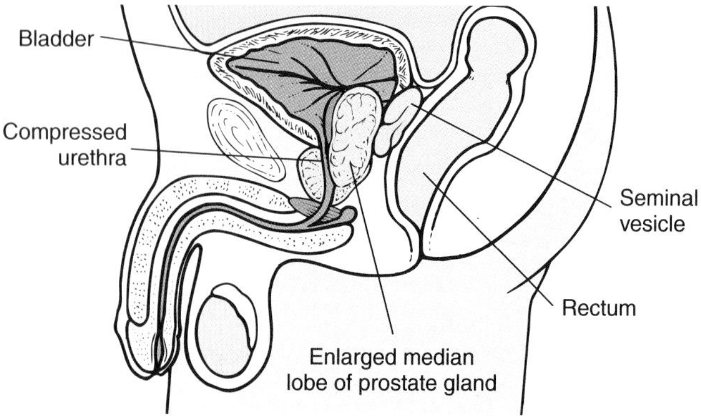

Figure 14-6 Benign prostatic hyperplasia. (From Shiland: Mastering Healthcare Terminology, ed 3, St. Louis, Mosby, 2010)

DISEASES OF MALE GENITAL ORGANS (N40-N53)

★ **(See Plate 5 of the Anatomy Illustrations.)**

● **N40 Benign prostatic hyperplasia**

Includes adenofibromatous hypertrophy of prostate
benign hypertrophy of the prostate
Enlargement of prostate gland usually occurring with age and causing obstructed urine flow
benign prostatic hypertrophy
BPH
enlarged prostate
nodular prostate
polyp of prostate

Excludes1 benign neoplasms of prostate (adenoma, benign) (fibroadenoma) (fibroma) (myoma) (D29.1)
malignant neoplasm of prostate (C61)

N40.0 Benign prostatic hyperplasia without lower urinary tract symptoms ♂ A
Enlarged prostate without LUTS
Enlarged prostate NOS

N40.1 Benign prostatic hyperplasia with lower urinary tract symptoms ♂ A
Enlarged prostate with LUTS
Use additional code for associated symptoms, when specified:
incomplete bladder emptying (R39.14)
nocturia (R35.1)
straining on urination (R39.16)
urinary frequency (R35.0)
urinary hesitancy (R39.11)
urinary incontinence (N39.4-)
urinary obstruction (N13.8)
urinary retention (R33.8)
urinary urgency (R39.15)
weak urinary stream (R39.12)
Coding Clinic: 2018, Q4, P55

N40.2 Nodular prostate without lower urinary tract symptoms ♂ A
Nodular prostate without LUTS

N40.3 Nodular prostate with lower urinary tract symptoms ♂ A
Use additional code for associated symptoms, when specified:
incomplete bladder emptying (R39.14)
nocturia (R35.1)
straining on urination (R39.16)
urinary frequency (R35.0)
urinary hesitancy (R39.11)
urinary incontinence (N39.4-)
urinary obstruction (N13.8)
urinary retention (R33.8)
urinary urgency (R39.15)
weak urinary stream (R39.12)

● **N41 Inflammatory diseases of prostate**
Use additional code (B95-B97), to identify infectious agent

N41.0 Acute prostatitis ♂ A
N41.1 Chronic prostatitis ♂ A
N41.2 Abscess of prostate ♂ A
N41.3 Prostatocystitis ♂ A
N41.4 Granulomatous prostatitis ♂ A
N41.8 Other inflammatory diseases of prostate ♂ A
N41.9 Inflammatory disease of prostate, unspecified ♂ A
Prostatitis NOS

● **N42 Other and unspecified disorders of prostate**

N42.0 Calculus of prostate ♂ A
Prostatic stone

N42.1 Congestion and hemorrhage of prostate ♂ A
Excludes1 enlarged prostate (N40.-)
hematuria (R31.-)
hyperplasia of prostate (N40.-)
inflammatory diseases of prostate (N41.-)

● **N42.3 Dysplasia of prostate**
Coding Clinic: 2016, Q4, P44

N42.30 Unspecified dysplasia of prostate ♂
N42.31 Prostatic intraepithelial neoplasia ♂
PIN
Prostatic intraepithelial neoplasia I (PIN I)
Prostatic intraepithelial neoplasia II (PIN II)
Excludes1 prostatic intraepithelial neoplasia III (PIN III) (D07.5)
N42.32 Atypical small acinar proliferation of prostate ♂
N42.39 Other dysplasia of prostate ♂

● **N42.8 Other specified disorders of prostate**

N42.81 Prostatodynia syndrome ♂ A
Painful prostate syndrome
N42.82 Prostatosis syndrome ♂ A
N42.83 Cyst of prostate ♂ A
N42.89 Other specified disorders of prostate ♂ A

N42.9 Disorder of prostate, unspecified ♂ A

● **N43 Hydrocele and spermatocele**

Includes hydrocele of spermatic cord, testis or tunica vaginalis

Excludes1 congenital hydrocele (P83.5)

N43.0 Encysted hydrocele ♂
N43.1 Infected hydrocele ♂
Use additional code (B95-B97), to identify infectious agent
N43.2 Other hydrocele ♂
N43.3 Hydrocele, unspecified ♂

● **N43.4 Spermatocele of epididymis**
Spermatic cyst

N43.40 Spermatocele of epididymis, unspecified ♂
N43.41 Spermatocele of epididymis, single ♂
N43.42 Spermatocele of epididymis, multiple ♂

Item 14–7 Hydrocele is a sac of fluid accumulating in the testes membrane.

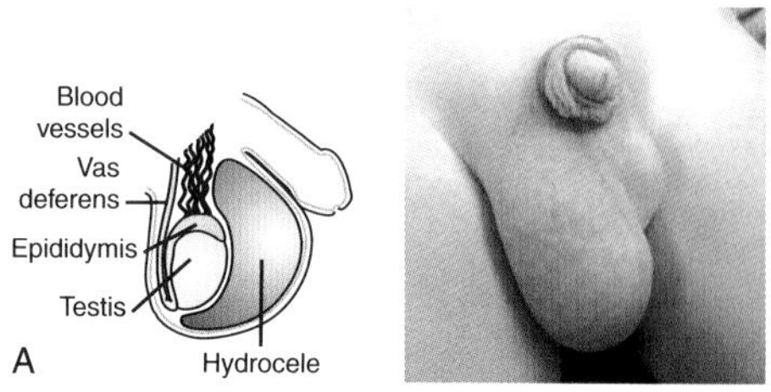

Figure 14-7 A. Hydrocele. **B.** Newborn with large right hydrocele. (**B** from Nelson WE, Kliegman R: Nelson Textbook of Pediatrics, Philadelphia, Saunders Elsevier, 2011)

N44 Noninflammatory disorders of testis

N44.0 Torsion of testis

N44.00 Torsion of testis, unspecified ♂

N44.01 Extravaginal torsion of spermatic cord ♂

N44.02 Intravaginal torsion of spermatic cord ♂
Torsion of spermatic cord NOS

N44.03 Torsion of appendix testis ♂

N44.04 Torsion of appendix epididymis ♂

N44.1 Cyst of tunica albuginea testis ♂

N44.2 Benign cyst of testis ♂

N44.8 Other noninflammatory disorders of the testis ♂

N45 Orchitis and epididymitis

Orchitis is inflammation of one or both of the testes as a result of mumps or other infection, trauma, or metastasis. Epididymitis is inflammation of the tubular structure that connects the testicle with the vas deferens.

Use additional code (B95-B97), to identify infectious agent

N45.1 Epididymitis ♂

N45.2 Orchitis ♂

N45.3 Epididymo-orchitis ♂

N45.4 Abscess of epididymis or testis ♂

N46 Male infertility

Excludes1 vasectomy status (Z98.52)

N46.0 Azoospermia
Absolute male infertility
Male infertility due to germinal (cell) aplasia
Male infertility due to spermatogenic arrest (complete)

N46.01 Organic azoospermia ♂ A
Azoospermia NOS

N46.02 Azoospermia due to extratesticular causes
Code also associated cause

N46.021 Azoospermia due to drug therapy ♂ A

N46.022 Azoospermia due to infection ♂ A

N46.023 Azoospermia due to obstruction of efferent ducts ♂ A

N46.024 Azoospermia due to radiation ♂ A

N46.025 Azoospermia due to systemic disease ♂ A

N46.029 Azoospermia due to other extratesticular causes ♂ A

N46.1 Oligospermia
Male infertility due to germinal cell desquamation
Male infertility due to hypospermatogenesis
Male infertility due to incomplete spermatogenic arrest

N46.11 Organic oligospermia ♂ A
Oligospermia NOS

N46.12 Oligospermia due to extratesticular causes
Code also associated cause

N46.121 Oligospermia due to drug therapy ♂ A

N46.122 Oligospermia due to infection ♂ A

N46.123 Oligospermia due to obstruction of efferent ducts ♂ A

N46.124 Oligospermia due to radiation ♂ A

N46.125 Oligospermia due to systemic disease ♂ A

N46.129 Oligospermia due to other extratesticular causes ♂ A

N46.8 Other male infertility ♂ A

N46.9 Male infertility, unspecified ♂ A

Item 14–8 Male infertility is the inability of the female sex partner to conceive after one year of unprotected intercourse.

Azoospermia is no sperm ejaculated and **oligospermia** is few sperm ejaculated—both resulting in infertility. Extratesticular causes such as injury, infections, radiation, and chemotherapy may also cause male infertility.

N47 Disorders of prepuce

N47.0 Adherent prepuce, newborn ♂ N

N47.1 Phimosis ♂

N47.2 Paraphimosis ♂

N47.3 Deficient foreskin ♂

N47.4 Benign cyst of prepuce ♂

N47.5 Adhesions of prepuce and glans penis ♂

N47.6 Balanoposthitis ♂
Use additional code (B95-B97), to identify infectious agent

Excludes1 balanitis (N48.1)

N47.7 Other inflammatory diseases of prepuce ♂
Use additional code (B95-B97), to identify infectious agent

N47.8 Other disorders of prepuce ♂

N48 Other disorders of penis

N48.0 Leukoplakia of penis ♂
Balanitis xerotica obliterans
Kraurosis of penis
Lichen sclerosus of external male genital organs

Excludes1 carcinoma in situ of penis (D07.4)

N48.1 Balanitis ♂
Use additional code (B95-B97), to identify infectious agent

Excludes1 amebic balanitis (A06.8)
balanitis xerotica obliterans (N48.0)
candidal balanitis (B37.42)
gonococcal balanitis (A54.23)
herpesviral [herpes simplex] balanitis (A60.01)

N48.2 Other inflammatory disorders of penis
Use additional code (B95-B97), to identify infectious agent

Excludes1 balanitis (N48.1)
balanitis xerotica obliterans (N48.0)
balanoposthitis (N47.6)

N48.21 Abscess of corpus cavernosum and penis ♂

N48.22 Cellulitis of corpus cavernosum and penis ♂

N48.29 Other inflammatory disorders of penis ♂

N48.3 Priapism
Painful erection
Code first underlying cause

N48.30 Priapism, unspecified ♂

N48.31 Priapism due to trauma ♂

N48.32 Priapism due to disease classified elsewhere ♂

N48.33 Priapism, drug-induced ♂

N48.39 Other priapism ♂

N48.5 Ulcer of penis ♂

N48.6 Induration penis plastica ♂
Peyronie's disease
Plastic induration of penis

N48.8 Other specified disorders of penis

N48.81 Thrombosis of superficial vein of penis ♂

N48.82 Acquired torsion of penis ♂
Acquired torsion of penis NOS

Excludes1 congenital torsion of penis (Q55.63)

N48.83 Acquired buried penis ♂

Excludes1 congenital hidden penis (Q55.64)

N48.89 Other specified disorders of penis ♂

N48.9 Disorder of penis, unspecified ♂

CHAPTER 14 (N00-N99)

N49 Inflammatory disorders of male genital organs, not elsewhere classified

Use additional code (B95-B97), to identify infectious agent

Excludes1 inflammation of penis (N48.1, N48.2-)
orchitis and epididymitis (N45.-)

N49.Ø Inflammatory disorders of seminal vesicle ♂
Vesiculitis NOS

N49.1 Inflammatory disorders of spermatic cord, tunica vaginalis and vas deferens ♂
Vasitis

N49.2 Inflammatory disorders of scrotum ♂

N49.3 Fournier gangrene ♂

N49.8 Inflammatory disorders of other specified male genital organs ♂
Inflammation of multiple sites in male genital organs

N49.9 Inflammatory disorder of unspecified male genital organ ♂
Abscess of unspecified male genital organ
Boil of unspecified male genital organ
Carbuncle of unspecified male genital organ
Cellulitis of unspecified male genital organ

N5Ø Other and unspecified disorders of male genital organs

Excludes2 torsion of testis (N44.Ø-)

N5Ø.Ø Atrophy of testis ♂

N5Ø.1 Vascular disorders of male genital organs ♂
Hematocele, NOS, of male genital organs
Hemorrhage of male genital organs
Thrombosis of male genital organs

N5Ø.3 Cyst of epididymis ♂

N5Ø.8 Other specified disorders of male genital organs
Coding Clinic: 2016, Q4, P45

N5Ø.81 Testicular pain

N5Ø.811 Right testicular pain ♂

N5Ø.812 Left testicular pain ♂

N5Ø.819 Testicular pain, unspecified ♂

N5Ø.82 Scrotal pain ♂

N5Ø.89 Other specified disorders of the male genital organs ♂
Atrophy of scrotum, seminal vesicle, spermatic cord, tunica vaginalis and vas deferens
Chylocele, tunica vaginalis (nonfilarial) NOS
Edema of scrotum, seminal vesicle, spermatic cord, tunica vaginalis and vas deferens
Hypertrophy of scrotum, seminal vesicle, spermatic cord, tunica vaginalis and vas deferens
Stricture of spermatic cord, tunica vaginalis, and vas deferens
Ulcer of scrotum, seminal vesicle, spermatic cord, testis, tunica vaginalis and vas deferens
Urethroscrotal fistula

N5Ø.9 Disorder of male genital organs, unspecified ♂

N51 Disorders of male genital organs in diseases classified elsewhere ♂

Code first underlying disease, such as:
filariasis (B74.Ø-B74.9)

Excludes1 amebic balanitis (AØ6.8)
candidal balanitis (B37.42)
gonococcal balanitis (A54.23)
gonococcal prostatitis (A54.22)
herpesviral [herpes simplex] balanitis (A6Ø.Ø1)
trichomonal prostatitis (A59.Ø2)
tuberculous prostatitis (A18.14)

Item 14–9 Seminal vesiculitis is an inflammation of the seminal vesicle. **Spermatocele** is a benign cystic accumulation of sperm arising from the head of the epididymis. **Torsion of the testis** is a medical emergency occurring most commonly in boys 7 to 12 years of age and results from a congenital abnormality of the covering of the testis allowing the testis to twist within its sac and cutting off the blood supply to the testis.

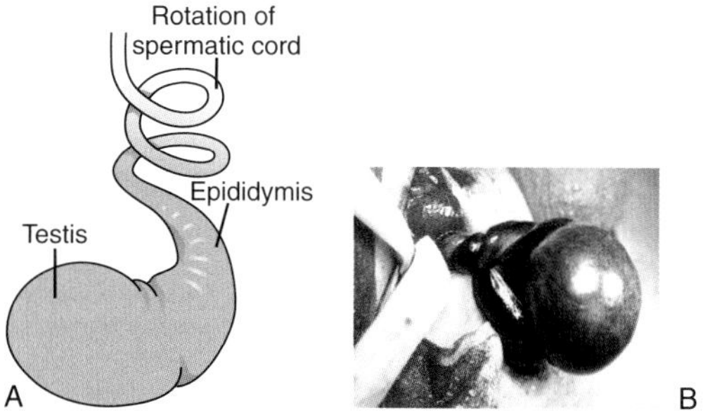

Figure 14-8 A. Torsion of testis. **B.** Torsion of the testis. (**B** from Kliegman R, Nelson WE: Nelson Textbook of Pediatrics, Philadelphia, Saunders, 2007)

N52 Male erectile dysfunction

Excludes1 psychogenic impotence (F52.21)

N52.Ø Vasculogenic erectile dysfunction

N52.Ø1 Erectile dysfunction due to arterial insufficiency ♂ A

N52.Ø2 Corporo-venous occlusive erectile dysfunction ♂ A

N52.Ø3 Combined arterial insufficiency and corporo-venous occlusive erectile dysfunction ♂ A

N52.1 Erectile dysfunction due to diseases classified elsewhere ♂ A
Code first underlying disease

N52.2 Drug-induced erectile dysfunction ♂ A

N52.3 Postprocedural erectile dysfunction

N52.31 Erectile dysfunction following radical prostatectomy ♂ A

N52.32 Erectile dysfunction following radical cystectomy ♂ A

N52.33 Erectile dysfunction following urethral surgery ♂ A

N52.34 Erectile dysfunction following simple prostatectomy ♂ A

N52.35 Erectile dysfunction following radiation therapy ♂ A
Coding Clinic: 2016, Q4, P45

N52.36 Erectile dysfunction following interstitial seed therapy ♂ A
Coding Clinic: 2016, Q4, P45

N52.37 Erectile dysfunction following prostate ablative therapy ♂ A
Erectile dysfunction following cryotherapy
Erectile dysfunction following other prostate ablative therapies
Erectile dysfunction following ultrasound ablative therapies
Coding Clinic: 2016, Q4, P45

N52.39 Other and unspecified postprocedural erectile dysfunction ♂ A

N52.8 Other male erectile dysfunction ♂ A

N52.9 Male erectile dysfunction, unspecified ♂ A
Impotence NOS

● N53 Other male sexual dysfunction
Excludes1 psychogenic sexual dysfunction (F52.-)
● N53.1 Ejaculatory dysfunction
Excludes1 premature ejaculation (F52.4)
N53.11 **Retarded ejaculation** ♂
N53.12 **Painful ejaculation** ♂
N53.13 **Anejaculatory orgasm** ♂
N53.14 **Retrograde ejaculation** ♂
N53.19 **Other ejaculatory dysfunction** ♂
Ejaculatory dysfunction NOS
N53.8 **Other male sexual dysfunction** ♂
N53.9 **Unspecified male sexual dysfunction** ♂

DISORDERS OF BREAST (N60-N65)

Excludes1 disorders of breast associated with childbirth (O91-O92)

● N60 Benign mammary dysplasia
Benign lumpiness of breast
Includes fibrocystic mastopathy
● N60.0 Solitary cyst of breast
Cyst of breast
N60.01 **Solitary cyst of right breast**
N60.02 **Solitary cyst of left breast**
N60.09 **Solitary cyst of unspecified breast**
● N60.1 Diffuse cystic mastopathy
Cystic breast
Fibrocystic disease of breast
Excludes1 diffuse cystic mastopathy with epithelial proliferation (N60.3-)
N60.11 **Diffuse cystic mastopathy of right breast** A
N60.12 **Diffuse cystic mastopathy of left breast** A
N60.19 **Diffuse cystic mastopathy of unspecified breast** A
● N60.2 Fibroadenosis of breast
Adenofibrosis of breast
Excludes2 fibroadenoma of breast (D24.-)
N60.21 **Fibroadenosis of right breast**
N60.22 **Fibroadenosis of left breast**
N60.29 **Fibroadenosis of unspecified breast**
● N60.3 Fibrosclerosis of breast
Cystic mastopathy with epithelial proliferation
N60.31 **Fibrosclerosis of right breast**
N60.32 **Fibrosclerosis of left breast**
N60.39 **Fibrosclerosis of unspecified breast**
● N60.4 Mammary duct ectasia
N60.41 **Mammary duct ectasia of right breast**
N60.42 **Mammary duct ectasia of left breast**
N60.49 **Mammary duct ectasia of unspecified breast**
● N60.8 Other benign mammary dysplasias
N60.81 **Other benign mammary dysplasias of right breast**
N60.82 **Other benign mammary dysplasias of left breast**
N60.89 **Other benign mammary dysplasias of unspecified breast**
● N60.9 Unspecified benign mammary dysplasia
N60.91 **Unspecified benign mammary dysplasia of right breast**
N60.92 **Unspecified benign mammary dysplasia of left breast**
N60.99 **Unspecified benign mammary dysplasia of unspecified breast**

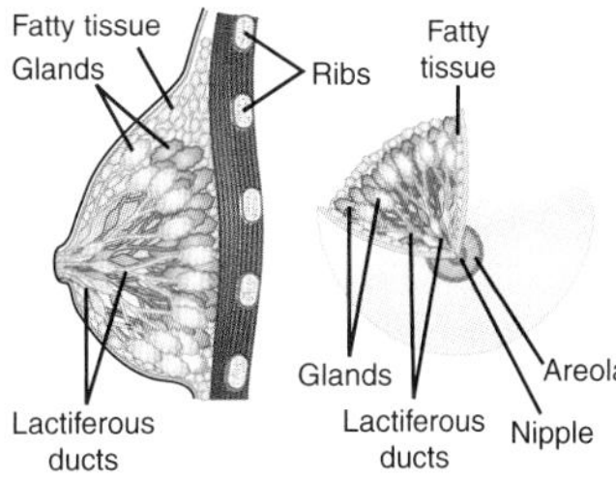

Figure 14-9 Breast.

● N61 Inflammatory disorders of breast
Excludes1 inflammatory carcinoma of breast (C50.9)
inflammatory disorder of breast associated with childbirth (O91.-)
neonatal infective mastitis (P39.0)
thrombophlebitis of breast [Mondor's disease] (I80.8)
N61.0 **Mastitis without abscess**
Infective mastitis (acute) (nonpuerperal) (subacute)
Mastitis (acute) (nonpuerperal) (subacute) NOS
Cellulitis (acute) (nonpuerperal) (subacute) of breast NOS
Cellulitis (acute) (nonpuerperal) (subacute) of nipple NOS
N61.1 **Abscess of the breast and nipple**
Abscess (acute) (chronic) (nonpuerperal) of areola
Abscess (acute) (chronic) (nonpuerperal) of breast
Carbuncle of breast
Mastitis with abscess

N62 Hypertrophy of breast
Gynecomastia
Hypertrophy of breast NOS
Massive pubertal hypertrophy of breast
Excludes1 breast engorgement of newborn (P83.4)
disproportion of reconstructed breast (N65.1)

● N63 Unspecified lump in breast
Nodule(s) NOS in breast
N63.0 **Unspecified lump in unspecified breast**
● N63.1 Unspecified lump in the right breast
N63.10 **Unspecified lump in the right breast, unspecified quadrant**
N63.11 **Unspecified lump in the right breast, upper outer quadrant**
Coding Clinic: 2017, Q4, P19
N63.12 **Unspecified lump in the right breast, upper inner quadrant**
N63.13 **Unspecified lump in the right breast, lower outer quadrant**
N63.14 **Unspecified lump in the right breast, lower inner quadrant**
▶ N63.15 **Unspecified lump in the right breast, overlapping quadrants**
● N63.2 Unspecified lump in the left breast
N63.20 **Unspecified lump in the left breast, unspecified quadrant**
N63.21 **Unspecified lump in the left breast, upper outer quadrant**
N63.22 **Unspecified lump in the left breast, upper inner quadrant**
N63.23 **Unspecified lump in the left breast, lower outer quadrant**
N63.24 **Unspecified lump in the left breast, lower inner quadrant**
▶ N63.25 **Unspecified lump in the left breast, overlapping quadrants**

● N63.3 **Unspecified lump in axillary tail**
- N63.31 **Unspecified lump in axillary tail of the right breast**
- N63.32 **Unspecified lump in axillary tail of the left breast**

● N63.4 **Unspecified lump in breast, subareolar**
- N63.41 **Unspecified lump in right breast, subareolar**
- N63.42 **Unspecified lump in left breast, subareolar**

● N64 **Other disorders of breast**

Excludes2 mechanical complication of breast prosthesis and implant (T85.4-)

N64.0 **Fissure and fistula of nipple**

N64.1 **Fat necrosis of breast**
Fat necrosis (segmental) of breast
Code first breast necrosis due to breast graft (T85.898)

N64.2 **Atrophy of breast**

N64.3 **Galactorrhea not associated with childbirth**
Excessive or spontaneous flow of milk

N64.4 **Mastodynia**

● N64.5 **Other signs and symptoms in breast**

Excludes2 abnormal findings on diagnostic imaging of breast (R92.-)

- N64.51 **Induration of breast**
- N64.52 **Nipple discharge**
  Excludes1 abnormal findings in nipple discharge (R89.-)
- N64.53 **Retraction of nipple**
- N64.59 **Other signs and symptoms in breast**

● N64.8 **Other specified disorders of breast**
- N64.81 **Ptosis of breast** A
  Excludes1 ptosis of native breast in relation to reconstructed breast (N65.1)
- N64.82 **Hypoplasia of breast** A
  Micromastia
  Excludes1 congenital absence of breast (Q83.0)
  hypoplasia of native breast in relation to reconstructed breast (N65.1)
- N64.89 **Other specified disorders of breast**
  Galactocele
  Subinvolution of breast (postlactational)
  Coding Clinic: 2019, Q1, P32; 2018, Q1, P4

N64.9 **Disorder of breast, unspecified**
Coding Clinic: 2018, Q1, P4

● N65 **Deformity and disproportion of reconstructed breast**

N65.0 **Deformity of reconstructed breast** A
Contour irregularity in reconstructed breast
Excess tissue in reconstructed breast
Misshapen reconstructed breast

N65.1 **Disproportion of reconstructed breast** A
Breast asymmetry between native breast and reconstructed breast
Disproportion between native breast and reconstructed breast

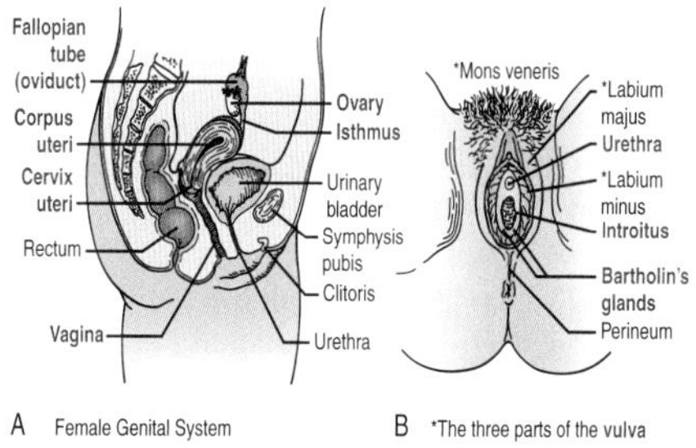

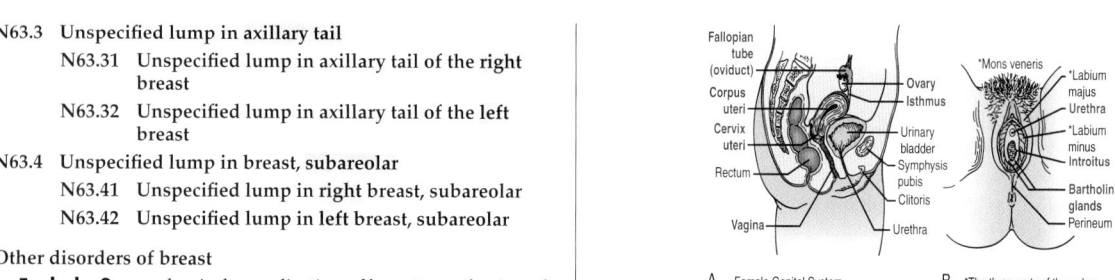

Figure 14-10 A. Female genital system. **B.** External female genital system. (From Buck CJ: Step-by-Step Medical Coding, ed 2016, St. Louis, Elsevier, 2016)

Item 14–10 Salpingitis is an infection of one or both fallopian tubes. **Oophoritis** is an infection of one or both ovaries.

INFLAMMATORY DISEASES OF FEMALE PELVIC ORGANS (N70-N77)

Excludes1 inflammatory diseases of female pelvic organs complicating:
abortion or ectopic or molar pregnancy (O00-O07, O08.0)
pregnancy, childbirth and the puerperium (O23.-, O75.3, O85, O86.-)

★**(See Plate 35 of the Anatomy Illustrations.)**

● N70 **Salpingitis and oophoritis**
Oophoritis = inflammation of ovary
Salpingitis = inflammation of falloplan tube

Includes abscess (of) fallopian tube
abscess (of) ovary
pyosalpinx
salpingo-oophoritis
tubo-ovarian abscess
tubo-ovarian inflammatory disease

Use additional code (B95-B97), to identify infectious agent

Excludes1 gonococcal infection (A54.24)
tuberculous infection (A18.17)

● N70.0 **Acute salpingitis and oophoritis**
- N70.01 **Acute salpingitis** ♀
- N70.02 **Acute oophoritis** ♀
- N70.03 **Acute salpingitis and oophoritis** ♀

● N70.1 **Chronic salpingitis and oophoritis**
Hydrosalpinx
- N70.11 **Chronic salpingitis** ♀
- N70.12 **Chronic oophoritis** ♀
- N70.13 **Chronic salpingitis and oophoritis** ♀

● N70.9 **Salpingitis and oophoritis, unspecified**
- N70.91 **Salpingitis, unspecified** ♀
- N70.92 **Oophoritis, unspecified** ♀
- N70.93 **Salpingitis and oophoritis, unspecified** ♀

● N71 **Inflammatory disease of uterus, except cervix**

Includes endo (myo) metritis
metritis
myometritis
pyometra
uterine abscess

Use additional code (B95-B97), to identify infectious agent

Excludes1 hyperplastic endometritis (N85.0-)
infection of uterus following delivery (O85, O86.-)

N71.0 **Acute inflammatory disease of uterus** ♀

N71.1 **Chronic inflammatory disease of uterus** ♀

N71.9 **Inflammatory disease of uterus, unspecified** ♀

N72 Inflammatory disease of cervix uteri ♀

Includes cervicitis (with or without erosion or ectropion)
endocervicitis (with or without erosion or ectropion)
exocervicitis (with or without erosion or ectropion)

Use additional code (B95-B97), to identify infectious agent

Excludes1 erosion and ectropion of cervix without cervicitis (N86)

N73 Other female pelvic inflammatory diseases

Use additional code (B95-B97), to identify infectious agent

N73.0 Acute parametritis and pelvic cellulitis ♀
Abscess of broad ligament
Abscess of parametrium
Pelvic cellulitis, female

N73.1 Chronic parametritis and pelvic cellulitis ♀
Any condition in N73.0 specified as chronic

Excludes1 tuberculous parametritis and pelvic cellultis (A18.17)

N73.2 Unspecified parametritis and pelvic cellulitis ♀
Any condition in N73.0 unspecified whether acute or chronic

N73.3 Female acute pelvic peritonitis ♀

N73.4 Female chronic pelvic peritonitis ♀

Excludes1 tuberculous pelvic (female) peritonitis (A18.17)

N73.5 Female pelvic peritonitis, unspecified ♀

N73.6 Female pelvic peritoneal adhesions (postinfective) ♀

Excludes2 postprocedural pelvic peritoneal adhesions (N99.4)

N73.8 Other specified female pelvic inflammatory diseases ♀

N73.9 Female pelvic inflammatory disease, unspecified ♀
Female pelvic infection or inflammation NOS

N74 Female pelvic inflammatory disorders in diseases classified elsewhere ♀

Code first underlying disease

Excludes1 chlamydial cervicitis (A56.02)
chlamydial pelvic inflammatory disease (A56.11)
gonococcal cervicitis (A54.03)
gonococcal pelvic inflammatory disease (A54.24)
herpesviral [herpes simplex] cervicitis (A60.03)
herpesviral [herpes simplex] pelvic inflammatory disease (A60.09)
syphilitic cervicitis (A52.76)
syphilitic pelvic inflammatory disease (A52.76)
trichomonal cervicitis (A59.09)
tuberculous cervicitis (A18.16)
tuberculous pelvic inflammatory disease (A18.17)

N75 Diseases of Bartholin's gland

N75.0 Cyst of Bartholin's gland ♀
Cysts filled with liquid or semisolid material

N75.1 Abscess of Bartholin's gland ♀
Localized collection of pus

N75.8 Other diseases of Bartholin's gland ♀
Bartholinitis

N75.9 Disease of Bartholin's gland, unspecified ♀

N76 Other inflammation of vagina and vulva

Use additional code (B95-B97), to identify infectious agent

Excludes2 senile (atrophic) vaginitis (N95.2)
vulvar vestibulitis (N94.810)

N76.0 Acute vaginitis ♀
Acute vulvovaginitis
Vaginitis NOS
Vulvovaginitis NOS

N76.1 Subacute and chronic vaginitis ♀
Chronic vulvovaginitis
Subacute vulvovaginitis

N76.2 Acute vulvitis ♀
Vulvitis NOS

N76.3 Subacute and chronic vulvitis ♀

N76.4 Abscess of vulva ♀
Furuncle of vulva

N76.5 Ulceration of vagina ♀

N76.6 Ulceration of vulva ♀

N76.8 Other specified inflammation of vagina and vulva

N76.81 Mucositis (ulcerative) of vagina and vulva ♀
Code also type of associated therapy, such as:
antineoplastic and immunosuppressive drugs (T45.1X-)
radiological procedure and radiotherapy (Y84.2)

Excludes2 gastrointestinal mucositis (ulcerative) (K92.81)
nasal mucositis (ulcerative) (J34.81)
oral mucositis (ulcerative) (K12.3-)

N76.89 Other specified inflammation of vagina and vulva ♀

N77 Vulvovaginal ulceration and inflammation in diseases classified elsewhere

N77.0 Ulceration of vulva in diseases classified elsewhere ♀

Code first underlying disease, such as:
Behçet's disease (M35.2)

Excludes1 ulceration of vulva in gonococcal infection (A54.02)
ulceration of vulva in herpesviral [herpes simplex] infection (A60.04)
ulceration of vulva in syphilis (A51.0)
ulceration of vulva in tuberculosis (A18.18)

N77.1 Vaginitis, vulvitis and vulvovaginitis in diseases classified elsewhere ♀

Code first underlying disease, such as:
pinworm (B80)

Excludes1 candidial vulvovaginitis (B37.3)
chlamydial vulvovaginitis (A56.02)
gonococcal vulvovaginitis (A54.02)
herpesviral [herpes simplex] vulvovaginitis (A60.04)
trichomonal vulvovaginitis (A59.01)
tuberculous vulvovaginitis (A18.18)
vulvovaginitis in early syphilis (A51.0)
vulvovaginitis in late syphilis (A52.76)

Item 14–11 Endometriosis is a condition for which no clear cause has been identified. Endometrial tissue is expelled from the uterus into the abdominal cavity and can implant onto a variety of organs. Classification is based on the site of implant of the endometrial tissue.

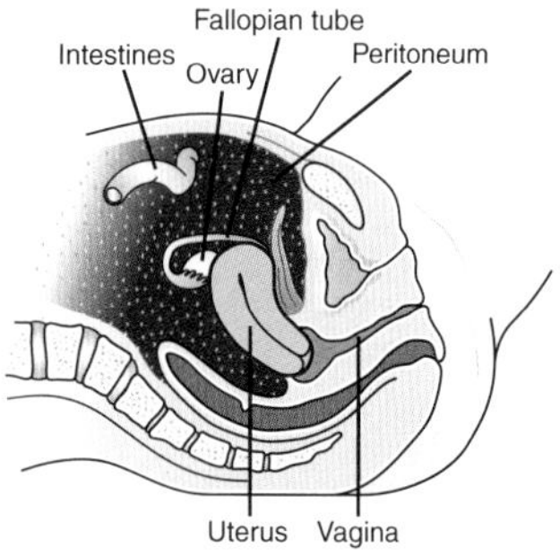

Figure 14-11 Sites of potential endometrial implants.

NONINFLAMMATORY DISORDERS OF FEMALE GENITAL TRACT (N8Ø-N98)

● **N8Ø Endometriosis**
- **N8Ø.Ø Endometriosis of uterus** ♀
  - Adenomyosis
  - **Excludes1** stromal endometriosis (D39.Ø)
- **N8Ø.1 Endometriosis of ovary** ♀
- **N8Ø.2 Endometriosis of fallopian tube** ♀
- **N8Ø.3 Endometriosis of pelvic peritoneum** ♀
- **N8Ø.4 Endometriosis of rectovaginal septum and vagina** ♀
- **N8Ø.5 Endometriosis of intestine** ♀
- **N8Ø.6 Endometriosis in cutaneous scar** ♀
- **N8Ø.8 Other endometriosis** ♀
  - Endometriosis of thorax
- **N8Ø.9 Endometriosis, unspecified** ♀

● **N81 Female genital prolapse**
- **Excludes1** genital prolapse complicating pregnancy, labor or delivery (O34.5-)
  - prolapse and hernia of ovary and fallopian tube (N83.4-)
  - prolapse of vaginal vault after hysterectomy (N99.3)
- **N81.Ø Urethrocele** ♀
  - **Excludes1** urethrocele with cystocele (N81.1-)
    - urethrocele with prolapse of uterus (N81.2-N81.4)
- ● **N81.1 Cystocele**
  - Cystocele with urethrocele
  - Cystourethrocele
  - **Excludes1** cystocele with prolapse of uterus (N81.2-N81.4)
  - **N81.1Ø Cystocele, unspecified** ♀
    - Prolapse of (anterior) vaginal wall NOS
  - **N81.11 Cystocele, midline** ♀
  - **N81.12 Cystocele, lateral** ♀
    - Paravaginal cystocele

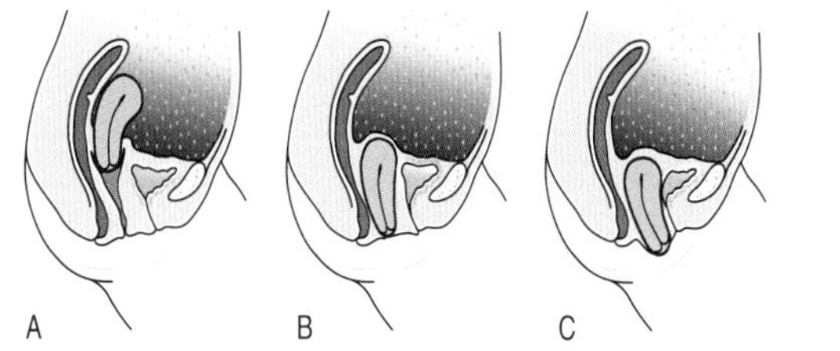

Figure 14-12 Three stages of uterine prolapse. **A.** Uterus is prolapsed. **B.** Vagina and uterus are prolapsed (incomplete uterovaginal prolapse). **C.** Vagina and uterus are completely prolapsed and are exposed through the external genitalia (complete uterovaginal prolapse).

- **N81.2 Incomplete uterovaginal prolapse** ♀
  - First degree uterine prolapse
  - Prolapse of cervix NOS
  - Second degree uterine prolapse
  - **Excludes1** cervical stump prolapse (N81.85)
- **N81.3 Complete uterovaginal prolapse** ♀
  - Procidentia (uteri) NOS
  - Third degree uterine prolapse
- **N81.4 Uterovaginal prolapse, unspecified** ♀
  - Prolapse of uterus NOS
- **N81.5 Vaginal enterocele** ♀
  - **Excludes1** enterocele with prolapse of uterus (N81.2-N81.4)
- **N81.6 Rectocele** ♀
  - Prolapse of posterior vaginal wall
  - Use additional code for any associated fecal incontinence, if applicable (R15.-)
  - **Excludes2** perineocele (N81.81)
    - rectal prolapse (K62.3)
    - rectocele with prolapse of uterus (N81.2-N81.4)
- ● **N81.8 Other female genital prolapse**
  - **N81.81 Perineocele** ♀
  - **N81.82 Incompetence or weakening of pubocervical tissue** ♀
  - **N81.83 Incompetence or weakening of rectovaginal tissue** ♀
  - **N81.84 Pelvic muscle wasting** ♀
    - Disuse atrophy of pelvic muscles and anal sphincter
  - **N81.85 Cervical stump prolapse** ♀
  - **N81.89 Other female genital prolapse** ♀
    - Deficient perineum
    - Old laceration of muscles of pelvic floor
- **N81.9 Female genital prolapse, unspecified** ♀

● **N82 Fistulae involving female genital tract**
- **Excludes1** vesicointestinal fistulae (N32.1)
- **N82.Ø Vesicovaginal fistula** ♀
- **N82.1 Other female urinary-genital tract fistulae** ♀
  - Cervicovesical fistula
  - Ureterovaginal fistula
  - Urethrovaginal fistula
  - Uteroureteric fistula
  - Uterovesical fistula
  - Coding Clinic: 2Ø17, Q3, P4
- **N82.2 Fistula of vagina to small intestine** ♀
- **N82.3 Fistula of vagina to large intestine** ♀
  - Rectovaginal fistula
- **N82.4 Other female intestinal-genital tract fistulae** ♀
  - Intestinouterine fistula
- **N82.5 Female genital tract-skin fistulae** ♀
  - Uterus to abdominal wall fistula
  - Vaginoperineal fistula
- **N82.8 Other female genital tract fistulae** ♀
- **N82.9 Female genital tract fistula, unspecified** ♀

● **N83 Noninflammatory disorders of ovary, fallopian tube and broad ligament**
- **Excludes2** hydrosalpinx (N7Ø.1-)
- ● **N83.Ø Follicular cyst of ovary**
  - Cyst of graafian follicle
  - Hemorrhagic follicular cyst (of ovary)
  - Coding Clinic: 2Ø16, Q4, P46
  - **N83.ØØ Follicular cyst of ovary, unspecified side** ♀
  - **N83.Ø1 Follicular cyst of right ovary** ♀
  - **N83.Ø2 Follicular cyst of left ovary** ♀

● N83.1 **Corpus luteum cyst**
Hemorrhagic corpus luteum cyst
Coding Clinic: 2016, Q4, P46
N83.10 **Corpus luteum cyst of ovary, unspecified side** ♀
N83.11 **Corpus luteum cyst of right ovary** ♀
N83.12 **Corpus luteum cyst of left ovary** ♀

● N83.2 **Other and unspecified ovarian cysts**
Excludes1 developmental ovarian cyst (Q50.1)
neoplastic ovarian cyst (D27.-)
polycystic ovarian syndrome (E28.2)
Stein-Leventhal syndrome (E28.2)
Coding Clinic: 2016, Q4, P46
● N83.20 **Unspecified ovarian cysts**
N83.201 **Unspecified ovarian cyst, right side** ♀
N83.202 **Unspecified ovarian cyst, left side** ♀
N83.209 **Unspecified ovarian cyst, unspecified side** ♀
Ovarian cyst, NOS
● N83.29 **Other ovarian cysts**
Retention cyst of ovary
Simple cyst of ovary
N83.291 **Other ovarian cyst, right side** ♀
N83.292 **Other ovarian cyst, left side** ♀
N83.299 **Other ovarian cyst, unspecified side** ♀

● N83.3 **Acquired atrophy of ovary and fallopian tube**
Coding Clinic: 2016, Q4, P46
● N83.31 **Acquired atrophy of ovary**
N83.311 **Acquired atrophy of right ovary** ♀
N83.312 **Acquired atrophy of left ovary** ♀
N83.319 **Acquired atrophy of ovary, unspecified side** ♀
Acquired atrophy of ovary, NOS
● N83.32 **Acquired atrophy of fallopian tube**
N83.321 **Acquired atrophy of right fallopian tube** ♀
N83.322 **Acquired atrophy of left fallopian tube** ♀
N83.329 **Acquired atrophy of fallopian tube, unspecified side** ♀
Acquired atrophy of fallopian tube, NOS
● N83.33 **Acquired atrophy of ovary and fallopian tube**
N83.331 **Acquired atrophy of right ovary and fallopian tube** ♀
N83.332 **Acquired atrophy of left ovary and fallopian tube** ♀
N83.339 **Acquired atrophy of ovary and fallopian tube, unspecified side** ♀
Acquired atrophy of ovary and fallopian tube, NOS

● N83.4 **Prolapse and hernia of ovary and fallopian tube**
Coding Clinic: 2016, Q4, P46
N83.40 **Prolapse and hernia of ovary and fallopian tube, unspecified side** ♀
Prolapse and hernia of ovary and fallopian tube, NOS
N83.41 **Prolapse and hernia of right ovary and fallopian tube** ♀
N83.42 **Prolapse and hernia of left ovary and fallopian tube** ♀

● N83.5 **Torsion of ovary, ovarian pedicle and fallopian tube**
Torsion of accessory tube
Coding Clinic: 2016, Q4, P46
● N83.51 **Torsion of ovary and ovarian pedicle**
N83.511 **Torsion of right ovary and ovarian pedicle** ♀
N83.512 **Torsion of left ovary and ovarian pedicle** ♀
N83.519 **Torsion of ovary and ovarian pedicle, unspecified side** ♀
Torsion of ovary and ovarian pedicle, NOS
● N83.52 **Torsion of fallopian tube**
Torsion of hydatid of Morgagni
N83.521 **Torsion of right fallopian tube** ♀
N83.522 **Torsion of left fallopian tube** ♀
N83.529 **Torsion of fallopian tube, unspecified side** ♀
Torsion of fallopian tube, NOS
N83.53 **Torsion of ovary, ovarian pedicle and fallopian tube** ♀

N83.6 **Hematosalpinx** ♀
Excludes1 hematosalpinx (with) (in):
hematocolpos (N89.7)
hematometra (N85.7)
tubal pregnancy (O00.1-)
N83.7 **Hematoma of broad ligament** ♀
N83.8 **Other noninflammatory disorders of ovary, fallopian tube and broad ligament** ♀
Broad ligament laceration syndrome [Allen-Masters]
N83.9 **Noninflammatory disorder of ovary, fallopian tube and broad ligament, unspecified** ♀

● N84 **Polyp of female genital tract**
Excludes1 adenomatous polyp (D28.-)
placental polyp (O90.89)
N84.0 **Polyp of corpus uteri** ♀
Polyp of endometrium
Polyp of uterus NOS
Excludes1 polypoid endometrial hyperplasia (N85.0-)
N84.1 **Polyp of cervix uteri** ♀
Mucous polyp of cervix
N84.2 **Polyp of vagina** ♀
N84.3 **Polyp of vulva** ♀
Polyp of labia
N84.8 **Polyp of other parts of female genital tract** ♀
N84.9 **Polyp of female genital tract, unspecified** ♀

● N85 **Other noninflammatory disorders of uterus, except cervix**
Excludes1 endometriosis (N80.-)
inflammatory diseases of uterus (N71.-)
noninflammatory disorders of cervix, except malposition (N86-N88)
polyp of corpus uteri (N84.0)
uterine prolapse (N81.-)
● N85.0 **Endometrial hyperplasia**
N85.00 **Endometrial hyperplasia, unspecified** ♀
Hyperplasia (adenomatous) (cystic) (glandular) of endometrium
Hyperplastic endometritis
N85.01 **Benign endometrial hyperplasia** ♀
Endometrial hyperplasia (complex) (simple) without atypia
N85.02 **Endometrial intraepithelial neoplasia [EIN]** ♀
Endometrial hyperplasia with atypia
Excludes1 malignant neoplasm of endometrium (with endometrial intraepithelial neoplasia [EIN]) (C54.1)

CHAPTER 14 (N00-N99)

N85.2 **Hypertrophy of uterus** ♀
Bulky or enlarged uterus
Excludes1 puerperal hypertrophy of uterus (O90.89)

N85.3 **Subinvolution of uterus** ♀
Excludes1 puerperal subinvolution of uterus (O90.89)

N85.4 **Malposition of uterus** ♀
Anteversion of uterus
Retroflexion of uterus
Retroversion of uterus
Excludes1 malposition of uterus complicating pregnancy, labor or delivery (O34.5-, O65.5)

N85.5 **Inversion of uterus** ♀
Excludes1 current obstetric trauma (O71.2)
postpartum inversion of uterus (O71.2)

N85.6 **Intrauterine synechiae** ♀

N85.7 **Hematometra** ♀
Hematosalpinx with hematometra
Excludes1 hematometra with hematocolpos (N89.7)

N85.8 **Other specified noninflammatory disorders of uterus** ♀
Atrophy of uterus, acquired
Fibrosis of uterus NOS

N85.9 **Noninflammatory disorder of uterus, unspecified** ♀
Disorder of uterus NOS

N86 **Erosion and ectropion of cervix uteri** ♀
Decubitus (trophic) ulcer of cervix
Eversion of cervix
Excludes1 erosion and ectropion of cervix with cervicitis (N72)

● N87 **Dysplasia of cervix uteri**
Excludes1 abnormal results from cervical cytologic examination without histologic confirmation (R87.61-)
carcinoma in situ of cervix uteri (D06.-)
cervical intraepithelial neoplasia III [CIN III] (D06.-)
HGSIL of cervix (R87.613)
severe dysplasia of cervix uteri (D06.-)

N87.0 **Mild cervical dysplasia** ♀
Cervical intraepithelial neoplasia I [CIN I]

N87.1 **Moderate cervical dysplasia** ♀
Cervical intraepithelial neoplasia II [CIN II]

N87.9 **Dysplasia of cervix uteri, unspecified** ♀
Anaplasia of cervix
Cervical atypism
Cervical dysplasia NOS

● N88 **Other noninflammatory disorders of cervix uteri**
Excludes2 inflammatory disease of cervix (N72)
polyp of cervix (N84.1)

N88.0 **Leukoplakia of cervix uteri** ♀

N88.1 **Old laceration of cervix uteri** ♀
Adhesions of cervix
Excludes1 current obstetric trauma (O71.3)

N88.2 **Stricture and stenosis of cervix uteri** ♀
Excludes1 stricture and stenosis of cervix uteri complicating labor (O65.5)

N88.3 **Incompetence of cervix uteri** ♀
Investigation and management of (suspected) cervical incompetence in a nonpregnant woman
Excludes1 cervical incompetence complicating pregnancy (O34.3-)

N88.4 **Hypertrophic elongation of cervix uteri** ♀

N88.8 **Other specified noninflammatory disorders of cervix uteri** ♀
Excludes1 current obstetric trauma (O71.3)

N88.9 **Noninflammatory disorder of cervix uteri, unspecified** ♀

● N89 **Other noninflammatory disorders of vagina**
Excludes1 abnormal results from vaginal cytologic examination without histologic confirmation (R87.62-)
carcinoma in situ of vagina (D07.2)
HGSIL of vagina (R87.623)
inflammation of vagina (N76.-)
senile (atrophic) vaginitis (N95.2)
severe dysplasia of vagina (D07.2)
trichomonal leukorrhea (A59.00)
vaginal intraepithelial neoplasia [VAIN], grade III (D07.2)

N89.0 **Mild vaginal dysplasia** ♀
Vaginal intraepithelial neoplasia [VAIN], grade I

N89.1 **Moderate vaginal dysplasia** ♀
Vaginal intraepithelial neoplasia [VAIN], grade II

N89.3 **Dysplasia of vagina, unspecified** ♀

N89.4 **Leukoplakia of vagina** ♀

N89.5 **Stricture and atresia of vagina** ♀
Vaginal adhesions
Vaginal stenosis
Excludes1 congenital atresia or stricture (Q52.4)
postprocedural adhesions of vagina (N99.2)

N89.6 **Tight hymenal ring** ♀
Rigid hymen
Tight introitus
Excludes1 imperforate hymen (Q52.3)

N89.7 **Hematocolpos** ♀
Hematocolpos with hematometra or hematosalpinx
Coding Clinic: 2016, Q4, P59

N89.8 **Other specified noninflammatory disorders of vagina** ♀
Leukorrhea NOS
Old vaginal laceration
Pessary ulcer of vagina
Excludes1 current obstetric trauma (O70.-, O71.4, O71.7-O71.8)
old laceration involving muscles of pelvic floor (N81.8)

N89.9 **Noninflammatory disorder of vagina, unspecified** ♀

● N90 **Other noninflammatory disorders of vulva and perineum**
Excludes1 anogenital (venereal) warts (A63.0)
carcinoma in situ of vulva (D07.1)
condyloma acuminatum (A63.0)
current obstetric trauma (O70.-, O71.7-O71.8)
inflammation of vulva (N76.-)
severe dysplasia of vulva (D07.1)
vulvar intraepithelial neoplasm III [VIN III] (D07.1)

N90.0 **Mild vulvar dysplasia** ♀
Vulvar intraepithelial neoplasia [VIN], grade I

N90.1 **Moderate vulvar dysplasia** ♀
Vulvar intraepithelial neoplasia [VIN], grade II

N90.3 **Dysplasia of vulva, unspecified** ♀

N90.4 **Leukoplakia of vulva** ♀
Dystrophy of vulva
Kraurosis of vulva
Lichen sclerosus of external female genital organs

N90.5 **Atrophy of vulva** ♀
Stenosis of vulva

● N90.6 **Hypertrophy of vulva**
Coding Clinic: 2016, Q4, P46

N90.60 **Unspecified hypertrophy of vulva** ♀
Unspecified hypertrophy of labia

N90.61 **Childhood asymmetric labium majus enlargement** ♀
CALME

N90.69 **Other specified hypertrophy of vulva** ♀
Other specified hypertrophy of labia

N90.7 Vulvar cyst ♀

● **N90.8 Other specified noninflammatory disorders of vulva and perineum**

● **N90.81 Female genital mutilation status**
Female genital cutting status

N90.810 Female genital mutilation status, unspecified ♀
Female genital cutting status, unspecified
Female genital mutilation status NOS

N90.811 Female genital mutilation Type I status ♀
Clitorectomy status
Female genital cutting Type I status

N90.812 Female genital mutilation Type II status ♀
Clitorectomy with excision of labia minora status
Female genital cutting Type II status

N90.813 Female genital mutilation Type III status ♀
Female genital cutting Type III status
Infibulation status

N90.818 Other female genital mutilation status ♀
Female genital cutting Type IV status
Female genital mutilation Type IV status
Other female genital cutting status

N90.89 Other specified noninflammatory disorders of vulva and perineum ♀
Adhesions of vulva
Hypertrophy of clitoris

N90.9 Noninflammatory disorder of vulva and perineum, unspecified ♀

● **N91 Absent, scanty and rare menstruation**
Excludes1 ovarian dysfunction (E28.-)

N91.0 Primary amenorrhea ♀
N91.1 Secondary amenorrhea ♀
N91.2 Amenorrhea, unspecified ♀
N91.3 Primary oligomenorrhea ♀
N91.4 Secondary oligomenorrhea ♀
N91.5 Oligomenorrhea, unspecified ♀
Hypomenorrhea NOS

● **N92 Excessive, frequent and irregular menstruation**
Excludes1 postmenopausal bleeding (N95.0)
precocious puberty (menstruation) (E30.1)

N92.0 Excessive and frequent menstruation with regular cycle ♀
Heavy periods NOS
Polymenorrhea
Menorrhagia NOS

N92.1 Excessive and frequent menstruation with irregular cycle ♀
Irregular intermenstrual bleeding
Irregular, shortened intervals between menstrual bleeding
Menometrorrhagia
Metrorrhagia

N92.2 Excessive menstruation at puberty ♀ P
Excessive bleeding associated with onset of menstrual periods
Pubertal menorrhagia
Puberty bleeding

N92.3 Ovulation bleeding ♀
Regular intermenstrual bleeding

N92.4 Excessive bleeding in the premenopausal period ♀
Climacteric menorrhagia or metrorrhagia
Menopausal menorrhagia or metrorrhagia
▶ Perimenopausal bleeding
▶ Perimenopausal menorrhagia or metrorrhagia
Preclimacteric menorrhagia or metrorrhagia
Premenopausal menorrhagia or metrorrhagia

N92.5 Other specified irregular menstruation ♀

N92.6 Irregular menstruation, unspecified ♀
Irregular bleeding NOS
Irregular periods NOS
Excludes1 irregular menstruation with:
lengthened intervals or scanty bleeding (N91.3-N91.5)
shortened intervals or excessive bleeding (N92.1)

● **N93 Other abnormal uterine and vaginal bleeding**
Excludes1 neonatal vaginal hemorrhage (P54.6)
precocious puberty (menstruation) (E30.1)
pseudomenses (P54.6)

N93.0 Postcoital and contact bleeding ♀

N93.1 Pre-pubertal vaginal bleeding ♀
Coding Clinic: 2016, Q4, P47

N93.8 Other specified abnormal uterine and vaginal bleeding ♀
Dysfunctional or functional uterine or vaginal bleeding NOS

N93.9 Abnormal uterine and vaginal bleeding, unspecified ♀

● **N94 Pain and other conditions associated with female genital organs and menstrual cycle**

N94.0 Mittelschmerz ♀
Ovulation pain

● **N94.1 Dyspareunia**
Painful intercourse/coitus
Excludes1 psychogenic dyspareunia (F52.6)
Coding Clinic: 2016, Q4, P47

N94.10 Unspecified dyspareunia ♀
N94.11 Superficial (introital) dyspareunia ♀
N94.12 Deep dyspareunia ♀
N94.19 Other specified dyspareunia ♀

N94.2 Vaginismus ♀
Vagina tightness
Excludes1 psychogenic vaginismus (F52.5)

N94.3 Premenstrual tension syndrome ♀
AKA: PMS
Code also associated menstrual migraine (G43.82-, G43.83-)
Excludes1 Premenstrual dysphoric disorder (F32.81)
Coding Clinic: 2016, Q4, P14

N94.4 Primary dysmenorrhea ♀
Lifelong painful menstruation

N94.5 Secondary dysmenorrhea ♀
Later onset of painful menstruation

N94.6 Dysmenorrhea, unspecified ♀
Excludes1 psychogenic dysmenorrhea (F45.8)

● **N94.8 Other specified conditions associated with female genital organs and menstrual cycle**

● **N94.81 Vulvodynia**
N94.810 Vulvar vestibulitis ♀
N94.818 Other vulvodynia ♀
N94.819 Vulvodynia, unspecified ♀
Vulvodynia NOS

N94.89 Other specified conditions associated with female genital organs and menstrual cycle ♀

N94.9 Unspecified condition associated with female genital organs and menstrual cycle ♀

CHAPTER 14 (N00-N99)

● **N95 Menopausal and other perimenopausal disorders**
Menopausal and other perimenopausal disorders due to naturally occurring (age-related) menopause and perimenopause
Excludes1 excessive bleeding in the premenopausal period (N92.4)
menopausal and perimenopausal disorders due to artificial or premature menopause (E89.4-, E28.31-)
premature menopause (E28.31-)
Excludes2 postmenopausal osteoporosis (M81.Ø-)
postmenopausal osteoporosis with current pathological fracture (M8Ø.Ø-)
postmenopausal urethritis (N34.2)

N95.Ø Postmenopausal bleeding ♀

N95.1 Menopausal and female climacteric states ♀
Symptoms such as flushing, sleeplessness, headache, lack of concentration, associated with natural (age-related) menopause
Use additional code for associated symptoms
Excludes1 asymptomatic menopausal state (Z78.Ø)
symptoms associated with artificial menopause (E89.41)
symptoms associated with premature menopause (E28.31Ø)

N95.2 Postmenopausal atrophic vaginitis ♀
Senile (atrophic) vaginitis

N95.8 Other specified menopausal and perimenopausal disorders ♀

N95.9 Unspecified menopausal and perimenopausal disorder ♀

N96 Recurrent pregnancy loss ♀
Investigation or care in a nonpregnant woman with history of recurrent pregnancy loss
Excludes1 recurrent pregnancy loss with current pregnancy (O26.2-)

● **N97 Female infertility**
Includes inability to achieve a pregnancy
sterility, female NOS
Excludes1 female infertility associated with:
hypopituitarism (E23.Ø)
Stein-Leventhal syndrome (E28.2)
Excludes2 incompetence of cervix uteri (N88.3)

N97.Ø Female infertility associated with anovulation ♀

N97.1 Female infertility of tubal origin ♀
Female infertility associated with congenital anomaly of tube
Female infertility due to tubal block
Female infertility due to tubal occlusion
Female infertility due to tubal stenosis

N97.2 Female infertility of uterine origin ♀
Female infertility associated with congenital anomaly of uterus
Female infertility due to nonimplantation of ovum

N97.8 Female infertility of other origin ♀

N97.9 Female infertility, unspecified ♀

● **N98 Complications associated with artificial fertilization**

N98.Ø Infection associated with artificial insemination ♀

N98.1 Hyperstimulation of ovaries ♀
Hyperstimulation of ovaries NOS
Hyperstimulation of ovaries associated with induced ovulation

N98.2 Complications of attempted introduction of fertilized ovum following in vitro fertilization ♀

N98.3 Complications of attempted introduction of embryo in embryo transfer ♀

N98.8 Other complications associated with artificial fertilization ♀

N98.9 Complication associated with artificial fertilization, unspecified ♀

INTRAOPERATIVE AND POSTPROCEDURAL COMPLICATIONS AND DISORDERS OF GENITOURINARY SYSTEM, NOT ELSEWHERE CLASSIFIED (N99)

● **N99 Intraoperative and postprocedural complications and disorders of genitourinary system, not elsewhere classified**
Excludes2 irradiation cystitis (N3Ø.4-)
postoophorectomy osteoporosis with current pathological fracture (M8Ø.8-)
postoophorectomy osteoporosis without current pathological fracture (M81.8)

N99.Ø Postprocedural (acute) (chronic) kidney failure
Use additional code to type of kidney disease

● **N99.1 Postprocedural urethral stricture**
Postcatheterization urethral stricture

● **N99.11 Postprocedural urethral stricture, male**

N99.11Ø Postprocedural urethral stricture, male, meatal ♂

N99.111 Postprocedural bulbous urethral stricture, male ♂

N99.112 Postprocedural membranous urethral stricture, male ♂

N99.113 Postprocedural anterior bulbous urethral stricture, male ♂
Coding Clinic: 2016, Q4, P48

N99.114 Postprocedural urethral stricture, male, unspecified ♂

N99.115 Postprocedural fossa navicularis urethral stricture ♂
Coding Clinic: 2016, Q4, P47

N99.116 Postprocedural urethral stricture, male, overlapping sites ♂

N99.12 Postprocedural urethral stricture, female ♀

N99.2 Postprocedural adhesions of vagina ♀

N99.3 Prolapse of vaginal vault after hysterectomy ♀

N99.4 Postprocedural pelvic peritoneal adhesions
Excludes2 pelvic peritoneal adhesions NOS (N73.6)
postinfective pelvic peritoneal adhesions (N73.6)

● **N99.5 Complications of stoma of urinary tract**
Excludes2 mechanical complication of urinary catheter (T83.Ø-)

● **N99.51 Complication of cystostomy**

N99.51Ø Cystostomy hemorrhage HCC

N99.511 Cystostomy infection HCC

N99.512 Cystostomy malfunction HCC

N99.518 Other cystostomy complication HCC

● **N99.52 Complication of incontinent external stoma of urinary tract**

N99.52Ø Hemorrhage of incontinent external stoma of urinary tract HCC

N99.521 Infection of incontinent external stoma of urinary tract HCC
Coding Clinic: 2016, Q4, P48

N99.522 Malfunction of incontinent external stoma of urinary tract HCC

N99.523 Herniation of incontinent stoma of urinary tract HCC
Coding Clinic: 2016, Q4, P48

N99.524 Stenosis of incontinent stoma of urinary tract HCC
Coding Clinic: 2016, Q4, P48

N99.528 Other complication of incontinent external stoma of urinary tract HCC

● **N99.53** Complication of **continent stoma** of urinary tract

    N99.530   **Hemorrhage** of continent stoma of urinary tract 🦠

    N99.531   **Infection** of continent stoma of urinary tract 🦠

    N99.532   **Malfunction** of continent stoma of urinary tract 🦠

    N99.533   **Herniation** of continent stoma of urinary tract 🦠
              Coding Clinic: 2016, Q4, P48

    N99.534   **Stenosis** of continent stoma of urinary tract 🦠
              Coding Clinic: 2016, Q4, P48

    N99.538   **Other** complication of continent stoma of urinary tract 🦠

● **N99.6** Intraoperative hemorrhage and hematoma of a genitourinary system organ or structure complicating a procedure

    Excludes1   intraoperative hemorrhage and hematoma of a genitourinary system organ or structure due to accidental puncture or laceration during a procedure (N99.7-)

    N99.61   Intraoperative hemorrhage and hematoma of a genitourinary system organ or structure complicating a **genitourinary system procedure**

    N99.62   Intraoperative hemorrhage and hematoma of a genitourinary system organ or structure complicating **other procedure**

● **N99.7** **Accidental puncture and laceration** of a genitourinary system organ or structure during a procedure

    N99.71   Accidental puncture and laceration of a genitourinary system organ or structure during a **genitourinary system procedure**

    N99.72   Accidental puncture and laceration of a genitourinary system organ or structure during **other procedure**

● **N99.8** **Other intraoperative and postprocedural** complications and disorders of genitourinary system
    Coding Clinic: 2016, Q4, P10

    N99.81   **Other** intraoperative complications of genitourinary system

●   N99.82   **Postprocedural hemorrhage** of a genitourinary system organ or structure following a procedure

    N99.820   Postprocedural hemorrhage of a genitourinary system organ or structure following a **genitourinary system procedure**

    N99.821   Postprocedural hemorrhage of a genitourinary system organ or structure following **other procedure**

    N99.83   Residual ovary syndrome ♀

●   N99.84   **Postprocedural hematoma and seroma** of a genitourinary system organ or structure following a procedure

    N99.840   Postprocedural **hematoma** of a genitourinary system organ or structure following a **genitourinary system procedure**

    N99.841   Postprocedural **hematoma** of a genitourinary system organ or structure following **other procedure**

    N99.842   Postprocedural **seroma** of a genitourinary system organ or structure following a **genitourinary system procedure**

    N99.843   Postprocedural **seroma** of a genitourinary system organ or structure following **other procedure**

▶ N99.85   Post endometrial ablation syndrome

    N99.89   **Other** postprocedural complications and disorders of genitourinary system

CHAPTER 14 (N00-N99)

CHAPTER 15

PREGNANCY, CHILDBIRTH, AND THE PUERPERIUM (O00-O9A)

OGCR Chapter-Specific Coding Guidelines

15. **Chapter 15: Pregnancy, Childbirth, and the Puerperium (O00-O9A)**
 a. **General Rules for Obstetric Cases**
 1) **Codes from Chapter 15 and sequencing priority**
 Obstetric cases require codes from Chapter 15, codes in the range O00-O9A, Pregnancy, Childbirth, and the Puerperium. Chapter 15 codes have sequencing priority over codes from other chapters. Additional codes from other chapters may be used in conjunction with Chapter 15 codes to further specify conditions. Should the provider document that the pregnancy is incidental to the encounter, then code Z33.1, Pregnant state, incidental, should be used in place of any Chapter 15 codes. It is the provider's responsibility to state that the condition being treated is not affecting the pregnancy.

 2) **Chapter 15 codes used only on the maternal record**
 Chapter 15 codes are to be used only on the maternal record, never on the record of the newborn.

 3) **Final character for trimester**
 The majority of codes in Chapter 15 have a final character indicating the trimester of pregnancy. The timeframes for the trimesters are indicated at the beginning of the chapter. If trimester is not a component of a code it is because the condition always occurs in a specific trimester, or the concept of trimester of pregnancy is not applicable. Certain codes have characters for only certain trimesters because the condition does not occur in all trimesters, but it may occur in more than just one.

 Assignment of the final character for trimester should be based on the provider's documentation of the trimester (or number of weeks) for the current admission/encounter. This applies to the assignment of trimester for pre-existing conditions as well as those that develop during or are due to the pregnancy. The provider's documentation of the number of weeks may be used to assign the appropriate code identifying the trimester.

 Whenever delivery occurs during the current admission, and there is an "in childbirth" option for the obstetric complication being coded, the "in childbirth" code should be assigned.

 4) **Selection of trimester for inpatient admissions that encompass more than one trimester**
 In instances when a patient is admitted to a hospital for complications of pregnancy during one trimester and remains in the hospital into a subsequent trimester, the trimester character for the antepartum complication code should be assigned on the basis of the trimester when the complication developed, not the trimester of the discharge. If the condition developed prior to the current admission/encounter or represents a pre-existing condition, the trimester character for the trimester at the time of the admission/encounter should be assigned.

 5) **Unspecified trimester**
 Each category that includes codes for trimester has a code for "unspecified trimester." The "unspecified trimester" code should rarely be used, such as when the documentation in the record is insufficient to determine the trimester and it is not possible to obtain clarification.

 6) **7th character for Fetus Identification**
 Where applicable, a 7th character is to be assigned for certain categories (O31, O32, O33.3 - O33.6, O35, O36, O40, O41, O60.1, O60.2, O64, and O69) to identify the fetus for which the complication code applies.
 Assign 7th character "0":
 • For single gestations
 • When the documentation in the record is insufficient to determine the fetus affected and it is not possible to obtain clarification.
 • When it is not possible to clinically determine which fetus is affected.

 b. **Selection of OB Principal or First-listed Diagnosis**
 1) **Routine outpatient prenatal visits**
 For routine outpatient prenatal visits when no complications are present, a code from category Z34, Encounter for supervision of normal pregnancy, should be used as the first-listed diagnosis. These codes should not be used in conjunction with Chapter 15 codes.

 2) **Supervision of High-Risk Pregnancy**
 Codes from category O09, Supervision of high-risk pregnancy, are intended for use only during the prenatal period. For complications during the labor or delivery episode as a result of a high-risk pregnancy, assign the applicable complication codes from Chapter 15. If there are no complications during the labor or delivery episode, assign code O80, Encounter for full-term uncomplicated delivery.

For routine prenatal outpatient visits for patients with high-risk pregnancies, a code from category O09, Supervision of high-risk pregnancy, should be used as the first-listed diagnosis. Secondary Chapter 15 codes may be used in conjunction with these codes if appropriate.

 3) **Episodes when no delivery occurs**
 In episodes when no delivery occurs, the principal diagnosis should correspond to the principal complication of the pregnancy which necessitated the encounter. Should more than one complication exist, all of which are treated or monitored, any of the complications codes may be sequenced first.

 4) **When a delivery occurs**
 When an obstetric patient is admitted and delivers during that admission, the condition that prompted the admission should be sequenced as the principal diagnosis. If multiple conditions prompted the admission, sequence the one most related to the delivery as the principal diagnosis. A code for any complication of the delivery should be assigned as an additional diagnosis. In cases of cesarean delivery, if the patient was admitted with a condition that resulted in the performance of a cesarean procedure, that condition should be selected as the principal diagnosis. If the reason for the admission was unrelated to the condition resulting in the cesarean delivery, the condition related to the reason for the admission should be selected as the principal diagnosis.

 5) **Outcome of delivery**
 A code from category Z37, Outcome of delivery, should be included on every maternal record when a delivery has occurred. These codes are not to be used on subsequent records or on the newborn record.

 c. **Pre-existing conditions versus conditions due to the pregnancy**
 Certain categories in Chapter 15 distinguish between conditions of the mother that existed prior to pregnancy (pre-existing) and those that are a direct result of pregnancy. When assigning codes from Chapter 15, it is important to assess if a condition was pre-existing prior to pregnancy or developed during or due to the pregnancy in order to assign the correct code.

 Categories that do not distinguish between pre-existing and pregnancy-related conditions may be used for either. It is acceptable to use codes specifically for the puerperium with codes complicating pregnancy and childbirth if a condition arises postpartum during the delivery encounter.

 d. **Pre-existing hypertension in pregnancy**
 Category O10, Pre-existing hypertension complicating pregnancy, childbirth and the puerperium, includes codes for hypertensive heart and hypertensive chronic kidney disease. When assigning one of the O10 codes that includes hypertensive heart disease or hypertensive chronic kidney disease, it is necessary to add a secondary code from the appropriate hypertension category to specify the type of heart failure or chronic kidney disease.
 See Section I.C.9. Hypertension.

 e. **Fetal Conditions Affecting the Management of the Mother**
 1) **Codes from categories O35 and O36**
 Codes from categories O35, Maternal care for known or suspected fetal abnormality and damage, and O36, Maternal care for other fetal problems, are assigned only when the fetal condition is actually responsible for modifying the management of the mother, i.e., by requiring diagnostic studies, additional observation, special care, or termination of pregnancy. The fact that the fetal condition exists does not justify assigning a code from this series to the mother's record.

 2) **In utero surgery**
 In cases when surgery is performed on the fetus, a diagnosis code from category O35, Maternal care for known or suspected fetal abnormality and damage, should be assigned identifying the fetal condition. Assign the appropriate procedure code for the procedure performed.

 No code from Chapter 16, the perinatal codes, should be used on the mother's record to identify fetal conditions. Surgery performed in utero on a fetus is still to be coded as an obstetric encounter.

 f. **HIV Infection in Pregnancy, Childbirth, and the Puerperium**
 During pregnancy, childbirth or the puerperium, a patient admitted because of an HIV-related illness should receive a principal diagnosis from subcategory O98.7-, Human immunodeficiency [HIV] disease complicating pregnancy, childbirth and the puerperium, followed by the code(s) for the HIV-related illness(es).

 Patients with asymptomatic HIV infection status admitted during pregnancy, childbirth, or the puerperium should receive codes of O98.7- and Z21, Asymptomatic human immunodeficiency virus [HIV] infection status.

 g. **Diabetes mellitus in pregnancy**
 Diabetes mellitus is a significant complicating factor in pregnancy. Pregnant women who are diabetic should be assigned a code from category O24, Diabetes mellitus in pregnancy, childbirth, and the puerperium, first, followed by the appropriate diabetes code(s) (E08-E13) from Chapter 4.

h. Long-term use of insulin and oral hypoglycemics
See Section I.C.4.a.3 for information on the long-term use of insulin and oral hypoglycemic.

i. Gestational (pregnancy induced) diabetes
Gestational (pregnancy induced) diabetes can occur during the second and third trimester of pregnancy in women who were not diabetic prior to pregnancy. Gestational diabetes can cause complications in the pregnancy similar to those of pre-existing diabetes mellitus. It also puts the woman at greater risk of developing diabetes after the pregnancy. Codes for gestational diabetes are in subcategory O24.4, Gestational diabetes mellitus. No other code from category O24, Diabetes mellitus in pregnancy, childbirth, and the puerperium, should be used with a code from O24.4.

The codes under subcategory O24.4 include diet controlled, insulin controlled, and controlled by oral hypoglycemic drugs. If a patient with gestational diabetes is treated with both diet and insulin, only the code for insulin-controlled is required. If a patient with gestational diabetes is treated with both diet and oral hypoglycemic medications, only the code for "controlled by oral hypoglycemic drugs" is required. Code Z79.4, Long-term (current) use of insulin or code Z79.84, Long-term (current) use of oral hypoglycemic drugs, should not be assigned with codes from subcategory O24.4.

An abnormal glucose tolerance in pregnancy is assigned a code from subcategory O99.81, Abnormal glucose complicating pregnancy, childbirth, and the puerperium.

j. Sepsis and septic shock complicating abortion, pregnancy, childbirth and the puerperium
When assigning a Chapter 15 code for sepsis complicating abortion, pregnancy, childbirth, and the puerperium, a code for the specific type of infection should be assigned as an additional diagnosis. If severe sepsis is present, a code from subcategory R65.2, Severe sepsis, and code(s) for associated organ dysfunction(s) should also be assigned as additional diagnoses.

k. Puerperal sepsis
Code O85, Puerperal sepsis, should be assigned with a secondary code to identify the causal organism (e.g., for a bacterial infection, assign a code from category B95-B96, Bacterial infections in conditions classified elsewhere). A code from category A40, Streptococcal sepsis, or A41, Other sepsis, should not be used for puerperal sepsis. If applicable, use additional codes to identify severe sepsis (R65.2-) and any associated acute organ dysfunction.

l. Alcohol, tobacco and drug use during pregnancy, childbirth and the puerperium

1) Alcohol use during pregnancy, childbirth and the puerperium
Codes under subcategory O99.31, Alcohol use complicating pregnancy, childbirth, and the puerperium, should be assigned for any pregnancy case when a mother uses alcohol during the pregnancy or postpartum. A secondary code from category F10, Alcohol-related disorders, should also be assigned to identify manifestations of the alcohol use.

2) Tobacco use during pregnancy, childbirth, and the puerperium
Codes under subcategory O99.33, Smoking (tobacco) complicating pregnancy, childbirth, and the puerperium, should be assigned for any pregnancy case when a mother uses any type of tobacco product during the pregnancy or postpartum. A secondary code from category F17, Nicotine dependence, should also be assigned to identify the type of nicotine dependence.

3) Drug use during pregnancy, childbirth and the puerperium
Codes under subcategory O99.32, Drug use complicating pregnancy, childbirth, and the puerperium, should be assigned for any pregnancy case when a mother uses drugs during the pregnancy or postpartum. This can involve illegal drugs, or inappropriate use or abuse of prescription drugs. Secondary code(s) from categories F11-F16 and F18-F19 should also be assigned to identify manifestations of the drug use.

m. Poisoning, toxic effects, adverse effects and underdosing in a pregnant patient
A code from subcategory O9A.2, Injury, poisoning and certain other consequences of external causes complicating pregnancy, childbirth, and the puerperium, should be sequenced first, followed by the appropriate injury, poisoning, toxic effect, adverse effect or underdosing code, and then the additional code(s) that specifies the condition caused by the poisoning, toxic effect, adverse effect or underdosing.
See Section I.C.19. Adverse effects, poisoning, underdosing and toxic effects.

n. Normal Delivery, Code O80

1) Encounter for full-term uncomplicated delivery
Code O80 should be assigned when a woman is admitted for a full-term normal delivery and delivers a single, healthy infant without any complications antepartum, during the delivery, or postpartum during the delivery episode. Code O80 is always a principal

diagnosis. It is not to be used if any other code from Chapter 15 is needed to describe a current complication of the antenatal, delivery, or perinatal period. Additional codes from other chapters may be used with code O80 if they are not related to or are in any way complicating the pregnancy.

2) Uncomplicated delivery with resolved antepartum complication
Code O80 may be used if the patient had a complication at some point during the pregnancy, but the complication is not present at the time of the admission for delivery.

3) Outcome of delivery for O80
Z37.0, Single live birth, is the only outcome of delivery code appropriate for use with O80.

o. The Peripartum and Postpartum Periods

1) Peripartum and Postpartum periods
The postpartum period begins immediately after delivery and continues for six weeks following delivery. The peripartum period is defined as the last month of pregnancy to five months postpartum.

2) Peripartum and postpartum complication
A postpartum complication is any complication occurring within the six-week period.

3) Pregnancy-related complications after 6 week period
Chapter 15 codes may also be used to describe pregnancy-related complications after the peripartum or postpartum period if the provider documents that a condition is pregnancy related.

4) Admission for routine postpartum care following delivery outside hospital
When the mother delivers outside the hospital prior to admission and is admitted for routine postpartum care and no complications are noted, code Z39.0, Encounter for care and examination of mother immediately after delivery, should be assigned as the principal diagnosis.

5) Pregnancy associated cardiomyopathy
Pregnancy associated cardiomyopathy, code O90.3, is unique in that it may be diagnosed in the third trimester of pregnancy but may continue to progress months after delivery. For this reason, it is referred to as peripartum cardiomyopathy. Code O90.3 is only for use when the cardiomyopathy develops as a result of pregnancy in a woman who did not have pre-existing heart disease.

p. Code O94, Sequelae of complication of pregnancy, childbirth, and the puerperium

1) Code O94
Code O94, Sequelae of complication of pregnancy, childbirth, and the puerperium, is for use in those cases when an initial complication of a pregnancy develops a sequelae requiring care or treatment at a future date.

2) After the initial postpartum period
This code may be used at any time after the initial postpartum period.

3) Sequencing of Code O94
This code, like all sequela codes, is to be sequenced following the code describing the sequelae of the complication.

q. Termination of Pregnancy and Spontaneous abortions

1) Abortion with Liveborn Fetus
When an attempted termination of pregnancy results in a liveborn fetus assign code Z33.2, Encounter for elective termination of pregnancy and a code from category Z37, Outcome of Delivery.

2) Retained Products of Conception following an abortion
Subsequent encounters for retained products of conception following a spontaneous abortion or elective termination of pregnancy, without complications are assigned O03.4, Incomplete spontaneous, abortion without complication, or codes O07.4, Failed attempted termination of pregnancy without complication. This advice is appropriate even when the patient was discharged previously with a discharge diagnosis of complete abortion. If the patient has a specific complication associated with the spontaneous abortion or elective termination of pregnancy in addition to retained products of conception, assign the appropriate complication in category O03 or O07 instead of code O03.4 or O07.4

3) Complications leading to abortion
Codes from Chapter 15 may be used as additional codes to identify any documented complications of the pregnancy in conjunction with codes in categories in O04, O07 and O08.

r. Abuse in a pregnant patient
For suspected or confirmed cases of abuse of a pregnant patient, a code(s) from subcategories O9A.3, Physical abuse complicating pregnancy, childbirth, and the puerperium, O9A.4, Sexual abuse complicating pregnancy, childbirth, and the puerperium, and O9A.5, Psychological abuse complicating pregnancy, childbirth, and the puerperium, should be sequenced first, followed by the appropriate codes (if applicable) to identify any associated current injury due to physical abuse, sexual abuse, and the perpetrator of abuse.
See Section I.C.19. Adult and child abuse, neglect and other maltreatment.

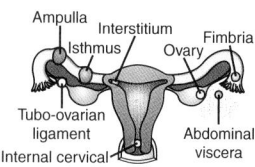

Figure 15-1   Implantation sites of ectopic pregnancy.

Item 15–1   **Ectopic** pregnancy most often occurs in the fallopian tube. Pregnancy outside the uterus may end in a lifethreatening rupture.

★ **(See Plate 4 of the Anatomy Illustrations.)**

CHAPTER 15

PREGNANCY, CHILDBIRTH, AND THE PUERPERIUM (O00-O9A)

Note: CODES FROM THIS CHAPTER ARE FOR USE ONLY ON MATERNAL RECORDS, NEVER ON NEWBORN RECORDS

Codes from this chapter are for use for conditions related to or aggravated by the pregnancy, childbirth, or by the puerperium (maternal causes or obstetric causes)

Trimesters are counted from the first day of the last menstrual period. They are defined as follows:

1st trimester - less than 14 weeks 0 days

2nd trimester - 14 weeks 0 days to less than 28 weeks 0 days

3rd trimester - 28 weeks 0 days until delivery

Use additional code from category Z3A, Weeks of gestation, to identify the specific week of the pregnancy, if known.

Excludes1   supervision of normal pregnancy (Z34.-)

Excludes2   mental and behavioral disorders associated with the puerperium (F53.-)
obstetrical tetanus (A34)
postpartum necrosis of pituitary gland (E23.0)
puerperal osteomalacia (M83.0)

This chapter contains the following blocks:

O00-O08	Pregnancy with abortive outcome
O09	Supervision of high risk pregnancy
O10-O16	Edema, proteinuria and hypertensive disorders in pregnancy, childbirth and the puerperium
O20-O29	Other maternal disorders predominantly related to pregnancy
O30-O48	Maternal care related to the fetus and amniotic cavity and possible delivery problems
O60-O77	Complications of labor and delivery
O80, O82	Encounter for delivery
O85-O92	Complications predominantly related to the puerperium
O94-O9A	Other obstetric conditions, not elsewhere classified

Excludes1   continuing pregnancy in multiple gestation after abortion of one fetus or more (O31.1-, O31.3-)

Coding Clinic: 2016, Q4, P130

● **O00**   **Ectopic pregnancy**

  Includes   ruptured ectopic pregnancy

  Use additional code from category O08 to identify any associated complication

● **O00.0**   **Abdominal pregnancy**

  Excludes1   maternal care for viable fetus in abdominal pregnancy (O36.7-)

  Coding Clinic: 2016, Q4, P49

  O00.00   **Abdominal pregnancy without intrauterine pregnancy** ♀   M
       Abdominal pregnancy NOS

  O00.01   **Abdominal pregnancy with intrauterine pregnancy** ♀   M

● **O00.1**   **Tubal pregnancy**
   Fallopian pregnancy
   Rupture of (fallopian) tube due to pregnancy
   Tubal abortion
   Coding Clinic: 2016, Q4, P49

  ● **O00.10**   **Tubal pregnancy without intrauterine pregnancy**
       Tubal pregnancy NOS

    O00.101   **Right tubal pregnancy without intrauterine pregnancy** ♀   M

    O00.102   **Left tubal pregnancy without intrauterine pregnancy** ♀   M

    O00.109   **Unspecified tubal pregnancy without intrauterine pregnancy** ♀   M

  ● **O00.11**   **Tubal pregnancy with intrauterine pregnancy**

    O00.111   **Right tubal pregnancy with intrauterine pregnancy** ♀   M

    O00.112   **Left tubal pregnancy with intrauterine pregnancy** ♀   M

    O00.119   **Unspecified tubal pregnancy with intrauterine pregnancy** ♀   M

● **O00.2**   **Ovarian pregnancy**
   Coding Clinic: 2016, Q4, P49

  ● **O00.20**   **Ovarian pregnancy without intrauterine pregnancy**
       Ovarian pregnancy NOS

    O00.201   **Right ovarian pregnancy without intrauterine pregnancy** ♀   M

    O00.202   **Left ovarian pregnancy without intrauterine pregnancy** ♀   M

    O00.209   **Unspecified ovarian pregnancy without intrauterine pregnancy** ♀   M

  ● **O00.21**   **Ovarian pregnancy with intrauterine pregnancy**

    O00.211   **Right ovarian pregnancy with intrauterine pregnancy** ♀   M

    O00.212   **Left ovarian pregnancy with intrauterine pregnancy** ♀   M

    O00.219   **Unspecified ovarian pregnancy with intrauterine pregnancy** ♀   M

● **O00.8**   **Other ectopic pregnancy**
   Cervical pregnancy
   Cornual pregnancy
   Intraligamentous pregnancy
   Mural pregnancy
   Coding Clinic: 2016, Q4, P49

  O00.80   **Other ectopic pregnancy without intrauterine pregnancy** ♀   M
       Other ectopic pregnancy NOS

  O00.81   **Other ectopic pregnancy with intrauterine pregnancy** ♀   M

▶ New   ⬛ Revised   ~~deleted~~ Deleted   Excludes 1   Excludes 2   Includes   Use additional   Code first   Code also   Key words

OGCR Official Guidelines   X Assign placeholder X   ● Use Additional Character(s)   ▷ Manifestation Code   🐾 Hierarchical Condition Category   Coding Clinic

● O00.9 **Ectopic pregnancy, unspecified**
Coding Clinic: 2016, Q4, P49
O00.90 **Unspecified ectopic pregnancy without intrauterine pregnancy ♀** M
Ectopic pregnancy NOS
O00.91 **Unspecified ectopic pregnancy with intrauterine pregnancy ♀** M

● O01 **Hydatidiform mole**
Use additional code from category O08 to identify any associated complication
Excludes1 chorioadenoma (destruens) (D39.2)
malignant hydatidiform mole (D39.2)
O01.0 **Classical hydatidiform mole ♀** M
Complete hydatidiform mole
O01.1 **Incomplete and partial hydatidiform mole ♀** M
O01.9 **Hydatidiform mole, unspecified ♀** M
Trophoblastic disease NOS
Vesicular mole NOS

● O02 **Other abnormal products of conception**
Use additional code from category O08 to identify any associated complication
Excludes1 papyraceous fetus (O31.0-)
O02.0 **Blighted ovum and nonhydatidiform mole ♀** M
Carneous mole
Fleshy mole
Intrauterine mole NOS
Molar pregnancy NEC
Pathological ovum
O02.1 **Missed abortion ♀** M
Early fetal death, before completion of 20 weeks of gestation, with retention of dead fetus
Excludes1 failed induced abortion (O07.-)
fetal death (intrauterine) (late) (O36.4)
missed abortion with blighted ovum (O02.0)
missed abortion with hydatidiform mole (O01.-)
missed abortion with nonhydatidiform (O02.0)
missed abortion with other abnormal products of conception (O02.8-)
missed delivery (O36.4)
stillbirth (P95)
● O02.8 **Other specified abnormal products of conception**
Excludes1 abnormal products of conception with blighted ovum (O02.0)
abnormal products of conception with hydatidiform mole (O01.-)
abnormal products of conception with nonhydatidiform mole (O02.0)
O02.81 **Inappropriate change in quantitative human chorionic gonadotropin (hCG) in early pregnancy ♀** M
Biochemical pregnancy
Chemical pregnancy
Inappropriate level of quantitative human chorionic gonadotropin (hCG) for gestational age in early pregnancy
O02.89 **Other abnormal products of conception ♀** M
O02.9 **Abnormal product of conception, unspecified ♀** M

Item 15–2 A **hydatidiform** mole is an overproduction of placental tissue. The tumor secretes a hormone, chorionic gonadotropic hormone (CGH), that indicates a positive pregnancy test. There is no viable fetus. More than 80% of hydatidiform moles are noncancerous.

● O03 **Spontaneous abortion**
Note: Incomplete abortion includes retained products of conception following spontaneous abortion.
Includes miscarriage
O03.0 **Genital tract and pelvic infection following incomplete spontaneous abortion ♀** M
Endometritis following incomplete spontaneous abortion
Oophoritis following incomplete spontaneous abortion
Parametritis following incomplete spontaneous abortion
Pelvic peritonitis following incomplete spontaneous abortion
Salpingitis following incomplete spontaneous abortion
Salpingo-oophoritis following incomplete spontaneous abortion
Excludes1 sepsis following incomplete spontaneous abortion (O03.37)
urinary tract infection following incomplete spontaneous abortion (O03.38)
O03.1 **Delayed or excessive hemorrhage following incomplete spontaneous abortion ♀** M
Afibrinogenemia following incomplete spontaneous abortion
Defibrination syndrome following incomplete spontaneous abortion
Hemolysis following incomplete spontaneous abortion
Intravascular coagulation following incomplete spontaneous abortion
O03.2 **Embolism following incomplete spontaneous abortion ♀** M
Air embolism following incomplete spontaneous abortion
Amniotic fluid embolism following incomplete spontaneous abortion
Blood-clot embolism following incomplete spontaneous abortion
Embolism NOS following incomplete spontaneous abortion
Fat embolism following incomplete spontaneous abortion
Pulmonary embolism following incomplete spontaneous abortion
Pyemic embolism following incomplete spontaneous abortion
Septic or septicopyemic embolism following incomplete spontaneous abortion
Soap embolism following incomplete spontaneous abortion
● O03.3 **Other and unspecified complications following incomplete spontaneous abortion**
O03.30 **Unspecified complication following incomplete spontaneous abortion ♀** M
O03.31 **Shock following incomplete spontaneous abortion ♀** M
Circulatory collapse following incomplete spontaneous abortion
Shock (postprocedural) following incomplete spontaneous abortion
Excludes1 shock due to infection following incomplete spontaneous abortion (O03.37)
O03.32 **Renal failure following incomplete spontaneous abortion ♀** M
Kidney failure (acute) following incomplete spontaneous abortion
Oliguria following incomplete spontaneous abortion
Renal shutdown following incomplete spontaneous abortion
Renal tubular necrosis following incomplete spontaneous abortion
Uremia following incomplete spontaneous abortion

CHAPTER 15 (O00-O9A)

O03.33 **Metabolic disorder following incomplete spontaneous abortion** ♀ M

O03.34 **Damage to pelvic organs following incomplete spontaneous abortion** ♀ M
- Laceration, perforation, tear or chemical damage of bladder following incomplete spontaneous abortion
- Laceration, perforation, tear or chemical damage of bowel following incomplete spontaneous abortion
- Laceration, perforation, tear or chemical damage of broad ligament following incomplete spontaneous abortion
- Laceration, perforation, tear or chemical damage of cervix following incomplete spontaneous abortion
- Laceration, perforation, tear or chemical damage of periurethral tissue following incomplete spontaneous abortion
- Laceration, perforation, tear or chemical damage of uterus following incomplete spontaneous abortion
- Laceration, perforation, tear or chemical damage of vagina following incomplete spontaneous abortion

O03.35 **Other venous complications following incomplete spontaneous abortion** ♀ M

O03.36 **Cardiac arrest following incomplete spontaneous abortion** ♀ M

O03.37 **Sepsis following incomplete spontaneous abortion** ♀ M

Use additional code to identify infectious agent (B95-B97)

Use additional code to identify severe sepsis, if applicable (R65.2-)

Excludes1 septic or septicopyemic embolism following incomplete spontaneous abortion (O03.2)

O03.38 **Urinary tract infection following incomplete spontaneous abortion** ♀ M
- Cystitis following incomplete spontaneous abortion

O03.39 **Incomplete spontaneous abortion with other complications** ♀ M

O03.4 **Incomplete spontaneous abortion without complication** ♀ M

O03.5 **Genital tract and pelvic infection following complete or unspecified spontaneous abortion** ♀ M
- Endometritis following complete or unspecified spontaneous abortion
- Oophoritis following complete or unspecified spontaneous abortion
- Parametritis following complete or unspecified spontaneous abortion
- Pelvic peritonitis following complete or unspecified spontaneous abortion
- Salpingitis following complete or unspecified spontaneous abortion
- Salpingo-oophoritis following complete or unspecified spontaneous abortion

Excludes1 sepsis following complete or unspecified spontaneous abortion (O03.87)
urinary tract infection following complete or unspecified spontaneous abortion (O03.88)

O03.6 **Delayed or excessive hemorrhage following complete or unspecified spontaneous abortion** ♀ M
- Afibrinogenemia following complete or unspecified spontaneous abortion
- Defibrination syndrome following complete or unspecified spontaneous abortion
- Hemolysis following complete or unspecified spontaneous abortion
- Intravascular coagulation following complete or unspecified spontaneous abortion

O03.7 **Embolism following complete or unspecified spontaneous abortion** ♀ M
- Air embolism following complete or unspecified spontaneous abortion
- Amniotic fluid embolism following complete or unspecified spontaneous abortion
- Blood-clot embolism following complete or unspecified spontaneous abortion
- Embolism NOS following complete or unspecified spontaneous abortion
- Fat embolism following complete or unspecified spontaneous abortion
- Pulmonary embolism following complete or unspecified spontaneous abortion
- Pyemic embolism following complete or unspecified spontaneous abortion
- Septic or septicopyemic embolism following complete or unspecified spontaneous abortion
- Soap embolism following complete or unspecified spontaneous abortion

● O03.8 **Other and unspecified complications following complete or unspecified spontaneous abortion**

O03.80 **Unspecified complication following complete or unspecified spontaneous abortion** ♀ M

O03.81 **Shock following complete or unspecified spontaneous abortion** ♀ M
- Circulatory collapse following complete or unspecified spontaneous abortion
- Shock (postprocedural) following complete or unspecified spontaneous abortion

Excludes1 shock due to infection following complete or unspecified spontaneous abortion (O03.87)

O03.82 **Renal failure following complete or unspecified spontaneous abortion** ♀ M
- Kidney failure (acute) following complete or unspecified spontaneous abortion
- Oliguria following complete or unspecified spontaneous abortion
- Renal shutdown following complete or unspecified spontaneous abortion
- Renal tubular necrosis following complete or unspecified spontaneous abortion
- Uremia following complete or unspecified spontaneous abortion

O03.83 **Metabolic disorder following complete or unspecified spontaneous abortion** ♀ M

O03.84 **Damage to pelvic organs following complete or unspecified spontaneous abortion** ♀ M
- Laceration, perforation, tear or chemical damage of bladder following complete or unspecified spontaneous abortion
- Laceration, perforation, tear or chemical damage of bowel following complete or unspecified spontaneous abortion
- Laceration, perforation, tear or chemical damage of broad ligament following complete or unspecified spontaneous abortion
- Laceration, perforation, tear or chemical damage of cervix following complete or unspecified spontaneous abortion
- Laceration, perforation, tear or chemical damage of periurethral tissue following complete or unspecified spontaneous abortion
- Laceration, perforation, tear or chemical damage of uterus following complete or unspecified spontaneous abortion
- Laceration, perforation, tear or chemical damage of vagina following complete or unspecified spontaneous abortion

CHAPTER 15 (O00-O9A)

O03.85 **Other venous complications following complete or unspecified spontaneous abortion ♀** M

O03.86 **Cardiac arrest following complete or unspecified spontaneous abortion ♀** M

O03.87 **Sepsis following complete or unspecified spontaneous abortion ♀** M
Use additional code to identify infectious agent (B95-B97)
Use additional code to identify severe sepsis, if applicable (R65.2-)
Excludes1 septic or septicopyemic embolism following complete or unspecified spontaneous abortion (O03.7)

O03.88 **Urinary tract infection following complete or unspecified spontaneous abortion ♀** M
Cystitis following complete or unspecified spontaneous abortion

O03.89 **Complete or unspecified spontaneous abortion with other complications ♀** M

O03.9 **Complete or unspecified spontaneous abortion without complication ♀** M
Miscarriage NOS
Spontaneous abortion NOS

● O04 **Complications following (induced) termination of pregnancy**
Includes complications following (induced) termination of pregnancy
Excludes1 encounter for elective termination of pregnancy, uncomplicated (Z33.2)
failed attempted termination of pregnancy (O07.-)

O04.5 **Genital tract and pelvic infection following (induced) termination of pregnancy ♀** M
Endometritis following (induced) termination of pregnancy
Oophoritis following (induced) termination of pregnancy
Parametritis following (induced) termination of pregnancy
Pelvic peritonitis following (induced) termination of pregnancy
Salpingitis following (induced) termination of pregnancy
Salpingo-oophoritis following (induced) termination of pregnancy
Excludes1 sepsis following (induced) termination of pregnancy (O04.87)
urinary tract infection following (induced) termination of pregnancy (O04.88)

O04.6 **Delayed or excessive hemorrhage following (induced) termination of pregnancy ♀** M
Afibrinogenemia following (induced) termination of pregnancy
Defibrination syndrome following (induced) termination of pregnancy
Hemolysis following (induced) termination of pregnancy
Intravascular coagulation following (induced) termination of pregnancy

O04.7 **Embolism following (induced) termination of pregnancy ♀** M
Air embolism following (induced) termination of pregnancy
Amniotic fluid embolism following (induced) termination of pregnancy
Blood-clot embolism following (induced) termination of pregnancy
Embolism NOS following (induced) termination of pregnancy
Fat embolism following (induced) termination of pregnancy
Pulmonary embolism following (induced) termination of pregnancy
Pyemic embolism following (induced) termination of pregnancy
Septic or septicopyemic embolism following (induced) termination of pregnancy
Soap embolism following (induced) termination of pregnancy

● O04.8 **(Induced) termination of pregnancy with other and unspecified complications**

O04.80 **(Induced) termination of pregnancy with unspecified complications ♀** M

O04.81 **Shock following (induced) termination of pregnancy ♀** M
Circulatory collapse following (induced) termination of pregnancy
Shock (postprocedural) following (induced) termination of pregnancy
Excludes1 shock due to infection following (induced) termination of pregnancy (O04.87)

O04.82 **Renal failure following (induced) termination of pregnancy ♀** M
Kidney failure (acute) following (induced) termination of pregnancy
Oliguria following (induced) termination of pregnancy
Renal shutdown following (induced) termination of pregnancy
Renal tubular necrosis following (induced) termination of pregnancy
Uremia following (induced) termination of pregnancy

O04.83 **Metabolic disorder following (induced) termination of pregnancy ♀** M

O04.84 **Damage to pelvic organs following (induced) termination of pregnancy ♀** M
Laceration, perforation, tear or chemical damage of bladder following (induced) termination of pregnancy
Laceration, perforation, tear or chemical damage of bowel following (induced) termination of pregnancy
Laceration, perforation, tear or chemical damage of broad ligament following (induced) termination of pregnancy
Laceration, perforation, tear or chemical damage of cervix following (induced) termination of pregnancy
Laceration, perforation, tear or chemical damage of periurethral tissue following (induced) termination of pregnancy
Laceration, perforation, tear or chemical damage of uterus following (induced) termination of pregnancy
Laceration, perforation, tear or chemical damage of vagina following (induced) termination of pregnancy

O04.85 Other venous complications following (induced) termination of pregnancy ♀ M

O04.86 Cardiac arrest following (induced) termination of pregnancy ♀ M

O04.87 Sepsis following (induced) termination of pregnancy ♀ M

Use additional code to identify infectious agent (B95-B97)

Use additional code to identify severe sepsis, if applicable (R65.2-)

Excludes1 septic or septicopyemic embolism following (induced) termination of pregnancy (O04.7)

O04.88 Urinary tract infection following (induced) termination of pregnancy ♀ M

Cystitis following (induced) termination of pregnancy

O04.89 (Induced) termination of pregnancy with other complications ♀ M

● **O07 Failed attempted termination of pregnancy**

Includes failure of attempted induction of termination of pregnancy
incomplete elective abortion

Excludes1 incomplete spontaneous abortion (O03.0-)

O07.0 Genital tract and pelvic infection following failed attempted termination of pregnancy ♀ M

Endometritis following failed attempted termination of pregnancy
Oophoritis following failed attempted termination of pregnancy
Parametritis following failed attempted termination of pregnancy
Pelvic peritonitis following failed attempted termination of pregnancy
Salpingitis following failed attempted termination of pregnancy
Salpingo-oophoritis following failed attempted termination of pregnancy

Excludes1 sepsis following failed attempted termination of pregnancy (O07.37)
urinary tract infection following failed attempted termination of pregnancy (O07.38)

O07.1 Delayed or excessive hemorrhage following failed attempted termination of pregnancy ♀ M

Afibrinogenemia following failed attempted termination of pregnancy
Defibrination syndrome following failed attempted termination of pregnancy
Hemolysis following failed attempted termination of pregnancy
Intravascular coagulation following failed attempted termination of pregnancy

O07.2 Embolism following failed attempted termination of pregnancy ♀ M

Air embolism following failed attempted termination of pregnancy
Amniotic fluid embolism following failed attempted termination of pregnancy
Blood-clot embolism following failed attempted termination of pregnancy
Embolism NOS following failed attempted termination of pregnancy
Fat embolism following failed attempted termination of pregnancy
Pulmonary embolism following failed attempted termination of pregnancy
Pyemic embolism following failed attempted termination of pregnancy
Septic or septicopyemic embolism following failed attempted termination of pregnancy
Soap embolism following failed attempted termination of pregnancy

● **O07.3 Failed attempted termination of pregnancy with other and unspecified complications**

O07.30 Failed attempted termination of pregnancy with unspecified complications ♀ M

O07.31 Shock following failed attempted termination of pregnancy ♀ M

Circulatory collapse following failed attempted termination of pregnancy
Shock (postprocedural) following failed attempted termination of pregnancy

Excludes1 shock due to infection following failed attempted termination of pregnancy (O07.37)

O07.32 Renal failure following failed attempted termination of pregnancy ♀ M

Kidney failure (acute) following failed attempted termination of pregnancy
Oliguria following failed attempted termination of pregnancy
Renal shutdown following failed attempted termination of pregnancy
Renal tubular necrosis following failed attempted termination of pregnancy
Uremia following failed attempted termination of pregnancy

O07.33 Metabolic disorder following failed attempted termination of pregnancy ♀ M

O07.34 Damage to pelvic organs following failed attempted termination of pregnancy ♀ M

Laceration, perforation, tear or chemical damage of bladder following failed attempted termination of pregnancy
Laceration, perforation, tear or chemical damage of bowel following failed attempted termination of pregnancy
Laceration, perforation, tear or chemical damage of broad ligament following failed attempted termination of pregnancy
Laceration, perforation, tear or chemical damage of cervix following failed attempted termination of pregnancy
Laceration, perforation, tear or chemical damage of periurethral tissue following failed attempted termination of pregnancy
Laceration, perforation, tear or chemical damage of uterus following failed attempted termination of pregnancy
Laceration, perforation, tear or chemical damage of vagina following failed attempted termination of pregnancy

O07.35 Other venous complications following failed attempted termination of pregnancy ♀ M

O07.36 Cardiac arrest following failed attempted termination of pregnancy ♀ M

O07.37 Sepsis following failed attempted termination of pregnancy ♀ M

Use additional code (B95-B97), to identify infectious agent

Use additional code (R65.2-) to identify severe sepsis, if applicable

Excludes1 septic or septicopyemic embolism following failed attempted termination of pregnancy (O07.2)

O07.38 Urinary tract infection following failed attempted termination of pregnancy ♀ M

Cystitis following failed attempted termination of pregnancy

O07.39 Failed attempted termination of pregnancy with other complications ♀ M

O07.4 Failed attempted termination of pregnancy without complication ♀ M

CHAPTER 15 (O00-O9A)

O08 Complications following ectopic and molar pregnancy
This category is for use with categories O00-O02 to identify any associated complications.

O08.0 Genital tract and pelvic infection following ectopic and molar pregnancy ♀ M
Endometritis following ectopic and molar pregnancy
Oophoritis following ectopic and molar pregnancy
Parametritis following ectopic and molar pregnancy
Pelvic peritonitis following ectopic and molar pregnancy
Salpingitis following ectopic and molar pregnancy
Salpingo-oophoritis following ectopic and molar pregnancy
Excludes1 sepsis following ectopic and molar pregnancy (O08.82)
urinary tract infection (O08.83)

O08.1 Delayed or excessive hemorrhage following ectopic and molar pregnancy ♀ M
Afibrinogenemia following ectopic and molar pregnancy
Defibrination syndrome following ectopic and molar pregnancy
Hemolysis following ectopic and molar pregnancy
Intravascular coagulation following ectopic and molar pregnancy
Excludes1 delayed or excessive hemorrhage due to incomplete abortion (O03.1)

O08.2 Embolism following ectopic and molar pregnancy ♀ M
Air embolism following ectopic and molar pregnancy
Amniotic fluid embolism following ectopic and molar pregnancy
Blood-clot embolism following ectopic and molar pregnancy
Embolism NOS following ectopic and molar pregnancy
Fat embolism following ectopic and molar pregnancy
Pulmonary embolism following ectopic and molar pregnancy
Pyemic embolism following ectopic and molar pregnancy
Septic or septicopyemic embolism following ectopic and molar pregnancy
Soap embolism following ectopic and molar pregnancy

O08.3 Shock following ectopic and molar pregnancy ♀ M
Circulatory collapse following ectopic and molar pregnancy
Shock (postprocedural) following ectopic and molar pregnancy
Excludes1 shock due to infection following ectopic and molar pregnancy (O08.82)

O08.4 Renal failure following ectopic and molar pregnancy ♀ M
Kidney failure (acute) following ectopic and molar pregnancy
Oliguria following ectopic and molar pregnancy
Renal shutdown following ectopic and molar pregnancy
Renal tubular necrosis following ectopic and molar pregnancy
Uremia following ectopic and molar pregnancy

O08.5 Metabolic disorders following an ectopic and molar pregnancy ♀ M

O08.6 Damage to pelvic organs and tissues following an ectopic and molar pregnancy ♀ M
Laceration, perforation, tear or chemical damage of bladder following an ectopic and molar pregnancy
Laceration, perforation, tear or chemical damage of bowel following an ectopic and molar pregnancy
Laceration, perforation, tear or chemical damage of broad ligament following an ectopic and molar pregnancy
Laceration, perforation, tear or chemical damage of cervix following an ectopic and molar pregnancy
Laceration, perforation, tear or chemical damage of periurethral tissue following an ectopic and molar pregnancy
Laceration, perforation, tear or chemical damage of uterus following an ectopic and molar pregnancy
Laceration, perforation, tear or chemical damage of vagina following an ectopic and molar pregnancy

O08.7 Other venous complications following an ectopic and molar pregnancy ♀ M

O08.8 Other complications following an ectopic and molar pregnancy

O08.81 Cardiac arrest following an ectopic and molar pregnancy ♀ M

O08.82 Sepsis following ectopic and molar pregnancy ♀ M
Use additional code (B95-B97), to identify infectious agent
Use additional code (R65.2-) to identify severe sepsis, if applicable
Excludes1 septic or septicopyemic embolism following ectopic and molar pregnancy (O08.2)

O08.83 Urinary tract infection following an ectopic and molar pregnancy ♀ M
Cystitis following an ectopic and molar pregnancy

O08.89 Other complications following an ectopic and molar pregnancy ♀ M

O08.9 Unspecified complication following an ectopic and molar pregnancy ♀ M

SUPERVISION OF HIGH RISK PREGNANCY (O09)

O09 Supervision of high risk pregnancy
Coding Clinic: 2016, Q4, P125, 150

O09.0 Supervision of pregnancy with history of infertility
O09.00 Supervision of pregnancy with history of infertility, unspecified trimester ♀ M
O09.01 Supervision of pregnancy with history of infertility, first trimester ♀ M
O09.02 Supervision of pregnancy with history of infertility, second trimester ♀ M
O09.03 Supervision of pregnancy with history of infertility, third trimester ♀ M

O09.1 Supervision of pregnancy with history of ectopic pregnancy
Coding Clinic: 2016, Q4, P49-50
O09.10 Supervision of pregnancy with history of ectopic pregnancy, unspecified trimester ♀ M
O09.11 Supervision of pregnancy with history of ectopic pregnancy, first trimester ♀ M
O09.12 Supervision of pregnancy with history of ectopic pregnancy, second trimester ♀ M
O09.13 Supervision of pregnancy with history of ectopic pregnancy, third trimester ♀ M

O09.A Supervision of pregnancy with history of molar pregnancy
Coding Clinic: 2016, Q4, P50
O09.A0 Supervision of pregnancy with history of molar pregnancy, unspecified trimester ♀ M
O09.A1 Supervision of pregnancy with history of molar pregnancy, first trimester ♀ M
O09.A2 Supervision of pregnancy with history of molar pregnancy, second trimester ♀ M
O09.A3 Supervision of pregnancy with history of molar pregnancy, third trimester ♀ M

● **O09.2** Supervision of pregnancy with other poor reproductive or obstetric history
Excludes2 pregnancy care for patient with history of recurrent pregnancy loss (O26.2-)

● **O09.21** Supervision of pregnancy with history of pre-term labor
- **O09.211** Supervision of pregnancy with history of pre-term labor, first trimester ♀ M
- **O09.212** Supervision of pregnancy with history of pre-term labor, second trimester ♀ M
- **O09.213** Supervision of pregnancy with history of pre-term labor, third trimester ♀ M
- **O09.219** Supervision of pregnancy with history of pre-term labor, unspecified trimester ♀ M

● **O09.29** Supervision of pregnancy with other poor reproductive or obstetric history
Supervision of pregnancy with history of neonatal death
Supervision of pregnancy with history of stillbirth
- **O09.291** Supervision of pregnancy with other poor reproductive or obstetric history, first trimester ♀ M
- **O09.292** Supervision of pregnancy with other poor reproductive or obstetric history, second trimester ♀ M
- **O09.293** Supervision of pregnancy with other poor reproductive or obstetric history, third trimester ♀ M
- **O09.299** Supervision of pregnancy with other poor reproductive or obstetric history, unspecified trimester ♀ M

● **O09.3** Supervision of pregnancy with insufficient antenatal care
Supervision of concealed pregnancy
Supervision of hidden pregnancy
- **O09.30** Supervision of pregnancy with insufficient antenatal care, unspecified trimester ♀ M
- **O09.31** Supervision of pregnancy with insufficient antenatal care, first trimester ♀ M
- **O09.32** Supervision of pregnancy with insufficient antenatal care, second trimester ♀ M
- **O09.33** Supervision of pregnancy with insufficient antenatal care, third trimester ♀ M

● **O09.4** Supervision of pregnancy with grand multiparity
- **O09.40** Supervision of pregnancy with grand multiparity, unspecified trimester ♀ M
- **O09.41** Supervision of pregnancy with grand multiparity, first trimester ♀ M
- **O09.42** Supervision of pregnancy with grand multiparity, second trimester ♀ M
- **O09.43** Supervision of pregnancy with grand multiparity, third trimester ♀ M

● **O09.5** Supervision of elderly primigravida and multigravida
Pregnancy for a female 35 years and older at expected date of delivery

● **O09.51** Supervision of elderly primigravida
- **O09.511** Supervision of elderly primigravida, first trimester ♀ M
- **O09.512** Supervision of elderly primigravida, second trimester ♀ M
- **O09.513** Supervision of elderly primigravida, third trimester ♀ M
- **O09.519** Supervision of elderly primigravida, unspecified trimester ♀ M

● **O09.52** Supervision of elderly multigravida
- **O09.521** Supervision of elderly multigravida, first trimester ♀ M
- **O09.522** Supervision of elderly multigravida, second trimester ♀ M
- **O09.523** Supervision of elderly multigravida, third trimester ♀ M
  Coding Clinic: 2016, Q4, P150
- **O09.529** Supervision of elderly multigravida, unspecified trimester ♀ M

● **O09.6** Supervision of young primigravida and multigravida
Supervision of pregnancy for a female less than 16 years old at expected date of delivery

● **O09.61** Supervision of young primigravida
- **O09.611** Supervision of young primigravida, first trimester ♀ M
- **O09.612** Supervision of young primigravida, second trimester ♀ M
- **O09.613** Supervision of young primigravida, third trimester ♀ M
- **O09.619** Supervision of young primigravida, unspecified trimester ♀ M

● **O09.62** Supervision of young multigravida
- **O09.621** Supervision of young multigravida, first trimester ♀ M
- **O09.622** Supervision of young multigravida, second trimester ♀ M
- **O09.623** Supervision of young multigravida, third trimester ♀ M
- **O09.629** Supervision of young multigravida, unspecified trimester ♀ M

● **O09.7** Supervision of high risk pregnancy due to social problems
- **O09.70** Supervision of high risk pregnancy due to social problems, unspecified trimester ♀ M
- **O09.71** Supervision of high risk pregnancy due to social problems, first trimester ♀ M
- **O09.72** Supervision of high risk pregnancy due to social problems, second trimester ♀ M
- **O09.73** Supervision of high risk pregnancy due to social problems, third trimester ♀ M

● **O09.8** Supervision of other high risk pregnancies

● **O09.81** Supervision of pregnancy resulting from assisted reproductive technology
Supervision of pregnancy resulting from in-vitro fertilization
Excludes2 gestational carrier status (Z33.3)
- **O09.811** Supervision of pregnancy resulting from assisted reproductive technology, first trimester ♀ M
- **O09.812** Supervision of pregnancy resulting from assisted reproductive technology, second trimester ♀ M
- **O09.813** Supervision of pregnancy resulting from assisted reproductive technology, third trimester ♀ M
- **O09.819** Supervision of pregnancy resulting from assisted reproductive technology, unspecified trimester ♀ M

● O09.82 **Supervision of pregnancy with history of in utero procedure during previous pregnancy**

O09.821 **Supervision of pregnancy with history of in utero procedure during previous pregnancy, first trimester** ♀ M

O09.822 **Supervision of pregnancy with history of in utero procedure during previous pregnancy, second trimester** ♀ M

O09.823 **Supervision of pregnancy with history of in utero procedure during previous pregnancy, third trimester** ♀ M

O09.829 **Supervision of pregnancy with history of in utero procedure during previous pregnancy, unspecified trimester** ♀ M

Excludes1 supervision of pregnancy affected by in utero procedure during current pregnancy (O35.7)

● O09.89 **Supervision of other high risk pregnancies**

O09.891 **Supervision of other high risk pregnancies, first trimester** ♀ M

O09.892 **Supervision of other high risk pregnancies, second trimester** ♀ M

O09.893 **Supervision of other high risk pregnancies, third trimester** ♀ M

O09.899 **Supervision of other high risk pregnancies, unspecified trimester** ♀ M

● O09.9 **Supervision of high risk pregnancy, unspecified**

O09.90 **Supervision of high risk pregnancy, unspecified, unspecified trimester** ♀ M

O09.91 **Supervision of high risk pregnancy, unspecified, first trimester** ♀ M

O09.92 **Supervision of high risk pregnancy, unspecified, second trimester** ♀ M

O09.93 **Supervision of high risk pregnancy, unspecified, third trimester** ♀ M

EDEMA, PROTEINURIA AND HYPERTENSIVE DISORDERS IN PREGNANCY, CHILDBIRTH AND THE PUERPERIUM (O10-O16)

● O10 **Pre-existing hypertension complicating pregnancy, childbirth and the puerperium**

Includes pre-existing hypertension with pre-existing proteinuria complicating pregnancy, childbirth and the puerperium

Excludes2 pre-existing hypertension with superimposed pre-eclampsia complicating pregnancy, childbirth and the puerperium (O11.-)

Coding Clinic: 2016, Q4, P50

● O10.0 **Pre-existing essential hypertension complicating pregnancy, childbirth and the puerperium**

Any condition in I10 specified as a reason for obstetric care during pregnancy, childbirth or the puerperium

● O10.01 **Pre-existing essential hypertension complicating pregnancy**

O10.011 **Pre-existing essential hypertension complicating pregnancy, first trimester** ♀ M

O10.012 **Pre-existing essential hypertension complicating pregnancy, second trimester** ♀ M

O10.013 **Pre-existing essential hypertension complicating pregnancy, third trimester** ♀ M

O10.019 **Pre-existing essential hypertension complicating pregnancy, unspecified trimester** ♀ M

O10.02 **Pre-existing essential hypertension complicating childbirth** ♀ M

O10.03 **Pre-existing essential hypertension complicating the puerperium** ♀ M

● O10.1 **Pre-existing hypertensive heart disease complicating pregnancy, childbirth and the puerperium**

Any condition in I11 specified as a reason for obstetric care during pregnancy, childbirth or the puerperium

Use additional code from I11 to identify the type of hypertensive heart disease

● O10.11 **Pre-existing hypertensive heart disease complicating pregnancy**

O10.111 **Pre-existing hypertensive heart disease complicating pregnancy, first trimester** ♀ M

O10.112 **Pre-existing hypertensive heart disease complicating pregnancy, second trimester** ♀ M

O10.113 **Pre-existing hypertensive heart disease complicating pregnancy, third trimester** ♀ M

O10.119 **Pre-existing hypertensive heart disease complicating pregnancy, unspecified trimester** ♀ M

O10.12 **Pre-existing hypertensive heart disease complicating childbirth** ♀ M

O10.13 **Pre-existing hypertensive heart disease complicating the puerperium** ♀ M

● O10.2 **Pre-existing hypertensive chronic kidney disease complicating pregnancy, childbirth and the puerperium**

Any condition in I12 specified as a reason for obstetric care during pregnancy, childbirth or the puerperium

Use additional code from I12 to identify the type of hypertensive chronic kidney disease

● O10.21 **Pre-existing hypertensive chronic kidney disease complicating pregnancy**

O10.211 **Pre-existing hypertensive chronic kidney disease complicating pregnancy, first trimester** ♀ M

O10.212 **Pre-existing hypertensive chronic kidney disease complicating pregnancy, second trimester** ♀ M

O10.213 **Pre-existing hypertensive chronic kidney disease complicating pregnancy, third trimester** ♀ M

O10.219 **Pre-existing hypertensive chronic kidney disease complicating pregnancy, unspecified trimester** ♀ M

O10.22 **Pre-existing hypertensive chronic kidney disease complicating childbirth** ♀ M

O10.23 **Pre-existing hypertensive chronic kidney disease complicating the puerperium** ♀ M

O10.3 Pre-existing hypertensive heart and chronic kidney disease complicating pregnancy, childbirth and the puerperium
Any condition in I13 specified as a reason for obstetric care during pregnancy, childbirth or the puerperium
Use additional code from I13 to identify the type of hypertensive heart and chronic kidney disease

O10.31 Pre-existing hypertensive heart and chronic kidney disease complicating pregnancy
- O10.311 Pre-existing hypertensive heart and chronic kidney disease complicating pregnancy, first trimester ♀ M
- O10.312 Pre-existing hypertensive heart and chronic kidney disease complicating pregnancy, second trimester ♀ M
- O10.313 Pre-existing hypertensive heart and chronic kidney disease complicating pregnancy, third trimester ♀ M
- O10.319 Pre-existing hypertensive heart and chronic kidney disease complicating pregnancy, unspecified trimester ♀ M

- O10.32 Pre-existing hypertensive heart and chronic kidney disease complicating childbirth ♀ M
- O10.33 Pre-existing hypertensive heart and chronic kidney disease complicating the puerperium ♀ M

O10.4 Pre-existing secondary hypertension complicating pregnancy, childbirth and the puerperium
Any condition in I15 specified as a reason for obstetric care during pregnancy, childbirth or the puerperium
Use additional code from I15 to identify the type of secondary hypertension

O10.41 Pre-existing secondary hypertension complicating pregnancy
- O10.411 Pre-existing secondary hypertension complicating pregnancy, first trimester ♀ M
- O10.412 Pre-existing secondary hypertension complicating pregnancy, second trimester ♀ M
- O10.413 Pre-existing secondary hypertension complicating pregnancy, third trimester ♀ M
- O10.419 Pre-existing secondary hypertension complicating pregnancy, unspecified trimester ♀ M

- O10.42 Pre-existing secondary hypertension complicating childbirth ♀ M
- O10.43 Pre-existing secondary hypertension complicating the puerperium ♀ M

O10.9 Unspecified pre-existing hypertension complicating pregnancy, childbirth and the puerperium

O10.91 Unspecified pre-existing hypertension complicating pregnancy
- O10.911 Unspecified pre-existing hypertension complicating pregnancy, first trimester ♀ M
- O10.912 Unspecified pre-existing hypertension complicating pregnancy, second trimester ♀ M
- O10.913 Unspecified pre-existing hypertension complicating pregnancy, third trimester ♀ M
- O10.919 Unspecified pre-existing hypertension complicating pregnancy, unspecified trimester ♀ M

- O10.92 Unspecified pre-existing hypertension complicating childbirth ♀ M
- O10.93 Unspecified pre-existing hypertension complicating the puerperium ♀ M

O11 Pre-existing hypertension with pre-eclampsia
Includes conditions in O10 complicated by pre-eclampsia
pre-eclampsia superimposed pre-existing hypertension
Use additional code from O10 to identify the type of hypertension
Coding Clinic: 2016, Q4, P50

- O11.1 Pre-existing hypertension with pre-eclampsia, first trimester ♀ M
- O11.2 Pre-existing hypertension with pre-eclampsia, second trimester ♀ M
- O11.3 Pre-existing hypertension with pre-eclampsia, third trimester ♀ M
- O11.4 Pre-existing hypertension with pre-eclampsia, complicating childbirth ♀ M
- O11.5 Pre-existing hypertension with pre-eclampsia, complicating the puerperium ♀ M
- O11.9 Pre-existing hypertension with pre-eclampsia, unspecified trimester ♀ M

O12 Gestational [pregnancy-induced] edema and proteinuria without hypertension
Coding Clinic: 2016, Q4, P50

O12.0 Gestational edema
- O12.00 Gestational edema, unspecified trimester ♀ M
- O12.01 Gestational edema, first trimester ♀ M
- O12.02 Gestational edema, second trimester ♀ M
- O12.03 Gestational edema, third trimester ♀ M
- O12.04 Gestational edema, complicating childbirth ♀ M
- O12.05 Gestational edema, complicating the puerperium ♀ M

O12.1 Gestational proteinuria
- O12.10 Gestational proteinuria, unspecified trimester ♀ M
- O12.11 Gestational proteinuria, first trimester ♀ M
- O12.12 Gestational proteinuria, second trimester ♀ M
- O12.13 Gestational proteinuria, third trimester ♀ M
- O12.14 Gestational proteinuria, complicating childbirth ♀ M
- O12.15 Gestational proteinuria, complicating the puerperium ♀ M

O12.2 Gestational edema with proteinuria
- O12.20 Gestational edema with proteinuria, unspecified trimester ♀ M
- O12.21 Gestational edema with proteinuria, first trimester ♀ M
- O12.22 Gestational edema with proteinuria, second trimester ♀ M
- O12.23 Gestational edema with proteinuria, third trimester ♀ M
- O12.24 Gestational edema with proteinuria, complicating childbirth ♀ M
- O12.25 Gestational edema with proteinuria, complicating the puerperium ♀ M

O13 Gestational [pregnancy-induced] hypertension without significant proteinuria

Includes gestational hypertension NOS
transient hypertension of pregnancy ♀

Coding Clinic: 2016, Q4, P50

O13.1 Gestational [pregnancy-induced] hypertension without significant proteinuria, **first trimester** ♀ M

O13.2 Gestational [pregnancy-induced] hypertension without significant proteinuria, **second trimester** ♀ M

O13.3 Gestational [pregnancy-induced] hypertension without significant proteinuria, **third trimester** ♀ M

O13.4 Gestational [pregnancy-induced] hypertension without significant proteinuria, complicating childbirth ♀ M

O13.5 Gestational [pregnancy-induced] hypertension without significant proteinuria, complicating the puerperium ♀ M

O13.9 Gestational [pregnancy-induced] hypertension without significant proteinuria, unspecified trimester ♀ M

O14 Pre-eclampsia

Excludes1 pre-existing hypertension with pre-eclampsia (O11)

Coding Clinic: 2016, Q4, P50

O14.0 Mild to moderate pre-eclampsia

O14.00 Mild to moderate pre-eclampsia, unspecified trimester ♀ M

O14.02 Mild to moderate pre-eclampsia, second trimester ♀ M

O14.03 Mild to moderate pre-eclampsia, third trimester ♀ M

O14.04 Mild to moderate pre-eclampsia, complicating childbirth ♀ M
Coding Clinic: 2019, Q2, P8

O14.05 Mild to moderate pre-eclampsia, complicating the puerperium ♀ M

O14.1 Severe pre-eclampsia

Excludes1 HELLP syndrome (O14.2-)

H=hemolysis, EL=elevated liver enzymes, LP=low platelet count

O14.10 Severe pre-eclampsia, unspecified trimester ♀ M

O14.12 Severe pre-eclampsia, second trimester ♀ M

O14.13 Severe pre-eclampsia, third trimester ♀ M

O14.14 Severe pre-eclampsia complicating childbirth ♀ M

O14.15 Severe pre-eclampsia, complicating the puerperium ♀ M

O14.2 HELLP syndrome

Severe pre-eclampsia with hemolysis, elevated liver enzymes and low platelet count (HELLP)

O14.20 HELLP syndrome (HELLP), unspecified trimester ♀ M

O14.22 HELLP syndrome (HELLP), second trimester ♀ M

O14.23 HELLP syndrome (HELLP), third trimester ♀ M

O14.24 HELLP syndrome, complicating childbirth ♀ M

O14.25 HELLP syndrome, complicating the puerperium ♀ M

O14.9 Unspecified pre-eclampsia

O14.90 Unspecified pre-eclampsia, unspecified trimester ♀ M

O14.92 Unspecified pre-eclampsia, second trimester ♀ M

O14.93 Unspecified pre-eclampsia, third trimester ♀ M

O14.94 Unspecified pre-eclampsia, complicating childbirth ♀ M

O14.95 Unspecified pre-eclampsia, complicating the puerperium ♀ M

O15 Eclampsia

Includes convulsions following conditions in O10-O14 and O16

O15.0 Eclampsia complicating pregnancy

Coding Clinic: 2016, Q4, P50

O15.00 Eclampsia complicating pregnancy, unspecified trimester ♀ M

O15.02 Eclampsia complicating pregnancy, second trimester ♀ M

O15.03 Eclampsia complicating pregnancy, third trimester ♀ M

O15.1 Eclampsia complicating labor ♀ M

O15.2 Eclampsia complicating the puerperium ♀ M

O15.9 Eclampsia, unspecified as to time period ♀ M
Eclampsia NOS

O16 Unspecified maternal hypertension

Coding Clinic: 2016, Q4, P50

O16.1 Unspecified maternal hypertension, first trimester ♀ M

O16.2 Unspecified maternal hypertension, second trimester ♀ M

O16.3 Unspecified maternal hypertension, third trimester ♀ M

O16.4 Unspecified maternal hypertension, complicating childbirth ♀ M

O16.5 Unspecified maternal hypertension, complicating the puerperium ♀ M

O16.9 Unspecified maternal hypertension, unspecified trimester ♀ M

OTHER MATERNAL DISORDERS PREDOMINANTLY RELATED TO PREGNANCY (O20-O29)

Excludes2 maternal care related to the fetus and amniotic cavity and possible delivery problems (O30-O48)
maternal diseases classifiable elsewhere but complicating pregnancy, labor and delivery, and the puerperium (O98-O99)

O20 Hemorrhage in early pregnancy

Includes hemorrhage before completion of 20 weeks gestation

Excludes1 pregnancy with abortive outcome (O00-O08)

O20.0 Threatened abortion ♀ M
Hemorrhage specified as due to threatened abortion

O20.8 Other hemorrhage in early pregnancy ♀ M

O20.9 Hemorrhage in early pregnancy, unspecified ♀ M

O21 Excessive vomiting in pregnancy

O21.0 Mild hyperemesis gravidarum ♀ M
Hyperemesis gravidarum, mild or unspecified, starting before the end of the 20th week of gestation

O21.1 Hyperemesis gravidarum with metabolic disturbance ♀ M
Hyperemesis gravidarum, starting before the end of the 20th week of gestation, with metabolic disturbance such as carbohydrate depletion
Hyperemesis gravidarum, starting before the end of the 20th week of gestation, with metabolic disturbance such as dehydration
Hyperemesis gravidarum, starting before the end of the 20th week of gestation, with metabolic disturbance such as electrolyte imbalance

O21.2 Late vomiting of pregnancy ♀ M
Excessive vomiting starting after 20 completed weeks of gestation

O21.8 Other vomiting complicating pregnancy ♀ M
Vomiting due to diseases classified elsewhere, complicating pregnancy
Use additional code, to identify cause

O21.9 Vomiting of pregnancy, unspecified ♀ M

CHAPTER 15 (O00-O9A)

● O22 Venous complications and hemorrhoids in pregnancy
Excludes1 venous complications of:
abortion NOS (O03.9)
ectopic or molar pregnancy (O08.7)
failed attempted abortion (O07.35)
induced abortion (O04.85)
spontaneous abortion (O03.89)
Excludes2 obstetric pulmonary embolism (O88.-)
venous complications and hemorrhoids of childbirth and the puerperium (O87.-)

● O22.0 **Varicose veins of lower extremity** in pregnancy
Varicose veins NOS in pregnancy
O22.00 Varicose veins of lower extremity in pregnancy, **unspecified trimester** ♀ M
O22.01 Varicose veins of lower extremity in pregnancy, **first trimester** ♀ M
O22.02 Varicose veins of lower extremity in pregnancy, **second trimester** ♀ M
O22.03 Varicose veins of lower extremity in pregnancy, **third trimester** ♀ M

● O22.1 **Genital varices** in pregnancy
Perineal varices in pregnancy
Vaginal varices in pregnancy
Vulval varices in pregnancy
O22.10 Genital varices in pregnancy, **unspecified trimester** ♀ M
O22.11 Genital varices in pregnancy, **first trimester** ♀ M
O22.12 Genital varices in pregnancy, **second trimester** ♀ M
O22.13 Genital varices in pregnancy, **third trimester** ♀ M

● O22.2 **Superficial thrombophlebitis** in pregnancy
Phlebitis in pregnancy NOS
Thrombophlebitis of legs in pregnancy
Thrombosis in pregnancy NOS
Use additional code to identify the superficial thrombophlebitis (I80.0-)
O22.20 Superficial thrombophlebitis in pregnancy, **unspecified trimester** ♀ M
O22.21 Superficial thrombophlebitis in pregnancy, **first trimester** ♀ M
O22.22 Superficial thrombophlebitis in pregnancy, **second trimester** ♀ M
O22.23 Superficial thrombophlebitis in pregnancy, **third trimester** ♀ M

● O22.3 **Deep phlebothrombosis** in pregnancy
Deep vein thrombosis, antepartum
Use additional code to identify the deep vein thrombosis (I82.4-, I82.5-, I82.62-. I82.72-)
Use additional code, if applicable, for associated long-term (current) use of anticoagulants (Z79.01)
O22.30 Deep phlebothrombosis in pregnancy, **unspecified trimester** ♀ M
O22.31 Deep phlebothrombosis in pregnancy, **first trimester** ♀ M
O22.32 Deep phlebothrombosis in pregnancy, **second trimester** ♀ M
O22.33 Deep phlebothrombosis in pregnancy, **third trimester** ♀ M

● O22.4 **Hemorrhoids** in pregnancy
O22.40 Hemorrhoids in pregnancy, **unspecified trimester** ♀ M
O22.41 Hemorrhoids in pregnancy, **first trimester** ♀ M
O22.42 Hemorrhoids in pregnancy, **second trimester** ♀ M
O22.43 Hemorrhoids in pregnancy, **third trimester** ♀ M

● O22.5 **Cerebral venous thrombosis** in pregnancy
Cerebrovenous sinus thrombosis in pregnancy
O22.50 Cerebral venous thrombosis in pregnancy, **unspecified trimester** ♀ M
O22.51 Cerebral venous thrombosis in pregnancy, **first trimester** ♀ M
O22.52 Cerebral venous thrombosis in pregnancy, **second trimester** ♀ M
O22.53 Cerebral venous thrombosis in pregnancy, **third trimester** ♀ M

● O22.8 **Other** venous complications in pregnancy
● O22.8X Other venous complications in pregnancy
O22.8X1 Other venous complications in pregnancy, **first trimester** ♀ M
O22.8X2 Other venous complications in pregnancy, **second trimester** ♀ M
O22.8X3 Other venous complications in pregnancy, **third trimester** ♀ M
O22.8X9 Other venous complications in pregnancy, **unspecified trimester** ♀ M

● O22.9 Venous complication in pregnancy, **unspecified**
Gestational phlebitis NOS
Gestational phlebopathy NOS
Gestational thrombosis NOS
O22.90 Venous complication in pregnancy, unspecified, **unspecified trimester** ♀ M
O22.91 Venous complication in pregnancy, unspecified, **first trimester** ♀ M
O22.92 Venous complication in pregnancy, unspecified, **second trimester** ♀ M
O22.93 Venous complication in pregnancy, unspecified, **third trimester** ♀ M

● O23 **Infections of genitourinary tract** in pregnancy
Use additional code to identify organism (B95.-, B96.-)
Excludes2 gonococcal infections complicating pregnancy, childbirth and the puerperium (O98.2)
infections with a predominantly sexual mode of transmission NOS complicating pregnancy, childbirth and the puerperium (O98.3)
syphilis complicating pregnancy, childbirth and the puerperium (O98.1)
tuberculosis of genitourinary system complicating pregnancy, childbirth and the puerperium (O98.0)
venereal disease NOS complicating pregnancy, childbirth and the puerperium (O98.3)

● O23.0 Infections of **kidney** in pregnancy
Pyelonephritis in pregnancy
O23.00 Infections of kidney in pregnancy, **unspecified trimester** ♀ M
O23.01 Infections of kidney in pregnancy, **first trimester** ♀ M
O23.02 Infections of kidney in pregnancy, **second trimester** ♀ M
O23.03 Infections of kidney in pregnancy, **third trimester** ♀ M

● O23.1 Infections of **bladder** in pregnancy
O23.10 Infections of bladder in pregnancy, **unspecified trimester** ♀ M
O23.11 Infections of bladder in pregnancy, **first trimester** ♀ M
O23.12 Infections of bladder in pregnancy, **second trimester** ♀ M
O23.13 Infections of bladder in pregnancy, **third trimester** ♀ M

● O23.2 Infections of **urethra** in pregnancy
- O23.20 Infections of urethra in pregnancy, **unspecified trimester** ♀ M
- O23.21 Infections of urethra in pregnancy, **first trimester** ♀ M
- O23.22 Infections of urethra in pregnancy, **second trimester** ♀ M
- O23.23 Infections of urethra in pregnancy, **third trimester** ♀ M

● O23.3 Infections of **other parts of urinary tract** in pregnancy
- O23.30 Infections of other parts of urinary tract in pregnancy, **unspecified trimester** ♀ M
- O23.31 Infections of other parts of urinary tract in pregnancy, **first trimester** ♀ M
- O23.32 Infections of other parts of urinary tract in pregnancy, **second trimester** ♀ M
- O23.33 Infections of other parts of urinary tract in pregnancy, **third trimester** ♀ M

● O23.4 **Unspecified** infection of urinary tract in pregnancy
- O23.40 Unspecified infection of urinary tract in pregnancy, **unspecified trimester** ♀ M
- O23.41 Unspecified infection of urinary tract in pregnancy, **first trimester** ♀ M
- O23.42 Unspecified infection of urinary tract in pregnancy, **second trimester** ♀ M
- O23.43 Unspecified infection of urinary tract in pregnancy, **third trimester** ♀ M

● O23.5 Infections of the **genital tract** in pregnancy

● O23.51 Infection of **cervix** in pregnancy
- O23.511 Infections of cervix in pregnancy, **first trimester** ♀ M
- O23.512 Infections of cervix in pregnancy, **second trimester** ♀ M
- O23.513 Infections of cervix in pregnancy, **third trimester** ♀ M
- O23.519 Infections of cervix in pregnancy, **unspecified trimester** ♀ M

● O23.52 **Salpingo-oophoritis** in pregnancy

Oophoritis = inflammation of ovary
Salpingitis = inflammation of fallopian tube

Oophoritis in pregnancy
Salpingitis in pregnancy
- O23.521 Salpingo-oophoritis in pregnancy, **first trimester** ♀ M
- O23.522 Salpingo-oophoritis in pregnancy, **second trimester** ♀ M
- O23.523 Salpingo-oophoritis in pregnancy, **third trimester** ♀ M
- O23.529 Salpingo-oophoritis in pregnancy, **unspecified trimester** ♀ M

● O23.59 Infection of **other part** of genital tract in pregnancy
- O23.591 Infection of other part of genital tract in pregnancy, **first trimester** ♀ M
- O23.592 Infection of other part of genital tract in pregnancy, **second trimester** ♀ M
- O23.593 Infection of other part of genital tract in pregnancy, **third trimester** ♀ M
- O23.599 Infection of other part of genital tract in pregnancy, **unspecified trimester** ♀ M

● O23.9 **Unspecified** genitourinary tract infection in pregnancy

Genitourinary tract infection in pregnancy NOS
- O23.90 Unspecified genitourinary tract infection in pregnancy, **unspecified trimester** ♀ M
- O23.91 Unspecified genitourinary tract infection in pregnancy, **first trimester** ♀ M
- O23.92 Unspecified genitourinary tract infection in pregnancy, **second trimester** ♀ M
- O23.93 Unspecified genitourinary tract infection in pregnancy, **third trimester** ♀ M

OGCR Section I.C.15.g.

Diabetes mellitus in pregnancy

Diabetes mellitus is a significant complicating factor in pregnancy. Pregnant women who are diabetic should be assigned a code from category O24, Diabetes mellitus in pregnancy, childbirth, and the puerperium, first, followed by the appropriate diabetes code(s) (E08-E13) from Chapter 4.

● O24 **Diabetes mellitus** in pregnancy, childbirth, and the puerperium

● O24.0 **Pre-existing type 1** diabetes mellitus, in pregnancy, childbirth and the puerperium

Juvenile onset diabetes mellitus, in pregnancy, childbirth and the puerperium
Ketosis-prone diabetes mellitus in pregnancy, childbirth and the puerperium

Use additional code from category E10 to further identify any manifestations

● O24.01 Pre-existing type 1 diabetes mellitus, in **pregnancy**
- O24.011 Pre-existing type 1 diabetes mellitus, in pregnancy, **first trimester** ♀ M
- O24.012 Pre-existing type 1 diabetes mellitus, in pregnancy, **second trimester** ♀ M
- O24.013 Pre-existing type 1 diabetes mellitus, in pregnancy, **third trimester** ♀ M
- O24.019 Pre-existing type 1 diabetes mellitus, in pregnancy, **unspecified trimester** ♀ M

O24.02 Pre-existing type 1 diabetes mellitus, in **childbirth** ♀ M

O24.03 Pre-existing type 1 diabetes mellitus, in the **puerperium** ♀ M

● O24.1 **Pre-existing type 2** diabetes mellitus, in pregnancy, childbirth and the puerperium

Insulin-resistant diabetes mellitus in pregnancy, childbirth and the puerperium

Use additional code (for):
- from category E11 to further identify any manifestations
- long-term (current) use of insulin (Z79.4)

● O24.11 Pre-existing type 2 diabetes mellitus, in **pregnancy**
- O24.111 Pre-existing type 2 diabetes mellitus, in pregnancy, **first trimester** ♀ M
- O24.112 Pre-existing type 2 diabetes mellitus, in pregnancy, **second trimester** ♀ M
- O24.113 Pre-existing type 2 diabetes mellitus, in pregnancy, **third trimester** ♀ M
- O24.119 Pre-existing type 2 diabetes mellitus, in pregnancy, **unspecified trimester** ♀ M

O24.12 Pre-existing type 2 diabetes mellitus, in **childbirth** ♀ M

O24.13 Pre-existing type 2 diabetes mellitus, in the **puerperium** ♀ M

CHAPTER 15 (O00-O9A)

● O24.3 **Unspecified pre-existing diabetes mellitus in pregnancy, childbirth and the puerperium**
Use additional code (for):
from category E11 to further identify any manifestation
long-term (current) use of insulin (Z79.4)

● O24.31 **Unspecified pre-existing diabetes mellitus in pregnancy**

O24.311 **Unspecified pre-existing diabetes mellitus in pregnancy, first trimester** ♀ M

O24.312 **Unspecified pre-existing diabetes mellitus in pregnancy, second trimester** ♀ M

O24.313 **Unspecified pre-existing diabetes mellitus in pregnancy, third trimester** ♀ M

O24.319 **Unspecified pre-existing diabetes mellitus in pregnancy, unspecified trimester** ♀ M

O24.32 **Unspecified pre-existing diabetes mellitus in childbirth** ♀ M

O24.33 **Unspecified pre-existing diabetes mellitus in the puerperium** ♀ M

● O24.4 **Gestational diabetes mellitus**
Diabetes mellitus arising in pregnancy
Gestational diabetes mellitus NOS
Coding Clinic: 2016, Q4, P50, 126

● O24.41 **Gestational diabetes mellitus in pregnancy**

O24.410 **Gestational diabetes mellitus in pregnancy, diet controlled** ♀ M

O24.414 **Gestational diabetes mellitus in pregnancy, insulin controlled** ♀ M

O24.415 **Gestational diabetes mellitus in pregnancy, controlled by oral hypoglycemic drugs** ♀ M
Gestational diabetes mellitus in pregnancy, controlled by oral antidiabetic drugs
Coding Clinic: 2016, Q4, P50

O24.419 **Gestational diabetes mellitus in pregnancy, unspecified control** ♀ M
Coding Clinic: 2015, Q4, P34

OGCR Section I.C.15.i.

Gestational (pregnancy induced) diabetes

Gestational (pregnancy induced) diabetes can occur during the second and third trimester of pregnancy in women who were not diabetic prior to pregnancy. Gestational diabetes can cause complications in the pregnancy similar to those of pre-existing diabetes mellitus. It also puts the woman at greater risk of developing diabetes after the pregnancy. Codes for gestational diabetes are in subcategory O24.4, Gestational diabetes mellitus. No other code from category O24, Diabetes mellitus in pregnancy, childbirth, and the puerperium, should be used with a code from O24.4

The codes under subcategory O24.4 include diet controlled, insulin controlled, **and controlled by oral hypoglycemic drugs.** If a patient with gestational diabetes is treated with both diet and insulin, only the code for insulin-controlled is required. **If a patient with gestational diabetes is treated with both diet and oral hypoglycemic medications, only the code for "controlled by oral hypoglycemic drugs" is required.** Code Z79.4, Long-term (current) use of insulin **or code Z79.84, Long-term (current) use of oral hypoglycemic drugs,** should not be assigned with codes from subcategory O24.4.

An abnormal glucose tolerance in pregnancy is assigned a code from subcategory O99.81, Abnormal glucose complicating pregnancy, childbirth, and the puerperium.

● O24.42 **Gestational diabetes mellitus in childbirth**

O24.420 **Gestational diabetes mellitus in childbirth, diet controlled** ♀ M

O24.424 **Gestational diabetes mellitus in childbirth, insulin controlled** ♀ M

O24.425 **Gestational diabetes mellitus in childbirth, controlled by oral hypoglycemic drugs** ♀ M
Gestational diabetes mellitus in childbirth, controlled by oral antidiabetic drugs
Coding Clinic: 2016, Q4, P50

O24.429 **Gestational diabetes mellitus in childbirth, unspecified control** ♀ M

● O24.43 **Gestational diabetes mellitus in the puerperium**

O24.430 **Gestational diabetes mellitus in the puerperium, diet controlled** ♀ M

O24.434 **Gestational diabetes mellitus in the puerperium, insulin controlled** ♀ M

O24.435 **Gestational diabetes mellitus in puerperium, controlled by oral hypoglycemic drugs** ♀ M
Gestational diabetes mellitus in puerperium, controlled by oral antidiabetic drugs
Coding Clinic: 2016, Q4, P50

O24.439 **Gestational diabetes mellitus in the puerperium, unspecified control** ♀ M

● O24.8 **Other pre-existing diabetes mellitus in pregnancy, childbirth, and the puerperium**
Use additional code (for):
from categories E08, E09 and E13 to further identify any manifestation
long-term (current) use of insulin (Z79.4)

● O24.81 **Other pre-existing diabetes mellitus in pregnancy**

O24.811 **Other pre-existing diabetes mellitus in pregnancy, first trimester** ♀ M

O24.812 **Other pre-existing diabetes mellitus in pregnancy, second trimester** ♀ M

O24.813 **Other pre-existing diabetes mellitus in pregnancy, third trimester** ♀ M

O24.819 **Other pre-existing diabetes mellitus in pregnancy, unspecified trimester** ♀ M

O24.82 **Other pre-existing diabetes mellitus in childbirth** ♀ M

O24.83 **Other pre-existing diabetes mellitus in the puerperium** ♀ M

● O24.9 **Unspecified diabetes mellitus in pregnancy, childbirth and the puerperium**
Use additional code for long-term (current) use of insulin (Z79.4)
Unknown whether patient was diabetic before pregnancy occurred

● O24.91 **Unspecified diabetes mellitus in pregnancy**

O24.911 **Unspecified diabetes mellitus in pregnancy, first trimester** ♀ M

O24.912 **Unspecified diabetes mellitus in pregnancy, second trimester** ♀ M

O24.913 **Unspecified diabetes mellitus in pregnancy, third trimester** ♀ M

O24.919 **Unspecified diabetes mellitus in pregnancy, unspecified trimester** ♀ M

O24.92 **Unspecified diabetes mellitus in childbirth** ♀ M

O24.93 **Unspecified diabetes mellitus in the puerperium** ♀ M

● **O25 Malnutrition in pregnancy, childbirth and the puerperium**

● **O25.1 Malnutrition in pregnancy**

O25.10 Malnutrition in pregnancy, unspecified trimester ♀ M

O25.11 Malnutrition in pregnancy, first trimester ♀ M

O25.12 Malnutrition in pregnancy, second trimester ♀ M

O25.13 Malnutrition in pregnancy, third trimester ♀ M

O25.2 Malnutrition in childbirth ♀ M

O25.3 Malnutrition in the puerperium ♀ M

● **O26 Maternal care for other conditions predominantly related to pregnancy**

● **O26.0 Excessive weight gain in pregnancy**

Excludes2 gestational edema (O12.0, O12.2)

O26.00 Excessive weight gain in pregnancy, unspecified trimester ♀ M

O26.01 Excessive weight gain in pregnancy, first trimester ♀ M

O26.02 Excessive weight gain in pregnancy, second trimester ♀ M

O26.03 Excessive weight gain in pregnancy, third trimester ♀ M

● **O26.1 Low weight gain in pregnancy**

O26.10 Low weight gain in pregnancy, unspecified trimester ♀ M

O26.11 Low weight gain in pregnancy, first trimester ♀ M

O26.12 Low weight gain in pregnancy, second trimester ♀ M

O26.13 Low weight gain in pregnancy, third trimester ♀ M

● **O26.2 Pregnancy care for patient with recurrent pregnancy loss**

O26.20 Pregnancy care for patient with recurrent pregnancy loss, unspecified trimester ♀ M

O26.21 Pregnancy care for patient with recurrent pregnancy loss, first trimester ♀ M

O26.22 Pregnancy care for patient with recurrent pregnancy loss, second trimester ♀ M

O26.23 Pregnancy care for patient with recurrent pregnancy loss, third trimester ♀ M

● **O26.3 Retained intrauterine contraceptive device in pregnancy**

O26.30 Retained intrauterine contraceptive device in pregnancy, unspecified trimester ♀ M

O26.31 Retained intrauterine contraceptive device in pregnancy, first trimester ♀ M

O26.32 Retained intrauterine contraceptive device in pregnancy, second trimester ♀ M

O26.33 Retained intrauterine contraceptive device in pregnancy, third trimester ♀ M

● **O26.4 Herpes gestationis**

O26.40 Herpes gestationis, unspecified trimester ♀ M

O26.41 Herpes gestationis, first trimester ♀ M

O26.42 Herpes gestationis, second trimester ♀ M

O26.43 Herpes gestationis, third trimester ♀ M

● **O26.5 Maternal hypotension syndrome**

Supine hypotensive syndrome

O26.50 Maternal hypotension syndrome, unspecified trimester ♀ M

O26.51 Maternal hypotension syndrome, first trimester ♀ M

O26.52 Maternal hypotension syndrome, second trimester ♀ M

O26.53 Maternal hypotension syndrome, third trimester ♀ M

● **O26.6 Liver and biliary tract disorders in pregnancy, childbirth and the puerperium**

Use additional code to identify the specific disorder

Excludes2 hepatorenal syndrome following labor and delivery (O90.4)

● **O26.61 Liver and biliary tract disorders in pregnancy**

O26.611 Liver and biliary tract disorders in pregnancy, first trimester ♀ M

O26.612 Liver and biliary tract disorders in pregnancy, second trimester ♀ M

O26.613 Liver and biliary tract disorders in pregnancy, third trimester ♀ M

O26.619 Liver and biliary tract disorders in pregnancy, unspecified trimester ♀ M

O26.62 Liver and biliary tract disorders in childbirth ♀ M

O26.63 Liver and biliary tract disorders in the puerperium ♀ M

● **O26.7 Subluxation of symphysis (pubis) in pregnancy, childbirth and the puerperium**

Excludes1 traumatic separation of symphysis (pubis) during childbirth (O71.6)

● **O26.71 Subluxation of symphysis (pubis) in pregnancy**

O26.711 Subluxation of symphysis (pubis) in pregnancy, first trimester ♀ M

O26.712 Subluxation of symphysis (pubis) in pregnancy, second trimester ♀ M

O26.713 Subluxation of symphysis (pubis) in pregnancy, third trimester ♀ M

O26.719 Subluxation of symphysis (pubis) in pregnancy, unspecified trimester ♀ M

O26.72 Subluxation of symphysis (pubis) in childbirth ♀ M

O26.73 Subluxation of symphysis (pubis) in the puerperium ♀ M

● **O26.8 Other specified pregnancy related conditions**

● **O26.81 Pregnancy related exhaustion and fatigue**

O26.811 Pregnancy related exhaustion and fatigue, first trimester ♀ M

O26.812 Pregnancy related exhaustion and fatigue, second trimester ♀ M

O26.813 Pregnancy related exhaustion and fatigue, third trimester ♀ M

O26.819 Pregnancy related exhaustion and fatigue, unspecified trimester ♀ M

● **O26.82 Pregnancy related peripheral neuritis**

O26.821 Pregnancy related peripheral neuritis, first trimester ♀ M

O26.822 Pregnancy related peripheral neuritis, second trimester ♀ M

O26.823 Pregnancy related peripheral neuritis, third trimester ♀ M

O26.829 Pregnancy related peripheral neuritis, unspecified trimester ♀ M

● **O26.83 Pregnancy related renal disease**

Use additional code to identify the specific disorder

O26.831 Pregnancy related renal disease, first trimester ♀ M

O26.832 Pregnancy related renal disease, second trimester ♀ M

O26.833 Pregnancy related renal disease, third trimester ♀ M

O26.839 Pregnancy related renal disease, unspecified trimester ♀ M

CHAPTER 15 (O00-O9A)

● O26.84 Uterine size-date discrepancy complicating pregnancy
Excludes1 encounter for suspected problem with fetal growth ruled out (Z03.74)
O26.841 Uterine size-date discrepancy, first trimester ♀ M
O26.842 Uterine size-date discrepancy, second trimester ♀ M
O26.843 Uterine size-date discrepancy, third trimester ♀ M
O26.849 Uterine size-date discrepancy, unspecified trimester ♀ M

● O26.85 Spotting complicating pregnancy
O26.851 Spotting complicating pregnancy, first trimester ♀ M
O26.852 Spotting complicating pregnancy, second trimester ♀ M
O26.853 Spotting complicating pregnancy, third trimester ♀ M
O26.859 Spotting complicating pregnancy, unspecified trimester ♀ M

O26.86 Pruritic urticarial papules and plaques of pregnancy (PUPPP) ♀ M
Polymorphic eruption of pregnancy

● O26.87 Cervical shortening
Excludes1 encounter for suspected cervical shortening ruled out (Z03.75)
O26.872 Cervical shortening, second trimester ♀ M
O26.873 Cervical shortening, third trimester ♀ M
O26.879 Cervical shortening, unspecified trimester ♀ M

● O26.89 Other specified pregnancy related conditions
O26.891 Other specified pregnancy related conditions, first trimester ♀ M
O26.892 Other specified pregnancy related conditions, second trimester ♀ M
O26.893 Other specified pregnancy related conditions, third trimester ♀ M
Coding Clinic: 2015, Q3, P40
O26.899 Other specified pregnancy related conditions, unspecified trimester ♀ M

● O26.9 Pregnancy related conditions, unspecified
O26.90 Pregnancy related conditions, unspecified, unspecified trimester ♀ M
O26.91 Pregnancy related conditions, unspecified, first trimester ♀ M
O26.92 Pregnancy related conditions, unspecified, second trimester ♀ M
O26.93 Pregnancy related conditions, unspecified, third trimester ♀ M

● O28 Abnormal findings on antenatal screening of mother
Excludes1 diagnostic findings classified elsewhere - see Alphabetical Index
O28.0 Abnormal hematological finding on antenatal screening of mother ♀ M
O28.1 Abnormal biochemical finding on antenatal screening of mother ♀ M
O28.2 Abnormal cytological finding on antenatal screening of mother ♀ M
O28.3 Abnormal ultrasonic finding on antenatal screening of mother ♀ M
Coding Clinic: 2016, Q4, P5
O28.4 Abnormal radiological finding on antenatal screening of mother ♀ M
O28.5 Abnormal chromosomal and genetic finding on antenatal screening of mother ♀ M
O28.8 Other abnormal findings on antenatal screening of mother ♀ M
O28.9 Unspecified abnormal findings on antenatal screening of mother ♀ M

● O29 Complications of anesthesia during pregnancy
Includes maternal complications arising from the administration of a general, regional or local anesthetic, analgesic or other sedation during pregnancy
Use additional code, if necessary, to identify the complication
Excludes2 complications of anesthesia during labor and delivery (O74.-)
complications of anesthesia during the puerperium (O89.-)

● O29.0 Pulmonary complications of anesthesia during pregnancy

● O29.01 Aspiration pneumonitis due to anesthesia during pregnancy
Inhalation of stomach contents or secretions NOS due to anesthesia during pregnancy
Mendelson's syndrome due to anesthesia during pregnancy
O29.011 Aspiration pneumonitis due to anesthesia during pregnancy, first trimester ♀ M
O29.012 Aspiration pneumonitis due to anesthesia during pregnancy, second trimester ♀ M
O29.013 Aspiration pneumonitis due to anesthesia during pregnancy, third trimester ♀ M
O29.019 Aspiration pneumonitis due to anesthesia during pregnancy, unspecified trimester ♀ M

● O29.02 Pressure collapse of lung due to anesthesia during pregnancy
O29.021 Pressure collapse of lung due to anesthesia during pregnancy, first trimester ♀ M
O29.022 Pressure collapse of lung due to anesthesia during pregnancy, second trimester ♀ M
O29.023 Pressure collapse of lung due to anesthesia during pregnancy, third trimester ♀ M
O29.029 Pressure collapse of lung due to anesthesia during pregnancy, unspecified trimester ♀ M

● O29.09 Other pulmonary complications of anesthesia during pregnancy
O29.091 Other pulmonary complications of anesthesia during pregnancy, first trimester ♀ M
O29.092 Other pulmonary complications of anesthesia during pregnancy, second trimester ♀ M
O29.093 Other pulmonary complications of anesthesia during pregnancy, third trimester ♀ M
O29.099 Other pulmonary complications of anesthesia during pregnancy, unspecified trimester ♀ M

O29.1 Cardiac complications of anesthesia during pregnancy
O29.11 Cardiac arrest due to anesthesia during pregnancy
O29.111 Cardiac arrest due to anesthesia during pregnancy, first trimester ♀ M
O29.112 Cardiac arrest due to anesthesia during pregnancy, second trimester ♀ M
O29.113 Cardiac arrest due to anesthesia during pregnancy, third trimester ♀ M
O29.119 Cardiac arrest due to anesthesia during pregnancy, unspecified trimester ♀ M
O29.12 Cardiac failure due to anesthesia during pregnancy
O29.121 Cardiac failure due to anesthesia during pregnancy, first trimester ♀ M
O29.122 Cardiac failure due to anesthesia during pregnancy, second trimester ♀ M
O29.123 Cardiac failure due to anesthesia during pregnancy, third trimester ♀ M
O29.129 Cardiac failure due to anesthesia during pregnancy, unspecified trimester ♀ M
O29.19 Other cardiac complications of anesthesia during pregnancy
O29.191 Other cardiac complications of anesthesia during pregnancy, first trimester ♀ M
O29.192 Other cardiac complications of anesthesia during pregnancy, second trimester ♀ M
O29.193 Other cardiac complications of anesthesia during pregnancy, third trimester ♀ M
O29.199 Other cardiac complications of anesthesia during pregnancy, unspecified trimester ♀ M
O29.2 Central nervous system complications of anesthesia during pregnancy
O29.21 Cerebral anoxia due to anesthesia during pregnancy
O29.211 Cerebral anoxia due to anesthesia during pregnancy, first trimester ♀ M
O29.212 Cerebral anoxia due to anesthesia during pregnancy, second trimester ♀ M
O29.213 Cerebral anoxia due to anesthesia during pregnancy, third trimester ♀ M
O29.219 Cerebral anoxia due to anesthesia during pregnancy, unspecified trimester ♀ M
O29.29 Other central nervous system complications of anesthesia during pregnancy
O29.291 Other central nervous system complications of anesthesia during pregnancy, first trimester ♀ M
O29.292 Other central nervous system complications of anesthesia during pregnancy, second trimester ♀ M
O29.293 Other central nervous system complications of anesthesia during pregnancy, third trimester ♀ M
O29.299 Other central nervous system complications of anesthesia during pregnancy, unspecified trimester ♀ M
O29.3 Toxic reaction to local anesthesia during pregnancy
O29.3X Toxic reaction to local anesthesia during pregnancy
O29.3X1 Toxic reaction to local anesthesia during pregnancy, first trimester ♀ M
O29.3X2 Toxic reaction to local anesthesia during pregnancy, second trimester ♀ M
O29.3X3 Toxic reaction to local anesthesia during pregnancy, third trimester ♀ M
O29.3X9 Toxic reaction to local anesthesia during pregnancy, unspecified trimester ♀ M
O29.4 Spinal and epidural anesthesia induced headache during pregnancy
O29.40 Spinal and epidural anesthesia induced headache during pregnancy, unspecified trimester ♀ M
O29.41 Spinal and epidural anesthesia induced headache during pregnancy, first trimester ♀ M
O29.42 Spinal and epidural anesthesia induced headache during pregnancy, second trimester ♀ M
O29.43 Spinal and epidural anesthesia induced headache during pregnancy, third trimester ♀ M
O29.5 Other complications of spinal and epidural anesthesia during pregnancy
O29.5X Other complications of spinal and epidural anesthesia during pregnancy
O29.5X1 Other complications of spinal and epidural anesthesia during pregnancy, first trimester ♀ M
O29.5X2 Other complications of spinal and epidural anesthesia during pregnancy, second trimester ♀ M
O29.5X3 Other complications of spinal and epidural anesthesia during pregnancy, third trimester ♀ M
O29.5X9 Other complications of spinal and epidural anesthesia during pregnancy, unspecified trimester ♀ M
O29.6 Failed or difficult intubation for anesthesia during pregnancy
O29.60 Failed or difficult intubation for anesthesia during pregnancy, unspecified trimester ♀ M
O29.61 Failed or difficult intubation for anesthesia during pregnancy, first trimester ♀ M
O29.62 Failed or difficult intubation for anesthesia during pregnancy, second trimester ♀ M
O29.63 Failed or difficult intubation for anesthesia during pregnancy, third trimester ♀ M
O29.8 Other complications of anesthesia during pregnancy
O29.8X Other complications of anesthesia during pregnancy
O29.8X1 Other complications of anesthesia during pregnancy, first trimester ♀ M
O29.8X2 Other complications of anesthesia during pregnancy, second trimester ♀ M
O29.8X3 Other complications of anesthesia during pregnancy, third trimester ♀ M
O29.8X9 Other complications of anesthesia during pregnancy, unspecified trimester ♀ M

O29.9 **Unspecified** complication of anesthesia during pregnancy
- O29.90 Unspecified complication of anesthesia during pregnancy, **unspecified trimester** ♀ M
- O29.91 Unspecified complication of anesthesia during pregnancy, **first trimester** ♀ M
- O29.92 Unspecified complication of anesthesia during pregnancy, **second trimester** ♀ M
- O29.93 Unspecified complication of anesthesia during pregnancy, **third trimester** ♀ M

MATERNAL CARE RELATED TO THE FETUS AND AMNIOTIC CAVITY AND POSSIBLE DELIVERY PROBLEMS (O30-O48)

O30 Multiple gestation

Code also any complications specific to multiple gestation

Coding Clinic: 2016, Q4, P51

O30.0 Twin pregnancy

O30.00 Twin pregnancy, **unspecified** number of placenta and **unspecified** number of amniotic sacs
- O30.001 Twin pregnancy, unspecified number of placenta and unspecified number of amniotic sacs, **first trimester** ♀ M
- O30.002 Twin pregnancy, unspecified number of placenta and unspecified number of amniotic sacs, **second trimester** ♀ M
- O30.003 Twin pregnancy, unspecified number of placenta and unspecified number of amniotic sacs, **third trimester** ♀ M
- O30.009 Twin pregnancy, unspecified number of placenta and unspecified number of amniotic sacs, **unspecified trimester** ♀ M

O30.01 Twin pregnancy, **monochorionic/monoamniotic**

Twin pregnancy, one placenta, one amniotic sac

Excludes1 conjoined twins (O30.02-)
- O30.011 Twin pregnancy, monochorionic/monoamniotic, **first trimester** ♀ M
- O30.012 Twin pregnancy, monochorionic/monoamniotic, **second trimester** ♀ M
- O30.013 Twin pregnancy, monochorionic/monoamniotic, **third trimester** ♀ M
- O30.019 Twin pregnancy, monochorionic/monoamniotic, **unspecified trimester** ♀ M

O30.02 **Conjoined** twin pregnancy
- O30.021 Conjoined twin pregnancy, **first trimester** ♀ M
- O30.022 Conjoined twin pregnancy, **second trimester** ♀ M
- O30.023 Conjoined twin pregnancy, **third trimester** ♀ M
- O30.029 Conjoined twin pregnancy, **unspecified trimester** ♀ M

O30.03 Twin pregnancy, **monochorionic/diamniotic**

Twin pregnancy, one placenta, two amniotic sacs
- O30.031 Twin pregnancy, monochorionic/diamniotic, **first trimester** ♀ M
- O30.032 Twin pregnancy, monochorionic/diamniotic, **second trimester** ♀ M
- O30.033 Twin pregnancy, monochorionic/diamniotic, **third trimester** ♀ M
- O30.039 Twin pregnancy, monochorionic/diamniotic, **unspecified trimester** ♀ M

O30.04 Twin pregnancy, **dichorionic/diamniotic**

Twin pregnancy, two placentae, two amniotic sacs
- O30.041 Twin pregnancy, dichorionic/diamniotic, **first trimester** ♀ M
- O30.042 Twin pregnancy, dichorionic/diamniotic, **second trimester** ♀ M
- O30.043 Twin pregnancy, dichorionic/diamniotic, **third trimester** ♀ M
- O30.049 Twin pregnancy, dichorionic/diamniotic, **unspecified trimester** ♀ M

O30.09 Twin pregnancy, **unable to determine** number of placenta and number of amniotic sacs
- O30.091 Twin pregnancy, unable to determine number of placenta and number of amniotic sacs, **first trimester** ♀ M
- O30.092 Twin pregnancy, unable to determine number of placenta and number of amniotic sacs, **second trimester** ♀ M
- O30.093 Twin pregnancy, unable to determine number of placenta and number of amniotic sacs, **third trimester** ♀ M
- O30.099 Twin pregnancy, unable to determine number of placenta and number of amniotic sacs, **unspecified trimester** ♀ M

O30.1 **Triplet** pregnancy

O30.10 Triplet pregnancy, **unspecified** number of placenta and **unspecified** number of amniotic sacs
- O30.101 Triplet pregnancy, unspecified number of placenta and unspecified number of amniotic sacs, **first trimester** ♀ M
- O30.102 Triplet pregnancy, unspecified number of placenta and unspecified number of amniotic sacs, **second trimester** ♀ M
- O30.103 Triplet pregnancy, unspecified number of placenta and unspecified number of amniotic sacs, **third trimester** ♀ M
  Coding Clinic: 2016, Q2, P8
- O30.109 Triplet pregnancy, unspecified number of placenta and unspecified number of amniotic sacs, **unspecified trimester** ♀ M

O30.11 Triplet pregnancy with **two or more monochorionic fetuses**
- O30.111 Triplet pregnancy with two or more monochorionic fetuses, **first trimester** ♀ M
- O30.112 Triplet pregnancy with two or more monochorionic fetuses, **second trimester** ♀ M
- O30.113 Triplet pregnancy with two or more monochorionic fetuses, **third trimester** ♀ M
- O30.119 Triplet pregnancy with two or more monochorionic fetuses, **unspecified trimester** ♀ M

O30.12 Triplet pregnancy with **two or more monoamniotic fetuses**
- O30.121 Triplet pregnancy with two or more monoamniotic fetuses, **first trimester** ♀ M
- O30.122 Triplet pregnancy with two or more monoamniotic fetuses, **second trimester** ♀ M
- O30.123 Triplet pregnancy with two or more monoamniotic fetuses, **third trimester** ♀ M
- O30.129 Triplet pregnancy with two or more monoamniotic fetuses, **unspecified trimester** ♀ M

● O30.13 Triplet pregnancy, trichorionic/triamniotic
- O30.131 Triplet pregnancy, trichorionic/triamniotic, first trimester ♀ M
- O30.132 Triplet pregnancy, trichorionic/triamniotic, second trimester ♀ M
- O30.133 Triplet pregnancy, trichorionic/triamniotic, third trimester ♀ M
- O30.139 Triplet pregnancy, trichorionic/triamniotic, unspecified trimester ♀ M

● O30.19 Triplet pregnancy, **unable to determine** number of placenta and number of amniotic sacs
- O30.191 Triplet pregnancy, unable to determine number of placenta and number of amniotic sacs, **first trimester** ♀ M
- O30.192 Triplet pregnancy, unable to determine number of placenta and number of amniotic sacs, **second trimester** ♀ M
- O30.193 Triplet pregnancy, unable to determine number of placenta and number of amniotic sacs, **third trimester** ♀ M
- O30.199 Triplet pregnancy, unable to determine number of placenta and number of amniotic sacs, **unspecified trimester** ♀ M

● O30.2 Quadruplet pregnancy

● O30.20 Quadruplet pregnancy, **unspecified** number of placenta and **unspecified** number of amniotic sacs
- O30.201 Quadruplet pregnancy, unspecified number of placenta and unspecified number of amniotic sacs, **first trimester** ♀ M
- O30.202 Quadruplet pregnancy, unspecified number of placenta and unspecified number of amniotic sacs, **second trimester** ♀ M
- O30.203 Quadruplet pregnancy, unspecified number of placenta and unspecified number of amniotic sacs, **third trimester** ♀ M
- O30.209 Quadruplet pregnancy, unspecified number of placenta and unspecified number of amniotic sacs, **unspecified trimester** ♀ M

● O30.21 Quadruplet pregnancy with two or more monochorionic fetuses
- O30.211 Quadruplet pregnancy with two or more monochorionic fetuses, first trimester ♀ M
- O30.212 Quadruplet pregnancy with two or more monochorionic fetuses, second trimester ♀ M
- O30.213 Quadruplet pregnancy with two or more monochorionic fetuses, third trimester ♀ M
- O30.219 Quadruplet pregnancy with two or more monochorionic fetuses, unspecified trimester ♀ M

● O30.22 Quadruplet pregnancy with two or more monoamniotic fetuses
- O30.221 Quadruplet pregnancy with two or more monoamniotic fetuses, first trimester ♀ M
- O30.222 Quadruplet pregnancy with two or more monoamniotic fetuses, second trimester ♀ M
- O30.223 Quadruplet pregnancy with two or more monoamniotic fetuses, third trimester ♀ M
- O30.229 Quadruplet pregnancy with two or more monoamniotic fetuses, unspecified trimester ♀ M

● O30.23 Quadruplet pregnancy, quadrachorionic/quadra-amniotic
- O30.231 Quadruplet pregnancy, quadrachorionic/quadra-amniotic, first trimester ♀ M
- O30.232 Quadruplet pregnancy, quadrachorionic/quadra-amniotic, second trimester ♀ M
- O30.233 Quadruplet pregnancy, quadrachorionic/quadra-amniotic, third trimester ♀ M
- O30.239 Quadruplet pregnancy, quadrachorionic/quadra-amniotic, unspecifiedtrimester ♀ M

● O30.29 Quadruplet pregnancy, **unable to determine** number of placenta and number of amniotic sacs
- O30.291 Quadruplet pregnancy, unable to determine number of placenta and number of amniotic sacs, **first trimester** ♀ M
- O30.292 Quadruplet pregnancy, unable to determine number of placenta and number of amniotic sacs, **second trimester** ♀ M
- O30.293 Quadruplet pregnancy, unable to determine number of placenta and number of amniotic sacs, **third trimester** ♀ M
- O30.299 Quadruplet pregnancy, unable to determine number of placenta and number of amniotic sacs, **unspecified trimester** ♀ M

● O30.8 Other specified multiple gestation

Multiple gestation pregnancy greater then quadruplets

● O30.80 Other specified multiple gestation, **unspecified** number of placenta and **unspecified** number of amniotic sacs
- O30.801 Other specified multiple gestation, unspecified number of placenta and unspecified number of amniotic sacs, **first trimester** ♀ M
- O30.802 Other specified multiple gestation, unspecified number of placenta and unspecified number of amniotic sacs, **second trimester** ♀ M
- O30.803 Other specified multiple gestation, unspecified number of placenta and unspecified number of amniotic sacs, **third trimester** ♀ M
- O30.809 Other specified multiple gestation, unspecified number of placenta and unspecified number of amniotic sacs, **unspecified trimester** ♀ M

● O30.81 Other specified multiple gestation with **two or more monochorionic fetuses**
- O30.811 Other specified multiple gestation with two or more monochorionic fetuses, **first trimester** ♀ M
- O30.812 Other specified multiple gestation with two or more monochorionic fetuses, **second trimester** ♀ M
- O30.813 Other specified multiple gestation with two or more monochorionic fetuses, **third trimester** ♀ M
- O30.819 Other specified multiple gestation with two or more monochorionic fetuses, **unspecified trimester** ♀ M

● **O30.82 Other specified multiple gestation with two or more monoamniotic fetuses**

O30.821 **Other specified multiple gestation with two or more monoamniotic fetuses, first trimester** ♀ M

O30.822 **Other specified multiple gestation with two or more monoamniotic fetuses, second trimester** ♀ M

O30.823 **Other specified multiple gestation with two or more monoamniotic fetuses, third trimester** ♀ M

O30.829 **Other specified multiple gestation with two or more monoamniotic fetuses, unspecified trimester** ♀ M

● **O30.83 Other specified multiple gestation, number of chorions and amnions are both equalto the number of fetuses**

Pentachorionic, penta-amniotic pregnancy (quintuplets)
Hexachorionic, hexa-amniotic pregnancy (sextuplets)
Heptachorionic, hepta-amniotic pregnancy (septuplets)

O30.831 Other specified multiple gestation, number of chorions and amnions are both equal to the number of fetuses, first trimester ♀ M

O30.832 Other specified multiple gestation, number of chorions and amnions are both equal to the number of fetuses, second trimester ♀ M

O30.833 Other specified multiple gestation, number of chorions and amnions are both equal to the number of fetuses, third trimester ♀ M

O30.839 Other specified multiple gestation, number of chorions and amnions are both equal to the number of fetuses, unspecified trimester ♀ M

● **O30.89 Other specified multiple gestation, unable to determine number of placenta and number of amniotic sacs**

O30.891 Other specified multiple gestation, unable to determine number of placenta and number of amniotic sacs, first trimester ♀ M

O30.892 Other specified multiple gestation, unable to determine number of placenta and number of amniotic sacs, second trimester ♀ M

O30.893 Other specified multiple gestation, unable to determine number of placenta and number of amniotic sacs, third trimester ♀ M

O30.899 Other specified multiple gestation, unable to determine number of placenta and number of amniotic sacs, unspecified trimester ♀ M

● **O30.9 Multiple gestation, unspecified**

Multiple pregnancy NOS

O30.90 Multiple gestation, unspecified, unspecified trimester ♀ M

O30.91 Multiple gestation, unspecified, first trimester ♀ M

O30.92 Multiple gestation, unspecified, second trimester ♀ M

O30.93 Multiple gestation, unspecified, third trimester ♀ M

● **O31 Complications specific to multiple gestation**

Excludes2 delayed delivery of second twin, triplet, etc. (O63.2)
malpresentation of one fetus or more (O32.9)
placental transfusion syndromes (O43.0-)

Coding Clinic: 2012, Q4, P107

One of the following 7th characters is to be assigned to each code under category O31. 7th character 0 is for single gestations and multiple gestations where the fetus is unspecified. 7th characters 1 through 9 are for cases of multiple gestations to identify the fetus for which the code applies. The appropriate code from category O30, Multiple gestation, must also be assigned when assigning a code from category O31 that has a 7th character of 1 through 9.

0	not applicable or unspecified
1	fetus 1
2	fetus 2
3	fetus 3
4	fetus 4
5	fetus 5
9	other fetus

● **O31.0 Papyraceous fetus**

Fetus compressus

X● O31.00 Papyraceous fetus, unspecified trimester ♀ M

X● O31.01 Papyraceous fetus, first trimester ♀ M

X● O31.02 Papyraceous fetus, second trimester ♀ M

X● O31.03 Papyraceous fetus, third trimester ♀ M

● **O31.1 Continuing pregnancy after spontaneous abortion of one fetus or more**

X● O31.10 Continuing pregnancy after spontaneous abortion of one fetus or more, unspecified trimester ♀ M

X● O31.11 Continuing pregnancy after spontaneous abortion of one fetus or more, first trimester ♀ M

X● O31.12 Continuing pregnancy after spontaneous abortion of one fetus or more, second trimester ♀ M

X● O31.13 Continuing pregnancy after spontaneous abortion of one fetus or more, third trimester ♀ M

● **O31.2 Continuing pregnancy after intrauterine death of one fetus or more**

X● O31.20 Continuing pregnancy after intrauterine death of one fetus or more, unspecified trimester ♀ M

X● O31.21 Continuing pregnancy after intrauterine death of one fetus or more, first trimester ♀ M

X● O31.22 Continuing pregnancy after intrauterine death of one fetus or more, second trimester ♀ M

X● O31.23 Continuing pregnancy after intrauterine death of one fetus or more, third trimester ♀ M

● **O31.3 Continuing pregnancy after elective fetal reduction of one fetus or more**

Continuing pregnancy after selective termination of one fetus or more

X● O31.30 Continuing pregnancy after elective fetal reduction of one fetus or more, unspecified trimester ♀ M

X● O31.31 Continuing pregnancy after elective fetal reduction of one fetus or more, first trimester ♀ M

X● O31.32 Continuing pregnancy after elective fetal reduction of one fetus or more, second trimester ♀ M

X● O31.33 Continuing pregnancy after elective fetal reduction of one fetus or more, third trimester ♀ M

● O31.8 **Other complications specific to multiple gestation**

● O31.8X **Other complications specific to multiple gestation**

● O31.8X1 **Other complications specific to multiple gestation, first trimester** ♀ M

● O31.8X2 **Other complications specific to multiple gestation, second trimester** ♀ M

● O31.8X3 **Other complications specific to multiple gestation, third trimester** ♀ M

● O31.8X9 **Other complications specific to multiple gestation, unspecified trimester** ♀ M

● O32 **Maternal care for malpresentation of fetus**

Includes the listed conditions as a reason for observation, hospitalization or other obstetric care of the mother, or for cesarean delivery before onset of labor

Excludes1 malpresentation of fetus with obstructed labor (O64.-)

Coding Clinic: 2012, Q4, P107

One of the following 7th characters is to be assigned to each code under category O32. 7th character Ø is for single gestations and multiple gestations where the fetus is unspecified. 7th characters 1 through 9 are for cases of multiple gestations to identify the fetus for which the code applies. The appropriate code from category O3Ø, Multiple gestation, must also be assigned when assigning a code from category O32 that has a 7th character of 1 through 9.

Ø	not applicable or unspecified
1	fetus 1
2	fetus 2
3	fetus 3
4	fetus 4
5	fetus 5
9	other fetus

X● O32.Ø **Maternal care for unstable lie** ♀ M

X● O32.1 **Maternal care for breech presentation** ♀ M
Maternal care for buttocks presentation
Maternal care for complete breech
Maternal care for frank breech

Excludes1 footling presentation (O32.8)
incomplete breech (O32.8)

X● O32.2 **Maternal care for transverse and oblique lie** ♀ M
Maternal care for oblique presentation
Maternal care for transverse presentation

X● O32.3 **Maternal care for face, brow and chin presentation** ♀ M

X● O32.4 **Maternal care for high head at term** ♀ M
Maternal care for failure of head to enter pelvic brim

X● O32.6 **Maternal care for compound presentation** ♀ M

X● O32.8 **Maternal care for other malpresentation of fetus** ♀ M
Maternal care for footling presentation
Maternal care for incomplete breech

X● O32.9 **Maternal care for malpresentation of fetus, unspecified** ♀ M

● O33 **Maternal care for disproportion**

Includes the listed conditions as a reason for observation, hospitalization or other obstetric care of the mother, or for cesarean delivery before onset of labor

Excludes1 disproportion with obstructed labor (O65-O66)

O33.Ø **Maternal care for disproportion due to deformity of maternal pelvic bones** ♀ M
Maternal care for disproportion due to pelvic deformity causing disproportion NOS

O33.1 **Maternal care for disproportion due to generally contracted pelvis** ♀ M
Maternal care for disproportion due to contracted pelvis NOS causing disproportion

O33.2 **Maternal care for disproportion due to inlet contraction of pelvis** ♀ M
Maternal care for disproportion due to inlet contraction (pelvis) causing disproportion

X● O33.3 **Maternal care for disproportion due to outlet contraction of pelvis** ♀ M
Maternal care for disproportion due to mid-cavity contraction (pelvis)
Maternal care for disproportion due to outlet contraction (pelvis)

One of the following 7th characters is to be assigned to code O33.3. 7th character Ø is for single gestations and multiple gestations where the fetus is unspecified. 7th characters 1 through 9 are for cases of multiple gestations to identify the fetus for which the code applies. The appropriate code from category O3Ø, Multiple gestation, must also be assigned when assigning code O33.3 with a 7th character of 1 through 9.

Ø	not applicable or unspecified
1	fetus 1
2	fetus 2
3	fetus 3
4	fetus 4
5	fetus 5
9	other fetus

X● O33.4 **Maternal care for disproportion of mixed maternal and fetal origin** ♀ M

One of the following 7th characters is to be assigned to code O33.4. 7th character Ø is for single gestations and multiple gestations where the fetus is unspecified. 7th characters 1 through 9 are for cases of multiple gestations to identify the fetus for which the code applies. The appropriate code from category O3Ø, Multiple gestation, must also be assigned when assigning code O33.4 with a 7th character of 1 through 9.

Ø	not applicable or unspecified
1	fetus 1
2	fetus 2
3	fetus 3
4	fetus 4
5	fetus 5
9	other fetus

X● O33.5 **Maternal care for disproportion due to unusually large fetus** ♀ M
Maternal care for disproportion due to disproportion of fetal origin with normally formed fetus
Maternal care for disproportion due to fetal disproportion NOS

One of the following 7th characters is to be assigned to code O33.5. 7th character Ø is for single gestations and multiple gestations where the fetus is unspecified. 7th characters 1 through 9 are for cases of multiple gestations to identify the fetus for which the code applies. The appropriate code from category O3Ø, Multiple gestation, must also be assigned when assigning code O33.5 with a 7th character of 1 through 9.

Ø	not applicable or unspecified
1	fetus 1
2	fetus 2
3	fetus 3
4	fetus 4
5	fetus 5
9	other fetus

X● O33.6 **Maternal care for disproportion due to hydrocephalic fetus ♀** M

One of the following 7th characters is to be assigned to code O33.6. 7th character Ø is for single gestations and multiple gestations where the fetus is unspecified. 7th characters 1 through 9 are for cases of multiple gestations to identify the fetus for which the code applies. The appropriate code from category O3Ø, Multiple gestation, must also be assigned when assigning code O33.6 with a 7th character of 1 through 9.

Ø	not applicable or unspecified
1	fetus 1
2	fetus 2
3	fetus 3
4	fetus 4
5	fetus 5
9	other fetus

X● O33.7 **Maternal care for disproportion due to other fetal deformities ♀** M

Maternal care for disproportion due to fetal ascites
Maternal care for disproportion due to fetal hydrops
Maternal care for disproportion due to fetal meningomyelocele
Maternal care for disproportion due to fetal sacral teratoma
Maternal care for disproportion due to fetal tumor

Excludes1 obstructed labor due to other fetal deformities (O66.3)

Coding Clinic: 2Ø16, Q4, P51

One of the following 7th characters is to be assigned to code O33.7. 7th character Ø is for single gestations and multiple gestations where the fetus is unspecified. 7th characters 1 through 9 are for cases of multiple gestations to identify the fetus for which the code applies. The appropriate code from category O3Ø, Multiple gestation, must also be assigned when assigning code O33.7 with a 7th character of 1 through 9.

Ø	not applicable or unspecified
1	fetus 1
2	fetus 2
3	fetus 3
4	fetus 4
5	fetus 5
9	other fetus

O33.8 **Maternal care for disproportion of other origin ♀** M

O33.9 **Maternal care for disproportion, unspecified ♀** M

Maternal care for disproportion due to cephalopelvic disproportion NOS
Maternal care for disproportion due to fetopelvic disproportion NOS

● O34 **Maternal care for abnormality of pelvic organs**

Includes the listed conditions as a reason for hospitalization or other obstetric care of the mother, or for cesarean delivery before onset of labor

Code first any associated obstructed labor (O65.5)

Use additional code for specific condition

● O34.Ø **Maternal care for congenital malformation of uterus**

Maternal care for double uterus
Maternal care for uterus bicornis

O34.ØØ **Maternal care for unspecified congenital malformation of uterus, unspecified trimester ♀** M

O34.Ø1 **Maternal care for unspecified congenital malformation of uterus, first trimester ♀** M

O34.Ø2 **Maternal care for unspecified congenital malformation of uterus, second trimester ♀** M

O34.Ø3 **Maternal care for unspecified congenital malformation of uterus, third trimester ♀** M

● O34.1 **Maternal care for benign tumor of corpus uteri**

Excludes2 maternal care for benign tumor of cervix (O34.4-)
maternal care for malignant neoplasm of uterus (O9A.1-)

O34.1Ø **Maternal care for benign tumor of corpus uteri, unspecified trimester ♀** M

O34.11 **Maternal care for benign tumor of corpus uteri, first trimester ♀** M

O34.12 **Maternal care for benign tumor of corpus uteri, second trimester ♀** M

O34.13 **Maternal care for benign tumor of corpus uteri, third trimester ♀** M

● O34.2 **Maternal care due to uterine scar from previous surgery**

Coding Clinic: 2Ø16, Q4, P76

● O34.21 **Maternal care for scar from previous cesarean delivery**

Coding Clinic: 2Ø16, Q4, P51

O34.211 **Maternal care for low transverse scar from previous cesarean delivery ♀** M

O34.212 **Maternal care for vertical scar from previous cesarean delivery ♀** M

Maternal care for classical scar from previous cesarean delivery

O34.219 **Maternal care for unspecified type scar from previous cesarean delivery ♀** M

O34.29 **Maternal care due to uterine scar from other previous surgery ♀** M

Maternal care due to uterine scar from other transmural uterine incision

● O34.3 **Maternal care for cervical incompetence**

Maternal care for cerclage with or without cervical incompetence
Maternal care for Shirodkar suture with or without cervical incompetence

O34.3Ø **Maternal care for cervical incompetence, unspecified trimester ♀** M

O34.31 **Maternal care for cervical incompetence, first trimester ♀** M

O34.32 **Maternal care for cervical incompetence, second trimester ♀** M

O34.33 **Maternal care for cervical incompetence, third trimester ♀** M

● O34.4 **Maternal care for other abnormalities of cervix**

O34.4Ø **Maternal care for other abnormalities of cervix, unspecified trimester ♀** M

O34.41 **Maternal care for other abnormalities of cervix, first trimester ♀** M

O34.42 **Maternal care for other abnormalities of cervix, second trimester ♀** M

O34.43 **Maternal care for other abnormalities of cervix, third trimester ♀** M

● O34.5 **Maternal care for other abnormalities of gravid uterus**

● O34.51 **Maternal care for incarceration of gravid uterus**

O34.511 **Maternal care for incarceration of gravid uterus, first trimester ♀** M

O34.512 **Maternal care for incarceration of gravid uterus, second trimester ♀** M

O34.513 **Maternal care for incarceration of gravid uterus, third trimester ♀** M

O34.519 **Maternal care for incarceration of gravid uterus, unspecified trimester ♀** M

O34.52 Maternal care for prolapse of gravid uterus
- O34.521 Maternal care for prolapse of gravid uterus, first trimester ♀ M
- O34.522 Maternal care for prolapse of gravid uterus, second trimester ♀ M
- O34.523 Maternal care for prolapse of gravid uterus, third trimester ♀ M
- O34.529 Maternal care for prolapse of gravid uterus, unspecified trimester ♀ M

O34.53 Maternal care for retroversion of gravid uterus
- O34.531 Maternal care for retroversion of gravid uterus, first trimester ♀ M
- O34.532 Maternal care for retroversion of gravid uterus, second trimester ♀ M
- O34.533 Maternal care for retroversion of gravid uterus, third trimester ♀ M
- O34.539 Maternal care for retroversion of gravid uterus, unspecified trimester ♀ M

O34.59 Maternal care for other abnormalities of gravid uterus
- O34.591 Maternal care for other abnormalities of gravid uterus, first trimester ♀ M
- O34.592 Maternal care for other abnormalities of gravid uterus, second trimester ♀ M
- O34.593 Maternal care for other abnormalities of gravid uterus, third trimester ♀ M
- O34.599 Maternal care for other abnormalities of gravid uterus, unspecified trimester ♀ M

O34.6 Maternal care for abnormality of vagina

Excludes2 maternal care for vaginal varices in pregnancy (O22.1-)

- O34.60 Maternal care for abnormality of vagina, unspecified trimester ♀ M
- O34.61 Maternal care for abnormality of vagina, first trimester ♀ M
- O34.62 Maternal care for abnormality of vagina, second trimester ♀ M
- O34.63 Maternal care for abnormality of vagina, third trimester ♀ M

O34.7 Maternal care for abnormality of vulva and perineum

Excludes2 maternal care for perineal and vulval varices in pregnancy (O22.1-)

- O34.70 Maternal care for abnormality of vulva and perineum, unspecified trimester ♀ M
- O34.71 Maternal care for abnormality of vulva and perineum, first trimester ♀ M
- O34.72 Maternal care for abnormality of vulva and perineum, second trimester ♀ M
- O34.73 Maternal care for abnormality of vulva and perineum, third trimester ♀ M

O34.8 Maternal care for other abnormalities of pelvic organs
- O34.80 Maternal care for other abnormalities of pelvic organs, unspecified trimester ♀ M
- O34.81 Maternal care for other abnormalities of pelvic organs, first trimester ♀ M
- O34.82 Maternal care for other abnormalities of pelvic organs, second trimester ♀ M
- O34.83 Maternal care for other abnormalities of pelvic organs, third trimester ♀ M

O34.9 Maternal care for abnormality of pelvic organ, unspecified
- O34.90 Maternal care for abnormality of pelvic organ, unspecified, unspecified trimester ♀ M
- O34.91 Maternal care for abnormality of pelvic organ, unspecified, first trimester ♀ M
- O34.92 Maternal care for abnormality of pelvic organ, unspecified, second trimester ♀ M
- O34.93 Maternal care for abnormality of pelvic organ, unspecified, third trimester ♀ M

O35 Maternal care for known or suspected fetal abnormality and damage

Includes the listed conditions in the fetus as a reason for hospitalization or other obstetric care to the mother, or for termination of pregnancy

Code also any associated maternal condition

Excludes1 encounter for suspected maternal and fetal conditions ruled out (Z03.7-)

One of the following 7th characters is to be assigned to each code under category O35. 7th character 0 is for single gestations and multiple gestations where the fetus is unspecified. 7th characters 1 through 9 are for cases of multiple gestations to identify the fetus for which the code applies. The appropriate code from category O30, Multiple gestation, must also be assigned when assigning a code from category O35 that has a 7th character of 1 through 9.

0	not applicable or unspecified
1	fetus 1
2	fetus 2
3	fetus 3
4	fetus 4
5	fetus 5
9	other fetus

X **O35.0 Maternal care for (suspected) central nervous system malformation in fetus** ♀ M
- Maternal care for fetal anencephaly
- Maternal care for fetal hydrocephalus
- Maternal care for fetal spina bifida

Excludes2 chromosomal abnormality in fetus (O35.1)

X **O35.1 Maternal care for (suspected) chromosomal abnormality in fetus** ♀ M

X **O35.2 Maternal care for (suspected) hereditary disease in fetus** ♀ M

Excludes2 chromosomal abnormality in fetus (O35.1)

X **O35.3 Maternal care for (suspected) damage to fetus from viral disease in mother** ♀ M
- Maternal care for damage to fetus from maternal cytomegalovirus infection
- Maternal care for damage to fetus from maternal rubella

Coding Clinic: 2016, Q4, P6

X **O35.4 Maternal care for (suspected) damage to fetus from alcohol** ♀ M

X **O35.5 Maternal care for (suspected) damage to fetus by drugs** ♀ M
- Maternal care for damage to fetus from drug addiction

X **O35.6 Maternal care for (suspected) damage to fetus by radiation** ♀ M

X **O35.7 Maternal care for (suspected) damage to fetus by other medical procedures** ♀ M
- Maternal care for damage to fetus by amniocentesis
- Maternal care for damage to fetus by biopsy procedures
- Maternal care for damage to fetus by hematological investigation
- Maternal care for damage to fetus by intrauterine contraceptive device
- Maternal care for damage to fetus by intrauterine surgery

X **O35.8 Maternal care for other (suspected) fetal abnormality and damage** ♀ M
- Maternal care for damage to fetus from maternal listeriosis
- Maternal care for damage to fetus from maternal toxoplasmosis

X **O35.9 Maternal care for (suspected) fetal abnormality and damage, unspecified** ♀ M

CHAPTER 15 (O00-O9A)

OGCR Section I.C.15.e.1.

Fetal Conditions Affecting the Management of the Mother

1) Code from categories O35 and O36

Codes from categories O35, Maternal care for known or suspected fetal abnormality and damage, and O36, Maternal care for other fetal problems, are assigned only when the fetal condition is actually responsible for modifying the management of the mother, i.e., by requiring diagnostic studies, additional observation, special care, or termination of pregnancy. The fact that the fetal condition exists does not justify assigning a code from this series to the mother's record.

2) In utero surgery

In cases when surgery is performed on the fetus, a diagnosis code from category O35, Maternal care for known or suspected fetal abnormality and damage, should be assigned identifying the fetal condition. Assign the appropriate procedure code for the procedure performed.

No code from Chapter 16, the perinatal codes, should be used on the mother's record to identify fetal conditions. Surgery performed in utero on a fetus is still to be coded as an obstetric encounter.

O36 Maternal care for other fetal problems

Includes the listed conditions in the fetus as a reason for hospitalization or other obstetric care of the mother, or for termination of pregnancy

Excludes1 encounter for suspected maternal and fetal conditions ruled out (Z03.7-)
placental transfusion syndromes (O43.0-)

Excludes2 labor and delivery complicated by fetal stress (O77.-)

One of the following 7th characters is to be assigned to each code under category O36. 7th character 0 is for single gestations and multiple gestations where the fetus is unspecified. 7th characters 1 through 9 are for cases of multiple gestations to identify the fetus for which the code applies. The appropriate code from category O30, Multiple gestation, must also be assigned when assigning a code from category O36 that has a 7th character of 1 through 9.

0	not applicable or unspecified
1	fetus 1
2	fetus 2
3	fetus 3
4	fetus 4
5	fetus 5
9	other fetus

Coding Clinic: 2015, Q3, P40

O36.0 Maternal care for rhesus isoimmunization
Maternal care for Rh incompatibility (with hydrops fetalis)

O36.01 Maternal care for anti-D [Rh] antibodies

O36.011 Maternal care for anti-D [Rh] antibodies, first trimester ♀ M

O36.012 Maternal care for anti-D [Rh] antibodies, second trimester ♀ M

O36.013 Maternal care for anti-D [Rh] antibodies, third trimester ♀ M

O36.019 Maternal care for anti-D [Rh] antibodies, unspecified trimester ♀ M

O36.09 Maternal care for other rhesus isoimmunization

O36.091 Maternal care for other rhesus isoimmunization, first trimester ♀ M

O36.092 Maternal care for other rhesus isoimmunization, second trimester ♀ M

O36.093 Maternal care for other rhesus isoimmunization, third trimester ♀ M
Coding Clinic: 2015, Q3, P40

O36.099 Maternal care for other rhesus isoimmunization, unspecified trimester ♀ M

O36.1 Maternal care for other isoimmunization
Maternal care for ABO isoimmunization

O36.11 Maternal care for Anti-A sensitization
Maternal care for isoimmunization NOS (with hydrops fetalis)

O36.111 Maternal care for Anti-A sensitization, first trimester ♀ M

O36.112 Maternal care for Anti-A sensitization, second trimester ♀ M

O36.113 Maternal care for Anti-A sensitization, third trimester ♀ M

O36.119 Maternal care for Anti-A sensitization, unspecified trimester ♀ M

O36.19 Maternal care for other isoimmunization
Maternal care for Anti-B sensitization

O36.191 Maternal care for other isoimmunization, first trimester ♀ M

O36.192 Maternal care for other isoimmunization, second trimester ♀ M

O36.193 Maternal care for other isoimmunization, third trimester ♀ M

O36.199 Maternal care for other isoimmunization, unspecified trimester ♀ M

O36.2 Maternal care for hydrops fetalis
Maternal care for hydrops fetalis NOS
Maternal care for hydrops fetalis not associated with isoimmunization

Excludes1 hydrops fetalis associated with ABO isoimmunization (O36.1-)
hydrops fetalis associated with rhesus isoimmunization (O36.0-)

O36.20 Maternal care for hydrops fetalis, unspecified trimester ♀ M

O36.21 Maternal care for hydrops fetalis, first trimester ♀ M

O36.22 Maternal care for hydrops fetalis, second trimester ♀ M

O36.23 Maternal care for hydrops fetalis, third trimester ♀ M

O36.4 Maternal care for intrauterine death ♀ M
Maternal care for intrauterine fetal death NOS
Maternal care for intrauterine fetal death after completion of 20 weeks of gestation
Maternal care for late fetal death
Maternal care for missed delivery

Excludes1 missed abortion (O02.1)
stillbirth (P95)

O36.5 Maternal care for known or suspected poor fetal growth

O36.51 Maternal care for known or suspected placental insufficiency

O36.511 Maternal care for known or suspected placental insufficiency, first trimester ♀ M

O36.512 Maternal care for known or suspected placental insufficiency, second trimester ♀ M

O36.513 Maternal care for known or suspected placental insufficiency, third trimester ♀ M

O36.519 Maternal care for known or suspected placental insufficiency, unspecified trimester ♀ M

O36.59 Maternal care for other known or suspected poor fetal growth
Maternal care for known or suspected light-for-dates NOS
Maternal care for known or suspected small-for-dates NOS

O36.591 Maternal care for other known or suspected poor fetal growth, first trimester ♀ M
O36.592 Maternal care for other known or suspected poor fetal growth, second trimester ♀ M
O36.593 Maternal care for other known or suspected poor fetal growth, third trimester ♀ M
O36.599 Maternal care for other known or suspected poor fetal growth, unspecified trimester ♀ M

O36.6 Maternal care for excessive fetal growth
Maternal care for known or suspected large-for-dates

X **O36.60 Maternal care for excessive fetal growth, unspecified trimester ♀** M
X **O36.61 Maternal care for excessive fetal growth, first trimester ♀** M
X **O36.62 Maternal care for excessive fetal growth, second trimester ♀** M
X **O36.63 Maternal care for excessive fetal growth, third trimester ♀** M

O36.7 Maternal care for viable fetus in abdominal pregnancy

X **O36.70 Maternal care for viable fetus in abdominal pregnancy, unspecified trimester ♀** M
X **O36.71 Maternal care for viable fetus in abdominal pregnancy, first trimester ♀** M
X **O36.72 Maternal care for viable fetus in abdominal pregnancy, second trimester ♀** M
X **O36.73 Maternal care for viable fetus in abdominal pregnancy, third trimester ♀** M

O36.8 Maternal care for other specified fetal problems

X **O36.80 Pregnancy with inconclusive fetal viability ♀** M
Encounter to determine fetal viability of pregnancy
Coding Clinic: 2019, Q2, P29

O36.81 Decreased fetal movements

O36.812 Decreased fetal movements, second trimester ♀ M
O36.813 Decreased fetal movements, third trimester ♀ M
O36.819 Decreased fetal movements, unspecified trimester ♀ M

O36.82 Fetal anemia and thrombocytopenia

O36.821 Fetal anemia and thrombocytopenia, first trimester ♀ M
O36.822 Fetal anemia and thrombocytopenia, second trimester ♀ M
O36.823 Fetal anemia and thrombocytopenia, third trimester ♀ M
O36.829 Fetal anemia and thrombocytopenia, unspecified trimester ♀ M

O36.83 Maternal care for abnormalities of the fetal heart rate or rhythm
▶Maternal care for depressed fetal heart rate tones
▶Maternal care for fetal bradycardia
▶Maternal care for fetal heart rate abnormal variability
▶Maternal care for fetal heart rate decelerations
▶Maternal care for fetal heart rate irregularity
▶Maternal care for fetal tachycardia
▶Maternal care for non-reassuring fetal heart rate or rhythm

O36.831 Maternal care for abnormalities of the fetal heart rate or rhythm, first trimester ♀ M
O36.832 Maternal care for abnormalities of the fetal heart rate or rhythm, second trimester ♀ M
O36.833 Maternal care for abnormalities of the fetal heart rate or rhythm, third trimester ♀ M
O36.839 Maternal care for abnormalities of the fetal heart rate or rhythm, unspecified trimester ♀ M

O36.89 Maternal care for other specified fetal problems

O36.891 Maternal care for other specified fetal problems, first trimester ♀ M
O36.892 Maternal care for other specified fetal problems, second trimester ♀ M
O36.893 Maternal care for other specified fetal problems, third trimester ♀ M
O36.899 Maternal care for other specified fetal problems, unspecified trimester ♀ M

O36.9 Maternal care for fetal problem, unspecified

X **O36.90 Maternal care for fetal problem, unspecified, unspecified trimester ♀** M
X **O36.91 Maternal care for fetal problem, unspecified, first trimester ♀** M
X **O36.92 Maternal care for fetal problem, unspecified, second trimester ♀** M
X **O36.93 Maternal care for fetal problem, unspecified, third trimester ♀** M

O40 Polyhydramnios

Overabundance of amniotic fluid

Includes hydramnios
Excludes1 encounter for suspected maternal and fetal conditions ruled out (Z03.7-)

One of the following 7th characters is to be assigned to each code under category O40. 7th character 0 is for single gestations and multiple gestations where the fetus is unspecified. 7th characters 1 through 9 are for cases of multiple gestations to identify the fetus for which the code applies. The appropriate code from category O30, Multiple gestation, must also be assigned when assigning a code from category O40 that has a 7th character of 1 through 9.

0	not applicable or unspecified
1	fetus 1
2	fetus 2
3	fetus 3
4	fetus 4
5	fetus 5
9	other fetus

X **O40.1 Polyhydramnios, first trimester ♀** M
X **O40.2 Polyhydramnios, second trimester ♀** M
X **O40.3 Polyhydramnios, third trimester ♀** M
X **O40.9 Polyhydramnios, unspecified trimester ♀** M

CHAPTER 15 (O00-O9A)

O41 Other disorders of amniotic fluid and membranes

Excludes1 encounter for suspected maternal and fetal conditions ruled out (Z03.7-)

One of the following 7th characters is to be assigned to each code under category O41. 7th character 0 is for single gestations and multiple gestations where the fetus is unspecified. 7th characters 1 through 9 are for cases of multiple gestations to identify the fetus for which the code applies. The appropriate code from category O30, Multiple gestation, must also be assigned when assigning a code from category O41 that has a 7th character of 1 through 9.

0	not applicable or unspecified
1	fetus 1
2	fetus 2
3	fetus 3
4	fetus 4
5	fetus 5
9	other fetus

O41.0 Oligohydramnios
Scant volume of amniotic fluid
Oligohydramnios without rupture of membranes
- X O41.00 Oligohydramnios, **unspecified trimester** ♀ M
- X O41.01 Oligohydramnios, **first trimester** ♀ M
- X O41.02 Oligohydramnios, **second trimester** ♀ M
- X O41.03 Oligohydramnios, **third trimester** ♀ M

O41.1 Infection of amniotic sac and membranes
- O41.10 Infection of amniotic sac and membranes, unspecified
  - O41.101 Infection of amniotic sac and membranes, unspecified, **first trimester** ♀ M
  - O41.102 Infection of amniotic sac and membranes, unspecified, **second trimester** ♀ M
  - O41.103 Infection of amniotic sac and membranes, unspecified, **third trimester** ♀ M
  - O41.109 Infection of amniotic sac and membranes, unspecified, **unspecified trimester** ♀ M
- O41.12 Chorioamnionitis
  Coding Clinic: 2019, Q2, P34-35
  - O41.121 Chorioamnionitis, **first trimester** ♀ M
  - O41.122 Chorioamnionitis, **second trimester** ♀ M
  - O41.123 Chorioamnionitis, **third trimester** ♀ M
  - O41.129 Chorioamnionitis, **unspecified trimester** ♀ M
- O41.14 Placentitis
  - O41.141 Placentitis, **first trimester** ♀ M
  - O41.142 Placentitis, **second trimester** ♀ M
  - O41.143 Placentitis, **third trimester** ♀ M
  - O41.149 Placentitis, **unspecified trimester** ♀ M

O41.8 Other specified disorders of amniotic fluid and membranes
- O41.8X Other specified disorders of amniotic fluid and membranes
  - O41.8X1 Other specified disorders of amniotic fluid and membranes, **first trimester** ♀ M
  - O41.8X2 Other specified disorders of amniotic fluid and membranes, **second trimester** ♀ M
  - O41.8X3 Other specified disorders of amniotic fluid and membranes, **third trimester** ♀ M
  - O41.8X9 Other specified disorders of amniotic fluid and membranes, **unspecified trimester** ♀ M

O41.9 Disorder of amniotic fluid and membranes, **unspecified**
- X O41.90 Disorder of amniotic fluid and membranes, unspecified, **unspecified trimester** ♀ M
- X O41.91 Disorder of amniotic fluid and membranes, unspecified, **first trimester** ♀ M
- X O41.92 Disorder of amniotic fluid and membranes, unspecified, **second trimester** ♀ M
- X O41.93 Disorder of amniotic fluid and membranes, unspecified, **third trimester** ♀ M

O42 Premature rupture of membranes

O42.0 Premature rupture of membranes, **onset of labor within 24 hours of rupture**
- O42.00 Premature rupture of membranes, onset of labor within 24 hours of rupture, **unspecified** weeks of gestation ♀ M
- O42.01 **Preterm** premature rupture of membranes, onset of labor within 24 hours of rupture
  Premature rupture of membranes before 37 completed weeks of gestation
  - O42.011 Preterm premature rupture of membranes, onset of labor within 24 hours of rupture, **first trimester** ♀ M
  - O42.012 Preterm premature rupture of membranes, onset of labor within 24 hours of rupture, **second trimester** ♀ M
  - O42.013 Preterm premature rupture of membranes, onset of labor within 24 hours of rupture, **third trimester** ♀ M
  - O42.019 Preterm premature rupture of membranes, onset of labor within 24 hours of rupture, **unspecified trimester** ♀ M
- O42.02 **Full-term** premature rupture of membranes, onset of labor within 24 hours of rupture ♀ M
  Premature rupture of membranes at or after 37 completed weeks of gestation, onset of labor within 24 hours of rupture

O42.1 Premature rupture of membranes, **onset of labor more than 24 hours following rupture**
- O42.10 Premature rupture of membranes, onset of labor more than 24 hours following rupture, **unspecified** weeks of gestation ♀ M
- O42.11 **Preterm** premature rupture of membranes, onset of labor more than 24 hours following rupture
  Premature rupture of membranes before 37 completed weeks of gestation
  - O42.111 Preterm premature rupture of membranes, onset of labor more than 24 hours following rupture, **first trimester** ♀ M
  - O42.112 Preterm premature rupture of membranes, onset of labor more than 24 hours following rupture, **second trimester** ♀ M
  - O42.113 Preterm premature rupture of membranes, onset of labor more than 24 hours following rupture, **third trimester** ♀ M
  - O42.119 Preterm premature rupture of membranes, onset of labor more than 24 hours following rupture, **unspecified trimester** ♀ M
- O42.12 **Full-term** premature rupture of membranes, onset of labor more than 24 hours following rupture ♀ M
  Premature rupture of membranes at or after 37 completed weeks of gestation, onset of labor more than 24 hours following rupture

● O42.9 Premature rupture of membranes, unspecified as to length of time between rupture and onset of labor
- O42.90 Premature rupture of membranes, unspecified as to length of time between rupture and onset of labor, unspecified weeks of gestation ♀ M
- ● O42.91 Preterm premature rupture of membranes, unspecified as to length of time between rupture and onset of labor
  - Premature rupture of membranes before 37 completed weeks of gestation
  - O42.911 Preterm premature rupture of membranes, unspecified as to length of time between rupture and onset of labor, first trimester ♀ M
  - O42.912 Preterm premature rupture of membranes, unspecified as to length of time between rupture and onset of labor, second trimester ♀ M
  - O42.913 Preterm premature rupture of membranes, unspecified as to length of time between rupture and onset of labor, third trimester ♀ M
  - O42.919 Preterm premature rupture of membranes, unspecified as to length of time between rupture and onset of labor, unspecified trimester ♀ M
- O42.92 Full-term premature rupture of membranes, unspecified as to length of time between rupture and onset of labor ♀ M
  - Premature rupture of membranes at or after 37 completed weeks of gestation, unspecified as to length of time between rupture and onset of labor

● O43 Placental disorders

Excludes2 maternal care for poor fetal growth due to placental insufficiency (O36.5-)
placenta previa (O44.-)
placental polyp (O90.89)
placentitis (O41.14-)
premature separation of placenta [abruptio placentae] (O45.-)

● O43.0 Placental transfusion syndromes
- ● O43.01 Fetomaternal placental transfusion syndrome
  - Maternofetal placental transfusion syndrome
  - O43.011 Fetomaternal placental transfusion syndrome, first trimester ♀ M
  - O43.012 Fetomaternal placental transfusion syndrome, second trimester ♀ M
  - O43.013 Fetomaternal placental transfusion syndrome, third trimester ♀ M
  - O43.019 Fetomaternal placental transfusion syndrome, unspecified trimester ♀ M
- ● O43.02 Fetus-to-fetus placental transfusion syndrome
  - O43.021 Fetus-to-fetus placental transfusion syndrome, first trimester ♀ M
  - O43.022 Fetus-to-fetus placental transfusion syndrome, second trimester ♀ M
  - O43.023 Fetus-to-fetus placental transfusion syndrome, third trimester ♀ M
  - O43.029 Fetus-to-fetus placental transfusion syndrome, unspecified trimester ♀ M

● O43.1 Malformation of placenta
- ● O43.10 Malformation of placenta, unspecified
  - Abnormal placenta NOS
  - O43.101 Malformation of placenta, unspecified, first trimester ♀ M
  - O43.102 Malformation of placenta, unspecified, second trimester ♀ M
  - O43.103 Malformation of placenta, unspecified, third trimester ♀ M
  - O43.109 Malformation of placenta, unspecified, unspecified trimester ♀ M
- ● O43.11 Circumvallate placenta
  - O43.111 Circumvallate placenta, first trimester ♀ M
  - O43.112 Circumvallate placenta, second trimester ♀ M
  - O43.113 Circumvallate placenta, third trimester ♀ M
  - O43.119 Circumvallate placenta, unspecified trimester ♀ M
- ● O43.12 Velamentous insertion of umbilical cord
  - O43.121 Velamentous insertion of umbilical cord, first trimester ♀ M
  - O43.122 Velamentous insertion of umbilical cord, second trimester ♀ M
  - O43.123 Velamentous insertion of umbilical cord, third trimester ♀ M
  - O43.129 Velamentous insertion of umbilical cord, unspecified trimester ♀ M
- ● O43.19 Other malformation of placenta
  - O43.191 Other malformation of placenta, first trimester ♀ M
  - O43.192 Other malformation of placenta, second trimester ♀ M
  - O43.193 Other malformation of placenta, third trimester ♀ M
  - O43.199 Other malformation of placenta, unspecified trimester ♀ M

● O43.2 Morbidly adherent placenta

Code also associated third stage postpartum hemorrhage, if applicable (O72.0)

Excludes1 retained placenta (O73.-)

- ● O43.21 Placenta accreta
  - O43.211 Placenta accreta, first trimester ♀ M
  - O43.212 Placenta accreta, second trimester ♀ M
  - O43.213 Placenta accreta, third trimester ♀ M
  - O43.219 Placenta accreta, unspecified trimester ♀ M
- ● O43.22 Placenta increta
  - O43.221 Placenta increta, first trimester ♀ M
  - O43.222 Placenta increta, second trimester ♀ M
  - O43.223 Placenta increta, third trimester ♀ M
  - O43.229 Placenta increta, unspecified trimester ♀ M
- ● O43.23 Placenta percreta
  - O43.231 Placenta percreta, first trimester ♀ M
  - O43.232 Placenta percreta, second trimester ♀ M
  - O43.233 Placenta percreta, third trimester ♀ M
  - O43.239 Placenta percreta, unspecified trimester ♀ M

● O43.8 Other placental disorders
- ● O43.81 Placental infarction
  - O43.811 Placental infarction, first trimester ♀ M
  - O43.812 Placental infarction, second trimester ♀ M
  - O43.813 Placental infarction, third trimester ♀ M
  - O43.819 Placental infarction, unspecified trimester ♀ M
- ● O43.89 Other placental disorders
  - Placental dysfunction
  - O43.891 Other placental disorders, first trimester ♀ M
  - O43.892 Other placental disorders, second trimester ♀ M
  - O43.893 Other placental disorders, third trimester ♀ M
  - O43.899 Other placental disorders, unspecified trimester ♀ M

O43.9 Unspecified placental disorder

O43.9Ø	**Unspecified placental disorder, unspecified trimester** ♀	M
O43.91	**Unspecified placental disorder, first trimester** ♀	M
O43.92	**Unspecified placental disorder, second trimester** ♀	M
O43.93	**Unspecified placental disorder, third trimester** ♀	M

O44 Placenta previa

Coding Clinic: 2Ø16, Q4, P52

O44.Ø Complete placenta previa NOS or without hemorrhage

Placenta previa NOS

O44.ØØ	**Complete placenta previa NOS or without hemorrhage, unspecified trimester** ♀	M
O44.Ø1	**Complete placenta previa NOS or without hemorrhage, first trimester** ♀	M
O44.Ø2	**Complete placenta previa NOS or without hemorrhage, second trimester** ♀	M
O44.Ø3	**Complete placenta previa NOS or without hemorrhage, third trimester** ♀	M

O44.1 Complete placenta previa with hemorrhage

Excludes1 labor and delivery complicated by hemorrhage from vasa previa (O69.4)

O44.1Ø	**Complete placenta previa with hemorrhage, unspecified trimester** ♀	M
O44.11	**Complete placenta previa with hemorrhage, first trimester** ♀	M
O44.12	**Complete placenta previa with hemorrhage, second trimester** ♀	M
O44.13	**Complete placenta previa with hemorrhage, third trimester** ♀	M

O44.2 Partial placenta previa without hemorrhage

Marginal placenta previa, NOS or without hemorrhage

O44.2Ø	**Partial placenta previa NOS or without hemorrhage, unspecified trimester** ♀	M
O44.21	**Partial placenta previa NOS or without hemorrhage, first trimester** ♀	M
O44.22	**Partial placenta previa NOS or without hemorrhage, second trimester** ♀	M
O44.23	**Partial placenta previa NOS or without hemorrhage, third trimester** ♀	M

O44.3 Partial placenta previa with hemorrhage

Marginal placenta previa with hemorrhage

O44.3Ø	**Partial placenta previa with hemorrhage, unspecified trimester** ♀	M
O44.31	**Partial placenta previa with hemorrhage, first trimester** ♀	M
O44.32	**Partial placenta previa with hemorrhage, second trimester** ♀	M
O44.33	**Partial placenta previa with hemorrhage, third trimester** ♀	M

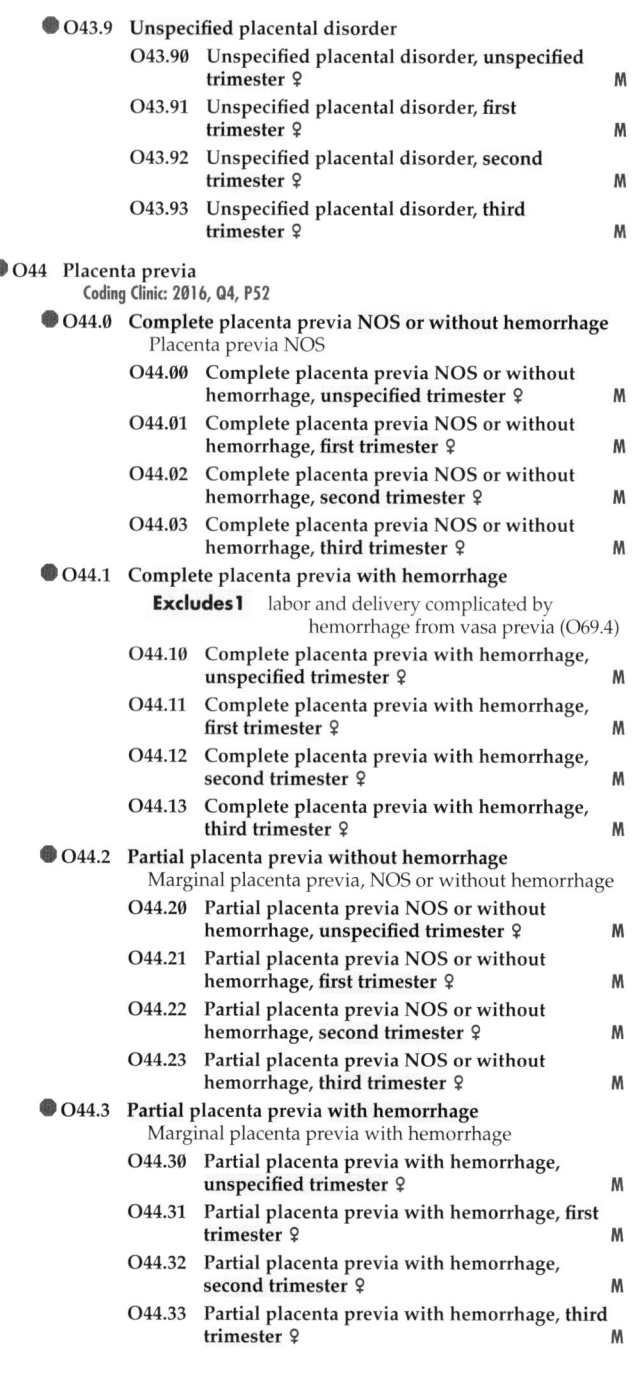

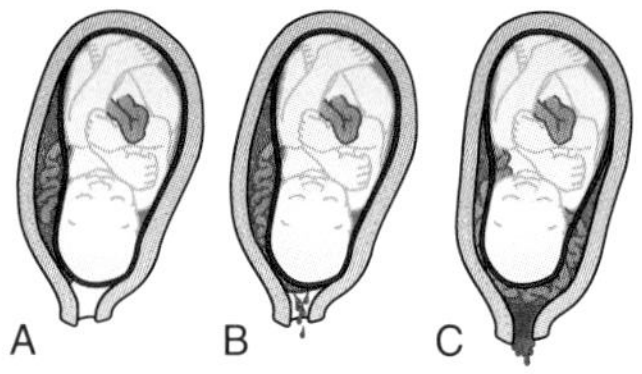

Figure 15-2 **A.** Marginal placento previa. **B.** Partial placenta previa. **C.** Total placento previa.

Item 15-3 **Placenta previa** is a condition in which the opening of the cervix is obstructed by the displaced placenta. The three types, marginal, partial, and total, are varying degrees of placenta displacement. Placenta abruption is the premature breaking away of the placenta from the site of the uterine implant before the delivery of the fetus.

O44.4 Low lying placenta NOS or without hemorrhage

Low implantation of placenta NOS or without hemorrhage

O44.4Ø	**Low lying placenta NOS or without hemorrhage, unspecified trimester** ♀	M
O44.41	**Low lying placenta NOS or without hemorrhage, first trimester** ♀	M
O44.42	**Low lying placenta NOS or without hemorrhage, second trimester** ♀	M
O44.43	**Low lying placenta NOS or without hemorrhage, third trimester** ♀	M

O44.5 Low lying placenta with hemorrhage

Low implantation of placenta with hemorrhage

O44.5Ø	**Low lying placenta with hemorrhage, unspecified trimester** ♀	M
O44.51	**Low lying placenta with hemorrhage, first trimester** ♀	M
O44.52	**Low lying placenta with hemorrhage, second trimester** ♀	M
O44.53	**Low lying placenta with hemorrhage, third trimester** ♀	M

O45 Premature separation of placenta [abruptio placentae]

O45.Ø Premature separation of placenta with coagulation defect

O45.ØØ Premature separation of placenta with coagulation defect, unspecified

O45.ØØ1	**Premature separation of placenta with coagulation defect, unspecified, first trimester** ♀	M
O45.ØØ2	**Premature separation of placenta with coagulation defect, unspecified, second trimester** ♀	M
O45.ØØ3	**Premature separation of placenta with coagulation defect, unspecified, third trimester** ♀	M
O45.ØØ9	**Premature separation of placenta with coagulation defect, unspecified, unspecified trimester** ♀	M

O45.Ø1 Premature separation of placenta with afibrinogenemia

Premature separation of placenta with hypofibrinogenemia

O45.Ø11	**Premature separation of placenta with afibrinogenemia, first trimester** ♀	M
O45.Ø12	**Premature separation of placenta with afibrinogenemia, second trimester** ♀	M
O45.Ø13	**Premature separation of placenta with afibrinogenemia, third trimester** ♀	M
O45.Ø19	**Premature separation of placenta with afibrinogenemia, unspecified trimester** ♀	M

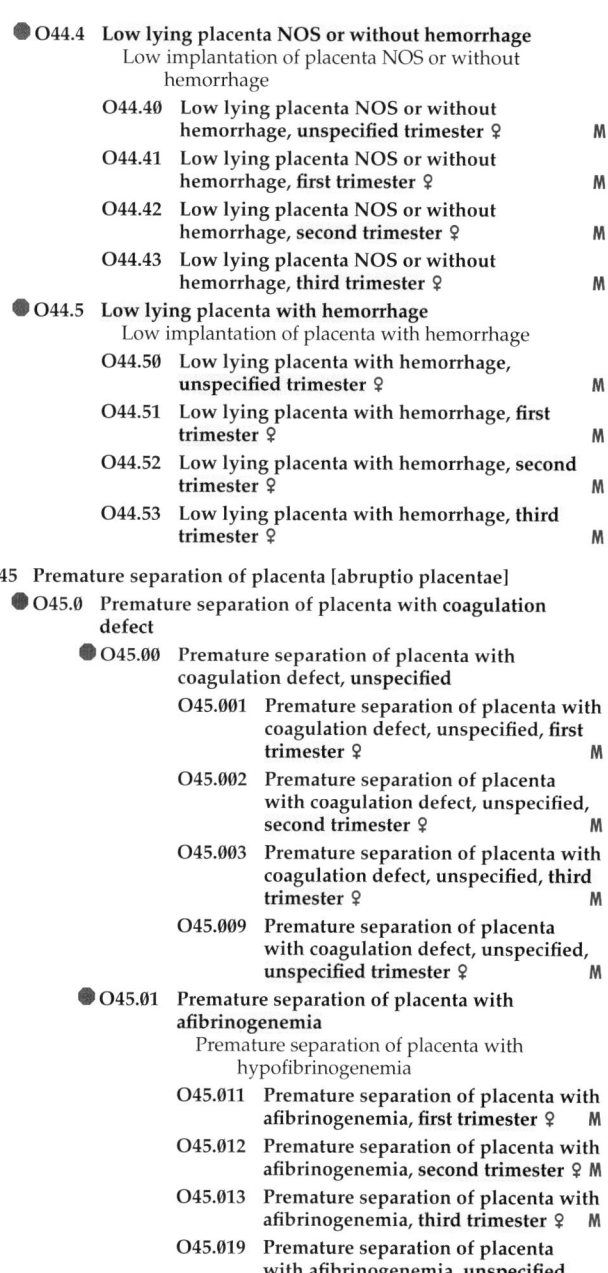

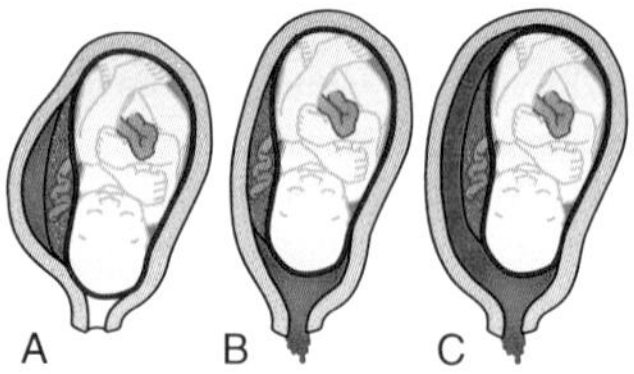

Figure 15-3 Abruptio placentae is classified according to the grade of separation of the placenta from the uterine wall. **A.** Mild separation in which hemorrhage is internal. **B.** Moderate separation in which there is external hemorrhage. **C.** Severe separation in which there is external hemorrhage and extreme separation.

- O45.02 Premature separation of placenta with disseminated intravascular coagulation
  - O45.021 Premature separation of placenta with disseminated intravascular coagulation, first trimester ♀ M
  - O45.022 Premature separation of placenta with disseminated intravascular coagulation, second trimester ♀ M
  - O45.023 Premature separation of placenta with disseminated intravascular coagulation, third trimester ♀ M
  - O45.029 Premature separation of placenta with disseminated intravascular coagulation, unspecified trimester ♀ M
- O45.09 Premature separation of placenta with other coagulation defect
  - O45.091 Premature separation of placenta with other coagulation defect, first trimester ♀ M
  - O45.092 Premature separation of placenta with other coagulation defect, second trimester ♀ M
  - O45.093 Premature separation of placenta with other coagulation defect, third trimester ♀ M
  - O45.099 Premature separation of placenta with other coagulation defect, unspecified trimester ♀ M

O45.8 Other premature separation of placenta
- O45.8X Other premature separation of placenta
  - O45.8X1 Other premature separation of placenta, first trimester ♀ M
  - O45.8X2 Other premature separation of placenta, second trimester ♀ M
  - O45.8X3 Other premature separation of placenta, third trimester ♀ M
  - O45.8X9 Other premature separation of placenta, unspecified trimester ♀ M

O45.9 Premature separation of placenta, unspecified
  Abruptio placentae NOS
- O45.90 Premature separation of placenta, unspecified, unspecified trimester ♀ M
- O45.91 Premature separation of placenta, unspecified, first trimester ♀ M
- O45.92 Premature separation of placenta, unspecified, second trimester ♀ M
- O45.93 Premature separation of placenta, unspecified, third trimester ♀ M

O46 Antepartum hemorrhage, not elsewhere classified

Excludes1 hemorrhage in early pregnancy (O2Ø.-)
intrapartum hemorrhage NEC (O67.-)
placenta previa (O44.-)
premature separation of placenta [abruptio placentae] (O45.-)

O46.Ø Antepartum hemorrhage with coagulation defect
- O46.ØØ Antepartum hemorrhage with coagulation defect, unspecified
  - O46.ØØ1 Antepartum hemorrhage with coagulation defect, unspecified, first trimester ♀ M
  - O46.ØØ2 Antepartum hemorrhage with coagulation defect, unspecified, second trimester ♀ M
  - O46.ØØ3 Antepartum hemorrhage with coagulation defect, unspecified, third trimester ♀ M
  - O46.ØØ9 Antepartum hemorrhage with coagulation defect, unspecified, unspecified trimester ♀ M
- O46.Ø1 Antepartum hemorrhage with afibrinogenemia
  Antepartum hemorrhage with hypofibrinogenemia
  - O46.Ø11 Antepartum hemorrhage with afibrinogenemia, first trimester ♀ M
  - O46.Ø12 Antepartum hemorrhage with afibrinogenemia, second trimester ♀ M
  - O46.Ø13 Antepartum hemorrhage with afibrinogenemia, third trimester ♀ M
  - O46.Ø19 Antepartum hemorrhage with afibrinogenemia, unspecified trimester ♀ M
- O46.Ø2 Antepartum hemorrhage with disseminated intravascular coagulation
  - O46.Ø21 Antepartum hemorrhage with disseminated intravascular coagulation, first trimester ♀ M
  - O46.Ø22 Antepartum hemorrhage with disseminated intravascular coagulation, second trimester ♀ M
  - O46.Ø23 Antepartum hemorrhage with disseminated intravascular coagulation, third trimester ♀ M
  - O46.Ø29 Antepartum hemorrhage with disseminated intravascular coagulation, unspecified trimester ♀ M
- O46.Ø9 Antepartum hemorrhage with other coagulation defect
  - O46.Ø91 Antepartum hemorrhage with other coagulation defect, first trimester ♀ M
  - O46.Ø92 Antepartum hemorrhage with other coagulation defect, second trimester ♀ M
  - O46.Ø93 Antepartum hemorrhage with other coagulation defect, third trimester ♀ M
  - O46.Ø99 Antepartum hemorrhage with other coagulation defect, unspecified trimester ♀ M

O46.8 Other antepartum hemorrhage
- O46.8x Other antepartum hemorrhage
  - O46.8x1 Other antepartum hemorrhage, first trimester ♀ M
  - O46.8x2 Other antepartum hemorrhage, second trimester ♀ M
  - O46.8x3 Other antepartum hemorrhage, third trimester ♀ M
  - O46.8x9 Other antepartum hemorrhage, unspecified trimester ♀ M

O46.9 Antepartum hemorrhage, unspecified
- O46.9Ø Antepartum hemorrhage, unspecified, unspecified trimester ♀ M
- O46.91 Antepartum hemorrhage, unspecified, first trimester ♀ M
- O46.92 Antepartum hemorrhage, unspecified, second trimester ♀ M
- O46.93 Antepartum hemorrhage, unspecified, third trimester ♀ M

O47 False labor

Includes Braxton Hicks contractions
threatened labor

Excludes1 preterm labor (O6Ø.-)

O47.Ø False labor before 37 completed weeks of gestation
- O47.ØØ False labor before 37 completed weeks of gestation, unspecified trimester ♀ M
- O47.Ø2 False labor before 37 completed weeks of gestation, second trimester ♀ M
- O47.Ø3 False labor before 37 completed weeks of gestation, third trimester ♀ M

O47.1 False labor at or after 37 completed weeks of gestation ♀ M

O47.9 False labor, unspecified ♀ M

CHAPTER 15 (OØØ-O9A)

● O48 Late pregnancy

O48.0 **Post-term pregnancy** ♀ M

Pregnancy over 40 completed weeks to 42 completed weeks gestation

O48.1 **Prolonged pregnancy** ♀ M

Pregnancy which has advanced beyond 42 completed weeks gestation

COMPLICATIONS OF LABOR AND DELIVERY (O60-O77)

● O60 Preterm labor

Includes onset (spontaneous) of labor before 37 completed weeks of gestation

Excludes1 false labor (O47.0-)
threatened labor NOS (O47.0-)

● O60.0 **Preterm labor without delivery**

O60.00 **Preterm labor without delivery, unspecified trimester** ♀ M

O60.02 **Preterm labor without delivery, second trimester** ♀ M

O60.03 **Preterm labor without delivery, third trimester** ♀ M

● O60.1 **Preterm labor with preterm delivery**

One of the following 7th characters is to be assigned to each code under subcategory O60.1. 7th character 0 is for single gestations and multiple gestations where the fetus is unspecified. 7th characters 1 through 9 are for cases of multiple gestations to identify the fetus for which the code applies. The appropriate code from category O30, Multiple gestation, must also be assigned when assigning a code from subcategory O60.1 that has a 7th character of 1 through 9.

0	not applicable or unspecified
1	fetus 1
2	fetus 2
3	fetus 3
4	fetus 4
5	fetus 5
9	other fetus

Coding Clinic: 2016, Q2, P11

X● O60.10 **Preterm labor with preterm delivery, unspecified trimester** ♀ M

Preterm labor with delivery NOS

X● O60.12 **Preterm labor second trimester with preterm delivery second trimester** ♀ M

X● O60.13 **Preterm labor second trimester with preterm delivery third trimester** ♀ M

X● O60.14 **Preterm labor third trimester with preterm delivery third trimester** ♀ M

Coding Clinic: 2016, Q2, P10

● O60.2 **Term delivery with preterm labor**

One of the following 7th characters is to be assigned to each code under subcategory O60.2. 7th character 0 is for single gestations and multiple gestations where the fetus is unspecified. 7th characters 1 through 9 are for cases of multiple gestations to identify the fetus for which the code applies. The appropriate code from category O30, Multiple gestation, must also be assigned when assigning a code from subcategory O60.2 that has a 7th character of 1 through 9.

0	not applicable or unspecified
1	fetus 1
2	fetus 2
3	fetus 3
4	fetus 4
5	fetus 5
9	other fetus

X● O60.20 **Term delivery with preterm labor, unspecified trimester** ♀ M

X● O60.22 **Term delivery with preterm labor, second trimester** ♀ M

X● O60.23 **Term delivery with preterm labor, third trimester** ♀ M

● O61 Failed induction of labor

O61.0 **Failed medical induction of labor** ♀ M

Failed induction (of labor) by oxytocin
Failed induction (of labor) by prostaglandins

O61.1 **Failed instrumental induction of labor** ♀ M

Failed mechanical induction (of labor)
Failed surgical induction (of labor)

O61.8 **Other failed induction of labor** ♀ M

O61.9 **Failed induction of labor, unspecified** ♀ M

● O62 Abnormalities of forces of labor

O62.0 **Primary inadequate contractions** ♀ M

Failure of cervical dilatation
Primary hypotonic uterine dysfunction
Uterine inertia during latent phase of labor

O62.1 **Secondary uterine inertia** ♀ M

Arrested active phase of labor
Secondary hypotonic uterine dysfunction

O62.2 **Other uterine inertia** ♀ M

Atony of uterus without hemorrhage
Atony of uterus NOS
Desultory labor
Hypotonic uterine dysfunction NOS
Irregular labor
Poor contractions
Slow slope active phase of labor
Uterine inertia NOS

Excludes1 atony of uterus with hemorrhage (postpartum) (O72.1)
postpartum atony of uterus without hemorrhage (O75.89)

O62.3 **Precipitate labor** ♀ M

O62.4 **Hypertonic, incoordinate, and prolonged uterine contractions** ♀ M

Cervical spasm
Contraction ring dystocia
Dyscoordinate labor
Hour-glass contraction of uterus
Hypertonic uterine dysfunction
Incoordinate uterine action
Tetanic contractions
Uterine dystocia NOS
Uterine spasm

Excludes1 dystocia (fetal) (maternal) NOS (O66.9)

O62.8 **Other abnormalities of forces of labor** ♀ M

O62.9 **Abnormality of forces of labor, unspecified** ♀ M

CHAPTER 15 (O00-O9A)

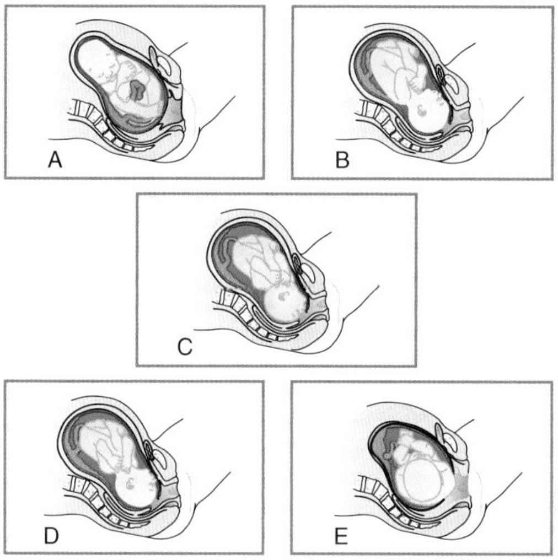

Figure 15-4 Five types of malposition and malpresentation of the fetus: **A.** Breech. **B.** Vertex. **C.** Face. **D.** Brow. **E.** Shoulder.

● O63 Long labor

- O63.Ø **Prolonged first stage (of labor)** ♀ M
- O63.1 **Prolonged second stage (of labor)** ♀ M
- O63.2 **Delayed delivery of second twin, triplet, etc.** ♀ M
- O63.9 **Long labor, unspecified** ♀ M
  - Prolonged labor NOS

● O64 **Obstructed labor due to malposition and malpresentation of fetus**

One of the following 7th characters is to be assigned to each code under category O64. 7th character Ø is for single gestations and multiple gestations where the fetus is unspecified. 7th characters 1 through 9 are for cases of multiple gestations to identify the fetus for which the code applies. The appropriate code from category O3Ø, Multiple gestation, must also be assigned when assigning a code from category O64 that has a 7th character of 1 through 9.

Ø	not applicable or unspecified
1	fetus 1
2	fetus 2
3	fetus 3
4	fetus 4
5	fetus 5
9	other fetus

X● O64.Ø **Obstructed labor due to incomplete rotation of fetal head** ♀ M
- Deep transverse arrest
- Obstructed labor due to persistent occipitoiliac (position)
- Obstructed labor due to persistent occipitoposterior (position)
- Obstructed labor due to persistent occipitosacral (position)
- Obstructed labor due to persistent occipitotransverse (position)

X● O64.1 **Obstructed labor due to breech presentation** ♀ M
- Obstructed labor due to buttocks presentation
- Obstructed labor due to complete breech presentation
- Obstructed labor due to frank breech presentation

X● O64.2 **Obstructed labor due to face presentation** ♀ M
- Obstructed labor due to chin presentation

X● O64.3 **Obstructed labor due to brow presentation** ♀ M

X● O64.4 **Obstructed labor due to shoulder presentation** ♀ M
- Prolapsed arm
- **Excludes1** impacted shoulders (O66.Ø)
  shoulder dystocia (O66.Ø)

X● O64.5 **Obstructed labor due to compound presentation** ♀ M

X● O64.8 **Obstructed labor due to other malposition and malpresentation** ♀ M
- Obstructed labor due to footling presentation
- Obstructed labor due to incomplete breech presentation

X● O64.9 **Obstructed labor due to malposition and malpresentation, unspecified** ♀ M

● O65 Obstructed labor due to maternal pelvic abnormality

- O65.Ø **Obstructed labor due to deformed pelvis** ♀ M
- O65.1 **Obstructed labor due to generally contracted pelvis** ♀ M
- O65.2 **Obstructed labor due to pelvic inlet contraction** ♀ M
- O65.3 **Obstructed labor due to pelvic outlet and mid-cavity contraction** ♀ M
- O65.4 **Obstructed labor due to fetopelvic disproportion, unspecified** ♀ M
  - **Excludes1** dystocia due to abnormality of fetus (O66.2-O66.3)
- O65.5 **Obstructed labor due to abnormality of maternal pelvic organs** ♀ M
  - Obstructed labor due to conditions listed in O34.-
  - Use additional code to identify abnormality of pelvic organs O34.-
- O65.8 **Obstructed labor due to other maternal pelvic abnormalities** ♀ M
- O65.9 **Obstructed labor due to maternal pelvic abnormality, unspecified** ♀ M

● O66 Other obstructed labor

- O66.Ø **Obstructed labor due to shoulder dystocia** ♀ M
  - Impacted shoulders
- O66.1 **Obstructed labor due to locked twins** ♀ M
- O66.2 **Obstructed labor due to unusually large fetus** ♀ M
- O66.3 **Obstructed labor due to other abnormalities of fetus** ♀ M
  - Dystocia due to fetal ascites
  - Dystocia due to fetal hydrops
  - Dystocia due to fetal meningomyelocele
  - Dystocia due to fetal sacral teratoma
  - Dystocia due to fetal tumor
  - Dystocia due to hydrocephalic fetus
  - Use additional code to identify cause of obstruction
- ● O66.4 Failed trial of labor
  - O66.4Ø **Failed trial of labor, unspecified** ♀ M
  - O66.41 **Failed attempted vaginal birth after previous cesarean delivery** ♀ M
    - *Code first rupture of uterus, if applicable (O71.Ø-, O71.1)*
- O66.5 **Attempted application of vacuum extractor and forceps** ♀ M
  - Attempted application of vacuum or forceps, with subsequent delivery by forceps or cesarean delivery
- O66.6 **Obstructed labor due to other multiple fetuses** ♀ M
- O66.8 **Other specified obstructed labor** ♀ M
  - Use additional code to identify cause of obstruction
- O66.9 **Obstructed labor, unspecified** ♀ M
  - Dystocia NOS
  - Fetal dystocia NOS
  - Maternal dystocia NOS

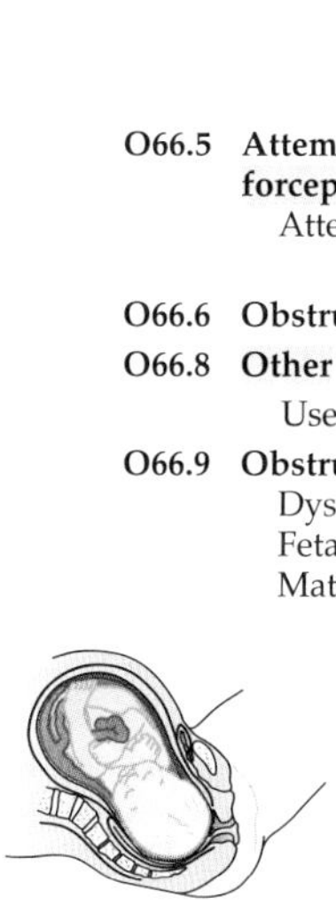

Figure 15-5 Hydrocephalic fetus causing disproportion.

CHAPTER 15 (OØØ-O9A)

● **O67 Labor and delivery complicated by intrapartum hemorrhage, not elsewhere classified**

Excludes1 antepartum hemorrhage NEC (O46.-)
placenta previa (O44.-)
premature separation of placenta [abruptio placentae] (O45.-)

Excludes2 postpartum hemorrhage (O72.-)

O67.0 Intrapartum hemorrhage with coagulation defect ♀ M
Intrapartum hemorrhage (excessive) associated with afibrinogenemia
Intrapartum hemorrhage (excessive) associated with disseminated intravascular coagulation
Intrapartum hemorrhage (excessive) associated with hyperfibrinolysis
Intrapartum hemorrhage (excessive) associated with hypofibrinogenemia

O67.8 Other intrapartum hemorrhage ♀ M
Excessive intrapartum hemorrhage

O67.9 Intrapartum hemorrhage, unspecified ♀ M

O68 Labor and delivery complicated by abnormality of fetal acid-base balance ♀ M
Fetal acidemia complicating labor and delivery
Fetal acidosis complicating labor and delivery
Fetal alkalosis complicating labor and delivery
Fetal metabolic acidemia complicating labor and delivery

Excludes1 fetal stress NOS (O77.9)
labor and delivery complicated by electrocardiographic evidence of fetal stress (O77.8)
labor and delivery complicated by ultrasonic evidence of fetal stress (O77.8)

Excludes2 abnormality in fetal heart rate or rhythm (O76)
labor and delivery complicated by meconium in amniotic fluid (O77.0)

● **O69 Labor and delivery complicated by umbilical cord complications**

One of the following 7th characters is to be assigned to each code under category O69. 7th character 0 is for single gestations and multiple gestations where the fetus is unspecified. 7th characters 1 through 9 are for cases of multiple gestations to identify the fetus for which the code applies. The appropriate code from category O30, Multiple gestation, must also be assigned when assigning a code from category O69 that has a 7th character of 1 through 9.

0	not applicable or unspecified
1	fetus 1
2	fetus 2
3	fetus 3
4	fetus 4
5	fetus 5
9	other fetus

X● **O69.0 Labor and delivery complicated by prolapse of cord ♀** M

X● **O69.1 Labor and delivery complicated by cord around neck, with compression ♀** M

Excludes1 labor and delivery complicated by cord around neck, without compression (O69.81)

X● **O69.2 Labor and delivery complicated by other cord entanglement, with compression ♀** M
Labor and delivery complicated by compression of cord NOS
Labor and delivery complicated by entanglement of cords of twins in monoamniotic sac
Labor and delivery complicated by knot in cord

Excludes1 labor and delivery complicated by other cord entanglement, without compression (O69.82)

X● **O69.3 Labor and delivery complicated by short cord ♀** M

X● **O69.4 Labor and delivery complicated by vasa previa ♀** M
Labor and delivery complicated by hemorrhage from vasa previa

X● **O69.5 Labor and delivery complicated by vascular lesion of cord ♀** M
Labor and delivery complicated by cord bruising
Labor and delivery complicated by cord hematoma
Labor and delivery complicated by thrombosis of umbilical vessels

● **O69.8 Labor and delivery complicated by other cord complications**

X● **O69.81 Labor and delivery complicated by cord around neck, without compression ♀** M

X● **O69.82 Labor and delivery complicated by other cord entanglement, without compression ♀** M

X● **O69.89 Labor and delivery complicated by other cord complications ♀** M

X● **O69.9 Labor and delivery complicated by cord complication, unspecified ♀** M

● **O70 Perineal laceration during delivery**

Includes episiotomy extended by laceration

Excludes1 obstetric high vaginal laceration alone (O71.4)

O70.0 First degree perineal laceration during delivery ♀ M
Perineal laceration, rupture or tear involving fourchette during delivery
Perineal laceration, rupture or tear involving labia during delivery
Perineal laceration, rupture or tear involving skin during delivery
Perineal laceration, rupture or tear involving vagina during delivery
Perineal laceration, rupture or tear involving vulva during delivery
Slight perineal laceration, rupture or tear during delivery

O70.1 Second degree perineal laceration during delivery ♀ M
Perineal laceration, rupture or tear during delivery as in O70.0, also involving pelvic floor
Perineal laceration, rupture or tear during delivery as in O70.0, also involving perineal muscles
Perineal laceration, rupture or tear during delivery as in O70.0, also involving vaginal muscles

Excludes1 perineal laceration involving anal sphincter (O70.2)

Coding Clinic: 2016, CODING CIQ4, P53, Q2, P34

● **O70.2 Third degree perineal laceration during delivery**
Perineal laceration, rupture or tear during delivery as in O70.1, also involving anal sphincter
Perineal laceration, rupture or tear during delivery as in O70.1, also involving rectovaginal septum
Perineal laceration, rupture or tear during delivery as in O70.1, also involving sphincter NOS

Excludes1 anal sphincter tear during delivery without third degree perineal laceration (O70.4)
perineal laceration involving anal or rectal mucosa (O70.3)

O70.20 Third degree perineal laceration during delivery, unspecified ♀ M

O70.21 Third degree perineal laceration during delivery, IIIa ♀ M
Third degree perineal laceration during delivery with less than 50% of external anal sphincter (EAS) thickness torn

O70.22 Third degree perineal laceration during delivery, IIIb ♀ M
Third degree perineal laceration during delivery with more than 50% external anal sphincter (EAS) thickness torn

O70.23 Third degree perineal laceration during delivery, IIIc ♀ M
Third degree perineal laceration during delivery with both external anal sphincter (EAS) and internal anal sphincter (IAS) torn

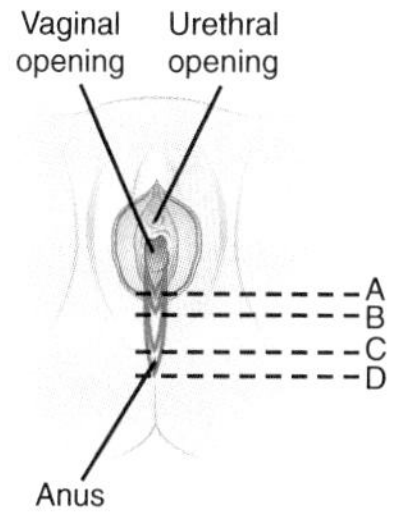

Figure 15-6 Perineal lacerations: **A.** First-degree is laceration of superficial tissues. **B.** Second-degree is limited to the pelvic floor and may involve the perineal or vaginal muscles. **C.** Third-degree involves the anal sphincter. **D.** Fourth-degree involves anal or rectal mucosa.

O7Ø.3 Fourth degree perineal laceration during delivery ♀ M
Perineal laceration, rupture or tear during delivery as in O7Ø.2, also involving anal mucosa
Perineal laceration, rupture or tear during delivery as in O7Ø.2, also involving rectal mucosa

O7Ø.4 Anal sphincter tear complicating delivery, not associated with third degree laceration ♀ M
Excludes1 anal sphincter tear with third degree perineal laceration (O7Ø.2)

O7Ø.9 Perineal laceration during delivery, unspecified ♀ M

O71 Other obstetric trauma
Includes obstetric damage from instruments

O71.Ø Rupture of uterus (spontaneous) before onset of labor
Excludes1 disruption of (current) cesarean delivery wound (O9Ø.Ø)
laceration of uterus, NEC (O71.81)

O71.ØØ Rupture of uterus before onset of labor, unspecified trimester ♀ M

O71.Ø2 Rupture of uterus before onset of labor, second trimester ♀ M

O71.Ø3 Rupture of uterus before onset of labor, third trimester ♀ M

O71.1 Rupture of uterus during labor ♀ M
Rupture of uterus not stated as occurring before onset of labor
Excludes1 disruption of cesarean delivery wound (O9Ø.Ø)
laceration of uterus, NEC (O71.81)

O71.2 Postpartum inversion of uterus ♀ M

O71.3 Obstetric laceration of cervix ♀ M
Annular detachment of cervix

O71.4 Obstetric high vaginal laceration alone ♀ M
Laceration of vaginal wall without perineal laceration
Excludes1 obstetric high vaginal laceration with perineal laceration (O7Ø.-)

O71.5 Other obstetric injury to pelvic organs ♀ M
Obstetric injury to bladder
Obstetric injury to urethra
Excludes2 obstetric periurethral trauma (O71.82)

O71.6 Obstetric damage to pelvic joints and ligaments ♀ M
Obstetric avulsion of inner symphyseal cartilage
Obstetric damage to coccyx
Obstetric traumatic separation of symphysis (pubis)

O71.7 Obstetric hematoma of pelvis ♀ M
Obstetric hematoma of perineum
Obstetric hematoma of vagina
Obstetric hematoma of vulva

O71.8 Other specified obstetric trauma

O71.81 Laceration of uterus, not elsewhere classified ♀ M

O71.82 Other specified trauma to perineum and vulva ♀ M
Obstetric periurethral trauma

O71.89 Other specified obstetric trauma ♀ M

O71.9 Obstetric trauma, unspecified ♀ M

O72 Postpartum hemorrhage
Includes hemorrhage after delivery of fetus or infant

O72.Ø Third-stage hemorrhage ♀ M
Hemorrhage associated with retained, trapped or adherent placenta
Retained placenta NOS
Code also type of adherent placenta (O43.2-)

O72.1 Other immediate postpartum hemorrhage ♀ M
Hemorrhage following delivery of placenta
Postpartum hemorrhage (atonic) NOS
Uterine atony with hemorrhage
Excludes1 uterine atony NOS (O62.2)
uterine atony without hemorrhage (O62.2)
postpartum atony of uterus without hemorrhage (O75.89)

O72.2 Delayed and secondary postpartum hemorrhage ♀ M
Hemorrhage associated with retained portions of placenta or membranes after the first 24 hours following delivery of placenta
Retained products of conception NOS, following delivery

O72.3 Postpartum coagulation defects ♀ M
Postpartum afibrinogenemia
Postpartum fibrinolysis

O73 Retained placenta and membranes, without hemorrhage
Excludes1 placenta accreta (O43.21-)
placenta increta (O43.22-)
placenta percreta (O43.23-)

O73.Ø Retained placenta without hemorrhage ♀ M
Adherent placenta, without hemorrhage
Trapped placenta without hemorrhage

O73.1 Retained portions of placenta and membranes, without hemorrhage ♀ M
Retained products of conception following delivery, without hemorrhage

O74 Complications of anesthesia during labor and delivery
Includes maternal complications arising from the administration of a general, regional or local anesthetic, analgesic or other sedation during labor and delivery
Use additional code, if applicable, to identify specific complication

O74.Ø Aspiration pneumonitis due to anesthesia during labor and delivery ♀ M
Inhalation of stomach contents or secretions NOS due to anesthesia during labor and delivery
Mendelson's syndrome due to anesthesia during labor and delivery

O74.1 Other pulmonary complications of anesthesia during labor and delivery ♀ M

O74.2 Cardiac complications of anesthesia during labor and delivery ♀ M

O74.3 Central nervous system complications of anesthesia during labor and delivery ♀ M

O74.4 Toxic reaction to local anesthesia during labor and delivery ♀ M

O74.5 Spinal and epidural anesthesia-induced headache during labor and delivery ♀ M

O74.6 Other complications of spinal and epidural anesthesia during labor and delivery ♀ M

O74.7 Failed or difficult intubation for anesthesia during labor and delivery ♀ M

O74.8 Other complications of anesthesia during labor and delivery ♀ M

O74.9 Complication of anesthesia during labor and delivery, unspecified ♀ M

● **O75 Other complications of labor and delivery, not elsewhere classified**

Excludes2 puerperal (postpartum) infection (O86.-)
puerperal (postpartum) sepsis (O85)

O75.0 Maternal distress during labor and delivery ♀ M

O75.1 Shock during or following labor and delivery ♀ M
Obstetric shock following labor and delivery

O75.2 Pyrexia during labor, not elsewhere classified ♀ M

O75.3 Other infection during labor ♀ M
Sepsis during labor
Use additional code (B95-B97), to identify infectious agent

O75.4 Other complications of obstetric surgery and procedures ♀ M
Cardiac arrest following obstetric surgery or procedures
Cardiac failure following obstetric surgery or procedures
Cerebral anoxia following obstetric surgery or procedures
Pulmonary edema following obstetric surgery or procedures
Use additional code to identify specific complication

Excludes2 complications of anesthesia during labor and delivery (O74.-)
disruption of obstetrical (surgical) wound (O90.0-O90.1)
hematoma of obstetrical (surgical) wound (O90.2)
infection of obstetrical (surgical) wound (O86.0-)

O75.5 Delayed delivery after artificial rupture of membranes ♀ M

● **O75.8 Other specified complications of labor and delivery**

O75.81 Maternal exhaustion complicating labor and delivery ♀ M

O75.82 Onset (spontaneous) of labor after 37 completed weeks of gestation but before 39 completed weeks gestation, with delivery by (planned) cesarean section ♀ M
Delivery by (planned) cesarean section occurring after 37 completed weeks of gestation but before 39 completed weeks gestation due to (spontaneous) onset of labor
Code first to specify reason for planned cesarean section such as:
cephalopelvic disproportion (normally formed fetus) (O33.9)
previous cesarean delivery (O34.21)

O75.89 Other specified complications of labor and delivery ♀ M

O75.9 Complication of labor and delivery, unspecified ♀ M

O76 Abnormality in fetal heart rate and rhythm complicating labor and delivery ♀ M
Depressed fetal heart rate tones complicating labor and delivery
Fetal bradycardia complicating labor and delivery
Fetal heart rate decelerations complicating labor and delivery
Fetal heart rate irregularity complicating labor and delivery
Fetal heart rate abnormal variability complicating labor and delivery
Fetal tachycardia complicating labor and delivery
Non-reassuring fetal heart rate or rhythm complicating labor and delivery

Excludes1 fetal stress NOS (O77.9)
labor and delivery complicated by electrocardiographic evidence of fetal stress (O77.8)
labor and delivery complicated by ultrasonic evidence of fetal stress (O77.8)

Excludes2 fetal metabolic acidemia (O68)
other fetal stress (O77.0-O77.1)

● **O77 Other fetal stress complicating labor and delivery**

O77.0 Labor and delivery complicated by meconium in amniotic fluid ♀ M

O77.1 Fetal stress in labor or delivery due to drug administration ♀ M

O77.8 Labor and delivery complicated by other evidence of fetal stress ♀ M
Labor and delivery complicated by electrocardiographic evidence of fetal stress
Labor and delivery complicated by ultrasonic evidence of fetal stress

Excludes1 abnormality of fetal acid-base balance (O68)
abnormality in fetal heart rate or rhythm (O76)
fetal metabolic acidemia (O68)

O77.9 Labor and delivery complicated by fetal stress, unspecified ♀ M

Excludes1 abnormality of fetal acid-base balance (O68)
abnormality in fetal heart rate or rhythm (O76)
fetal metabolic acidemia (O68)

OGCR Section I.C., Chapter 15.n.

Normal Delivery, Code O80

1) Encounter for full-term uncomplicated delivery

Code O80 should be assigned when a woman is admitted for a full-term normal delivery and delivers a single, healthy infant without any complications antepartum, during the delivery, or postpartum during the delivery episode. Code O80 is always a principal diagnosis. It is not to be used if any other code from Chapter 15 is needed to describe a current complication of the antenatal, delivery, or perinatal period. Additional codes from other chapters may be used with code O80 if they are not related to or are in any way complicating the pregnancy.

2) Uncomplicated delivery with resolved antepartum complication

Code O80 may be used if the patient had a complication at some point during the pregnancy, but the complication is not present at the time of the admission for delivery.

3) Outcome of delivery for O80

Z37.0, Single live brith, is the only outcome of delivery code appropriate for use with O80.

ENCOUNTER FOR DELIVERY (O80-O82)

O80 Encounter for full-term uncomplicated delivery ♀ M
Delivery requiring minimal or no assistance, with or without episiotomy, without fetal manipulation [e.g., rotation version] or instrumentation [forceps] of a spontaneous, cephalic, vaginal, full-term, single, live-born infant. This code is for use as a single diagnosis code and is not to be used with any other code from Chapter 15.
Use additional code to indicate outcome of delivery (Z37.0)
Coding Clinic: 2016, Q4, P124, 150

O82 Encounter for cesarean delivery without indication ♀ M
Use additional code to indicate outcome of delivery (Z37.0)

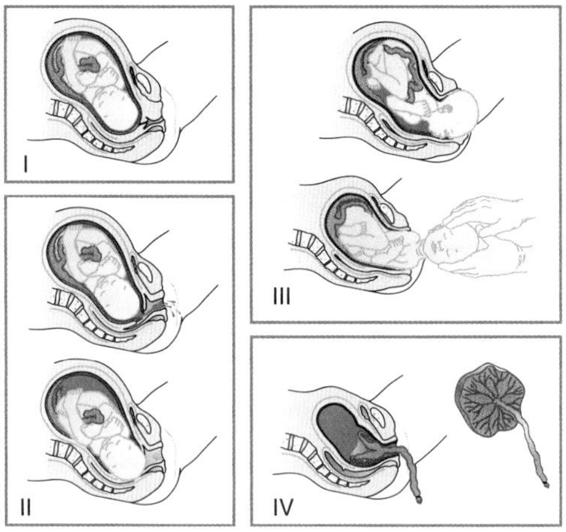

Figure 15-7 The four stages of normal delivery: **I.** Lightening, which occurs 2 to 4 weeks before birth, at which time the fetus turns with head toward the vagina. **II.** Regular contractions begin, the amniotic sac ruptures, and dilation is complete. **III.** Delivery of the head and rotation. **IV.** Expulsion of placenta.

COMPLICATIONS PREDOMINANTLY RELATED TO THE PUERPERIUM (O85-O92)

Excludes2 mental and behavioral disorders associated with the puerperium (F53.-)
obstetrical tetanus (A34)
puerperal osteomalacia (M83.0)

O85 Puerperal sepsis ♀ M
Postpartum sepsis
Puerperal peritonitis
Puerperal pyemia
Use additional code (B95-B97), to identify infectious agent
Use additional code (R65.2-) to identify severe sepsis, if applicable
Excludes1 fever of unknown origin following delivery (O86.4)
genital tract infection following delivery (O86.1-)
obstetric pyemic and septic embolism (O88.3-)
puerperal septic thrombophlebitis (O86.81)
urinary tract infection following delivery (O86.2-)
Excludes2 sepsis during labor (O75.3)
Coding Clinic: 2018, Q4, P23

● **O86 Other puerperal infections**
Use additional code (B95-B97), to identify infectious agent
Excludes2 infection during labor (O75.3)
obstetrical tetanus (A34)

● **O86.0 Infection of obstetric surgical wound**
Infected cesarean delivery wound following delivery
Infected perineal repair following delivery
Excludes1 complications of procedures, not elsewhere classified (T81.44)
postprocedural fever NOS (R50.82)
postprocedural retroperitoneal abscess (K68.11)

O86.00 Infection of obstetric surgical wound, unspecified ♀ M

O86.01 Infection of obstetric surgical wound, superficial incisional site ♀ M
Subcutaneous abscess following an obstetrical procedure
Stitch abscess following an obstetrical procedure

O86.02 Infection of obstetric surgical wound, deep incisional site ♀ M
Intramuscular abscess following an obstetrical procedure
Sub-fascial abscess following an obstetrical procedure
Coding Clinic: 2018, Q4, P23

O86.03 Infection of obstetric surgical wound, organ and space site ♀ M
Intraabdominal abscess following an obstetrical procedure
Subphrenic abscess following an obstetrical procedure

O86.04 Sepsis following an obstetrical procedure ♀ M
Use additional code to identify the sepsis

O86.09 Infection of obstetric surgical wound, other surgical site ♀ M

● **O86.1 Other infection of genital tract following delivery**

O86.11 Cervicitis following delivery ♀ M

O86.12 Endometritis following delivery ♀ M

O86.13 Vaginitis following delivery ♀ M

O86.19 Other infection of genital tract following delivery ♀ M

● **O86.2 Urinary tract infection following delivery**

O86.20 Urinary tract infection following delivery, unspecified ♀ M
Puerperal urinary tract infection NOS

O86.21 Infection of kidney following delivery ♀ M

O86.22 Infection of bladder following delivery ♀ M
Infection of urethra following delivery

O86.29 Other urinary tract infection following delivery ♀ M

O86.4 Pyrexia of unknown origin following delivery ♀ M
Puerperal infection NOS following delivery
Puerperal pyrexia NOS following delivery
Excludes2 pyrexia during labor (O75.2)

● **O86.8 Other specified puerperal infections**

O86.81 Puerperal septic thrombophlebitis ♀ M

O86.89 Other specified puerperal infections ♀ M

● **O87 Venous complications and hemorrhoids in the puerperium**
Includes venous complications in labor, delivery and the puerperium
Excludes2 obstetric embolism (O88.-)
puerperal septic thrombophlebitis (O86.81)
venous complications in pregnancy (O22.-)

O87.0 Superficial thrombophlebitis in the puerperium ♀ M
Puerperal phlebitis NOS
Puerperal thrombosis NOS

O87.1 Deep phlebothrombosis in the puerperium ♀ M
Deep vein thrombosis, postpartum
Pelvic thrombophlebitis, postpartum
Use additional code to identify the deep vein thrombosis (I82.4-, I82.5-, I82.62-. I82.72-)
Use additional code, if applicable, for associated long-term (current) use of anticoagulants (Z79.01)

O87.2 Hemorrhoids in the puerperium ♀ M

O87.3 Cerebral venous thrombosis in the puerperium ♀ M
Cerebrovenous sinus thrombosis in the puerperium

O87.4 Varicose veins of lower extremity in the puerperium ♀ M

O87.8 Other venous complications in the puerperium ♀ M
Genital varices in the puerperium

O87.9 Venous complication in the puerperium, unspecified ♀ M
Puerperal phlebopathy NOS

O88 Obstetric embolism
Excludes1 embolism complicating abortion NOS (O03.2)
embolism complicating ectopic or molar pregnancy (O08.2)
embolism complicating failed attempted abortion (O07.2)
embolism complicating induced abortion (O04.7)
embolism complicating spontaneous abortion (O03.2, O03.7)

● **O88.0 Obstetric air embolism**

● **O88.01 Obstetric air embolism in pregnancy**

O88.011 Air embolism in pregnancy, first trimester ♀ M

O88.012 Air embolism in pregnancy, second trimester ♀ M

O88.013 Air embolism in pregnancy, third trimester ♀ M

O88.019 Air embolism in pregnancy, unspecified trimester ♀ M

O88.02 Air embolism in childbirth ♀ M

O88.03 Air embolism in the puerperium ♀ M

CHAPTER 15 (O00-O9A)

● **O88.1 Amniotic fluid embolism**
Anaphylactoid syndrome in pregnancy

● **O88.11 Amniotic fluid embolism in pregnancy**

O88.111 **Amniotic fluid embolism in pregnancy, first trimester** ♀ M

O88.112 **Amniotic fluid embolism in pregnancy, second trimester** ♀ M

O88.113 **Amniotic fluid embolism in pregnancy, third trimester** ♀ M

O88.119 **Amniotic fluid embolism in pregnancy, unspecified trimester** ♀ M

O88.12 **Amniotic fluid embolism in childbirth** ♀ M

O88.13 **Amniotic fluid embolism in the puerperium** ♀ M

● **O88.2 Obstetric thromboembolism**

● **O88.21 Thromboembolism in pregnancy**
Obstetric (pulmonary) embolism NOS

O88.211 **Thromboembolism in pregnancy, first trimester** ♀ M

O88.212 **Thromboembolism in pregnancy, second trimester** ♀ M

O88.213 **Thromboembolism in pregnancy, third trimester** ♀ M

O88.219 **Thromboembolism in pregnancy, unspecified trimester** ♀ M

O88.22 **Thromboembolism in childbirth** ♀ M

O88.23 **Thromboembolism in the puerperium** ♀ M
Puerperal (pulmonary) embolism NOS

● **O88.3 Obstetric pyemic and septic embolism**

● **O88.31 Pyemic and septic embolism in pregnancy**

O88.311 **Pyemic and septic embolism in pregnancy, first trimester** ♀ M

O88.312 **Pyemic and septic embolism in pregnancy, second trimester** ♀ M

O88.313 **Pyemic and septic embolism in pregnancy, third trimester** ♀ M

O88.319 **Pyemic and septic embolism in pregnancy, unspecified trimester** ♀ M

O88.32 **Pyemic and septic embolism in childbirth** ♀ M

O88.33 **Pyemic and septic embolism in the puerperium** ♀ M

● **O88.8 Other obstetric embolism**
Obstetric fat embolism

● **O88.81 Other embolism in pregnancy**

O88.811 **Other embolism in pregnancy, first trimester** ♀ M

O88.812 **Other embolism in pregnancy, second trimester** ♀ M

O88.813 **Other embolism in pregnancy, third trimester** ♀ M

O88.819 **Other embolism in pregnancy, unspecified trimester** ♀ M

O88.82 **Other embolism in childbirth** ♀ M

O88.83 **Other embolism in the puerperium** ♀ M

● **O89 Complications of anesthesia during the puerperium**

Includes maternal complications arising from the administration of a general, regional or local anesthetic, analgesic or other sedation during the puerperium

Use additional code, if applicable, to identify specific complication

● **O89.Ø Pulmonary complications of anesthesia during the puerperium**

O89.Ø1 **Aspiration pneumonitis due to anesthesia during the puerperium** ♀ M
Inhalation of stomach contents or secretions NOS due to anesthesia during the puerperium
Mendelson's syndrome due to anesthesia during the puerperium

O89.Ø9 **Other pulmonary complications of anesthesia during the puerperium** ♀ M

O89.1 **Cardiac complications of anesthesia during the puerperium** ♀ M

O89.2 **Central nervous system complications of anesthesia during the puerperium** ♀ M

O89.3 **Toxic reaction to local anesthesia during the puerperium** ♀ M

O89.4 **Spinal and epidural anesthesia-induced headache during the puerperium** ♀ M

O89.5 **Other complications of spinal and epidural anesthesia during the puerperium** ♀ M

O89.6 **Failed or difficult intubation for anesthesia during the puerperium** ♀ M

O89.8 **Other complications of anesthesia during the puerperium** ♀ M

O89.9 **Complication of anesthesia during the puerperium, unspecified** ♀ M

● **O9Ø Complications of the puerperium, not elsewhere classified**

O9Ø.Ø **Disruption of cesarean delivery wound** ♀ M
Dehiscence of cesarean delivery wound

Excludes1 rupture of uterus (spontaneous) before onset of labor (O71.Ø-)
rupture of uterus during labor (O71.1)

O9Ø.1 **Disruption of perineal obstetric wound** ♀ M
Disruption of wound of episiotomy
Disruption of wound of perineal laceration
Secondary perineal tear

O9Ø.2 **Hematoma of obstetric wound** ♀ M

O9Ø.3 **Peripartum cardiomyopathy** ♀ M
Conditions in I42.- arising during pregnancy and the puerperium

Excludes1 pre-existing heart disease complicating pregnancy and the puerperium (O99.4-)

O9Ø.4 **Postpartum acute kidney failure** ♀ M
Hepatorenal syndrome following labor and delivery

O9Ø.5 **Postpartum thyroiditis** ♀ M

O9Ø.6 **Postpartum mood disturbance** ♀ M
Postpartum blues
Postpartum sadness
Postpartum dysphoria

Excludes1 postpartum depression (F53.Ø)
puerperal psychosis (F53.1)

● **O9Ø.8 Other complications of the puerperium, not elsewhere classified**

O9Ø.81 **Anemia of the puerperium** ♀ M
Postpartum anemia NOS

Excludes1 pre-existing anemia complicating the puerperium (O99.Ø3)

O9Ø.89 **Other complications of the puerperium, not elsewhere classified** ♀ M
Placental polyp

O9Ø.9 **Complication of the puerperium, unspecified** ♀ M

O91 Infections of breast associated with pregnancy, the puerperium and lactation
Use additional code to identify infection

O91.0 Infection of nipple associated with pregnancy, the puerperium and lactation

O91.01 Infection of nipple associated with pregnancy
Gestational abscess of nipple

O91.011 **Infection of nipple associated with pregnancy, first trimester** ♀ M
O91.012 **Infection of nipple associated with pregnancy, second trimester** ♀ M
O91.013 **Infection of nipple associated with pregnancy, third trimester** ♀ M
O91.019 **Infection of nipple associated with pregnancy, unspecified trimester** ♀ M

O91.02 **Infection of nipple associated with the puerperium** ♀ M
Puerperal abscess of nipple

O91.03 **Infection of nipple associated with lactation** ♀ M
Abscess of nipple associated with lactation

O91.1 Abscess of breast associated with pregnancy, the puerperium and lactation

O91.11 Abscess of breast associated with pregnancy
Gestational mammary abscess
Gestational purulent mastitis
Gestational subareolar abscess

O91.111 **Abscess of breast associated with pregnancy, first trimester** ♀ M
O91.112 **Abscess of breast associated with pregnancy, second trimester** ♀ M
O91.113 **Abscess of breast associated with pregnancy, third trimester** ♀ M
O91.119 **Abscess of breast associated with pregnancy, unspecified trimester** ♀ M

O91.12 **Abscess of breast associated with the puerperium** ♀ M
Puerperal mammary abscess
Puerperal purulent mastitis
Puerperal subareolar abscess

O91.13 **Abscess of breast associated with lactation** ♀ M
Mammary abscess associated with lactation
Purulent mastitis associated with lactation
Subareolar abscess associated with lactation

O91.2 Nonpurulent mastitis associated with pregnancy, the puerperium and lactation

O91.21 Nonpurulent mastitis associated with pregnancy
Gestational interstitial mastitis
Gestational lymphangitis of breast
Gestational mastitis NOS
Gestational parenchymatous mastitis

O91.211 **Nonpurulent mastitis associated with pregnancy, first trimester** ♀ M
O91.212 **Nonpurulent mastitis associated with pregnancy, second trimester** ♀ M
O91.213 **Nonpurulent mastitis associated with pregnancy, third trimester** ♀ M
O91.219 **Nonpurulent mastitis associated with pregnancy, unspecified trimester** ♀ M

O91.22 **Nonpurulent mastitis associated with the puerperium** ♀ M
Puerperal interstitial mastitis
Puerperal lymphangitis of breast
Puerperal mastitis NOS
Puerperal parenchymatous mastitis

O91.23 **Nonpurulent mastitis associated with lactation** ♀ M
Interstitial mastitis associated with lactation
Lymphangitis of breast associated with lactation
Mastitis NOS associated with lactation
Parenchymatous mastitis associated with lactation

O92 Other disorders of breast and disorders of lactation associated with pregnancy and the puerperium

O92.0 Retracted nipple associated with pregnancy, the puerperium, and lactation

O92.01 Retracted nipple associated with pregnancy

O92.011 **Retracted nipple associated with pregnancy, first trimester** ♀ M
O92.012 **Retracted nipple associated with pregnancy, second trimester** ♀ M
O92.013 **Retracted nipple associated with pregnancy, third trimester** ♀ M
O92.019 **Retracted nipple associated with pregnancy, unspecified trimester** ♀ M

O92.02 **Retracted nipple associated with the puerperium** ♀ M
O92.03 **Retracted nipple associated with lactation** ♀ M

O92.1 Cracked nipple associated with pregnancy, the puerperium, and lactation
Fissure of nipple, gestational or puerperal

O92.11 Cracked nipple associated with pregnancy

O92.111 **Cracked nipple associated with pregnancy, first trimester** ♀ M
O92.112 **Cracked nipple associated with pregnancy, second trimester** ♀ M
O92.113 **Cracked nipple associated with pregnancy, third trimester** ♀ M
O92.119 **Cracked nipple associated with pregnancy, unspecified trimester** ♀ M

O92.12 **Cracked nipple associated with the puerperium** ♀ M
O92.13 **Cracked nipple associated with lactation** ♀ M

O92.2 Other and unspecified disorders of breast associated with pregnancy and the puerperium

O92.20 **Unspecified disorder of breast associated with pregnancy and the puerperium** ♀ M
O92.29 **Other disorders of breast associated with pregnancy and the puerperium** ♀ M

O92.3 **Agalactia** ♀ M
Primary agalactia
Excludes1 elective agalactia (O92.5)
secondary agalactia (O92.5)
therapeutic agalactia (O92.5)

O92.4 **Hypogalactia** ♀ M

O92.5 **Suppressed lactation** ♀ M
Elective agalactia
Therapeutic agalactia
Secondary agalactia
Excludes1 primary agalactia (O92.3)

O92.6 **Galactorrhea** ♀ M

O92.7 Other and unspecified disorders of lactation

O92.70 **Unspecified disorders of lactation** ♀ M
O92.79 **Other disorders of lactation** ♀ M
Puerperal galactocele

OTHER OBSTETRIC CONDITIONS, NOT ELSEWHERE CLASSIFIED (O94-O9A)

O94 Sequelae of complication of pregnancy, childbirth, and the puerperium ♀ M
Note: This category is to be used to indicate conditions in O00-O77.-, O85-O94 and O98-O9A.- as the cause of late effects. The "sequelae" include conditions specified as such, or as late effects, which may occur at any time after the puerperium.
Code first condition resulting from (sequela) of complication of pregnancy, childbirth, and the puerperium

O98 Maternal infectious and parasitic diseases classifiable elsewhere but complicating pregnancy, childbirth and the puerperium

Includes the listed conditions when complicating the pregnant state, when aggravated by the pregnancy, or as a reason for obstetric care

Use additional code (Chapter 1), to identify specific infectious or parasitic disease

Excludes2 herpes gestationis (O26.4-)
infectious carrier state (O99.82-, O99.83-)
obstetrical tetanus (A34)
puerperal infection (O86.-)
puerperal sepsis (O85)
when the reason for maternal care is that the disease is known or suspected to have affected the fetus (O35-O36)

● O98.0 **Tuberculosis complicating pregnancy, childbirth and the puerperium**
Conditions in A15-A19

● O98.01 Tuberculosis complicating **pregnancy**
- O98.011 Tuberculosis complicating pregnancy, **first trimester** ♀ M
- O98.012 Tuberculosis complicating pregnancy, **second trimester** ♀ M
- O98.013 Tuberculosis complicating pregnancy, **third trimester** ♀ M
- O98.019 Tuberculosis complicating pregnancy, **unspecified trimester** ♀ M

O98.02 Tuberculosis complicating **childbirth** ♀ M

O98.03 Tuberculosis complicating the **puerperium** ♀ M

● O98.1 **Syphilis complicating pregnancy, childbirth and the puerperium**
Conditions in A50-A53

● O98.11 Syphilis complicating **pregnancy**
- O98.111 Syphilis complicating pregnancy, **first trimester** ♀ M
- O98.112 Syphilis complicating pregnancy, **second trimester** ♀ M
- O98.113 Syphilis complicating pregnancy, **third trimester** ♀ M
- O98.119 Syphilis complicating pregnancy, **unspecified trimester** ♀ M

O98.12 Syphilis complicating **childbirth** ♀ M

O98.13 Syphilis complicating the **puerperium** ♀ M

● O98.2 **Gonorrhea complicating pregnancy, childbirth and the puerperium**
Conditions in A54.-

● O98.21 Gonorrhea complicating **pregnancy**
- O98.211 Gonorrhea complicating pregnancy, **first trimester** ♀ M
- O98.212 Gonorrhea complicating pregnancy, **second trimester** ♀ M
- O98.213 Gonorrhea complicating pregnancy, **third trimester** ♀ M
- O98.219 Gonorrhea complicating pregnancy, **unspecified trimester** ♀ M

O98.22 Gonorrhea complicating **childbirth** ♀ M

O98.23 Gonorrhea complicating the **puerperium** ♀ M

● O98.3 **Other infections with a predominantly sexual mode of transmission complicating pregnancy, childbirth and the puerperium**
Conditions in A55-A64

● O98.31 Other infections with a predominantly sexual mode of transmission complicating **pregnancy**
- O98.311 Other infections with a predominantly sexual mode of transmission complicating pregnancy, **first trimester** ♀ M
- O98.312 Other infections with a predominantly sexual mode of transmission complicating pregnancy, **second trimester** ♀ M
- O98.313 Other infections with a predominantly sexual mode of transmission complicating pregnancy, **third trimester** ♀ M
- O98.319 Other infections with a predominantly sexual mode of transmission complicating pregnancy, **unspecified trimester** ♀ M

O98.32 Other infections with a predominantly sexual mode of transmission complicating **childbirth** ♀ M

O98.33 Other infections with a predominantly sexual mode of transmission complicating the **puerperium** ♀ M

● O98.4 **Viral hepatitis complicating pregnancy, childbirth and the puerperium**
Conditions in B15-B19

● O98.41 Viral hepatitis complicating **pregnancy**
- O98.411 Viral hepatitis complicating pregnancy, **first trimester** ♀ M
- O98.412 Viral hepatitis complicating pregnancy, **second trimester** ♀ M
- O98.413 Viral hepatitis complicating pregnancy, **third trimester** ♀ M
- O98.419 Viral hepatitis complicating pregnancy, **unspecified trimester** ♀ M

O98.42 Viral hepatitis complicating **childbirth** ♀ M

O98.43 Viral hepatitis complicating the **puerperium** ♀ M

● O98.5 **Other viral diseases complicating pregnancy, childbirth and the puerperium**
Conditions in A80-B09, B25-B34, R87.81-, R87.82-

Excludes:1 human immunodeficiency virus [HIV] disease complicating pregnancy, childbirth and the puerperium (O98.7-)

● O98.51 Other viral diseases complicating **pregnancy**
- O98.511 Other viral diseases complicating pregnancy, **first trimester** ♀ M
- O98.512 Other viral diseases complicating pregnancy, **second trimester** ♀ M
  Coding Clinic: 2016, Q4, P5-6
- O98.513 Other viral diseases complicating pregnancy, **third trimester** ♀ M
  Coding Clinic: 2016, Q4, P6
- O98.519 Other viral diseases complicating pregnancy, **unspecified trimester** ♀ M

O98.52 Other viral diseases complicating **childbirth** ♀ M

O98.53 Other viral diseases complicating the **puerperium** ♀ M

CHAPTER 15 (O00-O9A)

▶ New ▶ Revised ~~deleted~~ Deleted Excludes 1 Excludes 2 Includes Use additional Code first Code also Key words
OGCR Official Guidelines X Assign placeholder X ● Use Additional Character(s) Manifestation Code Hierarchical Condition Category Coding Clinic

● O98.6 **Protozoal diseases** complicating pregnancy, childbirth and the puerperium
Conditions in B5Ø-B64

● O98.61 Protozoal diseases complicating **pregnancy**
- O98.611 Protozoal diseases complicating pregnancy, **first trimester** ♀ M
- O98.612 Protozoal diseases complicating pregnancy, **second trimester** ♀ M
- O98.613 Protozoal diseases complicating pregnancy, **third trimester** ♀ M
- O98.619 Protozoal diseases complicating pregnancy, **unspecified trimester** ♀ M

O98.62 Protozoal diseases complicating **childbirth** ♀ M

O98.63 Protozoal diseases complicating the **puerperium** ♀ M

● O98.7 **Human immunodeficiency virus [HIV] disease** complicating pregnancy, childbirth and the puerperium
Use additional code to identify the type of HIV disease:
Acquired immune deficiency syndrome (AIDS) (B2Ø)
Asymptomatic HIV status (Z21)
HIV positive NOS (Z21)
Symptomatic HIV disease (B2Ø)

OGCR Section I.C.15.f.

HIV Infection in Pregnancy, Childbirth and the Puerperium

During pregnancy, childbirth or the puerperium, a patient admitted because of an HIV-related illness should receive a principal diagnosis from subcategory O98.7-, Human immunodeficiency [HIV] disease complicating pregnancy, childbirth and the puerperium, followed by the code(s) for the HIV-related illness(es).

Patients with asymptomatic HIV infection status admitted during pregnancy, childbirth, or the puerperium should receive codes of O98.7- and Z21, Asymptomatic human immunodeficiency virus [HIV] infection status.

● O98.71 Human immunodeficiency virus [HIV] disease complicating **pregnancy**
- O98.711 Human immunodeficiency virus [HIV] disease complicating pregnancy, **first trimester** ♀ M
- O98.712 Human immunodeficiency virus [HIV] disease complicating pregnancy, **second trimester** ♀ M
- O98.713 Human immunodeficiency virus [HIV] disease complicating pregnancy, **third trimester** ♀ M
- O98.719 Human immunodeficiency virus [HIV] disease complicating pregnancy, **unspecified trimester** ♀ M

O98.72 Human immunodeficiency virus [HIV] disease complicating **childbirth** ♀ M

O98.73 Human immunodeficiency virus [HIV] disease complicating the **puerperium** ♀ M

● O98.8 **Other maternal infectious** and parasitic diseases complicating pregnancy, childbirth and the puerperium

● O98.81 Other maternal infectious and parasitic diseases complicating **pregnancy**
- O98.811 Other maternal infectious and parasitic diseases complicating pregnancy, **first trimester** ♀ M
- O98.812 Other maternal infectious and parasitic diseases complicating pregnancy, **second trimester** ♀ M
- O98.813 Other maternal infectious and parasitic diseases complicating pregnancy, **third trimester** ♀ M
- O98.819 Other maternal infectious and parasitic diseases complicating pregnancy, **unspecified trimester** ♀ M

O98.82 Other maternal infectious and parasitic diseases complicating **childbirth** ♀ M

O98.83 Other maternal infectious and parasitic diseases complicating the **puerperium** ♀ M

● O98.9 **Unspecified maternal infectious and parasitic disease** complicating pregnancy, childbirth and the puerperium

● O98.91 **Unspecified** maternal infectious and parasitic disease complicating **pregnancy**
- O98.911 Unspecified maternal infectious and parasitic disease complicating pregnancy, **first trimester** ♀ M
- O98.912 Unspecified maternal infectious and parasitic disease complicating pregnancy, **second trimester** ♀ M
- O98.913 Unspecified maternal infectious and parasitic disease complicating pregnancy, **third trimester** ♀ M
- O98.919 Unspecified maternal infectious and parasitic disease complicating pregnancy, **unspecified trimester** ♀ M

O98.92 **Unspecified** maternal infectious and parasitic disease complicating **childbirth** ♀ M

O98.93 **Unspecified** maternal infectious and parasitic disease complicating the **puerperium** ♀ M

● O99 **Other maternal diseases** classifiable elsewhere but complicating pregnancy, childbirth and the puerperium

Includes: conditions which complicate the pregnant state, are aggravated by the pregnancy or are a main reason for obstetric care

Use additional code to identify specific condition

Excludes2 when the reason for maternal care is that the condition is known or suspected to have affected the fetus (O35-O36)

Coding Clinic: 2018, Q4, P8-9

● O99.Ø **Anemia** complicating pregnancy, childbirth and the puerperium
Conditions in D5Ø-D64

Excludes1 anemia arising in the puerperium (O9Ø.81)
postpartum anemia NOS (O9Ø.81)

● O99.Ø1 Anemia complicating **pregnancy**
- O99.Ø11 Anemia complicating pregnancy, **first trimester** ♀ M
- O99.Ø12 Anemia complicating pregnancy, **second trimester** ♀ M
- O99.Ø13 Anemia complicating pregnancy, **third trimester** ♀ M
- O99.Ø19 Anemia complicating pregnancy, **unspecified trimester** ♀ M

O99.Ø2 Anemia complicating **childbirth** ♀ M

O99.Ø3 Anemia complicating the **puerperium** ♀ M

Excludes1 postpartum anemia not pre-existing prior to delivery (O9Ø.81)

O99.1 Other diseases of the blood and blood-forming organs and certain disorders involving the immune mechanism complicating pregnancy, childbirth and the puerperium
Conditions in D65-D89
Excludes1 hemorrhage with coagulation defects (O45.-, O46.Ø-, O67.Ø, O72.3)

O99.11 Other diseases of the blood and blood-forming organs and certain disorders involving the immune mechanism complicating pregnancy

O99.111 Other diseases of the blood and blood-forming organs and certain disorders involving the immune mechanism complicating pregnancy, first trimester ♀ M

O99.112 Other diseases of the blood and blood-forming organs and certain disorders involving the immune mechanism complicating pregnancy, second trimester ♀ M

O99.113 Other diseases of the blood and blood-forming organs and certain disorders involving the immune mechanism complicating pregnancy, third trimester ♀ M

O99.119 Other diseases of the blood and blood-forming organs and certain disorders involving the immune mechanism complicating pregnancy, unspecified trimester ♀ M

O99.12 Other diseases of the blood and blood-forming organs and certain disorders involving the immune mechanism complicating childbirth ♀ M

O99.13 Other diseases of the blood and blood-forming organs and certain disorders involving the immune mechanism complicating the puerperium ♀ M

O99.2 Endocrine, nutritional and metabolic diseases complicating pregnancy, childbirth and the puerperium
Conditions in EØØ-E88
Excludes2 diabetes mellitus (O24.-)
malnutrition (O25.-)
postpartum thyroiditis (O9Ø.5)

O99.21 Obesity complicating pregnancy, childbirth, and the puerperium
Use additional code to identify the type of obesity (E66.-)

O99.21Ø Obesity complicating pregnancy, unspecified trimester ♀ M

O99.211 Obesity complicating pregnancy, first trimester ♀ M

O99.212 Obesity complicating pregnancy, second trimester ♀ M

O99.213 Obesity complicating pregnancy, third trimester ♀ M

O99.214 Obesity complicating childbirth ♀ M
Coding Clinic: 2018, Q4, P8Ø

O99.215 Obesity complicating the puerperium ♀ M

O99.28 Other endocrine, nutritional and metabolic diseases complicating pregnancy, childbirth and the puerperium

O99.28Ø Endocrine, nutritional and metabolic diseases complicating pregnancy, unspecified trimester ♀ M

O99.281 Endocrine, nutritional and metabolic diseases complicating pregnancy, first trimester ♀ M

O99.282 Endocrine, nutritional and metabolic diseases complicating pregnancy, second trimester ♀ M

O99.283 Endocrine, nutritional and metabolic diseases complicating pregnancy, third trimester ♀ M

O99.284 Endocrine, nutritional and metabolic diseases complicating childbirth ♀ M

O99.285 Endocrine, nutritional and metabolic diseases complicating the puerperium ♀ M

O99.3 Mental disorders and diseases of the nervous system complicating pregnancy, childbirth and the puerperium

O99.31 Alcohol use complicating pregnancy, childbirth, and the puerperium
Use additional code(s) from F1Ø to identify manifestations of the alcohol use

O99.31Ø Alcohol use complicating pregnancy, unspecified trimester ♀ M

O99.311 Alcohol use complicating pregnancy, first trimester ♀ M

O99.312 Alcohol use complicating pregnancy, second trimester ♀ M

O99.313 Alcohol use complicating pregnancy, third trimester ♀ M

O99.314 Alcohol use complicating childbirth ♀ M

O99.315 Alcohol use complicating the puerperium ♀ M

O99.32 Drug use complicating pregnancy, childbirth, and the puerperium
Use additional code(s) from F11-F16 and F18-F19 to identify manifestations of the drug use

O99.32Ø Drug use complicating pregnancy, unspecified trimester ♀ M

O99.321 Drug use complicating pregnancy, first trimester ♀ M

O99.322 Drug use complicating pregnancy, second trimester ♀ M

O99.323 Drug use complicating pregnancy, third trimester ♀ M

O99.324 Drug use complicating childbirth ♀ M

O99.325 Drug use complicating the puerperium ♀ M

O99.33 Tobacco use disorder complicating pregnancy, childbirth, and the puerperium
Smoking complicating pregnancy, childbirth, and the puerperium
Use additional code from category F17 to identify type of tobacco nicotine dependence

O99.33Ø Smoking (tobacco) complicating pregnancy, unspecified trimester ♀ M

O99.331 Smoking (tobacco) complicating pregnancy, first trimester ♀ M

O99.332 Smoking (tobacco) complicating pregnancy, second trimester ♀ M

O99.333 Smoking (tobacco) complicating pregnancy, third trimester ♀ M

O99.334 Smoking (tobacco) complicating childbirth ♀ M

O99.335 Smoking (tobacco) complicating the puerperium ♀ M

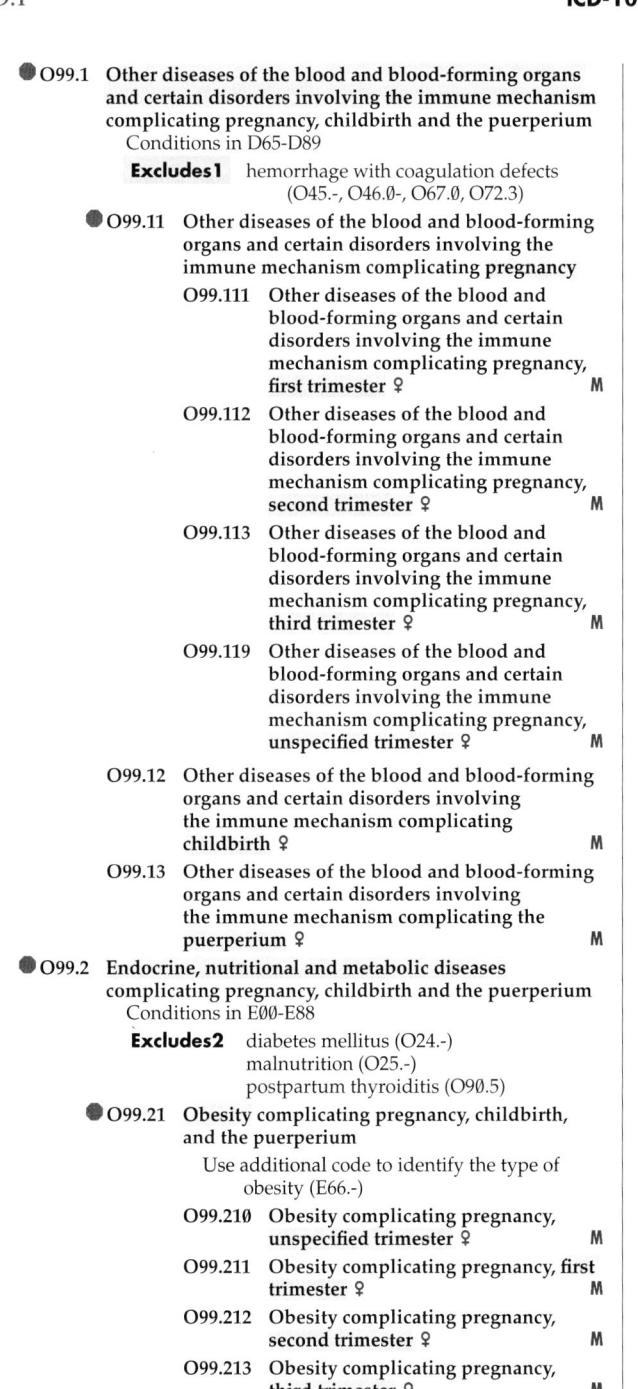

O99.34 Other mental disorders complicating pregnancy, childbirth, and the puerperium
Conditions in F01-F09, F20-F99 and F54-F99
Excludes2 postpartum mood disturbance (O90.6)
postnatal psychosis (F53.1)
puerperal psychosis (F53.1)
Coding Clinic: 2018, Q4, P9

O99.340 Other mental disorders complicating pregnancy, unspecified trimester ♀ M
O99.341 Other mental disorders complicating pregnancy, first trimester ♀ M
O99.342 Other mental disorders complicating pregnancy, second trimester ♀ M
O99.343 Other mental disorders complicating pregnancy, third trimester ♀ M
O99.344 Other mental disorders complicating childbirth ♀ M
O99.345 Other mental disorders complicating the puerperium ♀ M
Coding Clinic: 2018, Q4, P8-9

O99.35 Diseases of the nervous system complicating pregnancy, childbirth, and the puerperium
Conditions in G00-G99
Excludes2 pregnancy related peripheral neuritis (O26.8-)

O99.350 Diseases of the nervous system complicating pregnancy, unspecified trimester ♀ M
O99.351 Diseases of the nervous system complicating pregnancy, first trimester ♀ M
O99.352 Diseases of the nervous system complicating pregnancy, second trimester ♀ M
O99.353 Diseases of the nervous system complicating pregnancy, third trimester ♀ M
O99.354 Diseases of the nervous system complicating childbirth ♀ M
O99.355 Diseases of the nervous system complicating the puerperium ♀ M

O99.4 Diseases of the circulatory system complicating pregnancy, childbirth and the puerperium
Conditions in I00-I99
Excludes1 peripartum cardiomyopathy (O90.3)
Excludes2 hypertensive disorders (O10-O16)
obstetric embolism (O88.-)
venous complications and cerebrovenous sinus thrombosis in labor, childbirth and the puerperium (O87.-)
venous complications and cerebrovenous sinus thrombosis in pregnancy (O22.-)

O99.41 Diseases of the circulatory system complicating pregnancy
Coding Clinic: 2016, Q2, P8

O99.411 Diseases of the circulatory system complicating pregnancy, first trimester ♀ M
O99.412 Diseases of the circulatory system complicating pregnancy, second trimester ♀ M
O99.413 Diseases of the circulatory system complicating pregnancy, third trimester ♀ M
O99.419 Diseases of the circulatory system complicating pregnancy, unspecified trimester ♀ M

O99.42 Diseases of the circulatory system complicating childbirth ♀ M
O99.43 Diseases of the circulatory system complicating the puerperium ♀ M

O99.5 Diseases of the respiratory system complicating pregnancy, childbirth and the puerperium
Conditions in J00-J99

O99.51 Diseases of the respiratory system complicating pregnancy
O99.511 Diseases of the respiratory system complicating pregnancy, first trimester ♀ M
O99.512 Diseases of the respiratory system complicating pregnancy, second trimester ♀ M
O99.513 Diseases of the respiratory system complicating pregnancy, third trimester ♀ M
O99.519 Diseases of the respiratory system complicating pregnancy, unspecified trimester ♀ M

O99.52 Diseases of the respiratory system complicating childbirth ♀ M
O99.53 Diseases of the respiratory system complicating the puerperium ♀ M

O99.6 Diseases of the digestive system complicating pregnancy, childbirth and the puerperium
Conditions in K00-K93
Excludes2 hemorrhoids in pregnancy (O22.4-)
liver and biliary tract disorders in pregnancy, childbirth and the puerperium (O26.6-)

O99.61 Diseases of the digestive system complicating pregnancy
O99.611 Diseases of the digestive system complicating pregnancy, first trimester ♀ M
O99.612 Diseases of the digestive system complicating pregnancy, second trimester ♀ M
O99.613 Diseases of the digestive system complicating pregnancy, third trimester ♀ M
O99.619 Diseases of the digestive system complicating pregnancy, unspecified trimester ♀ M

O99.62 Diseases of the digestive system complicating childbirth ♀ M
O99.63 Diseases of the digestive system complicating the puerperium ♀ M

O99.7 Diseases of the skin and subcutaneous tissue complicating pregnancy, childbirth and the puerperium
Conditions in L00-L99
Excludes2 herpes gestationis (O26.4)
pruritic urticarial papules and plaques of pregnancy (PUPPP) (O26.86)

O99.71 Diseases of the skin and subcutaneous tissue complicating pregnancy
O99.711 Diseases of the skin and subcutaneous tissue complicating pregnancy, first trimester ♀ M
O99.712 Diseases of the skin and subcutaneous tissue complicating pregnancy, second trimester ♀ M
O99.713 Diseases of the skin and subcutaneous tissue complicating pregnancy, third trimester ♀ M
O99.719 Diseases of the skin and subcutaneous tissue complicating pregnancy, unspecified trimester ♀ M

O99.72 Diseases of the skin and subcutaneous tissue complicating childbirth ♀ M
O99.73 Diseases of the skin and subcutaneous tissue complicating the puerperium ♀ M

● O99.8 **Other specified diseases and conditions complicating pregnancy, childbirth and the puerperium**
Conditions in DØØ-D48, HØØ-H95, MØØ-N99, and QØØ-Q99
Use additional code to identify condition
Excludes2 genitourinary infections in pregnancy (O23.-)
infection of genitourinary tract following delivery (O86.1-O86.4)
malignant neoplasm complicating pregnancy, childbirth and the puerperium (O9A.1-)
maternal care for known or suspected abnormality of maternal pelvic organs (O34.-)
postpartum acute kidney failure (O9Ø.4)
traumatic injuries in pregnancy (O9A.2-)

● O99.81 **Abnormal glucose complicating pregnancy, childbirth and the puerperium**
Excludes1 gestational diabetes (O24.4-)
O99.81Ø **Abnormal glucose complicating pregnancy** ♀ M
O99.814 **Abnormal glucose complicating childbirth** ♀ M
O99.815 **Abnormal glucose complicating the puerperium** ♀ M

● O99.82 **Streptococcus B carrier state complicating pregnancy, childbirth and the puerperium**
Excludes1 Carrier of streptococcus group B (GBS) in a nonpregnant woman (Z22.33Ø)
O99.82Ø **Streptococcus B carrier state complicating pregnancy** ♀ M
O99.824 **Streptococcus B carrier state complicating childbirth** ♀ M
Coding Clinic: 2Ø19, Q2, P9
O99.825 **Streptococcus B carrier state complicating the puerperium** ♀ M

● O99.83 **Other infection carrier state complicating pregnancy, childbirth and the puerperium**
Use additional code to identify the carrier state (Z22.-)
O99.83Ø **Other infection carrier state complicating pregnancy** ♀ M
O99.834 **Other infection carrier state complicating childbirth** ♀ M
O99.835 **Other infection carrier state complicating the puerperium** ♀ M

● O99.84 **Bariatric surgery status complicating pregnancy, childbirth and the puerperium**
Gastric banding status complicating pregnancy, childbirth and the puerperium
Gastric bypass status for obesity complicating pregnancy, childbirth and the puerperium
Obesity surgery status complicating pregnancy, childbirth and the puerperium
O99.84Ø **Bariatric surgery status complicating pregnancy, unspecified trimester** ♀ M
O99.841 **Bariatric surgery status complicating pregnancy, first trimester** ♀ M
O99.842 **Bariatric surgery status complicating pregnancy, second trimester** ♀ M
O99.843 **Bariatric surgery status complicating pregnancy, third trimester** ♀ M
O99.844 **Bariatric surgery status complicating childbirth** ♀ M
O99.845 **Bariatric surgery status complicating the puerperium** ♀ M

O99.89 **Other specified diseases and conditions complicating pregnancy, childbirth and the puerperium** ♀ M

OGCR Section I.C.2.l.3.
Malignant neoplasm in a pregnant patient
When a pregnant woman has a malignant neoplasm, a code from subcategory O9A.1-, Malignant neoplasm complicating pregnancy, childbirth, and the puerperium, should be sequenced first, followed by the appropriate code from Chapter 2 to indicate the type of neoplasm.

● O9A **Maternal malignant neoplasms, traumatic injuries and abuse classifiable elsewhere but complicating pregnancy, childbirth and the puerperium**

● O9A.1 **Malignant neoplasm complicating pregnancy, childbirth and the puerperium**
Conditions in CØØ-C96
Use additional code to identify neoplasm
Excludes2 maternal care for benign tumor of corpus uteri (O34.1-)
maternal care for benign tumor of cervix (O34.4-)

● O9A.11 **Malignant neoplasm complicating pregnancy**
O9A.111 **Malignant neoplasm complicating pregnancy, first trimester** ♀ M
O9A.112 **Malignant neoplasm complicating pregnancy, second trimester** ♀ M
O9A.113 **Malignant neoplasm complicating pregnancy, third trimester** ♀ M
O9A.119 **Malignant neoplasm complicating pregnancy, unspecified trimester** ♀ M
O9A.12 **Malignant neoplasm complicating childbirth** ♀ M
O9A.13 **Malignant neoplasm complicating the puerperium** ♀ M
Coding Clinic: 2Ø15, Q3, P19

● O9A.2 **Injury, poisoning and certain other consequences of external causes complicating pregnancy, childbirth and the puerperium**
Conditions in SØØ-T88, except T74 and T76
Use additional code(s) to identify the injury or poisoning
Excludes2 physical, sexual and psychological abuse complicating pregnancy, childbirth and the puerperium (O9A.3-, O9A.4-, O9A.5-)

● O9A.21 **Injury, poisoning and certain other consequences of external causes complicating pregnancy**
O9A.211 **Injury, poisoning and certain other consequences of external causes complicating pregnancy, first trimester** ♀ M
O9A.212 **Injury, poisoning and certain other consequences of external causes complicating pregnancy, second trimester** ♀ M
O9A.213 **Injury, poisoning and certain other consequences of external causes complicating pregnancy, third trimester** ♀ M
O9A.219 **Injury, poisoning and certain other consequences of external causes complicating pregnancy, unspecified trimester** ♀ M
O9A.22 **Injury, poisoning and certain other consequences of external causes complicating childbirth** ♀ M
O9A.23 **Injury, poisoning and certain other consequences of external causes complicating the puerperium** ♀ M

● **O9A.3 Physical abuse complicating pregnancy, childbirth and the puerperium**
Conditions in T74.11 or T76.11

Use additional code (if applicable):
to identify any associated current injury due to physical abuse
to identify the perpetrator of abuse (Y07.-)

Excludes2 sexual abuse complicating pregnancy, childbirth and the puerperium (O9A.4)

● **O9A.31 Physical abuse complicating pregnancy**

O9A.311 Physical abuse complicating pregnancy, **first trimester** ♀ M

O9A.312 Physical abuse complicating pregnancy, **second trimester** ♀ M

O9A.313 Physical abuse complicating pregnancy, **third trimester** ♀ M

O9A.319 Physical abuse complicating pregnancy, **unspecified trimester** ♀ M

O9A.32 Physical abuse complicating **childbirth** ♀ M

O9A.33 Physical abuse complicating the **puerperium** ♀ M

● **O9A.4 Sexual abuse complicating pregnancy, childbirth and the puerperium**
Conditions in T74.21 or T76.21

Use additional code (if applicable):
to identify any associated current injury due to sexual abuse
to identify the perpetrator of abuse (Y07.-)

● **O9A.41 Sexual abuse complicating pregnancy**

O9A.411 Sexual abuse complicating pregnancy, **first trimester** ♀ M

O9A.412 Sexual abuse complicating pregnancy, **second trimester** ♀ M

O9A.413 Sexual abuse complicating pregnancy, **third trimester** ♀ M

O9A.419 Sexual abuse complicating pregnancy, **unspecified trimester** ♀ M

O9A.42 Sexual abuse complicating **childbirth** ♀ M

O9A.43 Sexual abuse complicating the **puerperium** ♀ M

● **O9A.5 Psychological abuse complicating pregnancy, childbirth and the puerperium**
Conditions in T74.31 or T76.31

Use additional code to identify the perpetrator of abuse (Y07.-)

● **O9A.51 Psychological abuse complicating pregnancy**

O9A.511 Psychological abuse complicating pregnancy, **first trimester** ♀ M

O9A.512 Psychological abuse complicating pregnancy, **second trimester** ♀ M

O9A.513 Psychological abuse complicating pregnancy, **third trimester** ♀ M

O9A.519 Psychological abuse complicating pregnancy, **unspecified trimester** ♀ M

O9A.52 Psychological abuse complicating **childbirth** ♀ M

O9A.53 Psychological abuse complicating the **puerperium** ♀ M

CHAPTER 15 (O0Ø-O9A)

CHAPTER 16

CERTAIN CONDITIONS ORIGINATING IN THE PERINATAL PERIOD (P00-P96)

OGCR Chapter-Specific Coding Guidelines

16. **Chapter 16: Certain Conditions Originating in the Perinatal Period (P00-P96)**

For coding and reporting purposes the perinatal period is defined as before birth through the 28th day following birth. The following guidelines are provided for reporting purposes

a. General Perinatal Rules

1) Use of Chapter 16 Codes

Codes in this chapter are <u>never</u> for use on the maternal record. Codes from Chapter 15, the obstetric chapter, are never permitted on the newborn record. Chapter 16 codes may be used throughout the life of the patient if the condition is still present.

2) Principal Diagnosis for Birth Record

When coding the birth episode in a newborn record, assign a code from category Z38, Liveborn infants according to place of birth and type of delivery, as the principal diagnosis. A code from category Z38 is assigned only once, to a newborn at the time of birth. If a newborn is transferred to another institution, a code from category Z38 should not be used at the receiving hospital.

A code from category Z38 is used only on the newborn record, not on the mother's record.

3) Use of Codes from other Chapters with Codes from Chapter 16

Codes from other chapters may be used with codes from chapter 16 if the codes from the other chapters provide more specific detail. Codes for signs and symptoms may be assigned when a definitive diagnosis has not been established. If the reason for the encounter is a perinatal condition, the code from Chapter 16 should be sequenced first.

4) Use of Chapter 16 Codes after the Perinatal Period

Should a condition originate in the perinatal period, and continue throughout the life of the patient, the perinatal code should continue to be used regardless of the patient's age.

5) Birth process or community acquired conditions

If a newborn has a condition that may be either due to the birth process or community acquired and the documentation does not indicate which it is, the default is due to the birth process and the code from Chapter 16 should be used. If the condition is community-acquired, a code from Chapter 16 should not be assigned.

6) Code all clinically significant conditions

All clinically significant conditions noted on routine newborn examination should be coded. A condition is clinically significant if it requires:

- clinical evaluation; or
- therapeutic treatment; or
- diagnostic procedures; or
- extended length of hospital stay; or
- increased nursing care and/or monitoring; or
- has implications for future health care needs

Note: The perinatal guidelines listed above are the same as the general coding guidelines for "additional diagnoses", except for the final point regarding implications for future health care needs. Codes should be assigned for conditions that have been specified by the provider as having implications for future health care needs.

b. Observation and Evaluation of Newborns for Suspected Conditions Not Found

1) Use of Z05 codes

Assign a code from category Z05, Observation and evaluation of newborns and infants for suspected conditions ruled out, to identify those instances when a healthy newborn is evaluated for a suspected condition that is determined after study not to be present. Do not use a code from category Z05 when the patient has identified signs or symptoms of a suspected problem; in such cases code the sign or symptom.

2) Z05 on Other than the Birth Record

A code from category Z05 may also be assigned as a principal or first-listed code for readmissions or encounters when the code from category Z38 code no longer applies. Codes from category Z05 are for use only for healthy newborns and infants for which no condition after study is found to be present.

3) Z05 on a birth record

A code from category Z05 is to be used as a secondary code after the code from category Z38, Liveborn infants according to place of birth and type of delivery.

c. Coding Additional Perinatal Diagnoses

1) Assigning codes for conditions that require treatment

Assign codes for conditions that require treatment or further investigation, prolong the length of stay, or require resource utilization.

2) Codes for conditions specified as having implications for future health care needs

Assign codes for conditions that have been specified by the provider as having implications for future health care needs.

Note: This guideline should not be used for adult patients.

d. Prematurity and Fetal Growth Retardation

Providers utilize different criteria in determining prematurity. A code for prematurity should not be assigned unless it is documented. Assignment of codes in categories P05, Disorders of newborn related to slow fetal growth and fetal malnutrition, and P07, Disorders of newborn related to short gestation and low birth weight, not elsewhere classified, should be based on the recorded birth weight and estimated gestational age.

When both birth weight and gestational age are available, two codes from category P07 should be assigned, with the code for birth weight sequenced before the code for gestational age.

e. Low birth weight and immaturity status

Codes from category P07, Disorders of newborn related to short gestation and low birth weight, not elsewhere classified, are for use for a child or adult who was premature or had a low birth weight as a newborn and this is affecting the patient's current health status.

See Section I.C.21. Factors influencing health status and contact with health services, Status.

f. Bacterial Sepsis of Newborn

Category P36, Bacterial sepsis of newborn, includes congenital sepsis. If a perinate is documented as having sepsis without documentation of congenital or community acquired, the default is congenital and a code from category P36 should be assigned. If the P36 code includes the causal organism, an additional code from category B95, Streptococcus, Staphylococcus, and Enterococcus as the cause of diseases classified elsewhere, or B96, Other bacterial agents as the cause of diseases classified elsewhere, should not be assigned. If the P36 code does not include the causal organism, assign an additional code from category B96. If applicable, use additional codes to identify severe sepsis (R65.2-) and any associated acute organ dysfunction.

g. Stillbirth

Code P95, Stillbirth, is only for use in institutions that maintain separate records for stillbirths. No other code should be used with P95. Code P95 should not be used on the mother's record.

CHAPTER 16

CERTAIN CONDITIONS ORIGINATING IN THE PERINATAL PERIOD (P00-P96)

Note: Codes from this chapter are for use on newborn records only, never on maternal records.

Includes	conditions that have their origin in the fetal or perinatal period (before birth through the first 28 days after birth) even if morbidity occurs later
Excludes2	congenital malformations, deformations and chromosomal abnormalities (Q00-Q99)
	endocrine, nutritional and metabolic diseases (E00-E88)
	injury, poisoning and certain other consequences of external causes (S00-T88)
	neoplasms (C00-D49)
	tetanus neonatorum (A33)

This chapter contains the following blocks:

P00-P04	Newborn affected by maternal factors and by complications of pregnancy, labor, and delivery
P05-P08	Disorders of newborns related to length of gestation and fetal growth
P09	Abnormal findings on neonatal screening
P10-P15	Birth trauma
P19-P29	Respiratory and cardiovascular disorders specific to the perinatal period
P35-P39	Infections specific to the perinatal period
P50-P61	Hemorrhagic and hematological disorders of newborn
P70-P74	Transitory endocrine and metabolic disorders specific to newborn
P76-P78	Digestive system disorders of newborn
P80-P83	Conditions involving the integument and temperature regulation of newborn
P84	Other problems with newborn
P90-P96	Other disorders originating in the perinatal period

NEWBORN AFFECTED BY MATERNAL FACTORS AND BY COMPLICATIONS OF PREGNANCY, LABOR, AND DELIVERY (P00–P04)

Note: These codes are for use when the listed maternal conditions are specified as the cause of confirmed morbidity or potential morbidity which have their origin in the perinatal period (before birth through the first 28 days after birth).

● **P00**   **Newborn affected by maternal conditions that may be unrelated to present pregnancy**

Code first any current condition in newborn

Excludes2	encounter for observation of newborn for suspected diseases and conditions ruled out (Z05.-)
	newborn affected by maternal complications of pregnancy (P01.-)
	newborn affected by maternal endocrine and metabolic disorders (P70–P74)
	newborn affected by noxious substances transmitted via placenta or breast milk (P04.-)

Coding Clinic: 2016, Q4, P54

P00.0   **Newborn affected by maternal hypertensive disorders**
Newborn affected by maternal conditions classifiable to O10-O11, O13-O16

P00.1   **Newborn affected by maternal renal and urinary tract diseases**
Newborn affected by maternal conditions classifiable to N00-N39

P00.2   **Newborn affected by maternal infectious and parasitic diseases**
Newborn affected by maternal infectious disease classifiable to A00-B99, J09 and J10

Excludes1	maternal genital tract or other localized infections (P00.8)
Excludes2	infections specific to the perinatal period (P35-P39)

Coding Clinic: 2019, Q2, P10; 2015, Q3, P21

P00.3   **Newborn affected by other maternal circulatory and respiratory diseases**
Newborn affected by maternal conditions classifiable to I00-I99, J00-J99, Q20-Q34 and not included in P00.0, P00.2

P00.4   **Newborn affected by maternal nutritional disorders**
Newborn affected by maternal disorders classifiable to E40-E64
Maternal malnutrition NOS

P00.5   **Newborn affected by maternal injury**
Newborn affected by maternal conditions classifiable to O9A.2-

P00.6   **Newborn affected by surgical procedure on mother**
Newborn affected by amniocentesis

Excludes1	Cesarean delivery for present delivery (P03.4)
	damage to placenta from amniocentesis, cesarean delivery or surgical induction (P02.1)
	previous surgery to uterus or pelvic organs (P03.89)
Excludes2	newborn affected by complication of (fetal) intrauterine procedure (P96.5)

P00.7   **Newborn affected by other medical procedures on mother, not elsewhere classified**
Newborn affected by radiation to mother

Excludes1	damage to placenta from amniocentesis, cesarean delivery or surgical induction (P02.1)
	newborn affected by other complications of labor and delivery (P03.-)

● **P00.8**   **Newborn affected by other maternal conditions**

P00.81   **Newborn affected by periodontal disease in mother**

P00.89   **Newborn affected by other maternal conditions**
Newborn affected by conditions classifiable to T80-T88
Newborn affected by maternal genital tract or other localized infections
Newborn affected by maternal systemic lupus erythematosus
Coding Clinic: 2019, Q2, P9

P00.9   **Newborn affected by unspecified maternal condition**

● **P01**   **Newborn affected by maternal complications of pregnancy**

Code first any current condition in newborn

Excludes2	encounter for observation of newborn for suspected diseases and conditions ruled out (Z05.-)

Coding Clinic: 2016, Q4, P54

P01.0   **Newborn affected by incompetent cervix**

P01.1   **Newborn affected by premature rupture of membranes**

P01.2   **Newborn affected by oligohydramnios**

Excludes1	oligohydramnios due to premature rupture of membranes (P01.1)

P01.3   **Newborn affected by polyhydramnios**
Excess of amniotic fluid, usually > 2000 mL
Newborn affected by hydramnios

P01.4   **Newborn affected by ectopic pregnancy**
Newborn affected by abdominal pregnancy

P01.5   **Newborn affected by multiple pregnancy**
Newborn affected by triplet (pregnancy)
Newborn affected by twin (pregnancy)

P01.6   **Newborn affected by maternal death**

P01.7   **Newborn affected by malpresentation before labor**
Newborn affected by breech presentation before labor
Newborn affected by external version before labor
Newborn affected by face presentation before labor
Newborn affected by transverse lie before labor
Newborn affected by unstable lie before labor

P01.8   **Newborn affected by other maternal complications of pregnancy**

P01.9   **Newborn affected by maternal complication of pregnancy, unspecified**

CHAPTER 16 (P00-P96)

P02 Newborn affected by complications of placenta, cord and membranes

Code first any current condition in newborn

Excludes2 encounter for observation of newborn for suspected diseases and conditions ruled out (Z05.-)

Coding Clinic: 2016, Q4, P54

P02.0 Newborn affected by placenta previa

P02.1 Newborn affected by other forms of placental separation and hemorrhage

Newborn affected by abruptio placenta
Newborn affected by accidental hemorrhage
Newborn affected by antepartum hemorrhage
Newborn affected by damage to placenta from amniocentesis, cesarean delivery or surgical induction
Newborn affected by maternal blood loss
Newborn affected by premature separation of placenta

P02.2 Newborn affected by other and unspecified morphological and functional abnormalities of placenta

P02.20 Newborn affected by unspecified morphological and functional abnormalities of placenta

P02.29 Newborn affected by other morphological and functional abnormalities of placenta

Newborn affected by placental dysfunction
Newborn affected by placental infarction
Newborn affected by placental insufficiency

P02.3 Newborn affected by placental transfusion syndromes

Newborn affected by placental and cord abnormalities resulting in twin-to-twin or other transplacental transfusion

P02.4 Newborn affected by prolapsed cord

P02.5 Newborn affected by other compression of umbilical cord

Newborn affected by umbilical cord (tightly) around neck
Newborn affected by entanglement of umbilical cord
Newborn affected by knot in umbilical cord

P02.6 Newborn affected by other and unspecified conditions of umbilical cord

P02.60 Newborn affected by unspecified conditions of umbilical cord

P02.69 Newborn affected by other conditions of umbilical cord

Newborn affected by short umbilical cord
Newborn affected by vasa previa

Excludes1 newborn affected by single umbilical artery (Q27.0)

P02.7 Newborn affected by chorioamnionitis

Inflammation of chorion and amnion

P02.70 Newborn affected by fetal inflammatory response syndrome HCC

Newborn affected by FIRS

P02.78 Newborn affected by other conditions from chorioamnionitis

Newborn affected by amnionitis
Newborn affected by membranitis
Newborn affected by placentitis

P02.8 Newborn affected by other abnormalities of membranes

P02.9 Newborn affected by abnormality of membranes, unspecified

P03 Newborn affected by other complications of labor and delivery

Code first any current condition in newborn

Excludes2 encounter for observation of newborn for suspected diseases and conditions ruled out (Z05.-)

Coding Clinic: 2016, Q4, P54

P03.0 Newborn affected by breech delivery and extraction

P03.1 Newborn affected by other malpresentation, malposition and disproportion during labor and delivery

Newborn affected by contracted pelvis
Newborn affected by conditions classifiable to O64-O66
Newborn affected by persistent occipitoposterior
Newborn affected by transverse lie

P03.2 Newborn affected by forceps delivery

P03.3 Newborn affected by delivery by vacuum extractor [ventouse]

P03.4 Newborn affected by Cesarean delivery

P03.5 Newborn affected by precipitate delivery

Newborn affected by rapid second stage

P03.6 Newborn affected by abnormal uterine contractions

Newborn affected by conditions classifiable to O62.-, except O62.3
Newborn affected by hypertonic labor
Newborn affected by uterine inertia

P03.8 Newborn affected by other specified complications of labor and delivery

P03.81 Newborn affected by abnormality in fetal (intrauterine) heart rate or rhythm

Excludes1 neonatal cardiac dysrhythmia (P29.1-)

P03.810 Newborn affected by abnormality in fetal (intrauterine) heart rate or rhythm before the onset of labor

P03.811 Newborn affected by abnormality in fetal (intrauterine) heart rate or rhythm during labor

P03.819 Newborn affected by abnormality in fetal (intrauterine) heart rate or rhythm, unspecified as to time of onset

P03.82 Meconium passage during delivery

Excludes1 meconium aspiration (P24.00, P24.01)
meconium staining (P96.83)

P03.89 Newborn affected by other specified complications of labor and delivery

Newborn affected by abnormality of maternal soft tissues
Newborn affected by conditions classifiable to O60-O75 and by procedures used in labor and delivery not included in P02.- and P03.0-P03.6
Newborn affected by induction of labor

P03.9 Newborn affected by complication of labor and delivery, unspecified

CHAPTER 16 (P00-P96)

P04 Newborn affected by noxious substances transmitted via placenta or breast milk

Includes nonteratogenic effects of substances transmitted via placenta

Excludes2 congenital malformations (Q00-Q99)
encounter for observation of newborn for suspected diseases and conditions ruled out (Z05.-)
neonatal jaundice from excessive hemolysis due to drugs or toxins transmitted from mother (P58.4)
newborn in contact with and (suspected) exposures hazardous to health not transmitted via placenta or breast milk (Z77.-)

Coding Clinic: 2016, Q4, P54

P04.0 Newborn affected by maternal anesthesia and analgesia in pregnancy, labor and delivery
Newborn affected by reactions and intoxications from maternal opiates and tranquilizers administered for procedures during pregnancy or labor and delivery

Excludes2 newborn affected by other maternal medication (P04.1-)

P04.1 Newborn affected by other maternal medication
Code first withdrawal symptoms from maternal use of drugs of addiction, if applicable (P96.1)

Excludes1 dysmorphism due to warfarin (Q86.2)
fetal hydantoin syndrome (Q86.1)

Excludes2 maternal anesthesia and analgesia in pregnancy, labor and delivery (P04.0)
maternal use of drugs of addiction (P04.4-)

P04.11 Newborn affected by maternal antineoplastic chemotherapy

P04.12 Newborn affected by maternal cytotoxic drugs

P04.13 Newborn affected by maternal use of anticonvulsants

P04.14 Newborn affected by maternal use of opiates

P04.15 Newborn affected by maternal use of antidepressants

P04.16 Newborn affected by maternal use of amphetamines

P04.17 Newborn affected by maternal use of sedative-hypnotics

P04.1A Newborn affected by maternal use of anxiolytics

P04.18 Newborn affected by other maternal medication

P04.19 Newborn affected by maternal use of unspecified medication

Coding Clinic: 2016, Q4, P55

P04.2 Newborn affected by maternal use of tobacco
Newborn affected by exposure in utero to tobacco smoke

Excludes2 newborn exposure to environmental tobacco smoke (P96.81)

P04.3 Newborn affected by maternal use of alcohol

Excludes1 fetal alcohol syndrome (Q86.0)

P04.4 Newborn affected by maternal use of drugs of addiction

P04.40 Newborn affected by maternal use of unspecified drugs of addiction

P04.41 Newborn affected by maternal use of cocaine
~~"Crack baby"~~

P04.42 Newborn affected by maternal use of hallucinogens

Excludes2 newborn affected by other maternal medication (P04.1-)

P04.49 Newborn affected by maternal use of other drugs of addiction

Excludes2 newborn affected by maternal anesthesia and analgesia (P04.0)
withdrawal symptoms from maternal use of drugs of addiction (P96.1)

P04.5 Newborn affected by maternal use of nutritional chemical substances

P04.6 Newborn affected by maternal exposure to environmental chemical substances

P04.8 Newborn affected by other maternal noxious substances

P04.81 Newborn affected by maternal use of cannabis

P04.89 Newborn affected by other maternal noxious substances

P04.9 Newborn affected by maternal noxious substance, unspecified

OGCR Section I.C.16.d.

Prematurity and Fetal Growth Retardation

Providers utilize different criteria in determining prematurity. A code for prematurity should not be assigned unless it is documented. Assignment of codes in categories P05, Disorders of newborn related to slow fetal growth and fetal malnutrition, and P07, Disorders of newborn related to short gestation and low birth weight, not elsewhere classified, should be based on the recorded birth weight and estimated gestational age.

When both birth weight and gestational age are available, two codes from category P07 should be assigned, with the code for birth weight sequenced before the code for gestational age.

DISORDERS OF NEWBORN RELATED TO LENGTH OF GESTATION AND FETAL GROWTH (P05-P08)

P05 Disorders of newborn related to slow fetal growth and fetal malnutrition

Coding Clinic: 2016, Q4, P56

P05.0 Newborn light for gestational age
Newborn light-for-dates
Weight below but length above 10th percentile for gestational age

P05.00 Newborn light for gestational age, unspecified weight

P05.01 Newborn light for gestational age, less than 500 grams

P05.02 Newborn light for gestational age, 500-749 grams

P05.03 Newborn light for gestational age, 750-999 grams

P05.04 Newborn light for gestational age, 1000-1249 grams

P05.05 Newborn light for gestational age, 1250-1499 grams

P05.06 Newborn light for gestational age, 1500-1749 grams

P05.07 Newborn light for gestational age, 1750-1999 grams

P05.08 Newborn light for gestational age, 2000-2499 grams

P05.09 Newborn light for gestational age, 2500 grams and over
Newborn light for gestational age, other
Coding Clinic: 2016, Q4, P55

● **P05.1 Newborn small for gestational age**
Newborn small-and-light-for-dates
Newborn small-for-dates
Weight and length below 10th percentile for gestational age

P05.10 Newborn small for gestational age, unspecified weight

P05.11 Newborn small for gestational age, less than 500 grams

P05.12 Newborn small for gestational age, 500-749 grams

P05.13 Newborn small for gestational age, 750-999 grams

P05.14 Newborn small for gestational age, 1000-1249 grams

P05.15 Newborn small for gestational age, 1250-1499 grams

P05.16 Newborn small for gestational age, 1500-1749 grams

P05.17 Newborn small for gestational age, 1750-1999 grams

P05.18 Newborn small for gestational age, 2000-2499 grams

P05.19 Newborn small for gestational age, other
Newborn small for gestational age, 2500 grams and over
Coding Clinic: 2016, Q4, P55

P05.2 Newborn affected by fetal (intrauterine) malnutrition not light or small for gestational age
Infant, not light or small for gestational age, showing signs of fetal malnutrition, such as dry, peeling skin and loss of subcutaneous tissue
Excludes1 newborn affected by fetal malnutrition with light for gestational age (P05.0-)
newborn affected by fetal malnutrition with small for gestational age (P05.1-)

P05.9 Newborn affected by slow intrauterine growth, unspecified
Newborn affected by fetal growth retardation NOS

● **P07 Disorders of newborn related to short gestation and low birth weight, not elsewhere classified**
Note: When both birth weight and gestational age of the newborn are available, both should be coded with birth weight sequenced before gestational age.
Includes the listed conditions, without further specification, as the cause of morbidity or additional care, in newborn

● **P07.0 Extremely low birth weight newborn**
Newborn birth weight 999 g. or less
Excludes1 low birth weight due to slow fetal growth and fetal malnutrition (P05.-)

P07.00 Extremely low birth weight newborn, unspecified weight

P07.01 Extremely low birth weight newborn, less than 500 grams

P07.02 Extremely low birth weight newborn, 500-749 grams

P07.03 Extremely low birth weight newborn, 750-999 grams

● **P07.1 Other low birth weight newborn**
Newborn birth weight 1000-2499 g.
Excludes1 low birth weight due to slow fetal growth and fetal malnutrition (P05.-)

P07.10 Other low birth weight newborn, unspecified weight

P07.14 Other low birth weight newborn, 1000-1249 grams

P07.15 Other low birth weight newborn, 1250-1499 grams

P07.16 Other low birth weight newborn, 1500-1749 grams

P07.17 Other low birth weight newborn, 1750-1999 grams

P07.18 Other low birth weight newborn, 2000-2499 grams

● **P07.2 Extreme immaturity of newborn**
Less than 28 completed weeks (less than 196 completed days) of gestation

P07.20 Extreme immaturity of newborn, unspecified weeks of gestation
Gestational age less than 28 completed weeks NOS

P07.21 Extreme immaturity of newborn, gestational age less than 23 completed weeks
Extreme immaturity of newborn, gestational age less than 23 weeks, 0 days

P07.22 Extreme immaturity of newborn, gestational age 23 completed weeks
Extreme immaturity of newborn, gestational age 23 weeks, 0 days through 23 weeks, 6 days

P07.23 Extreme immaturity of newborn, gestational age 24 completed weeks
Extreme immaturity of newborn, gestational age 24 weeks, 0 days through 24 weeks, 6 days

P07.24 Extreme immaturity of newborn, gestational age 25 completed weeks
Extreme immaturity of newborn, gestational age 25 weeks, 0 days through 25 weeks, 6 days

P07.25 Extreme immaturity of newborn, gestational age 26 completed weeks
Extreme immaturity of newborn, gestational age 26 weeks, 0 days through 26 weeks, 6 days

P07.26 Extreme immaturity of newborn, gestational age 27 completed weeks
Extreme immaturity of newborn, gestational age 27 weeks, 0 days through 27 weeks, 6 days

● **P07.3 Preterm [premature] newborn [other]**
28 completed weeks or more but less than 37 completed weeks (196 completed days but less than 259 completed days) of gestation
Prematurity NOS

P07.30 Preterm newborn, unspecified weeks of gestation

P07.31 Preterm newborn, gestational age 28 completed weeks
Preterm newborn, gestational age 28 weeks, 0 days through 28 weeks, 6 days

P07.32 Preterm newborn, gestational age 29 completed weeks
Preterm newborn, gestational age 29 weeks, 0 days through 29 weeks, 6 days

P07.33 Preterm newborn, gestational age 30 completed weeks
Preterm newborn, gestational age 30 weeks, 0 days through 30 weeks, 6 days

P07.34 Preterm newborn, gestational age 31 completed weeks
Preterm newborn, gestational age 31 weeks, 0 days through 31 weeks, 6 days

P07.35 Preterm newborn, gestational age 32 completed weeks
Preterm newborn, gestational age 32 weeks, 0 days through 32 weeks, 6 days

P07.36 Preterm newborn, gestational age 33 completed weeks
Preterm newborn, gestational age 33 weeks, 0 days through 33 weeks, 6 days

P07.37 Preterm newborn, gestational age 34 completed weeks
Preterm newborn, gestational age 34 weeks, 0 days through 34 weeks, 6 days
Coding Clinic: 2017, Q2, P7

P07.38 Preterm newborn, gestational age 35 completed weeks
Preterm newborn, gestational age 35 weeks, 0 days through 35 weeks, 6 days

P07.39 Preterm newborn, gestational age 36 completed weeks
Preterm newborn, gestational age 36 weeks, 0 days through 36 weeks, 6 days
Coding Clinic: 2017, Q3, P26

P08 Disorders of newborn related to long gestation and high birth weight
Note: When both birth weight and gestational age of the newborn are available, priority of assignment should be given to birth weight.
Includes the listed conditions, without further specification, as causes of morbidity or additional care, in newborn

P08.0 Exceptionally large newborn baby
Usually implies a birth weight of 4500 g. or more
Excludes1 syndrome of infant of diabetic mother (P70.1)
syndrome of infant of mother with gestational diabetes (P70.0)

P08.1 Other heavy for gestational age newborn
Other newborn heavy- or large-for-dates regardless of period of gestation
Usually implies a birth weight of 4000 g. to 4499 g.
Excludes1 newborn with a birth weight of 4500 or more (P08.0)
syndrome of infant of diabetic mother (P70.1)
syndrome of infant of mother with gestational diabetes (P70.0)

P08.2 Late newborn, not heavy for gestational age

P08.21 Post-term newborn
Newborn with gestation period over 40 completed weeks to 42 completed weeks

P08.22 Prolonged gestation of newborn
Newborn with gestation period over 42 completed weeks (294 days or more), not heavy- or large-for-dates
Postmaturity NOS

ABNORMAL FINDINGS ON NEONATAL SCREENING (P09)

P09 Abnormal findings on neonatal screening
Use additional code to identify signs, symptoms and conditions associated with the screening
Excludes2 nonspecific serologic evidence of human immunodeficiency virus [HIV] (R75)

BIRTH TRAUMA (P10-P15)

P10 Intracranial laceration and hemorrhage due to birth injury
Excludes1 intracranial hemorrhage of newborn NOS (P52.9)
intracranial hemorrhage of newborn due to anoxia or hypoxia (P52.-)
nontraumatic intracranial hemorrhage of newborn (P52.-)

P10.0 Subdural hemorrhage due to birth injury
Subdural hematoma (localized) due to birth injury
Excludes1 subdural hemorrhage accompanying tentorial tear (P10.4)

P10.1 Cerebral hemorrhage due to birth injury

P10.2 Intraventricular hemorrhage due to birth injury

P10.3 Subarachnoid hemorrhage due to birth injury

P10.4 Tentorial tear due to birth injury
Pertaining to tentorium of cerebellum (extension of dura mater that separates cerebellum from inferior portion of occipital lobes)

P10.8 Other intracranial lacerations and hemorrhages due to birth injury

P10.9 Unspecified intracranial laceration and hemorrhage due to birth injury

P11 Other birth injuries to central nervous system

P11.0 Cerebral edema due to birth injury

P11.1 Other specified brain damage due to birth injury

P11.2 Unspecified brain damage due to birth injury

P11.3 Birth injury to facial nerve
Facial palsy due to birth injury

P11.4 Birth injury to other cranial nerves

P11.5 Birth injury to spine and spinal cord
Fracture of spine due to birth injury

P11.9 Birth injury to central nervous system, unspecified

P12 Birth injury to scalp

P12.0 Cephalhematoma due to birth injury

P12.1 Chignon (from vacuum extraction) due to birth injury

P12.2 Epicranial subaponeurotic hemorrhage due to birth injury
Subgaleal hemorrhage

P12.3 Bruising of scalp due to birth injury

P12.4 Injury of scalp of newborn due to monitoring equipment
Sampling incision of scalp of newborn
Scalp clip (electrode) injury of newborn

P12.8 Other birth injuries to scalp

P12.81 Caput succedaneum

P12.89 Other birth injuries to scalp

P12.9 Birth injury to scalp, unspecified

P13 Birth injury to skeleton
Excludes2 birth injury to spine (P11.5)

P13.0 Fracture of skull due to birth injury

P13.1 Other birth injuries to skull
Excludes1 cephalhematoma (P12.0)

P13.2 Birth injury to femur

P13.3 Birth injury to other long bones

P13.4 Fracture of clavicle due to birth injury

P13.8 Birth injuries to other parts of skeleton

P13.9 Birth injury to skeleton, unspecified

P14 Birth injury to peripheral nervous system

P14.0 Erb's paralysis due to birth injury

P14.1 Klumpke's paralysis due to birth injury

P14.2 Phrenic nerve paralysis due to birth injury

P14.3 Other brachial plexus birth injuries

P14.8 Birth injuries to other parts of peripheral nervous system

P14.9 Birth injury to peripheral nervous system, unspecified

Item 16–1 The **peripheral nervous system** consists of 31 pairs of spinal nerves, 12 pairs of cranial nerves, and the autonomic nerves, which are divided into the parasympathetic and sympathetic nerves. The cranial nerves are: olfactory (I), optic (II), oculomotor (III), trochlear (IV), trigeminal (V), abducens (VI), facial (VII), vestibulocochlear (VIII), glossopharyngeal (IX), vagus (X), accessory (XI), and hypoglossal (XII).

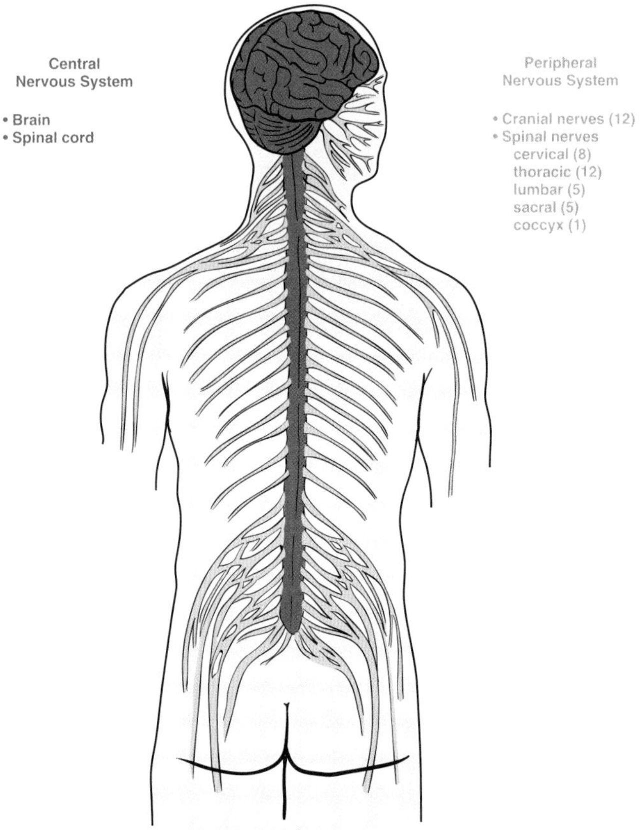

Figure 16-1 The central nervous system consists of the brain and spinal cord. The peripheral nervous system consists of nerves that lie outside the skull and spinal cord. (From Stoy: Mosby's EMT-Basic Textbook, ed 2, St. Louis, Mosby, 2007)

● **P15** Other birth injuries
- **P15.Ø** **Birth injury to liver**
  - Rupture of liver due to birth injury
- **P15.1** **Birth injury to spleen**
  - Rupture of spleen due to birth injury
- **P15.2** **Sternomastoid injury due to birth injury**
- **P15.3** **Birth injury to eye**
  - Subconjunctival hemorrhage due to birth injury
  - Traumatic glaucoma due to birth injury
- **P15.4** **Birth injury to face**
  - Facial congestion due to birth injury
- **P15.5** **Birth injury to external genitalia**
- **P15.6** **Subcutaneous fat necrosis due to birth injury**
- **P15.8** **Other specified birth injuries**
- **P15.9** **Birth injury, unspecified**

RESPIRATORY AND CARDIOVASCULAR DISORDERS SPECIFIC TO THE PERINATAL PERIOD (P19-P29)

● **P19** Metabolic acidemia in newborn
- **Includes** metabolic acidemia in newborn
- **P19.Ø** **Metabolic acidemia in newborn first noted before onset of labor**
- **P19.1** **Metabolic acidemia in newborn first noted during labor**
- **P19.2** **Metabolic acidemia noted at birth**
- **P19.9** **Metabolic acidemia, unspecified**

● **P22** Respiratory distress of newborn
- ~~**Excludes1** respiratory arrest of newborn (P28.81)~~
  - ~~respiratory failure of newborn NOS (P28.5)~~
- Coding Clinic: 2019, Q2, P29
- **P22.Ø** **Respiratory distress syndrome of newborn**
  - Cardiorespiratory distress syndrome of newborn
  - Hyaline membrane disease
  - Idiopathic respiratory distress syndrome [IRDS or RDS] of newborn
  - Pulmonary hypoperfusion syndrome
  - Respiratory distress syndrome, type I
  - ▶ **Excludes2** respiratory arrest of newborn (P28.81)
    - ▶respiratory failure of newborn NOS (P28.5)
  - Coding Clinic: 2019, Q2, P29
- **P22.1** **Transient tachypnea of newborn**
  - Idiopathic tachypnea of newborn
  - Respiratory distress syndrome, type II
  - Wet lung syndrome
- **P22.8** **Other respiratory distress of newborn**
  - ▶ **Excludes1** respiratory arrest of newborn (P28.81)
    - ▶respiratory failure of newborn NOS (P28.5)
- **P22.9** **Respiratory distress of newborn, unspecified**
  - ▶ **Excludes1** respiratory arrest of newborn (P28.81)
    - ▶respiratory failure of newborn NOS (P28.5)

● **P23** Congenital pneumonia
- **Includes** infective pneumonia acquired in utero or during birth
- **Excludes1** neonatal pneumonia resulting from aspiration (P24.-)
- **P23.Ø** **Congenital pneumonia due to viral agent**
  - Use additional code (B97) to identify organism
  - **Excludes1** congenital rubella pneumonitis (P35.Ø)
- **P23.1** **Congenital pneumonia due to Chlamydia**
- **P23.2** **Congenital pneumonia due to staphylococcus**
- **P23.3** **Congenital pneumonia due to streptococcus, group B**
- **P23.4** **Congenital pneumonia due to Escherichia coli**
- **P23.5** **Congenital pneumonia due to Pseudomonas**
- **P23.6** **Congenital pneumonia due to other bacterial agents**
  - Congenital pneumonia due to Hemophilus influenzae
  - Congenital pneumonia due to Klebsiella pneumoniae
  - Congenital pneumonia due to Mycoplasma
  - Congenital pneumonia due to Streptococcus, except group B
  - Use additional code (B95-B96) to identify organism
- **P23.8** **Congenital pneumonia due to other organisms**
- **P23.9** **Congenital pneumonia, unspecified**

P24 Neonatal aspiration
Includes aspiration in utero and during delivery

P24.0 **Meconium aspiration**
Excludes1 meconium passage (without aspiration) during delivery (P03.82)
meconium staining (P96.83)

P24.00 **Meconium aspiration without respiratory symptoms**
Meconium aspiration NOS

P24.01 **Meconium aspiration with respiratory symptoms**
Meconium aspiration pneumonia
Meconium aspiration pneumonitis
Meconium aspiration syndrome NOS
Use additional code to identify any secondary pulmonary hypertension, if applicable (I27.2-)

P24.1 Neonatal aspiration of (clear) **amniotic fluid and mucus**
Neonatal aspiration of liquor (amnii)

P24.10 **Neonatal aspiration of (clear) amniotic fluid and mucus without respiratory symptoms**
Neonatal aspiration of amniotic fluid and mucus NOS

P24.11 **Neonatal aspiration of (clear) amniotic fluid and mucus with respiratory symptoms**
Neonatal aspiration of amniotic fluid and mucus with pneumonia
Neonatal aspiration of amniotic fluid and mucus with pneumonitis
Use additional code to identify any secondary pulmonary hypertension, if applicable (I27.2-)

P24.2 Neonatal aspiration of **blood**

P24.20 **Neonatal aspiration of blood without respiratory symptoms**
Neonatal aspiration of blood NOS

P24.21 **Neonatal aspiration of blood with respiratory symptoms**
Neonatal aspiration of blood with pneumonia
Neonatal aspiration of blood with pneumonitis
Use additional code to identify any secondary pulmonary hypertension, if applicable (I27.2-)

P24.3 **Neonatal aspiration of milk and regurgitated food**
Neonatal aspiration of stomach contents

P24.30 **Neonatal aspiration of milk and regurgitated food without respiratory symptoms**
Neonatal aspiration of milk and regurgitated food NOS

P24.31 **Neonatal aspiration of milk and regurgitated food with respiratory symptoms**
Neonatal aspiration of milk and regurgitated food with pneumonia
Neonatal aspiration of milk and regurgitated food with pneumonitis
Use additional code to identify any secondary pulmonary hypertension, if applicable (I27.2-)

P24.8 Other neonatal aspiration

P24.80 **Other neonatal aspiration without respiratory symptoms**
Neonatal aspiration NEC

P24.81 **Other neonatal aspiration with respiratory symptoms**
Neonatal aspiration pneumonia NEC
Neonatal aspiration with pneumonitis NEC
Neonatal aspiration with pneumonia NOS
Neonatal aspiration with pneumonitis NOS
Use additional code to identify any secondary pulmonary hypertension, if applicable (I27.2-)

P24.9 Neonatal aspiration, **unspecified**

P25 Interstitial emphysema and related conditions originating in the perinatal period

P25.0 **Interstitial emphysema originating in the perinatal period**

P25.1 **Pneumothorax originating in the perinatal period**

P25.2 **Pneumomediastinum originating in the perinatal period**

P25.3 **Pneumopericardium originating in the perinatal period**

P25.8 **Other conditions related to interstitial emphysema originating in the perinatal period**

P26 Pulmonary hemorrhage originating in the perinatal period
Excludes1 acute idiopathic hemorrhage in infants over 28 days old (R04.81)

P26.0 **Tracheobronchial hemorrhage originating in the perinatal period**

P26.1 **Massive pulmonary hemorrhage originating in the perinatal period**

P26.8 **Other pulmonary hemorrhages originating in the perinatal period**

P26.9 **Unspecified pulmonary hemorrhage originating in the perinatal period**

P27 Chronic respiratory disease originating in the perinatal period
Excludes2 respiratory distress of newborn (P22.0-P22.9)

P27.0 **Wilson-Mikity syndrome**
Pulmonary dysmaturity

P27.1 **Bronchopulmonary dysplasia originating in the perinatal period**

P27.8 **Other chronic respiratory diseases originating in the perinatal period**
Congenital pulmonary fibrosis
Ventilator lung in newborn

P27.9 **Unspecified chronic respiratory disease originating in the perinatal period**

P28 Other respiratory conditions originating in the perinatal period
Excludes1 congenital malformations of the respiratory system (Q30-Q34)

P28.0 **Primary atelectasis of newborn**
Failure of lungs to expand properly at birth
Primary failure to expand terminal respiratory units
Pulmonary hypoplasia associated with short gestation
Pulmonary immaturity NOS

P28.1 Other and unspecified atelectasis of newborn

P28.10 **Unspecified atelectasis of newborn**
Atelectasis of newborn NOS

P28.11 **Resorption atelectasis without respiratory distress syndrome**
Excludes1 resorption atelectasis with respiratory distress syndrome (P22.0)

P28.19 **Other atelectasis of newborn**
Partial atelectasis of newborn
Secondary atelectasis of newborn

P28.2 **Cyanotic attacks of newborn**
Excludes1 apnea of newborn (P28.3-P28.4)

P28.3 **Primary sleep apnea of newborn**
Central sleep apnea of newborn
Obstructive sleep apnea of newborn
Sleep apnea of newborn NOS

P28.4 **Other apnea of newborn**
Apnea of prematurity
Obstructive apnea of newborn
Excludes1 obstructive sleep apnea of newborn (P28.3)

P28.5 **Respiratory failure of newborn**
Excludes1 respiratory arrest of newborn (P28.81)
respiratory distress of newborn (P22.0-)
Coding Clinic: 2019, Q2, P29

CHAPTER 16 (P00-P96)

P28.8 Other specified respiratory conditions of newborn
P28.81 **Respiratory arrest of newborn**
Coding Clinic: 2017, Q2, P6
P28.89 **Other specified respiratory conditions of newborn**
Congenital laryngeal stridor
Sniffles in newborn
Snuffles in newborn
Excludes1 early congenital syphilitic rhinitis (A50.05)
P28.9 **Respiratory condition of newborn, unspecified**
Respiratory depression in newborn

P29 Cardiovascular disorders originating in the perinatal period
Excludes1 congenital malformations of the circulatory system (Q20-Q28)
P29.0 **Neonatal cardiac failure**
P29.1 Neonatal cardiac dysrhythmia
P29.11 **Neonatal tachycardia**
P29.12 **Neonatal bradycardia**
P29.2 **Neonatal hypertension**
P29.3 Persistent fetal circulation
P29.30 **Pulmonary hypertension of newborn**
Persistent pulmonary hypertension of newborn
P29.38 **Other persistent fetal circulation**
Delayed closure of ductus arteriosus
P29.4 **Transient myocardial ischemia in newborn**
P29.8 Other cardiovascular disorders originating in the perinatal period
P29.81 **Cardiac arrest of newborn**
P29.89 **Other cardiovascular disorders originating in the perinatal period**
P29.9 **Cardiovascular disorder originating in the perinatal period, unspecified**

INFECTIONS SPECIFIC TO THE PERINATAL PERIOD (P35-P39)

Infections acquired in utero, during birth via the umbilicus, or during the first 28 days after birth
Excludes2 asymptomatic human immunodeficiency virus [HIV] infection status (Z21)
congenital gonococcal infection (A54.-)
congenital pneumonia (P23.-)
congenital syphilis (A50.-)
human immunodeficiency virus [HIV] disease (B20)
infant botulism (A48.51)
infectious diseases not specific to the perinatal period (A00-B99, J09, J10.-)
intestinal infectious disease (A00-A09)
laboratory evidence of human immunodeficiency virus [HIV] (R75)
tetanus neonatorum (A33)

P35 Congenital viral diseases
Includes infections acquired in utero or during birth
P35.0 **Congenital rubella syndrome**
Congenital rubella pneumonitis
P35.1 **Congenital cytomegalovirus infection**
Viruses transmitted by multiple routes that cause mild/subclinical infection
P35.2 **Congenital herpesviral [herpes simplex] infection**
P35.3 **Congenital viral hepatitis**
P35.4 **Congenital Zika virus disease**
Use additional code to identify manifestations of congenital Zika virus disease
Coding Clinic: 2018, Q4, P26
P35.8 **Other congenital viral diseases**
Congenital varicella [chickenpox]
Coding Clinic: 2016, Q4, P7
P35.9 **Congenital viral disease, unspecified**

P36 Bacterial sepsis of newborn
Includes congenital sepsis
Use additional code(s), if applicable, to identify severe sepsis (R65.2-) and associated acute organ dysfunction(s)
P36.0 **Sepsis of newborn due to streptococcus, group B**
P36.1 Sepsis of newborn due to other and unspecified streptococci
P36.10 **Sepsis of newborn due to unspecified streptococci**
P36.19 **Sepsis of newborn due to other streptococci**
P36.2 **Sepsis of newborn due to Staphylococcus aureus**
P36.3 Sepsis of newborn due to other and unspecified staphylococci
P36.30 **Sepsis of newborn due to unspecified staphylococci**
P36.39 **Sepsis of newborn due to other staphylococci**
P36.4 **Sepsis of newborn due to Escherichia coli**
P36.5 **Sepsis of newborn due to anaerobes**
P36.8 **Other bacterial sepsis of newborn**
Use additional code from category B96 to identify organism
P36.9 **Bacterial sepsis of newborn, unspecified**

P37 Other congenital infectious and parasitic diseases
Excludes2 congenital syphilis (A50.-)
infectious neonatal diarrhea (A00-A09)
necrotizing enterocolitis in newborn (P77.-)
noninfectious neonatal diarrhea (P78.3)
ophthalmia neonatorum due to gonococcus (A54.31)
tetanus neonatorum (A33)
P37.0 **Congenital tuberculosis**
P37.1 **Congenital toxoplasmosis**
Parasitic infection, often causing mild flu-like illness
Hydrocephalus due to congenital toxoplasmosis
P37.2 **Neonatal (disseminated) listeriosis**
Acquired transplacentally or during/after parturition in which symptoms are those of sepsis
P37.3 **Congenital falciparum malaria**
P37.4 **Other congenital malaria**
P37.5 **Neonatal candidiasis**
P37.8 **Other specified congenital infectious and parasitic diseases**
P37.9 **Congenital infectious or parasitic disease, unspecified**

P38 Omphalitis of newborn
Inflammation of umbilicus
Excludes1 omphalitis not of newborn (L08.82)
tetanus omphalitis (A33)
umbilical hemorrhage of newborn (P51.-)
P38.1 **Omphalitis with mild hemorrhage**
P38.9 **Omphalitis without hemorrhage**
Omphalitis of newborn NOS

P39 Other infections specific to the perinatal period
Use additional code to identify organism or specific infection
P39.0 **Neonatal infective mastitis**
Excludes1 breast engorgement of newborn (P83.4)
noninfective mastitis of newborn (P83.4)
P39.1 **Neonatal conjunctivitis and dacryocystitis**
Neonatal chlamydial conjunctivitis
Ophthalmia neonatorum NOS
Neonate = newborn
Excludes1 gonococcal conjunctivitis (A54.31)
P39.2 **Intra-amniotic infection affecting newborn, not elsewhere classified**
P39.3 **Neonatal urinary tract infection**
P39.4 **Neonatal skin infection**
Neonatal pyoderma
Excludes1 pemphigus neonatorum (L00)
staphylococcal scalded skin syndrome (L00)
P39.8 **Other specified infections specific to the perinatal period**
P39.9 **Infection specific to the perinatal period, unspecified**

HEMORRHAGIC AND HEMATOLOGICAL DISORDERS OF NEWBORN (P50-P61)

Excludes1 congenital stenosis and stricture of bile ducts (Q44.3)
Crigler-Najjar syndrome (E80.5)
Dubin-Johnson syndrome (E80.6)
Gilbert syndrome (E80.4)
hereditary hemolytic anemias (D55-D58)

● **P50 Newborn affected by intrauterine (fetal) blood loss**
Excludes1 congenital anemia from intrauterine (fetal) blood loss (P61.3)
P50.0 Newborn affected by intrauterine (fetal) blood loss from vasa previa
P50.1 Newborn affected by intrauterine (fetal) blood loss from ruptured cord
P50.2 Newborn affected by intrauterine (fetal) blood loss from placenta
P50.3 Newborn affected by hemorrhage into co-twin
P50.4 Newborn affected by hemorrhage into maternal circulation
P50.5 Newborn affected by intrauterine (fetal) blood loss from cut end of co-twin's cord
P50.8 Newborn affected by other intrauterine (fetal) blood loss
P50.9 Newborn affected by intrauterine (fetal) blood loss, unspecified
Newborn affected by fetal hemorrhage NOS

● **P51 Umbilical hemorrhage of newborn**
Excludes1 omphalitis with mild hemorrhage (P38.1)
umbilical hemorrhage from cut end of co-twins cord (P50.5)
P51.0 Massive umbilical hemorrhage of newborn
P51.8 Other umbilical hemorrhages of newborn
Slipped umbilical ligature NOS
P51.9 Umbilical hemorrhage of newborn, unspecified

● **P52 Intracranial nontraumatic hemorrhage of newborn**
Includes intracranial hemorrhage due to anoxia or hypoxia
Excludes1 intracranial hemorrhage due to birth injury (P10.-)
intracranial hemorrhage due to other injury (S06.-)
P52.0 Intraventricular (nontraumatic) hemorrhage, grade 1, of newborn
Subependymal hemorrhage (without intraventricular extension)
Bleeding into germinal matrix
P52.1 Intraventricular (nontraumatic) hemorrhage, grade 2, of newborn
Subependymal hemorrhage with intraventricular extension
Bleeding into ventricle
● **P52.2 Intraventricular (nontraumatic) hemorrhage, grade 3 and grade 4, of newborn**
P52.21 Intraventricular (nontraumatic) hemorrhage, grade 3, of newborn
Subependymal hemorrhage with intraventricular extension with enlargement of ventricle
P52.22 Intraventricular (nontraumatic) hemorrhage, grade 4, of newborn
Bleeding into cerebral cortex
Subependymal hemorrhage with intracerebral extension
P52.3 Unspecified intraventricular (nontraumatic) hemorrhage of newborn
P52.4 Intracerebral (nontraumatic) hemorrhage of newborn
P52.5 Subarachnoid (nontraumatic) hemorrhage of newborn
P52.6 Cerebellar (nontraumatic) and posterior fossa hemorrhage of newborn
P52.8 Other intracranial (nontraumatic) hemorrhages of newborn
P52.9 Intracranial (nontraumatic) hemorrhage of newborn, unspecified

P53 Hemorrhagic disease of newborn
Vitamin K deficiency of newborn

● **P54 Other neonatal hemorrhages**
Excludes1 newborn affected by (intrauterine) blood loss (P50.-)
pulmonary hemorrhage originating in the perinatal period (P26.-)
P54.0 Neonatal hematemesis
Vomiting of blood
Excludes1 neonatal hematemesis due to swallowed maternal blood (P78.2)
P54.1 Neonatal melena
Dark-colored feces stained with blood pigments
Excludes1 neonatal melena due to swallowed maternal blood (P78.2)
P54.2 Neonatal rectal hemorrhage
P54.3 Other neonatal gastrointestinal hemorrhage
P54.4 Neonatal adrenal hemorrhage
P54.5 Neonatal cutaneous hemorrhage
Neonatal bruising
Neonatal ecchymoses
Neonatal petechiae
Neonatal superficial hematomata
Excludes2 bruising of scalp due to birth injury (P12.3)
cephalhematoma due to birth injury (P12.0)
P54.6 Neonatal vaginal hemorrhage ♀
Neonatal pseudomenses
P54.8 Other specified neonatal hemorrhages
P54.9 Neonatal hemorrhage, unspecified

● **P55 Hemolytic disease of newborn**
AKA erythroblastosis fetalis and is due to Rh isoimmunization, result of Rh blood factor incompatibilities between mother (Rh negative) and fetus (Rh positive)
P55.0 Rh isoimmunization of newborn
P55.1 ABO isoimmunization of newborn
Coding Clinic: 2015, Q3, P20
P55.8 Other hemolytic diseases of newborn
P55.9 Hemolytic disease of newborn, unspecified

● **P56 Hydrops fetalis due to hemolytic disease**
Caused by maternal sensitization to fetal blood group antigen
Excludes1 hydrops fetalis NOS (P83.2)
P56.0 Hydrops fetalis due to isoimmunization
● **P56.9 Hydrops fetalis due to other and unspecified hemolytic disease**
P56.90 Hydrops fetalis due to unspecified hemolytic disease
P56.99 Hydrops fetalis due to other hemolytic disease

● **P57 Kernicterus**
High levels of bilirubin in blood, with severe neural symptoms
P57.0 Kernicterus due to isoimmunization
P57.8 Other specified kernicterus
Excludes1 Crigler-Najjar syndrome (E80.5)
P57.9 Kernicterus, unspecified

CHAPTER 16 (P00-P96)

● **P58** Neonatal jaundice due to other excessive hemolysis
Excludes1 jaundice due to isoimmunization (P55-P57)
P58.0 Neonatal jaundice due to **bruising**
P58.1 Neonatal jaundice due to **bleeding**
P58.2 Neonatal jaundice due to **infection**
P58.3 Neonatal jaundice due to **polycythemia**
● P58.4 Neonatal jaundice due to **drugs or toxins** transmitted from mother or given to newborn
Code first poisoning due to drug or toxin, if applicable (T36-T65 with fifth or sixth character 1-4 or 6)
Use additional code for adverse effect, if applicable, to identify drug (T36-T50 with fifth or sixth character 5)
P58.41 **Neonatal jaundice due to drugs or toxins transmitted from mother**
P58.42 **Neonatal jaundice due to drugs or toxins given to newborn**
P58.5 Neonatal jaundice due to **swallowed maternal blood**
P58.8 Neonatal jaundice due to **other** specified excessive hemolysis
P58.9 Neonatal jaundice due to excessive hemolysis, **unspecified**

● **P59** Neonatal jaundice from other and unspecified causes
Excludes1 jaundice due to inborn errors of metabolism (E70-E88)
kernicterus (P57.-)
P59.0 Neonatal jaundice associated with **preterm delivery**
Hyperbilirubinemia of prematurity
Jaundice due to delayed conjugation associated with preterm delivery
P59.1 **Inspissated bile syndrome**
● P59.2 **Neonatal jaundice from other and unspecified hepatocellular damage**
Excludes1 congenital viral hepatitis (P35.3)
P59.20 **Neonatal jaundice from unspecified hepatocellular damage**
P59.29 **Neonatal jaundice from other hepatocellular damage**
Neonatal giant cell hepatitis
Neonatal (idiopathic) hepatitis
P59.3 Neonatal jaundice from **breast milk inhibitor**
P59.8 Neonatal jaundice from **other** specified causes
P59.9 Neonatal jaundice, **unspecified**
Neonatal physiological jaundice (intense)(prolonged) NOS
Coding Clinic: 2015, Q3, P20

P60 Disseminated intravascular coagulation of newborn
Defibrination syndrome of newborn

● **P61** Other perinatal hematological disorders
Excludes1 transient hypogammaglobulinemia of infancy (D80.7)
P61.0 **Transient neonatal thrombocytopenia**
Lack of sufficient numbers of circulating thrombocytes (platelets)
Neonatal thrombocytopenia due to exchange transfusion
Neonatal thrombocytopenia due to idiopathic maternal thrombocytopenia
Neonatal thrombocytopenia due to isoimmunization
P61.1 **Polycythemia neonatorum**
Neonate = newborn
P61.2 **Anemia of prematurity**
P61.3 **Congenital anemia from fetal blood loss**
P61.4 **Other congenital anemias, not elsewhere classified**
Congenital anemia NOS
P61.5 **Transient neonatal neutropenia**
Low levels of granulocytic neutrophilic white blood cells
Excludes1 congenital neutropenia (nontransient) (D70.0)
P61.6 **Other transient neonatal disorders of coagulation**
P61.8 **Other specified perinatal hematological disorders**
P61.9 **Perinatal hematological disorder, unspecified**

TRANSITORY ENDOCRINE AND METABOLIC DISORDERS SPECIFIC TO NEWBORN (P70-P74)

Includes transitory endocrine and metabolic disturbances caused by the infant's response to maternal endocrine and metabolic factors, or its adjustment to extrauterine environment

● **P70** Transitory disorders of carbohydrate metabolism specific to newborn
P70.0 Syndrome of infant of mother with **gestational diabetes**
Newborn (with hypoglycemia) affected by maternal gestational diabetes
Excludes1 newborn (with hypoglycemia) affected by maternal (pre-existing) diabetes mellitus (P70.1)
syndrome of infant of a diabetic mother (P70.1)
P70.1 Syndrome of infant of a **diabetic mother**
Newborn (with hypoglycemia) affected by maternal (pre-existing) diabetes mellitus
Excludes1 newborn (with hypoglycemia) affected by maternal gestational diabetes (P70.0)
syndrome of infant of mother with gestational diabetes (P70.0)
P70.2 **Neonatal diabetes mellitus**
P70.3 **Iatrogenic neonatal hypoglycemia**
P70.4 **Other neonatal hypoglycemia**
Transitory neonatal hypoglycemia
P70.8 **Other transitory disorders of carbohydrate metabolism of newborn**
P70.9 **Transitory disorder of carbohydrate metabolism of newborn, unspecified**

● **P71** Transitory neonatal disorders of calcium and magnesium metabolism
P71.0 **Cow's milk hypocalcemia in newborn**
P71.1 **Other neonatal hypocalcemia**
Excludes1 neonatal hypoparathyroidism (P71.4)
P71.2 **Neonatal hypomagnesemia**
P71.3 **Neonatal tetany without calcium or magnesium deficiency**
Neonatal tetany NOS
P71.4 **Transitory neonatal hypoparathyroidism**
P71.8 **Other transitory neonatal disorders of calcium and magnesium metabolism**
Coding Clinic: 2016, Q4, P55
P71.9 **Transitory neonatal disorder of calcium and magnesium metabolism, unspecified**

● **P72** Other transitory neonatal endocrine disorders
Excludes1 congenital hypothyroidism with or without goiter (E03.0-E03.1)
dyshormogenetic goiter (E07.1)
Pendred's syndrome (E07.1)
P72.0 **Neonatal goiter, not elsewhere classified**
Transitory congenital goiter with normal functioning
P72.1 **Transitory neonatal hyperthyroidism**
Neonatal thyrotoxicosis
P72.2 **Other transitory neonatal disorders of thyroid function, not elsewhere classified**
Transitory neonatal hypothyroidism
P72.8 **Other specified transitory neonatal endocrine disorders**
P72.9 **Transitory neonatal endocrine disorder, unspecified**

● **P74** Other transitory neonatal electrolyte and metabolic disturbances
P74.0 **Late metabolic acidosis of newborn**
Excludes1 (fetal) metabolic acidosis of newborn (P19)
P74.1 **Dehydration of newborn**

● P74.2 **Disturbances of sodium balance of newborn**
Coding Clinic: 2018, Q2, P6
P74.21 **Hypernatremia of newborn**
P74.22 **Hyponatremia of newborn**

● P74.3 **Disturbances of potassium balance of newborn**
P74.31 **Hyperkalemia of newborn**
P74.32 **Hypokalemia of newborn**

● P74.4 **Other transitory electrolyte disturbances of newborn**
P74.41 **Alkalosis of newborn**
Hyperbicarbonatemia
● P74.42 **Disturbances of chlorine balance of newborn**
P74.421 **Hyperchloremia of newborn**
Hyperchloremic metabolic acidosis
Excludes2 late metabolic acidosis of the newborn (P74.Ø)
P74.422 **Hypochloremia of newborn**
P74.49 **Other transitory electrolyte disturbance of newborn**

P74.5 **Transitory tyrosinemia of newborn**
P74.6 **Transitory hyperammonemia of newborn**
P74.8 **Other transitory metabolic disturbances of newborn**
Amino-acid metabolic disorders described as transitory
P74.9 **Transitory metabolic disturbance of newborn, unspecified**

DIGESTIVE SYSTEM DISORDERS OF NEWBORN (P76-P78)

● P76 **Other intestinal obstruction of newborn**
P76.Ø **Meconium plug syndrome**
Fetal stool obstruction in large intestine, present at birth; may be symptom of organic disease.
Meconium ileus NOS
Excludes1 meconium ileus in cystic fibrosis (E84.11)
P76.1 **Transitory ileus of newborn**
Temporary obstruction of ileus (small intestine)
Excludes1 Hirschsprung's disease (Q43.1)
P76.2 **Intestinal obstruction due to inspissated milk**
Being thickened, dried, or made less fluid
P76.8 **Other specified intestinal obstruction of newborn**
Excludes1 intestinal obstruction classifiable to K56.-
P76.9 **Intestinal obstruction of newborn, unspecified**

● P77 **Necrotizing enterocolitis of newborn**
P77.1 **Stage 1 necrotizing enterocolitis in newborn**
Necrotizing enterocolitis without pneumatosis, without perforation
P77.2 **Stage 2 necrotizing enterocolitis in newborn**
Necrotizing enterocolitis with pneumatosis, without perforation
P77.3 **Stage 3 necrotizing enterocolitis in newborn**
Necrotizing enterocolitis with perforation
Necrotizing enterocolitis with pneumatosis and perforation
P77.9 **Necrotizing enterocolitis in newborn, unspecified**
Necrotizing enterocolitis in newborn, NOS

● P78 **Other perinatal digestive system disorders**
Excludes1 cystic fibrosis (E84.Ø-E84.9)
neonatal gastrointestinal hemorrhages (P54.Ø-P54.3)
P78.Ø **Perinatal intestinal perforation**
Meconium peritonitis
P78.1 **Other neonatal peritonitis**
Neonatal peritonitis NOS
P78.2 **Neonatal hematemesis and melena due to swallowed maternal blood**
P78.3 **Noninfective neonatal diarrhea**
Neonatal diarrhea NOS
● P78.8 **Other specified perinatal digestive system disorders**
P78.81 **Congenital cirrhosis (of liver)**
P78.82 **Peptic ulcer of newborn**
P78.83 **Newborn esophageal reflux**
Neonatal esophageal reflux
P78.84 **Gestational alloimmune liver disease**
GALD
Neonatal hemochromatosis
Excludes1 hemochromatosis (E83.11-)
P78.89 **Other specified perinatal digestive system disorders**
P78.9 **Perinatal digestive system disorder, unspecified**

CONDITIONS INVOLVING THE INTEGUMENT AND TEMPERATURE REGULATION OF NEWBORN (P8Ø-P83)

● P8Ø **Hypothermia of newborn**
P8Ø.Ø **Cold injury syndrome**
Severe and usually chronic hypothermia associated with a pink flushed appearance, edema and neurological and biochemical abnormalities.
Excludes1 mild hypothermia of newborn (P8Ø.8)
P8Ø.8 **Other hypothermia of newborn**
Mild hypothermia of newborn
P8Ø.9 **Hypothermia of newborn, unspecified**

● P81 **Other disturbances of temperature regulation of newborn**
P81.Ø **Environmental hyperthermia of newborn**
P81.8 **Other specified disturbances of temperature regulation of newborn**
P81.9 **Disturbance of temperature regulation of newborn, unspecified**
Fever of newborn NOS

● P83 **Other conditions of integument specific to newborn**
Excludes1 congenital malformations of skin and integument (Q8Ø-Q84)
hydrops fetalis due to hemolytic disease (P56.-)
neonatal skin infection (P39.4)
staphylococcal scalded skin syndrome (LØØ)
Excludes2 cradle cap (L21.Ø)
diaper [napkin] dermatitis (L22)
P83.Ø **Sclerema neonatorum**
Neonate = newborn
P83.1 **Neonatal erythema toxicum**
Benign, generalized, transient pustules that become firm vesicles
P83.2 **Hydrops fetalis not due to hemolytic disease**
Severe, life-threatening problem of severe edema (swelling) as a result of too much fluid leaving blood and entering tissue
Hydrops fetalis NOS
● P83.3 **Other and unspecified edema specific to newborn**
P83.3Ø **Unspecified edema specific to newborn**
P83.39 **Other edema specific to newborn**
P83.4 **Breast engorgement of newborn**
Noninfective mastitis of newborn
P83.5 **Congenital hydrocele** ♂
P83.6 **Umbilical polyp of newborn**
● P83.8 **Other specified conditions of integument specific to newborn**
P83.81 **Umbilical granuloma**
Excludes2 Granulomatous disorder of the skin and subcutaneous tissue, unspecified (L92.9)
P83.88 **Other specified conditions of integument specific to newborn**
Bronze baby syndrome
Neonatal scleroderma
Urticaria neonatorum
P83.9 **Condition of the integument specific to newborn, unspecified**

CHAPTER 16 (PØØ-P96)

OTHER PROBLEMS WITH NEWBORN (P84)

P84 Other problems with newborn
Acidemia of newborn
Acidosis of newborn
Anoxia of newborn NOS
Asphyxia of newborn NOS
Hypercapnia of newborn
Hypoxemia of newborn
Hypoxia of newborn NOS
Mixed metabolic and respiratory acidosis of newborn
Excludes1 intracranial hemorrhage due to anoxia or hypoxia (P52.-)
hypoxic ischemic encephalopathy [HIE] (P91.6-)
late metabolic acidosis of newborn (P74.Ø)

OTHER DISORDERS ORIGINATING IN THE PERINATAL PERIOD (P9Ø-P96)

P9Ø Convulsions of newborn
Excludes1 benign myoclonic epilepsy in infancy (G4Ø.3-)
benign neonatal convulsions (familial) (G4Ø.3-)

● **P91 Other disturbances of cerebral status of newborn**
P91.Ø Neonatal cerebral ischemia
P91.1 Acquired periventricular cysts of newborn
P91.2 Neonatal cerebral leukomalacia
Degeneration of white matter adjacent to cerebral ventricles following cerebral hypoxia or brain ischemia in neonates
Periventricular leukomalacia
P91.3 Neonatal cerebral irritability
P91.4 Neonatal cerebral depression
P91.5 Neonatal coma
● **P91.6 Hypoxic ischemic encephalopathy [HIE]**
Excludes1 Neonatal cerebral depression (P91.4)
Neonatal cerebral irritability (P91.3)
Neonatal coma (P91.5)
P91.6Ø Hypoxic ischemic encephalopathy [HIE], unspecified
P91.61 Mild hypoxic ischemic encephalopathy [HIE]
P91.62 Moderate hypoxic ischemic encephalopathy [HIE]
P91.63 Severe hypoxic ischemic encephalopathy [HIE]
● **P91.8 Other specified disturbances of cerebral status of newborn**
● **P91.81 Neonatal encephalopathy**
P91.811 Neonatal encephalopathy in diseases classified elsewhere
Code first underlying condition, if known, such as:
congenital cirrhosis (of liver) (P78.81)
intracranial nontraumatic hemorrhage of newborn (P52.-)
kernicterus (P57.-)
P91.819 Neonatal encephalopathy, unspecified
P91.88 Other specified disturbances of cerebral status of newborn
P91.9 Disturbance of cerebral status of newborn, unspecified

● **P92 Feeding problems of newborn**
Excludes1 eating disorders (F5Ø.-)
feeding problems in child over 28 days old (R63.3)
Coding Clinic: 2Ø17, Q1, P28; 2Ø16, Q3, P19

● **P92.Ø Vomiting of newborn**
Excludes1 vomiting of child over 28 days old (R11.-)
P92.Ø1 Bilious vomiting of newborn
Excludes1 bilious vomiting in child over 28 days old (R11.14)
P92.Ø9 Other vomiting of newborn
Excludes1 regurgitation of food in newborn (P92.1)
P92.1 Regurgitation and rumination of newborn
P92.2 Slow feeding of newborn
P92.3 Underfeeding of newborn
P92.4 Overfeeding of newborn
P92.5 Neonatal difficulty in feeding at breast
Coding Clinic: 2Ø17, Q1, P28; 2Ø16, Q3, P19
P92.6 Failure to thrive in newborn
Excludes1 failure to thrive in child over 28 days old (R62.51)
P92.8 Other feeding problems of newborn
P92.9 Feeding problem of newborn, unspecified

● **P93 Reactions and intoxications due to drugs administered to newborn**
Includes reactions and intoxications due to drugs administered to fetus affecting newborn
Excludes1 jaundice due to drugs or toxins transmitted from mother or given to newborn (P58.4-)
reactions and intoxications from maternal opiates, tranquilizers and other medication (PØ4.Ø-PØ4.1, PØ4.4-)
withdrawal symptoms from maternal use of drugs of addiction (P96.1)
withdrawal symptoms from therapeutic use of drugs in newborn (P96.2)
P93.Ø Grey baby syndrome
Grey syndrome from chloramphenicol administration in newborn
P93.8 Other reactions and intoxications due to drugs administered to newborn
Use additional code for adverse effect, if applicable, to identify drug (T36-T5Ø with fifth or sixth character 5)

● **P94 Disorders of muscle tone of newborn**
P94.Ø Transient neonatal myasthenia gravis
Excludes1 myasthenia gravis (G7Ø.Ø)
P94.1 Congenital hypertonia
P94.2 Congenital hypotonia
Floppy baby syndrome, unspecified
P94.8 Other disorders of muscle tone of newborn
P94.9 Disorder of muscle tone of newborn, unspecified

OGCR Section I.C.16.g.
Stillbirth
Code P95, Stillbirth, is only for use for institutions that maintain separate records for stillbirths. No other code should be used with P95. Code P95 should not be used on the mother's record.

P95 Stillbirth
Deadborn fetus NOS
Fetal death of unspecified cause
Stillbirth NOS
Excludes1 maternal care for intrauterine death (O36.4)
missed abortion (OØ2.1)
outcome of delivery, stillbirth (Z37.1, Z37.3, Z37.4, Z37.7)

P96 Other conditions originating in the perinatal period

P96.Ø Congenital renal failure
Uremia of newborn

P96.1 Neonatal withdrawal symptoms from maternal use of drugs of addiction
Drug withdrawal syndrome in infant of dependent mother
Neonatal abstinence syndrome
Excludes1 reactions and intoxications from maternal opiates and tranquilizers administered during labor and delivery (PØ4.Ø)

P96.2 Withdrawal symptoms from therapeutic use of drugs in newborn

P96.3 Wide cranial sutures of newborn
Neonatal craniotabes

P96.5 Complication to newborn due to (fetal) intrauterine procedure
Excludes2 newborn affected by amniocentesis (PØØ.6)

P96.8 Other specified conditions originating in the perinatal period

P96.81 Exposure to (parental) (environmental) tobacco smoke in the perinatal period
Excludes2 newborn affected by in utero exposure to tobacco (PØ4.2)
exposure to environmental tobacco smoke after the perinatal period (Z77.22)

P96.82 Delayed separation of umbilical cord

P96.83 Meconium staining
Excludes1 meconium aspiration (P24.ØØ, P24.Ø1)
meconium passage during delivery (PØ3.82)

P96.89 Other specified conditions originating in the perinatal period
Use additional code to specify condition

P96.9 Condition originating in the perinatal period, unspecified
Congenital debility NOS

CHAPTER 16 (PØØ-P96)

CHAPTER 17

CONGENITAL MALFORMATIONS, DEFORMATIONS, AND CHROMOSOMAL ABNORMALITIES (Q00-Q99)

OGCR Chapter-Specific Coding Guidelines

17. **Chapter 17: Congenital malformations, deformations, and chromosomal abnormalities (Q00-Q99)**
Assign an appropriate code(s) from categories Q00-Q99, Congenital malformations, deformations, and chromosomal abnormalities when a malformation/deformation or chromosomal abnormality is documented. A malformation/deformation/ or chromosomal abnormality may be the principal/first-listed diagnosis on a record or a secondary diagnosis.

When a malformation/deformation/or chromosomal abnormality does not have a unique code assignment, assign additional code(s) for any manifestations that may be present.

When the code assignment specifically identifies the malformation/deformation/or chromosomal abnormality, manifestations that are an inherent component of the anomaly should not be coded separately. Additional codes should be assigned for manifestations that are not an inherent component.

Codes from Chapter 17 may be used throughout the life of the patient. If a congenital malformation or deformity has been corrected, a personal history code should be used to identify the history of the malformation or deformity. Although present at birth, malformation/deformation/or chromosomal abnormality may not be identified until later in life. Whenever the condition is diagnosed by the physician, it is appropriate to assign a code from codes Q00-Q99.

For the birth admission, the appropriate code from category Z38, Liveborn infants, according to place of birth and type of delivery, should be sequenced as the principal diagnosis, followed by any congenital anomaly codes, Q00-Q99.

CHAPTER 17

CONGENITAL MALFORMATIONS, DEFORMATIONS, AND CHROMOSOMAL ABNORMALITIES (Q00-Q99)

Note: Codes from this chapter are not for use on maternal records

Excludes2 inborn errors of metabolism (E70-E88)

This chapter contains the following blocks:

Q00-Q07	Congenital malformations of the nervous system
Q10-Q18	Congenital malformations of eye, ear, face and neck
Q20-Q28	Congenital malformations of the circulatory system
Q30-Q34	Congenital malformations of the respiratory system
Q35-Q37	Cleft lip and cleft palate
Q38-Q45	Other congenital malformations of the digestive system
Q50-Q56	Congenital malformations of genital organs
Q60-Q64	Congenital malformations of the urinary system
Q65-Q79	Congenital malformations and deformations of the musculoskeletal system
Q80-Q89	Other congenital malformations
Q90-Q99	Chromosomal abnormalities, not elsewhere classified

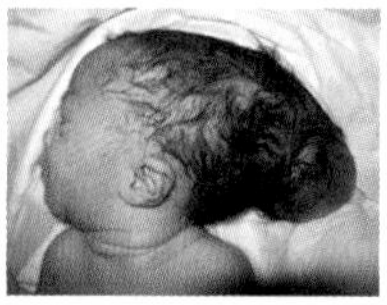

Figure 17-1 An infant with a large occipital encephalocele. The large skin-covered encephalocele is visible. (From Swaiman KF, Ashwal S, Ferriero DM: Pediatric Neurology: Principles and Practice, Philadelphia, Saunders, 2012)

CONGENITAL MALFORMATIONS OF THE NERVOUS SYSTEM (Q00–Q07)

● **Q00 Anencephaly and similar malformations**

Q00.0 Anencephaly

Absence of skull with cerebral hemispheres missing or reduced to small masses attached to base of cranium

Acephaly
Acrania
Amyelencephaly
Hemianencephaly
Hemicephaly

Q00.1 Craniorachischisis

Developmental anomaly consisting of fissure of cranium and vertebral column

Q00.2 Iniencephaly

Developmental anomaly characterized by enlargement of foramen magnum and absence of laminae and spinous processes of cervical, dorsal

● **Q01 Encephalocele**

Sac-like protrusions of brain and membranes visible through an opening in skull

Includes Arnold-Chiari syndrome, type III
encephalocystocele
encephalomyelocele
hydroencephalocele
hydromeningocele, cranial
meningocele, cerebral
meningoencephalocele

Excludes1 Meckel-Gruber syndrome (Q61.9)

Q01.0 Frontal encephalocele
Q01.1 Nasofrontal encephalocele
Q01.2 Occipital encephalocele
Q01.8 Encephalocele of other sites
Q01.9 Encephalocele, unspecified

Q02 Microcephaly

Head size measures significantly below normal based on standardized charts

Includes hydromicrocephaly
micrencephalon

~~Use additional code, if applicable, to identify congenital Zika virus disease~~

▶ *Code first, if applicable, congenital Zika virus disease*

Excludes1 Meckel-Gruber syndrome (Q61.9)

Coding Clinic: 2018, Q4, P26; 2016, Q4, P7

● **Q03 Congenital hydrocephalus**

Accumulation of cerebrospinal fluid in ventricles resulting in swelling and enlargement

Includes hydrocephalus in newborn

Excludes1 Arnold-Chiari syndrome, type II (Q07.0-)
acquired hydrocephalus (G91.-)
hydrocephalus due to congenital toxoplasmosis (P37.1)
hydrocephalus with spina bifida (Q05.0-Q05.4)

Q03.0 Malformations of aqueduct of Sylvius

Anomaly of aqueduct of Sylvius
Obstruction of aqueduct of Sylvius, congenital
Stenosis of aqueduct of Sylvius

Q03.1 Atresia of foramina of Magendie and Luschka

Dandy-Walker syndrome

Q03.8 Other congenital hydrocephalus
Q03.9 Congenital hydrocephalus, unspecified

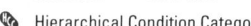

Q04 Other congenital malformations of brain
Excludes1 cyclopia (Q87.0)
macrocephaly (Q75.3)

Q04.0 Congenital malformations of corpus callosum
Agenesis of corpus callosum

Q04.1 Arhinencephaly
Congenital absence of olfactory bulbs, tract, or nerves

Q04.2 Holoprosencephaly
Failure of cleavage of forebrain (prosencephalon) resulting in incomplete or absent cortical separation and deficits in midline facial development

Q04.3 Other reduction deformities of brain
Absence of part of brain
Agenesis of part of brain
Cerebral cortex are not fully formed, brain surface is smooth
Agyria
Aplasia of part of brain
Hydranencephaly
Hypoplasia of part of brain
Lissencephaly
Congenital malformation or absence of convolutions of cerebral cortex
Microgyria
Malformation of brain characterized by excessive number of small convolutions (gyri) on surface
Pachygyria
Reduction in number of sulci of cerebrum
Excludes1 congenital malformations of corpus callosum (Q04.0)

Q04.4 Septo-optic dysplasia of brain

Q04.5 Megalencephaly
Abnormally large brain

Q04.6 Congenital cerebral cysts
Porencephaly
Schizencephaly
Excludes1 acquired porencephalic cyst (G93.0)

Q04.8 Other specified congenital malformations of brain
Arnold-Chiari syndrome, type IV
Macrogyria

Q04.9 Congenital malformation of brain, unspecified
Congenital anomaly NOS of brain
Congenital deformity NOS of brain
Congenital disease or lesion NOS of brain
Multiple anomalies NOS of brain, congenital

Q05 Spina bifida
Developmental anomaly characterized by defective closure of vertebral arch, through which spinal cord and meninges may protrude
Includes hydromeningocele (spinal)
meningocele (spinal)
meningomyelocele
myelocele
myelomeningocele
rachischisis
spina bifida (aperta)(cystica)
syringomyelocele

Use additional code for any associated paraplegia (paraparesis) (G82.2-)
Excludes1 Arnold-Chiari syndrome, type II (Q07.0-)
spina bifida occulta (Q76.0)

Q05.0 Cervical spina bifida with hydrocephalus

Q05.1 Thoracic spina bifida with hydrocephalus
Dorsal spina bifida with hydrocephalus
Thoracolumbar spina bifida with hydrocephalus

Q05.2 Lumbar spina bifida with hydrocephalus
Lumbosacral spina bifida with hydrocephalus

Q05.3 Sacral spina bifida with hydrocephalus

Q05.4 Unspecified spina bifida with hydrocephalus

Q05.5 Cervical spina bifida without hydrocephalus

Q05.6 Thoracic spina bifida without hydrocephalus
Dorsal spina bifida NOS
Thoracolumbar spina bifida NOS

Q05.7 Lumbar spina bifida without hydrocephalus
Lumbosacral spina bifida NOS

Q05.8 Sacral spina bifida without hydrocephalus

Q05.9 Spina bifida, unspecified

Q06 Other congenital malformations of spinal cord

Q06.0 Amyelia
Congenital absence of spinal cord

Q06.1 Hypoplasia and dysplasia of spinal cord
Underdevelopment of spinal cord
Atelomyelia
Congenitally incomplete development of spinal cord
Myelatelia
Myelodysplasia of spinal cord
Defective development of spinal cord, especially lower segments

Q06.2 Diastematomyelia
Congenital anomaly, associated with spina bifida, in which spinal cord is split into halves and surrounded by dural sac

Q06.3 Other congenital cauda equina malformations

Q06.4 Hydromyelia
Dilation of central canal of spinal cord with increased fluid accumulation
Hydrorachis

Q06.8 Other specified congenital malformations of spinal cord

Q06.9 Congenital malformation of spinal cord, unspecified
Congenital anomaly NOS of spinal cord
Congenital deformity NOS of spinal cord
Congenital disease or lesion NOS of spinal cord

Q07 Other congenital malformations of nervous system
Excludes2 congenital central alveolar hypoventilation syndrome (G47.35)
familial dysautonomia [Riley-Day] (G90.1)
neurofibromatosis (nonmalignant) (Q85.0-)

Q07.0 Arnold-Chiari syndrome
Herniation of cerebellar tonsils and vermis through foramen magnum into spinal canal
Arnold-Chiari syndrome, type II
Excludes1 Arnold-Chiari syndrome, type III (Q01.-)
Arnold-Chiari syndrome, type IV (Q04.8)

Q07.00 Arnold-Chiari syndrome without spina bifida or hydrocephalus

Q07.01 Arnold-Chiari syndrome with spina bifida

Q07.02 Arnold-Chiari syndrome with hydrocephalus

Q07.03 Arnold-Chiari syndrome with spina bifida and hydrocephalus

Q07.8 Other specified congenital malformations of nervous system
Agenesis of nerve
Displacement of brachial plexus
Jaw-winking syndrome
Marcus Gunn's syndrome

Q07.9 Congenital malformation of nervous system, unspecified
Congenital anomaly NOS of nervous system
Congenital deformity NOS of nervous system
Congenital disease or lesion NOS of nervous system

CHAPTER 17 (Q00-Q99)

CONGENITAL MALFORMATIONS OF EYE, EAR, FACE AND NECK (Q10-Q18)

Excludes2 cleft lip and cleft palate (Q35-Q37)
congenital malformation of cervical spine (Q05.0, Q05.5, Q67.5, Q76.0-Q76.4)
congenital malformation of larynx (Q31.-)
congenital malformation of lip NEC (Q38.0)
congenital malformation of nose (Q30.-)
congenital malformation of parathyroid gland (Q89.2)
congenital malformation of thyroid gland (Q89.2)

● **Q10 Congenital malformations of eyelid, lacrimal apparatus and orbit**

Excludes1 cryptophthalmos NOS (Q11.2)
cryptophthalmos syndrome (Q87.0)

Q10.0 Congenital ptosis
Prolapse or drooping of upper eyelid from paralysis of third nerve or from sympathetic innervations

Q10.1 Congenital ectropion
Outward turning of eyelid

Q10.2 Congenital entropion
Inward turning of eyelid

Q10.3 Other congenital malformations of eyelid
Ablepharon
Blepharophimosis, congenital
Coloboma of eyelid
Congenital absence or agenesis of cilia
Congenital absence or agenesis of eyelid
Congenital accessory eyelid
Congenital accessory eye muscle
Congenital malformation of eyelid NOS

Q10.4 Absence and agenesis of lacrimal apparatus
Congenital absence of punctum lacrimale

Q10.5 Congenital stenosis and stricture of lacrimal duct

Q10.6 Other congenital malformations of lacrimal apparatus
Congenital malformation of lacrimal apparatus NOS

Q10.7 Congenital malformation of orbit

● **Q11 Anophthalmos, microphthalmos and macrophthalmos**
Absence of eye and optic pit

Q11.0 Cystic eyeball

Q11.1 Other anophthalmos
Anophthalmos NOS
Agenesis of eye
Absence of eye
Aplasia of eye

Q11.2 Microphthalmos
Partial absence of eye and optic pit
Cryptophthalmos NOS
Dysplasia of eye
Hypoplasia of eye
Rudimentary eye
Excludes1 cryptophthalmos syndrome (Q87.0)

Q11.3 Macrophthalmos
Congenital enlargement of eyes
Excludes1 macrophthalmos in congenital glaucoma (Q15.0)

● **Q12 Congenital lens malformations**

Q12.0 Congenital cataract

Q12.1 Congenital displaced lens

Q12.2 Coloboma of lens

Q12.3 Congenital aphakia

Q12.4 Spherophakia
Smaller, more spherical optic lens than normal

Q12.8 Other congenital lens malformations
Microphakia

Q12.9 Congenital lens malformation, unspecified

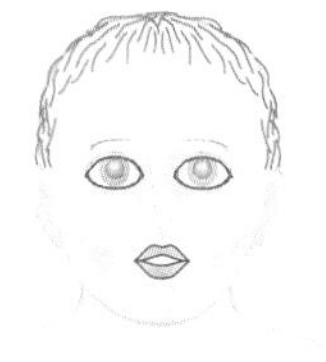

Figure 17-2 Bilateral congenital **hydrophthalmia,** in which the eyes are very large in comparison to the other facial features due to glaucoma.

● **Q13 Congenital malformations of anterior segment of eye**

Q13.0 Coloboma of iris
Coloboma NOS

Q13.1 Absence of iris
Aniridia
Use additional code for associated glaucoma (H42)

Q13.2 Other congenital malformations of iris
Anisocoria, congenital
Atresia of pupil
Congenital malformation of iris NOS
Corectopia

Q13.3 Congenital corneal opacity

Q13.4 Other congenital corneal malformations
Congenital malformation of cornea NOS
Microcornea
Peter's anomaly

Q13.5 Blue sclera
Condition of unusual blueness of sclera; not harmful

● **Q13.8 Other congenital malformations of anterior segment of eye**

Q13.81 Rieger's anomaly
Use additional code for associated glaucoma (H42)

Q13.89 Other congenital malformations of anterior segment of eye

Q13.9 Congenital malformation of anterior segment of eye, unspecified

● **Q14 Congenital malformations of posterior segment of eye**

Excludes2 optic nerve hypoplasia (H47.03-)

Q14.0 Congenital malformation of vitreous humor
Congenital vitreous opacity

Q14.1 Congenital malformation of retina
Congenital retinal aneurysm

Q14.2 Congenital malformation of optic disc
Coloboma of optic disc

Q14.3 Congenital malformation of choroid

Q14.8 Other congenital malformations of posterior segment of eye
Coloboma of the fundus

Q14.9 Congenital malformation of posterior segment of eye, unspecified

CHAPTER 17 (Q00-Q99)

Q15 Other congenital malformations of eye

Excludes1 congenital nystagmus (H55.01)
ocular albinism (E70.31-)
optic nerve hypoplasia (H47.03-)
retinitis pigmentosa (H35.52)

Q15.0 Congenital glaucoma
Axenfeld's anomaly
Buphthalmos
Congenital syndrome characterized by enlargement of the eye with symptoms of glaucoma.
Glaucoma of childhood
Glaucoma of newborn
Hydrophthalmos
Keratoglobus, congenital, with glaucoma
Macrocornea with glaucoma
Macrophthalmos in congenital glaucoma
Megalocornea with glaucoma

Q15.8 Other specified congenital malformations of eye

Q15.9 Congenital malformation of eye, unspecified
Congenital anomaly of eye
Congenital deformity of eye

Q16 Congenital malformations of ear causing impairment of hearing

Excludes1 congenital deafness (H90.-)

Q16.0 Congenital absence of (ear) auricle

Q16.1 Congenital absence, atresia and stricture of auditory canal (external)
Congenital atresia or stricture of osseous meatus

Q16.2 Absence of eustachian tube

Q16.3 Congenital malformation of ear ossicles
Congenital fusion of ear ossicles

Q16.4 Other congenital malformations of middle ear
Congenital malformation of middle ear NOS

Q16.5 Congenital malformation of inner ear
Congenital anomaly of membranous labyrinth
Congenital anomaly of organ of Corti

Q16.9 Congenital malformation of ear causing impairment of hearing, unspecified
Congenital absence of ear NOS

Q17 Other congenital malformations of ear

Excludes1 congenital malformations of ear with impairment of hearing (Q16.0-Q16.9)
preauricular sinus (Q18.1)

Q17.0 Accessory auricle
Accessory tragus
Polyotia
Preauricular appendage or tag
Supernumerary ear
Supernumerary lobule

Q17.1 Macrotia
Enlarged ears

Q17.2 Microtia
An abnormally small or underdeveloped external ear

Q17.3 Other misshapen ear
Pointed ear

Q17.4 Misplaced ear
Low-set ears
Excludes1 cervical auricle (Q18.2)

Q17.5 Prominent ear
Bat ear

Q17.8 Other specified congenital malformations of ear
Congenital absence of lobe of ear

Q17.9 Congenital malformation of ear, unspecified
Congenital anomaly of ear NOS

Q18 Other congenital malformations of face and neck

Excludes1 cleft lip and cleft palate (Q35-Q37)
conditions classified to Q67.0-Q67.4
congenital malformations of skull and face bones (Q75.-)
cyclopia (Q87.0)
dentofacial anomalies [including malocclusion] (M26.-)
malformation syndromes affecting facial appearance (Q87.0)
persistent thyroglossal duct (Q89.2)

Q18.0 Sinus, fistula and cyst of branchial cleft
Branchial vestige
Brachial remnants (cysts, fistula, skin tags) that are developmental anomalies

Q18.1 Preauricular sinus and cyst
Fistula of auricle, congenital
Cervicoaural fistula
Abnormal passage in neck originating from first branchial cleft

Q18.2 Other branchial cleft malformations
Branchial cleft malformation NOS
Cervical auricle
Otocephaly

Q18.3 Webbing of neck
Pterygium colli
Thick fold of skin on side of neck

Q18.4 Macrostomia
Results from failure of union of maxillary and mandibular processes, results in abnormally large mouth

Q18.5 Microstomia

Q18.6 Macrocheilia
Excessive size of lips
Hypertrophy of lip, congenital

Q18.7 Microcheilia
Abnormal smallness of lips

Q18.8 Other specified congenital malformations of face and neck
Medial cyst of face and neck
Medial fistula of face and neck
Medial sinus of face and neck

Q18.9 Congenital malformation of face and neck, unspecified
Congenital anomaly NOS of face and neck

CONGENITAL MALFORMATIONS OF THE CIRCULATORY SYSTEM (Q20-Q28)

Q20 Congenital malformations of cardiac chambers and connections

Excludes1 dextrocardia with situs inversus (Q89.3)
mirror-image atrial arrangement with situs inversus (Q89.3)

Q20.0 Common arterial trunk
Persistent truncus arteriosus
Excludes1 aortic septal defect (Q21.4)

Q20.1 Double outlet right ventricle
Taussig-Bing syndrome

Q20.2 Double outlet left ventricle

Q20.3 Discordant ventriculoarterial connection
Dextrotransposition of aorta
Transposition of great vessels (complete)

Q20.4 Double inlet ventricle
Common ventricle
Cor triloculare biatriatum
Single ventricle

Q20.5 Discordant atrioventricular connection
Corrected transposition
Levotransposition
Ventricular inversion

Q20.6 Isomerism of atrial appendages
Isomerism of atrial appendages with asplenia or polysplenia

Q20.8 Other congenital malformations of cardiac chambers and connections
Cor binoculare

Q20.9 Congenital malformation of cardiac chambers and connections, unspecified

● Q21 Congenital malformations of cardiac septa
Excludes1 acquired cardiac septal defect (I51.Ø)

Q21.Ø Ventricular septal defect
Roger's disease

Q21.1 Atrial septal defect
Coronary sinus defect
Patent or persistent foramen ovale
Patent or persistent ostium secundum defect (type II)
Patent or persistent sinus venosus defect

Q21.2 Atrioventricular septal defect
Common atrioventricular canal
Endocardial cushion defect
Ostium primum atrial septal defect (type I)

Q21.3 Tetralogy of Fallot
Ventricular septal defect with pulmonary stenosis or atresia, dextroposition of aorta and hypertrophy of right ventricle.

Q21.4 Aortopulmonary septal defect
Aortic septal defect
Aortopulmonary window

Q21.8 Other congenital malformations of cardiac septa
Eisenmenger's defect
Pentalogy of Fallot
Code also if applicable:
Eisenmenger's complex (I27.83)
Eisenmenger's syndrome (I27.83)

Q21.9 Congenital malformation of cardiac septum, unspecified
Septal (heart) defect NOS

● Q22 Congenital malformations of pulmonary and tricuspid valves

Q22.Ø Pulmonary valve atresia

Q22.1 Congenital pulmonary valve stenosis

Q22.2 Congenital pulmonary valve insufficiency
Congenital pulmonary valve regurgitation

Q22.3 Other congenital malformations of pulmonary valve
Congenital malformation of pulmonary valve NOS
Supernumerary cusps of pulmonary valve

Q22.4 Congenital tricuspid stenosis
Congenital tricuspid atresia

Q22.5 Ebstein's anomaly
Malformation of tricuspid valve

Q22.6 Hypoplastic right heart syndrome

Q22.8 Other congenital malformations of tricuspid valve

Q22.9 Congenital malformation of tricuspid valve, unspecified

● Q23 Congenital malformations of aortic and mitral valves

Q23.Ø Congenital stenosis of aortic valve
Congenital aortic atresia
Congenital aortic stenosis NOS
Excludes1 congenital stenosis of aortic valve in hypoplastic left heart syndrome (Q23.4)
congenital subaortic stenosis (Q24.4)
supravalvular aortic stenosis (congenital) (Q25.3)

Q23.1 Congenital insufficiency of aortic valve
Bicuspid aortic valve
Congenital aortic insufficiency

Q23.2 Congenital mitral stenosis
Congenital mitral atresia

Q23.3 Congenital mitral insufficiency

Q23.4 Hypoplastic left heart syndrome

Q23.8 Other congenital malformations of aortic and mitral valves

Q23.9 Congenital malformation of aortic and mitral valves, unspecified

● Q24 Other congenital malformations of heart
Excludes1 endocardial fibroelastosis (I42.4)

Q24.Ø Dextrocardia
Heart is located in right hemithorax
Excludes1 dextrocardia with situs inversus (Q89.3)
isomerism of atrial appendages (with asplenia or polysplenia) (Q2Ø.6)
mirror-image atrial arrangement with situs inversus (Q89.3)

Q24.1 Levocardia
Normal position of heart but related structures on wrong side

Q24.2 Cor triatriatum
Congenital heart defect; left atrium is subdivided

Q24.3 Pulmonary infundibular stenosis
Subvalvular pulmonic stenosis

Q24.4 Congenital subaortic stenosis

Q24.5 Malformation of coronary vessels
Congenital coronary (artery) aneurysm

Q24.6 Congenital heart block

Q24.8 Other specified congenital malformations of heart
Congenital diverticulum of left ventricle
Congenital malformation of myocardium
Congenital malformation of pericardium
Malposition of heart
Uhl's disease

Q24.9 Congenital malformation of heart, unspecified
Congenital anomaly of heart
Congenital disease of heart

● Q25 Congenital malformations of great arteries

Q25.Ø Patent ductus arteriosus
Fetal blood vessel connecting left pulmonary artery directly to descending aorta
Patent ductus Botallo
Persistent ductus arteriosus

Q25.1 Coarctation of aorta
Coarctation of aorta (preductal) (postductal)
Stenosis of aorta
Coding Clinic: 2Ø16, Q4, P56-57

● Q25.2 Atresia of aorta
Coding Clinic: 2Ø16, Q4, P56

Q25.21 Interruption of aortic arch
Atresia of aortic arch

Q25.29 Other atresia of aorta
Atresia of aorta

Q25.3 Supravalvular aortic stenosis
Excludes1 congenital aortic stenosis NOS (Q23.Ø)
congenital stenosis of aortic valve (Q23.Ø)

● Q25.4 Other congenital malformations of aorta
Excludes1 hypoplasia of aorta in hypoplastic left heart syndrome (Q23.4)
Coding Clinic: 2Ø16, Q4, P57

Q25.4Ø Congenital malformation of aorta unspecified

Q25.41 Absence and aplasia of aorta

Q25.42 Hypoplasia of aorta

Q25.43 Congenital aneurysm of aorta
Congenital aneurysm of aortic root
Congenital aneurysm of aortic sinus

Q25.44 Congenital dilation of aorta

Q25.45 Double aortic arch
Vascular ring of aorta

Q25.46 Tortuous aortic arch
Persistent convolutions of aortic arch

Q25.47 Right aortic arch
Persistent right aortic arch

Q25.48 Anomalous origin of subclavian artery

Q25.49 Other congenital malformations of aorta
Aortic arch
Bovine arch

Q25.5 **Atresia of pulmonary artery**

Q25.6 **Stenosis of pulmonary artery**
Supravalvular pulmonary stenosis

Q25.7 **Other congenital malformations of pulmonary artery**

Q25.71 **Coarctation of pulmonary artery**

Q25.72 **Congenital pulmonary arteriovenous malformation**
Congenital pulmonary arteriovenous aneurysm

Q25.79 **Other congenital malformations of pulmonary artery**
Aberrant pulmonary artery
Agenesis of pulmonary artery
Congenital aneurysm of pulmonary artery
Congenital anomaly of pulmonary artery
Hypoplasia of pulmonary artery

Q25.8 **Other congenital malformations of other great arteries**

Q25.9 **Congenital malformation of great arteries, unspecified**

Q26 **Congenital malformations of great veins**

Q26.0 **Congenital stenosis of vena cava**
Congenital stenosis of vena cava (inferior)(superior)

Q26.1 **Persistent left superior vena cava**

Q26.2 **Total anomalous pulmonary venous connection**
Total anomalous pulmonary venous return [TAPVR], subdiaphragmatic
Total anomalous pulmonary venous return [TAPVR], supradiaphragmatic

Q26.3 **Partial anomalous pulmonary venous connection**
Partial anomalous pulmonary venous return

Q26.4 **Anomalous pulmonary venous connection, unspecified**

Q26.5 **Anomalous portal venous connection**

Q26.6 **Portal vein-hepatic artery fistula**

Q26.8 **Other congenital malformations of great veins**
Absence of vena cava (inferior) (superior)
Azygos continuation of inferior vena cava
Persistent left posterior cardinal vein
Scimitar syndrome

Q26.9 **Congenital malformation of great vein, unspecified**
Congenital anomaly of vena cava (inferior) (superior) NOS

Q27 **Other congenital malformations of peripheral vascular system**
Excludes2 anomalies of cerebral and precerebral vessels (Q28.0-Q28.3)
anomalies of coronary vessels (Q24.5)
anomalies of pulmonary artery (Q25.5-Q25.7)
congenital retinal aneurysm (Q14.1)
hemangioma and lymphangioma (D18.-)

Q27.0 **Congenital absence and hypoplasia of umbilical artery**
Single umbilical artery

Q27.1 **Congenital renal artery stenosis**

Q27.2 **Other congenital malformations of renal artery**
Congenital malformation of renal artery NOS
Multiple renal arteries

Q27.3 **Arteriovenous malformation (peripheral)**
Arteriovenous aneurysm
Excludes1 acquired arteriovenous aneurysm (I77.0)
Excludes2 arteriovenous malformation of cerebral vessels (Q28.2)
arteriovenous malformation of precerebral vessels (Q28.0)

Q27.30 **Arteriovenous malformation, site unspecified**

Q27.31 **Arteriovenous malformation of vessel of upper limb**

Q27.32 **Arteriovenous malformation of vessel of lower limb**

Q27.33 **Arteriovenous malformation of digestive system vessel**

Q27.34 **Arteriovenous malformation of renal vessel**

Q27.39 **Arteriovenous malformation, other site**

Q27.4 **Congenital phlebectasia**

Q27.8 **Other specified congenital malformations of peripheral vascular system**
Absence of peripheral vascular system
Atresia of peripheral vascular system
Congenital aneurysm (peripheral)
Congenital stricture, artery
Congenital varix
Excludes1 arteriovenous malformation (Q27.3-)

Q27.9 **Congenital malformation of peripheral vascular system, unspecified**
Anomaly of artery or vein NOS

Q28 **Other congenital malformations of circulatory system**
Excludes1 congenital aneurysm NOS (Q27.8)
congenital coronary aneurysm (Q24.5)
ruptured cerebral arteriovenous malformation (I60.8)
ruptured malformation of precerebral vessels (I72.0)
Excludes2 congenital peripheral aneurysm (Q27.8)
congenital pulmonary aneurysm (Q25.79)
congenital retinal aneurysm (Q14.1)

Q28.0 **Arteriovenous malformation of precerebral vessels**
Congenital arteriovenous precerebral aneurysm (nonruptured)

Q28.1 **Other malformations of precerebral vessels**
Congenital malformation of precerebral vessels NOS
Congenital precerebral aneurysm (nonruptured)

Q28.2 **Arteriovenous malformation of cerebral vessels**
Arteriovenous malformation of brain NOS
Congenital arteriovenous cerebral aneurysm (nonruptured)

Q28.3 **Other malformations of cerebral vessels**
Congenital cerebral aneurysm (nonruptured)
Congenital malformation of cerebral vessels NOS
Developmental venous anomaly

Q28.8 **Other specified congenital malformations of circulatory system**
Congenital aneurysm, specified site NEC
Spinal vessel anomaly

Q28.9 **Congenital malformation of circulatory system, unspecified**

CONGENITAL MALFORMATIONS OF THE RESPIRATORY SYSTEM (Q30-Q34)

Q30 **Congenital malformations of nose**
Excludes1 congenital deviation of nasal septum (Q67.4)

Q30.0 **Choanal atresia**
Atresia of nares (anterior) (posterior)
Congenital stenosis of nares (anterior) (posterior)

Q30.1 **Agenesis and underdevelopment of nose**
Congenital absent of nose

Q30.2 **Fissured, notched and cleft nose**

Q30.3 **Congenital perforated nasal septum**

Q30.8 **Other congenital malformations of nose**
Accessory nose
Congenital anomaly of nasal sinus wall

Q30.9 **Congenital malformation of nose, unspecified**

● Q31 **Congenital malformations of larynx**
Excludes1 congenital laryngeal stridor NOS (P28.89)

Q31.0 **Web of larynx**
Glottic web of larynx
Subglottic web of larynx
Web of larynx NOS

Q31.1 **Congenital subglottic stenosis**

Q31.2 **Laryngeal hypoplasia**

Q31.3 **Laryngocele**

Q31.5 **Congenital laryngomalacia**

Q31.8 **Other congenital malformations of larynx**
Absence of larynx
Agenesis of larynx
Atresia of larynx
Congenital cleft thyroid cartilage
Congenital fissure of epiglottis
Congenital stenosis of larynx NEC
Posterior cleft of cricoid cartilage

Q31.9 **Congenital malformation of larynx, unspecified**

● Q32 **Congenital malformations of trachea and bronchus**
Excludes1 congenital bronchiectasis (Q33.4)

Q32.0 **Congenital tracheomalacia**

Q32.1 **Other congenital malformations of trachea**
Atresia of trachea
Congenital anomaly of tracheal cartilage
Congenital dilatation of trachea
Congenital malformation of trachea
Congenital stenosis of trachea
Congenital tracheocele

Q32.2 **Congenital bronchomalacia**

Q32.3 **Congenital stenosis of bronchus**

Q32.4 **Other congenital malformations of bronchus**
Absence of bronchus
Agenesis of bronchus
Atresia of bronchus
Congenital diverticulum of bronchus
Congenital malformation of bronchus NOS

● Q33 **Congenital malformations of lung**

Q33.0 **Congenital cystic lung**
Congenital cystic lung disease
Congenital honeycomb lung
Congenital polycystic lung disease
Excludes1 cystic fibrosis (E84.0)
cystic lung disease, acquired or unspecified (J98.4)

Q33.1 **Accessory lobe of lung**
Azygos lobe (fissured), lung

Q33.2 **Sequestration of lung**

Q33.3 **Agenesis of lung**
Congenital absence of lung (lobe)

Q33.4 **Congenital bronchiectasis**

Q33.5 **Ectopic tissue in lung**

Q33.6 **Congenital hypoplasia and dysplasia of lung**
Excludes1 pulmonary hypoplasia associated with short gestation (P28.0)

Q33.8 **Other congenital malformations of lung**

Q33.9 **Congenital malformation of lung, unspecified**

● Q34 **Other congenital malformations of respiratory system**
Excludes2 congenital central alveolar hypoventilation syndrome (G47.35)

Q34.0 **Anomaly of pleura**

Q34.1 **Congenital cyst of mediastinum**

Q34.8 **Other specified congenital malformations of respiratory system**
Atresia of nasopharynx

Q34.9 **Congenital malformation of respiratory system, unspecified**
Congenital absence of respiratory system
Congenital anomaly of respiratory system NOS

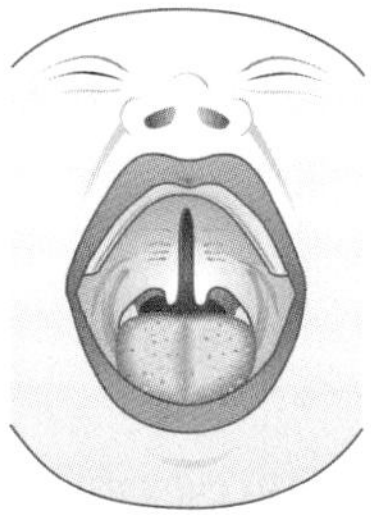

Figure 17-3 Cleft palate.

CLEFT LIP AND CLEFT PALATE (Q35-Q37)

Use additional code to identify associated malformation of the nose (Q30.2)
Excludes1 Robin's syndrome (Q87.0)

● Q35 **Cleft palate**
Includes fissure of palate
palatoschisis
Excludes1 cleft palate with cleft lip (Q37.-)

Q35.1 **Cleft hard palate**

Q35.3 **Cleft soft palate**

Q35.5 **Cleft hard palate with cleft soft palate**

Q35.7 **Cleft uvula**

Q35.9 **Cleft palate, unspecified**
Cleft palate NOS

● Q36 **Cleft lip**
Includes cheiloschisis
congenital fissure of lip
harelip
labium leporinum
Excludes1 cleft lip with cleft palate (Q37.-)

Q36.0 **Cleft lip, bilateral**

Q36.1 **Cleft lip, median**

Q36.9 **Cleft lip, unilateral**
Cleft lip NOS

● Q37 **Cleft palate with cleft lip**
Includes cheilopalatoschisis

Q37.0 **Cleft hard palate with bilateral cleft lip**

Q37.1 **Cleft hard palate with unilateral cleft lip**
Cleft hard palate with cleft lip NOS

Q37.2 **Cleft soft palate with bilateral cleft lip**

Q37.3 **Cleft soft palate with unilateral cleft lip**
Cleft soft palate with cleft lip NOS

Q37.4 **Cleft hard and soft palate with bilateral cleft lip**

Q37.5 **Cleft hard and soft palate with unilateral cleft lip**
Cleft hard and soft palate with cleft lip NOS

Q37.8 **Unspecified cleft palate with bilateral cleft lip**

Q37.9 **Unspecified cleft palate with unilateral cleft lip**
Cleft palate with cleft lip NOS

OTHER CONGENITAL MALFORMATIONS OF THE DIGESTIVE SYSTEM (Q38-Q45)

Q38 Other congenital malformations of tongue, mouth and pharynx

Excludes1 dentofacial anomalies (M26.-)
macrostomia (Q18.4)
microstomia (Q18.5)

Q38.0 Congenital malformations of lips, not elsewhere classified
Congenital fistula of lip
Congenital malformation of lip NOS
Van der Woude's syndrome
Excludes1 cleft lip (Q36.-)
cleft lip with cleft palate (Q37.-)
macrocheilia (Q18.6)
microcheilia (Q18.7)

Q38.1 Ankyloglossia
Restricted movement of tongue resulting in speech difficulty
Tongue tie

Q38.2 Macroglossia
Excessive size of tongue
Congenital hypertrophy of tongue

Q38.3 Other congenital malformations of tongue
Aglossia
Bifid tongue
Congenital adhesion of tongue
Congenital fissure of tongue
Congenital malformation of tongue NOS
Double tongue
Hypoglossia
Hypoplasia of tongue
Microglossia

Q38.4 Congenital malformations of salivary glands and ducts
Atresia of salivary glands and ducts
Congenital absence of salivary glands and ducts
Congenital accessory salivary glands and ducts
Congenital fistula of salivary gland

Q38.5 Congenital malformations of palate, not elsewhere classified
Congenital absence of uvula
Congenital malformation of palate NOS
Congenital high arched palate
Excludes1 cleft palate (Q35.-)
cleft palate with cleft lip (Q37.-)

Q38.6 Other congenital malformations of mouth
Congenital malformation of mouth NOS

Q38.7 Congenital pharyngeal pouch
Congenital diverticulum of pharynx
Excludes1 pharyngeal pouch syndrome (D82.1)

Q38.8 Other congenital malformations of pharynx
Congenital malformation of pharynx NOS
Imperforate pharynx

Q39 Congenital malformations of esophagus

Q39.Ø Atresia of esophagus without fistula
Atresia of esophagus NOS

Q39.1 Atresia of esophagus with tracheo-esophageal fistula
Atresia of esophagus with broncho-esophageal fistula

Q39.2 Congenital tracheo-esophageal fistula without atresia
Congenital tracheo-esophageal fistula NOS

Q39.3 Congenital stenosis and stricture of esophagus

Q39.4 Esophageal web

Q39.5 Congenital dilatation of esophagus
Congenital cardiospasm

Q39.6 Congenital diverticulum of esophagus
Congenital esophageal pouch

Q39.8 Other congenital malformations of esophagus
Congenital absence of esophagus
Congenital displacement of esophagus
Congenital duplication of esophagus

Q39.9 Congenital malformation of esophagus, unspecified

Q40 Other congenital malformations of upper alimentary tract

Q40.Ø Congenital hypertrophic pyloric stenosis
Congenital or infantile constriction
Congenital or infantile hypertrophy
Congenital or infantile spasm
Congenital or infantile stenosis
Congenital or infantile stricture

Q40.1 Congenital hiatus hernia
Congenital displacement of cardia through esophageal hiatus
Excludes1 congenital diaphragmatic hernia (Q79.Ø)

Q40.2 Other specified congenital malformations of stomach
Congenital displacement of stomach
Congenital diverticulum of stomach
Congenital hourglass stomach
Congenital duplication of stomach
Megalogastria
Microgastria

Q40.3 Congenital malformation of stomach, unspecified

Q40.8 Other specified congenital malformations of upper alimentary tract

Q40.9 Congenital malformation of upper alimentary tract, unspecified
Congenital anomaly of upper alimentary tract
Congenital deformity of upper alimentary tract

Q41 Congenital absence, atresia and stenosis of small intestine

Includes congenital obstruction, occlusion or stricture of small intestine or intestine NOS
Excludes1 cystic fibrosis with intestinal manifestation (E84.11)
meconium ileus NOS (without cystic fibrosis) (P76.Ø)

Q41.Ø Congenital absence, atresia and stenosis of duodenum

Q41.1 Congenital absence, atresia and stenosis of jejunum
Apple peel syndrome
Imperforate jejunum

Q41.2 Congenital absence, atresia and stenosis of ileum

Q41.8 Congenital absence, atresia and stenosis of other specified parts of small intestine

Q41.9 Congenital absence, atresia and stenosis of small intestine, part unspecified
Congenital absence, atresia and stenosis of intestine NOS

Q42 Congenital absence, atresia and stenosis of large intestine

Includes congenital obstruction, occlusion and stricture of large intestine

Q42.Ø Congenital absence, atresia and stenosis of rectum with fistula

Q42.1 Congenital absence, atresia and stenosis of rectum without fistula
Imperforate rectum

Q42.2 Congenital absence, atresia and stenosis of anus with fistula

Q42.3 Congenital absence, atresia and stenosis of anus without fistula
Imperforate anus

Q42.8 Congenital absence, atresia and stenosis of other parts of large intestine

Q42.9 Congenital absence, atresia and stenosis of large intestine, part unspecified

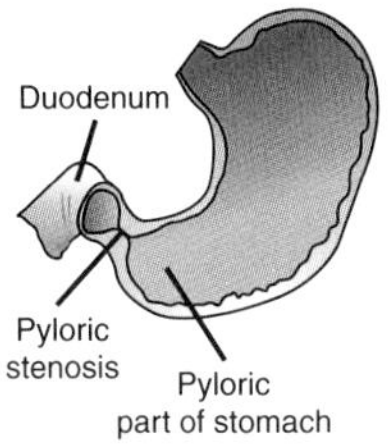

Figure 17-4 Pyloric stenosis.

CHAPTER 17 (QØØ-Q99)

Q43 Other congenital malformations of intestine

Q43.0 Meckel's diverticulum (displaced) (hypertrophic)
Congenital abnormality in which a pouch remains on the lower end of the small intestine
Persistent omphalomesenteric duct
Persistent vitelline duct

Q43.1 Hirschsprung's disease
Developmental disorder of enteric nervous system characterized by absence of ganglion cells in distal colon resulting in functional obstruction
Aganglionosis
Congenital (aganglionic) megacolon

Q43.2 Other congenital functional disorders of colon
Congenital dilatation of colon

Q43.3 Congenital malformations of intestinal fixation
Congenital omental, anomalous adhesions [bands]
Congenital peritoneal adhesions [bands]
Incomplete rotation of cecum and colon
Insufficient rotation of cecum and colon
Jackson's membrane
Malrotation of colon
Rotation failure of cecum and colon
Universal mesentery

Q43.4 Duplication of intestine

Q43.5 Ectopic anus
Anal opening in abnormal location

Q43.6 Congenital fistula of rectum and anus
Excludes1 congenital fistula of anus with absence, atresia and stenosis (Q42.2)
congenital fistula of rectum with absence, atresia and stenosis (Q42.0)
congenital rectovaginal fistula (Q52.2)
congenital urethrorectal fistula (Q64.73)
pilonidal fistula or sinus (L05.-)

Q43.7 Persistent cloaca
Malformation in which rectum, vagina, and urinary tract form one channel; AKA congenital cloaca
Cloaca NOS

Q43.8 Other specified congenital malformations of intestine
Congenital blind loop syndrome
Congenital diverticulitis, colon
Congenital diverticulum, intestine
Dolichocolon
Megaloappendix
Megaloduodenum
Microcolon
Transposition of appendix
Transposition of colon
Transposition of intestine

Q43.9 Congenital malformation of intestine, unspecified

Q44 Congenital malformations of gallbladder, bile ducts and liver

Q44.0 Agenesis, aplasia and hypoplasia of gallbladder
Congenital absence of gallbladder

Q44.1 Other congenital malformations of gallbladder
Congenital malformation of gallbladder NOS
Intrahepatic gallbladder

Q44.2 Atresia of bile ducts

Q44.3 Congenital stenosis and stricture of bile ducts

Q44.4 Choledochal cyst

Q44.5 Other congenital malformations of bile ducts
Accessory hepatic duct
Biliary duct duplication
Congenital malformation of bile duct NOS
Cystic duct duplication

Q44.6 Cystic disease of liver
Fibrocystic disease of liver

Q44.7 Other congenital malformations of liver
Accessory liver
Alagille's syndrome
Congenital absence of liver
Congenital hepatomegaly
Congenital malformation of liver NOS

Q45 Other congenital malformations of digestive system
Excludes2 congenital diaphragmatic hernia (Q79.0)
congenital hiatus hernia (Q40.1)

Q45.0 Agenesis, aplasia and hypoplasia of pancreas
Congenital absence of pancreas

Q45.1 Annular pancreas

Q45.2 Congenital pancreatic cyst

Q45.3 Other congenital malformations of pancreas and pancreatic duct
Accessory pancreas
Congenital malformation of pancreas or pancreatic duct NOS
Excludes1 congenital diabetes mellitus (E10.-)
cystic fibrosis (E84.0-E84.9)
fibrocystic disease of pancreas (E84.-)
neonatal diabetes mellitus (P70.2)

Q45.8 Other specified congenital malformations of digestive system
Absence (complete) (partial) of alimentary tract NOS
Duplication of digestive system
Malposition, congenital of digestive system

Q45.9 Congenital malformation of digestive system, unspecified
Congenital anomaly of digestive system
Congenital deformity of digestive system

CONGENITAL MALFORMATIONS OF GENITAL ORGANS (Q50-Q56)

Excludes1 androgen insensitivity syndrome (E34.5-)
syndromes associated with anomalies in the number and form of chromosomes (Q90-Q99)

Q50 Congenital malformations of ovaries, fallopian tubes and broad ligaments

Q50.0 Congenital absence of ovary
Excludes1 Turner's syndrome (Q96.-)

Q50.01 Congenital absence of ovary, unilateral ♀

Q50.02 Congenital absence of ovary, bilateral ♀

Q50.1 Developmental ovarian cyst ♀

Q50.2 Congenital torsion of ovary ♀

Q50.3 Other congenital malformations of ovary

Q50.31 Accessory ovary ♀

Q50.32 Ovarian streak ♀
Inadequate ovaries with absent follicular and hormonal function
46, XX with streak gonads

Q50.39 Other congenital malformation of ovary ♀
Congenital malformation of ovary NOS

Q50.4 Embryonic cyst of fallopian tube ♀
Fimbrial cyst

Q50.5 Embryonic cyst of broad ligament ♀
Epoophoron cyst
Parovarian cyst

Q50.6 Other congenital malformations of fallopian tube and broad ligament ♀
Absence of fallopian tube and broad ligament
Accessory fallopian tube and broad ligament
Atresia of fallopian tube and broad ligament
Congenital malformation of fallopian tube or broad ligament NOS

Q51 Congenital malformations of uterus and cervix

Q51.0 Agenesis and aplasia of uterus ♀
Congenital absence of uterus

Q51.1 Doubling of uterus with doubling of cervix and vagina

Q51.10 Doubling of uterus with doubling of cervix and vagina without obstruction ♀
Doubling of uterus with doubling of cervix and vagina NOS

Q51.11 Doubling of uterus with doubling of cervix and vagina with obstruction ♀

● Q51.2 **Other doubling of uterus**
Doubling of uterus NOS
Septate uterus
Q51.20 **Other doubling of uterus, unspecified** ♀
Septate uterus, unspecified
Q51.21 **Other complete doubling of uterus** ♀
Complete septate uterus
Q51.22 **Other partial doubling of uterus** ♀
Partial septate uterus
Q51.28 **Other doubling of uterus, other specified** ♀
Septate uterus, other specified
Q51.3 **Bicornate uterus** ♀
Bicornate uterus, complete or partial
Birth defect in which uterus has two separate "horns" that form top of uterus
Q51.4 **Unicornate uterus** ♀
Unicornate uterus with or without a separate uterine horn
Uterus with only one functioning horn
Uterus with half being undeveloped
Q51.5 **Agenesis and aplasia of cervix** ♀
Congenital absence of cervix
Q51.6 **Embryonic cyst of cervix** ♀
Q51.7 **Congenital fistulae between uterus and digestive and urinary tracts** ♀
● Q51.8 **Other congenital malformations of uterus and cervix**
● Q51.81 **Other congenital malformations of uterus**
Q51.810 **Arcuate uterus** ♀
Arcuatus uterus
Q51.811 **Hypoplasia of uterus** ♀
Q51.818 **Other congenital malformations of uterus** ♀
Müllerian anomaly of uterus NEC
● Q51.82 **Other congenital malformations of cervix**
Q51.820 **Cervical duplication** ♀
Q51.821 **Hypoplasia of cervix** ♀
Q51.828 **Other congenital malformations of cervix** ♀
Q51.9 **Congenital malformation of uterus and cervix, unspecified** ♀

● Q52 **Other congenital malformations of female genitalia**
Q52.0 **Congenital absence of vagina** ♀
Vaginal agenesis, total or partial
● Q52.1 **Doubling of vagina**
Excludes1 doubling of vagina with doubling of uterus and cervix (Q51.1-)
Q52.10 **Doubling of vagina, unspecified** ♀
Septate vagina NOS
Q52.11 **Transverse vaginal septum** ♀
● Q52.12 **Longitudinal vaginal septum**
Coding Clinic: 2016, Q4, P58
Q52.120 **Longitudinal vaginal septum, nonobstructing** ♀
Q52.121 **Longitudinal vaginal septum, obstructing, right side** ♀
Q52.122 **Longitudinal vaginal septum, obstructing, left side** ♀
Q52.123 **Longitudinal vaginal septum, microperforate, right side** ♀
Q52.124 **Longitudinal vaginal septum, microperforate, left side** ♀
Coding Clinic: 2016, Q4, P59
Q52.129 **Other and unspecified longitudinal vaginal septum** ♀
Q52.2 **Congenital rectovaginal fistula** ♀
Excludes1 cloaca (Q43.7)
Q52.3 **Imperforate hymen** ♀
Membrane (hymen) completely closes vaginal orifice
Q52.4 **Other congenital malformations of vagina** ♀
Canal of Nuck cyst, congenital
Congenital malformation of vagina NOS
Embryonic vaginal cyst
Gartner's duct cyst
Q52.5 **Fusion of labia** ♀
Q52.6 **Congenital malformation of clitoris** ♀
● Q52.7 **Other and unspecified congenital malformations of vulva**
Q52.70 **Unspecified congenital malformations of vulva** ♀
Congenital malformation of vulva NOS
Q52.71 **Congenital absence of vulva** ♀
Q52.79 **Other congenital malformations of vulva** ♀
Congenital cyst of vulva
Q52.8 **Other specified congenital malformations of female genitalia** ♀
Q52.9 **Congenital malformation of female genitalia, unspecified** ♀

● Q53 **Undescended and ectopic testicle**
● Q53.0 **Ectopic testis**
Q53.00 **Ectopic testis, unspecified** ♂
Q53.01 **Ectopic testis, unilateral** ♂
Q53.02 **Ectopic testes, bilateral** ♂
● Q53.1 **Undescended testicle, unilateral**
Q53.10 **Unspecified undescended testicle, unilateral** ♂
● Q53.11 **Abdominal testis, unilateral**
Q53.111 **Unilateral intraabdominal testis** ♂
Q53.112 **Unilateral inguinal testis** ♂
Q53.12 **Ectopic perineal testis, unilateral** ♂
Q53.13 **Unilateral high scrotal testis** ♂
● Q53.2 **Undescended testicle, bilateral**
Q53.20 **Undescended testicle, unspecified, bilateral** ♂
● Q53.21 **Abdominal testis, bilateral**
Q53.211 **Bilateral intraabdominal testes** ♂
Q53.212 **Bilateral inguinal testes** ♂
Q53.22 **Ectopic perineal testis, bilateral** ♂
Q53.23 **Bilateral high scrotal testes** ♂
Q53.9 **Undescended testicle, unspecified** ♂
Cryptorchism NOS

Item 17-1 Testes form in the abdomen of the male and only descend into the scrotum during normal embryonic development. "Ectopic" testes are out of their normal place or "retained" (left behind) in the abdomen. Crypto (hidden) orchism (testicle) is a major risk factor for testicular cancer.

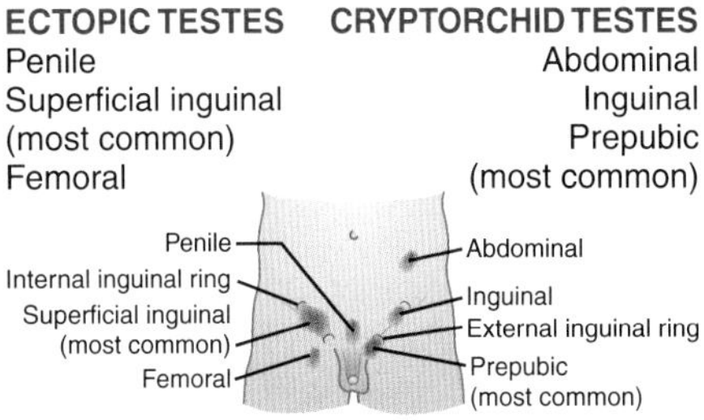

Figure 17-5 Undescended testes and the positions of the testes in various types of cryptorchidism or abnormal paths of descent.

CHAPTER 17 (Q00-Q99)

● **Q54 Hypospadias**
Birth defect of male; urethra opens in abnormal location on shaft
Excludes1 epispadias (Q64.Ø)

Q54.Ø Hypospadias, balanic ♂
Hypospadias, coronal
Hypospadias, glandular

Q54.1 Hypospadias, penile ♂

Q54.2 Hypospadias, penoscrotal ♂

Q54.3 Hypospadias, perineal ♂

Q54.4 Congenital chordee ♂
Chordee without hypospadias

Q54.8 Other hypospadias ♂
Hypospadias with intersex state

Q54.9 Hypospadias, unspecified ♂

● **Q55 Other congenital malformations of male genital organs**
Excludes1 congenital hydrocele (P83.5)
hypospadias (Q54.-)

Q55.Ø Absence and aplasia of testis ♂
Monorchism

Q55.1 Hypoplasia of testis and scrotum ♂
Fusion of testes

● **Q55.2 Other and unspecified congenital malformations of testis and scrotum**

Q55.2Ø Unspecified congenital malformations of testis and scrotum ♂
Congenital malformation of testis or scrotum NOS

Q55.21 Polyorchism ♂
Developmental anomaly characterized by presence of more than two testes

Q55.22 Retractile testis ♂

Q55.23 Scrotal transposition ♂

Q55.29 Other congenital malformations of testis and scrotum ♂

Q55.3 Atresia of vas deferens ♂
Code first any associated cystic fibrosis (E84.-)

Q55.4 Other congenital malformations of vas deferens, epididymis, seminal vesicles and prostate ♂
Absence or aplasia of prostate
Absence or aplasia of spermatic cord
Congenital malformation of vas deferens, epididymis, seminal vesicles or prostate NOS

Q55.5 Congenital absence and aplasia of penis ♂

● **Q55.6 Other congenital malformations of penis**

Q55.61 Curvature of penis (lateral) ♂

Q55.62 Hypoplasia of penis ♂
Underdevelopment penis
Micropenis

Q55.63 Congenital torsion of penis ♂
Excludes1 acquired torsion of penis (N48.82)

Q55.64 Hidden penis ♂
Buried penis
Concealed penis
Excludes1 acquired buried penis (N48.83)

Q55.69 Other congenital malformation of penis ♂
Congenital malformation of penis NOS

Q55.7 Congenital vasocutaneous fistula ♂
Abnormal opening between vas deferens and skin

Q55.8 Other specified congenital malformations of male genital organs ♂

Q55.9 Congenital malformation of male genital organ, unspecified ♂
Congenital anomaly of male genital organ
Congenital deformity of male genital organ

● **Q56 Indeterminate sex and pseudohermaphroditism**
Internal reproductive organs are opposite external physical characteristics.
Excludes1 46,XX true hermaphrodite (Q99.1)
androgen insensitivity syndrome (E34.5-)
chimera 46,XX/46,XY true hermaphrodite (Q99.Ø)
female pseudohermaphroditism with adrenocortical disorder (E25.-)
pseudohermaphroditism with specified chromosomal anomaly (Q96-Q99)
pure gonadal dysgenesis (Q99.1)

Q56.Ø Hermaphroditism, not elsewhere classified
Ovotestis

Q56.1 Male pseudohermaphroditism, not elsewhere classified ♂
46, XY with streak gonads
Male pseudohermaphroditism NOS

Q56.2 Female pseudohermaphroditism, not elsewhere classified ♀
Female pseudohermaphroditism NOS

Q56.3 Pseudohermaphroditism, unspecified

Q56.4 Indeterminate sex, unspecified
Ambiguous genitalia

CONGENITAL MALFORMATIONS OF THE URINARY SYSTEM (Q6Ø-Q64)

● **Q6Ø Renal agenesis and other reduction defects of kidney**
Includes congenital absence of kidney
congenital atrophy of kidney
infantile atrophy of kidney

Q6Ø.Ø Renal agenesis, unilateral

Q6Ø.1 Renal agenesis, bilateral

Q6Ø.2 Renal agenesis, unspecified

Q6Ø.3 Renal hypoplasia, unilateral

Q6Ø.4 Renal hypoplasia, bilateral

Q6Ø.5 Renal hypoplasia, unspecified

Q6Ø.6 Potter's syndrome

● **Q61 Cystic kidney disease**
Cysts that develop in failing kidney due to end-stage renal disease
Excludes1 acquired cyst of kidney (N28.1)
Potter's syndrome (Q6Ø.6)

● **Q61.Ø Congenital renal cyst**

Q61.ØØ Congenital renal cyst, unspecified
Cyst of kidney NOS (congenital)

Q61.Ø1 Congenital single renal cyst

Q61.Ø2 Congenital multiple renal cysts

● **Q61.1 Polycystic kidney, infantile type**
Polycystic kidney, autosomal recessive

Q61.11 Cystic dilatation of collecting ducts

Q61.19 Other polycystic kidney, infantile type

Q61.2 Polycystic kidney, adult type
Polycystic kidney, autosomal dominant

Q61.3 Polycystic kidney, unspecified
Coding Clinic: 2Ø16, Q3, P23

Q61.4 Renal dysplasia
Multicystic dysplastic kidney
Multicystic kidney (development)
Multicystic kidney disease
Multicystic renal dysplasia
Excludes1 polycystic kidney disease (Q61.11-Q61.3)

Q61.5 Medullary cystic kidney
Nephronopthisis
Sponge kidney NOS

Q61.8 Other cystic kidney diseases
Fibrocystic kidney
Fibrocystic renal degeneration or disease

Q61.9 Cystic kidney disease, unspecified
Meckel-Gruber syndrome

● Q62 **Congenital obstructive defects of renal pelvis and congenital malformations of ureter**
Q62.0 **Congenital hydronephrosis**
● Q62.1 **Congenital occlusion of ureter**
Atresia and stenosis of ureter
Q62.10 **Congenital occlusion of ureter, unspecified**
Q62.11 **Congenital occlusion of ureteropelvic junction**
Q62.12 **Congenital occlusion of ureterovesical orifice**
Q62.2 **Congenital megaureter**
Congenital dilatation of ureter
● Q62.3 **Other obstructive defects of renal pelvis and ureter**
Q62.31 **Congenital ureterocele, orthotopic**
Q62.32 **Cecoureterocele**
Ectopic ureterocele
Q62.39 **Other obstructive defects of renal pelvis and ureter**
Ureteropelvic junction obstruction NOS
Q62.4 **Agenesis of ureter**
Congenital absence ureter
Q62.5 **Duplication of ureter**
Accessory ureter
Double ureter
● Q62.6 **Malposition of ureter**
Q62.60 **Malposition of ureter, unspecified**
Q62.61 **Deviation of ureter**
Q62.62 **Displacement of ureter**
Q62.63 **Anomalous implantation of ureter**
Ectopia of ureter
Ectopic ureter
Q62.69 **Other malposition of ureter**
Q62.7 **Congenital vesico-uretero-renal reflux**
Q62.8 **Other congenital malformations of ureter**
Anomaly of ureter NOS

● Q63 **Other congenital malformations of kidney**
Excludes1 congenital nephrotic syndrome (N04.-)
Q63.0 **Accessory kidney**
Q63.1 **Lobulated, fused and horseshoe kidney**
Q63.2 **Ectopic kidney**
Congenital displaced kidney
Malrotation of kidney
Q63.3 **Hyperplastic and giant kidney**
Compensatory hypertrophy of kidney
Q63.8 **Other specified congenital malformations of kidney**
Congenital renal calculi
Q63.9 **Congenital malformation of kidney, unspecified**

● Q64 **Other congenital malformations of urinary system**
Q64.0 **Epispadias**
Urethral opening somewhere on dorsum of penis
Excludes1 hypospadias (Q54.-)
● Q64.1 **Exstrophy of urinary bladder**
Bladder is exposed, inside out, and protrudes through abdominal wall
Q64.10 **Exstrophy of urinary bladder, unspecified**
Ectopia vesicae
Q64.11 **Supravesical fissure of urinary bladder**
Q64.12 **Cloacal exstrophy of urinary bladder**
Q64.19 **Other exstrophy of urinary bladder**
Extroversion of bladder
Q64.2 **Congenital posterior urethral valves**
● Q64.3 **Other atresia and stenosis of urethra and bladder neck**
Q64.31 **Congenital bladder neck obstruction**
Congenital obstruction of vesicourethral orifice
Q64.32 **Congenital stricture of urethra**
Q64.33 **Congenital stricture of urinary meatus**
Q64.39 **Other atresia and stenosis of urethra and bladder neck**
Atresia and stenosis of urethra and bladder neck NOS
Q64.4 **Malformation of urachus**
Cyst of urachus
Patent urachus
Prolapse of urachus
Q64.5 **Congenital absence of bladder and urethra**
Q64.6 **Congenital diverticulum of bladder**
● Q64.7 **Other and unspecified congenital malformations of bladder and urethra**
Excludes1 congenital prolapse of bladder (mucosa) (Q79.4)
Q64.70 **Unspecified congenital malformation of bladder and urethra**
Malformation of bladder or urethra NOS
Q64.71 **Congenital prolapse of urethra**
Q64.72 **Congenital prolapse of urinary meatus**
Q64.73 **Congenital urethrorectal fistula**
Q64.74 **Double urethra**
Q64.75 **Double urinary meatus**
Q64.79 **Other congenital malformations of bladder and urethra**
Q64.8 **Other specified congenital malformations of urinary system**
Q64.9 **Congenital malformation of urinary system, unspecified**
Congenital anomaly NOS of urinary system
Congenital deformity NOS of urinary system

CONGENITAL MALFORMATIONS AND DEFORMATIONS OF THE MUSCULOSKELETAL SYSTEM (Q65-Q79)

● Q65 **Congenital deformities of hip**
Excludes1 clicking hip (R29.4)
● Q65.0 **Congenital dislocation of hip, unilateral**
Q65.00 **Congenital dislocation of unspecified hip, unilateral**
Q65.01 **Congenital dislocation of right hip, unilateral**
Q65.02 **Congenital dislocation of left hip, unilateral**
Q65.1 **Congenital dislocation of hip, bilateral**
Q65.2 **Congenital dislocation of hip, unspecified**
● Q65.3 **Congenital partial dislocation of hip, unilateral**
Q65.30 **Congenital partial dislocation of unspecified hip, unilateral**
Q65.31 **Congenital partial dislocation of right hip, unilateral**
Q65.32 **Congenital partial dislocation of left hip, unilateral**
Q65.4 **Congenital partial dislocation of hip, bilateral**
Q65.5 **Congenital partial dislocation of hip, unspecified**
Q65.6 **Congenital unstable hip**
Congenital dislocatable hip
● Q65.8 **Other congenital deformities of hip**
Q65.81 **Congenital coxa valga**
Q65.82 **Congenital coxa vara**
Q65.89 **Other specified congenital deformities of hip**
Anteversion of femoral neck
Congenital acetabular dysplasia
Q65.9 **Congenital deformity of hip, unspecified**

Item 17-2 **Equinus foot** is a term referring to the hoof of a horse. The deformity is usually congenital or spastic. **Talipes equinovarus** is referred to as clubfoot. The foot tends to be smaller than normal, with the heel pointing downward and the forefoot turning inward. The heel cord (Achilles tendon) is tight, causing the heel to be drawn up toward the leg.

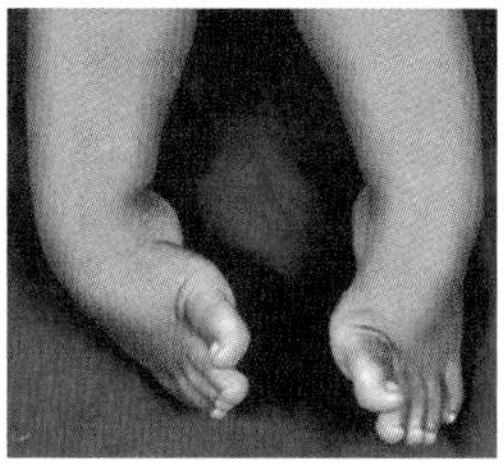

Figure 17-6 Supination and cavus deformity of forefoot. (From Kliegman R, Nelson WE: Nelson Textbook of Pediatrics, Philadelphia, Saunders, 2007)

● Q66 **Congenital deformities of feet**

Excludes1 reduction defects of feet (Q72.-)
valgus deformities (acquired) (M21.Ø-)
varus deformities (acquired) (M21.1-)

● Q66.Ø **Congenital talipes equinovarus**
Heel is turned inward from midline and foot is plantar flexed; AKA clubfoot

▶Q66.ØØ **Congenital talipes equinovarus, unspecified foot**

▶Q66.Ø1 **Congenital talipes equinovarus, right foot**

▶Q66.Ø2 **Congenital talipes equinovarus, left foot**

● Q66.1 **Congenital talipes calcaneovarus**
Deformity of foot in which heel is turned toward midline of body and anterior of foot is elevated

▶Q66.1Ø **Congenital talipes calcaneovarus, unspecified foot**

▶Q66.11 **Congenital talipes calcaneovarus, right foot**

▶Q66.12 **Congenital talipes calcaneovarus, left foot**

● Q66.2 **Congenital metatarsus (primus) varus**
Angulation of first metatarsal bone toward midline of body
Coding Clinic: 2Ø16, Q4, P59

● Q66.21 **Congenital metatarsus primus varus**

▶Q66.211 **Congenital metatarsus primus varus, right foot**

▶Q66.212 **Congenital metatarsus primus varus, left foot**

▶Q66.219 **Congenital metatarsus primus varus, unspecified foot**

● Q66.22 **Congenital metatarsus adductus**
Congenital metatarsus varus

▶Q66.221 **Congenital metatarsus adductus, right foot**

▶Q66.222 **Congenital metatarsus adductus, left foot**

▶Q66.229 **Congenital metatarsus adductus, unspecified foot**

● Q66.3 **Other congenital varus deformities of feet**
Hallux varus, congenital

▶Q66.3Ø **Other congenital varus deformities of feet, unspecified foot**

▶Q66.31 **Other congenital varus deformities of feet, right foot**

▶Q66.32 **Other congenital varus deformities of feet, left foot**

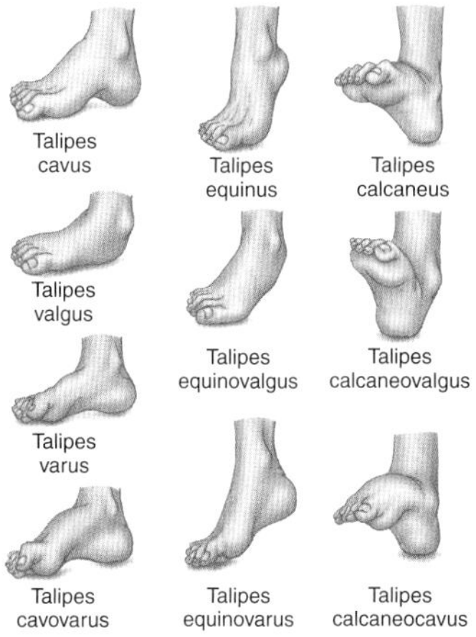

Figure 17-7 Talipes. (From Dorland: Dorland's Illustrated Medical Dictionary, ed 31, Saunders, 2007, p 1893)

● Q66.4 **Congenital talipes calcaneovalgus**

▶Q66.4Ø **Congenital talipes calcaneovalgus, unspecified foot**

▶Q66.41 **Congenital talipes calcaneovalgus, right foot**

▶Q66.42 **Congenital talipes calcaneovalgus, left foot**

● Q66.5 **Congenital pes planus**
Congenital flat foot
Congenital rigid flat foot
Congenital spastic (everted) flat foot

Excludes1 pes planus, acquired (M21.4)

Q66.5Ø **Congenital pes planus, unspecified foot**

Q66.51 **Congenital pes planus, right foot**

Q66.52 **Congenital pes planus, left foot**

Q66.6 **Other congenital valgus deformities of feet**
Inward angulation
Congenital metatarsus valgus

● Q66.7 **Congenital pes cavus**

▶Q66.7Ø **Congenital pes cavus, unspecified foot**

▶Q66.71 **Congenital pes cavus, right foot**

▶Q66.72 **Congenital pes cavus, left foot**

● Q66.8 **Other congenital deformities of feet**

Q66.8Ø **Congenital vertical talus deformity, unspecified foot**

Q66.81 **Congenital vertical talus deformity, right foot**

Q66.82 **Congenital vertical talus deformity, left foot**

Q66.89 **Other specified congenital deformities of feet**
Congenital asymmetric talipes
Congenital clubfoot NOS
Congenital talipes NOS
Congenital tarsal coalition
Hammer toe, congenital

● Q66.9 **Congenital deformity of feet, unspecified**

▶Q66.9Ø **Congenital deformity of feet, unspecified, unspecified foot**

▶Q66.91 **Congenital deformity of feet, unspecified, right foot**

▶Q66.92 **Congenital deformity of feet, unspecified, left foot**

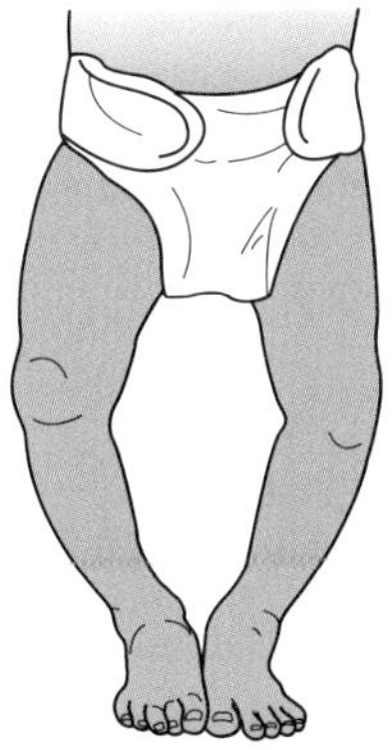

Figure 17-8 Mild to moderate inbowing of the lower leg. (From Lissauer T, Clayden G: Illustrated Textbook of Paediatrics, Edinburgh, Mosby, 2011)

● Q67 **Congenital musculoskeletal deformities of head, face, spine and chest**

Excludes1 congenital malformation syndromes classified to Q87.-
Potter's syndrome (Q60.6)

Q67.0 **Congenital facial asymmetry**

Q67.1 **Congenital compression facies**

Q67.2 **Dolichocephaly**
Long head dimension

Q67.3 **Plagiocephaly**
Asymmetric shape of head resulting from irregular closure of cranial sutures

Q67.4 **Other congenital deformities of skull, face and jaw**
Congenital depressions in skull
Congenital hemifacial atrophy or hypertrophy
Deviation of nasal septum, congenital
Squashed or bent nose, congenital
Excludes1 dentofacial anomalies [including malocclusion] (M26.-)
syphilitic saddle nose (A50.5)

Q67.5 **Congenital deformity of spine**
Congenital postural scoliosis
Congenital scoliosis NOS
Excludes1 infantile idiopathic scoliosis (M41.0)
scoliosis due to congenital bony malformation (Q76.3)

Q67.6 **Pectus excavatum**
Congenital funnel chest
Funnel-shaped chest depression

Q67.7 **Pectus carinatum**
Congenital pigeon chest

Q67.8 **Other congenital deformities of chest**
Congenital deformity of chest wall NOS

● Q68 **Other congenital musculoskeletal deformities**

Excludes1 reduction defects of limb(s) (Q71-Q73)
Excludes2 congenital myotonic chondrodystrophy (G71.13)

Q68.0 **Congenital deformity of sternocleidomastoid muscle**
Congenital contracture of sternocleidomastoid (muscle)
Congenital (sternomastoid) torticollis
Sternomastoid tumor (congenital)

Q68.1 **Congenital deformity of finger(s) and hand**
Congenital clubfinger
Spade-like hand (congenital)

Q68.2 **Congenital deformity of knee**
Congenital dislocation of knee
Congenital genu recurvatum
Hyperextension of knee resulting from hypermobility

Q68.3 **Congenital bowing of femur**
Excludes1 anteversion of femur (neck) (Q65.89)

Q68.4 **Congenital bowing of tibia and fibula**

Q68.5 **Congenital bowing of long bones of leg, unspecified**

Q68.6 **Discoid meniscus**

Q68.8 **Other specified congenital musculoskeletal deformities**
Congenital deformity of clavicle
Congenital deformity of elbow
Congenital deformity of forearm
Congenital deformity of scapula
Congenital deformity of wrist
Congenital dislocation of elbow
Congenital dislocation of shoulder
Congenital dislocation of wrist

● Q69 **Polydactyly**
AKA hyperdactyly, consists of supernumerary fingers or toes

Q69.0 **Accessory finger(s)**

Q69.1 **Accessory thumb(s)**

Q69.2 **Accessory toe(s)**
Accessory hallux

Q69.9 **Polydactyly, unspecified**
Supernumerary digit(s) NOS

● Q70 **Syndactyly**
Webbing between distal phalanges of adjacent digits

● Q70.0 **Fused fingers**
Complex syndactyly of fingers with synostosis
Q70.00 **Fused fingers, unspecified hand**
Q70.01 **Fused fingers, right hand**
Q70.02 **Fused fingers, left hand**
Q70.03 **Fused fingers, bilateral**

● Q70.1 **Webbed fingers**
Simple syndactyly of fingers without synostosis
Q70.10 **Webbed fingers, unspecified hand**
Q70.11 **Webbed fingers, right hand**
Q70.12 **Webbed fingers, left hand**
Q70.13 **Webbed fingers, bilateral**

● Q70.2 **Fused toes**
Complex syndactyly of toes with synostosis
Q70.20 **Fused toes, unspecified foot**
Q70.21 **Fused toes, right foot**
Q70.22 **Fused toes, left foot**
Q70.23 **Fused toes, bilateral**

● Q70.3 **Webbed toes**
Simple syndactyly of toes without synostosis
Q70.30 **Webbed toes, unspecified foot**
Q70.31 **Webbed toes, right foot**
Q70.32 **Webbed toes, left foot**
Q70.33 **Webbed toes, bilateral**

Q70.4 **Polysyndactyly, unspecified**
Excludes1 specified syndactyly of hand and feet - code to specified conditions (Q70.0- -Q70.3-)
Extra and webbed digits

Q70.9 **Syndactyly, unspecified**
Symphalangy NOS

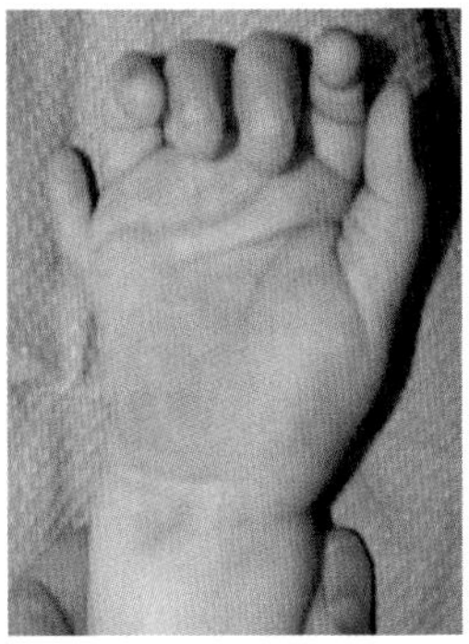

Figure 17-9 Thumb and index finger. (From Chung K: Hand and Upper Extremity Reconstruction, 1e, Saunders, 2008)

CHAPTER 17 (Q00-Q99)

- Q71 Reduction defects of **upper limb**
  - Q71.0 Congenital **complete absence** of upper limb
    - Q71.00 Congenital complete absence of **unspecified** upper limb
    - Q71.01 Congenital complete absence of **right** upper limb
    - Q71.02 Congenital complete absence of **left** upper limb
    - Q71.03 Congenital complete absence of upper limb, **bilateral**
  - Q71.1 Congenital absence **of upper arm and forearm with hand** present
    - Q71.10 Congenital absence of **unspecified** upper arm and forearm with hand present
    - Q71.11 Congenital absence of **right** upper arm and forearm with hand present
    - Q71.12 Congenital absence of **left** upper arm and forearm with hand present
    - Q71.13 Congenital absence of upper arm and forearm with hand present, **bilateral**
  - Q71.2 Congenital **absence of both forearm and hand**
    - Q71.20 Congenital absence of both forearm and hand, **unspecified** upper limb
    - Q71.21 Congenital absence of both forearm and hand, **right** upper limb
    - Q71.22 Congenital absence of both forearm and hand, **left** upper limb
    - Q71.23 Congenital absence of both forearm and hand, **bilateral**
  - Q71.3 Congenital **absence of hand and finger**
    - Q71.30 Congenital absence of **unspecified** hand and finger
    - Q71.31 Congenital absence of **right** hand and finger
    - Q71.32 Congenital absence of **left** hand and finger
    - Q71.33 Congenital absence of hand and finger, **bilateral**
  - Q71.4 Longitudinal reduction defect of **radius**
    - Clubhand (congenital)
    - Radial clubhand
    - Q71.40 Longitudinal reduction defect of **unspecified** radius
    - Q71.41 Longitudinal reduction defect of **right** radius
    - Q71.42 Longitudinal reduction defect of **left** radius
    - Q71.43 Longitudinal reduction defect of radius, **bilateral**
  - Q71.5 Longitudinal reduction defect of **ulna**
    - Q71.50 Longitudinal reduction defect of **unspecified** ulna
    - Q71.51 Longitudinal reduction defect of **right** ulna
    - Q71.52 Longitudinal reduction defect of **left** ulna
    - Q71.53 Longitudinal reduction defect of ulna, **bilateral**
  - Q71.6 **Lobster-claw hand**
    - Q71.60 Lobster-claw hand, **unspecified** hand
    - Q71.61 Lobster-claw **right** hand
    - Q71.62 Lobster-claw **left** hand
    - Q71.63 Lobster-claw hand, **bilateral**
  - Q71.8 **Other** reduction defects of upper limb
    - Q71.81 Congenital **shortening** of upper limb
      - Q71.811 Congenital shortening of **right** upper limb
      - Q71.812 Congenital shortening of **left** upper limb
      - Q71.813 Congenital shortening of upper limb, **bilateral**
      - Q71.819 Congenital shortening of **unspecified** upper limb
    - Q71.89 **Other** reduction defects of upper limb
      - Q71.891 Other reduction defects of **right** upper limb
      - Q71.892 Other reduction defects of **left** upper limb
      - Q71.893 Other reduction defects of upper limb, **bilateral**
      - Q71.899 Other reduction defects of **unspecified** upper limb
  - Q71.9 **Unspecified** reduction defect of upper limb
    - Q71.90 Unspecified reduction defect of **unspecified** upper limb
    - Q71.91 Unspecified reduction defect of **right** upper limb
    - Q71.92 Unspecified reduction defect of **left** upper limb
    - Q71.93 Unspecified reduction defect of upper limb, **bilateral**

- Q72 Reduction defects of **lower limb**
  - Q72.0 Congenital **complete absence** of lower limb
    - Q72.00 Congenital complete absence of **unspecified** lower limb
    - Q72.01 Congenital complete absence of **right** lower limb
    - Q72.02 Congenital complete absence of **left** lower limb
    - Q72.03 Congenital complete absence of lower limb, **bilateral**
  - Q72.1 Congenital absence of thigh and lower leg with foot present
    - Q72.10 Congenital absence of **unspecified** thigh and lower leg with foot present
    - Q72.11 Congenital absence of **right** thigh and lower leg with foot present
    - Q72.12 Congenital absence of **left** thigh and lower leg with foot present
    - Q72.13 Congenital absence of thigh and lower leg with foot present, **bilateral**
  - Q72.2 Congenital **absence of both lower leg and foot**
    - Q72.20 Congenital absence of both lower leg and foot, **unspecified** lower limb
    - Q72.21 Congenital absence of both lower leg and foot, **right** lower limb
    - Q72.22 Congenital absence of both left lower leg and foot, **left** lower limb
    - Q72.23 Congenital absence of both lower leg and foot, **bilateral**
  - Q72.3 Congenital **absence of foot and toe(s)**
    - Q72.30 Congenital absence of **unspecified** foot and toe(s)
    - Q72.31 Congenital absence of **right** foot and toe(s)
    - Q72.32 Congenital absence of **left** foot and toe(s)
    - Q72.33 Congenital absence of foot and toe(s), **bilateral**
  - Q72.4 Longitudinal reduction defect of **femur**
    - Proximal femoral focal deficiency
    - Q72.40 Longitudinal reduction defect of **unspecified** femur
    - Q72.41 Longitudinal reduction defect of **right** femur
    - Q72.42 Longitudinal reduction defect of **left** femur
    - Q72.43 Longitudinal reduction defect of femur, **bilateral**
  - Q72.5 Longitudinal reduction defect of **tibia**
    - Q72.50 Longitudinal reduction defect of **unspecified** tibia
    - Q72.51 Longitudinal reduction defect of **right** tibia
    - Q72.52 Longitudinal reduction defect of **left** tibia
    - Q72.53 Longitudinal reduction defect of tibia, **bilateral**

CHAPTER 17 (Q00-Q99)

● Q72.6 **Longitudinal reduction defect of fibula**
- Q72.60 **Longitudinal reduction defect of unspecified fibula**
- Q72.61 **Longitudinal reduction defect of right fibula**
- Q72.62 **Longitudinal reduction defect of left fibula**
- Q72.63 **Longitudinal reduction defect of fibula, bilateral**

● Q72.7 **Split foot**
- Q72.70 **Split foot, unspecified lower limb**
- Q72.71 **Split foot, right lower limb**
- Q72.72 **Split foot, left lower limb**
- Q72.73 **Split foot, bilateral**

● Q72.8 **Other reduction defects of lower limb**

● Q72.81 **Congenital shortening of lower limb**
- Q72.811 **Congenital shortening of right lower limb**
- Q72.812 **Congenital shortening of left lower limb**
- Q72.813 **Congenital shortening of lower limb, bilateral**
- Q72.819 **Congenital shortening of unspecified lower limb**

● Q72.89 **Other reduction defects of lower limb**
- Q72.891 **Other reduction defects of right lower limb**
- Q72.892 **Other reduction defects of left lower limb**
- Q72.893 **Other reduction defects of lower limb, bilateral**
- Q72.899 **Other reduction defects of unspecified lower limb**

● Q72.9 **Unspecified reduction defect of lower limb**
- Q72.90 **Unspecified reduction defect of unspecified lower limb**
- Q72.91 **Unspecified reduction defect of right lower limb**
- Q72.92 **Unspecified reduction defect of left lower limb**
- Q72.93 **Unspecified reduction defect of lower limb, bilateral**

● Q73 **Reduction defects of unspecified limb**

Q73.0 **Congenital absence of unspecified limb(s)**
Amelia NOS

Q73.1 **Phocomelia, unspecified limb(s)**
Phocomelia NOS
Absence/shortening of long bones primarily as a result of thalidomide

Q73.8 **Other reduction defects of unspecified limb(s)**
Longitudinal reduction deformity of unspecified limb(s)
Ectromelia of limb NOS
Gross hypoplasia or aplasia of one or more long bones of limb(s)
Hemimelia of limb NOS
Absence of one-half of long bone
Reduction defect of limb NOS

● Q74 **Other congenital malformations of limb(s)**

Excludes1 polydactyly (Q69.-)
reduction defect of limb (Q71-Q73)
syndactyly (Q70.-)

Q74.0 **Other congenital malformations of upper limb(s), including shoulder girdle**
Accessory carpal bones
Cleidocranial dysostosis
Congenital pseudarthrosis of clavicle
Macrodactylia (fingers)
Madelung's deformity
Radioulnar synostosis
Sprengel's deformity
Triphalangeal thumb

Q74.1 **Congenital malformation of knee**
Congenital absence of patella
Congenital dislocation of patella
Congenital genu valgum
Congenital genu varum
Rudimentary patella

Excludes1 congenital dislocation of knee (Q68.2)
congenital genu recurvatum (Q68.2)
nail patella syndrome (Q87.2)

Q74.2 **Other congenital malformations of lower limb(s), including pelvic girdle**
Congenital fusion of sacroiliac joint
Congenital malformation of ankle joint
Congenital malformation of sacroiliac joint

Excludes1 anteversion of femur (neck) (Q65.89)

Q74.3 **Arthrogryposis multiplex congenita**

Q74.8 **Other specified congenital malformations of limb(s)**

Q74.9 **Unspecified congenital malformation of limb(s)**
Congenital anomaly of limb(s) NOS

● Q75 **Other congenital malformations of skull and face bones**

Excludes1 congenital malformation of face NOS (Q18.-)
congenital malformation syndromes classified to Q87.-
dentofacial anomalies [including malocclusion] (M26.-)
musculoskeletal deformities of head and face (Q67.0-Q67.4)
skull defects associated with congenital anomalies of brain such as:
anencephaly (Q00.0)
encephalocele (Q01.-)
hydrocephalus (Q03.-)
microcephaly (Q02)

Q75.0 **Craniosynostosis**
Premature closure of sutures of skull
Acrocephaly
Imperfect fusion of skull
Oxycephaly
Trigonocephaly

Q75.1 **Craniofacial dysostosis**
Congential deformity of head
Crouzon's disease

Item 17-3 **Anencephalus** is a congenital deformity of the cranial vault. **Craniosynostosis,** also known as craniostenosis and stenocephaly, signifies any form of congenital deformity of the skull that results from the premature closing of the sutures of the skull. **Iniencephaly** is a deformity in which the head and neck are flexed backward to a great extent and the head is very large in comparison to the shortened body.

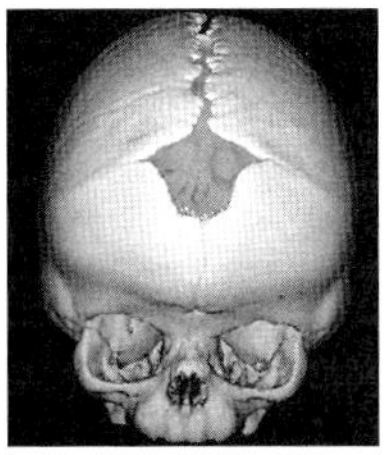

Figure 17-10 Generalized craniosynostosis without symptoms or signs of increased intracranial pressure. (From Goetz C: Textbook of Clinical Neurology, St. Louis, MO, Elsevier, 2007)

CHAPTER 17 (Q00-Q99)

Q75.2 Hypertelorism

Q75.3 Macrocephaly
Unusually large size of head; AKA megalocephaly

Q75.4 Mandibulofacial dysostosis
Franceschetti syndrome
Treacher Collins syndrome

Q75.5 Oculomandibular dysostosis
Ossification of occular and mandibular bones

Q75.8 Other specified congenital malformations of skull and face bones
Absence of skull bone, congenital
Congenital deformity of forehead
Platybasia

Q75.9 Congenital malformation of skull and face bones, unspecified
Congenital anomaly of face bones NOS
Congenital anomaly of skull NOS

● **Q76 Congenital malformations of spine and bony thorax**
Excludes1 congenital musculoskeletal deformities of spine and chest (Q67.5-Q67.8)

Q76.Ø Spina bifida occulta
Excludes1 meningocele (spinal) (QØ5.-)
spina bifida (aperta) (cystica) (QØ5.-)

Q76.1 Klippel-Feil syndrome
Cervical fusion syndrome

Q76.2 Congenital spondylolisthesis
Congenital spondylolysis
Excludes1 spondylolisthesis (acquired) (M43.1-)
spondylolysis (acquired) (M43.Ø-)

Q76.3 Congenital scoliosis due to congenital bony malformation
Hemivertebra fusion or failure of segmentation with scoliosis

● **Q76.4 Other congenital malformations of spine, not associated with scoliosis**

● **Q76.41 Congenital kyphosis**
Abnormal increase in convexity curvature of thoracic spinal column; AKA humpback

Q76.411 Congenital kyphosis, occipito-atlanto-axial region

Q76.412 Congenital kyphosis, cervical region

Q76.413 Congenital kyphosis, cervicothoracic region

Q76.414 Congenital kyphosis, thoracic region

Q76.415 Congenital kyphosis, thoracolumbar region

Q76.419 Congenital kyphosis, unspecified region

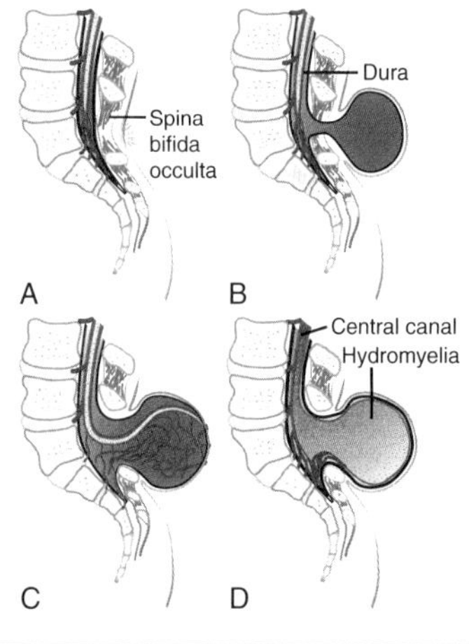

Figure 17-11 **A.** Spina bifida occulta. **B.** Meningocele. **C.** Myelomeningocele. **D.** Myelocystocele (syringomyelocele) or hydromyelia.

Item 17-4 Spina bifida is a midline spinal defect in which one or more vertebrae fail to fuse, leaving an opening in the vertebral canal. When the defect is not visible, it is called spina bifida occulta, and when it is visible, it is called spina bifida cystica.

● **Q76.42 Congenital lordosis**
An abnormal increase in curvature of lumbar spine (sway back)

Q76.425 Congenital lordosis, thoracolumbar region

Q76.426 Congenital lordosis, lumbar region

Q76.427 Congenital lordosis, lumbosacral region

Q76.428 Congenital lordosis, sacral and sacrococcygeal region

Q76.429 Congenital lordosis, unspecified region

Q76.49 Other congenital malformations of spine, not associated with scoliosis
Congenital absence of vertebra NOS
Congenital fusion of spine NOS
Congenital malformation of lumbosacral (joint) (region) NOS
Congenital malformation of spine NOS
Hemivertebra NOS
Malformation of spine NOS
Platyspondylisis NOS
Supernumerary vertebra NOS

Q76.5 Cervical rib
Supernumerary rib in cervical region

Q76.6 Other congenital malformations of ribs
Accessory rib
Congenital absence of rib
Congenital fusion of ribs
Congenital malformation of ribs NOS
Excludes1 short rib syndrome (Q77.2)

Q76.7 Congenital malformation of sternum
Congenital absence of sternum
Sternum bifidum

Q76.8 Other congenital malformations of bony thorax

Q76.9 Congenital malformation of bony thorax, unspecified

● **Q77 Osteochondrodysplasia with defects of growth of tubular bones and spine**
Excludes1 mucopolysaccharidosis (E76.Ø-E76.3)
Excludes2 congenital myotonic chondrodystrophy (G71.13)

Q77.Ø Achondrogenesis
Hypochondrogenesis

Q77.1 Thanatophoric short stature

Q77.2 Short rib syndrome
Asphyxiating thoracic dysplasia [Jeune]

Q77.3 Chondrodysplasia punctata
Benign cartilaginous neoplasms
Excludes1 rhizomelic chondrodysplasia punctata (E71.43)

Q77.4 Achondroplasia
Disturbance of epiphyseal chondroblastic growth and maturation, results in dwarfism
Hypochondroplasia
Osteosclerosis congenita

Q77.5 Diastrophic dysplasia

Q77.6 Chondroectodermal dysplasia
Defective development of skin, hair, teeth, with polydactyly and defect of cardiac septum
Ellis-van Creveld syndrome

Q77.7 Spondyloepiphyseal dysplasia

Q77.8 Other osteochondrodysplasia with defects of growth of tubular bones and spine

Q77.9 Osteochondrodysplasia with defects of growth of tubular bones and spine, unspecified

Q78 Other osteochondrodysplasias
Disorder of development of bone and cartilage; common cause of dwarfism
Excludes2 congenital myotonic chondrodystrophy (G71.13)

Q78.0 Osteogenesis imperfecta
Fragilitas ossium
Osteopsathyrosis

Q78.1 Polyostotic fibrous dysplasia
Albright(-McCune)(-Sternberg) syndrome

Q78.2 Osteopetrosis
Abnormally dense bone; AKA marble bones disease, ivory bones
Albers-Schönberg syndrome
Osteosclerosis NOS

Q78.3 Progressive diaphyseal dysplasia
Camurati-Engelmann syndrome

Q78.4 Enchondromatosis
Thinning of overlying cortex of bone and distorted length
Maffucci's syndrome
Ollier's disease

Q78.5 Metaphyseal dysplasia
Disturbance in enchondral bone growth, causing ends of shafts to remain larger than normal in circumference
Pyle's syndrome

Q78.6 Multiple congenital exostoses
Diaphyseal aclasis

Q78.8 Other specified osteochondrodysplasias
Osteopoikilosis

Q78.9 Osteochondrodysplasia, unspecified
Chondrodystrophy NOS
AKA skeletal dysplasia (dwarfism) caused by genetic mutations affecting hyaline cartilage capping long bones and vertebrae
Osteodystrophy NOS

Q79 Congenital malformations of musculoskeletal system, not elsewhere classified
Excludes2 congenital (sternomastoid) torticollis (Q68.0)

Q79.0 Congenital diaphragmatic hernia
Excludes1 congenital hiatus hernia (Q40.1)

Q79.1 Other congenital malformations of diaphragm
Absence of diaphragm
Congenital malformation of diaphragm NOS
Eventration of diaphragm

Q79.2 Exomphalos
Abdominal hernia in which part of intestine protrudes at umbilicus; AKA exomphalos and exumbilication
Omphalocele
Excludes1 umbilical hernia (K42.-)

Q79.3 Gastroschisis
Congenital fissure of anterior abdominal wall often with protrusion of small/large intestine

Q79.4 Prune belly syndrome
Congenital prolapse of bladder mucosa
Eagle-Barrett syndrome

Q79.5 Other congenital malformations of abdominal wall
Excludes1 umbilical hernia (K42.-)

Q79.51 Congenital hernia of bladder

Q79.59 Other congenital malformations of abdominal wall

Q79.6 Ehlers-Danlos syndromes
Group of inherited disorders of connective tissue; AKA cutis hyperelastica

▶**Q79.60 Ehlers-Danlos syndrome, unspecified**

▶**Q79.61 Classical Ehlers-Danlos syndrome**
▶Classical EDS (cEDS)

▶**Q79.62 Hypermobile Ehlers-Danlos syndrome**
▶Hypermobile EDS (hEDS)

▶**Q79.63 Vascular Ehlers-Danlos syndrome**
▶Vascular EDS (vEDS)

▶**Q79.69 Other Ehlers-Danlos syndromes**

Q79.8 Other congenital malformations of musculoskeletal system
Absence of muscle
Absence of tendon
Accessory muscle
Amyotrophia congenita
Congenital constricting bands
Congenital shortening of tendon
Poland syndrome

Q79.9 Congenital malformation of musculoskeletal system, unspecified
Congenital anomaly of musculoskeletal system NOS
Congenital deformity of musculoskeletal system NOS

OTHER CONGENITAL MALFORMATIONS (Q80-Q89)

Q80 Congenital ichthyosis
Characterized by increased keratinization, resulting in noninflammatory scaling of skin
Excludes1 Refsum's disease (G60.1)

Q80.0 Ichthyosis vulgaris

Q80.1 X-linked ichthyosis

Q80.2 Lamellar ichthyosis
Collodion baby

Q80.3 Congenital bullous ichthyosiform erythroderma

Q80.4 Harlequin fetus

Q80.8 Other congenital ichthyosis

Q80.9 Congenital ichthyosis, unspecified

Q81 Epidermolysis bullosa
Loosening of epidermis

Q81.0 Epidermolysis bullosa simplex
Excludes1 Cockayne's syndrome (Q87.19)

Q81.1 Epidermolysis bullosa letalis
Herlitz' syndrome

Q81.2 Epidermolysis bullosa dystrophica

Q81.8 Other epidermolysis bullosa

Q81.9 Epidermolysis bullosa, unspecified

Q82 Other congenital malformations of skin
Excludes1 acrodermatitis enteropathica (E83.2)
congenital erythropoietic porphyria (E80.0)
pilonidal cyst or sinus (L05.-)
Sturge-Weber (-Dimitri) syndrome (Q85.8)

Q82.0 Hereditary lymphedema
Characterized by swelling of subcutaneous tissue caused by obstruction of lymphatic vessels and resulting edema of lymph fluid

Q82.1 Xeroderma pigmentosum
Extreme sensitivity to ultraviolet rays that most commonly affects the eyes and skin, but may also involve the nervous system

Q82.2 Congenital cutaneous mastocytosis
Characterized by infiltrates of mast cells in tissues/organs
Congenital diffuse cutaneous mastocytosis
Congenital maculopapular cutaneous mastocytosis
Congenital urticaria pigmentosa
Excludes1 cutaneous mastocytosis NOS (D47.01)
diffuse cutaneous mastocytosis (with onset after newborn period) (D47.01)
malignant mastocytosis (C96.2-)
systemic mastocytosis (D47.02)
urticaria pigmentosa (non-congenital) (with onset after newborn period) (D47.01)

Q82.3 Incontinentia pigmenti
Characterized by hypopigmented cutaneous in adults and early childhood

Q82.4 Ectodermal dysplasia (anhidrotic)
Absence/deficiency of tissues/structures, including teeth, hair, nails, and certain glands
Excludes1 Ellis-van Creveld syndrome (Q77.6)

CHAPTER 17 (Q00-Q99)

Q82.5 **Congenital non-neoplastic nevus**
Birthmark NOS
Flammeus Nevus
Portwine Nevus
Sanguineous Nevus
Strawberry Nevus
Vascular Nevus NOS
Verrucous Nevus
Excludes2 Café au lait spots (L81.3)
lentigo (L81.4)
nevus NOS (D22.-)
araneus nevus (I78.1)
melanocytic nevus (D22.-)
pigmented nevus (D22.-)
spider nevus (I78.1)
stellar nevus (I78.1)

Q82.6 **Congenital sacral dimple**
Parasacral dimple
Excludes2 pilonidal cyst with abscess (LØ5.Ø1)
pilonidal cyst without abscess (LØ5.91)
Coding Clinic: 2Ø16, Q4, P6Ø

Q82.8 **Other specified congenital malformations of skin**
Abnormal palmar creases
Accessory skin tags
Benign familial pemphigus [Hailey-Hailey]
Congenital poikiloderma
Cutis laxa (hyperelastica)
Dermatoglyphic anomalies
Inherited keratosis palmaris et plantaris
Keratosis follicularis [Darier-White]
Excludes1 Ehlers-Danlos syndrome (Q79.6-)
Coding Clinic: 2Ø16, Q1, P17

Q82.9 **Congenital malformation of skin, unspecified**

● Q83 **Congenital malformations of breast**
Excludes2 absence of pectoral muscle (Q79.8)
hypoplasia of breast (N64.82)
micromastia (N64.82)

Q83.Ø **Congenital absence of breast with absent nipple**

Q83.1 **Accessory breast**
Supernumerary breast

Q83.2 **Absent nipple**

Q83.3 **Accessory nipple**
Supernumerary nipple

Q83.8 **Other congenital malformations of breast**

Q83.9 **Congenital malformation of breast, unspecified**

● Q84 **Other congenital malformations of integument**

Q84.Ø **Congenital alopecia**
Congenital atrichosis

Q84.1 **Congenital morphological disturbances of hair, not elsewhere classified**
Beaded hair
Monilethrix
Pili annulati
Excludes1 Menkes' kinky hair syndrome (E83.Ø)

Q84.2 **Other congenital malformations of hair**
Congenital hypertrichosis
Congenital malformation of hair NOS
Persistent lanugo

Q84.3 **Anonychia**
Absence of nail
Excludes1 nail patella syndrome (Q87.2)

Q84.4 **Congenital leukonychia**
Opaque, whitish discoloration of nails; AKA leukopathia unguium

Q84.5 **Enlarged and hypertrophic nails**
Congenital onychauxis
Pachyonychia

Q84.6 **Other congenital malformations of nails**
Congenital clubnail
Congenital koilonychia
Congenital malformation of nail NOS

Q84.8 **Other specified congenital malformations of integument**
Aplasia cutis congenita

Q84.9 **Congenital malformation of integument, unspecified**
Congenital anomaly of integument NOS
Congenital deformity of integument NOS

● Q85 **Phakomatoses, not elsewhere classified**
Excludes1 ataxia telangiectasia [Louis-Bar] (G11.3)
familial dysautonomia [Riley-Day] (G9Ø.1)

● Q85.Ø **Neurofibromatosis (nonmalignant)**
Developmental changes in nervous system and other structures, with formation of neurofibromas

Q85.ØØ **Neurofibromatosis, unspecified** (HCC)

Q85.Ø1 **Neurofibromatosis, type 1** (HCC)
Von Recklinghausen disease

Q85.Ø2 **Neurofibromatosis, type 2** (HCC)
Acoustic neurofibromatosis

Q85.Ø3 **Schwannomatosis** (HCC)

Q85.Ø9 **Other neurofibromatosis** (HCC)

Q85.1 **Tuberous sclerosis** (HCC)
Bourneville's disease
Epiloia

Q85.8 **Other phakomatoses, not elsewhere classified** (HCC)
Peutz-Jeghers Syndrome
Sturge-Weber(-Dimitri) syndrome
von Hippel-Lindau syndrome
Excludes1 Meckel-Gruber syndrome (Q61.9)

Q85.9 **Phakomatosis, unspecified** (HCC)
Hamartosis NOS

● Q86 **Congenital malformation syndromes due to known exogenous causes, not elsewhere classified**
Excludes2 iodine-deficiency-related hypothyroidism (EØØ-EØ2)
nonteratogenic effects of substances transmitted via placenta or breast milk (PØ4.-)

Q86.Ø **Fetal alcohol syndrome (dysmorphic)**

Q86.1 **Fetal hydantoin syndrome**
Meadow's syndrome

Q86.2 **Dysmorphism due to warfarin**

Q86.8 **Other congenital malformation syndromes due to known exogenous causes**

● Q87 **Other specified congenital malformation syndromes affecting multiple systems**
Use additional code(s) to identify all associated manifestations

Q87.Ø **Congenital malformation syndromes predominantly affecting facial appearance**
Acrocephalopolysyndactyly
Acrocephalosyndactyly [Apert]
Cryptophthalmos syndrome
Cyclopia
Goldenhar syndrome
Moebius syndrome
Oro-facial-digital syndrome
Robin syndrome
Whistling face

CHAPTER 17 (QØØ-Q99)

Q87.1 Congenital malformation syndromes predominantly associated with short stature

~~Aarskog syndrome~~
~~Cockayne syndrome~~
~~De Lange syndrome~~
~~Dubowitz syndrome~~
~~Noonan syndrome~~
~~Prader-Willi syndrome~~
~~Robinow-Silverman-Smith syndrome~~
~~Russell-Silver syndrome~~
~~Seckel syndrome~~

Q87.11 Prader-Willi syndrome

Q87.19 Other congenital malformation syndromes predominantly associated with short stature

Aarskog syndrome
Cockayne syndrome
De Lange syndrome
Dubowitz syndrome
Noonan syndrome
Robinow-Silverman-Smith syndrome
Russell-Silver syndrome
Seckel syndrome

Excludes1 Ellis-van Creveld syndrome (Q77.6)
Smith-Lemli-Opitz syndrome (E78.72)

Q87.2 Congenital malformation syndromes predominantly involving limbs

Holt-Oram syndrome
Klippel-Trenaunay-Weber syndrome
Nail patella syndrome
Rubinstein-Taybi syndrome
Sirenomelia syndrome
Thrombocytopenia with absent radius [TAR] syndrome
VATER syndrome

Q87.3 Congenital malformation syndromes involving early overgrowth

Beckwith-Wiedemann syndrome
Sotos' syndrome
Weaver syndrome

Q87.4 Marfan's syndrome

Q87.40 Marfan's syndrome, unspecified

Q87.41 Marfan's syndrome with cardiovascular manifestations

Q87.410 Marfan's syndrome with aortic dilation

Q87.418 Marfan's syndrome with other cardiovascular manifestations

Q87.42 Marfan's syndrome with ocular manifestations

Q87.43 Marfan's syndrome with skeletal manifestation

Q87.5 Other congenital malformation syndromes with other skeletal changes

Q87.8 Other specified congenital malformation syndromes, not elsewhere classified

Excludes1 Zellweger syndrome (E71.510)

Q87.81 Alport syndrome

Progressive sensorineural hearing loss, progressive pyelonephritis or glomerulonephritis, and ocular defects

Use additional code to identify stage of chronic kidney disease (N18.1-N18.6)

Q87.82 Arterial tortuosity syndrome

Coding Clinic: 2016, Q4, P60-61

Q87.89 Other specified congenital malformation syndromes, not elsewhere classified

Laurence-Moon (-Bardet)-Biedl syndrome

Q89 Other congenital malformations, not elsewhere classified

Q89.0 Congenital absence and malformations of spleen

Excludes1 isomerism of atrial appendages (with asplenia or polysplenia) (Q20.6)

Q89.01 Asplenia (congenital)

Q89.09 Congenital malformations of spleen

Congenital splenomegaly

Q89.1 Congenital malformations of adrenal gland

Excludes1 adrenogenital disorders (E25.-)
congenital adrenal hyperplasia (E25.0)

Q89.2 Congenital malformations of other endocrine glands

Congenital malformation of parathyroid or thyroid gland
Persistent thyroglossal duct
Thyroglossal cyst

Excludes1 congenital goiter (E03.0)
congenital hypothyroidism (E03.1)

Q89.3 Situs inversus

Lateral transposition of viscera of thorax and abdomen
Dextrocardia with situs inversus
Mirror-image atrial arrangement with situs inversus
Situs inversus or transversus abdominalis
Situs inversus or transversus thoracis
Transposition of abdominal viscera
Transposition of thoracic viscera

Excludes1 dextrocardia NOS (Q24.0)

Q89.4 Conjoined twins

Craniopagus
Dicephaly
Pygopagus
Thoracopagus

Q89.7 Multiple congenital malformations, not elsewhere classified

Multiple congenital anomalies NOS
Multiple congenital deformities NOS

Excludes1 congenital malformation syndromes affecting multiple systems (Q87.-)

Q89.8 Other specified congenital malformations

Use additional code(s) to identify all associated manifestations

Q89.9 Congenital malformation, unspecified

Congenital anomaly NOS
Congenital deformity NOS

CHROMOSOMAL ABNORMALITIES, NOT ELSEWHERE CLASSIFIED (Q90-Q99)

Excludes2 mitochondrial metabolic disorders (E88.4-)

Q90 Down syndrome

Use additional code(s) to identify any associated physical conditions and degree of intellectual disabilities (F70-F79)

Q90.0 Trisomy 21, nonmosaicism (meiotic nondisjunction)

Trisomy 21, nondisjunction, accounts for 95% of Downs syndrome cases

Q90.1 Trisomy 21, mosaicism (mitotic nondisjunction)

Q90.2 Trisomy 21, translocation

Q90.9 Down syndrome, unspecified

Trisomy 21 NOS

Q91 Trisomy 18 and Trisomy 13

Q91.0 Trisomy 18, nonmosaicism (meiotic nondisjunction)

Q91.1 Trisomy 18, mosaicism (mitotic nondisjunction)

Q91.2 Trisomy 18, translocation

Q91.3 Trisomy 18, unspecified

Q91.4 Trisomy 13, nonmosaicism (meiotic nondisjunction)

Q91.5 Trisomy 13, mosaicism (mitotic nondisjunction)

Q91.6 Trisomy 13, translocation

Q91.7 Trisomy 13, unspecified

CHAPTER 17 (Q00-Q99)

● **Q92** Other trisomies and partial trisomies of the autosomes, not elsewhere classified

> **Includes** unbalanced translocations and insertions
>
> **Excludes1** trisomies of chromosomes 13, 18, 21 (Q90-Q91)

Q92.0 Whole chromosome trisomy, nonmosaicism (meiotic nondisjunction)

Q92.1 Whole chromosome trisomy, mosaicism (mitotic nondisjunction)

Q92.2 Partial trisomy
> Less than whole arm duplicated
> Whole arm or more duplicated
>
> **Excludes1** partial trisomy due to unbalanced translocation (Q92.5)

Q92.5 Duplications with other complex rearrangements
> Partial trisomy due to unbalanced translocations
> Code also any associated deletions due to unbalanced translocations, inversions and insertions (Q93.7)

● **Q92.6** Marker chromosomes
> Trisomies due to dicentrics
> Trisomies due to extra rings
> Trisomies due to isochromosomes
> Individual with marker heterochromatin

Q92.61 Marker chromosomes in normal individual

Q92.62 Marker chromosomes in abnormal individual

Q92.7 Triploidy and polyploidy

Q92.8 Other specified trisomies and partial trisomies of autosomes
> Duplications identified by fluorescence in situ hybridization (FISH)
> Duplications identified by in situ hybridization (ISH)
> Duplications seen only at prometaphase

Q92.9 Trisomy and partial trisomy of autosomes, unspecified

● **Q93** Monosomies and deletions from the autosomes, not elsewhere classified

Q93.0 Whole chromosome monosomy, nonmosaicism (meiotic nondisjunction)

Q93.1 Whole chromosome monosomy, mosaicism (mitotic nondisjunction)

Q93.2 Chromosome replaced with ring, dicentric or isochromosome

Q93.3 Deletion of short arm of chromosome 4
> Wolff-Hirschorn syndrome

Q93.4 Deletion of short arm of chromosome 5
> Cri-du-chat syndrome

● **Q93.5** Other deletions of part of a chromosome

Q93.51 Angelman syndrome

Q93.59 Other deletions of part of a chromosome

Q93.7 Deletions with other complex rearrangements
> Deletions due to unbalanced translocations, inversions and insertions
> Code also any associated duplications due to unbalanced translocations, inversions and insertions (Q92.5)

● **Q93.8** Other deletions from the autosomes

Q93.81 Velo-cardio-facial syndrome
> Deletion 22q11.2

Q93.82 Williams syndrome

Q93.88 Other microdeletions Miller-Dieker syndrome
> Smith-Magenis syndrome

Q93.89 Other deletions from the autosomes
> Deletions identified by fluorescence in situ hybridization (FISH)
> Deletions identified by in situ hybridization (ISH)
> Deletions seen only at prometaphase

Q93.9 Deletion from autosomes, unspecified

● **Q95** Balanced rearrangements and structural markers, not elsewhere classified

> **Includes** Robertsonian and balanced reciprocal translocations and insertions

Q95.0 Balanced translocation and insertion in normal individual

Q95.1 Chromosome inversion in normal individual

Q95.2 Balanced autosomal rearrangement in abnormal individual

Q95.3 Balanced sex/autosomal rearrangement in abnormal individual

Q95.5 Individual with autosomal fragile site

Q95.8 Other balanced rearrangements and structural markers

Q95.9 Balanced rearrangement and structural marker, unspecified

● **Q96** Turner's syndrome
> *Caused by missing or incomplete X chromosome affecting growth and sexual development*
>
> ▶ **Excludes1** Noonan syndrome (Q87.19)

Q96.0 Karyotype 45, X ♀

Q96.1 Karyotype 46, X iso (Xq) ♀
> Karyotype 46, isochromosome Xq

Q96.2 Karyotype 46, X with abnormal sex chromosome, except iso (Xq) ♀
> Karyotype 46, X with abnormal sex chromosome, except isochromosome Xq

Q96.3 Mosaicism, 45, X/46, XX or XY ♀

Q96.4 Mosaicism, 45, X/other cell line(s) with abnormal sex chromosome ♀

Q96.8 Other variants of Turner's syndrome ♀

Q96.9 Turner's syndrome, unspecified ♀

● **Q97** Other sex chromosome abnormalities, female phenotype, not elsewhere classified

> **Excludes1** Turner's syndrome (Q96.-)

Q97.0 Karyotype 47, XXX ♀

Q97.1 Female with more than three X chromosomes ♀

Q97.2 Mosaicism, lines with various numbers of X chromosomes ♀

Q97.3 Female with 46, XY karyotype ♀

Q97.8 Other specified sex chromosome abnormalities, female phenotype ♀

Q97.9 Sex chromosome abnormality, female phenotype, unspecified ♀

● **Q98** Other sex chromosome abnormalities, male phenotype, not elsewhere classified

Q98.0 Klinefelter syndrome karyotype 47, XXY ♂

Q98.1 Klinefelter syndrome, male with more than two X chromosomes ♂

Q98.3 Other male with 46, XX karyotype ♂

Q98.4 Klinefelter syndrome, unspecified ♂

Q98.5 Karyotype 47, XYY ♂

Q98.6 Male with structurally abnormal sex chromosome ♂

Q98.7 Male with sex chromosome mosaicism ♂

Q98.8 Other specified sex chromosome abnormalities, male phenotype ♂

Q98.9 Sex chromosome abnormality, male phenotype, unspecified ♂

● **Q99** Other chromosome abnormalities, not elsewhere classified

Q99.0 Chimera 46, XX/46, XY
> Chimera 46, XX/46, XY true hermaphrodite

Q99.1 46, XX true hermaphrodite
> 46, XX with streak gonads
> 46, XY with streak gonads
> Pure gonadal dysgenesis

Q99.2 Fragile X chromosome
> Fragile X syndrome

Q99.8 Other specified chromosome abnormalities

Q99.9 Chromosomal abnormality, unspecified

▶ New　　▶ Revised　　~~deleted~~ Deleted　　Excludes 1　　Excludes 2　　Includes　　Use additional　　Code first　　Code also　　Key words

OGCR Official Guidelines　　X Assign placeholder X　　● Use Additional Character(s)　　▶ Manifestation Code　　🏷 Hierarchical Condition Category　　**Coding Clinic**

CHAPTER 18

SYMPTOMS, SIGNS, AND ABNORMAL CLINICAL AND LABORATORY FINDINGS, NOT ELSEWHERE CLASSIFIED (R00-R99)

OGCR Chapter-Specific Coding Guidelines

18. **Chapter 18: Symptoms, signs, and abnormal clinical and laboratory findings, not elsewhere classified (R00-R99)**
Chapter 18 includes symptoms, signs, abnormal results of clinical or other investigative procedures, and ill-defined conditions regarding which no diagnosis classifiable elsewhere is recorded. Signs and symptoms that point to a specific diagnosis have been assigned to a category in other chapters of the classification.

a. Use of symptom codes
Codes that describe symptoms and signs are acceptable for reporting purposes when a related definitive diagnosis has not been established (confirmed) by the provider.

b. Use of a symptom code with a definitive diagnosis code
Codes for signs and symptoms may be reported in addition to a related definitive diagnosis when the sign or symptom is not routinely associated with that diagnosis, such as the various signs and symptoms associated with complex syndromes. The definitive diagnosis code should be sequenced before the symptom code.

Signs or symptoms that are associated routinely with a disease process should not be assigned as additional codes, unless otherwise instructed by the classification.

c. Combination codes that include symptoms
ICD-10-CM contains a number of combination codes that identify both the definitive diagnosis and common symptoms of that diagnosis. When using one of these combination codes, an additional code should not be assigned for the symptom.

d. Repeated falls
Code R29.6, Repeated falls, is for use for encounters when a patient has recently fallen and the reason for the fall is being investigated.

Code Z91.81, History of falling, is for use when a patient has fallen in the past and is at risk for future falls. When appropriate, both codes R29.6 and Z91.81 may be assigned together.

e. Coma scale
The coma scale codes (R40.2-) can be used in conjunction with traumatic brain injury codes, acute cerebrovascular disease or sequelae of cerebrovascular disease codes. These codes are primarily for use by trauma registries, but they may be used in any setting where this information is collected. The coma scale may also be used to assess the status of the central nervous system for other non-trauma conditions, such as monitoring patients in the intensive care unit regardless of medical condition. The coma scale codes should be sequenced after the diagnosis code(s).

These codes, one from each subcategory, are needed to complete the scale. The 7th character indicates when the scale was recorded. The 7th character should match for all three codes.

At a minimum, report the initial score documented on presentation at your facility. This may be a score from the emergency medicine technician (EMT) or in the emergency department. If desired, a facility may choose to capture multiple coma scale scores.

Assign code R40.24, Glasgow coma scale, total score, when only the total score is documented in the medical record and not the individual score(s).

Do not report codes for individual or total Glasgow coma scale scores for a patient with a medically induced coma or a sedated patient.

See Section I.B.14 for coma scale documentation by clinicians other than patient's provider.

f. Functional quadriplegia
GUIDELINE HAS BEEN DELETED EFFECTIVE OCTOBER 1, 2017

g. SIRS due to Non-Infectious Process
The systemic inflammatory response syndrome (SIRS) can develop as a result of certain non-infectious disease processes, such as trauma, malignant neoplasm, or pancreatitis. When SIRS is documented with a noninfectious condition, and no subsequent infection is documented, the code for the underlying condition, such as an injury, should be assigned, followed by code R65.10, Systemic inflammatory response syndrome (SIRS) of non-infectious origin without acute organ dysfunction, or code R65.11, Systemic inflammatory response syndrome (SIRS) of non-infectious origin with acute organ dysfunction. If an associated acute organ dysfunction is documented, the appropriate code(s) for the specific type of organ dysfunction(s) should be assigned in addition to code R65.11. If acute organ dysfunction is documented, but it cannot be determined if the acute organ dysfunction is associated with SIRS or due to another condition (e.g., directly due to the trauma), the provider should be queried.

h. Death NOS
Code R99, Ill-defined and unknown cause of mortality, is only for use in the very limited circumstance when a patient who has already died is brought into an emergency department or other healthcare facility and is pronounced dead upon arrival. It does not represent the discharge disposition of death.

i. NIHSS Stroke Scale
The NIH stroke scale (NIHSS) codes (R29.7- -) can be used in conjunction with acute stroke codes (I63) to identify the patient's neurological status and the severity of the stroke. The stroke scale codes should be sequenced after the acute stroke diagnosis code(s).

At a minimum, report the initial score documented. If desired, a facility may choose to capture multiple stroke scale scores.

See Section I.B.14 for NIHSS stroke scale documentation by clinicians other than patient's provider.

OGCR Section I.B.4.

Signs and symptoms

Codes that describe symptoms and signs, as opposed to diagnoses, are acceptable for reporting purposes when a related definitive diagnosis has not been established (confirmed) by the provider. Chapter 18 of ICD-10-CM, Symptoms, Signs, and Abnormal Clinical and Laboratory Findings, Not Elsewhere Classified (codes RØØ.Ø-R99) contains many, but not all codes for symptoms.

CHAPTER 18

SYMPTOMS, SIGNS, AND ABNORMAL CLINICAL AND LABORATORY FINDINGS, NOT ELSEWHERE CLASSIFIED (RØØ-R99)

Note: This chapter includes symptoms, signs, abnormal results of clinical or other investigative procedures, and ill-defined conditions regarding which no diagnosis classifiable elsewhere is recorded.

Signs and symptoms that point rather definitely to a given diagnosis have been assigned to a category in other chapters of the classification. In general, categories in this chapter include the less well-defined conditions and symptoms that, without the necessary study of the case to establish a final diagnosis, point perhaps equally to two or more diseases or to two or more systems of the body. Practically all categories in the chapter could be designated "not otherwise specified", "unknown etiology" or "transient". The Alphabetical Index should be consulted to determine which symptoms and signs are to be allocated here and which to other chapters. The residual subcategories, numbered .8, are generally provided for other relevant symptoms that cannot be allocated elsewhere in the classification.

The conditions and signs or symptoms included in categories RØØ-R94 consist of:

(a) cases for which no more specific diagnosis can be made even after all the facts bearing on the case have been investigated;
(b) signs or symptoms existing at the time of initial encounter that proved to be transient and whose causes could not be determined;
(c) provisional diagnosis in a patient who failed to return for further investigation or care;
(d) cases referred elsewhere for investigation or treatment before the diagnosis was made;
(e) cases in which a more precise diagnosis was not available for any other reason;
(f) certain symptoms, for which supplementary information is provided, that represent important problems in medical care in their own right.

Excludes2 abnormal findings on antenatal screening of mother (O28.-)
certain conditions originating in the perinatal period (PØ4-P96)
signs and symptoms classified in the body system chapters
signs and symptoms of breast (N63, N64.5)

This chapter contains the following blocks:

RØØ-RØ9	Symptoms and signs involving the circulatory and respiratory systems
R1Ø-R19	Symptoms and signs involving the digestive system and abdomen
R2Ø-R23	Symptoms and signs involving the skin and subcutaneous tissue
R25-R29	Symptoms and signs involving the nervous and musculoskeletal systems
R3Ø-R39	Symptoms and signs involving the genitourinary system
R4Ø-R46	Symptoms and signs involving cognition, perception, emotional state and behavior
R47-R49	Symptoms and signs involving speech and voice
R5Ø-R69	General symptoms and signs
R7Ø-R79	Abnormal findings on examination of blood, without diagnosis
R8Ø-R82	Abnormal findings on examination of urine, without diagnosis
R83-R89	Abnormal findings on examination of other body fluids, substances and tissues, without diagnosis
R9Ø-R94	Abnormal findings on diagnostic imaging and in function studies, without diagnosis
R97	Abnormal tumor markers
R99	Ill-defined and unknown cause of mortality

SYMPTOMS AND SIGNS INVOLVING THE CIRCULATORY AND RESPIRATORY SYSTEMS (RØØ-RØ9)

● **RØØ Abnormalities of heart beat**

Excludes1 abnormalities originating in the perinatal period (P29.1-)

Excludes2 specified arrhythmias (I47-I49)

RØØ.Ø Tachycardia, unspecified

Rapid heart rate >1ØØ beats
Rapid heart beat
Sinoauricular tachycardia NOS
Sinus [sinusal] tachycardia NOS

Excludes1 neonatal tachycardia (P29.11)
paroxysmal tachycardia (I47.-)

RØØ.1 Bradycardia, unspecified

Slow heart rate, <6Ø
Sinoatrial bradycardia
Sinus bradycardia
Slow heart beat
Vagal bradycardia

Use additional code for adverse effect, if applicable, to identify drug (T36-T5Ø with fifth or sixth character 5)

Excludes1 neonatal bradycardia (P29.12)

RØØ.2 Palpitations

Awareness of heart beat

RØØ.8 Other abnormalities of heart beat

RØØ.9 Unspecified abnormalities of heart beat

CHAPTER 18 (RØØ-R99)

RØ1 Cardiac murmurs and other cardiac sounds
Excludes1 cardiac murmurs and sounds originating in the perinatal period (P29.8)
RØ1.Ø Benign and innocent cardiac murmurs
Functional cardiac murmur
RØ1.1 Cardiac murmur, unspecified
Cardiac bruit NOS
Heart murmur NOS
Systolic murmur NOS
RØ1.2 Other cardiac sounds
Cardiac dullness, increased or decreased
Precordial friction

OGCR Section I.C.9.a.7.
Hypertension, Transient
Assign code RØ3.Ø, Elevated blood pressure reading without diagnosis of hypertension, unless patient has an established diagnosis of hypertension. Assign code O13.-, Gestational [pregnancy-induced] hypertension with significant proteinuria, or O14.-, Pre-eclampsia, for transient hypertension of pregnancy.

RØ3 Abnormal blood-pressure reading, without diagnosis
RØ3.Ø Elevated blood-pressure reading, without diagnosis of hypertension
Note: This category is to be used to record an episode of elevated blood pressure in a patient in whom no formal diagnosis of hypertension has been made, or as an isolated incidental finding.
RØ3.1 Nonspecific low blood-pressure reading
Excludes1 hypotension (I95.-)
maternal hypotension syndrome (O26.5-)
neurogenic orthostatic hypotension (G9Ø.3)

RØ4 Hemorrhage from respiratory passages
RØ4.Ø Epistaxis
Hemorrhage from nose
Nosebleed
Coding Clinic: 2018, Q4, P38
RØ4.1 Hemorrhage from throat
Excludes2 hemoptysis (RØ4.2)
RØ4.2 Hemoptysis
Blood-stained sputum
Cough with hemorrhage
RØ4.8 Hemorrhage from other sites in respiratory passages
RØ4.81 Acute idiopathic pulmonary hemorrhage in infants P
AIPHI
Acute idiopathic hemorrhage in infants over 28 days old
Excludes1 perinatal pulmonary hemorrhage (P26.-)
von Willebrand's disease (D68.Ø)
RØ4.89 Hemorrhage from other sites in respiratory passages
Pulmonary hemorrhage NOS
RØ4.9 Hemorrhage from respiratory passages, unspecified

RØ5 Cough
Excludes1 cough with hemorrhage (RØ4.2)
smoker's cough (J41.Ø)

RØ6 Abnormalities of breathing
Excludes1 acute respiratory distress syndrome (J8Ø)
respiratory arrest (RØ9.2)
respiratory arrest of newborn (P28.81)
respiratory distress syndrome of newborn (P22.-)
respiratory failure (J96.-)
respiratory failure of newborn (P28.5)
RØ6.Ø Dyspnea
Excludes1 tachypnea NOS (RØ6.82)
transient tachypnea of newborn (P22.1)
RØ6.ØØ Dyspnea, unspecified
Coding Clinic: 2017, Q1, P26-27
RØ6.Ø1 Orthopnea
RØ6.Ø2 Shortness of breath
RØ6.Ø3 Acute respiratory distress
RØ6.Ø9 Other forms of dyspnea
RØ6.1 Stridor
Harsh, high-pitched breath sound
Excludes1 congenital laryngeal stridor (P28.89)
laryngismus (stridulus) (J38.5)
RØ6.2 Wheezing
Excludes1 Asthma (J45.-)
Coding Clinic: 2016, Q2, P34
RØ6.3 Periodic breathing
Cheyne-Stokes breathing
An abnormal pattern of breathing with gradually increasing and decreasing tidal volume with some periods of apnea
RØ6.4 Hyperventilation
Excludes1 psychogenic hyperventilation (F45.8)
RØ6.5 Mouth breathing
Excludes2 dry mouth NOS (R68.2)
RØ6.6 Hiccough
Excludes1 psychogenic hiccough (F45.8)
RØ6.7 Sneezing
RØ6.8 Other abnormalities of breathing
RØ6.81 Apnea, not elsewhere classified
Apnea NOS
Excludes1 apnea (of) newborn (P28.4)
sleep apnea (G47.3-)
sleep apnea of newborn (primary) (P28.3)
RØ6.82 Tachypnea, not elsewhere classified
Tachypnea NOS
Excludes1 transitory tachypnea of newborn (P22.1)
RØ6.83 Snoring
RØ6.89 Other abnormalities of breathing
Breath-holding (spells)
Sighing
RØ6.9 Unspecified abnormalities of breathing

RØ7 Pain in throat and chest
Excludes1 epidemic myalgia (B33.Ø)
Excludes2 jaw pain R68.84
pain in breast (N64.4)
RØ7.Ø Pain in throat
Excludes1 chronic sore throat (J31.2)
sore throat (acute) NOS (JØ2.9)
Excludes2 dysphagia (R13.1-)
pain in neck (M54.2)
RØ7.1 Chest pain on breathing
Painful respiration
RØ7.2 Precordial pain

CHAPTER 18 (RØØ-R99)

● RØ7.8 Other chest pain
  RØ7.81 **Pleurodynia**
    Pleurodynia NOS
    Excludes1 epidemic pleurodynia (B33.Ø)
  RØ7.82 **Intercostal pain**
  RØ7.89 **Other chest pain**
    Anterior chest-wall pain NOS
RØ7.9 Chest pain, **unspecified**

● **RØ9 Other symptoms and signs involving the circulatory and respiratory system**
Excludes1 acute respiratory distress syndrome (J8Ø)
respiratory arrest of newborn (P28.81)
respiratory distress syndrome of newborn (P22.Ø)
respiratory failure (J96.-)
respiratory failure of newborn (P28.5)

● **RØ9.Ø Asphyxia and hypoxemia**
Excludes1 asphyxia due to carbon monoxide (T58.-)
asphyxia due to foreign body in respiratory tract (T17.-)
birth (intrauterine) asphyxia (P84)
hyperventilation (RØ6.4)
traumatic asphyxia (T71.-)
Excludes2 hypercapnia (RØ6.89)
  RØ9.Ø1 **Asphyxia**
  RØ9.Ø2 **Hypoxemia**

RØ9.1 **Pleurisy**
Occurs when double membrane (pleura) lining chest cavity and lung surface becomes inflamed, causing sharp pain on inspiration/expiration
Excludes1 pleurisy with effusion (J9Ø)

RØ9.2 **Respiratory arrest** (HCC)
Cardiorespiratory failure
Excludes1 cardiac arrest (I46.-)
respiratory arrest of newborn (P28.81)
respiratory distress of newborn (P22.Ø)
respiratory failure (J96.-)
respiratory failure of newborn (P28.5)
respiratory insufficiency (RØ6.89)
respiratory insufficiency of newborn (P28.5)

RØ9.3 **Abnormal sputum**
Abnormal amount of sputum
Abnormal color of sputum
Abnormal odor of sputum
Excessive sputum
Excludes1 blood-stained sputum (RØ4.2)

● **RØ9.8 Other specified symptoms and signs involving the circulatory and respiratory systems**
  RØ9.81 **Nasal congestion**
  RØ9.82 **Postnasal drip**
  RØ9.89 **Other specified symptoms and signs involving the circulatory and respiratory systems**
    Bruit (arterial)
    Abnormal chest percussion
    Feeling of foreign body in throat
    Friction sounds in chest
    Chest tympany
    Choking sensation
    Rales
    Wet rattling, clicking, crackling sounds on auscultation
    Weak pulse
    Excludes2 foreign body in throat (T17.2-)
    wheezing (RØ6.2)

SYMPTOMS AND SIGNS INVOLVING THE DIGESTIVE SYSTEM AND ABDOMEN (R1Ø-R19)

Excludes2 congenital or infantile pylorospasm (Q4Ø.Ø)
gastrointestinal hemorrhage (K92.Ø-K92.2)
intestinal obstruction (K56.-)
newborn gastrointestinal hemorrhage (P54.Ø-P54.3)
newborn intestinal obstruction (P76.-)
pylorospasm (K31.3)
signs and symptoms involving the urinary system (R3Ø-R39)
symptoms referable to female genital organs (N94.-)
symptoms referable to male genital organs (N48-N5Ø)

● **R1Ø Abdominal and pelvic pain**
Excludes1 renal colic (N23)
Excludes2 dorsalgia (M54.-)
flatulence and related conditions (R14.-)

R1Ø.Ø **Acute abdomen**
Severe abdominal pain (generalized) (with abdominal rigidity)
Excludes1 abdominal rigidity NOS (R19.3)
generalized abdominal pain NOS (R1Ø.84)
localized abdominal pain (R1Ø.1-R1Ø.3-)

● R1Ø.1 **Pain localized to upper abdomen**
  R1Ø.1Ø **Upper abdominal pain, unspecified**
  R1Ø.11 **Right upper quadrant pain**
  R1Ø.12 **Left upper quadrant pain**
  R1Ø.13 **Epigastric pain**
    Dyspepsia
    Excludes1 functional dyspepsia (K3Ø)

R1Ø.2 **Pelvic and perineal pain**
Excludes1 vulvodynia (N94.81)

● R1Ø.3 **Pain localized to other parts of lower abdomen**
  R1Ø.3Ø **Lower abdominal pain, unspecified**
  R1Ø.31 **Right lower quadrant pain**
  R1Ø.32 **Left lower quadrant pain**
  R1Ø.33 **Periumbilical pain**

● R1Ø.8 **Other abdominal pain**
  ● R1Ø.81 **Abdominal tenderness**
    Abdominal tenderness NOS
    R1Ø.811 **Right upper quadrant abdominal tenderness**
    R1Ø.812 **Left upper quadrant abdominal tenderness**
    R1Ø.813 **Right lower quadrant abdominal tenderness**
    R1Ø.814 **Left lower quadrant abdominal tenderness**
    R1Ø.815 **Periumbilic abdominal tenderness**
    R1Ø.816 **Epigastric abdominal tenderness**
    R1Ø.817 **Generalized abdominal tenderness**
    R1Ø.819 **Abdominal tenderness, unspecified site**

● R10.82 **Rebound abdominal tenderness**
- R10.821 **Right upper quadrant rebound abdominal tenderness**
- R10.822 **Left upper quadrant rebound abdominal tenderness**
- R10.823 **Right lower quadrant rebound abdominal tenderness**
- R10.824 **Left lower quadrant rebound abdominal tenderness**
- R10.825 **Periumbilic rebound abdominal tenderness**
- R10.826 **Epigastric rebound abdominal tenderness**
- R10.827 **Generalized rebound abdominal tenderness**
- R10.829 **Rebound abdominal tenderness, unspecified site**

R10.83 **Colic** P
Colic NOS
Infantile colic
Excludes1 colic in adult and child over 12 months old (R10.84)

R10.84 **Generalized abdominal pain**
Excludes1 generalized abdominal pain associated with acute abdomen (R10.0)

R10.9 **Unspecified abdominal pain**

● R11 **Nausea and vomiting**
Excludes1 cyclical vomiting associated with migraine (G43.A-)
excessive vomiting in pregnancy (O21.-)
hematemesis (K92.0)
neonatal hematemesis (P54.0)
newborn vomiting (P92.0-)
psychogenic vomiting (F50.89)
vomiting associated with bulimia nervosa (F50.2)
vomiting following gastrointestinal surgery (K91.0)
Coding Clinic: 2017, Q1, P27

● R11.0 **Nausea**
Nausea NOS
Nausea without vomiting

● R11.1 **Vomiting**
- R11.10 **Vomiting, unspecified**
  Vomiting NOS
- R11.11 **Vomiting without nausea**
- R11.12 **Projectile vomiting**
- R11.13 **Vomiting of fecal matter**
- R11.14 **Bilious vomiting**
  Bilious emesis
- ▶R11.15 **Cyclical vomiting syndrome unrelated to migraine**
  ▶Cyclic vomiting syndrome NOS
  ▶Persistent vomiting
  ▶ **Excludes1** cyclical vomiting in migraine (G43.A-)
  ▶ **Excludes2** bulimia nervosa (F50.2)
  ▶diabetes mellitus due to underlying condition (E08.-)

R11.2 **Nausea with vomiting, unspecified**
Persistent nausea with vomiting NOS

R12 **Heartburn**
Excludes1 dyspepsia NOS (R10.13)
functional dyspepsia (K30)

● R13 **Aphagia and dysphagia**

R13.0 **Aphagia**
Inability to swallow
Excludes1 psychogenic aphagia (F50.9)

● R13.1 **Dysphagia**
Difficulty swallowing
Code first, if applicable, dysphagia following cerebrovascular disease (I69. with final characters -91)
Excludes1 psychogenic dysphagia (F45.8)
- R13.10 **Dysphagia, unspecified**
  Difficulty in swallowing NOS
- R13.11 **Dysphagia, oral phase**
- R13.12 **Dysphagia, oropharyngeal phase**
- R13.13 **Dysphagia, pharyngeal phase**
- R13.14 **Dysphagia, pharyngoesophageal phase**
- R13.19 **Other dysphagia**
  Cervical dysphagia
  Neurogenic dysphagia

● R14 **Flatulence and related conditions**
Excludes1 psychogenic aerophagy (F45.8)

R14.0 **Abdominal distension (gaseous)**
Bloating
Tympanites (abdominal) (intestinal)

R14.1 **Gas pain**

R14.2 **Eructation**
Belching air from stomach through mouth

R14.3 **Flatulence**

● R15 **Fecal incontinence**
Includes encopresis NOS
Excludes1 fecal incontinence of nonorganic origin (F98.1)

R15.0 **Incomplete defecation**
Excludes1 constipation (K59.0-)
fecal impaction (K56.41)

R15.1 **Fecal smearing**
Fecal soiling

R15.2 **Fecal urgency**

R15.9 **Full incontinence of feces**
Fecal incontinence NOS

● R16 **Hepatomegaly and splenomegaly, not elsewhere classified**
Enlargement of liver or spleen

R16.0 **Hepatomegaly, not elsewhere classified**
Hepatomegaly NOS

R16.1 **Splenomegaly, not elsewhere classified**
Splenomegaly NOS

R16.2 **Hepatomegaly with splenomegaly, not elsewhere classified**
Hepatosplenomegaly NOS

R17 **Unspecified jaundice**
Excludes1 neonatal jaundice (P55, P57-P59)

● R18 **Ascites**
Includes fluid in peritoneal cavity
Excludes1 ascites in alcoholic cirrhosis (K70.31)
ascites in alcoholic hepatitis (K70.11)
ascites in toxic liver disease with chronic active hepatitis (K71.51)

R18.0 **Malignant ascites**
Code first malignancy, such as:
malignant neoplasm of ovary (C56.-)
secondary malignant neoplasm of retroperitoneum and peritoneum (C78.6)

R18.8 **Other ascites**
Ascites NOS
Peritoneal effusion (chronic)
Coding Clinic: 2018, Q1, P4

CHAPTER 18 (R00-R99)

● **R19 Other symptoms and signs involving the digestive system and abdomen**
Excludes1 acute abdomen (R10.0)

● **R19.0 Intra-abdominal and pelvic swelling, mass and lump**
Excludes1 abdominal distension (gaseous) (R14.-)
ascites (R18.-)

R19.00 Intra-abdominal and pelvic swelling, mass and lump, unspecified site

R19.01 Right upper quadrant abdominal swelling, mass and lump

R19.02 Left upper quadrant abdominal swelling, mass and lump

R19.03 Right lower quadrant abdominal swelling, mass and lump

R19.04 Left lower quadrant abdominal swelling, mass and lump

R19.05 Periumbilic swelling, mass or lump
Diffuse or generalized umbilical swelling or mass

R19.06 Epigastric swelling, mass or lump

R19.07 Generalized intra-abdominal and pelvic swelling, mass and lump
Diffuse or generalized intra-abdominal swelling or mass NOS
Diffuse or generalized pelvic swelling or mass NOS

R19.09 Other intra-abdominal and pelvic swelling, mass and lump

● **R19.1 Abnormal bowel sounds**

R19.11 Absent bowel sounds

R19.12 Hyperactive bowel sounds

R19.15 Other abnormal bowel sounds
Abnormal bowel sounds NOS

R19.2 Visible peristalsis
Hyperperistalsis

● **R19.3 Abdominal rigidity**
Excludes1 abdominal rigidity with severe abdominal pain (R10.0)

R19.30 Abdominal rigidity, unspecified site

R19.31 Right upper quadrant abdominal rigidity

R19.32 Left upper quadrant abdominal rigidity

R19.33 Right lower quadrant abdominal rigidity

R19.34 Left lower quadrant abdominal rigidity

R19.35 Periumbilic abdominal rigidity

R19.36 Epigastric abdominal rigidity

R19.37 Generalized abdominal rigidity

R19.4 Change in bowel habit
Excludes1 constipation (K59.0-)
functional diarrhea (K59.1)

R19.5 Other fecal abnormalities
Abnormal stool color
Bulky stools
Mucus in stools
Occult blood in feces
Occult blood in stools
Excludes1 melena (K92.1)
neonatal melena (P54.1)
Coding Clinic: 2019, Q1, P32

R19.6 Halitosis

R19.7 Diarrhea, unspecified
Diarrhea NOS
Excludes1 functional diarrhea (K59.1)
neonatal diarrhea (P78.3)
psychogenic diarrhea (F45.8)

R19.8 Other specified symptoms and signs involving the digestive system and abdomen

SYMPTOMS AND SIGNS INVOLVING THE SKIN AND SUBCUTANEOUS TISSUE (R20-R23)

Excludes2 symptoms relating to breast (N64.4-N64.5)

● **R20 Disturbances of skin sensation**
Excludes1 dissociative anesthesia and sensory loss (F44.6)
psychogenic disturbances (F45.8)

R20.0 Anesthesia of skin
Loss of sensation

R20.1 Hypoesthesia of skin
Unpleasant abnormal sensation

R20.2 Paresthesia of skin
Abnormal touch sensation, including burning, prickling, often in absence of external stimulus
Formication
Tingling skin
Pins and needles
Excludes1 acroparesthesia (I73.8)

R20.3 Hyperesthesia

R20.8 Other disturbances of skin sensation

R20.9 Unspecified disturbances of skin sensation

R21 Rash and other nonspecific skin eruption
Includes rash NOS
Excludes1 specified type of rash- code to condition
vesicular eruption (R23.8)

● **R22 Localized swelling, mass and lump of skin and subcutaneous tissue**
Includes subcutaneous nodules (localized) (superficial)
Excludes1 abnormal findings on diagnostic imaging (R90-R93)
edema (R60.-)
enlarged lymph nodes (R59.-)
localized adiposity (E65)
swelling of joint (M25.4-)

R22.0 Localized swelling, mass and lump, head

R22.1 Localized swelling, mass and lump, neck

R22.2 Localized swelling, mass and lump, trunk
Excludes1 intra-abdominal or pelvic mass and lump (R19.0-)
intra-abdominal or pelvic swelling (R19.0-)
Excludes2 breast mass and lump (N63)

● **R22.3 Localized swelling, mass and lump, upper limb**

R22.30 Localized swelling, mass and lump, unspecified upper limb

R22.31 Localized swelling, mass and lump, right upper limb

R22.32 Localized swelling, mass and lump, left upper limb

R22.33 Localized swelling, mass and lump, upper limb, bilateral

● **R22.4 Localized swelling, mass and lump, lower limb**

R22.40 Localized swelling, mass and lump, unspecified lower limb

R22.41 Localized swelling, mass and lump, right lower limb

R22.42 Localized swelling, mass and lump, left lower limb

R22.43 Localized swelling, mass and lump, lower limb, bilateral

R22.9 Localized swelling, mass and lump, unspecified

CHAPTER 18 (R00-R99)

R23 Other skin changes

R23.0 Cyanosis

Excludes1 acrocyanosis (I73.8)
cyanotic attacks of newborn (P28.2)

R23.1 Pallor

Clammy skin

R23.2 Flushing

Excessive blushing

Code first, if applicable, menopausal and female climacteric states (N95.1)

R23.3 Spontaneous ecchymoses

Small hemorrhagic spot of skin; AKA black and blue spot

Petechiae

Excludes1 ecchymoses of newborn (P54.5)
purpura (D69.-)

R23.4 Changes in skin texture

Desquamation of skin
Scaling of skin
Induration of skin

Excludes1 epidermal thickening NOS (L85.9)

R23.8 Other skin changes

R23.9 Unspecified skin changes

SYMPTOMS AND SIGNS INVOLVING THE NERVOUS AND MUSCULOSKELETAL SYSTEMS (R25-R29)

R25 Abnormal involuntary movements

Excludes1 specific movement disorders (G20-G26)
stereotyped movement disorders (F98.4)
tic disorders (F95.-)

R25.0 Abnormal head movements

R25.1 Tremor, unspecified

Excludes1 chorea NOS (G25.5)
essential tremor (G25.0)
hysterical tremor (F44.4)
intention tremor (G25.2)

R25.2 Cramp and spasm

Excludes2 carpopedal spasm (R29.0)
charley-horse (M62.831)
infantile spasms (G40.4-)
muscle spasm of back (M62.830)
muscle spasm of calf (M62.831)

R25.3 Fasciculation

Twitching NOS

R25.8 Other abnormal involuntary movements

R25.9 Unspecified abnormal involuntary movements

R26 Abnormalities of gait and mobility

Excludes1 ataxia NOS (R27.0)
hereditary ataxia (G11.-)
locomotor (syphilitic) ataxia (A52.11)
immobility syndrome (paraplegic) (M62.3)

R26.0 Ataxic gait

Staggering gait

R26.1 Paralytic gait

Spastic gait

R26.2 Difficulty in walking, not elsewhere classified

Excludes1 falling (R29.6)
unsteadiness on feet (R26.81)

Coding Clinic: 2016, Q2, P7

R26.8 Other abnormalities of gait and mobility

R26.81 Unsteadiness on feet

R26.89 Other abnormalities of gait and mobility

R26.9 Unspecified abnormalities of gait and mobility

R27 Other lack of coordination

Excludes1 ataxic gait (R26.0)
hereditary ataxia (G11.-)
vertigo NOS (R42)

R27.0 Ataxia, unspecified

Excludes1 ataxia following cerebrovascular disease (I69. with final characters -93)

R27.8 Other lack of coordination

R27.9 Unspecified lack of coordination

R29 Other symptoms and signs involving the nervous and musculoskeletal systems

R29.0 Tetany

Hyperexcitability of nerves and muscles characterized by spasm, twitching, and cramps

Carpopedal spasm

Excludes1 hysterical tetany (F44.5)
neonatal tetany (P71.3)
parathyroid tetany (E20.9)
post-thyroidectomy tetany (E89.2)

R29.1 Meningismus

R29.2 Abnormal reflex

Excludes2 abnormal pupillary reflex (H57.0)
hyperactive gag reflex (J39.2)
vasovagal reaction or syncope (R55)

R29.3 Abnormal posture

R29.4 Clicking hip

Excludes1 congenital deformities of hip (Q65.-)

R29.5 Transient paralysis

Code first any associated spinal cord injury (S14.0, S14.1-, S24.0, S24.1-, S34.0-, S34.1-)

Excludes1 transient ischemic attack (G45.9)

R29.6 Repeated falls

Falling
Tendency to fall

Excludes2 at risk for falling (Z91.81)
history of falling (Z91.81)

OGCR Section I.C.18.d.

Repeated falls

Code R29.6, Repeated falls, is for use for encounters when a patient has recently fallen and the reason for the fall is being investigated.

Code Z91.81, History of falling, is for use when a patient has fallen in the past and is at risk for future falls.When appropriate, both codes R29.6 and Z91.81 may be assigned together.

Coding Clinic: 2016, Q2, P7

R29.7 National Institutes of Health Stroke Scale (NIHSS) score

Code first the type of cerebral infarction (I63-)

Coding Clinic: 2016, Q4, P61, 127

R29.70 NIHSS score 0-9

R29.700 NIHSS score 0
R29.701 NIHSS score 1
R29.702 NIHSS score 2
R29.703 NIHSS score 3
R29.704 NIHSS score 4
R29.705 NIHSS score 5
R29.706 NIHSS score 6
R29.707 NIHSS score 7
R29.708 NIHSS score 8
R29.709 NIHSS score 9

R29.71 NIHSS score 10-19

R29.710 NIHSS score 10
R29.711 NIHSS score 11
R29.712 NIHSS score 12
R29.713 NIHSS score 13
R29.714 NIHSS score 14
R29.715 NIHSS score 15
R29.716 NIHSS score 16
R29.717 NIHSS score 17
R29.718 NIHSS score 18
R29.719 NIHSS score 19

OGCR Section I.C.18.i.

NIHSS Stroke Scale

The NIH stroke scale (NIHSS) codes (R29.7- -) can be used in conjunction with acute stroke codes (I63) to identify the patient's neurological status and the severity of the stroke. The stroke scale codes should be sequenced after the acute stroke diagnosis code(s).

At a minimum, report the initial score documented. If desired, a facility may choose to capture multiple stroke scale scores.

● R29.72 **NIHSS score 2Ø-29**
- R29.72Ø NIHSS score 2Ø
- R29.721 NIHSS score 21
- R29.722 NIHSS score 22
- R29.723 NIHSS score 23
- R29.724 NIHSS score 24
- R29.725 NIHSS score 25
- R29.726 NIHSS score 26
- R29.727 NIHSS score 27
- R29.728 NIHSS score 28
- R29.729 NIHSS score 29

● R29.73 **NIHSS score 3Ø-39**
- R29.73Ø NIHSS score 3Ø
  Coding Clinic: 2Ø16, Q4, P62
- R29.731 NIHSS score 31
- R29.732 NIHSS score 32
- R29.733 NIHSS score 33
- R29.734 NIHSS score 34
- R29.735 NIHSS score 35
- R29.736 NIHSS score 36
- R29.737 NIHSS score 37
- R29.738 NIHSS score 38
- R29.739 NIHSS score 39

● R29.74 **NIHSS score 4Ø-42**
- R29.74Ø NIHSS score 4Ø
- R29.741 NIHSS score 41
- R29.742 NIHSS score 42

● R29.8 **Other symptoms and signs involving the nervous and musculoskeletal systems**

● R29.81 **Other symptoms and signs involving the nervous system**

R29.81Ø **Facial weakness**
Facial droop
Excludes1 Bell's palsy (G51.Ø)
facial weakness following cerebrovascular disease (I69. with final characters -92)

R29.818 **Other symptoms and signs involving the nervous system**

● R29.89 **Other symptoms and signs involving the musculoskeletal system**
Excludes2 pain in limb (M79.6-)

R29.89Ø **Loss of height**
Excludes1 osteoporosis (M8Ø-M81)

R29.891 **Ocular torticollis**
Excludes1 congenital (sternomastoid) torticollis Q68.Ø
psychogenic torticollis (F45.8)
spasmodic torticollis (G24.3)
torticollis due to birth injury (P15.8)
torticollis NOS M43.6

R29.898 **Other symptoms and signs involving the musculoskeletal system**

● R29.9 **Unspecified symptoms and signs involving the nervous and musculoskeletal systems**

R29.9Ø **Unspecified symptoms and signs involving the nervous system**

R29.91 **Unspecified symptoms and signs involving the musculoskeletal system**

SYMPTOMS AND SIGNS INVOLVING THE GENITOURINARY SYSTEM (R3Ø-R39)

● R3Ø **Pain associated with micturition**
Excludes1 psychogenic pain associated with micturition (F45.8)

R3Ø.Ø **Dysuria**
Painful urination
Strangury

R3Ø.1 **Vesical tenesmus**
Straining to urinate, with sensation of a full bladder even when empty

R3Ø.9 **Painful micturition, unspecified**
Painful urination NOS

● R31 **Hematuria**
Excludes1 hematuria included with underlying conditions, such as:
acute cystitis with hematuria (N3Ø.Ø1)
recurrent and persistent hematuria in glomerular diseases (NØ2.-)

R31.Ø **Gross hematuria**
Coding Clinic: 2Ø17, Q1, P17

R31.1 **Benign essential microscopic hematuria**

● R31.2 **Other microscopic hematuria**
Coding Clinic: 2Ø16, Q4, P62

R31.21 **Asymptomatic microscopic hematuria**
AMH

R31.29 **Other microscopic hematuria**

R31.9 **Hematuria, unspecified**
Coding Clinic: 2Ø17, Q1, P6

R32 **Unspecified urinary incontinence**
Enuresis NOS
Excludes1 functional urinary incontinence (R39.81)
nonorganic enuresis (F98.Ø)
stress incontinence and other specified urinary incontinence (N39.3-N39.4-)
urinary incontinence associated with cognitive impairment (R39.81)

● R33 **Retention of urine**
Excludes1 psychogenic retention of urine (F45.8)

R33.Ø **Drug induced retention of urine**
Use additional code for adverse effect, if applicable, to identify drug (T36-T5Ø with fifth or sixth character 5)

R33.8 **Other retention of urine**
Code first, if applicable, any causal condition, such as:
enlarged prostate (N4Ø.1)
Coding Clinic: 2Ø18, Q4, P55

R33.9 **Retention of urine, unspecified**

R34 **Anuria and oliguria**
Excludes1 anuria and oliguria complicating abortion or ectopic or molar pregnancy (OØØ-OØ7, OØ8.4)
anuria and oliguria complicating pregnancy (O26.83-)
anuria and oliguria complicating the puerperium (O9Ø.4)

R35 Polyuria
Passage of excessive volume of urine
Code first, if applicable, any causal condition, such as:
enlarged prostate (N40.1)
Excludes1 psychogenic polyuria (F45.8)

R35.0 Frequency of micturition
Discharge or passage of urine; AKA uresis

R35.1 Nocturia
Urinary frequency at night

R35.8 Other polyuria
Polyuria NOS

R36 Urethral discharge

R36.0 Urethral discharge without blood

R36.1 Hematospermia ♂
Presence of blood in semen

R36.9 Urethral discharge, unspecified
Penile discharge NOS
Urethrorrhea

R37 Sexual dysfunction, unspecified

R39 Other and unspecified symptoms and signs involving the genitourinary system

R39.0 Extravasation of urine
Leakage, discharge

R39.1 Other difficulties with micturition
Code first, if applicable, any causal condition, such as:
enlarged prostate (N40.1)

R39.11 Hesitancy of micturition

R39.12 Poor urinary stream
Weak urinary steam

R39.13 Splitting of urinary stream

R39.14 Feeling of incomplete bladder emptying

R39.15 Urgency of urination
Excludes1 urge incontinence (N39.41, N39.46)

R39.16 Straining to void

R39.19 Other difficulties with micturition
Coding Clinic: 2016, Q4, P63

R39.191 Need to immediately re-void

R39.192 Position dependent micturition

R39.198 Other difficulties with micturition

R39.2 Extrarenal uremia
Prerenal uremia
Excludes1 uremia NOS (N19)

R39.8 Other symptoms and signs involving the genitourinary system

R39.81 Functional urinary incontinence
Urinary incontinence due to cognitive impairment, or severe physical disability or immobility
Excludes1 stress incontinence and other specified urinary incontinence (N39.3-N39.4-)
urinary incontinence NOS (R32)

R39.82 Chronic bladder pain
Coding Clinic: 2016, Q4, P64

R39.83 Unilateral non-palpable testicle ♂

R39.84 Bilateral non-palpable testicles ♂

R39.89 Other symptoms and signs involving the genitourinary system
Coding Clinic: 2016, Q4, P64

R39.9 Unspecified symptoms and signs involving the genitourinary system

SYMPTOMS AND SIGNS INVOLVING COGNITION, PERCEPTION, EMOTIONAL STATE AND BEHAVIOR (R40-R46)

Excludes2 symptoms and signs constituting part of a pattern of mental disorder (F01-F99)
Coding Clinic: 2015, Q4, P40

R40 Somnolence, stupor and coma
Excludes1 neonatal coma (P91.5)
somnolence, stupor and coma in diabetes (E08-E13)
somnolence, stupor and coma in hepatic failure (K72.-)
somnolence, stupor and coma in hypoglycemia (nondiabetic) (E15)

R40.0 Somnolence
Drowsiness
Excludes1 coma (R40.2-)

R40.1 Stupor
Lowered level of consciousness
Catatonic stupor
Semicoma
Excludes1 catatonic schizophrenia (F20.2)
coma (R40.2-)
depressive stupor (F31-F33)
dissociative stupor (F44.2)
manic stupor (F30.2)

OGCR Section I.C.18.e.

Coma scale

The coma scale codes (R40.2-) can be used in conjunction with traumatic brain injury codes, acute cerebrovascular disease or sequelae of cerebrovascular disease codes. These codes are primarily for use by trauma registries, but they may be used in any setting where this information is collected. The coma scale may also be used to assess the status of the central nervous system for other non-trauma conditions, such as monitoring patients in the intensive care unit regardless of medical condition. The coma scale codes should be sequenced after the diagnosis code(s).

These codes, one from each subcategory, are needed to complete the scale. The 7th character indicates when the scale was recorded. The 7th character should match for all three codes.

At a minimum, report the initial score documented on presentation at your facility. This may be a score from the emergency medicine technician (EMT) or in the emergency department. If desired, a facility may choose to capture multiple coma scale scores.

Assign code R40.24, Glasgow coma scale, total score, when only the total score is documented in the medical record and not the individual score(s).

R40.2 Coma
Code first any associated:
fracture of skull (S02.-)
intracranial injury (S06.-)

Note: One code from each subcategory R40.21-R40-23 is required to complete the coma scale
Coding Clinic: 2016, Q4, P127

R40.20 Unspecified coma
Coma NOS
Unconsciousness NOS

R40.21 Coma scale, eyes open
The following appropriate 7th character is to be added to subcategory R40.21-:

0	unspecified time
1	in the field [EMT or ambulance]
2	at arrival to emergency department
3	at hospital admission
4	24 hours or more after hospital admission

Coding Clinic: 2017, Q4, P25; 2015, Q2, P18

R40.211 Coma scale, eyes open, never
Coma scale eye opening score of 1

CHAPTER 18 (R00-R99)

● **R40.212 Coma scale, eyes open, to pain** HCC
Coma scale eye opening score of 2

● **R40.213 Coma scale, eyes open, to sound**
Coma scale eye opening score of 3

● **R40.214 Coma scale, eyes open, spontaneous**
Coma scale eye opening score of 4

● **R40.22 Coma scale, best verbal response**

The following appropriate 7th character is to be added to subcategory R40.22-:

0	unspecified time
1	in the field [EMT or ambulance]
2	at arrival to emergency department
3	at hospital admission
4	24 hours or more after hospital admission

Coding Clinic: 2017, Q4, P25; 2015, Q2, P18

● **R40.221 Coma scale, best verbal response, none** HCC
Coma scale verbal score of 1

● **R40.222 Coma scale, best verbal response, incomprehensible words** HCC
Coma scale verbal score of 2
Incomprehensible sounds (2-5 years of age)
Moans/grunts to pain; restless (<2 years old)

● **R40.223 Coma scale, best verbal response, inappropriate words**
Coma scale verbal score of 3
Inappropriate crying or screaming (< 2 years of age)
Screaming (2-5 years of age)

● **R40.224 Coma scale, best verbal response, confused conversation**
Coma scale verbal score of 4
Inappropriate words (2-5 years of age)
Irritable cries (< 2 years of age)

● **R40.225 Coma scale, best verbal response, oriented**
Coma scale verbal score of 5
Cooing or babbling or crying appropriately (< 2 years of age)
Uses appropriate words (2- 5 years of age)

● **R40.23 Coma scale, best motor response**

The following appropriate 7th character is to be added to subcategory R40.23-:

0	unspecified time
1	in the field [EMT or ambulance]
2	at arrival to emergency department
3	at hospital admission
4	24 hours or more after hospital admission

Coding Clinic: 2017, Q4, P25; 2015, Q2, P18

● **R40.231 Coma scale, best motor response, none** HCC
Coma scale motor score of 1

● **R40.232 Coma scale, best motor response, extension** HCC
Abnormal extensor posturing to pain or noxious stimuli (< 2 years of age)
Coma scale motor score of 2
Extensor posturing to pain or noxious stimuli (2-5 years of age)

Glasgow Coma Scale

Eye Opening Response	
• Spontaneous--open with blinking at baseline	**4 points**
• To verbal stimuli, command, speech	**3 points**
• To pain only (not applied to face)	**2 points**
• No response	**1 point**
Verbal Response	
• Oriented	**5 points**
• Confused conversation, but able to answer questions	**4 points**
• Inappropriate words	**3 points**
• Incomprehensible speech	**2 points**
• No response	**1 point**
Motor Response	
• Obeys commands for movement	**6 points**
• Purposeful movement to painful stimulus	**5 points**
• Withdraws in response to pain	**4 points**
• Flexion in response to pain (decorticate posturing)	**3 points**
• Extension response in response to pain (decerebrate posturing)	**2 points**
• No response	**1 point**
Categorization: Coma: No eye opening, no ability to follow commands, no word verbalizations (3-8)	
Head Injury Classification: Severe Head Injury--GCS score of 8 or less; Moderate Head Injury--GCS score of 9 to 12; Mild head injury--GCS score of 13 to 15	
(Adapted from: Advanced Trauma Life Support: Course for Physicians, American College of Surgeons, 1993). http://www.bt.cdc.gov/masscasulatires/gscale.asp	

Figure 18-1

● **R40.233 Coma scale, best motor response, abnormal flexion**
Coma scale motor score of 3
Abnormal flexure posturing to pain or noxious stimuli (2-5 years of age)
Flexion/decorticate posturing (< 2 years of age)

● **R40.234 Coma scale, best motor response, flexion withdrawal** HCC
Coma scale motor score of 4
Withdraws from pain or noxious stimuli (2-5 years of age)

● **R40.235 Coma scale, best motor response, localizes pain**
Coma scale motor score of 5
Localizes pain (2-5 years of age)
Withdraws to touch (< 2 years of age)

● **R40.236 Coma scale, best motor response, obeys commands**
Coma scale motor score of 6
Normal or spontaneous movement (< 2 years of age)
Obeys commands (2-5 years of age)

● R40.24 **Glasgow coma scale, total score**
Note: Assign a code from subcategory R40.24, when only the total coma score is documented
The following appropriate 7th character is to be added to subcategory R40.24-:

0	unspecified time
1	in the field [EMT or ambulance]
2	at arrival to emergency department
3	at hospital admission
4	24 hours or more after hospital admission

Coding Clinic: 2016, Q4, P64; 2015, Q2, P18

● R40.241 **Glasgow coma scale score 13-15**
● R40.242 **Glasgow coma scale score 9-12**
● R40.243 **Glasgow coma scale score 3-8**
● R40.244 **Other coma, without documented Glasgow coma scale score, or with partial score reported**

R40.3 **Persistent vegetative state**
R40.4 **Transient alteration of awareness**

● R41 **Other symptoms and signs involving cognitive functions and awareness**
Excludes1 dissociative [conversion] disorders (F44.-)
mild cognitive impairment, so stated (G31.84)

R41.0 **Disorientation, unspecified**
Confusion NOS
Delirium NOS
Coding Clinic: 2019, Q2, P34; 2016, Q4, P71

R41.1 **Anterograde amnesia**
R41.2 **Retrograde amnesia**
R41.3 **Other amnesia**
Amnesia NOS
Memory loss NOS
Excludes1 amnestic disorder due to known physiologic condition (F04)
amnestic syndrome due to psychoactive substance use (F10-F19 with 5th character .6)
mild memory disturbance due to known physiological condition (F06.8)
transient global amnesia (G45.4)

R41.4 **Neurologic neglect syndrome**
Asomatognosia
Hemi-akinesia
Hemi-inattention
Hemispatial neglect
Left-sided neglect
Sensory neglect
Visuospatial neglect
Excludes1 visuospatial deficit (R41.842)

● R41.8 **Other symptoms and signs involving cognitive functions and awareness**
R41.81 **Age-related cognitive decline** A
Senility NOS
R41.82 **Altered mental status, unspecified**
Change in mental status NOS
Excludes1 altered level of consciousness (R40.-)
altered mental status due to known condition - code to condition
delirium NOS (R41.0)
Coding Clinic: 2012, Q4, P98
R41.83 **Borderline intellectual functioning**
IQ level 71 to 84
Excludes1 intellectual disabilities (F70-F79)

● R41.84 **Other specified cognitive deficit**
Excludes1 cognitive deficits as sequelae of cerebrovascular disease (I69.01-, I69.11-, I69.21-, I69.31-, I69.81-, I69.91-)
R41.840 **Attention and concentration deficit**
Excludes1 attention-deficit hyperactivity disorders (F90.-)
R41.841 **Cognitive communication deficit**
R41.842 **Visuospatial deficit**
R41.843 **Psychomotor deficit**
R41.844 **Frontal lobe and executive function deficit**
R41.89 **Other symptoms and signs involving cognitive functions and awareness**
Anosognosia

R41.9 **Unspecified symptoms and signs involving cognitive functions and awareness**
Unspecified neurocognitive disorder

R42 **Dizziness and giddiness**
Light-headedness
Vertigo NOS
Excludes1 vertiginous syndromes (H81.-)
vertigo from infrasound (T75.23)
Coding Clinic: 2015, Q4, P40

● R43 **Disturbances of smell and taste**
R43.0 **Anosmia**
Absence of sense of smell; AKA anosphresia and olfactory anesthesia
R43.1 **Parosmia**
R43.2 **Parageusia**
Perversion of sense of taste or bad taste in mouth; AKA dysgeusia
R43.8 **Other disturbances of smell and taste**
Mixed disturbance of smell and taste
R43.9 **Unspecified disturbances of smell and taste**

● R44 **Other symptoms and signs involving general sensations and perceptions**
Excludes1 alcoholic hallucinations (F1.5)
hallucinations in drug psychosis (F11-F19 with .5)
hallucinations in mood disorders with psychotic symptoms (F30.2, F31.5, F32.3, F33.3)
hallucinations in schizophrenia, schizotypal and delusional disorders (F20-F29)
Excludes2 disturbances of skin sensation (R20.-)
R44.0 **Auditory hallucinations**
R44.1 **Visual hallucinations**
R44.2 **Other hallucinations**
R44.3 **Hallucinations, unspecified**
R44.8 **Other symptoms and signs involving general sensations and perceptions**
R44.9 **Unspecified symptoms and signs involving general sensations and perceptions**

● R45 **Symptoms and signs involving emotional state**
R45.0 **Nervousness**
Nervous tension
R45.1 **Restlessness and agitation**
R45.2 **Unhappiness**
R45.3 **Demoralization and apathy**
Excludes1 anhedonia (R45.84)

CHAPTER 18 (R00-R99)

R45.4 **Irritability and anger**

R45.5 **Hostility**

R45.6 **Violent behavior**

R45.7 **State of emotional shock and stress, unspecified**

● R45.8 **Other symptoms and signs involving emotional state**

R45.81 **Low self-esteem**

R45.82 **Worries**

R45.83 **Excessive crying of child, adolescent or adult**

Excludes1 excessive crying of infant (baby) R68.11

R45.84 **Anhedonia**

Total loss of feeling of pleasure in pleasurable acts

● R45.85 **Homicidal and suicidal ideations**

Excludes1 suicide attempt (T14.91)

R45.850 **Homicidal ideations**

R45.851 **Suicidal ideations**

R45.86 **Emotional lability**

R45.87 **Impulsiveness**

R45.89 **Other symptoms and signs involving emotional state**

● R46 **Symptoms and signs involving appearance and behavior**

Excludes1 appearance and behavior in schizophrenia, schizotypal and delusional disorders (F20-F29)
mental and behavioral disorders (F01-F99)

R46.0 **Very low level of personal hygiene**

R46.1 **Bizarre personal appearance**

R46.2 **Strange and inexplicable behavior**

R46.3 **Overactivity**

R46.4 **Slowness and poor responsiveness**

Excludes1 stupor (R40.1)

R46.5 **Suspiciousness and marked evasiveness**

R46.6 **Undue concern and preoccupation with stressful events**

R46.7 **Verbosity and circumstantial detail obscuring reason for contact**

● R46.8 **Other symptoms and signs involving appearance and behavior**

R46.81 **Obsessive-compulsive behavior**

Excludes1 obsessive-compulsive disorder (F42-)

R46.89 **Other symptoms and signs involving appearance and behavior**

SYMPTOMS AND SIGNS INVOLVING SPEECH AND VOICE (R47-R49)

● R47 **Speech disturbances, not elsewhere classified**

Excludes1 autism (F84.0)
cluttering (F80.81)
specific developmental disorders of speech and language (F80.-)
stuttering (F80.81)

● R47.0 **Dysphasia and aphasia**

R47.01 **Aphasia**

Excludes1 aphasia following cerebrovascular disease (I69. with final characters -20)
progressive isolated aphasia (G31.01)

R47.02 **Dysphasia**

Impairment in comprehension of speech, caused by left-sided brain damage

Excludes1 dysphasia following cerebrovascular disease (I69. with final characters -21)

R47.1 **Dysarthria and anarthria**

Motor speech disorder

Excludes1 dysarthria following cerebrovascular disease (I69. with final characters -22)

● R47.8 **Other speech disturbances**

Excludes1 dysarthria following cerebrovascular disease (I69. with final characters -28)

R47.81 **Slurred speech**

R47.82 ***Fluency disorder in conditions classified elsewhere***

Stuttering in conditions classified elsewhere

Code first underlying disease or condition, such as:
Parkinson's disease (G20)

Excludes1 adult onset fluency disorder (F98.5)
childhood onset fluency disorder (F80.81)
fluency disorder (stuttering) following cerebrovascular disease (I69. with final characters -23)

R47.89 **Other speech disturbances**

R47.9 **Unspecified speech disturbances**

● R48 **Dyslexia and other symbolic dysfunctions, not elsewhere classified**

Excludes1 specific developmental disorders of scholastic skills (F81.-)

R48.0 **Dyslexia and alexia**

R48.1 **Agnosia**

Loss of ability to recognize objects, persons, sounds, shapes, or smells

Astereognosia (astereognosis)
Autotopagnosia

Excludes1 visual object agnosia (R48.3)

R48.2 **Apraxia**

Loss of ability to execute or carry out learned purposeful movements

Excludes1 apraxia following cerebrovascular disease (I69. with final characters -90)

R48.3 **Visual agnosia**

Prosopagnosia
Simultanagnosia (asimultagnosia)

R48.8 **Other symbolic dysfunctions**

Acalculia

Difficulty performing simple mathematical tasks resulting from neurological injury

Agraphia

Coding Clinic: 2017, Q1, P27

R48.9 **Unspecified symbolic dysfunctions**

● R49 **Voice and resonance disorders**

Excludes1 psychogenic voice and resonance disorders (F44.4)

R49.0 **Dysphonia**

Hoarseness

R49.1 **Aphonia**

Loss of voice

● R49.2 **Hypernasality and hyponasality**

R49.21 **Hypernasality**

R49.22 **Hyponasality**

R49.8 **Other voice and resonance disorders**

R49.9 **Unspecified voice and resonance disorder**

Change in voice NOS
Resonance disorder NOS

CHAPTER 18 (R00-R99)

GENERAL SYMPTOMS AND SIGNS (R50-R69)

R50 Fever of other and unknown origin
Excludes1 chills without fever (R68.83)
febrile convulsions (R56.0-)
fever of unknown origin during labor (O75.2)
fever of unknown origin in newborn (P81.9)
hypothermia due to illness (R68.0)
malignant hyperthermia due to anesthesia (T88.3)
puerperal pyrexia NOS (O86.4)

R50.2 Drug induced fever
Use additional code for adverse effect, if applicable, to identify drug (T36-T50 with fifth or sixth character 5)
Excludes1 postvaccination (postimmunization) fever (R50.83)

R50.8 Other specified fever

R50.81 Fever presenting with conditions classified elsewhere
Code first underlying condition when associated fever is present, such as with:
leukemia (C91-C95)
neutropenia (D70.-)
sickle-cell disease (D57.-)
Coding Clinic: 2019, Q2, P25

R50.82 Postprocedural fever
Excludes1 postprocedural infection (T81.44)
posttransfusion fever (R50.84)
postvaccination (postimmunization) fever (R50.83)

R50.83 Postvaccination fever
Postimmunization fever

R50.84 Febrile nonhemolytic transfusion reaction
FNHTR
Posttransfusion fever

R50.9 Fever, unspecified
Fever NOS
Fever of unknown origin [FUO]
Fever with chills
Fever with rigors
Hyperpyrexia NOS
Persistent fever
Pyrexia NOS

R51 Headache
Facial pain NOS
Excludes1 atypical face pain (G50.1)
migraine and other headache syndromes (G43-G44)
trigeminal neuralgia (G50.0)

R52 Pain, unspecified
Acute pain NOS
Pain NOS
Generalized pain NOS
Excludes1 acute and chronic pain, not elsewhere classified (G89.-)
localized pain, unspecified type - code to pain by site, such as:
abdomen pain (R10.-)
back pain (M54.9)
breast pain (N64.4)
chest pain (R07.1-R07.9)
ear pain (H92.0-)
eye pain (H57.1)
headache (R51)
joint pain (M25.5-)
limb pain (M79.6-)
lumbar region pain (M54.5)
pelvic and perineal pain (R10.2)
shoulder pain (M25.51-)
spine pain (M54.-)
throat pain (R07.0)
tongue pain (K14.6)
tooth pain (K08.8)
renal colic (N23)
pain disorders exclusively related to psychological factors (F45.41)

R53 Malaise and fatigue

R53.0 Neoplastic (malignant) related fatigue
Code first associated neoplasm

R53.1 Weakness
Asthenia NOS
Excludes1 age-related weakness (R54)
muscle weakness (M62.8-)
sarcopenia (M62.84)
senile asthenia (R54)
Coding Clinic: 2017, Q1, P7

R53.2 Functional quadriplegia
Complete immobility due to severe physical disability or frailty
Excludes1 frailty NOS (R54)
hysterical paralysis (F44.4)
immobility syndrome (M62.3)
neurologic quadriplegia (G82.5-)
quadriplegia (G82.50)
Coding Clinic: 2016, Q2, P6

R53.8 Other malaise and fatigue
Excludes1 combat exhaustion and fatigue (F43.0)
congenital debility (P96.9)
exhaustion and fatigue due to excessive exertion (T73.3)
exhaustion and fatigue due to exposure (T73.2)
exhaustion and fatigue due to heat (T67.-)
exhaustion and fatigue due to pregnancy (O26.8-)
exhaustion and fatigue due to recurrent depressive episode (F33)
exhaustion and fatigue due to senile debility (R54)

R53.81 Other malaise
Chronic debility
Debility NOS
General physical deterioration
Malaise NOS
Nervous debility
Excludes1 age-related physical debility (R54)

R53.82 Chronic fatigue, unspecified
Chronic fatigue syndrome NOS
Excludes1 postviral fatigue syndrome (G93.3)

R53.83 Other fatigue
Fatigue NOS
Lethargy
Lack of energy
Tiredness
Excludes2 exhaustion and fatigue due to depressive episode (F32.-)
Coding Clinic: 2017, Q1, P7

R54 Age-related physical debility A
Frailty
Senile asthenia
Old age
Senile debility
Senescence
Excludes1 age-related cognitive decline (R41.81)
sarcopenia (M62.84)
senile psychosis (F03)
senility NOS (R41.81)

CHAPTER 18 (R00-R99)

R55 Syncope and collapse
Blackout
Fainting
Vasovagal attack
Excludes1 cardiogenic shock (R57.Ø)
carotid sinus syncope (G9Ø.Ø1)
heat syncope (T67.1)
neurocirculatory asthenia (F45.8)
neurogenic orthostatic hypotension (G9Ø.3)
orthostatic hypotension (I95.1)
postprocedural shock (T81.1-)
psychogenic syncope (F48.8)
shock NOS (R57.9)
shock complicating or following abortion or ectopic or molar pregnancy (OØØ-OØ7, OØ8.3)
shock complicating or following labor and delivery (O75.1)
Stokes-Adams attack (I45.9)
unconsciousness NOS (R4Ø.2-)

● **R56 Convulsions, not elsewhere classified**
Excludes1 dissociative convulsions and seizures (F44.5)
epileptic convulsions and seizures (G4Ø.-)
newborn convulsions and seizures (P9Ø)

● **R56.Ø Febrile convulsions**
R56.ØØ Simple febrile convulsions HCC
Febrile convulsion NOS
Febrile seizure NOS
R56.Ø1 Complex febrile convulsions HCC
Atypical febrile seizure
Complex febrile seizure
Complicated febrile seizure
Excludes1 status epilepticus (G4Ø.9Ø1)
R56.1 Post traumatic seizures HCC
Excludes1 post traumatic epilepsy (G4Ø.-)
R56.9 Unspecified convulsions HCC
Convulsion disorder
Fit NOS
Recurrent convulsions
Seizure(s) (convulsive) NOS

● **R57 Shock, not elsewhere classified**
Excludes1 anaphylactic shock NOS (T78.2)
anaphylactic reaction or shock due to adverse food reaction (T78.Ø-)
anaphylactic shock due to adverse effect of correct drug or medicament properly administered (T88.6)
anaphylactic shock due to serum (T8Ø.5-)
anesthetic shock (T88.3)
electric shock (T75.4)
obstetric shock (O75.1)
postprocedural shock (T81.1-)
psychic shock (F43.Ø)
shock complicating or following ectopic or molar pregnancy (OØØ-OØ7, OØ8.3)
shock due to lightning (T75.Ø1)
traumatic shock (T79.4)
toxic shock syndrome (A48.3)
R57.Ø Cardiogenic shock HCC
Excludes2 septic shock (R65.21)
R57.1 Hypovolemic shock HCC
Decreased blood volume (loss)
Coding Clinic: 2019, Q2, P7-8
R57.8 Other shock HCC
R57.9 Shock, unspecified HCC
Failure of peripheral circulation NOS
Resulting in significant blood pressure drop

R58 Hemorrhage, not elsewhere classified
Hemorrhage NOS
Excludes1 hemorrhage included with underlying conditions, such as:
acute duodenal ulcer with hemorrhage (K26.Ø)
acute gastritis with bleeding (K29.Ø1)
ulcerative enterocolitis with rectal bleeding (K51.Ø1)

● **R59 Enlarged lymph nodes**
Includes swollen glands
Excludes1 lymphadenitis NOS (I88.9)
acute lymphadenitis (LØ4.-)
chronic lymphadenitis (I88.1)
mesenteric (acute) (chronic) lymphadenitis (I88.Ø)
R59.Ø Localized enlarged lymph nodes
R59.1 Generalized enlarged lymph nodes
Lymphadenopathy NOS
R59.9 Enlarged lymph nodes, unspecified

● **R6Ø Edema, not elsewhere classified**
Excludes1 angioneurotic edema (T78.3)
ascites (R18.-)
cerebral edema (G93.6)
cerebral edema due to birth injury (P11.Ø)
edema of larynx (J38.4)
edema of nasopharynx (J39.2)
edema of pharynx (J39.2)
gestational edema (O12.Ø-)
hereditary edema (Q82.Ø)
hydrops fetalis NOS (P83.2)
hydrothorax (J94.8)
hydrops fetalis NOS (P83.2)
newborn edema (P83.3)
pulmonary edema (J81.-)
R6Ø.Ø Localized edema
R6Ø.1 Generalized edema
Excludes2 nutritional edema (E4Ø-E46)
R6Ø.9 Edema, unspecified
Fluid retention NOS

R61 Generalized hyperhidrosis
Excessive sweating
Night sweats
Secondary hyperhidrosis
Code first, if applicable, menopausal and female climacteric states (N95.1)
Excludes1 focal (primary) (secondary) hyperhidrosis (L74.5-)
Frey's syndrome (L74.52)
localized (primary) (secondary) hyperhidrosis (L74.5-)

● **R62 Lack of expected normal physiological development in childhood and adults**
Excludes1 delayed puberty (E3Ø.Ø)
gonadal dysgenesis (Q99.1)
hypopituitarism (E23.Ø)
R62.Ø Delayed milestone in childhood P
Delayed attainment of expected physiological developmental stage
Late talker
Late walker
● **R62.5 Other and unspecified lack of expected normal physiological development in childhood**
Excludes1 HIV disease resulting in failure to thrive (B2Ø)
physical retardation due to malnutrition (E45)
R62.5Ø Unspecified lack of expected normal physiological development in childhood
Infantilism NOS
R62.51 Failure to thrive (child) P
Failure to gain weight
Excludes1 failure to thrive in child under 28 days old (P92.6)
Coding Clinic: 2018, Q4, P82
R62.52 Short stature (child)
Lack of growth
Physical retardation
Short stature NOS
Excludes1 short stature due to endocrine disorder (E34.3)
R62.59 Other lack of expected normal physiological development in childhood
R62.7 Adult failure to thrive A

R63 Symptoms and signs concerning food and fluid intake
Excludes1 bulimia NOS (F5Ø.2)
~~eating disorders of nonorganic origin (F5Ø.-)~~
~~malnutrition (E4Ø-E46)~~

R63.Ø Anorexia
Loss of appetite
Excludes1 anorexia nervosa (F5Ø.Ø-)
loss of appetite of nonorganic origin (F5Ø.89)

R63.1 Polydipsia
Excessive thirst

R63.2 Polyphagia
Excessive eating
Hyperalimentation NOS

R63.3 Feeding difficulties
Feeding problem (elderly) (infant) NOS
Picky eater
Excludes1 eating disorders (F5Ø.-)
feeding problems of newborn (P92.-)
infant feeding disorder of nonorganic origin (F98.2-)
Coding Clinic: 2017, Q1, P27; 2016, Q3, P19

R63.4 Abnormal weight loss

R63.5 Abnormal weight gain
Excludes1 excessive weight gain in pregnancy (O26.Ø-)
obesity (E66.-)

R63.6 Underweight
Use additional code to identify body mass index (BMI), if known (Z68.-)
Excludes1 abnormal weight loss (R63.4)
anorexia nervosa (F5Ø.Ø-)
malnutrition (E4Ø-E46)

R63.8 Other symptoms and signs concerning food and fluid intake

R64 Cachexia
Wasting syndrome
Code first underlying condition, if known
Excludes1 abnormal weight loss (R63.4)
nutritional marasmus (E41)
Coding Clinic: 2017, Q3, P25

R65 Symptoms and signs specifically associated with systemic inflammation and infection

R65.1 Systemic inflammatory response syndrome (SIRS) of non-infectious origin
Code first underlying condition, such as:
heatstroke (T67.Ø-)
injury and trauma (SØØ-T88)
Excludes1 sepsis - code to infection
severe sepsis (R65.2)
Coding Clinic: 2019, Q2, P38

R65.1Ø Systemic inflammatory response syndrome (SIRS) of non-infectious origin without acute organ dysfunction
Systemic inflammatory response syndrome (SIRS) NOS
Coding Clinic: 2019, Q2, P25, 38

R65.11 Systemic inflammatory response syndrome (SIRS) of non-infectious origin with acute organ dysfunction
Use additional code to identify specific acute organ dysfunction, such as:
acute kidney failure (N17.-)
acute respiratory failure (J96.Ø-)
critical illness myopathy (G72.81)
critical illness polyneuropathy (G62.81)
disseminated intravascular coagulopathy [DIC] (D65)
encephalopathy (metabolic) (septic) (G93.41)
hepatic failure (K72.Ø-)

OGCR Section I.C.18.g.
SIRS due to Non-Infectious Process
The systemic inflammatory response syndrome (SIRS) can develop as a result of certain non-infectious disease processes, such as trauma, malignant neoplasm, or pancreatitis. When SIRS is documented with a noninfectious condition, and no subsequent infection is documented, the code for the underlying condition, such as an injury, should be assigned, followed by code R65.1Ø, Systemic inflammatory response syndrome (SIRS) of non-infectious origin without acute organ dysfunction, or code R65.11, Systemic inflammatory response syndrome (SIRS) of non-infectious origin with acute organ dysfunction. If an associated acute organ dysfunction is documented, the appropriate code(s) for the specific type of organ dysfunction(s) should be assigned in addition to code R65.11. If acute organ dysfunction is documented, but it cannot be determined if the acute organ dysfunction is associated with SIRS or due to another condition (e.g., directly due to the trauma), the provider should be queried.

R65.2 Severe sepsis
Infection with associated acute organ dysfunction
Sepsis with acute organ dysfunction
Sepsis with multiple organ dysfunction
Systemic inflammatory response syndrome due to infectious process with acute organ dysfunction
Code first underlying infection, such as:
infection following a procedure (T81.44)
infections following infusion, transfusion and therapeutic injection (T8Ø.2-)
puerperal sepsis (O85)
sepsis following complete or unspecified spontaneous abortion (OØ3.87)
sepsis following ectopic and molar pregnancy (OØ8.82)
sepsis following incomplete spontaneous abortion (OØ3.37)
sepsis following (induced) termination of pregnancy (OØ4.87)
sepsis NOS (A41.9)
Use additional code to identify specific acute organ dysfunction, such as:
acute kidney failure (N17.-)
acute respiratory failure (J96.Ø-)
critical illness myopathy (G72.81)
critical illness polyneuropathy (G62.81)
disseminated intravascular coagulopathy [DIC] (D65)
encephalopathy (metabolic) (septic) (G93.41)
hepatic failure (K72.Ø-)
Coding Clinic: 2017, Q4, P99; 2016, Q3, P8

R65.2Ø Severe sepsis without septic shock
Severe sepsis NOS
Coding Clinic: 2019, Q1, P14; 2018, Q4, P9Ø; 2016, Q3, P14

R65.21 Severe sepsis with septic shock

R68 Other general symptoms and signs

R68.Ø Hypothermia, not associated with low environmental temperature
Excludes1 hypothermia NOS (accidental) (T68)
hypothermia due to anesthesia (T88.51)
hypothermia due to low environmental temperature (T68)
newborn hypothermia (P8Ø.-)

R68.1 Nonspecific symptoms peculiar to infancy
Excludes1 colic, infantile (R1Ø.83)
neonatal cerebral irritability (P91.3)
teething syndrome (KØØ.7)

R68.11 Excessive crying of infant (baby) P
Excludes1 excessive crying of child, adolescent, or adult (R45.83)

R68.12 Fussy infant (baby) P
Irritable infant

CHAPTER 18 (RØØ-R99)

R68.13 Apparent life threatening event in infant (ALTE) P
Apparent life threatening event in newborn
Brief resolved unexplained event (BRUE)
Code first confirmed diagnosis, if known
Use additional code(s) for associated signs and symptoms if no confirmed diagnosis established, or if signs and symptoms are not associated routinely with confirmed diagnosis, or provide additional information for cause of ALTE

R68.19 Other nonspecific symptoms peculiar to infancy P

R68.2 Dry mouth, unspecified
Excludes1 dry mouth due to dehydration (E86.0)
dry mouth due to sicca syndrome [Sjögren] (M35.0-)
salivary gland hyposecretion (K11.7)

R68.3 Clubbing of fingers
Clubbing of nails
Excludes1 congenital clubfinger (Q68.1)

● **R68.8 Other general symptoms and signs**

R68.81 Early satiety

R68.82 Decreased libido A
Decreased sexual desire

R68.83 Chills (without fever)
Chills NOS
Excludes1 chills with fever (R50.9)

R68.84 Jaw pain
Mandibular pain
Maxilla pain
Excludes1 temporomandibular joint arthralgia (M26.62-)

R68.89 Other general symptoms and signs

R69 Illness, unspecified
Unknown and unspecified cases of morbidity

ABNORMAL FINDINGS ON EXAMINATION OF BLOOD, WITHOUT DIAGNOSIS (R70-R79)

Excludes2 abnormal findings on antenatal screening of mother (O28.-)
abnormalities of lipids (E78.-)
abnormalities of platelets and thrombocytes (D69.-)
abnormalities of white blood cells classified elsewhere (D70-D72)
coagulation hemorrhagic disorders (D65-D68)
diagnostic abnormal findings classified elsewhere —*see* Alphabetical Index
hemorrhagic and hematological disorders of newborn (P50-P61)

● **R70 Elevated erythrocyte sedimentation rate and abnormality of plasma viscosity**

R70.0 Elevated erythrocyte sedimentation rate

R70.1 Abnormal plasma viscosity

● **R71 Abnormality of red blood cells**
Excludes1 anemias (D50-D64)
anemia of premature infant (P61.2)
benign (familial) polycythemia (D75.0)
congenital anemias (P61.2-P61.4)
newborn anemia due to isoimmunization (P55.-)
polycythemia neonatorum (P61.1)
polycythemia NOS (D75.1)
polycythemia vera (D45)
secondary polycythemia (D75.1)

R71.0 Precipitous drop in hematocrit
Drop (precipitous) in hemoglobin
Drop in hematocrit
Blood volume that has decreased red blood cells

R71.8 Other abnormality of red blood cells
Abnormal red-cell morphology NOS
Abnormal red-cell volume NOS
Anisocytosis
Red blood cells of unequal size
Poikilocytosis
Red blood cells of abnormal shape

● **R73 Elevated blood glucose level**
Excludes1 diabetes mellitus (E08-E13)
diabetes mellitus in pregnancy, childbirth and the puerperium (O24.-)
neonatal disorders (P70.0-P70.2)
postsurgical hypoinsulinemia (E89.1)

● **R73.0 Abnormal glucose**
Excludes1 abnormal glucose in pregnancy (O99.81-)
diabetes mellitus (E08-E13)
dysmetabolic syndrome X (E88.81)
gestational diabetes (O24.4-)
glycosuria (R81)
hypoglycemia (E16.2)

R73.01 Impaired fasting glucose
Elevated fasting glucose

R73.02 Impaired glucose tolerance (oral)
Elevated glucose tolerance

R73.03 Prediabetes
Latent diabetes
Coding Clinic: 2016, Q4, P65

R73.09 Other abnormal glucose
Abnormal glucose NOS
Abnormal non-fasting glucose tolerance
Coding Clinic: 2016, Q4, P65

R73.9 Hyperglycemia, unspecified

● **R74 Abnormal serum enzyme levels**

R74.0 Nonspecific elevation of levels of transaminase and lactic acid dehydrogenase [LDH]

R74.8 Abnormal levels of other serum enzymes
Abnormal level of acid phosphatase
Abnormal level of alkaline phosphatase
Abnormal level of amylase
Abnormal level of lipase [triacylglycerol lipase]
Coding Clinic: 2019, Q2, P6

R74.9 Abnormal serum enzyme level, unspecified

OGCR Section I.C.1.e and f.

Patients with inconclusive HIV serology

e. Patients with inconclusive HIV serology, but no definitive diagnosis or manifestations of the illness, may be assigned code R75, Inconclusive laboratory evidence of human immunodeficiency virus [HIV].

f. Previously diagnosed HIV-related illness

Patients with any known prior diagnosis of an HIV-related illness should be coded to B20. Once a patient has developed an HIV-related illness, the patient should always be assigned code B20 on every subsequent admission/encounter. Patients previously diagnosed with any HIV illness (B20) should never be assigned to R75 or Z21, Asymptomatic human immunodeficiency virus [HIV] infection status.

R75 Inconclusive laboratory evidence of human immunodeficiency virus [HIV]
Nonconclusive HIV-test finding in infants
Excludes1 asymptomatic human immunodeficiency virus [HIV] infection status (Z21)
human immunodeficiency virus [HIV] disease (B20)

● **R76 Other abnormal immunological findings in serum**

R76.0 Raised antibody titer
Excludes1 isoimmunization in pregnancy (O36.0-O36.1)
isoimmunization affecting newborn (P55.-)

New Revised ~~deleted~~ Deleted Excludes 1 Excludes 2 Includes Use additional Code first Code also Key words
OGCR Official Guidelines X Assign placeholder X ● Use Additional Character(s) Manifestation Code Hierarchical Condition Category Coding Clinic

CHAPTER 18 (R00-R99)

● R76.1 **Nonspecific reaction to test for tuberculosis**

R76.11 **Nonspecific reaction to tuberculin skin test without active tuberculosis**
Abnormal result of Mantoux test
PPD positive
Tuberculin (skin test) positive
Tuberculin (skin test) reactor
Excludes1 nonspecific reaction to cell mediated immunity measurement of gamma interferon antigen response without active tuberculosis (R76.12)

R76.12 **Nonspecific reaction to cell mediated immunity measurement of gamma interferon antigen response without active tuberculosis**
Nonspecific reaction to QuantiFERON-TB test (QFT) without active tuberculosis
Excludes1 nonspecific reaction to tuberculin skin test without active tuberculosis (R76.11)
positive tuberculin skin test (R76.11)

R76.8 **Other specified abnormal immunological findings in serum**
Raised level of immunoglobulins NOS

R76.9 **Abnormal immunological finding in serum, unspecified**

● R77 **Other abnormalities of plasma proteins**
Excludes1 disorders of plasma-protein metabolism (E88.0-)

R77.0 **Abnormality of albumin**

R77.1 **Abnormality of globulin**
Hyperglobulinemia NOS

R77.2 **Abnormality of alphafetoprotein**

R77.8 **Other specified abnormalities of plasma proteins**
Coding Clinic: 2019, Q2, P6

R77.9 **Abnormality of plasma protein, unspecified**
Coding Clinic: 2019, Q2, P6

● R78 **Findings of drugs and other substances, not normally found in blood**
Use additional code to identify any retained foreign body, if applicable (Z18.-)
Excludes1 mental or behavioral disorders due to psychoactive substance use (F10-F19)

R78.0 **Finding of alcohol in blood**
Use additional external cause code (Y90.-), for detail regarding alcohol level.

R78.1 **Finding of opiate drug in blood**

R78.2 **Finding of cocaine in blood**

R78.3 **Finding of hallucinogen in blood**

R78.4 **Finding of other drugs of addictive potential in blood**

R78.5 **Finding of other psychotropic drug in blood**

R78.6 **Finding of steroid agent in blood**

● R78.7 **Finding of abnormal level of heavy metals in blood**

R78.71 **Abnormal lead level in blood**
Excludes1 lead poisoning (T56.0-)

R78.79 **Finding of abnormal level of heavy metals in blood**

● R78.8 **Finding of other specified substances, not normally found in blood**

R78.81 **Bacteremia**
Blood poisoning/bacteremia
Excludes1 sepsis-code to specified infection

R78.89 **Finding of other specified substances, not normally found in blood**
Finding of abnormal level of lithium in blood

R78.9 **Finding of unspecified substance, not normally found in blood**

● R79 **Other abnormal findings of blood chemistry**
Use additional code to identify any retained foreign body, if applicable (Z18.-)
Excludes1 asymptomatic hyperuricemia (E79.0)
hyperglycemia NOS (R73.9)
hypoglycemia NOS (E16.2)
neonatal hypoglycemia (P70.3-P70.4)
specific findings indicating disorder of amino-acid metabolism (E70-E72)
specific findings indicating disorder of carbohydrate metabolism (E73-E74)
specific findings indicating disorder of lipid metabolism (E75.-)

R79.0 **Abnormal level of blood mineral**
Abnormal blood level of cobalt
Abnormal blood level of copper
Abnormal blood level of iron
Abnormal blood level of magnesium
Abnormal blood level of mineral NEC
Abnormal blood level of zinc
Excludes1 abnormal level of lithium (R78.89)
disorders of mineral metabolism (E83.-)
neonatal hypomagnesemia (P71.2)
nutritional mineral deficiency (E58-E61)

R79.1 **Abnormal coagulation profile**
Abnormal or prolonged bleeding time
Abnormal or prolonged coagulation time
Abnormal or prolonged partial thromboplastin time [PTT]
Abnormal or prolonged prothrombin time [PT]
Excludes1 coagulation defects (D68.-)
Excludes2 abnormality of fluid, electrolyte or acid-base balance (E86-E87)

● R79.8 **Other specified abnormal findings of blood chemistry**

R79.81 **Abnormal blood-gas level**

R79.82 **Elevated C-reactive protein (CRP)**

R79.89 **Other specified abnormal findings of blood chemistry**
Coding Clinic: 2019, Q2, P6

R79.9 **Abnormal finding of blood chemistry, unspecified**

ABNORMAL FINDINGS ON EXAMINATION OF URINE, WITHOUT DIAGNOSIS (R80-R82)

Excludes1 abnormal findings on antenatal screening of mother (O28.-)
diagnostic abnormal findings classified elsewhere - see Alphabetical Index
specific findings indicating disorder of amino-acid metabolism (E70-E72)
specific findings indicating disorder of carbohydrate metabolism (E73-E74)

● R80 **Proteinuria**
Excludes1 gestational proteinuria (O12.1-)

R80.0 **Isolated proteinuria**
Idiopathic proteinuria
Excludes1 isolated proteinuria with specific morphological lesion (N06.-)

R80.1 **Persistent proteinuria, unspecified**

R80.2 **Orthostatic proteinuria, unspecified**
Postural proteinuria

R80.3 **Bence Jones proteinuria**

R80.8 **Other proteinuria**

R80.9 **Proteinuria, unspecified**
Albuminuria NOS

R81 **Glycosuria**
Excludes1 renal glycosuria (E74.8)

CHAPTER 18 (R00-R99)

● **R82 Other and unspecified abnormal findings in urine**
Includes chromoabnormalities in urine
Use additional code to identify any retained foreign body, if applicable (Z18.-)
Excludes2 hematuria (R31.-)

R82.Ø Chyluria
White milky urine
Excludes1 filarial chyluria (B74.-)

R82.1 Myoglobinuria
Presence of myoglobin (iron containing protein) in urine

R82.2 Biliuria
Presence of bile pigments/salts in urine

R82.3 Hemoglobinuria
Presence of hemoglobin in urine
Excludes1 hemoglobinuria due to hemolysis from external causes NEC (D59.6)
hemoglobinuria due to paroxysmal nocturnal [Marchiafava-Micheli] (D59.5)

R82.4 Acetonuria
Ketonuria

R82.5 Elevated urine levels of drugs, medicaments and biological substances
Elevated urine levels of catecholamines
Elevated urine levels of indoleacetic acid
Elevated urine levels of 17-ketosteroids
Elevated urine levels of steroids

R82.6 Abnormal urine levels of substances chiefly nonmedicinal as to source
Abnormal urine level of heavy metals

● **R82.7 Abnormal findings on microbiological examination of urine**
Excludes1 colonization status (Z22.-)
Coding Clinic: 2016, Q4, P65

R82.71 Bacteriuria

R82.79 Other abnormal findings on microbiological examination of urine
Positive culture findings of urine

● **R82.8 Abnormal findings on cytological and histological examination of urine**

▶**R82.81 Pyuria**
▶Sterile pyuria

▶**R82.89 Other abnormal findings on cytological and histological examination of urine**

● **R82.9 Other and unspecified abnormal findings in urine**

R82.9Ø Unspecified abnormal findings in urine

R82.91 Other chromoabnormalities of urine
Chromoconversion (dipstick)
Idiopathic dipstick converts positive for blood with no cellular forms in sediment
Excludes1 hemoglobinuria (R82.3)
myoglobinuria (R82.1)

● **R82.99 Other abnormal findings in urine**

R82.991 Hypocitraturia

R82.992 Hyperoxaluria
Excludes1 Primary hyperoxaluria (E72.53)

R82.993 Hyperuricosuria

R82.994 Hypercalciuria
Idiopathic hypercalciuria

R82.998 Other abnormal findings in urine
Cells and casts in urine
Crystalluria
Melanuria

ABNORMAL FINDINGS ON EXAMINATION OF OTHER BODY FLUIDS, SUBSTANCES AND TISSUES, WITHOUT DIAGNOSIS (R83-R89)

Excludes1 abnormal findings on antenatal screening of mother (O28.-)
diagnostic abnormal findings classified elsewhere - see Alphabetical Index
Excludes2 abnormal findings on examination of blood, without diagnosis (R7Ø-R79)
abnormal findings on examination of urine, without diagnosis (R8Ø-R82)
abnormal tumor markers (R97.-)

● **R83 Abnormal findings in cerebrospinal fluid**

R83.Ø Abnormal level of enzymes in cerebrospinal fluid

R83.1 Abnormal level of hormones in cerebrospinal fluid

R83.2 Abnormal level of other drugs, medicaments and biological substances in cerebrospinal fluid

R83.3 Abnormal level of substances chiefly nonmedicinal as to source in cerebrospinal fluid

R83.4 Abnormal immunological findings in cerebrospinal fluid

R83.5 Abnormal microbiological findings in cerebrospinal fluid
Positive culture findings in cerebrospinal fluid
Excludes1 colonization status (Z22.-)

R83.6 Abnormal cytological findings in cerebrospinal fluid

R83.8 Other abnormal findings in cerebrospinal fluid
Abnormal chromosomal findings in cerebrospinal fluid

R83.9 Unspecified abnormal finding in cerebrospinal fluid

● **R84 Abnormal findings in specimens from respiratory organs and thorax**
Includes abnormal findings in bronchial washings
abnormal findings in nasal secretions
abnormal findings in pleural fluid
abnormal findings in sputum
abnormal findings in throat scrapings
Excludes1 blood-stained sputum (RØ4.2)

R84.Ø Abnormal level of enzymes in specimens from respiratory organs and thorax

R84.1 Abnormal level of hormones in specimens from respiratory organs and thorax

R84.2 Abnormal level of other drugs, medicaments and biological substances in specimens from respiratory organs and thorax

R84.3 Abnormal level of substances chiefly nonmedicinal as to source in specimens from respiratory organs and thorax

R84.4 Abnormal immunological findings in specimens from respiratory organs and thorax

R84.5 Abnormal microbiological findings in specimens from respiratory organs and thorax
Positive culture findings in specimens from respiratory organs and thorax
Excludes1 colonization status (Z22.-)

R84.6 Abnormal cytological findings in specimens from respiratory organs and thorax

R84.7 Abnormal histological findings in specimens from respiratory organs and thorax

R84.8 Other abnormal findings in specimens from respiratory organs and thorax
Abnormal chromosomal findings in specimens from respiratory organs and thorax

R84.9 Unspecified abnormal finding in specimens from respiratory organs and thorax

R85 Abnormal findings in specimens from digestive organs and abdominal cavity

Includes abnormal findings in peritoneal fluid
abnormal findings in saliva

Excludes1 cloudy peritoneal dialysis effluent (R88.Ø)
fecal abnormalities (R19.5)

R85.Ø Abnormal level of enzymes in specimens from digestive organs and abdominal cavity

R85.1 Abnormal level of hormones in specimens from digestive organs and abdominal cavity

R85.2 Abnormal level of other drugs, medicaments and biological substances in specimens from digestive organs and abdominal cavity

R85.3 Abnormal level of substances chiefly nonmedicinal as to source in specimens from digestive organs and abdominal cavity

R85.4 Abnormal immunological findings in specimens from digestive organs and abdominal cavity

R85.5 Abnormal microbiological findings in specimens from digestive organs and abdominal cavity

Positive culture findings in specimens from digestive organs and abdominal cavity

Excludes1 colonization status (Z22.-)

R85.6 Abnormal cytological findings in specimens from digestive organs and abdominal cavity

R85.61 Abnormal cytologic smear of anus

Excludes1 abnormal cytological findings in specimens from other digestive organs and abdominal cavity (R85.69)
carcinoma in situ of anus (histologically confirmed) (DØ1.3)
anal intraepithelial neoplasia I [AIN I] (K62.82)
anal intraepithelial neoplasia II [AIN II] (K62.82)
anal intraepithelial neoplasia III [AIN III] (DØ1.3)
dysplasia (mild) (moderate) of anus (histologically confirmed) (K62.82)
severe dysplasia of anus (histologically confirmed) (DØ1.3)

Excludes2 anal high risk human papillomavirus (HPV) DNA test positive (R85.81)
anal low risk human papillomavirus (HPV) DNA test positive (R85.82)

R85.61Ø Atypical squamous cells of undetermined significance on cytologic smear of anus (ASC-US)

R85.611 Atypical squamous cells cannot exclude high grade squamous intraepithelial lesion on cytologic smear of anus (ASC-H)

R85.612 Low grade squamous intraepithelial lesion on cytologic smear of anus (LGSIL)

R85.613 High grade squamous intraepithelial lesion on cytologic smear of anus (HGSIL)

R85.614 Cytologic evidence of malignancy on smear of anus

R85.615 Unsatisfactory cytologic smear of anus

Inadequate sample of cytologic smear of anus

R85.616 Satisfactory anal smear but lacking transformation zone

R85.618 Other abnormal cytological findings on specimens from anus

R85.619 Unspecified abnormal cytological findings in specimens from anus

Abnormal anal cytology NOS
Atypical glandular cells of anus NOS

R85.69 Abnormal cytological findings in specimens from other digestive organs and abdominal cavity

R85.7 Abnormal histological findings in specimens from digestive organs and abdominal cavity

R85.8 Other abnormal findings in specimens from digestive organs and abdominal cavity

R85.81 Anal high risk human papillomavirus (HPV) DNA test positive

Excludes1 anogenital warts due to human papillomavirus (HPV) (A63.Ø)
condyloma acuminatum (A63.Ø)

R85.82 Anal low risk human papillomavirus (HPV) DNA test positive

Use additional code for associated human papillomavirus (B97.7)

R85.89 Other abnormal findings in specimens from digestive organs and abdominal cavity

Abnormal chromosomal findings in specimens from digestive organs and abdominal cavity

R85.9 Unspecified abnormal finding in specimens from digestive organs and abdominal cavity

R86 Abnormal findings in specimens from male genital organs

Includes abnormal findings in prostatic secretions
abnormal findings in semen, seminal fluid
abnormal spermatozoa

Excludes1 azoospermia (N46.Ø-)
oligospermia (N46.1-)

R86.Ø Abnormal level of enzymes in specimens from male genital organs ♂

R86.1 Abnormal level of hormones in specimens from male genital organs ♂

R86.2 Abnormal level of other drugs, medicaments and biological substances in specimens from male genital organs ♂

R86.3 Abnormal level of substances chiefly nonmedicinal as to source in specimens from male genital organs ♂

R86.4 Abnormal immunological findings in specimens from male genital organs ♂

R86.5 Abnormal microbiological findings in specimens from male genital organs ♂

Positive culture findings in specimens from male genital organs

Excludes1 colonization status (Z22.-)

R86.6 Abnormal cytological findings in specimens from male genital organs ♂

R86.7 Abnormal histological findings in specimens from male genital organs ♂

R86.8 Other abnormal findings in specimens from male genital organs ♂

Abnormal chromosomal findings in specimens from male genital organs

R86.9 Unspecified abnormal finding in specimens from male genital organs ♂

● **R87 Abnormal findings in specimens from female genital organs**

Includes abnormal findings in secretion and smears from cervix uteri
abnormal findings in secretion and smears from vagina
abnormal findings in secretion and smears from vulva

R87.Ø **Abnormal level of enzymes in specimens from female genital organs** ♀

R87.1 **Abnormal level of hormones in specimens from female genital organs** ♀

R87.2 **Abnormal level of other drugs, medicaments and biological substances in specimens from female genital organs** ♀

R87.3 **Abnormal level of substances chiefly nonmedicinal as to source in specimens from female genital organs** ♀

R87.4 **Abnormal immunological findings in specimens from female genital organs** ♀

R87.5 **Abnormal microbiological findings in specimens from female genital organs** ♀
Positive culture findings in specimens from female genital organs
Excludes1 colonization status (Z22.-)

● R87.6 **Abnormal cytological findings in specimens from female genital organs**

● R87.61 **Abnormal cytological findings in specimens from cervix uteri**

Excludes1 abnormal cytological findings in specimens from other female genital organs (R87.69)
abnormal cytological findings in specimens from vagina (R87.62-)
carcinoma in situ of cervix uteri (histologically confirmed) (DØ6.-)
cervical intraepithelial neoplasia I [CIN I] (N87.Ø)
cervical intraepithelial neoplasia II [CIN II] (N87.1)
cervical intraepithelial neoplasia III [CIN III] (DØ6.-)
dysplasia (mild) (moderate) of cervix uteri (histologically confirmed) (N87.-)
severe dysplasia of cervix uteri (histologically confirmed) (DØ6.-)

Excludes2 cervical high risk human papillomavirus (HPV) DNA test positive (R87.81Ø)
cervical low risk human papillomavirus (HPV) DNA test positive (R87.82Ø)

R87.61Ø **Atypical squamous cells of undetermined significance on cytologic smear of cervix (ASC-US)** ♀

R87.611 **Atypical squamous cells cannot exclude high grade squamous intraepithelial lesion on cytologic smear of cervix (ASC-H)** ♀

R87.612 **Low grade squamous intraepithelial lesion on cytologic smear of cervix (LGSIL)** ♀

R87.613 **High grade squamous intraepithelial lesion on cytologic smear of cervix (HGSIL)** ♀

R87.614 **Cytologic evidence of malignancy on smear of cervix** ♀

R87.615 **Unsatisfactory cytologic smear of cervix** ♀
Inadequate sample of cytologic smear of cervix

R87.616 **Satisfactory cervical smear but lacking transformation zone** ♀

R87.618 **Other abnormal cytological findings on specimens from cervix uteri** ♀

R87.619 **Unspecified abnormal cytological findings in specimens from cervix uteri** ♀
Abnormal cervical cytology NOS
Abnormal Papanicolaou smear of cervix NOS
Abnormal thin preparation smear of cervix NOS
Atypical endocervial cells of cervix NOS
Atypical endometrial cells of cervix NOS
Atypical glandular cells of cervix NOS

● R87.62 **Abnormal cytological findings in specimens from vagina**

Use additional code to identify acquired absence of uterus and cervix, if applicable (Z9Ø.71-)

Excludes1 abnormal cytological findings in specimens from cervix uteri (R87.61-)
abnormal cytological findings in specimens from other female genital organs (R87.69)
carcinoma in situ of vagina (histologically confirmed) (DØ7.2)
vaginal intraepithelial neoplasia I [VAIN I] (N89.Ø)
vaginal intraepithelial neoplasia II [VAIN II] (N89.1)
vaginal intraepithelial neoplasia III [VAIN III] (DØ7.2)
dysplasia (mild) (moderate) of vagina (histologically confirmed) (N89.-)
severe dysplasia of vagina (histologically confirmed) (DØ7.2)

Excludes2 vaginal high risk human papillomavirus (HPV) DNA test positive (R87.811)
vaginal low risk human papillomavirus (HPV) DNA test positive (R87.821)

R87.62Ø **Atypical squamous cells of undetermined significance on cytologic smear of vagina (ASC-US)** ♀

R87.621 **Atypical squamous cells cannot exclude high grade squamous intraepithelial lesion on cytologic smear of vagina (ASC-H)** ♀

R87.622 **Low grade squamous intraepithelial lesion on cytologic smear of vagina (LGSIL)** ♀

R87.623 **High grade squamous intraepithelial lesion on cytologic smear of vagina (HGSIL)** ♀

R87.624 **Cytologic evidence of malignancy on smear of vagina** ♀

R87.625 **Unsatisfactory cytologic smear of vagina** ♀
Inadequate sample of cytologic smear of vagina

R87.628 **Other abnormal cytological findings on specimens from vagina** ♀

R87.629 **Unspecified abnormal cytological findings in specimens from vagina ♀**
Abnormal Papanicolaou smear of vagina NOS
Abnormal thin preparation smear of vagina NOS
Abnormal vaginal cytology NOS
Atypical endocervical cells of vagina NOS
Atypical endometrial cells of vagina NOS
Atypical glandular cells of vagina NOS

R87.69 **Abnormal cytological findings in specimens from other female genital organs ♀**
Abnormal cytological findings in specimens from female genital organs NOS
Excludes1 dysplasia of vulva (histologically confirmed) (N90.0-N90.3)

R87.7 **Abnormal histological findings in specimens from female genital organs ♀**
Excludes1 carcinoma in situ (histologically confirmed) of female genital organs (D06-D07.3)
cervical intraepithelial neoplasia I [CIN I] (N87.0)
cervical intraepithelial neoplasia II [CIN II] (N87.1)
cervical intraepithelial neoplasia III [CIN III] (D06.-)
dysplasia (mild) (moderate) of cervix uteri (histologically confirmed) (N87.-)
dysplasia (mild) (moderate) of vagina (histologically confirmed) (N89.-)
vaginal intraepithelial neoplasia I [VAIN I] (N89.0)
vaginal intraepithelial neoplasia II [VAIN II] (N89.1)
vaginal intraepithelial neoplasia III [VAIN III] (D07.2)
severe dysplasia of cervix uteri (histologically confirmed) (D06.-)
severe dysplasia of vagina (histologically confirmed) (D07.2)

● R87.8 **Other abnormal findings in specimens from female genital organs**

● R87.81 **High risk human papillomavirus (HPV) DNA test positive from female genital organs**
Excludes1 anogenital warts due to human papillomavirus (HPV) (A63.0)
condyloma acuminatum (A63.0)

R87.810 **Cervical high risk human papillomavirus (HPV) DNA test positive ♀**

R87.811 **Vaginal high risk human papillomavirus (HPV) DNA test positive ♀**

● R87.82 **Low risk human papillomavirus (HPV) DNA test positive from female genital organs**
Use additional code for associated human papillomavirus (B97.7)

R87.820 **Cervical low risk human papillomavirus (HPV) DNA test positive ♀**

R87.821 **Vaginal low risk human papillomavirus (HPV) DNA test positive ♀**

R87.89 **Other abnormal findings in specimens from female genital organs ♀**
Abnormal chromosomal findings in specimens from female genital organs

R87.9 **Unspecified abnormal finding in specimens from female genital organs ♀**

● R88 **Abnormal findings in other body fluids and substances**

R88.0 **Cloudy (hemodialysis) (peritoneal) dialysis effluent**

R88.8 **Abnormal findings in other body fluids and substances**

● R89 **Abnormal findings in specimens from other organs, systems and tissues**
Includes abnormal findings in nipple discharge
abnormal findings in synovial fluid
abnormal findings in wound secretions

R89.0 **Abnormal level of enzymes in specimens from other organs, systems and tissues**

R89.1 **Abnormal level of hormones in specimens from other organs, systems and tissues**

R89.2 **Abnormal level of other drugs, medicaments and biological substances in specimens from other organs, systems and tissues**

R89.3 **Abnormal level of substances chiefly nonmedicinal as to source in specimens from other organs, systems and tissues**

R89.4 **Abnormal immunological findings in specimens from other organs, systems and tissues**

R89.5 **Abnormal microbiological findings in specimens from other organs, systems and tissues**
Positive culture findings in specimens from other organs, systems and tissues
Excludes1 colonization status (Z22.-)

R89.6 **Abnormal cytological findings in specimens from other organs, systems and tissues**

R89.7 **Abnormal histological findings in specimens from other organs, systems and tissues**

R89.8 **Other abnormal findings in specimens from other organs, systems and tissues**
Abnormal chromosomal findings in specimens from other organs, systems and tissues

R89.9 **Unspecified abnormal finding in specimens from other organs, systems and tissues**

ABNORMAL FINDINGS ON DIAGNOSTIC IMAGING AND IN FUNCTION STUDIES, WITHOUT DIAGNOSIS (R90-R94)

Includes nonspecific abnormal findings on diagnostic imaging by computerized axial tomography [CAT scan]
nonspecific abnormal findings on diagnostic imaging by magnetic resonance imaging [MRI][NMR]
nonspecific abnormal findings on diagnostic imaging by positron emission tomography [PET scan]
nonspecific abnormal findings on diagnostic imaging by thermography
nonspecific abnormal findings on diagnostic imaging by ultrasound [echogram]
nonspecific abnormal findings on diagnostic imaging by X-ray examination
Excludes1 abnormal findings on antenatal screening of mother (O28.-)
diagnostic abnormal findings classified elsewhere - see Alphabetical Index

● R90 **Abnormal findings on diagnostic imaging of central nervous system**

R90.0 **Intracranial space-occupying lesion found on diagnostic imaging of central nervous system**

● R90.8 **Other abnormal findings on diagnostic imaging of central nervous system**

R90.81 **Abnormal echoencephalogram**

R90.82 **White matter disease, unspecified**

R90.89 **Other abnormal findings on diagnostic imaging of central nervous system**
Other cerebrovascular abnormality found on diagnostic imaging of central nervous system

● **R91 Abnormal findings on diagnostic imaging of lung**

R91.1 Solitary pulmonary nodule
Coin lesion lung
Solitary pulmonary nodule, subsegmental branch of the bronchial tree

R91.8 Other nonspecific abnormal finding of lung field
Lung mass NOS found on diagnostic imaging of lung
Pulmonary infiltrate NOS
Shadow, lung

● **R92 Abnormal and inconclusive findings on diagnostic imaging of breast**

R92.Ø Mammographic microcalcification found on diagnostic imaging of breast
Excludes2 mammographic calcification (calculus) found on diagnostic imaging of breast (R92.1)

R92.1 Mammographic calcification found on diagnostic imaging of breast
Mammographic calculus found on diagnostic imaging of breast

R92.2 Inconclusive mammogram
Dense breasts NOS
Inconclusive mammogram NEC
Inconclusive mammography due to dense breasts
Inconclusive mammography NEC
Coding Clinic: 2Ø15, Q1, P24

R92.8 Other abnormal and inconclusive findings on diagnostic imaging of breast

● **R93 Abnormal findings on diagnostic imaging of other body structures**

R93.Ø Abnormal findings on diagnostic imaging of skull and head, not elsewhere classified
Excludes1 intracranial space-occupying lesion found on diagnostic imaging (R9Ø.Ø)

R93.1 Abnormal findings on diagnostic imaging of heart and coronary circulation
Abnormal echocardiogram NOS
Abnormal heart shadow

R93.2 Abnormal findings on diagnostic imaging of liver and biliary tract
Nonvisualization of gallbladder

R93.3 Abnormal findings on diagnostic imaging of other parts of digestive tract

● **R93.4 Abnormal findings on diagnostic imaging of urinary organs**
Excludes2 hypertrophy of kidney (N28.81)
Coding Clinic: 2Ø16, Q4, P66

R93.41 Abnormal radiologic findings on diagnostic imaging of renal pelvis, ureter, or bladder
Filling defect of bladder found on diagnostic imaging
Filling defect of renal pelvis found on diagnostic imaging
Filling defect of ureter found on diagnostic imaging

● **R93.42 Abnormal radiologic findings on diagnostic imaging of kidney**

R93.421 Abnormal radiologic findings on diagnostic imaging of right kidney

R93.422 Abnormal radiologic findings on diagnostic imaging of left kidney

R93.429 Abnormal radiologic findings on diagnostic imaging of unspecified kidney

R93.49 Abnormal radiologic findings on diagnostic imaging of other urinary organs

R93.5 Abnormal findings on diagnostic imaging of other abdominal regions, including retroperitoneum

R93.6 Abnormal findings on diagnostic imaging of limbs
Excludes2 abnormal finding in skin and subcutaneous tissue (R93.8-)

R93.7 Abnormal findings on diagnostic imaging of other parts of musculoskeletal system
Excludes2 abnormal findings on diagnostic imaging of skull (R93.Ø)

● **R93.8 Abnormal findings on diagnostic imaging of other specified body structures**

● **R93.81 Abnormal radiologic findings on diagnostic imaging of testis**

R93.811 Abnormal radiologic findings on diagnostic imaging of right testicle ♂

R93.812 Abnormal radiologic findings on diagnostic imaging of left testicle ♂

R93.813 Abnormal radiologic findings on diagnostic imaging of testicles, bilateral ♂

R93.819 Abnormal radiologic findings on diagnostic imaging of unspecified testicle ♂

R93.89 Abnormal findings on diagnostic imaging of other specified body structures
Abnormal finding by radioisotope localization of placenta
Abnormal radiological finding in skin and subcutaneous tissue
Mediastinal shift

R93.9 Diagnostic imaging inconclusive due to excess body fat of patient

● **R94 Abnormal results of function studies**
Includes abnormal results of radionuclide [radioisotope] uptake studies
abnormal results of scintigraphy

● **R94.Ø Abnormal results of function studies of central nervous system**

R94.Ø1 Abnormal electroencephalogram [EEG]

R94.Ø2 Abnormal brain scan

R94.Ø9 Abnormal results of other function studies of central nervous system

● **R94.1 Abnormal results of function studies of peripheral nervous system and special senses**

● **R94.11 Abnormal results of function studies of eye**

R94.11Ø Abnormal electro-oculogram [EOG]

R94.111 Abnormal electroretinogram [ERG]
Abnormal retinal function study

R94.112 Abnormal visually evoked potential [VEP]

R94.113 Abnormal oculomotor study

R94.118 Abnormal results of other function studies of eye

● **R94.12 Abnormal results of function studies of ear and other special senses**

R94.12Ø Abnormal auditory function study
Coding Clinic: 2Ø16, Q3, P17

R94.121 Abnormal vestibular function study

R94.128 Abnormal results of other function studies of ear and other special senses

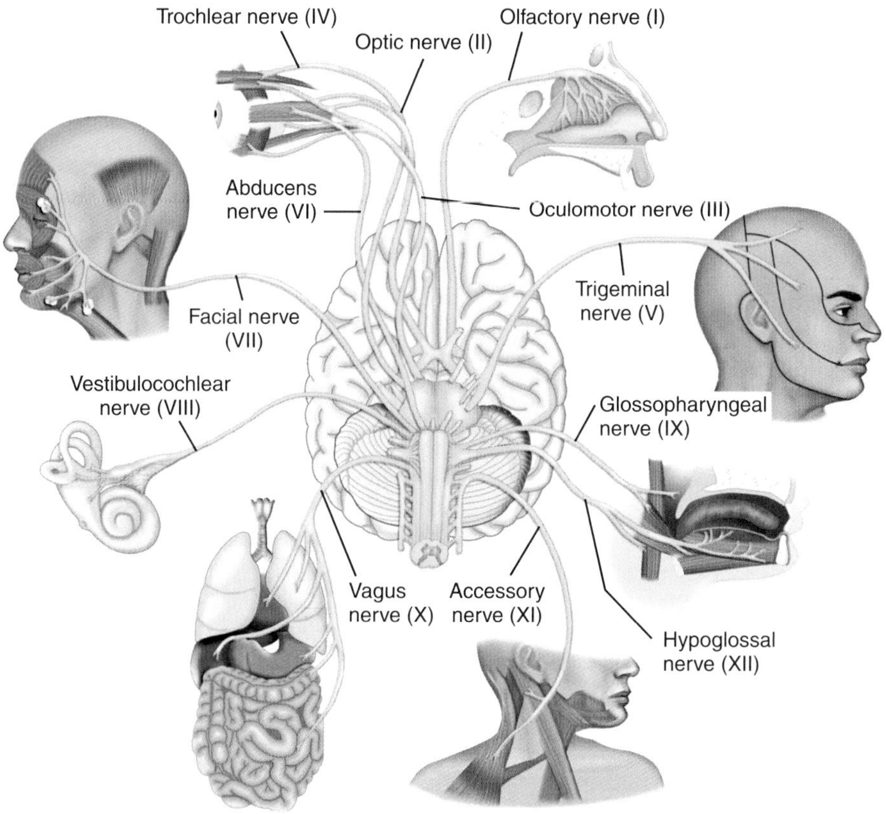

Figure 18-2 Cranial nerves. (From Patton and Thibodeau: Anatomy and physiology, ed 7, St. Louis, Mosby, 2009)

Item 18-1 The **peripheral nervous system** consists of 31 pairs of spinal nerves, 12 pairs of cranial nerves, and the autonomic nerves, which are divided into the parasympathetic and sympathetic nerves. The cranial nerves are: olfactory (I), optic (II), oculomotor (III), trochlear (IV), trigeminal (V), abducens (VI), facial (VII), vestibulocochlear (VIII), glossopharyngeal (IX), vagus (X), accessory (XI), and hypoglossal (XII).

● **R94.13 Abnormal results of function studies of peripheral nervous system**
- **R94.130 Abnormal response to nerve stimulation, unspecified**
- **R94.131 Abnormal electromyogram [EMG]**
  - **Excludes1** electromyogram of eye (R94.113)
- **R94.138 Abnormal results of other function studies of peripheral nervous system**

R94.2 Abnormal results of pulmonary function studies
Reduced ventilatory capacity
Reduced vital capacity

● **R94.3 Abnormal results of cardiovascular function studies**
- **R94.30 Abnormal result of cardiovascular function study, unspecified**
- **R94.31 Abnormal electrocardiogram [ECG] [EKG]**
  - **Excludes1** long QT syndrome (I45.81)
- **R94.39 Abnormal result of other cardiovascular function study**
  Abnormal electrophysiological intracardiac studies
  Abnormal phonocardiogram
  Abnormal vectorcardiogram

R94.4 Abnormal results of kidney function studies
Abnormal renal function test

R94.5 Abnormal results of liver function studies

R94.6 Abnormal results of thyroid function studies

R94.7 Abnormal results of other endocrine function studies
Excludes2 abnormal glucose (R73.Ø-)

R94.8 Abnormal results of function studies of other organs and systems
Abnormal basal metabolic rate [BMR]
Abnormal bladder function test
Abnormal splenic function test

ABNORMAL TUMOR MARKERS (R97)

● **R97 Abnormal tumor markers**
Elevated tumor associated antigens [TAA]
Elevated tumor specific antigens [TSA]
- **R97.Ø Elevated carcinoembryonic antigen [CEA]**
- **R97.1 Elevated cancer antigen 125 [CA 125]**
- ● **R97.2 Elevated prostate specific antigen [PSA]**
  Coding Clinic: 2016, Q4, P66
  - **R97.2Ø Elevated prostate specific antigen [PSA]** ♂ A
  - **R97.21 Rising PSA following treatment for malignant neoplasm of prostate** ♂ A
- **R97.8 Other abnormal tumor markers**

ILL-DEFINED AND UNKNOWN CAUSE OF MORTALITY (R99)

R99 Ill-defined and unknown cause of mortality
Death (unexplained) NOS
Unspecified cause of mortality

OGCR Section I.C.18.h.

Death NOS

Code R99, Ill-defined and unknown cause of mortality, is only for use in the very limited circumstance when a patient who has already died is brought into the emergency department or other healthcare facility and is pronounced dead upon arrival. It does not represent the discharge disposition of death.

CHAPTER 19

INJURY, POISONING AND CERTAIN OTHER CONSEQUENCES OF EXTERNAL CAUSES (SØØ-T88)

OGCR Chapter-Specific Coding Guidelines

19. Chapter 19: Injury, poisoning, and certain other consequences of external causes (SØØ-T88)

a. Application of 7th Characters in Chapter 19

Most categories in Chapter 19 have a 7th character requirement for each applicable code. Most categories in this chapter have three 7th character values (with the exception of fractures): A, initial encounter, D, subsequent encounter and S, sequela. Categories for traumatic fractures have additional 7th character values. While the patient may be seen by a new or different provider over the course of treatment for an injury, assignment of the 7th character is based on whether the patient is undergoing active treatment and not whether the provider is seeing the patient for the first time.

For complication codes, active treatment refers to treatment for the condition described by the code, even though it may be related to an earlier precipitating problem. For example, code T84.50XA, Infection and inflammatory reaction due to unspecified internal joint prosthesis, initial encounter, is used when active treatment is provided for the infection, even though the condition relates to the prosthetic device, implant or graft that was placed at a previous encounter.

7th character "A", initial encounter is used for each encounter where the patient is receiving active treatment for the condition.

7th character "D" subsequent encounter is used for encounters after the patient has completed active treatment of the condition and is receiving routine care for the condition during the healing or recovery phase.

The aftercare Z codes should not be used for aftercare for conditions such as injuries or poisonings, where 7th characters are provided to identify subsequent care. For example, for aftercare of an injury, assign the acute injury code with the 7th character "D" (subsequent encounter).

7th character "S", sequela, is for use for complications or conditions that arise as a direct result of a condition, such as scar formation after a burn. The scars are sequelae of the burn. When using 7th character "S", it is necessary to use both the injury code that precipitated the sequela and the code for the sequela itself. The "S" is added only to the injury code, not the sequela code. The 7th character "S" identifies the injury responsible for the sequela. The specific type of sequela (e.g. scar) is sequenced first, followed by the injury code.

See Section I.B.1Ø. Sequelae, (Late Effects).

b. Coding of Injuries

When coding injuries, assign separate codes for each injury unless a combination code is provided, in which case the combination code is assigned. Codes from category TØ7, Unspecified multiple injuries should not be assigned in the inpatient setting unless information for a more specific code is not available. Traumatic injury codes (SØØ-T14.9) are not to be used for normal, healing surgical wounds or to identify complications of surgical wounds.

The code for the most serious injury, as determined by the provider and the focus of treatment, is sequenced first.

1) Superficial injuries

Superficial injuries such as abrasions or contusions are not coded when associated with more severe injuries of the same site.

2) Primary injury with damage to nerves/blood vessels

When a primary injury results in minor damage to peripheral nerves or blood vessels, the primary injury is sequenced first with additional code(s) for injuries to nerves and spinal cord (such as category SØ4), and/or injury to blood vessels (such as category S15). When the primary injury is to the blood vessels or nerves, that injury should be sequenced first.

c. Coding of Traumatic Fractures

The principles of multiple coding of injuries should be followed in coding fractures. Fractures of specified sites are coded individually by site in accordance with both the provisions within categories SØ2, S12, S22, S32, S42, S49, S52, S59, S62, S72, S79, S82, S89, S92 and the level of detail furnished by medical record content.

A fracture not indicated as open or closed should be coded to closed. A fracture not indicated whether displaced or not displaced should be coded to displaced.

More specific guidelines are as follows:

1) Initial vs. Subsequent Encounter for Fractures

Traumatic fractures are coded using the appropriate 7th character for initial encounter (A, B, C) for each encounter where the patient is receiving active treatment for the fracture. The appropriate 7th character for initial encounter should also be assigned for a patient who delayed seeking treatment for the fracture or nonunion.

Fractures are coded using the appropriate 7th character for subsequent care for encounters after the patient has completed active treatment of the fracture and is receiving routine care for the fracture during the healing or recovery phase.

Care for complications of surgical treatment for fracture repairs during the healing or recovery phase should be coded with the appropriate complication codes.

Care of complications of fractures, such as malunion and nonunion, should be reported with the appropriate 7th character for subsequent care with nonunion (K, M, N,) or subsequent care with malunion (P, Q, R).

Malunion/nonunion: The appropriate 7th character for initial encounter should also be assigned for a patient who delayed seeking treatment for the fracture or nonunion.

The open fracture designations in the assignment of the 7th character for fractures of the forearm, femur and lower leg, including ankle are based on the Gustilo open fracture classification. When the Gustilo classification type is not specified for an open fracture, the 7th character for open fracture type I or II should be assigned (B, E, H, M, Q).

A code from category M8Ø, not a traumatic fracture code, should be used for any patient with known osteoporosis who suffers a fracture, even if the patient had a minor fall or trauma, if that fall or trauma would not usually break a normal, healthy bone.

See Section I.C.13. Osteoporosis.

The aftercare Z codes should not be used for aftercare for traumatic fractures. For aftercare of a traumatic fracture, assign the acute fracture code with the appropriate 7th character.

2) Multiple fractures sequencing

Multiple fractures are sequenced in accordance with the severity of the fracture.

d. Coding of Burns and Corrosions

The ICD-10-CM makes a distinction between burns and corrosions. The burn codes are for thermal burns, except sunburns, that come from a heat source, such as a fire or hot appliance. The burn codes are also for burns resulting from electricity and radiation. Corrosions are burns due to chemicals. The guidelines are the same for burns and corrosions.

Current burns (T2Ø-T25) are classified by depth, extent and by agent (X code). Burns are classified by depth as first degree (erythema), second degree (blistering), and third degree (full-thickness involvement). Burns of the eye and internal organs (T26-T28) are classified by site, but not by degree.

1) Sequencing of burn and related condition codes

Sequence first the code that reflects the highest degree of burn when more than one burn is present.

a. When the reason for the admission or encounter is for treatment of external multiple burns, sequence first the code that reflects the burn of the highest degree.

b. When a patient has both internal and external burns, the circumstances of admission govern the selection of the principal diagnosis or first-listed diagnosis.

c. When a patient is admitted for burn injuries and other related conditions such as smoke inhalation and/or respiratory failure, the circumstances of admission govern the selection of the principal or first-listed diagnosis.

2) Burns of the same *anatomic* site
Classify burns of the same anatomic site and on the same side but of different degrees to the subcategory identifying the highest degree recorded in the diagnosis (e.g., for second- and third-degree burns of right thigh, assign only code T24.311-).

3) Non-healing burns
Non-healing burns are coded as acute burns.
Necrosis of burned skin should be coded as a non-healed burn.

4) Infected Burn
For any documented infected burn site, use an additional code for the infection.

5) Assign separate codes for each burn site
When coding burns, assign separate codes for each burn site. Category T30, Burn and corrosion, body region unspecified is extremely vague and should rarely be used.
Codes for burns of "multiple sites" should only be assigned when the medical record documentation does not specify the individual sites.

6) Burns and Corrosions Classified According to Extent of Body Surface Involved
Assign codes from category T31, Burns classified according to extent of body surface involved, or T32, Corrosions classified according to extent of body surface involved, when the site of the burn is not specified or when there is a need for additional data. It is advisable to use category T31 as additional coding when needed to provide data for evaluating burn mortality, such as that needed by burn units. It is also advisable to use category T31 as an additional code for reporting purposes when there is mention of a third-degree burn involving 20 percent or more of the body surface.
Categories T31 and T32 are based on the classic "rule of nines" in estimating body surface involved: head and neck are assigned nine percent, each arm nine percent, each leg 18 percent, the anterior trunk 18 percent, posterior trunk 18 percent, and genitalia one percent. Providers may change these percentage assignments where necessary to accommodate infants and children who have proportionately larger heads than adults, and patients who have large buttocks, thighs, or abdomen that involve burns.

7) Encounters for treatment of sequela of burns
Encounters for the treatment of the late effects of burns or corrosions (i.e., scars or joint contractures) should be coded with a burn or corrosion code with the 7th character "S" for sequela.

8) Sequelae with a late effect code and current burn
When appropriate, both a code for a current burn or corrosion with 7th character "A" or "D" and a burn or corrosion code with 7th character "S" may be assigned on the same record (when both a current burn and sequelae of an old burn exist). Burns and corrosions do not heal at the same rate and a current healing wound may still exist with sequela of a healed burn or corrosion.
See Section I.B.10. Sequela, (Late Effects).

9) Use of an external cause code with burns and corrosions
An external cause code should be used with burns and corrosions to identify the source and intent of the burn, as well as the place where it occurred.

e. Adverse Effects, Poisoning , Underdosing and Toxic Effects
Codes in categories T36-T65 are combination codes that include the substance that was taken as well as the intent. No additional external cause code is required for poisonings, toxic effects, adverse effects and underdosing codes.

1) Do not code directly from the Table of Drugs
Do not code directly from the Table of Drugs and Chemicals. Always refer back to the Tabular List.

2) Use as many codes as necessary to describe
Use as many codes as necessary to describe completely all drugs, medicinal or biological substances.

3) If the same code would describe the causative agent
If the same code would describe the causative agent for more than one adverse reaction, poisoning, toxic effect or underdosing, assign the code only once.

4) If two or more drugs, medicinal or biological substances
If two or more drugs, medicinal or biological substances are reported, code each individually unless a combination code is listed in the Table of Drugs and Chemicals.

5) The occurrence of drug toxicity is classified in ICD-10-CM as follows:

(a) Adverse Effect
When coding an adverse effect of a drug that has been correctly prescribed and properly administered, assign the appropriate code for the nature of the adverse effect followed by the appropriate code for the adverse effect of the drug (T36-T50). The code for the drug should have a 5th or 6th character "5" (for example T36.0X5-) Examples of the nature of an adverse effect are tachycardia, delirium, gastrointestinal hemorrhaging, vomiting, hypokalemia, hepatitis, renal failure, or respiratory failure.

(b) Poisoning
When coding a poisoning or reaction to the improper use of a medication (e.g., overdose, wrong substance given or taken in error, wrong route of administration), first assign the appropriate code from categories T36-T50. The poisoning codes have an associated intent as their 5th or 6th character (accidental, intentional self-harm, assault and undetermined). If the intent of the poisoning is unknown or unspecified, code the intent as accidental intent. The undetermined intent is only for use if the documentation in the record specifies that the intent cannot be determined. Use additional code(s) for all manifestations of poisonings.
If there is also a diagnosis of abuse or dependence of the substance, the abuse or dependence is assigned as an additional code.
Examples of poisoning include:

(i) Error was made in drug prescription
Errors made in drug prescription or in the administration of the drug by provider, nurse, patient, or other person.

(ii) Overdose of a drug intentionally taken If an overdose of a drug was intentionally taken or administered and resulted in drug toxicity, it would be coded as a poisoning.

(iii) Nonprescribed drug taken with correctly prescribed and properly administered drug. If a nonprescribed drug or medicinal agent was taken in combination with a correctly prescribed and properly administered drug, any drug toxicity or other reaction resulting from the interaction of the two drugs would be classified as a poisoning.

(iv) Interaction of drug(s) and alcohol. When a reaction results from the interaction of a drug(s) and alcohol, this would be classified as poisoning.
See Section I.C.4. if poisoning is the result of insulin pump malfunctions.

(c) Underdosing
Underdosing refers to taking less of a medication than is prescribed by a provider or a manufacturer's instruction. Discontinuing the use of a prescribed medication on the patient's own initiative (not directed by the patient's provider) is also classified as an underdosing. For underdosing, assign the code from categories T36-T50 (fifth or sixth character "6").

CHAPTER 19 (S00-T88)

Codes for underdosing should never be assigned as principal or first-listed codes. If a patient has a relapse or exacerbation of the medical condition for which the drug is prescribed because of the reduction in dose, then the medical condition itself should be coded.

Noncompliance (Z91.12-, Z91.13- and Z91.14-) or complication of care (Y63.6-Y63.9) codes are to be used with an underdosing code to indicate intent, if known.

(d) Toxic Effects

When a harmful substance is ingested or comes in contact with a person, this is classified as a toxic effect. The toxic effect codes are in categories T51-T65.

Toxic effect codes have an associated intent: accidental, intentional self-harm, assault and undetermined.

f. Adult and child abuse, neglect and other maltreatment

Sequence first the appropriate code from categories T74 (Adult and child abuse, neglect and other maltreatment, confirmed) or T76 (Adult and child abuse, neglect and other maltreatment, suspected) for abuse, neglect and other maltreatment, followed by any accompanying mental health or injury code(s).

If the documentation in the medical record states abuse or neglect it is coded as confirmed (T74.-). It is coded as suspected if it is documented as suspected (T76.-).

For cases of confirmed abuse or neglect an external cause code from the assault section (X92-Y09) should be added to identify the cause of any physical injuries. A perpetrator code (Y07) should be added when the perpetrator of the abuse is known. For suspected cases of abuse or neglect, do not report external cause or perpetrator code.

If a suspected case of abuse, neglect or mistreatment is ruled out during an encounter code Z04.71, Encounter for examination and observation following alleged physical adult abuse, ruled out, or code Z04.72, Encounter for examination and observation following alleged child physical abuse, ruled out, should be used, not a code from T76.

If a suspected case of alleged rape or sexual abuse is ruled out during an encounter code Z04.41, Encounter for examination and observation following alleged adult rape or code Z04.42, Encounter for examination and observation following alleged child rape, should be used, not a code from T76.

If a suspected case of forced sexual exploitation or forced labor exploitation is ruled out during an encounter, code Z04.81, Encounter for examination and observation of victim following forced sexual exploitation, or code Z04.82, Encounter for examination and observation of victim following forced labor exploitation, should be used, not a code from T76.

See Section I.C.15. Abuse in a pregnant patient.

g. Complications of care

1) General guidelines for complications of care

(a) Documentation of complications of care

See Section I.B.16. for information on documentation of complications of care.

2) Pain due to medical devices

Pain associated with devices, implants or grafts left in a surgical site (for example painful hip prosthesis) is assigned to the appropriate code(s) found in Chapter 19, Injury, poisoning, and certain other consequences of external causes. Specific codes for pain due to medical devices are found in the T code section of the ICD-10-CM. Use additional code(s) from category G89 to identify acute or chronic pain due to presence of the device, implant or graft (G89.18 or G89.28).

3) Transplant complications

(a) Transplant complications other than kidney

Codes under category T86, Complications of transplanted organs and tissues, are for use for both complications and rejection of transplanted organs. A transplant complication code is only assigned if the complication affects the function of the transplanted organ. Two codes are required to fully describe a transplant complication: the appropriate code from category T86 and a secondary code that identifies the complication.

Pre-existing conditions or conditions that develop after the transplant are not coded as complications unless they affect the function of the transplanted organs.

See I.C.21. for transplant organ removal status.

See I.C.2. for malignant neoplasm associated with transplanted organ.

(b) Kidney transplant complications

Patients who have undergone kidney transplant may still have some form of chronic kidney disease (CKD) because the kidney transplant may not fully restore kidney function. Code T86.1- should be assigned for documented complications of a kidney transplant, such as transplant failure or rejection or other transplant complication. Code T86.1- should not be assigned for post kidney transplant patients who have chronic kidney (CKD) unless a transplant complication such as transplant failure or rejection is documented. If the documentation is unclear as to whether the patient has a complication of the transplant, query the provider.

Conditions that affect the function of the transplanted kidney, other than CKD, should be assigned a code from subcategory T86.1, Complications of transplanted organ, Kidney, and a secondary code that identifies the complication.

For patients with CKD following a kidney transplant, but who do not have a complication such as failure or rejection, *see Section I.C.14. Chronic kidney disease and kidney transplant status.*

4) Complication codes that include the external cause

As with certain other T codes, some of the complications of care codes have the external cause included in the code. The code includes the nature of the complication as well as the type of procedure that caused the complication. No external cause code indicating the type of procedure is necessary for these codes.

5) Complications of care codes within the body system chapters

Intraoperative and postprocedural complication codes are found within the body system chapters with codes specific to the organs and structures of that body system. These codes should be sequenced first, followed by a code(s) for the specific complication, if applicable.

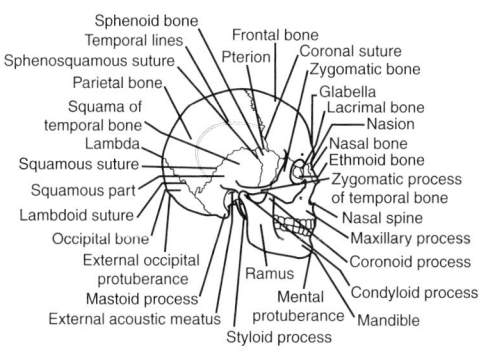

Figure 19-1 Lateral view of skull.

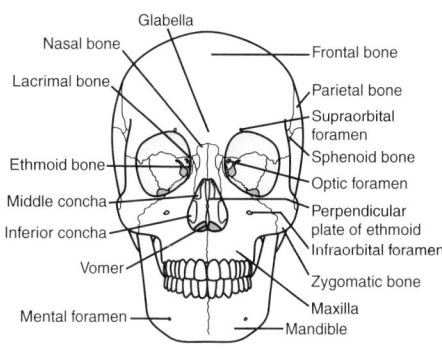

Figure 19-2 Frontal view of skull.

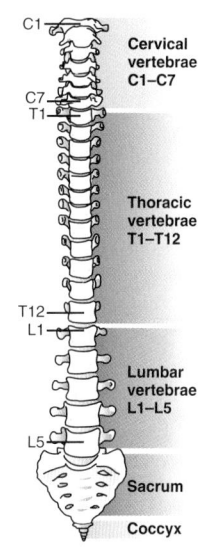

Figure 19-3 Anterior view of vertebral column.

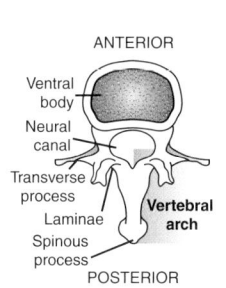

Figure 19-4 Vertebra viewed from above.

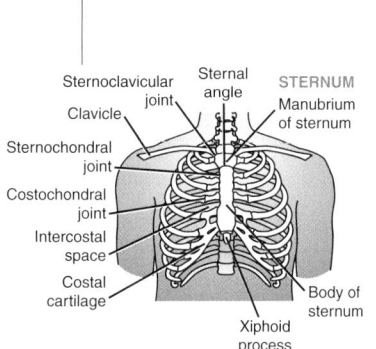

Figure 19-5 Anterior view of rib cage.

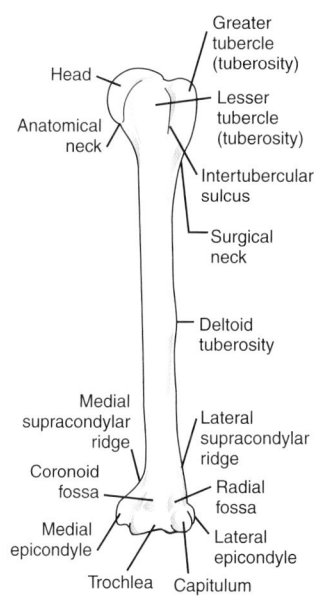

Figure 19-6 Anterior aspect of left humerus.

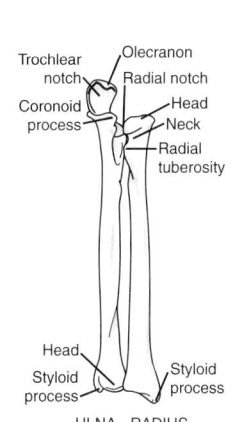

Figure 19-7 Anterior aspect of left radius and ulna.

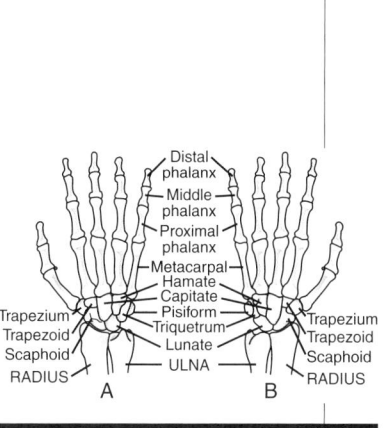

Figure 19-8 Right hand and wrist: **A.** Dorsal surface. **B.** Palmar surface.

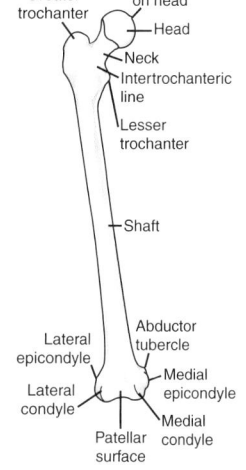

Figure 19-9 Anterior aspect of right femur.

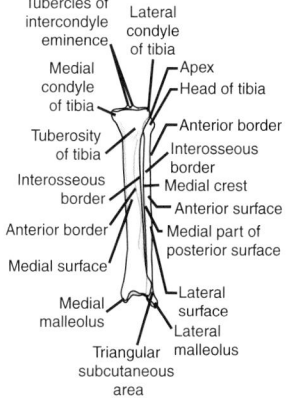

Figure 19-10 Anterior aspect of left tibia and fibula.

CHAPTER 19 (S00-T88)

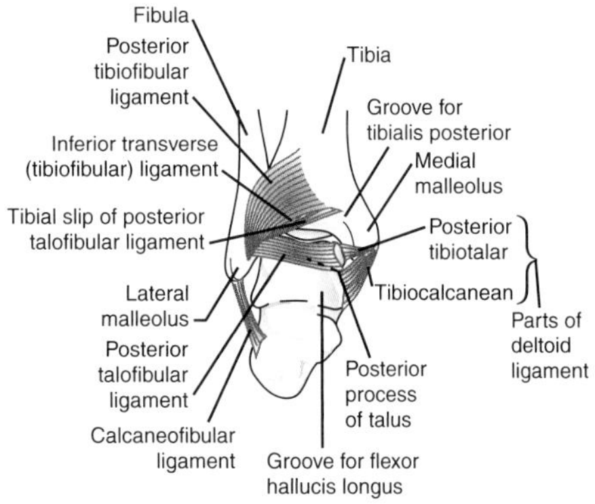

Figure 19-11 Posterior aspect of the left ankle joint.

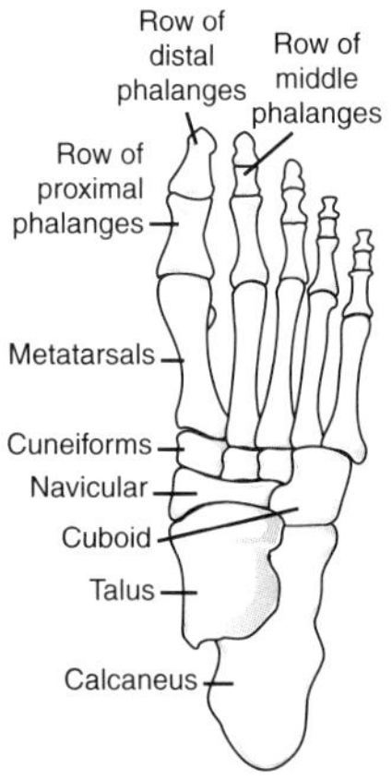

Figure 19-12 Right foot viewed from above.

CHAPTER 19

INJURY, POISONING AND CERTAIN OTHER CONSEQUENCES OF EXTERNAL CAUSES (SØØ-T88)

Note: Use secondary code(s) from Chapter 2Ø, External causes of morbidity, to indicate cause of injury. Codes within the T section that include the external cause do not require an additional external cause code.

Use additional code to identify any retained foreign body, if applicable (Z18.-)

Excludes1 birth trauma (P1Ø-P15)
obstetric trauma (O7Ø-O71)

Note: The chapter uses the S-section for coding different types of injuries related to single body regions and the T-section to cover injuries to unspecified body regions as well as poisoning and certain other consequences of external causes.

This chapter contains the following blocks:

SØØ-SØ9	Injuries to the head
S1Ø-S19	Injuries to the neck
S2Ø-S29	Injuries to the thorax
S3Ø-S39	Injuries to the abdomen, lower back, lumbar spine, pelvis and external genitals
S4Ø-S49	Injuries to the shoulder and upper arm
S5Ø-S59	Injuries to the elbow and forearm
S6Ø-S69	Injuries to the wrist, hand, and fingers
S7Ø-S79	Injuries to the hip and thigh
S8Ø-S89	Injuries to the knee and lower leg
S9Ø-S99	Injuries to the ankle and foot
TØ7	Injuries involving multiple body regions
T14	Injury of unspecified body region
T15-T19	Effects of foreign body entering through natural orifice
T2Ø-T25	Burns and corrosions of external body surface, specified by site
T26-T28	Burns and corrosions confined to eye and internal organs
T3Ø-T32	Burns and corrosions of multiple and unspecified body regions
T33-T34	Frostbite
T36-T5Ø	Poisoning by, adverse effect of and underdosing of drugs, medicaments and biological substances
T51-T65	Toxic effects of substances chiefly nonmedicinal as to source
T66-T78	Other and unspecified effects of external causes
T79	Certain early complications of trauma
T8Ø-T88	Complications of surgical and medical care, not elsewhere classified

INJURIES TO THE HEAD (SØØ-SØ9)

Includes injuries of ear
injuries of eye
injuries of face [any part]
injuries of gum
injuries of jaw
injuries of oral cavity
injuries of palate
injuries of periocular area
injuries of scalp
injuries of temporomandibular joint area
injuries of tongue
injuries of tooth

Code also for any associated infection

Excludes2 burns and corrosions (T2Ø-T32)
effects of foreign body in ear (T16)
effects of foreign body in larynx (T17.3)
effects of foreign body in mouth NOS (T18.Ø)
effects of foreign body in nose (T17.Ø-T17.1)
effects of foreign body in pharynx (T17.2)
effects of foreign body on external eye (T15.-)
frostbite (T33-T34)
insect bite or sting, venomous (T63.4)

● SØØ Superficial injury of head

Excludes1 diffuse cerebral contusion (SØ6.2-)
focal cerebral contusion (SØ6.3-)
injury of eye and orbit (SØ5.-)
open wound of head (SØ1.-)

The appropriate 7th character is to be added to each code from category SØØ

A	initial encounter *All encounters involving diagnosis and treatment*
D	subsequent encounter *Encounters during the healing phase*
S	sequela

● SØØ.Ø Superficial injury of scalp

X● **SØØ.ØØ Unspecified superficial injury of scalp**

X● **SØØ.Ø1 Abrasion of scalp**

X● **SØØ.Ø2 Blister (nonthermal) of scalp**

X● **SØØ.Ø3 Contusion of scalp**
Bruise of scalp
Hematoma of scalp

X● **SØØ.Ø4 External constriction of part of scalp**

X● **SØØ.Ø5 Superficial foreign body of scalp**
Splinter in the scalp

X● **SØØ.Ø6 Insect bite (nonvenomous) of scalp**

X● **SØØ.Ø7 Other superficial bite of scalp**
Excludes1 open bite of scalp (SØ1.Ø5)

- ● **S00.1** Contusion of eyelid and periocular area
  Black eye
  Excludes2 contusion of eyeball and orbital tissues (S05.1)
  - X● **S00.10** Contusion of unspecified eyelid and periocular area
  - X● **S00.11** Contusion of right eyelid and periocular area
  - X● **S00.12** Contusion of left eyelid and periocular area
- ● **S00.2** Other and unspecified superficial injuries of eyelid and periocular area
  Excludes2 superficial injury of conjunctiva and cornea (S05.0-)
  - ● **S00.20** Unspecified superficial injury of eyelid and periocular area
    - ● **S00.201** Unspecified superficial injury of right eyelid and periocular area
    - ● **S00.202** Unspecified superficial injury of left eyelid and periocular area
    - ● **S00.209** Unspecified superficial injury of unspecified eyelid and periocular area
  - ● **S00.21** Abrasion of eyelid and periocular area
    - ● **S00.211** Abrasion of right eyelid and periocular area
    - ● **S00.212** Abrasion of left eyelid and periocular area
    - ● **S00.219** Abrasion of unspecified eyelid and periocular area
  - ● **S00.22** Blister (nonthermal) of eyelid and periocular area
    - ● **S00.221** Blister (nonthermal) of right eyelid and periocular area
    - ● **S00.222** Blister (nonthermal) of left eyelid and periocular area
    - ● **S00.229** Blister (nonthermal) of unspecified eyelid and periocular area
  - ● **S00.24** External constriction of eyelid and periocular area
    - ● **S00.241** External constriction of right eyelid and periocular area
    - ● **S00.242** External constriction of left eyelid and periocular area
    - ● **S00.249** External constriction of unspecified eyelid and periocular area
  - ● **S00.25** Superficial foreign body of eyelid and periocular area
    Splinter of eyelid and periocular area
    Excludes2 retained foreign body in eyelid (H02.81-)
    - ● **S00.251** Superficial foreign body of right eyelid and periocular area
    - ● **S00.252** Superficial foreign body of left eyelid and periocular area
    - ● **S00.259** Superficial foreign body of unspecified eyelid and periocular area
  - ● **S00.26** Insect bite (nonvenomous) of eyelid and periocular area
    - ● **S00.261** Insect bite (nonvenomous) of right eyelid and periocular area
    - ● **S00.262** Insect bite (nonvenomous) of left eyelid and periocular area
    - ● **S00.269** Insect bite (nonvenomous) of unspecified eyelid and periocular area
  - ● **S00.27** Other superficial bite of eyelid and periocular area
    Excludes1 open bite of eyelid and periocular area (S01.15)
    - ● **S00.271** Other superficial bite of right eyelid and periocular area
    - ● **S00.272** Other superficial bite of left eyelid and periocular area
    - ● **S00.279** Other superficial bite of unspecified eyelid and periocular area
- ● **S00.3** Superficial injury of nose
  - X● **S00.30** Unspecified superficial injury of nose
  - X● **S00.31** Abrasion of nose
  - X● **S00.32** Blister (nonthermal) of nose
  - X● **S00.33** Contusion of nose
    Bruise of nose
    Hematoma of nose
  - X● **S00.34** External constriction of nose
  - X● **S00.35** Superficial foreign body of nose
    Splinter in the nose
  - X● **S00.36** Insect bite (nonvenomous) of nose
  - X● **S00.37** Other superficial bite of nose
    Excludes1 open bite of nose (S01.25)
- ● **S00.4** Superficial injury of ear
  - ● **S00.40** Unspecified superficial injury of ear
    - ● **S00.401** Unspecified superficial injury of right ear
    - ● **S00.402** Unspecified superficial injury of left ear
    - ● **S00.409** Unspecified superficial injury of unspecified ear
  - ● **S00.41** Abrasion of ear
    - ● **S00.411** Abrasion of right ear
    - ● **S00.412** Abrasion of left ear
    - ● **S00.419** Abrasion of unspecified ear
  - ● **S00.42** Blister (nonthermal) of ear
    - ● **S00.421** Blister (nonthermal) of right ear
    - ● **S00.422** Blister (nonthermal) of left ear
    - ● **S00.429** Blister (nonthermal) of unspecified ear
  - ● **S00.43** Contusion of ear
    Bruise of ear
    Hematoma of ear
    - ● **S00.431** Contusion of right ear
    - ● **S00.432** Contusion of left ear
    - ● **S00.439** Contusion of unspecified ear
  - ● **S00.44** External constriction of ear
    - ● **S00.441** External constriction of right ear
    - ● **S00.442** External constriction of left ear
    - ● **S00.449** External constriction of unspecified ear
  - ● **S00.45** Superficial foreign body of ear
    Splinter in the ear
    - ● **S00.451** Superficial foreign body of right ear
    - ● **S00.452** Superficial foreign body of left ear
    - ● **S00.459** Superficial foreign body of unspecified ear
  - ● **S00.46** Insect bite (nonvenomous) of ear
    - ● **S00.461** Insect bite (nonvenomous) of right ear
    - ● **S00.462** Insect bite (nonvenomous) of left ear
    - ● **S00.469** Insect bite (nonvenomous) of unspecified ear

S00.47 Other superficial bite of ear
Excludes1 open bite of ear (S01.35)
S00.471 Other superficial bite of right ear
S00.472 Other superficial bite of left ear
S00.479 Other superficial bite of unspecified ear

S00.5 Superficial injury of lip and oral cavity
S00.50 Unspecified superficial injury of lip and oral cavity
S00.501 Unspecified superficial injury of lip
S00.502 Unspecified superficial injury of oral cavity
S00.51 Abrasion of lip and oral cavity
S00.511 Abrasion of lip
S00.512 Abrasion of oral cavity
S00.52 Blister (nonthermal) of lip and oral cavity
S00.521 Blister (nonthermal) of lip
S00.522 Blister (nonthermal) of oral cavity
S00.53 Contusion of lip and oral cavity
S00.531 Contusion of lip
Bruise of lip
Hematoma of lip
S00.532 Contusion of oral cavity
Bruise of oral cavity
Hematoma of oral cavity
S00.54 External constriction of lip and oral cavity
S00.541 External constriction of lip
S00.542 External constriction of oral cavity
S00.55 Superficial foreign body of lip and oral cavity
S00.551 Superficial foreign body of lip
Splinter of lip and oral cavity
S00.552 Superficial foreign body of oral cavity
Splinter of lip and oral cavity
S00.56 Insect bite (nonvenomous) of lip and oral cavity
S00.561 Insect bite (nonvenomous) of lip
S00.562 Insect bite (nonvenomous) of oral cavity
S00.57 Other superficial bite of lip and oral cavity
S00.571 Other superficial bite of lip
Excludes1 open bite of lip (S01.551)
S00.572 Other superficial bite of oral cavity
Excludes1 open bite of oral cavity (S01.552)

S00.8 Superficial injury of other parts of head
Superficial injuries of face [any part]
X S00.80 Unspecified superficial injury of other part of head
X S00.81 Abrasion of other part of head
X S00.82 Blister (nonthermal) of other part of head
X S00.83 Contusion of other part of head
Bruise of other part of head
Hematoma of other part of head
X S00.84 External constriction of other part of head
X S00.85 Superficial foreign body of other part of head
Splinter in other part of head
X S00.86 Insect bite (nonvenomous) of other part of head
X S00.87 Other superficial bite of other part of head
Excludes1 open bite of other part of head (S01.85)

S00.9 Superficial injury of unspecified part of head
X S00.90 Unspecified superficial injury of unspecified part of head
X S00.91 Abrasion of unspecified part of head
X S00.92 Blister (nonthermal) of unspecified part of head
X S00.93 Contusion of unspecified part of head
Bruise of head
Hematoma of head
X S00.94 External constriction of unspecified part of head
X S00.95 Superficial foreign body of unspecified part of head
Splinter of head
X S00.96 Insect bite (nonvenomous) of unspecified part of head
X S00.97 Other superficial bite of unspecified part of head
Excludes1 open bite of head (S01.95)

S01 Open wound of head
Code also any associated:
injury of cranial nerve (S04.-)
injury of muscle and tendon of head (S09.1-)
intracranial injury (S06.-)
wound infection
Excludes1 open skull fracture (S02.- with 7th character B)
Excludes2 injury of eye and orbit (S05.-)
traumatic amputation of part of head (S08.-)

The appropriate 7th character is to be added to each code from category S01

A	initial encounter
D	subsequent encounter
S	sequela

S01.0 Open wound of scalp
Excludes1 avulsion of scalp (S08.0)
X S01.00 Unspecified open wound of scalp
X S01.01 Laceration without foreign body of scalp
X S01.02 Laceration with foreign body of scalp
Coding Clinic: 2015, Q1, P5-7
X S01.03 Puncture wound without foreign body of scalp
X S01.04 Puncture wound with foreign body of scalp
X S01.05 Open bite of scalp
Bite of scalp NOS
Excludes1 superficial bite of scalp (S00.06, S00.07-)

S01.1 Open wound of eyelid and periocular area
Open wound of eyelid and periocular area with or without involvement of lacrimal passages
S01.10 Unspecified open wound of eyelid and periocular area
S01.101 Unspecified open wound of right eyelid and periocular area
S01.102 Unspecified open wound of left eyelid and periocular area
S01.109 Unspecified open wound of unspecified eyelid and periocular area
S01.11 Laceration without foreign body of eyelid and periocular area
S01.111 Laceration without foreign body of right eyelid and periocular area
S01.112 Laceration without foreign body of left eyelid and periocular area
S01.119 Laceration without foreign body of unspecified eyelid and periocular area
S01.12 Laceration with foreign body of eyelid and periocular area
S01.121 Laceration with foreign body of right eyelid and periocular area
S01.122 Laceration with foreign body of left eyelid and periocular area
S01.129 Laceration with foreign body of unspecified eyelid and periocular area

S01.13 Puncture wound without foreign body of eyelid and periocular area
- S01.131 Puncture wound without foreign body of right eyelid and periocular area
- S01.132 Puncture wound without foreign body of left eyelid and periocular area
- S01.139 Puncture wound without foreign body of unspecified eyelid and periocular area

S01.14 Puncture wound with foreign body of eyelid and periocular area
- S01.141 Puncture wound with foreign body of right eyelid and periocular area
- S01.142 Puncture wound with foreign body of left eyelid and periocular area
- S01.149 Puncture wound with foreign body of unspecified eyelid and periocular area

S01.15 Open bite of eyelid and periocular area
Bite of eyelid and periocular area NOS
Excludes1 superficial bite of eyelid and periocular area (S00.26, S00.27)
- S01.151 Open bite of right eyelid and periocular area
- S01.152 Open bite of left eyelid and periocular area
- S01.159 Open bite of unspecified eyelid and periocular area

S01.2 Open wound of nose
- X S01.20 Unspecified open wound of nose
- X S01.21 Laceration without foreign body of nose
  Coding Clinic: 2015, Q1, P5-6
- X S01.22 Laceration with foreign body of nose
- X S01.23 Puncture wound without foreign body of nose
- X S01.24 Puncture wound with foreign body of nose
- X S01.25 Open bite of nose
  Bite of nose NOS
  Excludes1 superficial bite of nose (S00.36, S00.37)

S01.3 Open wound of ear

S01.30 Unspecified open wound of ear
- S01.301 Unspecified open wound of right ear
- S01.302 Unspecified open wound of left ear
- S01.309 Unspecified open wound of unspecified ear

S01.31 Laceration without foreign body of ear
- S01.311 Laceration without foreign body of right ear
- S01.312 Laceration without foreign body of left ear
- S01.319 Laceration without foreign body of unspecified ear

S01.32 Laceration with foreign body of ear
- S01.321 Laceration with foreign body of right ear
- S01.322 Laceration with foreign body of left ear
- S01.329 Laceration with foreign body of unspecified ear

S01.33 Puncture wound without foreign body of ear
- S01.331 Puncture wound without foreign body of right ear
- S01.332 Puncture wound without foreign body of left ear
- S01.339 Puncture wound without foreign body of unspecified ear

S01.34 Puncture wound with foreign body of ear
- S01.341 Puncture wound with foreign body of right ear
- S01.342 Puncture wound with foreign body of left ear
- S01.349 Puncture wound with foreign body of unspecified ear

S01.35 Open bite of ear
Bite of ear NOS
Excludes1 superficial bite of ear (S00.46, S00.47)
- S01.351 Open bite of right ear
- S01.352 Open bite of left ear
- S01.359 Open bite of unspecified ear

S01.4 Open wound of cheek and temporomandibular area

S01.40 Unspecified open wound of cheek and temporomandibular area
- S01.401 Unspecified open wound of right cheek and temporomandibular area
- S01.402 Unspecified open wound of left cheek and temporomandibular area
- S01.409 Unspecified open wound of unspecified cheek and temporomandibular area

S01.41 Laceration without foreign body of cheek and temporomandibular area
- S01.411 Laceration without foreign body of right cheek and temporomandibular area
  Coding Clinic: 2015, Q1, P5-7
- S01.412 Laceration without foreign body of left cheek and temporomandibular area
- S01.419 Laceration without foreign body of unspecified cheek and temporomandibular area

S01.42 Laceration with foreign body of cheek and temporomandibular area
- S01.421 Laceration with foreign body of right cheek and temporomandibular area
- S01.422 Laceration with foreign body of left cheek and temporomandibular area
- S01.429 Laceration with foreign body of unspecified cheek and temporomandibular area

S01.43 Puncture wound without foreign body of cheek and temporomandibular area
- S01.431 Puncture wound without foreign body of right cheek and temporomandibular area
- S01.432 Puncture wound without foreign body of left cheek and temporomandibular area
- S01.439 Puncture wound without foreign body of unspecified cheek and temporomandibular area

S01.44 Puncture wound with foreign body of cheek and temporomandibular area

S01.441 Puncture wound with foreign body of right cheek and temporomandibular area

S01.442 Puncture wound with foreign body of left cheek and temporomandibular area

S01.449 Puncture wound with foreign body of unspecified cheek and temporomandibular area

S01.45 Open bite of cheek and temporomandibular area

Bite of cheek and temporomandibular area NOS

Excludes2 superficial bite of cheek and temporomandibular area (S00.86, S00.87)

S01.451 Open bite of right cheek and temporomandibular area

S01.452 Open bite of left cheek and temporomandibular area

S01.459 Open bite of unspecified cheek and temporomandibular area

S01.5 Open wound of lip and oral cavity

Excludes2 tooth dislocation (S03.2)
tooth fracture (S02.5)

S01.50 Unspecified open wound of lip and oral cavity

S01.501 Unspecified open wound of lip

S01.502 Unspecified open wound of oral cavity

S01.51 Laceration of lip and oral cavity without foreign body

S01.511 Laceration without foreign body of lip

S01.512 Laceration without foreign body of oral cavity

S01.52 Laceration of lip and oral cavity with foreign body

S01.521 Laceration with foreign body of lip

S01.522 Laceration with foreign body of oral cavity

S01.53 Puncture wound of lip and oral cavity without foreign body

S01.531 Puncture wound without foreign body of lip

S01.532 Puncture wound without foreign body of oral cavity

S01.54 Puncture wound of lip and oral cavity with foreign body

S01.541 Puncture wound with foreign body of lip

S01.542 Puncture wound with foreign body of oral cavity

S01.55 Open bite of lip and oral cavity

S01.551 Open bite of lip

Bite of lip NOS

Excludes1 superficial bite of lip (S00.571)

S01.552 Open bite of oral cavity

Bite of oral cavity NOS

Excludes1 superficial bite of oral cavity (S00.572)

S01.8 Open wound of other parts of head

X **S01.80** Unspecified open wound of other part of head

X **S01.81** Laceration without foreign body of other part of head

X **S01.82** Laceration with foreign body of other part of head

X **S01.83** Puncture wound without foreign body of other part of head

X **S01.84** Puncture wound with foreign body of other part of head

X **S01.85** Open bite of other part of head

Bite of other part of head NOS

Excludes1 superficial bite of other part of head (S00.87)

S01.9 Open wound of unspecified part of head

X **S01.90** Unspecified open wound of unspecified part of head

X **S01.91** Laceration without foreign body of unspecified part of head

X **S01.92** Laceration with foreign body of unspecified part of head

X **S01.93** Puncture wound without foreign body of unspecified part of head

X **S01.94** Puncture wound with foreign body of unspecified part of head

X **S01.95** Open bite of unspecified part of head

Bite of head NOS

Excludes1 superficial bite of head NOS (S00.97)

S02 Fracture of skull and facial bones

Note: A fracture not indicated as open or closed should be coded to closed

The appropriate 7th character is to be added to each code from category S02

A	initial encounter for closed fracture
B	initial encounter for open fracture
D	subsequent encounter for fracture with routine healing
G	subsequent encounter for fracture with delayed healing
K	subsequent encounter for fracture with nonunion
S	sequela

Code also any associated intracranial injury (S06.-)

X **S02.0** Fracture of vault of skull A, B, S

Fracture of frontal bone
Fracture of parietal bone

S02.1 Fracture of base of skull

~~Excludes1 orbit NOS (S02.8)~~

▶ **Excludes2** lateral orbital wall (S02.84-)
▶medial orbital wall (S02.83-)
orbital floor (S02.3-)

Coding Clinic: 2016, Q4, P66

S02.10 Unspecified fracture of base of skull

S02.101 Fracture of base of skull, right side A, B, S

S02.102 Fracture of base of skull, left side A, B, S

S02.109 Fracture of base of skull, unspecified side A, B, S

S02.11 Fracture of occiput

S02.110 Type I occipital condyle fracture, unspecified side A, B, S

S02.111 Type II occipital condyle fracture, unspecified side A, B, S

S02.112 Type III occipital condyle fracture, unspecified side A, B, S

S02.113 Unspecified occipital condyle fracture A, B, S

S02.118 Other fracture of occiput, unspecified side A, B, S

S02.119 Unspecified fracture of occiput A, B, S

SØ2.11A Type I occipital condyle fracture, right side A, B, S

SØ2.11B Type I occipital condyle fracture, left side A, B, S

SØ2.11C Type II occipital condyle fracture, right side A, B, S

SØ2.11D Type II occipital condyle fracture, left side A, B, S

SØ2.11E Type III occipital condyle fracture, right side A, B, S

SØ2.11F Type III occipital condyle fracture, left side A, B, S

SØ2.11G Other fracture of occiput, right side A, B, S

SØ2.11H Other fracture of occiput, left side A, B, S

SØ2.12 Fracture of orbital roof

SØ2.121 Fracture of orbital roof, right side

SØ2.122 Fracture of orbital roof, left side

SØ2.129 Fracture of orbital roof, unspecified side

X SØ2.19 Other fracture of base of skull A, B, S
Fracture of anterior fossa of base of skull
Fracture of ethmoid sinus
Fracture of frontal sinus
Fracture of middle fossa of base of skull
~~Fracture of orbital roof~~
Fracture of posterior fossa of base of skull
Fracture of sphenoid
Fracture of temporal bone

X SØ2.2 Fracture of nasal bones

SØ2.3 Fracture of orbital floor
Fracture of inferior orbital wall
Excludes1 orbit NOS (SØ2.85)
Excludes2 lateral orbital wall (SØ2.84-)
medial orbital wall (SØ2.83-)
orbital roof (SØ2.1-)
Coding Clinic: 2016, Q4, P66

X SØ2.30 Fracture of orbital floor, unspecified side A, B, S

X SØ2.31 Fracture of orbital floor, right side A, B, S

X SØ2.32 Fracture of orbital floor, left side A, B, S

SØ2.4 Fracture of malar, maxillary and zygoma bones
Fracture of superior maxilla
Fracture of upper jaw (bone)
Fracture of zygomatic process of temporal bone
Coding Clinic: 2016, Q4, P66

SØ2.40 Fracture of malar, maxillary and zygoma bones, unspecified

SØ2.400 Malar fracture unspecified side A, B, S

SØ2.401 Maxillary fracture, unspecified side A, B, S

SØ2.402 Zygomatic fracture, unspecified side A, B, S

SØ2.40A Malar fracture, right side A, B, S

SØ2.40B Malar fracture, left side A, B, S

SØ2.40C Maxillary fracture, right side A, B, S

SØ2.40D Maxillary fracture, left side A, B, S

SØ2.40E Zygomatic fracture, right side A, B, S

SØ2.40F Zygomatic fracture, left side A, B, S

SØ2.41 LeFort fracture

SØ2.411 LeFort I fracture A, B, S

SØ2.412 LeFort II fracture A, B, S

SØ2.413 LeFort III fracture A, B, S

X SØ2.42 Fracture of alveolus of maxilla A, B, S

X SØ2.5 Fracture of tooth (traumatic) Broken tooth
Excludes1 cracked tooth (nontraumatic) (KØ3.81)

SØ2.6 Fracture of mandible
Fracture of lower jaw (bone)
Coding Clinic: 2016, Q4, P66

SØ2.60 Fracture of mandible of unspecified site

SØ2.600 Fracture of unspecified part of body of mandible, unspecified side A, B, S

SØ2.601 Fracture of unspecified part of body of right mandible A, B, S

SØ2.602 Fracture of unspecified part of body of left mandible A, B, S

SØ2.609 Fracture of mandible, unspecified A, B, S

SØ2.61 Fracture of condylar process of mandible

SØ2.610 Fracture of condylar process of mandible, unspecified side A, B, S

SØ2.611 Fracture of condylar process of right mandible A, B, S

SØ2.612 Fracture of condylar process of left mandible A, B, S

SØ2.62 Fracture of subcondylar process of mandible

SØ2.620 Fracture of subcondylar process of mandible, unspecified side A, B, S

SØ2.621 Fracture of subcondylar process of right mandible A, B, S

SØ2.622 Fracture of subcondylar process of left mandible A, B, S

SØ2.63 Fracture of coronoid process of mandible

SØ2.630 Fracture of coronoid process of mandible, unspecified side A, B, S

SØ2.631 Fracture of coronoid process of right mandible A, B, S

SØ2.632 Fracture of coronoid process of left mandible A, B, S

SØ2.64 Fracture of ramus of mandible

SØ2.640 Fracture of ramus of mandible, unspecified side A, B, S

SØ2.641 Fracture of ramus of right mandible A, B, S

SØ2.642 Fracture of ramus of left mandible A, B, S

SØ2.65 Fracture of angle of mandible

SØ2.650 Fracture of angle of mandible, unspecified side A, B, S

SØ2.651 Fracture of angle of right mandible A, B, S

SØ2.652 Fracture of angle of left mandible A, B, S

X SØ2.66 Fracture of symphysis of mandible A, B, S

SØ2.67 Fracture of alveolus of mandible

SØ2.670 Fracture of alveolus of mandible, unspecified side A, B, S

SØ2.671 Fracture of alveolus of right mandible A, B, S

SØ2.672 Fracture of alveolus of left mandible A, B, S

X SØ2.69 Fracture of mandible of other specified site A, B, S

S02.8 Fractures of other specified skull and facial bones
~~Fracture of orbit NOS~~
Fracture of palate
~~Excludes1 fracture of orbital floor (S02.3-)~~
~~fracture of orbital roof (S02.1-)~~
Excludes2 lateral orbital wall (S02.84-)
medial orbital wall (S02.83-)
Coding Clinic: 2016, Q4, P66

X S02.80 Fracture of other specified skull and facial bones, unspecified side A, B, S
X S02.81 Fracture of other specified skull and facial bones, right side A, B, S
X S02.82 Fracture of other specified skull and facial bones, left side A, B, S

S02.83 Fracture of medial orbital wall
Excludes2 orbital floor (S02.3-)
orbital roof (S02.12-)
S02.831 Fracture of medial orbital wall, right side
S02.832 Fracture of medial orbital wall, left side
S02.839 Fracture of medial orbital wall, unspecified side

S02.84 Fracture of lateral orbital wall
Excludes2 orbital floor (S02.3-)
orbital roof (S02.12-)
S02.841 Fracture of lateral orbital wall, right side
S02.842 Fracture of lateral orbital wall, left side
S02.849 Fracture of lateral orbital wall, unspecified side

S02.85 Fracture of orbit, unspecified
Fracture of orbit NOS
Fracture of orbit wall NOS
Excludes1 lateral orbital wall (S02.84-)
medial orbital wall (S02.83-)
orbital floor (S02.3-)
orbital roof (S02.12-)

S02.9 Fracture of unspecified skull and facial bones
X S02.91 Unspecified fracture of skull A, B, S
X S02.92 Unspecified fracture of facial bones A, B, S

S03 Dislocation and sprain of joints and ligaments of head

Includes avulsion of joint (capsule) or ligament of head
laceration of cartilage, joint (capsule) or ligament of head
sprain of cartilage, joint (capsule) or ligament of head
traumatic hemarthrosis of joint or ligament of head
traumatic rupture of joint or ligament of head
traumatic subluxation of joint or ligament of head
traumatic tear of joint or ligament of head

Code also any associated open wound

Excludes2 Strain of muscle or tendon of head (S09.1)

The appropriate 7th character is to be added to each code from category S03

A	initial encounter
D	subsequent encounter
S	sequela

S03.0 Dislocation of jaw
Dislocation of jaw (cartilage) (meniscus)
Dislocation of mandible
Dislocation of temporomandibular (joint)
Coding Clinic: 2016, Q4, P67
X S03.00 Dislocation of jaw, unspecified side
X S03.01 Dislocation of jaw, right side
X S03.02 Dislocation of jaw, left side
X S03.03 Dislocation of jaw, bilateral side

X S03.1 Dislocation of septal cartilage of nose
X S03.2 Dislocation of tooth

S03.4 Sprain of jaw
Sprain of temporomandibular (joint) (ligament)
Coding Clinic: 2016, Q4, P67
X S03.40 Sprain of jaw, unspecified side
X S03.41 Sprain of jaw, right side
X S03.42 Sprain of jaw, left side
X S03.43 Sprain of jaw, bilateral side

X S03.8 Sprain of joints and ligaments of other parts of head
X S03.9 Sprain of joints and ligaments of unspecified parts of head

S04 Injury of cranial nerve

The selection of side should be based on the side of the body being affected

Code first any associated intracranial injury (S06.-)

Code also any associated:
open wound of head (S01.-)
skull fracture (S02.-)

The appropriate 7th character is to be added to each code from category S04

A	initial encounter
D	subsequent encounter
S	sequela

S04.0 Injury of optic nerve and pathways
Use additional code to identify any visual field defect or blindness (H53.4-, H54.-)

S04.01 Injury of optic nerve
Injury of 2nd cranial nerve
S04.011 Injury of optic nerve, right eye
S04.012 Injury of optic nerve, left eye
S04.019 Injury of optic nerve, unspecified eye
Injury of optic nerve NOS

X S04.02 Injury of optic chiasm

S04.03 Injury of optic tract and pathways
Injury of optic radiation
S04.031 Injury of optic tract and pathways, right side
S04.032 Injury of optic tract and pathways, left side
S04.039 Injury of optic tract and pathways, unspecified side
Injury of optic tract and pathways NOS

S04.04 Injury of visual cortex
S04.041 Injury of visual cortex, right side
S04.042 Injury of visual cortex, left side
S04.049 Injury of visual cortex, unspecified side
Injury of visual cortex NOS

S04.1 Injury of oculomotor nerve
Injury of 3rd cranial nerve
X S04.10 Injury of oculomotor nerve, unspecified side
X S04.11 Injury of oculomotor nerve, right side
X S04.12 Injury of oculomotor nerve, left side

S04.2 Injury of trochlear nerve
Injury of 4th cranial nerve
X S04.20 Injury of trochlear nerve, unspecified side
X S04.21 Injury of trochlear nerve, right side
X S04.22 Injury of trochlear nerve, left side

S04.3 Injury of trigeminal nerve
Injury of 5th cranial nerve
X S04.30 Injury of trigeminal nerve, unspecified side
X S04.31 Injury of trigeminal nerve, right side
X S04.32 Injury of trigeminal nerve, left side

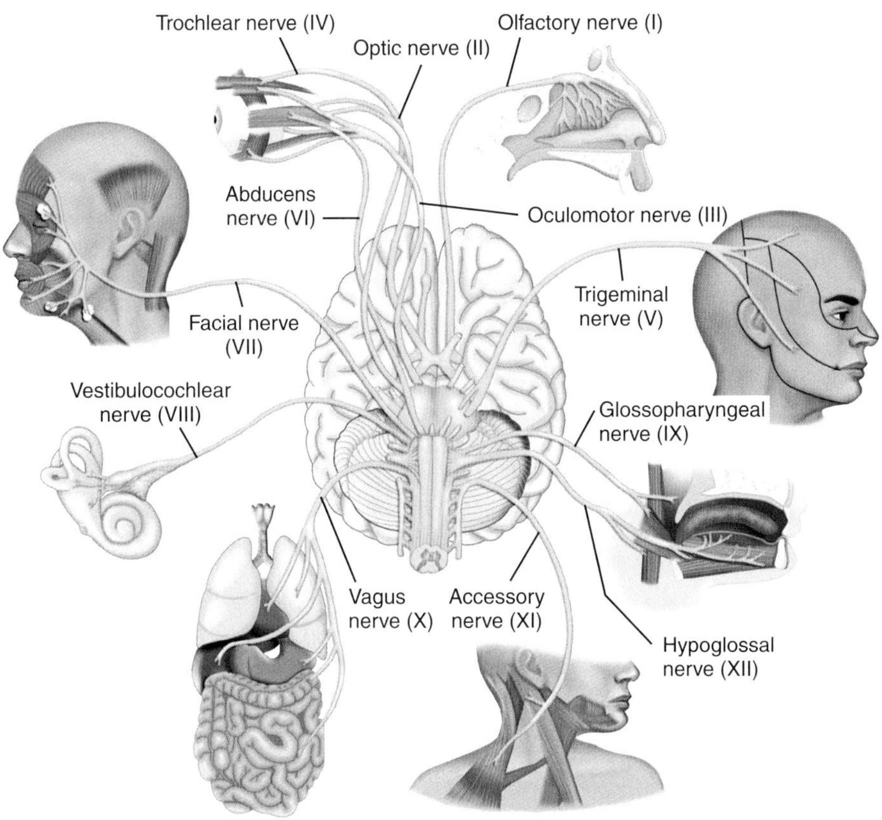

Figure 19-13 Cranial nerves. (From Patton and Thibodeau: Anatomy and physiology, ed 7, St. Louis, Mosby, 2009)

● **S04.4 Injury of abducent nerve**
Injury of 6th cranial nerve
X● **S04.40 Injury of abducent nerve, unspecified side**
X● **S04.41 Injury of abducent nerve, right side**
X● **S04.42 Injury of abducent nerve, left side**

● **S04.5 Injury of facial nerve**
Injury of 7th cranial nerve
X● **S04.50 Injury of facial nerve, unspecified side**
X● **S04.51 Injury of facial nerve, right side**
X● **S04.52 Injury of facial nerve, left side**

● **S04.6 Injury of acoustic nerve**
Injury of auditory nerve
Injury of 8th cranial nerve
X● **S04.60 Injury of acoustic nerve, unspecified side**
X● **S04.61 Injury of acoustic nerve, right side**
X● **S04.62 Injury of acoustic nerve, left side**

● **S04.7 Injury of accessory nerve**
Injury of 11th cranial nerve
X● **S04.70 Injury of accessory nerve, unspecified side**
X● **S04.71 Injury of accessory nerve, right side**
X● **S04.72 Injury of accessory nerve, left side**

● **S04.8 Injury of other cranial nerves**
● **S04.81 Injury of olfactory [1st] nerve**
● **S04.811 Injury of olfactory [1st] nerve, right side**
● **S04.812 Injury of olfactory [1st] nerve, left side**
● **S04.819 Injury of olfactory [1st] nerve, unspecified side**
● **S04.89 Injury of other cranial nerves**
Injury of vagus [10th] nerve
● **S04.891 Injury of other cranial nerves, right side**
● **S04.892 Injury of other cranial nerves, left side**
● **S04.899 Injury of other cranial nerves, unspecified side**

X● **S04.9 Injury of unspecified cranial nerve**

● **S05 Injury of eye and orbit**

Includes open wound of eye and orbit

Excludes2 2nd cranial [optic] nerve injury (S04.0-)
3rd cranial [oculomotor] nerve injury (S04.1-)
open wound of eyelid and periocular area (S01.1-)
orbital bone fracture (S02.1-, S02.3-, S02.8-)
superficial injury of eyelid (S00.1-S00.2)

The appropriate 7th character is to be added to each code from category S05

A	initial encounter
D	subsequent encounter
S	sequela

● **S05.0 Injury of conjunctiva and corneal abrasion without foreign body**

Excludes1 foreign body in conjunctival sac (T15.1)
foreign body in cornea (T15.0)

X● **S05.00 Injury of conjunctiva and corneal abrasion without foreign body, unspecified eye**
X● **S05.01 Injury of conjunctiva and corneal abrasion without foreign body, right eye**
X● **S05.02 Injury of conjunctiva and corneal abrasion without foreign body, left eye**

● **S05.1 Contusion of eyeball and orbital tissues**
Traumatic hyphema

Excludes2 black eye NOS (S00.1)
contusion of eyelid and periocular area (S00.1)

X● **S05.10 Contusion of eyeball and orbital tissues, unspecified eye**
X● **S05.11 Contusion of eyeball and orbital tissues, right eye**
X● **S05.12 Contusion of eyeball and orbital tissues, left eye**

S05.2 Ocular laceration and rupture with prolapse or loss of intraocular tissue
- X **S05.20** Ocular laceration and rupture with prolapse or loss of intraocular tissue, **unspecified** eye
- X **S05.21** Ocular laceration and rupture with prolapse or loss of intraocular tissue, **right** eye
- X **S05.22** Ocular laceration and rupture with prolapse or loss of intraocular tissue, **left** eye

S05.3 Ocular laceration without prolapse or loss of intraocular tissue
Laceration of eye NOS
- X **S05.30** Ocular laceration without prolapse or loss of intraocular tissue, **unspecified** eye
- X **S05.31** Ocular laceration without prolapse or loss of intraocular tissue, **right** eye
- X **S05.32** Ocular laceration without prolapse or loss of intraocular tissue, **left** eye

S05.4 **Penetrating wound of orbit** with or without foreign body
Excludes2 retained (old) foreign body following penetrating wound in orbit (H05.5-)
- X **S05.40** Penetrating wound of orbit with or without foreign body, **unspecified** eye
- X **S05.41** Penetrating wound of orbit with or without foreign body, **right** eye
- X **S05.42** Penetrating wound of orbit with or without foreign body, **left** eye

S05.5 Penetrating wound with foreign body of eyeball
Excludes2 retained (old) intraocular foreign body (H44.6-, H44.7)
- X **S05.50** Penetrating wound with foreign body of **unspecified** eyeball
- X **S05.51** Penetrating wound with foreign body of **right** eyeball
- X **S05.52** Penetrating wound with foreign body of **left** eyeball

S05.6 **Penetrating wound without foreign body of eyeball**
Ocular penetration NOS
- X **S05.60** Penetrating wound without foreign body of **unspecified** eyeball
- X **S05.61** Penetrating wound without foreign body of **right** eyeball
- X **S05.62** Penetrating wound without foreign body of **left** eyeball

S05.7 Avulsion of eye
Traumatic enucleation
- X **S05.70** Avulsion of **unspecified** eye
- X **S05.71** Avulsion of **right** eye
- X **S05.72** Avulsion of **left** eye

S05.8 Other injuries of eye and orbit
Lacrimal duct injury
- **S05.8X** Other injuries of eye and orbit
  - **S05.8X1** Other injuries of **right** eye and orbit
  - **S05.8X2** Other injuries of **left** eye and orbit
  - **S05.8X9** Other injuries of **unspecified** eye and orbit

S05.9 **Unspecified injury** of eye and orbit
Injury of eye NOS
- X **S05.90** Unspecified injury of **unspecified** eye and orbit
- X **S05.91** Unspecified injury of **right** eye and orbit
- X **S05.92** Unspecified injury of **left** eye and orbit

S06 Intracranial injury
Includes traumatic brain injury
Code also any associated:
open wound of head (S01.-)
skull fracture (S02.-)
Excludes1 head injury NOS (S09.90)
The appropriate 7th character is to be added to each code from category S06

A	initial encounter
D	subsequent encounter
S	sequela

Note: 7th characters D and S do not apply to codes in category S06 with 6th character 7 - death due to brain injury prior to regaining consciousness, or 8 - death due to other cause prior to regaining consciousness.
Coding Clinic: 2015, Q4, P40

S06.0 Concussion
Commotio cerebri
Excludes1 concussion with other intracranial injuries classified in subcategories S06.1- to S06.6-, S06.81- and S06.82- code to specified intracranial injury
Coding Clinic: 2016, Q4, P67
- **S06.0X** Concussion
  - **S06.0X0** Concussion without loss of consciousness S
  - **S06.0X1** Concussion with loss of consciousness of 30 minutes or less S
  - **S06.0X9** Concussion with loss of consciousness of unspecified duration S
    Concussion NOS
    Coding Clinic: 2016, Q4, P68

S06.1 Traumatic cerebral edema
Diffuse traumatic cerebral edema
Focal traumatic cerebral edema
Coding Clinic: 2016, Q4, P67
- **S06.1X** Traumatic cerebral edema
  - **S06.1X0** Traumatic cerebral edema without loss of consciousness A, S
    Coding Clinic: 2015, Q1, P12
  - **S06.1X1** Traumatic cerebral edema with loss of consciousness of 30 minutes or less A, S
  - **S06.1X2** Traumatic cerebral edema with loss of consciousness of 31 minutes to 59 minutes A, S
  - **S06.1X3** Traumatic cerebral edema with loss of consciousness of 1 hour to 5 hours 59 minutes A, S
  - **S06.1X4** Traumatic cerebral edema with loss of consciousness of 6 hours to 24 hours A, S
  - **S06.1X5** Traumatic cerebral edema with loss of consciousness greater than 24 hours with return to pre-existing conscious level A, S
  - **S06.1X6** Traumatic cerebral edema with loss of consciousness greater than 24 hours without return to pre-existing conscious level with patient surviving A, S

- **S06.1X7** Traumatic cerebral edema with loss of consciousness of any duration with death due to brain injury prior to regaining consciousness
- **S06.1X8** Traumatic cerebral edema with loss of consciousness of any duration with death due to other cause prior to regaining consciousness
- **S06.1X9** Traumatic cerebral edema with loss of consciousness of unspecified duration A, S
  Traumatic cerebral edema NOS

S06.2 Diffuse traumatic brain injury
Diffuse axonal brain injury
Excludes1 traumatic diffuse cerebral edema (S06.1X-)

S06.2X Diffuse traumatic brain injury
- **S06.2X0** Diffuse traumatic brain injury without loss of consciousness A, S
- **S06.2X1** Diffuse traumatic brain injury with loss of consciousness of 30 minutes or less A, S
- **S06.2X2** Diffuse traumatic brain injury with loss of consciousness of 31 minutes to 59 minutes A, S
- **S06.2X3** Diffuse traumatic brain injury with loss of consciousness of 1 hour to 5 hours 59 minutes A, S
- **S06.2X4** Diffuse traumatic brain injury with loss of consciousness of 6 hours to 24 hours A, S
- **S06.2X5** Diffuse traumatic brain injury with loss of consciousness greater than 24 hours with return to pre-existing conscious levels A, S
- **S06.2X6** Diffuse traumatic brain injury with loss of consciousness greater than 24 hours without return to pre-existing conscious level with patient surviving A, S
- **S06.2X7** Diffuse traumatic brain injury with loss of consciousness of any duration with death due to brain injury prior to regaining consciousness
- **S06.2X8** Diffuse traumatic brain injury with loss of consciousness of any duration with death due to other cause prior to regaining consciousness
- **S06.2X9** Diffuse traumatic brain injury with loss of consciousness of unspecified duration A, S
  Diffuse traumatic brain injury NOS

S06.3 Focal traumatic brain injury
Excludes1 any condition classifiable to S06.4-S06.6
focal cerebral edema (S06.1)

S06.30 Unspecified focal traumatic brain injury
- **S06.300** Unspecified focal traumatic brain injury without loss of consciousness A, S
- **S06.301** Unspecified focal traumatic brain injury with loss of consciousness of 30 minutes or less A, S
- **S06.302** Unspecified focal traumatic brain injury with loss of consciousness of 31 minutes to 59 minutes A, S
- **S06.303** Unspecified focal traumatic brain injury with loss of consciousness of 1 hour to 5 hours 59 minutes A, S
- **S06.304** Unspecified focal traumatic brain injury with loss of consciousness of 6 hours to 24 hours A, S
- **S06.305** Unspecified focal traumatic brain injury with loss of consciousness greater than 24 hours with return to pre-existing conscious level A, S
- **S06.306** Unspecified focal traumatic brain injury with loss of consciousness greater than 24 hours without return to pre-existing conscious level with patient surviving A, S
- **S06.307** Unspecified focal traumatic brain injury with loss of consciousness of any duration with death due to brain injury prior to regaining consciousness
- **S06.308** Unspecified focal traumatic brain injury with loss of consciousness of any duration with death due to other cause prior to regaining consciousness
- **S06.309** Unspecified focal traumatic brain injury with loss of consciousness of unspecified duration A, S
  Unspecified focal traumatic brain injury NOS

S06.31 Contusion and laceration of right cerebrum
- **S06.310** Contusion and laceration of right cerebrum without loss of consciousness A, S
- **S06.311** Contusion and laceration of right cerebrum with loss of consciousness of 30 minutes or less A, S
- **S06.312** Contusion and laceration of right cerebrum with loss of consciousness of 31 minutes to 59 minutes A, S
- **S06.313** Contusion and laceration of right cerebrum with loss of consciousness of 1 hour to 5 hours 59 minutes A, S
- **S06.314** Contusion and laceration of right cerebrum with loss of consciousness of 6 hours to 24 hours A, S
- **S06.315** Contusion and laceration of right cerebrum with loss of consciousness greater than 24 hours with return to pre-existing conscious level A, S
- **S06.316** Contusion and laceration of right cerebrum with loss of consciousness greater than 24 hours without return to pre-existing conscious level with patient surviving A, S
- **S06.317** Contusion and laceration of right cerebrum with loss of consciousness of any duration with death due to brain injury prior to regaining consciousness
- **S06.318** Contusion and laceration of right cerebrum with loss of consciousness of any duration with death due to other cause prior to regaining consciousness
- **S06.319** Contusion and laceration of right cerebrum with loss of consciousness of unspecified duration A, S
  Contusion and laceration of right cerebrum NOS

- S06.32 Contusion and laceration of left cerebrum
  - S06.320 Contusion and laceration of left cerebrum without loss of consciousness A, S
  - S06.321 Contusion and laceration of left cerebrum with loss of consciousness of 30 minutes or less A, S
  - S06.322 Contusion and laceration of left cerebrum with loss of consciousness of 31 minutes to 59 minutes A, S
  - S06.323 Contusion and laceration of left cerebrum with loss of consciousness of 1 hour to 5 hours 59 minutes A, S
  - S06.324 Contusion and laceration of left cerebrum with loss of consciousness of 6 hours to 24 hours A, S
  - S06.325 Contusion and laceration of left cerebrum with loss of consciousness greater than 24 hours with return to pre-existing conscious level A, S
  - S06.326 Contusion and laceration of left cerebrum with loss of consciousness greater than 24 hours without return to pre-existing conscious level with patient surviving A, S
  - S06.327 Contusion and laceration of left cerebrum with loss of consciousness of any duration with death due to brain injury prior to regaining consciousness
  - S06.328 Contusion and laceration of left cerebrum with loss of consciousness of any duration with death due to other cause prior to regaining consciousness
  - S06.329 Contusion and laceration of left cerebrum with loss of consciousness of unspecified duration A, S
    Contusion and laceration of left cerebrum NOS
- S06.33 Contusion and laceration of cerebrum, unspecified
  - S06.330 Contusion and laceration of cerebrum, unspecified, without loss of consciousness A, S
  - S06.331 Contusion and laceration of cerebrum, unspecified, with loss of consciousness of 30 minutes or less A, S
  - S06.332 Contusion and laceration of cerebrum, unspecified, with loss of consciousness of 31 minutes to 59 minutes A, S
  - S06.333 Contusion and laceration of cerebrum, unspecified, with loss of consciousness of 1 hour to 5 hours 59 minutes A, S
  - S06.334 Contusion and laceration of cerebrum, unspecified, with loss of consciousness of 6 hours to 24 hours A, S
  - S06.335 Contusion and laceration of cerebrum, unspecified, with loss of consciousness greater than 24 hours with return to pre-existing conscious level A, S
  - S06.336 Contusion and laceration of cerebrum, unspecified, with loss of consciousness greater than 24 hours without return to pre-existing conscious level with patient surviving A, S
  - S06.337 Contusion and laceration of cerebrum, unspecified, with loss of consciousness of any duration with death due to brain injury prior to regaining consciousness
  - S06.338 Contusion and laceration of cerebrum, unspecified, with loss of consciousness of any duration with death due to other cause prior to regaining consciousness
  - S06.339 Contusion and laceration of cerebrum, unspecified, with loss of consciousness of unspecified duration A, S
    Contusion and laceration of cerebrum NOS
- S06.34 Traumatic hemorrhage of right cerebrum
  Traumatic intracerebral hemorrhage and hematoma of right cerebrum
  - S06.340 Traumatic hemorrhage of right cerebrum without loss of consciousness A, S
    Coding Clinic: 2015, Q1, P12
  - S06.341 Traumatic hemorrhage of right cerebrum with loss of consciousness of 30 minutes or less A, S
  - S06.342 Traumatic hemorrhage of right cerebrum with loss of consciousness of 31 minutes to 59 minutes A, S
  - S06.343 Traumatic hemorrhage of right cerebrum with loss of consciousness of 1 hours to 5 hours 59 minutes A, S
  - S06.344 Traumatic hemorrhage of right cerebrum with loss of consciousness of 6 hours to 24 hours A, S
  - S06.345 Traumatic hemorrhage of right cerebrum with loss of consciousness greater than 24 hours with return to pre-existing conscious level A, S
  - S06.346 Traumatic hemorrhage of right cerebrum with loss of consciousness greater than 24 hours without return to pre-existing conscious level with patient surviving A, S
  - S06.347 Traumatic hemorrhage of right cerebrum with loss of consciousness of any duration with death due to brain injury prior to regaining consciousness
  - S06.348 Traumatic hemorrhage of right cerebrum with loss of consciousness of any duration with death due to other cause prior to regaining consciousness
  - S06.349 Traumatic hemorrhage of right cerebrum with loss of consciousness of unspecified duration A, S
    Traumatic hemorrhage of right cerebrum NOS

● **SØ6.35 Traumatic hemorrhage of left cerebrum**
Traumatic intracerebral hemorrhage and hematoma of left cerebrum

● **SØ6.350** Traumatic hemorrhage of left cerebrum **without loss of consciousness** A, S

● **SØ6.351** Traumatic hemorrhage of left cerebrum with loss of consciousness of **3Ø minutes or less** A, S

● **SØ6.352** Traumatic hemorrhage of left cerebrum with loss of consciousness of **31 minutes to 59 minutes** A, S

● **SØ6.353** Traumatic hemorrhage of left cerebrum with loss of consciousness of **1 hours to 5 hours 59 minutes** A, S

● **SØ6.354** Traumatic hemorrhage of left cerebrum with loss of consciousness of **6 hours to 24 hours** A, S

● **SØ6.355** Traumatic hemorrhage of left cerebrum with loss of consciousness **greater than 24 hours with return to pre-existing conscious level** A, S

● **SØ6.356** Traumatic hemorrhage of left cerebrum with loss of consciousness **greater than 24 hours without return to pre-existing conscious level with patient surviving** A, S

● **SØ6.357** Traumatic hemorrhage of left cerebrum with loss of consciousness of **any duration with death due to brain injury** prior to regaining consciousness

● **SØ6.358** Traumatic hemorrhage of left cerebrum with loss of consciousness of **any duration with death due to other cause** prior to regaining consciousness

● **SØ6.359** Traumatic hemorrhage of left cerebrum with loss of consciousness of **unspecified duration** A, S
Traumatic hemorrhage of left cerebrum NOS

● **SØ6.36 Traumatic hemorrhage of cerebrum, unspecified**
Traumatic intracerebral hemorrhage and hematoma, unspecified

● **SØ6.360** Traumatic hemorrhage of cerebrum, unspecified, **without loss of consciousness** A, S

● **SØ6.361** Traumatic hemorrhage of cerebrum, unspecified, with loss of consciousness of **3Ø minutes or less** A, S

● **SØ6.362** Traumatic hemorrhage of cerebrum, unspecified, with loss of consciousness of **31 minutes to 59 minutes** A, S

● **SØ6.363** Traumatic hemorrhage of cerebrum, unspecified, with loss of consciousness of **1 hours to 5 hours 59 minutes** A, S

● **SØ6.364** Traumatic hemorrhage of cerebrum, unspecified, with loss of consciousness of **6 hours to 24 hours** A, S

● **SØ6.365** Traumatic hemorrhage of cerebrum, unspecified, with loss of consciousness **greater than 24 hours with return to pre-existing conscious level** A, S

● **SØ6.366** Traumatic hemorrhage of cerebrum, unspecified, with loss of consciousness **greater than 24 hours without return to pre-existing conscious level with patient surviving** A, S

● **SØ6.367** Traumatic hemorrhage of cerebrum, unspecified, with loss of consciousness of **any duration with death due to brain injury** prior to regaining consciousness

● **SØ6.368** Traumatic hemorrhage of cerebrum, unspecified, with loss of consciousness of **any duration with death due to other cause** prior to regaining consciousness

● **SØ6.369** Traumatic hemorrhage of cerebrum, unspecified, with loss of consciousness of **unspecified duration** A, S
Traumatic hemorrhage of cerebrum NOS

● **SØ6.37 Contusion, laceration, and hemorrhage of cerebellum**

● **SØ6.370** Contusion, laceration, and hemorrhage of cerebellum **without loss of consciousness** A, S

● **SØ6.371** Contusion, laceration, and hemorrhage of cerebellum with loss of consciousness of **3Ø minutes or less** A, S

● **SØ6.372** Contusion, laceration, and hemorrhage of cerebellum with loss of consciousness of **31 minutes to 59 minutes** A, S

● **SØ6.373** Contusion, laceration, and hemorrhage of cerebellum with loss of consciousness of **1 hour to 5 hours 59 minutes** A, S

● **SØ6.374** Contusion, laceration, and hemorrhage of cerebellum with loss of consciousness of **6 hours to 24 hours** A, S

● **SØ6.375** Contusion, laceration, and hemorrhage of cerebellum with loss of consciousness **greater than 24 hours with return to pre-existing conscious level** A, S

● **SØ6.376** Contusion, laceration, and hemorrhage of cerebellum with loss of consciousness **greater than 24 hours without return to pre-existing conscious level with patient surviving** A, S

● **SØ6.377** Contusion, laceration, and hemorrhage of cerebellum with loss of consciousness of **any duration with death due to brain injury** prior to regaining consciousness

● **SØ6.378** Contusion, laceration, and hemorrhage of cerebellum with loss of consciousness of **any duration with death due to other cause** prior to regaining consciousness

● **SØ6.379** Contusion, laceration, and hemorrhage of cerebellum with loss of consciousness of **unspecified duration** A, S
Contusion, laceration, and hemorrhage of cerebellum NOS

SØ6.38 Contusion, laceration, and hemorrhage of brainstem

- **SØ6.38Ø** Contusion, laceration, and hemorrhage of brainstem without loss of consciousness A, S
- **SØ6.381** Contusion, laceration, and hemorrhage of brainstem with loss of consciousness of 3Ø minutes or less A, S
- **SØ6.382** Contusion, laceration, and hemorrhage of brainstem with loss of consciousness of 31 minutes to 59 minutes A, S
- **SØ6.383** Contusion, laceration, and hemorrhage of brainstem with loss of consciousness of 1 hour to 5 hours 59 minutes A, S
- **SØ6.384** Contusion, laceration, and hemorrhage of brainstem with loss of consciousness of 6 hours to 24 hours A, S
- **SØ6.385** Contusion, laceration, and hemorrhage of brainstem with loss of consciousness greater than 24 hours with return to pre-existing conscious level A, S
- **SØ6.386** Contusion, laceration, and hemorrhage of brainstem with loss of consciousness greater than 24 hours without return to pre-existing conscious level with patient surviving A, S
- **SØ6.387** Contusion, laceration, and hemorrhage of brainstem with loss of consciousness of any duration with death due to brain injury prior to regaining consciousness
- **SØ6.388** Contusion, laceration, and hemorrhage of brainstem with loss of consciousness of any duration with death due to other cause prior to regaining consciousness
- **SØ6.389** Contusion, laceration, and hemorrhage of brainstem with loss of consciousness of unspecified duration A, S
  Contusion, laceration, and hemorrhage of brainstem NOS

SØ6.4 Epidural hemorrhage
Situated outside dura mater
Extradural hemorrhage NOS
Intracranial hemorrhage due to trauma
Extradural hemorrhage (traumatic)

SØ6.4X Epidural hemorrhage

- **SØ6.4XØ** Epidural hemorrhage without loss of consciousness A, S
- **SØ6.4X1** Epidural hemorrhage with loss of consciousness of 3Ø minutes or less A, S
- **SØ6.4X2** Epidural hemorrhage with loss of consciousness of 31 minutes to 59 minutes A, S
- **SØ6.4X3** Epidural hemorrhage with loss of consciousness of 1 hour to 5 hours 59 minutes A, S
- **SØ6.4X4** Epidural hemorrhage with loss of consciousness of 6 hours to 24 hours A, S
- **SØ6.4X5** Epidural hemorrhage with loss of consciousness greater than 24 hours with return to pre-existing conscious level A, S
- **SØ6.4X6** Epidural hemorrhage with loss of consciousness greater than 24 hours without return to pre-existing conscious level with patient surviving A, S
- **SØ6.4X7** Epidural hemorrhage with loss of consciousness of any duration with death due to brain injury prior to regaining consciousness
- **SØ6.4X8** Epidural hemorrhage with loss of consciousness of any duration with death due to other causes prior to regaining consciousness
- **SØ6.4X9** Epidural hemorrhage with loss of consciousness of unspecified duration A, S
  Epidural hemorrhage NOS

SØ6.5 Traumatic subdural hemorrhage

SØ6.5X Traumatic subdural hemorrhage

- **SØ6.5XØ** Traumatic subdural hemorrhage without loss of consciousness A, S
  Coding Clinic: 2Ø18, Q2, P13; 2Ø15, Q3, P37
- **SØ6.5X1** Traumatic subdural hemorrhage with loss of consciousness of 3Ø minutes or less A, S
- **SØ6.5X2** Traumatic subdural hemorrhage with loss of consciousness of 31 minutes to 59 minutes A, S
- **SØ6.5X3** Traumatic subdural hemorrhage with loss of consciousness of 1 hour to 5 hours 59 minutes A, S
- **SØ6.5X4** Traumatic subdural hemorrhage with loss of consciousness of 6 hours to 24 hours A, S
- **SØ6.5X5** Traumatic subdural hemorrhage with loss of consciousness greater than 24 hours with return to pre-existing conscious level A, S
- **SØ6.5X6** Traumatic subdural hemorrhage with loss of consciousness greater than 24 hours without return to pre-existing conscious level with patient surviving A, S
- **SØ6.5X7** Traumatic subdural hemorrhage with loss of consciousness of any duration with death due to brain injury before regaining consciousness
- **SØ6.5X8** Traumatic subdural hemorrhage with loss of consciousness of any duration with death due to other cause before regaining consciousness
- **SØ6.5X9** Traumatic subdural hemorrhage with loss of consciousness of unspecified duration A, S
  Traumatic subdural hemorrhage NOS

SØ6.6 Traumatic subarachnoid hemorrhage
Between arachnoid and pia mater
Coding Clinic: 2016, Q4, P67

SØ6.6X Traumatic subarachnoid hemorrhage

- **SØ6.6XØ** Traumatic subarachnoid hemorrhage without loss of consciousness A, S
  Coding Clinic: 2Ø15, Q3, P37
- **SØ6.6X1** Traumatic subarachnoid hemorrhage with loss of consciousness of 3Ø minutes or less A, S
- **SØ6.6X2** Traumatic subarachnoid hemorrhage with loss of consciousness of 31 minutes to 59 minutes A, S
- **SØ6.6X3** Traumatic subarachnoid hemorrhage with loss of consciousness of 1 hour to 5 hours 59 minutes A, S

- **S06.6X4** Traumatic subarachnoid hemorrhage with loss of consciousness of **6 hours to 24 hours** A, S
- **S06.6X5** Traumatic subarachnoid hemorrhage with loss of consciousness **greater than 24 hours with return to pre-existing conscious level** A, S
- **S06.6X6** Traumatic subarachnoid hemorrhage with loss of consciousness **greater than 24 hours without return to pre-existing conscious level with patient surviving** A, S
- **S06.6X7** Traumatic subarachnoid hemorrhage with loss of consciousness of **any duration with death due to brain injury** prior to regaining consciousness
- **S06.6X8** Traumatic subarachnoid hemorrhage with loss of consciousness of **any duration with death due to other cause** prior to regaining consciousness
- **S06.6X9** Traumatic subarachnoid hemorrhage with loss of consciousness of **unspecified duration** A, S
  - Traumatic subarachnoid hemorrhage NOS

S06.8 Other specified intracranial injuries

S06.81 Injury of **right internal carotid artery**, intracranial portion, not elsewhere classified
Coding Clinic: 2016, Q4, P67

- **S06.810** Injury of right internal carotid artery, intracranial portion, not elsewhere classified **without loss of consciousness** A, S
- **S06.811** Injury of right internal carotid artery, intracranial portion, not elsewhere classified with loss of consciousness of **30 minutes or less** A, S
- **S06.812** Injury of right internal carotid artery, intracranial portion, not elsewhere classified with loss of consciousness of **31 minutes to 59 minutes** A, S
- **S06.813** Injury of right internal carotid artery, intracranial portion, not elsewhere classified with loss of consciousness of **1 hour to 5 hours 59 minutes** A, S
- **S06.814** Injury of right internal carotid artery, intracranial portion, not elsewhere classified with loss of consciousness of **6 hours to 24 hours** A, S
- **S06.815** Injury of right internal carotid artery, intracranial portion, not elsewhere classified with loss of consciousness **greater than 24 hours with return to pre-existing conscious level** A, S
- **S06.816** Injury of right internal carotid artery, intracranial portion, not elsewhere classified with loss of consciousness **greater than 24 hours without return to pre-existing conscious level with patient surviving** A, S
- **S06.817** Injury of right internal carotid artery, intracranial portion, not elsewhere classified with loss of consciousness **of any duration with death due to brain injury** prior to regaining consciousness
- **S06.818** Injury of right internal carotid artery, intracranial portion, not elsewhere classified with loss of consciousness **of any duration with death due to other cause** prior to regaining consciousness
- **S06.819** Injury of right internal carotid artery, intracranial portion, not elsewhere classified with loss of consciousness of **unspecified duration** A, S
  - Injury of right internal carotid artery, intracranial portion, not elsewhere classified NOS

S06.82 Injury of **left internal carotid artery**, intracranial portion, not elsewhere classified
Coding Clinic: 2016, Q4, P67

- **S06.820** Injury of left internal carotid artery, intracranial portion, not elsewhere classified **without loss of consciousness** A, S
- **S06.821** Injury of left internal carotid artery, intracranial portion, not elsewhere classified with loss of consciousness of **30 minutes or less** A, S
- **S06.822** Injury of left internal carotid artery, intracranial portion, not elsewhere classified with loss of consciousness **of 31 minutes to 59 minutes** A, S
- **S06.823** Injury of left internal carotid artery, intracranial portion, not elsewhere classified with loss of consciousness **of 1 hour to 5 hours 59 minutes** A, S
- **S06.824** Injury of left internal carotid artery, intracranial portion, not elsewhere classified with loss of consciousness of **6 hours to 24 hours** A, S
- **S06.825** Injury of left internal carotid artery, intracranial portion, not elsewhere classified with loss of consciousness **greater than 24 hours with return to pre-existing conscious level**
- **S06.826** Injury of left internal carotid artery, intracranial portion, not elsewhere classified with loss of consciousness **greater than 24 hours without return to pre-existing conscious level with patient surviving** A, S
- **S06.827** Injury of left internal carotid artery, intracranial portion, not elsewhere classified with loss of consciousness **of any duration with death due to brain injury** prior to regaining consciousness
- **S06.828** Injury of left internal carotid artery, intracranial portion, not elsewhere classified with loss of consciousness **of any duration with death due to other cause** prior to regaining consciousness
- **S06.829** Injury of left internal carotid artery, intracranial portion, not elsewhere classified with loss of consciousness **of unspecified duration** A, S
  - Injury of left internal carotid artery, intracranial portion, not elsewhere classified NOS

● S06.89 Other specified intracranial injury
  Excludes1 concussion (S06.0X-)
  ● S06.890 Other specified intracranial injury without loss of consciousness A, S
  ● S06.891 Other specified intracranial injury with loss of consciousness of 30 minutes or less A, S
  ● S06.892 Other specified intracranial injury with loss of consciousness of 31 minutes to 59 minutes A, S
  ● S06.893 Other specified intracranial injury with loss of consciousness of 1 hour to 5 hours 59 minutes A, S
  ● S06.894 Other specified intracranial injury with loss of consciousness of 6 hours to 24 hours A, S
  ● S06.895 Other specified intracranial injury with loss of consciousness greater than 24 hours with return to pre-existing conscious level A, S
  ● S06.896 Other specified intracranial injury with loss of consciousness greater than 24 hours without return to pre-existing conscious level with patient surviving A, S
  ● S06.897 Other specified intracranial injury with loss of consciousness of any duration with death due to brain injury prior to regaining consciousness
  ● S06.898 Other specified intracranial injury with loss of consciousness of any duration with death due to other cause prior to regaining consciousness
  ● S06.899 Other specified intracranial injury with loss of consciousness of unspecified duration A, S

● S06.9 Unspecified intracranial injury
  Brain injury NOS
  Head injury NOS with loss of consciousness
  Traumatic brain injury NOS
  Excludes1 conditions classifiable to S06.0- to S06.8- code to specified intracranial injury
  head injury NOS (S09.90)
● S06.9X Unspecified intracranial injury
  ● S06.9X0 Unspecified intracranial injury without loss of consciousness A, S
  ● S06.9X1 Unspecified intracranial injury with loss of consciousness of 30 minutes or less A, S
  ● S06.9X2 Unspecified intracranial injury with loss of consciousness of 31 minutes to 59 minutes A, S
  ● S06.9X3 Unspecified intracranial injury with loss of consciousness of 1 hour to 5 hours 59 minutes A, S
  ● S06.9X4 Unspecified intracranial injury with loss of consciousness of 6 hours to 24 hours A, S
  ● S06.9X5 Unspecified intracranial injury with loss of consciousness greater than 24 hours with return to pre-existing conscious level A, S
  ● S06.9X6 Unspecified intracranial injury with loss of consciousness greater than 24 hours without return to pre-existing conscious level with patient surviving A, S
  ● S06.9X7 Unspecified intracranial injury with loss of consciousness of any duration with death due to brain injury prior to regaining consciousness
  ● S06.9X8 Unspecified intracranial injury with loss of consciousness of any duration with death due to other cause prior to regaining consciousness
  ● S06.9X9 Unspecified intracranial injury with loss of consciousness of unspecified duration A, S

● S07 Crushing injury of head
  Use additional code for all associated injuries, such as:
  intracranial injuries (S06.-)
  skull fractures (S02.-)
  The appropriate 7th character is to be added to each code from category S07

A	initial encounter
D	subsequent encounter
S	sequela

X● S07.0 Crushing injury of face
X● S07.1 Crushing injury of skull
X● S07.8 Crushing injury of other parts of head
X● S07.9 Crushing injury of head, part unspecified

● S08 Avulsion and traumatic amputation of part of head
  An amputation not identified as partial or complete should be coded to complete
  The appropriate 7th character is to be added to each code from category S08

A	initial encounter
D	subsequent encounter
S	sequela

X● S08.0 Avulsion of scalp
● S08.1 Traumatic amputation of ear
  ● S08.11 Complete traumatic amputation of ear
    ● S08.111 Complete traumatic amputation of right ear
    ● S08.112 Complete traumatic amputation of left ear
    ● S08.119 Complete traumatic amputation of unspecified ear
  ● S08.12 Partial traumatic amputation of ear
    ● S08.121 Partial traumatic amputation of right ear
    ● S08.122 Partial traumatic amputation of left ear
    ● S08.129 Partial traumatic amputation of unspecified ear
● S08.8 Traumatic amputation of other parts of head
  ● S08.81 Traumatic amputation of nose
    ● S08.811 Complete traumatic amputation of nose
    ● S08.812 Partial traumatic amputation of nose
  X● S08.89 Traumatic amputation of other parts of head

● **S09 Other and unspecified injuries of head**

The appropriate 7th character is to be added to each code from category S09

A	initial encounter
D	subsequent encounter
S	sequela

X● **S09.0 Injury of blood vessels of head, not elsewhere classified**

Excludes1 injury of cerebral blood vessels (S06.-)
injury of precerebral blood vessels (S15.-)

● **S09.1 Injury of muscle and tendon of head**

Code also any associated open wound (S01.-)

Excludes2 sprain to joints and ligament of head (S03.9)

X● **S09.10 Unspecified injury of muscle and tendon of head**
Injury of muscle and tendon of head NOS

X● **S09.11 Strain of muscle and tendon of head**

X● **S09.12 Laceration of muscle and tendon of head**

X● **S09.19 Other specified injury of muscle and tendon of head**

● **S09.2 Traumatic rupture of ear drum**

Excludes1 traumatic rupture of ear drum due to blast injury (S09.31-)

X● **S09.20 Traumatic rupture of unspecified ear drum**

X● **S09.21 Traumatic rupture of right ear drum**

X● **S09.22 Traumatic rupture of left ear drum**

● **S09.3 Other specified and unspecified injury of middle and inner ear**

Excludes1 injury to ear NOS (S09.91-)

Excludes2 injury to external ear (S00.4-, S01.3-, S08.1-)

● **S09.30 Unspecified injury of middle and inner ear**

● **S09.301 Unspecified injury of right middle and inner ear**

● **S09.302 Unspecified injury of left middle and inner ear**

● **S09.309 Unspecified injury of unspecified middle and inner ear**

● **S09.31 Primary blast injury of ear**
Blast injury of ear NOS

● **S09.311 Primary blast injury of right ear**

● **S09.312 Primary blast injury of left ear**

● **S09.313 Primary blast injury of ear, bilateral**

● **S09.319 Primary blast injury of unspecified ear**

● **S09.39 Other specified injury of middle and inner ear**
Secondary blast injury to ear

● **S09.391 Other specified injury of right middle and inner ear**

● **S09.392 Other specified injury of left middle and inner ear**

● **S09.399 Other specified injury of unspecified middle and inner ear**

X● **S09.8 Other specified injuries of head**

● **S09.9 Unspecified injury of face and head**

X● **S09.90 Unspecified injury of head**
Head injury NOS

Excludes1 brain injury NOS (S06.9-)
head injury NOS with loss of consciousness (S06.9-)
intracranial injury NOS (S06.9-)

X● **S09.91 Unspecified injury of ear**
Injury of ear NOS

X● **S09.92 Unspecified injury of nose**
Injury of nose NOS

X● **S09.93 Unspecified injury of face**
Injury of face NOS

INJURIES TO THE NECK (S10-S19)

Includes injuries of nape
injuries of supraclavicular region
injuries of throat

Excludes2 burns and corrosions (T20-T32)
effects of foreign body in esophagus (T18.1)
effects of foreign body in larynx (T17.3)
effects of foreign body in pharynx (T17.2)
effects of foreign body in trachea (T17.4)
frostbite (T33-T34)
insect bite or sting, venomous (T63.4)

● **S10 Superficial injury of neck**

The appropriate 7th character is to be added to each code from category S10

A	initial encounter
D	subsequent encounter
S	sequela

X● **S10.0 Contusion of throat**
Contusion of cervical esophagus
Contusion of larynx
Contusion of pharynx
Contusion of trachea

● **S10.1 Other and unspecified superficial injuries of throat**

X● **S10.10 Unspecified superficial injuries of throat**

X● **S10.11 Abrasion of throat**

X● **S10.12 Blister (nonthermal) of throat**

X● **S10.14 External constriction of part of throat**

X● **S10.15 Superficial foreign body of throat**
Splinter in the throat

X● **S10.16 Insect bite (nonvenomous) of throat**

X● **S10.17 Other superficial bite of throat**

Excludes1 open bite of throat (S11.85)

● **S10.8 Superficial injury of other specified parts of neck**

X● **S10.80 Unspecified superficial injury of other specified part of neck**

X● **S10.81 Abrasion of other specified part of neck**

X● **S10.82 Blister (nonthermal) of other specified part of neck**

X● **S10.83 Contusion of other specified part of neck**

X● **S10.84 External constriction of other specified part of neck**

X● **S10.85 Superficial foreign body of other specified part of neck**
Splinter in other part of neck

X● **S10.86 Insect bite of other specified part of neck**

X● **S10.87 Other superficial bite of other specified part of neck**

Excludes1 open bite of other specified parts of neck (S11.85)

● **S10.9 Superficial injury of unspecified part of neck**

X● **S10.90 Unspecified superficial injury of unspecified part of neck**

X● **S10.91 Abrasion of unspecified part of neck**

X● **S10.92 Blister (nonthermal) of unspecified part of neck**

X● **S10.93 Contusion of unspecified part of neck**

X● **S10.94 External constriction of unspecified part of neck**

X● **S10.95 Superficial foreign body of unspecified part of neck**

X● **S10.96 Insect bite of unspecified part of neck**

X● **S10.97 Other superficial bite of unspecified part of neck**

S11 Open wound of neck

Code also any associated:
spinal cord injury (S14.0, S14.1-)
wound infection

Excludes2 open fracture of vertebra (S12.- with 7th character B)

The appropriate 7th character is to be added to each code from category S11

A	initial encounter
D	subsequent encounter
S	sequela

S11.0 Open wound of larynx and trachea

S11.01 Open wound of larynx

Excludes2 open wound of vocal cord (S11.03)

S11.011 Laceration without foreign body of larynx

S11.012 Laceration with foreign body of larynx

S11.013 Puncture wound without foreign body of larynx

S11.014 Puncture wound with foreign body of larynx

S11.015 Open bite of larynx
Bite of larynx NOS

S11.019 Unspecified open wound of larynx

S11.02 Open wound of trachea
Open wound of cervical trachea
Open wound of trachea NOS

Excludes2 open wound of thoracic trachea (S27.5-)

S11.021 Laceration without foreign body of trachea

S11.022 Laceration with foreign body of trachea

S11.023 Puncture wound without foreign body of trachea

S11.024 Puncture wound with foreign body of trachea

S11.025 Open bite of trachea
Bite of trachea NOS

S11.029 Unspecified open wound of trachea

S11.03 Open wound of vocal cord

S11.031 Laceration without foreign body of vocal cord

S11.032 Laceration with foreign body of vocal cord

S11.033 Puncture wound without foreign body of vocal cord

S11.034 Puncture wound with foreign body of vocal cord

S11.035 Open bite of vocal cord
Bite of vocal cord NOS

S11.039 Unspecified open wound of vocal cord

S11.1 Open wound of thyroid gland

X **S11.10 Unspecified open wound of thyroid gland**

X **S11.11 Laceration without foreign body of thyroid gland**

X **S11.12 Laceration with foreign body of thyroid gland**

X **S11.13 Puncture wound without foreign body of thyroid gland**

X **S11.14 Puncture wound with foreign body of thyroid gland**

X **S11.15 Open bite of thyroid gland**
Bite of thyroid gland NOS

S11.2 Open wound of pharynx and cervical esophagus

Excludes1 open wound of esophagus NOS (S27.8-)

X **S11.20 Unspecified open wound of pharynx and cervical esophagus**

X **S11.21 Laceration without foreign body of pharynx and cervical esophagus**

X **S11.22 Laceration with foreign body of pharynx and cervical esophagus**

X **S11.23 Puncture wound without foreign body of pharynx and cervical esophagus**

X **S11.24 Puncture wound with foreign body of pharynx and cervical esophagus**

X **S11.25 Open bite of pharynx and cervical esophagus**
Bite of pharynx and cervical esophagus NOS

S11.8 Open wound of other specified parts of neck

X **S11.80 Unspecified open specified wound of other part of neck**

X **S11.81 Laceration without foreign body of other specified part of neck**

X **S11.82 Laceration with foreign body of other specified part of neck**

X **S11.83 Puncture wound without foreign body of other specified part of neck**

X **S11.84 Puncture wound with foreign body of other specified part of neck**

X **S11.85 Open bite of other specified part of neck**
Bite of other part of neck NOS

Excludes1 superficial bite of other specified part of neck (S10.87)

X **S11.89 Other open wound of other part of neck**

S11.9 Open wound of unspecified part of neck

X **S11.90 Unspecified open wound of unspecified part of neck**

X **S11.91 Laceration without foreign body of unspecified part of neck**

X **S11.92 Laceration with foreign body of unspecified part of neck**

X **S11.93 Puncture wound without foreign body of unspecified part of neck**

X **S11.94 Puncture wound with foreign body of unspecified part of neck**

X **S11.95 Open bite of unspecified part of neck**
Bite of neck NOS

Excludes1 superficial bite of neck (S10.97)

S12 Fracture of cervical vertebra and other parts of neck

Note: A fracture not indicated as displaced or nondisplaced should be coded to displaced

A fracture not indicated as open or closed should be coded to closed

Includes fracture of cervical neural arch
fracture of cervical spine
fracture of cervical spinous process
fracture of cervical transverse process
fracture of cervical vertebral arch
fracture of neck

Code first any associated cervical spinal cord injury (S14.Ø, S14.1-)

The appropriate 7th character is to be added to all codes from subcategories S12.Ø-S12.6

A	initial encounter for closed fracture
B	initial encounter for open fracture
D	subsequent encounter for fracture with routine healing
G	subsequent encounter for fracture with delayed healing
K	subsequent encounter for fracture with nonunion
S	sequela

S12.Ø Fracture of first cervical vertebra
Atlas

S12.ØØ Unspecified fracture of first cervical vertebra

S12.ØØØ Unspecified displaced fracture of first cervical vertebra A, B

S12.ØØ1 Unspecified nondisplaced fracture of first cervical vertebra A, B

X **S12.Ø1 Stable burst fracture of first cervical vertebra** A, B

X **S12.Ø2 Unstable burst fracture of first cervical vertebra** A, B

S12.Ø3 Posterior arch fracture of first cervical vertebra

S12.Ø3Ø Displaced posterior arch fracture of first cervical vertebra A, B

S12.Ø31 Nondisplaced posterior arch fracture of first cervical vertebra A, B

S12.Ø4 Lateral mass fracture of first cervical vertebra

S12.Ø4Ø Displaced lateral mass fracture of first cervical vertebra A, B

S12.Ø41 Nondisplaced lateral mass fracture of first cervical vertebra A, B

S12.Ø9 Other fracture of first cervical vertebra

S12.Ø9Ø Other displaced fracture of first cervical vertebra A, B

S12.Ø91 Other nondisplaced fracture of first cervical vertebra A, B

S12.1 Fracture of second cervical vertebra
Axis

S12.1Ø Unspecified fracture of second cervical vertebra

S12.1ØØ Unspecified displaced fracture of second cervical vertebra A, B

S12.1Ø1 Unspecified nondisplaced fracture of second cervical vertebra A, B

S12.11 Type II dens fracture

S12.11Ø Anterior displaced Type II dens fracture A, B

S12.111 Posterior displaced Type II dens fracture A, B

S12.112 Nondisplaced Type II dens fracture A, B

S12.12 Other dens fracture

S12.12Ø Other displaced dens fracture A, B

S12.121 Other nondisplaced dens fracture A, B

S12.13 Unspecified traumatic spondylolisthesis of second cervical vertebra

S12.13Ø Unspecified traumatic displaced spondylolisthesis of second cervical vertebra A, B

S12.131 Unspecified traumatic nondisplaced spondylolisthesis of second cervical vertebra A, B

X **S12.14 Type III traumatic spondylolisthesis of second cervical vertebra** A, B

S12.15 Other traumatic spondylolisthesis of second cervical vertebra

S12.15Ø Other traumatic displaced spondylolisthesis of second cervical vertebra A, B

S12.151 Other traumatic nondisplaced spondylolisthesis of second cervical vertebra A, B

S12.19 Other fracture of second cervical vertebra

S12.19Ø Other displaced fracture of second cervical vertebra A, B

S12.191 Other nondisplaced fracture of second cervical vertebra A, B

S12.2 Fracture of third cervical vertebra

S12.2Ø Unspecified fracture of third cervical vertebra

S12.2ØØ Unspecified displaced fracture of third cervical vertebra A, B

S12.2Ø1 Unspecified nondisplaced fracture of third cervical vertebra A, B

S12.23 Unspecified traumatic spondylolisthesis of third cervical vertebra

S12.23Ø Unspecified traumatic displaced spondylolisthesis of third cervical vertebra A, B

S12.231 Unspecified traumatic nondisplaced spondylolisthesis of third cervical vertebra A, B

X **S12.24 Type III traumatic spondylolisthesis of third cervical vertebra** A, B

S12.25 Other traumatic spondylolisthesis of third cervical vertebra

S12.25Ø Other traumatic displaced spondylolisthesis of third cervical vertebra A, B

S12.251 Other traumatic nondisplaced spondylolisthesis of third cervical vertebra A, B

S12.29 Other fracture of third cervical vertebra

S12.29Ø Other displaced fracture of third cervical vertebra A, B

S12.291 Other nondisplaced fracture of third cervical vertebra A, B

S12.3 Fracture of fourth cervical vertebra

S12.3Ø Unspecified fracture of fourth cervical vertebra

S12.3ØØ Unspecified displaced fracture of fourth cervical vertebra A, B

S12.3Ø1 Unspecified nondisplaced fracture of fourth cervical vertebra A, B

S12.33 Unspecified traumatic spondylolisthesis of fourth cervical vertebra

S12.33Ø Unspecified traumatic displaced spondylolisthesis of fourth cervical vertebra A, B

S12.331 Unspecified traumatic nondisplaced spondylolisthesis of fourth cervical vertebra A, B

X **S12.34 Type III traumatic spondylolisthesis of fourth cervical vertebra** A, B

S12.35 Other traumatic spondylolisthesis of fourth cervical vertebra
S12.350 Other traumatic displaced spondylolisthesis of fourth cervical vertebra A, B
S12.351 Other traumatic nondisplaced spondylolisthesis of fourth cervical vertebra A, B
S12.39 Other fracture of fourth cervical vertebra
S12.390 Other displaced fracture of fourth cervical vertebra A, B
S12.391 Other nondisplaced fracture of fourth cervical vertebra A, B
S12.4 Fracture of fifth cervical vertebra
S12.40 Unspecified fracture of fifth cervical vertebra
S12.400 Unspecified displaced fracture of fifth cervical vertebra A, B
S12.401 Unspecified nondisplaced fracture of fifth cervical vertebra A, B
S12.43 Unspecified traumatic spondylolisthesis of fifth cervical vertebra
S12.430 Unspecified traumatic displaced spondylolisthesis of fifth cervical vertebra A, B
S12.431 Unspecified traumatic nondisplaced spondylolisthesis of fifth cervical vertebra A, B
X S12.44 Type III traumatic spondylolisthesis of fifth cervical vertebra A, B
S12.45 Other traumatic spondylolisthesis of fifth cervical vertebra
S12.450 Other traumatic displaced spondylolisthesis of fifth cervical vertebra A, B
S12.451 Other traumatic nondisplaced spondylolisthesis of fifth cervical vertebra A, B
S12.49 Other fracture of fifth cervical vertebra
S12.490 Other displaced fracture of fifth cervical vertebra A, B
S12.491 Other nondisplaced fracture of fifth cervical vertebra A, B
S12.5 Fracture of sixth cervical vertebra
S12.50 Unspecified fracture of sixth cervical vertebra
S12.500 Unspecified displaced fracture of sixth cervical vertebra A, B
S12.501 Unspecified nondisplaced fracture of sixth cervical vertebra A, B
S12.53 Unspecified traumatic spondylolisthesis of sixth cervical vertebra
S12.530 Unspecified traumatic displaced spondylolisthesis of sixth cervical vertebra A, B
S12.531 Unspecified traumatic nondisplaced spondylolisthesis of sixth cervical vertebra A, B
X S12.54 Type III traumatic spondylolisthesis of sixth cervical vertebra A, B
S12.55 Other traumatic spondylolisthesis of sixth cervical vertebra
S12.550 Other traumatic displaced spondylolisthesis of sixth cervical vertebra A, B
S12.551 Other traumatic nondisplaced spondylolisthesis of sixth cervical vertebra A, B
S12.59 Other fracture of sixth cervical vertebra
S12.590 Other displaced fracture of sixth cervical vertebra A, B
S12.591 Other nondisplaced fracture of sixth cervical vertebra A, B
S12.6 Fracture of seventh cervical vertebra
S12.60 Unspecified fracture of seventh cervical vertebra
S12.600 Unspecified displaced fracture of seventh cervical vertebra A, B
S12.601 Unspecified nondisplaced fracture of seventh cervical vertebra A, B
S12.63 Unspecified traumatic spondylolisthesis of seventh cervical vertebra
S12.630 Unspecified traumatic displaced spondylolisthesis of seventh cervical vertebra A, B
S12.631 Unspecified traumatic nondisplaced spondylolisthesis of seventh cervical vertebra A, B
X S12.64 Type III traumatic spondylolisthesis of seventh cervical vertebra A, B
S12.65 Other traumatic spondylolisthesis of seventh cervical vertebra
S12.650 Other traumatic displaced spondylolisthesis of seventh cervical vertebra A, B
S12.651 Other traumatic nondisplaced spondylolisthesis of seventh cervical vertebra A, B
S12.69 Other fracture of seventh cervical vertebra
S12.690 Other displaced fracture of seventh cervical vertebra A, B
S12.691 Other nondisplaced fracture of seventh cervical vertebra A, B
X S12.8 Fracture of other parts of neck A

Hyoid bone
Larynx
Thyroid cartilage
Trachea

The appropriate 7th character is to be added to code S12.8

A	initial encounter
D	subsequent encounter
S	sequela

X S12.9 Fracture of neck, unspecified A

Fracture of neck NOS
Fracture of cervical spine NOS
Fracture of cervical vertebra NOS

The appropriate 7th character is to be added to code S12.9

A	initial encounter
D	subsequent encounter
S	sequela

S13 Dislocation and sprain of joints and ligaments at neck level

Includes avulsion of joint or ligament at neck level
laceration of cartilage, joint or ligament at neck level
sprain of cartilage, joint or ligament at neck level
traumatic hemarthrosis of joint or ligament at neck level
traumatic rupture of joint or ligament at neck level
traumatic subluxation of joint or ligament at neck level
traumatic tear of joint or ligament at neck level

Code also any associated open wound

Excludes2 strain of muscle or tendon at neck level (S16.1)

The appropriate 7th character is to be added to each code from category S13

A	initial encounter
D	subsequent encounter
S	sequela

X **S13.0 Traumatic rupture of cervical intervertebral disc**

Excludes1 rupture or displacement (nontraumatic) of cervical intervertebral disc NOS (M50.-)

S13.1 Subluxation and dislocation of cervical vertebrae

Code also any associated:
open wound of neck (S11.-)
spinal cord injury (S14.1-)

Excludes2 fracture of cervical vertebrae (S12.0-S12.3-)

S13.10 Subluxation and dislocation of unspecified cervical vertebrae

S13.100 Subluxation of unspecified cervical vertebrae

S13.101 Dislocation of unspecified cervical vertebrae

S13.11 Subluxation and dislocation of C0/C1 cervical vertebrae

Subluxation and dislocation of atlantooccipital joint
Subluxation and dislocation of atloidooccipital joint
Subluxation and dislocation of occipitoatloid joint

S13.110 Subluxation of C0/C1 cervical vertebrae

S13.111 Dislocation of C0/C1 cervical vertebrae

S13.12 Subluxation and dislocation of C1/C2 cervical vertebrae

Subluxation and dislocation of atlantoaxial joint

S13.120 Subluxation of C1/C2 cervical vertebrae

S13.121 Dislocation of C1/C2 cervical vertebrae

S13.13 Subluxation and dislocation of C2/C3 cervical vertebrae

S13.130 Subluxation of C2/C3 cervical vertebrae

S13.131 Dislocation of C2/C3 cervical vertebrae

S13.14 Subluxation and dislocation of C3/C4 cervical vertebrae

S13.140 Subluxation of C3/C4 cervical vertebrae

S13.141 Dislocation of C3/C4 cervical vertebrae

S13.15 Subluxation and dislocation of C4/C5 cervical vertebrae

S13.150 Subluxation of C4/C5 cervical vertebrae

S13.151 Dislocation of C4/C5 cervical vertebrae

S13.16 Subluxation and dislocation of C5/C6 cervical vertebrae

S13.160 Subluxation of C5/C6 cervical vertebrae

S13.161 Dislocation of C5/C6 cervical vertebrae

S13.17 Subluxation and dislocation of C6/C7 cervical vertebrae

S13.170 Subluxation of C6/C7 cervical vertebrae

S13.171 Dislocation of C6/C7 cervical vertebrae

S13.18 Subluxation and dislocation of C7/T1 cervical vertebrae

S13.180 Subluxation of C7/T1 cervical vertebrae

S13.181 Dislocation of C7/T1 cervical vertebrae

S13.2 Dislocation of other and unspecified parts of neck

X **S13.20 Dislocation of unspecified parts of neck**

X **S13.29 Dislocation of other parts of neck**

X **S13.4 Sprain of ligaments of cervical spine**

Sprain of anterior longitudinal (ligament), cervical
Sprain of atlanto-axial (joints)
Sprain of atlanto-occipital (joints)
Whiplash injury of cervical spine

X **S13.5 Sprain of thyroid region**

Sprain of cricoarytenoid (joint) (ligament)
Sprain of cricothyroid (joint) (ligament)
Sprain of thyroid cartilage

X **S13.8 Sprain of joints and ligaments of other parts of neck**

X **S13.9 Sprain of joints and ligaments of unspecified parts of neck**

S14 Injury of nerves and spinal cord at neck level

Note: Code to highest level of cervical cord injury

Code also any associated:
fracture of cervical vertebra (S12.0--S12.6.-)
open wound of neck (S11.-)
transient paralysis (R29.5)

The appropriate 7th character is to be added to each code from category S14

A	initial encounter
D	subsequent encounter
S	sequela

X **S14.0 Concussion and edema of cervical spinal cord A, D, S**

S14.1 Other and unspecified injuries of cervical spinal cord

S14.10 Unspecified injury of cervical spinal cord

S14.101 Unspecified injury at C1 level of cervical spinal cord A, D, S

S14.102 Unspecified injury at C2 level of cervical spinal cord A, D, S

S14.103 Unspecified injury at C3 level of cervical spinal cord A, D, S

S14.104 Unspecified injury at C4 level of cervical spinal cord A, D, S

S14.105 Unspecified injury at C5 level of cervical spinal cord A, D, S

S14.106 Unspecified injury at C6 level of cervical spinal cord A, D, S

S14.107 Unspecified injury at C7 level of cervical spinal cord A, D, S

S14.108 Unspecified injury at C8 level of cervical spinal cord A, D, S

S14.109 Unspecified injury at unspecified level of cervical spinal cord A, D, S

Injury of cervical spinal cord NOS

S14.11 **Complete lesion** of cervical spinal cord
- S14.111 Complete lesion at **C1 level** of cervical spinal cord A, D, S
- S14.112 Complete lesion at **C2 level** of cervical spinal cord A, D, S
- S14.113 Complete lesion at **C3 level** of cervical spinal cord A, D, S
- S14.114 Complete lesion at **C4 level** of cervical spinal cord A, D, S
- S14.115 Complete lesion at **C5 level** of cervical spinal cord A, D, S
- S14.116 Complete lesion at **C6 level** of cervical spinal cord A, D, S
- S14.117 Complete lesion at **C7 level** of cervical spinal cord A, D, S
- S14.118 Complete lesion at **C8 level** of cervical spinal cord A, D, S
- S14.119 Complete lesion at **unspecified level** of cervical spinal cord A, D, S

S14.12 **Central cord syndrome** of cervical spinal cord
- S14.121 Central cord syndrome at **C1 level** of cervical spinal cord A, D, S
- S14.122 Central cord syndrome at **C2 level** of cervical spinal cord A, D, S
- S14.123 Central cord syndrome at **C3 level** of cervical spinal cord A, D, S
- S14.124 Central cord syndrome at **C4 level** of cervical spinal cord A, D, S
- S14.125 Central cord syndrome at **C5 level** of cervical spinal cord A, D, S
- S14.126 Central cord syndrome at **C6 level** of cervical spinal cord A, D, S
- S14.127 Central cord syndrome at **C7 level** of cervical spinal cord A, D, S
- S14.128 Central cord syndrome at **C8 level** of cervical spinal cord A, D, S
- S14.129 Central cord syndrome at **unspecified level** of cervical spinal cord A, D, S

S14.13 **Anterior cord syndrome** of cervical spinal cord
- S14.131 Anterior cord syndrome at **C1 level** of cervical spinal cord A, D, S
- S14.132 Anterior cord syndrome at **C2 level** of cervical spinal cord A, D, S
- S14.133 Anterior cord syndrome at **C3 level** of cervical spinal cord A, D, S
- S14.134 Anterior cord syndrome at **C4 level** of cervical spinal cord A, D, S
- S14.135 Anterior cord syndrome at **C5 level** of cervical spinal cord A, D, S
- S14.136 Anterior cord syndrome at **C6 level** of cervical spinal cord A, D, S
- S14.137 Anterior cord syndrome at **C7 level** of cervical spinal cord A, D, S
- S14.138 Anterior cord syndrome at **C8 level** of cervical spinal cord A, D, S
- S14.139 Anterior cord syndrome at **unspecified level** of cervical spinal cord A, D, S

S14.14 **Brown-Séquard syndrome** of cervical spinal cord
- S14.141 Brown-Séquard syndrome at **C1 level** of cervical spinal cord A, D, S
- S14.142 Brown-Séquard syndrome at **C2 level** of cervical spinal cord A, D, S
- S14.143 Brown-Séquard syndrome at **C3 level** of cervical spinal cord A, D, S
- S14.144 Brown-Séquard syndrome at **C4 level** of cervical spinal cord A, D, S
- S14.145 Brown-Séquard syndrome at **C5 level** of cervical spinal cord A, D, S
- S14.146 Brown-Séquard syndrome at **C6 level** of cervical spinal cord A, D, S
- S14.147 Brown-Séquard syndrome at **C7 level** of cervical spinal cord A, D, S
- S14.148 Brown-Séquard syndrome at **C8 level** of cervical spinal cord A, D, S
- S14.149 Brown-Séquard syndrome at **unspecified level** of cervical spinal cord A, D, S

S14.15 **Other incomplete lesions** of cervical spinal cord
Incomplete lesion of cervical spinal cord NOS
Posterior cord syndrome of cervical spinal cord
- S14.151 Other incomplete lesion at **C1 level** of cervical spinal cord A, D, S
- S14.152 Other incomplete lesion at **C2 level** of cervical spinal cord A, D, S
- S14.153 Other incomplete lesion at **C3 level** of cervical spinal cord A, D, S
- S14.154 Other incomplete lesion at **C4 level** of cervical spinal cord A, D, S
- S14.155 Other incomplete lesion at **C5 level** of cervical spinal cord A, D, S
- S14.156 Other incomplete lesion at **C6 level** of cervical spinal cord A, D, S
- S14.157 Other incomplete lesion at **C7 level** of cervical spinal cord A, D, S
- S14.158 Other incomplete lesion at **C8 level** of cervical spinal cord A, D, S
- S14.159 Other incomplete lesion at **unspecified level** of cervical spinal cord A, D, S

X S14.2 Injury of **nerve root** of cervical spine
X S14.3 Injury of **brachial plexus**
X S14.4 Injury of **peripheral nerves** of neck
X S14.5 Injury of **cervical sympathetic nerves**
X S14.8 Injury of **other specified** nerves of neck
X S14.9 Injury of **unspecified** nerves of neck

S15 Injury of blood vessels at neck level

Code also any associated open wound (S11.-)

The appropriate 7th character is to be added to each code from category S15

A	initial encounter
D	subsequent encounter
S	sequela

S15.Ø Injury of **carotid artery** of neck
Injury of carotid artery (common) (external) (internal, extracranial portion)
Injury of carotid artery NOS

Excludes1 injury of internal carotid artery, intracranial portion (SØ6.8)

S15.ØØ **Unspecified** injury of carotid artery
- S15.ØØ1 Unspecified injury of **right** carotid artery
- S15.ØØ2 Unspecified injury of **left** carotid artery
- S15.ØØ9 Unspecified injury of **unspecified** carotid artery

S15.Ø1 **Minor laceration** of carotid artery
Incomplete transection of carotid artery
Laceration of carotid artery NOS
Superficial laceration of carotid artery
- S15.Ø11 Minor laceration of **right** carotid artery
- S15.Ø12 Minor laceration of **left** carotid artery
- S15.Ø19 Minor laceration of **unspecified** carotid artery

S15.02 **Major laceration** of carotid artery
Complete transection of carotid artery
Traumatic rupture of carotid artery
S15.021 Major laceration of **right** carotid artery
S15.022 Major laceration of **left** carotid artery
S15.029 Major laceration of **unspecified** carotid artery
S15.09 **Other** specified injury of carotid artery
S15.091 Other specified injury of **right** carotid artery
S15.092 Other specified injury of **left** carotid artery
S15.099 Other specified injury of **unspecified** carotid artery
S15.1 Injury of **vertebral artery**
S15.10 **Unspecified** injury of vertebral artery
S15.101 Unspecified injury of **right** vertebral artery
S15.102 Unspecified injury of **left** vertebral artery
S15.109 Unspecified injury of **unspecified** vertebral artery
S15.11 **Minor laceration** of vertebral artery
Incomplete transection of vertebral artery
Laceration of vertebral artery NOS
Superficial laceration of vertebral artery
S15.111 Minor laceration of **right** vertebral artery
S15.112 Minor laceration of **left** vertebral artery
S15.119 Minor laceration of **unspecified** vertebral artery
S15.12 **Major laceration** of vertebral artery
Complete transection of vertebral artery
Traumatic rupture of vertebral artery
S15.121 Major laceration of **right** vertebral artery
S15.122 Major laceration of **left** vertebral artery
S15.129 Major laceration of **unspecified** vertebral artery
S15.19 **Other** specified injury of vertebral artery
S15.191 Other specified injury of **right** vertebral artery
S15.192 Other specified injury of **left** vertebral artery
S15.199 Other specified injury of **unspecified** vertebral artery
S15.2 Injury of **external jugular vein**
S15.20 **Unspecified** injury of external jugular vein
S15.201 Unspecified injury of **right** external jugular vein
S15.202 Unspecified injury of **left** external jugular vein
S15.209 Unspecified injury of **unspecified** external jugular vein
S15.21 **Minor laceration** of external jugular vein
Incomplete transection of external jugular vein
Laceration of external jugular vein NOS
Superficial laceration of external jugular vein
S15.211 Minor laceration of **right** external jugular vein
S15.212 Minor laceration of **left** external jugular vein
S15.219 Minor laceration of **unspecified** external jugular vein
S15.22 **Major laceration** of external jugular vein
Complete transection of external jugular vein
Traumatic rupture of external jugular vein
S15.221 Major laceration of **right** external jugular vein
S15.222 Major laceration of **left** external jugular vein
S15.229 Major laceration of **unspecified** external jugular vein
S15.29 **Other** specified injury of external jugular vein
S15.291 Other specified injury of **right** external jugular vein
S15.292 Other specified injury of **left** external jugular vein
S15.299 Other specified injury of **unspecified** external jugular vein
S15.3 Injury of **internal jugular vein**
S15.30 **Unspecified** injury of internal jugular vein
S15.301 Unspecified injury of **right** internal jugular vein
S15.302 Unspecified injury of **left** internal jugular vein
S15.309 Unspecified injury of **unspecified** internal jugular vein
S15.31 **Minor laceration** of internal jugular vein
Incomplete transection of internal jugular vein
Laceration of internal jugular vein NOS
Superficial laceration of internal jugular vein
S15.311 Minor laceration of **right** internal jugular vein
S15.312 Minor laceration of **left** internal jugular vein
S15.319 Minor laceration of **unspecified** internal jugular vein
S15.32 **Major laceration** of internal jugular vein
Complete transection of internal jugular vein
Traumatic rupture of internal jugular vein
S15.321 Major laceration of **right** internal jugular vein
S15.322 Major laceration of **left** internal jugular vein
S15.329 Major laceration of **unspecified** internal jugular vein
S15.39 **Other** specified injury of internal jugular vein
S15.391 Other specified injury of **right** internal jugular vein
S15.392 Other specified injury of **left** internal jugular vein
S15.399 Other specified injury of **unspecified** internal jugular vein
X S15.8 Injury of **other** specified blood vessels at neck level
X S15.9 Injury of **unspecified** blood vessel at neck level

S16 Injury of muscle, fascia and tendon at neck level
Code also any associated open wound (S11.-)
Excludes2 sprain of joint or ligament at neck level (S13.9)
The appropriate 7th character is to be added to each code from category S16

A	initial encounter
D	subsequent encounter
S	sequela

X S16.1 **Strain** of muscle, fascia and tendon at neck level
X S16.2 **Laceration** of muscle, fascia and tendon at neck level
X S16.8 **Other** specified injury of muscle, fascia and tendon at neck level
X S16.9 **Unspecified** injury of muscle, fascia and tendon at neck level

CHAPTER 19 (SØØ-T88)

● S17 Crushing injury of neck

Use additional code for all associated injuries, such as:
injury of blood vessels (S15.-)
open wound of neck (S11.-)
spinal cord injury (S14.0, S14.1-)
vertebral fracture (S12.0--S12.3-)

The appropriate 7th character is to be added to each code from category S17

A	initial encounter
D	subsequent encounter
S	sequela

X● S17.0 Crushing injury of larynx and trachea
X● S17.8 Crushing injury of other specified parts of neck
X● S17.9 Crushing injury of neck, part unspecified

● S19 Other and unspecified injuries of neck

The appropriate 7th character is to be added to each code from category S19

A	initial encounter
D	subsequent encounter
S	sequela

● S19.8 Other specified injuries of neck
X● S19.80 Other specified injuries of unspecified part of neck
X● S19.81 Other specified injuries of larynx
X● S19.82 Other specified injuries of cervical trachea
Excludes2 other specified injury of thoracic trachea (S27.5-)
X● S19.83 Other specified injuries of vocal cord
X● S19.84 Other specified injuries of thyroid gland
X● S19.85 Other specified injuries of pharynx and cervical esophagus
X● S19.89 Other specified injuries of other specified part of neck
X● S19.9 Unspecified injury of neck

INJURIES TO THE THORAX (S20-S29)

Includes injuries of breast
injuries of chest (wall)
injuries of interscapular area

Excludes2 burns and corrosions (T20-T32)
effects of foreign body in bronchus (T17.5)
effects of foreign body in esophagus (T18.1)
effects of foreign body in lung (T17.8)
effects of foreign body in trachea (T17.4)
frostbite (T33-T34)
injuries of axilla
injuries of clavicle
injuries of scapular region
injuries of shoulder
insect bite or sting, venomous (T63.4)

● S20 Superficial injury of thorax

The appropriate 7th character is to be added to each code from category S20

A	initial encounter
D	subsequent encounter
S	sequela

● S20.0 Contusion of breast
X● S20.00 Contusion of breast, unspecified breast
X● S20.01 Contusion of right breast
X● S20.02 Contusion of left breast

● S20.1 Other and unspecified superficial injuries of breast
● S20.10 Unspecified superficial injuries of breast
● S20.101 Unspecified superficial injuries of breast, right breast
● S20.102 Unspecified superficial injuries of breast, left breast
● S20.109 Unspecified superficial injuries of breast, unspecified breast
● S20.11 Abrasion of breast
● S20.111 Abrasion of breast, right breast
● S20.112 Abrasion of breast, left breast
● S20.119 Abrasion of breast, unspecified breast
● S20.12 Blister (nonthermal) of breast
● S20.121 Blister (nonthermal) of breast, right breast
● S20.122 Blister (nonthermal) of breast, left breast
● S20.129 Blister (nonthermal) of breast, unspecified breast
● S20.14 External constriction of part of breast
● S20.141 External constriction of part of breast, right breast
● S20.142 External constriction of part of breast, left breast
● S20.149 External constriction of part of breast, unspecified breast
● S20.15 Superficial foreign body of breast
Splinter in the breast
● S20.151 Superficial foreign body of breast, right breast
● S20.152 Superficial foreign body of breast, left breast
● S20.159 Superficial foreign body of breast, unspecified breast
● S20.16 Insect bite (nonvenomous) of breast
● S20.161 Insect bite (nonvenomous) of breast, right breast
● S20.162 Insect bite (nonvenomous) of breast, left breast
● S20.169 Insect bite (nonvenomous) of breast, unspecified breast
● S20.17 Other superficial bite of breast
Excludes1 open bite of breast (S21.05-)
● S20.171 Other superficial bite of breast, right breast
● S20.172 Other superficial bite of breast, left breast
● S20.179 Other superficial bite of breast, unspecified breast

● S20.2 Contusion of thorax
X● S20.20 Contusion of thorax, unspecified
● S20.21 Contusion of front wall of thorax
● S20.211 Contusion of right front wall of thorax
● S20.212 Contusion of left front wall of thorax
● S20.219 Contusion of unspecified front wall of thorax
● S20.22 Contusion of back wall of thorax
● S20.221 Contusion of right back wall of thorax
● S20.222 Contusion of left back wall of thorax
● S20.229 Contusion of unspecified back wall of thorax

S20.3 Other and unspecified superficial injuries of front wall of thorax
S20.30 Unspecified superficial injuries of front wall of thorax
S20.301 Unspecified superficial injuries of right front wall of thorax
S20.302 Unspecified superficial injuries of left front wall of thorax
S20.309 Unspecified superficial injuries of unspecified front wall of thorax
S20.31 Abrasion of front wall of thorax
S20.311 Abrasion of right front wall of thorax
S20.312 Abrasion of left front wall of thorax
S20.319 Abrasion of unspecified front wall of thorax
S20.32 Blister (nonthermal) of front wall of thorax
S20.321 Blister (nonthermal) of right front wall of thorax
S20.322 Blister (nonthermal) of left front wall of thorax
S20.329 Blister (nonthermal) of unspecified front wall of thorax
S20.34 External constriction of front wall of thorax
S20.341 External constriction of right front wall of thorax
S20.342 External constriction of left front wall of thorax
S20.349 External constriction of unspecified front wall of thorax
S20.35 Superficial foreign body of front wall of thorax
Splinter in front wall of thorax
S20.351 Superficial foreign body of right front wall of thorax
S20.352 Superficial foreign body of left front wall of thorax
S20.359 Superficial foreign body of unspecified front wall of thorax
S20.36 Insect bite (nonvenomous) of front wall of thorax
S20.361 Insect bite (nonvenomous) of right front wall of thorax
S20.362 Insect bite (nonvenomous) of left front wall of thorax
S20.369 Insect bite (nonvenomous) of unspecified front wall of thorax
S20.37 Other superficial bite of front wall of thorax
Excludes1 open bite of front wall of thorax (S21.14)
S20.371 Other superficial bite of right front wall of thorax
S20.372 Other superficial bite of left front wall of thorax
S20.379 Other superficial bite of unspecified front wall of thorax
S20.4 Other and unspecified superficial injuries of back wall of thorax
S20.40 Unspecified superficial injuries of back wall of thorax
S20.401 Unspecified superficial injuries of right back wall of thorax
S20.402 Unspecified superficial injuries of left back wall of thorax
S20.409 Unspecified superficial injuries of unspecified back wall of thorax
S20.41 Abrasion of back wall of thorax
S20.411 Abrasion of right back wall of thorax
S20.412 Abrasion of left back wall of thorax
S20.419 Abrasion of unspecified back wall of thorax
S20.42 Blister (nonthermal) of back wall of thorax
S20.421 Blister (nonthermal) of right back wall of thorax
S20.422 Blister (nonthermal) of left back wall of thorax
S20.429 Blister (nonthermal) of unspecified back wall of thorax
S20.44 External constriction of back wall of thorax
S20.441 External constriction of right back wall of thorax
S20.442 External constriction of left back wall of thorax
S20.449 External constriction of unspecified back wall of thorax
S20.45 Superficial foreign body of back wall of thorax
Splinter of back wall of thorax
S20.451 Superficial foreign body of right back wall of thorax
S20.452 Superficial foreign body of left back wall of thorax
S20.459 Superficial foreign body of unspecified back wall of thorax
S20.46 Insect bite (nonvenomous) of back wall of thorax
S20.461 Insect bite (nonvenomous) of right back wall of thorax
S20.462 Insect bite (nonvenomous) of left back wall of thorax
S20.469 Insect bite (nonvenomous) of unspecified back wall of thorax
S20.47 Other superficial bite of back wall of thorax
Excludes1 open bite of back wall of thorax (S21.24)
S20.471 Other superficial bite of right back wall of thorax
S20.472 Other superficial bite of left back wall of thorax
S20.479 Other superficial bite of unspecified back wall of thorax
S20.9 Superficial injury of unspecified parts of thorax
Excludes1 contusion of thorax NOS (S20.20)
X S20.90 Unspecified superficial injury of unspecified parts of thorax
Superficial injury of thoracic wall NOS
X S20.91 Abrasion of unspecified parts of thorax
X S20.92 Blister (nonthermal) of unspecified parts of thorax
X S20.94 External constriction of unspecified parts of thorax
X S20.95 Superficial foreign body of unspecified parts of thorax
Splinter in thorax NOS
X S20.96 Insect bite (nonvenomous) of unspecified parts of thorax
X S20.97 Other superficial bite of unspecified parts of thorax
Excludes1 open bite of thorax NOS (S21.95)

Item 19–1 Pneumothorax is a collection of gas (positive air pressure) in the pleural space, resulting in the lung collapsing. A **tension pneumothorax** is life-threatening and is a result of air in the pleural space causing a displacement in the mediastinal structures and cardiopulmonary function compromise. A **traumatic pneumothorax** results from blunt or penetrating injury that disrupts the parietal/visceral pleura. **Hemothorax** is blood or bloody fluid in the pleural cavity as a result of traumatic blood vessel rupture or inflammation of the lungs from pneumonia.

● S21 Open wound of thorax

Code also any associated injury such as:
- injury of heart (S26.-)
- injury of intrathoracic organs (S27.-)
- rib fracture (S22.3-, S22.4-)
- spinal cord injury (S24.Ø-, S24.1-)
- traumatic hemothorax (S27.1)
- traumatic hemopneumothorax (S27.3)
- traumatic pneumothorax (S27.Ø)
- wound infection

Excludes1 traumatic amputation (partial) of thorax (S28.1)

The appropriate 7th character is to be added to each code from category S21

A	initial encounter
D	subsequent encounter
S	sequela

● S21.Ø Open wound of breast
- ● S21.ØØ **Unspecified** open wound of breast
  - ● S21.ØØ1 **Unspecified** open wound of **right** breast
  - ● S21.ØØ2 **Unspecified** open wound of **left** breast
  - ● S21.ØØ9 **Unspecified** open wound of **unspecified** breast
- ● S21.Ø1 **Laceration without foreign body** of breast
  - ● S21.Ø11 Laceration without foreign body of **right** breast
  - ● S21.Ø12 Laceration without foreign body of **left** breast
  - ● S21.Ø19 Laceration without foreign body of **unspecified** breast
- ● S21.Ø2 **Laceration with foreign body** of breast
  - ● S21.Ø21 Laceration with foreign body of **right** breast
  - ● S21.Ø22 Laceration with foreign body of **left** breast
  - ● S21.Ø29 Laceration with foreign body of **unspecified** breast
- ● S21.Ø3 **Puncture wound without foreign body** of breast
  - ● S21.Ø31 Puncture wound without foreign body of **right** breast
  - ● S21.Ø32 Puncture wound without foreign body of **left** breast
  - ● S21.Ø39 Puncture wound without foreign body of **unspecified** breast
- ● S21.Ø4 **Puncture wound with foreign body** of breast
  - ● S21.Ø41 Puncture wound with foreign body of **right** breast
  - ● S21.Ø42 Puncture wound with foreign body of **left** breast
  - ● S21.Ø49 Puncture wound with foreign body of **unspecified** breast
- ● S21.Ø5 **Open bite** of breast

  Bite of breast NOS

  Excludes1 superficial bite of breast (S2Ø.17)
  - ● S21.Ø51 Open bite of **right** breast
  - ● S21.Ø52 Open bite of **left** breast
  - ● S21.Ø59 Open bite of **unspecified** breast

● S21.1 **Open wound of front wall of thorax without penetration into thoracic cavity**

Open wound of chest without penetration into thoracic cavity
- ● S21.1Ø **Unspecified open wound of front wall of thorax without penetration into thoracic cavity**
  - ● S21.1Ø1 **Unspecified** open wound of **right** front wall of thorax without penetration into thoracic cavity
  - ● S21.1Ø2 **Unspecified** open wound of **left** front wall of thorax without penetration into thoracic cavity
  - ● S21.1Ø9 **Unspecified** open wound of **unspecified** front wall of thorax without penetration into thoracic cavity
- ● S21.11 **Laceration without foreign body** of front wall of thorax without penetration into thoracic cavity
  - ● S21.111 Laceration without foreign body of **right** front wall of thorax without penetration into thoracic cavity
  - ● S21.112 Laceration without foreign body of **left** front wall of thorax without penetration into thoracic cavity
  - ● S21.119 Laceration without foreign body of **unspecified** front wall of thorax without penetration into thoracic cavity
- ● S21.12 **Laceration with foreign body** of front wall of thorax without penetration into thoracic cavity
  - ● S21.121 Laceration with foreign body of **right** front wall of thorax without penetration into thoracic cavity
  - ● S21.122 Laceration with foreign body of **left** front wall of thorax without penetration into thoracic cavity
  - ● S21.129 Laceration with foreign body of **unspecified** front wall of thorax without penetration into thoracic cavity
- ● S21.13 **Puncture wound without foreign body** of front wall of thorax without penetration into thoracic cavity
  - ● S21.131 Puncture wound without foreign body of **right** front wall of thorax without penetration into thoracic cavity
  - ● S21.132 Puncture wound without foreign body of **left** front wall of thorax without penetration into thoracic cavity
  - ● S21.139 Puncture wound without foreign body of **unspecified** front wall of thorax without penetration into thoracic cavity
- ● S21.14 **Puncture wound with foreign body** of front wall of thorax without penetration into thoracic cavity
  - ● S21.141 Puncture wound with foreign body of **right** front wall of thorax without penetration into thoracic cavity
  - ● S21.142 Puncture wound with foreign body of **left** front wall of thorax without penetration into thoracic cavity
  - ● S21.149 Puncture wound with foreign body of **unspecified** front wall of thorax without penetration into thoracic cavity

S21.15 **Open bite of front wall of thorax without penetration into thoracic cavity**
Bite of front wall of thorax NOS
Excludes1 superficial bite of front wall of thorax (S20.37)

S21.151 Open bite of **right** front wall of thorax without penetration into thoracic cavity

S21.152 Open bite of **left** front wall of thorax without penetration into thoracic cavity

S21.159 Open bite of **unspecified** front wall of thorax without penetration into thoracic cavity

S21.2 Open wound of **back wall** of thorax without penetration into thoracic cavity

S21.20 **Unspecified** open wound of back wall of thorax without penetration into thoracic cavity

S21.201 Unspecified open wound of **right** back wall of thorax without penetration into thoracic cavity

S21.202 Unspecified open wound of **left** back wall of thorax without penetration into thoracic cavity

S21.209 Unspecified open wound of **unspecified** back wall of thorax without penetration into thoracic cavity

S21.21 **Laceration without foreign body** of back wall of thorax without penetration into thoracic cavity

S21.211 Laceration without foreign body of **right** back wall of thorax without penetration into thoracic cavity

S21.212 Laceration without foreign body of **left** back wall of thorax without penetration into thoracic cavity

S21.219 Laceration without foreign body of **unspecified** back wall of thorax without penetration into thoracic cavity

S21.22 **Laceration with foreign body** of back wall of thorax without penetration into thoracic cavity

S21.221 Laceration with foreign body of **right** back wall of thorax without penetration into thoracic cavity

S21.222 Laceration with foreign body of **left** back wall of thorax without penetration into thoracic cavity

S21.229 Laceration with foreign body of **unspecified** back wall of thorax without penetration into thoracic cavity

S21.23 **Puncture wound without foreign body** of back wall of thorax without penetration into thoracic cavity

S21.231 Puncture wound without foreign body of **right** back wall of thorax without penetration into thoracic cavity

S21.232 Puncture wound without foreign body of **left** back wall of thorax without penetration into thoracic cavity

S21.239 Puncture wound without foreign body of **unspecified** back wall of thorax without penetration into thoracic cavity

S21.24 **Puncture wound with foreign body** of back wall of thorax without penetration into thoracic cavity

S21.241 Puncture wound with foreign body of **right** back wall of thorax without penetration into thoracic cavity

S21.242 Puncture wound with foreign body of **left** back wall of thorax without penetration into thoracic cavity

S21.249 Puncture wound with foreign body of **unspecified** back wall of thorax without penetration into thoracic cavity

S21.25 **Open bite** of back wall of thorax without penetration into thoracic cavity
Bite of back wall of thorax NOS
Excludes1 superficial bite of back wall of thorax (S20.47)

S21.251 Open bite of **right** back wall of thorax without penetration into thoracic cavity

S21.252 Open bite of **left** back wall of thorax without penetration into thoracic cavity

S21.259 Open bite of **unspecified** back wall of thorax without penetration into thoracic cavity

S21.3 Open wound of **front wall** of thorax **with penetration** into thoracic cavity
Open wound of chest with penetration into thoracic cavity

S21.30 **Unspecified** open wound of front wall of thorax with penetration into thoracic cavity

S21.301 Unspecified open wound of **right** front wall of thorax with penetration into thoracic cavity

S21.302 Unspecified open wound of **left** front wall of thorax with penetration into thoracic cavity

S21.309 Unspecified open wound of **unspecified** front wall of thorax with penetration into thoracic cavity

S21.31 **Laceration without foreign body** of front wall of thorax with penetration into thoracic cavity

S21.311 Laceration without foreign body of **right** front wall of thorax with penetration into thoracic cavity

S21.312 Laceration without foreign body of **left** front wall of thorax with penetration into thoracic cavity

S21.319 Laceration without foreign body of **unspecified** front wall of thorax with penetration into thoracic cavity

S21.32 **Laceration with foreign body** of front wall of thorax with penetration into thoracic cavity

S21.321 Laceration with foreign body of **right** front wall of thorax with penetration into thoracic cavity

S21.322 Laceration with foreign body of **left** front wall of thorax with penetration into thoracic cavity

S21.329 Laceration with foreign body of **unspecified** front wall of thorax with penetration into thoracic cavity

● S21.33 **Puncture wound without foreign body** of front wall of thorax with penetration into thoracic cavity
● S21.331 Puncture wound without foreign body of **right** front wall of thorax with penetration into thoracic cavity
● S21.332 Puncture wound without foreign body of **left** front wall of thorax with penetration into thoracic cavity
● S21.339 Puncture wound without foreign body of **unspecified** front wall of thorax with penetration into thoracic cavity
● S21.34 **Puncture wound with foreign body** of front wall of thorax with penetration into thoracic cavity
● S21.341 Puncture wound with foreign body of **right** front wall of thorax with penetration into thoracic cavity
● S21.342 Puncture wound with foreign body of **left** front wall of thorax with penetration into thoracic cavity
● S21.349 Puncture wound with foreign body of **unspecified** front wall of thorax with penetration into thoracic cavity
● S21.35 **Open bite** of front wall of thorax with penetration into thoracic cavity
Excludes1 superficial bite of front wall of thorax (S2Ø.37)
● S21.351 Open bite of **right** front wall of thorax with penetration into thoracic cavity
● S21.352 Open bite of **left** front wall of thorax with penetration into thoracic cavity
● S21.359 Open bite of **unspecified** front wall of thorax with penetration into thoracic cavity
● S21.4 Open wound of **back wall** of thorax with **penetration into thoracic cavity**
● S21.4Ø **Unspecified** open wound of back wall of thorax with penetration into thoracic cavity
● S21.4Ø1 Unspecified open wound of **right** back wall of thorax with penetration into thoracic cavity
● S21.4Ø2 Unspecified open wound of **left** back wall of thorax with penetration into thoracic cavity
● S21.4Ø9 Unspecified open wound of **unspecified** back wall of thorax with penetration into thoracic cavity
● S21.41 **Laceration without foreign body** of back wall of thorax with penetration into thoracic cavity
● S21.411 Laceration without foreign body of **right** back wall of thorax with penetration into thoracic cavity
● S21.412 Laceration without foreign body of **left** back wall of thorax with penetration into thoracic cavity
● S21.419 Laceration without foreign body of **unspecified** back wall of thorax with penetration into thoracic cavity
● S21.42 **Laceration with foreign body** of back wall of thorax with penetration into thoracic cavity
● S21.421 Laceration with foreign body of **right** back wall of thorax with penetration into thoracic cavity
● S21.422 Laceration with foreign body of **left** back wall of thorax with penetration into thoracic cavity
● S21.429 Laceration with foreign body of **unspecified** back wall of thorax with penetration into thoracic cavity
● S21.43 **Puncture wound without foreign body** of back wall of thorax with penetration into thoracic cavity
● S21.431 Puncture wound without foreign body of **right** back wall of thorax with penetration into thoracic cavity
● S21.432 Puncture wound without foreign body of **left** back wall of thorax with penetration into thoracic cavity
● S21.439 Puncture wound without foreign body of **unspecified** back wall of thorax with penetration into thoracic cavity
● S21.44 **Puncture wound with foreign body** of back wall of thorax with penetration into thoracic cavity
● S21.441 Puncture wound with foreign body of **right** back wall of thorax with penetration into thoracic cavity
● S21.442 Puncture wound with foreign body of **left** back wall of thorax with penetration into thoracic cavity
● S21.449 Puncture wound with foreign body of **unspecified** back wall of thorax with penetration into thoracic cavity
● S21.45 **Open bite** of back wall of thorax with penetration into thoracic cavity
Bite of back wall of thorax NOS
Excludes1 superficial bite of back wall of thorax (S2Ø.47)
● S21.451 Open bite of **right** back wall of thorax with penetration into thoracic cavity
● S21.452 Open bite of **left** back wall of thorax with penetration into thoracic cavity
● S21.459 Open bite of **unspecified** back wall of thorax with penetration into thoracic cavity
● S21.9 Open wound of **unspecified part** of thorax
Open wound of thoracic wall NOS
X● S21.9Ø **Unspecified** open wound of unspecified part of thorax
X● S21.91 **Laceration without foreign body** of unspecified part of thorax
X● S21.92 **Laceration with foreign body** of unspecified part of thorax
X● S21.93 **Puncture wound without foreign body** of unspecified part of thorax
X● S21.94 **Puncture wound with foreign body** of unspecified part of thorax
X● S21.95 **Open bite** of unspecified part of thorax
Excludes1 superficial bite of thorax (S2Ø.97)

S22 Fracture of rib(s), sternum and thoracic spine

Note: A fracture not indicated as displaced or nondisplaced should be coded to displaced

A fracture not indicated as open or closed should be coded to closed

Includes fracture of thoracic neural arch
fracture of thoracic spinous process
fracture of thoracic transverse process
fracture of thoracic vertebra
fracture of thoracic vertebral arch

Code first any associated:
injury of intrathoracic organ (S27.-)
spinal cord injury (S24.Ø-, S24.1-)

Excludes1 transection of thorax (S28.1)

Excludes2 fracture of clavicle (S42.Ø-)
fracture of scapula (S42.1-)

The appropriate 7th character is to be added to each code from category S22

A	initial encounter for closed fracture
B	initial encounter for open fracture
D	subsequent encounter for fracture with routine healing
G	subsequent encounter for fracture with delayed healing
K	subsequent encounter for fracture with nonunion
S	sequela

S22.Ø Fracture of thoracic vertebra

S22.ØØ Fracture of unspecified thoracic vertebra
- **S22.ØØØ Wedge compression fracture of unspecified thoracic vertebra** A, B
- **S22.ØØ1 Stable burst fracture of unspecified thoracic vertebra** A, B
- **S22.ØØ2 Unstable burst fracture of unspecified thoracic vertebra** A, B
- **S22.ØØ8 Other fracture of unspecified thoracic vertebra** A, B
- **S22.ØØ9 Unspecified fracture of unspecified thoracic vertebra** A, B

S22.Ø1 Fracture of first thoracic vertebra
- **S22.Ø1Ø Wedge compression fracture of first thoracic vertebra** A, B
- **S22.Ø11 Stable burst fracture of first thoracic vertebra** A, B
- **S22.Ø12 Unstable burst fracture of first thoracic vertebra** A, B
- **S22.Ø18 Other fracture of first thoracic vertebra** A, B
- **S22.Ø19 Unspecified fracture of first thoracic vertebra** A, B

S22.Ø2 Fracture of second thoracic vertebra
- **S22.Ø2Ø Wedge compression fracture of second thoracic vertebra** A, B
- **S22.Ø21 Stable burst fracture of second thoracic vertebra** A, B
- **S22.Ø22 Unstable burst fracture of second thoracic vertebra** A, B
- **S22.Ø28 Other fracture of second thoracic vertebra** A, B
- **S22.Ø29 Unspecified fracture of second thoracic vertebra** A, B

S22.Ø3 Fracture of third thoracic vertebra
- **S22.Ø3Ø Wedge compression fracture of third thoracic vertebra** A, B
- **S22.Ø31 Stable burst fracture of third thoracic vertebra** A, B
- **S22.Ø32 Unstable burst fracture of third thoracic vertebra** A, B
- **S22.Ø38 Other fracture of third thoracic vertebra** A, B
- **S22.Ø39 Unspecified fracture of third thoracic vertebra** A, B

S22.Ø4 Fracture of fourth thoracic vertebra
- **S22.Ø4Ø Wedge compression fracture of fourth thoracic vertebra** A, B
- **S22.Ø41 Stable burst fracture of fourth thoracic vertebra** A, B
- **S22.Ø42 Unstable burst fracture of fourth thoracic vertebra** A, B
- **S22.Ø48 Other fracture of fourth thoracic vertebra** A, B
- **S22.Ø49 Unspecified fracture of fourth thoracic vertebra** A, B

S22.Ø5 Fracture of T5-T6 vertebra
- **S22.Ø5Ø Wedge compression fracture of T5-T6 vertebra** A, B
- **S22.Ø51 Stable burst fracture of T5-T6 vertebra** A, B
- **S22.Ø52 Unstable burst fracture of T5-T6 vertebra** A, B
- **S22.Ø58 Other fracture of T5-T6 vertebra** A, B
- **S22.Ø59 Unspecified fracture of T5-T6 vertebra** A, B

S22.Ø6 Fracture of T7-T8 vertebra
- **S22.Ø6Ø Wedge compression fracture of T7-T8 vertebra** A, B
- **S22.Ø61 Stable burst fracture of T7-T8 vertebra** A, B
- **S22.Ø62 Unstable burst fracture of T7-T8 vertebra** A, B
- **S22.Ø68 Other fracture of T7-T8 thoracic vertebra** A, B
- **S22.Ø69 Unspecified fracture of T7-T8 vertebra** A, B

S22.Ø7 Fracture of T9-T1Ø vertebra
- **S22.Ø7Ø Wedge compression fracture of T9-T1Ø vertebra** A, B
- **S22.Ø71 Stable burst fracture of T9-T1Ø vertebra** A, B
- **S22.Ø72 Unstable burst fracture of T9-T1Ø vertebra** A, B
- **S22.Ø78 Other fracture of T9-T1Ø vertebra** A, B
- **S22.Ø79 Unspecified fracture of T9-T1Ø vertebra** A, B

S22.Ø8 Fracture of T11-T12 vertebra
- **S22.Ø8Ø Wedge compression fracture of T11-T12 vertebra** A, B
- **S22.Ø81 Stable burst fracture of T11-T12 vertebra** A, B
- **S22.Ø82 Unstable burst fracture of T11-T12 vertebra** A, B
- **S22.Ø88 Other fracture of T11-T12 vertebra** A, B
- **S22.Ø89 Unspecified fracture of T11-T12 vertebra** A, B

S22.2 Fracture of sternum
- X **S22.2Ø Unspecified fracture of sternum**
- X **S22.21 Fracture of manubrium**
- X **S22.22 Fracture of body of sternum**
- X **S22.23 Sternal manubrial dissociation**
- X **S22.24 Fracture of xiphoid process**

● S22.3 Fracture of one rib

X● S22.31 Fracture of one rib, right side

X● S22.32 Fracture of one rib, left side

X● S22.39 Fracture of one rib, unspecified side

● S22.4 Multiple fractures of ribs

Fractures of two or more ribs

Excludes1 flail chest (S22.5-)

X● S22.41 Multiple fractures of ribs, right side

X● S22.42 Multiple fractures of ribs, left side

X● S22.43 Multiple fractures of ribs, bilateral

X● S22.49 Multiple fractures of ribs, unspecified side

X● S22.5 Flail chest

Unstable chest due to sternum and/or rib fracture

X● S22.9 Fracture of bony thorax, part unspecified

● S23 Dislocation and sprain of joints and ligaments of thorax

Includes avulsion of joint or ligament of thorax
laceration of cartilage, joint or ligament of thorax
sprain of cartilage, joint or ligament of thorax
traumatic hemarthrosis of joint or ligament of thorax
traumatic rupture of joint or ligament of thorax
traumatic subluxation of joint or ligament of thorax
traumatic tear of joint or ligament of thorax

Code also any associated open wound

Excludes2 dislocation, sprain of sternoclavicular joint (S43.2, S43.6)
strain of muscle or tendon of thorax (S29.Ø1-)

The appropriate 7th character is to be added to each code from category S23

A	initial encounter
D	subsequent encounter
S	sequela

X● S23.Ø Traumatic rupture of thoracic intervertebral disc

Excludes1 rupture or displacement (nontraumatic) of thoracic intervertebral disc NOS (M51.- with fifth character 4)

● S23.1 Subluxation and dislocation of thoracic vertebra

Code also any associated
open wound of thorax (S21.-)
spinal cord injury (S24.Ø-, S24.1-)

Excludes2 fracture of thoracic vertebrae (S22.Ø-)

● S23.10 Subluxation and dislocation of unspecified thoracic vertebra

● S23.1ØØ Subluxation of unspecified thoracic vertebra

● S23.1Ø1 Dislocation of unspecified thoracic vertebra

● S23.11 Subluxation and dislocation of T1/T2 thoracic vertebra

● S23.11Ø Subluxation of T1/T2 thoracic vertebra

● S23.111 Dislocation of T1/T2 thoracic vertebra

● S23.12 Subluxation and dislocation of T2/T3-T3/T4 thoracic vertebra

● S23.12Ø Subluxation of T2/T3 thoracic vertebra

● S23.121 Dislocation of T2/T3 thoracic vertebra

● S23.122 Subluxation of T3/T4 thoracic vertebra

● S23.123 Dislocation of T3/T4 thoracic vertebra

● S23.13 Subluxation and dislocation of T4/T5-T5/T6 thoracic vertebra

● S23.13Ø Subluxation of T4/T5 thoracic vertebra

● S23.131 Dislocation of T4/T5 thoracic vertebra

● S23.132 Subluxation of T5/T6 thoracic vertebra

● S23.133 Dislocation of T5/T6 thoracic vertebra

● S23.14 Subluxation and dislocation of T6/T7-T7/T8 thoracic vertebra

● S23.14Ø Subluxation of T6/T7 thoracic vertebra

● S23.141 Dislocation of T6/T7 thoracic vertebra

● S23.142 Subluxation of T7/T8 thoracic vertebra

● S23.143 Dislocation of T7/T8 thoracic vertebra

● S23.15 Subluxation and dislocation of T8/T9-T9/T1Ø thoracic vertebra

● S23.15Ø Subluxation of T8/T9 thoracic vertebra

● S23.151 Dislocation of T8/T9 thoracic vertebra

● S23.152 Subluxation of T9/T1Ø thoracic vertebra

● S23.153 Dislocation of T9/T1Ø thoracic vertebra

● S23.16 Subluxation and dislocation of T1Ø/T11-T11/T12 thoracic vertebra

● S23.16Ø Subluxation of T1Ø/T11 thoracic vertebra

● S23.161 Dislocation of T1Ø/T11 thoracic vertebra

● S23.162 Subluxation of T11/T12 thoracic vertebra

● S23.163 Dislocation of T11/T12 thoracic vertebra

● S23.17 Subluxation and dislocation of T12/L1 thoracic vertebra

● S23.17Ø Subluxation of T12/L1 thoracic vertebra

● S23.171 Dislocation of T12/L1 thoracic vertebra

● S23.2 Dislocation of other and unspecified parts of thorax

X● S23.2Ø Dislocation of unspecified part of thorax

X● S23.29 Dislocation of other parts of thorax

X● S23.3 Sprain of ligaments of thoracic spine

● S23.4 Sprain of ribs and sternum

X● S23.41 Sprain of ribs

● S23.42 Sprain of sternum

● S23.42Ø Sprain of sternoclavicular (joint) (ligament)

● S23.421 Sprain of chondrosternal joint

● S23.428 Other sprain of sternum

● S23.429 Unspecified sprain of sternum

X● S23.8 Sprain of other specified parts of thorax

X● S23.9 Sprain of unspecified parts of thorax

S24 Injury of nerves and spinal cord at thorax level

Note: Code to highest level of thoracic spinal cord injury.

Injuries to the spinal cord (S24.0 and S24.1) refer to the cord level and not bone level injury, and can affect nerve roots at and below the level given.

Code also any associated:
- fracture of thoracic vertebra (S22.0-)
- open wound of thorax (S21.-)
- transient paralysis (R29.5)

Excludes2 injury of brachial plexus (S14.3)

The appropriate 7th character is to be added to each code from category S24

A	initial encounter
D	subsequent encounter
S	sequela

X **S24.0** Concussion and edema of thoracic spinal cord A, D, S

S24.1 Other and unspecified injuries of thoracic spinal cord

S24.10 Unspecified injury of thoracic spinal cord
- **S24.101** Unspecified injury at T1 level of thoracic spinal cord A, D, S
- **S24.102** Unspecified injury at T2-T6 level of thoracic spinal cord A, D, S
- **S24.103** Unspecified injury at T7-T10 level of thoracic spinal cord A, D, S
- **S24.104** Unspecified injury at T11-T12 level of thoracic spinal cord A, D, S
- **S24.109** Unspecified injury at unspecified level of thoracic spinal cord A, D, S
  Injury of thoracic spinal cord NOS

S24.11 Complete lesion of thoracic spinal cord
- **S24.111** Complete lesion at T1 level of thoracic spinal cord A, D, S
- **S24.112** Complete lesion at T2-T6 level of thoracic spinal cord A, D, S
- **S24.113** Complete lesion at T7-T10 level of thoracic spinal cord A, D, S
- **S24.114** Complete lesion at T11-T12 level of thoracic spinal cord A, D, S
- **S24.119** Complete lesion at unspecified level of thoracic spinal cord A, D, S

S24.13 Anterior cord syndrome of thoracic spinal cord
- **S24.131** Anterior cord syndrome at T1 level of thoracic spinal cord A, D, S
- **S24.132** Anterior cord syndrome at T2-T6 level of thoracic spinal cord A, D, S
- **S24.133** Anterior cord syndrome at T7-T10 level of thoracic spinal cord A, D, S
- **S24.134** Anterior cord syndrome at T11-T12 level of thoracic spinal cord A, D, S
- **S24.139** Anterior cord syndrome at unspecified level of thoracic spinal cord A, D, S

S24.14 Brown-Séquard syndrome of thoracic spinal cord
- **S24.141** Brown-Séquard syndrome at T1 level of thoracic spinal cord A, D, S
- **S24.142** Brown-Séquard syndrome at T2-T6 level of thoracic spinal cord A, D, S
- **S24.143** Brown-Séquard syndrome at T7-T10 level of thoracic spinal cord A, D, S
- **S24.144** Brown-Séquard syndrome at T11-T12 level of thoracic spinal cord A, D, S
- **S24.149** Brown-Séquard syndrome at unspecified level of thoracic spinal cord A, D, S

S24.15 Other incomplete lesions of thoracic spinal cord
Incomplete lesion of thoracic spinal cord NOS
Posterior cord syndrome of thoracic spinal cord
- **S24.151** Other incomplete lesion at T1 level of thoracic spinal cord A, D, S
- **S24.152** Other incomplete lesion at T2-T6 level of thoracic spinal cord A, D, S
- **S24.153** Other incomplete lesion at T7-T10 level of thoracic spinal cord A, D, S
- **S24.154** Other incomplete lesion at T11-T12 level of thoracic spinal cord A, D, S
- **S24.159** Other incomplete lesion at unspecified level of thoracic spinal cord A, D, S

X **S24.2** Injury of nerve root of thoracic spine

X **S24.3** Injury of peripheral nerves of thorax

X **S24.4** Injury of thoracic sympathetic nervous system
Injury of cardiac plexus
Injury of esophageal plexus
Injury of pulmonary plexus
Injury of stellate ganglion
Injury of thoracic sympathetic ganglion

X **S24.8** Injury of other specified nerves of thorax

X **S24.9** Injury of unspecified nerve of thorax

S25 Injury of blood vessels of thorax

The appropriate 7th character is to be added to each code from category S25

A	initial encounter
D	subsequent encounter
S	sequela

Code also any associated open wound (S21.-)

S25.0 Injury of thoracic aorta
Injury of aorta NOS
- X **S25.00** Unspecified injury of thoracic aorta
- X **S25.01** Minor laceration of thoracic aorta
  Incomplete transection of thoracic aorta
  Laceration of thoracic aorta NOS
  Superficial laceration of thoracic aorta
- X **S25.02** Major laceration of thoracic aorta
  Complete transection of thoracic aorta
  Traumatic rupture of thoracic aorta
- X **S25.09** Other specified injury of thoracic aorta

S25.1 Injury of innominate or subclavian artery

S25.10 Unspecified injury of innominate or subclavian artery
- **S25.101** Unspecified injury of right innominate or subclavian artery
- **S25.102** Unspecified injury of left innominate or subclavian artery
- **S25.109** Unspecified injury of unspecified innominate or subclavian artery

S25.11 Minor laceration of innominate or subclavian artery
Incomplete transection of innominate or subclavian artery
Laceration of innominate or subclavian artery NOS
Superficial laceration of innominate or subclavian artery
- **S25.111** Minor laceration of right innominate or subclavian artery
- **S25.112** Minor laceration of left innominate or subclavian artery
- **S25.119** Minor laceration of unspecified innominate or subclavian artery

CHAPTER 19 (S00-T88)

S25.12 **Major laceration of innominate or subclavian artery**
Complete transection of innominate or subclavian artery
Traumatic rupture of innominate or subclavian artery
S25.121 **Major laceration of right innominate or subclavian artery**
S25.122 **Major laceration of left innominate or subclavian artery**
S25.129 **Major laceration of unspecified innominate or subclavian artery**
S25.19 **Other specified injury of innominate or subclavian artery**
S25.191 **Other specified injury of right innominate or subclavian artery**
S25.192 **Other specified injury of left innominate or subclavian artery**
S25.199 **Other specified injury of unspecified innominate or subclavian artery**
S25.2 **Injury of superior vena cava**
Injury of vena cava NOS
X S25.20 **Unspecified injury of superior vena cava**
X S25.21 **Minor laceration of superior vena cava**
Incomplete transection of superior vena cava
Laceration of superior vena cava NOS
Superficial laceration of superior vena cava
X S25.22 **Major laceration of superior vena cava**
Complete transection of superior vena cava
Traumatic rupture of superior vena cava
X S25.29 **Other specified injury of superior vena cava**
S25.3 **Injury of innominate or subclavian vein**
S25.30 **Unspecified injury of innominate or subclavian vein**
S25.301 **Unspecified injury of right innominate or subclavian vein**
S25.302 **Unspecified injury of left innominate or subclavian vein**
S25.309 **Unspecified injury of unspecified innominate or subclavian vein**
S25.31 **Minor laceration of innominate or subclavian vein**
Incomplete transection of innominate or subclavian vein
Laceration of innominate or subclavian vein NOS
Superficial laceration of innominate or subclavian vein
S25.311 **Minor laceration of right innominate or subclavian vein**
S25.312 **Minor laceration of left innominate or subclavian vein**
S25.319 **Minor laceration of unspecified innominate or subclavian vein**
S25.32 **Major laceration of innominate or subclavian vein**
Complete transection of innominate or subclavian vein
Traumatic rupture of innominate or subclavian vein
S25.321 **Major laceration of right innominate or subclavian vein**
S25.322 **Major laceration of left innominate or subclavian vein**
S25.329 **Major laceration of unspecified innominate or subclavian vein**
S25.39 **Other specified injury of innominate or subclavian vein**
S25.391 **Other specified injury of right innominate or subclavian vein**
S25.392 **Other specified injury of left innominate or subclavian vein**
S25.399 **Other specified injury of unspecified innominate or subclavian vein**
S25.4 **Injury of pulmonary blood vessels**
S25.40 **Unspecified injury of pulmonary blood vessels**
S25.401 **Unspecified injury of right pulmonary blood vessels**
S25.402 **Unspecified injury of left pulmonary blood vessels**
S25.409 **Unspecified injury of unspecified pulmonary blood vessels**
S25.41 **Minor laceration of pulmonary blood vessels**
Incomplete transection of pulmonary blood vessels
Laceration of pulmonary blood vessels NOS
Superficial laceration of pulmonary blood vessels
S25.411 **Minor laceration of right pulmonary blood vessels**
S25.412 **Minor laceration of left pulmonary blood vessels**
S25.419 **Minor laceration of unspecified pulmonary blood vessels**
S25.42 **Major laceration of pulmonary blood vessels**
Complete transection of pulmonary blood vessels
Traumatic rupture of pulmonary blood vessels
S25.421 **Major laceration of right pulmonary blood vessels**
S25.422 **Major laceration of left pulmonary blood vessels**
S25.429 **Major laceration of unspecified pulmonary blood vessels**
S25.49 **Other specified injury of pulmonary blood vessels**
S25.491 **Other specified injury of right pulmonary blood vessels**
S25.492 **Other specified injury of left pulmonary blood vessels**
S25.499 **Other specified injury of unspecified pulmonary blood vessels**
S25.5 **Injury of intercostal blood vessels**
S25.50 **Unspecified injury of intercostal blood vessels**
S25.501 **Unspecified injury of intercostal blood vessels, right side**
S25.502 **Unspecified injury of intercostal blood vessels, left side**
S25.509 **Unspecified injury of intercostal blood vessels, unspecified side**
S25.51 **Laceration of intercostal blood vessels**
S25.511 **Laceration of intercostal blood vessels, right side**
S25.512 **Laceration of intercostal blood vessels, left side**
S25.519 **Laceration of intercostal blood vessels, unspecified side**
S25.59 **Other specified injury of intercostal blood vessels**
S25.591 **Other specified injury of intercostal blood vessels, right side**
S25.592 **Other specified injury of intercostal blood vessels, left side**
S25.599 **Other specified injury of intercostal blood vessels, unspecified side**

S25.8 **Injury of other blood vessels of thorax**
Injury of azygos vein
Injury of mammary artery or vein

S25.80 **Unspecified injury of other blood vessels of thorax**

S25.801 **Unspecified injury of other blood vessels of thorax, right side**

S25.802 **Unspecified injury of other blood vessels of thorax, left side**

S25.809 **Unspecified injury of other blood vessels of thorax, unspecified side**

S25.81 **Laceration of other blood vessels of thorax**

S25.811 **Laceration of other blood vessels of thorax, right side**

S25.812 **Laceration of other blood vessels of thorax, left side**

S25.819 **Laceration of other blood vessels of thorax, unspecified side**

S25.89 **Other specified injury of other blood vessels of thorax**

S25.891 **Other specified injury of other blood vessels of thorax, right side**

S25.892 **Other specified injury of other blood vessels of thorax, left side**

S25.899 **Other specified injury of other blood vessels of thorax, unspecified side**

S25.9 **Injury of unspecified blood vessel of thorax**

X **S25.90** **Unspecified injury of unspecified blood vessel of thorax**

X **S25.91** **Laceration of unspecified blood vessel of thorax**

X **S25.99** **Other specified injury of unspecified blood vessel of thorax**

S26 **Injury of heart**
The appropriate 7th character is to be added to each code from category S26

A	initial encounter
D	subsequent encounter
S	sequela

Code also any associated:
open wound of thorax (S21.-)
traumatic hemopneumothorax (S27.2)
traumatic hemothorax (S27.1)
traumatic pneumothorax (S27.Ø)

S26.Ø **Injury of heart with hemopericardium**
Hemopericardium: effusion of blood within pericardium

X **S26.ØØ** **Unspecified injury of heart with hemopericardium**

X **S26.Ø1** **Contusion of heart with hemopericardium**

S26.Ø2 **Laceration of heart with hemopericardium**

S26.Ø2Ø **Mild laceration of heart with hemopericardium**
Laceration of heart without penetration of heart chamber

S26.Ø21 **Moderate laceration of heart with hemopericardium**
Laceration of heart with penetration of heart chamber

S26.Ø22 **Major laceration of heart with hemopericardium**
Laceration of heart with penetration of multiple heart chambers

X **S26.Ø9** **Other injury of heart with hemopericardium**

S26.1 **Injury of heart without hemopericardium**
Hemopericardium: effusion of blood within pericardium

X **S26.1Ø** **Unspecified injury of heart without hemopericardium**

X **S26.11** **Contusion of heart without hemopericardium**

X **S26.12** **Laceration of heart without hemopericardium**

X **S26.19** **Other injury of heart without hemopericardium**

Item 19-2 Pneumothorax is a collection of gas (positive air pressure) in the pleural space resulting in the lung collapsing. A **tension pneumothorax** is life-threatening and is a result of air in the pleural space causing a displacement in the mediastinal structures and cardiopulmonary function compromise. A **traumatic pneumothorax** results from blunt or penetrating injury that disrupts the parietal/visceral pleura. **Hemothorax** is blood or bloody fluid in the pleural cavity as a result of traumatic blood vessel rupture or inflammation of the lungs from pneumonia.

S26.9 **Injury of heart, unspecified with or without hemopericardium**
Hemopericardium: effusion of blood within pericardium

X **S26.9Ø** **Unspecified injury of heart, unspecified with or without hemopericardium**

X **S26.91** **Contusion of heart, unspecified with or without hemopericardium**

X **S26.92** **Laceration of heart, unspecified with or without hemopericardium**
Laceration of heart NOS

X **S26.99** **Other injury of heart, unspecified with or without hemopericardium**

S27 **Injury of other and unspecified intrathoracic organs**
Code also any associated open wound of thorax (S21.-)
Excludes2 injury of cervical esophagus (S1Ø-S19)
injury of trachea (cervical) (S1Ø-S19)
The appropriate 7th character is to be added to each code from category S27

A	initial encounter
D	subsequent encounter
S	sequela

X **S27.Ø** Traumatic **pneumothorax**
Excludes1 spontaneous pneumothorax (J93.-)

X **S27.1** Traumatic **hemothorax**

X **S27.2** Traumatic **hemopneumothorax**

S27.3 Other and unspecified injuries of **lung**

S27.3Ø Unspecified injury of lung

S27.3Ø1 Unspecified injury of lung, **unilateral**

S27.3Ø2 Unspecified injury of lung, **bilateral**

S27.3Ø9 Unspecified injury of lung, **unspecified**

S27.31 Primary blast injury of lung
Blast injury of lung NOS

S27.311 Primary blast injury of lung, **unilateral**

S27.312 Primary blast injury of lung, **bilateral**

S27.319 Primary blast injury of lung, **unspecified**

S27.32 Contusion of lung

S27.321 Contusion of lung, **unilateral**

S27.322 Contusion of lung, **bilateral**

S27.329 Contusion of lung, **unspecified**

S27.33 Laceration of lung

S27.331 Laceration of lung, **unilateral**

S27.332 Laceration of lung, **bilateral**

S27.339 Laceration of lung, **unspecified**

S27.39 Other injuries of lung
Secondary blast injury of lung

S27.391 Other injuries of lung, **unilateral**

S27.392 Other injuries of lung, **bilateral**

S27.399 Other injuries of lung, **unspecified**

CHAPTER 19 (SØØ-T88)

- S27.4 Injury of bronchus
  - S27.40 Unspecified injury of bronchus
    - S27.401 Unspecified injury of bronchus, unilateral
    - S27.402 Unspecified injury of bronchus, bilateral
    - S27.409 Unspecified injury of bronchus, unspecified
  - S27.41 Primary blast injury of bronchus
    Blast injury of bronchus NOS
    - S27.411 Primary blast injury of bronchus, unilateral
    - S27.412 Primary blast injury of bronchus, bilateral
    - S27.419 Primary blast injury of bronchus, unspecified
  - S27.42 Contusion of bronchus
    - S27.421 Contusion of bronchus, unilateral
    - S27.422 Contusion of bronchus, bilateral
    - S27.429 Contusion of bronchus, unspecified
  - S27.43 Laceration of bronchus
    - S27.431 Laceration of bronchus, unilateral
    - S27.432 Laceration of bronchus, bilateral
    - S27.439 Laceration of bronchus, unspecified
  - S27.49 Other injury of bronchus
    Secondary blast injury of bronchus
    - S27.491 Other injury of bronchus, unilateral
    - S27.492 Other injury of bronchus, bilateral
    - S27.499 Other injury of bronchus, unspecified
- S27.5 Injury of thoracic trachea
  - X S27.50 Unspecified injury of thoracic trachea
  - X S27.51 Primary blast injury of thoracic trachea
    Blast injury of thoracic trachea NOS
  - X S27.52 Contusion of thoracic trachea
  - X S27.53 Laceration of thoracic trachea
  - X S27.59 Other injury of thoracic trachea
    Secondary blast injury of thoracic trachea
- S27.6 Injury of pleura
  - X S27.60 Unspecified injury of pleura
  - X S27.63 Laceration of pleura
  - X S27.69 Other injury of pleura
- S27.8 Injury of other specified intrathoracic organs
  - S27.80 Injury of diaphragm
    - S27.802 Contusion of diaphragm
    - S27.803 Laceration of diaphragm
    - S27.808 Other injury of diaphragm
    - S27.809 Unspecified injury of diaphragm
  - S27.81 Injury of esophagus (thoracic part)
    - S27.812 Contusion of esophagus (thoracic part)
    - S27.813 Laceration of esophagus (thoracic part)
    - S27.818 Other injury of esophagus (thoracic part)
    - S27.819 Unspecified injury of esophagus (thoracic part)
  - S27.89 Injury of other specified intrathoracic organs
    Injury of lymphatic thoracic duct
    Injury of thymus gland
    - S27.892 Contusion of other specified intrathoracic organs
    - S27.893 Laceration of other specified intrathoracic organs
    - S27.898 Other injury of other specified intrathoracic organs
    - S27.899 Unspecified injury of other specified intrathoracic organs
- X S27.9 Injury of unspecified intrathoracic organ

S28 Crushing injury of thorax, and traumatic amputation of part of thorax

The appropriate 7th character is to be added to each code from category S28

A	initial encounter
D	subsequent encounter
S	sequela

- X S28.0 Crushed chest
  Use additional code for all associated injuries
  Excludes1 flail chest (S22.5)
- X S28.1 Traumatic amputation (partial) of part of thorax, except breast
- S28.2 Traumatic amputation of breast
  - S28.21 Complete traumatic amputation of breast
    Traumatic amputation of breast NOS
    - S28.211 Complete traumatic amputation of right breast
    - S28.212 Complete traumatic amputation of left breast
    - S28.219 Complete traumatic amputation of unspecified breast
  - S28.22 Partial traumatic amputation of breast
    - S28.221 Partial traumatic amputation of right breast
    - S28.222 Partial traumatic amputation of left breast
    - S28.229 Partial traumatic amputation of unspecified breast

S29 Other and unspecified injuries of thorax

Code also any associated open wound (S21.-)

The appropriate 7th character is to be added to each code from category S29

A	initial encounter
D	subsequent encounter
S	sequela

- S29.0 Injury of muscle and tendon at thorax level
  - S29.00 Unspecified injury of muscle and tendon of thorax
    - S29.001 Unspecified injury of muscle and tendon of front wall of thorax
    - S29.002 Unspecified injury of muscle and tendon of back wall of thorax
    - S29.009 Unspecified injury of muscle and tendon of unspecified wall of thorax
  - S29.01 Strain of muscle and tendon of thorax
    - S29.011 Strain of muscle and tendon of front wall of thorax
    - S29.012 Strain of muscle and tendon of back wall of thorax
    - S29.019 Strain of muscle and tendon of unspecified wall of thorax
  - S29.02 Laceration of muscle and tendon of thorax
    - S29.021 Laceration of muscle and tendon of front wall of thorax
    - S29.022 Laceration of muscle and tendon of back wall of thorax
    - S29.029 Laceration of muscle and tendon of unspecified wall of thorax
  - S29.09 Other injury of muscle and tendon of thorax
    - S29.091 Other injury of muscle and tendon of front wall of thorax
    - S29.092 Other injury of muscle and tendon of back wall of thorax
    - S29.099 Other injury of muscle and tendon of unspecified wall of thorax
- X S29.8 Other specified injuries of thorax
- X S29.9 Unspecified injury of thorax

INJURIES TO THE ABDOMEN, LOWER BACK, LUMBAR SPINE PELVIS AND EXTERNAL GENITALS (S30-S39)

Includes injuries to the abdominal wall
injuries to the anus
injuries to the buttock
injuries to the external genitalia
injuries to the flank
injuries to the groin

Excludes2 burns and corrosions (T20-T32)
effects of foreign body in anus and rectum (T18.5)
effects of foreign body in genitourinary tract (T19.-)
effects of foreign body in stomach, small intestine and colon (T18.2-T18.4)
frostbite (T33-T34)
insect bite or sting, venomous (T63.4)

● **S30 Superficial injury of abdomen, lower back, pelvis and external genitals**

Excludes2 superficial injury of hip (S70.-)

The appropriate 7th character is to be added to each code from category S30

A	initial encounter
D	subsequent encounter
S	sequela

X● **S30.0 Contusion of lower back and pelvis**
Contusion of buttock

X● **S30.1 Contusion of abdominal wall**
Contusion of flank
Contusion of groin

● **S30.2 Contusion of external genital organs**

● **S30.20 Contusion of unspecified external genital organ**

● **S30.201 Contusion of unspecified external genital organ, male ♂**

● **S30.202 Contusion of unspecified external genital organ, female ♀**

X● **S30.21 Contusion of penis ♂**

X● **S30.22 Contusion of scrotum and testes ♂**

X● **S30.23 Contusion of vagina and vulva ♀**

X● **S30.3 Contusion of anus**

● **S30.8 Other superficial injuries of abdomen, lower back, pelvis and external genitals**

● **S30.81 Abrasion of abdomen, lower back, pelvis and external genitals**

● **S30.810 Abrasion of lower back and pelvis**

● **S30.811 Abrasion of abdominal wall**

● **S30.812 Abrasion of penis ♂**

● **S30.813 Abrasion of scrotum and testes ♂**

● **S30.814 Abrasion of vagina and vulva ♀**

● **S30.815 Abrasion of unspecified external genital organs, male ♂**

● **S30.816 Abrasion of unspecified external genital organs, female ♀**

● **S30.817 Abrasion of anus**

● **S30.82 Blister (nonthermal) of abdomen, lower back, pelvis and external genitals**

● **S30.820 Blister (nonthermal) of lower back and pelvis**

● **S30.821 Blister (nonthermal) of abdominal wall**

● **S30.822 Blister (nonthermal) of penis ♂**

● **S30.823 Blister (nonthermal) of scrotum and testes ♂**

● **S30.824 Blister (nonthermal) of vagina and vulva ♀**

● **S30.825 Blister (nonthermal) of unspecified external genital organs, male ♂**

● **S30.826 Blister (nonthermal) of unspecified external genital organs, female ♀**

● **S30.827 Blister (nonthermal) of anus**

● **S30.84 External constriction of abdomen, lower back, pelvis and external genitals**

● **S30.840 External constriction of lower back and pelvis**

● **S30.841 External constriction of abdominal wall**

● **S30.842 External constriction of penis ♂**
Hair tourniquet syndrome of penis
Use additional cause code to identify the constricting item (W49.0-)

● **S30.843 External constriction of scrotum and testes ♂**

● **S30.844 External constriction of vagina and vulva ♀**

● **S30.845 External constriction of unspecified external genital organs, male ♂**

● **S30.846 External constriction of unspecified external genital organs, female ♀**

● **S30.85 Superficial foreign body of abdomen, lower back, pelvis and external genitals**
Splinter in the abdomen, lower back, pelvis and external genitals

● **S30.850 Superficial foreign body of lower back and pelvis**

● **S30.851 Superficial foreign body of abdominal wall**

● **S30.852 Superficial foreign body of penis ♂**

● **S30.853 Superficial foreign body of scrotum and testes ♂**

● **S30.854 Superficial foreign body of vagina and vulva ♀**

● **S30.855 Superficial foreign body of unspecified external genital organs, male ♂**

● **S30.856 Superficial foreign body of unspecified external genital organs, female ♀**

● **S30.857 Superficial foreign body of anus**

● **S30.86 Insect bite (nonvenomous) of abdomen, lower back, pelvis and external genitals**

● **S30.860 Insect bite (nonvenomous) of lower back and pelvis**

● **S30.861 Insect bite (nonvenomous) of abdominal wall**

● **S30.862 Insect bite (nonvenomous) of penis ♂**

● **S30.863 Insect bite (nonvenomous) of scrotum and testes ♂**

● **S30.864 Insect bite (nonvenomous) of vagina and vulva ♀**

● **S30.865 Insect bite (nonvenomous) of unspecified external genital organs, male ♂**

● **S30.866 Insect bite (nonvenomous) of unspecified external genital organs, female ♀**

● **S30.867 Insect bite (nonvenomous) of anus**

● S30.87 **Other superficial bite** of abdomen, lower back, pelvis and external genitals
Excludes1 open bite of abdomen, lower back, pelvis and external genitals (S31.05, S31.15, S31.25, S31.35, S31.45, S31.55)
● S30.870 Other superficial bite of **lower back and pelvis**
● S30.871 Other superficial bite of **abdominal wall**
● S30.872 Other superficial bite of **penis** ♂
● S30.873 Other superficial bite of **scrotum and testes** ♂
● S30.874 Other superficial bite of **vagina and vulva** ♀
● S30.875 Other superficial bite of **unspecified** external genital organs, **male** ♂
● S30.876 Other superficial bite of **unspecified** external genital organs, **female** ♀
● S30.877 Other superficial bite of **anus**
● S30.9 **Unspecified** superficial injury of abdomen, lower back, pelvis and external genitals
X● S30.91 Unspecified superficial injury of **lower back and pelvis**
X● S30.92 Unspecified superficial injury of **abdominal wall**
X● S30.93 Unspecified superficial injury of **penis** ♂
X● S30.94 Unspecified superficial injury of **scrotum and testes** ♂
X● S30.95 Unspecified superficial injury of **vagina and vulva** ♀
X● S30.96 Unspecified superficial injury of **unspecified** external genital organs, **male** ♂
X● S30.97 Unspecified superficial injury of **unspecified** external genital organs, **female** ♀
X● S30.98 Unspecified superficial injury of **anus**

● S31 Open wound of abdomen, lower back, pelvis and external genitals
Code also any associated:
spinal cord injury (S24.0, S24.1-, S34.0-, S34.1-)
wound infection
Excludes1 traumatic amputation of part of abdomen, lower back and pelvis (S38.2-, S38.3)
Excludes2 open wound of hip (S71.00-S71.02)
open fracture of pelvis (S32.1--S32.9 with 7th character B)
The appropriate 7th character is to be added to each code from category S31

A	initial encounter
D	subsequent encounter
S	sequela

● S31.0 Open wound of **lower back and pelvis**
● S31.00 **Unspecified** open wound of lower back and pelvis
● S31.000 Unspecified open wound of lower back and pelvis **without penetration** into retroperitoneum
Unspecified open wound of lower back and pelvis NOS
● S31.001 Unspecified open wound of lower back and pelvis **with penetration** into retroperitoneum
● S31.01 **Laceration without foreign body** of lower back and pelvis
● S31.010 Laceration without foreign body of lower back and pelvis **without penetration** into retroperitoneum
Laceration without foreign body of lower back and pelvis NOS
● S31.011 Laceration without foreign body of lower back and pelvis **with penetration** into retroperitoneum
● S31.02 **Laceration with foreign body** of lower back and pelvis
● S31.020 Laceration with foreign body of lower back and pelvis **without penetration** into retroperitoneum
Laceration with foreign body of lower back and pelvis NOS
● S31.021 Laceration with foreign body of lower back and pelvis **with penetration** into retroperitoneum
● S31.03 **Puncture wound without foreign body** of lower back and pelvis
● S31.030 Puncture wound without foreign body of lower back and pelvis **without penetration** into retroperitoneum
Puncture wound without foreign body of lower back and pelvis NOS
● S31.031 Puncture wound without foreign body of lower back and pelvis **with penetration** into retroperitoneum
● S31.04 **Puncture wound with foreign body** of lower back and pelvis
● S31.040 Puncture wound with foreign body of lower back and pelvis **without penetration** into retroperitoneum
Puncture wound with foreign body of lower back and pelvis NOS
● S31.041 Puncture wound with foreign body of lower back and pelvis **with penetration** into retroperitoneum
● S31.05 **Open bite** of lower back and pelvis
Bite of lower back and pelvis NOS
Excludes1 superficial bite of lower back and pelvis (S30.860, S30.870)
● S31.050 Open bite of lower back and pelvis **without penetration** into retroperitoneum
Open bite of lower back and pelvis NOS
● S31.051 Open bite of lower back and pelvis **with penetration** into retroperitoneum
● S31.1 Open wound of **abdominal wall without penetration** into peritoneal cavity
Open wound of abdominal wall NOS
Excludes2 open wound of abdominal wall with penetration into peritoneal cavity (S31.6-)
● S31.10 **Unspecified** open wound of abdominal wall without penetration into peritoneal cavity
● S31.100 Unspecified open wound of abdominal wall, **right upper** quadrant without penetration into peritoneal cavity
● S31.101 Unspecified open wound of abdominal wall, **left upper** quadrant without penetration into peritoneal cavity

- S31.102 **Unspecified** open wound of abdominal wall, **epigastric region** without penetration into peritoneal cavity
- S31.103 **Unspecified** open wound of abdominal wall, **right lower** quadrant without penetration into peritoneal cavity
- S31.104 **Unspecified** open wound of abdominal wall, **left lower** quadrant without penetration into peritoneal cavity
- S31.105 **Unspecified** open wound of abdominal wall, **periumbilic region** without penetration into peritoneal cavity
- S31.109 **Unspecified** open wound of abdominal wall, **unspecified** quadrant without penetration into peritoneal cavity
  Unspecified open wound of abdominal wall NOS

S31.11 **Laceration without foreign** body of abdominal wall without penetration into peritoneal cavity

- S31.110 Laceration without foreign body of abdominal wall, **right upper** quadrant without penetration into peritoneal cavity
- S31.111 Laceration without foreign body of abdominal wall, **left upper** quadrant without penetration into peritoneal cavity
- S31.112 Laceration without foreign body of abdominal wall, **epigastric region** without penetration into peritoneal cavity
- S31.113 Laceration without foreign body of abdominal wall, **right lower** quadrant without penetration into peritoneal cavity
- S31.114 Laceration without foreign body of abdominal wall, **left lower** quadrant without penetration into peritoneal cavity
- S31.115 Laceration without foreign body of abdominal wall, **periumbilic region** without penetration into peritoneal cavity
- S31.119 Laceration without foreign body of abdominal wall, **unspecified** quadrant without penetration into peritoneal cavity

S31.12 **Laceration with foreign body** of abdominal wall without penetration into peritoneal cavity

- S31.120 Laceration of abdominal wall with foreign body, **right upper** quadrant without penetration into peritoneal cavity
- S31.121 Laceration of abdominal wall with foreign body, **left upper** quadrant without penetration into peritoneal cavity
- S31.122 Laceration of abdominal wall with foreign body, **epigastric region** without penetration into peritoneal cavity
- S31.123 Laceration of abdominal wall with foreign body, **right lower** quadrant without penetration into peritoneal cavity
- S31.124 Laceration of abdominal wall with foreign body, **left lower** quadrant without penetration into peritoneal cavity
- S31.125 Laceration of abdominal wall with foreign body, **periumbilic region** without penetration into peritoneal cavity
- S31.129 Laceration of abdominal wall with foreign body, **unspecified** quadrant without penetration into peritoneal cavity

S31.13 **Puncture wound** of abdominal wall **without foreign body** without penetration into peritoneal cavity

- S31.130 Puncture wound of abdominal wall without foreign body, **right upper** quadrant without penetration into peritoneal cavity
- S31.131 Puncture wound of abdominal wall without foreign body, **left upper** quadrant without penetration into peritoneal cavity
- S31.132 Puncture wound of abdominal wall without foreign body, **epigastric region** without penetration into peritoneal cavity
- S31.133 Puncture wound of abdominal wall without foreign body, **right lower** quadrant without penetration into peritoneal cavity
- S31.134 Puncture wound of abdominal wall without foreign body, **left lower** quadrant without penetration into peritoneal cavity
- S31.135 Puncture wound of abdominal wall without foreign body, **periumbilic region** without penetration into peritoneal cavity
- S31.139 Puncture wound of abdominal wall without foreign body, **unspecified** quadrant without penetration into peritoneal cavity

S31.14 **Puncture wound** of abdominal wall **with foreign body** without penetration into peritoneal cavity

- S31.140 Puncture wound of abdominal wall with foreign body, **right upper** quadrant without penetration into peritoneal cavity
- S31.141 Puncture wound of abdominal wall with foreign body, **left upper** quadrant without penetration into peritoneal cavity
- S31.142 Puncture wound of abdominal wall with foreign body, **epigastric region** without penetration into peritoneal cavity
- S31.143 Puncture wound of abdominal wall with foreign body, **right lower** quadrant without penetration into peritoneal cavity
- S31.144 Puncture wound of abdominal wall with foreign body, **left lower** quadrant without penetration into peritoneal cavity
- S31.145 Puncture wound of abdominal wall with foreign body, **periumbilic region** without penetration into peritoneal cavity
- S31.149 Puncture wound of abdominal wall with foreign body, **unspecified** quadrant without penetration into peritoneal cavity

CHAPTER 19 (SØ-T88)

● S31.15 **Open bite of abdominal wall without penetration into peritoneal cavity**
Bite of abdominal wall NOS
Excludes1 superficial bite of abdominal wall (S30.871)

● S31.150 **Open bite of abdominal wall, right upper quadrant without penetration into peritoneal cavity**

● S31.151 **Open bite of abdominal wall, left upper quadrant without penetration into peritoneal cavity**

● S31.152 **Open bite of abdominal wall, epigastric region without penetration into peritoneal cavity**

● S31.153 **Open bite of abdominal wall, right lower quadrant without penetration into peritoneal cavity**

● S31.154 **Open bite of abdominal wall, left lower quadrant without penetration into peritoneal cavity**

● S31.155 **Open bite of abdominal wall, periumbilic region without penetration into peritoneal cavity**

● S31.159 **Open bite of abdominal wall, unspecified quadrant without penetration into peritoneal cavity**

● S31.2 Open wound of penis

X● S31.20 **Unspecified open wound of penis** ♂

X● S31.21 **Laceration without foreign body of penis** ♂

X● S31.22 **Laceration with foreign body of penis** ♂

X● S31.23 **Puncture wound without foreign body of penis** ♂

X● S31.24 **Puncture wound with foreign body of penis** ♂

X● S31.25 **Open bite of penis** ♂
Bite of penis NOS
Excludes1 superficial bite of penis (S30.862, S30.872)

● S31.3 Open wound of scrotum and testes

X● S31.30 **Unspecified open wound of scrotum and testes** ♂

X● S31.31 **Laceration without foreign body of scrotum and testes** ♂

X● S31.32 **Laceration with foreign body of scrotum and testes** ♂

X● S31.33 **Puncture wound without foreign body of scrotum and testes** ♂

X● S31.34 **Puncture wound with foreign body of scrotum and testes** ♂

X● S31.35 **Open bite of scrotum and testes** ♂
Bite of scrotum and testes NOS
Excludes1 superficial bite of scrotum and testes (S30.863, S30.873)

● S31.4 Open wound of vagina and vulva
Excludes1 injury to vagina and vulva during delivery (O70.-, O71.4)

X● S31.40 **Unspecified open wound of vagina and vulva** ♀

X● S31.41 **Laceration without foreign body of vagina and vulva** ♀

X● S31.42 **Laceration with foreign body of vagina and vulva** ♀

X● S31.43 **Puncture wound without foreign body of vagina and vulva** ♀

X● S31.44 **Puncture wound with foreign body of vagina and vulva** ♀

X● S31.45 **Open bite of vagina and vulva** ♀
Bite of vagina and vulva NOS
Excludes1 superficial bite of vagina and vulva (S30.864, S30.874)

● S31.5 Open wound of unspecified external genital organs
Excludes1 traumatic amputation of external genital organs (S38.21, S38.22)

● S31.50 **Unspecified open wound of unspecified external genital organs**

● S31.501 **Unspecified open wound of unspecified external genital organs, male** ♂

● S31.502 **Unspecified open wound of unspecified external genital organs, female** ♀

● S31.51 **Laceration without foreign body of unspecified external genital organs**

● S31.511 **Laceration without foreign body of unspecified external genital organs, male** ♂

● S31.512 **Laceration without foreign body of unspecified external genital organs, female** ♀

● S31.52 **Laceration with foreign body of unspecified external genital organs**

● S31.521 **Laceration with foreign body of unspecified external genital organs, male** ♂

● S31.522 **Laceration with foreign body of unspecified external genital organs, female** ♀

● S31.53 **Puncture wound without foreign body of unspecified external genital organs**

● S31.531 **Puncture wound without foreign body of unspecified external genital organs, male** ♂

● S31.532 **Puncture wound without foreign body of unspecified external genital organs, female** ♀

● S31.54 **Puncture wound with foreign body of unspecified external genital organs**

● S31.541 **Puncture wound with foreign body of unspecified external genital organs, male** ♂

● S31.542 **Puncture wound with foreign body of unspecified external genital organs, female** ♀

● S31.55 **Open bite of unspecified external genital organs**
Bite of unspecified external genital organs NOS
Excludes1 superficial bite of unspecified external genital organs (S30.865, S30.866, S30.875, S30.876)

● S31.551 **Open bite of unspecified external genital organs, male** ♂

● S31.552 **Open bite of unspecified external genital organs, female** ♀

● S31.6 Open wound of abdominal wall with penetration into peritoneal cavity

● S31.60 **Unspecified open wound of abdominal wall with penetration into peritoneal cavity**

● S31.600 **Unspecified open wound of abdominal wall, right upper quadrant with penetration into peritoneal cavity**

● S31.601 **Unspecified open wound of abdominal wall, left upper quadrant with penetration into peritoneal cavity**

● S31.602 **Unspecified open wound of abdominal wall, epigastric region with penetration into peritoneal cavity**

- S31.6Ø3 Unspecified open wound of abdominal wall, **right lower** quadrant with penetration into peritoneal cavity
- S31.6Ø4 Unspecified open wound of abdominal wall, **left lower** quadrant with penetration into peritoneal cavity
- S31.6Ø5 Unspecified open wound of abdominal wall, **periumbilic region** with penetration into peritoneal cavity
- S31.6Ø9 Unspecified open wound of abdominal wall, **unspecified** quadrant with penetration into peritoneal cavity

S31.61 **Laceration without foreign body** of abdominal wall with penetration into peritoneal cavity

- S31.61Ø Laceration without foreign body of abdominal wall, **right upper** quadrant with penetration into peritoneal cavity
- S31.611 Laceration without foreign body of abdominal wall, **left upper** quadrant with penetration into peritoneal cavity
- S31.612 Laceration without foreign body of abdominal wall, **epigastric region** with penetration into peritoneal cavity
- S31.613 Laceration without foreign body of abdominal wall, **right lower** quadrant with penetration into peritoneal cavity
  Coding Clinic: 2Ø15, Q4, P37
- S31.614 Laceration without foreign body of abdominal wall, **left lower** quadrant with penetration into peritoneal cavity
- S31.615 Laceration without foreign body of abdominal wall, **periumbilic region** with penetration into peritoneal cavity
- S31.619 Laceration without foreign body of abdominal wall, **unspecified** quadrant with penetration into peritoneal cavity

S31.62 **Laceration with foreign body** of abdominal wall with penetration into peritoneal cavity

- S31.62Ø Laceration with foreign body of abdominal wall, **right upper** quadrant with penetration into peritoneal cavity
- S31.621 Laceration with foreign body of abdominal wall, **left upper** quadrant with penetration into peritoneal cavity
- S31.622 Laceration with foreign body of abdominal wall, **epigastric region** with penetration into peritoneal cavity
- S31.623 Laceration with foreign body of abdominal wall, **right lower** quadrant with penetration into peritoneal cavity
- S31.624 Laceration with foreign body of abdominal wall, **left lower** quadrant with penetration into peritoneal cavity
- S31.625 Laceration with foreign body of abdominal wall, **periumbilic region** with penetration into peritoneal cavity
- S31.629 Laceration with foreign body of abdominal wall, **unspecified** quadrant with penetration into peritoneal cavity

S31.63 **Puncture wound without foreign body** of abdominal wall with penetration into peritoneal cavity

- S31.63Ø Puncture wound without foreign body of abdominal wall, **right upper** quadrant with penetration into peritoneal cavity
- S31.631 Puncture wound without foreign body of abdominal wall, **left upper** quadrant with penetration into peritoneal cavity
- S31.632 Puncture wound without foreign body of abdominal wall, **epigastric region** with penetration into peritoneal cavity
- S31.633 Puncture wound without foreign body of abdominal wall, **right lower** quadrant with penetration into peritoneal cavity
- S31.634 Puncture wound without foreign body of abdominal wall, **left lower** quadrant with penetration into peritoneal cavity
- S31.635 Puncture wound without foreign body of abdominal wall, **periumbilic region** with penetration into peritoneal cavity
- S31.639 Puncture wound without foreign body of abdominal wall, **unspecified** quadrant with penetration into peritoneal cavity

S31.64 **Puncture wound with foreign body** of abdominal wall with penetration into peritoneal cavity

- S31.64Ø Puncture wound with foreign body of abdominal wall, **right upper** quadrant with penetration into peritoneal cavity
- S31.641 Puncture wound with foreign body of abdominal wall, **left upper** quadrant with penetration into peritoneal cavity
- S31.642 Puncture wound with foreign body of abdominal wall, **epigastric region** with penetration into peritoneal cavity
- S31.643 Puncture wound with foreign body of abdominal wall, **right lower** quadrant with penetration into peritoneal cavity
- S31.644 Puncture wound with foreign body of abdominal wall, **left lower** quadrant with penetration into peritoneal cavity
- S31.645 Puncture wound with foreign body of abdominal wall, **periumbilic region** with penetration into peritoneal cavity
- S31.649 Puncture wound with foreign body of abdominal wall, **unspecified** quadrant with penetration into peritoneal cavity

- S31.65 Open bite of abdominal wall with penetration into peritoneal cavity
  - **Excludes1** superficial bite of abdominal wall (S30.861, S30.871)
  - S31.650 Open bite of abdominal wall, right upper quadrant with penetration into peritoneal cavity
  - S31.651 Open bite of abdominal wall, left upper quadrant with penetration into peritoneal cavity
  - S31.652 Open bite of abdominal wall, epigastric region with penetration into peritoneal cavity
  - S31.653 Open bite of abdominal wall, right lower quadrant with penetration into peritoneal cavity
  - S31.654 Open bite of abdominal wall, left lower quadrant with penetration into peritoneal cavity
  - S31.655 Open bite of abdominal wall, periumbilic region with penetration into peritoneal cavity
  - S31.659 Open bite of abdominal wall, unspecified quadrant with penetration into peritoneal cavity

S31.8 Open wound of other parts of abdomen, lower back and pelvis

- S31.80 Open wound of unspecified buttock
  - S31.801 Laceration without foreign body of unspecified buttock
  - S31.802 Laceration with foreign body of unspecified buttock
  - S31.803 Puncture wound without foreign body of unspecified buttock
  - S31.804 Puncture wound with foreign body of unspecified buttock
  - S31.805 Open bite of unspecified buttock
    - Bite of buttock NOS
    - **Excludes1** superficial bite of buttock (S30.870)
  - S31.809 Unspecified open wound of unspecified buttock
- S31.81 Open wound of right buttock
  - S31.811 Laceration without foreign body of right buttock
  - S31.812 Laceration with foreign body of right buttock
  - S31.813 Puncture wound without foreign body of right buttock
  - S31.814 Puncture wound with foreign body of right buttock
  - S31.815 Open bite of right buttock
    - Bite of right buttock NOS
    - **Excludes1** superficial bite of buttock (S30.870)
  - S31.819 Unspecified open wound of right buttock
- S31.82 Open wound of left buttock
  - S31.821 Laceration without foreign body of left buttock
  - S31.822 Laceration with foreign body of left buttock
  - S31.823 Puncture wound without foreign body of left buttock
  - S31.824 Puncture wound with foreign body of left buttock
  - S31.825 Open bite of left buttock
    - Bite of left buttock NOS
    - **Excludes1** superficial bite of buttock (S30.870)
  - S31.829 Unspecified open wound of left buttock
- S31.83 Open wound of anus
  - S31.831 Laceration without foreign body of anus
  - S31.832 Laceration with foreign body of anus
  - S31.833 Puncture wound without foreign body of anus
  - S31.834 Puncture wound with foreign body of anus
  - S31.835 Open bite of anus
    - Bite of anus NOS
    - **Excludes1** superficial bite of anus (S30.877)
  - S31.839 Unspecified open wound of anus

S32 Fracture of lumbar spine and pelvis

Note: A fracture not indicated as displaced or nondisplaced should be coded to displaced

A fracture not indicated as opened or closed should be coded to closed

Includes fracture of lumbosacral neural arch
fracture of lumbosacral spinous process
fracture of lumbosacral transverse process
fracture of lumbosacral vertebra
fracture of lumbosacral vertebral arch

Code first any associated spinal cord and spinal nerve injury (S34.-)

Excludes1 transection of abdomen (S38.3)

Excludes2 fracture of hip NOS (S72.0-)

The appropriate 7th character is to be added to each code from category S32

A	initial encounter for closed fracture
B	initial encounter for open fracture
D	subsequent encounter for fracture with routine healing
G	subsequent encounter for fracture with delayed healing
K	subsequent encounter for fracture with nonunion
S	sequela

S32.0 Fracture of lumbar vertebra

Fracture of lumbar spine NOS

- S32.00 Fracture of unspecified lumbar vertebra
  - S32.000 Wedge compression fracture of unspecified lumbar vertebra A, B
  - S32.001 Stable burst fracture of unspecified lumbar vertebra A, B
  - S32.002 Unstable burst fracture of unspecified lumbar vertebra A, B
  - S32.008 Other fracture of unspecified lumbar vertebra A, B
  - S32.009 Unspecified fracture of unspecified lumbar vertebra A, B
- S32.01 Fracture of first lumbar vertebra
  - S32.010 Wedge compression fracture of first lumbar vertebra A, B
  - S32.011 Stable burst fracture of first lumbar vertebra A, B
  - S32.012 Unstable burst fracture of first lumbar vertebra A, B
  - S32.018 Other fracture of first lumbar vertebra A, B
  - S32.019 Unspecified fracture of first lumbar vertebra A, B
- S32.02 Fracture of second lumbar vertebra
  - S32.020 Wedge compression fracture of second lumbar vertebra A, B
  - S32.021 Stable burst fracture of second lumbar vertebra A, B
  - S32.022 Unstable burst fracture of second lumbar vertebra A, B
  - S32.028 Other fracture of second lumbar vertebra A, B
  - S32.029 Unspecified fracture of second lumbar vertebra A, B

S32.03 Fracture of third lumbar vertebra
- S32.030 Wedge compression fracture of third lumbar vertebra A, B
- S32.031 Stable burst fracture of third lumbar vertebra A, B
- S32.032 Unstable burst fracture of third lumbar vertebra A, B
- S32.038 Other fracture of third lumbar vertebra A, B
- S32.039 Unspecified fracture of third lumbar vertebra A, B

S32.04 Fracture of fourth lumbar vertebra
- S32.040 Wedge compression fracture of fourth lumbar vertebra A, B
- S32.041 Stable burst fracture of fourth lumbar vertebra A, B
- S32.042 Unstable burst fracture of fourth lumbar vertebra A, B
- S32.048 Other fracture of fourth lumbar vertebra A, B
- S32.049 Unspecified fracture of fourth lumbar vertebra A, B

S32.05 Fracture of fifth lumbar vertebra
- S32.050 Wedge compression fracture of fifth lumbar vertebra A, B
- S32.051 Stable burst fracture of fifth lumbar vertebra A, B
- S32.052 Unstable burst fracture of fifth lumbar vertebra A, B
- S32.058 Other fracture of fifth lumbar vertebra A, B
- S32.059 Unspecified fracture of fifth lumbar vertebra A, B

S32.1 Fracture of sacrum

For vertical fractures, code to most medial fracture extension

Use two codes if both a vertical and transverse fracture are present

Code also any associated fracture of pelvic ring (S32.8-)

X S32.10 Unspecified fracture of sacrum A, B

S32.11 Zone I fracture of sacrum

Vertical sacral ala fracture of sacrum
- S32.110 Nondisplaced Zone I fracture of sacrum A, B
- S32.111 Minimally displaced Zone I fracture of sacrum A, B
- S32.112 Severely displaced Zone I fracture of sacrum A, B
- S32.119 Unspecified Zone I fracture of sacrum A, B

S32.12 Zone II fracture of sacrum

Vertical foraminal region fracture of sacrum
- S32.120 Nondisplaced Zone II fracture of sacrum A, B
- S32.121 Minimally displaced Zone II fracture of sacrum A, B
- S32.122 Severely displaced Zone II fracture of sacrum A, B
- S32.129 Unspecified Zone II fracture of sacrum A, B

S32.13 Zone III fracture of sacrum

Vertical fracture into spinal canal region of sacrum
- S32.130 Nondisplaced Zone III fracture of sacrum A, B
- S32.131 Minimally displaced Zone III fracture of sacrum A, B
- S32.132 Severely displaced Zone III fracture of sacrum A, B
- S32.139 Unspecified Zone III fracture of sacrum A, B

X S32.14 Type 1 fracture of sacrum A, B

Transverse flexion fracture of sacrum without displacement

X S32.15 Type 2 fracture of sacrum A, B

Transverse flexion fracture of sacrum with posterior displacement

X S32.16 Type 3 fracture of sacrum A, B

Transverse extension fracture of sacrum with anterior displacement

X S32.17 Type 4 fracture of sacrum A, B

Transverse segmental comminution of upper sacrum

X S32.19 Other fracture of sacrum A, B

X S32.2 Fracture of coccyx A, B

S32.3 Fracture of ilium

Excludes1 fracture of ilium with associated disruption of pelvic ring (S32.8-)

S32.30 Unspecified fracture of ilium
- S32.301 Unspecified fracture of right ilium A, B
- S32.302 Unspecified fracture of left ilium A, B
- S32.309 Unspecified fracture of unspecified ilium A, B

S32.31 Avulsion fracture of ilium
- S32.311 Displaced avulsion fracture of right ilium A, B
- S32.312 Displaced avulsion fracture of left ilium A, B
- S32.313 Displaced avulsion fracture of unspecified ilium A, B
- S32.314 Nondisplaced avulsion fracture of right ilium A, B
- S32.315 Nondisplaced avulsion fracture of left ilium A, B
- S32.316 Nondisplaced avulsion fracture of unspecified ilium A, B

S32.39 Other fracture of ilium
- S32.391 Other fracture of right ilium A, B
- S32.392 Other fracture of left ilium A, B
- S32.399 Other fracture of unspecified ilium A, B

S32.4 Fracture of acetabulum

Code also any associated fracture of pelvic ring (S32.8-)

S32.40 Unspecified fracture of acetabulum
- S32.401 Unspecified fracture of right acetabulum A, B
- S32.402 Unspecified fracture of left acetabulum A, B
- S32.409 Unspecified fracture of unspecified acetabulum A, B

S32.41 Fracture of anterior wall of acetabulum
- S32.411 Displaced fracture of anterior wall of right acetabulum A, B
- S32.412 Displaced fracture of anterior wall of left acetabulum A, B
- S32.413 Displaced fracture of anterior wall of unspecified acetabulum A, B
- S32.414 Nondisplaced fracture of anterior wall of right acetabulum A, B
- S32.415 Nondisplaced fracture of anterior wall of left acetabulum A, B
- S32.416 Nondisplaced fracture of anterior wall of unspecified acetabulum A, B

- S32.42 Fracture of **posterior wall** of acetabulum
  - S32.421 **Displaced** fracture of posterior wall of **right** acetabulum A, B
  - S32.422 **Displaced** fracture of posterior wall of **left** acetabulum A, B
  - S32.423 **Displaced** fracture of posterior wall of **unspecified** acetabulum A, B
  - S32.424 **Nondisplaced** fracture of posterior wall of **right** acetabulum A, B
  - S32.425 **Nondisplaced** fracture of posterior wall of **left** acetabulum A, B
  - S32.426 **Nondisplaced** fracture of posterior wall of **unspecified** acetabulum A, B
- S32.43 Fracture of **anterior column** [iliopubic] of acetabulum
  - S32.431 **Displaced** fracture of anterior column [iliopubic] of **right** acetabulum A, B
  - S32.432 **Displaced** fracture of anterior column [iliopubic] of **left** acetabulum A, B
  - S32.433 **Displaced** fracture of anterior column [iliopubic] of **unspecified** acetabulum A, B
  - S32.434 **Nondisplaced** fracture of anterior column [iliopubic] of **right** acetabulum A, B
  - S32.435 **Nondisplaced** fracture of anterior column [iliopubic] of **left** acetabulum A, B
  - S32.436 **Nondisplaced** fracture of anterior column [iliopubic] of **unspecified** acetabulum A, B
- S32.44 Fracture of **posterior column** [ilioischial] of acetabulum
  - S32.441 **Displaced** fracture of posterior column [ilioischial] of **right** acetabulum A, B
  - S32.442 **Displaced** fracture of posterior column [ilioischial] of **left** acetabulum A, B
  - S32.443 **Displaced** fracture of posterior column [ilioischial] of **unspecified** acetabulum A, B
  - S32.444 **Nondisplaced** fracture of posterior column [ilioischial] of **right** acetabulum A, B
  - S32.445 **Nondisplaced** fracture of posterior column [ilioischial] of **left** acetabulum A, B
  - S32.446 **Nondisplaced** fracture of posterior column [ilioischial] of **unspecified** acetabulum A, B
- S32.45 **Transverse** fracture of acetabulum
  - S32.451 **Displaced** transverse fracture of **right** acetabulum A, B
  - S32.452 **Displaced** transverse fracture of **left** acetabulum A, B
  - S32.453 **Displaced** transverse fracture of **unspecified** acetabulum A, B
  - S32.454 **Nondisplaced** transverse fracture of **right** acetabulum A, B
  - S32.455 **Nondisplaced** transverse fracture of **left** acetabulum A, B
  - S32.456 **Nondisplaced** transverse fracture of **unspecified** acetabulum A, B
- S32.46 **Associated transverse-posterior** fracture of acetabulum
  - S32.461 **Displaced** associated transverse-posterior fracture of **right** acetabulum A, B
  - S32.462 **Displaced** associated transverse-posterior fracture of **left** acetabulum A, B
  - S32.463 **Displaced** associated transverse-posterior fracture of **unspecified** acetabulum A, B
  - S32.464 **Nondisplaced** associated transverse-posterior fracture of **right** acetabulum A, B
  - S32.465 **Nondisplaced** associated transverse-posterior fracture of **left** acetabulum A, B
  - S32.466 **Nondisplaced** associated transverse-posterior fracture of **unspecified** acetabulum A, B
- S32.47 Fracture of **medial wall** of acetabulum
  - S32.471 **Displaced** fracture of medial wall of **right** acetabulum A, B
  - S32.472 **Displaced** fracture of medial wall of **left** acetabulum A, B
  - S32.473 **Displaced** fracture of medial wall of **unspecified** acetabulum A, B
  - S32.474 **Nondisplaced** fracture of medial wall of **right** acetabulum A, B
  - S32.475 **Nondisplaced** fracture of medial wall of **left** acetabulum A, B
  - S32.476 **Nondisplaced** fracture of medial wall of **unspecified** acetabulum A, B
- S32.48 **Dome** fracture of acetabulum
  - S32.481 **Displaced** dome fracture of **right** acetabulum A, B
  - S32.482 **Displaced** dome fracture of **left** acetabulum A, B
  - S32.483 **Displaced** dome fracture of **unspecified** acetabulum A, B
  - S32.484 **Nondisplaced** dome fracture of **right** acetabulum A, B
  - S32.485 **Nondisplaced** dome fracture of **left** acetabulum A, B
  - S32.486 **Nondisplaced** dome fracture of **unspecified** acetabulum A, B
- S32.49 **Other** fracture of acetabulum
  - S32.491 Other fracture of **right** acetabulum A, B
  - S32.492 Other fracture of **left** acetabulum A, B
  - S32.499 Other fracture of **unspecified** acetabulum A, B

S32.5 Fracture of **pubis**

Excludes1 fracture of pubis with associated disruption of pelvic ring (S32.8-)

- S32.5Ø **Unspecified** fracture of pubis
  - S32.5Ø1 Unspecified fracture of **right** pubis A, B
  - S32.5Ø2 Unspecified fracture of **left** pubis A, B
  - S32.5Ø9 Unspecified fracture of **unspecified** pubis A, B
- S32.51 Fracture of superior **rim** of pubis
  - S32.511 Fracture of superior rim of **right** pubis A, B
  - S32.512 Fracture of superior rim of **left** pubis A, B
  - S32.519 Fracture of superior rim of **unspecified** pubis A, B

S32.59 Other specified fracture of pubis

S32.591 Other specified fracture of right pubis A, B

S32.592 Other specified fracture of left pubis A, B

S32.599 Other specified fracture of unspecified pubis A, B

S32.6 Fracture of ischium

Excludes1 fracture of ischium with associated disruption of pelvic ring (S32.8-)

S32.60 Unspecified fracture of ischium

S32.601 Unspecified fracture of right ischium A, B

S32.602 Unspecified fracture of left ischium A, B

S32.609 Unspecified fracture of unspecified ischium A, B

S32.61 Avulsion fracture of ischium

S32.611 Displaced avulsion fracture of right ischium A, B

S32.612 Displaced avulsion fracture of left ischium A, B

S32.613 Displaced avulsion fracture of unspecified ischium A, B

S32.614 Nondisplaced avulsion fracture of right ischium A, B

S32.615 Nondisplaced avulsion fracture of left ischium A, B

S32.616 Nondisplaced avulsion fracture of unspecified ischium A, B

S32.69 Other specified fracture of ischium

S32.691 Other specified fracture of right ischium A, B

S32.692 Other specified fracture of left ischium A, B

S32.699 Other specified fracture of unspecified ischium A, B

S32.8 Fracture of other parts of pelvis

Code also any associated:
fracture of acetabulum (S32.4-)
sacral fracture (S32.1-)

S32.81 **Multiple fractures of pelvis with disruption of pelvic ring**

Multiple pelvic fractures with disruption of pelvic circle

S32.810 **Multiple fractures of pelvis with stable disruption of pelvic ring** A, B

S32.811 **Multiple fractures of pelvis with unstable disruption of pelvic ring** A, B

X S32.82 **Multiple fractures of pelvis without disruption of pelvic ring** A, B

Multiple pelvic fractures without disruption of pelvic circle

X S32.89 Fracture of other parts of pelvis A, B

X S32.9 Fracture of unspecified parts of lumbosacral spine and pelvis A, B

Fracture of lumbosacral spine NOS
Fracture of pelvis NOS
Coding Clinic: 2012, Q4, P93

S33 **Dislocation and sprain of joints and ligaments of lumbar spine and pelvis**

Includes avulsion of joint or ligament of lumbar spine and pelvis
laceration of cartilage, joint or ligament of lumbar spine and pelvis
sprain of cartilage, joint or ligament of lumbar spine and pelvis
traumatic hemarthrosis of joint or ligament of lumbar spine and pelvis
traumatic rupture of joint or ligament of lumbar spine and pelvis
traumatic subluxation of joint or ligament of lumbar spine and pelvis
traumatic tear of joint or ligament of lumbar spine and pelvis

Code also any associated open wound

Excludes1 nontraumatic rupture or displacement of lumbar intervertebral disc NOS (M51.-)
obstetric damage to pelvic joints and ligaments (O71.6)

Excludes2 dislocation and sprain of joints and ligaments of hip (S73.-)
strain of muscle of lower back and pelvis (S39.01-)

The appropriate 7th character is to be added to each code from category S33

A	initial encounter
D	subsequent encounter
S	sequela

X S33.0 **Traumatic rupture of lumbar intervertebral disc**

Excludes1 rupture or displacement (nontraumatic) of lumbar intervertebral disc NOS (M51.- with fifth character 6)

S33.1 **Subluxation and dislocation of lumbar vertebra**

Code also any associated:
open wound of abdomen, lower back and pelvis (S31)
spinal cord injury (S24.0, S24.1-, S34.0-, S34.1-)

Excludes2 fracture of lumbar vertebrae (S32.0-)

S33.10 **Subluxation and dislocation of unspecified lumbar vertebra**

S33.100 **Subluxation of unspecified lumbar vertebra**

S33.101 **Dislocation of unspecified lumbar vertebra**

S33.11 **Subluxation and dislocation of L1/L2 lumbar vertebra**

S33.110 **Subluxation of L1/L2 lumbar vertebra**

S33.111 **Dislocation of L1/L2 lumbar vertebra**

S33.12 **Subluxation and dislocation of L2/L3 lumbar vertebra**

S33.120 **Subluxation of L2/L3 lumbar vertebra**

S33.121 **Dislocation of L2/L3 lumbar vertebra**

S33.13 **Subluxation and dislocation of L3/L4 lumbar vertebra**

S33.130 **Subluxation of L3/L4 lumbar vertebra**

S33.131 **Dislocation of L3/L4 lumbar vertebra**

S33.14 **Subluxation and dislocation of L4/L5 lumbar vertebra**

S33.140 **Subluxation of L4/L5 lumbar vertebra**

S33.141 **Dislocation of L4/L5 lumbar vertebra**

X S33.2 Dislocation of sacroiliac and sacrococcygeal joint

● S33.3 Dislocation of other and unspecified parts of lumbar spine and pelvis
- X● S33.30 **Dislocation of unspecified parts of lumbar spine and pelvis**
- X● S33.39 **Dislocation of other parts of lumbar spine and pelvis**

X● S33.4 Traumatic rupture of **symphysis pubis**
X● S33.5 Sprain of ligaments of **lumbar spine**
X● S33.6 Sprain of **sacroiliac** joint
X● S33.8 Sprain of **other parts** of lumbar spine and pelvis
X● S33.9 Sprain of **unspecified** parts of lumbar spine and pelvis

● S34 **Injury of lumbar and sacral spinal cord and nerves at abdomen, lower back and pelvis level**

Note: Code to highest level of lumbar cord injury

Injuries to the spinal cord (S34.Ø and S34.1) refer to the cord level and not bone level injury, and can affect nerve roots at and below the level given.

The appropriate 7th character is to be added to each code from category S34

A	initial encounter
D	subsequent encounter
S	sequela

Code also any associated:
fracture of vertebra (S22.Ø-, S32.Ø-)
open wound of abdomen, lower back and pelvis (S31.-)
transient paralysis (R29.5)

● S34.Ø **Concussion and edema** of lumbar and sacral spinal cord
- X● S34.Ø1 Concussion and edema of **lumbar** spinal cord A, D, S HCC
- X● S34.Ø2 Concussion and edema of **sacral** spinal cord A, D, S HCC
  Concussion and edema of conus medullaris

● S34.1 Other and unspecified injury of lumbar and sacral spinal cord
- ● S34.1Ø **Unspecified** injury to lumbar spinal cord
  - ● S34.1Ø1 Unspecified injury to L_1 level of lumbar spinal cord A, D, S HCC
    Unspecified injury to lumbar spinal cord level 1
  - ● S34.1Ø2 Unspecified injury to L_2 level of lumbar spinal cord A, D, S HCC
    Unspecified injury to lumbar spinal cord level 2
  - ● S34.1Ø3 Unspecified injury to L_3 level of lumbar spinal cord A, D, S HCC
    Unspecified injury to lumbar spinal cord level 3
  - ● S34.1Ø4 Unspecified injury to L_4 level of lumbar spinal cord A, D, S HCC
    Unspecified injury to lumbar spinal cord level 4
  - ● S34.1Ø5 Unspecified injury to L_5 level of lumbar spinal cord A, D, S HCC
    Unspecified injury to lumbar spinal cord level 5
  - ● S34.1Ø9 Unspecified injury to **unspecified level** of lumbar spinal cord A, D, S HCC
- ● S34.11 **Complete lesion** of lumbar spinal cord
  - ● S34.111 Complete lesion of L_1 level of lumbar spinal cord A, D, S HCC
    Complete lesion of lumbar spinal cord level 1
  - ● S34.112 Complete lesion of L_2 level of lumbar spinal cord A, D, S HCC
    Complete lesion of lumbar spinal cord level 2
  - ● S34.113 Complete lesion of L_3 level of lumbar spinal cord A, D, S HCC
    Complete lesion of lumbar spinal cord level 3
  - ● S34.114 Complete lesion of L_4 level of lumbar spinal cord A, D, S HCC
    Complete lesion of lumbar spinal cord level 4
  - ● S34.115 Complete lesion of L_5 level of lumbar spinal cord A, D, S HCC
    Complete lesion of lumbar spinal cord level 5
  - ● S34.119 Complete lesion of **unspecified level** of lumbar spinal cord A, D, S HCC
- ● S34.12 **Incomplete lesion** of lumbar spinal cord
  - ● S34.121 Incomplete lesion of L_1 level of lumbar spinal cord A, D, S HCC
    Incomplete lesion of lumbar spinal cord level 1
  - ● S34.122 Incomplete lesion of L_2 level of lumbar spinal cord A, D, S HCC
    Incomplete lesion of lumbar spinal cord level 2
  - ● S34.123 Incomplete lesion of L_3 level of lumbar spinal cord A, D, S HCC
    Incomplete lesion of lumbar spinal cord level 3
  - ● S34.124 Incomplete lesion of L_4 level of lumbar spinal cord A, D, S HCC
    Incomplete lesion of lumbar spinal cord level 4
  - ● S34.125 Incomplete lesion of L_5 level of lumbar spinal cord A, D, S HCC
    Incomplete lesion of lumbar spinal cord level 5
  - ● S34.129 Incomplete lesion of **unspecified level** of lumbar spinal cord A, D, S HCC
- ● S34.13 Other and unspecified injury to **sacral** spinal cord
  Other injury to conus medullaris
  - ● S34.131 **Complete lesion** of sacral spinal cord A, D, S HCC
    Complete lesion of conus medullaris
  - ● S34.132 **Incomplete lesion** of sacral spinal cord A, D, S HCC
    Incomplete lesion of conus medullaris
  - ● S34.139 **Unspecified injury** to sacral spinal cord A, D, S HCC
    Unspecified injury of conus medullaris

● S34.2 Injury of **nerve root** of lumbar and sacral spine
- X● S34.21 Injury of nerve root of **lumbar** spine
- X● S34.22 Injury of nerve root of **sacral** spine

X● S34.3 Injury of cauda equina A, D, S HCC
X● S34.4 Injury of lumbosacral plexus
X● S34.5 Injury of lumbar, sacral and pelvic sympathetic nerves
Injury of celiac ganglion or plexus
Injury of hypogastric plexus
Injury of mesenteric plexus (inferior) (superior)
Injury of splanchnic nerve
X● S34.6 Injury of peripheral nerve(s) at abdomen, lower back and pelvis level
X● S34.8 Injury of other nerves at abdomen, lower back and pelvis level
X● S34.9 Injury of **unspecified** nerves at abdomen, lower back and pelvis level

CHAPTER 19 (SØØ-T88)

S35 Injury of blood vessels at abdomen, lower back and pelvis level

The appropriate 7th character is to be added to each code from category S35

A	initial encounter
D	subsequent encounter
S	sequela

Code also any associated open wound (S31.-)

S35.0 Injury of abdominal aorta

Excludes1 injury of aorta NOS (S25.0)

X **S35.00 Unspecified injury of abdominal aorta**

X **S35.01 Minor laceration of abdominal aorta**

Incomplete transection of abdominal aorta
Laceration of abdominal aorta NOS
Superficial laceration of abdominal aorta

X **S35.02 Major laceration of abdominal aorta**

Complete transection of abdominal aorta
Traumatic rupture of abdominal aorta

X **S35.09 Other injury of abdominal aorta**

S35.1 Injury of inferior vena cava

Injury of hepatic vein

Excludes1 injury of vena cava NOS (S25.2)

X **S35.10 Unspecified injury of inferior vena cava**

X **S35.11 Minor laceration of inferior vena cava**

Incomplete transection of inferior vena cava
Laceration of inferior vena cava NOS
Superficial laceration of inferior vena cava

X **S35.12 Major laceration of inferior vena cava**

Complete transection of inferior vena cava
Traumatic rupture of inferior vena cava

X **S35.19 Other injury of inferior vena cava**

S35.2 Injury of celiac or mesenteric artery and branches

S35.21 Injury of celiac artery

S35.211 Minor laceration of celiac artery

Incomplete transection of celiac artery
Laceration of celiac artery NOS
Superficial laceration of celiac artery

S35.212 Major laceration of celiac artery

Complete transection of celiac artery
Traumatic rupture of celiac artery

S35.218 Other injury of celiac artery

S35.219 Unspecified injury of celiac artery

S35.22 Injury of superior mesenteric artery

S35.221 Minor laceration of superior mesenteric artery

Incomplete transection of superior mesenteric artery
Laceration of superior mesenteric artery NOS
Superficial laceration of superior mesenteric artery

S35.222 Major laceration of superior mesenteric artery

Complete transection of superior mesenteric artery
Traumatic rupture of superior mesenteric artery

S35.228 Other injury of superior mesenteric artery

S35.229 Unspecified injury of superior mesenteric artery

S35.23 Injury of inferior mesenteric artery

S35.231 Minor laceration of inferior mesenteric artery

Incomplete transection of inferior mesenteric artery
Laceration of inferior mesenteric artery NOS
Superficial laceration of inferior mesenteric artery

S35.232 Major laceration of inferior mesenteric artery

Complete transection of inferior mesenteric artery
Traumatic rupture of inferior mesenteric artery

S35.238 Other injury of inferior mesenteric artery

S35.239 Unspecified injury of inferior mesenteric artery

S35.29 Injury of branches of celiac and mesenteric artery

Injury of gastric artery
Injury of gastroduodenal artery
Injury of hepatic artery
Injury of splenic artery

S35.291 Minor laceration of branches of celiac and mesenteric artery

Incomplete transection of branches of celiac and mesenteric artery
Laceration of branches of celiac and mesenteric artery NOS
Superficial laceration of branches of celiac and mesenteric artery

S35.292 Major laceration of branches of celiac and mesenteric artery

Complete transection of branches of celiac and mesenteric artery
Traumatic rupture of branches of celiac and mesenteric artery

S35.298 Other injury of branches of celiac and mesenteric artery

S35.299 Unspecified injury of branches of celiac and mesenteric artery

S35.3 Injury of portal or splenic vein and branches

S35.31 Injury of portal vein

S35.311 Laceration of portal vein

S35.318 Other specified injury of portal vein

S35.319 Unspecified injury of portal vein

S35.32 Injury of splenic vein

S35.321 Laceration of splenic vein

S35.328 Other specified injury of splenic vein

S35.329 Unspecified injury of splenic vein

S35.33 Injury of superior mesenteric vein

S35.331 Laceration of superior mesenteric vein

S35.338 Other specified injury of superior mesenteric vein

S35.339 Unspecified injury of superior mesenteric vein

S35.34 Injury of inferior mesenteric vein

S35.341 Laceration of inferior mesenteric vein

S35.348 Other specified injury of inferior mesenteric vein

S35.349 Unspecified injury of inferior mesenteric vein

● S35.4 Injury of renal blood vessels
● S35.40 Unspecified injury of renal blood vessel
● S35.401 Unspecified injury of right renal artery
● S35.402 Unspecified injury of left renal artery
● S35.403 Unspecified injury of unspecified renal artery
● S35.404 Unspecified injury of right renal vein
● S35.405 Unspecified injury of left renal vein
● S35.406 Unspecified injury of unspecified renal vein
● S35.41 Laceration of renal blood vessel
● S35.411 Laceration of right renal artery
● S35.412 Laceration of left renal artery
● S35.413 Laceration of unspecified renal artery
● S35.414 Laceration of right renal vein
● S35.415 Laceration of left renal vein
● S35.416 Laceration of unspecified renal vein
● S35.49 Other specified injury of renal blood vessel
● S35.491 Other specified injury of right renal artery
● S35.492 Other specified injury of left renal artery
● S35.493 Other specified injury of unspecified renal artery
● S35.494 Other specified injury of right renal vein
● S35.495 Other specified injury of left renal vein
● S35.496 Other specified injury of unspecified renal vein
● S35.5 Injury of iliac blood vessels
X● S35.50 Injury of unspecified iliac blood vessel(s)
● S35.51 Injury of iliac artery or vein
Injury of hypogastric artery or vein
● S35.511 Injury of right iliac artery
● S35.512 Injury of left iliac artery
● S35.513 Injury of unspecified iliac artery
● S35.514 Injury of right iliac vein
● S35.515 Injury of left iliac vein
● S35.516 Injury of unspecified iliac vein
● S35.53 Injury of uterine artery or vein
● S35.531 Injury of right uterine artery ♀
● S35.532 Injury of left uterine artery ♀
● S35.533 Injury of unspecified uterine artery ♀
● S35.534 Injury of right uterine vein ♀
● S35.535 Injury of left uterine vein ♀
● S35.536 Injury of unspecified uterine vein ♀
X● S35.59 Injury of other iliac blood vessels
● S35.8 Injury of other blood vessels at abdomen, lower back and pelvis level
Injury of ovarian artery or vein
● S35.8X Injury of other blood vessels at abdomen, lower back and pelvis level
● S35.8X1 Laceration of other blood vessels at abdomen, lower back and pelvis level
● S35.8X8 Other specified injury of other blood vessels at abdomen, lower back and pelvis level
● S35.8X9 Unspecified injury of other blood vessels at abdomen, lower back and pelvis level
● S35.9 Injury of unspecified blood vessel at abdomen, lower back and pelvis level
X● S35.90 Unspecified injury of unspecified blood vessel at abdomen, lower back and pelvis level
X● S35.91 Laceration of unspecified blood vessel at abdomen, lower back and pelvis level
X● S35.99 Other specified injury of unspecified blood vessel at abdomen, lower back and pelvis level

● S36 Injury of intra-abdominal organs
The appropriate 7th character is to be added to each code from category S36

A	initial encounter
D	subsequent encounter
S	sequela

Code also any associated open wound (S31.-)
● S36.0 Injury of spleen
X● S36.00 Unspecified injury of spleen
● S36.02 Contusion of spleen
● S36.020 Minor contusion of spleen
Contusion of spleen less than 2 cm
● S36.021 Major contusion of spleen
Contusion of spleen greater than 2 cm
● S36.029 Unspecified contusion of spleen
Coding Clinic: 2015, Q2, P36, Q1, P11
● S36.03 Laceration of spleen
● S36.030 Superficial (capsular) laceration of spleen
Laceration of spleen less than 1 cm
Minor laceration of spleen
● S36.031 Moderate laceration of spleen
Laceration of spleen 1 to 3 cm
Coding Clinic: 2015, Q2, P36, Q1, P11
● S36.032 Major laceration of spleen
Avulsion of spleen
Laceration of spleen greater than 3 cm
Massive laceration of spleen
Multiple moderate lacerations of spleen
Stellate laceration of spleen
● S36.039 Unspecified laceration of spleen
X● S36.09 Other injury of spleen
● S36.1 Injury of liver and gallbladder and bile duct
● S36.11 Injury of liver
● S36.112 Contusion of liver
● S36.113 Laceration of liver, unspecified degree
● S36.114 Minor laceration of liver
Laceration involving capsule only, or, without significant involvement of hepatic parenchyma [i.e., less than 1 cm deep]
● S36.115 Moderate laceration of liver
Laceration involving parenchyma but without major disruption of parenchyma [i.e., less than 10 cm long and less than 3 cm deep]
● S36.116 Major laceration of liver
Laceration with significant disruption of hepatic parenchyma [i.e., greater than 10 cm long and 3 cm deep]
Multiple moderate lacerations, with or without hematoma
Stellate laceration of liver
● S36.118 Other injury of liver
● S36.119 Unspecified injury of liver
Coding Clinic: 2015, Q2, P17
● S36.12 Injury of gallbladder
● S36.122 Contusion of gallbladder
● S36.123 Laceration of gallbladder
● S36.128 Other injury of gallbladder
● S36.129 Unspecified injury of gallbladder
X● S36.13 Injury of bile duct

- S36.2 Injury of pancreas
  - S36.20 Unspecified injury of pancreas
    - S36.200 Unspecified injury of head of pancreas
    - S36.201 Unspecified injury of body of pancreas
    - S36.202 Unspecified injury of tail of pancreas
    - S36.209 Unspecified injury of unspecified part of pancreas
  - S36.22 Contusion of pancreas
    - S36.220 Contusion of head of pancreas
    - S36.221 Contusion of body of pancreas
    - S36.222 Contusion of tail of pancreas
    - S36.229 Contusion of unspecified part of pancreas
  - S36.23 Laceration of pancreas, unspecified degree
    - S36.230 Laceration of head of pancreas, unspecified degree
    - S36.231 Laceration of body of pancreas, unspecified degree
    - S36.232 Laceration of tail of pancreas, unspecified degree
    - S36.239 Laceration of unspecified part of pancreas, unspecified degree
  - S36.24 Minor laceration of pancreas
    - S36.240 Minor laceration of head of pancreas
    - S36.241 Minor laceration of body of pancreas
    - S36.242 Minor laceration of tail of pancreas
    - S36.249 Minor laceration of unspecified part of pancreas
  - S36.25 Moderate laceration of pancreas
    - S36.250 Moderate laceration of head of pancreas
    - S36.251 Moderate laceration of body of pancreas
    - S36.252 Moderate laceration of tail of pancreas
    - S36.259 Moderate laceration of unspecified part of pancreas
  - S36.26 Major laceration of pancreas
    - S36.260 Major laceration of head of pancreas
    - S36.261 Major laceration of body of pancreas
    - S36.262 Major laceration of tail of pancreas
    - S36.269 Major laceration of unspecified part of pancreas
  - S36.29 Other injury of pancreas
    - S36.290 Other injury of head of pancreas
    - S36.291 Other injury of body of pancreas
    - S36.292 Other injury of tail of pancreas
    - S36.299 Other injury of unspecified part of pancreas
- S36.3 Injury of stomach
  - X S36.30 Unspecified injury of stomach
  - X S36.32 Contusion of stomach
  - X S36.33 Laceration of stomach
  - X S36.39 Other injury of stomach
- S36.4 Injury of small intestine
  - S36.40 Unspecified injury of small intestine
    - S36.400 Unspecified injury of duodenum
    - S36.408 Unspecified injury of other part of small intestine
    - S36.409 Unspecified injury of unspecified part of small intestine
  - S36.41 Primary blast injury of small intestine
    Blast injury of small intestine NOS
    - S36.410 Primary blast injury of duodenum
    - S36.418 Primary blast injury of other part of small intestine
    - S36.419 Primary blast injury of unspecified part of small intestine
  - S36.42 Contusion of small intestine
    - S36.420 Contusion of duodenum
    - S36.428 Contusion of other part of small intestine
    - S36.429 Contusion of unspecified part of small intestine
  - S36.43 Laceration of small intestine
    - S36.430 Laceration of duodenum
    - S36.438 Laceration of other part of small intestine
    - S36.439 Laceration of unspecified part of small intestine
  - S36.49 Other injury of small intestine
    - S36.490 Other injury of duodenum
    - S36.498 Other injury of other part of small intestine
    - S36.499 Other injury of unspecified part of small intestine
- S36.5 Injury of colon
  Excludes2 injury of rectum (S36.6-)
  - S36.50 Unspecified injury of colon
    - S36.500 Unspecified injury of ascending [right] colon
    - S36.501 Unspecified injury of transverse colon
    - S36.502 Unspecified injury of descending [left] colon
    - S36.503 Unspecified injury of sigmoid colon
    - S36.508 Unspecified injury of other part of colon
    - S36.509 Unspecified injury of unspecified part of colon
  - S36.51 Primary blast injury of colon
    Blast injury of colon NOS
    - S36.510 Primary blast injury of ascending [right] colon
    - S36.511 Primary blast injury of transverse colon
    - S36.512 Primary blast injury of descending [left] colon
    - S36.513 Primary blast injury of sigmoid colon
    - S36.518 Primary blast injury of other part of colon
    - S36.519 Primary blast injury of unspecified part of colon
  - S36.52 Contusion of colon
    - S36.520 Contusion of ascending [right] colon
    - S36.521 Contusion of transverse colon
    - S36.522 Contusion of descending [left] colon
    - S36.523 Contusion of sigmoid colon
    - S36.528 Contusion of other part of colon
    - S36.529 Contusion of unspecified part of colon
  - S36.53 Laceration of colon
    - S36.530 Laceration of ascending [right] colon
    - S36.531 Laceration of transverse colon
    - S36.532 Laceration of descending [left] colon
    - S36.533 Laceration of sigmoid colon
    - S36.538 Laceration of other part of colon
    - S36.539 Laceration of unspecified part of colon

CHAPTER 19 (S00-T88)

- S36.59 **Other injury of colon**
  Secondary blast injury of colon
  - S36.590 Other injury of **ascending [right]** colon
  - S36.591 Other injury of **transverse** colon
  - S36.592 Other injury of **descending [left]** colon
  - S36.593 Other injury of **sigmoid** colon
  - S36.598 Other injury of **other** part of colon
  - S36.599 Other injury of **unspecified** part of colon
- S36.6 **Injury of rectum**
  - X S36.60 **Unspecified** injury of rectum
  - X S36.61 **Primary blast** injury of rectum
    Blast injury of rectum NOS
  - X S36.62 **Contusion** of rectum
  - X S36.63 **Laceration** of rectum
  - X S36.69 **Other** injury of rectum
    Secondary blast injury of rectum
- S36.8 Injury of other intra-abdominal organs
  - X S36.81 Injury of **peritoneum**
  - S36.89 Injury of **other intra-abdominal organs**
    Injury of retroperitoneum
    - S36.892 **Contusion** of other intra-abdominal organs
    - S36.893 **Laceration** of other intra-abdominal organs
    - S36.898 **Other** injury of other intra-abdominal organs
    - S36.899 **Unspecified** injury of other intra-abdominal organs
- S36.9 Injury of **unspecified intra-abdominal organ**
  - X S36.90 **Unspecified** injury of unspecified intra-abdominal organ
  - X S36.92 **Contusion** of unspecified intra-abdominal organ
  - X S36.93 **Laceration** of unspecified intra-abdominal organ
  - X S36.99 **Other** injury of unspecified intra-abdominal organ

S37 Injury of urinary and pelvic organs

Code also any associated open wound (S31.-)

Excludes1 obstetric trauma to pelvic organs (O71.-)

Excludes2 injury of peritoneum (S36.81)
injury of retroperitoneum (S36.89-)

The appropriate 7th character is to be added to each code from category S37

A	initial encounter
D	subsequent encounter
S	sequela

- S37.0 Injury of **kidney**
  Excludes2 acute kidney injury (nontraumatic) (N17.9)
  - S37.00 **Unspecified** injury of kidney
    - S37.001 Unspecified injury of **right** kidney
    - S37.002 Unspecified injury of **left** kidney
    - S37.009 Unspecified injury of **unspecified** kidney
  - S37.01 **Minor contusion** of kidney
    Contusion of kidney less than 2 cm
    Contusion of kidney NOS
    - S37.011 Minor contusion of **right** kidney
    - S37.012 Minor contusion of **left** kidney
    - S37.019 Minor contusion of **unspecified** kidney
  - S37.02 **Major contusion** of kidney
    Contusion of kidney greater than 2 cm
    - S37.021 Major contusion of **right** kidney
    - S37.022 Major contusion of **left** kidney
    - S37.029 Major contusion of **unspecified** kidney
  - S37.03 **Laceration** of kidney, **unspecified degree**
    - S37.031 Laceration of **right** kidney, unspecified degree
    - S37.032 Laceration of **left** kidney, unspecified degree
    - S37.039 Laceration of **unspecified** kidney, unspecified degree
  - S37.04 **Minor laceration** of kidney
    Laceration of kidney less than 1 cm
    - S37.041 Minor laceration of **right** kidney
    - S37.042 Minor laceration of **left** kidney
    - S37.049 Minor laceration of **unspecified** kidney
  - S37.05 **Moderate laceration** of kidney
    Laceration of kidney 1 to 3 cm
    - S37.051 Moderate laceration of **right** kidney
    - S37.052 Moderate laceration of **left** kidney
    - S37.059 Moderate laceration of **unspecified** kidney
  - S37.06 **Major laceration** of kidney
    Avulsion of kidney
    Laceration of kidney greater than 3 cm
    Massive laceration of kidney
    Multiple moderate lacerations of kidney
    Stellate laceration of kidney
    - S37.061 Major laceration of **right** kidney
    - S37.062 Major laceration of **left** kidney
    - S37.069 Major laceration of **unspecified** kidney
  - S37.09 **Other** injury of kidney
    - S37.091 Other injury of **right** kidney
    - S37.092 Other injury of **left** kidney
    - S37.099 Other injury of **unspecified** kidney
- S37.1 Injury of **ureter**
  - X S37.10 **Unspecified** injury of ureter
  - X S37.12 **Contusion** of ureter
  - X S37.13 **Laceration** of ureter
  - X S37.19 **Other** injury of ureter
- S37.2 Injury of **bladder**
  - X S37.20 **Unspecified** injury of bladder
  - X S37.22 **Contusion** of bladder
  - X S37.23 **Laceration** of bladder
  - X S37.29 **Other** injury of bladder
- S37.3 Injury of **urethra**
  - X S37.30 **Unspecified** injury of urethra
  - X S37.32 **Contusion** of urethra
  - X S37.33 **Laceration** of urethra
  - X S37.39 **Other** injury of urethra
- S37.4 Injury of **ovary**
  - S37.40 **Unspecified** injury of ovary
    - S37.401 Unspecified injury of ovary, **unilateral** ♀
    - S37.402 Unspecified injury of ovary, **bilateral** ♀
    - S37.409 Unspecified injury of ovary, **unspecified** ♀
  - S37.42 **Contusion** of ovary
    - S37.421 Contusion of ovary, **unilateral** ♀
    - S37.422 Contusion of ovary, **bilateral** ♀
    - S37.429 Contusion of ovary, **unspecified** ♀

CHAPTER 19 (S00-T88)

- S37.43 Laceration of ovary
  - S37.431 Laceration of ovary, unilateral ♀
  - S37.432 Laceration of ovary, bilateral ♀
  - S37.439 Laceration of ovary, unspecified ♀
- S37.49 Other injury of ovary
  - S37.491 Other injury of ovary, unilateral ♀
  - S37.492 Other injury of ovary, bilateral ♀
  - S37.499 Other injury of ovary, unspecified ♀

S37.5 Injury of fallopian tube
- S37.50 Unspecified injury of fallopian tube
  - S37.501 Unspecified injury of fallopian tube, unilateral ♀
  - S37.502 Unspecified injury of fallopian tube, bilateral ♀
  - S37.509 Unspecified injury of fallopian tube, unspecified ♀
- S37.51 Primary blast injury of fallopian tube
  Blast injury of fallopian tube NOS
  - S37.511 Primary blast injury of fallopian tube, unilateral ♀
  - S37.512 Primary blast injury of fallopian tube, bilateral ♀
  - S37.519 Primary blast injury of fallopian tube, unspecified ♀
- S37.52 Contusion of fallopian tube
  - S37.521 Contusion of fallopian tube, unilateral ♀
  - S37.522 Contusion of fallopian tube, bilateral ♀
  - S37.529 Contusion of fallopian tube, unspecified ♀
- S37.53 Laceration of fallopian tube
  - S37.531 Laceration of fallopian tube, unilateral ♀
  - S37.532 Laceration of fallopian tube, bilateral ♀
  - S37.539 Laceration of fallopian tube, unspecified ♀
- S37.59 Other injury of fallopian tube
  Secondary blast injury of fallopian tube
  - S37.591 Other injury of fallopian tube, unilateral ♀
  - S37.592 Other injury of fallopian tube, bilateral ♀
  - S37.599 Other injury of fallopian tube, unspecified ♀

S37.6 Injury of uterus
  Excludes1 injury to gravid uterus (O9A.2-)
  injury to uterus during delivery (O71.-)
- X S37.60 Unspecified injury of uterus ♀
- X S37.62 Contusion of uterus ♀
- X S37.63 Laceration of uterus ♀
- X S37.69 Other injury of uterus ♀

S37.8 Injury of other urinary and pelvic organs
- S37.81 Injury of adrenal gland
  - S37.812 Contusion of adrenal gland
  - S37.813 Laceration of adrenal gland
  - S37.818 Other injury of adrenal gland
  - S37.819 Unspecified injury of adrenal gland
- S37.82 Injury of prostate
  - S37.822 Contusion of prostate ♂
  - S37.823 Laceration of prostate ♂
  - S37.828 Other injury of prostate ♂
  - S37.829 Unspecified injury of prostate ♂
- S37.89 Injury of other urinary and pelvic organ
  - S37.892 Contusion of other urinary and pelvic organ
  - S37.893 Laceration of other urinary and pelvic organ
  - S37.898 Other injury of other urinary and pelvic organ
  - S37.899 Unspecified injury of other urinary and pelvic organ

S37.9 Injury of unspecified urinary and pelvic organ
- X S37.90 Unspecified injury of unspecified urinary and pelvic organ
- X S37.92 Contusion of unspecified urinary and pelvic organ
- X S37.93 Laceration of unspecified urinary and pelvic organ
- X S37.99 Other injury of unspecified urinary and pelvic organ

S38 Crushing injury and traumatic amputation of abdomen, lower back, pelvis and external genitals

An amputation not identified as partial or complete should be coded to complete

The appropriate 7th character is to be added to each code from category S38

A	initial encounter
D	subsequent encounter
S	sequela

S38.0 Crushing injury of external genital organs
  Use additional code for any associated injuries
- S38.00 Crushing injury of unspecified external genital organs
  - S38.001 Crushing injury of unspecified external genital organs, male ♂
  - S38.002 Crushing injury of unspecified external genital organs, female ♀
- X S38.01 Crushing injury of penis ♂
- X S38.02 Crushing injury of scrotum and testis ♂
- X S38.03 Crushing injury of vulva ♀

X S38.1 Crushing injury of abdomen, lower back, and pelvis
  Use additional code for all associated injuries, such as:
  fracture of thoracic or lumbar spine and pelvis (S22.0-, S32.-)
  injury to intra-abdominal organs (S36.-)
  injury to urinary and pelvic organs (S37.-)
  open wound of abdominal wall (S31.-)
  spinal cord injury (S34.0, S34.1-)
  Excludes2 crushing injury of external genital organs (S38.0-)

S38.2 Traumatic amputation of external genital organs
- S38.21 Traumatic amputation of female external genital organs
  Traumatic amputation of clitoris
  Traumatic amputation of labium (majus) (minus)
  Traumatic amputation of vulva
  - S38.211 Complete traumatic amputation of female external genital organs ♀
  - S38.212 Partial traumatic amputation of female external genital organs ♀
- S38.22 Traumatic amputation of penis
  - S38.221 Complete traumatic amputation of penis ♂
  - S38.222 Partial traumatic amputation of penis ♂
- S38.23 Traumatic amputation of scrotum and testis
  - S38.231 Complete traumatic amputation of scrotum and testis ♂
  - S38.232 Partial traumatic amputation of scrotum and testis ♂

X S38.3 Transection (partial) of abdomen

S39 Other and unspecified injuries of abdomen, lower back, pelvis and external genitals

Code also any associated open wound (S31.-)

Excludes2 sprain of joints and ligaments of lumbar spine and pelvis (S33.-)

The appropriate 7th character is to be added to each code from category S39

A	initial encounter
D	subsequent encounter
S	sequela

- **S39.0** Injury of **muscle, fascia and tendon** of abdomen, lower back and pelvis
  - **S39.00** **Unspecified** injury of muscle, fascia and tendon of abdomen, lower back and pelvis
    - S39.001 Unspecified injury of muscle, fascia and tendon of **abdomen**
    - S39.002 Unspecified injury of muscle, fascia and tendon of **lower back**
    - S39.003 Unspecified injury of muscle, fascia and tendon of **pelvis**
  - **S39.01** **Strain** of muscle, fascia and tendon of abdomen, lower back and pelvis
    - S39.011 Strain of muscle, fascia and tendon of **abdomen**
    - S39.012 Strain of muscle, fascia and tendon of **lower back**
      Coding Clinic: 2016, Q4, P74
    - S39.013 Strain of muscle, fascia and tendon of **pelvis**
  - **S39.02** **Laceration** of muscle, fascia and tendon of abdomen, lower back and pelvis
    - S39.021 Laceration of muscle, fascia and tendon of **abdomen**
    - S39.022 Laceration of muscle, fascia and tendon of **lower back**
    - S39.023 Laceration of muscle, fascia and tendon of **pelvis**
  - **S39.09** **Other** injury of muscle, fascia and tendon of abdomen, lower back and pelvis
    - S39.091 Other injury of muscle, fascia and tendon of **abdomen**
    - S39.092 Other injury of muscle, fascia and tendon of **lower back**
    - S39.093 Other injury of muscle, fascia and tendon of **pelvis**
- **S39.8** **Other** specified injuries of abdomen, lower back, pelvis and external genitals
  - X S39.81 Other specified injuries of **abdomen**
  - X S39.82 Other specified injuries of **lower back**
  - X S39.83 Other specified injuries of **pelvis**
  - S39.84 Other specified injuries of **external genitals**
    - S39.840 Fracture of **corpus cavernosum penis** ♂
    - S39.848 **Other** specified injuries of external genitals
- **S39.9** **Unspecified** injury of abdomen, lower back, pelvis and external genitals
  - X S39.91 Unspecified injury of **abdomen**
  - X S39.92 Unspecified injury of **lower back**
  - X S39.93 Unspecified injury of **pelvis**
  - X S39.94 Unspecified injury of **external genitals**

INJURIES TO THE SHOULDER AND UPPER ARM (S40-S49)

Includes injuries of axilla injuries of scapular region

Excludes2 burns and corrosions (T20-T32)
frostbite (T33-T34)
injuries of elbow (S50-S59)
insect bite or sting, venomous (T63.4)

S40 Superficial injury of shoulder and upper arm

The appropriate 7th character is to be added to each code from category S40

A	initial encounter
D	subsequent encounter
S	sequela

- **S40.0** **Contusion** of shoulder and upper arm
  - S40.01 Contusion of **shoulder**
    - S40.011 Contusion of **right** shoulder
    - S40.012 Contusion of **left** shoulder
    - S40.019 Contusion of **unspecified** shoulder
  - S40.02 Contusion of **upper arm**
    - S40.021 Contusion of **right** upper arm
    - S40.022 Contusion of **left** upper arm
    - S40.029 Contusion of **unspecified** upper arm
- **S40.2** Other superficial injuries of **shoulder**
  - S40.21 **Abrasion** of shoulder
    - S40.211 Abrasion of **right** shoulder
    - S40.212 Abrasion of **left** shoulder
    - S40.219 Abrasion of **unspecified** shoulder
  - S40.22 **Blister** (nonthermal) of shoulder
    - S40.221 Blister (nonthermal) of **right** shoulder
    - S40.222 Blister (nonthermal) of **left** shoulder
    - S40.229 Blister (nonthermal) of **unspecified** shoulder
  - S40.24 **External constriction** of shoulder
    - S40.241 External constriction of **right** shoulder
    - S40.242 External constriction of **left** shoulder
    - S40.249 External constriction of **unspecified** shoulder
  - S40.25 **Superficial foreign body** of shoulder
    Splinter in the shoulder
    - S40.251 Superficial foreign body of **right** shoulder
    - S40.252 Superficial foreign body of **left** shoulder
    - S40.259 Superficial foreign body of **unspecified** shoulder
  - S40.26 **Insect bite** (nonvenomous) of shoulder
    - S40.261 Insect bite (nonvenomous) of **right** shoulder
    - S40.262 Insect bite (nonvenomous) of **left** shoulder
    - S40.269 Insect bite (nonvenomous) of **unspecified** shoulder
  - S40.27 **Other superficial bite** of shoulder
    Excludes1 open bite of shoulder (S41.05)
    - S40.271 Other superficial bite of **right** shoulder
    - S40.272 Other superficial bite of **left** shoulder
    - S40.279 Other superficial bite of **unspecified** shoulder

CHAPTER 19 (S00-T88)

▶ New ➡ Revised ~~deleted~~ Deleted Excludes 1 Excludes 2 Includes Use additional Code first Code also Key words
OGCR Official Guidelines X Assign placeholder X ● Use Additional Character(s) ▶ Manifestation Code Hierarchical Condition Category Coding Clinic

S40.8 Other superficial injuries of upper arm
S40.81 Abrasion of upper arm
S40.811 Abrasion of right upper arm
S40.812 Abrasion of left upper arm
S40.819 Abrasion of unspecified upper arm
S40.82 Blister (nonthermal) of upper arm
S40.821 Blister (nonthermal) of right upper arm
S40.822 Blister (nonthermal) of left upper arm
S40.829 Blister (nonthermal) of unspecified upper arm
S40.84 External constriction of upper arm
S40.841 External constriction of right upper arm
S40.842 External constriction of left upper arm
S40.849 External constriction of unspecified upper arm
S40.85 Superficial foreign body of upper arm
Splinter in the upper arm
S40.851 Superficial foreign body of right upper arm
S40.852 Superficial foreign body of left upper arm
S40.859 Superficial foreign body of unspecified upper arm
S40.86 Insect bite (nonvenomous) of upper arm
S40.861 Insect bite (nonvenomous) of right upper arm
S40.862 Insect bite (nonvenomous) of left upper arm
S40.869 Insect bite (nonvenomous) of unspecified upper arm
S40.87 Other superficial bite of upper arm
Excludes1 open bite of upper arm (S41.14)
Excludes2 other superficial bite of shoulder (S40.27-)
S40.871 Other superficial bite of right upper arm
S40.872 Other superficial bite of left upper arm
S40.879 Other superficial bite of unspecified upper arm
S40.9 Unspecified superficial injury of shoulder and upper arm
S40.91 Unspecified superficial injury of shoulder
S40.911 Unspecified superficial injury of right shoulder
S40.912 Unspecified superficial injury of left shoulder
S40.919 Unspecified superficial injury of unspecified shoulder
S40.92 Unspecified superficial injury of upper arm
S40.921 Unspecified superficial injury of right upper arm
S40.922 Unspecified superficial injury of left upper arm
S40.929 Unspecified superficial injury of unspecified upper arm

S41 Open wound of shoulder and upper arm
Code also any associated wound infection
Excludes1 traumatic amputation of shoulder and upper arm (S48.-)
Excludes2 open fracture of shoulder and upper arm (S42.- with 7th character B or C)
The appropriate 7th character is to be added to each code from category S41

A	initial encounter
D	subsequent encounter
S	sequela

S41.0 Open wound of shoulder
S41.00 Unspecified open wound of shoulder
S41.001 Unspecified open wound of right shoulder
S41.002 Unspecified open wound of left shoulder
S41.009 Unspecified open wound of unspecified shoulder
S41.01 Laceration without foreign body of shoulder
S41.011 Laceration without foreign body of right shoulder
S41.012 Laceration without foreign body of left shoulder
S41.019 Laceration without foreign body of unspecified shoulder
S41.02 Laceration with foreign body of shoulder
S41.021 Laceration with foreign body of right shoulder
S41.022 Laceration with foreign body of left shoulder
S41.029 Laceration with foreign body of unspecified shoulder
S41.03 Puncture wound without foreign body of shoulder
S41.031 Puncture wound without foreign body of right shoulder
S41.032 Puncture wound without foreign body of left shoulder
S41.039 Puncture wound without foreign body of unspecified shoulder
S41.04 Puncture wound with foreign body of shoulder
S41.041 Puncture wound with foreign body of right shoulder
S41.042 Puncture wound with foreign body of left shoulder
S41.049 Puncture wound with foreign body of unspecified shoulder
S41.05 Open bite of shoulder
Bite of shoulder NOS
Excludes1 superficial bite of shoulder (S40.27)
S41.051 Open bite of right shoulder
S41.052 Open bite of left shoulder
S41.059 Open bite of unspecified shoulder
S41.1 Open wound of upper arm
S41.10 Unspecified open wound of upper arm
S41.101 Unspecified open wound of right upper arm
S41.102 Unspecified open wound of left upper arm
S41.109 Unspecified open wound of unspecified upper arm

CHAPTER 19 (S00-T88)

● S41.11 Laceration without foreign body of upper arm
- ● S41.111 Laceration without foreign body of right upper arm
- ● S41.112 Laceration without foreign body of left upper arm
- ● S41.119 Laceration without foreign body of unspecified upper arm

● S41.12 Laceration with foreign body of upper arm
- ● S41.121 Laceration with foreign body of right upper arm
- ● S41.122 Laceration with foreign body of left upper arm
- ● S41.129 Laceration with foreign body of unspecified upper arm

● S41.13 Puncture wound without foreign body of upper arm
- ● S41.131 Puncture wound without foreign body of right upper arm
- ● S41.132 Puncture wound without foreign body of left upper arm
- ● S41.139 Puncture wound without foreign body of unspecified upper arm

● S41.14 Puncture wound with foreign body of upper arm
- ● S41.141 Puncture wound with foreign body of right upper arm
- ● S41.142 Puncture wound with foreign body of left upper arm
- ● S41.149 Puncture wound with foreign body of unspecified upper arm

● S41.15 Open bite of upper arm

Bite of upper arm NOS

Excludes1 superficial bite of upper arm (S4Ø.87)
- ● S41.151 Open bite of right upper arm
- ● S41.152 Open bite of left upper arm
- ● S41.159 Open bite of unspecified upper arm

● S42 Fracture of shoulder and upper arm

Note: A fracture not indicated as displaced or nondisplaced should be coded to displaced

A fracture not indicated as open or closed should be coded to closed

Excludes1 traumatic amputation of shoulder and upper arm (S48.-)

The appropriate 7th character is to be added to all codes from category S42

A	initial encounter for closed fracture
B	initial encounter for open fracture
D	subsequent encounter for fracture with routine healing
G	subsequent encounter for fracture with delayed healing
K	subsequent encounter for fracture with nonunion
P	subsequent encounter for fracture with malunion
S	sequela

● S42.Ø Fracture of clavicle

● S42.ØØ Fracture of unspecified part of clavicle
- ● S42.ØØ1 Fracture of unspecified part of right clavicle
- ● S42.ØØ2 Fracture of unspecified part of left clavicle
- ● S42.ØØ9 Fracture of unspecified part of unspecified clavicle
  Coding Clinic: 2Ø12, Q4, P3

● S42.Ø1 Fracture of sternal end of clavicle
- ● S42.Ø11 Anterior displaced fracture of sternal end of right clavicle
- ● S42.Ø12 Anterior displaced fracture of sternal end of left clavicle
- ● S42.Ø13 Anterior displaced fracture of sternal end of unspecified clavicle
  Displaced fracture of sternal end of clavicle NOS
- ● S42.Ø14 Posterior displaced fracture of sternal end of right clavicle
- ● S42.Ø15 Posterior displaced fracture of sternal end of left clavicle
- ● S42.Ø16 Posterior displaced fracture of sternal end of unspecified clavicle
- ● S42.Ø17 Nondisplaced fracture of sternal end of right clavicle
- ● S42.Ø18 Nondisplaced fracture of sternal end of left clavicle
- ● S42.Ø19 Nondisplaced fracture of sternal end of unspecified clavicle

● S42.Ø2 Fracture of shaft of clavicle
- ● S42.Ø21 Displaced fracture of shaft of right clavicle
- ● S42.Ø22 Displaced fracture of shaft of left clavicle
- ● S42.Ø23 Displaced fracture of shaft of unspecified clavicle
- ● S42.Ø24 Nondisplaced fracture of shaft of right clavicle
- ● S42.Ø25 Nondisplaced fracture of shaft of left clavicle
- ● S42.Ø26 Nondisplaced fracture of shaft of unspecified clavicle

● S42.Ø3 Fracture of lateral end of clavicle

Fracture of acromial end of clavicle
- ● S42.Ø31 Displaced fracture of lateral end of right clavicle
- ● S42.Ø32 Displaced fracture of lateral end of left clavicle
- ● S42.Ø33 Displaced fracture of lateral end of unspecified clavicle
- ● S42.Ø34 Nondisplaced fracture of lateral end of right clavicle
- ● S42.Ø35 Nondisplaced fracture of lateral end of left clavicle
- ● S42.Ø36 Nondisplaced fracture of lateral end of unspecified clavicle

● S42.1 Fracture of scapula

● S42.1Ø Fracture of unspecified part of scapula
- ● S42.1Ø1 Fracture of unspecified part of scapula, right shoulder
- ● S42.1Ø2 Fracture of unspecified part of scapula, left shoulder
- ● S42.1Ø9 Fracture of unspecified part of scapula, unspecified shoulder

● S42.11 Fracture of body of scapula
- ● S42.111 Displaced fracture of body of scapula, right shoulder
- ● S42.112 Displaced fracture of body of scapula, left shoulder
- ● S42.113 Displaced fracture of body of scapula, unspecified shoulder
- ● S42.114 Nondisplaced fracture of body of scapula, right shoulder
- ● S42.115 Nondisplaced fracture of body of scapula, left shoulder
- ● S42.116 Nondisplaced fracture of body of scapula, unspecified shoulder

S42.12 Fracture of acromial process
- S42.121 Displaced fracture of acromial process, right shoulder
- S42.122 Displaced fracture of acromial process, left shoulder
- S42.123 Displaced fracture of acromial process, unspecified shoulder
- S42.124 Nondisplaced fracture of acromial process, right shoulder
- S42.125 Nondisplaced fracture of acromial process, left shoulder
- S42.126 Nondisplaced fracture, of acromial process, unspecified shoulder

S42.13 Fracture of coracoid process
- S42.131 Displaced fracture of coracoid process, right shoulder
- S42.132 Displaced fracture of coracoid process, left shoulder
- S42.133 Displaced fracture of coracoid process, unspecified shoulder
- S42.134 Nondisplaced fracture of coracoid process, right shoulder
- S42.135 Nondisplaced fracture of coracoid process, left shoulder
- S42.136 Nondisplaced fracture of coracoid process, unspecified shoulder

S42.14 Fracture of glenoid cavity of scapula
- S42.141 Displaced fracture of glenoid cavity of scapula, right shoulder
- S42.142 Displaced fracture of glenoid cavity of scapula, left shoulder
- S42.143 Displaced fracture of glenoid cavity of scapula, unspecified shoulder
- S42.144 Nondisplaced fracture of glenoid cavity of scapula, right shoulder
- S42.145 Nondisplaced fracture of glenoid cavity of scapula, left shoulder
- S42.146 Nondisplaced fracture of glenoid cavity of scapula, unspecified shoulder

S42.15 Fracture of neck of scapula
- S42.151 Displaced fracture of neck of scapula, right shoulder
- S42.152 Displaced fracture of neck of scapula, left shoulder
- S42.153 Displaced fracture of neck of scapula, unspecified shoulder
- S42.154 Nondisplaced fracture of neck of scapula, right shoulder
- S42.155 Nondisplaced fracture of neck of scapula, left shoulder
- S42.156 Nondisplaced fracture of neck of scapula, unspecified shoulder

S42.19 Fracture of other part of scapula
- S42.191 Fracture of other part of scapula, right shoulder
- S42.192 Fracture of other part of scapula, left shoulder
- S42.199 Fracture of other part of scapula, unspecified shoulder

S42.2 Fracture of upper end of humerus

Fracture of proximal end of humerus

Excludes2 fracture of shaft of humerus (S42.3-)
physeal fracture of upper end of humerus (S49.Ø-)

S42.2Ø Unspecified fracture of upper end of humerus
- S42.2Ø1 Unspecified fracture of upper end of right humerus
- S42.2Ø2 Unspecified fracture of upper end of left humerus
- S42.2Ø9 Unspecified fracture of upper end of unspecified humerus

S42.21 Unspecified fracture of surgical neck of humerus

Fracture of neck of humerus NOS
- S42.211 Unspecified displaced fracture of surgical neck of right humerus
- S42.212 Unspecified displaced fracture of surgical neck of left humerus
- S42.213 Unspecified displaced fracture of surgical neck of unspecified humerus
- S42.214 Unspecified nondisplaced fracture of surgical neck of right humerus
- S42.215 Unspecified nondisplaced fracture of surgical neck of left humerus
- S42.216 Unspecified nondisplaced fracture of surgical neck of unspecified humerus

S42.22 2-part fracture of surgical neck of humerus
- S42.221 2-part displaced fracture of surgical neck of right humerus
- S42.222 2-part displaced fracture of surgical neck of left humerus
- S42.223 2-part displaced fracture of surgical neck of unspecified humerus
- S42.224 2-part nondisplaced fracture of surgical neck of right humerus
- S42.225 2-part nondisplaced fracture of surgical neck of left humerus
- S42.226 2-part nondisplaced fracture of surgical neck of unspecified humerus

S42.23 3-part fracture of surgical neck of humerus
- S42.231 3-part fracture of surgical neck of right humerus
- S42.232 3-part fracture of surgical neck of left humerus
- S42.239 3-part fracture of surgical neck of unspecified humerus

S42.24 4-part fracture of surgical neck of humerus
- S42.241 4-part fracture of surgical neck of right humerus
- S42.242 4-part fracture of surgical neck of left humerus
- S42.249 4-part fracture of surgical neck of unspecified humerus

S42.25 Fracture of greater tuberosity of humerus
- S42.251 Displaced fracture of greater tuberosity of right humerus
- S42.252 Displaced fracture of greater tuberosity of left humerus
- S42.253 Displaced fracture of greater tuberosity of unspecified humerus
- S42.254 Nondisplaced fracture of greater tuberosity of right humerus
- S42.255 Nondisplaced fracture of greater tuberosity of left humerus
- S42.256 Nondisplaced fracture of greater tuberosity of unspecified humerus

S42.26 Fracture of lesser tuberosity of humerus
- S42.261 Displaced fracture of lesser tuberosity of right humerus
- S42.262 Displaced fracture of lesser tuberosity of left humerus
- S42.263 Displaced fracture of lesser tuberosity of unspecified humerus
- S42.264 Nondisplaced fracture of lesser tuberosity of right humerus
- S42.265 Nondisplaced fracture of lesser tuberosity of left humerus
- S42.266 Nondisplaced fracture of lesser tuberosity of unspecified humerus

● S42.27 **Torus fracture of upper end of humerus**
The appropriate 7th character is to be added to all codes in subcategory S42.27

A	initial encounter for closed fracture
D	subsequent encounter for fracture with routine healing
G	subsequent encounter for fracture with delayed healing
K	subsequent encounter for fracture with nonunion
P	subsequent encounter for fracture with malunion
S	sequela

● S42.271 **Torus fracture of upper end of right humerus**
● S42.272 **Torus fracture of upper end of left humerus**
● S42.279 **Torus fracture of upper end of unspecified humerus**

● S42.29 **Other fracture of upper end of humerus**
Fracture of anatomical neck of humerus
Fracture of articular head of humerus
● S42.291 **Other displaced fracture of upper end of right humerus**
● S42.292 **Other displaced fracture of upper end of left humerus**
● S42.293 **Other displaced fracture of upper end of unspecified humerus**
● S42.294 **Other nondisplaced fracture of upper end of right humerus**
● S42.295 **Other nondisplaced fracture of upper end of left humerus**
Coding Clinic: 2019, Q1, P19
● S42.296 **Other nondisplaced fracture of upper end of unspecified humerus**

● S42.3 **Fracture of shaft of humerus**
Fracture of humerus NOS
Fracture of upper arm NOS
Excludes2 physeal fractures of upper end of humerus (S49.0-)
physeal fractures of lower end of humerus (S49.1-)

● S42.30 **Unspecified fracture of shaft of humerus**
● S42.301 **Unspecified fracture of shaft of humerus, right arm**
● S42.302 **Unspecified fracture of shaft of humerus, left arm**
● S42.309 **Unspecified fracture of shaft of humerus, unspecified arm**

● S42.31 **Greenstick fracture of shaft of humerus**
The appropriate 7th character is to be added to all codes in subcategory S42.31

A	initial encounter for closed fracture
D	subsequent encounter for fracture with routine healing
G	subsequent encounter for fracture with delayed healing
K	subsequent encounter for fracture with nonunion
P	subsequent encounter for fracture with malunion
S	sequela

● S42.311 **Greenstick fracture of shaft of humerus, right arm**
● S42.312 **Greenstick fracture of shaft of humerus, left arm**
● S42.319 **Greenstick fracture of shaft of humerus, unspecified arm**

● S42.32 **Transverse fracture of shaft of humerus**
● S42.321 **Displaced transverse fracture of shaft of humerus, right arm**
● S42.322 **Displaced transverse fracture of shaft of humerus, left arm**
● S42.323 **Displaced transverse fracture of shaft of humerus, unspecified arm**
● S42.324 **Nondisplaced transverse fracture of shaft of humerus, right arm**
● S42.325 **Nondisplaced transverse fracture of shaft of humerus, left arm**
● S42.326 **Nondisplaced transverse fracture of shaft of humerus, unspecified arm**

● S42.33 **Oblique fracture of shaft of humerus**
● S42.331 **Displaced oblique fracture of shaft of humerus, right arm**
● S42.332 **Displaced oblique fracture of shaft of humerus, left arm**
● S42.333 **Displaced oblique fracture of shaft of humerus, unspecified arm**
● S42.334 **Nondisplaced oblique fracture of shaft of humerus, right arm**
● S42.335 **Nondisplaced oblique fracture of shaft of humerus, left arm**
● S42.336 **Nondisplaced oblique fracture of shaft of humerus, unspecified arm**

● S42.34 **Spiral fracture of shaft of humerus**
● S42.341 **Displaced spiral fracture of shaft of humerus, right arm**
● S42.342 **Displaced spiral fracture of shaft of humerus, left arm**
● S42.343 **Displaced spiral fracture of shaft of humerus, unspecified arm**
● S42.344 **Nondisplaced spiral fracture of shaft of humerus, right arm**
● S42.345 **Nondisplaced spiral fracture of shaft of humerus, left arm**
● S42.346 **Nondisplaced spiral fracture of shaft of humerus, unspecified arm**

● S42.35 **Comminuted fracture of shaft of humerus**
● S42.351 **Displaced comminuted fracture of shaft of humerus, right arm**
● S42.352 **Displaced comminuted fracture of shaft of humerus, left arm**
● S42.353 **Displaced comminuted fracture of shaft of humerus, unspecified arm**
● S42.354 **Nondisplaced comminuted fracture of shaft of humerus, right arm**
● S42.355 **Nondisplaced comminuted fracture of shaft of humerus, left arm**
● S42.356 **Nondisplaced comminuted fracture of shaft of humerus, unspecified arm**

● S42.36 **Segmental fracture of shaft of humerus**
● S42.361 **Displaced segmental fracture of shaft of humerus, right arm**
● S42.362 **Displaced segmental fracture of shaft of humerus, left arm**
● S42.363 **Displaced segmental fracture of shaft of humerus, unspecified arm**
● S42.364 **Nondisplaced segmental fracture of shaft of humerus, right arm**
● S42.365 **Nondisplaced segmental fracture of shaft of humerus, left arm**
● S42.366 **Nondisplaced segmental fracture of shaft of humerus, unspecified arm**

● S42.39 Other fracture of shaft of humerus

● S42.391 Other fracture of shaft of **right** humerus

● S42.392 Other fracture of shaft of **left** humerus

● S42.399 Other fracture of shaft of **unspecified** humerus

● S42.4 Fracture of **lower end** of humerus
Fracture of distal end of humerus

Excludes2 fracture of shaft of humerus (S42.3-)
physeal fracture of lower end of humerus (S49.1-)

● S42.40 **Unspecified** fracture of lower end of humerus
Fracture of elbow NOS

● S42.401 Unspecified fracture of lower end of **right** humerus

● S42.402 Unspecified fracture of lower end of **left** humerus

● S42.409 Unspecified fracture of lower end of **unspecified** humerus

● S42.41 **Simple supracondylar** fracture **without intercondylar fracture** of humerus

● S42.411 **Displaced** simple supracondylar fracture without intercondylar fracture of **right** humerus

● S42.412 **Displaced** simple supracondylar fracture without intercondylar fracture of **left** humerus

● S42.413 **Displaced** simple supracondylar fracture without intercondylar fracture of **unspecified** humerus

● S42.414 **Nondisplaced** simple supracondylar fracture without intercondylar fracture of **right** humerus

● S42.415 **Nondisplaced** simple supracondylar fracture without intercondylar fracture of **left** humerus

● S42.416 **Nondisplaced** simple supracondylar fracture without intercondylar fracture of **unspecified** humerus

● S42.42 **Comminuted supracondylar** fracture **without intercondylar fracture** of humerus

● S42.421 **Displaced** comminuted supracondylar fracture without intercondylar fracture of **right** humerus

● S42.422 **Displaced** comminuted supracondylar fracture without intercondylar fracture of **left** humerus

● S42.423 **Displaced** comminuted supracondylar fracture without intercondylar fracture of **unspecified** humerus

● S42.424 **Nondisplaced** comminuted supracondylar fracture without intercondylar fracture of **right** humerus

● S42.425 **Nondisplaced** comminuted supracondylar fracture without intercondylar fracture of **left** humerus

● S42.426 **Nondisplaced** comminuted supracondylar fracture without intercondylar fracture of **unspecified** humerus

● S42.43 Fracture (avulsion) of **lateral epicondyle** of humerus

● S42.431 **Displaced** fracture (avulsion) of lateral epicondyle of **right** humerus

● S42.432 **Displaced** fracture (avulsion) of lateral epicondyle of **left** humerus

● S42.433 **Displaced** fracture (avulsion) of lateral epicondyle of **unspecified** humerus

● S42.434 **Nondisplaced** fracture (avulsion) of lateral epicondyle of **right** humerus

● S42.435 **Nondisplaced** fracture (avulsion) of lateral epicondyle of **left** humerus

● S42.436 **Nondisplaced** fracture (avulsion) of lateral epicondyle of **unspecified** humerus

● S42.44 Fracture (avulsion) of **medial epicondyle** of humerus

● S42.441 **Displaced** fracture (avulsion) of medial epicondyle of **right** humerus

● S42.442 **Displaced** fracture (avulsion) of medial epicondyle of **left** humerus

● S42.443 **Displaced** fracture (avulsion) of medial epicondyle of **unspecified** humerus

● S42.444 **Nondisplaced** fracture (avulsion) of medial epicondyle of **right** humerus

● S42.445 **Nondisplaced** fracture (avulsion) of medial epicondyle of **left** humerus

● S42.446 **Nondisplaced** fracture (avulsion) of medial epicondyle of **unspecified** humerus

● S42.447 **Incarcerated** fracture (avulsion) of medial epicondyle of **right** humerus

● S42.448 **Incarcerated** fracture (avulsion) of medial epicondyle of **left** humerus

● S42.449 **Incarcerated** fracture (avulsion) of medial epicondyle of **unspecified** humerus

● S42.45 Fracture of **lateral condyle** of humerus
Fracture of capitellum of humerus

● S42.451 **Displaced** fracture of lateral condyle of **right** humerus

● S42.452 **Displaced** fracture of lateral condyle of **left** humerus

● S42.453 **Displaced** fracture of lateral condyle of **unspecified** humerus

● S42.454 **Nondisplaced** fracture of lateral condyle of **right** humerus

● S42.455 **Nondisplaced** fracture of lateral condyle of **left** humerus

● S42.456 **Nondisplaced** fracture of lateral condyle of **unspecified** humerus

● S42.46 Fracture of **medial condyle** of humerus
Trochlea fracture of humerus

● S42.461 **Displaced** fracture of medial condyle of **right** humerus

● S42.462 **Displaced** fracture of medial condyle of **left** humerus

● S42.463 **Displaced** fracture of medial condyle of **unspecified** humerus

● S42.464 **Nondisplaced** fracture of medial condyle of **right** humerus

● S42.465 **Nondisplaced** fracture of medial condyle of **left** humerus

● S42.466 **Nondisplaced** fracture of medial condyle of **unspecified** humerus

S42.47 **Transcondylar fracture of humerus**
- S42.471 **Displaced transcondylar fracture of right humerus**
- S42.472 **Displaced transcondylar fracture of left humerus**
- S42.473 **Displaced transcondylar fracture of unspecified humerus**
- S42.474 **Nondisplaced transcondylar fracture of right humerus**
- S42.475 **Nondisplaced transcondylar fracture of left humerus**
- S42.476 **Nondisplaced transcondylar fracture of unspecified humerus**

S42.48 **Torus fracture of lower end of humerus**

The appropriate 7th character is to be added to all codes in subcategory S42.48

A	initial encounter for closed fracture
D	subsequent encounter for fracture with routine healing
G	subsequent encounter for fracture with delayed healing
K	subsequent encounter for fracture with nonunion
P	subsequent encounter for fracture with malunion
S	sequela

- S42.481 **Torus fracture of lower end of right humerus**
- S42.482 **Torus fracture of lower end of left humerus**
- S42.489 **Torus fracture of lower end of unspecified humerus**

S42.49 **Other fracture of lower end of humerus**
- S42.491 **Other displaced fracture of lower end of right humerus**
- S42.492 **Other displaced fracture of lower end of left humerus**
- S42.493 **Other displaced fracture of lower end of unspecified humerus**
- S42.494 **Other nondisplaced fracture of lower end of right humerus**
- S42.495 **Other nondisplaced fracture of lower end of left humerus**
- S42.496 **Other nondisplaced fracture of lower end of unspecified humerus**

S42.9 **Fracture of shoulder girdle, part unspecified**

Fracture of shoulder NOS
- X S42.90 **Fracture of unspecified shoulder girdle, part unspecified**
- X S42.91 **Fracture of right shoulder girdle, part unspecified**
- X S42.92 **Fracture of left shoulder girdle, part unspecified**

S43 **Dislocation and sprain of joints and ligaments of shoulder girdle**

Includes avulsion of joint or ligament of shoulder girdle
laceration of cartilage, joint or ligament of shoulder girdle
sprain of cartilage, joint or ligament of shoulder girdle
traumatic hemarthrosis of joint or ligament of shoulder girdle
traumatic rupture of joint or ligament of shoulder girdle
traumatic subluxation of joint or ligament of shoulder girdle
traumatic tear of joint or ligament of shoulder girdle

Code also any associated open wound

Excludes2 strain of muscle, fascia and tendon of shoulder and upper arm (S46.-)

The appropriate 7th character is to be added to each code from category S43

A	initial encounter
D	subsequent encounter
S	sequela

S43.Ø **Subluxation and dislocation of shoulder joint**

Dislocation of glenohumeral joint
Subluxation of glenohumeral joint

S43.ØØ **Unspecified subluxation and dislocation of shoulder joint**

Dislocation of humerus NOS
Subluxation of humerus NOS
- S43.ØØ1 **Unspecified subluxation of right shoulder joint**
- S43.ØØ2 **Unspecified subluxation of left shoulder joint**
- S43.ØØ3 **Unspecified subluxation of unspecified shoulder joint**
- S43.ØØ4 **Unspecified dislocation of right shoulder joint**
- S43.ØØ5 **Unspecified dislocation of left shoulder joint**
- S43.ØØ6 **Unspecified dislocation of unspecified shoulder joint**

S43.Ø1 **Anterior subluxation and dislocation of humerus**
- S43.Ø11 **Anterior subluxation of right humerus**
- S43.Ø12 **Anterior subluxation of left humerus**
- S43.Ø13 **Anterior subluxation of unspecified humerus**
- S43.Ø14 **Anterior dislocation of right humerus**
- S43.Ø15 **Anterior dislocation of left humerus**
- S43.Ø16 **Anterior dislocation of unspecified humerus**

S43.Ø2 **Posterior subluxation and dislocation of humerus**
- S43.Ø21 **Posterior subluxation of right humerus**
- S43.Ø22 **Posterior subluxation of left humerus**
- S43.Ø23 **Posterior subluxation of unspecified humerus**
- S43.Ø24 **Posterior dislocation of right humerus**
- S43.Ø25 **Posterior dislocation of left humerus**
- S43.Ø26 **Posterior dislocation of unspecified humerus**

S43.03 Inferior subluxation and dislocation of humerus
- S43.031 Inferior subluxation of right humerus
- S43.032 Inferior subluxation of left humerus
- S43.033 Inferior subluxation of unspecified humerus
- S43.034 Inferior dislocation of right humerus
- S43.035 Inferior dislocation of left humerus
- S43.036 Inferior dislocation of unspecified humerus

S43.08 Other subluxation and dislocation of shoulder joint
- S43.081 Other subluxation of right shoulder joint
- S43.082 Other subluxation of left shoulder joint
- S43.083 Other subluxation of unspecified shoulder joint
- S43.084 Other dislocation of right shoulder joint
- S43.085 Other dislocation of left shoulder joint
- S43.086 Other dislocation of unspecified shoulder joint

S43.1 Subluxation and dislocation of acromioclavicular joint

S43.10 Unspecified dislocation of acromioclavicular joint
- S43.101 Unspecified dislocation of right acromioclavicular joint
- S43.102 Unspecified dislocation of left acromioclavicular joint
- S43.109 Unspecified dislocation of unspecified acromioclavicular joint

S43.11 Subluxation of acromioclavicular joint
- S43.111 Subluxation of right acromioclavicular joint
- S43.112 Subluxation of left acromioclavicular joint
- S43.119 Subluxation of unspecified acromioclavicular joint

S43.12 Dislocation of acromioclavicular joint, 100%-200% displacement
- S43.121 Dislocation of right acromioclavicular joint, 100%-200% displacement
- S43.122 Dislocation of left acromioclavicular joint, 100%-200% displacement
- S43.129 Dislocation of unspecified acromioclavicular joint, 100%-200% displacement

S43.13 Dislocation of acromioclavicular joint, greater than 200% displacement
- S43.131 Dislocation of right acromioclavicular joint, greater than 200% displacement
- S43.132 Dislocation of left acromioclavicular joint, greater than 200% displacement
- S43.139 Dislocation of unspecified acromioclavicular joint, greater than 200% displacement

S43.14 Inferior dislocation of acromioclavicular joint
- S43.141 Inferior dislocation of right acromioclavicular joint
- S43.142 Inferior dislocation of left acromioclavicular joint
- S43.149 Inferior dislocation of unspecified acromioclavicular joint

S43.15 Posterior dislocation of acromioclavicular joint
- S43.151 Posterior dislocation of right acromioclavicular joint
- S43.152 Posterior dislocation of left acromioclavicular joint
- S43.159 Posterior dislocation of unspecified acromioclavicular joint

S43.2 Subluxation and dislocation of sternoclavicular joint

S43.20 Unspecified subluxation and dislocation of sternoclavicular joint
- S43.201 Unspecified subluxation of right sternoclavicular joint
- S43.202 Unspecified subluxation of left sternoclavicular joint
- S43.203 Unspecified subluxation of unspecified sternoclavicular joint
- S43.204 Unspecified dislocation of right sternoclavicular joint
- S43.205 Unspecified dislocation of left sternoclavicular joint
- S43.206 Unspecified dislocation of unspecified sternoclavicular joint

S43.21 Anterior subluxation and dislocation of sternoclavicular joint
- S43.211 Anterior subluxation of right sternoclavicular joint
- S43.212 Anterior subluxation of left sternoclavicular joint
- S43.213 Anterior subluxation of unspecified sternoclavicular joint
- S43.214 Anterior dislocation of right sternoclavicular joint
- S43.215 Anterior dislocation of left sternoclavicular joint
- S43.216 Anterior dislocation of unspecified sternoclavicular joint

S43.22 Posterior subluxation and dislocation of sternoclavicular joint
- S43.221 Posterior subluxation of right sternoclavicular joint
- S43.222 Posterior subluxation of left sternoclavicular joint
- S43.223 Posterior subluxation of unspecified sternoclavicular joint
- S43.224 Posterior dislocation of right sternoclavicular joint
- S43.225 Posterior dislocation of left sternoclavicular joint
- S43.226 Posterior dislocation of unspecified sternoclavicular joint

S43.3 Subluxation and dislocation of other and unspecified parts of shoulder girdle

S43.30 Subluxation and dislocation of unspecified parts of shoulder girdle

Dislocation of shoulder girdle NOS
Subluxation of shoulder girdle NOS
- S43.301 Subluxation of unspecified parts of right shoulder girdle
- S43.302 Subluxation of unspecified parts of left shoulder girdle
- S43.303 Subluxation of unspecified parts of unspecified shoulder girdle
- S43.304 Dislocation of unspecified parts of right shoulder girdle
- S43.305 Dislocation of unspecified parts of left shoulder girdle
- S43.306 Dislocation of unspecified parts of unspecified shoulder girdle

● S43.31 Subluxation and dislocation of scapula
● S43.311 Subluxation of right scapula
● S43.312 Subluxation of left scapula
● S43.313 Subluxation of unspecified scapula
● S43.314 Dislocation of right scapula
● S43.315 Dislocation of left scapula
● S43.316 Dislocation of unspecified scapula
● S43.39 Subluxation and dislocation of other parts of shoulder girdle
● S43.391 Subluxation of other parts of right shoulder girdle
● S43.392 Subluxation of other parts of left shoulder girdle
● S43.393 Subluxation of other parts of unspecified shoulder girdle
● S43.394 Dislocation of other parts of right shoulder girdle
● S43.395 Dislocation of other parts of left shoulder girdle
● S43.396 Dislocation of other parts of unspecified shoulder girdle
● S43.4 Sprain of shoulder joint
● S43.40 Unspecified sprain of shoulder joint
● S43.401 Unspecified sprain of right shoulder joint
● S43.402 Unspecified sprain of left shoulder joint
● S43.409 Unspecified sprain of unspecified shoulder joint
● S43.41 Sprain of coracohumeral (ligament)
● S43.411 Sprain of right coracohumeral (ligament)
● S43.412 Sprain of left coracohumeral (ligament)
● S43.419 Sprain of unspecified coracohumeral (ligament)
● S43.42 Sprain of rotator cuff capsule
Encounters during the healing phase
Excludes1 rotator cuff syndrome (complete) (incomplete), not specified as traumatic (M75.1-)
Excludes2 injury of tendon of rotator cuff (S46.Ø-)
● S43.421 Sprain of right rotator cuff capsule
● S43.422 Sprain of left rotator cuff capsule
● S43.429 Sprain of unspecified rotator cuff capsule
● S43.43 Superior glenoid labrum lesion
SLAP lesion
Coding Clinic: 2Ø19, Q2, P27
● S43.431 Superior glenoid labrum lesion of right shoulder
● S43.432 Superior glenoid labrum lesion of left shoulder
● S43.439 Superior glenoid labrum lesion of unspecified shoulder
● S43.49 Other sprain of shoulder joint
● S43.491 Other sprain of right shoulder joint
● S43.492 Other sprain of left shoulder joint
● S43.499 Other sprain of unspecified shoulder joint
● S43.5 Sprain of acromioclavicular joint
Sprain of acromioclavicular ligament
X● S43.5Ø Sprain of unspecified acromioclavicular joint
X● S43.51 Sprain of right acromioclavicular joint
X● S43.52 Sprain of left acromioclavicular joint
● S43.6 Sprain of sternoclavicular joint
X● S43.6Ø Sprain of unspecified sternoclavicular joint
X● S43.61 Sprain of right sternoclavicular joint
X● S43.62 Sprain of left sternoclavicular joint
● S43.8 Sprain of other specified parts of shoulder girdle
X● S43.8Ø Sprain of other specified parts of unspecified shoulder girdle
X● S43.81 Sprain of other specified parts of right shoulder girdle
X● S43.82 Sprain of other specified parts of left shoulder girdle
● S43.9 Sprain of unspecified parts of shoulder girdle
X● S43.9Ø Sprain of unspecified parts of unspecified shoulder girdle
Sprain of shoulder girdle NOS
X● S43.91 Sprain of unspecified parts of right shoulder girdle
X● S43.92 Sprain of unspecified parts of left shoulder girdle

● S44 Injury of nerves at shoulder and upper arm level
Code also any associated open wound (S41.-)
Excludes2 injury of brachial plexus (S14.3-)
The appropriate 7th character is to be added to each code from category S44

A	initial encounter
D	subsequent encounter
S	sequela

● S44.Ø Injury of ulnar nerve at upper arm level
Excludes1 ulnar nerve NOS (S54.Ø)
X● S44.ØØ Injury of ulnar nerve at upper arm level, unspecified arm
X● S44.Ø1 Injury of ulnar nerve at upper arm level, right arm
X● S44.Ø2 Injury of ulnar nerve at upper arm level, left arm
● S44.1 Injury of median nerve at upper arm level
Excludes1 median nerve NOS (S54.1)
X● S44.1Ø Injury of median nerve at upper arm level, unspecified arm
X● S44.11 Injury of median nerve at upper arm level, right arm
X● S44.12 Injury of median nerve at upper arm level, left arm
● S44.2 Injury of radial nerve at upper arm level
Excludes1 radial nerve NOS (S54.2)
X● S44.2Ø Injury of radial nerve at upper arm level, unspecified arm
X● S44.21 Injury of radial nerve at upper arm level, right arm
X● S44.22 Injury of radial nerve at upper arm level, left arm
● S44.3 Injury of axillary nerve
X● S44.3Ø Injury of axillary nerve, unspecified arm
X● S44.31 Injury of axillary nerve, right arm
X● S44.32 Injury of axillary nerve, left arm
● S44.4 Injury of musculocutaneous nerve
X● S44.4Ø Injury of musculocutaneous nerve, unspecified arm
X● S44.41 Injury of musculocutaneous nerve, right arm
X● S44.42 Injury of musculocutaneous nerve, left arm

- S44.5 Injury of cutaneous sensory nerve at shoulder and upper arm level
  - X S44.50 Injury of cutaneous sensory nerve at shoulder and upper arm level, unspecified arm
  - X S44.51 Injury of cutaneous sensory nerve at shoulder and upper arm level, right arm
  - X S44.52 Injury of cutaneous sensory nerve at shoulder and upper arm level, left arm
- S44.8 Injury of other nerves at shoulder and upper arm level
  - S44.8X Injury of other nerves at shoulder and upper arm level
    - S44.8X1 Injury of other nerves at shoulder and upper arm level, right arm
    - S44.8X2 Injury of other nerves at shoulder and upper arm level, left arm
    - S44.8X9 Injury of other nerves at shoulder and upper arm level, unspecified arm
- S44.9 Injury of unspecified nerve at shoulder and upper arm level
  - X S44.90 Injury of unspecified nerve at shoulder and upper arm level, unspecified arm
  - X S44.91 Injury of unspecified nerve at shoulder and upper arm level, right arm
  - X S44.92 Injury of unspecified nerve at shoulder and upper arm level, left arm

S45 Injury of blood vessels at shoulder and upper arm level

Code also any associated open wound (S41.-)

Excludes2 injury of subclavian artery (S25.1)
injury of subclavian vein (S25.3)

The appropriate 7th character is to be added to each code from category S45

A	initial encounter
D	subsequent encounter
S	sequela

- S45.Ø Injury of axillary artery
  - S45.ØØ Unspecified injury of axillary artery
    - S45.ØØ1 Unspecified injury of axillary artery, right side
    - S45.ØØ2 Unspecified injury of axillary artery, left side
    - S45.ØØ9 Unspecified injury of axillary artery, unspecified side
  - S45.Ø1 Laceration of axillary artery
    - S45.Ø11 Laceration of axillary artery, right side
    - S45.Ø12 Laceration of axillary artery, left side
    - S45.Ø19 Laceration of axillary artery, unspecified side
  - S45.Ø9 Other specified injury of axillary artery
    - S45.Ø91 Other specified injury of axillary artery, right side
    - S45.Ø92 Other specified injury of axillary artery, left side
    - S45.Ø99 Other specified injury of axillary artery, unspecified side
- S45.1 Injury of brachial artery
  - S45.1Ø Unspecified injury of brachial artery
    - S45.1Ø1 Unspecified injury of brachial artery, right side
    - S45.1Ø2 Unspecified injury of brachial artery, left side
    - S45.1Ø9 Unspecified injury of brachial artery, unspecified side
  - S45.11 Laceration of brachial artery
    - S45.111 Laceration of brachial artery, right side
    - S45.112 Laceration of brachial artery, left side
    - S45.119 Laceration of brachial artery, unspecified side
  - S45.19 Other specified injury of brachial artery
    - S45.191 Other specified injury of brachial artery, right side
    - S45.192 Other specified injury of brachial artery, left side
    - S45.199 Other specified injury of brachial artery, unspecified side
- S45.2 Injury of axillary or brachial vein
  - S45.2Ø Unspecified injury of axillary or brachial vein
    - S45.2Ø1 Unspecified injury of axillary or brachial vein, right side
    - S45.2Ø2 Unspecified injury of axillary or brachial vein, left side
    - S45.2Ø9 Unspecified injury of axillary or brachial vein, unspecified side
  - S45.21 Laceration of axillary or brachial vein
    - S45.211 Laceration of axillary or brachial vein, right side
    - S45.212 Laceration of axillary or brachial vein, left side
    - S45.219 Laceration of axillary or brachial vein, unspecified side
  - S45.29 Other specified injury of axillary or brachial vein
    - S45.291 Other specified injury of axillary or brachial vein, right side
    - S45.292 Other specified injury of axillary or brachial vein, left side
    - S45.299 Other specified injury of axillary or brachial vein, unspecified side
- S45.3 Injury of superficial vein at shoulder and upper arm level
  - S45.3Ø Unspecified injury of superficial vein at shoulder and upper arm level
    - S45.3Ø1 Unspecified injury of superficial vein at shoulder and upper arm level, right arm
    - S45.3Ø2 Unspecified injury of superficial vein at shoulder and upper arm level, left arm
    - S45.3Ø9 Unspecified injury of superficial vein at shoulder and upper arm level, unspecified arm
  - S45.31 Laceration of superficial vein at shoulder and upper arm level
    - S45.311 Laceration of superficial vein at shoulder and upper arm level, right arm
    - S45.312 Laceration of superficial vein at shoulder and upper arm level, left arm
    - S45.319 Laceration of superficial vein at shoulder and upper arm level, unspecified arm
  - S45.39 Other specified injury of superficial vein at shoulder and upper arm level
    - S45.391 Other specified injury of superficial vein at shoulder and upper arm level, right arm
    - S45.392 Other specified injury of superficial vein at shoulder and upper arm level, left arm
    - S45.399 Other specified injury of superficial vein at shoulder and upper arm level, unspecified arm

- S45.8 Injury of other specified blood vessels at shoulder and upper arm level
  - S45.80 Unspecified injury of other specified blood vessels at shoulder and upper arm level
    - S45.801 Unspecified injury of other specified blood vessels at shoulder and upper arm level, right arm
    - S45.802 Unspecified injury of other specified blood vessels at shoulder and upper arm level, left arm
    - S45.809 Unspecified injury of other specified blood vessels at shoulder and upper arm level, unspecified arm
  - S45.81 Laceration of other specified blood vessels at shoulder and upper arm level
    - S45.811 Laceration of other specified blood vessels at shoulder and upper arm level, right arm
    - S45.812 Laceration of other specified blood vessels at shoulder and upper arm level, left arm
    - S45.819 Laceration of other specified blood vessels at shoulder and upper arm level, unspecified arm
  - S45.89 Other specified injury of other specified blood vessels at shoulder and upper arm level
    - S45.891 Other specified injury of other specified blood vessels at shoulder and upper arm level, right arm
    - S45.892 Other specified injury of other specified blood vessels at shoulder and upper arm level, left arm
    - S45.899 Other specified injury of other specified blood vessels at shoulder and upper arm level, unspecified arm
- S45.9 Injury of unspecified blood vessel at shoulder and upper arm level
  - S45.90 Unspecified injury of unspecified blood vessel at shoulder and upper arm level
    - S45.901 Unspecified injury of unspecified blood vessel at shoulder and upper arm level, right arm
    - S45.902 Unspecified injury of unspecified blood vessel at shoulder and upper arm level, left arm
    - S45.909 Unspecified injury of unspecified blood vessel at shoulder and upper arm level, unspecified arm
  - S45.91 Laceration of unspecified blood vessel at shoulder and upper arm level
    - S45.911 Laceration of unspecified blood vessel at shoulder and upper arm level, right arm
    - S45.912 Laceration of unspecified blood vessel at shoulder and upper arm level, left arm
    - S45.919 Laceration of unspecified blood vessel at shoulder and upper arm level, unspecified arm
  - S45.99 Other specified injury of unspecified blood vessel at shoulder and upper arm level
    - S45.991 Other specified injury of unspecified blood vessel at shoulder and upper arm level, right arm
    - S45.992 Other specified injury of unspecified blood vessel at shoulder and upper arm level, left arm
    - S45.999 Other specified injury of unspecified blood vessel at shoulder and upper arm level, unspecified arm

S46 Injury of muscle, fascia and tendon at shoulder and upper arm level

Code also any associated open wound (S41.-)

Excludes2 injury of muscle, fascia and tendon at elbow (S56.-)
sprain of joints and ligaments of shoulder girdle (S43.9)

The appropriate 7th character is to be added to each code from category S46

A	initial encounter
D	subsequent encounter
S	sequela

- S46.0 Injury of muscle(s) and tendon(s) of the rotator cuff of shoulder
  - S46.00 Unspecified injury of muscle(s) and tendon(s) of the rotator cuff of shoulder
    - S46.001 Unspecified injury of muscle(s) and tendon(s) of the rotator cuff of right shoulder
    - S46.002 Unspecified injury of muscle(s) and tendon(s) of the rotator cuff of left shoulder
    - S46.009 Unspecified injury of muscle(s) and tendon(s) of the rotator cuff of unspecified shoulder
  - S46.01 Strain of muscle(s) and tendon(s) of the rotator cuff of shoulder
    Acute onset due to trauma to rotator cuff muscle/tendon
    - S46.011 Strain of muscle(s) and tendon(s) of the rotator cuff of right shoulder
    - S46.012 Strain of muscle(s) and tendon(s) of the rotator cuff of left shoulder
    - S46.019 Strain of muscle(s) and tendon(s) of the rotator cuff of unspecified shoulder
  - S46.02 Laceration of muscle(s) and tendon(s) of the rotator cuff of shoulder
    - S46.021 Laceration of muscle(s) and tendon(s) of the rotator cuff of right shoulder
    - S46.022 Laceration of muscle(s) and tendon(s) of the rotator cuff of left shoulder
    - S46.029 Laceration of muscle(s) and tendon(s) of the rotator cuff of unspecified shoulder
  - S46.09 Other injury of muscle(s) and tendon(s) of the rotator cuff of shoulder
    - S46.091 Other injury of muscle(s) and tendon(s) of the rotator cuff of right shoulder
    - S46.092 Other injury of muscle(s) and tendon(s) of the rotator cuff of left shoulder
    - S46.099 Other injury of muscle(s) and tendon(s) of the rotator cuff of unspecified shoulder
- S46.1 Injury of muscle, fascia and tendon of long head of biceps
  - S46.10 Unspecified injury of muscle, fascia and tendon of long head of biceps
    - S46.101 Unspecified injury of muscle, fascia and tendon of long head of biceps, right arm
    - S46.102 Unspecified injury of muscle, fascia and tendon of long head of biceps, left arm
    - S46.109 Unspecified injury of muscle, fascia and tendon of long head of biceps, unspecified arm

- S46.11 Strain of muscle, fascia and tendon of long head of biceps
  Coding Clinic: 2019, Q2, P27
  - S46.111 Strain of muscle, fascia and tendon of long head of biceps, right arm
  - S46.112 Strain of muscle, fascia and tendon of long head of biceps, left arm
  - S46.119 Strain of muscle, fascia and tendon of long head of biceps, unspecified arm
- S46.12 Laceration of muscle, fascia and tendon of long head of biceps
  - S46.121 Laceration of muscle, fascia and tendon of long head of biceps, right arm
  - S46.122 Laceration of muscle, fascia and tendon of long head of biceps, left arm
  - S46.129 Laceration of muscle, fascia and tendon of long head of biceps, unspecified arm
- S46.19 Other injury of muscle, fascia and tendon of long head of biceps
  - S46.191 Other injury of muscle, fascia and tendon of long head of biceps, right arm
  - S46.192 Other injury of muscle, fascia and tendon of long head of biceps, left arm
  - S46.199 Other injury of muscle, fascia and tendon of long head of biceps, unspecified arm

S46.2 Injury of muscle, fascia and tendon of other parts of biceps
- S46.20 Unspecified injury of muscle, fascia and tendon of other parts of biceps
  - S46.201 Unspecified injury of muscle, fascia and tendon of other parts of biceps, right arm
  - S46.202 Unspecified injury of muscle, fascia and tendon of other parts of biceps, left arm
  - S46.209 Unspecified injury of muscle, fascia and tendon of other parts of biceps, unspecified arm
- S46.21 Strain of muscle, fascia and tendon of other parts of biceps
  - S46.211 Strain of muscle, fascia and tendon of other parts of biceps, right arm
  - S46.212 Strain of muscle, fascia and tendon of other parts of biceps, left arm
  - S46.219 Strain of muscle, fascia and tendon of other parts of biceps, unspecified arm
- S46.22 Laceration of muscle, fascia and tendon of other parts of biceps
  - S46.221 Laceration of muscle, fascia and tendon of other parts of biceps, right arm
  - S46.222 Laceration of muscle, fascia and tendon of other parts of biceps, left arm
  - S46.229 Laceration of muscle, fascia and tendon of other parts of biceps, unspecified arm
- S46.29 Other injury of muscle, fascia and tendon of other parts of biceps
  - S46.291 Other injury of muscle, fascia and tendon of other parts of biceps, right arm
  - S46.292 Other injury of muscle, fascia and tendon of other parts of biceps, left arm
  - S46.299 Other injury of muscle, fascia and tendon of other parts of biceps, unspecified arm

S46.3 Injury of muscle, fascia and tendon of triceps
- S46.30 Unspecified injury of muscle, fascia and tendon of triceps
  - S46.301 Unspecified injury of muscle, fascia and tendon of triceps, right arm
  - S46.302 Unspecified injury of muscle, fascia and tendon of triceps, left arm
  - S46.309 Unspecified injury of muscle, fascia and tendon of triceps, unspecified arm
- S46.31 Strain of muscle, fascia and tendon of triceps
  - S46.311 Strain of muscle, fascia and tendon of triceps, right arm
  - S46.312 Strain of muscle, fascia and tendon of triceps, left arm
  - S46.319 Strain of muscle, fascia and tendon of triceps, unspecified arm
- S46.32 Laceration of muscle, fascia and tendon of triceps
  - S46.321 Laceration of muscle, fascia and tendon of triceps, right arm
  - S46.322 Laceration of muscle, fascia and tendon of triceps, left arm
  - S46.329 Laceration of muscle, fascia and tendon of triceps, unspecified arm
- S46.39 Other injury of muscle, fascia and tendon of triceps
  - S46.391 Other injury of muscle, fascia and tendon of triceps, right arm
  - S46.392 Other injury of muscle, fascia and tendon of triceps, left arm
  - S46.399 Other injury of muscle, fascia and tendon of triceps, unspecified arm

S46.8 Injury of other muscles, fascia and tendons at shoulder and upper arm level
- S46.80 Unspecified injury of other muscles, fascia and tendons at shoulder and upper arm level
  - S46.801 Unspecified injury of other muscles, fascia and tendons at shoulder and upper arm level, right arm
  - S46.802 Unspecified injury of other muscles, fascia and tendons at shoulder and upper arm level, left arm
  - S46.809 Unspecified injury of other muscles, fascia and tendons at shoulder and upper arm level, unspecified arm
- S46.81 Strain of other muscles, fascia and tendons at shoulder and upper arm level
  - S46.811 Strain of other muscles, fascia and tendons at shoulder and upper arm level, right arm
  - S46.812 Strain of other muscles, fascia and tendons at shoulder and upper arm level, left arm
  - S46.819 Strain of other muscles, fascia and tendons at shoulder and upper arm level, unspecified arm
- S46.82 Laceration of other muscles, fascia and tendons at shoulder and upper arm level
  - S46.821 Laceration of other muscles, fascia and tendons at shoulder and upper arm level, right arm
  - S46.822 Laceration of other muscles, fascia and tendons at shoulder and upper arm level, left arm
  - S46.829 Laceration of other muscles, fascia and tendons at shoulder and upper arm level, unspecified arm

● S46.89 **Other** injury of other muscles, fascia and tendons at shoulder and upper arm level
● S46.891 Other injury of other muscles, fascia and tendons at shoulder and upper arm level, **right** arm
● S46.892 Other injury of other muscles, fascia and tendons at shoulder and upper arm level, **left** arm
● S46.899 Other injury of other muscles, fascia and tendons at shoulder and upper arm level, **unspecified** arm

● S46.9 Injury of **unspecified** muscle, fascia and tendon at shoulder and upper arm level
● S46.90 **Unspecified** injury of unspecified muscle, fascia and tendon at shoulder and upper arm level
● S46.901 Unspecified injury of unspecified muscle, fascia and tendon at shoulder and upper arm level, **right** arm
● S46.902 Unspecified injury of unspecified muscle, fascia and tendon at shoulder and upper arm level, **left** arm
● S46.909 Unspecified injury of unspecified muscle, fascia and tendon at shoulder and upper arm level, **unspecified** arm
● S46.91 **Strain** of unspecified muscle, fascia and tendon at shoulder and upper arm level
● S46.911 Strain of unspecified muscle, fascia and tendon at shoulder and upper arm level, **right** arm
● S46.912 Strain of unspecified muscle, fascia and tendon at shoulder and upper arm level, **left** arm
● S46.919 Strain of unspecified muscle, fascia and tendon at shoulder and upper arm level, **unspecified** arm
● S46.92 **Laceration** of unspecified muscle, fascia and tendon at shoulder and upper arm level
● S46.921 Laceration of unspecified muscle, fascia and tendon at shoulder and upper arm level, **right** arm
● S46.922 Laceration of unspecified muscle, fascia and tendon at shoulder and upper arm level, **left** arm
● S46.929 Laceration of unspecified muscle, fascia and tendon at shoulder and upper arm level, **unspecified** arm
● S46.99 **Other** injury of unspecified muscle, fascia and tendon at shoulder and upper arm level
● S46.991 Other injury of unspecified muscle, fascia and tendon at shoulder and upper arm level, **right** arm
● S46.992 Other injury of unspecified muscle, fascia and tendon at shoulder and upper arm level, **left** arm
● S46.999 Other injury of unspecified muscle, fascia and tendon at shoulder and upper arm level, **unspecified** arm

● S47 **Crushing injury** of shoulder and upper arm

Use additional code for all associated injuries

Excludes2 crushing injury of elbow (S57.Ø-)

The appropriate 7th character is to be added to each code from category S47

A	initial encounter
D	subsequent encounter
S	sequela

X● S47.1 Crushing injury of **right** shoulder and upper arm
X● S47.2 Crushing injury of **left** shoulder and upper arm
X● S47.9 Crushing injury of shoulder and upper arm, **unspecified** arm

● S48 **Traumatic amputation** of shoulder and upper arm

An amputation not identified as partial or complete should be coded to complete

Excludes1 traumatic amputation at elbow level (S58.Ø)

The appropriate 7th character is to be added to each code from category S48

A	initial encounter
D	subsequent encounter
S	sequela

● S48.Ø Traumatic amputation at **shoulder joint**
● S48.Ø1 **Complete** traumatic amputation at shoulder joint
● S48.Ø11 Complete traumatic amputation at **right** shoulder joint A, S
● S48.Ø12 Complete traumatic amputation at **left** shoulder joint A, S
● S48.Ø19 Complete traumatic amputation at **unspecified** shoulder joint A, S
● S48.Ø2 **Partial** traumatic amputation at shoulder joint
● S48.Ø21 Partial traumatic amputation at **right** shoulder joint A, S
● S48.Ø22 Partial traumatic amputation at **left** shoulder joint A, S
● S48.Ø29 Partial traumatic amputation at **unspecified** shoulder joint A, S

● S48.1 Traumatic amputation at level **between shoulder and elbow**
● S48.11 **Complete** traumatic amputation at level between shoulder and elbow
● S48.111 Complete traumatic amputation at level between **right** shoulder and elbow A, S
● S48.112 Complete traumatic amputation at level between **left** shoulder and elbow A, S
● S48.119 Complete traumatic amputation at level between **unspecified** shoulder and elbow A, S
● S48.12 **Partial** traumatic amputation at level between shoulder and elbow
● S48.121 Partial traumatic amputation at level between **right** shoulder and elbow A, S
● S48.122 Partial traumatic amputation at level between **left** shoulder and elbow A, S
● S48.129 Partial traumatic amputation at level between **unspecified** shoulder and elbow A, S

● S48.9 Traumatic amputation of shoulder and upper arm, level **unspecified**
● S48.91 **Complete** traumatic amputation of shoulder and upper arm, level unspecified
● S48.911 Complete traumatic amputation of **right** shoulder and upper arm, level unspecified A, S
● S48.912 Complete traumatic amputation of **left** shoulder and upper arm, level unspecified A, S
● S48.919 Complete traumatic amputation of **unspecified** shoulder and upper arm, level unspecified A, S
● S48.92 **Partial** traumatic amputation of shoulder and upper arm, level unspecified
● S48.921 Partial traumatic amputation of **right** shoulder and upper arm, level unspecified A, S
● S48.922 Partial traumatic amputation of **left** shoulder and upper arm, level unspecified A, S
● S48.929 Partial traumatic amputation of **unspecified** shoulder and upper arm, level unspecified A, S

Item 19–3 SALTER-HARRIS TYPE 1: epiphysis is completely separated from end of bone, or metaphysic growth plate remains attached to epiphysis

SALTER-HARRIS TYPE 2: epiphysis and growth plate are partially separated from metaphysis, which is cracked—most common type

SALTER-HARRIS TYPE 3: fracture occurring through epiphysis and separates part of epiphysis and growth plate from metaphysis fracture, usually at distal end of tibia

SALTER-HARRIS TYPE 4: fracture runs through epiphysis, across growth plate, into metaphysic, surgery is required to restore joint surface to normal and align growth plate

● **S49 Other and unspecified injuries of shoulder and upper arm**

The appropriate 7th character is to be added to each code from subcategories S49.0 and S49.1

A	initial encounter for closed fracture
D	subsequent encounter for fracture with routine healing
G	subsequent encounter for fracture with delayed healing
K	subsequent encounter for fracture with nonunion
P	subsequent encounter for fracture with malunion
S	sequela

● **S49.0 Physeal fracture of upper end of humerus**
- ● S49.00 **Unspecified** physeal fracture of upper end of humerus
  - ● S49.001 Unspecified physeal fracture of upper end of humerus, **right arm**
  - ● S49.002 Unspecified physeal fracture of upper end of humerus, **left arm**
  - ● S49.009 Unspecified physeal fracture of upper end of humerus, **unspecified** arm
- ● S49.01 **Salter-Harris Type I** physeal fracture of upper end of humerus
  - ● S49.011 Salter-Harris Type I physeal fracture of upper end of humerus, **right arm**
  - ● S49.012 Salter-Harris Type I physeal fracture of upper end of humerus, **left arm**
  - ● S49.019 Salter-Harris Type I physeal fracture of upper end of humerus, **unspecified** arm
- ● S49.02 **Salter-Harris Type II** physeal fracture of upper end of humerus
  - ● S49.021 Salter-Harris Type II physeal fracture of upper end of humerus, **right arm**
  - ● S49.022 Salter-Harris Type II physeal fracture of upper end of humerus, **left arm**
  - ● S49.029 Salter-Harris Type II physeal fracture of upper end of humerus, **unspecified** arm
- ● S49.03 **Salter-Harris Type III** physeal fracture of upper end of humerus
  - ● S49.031 Salter-Harris Type III physeal fracture of upper end of humerus, **right arm**
  - ● S49.032 Salter-Harris Type III physeal fracture of upper end of humerus, **left arm**
  - ● S49.039 Salter-Harris Type III physeal fracture of upper end of humerus, **unspecified** arm
- ● S49.04 **Salter-Harris Type IV** physeal fracture of upper end of humerus
  - ● S49.041 Salter-Harris Type IV physeal fracture of upper end of humerus, **right arm**
  - ● S49.042 Salter-Harris Type IV physeal fracture of upper end of humerus, **left arm**
  - ● S49.049 Salter-Harris Type IV physeal fracture of upper end of humerus, **unspecified** arm
- ● S49.09 **Other** physeal fracture of upper end of humerus
  - ● S49.091 Other physeal fracture of upper end of humerus, **right arm**
  - ● S49.092 Other physeal fracture of upper end of humerus, **left arm**
  - ● S49.099 Other physeal fracture of upper end of humerus, **unspecified** arm

● **S49.1 Physeal fracture of lower end of humerus**
- ● S49.10 **Unspecified** physeal fracture of lower end of humerus
  - ● S49.101 Unspecified physeal fracture of lower end of humerus, **right arm**
  - ● S49.102 Unspecified physeal fracture of lower end of humerus, **left arm**
  - ● S49.109 Unspecified physeal fracture of lower end of humerus, **unspecified** arm
- ● S49.11 **Salter-Harris Type I** physeal fracture of lower end of humerus
  - ● S49.111 Salter-Harris Type I physeal fracture of lower end of humerus, **right arm**
  - ● S49.112 Salter-Harris Type I physeal fracture of lower end of humerus, **left arm**
  - ● S49.119 Salter-Harris Type I physeal fracture of lower end of humerus, **unspecified** arm
- ● S49.12 **Salter-Harris Type II** physeal fracture of lower end of humerus
  - ● S49.121 Salter-Harris Type II physeal fracture of lower end of humerus, **right arm**
  - ● S49.122 Salter-Harris Type II physeal fracture of lower end of humerus, **left arm**
  - ● S49.129 Salter-Harris Type II physeal fracture of lower end of humerus, **unspecified** arm
- ● S49.13 **Salter-Harris Type III** physeal fracture of lower end of humerus
  - ● S49.131 Salter-Harris Type III physeal fracture of lower end of humerus, **right arm**
  - ● S49.132 Salter-Harris Type III physeal fracture of lower end of humerus, **left arm**
  - ● S49.139 Salter-Harris Type III physeal fracture of lower end of humerus, **unspecified** arm
- ● S49.14 **Salter-Harris Type IV** physeal fracture of lower end of humerus
  - ● S49.141 Salter-Harris Type IV physeal fracture of lower end of humerus, **right arm**
  - ● S49.142 Salter-Harris Type IV physeal fracture of lower end of humerus, **left arm**
  - ● S49.149 Salter-Harris Type IV physeal fracture of lower end of humerus, **unspecified** arm
- ● S49.19 **Other** physeal fracture of lower end of humerus
  - ● S49.191 Other physeal fracture of lower end of humerus, **right arm**
  - ● S49.192 Other physeal fracture of lower end of humerus, **left arm**
  - ● S49.199 Other physeal fracture of lower end of humerus, **unspecified** arm

● S49.8 Other specified injuries of shoulder and upper arm
The appropriate 7th character is to be added to each code in subcategory S49.8

A	initial encounter
D	subsequent encounter
S	sequela

X● S49.80 Other specified injuries of shoulder and upper arm, unspecified arm
X● S49.81 Other specified injuries of right shoulder and upper arm
X● S49.82 Other specified injuries of left shoulder and upper arm

● S49.9 Unspecified injury of shoulder and upper arm
The appropriate 7th character is to be added to each code in subcategory S49.9

A	initial encounter
D	subsequent encounter
S	sequela

X● S49.90 Unspecified injury of shoulder and upper arm, unspecified arm
X● S49.91 Unspecified injury of right shoulder and upper arm
X● S49.92 Unspecified injury of left shoulder and upper arm

INJURIES TO THE ELBOW AND FOREARM (S50-S59)

Excludes2 burns and corrosions (T20-T32)
frostbite (T33-T34)
injuries of wrist and hand (S60-S69)
insect bite or sting, venomous (T63.4)

● S50 Superficial injury of elbow and forearm
Excludes2 superficial injury of wrist and hand (S60.-)
The appropriate 7th character is to be added to each code from category S50

A	initial encounter
D	subsequent encounter
S	sequela

● S50.0 Contusion of elbow
X● S50.00 Contusion of unspecified elbow
X● S50.01 Contusion of right elbow
X● S50.02 Contusion of left elbow

● S50.1 Contusion of forearm
X● S50.10 Contusion of unspecified forearm
X● S50.11 Contusion of right forearm
X● S50.12 Contusion of left forearm

● S50.3 Other superficial injuries of elbow
● S50.31 Abrasion of elbow
● S50.311 Abrasion of right elbow
● S50.312 Abrasion of left elbow
● S50.319 Abrasion of unspecified elbow
● S50.32 Blister (nonthermal) of elbow
● S50.321 Blister (nonthermal) of right elbow
● S50.322 Blister (nonthermal) of left elbow
● S50.329 Blister (nonthermal) of unspecified elbow
● S50.34 External constriction of elbow
● S50.341 External constriction of right elbow
● S50.342 External constriction of left elbow
● S50.349 External constriction of unspecified elbow
● S50.35 Superficial foreign body of elbow
Splinter in the elbow
● S50.351 Superficial foreign body of right elbow
● S50.352 Superficial foreign body of left elbow
● S50.359 Superficial foreign body of unspecified elbow
● S50.36 Insect bite (nonvenomous) of elbow
● S50.361 Insect bite (nonvenomous) of right elbow
● S50.362 Insect bite (nonvenomous) of left elbow
● S50.369 Insect bite (nonvenomous) of unspecified elbow
● S50.37 Other superficial bite of elbow
Excludes1 open bite of elbow (S51.04)
● S50.371 Other superficial bite of right elbow
● S50.372 Other superficial bite of left elbow
● S50.379 Other superficial bite of unspecified elbow

● S50.8 Other superficial injuries of forearm
● S50.81 Abrasion of forearm
● S50.811 Abrasion of right forearm
● S50.812 Abrasion of left forearm
● S50.819 Abrasion of unspecified forearm
● S50.82 Blister (nonthermal) of forearm
● S50.821 Blister (nonthermal) of right forearm
● S50.822 Blister (nonthermal) of left forearm
● S50.829 Blister (nonthermal) of unspecified forearm
● S50.84 External constriction of forearm
● S50.841 External constriction of right forearm
● S50.842 External constriction of left forearm
● S50.849 External constriction of unspecified forearm
● S50.85 Superficial foreign body of forearm
Splinter in the forearm
● S50.851 Superficial foreign body of right forearm
● S50.852 Superficial foreign body of left forearm
● S50.859 Superficial foreign body of unspecified forearm
● S50.86 Insect bite (nonvenomous) of forearm
● S50.861 Insect bite (nonvenomous) of right forearm
● S50.862 Insect bite (nonvenomous) of left forearm
● S50.869 Insect bite (nonvenomous) of unspecified forearm
● S50.87 Other superficial bite of forearm
Excludes1 open bite of forearm (S51.84)
● S50.871 Other superficial bite of right forearm
● S50.872 Other superficial bite of left forearm
● S50.879 Other superficial bite of unspecified forearm

● S50.9 Unspecified superficial injury of elbow and forearm
● S50.90 Unspecified superficial injury of elbow
● S50.901 Unspecified superficial injury of right elbow
● S50.902 Unspecified superficial injury of left elbow
● S50.909 Unspecified superficial injury of unspecified elbow

S50.91 Unspecified superficial injury of forearm
- **S50.911 Unspecified superficial injury of right forearm**
- **S50.912 Unspecified superficial injury of left forearm**
- **S50.919 Unspecified superficial injury of unspecified forearm**

S51 Open wound of elbow and forearm

Code also any associated wound infection

Excludes1 open fracture of elbow and forearm (S52.- with open fracture 7th character)
traumatic amputation of elbow and forearm (S58.-)

Excludes2 open wound of wrist and hand (S61.-)

The appropriate 7th character is to be added to each code from category S51

A	initial encounter
D	subsequent encounter
S	sequela

S51.0 Open wound of elbow

S51.00 Unspecified open wound of elbow
- **S51.001 Unspecified open wound of right elbow**
  Coding Clinic: 2012, Q4, P108
- **S51.002 Unspecified open wound of left elbow**
- **S51.009 Unspecified open wound of unspecified elbow**
  Open wound of elbow NOS

S51.01 Laceration without foreign body of elbow
- **S51.011 Laceration without foreign body of right elbow**
- **S51.012 Laceration without foreign body of left elbow**
- **S51.019 Laceration without foreign body of unspecified elbow**

S51.02 Laceration with foreign body of elbow
- **S51.021 Laceration with foreign body of right elbow**
- **S51.022 Laceration with foreign body of left elbow**
- **S51.029 Laceration with foreign body of unspecified elbow**

S51.03 Puncture wound without foreign body of elbow
- **S51.031 Puncture wound without foreign body of right elbow**
- **S51.032 Puncture wound without foreign body of left elbow**
- **S51.039 Puncture wound without foreign body of unspecified elbow**

S51.04 Puncture wound with foreign body of elbow
- **S51.041 Puncture wound with foreign body of right elbow**
- **S51.042 Puncture wound with foreign body of left elbow**
- **S51.049 Puncture wound with foreign body of unspecified elbow**

S51.05 Open bite of elbow

Bite of elbow NOS

Excludes1 superficial bite of elbow (S50.36, S50.37)
- **S51.051 Open bite, right elbow**
- **S51.052 Open bite, left elbow**
- **S51.059 Open bite, unspecified elbow**

S51.8 Open wound of forearm

Excludes2 open wound of elbow (S51.0-)

S51.80 Unspecified open wound of forearm
- **S51.801 Unspecified open wound of right forearm**
- **S51.802 Unspecified open wound of left forearm**
- **S51.809 Unspecified open wound of unspecified forearm**
  Open wound of forearm NOS

S51.81 Laceration without foreign body of forearm
- **S51.811 Laceration without foreign body of right forearm**
- **S51.812 Laceration without foreign body of left forearm**
- **S51.819 Laceration without foreign body of unspecified forearm**

S51.82 Laceration with foreign body of forearm
- **S51.821 Laceration with foreign body of right forearm**
- **S51.822 Laceration with foreign body of left forearm**
- **S51.829 Laceration with foreign body of unspecified forearm**

S51.83 Puncture wound without foreign body of forearm
- **S51.831 Puncture wound without foreign body of right forearm**
- **S51.832 Puncture wound without foreign body of left forearm**
- **S51.839 Puncture wound without foreign body of unspecified forearm**

S51.84 Puncture wound with foreign body of forearm
- **S51.841 Puncture wound with foreign body of right forearm**
- **S51.842 Puncture wound with foreign body of left forearm**
- **S51.849 Puncture wound with foreign body of unspecified forearm**

S51.85 Open bite of forearm

Bite of forearm NOS

Excludes1 superficial bite of forearm (S50.86, S50.87)
- **S51.851 Open bite of right forearm**
- **S51.852 Open bite of left forearm**
- **S51.859 Open bite of unspecified forearm**

S52 Fracture of forearm

Note: A fracture not identified as displaced or nondisplaced should be coded to displaced

A fracture not designated as open or closed should be coded to closed

The open fracture designations are based on the Gustilo open fracture classification

Excludes1 traumatic amputation of forearm (S58.-)

Excludes2 fracture at wrist and hand level (S62.-)

The appropriate 7th character is to be added to all codes from category S52

A	initial encounter for closed fracture
B	initial encounter for open fracture type I or II initial encounter for open fracture NOS
C	initial encounter for open fracture type IIIA, IIIB, or IIIC
D	subsequent encounter for closed fracture with routine healing
E	subsequent encounter for open fracture type I or II with routine healing
F	subsequent encounter for open fracture type IIIA, IIIB, or IIIC with routine healing
G	subsequent encounter for closed fracture with delayed healing
H	subsequent encounter for open fracture type I or II with delayed healing
J	subsequent encounter for open fracture type IIIA, IIIB, or IIIC with delayed healing
K	subsequent encounter for closed fracture with nonunion
M	subsequent encounter for open fracture type I or II with nonunion
N	subsequent encounter for open fracture type IIIA, IIIB, or IIIC with nonunion
P	subsequent encounter for closed fracture with malunion
Q	subsequent encounter for open fracture type I or II with malunion
R	subsequent encounter for open fracture type IIIA, IIIB, or IIIC with malunion
S	sequela

Coding Clinic: 2016, Q1, P33

S52.0 Fracture of upper end of ulna

Fracture of proximal end of ulna

Excludes2 fracture of elbow NOS (S42.40-)
fractures of shaft of ulna (S52.2-)

S52.00 Unspecified fracture of upper end of ulna

S52.001 Unspecified fracture of upper end of right ulna

S52.002 Unspecified fracture of upper end of left ulna

S52.009 Unspecified fracture of upper end of unspecified ulna

S52.01 Torus fracture of upper end of ulna

The appropriate 7th character is to be added to all codes in subcategory S52.01

A	initial encounter for closed fracture
D	subsequent encounter for fracture with routine healing
G	subsequent encounter for fracture with delayed healing
K	subsequent encounter for fracture with nonunion
P	subsequent encounter for fracture with malunion
S	sequela

S52.011 Torus fracture of upper end of right ulna

S52.012 Torus fracture of upper end of left ulna

S52.019 Torus fracture of upper end of unspecified ulna

S52.02 Fracture of olecranon process without intraarticular extension of ulna

S52.021 Displaced fracture of olecranon process without intraarticular extension of right ulna

S52.022 Displaced fracture of olecranon process without intraarticular extension of left ulna

S52.023 Displaced fracture of olecranon process without intraarticular extension of unspecified ulna

S52.024 Nondisplaced fracture of olecranon process without intraarticular extension of right ulna

S52.025 Nondisplaced fracture of olecranon process without intraarticular extension of left ulna

S52.026 Nondisplaced fracture of olecranon process without intraarticular extension of unspecified ulna

S52.03 Fracture of olecranon process with intraarticular extension of ulna

S52.031 Displaced fracture of olecranon process with intraarticular extension of right ulna

S52.032 Displaced fracture of olecranon process with intraarticular extension of left ulna

S52.033 Displaced fracture of olecranon process with intraarticular extension of unspecified ulna

S52.034 Nondisplaced fracture of olecranon process with intraarticular extension of right ulna

S52.035 Nondisplaced fracture of olecranon process with intraarticular extension of left ulna

S52.036 Nondisplaced fracture of olecranon process with intraarticular extension of unspecified ulna

S52.04 Fracture of coronoid process of ulna

S52.041 Displaced fracture of coronoid process of right ulna

S52.042 Displaced fracture of coronoid process of left ulna

S52.043 Displaced fracture of coronoid process of unspecified ulna

S52.044 Nondisplaced fracture of coronoid process of right ulna

S52.045 Nondisplaced fracture of coronoid process of left ulna

S52.046 Nondisplaced fracture of coronoid process of unspecified ulna

S52.09 Other fracture of upper end of ulna

S52.091 Other fracture of upper end of right ulna

S52.092 Other fracture of upper end of left ulna

S52.099 Other fracture of upper end of unspecified ulna

S52.1 Fracture of upper end of radius

Fracture of proximal end of radius

Excludes2 physeal fractures of upper end of radius (S59.2-)
fracture of shaft of radius (S52.3-)

S52.10 Unspecified fracture of upper end of radius

S52.101 Unspecified fracture of upper end of right radius

S52.102 Unspecified fracture of upper end of left radius

S52.109 Unspecified fracture of upper end of unspecified radius

S52.11 Torus fracture of upper end of radius

The appropriate 7th character is to be added to all codes in subcategory S52.11

A	initial encounter for closed fracture
D	subsequent encounter for fracture with routine healing
G	subsequent encounter for fracture with delayed healing
K	subsequent encounter for fracture with nonunion
P	subsequent encounter for fracture with malunion
S	sequela

S52.111 Torus fracture of upper end of right radius
S52.112 Torus fracture of upper end of left radius
S52.119 Torus fracture of upper end of unspecified radius

S52.12 Fracture of head of radius
S52.121 Displaced fracture of head of right radius
S52.122 Displaced fracture of head of left radius
S52.123 Displaced fracture of head of unspecified radius
S52.124 Nondisplaced fracture of head of right radius
S52.125 Nondisplaced fracture of head of left radius
S52.126 Nondisplaced fracture of head of unspecified radius

S52.13 Fracture of neck of radius
S52.131 Displaced fracture of neck of right radius
S52.132 Displaced fracture of neck of left radius
S52.133 Displaced fracture of neck of unspecified radius
S52.134 Nondisplaced fracture of neck of right radius
S52.135 Nondisplaced fracture of neck of left radius
S52.136 Nondisplaced fracture of neck of unspecified radius

S52.18 Other fracture of upper end of radius
S52.181 Other fracture of upper end of right radius
S52.182 Other fracture of upper end of left radius
S52.189 Other fracture of upper end of unspecified radius

S52.2 Fracture of shaft of ulna

S52.20 Unspecified fracture of shaft of ulna

Fracture of ulna NOS

S52.201 Unspecified fracture of shaft of right ulna
S52.202 Unspecified fracture of shaft of left ulna
S52.209 Unspecified fracture of shaft of unspecified ulna

S52.21 Greenstick fracture of shaft of ulna

The appropriate 7th character is to be added to all codes in subcategory S52.21

A	initial encounter for closed fracture
D	subsequent encounter for fracture with routine healing
G	subsequent encounter for fracture with delayed healing
K	subsequent encounter for fracture with nonunion
P	subsequent encounter for fracture with malunion
S	sequela

S52.211 Greenstick fracture of shaft of right ulna
S52.212 Greenstick fracture of shaft of left ulna
S52.219 Greenstick fracture of shaft of unspecified ulna

S52.22 Transverse fracture of shaft of ulna
S52.221 Displaced transverse fracture of shaft of right ulna
S52.222 Displaced transverse fracture of shaft of left ulna
S52.223 Displaced transverse fracture of shaft of unspecified ulna
S52.224 Nondisplaced transverse fracture of shaft of right ulna
S52.225 Nondisplaced transverse fracture of shaft of left ulna
S52.226 Nondisplaced transverse fracture of shaft of unspecified ulna

S52.23 Oblique fracture of shaft of ulna
S52.231 Displaced oblique fracture of shaft of right ulna
S52.232 Displaced oblique fracture of shaft of left ulna
S52.233 Displaced oblique fracture of shaft of unspecified ulna
S52.234 Nondisplaced oblique fracture of shaft of right ulna
S52.235 Nondisplaced oblique fracture of shaft of left ulna
S52.236 Nondisplaced oblique fracture of shaft of unspecified ulna

S52.24 Spiral fracture of shaft of ulna
S52.241 Displaced spiral fracture of shaft of ulna, right arm
S52.242 Displaced spiral fracture of shaft of ulna, left arm
S52.243 Displaced spiral fracture of shaft of ulna, unspecified arm
S52.244 Nondisplaced spiral fracture of shaft of ulna, right arm
S52.245 Nondisplaced spiral fracture of shaft of ulna, left arm
S52.246 Nondisplaced spiral fracture of shaft of ulna, unspecified arm

S52.25 Comminuted fracture of shaft of ulna
S52.251 Displaced comminuted fracture of shaft of ulna, right arm
S52.252 Displaced comminuted fracture of shaft of ulna, left arm
S52.253 Displaced comminuted fracture of shaft of ulna, unspecified arm
S52.254 Nondisplaced comminuted fracture of shaft of ulna, right arm
S52.255 Nondisplaced comminuted fracture of shaft of ulna, left arm
S52.256 Nondisplaced comminuted fracture of shaft of ulna, unspecified arm

S52.26 Segmental fracture of shaft of ulna
S52.261 Displaced segmental fracture of shaft of ulna, right arm
S52.262 Displaced segmental fracture of shaft of ulna, left arm
S52.263 Displaced segmental fracture of shaft of ulna, unspecified arm
S52.264 Nondisplaced segmental fracture of shaft of ulna, right arm
S52.265 Nondisplaced segmental fracture of shaft of ulna, left arm
S52.266 Nondisplaced segmental fracture of shaft of ulna, unspecified arm
S52.27 Monteggia's fracture of ulna
Fracture of upper shaft of ulna with dislocation of radial head
S52.271 Monteggia's fracture of right ulna
S52.272 Monteggia's fracture of left ulna
S52.279 Monteggia's fracture of unspecified ulna
S52.28 Bent bone of ulna
S52.281 Bent bone of right ulna
S52.282 Bent bone of left ulna
S52.283 Bent bone of unspecified ulna
S52.29 Other fracture of shaft of ulna
S52.291 Other fracture of shaft of right ulna
S52.292 Other fracture of shaft of left ulna
S52.299 Other fracture of shaft of unspecified ulna
S52.3 Fracture of shaft of radius
S52.30 Unspecified fracture of shaft of radius
S52.301 Unspecified fracture of shaft of right radius
S52.302 Unspecified fracture of shaft of left radius
S52.309 Unspecified fracture of shaft of unspecified radius
S52.31 Greenstick fracture of shaft of radius
The appropriate 7th character is to be added to all codes in subcategory S52.31

A	initial encounter for closed fracture
D	subsequent encounter for fracture with routine healing
G	subsequent encounter for fracture with delayed healing
K	subsequent encounter for fracture with nonunion
P	subsequent encounter for fracture with malunion
S	sequela

S52.311 Greenstick fracture of shaft of radius, right arm
S52.312 Greenstick fracture of shaft of radius, left arm
S52.319 Greenstick fracture of shaft of radius, unspecified arm
S52.32 Transverse fracture of shaft of radius
S52.321 Displaced transverse fracture of shaft of right radius
S52.322 Displaced transverse fracture of shaft of left radius
S52.323 Displaced transverse fracture of shaft of unspecified radius
S52.324 Nondisplaced transverse fracture of shaft of right radius
S52.325 Nondisplaced transverse fracture of shaft of left radius
S52.326 Nondisplaced transverse fracture of shaft of unspecified radius
S52.33 Oblique fracture of shaft of radius
S52.331 Displaced oblique fracture of shaft of right radius
S52.332 Displaced oblique fracture of shaft of left radius
S52.333 Displaced oblique fracture of shaft of unspecified radius
S52.334 Nondisplaced oblique fracture of shaft of right radius
S52.335 Nondisplaced oblique fracture of shaft of left radius
S52.336 Nondisplaced oblique fracture of shaft of unspecified radius
S52.34 Spiral fracture of shaft of radius
S52.341 Displaced spiral fracture of shaft of radius, right arm
S52.342 Displaced spiral fracture of shaft of radius, left arm
S52.343 Displaced spiral fracture of shaft of radius, unspecified arm
S52.344 Nondisplaced spiral fracture of shaft of radius, right arm
S52.345 Nondisplaced spiral fracture of shaft of radius, left arm
S52.346 Nondisplaced spiral fracture of shaft of radius, unspecified arm
S52.35 Comminuted fracture of shaft of radius
S52.351 Displaced comminuted fracture of shaft of radius, right arm
S52.352 Displaced comminuted fracture of shaft of radius, left arm
S52.353 Displaced comminuted fracture of shaft of radius, unspecified arm
S52.354 Nondisplaced comminuted fracture of shaft of radius, right arm
S52.355 Nondisplaced comminuted fracture of shaft of radius, left arm
S52.356 Nondisplaced comminuted fracture of shaft of radius, unspecified arm
S52.36 Segmental fracture of shaft of radius
S52.361 Displaced segmental fracture of shaft of radius, right arm
S52.362 Displaced segmental fracture of shaft of radius, left arm
S52.363 Displaced segmental fracture of shaft of radius, unspecified arm
S52.364 Nondisplaced segmental fracture of shaft of radius, right arm
S52.365 Nondisplaced segmental fracture of shaft of radius, left arm
S52.366 Nondisplaced segmental fracture of shaft of radius, unspecified arm
S52.37 Galeazzi's fracture
Fracture of lower shaft of radius with radioulnar joint dislocation
S52.371 Galeazzi's fracture of right radius
S52.372 Galeazzi's fracture of left radius
S52.379 Galeazzi's fracture of unspecified radius
S52.38 Bent bone of radius
S52.381 Bent bone of right radius
S52.382 Bent bone of left radius
S52.389 Bent bone of unspecified radius
S52.39 Other fracture of shaft of radius
S52.391 Other fracture of shaft of radius, right arm
S52.392 Other fracture of shaft of radius, left arm
S52.399 Other fracture of shaft of radius, unspecified arm

CHAPTER 19 (SØØ-T88)

S52.5 Fracture of lower end of radius
Fracture of distal end of radius
Excludes2 physeal fractures of lower end of radius (S59.2-)

S52.50 Unspecified fracture of the lower end of radius
S52.501 Unspecified fracture of the lower end of right radius
S52.502 Unspecified fracture of the lower end of left radius
S52.509 Unspecified fracture of the lower end of unspecified radius

S52.51 Fracture of radial styloid process
S52.511 Displaced fracture of right radial styloid process
S52.512 Displaced fracture of left radial styloid process
S52.513 Displaced fracture of unspecified radial styloid process
S52.514 Nondisplaced fracture of right radial styloid process
S52.515 Nondisplaced fracture of left radial styloid process
S52.516 Nondisplaced fracture of unspecified radial styloid process

S52.52 Torus fracture of lower end of radius
The appropriate 7th character is to be added to all codes in subcategory S52.52

A	initial encounter for closed fracture
D	subsequent encounter for fracture with routine healing
G	subsequent encounter for fracture with delayed healing
K	subsequent encounter for fracture with nonunion
P	subsequent encounter for fracture with malunion
S	sequela

S52.521 Torus fracture of lower end of right radius
S52.522 Torus fracture of lower end of left radius
S52.529 Torus fracture of lower end of unspecified radius

S52.53 Colles' fracture
S52.531 Colles' fracture of right radius
S52.532 Colles' fracture of left radius
Coding Clinic: 2016, Q2, P5
S52.539 Colles' fracture of unspecified radius

S52.54 Smith's fracture
S52.541 Smith's fracture of right radius
S52.542 Smith's fracture of left radius
S52.549 Smith's fracture of unspecified radius

S52.55 Other extraarticular fracture of lower end of radius
S52.551 Other extraarticular fracture of lower end of right radius
S52.552 Other extraarticular fracture of lower end of left radius
S52.559 Other extraarticular fracture of lower end of unspecified radius

S52.56 Barton's fracture
S52.561 Barton's fracture of right radius
S52.562 Barton's fracture of left radius
S52.569 Barton's fracture of unspecified radius

S52.57 Other intraarticular fracture of lower end of radius
S52.571 Other intraarticular fracture of lower end of right radius
S52.572 Other intraarticular fracture of lower end of left radius
S52.579 Other intraarticular fracture of lower end of unspecified radius

S52.59 Other fractures of lower end of radius
S52.591 Other fractures of lower end of right radius
S52.592 Other fractures of lower end of left radius
S52.599 Other fractures of lower end of unspecified radius

S52.6 Fracture of lower end of ulna

S52.60 Unspecified fracture of lower end of ulna
S52.601 Unspecified fracture of lower end of right ulna
S52.602 Unspecified fracture of lower end of left ulna
S52.609 Unspecified fracture of lower end of unspecified ulna

S52.61 Fracture of ulna styloid process
S52.611 Displaced fracture of right ulna styloid process
S52.612 Displaced fracture of left ulna styloid process
S52.613 Displaced fracture of unspecified ulna styloid process
S52.614 Nondisplaced fracture of right ulna styloid process
S52.615 Nondisplaced fracture of left ulna styloid process
S52.616 Nondisplaced fracture of unspecified ulna styloid process

S52.62 Torus fracture of lower end of ulna
The appropriate 7th character is to be added to all codes in subcategory S52.62

A	initial encounter for closed fracture
D	subsequent encounter for fracture with routine healing
G	subsequent encounter for fracture with delayed healing
K	subsequent encounter for fracture with nonunion
P	subsequent encounter for fracture with malunion
S	sequela

S52.621 Torus fracture of lower end of right ulna
S52.622 Torus fracture of lower end of left ulna
S52.629 Torus fracture of lower end of unspecified ulna

S52.69 Other fracture of lower end of ulna
S52.691 Other fracture of lower end of right ulna
S52.692 Other fracture of lower end of left ulna
S52.699 Other fracture of lower end of unspecified ulna

S52.9 Unspecified fracture of forearm
X S52.90 Unspecified fracture of unspecified forearm
X S52.91 Unspecified fracture of right forearm
X S52.92 Unspecified fracture of left forearm

S53 Dislocation and sprain of joints and ligaments of elbow

Includes avulsion of joint or ligament of elbow
laceration of cartilage, joint or ligament of elbow
sprain of cartilage, joint or ligament of elbow
traumatic hemarthrosis of joint or ligament of elbow
traumatic rupture of joint or ligament of elbow
traumatic subluxation of joint or ligament of elbow
traumatic tear of joint or ligament of elbow

Code also any associated open wound

Excludes2 strain of muscle, fascia and tendon at forearm level (S56.-)

The appropriate 7th character is to be added to each code from category S53

A	initial encounter
D	subsequent encounter
S	sequela

S53.0 **Subluxation and dislocation of radial head**
Dislocation of radiohumeral joint
Subluxation of radiohumeral joint
Excludes1 Monteggia's fracture-dislocation (S52.27-)

S53.00 **Unspecified subluxation and dislocation of radial head**
- S53.001 **Unspecified subluxation of right radial head**
- S53.002 **Unspecified subluxation of left radial head**
- S53.003 **Unspecified subluxation of unspecified radial head**
- S53.004 **Unspecified dislocation of right radial head**
- S53.005 **Unspecified dislocation of left radial head**
- S53.006 **Unspecified dislocation of unspecified radial head**

S53.01 **Anterior** subluxation and dislocation of radial head
Anteriomedial subluxation and dislocation of radial head
- S53.011 **Anterior subluxation of right radial head**
- S53.012 **Anterior subluxation of left radial head**
- S53.013 **Anterior subluxation of unspecified radial head**
- S53.014 **Anterior dislocation of right radial head**
- S53.015 **Anterior dislocation of left radial head**
- S53.016 **Anterior dislocation of unspecified radial head**

S53.02 **Posterior** subluxation and dislocation of radial head
Posteriolateral subluxation and dislocation of radial head
- S53.021 **Posterior subluxation of right radial head**
- S53.022 **Posterior subluxation of left radial head**
- S53.023 **Posterior subluxation of unspecified radial head**
- S53.024 **Posterior dislocation of right radial head**
- S53.025 **Posterior dislocation of left radial head**
- S53.026 **Posterior dislocation of unspecified radial head**

S53.03 **Nursemaid's elbow**
- S53.031 **Nursemaid's elbow, right elbow**
  Coding Clinic: 2015, Q1, P7-8
- S53.032 **Nursemaid's elbow, left elbow**
- S53.033 **Nursemaid's elbow, unspecified elbow**

S53.09 **Other** subluxation and dislocation of radial head
- S53.091 **Other subluxation of right radial head**
- S53.092 **Other subluxation of left radial head**
- S53.093 **Other subluxation of unspecified radial head**
- S53.094 **Other dislocation of right radial head**
- S53.095 **Other dislocation of left radial head**
- S53.096 **Other dislocation of unspecified radial head**

S53.1 **Subluxation and dislocation of ulnohumeral joint**
Subluxation and dislocation of elbow NOS
Excludes1 dislocation of radial head alone (S53.0-)

S53.10 **Unspecified** subluxation and dislocation of ulnohumeral joint
- S53.101 **Unspecified subluxation of right ulnohumeral joint**
- S53.102 **Unspecified subluxation of left ulnohumeral joint**
- S53.103 **Unspecified subluxation of unspecified ulnohumeral joint**
- S53.104 **Unspecified dislocation of right ulnohumeral joint**
- S53.105 **Unspecified dislocation of left ulnohumeral joint**
- S53.106 **Unspecified dislocation of unspecified ulnohumeral joint**

S53.11 **Anterior** subluxation and dislocation of ulnohumeral joint
- S53.111 **Anterior subluxation of right ulnohumeral joint**
- S53.112 **Anterior subluxation of left ulnohumeral joint**
- S53.113 **Anterior subluxation of unspecified ulnohumeral joint**
- S53.114 **Anterior dislocation of right ulnohumeral joint**
  Coding Clinic: 2012, Q4, P108
- S53.115 **Anterior dislocation of left ulnohumeral joint**
- S53.116 **Anterior dislocation of unspecified ulnohumeral joint**

S53.12 **Posterior** subluxation and dislocation of ulnohumeral joint
- S53.121 **Posterior subluxation of right ulnohumeral joint**
- S53.122 **Posterior subluxation of left ulnohumeral joint**
- S53.123 **Posterior subluxation of unspecified ulnohumeral joint**
- S53.124 **Posterior dislocation of right ulnohumeral joint**
- S53.125 **Posterior dislocation of left ulnohumeral joint**
- S53.126 **Posterior dislocation of unspecified ulnohumeral joint**

- S53.13 **Medial** subluxation and dislocation of ulnohumeral joint
  - S53.131 Medial subluxation of right ulnohumeral joint
  - S53.132 Medial subluxation of left ulnohumeral joint
  - S53.133 Medial subluxation of unspecified ulnohumeral joint
  - S53.134 Medial dislocation of right ulnohumeral joint
  - S53.135 Medial dislocation of left ulnohumeral joint
  - S53.136 Medial dislocation of unspecified ulnohumeral joint
- S53.14 **Lateral** subluxation and dislocation of ulnohumeral joint
  - S53.141 Lateral subluxation of right ulnohumeral joint
  - S53.142 Lateral subluxation of left ulnohumeral joint
  - S53.143 Lateral subluxation of unspecified ulnohumeral joint
  - S53.144 Lateral dislocation of right ulnohumeral joint
  - S53.145 Lateral dislocation of left ulnohumeral joint
  - S53.146 Lateral dislocation of unspecified ulnohumeral joint
- S53.19 **Other** subluxation and dislocation of ulnohumeral joint
  - S53.191 Other subluxation of right ulnohumeral joint
  - S53.192 Other subluxation of left ulnohumeral joint
  - S53.193 Other subluxation of unspecified ulnohumeral joint
  - S53.194 Other dislocation of right ulnohumeral joint
  - S53.195 Other dislocation of left ulnohumeral joint
  - S53.196 Other dislocation of unspecified ulnohumeral joint

S53.2 **Traumatic rupture of radial collateral ligament**

Excludes1 sprain of radial collateral ligament NOS (S53.43-)

- X S53.20 Traumatic rupture of unspecified radial collateral ligament
- X S53.21 Traumatic rupture of right radial collateral ligament
- X S53.22 Traumatic rupture of left radial collateral ligament

S53.3 **Traumatic rupture of ulnar collateral ligament**

Excludes1 sprain of ulnar collateral ligament (S53.44-)

- X S53.30 Traumatic rupture of unspecified ulnar collateral ligament
- X S53.31 Traumatic rupture of right ulnar collateral ligament
- X S53.32 Traumatic rupture of left ulnar collateral ligament

S53.4 **Sprain of elbow**

Excludes2 traumatic rupture of radial collateral ligament (S53.2-)
traumatic rupture of ulnar collateral ligament (S53.3-)

- S53.40 **Unspecified** sprain of elbow
  - S53.401 Unspecified sprain of right elbow
  - S53.402 Unspecified sprain of left elbow
  - S53.409 Unspecified sprain of unspecified elbow
    Sprain of elbow NOS
- S53.41 **Radiohumeral** (joint) sprain
  - S53.411 Radiohumeral (joint) sprain of right elbow
  - S53.412 Radiohumeral (joint) sprain of left elbow
  - S53.419 Radiohumeral (joint) sprain of unspecified elbow
- S53.42 **Ulnohumeral** (joint) sprain
  - S53.421 Ulnohumeral (joint) sprain of right elbow
  - S53.422 Ulnohumeral (joint) sprain of left elbow
  - S53.429 Ulnohumeral (joint) sprain of unspecified elbow
- S53.43 **Radial collateral ligament** sprain
  - S53.431 Radial collateral ligament sprain of right elbow
  - S53.432 Radial collateral ligament sprain of left elbow
  - S53.439 Radial collateral ligament sprain of unspecified elbow
- S53.44 **Ulnar collateral ligament** sprain
  - S53.441 Ulnar collateral ligament sprain of right elbow
  - S53.442 Ulnar collateral ligament sprain of left elbow
  - S53.449 Ulnar collateral ligament sprain of unspecified elbow
- S53.49 **Other** sprain of elbow
  - S53.491 Other sprain of right elbow
  - S53.492 Other sprain of left elbow
  - S53.499 Other sprain of unspecified elbow

S54 Injury of nerves at forearm level

Code also any associated open wound (S51.-)

Excludes2 injury of nerves at wrist and hand level (S64.-)

The appropriate 7th character is to be added to each code from category S54

A	initial encounter
D	subsequent encounter
S	sequela

S54.0 **Injury of ulnar nerve** at forearm level
Injury of ulnar nerve NOS

- X S54.00 Injury of ulnar nerve at forearm level, unspecified arm
- X S54.01 Injury of ulnar nerve at forearm level, right arm
- X S54.02 Injury of ulnar nerve at forearm level, left arm

S54.1 **Injury of median nerve** at forearm level
Injury of median nerve NOS

- X S54.10 Injury of median nerve at forearm level, unspecified arm
- X S54.11 Injury of median nerve at forearm level, right arm
- X S54.12 Injury of median nerve at forearm level, left arm

S54.2 **Injury of radial nerve** at forearm level
Injury of radial nerve NOS

- X S54.20 Injury of radial nerve at forearm level, unspecified arm
- X S54.21 Injury of radial nerve at forearm level, right arm
- X S54.22 Injury of radial nerve at forearm level, left arm

S54.3 **Injury of cutaneous sensory nerve** at forearm level

- X S54.30 Injury of cutaneous sensory nerve at forearm level, unspecified arm
- X S54.31 Injury of cutaneous sensory nerve at forearm level, right arm
- X S54.32 Injury of cutaneous sensory nerve at forearm level, left arm

CHAPTER 19 (S00-T88)

- S54.8 Injury of other nerves at forearm level
  - S54.8X Injury of other nerves at forearm level
    - S54.8X1 Injury of other nerves at forearm level, **right** arm
    - S54.8X2 Injury of other nerves at forearm level, **left** arm
    - S54.8X9 Injury of other nerves at forearm level, **unspecified** arm
- S54.9 Injury of **unspecified** nerve at forearm level
  - X S54.90 Injury of unspecified nerve at forearm level, **unspecified** arm
  - X S54.91 Injury of unspecified nerve at forearm level, **right** arm
  - X S54.92 Injury of unspecified nerve at forearm level, **left** arm

S55 Injury of blood vessels at forearm level

Code also any associated open wound (S51.-)

Excludes2 injury of blood vessels at wrist and hand level (S65.-)
injury of brachial vessels (S45.1-S45.2)

The appropriate 7th character is to be added to each code from category S55

A	initial encounter
D	subsequent encounter
S	sequela

- S55.0 Injury of **ulnar artery** at forearm level
  - S55.00 **Unspecified** injury of ulnar artery at forearm level
    - S55.001 Unspecified injury of ulnar artery at forearm level, **right** arm
    - S55.002 Unspecified injury of ulnar artery at forearm level, **left** arm
    - S55.009 Unspecified injury of ulnar artery at forearm level, **unspecified** arm
  - S55.01 **Laceration** of ulnar artery at forearm level
    - S55.011 Laceration of ulnar artery at forearm level, **right** arm
    - S55.012 Laceration of ulnar artery at forearm level, **left** arm
    - S55.019 Laceration of ulnar artery at forearm level, **unspecified** arm
  - S55.09 **Other** specified injury of ulnar artery at forearm level
    - S55.091 Other specified injury of ulnar artery at forearm level, **right** arm
    - S55.092 Other specified injury of ulnar artery at forearm level, **left** arm
    - S55.099 Other specified injury of ulnar artery at forearm level, **unspecified** arm
- S55.1 Injury of **radial artery** at forearm level
  - S55.10 **Unspecified** injury of radial artery at forearm level
    - S55.101 Unspecified injury of radial artery at forearm level, **right** arm
    - S55.102 Unspecified injury of radial artery at forearm level, **left** arm
    - S55.109 Unspecified injury of radial artery at forearm level, **unspecified** arm
  - S55.11 **Laceration** of radial artery at forearm level
    - S55.111 Laceration of radial artery at forearm level, **right** arm
    - S55.112 Laceration of radial artery at forearm level, **left** arm
    - S55.119 Laceration of radial artery at forearm level, **unspecified** arm
  - S55.19 **Other** specified injury of radial artery at forearm level
    - S55.191 Other specified injury of radial artery at forearm level, **right** arm
    - S55.192 Other specified injury of radial artery at forearm level, **left** arm
    - S55.199 Other specified injury of radial artery at forearm level, **unspecified** arm
- S55.2 Injury of **vein** at forearm level
  - S55.20 **Unspecified** injury of vein at forearm level
    - S55.201 Unspecified injury of vein at forearm level, **right** arm
    - S55.202 Unspecified injury of vein at forearm level, **left** arm
    - S55.209 Unspecified injury of vein at forearm level, **unspecified** arm
  - S55.21 **Laceration** of vein at forearm level
    - S55.211 Laceration of vein at forearm level, **right** arm
    - S55.212 Laceration of vein at forearm level, **left** arm
    - S55.219 Laceration of vein at forearm level, **unspecified** arm
  - S55.29 **Other** specified injury of vein at forearm level
    - S55.291 Other specified injury of vein at forearm level, **right** arm
    - S55.292 Other specified injury of vein at forearm level, **left** arm
    - S55.299 Other specified injury of vein at forearm level, **unspecified** arm
- S55.8 Injury of **other blood vessels** at forearm level
  - S55.80 **Unspecified** injury of other blood vessels at forearm level
    - S55.801 Unspecified injury of other blood vessels at forearm level, **right** arm
    - S55.802 Unspecified injury of other blood vessels at forearm level, **left** arm
    - S55.809 Unspecified injury of other blood vessels at forearm level, **unspecified** arm
  - S55.81 **Laceration** of other blood vessels at forearm level
    - S55.811 Laceration of other blood vessels at forearm level, **right** arm
    - S55.812 Laceration of other blood vessels at forearm level, **left** arm
    - S55.819 Laceration of other blood vessels at forearm level, **unspecified** arm
  - S55.89 **Other** specified injury of other blood vessels at forearm level
    - S55.891 Other specified injury of other blood vessels at forearm level, **right** arm
    - S55.892 Other specified injury of other blood vessels at forearm level, **left** arm
    - S55.899 Other specified injury of other blood vessels at forearm level, **unspecified** arm
- S55.9 Injury of **unspecified blood vessel** at forearm level
  - S55.90 **Unspecified** injury of unspecified blood vessel at forearm level
    - S55.901 Unspecified injury of unspecified blood vessel at forearm level, **right** arm
    - S55.902 Unspecified injury of unspecified blood vessel at forearm level, **left** arm
    - S55.909 Unspecified injury of unspecified blood vessel at forearm level, **unspecified** arm

- S55.91 **Laceration** of unspecified blood vessel at forearm level
  - S55.911 Laceration of **unspecified** blood vessel at forearm level, **right** arm
  - S55.912 Laceration of **unspecified** blood vessel at forearm level, **left** arm
  - S55.919 Laceration of **unspecified** blood vessel at forearm level, unspecified arm
- S55.99 **Other** specified injury of unspecified blood vessel at forearm level
  - S55.991 Other specified injury of **unspecified** blood vessel at forearm level, **right** arm
  - S55.992 Other specified injury of **unspecified** blood vessel at forearm level, **left** arm
  - S55.999 Other specified injury of **unspecified** blood vessel at forearm level, **unspecified** arm

S56 Injury of muscle, fascia and tendon at forearm level

Code also any associated open wound (S51.-)

Excludes2 injury of muscle, fascia and tendon at or below wrist (S66.-)
sprain of joints and ligaments of elbow (S53.4-)

The appropriate 7th character is to be added to each code from category S56

A	initial encounter
D	subsequent encounter
S	sequela

- S56.Ø Injury of **flexor** muscle, fascia and tendon of **thumb** at forearm level
  - S56.ØØ **Unspecified** injury of flexor muscle, fascia and tendon of thumb at forearm level
    - S56.ØØ1 Unspecified injury of flexor muscle, fascia and tendon of **right** thumb at forearm level
    - S56.ØØ2 Unspecified injury of flexor muscle, fascia and tendon of **left** thumb at forearm level
    - S56.ØØ9 Unspecified injury of flexor muscle, fascia and tendon of **unspecified** thumb at forearm level
  - S56.Ø1 **Strain** of flexor muscle, fascia and tendon of thumb at forearm level
    - S56.Ø11 Strain of flexor muscle, fascia and tendon of **right** thumb at forearm level
    - S56.Ø12 Strain of flexor muscle, fascia and tendon of **left** thumb at forearm level
    - S56.Ø19 Strain of flexor muscle, fascia and tendon of **unspecified** thumb at forearm level
  - S56.Ø2 **Laceration** of flexor muscle, fascia and tendon of thumb at forearm level
    - S56.Ø21 Laceration of flexor muscle, fascia and tendon of **right** thumb at forearm level
    - S56.Ø22 Laceration of flexor muscle, fascia and tendon of **left** thumb at forearm level
    - S56.Ø29 Laceration of flexor muscle, fascia and tendon of **unspecified** thumb at forearm level
  - S56.Ø9 **Other** injury of flexor muscle, fascia and tendon of thumb at forearm level
    - S56.Ø91 Other injury of flexor muscle, fascia and tendon of **right** thumb at forearm level
    - S56.Ø92 Other injury of flexor muscle, fascia and tendon of **left** thumb at forearm level
    - S56.Ø99 Other injury of flexor muscle, fascia and tendon of **unspecified** thumb at forearm level
- S56.1 Injury of **flexor** muscle, fascia and tendon of **other and unspecified finger** at forearm level
  - S56.1Ø **Unspecified** injury of flexor muscle, fascia and tendon of other and unspecified finger at forearm level
    - S56.1Ø1 Unspecified injury of flexor muscle, fascia and tendon of **right index** finger at forearm level
    - S56.1Ø2 Unspecified injury of flexor muscle, fascia and tendon of **left index** finger at forearm level
    - S56.1Ø3 Unspecified injury of flexor muscle, fascia and tendon of **right middle** finger at forearm level
    - S56.1Ø4 Unspecified injury of flexor muscle, fascia and tendon of **left middle** finger at forearm level
    - S56.1Ø5 Unspecified injury of flexor muscle, fascia and tendon of **right ring** finger at forearm level
    - S56.1Ø6 Unspecified injury of flexor muscle, fascia and tendon of **left ring** finger at forearm level
    - S56.1Ø7 Unspecified injury of flexor muscle, fascia and tendon of **right little** finger at forearm level
    - S56.1Ø8 Unspecified injury of flexor muscle, fascia and tendon of **left little** finger at forearm level
    - S56.1Ø9 Unspecified injury of flexor muscle, fascia and tendon of **unspecified** finger at forearm level
  - S56.11 **Strain** of flexor muscle, fascia and tendon of other and unspecified finger at forearm level
    - S56.111 Strain of flexor muscle, fascia and tendon of **right index** finger at forearm level
    - S56.112 Strain of flexor muscle, fascia and tendon of **left index** finger at forearm level
    - S56.113 Strain of flexor muscle, fascia and tendon of **right middle** finger at forearm level
    - S56.114 Strain of flexor muscle, fascia and tendon of **left middle** finger at forearm level
    - S56.115 Strain of flexor muscle, fascia and tendon of **right ring** finger at forearm level
    - S56.116 Strain of flexor muscle, fascia and tendon of **left ring** finger at forearm level
    - S56.117 Strain of flexor muscle, fascia and tendon of **right little** finger at forearm level
    - S56.118 Strain of flexor muscle, fascia and tendon of **left little** finger at forearm level
    - S56.119 Strain of flexor muscle, fascia and tendon of finger of **unspecified** finger at forearm level

CHAPTER 19 (SØØ-T88)

● S56.12 **Laceration** of flexor muscle, fascia and tendon of other and unspecified finger at forearm level
- ● S56.121 Laceration of flexor muscle, fascia and tendon of **right index** finger at forearm level
- ● S56.122 Laceration of flexor muscle, fascia and tendon of **left index** finger at forearm level
- ● S56.123 Laceration of flexor muscle, fascia and tendon of **right middle** finger at forearm level
- ● S56.124 Laceration of flexor muscle, fascia and tendon of **left middle** finger at forearm level
- ● S56.125 Laceration of flexor muscle, fascia and tendon of **right ring** finger at forearm level
- ● S56.126 Laceration of flexor muscle, fascia and tendon of **left ring** finger at forearm level
- ● S56.127 Laceration of flexor muscle, fascia and tendon of **right little** finger at forearm level
- ● S56.128 Laceration of flexor muscle, fascia and tendon of **left little** finger at forearm level
- ● S56.129 Laceration of flexor muscle, fascia and tendon of **unspecified** finger at forearm level

● S56.19 **Other** injury of flexor muscle, fascia and tendon of other and unspecified finger at forearm level
- ● S56.191 Other injury of flexor muscle, fascia and tendon of **right index** finger at forearm level
- ● S56.192 Other injury of flexor muscle, fascia and tendon of **left index** finger at forearm level
- ● S56.193 Other injury of flexor muscle, fascia and tendon of **right middle** finger at forearm level
- ● S56.194 Other injury of flexor muscle, fascia and tendon of **left middle** finger at forearm level
- ● S56.195 Other injury of flexor muscle, fascia and tendon of **right ring** finger at forearm level
- ● S56.196 Other injury of flexor muscle, fascia and tendon of **left ring** finger at forearm level
- ● S56.197 Other injury of flexor muscle, fascia and tendon of **right little** finger at forearm level
- ● S56.198 Other injury of flexor muscle, fascia and tendon of **left little** finger at forearm level
- ● S56.199 Other injury of flexor muscle, fascia and tendon of **unspecified** finger at forearm level

● S56.2 Injury of **other flexor** muscle, fascia and tendon at forearm level

● S56.20 **Unspecified** injury of other flexor muscle, fascia and tendon at forearm level
- ● S56.201 Unspecified injury of other flexor muscle, fascia and tendon at forearm level, **right** arm
- ● S56.202 Unspecified injury of other flexor muscle, fascia and tendon at forearm level, **left** arm
- ● S56.209 Unspecified injury of other flexor muscle, fascia and tendon at forearm level, **unspecified** arm

● S56.21 **Strain** of other flexor muscle, fascia and tendon at forearm level
- ● S56.211 Strain of other flexor muscle, fascia and tendon at forearm level, **right** arm
- ● S56.212 Strain of other flexor muscle, fascia and tendon at forearm level, **left** arm
- ● S56.219 Strain of other flexor muscle, fascia and tendon at forearm level, **unspecified** arm

● S56.22 **Laceration** of other flexor muscle, fascia and tendon at forearm level
- ● S56.221 Laceration of other flexor muscle, fascia and tendon at forearm level, **right** arm
- ● S56.222 Laceration of other flexor muscle, fascia and tendon at forearm level, **left** arm
- ● S56.229 Laceration of other flexor muscle, fascia and tendon at forearm level, **unspecified** arm

● S56.29 **Other** injury of other flexor muscle, fascia and tendon at forearm level
- ● S56.291 Other injury of other flexor muscle, fascia and tendon at forearm level, **right** arm
- ● S56.292 Other injury of other flexor muscle, fascia and tendon at forearm level, **left** arm
- ● S56.299 Other injury of other flexor muscle, fascia and tendon at forearm level, **unspecified** arm

● S56.3 Injury of **extensor or abductor** muscles, fascia and tendons of **thumb** at forearm level

● S56.30 **Unspecified** injury of extensor or abductor muscles, fascia and tendons of thumb at forearm level
- ● S56.301 Unspecified injury of extensor or abductor muscles, fascia and tendons of **right** thumb at forearm level
- ● S56.302 Unspecified injury of extensor or abductor muscles, fascia and tendons of **left** thumb at forearm level
- ● S56.309 Unspecified injury of extensor or abductor muscles, fascia and tendons of **unspecified** thumb at forearm level

● S56.31 **Strain** of extensor or abductor muscles, fascia and tendons of thumb at forearm level
- ● S56.311 Strain of extensor or abductor muscles, fascia and tendons of **right** thumb at forearm level
- ● S56.312 Strain of extensor or abductor muscles, fascia and tendons of **left** thumb at forearm level
- ● S56.319 Strain of extensor or abductor muscles, fascia and tendons of **unspecified** thumb at forearm level

● S56.32 **Laceration** of extensor or abductor muscles, fascia and tendons of thumb at forearm level
- ● S56.321 Laceration of extensor or abductor muscles, fascia and tendons of **right** thumb at forearm level
- ● S56.322 Laceration of extensor or abductor muscles, fascia and tendons of **left** thumb at forearm level
- ● S56.329 Laceration of extensor or abductor muscles, fascia and tendons of **unspecified** thumb at forearm level

S56.39 **Other** injury of extensor or abductor muscles, fascia and tendons of thumb at forearm level

S56.391 Other injury of extensor or abductor muscles, fascia and tendons of **right** thumb at forearm level

S56.392 Other injury of extensor or abductor muscles, fascia and tendons of **left** thumb at forearm level

S56.399 Other injury of extensor or abductor muscles, fascia and tendons of **unspecified** thumb at forearm level

S56.4 Injury of **extensor** muscle, fascia and tendon of **other and unspecified finger** at forearm level

S56.40 **Unspecified** injury of extensor muscle, fascia and tendon of other and unspecified finger at forearm level

S56.401 Unspecified injury of extensor muscle, fascia and tendon of **right index** finger at forearm level

S56.402 Unspecified injury of extensor muscle, fascia and tendon of **left index** finger at forearm level

S56.403 Unspecified injury of extensor muscle, fascia and tendon of **right middle** finger at forearm level

S56.404 Unspecified injury of extensor muscle, fascia and tendon of **left middle** finger at forearm level

S56.405 Unspecified injury of extensor muscle, fascia and tendon of **right ring** finger at forearm level

S56.406 Unspecified injury of extensor muscle, fascia and tendon of **left ring** finger at forearm level

S56.407 Unspecified injury of extensor muscle, fascia and tendon of **right little** finger at forearm level

S56.408 Unspecified injury of extensor muscle, fascia and tendon of **left little** finger at forearm level

S56.409 Unspecified injury of extensor muscle, fascia and tendon of **unspecified** finger at forearm level

S56.41 **Strain** of extensor muscle, fascia and tendon of other and unspecified finger at forearm level

S56.411 Strain of extensor muscle, fascia and tendon of **right index** finger at forearm level

S56.412 Strain of extensor muscle, fascia and tendon of **left index** finger at forearm level

S56.413 Strain of extensor muscle, fascia and tendon of **right middle** finger at forearm level

S56.414 Strain of extensor muscle, fascia and tendon of **left middle** finger at forearm level

S56.415 Strain of extensor muscle, fascia and tendon of **right ring** finger at forearm level

S56.416 Strain of extensor muscle, fascia and tendon of **left ring** finger at forearm level

S56.417 Strain of extensor muscle, fascia and tendon of **right little** finger at forearm level

S56.418 Strain of extensor muscle, fascia and tendon of **left little** finger at forearm level

S56.419 Strain of extensor muscle, fascia and tendon of finger, **unspecified** finger at forearm level

S56.42 **Laceration** of extensor muscle, fascia and tendon of other and unspecified finger at forearm level

S56.421 Laceration of extensor muscle, fascia and tendon of **right index** finger at forearm level

S56.422 Laceration of extensor muscle, fascia and tendon of **left index** finger at forearm level

S56.423 Laceration of extensor muscle, fascia and tendon of **right middle** finger at forearm level

S56.424 Laceration of extensor muscle, fascia and tendon of **left middle** finger at forearm level

S56.425 Laceration of extensor muscle, fascia and tendon of **right ring** finger at forearm level

S56.426 Laceration of extensor muscle, fascia and tendon of **left ring** finger at forearm level

S56.427 Laceration of extensor muscle, fascia and tendon of **right little** finger at forearm level

S56.428 Laceration of extensor muscle, fascia and tendon of **left little** finger at forearm level

S56.429 Laceration of extensor muscle, fascia and tendon of **unspecified** finger at forearm level

S56.49 **Other** injury of extensor muscle, fascia and tendon of other and unspecified finger at forearm level

S56.491 Other injury of extensor muscle, fascia and tendon of **right index** finger at forearm level

S56.492 Other injury of extensor muscle, fascia and tendon of **left index** finger at forearm level

S56.493 Other injury of extensor muscle, fascia and tendon of **right middle** finger at forearm level

S56.494 Other injury of extensor muscle, fascia and tendon of **left middle** finger at forearm level

S56.495 Other injury of extensor muscle, fascia and tendon of **right ring** finger at forearm level

S56.496 Other injury of extensor muscle, fascia and tendon of **left ring** finger at forearm level

S56.497 Other injury of extensor muscle, fascia and tendon of **right little** finger at forearm level

S56.498 Other injury of extensor muscle, fascia and tendon of **left little** finger at forearm level

S56.499 Other injury of extensor muscle, fascia and tendon of **unspecified** finger at forearm level

S56.5 Injury of **other extensor** muscle, fascia and tendon at forearm level

S56.50 **Unspecified** injury of other extensor muscle, fascia and tendon at forearm level

S56.501 Unspecified injury of other extensor muscle, fascia and tendon at forearm level, **right arm**

S56.502 Unspecified injury of other extensor muscle, fascia and tendon at forearm level, **left arm**

S56.509 Unspecified injury of other extensor muscle, fascia and tendon at forearm level, **unspecified arm**

S56.51 Strain of other extensor muscle, fascia and tendon at forearm level
S56.511 Strain of other extensor muscle, fascia and tendon at forearm level, right arm
S56.512 Strain of other extensor muscle, fascia and tendon at forearm level, left arm
S56.519 Strain of other extensor muscle, fascia and tendon at forearm level, unspecified arm
S56.52 Laceration of other extensor muscle, fascia and tendon at forearm level
S56.521 Laceration of other extensor muscle, fascia and tendon at forearm level, right arm
S56.522 Laceration of other extensor muscle, fascia and tendon at forearm level, left arm
S56.529 Laceration of other extensor muscle, fascia and tendon at forearm level, unspecified arm
S56.59 Other injury of other extensor muscle, fascia and tendon at forearm level
S56.591 Other injury of other extensor muscle, fascia and tendon at forearm level, right arm
S56.592 Other injury of other extensor muscle, fascia and tendon at forearm level, left arm
S56.599 Other injury of other extensor muscle, fascia and tendon at forearm level, unspecified arm
S56.8 Injury of other muscles, fascia and tendons at forearm level
S56.80 Unspecified injury of other muscles, fascia and tendons at forearm level
S56.801 Unspecified injury of other muscles, fascia and tendons at forearm level, right arm
S56.802 Unspecified injury of other muscles, fascia and tendons at forearm level, left arm
S56.809 Unspecified injury of other muscles, fascia and tendons at forearm level, unspecified arm
S56.81 Strain of other muscles, fascia and tendons at forearm level
S56.811 Strain of other muscles, fascia and tendons at forearm level, right arm
S56.812 Strain of other muscles, fascia and tendons at forearm level, left arm
S56.819 Strain of other muscles, fascia and tendons at forearm level, unspecified arm
S56.82 Laceration of other muscles, fascia and tendons at forearm level
S56.821 Laceration of other muscles, fascia and tendons at forearm level, right arm
S56.822 Laceration of other muscles, fascia and tendons at forearm level, left arm
S56.829 Laceration of other muscles, fascia and tendons at forearm level, unspecified arm
S56.89 Other injury of other muscles, fascia and tendons at forearm level
S56.891 Other injury of other muscles, fascia and tendons at forearm level, right arm
S56.892 Other injury of other muscles, fascia and tendons at forearm level, left arm
S56.899 Other injury of other muscles, fascia and tendons at forearm level, unspecified arm
S56.9 Injury of unspecified muscles, fascia and tendons at forearm level
S56.90 Unspecified injury of unspecified muscles, fascia and tendons at forearm level
S56.901 Unspecified injury of unspecified muscles, fascia and tendons at forearm level, right arm
S56.902 Unspecified injury of unspecified muscles, fascia and tendons at forearm level, left arm
S56.909 Unspecified injury of unspecified muscles, fascia and tendons at forearm level, unspecified arm
S56.91 Strain of unspecified muscles, fascia and tendons at forearm level
S56.911 Strain of unspecified muscles, fascia and tendons at forearm level, right arm
S56.912 Strain of unspecified muscles, fascia and tendons at forearm level, left arm
S56.919 Strain of unspecified muscles, fascia and tendons at forearm level, unspecified arm
S56.92 Laceration of unspecified muscles, fascia and tendons at forearm level
S56.921 Laceration of unspecified muscles, fascia and tendons at forearm level, right arm
S56.922 Laceration of unspecified muscles, fascia and tendons at forearm level, left arm
S56.929 Laceration of unspecified muscles, fascia and tendons at forearm level, unspecified arm
S56.99 Other injury of unspecified muscles, fascia and tendons at forearm level
S56.991 Other injury of unspecified muscles, fascia and tendons at forearm level, right arm
S56.992 Other injury of unspecified muscles, fascia and tendons at forearm level, left arm
S56.999 Other injury of unspecified muscles, fascia and tendons at forearm level, unspecified arm

S57 Crushing injury of elbow and forearm

Use additional code(s) for all associated injuries

Excludes2 crushing injury of wrist and hand (S67.-)

The appropriate 7th character is to be added to each code from category S57

A	initial encounter
D	subsequent encounter
S	sequela

S57.0 Crushing injury of elbow
X S57.00 Crushing injury of unspecified elbow
X S57.01 Crushing injury of right elbow
X S57.02 Crushing injury of left elbow
S57.8 Crushing injury of forearm
X S57.80 Crushing injury of unspecified forearm
X S57.81 Crushing injury of right forearm
X S57.82 Crushing injury of left forearm

S58 Traumatic amputation of elbow and forearm

An amputation not identified as partial or complete should be coded to complete

Excludes1 traumatic amputation of wrist and hand (S68.-)

The appropriate 7th character is to be added to each code from category S58

A	initial encounter
D	subsequent encounter
S	sequela

S58.Ø Traumatic amputation **at elbow level**

- **S58.Ø1** **Complete** traumatic amputation at elbow level
  - **S58.Ø11** Complete traumatic amputation at elbow level, **right** arm A, S
  - **S58.Ø12** Complete traumatic amputation at elbow level, **left** arm A, S
  - **S58.Ø19** Complete traumatic amputation at elbow level, **unspecified** arm A, S
- **S58.Ø2** **Partial** traumatic amputation at elbow level
  - **S58.Ø21** Partial traumatic amputation at elbow level, **right** arm A, S
  - **S58.Ø22** Partial traumatic amputation at elbow level, **left** arm A, S
  - **S58.Ø29** Partial traumatic amputation at elbow level, **unspecified** arm A, S

S58.1 Traumatic amputation at level **between elbow and wrist**

- **S58.11** **Complete** traumatic amputation at level between elbow and wrist
  - **S58.111** Complete traumatic amputation at level between elbow and wrist, **right** arm A, S
  - **S58.112** Complete traumatic amputation at level between elbow and wrist, **left** arm A, S
  - **S58.119** Complete traumatic amputation at level between elbow and wrist, **unspecified** arm A, S
- **S58.12** **Partial** traumatic amputation at level between elbow and wrist
  - **S58.121** Partial traumatic amputation at level between elbow and wrist, **right** arm A, S
  - **S58.122** Partial traumatic amputation at level between elbow and wrist, **left** arm A, S
  - **S58.129** Partial traumatic amputation at level between elbow and wrist, **unspecified** arm A, S

S58.9 Traumatic amputation of forearm, **level unspecified**

Excludes1 traumatic amputation of wrist (S68.-)

- **S58.91** **Complete** traumatic amputation of forearm, level unspecified
  - **S58.911** Complete traumatic amputation of **right** forearm, level unspecified A, S
  - **S58.912** Complete traumatic amputation of **left** forearm, level unspecified A, S
  - **S58.919** Complete traumatic amputation of **unspecified** forearm, level unspecified A, S
- **S58.92** **Partial** traumatic amputation of forearm, level unspecified
  - **S58.921** Partial traumatic amputation of **right** forearm, level unspecified A, S
  - **S58.922** Partial traumatic amputation of **left** forearm, level unspecified A, S
  - **S58.929** Partial traumatic amputation of **unspecified** forearm, level unspecified A, S

Item 19–4 **SALTER-HARRIS TYPE 1:** epiphysis is completely separated from end of bone, or metaphysic growth plate remains attached to epiphysis

SALTER-HARRIS TYPE 2: epiphysis and growth plate are partially separated from metaphysis, which is cracked—most common type

SALTER-HARRIS TYPE 3: fracture occurring through epiphysis and separates part of epiphysis and growth plate from metaphysis fracture, usually at distal end of tibia

SALTER-HARRIS TYPE 4: fracture runs through epiphysis, across growth plate, into metaphysic, surgery is required to restore joint surface to normal and align growth plate

S59 Other and unspecified injuries of elbow and forearm

Excludes2 other and unspecified injuries of wrist and hand (S69.-)

The appropriate 7th character is to be added to each code from subcategories S59.Ø, S59.1, and S59.2

A	initial encounter for closed fracture
D	subsequent encounter for fracture with routine healing
G	subsequent encounter for fracture with delayed healing
K	subsequent encounter for fracture with nonunion
P	subsequent encounter for fracture with malunion
S	sequela

S59.Ø **Physeal fracture of lower end of ulna**

- **S59.ØØ** **Unspecified** physeal fracture of lower end of ulna
  - **S59.ØØ1** Unspecified physeal fracture of lower end of ulna, **right** arm
  - **S59.ØØ2** Unspecified physeal fracture of lower end of ulna, **left** arm
  - **S59.ØØ9** Unspecified physeal fracture of lower end of ulna, **unspecified** arm
- **S59.Ø1** **Salter-Harris Type I** physeal fracture of lower end of ulna
  - **S59.Ø11** Salter-Harris Type I physeal fracture of lower end of ulna, **right** arm
  - **S59.Ø12** Salter-Harris Type I physeal fracture of lower end of ulna, **left** arm
  - **S59.Ø19** Salter-Harris Type I physeal fracture of lower end of ulna, **unspecified** arm
- **S59.Ø2** **Salter-Harris Type II** physeal fracture of lower end of ulna
  - **S59.Ø21** Salter-Harris Type II physeal fracture of lower end of ulna, **right** arm
  - **S59.Ø22** Salter-Harris Type II physeal fracture of lower end of ulna, **left** arm
  - **S59.Ø29** Salter-Harris Type II physeal fracture of lower end of ulna, **unspecified** arm
- **S59.Ø3** **Salter-Harris Type III** physeal fracture of lower end of ulna
  - **S59.Ø31** Salter-Harris Type III physeal fracture of lower end of ulna, **right** arm
  - **S59.Ø32** Salter-Harris Type III physeal fracture of lower end of ulna, **left** arm
  - **S59.Ø39** Salter-Harris Type III physeal fracture of lower end of ulna, **unspecified** arm
- **S59.Ø4** **Salter-Harris Type IV** physeal fracture of lower end of ulna
  - **S59.Ø41** Salter-Harris Type IV physeal fracture of lower end of ulna, **right** arm
  - **S59.Ø42** Salter-Harris Type IV physeal fracture of lower end of ulna, **left** arm
  - **S59.Ø49** Salter-Harris Type IV physeal fracture of lower end of ulna, **unspecified** arm

- S59.09 Other physeal fracture of lower end of ulna
  - S59.091 Other physeal fracture of lower end of ulna, **right** arm
  - S59.092 Other physeal fracture of lower end of ulna, **left** arm
  - S59.099 Other physeal fracture of lower end of ulna, **unspecified** arm
- S59.1 Physeal fracture of upper end of radius
  - S59.10 Unspecified physeal fracture of upper end of radius
    - S59.101 Unspecified physeal fracture of upper end of radius, **right** arm
    - S59.102 Unspecified physeal fracture of upper end of radius, **left** arm
    - S59.109 Unspecified physeal fracture of upper end of radius, **unspecified** arm
  - S59.11 Salter-Harris Type I physeal fracture of upper end of radius
    - S59.111 Salter-Harris Type I physeal fracture of upper end of radius, **right** arm
    - S59.112 Salter-Harris Type I physeal fracture of upper end of radius, **left** arm
    - S59.119 Salter-Harris Type I physeal fracture of upper end of radius, **unspecified** arm
  - S59.12 Salter-Harris Type II physeal fracture of upper end of radius
    - S59.121 Salter-Harris Type II physeal fracture of upper end of radius, **right** arm
    - S59.122 Salter-Harris Type II physeal fracture of upper end of radius, **left** arm
    - S59.129 Salter-Harris Type II physeal fracture of upper end of radius, **unspecified** arm
  - S59.13 Salter-Harris Type III physeal fracture of upper end of radius
    - S59.131 Salter-Harris Type III physeal fracture of upper end of radius, **right** arm
    - S59.132 Salter-Harris Type III physeal fracture of upper end of radius, **left** arm
    - S59.139 Salter-Harris Type III physeal fracture of upper end of radius, **unspecified** arm
  - S59.14 Salter-Harris Type IV physeal fracture of upper end of radius
    - S59.141 Salter-Harris Type IV physeal fracture of upper end of radius, **right** arm
    - S59.142 Salter-Harris Type IV physeal fracture of upper end of radius, **left** arm
    - S59.149 Salter-Harris Type IV physeal fracture of upper end of radius, **unspecified** arm
  - S59.19 Other physeal fracture of upper end of radius
    - S59.191 Other physeal fracture of upper end of radius, **right** arm
    - S59.192 Other physeal fracture of upper end of radius, **left** arm
    - S59.199 Other physeal fracture of upper end of radius, **unspecified** arm
- S59.2 Physeal fracture of lower end of radius
  - S59.20 Unspecified physeal fracture of lower end of radius
    - S59.201 Unspecified physeal fracture of lower end of radius, **right** arm
    - S59.202 Unspecified physeal fracture of lower end of radius, **left** arm
    - S59.209 Unspecified physeal fracture of lower end of radius, **unspecified** arm
  - S59.21 Salter-Harris Type I physeal fracture of lower end of radius
    - S59.211 Salter-Harris Type I physeal fracture of lower end of radius, **right** arm
    - S59.212 Salter-Harris Type I physeal fracture of lower end of radius, **left** arm
    - S59.219 Salter-Harris Type I physeal fracture of lower end of radius, **unspecified** arm
  - S59.22 Salter-Harris Type II physeal fracture of lower end of radius
    - S59.221 Salter-Harris Type II physeal fracture of lower end of radius, **right** arm
    - S59.222 Salter-Harris Type II physeal fracture of lower end of radius, **left** arm
    - S59.229 Salter-Harris Type II physeal fracture of lower end of radius, **unspecified** arm
  - S59.23 Salter-Harris Type III physeal fracture of lower end of radius
    - S59.231 Salter-Harris Type III physeal fracture of lower end of radius, **right** arm
    - S59.232 Salter-Harris Type III physeal fracture of lower end of radius, **left** arm
    - S59.239 Salter-Harris Type III physeal fracture of lower end of radius, **unspecified** arm
  - S59.24 Salter-Harris Type IV physeal fracture of lower end of radius
    - S59.241 Salter-Harris Type IV physeal fracture of lower end of radius, **right** arm
    - S59.242 Salter-Harris Type IV physeal fracture of lower end of radius, **left** arm
    - S59.249 Salter-Harris Type IV physeal fracture of lower end of radius, **unspecified** arm
  - S59.29 Other physeal fracture of lower end of radius
    - S59.291 Other physeal fracture of lower end of radius, **right** arm
    - S59.292 Other physeal fracture of lower end of radius, **left** arm
    - S59.299 Other physeal fracture of lower end of radius, **unspecified** arm
- S59.8 Other specified injuries of elbow and forearm

  The appropriate 7th character is to be added to each code in subcategory S59.8

A	initial encounter
D	subsequent encounter
S	sequela

  - S59.80 Other specified injuries of **elbow**
    - S59.801 Other specified injuries of **right** elbow
    - S59.802 Other specified injuries of **left** elbow
    - S59.809 Other specified injuries of **unspecified** elbow
  - S59.81 Other specified injuries of **forearm**
    - S59.811 Other specified injuries **right** forearm
    - S59.812 Other specified injuries **left** forearm
    - S59.819 Other specified injuries **unspecified** forearm

S59.9 Unspecified injury of elbow and forearm

The appropriate 7th character is to be added to each code in subcategory S59.9

A	initial encounter
D	subsequent encounter
S	sequela

S59.90 Unspecified injury of elbow
- **S59.901 Unspecified injury of right elbow**
- **S59.902 Unspecified injury of left elbow**
- **S59.909 Unspecified injury of unspecified elbow**

S59.91 Unspecified injury of forearm
- **S59.911 Unspecified injury of right forearm**
- **S59.912 Unspecified injury of left forearm**
- **S59.919 Unspecified injury of unspecified forearm**

INJURIES TO THE WRIST, HAND AND FINGERS (S60-S69)

Excludes2 burns and corrosions (T20-T32)
frostbite (T33-T34)
insect bite or sting, venomous (T63.4)

S60 Superficial injury of wrist, hand and fingers

The appropriate 7th character is to be added to each code from category S60

A	initial encounter
D	subsequent encounter
S	sequela

S60.0 Contusion of finger without damage to nail

Excludes1 contusion involving nail (matrix) (S60.1)

X **S60.00 Contusion of unspecified finger without damage to nail**
Contusion of finger(s) NOS

S60.01 Contusion of thumb without damage to nail
- **S60.011 Contusion of right thumb without damage to nail**
- **S60.012 Contusion of left thumb without damage to nail**
- **S60.019 Contusion of unspecified thumb without damage to nail**

S60.02 Contusion of index finger without damage to nail
- **S60.021 Contusion of right index finger without damage to nail**
- **S60.022 Contusion of left index finger without damage to nail**
- **S60.029 Contusion of unspecified index finger without damage to nail**

S60.03 Contusion of middle finger without damage to nail
- **S60.031 Contusion of right middle finger without damage to nail**
- **S60.032 Contusion of left middle finger without damage to nail**
- **S60.039 Contusion of unspecified middle finger without damage to nail**

S60.04 Contusion of ring finger without damage to nail
- **S60.041 Contusion of right ring finger without damage to nail**
- **S60.042 Contusion of left ring finger without damage to nail**
- **S60.049 Contusion of unspecified ring finger without damage to nail**

S60.05 Contusion of little finger without damage to nail
- **S60.051 Contusion of right little finger without damage to nail**
- **S60.052 Contusion of left little finger without damage to nail**
- **S60.059 Contusion of unspecified little finger without damage to nail**

S60.1 Contusion of finger with damage to nail

X **S60.10 Contusion of unspecified finger with damage to nail**

S60.11 Contusion of thumb with damage to nail
- **S60.111 Contusion of right thumb with damage to nail**
- **S60.112 Contusion of left thumb with damage to nail**
- **S60.119 Contusion of unspecified thumb with damage to nail**

S60.12 Contusion of index finger with damage to nail
- **S60.121 Contusion of right index finger with damage to nail**
- **S60.122 Contusion of left index finger with damage to nail**
- **S60.129 Contusion of unspecified index finger with damage to nail**

S60.13 Contusion of middle finger with damage to nail
- **S60.131 Contusion of right middle finger with damage to nail**
- **S60.132 Contusion of left middle finger with damage to nail**
- **S60.139 Contusion of unspecified middle finger with damage to nail**

S60.14 Contusion of ring finger with damage to nail
- **S60.141 Contusion of right ring finger with damage to nail**
- **S60.142 Contusion of left ring finger with damage to nail**
- **S60.149 Contusion of unspecified ring finger with damage to nail**

S60.15 Contusion of little finger with damage to nail
- **S60.151 Contusion of right little finger with damage to nail**
- **S60.152 Contusion of left little finger with damage to nail**
- **S60.159 Contusion of unspecified little finger with damage to nail**

S60.2 Contusion of wrist and hand

Excludes2 contusion of fingers (S60.0-, S60.1-)

S60.21 Contusion of wrist
- **S60.211 Contusion of right wrist**
- **S60.212 Contusion of left wrist**
- **S60.219 Contusion of unspecified wrist**

S60.22 Contusion of hand
- **S60.221 Contusion of right hand**
- **S60.222 Contusion of left hand**
- **S60.229 Contusion of unspecified hand**

S60.3 Other superficial injuries of thumb

S60.31 Abrasion of thumb
- **S60.311 Abrasion of right thumb**
- **S60.312 Abrasion of left thumb**
- **S60.319 Abrasion of unspecified thumb**

S60.32 Blister (nonthermal) of thumb
- **S60.321 Blister (nonthermal) of right thumb**
- **S60.322 Blister (nonthermal) of left thumb**
- **S60.329 Blister (nonthermal) of unspecified thumb**

S60.34 External constriction of thumb
Hair tourniquet syndrome of thumb
Use additional cause code to identify the constricting item (W49.0-)
S60.341 External constriction of right thumb
S60.342 External constriction of left thumb
S60.349 External constriction of unspecified thumb
S60.35 Superficial foreign body of thumb
Splinter in the thumb
S60.351 Superficial foreign body of right thumb
S60.352 Superficial foreign body of left thumb
S60.359 Superficial foreign body of unspecified thumb
S60.36 Insect bite (nonvenomous) of thumb
S60.361 Insect bite (nonvenomous) of right thumb
S60.362 Insect bite (nonvenomous) of left thumb
S60.369 Insect bite (nonvenomous) of unspecified thumb
S60.37 Other superficial bite of thumb
Excludes1 open bite of thumb (S61.05-, S61.15-)
S60.371 Other superficial bite of right thumb
S60.372 Other superficial bite of left thumb
S60.379 Other superficial bite of unspecified thumb
S60.39 Other superficial injuries of thumb
S60.391 Other superficial injuries of right thumb
S60.392 Other superficial injuries of left thumb
S60.399 Other superficial injuries of unspecified thumb
S60.4 Other superficial injuries of other fingers
S60.41 Abrasion of fingers
S60.410 Abrasion of right index finger
S60.411 Abrasion of left index finger
S60.412 Abrasion of right middle finger
S60.413 Abrasion of left middle finger
S60.414 Abrasion of right ring finger
S60.415 Abrasion of left ring finger
S60.416 Abrasion of right little finger
S60.417 Abrasion of left little finger
S60.418 Abrasion of other finger
Abrasion of specified finger with unspecified laterality
S60.419 Abrasion of unspecified finger
S60.42 Blister (nonthermal) of fingers
S60.420 Blister (nonthermal) of right index finger
S60.421 Blister (nonthermal) of left index finger
S60.422 Blister (nonthermal) of right middle finger
S60.423 Blister (nonthermal) of left middle finger
S60.424 Blister (nonthermal) of right ring finger
S60.425 Blister (nonthermal) of left ring finger
S60.426 Blister (nonthermal) of right little finger
S60.427 Blister (nonthermal) of left little finger
S60.428 Blister (nonthermal) of other finger
Blister (nonthermal) of specified finger with unspecified laterality
S60.429 Blister (nonthermal) of unspecified finger
S60.44 External constriction of fingers
Hair tourniquet syndrome of finger
Use additional cause code to identify the constricting item (W49.0-)
S60.440 External constriction of right index finger
S60.441 External constriction of left index finger
S60.442 External constriction of right middle finger
S60.443 External constriction of left middle finger
S60.444 External constriction of right ring finger
S60.445 External constriction of left ring finger
S60.446 External constriction of right little finger
S60.447 External constriction of left little finger
S60.448 External constriction of other finger
External constriction of specified finger with unspecified laterality
S60.449 External constriction of unspecified finger
S60.45 Superficial foreign body of fingers
Splinter in the finger(s)
S60.450 Superficial foreign body of right index finger
S60.451 Superficial foreign body of left index finger
S60.452 Superficial foreign body of right middle finger
S60.453 Superficial foreign body of left middle finger
S60.454 Superficial foreign body of right ring finger
S60.455 Superficial foreign body of left ring finger
S60.456 Superficial foreign body of right little finger
S60.457 Superficial foreign body of left little finger
S60.458 Superficial foreign body of other finger
Superficial foreign body of specified finger with unspecified laterality
S60.459 Superficial foreign body of unspecified finger

- S60.46 **Insect bite (nonvenomous) of fingers**
  - S60.460 Insect bite (nonvenomous) of right index finger
  - S60.461 Insect bite (nonvenomous) of left index finger
  - S60.462 Insect bite (nonvenomous) of right middle finger
  - S60.463 Insect bite (nonvenomous) of left middle finger
  - S60.464 Insect bite (nonvenomous) of right ring finger
  - S60.465 Insect bite (nonvenomous) of left ring finger
  - S60.466 Insect bite (nonvenomous) of right little finger
  - S60.467 Insect bite (nonvenomous) of left little finger
  - S60.468 Insect bite (nonvenomous) of other finger
    Insect bite (nonvenomous) of specified finger with unspecified laterality
  - S60.469 Insect bite (nonvenomous) of unspecified finger
- S60.47 **Other superficial bite of fingers**
  Excludes1 open bite of fingers (S61.25-, S61.35-)
  - S60.470 Other superficial bite of right index finger
  - S60.471 Other superficial bite of left index finger
  - S60.472 Other superficial bite of right middle finger
  - S60.473 Other superficial bite of left middle finger
  - S60.474 Other superficial bite of right ring finger
  - S60.475 Other superficial bite of left ring finger
  - S60.476 Other superficial bite of right little finger
  - S60.477 Other superficial bite of left little finger
  - S60.478 Other superficial bite of other finger
    Other superficial bite of specified finger with unspecified laterality
  - S60.479 Other superficial bite of unspecified finger

S60.5 Other superficial injuries of hand
Excludes2 superficial injuries of fingers (S60.3-, S60.4-)

- S60.51 **Abrasion of hand**
  - S60.511 Abrasion of right hand
  - S60.512 Abrasion of left hand
  - S60.519 Abrasion of unspecified hand
- S60.52 **Blister (nonthermal) of hand**
  - S60.521 Blister (nonthermal) of right hand
  - S60.522 Blister (nonthermal) of left hand
  - S60.529 Blister (nonthermal) of unspecified hand
- S60.54 **External constriction of hand**
  - S60.541 External constriction of right hand
  - S60.542 External constriction of left hand
  - S60.549 External constriction of unspecified hand
- S60.55 **Superficial foreign body of hand**
  Splinter in the hand
  - S60.551 Superficial foreign body of right hand
  - S60.552 Superficial foreign body of left hand
  - S60.559 Superficial foreign body of unspecified hand
- S60.56 **Insect bite (nonvenomous) of hand**
  - S60.561 Insect bite (nonvenomous) of right hand
  - S60.562 Insect bite (nonvenomous) of left hand
  - S60.569 Insect bite (nonvenomous) of unspecified hand
- S60.57 **Other superficial bite of hand**
  Excludes1 open bite of hand (S61.45-)
  - S60.571 Other superficial bite of hand of right hand
  - S60.572 Other superficial bite of hand of left hand
  - S60.579 Other superficial bite of hand of unspecified hand

S60.8 Other superficial injuries of wrist

- S60.81 **Abrasion of wrist**
  - S60.811 Abrasion of right wrist
  - S60.812 Abrasion of left wrist
  - S60.819 Abrasion of unspecified wrist
- S60.82 **Blister (nonthermal) of wrist**
  - S60.821 Blister (nonthermal) of right wrist
  - S60.822 Blister (nonthermal) of left wrist
  - S60.829 Blister (nonthermal) of unspecified wrist
- S60.84 **External constriction of wrist**
  - S60.841 External constriction of right wrist
  - S60.842 External constriction of left wrist
  - S60.849 External constriction of unspecified wrist
- S60.85 **Superficial foreign body of wrist**
  Splinter in the wrist
  - S60.851 Superficial foreign body of right wrist
  - S60.852 Superficial foreign body of left wrist
  - S60.859 Superficial foreign body of unspecified wrist
- S60.86 **Insect bite (nonvenomous) of wrist**
  - S60.861 Insect bite (nonvenomous) of right wrist
  - S60.862 Insect bite (nonvenomous) of left wrist
  - S60.869 Insect bite (nonvenomous) of unspecified wrist
- S60.87 **Other superficial bite of wrist**
  Excludes1 open bite of wrist (S61.55)
  - S60.871 Other superficial bite of right wrist
  - S60.872 Other superficial bite of left wrist
  - S60.879 Other superficial bite of unspecified wrist

S60.9 Unspecified superficial injury of wrist, hand and fingers

- S60.91 **Unspecified superficial injury of wrist**
  - S60.911 Unspecified superficial injury of right wrist
  - S60.912 Unspecified superficial injury of left wrist
  - S60.919 Unspecified superficial injury of unspecified wrist

S60.92 **Unspecified** superficial injury of **hand**
S60.921 Unspecified superficial injury of **right** hand
S60.922 Unspecified superficial injury of **left** hand
S60.929 Unspecified superficial injury of **unspecified** hand
S60.93 **Unspecified** superficial injury of **thumb**
S60.931 Unspecified superficial injury of **right** thumb
S60.932 Unspecified superficial injury of **left** thumb
S60.939 Unspecified superficial injury of **unspecified** thumb
S60.94 **Unspecified** superficial injury of **other fingers**
S60.940 Unspecified superficial injury of **right index** finger
S60.941 Unspecified superficial injury of **left index** finger
S60.942 Unspecified superficial injury of **right middle** finger
S60.943 Unspecified superficial injury of **left middle** finger
S60.944 Unspecified superficial injury of **right ring** finger
S60.945 Unspecified superficial injury of **left ring** finger
S60.946 Unspecified superficial injury of **right little** finger
S60.947 Unspecified superficial injury of **left little** finger
S60.948 Unspecified superficial injury of **other** finger
Unspecified superficial injury of specified finger with unspecified laterality
S60.949 Unspecified superficial injury of **unspecified** finger

S61 **Open wound of wrist, hand and fingers**
Code also any associated wound infection
Excludes1 open fracture of wrist, hand and finger (S62.- with 7th character B)
traumatic amputation of wrist and hand (S68.-)
The appropriate 7th character is to be added to each code from category S61

A	initial encounter
D	subsequent encounter
S	sequela

S61.0 Open wound of **thumb without damage to nail**
Excludes1 open wound of thumb with damage to nail (S61.1-)
S61.00 **Unspecified** open wound of thumb without damage to nail
S61.001 Unspecified open wound of **right** thumb without damage to nail
S61.002 Unspecified open wound of **left** thumb without damage to nail
S61.009 Unspecified open wound of **unspecified** thumb without damage to nail
S61.01 **Laceration without foreign body** of thumb without damage to nail
S61.011 Laceration without foreign body of **right** thumb without damage to nail
S61.012 Laceration without foreign body of **left** thumb without damage to nail
S61.019 Laceration without foreign body of **unspecified** thumb without damage to nail
S61.02 **Laceration with foreign body** of thumb without damage to nail
S61.021 Laceration with foreign body of **right** thumb without damage to nail
S61.022 Laceration with foreign body of **left** thumb without damage to nail
S61.029 Laceration with foreign body of **unspecified** thumb without damage to nail
S61.03 **Puncture wound without foreign body** of thumb without damage to nail
S61.031 Puncture wound without foreign body of **right** thumb without damage to nail
S61.032 Puncture wound without foreign body of **left** thumb without damage to nail
S61.039 Puncture wound without foreign body of **unspecified** thumb without damage to nail
S61.04 **Puncture wound with foreign body** of thumb without damage to nail
S61.041 Puncture wound with foreign body of **right** thumb without damage to nail
S61.042 Puncture wound with foreign body of **left** thumb without damage to nail
S61.049 Puncture wound with foreign body of **unspecified** thumb without damage to nail
S61.05 **Open bite** of thumb without damage to nail
Bite of thumb NOS
Excludes1 superficial bite of thumb (S60.36-, S60.37-)
S61.051 Open bite of **right** thumb without damage to nail
S61.052 Open bite of **left** thumb without damage to nail
S61.059 Open bite of **unspecified** thumb without damage to nail
S61.1 Open wound of **thumb with damage to nail**
S61.10 **Unspecified** open wound of thumb with damage to nail
S61.101 Unspecified open wound of **right** thumb with damage to nail
S61.102 Unspecified open wound of **left** thumb with damage to nail
S61.109 Unspecified open wound of **unspecified** thumb with damage to nail
S61.11 **Laceration without foreign body** of thumb with damage to nail
S61.111 Laceration without foreign body of **right** thumb with damage to nail
S61.112 Laceration without foreign body of **left** thumb with damage to nail
S61.119 Laceration without foreign body of **unspecified** thumb with damage to nail
S61.12 **Laceration with foreign body** of thumb with damage to nail
S61.121 Laceration with foreign body of **right** thumb with damage to nail
S61.122 Laceration with foreign body of **left** thumb with damage to nail
S61.129 Laceration with foreign body of **unspecified** thumb with damage to nail

CHAPTER 19 (S00-T88)

- S61.13 **Puncture wound without foreign body of thumb with damage to nail**
  - S61.131 Puncture wound without foreign body of right thumb with damage to nail
  - S61.132 Puncture wound without foreign body of left thumb with damage to nail
  - S61.139 Puncture wound without foreign body of unspecified thumb with damage to nail
- S61.14 **Puncture wound with foreign body of thumb with damage to nail**
  - S61.141 Puncture wound with foreign body of right thumb with damage to nail
  - S61.142 Puncture wound with foreign body of left thumb with damage to nail
  - S61.149 Puncture wound with foreign body of unspecified thumb with damage to nail
- S61.15 **Open bite of thumb with damage to nail**
  Bite of thumb with damage to nail NOS
  Excludes1 superficial bite of thumb (S6Ø.36-, S6Ø.37-)
  - S61.151 Open bite of right thumb with damage to nail
  - S61.152 Open bite of left thumb with damage to nail
  - S61.159 Open bite of unspecified thumb with damage to nail

S61.2 Open wound of other finger without damage to nail

Excludes1 open wound of finger involving nail (matrix) (S61.3-)

Excludes2 open wound of thumb without damage to nail (S61.Ø-)

- S61.2Ø **Unspecified open wound of other finger without damage to nail**
  - S61.2ØØ Unspecified open wound of right index finger without damage to nail
  - S61.2Ø1 Unspecified open wound of left index finger without damage to nail
  - S61.2Ø2 Unspecified open wound of right middle finger without damage to nail
  - S61.2Ø3 Unspecified open wound of left middle finger without damage to nail
  - S61.2Ø4 Unspecified open wound of right ring finger without damage to nail
  - S61.2Ø5 Unspecified open wound of left ring finger without damage to nail
  - S61.2Ø6 Unspecified open wound of right little finger without damage to nail
  - S61.2Ø7 Unspecified open wound of left little finger without damage to nail
  - S61.2Ø8 Unspecified open wound of other finger without damage to nail
    Unspecified open wound of specified finger with unspecified laterality without damage to nail
  - S61.2Ø9 Unspecified open wound of unspecified finger without damage to nail
- S61.21 **Laceration without foreign body of finger without damage to nail**
  - S61.21Ø Laceration without foreign body of right index finger without damage to nail
  - S61.211 Laceration without foreign body of left index finger without damage to nail
  - S61.212 Laceration without foreign body of right middle finger without damage to nail
  - S61.213 Laceration without foreign body of left middle finger without damage to nail
  - S61.214 Laceration without foreign body of right ring finger without damage to nail
  - S61.215 Laceration without foreign body of left ring finger without damage to nail
  - S61.216 Laceration without foreign body of right little finger without damage to nail
  - S61.217 Laceration without foreign body of left little finger without damage to nail
  - S61.218 Laceration without foreign body of other finger without damage to nail
    Laceration without foreign body of specified finger with unspecified laterality without damage to nail
  - S61.219 Laceration without foreign body of unspecified finger without damage to nail
- S61.22 **Laceration with foreign body of finger without damage to nail**
  - S61.22Ø Laceration with foreign body of right index finger without damage to nail
  - S61.221 Laceration with foreign body of left index finger without damage to nail
  - S61.222 Laceration with foreign body of right middle finger without damage to nail
  - S61.223 Laceration with foreign body of left middle finger without damage to nail
  - S61.224 Laceration with foreign body of right ring finger without damage to nail
  - S61.225 Laceration with foreign body of left ring finger without damage to nail
  - S61.226 Laceration with foreign body of right little finger without damage to nail
  - S61.227 Laceration with foreign body of left little finger without damage to nail
  - S61.228 Laceration with foreign body of other finger without damage to nail
    Laceration with foreign body of specified finger with unspecified laterality without damage to nail
  - S61.229 Laceration with foreign body of unspecified finger without damage to nail

S61.23 **Puncture wound without foreign body of finger without damage to nail**
- S61.230 Puncture wound without foreign body of **right index** finger without damage to nail
- S61.231 Puncture wound without foreign body of **left index** finger without damage to nail
- S61.232 Puncture wound without foreign body of **right middle** finger without damage to nail
- S61.233 Puncture wound without foreign body of **left middle** finger without damage to nail
- S61.234 Puncture wound without foreign body of **right ring** finger without damage to nail
- S61.235 Puncture wound without foreign body of **left ring** finger without damage to nail
- S61.236 Puncture wound without foreign body of **right little** finger without damage to nail
- S61.237 Puncture wound without foreign body of **left little** finger without damage to nail
- S61.238 Puncture wound without foreign body of **other** finger without damage to nail
  Puncture wound without foreign body of specified finger with unspecified laterality without damage to nail
- S61.239 Puncture wound without foreign body of **unspecified** finger without damage to nail

S61.24 **Puncture wound with foreign body of finger without damage to nail**
- S61.240 Puncture wound with foreign body of **right index** finger without damage to nail
- S61.241 Puncture wound with foreign body of **left index** finger without damage to nail
- S61.242 Puncture wound with foreign body of **right middle** finger without damage to nail
- S61.243 Puncture wound with foreign body of **left middle** finger without damage to nail
- S61.244 Puncture wound with foreign body of **right ring** finger without damage to nail
- S61.245 Puncture wound with foreign body of **left ring** finger without damage to nail
- S61.246 Puncture wound with foreign body of **right little** finger without damage to nail
- S61.247 Puncture wound with foreign body of **left little** finger without damage to nail
- S61.248 Puncture wound with foreign body of **other** finger without damage to nail
  Puncture wound with foreign body of specified finger with unspecified laterality without damage to nail
- S61.249 Puncture wound with foreign body of **unspecified** finger without damage to nail

S61.25 **Open bite of finger without damage to nail**
Bite of finger without damage to nail NOS
Excludes1 superficial bite of finger (S6Ø.46-, S6Ø.47-)
- S61.25Ø Open bite of **right index** finger without damage to nail
- S61.251 Open bite of **left index** finger without damage to nail
- S61.252 Open bite of **right middle** finger without damage to nail
- S61.253 Open bite of **left middle** finger without damage to nail
- S61.254 Open bite of **right ring** finger without damage to nail
- S61.255 Open bite of **left ring** finger without damage to nail
- S61.256 Open bite of **right little** finger without damage to nail
- S61.257 Open bite of **left little** finger without damage to nail
- S61.258 Open bite of **other** finger without damage to nail
  Open bite of specified finger with unspecified laterality without damage to nail
- S61.259 Open bite of **unspecified** finger without damage to nail

S61.3 Open wound of other finger with damage to nail

S61.3Ø **Unspecified open wound of finger with damage to nail**
- S61.3ØØ Unspecified open wound of **right index** finger with damage to nail
- S61.3Ø1 Unspecified open wound of **left index** finger with damage to nail
- S61.3Ø2 Unspecified open wound of **right middle** finger with damage to nail
- S61.3Ø3 Unspecified open wound of **left middle** finger with damage to nail
- S61.3Ø4 Unspecified open wound of **right ring** finger with damage to nail
- S61.3Ø5 Unspecified open wound of **left ring** finger with damage to nail
- S61.3Ø6 Unspecified open wound of **right little** finger with damage to nail
- S61.3Ø7 Unspecified open wound of **left little** finger with damage to nail
- S61.3Ø8 Unspecified open wound of **other** finger with damage to nail
  Unspecified open wound of specified finger with unspecified laterality with damage to nail
- S61.3Ø9 Unspecified open wound of **unspecified** finger with damage to nail

S61.31 **Laceration without foreign body of finger with damage to nail**
- S61.31Ø Laceration without foreign body of **right index** finger with damage to nail
- S61.311 Laceration without foreign body of **left index** finger with damage to nail
- S61.312 Laceration without foreign body of **right middle** finger with damage to nail
- S61.313 Laceration without foreign body of **left middle** finger with damage to nail
- S61.314 Laceration without foreign body of **right ring** finger with damage to nail

- S61.315 Laceration without foreign body of left ring finger with damage to nail
- S61.316 Laceration without foreign body of right little finger with damage to nail
- S61.317 Laceration without foreign body of left little finger with damage to nail
- S61.318 Laceration without foreign body of other finger with damage to nail
  Laceration without foreign body of specified finger with unspecified laterality with damage to nail
- S61.319 Laceration without foreign body of unspecified finger with damage to nail

S61.32 Laceration with foreign body of finger with damage to nail

- S61.320 Laceration with foreign body of right index finger with damage to nail
- S61.321 Laceration with foreign body of left index finger with damage to nail
- S61.322 Laceration with foreign body of right middle finger with damage to nail
- S61.323 Laceration with foreign body of left middle finger with damage to nail
- S61.324 Laceration with foreign body of right ring finger with damage to nail
- S61.325 Laceration with foreign body of left ring finger with damage to nail
- S61.326 Laceration with foreign body of right little finger with damage to nail
- S61.327 Laceration with foreign body of left little finger with damage to nail
- S61.328 Laceration with foreign body of other finger with damage to nail
  Laceration with foreign body of specified finger with unspecified laterality with damage to nail
- S61.329 Laceration with foreign body of unspecified finger with damage to nail

S61.33 Puncture wound without foreign body of finger with damage to nail

- S61.330 Puncture wound without foreign body of right index finger with damage to nail
- S61.331 Puncture wound without foreign body of left index finger with damage to nail
- S61.332 Puncture wound without foreign body of right middle finger with damage to nail
- S61.333 Puncture wound without foreign body of left middle finger with damage to nail
- S61.334 Puncture wound without foreign body of right ring finger with damage to nail
- S61.335 Puncture wound without foreign body of left ring finger with damage to nail
- S61.336 Puncture wound without foreign body of right little finger with damage to nail
- S61.337 Puncture wound without foreign body of left little finger with damage to nail
- S61.338 Puncture wound without foreign body of other finger with damage to nail
  Puncture wound without foreign body of specified finger with unspecified laterality with damage to nail
- S61.339 Puncture wound without foreign body of unspecified finger with damage to nail

S61.34 Puncture wound with foreign body of finger with damage to nail

- S61.340 Puncture wound with foreign body of right index finger with damage to nail
- S61.341 Puncture wound with foreign body of left index finger with damage to nail
- S61.342 Puncture wound with foreign body of right middle finger with damage to nail
- S61.343 Puncture wound with foreign body of left middle finger with damage to nail
- S61.344 Puncture wound with foreign body of right ring finger with damage to nail
- S61.345 Puncture wound with foreign body of left ring finger with damage to nail
- S61.346 Puncture wound with foreign body of right little finger with damage to nail
- S61.347 Puncture wound with foreign body of left little finger with damage to nail
- S61.348 Puncture wound with foreign body of other finger with damage to nail
  Puncture wound with foreign body of specified finger with unspecified laterality with damage to nail
- S61.349 Puncture wound with foreign body of unspecified finger with damage to nail

S61.35 Open bite of finger with damage to nail

Bite of finger with damage to nail NOS

Excludes1 superficial bite of finger (S60.46-, S60.47-)

- S61.350 Open bite of right index finger with damage to nail
- S61.351 Open bite of left index finger with damage to nail
- S61.352 Open bite of right middle finger with damage to nail
- S61.353 Open bite of left middle finger with damage to nail
- S61.354 Open bite of right ring finger with damage to nail
- S61.355 Open bite of left ring finger with damage to nail
- S61.356 Open bite of right little finger with damage to nail
- S61.357 Open bite of left little finger with damage to nail
- S61.358 Open bite of other finger with damage to nail
  Open bite of specified finger with unspecified laterality with damage to nail
- S61.359 Open bite of unspecified finger with damage to nail

- S61.4 Open wound of hand
  - S61.40 Unspecified open wound of hand
    - S61.401 Unspecified open wound of right hand
    - S61.402 Unspecified open wound of left hand
    - S61.409 Unspecified open wound of unspecified hand
  - S61.41 Laceration without foreign body of hand
    - S61.411 Laceration without foreign body of right hand
    - S61.412 Laceration without foreign body of left hand
    - S61.419 Laceration without foreign body of unspecified hand
  - S61.42 Laceration with foreign body of hand
    - S61.421 Laceration with foreign body of right hand
    - S61.422 Laceration with foreign body of left hand
    - S61.429 Laceration with foreign body of unspecified hand
  - S61.43 Puncture wound without foreign body of hand
    - S61.431 Puncture wound without foreign body of right hand
    - S61.432 Puncture wound without foreign body of left hand
    - S61.439 Puncture wound without foreign body of unspecified hand
  - S61.44 Puncture wound with foreign body of hand
    - S61.441 Puncture wound with foreign body of right hand
    - S61.442 Puncture wound with foreign body of left hand
    - S61.449 Puncture wound with foreign body of unspecified hand
  - S61.45 Open bite of hand
    Bite of hand NOS
    Excludes1 superficial bite of hand (S60.56-, S60.57-)
    - S61.451 Open bite of right hand
    - S61.452 Open bite of left hand
    - S61.459 Open bite of unspecified hand
- S61.5 Open wound of wrist
  - S61.50 Unspecified open wound of wrist
    - S61.501 Unspecified open wound of right wrist
    - S61.502 Unspecified open wound of left wrist
    - S61.509 Unspecified open wound of unspecified wrist
  - S61.51 Laceration without foreign body of wrist
    - S61.511 Laceration without foreign body of right wrist
    - S61.512 Laceration without foreign body of left wrist
    - S61.519 Laceration without foreign body of unspecified wrist
  - S61.52 Laceration with foreign body of wrist
    - S61.521 Laceration with foreign body of right wrist
    - S61.522 Laceration with foreign body of left wrist
    - S61.529 Laceration with foreign body of unspecified wrist
  - S61.53 Puncture wound without foreign body of wrist
    - S61.531 Puncture wound without foreign body of right wrist
    - S61.532 Puncture wound without foreign body of left wrist
    - S61.539 Puncture wound without foreign body of unspecified wrist
  - S61.54 Puncture wound with foreign body of wrist
    - S61.541 Puncture wound with foreign body of right wrist
    - S61.542 Puncture wound with foreign body of left wrist
    - S61.549 Puncture wound with foreign body of unspecified wrist
  - S61.55 Open bite of wrist
    Bite of wrist NOS
    Excludes1 superficial bite of wrist (S60.86-, S60.87-)
    - S61.551 Open bite of right wrist
    - S61.552 Open bite of left wrist
    - S61.559 Open bite of unspecified wrist

- S62 Fracture at wrist and hand level
  Note: A fracture not indicated as displaced or nondisplaced should be coded to displaced
  A fracture not indicated as open or closed should be coded to closed
  Excludes1 traumatic amputation of wrist and hand (S68.-)
  Excludes2 fracture of distal parts of ulna and radius (S52.-)
  The appropriate 7th character is to be added to each code from category S62

A	initial encounter for closed fracture
B	initial encounter for open fracture
D	subsequent encounter for fracture with routine healing
G	subsequent encounter for fracture with delayed healing
K	subsequent encounter for fracture with nonunion
P	subsequent encounter for fracture with malunion
S	sequela

- S62.0 Fracture of navicular [scaphoid] bone of wrist
  - S62.00 Unspecified fracture of navicular [scaphoid] bone of wrist
    - S62.001 Unspecified fracture of navicular [scaphoid] bone of right wrist
    - S62.002 Unspecified fracture of navicular [scaphoid] bone of left wrist
      Coding Clinic: 2012, Q4, P106
    - S62.009 Unspecified fracture of navicular [scaphoid] bone of unspecified wrist
  - S62.01 Fracture of distal pole of navicular [scaphoid] bone of wrist
    Fracture of volar tuberosity of navicular [scaphoid] bone of wrist
    - S62.011 Displaced fracture of distal pole of navicular [scaphoid] bone of right wrist
    - S62.012 Displaced fracture of distal pole of navicular [scaphoid] bone of left wrist
    - S62.013 Displaced fracture of distal pole of navicular [scaphoid] bone of unspecified wrist
    - S62.014 Nondisplaced fracture of distal pole of navicular [scaphoid] bone of right wrist
    - S62.015 Nondisplaced fracture of distal pole of navicular [scaphoid] bone of left wrist
    - S62.016 Nondisplaced fracture of distal pole of navicular [scaphoid] bone of unspecified wrist

CHAPTER 19 (S00-T88)

New Revised ~~deleted~~ Deleted Excludes 1 Excludes 2 Includes Use additional Code first Code also Key words
OGCR Official Guidelines X Assign placeholder X ● Use Additional Character(s) Manifestation Code Hierarchical Condition Category Coding Clinic

- S62.02 Fracture of **middle third** of navicular [scaphoid] bone of wrist
  - S62.021 **Displaced** fracture of middle third of navicular [scaphoid] bone of **right** wrist
  - S62.022 **Displaced** fracture of middle third of navicular [scaphoid] bone of **left** wrist
  - S62.023 **Displaced** fracture of middle third of navicular [scaphoid] bone of **unspecified** wrist
  - S62.024 **Nondisplaced** fracture of middle third of navicular [scaphoid] bone of **right** wrist
  - S62.025 **Nondisplaced** fracture of middle third of navicular [scaphoid] bone of **left** wrist
  - S62.026 **Nondisplaced** fracture of middle third of navicular [scaphoid] bone of **unspecified** wrist
- S62.03 Fracture of **proximal third** of navicular [scaphoid] bone of wrist
  - S62.031 **Displaced** fracture of proximal third of navicular [scaphoid] bone of **right** wrist
  - S62.032 **Displaced** fracture of proximal third of navicular [scaphoid] bone of **left** wrist
  - S62.033 **Displaced** fracture of proximal third of navicular [scaphoid] bone of **unspecified** wrist
  - S62.034 **Nondisplaced** fracture of proximal third of navicular [scaphoid] bone of **right** wrist
  - S62.035 **Nondisplaced** fracture of proximal third of navicular [scaphoid] bone of **left** wrist
  - S62.036 **Nondisplaced** fracture of proximal third of navicular [scaphoid] bone of **unspecified** wrist

S62.1 Fracture of other and unspecified **carpal bone(s)**

Excludes2 fracture of scaphoid of wrist (S62.0-)

- S62.10 Fracture of **unspecified** carpal bone
  Fracture of wrist NOS
  - S62.101 Fracture of unspecified carpal bone, **right** wrist
  - S62.102 Fracture of unspecified carpal bone, **left** wrist
    Coding Clinic: 2012, Q4, P95
  - S62.109 Fracture of unspecified carpal bone, **unspecified** wrist
- S62.11 Fracture of **triquetrum** [cuneiform] bone of wrist
  - S62.111 **Displaced** fracture of triquetrum [cuneiform] bone, **right** wrist
  - S62.112 **Displaced** fracture of triquetrum [cuneiform] bone, **left** wrist
  - S62.113 **Displaced** fracture of triquetrum [cuneiform] bone, **unspecified** wrist
  - S62.114 **Nondisplaced** fracture of triquetrum [cuneiform] bone, **right** wrist
  - S62.115 **Nondisplaced** fracture of triquetrum [cuneiform] bone, **left** wrist
  - S62.116 **Nondisplaced** fracture of triquetrum [cuneiform] bone, **unspecified** wrist
- S62.12 Fracture of **lunate** [semilunar]
  - S62.121 **Displaced** fracture of lunate [semilunar], **right** wrist
  - S62.122 **Displaced** fracture of lunate [semilunar], **left** wrist
  - S62.123 **Displaced** fracture of lunate [semilunar], **unspecified** wrist
  - S62.124 **Nondisplaced** fracture of lunate [semilunar], **right** wrist
  - S62.125 **Nondisplaced** fracture of lunate [semilunar], **left** wrist
  - S62.126 **Nondisplaced** fracture of lunate [semilunar], **unspecified** wrist
- S62.13 Fracture of **capitate** [os magnum] bone
  - S62.131 **Displaced** fracture of capitate [os magnum] bone, **right** wrist
  - S62.132 **Displaced** fracture of capitate [os magnum] bone, **left** wrist
  - S62.133 **Displaced** fracture of capitate [os magnum] bone, **unspecified** wrist
  - S62.134 **Nondisplaced** fracture of capitate [os magnum] bone, **right** wrist
  - S62.135 **Nondisplaced** fracture of capitate [os magnum] bone, **left** wrist
  - S62.136 **Nondisplaced** fracture of capitate [os magnum] bone, **unspecified** wrist
- S62.14 Fracture of **body of hamate** [unciform] bone
  Fracture of hamate [unciform] bone NOS
  - S62.141 **Displaced** fracture of body of hamate [unciform] bone, **right** wrist
  - S62.142 **Displaced** fracture of body of hamate [unciform] bone, **left** wrist
  - S62.143 **Displaced** fracture of body of hamate [unciform] bone, **unspecified** wrist
  - S62.144 **Nondisplaced** fracture of body of hamate [unciform] bone, **right** wrist
  - S62.145 **Nondisplaced** fracture of body of hamate [unciform] bone, **left** wrist
  - S62.146 **Nondisplaced** fracture of body of hamate [unciform] bone, **unspecified** wrist
- S62.15 Fracture of **hook process of hamate** [unciform] bone
  Fracture of unciform process of hamate [unciform] bone
  - S62.151 **Displaced** fracture of hook process of hamate [unciform] bone, **right** wrist
  - S62.152 **Displaced** fracture of hook process of hamate [unciform] bone, **left** wrist
  - S62.153 **Displaced** fracture of hook process of hamate [unciform] bone, **unspecified** wrist
  - S62.154 **Nondisplaced** fracture of hook process of hamate [unciform] bone, **right** wrist
  - S62.155 **Nondisplaced** fracture of hook process of hamate [unciform] bone, **left** wrist
  - S62.156 **Nondisplaced** fracture of hook process of hamate [unciform] bone, **unspecified** wrist
- S62.16 Fracture of **pisiform**
  - S62.161 **Displaced** fracture of pisiform, **right** wrist
  - S62.162 **Displaced** fracture of pisiform, **left** wrist
  - S62.163 **Displaced** fracture of pisiform, **unspecified** wrist
  - S62.164 **Nondisplaced** fracture of pisiform, **right** wrist
  - S62.165 **Nondisplaced** fracture of pisiform, **left** wrist
  - S62.166 **Nondisplaced** fracture of pisiform, **unspecified** wrist

CHAPTER 19 (SØØ-T88)

- S62.17 Fracture of trapezium [larger multangular]
  - S62.171 Displaced fracture of trapezium [larger multangular], right wrist
  - S62.172 Displaced fracture of trapezium [larger multangular], left wrist
  - S62.173 Displaced fracture of trapezium [larger multangular], unspecified wrist
  - S62.174 Nondisplaced fracture of trapezium [larger multangular], right wrist
  - S62.175 Nondisplaced fracture of trapezium [larger multangular], left wrist
  - S62.176 Nondisplaced fracture of trapezium [larger multangular], unspecified wrist
- S62.18 Fracture of trapezoid [smaller multangular]
  - S62.181 Displaced fracture of trapezoid [smaller multangular], right wrist
  - S62.182 Displaced fracture of trapezoid [smaller multangular], left wrist
  - S62.183 Displaced fracture of trapezoid [smaller multangular], unspecified wrist
  - S62.184 Nondisplaced fracture of trapezoid [smaller multangular], right wrist
  - S62.185 Nondisplaced fracture of trapezoid [smaller multangular], left wrist
  - S62.186 Nondisplaced fracture of trapezoid [smaller multangular], unspecified wrist

S62.2 Fracture of first metacarpal bone

- S62.2Ø Unspecified fracture of first metacarpal bone
  - S62.2Ø1 Unspecified fracture of first metacarpal bone, right hand
  - S62.2Ø2 Unspecified fracture of first metacarpal bone, left hand
  - S62.2Ø9 Unspecified fracture of first metacarpal bone, unspecified hand
- S62.21 Bennett's fracture
  - S62.211 Bennett's fracture, right hand
  - S62.212 Bennett's fracture, left hand
  - S62.213 Bennett's fracture, unspecified hand
- S62.22 Rolando's fracture
  - S62.221 Displaced Rolando's fracture, right hand
  - S62.222 Displaced Rolando's fracture, left hand
  - S62.223 Displaced Rolando's fracture, unspecified hand
  - S62.224 Nondisplaced Rolando's fracture, right hand
  - S62.225 Nondisplaced Rolando's fracture, left hand
  - S62.226 Nondisplaced Rolando's fracture, unspecified hand
- S62.23 Other fracture of base of first metacarpal bone
  - S62.231 Other displaced fracture of base of first metacarpal bone, right hand
  - S62.232 Other displaced fracture of base of first metacarpal bone, left hand
  - S62.233 Other displaced fracture of base of first metacarpal bone, unspecified hand
  - S62.234 Other nondisplaced fracture of base of first metacarpal bone, right hand
  - S62.235 Other nondisplaced fracture of base of first metacarpal bone, left hand
  - S62.236 Other nondisplaced fracture of base of first metacarpal bone, unspecified hand
- S62.24 Fracture of shaft of first metacarpal bone
  - S62.241 Displaced fracture of shaft of first metacarpal bone, right hand
  - S62.242 Displaced fracture of shaft of first metacarpal bone, left hand
  - S62.243 Displaced fracture of shaft of first metacarpal bone, unspecified hand
  - S62.244 Nondisplaced fracture of shaft of first metacarpal bone, right hand
  - S62.245 Nondisplaced fracture of shaft of first metacarpal bone, left hand
  - S62.246 Nondisplaced fracture of shaft of first metacarpal bone, unspecified hand
- S62.25 Fracture of neck of first metacarpal bone
  - S62.251 Displaced fracture of neck of first metacarpal bone, right hand
  - S62.252 Displaced fracture of neck of first metacarpal bone, left hand
  - S62.253 Displaced fracture of neck of first metacarpal bone, unspecified hand
  - S62.254 Nondisplaced fracture of neck of first metacarpal bone, right hand
  - S62.255 Nondisplaced fracture of neck of first metacarpal bone, left hand
  - S62.256 Nondisplaced fracture of neck of first metacarpal bone, unspecified hand
- S62.29 Other fracture of first metacarpal bone
  - S62.291 Other fracture of first metacarpal bone, right hand
  - S62.292 Other fracture of first metacarpal bone, left hand
  - S62.299 Other fracture of first metacarpal bone, unspecified hand

S62.3 Fracture of other and unspecified metacarpal bone

Excludes2 fracture of first metacarpal bone (S62.2-)

- S62.3Ø Unspecified fracture of other metacarpal bone
  - S62.3ØØ Unspecified fracture of second metacarpal bone, right hand
  - S62.3Ø1 Unspecified fracture of second metacarpal bone, left hand
  - S62.3Ø2 Unspecified fracture of third metacarpal bone, right hand
  - S62.3Ø3 Unspecified fracture of third metacarpal bone, left hand
  - S62.3Ø4 Unspecified fracture of fourth metacarpal bone, right hand
  - S62.3Ø5 Unspecified fracture of fourth metacarpal bone, left hand
  - S62.3Ø6 Unspecified fracture of fifth metacarpal bone, right hand
  - S62.3Ø7 Unspecified fracture of fifth metacarpal bone, left hand
  - S62.3Ø8 Unspecified fracture of other metacarpal bone
    - Unspecified fracture of specified metacarpal bone with unspecified laterality
  - S62.3Ø9 Unspecified fracture of unspecified metacarpal bone
- S62.31 Displaced fracture of base of other metacarpal bone
  - S62.31Ø Displaced fracture of base of second metacarpal bone, right hand
  - S62.311 Displaced fracture of base of second metacarpal bone, left hand
  - S62.312 Displaced fracture of base of third metacarpal bone, right hand
  - S62.313 Displaced fracture of base of third metacarpal bone, left hand

S62.314 Displaced fracture of base of fourth metacarpal bone, right hand

S62.315 Displaced fracture of base of fourth metacarpal bone, left hand

S62.316 Displaced fracture of base of fifth metacarpal bone, right hand

S62.317 Displaced fracture of base of fifth metacarpal bone, left hand

S62.318 Displaced fracture of base of other metacarpal bone
Displaced fracture of base of specified metacarpal bone with unspecified laterality

S62.319 Displaced fracture of base of unspecified metacarpal bone

S62.32 Displaced fracture of shaft of other metacarpal bone

S62.320 Displaced fracture of shaft of second metacarpal bone, right hand

S62.321 Displaced fracture of shaft of second metacarpal bone, left hand

S62.322 Displaced fracture of shaft of third metacarpal bone, right hand

S62.323 Displaced fracture of shaft of third metacarpal bone, left hand

S62.324 Displaced fracture of shaft of fourth metacarpal bone, right hand

S62.325 Displaced fracture of shaft of fourth metacarpal bone, left hand

S62.326 Displaced fracture of shaft of fifth metacarpal bone, right hand

S62.327 Displaced fracture of shaft of fifth metacarpal bone, left hand

S62.328 Displaced fracture of shaft of other metacarpal bone
Displaced fracture of shaft of specified metacarpal bone with unspecified laterality

S62.329 Displaced fracture of shaft of unspecified metacarpal bone

S62.33 Displaced fracture of neck of other metacarpal bone

S62.330 Displaced fracture of neck of second metacarpal bone, right hand

S62.331 Displaced fracture of neck of second metacarpal bone, left hand

S62.332 Displaced fracture of neck of third metacarpal bone, right hand

S62.333 Displaced fracture of neck of third metacarpal bone, left hand

S62.334 Displaced fracture of neck of fourth metacarpal bone, right hand

S62.335 Displaced fracture of neck of fourth metacarpal bone, left hand

S62.336 Displaced fracture of neck of fifth metacarpal bone, right hand

S62.337 Displaced fracture of neck of fifth metacarpal bone, left hand

S62.338 Displaced fracture of neck of other metacarpal bone
Displaced fracture of neck of specified metacarpal bone with unspecified laterality

S62.339 Displaced fracture of neck of unspecified metacarpal bone

S62.34 Nondisplaced fracture of base of other metacarpal bone

S62.340 Nondisplaced fracture of base of second metacarpal bone, right hand

S62.341 Nondisplaced fracture of base of second metacarpal bone, left hand

S62.342 Nondisplaced fracture of base of third metacarpal bone, right hand

S62.343 Nondisplaced fracture of base of third metacarpal bone, left hand

S62.344 Nondisplaced fracture of base of fourth metacarpal bone, right hand

S62.345 Nondisplaced fracture of base of fourth metacarpal bone, left hand

S62.346 Nondisplaced fracture of base of fifth metacarpal bone, right hand

S62.347 Nondisplaced fracture of base of fifth metacarpal bone, left hand

S62.348 Nondisplaced fracture of base of other metacarpal bone
Nondisplaced fracture of base of specified metacarpal bone with unspecified laterality

S62.349 Nondisplaced fracture of base of unspecified metacarpal bone

S62.35 Nondisplaced fracture of shaft of other metacarpal bone

S62.350 Nondisplaced fracture of shaft of second metacarpal bone, right hand

S62.351 Nondisplaced fracture of shaft of second metacarpal bone, left hand

S62.352 Nondisplaced fracture of shaft of third metacarpal bone, right hand

S62.353 Nondisplaced fracture of shaft of third metacarpal bone, left hand

S62.354 Nondisplaced fracture of shaft of fourth metacarpal bone, right hand

S62.355 Nondisplaced fracture of shaft of fourth metacarpal bone, left hand

S62.356 Nondisplaced fracture of shaft of fifth metacarpal bone, right hand

S62.357 Nondisplaced fracture of shaft of fifth metacarpal bone, left hand

S62.358 Nondisplaced fracture of shaft of other metacarpal bone
Nondisplaced fracture of shaft of specified metacarpal bone with unspecified laterality

S62.359 Nondisplaced fracture of shaft of unspecified metacarpal bone

S62.36 Nondisplaced fracture of neck of other metacarpal bone

S62.360 Nondisplaced fracture of neck of second metacarpal bone, right hand

S62.361 Nondisplaced fracture of neck of second metacarpal bone, left hand

S62.362 Nondisplaced fracture of neck of third metacarpal bone, right hand

S62.363 Nondisplaced fracture of neck of third metacarpal bone, left hand

S62.364 Nondisplaced fracture of neck of fourth metacarpal bone, right hand

S62.365 Nondisplaced fracture of neck of fourth metacarpal bone, left hand

S62.366 Nondisplaced fracture of neck of fifth metacarpal bone, right hand

S62.367 Nondisplaced fracture of neck of fifth metacarpal bone, left hand

S62.368 Nondisplaced fracture of neck of other metacarpal bone
Nondisplaced fracture of neck of specified metacarpal bone with unspecified laterality

S62.369 Nondisplaced fracture of neck of unspecified metacarpal bone

S62.39 Other fracture of other metacarpal bone
- S62.390 Other fracture of second metacarpal bone, right hand
- S62.391 Other fracture of second metacarpal bone, left hand
- S62.392 Other fracture of third metacarpal bone, right hand
- S62.393 Other fracture of third metacarpal bone, left hand
- S62.394 Other fracture of fourth metacarpal bone, right hand
- S62.395 Other fracture of fourth metacarpal bone, left hand
- S62.396 Other fracture of fifth metacarpal bone, right hand
- S62.397 Other fracture of fifth metacarpal bone, left hand
- S62.398 Other fracture of other metacarpal bone
  Other fracture of specified metacarpal bone with unspecified laterality
- S62.399 Other fracture of unspecified metacarpal bone

S62.5 Fracture of thumb

S62.50 Fracture of unspecified phalanx of thumb
- S62.501 Fracture of unspecified phalanx of right thumb
- S62.502 Fracture of unspecified phalanx of left thumb
- S62.509 Fracture of unspecified phalanx of unspecified thumb

S62.51 Fracture of proximal phalanx of thumb
- S62.511 Displaced fracture of proximal phalanx of right thumb
- S62.512 Displaced fracture of proximal phalanx of left thumb
- S62.513 Displaced fracture of proximal phalanx of unspecified thumb
- S62.514 Nondisplaced fracture of proximal phalanx of right thumb
- S62.515 Nondisplaced fracture of proximal phalanx of left thumb
- S62.516 Nondisplaced fracture of proximal phalanx of unspecified thumb

S62.52 Fracture of distal phalanx of thumb
- S62.521 Displaced fracture of distal phalanx of right thumb
- S62.522 Displaced fracture of distal phalanx of left thumb
- S62.523 Displaced fracture of distal phalanx of unspecified thumb
- S62.524 Nondisplaced fracture of distal phalanx of right thumb
- S62.525 Nondisplaced fracture of distal phalanx of left thumb
- S62.526 Nondisplaced fracture of distal phalanx of unspecified thumb

S62.6 Fracture of other and unspecified finger(s)

Excludes2 fracture of thumb (S62.5-)

S62.60 Fracture of unspecified phalanx of finger
- S62.600 Fracture of unspecified phalanx of right index finger
- S62.601 Fracture of unspecified phalanx of left index finger
- S62.602 Fracture of unspecified phalanx of right middle finger
- S62.603 Fracture of unspecified phalanx of left middle finger
- S62.604 Fracture of unspecified phalanx of right ring finger
- S62.605 Fracture of unspecified phalanx of left ring finger
- S62.606 Fracture of unspecified phalanx of right little finger
- S62.607 Fracture of unspecified phalanx of left little finger
- S62.608 Fracture of unspecified phalanx of other finger
  Fracture of unspecified phalanx of specified finger with unspecified laterality
- S62.609 Fracture of unspecified phalanx of unspecified finger

S62.61 Displaced fracture of proximal phalanx of finger
- S62.610 Displaced fracture of proximal phalanx of right index finger
- S62.611 Displaced fracture of proximal phalanx of left index finger
- S62.612 Displaced fracture of proximal phalanx of right middle finger
- S62.613 Displaced fracture of proximal phalanx of left middle finger
- S62.614 Displaced fracture of proximal phalanx of right ring finger
- S62.615 Displaced fracture of proximal phalanx of left ring finger
- S62.616 Displaced fracture of proximal phalanx of right little finger
- S62.617 Displaced fracture of proximal phalanx of left little finger
- S62.618 Displaced fracture of proximal phalanx of other finger
  Displaced fracture of proximal phalanx of specified finger with unspecified laterality
- S62.619 Displaced fracture of proximal phalanx of unspecified finger

S62.62 Displaced fracture of middle phalanx of finger
- S62.620 Displaced fracture of middle phalanx of right index finger
- S62.621 Displaced fracture of middle phalanx of left index finger
- S62.622 Displaced fracture of middle phalanx of right middle finger
- S62.623 Displaced fracture of middle phalanx of left middle finger
- S62.624 Displaced fracture of middle phalanx of right ring finger
- S62.625 Displaced fracture of middle phalanx of left ring finger
- S62.626 Displaced fracture of middle phalanx of right little finger
- S62.627 Displaced fracture of middle phalanx of left little finger
- S62.628 Displaced fracture of middle phalanx of other finger
  Displaced fracture of middle phalanx of specified finger with unspecified laterality
- S62.629 Displaced fracture of middle phalanx of unspecified finger

● S62.63 Displaced fracture of distal phalanx of finger
● S62.630 Displaced fracture of distal phalanx of right index finger
● S62.631 Displaced fracture of distal phalanx of left index finger
● S62.632 Displaced fracture of distal phalanx of right middle finger
● S62.633 Displaced fracture of distal phalanx of left middle finger
● S62.634 Displaced fracture of distal phalanx of right ring finger
● S62.635 Displaced fracture of distal phalanx of left ring finger
● S62.636 Displaced fracture of distal phalanx of right little finger
● S62.637 Displaced fracture of distal phalanx of left little finger
● S62.638 Displaced fracture of distal phalanx of other finger
Displaced fracture of distal phalanx of specified finger with unspecified laterality
● S62.639 Displaced fracture of distal phalanx of unspecified finger
● S62.64 Nondisplaced fracture of proximal phalanx of finger
● S62.640 Nondisplaced fracture of proximal phalanx of right index finger
● S62.641 Nondisplaced fracture of proximal phalanx of left index finger
● S62.642 Nondisplaced fracture of proximal phalanx of right middle finger
● S62.643 Nondisplaced fracture of proximal phalanx of left middle finger
● S62.644 Nondisplaced fracture of proximal phalanx of right ring finger
● S62.645 Nondisplaced fracture of proximal phalanx of left ring finger
● S62.646 Nondisplaced fracture of proximal phalanx of right little finger
● S62.647 Nondisplaced fracture of proximal phalanx of left little finger
● S62.648 Nondisplaced fracture of proximal phalanx of other finger
Nondisplaced fracture of proximal phalanx of specified finger with unspecified laterality
● S62.649 Nondisplaced fracture of proximal phalanx of unspecified finger
● S62.65 Nondisplaced fracture of middle phalanx of finger
● S62.650 Nondisplaced fracture of middle phalanx of right index finger
● S62.651 Nondisplaced fracture of middle phalanx of left index finger
● S62.652 Nondisplaced fracture of middle phalanx of right middle finger
● S62.653 Nondisplaced fracture of middle phalanx of left middle finger
● S62.654 Nondisplaced fracture of middle phalanx of right ring finger
● S62.655 Nondisplaced fracture of middle phalanx of left ring finger
● S62.656 Nondisplaced fracture of middle phalanx of right little finger

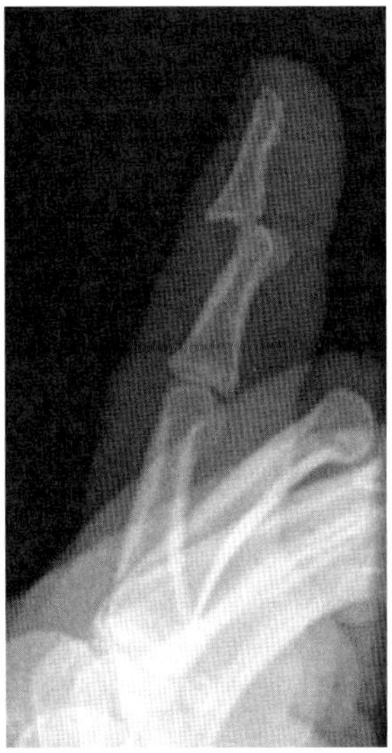

Figure 19-14 Dorsal dislocation of the distal phalanx of the index finger. (From Hardy M, Snaith B: Musculoskeletal Trauma: A Guide to Assessment and Diagnosis, 1e, Elsevier, 2011)

● S62.657 Nondisplaced fracture of middle phalanx of left little finger
● S62.658 Nondisplaced fracture of middle phalanx of other finger
Nondisplaced fracture of middle phalanx of specified finger with unspecified laterality
● S62.659 Nondisplaced fracture of middle phalanx of unspecified finger
● S62.66 Nondisplaced fracture of distal phalanx of finger
● S62.660 Nondisplaced fracture of distal phalanx of right index finger
● S62.661 Nondisplaced fracture of distal phalanx of left index finger
● S62.662 Nondisplaced fracture of distal phalanx of right middle finger
● S62.663 Nondisplaced fracture of distal phalanx of left middle finger
● S62.664 Nondisplaced fracture of distal phalanx of right ring finger
● S62.665 Nondisplaced fracture of distal phalanx of left ring finger
● S62.666 Nondisplaced fracture of distal phalanx of right little finger
● S62.667 Nondisplaced fracture of distal phalanx of left little finger
● S62.668 Nondisplaced fracture of distal phalanx of other finger
Nondisplaced fracture of distal phalanx of specified finger with unspecified laterality
● S62.669 Nondisplaced fracture of distal phalanx of unspecified finger
● S62.9 Unspecified fracture of wrist and hand
X● S62.90 Unspecified fracture of unspecified wrist and hand
X● S62.91 Unspecified fracture of right wrist and hand
X● S62.92 Unspecified fracture of left wrist and hand

S63 Dislocation and sprain of joints and ligaments at wrist and hand level

Includes avulsion of joint or ligament at wrist and hand level
laceration of cartilage, joint or ligament at wrist and hand level
sprain of cartilage, joint or ligament at wrist and hand level
traumatic hemarthrosis of joint or ligament at wrist and hand level
traumatic rupture of joint or ligament at wrist and hand level
traumatic subluxation of joint or ligament at wrist and hand level
traumatic tear of joint or ligament at wrist and hand level

Code also any associated open wound

Excludes2 strain of muscle, fascia and tendon of wrist and hand (S66.-)

The appropriate 7th character is to be added to each code from category S63

A	initial encounter
D	subsequent encounter
S	sequela

S63.Ø Subluxation and dislocation of wrist and hand joints

- **S63.ØØ Unspecified subluxation and dislocation of wrist and hand**
  Dislocation of carpal bone NOS
  Dislocation of distal end of radius NOS
  Subluxation of carpal bone NOS
  Subluxation of distal end of radius NOS
  - S63.ØØ1 Unspecified subluxation of right wrist and hand
  - S63.ØØ2 Unspecified subluxation of left wrist and hand
  - S63.ØØ3 Unspecified subluxation of unspecified wrist and hand
  - S63.ØØ4 Unspecified dislocation of right wrist and hand
  - S63.ØØ5 Unspecified dislocation of left wrist and hand
  - S63.ØØ6 Unspecified dislocation of unspecified wrist and hand
- **S63.Ø1 Subluxation and dislocation of distal radioulnar joint**
  - S63.Ø11 Subluxation of distal radioulnar joint of right wrist
  - S63.Ø12 Subluxation of distal radioulnar joint of left wrist
  - S63.Ø13 Subluxation of distal radioulnar joint of unspecified wrist
  - S63.Ø14 Dislocation of distal radioulnar joint of right wrist
  - S63.Ø15 Dislocation of distal radioulnar joint of left wrist
  - S63.Ø16 Dislocation of distal radioulnar joint of unspecified wrist
- **S63.Ø2 Subluxation and dislocation of radiocarpal joint**
  - S63.Ø21 Subluxation of radiocarpal joint of right wrist
  - S63.Ø22 Subluxation of radiocarpal joint of left wrist
  - S63.Ø23 Subluxation of radiocarpal joint of unspecified wrist
  - S63.Ø24 Dislocation of radiocarpal joint of right wrist
  - S63.Ø25 Dislocation of radiocarpal joint of left wrist
  - S63.Ø26 Dislocation of radiocarpal joint of unspecified wrist
- **S63.Ø3 Subluxation and dislocation of midcarpal joint**
  - S63.Ø31 Subluxation of midcarpal joint of right wrist
  - S63.Ø32 Subluxation of midcarpal joint of left wrist
  - S63.Ø33 Subluxation of midcarpal joint of unspecified wrist
  - S63.Ø34 Dislocation of midcarpal joint of right wrist
  - S63.Ø35 Dislocation of midcarpal joint of left wrist
  - S63.Ø36 Dislocation of midcarpal joint of unspecified wrist
- **S63.Ø4 Subluxation and dislocation of carpometacarpal joint of thumb**
  Excludes2 interphalangeal subluxation and dislocation of thumb (S63.1-)
  - S63.Ø41 Subluxation of carpometacarpal joint of right thumb
  - S63.Ø42 Subluxation of carpometacarpal joint of left thumb
  - S63.Ø43 Subluxation of carpometacarpal joint of unspecified thumb
  - S63.Ø44 Dislocation of carpometacarpal joint of right thumb
  - S63.Ø45 Dislocation of carpometacarpal joint of left thumb
  - S63.Ø46 Dislocation of carpometacarpal joint of unspecified thumb
- **S63.Ø5 Subluxation and dislocation of other carpometacarpal joint**
  Excludes2 subluxation and dislocation of carpometacarpal joint of thumb (S63.Ø4-)
  - S63.Ø51 Subluxation of other carpometacarpal joint of right hand
  - S63.Ø52 Subluxation of other carpometacarpal joint of left hand
  - S63.Ø53 Subluxation of other carpometacarpal joint of unspecified hand
  - S63.Ø54 Dislocation of other carpometacarpal joint of right hand
  - S63.Ø55 Dislocation of other carpometacarpal joint of left hand
  - S63.Ø56 Dislocation of other carpometacarpal joint of unspecified hand
- **S63.Ø6 Subluxation and dislocation of metacarpal (bone), proximal end**
  - S63.Ø61 Subluxation of metacarpal (bone), proximal end of right hand
  - S63.Ø62 Subluxation of metacarpal (bone), proximal end of left hand
  - S63.Ø63 Subluxation of metacarpal (bone), proximal end of unspecified hand
  - S63.Ø64 Dislocation of metacarpal (bone), proximal end of right hand
  - S63.Ø65 Dislocation of metacarpal (bone), proximal end of left hand
  - S63.Ø66 Dislocation of metacarpal (bone), proximal end of unspecified hand
- **S63.Ø7 Subluxation and dislocation of distal end of ulna**
  - S63.Ø71 Subluxation of distal end of right ulna
  - S63.Ø72 Subluxation of distal end of left ulna
  - S63.Ø73 Subluxation of distal end of unspecified ulna
  - S63.Ø74 Dislocation of distal end of right ulna
  - S63.Ø75 Dislocation of distal end of left ulna
  - S63.Ø76 Dislocation of distal end of unspecified ulna

- S63.09 Other subluxation and dislocation of wrist and hand
  - S63.091 Other subluxation of right wrist and hand
  - S63.092 Other subluxation of left wrist and hand
  - S63.093 Other subluxation of unspecified wrist and hand
  - S63.094 Other dislocation of right wrist and hand
  - S63.095 Other dislocation of left wrist and hand
  - S63.096 Other dislocation of unspecified wrist and hand

S63.1 Subluxation and dislocation of thumb

- S63.10 Unspecified subluxation and dislocation of thumb
  - S63.101 Unspecified subluxation of right thumb
  - S63.102 Unspecified subluxation of left thumb
  - S63.103 Unspecified subluxation of unspecified thumb
  - S63.104 Unspecified dislocation of right thumb
  - S63.105 Unspecified dislocation of left thumb
  - S63.106 Unspecified dislocation of unspecified thumb
- S63.11 Subluxation and dislocation of metacarpophalangeal joint of thumb
  - S63.111 Subluxation of metacarpophalangeal joint of right thumb
  - S63.112 Subluxation of metacarpophalangeal joint of left thumb
  - S63.113 Subluxation of metacarpophalangeal joint of unspecified thumb
  - S63.114 Dislocation of metacarpophalangeal joint of right thumb
  - S63.115 Dislocation of metacarpophalangeal joint of left thumb
  - S63.116 Dislocation of metacarpophalangeal joint of unspecified thumb
- S63.12 Subluxation and dislocation of interphalangeal joint of thumb
  - S63.121 Subluxation of interphalangeal joint of right thumb
  - S63.122 Subluxation of interphalangeal joint of left thumb
  - S63.123 Subluxation of interphalangeal joint of unspecified thumb
  - S63.124 Dislocation of interphalangeal joint of right thumb
  - S63.125 Dislocation of interphalangeal joint of left thumb
  - S63.126 Dislocation of interphalangeal joint of unspecified thumb

S63.2 Subluxation and dislocation of other finger(s)

Excludes2 subluxation and dislocation of thumb (S63.1-)

- S63.20 Unspecified subluxation of other finger
  - S63.200 Unspecified subluxation of right index finger
  - S63.201 Unspecified subluxation of left index finger
  - S63.202 Unspecified subluxation of right middle finger
  - S63.203 Unspecified subluxation of left middle finger
  - S63.204 Unspecified subluxation of right ring finger
  - S63.205 Unspecified subluxation of left ring finger
  - S63.206 Unspecified subluxation of right little finger
  - S63.207 Unspecified subluxation of left little finger
  - S63.208 Unspecified subluxation of other finger
    Unspecified subluxation of specified finger with unspecified laterality
  - S63.209 Unspecified subluxation of unspecified finger
- S63.21 Subluxation of metacarpophalangeal joint of finger
  - S63.210 Subluxation of metacarpophalangeal joint of right index finger
  - S63.211 Subluxation of metacarpophalangeal joint of left index finger
  - S63.212 Subluxation of metacarpophalangeal joint of right middle finger
  - S63.213 Subluxation of metacarpophalangeal joint of left middle finger
  - S63.214 Subluxation of metacarpophalangeal joint of right ring finger
  - S63.215 Subluxation of metacarpophalangeal joint of left ring finger
  - S63.216 Subluxation of metacarpophalangeal joint of right little finger
  - S63.217 Subluxation of metacarpophalangeal joint of left little finger
  - S63.218 Subluxation of metacarpophalangeal joint of other finger
    Subluxation of metacarpophalangeal joint of specified finger with unspecified laterality
  - S63.219 Subluxation of metacarpophalangeal joint of unspecified finger
- S63.22 Subluxation of unspecified interphalangeal joint of finger
  - S63.220 Subluxation of unspecified interphalangeal joint of right index finger
  - S63.221 Subluxation of unspecified interphalangeal joint of left index finger
  - S63.222 Subluxation of unspecified interphalangeal joint of right middle finger
  - S63.223 Subluxation of unspecified interphalangeal joint of left middle finger
  - S63.224 Subluxation of unspecified interphalangeal joint of right ring finger
  - S63.225 Subluxation of unspecified interphalangeal joint of left ring finger
  - S63.226 Subluxation of unspecified interphalangeal joint of right little finger
  - S63.227 Subluxation of unspecified interphalangeal joint of left little finger
  - S63.228 Subluxation of unspecified interphalangeal joint of other finger
    Subluxation of unspecified interphalangeal joint of specified finger with unspecified laterality
  - S63.229 Subluxation of unspecified interphalangeal joint of unspecified finger

S63.23 **Subluxation of proximal interphalangeal joint of finger**

S63.230 Subluxation of proximal interphalangeal joint of **right index** finger

S63.231 Subluxation of proximal interphalangeal joint of **left index** finger

S63.232 Subluxation of proximal interphalangeal joint of **right middle** finger

S63.233 Subluxation of proximal interphalangeal joint of **left middle** finger

S63.234 Subluxation of proximal interphalangeal joint of **right ring** finger

S63.235 Subluxation of proximal interphalangeal joint of **left ring** finger

S63.236 Subluxation of proximal interphalangeal joint of **right little** finger

S63.237 Subluxation of proximal interphalangeal joint of **left little** finger

S63.238 Subluxation of proximal interphalangeal joint of **other** finger
Subluxation of proximal interphalangeal joint of specified finger with unspecified laterality

S63.239 Subluxation of proximal interphalangeal joint of **unspecified** finger

S63.24 **Subluxation of distal interphalangeal joint of finger**

S63.240 Subluxation of distal interphalangeal joint of **right index** finger

S63.241 Subluxation of distal interphalangeal joint of **left index** finger

S63.242 Subluxation of distal interphalangeal joint of **right middle** finger

S63.243 Subluxation of distal interphalangeal joint of **left middle** finger

S63.244 Subluxation of distal interphalangeal joint of **right ring** finger

S63.245 Subluxation of distal interphalangeal joint of **left ring** finger

S63.246 Subluxation of distal interphalangeal joint of **right little** finger

S63.247 Subluxation of distal interphalangeal joint of **left little** finger

S63.248 Subluxation of distal interphalangeal joint of **other** finger
Subluxation of distal interphalangeal joint of specified finger with unspecified laterality

S63.249 Subluxation of distal interphalangeal joint of **unspecified** finger

S63.25 **Unspecified dislocation of other finger**

S63.250 Unspecified dislocation of **right index** finger

S63.251 Unspecified dislocation of **left index** finger

S63.252 Unspecified dislocation of **right middle** finger

S63.253 Unspecified dislocation of **left middle** finger

S63.254 Unspecified dislocation of **right ring** finger

S63.255 Unspecified dislocation of **left ring** finger

S63.256 Unspecified dislocation of **right little** finger

S63.257 Unspecified dislocation of **left little** finger

S63.258 Unspecified dislocation of **other** finger
Unspecified dislocation of specified finger with unspecified laterality

S63.259 Unspecified dislocation of **unspecified** finger
Unspecified dislocation of unspecified finger with unspecified laterality

S63.26 **Dislocation of metacarpophalangeal joint of finger**

S63.260 Dislocation of metacarpophalangeal joint of **right index** finger

S63.261 Dislocation of metacarpophalangeal joint of **left index** finger

S63.262 Dislocation of metacarpophalangeal joint of **right middle** finger

S63.263 Dislocation of metacarpophalangeal joint of **left middle** finger

S63.264 Dislocation of metacarpophalangeal joint of **right ring** finger

S63.265 Dislocation of metacarpophalangeal joint of **left ring** finger

S63.266 Dislocation of metacarpophalangeal joint of **right little** finger

S63.267 Dislocation of metacarpophalangeal joint of **left little** finger

S63.268 Dislocation of metacarpophalangeal joint of **other** finger
Dislocation of metacarpophalangeal joint of specified finger with unspecified laterality

S63.269 Dislocation of metacarpophalangeal joint of **unspecified** finger

S63.27 **Dislocation of unspecified interphalangeal joint of finger**

S63.270 Dislocation of unspecified interphalangeal joint of **right index** finger

S63.271 Dislocation of unspecified interphalangeal joint of **left index** finger

S63.272 Dislocation of unspecified interphalangeal joint of **right middle** finger

- S63.273 Dislocation of unspecified interphalangeal joint of **left middle** finger
- S63.274 Dislocation of unspecified interphalangeal joint of **right ring** finger
- S63.275 Dislocation of unspecified interphalangeal joint of **left ring** finger
- S63.276 Dislocation of unspecified interphalangeal joint of **right little** finger
- S63.277 Dislocation of unspecified interphalangeal joint of **left little** finger
- S63.278 Dislocation of unspecified interphalangeal joint of **other** finger
  Dislocation of unspecified interphalangeal joint of specified finger with unspecified laterality
- S63.279 Dislocation of unspecified interphalangeal joint of **unspecified** finger
  Dislocation of unspecified interphalangeal joint of unspecified finger without specified laterality

S63.28 **Dislocation of proximal interphalangeal** joint of finger
- S63.280 Dislocation of proximal interphalangeal joint of **right index** finger
- S63.281 Dislocation of proximal interphalangeal joint of **left index** finger
- S63.282 Dislocation of proximal interphalangeal joint of **right middle** finger
- S63.283 Dislocation of proximal interphalangeal joint of **left middle** finger
- S63.284 Dislocation of proximal interphalangeal joint of **right ring** finger
- S63.285 Dislocation of proximal interphalangeal joint of **left ring** finger
- S63.286 Dislocation of proximal interphalangeal joint of **right little** finger
- S63.287 Dislocation of proximal interphalangeal joint of **left little** finger
- S63.288 Dislocation of proximal interphalangeal joint of **other** finger
  Dislocation of proximal interphalangeal joint of specified finger with unspecified laterality
- S63.289 Dislocation of proximal interphalangeal joint of **unspecified** finger

S63.29 **Dislocation** of **distal interphalangeal** joint of finger
- S63.290 Dislocation of distal interphalangeal joint of **right index** finger
- S63.291 Dislocation of distal interphalangeal joint of **left index** finger
- S63.292 Dislocation of distal interphalangeal joint of **right middle** finger
- S63.293 Dislocation of distal interphalangeal joint of **left middle** finger
- S63.294 Dislocation of distal interphalangeal joint of **right ring** finger
- S63.295 Dislocation of distal interphalangeal joint of **left ring** finger
- S63.296 Dislocation of distal interphalangeal joint of **right little** finger
- S63.297 Dislocation of distal interphalangeal joint of **left little** finger
- S63.298 Dislocation of distal interphalangeal joint of **other** finger
  Dislocation of distal interphalangeal joint of specified finger with unspecified laterality
- S63.299 Dislocation of distal interphalangeal joint of **unspecified** finger

S63.3 Traumatic rupture of **ligament of wrist**

S63.30 Traumatic rupture of **unspecified** ligament of wrist
- S63.301 Traumatic rupture of unspecified ligament of **right** wrist
- S63.302 Traumatic rupture of unspecified ligament of **left** wrist
- S63.309 Traumatic rupture of unspecified ligament of **unspecified** wrist

S63.31 Traumatic rupture of **collateral** ligament of wrist
- S63.311 Traumatic rupture of collateral ligament of **right** wrist
- S63.312 Traumatic rupture of collateral ligament of **left** wrist
- S63.319 Traumatic rupture of collateral ligament of **unspecified** wrist

S63.32 Traumatic rupture of **radiocarpal** ligament
- S63.321 Traumatic rupture of **right** radiocarpal ligament
- S63.322 Traumatic rupture of **left** radiocarpal ligament
- S63.329 Traumatic rupture of **unspecified** radiocarpal ligament

S63.33 Traumatic rupture of **ulnocarpal** (palmar) ligament
- S63.331 Traumatic rupture of **right** ulnocarpal (palmar) ligament
- S63.332 Traumatic rupture of **left** ulnocarpal (palmar) ligament
- S63.339 Traumatic rupture of **unspecified** ulnocarpal (palmar) ligament

S63.39 Traumatic rupture of **other** ligament of wrist
- S63.391 Traumatic rupture of other ligament of **right** wrist
- S63.392 Traumatic rupture of other ligament of **left** wrist
- S63.399 Traumatic rupture of other ligament of **unspecified** wrist

CHAPTER 19 (S00-T88)

● S63.4 Traumatic rupture of **ligament of finger at metacarpophalangeal and interphalangeal** joint(s)

● S63.4Ø Traumatic rupture of **unspecified** ligament of finger at metacarpophalangeal and interphalangeal joint

● S63.4ØØ Traumatic rupture of unspecified ligament of **right index** finger at metacarpophalangeal and interphalangeal joint

● S63.4Ø1 Traumatic rupture of unspecified ligament of **left index** finger at metacarpophalangeal and interphalangeal joint

● S63.4Ø2 Traumatic rupture of unspecified ligament of **right middle** finger at metacarpophalangeal and interphalangeal joint

● S63.4Ø3 Traumatic rupture of unspecified ligament of **left middle** finger at metacarpophalangeal and interphalangeal joint

● S63.4Ø4 Traumatic rupture of unspecified ligament of **right ring** finger at metacarpophalangeal and interphalangeal joint

● S63.4Ø5 Traumatic rupture of unspecified ligament of **left ring** finger at metacarpophalangeal and interphalangeal joint

● S63.4Ø6 Traumatic rupture of unspecified ligament of **right little** finger at metacarpophalangeal and interphalangeal joint

● S63.4Ø7 Traumatic rupture of unspecified ligament of **left little** finger at metacarpophalangeal and interphalangeal joint

● S63.4Ø8 Traumatic rupture of unspecified ligament of **other** finger at metacarpophalangeal and interphalangeal joint

Traumatic rupture of unspecified ligament of specified finger with unspecified laterality at metacarpophalangeal and interphalangeal joint

● S63.4Ø9 Traumatic rupture of unspecified ligament of **unspecified** finger at metacarpophalangeal and interphalangeal joint

● S63.41 Traumatic rupture of **collateral ligament** of finger at metacarpophalangeal and interphalangeal joint

● S63.41Ø Traumatic rupture of collateral ligament of **right index** finger at metacarpophalangeal and interphalangeal joint

● S63.411 Traumatic rupture of collateral ligament of **left index** finger at metacarpophalangeal and interphalangeal joint

● S63.412 Traumatic rupture of collateral ligament of **right middle** finger at metacarpophalangeal and interphalangeal joint

● S63.413 Traumatic rupture of collateral ligament of **left middle** finger at metacarpophalangeal and interphalangeal joint

● S63.414 Traumatic rupture of collateral ligament of **right ring** finger at metacarpophalangeal and interphalangeal joint

● S63.415 Traumatic rupture of collateral ligament of **left ring** finger at metacarpophalangeal and interphalangeal joint

● S63.416 Traumatic rupture of collateral ligament of **right little** finger at metacarpophalangeal and interphalangeal joint

● S63.417 Traumatic rupture of collateral ligament of **left little** finger at metacarpophalangeal and interphalangeal joint

● S63.418 Traumatic rupture of collateral ligament of **other** finger at metacarpophalangeal and interphalangeal joint

Traumatic rupture of collateral ligament of specified finger with unspecified laterality at metacarpophalangeal and interphalangeal joint

● S63.419 Traumatic rupture of collateral ligament of **unspecified** finger at metacarpophalangeal and interphalangeal joint

● S63.42 Traumatic rupture of **palmar ligament** of finger at metacarpophalangeal and interphalangeal joint

● S63.42Ø Traumatic rupture of palmar ligament of **right index** finger at metacarpophalangeal and interphalangeal joint

● S63.421 Traumatic rupture of palmar ligament of **left index** finger at metacarpophalangeal and interphalangeal joint

● S63.422 Traumatic rupture of palmar ligament of **right middle** finger at metacarpophalangeal and interphalangeal joint

● S63.423 Traumatic rupture of palmar ligament of **left middle** finger at metacarpophalangeal and interphalangeal joint

● S63.424 Traumatic rupture of palmar ligament of **right ring** finger at metacarpophalangeal and interphalangeal joint

● S63.425 Traumatic rupture of palmar ligament of **left ring** finger at metacarpophalangeal and interphalangeal joint

● S63.426 Traumatic rupture of palmar ligament of **right little** finger at metacarpophalangeal and interphalangeal joint

● S63.427 Traumatic rupture of palmar ligament of **left little** finger at metacarpophalangeal and interphalangeal joint

● S63.428 Traumatic rupture of palmar ligament of **other** finger at metacarpophalangeal and interphalangeal joint

Traumatic rupture of palmar ligament of specified finger with unspecified laterality at metacarpophalangeal and interphalangeal joint

● S63.429 Traumatic rupture of palmar ligament of **unspecified** finger at metacarpophalangeal and interphalangeal joint

- S63.43 Traumatic rupture of volar plate of finger at metacarpophalangeal and interphalangeal joint
  - S63.430 Traumatic rupture of volar plate of **right index** finger at metacarpophalangeal and interphalangeal joint
  - S63.431 Traumatic rupture of volar plate of **left index** finger at metacarpophalangeal and interphalangeal joint
  - S63.432 Traumatic rupture of volar plate of **right middle** finger at metacarpophalangeal and interphalangeal joint
  - S63.433 Traumatic rupture of volar plate of **left middle** finger at metacarpophalangeal and interphalangeal joint
  - S63.434 Traumatic rupture of volar plate of **right ring** finger at metacarpophalangeal and interphalangeal joint
  - S63.435 Traumatic rupture of volar plate of **left ring** finger at metacarpophalangeal and interphalangeal joint
  - S63.436 Traumatic rupture of volar plate of **right little** finger at metacarpophalangeal and interphalangeal joint
  - S63.437 Traumatic rupture of volar plate of **left little** finger at metacarpophalangeal and interphalangeal joint
  - S63.438 Traumatic rupture of volar plate of **other** finger at metacarpophalangeal and interphalangeal joint
    Traumatic rupture of volar plate of specified finger with unspecified laterality at metacarpophalangeal and interphalangeal joint
  - S63.439 Traumatic rupture of volar plate of **unspecified** finger at metacarpophalangeal and interphalangeal joint
- S63.49 Traumatic rupture of **other** ligament of finger at metacarpophalangeal and interphalangeal joint
  - S63.490 Traumatic rupture of other ligament of **right index** finger at metacarpophalangeal and interphalangeal joint
  - S63.491 Traumatic rupture of other ligament of **left index** finger at metacarpophalangeal and interphalangeal joint
  - S63.492 Traumatic rupture of other ligament of **right middle** finger at metacarpophalangeal and interphalangeal joint
  - S63.493 Traumatic rupture of other ligament of **left middle** finger at metacarpophalangeal and interphalangeal joint
  - S63.494 Traumatic rupture of other ligament of **right ring** finger at metacarpophalangeal and interphalangeal joint
  - S63.495 Traumatic rupture of other ligament of **left ring** finger at metacarpophalangeal and interphalangeal joint
  - S63.496 Traumatic rupture of other ligament of **right little** finger at metacarpophalangeal and interphalangeal joint
  - S63.497 Traumatic rupture of other ligament of **left little** finger at metacarpophalangeal and interphalangeal joint
  - S63.498 Traumatic rupture of other ligament of **other** finger at metacarpophalangeal and interphalangeal joint
    Traumatic rupture of ligament of specified finger with unspecified laterality at metacarpophalangeal and interphalangeal joint
  - S63.499 Traumatic rupture of other ligament of **unspecified** finger at metacarpophalangeal and interphalangeal joint

- S63.5 Other and unspecified sprain of **wrist**
  - S63.50 Unspecified sprain of wrist
    - S63.501 Unspecified sprain of **right** wrist
    - S63.502 Unspecified sprain of **left** wrist
    - S63.509 Unspecified sprain of **unspecified** wrist
  - S63.51 Sprain of **carpal** (joint)
    - S63.511 Sprain of carpal joint of **right** wrist
    - S63.512 Sprain of carpal joint of **left** wrist
    - S63.519 Sprain of carpal joint of **unspecified** wrist
  - S63.52 Sprain of **radiocarpal** joint
    Excludes1 traumatic rupture of radiocarpal ligament (S63.32-)
    - S63.521 Sprain of radiocarpal joint of **right** wrist
    - S63.522 Sprain of radiocarpal joint of **left** wrist
    - S63.529 Sprain of radiocarpal joint of **unspecified** wrist
  - S63.59 Other specified sprain of wrist
    - S63.591 Other specified sprain of **right** wrist
    - S63.592 Other specified sprain of **left** wrist
    - S63.599 Other specified sprain of **unspecified** wrist
- S63.6 Other and unspecified sprain of **finger(s)**
  Excludes1 traumatic rupture of ligament of finger at metacarpophalangeal and interphalangeal joint(s) (S63.4-)
  - S63.60 Unspecified sprain of thumb
    - S63.601 Unspecified sprain of **right** thumb
    - S63.602 Unspecified sprain of **left** thumb
    - S63.609 Unspecified sprain of **unspecified** thumb
  - S63.61 Unspecified sprain of other and unspecified finger(s)
    - S63.610 Unspecified sprain of **right index** finger
    - S63.611 Unspecified sprain of **left index** finger
    - S63.612 Unspecified sprain of **right middle** finger
    - S63.613 Unspecified sprain of **left middle** finger
    - S63.614 Unspecified sprain of **right ring** finger
    - S63.615 Unspecified sprain of **left ring** finger
    - S63.616 Unspecified sprain of **right little** finger
    - S63.617 Unspecified sprain of **left little** finger
    - S63.618 Unspecified sprain of **other** finger
      Unspecified sprain of specified finger with unspecified laterality
    - S63.619 Unspecified sprain of **unspecified** finger

S63.62 Sprain of interphalangeal joint of thumb
- S63.621 Sprain of interphalangeal joint of right thumb
- S63.622 Sprain of interphalangeal joint of left thumb
- S63.629 Sprain of interphalangeal joint of unspecified thumb

S63.63 Sprain of interphalangeal joint of other and unspecified finger(s)
- S63.630 Sprain of interphalangeal joint of right index finger
- S63.631 Sprain of interphalangeal joint of left index finger
- S63.632 Sprain of interphalangeal joint of right middle finger
- S63.633 Sprain of interphalangeal joint of left middle finger
- S63.634 Sprain of interphalangeal joint of right ring finger
- S63.635 Sprain of interphalangeal joint of left ring finger
- S63.636 Sprain of interphalangeal joint of right little finger
- S63.637 Sprain of interphalangeal joint of left little finger
- S63.638 Sprain of interphalangeal joint of other finger
- S63.639 Sprain of interphalangeal joint of unspecified finger

S63.64 Sprain of metacarpophalangeal joint of thumb
- S63.641 Sprain of metacarpophalangeal joint of right thumb
- S63.642 Sprain of metacarpophalangeal joint of left thumb
- S63.649 Sprain of metacarpophalangeal joint of unspecified thumb

S63.65 Sprain of metacarpophalangeal joint of other and unspecified finger(s)
- S63.650 Sprain of metacarpophalangeal joint of right index finger
- S63.651 Sprain of metacarpophalangeal joint of left index finger
- S63.652 Sprain of metacarpophalangeal joint of right middle finger
- S63.653 Sprain of metacarpophalangeal joint of left middle finger
- S63.654 Sprain of metacarpophalangeal joint of right ring finger
- S63.655 Sprain of metacarpophalangeal joint of left ring finger
- S63.656 Sprain of metacarpophalangeal joint of right little finger
- S63.657 Sprain of metacarpophalangeal joint of left little finger
- S63.658 Sprain of metacarpophalangeal joint of other finger
  - Sprain of metacarpophalangeal joint of specified finger with unspecified laterality
- S63.659 Sprain of metacarpophalangeal joint of unspecified finger

S63.68 Other sprain of thumb
- S63.681 Other sprain of right thumb
- S63.682 Other sprain of left thumb
- S63.689 Other sprain of unspecified thumb

S63.69 Other sprain of other and unspecified finger(s)
- S63.690 Other sprain of right index finger
- S63.691 Other sprain of left index finger
- S63.692 Other sprain of right middle finger
- S63.693 Other sprain of left middle finger
- S63.694 Other sprain of right ring finger
- S63.695 Other sprain of left ring finger
- S63.696 Other sprain of right little finger
- S63.697 Other sprain of left little finger
- S63.698 Other sprain of other finger
  - Other sprain of specified finger with unspecified laterality
- S63.699 Other sprain of unspecified finger

S63.8 Sprain of other part of wrist and hand
- S63.8X Sprain of other part of wrist and hand
  - S63.8X1 Sprain of other part of right wrist and hand
  - S63.8X2 Sprain of other part of left wrist and hand
  - S63.8X9 Sprain of other part of unspecified wrist and hand

S63.9 Sprain of unspecified part of wrist and hand
- X S63.90 Sprain of unspecified part of unspecified wrist and hand
- X S63.91 Sprain of unspecified part of right wrist and hand
- X S63.92 Sprain of unspecified part of left wrist and hand

S64 Injury of nerves at wrist and hand level

The appropriate 7th character is to be added to each code from category S64

A	initial encounter
D	subsequent encounter
S	sequela

Code also any associated open wound (S61.-)

S64.0 Injury of ulnar nerve at wrist and hand level
- X S64.00 Injury of ulnar nerve at wrist and hand level of unspecified arm
- X S64.01 Injury of ulnar nerve at wrist and hand level of right arm
- X S64.02 Injury of ulnar nerve at wrist and hand level of left arm

S64.1 Injury of median nerve at wrist and hand level
- X S64.10 Injury of median nerve at wrist and hand level of unspecified arm
- X S64.11 Injury of median nerve at wrist and hand level of right arm
- X S64.12 Injury of median nerve at wrist and hand level of left arm

S64.2 Injury of radial nerve at wrist and hand level
- X S64.20 Injury of radial nerve at wrist and hand level of unspecified arm
- X S64.21 Injury of radial nerve at wrist and hand level of right arm
- X S64.22 Injury of radial nerve at wrist and hand level of left arm

S64.3 Injury of digital nerve of thumb
- X S64.30 Injury of digital nerve of unspecified thumb
- X S64.31 Injury of digital nerve of right thumb
- X S64.32 Injury of digital nerve of left thumb

S64.4 Injury of **digital nerve** of other and unspecified **finger**
- X S64.40 Injury of digital nerve of **unspecified** finger
- S64.49 Injury of digital nerve of other finger
  - S64.490 Injury of digital nerve of **right index** finger
  - S64.491 Injury of digital nerve of **left index** finger
  - S64.492 Injury of digital nerve of **right middle** finger
  - S64.493 Injury of digital nerve of **left middle** finger
  - S64.494 Injury of digital nerve of **right ring** finger
  - S64.495 Injury of digital nerve of **left ring** finger
  - S64.496 Injury of digital nerve of **right little** finger
  - S64.497 Injury of digital nerve of **left little** finger
  - S64.498 Injury of digital nerve of **other** finger
    Injury of digital nerve of specified finger with unspecified laterality

S64.8 Injury of **other nerves** at wrist and hand level
- S64.8X Injury of other nerves at wrist and hand level
  - S64.8X1 Injury of other nerves at wrist and hand level of **right** arm
  - S64.8X2 Injury of other nerves at wrist and hand level of **left** arm
  - S64.8X9 Injury of other nerves at wrist and hand level of **unspecified** arm

S64.9 Injury of **unspecified nerve** at wrist and hand level
- X S64.90 Injury of unspecified nerve at wrist and hand level of **unspecified** arm
- X S64.91 Injury of unspecified nerve at wrist and hand level of **right** arm
- X S64.92 Injury of unspecified nerve at wrist and hand level of **left** arm

S65 Injury of blood vessels at wrist and hand level

The appropriate 7th character is to be added to each code from category S65

A	initial encounter
D	subsequent encounter
S	sequela

Code also any associated open wound (S61.-)

S65.0 Injury of **ulnar artery** at wrist and hand level
- S65.00 **Unspecified** injury of ulnar artery at wrist and hand level
  - S65.001 Unspecified injury of ulnar artery at wrist and hand level of **right** arm
  - S65.002 Unspecified injury of ulnar artery at wrist and hand level of **left** arm
  - S65.009 Unspecified injury of ulnar artery at wrist and hand level of **unspecified** arm
- S65.01 **Laceration** of ulnar artery at wrist and hand level
  - S65.011 Laceration of ulnar artery at wrist and hand level of **right** arm
  - S65.012 Laceration of ulnar artery at wrist and hand level of **left** arm
  - S65.019 Laceration of ulnar artery at wrist and hand level of **unspecified** arm
- S65.09 **Other** specified injury of ulnar artery at wrist and hand level
  - S65.091 Other specified injury of ulnar artery at wrist and hand level of **right** arm
  - S65.092 Other specified injury of ulnar artery at wrist and hand level of **left** arm
  - S65.099 Other specified injury of ulnar artery at wrist and hand level of **unspecified** arm

S65.1 Injury of **radial artery** at wrist and hand level
- S65.10 **Unspecified** injury of radial artery at wrist and hand level
  - S65.101 Unspecified injury of radial artery at wrist and hand level of **right** arm
  - S65.102 Unspecified injury of radial artery at wrist and hand level of **left** arm
  - S65.109 Unspecified injury of radial artery at wrist and hand level of **unspecified** arm
- S65.11 **Laceration** of radial artery at wrist and hand level
  - S65.111 Laceration of radial artery at wrist and hand level of **right** arm
  - S65.112 Laceration of radial artery at wrist and hand level of **left** arm
  - S65.119 Laceration of radial artery at wrist and hand level of **unspecified** arm
- S65.19 **Other** specified injury of radial artery at wrist and hand level
  - S65.191 Other specified injury of radial artery at wrist and hand level of **right** arm
  - S65.192 Other specified injury of radial artery at wrist and hand level of **left** arm
  - S65.199 Other specified injury of radial artery at wrist and hand level of **unspecified** arm

S65.2 Injury of **superficial palmar arch**
- S65.20 **Unspecified** injury of superficial palmar arch
  - S65.201 Unspecified injury of superficial palmar arch of **right** hand
  - S65.202 Unspecified injury of superficial palmar arch of **left** hand
  - S65.209 Unspecified injury of superficial palmar arch of **unspecified** hand
- S65.21 **Laceration** of superficial palmar arch
  - S65.211 Laceration of superficial palmar arch of **right** hand
  - S65.212 Laceration of superficial palmar arch of **left** hand
  - S65.219 Laceration of superficial palmar arch of **unspecified** hand
- S65.29 **Other** specified injury of superficial palmar arch
  - S65.291 Other specified injury of superficial palmar arch of **right** hand
  - S65.292 Other specified injury of superficial palmar arch of **left** hand
  - S65.299 Other specified injury of superficial palmar arch of **unspecified** hand

S65.3 Injury of **deep palmar arch**
- S65.30 **Unspecified** injury of deep palmar arch
  - S65.301 Unspecified injury of deep palmar arch of **right** hand
  - S65.302 Unspecified injury of deep palmar arch of **left** hand
  - S65.309 Unspecified injury of deep palmar arch of **unspecified** hand

- S65.31 Laceration of deep palmar arch
  - S65.311 Laceration of deep palmar arch of right hand
  - S65.312 Laceration of deep palmar arch of left hand
  - S65.319 Laceration of deep palmar arch of unspecified hand
- S65.39 Other specified injury of deep palmar arch
  - S65.391 Other specified injury of deep palmar arch of right hand
  - S65.392 Other specified injury of deep palmar arch of left hand
  - S65.399 Other specified injury of deep palmar arch of unspecified hand

S65.4 Injury of blood vessel of thumb
- S65.40 Unspecified injury of blood vessel of thumb
  - S65.401 Unspecified injury of blood vessel of right thumb
  - S65.402 Unspecified injury of blood vessel of left thumb
  - S65.409 Unspecified injury of blood vessel of unspecified thumb
- S65.41 Laceration of blood vessel of thumb
  - S65.411 Laceration of blood vessel of right thumb
  - S65.412 Laceration of blood vessel of left thumb
  - S65.419 Laceration of blood vessel of unspecified thumb
- S65.49 Other specified injury of blood vessel of thumb
  - S65.491 Other specified injury of blood vessel of right thumb
  - S65.492 Other specified injury of blood vessel of left thumb
  - S65.499 Other specified injury of blood vessel of unspecified thumb

S65.5 Injury of blood vessel of other and unspecified finger
- S65.50 Unspecified injury of blood vessel of other and unspecified finger
  - S65.500 Unspecified injury of blood vessel of right index finger
  - S65.501 Unspecified injury of blood vessel of left index finger
  - S65.502 Unspecified injury of blood vessel of right middle finger
  - S65.503 Unspecified injury of blood vessel of left middle finger
  - S65.504 Unspecified injury of blood vessel of right ring finger
  - S65.505 Unspecified injury of blood vessel of left ring finger
  - S65.506 Unspecified injury of blood vessel of right little finger
  - S65.507 Unspecified injury of blood vessel of left little finger
  - S65.508 Unspecified injury of blood vessel of other finger
    - Unspecified injury of blood vessel of specified finger with unspecified laterality
  - S65.509 Unspecified injury of blood vessel of unspecified finger
- S65.51 Laceration of blood vessel of other and unspecified finger
  - S65.510 Laceration of blood vessel of right index finger
  - S65.511 Laceration of blood vessel of left index finger
  - S65.512 Laceration of blood vessel of right middle finger
  - S65.513 Laceration of blood vessel of left middle finger
  - S65.514 Laceration of blood vessel of right ring finger
  - S65.515 Laceration of blood vessel of left ring finger
  - S65.516 Laceration of blood vessel of right little finger
  - S65.517 Laceration of blood vessel of left little finger
  - S65.518 Laceration of blood vessel of other finger
    - Laceration of blood vessel of specified finger with unspecified laterality
  - S65.519 Laceration of blood vessel of unspecified finger
- S65.59 Other specified injury of blood vessel of other and unspecified finger
  - S65.590 Other specified injury of blood vessel of right index finger
  - S65.591 Other specified injury of blood vessel of left index finger
  - S65.592 Other specified injury of blood vessel of right middle finger
  - S65.593 Other specified injury of blood vessel of left middle finger
  - S65.594 Other specified injury of blood vessel of right ring finger
  - S65.595 Other specified injury of blood vessel of left ring finger
  - S65.596 Other specified injury of blood vessel of right little finger
  - S65.597 Other specified injury of blood vessel of left little finger
  - S65.598 Other specified injury of blood vessel of other finger
    - Other specified injury of blood vessel of specified finger with unspecified laterality
  - S65.599 Other specified injury of blood vessel of unspecified finger

S65.8 Injury of other blood vessels at wrist and hand level
- S65.80 Unspecified injury of other blood vessels at wrist and hand level
  - S65.801 Unspecified injury of other blood vessels at wrist and hand level of right arm
  - S65.802 Unspecified injury of other blood vessels at wrist and hand level of left arm
  - S65.809 Unspecified injury of other blood vessels at wrist and hand level of unspecified arm

- S65.81 **Laceration** of other blood vessels at wrist and hand level
  - S65.811 Laceration of other blood vessels at wrist and hand level of **right** arm
  - S65.812 Laceration of other blood vessels at wrist and hand level of **left** arm
  - S65.819 Laceration of other blood vessels at wrist and hand level of **unspecified** arm
- S65.89 **Other** specified injury of other blood vessels at wrist and hand level
  - S65.891 Other specified injury of other blood vessels at wrist and hand level of **right** arm
  - S65.892 Other specified injury of other blood vessels at wrist and hand level of **left** arm
  - S65.899 Other specified injury of other blood vessels at wrist and hand level of **unspecified** arm

S65.9 Injury of **unspecified blood vessel** at wrist and hand level

- S65.90 **Unspecified** injury of unspecified blood vessel at wrist and hand level
  - S65.901 Unspecified injury of unspecified blood vessel at wrist and hand level of **right** arm
  - S65.902 Unspecified injury of unspecified blood vessel at wrist and hand level of **left** arm
  - S65.909 Unspecified injury of unspecified blood vessel at wrist and hand level of **unspecified** arm
- S65.91 **Laceration** of **unspecified** blood vessel at wrist and hand level
  - S65.911 Laceration of unspecified blood vessel at wrist and hand level of **right** arm
  - S65.912 Laceration of unspecified blood vessel at wrist and hand level of **left** arm
  - S65.919 Laceration of unspecified blood vessel at wrist and hand level of **unspecified** arm
- S65.99 **Other** specified injury of unspecified blood vessel at wrist and hand level
  - S65.991 Other specified injury of **unspecified** blood vessel at wrist and hand of **right** arm
  - S65.992 Other specified injury of **unspecified** blood vessel at wrist and hand of **left** arm
  - S65.999 Other specified injury of **unspecified** blood vessel at wrist and hand of **unspecified** arm

S66 Injury of muscle, fascia and tendon at wrist and hand level

Code also any associated open wound (S61.-)

Excludes2 sprain of joints and ligaments of wrist and hand (S63.-)

The appropriate 7th character is to be added to each code from category S66

A	initial encounter
D	subsequent encounter
S	sequela

S66.Ø Injury of **long flexor** muscle, fascia and tendon of **thumb** at wrist and hand level

- S66.ØØ **Unspecified** injury of long flexor muscle, fascia and tendon of thumb at wrist and hand level
  - S66.ØØ1 Unspecified injury of long flexor muscle, fascia and tendon of **right** thumb at wrist and hand level
  - S66.ØØ2 Unspecified injury of long flexor muscle, fascia and tendon of **left** thumb at wrist and hand level
  - S66.ØØ9 Unspecified injury of long flexor muscle, fascia and tendon of **unspecified** thumb at wrist and hand level
- S66.Ø1 **Strain** of long flexor muscle, fascia and tendon of thumb at wrist and hand level
  - S66.Ø11 Strain of long flexor muscle, fascia and tendon of **right** thumb at wrist and hand level
  - S66.Ø12 Strain of long flexor muscle, fascia and tendon of **left** thumb at wrist and hand level
  - S66.Ø19 Strain of long flexor muscle, fascia and tendon of **unspecified** thumb at wrist and hand level
- S66.Ø2 **Laceration** of long flexor muscle, fascia and tendon of thumb at wrist and hand level
  - S66.Ø21 Laceration of long flexor muscle, fascia and tendon of **right** thumb at wrist and hand level
  - S66.Ø22 Laceration of long flexor muscle, fascia and tendon of **left** thumb at wrist and hand level
  - S66.Ø29 Laceration of long flexor muscle, fascia and tendon of **unspecified** thumb at wrist and hand level
- S66.Ø9 **Other** specified injury of long flexor muscle, fascia and tendon of thumb at wrist and hand level
  - S66.Ø91 Other specified injury of long flexor muscle, fascia and tendon of **right** thumb at wrist and hand level
  - S66.Ø92 Other specified injury of long flexor muscle, fascia and tendon of **left** thumb at wrist and hand level
  - S66.Ø99 Other specified injury of long flexor muscle, fascia and tendon of **unspecified** thumb at wrist and hand level

● S66.1 Injury of **flexor** muscle, fascia and tendon of other and unspecified **finger** at wrist and hand level

Excludes2 injury of long flexor muscle, fascia and tendon of thumb at wrist and hand level (S66.Ø-)

● S66.1Ø **Unspecified** injury of flexor muscle, fascia and tendon of other and unspecified finger at wrist and hand level

● S66.1ØØ Unspecified injury of flexor muscle, fascia and tendon of **right index** finger at wrist and hand level

● S66.1Ø1 Unspecified injury of flexor muscle, fascia and tendon of **left index** finger at wrist and hand level

● S66.1Ø2 Unspecified injury of flexor muscle, fascia and tendon of **right middle** finger at wrist and hand level

● S66.1Ø3 Unspecified injury of flexor muscle, fascia and tendon of **left middle** finger at wrist and hand level

● S66.1Ø4 Unspecified injury of flexor muscle, fascia and tendon of **right ring** finger at wrist and hand level

● S66.1Ø5 Unspecified injury of flexor muscle, fascia and tendon of **left ring** finger at wrist and hand level

● S66.1Ø6 Unspecified injury of flexor muscle, fascia and tendon of **right little** finger at wrist and hand level

● S66.1Ø7 Unspecified injury of flexor muscle, fascia and tendon of **left little** finger at wrist and hand level

● S66.1Ø8 Unspecified injury of flexor muscle, fascia and tendon of **other** finger at wrist and hand level

Unspecified injury of flexor muscle, fascia and tendon of specified finger with unspecified laterality at wrist and hand level

● S66.1Ø9 Unspecified injury of flexor muscle, fascia and tendon of **unspecified** finger at wrist and hand level

● S66.11 **Strain** of flexor muscle, fascia and tendon of other and unspecified finger at wrist and hand level

● S66.11Ø Strain of flexor muscle, fascia and tendon of **right index** finger at wrist and hand level

● S66.111 Strain of flexor muscle, fascia and tendon of **left index** finger at wrist and hand level

● S66.112 Strain of flexor muscle, fascia and tendon of **right middle** finger at wrist and hand level

● S66.113 Strain of flexor muscle, fascia and tendon of **left middle** finger at wrist and hand level

● S66.114 Strain of flexor muscle, fascia and tendon of **right ring** finger at wrist and hand level

● S66.115 Strain of flexor muscle, fascia and tendon of **left ring** finger at wrist and hand level

● S66.116 Strain of flexor muscle, fascia and tendon of **right little** finger at wrist and hand level

● S66.117 Strain of flexor muscle, fascia and tendon of **left little** finger at wrist and hand level

● S66.118 Strain of flexor muscle, fascia and tendon of **other** finger at wrist and hand level

Strain of flexor muscle, fascia and tendon of specified finger with unspecified laterality at wrist and hand level

● S66.119 Strain of flexor muscle, fascia and tendon of **unspecified** finger at wrist and hand level

● S66.12 **Laceration** of flexor muscle, fascia and tendon of other and unspecified finger at wrist and hand level

● S66.12Ø Laceration of flexor muscle, fascia and tendon of **right index** finger at wrist and hand level

● S66.121 Laceration of flexor muscle, fascia and tendon of **left index** finger at wrist and hand level

● S66.122 Laceration of flexor muscle, fascia and tendon of **right middle** finger at wrist and hand level

● S66.123 Laceration of flexor muscle, fascia and tendon of **left middle** finger at wrist and hand level

● S66.124 Laceration of flexor muscle, fascia and tendon of **right ring** finger at wrist and hand level

● S66.125 Laceration of flexor muscle, fascia and tendon of **left ring** finger at wrist and hand level

● S66.126 Laceration of flexor muscle, fascia and tendon of **right little** finger at wrist and hand level

● S66.127 Laceration of flexor muscle, fascia and tendon of **left little** finger at wrist and hand level

● S66.128 Laceration of flexor muscle, fascia and tendon of **other** finger at wrist and hand level

Laceration of flexor muscle, fascia and tendon of specified finger with unspecified laterality at wrist and hand level

● S66.129 Laceration of flexor muscle, fascia and tendon of **unspecified** finger at wrist and hand level

● S66.19 **Other** injury of flexor muscle, fascia and tendon of other and unspecified finger at wrist and hand level

● S66.19Ø Other injury of flexor muscle, fascia and tendon of **right index** finger at wrist and hand level

● S66.191 Other injury of flexor muscle, fascia and tendon of **left index** finger at wrist and hand level

● S66.192 Other injury of flexor muscle, fascia and tendon of **right middle** finger at wrist and hand level

● S66.193 Other injury of flexor muscle, fascia and tendon of **left middle** finger at wrist and hand level

● S66.194 Other injury of flexor muscle, fascia and tendon of **right ring** finger at wrist and hand level

● S66.195 Other injury of flexor muscle, fascia and tendon of **left ring** finger at wrist and hand level

● S66.196 Other injury of flexor muscle, fascia and tendon of **right little** finger at wrist and hand level

● S66.197 Other injury of flexor muscle, fascia and tendon of **left little** finger at wrist and hand level

S66.198 **Other injury of flexor muscle, fascia and tendon of other finger at wrist and hand level**
Other injury of flexor muscle, fascia and tendon of specified finger with unspecified laterality at wrist and hand level

S66.199 **Other injury of flexor muscle, fascia and tendon of unspecified finger at wrist and hand level**

S66.2 **Injury of extensor muscle, fascia and tendon of thumb at wrist and hand level**

S66.20 **Unspecified injury of extensor muscle, fascia and tendon of thumb at wrist and hand level**

S66.201 **Unspecified injury of extensor muscle, fascia and tendon of right thumb at wrist and hand level**

S66.202 **Unspecified injury of extensor muscle, fascia and tendon of left thumb at wrist and hand level**

S66.209 **Unspecified injury of extensor muscle, fascia and tendon of unspecified thumb at wrist and hand level**

S66.21 **Strain of extensor muscle, fascia and tendon of thumb at wrist and hand level**

S66.211 **Strain of extensor muscle, fascia and tendon of right thumb at wrist and hand level**

S66.212 **Strain of extensor muscle, fascia and tendon of left thumb at wrist and hand level**

S66.219 **Strain of extensor muscle, fascia and tendon of unspecified thumb at wrist and hand level**

S66.22 **Laceration of extensor muscle, fascia and tendon of thumb at wrist and hand level**

S66.221 **Laceration of extensor muscle, fascia and tendon of right thumb at wrist and hand level**

S66.222 **Laceration of extensor muscle, fascia and tendon of left thumb at wrist and hand level**

S66.229 **Laceration of extensor muscle, fascia and tendon of unspecified thumb at wrist and hand level**

S66.29 **Other specified injury of extensor muscle, fascia and tendon of thumb at wrist and hand level**

S66.291 **Other specified injury of extensor muscle, fascia and tendon of right thumb at wrist and hand level**

S66.292 **Other specified injury of extensor muscle, fascia and tendon of left thumb at wrist and hand level**

S66.299 **Other specified injury of extensor muscle, fascia and tendon of unspecified thumb at wrist and hand level**

S66.3 **Injury of extensor muscle, fascia and tendon of other and unspecified finger at wrist and hand level**

Excludes2 injury of extensor muscle, fascia and tendon of thumb at wrist and hand level (S66.2-)

S66.30 **Unspecified injury of extensor muscle, fascia and tendon of other and unspecified finger at wrist and hand level**

S66.300 **Unspecified injury of extensor muscle, fascia and tendon of right index finger at wrist and hand level**

S66.301 **Unspecified injury of extensor muscle, fascia and tendon of left index finger at wrist and hand level**

S66.302 **Unspecified injury of extensor muscle, fascia and tendon of right middle finger at wrist and hand level**

S66.303 **Unspecified injury of extensor muscle, fascia and tendon of left middle finger at wrist and hand level**

S66.304 **Unspecified injury of extensor muscle, fascia and tendon of right ring finger at wrist and hand level**

S66.305 **Unspecified injury of extensor muscle, fascia and tendon of left ring finger at wrist and hand level**

S66.306 **Unspecified injury of extensor muscle, fascia and tendon of right little finger at wrist and hand level**

S66.307 **Unspecified injury of extensor muscle, fascia and tendon of left little finger at wrist and hand level**

S66.308 **Unspecified injury of extensor muscle, fascia and tendon of other finger at wrist and hand level**
Unspecified injury of extensor muscle, fascia and tendon of specified finger with unspecified laterality at wrist and hand level

S66.309 **Unspecified injury of extensor muscle, fascia and tendon of unspecified finger at wrist and hand level**

S66.31 **Strain of extensor muscle, fascia and tendon of other and unspecified finger at wrist and hand level**

S66.310 **Strain of extensor muscle, fascia and tendon of right index finger at wrist and hand level**

S66.311 **Strain of extensor muscle, fascia and tendon of left index finger at wrist and hand level**

S66.312 **Strain of extensor muscle, fascia and tendon of right middle finger at wrist and hand level**

S66.313 **Strain of extensor muscle, fascia and tendon of left middle finger at wrist and hand level**

S66.314 **Strain of extensor muscle, fascia and tendon of right ring finger at wrist and hand level**

S66.315 **Strain of extensor muscle, fascia and tendon of left ring finger at wrist and hand level**

S66.316 **Strain of extensor muscle, fascia and tendon of right little finger at wrist and hand level**

S66.317 **Strain of extensor muscle, fascia and tendon of left little finger at wrist and hand level**

S66.318 **Strain of extensor muscle, fascia and tendon of other finger at wrist and hand level**
Strain of extensor muscle, fascia and tendon of specified finger with unspecified laterality at wrist and hand level

S66.319 **Strain of extensor muscle, fascia and tendon of unspecified finger at wrist and hand level**

● S66.32 **Laceration** of extensor muscle, fascia and tendon of other and unspecified finger at wrist and hand level
- ● S66.320 Laceration of extensor muscle, fascia and tendon of **right index** finger at wrist and hand level
- ● S66.321 Laceration of extensor muscle, fascia and tendon of **left index** finger at wrist and hand level
- ● S66.322 Laceration of extensor muscle, fascia and tendon of **right middle** finger at wrist and hand level
- ● S66.323 Laceration of extensor muscle, fascia and tendon of **left middle** finger at wrist and hand level
- ● S66.324 Laceration of extensor muscle, fascia and tendon of **right ring** finger at wrist and hand level
- ● S66.325 Laceration of extensor muscle, fascia and tendon of **left ring** finger at wrist and hand level
- ● S66.326 Laceration of extensor muscle, fascia and tendon of **right little** finger at wrist and hand level
- ● S66.327 Laceration of extensor muscle, fascia and tendon of **left little** finger at wrist and hand level
- ● S66.328 Laceration of extensor muscle, fascia and tendon of **other** finger at wrist and hand level
  - Laceration of extensor muscle, fascia and tendon of specified finger with unspecified laterality at wrist and hand level
- ● S66.329 Laceration of extensor muscle, fascia and tendon of **unspecified** finger at wrist and hand level

● S66.39 **Other** injury of extensor muscle, fascia and tendon of other and unspecified finger at wrist and hand level
- ● S66.390 Other injury of extensor muscle, fascia and tendon of **right index** finger at wrist and hand level
- ● S66.391 Other injury of extensor muscle, fascia and tendon of **left index** finger at wrist and hand level
- ● S66.392 Other injury of extensor muscle, fascia and tendon of **right middle** finger at wrist and hand level
- ● S66.393 Other injury of extensor muscle, fascia and tendon of **left middle** finger at wrist and hand level
- ● S66.394 Other injury of extensor muscle, fascia and tendon of **right ring** finger at wrist and hand level
- ● S66.395 Other injury of extensor muscle, fascia and tendon of **left ring** finger at wrist and hand level
- ● S66.396 Other injury of extensor muscle, fascia and tendon of **right little** finger at wrist and hand level
- ● S66.397 Other injury of extensor muscle, fascia and tendon of **left little** finger at wrist and hand level
- ● S66.398 Other injury of extensor muscle, fascia and tendon of **other** finger at wrist and hand level
  - Other injury of extensor muscle, fascia and tendon of specified finger with unspecified laterality at wrist and hand level
- ● S66.399 Other injury of extensor muscle, fascia and tendon of **unspecified** finger at wrist and hand level

● S66.4 Injury of **intrinsic** muscle, fascia and tendon of **thumb** at wrist and hand level

● S66.40 **Unspecified** injury of intrinsic muscle, fascia and tendon of thumb at wrist and hand level
- ● S66.401 Unspecified injury of intrinsic muscle, fascia and tendon of **right** thumb at wrist and hand level
- ● S66.402 Unspecified injury of intrinsic muscle, fascia and tendon of **left** thumb at wrist and hand level
- ● S66.409 Unspecified injury of intrinsic muscle, fascia and tendon of **unspecified** thumb at wrist and hand level

● S66.41 **Strain** of intrinsic muscle, fascia and tendon of thumb at wrist and hand level
- ● S66.411 Strain of intrinsic muscle, fascia and tendon of **right** thumb at wrist and hand level
- ● S66.412 Strain of intrinsic muscle, fascia and tendon of **left** thumb at wrist and hand level
- ● S66.419 Strain of intrinsic muscle, fascia and tendon of **unspecified** thumb at wrist and hand level

● S66.42 **Laceration** of intrinsic muscle, fascia and tendon of thumb at wrist and hand level
- ● S66.421 Laceration of intrinsic muscle, fascia and tendon of **right** thumb at wrist and hand level
- ● S66.422 Laceration of intrinsic muscle, fascia and tendon of **left** thumb at wrist and hand level
- ● S66.429 Laceration of intrinsic muscle, fascia and tendon of **unspecified** thumb at wrist and hand level

● S66.49 **Other** specified injury of intrinsic muscle, fascia and tendon of thumb at wrist and hand level
- ● S66.491 Other specified injury of intrinsic muscle, fascia and tendon of **right** thumb at wrist and hand level
- ● S66.492 Other specified injury of intrinsic muscle, fascia and tendon of **left** thumb at wrist and hand level
- ● S66.499 Other specified injury of intrinsic muscle, fascia and tendon of **unspecified** thumb at wrist and hand level

● S66.5 Injury of **intrinsic** muscle, fascia and tendon of other and unspecified **finger** at wrist and hand level

Excludes2 injury of intrinsic muscle, fascia and tendon of thumb at wrist and hand level (S66.4-)

● S66.50 **Unspecified** injury of intrinsic muscle, fascia and tendon of other and unspecified finger at wrist and hand level
- ● S66.500 Unspecified injury of intrinsic muscle, fascia and tendon of **right index** finger at wrist and hand level
- ● S66.501 Unspecified injury of intrinsic muscle, fascia and tendon of **left index** finger at wrist and hand level
- ● S66.502 Unspecified injury of intrinsic muscle, fascia and tendon of **right middle** finger at wrist and hand level

S66.503 **Unspecified injury of intrinsic muscle, fascia and tendon of left middle finger at wrist and hand level**

S66.504 **Unspecified injury of intrinsic muscle, fascia and tendon of right ring finger at wrist and hand level**

S66.505 **Unspecified injury of intrinsic muscle, fascia and tendon of left ring finger at wrist and hand level**

S66.506 **Unspecified injury of intrinsic muscle, fascia and tendon of right little finger at wrist and hand level**

S66.507 **Unspecified injury of intrinsic muscle, fascia and tendon of left little finger at wrist and hand level**

S66.508 **Unspecified injury of intrinsic muscle, fascia and tendon of other finger at wrist and hand level**
Unspecified injury of intrinsic muscle, fascia and tendon of specified finger with unspecified laterality at wrist and hand level

S66.509 **Unspecified injury of intrinsic muscle, fascia and tendon of unspecified finger at wrist and hand level**

S66.51 **Strain of intrinsic muscle, fascia and tendon of other and unspecified finger at wrist and hand level**

S66.510 **Strain of intrinsic muscle, fascia and tendon of right index finger at wrist and hand level**

S66.511 **Strain of intrinsic muscle, fascia and tendon of left index finger at wrist and hand level**

S66.512 **Strain of intrinsic muscle, fascia and tendon of right middle finger at wrist and hand level**

S66.513 **Strain of intrinsic muscle, fascia and tendon of left middle finger at wrist and hand level**

S66.514 **Strain of intrinsic muscle, fascia and tendon of right ring finger at wrist and hand level**

S66.515 **Strain of intrinsic muscle, fascia and tendon of left ring finger at wrist and hand level**

S66.516 **Strain of intrinsic muscle, fascia and tendon of right little finger at wrist and hand level**

S66.517 **Strain of intrinsic muscle, fascia and tendon of left little finger at wrist and hand level**

S66.518 **Strain of intrinsic muscle, fascia and tendon of other finger at wrist and hand level**
Strain of intrinsic muscle, fascia and tendon of specified finger with unspecified laterality at wrist and hand level

S66.519 **Strain of intrinsic muscle, fascia and tendon of unspecified finger at wrist and hand level**

S66.52 **Laceration of intrinsic muscle, fascia and tendon of other and unspecified finger at wrist and hand level**

S66.520 **Laceration of intrinsic muscle, fascia and tendon of right index finger at wrist and hand level**

S66.521 **Laceration of intrinsic muscle, fascia and tendon of left index finger at wrist and hand level**

S66.522 **Laceration of intrinsic muscle, fascia and tendon of right middle finger at wrist and hand level**

S66.523 **Laceration of intrinsic muscle, fascia and tendon of left middle finger at wrist and hand level**

S66.524 **Laceration of intrinsic muscle, fascia and tendon of right ring finger at wrist and hand level**

S66.525 **Laceration of intrinsic muscle, fascia and tendon of left ring finger at wrist and hand level**

S66.526 **Laceration of intrinsic muscle, fascia and tendon of right little finger at wrist and hand level**

S66.527 **Laceration of intrinsic muscle, fascia and tendon of left little finger at wrist and hand level**

S66.528 **Laceration of intrinsic muscle, fascia and tendon of other finger at wrist and hand level**
Laceration of intrinsic muscle, fascia and tendon of specified finger with unspecified laterality at wrist and hand level

S66.529 **Laceration of intrinsic muscle, fascia and tendon of unspecified finger at wrist and hand level**

S66.59 **Other injury of intrinsic muscle, fascia and tendon of other and unspecified finger at wrist and hand level**

S66.590 **Other injury of intrinsic muscle, fascia and tendon of right index finger at wrist and hand level**

S66.591 **Other injury of intrinsic muscle, fascia and tendon of left index finger at wrist and hand level**

S66.592 **Other injury of intrinsic muscle, fascia and tendon of right middle finger at wrist and hand level**

S66.593 **Other injury of intrinsic muscle, fascia and tendon of left middle finger at wrist and hand level**

S66.594 **Other injury of intrinsic muscle, fascia and tendon of right ring finger at wrist and hand level**

S66.595 **Other injury of intrinsic muscle, fascia and tendon of left ring finger at wrist and hand level**

S66.596 **Other injury of intrinsic muscle, fascia and tendon of right little finger at wrist and hand level**

S66.597 **Other injury of intrinsic muscle, fascia and tendon of left little finger at wrist and hand level**

S66.598 **Other injury of intrinsic muscle, fascia and tendon of other finger at wrist and hand level**
Other injury of intrinsic muscle, fascia and tendon of specified finger with unspecified laterality at wrist and hand level

S66.599 **Other injury of intrinsic muscle, fascia and tendon of unspecified finger at wrist and hand level**

- S66.8 Injury of **other specified** muscles, fascia and tendons at wrist and hand level
  - S66.80 **Unspecified** injury of other specified muscles, fascia and tendons at wrist and hand level
    - S66.801 Unspecified injury of other specified muscles, fascia and tendons at wrist and hand level, **right** hand
    - S66.802 Unspecified injury of other specified muscles, fascia and tendons at wrist and hand level, **left** hand
    - S66.809 Unspecified injury of other specified muscles, fascia and tendons at wrist and hand level, **unspecified** hand
  - S66.81 **Strain** of other specified muscles, fascia and tendons at wrist and hand level
    - S66.811 Strain of other specified muscles, fascia and tendons at wrist and hand level, **right** hand
    - S66.812 Strain of other specified muscles, fascia and tendons at wrist and hand level, **left** hand
    - S66.819 Strain of other specified muscles, fascia and tendons at wrist and hand level, **unspecified** hand
  - S66.82 **Laceration** of other specified muscles, fascia and tendons at wrist and hand level
    - S66.821 Laceration of other specified muscles, fascia and tendons at wrist and hand level, **right** hand
    - S66.822 Laceration of other specified muscles, fascia and tendons at wrist and hand level, **left** hand
    - S66.829 Laceration of other specified muscles, fascia and tendons at wrist and hand level, **unspecified** hand
  - S66.89 **Other** injury of other specified muscles, fascia and tendons at wrist and hand level
    - S66.891 Other injury of other specified muscles, fascia and tendons at wrist and hand level, **right** hand
    - S66.892 Other injury of other specified muscles, fascia and tendons at wrist and hand level, **left** hand
    - S66.899 Other injury of other specified muscles, fascia and tendons at wrist and hand level, **unspecified** hand
- S66.9 Injury of **unspecified** muscle, fascia and tendon at wrist and hand level
  - S66.90 **Unspecified** injury of unspecified muscle, fascia and tendon at wrist and hand level
    - S66.901 Unspecified injury of unspecified muscle, fascia and tendon at wrist and hand level, **right** hand
    - S66.902 Unspecified injury of unspecified muscle, fascia and tendon at wrist and hand level, **left** hand
    - S66.909 Unspecified injury of unspecified muscle, fascia and tendon at wrist and hand level, **unspecified** hand
  - S66.91 **Strain** of unspecified muscle, fascia and tendon at wrist and hand level
    - S66.911 Strain of unspecified muscle, fascia and tendon at wrist and hand level, **right** hand
    - S66.912 Strain of unspecified muscle, fascia and tendon at wrist and hand level, **left** hand
    - S66.919 Strain of unspecified muscle, fascia and tendon at wrist and hand level, **unspecified** hand
  - S66.92 **Laceration** of unspecified muscle, fascia and tendon at wrist and hand level
    - S66.921 Laceration of unspecified muscle, fascia and tendon at wrist and hand level, **right** hand
    - S66.922 Laceration of unspecified muscle, fascia and tendon at wrist and hand level, **left** hand
    - S66.929 Laceration of unspecified muscle, fascia and tendon at wrist and hand level, **unspecified** hand
  - S66.99 **Other** injury of unspecified muscle, fascia and tendon at wrist and hand level
    - S66.991 Other injury of unspecified muscle, fascia and tendon at wrist and hand level, **right** hand
    - S66.992 Other injury of unspecified muscle, fascia and tendon at wrist and hand level, **left** hand
    - S66.999 Other injury of unspecified muscle, fascia and tendon at wrist and hand level, **unspecified** hand

S67 Crushing injury of wrist, hand and fingers

Use additional code for all associated injuries, such as:
fracture of wrist and hand (S62.-)
open wound of wrist and hand (S61.-)

The appropriate 7th character is to be added to each code from category S67

A	initial encounter
D	subsequent encounter
S	sequela

- S67.Ø Crushing injury of **thumb**
  - X S67.ØØ Crushing injury of **unspecified** thumb
  - X S67.Ø1 Crushing injury of **right** thumb
  - X S67.Ø2 Crushing injury of **left** thumb
- S67.1 Crushing injury of other and unspecified **finger(s)**
  - **Excludes2** crushing injury of thumb (S67.Ø-)
  - X S67.1Ø Crushing injury of **unspecified** finger(s)
  - S67.19 Crushing injury of other finger(s)
    - S67.19Ø Crushing injury of **right index** finger
    - S67.191 Crushing injury of **left index** finger
    - S67.192 Crushing injury of **right middle** finger
    - S67.193 Crushing injury of **left middle** finger
    - S67.194 Crushing injury of **right ring** finger
    - S67.195 Crushing injury of **left ring** finger
    - S67.196 Crushing injury of **right little** finger
    - S67.197 Crushing injury of **left little** finger
    - S67.198 Crushing injury of **other** finger
      Crushing injury of specified finger with unspecified laterality
- S67.2 Crushing injury of **hand**
  - **Excludes2** crushing injury of fingers (S67.1-)
    crushing injury of thumb (S67.Ø-)
  - X S67.2Ø Crushing injury of **unspecified** hand
  - X S67.21 Crushing injury of **right** hand
  - X S67.22 Crushing injury of **left** hand
- S67.3 Crushing injury of **wrist**
  - X S67.3Ø Crushing injury of **unspecified** wrist
  - X S67.31 Crushing injury of **right** wrist
  - X S67.32 Crushing injury of **left** wrist

CHAPTER 19 (SØØ-T88)

● S67.4 Crushing injury of wrist and hand
Excludes1 crushing injury of hand alone (S67.2-)
crushing injury of wrist alone (S67.3-)
Excludes2 crushing injury of fingers (S67.1-)
crushing injury of thumb (S67.Ø-)
X● S67.4Ø Crushing injury of unspecified wrist and hand
X● S67.41 Crushing injury of right wrist and hand
X● S67.42 Crushing injury of left wrist and hand
● S67.9 Crushing injury of unspecified part(s) of wrist, hand and fingers
X● S67.9Ø Crushing injury of unspecified part(s) of unspecified wrist, hand and fingers
X● S67.91 Crushing injury of unspecified part(s) of right wrist, hand and fingers
X● S67.92 Crushing injury of unspecified part(s) of left wrist, hand and fingers

● S68 Traumatic amputation of wrist, hand and fingers
An amputation not identified as partial or complete should be coded to complete
The appropriate 7th character is to be added to each code from category S68

A	initial encounter
D	subsequent encounter
S	sequela

● S68.Ø Traumatic metacarpophalangeal amputation of thumb
Traumatic amputation of thumb NOS
● S68.Ø1 Complete traumatic metacarpophalangeal amputation of thumb
● S68.Ø11 Complete traumatic metacarpophalangeal amputation of right thumb S
● S68.Ø12 Complete traumatic metacarpophalangeal amputation of left thumb S
● S68.Ø19 Complete traumatic metacarpophalangeal amputation of unspecified thumb S
● S68.Ø2 Partial traumatic metacarpophalangeal amputation of thumb
● S68.Ø21 Partial traumatic metacarpophalangeal amputation of right thumb S
● S68.Ø22 Partial traumatic metacarpophalangeal amputation of left thumb S
● S68.Ø29 Partial traumatic metacarpophalangeal amputation of unspecified thumb S
● S68.1 Traumatic metacarpophalangeal amputation of other and unspecified finger
Traumatic amputation of finger NOS
Excludes2 traumatic metacarpophalangeal amputation of thumb (S68.Ø-)
● S68.11 Complete traumatic metacarpophalangeal amputation of other and unspecified finger
● S68.11Ø Complete traumatic metacarpophalangeal amputation of right index finger S
● S68.111 Complete traumatic metacarpophalangeal amputation of left index finger S
● S68.112 Complete traumatic metacarpophalangeal amputation of right middle finger S
● S68.113 Complete traumatic metacarpophalangeal amputation of left middle finger S
● S68.114 Complete traumatic metacarpophalangeal amputation of right ring finger S
● S68.115 Complete traumatic metacarpophalangeal amputation of left ring finger S
● S68.116 Complete traumatic metacarpophalangeal amputation of right little finger S
● S68.117 Complete traumatic metacarpophalangeal amputation of left little finger S
● S68.118 Complete traumatic metacarpophalangeal amputation of other finger S
Complete traumatic metacarpophalangeal amputation of specified finger with unspecified laterality
● S68.119 Complete traumatic metacarpophalangeal amputation of unspecified finger S
● S68.12 Partial traumatic metacarpophalangeal amputation of other and unspecified finger
● S68.12Ø Partial traumatic metacarpophalangeal amputation of right index finger S
● S68.121 Partial traumatic metacarpophalangeal amputation of left index finger S
● S68.122 Partial traumatic metacarpophalangeal amputation of right middle finger S
● S68.123 Partial traumatic metacarpophalangeal amputation of left middle finger S
● S68.124 Partial traumatic metacarpophalangeal amputation of right ring finger S
● S68.125 Partial traumatic metacarpophalangeal amputation of left ring finger S
● S68.126 Partial traumatic metacarpophalangeal amputation of right little finger S
● S68.127 Partial traumatic metacarpophalangeal amputation of left little finger S
● S68.128 Partial traumatic metacarpophalangeal amputation of other finger S
Partial traumatic metacarpophalangeal amputation of specified finger with unspecified laterality
● S68.129 Partial traumatic metacarpophalangeal amputation of unspecified finger S
● S68.4 Traumatic amputation of hand at wrist level
Traumatic amputation of hand NOS
Traumatic amputation of wrist
● S68.41 Complete traumatic amputation of hand at wrist level
● S68.411 Complete traumatic amputation of right hand at wrist level A, S
● S68.412 Complete traumatic amputation of left hand at wrist level A, S
● S68.419 Complete traumatic amputation of unspecified hand at wrist level A, S

CHAPTER 19 (SØØ-T88)

S68.42 Partial traumatic amputation of hand at wrist level
- S68.421 Partial traumatic amputation of right hand at wrist level A, S
- S68.422 Partial traumatic amputation of left hand at wrist level A, S
- S68.429 Partial traumatic amputation of unspecified hand at wrist level A, S

S68.5 Traumatic transphalangeal amputation of thumb
Traumatic interphalangeal joint amputation of thumb

S68.51 Complete traumatic transphalangeal amputation of thumb
- S68.511 Complete traumatic transphalangeal amputation of right thumb S
- S68.512 Complete traumatic transphalangeal amputation of left thumb S
- S68.519 Complete traumatic transphalangeal amputation of unspecified thumb S

S68.52 Partial traumatic transphalangeal amputation of thumb
- S68.521 Partial traumatic transphalangeal amputation of right thumb S
- S68.522 Partial traumatic transphalangeal amputation of left thumb S
- S68.529 Partial traumatic transphalangeal amputation of unspecified thumb S

S68.6 Traumatic transphalangeal amputation of other and unspecified finger

S68.61 Complete traumatic transphalangeal amputation of other and unspecified finger(s)
- S68.610 Complete traumatic transphalangeal amputation of right index finger S
- S68.611 Complete traumatic transphalangeal amputation of left index finger S
- S68.612 Complete traumatic transphalangeal amputation of right middle finger S
- S68.613 Complete traumatic transphalangeal amputation of left middle finger S
- S68.614 Complete traumatic transphalangeal amputation of right ring finger S
- S68.615 Complete traumatic transphalangeal amputation of left ring finger S
- S68.616 Complete traumatic transphalangeal amputation of right little finger S
- S68.617 Complete traumatic transphalangeal amputation of left little finger S
- S68.618 Complete traumatic transphalangeal amputation of other finger S
  Complete traumatic transphalangeal amputation of specified finger with unspecified laterality
- S68.619 Complete traumatic transphalangeal amputation of unspecified finger S

S68.62 Partial traumatic transphalangeal amputation of other and unspecified finger
- S68.620 Partial traumatic transphalangeal amputation of right index finger S
- S68.621 Partial traumatic transphalangeal amputation of left index finger S
- S68.622 Partial traumatic transphalangeal amputation of right middle finger S
- S68.623 Partial traumatic transphalangeal amputation of left middle finger S
- S68.624 Partial traumatic transphalangeal amputation of right ring finger S
- S68.625 Partial traumatic transphalangeal amputation of left ring finger S
- S68.626 Partial traumatic transphalangeal amputation of right little finger S
- S68.627 Partial traumatic transphalangeal amputation of left little finger S
- S68.628 Partial traumatic transphalangeal amputation of other finger S
  Partial traumatic transphalangeal amputation of specified finger with unspecified laterality
- S68.629 Partial traumatic transphalangeal amputation of unspecified finger S

S68.7 Traumatic transmetacarpal amputation of hand

S68.71 Complete traumatic transmetacarpal amputation of hand
- S68.711 Complete traumatic transmetacarpal amputation of right hand A, S
- S68.712 Complete traumatic transmetacarpal amputation of left hand A, S
- S68.719 Complete traumatic transmetacarpal amputation of unspecified hand A, S

S68.72 Partial traumatic transmetacarpal amputation of hand
- S68.721 Partial traumatic transmetacarpal amputation of right hand A, S
- S68.722 Partial traumatic transmetacarpal amputation of left hand A, S
- S68.729 Partial traumatic transmetacarpal amputation of unspecified hand A, S

S69 Other and unspecified injuries of wrist, hand and finger(s)

The appropriate 7th character is to be added to each code from category S69

A	initial encounter
D	subsequent encounter
S	sequela

S69.8 Other specified injuries of wrist, hand and finger(s)
- X S69.80 Other specified injuries of unspecified wrist, hand and finger(s)
- X S69.81 Other specified injuries of right wrist, hand and finger(s)
- X S69.82 Other specified injuries of left wrist, hand and finger(s)

S69.9 Unspecified injury of wrist, hand and finger(s)
- X S69.90 Unspecified injury of unspecified wrist, hand and finger(s)
- X S69.91 Unspecified injury of right wrist, hand and finger(s)
- X S69.92 Unspecified injury of left wrist, hand and finger(s)

INJURIES TO THE HIP AND THIGH (S70-S79)

Excludes2 burns and corrosions (T20-T32)
frostbite (T33-T34)
snake bite (T63.0-)
venomous insect bite or sting (T63.4-)

S70 Superficial injury of hip and thigh
The appropriate 7th character is to be added to each code from category S70

A	initial encounter
D	subsequent encounter
S	sequela

- S70.0 Contusion of hip
  - X S70.00 Contusion of unspecified hip
  - X S70.01 Contusion of right hip
  - X S70.02 Contusion of left hip
- S70.1 Contusion of thigh
  - X S70.10 Contusion of unspecified thigh
  - X S70.11 Contusion of right thigh
  - X S70.12 Contusion of left thigh
- S70.2 Other superficial injuries of hip
  - S70.21 Abrasion of hip
    - S70.211 Abrasion, right hip
    - S70.212 Abrasion, left hip
    - S70.219 Abrasion, unspecified hip
  - S70.22 Blister (nonthermal) of hip
    - S70.221 Blister (nonthermal), right hip
    - S70.222 Blister (nonthermal), left hip
    - S70.229 Blister (nonthermal), unspecified hip
  - S70.24 External constriction of hip
    - S70.241 External constriction, right hip
    - S70.242 External constriction, left hip
    - S70.249 External constriction, unspecified hip
  - S70.25 Superficial foreign body of hip
    Splinter in the hip
    - S70.251 Superficial foreign body, right hip
    - S70.252 Superficial foreign body, left hip
    - S70.259 Superficial foreign body, unspecified hip
  - S70.26 Insect bite (nonvenomous) of hip
    - S70.261 Insect bite (nonvenomous), right hip
    - S70.262 Insect bite (nonvenomous), left hip
    - S70.269 Insect bite (nonvenomous), unspecified hip
  - S70.27 Other superficial bite of hip
    Excludes1 open bite of hip (S71.05-)
    - S70.271 Other superficial bite of hip, right hip
    - S70.272 Other superficial bite of hip, left hip
    - S70.279 Other superficial bite of hip, unspecified hip
- S70.3 Other superficial injuries of thigh
  - S70.31 Abrasion of thigh
    - S70.311 Abrasion, right thigh
    - S70.312 Abrasion, left thigh
    - S70.319 Abrasion, unspecified thigh
  - S70.32 Blister (nonthermal) of thigh
    - S70.321 Blister (nonthermal), right thigh
    - S70.322 Blister (nonthermal), left thigh
    - S70.329 Blister (nonthermal), unspecified thigh
  - S70.34 External constriction of thigh
    - S70.341 External constriction, right thigh
    - S70.342 External constriction, left thigh
    - S70.349 External constriction, unspecified thigh
  - S70.35 Superficial foreign body of thigh
    Splinter in the thigh
    - S70.351 Superficial foreign body, right thigh
    - S70.352 Superficial foreign body, left thigh
    - S70.359 Superficial foreign body, unspecified thigh
  - S70.36 Insect bite (nonvenomous) of thigh
    - S70.361 Insect bite (nonvenomous), right thigh
    - S70.362 Insect bite (nonvenomous), left thigh
    - S70.369 Insect bite (nonvenomous), unspecified thigh
  - S70.37 Other superficial bite of thigh
    Excludes1 open bite of thigh (S71.15)
    - S70.371 Other superficial bite of right thigh
    - S70.372 Other superficial bite of left thigh
    - S70.379 Other superficial bite of unspecified thigh
- S70.9 Unspecified superficial injury of hip and thigh
  - S70.91 Unspecified superficial injury of hip
    - S70.911 Unspecified superficial injury of right hip
    - S70.912 Unspecified superficial injury of left hip
    - S70.919 Unspecified superficial injury of unspecified hip
  - S70.92 Unspecified superficial injury of thigh
    - S70.921 Unspecified superficial injury of right thigh
    - S70.922 Unspecified superficial injury of left thigh
    - S70.929 Unspecified superficial injury of unspecified thigh

S71 Open wound of hip and thigh
Code also any associated wound infection
Excludes1 open fracture of hip and thigh (S72.-)
traumatic amputation of hip and thigh (S78.-)
Excludes2 bite of venomous animal (T63.-)
open wound of ankle, foot and toes (S91.-)
open wound of knee and lower leg (S81.-)
The appropriate 7th character is to be added to each code from category S71

A	initial encounter
D	subsequent encounter
S	sequela

- S71.0 Open wound of hip
  - S71.00 Unspecified open wound of hip
    - S71.001 Unspecified open wound, right hip
    - S71.002 Unspecified open wound, left hip
    - S71.009 Unspecified open wound, unspecified hip
  - S71.01 Laceration without foreign body of hip
    - S71.011 Laceration without foreign body, right hip
    - S71.012 Laceration without foreign body, left hip
    - S71.019 Laceration without foreign body, unspecified hip

- S71.02 **Laceration with foreign body of hip**
  - S71.021 Laceration with foreign body, right hip
  - S71.022 Laceration with foreign body, left hip
  - S71.029 Laceration with foreign body, unspecified hip
- S71.03 **Puncture wound without foreign body of hip**
  - S71.031 Puncture wound without foreign body, right hip
  - S71.032 Puncture wound without foreign body, left hip
  - S71.039 Puncture wound without foreign body, unspecified hip
- S71.04 **Puncture wound with foreign body of hip**
  - S71.041 Puncture wound with foreign body, right hip
  - S71.042 Puncture wound with foreign body, left hip
  - S71.049 Puncture wound with foreign body, unspecified hip
- S71.05 **Open bite of hip**
  Bite of hip NOS
  Excludes1 superficial bite of hip (S70.26, S70.27)
  - S71.051 Open bite, right hip
  - S71.052 Open bite, left hip
  - S71.059 Open bite, unspecified hip

S71.1 **Open wound of thigh**

- S71.10 **Unspecified open wound of thigh**
  - S71.101 Unspecified open wound, right thigh
  - S71.102 Unspecified open wound, left thigh
  - S71.109 Unspecified open wound, unspecified thigh
- S71.11 **Laceration without foreign body of thigh**
  - S71.111 Laceration without foreign body, right thigh
  - S71.112 Laceration without foreign body, left thigh
  - S71.119 Laceration without foreign body, unspecified thigh
- S71.12 **Laceration with foreign body of thigh**
  - S71.121 Laceration with foreign body, right thigh
  - S71.122 Laceration with foreign body, left thigh
  - S71.129 Laceration with foreign body, unspecified thigh
- S71.13 **Puncture wound without foreign body of thigh**
  - S71.131 Puncture wound without foreign body, right thigh
  - S71.132 Puncture wound without foreign body, left thigh
  - S71.139 Puncture wound without foreign body, unspecified thigh
- S71.14 **Puncture wound with foreign body of thigh**
  - S71.141 Puncture wound with foreign body, right thigh
  - S71.142 Puncture wound with foreign body, left thigh
  - S71.149 Puncture wound with foreign body, unspecified thigh
- S71.15 **Open bite of thigh**
  Bite of thigh NOS
  Excludes1 superficial bite of thigh (S70.37-)
  - S71.151 Open bite, right thigh
  - S71.152 Open bite, left thigh
  - S71.159 Open bite, unspecified thigh

S72 **Fracture of femur**

Note: A fracture not indicated as displaced or nondisplaced should be coded to displaced

A fracture not indicated as open or closed should be coded to closed

The open fracture designations are based on the Gustilo open fracture classification

Excludes1 traumatic amputation of hip and thigh (S78.-)

Excludes2 fracture of lower leg and ankle (S82.-)
fracture of foot (S92.-)
periprosthetic fracture of prosthetic implant of hip (M97.0-)

The appropriate 7th character is to be added to all codes from category S72

A	initial encounter for closed fracture
B	initial encounter for open fracture type I or II initial encounter for open fracture NOS
C	initial encounter for open fracture type IIIA, IIIB, or IIIC
D	subsequent encounter for closed fracture with routine healing
E	subsequent encounter for open fracture type I or II with routine healing
F	subsequent encounter for open fracture type IIIA, IIIB, or IIIC with routine healing
G	subsequent encounter for closed fracture with delayed healing
H	subsequent encounter for open fracture type I or II with delayed healing
J	subsequent encounter for open fracture type IIIA, IIIB, or IIIC with delayed healing
K	subsequent encounter for closed fracture with nonunion
M	subsequent encounter for open fracture type I or II with nonunion
N	subsequent encounter for open fracture type IIIA, IIIB, or IIIC with nonunion
P	subsequent encounter for closed fracture with malunion
Q	subsequent encounter for open fracture type I or II with malunion
R	subsequent encounter for open fracture type IIIA, IIIB, or IIIC with malunion
S	sequela

S72.0 **Fracture of head and neck of femur**
Excludes2 physeal fracture of upper end of femur (S79.0-)

- S72.00 **Fracture of unspecified part of neck of femur**
  Fracture of hip NOS
  Fracture of neck of femur NOS
  - S72.001 Fracture of unspecified part of neck of right femur A, B, C
  - S72.002 Fracture of unspecified part of neck of left femur A, B, C
    Coding Clinic: 2015, Q4, P37, Q1, P17
  - S72.009 Fracture of unspecified part of neck of unspecified femur A, B, C
- S72.01 **Unspecified intracapsular fracture of femur**
  Subcapital fracture of femur
  - S72.011 Unspecified intracapsular fracture of right femur A, B, C
  - S72.012 Unspecified intracapsular fracture of left femur A, B, C
  - S72.019 Unspecified intracapsular fracture of unspecified femur A, B, C

CHAPTER 19 (S00-T88)

S72.02 Fracture of **epiphysis** (separation) (upper) of femur
Transepiphyseal fracture of femur
Fracture and separation across growth plate
Excludes1 capital femoral epiphyseal fracture (pediatric) of femur (S79.01-)
Salter-Harris Type I physeal fracture of upper end of femur (S79.01-)

S72.021 **Displaced** fracture of epiphysis (separation) (upper) of **right** femur A, B, C
S72.022 **Displaced** fracture of epiphysis (separation) (upper) of **left** femur A, B, C
S72.023 **Displaced** fracture of epiphysis (separation) (upper) of **unspecified** femur A, B, C
S72.024 **Nondisplaced** fracture of epiphysis (separation) (upper) of **right** femur A, B, C
S72.025 **Nondisplaced** fracture of epiphysis (separation) (upper) of **left** femur A, B, C
S72.026 **Nondisplaced** fracture of epiphysis (separation) (upper) of **unspecified** femur A, B, C

S72.03 **Midcervical** fracture of femur
Transcervical fracture of femur NOS

S72.031 **Displaced** midcervical fracture of **right** femur A, B, C
S72.032 **Displaced** midcervical fracture of **left** femur A, B, C
S72.033 **Displaced** midcervical fracture of **unspecified** femur A, B, C
S72.034 **Nondisplaced** midcervical fracture of **right** femur A, B, C
S72.035 **Nondisplaced** midcervical fracture of **left** femur A, B, C
S72.036 **Nondisplaced** midcervical fracture of **unspecified** femur A, B, C

S72.04 Fracture of **base of neck** of femur
Cervicotrochanteric fracture of femur

S72.041 **Displaced** fracture of base of neck of **right** femur A, B, C
S72.042 **Displaced** fracture of base of neck of **left** femur A, B, C
S72.043 **Displaced** fracture of base of neck of **unspecified** femur A, B, C
S72.044 **Nondisplaced** fracture of base of neck of **right** femur A, B, C
S72.045 **Nondisplaced** fracture of base of neck of **left** femur A, B, C
S72.046 **Nondisplaced** fracture of base of neck of **unspecified** femur A, B, C

S72.05 **Unspecified** fracture of **head** of femur
Fracture of head of femur NOS

S72.051 **Unspecified** fracture of head of **right** femur A, B, C
S72.052 **Unspecified** fracture of head of **left** femur A, B, C
S72.059 **Unspecified** fracture of head of **unspecified** femur A, B, C

S72.06 **Articular** fracture of head of femur

S72.061 **Displaced** articular fracture of head of **right** femur A, B, C
S72.062 **Displaced** articular fracture of head of **left** femur A, B, C
S72.063 **Displaced** articular fracture of head of **unspecified** femur A, B, C
S72.064 **Nondisplaced** articular fracture of head of **right** femur A, B, C
S72.065 **Nondisplaced** articular fracture of head of **left** femur A, B, C
S72.066 **Nondisplaced** articular fracture of head of **unspecified** femur A, B, C

S72.09 **Other** fracture of **head and neck** of femur

S72.091 **Other** fracture of head and neck of **right** femur A, B, C
S72.092 **Other** fracture of head and neck of **left** femur A, B, C
S72.099 **Other** fracture of head and neck of **unspecified** femur A, B, C

S72.1 **Pertrochanteric** fracture
Fracture extending close to, but not into, joint

S72.10 **Unspecified trochanteric** fracture of femur
Fracture of trochanter NOS

S72.101 Unspecified trochanteric fracture of **right** femur A, B, C
S72.102 Unspecified trochanteric fracture of **left** femur A, B, C
S72.109 Unspecified trochanteric fracture of **unspecified** femur A, B, C

S72.11 Fracture of **greater trochanter** of femur

S72.111 **Displaced** fracture of greater trochanter of **right** femur A, B, C
S72.112 **Displaced** fracture of greater trochanter of **left** femur A, B, C
S72.113 **Displaced** fracture of greater trochanter of **unspecified** femur A, B, C
S72.114 **Nondisplaced** fracture of greater trochanter of **right** femur A, B, C
S72.115 **Nondisplaced** fracture of greater trochanter of **left** femur A, B, C
S72.116 **Nondisplaced** fracture of greater trochanter of **unspecified** femur A, B, C

S72.12 Fracture of **lesser trochanter** of femur

S72.121 **Displaced** fracture of lesser trochanter of **right** femur A, B, C
S72.122 **Displaced** fracture of lesser trochanter of **left** femur A, B, C
S72.123 **Displaced** fracture of lesser trochanter of **unspecified** femur A, B, C
S72.124 **Nondisplaced** fracture of lesser trochanter of **right** femur A, B, C
S72.125 **Nondisplaced** fracture of lesser trochanter of **left** femur A, B, C
S72.126 **Nondisplaced** fracture of lesser trochanter of **unspecified** femur A, B, C

S72.13 **Apophyseal** fracture of femur
Pertaining to articulations between articular facets of adjacent vertebrae
Excludes1 chronic (nontraumatic) slipped upper femoral epiphysis (M93.0-)

S72.131 **Displaced** apophyseal fracture of **right** femur A, B, C
S72.132 **Displaced** apophyseal fracture of **left** femur A, B, C
S72.133 **Displaced** apophyseal fracture of **unspecified** femur A, B, C
S72.134 **Nondisplaced** apophyseal fracture of **right** femur A, B, C
S72.135 **Nondisplaced** apophyseal fracture of **left** femur A, B, C
S72.136 **Nondisplaced** apophyseal fracture of **unspecified** femur A, B, C

S72.14 Intertrochanteric fracture of femur
S72.141 Displaced intertrochanteric fracture of right femur A, B, C
Coding Clinic: 2016, Q3, P17
S72.142 Displaced intertrochanteric fracture of left femur A, B, C
S72.143 Displaced intertrochanteric fracture of unspecified femur A, B, C
S72.144 Nondisplaced intertrochanteric fracture of right femur A, B, C
S72.145 Nondisplaced intertrochanteric fracture of left femur A, B, C
S72.146 Nondisplaced intertrochanteric fracture of unspecified femur A, B, C

S72.2 Subtrochanteric fracture of femur
Subtrochanteric: inferior to trochanter
X S72.21 Displaced subtrochanteric fracture of right femur A, B, C
X S72.22 Displaced subtrochanteric fracture of left femur A, B, C
X S72.23 Displaced subtrochanteric fracture of unspecified femur A, B, C
X S72.24 Nondisplaced subtrochanteric fracture of right femur A, B, C
X S72.25 Nondisplaced subtrochanteric fracture of left femur A, B, C
X S72.26 Nondisplaced subtrochanteric fracture of unspecified femur A, B, C

S72.3 Fracture of shaft of femur
S72.30 Unspecified fracture of shaft of femur
S72.301 Unspecified fracture of shaft of right femur A, B, C
Coding Clinic: 2018, Q2, P12
S72.302 Unspecified fracture of shaft of left femur A, B, C
S72.309 Unspecified fracture of shaft of unspecified femur A, B, C
S72.32 Transverse fracture of shaft of femur
S72.321 Displaced transverse fracture of shaft of right femur A, B, C
S72.322 Displaced transverse fracture of shaft of left femur A, B, C
S72.323 Displaced transverse fracture of shaft of unspecified femur A, B, C
S72.324 Nondisplaced transverse fracture of shaft of right femur A, B, C
S72.325 Nondisplaced transverse fracture of shaft of left femur A, B, C
S72.326 Nondisplaced transverse fracture of shaft of unspecified femur A, B, C
S72.33 Oblique fracture of shaft of femur
S72.331 Displaced oblique fracture of shaft of right femur A, B, C
S72.332 Displaced oblique fracture of shaft of left femur A, B, C
S72.333 Displaced oblique fracture of shaft of unspecified femur A, B, C
S72.334 Nondisplaced oblique fracture of shaft of right femur A, B, C
S72.335 Nondisplaced oblique fracture of shaft of left femur A, B, C
S72.336 Nondisplaced oblique fracture of shaft of unspecified femur A, B, C
S72.34 Spiral fracture of shaft of femur
S72.341 Displaced spiral fracture of shaft of right femur A, B, C
S72.342 Displaced spiral fracture of shaft of left femur A, B, C
S72.343 Displaced spiral fracture of shaft of unspecified femur A, B, C
S72.344 Nondisplaced spiral fracture of shaft of right femur A, B, C
S72.345 Nondisplaced spiral fracture of shaft of left femur A, B, C
S72.346 Nondisplaced spiral fracture of shaft of unspecified femur A, B, C
S72.35 Comminuted fracture of shaft of femur
S72.351 Displaced comminuted fracture of shaft of right femur A, B, C
S72.352 Displaced comminuted fracture of shaft of left femur A, B, C
S72.353 Displaced comminuted fracture of shaft of unspecified femur A, B, C
S72.354 Nondisplaced comminuted fracture of shaft of right femur A, B, C
S72.355 Nondisplaced comminuted fracture of shaft of left femur A, B, C
S72.356 Nondisplaced comminuted fracture of shaft of unspecified femur A, B, C
S72.36 Segmental fracture of shaft of femur
S72.361 Displaced segmental fracture of shaft of right femur A, B, C
S72.362 Displaced segmental fracture of shaft of left femur A, B, C
S72.363 Displaced segmental fracture of shaft of unspecified femur A, B, C
S72.364 Nondisplaced segmental fracture of shaft of right femur A, B, C
S72.365 Nondisplaced segmental fracture of shaft of left femur A, B, C
S72.366 Nondisplaced segmental fracture of shaft of unspecified femur A, B, C
S72.39 Other fracture of shaft of femur
S72.391 Other fracture of shaft of right femur A, B, C
S72.392 Other fracture of shaft of left femur A, B, C
S72.399 Other fracture of shaft of unspecified femur A, B, C

S72.4 Fracture of lower end of femur
Fracture of distal end of femur
Excludes2 fracture of shaft of femur (S72.3-)
physeal fracture of lower end of femur (S79.1-)
S72.40 Unspecified fracture of lower end of femur
S72.401 Unspecified fracture of lower end of right femur A, B, C
Coding Clinic: 2016, Q4, P43
S72.402 Unspecified fracture of lower end of left femur A, B, C
S72.409 Unspecified fracture of lower end of unspecified femur A, B, C

CHAPTER 19 (SØØ-T88)

S72.41 Unspecified condyle fracture of lower end of femur
Condyle fracture of femur NOS

- **S72.411 Displaced unspecified condyle fracture of lower end of right femur** A, B, C
- **S72.412 Displaced unspecified condyle fracture of lower end of left femur** A, B, C
- **S72.413 Displaced unspecified condyle fracture of lower end of unspecified femur** A, B, C
- **S72.414 Nondisplaced unspecified condyle fracture of lower end of right femur** A, B, C
- **S72.415 Nondisplaced unspecified condyle fracture of lower end of left femur** A, B, C
- **S72.416 Nondisplaced unspecified condyle fracture of lower end of unspecified femur** A, B, C

S72.42 Fracture of lateral condyle of femur

- **S72.421 Displaced fracture of lateral condyle of right femur** A, B, C
- **S72.422 Displaced fracture of lateral condyle of left femur** A, B, C
- **S72.423 Displaced fracture of lateral condyle of unspecified femur** A, B, C
- **S72.424 Nondisplaced fracture of lateral condyle of right femur** A, B, C
- **S72.425 Nondisplaced fracture of lateral condyle of left femur** A, B, C
- **S72.426 Nondisplaced fracture of lateral condyle of unspecified femur** A, B, C

S72.43 Fracture of medial condyle of femur

- **S72.431 Displaced fracture of medial condyle of right femur** A, B, C
- **S72.432 Displaced fracture of medial condyle of left femur** A, B, C
- **S72.433 Displaced fracture of medial condyle of unspecified femur** A, B, C
- **S72.434 Nondisplaced fracture of medial condyle of right femur** A, B, C
- **S72.435 Nondisplaced fracture of medial condyle of left femur** A, B, C
- **S72.436 Nondisplaced fracture of medial condyle of unspecified femur** A, B, C

S72.44 Fracture of lower epiphysis (separation) of femur

Excludes1 Salter-Harris Type I physeal fracture of lower end of femur (S79.11-)

- **S72.441 Displaced fracture of lower epiphysis (separation) of right femur** A, B, C
- **S72.442 Displaced fracture of lower epiphysis (separation) of left femur** A, B, C
- **S72.443 Displaced fracture of lower epiphysis (separation) of unspecified femur** A, B, C
- **S72.444 Nondisplaced fracture of lower epiphysis (separation) of right femur** A, B, C
- **S72.445 Nondisplaced fracture of lower epiphysis (separation) of left femur** A, B, C
- **S72.446 Nondisplaced fracture of lower epiphysis (separation) of unspecified femur** A, B, C

S72.45 Supracondylar fracture without intracondylar extension of lower end of femur
Supracondylar fracture of lower end of femur NOS

Excludes1 supracondylar fracture with intracondylar extension of lower end of femur (S72.46-)

- **S72.451 Displaced supracondylar fracture without intracondylar extension of lower end of right femur** A, B, C
- **S72.452 Displaced supracondylar fracture without intracondylar extension of lower end of left femur** A, B, C
- **S72.453 Displaced supracondylar fracture without intracondylar extension of lower end of unspecified femur** A, B, C
- **S72.454 Nondisplaced supracondylar fracture without intracondylar extension of lower end of right femur** A, B, C
- **S72.455 Nondisplaced supracondylar fracture without intracondylar extension of lower end of left femur** A, B, C
- **S72.456 Nondisplaced supracondylar fracture without intracondylar extension of lower end of unspecified femur** A, B, C

S72.46 Supracondylar fracture with intracondylar extension of lower end of femur

Excludes1 supracondylar fracture without intracondylar extension of lower end of femur (S72.45-)

- **S72.461 Displaced supracondylar fracture with intracondylar extension of lower end of right femur** A, B, C
- **S72.462 Displaced supracondylar fracture with intracondylar extension of lower end of left femur** A, B, C
- **S72.463 Displaced supracondylar fracture with intracondylar extension of lower end of unspecified femur** A, B, C
- **S72.464 Nondisplaced supracondylar fracture with intracondylar extension of lower end of right femur** A, B, C
- **S72.465 Nondisplaced supracondylar fracture with intracondylar extension of lower end of left femur** A, B, C
- **S72.466 Nondisplaced supracondylar fracture with intracondylar extension of lower end of unspecified femur** A, B, C

S72.47 Torus fracture of lower end of femur
The appropriate 7th character is to be added to all codes in subcategory S72.47

A	initial encounter for closed fracture
D	subsequent encounter for fracture with routine healing
G	subsequent encounter for fracture with delayed healing
K	subsequent encounter for fracture with nonunion
P	subsequent encounter for fracture with malunion
S	sequela

- **S72.471 Torus fracture of lower end of right femur** A
- **S72.472 Torus fracture of lower end of left femur** A
- **S72.479 Torus fracture of lower end of unspecified femur** A

S72.49 Other fracture of lower end of femur
S72.491 Other fracture of lower end of right femur A, B, C
S72.492 Other fracture of lower end of left femur A, B, C
S72.499 Other fracture of lower end of unspecified femur A, B, C
S72.8 Other fracture of femur
S72.8X Other fracture of femur
S72.8X1 Other fracture of right femur A, B, C
S72.8X2 Other fracture of left femur A, B, C
S72.8X9 Other fracture of unspecified femur A, B, C
S72.9 Unspecified fracture of femur
Fracture of thigh NOS
Fracture of upper leg NOS
Excludes1 fracture of hip NOS (S72.00-, S72.01-)
X S72.90 Unspecified fracture of unspecified femur A, B, C
Coding Clinic: 2012, Q4, P94
X S72.91 Unspecified fracture of right femur A, B, C
X S72.92 Unspecified fracture of left femur A, B, C

S73 Dislocation and sprain of joint and ligaments of hip
Includes avulsion of joint or ligament of hip
laceration of cartilage, joint or ligament of hip
sprain of cartilage, joint or ligament of hip
traumatic hemarthrosis of joint or ligament of hip
traumatic rupture of joint or ligament of hip
traumatic subluxation of joint or ligament of hip
traumatic tear of joint or ligament of hip
Code also any associated open wound
Excludes2 strain of muscle, fascia and tendon of hip and thigh (S76.-)
The appropriate 7th character is to be added to each code from category S73

A	initial encounter
D	subsequent encounter
S	sequela

S73.0 Subluxation and dislocation of hip
Out of position
Excludes2 dislocation and subluxation of hip prosthesis (T84.020, T84.021)
S73.00 Unspecified subluxation and dislocation of hip
Dislocation of hip NOS
Subluxation of hip NOS
S73.001 Unspecified subluxation of right hip A
S73.002 Unspecified subluxation of left hip A
S73.003 Unspecified subluxation of unspecified hip A
S73.004 Unspecified dislocation of right hip A
S73.005 Unspecified dislocation of left hip A
S73.006 Unspecified dislocation of unspecified hip A
S73.01 Posterior subluxation and dislocation of hip
S73.011 Posterior subluxation of right hip A
S73.012 Posterior subluxation of left hip A
S73.013 Posterior subluxation of unspecified hip A
S73.014 Posterior dislocation of right hip A
S73.015 Posterior dislocation of left hip A
S73.016 Posterior dislocation of unspecified hip A
S73.02 Obturator subluxation and dislocation of hip
S73.021 Obturator subluxation of right hip A
S73.022 Obturator subluxation of left hip A
S73.023 Obturator subluxation of unspecified hip A
S73.024 Obturator dislocation of right hip A
S73.025 Obturator dislocation of left hip A
S73.026 Obturator dislocation of unspecified hip A
S73.03 Other anterior subluxation and dislocation of hip
S73.031 Other anterior subluxation of right hip A
S73.032 Other anterior subluxation of left hip A
S73.033 Other anterior subluxation of unspecified hip A
S73.034 Other anterior dislocation of right hip A
S73.035 Other anterior dislocation of left hip A
S73.036 Other anterior dislocation of unspecified hip A
S73.04 Central subluxation and dislocation of hip
S73.041 Central subluxation of right hip A
S73.042 Central subluxation of left hip A
S73.043 Central subluxation of unspecified hip A
S73.044 Central dislocation of right hip A
S73.045 Central dislocation of left hip A
S73.046 Central dislocation of unspecified hip A
S73.1 Sprain of hip
S73.10 Unspecified sprain of hip
S73.101 Unspecified sprain of right hip
S73.102 Unspecified sprain of left hip
S73.109 Unspecified sprain of unspecified hip
S73.11 Iliofemoral ligament sprain of hip
S73.111 Iliofemoral ligament sprain of right hip
S73.112 Iliofemoral ligament sprain of left hip
S73.119 Iliofemoral ligament sprain of unspecified hip
S73.12 Ischiocapsular (ligament) sprain of hip
S73.121 Ischiocapsular ligament sprain of right hip
S73.122 Ischiocapsular ligament sprain of left hip
S73.129 Ischiocapsular ligament sprain of unspecified hip
S73.19 Other sprain of hip
S73.191 Other sprain of right hip
S73.192 Other sprain of left hip
S73.199 Other sprain of unspecified hip

S74 Injury of nerves at hip and thigh level

Code also any associated open wound (S71.-)

Excludes2 injury of nerves at ankle and foot level (S94.-)
injury of nerves at lower leg level (S84.-)

The appropriate 7th character is to be added to each code from category S74

A	initial encounter
D	subsequent encounter
S	sequela

S74.0 Injury of **sciatic nerve** at hip and thigh level

X **S74.00** Injury of sciatic nerve at hip and thigh level, **unspecified** leg

X **S74.01** Injury of sciatic nerve at hip and thigh level, **right** leg

X **S74.02** Injury of sciatic nerve at hip and thigh level, **left** leg

S74.1 Injury of **femoral nerve** at hip and thigh level

X **S74.10** Injury of femoral nerve at hip and thigh level, **unspecified** leg

X **S74.11** Injury of femoral nerve at hip and thigh level, **right** leg

X **S74.12** Injury of femoral nerve at hip and thigh level, **left** leg

S74.2 Injury of **cutaneous sensory nerve** at hip and thigh level

X **S74.20** Injury of cutaneous sensory nerve at hip and thigh level, **unspecified** leg

X **S74.21** Injury of cutaneous sensory nerve at hip and high level, **right** leg

X **S74.22** Injury of cutaneous sensory nerve at hip and thigh level, **left** leg

S74.8 Injury of **other nerves** at hip and thigh level

S74.8X Injury of other nerves at hip and thigh level

S74.8X1 Injury of other nerves at hip and thigh level, **right** leg

S74.8X2 Injury of other nerves at hip and thigh level, **left** leg

S74.8X9 Injury of other nerves at hip and thigh level, **unspecified** leg

S74.9 Injury of **unspecified nerve** at hip and thigh level

X **S74.90** Injury of unspecified nerve at hip and thigh level, **unspecified** leg

X **S74.91** Injury of unspecified nerve at hip and thigh level, **right** leg

X **S74.92** Injury of unspecified nerve at hip and thigh level, **left** leg

S75 Injury of blood vessels at hip and thigh level

Code also any associated open wound (S71.-)

Excludes2 injury of blood vessels at lower leg level (S85.-)
injury of popliteal artery (S85.0)

The appropriate 7th character is to be added to each code from category S75

A	initial encounter
D	subsequent encounter
S	sequela

S75.0 Injury of **femoral artery**

S75.00 **Unspecified** injury of femoral artery

S75.001 Unspecified injury of femoral artery, **right** leg

S75.002 Unspecified injury of femoral artery, **left** leg

S75.009 Unspecified injury of femoral artery, **unspecified** leg

S75.01 **Minor laceration** of femoral artery
Incomplete transection of femoral artery
Laceration of femoral artery NOS
Superficial laceration of femoral artery

S75.011 Minor laceration of femoral artery, **right** leg

S75.012 Minor laceration of femoral artery, **left** leg

S75.019 Minor laceration of femoral artery, **unspecified** leg

S75.02 **Major laceration** of femoral artery
Complete transection of femoral artery
Traumatic rupture of femoral artery

S75.021 Major laceration of femoral artery, **right** leg

S75.022 Major laceration of femoral artery, **left** leg

S75.029 Major laceration of femoral artery, **unspecified** leg

S75.09 **Other specified** injury of femoral artery

S75.091 Other specified injury of femoral artery, **right** leg

S75.092 Other specified injury of femoral artery, **left** leg

S75.099 Other specified injury of femoral artery, **unspecified** leg

S75.1 Injury of **femoral vein** at hip and thigh level

S75.10 **Unspecified** injury of femoral vein at hip and thigh level

S75.101 Unspecified injury of femoral vein at hip and thigh level, **right** leg

S75.102 Unspecified injury of femoral vein at hip and thigh level, **left** leg

S75.109 Unspecified injury of femoral vein at hip and thigh level, **unspecified** leg

S75.11 **Minor laceration** of femoral vein at hip and thigh level
Incomplete transection of femoral vein at hip and thigh level
Laceration of femoral vein at hip and thigh level NOS
Superficial laceration of femoral vein at hip and thigh level

S75.111 Minor laceration of femoral vein at hip and thigh level, **right** leg

S75.112 Minor laceration of femoral vein at hip and thigh level, **left** leg

S75.119 Minor laceration of femoral vein at hip and thigh level, **unspecified** leg

S75.12 **Major laceration** of femoral vein at hip and thigh level
Complete transection of femoral vein at hip and thigh level
Traumatic rupture of femoral vein at hip and thigh level

S75.121 Major laceration of femoral vein at hip and thigh level, **right** leg

S75.122 Major laceration of femoral vein at hip and thigh level, **left** leg

S75.129 Major laceration of femoral vein at hip and thigh level, **unspecified** leg

S75.19 **Other specified** injury of femoral vein at hip and thigh level

S75.191 Other specified injury of femoral vein at hip and thigh level, **right** leg

S75.192 Other specified injury of femoral vein at hip and thigh level, **left** leg

S75.199 Other specified injury of femoral vein at hip and thigh level, **unspecified** leg

- S75.2 Injury of **greater saphenous vein** at hip and thigh level
  - **Excludes1** greater saphenous vein NOS (S85.3)
  - S75.20 **Unspecified** injury of greater saphenous vein at hip and thigh level
    - S75.201 Unspecified injury of greater saphenous vein at hip and thigh level, **right** leg
    - S75.202 Unspecified injury of greater saphenous vein at hip and thigh level, **left** leg
    - S75.209 Unspecified injury of greater saphenous vein at hip and thigh level, **unspecified** leg
  - S75.21 **Minor laceration** of greater saphenous vein at hip and thigh level
    - Incomplete transection of greater saphenous vein at hip and thigh level
    - Laceration of greater saphenous vein at hip and thigh level NOS
    - Superficial laceration of greater saphenous vein at hip and thigh level
    - S75.211 Minor laceration of greater saphenous vein at hip and thigh level, **right** leg
    - S75.212 Minor laceration of greater saphenous vein at hip and thigh level, **left** leg
    - S75.219 Minor laceration of greater saphenous vein at hip and thigh level, **unspecified** leg
  - S75.22 **Major laceration** of greater saphenous vein at hip and thigh level
    - Complete transection of greater saphenous vein at hip and thigh level
    - Traumatic rupture of greater saphenous vein at hip and thigh level
    - S75.221 Major laceration of greater saphenous vein at hip and thigh level, **right** leg
    - S75.222 Major laceration of greater saphenous vein at hip and thigh level, **left** leg
    - S75.229 Major laceration of greater saphenous vein at hip and thigh level, **unspecified** leg
  - S75.29 **Other specified** injury of greater saphenous vein at hip and thigh level
    - S75.291 Other specified injury of greater saphenous vein at hip and thigh level, **right** leg
    - S75.292 Other specified injury of greater saphenous vein at hip and thigh level, **left** leg
    - S75.299 Other specified injury of greater saphenous vein at hip and thigh level, **unspecified** leg
- S75.8 Injury of **other blood vessels** at hip and thigh level
  - S75.80 **Unspecified** injury of other blood vessels at hip and thigh level
    - S75.801 Unspecified injury of other blood vessels at hip and thigh level, **right** leg
    - S75.802 Unspecified injury of other blood vessels at hip and thigh level, **left** leg
    - S75.809 Unspecified injury of other blood vessels at hip and thigh level, **unspecified** leg
  - S75.81 **Laceration** of other blood vessels at hip and thigh level
    - S75.811 Laceration of other blood vessels at hip and thigh level, **right** leg
    - S75.812 Laceration of other blood vessels at hip and thigh level, **left** leg
    - S75.819 Laceration of other blood vessels at hip and thigh level, **unspecified** leg
  - S75.89 **Other specified** injury of other blood vessels at hip and thigh level
    - S75.891 Other specified injury of other blood vessels at hip and thigh level, **right** leg
    - S75.892 Other specified injury of other blood vessels at hip and thigh level, **left** leg
    - S75.899 Other specified injury of other blood vessels at hip and thigh level, **unspecified** leg
- S75.9 Injury of **unspecified blood vessel** at hip and thigh level
  - S75.90 **Unspecified** injury of unspecified blood vessel at hip and thigh level
    - S75.901 Unspecified injury of unspecified blood vessel at hip and thigh level, **right** leg
    - S75.902 Unspecified injury of unspecified blood vessel at hip and thigh level, **left** leg
    - S75.909 Unspecified injury of unspecified blood vessel at hip and thigh level, **unspecified** leg
  - S75.91 **Laceration** of unspecified blood vessel at hip and thigh level
    - S75.911 Laceration of unspecified blood vessel at hip and thigh level, **right** leg
    - S75.912 Laceration of unspecified blood vessel at hip and thigh level, **left** leg
    - S75.919 Laceration of unspecified blood vessel at hip and thigh level, **unspecified** leg
  - S75.99 **Other specified** injury of unspecified blood vessel at hip and thigh level
    - S75.991 Other specified injury of unspecified blood vessel at hip and thigh level, **right** leg
    - S75.992 Other specified injury of unspecified blood vessel at hip and thigh level, **left** leg
    - S75.999 Other specified injury of unspecified blood vessel at hip and thigh level, **unspecified** leg

- S76 Injury of muscle, fascia and tendon at hip and thigh level
  - Code also any associated open wound (S71.-)
  - **Excludes2** injury of muscle, fascia and tendon at lower leg level (S86)
    - sprain of joint and ligament of hip (S73.1)
  - The appropriate 7th character is to be added to each code from category S76

A	initial encounter
D	subsequent encounter
S	sequela

- S76.0 Injury of muscle, fascia and tendon of hip
  - S76.00 **Unspecified** injury of muscle, fascia and tendon of hip
    - S76.001 Unspecified injury of muscle, fascia and tendon of **right** hip
    - S76.002 Unspecified injury of muscle, fascia and tendon of **left** hip
    - S76.009 Unspecified injury of muscle, fascia and tendon of **unspecified** hip
  - S76.01 **Strain** of muscle, fascia and tendon of hip
    - S76.011 Strain of muscle, fascia and tendon of **right** hip
    - S76.012 Strain of muscle, fascia and tendon of **left** hip
    - S76.019 Strain of muscle, fascia and tendon of **unspecified** hip

- S76.Ø2 **Laceration** of muscle, fascia and tendon of hip
  - S76.Ø21 Laceration of muscle, fascia and tendon of **right** hip
  - S76.Ø22 Laceration of muscle, fascia and tendon of **left** hip
  - S76.Ø29 Laceration of muscle, fascia and tendon of **unspecified** hip
- S76.Ø9 **Other** specified injury of muscle, fascia and tendon of hip
  - S76.Ø91 Other specified injury of muscle, fascia and tendon of **right** hip
  - S76.Ø92 Other specified injury of muscle, fascia and tendon of **left** hip
  - S76.Ø99 Other specified injury of muscle, fascia and tendon of **unspecified** hip

S76.1 Injury of **quadriceps** muscle, fascia and tendon
Injury of patellar ligament (tendon)

- S76.1Ø **Unspecified** injury of quadriceps muscle, fascia and tendon
  - S76.1Ø1 Unspecified injury of **right** quadriceps muscle, fascia and tendon
  - S76.1Ø2 Unspecified injury of **left** quadriceps muscle, fascia and tendon
  - S76.1Ø9 Unspecified injury of **unspecified** quadriceps muscle, fascia and tendon
- S76.11 **Strain** of quadriceps muscle, fascia and tendon
  - S76.111 Strain of **right** quadriceps muscle, fascia and tendon
  - S76.112 Strain of **left** quadriceps muscle, fascia and tendon
  - S76.119 Strain of **unspecified** quadriceps muscle, fascia and tendon
- S76.12 **Laceration** of quadriceps muscle, fascia and tendon
  - S76.121 Laceration of **right** quadriceps muscle, fascia and tendon
  - S76.122 Laceration of **left** quadriceps muscle, fascia and tendon
  - S76.129 Laceration of **unspecified** quadriceps muscle, fascia and tendon
- S76.19 **Other** specified injury of quadriceps muscle, fascia and tendon
  - S76.191 Other specified injury of **right** quadriceps muscle, fascia and tendon
  - S76.192 Other specified injury of **left** quadriceps muscle, fascia and tendon
  - S76.199 Other specified injury of **unspecified** quadriceps muscle, fascia and tendon

S76.2 Injury of **adductor** muscle, fascia and tendon of thigh

- S76.2Ø **Unspecified** injury of adductor muscle, fascia and tendon of thigh
  - S76.2Ø1 Unspecified injury of adductor muscle, fascia and tendon of **right** thigh
  - S76.2Ø2 Unspecified injury of adductor muscle, fascia and tendon of **left** thigh
  - S76.2Ø9 Unspecified injury of adductor muscle, fascia and tendon of **unspecified** thigh
- S76.21 **Strain** of adductor muscle, fascia and tendon of thigh
  - S76.211 Strain of adductor muscle, fascia and tendon of **right** thigh
  - S76.212 Strain of adductor muscle, fascia and tendon of **left** thigh
  - S76.219 Strain of adductor muscle, fascia and tendon of **unspecified** thigh
- S76.22 **Laceration** of adductor muscle, fascia and tendon of thigh
  - S76.221 Laceration of adductor muscle, fascia and tendon of **right** thigh
  - S76.222 Laceration of adductor muscle, fascia and tendon of **left** thigh
  - S76.229 Laceration of adductor muscle, fascia and tendon of **unspecified** thigh
- S76.29 **Other** injury of adductor muscle, fascia and tendon of thigh
  - S76.291 Other injury of adductor muscle, fascia and tendon of **right** thigh
  - S76.292 Other injury of adductor muscle, fascia and tendon of **left** thigh
  - S76.299 Other injury of adductor muscle, fascia and tendon of **unspecified** thigh

S76.3 Injury of muscle, fascia and tendon of the **posterior muscle group** at thigh level

- S76.3Ø **Unspecified** injury of muscle, fascia and tendon of the posterior muscle group at thigh level
  - S76.3Ø1 Unspecified injury of muscle, fascia and tendon of the posterior muscle group at thigh level, **right** thigh
  - S76.3Ø2 Unspecified injury of muscle, fascia and tendon of the posterior muscle group at thigh level, **left** thigh
  - S76.3Ø9 Unspecified injury of muscle, fascia and tendon of the posterior muscle group at thigh level, **unspecified** thigh
- S76.31 **Strain** of muscle, fascia and tendon of the posterior muscle group at thigh level
  - S76.311 Strain of muscle, fascia and tendon of the posterior muscle group at thigh level, **right** thigh
  - S76.312 Strain of muscle, fascia and tendon of the posterior muscle group at thigh level, **left** thigh
  - S76.319 Strain of muscle, fascia and tendon of the posterior muscle group at thigh level, **unspecified** thigh
- S76.32 **Laceration** of muscle, fascia and tendon of the posterior muscle group at thigh level
  - S76.321 Laceration of muscle, fascia and tendon of the posterior muscle group at thigh level, **right** thigh
  - S76.322 Laceration of muscle, fascia and tendon of the posterior muscle group at thigh level, **left** thigh
  - S76.329 Laceration of muscle, fascia and tendon of the posterior muscle group at thigh level, **unspecified** thigh
- S76.39 **Other** specified injury of muscle, fascia and tendon of the posterior muscle group at thigh level
  - S76.391 Other specified injury of muscle, fascia and tendon of the posterior muscle group at thigh level, **right** thigh
  - S76.392 Other specified injury of muscle, fascia and tendon of the posterior muscle group at thigh level, **left** thigh
  - S76.399 Other specified injury of muscle, fascia and tendon of the posterior muscle group at thigh level, **unspecified** thigh

S76.8 Injury of other specified muscles, fascia and tendons at thigh level
- S76.80 Unspecified injury of other specified muscles, fascia and tendons at thigh level
  - S76.801 Unspecified injury of other specified muscles, fascia and tendons at thigh level, right thigh
  - S76.802 Unspecified injury of other specified muscles, fascia and tendons at thigh level, left thigh
  - S76.809 Unspecified injury of other specified muscles, fascia and tendons at thigh level, unspecified thigh
- S76.81 Strain of other specified specified muscles, fascia and tendons at thigh level
  - S76.811 Strain of other specified muscles, fascia and tendons at thigh level, right thigh
  - S76.812 Strain of other specified muscles, fascia and tendons at thigh level, left thigh
  - S76.819 Strain of other specified muscles, fascia and tendons at thigh level, unspecified thigh
- S76.82 Laceration of other specified muscles, fascia and tendons at thigh level
  - S76.821 Laceration of other specified muscles, fascia and tendons at thigh level, right thigh
  - S76.822 Laceration of other specified muscles, fascia and tendons at thigh level, left thigh
  - S76.829 Laceration of other specified muscles, fascia and tendons at thigh level, unspecified thigh
- S76.89 Other injury of other specified muscles, fascia and tendons at thigh level
  - S76.891 Other injury of other specified muscles, fascia and tendons at thigh level, right thigh
  - S76.892 Other injury of other specified muscles, fascia and tendons at thigh level, left thigh
  - S76.899 Other injury of other specified muscles, fascia and tendons at thigh level, unspecified thigh

S76.9 Injury of unspecified muscles, fascia and tendons at thigh level
- S76.90 Unspecified injury of unspecified muscles, fascia and tendons at thigh level
  - S76.901 Unspecified injury of unspecified muscles, fascia and tendons at thigh level, right thigh
  - S76.902 Unspecified injury of unspecified muscles, fascia and tendons at thigh level, left thigh
  - S76.909 Unspecified injury of unspecified muscles, fascia and tendons at thigh level, unspecified thigh
- S76.91 Strain of unspecified muscles, fascia and tendons at thigh level
  - S76.911 Strain of unspecified muscles, fascia and tendons at thigh level, right thigh
  - S76.912 Strain of unspecified muscles, fascia and tendons at thigh level, left thigh
  - S76.919 Strain of unspecified muscles fascia and tendons at thigh level, unspecified thigh
- S76.92 Laceration of unspecified muscles, fascia and tendons at thigh level
  - S76.921 Laceration of unspecified muscles, fascia and tendons at thigh level, right thigh
  - S76.922 Laceration of unspecified muscles, fascia and tendons at thigh level, left thigh
  - S76.929 Laceration of unspecified muscles, fascia and tendons at thigh level, unspecified thigh
- S76.99 Other specified injury of unspecified muscles, fascia and tendons at thigh level
  - S76.991 Other specified injury of unspecified muscles, fascia and tendons at thigh level, right thigh
  - S76.992 Other specified injury of unspecified muscles, fascia and tendons at thigh level, left thigh
  - S76.999 Other specified injury of unspecified muscles, fascia and tendons at thigh level, unspecified thigh

S77 Crushing injury of hip and thigh

Use additional code(s) for all associated injuries

Excludes2 crushing injury of ankle and foot (S97.-)
crushing injury of lower leg (S87.-)

The appropriate 7th character is to be added to each code from category S77

A	initial encounter
D	subsequent encounter
S	sequela

- S77.0 Crushing injury of hip
  - X S77.00 Crushing injury of unspecified hip
  - X S77.01 Crushing injury of right hip
  - X S77.02 Crushing injury of left hip
- S77.1 Crushing injury of thigh
  - X S77.10 Crushing injury of unspecified thigh
  - X S77.11 Crushing injury of right thigh
  - X S77.12 Crushing injury of left thigh
- S77.2 Crushing injury of hip with thigh
  - X S77.20 Crushing injury of unspecified hip with thigh
  - X S77.21 Crushing injury of right hip with thigh
  - X S77.22 Crushing injury of left hip with thigh

S78 Traumatic amputation of hip and thigh

An amputation not identified as partial or complete should be coded to complete

Excludes1 traumatic amputation of knee (S88.0-)

The appropriate 7th character is to be added to each code from category S78

A	initial encounter
D	subsequent encounter
S	sequela

- S78.0 Traumatic amputation at hip joint
  - S78.01 Complete traumatic amputation at hip joint
    - S78.011 Complete traumatic amputation at right hip joint A, D, S
    - S78.012 Complete traumatic amputation at left hip joint A, D, S
    - S78.019 Complete traumatic amputation at unspecified hip joint A, D, S
  - S78.02 Partial traumatic amputation at hip joint
    - S78.021 Partial traumatic amputation at right hip joint A, D, S
    - S78.022 Partial traumatic amputation at left hip joint A, D, S
    - S78.029 Partial traumatic amputation at unspecified hip joint A, D, S

S78.1 Traumatic amputation at level **between hip and knee**

Excludes1 traumatic amputation of knee (S88.Ø-)

S78.11 **Complete** traumatic amputation at level between hip and knee

S78.111 Complete traumatic amputation at level between **right** hip and knee A, D, S

S78.112 Complete traumatic amputation at level between **left** hip and knee A, D, S

S78.119 Complete traumatic amputation at level between **unspecified** hip and knee A, D, S

S78.12 **Partial** traumatic amputation at level between hip and knee

S78.121 Partial traumatic amputation at level between **right** hip and knee A, D, S

S78.122 Partial traumatic amputation at level between **left** hip and knee A, D, S

S78.129 Partial traumatic amputation at level between **unspecified** hip and knee A, D, S

S78.9 Traumatic amputation of hip and thigh, **level unspecified**

S78.91 **Complete** traumatic amputation of hip and thigh, level unspecified

S78.911 Complete traumatic amputation of **right** hip and thigh, level unspecified A, D, S

S78.912 Complete traumatic amputation of **left** hip and thigh, level unspecified A, D, S

S78.919 Complete traumatic amputation of **unspecified** hip and thigh, level unspecified A, D, S

S78.92 **Partial** traumatic amputation of hip and thigh, level unspecified

S78.921 Partial traumatic amputation of **right** hip and thigh, level unspecified A, D, S

S78.922 Partial traumatic amputation of **left** hip and thigh, level unspecified A, D, S

S78.929 Partial traumatic amputation of **unspecified** hip and thigh, level unspecified A, D, S

S79 Other and unspecified injuries of hip and thigh

Note: A fracture not indicated as open or closed should be coded to closed

The appropriate 7th character is to be added to each code from subcategories S79.Ø and S79.1

A	initial encounter for closed fracture
D	subsequent encounter for fracture with routine healing
G	subsequent encounter for fracture with delayed healing
K	subsequent encounter for fracture with nonunion
P	subsequent encounter for fracture with malunion
S	sequela

S79.Ø Physeal fracture of **upper end** of femur

Excludes1 apophyseal fracture of upper end of femur (S72.13-)
nontraumatic slipped upper femoral epiphysis (M93.Ø-)

S79.ØØ **Unspecified** physeal fracture of upper end of femur

S79.ØØ1 Unspecified physeal fracture of upper end of **right** femur A

S79.ØØ2 Unspecified physeal fracture of upper end of **left** femur A

S79.ØØ9 Unspecified physeal fracture of upper end of **unspecified** femur A

Item 19–5 SALTER-HARRIS TYPE 1: epiphysis is completely separated from end of bone, or metaphysic growth plate remains attached to epiphysis
SALTER-HARRIS TYPE 2: epiphysis and growth plate are partially separated from metaphysis, which is cracked—most common type
SALTER-HARRIS TYPE 3: fracture occurring through epiphysis and separates part of epiphysis and growth plate from metaphysis fracture, usually at distal end of tibia
SALTER-HARRIS TYPE 4: fracture runs through epiphysis, across growth plate, into metaphysic; surgery is required to restore joint surface to normal and align growth plate

S79.Ø1 Salter-Harris Type I physeal fracture of upper end of femur

Acute on chronic slipped capital femoral epiphysis (traumatic)
Acute slipped capital femoral epiphysis (traumatic)
Capital femoral epiphyseal fracture

Excludes1 chronic slipped upper femoral epiphysis (nontraumatic) (M93.Ø2-)

S79.Ø11 Salter-Harris Type I physeal fracture of upper end of **right** femur A

S79.Ø12 Salter-Harris Type I physeal fracture of upper end of **left** femur A

S79.Ø19 Salter-Harris Type I physeal fracture of upper end of **unspecified** femur A

S79.Ø9 Other physeal fracture of upper end of femur

S79.Ø91 Other physeal fracture of upper end of **right** femur A

S79.Ø92 Other physeal fracture of upper end of **left** femur A

S79.Ø99 Other physeal fracture of upper end of **unspecified** femur A

S79.1 Physeal fracture of **lower end** of femur

S79.1Ø **Unspecified** physeal fracture of lower end of femur

S79.1Ø1 Unspecified physeal fracture of lower end of **right** femur A

S79.1Ø2 Unspecified physeal fracture of lower end of **left** femur A

S79.1Ø9 Unspecified physeal fracture of lower end of **unspecified** femur A

S79.11 Salter-Harris Type I physeal fracture of lower end of femur

S79.111 Salter-Harris Type I physeal fracture of lower end of **right** femur A

S79.112 Salter-Harris Type I physeal fracture of lower end of **left** femur A

S79.119 Salter-Harris Type I physeal fracture of lower end of **unspecified** femur A

S79.12 Salter-Harris Type II physeal fracture of lower end of femur

S79.121 Salter-Harris Type II physeal fracture of lower end of **right** femur A

S79.122 Salter-Harris Type II physeal fracture of lower end of **left** femur A

S79.129 Salter-Harris Type II physeal fracture of lower end of **unspecified** femur A

S79.13 Salter-Harris Type III physeal fracture of lower end of femur

S79.131 Salter-Harris Type III physeal fracture of lower end of **right** femur A

S79.132 Salter-Harris Type III physeal fracture of lower end of **left** femur A

S79.139 Salter-Harris Type III physeal fracture of lower end of **unspecified** femur A

- S79.14 Salter-Harris Type IV physeal fracture of lower end of femur
  - S79.141 Salter-Harris Type IV physeal fracture of lower end of right femur A
  - S79.142 Salter-Harris Type IV physeal fracture of lower end of left femur A
  - S79.149 Salter-Harris Type IV physeal fracture of lower end of unspecified femur A
- S79.19 Other physeal fracture of lower end of femur
  - S79.191 Other physeal fracture of lower end of right femur A
  - S79.192 Other physeal fracture of lower end of left femur A
  - S79.199 Other physeal fracture of lower end of unspecified femur A

S79.8 Other specified injuries of hip and thigh

The appropriate 7th character is to be added to each code in subcategory S79.8

A	initial encounter
D	subsequent encounter
S	sequela

- S79.81 Other specified injuries of hip
  - S79.811 Other specified injuries of right hip
  - S79.812 Other specified injuries of left hip
  - S79.819 Other specified injuries of unspecified hip
- S79.82 Other specified injuries of thigh
  - S79.821 Other specified injuries of right thigh
  - S79.822 Other specified injuries of left thigh
  - S79.829 Other specified injuries of unspecified thigh

S79.9 Unspecified injury of hip and thigh

The appropriate 7th character is to be added to each code in subcategory S79.9

A	initial encounter
D	subsequent encounter
S	sequela

- S79.91 Unspecified injury of hip
  - S79.911 Unspecified injury of right hip
  - S79.912 Unspecified injury of left hip
  - S79.919 Unspecified injury of unspecified hip
- S79.92 Unspecified injury of thigh
  - S79.921 Unspecified injury of right thigh
  - S79.922 Unspecified injury of left thigh
  - S79.929 Unspecified injury of unspecified thigh

INJURIES TO THE KNEE AND LOWER LEG (S80-S89)

Excludes2 burns and corrosions (T20-T32)
frostbite (T33-T34)
injuries of ankle and foot, except fracture of ankle and malleolus (S90-S99)
insect bite or sting, venomous (T63.4)

S80 Superficial injury of knee and lower leg

Excludes2 superficial injury of ankle and foot (S90.-)

The appropriate 7th character is to be added to each code from category S80

A	initial encounter
D	subsequent encounter
S	sequela

- S80.0 Contusion of knee
  - X S80.00 Contusion of unspecified knee
  - X S80.01 Contusion of right knee
  - X S80.02 Contusion of left knee
- S80.1 Contusion of lower leg
  - X S80.10 Contusion of unspecified lower leg
  - X S80.11 Contusion of right lower leg
  - X S80.12 Contusion of left lower leg
- S80.2 Other superficial injuries of knee
  - S80.21 Abrasion of knee
    - S80.211 Abrasion, right knee
    - S80.212 Abrasion, left knee
    - S80.219 Abrasion, unspecified knee
  - S80.22 Blister (nonthermal) of knee
    - S80.221 Blister (nonthermal), right knee
    - S80.222 Blister (nonthermal), left knee
    - S80.229 Blister (nonthermal), unspecified knee
  - S80.24 External constriction of knee
    - S80.241 External constriction, right knee
    - S80.242 External constriction, left knee
    - S80.249 External constriction, unspecified knee
  - S80.25 Superficial foreign body of knee
    Splinter in the knee
    - S80.251 Superficial foreign body, right knee
    - S80.252 Superficial foreign body, left knee
    - S80.259 Superficial foreign body, unspecified knee
  - S80.26 Insect bite (nonvenomous) of knee
    - S80.261 Insect bite (nonvenomous), right knee
    - S80.262 Insect bite (nonvenomous), left knee
    - S80.269 Insect bite (nonvenomous), unspecified knee
  - S80.27 Other superficial bite of knee
    Excludes1 open bite of knee (S81.05-)
    - S80.271 Other superficial bite of right knee
    - S80.272 Other superficial bite of left knee
    - S80.279 Other superficial bite of unspecified knee
- S80.8 Other superficial injuries of lower leg
  - S80.81 Abrasion of lower leg
    - S80.811 Abrasion, right lower leg
    - S80.812 Abrasion, left lower leg
    - S80.819 Abrasion, unspecified lower leg
  - S80.82 Blister (nonthermal) of lower leg
    - S80.821 Blister (nonthermal), right lower leg
    - S80.822 Blister (nonthermal), left lower leg
    - S80.829 Blister (nonthermal), unspecified lower leg
  - S80.84 External constriction of lower leg
    - S80.841 External constriction, right lower leg
    - S80.842 External constriction, left lower leg
    - S80.849 External constriction, unspecified lower leg
  - S80.85 Superficial foreign body of lower leg
    Splinter in the lower leg
    - S80.851 Superficial foreign body, right lower leg
    - S80.852 Superficial foreign body, left lower leg
    - S80.859 Superficial foreign body, unspecified lower leg

S80.86 **Insect bite (nonvenomous) of lower leg**
- S80.861 Insect bite (nonvenomous), **right lower leg**
- S80.862 Insect bite (nonvenomous), **left lower leg**
- S80.869 Insect bite (nonvenomous), **unspecified lower leg**

S80.87 **Other superficial bite of lower leg**
Excludes1 open bite of lower leg (S81.85-)
- S80.871 Other superficial bite, **right lower leg**
- S80.872 Other superficial bite, **left lower leg**
- S80.879 Other superficial bite, **unspecified lower leg**

S80.9 **Unspecified superficial injury of knee and lower leg**

S80.91 **Unspecified superficial injury of knee**
- S80.911 Unspecified superficial injury of **right knee**
- S80.912 Unspecified superficial injury of **left knee**
- S80.919 Unspecified superficial injury of **unspecified knee**

S80.92 **Unspecified superficial injury of lower leg**
- S80.921 Unspecified superficial injury of **right lower leg**
- S80.922 Unspecified superficial injury of **left lower leg**
- S80.929 Unspecified superficial injury of **unspecified lower leg**

S81 Open wound of knee and lower leg
Code also any associated wound infection
Excludes1 open fracture of knee and lower leg (S82.-)
traumatic amputation of lower leg (S88.-)
Excludes2 open wound of ankle and foot (S91.-)
The appropriate 7th character is to be added to each code from category S81

A	initial encounter
D	subsequent encounter
S	sequela

S81.0 **Open wound of knee**

S81.00 **Unspecified open wound of knee**
- S81.001 Unspecified open wound, **right knee**
- S81.002 Unspecified open wound, **left knee**
- S81.009 Unspecified open wound, **unspecified knee**

S81.01 **Laceration without foreign body of knee**
- S81.011 Laceration without foreign body, **right knee**
- S81.012 Laceration without foreign body, **left knee**
- S81.019 Laceration without foreign body, **unspecified knee**

S81.02 **Laceration with foreign body of knee**
- S81.021 Laceration with foreign body, **right knee**
- S81.022 Laceration with foreign body, **left knee**
- S81.029 Laceration with foreign body, **unspecified knee**

S81.03 **Puncture wound without foreign body of knee**
- S81.031 Puncture wound without foreign body, **right knee**
- S81.032 Puncture wound without foreign body, **left knee**
- S81.039 Puncture wound without foreign body, **unspecified knee**

S81.04 **Puncture wound with foreign body of knee**
- S81.041 Puncture wound with foreign body, **right knee**
- S81.042 Puncture wound with foreign body, **left knee**
- S81.049 Puncture wound with foreign body, **unspecified knee**

S81.05 **Open bite of knee**
Bite of knee NOS
Excludes1 superficial bite of knee (S80.27-)
- S81.051 Open bite, **right knee**
- S81.052 Open bite, **left knee**
- S81.059 Open bite, **unspecified knee**

S81.8 **Open wound of lower leg**

S81.80 **Unspecified open wound of lower leg**
- S81.801 Unspecified open wound, **right lower leg**
- S81.802 Unspecified open wound, **left lower leg**
- S81.809 Unspecified open wound, **unspecified lower leg**

S81.81 **Laceration without foreign body of lower leg**
- S81.811 Laceration without foreign body, **right lower leg**
- S81.812 Laceration without foreign body, **left lower leg**
- S81.819 Laceration without foreign body, **unspecified lower leg**

S81.82 **Laceration with foreign body of lower leg**
- S81.821 Laceration with foreign body, **right lower leg**
- S81.822 Laceration with foreign body, **left lower leg**
- S81.829 Laceration with foreign body, **unspecified lower leg**

S81.83 **Puncture wound without foreign body of lower leg**
- S81.831 Puncture wound without foreign body, **right lower leg**
- S81.832 Puncture wound without foreign body, **left lower leg**
- S81.839 Puncture wound without foreign body, **unspecified lower leg**

S81.84 **Puncture wound with foreign body of lower leg**
- S81.841 Puncture wound with foreign body, **right lower leg**
  Coding Clinic: 2016, Q3, P46
- S81.842 Puncture wound with foreign body, **left lower leg**
- S81.849 Puncture wound with foreign body, **unspecified lower leg**

S81.85 **Open bite of lower leg**
Bite of lower leg NOS
Excludes1 superficial bite of lower leg (S80.86-, S80.87-)
- S81.851 Open bite, **right lower leg**
- S81.852 Open bite, **left lower leg**
- S81.859 Open bite, **unspecified lower leg**

S82 Fracture of lower leg, including ankle

Note: A fracture not indicated as displaced or nondisplaced should be coded to displaced

A fracture not indicated as open or closed should be coded to closed

The open fracture designations are based on the Gustilo open fracture classification

Includes fracture of malleolus

Excludes1 traumatic amputation of lower leg (S88.-)

Excludes2 fracture of foot, except ankle (S92.-)
periprosthetic fracture of prosthetic implant of knee (M97.Ø-)

The appropriate 7th character is to be added to all codes from category S82

A	initial encounter for closed fracture
B	initial encounter for open fracture type I or II initial encounter for open fracture NOS
C	initial encounter for open fracture type IIIA, IIIB, or IIIC
D	subsequent encounter for closed fracture with routine healing
E	subsequent encounter for open fracture type I or II with routine healing
F	subsequent encounter for open fracture type IIIA, IIIB, or IIIC with routine healing
G	subsequent encounter for closed fracture with delayed healing
H	subsequent encounter for open fracture type I or II with delayed healing
J	subsequent encounter for open fracture type IIIA, IIIB, or IIIC with delayed healing
K	subsequent encounter for closed fracture with nonunion
M	subsequent encounter for open fracture type I or II with nonunion
N	subsequent encounter for open fracture type IIIA, IIIB, or IIIC with nonunion
P	subsequent encounter for closed fracture with malunion
Q	subsequent encounter for open fracture type I or II with malunion
R	subsequent encounter for open fracture type IIIA, IIIB, or IIIC with malunion
S	sequela

S82.Ø Fracture of patella
Knee cap

S82.ØØ Unspecified fracture of patella
- **S82.ØØ1 Unspecified fracture of right patella**
- **S82.ØØ2 Unspecified fracture of left patella**
- **S82.ØØ9 Unspecified fracture of unspecified patella**

S82.Ø1 Osteochondral fracture of patella
- **S82.Ø11 Displaced osteochondral fracture of right patella**
- **S82.Ø12 Displaced osteochondral fracture of left patella**
- **S82.Ø13 Displaced osteochondral fracture of unspecified patella**
- **S82.Ø14 Nondisplaced osteochondral fracture of right patella**
- **S82.Ø15 Nondisplaced osteochondral fracture of left patella**
- **S82.Ø16 Nondisplaced osteochondral fracture of unspecified patella**

S82.Ø2 Longitudinal fracture of patella
- **S82.Ø21 Displaced longitudinal fracture of right patella**
- **S82.Ø22 Displaced longitudinal fracture of left patella**
- **S82.Ø23 Displaced longitudinal fracture of unspecified patella**
- **S82.Ø24 Nondisplaced longitudinal fracture of right patella**
- **S82.Ø25 Nondisplaced longitudinal fracture of left patella**
- **S82.Ø26 Nondisplaced longitudinal fracture of unspecified patella**

S82.Ø3 Transverse fracture of patella
- **S82.Ø31 Displaced transverse fracture of right patella**
- **S82.Ø32 Displaced transverse fracture of left patella**
- **S82.Ø33 Displaced transverse fracture of unspecified patella**
- **S82.Ø34 Nondisplaced transverse fracture of right patella**
- **S82.Ø35 Nondisplaced transverse fracture of left patella**
- **S82.Ø36 Nondisplaced transverse fracture of unspecified patella**

S82.Ø4 Comminuted fracture of patella
- **S82.Ø41 Displaced comminuted fracture of right patella**
- **S82.Ø42 Displaced comminuted fracture of left patella**
- **S82.Ø43 Displaced comminuted fracture of unspecified patella**
- **S82.Ø44 Nondisplaced comminuted fracture of right patella**
- **S82.Ø45 Nondisplaced comminuted fracture of left patella**
- **S82.Ø46 Nondisplaced comminuted fracture of unspecified patella**

S82.Ø9 Other fracture of patella
- **S82.Ø91 Other fracture of right patella**
- **S82.Ø92 Other fracture of left patella**
- **S82.Ø99 Other fracture of unspecified patella**

S82.1 Fracture of upper end of tibia
Fracture of proximal end of tibia

Excludes2 fracture of shaft of tibia (S82.2-)
physeal fracture of upper end of tibia (S89.Ø-)

S82.1Ø Unspecified fracture of upper end of tibia
- **S82.1Ø1 Unspecified fracture of upper end of right tibia**
- **S82.1Ø2 Unspecified fracture of upper end of left tibia**
- **S82.1Ø9 Unspecified fracture of upper end of unspecified tibia**

S82.11 Fracture of tibial spine
- **S82.111 Displaced fracture of right tibial spine**
- **S82.112 Displaced fracture of left tibial spine**
- **S82.113 Displaced fracture of unspecified tibial spine**
- **S82.114 Nondisplaced fracture of right tibial spine**
- **S82.115 Nondisplaced fracture of left tibial spine**
- **S82.116 Nondisplaced fracture of unspecified tibial spine**

CHAPTER 19 (SØØ-T88)

S82.12 Fracture of lateral condyle of tibia
- S82.121 Displaced fracture of lateral condyle of right tibia
- S82.122 Displaced fracture of lateral condyle of left tibia
- S82.123 Displaced fracture of lateral condyle of unspecified tibia
- S82.124 Nondisplaced fracture of lateral condyle of right tibia
- S82.125 Nondisplaced fracture of lateral condyle of left tibia
- S82.126 Nondisplaced fracture of lateral condyle of unspecified tibia

S82.13 Fracture of medial condyle of tibia
- S82.131 Displaced fracture of medial condyle of right tibia
- S82.132 Displaced fracture of medial condyle of left tibia
- S82.133 Displaced fracture of medial condyle of unspecified tibia
- S82.134 Nondisplaced fracture of medial condyle of right tibia
- S82.135 Nondisplaced fracture of medial condyle of left tibia
- S82.136 Nondisplaced fracture of medial condyle of unspecified tibia

S82.14 Bicondylar fracture of tibia
Fracture of tibial plateau NOS
- S82.141 Displaced bicondylar fracture of right tibia
- S82.142 Displaced bicondylar fracture of left tibia
- S82.143 Displaced bicondylar fracture of unspecified tibia
- S82.144 Nondisplaced bicondylar fracture of right tibia
- S82.145 Nondisplaced bicondylar fracture of left tibia
- S82.146 Nondisplaced bicondylar fracture of unspecified tibia

S82.15 Fracture of tibial tuberosity
- S82.151 Displaced fracture of right tibial tuberosity
- S82.152 Displaced fracture of left tibial tuberosity
- S82.153 Displaced fracture of unspecified tibial tuberosity
- S82.154 Nondisplaced fracture of right tibial tuberosity
- S82.155 Nondisplaced fracture of left tibial tuberosity
- S82.156 Nondisplaced fracture of unspecified tibial tuberosity

S82.16 **Torus fracture of upper end of tibia**

The appropriate 7th character is to be added to all codes in subcategory S82.16

A	initial encounter for closed fracture
D	subsequent encounter for fracture with routine healing
G	subsequent encounter for fracture with delayed healing
K	subsequent encounter for fracture with nonunion
P	subsequent encounter for fracture with malunion
S	sequela

- S82.161 Torus fracture of upper end of right tibia
- S82.162 Torus fracture of upper end of left tibia
- S82.169 Torus fracture of upper end of unspecified tibia

S82.19 Other fracture of upper end of tibia
- S82.191 Other fracture of upper end of right tibia
- S82.192 Other fracture of upper end of left tibia
- S82.199 Other fracture of upper end of unspecified tibia

S82.2 Fracture of shaft of tibia

S82.20 Unspecified fracture of shaft of tibia
Fracture of tibia NOS
- S82.201 Unspecified fracture of shaft of right tibia
- S82.202 Unspecified fracture of shaft of left tibia
- S82.209 Unspecified fracture of shaft of unspecified tibia

S82.22 Transverse fracture of shaft of tibia
- S82.221 Displaced transverse fracture of shaft of right tibia
- S82.222 Displaced transverse fracture of shaft of left tibia
- S82.223 Displaced transverse fracture of shaft of unspecified tibia
- S82.224 Nondisplaced transverse fracture of shaft of right tibia
- S82.225 Nondisplaced transverse fracture of shaft of left tibia
- S82.226 Nondisplaced transverse fracture of shaft of unspecified tibia

S82.23 Oblique fracture of shaft of tibia
- S82.231 Displaced oblique fracture of shaft of right tibia
- S82.232 Displaced oblique fracture of shaft of left tibia
- S82.233 Displaced oblique fracture of shaft of unspecified tibia
- S82.234 Nondisplaced oblique fracture of shaft of right tibia
  Coding Clinic: 2015, Q1, P9-10
- S82.235 Nondisplaced oblique fracture of shaft of left tibia
- S82.236 Nondisplaced oblique fracture of shaft of unspecified tibia

S82.24 **Spiral** fracture of shaft of tibia
Toddler fracture
- S82.241 **Displaced** spiral fracture of shaft of **right** tibia
- S82.242 **Displaced** spiral fracture of shaft of **left** tibia
- S82.243 **Displaced** spiral fracture of shaft of **unspecified** tibia
- S82.244 **Nondisplaced** spiral fracture of shaft of **right** tibia
- S82.245 **Nondisplaced** spiral fracture of shaft of **left** tibia
- S82.246 **Nondisplaced** spiral fracture of shaft of **unspecified** tibia

S82.25 **Comminuted** fracture of shaft of tibia
- S82.251 **Displaced** comminuted fracture of shaft of **right** tibia
  Coding Clinic: 2015, Q2, P6
- S82.252 **Displaced** comminuted fracture of shaft of **left** tibia
- S82.253 **Displaced** comminuted fracture of shaft of **unspecified** tibia
- S82.254 **Nondisplaced** comminuted fracture of shaft of **right** tibia
- S82.255 **Nondisplaced** comminuted fracture of shaft of **left** tibia
- S82.256 **Nondisplaced** comminuted fracture of shaft of **unspecified** tibia

S82.26 **Segmental** fracture of shaft of tibia
- S82.261 **Displaced** segmental fracture of shaft of **right** tibia
- S82.262 **Displaced** segmental fracture of shaft of **left** tibia
- S82.263 **Displaced** segmental fracture of shaft of **unspecified** tibia
- S82.264 **Nondisplaced** segmental fracture of shaft of **right** tibia
- S82.265 **Nondisplaced** segmental fracture of shaft of **left** tibia
- S82.266 **Nondisplaced** segmental fracture of shaft of **unspecified** tibia

S82.29 **Other** fracture of shaft of tibia
- S82.291 Other fracture of shaft of **right** tibia
- S82.292 Other fracture of shaft of **left** tibia
- S82.299 Other fracture of shaft of **unspecified** tibia

S82.3 Fracture of **lower end** of tibia
Excludes1 bimalleolar fracture of lower leg (S82.84-)
fracture of medial malleolus alone (S82.5-)
Maisonneuve's fracture (S82.86-)
pilon fracture of distal tibia (S82.87-)
trimalleolar fractures of lower leg (S82.85-)

S82.30 **Unspecified** fracture of lower end of tibia
- S82.301 Unspecified fracture of lower end of **right** tibia
- S82.302 Unspecified fracture of lower end of **left** tibia
- S82.309 Unspecified fracture of lower end of **unspecified** tibia

S82.31 **Torus** fracture of lower end of tibia
The appropriate 7th character is to be added to all codes in subcategory S82.31

A	initial encounter for closed fracture
D	subsequent encounter for fracture with routine healing
G	subsequent encounter for fracture with delayed healing
K	subsequent encounter for fracture with nonunion
P	subsequent encounter for fracture with malunion
S	sequela

- S82.311 Torus fracture of lower end of **right** tibia
- S82.312 Torus fracture of lower end of **left** tibia
- S82.319 Torus fracture of lower end of **unspecified** tibia

S82.39 **Other** fracture of lower end of tibia
- S82.391 Other fracture of lower end of **right** tibia
- S82.392 Other fracture of lower end of **left** tibia
  Coding Clinic: 2015, Q1, P25
- S82.399 Other fracture of lower end of **unspecified** tibia

S82.4 Fracture of shaft of fibula
Excludes2 fracture of lateral malleolus alone (S82.6-)

S82.40 **Unspecified** fracture of shaft of fibula
- S82.401 Unspecified fracture of shaft of **right** fibula
- S82.402 Unspecified fracture of shaft of **left** fibula
- S82.409 Unspecified fracture of shaft of **unspecified** fibula

S82.42 **Transverse** fracture of shaft of fibula
- S82.421 **Displaced** transverse fracture of shaft of **right** fibula
- S82.422 **Displaced** transverse fracture of shaft of **left** fibula
- S82.423 **Displaced** transverse fracture of shaft of **unspecified** fibula
- S82.424 **Nondisplaced** transverse fracture of shaft of **right** fibula
- S82.425 **Nondisplaced** transverse fracture of shaft of **left** fibula
- S82.426 **Nondisplaced** transverse fracture of shaft of **unspecified** fibula

S82.43 **Oblique** fracture of shaft of fibula
- S82.431 **Displaced** oblique fracture of shaft of **right** fibula
- S82.432 **Displaced** oblique fracture of shaft of **left** fibula
- S82.433 **Displaced** oblique fracture of shaft of **unspecified** fibula
- S82.434 **Nondisplaced** oblique fracture of shaft of **right** fibula
- S82.435 **Nondisplaced** oblique fracture of shaft of **left** fibula
- S82.436 **Nondisplaced** oblique fracture of shaft of **unspecified** fibula

S82.44 Spiral fracture of shaft of fibula
- S82.441 Displaced spiral fracture of shaft of right fibula
- S82.442 Displaced spiral fracture of shaft of left fibula
- S82.443 Displaced spiral fracture of shaft of unspecified fibula
- S82.444 Nondisplaced spiral fracture of shaft of right fibula
- S82.445 Nondisplaced spiral fracture of shaft of left fibula
- S82.446 Nondisplaced spiral fracture of shaft of unspecified fibula

S82.45 Comminuted fracture of shaft of fibula
- S82.451 Displaced comminuted fracture of shaft of right fibula
- S82.452 Displaced comminuted fracture of shaft of left fibula
- S82.453 Displaced comminuted fracture of shaft of unspecified fibula
- S82.454 Nondisplaced comminuted fracture of shaft of right fibula
- S82.455 Nondisplaced comminuted fracture of shaft of left fibula
- S82.456 Nondisplaced comminuted fracture of shaft of unspecified fibula

S82.46 Segmental fracture of shaft of fibula
- S82.461 Displaced segmental fracture of shaft of right fibula
- S82.462 Displaced segmental fracture of shaft of left fibula
- S82.463 Displaced segmental fracture of shaft of unspecified fibula
- S82.464 Nondisplaced segmental fracture of shaft of right fibula
- S82.465 Nondisplaced segmental fracture of shaft of left fibula
- S82.466 Nondisplaced segmental fracture of shaft of unspecified fibula

S82.49 Other fracture of shaft of fibula
- S82.491 Other fracture of shaft of right fibula
- S82.492 Other fracture of shaft of left fibula
- S82.499 Other fracture of shaft of unspecified fibula

S82.5 Fracture of medial malleolus

Excludes1 pilon fracture of distal tibia (S82.87-)
Salter-Harris type III of lower end of tibia (S89.13-)
Salter-Harris type IV of lower end of tibia (S89.14-)

- X S82.51 Displaced fracture of medial malleolus of right tibia
- X S82.52 Displaced fracture of medial malleolus of left tibia
- X S82.53 Displaced fracture of medial malleolus of unspecified tibia
- X S82.54 Nondisplaced fracture of medial malleolus of right tibia
- X S82.55 Nondisplaced fracture of medial malleolus of left tibia
- X S82.56 Nondisplaced fracture of medial malleolus of unspecified tibia

S82.6 Fracture of lateral malleolus

Excludes1 pilon fracture of distal tibia (S82.87-)

- X S82.61 Displaced fracture of lateral malleolus of right fibula
- X S82.62 Displaced fracture of lateral malleolus of left fibula
- X S82.63 Displaced fracture of lateral malleolus of unspecified fibula
- X S82.64 Nondisplaced fracture of lateral malleolus of right fibula
- X S82.65 Nondisplaced fracture of lateral malleolus of left fibula
- X S82.66 Nondisplaced fracture of lateral malleolus of unspecified fibula

S82.8 Other fractures of lower leg

S82.81 Torus fracture of upper end of fibula

The appropriate 7th character is to be added to all codes in subcategory S82.81

A	initial encounter for closed fracture
D	subsequent encounter for fracture with routine healing
G	subsequent encounter for fracture with delayed healing
K	subsequent encounter for fracture with nonunion
P	subsequent encounter for fracture with malunion
S	sequela

- S82.811 Torus fracture of upper end of right fibula
- S82.812 Torus fracture of upper end of left fibula
- S82.819 Torus fracture of upper end of unspecified fibula

S82.82 Torus fracture of lower end of fibula

The appropriate 7th character is to be added to all codes in subcategory S82.82

A	initial encounter for closed fracture
D	subsequent encounter for fracture with routine healing
G	subsequent encounter for fracture with delayed healing
K	subsequent encounter for fracture with nonunion
P	subsequent encounter for fracture with malunion
S	sequela

- S82.821 Torus fracture of lower end of right fibula
- S82.822 Torus fracture of lower end of left fibula
- S82.829 Torus fracture of lower end of unspecified fibula

S82.83 Other fracture of upper and lower end of fibula
- S82.831 Other fracture of upper and lower end of right fibula
- S82.832 Other fracture of upper and lower end of left fibula
  Coding Clinic: 2015, Q1, P9-10
- S82.839 Other fracture of upper and lower end of unspecified fibula

- S82.84 Bimalleolar fracture of lower leg
  - S82.841 Displaced bimalleolar fracture of right lower leg
  - S82.842 Displaced bimalleolar fracture of left lower leg
  - S82.843 Displaced bimalleolar fracture of unspecified lower leg
  - S82.844 Nondisplaced bimalleolar fracture of right lower leg
  - S82.845 Nondisplaced bimalleolar fracture of left lower leg
  - S82.846 Nondisplaced bimalleolar fracture of unspecified lower leg
- S82.85 Trimalleolar fracture of lower leg
  - S82.851 Displaced trimalleolar fracture of right lower leg
  - S82.852 Displaced trimalleolar fracture of left lower leg
  - S82.853 Displaced trimalleolar fracture of unspecified lower leg
  - S82.854 Nondisplaced trimalleolar fracture of right lower leg
  - S82.855 Nondisplaced trimalleolar fracture of left lower leg
  - S82.856 Nondisplaced trimalleolar fracture of unspecified lower leg
- S82.86 Maisonneuve's fracture
  - S82.861 Displaced Maisonneuve's fracture of right leg
  - S82.862 Displaced Maisonneuve's fracture of left leg
  - S82.863 Displaced Maisonneuve's fracture of unspecified leg
  - S82.864 Nondisplaced Maisonneuve's fracture of right leg
  - S82.865 Nondisplaced Maisonneuve's fracture of left leg
  - S82.866 Nondisplaced Maisonneuve's fracture of unspecified leg
- S82.87 Pilon fracture of tibia
  - S82.871 Displaced pilon fracture of right tibia
  - S82.872 Displaced pilon fracture of left tibia
  - S82.873 Displaced pilon fracture of unspecified tibia
  - S82.874 Nondisplaced pilon fracture of right tibia
  - S82.875 Nondisplaced pilon fracture of left tibia
  - S82.876 Nondisplaced pilon fracture of unspecified tibia
- S82.89 Other fractures of lower leg
  Fracture of ankle NOS
  - S82.891 Other fracture of right lower leg
  - S82.892 Other fracture of left lower leg
  - S82.899 Other fracture of unspecified lower leg

S82.9 Unspecified fracture of lower leg
- X S82.90 Unspecified fracture of unspecified lower leg
- X S82.91 Unspecified fracture of right lower leg
- X S82.92 Unspecified fracture of left lower leg

S83 Dislocation and sprain of joints and ligaments of knee

Includes avulsion of joint or ligament of knee
laceration of cartilage, joint or ligament of knee
sprain of cartilage, joint or ligament of knee
traumatic hemarthrosis of joint or ligament of knee
traumatic rupture of joint or ligament of knee
traumatic subluxation of joint or ligament of knee
traumatic tear of joint or ligament of knee

Code also any associated open wound

Excludes1 derangement of patella (M22.Ø-M22.3)
injury of patellar ligament (tendon) (S76.1-)
internal derangement of knee (M23.-)
old dislocation of knee (M24.36)
pathological dislocation of knee (M24.36)
recurrent dislocation of knee (M22.Ø)

Excludes2 strain of muscle, fascia and tendon of lower leg (S86.-)

Coding Clinic: 2Ø19, Q2, P26

The appropriate 7th character is to be added to each code from category S83

A	initial encounter
D	subsequent encounter
S	sequela

S83.Ø Subluxation and dislocation of patella
- S83.ØØ Unspecified subluxation and dislocation of patella
  - S83.ØØ1 Unspecified subluxation of right patella
  - S83.ØØ2 Unspecified subluxation of left patella
  - S83.ØØ3 Unspecified subluxation of unspecified patella
  - S83.ØØ4 Unspecified dislocation of right patella
  - S83.ØØ5 Unspecified dislocation of left patella
  - S83.ØØ6 Unspecified dislocation of unspecified patella
- S83.Ø1 Lateral subluxation and dislocation of patella
  - S83.Ø11 Lateral subluxation of right patella
  - S83.Ø12 Lateral subluxation of left patella
  - S83.Ø13 Lateral subluxation of unspecified patella
  - S83.Ø14 Lateral dislocation of right patella
  - S83.Ø15 Lateral dislocation of left patella
  - S83.Ø16 Lateral dislocation of unspecified patella
- S83.Ø9 Other subluxation and dislocation of patella
  - S83.Ø91 Other subluxation of right patella
  - S83.Ø92 Other subluxation of left patella
  - S83.Ø93 Other subluxation of unspecified patella
  - S83.Ø94 Other dislocation of right patella
  - S83.Ø95 Other dislocation of left patella
  - S83.Ø96 Other dislocation of unspecified patella

CHAPTER 19 (SØØ-T88)

● S83.1 Subluxation and dislocation of **knee**
  Excludes2 instability of knee prosthesis (T84.022, T84.023)
 ● S83.10 **Unspecified** subluxation and dislocation of knee
  ● S83.101 Unspecified **subluxation of right knee**
  ● S83.102 Unspecified **subluxation of left knee**
  ● S83.103 Unspecified **subluxation of unspecified** knee
  ● S83.104 Unspecified **dislocation of right knee**
  ● S83.105 Unspecified **dislocation of left knee**
  ● S83.106 Unspecified **dislocation of unspecified** knee
 ● S83.11 **Anterior** subluxation and dislocation of **proximal end of tibia**
  Posterior subluxation and dislocation of distal end of femur
  ● S83.111 Anterior **subluxation** of proximal end of tibia, **right knee**
  ● S83.112 Anterior **subluxation** of proximal end of tibia, **left knee**
  ● S83.113 Anterior **subluxation** of proximal end of tibia, **unspecified** knee
  ● S83.114 Anterior **dislocation** of proximal end of tibia, **right knee**
  ● S83.115 Anterior **dislocation** of proximal end of tibia, **left knee**
  ● S83.116 Anterior **dislocation** of proximal end of tibia, **unspecified** knee
 ● S83.12 **Posterior** subluxation and dislocation of **proximal end of tibia**
  Anterior dislocation of distal end of femur
  ● S83.121 Posterior **subluxation** of proximal end of tibia, **right knee**
  ● S83.122 Posterior **subluxation** of proximal end of tibia, **left knee**
  ● S83.123 Posterior **subluxation** of proximal end of tibia, **unspecified** knee
  ● S83.124 Posterior **dislocation** of proximal end of tibia, **right knee**
  ● S83.125 Posterior **dislocation** of proximal end of tibia, **left knee**
  ● S83.126 Posterior **dislocation** of proximal end of tibia, **unspecified** knee
 ● S83.13 **Medial** subluxation and dislocation of **proximal end of tibia**
  ● S83.131 Medial **subluxation** of proximal end of tibia, **right knee**
  ● S83.132 Medial **subluxation** of proximal end of tibia, **left knee**
  ● S83.133 Medial **subluxation** of proximal end of tibia, **unspecified** knee
  ● S83.134 Medial **dislocation** of proximal end of tibia, **right knee**
  ● S83.135 Medial **dislocation** of proximal end of tibia, **left knee**
  ● S83.136 Medial **dislocation** of proximal end of tibia, **unspecified** knee
 ● S83.14 **Lateral** subluxation and dislocation of **proximal end of tibia**
  ● S83.141 Lateral **subluxation** of proximal end of tibia, **right knee**
  ● S83.142 Lateral **subluxation** of proximal end of tibia, **left knee**
  ● S83.143 Lateral **subluxation** of proximal end of tibia, **unspecified** knee
  ● S83.144 Lateral **dislocation** of proximal end of tibia, **right knee**
  ● S83.145 Lateral **dislocation** of proximal end of tibia, **left knee**
  ● S83.146 Lateral **dislocation** of proximal end of tibia, **unspecified** knee
 ● S83.19 **Other** subluxation and dislocation of knee
  ● S83.191 Other **subluxation of right knee**
  ● S83.192 Other **subluxation of left knee**
  ● S83.193 Other **subluxation of unspecified** knee
  ● S83.194 Other **dislocation of right knee**
  ● S83.195 Other **dislocation of left knee**
  ● S83.196 Other **dislocation of unspecified** knee
● S83.2 **Tear of meniscus**, current injury
  Excludes1 old bucket-handle tear (M23.2)
 ● S83.20 Tear of **unspecified** meniscus, current injury
  Tear of meniscus of knee NOS
  ● S83.200 **Bucket-handle** tear of unspecified meniscus, current injury, **right knee**
  ● S83.201 **Bucket-handle** tear of unspecified meniscus, current injury, **left knee**
  ● S83.202 **Bucket-handle** tear of unspecified meniscus, current injury, **unspecified** knee
  ● S83.203 **Other** tear of unspecified meniscus, current injury, **right knee**
  ● S83.204 **Other** tear of unspecified meniscus, current injury, **left knee**
  ● S83.205 **Other** tear of unspecified meniscus, current injury, **unspecified** knee
  ● S83.206 **Unspecified** tear of unspecified meniscus, current injury, **right knee**
  ● S83.207 **Unspecified** tear of unspecified meniscus, current injury, **left knee**
  ● S83.209 **Unspecified** tear of unspecified meniscus, current injury, **unspecified** knee
 ● S83.21 **Bucket-handle** tear of **medial** meniscus, current injury
  ● S83.211 Bucket-handle tear of medial meniscus, current injury, **right knee**
  ● S83.212 Bucket-handle tear of medial meniscus, current injury, **left knee**
  ● S83.219 Bucket-handle tear of medial meniscus, current injury, **unspecified** knee
 ● S83.22 **Peripheral** tear of **medial** meniscus, current injury
  ● S83.221 Peripheral tear of medial meniscus, current injury, **right knee**
  ● S83.222 Peripheral tear of medial meniscus, current injury, **left knee**
  ● S83.229 Peripheral tear of medial meniscus, current injury, **unspecified** knee

S83.23 Complex tear of medial meniscus, current injury
- S83.231 Complex tear of medial meniscus, current injury, right knee
- S83.232 Complex tear of medial meniscus, current injury, left knee
  - Coding Clinic: 2019, Q2, P26
- S83.239 Complex tear of medial meniscus, current injury, unspecified knee

S83.24 Other tear of medial meniscus, current injury
- S83.241 Other tear of medial meniscus, current injury, right knee
- S83.242 Other tear of medial meniscus, current injury, left knee
- S83.249 Other tear of medial meniscus, current injury, unspecified knee

S83.25 Bucket-handle tear of lateral meniscus, current injury
- S83.251 Bucket-handle tear of lateral meniscus, current injury, right knee
- S83.252 Bucket-handle tear of lateral meniscus, current injury, left knee
- S83.259 Bucket-handle tear of lateral meniscus, current injury, unspecified knee

S83.26 Peripheral tear of lateral meniscus, current injury
- S83.261 Peripheral tear of lateral meniscus, current injury, right knee
- S83.262 Peripheral tear of lateral meniscus, current injury, left knee
- S83.269 Peripheral tear of lateral meniscus, current injury, unspecified knee

S83.27 Complex tear of lateral meniscus, current injury
- S83.271 Complex tear of lateral meniscus, current injury, right knee
- S83.272 Complex tear of lateral meniscus, current injury, left knee
- S83.279 Complex tear of lateral meniscus, current injury, unspecified knee

S83.28 Other tear of lateral meniscus, current injury
- S83.281 Other tear of lateral meniscus, current injury, right knee
- S83.282 Other tear of lateral meniscus, current injury, left knee
- S83.289 Other tear of lateral meniscus, current injury, unspecified knee

S83.3 Tear of articular cartilage of knee, current
- X S83.30 Tear of articular cartilage of unspecified knee, current
- X S83.31 Tear of articular cartilage of right knee, current
- X S83.32 Tear of articular cartilage of left knee, current

S83.4 Sprain of collateral ligament of knee

S83.40 Sprain of unspecified collateral ligament of knee
- S83.401 Sprain of unspecified collateral ligament of right knee
- S83.402 Sprain of unspecified collateral ligament of left knee
- S83.409 Sprain of unspecified collateral ligament of unspecified knee

S83.41 Sprain of medial collateral ligament of knee
Sprain of tibial collateral ligament
- S83.411 Sprain of medial collateral ligament of right knee
- S83.412 Sprain of medial collateral ligament of left knee
- S83.419 Sprain of medial collateral ligament of unspecified knee

S83.42 Sprain of lateral collateral ligament of knee
Sprain of fibular collateral ligament
- S83.421 Sprain of lateral collateral ligament of right knee
- S83.422 Sprain of lateral collateral ligament of left knee
- S83.429 Sprain of lateral collateral ligament of unspecified knee

S83.5 Sprain of cruciate ligament of knee

S83.50 Sprain of unspecified cruciate ligament of knee
- S83.501 Sprain of unspecified cruciate ligament of right knee
- S83.502 Sprain of unspecified cruciate ligament of left knee
- S83.509 Sprain of unspecified cruciate ligament of unspecified knee

S83.51 Sprain of anterior cruciate ligament of knee
- S83.511 Sprain of anterior cruciate ligament of right knee
  - Coding Clinic: 2016, Q2, P4
- S83.512 Sprain of anterior cruciate ligament of left knee
- S83.519 Sprain of anterior cruciate ligament of unspecified knee

S83.52 Sprain of posterior cruciate ligament of knee
- S83.521 Sprain of posterior cruciate ligament of right knee
- S83.522 Sprain of posterior cruciate ligament of left knee
- S83.529 Sprain of posterior cruciate ligament of unspecified knee

S83.6 Sprain of the superior tibiofibular joint and ligament
- X S83.60 Sprain of the superior tibiofibular joint and ligament, unspecified knee
- X S83.61 Sprain of the superior tibiofibular joint and ligament, right knee
- X S83.62 Sprain of the superior tibiofibular joint and ligament, left knee

S83.8 Sprain of other specified parts of knee

S83.8X Sprain of other specified parts of knee
- S83.8X1 Sprain of other specified parts of right knee
- S83.8X2 Sprain of other specified parts of left knee
- S83.8X9 Sprain of other specified parts of unspecified knee

S83.9 Sprain of unspecified site of knee
- X S83.90 Sprain of unspecified site of unspecified knee
- X S83.91 Sprain of unspecified site of right knee
- X S83.92 Sprain of unspecified site of left knee

S84 Injury of nerves at lower leg level

Code also any associated open wound (S81.-)

Excludes2 injury of nerves at ankle and foot level (S94.-)

The appropriate 7th character is to be added to each code from category S84

A	initial encounter
D	subsequent encounter
S	sequela

S84.0 Injury of tibial nerve at lower leg level
- X S84.00 Injury of tibial nerve at lower leg level, unspecified leg
- X S84.01 Injury of tibial nerve at lower leg level, right leg
- X S84.02 Injury of tibial nerve at lower leg level, left leg

- S84.1 Injury of peroneal nerve at lower leg level
  - X S84.1Ø Injury of peroneal nerve at lower leg level, unspecified leg
  - X S84.11 Injury of peroneal nerve at lower leg level, right leg
  - X S84.12 Injury of peroneal nerve at lower leg level, left leg
- S84.2 Injury of cutaneous sensory nerve at lower leg level
  - X S84.2Ø Injury of cutaneous sensory nerve at lower leg level, unspecified leg
  - X S84.21 Injury of cutaneous sensory nerve at lower leg level, right leg
  - X S84.22 Injury of cutaneous sensory nerve at lower leg level, left leg
- S84.8 Injury of other nerves at lower leg level
  - S84.8Ø Injury of other nerves at lower leg level
    - S84.8Ø1 Injury of other nerves at lower leg level, right leg
    - S84.8Ø2 Injury of other nerves at lower leg level, left leg
    - S84.8Ø9 Injury of other nerves at lower leg level, unspecified leg
- S84.9 Injury of unspecified nerve at lower leg level
  - X S84.9Ø Injury of unspecified nerve at lower leg level, unspecified leg
  - X S84.91 Injury of unspecified nerve at lower leg level, right leg
  - X S84.92 Injury of unspecified nerve at lower leg level, left leg

S85 Injury of blood vessels at lower leg level

Code also any associated open wound (S81.-)

Excludes2 injury of blood vessels at ankle and foot level (S95.-)

The appropriate 7th character is to be added to each code from category S85

A	initial encounter
D	subsequent encounter
S	sequela

- S85.Ø Injury of popliteal artery
  - S85.ØØ Unspecified injury of popliteal artery
    - S85.ØØ1 Unspecified injury of popliteal artery, right leg
    - S85.ØØ2 Unspecified injury of popliteal artery, left leg
    - S85.ØØ9 Unspecified injury of popliteal artery, unspecified leg
  - S85.Ø1 Laceration of popliteal artery
    - S85.Ø11 Laceration of popliteal artery, right leg
    - S85.Ø12 Laceration of popliteal artery, left leg
    - S85.Ø19 Laceration of popliteal artery, unspecified leg
  - S85.Ø9 Other specified injury of popliteal artery
    - S85.Ø91 Other specified injury of popliteal artery, right leg
    - S85.Ø92 Other specified injury of popliteal artery, left leg
    - S85.Ø99 Other specified injury of popliteal artery, unspecified leg
- S85.1 Injury of tibial artery
  - S85.1Ø Unspecified injury of unspecified tibial artery
    Injury of tibial artery NOS
    - S85.1Ø1 Unspecified injury of unspecified tibial artery, right leg
    - S85.1Ø2 Unspecified injury of unspecified tibial artery, left leg
    - S85.1Ø9 Unspecified injury of unspecified tibial artery, unspecified leg
  - S85.11 Laceration of unspecified tibial artery
    - S85.111 Laceration of unspecified tibial artery, right leg
    - S85.112 Laceration of unspecified tibial artery, left leg
    - S85.119 Laceration of unspecified tibial artery, unspecified leg
  - S85.12 Other specified injury of unspecified tibial artery
    - S85.121 Other specified injury of unspecified tibial artery, right leg
    - S85.122 Other specified injury of unspecified tibial artery, left leg
    - S85.129 Other specified injury of unspecified tibial artery, unspecified leg
  - S85.13 Unspecified injury of anterior tibial artery
    - S85.131 Unspecified injury of anterior tibial artery, right leg
    - S85.132 Unspecified injury of anterior tibial artery, left leg
    - S85.139 Unspecified injury of anterior tibial artery, unspecified leg
  - S85.14 Laceration of anterior tibial artery
    - S85.141 Laceration of anterior tibial artery, right leg
    - S85.142 Laceration of anterior tibial artery, left leg
    - S85.149 Laceration of anterior tibial artery, unspecified leg
  - S85.15 Other specified injury of anterior tibial artery
    - S85.151 Other specified injury of anterior tibial artery, right leg
    - S85.152 Other specified injury of anterior tibial artery, left leg
    - S85.159 Other specified injury of anterior tibial artery, unspecified leg
  - S85.16 Unspecified injury of posterior tibial artery
    - S85.161 Unspecified injury of posterior tibial artery, right leg
    - S85.162 Unspecified injury of posterior tibial artery, left leg
    - S85.169 Unspecified injury of posterior tibial artery, unspecified leg
  - S85.17 Laceration of posterior tibial artery
    - S85.171 Laceration of posterior tibial artery, right leg
    - S85.172 Laceration of posterior tibial artery, left leg
    - S85.179 Laceration of posterior tibial artery, unspecified leg
  - S85.18 Other specified injury of posterior tibial artery
    - S85.181 Other specified injury of posterior tibial artery, right leg
    - S85.182 Other specified injury of posterior tibial artery, left leg
    - S85.189 Other specified injury of posterior tibial artery, unspecified leg
- S85.2 Injury of peroneal artery
  - S85.2Ø Unspecified injury of peroneal artery
    - S85.2Ø1 Unspecified injury of peroneal artery, right leg
    - S85.2Ø2 Unspecified injury of peroneal artery, left leg
    - S85.2Ø9 Unspecified injury of peroneal artery, unspecified leg

- S85.21 Laceration of peroneal artery
  - S85.211 Laceration of peroneal artery, right leg
  - S85.212 Laceration of peroneal artery, left leg
  - S85.219 Laceration of peroneal artery, unspecified leg
- S85.29 Other specified injury of peroneal artery
  - S85.291 Other specified injury of peroneal artery, right leg
  - S85.292 Other specified injury of peroneal artery, left leg
  - S85.299 Other specified injury of peroneal artery, unspecified leg

S85.3 Injury of greater saphenous vein at lower leg level
Injury of greater saphenous vein NOS
Injury of saphenous vein NOS

- S85.30 Unspecified injury of greater saphenous vein at lower leg level
  - S85.301 Unspecified injury of greater saphenous vein at lower leg level, right leg
  - S85.302 Unspecified injury of greater saphenous vein at lower leg level, left leg
  - S85.309 Unspecified injury of greater saphenous vein at lower leg level, unspecified leg
- S85.31 Laceration of greater saphenous vein at lower leg level
  - S85.311 Laceration of greater saphenous vein at lower leg level, right leg
  - S85.312 Laceration of greater saphenous vein at lower leg level, left leg
  - S85.319 Laceration of greater saphenous vein at lower leg level, unspecified leg
- S85.39 Other specified injury of greater saphenous vein at lower leg level
  - S85.391 Other specified injury of greater saphenous vein at lower leg level, right leg
  - S85.392 Other specified injury of greater saphenous vein at lower leg level, left leg
  - S85.399 Other specified injury of greater saphenous vein at lower leg level, unspecified leg

S85.4 Injury of lesser saphenous vein at lower leg level

- S85.40 Unspecified injury of lesser saphenous vein at lower leg level
  - S85.401 Unspecified injury of lesser saphenous vein at lower leg level, right leg
  - S85.402 Unspecified injury of lesser saphenous vein at lower leg level, left leg
  - S85.409 Unspecified injury of lesser saphenous vein at lower leg level, unspecified leg
- S85.41 Laceration of lesser saphenous vein at lower leg level
  - S85.411 Laceration of lesser saphenous vein at lower leg level, right leg
  - S85.412 Laceration of lesser saphenous vein at lower leg level, left leg
  - S85.419 Laceration of lesser saphenous vein at lower leg level, unspecified leg
- S85.49 Other specified injury of lesser saphenous vein at lower leg level
  - S85.491 Other specified injury of lesser saphenous vein at lower leg level, right leg
  - S85.492 Other specified injury of lesser saphenous vein at lower leg level, left leg
  - S85.499 Other specified injury of lesser saphenous vein at lower leg level, unspecified leg

S85.5 Injury of popliteal vein

- S85.50 Unspecified injury of popliteal vein
  - S85.501 Unspecified injury of popliteal vein, right leg
  - S85.502 Unspecified injury of popliteal vein, left leg
  - S85.509 Unspecified injury of popliteal vein, unspecified leg
- S85.51 Laceration of popliteal vein
  - S85.511 Laceration of popliteal vein, right leg
  - S85.512 Laceration of popliteal vein, left leg
  - S85.519 Laceration of popliteal vein, unspecified leg
- S85.59 Other specified injury of popliteal vein
  - S85.591 Other specified injury of popliteal vein, right leg
  - S85.592 Other specified injury of popliteal vein, left leg
  - S85.599 Other specified injury of popliteal vein, unspecified leg

S85.8 Injury of other blood vessels at lower leg level

- S85.80 Unspecified injury of other blood vessels at lower leg level
  - S85.801 Unspecified injury of other blood vessels at lower leg level, right leg
  - S85.802 Unspecified injury of other blood vessels at lower leg level, left leg
  - S85.809 Unspecified injury of other blood vessels at lower leg level, unspecified leg
- S85.81 Laceration of other blood vessels at lower leg level
  - S85.811 Laceration of other blood vessels at lower leg level, right leg
  - S85.812 Laceration of other blood vessels at lower leg level, left leg
  - S85.819 Laceration of other blood vessels at lower leg level, unspecified leg
- S85.89 Other specified injury of other blood vessels at lower leg level
  - S85.891 Other specified injury of other blood vessels at lower leg level, right leg
  - S85.892 Other specified injury of other blood vessels at lower leg level, left leg
  - S85.899 Other specified injury of other blood vessels at lower leg level, unspecified leg

S85.9 Injury of unspecified blood vessel at lower leg level

- S85.90 Unspecified injury of unspecified blood vessel at lower leg level
  - S85.901 Unspecified injury of unspecified blood vessel at lower leg level, right leg
  - S85.902 Unspecified injury of unspecified blood vessel at lower leg level, left leg
  - S85.909 Unspecified injury of unspecified blood vessel at lower leg level, unspecified leg

- S85.91 Laceration of unspecified blood vessel at lower leg level
  - S85.911 Laceration of unspecified blood vessel at lower leg level, **right leg**
  - S85.912 Laceration of unspecified blood vessel at lower leg level, **left leg**
  - S85.919 Laceration of unspecified blood vessel at lower leg level, **unspecified** leg
- S85.99 Other specified injury of unspecified blood vessel at lower leg level
  - S85.991 Other specified injury of unspecified blood vessel at lower leg level, **right** leg
  - S85.992 Other specified injury of unspecified blood vessel at lower leg level, **left** leg
  - S85.999 Other specified injury of unspecified blood vessel at lower leg level, **unspecified** leg

S86 Injury of muscle, fascia and tendon at lower leg level

Code also any associated open wound (S81.-)

Excludes2 injury of muscle, fascia and tendon at ankle (S96.-)
injury of patellar ligament (tendon) (S76.1-)
sprain of joints and ligaments of knee (S83.-)

The appropriate 7th character is to be added to each code from category S86

A	initial encounter
D	subsequent encounter
S	sequela

- S86.Ø Injury of Achilles tendon
  - S86.ØØ Unspecified injury of Achilles tendon
    - S86.ØØ1 Unspecified injury of **right** Achilles tendon
    - S86.ØØ2 Unspecified injury of **left** Achilles tendon
    - S86.ØØ9 Unspecified injury of **unspecified** Achilles tendon
  - S86.Ø1 Strain of Achilles tendon
    - S86.Ø11 Strain of **right** Achilles tendon
    - S86.Ø12 Strain of **left** Achilles tendon
    - S86.Ø19 Strain of **unspecified** Achilles tendon
  - S86.Ø2 Laceration of Achilles tendon
    - S86.Ø21 Laceration of **right** Achilles tendon
    - S86.Ø22 Laceration of **left** Achilles tendon
    - S86.Ø29 Laceration of **unspecified** Achilles tendon
  - S86.Ø9 Other specified injury of Achilles tendon
    - S86.Ø91 Other specified injury of **right** Achilles tendon
    - S86.Ø92 Other specified injury of **left** Achilles tendon
    - S86.Ø99 Other specified injury of **unspecified** Achilles tendon
- S86.1 Injury of other muscle(s) and tendon(s) of **posterior muscle group** at lower leg level
  - S86.1Ø Unspecified injury of other muscle(s) and tendon(s) of posterior muscle group at lower leg level
    - S86.1Ø1 Unspecified injury of other muscle(s) and tendon(s) of posterior muscle group at lower leg level, **right leg**
    - S86.1Ø2 Unspecified injury of other muscle(s) and tendon(s) of posterior muscle group at lower leg level, **left leg**
    - S86.1Ø9 Unspecified injury of other muscle(s) and tendon(s) of posterior muscle group at lower leg level, **unspecified** leg
  - S86.11 Strain of other muscle(s) and tendon(s) of posterior muscle group at lower leg level
    - S86.111 Strain of other muscle(s) and tendon(s) of posterior muscle group at lower leg level, **right leg**
    - S86.112 Strain of other muscle(s) and tendon(s) of posterior muscle group at lower leg level, **left leg**
    - S86.119 Strain of other muscle(s) and tendon(s) of posterior muscle group at lower leg level, **unspecified** leg
  - S86.12 Laceration of other muscle(s) and tendon(s) of posterior muscle group at lower leg level
    - S86.121 Laceration of other muscle(s) and tendon(s) of posterior muscle group at lower leg level, **right leg**
    - S86.122 Laceration of other muscle(s) and tendon(s) of posterior muscle group at lower leg level, **left leg**
    - S86.129 Laceration of other muscle(s) and tendon(s) of posterior muscle group at lower leg level, **unspecified** leg
  - S86.19 Other injury of other muscle(s) and tendon(s) of posterior muscle group at lower leg level
    - S86.191 Other injury of other muscle(s) and tendon(s) of posterior muscle group at lower leg level, **right leg**
    - S86.192 Other injury of other muscle(s) and tendon(s) of posterior muscle group at lower leg level, **left leg**
    - S86.199 Other injury of other muscle(s) and tendon(s) of posterior muscle group at lower leg level, **unspecified** leg
- S86.2 Injury of muscle(s) and tendon(s) of **anterior muscle group** at lower leg level
  - S86.2Ø Unspecified injury of muscle(s) and tendon(s) of anterior muscle group at lower leg level
    - S86.2Ø1 Unspecified injury of muscle(s) and tendon(s) of anterior muscle group at lower leg level, **right leg**
    - S86.2Ø2 Unspecified injury of muscle(s) and tendon(s) of anterior muscle group at lower leg level, **left leg**
    - S86.2Ø9 Unspecified injury of muscle(s) and tendon(s) of anterior muscle group at lower leg level, **unspecified** leg
  - S86.21 Strain of muscle(s) and tendon(s) of anterior muscle group at lower leg level
    - S86.211 Strain of muscle(s) and tendon(s) of anterior muscle group at lower leg level, **right leg**
    - S86.212 Strain of muscle(s) and tendon(s) of anterior muscle group at lower leg level, **left leg**
    - S86.219 Strain of muscle(s) and tendon(s) of anterior muscle group at lower leg level, **unspecified** leg
  - S86.22 Laceration of muscle(s) and tendon(s) of anterior muscle group at lower leg level
    - S86.221 Laceration of muscle(s) and tendon(s) of anterior muscle group at lower leg level, **right leg**
    - S86.222 Laceration of muscle(s) and tendon(s) of anterior muscle group at lower leg level, **left leg**
    - S86.229 Laceration of muscle(s) and tendon(s) of anterior muscle group at lower leg level, **unspecified** leg

- S86.29 **Other** injury of muscle(s) and tendon(s) of anterior muscle group at lower leg level
  - S86.291 Other injury of muscle(s) and tendon(s) of anterior muscle group at lower leg level, **right** leg
  - S86.292 Other injury of muscle(s) and tendon(s) of anterior muscle group at lower leg level, **left** leg
  - S86.299 Other injury of muscle(s) and tendon(s) of anterior muscle group at lower leg level, **unspecified** leg
- S86.3 Injury of muscle(s) and tendon(s) of **peroneal muscle group** at lower leg level
  - S86.30 **Unspecified** injury of muscle(s) and tendon(s) of peroneal muscle group at lower leg level
    - S86.301 Unspecified injury of muscle(s) and tendon(s) of peroneal muscle group at lower leg level, **right** leg
    - S86.302 Unspecified injury of muscle(s) and tendon(s) of peroneal muscle group at lower leg level, **left** leg
    - S86.309 Unspecified injury of muscle(s) and tendon(s) of peroneal muscle group at lower leg level, **unspecified** leg
  - S86.31 **Strain** of muscle(s) and tendon(s) of peroneal muscle group at lower leg level
    - S86.311 Strain of muscle(s) and tendon(s) of peroneal muscle group at lower leg level, **right** leg
    - S86.312 Strain of muscle(s) and tendon(s) of peroneal muscle group at lower leg level, **left** leg
    - S86.319 Strain of muscle(s) and tendon(s) of peroneal muscle group at lower leg level, **unspecified** leg
  - S86.32 **Laceration** of muscle(s) and tendon(s) of peroneal muscle group at lower leg level
    - S86.321 Laceration of muscle(s) and tendon(s) of peroneal muscle group at lower leg level, **right** leg
    - S86.322 Laceration of muscle(s) and tendon(s) of peroneal muscle group at lower leg level, **left** leg
    - S86.329 Laceration of muscle(s) and tendon(s) of peroneal muscle group at lower leg level, **unspecified** leg
  - S86.39 **Other** injury of muscle(s) and tendon(s) of peroneal muscle group at lower leg level
    - S86.391 Other injury of muscle(s) and tendon(s) of peroneal muscle group at lower leg level, **right** leg
    - S86.392 Other injury of muscle(s) and tendon(s) of peroneal muscle group at lower leg level, **left** leg
    - S86.399 Other injury of muscle(s) and tendon(s) of peroneal muscle group at lower leg level, **unspecified** leg
- S86.8 Injury of **other** muscles and tendons at lower leg level
  - S86.80 **Unspecified** injury of other muscles and tendons at lower leg level
    - S86.801 Unspecified injury of other muscle(s) and tendon(s) at lower leg level, **right** leg
    - S86.802 Unspecified injury of other muscle(s) and tendon(s) at lower leg level, **left** leg
    - S86.809 Unspecified injury of other muscle(s) and tendon(s) at lower leg level, **unspecified** leg
  - S86.81 **Strain** of other muscles and tendons at lower leg level
    - S86.811 Strain of other muscle(s) and tendon(s) at lower leg level, **right** leg
    - S86.812 Strain of other muscle(s) and tendon(s) at lower leg level, **left** leg
    - S86.819 Strain of other muscle(s) and tendon(s) at lower leg level, **unspecified** leg
  - S86.82 **Laceration** of other muscles and tendons at lower leg level
    - S86.821 Laceration of other muscle(s) and tendon(s) at lower leg level, **right** leg
    - S86.822 Laceration of other muscle(s) and tendon(s) at lower leg level, **left** leg
    - S86.829 Laceration of other muscle(s) and tendon(s) at lower leg level, **unspecified** leg
  - S86.89 **Other** injury of other muscles and tendons at lower leg level
    - S86.891 Other injury of other muscle(s) and tendon(s) at lower leg level, **right** leg
    - S86.892 Other injury of other muscle(s) and tendon(s) at lower leg level, **left** leg
    - S86.899 Other injury of other muscle(s) and tendon(s) at lower leg level, **unspecified** leg
- S86.9 Injury of **unspecified** muscle and tendon at lower leg level
  - S86.90 **Unspecified** injury of unspecified muscle and tendon at lower leg level
    - S86.901 Unspecified injury of unspecified muscle(s) and tendon(s) at lower leg level, **right** leg
    - S86.902 Unspecified injury of unspecified muscle(s) and tendon(s) at lower leg level, **left** leg
    - S86.909 Unspecified injury of unspecified muscle(s) and tendon(s) at lower leg level, **unspecified** leg
  - S86.91 **Strain** of unspecified muscle and tendon at lower leg level
    - S86.911 Strain of unspecified muscle(s) and tendon(s) at lower leg level, **right** leg
    - S86.912 Strain of unspecified muscle(s) and tendon(s) at lower leg level, **left** leg
    - S86.919 Strain of unspecified muscle(s) and tendon(s) at lower leg level, **unspecified** leg
  - S86.92 **Laceration** of unspecified muscle and tendon at lower leg level
    - S86.921 Laceration of unspecified muscle(s) and tendon(s) at lower leg level, **right** leg
    - S86.922 Laceration of unspecified muscle(s) and tendon(s) at lower leg level, **left** leg
    - S86.929 Laceration of unspecified muscle(s) and tendon(s) at lower leg level, **unspecified** leg
  - S86.99 **Other** injury of unspecified muscle and tendon at lower leg level
    - S86.991 Other injury of unspecified muscle(s) and tendon(s) at lower leg level, **right** leg
    - S86.992 Other injury of unspecified muscle(s) and tendon(s) at lower leg level, **left** leg
    - S86.999 Other injury of unspecified muscle(s) and tendon(s) at lower leg level, **unspecified** leg

S87 Crushing injury of lower leg
Use additional code(s) for all associated injuries
Excludes2 crushing injury of ankle and foot (S97.-)
The appropriate 7th character is to be added to each code from category S87

A	initial encounter
D	subsequent encounter
S	sequela

S87.0 Crushing injury of **knee**
X S87.00 Crushing injury of **unspecified** knee
X S87.01 Crushing injury of **right** knee
X S87.02 Crushing injury of **left** knee
S87.8 Crushing injury of **lower leg**
X S87.80 Crushing injury of **unspecified** lower leg
X S87.81 Crushing injury of **right** lower leg
X S87.82 Crushing injury of **left** lower leg

S88 Traumatic amputation of lower leg
An amputation not identified as partial or complete should be coded to complete
Excludes1 traumatic amputation of ankle and foot (S98.-)
The appropriate 7th character is to be added to each code from category S88

A	initial encounter
D	subsequent encounter
S	sequela

S88.0 Traumatic amputation at **knee level**
S88.01 **Complete** traumatic amputation at knee level
S88.011 Complete traumatic amputation at knee level, **right** lower leg A, D, S
S88.012 Complete traumatic amputation at knee level, **left** lower leg A, D, S
S88.019 Complete traumatic amputation at knee level, **unspecified** lower leg A, D, S
S88.02 **Partial** traumatic amputation at knee level
S88.021 Partial traumatic amputation at knee level, **right** lower leg A, D, S
S88.022 Partial traumatic amputation at knee level, **left** lower leg A, D, S
S88.029 Partial traumatic amputation at knee level, **unspecified** lower leg A, D, S
S88.1 Traumatic amputation at level **between knee and ankle**
S88.11 **Complete** traumatic amputation at level between knee and ankle
S88.111 Complete traumatic amputation at level between knee and ankle, **right** lower leg A, D, S
S88.112 Complete traumatic amputation at level between knee and ankle, **left** lower leg A, D, S
S88.119 Complete traumatic amputation at level between knee and ankle, **unspecified** lower leg A, D, S
S88.12 **Partial** traumatic amputation at level between knee and ankle
S88.121 Partial traumatic amputation at level between knee and ankle, **right** lower leg A, D, S
S88.122 Partial traumatic amputation at level between knee and ankle, **left** lower leg A, D, S
S88.129 Partial traumatic amputation at level between knee and ankle, **unspecified** lower leg A, D, S
S88.9 Traumatic amputation of lower leg, **level unspecified**
S88.91 **Complete** traumatic amputation of lower leg, level unspecified
S88.911 Complete traumatic amputation of **right** lower leg, level unspecified A, D, S
S88.912 Complete traumatic amputation of **left** lower leg, level unspecified A, D, S
S88.919 Complete traumatic amputation of **unspecified** lower leg, level unspecified A, D, S
S88.92 **Partial** traumatic amputation of lower leg, level unspecified
S88.921 Partial traumatic amputation of **right** lower leg, level **unspecified** A, D, S
S88.922 Partial traumatic amputation of **left** lower leg, level **unspecified** A, D, S
S88.929 Partial traumatic amputation of unspecified lower leg, level **unspecified** A, D, S

S89 Other and unspecified injuries of lower leg
Note: A fracture not indicated as open or closed should be coded to closed
Excludes2 other and unspecified injuries of ankle and foot (S99.-)
The appropriate 7th character is to be added to each code from subcategories S89.0, S89.1, S89.2, and S89.3

A	initial encounter for closed fracture
D	subsequent encounter for fracture with routine healing
G	subsequent encounter for fracture with delayed healing
K	subsequent encounter for fracture with nonunion
P	subsequent encounter for fracture with malunion
S	sequela

S89.0 **Physeal** fracture of **upper end of tibia**
S89.00 **Unspecified** physeal fracture of upper end of tibia
S89.001 Unspecified physeal fracture of upper end of **right** tibia
S89.002 Unspecified physeal fracture of upper end of **left** tibia
S89.009 Unspecified physeal fracture of upper end of **unspecified** tibia
S89.01 **Salter-Harris Type I** physeal fracture of upper end of tibia
S89.011 Salter-Harris Type I physeal fracture of upper end of **right** tibia
S89.012 Salter-Harris Type I physeal fracture of upper end of **left** tibia
S89.019 Salter-Harris Type I physeal fracture of upper end of **unspecified** tibia
S89.02 **Salter-Harris Type II** physeal fracture of upper end of tibia
S89.021 Salter-Harris Type II physeal fracture of upper end of **right** tibia
S89.022 Salter-Harris Type II physeal fracture of upper end of **left** tibia
S89.029 Salter-Harris Type II physeal fracture of upper end of **unspecified** tibia
S89.03 **Salter-Harris Type III** physeal fracture of upper end of tibia
S89.031 Salter-Harris Type III physeal fracture of upper end of **right** tibia
S89.032 Salter-Harris Type III physeal fracture of upper end of **left** tibia
S89.039 Salter-Harris Type III physeal fracture of upper end of **unspecified** tibia

CHAPTER 19 (S00-T88)

S89.04 Salter-Harris Type IV physeal fracture of upper end of tibia
- S89.041 Salter-Harris Type IV physeal fracture of upper end of **right** tibia
- S89.042 Salter-Harris Type IV physeal fracture of upper end of **left** tibia
- S89.049 Salter-Harris Type IV physeal fracture of upper end of **unspecified** tibia

S89.09 Other physeal fracture of upper end of tibia
- S89.091 Other physeal fracture of upper end of **right** tibia
- S89.092 Other physeal fracture of upper end of **left** tibia
- S89.099 Other physeal fracture of upper end of **unspecified** tibia

S89.1 Physeal fracture of lower end of tibia

S89.10 **Unspecified** physeal fracture of lower end of tibia
- S89.101 Unspecified physeal fracture of lower end of **right** tibia
- S89.102 Unspecified physeal fracture of lower end of **left** tibia
- S89.109 Unspecified physeal fracture of lower end of **unspecified** tibia

S89.11 **Salter-Harris Type I** physeal fracture of lower end of tibia
- S89.111 Salter-Harris Type I physeal fracture of lower end of **right** tibia
- S89.112 Salter-Harris Type I physeal fracture of lower end of **left** tibia
- S89.119 Salter-Harris Type I physeal fracture of lower end of **unspecified** tibia

S89.12 **Salter-Harris Type II** physeal fracture of lower end of tibia
- S89.121 Salter-Harris Type II physeal fracture of lower end of **right** tibia
- S89.122 Salter-Harris Type II physeal fracture of lower end of **left** tibia
- S89.129 Salter-Harris Type II physeal fracture of lower end of **unspecified** tibia

S89.13 **Salter-Harris Type III** physeal fracture of lower end of tibia

Excludes1 fracture of medial malleolus (adult) (S82.5-)

- S89.131 Salter-Harris Type III physeal fracture of lower end of **right** tibia
- S89.132 Salter-Harris Type III physeal fracture of lower end of **left** tibia
- S89.139 Salter-Harris Type III physeal fracture of lower end of **unspecified** tibia

S89.14 **Salter-Harris Type IV** physeal fracture of lower end of tibia

Excludes1 fracture of medial malleolus (adult) (S82.5-)

- S89.141 Salter-Harris Type IV physeal fracture of lower end of **right** tibia
- S89.142 Salter-Harris Type IV physeal fracture of lower end of **left** tibia
- S89.149 Salter-Harris Type IV physeal fracture of lower end of **unspecified** tibia

S89.19 **Other** physeal fracture of lower end of tibia
- S89.191 Other physeal fracture of lower end of **right** tibia
- S89.192 Other physeal fracture of lower end of **left** tibia
- S89.199 Other physeal fracture of lower end of **unspecified** tibia

S89.2 Physeal fracture of upper end of fibula

S89.20 **Unspecified** physeal fracture of upper end of fibula
- S89.201 Unspecified physeal fracture of upper end of **right** fibula
- S89.202 Unspecified physeal fracture of upper end of **left** fibula
- S89.209 Unspecified physeal fracture of upper end of **unspecified** fibula

S89.21 **Salter-Harris Type I** physeal fracture of upper end of fibula
- S89.211 Salter-Harris Type I physeal fracture of upper end of **right** fibula
- S89.212 Salter-Harris Type I physeal fracture of upper end of **left** fibula
- S89.219 Salter-Harris Type I physeal fracture of upper end of **unspecified** fibula

S89.22 **Salter-Harris Type II** physeal fracture of upper end of fibula
- S89.221 Salter-Harris Type II physeal fracture of upper end of **right** fibula
- S89.222 Salter-Harris Type II physeal fracture of upper end of **left** fibula
- S89.229 Salter-Harris Type II physeal fracture of upper end of **unspecified** fibula

S89.29 **Other** physeal fracture of upper end of fibula
- S89.291 Other physeal fracture of upper end of **right** fibula
- S89.292 Other physeal fracture of upper end of **left** fibula
- S89.299 Other physeal fracture of upper end of **unspecified** fibula

S89.3 Physeal fracture of lower end of fibula

S89.30 **Unspecified** physeal fracture of lower end of fibula
- S89.301 Unspecified physeal fracture of lower end of **right** fibula
- S89.302 Unspecified physeal fracture of lower end of **left** fibula
- S89.309 Unspecified physeal fracture of lower end of **unspecified** fibula

S89.31 **Salter-Harris Type I** physeal fracture of lower end of fibula
- S89.311 Salter-Harris Type I physeal fracture of lower end of **right** fibula
- S89.312 Salter-Harris Type I physeal fracture of lower end of **left** fibula
- S89.319 Salter-Harris Type I physeal fracture of lower end of **unspecified** fibula

S89.32 **Salter-Harris Type II** physeal fracture of lower end of fibula
- S89.321 Salter-Harris Type II physeal fracture of lower end of **right** fibula
- S89.322 Salter-Harris Type II physeal fracture of lower end of **left** fibula
- S89.329 Salter-Harris Type II physeal fracture of lower end of **unspecified** fibula

S89.39 **Other** physeal fracture of lower end of fibula
- S89.391 Other physeal fracture of lower end of **right** fibula
- S89.392 Other physeal fracture of lower end of **left** fibula
- S89.399 Other physeal fracture of lower end of **unspecified** fibula

● **S89.8 Other specified injuries of lower leg**

The appropriate 7th character is to be added to each code in subcategory S89.8

A	initial encounter
D	subsequent encounter
S	sequela

X● **S89.80** Other specified injuries of unspecified lower leg

X● **S89.81** Other specified injuries of right lower leg

X● **S89.82** Other specified injuries of left lower leg

● **S89.9 Unspecified injury of lower leg**

The appropriate 7th character is to be added to each code in subcategory S89.9

A	initial encounter
D	subsequent encounter
S	sequela

X● **S89.90** Unspecified injury of unspecified lower leg

X● **S89.91** Unspecified injury of right lower leg

X● **S89.92** Unspecified injury of left lower leg

INJURIES TO THE ANKLE AND FOOT (S90-S99)

Excludes2 burns and corrosions (T20-T32)
fracture of ankle and malleolus (S82.-)
frostbite (T33-T34)
insect bite or sting, venomous (T63.4)

● **S90 Superficial injury of ankle, foot and toes**

The appropriate 7th character is to be added to each code from category S90

A	initial encounter
D	subsequent encounter
S	sequela

● **S90.0** Contusion of ankle

X● **S90.00** Contusion of unspecified ankle

X● **S90.01** Contusion of right ankle

X● **S90.02** Contusion of left ankle

● **S90.1** Contusion of toe without damage to nail

● **S90.11** Contusion of great toe without damage to nail

● **S90.111** Contusion of right great toe without damage to nail

● **S90.112** Contusion of left great toe without damage to nail

● **S90.119** Contusion of unspecified great toe without damage to nail

● **S90.12** Contusion of lesser toe without damage to nail

● **S90.121** Contusion of right lesser toe(s) without damage to nail

● **S90.122** Contusion of left lesser toe(s) without damage to nail

● **S90.129** Contusion of unspecified lesser toe(s) without damage to nail
Contusion of toe NOS

● **S90.2** Contusion of toe with damage to nail

● **S90.21** Contusion of great toe with damage to nail

● **S90.211** Contusion of right great toe with damage to nail

● **S90.212** Contusion of left great toe with damage to nail

● **S90.219** Contusion of unspecified great toe with damage to nail

● **S90.22** Contusion of lesser toe with damage to nail

● **S90.221** Contusion of right lesser toe(s) with damage to nail

● **S90.222** Contusion of left lesser toe(s) with damage to nail

● **S90.229** Contusion of unspecified lesser toe(s) with damage to nail

● **S90.3** Contusion of foot

Excludes2 contusion of toes (S90.1-, S90.2-)

X● **S90.30** Contusion of unspecified foot
Contusion of foot NOS

X● **S90.31** Contusion of right foot

X● **S90.32** Contusion of left foot

● **S90.4** Other superficial injuries of toe

● **S90.41** Abrasion of toe

● **S90.411** Abrasion, right great toe

● **S90.412** Abrasion, left great toe

● **S90.413** Abrasion, unspecified great toe

● **S90.414** Abrasion, right lesser toe(s)

● **S90.415** Abrasion, left lesser toe(s)

● **S90.416** Abrasion, unspecified lesser toe(s)

● **S90.42** Blister (nonthermal) of toe

● **S90.421** Blister (nonthermal), right great toe

● **S90.422** Blister (nonthermal), left great toe

● **S90.423** Blister (nonthermal), unspecified great toe

● **S90.424** Blister (nonthermal), right lesser toe(s)

● **S90.425** Blister (nonthermal), left lesser toe(s)

● **S90.426** Blister (nonthermal), unspecified lesser toe(s)

● **S90.44** External constriction of toe
Hair tourniquet syndrome of toe

● **S90.441** External constriction, right great toe

● **S90.442** External constriction, left great toe

● **S90.443** External constriction, unspecified great toe

● **S90.444** External constriction, right lesser toe(s)

● **S90.445** External constriction, left lesser toe(s)

● **S90.446** External constriction, unspecified lesser toe(s)

● **S90.45** Superficial foreign body of toe
Splinter in the toe

● **S90.451** Superficial foreign body, right great toe

● **S90.452** Superficial foreign body, left great toe

● **S90.453** Superficial foreign body, unspecified great toe

● **S90.454** Superficial foreign body, right lesser toe(s)

● **S90.455** Superficial foreign body, left lesser toe(s)

● **S90.456** Superficial foreign body, unspecified lesser toe(s)

● **S90.46** Insect bite (nonvenomous) of toe

● **S90.461** Insect bite (nonvenomous), right great toe

● **S90.462** Insect bite (nonvenomous), left great toe

● **S90.463** Insect bite (nonvenomous), unspecified great toe

● **S90.464** Insect bite (nonvenomous), right lesser toe(s)

● **S90.465** Insect bite (nonvenomous), left lesser toe(s)

● **S90.466** Insect bite (nonvenomous), unspecified lesser toe(s)

- S90.47 Other superficial bite of toe
  - **Excludes1** open bite of toe (S91.15-, S91.25-)
  - S90.471 Other superficial bite of right great toe
  - S90.472 Other superficial bite of left great toe
  - S90.473 Other superficial bite of unspecified great toe
  - S90.474 Other superficial bite of right lesser toe(s)
  - S90.475 Other superficial bite of left lesser toe(s)
  - S90.476 Other superficial bite of unspecified lesser toe(s)
- S90.5 Other superficial injuries of ankle
  - S90.51 Abrasion of ankle
    - S90.511 Abrasion, right ankle
    - S90.512 Abrasion, left ankle
    - S90.519 Abrasion, unspecified ankle
  - S90.52 Blister (nonthermal) of ankle
    - S90.521 Blister (nonthermal), right ankle
    - S90.522 Blister (nonthermal), left ankle
    - S90.529 Blister (nonthermal), unspecified ankle
  - S90.54 External constriction of ankle
    - S90.541 External constriction, right ankle
    - S90.542 External constriction, left ankle
    - S90.549 External constriction, unspecified ankle
  - S90.55 Superficial foreign body of ankle
    - Splinter in the ankle
    - S90.551 Superficial foreign body, right ankle
    - S90.552 Superficial foreign body, left ankle
    - S90.559 Superficial foreign body, unspecified ankle
  - S90.56 Insect bite (nonvenomous) of ankle
    - S90.561 Insect bite (nonvenomous), right ankle
    - S90.562 Insect bite (nonvenomous), left ankle
    - S90.569 Insect bite (nonvenomous), unspecified ankle
  - S90.57 Other superficial bite of ankle
    - **Excludes1** open bite of ankle (S91.05-)
    - S90.571 Other superficial bite of ankle, right ankle
    - S90.572 Other superficial bite of ankle, left ankle
    - S90.579 Other superficial bite of ankle, unspecified ankle
- S90.8 Other superficial injuries of foot
  - S90.81 Abrasion of foot
    - S90.811 Abrasion, right foot
    - S90.812 Abrasion, left foot
    - S90.819 Abrasion, unspecified foot
  - S90.82 Blister (nonthermal) of foot
    - S90.821 Blister (nonthermal), right foot
    - S90.822 Blister (nonthermal), left foot
    - S90.829 Blister (nonthermal), unspecified foot
  - S90.84 External constriction of foot
    - S90.841 External constriction, right foot
    - S90.842 External constriction, left foot
    - S90.849 External constriction, unspecified foot
  - S90.85 Superficial foreign body of foot
    - Splinter in the foot
    - S90.851 Superficial foreign body, right foot
    - S90.852 Superficial foreign body, left foot
    - S90.859 Superficial foreign body, unspecified foot
  - S90.86 Insect bite (nonvenomous) of foot
    - S90.861 Insect bite (nonvenomous), right foot
    - S90.862 Insect bite (nonvenomous), left foot
    - S90.869 Insect bite (nonvenomous), unspecified foot
  - S90.87 Other superficial bite of foot
    - **Excludes1** open bite of foot (S91.35-)
    - S90.871 Other superficial bite of right foot
    - S90.872 Other superficial bite of left foot
    - S90.879 Other superficial bite of unspecified foot
- S90.9 Unspecified superficial injury of ankle, foot and toe
  - S90.91 Unspecified superficial injury of ankle
    - S90.911 Unspecified superficial injury of right ankle
    - S90.912 Unspecified superficial injury of left ankle
    - S90.919 Unspecified superficial injury of unspecified ankle
  - S90.92 Unspecified superficial injury of foot
    - S90.921 Unspecified superficial injury of right foot
    - S90.922 Unspecified superficial injury of left foot
    - S90.929 Unspecified superficial injury of unspecified foot
  - S90.93 Unspecified superficial injury of toes
    - S90.931 Unspecified superficial injury of right great toe
    - S90.932 Unspecified superficial injury of left great toe
    - S90.933 Unspecified superficial injury of unspecified great toe
    - S90.934 Unspecified superficial injury of right lesser toe(s)
    - S90.935 Unspecified superficial injury of left lesser toe(s)
    - S90.936 Unspecified superficial injury of unspecified lesser toe(s)

S91 Open wound of ankle, foot and toes

Code also any associated wound infection

Excludes1 open fracture of ankle, foot and toes (S92.-with 7th character B)
traumatic amputation of ankle and foot (S98.-)

The appropriate 7th character is to be added to each code from category S91

A	initial encounter
D	subsequent encounter
S	sequela

- S91.0 Open wound of ankle
  - S91.00 Unspecified open wound of ankle
    - S91.001 Unspecified open wound, right ankle
    - S91.002 Unspecified open wound, left ankle
    - S91.009 Unspecified open wound, unspecified ankle
  - S91.01 Laceration without foreign body of ankle
    - S91.011 Laceration without foreign body, right ankle
    - S91.012 Laceration without foreign body, left ankle
    - S91.019 Laceration without foreign body, unspecified ankle

CHAPTER 19 (S00-T88)

- S91.02 Laceration with foreign body of ankle
  - S91.021 Laceration with foreign body, right ankle
  - S91.022 Laceration with foreign body, left ankle
  - S91.029 Laceration with foreign body, unspecified ankle
- S91.03 Puncture wound without foreign body of ankle
  - S91.031 Puncture wound without foreign body, right ankle
  - S91.032 Puncture wound without foreign body, left ankle
  - S91.039 Puncture wound without foreign body, unspecified ankle
- S91.04 Puncture wound with foreign body of ankle
  - S91.041 Puncture wound with foreign body, right ankle
  - S91.042 Puncture wound with foreign body, left ankle
  - S91.049 Puncture wound with foreign body, unspecified ankle
- S91.05 Open bite of ankle

  Excludes1 superficial bite of ankle (S90.56-, S90.57-)
  - S91.051 Open bite, right ankle
  - S91.052 Open bite, left ankle
  - S91.059 Open bite, unspecified ankle

S91.1 Open wound of toe without damage to nail
- S91.10 Unspecified open wound of toe without damage to nail
  - S91.101 Unspecified open wound of right great toe without damage to nail
  - S91.102 Unspecified open wound of left great toe without damage to nail
  - S91.103 Unspecified open wound of unspecified great toe without damage to nail
  - S91.104 Unspecified open wound of right lesser toe(s) without damage to nail
  - S91.105 Unspecified open wound of left lesser toe(s) without damage to nail
  - S91.106 Unspecified open wound of unspecified lesser toe(s) without damage to nail
  - S91.109 Unspecified open wound of unspecified toe(s) without damage to nail
- S91.11 Laceration without foreign body of toe without damage to nail
  - S91.111 Laceration without foreign body of right great toe without damage to nail
  - S91.112 Laceration without foreign body of left great toe without damage to nail
  - S91.113 Laceration without foreign body of unspecified great toe without damage to nail
  - S91.114 Laceration without foreign body of right lesser toe(s) without damage to nail
  - S91.115 Laceration without foreign body of left lesser toe(s) without damage to nail
  - S91.116 Laceration without foreign body of unspecified lesser toe(s) without damage to nail
  - S91.119 Laceration without foreign body of unspecified toe without damage to nail
- S91.12 Laceration with foreign body of toe without damage to nail
  - S91.121 Laceration with foreign body of right great toe without damage to nail
  - S91.122 Laceration with foreign body of left great toe without damage to nail
  - S91.123 Laceration with foreign body of unspecified great toe without damage to nail
  - S91.124 Laceration with foreign body of right lesser toe(s) without damage to nail
  - S91.125 Laceration with foreign body of left lesser toe(s) without damage to nail
  - S91.126 Laceration with foreign body of unspecified lesser toe(s) without damage to nail
  - S91.129 Laceration with foreign body of unspecified toe(s) without damage to nail
- S91.13 Puncture wound without foreign body of toe without damage to nail
  - S91.131 Puncture wound without foreign body of right great toe without damage to nail
  - S91.132 Puncture wound without foreign body of left great toe without damage to nail
  - S91.133 Puncture wound without foreign body of unspecified great toe without damage to nail
  - S91.134 Puncture wound without foreign body of right lesser toe(s) without damage to nail
  - S91.135 Puncture wound without foreign body of left lesser toe(s) without damage to nail
  - S91.136 Puncture wound without foreign body of unspecified lesser toe(s) without damage to nail
  - S91.139 Puncture wound without foreign body of unspecified toe(s) without damage to nail
- S91.14 Puncture wound with foreign body of toe without damage to nail
  - S91.141 Puncture wound with foreign body of right great toe without damage to nail
  - S91.142 Puncture wound with foreign body of left great toe without damage to nail
  - S91.143 Puncture wound with foreign body of unspecified great toe without damage to nail
  - S91.144 Puncture wound with foreign body of right lesser toe(s) without damage to nail
  - S91.145 Puncture wound with foreign body of left lesser toe(s) without damage to nail
  - S91.146 Puncture wound with foreign body of unspecified lesser toe(s) without damage to nail
  - S91.149 Puncture wound with foreign body of unspecified toe(s) without damage to nail

- S91.15 **Open bite** of toe without damage to nail
  Bite of toe NOS
  Excludes1 superficial bite of toe (S90.46-, S90.47-)
  - S91.151 Open bite of **right great** toe without damage to nail
  - S91.152 Open bite of **left great** toe without damage to nail
  - S91.153 Open bite of **unspecified great** toe without damage to nail
  - S91.154 Open bite of **right lesser** toe(s) without damage to nail
  - S91.155 Open bite of **left lesser** toe(s) without damage to nail
  - S91.156 Open bite of **unspecified lesser** toe(s) without damage to nail
  - S91.159 Open bite of **unspecified toe**(s) without damage to nail
- S91.2 Open wound of **toe with damage to nail**
- S91.20 **Unspecified** open wound of toe with damage to nail
  - S91.201 Unspecified open wound of **right great** toe with damage to nail
  - S91.202 Unspecified open wound of **left great** toe with damage to nail
  - S91.203 Unspecified open wound of **unspecified great** toe with damage to nail
  - S91.204 Unspecified open wound of **right lesser** toe(s) with damage to nail
  - S91.205 Unspecified open wound of **left lesser** toe(s) with damage to nail
  - S91.206 Unspecified open wound of **unspecified lesser** toe(s) with damage to nail
  - S91.209 Unspecified open wound of **unspecified toe**(s) with damage to nail
- S91.21 **Laceration without foreign body** of toe with damage to nail
  - S91.211 Laceration without foreign body of **right great** toe with damage to nail
  - S91.212 Laceration without foreign body of **left great** toe with damage to nail
  - S91.213 Laceration without foreign body of **unspecified great** toe with damage to nail
  - S91.214 Laceration without foreign body of **right lesser** toe(s) with damage to nail
  - S91.215 Laceration without foreign body of **left lesser** toe(s) with damage to nail
  - S91.216 Laceration without foreign body of **unspecified lesser** toe(s) with damage to nail
  - S91.219 Laceration without foreign body of **unspecified toe**(s) with damage to nail
- S91.22 **Laceration with foreign body** of toe with damage to nail
  - S91.221 Laceration with foreign body of **right great** toe with damage to nail
  - S91.222 Laceration with foreign body of **left great** toe with damage to nail
  - S91.223 Laceration with foreign body of **unspecified great** toe with damage to nail
  - S91.224 Laceration with foreign body of **right lesser** toe(s) with damage to nail
  - S91.225 Laceration with foreign body of **left lesser** toe(s) with damage to nail
  - S91.226 Laceration with foreign body of **unspecified lesser** toe(s) with damage to nail
  - S91.229 Laceration with foreign body of **unspecified toe**(s) with damage to nail
- S91.23 **Puncture wound without foreign body** of toe with damage to nail
  - S91.231 Puncture wound without foreign body of **right great** toe with damage to nail
  - S91.232 Puncture wound without foreign body of **left great** toe with damage to nail
  - S91.233 Puncture wound without foreign body of **unspecified great** toe with damage to nail
  - S91.234 Puncture wound without foreign body of **right lesser** toe(s) with damage to nail
  - S91.235 Puncture wound without foreign body of **left lesser** toe(s) with damage to nail
  - S91.236 Puncture wound without foreign body of **unspecified lesser** toe(s) with damage to nail
  - S91.239 Puncture wound without foreign body of **unspecified toe**(s) with damage to nail
- S91.24 **Puncture wound with foreign body** of toe with damage to nail
  - S91.241 Puncture wound with foreign body of **right great** toe with damage to nail
  - S91.242 Puncture wound with foreign body of **left great** toe with damage to nail
  - S91.243 Puncture wound with foreign body of **unspecified great** toe with damage to nail
  - S91.244 Puncture wound with foreign body of **right lesser** toe(s) with damage to nail
  - S91.245 Puncture wound with foreign body of **left lesser** toe(s) with damage to nail
  - S91.246 Puncture wound with foreign body of **unspecified lesser** toe(s) with damage to nail
  - S91.249 Puncture wound with foreign body of **unspecified toe**(s) with damage to nail
- S91.25 **Open bite** of toe with damage to nail
  Bite of toe with damage to nail NOS
  Excludes1 superficial bite of toe (S90.46-, S90.47-)
  - S91.251 Open bite of **right great** toe with damage to nail
  - S91.252 Open bite of **left great** toe with damage to nail
  - S91.253 Open bite of **unspecified great** toe with damage to nail
  - S91.254 Open bite of **right lesser** toe(s) with damage to nail
  - S91.255 Open bite of **left lesser** toe(s) with damage to nail
  - S91.256 Open bite of **unspecified lesser** toe(s) with damage to nail
  - S91.259 Open bite of **unspecified toe**(s) with damage to nail

S91.3 Open wound of foot
S91.30 Unspecified open wound of foot
S91.301 Unspecified open wound, right foot
S91.302 Unspecified open wound, left foot
S91.309 Unspecified open wound, unspecified foot
S91.31 Laceration without foreign body of foot
S91.311 Laceration without foreign body, right foot
S91.312 Laceration without foreign body, left foot
S91.319 Laceration without foreign body, unspecified foot
S91.32 Laceration with foreign body of foot
S91.321 Laceration with foreign body, right foot
S91.322 Laceration with foreign body, left foot
S91.329 Laceration with foreign body, unspecified foot
S91.33 Puncture wound without foreign body of foot
S91.331 Puncture wound without foreign body, right foot
S91.332 Puncture wound without foreign body, left foot
S91.339 Puncture wound without foreign body, unspecified foot
S91.34 Puncture wound with foreign body of foot
S91.341 Puncture wound with foreign body, right foot
S91.342 Puncture wound with foreign body, left foot
S91.349 Puncture wound with foreign body, unspecified foot
S91.35 Open bite of foot
Excludes1 superficial bite of foot (S90.86-, S90.87-)
S91.351 Open bite, right foot
S91.352 Open bite, left foot
S91.359 Open bite, unspecified foot

S92 Fracture of foot and toe, except ankle
Note: A fracture not indicated as displaced or nondisplaced should be coded to displaced
A fracture not indicated as open or closed should be coded to closed
Excludes1 traumatic amputation of ankle and foot (S98.-)
Excludes2 fracture of ankle (S82.-)
fracture of malleolus (S82.-)
The appropriate 7th character is to be added to each code from category S92

A	initial encounter for closed fracture
B	initial encounter for open fracture
D	subsequent encounter for fracture with routine healing
G	subsequent encounter for fracture with delayed healing
K	subsequent encounter for fracture with nonunion
P	subsequent encounter for fracture with malunion
S	sequela

S92.0 Fracture of calcaneus
Heel bone Os calcis
Excludes2 Physeal fracture of calcaneus (S99.0-)
S92.00 Unspecified fracture of calcaneus
S92.001 Unspecified fracture of right calcaneus
S92.002 Unspecified fracture of left calcaneus
S92.009 Unspecified fracture of unspecified calcaneus
S92.01 Fracture of body of calcaneus
S92.011 Displaced fracture of body of right calcaneus
S92.012 Displaced fracture of body of left calcaneus
S92.013 Displaced fracture of body of unspecified calcaneus
S92.014 Nondisplaced fracture of body of right calcaneus
S92.015 Nondisplaced fracture of body of left calcaneus
S92.016 Nondisplaced fracture of body of unspecified calcaneus
S92.02 Fracture of anterior process of calcaneus
S92.021 Displaced fracture of anterior process of right calcaneus
S92.022 Displaced fracture of anterior process of left calcaneus
S92.023 Displaced fracture of anterior process of unspecified calcaneus
S92.024 Nondisplaced fracture of anterior process of right calcaneus
S92.025 Nondisplaced fracture of anterior process of left calcaneus
S92.026 Nondisplaced fracture of anterior process of unspecified calcaneus
S92.03 Avulsion fracture of tuberosity of calcaneus
S92.031 Displaced avulsion fracture of tuberosity of right calcaneus
S92.032 Displaced avulsion fracture of tuberosity of left calcaneus
S92.033 Displaced avulsion fracture of tuberosity of unspecified calcaneus
S92.034 Nondisplaced avulsion fracture of tuberosity of right calcaneus
S92.035 Nondisplaced avulsion fracture of tuberosity of left calcaneus
S92.036 Nondisplaced avulsion fracture of tuberosity of unspecified calcaneus
S92.04 Other fracture of tuberosity of calcaneus
S92.041 Displaced other fracture of tuberosity of right calcaneus
S92.042 Displaced other fracture of tuberosity of left calcaneus
S92.043 Displaced other fracture of tuberosity of unspecified calcaneus
S92.044 Nondisplaced other fracture of tuberosity of right calcaneus
S92.045 Nondisplaced other fracture of tuberosity of left calcaneus
S92.046 Nondisplaced other fracture of tuberosity of unspecified calcaneus
S92.05 Other extraarticular fracture of calcaneus
S92.051 Displaced other extraarticular fracture of right calcaneus
S92.052 Displaced other extraarticular fracture of left calcaneus
S92.053 Displaced other extraarticular fracture of unspecified calcaneus
S92.054 Nondisplaced other extraarticular fracture of right calcaneus
S92.055 Nondisplaced other extraarticular fracture of left calcaneus
S92.056 Nondisplaced other extraarticular fracture of unspecified calcaneus

- S92.06 Intraarticular fracture of calcaneus
  - S92.061 Displaced intraarticular fracture of right calcaneus
  - S92.062 Displaced intraarticular fracture of left calcaneus
  - S92.063 Displaced intraarticular fracture of unspecified calcaneus
  - S92.064 Nondisplaced intraarticular fracture of right calcaneus
  - S92.065 Nondisplaced intraarticular fracture of left calcaneus
  - S92.066 Nondisplaced intraarticular fracture of unspecified calcaneus
- S92.1 Fracture of talus
  Astragalus
  - S92.10 Unspecified fracture of talus
    - S92.101 Unspecified fracture of right talus
    - S92.102 Unspecified fracture of left talus
    - S92.109 Unspecified fracture of unspecified talus
  - S92.11 Fracture of neck of talus
    - S92.111 Displaced fracture of neck of right talus
    - S92.112 Displaced fracture of neck of left talus
    - S92.113 Displaced fracture of neck of unspecified talus
    - S92.114 Nondisplaced fracture of neck of right talus
    - S92.115 Nondisplaced fracture of neck of left talus
    - S92.116 Nondisplaced fracture of neck of unspecified talus
  - S92.12 Fracture of body of talus
    - S92.121 Displaced fracture of body of right talus
    - S92.122 Displaced fracture of body of left talus
    - S92.123 Displaced fracture of body of unspecified talus
    - S92.124 Nondisplaced fracture of body of right talus
    - S92.125 Nondisplaced fracture of body of left talus
    - S92.126 Nondisplaced fracture of body of unspecified talus
  - S92.13 Fracture of posterior process of talus
    - S92.131 Displaced fracture of posterior process of right talus
    - S92.132 Displaced fracture of posterior process of left talus
    - S92.133 Displaced fracture of posterior process of unspecified talus
    - S92.134 Nondisplaced fracture of posterior process of right talus
    - S92.135 Nondisplaced fracture of posterior process of left talus
    - S92.136 Nondisplaced fracture of posterior process of unspecified talus
  - S92.14 Dome fracture of talus
    Excludes1 osteochondritis dissecans (M93.2)
    - S92.141 Displaced dome fracture of right talus
    - S92.142 Displaced dome fracture of left talus
    - S92.143 Displaced dome fracture of unspecified talus
    - S92.144 Nondisplaced dome fracture of right talus
    - S92.145 Nondisplaced dome fracture of left talus
    - S92.146 Nondisplaced dome fracture of unspecified talus
  - S92.15 Avulsion fracture (chip fracture) of talus
    - S92.151 Displaced avulsion fracture (chip fracture) of right talus
    - S92.152 Displaced avulsion fracture (chip fracture) of left talus
    - S92.153 Displaced avulsion fracture (chip fracture) of unspecified talus
    - S92.154 Nondisplaced avulsion fracture (chip fracture) of right talus
    - S92.155 Nondisplaced avulsion fracture (chip fracture) of left talus
    - S92.156 Nondisplaced avulsion fracture (chip fracture) of unspecified talus
  - S92.19 Other fracture of talus
    - S92.191 Other fracture of right talus
    - S92.192 Other fracture of left talus
    - S92.199 Other fracture of unspecified talus
- S92.2 Fracture of other and unspecified tarsal bone(s)
  - S92.20 Fracture of unspecified tarsal bone(s)
    - S92.201 Fracture of unspecified tarsal bone(s) of right foot
    - S92.202 Fracture of unspecified tarsal bone(s) of left foot
    - S92.209 Fracture of unspecified tarsal bone(s) of unspecified foot
  - S92.21 Fracture of cuboid bone
    - S92.211 Displaced fracture of cuboid bone of right foot
    - S92.212 Displaced fracture of cuboid bone of left foot
    - S92.213 Displaced fracture of cuboid bone of unspecified foot
    - S92.214 Nondisplaced fracture of cuboid bone of right foot
    - S92.215 Nondisplaced fracture of cuboid bone of left foot
    - S92.216 Nondisplaced fracture of cuboid bone of unspecified foot
  - S92.22 Fracture of lateral cuneiform
    - S92.221 Displaced fracture of lateral cuneiform of right foot
    - S92.222 Displaced fracture of lateral cuneiform of left foot
    - S92.223 Displaced fracture of lateral cuneiform of unspecified foot
    - S92.224 Nondisplaced fracture of lateral cuneiform of right foot
    - S92.225 Nondisplaced fracture of lateral cuneiform of left foot
    - S92.226 Nondisplaced fracture of lateral cuneiform of unspecified foot
  - S92.23 Fracture of intermediate cuneiform
    - S92.231 Displaced fracture of intermediate cuneiform of right foot
    - S92.232 Displaced fracture of intermediate cuneiform of left foot
    - S92.233 Displaced fracture of intermediate cuneiform of unspecified foot
    - S92.234 Nondisplaced fracture of intermediate cuneiform of right foot
    - S92.235 Nondisplaced fracture of intermediate cuneiform of left foot
    - S92.236 Nondisplaced fracture of intermediate cuneiform of unspecified foot

S92.24 Fracture of medial cuneiform
- S92.241 Displaced fracture of medial cuneiform of right foot
- S92.242 Displaced fracture of medial cuneiform of left foot
- S92.243 Displaced fracture of medial cuneiform of unspecified foot
- S92.244 Nondisplaced fracture of medial cuneiform of right foot
- S92.245 Nondisplaced fracture of medial cuneiform of left foot
- S92.246 Nondisplaced fracture of medial cuneiform of unspecified foot

S92.25 Fracture of navicular [scaphoid] of foot
- S92.251 Displaced fracture of navicular [scaphoid] of right foot
- S92.252 Displaced fracture of navicular [scaphoid] of left foot
- S92.253 Displaced fracture of navicular [scaphoid] of unspecified foot
- S92.254 Nondisplaced fracture of navicular [scaphoid] of right foot
- S92.255 Nondisplaced fracture of navicular [scaphoid] of left foot
- S92.256 Nondisplaced fracture of navicular [scaphoid] of unspecified foot

S92.3 Fracture of metatarsal bone(s)

Excludes2 Physeal fracture of metatarsal (S99.1-)

S92.30 Fracture of unspecified metatarsal bone(s)
- S92.301 Fracture of unspecified metatarsal bone(s), right foot
- S92.302 Fracture of unspecified metatarsal bone(s), left foot
- S92.309 Fracture of unspecified metatarsal bone(s), unspecified foot

S92.31 Fracture of first metatarsal bone
- S92.311 Displaced fracture of first metatarsal bone, right foot
- S92.312 Displaced fracture of first metatarsal bone, left foot
- S92.313 Displaced fracture of first metatarsal bone, unspecified foot
- S92.314 Nondisplaced fracture of first metatarsal bone, right foot
- S92.315 Nondisplaced fracture of first metatarsal bone, left foot
- S92.316 Nondisplaced fracture of first metatarsal bone, unspecified foot

S92.32 Fracture of second metatarsal bone
- S92.321 Displaced fracture of second metatarsal bone, right foot
- S92.322 Displaced fracture of second metatarsal bone, left foot
- S92.323 Displaced fracture of second metatarsal bone, unspecified foot
- S92.324 Nondisplaced fracture of second metatarsal bone, right foot
- S92.325 Nondisplaced fracture of second metatarsal bone, left foot
- S92.326 Nondisplaced fracture of second metatarsal bone, unspecified foot

S92.33 Fracture of third metatarsal bone

Coding Clinic: 2018, Q1, P3
- S92.331 Displaced fracture of third metatarsal bone, right foot
- S92.332 Displaced fracture of third metatarsal bone, left foot
- S92.333 Displaced fracture of third metatarsal bone, unspecified foot
- S92.334 Nondisplaced fracture of third metatarsal bone, right foot
- S92.335 Nondisplaced fracture of third metatarsal bone, left foot
- S92.336 Nondisplaced fracture of third metatarsal bone, unspecified foot

S92.34 Fracture of fourth metatarsal bone
- S92.341 Displaced fracture of fourth metatarsal bone, right foot
- S92.342 Displaced fracture of fourth metatarsal bone, left foot
- S92.343 Displaced fracture of fourth metatarsal bone, unspecified foot
- S92.344 Nondisplaced fracture of fourth metatarsal bone, right foot
- S92.345 Nondisplaced fracture of fourth metatarsal bone, left foot
- S92.346 Nondisplaced fracture of fourth metatarsal bone, unspecified foot

S92.35 Fracture of fifth metatarsal bone
- S92.351 Displaced fracture of fifth metatarsal bone, right foot
- S92.352 Displaced fracture of fifth metatarsal bone, left foot
- S92.353 Displaced fracture of fifth metatarsal bone, unspecified foot
- S92.354 Nondisplaced fracture of fifth metatarsal bone, right foot
- S92.355 Nondisplaced fracture of fifth metatarsal bone, left foot
- S92.356 Nondisplaced fracture of fifth metatarsal bone, unspecified foot

S92.4 Fracture of great toe

Excludes2 Physeal fracture of phalanx of toe (S99.2-)

S92.40 Unspecified fracture of great toe
- S92.401 Displaced unspecified fracture of right great toe
- S92.402 Displaced unspecified fracture of left great toe
- S92.403 Displaced unspecified fracture of unspecified great toe
- S92.404 Nondisplaced unspecified fracture of right great toe
- S92.405 Nondisplaced unspecified fracture of left great toe
- S92.406 Nondisplaced unspecified fracture of unspecified great toe

S92.41 Fracture of proximal phalanx of great toe
- S92.411 Displaced fracture of proximal phalanx of right great toe
- S92.412 Displaced fracture of proximal phalanx of left great toe
- S92.413 Displaced fracture of proximal phalanx of unspecified great toe
- S92.414 Nondisplaced fracture of proximal phalanx of right great toe
- S92.415 Nondisplaced fracture of proximal phalanx of left great toe
- S92.416 Nondisplaced fracture of proximal phalanx of unspecified great toe

- S92.42 Fracture of distal phalanx of great toe
  - S92.421 Displaced fracture of distal phalanx of right great toe
  - S92.422 Displaced fracture of distal phalanx of left great toe
  - S92.423 Displaced fracture of distal phalanx of unspecified great toe
  - S92.424 Nondisplaced fracture of distal phalanx of right great toe
  - S92.425 Nondisplaced fracture of distal phalanx of left great toe
  - S92.426 Nondisplaced fracture of distal phalanx of unspecified great toe
- S92.49 Other fracture of great toe
  - S92.491 Other fracture of right great toe
  - S92.492 Other fracture of left great toe
  - S92.499 Other fracture of unspecified great toe

S92.5 Fracture of lesser toe(s)

Excludes2 Physeal fracture of phalanx of toe (S99.2-)

- S92.50 Unspecified fracture of lesser toe(s)
  - S92.501 Displaced unspecified fracture of right lesser toe(s)
  - S92.502 Displaced unspecified fracture of left lesser toe(s)
  - S92.503 Displaced unspecified fracture of unspecified lesser toe(s)
  - S92.504 Nondisplaced unspecified fracture of right lesser toe(s)
  - S92.505 Nondisplaced unspecified fracture of left lesser toe(s)
  - S92.506 Nondisplaced unspecified fracture of unspecified lesser toe(s)
- S92.51 Fracture of proximal phalanx of lesser toe(s)
  - S92.511 Displaced fracture of proximal phalanx of right lesser toe(s)
  - S92.512 Displaced fracture of proximal phalanx of left lesser toe(s)
  - S92.513 Displaced fracture of proximal phalanx of unspecified lesser toe(s)
  - S92.514 Nondisplaced fracture of proximal phalanx of right lesser toe(s)
  - S92.515 Nondisplaced fracture of proximal phalanx of left lesser toe(s)
  - S92.516 Nondisplaced fracture of proximal phalanx of unspecified lesser toe(s)
- S92.52 Fracture of middle phalanx of lesser toe(s)
  - S92.521 Displaced fracture of middle phalanx of right lesser toe(s)
  - S92.522 Displaced fracture of middle phalanx of left lesser toe(s)
  - S92.523 Displaced fracture of middle phalanx of unspecified lesser toe(s)
  - S92.524 Nondisplaced fracture of middle phalanx of right lesser toe(s)
  - S92.525 Nondisplaced fracture of middle phalanx of left lesser toe(s)
  - S92.526 Nondisplaced fracture of middle phalanx of unspecified lesser toe(s)
- S92.53 Fracture of distal phalanx of lesser toe(s)
  - S92.531 Displaced fracture of distal phalanx of right lesser toe(s)
  - S92.532 Displaced fracture of distal phalanx of left lesser toe(s)
  - S92.533 Displaced fracture of distal phalanx of unspecified lesser toe(s)
  - S92.534 Nondisplaced fracture of distal phalanx of right lesser toe(s)
  - S92.535 Nondisplaced fracture of distal phalanx of left lesser toe(s)
  - S92.536 Nondisplaced fracture of distal phalanx of unspecified lesser toe(s)
- S92.59 Other fracture of lesser toe(s)
  - S92.591 Other fracture of right lesser toe(s)
  - S92.592 Other fracture of left lesser toe(s)
  - S92.599 Other fracture of unspecified lesser toe(s)

S92.8 Other fracture of foot, except ankle

- S92.81 Other fracture of foot

  Sesamoid fracture of foot

  Coding Clinic: 2016, Q4, P68
  - S92.811 Other fracture of right foot
  - S92.812 Other fracture of left foot
  - S92.819 Other fracture of unspecified foot

S92.9 Unspecified fracture of foot and toe

- S92.90 Unspecified fracture of foot
  - S92.901 Unspecified fracture of right foot
  - S92.902 Unspecified fracture of left foot
  - S92.909 Unspecified fracture of unspecified foot
- S92.91 Unspecified fracture of toe
  - S92.911 Unspecified fracture of right toe(s)
  - S92.912 Unspecified fracture of left toe(s)
  - S92.919 Unspecified fracture of unspecified toe(s)

S93 Dislocation and sprain of joints and ligaments at ankle, foot and toe level

Includes avulsion of joint or ligament of ankle, foot and toe
laceration of cartilage, joint or ligament of ankle, foot and toe
sprain of cartilage, joint or ligament of ankle, foot and toe
traumatic hemarthrosis of joint or ligament of ankle, foot and toe
traumatic rupture of joint or ligament of ankle, foot and toe
traumatic subluxation of joint or ligament of ankle, foot and toe
traumatic tear of joint or ligament of ankle, foot and toe

Code also any associated open wound

Excludes2 strain of muscle and tendon of ankle and foot (S96.-)

The appropriate 7th character is to be added to each code from category S93

A	initial encounter
D	subsequent encounter
S	sequela

S93.0 Subluxation and dislocation of ankle joint

Subluxation and dislocation of astragalus
Subluxation and dislocation of fibula, lower end
Subluxation and dislocation of talus
Subluxation and dislocation of tibia, lower end

- X S93.01 Subluxation of right ankle joint
- X S93.02 Subluxation of left ankle joint
- X S93.03 Subluxation of unspecified ankle joint
- X S93.04 Dislocation of right ankle joint
- X S93.05 Dislocation of left ankle joint
- X S93.06 Dislocation of unspecified ankle joint

CHAPTER 19 (S00-T88)

S93.1 Subluxation and dislocation of toe

S93.10 Unspecified subluxation and dislocation of toe
Dislocation of toe NOS
Subluxation of toe NOS

- **S93.101** Unspecified subluxation of right toe(s)
- **S93.102** Unspecified subluxation of left toe(s)
- **S93.103** Unspecified subluxation of unspecified toe(s)
- **S93.104** Unspecified dislocation of right toe(s)
- **S93.105** Unspecified dislocation of left toe(s)
- **S93.106** Unspecified dislocation of unspecified toe(s)

S93.11 Dislocation of interphalangeal joint

- **S93.111** Dislocation of interphalangeal joint of right great toe
- **S93.112** Dislocation of interphalangeal joint of left great toe
- **S93.113** Dislocation of interphalangeal joint of unspecified great toe
- **S93.114** Dislocation of interphalangeal joint of right lesser toe(s)
- **S93.115** Dislocation of interphalangeal joint of left lesser toe(s)
- **S93.116** Dislocation of interphalangeal joint of unspecified lesser toe(s)
- **S93.119** Dislocation of interphalangeal joint of unspecified toe(s)

S93.12 Dislocation of metatarsophalangeal joint

- **S93.121** Dislocation of metatarsophalangeal joint of right great toe
- **S93.122** Dislocation of metatarsophalangeal joint of left great toe
- **S93.123** Dislocation of metatarsophalangeal joint of unspecified great toe
- **S93.124** Dislocation of metatarsophalangeal joint of right lesser toe(s)
- **S93.125** Dislocation of metatarsophalangeal joint of left lesser toe(s)
- **S93.126** Dislocation of metatarsophalangeal joint of unspecified lesser toe(s)
- **S93.129** Dislocation of metatarsophalangeal joint of unspecified toe(s)

S93.13 Subluxation of interphalangeal joint

- **S93.131** Subluxation of interphalangeal joint of right great toe
- **S93.132** Subluxation of interphalangeal joint of left great toe
- **S93.133** Subluxation of interphalangeal joint of unspecified great toe
- **S93.134** Subluxation of interphalangeal joint of right lesser toe(s)
- **S93.135** Subluxation of interphalangeal joint of left lesser toe(s)
- **S93.136** Subluxation of interphalangeal joint of unspecified lesser toe(s)
- **S93.139** Subluxation of interphalangeal joint of unspecified toe(s)

S93.14 Subluxation of metatarsophalangeal joint

- **S93.141** Subluxation of metatarsophalangeal joint of right great toe
- **S93.142** Subluxation of metatarsophalangeal joint of left great toe
- **S93.143** Subluxation of metatarsophalangeal joint of unspecified great toe
- **S93.144** Subluxation of metatarsophalangeal joint of right lesser toe(s)
- **S93.145** Subluxation of metatarsophalangeal joint of left lesser toe(s)
- **S93.146** Subluxation of metatarsophalangeal joint of unspecified lesser toe(s)
- **S93.149** Subluxation of metatarsophalangeal joint of unspecified toe(s)

S93.3 Subluxation and dislocation of foot

Excludes2 dislocation of toe (S93.1-)

S93.30 Unspecified subluxation and dislocation of foot
Dislocation of foot NOS
Subluxation of foot NOS

- **S93.301** Unspecified subluxation of right foot
- **S93.302** Unspecified subluxation of left foot
- **S93.303** Unspecified subluxation of unspecified foot
- **S93.304** Unspecified dislocation of right foot
- **S93.305** Unspecified dislocation of left foot
- **S93.306** Unspecified dislocation of unspecified foot

S93.31 Subluxation and dislocation of tarsal joint

- **S93.311** Subluxation of tarsal joint of right foot
- **S93.312** Subluxation of tarsal joint of left foot
- **S93.313** Subluxation of tarsal joint of unspecified foot
- **S93.314** Dislocation of tarsal joint of right foot
- **S93.315** Dislocation of tarsal joint of left foot
- **S93.316** Dislocation of tarsal joint of unspecified foot

S93.32 Subluxation and dislocation of tarsometatarsal joint

- **S93.321** Subluxation of tarsometatarsal joint of right foot
- **S93.322** Subluxation of tarsometatarsal joint of left foot
- **S93.323** Subluxation of tarsometatarsal joint of unspecified foot
- **S93.324** Dislocation of tarsometatarsal joint of right foot
- **S93.325** Dislocation of tarsometatarsal joint of left foot
- **S93.326** Dislocation of tarsometatarsal joint of unspecified foot

S93.33 Other subluxation and dislocation of foot

- **S93.331** Other subluxation of right foot
- **S93.332** Other subluxation of left foot
- **S93.333** Other subluxation of unspecified foot
- **S93.334** Other dislocation of right foot
- **S93.335** Other dislocation of left foot
- **S93.336** Other dislocation of unspecified foot

S93.4 Sprain of ankle
Injury to ligaments when one or more is stretched/torn

Excludes2 injury of Achilles tendon (S86.0-)

S93.40 Sprain of unspecified ligament of ankle
Sprain of ankle NOS
Sprained ankle NOS

- **S93.401** Sprain of unspecified ligament of right ankle
- **S93.402** Sprain of unspecified ligament of left ankle
- **S93.409** Sprain of unspecified ligament of unspecified ankle

S93.41 Sprain of calcaneofibular ligament

- **S93.411** Sprain of calcaneofibular ligament of right ankle
- **S93.412** Sprain of calcaneofibular ligament of left ankle
- **S93.419** Sprain of calcaneofibular ligament of unspecified ankle

CHAPTER 19 (S00-T88)

- S93.42 Sprain of deltoid ligament
  - S93.421 Sprain of deltoid ligament of right ankle
  - S93.422 Sprain of deltoid ligament of left ankle
  - S93.429 Sprain of deltoid ligament of unspecified ankle
- S93.43 Sprain of tibiofibular ligament
  - S93.431 Sprain of tibiofibular ligament of right ankle
  - S93.432 Sprain of tibiofibular ligament of left ankle
  - S93.439 Sprain of tibiofibular ligament of unspecified ankle
- S93.49 Sprain of other ligament of ankle
  Sprain of internal collateral ligament
  Sprain of talofibular ligament
  - S93.491 Sprain of other ligament of right ankle
  - S93.492 Sprain of other ligament of left ankle
  - S93.499 Sprain of other ligament of unspecified ankle

S93.5 Sprain of toe
- S93.50 Unspecified sprain of toe
  - S93.501 Unspecified sprain of right great toe
  - S93.502 Unspecified sprain of left great toe
  - S93.503 Unspecified sprain of unspecified great toe
  - S93.504 Unspecified sprain of right lesser toe(s)
  - S93.505 Unspecified sprain of left lesser toe(s)
  - S93.506 Unspecified sprain of unspecified lesser toe(s)
  - S93.509 Unspecified sprain of unspecified toe(s)
- S93.51 Sprain of interphalangeal joint of toe
  - S93.511 Sprain of interphalangeal joint of right great toe
  - S93.512 Sprain of interphalangeal joint of left great toe
  - S93.513 Sprain of interphalangeal joint of unspecified great toe
  - S93.514 Sprain of interphalangeal joint of right lesser toe(s)
  - S93.515 Sprain of interphalangeal joint of left lesser toe(s)
  - S93.516 Sprain of interphalangeal joint of unspecified lesser toe(s)
  - S93.519 Sprain of interphalangeal joint of unspecified toe(s)
- S93.52 Sprain of metatarsophalangeal joint of toe
  - S93.521 Sprain of metatarsophalangeal joint of right great toe
  - S93.522 Sprain of metatarsophalangeal joint of left great toe
  - S93.523 Sprain of metatarsophalangeal joint of unspecified great toe
  - S93.524 Sprain of metatarsophalangeal joint of right lesser toe(s)
  - S93.525 Sprain of metatarsophalangeal joint of left lesser toe(s)
  - S93.526 Sprain of metatarsophalangeal joint of unspecified lesser toe(s)
  - S93.529 Sprain of metatarsophalangeal joint of unspecified toe(s)

S93.6 Sprain of foot

Excludes2 sprain of metatarsophalangeal joint of toe (S93.52-)
sprain of toe (S93.5-)

- S93.60 Unspecified sprain of foot
  - S93.601 Unspecified sprain of right foot
  - S93.602 Unspecified sprain of left foot
  - S93.609 Unspecified sprain of unspecified foot
- S93.61 Sprain of tarsal ligament of foot
  - S93.611 Sprain of tarsal ligament of right foot
  - S93.612 Sprain of tarsal ligament of left foot
  - S93.619 Sprain of tarsal ligament of unspecified foot
- S93.62 Sprain of tarsometatarsal ligament of foot
  - S93.621 Sprain of tarsometatarsal ligament of right foot
  - S93.622 Sprain of tarsometatarsal ligament of left foot
  - S93.629 Sprain of tarsometatarsal ligament of unspecified foot
- S93.69 Other sprain of foot
  - S93.691 Other sprain of right foot
  - S93.692 Other sprain of left foot
  - S93.699 Other sprain of unspecified foot

S94 Injury of nerves at ankle and foot level

The appropriate 7th character is to be added to each code from category S94

A	initial encounter
D	subsequent encounter
S	sequela

Code also any associated open wound (S91.-)

- S94.0 Injury of lateral plantar nerve
  - X S94.00 Injury of lateral plantar nerve, unspecified leg
  - X S94.01 Injury of lateral plantar nerve, right leg
  - X S94.02 Injury of lateral plantar nerve, left leg
- S94.1 Injury of medial plantar nerve
  - X S94.10 Injury of medial plantar nerve, unspecified leg
  - X S94.11 Injury of medial plantar nerve, right leg
  - X S94.12 Injury of medial plantar nerve, left leg
- S94.2 Injury of deep peroneal nerve at ankle and foot level
  Injury of terminal, lateral branch of deep peroneal nerve
  - X S94.20 Injury of deep peroneal nerve at ankle and foot level, unspecified leg
  - X S94.21 Injury of deep peroneal nerve at ankle and foot level, right leg
  - X S94.22 Injury of deep peroneal nerve at ankle and foot level, left leg
- S94.3 Injury of cutaneous sensory nerve at ankle and foot level
  - X S94.30 Injury of cutaneous sensory nerve at ankle and foot level, unspecified leg
  - X S94.31 Injury of cutaneous sensory nerve at ankle and foot level, right leg
  - X S94.32 Injury of cutaneous sensory nerve at ankle and foot level, left leg
- S94.8 Injury of other nerves at ankle and foot level
  - S94.8X Injury of other nerves at ankle and foot level
    - S94.8X1 Injury of other nerves at ankle and foot level, right leg
    - S94.8X2 Injury of other nerves at ankle and foot level, left leg
    - S94.8X9 Injury of other nerves at ankle and foot level, unspecified leg

- S94.9 Injury of **unspecified nerve** at ankle and foot level
  - X S94.90 Injury of unspecified nerve at ankle and foot level, **unspecified** leg
  - X S94.91 Injury of unspecified nerve at ankle and foot level, **right** leg
  - X S94.92 Injury of unspecified nerve at ankle and foot level, **left** leg

S95 Injury of blood vessels at ankle and foot level

Code also any associated open wound (S91.-)

Excludes2 injury of posterior tibial artery and vein (S85.1-, S85.8-)

The appropriate 7th character is to be added to each code from category S95

A	initial encounter
D	subsequent encounter
S	sequela

- S95.Ø Injury of **dorsal artery** of foot
  - S95.ØØ **Unspecified** injury of dorsal artery of foot
    - S95.ØØ1 Unspecified injury of dorsal artery of **right** foot
    - S95.ØØ2 Unspecified injury of dorsal artery of **left** foot
    - S95.ØØ9 Unspecified injury of dorsal artery of **unspecified** foot
  - S95.Ø1 **Laceration** of dorsal artery of foot
    - S95.Ø11 Laceration of dorsal artery of **right** foot
    - S95.Ø12 Laceration of dorsal artery of **left** foot
    - S95.Ø19 Laceration of dorsal artery of **unspecified** foot
  - S95.Ø9 **Other** specified injury of dorsal artery of foot
    - S95.Ø91 Other specified injury of dorsal artery of **right** foot
    - S95.Ø92 Other specified injury of dorsal artery of **left** foot
    - S95.Ø99 Other specified injury of dorsal artery of **unspecified** foot
- S95.1 Injury of **plantar artery** of foot
  - S95.1Ø **Unspecified** injury of plantar artery of foot
    - S95.1Ø1 Unspecified injury of plantar artery of **right** foot
    - S95.1Ø2 Unspecified injury of plantar artery of **left** foot
    - S95.1Ø9 Unspecified injury of plantar artery of **unspecified** foot
  - S95.11 **Laceration** of plantar artery of foot
    - S95.111 Laceration of plantar artery of **right** foot
    - S95.112 Laceration of plantar artery of **left** foot
    - S95.119 Laceration of plantar artery of **unspecified** foot
  - S95.19 **Other** specified injury of plantar artery of foot
    - S95.191 Other specified injury of plantar artery of **right** foot
    - S95.192 Other specified injury of plantar artery of **left** foot
    - S95.199 Other specified injury of plantar artery of **unspecified** foot
- S95.2 Injury of **dorsal vein** of foot
  - S95.2Ø Unspecified injury of dorsal vein of foot
    - S95.2Ø1 **Unspecified** injury of dorsal vein of **right** foot
    - S95.2Ø2 **Unspecified** injury of dorsal vein of **left** foot
    - S95.2Ø9 **Unspecified** injury of dorsal vein of **unspecified** foot
  - S95.21 **Laceration** of dorsal vein of foot
    - S95.211 Laceration of dorsal vein of **right** foot
    - S95.212 Laceration of dorsal vein of **left** foot
    - S95.219 Laceration of dorsal vein of **unspecified** foot
  - S95.29 **Other** specified injury of dorsal vein of foot
    - S95.291 Other specified injury of dorsal vein of **right** foot
    - S95.292 Other specified injury of dorsal vein of **left** foot
    - S95.299 Other specified injury of dorsal vein of **unspecified** foot
- S95.8 Injury of **other blood vessels** at ankle and foot level
  - S95.8Ø **Unspecified** injury of other blood vessels at ankle and foot level
    - S95.8Ø1 Unspecified injury of other blood vessels at ankle and foot level, **right** leg
    - S95.8Ø2 Unspecified injury of other blood vessels at ankle and foot level, **left** leg
    - S95.8Ø9 Unspecified injury of other blood vessels at ankle and foot level, **unspecified** leg
  - S95.81 **Laceration** of other blood vessels at ankle and foot level
    - S95.811 Laceration of other blood vessels at ankle and foot level, **right** leg
    - S95.812 Laceration of other blood vessels at ankle and foot level, **left** leg
    - S95.819 Laceration of other blood vessels at ankle and foot level, **unspecified** leg
  - S95.89 **Other** specified injury of other blood vessels at ankle and foot level
    - S95.891 Other specified injury of other blood vessels at ankle and foot level, **right** leg
    - S95.892 Other specified injury of other blood vessels at ankle and foot level, **left** leg
    - S95.899 Other specified injury of other blood vessels at ankle and foot level, **unspecified** leg
- S95.9 Injury of **unspecified blood vessel** at ankle and foot level
  - S95.9Ø **Unspecified** injury of unspecified blood vessel at ankle and foot level
    - S95.9Ø1 Unspecified injury of unspecified blood vessel at ankle and foot level, **right** leg
    - S95.9Ø2 Unspecified injury of unspecified blood vessel at ankle and foot level, **left** leg
    - S95.9Ø9 Unspecified injury of unspecified blood vessel at ankle and foot level, **unspecified** leg
  - S95.91 **Laceration** of unspecified blood vessel at ankle and foot level
    - S95.911 Laceration of unspecified blood vessel at ankle and foot level, **right** leg
    - S95.912 Laceration of unspecified blood vessel at ankle and foot level, **left** leg
    - S95.919 Laceration of unspecified blood vessel at ankle and foot level, **unspecified** leg

● S95.99 Other specified injury of unspecified blood vessel at ankle and foot level
● S95.991 Other specified injury of unspecified blood vessel at ankle and foot level, right leg
● S95.992 Other specified injury of unspecified blood vessel at ankle and foot level, left leg
● S95.999 Other specified injury of unspecified blood vessel at ankle and foot level, unspecified leg

● S96 Injury of muscle and tendon at ankle and foot level
Code also any associated open wound (S91.-)
Excludes2 injury of Achilles tendon (S86.Ø-)
sprain of joints and ligaments of ankle and foot (S93.-)
The appropriate 7th character is to be added to each code from category S96

A	initial encounter
D	subsequent encounter
S	sequela

● S96.Ø Injury of muscle and tendon of long flexor muscle of toe at ankle and foot level
● S96.ØØ Unspecified injury of muscle and tendon of long flexor muscle of toe at ankle and foot level
● S96.ØØ1 Unspecified injury of muscle and tendon of long flexor muscle of toe at ankle and foot level, right foot
● S96.ØØ2 Unspecified injury of muscle and tendon of long flexor muscle of toe at ankle and foot level, left foot
● S96.ØØ9 Unspecified injury of muscle and tendon of long flexor muscle of toe at ankle and foot level, unspecified foot
● S96.Ø1 Strain of muscle and tendon of long flexor muscle of toe at ankle and foot level
● S96.Ø11 Strain of muscle and tendon of long flexor muscle of toe at ankle and foot level, right foot
● S96.Ø12 Strain of muscle and tendon of long flexor muscle of toe at ankle and foot level, left foot
● S96.Ø19 Strain of muscle and tendon of long flexor muscle of toe at ankle and foot level, unspecified foot
● S96.Ø2 Laceration of muscle and tendon of long flexor muscle of toe at ankle and foot level
● S96.Ø21 Laceration of muscle and tendon of long flexor muscle of toe at ankle and foot level, right foot
● S96.Ø22 Laceration of muscle and tendon of long flexor muscle of toe at ankle and foot level, left foot
● S96.Ø29 Laceration of muscle and tendon of long flexor muscle of toe at ankle and foot level, unspecified foot
● S96.Ø9 Other injury of muscle and tendon of long flexor muscle of toe at ankle and foot level
● S96.Ø91 Other injury of muscle and tendon of long flexor muscle of toe at ankle and foot level, right foot
● S96.Ø92 Other injury of muscle and tendon of long flexor muscle of toe at ankle and foot level, left foot
● S96.Ø99 Other injury of muscle and tendon of long flexor muscle of toe at ankle and foot level, unspecified foot

● S96.1 Injury of muscle and tendon of long extensor muscle of toe at ankle and foot level
● S96.1Ø Unspecified injury of muscle and tendon of long extensor muscle of toe at ankle and foot level
● S96.1Ø1 Unspecified injury of muscle and tendon of long extensor muscle of toe at ankle and foot level, right foot
● S96.1Ø2 Unspecified injury of muscle and tendon of long extensor muscle of toe at ankle and foot level, left foot
● S96.1Ø9 Unspecified injury of muscle and tendon of long extensor muscle of toe at ankle and foot level, unspecified foot
● S96.11 Strain of muscle and tendon of long extensor muscle of toe at ankle and foot level
● S96.111 Strain of muscle and tendon of long extensor muscle of toe at ankle and foot level, right foot
● S96.112 Strain of muscle and tendon of long extensor muscle of toe at ankle and foot level, left foot
● S96.119 Strain of muscle and tendon of long extensor muscle of toe at ankle and foot level, unspecified foot
● S96.12 Laceration of muscle and tendon of long extensor muscle of toe at ankle and foot level
● S96.121 Laceration of muscle and tendon of long extensor muscle of toe at ankle and foot level, right foot
● S96.122 Laceration of muscle and tendon of long extensor muscle of toe at ankle and foot level, left foot
● S96.129 Laceration of muscle and tendon of long extensor muscle of toe at ankle and foot level, unspecified foot
● S96.19 Other specified injury of muscle and tendon of long extensor muscle of toe at ankle and foot level
● S96.191 Other specified injury of muscle and tendon of long extensor muscle of toe at ankle and foot level, right foot
● S96.192 Other specified injury of muscle and tendon of long extensor muscle of toe at ankle and foot level, left foot
● S96.199 Other specified injury of muscle and tendon of long extensor muscle of toe at ankle and foot level, unspecified foot

● S96.2 Injury of intrinsic muscle and tendon at ankle and foot level
● S96.2Ø Unspecified injury of intrinsic muscle and tendon at ankle and foot level
● S96.2Ø1 Unspecified injury of intrinsic muscle and tendon at ankle and foot level, right foot
● S96.2Ø2 Unspecified injury of intrinsic muscle and tendon at ankle and foot level, left foot
● S96.2Ø9 Unspecified injury of intrinsic muscle and tendon at ankle and foot level, unspecified foot
● S96.21 Strain of intrinsic muscle and tendon at ankle and foot level
● S96.211 Strain of intrinsic muscle and tendon at ankle and foot level, right foot
● S96.212 Strain of intrinsic muscle and tendon at ankle and foot level, left foot
● S96.219 Strain of intrinsic muscle and tendon at ankle and foot level, unspecified foot

S96.22 **Laceration** of intrinsic muscle and tendon at ankle and foot level
- S96.221 Laceration of intrinsic muscle and tendon at ankle and foot level, **right** foot
- S96.222 Laceration of intrinsic muscle and tendon at left ankle and foot level, **left** foot
- S96.229 Laceration of intrinsic muscle and tendon at ankle and foot level, **unspecified** foot

S96.29 **Other** specified injury of intrinsic muscle and tendon at ankle and foot level
- S96.291 Other specified injury of intrinsic muscle and tendon at ankle and foot level, **right** foot
- S96.292 Other specified injury of intrinsic muscle and tendon at ankle and foot level, **left** foot
- S96.299 Other specified injury of intrinsic muscle and tendon at ankle and foot level, **unspecified** foot

S96.8 Injury of **other** specified muscles and tendons at ankle and foot level

S96.80 **Unspecified** injury of other specified muscles and tendons at ankle and foot level
- S96.801 Unspecified injury of other specified muscles and tendons at ankle and foot level, **right** foot
- S96.802 Unspecified injury of other specified muscles and tendons at ankle and foot level, **left** foot
- S96.809 Unspecified injury of other specified muscles and tendons at ankle and foot level, **unspecified** foot

S96.81 **Strain** of other specified muscles and tendons at ankle and foot level
- S96.811 Strain of other specified muscles and tendons at ankle and foot level, **right** foot
- S96.812 Strain of other specified muscles and tendons at ankle and foot level, **left** foot
- S96.819 Strain of other specified muscles and tendons at ankle and foot level, **unspecified** foot

S96.82 **Laceration** of other specified muscles and tendons at ankle and foot level
- S96.821 Laceration of other specified muscles and tendons at ankle and foot level, **right** foot
- S96.822 Laceration of other specified muscles and tendons at ankle and foot level, **left** foot
- S96.829 Laceration of other specified muscles and tendons at ankle and foot level, **unspecified** foot

S96.89 **Other** specified injury of other specified muscles and tendons at ankle and foot level
- S96.891 Other specified injury of other specified muscles and tendons at ankle and foot level, **right** foot
- S96.892 Other specified injury of other specified muscles and tendons at ankle and foot level, **left** foot
- S96.899 Other specified injury of other specified muscles and tendons at ankle and foot level, **unspecified** foot

S96.9 Injury of **unspecified** muscle and tendon at ankle and foot level

S96.90 **Unspecified** injury of unspecified muscle and tendon at ankle and foot level
- S96.901 Unspecified injury of unspecified muscle and tendon at ankle and foot level, **right** foot
- S96.902 Unspecified injury of unspecified muscle and tendon at ankle and foot level, **left** foot
- S96.909 Unspecified injury of unspecified muscle and tendon at ankle and foot level, **unspecified** foot

S96.91 **Strain** of unspecified muscle and tendon at ankle and foot level
- S96.911 Strain of unspecified muscle and tendon at ankle and foot level, **right** foot
- S96.912 Strain of unspecified muscle and tendon at ankle and foot level, **left** foot
- S96.919 Strain of unspecified muscle and tendon at ankle and foot level, **unspecified** foot

S96.92 **Laceration** of unspecified muscle and tendon at ankle and foot level
- S96.921 Laceration of unspecified muscle and tendon at ankle and foot level, **right** foot
- S96.922 Laceration of unspecified muscle and tendon at ankle and foot level, **left** foot
- S96.929 Laceration of unspecified muscle and tendon at ankle and foot level, **unspecified** foot

S96.99 **Other** specified injury of unspecified muscle and tendon at ankle and foot level
- S96.991 Other specified injury of unspecified muscle and tendon at ankle and foot level, **right** foot
- S96.992 Other specified injury of unspecified muscle and tendon at ankle and foot level, **left** foot
- S96.999 Other specified injury of unspecified muscle and tendon at ankle and foot level, **unspecified** foot

S97 **Crushing injury** of ankle and foot

Use additional code(s) for all associated injuries

The appropriate 7th character is to be added to each code from category S97

A	initial encounter
D	subsequent encounter
S	sequela

S97.0 Crushing injury of **ankle**
- X S97.00 Crushing injury of **unspecified** ankle
- X S97.01 Crushing injury of **right** ankle
- X S97.02 Crushing injury of **left** ankle

S97.1 Crushing injury of **toe**

S97.10 Crushing injury of **unspecified** toe(s)
- S97.101 Crushing injury of unspecified **right** toe(s)
- S97.102 Crushing injury of unspecified **left** toe(s)
- S97.109 Crushing injury of **unspecified** toe(s)
  Crushing injury of toe NOS

S97.11 Crushing injury of great toe
- S97.111 Crushing injury of right great toe
- S97.112 Crushing injury of left great toe
- S97.119 Crushing injury of unspecified great toe

S97.12 Crushing injury of lesser toe(s)
- S97.121 Crushing injury of right lesser toe(s)
- S97.122 Crushing injury of left lesser toe(s)
- S97.129 Crushing injury of lesser toe(s), unspecified toe(s)

S97.8 Crushing injury of foot
- X S97.80 Crushing injury of foot, unspecified side
  Crushing injury of foot NOS
- X S97.81 Crushing injury of right foot
- X S97.82 Crushing injury of left foot

S98 Traumatic amputation of ankle and foot

An amputation not identified as partial or complete should be coded to complete

The appropriate 7th character is to be added to each code from category S98

A	initial encounter
D	subsequent encounter
S	sequela

S98.Ø Traumatic amputation of foot at ankle level

S98.Ø1 Complete traumatic amputation of foot at ankle level
- S98.Ø11 Complete traumatic amputation of right foot at ankle level A, D, S
- S98.Ø12 Complete traumatic amputation of left foot at ankle level A, D, S
- S98.Ø19 Complete traumatic amputation of unspecified foot at ankle level A, D, S

S98.Ø2 Partial traumatic amputation of foot at ankle level
- S98.Ø21 Partial traumatic amputation of right foot at ankle level A, D, S
- S98.Ø22 Partial traumatic amputation of left foot at ankle level A, D, S
- S98.Ø29 Partial traumatic amputation of unspecified foot at ankle level A, D, S

S98.1 Traumatic amputation of one toe

S98.11 Complete traumatic amputation of great toe
- S98.111 Complete traumatic amputation of right great toe A, D, S
- S98.112 Complete traumatic amputation of left great toe A, D, S
- S98.119 Complete traumatic amputation of unspecified great toe A, D, S

S98.12 Partial traumatic amputation of great toe
- S98.121 Partial traumatic amputation of right great toe A, D, S
- S98.122 Partial traumatic amputation of left great toe A, D, S
- S98.129 Partial traumatic amputation of unspecified great toe A, D, S

S98.13 Complete traumatic amputation of one lesser toe
Traumatic amputation of toe NOS
- S98.131 Complete traumatic amputation of one right lesser toe A, D, S
- S98.132 Complete traumatic amputation of one left lesser toe A, D, S
- S98.139 Complete traumatic amputation of one unspecified lesser toe A, D, S

S98.14 Partial traumatic amputation of one lesser toe
- S98.141 Partial traumatic amputation of one right lesser toe A, D, S
- S98.142 Partial traumatic amputation of one left lesser toe A, D, S
- S98.149 Partial traumatic amputation of one unspecified lesser toe A, D, S

S98.2 Traumatic amputation of two or more lesser toes

S98.21 Complete traumatic amputation of two or more lesser toes
- S98.211 Complete traumatic amputation of two or more right lesser toes A, D, S
- S98.212 Complete traumatic amputation of two or more left lesser toes A, D, S
- S98.219 Complete traumatic amputation of two or more unspecified lesser toes A, D, S

S98.22 Partial traumatic amputation of two or more lesser toes
- S98.221 Partial traumatic amputation of two or more right lesser toes A, D, S
- S98.222 Partial traumatic amputation of two or more left lesser toes A, D, S
- S98.229 Partial traumatic amputation of two or more unspecified lesser toes A, D, S

S98.3 Traumatic amputation of midfoot

S98.31 Complete traumatic amputation of midfoot
- S98.311 Complete traumatic amputation of right midfoot A, D, S
- S98.312 Complete traumatic amputation of left midfoot A, D, S
- S98.319 Complete traumatic amputation of unspecified midfoot A, D, S

S98.32 Partial traumatic amputation of midfoot
- S98.321 Partial traumatic amputation of right midfoot A, D, S
- S98.322 Partial traumatic amputation of left midfoot A, D, S
- S98.329 Partial traumatic amputation of unspecified midfoot A, D, S

S98.9 Traumatic amputation of foot, level unspecified

S98.91 Complete traumatic amputation of foot, level unspecified
- S98.911 Complete traumatic amputation of right foot, level unspecified A, D, S
- S98.912 Complete traumatic amputation of left foot, level unspecified A, D, S
- S98.919 Complete traumatic amputation of unspecified foot, level unspecified A, D, S

S98.92 Partial traumatic amputation of foot, level unspecified
- S98.921 Partial traumatic amputation of right foot, level unspecified A, D, S
- S98.922 Partial traumatic amputation of left foot, level unspecified A, D, S
- S98.929 Partial traumatic amputation of unspecified foot, level unspecified A, D, S

● S99 **Other and unspecified injuries of ankle and foot**
Coding Clinic: 2016, Q4, P68

● S99.0 **Physeal fracture of calcaneus**

The appropriate 7th character is to be added to each code from subcategories S99.0

A	initial encounter for closed fracture
B	initial encounter for open fracture
D	subsequent encounter for fracture with routine healing
G	subsequent encounter for fracture with delayed healing
K	subsequent encounter for fracture with nonunion
P	subsequent encounter for fracture with malunion
S	sequela

● S99.00 **Unspecified physeal fracture of calcaneus**
● S99.001 Unspecified physeal fracture of right calcaneus
● S99.002 Unspecified physeal fracture of left calcaneus
● S99.009 Unspecified physeal fracture of unspecified calcaneus

● S99.01 **Salter-Harris Type I physeal fracture of calcaneus**
Coding Clinic: 2016, Q4, P69
● S99.011 Salter-Harris Type I physeal fracture of right calcaneus
● S99.012 Salter-Harris Type I physeal fracture of left calcaneus
● S99.019 Salter-Harris Type I physeal fracture of unspecified calcaneus

● S99.02 **Salter-Harris Type II physeal fracture of calcaneus**
Coding Clinic: 2016, Q4, P69
● S99.021 Salter-Harris Type II physeal fracture of right calcaneus
● S99.022 Salter-Harris Type II physeal fracture of left calcaneus
● S99.029 Salter-Harris Type II physeal fracture of unspecified calcaneus

● S99.03 **Salter-Harris Type III physeal fracture of calcaneus**
Coding Clinic: 2016, Q4, P69
● S99.031 Salter-Harris Type III physeal fracture of right calcaneus
● S99.032 Salter-Harris Type III physeal fracture of left calcaneus
● S99.039 Salter-Harris Type III physeal fracture of unspecified calcaneus

● S99.04 **Salter-Harris Type IV physeal fracture of calcaneus**
Coding Clinic: 2016, Q4, P69
● S99.041 Salter-Harris Type IV physeal fracture of right calcaneus
● S99.042 Salter-Harris Type IV physeal fracture of left calcaneus
● S99.049 Salter-Harris Type IV physeal fracture of unspecified calcaneus

● S99.09 **Other physeal fracture of calcaneus**
Coding Clinic: 2016, Q4, P69
● S99.091 Other physeal fracture of right calcaneus
● S99.092 Other physeal fracture of left calcaneus
● S99.099 Other physeal fracture of unspecified calcaneus

● S99.1 **Physeal fracture of metatarsal**

The appropriate 7th character is to be added to each code from subcategories S99.1

A	initial encounter for closed fracture
B	initial encounter for open fracture
D	subsequent encounter for fracture with routine healing
G	subsequent encounter for fracture with delayed healing
K	subsequent encounter for fracture with nonunion
P	subsequent encounter for fracture with malunion
S	sequela

● S99.10 **Unspecified physeal fracture of metatarsal**
● S99.101 Unspecified physeal fracture of right metatarsal
● S99.102 Unspecified physeal fracture of left metatarsal
● S99.109 Unspecified physeal fracture of unspecified metatarsal

● S99.11 **Salter-Harris Type I physeal fracture of metatarsal**
Coding Clinic: 2016, Q4, P69
● S99.111 Salter-Harris Type I physeal fracture of right metatarsal
● S99.112 Salter-Harris Type I physeal fracture of left metatarsal
Coding Clinic: 2018, Q1, P3
● S99.119 Salter-Harris Type I physeal fracture of unspecified metatarsal

● S99.12 **Salter-Harris Type II physeal fracture of metatarsal**
Coding Clinic: 2016, Q4, P69
● S99.121 Salter-Harris Type II physeal fracture of right metatarsal
● S99.122 Salter-Harris Type II physeal fracture of left metatarsal
● S99.129 Salter-Harris Type II physeal fracture of unspecified metatarsal

● S99.13 **Salter-Harris Type III physeal fracture of metatarsal**
Coding Clinic: 2016, Q4, P69
● S99.131 Salter-Harris Type III physeal fracture of right metatarsal
● S99.132 Salter-Harris Type III physeal fracture of left metatarsal
● S99.139 Salter-Harris Type III physeal fracture of unspecified metatarsal

● S99.14 **Salter-Harris Type IV physeal fracture of metatarsal**
Coding Clinic: 2016, Q4, P69
● S99.141 Salter-Harris Type IV physeal fracture of right metatarsal
● S99.142 Salter-Harris Type IV physeal fracture of left metatarsal
● S99.149 Salter-Harris Type IV physeal fracture of unspecified metatarsal

● S99.19 **Other physeal fracture of metatarsal**
Coding Clinic: 2016, Q4, P69
● S99.191 Other physeal fracture of right metatarsal
● S99.192 Other physeal fracture of left metatarsal
● S99.199 Other physeal fracture of unspecified metatarsal

● S99.2 **Physeal fracture of phalanx of toe**

The appropriate 7th character is to be added to each code from subcategories S99.2

A	initial encounter for closed fracture
B	initial encounter for open fracture
D	subsequent encounter for fracture with routine healing
G	subsequent encounter for fracture with delayed healing
K	subsequent encounter for fracture with nonunion
P	subsequent encounter for fracture with malunion
S	sequela

● S99.20 **Unspecified physeal fracture of phalanx of toe**

● S99.201 **Unspecified physeal fracture of phalanx of right toe**

● S99.202 **Unspecified physeal fracture of phalanx of right toe**

● S99.209 **Unspecified physeal fracture of phalanx of unspecified toe**

● S99.21 **Salter-Harris Type I physeal fracture of phalanx of toe**

Coding Clinic: 2016, Q4, P69

● S99.211 **Salter-Harris Type I physeal fracture of phalanx of right toe**

● S99.212 **Salter-Harris Type I physeal fracture of phalanx of left toe**

● S99.219 **Salter-Harris Type I physeal fracture of phalanx of unspecified toe**

● S99.22 **Salter-Harris Type II physeal fracture of phalanx of toe**

Coding Clinic: 2016, Q4, P69

● S99.221 **Salter-Harris Type II physeal fracture of phalanx of right toe**

● S99.222 **Salter-Harris Type II physeal fracture of phalanx of left toe**

● S99.229 **Salter-Harris Type II physeal fracture of phalanx of unspecified toe**

● S99.23 **Salter-Harris Type III physeal fracture of phalanx of toe**

Coding Clinic: 2016, Q4, P69

● S99.231 **Salter-Harris Type III physeal fracture of phalanx of right toe**

● S99.232 **Salter-Harris Type III physeal fracture of phalanx of left toe**

● S99.239 **Salter-Harris Type III physeal fracture of phalanx of unspecified toe**

● S99.24 **Salter-Harris Type IV physeal fracture of phalanx of toe**

Coding Clinic: 2016, Q4, P69

● S99.241 **Salter-Harris Type IV physeal fracture of phalanx of right toe**

● S99.242 **Salter-Harris Type IV physeal fracture of phalanx of left toe**

● S99.249 **Salter-Harris Type IV physeal fracture of phalanx of unspecified toe**

● S99.29 **Other physeal fracture of phalanx of toe**

Coding Clinic: 2016, Q4, P69

● S99.291 **Other physeal fracture of phalanx of right toe**

● S99.292 **Other physeal fracture of phalanx of left toe**

● S99.299 **Other physeal fracture of phalanx of unspecified toe**

● S99.8 **Other specified injuries of ankle and foot**

The appropriate 7th character is to be added to each code from subcategory S99.8

A	initial encounter
D	subsequent encounter
S	sequela

● S99.81 **Other specified injuries of ankle**

● S99.811 **Other specified injuries of right ankle**

● S99.812 **Other specified injuries of left ankle**

● S99.819 **Other specified injuries of unspecified ankle**

● S99.82 **Other specified injuries of foot**

● S99.821 **Other specified injuries of right foot**

● S99.822 **Other specified injuries of left foot**

● S99.829 **Other specified injuries of unspecified foot**

● S99.9 **Unspecified injury of ankle and foot**

The appropriate 7th character is to be added to each code from subcategory S99.9

A	initial encounter
D	subsequent encounter
S	sequela

● S99.91 **Unspecified injury of ankle**

● S99.911 **Unspecified injury of right ankle**

● S99.912 **Unspecified injury of left ankle**

● S99.919 **Unspecified injury of unspecified ankle**

● S99.92 **Unspecified injury of foot**

● S99.921 **Unspecified injury of right foot**

● S99.922 **Unspecified injury of left foot**

● S99.929 **Unspecified injury of unspecified foot**

INJURY, POISONING AND CERTAIN OTHER CONSEQUENCES OF EXTERNAL CAUSES (T07-T88)

INJURIES INVOLVING MULTIPLE BODY REGIONS (T07)

Excludes1 burns and corrosions (T20-T32)
frostbite (T33-T34)
insect bite or sting, venomous (T63.4)
sunburn (L55.-)

X● T07 **Unspecified multiple injuries**

The appropriate 7th character is to be added to code T07

A	initial encounter
D	subsequent encounter
S	sequela

Excludes1 injury NOS (T14.90)

INJURY OF UNSPECIFIED BODY REGION (T14)

● T14 **Injury of unspecified body region**

The appropriate 7th character is to be added to each code from category T14

A	initial encounter
D	subsequent encounter
S	sequela

Excludes1 multiple unspecified injuries (T07)

X● T14.8 **Other injury of unspecified body region**

Abrasion NOS
Contusion NOS
Crush injury NOS
Fracture NOS
Skin injury NOS
Vascular injury NOS
Wound NOS

● T14.9 **Unspecified injury**

X● T14.90 **Injury, unspecified**

Injury NOS

X● T14.91 **Suicide attempt A, D, S** HCC

Attempted suicide NOS

EFFECTS OF FOREIGN BODY ENTERING THROUGH NATURAL ORIFICE (T15-T19)

Excludes2 foreign body accidentally left in operation wound (T81.5-)
foreign body in penetrating wound - see open wound by body region
residual foreign body in soft tissue (M79.5)
splinter, without open wound - see superficial injury by body region

● **T15 Foreign body on external eye**

Excludes2 foreign body in penetrating wound of orbit and eye ball (S05.4-, S05.5-)
open wound of eyelid and periocular area (S01.1-)
retained foreign body in eyelid (H02.8-)
retained (old) foreign body in penetrating wound of orbit and eye ball (H05.5-, H44.6-, H44.7-)
superficial foreign body of eyelid and periocular area (S00.25-)

The appropriate 7th character is to be added to each code from category T15

A	initial encounter
D	subsequent encounter
S	sequela

● **T15.0 Foreign body in cornea**
X● **T15.00 Foreign body in cornea, unspecified eye**
X● **T15.01 Foreign body in cornea, right eye**
X● **T15.02 Foreign body in cornea, left eye**
● **T15.1 Foreign body in conjunctival sac**
X● **T15.10 Foreign body in conjunctival sac, unspecified eye**
X● **T15.11 Foreign body in conjunctival sac, right eye**
X● **T15.12 Foreign body in conjunctival sac, left eye**
● **T15.8 Foreign body in other and multiple parts of external eye**
Foreign body in lacrimal punctum
X● **T15.80 Foreign body in other and multiple parts of external eye, unspecified eye**
X● **T15.81 Foreign body in other and multiple parts of external eye, right eye**
X● **T15.82 Foreign body in other and multiple parts of external eye, left eye**
● **T15.9 Foreign body on external eye, part unspecified**
X● **T15.90 Foreign body on external eye, part unspecified, unspecified eye**
X● **T15.91 Foreign body on external eye, part unspecified, right eye**
X● **T15.92 Foreign body on external eye, part unspecified, left eye**

● **T16 Foreign body in ear**

Includes foreign body in auditory canal

The appropriate 7th character is to be added to each code from category T16

A	initial encounter
D	subsequent encounter
S	sequela

X● **T16.1 Foreign body in right ear**
X● **T16.2 Foreign body in left ear**
X● **T16.9 Foreign body in ear, unspecified ear**

● **T17 Foreign body in respiratory tract**

The appropriate 7th character is to be added to each code from category T17

A	initial encounter
D	subsequent encounter
S	sequela

X● **T17.0 Foreign body in nasal sinus**
X● **T17.1 Foreign body in nostril**
Foreign body in nose NOS
● **T17.2 Foreign body in pharynx**
Foreign body in nasopharynx
Foreign body in throat NOS
● **T17.20 Unspecified foreign body in pharynx**
● **T17.200 Unspecified foreign body in pharynx causing asphyxiation**
● **T17.208 Unspecified foreign body in pharynx causing other injury**
● **T17.21 Gastric contents in pharynx**
Aspiration of gastric contents into pharynx
Vomitus in pharynx
● **T17.210 Gastric contents in pharynx causing asphyxiation**
● **T17.218 Gastric contents in pharynx causing other injury**
● **T17.22 Food in pharynx**
Bones in pharynx
Seeds in pharynx
● **T17.220 Food in pharynx causing asphyxiation**
● **T17.228 Food in pharynx causing other injury**
● **T17.29 Other foreign object in pharynx**
● **T17.290 Other foreign object in pharynx causing asphyxiation**
● **T17.298 Other foreign object in pharynx causing other injury**
● **T17.3 Foreign body in larynx**
● **T17.30 Unspecified foreign body in larynx**
● **T17.300 Unspecified foreign body in larynx causing asphyxiation**
● **T17.308 Unspecified foreign body in larynx causing other injury**
● **T17.31 Gastric contents in larynx**
Aspiration of gastric contents into larynx
Vomitus in larynx
● **T17.310 Gastric contents in larynx causing asphyxiation**
● **T17.318 Gastric contents in larynx causing other injury**
● **T17.32 Food in larynx**
Bones in larynx
Seeds in larynx
● **T17.320 Food in larynx causing asphyxiation**
● **T17.328 Food in larynx causing other injury**
● **T17.39 Other foreign object in larynx**
● **T17.390 Other foreign object in larynx causing asphyxiation**
● **T17.398 Other foreign object in larynx causing other injury**
● **T17.4 Foreign body in trachea**
● **T17.40 Unspecified foreign body in trachea**
● **T17.400 Unspecified foreign body in trachea causing asphyxiation**
● **T17.408 Unspecified foreign body in trachea causing other injury**

- T17.41 **Gastric contents in trachea**
  - Aspiration of gastric contents into trachea
  - Vomitus in trachea
  - T17.410 **Gastric contents in trachea causing asphyxiation**
  - T17.418 **Gastric contents in trachea causing other injury**
- T17.42 **Food in trachea**
  - Bones in trachea
  - Seeds in trachea
  - T17.420 **Food in trachea causing asphyxiation**
  - T17.428 **Food in trachea causing other injury**
- T17.49 **Other foreign object in trachea**
  - T17.490 **Other foreign object in trachea causing asphyxiation**
  - T17.498 **Other foreign object in trachea causing other injury**

T17.5 **Foreign body in bronchus**
- T17.50 **Unspecified foreign body in bronchus**
  - T17.500 **Unspecified foreign body in bronchus causing asphyxiation**
  - T17.508 **Unspecified foreign body in bronchus causing other injury**
- T17.51 **Gastric contents in bronchus**
  - Aspiration of gastric contents into bronchus
  - Vomitus in bronchus
  - T17.510 **Gastric contents in bronchus causing asphyxiation**
  - T17.518 **Gastric contents in bronchus causing other injury**
- T17.52 **Food in bronchus**
  - Bones in bronchus
  - Seeds in bronchus
  - T17.520 **Food in bronchus causing asphyxiation**
  - T17.528 **Food in bronchus causing other injury**
- T17.59 **Other foreign object in bronchus**
  - T17.590 **Other foreign object in bronchus causing asphyxiation**
  - T17.598 **Other foreign object in bronchus causing other injury**

T17.8 **Foreign body in other parts of respiratory tract**
- Foreign body in bronchioles
- Foreign body in lung
- T17.80 **Unspecified foreign body in other parts of respiratory tract**
  - T17.800 **Unspecified foreign body in other parts of respiratory tract causing asphyxiation**
  - T17.808 **Unspecified foreign body in other parts of respiratory tract causing other injury**
- T17.81 **Gastric contents in other parts of respiratory tract**
  - Aspiration of gastric contents into other parts of respiratory tract
  - Vomitus in other parts of respiratory tract
  - T17.810 **Gastric contents in other parts of respiratory tract causing asphyxiation**
  - T17.818 **Gastric contents in other parts of respiratory tract causing other injury**
- T17.82 **Food in other parts of respiratory tract**
  - Bones in other parts of respiratory tract
  - Seeds in other parts of respiratory tract
  - T17.820 **Food in other parts of respiratory tract causing asphyxiation**
  - T17.828 **Food in other parts of respiratory tract causing other injury**
- T17.89 **Other foreign object in other parts of respiratory tract**
  - T17.890 **Other foreign object in other parts of respiratory tract causing asphyxiation**
  - T17.898 **Other foreign object in other parts of respiratory tract causing other injury**

T17.9 **Foreign body in respiratory tract, part unspecified**
- T17.90 **Unspecified foreign body in respiratory tract, part unspecified**
  - T17.900 **Unspecified foreign body in respiratory tract, part unspecified causing asphyxiation**
  - T17.908 **Unspecified foreign body in respiratory tract, part unspecified causing other injury**
- T17.91 **Gastric contents in respiratory tract, part unspecified**
  - Aspiration of gastric contents into respiratory tract, part unspecified
  - Vomitus in trachea respiratory tract, part unspecified
  - T17.910 **Gastric contents in respiratory tract, part unspecified causing asphyxiation**
  - T17.918 **Gastric contents in respiratory tract, part unspecified causing other injury**
- T17.92 **Food in respiratory tract, part unspecified**
  - Bones in respiratory tract, part unspecified
  - Seeds in respiratory tract, part unspecified
  - T17.920 **Food in respiratory tract, part unspecified causing asphyxiation**
  - T17.928 **Food in respiratory tract, part unspecified causing other injury**
- T17.99 **Other foreign object in respiratory tract, part unspecified**
  - T17.990 **Other foreign object in respiratory tract, part unspecified in causing asphyxiation**
  - T17.998 **Other foreign object in respiratory tract, part unspecified causing other injury**

T18 Foreign body in alimentary tract

Excludes2 foreign body in pharynx (T17.2-)

The appropriate 7th character is to be added to each code from category T18

A	initial encounter
D	subsequent encounter
S	sequela

X T18.0 **Foreign body in mouth**

X T18.1 **Foreign body in esophagus**

Excludes2 foreign body in respiratory tract (T17.-)

- T18.10 **Unspecified foreign body in esophagus**
  - T18.100 **Unspecified foreign body in esophagus causing compression of trachea**
    - Unspecified foreign body in esophagus causing obstruction of respiration
  - T18.108 **Unspecified foreign body in esophagus causing other injury**
- T18.11 **Gastric contents in esophagus**
  - Vomitus in esophagus
  - T18.110 **Gastric contents in esophagus causing compression of trachea**
    - Gastric contents in esophagus causing obstruction of respiration
  - T18.118 **Gastric contents in esophagus causing other injury**

CHAPTER 19 (S00-T88)

● **T18.12 Food in esophagus**
Bones in esophagus
Seeds in esophagus

● **T18.120 Food in esophagus causing compression of trachea**
Food in esophagus causing obstruction of respiration

● **T18.128 Food in esophagus causing other injury**

● **T18.19 Other foreign object in esophagus**

● **T18.190 Other foreign object in esophagus causing compression of trachea**
Other foreign body in esophagus causing obstruction of respiration
Coding Clinic: 2015, Q1, P24

● **T18.198 Other foreign object in esophagus causing other injury**
Coding Clinic: 2015, Q1, P24

X● **T18.2 Foreign body in stomach**

X● **T18.3 Foreign body in small intestine**

X● **T18.4 Foreign body in colon**

X● **T18.5 Foreign body in anus and rectum**
Foreign body in rectosigmoid (junction)

X● **T18.8 Foreign body in other parts of alimentary tract**

X● **T18.9 Foreign body of alimentary tract, part unspecified**
Foreign body in digestive system NOS
Swallowed foreign body NOS

● **T19 Foreign body in genitourinary tract**

Excludes2 complications due to implanted mesh (T83.7-)
mechanical complications of contraceptive device (intrauterine) (vaginal) (T83.3-)
presence of contraceptive device (intrauterine) (vaginal) (Z97.5)

The appropriate 7th character is to be added to each code from category T19

A	initial encounter
D	subsequent encounter
S	sequela

X● **T19.0 Foreign body in urethra**

X● **T19.1 Foreign body in bladder**

X● **T19.2 Foreign body in vulva and vagina** ♀

X● **T19.3 Foreign body in uterus** ♀

X● **T19.4 Foreign body in penis** ♂

X● **T19.8 Foreign body in other parts of genitourinary tract**

X● **T19.9 Foreign body in genitourinary tract, part unspecified**

BURNS AND CORROSIONS (T20-T32)

Includes burns (thermal) from electrical heating appliances
burns (thermal) from electricity
burns (thermal) from flame
burns (thermal) from friction
burns (thermal) from hot air and hot gases
burns (thermal) from hot objects
burns (thermal) from lightning
burns (thermal) from radiation chemical
burn [corrosion] (external) (internal) scalds

Excludes2 erythema [dermatitis] ab igne (L59.0)
radiation-related disorders of the skin and subcutaneous tissue (L55-L59)
sunburn (L55.-)

OGCR Section I.C.19.d.

Burns and Corrosions

The ICD-10-CM makes a distinction between burn and corrosions. The burn codes are for thermal burns, except sunburns, that come from a heat source, such as a fire or hot appliance. The burn codes are also for burns resulting from electricity and radiation. Corrosions are burns due to chemicals. The guidelines for burns and corrosions are the same.

Current burns (T20-T25) are classified by depth, extent and by agent (X code). Burns are classified by depth as first degree (erythema), second degree (blistering), and third degree (full-thickness involvement). Burns of the eye and internal organs (T26-T28) are classified by site, but not by degree.

1) Sequencing of burn and related condition codes

Sequence first the code that reflects the highest degree of burn when more than one burn is present.

a. When the reason for the admission or encounter is for treatment of external multiple burns, sequence first the code that reflects the burn of the highest degree.

b. When a patient has both internal and external burns, the circumstances of admission govern the selection of the principal diagnosis or first-listed diagnosis.

c. When a patient is admitted for burn injuries and other related conditions such as smoke inhalation and/or respiratory failure, the circumstances of admission govern the selection of the principal or first-listed diagnosis.

2) Burns of the same local site

Classify burns of the same local site (three-character category level, T20-T28) but of different degrees to the subcategory identifying the highest degree recorded in the diagnosis.

BURNS AND CORROSIONS OF EXTERNAL BODY SURFACE, SPECIFIED BY SITE (T20-T25)

Includes burns and corrosions of first degree [erythema]
burns and corrosions of second degree [blisters] [epidermal loss]
burns and corrosions of third degree [deep necrosis of underlying tissue] [full-thickness skin loss]

Use additional code from category T31 or T32 to identify extent of body surface involved

● **T20 Burn and corrosion of head, face, and neck**

Excludes2 burn and corrosion of ear drum (T28.41, T28.91)
burn and corrosion of eye and adnexa (T26.-)
burn and corrosion of mouth and pharynx (T28.0)

The appropriate 7th character is to be added to each code from category T20

A	initial encounter
D	subsequent encounter
S	sequela

● **T20.0 Burn of unspecified degree of head, face, and neck**
Use additional external cause code to identify the source, place and intent of the burn (X00-X19, X75-X77, X96-X98, Y92)

X● **T20.00 Burn of unspecified degree of head, face, and neck, unspecified site**

● **T20.01 Burn of unspecified degree of ear [any part, except ear drum]**

Excludes2 burn of ear drum (T28.41-)

● **T20.011 Burn of unspecified degree of right ear [any part, except ear drum]**

● **T20.012 Burn of unspecified degree of left ear [any part, except ear drum]**

● **T20.019 Burn of unspecified degree of unspecified ear [any part, except ear drum]**

CHAPTER 19 (S00-T88)

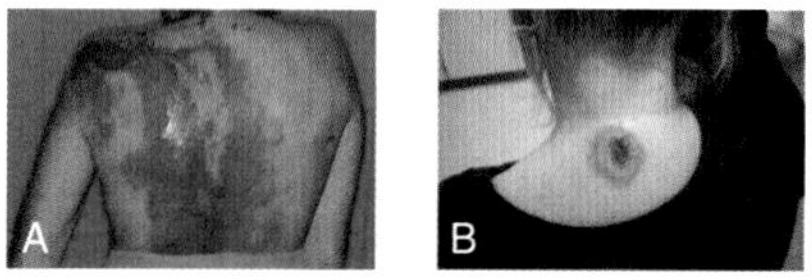

Figure 19-15 **A.** Second-degree burn. **B.** Third-degree burn. (A. From Black J, Hawks J: Medical-Surgical Nursing: Clinical Management for Positive Outcomes, 8e, Saunders, 2008. B. From Marx J, Hockberger R, Walls R: Rosen's Emergency Medicine - Concepts and Clinical Practice, 7e, Mosby, 2009)

X● **T20.02** Burn of unspecified degree of **lip(s)**
X● **T20.03** Burn of unspecified degree of **chin**
X● **T20.04** Burn of unspecified degree of **nose** (septum)
X● **T20.05** Burn of unspecified degree of **scalp** [any part]
X● **T20.06** Burn of unspecified degree of **forehead and cheek**
X● **T20.07** Burn of unspecified degree of **neck**
X● **T20.09** Burn of unspecified degree of **multiple sites** of head, face, and neck

● **T20.1** Burn of **first degree** of head, face, and neck
Use additional external cause code to identify the source, place and intent of the burn (X00-X19, X75-X77, X96-X98, Y92)
X● **T20.10** Burn of first degree of head, face, and neck, **unspecified** site
● **T20.11** Burn of first degree of **ear** [any part, except ear drum]
Excludes2 burn of ear drum (T28.41-)
● **T20.111** Burn of first degree of **right** ear [any part, except ear drum]
● **T20.112** Burn of first degree of **left** ear [any part, except ear drum]
● **T20.119** Burn of first degree of **unspecified** ear [any part, except ear drum]
X● **T20.12** Burn of first degree of **lip(s)**
X● **T20.13** Burn of first degree of **chin**
X● **T20.14** Burn of first degree of **nose** (septum)
X● **T20.15** Burn of first degree of **scalp** [any part]
X● **T20.16** Burn of first degree of **forehead and cheek**
X● **T20.17** Burn of first degree of **neck**
X● **T20.19** Burn of first degree of **multiple sites** of head, face, and neck

● **T20.2** Burn of **second degree** of head, face, and neck
Use additional external cause code to identify the source, place and intent of the burn (X00-X19, X75-X77, X96-X98, Y92)
X● **T20.20** Burn of second degree of head, face, and neck, **unspecified** site
● **T20.21** Burn of second degree of **ear** [any part, except ear drum]
Excludes2 burn of ear drum (T28.41-)
● **T20.211** Burn of second degree of **right** ear [any part, except ear drum]
● **T20.212** Burn of second degree of **left** ear [any part, except ear drum]
● **T20.219** Burn of second degree of **unspecified** ear [any part, except ear drum]
X● **T20.22** Burn of second degree of **lip(s)**
X● **T20.23** Burn of second degree of **chin**
X● **T20.24** Burn of second degree of **nose** (septum)
X● **T20.25** Burn of second degree of **scalp** [any part]
Coding Clinic: 2015, Q1, P19
X● **T20.26** Burn of second degree of **forehead and cheek**
X● **T20.27** Burn of second degree of **neck**
X● **T20.29** Burn of second degree of **multiple sites** of head, face, and neck

● **T20.3** Burn of **third degree** of head, face, and neck
Use additional external cause code to identify the source, place and intent of the burn (X00-X19, X75-X77, X96-X98, Y92)
X● **T20.30** Burn of third degree of head, face, and neck, **unspecified** site
● **T20.31** Burn of third degree of **ear** [any part, except ear drum]
Excludes2 burn of ear drum (T28.41-)
● **T20.311** Burn of third degree of **right** ear [any part, except ear drum]
● **T20.312** Burn of third degree of **left** ear [any part, except ear drum]
Coding Clinic: 2015, Q1, P18
● **T20.319** Burn of third degree of **unspecified** ear [any part, except ear drum]
X● **T20.32** Burn of third degree of **lip(s)**
X● **T20.33** Burn of third degree of **chin**
X● **T20.34** Burn of third degree of **nose** (septum)
X● **T20.35** Burn of third degree of **scalp** [any part]
X● **T20.36** Burn of third degree of **forehead and cheek**
X● **T20.37** Burn of third degree of **neck**
X● **T20.39** Burn of third degree of **multiple sites** of head, face, and neck

● **T20.4** Corrosion of **unspecified degree** of head, face, and neck
Code first (T51-T65) to identify chemical and intent
Use additional external cause code to identify place (Y92)
X● **T20.40** Corrosion of unspecified degree of head, face, and neck, **unspecified** site
● **T20.41** Corrosion of unspecified degree of **ear** [any part, except ear drum]
Excludes2 corrosion of ear drum (T28.91-)
● **T20.411** Corrosion of unspecified degree of **right** ear [any part, except ear drum]
● **T20.412** Corrosion of unspecified degree of **left** ear [any part, except ear drum]
● **T20.419** Corrosion of unspecified degree of **unspecified** ear [any part, except ear drum]
X● **T20.42** Corrosion of unspecified degree of **lip(s)**
X● **T20.43** Corrosion of unspecified degree of **chin**
X● **T20.44** Corrosion of unspecified degree of **nose** (septum)
X● **T20.45** Corrosion of unspecified degree of **scalp** [any part]
X● **T20.46** Corrosion of unspecified degree of **forehead and cheek**
X● **T20.47** Corrosion of unspecified degree of **neck**
X● **T20.49** Corrosion of unspecified degree of **multiple sites** of head, face, and neck

● **T20.5** Corrosion of **first degree** of head, face, and neck
Code first (T51-T65) to identify chemical and intent
Use additional external cause code to identify place (Y92)
X● **T20.50** Corrosion of first degree of head, face, and neck, **unspecified** site
● **T20.51** Corrosion of first degree of **ear** [any part, except ear drum]
Excludes2 corrosion of ear drum (T28.91-)
● **T20.511** Corrosion of first degree of **right** ear [any part, except ear drum]
● **T20.512** Corrosion of first degree of **left** ear [any part, except ear drum]
● **T20.519** Corrosion of first degree of **unspecified** ear [any part, except ear drum]

CHAPTER 19 (S00-T88)

X● **T20.52** Corrosion of first degree of **lip(s)**

X● **T20.53** Corrosion of first degree of **chin**

X● **T20.54** Corrosion of first degree of **nose** (septum)

X● **T20.55** Corrosion of first degree of **scalp** [any part]

X● **T20.56** Corrosion of first degree of **forehead and cheek**

X● **T20.57** Corrosion of first degree of **neck**

X● **T20.59** Corrosion of first degree of **multiple sites** of head, face, and neck

● **T20.6** Corrosion of **second degree** of head, face, and neck

Code first (T51-T65) *to identify chemical and intent*

Use additional external cause code to identify place (Y92)

X● **T20.60** Corrosion of second degree of head, face, and neck, **unspecified** site

● **T20.61** Corrosion of second degree of **ear** [any part, except ear drum]

Excludes2 corrosion of ear drum (T28.91-)

● **T20.611** Corrosion of second degree of right ear [any part, except ear drum]

● **T20.612** Corrosion of second degree of left ear [any part, except ear drum]

● **T20.619** Corrosion of second degree of **unspecified** ear [any part, except ear drum]

X● **T20.62** Corrosion of second degree of **lip(s)**

X● **T20.63** Corrosion of second degree of **chin**

X● **T20.64** Corrosion of second degree of **nose** (septum)

X● **T20.65** Corrosion of second degree of **scalp** [any part]

X● **T20.66** Corrosion of second degree of **forehead and cheek**

X● **T20.67** Corrosion of second degree of **neck**

X● **T20.69** Corrosion of second degree of **multiple sites** of head, face, and neck

● **T20.7** Corrosion of **third degree** of head, face, and neck

Code first (T51-T65) *to identify chemical and intent*

Use additional external cause code to identify place (Y92)

X● **T20.70** Corrosion of third degree of head, face, and neck, **unspecified** site

● **T20.71** Corrosion of third degree of **ear** [any part, except ear drum]

Excludes2 corrosion of ear drum (T28.91-)

● **T20.711** Corrosion of third degree of right ear [any part, except ear drum]

● **T20.712** Corrosion of third degree of left ear [any part, except ear drum]

● **T20.719** Corrosion of third degree of **unspecified** ear [any part, except ear drum]

X● **T20.72** Corrosion of third degree of **lip(s)**

X● **T20.73** Corrosion of third degree of **chin**

X● **T20.74** Corrosion of third degree of **nose** (septum)

X● **T20.75** Corrosion of third degree of **scalp** [any part]

X● **T20.76** Corrosion of third degree of **forehead and cheek**

X● **T20.77** Corrosion of third degree of **neck**

X● **T20.79** Corrosion of third degree of **multiple sites** of head, face, and neck

● **T21** **Burn and corrosion of trunk**

Includes burns and corrosion of hip region

Excludes2 burns and corrosion of axilla (T22.- with fifth character 4)
burns and corrosion of scapular region (T22.- with fifth character 6)
burns and corrosion of shoulder (T22.- with fifth character 5)

The appropriate 7th character is to be added to each code from category T21

A	initial encounter
D	subsequent encounter
S	sequela

● **T21.0** Burn of **unspecified degree** of trunk

Use additional external cause code to identify the source, place and intent of the burn (X00-X19, X75-X77, X96-X98, Y92)

X● **T21.00** Burn of unspecified degree of trunk, **unspecified** site

X● **T21.01** Burn of unspecified degree of **chest wall**
Burn of unspecified degree of breast

X● **T21.02** Burn of unspecified degree of **abdominal wall**
Burn of unspecified degree of flank
Burn of unspecified degree of groin

X● **T21.03** Burn of unspecified degree of **upper back**
Burn of unspecified degree of interscapular region

X● **T21.04** Burn of unspecified degree of **lower back**

X● **T21.05** Burn of unspecified degree of **buttock**
Burn of unspecified degree of anus

X● **T21.06** Burn of unspecified degree of **male genital region** ♂
Burn of unspecified degree of penis
Burn of unspecified degree of scrotum
Burn of unspecified degree of testis

X● **T21.07** Burn of unspecified degree of **female genital region** ♀
Burn of unspecified degree of labium (majus) (minus)
Burn of unspecified degree of perineum
Burn of unspecified degree of vulva

Excludes2 burn of vagina (T28.3)

X● **T21.09** Burn of unspecified degree of **other site** of trunk

● **T21.1** Burn of **first degree** of trunk

Use additional external cause code to identify the source, place and intent of the burn (X00-X19, X75-X77, X96-X98, Y92)

X● **T21.10** Burn of first degree of trunk, **unspecified** site

X● **T21.11** Burn of first degree of **chest wall**
Burn of first degree of breast

X● **T21.12** Burn of first degree of **abdominal wall**
Burn of first degree of flank
Burn of first degree of groin

X● **T21.13** Burn of first degree of **upper back**
Burn of first degree of interscapular region

X● **T21.14** Burn of first degree of **lower back**

X● **T21.15** Burn of first degree of **buttock**
Burn of first degree of anus

X● **T21.16** Burn of first degree of **male genital region** ♂
Burn of first degree of penis
Burn of first degree of scrotum
Burn of first degree of testis

X● **T21.17** Burn of first degree of **female genital region** ♀
Burn of first degree of labium (majus) (minus)
Burn of first degree of perineum
Burn of first degree of vulva

Excludes2 burn of vagina (T28.3)

X● **T21.19** Burn of first degree of **other site** of trunk

● **T21.2 Burn of second degree of trunk**
Use additional external cause code to identify the source, place and intent of the burn (XØØ-X19, X75-X77, X96-X98, Y92)

X● **T21.20 Burn of second degree of trunk, unspecified site**

X● **T21.21 Burn of second degree of chest wall**
Burn of second degree of breast

X● **T21.22 Burn of second degree of abdominal wall**
Burn of second degree of flank
Burn of second degree of groin

X● **T21.23 Burn of second degree of upper back**
Burn of second degree of interscapular region

X● **T21.24 Burn of second degree of lower back**

X● **T21.25 Burn of second degree of buttock**
Burn of second degree of anus

X● **T21.26 Burn of second degree of male genital region** ♂
Burn of second degree of penis
Burn of second degree of scrotum
Burn of second degree of testis

X● **T21.27 Burn of second degree of female genital region** ♀
Burn of second degree of labium (majus) (minus)
Burn of second degree of perineum
Burn of second degree of vulva
Excludes2 burn of vagina (T28.3)

X● **T21.29 Burn of second degree of other site of trunk**

● **T21.3 Burn of third degree of trunk**
Use additional external cause code to identify the source, place and intent of the burn (XØØ-X19, X75-X77, X96-X98, Y92)

X● **T21.30 Burn of third degree of trunk, unspecified site**

X● **T21.31 Burn of third degree of chest wall**
Burn of third degree of breast
Coding Clinic: 2Ø16, Q2, P6

X● **T21.32 Burn of third degree of abdominal wall**
Burn of third degree of flank
Burn of third degree of groin

X● **T21.33 Burn of third degree of upper back**
Burn of third degree of interscapular region

X● **T21.34 Burn of third degree of lower back**

X● **T21.35 Burn of third degree of buttock**
Burn of third degree of anus

X● **T21.36 Burn of third degree of male genital region** ♂
Burn of third degree of penis
Burn of third degree of scrotum
Burn of third degree of testis

X● **T21.37 Burn of third degree of female genital region** ♀
Burn of third degree of labium (majus) (minus)
Burn of third degree of perineum
Burn of third degree of vulva
Excludes2 burn of vagina (T28.3)

X● **T21.39 Burn of third degree of other site of trunk**

● **T21.4 Corrosion of unspecified degree of trunk**
Code first (T51-T65) to identify chemical and intent
Use additional external cause code to identify place (Y92)

X● **T21.40 Corrosion of unspecified degree of trunk, unspecified site**

X● **T21.41 Corrosion of unspecified degree of chest wall**
Corrosion of unspecified degree of breast

X● **T21.42 Corrosion of unspecified degree of abdominal wall**
Corrosion of unspecified degree of flank
Corrosion of unspecified degree of groin

X● **T21.43 Corrosion of unspecified degree of upper back**
Corrosion of unspecified degree of interscapular region

X● **T21.44 Corrosion of unspecified degree of lower back**

X● **T21.45 Corrosion of unspecified degree of buttock**
Corrosion of unspecified degree of anus

X● **T21.46 Corrosion of unspecified degree of male genital region** ♂
Corrosion of unspecified degree of penis
Corrosion of unspecified degree of scrotum
Corrosion of unspecified degree of testis

X● **T21.47 Corrosion of unspecified degree of female genital region** ♀
Corrosion of unspecified degree of labium (majus) (minus)
Corrosion of unspecified degree of perineum
Corrosion of unspecified degree of vulva
Excludes2 corrosion of vagina (T28.8)

X● **T21.49 Corrosion of unspecified degree of other site of trunk**

● **T21.5 Corrosion of first degree of trunk**
Code first (T51-T65) to identify chemical and intent
Use additional external cause code to identify place (Y92)

X● **T21.50 Corrosion of first degree of trunk, unspecified site**

X● **T21.51 Corrosion of first degree of chest wall**
Corrosion of first degree of breast

X● **T21.52 Corrosion of first degree of abdominal wall**
Corrosion of first degree of flank
Corrosion of first degree of groin

X● **T21.53 Corrosion of first degree of upper back**
Corrosion of first degree of interscapular region

X● **T21.54 Corrosion of first degree of lower back**

X● **T21.55 Corrosion of first degree of buttock**
Corrosion of first degree of anus

X● **T21.56 Corrosion of first degree of male genital region** ♂
Corrosion of first degree of penis
Corrosion of first degree of scrotum
Corrosion of first degree of testis

X● **T21.57 Corrosion of first degree of female genital region** ♀
Corrosion of first degree of labium (majus) (minus)
Corrosion of first degree of perineum
Corrosion of first degree of vulva
Excludes2 corrosion of vagina (T28.8)

X● **T21.59 Corrosion of first degree of other site of trunk**

● **T21.6 Corrosion of second degree of trunk**
Code first (T51-T65) to identify chemical and intent
Use additional external cause code to identify place (Y92)

X● **T21.60 Corrosion of second degree of trunk, unspecified site**

X● **T21.61 Corrosion of second degree of chest wall**
Corrosion of second degree of breast

X● **T21.62 Corrosion of second degree of abdominal wall**
Corrosion of second degree of flank
Corrosion of second degree of groin

X● **T21.63 Corrosion of second degree of upper back**
Corrosion of second degree of interscapular region

X● **T21.64 Corrosion of second degree of lower back**

X● **T21.65 Corrosion of second degree of buttock**
Corrosion of second degree of anus

X● **T21.66 Corrosion of second degree of male genital region** ♂
Corrosion of second degree of penis
Corrosion of second degree of scrotum
Corrosion of second degree of testis

X● T21.67 **Corrosion of second degree of female genital region** ♀
Corrosion of second degree of labium (majus) (minus)
Corrosion of second degree of perineum
Corrosion of second degree of vulva
Excludes2 corrosion of vagina (T28.8)

X● T21.69 **Corrosion of second degree of other site of trunk**

● T21.7 **Corrosion of third degree of trunk**
Code first (T51-T65) to identify chemical and intent
Use additional external cause code to identify place (Y92)

X● T21.70 **Corrosion of third degree of trunk, unspecified site**

X● T21.71 **Corrosion of third degree of chest wall**
Corrosion of third degree of breast

X● T21.72 **Corrosion of third degree of abdominal wall**
Corrosion of third degree of flank
Corrosion of third degree of groin

X● T21.73 **Corrosion of third degree of upper back**
Corrosion of third degree of interscapular region

X● T21.74 **Corrosion of third degree of lower back**

X● T21.75 **Corrosion of third degree of buttock**
Corrosion of third degree of anus

X● T21.76 **Corrosion of third degree of male genital region** ♂
Corrosion of third degree of penis
Corrosion of third degree of scrotum
Corrosion of third degree of testis

X● T21.77 **Corrosion of third degree of female genital region** ♀
Corrosion of third degree of labium (majus) (minus)
Corrosion of third degree of perineum
Corrosion of third degree of vulva
Excludes2 corrosion of vagina (T28.8)

X● T21.79 **Corrosion of third degree of other site of trunk**

● T22 **Burn and corrosion of shoulder and upper limb, except wrist and hand**
Excludes2 burn and corrosion of interscapular region (T21.-)
burn and corrosion of wrist and hand (T23.-)

The appropriate 7th character is to be added to each code from category T22

A	initial encounter
D	subsequent encounter
S	sequela

● T22.0 **Burn of unspecified degree of shoulder and upper limb, except wrist and hand**
Use additional external cause code to identify the source, place and intent of the burn (X00-X19, X75-X77, X96-X98, Y92)

X● T22.00 **Burn of unspecified degree of shoulder and upper limb, except wrist and hand, unspecified site**

● T22.01 **Burn of unspecified degree of forearm**
● T22.011 **Burn of unspecified degree of right forearm**
● T22.012 **Burn of unspecified degree of left forearm**
● T22.019 **Burn of unspecified degree of unspecified forearm**

● T22.02 **Burn of unspecified degree of elbow**
● T22.021 **Burn of unspecified degree of right elbow**
● T22.022 **Burn of unspecified degree of left elbow**
● T22.029 **Burn of unspecified degree of unspecified elbow**

● T22.03 **Burn of unspecified degree of upper arm**
● T22.031 **Burn of unspecified degree of right upper arm**
● T22.032 **Burn of unspecified degree of left upper arm**
● T22.039 **Burn of unspecified degree of unspecified upper arm**

● T22.04 **Burn of unspecified degree of axilla**
● T22.041 **Burn of unspecified degree of right axilla**
● T22.042 **Burn of unspecified degree of left axilla**
● T22.049 **Burn of unspecified degree of unspecified axilla**

● T22.05 **Burn of unspecified degree of shoulder**
● T22.051 **Burn of unspecified degree of right shoulder**
● T22.052 **Burn of unspecified degree of left shoulder**
● T22.059 **Burn of unspecified degree of unspecified shoulder**

● T22.06 **Burn of unspecified degree of scapular region**
● T22.061 **Burn of unspecified degree of right scapular region**
● T22.062 **Burn of unspecified degree of left scapular region**
● T22.069 **Burn of unspecified degree of unspecified scapular region**

● T22.09 **Burn of unspecified degree of multiple sites of shoulder and upper limb, except wrist and hand**
● T22.091 **Burn of unspecified degree of multiple sites of right shoulder and upper limb, except wrist and hand**
● T22.092 **Burn of unspecified degree of multiple sites of left shoulder and upper limb, except wrist and hand**
● T22.099 **Burn of unspecified degree of multiple sites of unspecified shoulder and upper limb, except wrist and hand**

● T22.1 **Burn of first degree of shoulder and upper limb, except wrist and hand**
Use additional external cause code to identify the source, place and intent of the burn (X00-X19, X75-X77, X96-X98, Y92)

X● T22.10 **Burn of first degree of shoulder and upper limb, except wrist and hand, unspecified site**

● T22.11 **Burn of first degree of forearm**
● T22.111 **Burn of first degree of right forearm**
● T22.112 **Burn of first degree of left forearm**
● T22.119 **Burn of first degree of unspecified forearm**

● T22.12 **Burn of first degree of elbow**
● T22.121 **Burn of first degree of right elbow**
● T22.122 **Burn of first degree of left elbow**
● T22.129 **Burn of first degree of unspecified elbow**

● T22.13 **Burn of first degree of upper arm**
● T22.131 **Burn of first degree of right upper arm**
● T22.132 **Burn of first degree of left upper arm**
● T22.139 **Burn of first degree of unspecified upper arm**

● T22.14 **Burn of first degree of axilla**
● T22.141 **Burn of first degree of right axilla**
● T22.142 **Burn of first degree of left axilla**
● T22.149 **Burn of first degree of unspecified axilla**

- T22.15 Burn of first degree of shoulder
  - T22.151 Burn of first degree of right shoulder
  - T22.152 Burn of first degree of left shoulder
  - T22.159 Burn of first degree of unspecified shoulder
- T22.16 Burn of first degree of scapular region
  - T22.161 Burn of first degree of right scapular region
  - T22.162 Burn of first degree of left scapular region
  - T22.169 Burn of first degree of unspecified scapular region
- T22.19 Burn of first degree of multiple sites of shoulder and upper limb, except wrist and hand
  - T22.191 Burn of first degree of multiple sites of right shoulder and upper limb, except wrist and hand
  - T22.192 Burn of first degree of multiple sites of left shoulder and upper limb, except wrist and hand
  - T22.199 Burn of first degree of multiple sites of unspecified shoulder and upper limb, except wrist and hand

T22.2 Burn of second degree of shoulder and upper limb, except wrist and hand

Use additional external cause code to identify the source, place and intent of the burn (XØØ-X19, X75-X77, X96-X98, Y92)

- X T22.2Ø Burn of second degree of shoulder and upper limb, except wrist and hand, unspecified site
- T22.21 Burn of second degree of forearm
  - T22.211 Burn of second degree of right forearm
  - T22.212 Burn of second degree of left forearm
  - T22.219 Burn of second degree of unspecified forearm
- T22.22 Burn of second degree of elbow
  - T22.221 Burn of second degree of right elbow
  - T22.222 Burn of second degree of left elbow
  - T22.229 Burn of second degree of unspecified elbow
- T22.23 Burn of second degree of upper arm
  - T22.231 Burn of second degree of right upper arm
  - T22.232 Burn of second degree of left upper arm
  - T22.239 Burn of second degree of unspecified upper arm
- T22.24 Burn of second degree of axilla
  - T22.241 Burn of second degree of right axilla
  - T22.242 Burn of second degree of left axilla
  - T22.249 Burn of second degree of unspecified axilla
- T22.25 Burn of second degree of shoulder
  - T22.251 Burn of second degree of right shoulder
  - T22.252 Burn of second degree of left shoulder
  - T22.259 Burn of second degree of unspecified shoulder
- T22.26 Burn of second degree of scapular region
  - T22.261 Burn of second degree of right scapular region
  - T22.262 Burn of second degree of left scapular region
  - T22.269 Burn of second degree of unspecified scapular region
- T22.29 Burn of second degree of multiple sites of shoulder and upper limb, except wrist and hand
  - T22.291 Burn of second degree of multiple sites of right shoulder and upper limb, except wrist and hand
  - T22.292 Burn of second degree of multiple sites of left shoulder and upper limb, except wrist and hand
  - T22.299 Burn of second degree of multiple sites of unspecified shoulder and upper limb, except wrist and hand

T22.3 Burn of third degree of shoulder and upper limb, except wrist and hand

Use additional external cause code to identify the source, place and intent of the burn (XØØ-X19, X75-X77, X96-X98, Y92)

- X T22.3Ø Burn of third degree of shoulder and upper limb, except wrist and hand, unspecified site
- T22.31 Burn of third degree of forearm
  - T22.311 Burn of third degree of right forearm
  - T22.312 Burn of third degree of left forearm
  - T22.319 Burn of third degree of unspecified forearm
- T22.32 Burn of third degree of elbow
  - T22.321 Burn of third degree of right elbow
  - T22.322 Burn of third degree of left elbow
  - T22.329 Burn of third degree of unspecified elbow
- T22.33 Burn of third degree of upper arm
  - T22.331 Burn of third degree of right upper arm
  - T22.332 Burn of third degree of left upper arm
  - T22.339 Burn of third degree of unspecified upper arm
- T22.34 Burn of third degree of axilla
  - T22.341 Burn of third degree of right axilla
  - T22.342 Burn of third degree of left axilla
  - T22.349 Burn of third degree of unspecified axilla
- T22.35 Burn of third degree of shoulder
  - T22.351 Burn of third degree of right shoulder
  - T22.352 Burn of third degree of left shoulder
  - T22.359 Burn of third degree of unspecified shoulder
- T22.36 Burn of third degree of scapular region
  - T22.361 Burn of third degree of right scapular region
  - T22.362 Burn of third degree of left scapular region
  - T22.369 Burn of third degree of unspecified scapular region
- T22.39 Burn of third degree of multiple sites of shoulder and upper limb, except wrist and hand
  - T22.391 Burn of third degree of multiple sites of right shoulder and upper limb, except wrist and hand
  - T22.392 Burn of third degree of multiple sites of left shoulder and upper limb, except wrist and hand
  - T22.399 Burn of third degree of multiple sites of unspecified shoulder and upper limb, except wrist and hand

● T22.4 Corrosion of **unspecified degree** of shoulder and upper limb, except wrist and hand

Code first (*T51-T65*) *to identify chemical and intent*

Use additional external cause code to identify place (Y92)

X● T22.40 Corrosion of unspecified degree of shoulder and upper limb, except wrist and hand, **unspecified** site

● T22.41 Corrosion of unspecified degree of **forearm**

● T22.411 Corrosion of unspecified degree of **right** forearm

● T22.412 Corrosion of unspecified degree of **left** forearm

● T22.419 Corrosion of unspecified degree of **unspecified** forearm

● T22.42 Corrosion of unspecified degree of **elbow**

● T22.421 Corrosion of unspecified degree of **right** elbow

● T22.422 Corrosion of unspecified degree of **left** elbow

● T22.429 Corrosion of unspecified degree of **unspecified** elbow

● T22.43 Corrosion of unspecified degree of **upper arm**

● T22.431 Corrosion of unspecified degree of **right** upper arm

● T22.432 Corrosion of unspecified degree of **left** upper arm

● T22.439 Corrosion of unspecified degree of **unspecified** upper arm

● T22.44 Corrosion of unspecified degree of **axilla**

● T22.441 Corrosion of unspecified degree of **right** axilla

● T22.442 Corrosion of unspecified degree of **left** axilla

● T22.449 Corrosion of unspecified degree of **unspecified** axilla

● T22.45 Corrosion of unspecified degree of **shoulder**

● T22.451 Corrosion of unspecified degree of **right** shoulder

● T22.452 Corrosion of unspecified degree of **left** shoulder

● T22.459 Corrosion of unspecified degree of **unspecified** shoulder

● T22.46 Corrosion of unspecified degree of **scapular region**

● T22.461 Corrosion of unspecified degree of **right** scapular region

● T22.462 Corrosion of unspecified degree of **left** scapular region

● T22.469 Corrosion of unspecified degree of **unspecified** scapular region

● T22.49 Corrosion of unspecified degree of **multiple sites** of shoulder and upper limb, except wrist and hand

● T22.491 Corrosion of unspecified degree of multiple sites of **right** shoulder and upper limb, except wrist and hand

● T22.492 Corrosion of unspecified degree of multiple sites of **left** shoulder and upper limb, except wrist and hand

● T22.499 Corrosion of unspecified degree of multiple sites of **unspecified** shoulder and upper limb, except wrist and hand

● T22.5 Corrosion of **first degree** of shoulder and upper limb, except wrist and hand

Code first (*T51-T65*) *to identify chemical and intent*

Use additional external cause code to identify place (Y92)

X● T22.50 Corrosion of first degree of shoulder and upper limb, except wrist and hand **unspecified** site

● T22.51 Corrosion of first degree of **forearm**

● T22.511 Corrosion of first degree of **right** forearm

● T22.512 Corrosion of first degree of **left** forearm

● T22.519 Corrosion of first degree of **unspecified** forearm

● T22.52 Corrosion of first degree of **elbow**

● T22.521 Corrosion of first degree of **right** elbow

● T22.522 Corrosion of first degree of **left** elbow

● T22.529 Corrosion of first degree of **unspecified** elbow

● T22.53 Corrosion of first degree of **upper arm**

● T22.531 Corrosion of first degree of **right** upper arm

● T22.532 Corrosion of first degree of **left** upper arm

● T22.539 Corrosion of first degree of **unspecified** upper arm

● T22.54 Corrosion of first degree of **axilla**

● T22.541 Corrosion of first degree of **right** axilla

● T22.542 Corrosion of first degree of **left** axilla

● T22.549 Corrosion of first degree of **unspecified** axilla

● T22.55 Corrosion of first degree of **shoulder**

● T22.551 Corrosion of first degree of **right** shoulder

● T22.552 Corrosion of first degree of **left** shoulder

● T22.559 Corrosion of first degree of **unspecified** shoulder

● T22.56 Corrosion of first degree of **scapular region**

● T22.561 Corrosion of first degree of **right** scapular region

● T22.562 Corrosion of first degree of **left** scapular region

● T22.569 Corrosion of first degree of **unspecified** scapular region

● T22.59 Corrosion of first degree of **multiple sites** of shoulder and upper limb, except wrist and hand

● T22.591 Corrosion of first degree of multiple sites of **right** shoulder and upper limb, except wrist and hand

● T22.592 Corrosion of first degree of multiple sites of **left** shoulder and upper limb, except wrist and hand

● T22.599 Corrosion of first degree of multiple sites of **unspecified** shoulder and upper limb, except wrist and hand

T22.6 Corrosion of **second degree** of shoulder and upper limb, except wrist and hand
Code first (T51-T65) to identify chemical and intent
Use additional external cause code to identify place (Y92)

- T22.60 Corrosion of second degree of shoulder and upper limb, except wrist and hand, **unspecified** site
- T22.61 Corrosion of second degree of **forearm**
  - T22.611 Corrosion of second degree of **right** forearm
  - T22.612 Corrosion of second degree of **left** forearm
  - T22.619 Corrosion of second degree of **unspecified** forearm
- T22.62 Corrosion of second degree of **elbow**
  - T22.621 Corrosion of second degree of **right** elbow
  - T22.622 Corrosion of second degree of **left** elbow
  - T22.629 Corrosion of second degree of **unspecified** elbow
- T22.63 Corrosion of second degree of **upper arm**
  - T22.631 Corrosion of second degree of **right** upper arm
  - T22.632 Corrosion of second degree of **left** upper arm
  - T22.639 Corrosion of second degree of **unspecified** upper arm
- T22.64 Corrosion of second degree of **axilla**
  - T22.641 Corrosion of second degree of **right** axilla
  - T22.642 Corrosion of second degree of **left** axilla
  - T22.649 Corrosion of second degree of **unspecified** axilla
- T22.65 Corrosion of second degree of **shoulder**
  - T22.651 Corrosion of second degree of **right** shoulder
  - T22.652 Corrosion of second degree of **left** shoulder
  - T22.659 Corrosion of second degree of **unspecified** shoulder
- T22.66 Corrosion of second degree of **scapular region**
  - T22.661 Corrosion of second degree of **right** scapular region
  - T22.662 Corrosion of second degree of **left** scapular region
  - T22.669 Corrosion of second degree of **unspecified** scapular region
- T22.69 Corrosion of second degree of **multiple sites** of shoulder and upper limb, except wrist and hand
  - T22.691 Corrosion of second degree of multiple sites of **right** shoulder and upper limb, except wrist and hand
  - T22.692 Corrosion of second degree of multiple sites of **left** shoulder and upper limb, except wrist and hand
  - T22.699 Corrosion of second degree of multiple sites of **unspecified** shoulder and upper limb, except wrist and hand

T22.7 Corrosion of **third degree** of shoulder and upper limb, except wrist and hand
Code first (T51-T65) to identify chemical and intent
Use additional external cause code to identify place (Y92)

- T22.70 Corrosion of third degree of shoulder and upper limb, except wrist and hand, **unspecified** site
- T22.71 Corrosion of third degree of **forearm**
  - T22.711 Corrosion of third degree of **right** forearm
  - T22.712 Corrosion of third degree of **left** forearm
  - T22.719 Corrosion of third degree of **unspecified** forearm
- T22.72 Corrosion of third degree of **elbow**
  - T22.721 Corrosion of third degree of **right** elbow
  - T22.722 Corrosion of third degree of **left** elbow
  - T22.729 Corrosion of third degree of **unspecified** elbow
- T22.73 Corrosion of third degree of **upper arm**
  - T22.731 Corrosion of third degree of **right** upper arm
  - T22.732 Corrosion of third degree of **left** upper arm
  - T22.739 Corrosion of third degree of **unspecified** upper arm
- T22.74 Corrosion of third degree of **axilla**
  - T22.741 Corrosion of third degree of **right** axilla
  - T22.742 Corrosion of third degree of **left** axilla
  - T22.749 Corrosion of third degree of **unspecified** axilla
- T22.75 Corrosion of third degree of **shoulder**
  - T22.751 Corrosion of third degree of **right** shoulder
  - T22.752 Corrosion of third degree of **left** shoulder
  - T22.759 Corrosion of third degree of **unspecified** shoulder
- T22.76 Corrosion of third degree of **scapular region**
  - T22.761 Corrosion of third degree of **right** scapular region
  - T22.762 Corrosion of third degree of **left** scapular region
  - T22.769 Corrosion of third degree of **unspecified** scapular region
- T22.79 Corrosion of third degree of **multiple sites** of shoulder and upper limb, except wrist and hand
  - T22.791 Corrosion of third degree of multiple sites of **right** shoulder and upper limb, except wrist and hand
  - T22.792 Corrosion of third degree of multiple sites of **left** shoulder and upper limb, except wrist and hand
  - T22.799 Corrosion of third degree of multiple sites of **unspecified** shoulder and upper limb, except wrist and hand

● **T23 Burn and corrosion of wrist and hand**

The appropriate 7th character is to be added to each code from category T23

A	initial encounter
D	subsequent encounter
S	sequela

● **T23.0** Burn of **unspecified degree** of wrist and hand

Use additional external cause code to identify the source, place and intent of the burn (X00-X19, X75-X77, X96-X98, Y92)

● **T23.00** Burn of unspecified degree of hand, **unspecified site**

● **T23.001** Burn of unspecified degree of **right** hand, unspecified site

● **T23.002** Burn of unspecified degree of **left** hand, unspecified site

● **T23.009** Burn of unspecified degree of **unspecified** hand, unspecified site

● **T23.01** Burn of unspecified degree of **thumb** (nail)

● **T23.011** Burn of unspecified degree of **right** thumb (nail)

● **T23.012** Burn of unspecified degree of **left** thumb (nail)

● **T23.019** Burn of unspecified degree of **unspecified** thumb (nail)

● **T23.02** Burn of unspecified degree of **single finger** (nail) **except thumb**

● **T23.021** Burn of unspecified degree of single **right** finger (nail) except thumb

● **T23.022** Burn of unspecified degree of single **left** finger (nail) except thumb

● **T23.029** Burn of unspecified degree of **unspecified** single finger (nail) except thumb

● **T23.03** Burn of unspecified degree of **multiple fingers** (nail), **not including thumb**

● **T23.031** Burn of unspecified degree of multiple **right** fingers (nail), not including thumb

● **T23.032** Burn of unspecified degree of multiple **left** fingers (nail), not including thumb

● **T23.039** Burn of unspecified degree of **unspecified** multiple fingers (nail), not including thumb

● **T23.04** Burn of unspecified degree of **multiple fingers** (nail), **including thumb**

● **T23.041** Burn of unspecified degree of multiple **right** fingers (nail), including thumb

● **T23.042** Burn of unspecified degree of multiple **left** fingers (nail), including thumb

● **T23.049** Burn of unspecified degree of **unspecified** multiple fingers (nail), including thumb

● **T23.05** Burn of unspecified degree of **palm**

● **T23.051** Burn of unspecified degree of **right** palm

● **T23.052** Burn of unspecified degree of **left** palm

● **T23.059** Burn of unspecified degree of **unspecified** palm

● **T23.06** Burn of unspecified degree of **back of hand**

● **T23.061** Burn of unspecified degree of back of **right** hand

● **T23.062** Burn of unspecified degree of back of **left** hand

● **T23.069** Burn of unspecified degree of back of **unspecified** hand

● **T23.07** Burn of unspecified degree of **wrist**

● **T23.071** Burn of unspecified degree of **right** wrist

● **T23.072** Burn of unspecified degree of **left** wrist

● **T23.079** Burn of unspecified degree of **unspecified** wrist

● **T23.09** Burn of unspecified degree of **multiple sites** of wrist and hand

● **T23.091** Burn of unspecified degree of multiple sites of **right** wrist and hand

● **T23.092** Burn of unspecified degree of multiple sites of **left** wrist and hand

● **T23.099** Burn of unspecified degree of multiple sites of **unspecified** wrist and hand

● **T23.1** Burn of **first degree** of wrist and hand

Use additional external cause code to identify the source, place and intent of the burn (X00-X19, X75-X77, X96-X98, Y92)

● **T23.10** Burn of first degree of hand, **unspecified site**

● **T23.101** Burn of first degree of **right** hand, unspecified site

● **T23.102** Burn of first degree of **left** hand, unspecified site

● **T23.109** Burn of first degree of **unspecified** hand, unspecified site

● **T23.11** Burn of first degree of **thumb** (nail)

● **T23.111** Burn of first degree of **right** thumb (nail)

● **T23.112** Burn of first degree of **left** thumb (nail)

● **T23.119** Burn of first degree of **unspecified** thumb (nail)

● **T23.12** Burn of first degree of **single finger** (nail) **except thumb**

● **T23.121** Burn of first degree of single **right** finger (nail) except thumb

● **T23.122** Burn of first degree of single **left** finger (nail) except thumb

● **T23.129** Burn of first degree of **unspecified** single finger (nail) except thumb

● **T23.13** Burn of first degree of **multiple fingers** (nail), **not including thumb**

● **T23.131** Burn of first degree of multiple **right** fingers (nail), not including thumb

● **T23.132** Burn of first degree of multiple **left** fingers (nail), not including thumb

● **T23.139** Burn of first degree of **unspecified** multiple fingers (nail), not including thumb

● **T23.14** Burn of first degree of **multiple fingers** (nail), **including thumb**

● **T23.141** Burn of first degree of multiple **right** fingers (nail), including thumb

● **T23.142** Burn of first degree of multiple **left** fingers (nail), including thumb

● **T23.149** Burn of first degree of **unspecified** multiple fingers (nail), including thumb

CHAPTER 19 (S00-T88)

T23.15 Burn of first degree of palm
- T23.151 Burn of first degree of right palm
- T23.152 Burn of first degree of left palm
- T23.159 Burn of first degree of unspecified palm

T23.16 Burn of first degree of back of hand
- T23.161 Burn of first degree of back of right hand
- T23.162 Burn of first degree of back of left hand
- T23.169 Burn of first degree of back of unspecified hand

T23.17 Burn of first degree of wrist
- T23.171 Burn of first degree of right wrist
- T23.172 Burn of first degree of left wrist
- T23.179 Burn of first degree of unspecified wrist

T23.19 Burn of first degree of multiple sites of wrist and hand
- T23.191 Burn of first degree of multiple sites of right wrist and hand
- T23.192 Burn of first degree of multiple sites of left wrist and hand
- T23.199 Burn of first degree of multiple sites of unspecified wrist and hand

T23.2 Burn of second degree of wrist and hand

Use additional external cause code to identify the source, place and intent of the burn (XØØ-X19, X75-X77, X96-X98, Y92)

T23.2Ø Burn of second degree of hand, unspecified site
- T23.2Ø1 Burn of second degree of right hand, unspecified site
- T23.2Ø2 Burn of second degree of left hand, unspecified site
- T23.2Ø9 Burn of second degree of unspecified hand, unspecified site

T23.21 Burn of second degree of thumb (nail)
- T23.211 Burn of second degree of right thumb (nail)
- T23.212 Burn of second degree of left thumb (nail)
- T23.219 Burn of second degree of unspecified thumb (nail)

T23.22 Burn of second degree of single finger (nail) except thumb
- T23.221 Burn of second degree of single right finger (nail) except thumb
- T23.222 Burn of second degree of single left finger (nail) except thumb
- T23.229 Burn of second degree of unspecified single finger (nail) except thumb

T23.23 Burn of second degree of multiple fingers (nail), not including thumb
- T23.231 Burn of second degree of multiple right fingers (nail), not including thumb
- T23.232 Burn of second degree of multiple left fingers (nail), not including thumb
- T23.239 Burn of second degree of unspecified multiple fingers (nail), not including thumb

T23.24 Burn of second degree of multiple fingers (nail), including thumb
- T23.241 Burn of second degree of multiple right fingers (nail), including thumb
- T23.242 Burn of second degree of multiple left fingers (nail), including thumb
- T23.249 Burn of second degree of unspecified multiple fingers (nail), including thumb

T23.25 Burn of second degree of palm
- T23.251 Burn of second degree of right palm
- T23.252 Burn of second degree of left palm
- T23.259 Burn of second degree of unspecified palm

T23.26 Burn of second degree of back of hand
- T23.261 Burn of second degree of back of right hand
- T23.262 Burn of second degree of back of left hand
- T23.269 Burn of second degree of back of unspecified hand

T23.27 Burn of second degree of wrist
- T23.271 Burn of second degree of right wrist
- T23.272 Burn of second degree of left wrist
- T23.279 Burn of second degree of unspecified wrist

T23.29 Burn of second degree of multiple sites of wrist and hand
- T23.291 Burn of second degree of multiple sites of right wrist and hand
- T23.292 Burn of second degree of multiple sites of left wrist and hand
- T23.299 Burn of second degree of multiple sites of unspecified wrist and hand

T23.3 Burn of third degree of wrist and hand

Use additional external cause code to identify the source, place and intent of the burn (XØØ-X19, X75-X77, X96-X98, Y92)

T23.3Ø Burn of third degree of hand, unspecified site
- T23.3Ø1 Burn of third degree of right hand, unspecified site
  Coding Clinic: 2Ø15, Q1, P19
- T23.3Ø2 Burn of third degree of left hand, unspecified site
  Coding Clinic: 2Ø16, Q2, P5
- T23.3Ø9 Burn of third degree of unspecified hand, unspecified site

T23.31 Burn of third degree of thumb (nail)
- T23.311 Burn of third degree of right thumb (nail)
- T23.312 Burn of third degree of left thumb (nail)
- T23.319 Burn of third degree of unspecified thumb (nail)

T23.32 Burn of third degree of single finger (nail) except thumb
- T23.321 Burn of third degree of single right finger (nail) except thumb
- T23.322 Burn of third degree of single left finger (nail) except thumb
- T23.329 Burn of third degree of unspecified single finger (nail) except thumb

T23.33 Burn of third degree of multiple fingers (nail), not including thumb
- T23.331 Burn of third degree of multiple right fingers (nail), not including thumb
- T23.332 Burn of third degree of multiple left fingers (nail), not including thumb
- T23.339 Burn of third degree of unspecified multiple fingers (nail), not including thumb

- T23.34 Burn of third degree of **multiple fingers** (nail), **including thumb**
  - T23.341 Burn of third degree of multiple **right** fingers (nail), including thumb
  - T23.342 Burn of third degree of multiple **left** fingers (nail), including thumb
  - T23.349 Burn of third degree of **unspecified** multiple fingers (nail), including thumb
- T23.35 Burn of third degree of **palm**
  - T23.351 Burn of third degree of **right** palm
  - T23.352 Burn of third degree of **left** palm
  - T23.359 Burn of third degree of **unspecified** palm
- T23.36 Burn of third degree of **back of hand**
  - T23.361 Burn of third degree of back of **right** hand
  - T23.362 Burn of third degree of back of **left** hand
  - T23.369 Burn of third degree of back of **unspecified** hand
- T23.37 Burn of third degree of **wrist**
  - T23.371 Burn of third degree of **right** wrist
  - T23.372 Burn of third degree of **left** wrist
  - T23.379 Burn of third degree of **unspecified** wrist
- T23.39 Burn of third degree of **multiple sites** of wrist and hand
  - T23.391 Burn of third degree of multiple sites of **right** wrist and hand
  - T23.392 Burn of third degree of multiple sites of **left** wrist and hand
  - T23.399 Burn of third degree of multiple sites of **unspecified** wrist and hand

T23.4 Corrosion of **unspecified degree** of wrist and hand

Code first *(T51-T65) to identify chemical and intent*

Use additional external cause code to identify place (Y92)

- T23.40 Corrosion of unspecified degree of hand, **unspecified site**
  - T23.401 Corrosion of unspecified degree of **right** hand, unspecified site
  - T23.402 Corrosion of unspecified degree of **left** hand, unspecified site
  - T23.409 Corrosion of unspecified degree of **unspecified** hand, unspecified site
- T23.41 Corrosion of unspecified degree of **thumb** (nail)
  - T23.411 Corrosion of unspecified degree of **right** thumb (nail)
  - T23.412 Corrosion of unspecified degree of **left** thumb (nail)
  - T23.419 Corrosion of unspecified degree of **unspecified** thumb (nail)
- T23.42 Corrosion of unspecified degree of **single finger** (nail) except thumb
  - T23.421 Corrosion of unspecified degree of single **right** finger (nail) except thumb
  - T23.422 Corrosion of unspecified degree of single **left** finger (nail) except thumb
  - T23.429 Corrosion of unspecified degree of **unspecified** single finger (nail) except thumb
- T23.43 Corrosion of unspecified degree of **multiple fingers** (nail), **not including thumb**
  - T23.431 Corrosion of unspecified degree of multiple **right** fingers (nail), not including thumb
  - T23.432 Corrosion of unspecified degree of multiple **left** fingers (nail), not including thumb
  - T23.439 Corrosion of unspecified degree of **unspecified** multiple fingers (nail), not including thumb
- T23.44 Corrosion of unspecified degree of **multiple fingers** (nail), **including thumb**
  - T23.441 Corrosion of unspecified degree of multiple **right** fingers (nail), including thumb
  - T23.442 Corrosion of unspecified degree of multiple **left** fingers (nail), including thumb
  - T23.449 Corrosion of unspecified degree of **unspecified** multiple fingers (nail), including thumb
- T23.45 Corrosion of unspecified degree of **palm**
  - T23.451 Corrosion of unspecified degree of **right** palm
  - T23.452 Corrosion of unspecified degree of **left** palm
  - T23.459 Corrosion of unspecified degree of **unspecified** palm
- T23.46 Corrosion of unspecified degree of **back of hand**
  - T23.461 Corrosion of unspecified degree of back of **right** hand
  - T23.462 Corrosion of unspecified degree of back of **left** hand
  - T23.469 Corrosion of unspecified degree of back of **unspecified** hand
- T23.47 Corrosion of unspecified degree of **wrist**
  - T23.471 Corrosion of unspecified degree of **right** wrist
  - T23.472 Corrosion of unspecified degree of **left** wrist
  - T23.479 Corrosion of unspecified degree of **unspecified** wrist
- T23.49 Corrosion of unspecified degree of **multiple sites** of wrist and hand
  - T23.491 Corrosion of unspecified degree of multiple sites of **right** wrist and hand
  - T23.492 Corrosion of unspecified degree of multiple sites of **left** wrist and hand
  - T23.499 Corrosion of unspecified degree of multiple sites of **unspecified** wrist and hand

T23.5 Corrosion of **first degree** of wrist and hand

Code first *(T51-T65) to identify chemical and intent*

Use additional external cause code to identify place (Y92)

- T23.50 Corrosion of first degree of hand, **unspecified site**
  - T23.501 Corrosion of first degree of **right** hand, unspecified site
  - T23.502 Corrosion of first degree of **left** hand, unspecified site
  - T23.509 Corrosion of first degree of **unspecified** hand, unspecified site

CHAPTER 19 (SØØ-T88)

- T23.51 Corrosion of first degree of **thumb** (nail)
  - T23.511 Corrosion of first degree of **right** thumb (nail)
  - T23.512 Corrosion of first degree of **left** thumb (nail)
  - T23.519 Corrosion of first degree of **unspecified** thumb (nail)
- T23.52 Corrosion of first degree of **single finger** (nail) **except thumb**
  - T23.521 Corrosion of first degree of single **right** finger (nail) except thumb
  - T23.522 Corrosion of first degree of single **left** finger (nail) except thumb
  - T23.529 Corrosion of first degree of **unspecified** single finger (nail) except thumb
- T23.53 Corrosion of first degree of **multiple fingers** (nail), **not including thumb**
  - T23.531 Corrosion of first degree of multiple **right** fingers (nail), not including thumb
  - T23.532 Corrosion of first degree of multiple **left** fingers (nail), not including thumb
  - T23.539 Corrosion of first degree of **unspecified** multiple fingers (nail), not including thumb
- T23.54 Corrosion of first degree of **multiple fingers** (nail), **including thumb**
  - T23.541 Corrosion of first degree of multiple **right** fingers (nail), including thumb
  - T23.542 Corrosion of first degree of multiple **left** fingers (nail), including thumb
  - T23.549 Corrosion of first degree of **unspecified** multiple fingers (nail), including thumb
- T23.55 Corrosion of first degree of **palm**
  - T23.551 Corrosion of first degree of **right** palm
  - T23.552 Corrosion of first degree of **left** palm
  - T23.559 Corrosion of first degree of **unspecified** palm
- T23.56 Corrosion of first degree of **back of hand**
  - T23.561 Corrosion of first degree of back of **right** hand
  - T23.562 Corrosion of first degree of back of **left** hand
  - T23.569 Corrosion of first degree of back of **unspecified** hand
- T23.57 Corrosion of first degree of **wrist**
  - T23.571 Corrosion of first degree of **right** wrist
  - T23.572 Corrosion of first degree of **left** wrist
  - T23.579 Corrosion of first degree of **unspecified** wrist
- T23.59 Corrosion of first degree of **multiple sites** of wrist and hand
  - T23.591 Corrosion of first degree of multiple sites of **right** wrist and hand
  - T23.592 Corrosion of first degree of multiple sites of **left** wrist and hand
  - T23.599 Corrosion of first degree of multiple sites of **unspecified** wrist and hand

- T23.6 Corrosion of **second degree** of wrist and hand

  Code first (T51-T65) to identify chemical and intent

  Use additional external cause code to identify place (Y92)
  - T23.60 Corrosion of second degree of hand, **unspecified site**
    - T23.601 Corrosion of second degree of **right** hand, unspecified site
    - T23.602 Corrosion of second degree of **left** hand, unspecified site
    - T23.609 Corrosion of second degree of **unspecified** hand, unspecified site
  - T23.61 Corrosion of second degree of **thumb** (nail)
    - T23.611 Corrosion of second degree of **right** thumb (nail)
    - T23.612 Corrosion of second degree of **left** thumb (nail)
    - T23.619 Corrosion of second degree of **unspecified** thumb (nail)
  - T23.62 Corrosion of second degree of **single finger** (nail) **except thumb**
    - T23.621 Corrosion of second degree of single **right** finger (nail) except thumb
    - T23.622 Corrosion of second degree of single **left** finger (nail) except thumb
    - T23.629 Corrosion of second degree of **unspecified** single finger (nail) except thumb
  - T23.63 Corrosion of second degree of **multiple fingers** (nail), **not including thumb**
    - T23.631 Corrosion of second degree of multiple **right** fingers (nail), not including thumb
    - T23.632 Corrosion of second degree of multiple **left** fingers (nail), not including thumb
    - T23.639 Corrosion of second degree of **unspecified** multiple fingers (nail), not including thumb
  - T23.64 Corrosion of second degree of **multiple fingers** (nail), **including thumb**
    - T23.641 Corrosion of second degree of multiple **right** fingers (nail), including thumb
    - T23.642 Corrosion of second degree of multiple **left** fingers (nail), including thumb
    - T23.649 Corrosion of second degree of **unspecified** multiple fingers (nail), including thumb
  - T23.65 Corrosion of second degree of **palm**
    - T23.651 Corrosion of second degree of **right** palm
    - T23.652 Corrosion of second degree of **left** palm
    - T23.659 Corrosion of second degree of **unspecified** palm
  - T23.66 Corrosion of second degree of **back of hand**
    - T23.661 Corrosion of second degree back of **right** hand
    - T23.662 Corrosion of second degree back of **left** hand
    - T23.669 Corrosion of second degree back of **unspecified** hand

T23.67 Corrosion of second degree of **wrist**

T23.671 Corrosion of second degree of **right** wrist

T23.672 Corrosion of second degree of **left** wrist

T23.679 Corrosion of second degree of **unspecified** wrist

T23.69 Corrosion of second degree of **multiple sites** of wrist and hand

T23.691 Corrosion of second degree of multiple sites of **right** wrist and hand

T23.692 Corrosion of second degree of multiple sites of **left** wrist and hand

T23.699 Corrosion of second degree of multiple sites of **unspecified** wrist and hand

T23.7 Corrosion of third degree of wrist and hand

Code first (T51-T65) to identify chemical and intent

Use additional external cause code to identify place (Y92)

T23.70 Corrosion of third degree of hand, **unspecified** site

T23.701 Corrosion of third degree of **right** hand, unspecified site

T23.702 Corrosion of third degree of **left** hand, unspecified site

T23.709 Corrosion of third degree of **unspecified** hand, unspecified site

T23.71 Corrosion of third degree of **thumb** (nail)

T23.711 Corrosion of third degree of **right** thumb (nail)

T23.712 Corrosion of third degree of **left** thumb (nail)

T23.719 Corrosion of third degree of **unspecified** thumb (nail)

T23.72 Corrosion of third degree of **single finger** (nail) except thumb

T23.721 Corrosion of third degree of single **right** finger (nail) except thumb

T23.722 Corrosion of third degree of single **left** finger (nail) except thumb

T23.729 Corrosion of third degree of **unspecified** single finger (nail) except thumb

T23.73 Corrosion of third degree of **multiple fingers** (nail), **not including thumb**

T23.731 Corrosion of third degree of multiple **right** fingers (nail), not including thumb

T23.732 Corrosion of third degree of multiple **left** fingers (nail), not including thumb

T23.739 Corrosion of third degree of **unspecified** multiple fingers (nail), not including thumb

T23.74 Corrosion of third degree of **multiple fingers** (nail), **including thumb**

T23.741 Corrosion of third degree of multiple **right** fingers (nail), including thumb

T23.742 Corrosion of third degree of multiple **left** fingers (nail), including thumb

T23.749 Corrosion of third degree of **unspecified** multiple fingers (nail), including thumb

T23.75 Corrosion of third degree of **palm**

T23.751 Corrosion of third degree of **right** palm

T23.752 Corrosion of third degree of **left** palm

T23.759 Corrosion of third degree of **unspecified** palm

T23.76 Corrosion of third degree of **back of hand**

T23.761 Corrosion of third degree of back of **right** hand

T23.762 Corrosion of third degree of back of **left** hand

T23.769 Corrosion of third degree of back of **unspecified** hand

T23.77 Corrosion of third degree of **wrist**

T23.771 Corrosion of third degree of **right** wrist

T23.772 Corrosion of third degree of **left** wrist

T23.779 Corrosion of third degree of **unspecified** wrist

T23.79 Corrosion of third degree of **multiple sites** of wrist and hand

T23.791 Corrosion of third degree of multiple sites of **right** wrist and hand

T23.792 Corrosion of third degree of multiple sites of **left** wrist and hand

T23.799 Corrosion of third degree of multiple sites of **unspecified** wrist and hand

T24 Burn and corrosion of lower limb, except ankle and foot

Excludes2 burn and corrosion of ankle and foot (T25.-)
burn and corrosion of hip region (T21.-)

The appropriate 7th character is to be added to each code from category T24

A	initial encounter
D	subsequent encounter
S	sequela

T24.Ø Burn of **unspecified degree** of lower limb, except ankle and foot

Use additional external cause code to identify the source, place and intent of the burn (XØØ-X19, X75-X77, X96-X98, Y92)

T24.ØØ Burn of unspecified degree of **unspecified site** of lower limb, except ankle and foot

T24.ØØ1 Burn of unspecified degree of unspecified site of **right** lower limb, except ankle and foot

T24.ØØ2 Burn of unspecified degree of unspecified site of **left** lower limb, except ankle and foot

T24.ØØ9 Burn of unspecified degree of unspecified site of **unspecified** lower limb, except ankle and foot

T24.Ø1 Burn of unspecified degree of **thigh**

T24.Ø11 Burn of unspecified degree of **right** thigh

T24.Ø12 Burn of unspecified degree of **left** thigh

T24.Ø19 Burn of unspecified degree of **unspecified** thigh

CHAPTER 19 (SØØ-T88)

T24.Ø2 Burn of unspecified degree of knee
- T24.Ø21 Burn of unspecified degree of right knee
- T24.Ø22 Burn of unspecified degree of left knee
- T24.Ø29 Burn of unspecified degree of unspecified knee

T24.Ø3 Burn of unspecified degree of lower leg
- T24.Ø31 Burn of unspecified degree of right lower leg
- T24.Ø32 Burn of unspecified degree of left lower leg
- T24.Ø39 Burn of unspecified degree of unspecified lower leg

T24.Ø9 Burn of unspecified degree of multiple sites of lower limb, except ankle and foot
- T24.Ø91 Burn of unspecified degree of multiple sites of right lower limb, except ankle and foot
- T24.Ø92 Burn of unspecified degree of multiple sites of left lower limb, except ankle and foot
- T24.Ø99 Burn of unspecified degree of multiple sites of unspecified lower limb, except ankle and foot

T24.1 Burn of first degree of lower limb, except ankle and foot

Use additional external cause code to identify the source, place and intent of the burn (XØØ-X19, X75-X77, X96-X98, Y92)

T24.1Ø Burn of first degree of unspecified site of lower limb, except ankle and foot
- T24.1Ø1 Burn of first degree of unspecified site of right lower limb, except ankle and foot
- T24.1Ø2 Burn of first degree of unspecified site of left lower limb, except ankle and foot
- T24.1Ø9 Burn of first degree of unspecified site of unspecified lower limb, except ankle and foot

T24.11 Burn of first degree of thigh
- T24.111 Burn of first degree of right thigh
- T24.112 Burn of first degree of left thigh
- T24.119 Burn of first degree of unspecified thigh

T24.12 Burn of first degree of knee
- T24.121 Burn of first degree of right knee
- T24.122 Burn of first degree of left knee
- T24.129 Burn of first degree of unspecified knee

T24.13 Burn of first degree of lower leg
- T24.131 Burn of first degree of right lower leg
- T24.132 Burn of first degree of left lower leg
- T24.139 Burn of first degree of unspecified lower leg

T24.19 Burn of first degree of multiple sites of lower limb, except ankle and foot
- T24.191 Burn of first degree of multiple sites of right lower limb, except ankle and foot
- T24.192 Burn of first degree of multiple sites of left lower limb, except ankle and foot
- T24.199 Burn of first degree of multiple sites of unspecified lower limb, except ankle and foot

T24.2 Burn of second degree of lower limb, except ankle and foot

Use additional external cause code to identify the source, place and intent of the burn (XØØ-X19, X75-X77, X96-X98, Y92)

T24.2Ø Burn of second degree of unspecified site of lower limb, except ankle and foot
- T24.2Ø1 Burn of second degree of unspecified site of right lower limb, except ankle and foot
- T24.2Ø2 Burn of second degree of unspecified site of left lower limb, except ankle and foot
- T24.2Ø9 Burn of second degree of unspecified site of unspecified lower limb, except ankle and foot

T24.21 Burn of second degree of thigh
- T24.211 Burn of second degree of right thigh
- T24.212 Burn of second degree of left thigh
- T24.219 Burn of second degree of unspecified thigh

T24.22 Burn of second degree of knee
- T24.221 Burn of second degree of right knee
- T24.222 Burn of second degree of left knee
- T24.229 Burn of second degree of unspecified knee

T24.23 Burn of second degree of lower leg
- T24.231 Burn of second degree of right lower leg
- T24.232 Burn of second degree of left lower leg
- T24.239 Burn of second degree of unspecified lower leg

T24.29 Burn of second degree of multiple sites of lower limb, except ankle and foot
- T24.291 Burn of second degree of multiple sites of right lower limb, except ankle and foot
- T24.292 Burn of second degree of multiple sites of left lower limb, except ankle and foot
- T24.299 Burn of second degree of multiple sites of unspecified lower limb, except ankle and foot

T24.3 Burn of third degree of lower limb, except ankle and foot

Use additional external cause code to identify the source, place and intent of the burn (XØØ-X19, X75-X77, X96-X98, Y92)

T24.3Ø Burn of third degree of unspecified site of lower limb, except ankle and foot
- T24.3Ø1 Burn of third degree of unspecified site of right lower limb, except ankle and foot
- T24.3Ø2 Burn of third degree of unspecified site of left lower limb, except ankle and foot
- T24.3Ø9 Burn of third degree of unspecified site of unspecified lower limb, except ankle and foot

T24.31 Burn of third degree of thigh
- T24.311 Burn of third degree of right thigh
- T24.312 Burn of third degree of left thigh
- T24.319 Burn of third degree of unspecified thigh

T24.32 Burn of third degree of **knee**
- T24.321 Burn of third degree of **right** knee
- T24.322 Burn of third degree of **left** knee
- T24.329 Burn of third degree of **unspecified** knee

T24.33 Burn of third degree of **lower leg**
- T24.331 Burn of third degree of **right** lower leg
- T24.332 Burn of third degree of **left** lower leg
- T24.339 Burn of third degree of **unspecified** lower leg

T24.39 Burn of third degree of **multiple sites** of lower limb, except ankle and foot
- T24.391 Burn of third degree of multiple sites of **right** lower limb, except ankle and foot
  Coding Clinic: 2016, Q2, P5
- T24.392 Burn of third degree of multiple sites of **left** lower limb, except ankle and foot
- T24.399 Burn of third degree of multiple sites of **unspecified** lower limb, except ankle and foot

T24.4 Corrosion of **unspecified degree** of lower limb, except ankle and foot
Code first (T51-T65) to identify chemical and intent
Use additional external cause code to identify place (Y92)

T24.40 Corrosion of unspecified degree of **unspecified** site of lower limb, except ankle and foot
- T24.401 Corrosion of unspecified degree of unspecified site of **right** lower limb, except ankle and foot
- T24.402 Corrosion of unspecified degree of unspecified site of **left** lower limb, except ankle and foot
- T24.409 Corrosion of unspecified degree of unspecified site of **unspecified** lower limb, except ankle and foot

T24.41 Corrosion of unspecified degree of **thigh**
- T24.411 Corrosion of unspecified degree of **right** thigh
- T24.412 Corrosion of unspecified degree of **left** thigh
- T24.419 Corrosion of unspecified degree of **unspecified** thigh

T24.42 Corrosion of unspecified degree of **knee**
- T24.421 Corrosion of unspecified degree of **right** knee
- T24.422 Corrosion of unspecified degree of **left** knee
- T24.429 Corrosion of unspecified degree of **unspecified** knee

T24.43 Corrosion of unspecified degree of **lower leg**
- T24.431 Corrosion of unspecified degree of **right** lower leg
- T24.432 Corrosion of unspecified degree of **left** lower leg
- T24.439 Corrosion of unspecified degree of **unspecified** lower leg

T24.49 Corrosion of unspecified degree of **multiple sites** of lower limb, except ankle and foot
- T24.491 Corrosion of unspecified degree of multiple sites of **right** lower limb, except ankle and foot
- T24.492 Corrosion of unspecified degree of multiple sites of **left** lower limb, except ankle and foot
- T24.499 Corrosion of unspecified degree of multiple sites of **unspecified** lower limb, except ankle and foot

T24.5 Corrosion of **first degree** of lower limb, except ankle and foot
Code first (T51-T65) to identify chemical and intent
Use additional external cause code to identify place (Y92)

T24.50 Corrosion of first degree of **unspecified site** of lower limb, except ankle and foot
- T24.501 Corrosion of first degree of unspecified site of **right** lower limb, except ankle and foot
- T24.502 Corrosion of first degree of unspecified site of **left** lower limb, except ankle and foot
- T24.509 Corrosion of first degree of unspecified site of **unspecified** lower limb, except ankle and foot

T24.51 Corrosion of first degree of **thigh**
- T24.511 Corrosion of first degree of **right** thigh
- T24.512 Corrosion of first degree of **left** thigh
- T24.519 Corrosion of first degree of **unspecified** thigh

T24.52 Corrosion of first degree of **knee**
- T24.521 Corrosion of first degree of **right** knee
- T24.522 Corrosion of first degree of **left** knee
- T24.529 Corrosion of first degree of **unspecified** knee

T24.53 Corrosion of first degree of **lower leg**
- T24.531 Corrosion of first degree of **right** lower leg
- T24.532 Corrosion of first degree of **left** lower leg
- T24.539 Corrosion of first degree of **unspecified** lower leg

T24.59 Corrosion of first degree of **multiple sites** of lower limb, except ankle and foot
- T24.591 Corrosion of first degree of multiple sites of **right** lower limb, except ankle and foot
- T24.592 Corrosion of first degree of multiple sites of **left** lower limb, except ankle and foot
- T24.599 Corrosion of first degree of multiple sites of **unspecified** lower limb, except ankle and foot

T24.6 Corrosion of **second degree** of lower limb, except ankle and foot
Code first (T51-T65) to identify chemical and intent
Use additional external cause code to identify place (Y92)

T24.60 Corrosion of second degree of **unspecified site** of lower limb, except ankle and foot
- T24.601 Corrosion of second degree of unspecified site of **right** lower limb, except ankle and foot
- T24.602 Corrosion of second degree of unspecified site of **left** lower limb, except ankle and foot
- T24.609 Corrosion of second degree of unspecified site of **unspecified** lower limb, except ankle and foot

T24.61 Corrosion of second degree of **thigh**
- T24.611 Corrosion of second degree of **right** thigh
- T24.612 Corrosion of second degree of **left** thigh
- T24.619 Corrosion of second degree of **unspecified** thigh

- T24.62 Corrosion of second degree of **knee**
  - T24.621 Corrosion of second degree of **right** knee
  - T24.622 Corrosion of second degree of **left** knee
  - T24.629 Corrosion of second degree of **unspecified** knee
- T24.63 Corrosion of second degree of **lower leg**
  - T24.631 Corrosion of second degree of **right** lower leg
  - T24.632 Corrosion of second degree of **left** lower leg
  - T24.639 Corrosion of second degree of **unspecified** lower leg
- T24.69 Corrosion of second degree of **multiple sites** of lower limb, except ankle and foot
  - T24.691 Corrosion of second degree of multiple sites of **right** lower limb, except ankle and foot
  - T24.692 Corrosion of second degree of multiple sites of **left** lower limb, except ankle and foot
  - T24.699 Corrosion of second degree of multiple sites of **unspecified** lower limb, except ankle and foot

T24.7 Corrosion of third degree of lower limb, except ankle and foot

Code first (T51-T65) to identify chemical and intent

Use additional external cause code to identify place (Y92)

- T24.70 Corrosion of third degree of **unspecified site** of lower limb, except ankle and foot
  - T24.701 Corrosion of third degree of unspecified site of **right** lower limb, except ankle and foot
  - T24.702 Corrosion of third degree of unspecified site of **left** lower limb, except ankle and foot
  - T24.709 Corrosion of third degree of unspecified site of **unspecified** lower limb, except ankle and foot
- T24.71 Corrosion of third degree of **thigh**
  - T24.711 Corrosion of third degree of **right** thigh
  - T24.712 Corrosion of third degree of **left** thigh
  - T24.719 Corrosion of third degree of **unspecified** thigh
- T24.72 Corrosion of third degree of **knee**
  - T24.721 Corrosion of third degree of **right** knee
  - T24.722 Corrosion of third degree of **left** knee
  - T24.729 Corrosion of third degree of **unspecified** knee
- T24.73 Corrosion of third degree of **lower leg**
  - T24.731 Corrosion of third degree of **right** lower leg
  - T24.732 Corrosion of third degree of **left** lower leg
  - T24.739 Corrosion of third degree of **unspecified** lower leg
- T24.79 Corrosion of third degree of **multiple sites** of lower limb, except ankle and foot
  - T24.791 Corrosion of third degree of multiple sites of **right** lower limb, except ankle and foot
  - T24.792 Corrosion of third degree of multiple sites of **left** lower limb, except ankle and foot
  - T24.799 Corrosion of third degree of multiple sites of **unspecified** lower limb, except ankle and foot

T25 Burn and corrosion of ankle and foot

The appropriate 7th character is to be added to each code from category T25

A	initial encounter
D	subsequent encounter
S	sequela

T25.0 Burn of unspecified degree of ankle and foot

Use additional external cause code to identify the source, place and intent of the burn (X00-X19, X75-X77, X96-X98, Y92)

- T25.01 Burn of unspecified degree of **ankle**
  - T25.011 Burn of unspecified degree of **right** ankle
  - T25.012 Burn of unspecified degree of **left** ankle
  - T25.019 Burn of unspecified degree of **unspecified** ankle
- T25.02 Burn of unspecified degree of **foot**
  - **Excludes2** burn of unspecified degree of toe(s) (nail) (T25.03-)
  - T25.021 Burn of unspecified degree of **right** foot
  - T25.022 Burn of unspecified degree of **left** foot
  - T25.029 Burn of unspecified degree of unspecified foot
- T25.03 Burn of unspecified degree of **toe(s) (nail)**
  - T25.031 Burn of unspecified degree of **right** toe(s) (nail)
  - T25.032 Burn of unspecified degree of **left** toe(s) (nail)
  - T25.039 Burn of unspecified degree of **unspecified** toe(s) (nail)
- T25.09 Burn of unspecified degree of **multiple sites** of ankle and foot
  - T25.091 Burn of unspecified degree of multiple sites of **right** ankle and foot
  - T25.092 Burn of unspecified degree of multiple sites of **left** ankle and foot
  - T25.099 Burn of unspecified degree of multiple sites of **unspecified** ankle and foot

T25.1 Burn of first degree of ankle and foot

Use additional external cause code to identify the source, place and intent of the burn (X00-X19, X75-X77, X96-X98, Y92)

- T25.11 Burn of first degree of **ankle**
  - T25.111 Burn of first degree of **right** ankle
  - T25.112 Burn of first degree of **left** ankle
  - T25.119 Burn of first degree of **unspecified** ankle
- T25.12 Burn of first degree of **foot**
  - **Excludes2** burn of first degree of toe(s) (nail) (T25.13-)
  - T25.121 Burn of first degree of **right** foot
  - T25.122 Burn of first degree of **left** foot
  - T25.129 Burn of first degree of **unspecified** foot
- T25.13 Burn of first degree of **toe(s) (nail)**
  - T25.131 Burn of first degree of **right** toe(s) (nail)
  - T25.132 Burn of first degree of **left** toe(s) (nail)
  - T25.139 Burn of first degree of **unspecified** toe(s) (nail)

T25.19 Burn of first degree of multiple sites of ankle and foot
- T25.191 Burn of first degree of multiple sites of right ankle and foot
- T25.192 Burn of first degree of multiple sites of left ankle and foot
- T25.199 Burn of first degree of multiple sites of unspecified ankle and foot

T25.2 Burn of second degree of ankle and foot

Use additional external cause code to identify the source, place and intent of the burn (XØØ-X19, X75-X77, X96-X98, Y92)

T25.21 Burn of second degree of ankle
- T25.211 Burn of second degree of right ankle
- T25.212 Burn of second degree of left ankle
- T25.219 Burn of second degree of unspecified ankle

T25.22 Burn of second degree of foot

Excludes2 burn of second degree of toe(s) (nail) (T25.23-)

- T25.221 Burn of second degree of right foot
- T25.222 Burn of second degree of left foot
- T25.229 Burn of second degree of unspecified foot

T25.23 Burn of second degree of toe(s) (nail)
- T25.231 Burn of second degree of right toe(s) (nail)
- T25.232 Burn of second degree of left toe(s) (nail)
- T25.239 Burn of second degree of unspecified toe(s) (nail)

T25.29 Burn of second degree of multiple sites of ankle and foot
- T25.291 Burn of second degree of multiple sites of right ankle and foot
- T25.292 Burn of second degree of multiple sites of left ankle and foot
- T25.299 Burn of second degree of multiple sites of unspecified ankle and foot

T25.3 Burn of third degree of ankle and foot

Use additional external cause code to identify the source, place and intent of the burn (XØØ-X19, X75-X77, X96-X98, Y92)

T25.31 Burn of third degree of ankle
- T25.311 Burn of third degree of right ankle
- T25.312 Burn of third degree of left ankle
- T25.319 Burn of third degree of unspecified ankle

T25.32 Burn of third degree of foot

Excludes2 burn of third degree of toe(s) (nail) (T25.33-)

- T25.321 Burn of third degree of right foot
- T25.322 Burn of third degree of left foot
- T25.329 Burn of third degree of unspecified foot

T25.33 Burn of third degree of toe(s) (nail)
- T25.331 Burn of third degree of right toe(s) (nail)
- T25.332 Burn of third degree of left toe(s) (nail)
- T25.339 Burn of third degree of unspecified toe(s) (nail)

T25.39 Burn of third degree of multiple sites of ankle and foot
- T25.391 Burn of third degree of multiple sites of right ankle and foot
- T25.392 Burn of third degree of multiple sites of left ankle and foot
- T25.399 Burn of third degree of multiple sites of unspecified ankle and foot

T25.4 Corrosion of unspecified degree of ankle and foot

Code first (T51-T65) to identify chemical and intent

Use additional external cause code to identify place (Y92)

T25.41 Corrosion of unspecified degree of ankle
- T25.411 Corrosion of unspecified degree of right ankle
- T25.412 Corrosion of unspecified degree of left ankle
- T25.419 Corrosion of unspecified degree of unspecified ankle

T25.42 Corrosion of unspecified degree of foot

Excludes2 corrosion of unspecified degree of toe(s) (nail) (T25.43-)

- T25.421 Corrosion of unspecified degree of right foot
- T25.422 Corrosion of unspecified degree of left foot
- T25.429 Corrosion of unspecified degree of unspecified foot

T25.43 Corrosion of unspecified degree of toe(s) (nail)
- T25.431 Corrosion of unspecified degree of right toe(s) (nail)
- T25.432 Corrosion of unspecified degree of left toe(s) (nail)
- T25.439 Corrosion of unspecified degree of unspecified toe(s) (nail)

T25.49 Corrosion of unspecified degree of multiple sites of ankle and foot
- T25.491 Corrosion of unspecified degree of multiple sites of right ankle and foot
- T25.492 Corrosion of unspecified degree of multiple sites of left ankle and foot
- T25.499 Corrosion of unspecified degree of multiple sites of unspecified ankle and foot

T25.5 Corrosion of first degree of ankle and foot

Code first (T51-T65) to identify chemical and intent

Use additional external cause code to identify place (Y92)

T25.51 Corrosion of first degree of ankle
- T25.511 Corrosion of first degree of right ankle
- T25.512 Corrosion of first degree of left ankle
- T25.519 Corrosion of first degree of unspecified ankle

T25.52 Corrosion of first degree of foot

Excludes2 corrosion of first degree of toe(s) (nail) (T25.53-)

- T25.521 Corrosion of first degree of right foot
- T25.522 Corrosion of first degree of left foot
- T25.529 Corrosion of first degree of unspecified foot

- T25.53 Corrosion of first degree of **toe(s)** (nail)
  - T25.531 Corrosion of first degree of **right** toe(s) (nail)
  - T25.532 Corrosion of first degree of **left** toe(s) (nail)
  - T25.539 Corrosion of first degree of **unspecified** toe(s) (nail)
- T25.59 Corrosion of first degree of **multiple sites** of ankle and foot
  - T25.591 Corrosion of first degree of multiple sites of **right** ankle and foot
  - T25.592 Corrosion of first degree of multiple sites of **left** ankle and foot
  - T25.599 Corrosion of first degree of multiple sites of **unspecified** ankle and foot

T25.6 Corrosion of **second degree** of ankle and foot

Code first (T51-T65) to identify chemical and intent

Use additional external cause code to identify place (Y92)

- T25.61 Corrosion of second degree of **ankle**
  - T25.611 Corrosion of second degree of **right** ankle
  - T25.612 Corrosion of second degree of **left** ankle
  - T25.619 Corrosion of second degree of **unspecified** ankle
- T25.62 Corrosion of second degree of **foot**

  Excludes2 corrosion of second degree of toe(s) (nail) (T25.63-)

  - T25.621 Corrosion of second degree of **right** foot
  - T25.622 Corrosion of second degree of **left** foot
  - T25.629 Corrosion of second degree of **unspecified** foot
- T25.63 Corrosion of second degree of **toe(s)** (nail)
  - T25.631 Corrosion of second degree of **right** toe(s) (nail)
  - T25.632 Corrosion of second degree of **left** toe(s) (nail)
  - T25.639 Corrosion of second degree of **unspecified** toe(s) (nail)
- T25.69 Corrosion of second degree of **multiple sites** of ankle and foot
  - T25.691 Corrosion of second degree of **right** ankle and foot
  - T25.692 Corrosion of second degree of **left** ankle and foot
  - T25.699 Corrosion of second degree of **unspecified** ankle and foot

T25.7 Corrosion of **third degree** of ankle and foot

Code first (T51-T65) to identify chemical and intent

Use additional external cause code to identify place (Y92)

- T25.71 Corrosion of third degree of **ankle**
  - T25.711 Corrosion of third degree of **right** ankle
  - T25.712 Corrosion of third degree of **left** ankle
  - T25.719 Corrosion of third degree of **unspecified** ankle
- T25.72 Corrosion of third degree of **foot**

  Excludes2 corrosion of third degree of toe(s) (nail) (T25.73-)

  - T25.721 Corrosion of third degree of **right** foot
  - T25.722 Corrosion of third degree of **left** foot
  - T25.729 Corrosion of third degree of **unspecified** foot
- T25.73 Corrosion of third degree of **toe(s)** (nail)
  - T25.731 Corrosion of third degree of **right** toe(s) (nail)
  - T25.732 Corrosion of third degree of **left** toe(s) (nail)
  - T25.739 Corrosion of third degree of **unspecified** toe(s) (nail)
- T25.79 Corrosion of third degree of **multiple sites** of ankle and foot
  - T25.791 Corrosion of third degree of multiple sites of **right** ankle and foot
  - T25.792 Corrosion of third degree of multiple sites of **left** ankle and foot
  - T25.799 Corrosion of third degree of multiple sites of **unspecified** ankle and foot

BURNS AND CORROSIONS CONFINED TO EYE AND INTERNAL ORGANS (T26-T28)

T26 Burn and corrosion confined to eye and adnexa

The appropriate 7th character is to be added to each code from category T26

A	initial encounter
D	subsequent encounter
S	sequela

- T26.0 Burn of **eyelid and periocular area**

  Use additional external cause code to identify the source, place and intent of the burn (X00-X19, X75-X77, X96-X98, Y92)

  - X T26.00 Burn of **unspecified** eyelid and periocular area
  - X T26.01 Burn of **right** eyelid and periocular area
  - X T26.02 Burn of **left** eyelid and periocular area
- T26.1 Burn of **cornea and conjunctival sac**

  Use additional external cause code to identify the source, place and intent of the burn (X00-X19, X75-X77, X96-X98, Y92)

  - X T26.10 Burn of cornea and conjunctival sac, **unspecified** eye
  - X T26.11 Burn of cornea and conjunctival sac, **right** eye
  - X T26.12 Burn of cornea and conjunctival sac, **left** eye
- T26.2 Burn with resulting **rupture and destruction of eyeball**

  Use additional external cause code to identify the source, place and intent of the burn (X00-X19, X75-X77, X96-X98, Y92)

  - X T26.20 Burn with resulting rupture and destruction of **unspecified** eyeball
  - X T26.21 Burn with resulting rupture and destruction of **right** eyeball
  - X T26.22 Burn with resulting rupture and destruction of **left** eyeball
- T26.3 Burns of **other specified parts** of eye and adnexa

  Use additional external cause code to identify the source, place and intent of the burn (X00-X19, X75-X77, X96-X98, Y92)

  - X T26.30 Burns of other specified parts of **unspecified** eye and adnexa
  - X T26.31 Burns of other specified parts of **right** eye and adnexa
  - X T26.32 Burns of other specified parts of **left** eye and adnexa

T26.4 Burn of eye and adnexa, part unspecified

Use additional external cause code to identify the source, place and intent of the burn (XØØ-X19, X75-X77, X96-X98, Y92)

X **T26.4Ø Burn of unspecified eye and adnexa, part unspecified**

X **T26.41 Burn of right eye and adnexa, part unspecified**

X **T26.42 Burn of left eye and adnexa, part unspecified**

T26.5 Corrosion of eyelid and periocular area

Code first (T51-T65) to identify chemical and intent

Use additional external cause code to identify place (Y92)

X **T26.5Ø Corrosion of unspecified eyelid and periocular area**

X **T26.51 Corrosion of right eyelid and periocular area**

X **T26.52 Corrosion of left eyelid and periocular area**

T26.6 Corrosion of cornea and conjunctival sac

Code first (T51-T65) to identify chemical and intent

Use additional external cause code to identify place (Y92)

X **T26.6Ø Corrosion of cornea and conjunctival sac, unspecified eye**

X **T26.61 Corrosion of cornea and conjunctival sac, right eye**

X **T26.62 Corrosion of cornea and conjunctival sac, left eye**

T26.7 Corrosion with resulting rupture and destruction of eyeball

Code first (T51-T65) to identify chemical and intent

Use additional external cause code to identify place (Y92)

X **T26.7Ø Corrosion with resulting rupture and destruction of unspecified eyeball**

X **T26.71 Corrosion with resulting rupture and destruction of right eyeball**

X **T26.72 Corrosion with resulting rupture and destruction of left eyeball**

T26.8 Corrosions of other specified parts of eye and adnexa

Code first (T51-T65) to identify chemical and intent

Use additional external cause code to identify place (Y92)

X **T26.8Ø Corrosions of other specified parts of unspecified eye and adnexa**

X **T26.81 Corrosions of other specified parts of right eye and adnexa**

X **T26.82 Corrosions of other specified parts of left eye and adnexa**

T26.9 Corrosion of eye and adnexa, part unspecified

Code first (T51-T65) to identify chemical and intent

Use additional external cause code to identify place (Y92)

X **T26.9Ø Corrosion of unspecified eye and adnexa, part unspecified**

X **T26.91 Corrosion of right eye and adnexa, part unspecified**

X **T26.92 Corrosion of left eye and adnexa, part unspecified**

T27 Burn and corrosion of respiratory tract

Use additional external cause code to identify the source and intent of the burn (XØØ-X19, X75-X77, X96-X98)

Use additional external cause code to identify place (Y92)

The appropriate 7th character is to be added to each code from category T27

A	initial encounter
D	subsequent encounter
S	sequela

X **T27.Ø Burn of larynx and trachea**

X **T27.1 Burn involving larynx and trachea with lung**

X **T27.2 Burn of other parts of respiratory tract**

Burn of thoracic cavity

X **T27.3 Burn of respiratory tract, part unspecified**

X **T27.4 Corrosion of larynx and trachea**

Code first (T51-T65) to identify chemical and intent

X **T27.5 Corrosion involving larynx and trachea with lung**

▶ *Code first (T51-T65) to identify chemical and intent*

X **T27.6 Corrosion of other parts of respiratory tract**

Code first (T51-T65) to identify chemical and intent

X **T27.7 Corrosion of respiratory tract, part unspecified**

Code first (T51-T65) to identify chemical and intent

T28 Burn and corrosion of other internal organs

Use additional external cause code to identify the source and intent of the burn (XØØ-X19, X75-X77, X96-X98)

Use additional external cause code to identify place (Y92)

The appropriate 7th character is to be added to each code from category T28

A	initial encounter
D	subsequent encounter
S	sequela

X **T28.Ø Burn of mouth and pharynx**

X **T28.1 Burn of esophagus**

X **T28.2 Burn of other parts of alimentary tract**

X **T28.3 Burn of internal genitourinary organs**

X **T28.4 Burns of other and unspecified internal organs**

~~*Code first (T51-T65) to identify chemical and intent*~~

X **T28.4Ø Burn of unspecified internal organ**

T28.41 Burn of ear drum

T28.411 Burn of right ear drum

T28.412 Burn of left ear drum

T28.419 Burn of unspecified ear drum

X **T28.49 Burn of other internal organ**

X **T28.5 Corrosion of mouth and pharynx**

Code first (T51-T65) to identify chemical and intent

X **T28.6 Corrosion of esophagus**

Code first (T51-T65) to identify chemical and intent

X **T28.7 Corrosion of other parts of alimentary tract**

Code first (T51-T65) to identify chemical and intent

X **T28.8 Corrosion of internal genitourinary organs**

Code first (T51-T65) to identify chemical and intent

T28.9 Corrosions of other and unspecified internal organs

Code first (T51-T65) to identify chemical and intent

X **T28.9Ø Corrosions of unspecified internal organs**

T28.91 Corrosions of ear drum

T28.911 Corrosions of right ear drum

T28.912 Corrosions of left ear drum

T28.919 Corrosions of unspecified ear drum

X **T28.99 Corrosions of other internal organs**

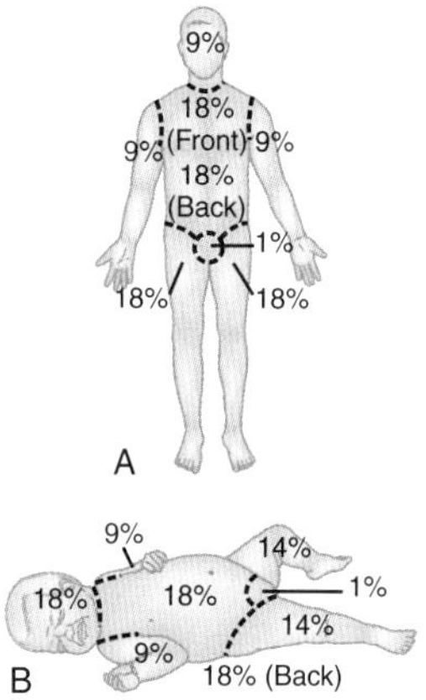

Figure 19-16 Rule of nines: percentages of total body area. (From Marx: Rosen's Emergency Medicine: Concepts and Clinical Practice, ed 6, Mosby, 2006)

OGCR Section I.C.19.d.5.

Assign separate code for each burn site

When coding burns, assign separate codes for each burn site. Category T30, Burn and corrosion, body region unspecified is extremely vague and should rarely be used.

BURNS AND CORROSIONS OF MULTIPLE AND UNSPECIFIED BODY REGIONS (T30-T32)

● **T30** Burn and corrosion, **body region unspecified**

- **T30.0** **Burn of unspecified body region, unspecified degree**
  - This code is not for inpatient use. Code to specified site and degree of burns
  - Burn NOS
  - Multiple burns NOS
- **T30.4** **Corrosion of unspecified body region, unspecified degree**
  - This code is not for inpatient use. Code to specified site and degree of corrosion
  - Corrosion NOS
  - Multiple corrosion NOS

● **T31** **Burns classified according to extent of body surface involved**

Note: This category is to be used as the primary code only when the site of the burn is unspecified. It should be used as a supplementary code with categories T20-T25 when the site is specified.

- **T31.0** Burns involving **less than 10%** of body surface
- ● **T31.1** Burns involving **10-19%** of body surface
  - **T31.10** **Burns involving 10-19% of body surface with 0% to 9% third degree burns**
    - Burns involving 10-19% of body surface NOS
  - **T31.11** **Burns involving 10-19% of body surface with 10-19% third degree burns**
- ● **T31.2** Burns involving **20-29%** of body surface
  - **T31.20** **Burns involving 20-29% of body surface with 0% to 9% third degree burns**
    - Burns involving 20-29% of body surface NOS
  - **T31.21** **Burns involving 20-29% of body surface with 10-19% third degree burns**
  - **T31.22** **Burns involving 20-29% of body surface with 20-29% third degree burns**
- ● **T31.3** Burns involving **30-39%** of body surface
  - **T31.30** **Burns involving 30-39% of body surface with 0% to 9% third degree burns**
    - Burns involving 30-39% of body surface NOS
  - **T31.31** **Burns involving 30-39% of body surface with 10-19% third degree burns**
  - **T31.32** **Burns involving 30-39% of body surface with 20-29% third degree burns**
  - **T31.33** **Burns involving 30-39% of body surface with 30-39% third degree burns**
- ● **T31.4** Burns involving **40-49%** of body surface
  - **T31.40** **Burns involving 40-49% of body surface with 0% to 9% third degree burns**
    - Burns involving 40-49% of body surface NOS
  - **T31.41** **Burns involving 40-49% of body surface with 10-19% third degree burns**
  - **T31.42** **Burns involving 40-49% of body surface with 20-29% third degree burns**
  - **T31.43** **Burns involving 40-49% of body surface with 30-39% third degree burns**
  - **T31.44** **Burns involving 40-49% of body surface with 40-49% third degree burns**
- ● **T31.5** Burns involving **50-59%** of body surface
  - **T31.50** **Burns involving 50-59% of body surface with 0% to 9% third degree burns**
    - Burns involving 50-59% of body surface NOS
  - **T31.51** **Burns involving 50-59% of body surface with 10-19% third degree burns**
  - **T31.52** **Burns involving 50-59% of body surface with 20-29% third degree burns**
  - **T31.53** **Burns involving 50-59% of body surface with 30-39% third degree burns**
  - **T31.54** **Burns involving 50-59% of body surface with 40-49% third degree burns**
  - **T31.55** **Burns involving 50-59% of body surface with 50-59% third degree burns**
- ● **T31.6** Burns involving **60-69%** of body surface
  - **T31.60** **Burns involving 60-69% of body surface with 0% to 9% third degree burns**
    - Burns involving 60-69% of body surface NOS
  - **T31.61** **Burns involving 60-69% of body surface with 10-19% third degree burns**
  - **T31.62** **Burns involving 60-69% of body surface with 20-29% third degree burns**
  - **T31.63** **Burns involving 60-69% of body surface with 30-39% third degree burns**
  - **T31.64** **Burns involving 60-69% of body surface with 40-49% third degree burns**
  - **T31.65** **Burns involving 60-69% of body surface with 50-59% third degree burns**
  - **T31.66** **Burns involving 60-69% of body surface with 60-69% third degree burns**
- ● **T31.7** Burns involving **70-79%** of body surface
  - **T31.70** **Burns involving 70-79% of body surface with 0% to 9% third degree burns**
    - Burns involving 70-79% of body surface NOS
  - **T31.71** **Burns involving 70-79% of body surface with 10-19% third degree burns**
  - **T31.72** **Burns involving 70-79% of body surface with 20-29% third degree burns**
  - **T31.73** **Burns involving 70-79% of body surface with 30-39% third degree burns**
  - **T31.74** **Burns involving 70-79% of body surface with 40-49% third degree burns**
  - **T31.75** **Burns involving 70-79% of body surface with 50-59% third degree burns**
  - **T31.76** **Burns involving 70-79% of body surface with 60-69% third degree burns**
  - **T31.77** **Burns involving 70-79% of body surface with 70-79% third degree burns**
- ● **T31.8** Burns involving **80-89%** of body surface
  - **T31.80** **Burns involving 80-89% of body surface with 0% to 9% third degree burns**
    - Burns involving 80-89% of body surface NOS
  - **T31.81** **Burns involving 80-89% of body surface with 10-19% third degree burns**
  - **T31.82** **Burns involving 80-89% of body surface with 20-29% third degree burns**
  - **T31.83** **Burns involving 80-89% of body surface with 30-39% third degree burns**

T31.84 Burns involving 80-89% of body surface with 40-49% third degree burns
T31.85 Burns involving 80-89% of body surface with 50-59% third degree burns
T31.86 Burns involving 80-89% of body surface with 60-69% third degree burns
T31.87 Burns involving 80-89% of body surface with 70-79% third degree burns
T31.88 Burns involving 80-89% of body surface with 80-89% third degree burns

T31.9 Burns involving 90% or more of body surface
T31.90 Burns involving 90% or more of body surface with 0% to 9% third degree burns
Burns involving 90% or more of body surface NOS
T31.91 Burns involving 90% or more of body surface with 10-19% third degree burns
T31.92 Burns involving 90% or more of body surface with 20-29% third degree burns
T31.93 Burns involving 90% or more of body surface with 30-39% third degree burns
T31.94 Burns involving 90% or more of body surface with 40-49% third degree burns
T31.95 Burns involving 90% or more of body surface with 50-59% third degree burns
T31.96 Burns involving 90% or more of body surface with 60-69% third degree burns
T31.97 Burns involving 90% or more of body surface with 70-79% third degree burns
T31.98 Burns involving 90% or more of body surface with 80-89% third degree burns
T31.99 Burns involving 90% or more of body surface with 90% or more third degree burns

T32 Corrosions classified according to extent of body surface involved

Note: This category is to be used as the primary code only when the site of the corrosion is unspecified. It may be used as a supplementary code with categories T20-T25 when the site is specified.

T32.0 Corrosions involving less than 10% of body surface

T32.1 Corrosions involving 10-19% of body surface
T32.10 Corrosions involving 10-19% of body surface with 0% to 9% third degree corrosion
Corrosions involving 10-19% of body surface NOS
T32.11 Corrosions involving 10-19% of body surface with 10-19% third degree corrosion

T32.2 Corrosions involving 20-29% of body surface
T32.20 Corrosions involving 20-29% of body surface with 0% to 9% third degree corrosion
T32.21 Corrosions involving 20-29% of body surface with 10-19% third degree corrosion
T32.22 Corrosions involving 20-29% of body surface with 20-29% third degree corrosion

T32.3 Corrosions involving 30-39% of body surface
T32.30 Corrosions involving 30-39% of body surface with 0% to 9% third degree corrosion
T32.31 Corrosions involving 30-39% of body surface with 10-19% third degree corrosion
T32.32 Corrosions involving 30-39% of body surface with 20-29% third degree corrosion
T32.33 Corrosions involving 30-39% of body surface with 30-39% third degree corrosion

T32.4 Corrosions involving 40-49% of body surface
T32.40 Corrosions involving 40-49% of body surface with 0% to 9% third degree corrosion
T32.41 Corrosions involving 40-49% of body surface with 10-19% third degree corrosion
T32.42 Corrosions involving 40-49% of body surface with 20-29% third degree corrosion
T32.43 Corrosions involving 40-49% of body surface with 30-39% third degree corrosion
T32.44 Corrosions involving 40-49% of body surface with 40-49% third degree corrosion

T32.5 Corrosions involving 50-59% of body surface
T32.50 Corrosions involving 50-59% of body surface with 0% to 9% third degree corrosion
T32.51 Corrosions involving 50-59% of body surface with 10-19% third degree corrosion
T32.52 Corrosions involving 50-59% of body surface with 20-29% third degree corrosion
T32.53 Corrosions involving 50-59% of body surface with 30-39% third degree corrosion
T32.54 Corrosions involving 50-59% of body surface with 40-49% third degree corrosion
T32.55 Corrosions involving 50-59% of body surface with 50-59% third degree corrosion

T32.6 Corrosions involving 60-69% of body surface
T32.60 Corrosions involving 60-69% of body surface with 0% to 9% third degree corrosion
T32.61 Corrosions involving 60-69% of body surface with 10-19% third degree corrosion
T32.62 Corrosions involving 60-69% of body surface with 20-29% third degree corrosion
T32.63 Corrosions involving 60-69% of body surface with 30-39% third degree corrosion
T32.64 Corrosions involving 60-69% of body surface with 40-49% third degree corrosion
T32.65 Corrosions involving 60-69% of body surface with 50-59% third degree corrosion
T32.66 Corrosions involving 60-69% of body surface with 60-69% third degree corrosion

T32.7 Corrosions involving 70-79% of body surface
T32.70 Corrosions involving 70-79% of body surface with 0% to 9% third degree corrosion
T32.71 Corrosions involving 70-79% of body surface with 10-19% third degree corrosion
T32.72 Corrosions involving 70-79% of body surface with 20-29% third degree corrosion
T32.73 Corrosions involving 70-79% of body surface with 30-39% third degree corrosion
T32.74 Corrosions involving 70-79% of body surface with 40-49% third degree corrosion
T32.75 Corrosions involving 70-79% of body surface with 50-59% third degree corrosion
T32.76 Corrosions involving 70-79% of body surface with 60-69% third degree corrosion
T32.77 Corrosions involving 70-79% of body surface with 70-79% third degree corrosion

T32.8 Corrosions involving 80-89% of body surface
T32.80 Corrosions involving 80-89% of body surface with 0% to 9% third degree corrosion
T32.81 Corrosions involving 80-89% of body surface with 10-19% third degree corrosion
T32.82 Corrosions involving 80-89% of body surface with 20-29% third degree corrosion
T32.83 Corrosions involving 80-89% of body surface with 30-39% third degree corrosion
T32.84 Corrosions involving 80-89% of body surface with 40-49% third degree corrosion
T32.85 Corrosions involving 80-89% of body surface with 50-59% third degree corrosion
T32.86 Corrosions involving 80-89% of body surface with 60-69% third degree corrosion
T32.87 Corrosions involving 80-89% of body surface with 70-79% third degree corrosion
T32.88 Corrosions involving 80-89% of body surface with 80-89% third degree corrosion

- T32.9 Corrosions involving 90% or more of body surface
  - T32.90 Corrosions involving 90% or more of body surface with 0% to 9% third degree corrosion
  - T32.91 Corrosions involving 90% or more of body surface with 10-19% third degree corrosion
  - T32.92 Corrosions involving 90% or more of body surface with 20-29% third degree corrosion
  - T32.93 Corrosions involving 90% or more of body surface with 30-39% third degree corrosion
  - T32.94 Corrosions involving 90% or more of body surface with 40-49% third degree corrosion
  - T32.95 Corrosions involving 90% or more of body surface with 50-59% third degree corrosion
  - T32.96 Corrosions involving 90% or more of body surface with 60-69% third degree corrosion
  - T32.97 Corrosions involving 90% or more of body surface with 70-79% third degree corrosion
  - T32.98 Corrosions involving 90% or more of body surface with 80-89% third degree corrosion
  - T32.99 Corrosions involving 90% or more of body surface with 90% or more third degree corrosion

FROSTBITE (T33-T34)

Excludes2 hypothermia and other effects of reduced temperature (T68, T69.-)

T33 Superficial frostbite

Includes frostbite with partial thickness skin loss

The appropriate 7th character is to be added to each code from category T33

A	initial encounter
D	subsequent encounter
S	sequela

- T33.0 Superficial frostbite of head
  - T33.01 Superficial frostbite of ear
    - T33.011 Superficial frostbite of right ear
    - T33.012 Superficial frostbite of left ear
    - T33.019 Superficial frostbite of unspecified ear
  - X T33.02 Superficial frostbite of nose
  - X T33.09 Superficial frostbite of other part of head
- X T33.1 Superficial frostbite of neck
- X T33.2 Superficial frostbite of thorax
- X T33.3 Superficial frostbite of abdominal wall, lower back and pelvis
- T33.4 Superficial frostbite of arm

  Excludes2 superficial frostbite of wrist and hand (T33.5-)
  - X T33.40 Superficial frostbite of unspecified arm
  - X T33.41 Superficial frostbite of right arm
  - X T33.42 Superficial frostbite of left arm
- T33.5 Superficial frostbite of wrist, hand, and fingers
  - T33.51 Superficial frostbite of wrist
    - T33.511 Superficial frostbite of right wrist
    - T33.512 Superficial frostbite of left wrist
    - T33.519 Superficial frostbite of unspecified wrist
  - T33.52 Superficial frostbite of hand

    Excludes2 superficial frostbite of fingers (T33.53-)
    - T33.521 Superficial frostbite of right hand
    - T33.522 Superficial frostbite of left hand
    - T33.529 Superficial frostbite of unspecified hand
  - T33.53 Superficial frostbite of finger(s)
    - T33.531 Superficial frostbite of right finger(s)
    - T33.532 Superficial frostbite of left finger(s)
    - T33.539 Superficial frostbite of unspecified finger(s)
- T33.6 Superficial frostbite of hip and thigh
  - X T33.60 Superficial frostbite of unspecified hip and thigh
  - X T33.61 Superficial frostbite of right hip and thigh
  - X T33.62 Superficial frostbite of left hip and thigh
- T33.7 Superficial frostbite of knee and lower leg

  Excludes2 superficial frostbite of ankle and foot (T33.8-)
  - X T33.70 Superficial frostbite of unspecified knee and lower leg
  - X T33.71 Superficial frostbite of right knee and lower leg
  - X T33.72 Superficial frostbite of left knee and lower leg
- T33.8 Superficial frostbite of ankle, foot, and toe(s)
  - T33.81 Superficial frostbite of ankle
    - T33.811 Superficial frostbite of right ankle
    - T33.812 Superficial frostbite of left ankle
    - T33.819 Superficial frostbite of unspecified ankle
  - T33.82 Superficial frostbite of foot
    - T33.821 Superficial frostbite of right foot
    - T33.822 Superficial frostbite of left foot
    - T33.829 Superficial frostbite of unspecified foot
  - T33.83 Superficial frostbite of toe(s)
    - T33.831 Superficial frostbite of right toe(s)
    - T33.832 Superficial frostbite of left toe(s)
    - T33.839 Superficial frostbite of unspecified toe(s)
- T33.9 Superficial frostbite of other and unspecified sites
  - X T33.90 Superficial frostbite of unspecified sites
    Superficial frostbite NOS
  - X T33.99 Superficial frostbite of other sites
    Superficial frostbite of leg NOS
    Superficial frostbite of trunk NOS

T34 Frostbite with tissue necrosis

The appropriate 7th character is to be added to each code from category T34

A	initial encounter
D	subsequent encounter
S	sequela

- T34.0 Frostbite with tissue necrosis of head
  - T34.01 Frostbite with tissue necrosis of ear
    - T34.011 Frostbite with tissue necrosis of right ear
    - T34.012 Frostbite with tissue necrosis of left ear
    - T34.019 Frostbite with tissue necrosis of unspecified ear
  - X T34.02 Frostbite with tissue necrosis of nose
  - X T34.09 Frostbite with tissue necrosis of other part of head
- X T34.1 Frostbite with tissue necrosis of neck
- X T34.2 Frostbite with tissue necrosis of thorax
- X T34.3 Frostbite with tissue necrosis of abdominal wall, lower back and pelvis
- T34.4 Frostbite with tissue necrosis of arm

  Excludes2 frostbite with tissue necrosis of wrist and hand (T34.5-)
  - X T34.40 Frostbite with tissue necrosis of unspecified arm
  - X T34.41 Frostbite with tissue necrosis of right arm
  - X T34.42 Frostbite with tissue necrosis of left arm

T34.5 Frostbite with tissue necrosis of wrist, hand, and finger(s)
- **T34.51 Frostbite with tissue necrosis of wrist**
  - **T34.511 Frostbite with tissue necrosis of right wrist**
  - **T34.512 Frostbite with tissue necrosis of left wrist**
  - **T34.519 Frostbite with tissue necrosis of unspecified wrist**
- **T34.52 Frostbite with tissue necrosis of hand**
  - **Excludes2** frostbite with tissue necrosis of finger(s) (T34.53-)
  - **T34.521 Frostbite with tissue necrosis of right hand**
  - **T34.522 Frostbite with tissue necrosis of left hand**
  - **T34.529 Frostbite with tissue necrosis of unspecified hand**
- **T34.53 Frostbite with tissue necrosis of finger(s)**
  - **T34.531 Frostbite with tissue necrosis of right finger(s)**
  - **T34.532 Frostbite with tissue necrosis of left finger(s)**
  - **T34.539 Frostbite with tissue necrosis of unspecified finger(s)**

T34.6 Frostbite with tissue necrosis of hip and thigh
- X **T34.60 Frostbite with tissue necrosis of unspecified hip and thigh**
- X **T34.61 Frostbite with tissue necrosis of right hip and thigh**
- X **T34.62 Frostbite with tissue necrosis of left hip and thigh**

T34.7 Frostbite with tissue necrosis of knee and lower leg
- **Excludes2** frostbite with tissue necrosis of ankle and foot (T34.8-)
- X **T34.70 Frostbite with tissue necrosis of unspecified knee and lower leg**
- X **T34.71 Frostbite with tissue necrosis of right knee and lower leg**
- X **T34.72 Frostbite with tissue necrosis of left knee and lower leg**

T34.8 Frostbite with tissue necrosis of ankle, foot, and toe(s)
- **T34.81 Frostbite with tissue necrosis of ankle**
  - **T34.811 Frostbite with tissue necrosis of right ankle**
  - **T34.812 Frostbite with tissue necrosis of left ankle**
  - **T34.819 Frostbite with tissue necrosis of unspecified ankle**
- **T34.82 Frostbite with tissue necrosis of foot**
  - **T34.821 Frostbite with tissue necrosis of right foot**
  - **T34.822 Frostbite with tissue necrosis of left foot**
  - **T34.829 Frostbite with tissue necrosis of unspecified foot**
- **T34.83 Frostbite with tissue necrosis of toe(s)**
  - **T34.831 Frostbite with tissue necrosis of right toe(s)**
  - **T34.832 Frostbite with tissue necrosis of left toe(s)**
  - **T34.839 Frostbite with tissue necrosis of unspecified toe(s)**

T34.9 Frostbite with tissue necrosis of other and unspecified sites
- X **T34.90 Frostbite with tissue necrosis of unspecified sites**
  - Frostbite with tissue necrosis NOS
- X **T34.99 Frostbite with tissue necrosis of other sites**
  - Frostbite with tissue necrosis of leg NOS
  - Frostbite with tissue necrosis of trunk NOS

OGCR See Section I.C.19.e.

Adverse Effects, Poisoning, Underdosing and Toxic Effects

Codes in categories T36-T65 are combination codes that include the substance that was taken as well as the intent. No additional external cause code is required for poisonings, toxic effects, adverse effects and underdosing codes.

POISONING BY, ADVERSE EFFECTS OF AND UNDERDOSING OF DRUGS MEDICAMENTS AND BIOLOGICAL SUBSTANCES (T36-T5Ø)

Includes adverse effect of correct substance properly administered
poisoning by overdose of substance
poisoning by wrong substance given or taken in error
underdosing by (inadvertently) (deliberately) taking less substance than prescribed or instructed

Code first, for adverse effects, the nature of the adverse effect, such as:
- adverse effect NOS (T88.7)
- aspirin gastritis (K29.-)
- blood disorders (D56-D76)
- contact dermatitis (L23-L25)
- dermatitis due to substances taken internally (L27.-)
- nephropathy (N14.Ø-N14.2)

Note: The drug giving rise to the adverse effect should be identified by use of codes from categories T36-T5Ø with fifth or sixth character 5.

Use additional code(s) to specify:
- manifestations of poisoning
- underdosing or failure in dosage during medical and surgical care (Y63.6, Y63.8-Y63.9)
- underdosing of medication regimen (Z91.12-, Z91.13-)

Excludes1 toxic reaction to local anesthesia in pregnancy (O29.3-)

Excludes2 abuse and dependence of psychoactive substances (F1Ø-F19)
abuse of non-dependence-producing substances (F55.-)
drug reaction and poisoning affecting newborn (PØØ-P96)
pathological drug intoxication (inebriation) (F1Ø-F19)

T36 Poisoning by, adverse effect of and underdosing of systemic antibiotics

Excludes1 antineoplastic antibiotics (T45.1-)
locally applied antibiotic NEC (T49.Ø)
topically used antibiotic for ear, nose and throat (T49.6)
topically used antibiotic for eye (T49.5)

The appropriate 7th character is to be added to each code from category T36

A	initial encounter
D	subsequent encounter
S	sequela

- **T36.Ø Poisoning by, adverse effect of and underdosing of penicillins**
  - **T36.ØX Poisoning by, adverse effect of and underdosing of penicillins**
    - **T36.ØX1 Poisoning by penicillins, accidental (unintentional)**
      - Poisoning by penicillins NOS
    - **T36.ØX2 Poisoning by penicillins, intentional self-harm** A, S
    - **T36.ØX3 Poisoning by penicillins, assault**
    - **T36.ØX4 Poisoning by penicillins, undetermined**
    - **T36.ØX5 Adverse effect of penicillins**
    - **T36.ØX6 Underdosing of penicillins**

CHAPTER 19 (SØØ-T88)

● T36.1 Poisoning by, adverse effect of and underdosing of cephalosporins and other betalactam antibiotics

● T36.1X Poisoning by, adverse effect of and underdosing of **cephalosporins and other beta-lactam antibiotics**

● T36.1X1 Poisoning by cephalosporins and other beta-lactam antibiotics, **accidental** (unintentional)
Poisoning by cephalosporins and other beta-lactam antibiotics NOS

● T36.1X2 Poisoning by cephalosporins and other beta-lactam antibiotics, **intentional** self-harm A, S

● T36.1X3 Poisoning by cephalosporins and other beta-lactam antibiotics, **assault**

● T36.1X4 Poisoning by cephalosporins and other beta-lactam antibiotics, **undetermined**

● T36.1X5 **Adverse effect** of cephalosporins and other beta-lactam antibiotics

● T36.1X6 **Underdosing** of cephalosporins and other beta-lactam antibiotics

● T36.2 Poisoning by, adverse effect of and underdosing of chloramphenicol group

● T36.2X Poisoning by, adverse effect of and underdosing of **chloramphenicol group**

● T36.2X1 Poisoning by chloramphenicol group, **accidental** (unintentional)
Poisoning by chloramphenicol group NOS

● T36.2X2 Poisoning by chloramphenicol group, **intentional** self-harm A, S

● T36.2X3 Poisoning by chloramphenicol group, **assault**

● T36.2X4 Poisoning by chloramphenicol group, **undetermined**

● T36.2X5 **Adverse effect** of chloramphenicol group

● T36.2X6 **Underdosing** of chloramphenicol group

● T36.3 Poisoning by, adverse effect of and underdosing of macrolides

● T36.3X Poisoning by, adverse effect of and underdosing of **macrolides**

● T36.3X1 Poisoning by macrolides, **accidental** (unintentional)
Poisoning by macrolides NOS

● T36.3X2 Poisoning by macrolides, **intentional** self-harm A, S

● T36.3X3 Poisoning by macrolides, **assault**

● T36.3X4 Poisoning by macrolides, **undetermined**

● T36.3X5 **Adverse effect** of macrolides

● T36.3X6 **Underdosing** of macrolides

● T36.4 Poisoning by, adverse effect of and underdosing of tetracyclines

● T36.4X Poisoning by, adverse effect of and underdosing of **tetracyclines**

● T36.4X1 Poisoning by tetracyclines, **accidental** (unintentional)
Poisoning by tetracyclines NOS

● T36.4X2 Poisoning by tetracyclines, **intentional** self-harm A, S

● T36.4X3 Poisoning by tetracyclines, **assault**

● T36.4X4 Poisoning by tetracyclines, **undetermined**

● T36.4X5 **Adverse effect** of tetracyclines

● T36.4X6 **Underdosing** of tetracyclines

● T36.5 Poisoning by, adverse effect of and underdosing of aminoglycosides
Poisoning by, adverse effect of and underdosing of streptomycin

● T36.5X Poisoning by, adverse effect of and underdosing of **aminoglycosides**

● T36.5X1 Poisoning by aminoglycosides, **accidental** (unintentional)
Poisoning by aminoglycosides NOS

● T36.5X2 Poisoning by aminoglycosides, **intentional** self-harm A, S

● T36.5X3 Poisoning by aminoglycosides, **assault**

● T36.5X4 Poisoning by aminoglycosides, **undetermined**

● T36.5X5 **Adverse effect** of aminoglycosides

● T36.5X6 **Underdosing** of aminoglycosides

● T36.6 Poisoning by, adverse effect of and underdosing of rifampicins

● T36.6X Poisoning by, adverse effect of and underdosing of **rifampicins**

● T36.6X1 Poisoning by rifampicins, **accidental** (unintentional)
Poisoning by rifampicins NOS

● T36.6X2 Poisoning by rifampicins, **intentional** self-harm A, S

● T36.6X3 Poisoning by rifampicins, **assault**

● T36.6X4 Poisoning by rifampicins, **undetermined**

● T36.6X5 **Adverse effect** of rifampicins

● T36.6X6 **Underdosing** of rifampicins

● T36.7 Poisoning by, adverse effect of and underdosing of antifungal antibiotics, systemically used

● T36.7X Poisoning by, adverse effect of and underdosing of **antifungal antibiotics, systemically used**

● T36.7X1 Poisoning by antifungal antibiotics, systemically used, **accidental** (unintentional)
Poisoning by antifungal antibiotics, systemically used NOS

● T36.7X2 Poisoning by antifungal antibiotics, systemically used, **intentional** self-harm A, S

● T36.7X3 Poisoning by antifungal antibiotics, systemically used, **assault**

● T36.7X4 Poisoning by antifungal antibiotics, systemically used, **undetermined**

● T36.7X5 **Adverse effect** of antifungal antibiotics, systemically used

● T36.7X6 **Underdosing** of antifungal antibiotics, systemically used

● T36.8 Poisoning by, adverse effect of and underdosing of other systemic antibiotics

● T36.8X Poisoning by, adverse effect of and underdosing of **other systemic antibiotics**

● T36.8X1 Poisoning by other systemic antibiotics, **accidental** (unintentional)
Poisoning by other systemic antibiotics NOS

● T36.8X2 Poisoning by other systemic antibiotics, **intentional** self-harm A, S

● T36.8X3 Poisoning by other systemic antibiotics, **assault**

● T36.8X4 Poisoning by other systemic antibiotics, **undetermined**

● T36.8X5 **Adverse effect** of other systemic antibiotics
Coding Clinic: 2017, Q1, P39

● T36.8X6 **Underdosing** of other systemic antibiotics

T36.9 Poisoning by, adverse effect of and underdosing of **unspecified systemic antibiotic**

X **T36.91** Poisoning by unspecified systemic antibiotic, **accidental** (unintentional)
Poisoning by systemic antibiotic NOS

X **T36.92** Poisoning by unspecified systemic antibiotic, **intentional** self-harm A, S

X **T36.93** Poisoning by unspecified systemic antibiotic, **assault**

X **T36.94** Poisoning by unspecified systemic antibiotic, **undetermined**

X **T36.95** **Adverse effect** of unspecified systemic antibiotic

X **T36.96** **Underdosing** of unspecified systemic antibiotic

T37 Poisoning by, adverse effect of and underdosing of other systemic anti-infectives and antiparasitics

Excludes1 anti-infectives topically used for ear, nose and throat (T49.6-)
anti-infectives topically used for eye (T49.5-)
locally applied anti-infectives NEC (T49.Ø-)

The appropriate 7th character is to be added to each code from category T37

A	initial encounter
D	subsequent encounter
S	sequela

T37.Ø Poisoning by, adverse effect of and underdosing of **sulfonamides**

T37.ØX Poisoning by, adverse effect of and underdosing of **sulfonamides**

T37.ØX1 Poisoning by sulfonamides, **accidental** (unintentional)
Poisoning by sulfonamides NOS

T37.ØX2 Poisoning by sulfonamides, **intentional** self-harm A, S

T37.ØX3 Poisoning by sulfonamides, **assault**

T37.ØX4 Poisoning by sulfonamides, **undetermined**

T37.ØX5 **Adverse effect** of sulfonamides

T37.ØX6 **Underdosing** of sulfonamides

T37.1 Poisoning by, adverse effect of and underdosing of **antimycobacterial drugs**

Excludes1 rifampicins (T36.6-) streptomycin (T36.5-)

T37.1X Poisoning by, adverse effect of and underdosing of **antimycobacterial drugs**

T37.1X1 Poisoning by antimycobacterial drugs, **accidental** (unintentional)
Poisoning by antimycobacterial drugs NOS

T37.1X2 Poisoning by antimycobacterial drugs, **intentional** self-harm A, S

T37.1X3 Poisoning by antimycobacterial drugs, **assault**

T37.1X4 Poisoning by antimycobacterial drugs, **undetermined**

T37.1X5 **Adverse effect** of antimycobacterial drugs

T37.1X6 **Underdosing** of antimycobacterial drugs

T37.2 Poisoning by, adverse effect of and underdosing of **antimalarials and drugs acting on other blood protozoa**

Excludes1 hydroxyquinoline derivatives (T37.8-)

T37.2X Poisoning by, adverse effect of and underdosing of **antimalarials and drugs acting on other blood protozoa**

T37.2X1 Poisoning by antimalarials and drugs acting on other blood protozoa, **accidental** (unintentional)
Poisoning by antimalarials and drugs acting on other blood protozoa NOS

T37.2X2 Poisoning by antimalarials and drugs acting on other blood protozoa, **intentional** self-harm A, S

T37.2X3 Poisoning by antimalarials and drugs acting on other blood protozoa, **assault**

T37.2X4 Poisoning by antimalarials and drugs acting on other blood protozoa, **undetermined**

T37.2X5 **Adverse effect** of antimalarials and drugs acting on other blood protozoa

T37.2X6 **Underdosing** of antimalarials and drugs acting on other blood protozoa

T37.3 Poisoning by, adverse effect of and underdosing of **other antiprotozoal drugs**

T37.3X Poisoning by, adverse effect of and underdosing of **other antiprotozoal drugs**

T37.3X1 Poisoning by other antiprotozoal drugs, **accidental** (unintentional)
Poisoning by other antiprotozoal drugs NOS

T37.3X2 Poisoning by other antiprotozoal drugs, **intentional** self-harm A, S

T37.3X3 Poisoning by other antiprotozoal drugs, **assault**

T37.3X4 Poisoning by other antiprotozoal drugs, **undetermined**

T37.3X5 **Adverse effect** of other antiprotozoal drugs

T37.3X6 **Underdosing** of other antiprotozoal drugs

T37.4 Poisoning by, adverse effect of and underdosing of **anthelminthics**

T37.4X Poisoning by, adverse effect of and underdosing of **anthelminthics**

T37.4X1 Poisoning by anthelminthics, **accidental** (unintentional)
Poisoning by anthelminthics NOS

T37.4X2 Poisoning by anthelminthics, **intentional** self-harm A, S

T37.4X3 Poisoning by anthelminthics, **assault**

T37.4X4 Poisoning by anthelminthics, **undetermined**

T37.4X5 **Adverse effect** of anthelminthics

T37.4X6 **Underdosing** of anthelminthics

T37.5 Poisoning by, adverse effect of and underdosing of antiviral drugs
Excludes1 amantadine (T42.8-)
cytarabine (T45.1-)
T37.5X Poisoning by, adverse effect of and underdosing of antiviral drugs
T37.5X1 Poisoning by antiviral drugs, accidental (unintentional)
Poisoning by antiviral drugs NOS
T37.5X2 Poisoning by antiviral drugs, intentional self-harm A, S
T37.5X3 Poisoning by antiviral drugs, assault
T37.5X4 Poisoning by antiviral drugs, undetermined
T37.5X5 Adverse effect of antiviral drugs
T37.5X6 Underdosing of antiviral drugs
T37.8 Poisoning by, adverse effect of and underdosing of other specified systemic anti-infectives and antiparasitics
Poisoning by, adverse effect of and underdosing of hydroxyquinoline derivatives
Excludes1 antimalarial drugs (T37.2-)
T37.8X Poisoning by, adverse effect of and underdosing of other specified systemic anti-infectives and antiparasitics
T37.8X1 Poisoning by other specified systemic anti-infectives and antiparasitics, accidental (unintentional)
Poisoning by other specified systemic anti-infectives and antiparasitics NOS
T37.8X2 Poisoning by other specified systemic anti-infectives and antiparasitics, intentional self-harm A, S
T37.8X3 Poisoning by other specified systemic anti-infectives and antiparasitics, assault
T37.8X4 Poisoning by other specified systemic anti-infectives and antiparasitics, undetermined
T37.8X5 Adverse effect of other specified systemic anti-infectives and antiparasitics
T37.8X6 Underdosing of other specified systemic anti-infectives and antiparasitics
T37.9 Poisoning by, adverse effect of and underdosing of unspecified systemic anti-infective and antiparasitics
X T37.91 Poisoning by unspecified systemic anti-infective and antiparasitics, accidental (unintentional)
Poisoning by, adverse effect of and underdosing of systemic anti-infective and antiparasitics NOS
X T37.92 Poisoning by unspecified systemic anti-infective and antiparasitics, intentional self-harm A, S
X T37.93 Poisoning by unspecified systemic anti-infective and antiparasitics, assault
X T37.94 Poisoning by unspecified systemic anti-infective and antiparasitics, undetermined
X T37.95 Adverse effect of unspecified systemic anti-infective and antiparasitic
X T37.96 Underdosing of unspecified systemic anti-infectives and antiparasitics

T38 Poisoning by, adverse effect of and underdosing of hormones and their synthetic substitutes and antagonists, not elsewhere classified
Excludes1 mineralocorticoids and their antagonists (T50.0-)
oxytocic hormones (T48.0-)
parathyroid hormones and derivatives (T50.9-)
The appropriate 7th character is to be added to each code from category T38

A	initial encounter
D	subsequent encounter
S	sequela

T38.0 Poisoning by, adverse effect of and underdosing of glucocorticoids and synthetic analogues
Excludes1 glucocorticoids, topically used (T49.-)
T38.0X Poisoning by, adverse effect of and underdosing of glucocorticoids and synthetic analogues
T38.0X1 Poisoning by glucocorticoids and synthetic analogues, accidental (unintentional)
Poisoning by glucocorticoids and synthetic analogues NOS
T38.0X2 Poisoning by glucocorticoids and synthetic analogues, intentional self-harm A, S
T38.0X3 Poisoning by glucocorticoids and synthetic analogues, assault
T38.0X4 Poisoning by glucocorticoids and synthetic analogues, undetermined
T38.0X5 Adverse effect of glucocorticoids and synthetic analogues
T38.0X6 Underdosing of glucocorticoids and synthetic analogues
T38.1 Poisoning by, adverse effect of and underdosing of thyroid hormones and substitutes
T38.1X Poisoning by, adverse effect of and underdosing of thyroid hormones and substitutes
T38.1X1 Poisoning by thyroid hormones and substitutes, accidental (unintentional)
Poisoning by thyroid hormones and substitutes NOS
T38.1X2 Poisoning by thyroid hormones and substitutes, intentional self-harm A, S
T38.1X3 Poisoning by thyroid hormones and substitutes, assault
T38.1X4 Poisoning by thyroid hormones and substitutes, undetermined
T38.1X5 Adverse effect of thyroid hormones and substitutes
T38.1X6 Underdosing of thyroid hormones and substitutes
T38.2 Poisoning by, adverse effect of and underdosing of antithyroid drugs
T38.2X Poisoning by, adverse effect of and underdosing of antithyroid drugs
T38.2X1 Poisoning by antithyroid drugs, accidental (unintentional)
Poisoning by antithyroid drugs NOS
T38.2X2 Poisoning by antithyroid drugs, intentional self-harm A, S
T38.2X3 Poisoning by antithyroid drugs, assault
T38.2X4 Poisoning by antithyroid drugs, undetermined
T38.2X5 Adverse effect of antithyroid drugs
T38.2X6 Underdosing of antithyroid drugs

T38.3 Poisoning by, adverse effect of and underdosing of insulin and oral hypoglycemic [antidiabetic] drugs

T38.3X Poisoning by, adverse effect of and underdosing of insulin and oral hypoglycemic [antidiabetic] drugs

T38.3X1 Poisoning by insulin and oral hypoglycemic [antidiabetic] drugs, accidental (unintentional)
Poisoning by insulin and oral hypoglycemic [antidiabetic] drugs NOS

T38.3X2 Poisoning by insulin and oral hypoglycemic [antidiabetic] drugs, intentional self-harm

T38.3X3 Poisoning by insulin and oral hypoglycemic [antidiabetic] drugs, assault A, S

T38.3X4 Poisoning by insulin and oral hypoglycemic [antidiabetic] drugs, undetermined

T38.3X5 Adverse effect of insulin and oral hypoglycemic [antidiabetic] drugs

T38.3X6 Underdosing of insulin and oral hypoglycemic [antidiabetic] drugs

T38.4 Poisoning by, adverse effect of and underdosing of oral contraceptives
Poisoning by, adverse effect of and underdosing of multiple- and single-ingredient oral contraceptive preparations

T38.4X Poisoning by, adverse effect of and underdosing of oral contraceptives

T38.4X1 Poisoning by oral contraceptives, accidental (unintentional)
Poisoning by oral contraceptives NOS

T38.4X2 Poisoning by oral contraceptives, intentional self-harm A, S

T38.4X3 Poisoning by oral contraceptives, assault

T38.4X4 Poisoning by oral contraceptives, undetermined

T38.4X5 Adverse effect of oral contraceptives

T38.4X6 Underdosing of oral contraceptives

T38.5 Poisoning by, adverse effect of and underdosing of other estrogens and progestogens
Poisoning by, adverse effect of and underdosing of estrogens and progestogens mixtures and substitutes

T38.5X Poisoning by, adverse effect of and underdosing of other estrogens and progestogens

T38.5X1 Poisoning by other estrogens and progestogens, accidental (unintentional)
Poisoning by other estrogens and progestogens NOS

T38.5X2 Poisoning by other estrogens and progestogens, intentional self-harm A, S

T38.5X3 Poisoning by other estrogens and progestogens, assault

T38.5X4 Poisoning by other estrogens and progestogens, undetermined

T38.5X5 Adverse effect of other estrogens and progestogens

T38.5X6 Underdosing of other estrogens and progestogens

T38.6 Poisoning by, adverse effect of and underdosing of antigonadotrophins, antiestrogens, antiandrogens, not elsewhere classified
Poisoning by, adverse effect of and underdosing of tamoxifen

T38.6X Poisoning by, adverse effect of and underdosing of antigonadotrophins, antiestrogens, antiandrogens, not elsewhere classified

T38.6X1 Poisoning by antigonadotrophins, antiestrogens, antiandrogens, not elsewhere classified, accidental (unintentional)
Poisoning by antigonadotrophins, antiestrogens, antiandrogens, not elsewhere classified NOS

T38.6X2 Poisoning by antigonadotrophins, antiestrogens, antiandrogens, not elsewhere classified, intentional self-harm A, S

T38.6X3 Poisoning by antigonadotrophins, antiestrogens, antiandrogens, not elsewhere classified, assault

T38.6X4 Poisoning by antigonadotrophins, antiestrogens, antiandrogens, not elsewhere classified, undetermined

T38.6X5 Adverse effect of antigonadotrophins, antiestrogens, antiandrogens, not elsewhere classified

T38.6X6 Underdosing of antigonadotrophins, antiestrogens, antiandrogens, not elsewhere classified

T38.7 Poisoning by, adverse effect of and underdosing of androgens and anabolic congeners

T38.7X Poisoning by, adverse effect of and underdosing of androgens and anabolic congeners

T38.7X1 Poisoning by androgens and anabolic congeners, accidental (unintentional)
Poisoning by androgens and anabolic congeners NOS

T38.7X2 Poisoning by androgens and anabolic congeners, intentional self-harm A, S

T38.7X3 Poisoning by androgens and anabolic congeners, assault

T38.7X4 Poisoning by androgens and anabolic congeners, undetermined

T38.7X5 Adverse effect of androgens and anabolic congeners

T38.7X6 Underdosing of androgens and anabolic congeners

T38.8 Poisoning by, adverse effect of and underdosing of other and unspecified hormones and synthetic substitutes

T38.80 Poisoning by, adverse effect of and underdosing of unspecified hormones and synthetic substitutes

T38.801 Poisoning by unspecified hormones and synthetic substitutes, accidental (unintentional)
Poisoning by unspecified hormones and synthetic substitutes NOS

T38.802 Poisoning by unspecified hormones and synthetic substitutes, intentional self-harm A, S

T38.803 Poisoning by unspecified hormones and synthetic substitutes, assault

T38.804 Poisoning by unspecified hormones and synthetic substitutes, undetermined

T38.805 Adverse effect of unspecified hormones and synthetic substitutes

T38.806 Underdosing of unspecified hormones and synthetic substitutes

● T38.81 Poisoning by, adverse effect of and underdosing of anterior pituitary [adenohypophyseal] hormones
- ● T38.811 Poisoning by anterior pituitary [adenohypophyseal] hormones, accidental (unintentional)
  - Poisoning by anterior pituitary [adenohypophyseal] hormones NOS
- ● T38.812 Poisoning by anterior pituitary [adenohypophyseal] hormones, intentional self-harm A, S HCC
- ● T38.813 Poisoning by anterior pituitary [adenohypophyseal] hormones, assault
- ● T38.814 Poisoning by anterior pituitary [adenohypophyseal] hormones, undetermined
- ● T38.815 Adverse effect of anterior pituitary [adenohypophyseal] hormones
- ● T38.816 Underdosing of anterior pituitary [adenohypophyseal] hormones

● T38.89 Poisoning by, adverse effect of and underdosing of other hormones and synthetic substitutes
- ● T38.891 Poisoning by other hormones and synthetic substitutes, accidental (unintentional)
  - Poisoning by other hormones and synthetic substitutes NOS
- ● T38.892 Poisoning by other hormones and synthetic substitutes, intentional self-harm A, S HCC
- ● T38.893 Poisoning by other hormones and synthetic substitutes, assault
- ● T38.894 Poisoning by other hormones and synthetic substitutes, undetermined
- ● T38.895 Adverse effect of other hormones and synthetic substitutes
- ● T38.896 Underdosing of other hormones and synthetic substitutes

● T38.9 Poisoning by, adverse effect of and underdosing of other and unspecified hormone antagonists

● T38.90 Poisoning by, adverse effect of and underdosing of unspecified hormone antagonists
- ● T38.901 Poisoning by unspecified hormone antagonists, accidental (unintentional)
  - Poisoning by unspecified hormone antagonists NOS
- ● T38.902 Poisoning by unspecified hormone antagonists, intentional self-harm A, S HCC
- ● T38.903 Poisoning by unspecified hormone antagonists, assault
- ● T38.904 Poisoning by unspecified hormone antagonists, undetermined
- ● T38.905 Adverse effect of unspecified hormone antagonists
- ● T38.906 Underdosing of unspecified hormone antagonists

● T38.99 Poisoning by, adverse effect of and underdosing of other hormone antagonists
- ● T38.991 Poisoning by other hormone antagonists, accidental (unintentional)
  - Poisoning by other hormone antagonists NOS
- ● T38.992 Poisoning by other hormone antagonists, intentional self-harm A, S HCC
- ● T38.993 Poisoning by other hormone antagonists, assault
- ● T38.994 Poisoning by other hormone antagonists, undetermined
- ● T38.995 Adverse effect of other hormone antagonists
- ● T38.996 Underdosing of other hormone antagonists

● T39 Poisoning by, adverse effect of and underdosing of nonopioid analgesics, antipyretics and antirheumatics

The appropriate 7th character is to be added to each code from category T39

A	initial encounter
D	subsequent encounter
S	sequela

● T39.0 Poisoning by, adverse effect of and underdosing of salicylates

● T39.01 Poisoning by, adverse effect of and underdosing of aspirin
- Poisoning by, adverse effect of and underdosing of acetylsalicylic acid
- ● T39.011 Poisoning by aspirin, accidental (unintentional)
- ● T39.012 Poisoning by aspirin, intentional self-harm A, S HCC
- ● T39.013 Poisoning by aspirin, assault
- ● T39.014 Poisoning by aspirin, undetermined
- ● T39.015 Adverse effect of aspirin
  - Coding Clinic: 2016, Q1, P15
- ● T39.016 Underdosing of aspirin

● T39.09 Poisoning by, adverse effect of and underdosing of other salicylates
- ● T39.091 Poisoning by salicylates, accidental (unintentional)
  - Poisoning by salicylates NOS
- ● T39.092 Poisoning by salicylates, intentional self-harm A, S HCC
- ● T39.093 Poisoning by salicylates, assault
- ● T39.094 Poisoning by salicylates, undetermined
- ● T39.095 Adverse effect of salicylates
- ● T39.096 Underdosing of salicylates

● T39.1 Poisoning by, adverse effect of and underdosing of 4-Aminophenol derivatives

● T39.1X Poisoning by, adverse effect of and underdosing of 4-Aminophenol derivatives
- ● T39.1X1 Poisoning by 4-Aminophenol derivatives, accidental (unintentional)
  - Poisoning by 4-Aminophenol derivatives NOS
- ● T39.1X2 Poisoning by 4-Aminophenol derivatives, intentional self-harm A, S HCC
- ● T39.1X3 Poisoning by 4-Aminophenol derivatives, assault
- ● T39.1X4 Poisoning by 4-Aminophenol derivatives, undetermined
- ● T39.1X5 Adverse effect of 4-Aminophenol derivatives
- ● T39.1X6 Underdosing of 4-Aminophenol derivatives

T39.2 Poisoning by, adverse effect of and underdosing of pyrazolone derivatives

T39.2X Poisoning by, adverse effect of and underdosing of **pyrazolone derivatives**

T39.2X1 **Poisoning by pyrazolone derivatives, accidental (unintentional)**
Poisoning by pyrazolone derivatives NOS

T39.2X2 **Poisoning by pyrazolone derivatives, intentional self-harm** A, S

T39.2X3 **Poisoning by pyrazolone derivatives, assault**

T39.2X4 **Poisoning by pyrazolone derivatives, undetermined**

T39.2X5 **Adverse effect of pyrazolone derivatives**

T39.2X6 **Underdosing of pyrazolone derivatives**

T39.3 Poisoning by, adverse effect of and underdosing of other nonsteroidal anti-inflammatory drugs [NSAID]

T39.31 Poisoning by, adverse effect of and underdosing of **propionic acid derivatives**
Poisoning by, adverse effect of and underdosing of fenoprofen
Poisoning by, adverse effect of and underdosing of flurbiprofen
Poisoning by, adverse effect of and underdosing of ibuprofen
Poisoning by, adverse effect of and underdosing of ketoprofen
Poisoning by, adverse effect of and underdosing of naproxen
Poisoning by, adverse effect of and underdosing of oxaprozin

T39.311 **Poisoning by propionic acid derivatives, accidental (unintentional)**

T39.312 **Poisoning by propionic acid derivatives, intentional self-harm** A, S

T39.313 **Poisoning by propionic acid derivatives, assault**

T39.314 **Poisoning by propionic acid derivatives, undetermined**

T39.315 **Adverse effect of propionic acid derivatives**

T39.316 **Underdosing of propionic acid derivatives**

T39.39 Poisoning by, adverse effect of and underdosing of **other nonsteroidal anti-inflammatory drugs [NSAID]**

T39.391 **Poisoning by other nonsteroidal anti-inflammatory drugs [NSAID], accidental (unintentional)**
Poisoning by other nonsteroidal anti-inflammatory drugs NOS

T39.392 **Poisoning by other nonsteroidal anti-inflammatory drugs [NSAID], intentional self-harm** A, S

T39.393 **Poisoning by other nonsteroidal anti-inflammatory drugs [NSAID], assault**

T39.394 **Poisoning by other nonsteroidal anti-inflammatory drugs [NSAID], undetermined**

T39.395 **Adverse effect of other nonsteroidal anti-inflammatory drugs [NSAID]**

T39.396 **Underdosing of other nonsteroidal anti-inflammatory drugs [NSAID]**

T39.4 Poisoning by, adverse effect of and underdosing of antirheumatics, not elsewhere classified

Excludes1 poisoning by, adverse effect of and underdosing of glucocorticoids (T38.0-)
poisoning by, adverse effect of and underdosing of salicylates (T39.0-)

T39.4X Poisoning by, adverse effect of and underdosing of **antirheumatics, not elsewhere classified**

T39.4X1 **Poisoning by antirheumatics, not elsewhere classified, accidental (unintentional)**
Poisoning by antirheumatics, not elsewhere classified NOS

T39.4X2 **Poisoning by antirheumatics, not elsewhere classified, intentional self-harm** A, S

T39.4X3 **Poisoning by antirheumatics, not elsewhere classified, assault**

T39.4X4 **Poisoning by antirheumatics, not elsewhere classified, undetermined**

T39.4X5 **Adverse effect of antirheumatics, not elsewhere classified**

T39.4X6 **Underdosing of antirheumatics, not elsewhere classified**

T39.8 Poisoning by, adverse effect of and underdosing of other nonopioid analgesics and antipyretics, not elsewhere classified

T39.8X Poisoning by, adverse effect of and underdosing of **other nonopioid analgesics and antipyretics, not elsewhere classified**

T39.8X1 **Poisoning by other nonopioid analgesics and antipyretics, not elsewhere classified, accidental (unintentional)**
Poisoning by other nonopioid analgesics and antipyretics, not elsewhere classified NOS

T39.8X2 **Poisoning by other nonopioid analgesics and antipyretics, not elsewhere classified, intentional self-harm** A, S

T39.8X3 **Poisoning by other nonopioid analgesics and antipyretics, not elsewhere classified, assault**

T39.8X4 **Poisoning by other nonopioid analgesics and antipyretics, not elsewhere classified, undetermined**

T39.8X5 **Adverse effect of other nonopioid analgesics and antipyretics, not elsewhere classified**

T39.8X6 **Underdosing of other nonopioid analgesics and antipyretics, not elsewhere classified**

T39.9 Poisoning by, adverse effect of and underdosing of **unspecified** nonopioid analgesic, antipyretic and antirheumatic

X T39.91 **Poisoning by unspecified nonopioid analgesic, antipyretic and antirheumatic, accidental (unintentional)**
Poisoning by nonopioid analgesic, antipyretic and antirheumatic NOS

X T39.92 **Poisoning by unspecified nonopioid analgesic, antipyretic and antirheumatic, intentional self-harm** A, S

X T39.93 **Poisoning by unspecified nonopioid analgesic, antipyretic and antirheumatic, assault**

X T39.94 **Poisoning by unspecified nonopioid analgesic, antipyretic and antirheumatic, undetermined**

X T39.95 **Adverse effect of unspecified nonopioid analgesic, antipyretic and antirheumatic**

X T39.96 **Underdosing of unspecified nonopioid analgesic, antipyretic and antirheumatic**

T40 Poisoning by, adverse effect of and underdosing of narcotics and psychodysleptics [hallucinogens]

Excludes2 drug dependence and related mental and behavioral disorders due to psychoactive substance use (F10.-F19.-)

The appropriate 7th character is to be added to each code from category T40

A	initial encounter
D	subsequent encounter
S	sequela

T40.0 Poisoning by, adverse effect of and underdosing of opium
T40.0X Poisoning by, adverse effect of and underdosing of **opium**
T40.0X1 Poisoning by opium, **accidental** (unintentional)
Poisoning by opium NOS
T40.0X2 Poisoning by opium, **intentional** self-harm A, S
T40.0X3 Poisoning by opium, **assault**
T40.0X4 Poisoning by opium, **undetermined**
T40.0X5 **Adverse effect** of opium
T40.0X6 **Underdosing** of opium
T40.1 Poisoning by and adverse effect of heroin
T40.1X Poisoning by and adverse effect of **heroin**
T40.1X1 Poisoning by heroin, **accidental** (unintentional)
Poisoning by heroin NOS
T40.1X2 Poisoning by heroin, **intentional** self-harm A, S
T40.1X3 Poisoning by heroin, **assault**
T40.1X4 Poisoning by heroin, **undetermined**
T40.2 Poisoning by, adverse effect of and underdosing of other opioids
T40.2X Poisoning by, adverse effect of and underdosing of **other opioids**
T40.2X1 Poisoning by other opioids, **accidental** (unintentional)
Poisoning by other opioids NOS
T40.2X2 Poisoning by other opioids, **intentional** self-harm A, S
T40.2X3 Poisoning by other opioids, **assault**
T40.2X4 Poisoning by other opioids, **undetermined**
T40.2X5 **Adverse effect** of other opioids
T40.2X6 **Underdosing** of other opioids
T40.3 Poisoning by, adverse effect of and underdosing of methadone
T40.3X Poisoning by, adverse effect of and underdosing of **methadone**
T40.3X1 Poisoning by methadone, **accidental** (unintentional)
Poisoning by methadone NOS
T40.3X2 Poisoning by methadone, **intentional** self-harm A, S
T40.3X3 Poisoning by methadone, **assault**
T40.3X4 Poisoning by methadone, **undetermined**
T40.3X5 **Adverse effect** of methadone
T40.3X6 **Underdosing** of methadone
T40.4 Poisoning by, adverse effect of and underdosing of other synthetic narcotics
T40.4X Poisoning by, adverse effect of and underdosing of **other synthetic narcotics**
T40.4X1 Poisoning by other synthetic narcotics, **accidental** (unintentional)
Poisoning by other synthetic narcotics NOS
T40.4X2 Poisoning by other synthetic narcotics, **intentional** self-harm A, S
T40.4X3 Poisoning by other synthetic narcotics, **assault**
T40.4X4 Poisoning by other synthetic narcotics, **undetermined**
T40.4X5 **Adverse effect** of other synthetic narcotics
T40.4X6 **Underdosing** of other synthetic narcotics
T40.5 Poisoning by, adverse effect of and underdosing of cocaine
T40.5X Poisoning by, adverse effect of and underdosing of **cocaine**
T40.5X1 Poisoning by cocaine, **accidental** (unintentional)
Poisoning by cocaine NOS
Coding Clinic: 2016, Q2, P9
T40.5X2 Poisoning by cocaine, **intentional** self-harm A, S
T40.5X3 Poisoning by cocaine, **assault**
T40.5X4 Poisoning by cocaine, **undetermined**
T40.5X5 **Adverse effect** of cocaine
T40.5X6 **Underdosing** of cocaine
T40.6 Poisoning by, adverse effect of and underdosing of other and unspecified narcotics
T40.60 Poisoning by, adverse effect of and underdosing of **unspecified narcotics**
T40.601 Poisoning by unspecified narcotics, **accidental** (unintentional)
Poisoning by narcotics NOS
T40.602 Poisoning by unspecified narcotics, **intentional** self-harm A, S
T40.603 Poisoning by unspecified narcotics, **assault**
T40.604 Poisoning by unspecified narcotics, **undetermined**
T40.605 **Adverse effect** of unspecified narcotics
T40.606 **Underdosing** of unspecified narcotics
T40.69 Poisoning by, adverse effect of and underdosing of **other narcotics**
T40.691 Poisoning by other narcotics, **accidental** (unintentional)
Poisoning by other narcotics NOS
T40.692 Poisoning by other narcotics, **intentional** self-harm A, S
T40.693 Poisoning by other narcotics, **assault**
T40.694 Poisoning by other narcotics, **undetermined**
T40.695 **Adverse effect** of other narcotics
T40.696 **Underdosing** of other narcotics

- T40.7 Poisoning by, adverse effect of and underdosing of cannabis (derivatives)
  - T40.7X Poisoning by, adverse effect of and underdosing of **cannabis** (derivatives)
    - T40.7X1 Poisoning by cannabis (derivatives), **accidental** (unintentional)
      Poisoning by cannabis NOS
    - T40.7X2 Poisoning by cannabis (derivatives), **intentional** self-harm A, S
    - T40.7X3 Poisoning by cannabis (derivatives), **assault**
    - T40.7X4 Poisoning by cannabis (derivatives), **undetermined**
    - T40.7X5 **Adverse effect** of cannabis (derivatives)
    - T40.7X6 **Underdosing** of cannabis (derivatives)
- T40.8 Poisoning by and adverse effect of lysergide [LSD]
  - T40.8X Poisoning by and adverse effect of **lysergide** [LSD]
    - T40.8X1 Poisoning by lysergide [LSD], **accidental** (unintentional)
      Poisoning by lysergide [LSD] NOS
    - T40.8X2 Poisoning by lysergide [LSD], **intentional** self-harm A, S
    - T40.8X3 Poisoning by lysergide [LSD], **assault**
    - T40.8X4 Poisoning by lysergide [LSD], **undetermined**
- T40.9 Poisoning by, adverse effect of and underdosing of other and unspecified psychodysleptics [hallucinogens]
  - T40.90 Poisoning by, adverse effect of and underdosing of **unspecified psychodysleptics** [hallucinogens]
    - T40.901 Poisoning by unspecified psychodysleptics [hallucinogens], **accidental** (unintentional)
    - T40.902 Poisoning by unspecified psychodysleptics [hallucinogens], **intentional** self-harm A, S
    - T40.903 Poisoning by unspecified psychodysleptics [hallucinogens], **assault**
    - T40.904 Poisoning by unspecified psychodysleptics [hallucinogens], **undetermined**
    - T40.905 **Adverse effect** of unspecified psychodysleptics [hallucinogens]
    - T40.906 **Underdosing** of unspecified psychodysleptics [hallucinogens]
  - T40.99 Poisoning by, adverse effect of and underdosing of **other psychodysleptics** [hallucinogens]
    - T40.991 Poisoning by other psychodysleptics [hallucinogens], **accidental** (unintentional)
      Poisoning by other psychodysleptics [hallucinogens] NOS
    - T40.992 Poisoning by other psychodysleptics [hallucinogens], **intentional** self-harm A, S
    - T40.993 Poisoning by other psychodysleptics [hallucinogens], **assault**
    - T40.994 Poisoning by other psychodysleptics [hallucinogens], **undetermined**
    - T40.995 **Adverse effect** of other psychodysleptics [hallucinogens]
    - T40.996 **Underdosing** of other psychodysleptics [hallucinogens]

- T41 Poisoning by, adverse effect of and underdosing of anesthetics and therapeutic gases

  Excludes1 benzodiazepines (T42.4-)
  cocaine (T40.5-)
  complications of anesthesia during pregnancy (O29.-)
  complications of anesthesia during labor and delivery (O74.-)
  complications of anesthesia during the puerperium (O89.-) opioids (T40.0-T40.2-)

  The appropriate 7th character is to be added to each code from category T41

A	initial encounter
D	subsequent encounter
S	sequela

- T41.0 Poisoning by, adverse effect of and underdosing of inhaled anesthetics
  Excludes1 oxygen (T41.5-)
  - T41.0X Poisoning by, adverse effect of and underdosing of **inhaled anesthetics**
    - T41.0X1 Poisoning by inhaled anesthetics, **accidental** (unintentional)
      Poisoning by inhaled anesthetics NOS
    - T41.0X2 Poisoning by inhaled anesthetics, **intentional** self-harm A, S
    - T41.0X3 Poisoning by inhaled anesthetics, **assault**
    - T41.0X4 **Poisoning** by inhaled anesthetics, undetermined
    - T41.0X5 **Adverse effect** of inhaled anesthetics
    - T41.0X6 **Underdosing** of inhaled anesthetics
- T41.1 Poisoning by, adverse effect of and underdosing of intravenous anesthetics
  Poisoning by, adverse effect of and underdosing of thiobarbiturates
  - T41.1X Poisoning by, adverse effect of and underdosing of **intravenous anesthetics**
    - T41.1X1 Poisoning by intravenous anesthetics, **accidental** (unintentional)
      Poisoning by intravenous anesthetics NOS
    - T41.1X2 Poisoning by intravenous anesthetics, **intentional** self-harm A, S
    - T41.1X3 Poisoning by intravenous anesthetics, **assault**
    - T41.1X4 Poisoning by intravenous anesthetics, **undetermined**
    - T41.1X5 **Adverse effect** of intravenous anesthetics
    - T41.1X6 **Underdosing** of intravenous anesthetics
- T41.2 Poisoning by, adverse effect of and underdosing of other and unspecified general anesthetics
  - T41.20 Poisoning by, adverse effect of and underdosing of **unspecified general anesthetics**
    - T41.201 Poisoning by unspecified general anesthetics, **accidental** (unintentional)
      Poisoning by general anesthetics NOS
    - T41.202 Poisoning by unspecified general anesthetics, **intentional** self-harm A, S
    - T41.203 Poisoning by unspecified general anesthetics, **assault**
    - T41.204 Poisoning by unspecified general anesthetics, **undetermined**
    - T41.205 **Adverse effect** of unspecified general anesthetics
      Coding Clinic: 2016, Q4, P73
    - T41.206 **Underdosing** of unspecified general anesthetics

T41.29 **Poisoning by, adverse effect of and underdosing of other general anesthetics**
- T41.291 **Poisoning by other general anesthetics, accidental (unintentional)**
  Poisoning by other general anesthetics NOS
- T41.292 **Poisoning by other general anesthetics, intentional self-harm** A, S
- T41.293 **Poisoning by other general anesthetics, assault**
- T41.294 **Poisoning by other general anesthetics, undetermined**
- T41.295 **Adverse effect of other general anesthetics**
- T41.296 **Underdosing of other general anesthetics**

T41.3 **Poisoning by, adverse effect of and underdosing of local anesthetics**
Cocaine (topical)
Excludes2 poisoning by cocaine used as a central nervous system stimulant (T40.5X1-T40.5X4)

T41.3X **Poisoning by, adverse effect of and underdosing of local anesthetics**
- T41.3X1 **Poisoning by local anesthetics, accidental (unintentional)**
  Poisoning by local anesthetics NOS
- T41.3X2 **Poisoning by local anesthetics, intentional self-harm** A, S
- T41.3X3 **Poisoning by local anesthetics, assault**
- T41.3X4 **Poisoning by local anesthetics, undetermined**
- T41.3X5 **Adverse effect of local anesthetics**
- T41.3X6 **Underdosing of local anesthetics**

T41.4 **Poisoning by, adverse effect of and underdosing of unspecified anesthetic**
- X T41.41 **Poisoning by unspecified anesthetic, accidental (unintentional)**
  Poisoning by anesthetic NOS
- X T41.42 **Poisoning by unspecified anesthetic, intentional self-harm** A, S
- X T41.43 **Poisoning by unspecified anesthetic, assault**
- X T41.44 **Poisoning by unspecified anesthetic, undetermined**
- X T41.45 **Adverse effect of unspecified anesthetic**
- X T41.46 **Underdosing of unspecified anesthetics**

T41.5 **Poisoning by, adverse effect of and underdosing of therapeutic gases**

T41.5X **Poisoning by, adverse effect of and underdosing of therapeutic gases**
- T41.5X1 **Poisoning by therapeutic gases, accidental (unintentional)**
  Poisoning by therapeutic gases NOS
- T41.5X2 **Poisoning by therapeutic gases, intentional self-harm** A, S
- T41.5X3 **Poisoning by therapeutic gases, assault**
- T41.5X4 **Poisoning by therapeutic gases, undetermined**
- T41.5X5 **Adverse effect of therapeutic gases**
- T41.5X6 **Underdosing of therapeutic gases**

T42 **Poisoning by, adverse effect of and underdosing of antiepileptic, sedative-hypnotic and antiparkinsonism drugs**
Excludes2 drug dependence and related mental and behavioral disorders due to psychoactive substance use (F10.--F19.-)

The appropriate 7th character is to be added to each code from category T42

A	initial encounter
D	subsequent encounter
S	sequela

T42.0 **Poisoning by, adverse effect of and underdosing of hydantoin derivatives**

T42.0X **Poisoning by, adverse effect of and underdosing of hydantoin derivatives**
- T42.0X1 **Poisoning by hydantoin derivatives, accidental (unintentional)**
  Poisoning by hydantoin derivatives NOS
- T42.0X2 **Poisoning by hydantoin derivatives, intentional self-harm** A, S
- T42.0X3 **Poisoning by hydantoin derivatives, assault**
- T42.0X4 **Poisoning by hydantoin derivatives, undetermined**
- T42.0X5 **Adverse effect of hydantoin derivatives**
- T42.0X6 **Underdosing of hydantoin derivatives**

T42.1 **Poisoning by, adverse effect of and underdosing of iminostilbenes**
Poisoning by, adverse effect of and underdosing of carbamazepine

T42.1X **Poisoning by, adverse effect of and underdosing of iminostilbenes**
- T42.1X1 **Poisoning by iminostilbenes, accidental (unintentional)**
  Poisoning by iminostilbenes NOS
- T42.1X2 **Poisoning by iminostilbenes, intentional self-harm** A, S
- T42.1X3 **Poisoning by iminostilbenes, assault**
- T42.1X4 **Poisoning by iminostilbenes, undetermined**
- T42.1X5 **Adverse effect of iminostilbenes**
- T42.1X6 **Underdosing of iminostilbenes**

T42.2 **Poisoning by, adverse effect of and underdosing of succinimides and oxazolidinediones**

T42.2X **Poisoning by, adverse effect of and underdosing of succinimides and oxazolidinediones**
- T42.2X1 **Poisoning by succinimides and oxazolidinediones, accidental (unintentional)**
  Poisoning by succinimides and oxazolidinediones NOS
- T42.2X2 **Poisoning by succinimides and oxazolidinediones, intentional self-harm** A, S
- T42.2X3 **Poisoning by succinimides and oxazolidinediones, assault**
- T42.2X4 **Poisoning by succinimides and oxazolidinediones, undetermined**
- T42.2X5 **Adverse effect of succinimides and oxazolidinediones**
- T42.2X6 **Underdosing of succinimides and oxazolidinediones**

T42.3 Poisoning by, adverse effect of and underdosing of barbiturates

Excludes1 poisoning by, adverse effect of and underdosing of thiobarbiturates (T41.1-)

T42.3X Poisoning by, adverse effect of and underdosing of barbiturates

T42.3X1 Poisoning by barbiturates, accidental (unintentional)
Poisoning by barbiturates NOS

T42.3X2 Poisoning by barbiturates, intentional self-harm A, S

T42.3X3 Poisoning by barbiturates, assault

T42.3X4 Poisoning by barbiturates, undetermined

T42.3X5 Adverse effect of barbiturates

T42.3X6 Underdosing of barbiturates

T42.4 Poisoning by, adverse effect of and underdosing of benzodiazepines

T42.4X Poisoning by, adverse effect of and underdosing of benzodiazepines

T42.4X1 Poisoning by benzodiazepines, accidental (unintentional)
Poisoning by benzodiazepines NOS

T42.4X2 Poisoning by benzodiazepines, intentional self-harm A, S

T42.4X3 Poisoning by benzodiazepines, assault

T42.4X4 Poisoning by benzodiazepines, undetermined

T42.4X5 Adverse effect of benzodiazepines

T42.4X6 Underdosing of benzodiazepines

T42.5 Poisoning by, adverse effect of and underdosing of mixed antiepileptics

T42.5X Poisoning by, adverse effect of and underdosing of antiepileptics

T42.5X1 Poisoning by mixed antiepileptics, accidental (unintentional)
Poisoning by mixed antiepileptics NOS

T42.5X2 Poisoning by mixed antiepileptics, intentional self-harm A, S

T42.5X3 Poisoning by mixed antiepileptics, assault

T42.5X4 Poisoning by mixed antiepileptics, undetermined

T42.5X5 Adverse effect of mixed antiepileptics

T42.5X6 Underdosing of mixed antiepileptics

T42.6 Poisoning by, adverse effect of and underdosing of other antiepileptic and sedative-hypnotic drugs
Poisoning by, adverse effect of and underdosing of methaqualone
Poisoning by, adverse effect of and underdosing of valproic acid

Excludes1 poisoning by, adverse effect of and underdosing of carbamazepine (T42.1-)

T42.6X Poisoning by, adverse effect of and underdosing of other antiepileptic and sedative-hypnotic drugs

T42.6X1 Poisoning by other antiepileptic and sedative-hypnotic drugs, accidental (unintentional)
Poisoning by other antiepileptic and sedative-hypnotic drugs NOS

T42.6X2 Poisoning by other antiepileptic and sedative-hypnotic drugs, intentional self-harm A, S

T42.6X3 Poisoning by other antiepileptic and sedative-hypnotic drugs, assault

T42.6X4 Poisoning by other antiepileptic and sedative-hypnotic drugs, undetermined

T42.6X5 Adverse effect of other antiepileptic and sedative-hypnotic drugs

T42.6X6 Underdosing of other antiepileptic and sedative-hypnotic drugs

T42.7 Poisoning by, adverse effect of and underdosing of unspecified antiepileptic and sedative-hypnotic drugs

X **T42.71 Poisoning by unspecified antiepileptic and sedative-hypnotic drugs, accidental (unintentional)**
Poisoning by antiepileptic and sedative-hypnotic drugs NOS

X **T42.72 Poisoning by unspecified antiepileptic and sedative-hypnotic drugs, intentional self-harm** A, S

X **T42.73 Poisoning by unspecified antiepileptic and sedative-hypnotic drugs, assault**

X **T42.74 Poisoning by unspecified antiepileptic and sedative-hypnotic drugs, undetermined**

X **T42.75 Adverse effect of unspecified antiepileptic and sedative-hypnotic drugs**

X **T42.76 Underdosing of unspecified antiepileptic and sedative-hypnotic drugs**

T42.8 Poisoning by, adverse effect of and underdosing of antiparkinsonism drugs and other central muscle-tone depressants
Poisoning by, adverse effect of and underdosing of amantadine

T42.8X Poisoning by, adverse effect of and underdosing of antiparkinsonism drugs and other central muscle-tone depressants

T42.8X1 Poisoning by antiparkinsonism drugs and other central muscle-tone depressants, accidental (unintentional)
Poisoning by antiparkinsonism drugs and other central muscle-tone depressants NOS

T42.8X2 Poisoning by antiparkinsonism drugs and other central muscle-tone depressants, intentional self-harm A, S

T42.8X3 Poisoning by antiparkinsonism drugs and other central muscle-tone depressants, assault

T42.8X4 Poisoning by antiparkinsonism drugs and other central muscle-tone depressants, undetermined

T42.8X5 Adverse effect of antiparkinsonism drugs and other central muscle-tone depressants

T42.8X6 Underdosing of antiparkinsonism drugs and other central muscle-tone depressants

CHAPTER 19 (SØ0-T88)

● T43 Poisoning by, adverse effect of and underdosing of psychotropic drugs, not elsewhere classified

Excludes1 appetite depressants (T50.5-)
barbiturates (T42.3-)
benzodiazepines (T42.4-)
methaqualone (T42.6-)
psychodysleptics [hallucinogens] (T40.7-T40.9-)

Excludes2 drug dependence and related mental and behavioral disorders due to psychoactive substance use (F10.--F19.-)

The appropriate 7th character is to be added to each code from category T43

A	initial encounter
D	subsequent encounter
S	sequela

● T43.0 Poisoning by, adverse effect of and underdosing of tricyclic and tetracyclic antidepressants

● T43.01 Poisoning by, adverse effect of and underdosing of **tricyclic antidepressants**

● T43.011 Poisoning by tricyclic antidepressants, **accidental** (unintentional)
Poisoning by tricyclic antidepressants NOS

● T43.012 Poisoning by tricyclic antidepressants, **intentional** self-harm A, S

● T43.013 Poisoning by tricyclic antidepressants, **assault**

● T43.014 Poisoning by tricyclic antidepressants, **undetermined**

● T43.015 **Adverse effect** of tricyclic antidepressants

● T43.016 **Underdosing** of tricyclic antidepressants

● T43.02 Poisoning by, adverse effect of and underdosing of **tetracyclic antidepressants**

● T43.021 Poisoning by tetracyclic antidepressants, **accidental** (unintentional)
Poisoning by tetracyclic antidepressants NOS

● T43.022 Poisoning by tetracyclic antidepressants, **intentional** self-harm A, S

● T43.023 Poisoning by tetracyclic antidepressants, **assault**

● T43.024 Poisoning by tetracyclic antidepressants, **undetermined**

● T43.025 **Adverse effect** of tetracyclic antidepressants

● T43.026 **Underdosing** of tetracyclic antidepressants

● T43.1 Poisoning by, adverse effect of and underdosing of monoamine-oxidase-inhibitor antidepressants

● T43.1X Poisoning by, adverse effect of and underdosing of **monoamine-oxidase-inhibitor antidepressants**

● T43.1X1 Poisoning by monoamine-oxidase-inhibitor antidepressants, **accidental** (unintentional)
Poisoning by monoamine-oxidase-inhibitor antidepressants NOS

● T43.1X2 Poisoning by monoamine-oxidase-inhibitor antidepressants, **intentional** self-harm A, S

● T43.1X3 Poisoning by monoamine-oxidase-inhibitor antidepressants, **assault**

● T43.1X4 Poisoning by monoamine-oxidase-inhibitor antidepressants, **undetermined**

● T43.1X5 **Adverse effect** of monoamine-oxidase-inhibitor antidepressants

● T43.1X6 **Underdosing** of monoamine-oxidase-inhibitor antidepressants

● T43.2 Poisoning by, adverse effect of and underdosing of other and unspecified antidepressants

● T43.20 Poisoning by, adverse effect of and underdosing of **unspecified antidepressants**

● T43.201 Poisoning by unspecified antidepressants, **accidental** (unintentional)
Poisoning by antidepressants NOS

● T43.202 Poisoning by unspecified antidepressants, **intentional** self-harm A, S

● T43.203 Poisoning by unspecified antidepressants, **assault**

● T43.204 Poisoning by unspecified antidepressants, **undetermined**

● T43.205 **Adverse effect** of unspecified antidepressants
Antidepressant discontinuation syndrome

● T43.206 **Underdosing** of unspecified antidepressants

● T43.21 Poisoning by, adverse effect of and underdosing of **selective serotonin and norepinephrine reuptake inhibitors**
Poisoning by, adverse effect of and underdosing of SSNRI antidepressants

● T43.211 Poisoning by selective serotonin and norepinephrine reuptake inhibitors, **accidental** (unintentional)

● T43.212 Poisoning by selective serotonin and norepinephrine reuptake inhibitors, **intentional** self-harm A, S

● T43.213 Poisoning by selective serotonin and norepinephrine reuptake inhibitors, **assault**

● T43.214 Poisoning by selective serotonin and norepinephrine reuptake inhibitors, **undetermined**

● T43.215 **Adverse effect** of selective serotonin and norepinephrine reuptake inhibitors

● T43.216 **Underdosing** of selective serotonin and norepinephrine reuptake inhibitors

● T43.22 Poisoning by, adverse effect of and underdosing of **selective serotonin reuptake inhibitors**
Poisoning by, adverse effect of and underdosing of SSRI antidepressants

● T43.221 Poisoning by selective serotonin reuptake inhibitors, **accidental** (unintentional)

● T43.222 Poisoning by selective serotonin reuptake inhibitors, **intentional** self-harm A, S

● T43.223 Poisoning by selective serotonin reuptake inhibitors, **assault**

● T43.224 Poisoning by selective serotonin reuptake inhibitors, undetermined

● T43.225 **Adverse effect** of selective serotonin reuptake inhibitors

● T43.226 **Underdosing** of selective serotonin reuptake inhibitors

● T43.29 Poisoning by, adverse effect of and underdosing of **other antidepressants**

● T43.291 Poisoning by other antidepressants, **accidental** (unintentional)
Poisoning by other antidepressants NOS

● T43.292 Poisoning by other antidepressants, **intentional** self-harm A, S

● T43.293 Poisoning by other antidepressants, **assault**

● T43.294 Poisoning by other antidepressants, **undetermined**

● T43.295 **Adverse effect** of other antidepressants

● T43.296 **Underdosing** of other antidepressants

● T43.3 Poisoning by, adverse effect of and underdosing of phenothiazine antipsychotics and neuroleptics

● T43.3X Poisoning by, adverse effect of and underdosing of **phenothiazine antipsychotics and neuroleptics**

● T43.3X1 Poisoning by phenothiazine antipsychotics and neuroleptics, **accidental** (unintentional)
Poisoning by phenothiazine antipsychotics and neuroleptics NOS

● T43.3X2 Poisoning by phenothiazine antipsychotics and neuroleptics, **intentional** self-harm A, S

● T43.3X3 Poisoning by phenothiazine antipsychotics and neuroleptics, **assault**

● T43.3X4 Poisoning by phenothiazine antipsychotics and neuroleptics, **undetermined**

● T43.3X5 **Adverse effect** of phenothiazine antipsychotics and neuroleptics

● T43.3X6 **Underdosing** of phenothiazine antipsychotics and neuroleptics

● T43.4 Poisoning by, adverse effect of and underdosing of butyrophenone and thiothixene neuroleptics

● T43.4X Poisoning by, adverse effect of and underdosing of **butyrophenone and thiothixene neuroleptics**

● T43.4X1 Poisoning by butyrophenone and thiothixene neuroleptics, **accidental** (unintentional)
Poisoning by butyrophenone and thiothixene neuroleptics NOS

● T43.4X2 Poisoning by butyrophenone and thiothixene neuroleptics, **intentional** self-harm A, S

● T43.4X3 Poisoning by butyrophenone and thiothixene neuroleptics, **assault**

● T43.4X4 Poisoning by butyrophenone and thiothixene neuroleptics, **undetermined**

● T43.4X5 **Adverse effect** of butyrophenone and thiothixene neuroleptics

● T43.4X6 **Underdosing** of butyrophenone and thiothixene neuroleptics

● T43.5 Poisoning by, adverse effect of and underdosing of other and unspecified antipsychotics and neuroleptics
Excludes1 poisoning by, adverse effect of and underdosing of rauwolfia (T46.5-)

● T43.5Ø Poisoning by, adverse effect of and underdosing of **unspecified antipsychotics and neuroleptics**

● T43.5Ø1 Poisoning by unspecified antipsychotics and neuroleptics, **accidental** (unintentional)
Poisoning by antipsychotics and neuroleptics NOS

● T43.5Ø2 Poisoning by unspecified antipsychotics and neuroleptics, **intentional** self-harm A, S

● T43.5Ø3 Poisoning by unspecified antipsychotics and neuroleptics, **assault**

● T43.5Ø4 Poisoning by unspecified antipsychotics and neuroleptics, **undetermined**

● T43.5Ø5 **Adverse effect** of unspecified antipsychotics and neuroleptics

● T43.5Ø6 **Underdosing** of unspecified antipsychotics and neuroleptics

● T43.59 Poisoning by, adverse effect of and underdosing of **other antipsychotics and neuroleptics**

● T43.591 Poisoning by other antipsychotics and neuroleptics, **accidental** (unintentional)
Poisoning by other antipsychotics and neuroleptics NOS

● T43.592 Poisoning by other antipsychotics and neuroleptics, **intentional** self-harm A, S
Coding Clinic: 2Ø17, Q1, P4Ø

● T43.593 Poisoning by other antipsychotics and neuroleptics, **assault**

● T43.594 Poisoning by other antipsychotics and neuroleptics, **undetermined**

● T43.595 **Adverse effect** of other antipsychotics and neuroleptics

● T43.596 **Underdosing** of other antipsychotics and neuroleptics

● T43.6 Poisoning by, adverse effect of and underdosing of psychostimulants
Excludes1 poisoning by, adverse effect of and underdosing of cocaine (T4Ø.5-)

● T43.6Ø Poisoning by, adverse effect of and underdosing of **unspecified psychostimulant**

● T43.6Ø1 Poisoning by unspecified psychostimulants, **accidental** (unintentional)
Poisoning by psychostimulants NOS

● T43.6Ø2 Poisoning by unspecified psychostimulants, **intentional** self-harm A, S

● T43.6Ø3 Poisoning by unspecified psychostimulants, **assault**

● T43.6Ø4 Poisoning by unspecified psychostimulants, **undetermined**

● T43.6Ø5 **Adverse effect** of unspecified psychostimulants

● T43.6Ø6 **Underdosing** of unspecified psychostimulants

- T43.61 Poisoning by, adverse effect of and underdosing of **caffeine**
  - T43.611 Poisoning by caffeine, **accidental** (unintentional)
    - Poisoning by caffeine NOS
  - T43.612 Poisoning by caffeine, **intentional** self-harm A, S
  - T43.613 Poisoning by caffeine, **assault**
  - T43.614 Poisoning by caffeine, **undetermined**
  - T43.615 **Adverse effect** of caffeine
  - T43.616 **Underdosing** of caffeine
- T43.62 Poisoning by, adverse effect of and underdosing of **amphetamines**
  - Poisoning by, adverse effect of and underdosing of methamphetamines
  - T43.621 Poisoning by amphetamines, **accidental** (unintentional)
    - Poisoning by amphetamines NOS
  - T43.622 Poisoning by amphetamines, **intentional** self-harm A, S
  - T43.623 Poisoning by amphetamines, **assault**
  - T43.624 Poisoning by amphetamines, **undetermined**
  - T43.625 **Adverse effect** of amphetamines
  - T43.626 **Underdosing** of amphetamines
- T43.63 Poisoning by, adverse effect of and underdosing of **methylphenidate**
  - T43.631 Poisoning by methylphenidate, **accidental** (unintentional)
    - Poisoning by methylphenidate NOS
  - T43.632 Poisoning by methylphenidate, **intentional** self-harm A, S
  - T43.633 Poisoning by methylphenidate, **assault**
  - T43.634 Poisoning by methylphenidate, **undetermined**
  - T43.635 **Adverse effect** of methylphenidate
  - T43.636 **Underdosing** of methylphenidate
- T43.64 Poisoning by ecstasy
  - Poisoning by MDMA
  - Poisoning by 3,4-methylenedioxymethamphetamine
  - T43.641 Poisoning by ecstasy, accidental (unintentional)
    - Poisoning by ecstasy NOS
    - Coding Clinic: 2018, Q4, P31
  - T43.642 Poisoning by ecstasy, intentional self-harm A, S
  - T43.643 Poisoning by ecstasy, assault
  - T43.644 Poisoning by ecstasy, undetermined
- T43.69 Poisoning by, adverse effect of and underdosing of **other psychostimulants**
  - T43.691 Poisoning by other psychostimulants, **accidental** (unintentional)
    - Poisoning by other psychostimulants NOS
  - T43.692 Poisoning by other psychostimulants, **intentional** self-harm A, S
  - T43.693 Poisoning by other psychostimulants, **assault**
  - T43.694 Poisoning by other psychostimulants, **undetermined**
  - T43.695 **Adverse effect** of other psychostimulants
  - T43.696 **Underdosing** of other psychostimulants
- T43.8 Poisoning by, adverse effect of and underdosing of other psychotropic drugs
  - T43.8X Poisoning by, adverse effect of and underdosing of **other psychotropic drugs**
    - T43.8X1 Poisoning by other psychotropic drugs, **accidental** (unintentional)
      - Poisoning by other psychotropic drugs NOS
    - T43.8X2 Poisoning by other psychotropic drugs, **intentional** self-harm A, S
    - T43.8X3 Poisoning by other psychotropic drugs, **assault**
    - T43.8X4 Poisoning by other psychotropic drugs, **undetermined**
    - T43.8X5 **Adverse effect** of other psychotropic drugs
    - T43.8X6 **Underdosing** of other psychotropic drugs
- T43.9 Poisoning by, adverse effect of and underdosing of **unspecified psychotropic drug**
  - X T43.91 Poisoning by unspecified psychotropic drug, **accidental** (unintentional)
    - Poisoning by psychotropic drug NOS
  - X T43.92 Poisoning by unspecified psychotropic drug, **intentional** self-harm A, S
  - X T43.93 Poisoning by unspecified psychotropic drug, **assault**
  - X T43.94 Poisoning by unspecified psychotropic drug, **undetermined**
  - X T43.95 **Adverse effect** of unspecified psychotropic drug
  - X T43.96 **Underdosing** of unspecified psychotropic drug

T44 Poisoning by, adverse effect of and underdosing of drugs primarily affecting the autonomic nervous system

The appropriate 7th character is to be added to each code from category T44

A	initial encounter
D	subsequent encounter
S	sequela

- T44.Ø Poisoning by, adverse effect of and underdosing of anticholinesterase agents
  - T44.ØX Poisoning by, adverse effect of and underdosing of **anticholinesterase agents**
    - T44.ØX1 Poisoning by anticholinesterase agents, **accidental** (unintentional)
      - Poisoning by anticholinesterase agents NOS
    - T44.ØX2 Poisoning by anticholinesterase agents, **intentional** self-harm A, S
    - T44.ØX3 Poisoning by anticholinesterase agents, **assault**
    - T44.ØX4 Poisoning by anticholinesterase agents, **undetermined**
    - T44.ØX5 **Adverse effect** of anticholinesterase agents
    - T44.ØX6 **Underdosing** of anticholinesterase agents
- T44.1 Poisoning by, adverse effect of and underdosing of other parasympathomimetics [cholinergics]
  - T44.1X Poisoning by, adverse effect of and underdosing of **other parasympathomimetics** [cholinergics]
    - T44.1X1 Poisoning by other parasympathomimetics [cholinergics], **accidental** (unintentional)
      - Poisoning by other parasympathomimetics [cholinergics] NOS
    - T44.1X2 Poisoning by other parasympathomimetics [cholinergics], **intentional** self-harm A, S

T44.1X3 Poisoning by other parasympathomimetics [cholinergics], **assault**

T44.1X4 Poisoning by other parasympathomimetics [cholinergics], **undetermined**

T44.1X5 **Adverse effect** of other parasympathomimetics [cholinergics]

T44.1X6 **Underdosing** of other parasympathomimetics [cholinergics]

T44.2 Poisoning by, adverse effect of and underdosing of ganglionic blocking drugs

T44.2X Poisoning by, adverse effect of and underdosing of ganglionic blocking drugs

T44.2X1 Poisoning by ganglionic blocking drugs, **accidental (unintentional)**
Poisoning by ganglionic blocking drugs NOS

T44.2X2 Poisoning by ganglionic blocking drugs, **intentional self-harm** A, S

T44.2X3 Poisoning by ganglionic blocking drugs, **assault**

T44.2X4 Poisoning by ganglionic blocking drugs, **undetermined**

T44.2X5 **Adverse effect** of ganglionic blocking drugs

T44.2X6 **Underdosing** of ganglionic blocking drugs

T44.3 Poisoning by, adverse effect of and underdosing of other parasympatholytics [anticholinergics and antimuscarinics] and spasmolytics
Poisoning by, adverse effect of and underdosing of papaverine

T44.3X Poisoning by, adverse effect of and underdosing of other parasympatholytics [anticholinergics and antimuscarinics] and spasmolytics

T44.3X1 Poisoning by other parasympatholytics [anticholinergics and antimuscarinics] and spasmolytics, **accidental (unintentional)**
Poisoning by other parasympatholytics [anticholinergics and antimuscarinics] and spasmolytics NOS

T44.3X2 Poisoning by other parasympatholytics [anticholinergics and antimuscarinics] and spasmolytics, **intentional self-harm** A, S

T44.3X3 Poisoning by other parasympatholytics [anticholinergics and antimuscarinics] and spasmolytics, **assault**

T44.3X4 Poisoning by other parasympatholytics [anticholinergics and antimuscarinics] and spasmolytics, **undetermined**

T44.3X5 **Adverse effect** of other parasympatholytics [anticholinergics and antimuscarinics] and spasmolytics

T44.3X6 **Underdosing** of other parasympatholytics [anticholinergics and antimuscarinics] and spasmolytics

T44.4 Poisoning by, adverse effect of and underdosing of predominantly alpha-adrenoreceptor agonists
Poisoning by, adverse effect of and underdosing of metaraminol

T44.4X Poisoning by, adverse effect of and underdosing of predominantly alpha-adrenoreceptor agonists

T44.4X1 Poisoning by predominantly alpha-adrenoreceptor agonists, **accidental (unintentional)**
Poisoning by predominantly alpha-adrenoreceptor agonists NOS

T44.4X2 Poisoning by predominantly alpha-adrenoreceptor agonists, **intentional self-harm** A, S

T44.4X3 Poisoning by predominantly alpha-adrenoreceptor agonists, **assault**

T44.4X4 Poisoning by predominantly alpha-adrenoreceptor agonists, **undetermined**

T44.4X5 **Adverse effect** of predominantly alpha-adrenoreceptor agonists

T44.4X6 **Underdosing** of predominantly alpha-adrenoreceptor agonists

T44.5 Poisoning by, adverse effect of and underdosing of predominantly beta-adrenoreceptor agonists
Excludes1 poisoning by, adverse effect of and underdosing of beta-adrenoreceptor agonists used in asthma therapy (T48.6-)

T44.5X Poisoning by, adverse effect of and underdosing of predominantly beta-adrenoreceptor agonists

T44.5X1 Poisoning by predominantly beta-adrenoreceptor agonists, **accidental (unintentional)**
Poisoning by predominantly beta-adrenoreceptor agonists NOS

T44.5X2 Poisoning by predominantly beta-adrenoreceptor agonists, **intentional self-harm** A, S

T44.5X3 Poisoning by predominantly beta-adrenoreceptor agonists, **assault**

T44.5X4 Poisoning by predominantly beta-adrenoreceptor agonists, **undetermined**

T44.5X5 **Adverse effect** of predominantly beta-adrenoreceptor agonists

T44.5X6 **Underdosing** of predominantly beta-adrenoreceptor agonists

T44.6 Poisoning by, adverse effect of and underdosing of alpha-adrenoreceptor antagonists
Excludes1 poisoning by, adverse effect of and underdosing of ergot alkaloids (T48.Ø)

T44.6X Poisoning by, adverse effect of and underdosing of alpha-adrenoreceptor antagonists

T44.6X1 Poisoning by alpha-adrenoreceptor antagonists, **accidental (unintentional)**
Poisoning by alpha-adrenoreceptor antagonists NOS

T44.6X2 Poisoning by alpha-adrenoreceptor antagonists, **intentional self-harm** A, S

T44.6X3 Poisoning by alpha-adrenoreceptor antagonists, **assault**

T44.6X4 Poisoning by alpha-adrenoreceptor antagonists, **undetermined**

T44.6X5 **Adverse effect** of alpha-adrenoreceptor antagonists

T44.6X6 **Underdosing** of alpha-adrenoreceptor antagonists

● T44.7 Poisoning by, adverse effect of and underdosing of beta-adrenoreceptor antagonists

● T44.7X Poisoning by, adverse effect of and underdosing of **beta-adrenoreceptor antagonists**

● T44.7X1 Poisoning by beta-adrenoreceptor antagonists, **accidental** (unintentional)
Poisoning by beta-adrenoreceptor antagonists NOS

● T44.7X2 Poisoning by beta-adrenoreceptor antagonists, **intentional** self-harm A, S

● T44.7X3 Poisoning by beta-adrenoreceptor antagonists, **assault**

● T44.7X4 Poisoning by beta-adrenoreceptor antagonists, **undetermined**

● T44.7X5 **Adverse effect** of beta-adrenoreceptor antagonists

● T44.7X6 **Underdosing** of beta-adrenoreceptor antagonists

● T44.8 Poisoning by, adverse effect of and underdosing of centrally-acting and adrenergic-neuron-blocking agents

Excludes1 poisoning by, adverse effect of and underdosing of clonidine (T46.5)
poisoning by, adverse effect of and underdosing of guanethidine (T46.5)

● T44.8X Poisoning by, adverse effect of and underdosing of **centrally-acting and adrenergic-neuron-blocking agents**

● T44.8X1 Poisoning by centrally-acting and adrenergic-neuron-blocking agents, **accidental** (unintentional)
Poisoning by centrally-acting and adrenergic-neuron-blocking agents NOS

● T44.8X2 Poisoning by centrally-acting and adrenergic-neuron-blocking agents, **intentional** self-harm A, S

● T44.8X3 Poisoning by centrally-acting and adrenergic-neuron-blocking agents, **assault**

● T44.8X4 Poisoning by centrally-acting and adrenergic-neuron-blocking agents, **undetermined**

● T44.8X5 **Adverse effect** of centrally-acting and adrenergic-neuron-blocking agents

● T44.8X6 **Underdosing** of centrally-acting and adrenergic-neuron-blocking agents

● T44.9 Poisoning by, adverse effect of and underdosing of other and unspecified drugs primarily affecting the autonomic nervous system
Poisoning by, adverse effect of and underdosing of drug stimulating both alpha and beta-adrenoreceptors

● T44.90 Poisoning by, adverse effect of and underdosing of **unspecified drugs primarily affecting the autonomic nervous system**

● T44.901 Poisoning by unspecified drugs primarily affecting the autonomic nervous system, **accidental** (unintentional)
Poisoning by unspecified drugs primarily affecting the autonomic nervous system NOS

● T44.902 Poisoning by unspecified drugs primarily affecting the autonomic nervous system, **intentional** self-harm A, S

● T44.903 Poisoning by unspecified drugs primarily affecting the autonomic nervous system, **assault**

● T44.904 Poisoning by unspecified drugs primarily affecting the autonomic nervous system, **undetermined**

● T44.905 **Adverse effect** of unspecified drugs primarily affecting the autonomic nervous system

● T44.906 **Underdosing** of unspecified drugs primarily affecting the autonomic nervous system

● T44.99 Poisoning by, adverse effect of and underdosing of **other drugs primarily affecting the autonomic nervous system**

● T44.991 Poisoning by other drug primarily affecting the autonomic nervous system, **accidental** (unintentional)
Poisoning by other drugs primarily affecting the autonomic nervous system NOS

● T44.992 Poisoning by other drug primarily affecting the autonomic nervous system, **intentional** self-harm A, S

● T44.993 Poisoning by other drug primarily affecting the autonomic nervous system, **assault**

● T44.994 Poisoning by other drug primarily affecting the autonomic nervous system, **undetermined**

● T44.995 **Adverse effect** of other drug primarily affecting the autonomic nervous system

● T44.996 **Underdosing** of other drug primarily affecting the autonomic nervous system

● T45 Poisoning by, adverse effect of and underdosing of primarily systemic and hematological agents, not elsewhere classified

The appropriate 7th character is to be added to each code from category T45

A	initial encounter
D	subsequent encounter
S	sequela

● T45.Ø Poisoning by, adverse effect of and underdosing of antiallergic and antiemetic drugs

Excludes1 poisoning by, adverse effect of and underdosing of phenothiazine-based neuroleptics (T43.3)

● T45.ØX Poisoning by, adverse effect of and underdosing of **antiallergic and antiemetic drugs**

● T45.ØX1 Poisoning by antiallergic and antiemetic drugs, **accidental** (unintentional)
Poisoning by antiallergic and antiemetic drugs NOS

● T45.ØX2 Poisoning by antiallergic and antiemetic drugs, **intentional** self-harm A, S

● T45.ØX3 Poisoning by antiallergic and antiemetic drugs, **assault**

● T45.ØX4 Poisoning by antiallergic and antiemetic drugs, **undetermined**

● T45.ØX5 **Adverse effect** of antiallergic and antiemetic drugs

● T45.ØX6 **Underdosing** of antiallergic and antiemetic drugs

T45.1 Poisoning by, adverse effect of and underdosing of antineoplastic and immunosuppressive drugs

Excludes1 poisoning by, adverse effect of and underdosing of tamoxifen (T38.6)

T45.1X Poisoning by, adverse effect of and underdosing of antineoplastic and immunosuppressive drugs

T45.1X1 Poisoning by antineoplastic and immunosuppressive drugs, accidental (unintentional)
Poisoning by antineoplastic and immunosuppressive drugs NOS

T45.1X2 Poisoning by antineoplastic and immunosuppressive drugs, intentional self-harm A, S

T45.1X3 Poisoning by antineoplastic and immunosuppressive drugs, assault

T45.1X4 Poisoning by antineoplastic and immunosuppressive drugs, undetermined

T45.1X5 Adverse effect of antineoplastic and immunosuppressive drugs
Coding Clinic: 2019, Q2, P25, 28; Q1, P17, 21

T45.1X6 Underdosing of antineoplastic and immunosuppressive drugs

T45.2 Poisoning by, adverse effect of and underdosing of vitamins

Excludes2 poisoning by, adverse effect of and underdosing of nicotinic acid (derivatives) (T46.7)
poisoning by, adverse effect of and underdosing of iron (T45.4)
poisoning by, adverse effect of and underdosing of vitamin K (T45.7)

T45.2X Poisoning by, adverse effect of and underdosing of vitamins

T45.2X1 Poisoning by vitamins, accidental (unintentional)
Poisoning by vitamins NOS

T45.2X2 Poisoning by vitamins, intentional self-harm A, S

T45.2X3 Poisoning by vitamins, assault

T45.2X4 Poisoning by vitamins, undetermined

T45.2X5 Adverse effect of vitamins

T45.2X6 Underdosing of vitamins

Excludes1 vitamin deficiencies (E50-E56)

T45.3 Poisoning by, adverse effect of and underdosing of enzymes

T45.3X Poisoning by, adverse effect of and underdosing of enzymes

T45.3X1 Poisoning by enzymes, accidental (unintentional)
Poisoning by enzymes NOS

T45.3X2 Poisoning by enzymes, intentional self-harm A, S

T45.3X3 Poisoning by enzymes, assault

T45.3X4 Poisoning by enzymes, undetermined

T45.3X5 Adverse effect of enzymes

T45.3X6 Underdosing of enzymes

T45.4 Poisoning by, adverse effect of and underdosing of iron and its compounds

T45.4X Poisoning by, adverse effect of and underdosing of iron and its compounds

T45.4X1 Poisoning by iron and its compounds, accidental (unintentional)
Poisoning by iron and its compounds NOS

T45.4X2 Poisoning by iron and its compounds, intentional self-harm A, S

T45.4X3 Poisoning by iron and its compounds, assault

T45.4X4 Poisoning by iron and its compounds, undetermined

T45.4X5 Adverse effect of iron and its compounds

T45.4X6 Underdosing of iron and its compounds

Excludes1 iron deficiency (E61.1)

T45.5 Poisoning by, adverse effect of and underdosing of anticoagulants and antithrombotic drugs

T45.51 Poisoning by, adverse effect of and underdosing of anticoagulants

T45.511 Poisoning by anticoagulants, accidental (unintentional)
Poisoning by anticoagulants NOS

T45.512 Poisoning by anticoagulants, intentional self-harm A, S

T45.513 Poisoning by anticoagulants, assault

T45.514 Poisoning by anticoagulants, undetermined

T45.515 Adverse effect of anticoagulants
Coding Clinic: 2016, Q1, P14; 2013, Q2, P35

T45.516 Underdosing of anticoagulants

T45.52 Poisoning by, adverse effect of and underdosing of antithrombotic drugs
Poisoning by, adverse effect of and underdosing of antiplatelet drugs

Excludes2 poisoning by, adverse effect of and underdosing of aspirin (T39.01-)
poisoning by, adverse effect of and underdosing of acetylsalicylic acid (T39.01-)

T45.521 Poisoning by antithrombotic drugs, accidental (unintentional)
Poisoning by antithrombotic drug NOS

T45.522 Poisoning by antithrombotic drugs, intentional self-harm A, S

T45.523 Poisoning by antithrombotic drugs, assault

T45.524 Poisoning by antithrombotic drugs, undetermined

T45.525 Adverse effect of antithrombotic drugs
Coding Clinic: 2016, Q1, P15

T45.526 Underdosing of antithrombotic drugs

T45.6 Poisoning by, adverse effect of and underdosing of fibrinolysis-affecting drugs

T45.60 Poisoning by, adverse effect of and underdosing of unspecified fibrinolysis-affecting drugs

T45.601 Poisoning by unspecified fibrinolysis-affecting drugs, accidental (unintentional)
Poisoning by fibrinolysis-affecting drug NOS

T45.602 Poisoning by unspecified fibrinolysis-affecting drugs, intentional self-harm A, S

T45.603 Poisoning by unspecified fibrinolysis-affecting drugs, assault

T45.604 Poisoning by unspecified fibrinolysis-affecting drugs, undetermined

T45.605 Adverse effect of unspecified fibrinolysis-affecting drugs

T45.606 Underdosing of unspecified fibrinolysis-affecting drugs

T45.61 Poisoning by, adverse effect of and underdosing of **thrombolytic drugs**

T45.611 Poisoning by thrombolytic drug, **accidental** (unintentional)
Poisoning by thrombolytic drug NOS

T45.612 Poisoning by thrombolytic drug, **intentional** self-harm A, S

T45.613 Poisoning by thrombolytic drug, **assault**

T45.614 Poisoning by thrombolytic drug, **undetermined**

T45.615 **Adverse effect** of thrombolytic drugs
Coding Clinic: 2017, Q2, P10

T45.616 **Underdosing** of thrombolytic drugs

T45.62 Poisoning by, adverse effect of and underdosing of **hemostatic drugs**

T45.621 Poisoning by hemostatic drug, **accidental** (unintentional)
Poisoning by hemostatic drug NOS

T45.622 Poisoning by hemostatic drug, **intentional** self-harm A, S

T45.623 Poisoning by hemostatic drug, **assault**

T45.624 Poisoning by hemostatic drug, **undetermined**

T45.625 **Adverse effect** of hemostatic drug

T45.626 **Underdosing** of hemostatic drugs

T45.69 Poisoning by, adverse effect of and underdosing of **other fibrinolysis-affecting drugs**

T45.691 Poisoning by other fibrinolysis-affecting drugs, **accidental** (unintentional)
Poisoning by other fibrinolysis-affecting drug NOS

T45.692 Poisoning by other fibrinolysis-affecting drugs, **intentional** self-harm A, S

T45.693 Poisoning by other fibrinolysis-affecting drugs, **assault**

T45.694 Poisoning by other fibrinolysis-affecting drugs, **undetermined**

T45.695 **Adverse effect** of other fibrinolysis-affecting drugs

T45.696 **Underdosing** of other fibrinolysis-affecting drugs

T45.7 Poisoning by, adverse effect of and underdosing of anticoagulant antagonists, vitamin K and other coagulants

T45.7X Poisoning by, adverse effect of and underdosing of **anticoagulant antagonists, vitamin K and other coagulants**

T45.7X1 Poisoning by anticoagulant antagonists, vitamin K and other coagulants, **accidental** (unintentional)
Poisoning by anticoagulant antagonists, vitamin K and other coagulants NOS

T45.7X2 Poisoning by anticoagulant antagonists, vitamin K and other coagulants, **intentional** self-harm A, S

T45.7X3 Poisoning by anticoagulant antagonists, vitamin K and other coagulants, **assault**

T45.7X4 Poisoning by anticoagulant antagonists, vitamin K and other coagulants, **undetermined**

T45.7X5 **Adverse effect** of anticoagulant antagonists, vitamin K and other coagulants

T45.7X6 **Underdosing** of anticoagulant antagonist, vitamin K and other coagulants
Excludes1 vitamin K deficiency (E56.1)

T45.8 Poisoning by, adverse effect of and underdosing of other primarily systemic and hematological agents
Poisoning by, adverse effect of and underdosing of liver preparations and other antianemic agents
Poisoning by, adverse effect of and underdosing of natural blood and blood products
Poisoning by, adverse effect of and underdosing of plasma substitute
Excludes2 poisoning by, adverse effect of and underdosing of immunoglobulin (T50.Z1)
poisoning by, adverse effect of and underdosing of iron (T45.4)
transfusion reactions (T80.-)

T45.8X Poisoning by, adverse effect of and underdosing of other primarily systemic and hematological agents

T45.8X1 Poisoning by other primarily systemic and hematological agents, **accidental** (unintentional)
Poisoning by other primarily systemic and hematological agents NOS

T45.8X2 Poisoning by other primarily systemic and hematological agents, **intentional** self-harm A, S

T45.8X3 Poisoning by other primarily systemic and hematological agents, **assault**

T45.8X4 Poisoning by other primarily systemic and hematological agents, **undetermined**

T45.8X5 **Adverse effect** of other primarily systemic and hematological agents
Coding Clinic: 2016, Q4, P42

T45.8X6 **Underdosing** of other primarily systemic and hematological agents

T45.9 Poisoning by, adverse effect of and underdosing of **unspecified primarily systemic and hematological agent**

X T45.91 Poisoning by unspecified primarily systemic and hematological agent, **accidental** (unintentional)
Poisoning by primarily systemic and hematological agent NOS

X T45.92 Poisoning by unspecified primarily systemic and hematological agent, **intentional** self-harm A, S

X T45.93 Poisoning by unspecified primarily systemic and hematological agent, **assault**

X T45.94 Poisoning by unspecified primarily systemic and hematological agent, **undetermined**

X T45.95 **Adverse effect** of unspecified primarily systemic and hematological agent

X T45.96 **Underdosing** of unspecified primarily systemic and hematological agent

T46 Poisoning by, adverse effect of and underdosing of agents primarily affecting the cardiovascular system

Excludes1 poisoning by, adverse effect of and underdosing of metaraminol (T44.4)

The appropriate 7th character is to be added to each code from category T46

A	initial encounter
D	subsequent encounter
S	sequela

T46.0 Poisoning by, adverse effect of and underdosing of cardiac-stimulant glycosides and drugs of similar action

T46.0X Poisoning by, adverse effect of and underdosing of cardiac-stimulant glycosides and drugs of similar action

T46.0X1 Poisoning by cardiac-stimulant glycosides and drugs of similar action, accidental (unintentional)
Poisoning by cardiac-stimulant glycosides and drugs of similar action NOS

T46.0X2 Poisoning by cardiac-stimulant glycosides and drugs of similar action, intentional self-harm A, S

T46.0X3 Poisoning by cardiac-stimulant glycosides and drugs of similar action, assault

T46.0X4 Poisoning by cardiac-stimulant glycosides and drugs of similar action, undetermined

T46.0X5 Adverse effect of cardiac-stimulant glycosides and drugs of similar action

T46.0X6 Underdosing of cardiac-stimulant glycosides and drugs of similar action

T46.1 Poisoning by, adverse effect of and underdosing of calcium-channel blockers

T46.1X Poisoning by, adverse effect of and underdosing of calcium-channel blockers

T46.1X1 Poisoning by calcium-channel blockers, accidental (unintentional)
Poisoning by calcium-channel blockers NOS

T46.1X2 Poisoning by calcium-channel blockers, intentional self-harm A, S

T46.1X3 Poisoning by calcium-channel blockers, assault

T46.1X4 Poisoning by calcium-channel blockers, undetermined

T46.1X5 Adverse effect of calcium-channel blockers

T46.1X6 Underdosing of calcium-channel blockers

T46.2 Poisoning by, adverse effect of and underdosing of other antidysrhythmic drugs, not elsewhere classified

Excludes1 poisoning by, adverse effect of and underdosing of beta-adrenoreceptor antagonists (T44.7-)

T46.2X Poisoning by, adverse effect of and underdosing of other antidysrhythmic drugs

T46.2X1 Poisoning by other antidysrhythmic drugs, accidental (unintentional)
Poisoning by other antidysrhythmic drugs NOS

T46.2X2 Poisoning by other antidysrhythmic drugs, intentional self-harm A, S

T46.2X3 Poisoning by other antidysrhythmic drugs, assault

T46.2X4 Poisoning by other antidysrhythmic drugs, undetermined

T46.2X5 Adverse effect of other antidysrhythmic drugs

T46.2X6 Underdosing of other antidysrhythmic drugs

T46.3 Poisoning by, adverse effect of and underdosing of coronary vasodilators
Poisoning by, adverse effect of and underdosing of dipyridamole

Excludes1 poisoning by, adverse effect of and underdosing of calcium-channel blockers (T46.1)

T46.3X Poisoning by, adverse effect of and underdosing of coronary vasodilators

T46.3X1 Poisoning by coronary vasodilators, accidental (unintentional)
Poisoning by coronary vasodilators NOS

T46.3X2 Poisoning by coronary vasodilators, intentional self-harm A, S

T46.3X3 Poisoning by coronary vasodilators, assault

T46.3X4 Poisoning by coronary vasodilators, undetermined

T46.3X5 Adverse effect of coronary vasodilators

T46.3X6 Underdosing of coronary vasodilators

T46.4 Poisoning by, adverse effect of and underdosing of angiotensin-converting-enzyme inhibitors

T46.4X Poisoning by, adverse effect of and underdosing of angiotensin-converting-enzyme inhibitors

T46.4X1 Poisoning by angiotensin-converting-enzyme inhibitors, accidental (unintentional)
Poisoning by angiotensin-converting-enzyme inhibitors NOS

T46.4X2 Poisoning by angiotensin-converting-enzyme inhibitors, intentional self-harm A, S

T46.4X3 Poisoning by angiotensin-converting-enzyme inhibitors, assault

T46.4X4 Poisoning by angiotensin-converting-enzyme inhibitors, undetermined

T46.4X5 Adverse effect of angiotensin-converting-enzyme inhibitors

T46.4X6 Underdosing of angiotensin-converting-enzyme inhibitors

T46.5 Poisoning by, adverse effect of and underdosing of other antihypertensive drugs

Excludes2 poisoning by, adverse effect of and underdosing of beta-adrenoreceptor antagonists (T44.7)
poisoning by, adverse effect of and underdosing of calcium-channel blockers (T46.1)
poisoning by, adverse effect of and underdosing of diuretics (T50.0-T50.2)

T46.5X Poisoning by, adverse effect of and underdosing of other antihypertensive drugs

T46.5X1 Poisoning by other antihypertensive drugs, accidental (unintentional)
Poisoning by other antihypertensive drugs NOS

T46.5X2 Poisoning by other antihypertensive drugs, intentional self-harm A, S

T46.5X3 Poisoning by other antihypertensive drugs, assault

T46.5X4 Poisoning by other antihypertensive drugs, undetermined

T46.5X5 Adverse effect of other antihypertensive drugs

T46.5X6 Underdosing of other antihypertensive drugs

CHAPTER 19 (S00-T88)

- T46.6 Poisoning by, adverse effect of and underdosing of antihyperlipidemic and antiarteriosclerotic drugs
  - T46.6X Poisoning by, adverse effect of and underdosing of **antihyperlipidemic and antiarteriosclerotic drugs**
    - T46.6X1 Poisoning by antihyperlipidemic and antiarteriosclerotic drugs, **accidental** (unintentional)
      Poisoning by antihyperlipidemic and antiarteriosclerotic drugs NOS
    - T46.6X2 Poisoning by antihyperlipidemic and antiarteriosclerotic drugs, **intentional** self-harm A, S
    - T46.6X3 Poisoning by antihyperlipidemic and antiarteriosclerotic drugs, **assault**
    - T46.6X4 Poisoning by antihyperlipidemic and antiarteriosclerotic drugs, **undetermined**
    - T46.6X5 **Adverse effect** of antihyperlipidemic and antiarteriosclerotic drugs
    - T46.6X6 **Underdosing** of antihyperlipidemic and antiarteriosclerotic drugs
- T46.7 Poisoning by, adverse effect of and underdosing of peripheral vasodilators
  Poisoning by, adverse effect of and underdosing of nicotinic acid (derivatives)
  Excludes1 poisoning by, adverse effect of and underdosing of papaverine (T44.3)
  - T46.7X Poisoning by, adverse effect of and underdosing of **peripheral vasodilators**
    - T46.7X1 Poisoning by peripheral vasodilators, **accidental** (unintentional)
      Poisoning by peripheral vasodilators NOS
    - T46.7X2 Poisoning by peripheral vasodilators, **intentional** self-harm A, S
    - T46.7X3 Poisoning by peripheral vasodilators, **assault**
    - T46.7X4 Poisoning by peripheral vasodilators, **undetermined**
    - T46.7X5 **Adverse effect** of peripheral vasodilators
    - T46.7X6 **Underdosing** of peripheral vasodilators
- T46.8 Poisoning by, adverse effect of and underdosing of antivaricose drugs, including sclerosing agents
  - T46.8X Poisoning by, adverse effect of and underdosing of **antivaricose drugs, including sclerosing agents**
    - T46.8X1 Poisoning by antivaricose drugs, including sclerosing agents, **accidental** (unintentional)
      Poisoning by antivaricose drugs, including sclerosing agents NOS
    - T46.8X2 Poisoning by antivaricose drugs, including sclerosing agents, **intentional** self-harm A, S
    - T46.8X3 Poisoning by antivaricose drugs, including sclerosing agents, **assault**
    - T46.8X4 Poisoning by antivaricose drugs, including sclerosing agents, **undetermined**
    - T46.8X5 **Adverse effect** of antivaricose drugs, including sclerosing agents
    - T46.8X6 **Underdosing** of antivaricose drugs, including sclerosing agents
- T46.9 Poisoning by, adverse effect of and underdosing of other and unspecified agents primarily affecting the cardiovascular system
  - T46.9Ø Poisoning by, adverse effect of and underdosing of **unspecified agents primarily affecting the cardiovascular system**
    - T46.9Ø1 Poisoning by unspecified agents primarily affecting the cardiovascular system, **accidental** (unintentional)
    - T46.9Ø2 Poisoning by unspecified agents primarily affecting the cardiovascular system, **intentional** self-harm A, S
    - T46.9Ø3 Poisoning by unspecified agents primarily affecting the cardiovascular system, **assault**
    - T46.9Ø4 Poisoning by unspecified agents primarily affecting the cardiovascular system, **undetermined**
    - T46.9Ø5 **Adverse effect** of unspecified agents primarily affecting the cardiovascular system
    - T46.9Ø6 **Underdosing** of unspecified agents primarily affecting the cardiovascular system
  - T46.99 Poisoning by, adverse effect of and underdosing of **other agents primarily affecting the cardiovascular system**
    - T46.991 Poisoning by other agents primarily affecting the cardiovascular system, **accidental** (unintentional)
    - T46.992 Poisoning by other agents primarily affecting the cardiovascular system, **intentional** self-harm A, S
    - T46.993 Poisoning by other agents primarily affecting the cardiovascular system, **assault**
    - T46.994 Poisoning by other agents primarily affecting the cardiovascular system, **undetermined**
    - T46.995 **Adverse effect** of other agents primarily affecting the cardiovascular system
    - T46.996 **Underdosing** of other agents primarily affecting the cardiovascular system

- T47 Poisoning by, adverse effect of and underdosing of agents primarily affecting the gastrointestinal system
  The appropriate 7th character is to be added to each code from category T47

A	initial encounter
D	subsequent encounter
S	sequela

- T47.Ø Poisoning by, adverse effect of and underdosing of histamine H2-receptor blockers
  - T47.ØX Poisoning by, adverse effect of and underdosing of **histamine H2-receptor blockers**
    - T47.ØX1 Poisoning by histamine H2-receptor blockers, **accidental** (unintentional)
      Poisoning by histamine H2-receptor blockers NOS
    - T47.ØX2 Poisoning by histamine H2-receptor blockers, **intentional** self-harm A, S
    - T47.ØX3 Poisoning by histamine H2-receptor blockers, **assault**
    - T47.ØX4 Poisoning by histamine H2-receptor blockers, **undetermined**
    - T47.ØX5 **Adverse effect** of histamine H2-receptor blockers
    - T47.ØX6 **Underdosing** of histamine H2-receptor blockers

T47.1 Poisoning by, adverse effect of and underdosing of other antacids and anti-gastric-secretion drugs
T47.1X Poisoning by, adverse effect of and underdosing of **other antacids and anti-gastric-secretion drugs**
T47.1X1 Poisoning by other antacids and anti-gastric-secretion drugs, **accidental** (unintentional)
Poisoning by other antacids and anti-gastric-secretion drugs NOS
T47.1X2 Poisoning by other antacids and anti-gastric-secretion drugs, **intentional** self-harm A, S
T47.1X3 Poisoning by other antacids and anti-gastric-secretion drugs, **assault**
T47.1X4 Poisoning by other antacids and anti-gastric-secretion drugs, **undetermined**
T47.1X5 **Adverse effect** of other antacids and anti-gastric-secretion drugs
T47.1X6 **Underdosing** of other antacids and anti-gastric-secretion drugs

T47.2 Poisoning by, adverse effect of and underdosing of stimulant laxatives
T47.2X Poisoning by, adverse effect of and underdosing of **stimulant laxatives**
T47.2X1 Poisoning by stimulant laxatives, **accidental** (unintentional)
Poisoning by stimulant laxatives NOS
T47.2X2 Poisoning by stimulant laxatives, **intentional** self-harm A, S
T47.2X3 Poisoning by stimulant laxatives, **assault**
T47.2X4 Poisoning by stimulant laxatives, **undetermined**
T47.2X5 **Adverse effect** of stimulant laxatives
T47.2X6 **Underdosing** of stimulant laxatives

T47.3 Poisoning by, adverse effect of and underdosing of saline and osmotic laxatives
T47.3X Poisoning by and adverse effect of **saline and osmotic laxatives**
T47.3X1 Poisoning by saline and osmotic laxatives, **accidental** (unintentional)
Poisoning by saline and osmotic laxatives NOS
T47.3X2 Poisoning by saline and osmotic laxatives, **intentional** self-harm
T47.3X3 Poisoning by saline and osmotic laxatives, **assault** A, S
T47.3X4 Poisoning by saline and osmotic laxatives, **undetermined**
T47.3X5 **Adverse effect** of saline and osmotic laxatives
T47.3X6 **Underdosing** of saline and osmotic laxatives

T47.4 Poisoning by, adverse effect of and underdosing of other laxatives
T47.4X Poisoning by, adverse effect of and underdosing of **other laxatives**
T47.4X1 Poisoning by other laxatives, **accidental** (unintentional)
Poisoning by other laxatives NOS
T47.4X2 Poisoning by other laxatives, **intentional** self-harm A, S
T47.4X3 Poisoning by other laxatives, **assault**
T47.4X4 Poisoning by other laxatives, **undetermined**
T47.4X5 **Adverse effect** of other laxatives
T47.4X6 **Underdosing** of other laxatives

T47.5 Poisoning by, adverse effect of and underdosing of **digestants**
T47.5X Poisoning by, adverse effect of and underdosing of digestants
T47.5X1 Poisoning by digestants, **accidental** (unintentional)
Poisoning by digestants NOS
T47.5X2 Poisoning by digestants, **intentional** self-harm A, S
T47.5X3 Poisoning by digestants, **assault**
T47.5X4 Poisoning by digestants, **undetermined**
T47.5X5 **Adverse effect** of digestants
T47.5X6 **Underdosing** of digestants

T47.6 Poisoning by, adverse effect of and underdosing of antidiarrheal drugs
Excludes2 poisoning by, adverse effect of and underdosing of systemic antibiotics and other anti-infectives (T36-T37)
T47.6X Poisoning by, adverse effect of and underdosing of **antidiarrheal drugs**
T47.6X1 Poisoning by antidiarrheal drugs, **accidental** (unintentional)
Poisoning by antidiarrheal drugs NOS
T47.6X2 Poisoning by antidiarrheal drugs, **intentional** self-harm A, S
T47.6X3 Poisoning by antidiarrheal drugs, **assault**
T47.6X4 Poisoning by antidiarrheal drugs, undetermined
T47.6X5 **Adverse effect** of antidiarrheal drugs
T47.6X6 **Underdosing** of antidiarrheal drugs

T47.7 Poisoning by, adverse effect of and underdosing of emetics
T47.7X Poisoning by, adverse effect of and underdosing of **emetics**
T47.7X1 Poisoning by emetics, **accidental** (unintentional)
Poisoning by emetics NOS
T47.7X2 Poisoning by emetics, **intentional** self-harm A, S
T47.7X3 Poisoning by emetics, **assault**
T47.7X4 Poisoning by emetics, **undetermined**
T47.7X5 **Adverse effect** of emetics
T47.7X6 **Underdosing** of emetics

T47.8 Poisoning by, adverse effect of and underdosing of other agents primarily affecting gastrointestinal system
T47.8X Poisoning by, adverse effect of and underdosing of **other agents primarily affecting gastrointestinal system**
T47.8X1 Poisoning by other agents primarily affecting gastrointestinal system, **accidental** (unintentional)
Poisoning by other agents primarily affecting gastrointestinal system NOS
T47.8X2 Poisoning by other agents primarily affecting gastrointestinal system, **intentional** self-harm A, S
T47.8X3 Poisoning by other agents primarily affecting gastrointestinal system, **assault**
T47.8X4 Poisoning by other agents primarily affecting gastrointestinal system, **undetermined**
T47.8X5 **Adverse effect** of other agents primarily affecting gastrointestinal system
T47.8X6 **Underdosing** of other agents primarily affecting gastrointestinal system

T47.9 Poisoning by, adverse effect of and underdosing of **unspecified agents primarily affecting the gastrointestinal system**

X T47.91 Poisoning by unspecified agents primarily affecting the gastrointestinal system, **accidental** (unintentional)
Poisoning by agents primarily affecting the gastrointestinal system NOS

X T47.92 Poisoning by unspecified agents primarily affecting the gastrointestinal system, **intentional** self-harm A, S

X T47.93 Poisoning by unspecified agents primarily affecting the gastrointestinal system, **assault**

X T47.94 Poisoning by unspecified agents primarily affecting the gastrointestinal system, **undetermined**

X T47.95 **Adverse effect** of unspecified agents primarily affecting the gastrointestinal system

X T47.96 **Underdosing** of unspecified agents primarily affecting the gastrointestinal system

T48 Poisoning by, adverse effect of and underdosing of agents primarily acting on smooth and skeletal muscles and the respiratory system

The appropriate 7th character is to be added to each code from category T48

A	initial encounter
D	subsequent encounter
S	sequela

T48.0 Poisoning by, adverse effect of and underdosing of oxytocic drugs

Excludes1 poisoning by, adverse effect of and underdosing of estrogens, progestogens and antagonists (T38.4-T38.6)

T48.0X Poisoning by, adverse effect of and underdosing of **oxytocic drugs**

T48.0X1 Poisoning by oxytocic drugs, **accidental** (unintentional)
Poisoning by oxytocic drugs NOS

T48.0X2 Poisoning by oxytocic drugs, **intentional** self-harm A, S

T48.0X3 Poisoning by oxytocic drugs, **assault**

T48.0X4 Poisoning by oxytocic drugs, **undetermined**

T48.0X5 **Adverse effect** of oxytocic drugs

T48.0X6 **Underdosing** of oxytocic drugs

T48.1 Poisoning by, adverse effect of and underdosing of skeletal muscle relaxants [neuromuscular blocking agents]

T48.1X Poisoning by, adverse effect of and underdosing of **skeletal muscle relaxants** [neuromuscular blocking agents]

T48.1X1 Poisoning by skeletal muscle relaxants [neuromuscular blocking agents], **accidental** (unintentional)
Poisoning by skeletal muscle relaxants [neuromuscular blocking agents] NOS

T48.1X2 Poisoning by skeletal muscle relaxants [neuromuscular blocking agents], **intentional** self-harm A, S

T48.1X3 Poisoning by skeletal muscle relaxants [neuromuscular blocking agents], **assault**

T48.1X4 Poisoning by skeletal muscle relaxants [neuromuscular blocking agents], **undetermined**

T48.1X5 **Adverse effect** of skeletal muscle relaxants [neuromuscular blocking agents]

T48.1X6 **Underdosing** of skeletal muscle relaxants [neuromuscular blocking agents]

T48.2 Poisoning by, adverse effect of and underdosing of other and unspecified drugs acting on muscles

T48.20 Poisoning by, adverse effect of and underdosing of **unspecified drugs acting on muscles**

T48.201 Poisoning by unspecified drugs acting on muscles, **accidental** (unintentional)
Poisoning by unspecified drugs acting on muscles NOS

T48.202 Poisoning by unspecified drugs acting on muscles, **intentional** self-harm A, S

T48.203 Poisoning by unspecified drugs acting on muscles, **assault**

T48.204 Poisoning by unspecified drugs acting on muscles, **undetermined**

T48.205 **Adverse effect** of unspecified drugs acting on muscles

T48.206 **Underdosing** of unspecified drugs acting on muscles

T48.29 Poisoning by, adverse effect of and underdosing of **other drugs acting on muscles**

T48.291 Poisoning by other drugs acting on muscles, **accidental** (unintentional)
Poisoning by other drugs acting on muscles NOS

T48.292 Poisoning by other drugs acting on muscles, **intentional** self-harm A, S

T48.293 Poisoning by other drugs acting on muscles, **assault**

T48.294 Poisoning by other drugs acting on muscles, **undetermined**

T48.295 **Adverse effect** of other drugs acting on muscles

T48.296 **Underdosing** of other drugs acting on muscles

T48.3 Poisoning by, adverse effect of and underdosing of antitussives

T48.3X Poisoning by, adverse effect of and underdosing of **antitussives**

T48.3X1 Poisoning by antitussives, **accidental** (unintentional)
Poisoning by antitussives NOS

T48.3X2 Poisoning by antitussives, **intentional** self-harm A, S

T48.3X3 Poisoning by antitussives, **assault**

T48.3X4 Poisoning by antitussives, **undetermined**

T48.3X5 **Adverse effect** of antitussives

T48.3X6 **Underdosing** of antitussives

T48.4 Poisoning by, adverse effect of and underdosing of expectorants

T48.4X Poisoning by, adverse effect of and underdosing of **expectorants**

T48.4X1 Poisoning by expectorants, **accidental** (unintentional)
Poisoning by expectorants NOS

T48.4X2 Poisoning by expectorants, **intentional** self-harm A, S

T48.4X3 Poisoning by expectorants, **assault**

T48.4X4 Poisoning by expectorants, **undetermined**

T48.4X5 **Adverse effect** of expectorants

T48.4X6 **Underdosing** of expectorants

T48.5 Poisoning by, adverse effect of and underdosing of other anti-common-cold drugs
Poisoning by, adverse effect of and underdosing of decongestants
Excludes2 poisoning by, adverse effect of and underdosing of antipyretics, NEC (T39.9-)
poisoning by, adverse effect of and underdosing of non-steroidal antiinflammatory drugs (T39.3-)
poisoning by, adverse effect of and underdosing of salicylates (T39.Ø-)

T48.5X Poisoning by, adverse effect of and underdosing of other anti-common-cold drugs

T48.5X1 Poisoning by other anti-common-cold drugs, accidental (unintentional)
Poisoning by other anti-common-cold drugs NOS

T48.5X2 Poisoning by other anti-common-cold drugs, intentional self-harm A, S

T48.5X3 Poisoning by other anti-common-cold drugs, assault

T48.5X4 Poisoning by other anti-common-cold drugs, undetermined

T48.5X5 Adverse effect of other anti-common-cold drugs

T48.5X6 Underdosing of other anti-common-cold drugs

T48.6 Poisoning by, adverse effect of and underdosing of antiasthmatics, not elsewhere classified
Poisoning by, adverse effect of and underdosing of beta-adrenoreceptor agonists used in asthma therapy
Excludes1 poisoning by, adverse effect of and underdosing of beta-adrenoreceptor agonists not used in asthma therapy (T44.5)
poisoning by, adverse effect of and underdosing of anterior pituitary [adenohypophyseal] hormones (T38.8)

T48.6X Poisoning by, adverse effect of and underdosing of antiasthmatics

T48.6X1 Poisoning by antiasthmatics, accidental (unintentional)
Poisoning by antiasthmatics NOS

T48.6X2 Poisoning by antiasthmatics, intentional self-harm A, S

T48.6X3 Poisoning by antiasthmatics, assault

T48.6X4 Poisoning by antiasthmatics, undetermined

T48.6X5 Adverse effect of antiasthmatics

T48.6X6 Underdosing of antiasthmatics

T48.9 Poisoning by, adverse effect of and underdosing of other and unspecified agents primarily acting on the respiratory system

T48.9Ø Poisoning by, adverse effect of and underdosing of unspecified agents primarily acting on the respiratory system

T48.9Ø1 Poisoning by unspecified agents primarily acting on the respiratory system, accidental (unintentional)

T48.9Ø2 Poisoning by unspecified agents primarily acting on the respiratory system, intentional self-harm A, S

T48.9Ø3 Poisoning by unspecified agents primarily acting on the respiratory system, assault

T48.9Ø4 Poisoning by unspecified agents primarily acting on the respiratory system, undetermined

T48.9Ø5 Adverse effect of unspecified agents primarily acting on the respiratory system

T48.9Ø6 Underdosing of unspecified agents primarily acting on the respiratory system

T48.99 Poisoning by, adverse effect of and underdosing of other agents primarily acting on the respiratory system

T48.991 Poisoning by other agents primarily acting on the respiratory system, accidental (unintentional)

T48.992 Poisoning by other agents primarily acting on the respiratory system, intentional self-harm A, S

T48.993 Poisoning by other agents primarily acting on the respiratory system, assault

T48.994 Poisoning by other agents primarily acting on the respiratory system, undetermined

T48.995 Adverse effect of other agents primarily acting on the respiratory system

T48.996 Underdosing of other agents primarily acting on the respiratory system

T49 Poisoning by, adverse effect of and underdosing of topical agents primarily affecting skin and mucous membrane and by ophthalmological, otorhinorlaryngological and dental drugs
Includes poisoning by, adverse effect of and underdosing of glucocorticoids, topically used
The appropriate 7th character is to be added to each code from category T49

A	initial encounter
D	subsequent encounter
S	sequela

T49.Ø Poisoning by, adverse effect of and underdosing of local antifungal, anti-infective and anti-inflammatory drugs

T49.ØX Poisoning by, adverse effect of and underdosing of local antifungal, anti-infective and anti-inflammatory drugs

T49.ØX1 Poisoning by local antifungal, anti-infective and anti-inflammatory drugs, accidental (unintentional)
Poisoning by local antifungal, anti-infective and anti-inflammatory drugs NOS

T49.ØX2 Poisoning by local antifungal, anti-infective and anti-inflammatory drugs, intentional self-harm A, S

T49.ØX3 Poisoning by local antifungal, anti-infective and anti-inflammatory drugs, assault

T49.ØX4 Poisoning by local antifungal, anti-infective and anti-inflammatory drugs, undetermined

T49.ØX5 Adverse effect of local antifungal, anti-infective and anti-inflammatory drugs

T49.ØX6 Underdosing of local antifungal, anti-infective and anti-inflammatory drugs

- T49.1 Poisoning by, adverse effect of and underdosing of antipruritics
  - T49.1X Poisoning by, adverse effect of and underdosing of **antipruritics**
    - T49.1X1 Poisoning by antipruritics, **accidental** (unintentional)
      Poisoning by antipruritics NOS
    - T49.1X2 Poisoning by antipruritics, **intentional** self-harm A, S
    - T49.1X3 Poisoning by antipruritics, **assault**
    - T49.1X4 Poisoning by antipruritics, **undetermined**
    - T49.1X5 **Adverse effect** of antipruritics
    - T49.1X6 **Underdosing** of antipruritics
- T49.2 Poisoning by, adverse effect of and underdosing of local astringents and local detergents
  - T49.2X Poisoning by, adverse effect of and underdosing of **local astringents and local detergents**
    - T49.2X1 Poisoning by local astringents and local detergents, **accidental** (unintentional)
      Poisoning by local astringents and local detergents NOS
    - T49.2X2 Poisoning by local astringents and local detergents, **intentional** self-harm A, S
    - T49.2X3 Poisoning by local astringents and local detergents, **assault**
    - T49.2X4 Poisoning by local astringents and local detergents, **undetermined**
    - T49.2X5 **Adverse effect** of local astringents and local detergents
    - T49.2X6 **Underdosing** of local astringents and local detergents
- T49.3 Poisoning by, adverse effect of and underdosing of emollients, demulcents and protectants
  - T49.3X Poisoning by, adverse effect of and underdosing of **emollients, demulcents and protectants**
    - T49.3X1 Poisoning by emollients, demulcents and protectants, **accidental** (unintentional)
      Poisoning by emollients, demulcents and protectants NOS
    - T49.3X2 Poisoning by emollients, demulcents and protectants, **intentional** self-harm A, S
    - T49.3X3 Poisoning by emollients, demulcents and protectants, **assault**
    - T49.3X4 Poisoning by emollients, demulcents and protectants, **undetermined**
    - T49.3X5 **Adverse effect** of emollients, demulcents and protectants
    - T49.3X6 **Underdosing** of emollients, demulcents and protectants
- T49.4 Poisoning by, adverse effect of and underdosing of keratolytics, keratoplastics, and other hair treatment drugs and preparations
  - T49.4X Poisoning by, adverse effect of and underdosing of **keratolytics, keratoplastics, and other hair treatment drugs and preparations**
    - T49.4X1 Poisoning by keratolytics, keratoplastics, and other hair treatment drugs and preparations, **accidental** (unintentional)
      Poisoning by keratolytics, keratoplastics, and other hair treatment drugs and preparations NOS
    - T49.4X2 Poisoning by keratolytics, keratoplastics, and other hair treatment drugs and preparations, **intentional** self-harm A, S
    - T49.4X3 Poisoning by keratolytics, keratoplastics, and other hair treatment drugs and preparations, **assault**
    - T49.4X4 Poisoning by keratolytics, keratoplastics, and other hair treatment drugs and preparations, **undetermined**
    - T49.4X5 **Adverse effect** of keratolytics, keratoplastics, and other hair treatment drugs and preparations
    - T49.4X6 **Underdosing** of keratolytics, keratoplastics, and other hair treatment drugs and preparations
- T49.5 Poisoning by, adverse effect of and underdosing of ophthalmological drugs and preparations
  - T49.5X Poisoning by, adverse effect of and underdosing of **ophthalmological drugs and preparations**
    - T49.5X1 Poisoning by ophthalmological drugs and preparations, **accidental** (unintentional)
      Poisoning by ophthalmological drugs and preparations NOS
    - T49.5X2 Poisoning by ophthalmological drugs and preparations, **intentional** self-harm A, S
    - T49.5X3 Poisoning by ophthalmological drugs and preparations, **assault**
    - T49.5X4 Poisoning by ophthalmological drugs and preparations, **undetermined**
    - T49.5X5 **Adverse effect** of ophthalmological drugs and preparations
    - T49.5X6 **Underdosing** of ophthalmological drugs and preparations
- T49.6 Poisoning by, adverse effect of and underdosing of otorhinolaryngological drugs and preparations
  - T49.6X Poisoning by, adverse effect of and underdosing of **otorhinolaryngological drugs and preparations**
    - T49.6X1 Poisoning by otorhinolaryngological drugs and preparations, **accidental** (unintentional)
      Poisoning by otorhinolaryngological drugs and preparations NOS
    - T49.6X2 Poisoning by otorhinolaryngological drugs and preparations, **intentional** self-harm A, S
    - T49.6X3 Poisoning by otorhinolaryngological drugs and preparations, **assault**
    - T49.6X4 Poisoning by otorhinolaryngological drugs and preparations, **undetermined**
    - T49.6X5 **Adverse effect** of otorhinolaryngological drugs and preparations
    - T49.6X6 **Underdosing** of otorhinolaryngological drugs and preparations
- T49.7 Poisoning by, adverse effect of and underdosing of dental drugs, topically applied
  - T49.7X Poisoning by, adverse effect of and underdosing of **dental drugs, topically applied**
    - T49.7X1 Poisoning by dental drugs, topically applied, **accidental** (unintentional)
      Poisoning by dental drugs, topically applied NOS
    - T49.7X2 Poisoning by dental drugs, topically applied, **intentional** self-harm A, S

T49.7X3 Poisoning by dental drugs, topically applied, **assault**

T49.7X4 Poisoning by dental drugs, topically applied, **undetermined**

T49.7X5 **Adverse effect** of dental drugs, topically applied

T49.7X6 **Underdosing** of dental drugs, topically applied

T49.8 Poisoning by, adverse effect of and underdosing of other topical agents

Poisoning by, adverse effect of and underdosing of spermicides

T49.8X Poisoning by, adverse effect of and underdosing of **other topical agents**

T49.8X1 Poisoning by other topical agents, **accidental** (unintentional)

Poisoning by other topical agents NOS

T49.8X2 Poisoning by other topical agents, **intentional** self-harm A, S

T49.8X3 Poisoning by other topical agents, **assault**

T49.8X4 Poisoning by other topical agents, **undetermined**

T49.8X5 **Adverse effect** of other topical agents

T49.8X6 **Underdosing** of other topical agents

T49.9 Poisoning by, adverse effect of and underdosing of **unspecified topical agent**

X T49.91 Poisoning by unspecified topical agent, **accidental** (unintentional)

X T49.92 Poisoning by unspecified topical agent, **intentional** self-harm A, S

X T49.93 Poisoning by unspecified topical agent, **assault**

X T49.94 Poisoning by unspecified topical agent, **undetermined**

X T49.95 **Adverse effect** of unspecified topical agent

X T49.96 **Underdosing** of unspecified topical agent

T50 Poisoning by, adverse effect of and underdosing of diuretics and other and unspecified drugs, medicaments and biological substances

The appropriate 7th character is to be added to each code from category T50

A	initial encounter
D	subsequent encounter
S	sequela

T50.0 Poisoning by, adverse effect of and underdosing of mineralocorticoids and their antagonists

T50.0X Poisoning by, adverse effect of and underdosing of **mineralocorticoids and their antagonists**

T50.0X1 Poisoning by mineralocorticoids and their antagonists, **accidental** (unintentional)

Poisoning by mineralocorticoids and their antagonists NOS

T50.0X2 Poisoning by mineralocorticoids and their antagonists, **intentional** self-harm A, S

T50.0X3 Poisoning by mineralocorticoids and their antagonists, **assault**

T50.0X4 Poisoning by mineralocorticoids and their antagonists, **undetermined**

T50.0X5 **Adverse effect** of mineralocorticoids and their antagonists

T50.0X6 **Underdosing** of mineralocorticoids and their antagonists

T50.1 Poisoning by, adverse effect of and underdosing of loop [high-ceiling] diuretics

T50.1X Poisoning by, adverse effect of and underdosing of **loop** [high-ceiling] **diuretics**

T50.1X1 Poisoning by loop [high-ceiling] diuretics, **accidental** (unintentional)

Poisoning by loop [high-ceiling] diuretics NOS

T50.1X2 Poisoning by loop [high-ceiling] diuretics, **intentional** self-harm A, S

T50.1X3 Poisoning by loop [high-ceiling] diuretics, **assault**

T50.1X4 Poisoning by loop [high-ceiling] diuretics, **undetermined**

T50.1X5 **Adverse effect** of loop [high-ceiling] diuretics

T50.1X6 **Underdosing** of loop [high-ceiling] diuretics

T50.2 Poisoning by, adverse effect of and underdosing of carbonic-anhydrase inhibitors, benzothiadiazides and other diuretics

Poisoning by, adverse effect of and underdosing of acetazolamide

T50.2X Poisoning by, adverse effect of and underdosing of **carbonic-anhydrase inhibitors, benzothiadiazides and other diuretics**

T50.2X1 Poisoning by carbonic-anhydrase inhibitors, benzothiadiazides and other diuretics, **accidental** (unintentional)

Poisoning by carbonic-anhydrase inhibitors, benzothiadiazides and other diuretics NOS

T50.2X2 Poisoning by carbonic-anhydrase inhibitors, benzothiadiazides and other diuretics, **intentional** self-harm A, S

T50.2X3 Poisoning by carbonic-anhydrase inhibitors, benzothiadiazides and other diuretics, **assault**

T50.2X4 Poisoning by carbonic-anhydrase inhibitors, benzothiadiazides and other diuretics, **undetermined**

T50.2X5 **Adverse effect** of carbonic-anhydrase inhibitors, benzothiadiazides and other diuretics

T50.2X6 **Underdosing** of carbonic-anhydrase inhibitors, benzothiadiazides and other diuretics

T50.3 Poisoning by, adverse effect of and underdosing of electrolytic, caloric and water-balance agents

Poisoning by, adverse effect of and underdosing of oral rehydration salts

T50.3X Poisoning by, adverse effect of and underdosing of **electrolytic, caloric and water-balance agents**

T50.3X1 Poisoning by electrolytic, caloric and water-balance agents, **accidental** (unintentional)

Poisoning by electrolytic, caloric and water-balance agents NOS

T50.3X2 Poisoning by electrolytic, caloric and water-balance agents, **intentional** self-harm A, S

T50.3X3 Poisoning by electrolytic, caloric and water-balance agents, **assault**

T50.3X4 Poisoning by electrolytic, caloric and water-balance agents, **undetermined**

T50.3X5 **Adverse effect** of electrolytic, caloric and water-balance agents

T50.3X6 **Underdosing** of electrolytic, caloric and water-balance agents

- **T50.4** Poisoning by, adverse effect of and underdosing of drugs affecting uric acid metabolism
  - **T50.4X** Poisoning by, adverse effect of and underdosing of **drugs affecting uric acid metabolism**
    - **T50.4X1** Poisoning by drugs affecting uric acid metabolism, **accidental** (unintentional)
      Poisoning by drugs affecting uric acid metabolism NOS
    - **T50.4X2** Poisoning by drugs affecting uric acid metabolism, **intentional** self-harm A, S
    - **T50.4X3** Poisoning by drugs affecting uric acid metabolism, **assault**
    - **T50.4X4** Poisoning by drugs affecting uric acid metabolism, **undetermined**
    - **T50.4X5** **Adverse effect** of drugs affecting uric acid metabolism
    - **T50.4X6** **Underdosing** of drugs affecting uric acid metabolism
- **T50.5** Poisoning by, adverse effect of and underdosing of appetite depressants
  - **T50.5X** Poisoning by, adverse effect of and underdosing of **appetite depressants**
    - **T50.5X1** Poisoning by appetite depressants, **accidental** (unintentional)
      Poisoning by appetite depressants NOS
    - **T50.5X2** Poisoning by appetite depressants, **intentional** self-harm A, S
    - **T50.5X3** Poisoning by appetite depressants, **assault**
    - **T50.5X4** Poisoning by appetite depressants, **undetermined**
    - **T50.5X5** **Adverse effect** of appetite depressants
    - **T50.5X6** **Underdosing** of appetite depressants
- **T50.6** Poisoning by, adverse effect of and underdosing of antidotes and chelating agents
  Poisoning by, adverse effect of and underdosing of alcohol deterrents
  - **T50.6X** Poisoning by, adverse effect of and underdosing of **antidotes and chelating agents**
    - **T50.6X1** Poisoning by antidotes and chelating agents, **accidental** (unintentional)
      Poisoning by antidotes and chelating agents NOS
    - **T50.6X2** Poisoning by antidotes and chelating agents, **intentional** self-harm A, S
    - **T50.6X3** Poisoning by antidotes and chelating agents, **assault**
    - **T50.6X4** Poisoning by antidotes and chelating agents, **undetermined**
    - **T50.6X5** **Adverse effect** of antidotes and chelating agents
    - **T50.6X6** **Underdosing** of antidotes and chelating agents
- **T50.7** Poisoning by, adverse effect of and underdosing of analeptics and opioid receptor antagonists
  - **T50.7X** Poisoning by, adverse effect of and underdosing of **analeptics and opioid receptor antagonists**
    - **T50.7X1** Poisoning by analeptics and opioid receptor antagonists, **accidental** (unintentional)
      Poisoning by analeptics and opioid receptor antagonists NOS
    - **T50.7X2** Poisoning by analeptics and opioid receptor antagonists, **intentional** self-harm A, S
    - **T50.7X3** Poisoning by analeptics and opioid receptor antagonists, **assault**
    - **T50.7X4** Poisoning by analeptics and opioid receptor antagonists, **undetermined**
    - **T50.7X5** **Adverse effect** of analeptics and opioid receptor antagonists
    - **T50.7X6** **Underdosing** of analeptics and opioid receptor antagonists
- **T50.8** Poisoning by, adverse effect of and underdosing of diagnostic agents
  - **T50.8X** Poisoning by, adverse effect of and underdosing of **diagnostic agents**
    - **T50.8X1** Poisoning by diagnostic agents, **accidental** (unintentional)
      Poisoning by diagnostic agents NOS
    - **T50.8X2** Poisoning by diagnostic agents, **intentional** self-harm A, S
    - **T50.8X3** Poisoning by diagnostic agents, **assault**
    - **T50.8X4** Poisoning by diagnostic agents, **undetermined**
    - **T50.8X5** **Adverse effect** of diagnostic agents
    - **T50.8X6** **Underdosing** of diagnostic agents
- **T50.A** Poisoning by, adverse effect of and underdosing of bacterial vaccines
  - **T50.A1** Poisoning by, adverse effect of and underdosing of **pertussis vaccine, including combinations with a pertussis component**
    - **T50.A11** Poisoning by pertussis vaccine, including combinations with a pertussis component, **accidental** (unintentional)
    - **T50.A12** Poisoning by pertussis vaccine, including combinations with a pertussis component, **intentional** self-harm A, S
    - **T50.A13** Poisoning by pertussis vaccine, including combinations with a pertussis component, **assault**
    - **T50.A14** Poisoning by pertussis vaccine, including combinations with a pertussis component, **undetermined**
    - **T50.A15** **Adverse effect** of pertussis vaccine, including combinations with a pertussis component
    - **T50.A16** **Underdosing** of pertussis vaccine, including combinations with a pertussis component
  - **T50.A2** Poisoning by, adverse effect of and underdosing of **mixed bacterial vaccines without a pertussis component**
    - **T50.A21** Poisoning by mixed bacterial vaccines without a pertussis component, **accidental** (unintentional)
    - **T50.A22** Poisoning by mixed bacterial vaccines without a pertussis component, **intentional** self-harm A, S
    - **T50.A23** Poisoning by mixed bacterial vaccines without a pertussis component, **assault**
    - **T50.A24** Poisoning by mixed bacterial vaccines without a pertussis component, **undetermined**
    - **T50.A25** **Adverse effect** of mixed bacterial vaccines without a pertussis component
    - **T50.A26** **Underdosing** of mixed bacterial vaccines without a pertussis component

T50.A9 Poisoning by, adverse effect of and underdosing of other bacterial vaccines
- T50.A91 Poisoning by other bacterial vaccines, accidental (unintentional)
- T50.A92 Poisoning by other bacterial vaccines, intentional self-harm A, S
- T50.A93 Poisoning by other bacterial vaccines, assault
- T50.A94 Poisoning by other bacterial vaccines, undetermined
- T50.A95 Adverse effect of other bacterial vaccines
- T50.A96 Underdosing of other bacterial vaccines

T50.B Poisoning by, adverse effect of and underdosing of viral vaccines

T50.B1 Poisoning by, adverse effect of and underdosing of smallpox vaccines
- T50.B11 Poisoning by smallpox vaccines, accidental (unintentional)
- T50.B12 Poisoning by smallpox vaccines, intentional self-harm A, S
- T50.B13 Poisoning by smallpox vaccines, assault
- T50.B14 Poisoning by smallpox vaccines, undetermined
- T50.B15 Adverse effect of smallpox vaccines
- T50.B16 Underdosing of smallpox vaccines

T50.B9 Poisoning by, adverse effect of and underdosing of other viral vaccines
- T50.B91 Poisoning by other viral vaccines, accidental (unintentional)
- T50.B92 Poisoning by other viral vaccines, intentional self-harm A, S
- T50.B93 Poisoning by other viral vaccines, assault
- T50.B94 Poisoning by other viral vaccines, undetermined
- T50.B95 Adverse effect of other viral vaccines
- T50.B96 Underdosing of other viral vaccines

T50.Z Poisoning by, adverse effect of and underdosing of other vaccines and biological substances

T50.Z1 Poisoning by, adverse effect of and underdosing of immunoglobulin
- T50.Z11 Poisoning by immunoglobulin, accidental (unintentional)
- T50.Z12 Poisoning by immunoglobulin, intentional self-harm A, S
- T50.Z13 Poisoning by immunoglobulin, assault
- T50.Z14 Poisoning by immunoglobulin, undetermined
- T50.Z15 Adverse effect of immunoglobulin
- T50.Z16 Underdosing of immunoglobulin

T50.Z9 Poisoning by, adverse effect of and underdosing of other vaccines and biological substances
- T50.Z91 Poisoning by other vaccines and biological substances, accidental (unintentional)
- T50.Z92 Poisoning by other vaccines and biological substances, intentional self-harm A, S
- T50.Z93 Poisoning by other vaccines and biological substances, assault
- T50.Z94 Poisoning by other vaccines and biological substances, undetermined
- T50.Z95 Adverse effect of other vaccines and biological substances
- T50.Z96 Underdosing of other vaccines and biological substances

T50.9 Poisoning by, adverse effect of and underdosing of other and unspecified drugs, medicaments and biological substances

T50.90 Poisoning by, adverse effect of and underdosing of unspecified drugs, medicaments and biological substances
- T50.901 Poisoning by unspecified drugs, medicaments and biological substances, accidental (unintentional)
  Coding Clinic: 2015, Q1, P21
- T50.902 Poisoning by unspecified drugs, medicaments and biological substances, intentional self-harm A, S
- T50.903 Poisoning by unspecified drugs, medicaments and biological substances, assault
- T50.904 Poisoning by unspecified drugs, medicaments and biological substances, undetermined
- T50.905 Adverse effect of unspecified drugs, medicaments and biological substances
- T50.906 Underdosing of unspecified drugs, medicaments and biological substances

▶T50.91 Poisoning by, adverse effect of and underdosing of multiple unspecified drugs, medicaments and biological substances
▶Multiple drug ingestion NOS
▶Code also any specific drugs, medicaments and biological substances
- ▶T50.911 Poisoning by multiple unspecified drugs, medicaments and biological substances, accidental (unintentional)
- ▶T50.912 Poisoning by multiple unspecified drugs, medicaments and biological substances, intentional self-harm
- ▶T50.913 Poisoning by multiple unspecified drugs, medicaments and biological substances, assault
- ▶T50.914 Poisoning by multiple unspecified drugs, medicaments and biological substances, undetermined
- ▶T50.915 Adverse effect of multiple unspecified drugs, medicaments and biological substances
- ▶T50.916 Underdosing of multiple unspecified drugs, medicaments and biological substances

T50.99 Poisoning by, adverse effect of and underdosing of other drugs, medicaments and biological substances
- T50.991 Poisoning by other drugs, medicaments and biological substances, accidental (unintentional)
- T50.992 Poisoning by other drugs, medicaments and biological substances, intentional self-harm A, S
- T50.993 Poisoning by other drugs, medicaments and biological substances, assault
- T50.994 Poisoning by other drugs, medicaments and biological substances, undetermined
- T50.995 Adverse effect of other drugs, medicaments and biological substances
- T50.996 Underdosing of other drugs, medicaments and biological substances

TOXIC EFFECTS OF SUBSTANCES CHIEFLY NONMEDICINAL AS TO SOURCE (T51-T65)

Note: When no intent is indicated code to accidental. Undetermined intent is only for use when there is specific documentation in the record that the intent of the toxic effect cannot be determined.

Use additional code(s): for all associated manifestations of toxic effect, such as:
respiratory conditions due to external agents (J6Ø-J7Ø)
personal history of foreign body fully removed (Z87.821)
to identify any retained foreign body, if applicable (Z18.-)

Excludes1 contact with and (suspected) exposure to toxic substances (Z77.-)

● **T51 Toxic effect of alcohol**

The appropriate 7th character is to be added to each code from category T51

A	initial encounter
D	subsequent encounter
S	sequela

● T51.Ø Toxic effect of ethanol
Toxic effect of ethyl alcohol
Excludes2 acute alcohol intoxication or 'hangover' effects (F1Ø.129, F1Ø.229, F1Ø.929)
drunkenness (F1Ø.129, F1Ø.229, F1Ø.929)
pathological alcohol intoxication (F1Ø.129, F1Ø.229, F1Ø.929)

● T51.ØX Toxic effect of ethanol
● T51.ØX1 Toxic effect of ethanol, accidental (unintentional)
Toxic effect of ethanol NOS
● T51.ØX2 Toxic effect of ethanol, intentional self-harm A, S
● T51.ØX3 Toxic effect of ethanol, assault
● T51.ØX4 Toxic effect of ethanol, undetermined

● T51.1 Toxic effect of methanol
Toxic effect of methyl alcohol
● T51.1X Toxic effect of methanol
● T51.1X1 Toxic effect of methanol, accidental (unintentional)
Toxic effect of methanol NOS
● T51.1X2 Toxic effect of methanol, intentional self-harm A, S
● T51.1X3 Toxic effect of methanol, assault
● T51.1X4 Toxic effect of methanol, undetermined

● T51.2 Toxic effect of 2-Propanol
Toxic effect of isopropyl alcohol
● T51.2X Toxic effect of 2-Propanol
● T51.2X1 Toxic effect of 2-Propanol, accidental (unintentional)
Toxic effect of 2-Propanol NOS
● T51.2X2 Toxic effect of 2-Propanol, intentional self-harm A, S
● T51.2X3 Toxic effect of 2-Propanol, assault
● T51.2X4 Toxic effect of 2-Propanol, undetermined

● T51.3 Toxic effect of fusel oil
Toxic effect of amyl alcohol
Toxic effect of butyl [1-butanol] alcohol
Toxic effect of propyl [1-propanol] alcohol
● T51.3X Toxic effect of fusel oil
● T51.3X1 Toxic effect of fusel oil, accidental (unintentional)
Toxic effect of fusel oil NOS
● T51.3X2 Toxic effect of fusel oil, intentional self-harm A, S
● T51.3X3 Toxic effect of fusel oil, assault
● T51.3X4 Toxic effect of fusel oil, undetermined

● T51.8 Toxic effect of other alcohols
● T51.8X Toxic effect of other alcohols
● T51.8X1 Toxic effect of other alcohols, accidental (unintentional)
Toxic effect of other alcohols NOS
● T51.8X2 Toxic effect of other alcohols, intentional self-harm A, S
● T51.8X3 Toxic effect of other alcohols, assault
● T51.8X4 Toxic effect of other alcohols, undetermined

● T51.9 Toxic effect of unspecified alcohol
X● T51.91 Toxic effect of unspecified alcohol, accidental (unintentional)
X● T51.92 Toxic effect of unspecified alcohol, intentional self-harm A, S
X● T51.93 Toxic effect of unspecified alcohol, assault
X● T51.94 Toxic effect of unspecified alcohol, undetermined

● **T52 Toxic effect of organic solvents**

Excludes1 halogen derivatives of aliphatic and aromatic hydrocarbons (T53.-)

The appropriate 7th character is to be added to each code from category T52

A	initial encounter
D	subsequent encounter
S	sequela

● T52.Ø Toxic effects of petroleum products
Toxic effects of gasoline [petrol]
Toxic effects of kerosene [paraffin oil]
Toxic effects of paraffin wax
Toxic effects of ether petroleum
Toxic effects of naphtha petroleum
Toxic effects of spirit petroleum
● T52.ØX Toxic effects of petroleum products
● T52.ØX1 Toxic effect of petroleum products, accidental (unintentional)
Toxic effects of petroleum products NOS
● T52.ØX2 Toxic effect of petroleum products, intentional self-harm A, S
● T52.ØX3 Toxic effect of petroleum products, assault
● T52.ØX4 Toxic effect of petroleum products, undetermined

● T52.1 Toxic effects of benzene
Excludes1 homologues of benzene (T52.2)
nitroderivatives and aminoderivatives of benzene and its homologues (T65.3)
● T52.1X Toxic effects of benzene
● T52.1X1 Toxic effect of benzene, accidental (unintentional)
Toxic effects of benzene NOS
● T52.1X2 Toxic effect of benzene, intentional self-harm A, S
● T52.1X3 Toxic effect of benzene, assault
● T52.1X4 Toxic effect of benzene, undetermined

● T52.2 Toxic effects of homologues of benzene
Toxic effects of toluene [methylbenzene]
Toxic effects of xylene [dimethylbenzene]
● T52.2X Toxic effects of homologues of benzene
● T52.2X1 Toxic effect of homologues of benzene, accidental (unintentional)
Toxic effects of homologues of benzene NOS
● T52.2X2 Toxic effect of homologues of benzene, intentional self-harm A, S
● T52.2X3 Toxic effect of homologues of benzene, assault
● T52.2X4 Toxic effect of homologues of benzene, undetermined

T52.3 Toxic effects of glycols
T52.3X Toxic effects of glycols
T52.3X1 Toxic effect of glycols, accidental (unintentional)
Toxic effects of glycols NOS
T52.3X2 Toxic effect of glycols, intentional self-harm A, S
T52.3X3 Toxic effect of glycols, assault
T52.3X4 Toxic effect of glycols, undetermined
T52.4 Toxic effects of ketones
T52.4X Toxic effects of ketones
T52.4X1 Toxic effect of ketones, accidental (unintentional)
Toxic effects of ketones NOS
T52.4X2 Toxic effect of ketones, intentional self-harm A, S
T52.4X3 Toxic effect of ketones, assault
T52.4X4 Toxic effect of ketones, undetermined
T52.8 Toxic effects of other organic solvents
T52.8X Toxic effects of other organic solvents
T52.8X1 Toxic effect of other organic solvents, accidental (unintentional)
Toxic effects of other organic solvents NOS
T52.8X2 Toxic effect of other organic solvents, intentional self-harm A, S
T52.8X3 Toxic effect of other organic solvents, assault
T52.8X4 Toxic effect of other organic solvents, undetermined
T52.9 Toxic effects of unspecified organic solvent
X T52.91 Toxic effect of unspecified organic solvent, accidental (unintentional)
X T52.92 Toxic effect of unspecified organic solvent, intentional self-harm A, S
X T52.93 Toxic effect of unspecified organic solvent, assault
X T52.94 Toxic effect of unspecified organic solvent, undetermined

T53 Toxic effect of halogen derivatives of aliphatic and aromatic hydrocarbons
The appropriate 7th character is to be added to each code from category T53

A	initial encounter
D	subsequent encounter
S	sequela

T53.Ø Toxic effects of carbon tetrachloride
Toxic effects of tetrachloromethane
T53.ØX Toxic effects of carbon tetrachloride
T53.ØX1 Toxic effect of carbon tetrachloride, accidental (unintentional)
Toxic effects of carbon tetrachloride NOS
T53.ØX2 Toxic effect of carbon tetrachloride, intentional self-harm A, S
T53.ØX3 Toxic effect of carbon tetrachloride, assault
T53.ØX4 Toxic effect of carbon tetrachloride, undetermined
T53.1 Toxic effects of chloroform
Toxic effects of trichloromethane
T53.1X Toxic effects of chloroform
T53.1X1 Toxic effect of chloroform, accidental (unintentional)
Toxic effects of chloroform NOS
T53.1X2 Toxic effect of chloroform, intentional self-harm A, S
T53.1X3 Toxic effect of chloroform, assault
T53.1X4 Toxic effect of chloroform, undetermined
T53.2 Toxic effects of trichloroethylene
Toxic effects of trichloroethene
T53.2X Toxic effects of trichloroethylene
T53.2X1 Toxic effect of trichloroethylene, accidental (unintentional)
Toxic effects of trichloroethylene NOS
T53.2X2 Toxic effect of trichloroethylene, intentional self-harm A, S
T53.2X3 Toxic effect of trichloroethylene, assault
T53.2X4 Toxic effect of trichloroethylene, undetermined
T53.3 Toxic effects of tetrachloroethylene
Toxic effects of perchloroethylene
Toxic effect of tetrachloroethene
T53.3X Toxic effects of tetrachloroethylene
T53.3X1 Toxic effect of tetrachloroethylene, accidental (unintentional)
Toxic effects of tetrachloroethylene NOS
T53.3X2 Toxic effect of tetrachloroethylene, intentional self-harm A, S
T53.3X3 Toxic effect of tetrachloroethylene, assault
T53.3X4 Toxic effect of tetrachloroethylene, undetermined
T53.4 Toxic effects of dichloromethane
Toxic effects of methylene chloride
T53.4X Toxic effects of dichloromethane
T53.4X1 Toxic effect of dichloromethane, accidental (unintentional)
Toxic effects of dichloromethane NOS
T53.4X2 Toxic effect of dichloromethane, intentional self-harm A, S
T53.4X3 Toxic effect of dichloromethane, assault
T53.4X4 Toxic effect of dichloromethane, undetermined
T53.5 Toxic effects of chlorofluorocarbons
T53.5X Toxic effects of chlorofluorocarbons
T53.5X1 Toxic effect of chlorofluorocarbons, accidental (unintentional)
Toxic effects of chlorofluorocarbons NOS
T53.5X2 Toxic effect of chlorofluorocarbons, intentional self-harm A, S
T53.5X3 Toxic effect of chlorofluorocarbons, assault
T53.5X4 Toxic effect of chlorofluorocarbons, undetermined

T53.6 Toxic effects of other halogen derivatives of aliphatic hydrocarbons

T53.6X Toxic effects of **other halogen derivatives of aliphatic hydrocarbons**

T53.6X1 Toxic effect of other halogen derivatives of aliphatic hydrocarbons, **accidental** (unintentional)
Toxic effects of other halogen derivatives of aliphatic hydrocarbons NOS

T53.6X2 Toxic effect of other halogen derivatives of aliphatic hydrocarbons, **intentional** self-harm A, S

T53.6X3 Toxic effect of other halogen derivatives of aliphatic hydrocarbons, **assault**

T53.6X4 Toxic effect of other halogen derivatives of aliphatic hydrocarbons, **undetermined**

T53.7 Toxic effects of other halogen derivatives of aromatic hydrocarbons

T53.7X Toxic effects of **other halogen derivatives of aromatic hydrocarbons**

T53.7X1 Toxic effect of other halogen derivatives of aromatic hydrocarbons, **accidental** (unintentional)
Toxic effects of other halogen derivatives of aromatic hydrocarbons NOS

T53.7X2 Toxic effect of other halogen derivatives of aromatic hydrocarbons, **intentional** self-harm A, S

T53.7X3 Toxic effect of other halogen derivatives of aromatic hydrocarbons, **assault**

T53.7X4 Toxic effect of other halogen derivatives of aromatic hydrocarbons, **undetermined**

T53.9 Toxic effects of **unspecified halogen derivatives of aliphatic and aromatic hydrocarbons**

X T53.91 Toxic effect of unspecified halogen derivatives of aliphatic and aromatic hydrocarbons, **accidental** (unintentional)

X T53.92 Toxic effect of unspecified halogen derivatives of aliphatic and aromatic hydrocarbons, **intentional** self-harm A, S

X T53.93 Toxic effect of unspecified halogen derivatives of aliphatic and aromatic hydrocarbons, **assault**

X T53.94 Toxic effect of unspecified halogen derivatives of aliphatic and aromatic hydrocarbons, **undetermined**

T54 Toxic effect of corrosive substances

The appropriate 7th character is to be added to each code from category T54

A	initial encounter
D	subsequent encounter
S	sequela

T54.Ø Toxic effects of phenol and phenol homologues

T54.ØX Toxic effects of **phenol and phenol homologues**

T54.ØX1 Toxic effect of phenol and **phenol homologues, accidental** (unintentional)
Toxic effects of phenol and phenol homologues NOS

T54.ØX2 Toxic effect of phenol and phenol homologues, **intentional self-harm** A, S

T54.ØX3 Toxic effect of phenol and phenol homologues, **assault**

T54.ØX4 Toxic effect of phenol and phenol homologues, **undetermined**

T54.1 Toxic effects of other corrosive organic compounds

T54.1X Toxic effects of **other corrosive organic compounds**

T54.1X1 Toxic effect of other corrosive **organic compounds, accidental** (unintentional)
Toxic effects of other corrosive organic compounds NOS

T54.1X2 Toxic effect of other corrosive organic compounds, **intentional self-harm** A, S

T54.1X3 Toxic effect of other corrosive organic compounds, **assault**

T54.1X4 Toxic effect of other corrosive organic compounds, **undetermined**

T54.2 Toxic effects of corrosive acids and acid-like substances
Toxic effects of hydrochloric acid
Toxic effects of sulfuric acid

T54.2X Toxic effects of **corrosive acids and acid-like substances**

T54.2X1 Toxic effect of corrosive acids and acid-like substances, **accidental** (unintentional)
Toxic effects of corrosive acids and acid-like substances NOS

T54.2X2 Toxic effect of corrosive acids and acid-like substances, **intentional** self-harm A, S

T54.2X3 Toxic effect of corrosive acids and acid-like substances, **assault**

T54.2X4 Toxic effect of corrosive acids and acid-like substances, **undetermined**

T54.3 Toxic effects of corrosive alkalis and alkali-like substances
Toxic effects of potassium hydroxide
Toxic effects of sodium hydroxide

T54.3X Toxic effects of **corrosive alkalis and alkali-like substances**

T54.3X1 Toxic effect of corrosive alkalis and alkali-like substances, **accidental** (unintentional)
Toxic effects of corrosive alkalis and alkali-like substances NOS

T54.3X2 Toxic effect of corrosive alkalis and alkali-like substances, **intentional** self-harm A, S

T54.3X3 Toxic effect of corrosive alkalis and alkali-like substances, **assault**

T54.3X4 Toxic effect of corrosive alkalis and alkali-like substances, **undetermined**

T54.9 Toxic effects of **unspecified corrosive substance**

X T54.91 Toxic effect of unspecified corrosive substance, **accidental** (unintentional)

X T54.92 Toxic effect of unspecified corrosive substance, **intentional** self-harm A, S

X T54.93 Toxic effect of unspecified corrosive substance, **assault**

X T54.94 Toxic effect of unspecified corrosive substance, **undetermined**

CHAPTER 19 (SØØ-T88)

T55 Toxic effect of soaps and detergents

The appropriate 7th character is to be added to each code from category T55

A	initial encounter
D	subsequent encounter
S	sequela

T55.Ø Toxic effect of soaps

T55.ØX Toxic effect of soaps

T55.ØX1 Toxic effect of soaps, accidental (unintentional)
Toxic effect of soaps NOS

T55.ØX2 Toxic effect of soaps, intentional self-harm A, S

T55.ØX3 Toxic effect of soaps, assault

T55.ØX4 Toxic effect of soaps, undetermined

T55.1 Toxic effect of detergents

T55.1X Toxic effect of detergents

T55.1X1 Toxic effect of detergents, accidental (unintentional)
Toxic effect of detergents NOS

T55.1X2 Toxic effect of detergents, intentional self-harm A, S

T55.1X3 Toxic effect of detergents, assault

T55.1X4 Toxic effect of detergents, undetermined

T56 Toxic effect of metals

Includes toxic effects of fumes and vapors of metals
toxic effects of metals from all sources, except medicinal substances

Use additional code to identify any retained metal foreign body, if applicable (Z18.Ø-, T18.1-)

Excludes1 arsenic and its compounds (T57.Ø)
manganese and its compounds (T57.2)

The appropriate 7th character is to be added to each code from category T56

A	initial encounter
D	subsequent encounter
S	sequela

T56.Ø Toxic effects of lead and its compounds

T56.ØX Toxic effects of lead and its compounds

T56.ØX1 Toxic effect of lead and its compounds, accidental (unintentional)
Toxic effects of lead and its compounds NOS

T56.ØX2 Toxic effect of lead and its compounds, intentional self-harm A, S

T56.ØX3 Toxic effect of lead and its compounds, assault

T56.ØX4 Toxic effect of lead and its compounds, undetermined

T56.1 Toxic effects of mercury and its compounds

T56.1X Toxic effects of mercury and its compounds

T56.1X1 Toxic effect of mercury and its compounds, accidental (unintentional)
Toxic effects of mercury and its compounds NOS

T56.1X2 Toxic effect of mercury and its compounds, intentional self-harm A, S

T56.1X3 Toxic effect of mercury and its compounds, assault

T56.1X4 Toxic effect of mercury and its compounds, undetermined

T56.2 Toxic effects of chromium and its compounds

T56.2X Toxic effects of chromium and its compounds

T56.2X1 Toxic effect of chromium and its compounds, accidental (unintentional)
Toxic effects of chromium and its compounds NOS

T56.2X2 Toxic effect of chromium and its compounds, intentional self-harm A, S

T56.2X3 Toxic effect of chromium and its compounds, assault

T56.2X4 Toxic effect of chromium and its compounds, undetermined

T56.3 Toxic effects of cadmium and its compounds

T56.3X Toxic effects of cadmium and its compounds

T56.3X1 Toxic effect of cadmium and its compounds, accidental (unintentional)
Toxic effects of cadmium and its compounds NOS

T56.3X2 Toxic effect of cadmium and its compounds, intentional self-harm A, S

T56.3X3 Toxic effect of cadmium and its compounds, assault

T56.3X4 Toxic effect of cadmium and its compounds, undetermined

T56.4 Toxic effects of copper and its compounds

T56.4X Toxic effects of copper and its compounds

T56.4X1 Toxic effect of copper and its compounds, accidental (unintentional)
Toxic effects of copper and its compounds NOS

T56.4X2 Toxic effect of copper and its compounds, intentional self-harm A, S

T56.4X3 Toxic effect of copper and its compounds, assault

T56.4X4 Toxic effect of copper and its compounds, undetermined

T56.5 Toxic effects of zinc and its compounds

T56.5X Toxic effects of zinc and its compounds

T56.5X1 Toxic effect of zinc and its compounds, accidental (unintentional)
Toxic effects of zinc and its compounds NOS

T56.5X2 Toxic effect of zinc and its compounds, intentional self-harm A, S

T56.5X3 Toxic effect of zinc and its compounds, assault

T56.5X4 Toxic effect of zinc and its compounds, undetermined

T56.6 Toxic effects of tin and its compounds

T56.6X Toxic effects of tin and its compounds

T56.6X1 Toxic effect of tin and its compounds, accidental (unintentional)
Toxic effects of tin and its compounds NOS

T56.6X2 Toxic effect of tin and its compounds, intentional self-harm A, S

T56.6X3 Toxic effect of tin and its compounds, assault

T56.6X4 Toxic effect of tin and its compounds, undetermined

● T56.7 Toxic effects of beryllium and its compounds
● T56.7X Toxic effects of **beryllium** and its compounds
● T56.7X1 Toxic effect of beryllium and its compounds, **accidental** (unintentional)
Toxic effects of beryllium and its compounds NOS
● T56.7X2 Toxic effect of beryllium and its compounds, **intentional** self-harm A, S
● T56.7X3 Toxic effect of beryllium and its compounds, **assault**
● T56.7X4 Toxic effect of beryllium and its compounds, **undetermined**
● T56.8 Toxic effects of other metals
● T56.81 Toxic effect of **thallium**
● T56.811 Toxic effect of thallium, **accidental** (unintentional)
Toxic effect of thallium NOS
● T56.812 Toxic effect of thallium, **intentional** self-harm A, S
● T56.813 Toxic effect of thallium, **assault**
● T56.814 Toxic effect of thallium, **undetermined**
● T56.89 Toxic effects of **other metals**
● T56.891 Toxic effect of other metals, **accidental** (unintentional)
Toxic effects of other metals NOS
● T56.892 Toxic effect of other metals, **intentional** self-harm A, S
● T56.893 Toxic effect of other metals, **assault**
● T56.894 Toxic effect of other metals, **undetermined**
● T56.9 Toxic effects of **unspecified** metal
X● T56.91 Toxic effect of unspecified metal, **accidental** (unintentional)
X● T56.92 Toxic effect of unspecified metal, **intentional** self-harm A, S
X● T56.93 Toxic effect of unspecified metal, **assault**
X● T56.94 Toxic effect of unspecified metal, **undetermined**

● T57 Toxic effect of other inorganic substances
The appropriate 7th character is to be added to each code from category T57

A	initial encounter
D	subsequent encounter
S	sequela

● T57.Ø Toxic effect of arsenic and its compounds
● T57.ØX Toxic effect of **arsenic** and its compounds
● T57.ØX1 Toxic effect of arsenic and its compounds, **accidental** (unintentional)
Toxic effect of arsenic and its compounds NOS
● T57.ØX2 Toxic effect of arsenic and its compounds, **intentional** self-harm A, S
● T57.ØX3 Toxic effect of arsenic and its compounds, **assault**
● T57.ØX4 Toxic effect of arsenic and its compounds, **undetermined**
● T57.1 Toxic effect of phosphorus and its compounds
Excludes1 organophosphate insecticides (T6Ø.Ø)
● T57.1X Toxic effect of **phosphorus** and its compounds
● T57.1X1 Toxic effect of phosphorus and its compounds, **accidental** (unintentional)
Toxic effect of phosphorus and its compounds NOS
● T57.1X2 Toxic effect of phosphorus and its compounds, **intentional** self-harm A, S
● T57.1X3 Toxic effect of phosphorus and its compounds, **assault**
● T57.1X4 Toxic effect of phosphorus and its compounds, **undetermined**
● T57.2 Toxic effect of manganese and its compounds
● T57.2X Toxic effect of **manganese** and its compounds
● T57.2X1 Toxic effect of manganese and its compounds, **accidental** (unintentional)
Toxic effect of manganese and its compounds NOS
● T57.2X2 Toxic effect of manganese and its compounds, **intentional** self-harm A, S
● T57.2X3 Toxic effect of manganese and its compounds, **assault**
● T57.2X4 Toxic effect of manganese and its compounds, **undetermined**
● T57.3 Toxic effect of hydrogen cyanide
● T57.3X Toxic effect of **hydrogen cyanide**
● T57.3X1 Toxic effect of hydrogen cyanide, **accidental** (unintentional)
Toxic effect of hydrogen cyanide NOS
● T57.3X2 Toxic effect of hydrogen cyanide, **intentional** self-harm A, S
● T57.3X3 Toxic effect of hydrogen cyanide, **assault**
● T57.3X4 Toxic effect of hydrogen cyanide, **undetermined**
● T57.8 Toxic effect of other specified inorganic substances
● T57.8X Toxic effect of **other specified inorganic substances**
● T57.8X1 Toxic effect of other specified inorganic substances, **accidental** (unintentional)
Toxic effect of other specified inorganic substances NOS
● T57.8X2 Toxic effect of other specified inorganic substances, **intentional** self-harm A, S
● T57.8X3 Toxic effect of other specified inorganic substances, **assault**
● T57.8X4 Toxic effect of other specified inorganic substances, **undetermined**
● T57.9 Toxic effect of **unspecified inorganic substance**
X● T57.91 Toxic effect of unspecified inorganic substance, **accidental** (unintentional)
X● T57.92 Toxic effect of unspecified inorganic substance, **intentional** self-harm A, S
X● T57.93 Toxic effect of unspecified inorganic substance, **assault**
X● T57.94 Toxic effect of unspecified inorganic substance, **undetermined**

● **T58 Toxic effect of carbon monoxide**

Includes asphyxiation from carbon monoxide
toxic effect of carbon monoxide from all sources

The appropriate 7th character is to be added to each code from category T58

A	initial encounter
D	subsequent encounter
S	sequela

● T58.Ø Toxic effect of **carbon monoxide from motor vehicle exhaust**
Toxic effect of exhaust gas from gas engine
Toxic effect of exhaust gas from motor pump

X● T58.Ø1 Toxic effect of carbon monoxide from motor vehicle exhaust, **accidental** (unintentional)

X● T58.Ø2 Toxic effect of carbon monoxide from motor vehicle exhaust, **intentional** self-harm A, S

X● T58.Ø3 Toxic effect of carbon monoxide from motor vehicle exhaust, **assault**

X● T58.Ø4 Toxic effect of carbon monoxide from motor vehicle exhaust, **undetermined**

● T58.1 Toxic effect of **carbon monoxide from utility gas**
Toxic effect of acetylene
Toxic effect of gas NOS used for lighting, heating, cooking
Toxic effect of water gas

X● T58.11 Toxic effect of carbon monoxide from utility gas, **accidental** (unintentional)

X● T58.12 Toxic effect of carbon monoxide from utility gas, **intentional** self-harm A, S

X● T58.13 Toxic effect of carbon monoxide from utility gas, **assault**

X● T58.14 Toxic effect of carbon monoxide from utility gas, **undetermined**

● T58.2 Toxic effect of carbon monoxide from incomplete combustion of other domestic fuels
Toxic effect of carbon monoxide from incomplete combustion of coal, coke, kerosene, wood

● T58.2X Toxic effect of carbon monoxide from incomplete combustion of other domestic fuels

● T58.2X1 Toxic effect of carbon monoxide from incomplete combustion of other domestic fuels, **accidental** (unintentional)

● T58.2X2 Toxic effect of carbon monoxide from incomplete combustion of other domestic fuels, **intentional** self-harm A, S

● T58.2X3 Toxic effect of carbon monoxide from incomplete combustion of other domestic fuels, **assault**

● T58.2X4 Toxic effect of carbon monoxide from incomplete combustion of other domestic fuels, **undetermined**

● T58.8 Toxic effect of carbon monoxide from other source
Toxic effect of carbon monoxide from blast furnace gas
Toxic effect of carbon monoxide from fuels in industrial use
Toxic effect of carbon monoxide from kiln vapor

● T58.8X Toxic effect of carbon monoxide from other source

● T58.8X1 Toxic effect of carbon monoxide from other source, **accidental** (unintentional)

● T58.8X2 Toxic effect of carbon monoxide from other source, **intentional** self-harm A, S

● T58.8X3 Toxic effect of carbon monoxide from other source, **assault**

● T58.8X4 Toxic effect of carbon monoxide from other source, **undetermined**

● T58.9 Toxic effect of **carbon monoxide from unspecified source**

X● T58.91 Toxic effect of carbon monoxide from unspecified source, **accidental** (unintentional)

X● T58.92 Toxic effect of carbon monoxide from unspecified source, **intentional** self-harm A, S

X● T58.93 Toxic effect of carbon monoxide from unspecified source, **assault**

X● T58.94 Toxic effect of carbon monoxide from unspecified source, **undetermined**

● **T59 Toxic effect of other gases, fumes and vapors**

Includes aerosol propellants

Excludes1 chlorofluorocarbons (T53.5)

The appropriate 7th character is to be added to each code from category T59

A	initial encounter
D	subsequent encounter
S	sequela

● T59.Ø Toxic effect of nitrogen oxides

● T59.ØX Toxic effect of **nitrogen oxides**

● T59.ØX1 Toxic effect of nitrogen oxides, **accidental** (unintentional)
Toxic effect of nitrogen oxides NOS

● T59.ØX2 Toxic effect of nitrogen oxides, **intentional** self-harm A, S

● T59.ØX3 Toxic effect of nitrogen oxides, **assault**

● T59.ØX4 Toxic effect of nitrogen oxides, **undetermined**

● T59.1 Toxic effect of sulfur dioxide

● T59.1X Toxic effect of **sulfur dioxide**

● T59.1X1 Toxic effect of sulfur dioxide, **accidental** (unintentional)
Toxic effect of sulfur dioxide NOS

● T59.1X2 Toxic effect of sulfur dioxide, **intentional** self-harm A, S

● T59.1X3 Toxic effect of sulfur dioxide, **assault**

● T59.1X4 Toxic effect of sulfur dioxide, **undetermined**

● T59.2 Toxic effect of formaldehyde

● T59.2X Toxic effect of **formaldehyde**

● T59.2X1 Toxic effect of formaldehyde, **accidental** (unintentional)
Toxic effect of formaldehyde NOS

● T59.2X2 Toxic effect of formaldehyde, **intentional** self-harm A, S

● T59.2X3 Toxic effect of formaldehyde, **assault**

● T59.2X4 Toxic effect of formaldehyde, **undetermined**

● T59.3 Toxic effect of lacrimogenic gas
Toxic effect of tear gas

● T59.3X Toxic effect of **lacrimogenic gas**

● T59.3X1 Toxic effect of lacrimogenic gas, **accidental** (unintentional)
Toxic effect of lacrimogenic gas NOS

● T59.3X2 Toxic effect of lacrimogenic gas, **intentional** self-harm A, S

● T59.3X3 Toxic effect of lacrimogenic gas, **assault**

● T59.3X4 Toxic effect of lacrimogenic gas, **undetermined**

- T59.4 Toxic effect of chlorine gas
  - T59.4X Toxic effect of **chlorine gas**
    - T59.4X1 Toxic effect of chlorine gas, **accidental** (unintentional)
      Toxic effect of chlorine gas NOS
    - T59.4X2 Toxic effect of chlorine gas, **intentional self-harm** A, S
    - T59.4X3 Toxic effect of chlorine gas, **assault**
    - T59.4X4 Toxic effect of chlorine gas, **undetermined**
- T59.5 Toxic effect of fluorine gas and hydrogen fluoride
  - T59.5X Toxic effect of **fluorine gas and hydrogen fluoride**
    - T59.5X1 Toxic effect of fluorine gas and hydrogen fluoride, **accidental** (unintentional)
      Toxic effect of fluorine gas and hydrogen fluoride NOS
    - T59.5X2 Toxic effect of fluorine gas and hydrogen fluoride, **intentional** self-harm A, S
    - T59.5X3 Toxic effect of fluorine gas and hydrogen fluoride, **assault**
    - T59.5X4 Toxic effect of fluorine gas and hydrogen fluoride, **undetermined**
- T59.6 Toxic effect of hydrogen sulfide
  - T59.6X Toxic effect of **hydrogen sulfide**
    - T59.6X1 Toxic effect of hydrogen sulfide, **accidental** (unintentional)
      Toxic effect of hydrogen sulfide NOS
    - T59.6X2 Toxic effect of hydrogen sulfide, **intentional self-harm** A, S
    - T59.6X3 Toxic effect of hydrogen sulfide, **assault**
    - T59.6X4 Toxic effect of hydrogen sulfide, **undetermined**
- T59.7 Toxic effect of carbon dioxide
  - T59.7X Toxic effect of **carbon dioxide**
    - T59.7X1 Toxic effect of carbon dioxide, **accidental** (unintentional)
      Toxic effect of carbon dioxide NOS
    - T59.7X2 Toxic effect of carbon dioxide, **intentional self-harm** A, S
    - T59.7X3 Toxic effect of carbon dioxide, **assault**
    - T59.7X4 Toxic effect of carbon dioxide, **undetermined**
- T59.8 Toxic effect of other specified gases, fumes and vapors
  - T59.81 Toxic effect of **smoke**
    Smoke inhalation
    Excludes2 toxic effect of cigarette (tobacco) smoke (T65.22-)
    - T59.811 Toxic effect of smoke, **accidental** (unintentional)
      Toxic effect of smoke NOS
    - T59.812 Toxic effect of smoke, **intentional** self-harm A, S
    - T59.813 Toxic effect of smoke, **assault**
    - T59.814 Toxic effect of smoke, **undetermined**
  - T59.89 Toxic effect of **other specified gases, fumes and vapors**
    - T59.891 Toxic effect of other specified gases, fumes and vapors, **accidental** (unintentional)
    - T59.892 Toxic effect of other specified gases, fumes and vapors, **intentional** self-harm A, S
    - T59.893 Toxic effect of other specified gases, fumes and vapors, **assault**
    - T59.894 Toxic effect of other specified gases, fumes and vapors, **undetermined**
- T59.9 Toxic effect of **unspecified gases, fumes and vapors**
  - X T59.91 Toxic effect of unspecified gases, fumes and vapors, **accidental** (unintentional)
  - X T59.92 Toxic effect of unspecified gases, fumes and vapors, **intentional** self-harm A, S
  - X T59.93 Toxic effect of unspecified gases, fumes and vapors, **assault**
  - X T59.94 Toxic effect of unspecified gases, fumes and vapors, **undetermined**

T60 Toxic effect of pesticides

Includes toxic effect of wood preservatives

The appropriate 7th character is to be added to each code from category T60

A	initial encounter
D	subsequent encounter
S	sequela

- T60.0 Toxic effect of organophosphate and carbamate insecticides
  - T60.0X Toxic effect of **organophosphate and carbamate insecticides**
    - T60.0X1 Toxic effect of organophosphate and carbamate insecticides, **accidental** (unintentional)
      Toxic effect of organophosphate and carbamate insecticides NOS
    - T60.0X2 Toxic effect of organophosphate and carbamate insecticides, **intentional** self-harm A, S
    - T60.0X3 Toxic effect of organophosphate and carbamate insecticides, **assault**
    - T60.0X4 Toxic effect of organophosphate and carbamate insecticides, **undetermined**
- T60.1 Toxic effect of halogenated insecticides
  Excludes1 chlorinated hydrocarbon (T53.-)
  - T60.1X Toxic effect of **halogenated insecticides**
    - T60.1X1 Toxic effect of halogenated insecticides, **accidental** (unintentional)
      Toxic effect of halogenated insecticides NOS
    - T60.1X2 Toxic effect of halogenated insecticides, **intentional** self-harm A, S
    - T60.1X3 Toxic effect of halogenated insecticides, **assault**
    - T60.1X4 Toxic effect of halogenated insecticides, **undetermined**
- T60.2 Toxic effect of other insecticides
  - T60.2X Toxic effect of **other insecticides**
    - T60.2X1 Toxic effect of other insecticides, **accidental** (unintentional)
      Toxic effect of other insecticides NOS
    - T60.2X2 Toxic effect of other insecticides, **intentional** self-harm A, S
    - T60.2X3 Toxic effect of other insecticides, **assault**
    - T60.2X4 Toxic effect of other insecticides, **undetermined**
- T60.3 Toxic effect of herbicides and fungicides
  - T60.3X Toxic effect of **herbicides and fungicides**
    - T60.3X1 Toxic effect of herbicides and fungicides, **accidental** (unintentional)
      Toxic effect of herbicides and fungicides NOS
    - T60.3X2 Toxic effect of herbicides and fungicides, **intentional** self-harm A, S
    - T60.3X3 Toxic effect of herbicides and fungicides, **assault**
    - T60.3X4 Toxic effect of herbicides and fungicides, **undetermined**

T60.4 Toxic effect of rodenticides

Excludes1 strychnine and its salts (T65.1)
thallium (T56.81-)

T60.4X Toxic effect of rodenticides

T60.4X1 Toxic effect of rodenticides, accidental (unintentional)
Toxic effect of rodenticides NOS

T60.4X2 Toxic effect of rodenticides, intentional self-harm A, S

T60.4X3 Toxic effect of rodenticides, assault

T60.4X4 Toxic effect of rodenticides, undetermined

T60.8 Toxic effect of other pesticides

T60.8X Toxic effect of other pesticides

T60.8X1 Toxic effect of other pesticides, accidental (unintentional)
Toxic effect of other pesticides NOS

T60.8X2 Toxic effect of other pesticides, intentional self-harm A, S

T60.8X3 Toxic effect of other pesticides, assault

T60.8X4 Toxic effect of other pesticides, undetermined

T60.9 Toxic effect of unspecified pesticide

X **T60.91 Toxic effect of unspecified pesticide, accidental (unintentional)**

X **T60.92 Toxic effect of unspecified pesticide, intentional self-harm A, S**

X **T60.93 Toxic effect of unspecified pesticide, assault**

X **T60.94 Toxic effect of unspecified pesticide, undetermined**

T61 Toxic effect of noxious substances eaten as seafood

Excludes1 allergic reaction to food, such as:
anaphylactic reaction or shock due to adverse food reaction (T78.0-)
bacterial foodborne intoxications (A05.-)
dermatitis (L23.6, L25.4, L27.2)
food protein-induced enterocolitis syndrome (K52.21)
food protein-induced enteropathy (K52.22)
gastroenteritis (noninfective) (K52.29)
toxic effect of aflatoxin and other mycotoxins (T64)
toxic effect of cyanides (T65.0-)
toxic effect of harmful algae bloom (T65.82-)
toxic effect of hydrogen cyanide (T57.3-)
toxic effect of mercury (T56.1-)
toxic effect of red tide (T65.82-)

The appropriate 7th character is to be added to each code from category T61

A	initial encounter
D	subsequent encounter
S	sequela

T61.0 Ciguatera fish poisoning

X **T61.01 Ciguatera fish poisoning, accidental (unintentional)**

X **T61.02 Ciguatera fish poisoning, intentional self-harm A, S**

X **T61.03 Ciguatera fish poisoning, assault**

X **T61.04 Ciguatera fish poisoning, undetermined**

T61.1 Scombroid fish poisoning
Histamine-like syndrome

X **T61.11 Scombroid fish poisoning, accidental (unintentional)**

X **T61.12 Scombroid fish poisoning, intentional self-harm A, S**

X **T61.13 Scombroid fish poisoning, assault**

X **T61.14 Scombroid fish poisoning, undetermined**

T61.7 Other fish and shellfish poisoning

T61.77 Other fish poisoning

T61.771 Other fish poisoning, accidental (unintentional)

T61.772 Other fish poisoning, intentional self-harm A, S

T61.773 Other fish poisoning, assault

T61.774 Other fish poisoning, undetermined

T61.78 Other shellfish poisoning

T61.781 Other shellfish poisoning, accidental (unintentional)

T61.782 Other shellfish poisoning, intentional self-harm A, S

T61.783 Other shellfish poisoning, assault

T61.784 Other shellfish poisoning, undetermined

T61.8 Toxic effect of other seafood

T61.8X Toxic effect of other seafood

T61.8X1 Toxic effect of other seafood, accidental (unintentional)

T61.8X2 Toxic effect of other seafood, intentional self-harm A, S

T61.8X3 Toxic effect of other seafood, assault

T61.8X4 Toxic effect of other seafood, undetermined

T61.9 Toxic effect of unspecified seafood

X **T61.91 Toxic effect of unspecified seafood, accidental (unintentional)**

X **T61.92 Toxic effect of unspecified seafood, intentional self-harm A, S**

X **T61.93 Toxic effect of unspecified seafood, assault**

X **T61.94 Toxic effect of unspecified seafood, undetermined**

T62 Toxic effect of other noxious substances eaten as food

Excludes1 allergic reaction to food, such as:
anaphylactic shock (reaction) due to adverse food reaction (T78.0-)
dermatitis (L23.6, L25.4, L27.2)
food protein-induced enterocolitis syndrome (K52.21)
food protein-induced enteropathy (K52.22)
gastroenteritis (noninfective) (K52.29)
bacterial food borne intoxications (A05.-)
toxic effect of aflatoxin and other mycotoxins (T64)
toxic effect of cyanides (T65.0-)
toxic effect of hydrogen cyanide (T57.3-)
toxic effect of mercury (T56.1-)

The appropriate 7th character is to be added to each code from category T62

A	initial encounter
D	subsequent encounter
S	sequela

T62.0 Toxic effect of ingested mushrooms

T62.0X Toxic effect of ingested mushrooms

T62.0X1 Toxic effect of ingested mushrooms, accidental (unintentional)
Toxic effect of ingested mushrooms NOS

T62.0X2 Toxic effect of ingested mushrooms, intentional self-harm A, S

T62.0X3 Toxic effect of ingested mushrooms, assault

T62.0X4 Toxic effect of ingested mushrooms, undetermined

T62.1 Toxic effect of ingested berries

T62.1X Toxic effect of **ingested berries**

T62.1X1 Toxic effect of ingested berries, **accidental** (unintentional)
Toxic effect of ingested berries NOS

T62.1X2 Toxic effect of ingested berries, **intentional** self-harm A, S

T62.1X3 Toxic effect of ingested berries, **assault**

T62.1X4 Toxic effect of ingested berries, **undetermined**

T62.2 Toxic effect of other ingested (parts of) plant(s)

T62.2X Toxic effect of **other ingested** (parts of) **plant(s)**

T62.2X1 Toxic effect of other ingested (parts of) plant(s), **accidental** (unintentional)
Toxic effect of other ingested (parts of) plant(s) NOS

T62.2X2 Toxic effect of other ingested (parts of) plant(s), **intentional** self-harm A, S

T62.2X3 Toxic effect of other ingested (parts of) plant(s), **assault**

T62.2X4 Toxic effect of other ingested (parts of) plant(s), **undetermined**

T62.8 Toxic effect of other specified noxious substances eaten as food

T62.8X Toxic effect of **other specified noxious substances eaten as food**

T62.8X1 Toxic effect of other specified noxious substances eaten as food, **accidental** (unintentional)
Toxic effect of other specified noxious substances eaten as food NOS

T62.8X2 Toxic effect of other specified noxious substances eaten as food, **intentional** self-harm A, S

T62.8X3 Toxic effect of other specified noxious substances eaten as food, **assault**

T62.8X4 Toxic effect of other specified noxious substances eaten as food, **undetermined**

T62.9 Toxic effect of **unspecified noxious substance eaten as food**

X T62.91 Toxic effect of unspecified noxious substance eaten as food, **accidental** (unintentional)
Toxic effect of unspecified noxious substance eaten as food NOS

X T62.92 Toxic effect of unspecified noxious substance eaten as food, **intentional** self-harm A, S

X T62.93 Toxic effect of unspecified noxious substance eaten as food, **assault**

X T62.94 Toxic effect of unspecified noxious substance eaten as food, **undetermined**

T63 Toxic effect of contact with venomous animals and plants

Includes bite or touch of venomous animal
pricked or stuck by thorn or leaf

Excludes2 ingestion of toxic animal or plant (T61.-, T62.-)

The appropriate 7th character is to be added to each code from category T63

A	initial encounter
D	subsequent encounter
S	sequela

T63.Ø Toxic effect of snake venom

T63.ØØ Toxic effect of **unspecified snake venom**

T63.ØØ1 Toxic effect of unspecified snake venom, **accidental** (unintentional)
Toxic effect of unspecified snake venom NOS

T63.ØØ2 Toxic effect of unspecified snake venom, **intentional** self-harm A, S

T63.ØØ3 Toxic effect of **unspecified** snake venom, **assault**

T63.ØØ4 Toxic effect of **unspecified** snake venom, **undetermined**

T63.Ø1 Toxic effect of **rattlesnake venom**

T63.Ø11 Toxic effect of rattlesnake venom, **accidental** (unintentional)
Toxic effect of rattlesnake venom NOS

T63.Ø12 Toxic effect of rattlesnake venom, **intentional** self-harm A, S

T63.Ø13 Toxic effect of rattlesnake venom, **assault**

T63.Ø14 Toxic effect of rattlesnake venom, **undetermined**

T63.Ø2 Toxic effect of **coral snake venom**

T63.Ø21 Toxic effect of coral snake venom, **accidental** (unintentional)
Toxic effect of coral snake venom NOS

T63.Ø22 Toxic effect of coral snake venom, **intentional** self-harm A, S

T63.Ø23 Toxic effect of coral snake venom, **assault**

T63.Ø24 Toxic effect of coral snake venom, **undetermined**

T63.Ø3 Toxic effect of **taipan venom**

T63.Ø31 Toxic effect of taipan venom, **accidental** (unintentional)
Toxic effect of taipan venom NOS

T63.Ø32 Toxic effect of taipan venom, **intentional** self-harm A, S

T63.Ø33 Toxic effect of taipan venom, **assault**

T63.Ø34 Toxic effect of taipan venom, **undetermined**

T63.Ø4 Toxic effect of **cobra venom**

T63.Ø41 Toxic effect of cobra venom, **accidental** (unintentional)
Toxic effect of cobra venom NOS

T63.Ø42 Toxic effect of cobra venom, **intentional** self-harm A, S

T63.Ø43 Toxic effect of cobra venom, **assault**

T63.Ø44 Toxic effect of cobra venom, **undetermined**

T63.06 Toxic effect of venom of **other North and South American snake**
- T63.061 Toxic effect of venom of other North and South American snake, **accidental** (unintentional)
  - Toxic effect of venom of other North and South American snake NOS
- T63.062 Toxic effect of venom of other North and South American snake, **intentional self-harm** A, S
- T63.063 Toxic effect of venom of other North and South American snake, **assault**
- T63.064 Toxic effect of venom of other North and South American snake, **undetermined**

T63.07 Toxic effect of venom of **other Australian snake**
- T63.071 Toxic effect of venom of other Australian snake, **accidental** (unintentional)
  - Toxic effect of venom of other Australian snake NOS
- T63.072 Toxic effect of venom of other Australian snake, **intentional self-harm** A, S
- T63.073 Toxic effect of venom of other Australian snake, **assault**
- T63.074 Toxic effect of venom of other Australian snake, **undetermined**

T63.08 Toxic effect of venom of **other African and Asian snake**
- T63.081 Toxic effect of venom of other African and Asian snake, **accidental** (unintentional)
  - Toxic effect of venom of other African and Asian snake NOS
- T63.082 Toxic effect of venom of other African and Asian snake, **intentional self-harm** A, S
- T63.083 Toxic effect of venom of other African and Asian snake, **assault**
- T63.084 Toxic effect of venom of other African and Asian snake, **undetermined**

T63.09 Toxic effect of venom of **other snake**
- T63.091 Toxic effect of venom of other snake, **accidental** (unintentional)
  - Toxic effect of venom of other snake NOS
- T63.092 Toxic effect of venom of other snake, **intentional self-harm** A, S
- T63.093 Toxic effect of venom of other snake, **assault**
- T63.094 Toxic effect of venom of other snake, **undetermined**

T63.1 Toxic effect of venom of other reptiles

T63.11 Toxic effect of venom of **gila monster**
- T63.111 Toxic effect of venom of gila monster, **accidental** (unintentional)
  - Toxic effect of venom of gila monster NOS
- T63.112 Toxic effect of venom of gila monster, **intentional self-harm** A, S
- T63.113 Toxic effect of venom of gila monster, **assault**
- T63.114 Toxic effect of venom of gila monster, **undetermined**

T63.12 Toxic effect of venom of **other venomous lizard**
- T63.121 Toxic effect of venom of other venomous lizard, **accidental** (unintentional)
  - Toxic effect of venom of other venomous lizard NOS
- T63.122 Toxic effect of venom of other venomous lizard, **intentional self-harm** A, S
- T63.123 Toxic effect of venom of other venomous lizard, **assault**
- T63.124 Toxic effect of venom of other venomous lizard, **undetermined**

T63.19 Toxic effect of venom of **other reptiles**
- T63.191 Toxic effect of venom of other reptiles, **accidental** (unintentional)
  - Toxic effect of venom of other reptiles NOS
- T63.192 Toxic effect of venom of other reptiles, **intentional self-harm** A, S
- T63.193 Toxic effect of venom of other reptiles, **assault**
- T63.194 Toxic effect of venom of other reptiles, **undetermined**

T63.2 Toxic effect of venom of scorpion

T63.2X Toxic effect of venom of scorpion
- T63.2X1 Toxic effect of venom of scorpion, **accidental** (unintentional)
  - Toxic effect of venom of scorpion NOS
- T63.2X2 Toxic effect of venom of scorpion, **intentional self-harm** A, S
- T63.2X3 Toxic effect of venom of scorpion, **assault**
- T63.2X4 Toxic effect of venom of scorpion, **undetermined**

T63.3 Toxic effect of venom of spider

T63.30 Toxic effect of **unspecified spider venom**
- T63.301 Toxic effect of unspecified spider venom, **accidental** (unintentional)
- T63.302 Toxic effect of unspecified spider venom, **intentional self-harm** A, S
- T63.303 Toxic effect of unspecified spider venom, **assault**
- T63.304 Toxic effect of unspecified spider venom, **undetermined**

T63.31 Toxic effect of venom of **black widow spider**
- T63.311 Toxic effect of venom of black widow spider, **accidental** (unintentional)
- T63.312 Toxic effect of venom of black widow spider, **intentional self-harm** A, S
- T63.313 Toxic effect of venom of black widow spider, **assault**
- T63.314 Toxic effect of venom of black widow spider, **undetermined**

T63.32 Toxic effect of venom of **tarantula**
- T63.321 Toxic effect of venom of tarantula, **accidental** (unintentional)
- T63.322 Toxic effect of venom of tarantula, **intentional self-harm** A, S
- T63.323 Toxic effect of venom of tarantula, **assault**
- T63.324 Toxic effect of venom of tarantula, **undetermined**

T63.33 Toxic effect of **venom of brown recluse spider**
- T63.331 Toxic effect of venom of brown recluse spider, **accidental** (unintentional)
- T63.332 Toxic effect of venom of brown recluse spider, **intentional** self-harm A, S
- T63.333 Toxic effect of venom of brown recluse spider, **assault**
- T63.334 Toxic effect of venom of brown recluse spider, **undetermined**

T63.39 Toxic effect of **venom of other spider**
- T63.391 Toxic effect of venom of other spider, **accidental** (unintentional)
- T63.392 Toxic effect of venom of other spider, **intentional** self-harm A, S
- T63.393 Toxic effect of venom of other spider, **assault**
- T63.394 Toxic effect of venom of other spider, **undetermined**

T63.4 Toxic effect of venom of other arthropods

T63.41 Toxic effect of **venom of centipedes and venomous millipedes**
- T63.411 Toxic effect of venom of centipedes and venomous millipedes, **accidental** (unintentional)
- T63.412 Toxic effect of venom of centipedes and venomous millipedes, **intentional** self-harm A, S
- T63.413 Toxic effect of venom of centipedes and venomous millipedes, **assault**
- T63.414 Toxic effect of venom of centipedes and venomous millipedes, **undetermined**

T63.42 Toxic effect of **venom of ants**
- T63.421 Toxic effect of venom of ants, **accidental** (unintentional)
- T63.422 Toxic effect of venom of ants, **intentional** self-harm A, S
- T63.423 Toxic effect of venom of ants, **assault**
- T63.424 Toxic effect of venom of ants, **undetermined**

T63.43 Toxic effect of **venom of caterpillars**
- T63.431 Toxic effect of venom of caterpillars, **accidental** (unintentional)
- T63.432 Toxic effect of venom of caterpillars, **intentional** self-harm A, S
- T63.433 Toxic effect of venom of caterpillars, **assault**
- T63.434 Toxic effect of venom of caterpillars, **undetermined**

T63.44 Toxic effect of **venom of bees**
- T63.441 Toxic effect of venom of bees, **accidental** (unintentional)
- T63.442 Toxic effect of venom of bees, **intentional** self-harm A, S
- T63.443 Toxic effect of venom of bees, **assault**
- T63.444 Toxic effect of venom of bees, **undetermined**

T63.45 Toxic effect of **venom of hornets**
- T63.451 Toxic effect of venom of hornets, **accidental** (unintentional)
- T63.452 Toxic effect of venom of hornets, **intentional** self-harm A, S
- T63.453 Toxic effect of venom of hornets, **assault**
- T63.454 Toxic effect of venom of hornets, **undetermined**

T63.46 Toxic effect of **venom of wasps**

Toxic effect of yellow jacket
- T63.461 Toxic effect of venom of wasps, **accidental** (unintentional)
- T63.462 Toxic effect of venom of wasps, **intentional** self-harm A, S
- T63.463 Toxic effect of venom of wasps, **assault**
- T63.464 Toxic effect of venom of wasps, **undetermined**

T63.48 Toxic effect of **venom of other arthropod**
- T63.481 Toxic effect of venom of other arthropod, **accidental** (unintentional)
- T63.482 Toxic effect of venom of other arthropod, **intentional** self-harm A, S
- T63.483 Toxic effect of venom of other arthropod, **assault**
- T63.484 Toxic effect of venom of other arthropod, **undetermined**

T63.5 Toxic effect of contact with venomous fish

Excludes2 poisoning by ingestion of fish (T61.-)

T63.51 Toxic effect of **contact with stingray**
- T63.511 Toxic effect of contact with stingray, **accidental** (unintentional)
- T63.512 Toxic effect of contact with stingray, **intentional** self-harm A, S
- T63.513 Toxic effect of contact with stingray, **assault**
- T63.514 Toxic effect of contact with stingray, **undetermined**

T63.59 Toxic effect of **contact with other venomous fish**
- T63.591 Toxic effect of contact with other venomous fish, **accidental** (unintentional)
- T63.592 Toxic effect of contact with other venomous fish, **intentional** self-harm A, S
- T63.593 Toxic effect of contact with other venomous fish, **assault**
- T63.594 Toxic effect of contact with other venomous fish, **undetermined**

T63.6 Toxic effect of contact with other venomous marine animals

Excludes1 sea-snake venom (T63.Ø9)

Excludes2 poisoning by ingestion of shellfish (T61.78-)

T63.61 Toxic effect of **contact with Portugese Man-o-war**

Toxic effect of contact with bluebottle
- T63.611 Toxic effect of contact with Portugese Man-o-war, **accidental** (unintentional)
- T63.612 Toxic effect of contact with Portugese Man-o-war, **intentional** self-harm A, S
- T63.613 Toxic effect of contact with Portugese Man-o-war, **assault**
- T63.614 Toxic effect of contact with Portugese Man-o-war, **undetermined**

T63.62 Toxic effect of **contact with other jellyfish**
- T63.621 Toxic effect of contact with other jellyfish, **accidental** (unintentional)
- T63.622 Toxic effect of contact with other jellyfish, **intentional** self-harm A, S
- T63.623 Toxic effect of contact with other jellyfish, **assault**
- T63.624 Toxic effect of contact with other jellyfish, **undetermined**

- T63.63 Toxic effect of contact with sea anemone
  - T63.631 Toxic effect of contact with sea anemone, accidental (unintentional)
  - T63.632 Toxic effect of contact with sea anemone, intentional self-harm A, S
  - T63.633 Toxic effect of contact with sea anemone, assault
  - T63.634 Toxic effect of contact with sea anemone, undetermined
- T63.69 Toxic effect of contact with other venomous marine animals
  - T63.691 Toxic effect of contact with other venomous marine animals, accidental (unintentional)
  - T63.692 Toxic effect of contact with other venomous marine animals, intentional self-harm A, S
  - T63.693 Toxic effect of contact with other venomous marine animals, assault
  - T63.694 Toxic effect of contact with other venomous marine animals, undetermined

T63.7 Toxic effect of contact with venomous plant

- T63.71 Toxic effect of contact with venomous marine plant
  - T63.711 Toxic effect of contact with venomous marine plant, accidental (unintentional)
  - T63.712 Toxic effect of contact with venomous marine plant, intentional self-harm A, S
  - T63.713 Toxic effect of contact with venomous marine plant, assault
  - T63.714 Toxic effect of contact with venomous marine plant, undetermined
- T63.79 Toxic effect of contact with other venomous plant
  - T63.791 Toxic effect of contact with other venomous plant, accidental (unintentional)
  - T63.792 Toxic effect of contact with other venomous plant, intentional self-harm A, S
  - T63.793 Toxic effect of contact with other venomous plant, assault
  - T63.794 Toxic effect of contact with other venomous plant, undetermined

T63.8 Toxic effect of contact with other venomous animals

- T63.81 Toxic effect of contact with venomous frog
  - **Excludes1** contact with nonvenomous frog (W62.0)
  - T63.811 Toxic effect of contact with venomous frog, accidental (unintentional)
  - T63.812 Toxic effect of contact with venomous frog, intentional self-harm A, S
  - T63.813 Toxic effect of contact with venomous frog, assault
  - T63.814 Toxic effect of contact with venomous frog, undetermined
- T63.82 Toxic effect of contact with venomous toad
  - **Excludes1** contact with nonvenomous toad (W62.1)
  - T63.821 Toxic effect of contact with venomous toad, accidental (unintentional)
  - T63.822 Toxic effect of contact with venomous toad, intentional self-harm A, S
  - T63.823 Toxic effect of contact with venomous toad, assault
  - T63.824 Toxic effect of contact with venomous toad, undetermined
- T63.83 Toxic effect of contact with other venomous amphibian
  - **Excludes1** contact with nonvenomous amphibian (W62.9)
  - T63.831 Toxic effect of contact with other venomous amphibian, accidental (unintentional)
  - T63.832 Toxic effect of contact with other venomous amphibian, intentional self-harm A, S
  - T63.833 Toxic effect of contact with other venomous amphibian, assault
  - T63.834 Toxic effect of contact with other venomous amphibian, undetermined
- T63.89 Toxic effect of contact with other venomous animals
  - T63.891 Toxic effect of contact with other venomous animals, accidental (unintentional)
  - T63.892 Toxic effect of contact with other venomous animals, intentional self-harm A, S
  - T63.893 Toxic effect of contact with other venomous animals, assault
  - T63.894 Toxic effect of contact with other venomous animals, undetermined

T63.9 Toxic effect of contact with unspecified venomous animal

- X T63.91 Toxic effect of contact with unspecified venomous animal, accidental (unintentional)
- X T63.92 Toxic effect of contact with unspecified venomous animal, intentional self-harm A, S
- X T63.93 Toxic effect of contact with unspecified venomous animal, assault
- X T63.94 Toxic effect of contact with unspecified venomous animal, undetermined

T64 Toxic effect of aflatoxin and other mycotoxin food contaminants

The appropriate 7th character is to be added to each code from category T64

A	initial encounter
D	subsequent encounter
S	sequela

T64.0 Toxic effect of aflatoxin

- X T64.01 Toxic effect of aflatoxin, accidental (unintentional)
- X T64.02 Toxic effect of aflatoxin, intentional self-harm A, S
- X T64.03 Toxic effect of aflatoxin, assault
- X T64.04 Toxic effect of aflatoxin, undetermined

T64.8 Toxic effect of other mycotoxin food contaminants

- X T64.81 Toxic effect of other mycotoxin food contaminants, accidental (unintentional)
- X T64.82 Toxic effect of other mycotoxin food contaminants, intentional self-harm A, S
- X T64.83 Toxic effect of other mycotoxin food contaminants, assault
- X T64.84 Toxic effect of other mycotoxin food contaminants, undetermined

CHAPTER 19 (S00-T88)

● T65 Toxic effect of other and unspecified substances

The appropriate 7th character is to be added to each code from category T65

A	initial encounter
D	subsequent encounter
S	sequela

● T65.0 Toxic effect of cyanides

Excludes1 hydrogen cyanide (T57.3-)

● T65.0X Toxic effect of cyanides

● T65.0X1 **Toxic effect of cyanides, accidental (unintentional)**
Toxic effect of cyanides NOS

● T65.0X2 **Toxic effect of cyanides, intentional self-harm** A, S

● T65.0X3 **Toxic effect of cyanides, assault**

● T65.0X4 **Toxic effect of cyanides, undetermined**

● T65.1 Toxic effect of strychnine and its salts

● T65.1X Toxic effect of strychnine and its salts

● T65.1X1 **Toxic effect of strychnine and its salts, accidental (unintentional)**
Toxic effect of strychnine and its salts NOS

● T65.1X2 **Toxic effect of strychnine and its salts, intentional self-harm** A, S

● T65.1X3 **Toxic effect of strychnine and its salts, assault**

● T65.1X4 **Toxic effect of strychnine and its salts, undetermined**

● T65.2 Toxic effect of tobacco and nicotine

Excludes2 nicotine dependence (F17.-)

● T65.21 Toxic effect of chewing tobacco

● T65.211 **Toxic effect of chewing tobacco, accidental (unintentional)**
Toxic effect of chewing tobacco NOS

● T65.212 **Toxic effect of chewing tobacco, intentional self-harm** A, S

● T65.213 **Toxic effect of chewing tobacco, assault**

● T65.214 **Toxic effect of chewing tobacco, undetermined**

● T65.22 Toxic effect of tobacco cigarettes
Toxic effect of tobacco smoke

Use additional code for exposure to second hand tobacco smoke (Z57.31, Z77.22)

● T65.221 **Toxic effect of tobacco cigarettes, accidental (unintentional)**
Toxic effect of tobacco cigarettes NOS

● T65.222 **Toxic effect of tobacco cigarettes, intentional self-harm** A, S

● T65.223 **Toxic effect of tobacco cigarettes, assault**

● T65.224 **Toxic effect of tobacco cigarettes, undetermined**

● T65.29 Toxic effect of other tobacco and nicotine

● T65.291 **Toxic effect of other tobacco and nicotine, accidental (unintentional)**
Toxic effect of other tobacco and nicotine NOS

● T65.292 **Toxic effect of other tobacco and nicotine, intentional self-harm** A, S

● T65.293 **Toxic effect of other tobacco and nicotine, assault**

● T65.294 **Toxic effect of other tobacco and nicotine, undetermined**

● T65.3 Toxic effect of nitroderivatives and aminoderivatives of benzene and its homologues
Toxic effect of anilin [benzenamine]
Toxic effect of nitrobenzene
Toxic effect of trinitrotoluene

● T65.3X Toxic effect of nitroderivatives and aminoderivatives of benzene and its homologues

● T65.3X1 **Toxic effect of nitroderivatives and aminoderivatives of benzene and its homologues, accidental (unintentional)**
Toxic effect of nitroderivatives and aminoderivatives of benzene and its homologues NOS

● T65.3X2 **Toxic effect of nitroderivatives and aminoderivatives of benzene and its homologues, intentional self-harm** A, S

● T65.3X3 **Toxic effect of nitroderivatives and aminoderivatives of benzene and its homologues, assault**

● T65.3X4 **Toxic effect of nitroderivatives and aminoderivatives of benzene and its homologues, undetermined**

● T65.4 Toxic effect of carbon disulfide

● T65.4X Toxic effect of carbon disulfide

● T65.4X1 **Toxic effect of carbon disulfide, accidental (unintentional)**
Toxic effect of carbon disulfide NOS

● T65.4X2 **Toxic effect of carbon disulfide, intentional self-harm** A, S

● T65.4X3 **Toxic effect of carbon disulfide, assault**

● T65.4X4 **Toxic effect of carbon disulfide, undetermined**

● T65.5 Toxic effect of nitroglycerin and other nitric acids and esters
Toxic effect of 1,2,3-Propanetriol trinitrate

● T65.5X Toxic effect of nitroglycerin and other nitric acids and esters

● T65.5X1 **Toxic effect of nitroglycerin and other nitric acids and esters, accidental (unintentional)**
Toxic effect of nitroglycerin and other nitric acids and esters NOS

● T65.5X2 **Toxic effect of nitroglycerin and other nitric acids and esters, intentional self-harm** A, S

● T65.5X3 **Toxic effect of nitroglycerin and other nitric acids and esters, assault**

● T65.5X4 **Toxic effect of nitroglycerin and other nitric acids and esters, undetermined**

● T65.6 Toxic effect of paints and dyes, not elsewhere classified

● T65.6X Toxic effect of paints and dyes, not elsewhere classified

● T65.6X1 **Toxic effect of paints and dyes, not elsewhere classified, accidental (unintentional)**
Toxic effect of paints and dyes NOS

● T65.6X2 **Toxic effect of paints and dyes, not elsewhere classified, intentional self-harm** A, S

● T65.6X3 **Toxic effect of paints and dyes, not elsewhere classified, assault**

● T65.6X4 **Toxic effect of paints and dyes, not elsewhere classified, undetermined**

● T65.8 Toxic effect of other specified substances

● T65.81 Toxic effect of latex

● T65.811 Toxic effect of latex, **accidental (unintentional)**
Toxic effect of latex NOS

● T65.812 Toxic effect of latex, **intentional** self-harm A, S

● T65.813 Toxic effect of latex, **assault**

● T65.814 Toxic effect of latex, **undetermined**

● T65.82 **Toxic effect of harmful algae and algae toxins**
Toxic effect of (harmful) algae bloom NOS
Toxic effect of blue-green algae bloom
Toxic effect of brown tide
Toxic effect of cyanobacteria bloom
Toxic effect of Florida red tide
Toxic effect of pfiesteria piscicida
Toxic effect of red tide

● T65.821 Toxic effect of harmful algae and algae toxins, **accidental (unintentional)**
Toxic effect of harmful algae and algae toxins NOS

● T65.822 Toxic effect of harmful algae and algae toxins, **intentional** self-harm A, S

● T65.823 Toxic effect of harmful algae and algae toxins, **assault**

● T65.824 Toxic effect of harmful algae and algae toxins, **undetermined**

● T65.83 Toxic effect of **fiberglass**

● T65.831 Toxic effect of fiberglass, **accidental (unintentional)**
Toxic effect of fiberglass NOS

● T65.832 Toxic effect of fiberglass, **intentional** self-harm A, S

● T65.833 Toxic effect of fiberglass, **assault**

● T65.834 Toxic effect of fiberglass, **undetermined**

● T65.89 Toxic effect of **other specified substances**

● T65.891 Toxic effect of other specified substances, **accidental** (unintentional)
Toxic effect of other specified substances NOS
Coding Clinic: 2018, Q1, P5

● T65.892 Toxic effect of other specified substances, **intentional** self-harm A, S

● T65.893 Toxic effect of other specified substances, **assault**

● T65.894 Toxic effect of other specified substances, **undetermined**

● T65.9 Toxic effect of **unspecified substance**

X● T65.91 Toxic effect of unspecified substance, **accidental (unintentional)**
Poisoning NOS

X● T65.92 Toxic effect of unspecified substance, **intentional** self-harm A, S

X● T65.93 Toxic effect of unspecified substance, **assault**

X● T65.94 Toxic effect of unspecified substance, **undetermined**

OTHER AND UNSPECIFIED EFFECTS OF EXTERNAL CAUSES (T66-T78)

● T66 Radiation sickness, **unspecified**

Excludes1 specified adverse effects of radiation, such as:
burns (T20-T31)
leukemia (C91-C95)
radiation gastroenteritis and colitis (K52.0)
radiation pneumonitis (J70.0)
radiation related disorders of the skin and subcutaneous tissue (L55-L59)
sunburn (L55.-)

The appropriate 7th character is to be added to code T66

A	initial encounter
D	subsequent encounter
S	sequela

● T67 Effects of heat and light

Excludes1 erythema [dermatitis] ab igne (L59.0)
malignant hyperpyrexia due to anesthesia (T88.3)
radiation-related disorders of the skin and subcutaneous tissue (L55-L59)

Excludes2 burns (T20-T31)
sunburn (L55.-)
sweat disorder due to heat (L74-L75)

The appropriate 7th character is to be added to each code from category T67

A	initial encounter
D	subsequent encounter
S	sequela

X● T67.0 Heatstroke and sunstroke
~~Heat apoplexy~~
~~Heat pyrexia~~
~~Siriasis~~
~~Thermoplegia~~
Use additional code(s) to identify any associated complications of heatstroke, such as:
coma and stupor (R40.-)
▶rhabdomyolysis (M62.82)
systemic inflammatory response syndrome (R65.1-)

▶X● T67.01 Heatstroke and sunstroke
▶Heat apoplexy
▶Heat pyrexia
▶Siriasis
▶Thermoplegia

▶X● T67.02 Exertional heatstroke

▶X● T67.09 Other heatstroke and sunstroke

X● T67.1 Heat **syncope**
Heat collapse

X● T67.2 Heat **cramp**

X● T67.3 Heat **exhaustion**, anhydrotic
Heat prostration due to water depletion
Excludes1 heat exhaustion due to salt depletion (T67.4)

X● T67.4 **Heat exhaustion due to salt depletion**
Heat prostration due to salt (and water) depletion

X● T67.5 Heat exhaustion, **unspecified**
Heat prostration NOS

X● T67.6 Heat **fatigue**, transient

X● T67.7 Heat **edema**

X● T67.8 **Other** effects of heat and light

X● T67.9 Effect of heat and light, **unspecified**

CHAPTER 19 (S00-T88)

X● **T68 Hypothermia**
Accidental hypothermia
Hypothermia NOS
Use additional code to identify source of exposure:
Exposure to excessive cold of man-made origin (W93)
Exposure to excessive cold of natural origin (X31)
Excludes1 hypothermia following anesthesia (T88.51)
hypothermia not associated with low environmental temperature (R68.Ø)
hypothermia of newborn (P8Ø.-)
Excludes2 frostbite (T33-T34)
The appropriate 7th character is to be added to code T68

A	initial encounter
D	subsequent encounter
S	sequela

● **T69 Other effects of reduced temperature**
Use additional code to identify source of exposure:
Exposure to excessive cold of man-made origin (W93)
Exposure to excessive cold of natural origin (X31)
Excludes2 frostbite (T33-T34)
The appropriate 7th character is to be added to each code from category T69

A	initial encounter
D	subsequent encounter
S	sequela

● **T69.Ø Immersion hand and foot**
● **T69.Ø1 Immersion hand**
● **T69.Ø11 Immersion hand, right hand**
● **T69.Ø12 Immersion hand, left hand**
● **T69.Ø19 Immersion hand, unspecified hand**
● **T69.Ø2 Immersion foot**
Trench foot
● **T69.Ø21 Immersion foot, right foot**
● **T69.Ø22 Immersion foot, left foot**
● **T69.Ø29 Immersion foot, unspecified foot**
X● **T69.1 Chilblains**
X● **T69.8 Other specified effects of reduced temperature**
X● **T69.9 Effect of reduced temperature, unspecified**

● **T7Ø Effects of air pressure and water pressure**
The appropriate 7th character is to be added to each code from category T7Ø

A	initial encounter
D	subsequent encounter
S	sequela

X● **T7Ø.Ø Otitic barotrauma**
Aero-otitis media
Effects of change in ambient atmospheric pressure or water pressure on ears
X● **T7Ø.1 Sinus barotrauma**
Aerosinusitis
Effects of change in ambient atmospheric pressure on sinuses
● **T7Ø.2 Other and unspecified effects of high altitude**
Excludes2 polycythemia due to high altitude (D75.1)
X● **T7Ø.2Ø Unspecified effects of high altitude**
X● **T7Ø.29 Other effects of high altitude**
Alpine sickness
Anoxia due to high altitude
Barotrauma NOS
Hypobaropathy
Mountain sickness
X● **T7Ø.3 Caisson disease [decompression sickness]**
Compressed-air disease
Diver's palsy or paralysis
X● **T7Ø.4 Effects of high-pressure fluids**
Hydraulic jet injection (industrial)
Pneumatic jet injection (industrial)
Traumatic jet injection (industrial)
X● **T7Ø.8 Other effects of air pressure and water pressure**
X● **T7Ø.9 Effect of air pressure and water pressure, unspecified**

● **T71 Asphyxiation**
Mechanical suffocation
Traumatic suffocation
Excludes1 acute respiratory distress (syndrome) (J8Ø)
anoxia due to high altitude (T7Ø.2)
asphyxia NOS (RØ9.Ø1)
asphyxia from carbon monoxide (T58.-)
asphyxia from inhalation of food or foreign body (T17.-)
asphyxia from other gases, fumes and vapors (T59.-)
respiratory distress (syndrome) in newborn (P22.-)
The appropriate 7th character is to be added to each code from category T71

A	initial encounter
D	subsequent encounter
S	sequela

● **T71.1 Asphyxiation due to mechanical threat to breathing**
Suffocation due to mechanical threat to breathing
● **T71.11 Asphyxiation due to smothering under pillow**
● **T71.111 Asphyxiation due to smothering under pillow, accidental**
Asphyxiation due to smothering under pillow NOS
● **T71.112 Asphyxiation due to smothering under pillow, intentional self-harm** A, S HCC
● **T71.113 Asphyxiation due to smothering under pillow, assault**
● **T71.114 Asphyxiation due to smothering under pillow, undetermined**
● **T71.12 Asphyxiation due to plastic bag**
● **T71.121 Asphyxiation due to plastic bag, accidental**
Asphyxiation due to plastic bag NOS
● **T71.122 Asphyxiation due to plastic bag, intentional self-harm** A, S HCC
● **T71.123 Asphyxiation due to plastic bag, assault**
● **T71.124 Asphyxiation due to plastic bag, undetermined**
● **T71.13 Asphyxiation due to being trapped in bed linens**
● **T71.131 Asphyxiation due to being trapped in bed linens, accidental**
Asphyxiation due to being trapped in bed linens NOS
● **T71.132 Asphyxiation due to being trapped in bed linens, intentional self-harm** A, S HCC
● **T71.133 Asphyxiation due to being trapped in bed linens, assault**
● **T71.134 Asphyxiation due to being trapped in bed linens, undetermined**

T71.14 Asphyxiation due to smothering under another person's body (in bed)

T71.141 Asphyxiation due to smothering under another person's body (in bed), accidental
Asphyxiation due to smothering under another person's body (in bed) NOS

T71.143 Asphyxiation due to smothering under another person's body (in bed), assault

T71.144 Asphyxiation due to smothering under another person's body (in bed), undetermined

T71.15 Asphyxiation due to smothering in furniture

T71.151 Asphyxiation due to smothering in furniture, accidental
Asphyxiation due to smothering in furniture NOS

T71.152 Asphyxiation due to smothering in furniture, intentional self-harm A, S

T71.153 Asphyxiation due to smothering in furniture, assault

T71.154 Asphyxiation due to smothering in furniture, undetermined

T71.16 Asphyxiation due to hanging
Hanging by window shade cord
Use additional code for any associated injuries, such as:
crushing injury of neck (S17.-)
fracture of cervical vertebrae (S12.Ø-S12.2-)
open wound of neck (S11.-)

T71.161 Asphyxiation due to hanging, accidental
Asphyxiation due to hanging NOS
Hanging NOS

T71.162 Asphyxiation due to hanging, intentional self-harm A, S

T71.163 Asphyxiation due to hanging, assault

T71.164 Asphyxiation due to hanging, undetermined

T71.19 Asphyxiation due to mechanical
Threat to breathing due to other causes

T71.191 Asphyxiation due to mechanical threat to breathing due to other causes, accidental
Asphyxiation due to other causes NOS
Coding Clinic: 2Ø16, Q4, P76

T71.192 Asphyxiation due to mechanical threat to breathing due to other causes, intentional self-harm A, S

T71.193 Asphyxiation due to mechanical threat to breathing due to other causes, assault

T71.194 Asphyxiation due to mechanical threat to breathing due to other causes, undetermined

T71.2 Asphyxiation due to systemic oxygen deficiency due to low oxygen content in ambient air
Suffocation due to systemic oxygen deficiency due to low oxygen content in ambient air

X **T71.2Ø Asphyxiation due to systemic oxygen deficiency due to low oxygen content in ambient air due to unspecified cause**

X **T71.21 Asphyxiation due to cave-in or falling earth**
Use additional code for any associated cataclysm (X34-X38)

T71.22 Asphyxiation due to being trapped in a car trunk

T71.221 Asphyxiation due to being trapped in a car trunk, accidental

T71.222 Asphyxiation due to being trapped in a car trunk, intentional self-harm A, S

T71.223 Asphyxiation due to being trapped in a car trunk, assault

T71.224 Asphyxiation due to being trapped in a car trunk, undetermined

T71.23 Asphyxiation due to being trapped in a (discarded) refrigerator

T71.231 Asphyxiation due to being trapped in a (discarded) refrigerator, accidental

T71.232 Asphyxiation due to being trapped in a (discarded) refrigerator, intentional self-harm A, S

T71.233 Asphyxiation due to being trapped in a (discarded) refrigerator, assault

T71.234 Asphyxiation due to being trapped in a (discarded) refrigerator, undetermined

X **T71.29 Asphyxiation due to being trapped in other low oxygen environment**

X **T71.9 Asphyxiation due to unspecified cause**
Suffocation (by strangulation) due to unspecified cause
Suffocation NOS
Systemic oxygen deficiency due to low oxygen content in ambient air due to unspecified cause
Systemic oxygen deficiency due to mechanical threat to breathing due to unspecified cause
Traumatic asphyxia NOS

T73 Effects of other deprivation
The appropriate 7th character is to be added to each code from category T73

A	initial encounter
D	subsequent encounter
S	sequela

X **T73.Ø Starvation**
Deprivation of food

X **T73.1 Deprivation of water**

X **T73.2 Exhaustion due to exposure**

X **T73.3 Exhaustion due to excessive exertion**
Exhaustion due to overexertion

X **T73.8 Other effects of deprivation**

X **T73.9 Effect of deprivation, unspecified**

T74 Adult and child abuse, neglect and other maltreatment, confirmed
Use additional code, if applicable, to identify any associated current injury
Use additional external cause code to identify perpetrator, if known (YØ7.-)
Excludes1 abuse and maltreatment in pregnancy (O9A.3-, O9A.4-, O9A.5-)
adult and child maltreatment, suspected (T76.-)
The appropriate 7th character is to be added to each code from category T74

A	initial encounter
D	subsequent encounter
S	sequela

T74.Ø Neglect or abandonment, confirmed

X **T74.Ø1 Adult neglect or abandonment, confirmed** A

X **T74.Ø2 Child neglect or abandonment, confirmed** P

T74.1 Physical abuse, confirmed
Excludes2 sexual abuse (T74.2-)
X T74.11 **Adult physical abuse, confirmed** A
X T74.12 **Child physical abuse, confirmed** P
Excludes2 shaken infant syndrome (T74.4)
T74.2 Sexual abuse, confirmed
Rape, confirmed
Sexual assault, confirmed
X T74.21 **Adult sexual abuse, confirmed** A
X T74.22 **Child sexual abuse, confirmed** P
T74.3 Psychological abuse, confirmed
Bullying and intimidation, confirmed
Intimidation through social media, confirmed
X T74.31 **Adult psychological abuse, confirmed** A
X T74.32 **Child psychological abuse, confirmed** P
X T74.4 Shaken infant syndrome P
T74.5 Forced sexual exploitation, confirmed
X T74.51 Adult forced sexual exploitation, confirmed P
X T74.52 Child sexual exploitation, confirmed P
T74.6 Forced labor exploitation, confirmed
X T74.61 Adult forced labor exploitation, confirmed P
X T74.62 Child forced labor exploitation, confirmed P
T74.9 Unspecified maltreatment, confirmed
X T74.91 Unspecified adult maltreatment, confirmed A
X T74.92 Unspecified child maltreatment, confirmed P

T75 Other and unspecified effects of other external causes
Excludes1 adverse effects NEC (T78.-)
Excludes2 burns (electric) (T20-T31)
The appropriate 7th character is to be added to each code from category T75

A	initial encounter
D	subsequent encounter
S	sequela

T75.0 Effects of lightning
Struck by lightning
X T75.00 Unspecified effects of lightning
Struck by lightning NOS
X T75.01 Shock due to being struck by lightning
X T75.09 Other effects of lightning
Use additional code for other effects of lightning
X T75.1 Unspecified effects of drowning and nonfatal submersion
Immersion
Excludes1 specified effects of drowning code to effects
T75.2 Effects of vibration
X T75.20 Unspecified effects of vibration
X T75.21 Pneumatic hammer syndrome
X T75.22 Traumatic vasospastic syndrome
X T75.23 Vertigo from infrasound
Excludes1 vertigo NOS (R42)
X T75.29 Other effects of vibration
X T75.3 Motion sickness
Airsickness
Seasickness
Travel sickness
Use additional external cause code to identify vehicle or type of motion (Y92.81-, Y93.5-)
X T75.4 Electrocution
Shock from electric current
Shock from electroshock gun (taser)
T75.8 Other specified effects of external causes
X T75.81 Effects of abnormal gravitation [G] forces
X T75.82 Effects of weightlessness
X T75.89 Other specified effects of external causes

T76 Adult and child abuse, neglect and other maltreatment, suspected
Use additional code, if applicable, to identify any associated current injury
Excludes1 adult and child maltreatment, confirmed (T74.-)
suspected abuse and maltreatment in pregnancy (O9A.3-, O9A.4-, O9A.5-)
suspected adult physical abuse, ruled out (Z04.71)
suspected adult sexual abuse, ruled out (Z04.41)
suspected child physical abuse, ruled out (Z04.72)
suspected child sexual abuse, ruled out (Z04.42)
The appropriate 7th character is to be added to each code from category T76

A	initial encounter
D	subsequent encounter
S	sequela

Coding Clinic: 2016, Q4, P129
T76.0 Neglect or abandonment, suspected
X T76.01 **Adult neglect or abandonment, suspected** A
X T76.02 **Child neglect or abandonment, suspected** P
T76.1 Physical abuse, suspected
X T76.11 **Adult physical abuse, suspected** A
X T76.12 **Child physical abuse, suspected** P
Coding Clinic: 2019, Q2, P12
T76.2 Sexual abuse, suspected
Rape, suspected
Excludes1 alleged abuse, ruled out (Z04.7)
X T76.21 **Adult sexual abuse, suspected** A
X T76.22 **Child sexual abuse, suspected** P
T76.3 Psychological abuse, suspected
Bullying and intimidation, suspected
Intimidation through social media, suspected
X T76.31 **Adult psychological abuse, suspected** A
X T76.32 **Child psychological abuse, suspected** P
T76.5 Forced sexual exploitation, suspected
X T76.51 Adult forced sexual exploitation, suspected P
X T76.52 Child sexual exploitation, suspected P
T76.6 Forced labor exploitation, suspected
X T76.61 Adult forced labor exploitation, suspected P
X T76.62 Child forced labor exploitation, suspected P
T76.9 Unspecified maltreatment, suspected
X T76.91 Unspecified adult maltreatment, suspected A
X T76.92 Unspecified child maltreatment, suspected P

T78 Adverse effects, not elsewhere classified

Excludes2 complications of surgical and medical care NEC (T80-T88)

The appropriate 7th character is to be added to each code from category T78

A	initial encounter
D	subsequent encounter
S	sequela

T78.0 Anaphylactic reaction due to food
Anaphylactic reaction due to adverse food reaction
Anaphylactic shock or reaction due to nonpoisonous foods
Anaphylactoid reaction due to food

X **T78.00 Anaphylactic reaction due to unspecified food**

X **T78.01 Anaphylactic reaction due to peanuts**

X **T78.02 Anaphylactic reaction due to shellfish (crustaceans)**

X **T78.03 Anaphylactic reaction due to other fish**

X **T78.04 Anaphylactic reaction due to fruits and vegetables**

X **T78.05 Anaphylactic reaction due to tree nuts and seeds**
Excludes2 anaphylactic reaction due to peanuts (T78.01)

X **T78.06 Anaphylactic reaction due to food additives**

X **T78.07 Anaphylactic reaction due to milk and dairy products**

X **T78.08 Anaphylactic reaction due to eggs**

X **T78.09 Anaphylactic reaction due to other food products**

X **T78.1 Other adverse food reactions, not elsewhere classified**
Use additional code to identify the type of reaction, if applicable
Excludes1 anaphylactic reaction or shock due to adverse food reaction (T78.0-)
anaphylactic reaction due to food (T78.0-)
bacterial food borne intoxications (A05.-)
Excludes2 allergic and dietetic gastroenteritis and colitis (K52.29)
allergic rhinitis due to food (J30.5)
dermatitis due to food in contact with skin (L23.6, L24.6, L25.4)
dermatitis due to ingested food (L27.2)
food protein-induced enterocolitis syndrome (K52.21)
food protein-induced enteropathy (K52.22)

X **T78.2 Anaphylactic shock, unspecified**
Occurs when allergic response triggers large quantities of histamines, prostaglandins, leukotrienes resulting in systemic vasodilation
Allergic shock
Anaphylactic reaction
Anaphylaxis
Excludes1 anaphylactic reaction or shock due to adverse effect of correct medicinal substance properly administered (T88.6)
anaphylactic reaction or shock due to adverse food reaction (T78.0-)
anaphylactic reaction or shock due to serum (T80.5-)

X **T78.3 Angioneurotic edema**
Allergic angioedema
Giant urticaria
Vascular disorder resulting from abnormalities of autonomic nervous system fibers supplying blood vessels
Quincke's edema
Excludes1 serum urticaria (T80.6-)
urticaria (L50.-)

T78.4 Other and unspecified allergy
Excludes1 specified types of allergic reaction such as:
allergic diarrhea (K52.29)
allergic gastroenteritis and colitis (K52.29)
dermatitis (L23-L25, L27.-)
food protein-induced enterocolitis syndrome (K52.21)
food protein-induced enteropathy (K52.22)
hay fever (J30.1)

X **T78.40 Allergy, unspecified**
Allergic reaction NOS
Hypersensitivity NOS

X **T78.41 Arthus phenomenon**
Arthus reaction

X **T78.49 Other allergy**

X **T78.8 Other adverse effects, not elsewhere classified**

CERTAIN EARLY COMPLICATIONS OF TRAUMA (T79)

T79 Certain early complications of trauma, not elsewhere classified
Excludes2 acute respiratory distress syndrome (J80)
complications occurring during or following medical procedures (T80-T88)
complications of surgical and medical care NEC (T80-T88)
newborn respiratory distress syndrome (P22.0)

The appropriate 7th character is to be added to each code from category T79

A	initial encounter
D	subsequent encounter
S	sequela

X **T79.0 Air embolism (traumatic)** A
Excludes1 air embolism complicating abortion or ectopic or molar pregnancy (O00-O07, O08.2)
air embolism complicating pregnancy, childbirth and the puerperium (O88.0)
air embolism following infusion, transfusion, and therapeutic injection (T80.0)
air embolism following procedure NEC (T81.7-)

X **T79.1 Fat embolism (traumatic)** A
Excludes1 fat embolism complicating:
abortion or ectopic or molar pregnancy (O00-O07, O08.2)
pregnancy, childbirth and the puerperium (O88.8)

X **T79.2 Traumatic secondary and recurrent hemorrhage and seroma** A

X● **T79.4 Traumatic shock** A

Shock (immediate) (delayed) following injury

Excludes1 anaphylactic shock due to adverse food reaction (T78.Ø-)
anaphylactic shock due to correct medicinal substance properly administered (T88.6)
anaphylactic shock due to serum (T8Ø.5-)
anaphylactic shock NOS (T78.2)
anesthetic shock (T88.2)
electric shock (T75.4)
nontraumatic shock NEC (R57.-)
obstetric shock (O75.1)
postprocedural shock (T81.1-)
septic shock (R65.21)
shock complicating abortion or ectopic or molar pregnancy (OØØ-OØ7, OØ8.3)
shock due to lightning (T75.Ø1)
shock NOS (R57.9)

X● **T79.5 Traumatic anuria** A

Crush syndrome
Renal failure following crushing

X● **T79.6 Traumatic ischemia of muscle** A

Traumatic rhabdomyolysis
Volkmann's ischemic contracture

Excludes2 anterior tibial syndrome (M76.8)
compartment syndrome (traumatic) (T79.A-)
nontraumatic ischemia of muscle (M62.2-)

X● **T79.7 Traumatic subcutaneous emphysema** A

Excludes1 emphysema NOS (J43)
emphysema (subcutaneous) resulting from a procedure (T81.82)

● **T79.A Traumatic compartment syndrome**

Excludes1 fibromyalgia (M79.7)
nontraumatic compartment syndrome (M79.A-)
~~traumatic ischemic infarction of muscle (T79.6)~~

▶ **Excludes2** traumatic ischemic infarction of muscle (T79.6)

X● **T79.AØ Compartment syndrome, unspecified**

Compartment syndrome NOS

● **T79.A1 Traumatic compartment syndrome of upper extremity**

Traumatic compartment syndrome of shoulder, arm, forearm, wrist, hand, and fingers

● **T79.A11 Traumatic compartment syndrome of right upper extremity** A

● **T79.A12 Traumatic compartment syndrome of left upper extremity** A

● **T79.A19 Traumatic compartment syndrome of unspecified upper extremity** A

● **T79.A2 Traumatic compartment syndrome of lower extremity**

Traumatic compartment syndrome of hip, buttock, thigh, leg, foot, and toes

● **T79.A21 Traumatic compartment syndrome of right lower extremity** A

● **T79.A22 Traumatic compartment syndrome of left lower extremity** A

● **T79.A29 Traumatic compartment syndrome of unspecified lower extremity**

X● **T79.A3 Traumatic compartment syndrome of abdomen** A

X● **T79.A9 Traumatic compartment syndrome of other sites** A

X● **T79.8 Other early complications of trauma** A

X● **T79.9 Unspecified early complication of trauma** A

COMPLICATIONS OF SURGICAL AND MEDICAL CARE NOT ELSEWHERE CLASSIFIED (T8Ø-T88)

Use additional code for adverse effect, if applicable, to identify drug (T36-T5Ø with fifth or sixth character 5)

Use additional code(s) to identify the specified condition resulting from the complication.

Use additional code to identify devices involved and details of circumstances (Y62-Y82)

Excludes2 any encounters with medical care for postprocedural conditions in which no complications are present, such as:
artificial opening status (Z93.-)
closure of external stoma (Z43.-)
fitting and adjustment of external prosthetic device (Z44.-)
burns and corrosions from local applications and irradiation (T2Ø-T32)
complications of surgical procedures during pregnancy, childbirth and the puerperium (OØØ-O9A)
mechanical complication of respirator [ventilator] (J95.85Ø)
poisoning and toxic effects of drugs and chemicals (T36-T65 with fifth or sixth character 1-4 or 6)
postprocedural fever (R5Ø.82)
specified complications classified elsewhere, such as:
cerebrospinal fluid leak from spinal puncture (G97.Ø)
colostomy malfunction (K94.Ø-)
disorders of fluid and electrolyte imbalance (E86-E87)
functional disturbances following cardiac surgery (I97.Ø-I97.1)
intraoperative and postprocedural complications of specified body systems (D78.-, E36.-, E89.-, G97.3-, G97.4, H59.3-, H59.-, H95.2-, H95.3, I97.4-, I97.5, J95.6-, J95.7, K91.6-, L76.-, M96.-, N99.-)
ostomy complications (J95.Ø-, K94.-, N99.5-)
postgastric surgery syndromes (K91.1)
postlaminectomy syndrome NEC (M96.1)
postmastectomy lymphedema syndrome (I97.2)
postsurgical blind-loop syndrome (K91.2)
ventilator associated pneumonia (J95.851)

● **T8Ø Complications following infusion, transfusion and therapeutic injection**

Includes complications following perfusion

Excludes2 bone marrow transplant rejection (T86.Ø1)
febrile nonhemolytic transfusion reaction (R5Ø.84)
fluid overload due to transfusion (E87.71)
posttransfusion purpura (D69.51)
transfusion associated circulatory overload (TACO) (E87.71)
transfusion (red blood cell) associated hemochromatosis (E83.111)
transfusion related acute lung injury (TRALI) (J95.84)

The appropriate 7th character is to be added to each code from category T8Ø

A	initial encounter
D	subsequent encounter
S	sequela

X● **T8Ø.Ø Air embolism following infusion, transfusion and therapeutic injection**

X● **T8Ø.1 Vascular complications following infusion, transfusion and therapeutic injection**

Use additional code to identify the vascular complication

Excludes2 extravasation of vesicant agent (T8Ø.81-)
infiltration of vesicant agent (T8Ø.81-)
vascular complications specified as due to prosthetic devices, implants and grafts (T82.8- T83.8-, T84.8-, T85.8-)
postprocedural vascular complications (T81.7-)

T80.2 Infections following infusion, transfusion and therapeutic injection
Use additional code to identify the specific infection, such as:
sepsis (A41.9)
Use additional code (R65.2-) to identify severe sepsis, if applicable
Excludes2 infections specified as due to prosthetic devices, implants and grafts (T82.6-T82.7, T83.5-T83.6, T84.5-T84.7, T85.7)
postprocedural infections (T81.44)
Coding Clinic: 2018, Q4, P89

T80.21 Infection due to central venous catheter
Infection due to pulmonary artery catheter (Swan-Ganz catheter)
Coding Clinic: 2019, Q1, P13-14; 2018, Q4, P89

T80.211 Bloodstream infection due to central venous catheter
Catheter-related bloodstream infection (CRBSI) NOS
Central line-associated bloodstream infection (CLABSI)
Bloodstream infection due to Hickman catheter
Bloodstream infection due to peripherally inserted central catheter (PICC)
Bloodstream infection due to portacath (port-a-cath)
Bloodstream infection due to pulmonary artery catheter
Bloodstream infection due to triple lumen catheter
Bloodstream infection due to umbilical venous catheter
Coding Clinic: 2018, Q4, P89

T80.212 Local infection due to central venous catheter
Exit or insertion site infection
Local infection due to Hickman catheter
Local infection due to peripherally inserted central catheter (PICC)
Local infection due to portacath (port-a-cath)
Local infection due to pulmonary artery catheter
Local infection due to triple lumen catheter
Local infection due to umbilical venous catheter
Port or reservoir infection
Tunnel infection

T80.218 Other infection due to central venous catheter
Other central line-associated infection
Other infection due to Hickman catheter
Other infection due to peripherally inserted central catheter (PICC)
Other infection due to portacath (port-a-cath)
Other infection due to pulmonary artery catheter
Other infection due to triple lumen catheter
Other infection due to umbilical venous catheter

T80.219 Unspecified infection due to central venous catheter
Central line-associated infection NOS
Unspecified infection due to Hickman catheter
Unspecified infection due to peripherally inserted central catheter (PICC)
Unspecified infection due to portacath (port-a-cath)
Unspecified infection due to pulmonary artery catheter
Unspecified infection due to triple lumen catheter
Unspecified infection due to umbilical venous catheter

X **T80.22 Acute infection following transfusion, infusion, or injection of blood and blood products**

X **T80.29 Infection following other infusion, transfusion and therapeutic injection**

T80.3 ABO incompatibility reaction due to transfusion of blood or blood products
Excludes1 minor blood group antigens reactions (Duffy) (E) (K) (Kell) (Kidd) (Lewis) (M) (N) (P) (S) (T80.A-)

X **T80.30 ABO incompatibility reaction due to transfusion of blood or blood products, unspecified**
ABO incompatibility blood transfusion NOS
Reaction to ABO incompatibility from transfusion NOS

T80.31 ABO incompatibility with hemolytic transfusion reaction

T80.310 ABO incompatibility with acute hemolytic transfusion reaction
ABO incompatibility with hemolytic transfusion reaction less than 24 hours after transfusion
Acute hemolytic transfusion reaction (AHTR) due to ABO incompatibility

T80.311 ABO incompatibility with delayed hemolytic transfusion reaction
ABO incompatibility with hemolytic transfusion reaction 24 hours or more after transfusion
Delayed hemolytic transfusion reaction (DHTR) due to ABO incompatibility

T80.319 ABO incompatibility with hemolytic transfusion reaction, unspecified
ABO incompatibility with hemolytic transfusion reaction at unspecified time after transfusion
Hemolytic transfusion reaction (HTR) due to ABO incompatibility NOS

X **T80.39 Other ABO incompatibility reaction due to transfusion of blood or blood products**
Delayed serologic transfusion reaction (DSTR) from ABO incompatibility
Other ABO incompatible blood transfusion
Other reaction to ABO incompatible blood transfusion

T80.4 Rh incompatibility reaction due to transfusion of blood or blood products
Reaction due to incompatibility of Rh antigens (C) (c) (D) (E) (e)

X **T80.40 Rh incompatibility reaction due to transfusion of blood or blood products, unspecified**
Reaction due to Rh factor in transfusion NOS
Rh incompatible blood transfusion NOS

CHAPTER 19 (S00-T88)

T80.41 **Rh incompatibility with hemolytic transfusion reaction**

T80.410 **Rh incompatibility with acute hemolytic transfusion reaction**
Acute hemolytic transfusion reaction (AHTR) due to Rh incompatibility
Rh incompatibility with hemolytic transfusion reaction less than 24 hours after transfusion

T80.411 **Rh incompatibility with delayed hemolytic transfusion reaction**
Delayed hemolytic transfusion reaction (DHTR) due to Rh incompatibility
Rh incompatibility with hemolytic transfusion reaction 24 hours or more after transfusion

T80.419 **Rh incompatibility with hemolytic transfusion reaction, unspecified**
Rh incompatibility with hemolytic transfusion reaction at unspecified time after transfusion
Hemolytic transfusion reaction (HTR) due to Rh incompatibility NOS

X T80.49 **Other Rh incompatibility reaction due to transfusion of blood or blood products**
Delayed serologic transfusion reaction (DSTR) from Rh incompatibility
Other reaction to Rh incompatible blood transfusion

T80.A **Non-ABO incompatibility reaction due to transfusion of blood or blood products**
Reaction due to incompatibility of minor antigens (Duffy) (Kell) (Kidd) (Lewis) (M) (N) (P) (S)

X T80.A0 **Non-ABO incompatibility reaction due to transfusion of blood or blood products, unspecified**
Non-ABO antigen incompatibility reaction from transfusion NOS

T80.A1 **Non-ABO incompatibility with hemolytic transfusion reaction**

T80.A10 **Non-ABO incompatibility with acute hemolytic transfusion reaction**
Acute hemolytic transfusion reaction (AHTR) due to non-ABO incompatibility
Non-ABO incompatibility with hemolytic transfusion reaction less than 24 hours after transfusion

T80.A11 **Non-ABO incompatibility with delayed hemolytic transfusion reaction**
Delayed hemolytic transfusion reaction (DHTR) due to non-ABO incompatibility
Non-ABO incompatibility with hemolytic transfusion reaction 24 or more hours after transfusion

T80.A19 **Non-ABO incompatibility with hemolytic transfusion reaction, unspecified**
Hemolytic transfusion reaction (HTR) due to non-ABO incompatibility NOS
Non-ABO incompatibility with hemolytic transfusion reaction at unspecified time after transfusion

X T80.A9 **Other non-ABO incompatibility reaction due to transfusion of blood or blood products**
Delayed serologic transfusion reaction (DSTR) from non-ABO incompatibility
Other reaction to non-ABO incompatible blood transfusion

T80.5 **Anaphylactic reaction due to serum**
Allergic reaction due to serum
Anaphylactic shock due to serum
Anaphylactoid reaction due to serum
Anaphylaxis due to serum
Excludes1 ABO incompatibility reaction due to transfusion of blood or blood products (T80.3-)
allergic reaction or shock NOS (T78.2)
anaphylactic reaction or shock NOS (T78.2)
anaphylactic reaction or shock due to adverse effect of correct medicinal substance properly administered (T88.6)
other serum reaction (T80.6-)

X T80.51 **Anaphylactic reaction due to administration of blood and blood products**

X T80.52 **Anaphylactic reaction due to vaccination**

X T80.59 **Anaphylactic reaction due to other serum**

T80.6 **Other serum reactions**
Intoxication by serum
Protein sickness
Serum rash
Serum sickness
Serum urticaria
Excludes2 serum hepatitis (B16-B19)

X T80.61 **Other serum reaction due to administration of blood and blood products**

X T80.62 **Other serum reaction due to vaccination**

X T80.69 **Other serum reaction due to other serum**
Code also, if applicable, arthropathy in hypersensitivity reactions classified elsewhere (M36.4)

T80.8 **Other complications following infusion, transfusion and therapeutic injection**

T80.81 **Extravasation of vesicant agent**
Infiltration of vesicant agent

T80.810 **Extravasation of vesicant antineoplastic chemotherapy**
Infiltration of vesicant antineoplastic chemotherapy

T80.818 **Extravasation of other vesicant agent**
Infiltration of other vesicant agent

X T80.89 **Other complications following infusion, transfusion and therapeutic injection**
Delayed serologic transfusion reaction (DSTR), unspecified incompatibility
Use additional code to identify graft-versus-host reaction, if applicable, (D89.81-)

T80.9 **Unspecified complication following infusion, transfusion and therapeutic injection**

X T80.90 **Unspecified complication following infusion and therapeutic injection**

T80.91 **Hemolytic transfusion reaction, unspecified incompatibility**
Excludes1 ABO incompatibility with hemolytic transfusion reaction (T80.31-)
Non-ABO incompatibility with hemolytic transfusion reaction (T80.A1-)
Rh incompatibility with hemolytic transfusion reaction (T80.41-)

T80.910 **Acute hemolytic transfusion reaction, unspecified incompatibility**

T80.911 **Delayed hemolytic transfusion reaction, unspecified incompatibility**

T80.919 Hemolytic transfusion reaction, unspecified incompatibility, unspecified as acute or delayed
Hemolytic transfusion reaction NOS

X **T80.92 Unspecified transfusion reaction**
Transfusion reaction NOS

T81 Complications of procedures, not elsewhere classified
Use additional code for adverse effect, if applicable, to identify drug (T36-T50 with fifth or sixth character 5)

Excludes2 complications following immunization (T88.0-T88.1)
complications following infusion, transfusion and therapeutic injection (T80.-)
complications of transplanted organs and tissue (T86.-)
poisoning and toxic effects of drugs and chemicals (T36-T65 with fifth or sixth character 1-4 or 6)
specified complications classified elsewhere, such as:
complication of prosthetic devices, implants and grafts (T82-T85)
dermatitis due to drugs and medicaments (L23.3, L24.4, L25.1, L27.0-L27.1)
endosseous dental implant failure (M27.6-)
floppy iris syndrome (IFIS) (intraoperative) H21.81
intraoperative and postprocedural complications of specific body system (D78.-, E36.-, E89.-, G97.3-, G97.4, H59.3-, H59.-, H95.2-, H95.3, I97.4-, I97.5, J95, K91.-, L76.-, M96.-, N99.-)
ostomy complications (J95.0-, K94.-, N99.5-)
plateau iris syndrome (post-iridectomy) (postprocedural) H21.82

Coding Clinic: 2019, Q2, P21-22; 2016, Q4, P29

The appropriate 7th character is to be added to each code from category T81

A	initial encounter
D	subsequent encounter
S	sequela

T81.1 Postprocedural shock
Shock during or resulting from a procedure, not elsewhere classified

Excludes1 anaphylactic shock NOS (T78.2)
anaphylactic shock due to correct substance properly administered (T88.6)
anaphylactic shock due to serum (T80.5-)
anesthetic shock (T88.2)
electric shock (T75.4)
obstetric shock (O75.1)
septic shock (R65.21)
shock following abortion or ectopic or molar pregnancy (O00-O07, O08.3)
traumatic shock (T79.4)

X **T81.10 Postprocedural shock unspecified**
Collapse NOS during or resulting from a procedure, not elsewhere classified
Postprocedural failure of peripheral circulation
Postprocedural shock NOS

X **T81.11 Postprocedural cardiogenic shock** A

X **T81.12 Postprocedural septic shock** A
Postprocedural endotoxic shock resulting from a procedure, not elsewhere classified
Postprocedural gram-negative shock resulting from a procedure, not elsewhere classified

Code first underlying infection

Use additional code, to identify any associated acute organ dysfunction, if applicable

X **T81.19 Other postprocedural shock**
Postprocedural hypovolemic shock

T81.3 Disruption of wound, not elsewhere classified
Disruption of any suture materials or other closure methods

Excludes1 breakdown (mechanical) of permanent sutures (T85.612)
displacement of permanent sutures (T85.622)
disruption of cesarean delivery wound (O90.0)
disruption of perineal obstetric wound (O90.1)
mechanical complication of permanent sutures NEC (T85.692)

X **T81.30 Disruption of wound, unspecified**
Disruption of wound NOS

X **T81.31 Disruption of external operation (surgical) wound, not elsewhere classified**

Excludes1 dehiscence of amputation stump (T87.81)

Dehiscence of operation wound NOS
Disruption of operation wound NOS
Disruption or dehiscence of closure of cornea
Disruption or dehiscence of closure of mucosa
Disruption or dehiscence of closure of skin and subcutaneous tissue
Full-thickness skin disruption or dehiscence
Superficial disruption or dehiscence of operation wound

Coding Clinic: 2015, Q1, P20

X **T81.32 Disruption of internal operation (surgical) wound, not elsewhere classified**
Deep disruption or dehiscence of operation wound NOS
Disruption or dehiscence of closure of internal organ or other internal tissue
Disruption or dehiscence of closure of muscle or muscle flap
Disruption or dehiscence of closure of ribs or rib cage
Disruption or dehiscence of closure of skull or craniotomy
Disruption or dehiscence of closure of sternum or sternotomy
Disruption or dehiscence of closure of tendon or ligament
Disruption or dehiscence of closure of superficial or muscular fascia

Coding Clinic: 2017, Q3, P4

X **T81.33 Disruption of traumatic injury wound repair**
Disruption or dehiscence of closure of traumatic laceration (external) (internal)

T81.4 Infection following a procedure
Use additional code to identify infection
Use additional code (R65.2-) to identify severe sepsis, if applicable

Excludes2 bleb associated endophthalmitis (H59.4-)
infection due to infusion, transfusion and therapeutic injection (T80.2-)
infection due to prosthetic devices, implants and grafts (T82.6-T82.7, T83.5-T83.6, T84.5-T84.7, T85.7)
obstetric surgical wound infection (O86.0-)
postprocedural fever NOS (R50.82)
postprocedural retroperitoneal abscess (K68.11)

X **T81.40 Infection following a procedure, unspecified**

X **T81.41 Infection following a procedure, superficial incisional surgical site**
Subcutaneous abscess following a procedure
Stitch abscess following a procedure

Coding Clinic: 2018, Q4, P34

X **T81.42 Infection following a procedure, deep incisional surgical site**
Intra-muscular abscess following a procedure

X ● T81.43 Infection following a procedure, organ and space surgical site
Intra-abdominal abscess following a procedure
Subphrenic abscess following a procedure

X ● T81.44 Sepsis following a procedure A
Use additional code to identify the sepsis

X ● T81.49 Infection following a procedure, other surgical site
Coding Clinic: 2015, Q4, P37

● T81.5 Complications of foreign body accidentally left in body following procedure

● T81.50 Unspecified complication of foreign body accidentally left in body following procedure

● T81.500 Unspecified complication of foreign body accidentally left in body following surgical operation

● T81.501 Unspecified complication of foreign body accidentally left in body following infusion or transfusion

● T81.502 Unspecified complication of foreign body accidentally left in body following kidney dialysis A, D, S

● T81.503 Unspecified complication of foreign body accidentally left in body following injection or immunization

● T81.504 Unspecified complication of foreign body accidentally left in body following endoscopic examination

● T81.505 Unspecified complication of foreign body accidentally left in body following heart catheterization

● T81.506 Unspecified complication of foreign body accidentally left in body following aspiration, puncture or other catheterization

● T81.507 Unspecified complication of foreign body accidentally left in body following removal of catheter or packing

● T81.508 Unspecified complication of foreign body accidentally left in body following other procedure

● T81.509 Unspecified complication of foreign body accidentally left in body following unspecified procedure

● T81.51 Adhesions due to foreign body accidentally left in body following procedure

● T81.510 Adhesions due to foreign body accidentally left in body following surgical operation

● T81.511 Adhesions due to foreign body accidentally left in body following infusion or transfusion

● T81.512 Adhesions due to foreign body accidentally left in body following kidney dialysis A, D, S

● T81.513 Adhesions due to foreign body accidentally left in body following injection or immunization

● T81.514 Adhesions due to foreign body accidentally left in body following endoscopic examination

● T81.515 Adhesions due to foreign body accidentally left in body following heart catheterization

● T81.516 Adhesions due to foreign body accidentally left in body following aspiration, puncture or other catheterization

● T81.517 Adhesions due to foreign body accidentally left in body following removal of catheter or packing

● T81.518 Adhesions due to foreign body accidentally left in body following other procedure

● T81.519 Adhesions due to foreign body accidentally left in body following unspecified procedure

● T81.52 Obstruction due to foreign body accidentally left in body following procedure

● T81.520 Obstruction due to foreign body accidentally left in body following surgical operation

● T81.521 Obstruction due to foreign body accidentally left in body following infusion or transfusion

● T81.522 Obstruction due to foreign body accidentally left in body following kidney dialysis A, D, S

● T81.523 Obstruction due to foreign body accidentally left in body following injection or immunization

● T81.524 Obstruction due to foreign body accidentally left in body following endoscopic examination

● T81.525 Obstruction due to foreign body accidentally left in body following heart catheterization

● T81.526 Obstruction due to foreign body accidentally left in body following aspiration, puncture or other catheterization

● T81.527 Obstruction due to foreign body accidentally left in body following removal of catheter or packing

● T81.528 Obstruction due to foreign body accidentally left in body following other procedure

● T81.529 Obstruction due to foreign body accidentally left in body following unspecified procedure

● T81.53 Perforation due to foreign body accidentally left in body following procedure

● T81.530 Perforation due to foreign body accidentally left in body following surgical operation

● T81.531 Perforation due to foreign body accidentally left in body following infusion or transfusion

● T81.532 Perforation due to foreign body accidentally left in body following kidney dialysis A, D, S

● T81.533 Perforation due to foreign body accidentally left in body following injection or immunization

● T81.534 Perforation due to foreign body accidentally left in body following endoscopic examination

● T81.535 Perforation due to foreign body accidentally left in body following heart catheterization

T81.536 Perforation due to foreign body accidentally left in body following aspiration, puncture or other catheterization

T81.537 Perforation due to foreign body accidentally left in body following removal of catheter or packing

T81.538 Perforation due to foreign body accidentally left in body following other procedure

T81.539 Perforation due to foreign body accidentally left in body following unspecified procedure

T81.59 Other complications of foreign body accidentally left in body following procedure

Excludes2 obstruction or perforation due to prosthetic devices and implants intentionally left in body (T82.Ø-T82.5, T83.Ø-T83.4, T83.7, T84.Ø-T84.4, T85.Ø-T85.6)

T81.59Ø Other complications of foreign body accidentally left in body following surgical operation

T81.591 Other complications of foreign body accidentally left in body following infusion or transfusion

T81.592 Other complications of foreign body accidentally left in body following kidney dialysis A, D, S

T81.593 Other complications of foreign body accidentally left in body following injection or immunization

T81.594 Other complications of foreign body accidentally left in body following endoscopic examination

T81.595 Other complications of foreign body accidentally left in body following heart catheterization

T81.596 Other complications of foreign body accidentally left in body following aspiration, puncture or other catheterization

T81.597 Other complications of foreign body accidentally left in body following removal of catheter or packing

T81.598 Other complications of foreign body accidentally left in body following other procedure

T81.599 Other complications of foreign body accidentally left in body following unspecified procedure

T81.6 Acute reaction to foreign substance accidentally left during a procedure

Excludes2 complications of foreign body accidentally left in body cavity or operation wound following procedure (T81.5-)

X T81.6Ø Unspecified acute reaction to foreign substance accidentally left during a procedure

X T81.61 Aseptic peritonitis due to foreign substance accidentally left during a procedure
Chemical peritonitis

X T81.69 Other acute reaction to foreign substance accidentally left during a procedure

T81.7 Vascular complications following a procedure, not elsewhere classified
Air embolism following procedure NEC
Phlebitis or thrombophlebitis resulting from a procedure

Excludes1 embolism complicating abortion or ectopic or molar pregnancy (OØØ-OØ7, OØ8.2)
embolism complicating pregnancy, childbirth and the puerperium (O88.-)
traumatic embolism (T79.Ø)

Excludes2 embolism due to prosthetic devices, implants and grafts (T82.8, T83.81, T84.8-, T85.1-)
embolism following infusion, transfusion and therapeutic injection (T8Ø.Ø)

Coding Clinic: 2Ø19, Q2, P23

T81.71 Complication of artery following a procedure, not elsewhere classified
Coding Clinic: 2Ø19, Q2, P22

T81.71Ø Complication of mesenteric artery following a procedure, not elsewhere classified

T81.711 Complication of renal artery following a procedure, not elsewhere classified

T81.718 Complication of other artery following a procedure, not elsewhere classified
Coding Clinic: 2Ø19, Q2, P22-23

T81.719 Complication of unspecified artery following a procedure, not elsewhere classified

X T81.72 Complication of vein following a procedure, not elsewhere classified
Coding Clinic: 2Ø19, Q2, P22

T81.8 Other complications of procedures, not elsewhere classified

Excludes2 hypothermia following anesthesia (T88.51)
malignant hyperpyrexia due to anesthesia (T88.3)

X T81.81 Complication of inhalation therapy

X T81.82 Emphysema (subcutaneous) resulting from a procedure

X T81.83 Persistent postprocedural fistula
Coding Clinic: 2Ø17, Q3, P3-5

X T81.89 Other complications of procedures, not elsewhere classified
Use additional code to specify complication, such as:
postprocedural delirium (FØ5)

X T81.9 Unspecified complication of procedure

● T82 **Complications of cardiac and vascular prosthetic devices, implants and grafts**

Excludes2 failure and rejection of transplanted organs and tissue (T86.-)

The appropriate 7th character is to be added to each code from category T82

A	initial encounter
D	subsequent encounter
S	sequela

● T82.0 **Mechanical complication of heart valve prosthesis**
Mechanical complication of artificial heart valve
Excludes1 mechanical complication of biological heart valve graft (T82.22-)

X● T82.01 **Breakdown (mechanical) of heart valve prosthesis**

X● T82.02 **Displacement of heart valve prosthesis**
Malposition of heart valve prosthesis

X● T82.03 **Leakage of heart valve prosthesis**

X● T82.09 **Other mechanical complication of heart valve prosthesis**
Obstruction (mechanical) of heart valve prosthesis
Perforation of heart valve prosthesis
Protrusion of heart valve prosthesis

● T82.1 **Mechanical complication of cardiac electronic device**

● T82.11 **Breakdown (mechanical) of cardiac electronic device**

● T82.110 **Breakdown (mechanical) of cardiac electrode**

● T82.111 **Breakdown (mechanical) of cardiac pulse generator (battery)**

● T82.118 **Breakdown (mechanical) of other cardiac electronic device**

● T82.119 **Breakdown (mechanical) of unspecified cardiac electronic device**

● T82.12 **Displacement of cardiac electronic device**
Malposition of cardiac electronic device

● T82.120 **Displacement of cardiac electrode**

● T82.121 **Displacement of cardiac pulse generator (battery)**

● T82.128 **Displacement of other cardiac electronic device**

● T82.129 **Displacement of unspecified cardiac electronic device**

● T82.19 **Other mechanical complication of cardiac electronic device**
Leakage of cardiac electronic device
Obstruction of cardiac electronic device
Perforation of cardiac electronic device
Protrusion of cardiac electronic device

● T82.190 **Other mechanical complication of cardiac electrode**

● T82.191 **Other mechanical complication of cardiac pulse generator (battery)**

● T82.198 **Other mechanical complication of other cardiac electronic device**

● T82.199 **Other mechanical complication of unspecified cardiac device**

● T82.2 **Mechanical complication of coronary artery bypass graft and biological heart valve graft**
Excludes1 mechanical complication of artificial heart valve prosthesis (T82.0-)

● T82.21 **Mechanical complication of coronary artery bypass graft**

● T82.211 **Breakdown (mechanical) of coronary artery bypass graft**

● T82.212 **Displacement of coronary artery bypass graft**
Malposition of coronary artery bypass graft

● T82.213 **Leakage of coronary artery bypass graft**

● T82.218 **Other mechanical complication of coronary artery bypass graft**
Obstruction, mechanical of coronary artery bypass graft
Perforation of coronary artery bypass graft
Protrusion of coronary artery bypass graft

● T82.22 **Mechanical complication of biological heart valve graft**

● T82.221 **Breakdown (mechanical) of biological heart valve graft**

● T82.222 **Displacement of biological heart valve graft**
Malposition of biological heart valve graft

● T82.223 **Leakage of biological heart valve graft**

● T82.228 **Other mechanical complication of biological heart valve graft**
Obstruction of biological heart valve graft
Perforation of biological heart valve graft
Protrusion of biological heart valve graft

● T82.3 **Mechanical complication of other vascular grafts**

● T82.31 **Breakdown (mechanical) of other vascular grafts**

● T82.310 **Breakdown (mechanical) of aortic (bifurcation) graft (replacement)** A HCC

● T82.311 **Breakdown (mechanical) of carotid arterial graft (bypass)** A HCC

● T82.312 **Breakdown (mechanical) of femoral arterial graft (bypass)** A HCC

● T82.318 **Breakdown (mechanical) of other vascular grafts** A HCC

● T82.319 **Breakdown (mechanical) of unspecified vascular grafts** A HCC

● T82.32 **Displacement of other vascular grafts**
Malposition of other vascular grafts

● T82.320 **Displacement of aortic (bifurcation) graft (replacement)** A HCC

● T82.321 **Displacement of carotid arterial graft (bypass)** A HCC

● T82.322 **Displacement of femoral arterial graft (bypass)** A HCC

● T82.328 **Displacement of other vascular grafts** A HCC

● T82.329 **Displacement of unspecified vascular grafts** A HCC

● T82.33 **Leakage** of other vascular grafts
- ● T82.330 **Leakage of aortic (bifurcation) graft (replacement)** A
- ● T82.331 **Leakage of carotid arterial graft (bypass)** A
- ● T82.332 **Leakage of femoral arterial graft (bypass)** A
- ● T82.338 **Leakage of other vascular grafts** A
- ● T82.339 **Leakage of unspecified vascular graft** A

● T82.39 **Other mechanical complication of other vascular grafts**
Obstruction (mechanical) of other vascular grafts
Perforation of other vascular grafts
Protrusion of other vascular grafts
- ● T82.390 **Other mechanical complication of aortic (bifurcation) graft (replacement)** A
- ● T82.391 **Other mechanical complication of carotid arterial graft (bypass)** A
- ● T82.392 **Other mechanical complication of femoral arterial graft (bypass)** A
- ● T82.398 **Other mechanical complication of other vascular grafts** A
- ● T82.399 **Other mechanical complication of unspecified vascular grafts** A

● T82.4 **Mechanical complication of vascular dialysis catheter**
Mechanical complication of hemodialysis catheter
Excludes1 mechanical complication of intraperitoneal dialysis catheter (T85.62)
- X● T82.41 **Breakdown (mechanical) of vascular dialysis catheter** A, D, S
- X● T82.42 **Displacement of vascular dialysis catheter** A, D, S
  Malposition of vascular dialysis catheter
- X● T82.43 **Leakage of vascular dialysis catheter** A, D, S
- X● T82.49 **Other complication of vascular dialysis catheter** A, D, S
  Obstruction (mechanical) of vascular dialysis catheter
  Perforation of vascular dialysis catheter
  Protrusion of vascular dialysis catheter

● T82.5 **Mechanical complication of other cardiac and vascular devices and implants**
Excludes2 mechanical complication of epidural and subdural infusion catheter (T85.61)

● T82.51 **Breakdown (mechanical) of other cardiac and vascular devices and implants**
- ● T82.510 **Breakdown (mechanical) of surgically created arteriovenous fistula** A
- ● T82.511 **Breakdown (mechanical) of surgically created arteriovenous shunt** A
- ● T82.512 **Breakdown (mechanical) of artificial heart**
- ● T82.513 **Breakdown (mechanical) of balloon (counterpulsation) device** A
- ● T82.514 **Breakdown (mechanical) of infusion catheter** A
- ● T82.515 **Breakdown (mechanical) of umbrella device** A
- ● T82.518 **Breakdown (mechanical) of other cardiac and vascular devices and implants** A
- ● T82.519 **Breakdown (mechanical) of unspecified cardiac and vascular devices and implants**

● T82.52 **Displacement of other cardiac and vascular devices and implants**
Malposition of other cardiac and vascular devices and implants
- ● T82.520 **Displacement of surgically created arteriovenous fistula** A
- ● T82.521 **Displacement of surgically created arteriovenous shunt** A
- ● T82.522 **Displacement of artificial heart**
- ● T82.523 **Displacement of balloon (counterpulsation) device** A
- ● T82.524 **Displacement of infusion catheter** A
- ● T82.525 **Displacement of umbrella device** A
- ● T82.528 **Displacement of other cardiac and vascular devices and implants** A
- ● T82.529 **Displacement of unspecified cardiac and vascular devices and implants**

● T82.53 **Leakage of other cardiac and vascular devices and implants**
- ● T82.530 **Leakage of surgically created arteriovenous fistula** A
- ● T82.531 **Leakage of surgically created arteriovenous shunt** A
- ● T82.532 **Leakage of artificial heart**
- ● T82.533 **Leakage of balloon (counterpulsation) device** A
- ● T82.534 **Leakage of infusion catheter** A
- ● T82.535 **Leakage of umbrella device** A
- ● T82.538 **Leakage of other cardiac and vascular devices and implants** A
- ● T82.539 **Leakage of unspecified cardiac and vascular devices and implants**

● T82.59 **Other mechanical complication of other cardiac and vascular devices and implants**
Obstruction (mechanical) of other cardiac and vascular devices and implants
Perforation of other cardiac and vascular devices and implants
Protrusion of other cardiac and vascular devices and implants
- ● T82.590 **Other mechanical complication of surgically created arteriovenous fistula** A
- ● T82.591 **Other mechanical complication of surgically created arteriovenous shunt** A
- ● T82.592 **Other mechanical complication of artificial heart**
- ● T82.593 **Other mechanical complication of balloon (counterpulsation) device** A
- ● T82.594 **Other mechanical complication of infusion catheter** A
- ● T82.595 **Other mechanical complication of umbrella device** A
- ● T82.598 **Other mechanical complication of other cardiac and vascular devices and implants** A
- ● T82.599 **Other mechanical complication of unspecified cardiac and vascular devices and implants**

X● T82.6 **Infection and inflammatory reaction due to cardiac valve prosthesis** A
Use additional code to identify infection

X● T82.7 **Infection and inflammatory reaction due to other cardiac and vascular devices, implants and grafts** A
Use additional code to identify infection
Coding Clinic: 2019, Q1, P13-14; 2018, Q4, P89

● T82.8 **Other specified complications** of cardiac and vascular prosthetic devices, implants and grafts

● T82.81 **Embolism** due to cardiac and vascular prosthetic devices, implants and grafts
Coding Clinic: 2016, Q4, P70

● T82.817 Embolism due to **cardiac** prosthetic devices, implants and grafts
Coding Clinic: 2016, Q4, P70; 2015, Q1, P20

● T82.818 Embolism due to **vascular** prosthetic devices, implants and grafts A

● T82.82 **Fibrosis** due to cardiac and vascular prosthetic devices, implants and grafts
Coding Clinic: 2016, Q4, P70

● T82.827 Fibrosis due to **cardiac** prosthetic devices, implants and grafts

● T82.828 Fibrosis due to **vascular** prosthetic devices, implants and grafts A

● T82.83 **Hemorrhage** due to cardiac and vascular prosthetic devices, implants and grafts
Coding Clinic: 2016, Q4, P70

● T82.837 Hemorrhage due to **cardiac** prosthetic devices, implants and grafts

● T82.838 Hemorrhage due to **vascular** prosthetic devices, implants and grafts A

● T82.84 **Pain** due to cardiac and vascular prosthetic devices, implants and grafts
Coding Clinic: 2016, Q4, P70

● T82.847 Pain due to **cardiac** prosthetic devices, implants and grafts

● T82.848 Pain due to **vascular** prosthetic devices, implants and grafts A

● T82.85 **Stenosis** due to cardiac and vascular prosthetic devices, implants and grafts

● T82.855 Stenosis of **coronary artery stent**
In-stent stenosis (restenosis) of coronary artery stent
Restenosis of coronary artery stent
Coding Clinic: 2016, Q4, P70

● T82.856 Stenosis of **peripheral vascular stent** A
In-stent stenosis (restenosis) of peripheral vascular stent
Restenosis of peripheral vascular stent
Coding Clinic: 2016, Q4, P70

● T82.857 Stenosis of other **cardiac** prosthetic devices, implants and grafts
Coding Clinic: 2016, Q4, P70

● T82.858 Stenosis of other **vascular** prosthetic devices, implants and grafts A
Coding Clinic: 2016, Q4, P70

● T82.86 **Thrombosis** of cardiac and vascular prosthetic devices, implants and grafts

● T82.867 Thrombosis due to **cardiac** prosthetic devices, implants and grafts

● T82.868 Thrombosis due to **vascular** prosthetic devices, implants and grafts A

● T82.89 **Other specified complication** of cardiac and vascular prosthetic devices, implants and grafts

● T82.897 Other specified complication of **cardiac** prosthetic devices, implants and grafts
Coding Clinic: 2019, Q2, P32-33

● T82.898 Other specified complication of **vascular** prosthetic devices, implants and grafts A

X● T82.9 **Unspecified** complication of cardiac and vascular prosthetic device, implant and graft

● T83 **Complications of genitourinary prosthetic devices, implants and grafts**

Excludes2 failure and rejection of transplanted organs and tissue (T86.-)

The appropriate 7th character is to be added to each code from category T83

A	initial encounter
D	subsequent encounter
S	sequela

Coding Clinic: 2016, Q4, P70-71

● T83.0 Mechanical complication of **urinary catheter**

Excludes2 complications of stoma of urinary tract (N99.5-)

Coding Clinic: 2016, Q4, P70

● T83.01 **Breakdown** (mechanical) of urinary catheter

● T83.010 Breakdown (mechanical) of **cystostomy** catheter A

● T83.011 Breakdown (mechanical) of **indwelling** urethral catheter A

● T83.012 Breakdown (mechanical) of **nephrostomy** catheter A

● T83.018 Breakdown (mechanical) of **other** urinary catheter A
Breakdown (mechanical) of Hopkins catheter
Breakdown (mechanical) of ileostomy catheter
Breakdown (mechanical) urostomy catheter

● T83.02 **Displacement** of urinary catheter
Malposition of urinary catheter

● T83.020 Displacement of **cystostomy** catheter A

● T83.021 Displacement of **indwelling** urethral catheter A

● T83.022 Displacement of **nephrostomy** catheter A

● T83.028 Displacement of **other** urinary catheter A
Displacement of Hopkins catheter
Displacement of ileostomy catheter
Displacement of urostomy catheter

● T83.03 **Leakage** of urinary catheter

● T83.030 Leakage of **cystostomy** catheter A

● T83.031 Leakage of **indwelling** urethral catheter A

● T83.032 Leakage of **nephrostomy** catheter A

● T83.038 Leakage of **other** urinary catheter A
Leakage of Hopkins catheter
Leakage of ileostomy catheter
Leakage of urostomy catheter

● T83.09 **Other** mechanical complication of urinary catheter
Obstruction (mechanical) of urinary catheter
Perforation of urinary catheter
Protrusion of urinary catheter

● T83.090 Other mechanical complication of **cystostomy** catheter A

● T83.091 Other mechanical complication of **indwelling** urethral catheter A

● T83.092 Other mechanical complication of **nephrostomy** catheter A

● T83.098 Other mechanical complication of **other** urinary catheter A
Other mechanical complication of Hopkins catheter
Other mechanical complication of ileostomy catheter
Other mechanical complication of urostomy catheter

T83.1 Mechanical complication of other urinary devices and implants
Coding Clinic: 2016, Q4, P70

T83.11 Breakdown (mechanical) of other urinary devices and implants

T83.110 Breakdown (mechanical) of urinary electronic stimulator device A

Excludes2 Breakdown (mechanical) of electrode (lead) for sacral nerve neurostimulator (T85.111)
Breakdown (mechanical) of implanted electronic sacral neurostimulator, pulse generator or receiver (T85.113)

T83.111 Breakdown (mechanical) of implanted urinary sphincter A

T83.112 Breakdown (mechanical) of indwelling ureteral stent A

T83.113 Breakdown (mechanical) of other urinary stents A
Breakdown (mechanical) of ileal conduit stent
Breakdown (mechanical) of nephroureteral stent

T83.118 Breakdown (mechanical) of other urinary devices and implants A

T83.12 Displacement of other urinary devices and implants
Malposition of other urinary devices and implants

T83.120 Displacement of urinary electronic stimulator device A

Excludes2 Displacement of electrode (lead) for sacral nerve neurostimulator (T85.121)
Displacement of implanted electronic sacral neurostimulator, pulse generator or receiver (T85.123)

T83.121 Displacement of implanted urinary sphincter A

T83.122 Displacement of indwelling ureteral stent A

T83.123 Displacement of other urinary stents A
Displacement of ileal conduit stent
Displacement of nephroureteral stent

T83.128 Displacement of other urinary devices and implants A

T83.19 Other mechanical complication of other urinary devices and implants
Leakage of other urinary devices and implants
Obstruction (mechanical) of other urinary devices and implants
Perforation of other urinary devices and implants
Protrusion of other urinary devices and implants

T83.190 Other mechanical complication of urinary electronic stimulator device A

Excludes2 Other mechanical complication of electrode (lead) for sacral nerve neurostimulator (T85.191)
Other mechanical complication of implanted electronic sacral neurostimulator, pulse generator or receiver (T85.193)

T83.191 Other mechanical complication of implanted urinary sphincter A

T83.192 Other mechanical complication of indwelling ureteral stent A

T83.193 Other mechanical complication of other urinary stent A
Other mechanical complication of ileal conduit stent
Other mechanical complication of nephroureteral stent

T83.198 Other mechanical complication of other urinary devices and implants A

T83.2 Mechanical complication of graft of urinary organ
Coding Clinic: 2016, Q4, P70

X **T83.21 Breakdown (mechanical) of graft of urinary organ** A

X **T83.22 Displacement of graft of urinary organ** A
Malposition of graft of urinary organ

X **T83.23 Leakage of graft of urinary organ** A

X **T83.24 Erosion of graft of urinary organ** A
Coding Clinic: 2016, Q4, P70

X **T83.25 Exposure of graft of urinary organ** A
Coding Clinic: 2016, Q4, P70

X **T83.29 Other mechanical complication of graft of urinary organ** A
Obstruction (mechanical) of graft of urinary organ
Perforation of graft of urinary organ
Protrusion of graft of urinary organ

T83.3 Mechanical complication of intrauterine contraceptive device

X **T83.31 Breakdown (mechanical) of intrauterine contraceptive device** ♀

X **T83.32 Displacement of intrauterine contraceptive device** ♀
Malposition of intrauterine contraceptive device
Missing string of intrauterine contraceptive device

X **T83.39 Other mechanical complication of intrauterine contraceptive device** ♀
Leakage of intrauterine contraceptive device
Obstruction (mechanical) of intrauterine contraceptive device
Perforation of intrauterine contraceptive device
Protrusion of intrauterine contraceptive device

CHAPTER 19 (S00-T88)

● T83.4 **Mechanical complication of other prosthetic devices, implants and grafts of genital tract**
Coding Clinic: 2016, Q4, P71

● T83.41 **Breakdown (mechanical) of other prosthetic devices, implants and grafts of genital tract**

● T83.410 **Breakdown (mechanical) of implanted penile prosthesis** ♂ A
Breakdown (mechanical) of penile prosthesis cylinder
Breakdown (mechanical) of penile prosthesis pump
Breakdown (mechanical) of penile prosthesis reservoir

● T83.411 **Breakdown (mechanical) of implanted testicular prosthesis** A

● T83.418 **Breakdown (mechanical) of other prosthetic devices, implants and grafts of genital tract** A

● T83.42 **Displacement of other prosthetic devices, implants and grafts of genital tract**
Malposition of other prosthetic devices, implants and grafts of genital tract

● T83.420 **Displacement of implanted penile prosthesis** ♂ A
Displacement of penile prosthesis cylinder
Displacement of penile prosthesis pump
Displacement of penile prosthesis reservoir

● T83.421 **Displacement of implanted testicular prosthesis** A

● T83.428 **Displacement of other prosthetic devices, implants and grafts of genital tract** A
Coding Clinic: 2018, Q1, P6

● T83.49 **Other mechanical complication of other prosthetic devices, implants and grafts of genital tract**
Leakage of other prosthetic devices, implants and grafts of genital tract
Obstruction, mechanical of other prosthetic devices, implants and grafts of genital tract
Perforation of other prosthetic devices, implants and grafts of genital tract
Protrusion of other prosthetic devices, implants and grafts of genital tract

● T83.490 **Other mechanical complication of implanted penile prosthesis** ♂ A
Other mechanical complication of penile prosthesis cylinder
Other mechanical complication of penile prosthesis pump
Other mechanical complication of penile prosthesis reservoir

● T83.491 **Other mechanical complication of implanted testicular prosthesis** A

● T83.498 **Other mechanical complication of other prosthetic devices, implants and grafts of genital tract** A

● T83.5 **Infection and inflammatory reaction due to prosthetic device, implant and graft in urinary system**
Use additional code to identify infection
Coding Clinic: 2016, Q4, P71

● T83.51 **Infection and inflammatory reaction due to urinary catheter**
Excludes2 complications of stoma of urinary tract (N99.5-)

● T83.510 **Infection and inflammatory reaction due to cystostomy catheter** A

● T83.511 **Infection and inflammatory reaction due to indwelling urethral catheter** A

● T83.512 **Infection and inflammatory reaction due to nephrostomy catheter** A

● T83.518 **Infection and inflammatory reaction due to other urinary catheter** A
Infection and inflammatory reaction due to Hopkins catheter
Infection and inflammatory reaction due to ileostomy catheter
Infection and inflammatory reaction due to urostomy catheter

● T83.59 **Infection and inflammatory reaction due to prosthetic device, implant and graft in urinary system**

● T83.590 **Infection and inflammatory reaction due to implanted urinary neurostimulation device** A
Excludes2 Infection and inflammatory reaction due to electrode lead of sacral nerve neurostimulator (T85.732)
Infection and inflammatory reaction due to pulse generator or receiver of sacral nerve neurostimulator (T85.734)

● T83.591 **Infection and inflammatory reaction due to implanted urinary sphincter** A

● T83.592 **Infection and inflammatory reaction due to indwelling ureteral stent** A

● T83.593 **Infection and inflammatory reaction due to other urinary stents** A
Infection and inflammatory reaction due to ileal conduit stents
Infection and inflammatory reaction due to nephroureteral stent

● T83.598 **Infection and inflammatory reaction due to other prosthetic device, implant and graft in urinary system** A

● T83.6 **Infection and inflammatory reaction due to prosthetic device, implant and graft in genital tract**
Use additional code to identify infection
Coding Clinic: 2016, Q4, P71

● T83.61 **Infection and inflammatory reaction due to implanted penile prosthesis** A
Infection and inflammatory reaction due to penile prosthesis cylinder
Infection and inflammatory reaction due to penile prosthesis pump
Infection and inflammatory reaction due to penile prosthesis reservoir

● T83.62 **Infection and inflammatory reaction due to implanted testicular prosthesis** A

● T83.69 **Infection and inflammatory reaction due to other prosthetic device, implant and graft in genital tract** A

● T83.7 **Complications due to implanted mesh and other prosthetic materials**
Coding Clinic: 2016, Q4, P71

● T83.71 **Erosion of implanted mesh and other prosthetic materials to surrounding organ or tissue**
Coding Clinic: 2016, Q4, P71

● T83.711 **Erosion of implanted vaginal mesh to surrounding organ or tissue** ♀ A
Erosion of implanted vaginal mesh into pelvic floor muscles
Coding Clinic: 2016, Q4, P71

● T83.712 **Erosion of implanted urethral mesh to surrounding organ or tissue** A
Erosion of implanted female urethral sling
Erosion of implanted male urethral sling
Erosion of implanted urethral mesh into pelvic floor muscles

● T83.713 **Erosion of implanted urethral bulking agent to surrounding organ or tissue** A

● T83.714 **Erosion of implanted ureteral bulking agent to surrounding organ or tissue** A

● T83.718 **Erosion of other implanted mesh to organ or tissue** A
Coding Clinic: 2016, Q4, P71

● T83.719 **Erosion of other prosthetic materials to surrounding organ or tissue** A
Coding Clinic: 2016, Q4, P71

● T83.72 **Exposure of implanted mesh and other prosthetic materials into surrounding organ or tissue**
Extrusion of implanted mesh
Coding Clinic: 2016, Q4, P71

● T83.721 **Exposure of implanted vaginal mesh into vagina** ♀ A
Exposure of implanted vaginal mesh through vaginal wall

● T83.722 **Exposure of implanted urethral mesh into urethra** A
Exposure of implanted female urethral sling
Exposure of implanted male urethral sling
Exposure of implanted urethral mesh through urethral wall

● T83.723 **Exposure of implanted urethral bulking agent into urethra** A

● T83.724 **Exposure of implanted ureteral bulking agent into ureter** A

● T83.728 **Exposure of other implanted mesh into organ or tissue** A
Coding Clinic: 2016, Q4, P71

● T83.729 **Exposure of other prosthetic materials into organ or tissue** A
Coding Clinic: 2016, Q4, P71

X● T83.79 **Other specified complications due to other genitourinary prosthetic materials** A

● T83.8 **Other specified complications of genitourinary prosthetic devices, implants and grafts**

X● T83.81 **Embolism due to genitourinary prosthetic devices, implants and grafts** A

X● T83.82 **Fibrosis due to genitourinary prosthetic devices, implants and grafts** A

X● T83.83 **Hemorrhage due to genitourinary prosthetic devices, implants and grafts** A

X● T83.84 **Pain due to genitourinary prosthetic devices, implants and grafts** A

X● T83.85 **Stenosis due to genitourinary prosthetic devices, implants and grafts** A

X● T83.86 **Thrombosis due to genitourinary prosthetic devices, implants and grafts** A

X● T83.89 **Other specified complication of genitourinary prosthetic devices, implants and grafts** A

X● T83.9 **Unspecified complication of genitourinary prosthetic device, implant and graft** A

● T84 **Complications of internal orthopedic prosthetic devices, implants and grafts**
Excludes2 failure and rejection of transplanted organs and tissues (T86.-)
fracture of bone following insertion of orthopedic implant, joint prosthesis or bone plate (M96.6)

The appropriate 7th character is to be added to each code from category T84

A	initial encounter
D	subsequent encounter
S	sequela

● T84.0 **Mechanical complication of internal joint prosthesis**

● T84.01 **Broken internal joint prosthesis**
Breakage (fracture) of prosthetic joint
Broken prosthetic joint implant
Excludes1 periprosthetic joint implant fracture (M97-)
Coding Clinic: 2016, Q4, P42

● T84.010 **Broken internal right hip prosthesis** A

● T84.011 **Broken internal left hip prosthesis** A

● T84.012 **Broken internal right knee prosthesis** A

● T84.013 **Broken internal left knee prosthesis** A

● T84.018 **Broken internal joint prosthesis, other site** A
Use additional code to identify the joint (Z96.6-)

● T84.019 **Broken internal joint prosthesis, unspecified site** A

CHAPTER 19 (S00-T88)

T84.02 **Dislocation** of internal joint prosthesis
Instability of internal joint prosthesis
Subluxation of internal joint prosthesis
- T84.020 Dislocation of internal **right hip** prosthesis A
- T84.021 Dislocation of internal **left hip** prosthesis A
  Coding Clinic: 2019, Q2, P27
- T84.022 Instability of internal **right knee** prosthesis A
- T84.023 Instability of internal **left knee** prosthesis A
- T84.028 Dislocation of **other** internal joint prosthesis A
  Use additional code to identify the joint (Z96.6-)
- T84.029 Dislocation of **unspecified** internal joint prosthesis A

T84.03 Mechanical **loosening** of internal prosthetic joint
Aseptic loosening of prosthetic joint
- T84.030 Mechanical loosening of internal **right hip** prosthetic joint A
- T84.031 Mechanical loosening of internal left **hip** prosthetic joint A
- T84.032 Mechanical loosening of internal **right knee** prosthetic joint A
- T84.033 Mechanical loosening of internal left **knee** prosthetic joint A
- T84.038 Mechanical loosening of **other** internal prosthetic joint A
  Use additional code to identify the joint (Z96.6-)
- T84.039 Mechanical loosening of **unspecified** internal prosthetic joint A

T84.05 **Periprosthetic osteolysis** of internal prosthetic joint
Use additional code to identify major osseous defect, if applicable (M89.7-)
- T84.050 Periprosthetic osteolysis of internal prosthetic **right hip** joint A
- T84.051 Periprosthetic osteolysis of internal prosthetic **left hip** joint A
- T84.052 Periprosthetic osteolysis of internal prosthetic **right knee** joint A
- T84.053 Periprosthetic osteolysis of internal prosthetic **left knee** joint A
- T84.058 Periprosthetic osteolysis of **other** internal prosthetic joint A
  Use additional code to identify the joint (Z96.6-)
- T84.059 Periprosthetic osteolysis of **unspecified** internal prosthetic joint A

T84.06 **Wear of articular bearing surface** of internal prosthetic joint
- T84.060 Wear of articular bearing surface of internal prosthetic **right hip** joint A
- T84.061 Wear of articular bearing surface of internal prosthetic **left hip** joint A
- T84.062 Wear of articular bearing surface of internal prosthetic **right knee** joint A
- T84.063 Wear of articular bearing surface of internal prosthetic **left knee** joint A
- T84.068 Wear of articular bearing surface of **other** internal prosthetic joint A
  Use additional code to identify the joint (Z96.6-)
- T84.069 Wear of articular bearing surface of **unspecified** internal prosthetic joint A

T84.09 **Other mechanical complication** of internal joint prosthesis
Prosthetic joint implant failure NOS
- T84.090 Other mechanical complication of internal **right hip** prosthesis A
  Coding Clinic: 2019, Q1, P20
- T84.091 Other mechanical complication of internal **left hip** prosthesis A
- T84.092 Other mechanical complication of internal **right knee** prosthesis A
- T84.093 Other mechanical complication of internal **left knee** prosthesis A
- T84.098 Other mechanical complication of **other** internal joint prosthesis A
  Use additional code to identify the joint (Z96.6-)
- T84.099 Other mechanical complication of **unspecified** internal joint prosthesis A

T84.1 Mechanical complication of **internal fixation device** of **bones of limb**
Excludes2 mechanical complication of internal fixation device of bones of feet (T84.2-)
mechanical complication of internal fixation device of bones of fingers (T84.2-)
mechanical complication of internal fixation device of bones of hands (T84.2-)
mechanical complication of internal fixation device of bones of toes (T84.2-)

T84.11 **Breakdown** (mechanical) of internal fixation device of bones of limb
- T84.110 Breakdown (mechanical) of internal fixation device of **right humerus** A
- T84.111 Breakdown (mechanical) of internal fixation device of **left humerus** A
- T84.112 Breakdown (mechanical) of internal fixation device of bone of **right forearm** A
- T84.113 Breakdown (mechanical) of internal fixation device of bone of **left forearm** A
- T84.114 Breakdown (mechanical) of internal fixation device of **right femur** A
- T84.115 Breakdown (mechanical) of internal fixation device of **left femur** A
- T84.116 Breakdown (mechanical) of internal fixation device of bone of **right lower leg** A
- T84.117 Breakdown (mechanical) of internal fixation device of bone of **left lower leg** A
- T84.119 Breakdown (mechanical) of internal fixation device of **unspecified** bone of limb A

T84.12 **Displacement** of internal fixation device of bones of limb
Malposition of internal fixation device of bones of limb
- T84.120 Displacement of internal fixation device of **right humerus** A
- T84.121 Displacement of internal fixation device of **left humerus** A
- T84.122 Displacement of internal fixation device of bone of **right forearm** A
- T84.123 Displacement of internal fixation device of bone of **left forearm** A
- T84.124 Displacement of internal fixation device of **right femur** A

T84.125 Displacement of internal fixation device of **left femur** A
T84.126 Displacement of internal fixation device of bone of **right lower leg** A
T84.127 Displacement of internal fixation device of bone of **left lower leg** A
T84.129 Displacement of internal fixation device of **unspecified** bone of limb A

T84.19 **Other mechanical complication** of internal **fixation device of bones of limb**
Obstruction (mechanical) of internal fixation device of bones of limb
Perforation of internal fixation device of bones of limb
Protrusion of internal fixation device of bones of limb

T84.190 Other mechanical complication of internal fixation device of **right humerus** A
T84.191 Other mechanical complication of internal fixation device of **left humerus** A
T84.192 Other mechanical complication of internal fixation device of bone of **right forearm** A
T84.193 Other mechanical complication of internal fixation device of bone of **left forearm** A
T84.194 Other mechanical complication of internal fixation device of **right femur** A
T84.195 Other mechanical complication of internal fixation device of **left femur** A
T84.196 Other mechanical complication of internal fixation device of bone of **right lower leg** A
T84.197 Other mechanical complication of internal fixation device of bone of **left lower leg** A
T84.199 Other mechanical complication of internal fixation device of **unspecified** bone of limb A

T84.2 Mechanical complication of **internal fixation device** of **other bones**

T84.21 **Breakdown** (mechanical) of internal fixation device of other bones
T84.210 Breakdown (mechanical) of internal fixation device of bones of **hand and fingers** A
T84.213 Breakdown (mechanical) of internal fixation device of bones of **foot and toes** A
T84.216 Breakdown (mechanical) of internal fixation device of **vertebrae** A
T84.218 Breakdown (mechanical) of internal fixation device of **other bones** A

T84.22 **Displacement** of internal fixation device of other bones
Malposition of internal fixation device of other bones
T84.220 Displacement of internal fixation device of bones of **hand and fingers** A
T84.223 Displacement of internal fixation device of bones of **foot and toes** A
T84.226 Displacement of internal fixation device of **vertebrae** A
T84.228 Displacement of internal fixation device of **other bones** A

T84.29 **Other mechanical complication** of internal **fixation device of other bones**
Obstruction (mechanical) of internal fixation device of other bones
Perforation of internal fixation device of other bones
Protrusion of internal fixation device of other bones
T84.290 Other mechanical complication of internal fixation device of bones of **hand and fingers** A
T84.293 Other mechanical complication of internal fixation device of bones of **foot and toes** A
T84.296 Other mechanical complication of internal fixation device of **vertebrae** A
T84.298 Other mechanical complication of internal fixation device of **other bones** A

T84.3 Mechanical complication of **other bone devices, implants and grafts**
Excludes2 other complications of bone graft (T86.83-)

T84.31 **Breakdown** (mechanical) of other bone devices, implants and grafts
T84.310 Breakdown (mechanical) of **electronic bone stimulator** A
T84.318 Breakdown (mechanical) of **other** bone devices, implants and grafts A

T84.32 **Displacement** of other bone devices, implants and grafts
Malposition of other bone devices, implants and grafts
T84.320 Displacement of **electronic bone stimulator** A
T84.328 Displacement of **other** bone devices, implants and grafts A

T84.39 **Other mechanical complication** of other bone devices, implants and grafts
Obstruction (mechanical) of other bone devices, implants and grafts
Perforation of other bone devices, implants and grafts
Protrusion of other bone devices, implants and grafts
T84.390 Other mechanical complication of **electronic bone stimulator** A
T84.398 Other mechanical complication of **other** bone devices, implants and grafts A

T84.4 Mechanical complication of **other internal orthopedic devices, implants and grafts**

T84.41 **Breakdown** (mechanical) of other internal orthopedic devices, implants and grafts
T84.410 Breakdown (mechanical) of **muscle and tendon graft** A
T84.418 Breakdown (mechanical) of **other** internal orthopedic devices, implants and grafts A

T84.42 **Displacement** of other internal orthopedic devices, implants and grafts
Malposition of other internal orthopedic devices, implants and grafts
T84.420 Displacement of **muscle and tendon graft** A
T84.428 Displacement of **other** internal orthopedic devices, implants and grafts A

CHAPTER 19 (SØØ-T88)

● T84.49 Other mechanical complication of other internal orthopedic devices, implants and grafts
Mechanical complication of other internal orthopedic devices, implants and grafts NOS
Obstruction (mechanical) of other internal orthopedic devices, implants and grafts
Perforation of other internal orthopedic devices, implants and grafts
Protrusion of other internal orthopedic devices, implants and grafts

● T84.49Ø Other mechanical complication of muscle and tendon graft A

● T84.498 Other mechanical complication of other internal orthopedic devices, implants and grafts A

● T84.5 Infection and inflammatory reaction due to internal joint prosthesis
Use additional code to identify infection
Coding Clinic: 2015, Q1, P16

X● T84.5Ø Infection and inflammatory reaction due to unspecified internal joint prosthesis A
Coding Clinic: 2Ø15, Q1, P3

X● T84.51 Infection and inflammatory reaction due to internal right hip prosthesis A
Coding Clinic: 2Ø15, Q4, P36

X● T84.52 Infection and inflammatory reaction due to internal left hip prosthesis A
Coding Clinic: 2Ø15, Q1, P16-17

X● T84.53 Infection and inflammatory reaction due to internal right knee prosthesis A

X● T84.54 Infection and inflammatory reaction due to internal left knee prosthesis A

X● T84.59 Infection and inflammatory reaction due to other internal joint prosthesis A

● T84.6 Infection and inflammatory reaction due to internal fixation device
Use additional code to identify infection

X● T84.6Ø Infection and inflammatory reaction due to internal fixation device of unspecified site A

● T84.61 Infection and inflammatory reaction due to internal fixation device of arm

● T84.61Ø Infection and inflammatory reaction due to internal fixation device of right humerus A

● T84.611 Infection and inflammatory reaction due to internal fixation device of left humerus A

● T84.612 Infection and inflammatory reaction due to internal fixation device of right radius A

● T84.613 Infection and inflammatory reaction due to internal fixation device of left radius A

● T84.614 Infection and inflammatory reaction due to internal fixation device of right ulna A

● T84.615 Infection and inflammatory reaction due to internal fixation device of left ulna A

● T84.619 Infection and inflammatory reaction due to internal fixation device of unspecified bone of arm A

● T84.62 Infection and inflammatory reaction due to internal fixation device of leg

● T84.62Ø Infection and inflammatory reaction due to internal fixation device of right femur A

● T84.621 Infection and inflammatory reaction due to internal fixation device of left femur A

● T84.622 Infection and inflammatory reaction due to internal fixation device of right tibia A

● T84.623 Infection and inflammatory reaction due to internal fixation device of left tibia A

● T84.624 Infection and inflammatory reaction due to internal fixation device of right fibula A

● T84.625 Infection and inflammatory reaction due to internal fixation device of left fibula A

● T84.629 Infection and inflammatory reaction due to internal fixation device of unspecified bone of leg A

X● T84.63 Infection and inflammatory reaction due to internal fixation device of spine A

X● T84.69 Infection and inflammatory reaction due to internal fixation device of other site A

● T84.7 Infection and inflammatory reaction due to other internal orthopedic prosthetic devices, implants and grafts A
Use additional code to identify infection

● T84.8 Other specified complications of internal orthopedic prosthetic devices, implants and grafts

X● T84.81 Embolism due to internal orthopedic prosthetic devices, implants and grafts A

X● T84.82 Fibrosis due to internal orthopedic prosthetic devices, implants and grafts A

X● T84.83 Hemorrhage due to internal orthopedic prosthetic devices, implants and grafts A

X● T84.84 Pain due to internal orthopedic prosthetic devices, implants and grafts A

X● T84.85 Stenosis due to internal orthopedic prosthetic devices, implants and grafts A

X● T84.86 Thrombosis due to internal orthopedic prosthetic devices, implants and grafts A

X● T84.89 Other specified complication of internal orthopedic prosthetic devices, implants and grafts A

X● T84.9 Unspecified complication of internal orthopedic prosthetic device, implant and graft A

● T85 Complications of other internal prosthetic devices, implants and grafts
Excludes2 failure and rejection of transplanted organs and tissue (T86.-)
The appropriate 7th character is to be added to each code from category T85

A	initial encounter
D	subsequent encounter
S	sequela

Coding Clinic: 2Ø16, Q4, P71

● T85.Ø Mechanical complication of ventricular intracranial (communicating) shunt

X● T85.Ø1 Breakdown (mechanical) of ventricular intracranial (communicating) shunt A

X● T85.Ø2 Displacement of ventricular intracranial (communicating) shunt A
Malposition of ventricular intracranial (communicating) shunt

X● T85.03 **Leakage of ventricular intracranial (communicating) shunt** A

X● T85.09 **Other mechanical complication of ventricular intracranial (communicating) shunt** A
Obstruction (mechanical) of ventricular intracranial (communicating) shunt
Perforation of ventricular intracranial (communicating) shunt
Protrusion of ventricular intracranial (communicating) shunt

● T85.1 **Mechanical complication of implanted electronic stimulator of nervous system**
Coding Clinic: 2016, Q4, P71

● T85.11 **Breakdown (mechanical) of implanted electronic stimulator of nervous system**

● T85.110 **Breakdown (mechanical) of implanted electronic neurostimulator of brain electrode (lead)** A

● T85.111 **Breakdown (mechanical) of implanted electronic neurostimulator of peripheral nerve electrode (lead)** A
Breakdown of electrode (lead) for cranial nerve neurostimulators
Breakdown of electrode (lead) for gastric neurostimulator
Breakdown of electrode (lead) for sacral nerve neurostimulator
Breakdown of electrode (lead) for vagal nerve neurostimulators

● T85.112 **Breakdown (mechanical) of implanted electronic neurostimulator of spinal cord electrode (lead)** A

● T85.113 **Breakdown (mechanical) of implanted electronic neurostimulator, generator** A
Breakdown (mechanical) of implanted electronic neurostimulator generator, brain, peripheral, gastric, spinal
Breakdown (mechanical) of implanted electronic sacral neurostimulator, pulse generator or receiver

● T85.118 **Breakdown (mechanical) of other implanted electronic stimulator of nervous system** A

● T85.12 **Displacement of implanted electronic stimulator of nervous system**
Malposition of implanted electronic stimulator of nervous system

● T85.120 **Displacement of implanted electronic neurostimulator of brain electrode (lead)** A

● T85.121 **Displacement of implanted electronic neurostimulator of peripheral nerve electrode (lead)** A
Displacement of electrode (lead) for cranial nerve neurostimulators
Displacement of electrode (lead) for gastric neurostimulator
Displacement of electrode (lead) for sacral nerve neurostimulator
Displacement of electrode (lead) for vagal nerve neurostimulators

● T85.122 **Displacement of implanted electronic neurostimulator of spinal cord electrode (lead)** A

● T85.123 **Displacement of implanted electronic neurostimulator, generator** A
Displacement of implanted electronic neurostimulator generator, brain, peripheral, gastric, spinal
Displacement of implanted electronic sacral neurostimulator, pulse generator or receiver

● T85.128 **Displacement of other implanted electronic stimulator of nervous system** A

● T85.19 **Other mechanical complication of implanted electronic stimulator of nervous system**
Leakage of implanted electronic stimulator of nervous system
Obstruction (mechanical) of implanted electronic stimulator of nervous system
Perforation of implanted electronic stimulator of nervous system
Protrusion of implanted electronic stimulator of nervous system

● T85.190 **Other mechanical complication of implanted electronic neurostimulator of brain electrode (lead)** A

● T85.191 **Other mechanical complication of implanted electronic neurostimulator of peripheral nerve electrode (lead)** A
Other mechanical complication of electrode (lead) for cranial nerve neurostimulators
Other mechanical complication of electrode (lead) for gastric neurostimulator
Other mechanical complication of electrode (lead) for sacral nerve neurostimulator
Other mechanical complication of electrode (lead) for vagal nerve neurostimulators

● T85.192 **Other mechanical complication of implanted electronic neurostimulator of spinal cord electrode (lead)** A

● T85.193 **Other mechanical complication of implanted electronic neurostimulator, generator** A
Other mechanical complication of implanted electronic neurostimulator generator, brain, peripheral, gastric, spinal
Other mechanical complication of implanted electronic sacral neurostimulator, pulse generator or receiver

● T85.199 **Other mechanical complication of other implanted electronic stimulator of nervous system** A

● T85.2 **Mechanical complication of intraocular lens**

X● T85.21 **Breakdown (mechanical) of intraocular lens**

X● T85.22 **Displacement of intraocular lens**
Malposition of intraocular lens

X● T85.29 **Other mechanical complication of intraocular lens**
Obstruction (mechanical) of intraocular lens
Perforation of intraocular lens
Protrusion of intraocular lens

● T85.3 **Mechanical complication of other ocular prosthetic devices, implants and grafts**
Excludes2 other complications of corneal graft (T86.84-)
● T85.31 **Breakdown (mechanical) of other ocular prosthetic devices, implants and grafts**
● T85.310 **Breakdown (mechanical) of prosthetic orbit of right eye**
● T85.311 **Breakdown (mechanical) of prosthetic orbit of left eye**
● T85.318 **Breakdown (mechanical) of other ocular prosthetic devices, implants and grafts**
● T85.32 **Displacement of other ocular prosthetic devices, implants and grafts**
Malposition of other ocular prosthetic devices, implants and grafts
● T85.320 **Displacement of prosthetic orbit of right eye**
● T85.321 **Displacement of prosthetic orbit of left eye**
● T85.328 **Displacement of other ocular prosthetic devices, implants and grafts**
● T85.39 **Other mechanical complication of other ocular prosthetic devices, implants and grafts**
Obstruction (mechanical) of other ocular prosthetic devices, implants and grafts
Perforation of other ocular prosthetic devices, implants and grafts
Protrusion of other ocular prosthetic devices, implants and grafts
● T85.390 **Other mechanical complication of prosthetic orbit of right eye**
● T85.391 **Other mechanical complication of prosthetic orbit of left eye**
● T85.398 **Other mechanical complication of other ocular prosthetic devices, implants and grafts**
● T85.4 **Mechanical complication of breast prosthesis and implant**
X● T85.41 **Breakdown (mechanical) of breast prosthesis and implant**
X● T85.42 **Displacement of breast prosthesis and implant**
Malposition of breast prosthesis and implant
X● T85.43 **Leakage of breast prosthesis and implant**
X● T85.44 **Capsular contracture of breast implant**
X● T85.49 **Other mechanical complication of breast prosthesis and implant**
Obstruction (mechanical) of breast prosthesis and implant
Perforation of breast prosthesis and implant
Protrusion of breast prosthesis and implant
● T85.5 **Mechanical complication of gastrointestinal prosthetic devices, implants and grafts**
● T85.51 **Breakdown (mechanical) of gastrointestinal prosthetic devices, implants and grafts**
● T85.510 **Breakdown (mechanical) of bile duct prosthesis**
● T85.511 **Breakdown (mechanical) of esophageal anti-reflux device**
● T85.518 **Breakdown (mechanical) of other gastrointestinal prosthetic devices, implants and grafts**
● T85.52 **Displacement of gastrointestinal prosthetic devices, implants and grafts**
Malposition of gastrointestinal prosthetic devices, implants and grafts
● T85.520 **Displacement of bile duct prosthesis**
● T85.521 **Displacement of esophageal anti-reflux device**
● T85.528 **Displacement of other gastrointestinal prosthetic devices, implants and grafts**
● T85.59 **Other mechanical complication of gastrointestinal prosthetic devices, implants and**
Obstruction, mechanical of gastrointestinal prosthetic devices, implants and grafts
Perforation of gastrointestinal prosthetic devices, implants and grafts
Protrusion of gastrointestinal prosthetic devices, implants and grafts
● T85.590 **Other mechanical complication of bile duct prosthesis**
● T85.591 **Other mechanical complication of esophageal anti-reflux device**
● T85.598 **Other mechanical complication of other gastrointestinal prosthetic devices, implants and grafts**
● T85.6 **Mechanical complication of other specified internal and external prosthetic devices, implants and grafts**
Coding Clinic: 2016, Q4, P71
● T85.61 **Breakdown (mechanical) of other specified internal prosthetic devices, implants and grafts**
● T85.610 **Breakdown (mechanical) of cranial or spinal infusion catheter**
Breakdown (mechanical) of epidural infusion catheter
Breakdown (mechanical) of intrathecal infusion catheter
Breakdown (mechanical) of subarachnoid infusion catheter
Breakdown (mechanical) of subdural infusion catheter
● T85.611 **Breakdown (mechanical) of intraperitoneal dialysis catheter** A, D, S ⓒ
Excludes1 mechanical complication of vascular dialysis catheter (T82.4-)
● T85.612 **Breakdown (mechanical) of permanent sutures**
Excludes1 mechanical complication of permanent (wire) suture used in bone repair (T84.1-T84.2)
● T85.613 **Breakdown (mechanical) of artificial skin graft and decellularized allodermis**
Failure of artificial skin graft and decellularized allodermis
Non-adherence of artificial skin graft and decellularized allodermis
Poor incorporation of artificial skin graft and decellularized allodermis
Shearing of artificial skin graft and decellularized allodermis
● T85.614 **Breakdown (mechanical) of insulin pump**
● T85.615 **Breakdown (mechanical) of other nervous system device, implant or graft** A ⓒ
Breakdown (mechanical) of intrathecal infusion pump
● T85.618 **Breakdown (mechanical) of other specified internal prosthetic devices, implants and grafts**

● T85.62 **Displacement of other specified internal prosthetic devices, implants and grafts**
Malposition of other specified internal prosthetic devices, implants and grafts

● T85.620 **Displacement of cranial or spinal infusion catheter**
Displacement of epidural infusion catheter
Displacement of intrathecal infusion catheter
Displacement of subarachnoid infusion catheter
Displacement of subdural infusion catheter

● T85.621 **Displacement of intraperitoneal dialysis catheter** A, D, S
Excludes1 mechanical complication of vascular dialysis catheter (T82.4-)

● T85.622 **Displacement of permanent sutures**
Excludes1 mechanical complication of permanent (wire) suture used in bone repair (T84.1-T84.2)

● T85.623 **Displacement of artificial skin graft and decellularized allodermis**
Dislodgement of artificial skin graft and decellularized allodermis

● T85.624 **Displacement of insulin pump**

● T85.625 **Displacement of other nervous system device, implant or graft** A
Displacement of intrathecal infusion pump

● T85.628 **Displacement of other specified internal prosthetic devices, implants and grafts**
Coding Clinic: 2015, Q1, P15

● T85.63 **Leakage of other specified internal prosthetic devices, implants and grafts**

● T85.630 **Leakage of cranial or spinal infusion catheter**
Leakage of epidural infusion catheter
Leakage of intrathecal infusion catheter
Leakage of subdural infusion catheter
Leakage of subarachnoid infusion catheter

● T85.631 **Leakage of intraperitoneal dialysis catheter** A, D, S
Excludes1 mechanical complication of vascular dialysis catheter (T82.4)

● T85.633 **Leakage of insulin pump**

● T85.635 **Leakage of other nervous system device, implant or graft** A
Leakage of intrathecal infusion pump

● T85.638 **Leakage of other specified internal prosthetic devices, implants and grafts**

● T85.69 **Other mechanical complication of other specified internal prosthetic devices, implants and grafts**
Obstruction, mechanical of other specified internal prosthetic devices, implants and grafts
Perforation of other specified internal prosthetic devices, implants and grafts
Protrusion of other specified internal prosthetic devices, implants and grafts

● T85.690 **Other mechanical complication of cranial or spinal infusion catheter**
Other mechanical complication of epidural infusion catheter
Other mechanical complication of intrathecal infusion catheter
Other mechanical complication of subarachnoid infusion catheter
Other mechanical complication of subdural infusion catheter

● T85.691 **Other mechanical complication of intraperitoneal dialysis catheter** A, D, S
Excludes1 mechanical complication of vascular dialysis catheter (T82.4)

● T85.692 **Other mechanical complication of permanent sutures**
Excludes1 mechanical complication of permanent (wire) suture used in bone repair (T84.1-T84.2)

● T85.693 **Other mechanical complication of artificial skin graft and decellularized allodermis**

● T85.694 **Other mechanical complication of insulin pump**

● T85.695 **Other mechanical complication of other nervous system device, implant or graft** A
Other mechanical complication of intrathecal infusion pump

● T85.698 **Other mechanical complication of other specified internal prosthetic devices, implants and grafts**
Mechanical complication of nonabsorbable surgical material NOS

● T85.7 **Infection and inflammatory reaction due to other internal prosthetic devices, implants and grafts**
Use additional code to identify infection
Coding Clinic: 2016, Q4, P72

X● T85.71 **Infection and inflammatory reaction due to peritoneal dialysis catheter** A, D, S

X● T85.72 **Infection and inflammatory reaction due to insulin pump** A

● T85.73 **Infection and inflammatory reaction due to nervous system devices, implants and graft**

● T85.730 **Infection and inflammatory reaction due to ventricular intracranial (communicating) shunt** A

● T85.731 **Infection and inflammatory reaction due to implanted electronic neurostimulator of brain, electrode (lead)** A

CHAPTER 19 (S00-T88)

T85.732 **Infection and inflammatory reaction due to implanted electronic neurostimulator of peripheral nerve, electrode (lead)** A
Infection and inflammatory reaction due to electrode (lead) for cranial nerve neurostimulators
Infection and inflammatory reaction due to electrode (lead) for gastric neurostimulator
Infection and inflammatory reaction due to electrode (lead) for sacral nerve neurostimulator
Infection and inflammatory reaction due to electrode (lead) for vagal nerve neurostimulators

T85.733 **Infection and inflammatory reaction due to implanted electronic neurostimulator of spinal cord, electrode (lead)** A

T85.734 **Infection and inflammatory reaction due to implanted electronic neurostimulator, generator** A
Generator pocket infection

T85.735 **Infection and inflammatory reaction due to cranial or spinal infusion catheter** A
Infection and inflammatory reaction due to epidural catheter
Infection and inflammatory reaction due to intrathecal infusion catheter
Infection and inflammatory reaction due to subarachnoid catheter
Infection and inflammatory reaction due to subdural catheter

T85.738 **Infection and inflammatory reaction due to other nervous system device, implant or graft** A
Infection and inflammatory reaction due to intrathecal infusion pump

X T85.79 **Infection and inflammatory reaction due to other internal prosthetic devices, implants and grafts** A
Coding Clinic: 2016, Q4, P72

T85.8 **Other specified complications of internal prosthetic devices, implants and grafts, not elsewhere classified**
Coding Clinic: 2016, Q4, P72

T85.81 **Embolism due to internal prosthetic devices, implants and grafts, not elsewhere classified**

T85.810 **Embolism due to nervous system prosthetic devices, implants and grafts** A

T85.818 **Embolism due to other internal prosthetic devices, implants and grafts**

T85.82 **Fibrosis due to internal prosthetic devices, implants and grafts, not elsewhere classified**

T85.820 **Fibrosis due to nervous system prosthetic devices, implants and grafts** A

T85.828 **Fibrosis due to other internal prosthetic devices, implants and grafts**

T85.83 **Hemorrhage due to internal prosthetic devices, implants and grafts, not elsewhere classified**

T85.830 **Hemorrhage due to nervous system prosthetic devices, implants and grafts** A

T85.838 **Hemorrhage due to other internal prosthetic devices, implants and grafts**

T85.84 **Pain due to internal prosthetic devices, implants and grafts, not elsewhere classified**

T85.840 **Pain due to nervous system prosthetic devices, implants and grafts** A

T85.848 **Pain due to other internal prosthetic devices, implants and grafts**

T85.85 **Stenosis due to internal prosthetic devices, implants and grafts, not elsewhere classified**

T85.850 **Stenosis due to nervous system prosthetic devices, implants and grafts** A

T85.858 **Stenosis due to other internal prosthetic devices, implants and grafts**

T85.86 **Thrombosis due to internal prosthetic devices, implants and grafts, not elsewhere classified**

T85.860 **Thrombosis due to nervous system prosthetic devices, implants and grafts** A

T85.868 **Thrombosis due to other internal prosthetic devices, implants and grafts**

T85.89 **Other specified complication of internal prosthetic devices, implants and grafts, not elsewhere classified**
Coding Clinic: 2016, Q4, P72

T85.890 **Other specified complication of nervous system prosthetic devices, implants and grafts** A

T85.898 **Other specified complication of other internal prosthetic devices, implants and grafts**

X T85.9 **Unspecified complication of internal prosthetic device, implant and graft**
Complication of internal prosthetic device, implant and graft NOS

OGCR Section I.C.19.g.3.

Organ Transplant Complications

Transplant Complications

(a) Transplant complications other than kidney

Codes under category T86, Complications of transplanted organs and tissues, are for use for both complications and rejection of transplanted organs. A transplant complication code is only assigned if the complication affects the function of the transplanted organ. Two codes are required to fully describe a transplant complication: the appropriate code from category T86 and a secondary code that identifies the complication.

Pre-existing conditions or conditions that develop after the transplant are not coded as complications unless they affect the function of the transplanted organs.

See I.C.21 for transplant organ removal status.

See I.C.2 for malignant neoplasm associated with transplanted organ.

T86 **Complications of transplanted organs and tissue**
Use additional code to identify other transplant complications, such as:
graft-versus-host disease (D89.81-)
malignancy associated with organ transplant (C80.2)
post-transplant lymphoproliferative disorders (PTLD) (D47.Z1)

T86.0 **Complications of bone marrow transplant**

T86.00 **Unspecified complication of bone marrow transplant**

T86.01 **Bone marrow transplant rejection**

T86.02 **Bone marrow transplant failure**

T86.03 **Bone marrow transplant infection**

T86.09 **Other complications of bone marrow transplant**

- T86.1 Complications of kidney transplant
  - T86.10 Unspecified complication of kidney transplant
  - T86.11 Kidney transplant rejection
  - T86.12 Kidney transplant failure
    Coding Clinic: 2013, Q1, P24
  - T86.13 Kidney transplant infection
    Use additional code to specify infection
  - T86.19 Other complication of kidney transplant
    Coding Clinic: 2019, Q2, P7
- T86.2 Complications of heart transplant
  Excludes1 complication of:
  artificial heart device (T82.5)
  heart-lung transplant (T86.3)
  - T86.20 Unspecified complication of heart transplant
  - T86.21 Heart transplant rejection
  - T86.22 Heart transplant failure
  - T86.23 Heart transplant infection
    Use additional code to specify infection
  - T86.29 Other complications of heart transplant
    - T86.290 Cardiac allograft vasculopathy
      Excludes1 atherosclerosis of coronary arteries (I25.75-, I25.76-, I25.81-)
    - T86.298 Other complications of heart transplant
- T86.3 Complications of heart-lung transplant
  - T86.30 Unspecified complication of heart-lung transplant
  - T86.31 Heart-lung transplant rejection
  - T86.32 Heart-lung transplant failure
  - T86.33 Heart-lung transplant infection
    Use additional code to specify infection
  - T86.39 Other complications of heart-lung transplant
- T86.4 Complications of liver transplant
  - T86.40 Unspecified complication of liver transplant
  - T86.41 Liver transplant rejection
  - T86.42 Liver transplant failure
  - T86.43 Liver transplant infection
    Use additional code to identify infection, such as:
    Cytomegalovirus (CMV) infection (B25.-)
  - T86.49 Other complications of liver transplant
- T86.5 Complications of stem cell transplant
  Complications from stem cells from peripheral blood
  Complications from stem cells from umbilical cord
- T86.8 Complications of other transplanted organs and tissues
  - T86.81 Complications of lung transplant
    Excludes1 complication of heart-lung transplant (T86.3-)
    - T86.810 Lung transplant rejection
    - T86.811 Lung transplant failure
    - T86.812 Lung transplant infection
      Use additional code to specify infection
    - T86.818 Other complications of lung transplant
      Coding Clinic: 2019, Q2, P7
    - T86.819 Unspecified complication of lung transplant
  - T86.82 Complications of skin graft (allograft) (autograft)
    Excludes2 complication of artificial skin graft (T85.693)
    - T86.820 Skin graft (allograft) rejection
    - T86.821 Skin graft (allograft) (autograft) failure
    - T86.822 Skin graft (allograft) (autograft) infection
      Use additional code to specify infection
    - T86.828 Other complications of skin graft (allograft) (autograft)
    - T86.829 Unspecified complication of skin graft (allograft) (autograft)
  - T86.83 Complications of bone graft
    Excludes2 mechanical complications of bone graft (T84.3-)
    - T86.830 Bone graft rejection
    - T86.831 Bone graft failure
    - T86.832 Bone graft infection
      Use additional code to specify infection
    - T86.838 Other complications of bone graft
    - T86.839 Unspecified complication of bone graft
  - T86.84 Complications of corneal transplant
    Excludes2 mechanical complications of corneal graft (T85.3-)
    - T86.840 Corneal transplant rejection
    - T86.841 Corneal transplant failure
    - T86.842 Corneal transplant infection
      Use additional code to specify infection
    - T86.848 Other complications of corneal transplant
    - T86.849 Unspecified complication of corneal transplant
  - T86.85 Complication of intestine transplant
    - T86.850 Intestine transplant rejection
    - T86.851 Intestine transplant failure
    - T86.852 Intestine transplant infection
      Use additional code to specify infection
    - T86.858 Other complications of intestine transplant
    - T86.859 Unspecified complication of intestine transplant
  - T86.89 Complications of other transplanted tissue
    Transplant failure or rejection of pancreas
    - T86.890 Other transplanted tissue rejection
    - T86.891 Other transplanted tissue failure
    - T86.892 Other transplanted tissue infection
      Use additional code to specify infection
    - T86.898 Other complications of other transplanted tissue
    - T86.899 Unspecified complication of other transplanted tissue

● T86.9 Complication of unspecified transplanted organ and tissue
- T86.90 Unspecified complication of unspecified transplanted organ and tissue
- T86.91 Unspecified transplanted organ and tissue rejection
- T86.92 Unspecified transplanted organ and tissue failure
- T86.93 Unspecified transplanted organ and tissue infection
  - Use additional code to specify infection
- T86.99 Other complications of unspecified transplanted organ and tissue

● T87 Complications peculiar to reattachment and amputation

● T87.0 Complications of reattached (part of) upper extremity
- ● T87.0X Complications of reattached (part of) upper extremity
  - T87.0X1 Complications of reattached (part of) right upper extremity
  - T87.0X2 Complications of reattached (part of) left upper extremity
  - T87.0X9 Complications of reattached (part of) unspecified upper extremity

● T87.1 Complications of reattached (part of) lower extremity
- ● T87.1X Complications of reattached (part of) lower extremity
  - T87.1X1 Complications of reattached (part of) right lower extremity
  - T87.1X2 Complications of reattached (part of) left lower extremity
  - T87.1X9 Complications of reattached (part of) unspecified lower extremity

T87.2 Complications of other reattached body part

● T87.3 Neuroma of amputation stump
- T87.30 Neuroma of amputation stump, unspecified extremity
- T87.31 Neuroma of amputation stump, right upper extremity
- T87.32 Neuroma of amputation stump, left upper extremity
- T87.33 Neuroma of amputation stump, right lower extremity
- T87.34 Neuroma of amputation stump, left lower extremity

● T87.4 Infection of amputation stump
- T87.40 Infection of amputation stump, unspecified extremity
- T87.41 Infection of amputation stump, right upper extremity
- T87.42 Infection of amputation stump, left upper extremity
- T87.43 Infection of amputation stump, right lower extremity
- T87.44 Infection of amputation stump, left lower extremity

● T87.5 Necrosis of amputation stump
- T87.50 Necrosis of amputation stump, unspecified extremity
- T87.51 Necrosis of amputation stump, right upper extremity
- T87.52 Necrosis of amputation stump, left upper extremity
- T87.53 Necrosis of amputation stump, right lower extremity
- T87.54 Necrosis of amputation stump, left lower extremity

● T87.8 Other complications of amputation stump
- T87.81 Dehiscence of amputation stump
- T87.89 Other complications of amputation stump
  - Amputation stump contracture
  - Amputation stump contracture of next proximal joint
  - Amputation stump flexion
  - Amputation stump edema
  - Amputation stump hematoma
  - **Excludes2** phantom limb syndrome (G54.6-G54.7)

T87.9 Unspecified complications of amputation stump

● T88 Other complications of surgical and medical care, not elsewhere classified

Excludes2
- complication following infusion, transfusion and therapeutic injection (T80.-)
- complication following procedure NEC (T81.-)
- complications of anesthesia in labor and delivery (O74.-)
- complications of anesthesia in pregnancy (O29.-)
- complications of anesthesia in puerperium (O89.-)
- complications of devices, implants and grafts (T82-T85)
- complications of obstetric surgery and procedure (O75.4)
- dermatitis due to drugs and medicaments (L23.3, L24.4, L25.1, L27.0-L27.1)
- poisoning and toxic effects of drugs and chemicals (T36-T65 with fifth or sixth character 1-4 or 6)
- specified complications classified elsewhere

The appropriate 7th character is to be added to each code from category T88

A	initial encounter
D	subsequent encounter
S	sequela

X● T88.0 Infection following immunization
- Sepsis following immunization
- Coding Clinic: 2019, Q1, P14;2018, Q4, P90

X● T88.1 Other complications following immunization, not elsewhere classified
- Generalized vaccinia
- Rash following immunization
- **Excludes1** vaccinia not from vaccine (B08.011)
- **Excludes2** anaphylactic shock due to serum (T80.5-)
  - other serum reactions (T80.6-)
  - postimmunization arthropathy (M02.2)
  - postimmunization encephalitis (G04.02)
  - postimmunization fever (R50.83)

X● T88.2 Shock due to anesthesia
- Use additional code for adverse effect, if applicable, to identify drug (T41.- with fifth or sixth character 5)
- **Excludes1** complications of anesthesia (in):
  - labor and delivery (O74.-)
  - pregnancy (O29.-)
  - puerperium (O89.-)
  - postprocedural shock NOS (T81.1-)

X● T88.3 Malignant hyperthermia due to anesthesia
- Use additional code for adverse effect, if applicable, to identify drug (T41.- with fifth or sixth character 5)

X● T88.4 Failed or difficult intubation

● T88.5   **Other complications of anesthesia**

> Use additional code for adverse effect, if applicable, to identify drug (T41.- with fifth or sixth character 5)
> Coding Clinic: 2016, Q4, P72

X● T88.51   **Hypothermia following anesthesia**

X● T88.52   **Failed moderate sedation during procedure**

> Failed conscious sedation during procedure
>
> **Excludes2**   personal history of failed moderate sedation (Z92.83)

X● T88.53   **Unintended awareness under general anesthesia during procedure**

> **Excludes2**   personal history of unintended awareness under general anesthesia (Z92.84)
> Coding Clinic: 2016, Q4, P72-73

X● T88.59   **Other complications of anesthesia**

X● T88.6   **Anaphylactic reaction due to adverse effect of correct drug or medicament properly administered**

> Anaphylactic shock due to adverse effect of correct drug or medicament properly administered
> Anaphylactoid reaction NOS
>
> Use additional code for adverse effect, if applicable, to identify drug (T36-T50 with fifth or sixth character 5)
>
> **Excludes1**   anaphylactic reaction due to serum (T80.5-)
> anaphylactic shock or reaction due to adverse food reaction (T78.0-)

X● T88.7   **Unspecified adverse effect of drug or medicament**

> Drug hypersensitivity NOS
> Drug reaction NOS
>
> Use additional code for adverse effect, if applicable, to identify drug (T36-T50 with fifth or sixth character 5)
>
> **Excludes1**   specified adverse effects of drugs and medicaments (A00-R94 and T80-T88.6, T88.8)

X● T88.8   **Other specified complications of surgical and medical care, not elsewhere classified**

> Use additional code to identify the complication

X● T88.9   **Complication of surgical and medical care, unspecified**

CHAPTER 19 (S00-T88)

CHAPTER 20

EXTERNAL CAUSES OF MORBIDITY
(V00-Y99)

OGCR Chapter-Specific Coding Guidelines

20. **Chapter 20: External Causes of Morbidity (V00-Y99)**
The external causes of morbidity codes should never be sequenced as the first-listed or principal diagnosis.

External cause codes are intended to provide data for injury research and evaluation of injury prevention strategies. These codes capture how the injury or health condition happened (cause), the intent (unintentional or accidental; or intentional, such as suicide or assault), the place where the event occurred the activity of the patient at the time of the event, and the person's status (e.g., civilian, military).

There is no national requirement for mandatory ICD-10-CM external cause code reporting. Unless a provider is subject to a state-based external cause code reporting mandate or these codes are required by a particular payer, reporting of ICD-10-CM codes in Chapter 20, External Causes of Morbidity, is not required. In the absence of a mandatory reporting requirement, providers are encouraged to voluntarily report external cause codes, as they provide valuable data for injury research and evaluation of injury prevention strategies.

a. General External Cause Coding Guidelines

1) Used with any code in the range of A00.0-T88.9, Z00-Z99
An external cause code may be used with any code in the range of A00.0-T88.9, Z00-Z99, classification that represents a health condition due to an external cause. Though they are most applicable to injuries, they are also valid for use with such things as infections or diseases due to an external source, and other health conditions, such as a heart attack that occurs during strenuous physical activity.

2) External cause code used for length of treatment
Assign the external cause code, with the appropriate 7th character (initial encounter, subsequent encounter or sequela) for each encounter for which the injury or condition is being treated.

Most categories in Chapter 20 have a 7th character requirement for each applicable code. Most categories in this chapter have three 7th character values: A, initial encounter, D, subsequent encounter and S, sequela. While the patient may be seen by a new or different provider over the course of treatment for an injury or condition, assignment of the 7th character for external cause should match the 7th character of the code assigned for the associated injury or condition for the encounter.

3) Use the full range of external cause codes
Use the full range of external cause codes to completely describe the cause, the intent, the place of occurrence and if applicable, the activity of the patient at the time of the event, and the patient's status, for all injuries, and other health conditions due to an external cause.

4) Assign as many external cause codes as necessary
Assign as many external cause codes as necessary to fully explain each cause. If only one external code can be recorded, assign the code most related to the principal diagnosis.

5) The selection of the appropriate external cause code
The selection of the appropriate external cause code is guided by the Alphabetic Index of External Causes and by Inclusion and Exclusion notes in the Tabular List.

6) External cause code can never be a principal diagnosis
An external cause code can never be a principal (first-listed) diagnosis.

7) Combination external cause codes
Certain of the external cause codes are combination codes that identify sequential events that result in an injury, such as a fall which results in striking against an object. The injury may be due to either event or both. The combination external cause code used should correspond to the sequence of events regardless of which caused the most serious injury.

8) No external cause code needed in certain circumstances
No external cause code from Chapter 20 is needed if the external cause and intent are included in a code from another chapter (e.g., T36.0X1- Poisoning by penicillins, accidental (unintentional)).

b. Place of Occurrence Guideline
Codes from category Y92, Place of occurrence of the external cause, are secondary codes for use after other external cause codes to identify the location of the patient at the time of injury or other condition.

Generally, a place of occurrence code is assigned only once, at the initial encounter for treatment. However, in the rare instance that a new injury occurs during hospitalization, an additional place of occurrence code may be assigned. No 7th characters are used for Y92. Only one code from Y92 should be recorded on a medical record.

Do not use place of occurrence code Y92.9 if the place is not stated or is not applicable.

c. Activity Code
Assign a code from category Y93, Activity code, to describe the activity of the patient at the time the injury or other health condition occurred.

An activity code is used only once, at the initial encounter for treatment. Only one code from Y93 should be recorded on a medical record.

The activity codes are not applicable to poisonings, adverse effects, misadventures or sequela.

Do not assign Y93.9, Unspecified activity, if the activity is not stated.

A code from category Y93 is appropriate for use with external cause and intent codes if identifying the activity provides additional information about the event.

d. Place of Occurrence, Activity, and Status Codes Used with Other External Cause Code
When applicable, place of occurrence, activity, and external cause status codes are sequenced after the main external cause code(s). Regardless of the number of external cause codes assigned, there should be only one place of occurrence code, one activity code, and one external cause status code assigned to an encounter.

e. If the Reporting Format Limits the Number of External Cause Codes

If the reporting format limits the number of external cause codes that can be used in reporting clinical data, report the code for the cause/intent most related to the principal diagnosis. If the format permits capture of additional external cause codes, the cause/intent, including medical misadventures, of the additional events should be reported rather than the codes for place, activity, or external status.

f. Multiple External Cause Coding Guidelines

More than one external cause code is required to fully describe the external cause of an illness or injury. The assignment of external cause codes should be sequenced in the following priority:

If two or more events cause separate injuries, an external cause code should be assigned for each cause. The first-listed external cause code will be selected in the following order:

External codes for child and adult abuse take priority over all other external cause codes.

See Section I.C.19., Child and Adult abuse guidelines.

External codes for terrorism events take priority over all other external cause codes except child and adult abuse.

External cause codes for cataclysmic events take priority over all other external cause codes except child and adult abuse and terrorism.

External cause codes for transport accidents take priority over all other external cause codes except cataclysmic events, child and adult abuse and terrorism.

Activity and external cause status codes are assigned following all causal (intent) external cause codes.

The first-listed external cause code should correspond to the cause of the most serious diagnosis due to an assault, accident, or self-harm, following the order of hierarchy listed above.

g. Child and Adult Abuse Guideline

Adult and child abuse, neglect and maltreatment are classified as assault. Any of the assault codes may be used to indicate the external cause of any injury resulting from the confirmed abuse.

For confirmed cases of abuse, neglect and maltreatment, when the perpetrator is known, a code from Y07, Perpetrator of maltreatment and neglect, should accompany any other assault codes.

See Section I.C.19. Adult and child abuse, neglect and other maltreatment

h. Unknown or Undetermined Intent Guideline

If the intent (accident, self-harm, assault) of the cause of an injury or other condition is unknown or unspecified, code the intent as accidental intent. All transport accident categories assume accidental intent.

1) Use of undetermined intent

External cause codes for events of undetermined intent are only for use if the documentation in the record specifies that the intent cannot be determined.

i. Sequelae (Late Effects) of External Cause Guidelines

1) Sequelae external cause codes

Sequela are reported using the external cause code with the 7th character "S" for sequela. These codes should be used with any report of a late effect or sequela resulting from a previous injury.

See Section I.B.10. Sequela, (Late Effects).

2) Sequela external cause code with a related current injury

A sequela external cause code should never be used with a related current nature of injury code.

3) Use of sequela external cause codes for subsequent visits

Use a late effect external cause code for subsequent visits when a late effect of the initial injury is being treated. Do not use a late effect external cause code for subsequent visits for follow-up care (e.g., to assess healing, to receive rehabilitative therapy) of the injury when no late effect of the injury has been documented.

j. Terrorism Guidelines

1) Cause of injury identified by the Federal Government (FBI) as terrorism

When the cause of an injury is identified by the Federal Government (FBI) as terrorism, the first-listed external cause code should be a code from category Y38, Terrorism. The definition of terrorism employed by the FBI is found at the inclusion note at the beginning of category Y38. Use additional code for place of occurrence (Y92.-). More than one Y38 code may be assigned if the injury is the result of more than one mechanism of terrorism.

2) Cause of an injury is suspected to be the result of terrorism

When the cause of an injury is suspected to be the result of terrorism a code from category Y38 should not be assigned. Suspected cases should be classified as assault.

3) Code Y38.9, Terrorism, secondary effects

Assign code Y38.9, Terrorism, secondary effects, for conditions occurring subsequent to the terrorist event. This code should not be assigned for conditions that are due to the initial terrorist act.

It is acceptable to assign code Y38.9 with another code from Y38 if there is an injury due to the initial terrorist event and an injury that is a subsequent result of the terrorist event.

k. External cause status

A code from category Y99, External cause status, should be assigned whenever any other external cause code is assigned for an encounter, including an Activity code, except for the events noted below. Assign a code from category Y99, External cause status, to indicate the work status of the person at the time the event occurred. The status code indicates whether the event occurred during military activity, whether a non-military person was at work, whether an individual including a student or volunteer was involved in a non-work activity at the time of the causal event.

A code from Y99, External cause status, should be assigned, when applicable, with other external cause codes, such as transport accidents and falls. The external cause status codes are not applicable to poisonings, adverse effects, misadventures or late effects.

Do not assign a code from category Y99 if no other external cause codes (cause, activity) are applicable for the encounter.

An external cause status code is used only once, at the initial encounter for treatment. Only one code from Y99 should be recorded on a medical record.

Do not assign code Y99.9, Unspecified external cause status, if the status is not stated.

CHAPTER 2Ø

EXTERNAL CAUSES OF MORBIDITY (VØØ-Y99)

Note: This chapter permits the classification of environmental events and circumstances as the cause of injury, and other adverse effects. Where a code from this section is applicable, it is intended that it shall be used secondary to a code from another chapter of the Classification indicating the nature of the condition. Most often, the condition will be classifiable to Chapter 19, Injury, poisoning and certain other consequences of external causes (SØØ-T88). Other conditions that may be stated to be due to external causes are classified in Chapters 1 to 18. For these conditions, codes from Chapter 2Ø should be used to provide additional information as to the cause of the condition.

This chapter contains the following blocks:

VØØ-X58	Accidents
VØØ-V99	Transport accidents
VØØ-VØ9	Pedestrian injured in transport accident
V1Ø-V19	Pedal cycle rider injured in transport accident
V2Ø-V29	Motorcycle rider injured in transport accident
V3Ø-V39	Occupant of three-wheeled motor vehicle injured in transport accident
V4Ø-V49	Car occupant injured in transport accident
V5Ø-V59	Occupant of pick-up truck or van injured in transport accident
V6Ø-V69	Occupant of heavy transport vehicle injured in transport accident
V7Ø-V79	Bus occupant injured in transport accident
V8Ø-V89	Other land transport accidents
V9Ø-V94	Water transport accidents
V95-V97	Air and space transport accidents
V98-V99	Other and unspecified transport accidents
WØØ-X58	Other external causes of accidental injury
WØØ-W19	Slipping, tripping, stumbling and falls
W2Ø-W49	Exposure to inanimate mechanical forces
W5Ø-W64	Exposure to animate mechanical forces
W65-W74	Accidental non-transport drowning and submersion
W85-W99	Exposure to electric current, radiation and extreme ambient air temperature and pressure
XØØ-XØ8	Exposure to smoke, fire and flames
X1Ø-X19	Contact with heat and hot substances
X3Ø-X39	Exposure to forces of nature
X5Ø	Overexertion and strenuous or repetitive movements
X52, X58	Accidental exposure to other specified factors
X71-X83	Intentional self-harm
X92-YØ9	Assault
Y21-Y33	Event of undetermined intent
Y35-Y38	Legal intervention, operations of war, military operations, and terrorism
Y62-Y84	Complications of medical and surgical care
Y62-Y69	Misadventures to patients during surgical and medical care
Y7Ø-Y82	Medical devices associated with adverse incidents in diagnostic and therapeutic use
Y83-Y84	Surgical and other medical procedures as the cause of abnormal reaction of the patient, or of later complication, without mention of misadventure at the time of the procedure
Y9Ø-Y99	Supplementary factors related to causes of morbidity classified elsewhere

ACCIDENTS (VØØ-X58)

TRANSPORT ACCIDENTS (VØØ-V99)

Note: This section is structured in 12 groups. Those relating to land transport accidents (VØØ-V89) reflect the victim's mode of transport and are subdivided to identify the victim's 'counterpart' or the type of event. The vehicle of which the injured person is an occupant is identified in the first two characters since it is seen as the most important factor to identify for prevention purposes. A transport accident is one in which the vehicle involved must be moving or running or in use for transport purposes at the time of the accident.

Use additional code to identify:
Airbag injury (W22.1)
Type of street or road (Y92.4-)
Use of cellular telephone and other electronic equipment at the time of the transport accident (Y93.C-)

Excludes1 agricultural vehicles in stationary use or maintenance (W31.-)
assault by crashing of motor vehicle (YØ3.-)
automobile or motor cycle in stationary use or maintenance - code to type of accident
crashing of motor vehicle, undetermined intent (Y32)
intentional self-harm by crashing of motor vehicle (X82)

Excludes2 transport accidents due to cataclysm (X34-X38)

Note: Definitions related to transport accidents:

(a) A transport accident (VØØ-V99) is any accident involving a device designed primarily for, or used at the time primarily for, conveying persons or good from one place to another.

(b) A public highway [trafficway] or street is the entire width between property lines (or other boundary lines) of land open to the public as a matter of right or custom for purposes of moving persons or property from one place to another. A roadway is that part of the public highway designed, improved and customarily used for vehicular traffic.

(c) A traffic accident is any vehicle accident occurring on the public highway [i.e., originating on, terminating on, or involving a vehicle partially on the highway]. A vehicle accident is assumed to have occurred on the public highway unless another place is specified, except in the case of accidents involving only off-road motor vehicles, which are classified as nontraffic accidents unless the contrary is stated.

(d) A nontraffic accident is any vehicle accident that occurs entirely in any place other than a public highway.

(e) A pedestrian is any person involved in an accident who was not at the time of the accident riding in or on a motor vehicle, railway train, streetcar or animal-drawn or other vehicle, or on a pedal cycle or animal. This includes, a person changing a tire, working on a parked car, or a person on foot. It also includes the user of a pedestrian conveyance such as a baby stroller, ice-skates, skis, sled, roller skates, a skateboard, nonmotorized or motorized wheelchair, motorized mobility scooter, or nonmotorized scooter.

(f) A driver is an occupant of a transport vehicle who is operating or intending to operate it.

(g) A passenger is any occupant of a transport vehicle other than the driver, except a person traveling on the outside of the vehicle.

(h) A person on the outside of a vehicle is any person being transported by a vehicle but not occupying the space normally reserved for the driver or passengers, or the space intended for the transport of property. This includes a person travelling on the bodywork, bumper, fender, roof, running board or step of a vehicle, as well as, hanging on the outside of the vehicle.

(i) A pedal cycle is any land transport vehicle operated solely by nonmotorized pedals including a bicycle or tricycle.

(j) A pedal cyclist is any person riding a pedal cycle or in a sidecar or trailer attached to a pedal cycle.

(k) A motorcycle is a two-wheeled motor vehicle with one or two riding saddles and sometimes with a third wheel for the support of a sidecar. The sidecar is considered part of the motorcycle. This includes a moped, motor scooter, or motorized bicycle.

(l) A motorcycle rider is any person riding a motorcycle or in a sidecar or trailer attached to the motorcycle.

(m) A three-wheeled motor vehicle is a motorized tricycle designed primarily for on-road use. This includes a motor-driven tricycle, a motorized rickshaw, or a three-wheeled motor car.

(n) A car [automobile] is a four-wheeled motor vehicle designed primarily for carrying up to 7 persons. A trailer being towed by the car is considered part of the car. It does not include a van or minivan—see definition (o)

(o) A pick-up truck or van is a four or six-wheeled motor vehicle designed for carrying passengers as well as property or cargo weighing less than the local limit for classification as a heavy goods vehicle, and not requiring a special driver's license. This includes a minivan and a sport-utility vehicle (SUV).

(p) A heavy transport vehicle is a motor vehicle designed primarily for carrying property, meeting local criteria for classification as a heavy goods vehicle in terms of weight and requiring a special driver's license.

(q) A bus (coach) is a motor vehicle designed or adapted primarily for carrying more than 10 passengers, and requiring a special driver's license.

(r) A railway train or railway vehicle is any device, with or without freight or passenger cars coupled to it, designed for traffic on a railway track. This includes subterranean (subways) or elevated trains.

(s) A streetcar is a device designed and used primarily for transporting passengers within a municipality, running on rails, usually subject to normal traffic control signals, and operated principally on a right-of-way that forms part of the roadway. This includes a tram or trolley that runs on rails. A trailer being towed by a streetcar is considered part of the streetcar.

(t) A special vehicle mainly used on industrial premises is a motor vehicle designed primarily for use within the buildings and premises of industrial or commercial establishments. This includes battery-powered airport passenger vehicles or baggage/mail trucks, forklifts, coal-cars in a coal mine, logging cars and trucks used in mines or quarries.

(u) A special vehicle mainly used in agriculture is a motor vehicle designed specifically for use in farming and agriculture (horticulture), to work the land, tend and harvest crops and transport materials on the farm. This includes harvesters, farm machinery and tractor and trailers.

(v) A special construction vehicle is a motor vehicle designed specifically for use on construction and demolition sites. This includes bulldozers, diggers, earth levellers, dump trucks, backhoes, front-end loaders, pavers, and mechanical shovels.

(w) A special all-terrain vehicle is a motor vehicle of special design to enable it to negotiate over rough or soft terrain, snow or sand. Examples of special design are high construction, special wheels and tires, tracks, and support on a cushion of air. This includes snow mobiles, all-terrain vehicles (ATV), and dune buggies. It does not include passenger vehicle designated as sport utility vehicles (SUV).

(x) A watercraft is any device designed for transporting passengers or goods on water. This includes motor or sail boats, ships, and hovercraft.

(y) An aircraft is any device for transporting passengers or goods in the air. This includes hot-air balloons, gliders, helicopters and airplanes.

(z) A military vehicle is any motorized vehicle operating on a public roadway owned by the military and being operated by a member of the military.

PEDESTRIAN INJURED IN TRANSPORT ACCIDENT (V00-V09)

Includes person changing tire on transport vehicle
person examining engine of vehicle broken down in (on side of) road

Excludes1 fall due to non-transport collision with other person (W03)
pedestrian on foot falling (slipping) on ice and snow (W00.-)
struck or bumped by another person (W51)

● **V00 Pedestrian conveyance accident**

Use additional place of occurrence and activity external cause codes, if known (Y92.-, Y93.-)

Excludes1 collision with another person without fall (W51)
fall due to person on foot colliding with another person on foot (W03)
fall from non-moving wheelchair, nonmotorized scooter and motorized mobility scooter without collision (W05.-)
pedestrian (conveyance) collision with other land transport vehicle (V01-V09)
pedestrian on foot falling (slipping) on ice and snow (W00.-)

The appropriate 7th character is to be added to each code from category V00

A	initial encounter
D	subsequent encounter
S	sequela

● **V00.0 Pedestrian on foot injured in collision with pedestrian conveyance**

X● **V00.01 Pedestrian on foot injured in collision with roller-skater**

X● **V00.02 Pedestrian on foot injured in collision with skateboarder**

X● **V00.09 Pedestrian on foot injured in collision with other pedestrian conveyance**

● **V00.1 Rolling-type pedestrian conveyance accident**

Excludes1 accident with baby stroller (V00.82-)
accident with wheelchair (powered) (V00.81-)
accident with motorized mobility scooter (V00.83-)

● **V00.11 In-line roller-skate accident**

● **V00.111 Fall from in-line roller-skates**

● **V00.112 In-line roller-skater colliding with stationary object**

● **V00.118 Other in-line roller-skate accident**

Excludes1 roller-skater collision with other land transport vehicle (V01-V09 with 5th character 1)

● **V00.12 Non-in-line roller-skate accident**

● **V00.121 Fall from non-in-line roller-skates**

● **V00.122 Non-in-line roller-skater colliding with stationary object**

● **V00.128 Other non-in-line roller-skating accident**

Excludes1 roller-skater collision with other land transport vehicle (V01-V09 with 5th character 1)

CHAPTER 20 (V00-Y99)

V00.13 Skateboard accident
- V00.131 Fall from skateboard
- V00.132 Skateboarder colliding with stationary object
- V00.138 Other skateboard accident
  - **Excludes1** skateboarder collision with other land transport vehicle (V01-V09 with 5th character 2)

V00.14 Scooter (nonmotorized) accident
- **Excludes1** motor scooter accident (V20-V29)
- V00.141 Fall from scooter (nonmotorized)
- V00.142 Scooter (nonmotorized) colliding with stationary object
- V00.148 Other scooter (nonmotorized) accident
  - **Excludes1** scooter (non-motorized) collision with other land transport vehicle (V01-V09 with fifth character 9)

V00.15 Heelies accident
- Rolling shoe
- Wheeled shoe
- Wheelies accident
- V00.151 Fall from heelies
- V00.152 Heelies colliding with stationary object
- V00.158 Other heelies accident

V00.18 Accident on other rolling-type pedestrian conveyance
- V00.181 Fall from other rolling-type pedestrian conveyance
- V00.182 Pedestrian on other rolling-type pedestrian conveyance colliding with stationary object
- V00.188 Other accident on other rolling-type pedestrian conveyance

V00.2 Gliding-type pedestrian conveyance accident

V00.21 Ice-skates accident
- V00.211 Fall from ice-skates
- V00.212 Ice-skater colliding with stationary object
- V00.218 Other ice-skates accident
  - **Excludes1** ice-skater collision with other land transport vehicle (V01-V09 with 5th character 9)

V00.22 Sled accident
- V00.221 Fall from sled
- V00.222 Sledder colliding with stationary object
- V00.228 Other sled accident
  - **Excludes1** sled collision with other land transport vehicle (V01-V09 with 5th character 9)

V00.28 Other gliding-type pedestrian conveyance accident
- V00.281 Fall from other gliding-type pedestrian conveyance
- V00.282 Pedestrian on other gliding-type pedestrian conveyance colliding with stationary object
- V00.288 Other accident on other gliding-type pedestrian conveyance
  - **Excludes1** gliding-type pedestrian conveyance collision with other land transport vehicle (V01-V09 with 5th character 9)

V00.3 Flat-bottomed pedestrian conveyance accident

V00.31 Snowboard accident
- V00.311 Fall from snowboard
- V00.312 Snowboarder colliding with stationary object
- V00.318 Other snowboard accident
  - **Excludes1** snowboarder collision with other land transport vehicle (V01-V09 with 5th character 9)

V00.32 Snow-ski accident
- V00.321 Fall from snow-skis
  - Coding Clinic: 2015, Q1, P12
- V00.322 Snow-skier colliding with stationary object
- V00.328 Other snow-ski accident
  - **Excludes1** snow-skier collision with other land transport vehicle (V01-V09 with 5th character 9)

V00.38 Other flat-bottomed pedestrian conveyance accident
- V00.381 Fall from other flat-bottomed pedestrian conveyance
- V00.382 Pedestrian on other flat-bottomed pedestrian conveyance colliding with stationary object
- V00.388 Other accident on other flat-bottomed pedestrian conveyance

V00.8 Accident on other pedestrian conveyance

V00.81 Accident with wheelchair (powered)
- V00.811 Fall from moving wheelchair (powered)
  - **Excludes1** fall from non-moving wheelchair (W05.0)
- V00.812 Wheelchair (powered) colliding with stationary object
- V00.818 Other accident with wheelchair (powered)

V00.82 Accident with baby stroller
- V00.821 Fall from baby stroller
- V00.822 Baby stroller colliding with stationary object
- V00.828 Other accident with baby stroller

● V00.83 Accident with motorized mobility scooter
● V00.831 **Fall from motorized mobility scooter**
Excludes1 fall from non-moving motorized mobility scooter (W05.2)
● V00.832 **Motorized mobility scooter colliding with stationary object**
● V00.838 **Other accident with motorized mobility scooter**
● V00.89 Accident on other pedestrian conveyance
● V00.891 **Fall from other pedestrian conveyance**
● V00.892 **Pedestrian on other pedestrian conveyance colliding with stationary object**
● V00.898 **Other accident on other pedestrian conveyance**
Excludes1 other pedestrian (conveyance) collision with other land transport vehicle (V01-V09 with 5th character 9)

● **V01 Pedestrian injured in collision with pedal cycle**
The appropriate 7th character is to be added to each code from category V01

A	initial encounter
D	subsequent encounter
S	sequela

● **V01.0 Pedestrian injured in collision with pedal cycle in nontraffic accident**
X● **V01.00 Pedestrian on foot injured in collision with pedal cycle in nontraffic accident**
Pedestrian NOS injured in collision with pedal cycle in nontraffic accident
X● **V01.01 Pedestrian on roller-skates injured in collision with pedal cycle in nontraffic accident**
X● **V01.02 Pedestrian on skateboard injured in collision with pedal cycle in nontraffic accident**
X● **V01.09 Pedestrian with other conveyance injured in collision with pedal cycle in nontraffic accident**
Pedestrian with baby stroller injured in collision with pedal cycle in nontraffic accident
Pedestrian in wheelchair (powered) injured in collision with pedal cycle in nontraffic accident
Pedestrian in motorized mobility scooter injured in collision with pedal cycle in nontraffic accident
Pedestrian on ice-skates injured in collision with pedal cycle in nontraffic accident
Pedestrian on nonmotorized scooter injured in collision with pedal cycle in nontraffic accident
Pedestrian on sled injured in collision with pedal cycle in nontraffic accident
Pedestrian on snowboard injured in collision with pedal cycle in nontraffic accident
Pedestrian on snow-skis injured in collision with pedal cycle in nontraffic accident

● **V01.1 Pedestrian injured in collision with pedal cycle in traffic accident**
X● **V01.10 Pedestrian on foot injured in collision with pedal cycle in traffic accident**
Pedestrian NOS injured in collision with pedal cycle in traffic accident
X● **V01.11 Pedestrian on roller-skates injured in collision with pedal cycle in traffic accident**
X● **V01.12 Pedestrian on skateboard injured in collision with pedal cycle in traffic accident**
X● **V01.19 Pedestrian with other conveyance injured in collision with pedal cycle in traffic accident**
Pedestrian with baby stroller injured in collision with pedal cycle in traffic accident
Pedestrian in wheelchair (powered) injured in collision with pedal cycle in traffic accident
Pedestrian in motorized mobility scooter injured in collision with pedal cycle in traffic accident
Pedestrian on ice-skates injured in collision with pedal cycle in traffic accident
Pedestrian on nonmotorized scooter injured in collision with pedal cycle in traffic accident
Pedestrian on sled injured in collision with pedal cycle in traffic accident
Pedestrian on snowboard injured in collision with pedal cycle in traffic accident
Pedestrian on snow-skis injured in collision with pedal cycle in traffic accident

● **V01.9 Pedestrian injured in collision with pedal cycle, unspecified whether traffic or nontraffic accident**
X● **V01.90 Pedestrian on foot injured in collision with pedal cycle, unspecified whether traffic or nontraffic accident**
Pedestrian NOS injured in collision with pedal cycle, unspecified whether traffic or nontraffic accident
X● **V01.91 Pedestrian on roller-skates injured in collision with pedal cycle, unspecified whether traffic or nontraffic accident**
X● **V01.92 Pedestrian on skateboard injured in collision with pedal cycle, unspecified whether traffic or nontraffic accident**
X● **V01.99 Pedestrian with other conveyance injured in collision with pedal cycle, unspecified whether traffic or nontraffic accident**
Pedestrian with baby stroller injured in collision with pedal cycle, unspecified whether traffic or nontraffic accident
Pedestrian in wheelchair (powered) injured in collision with pedal cycle, unspecified whether traffic or nontraffic accident
Pedestrian in motorized mobility scooter injured in collision with pedal cycle, unspecified whether traffic or nontraffic accident
Pedestrian on ice-skates injured in collision with pedal cycle unspecified, whether traffic or nontraffic accident
Pedestrian on nonmotorized scooter injured in collision with pedal cycle, unspecified whether traffic or nontraffic accident
Pedestrian on sled injured in collision with pedal cycle unspecified, whether traffic or nontraffic accident
Pedestrian on snowboard injured in collision with pedal cycle, unspecified whether traffic or nontraffic accident
Pedestrian on snow-skis injured in collision with pedal cycle, unspecified whether traffic or nontraffic accident

● VØ2 **Pedestrian injured in collision with two- or three-wheeled motor vehicle**

The appropriate 7th character is to be added to each code from category VØ2

A	initial encounter
D	subsequent encounter
S	sequela

● VØ2.Ø **Pedestrian injured in collision with two- or three-wheeled motor vehicle in nontraffic accident**

X● VØ2.ØØ **Pedestrian on foot injured in collision with two- or three-wheeled motor vehicle in nontraffic accident**

Pedestrian NOS injured in collision with two- or three-wheeled motor vehicle in nontraffic accident

X● VØ2.Ø1 **Pedestrian on roller-skates injured in collision with two- or three-wheeled motor vehicle in nontraffic accident**

X● VØ2.Ø2 **Pedestrian on skateboard injured in collision with two- or three-wheeled motor vehicle in nontraffic accident**

X● VØ2.Ø9 **Pedestrian with other conveyance injured in collision with two- or three-wheeled motor vehicle in nontraffic accident**

Pedestrian with baby stroller injured in collision with two- or three-wheeled motor vehicle in nontraffic accident

Pedestrian on ice-skates injured in collision with two- or three-wheeled motor vehicle in nontraffic accident

Pedestrian in wheelchair (powered) injured in collision with two- or three-wheeled motor vehicle in nontraffic accident

Pedestrian in motorized mobility scooter injured in collision with two- or three-wheeled motor vehicle in nontraffic accident

Pedestrian on nonmotorized scooter injured in collision with two- or three-wheeled motor vehicle in nontraffic accident

Pedestrian on sled injured in collision with two- or three-wheeled motor vehicle in nontraffic accident

Pedestrian on snowboard injured in collision with two- or three-wheeled motor vehicle in nontraffic accident

Pedestrian on snow-skis injured in collision with two- or three-wheeled motor vehicle in nontraffic accident

● VØ2.1 **Pedestrian injured in collision with two- or three-wheeled motor vehicle in traffic accident**

X● VØ2.1Ø **Pedestrian on foot injured in collision with two- or three-wheeled motor vehicle in traffic accident**

Pedestrian NOS injured in collision with two- or three-wheeled motor vehicle in traffic accident

X● VØ2.11 **Pedestrian on roller-skates injured in collision with two- or three-wheeled motor vehicle in traffic accident**

X● VØ2.12 **Pedestrian on skateboard injured in collision with two- or three-wheeled motor vehicle in traffic accident**

X● VØ2.19 **Pedestrian with other conveyance injured in collision with two- or three-wheeled motor vehicle in traffic accident**

Pedestrian with baby stroller injured in collision with two- or three-wheeled motor vehicle in traffic accident

Pedestrian in wheelchair (powered) injured in collision with two- or three-wheeled motor vehicle in traffic accident

Pedestrian in motorized mobility scooter injured in collision with two- or three-wheeled motor vehicle in traffic accident

Pedestrian on ice-skates injured in collision with two- or three-wheeled motor vehicle in traffic accident

Pedestrian on nonmotorized scooter injured in collision with two- or three-wheeled motor vehicle in traffic accident

Pedestrian on sled injured in collision with two- or three-wheeled motor vehicle in traffic accident

Pedestrian on snowboard injured in collision with two- or three-wheeled motor vehicle in traffic accident

Pedestrian on snow-skis injured in collision with two- or three-wheeled motor vehicle in traffic accident

● VØ2.9 **Pedestrian injured in collision with two- or three-wheeled motor vehicle, unspecified whether traffic or nontraffic accident**

X● VØ2.9Ø **Pedestrian on foot injured in collision with two- or three-wheeled motor vehicle, unspecified whether traffic or nontraffic accident**

Pedestrian NOS injured in collision with two- or three-wheeled motor vehicle, unspecified whether traffic or nontraffic accident

X● VØ2.91 **Pedestrian on roller-skates injured in collision with two- or three-wheeled motor vehicle, unspecified whether traffic or nontraffic accident**

X● VØ2.92 **Pedestrian on skateboard injured in collision with two- or three-wheeled motor vehicle, unspecified whether traffic or nontraffic accident**

X● **VØ2.99 Pedestrian with other conveyance injured in collision with two- or three-wheeled motor vehicle, unspecified whether traffic or nontraffic accident**
Pedestrian with baby stroller injured in collision with two- or three-wheeled motor vehicle, unspecified whether traffic or nontraffic accident
Pedestrian in wheelchair (powered) injured in collision with two- or three-wheeled motor vehicle, unspecified whether traffic or nontraffic accident
Pedestrian in motorized mobility scooter injured in collision with two- or three-wheeled motor vehicle, unspecified whether traffic or nontraffic accident
Pedestrian on ice-skates injured in collision with two- or three-wheeled motor vehicle, unspecified whether traffic or nontraffic accident
Pedestrian on nonmotorized scooter injured in collision with two- or three-wheeled motor vehicle, unspecified whether traffic or nontraffic accident
Pedestrian on sled injured in collision with two- or three-wheeled motor vehicle, unspecified whether traffic or nontraffic accident
Pedestrian on snowboard injured in collision with two- or three-wheeled motor vehicle, unspecified whether traffic or nontraffic accident
Pedestrian on snow-skis injured in collision with two- or three-wheeled motor vehicle, unspecified whether traffic or nontraffic accident

● **VØ3 Pedestrian injured in collision with car, pick-up truck or van**
The appropriate 7th character is to be added to each code from category VØ3

A	initial encounter
D	subsequent encounter
S	sequela

● **VØ3.Ø Pedestrian injured in collision with car, pick-up truck or van in nontraffic accident**

X● **VØ3.ØØ Pedestrian on foot injured in collision with car, pick-up truck or van in nontraffic accident**
Pedestrian NOS injured in collision with car, pick-up truck or van in nontraffic accident

X● **VØ3.Ø1 Pedestrian on roller-skates injured in collision with car, pick-up truck or van in nontraffic accident**

X● **VØ3.Ø2 Pedestrian on skateboard injured in collision with car, pick-up truck or van in nontraffic accident**

X● **VØ3.Ø9 Pedestrian with other conveyance injured in collision with car, pick-up truck or van in nontraffic accident**
Pedestrian with baby stroller injured in collision with car, pick-up truck or van in nontraffic accident
Pedestrian in wheelchair (powered) injured in collision with car, pick-up truck or van in nontraffic accident
Pedestrian in motorized mobility scooter injured in collision with car, pick-up truck or van in nontraffic accident
Pedestrian on ice-skates injured in collision with car, pick-up truck or van in nontraffic accident
Pedestrian on nonmotorized scooter injured in collision with car, pick-up truck or van in nontraffic accident
Pedestrian on sled injured in collision with car, pick-up truck or van in nontraffic accident
Pedestrian on snowboard injured in collision with car, pick-up truck or van in nontraffic accident
Pedestrian on snow-skis injured in collision with car, pick-up truck or van in nontraffic accident

● **VØ3.1 Pedestrian injured in collision with car, pick-up truck or van in traffic accident**

X● **VØ3.1Ø Pedestrian on foot injured in collision with car, pick-up truck or van in traffic accident**
Pedestrian NOS injured in collision with car, pick-up truck or van in traffic accident

X● **VØ3.11 Pedestrian on roller-skates injured in collision with car, pick-up truck or van in traffic accident**

X● **VØ3.12 Pedestrian on skateboard injured in collision with car, pick-up truck or van in traffic accident**

X● **VØ3.19 Pedestrian with other conveyance injured in collision with car, pick-up truck or van in traffic accident**
Pedestrian with baby stroller injured in collision with car, pick-up truck or van in traffic accident
Pedestrian in wheelchair (powered) injured in collision with car, pick-up truck or van in traffic accident
Pedestrian in motorized mobility scooter injured in collision with car, pick-up truck or van in traffic accident
Pedestrian on ice-skates injured in collision with car, pick-up truck or van in traffic accident
Pedestrian on nonmotorized scooter injured in collision with car, pick-up truck or van in traffic accident
Pedestrian on sled injured in collision with car, pick-up truck or van in traffic accident
Pedestrian on snowboard injured in collision with car, pick-up truck or van in traffic accident
Pedestrian on snow-skis injured in collision with car, pick-up truck or van in traffic accident

V03.9 Pedestrian injured in collision with car, pick-up truck or van, unspecified whether traffic or nontraffic accident

X **V03.90 Pedestrian on foot injured in collision with car, pick-up truck or van, unspecified whether traffic or nontraffic accident**
Pedestrian NOS injured in collision with car, pick-up truck or van, unspecified whether traffic or nontraffic accident

X **V03.91 Pedestrian on roller-skates injured in collision with car, pick-up truck or van, unspecified whether traffic or nontraffic accident**

X **V03.92 Pedestrian on skateboard injured in collision with car, pick-up truck or van, unspecified whether traffic or nontraffic accident**

X **V03.99 Pedestrian with other conveyance injured in collision with car, pick-up truck or van, unspecified whether traffic or nontraffic accident**
Pedestrian with baby stroller injured in collision with car, pick-up truck or van, unspecified whether traffic or nontraffic accident
Pedestrian in wheelchair (powered) injured in collision with car, pick-up truck or van, unspecified whether traffic or nontraffic accident
Pedestrian in motorized mobility scooter injured in collision with car, pick-up truck or van, unspecified whether traffic or nontraffic accident
Pedestrian on ice-skates injured in collision with car, pick-up truck or van, unspecified whether traffic or nontraffic accident
Pedestrian on nonmotorized scooter injured in collision with car, pick-up truck or van, unspecified whether traffic or nontraffic accident
Pedestrian on sled injured in collision with car, pick-up truck or van in nontraffic accident
Pedestrian on snowboard injured in collision with car, pick-up truck or van, unspecified whether traffic or nontraffic accident
Pedestrian on snow-skis injured in collision with car, pick-up truck or van, unspecified whether traffic or nontraffic accident

V04 Pedestrian injured in collision with heavy transport vehicle or bus

Excludes1 pedestrian injured in collision with military vehicle (V09.01, V09.21)

The appropriate 7th character is to be added to each code from category V04

A	initial encounter
D	subsequent encounter
S	sequela

V04.0 Pedestrian injured in collision with heavy transport vehicle or bus in nontraffic accident

X **V04.00 Pedestrian on foot injured in collision with heavy transport vehicle or bus in nontraffic accident**
Pedestrian NOS injured in collision with heavy transport vehicle or bus in nontraffic accident

X **V04.01 Pedestrian on roller-skates injured in collision with heavy transport vehicle or bus in nontraffic accident**

X **V04.02 Pedestrian on skateboard injured in collision with heavy transport vehicle or bus in nontraffic accident**

X **V04.09 Pedestrian with other conveyance injured in collision with heavy transport vehicle or bus in nontraffic accident**
Pedestrian with baby stroller injured in collision with heavy transport vehicle or bus in nontraffic accident
Pedestrian in wheelchair (powered) injured in collision with heavy transport vehicle or bus in nontraffic accident
Pedestrian in motorized mobility scooter injured in collision with heavy transport vehicle or bus in nontraffic accident
Pedestrian on ice-skates injured in collision with heavy transport vehicle or bus in nontraffic accident
Pedestrian on nonmotorized scooter injured in collision with heavy transport vehicle or bus in nontraffic accident
Pedestrian on sled injured in collision with heavy transport vehicle or bus in nontraffic accident
Pedestrian on snowboard injured in collision with heavy transport vehicle or bus in nontraffic accident
Pedestrian on snow-skis injured in collision with heavy transport vehicle or bus in nontraffic accident

V04.1 Pedestrian injured in collision with heavy transport vehicle or bus in traffic accident

X **V04.10 Pedestrian on foot injured in collision with heavy transport vehicle or bus in traffic accident**
Pedestrian NOS injured in collision with heavy transport vehicle or bus in traffic accident

X **V04.11 Pedestrian on roller-skates injured in collision with heavy transport vehicle or bus in traffic accident**

X **V04.12 Pedestrian on skateboard injured in collision with heavy transport vehicle or bus in traffic accident**

X **V04.19 Pedestrian with other conveyance injured in collision with heavy transport vehicle or bus in traffic accident**
Pedestrian with baby stroller injured in collision with heavy transport vehicle or bus in traffic accident
Pedestrian in wheelchair (powered) injured in collision with heavy transport vehicle or bus in traffic accident
Pedestrian in motorized mobility scooter injured in collision with heavy transport vehicle or bus in traffic accident
Pedestrian on ice-skates injured in collision with heavy transport vehicle or bus in traffic accident
Pedestrian on nonmotorized scooter injured in collision with heavy transport vehicle or bus in traffic accident
Pedestrian on sled injured in collision with heavy transport vehicle or bus in traffic accident
Pedestrian on snowboard injured in collision with heavy transport vehicle or bus in traffic accident
Pedestrian on snow-skis injured in collision with heavy transport vehicle or bus in traffic accident

VØ4.9 Pedestrian injured in collision with heavy transport vehicle or bus, unspecified whether traffic or nontraffic accident

X **VØ4.90 Pedestrian on foot injured in collision with heavy transport vehicle or bus, unspecified whether traffic or nontraffic accident**

Pedestrian NOS injured in collision with heavy transport vehicle or bus, unspecified whether traffic or nontraffic accident

X **VØ4.91 Pedestrian on roller-skates injured in collision with heavy transport vehicle or bus, unspecified whether traffic or nontraffic accident**

X **VØ4.92 Pedestrian on skateboard injured in collision with heavy transport vehicle or bus, unspecified whether traffic or nontraffic accident**

X **VØ4.99 Pedestrian with other conveyance injured in collision with heavy transport vehicle or bus, unspecified whether traffic or nontraffic accident**

Pedestrian with baby stroller injured in collision with heavy transport vehicle or bus, unspecified whether traffic or nontraffic accident
Pedestrian in wheelchair (powered) injured in collision with heavy transport vehicle or bus, unspecified whether traffic or nontraffic accident
Pedestrian in motorized mobility scooter injured in collision with heavy transport vehicle or bus, unspecified whether traffic or nontraffic accident
Pedestrian on ice-skates injured in collision with heavy transport vehicle or bus, unspecified whether traffic or nontraffic accident
Pedestrian on nonmotorized scooter injured in collision with heavy transport vehicle or bus, unspecified whether traffic or nontraffic accident
Pedestrian on sled injured in collision with heavy transport vehicle or bus, unspecified whether traffic or nontraffic accident
Pedestrian on snowboard injured in collision with heavy transport vehicle or bus, unspecified whether traffic or nontraffic accident
Pedestrian on snow-skis injured in collision with heavy transport vehicle or bus, unspecified whether traffic or nontraffic accident

VØ5 Pedestrian injured in collision with railway train or railway vehicle

The appropriate 7th character is to be added to each code from category VØ5

A	initial encounter
D	subsequent encounter
S	sequela

VØ5.Ø Pedestrian injured in collision with railway train or railway vehicle in nontraffic accident

X **VØ5.ØØ Pedestrian on foot injured in collision with railway train or railway vehicle in nontraffic accident**

Pedestrian NOS injured in collision with railway train or railway vehicle in nontraffic accident

X **VØ5.Ø1 Pedestrian on roller-skates injured in collision with railway train or railway vehicle in nontraffic accident**

X **VØ5.Ø2 Pedestrian on skateboard injured in collision with railway train or railway vehicle in nontraffic accident**

X **VØ5.Ø9 Pedestrian with other conveyance injured in collision with railway train or railway vehicle in nontraffic accident**

Pedestrian with baby stroller injured in collision with railway train or railway vehicle in nontraffic accident
Pedestrian in wheelchair (powered) injured in collision with railway train or railway vehicle in nontraffic accident
Pedestrian in motorized mobility scooter injured in collision with railway train or railway vehicle in nontraffic accident
Pedestrian on ice-skates injured in collision with railway train or railway vehicle in nontraffic accident
Pedestrian on nonmotorized scooter injured in collision with railway train or railway vehicle in nontraffic accident
Pedestrian on sled injured in collision with railway train or railway vehicle in nontraffic accident
Pedestrian on snowboard injured in collision with railway train or railway vehicle in nontraffic accident
Pedestrian on snow-skis injured in collision with railway train or railway vehicle in nontraffic accident

VØ5.1 Pedestrian injured in collision with railway train or railway vehicle in traffic accident

X **VØ5.1Ø Pedestrian on foot injured in collision with railway train or railway vehicle in traffic accident**

Pedestrian NOS injured in collision with railway train or railway vehicle in traffic accident

X **VØ5.11 Pedestrian on roller-skates injured in collision with railway train or railway vehicle in traffic accident**

X **VØ5.12 Pedestrian on skateboard injured in collision with railway train or railway vehicle in traffic accident**

X **VØ5.19 Pedestrian with other conveyance injured in collision with railway train or railway vehicle in traffic accident**

Pedestrian with baby stroller injured in collision with railway train or railway vehicle in traffic accident
Pedestrian in wheelchair (powered) injured in collision with railway train or railway vehicle in traffic accident
Pedestrian in motorized mobility scooter injured in collision with railway train or railway vehicle in traffic accident
Pedestrian on ice-skates injured in collision with railway train or railway vehicle in traffic accident
Pedestrian on nonmotorized scooter injured in collision with railway train or railway vehicle in traffic accident
Pedestrian on sled injured in collision with railway train or railway vehicle in traffic accident
Pedestrian on snowboard injured in collision with railway train or railway vehicle in traffic accident
Pedestrian on snow-skis injured in collision with railway train or railway vehicle in traffic accident

● **V05.9 Pedestrian injured in collision with railway train or railway vehicle, unspecified whether traffic or nontraffic accident**

X● **V05.90 Pedestrian on foot injured in collision with railway train or railway vehicle, unspecified whether traffic or nontraffic accident**

Pedestrian NOS injured in collision with railway train or railway vehicle, unspecified whether traffic or nontraffic accident

X● **V05.91 Pedestrian on roller-skates injured in collision with railway train or railway vehicle, unspecified whether traffic or nontraffic accident**

X● **V05.92 Pedestrian on skateboard injured in collision with railway train or railway vehicle, unspecified whether traffic or nontraffic accident**

X● **V05.99 Pedestrian with other conveyance injured in collision with railway train or railway vehicle, unspecified whether traffic or nontraffic accident**

Pedestrian with baby stroller injured in collision with railway train or railway vehicle, unspecified whether traffic or nontraffic

Pedestrian in wheelchair (powered) injured in collision with railway train or railway vehicle, unspecified whether traffic or nontraffic

Pedestrian in motorized mobility scooter injured in collision with railway train or railway vehicle, unspecified whether traffic or nontraffic

Pedestrian on ice-skates injured in collision with railway train or railway vehicle, unspecified whether traffic or nontraffic

Pedestrian on nonmotorized scooter injured in collision with railway train or railway vehicle, unspecified whether traffic or nontraffic

Pedestrian on sled injured in collision with railway train or railway vehicle, unspecified whether traffic or nontraffic

Pedestrian on snowboard injured in collision with railway train or railway vehicle, unspecified whether traffic or nontraffic

Pedestrian on snow-skis injured in collision with railway train or railway vehicle, unspecified whether traffic or nontraffic

● **V06 Pedestrian injured in collision with other nonmotor vehicle**

Includes collision with animal-drawn vehicle, animal being ridden, nonpowered streetcar

Excludes1 pedestrian injured in collision with pedestrian conveyance (V00.0-)

The appropriate 7th character is to be added to each code from category V06

A	initial encounter
D	subsequent encounter
S	sequela

● **V06.0 Pedestrian injured in collision with other nonmotor vehicle in nontraffic accident**

X● **V06.00 Pedestrian on foot injured in collision with other nonmotor vehicle in nontraffic accident**

Pedestrian NOS injured in collision with other nonmotor vehicle in nontraffic accident

X● **V06.01 Pedestrian on roller-skates injured in collision with other nonmotor vehicle in nontraffic accident**

X● **V06.02 Pedestrian on skateboard injured in collision with other nonmotor vehicle in nontraffic accident**

X● **V06.09 Pedestrian with other conveyance injured in collision with other nonmotor vehicle in nontraffic accident**

Pedestrian with baby stroller injured in collision with other nonmotor vehicle in nontraffic accident

Pedestrian in wheelchair (powered) injured in collision with other nonmotor vehicle in nontraffic accident

Pedestrian in motorized mobility scooter injured in collision with other nonmotor vehicle in nontraffic accident

Pedestrian on ice-skates injured in collision with other nonmotor vehicle in nontraffic accident

Pedestrian on nonmotorized scooter injured in collision with other nonmotor vehicle in nontraffic accident

Pedestrian on sled injured in collision with other nonmotor vehicle in nontraffic accident

Pedestrian on snowboard injured in collision with other nonmotor vehicle in nontraffic accident

Pedestrian on snow-skis injured in collision with other nonmotor vehicle in nontraffic accident

● **V06.1 Pedestrian injured in collision with other nonmotor vehicle in traffic accident**

X● **V06.10 Pedestrian on foot injured in collision with other nonmotor vehicle in traffic accident**

Pedestrian NOS injured in collision with other nonmotor vehicle in traffic accident

X● **V06.11 Pedestrian on roller-skates injured in collision with other nonmotor vehicle in traffic accident**

X● **V06.12 Pedestrian on skateboard injured in collision with other nonmotor vehicle in traffic accident**

X● **V06.19 Pedestrian with other conveyance injured in collision with other nonmotor vehicle in traffic accident**

Pedestrian with baby stroller injured in collision with other nonmotor vehicle in nontraffic accident

Pedestrian in wheelchair (powered) injured in collision with other nonmotor vehicle in traffic accident

Pedestrian in motorized mobility scooter injured in collision with other nonmotor vehicle in traffic accident

Pedestrian on ice-skates injured in collision with other nonmotor vehicle in traffic accident

Pedestrian on nonmotorized scooter injured in collision with other nonmotor vehicle in traffic accident

Pedestrian on sled injured in collision with other nonmotor vehicle in traffic accident

Pedestrian on snowboard injured in collision with other nonmotor vehicle in traffic accident

Pedestrian on snow-skis injured in collision with other nonmotor vehicle in traffic accident

● **V06.9 Pedestrian injured in collision with other nonmotor vehicle, unspecified whether traffic or nontraffic accident**

X● **V06.90 Pedestrian on foot injured in collision with other nonmotor vehicle, unspecified whether traffic or nontraffic accident**

Pedestrian NOS injured in collision with other nonmotor vehicle, unspecified whether traffic or nontraffic accident

X● **V06.91 Pedestrian on roller-skates injured in collision with other nonmotor vehicle, unspecified whether traffic or nontraffic accident**

X● **VØ6.92 Pedestrian on skateboard injured in collision with other nonmotor vehicle, unspecified whether traffic or nontraffic accident**

X● **VØ6.99 Pedestrian with other conveyance injured in collision with other nonmotor vehicle, unspecified whether traffic or nontraffic accident**

Pedestrian with baby stroller injured in collision with other nonmotor vehicle, unspecified whether traffic or nontraffic accident

Pedestrian in wheelchair (powered) injured in collision with other nonmotor vehicle, unspecified whether traffic or nontraffic accident

Pedestrian in motorized mobility scooter injured in collision with other nonmotor vehicle, unspecified whether traffic or nontraffic accident

Pedestrian on ice-skates injured in collision with other nonmotor vehicle, unspecified whether traffic or nontraffic accident

Pedestrian on nonmotorized scooter injured in collision with other nonmotor vehicle, unspecified whether traffic or nontraffic accident

Pedestrian on sled injured in collision with other nonmotor vehicle, unspecified whether traffic or nontraffic accident

Pedestrian on snowboard injured in collision with other nonmotor vehicle, unspecified whether traffic or nontraffic accident

Pedestrian on snow-skis injured in collision with other nonmotor vehicle, unspecified whether traffic or nontraffic accident

● **VØ9 Pedestrian injured in other and unspecified transport accidents**

The appropriate 7th character is to be added to each code from category VØ9

A	initial encounter
D	subsequent encounter
S	sequela

● **VØ9.Ø Pedestrian injured in nontraffic accident involving other and unspecified motor vehicles**

X● **VØ9.ØØ Pedestrian injured in nontraffic accident involving unspecified motor vehicles**

X● **VØ9.Ø1 Pedestrian injured in nontraffic accident involving military vehicle**

X● **VØ9.Ø9 Pedestrian injured in nontraffic accident involving other motor vehicles**

Pedestrian injured in nontraffic accident by special vehicle

X● **VØ9.1 Pedestrian injured in unspecified nontraffic accident**

● **VØ9.2 Pedestrian injured in traffic accident involving other and unspecified motor vehicles**

X● **VØ9.2Ø Pedestrian injured in traffic accident involving unspecified motor vehicles**

X● **VØ9.21 Pedestrian injured in traffic accident involving military vehicle**

X● **VØ9.29 Pedestrian injured in traffic accident involving other motor vehicles**

X● **VØ9.3 Pedestrian injured in unspecified traffic accident**

X● **VØ9.9 Pedestrian injured in unspecified transport accident**

PEDAL CYCLE RIDER INJURED IN TRANSPORT ACCIDENT (V1Ø-V19)

Includes any non-motorized vehicle, excluding an animal-drawn vehicle, or a sidecar or trailer attached to the pedal cycle

Excludes2 rupture of pedal cycle tire (W37.Ø)

● **V1Ø Pedal cycle rider injured in collision with pedestrian or animal**

Excludes1 pedal cycle rider collision with animal-drawn vehicle or animal being ridden (V16.-)

The appropriate 7th character is to be added to each code from category V1Ø

A	initial encounter
D	subsequent encounter
S	sequela

X● **V1Ø.Ø Pedal cycle driver injured in collision with pedestrian or animal in nontraffic accident**

X● **V1Ø.1 Pedal cycle passenger injured in collision with pedestrian or animal in nontraffic accident**

X● **V1Ø.2 Unspecified pedal cyclist injured in collision with pedestrian or animal in nontraffic accident**

X● **V1Ø.3 Person boarding or alighting a pedal cycle injured in collision with pedestrian or animal**

X● **V1Ø.4 Pedal cycle driver injured in collision with pedestrian or animal in traffic accident**

X● **V1Ø.5 Pedal cycle passenger injured in collision with pedestrian or animal in traffic accident**

X● **V1Ø.9 Unspecified pedal cyclist injured in collision with pedestrian or animal in traffic accident**

● **V11 Pedal cycle rider injured in collision with other pedal cycle**

The appropriate 7th character is to be added to each code from category V11

A	initial encounter
D	subsequent encounter
S	sequela

X● **V11.Ø Pedal cycle driver injured in collision with other pedal cycle in nontraffic accident**

X● **V11.1 Pedal cycle passenger injured in collision with other pedal cycle in nontraffic accident**

X● **V11.2 Unspecified pedal cyclist injured in collision with other pedal cycle in nontraffic accident**

X● **V11.3 Person boarding or alighting a pedal cycle injured in collision with other pedal cycle**

X● **V11.4 Pedal cycle driver injured in collision with other pedal cycle in traffic accident**

X● **V11.5 Pedal cycle passenger injured in collision with other pedal cycle in traffic accident**

X● **V11.9 Unspecified pedal cyclist injured in collision with other pedal cycle in traffic accident**

● **V12 Pedal cycle rider injured in collision with two- or three-wheeled motor vehicle**

The appropriate 7th character is to be added to each code from category V12

A	initial encounter
D	subsequent encounter
S	sequela

X● **V12.0 Pedal cycle driver injured in collision with two- or three-wheeled motor vehicle in nontraffic accident**

X● **V12.1 Pedal cycle passenger injured in collision with two- or three-wheeled motor vehicle in nontraffic accident**

X● **V12.2 Unspecified pedal cyclist injured in collision with two- or three-wheeled motor vehicle in nontraffic accident**

X● **V12.3 Person boarding or alighting a pedal cycle injured in collision with two- or three-wheeled motor vehicle**

X● **V12.4 Pedal cycle driver injured in collision with two- or three-wheeled motor vehicle in traffic accident**

X● **V12.5 Pedal cycle passenger injured in collision with two- or three-wheeled motor vehicle in traffic accident**

X● **V12.9 Unspecified pedal cyclist injured in collision with two- or three-wheeled motor vehicle in traffic accident**

● **V13 Pedal cycle rider injured in collision with car, pick-up truck or van**

The appropriate 7th character is to be added to each code from category V13

A	initial encounter
D	subsequent encounter
S	sequela

X● **V13.0 Pedal cycle driver injured in collision with car, pick-up truck or van in nontraffic accident**

X● **V13.1 Pedal cycle passenger injured in collision with car, pick-up truck or van in nontraffic accident**

X● **V13.2 Unspecified pedal cyclist injured in collision with car, pick-up truck or van in nontraffic accident**

X● **V13.3 Person boarding or alighting a pedal cycle injured in collision with car, pick-up truck or van**

X● **V13.4 Pedal cycle driver injured in collision with car, pick-up truck or van in traffic accident**

X● **V13.5 Pedal cycle passenger injured in collision with car, pick-up truck or van in traffic accident**

X● **V13.9 Unspecified pedal cyclist injured in collision with car, pick-up truck or van in traffic accident**

● **V14 Pedal cycle rider injured in collision with heavy transport vehicle or bus**

Excludes1 pedal cycle rider injured in collision with military vehicle (V19.81)

The appropriate 7th character is to be added to each code from category V14

A	initial encounter
D	subsequent encounter
S	sequela

X● **V14.0 Pedal cycle driver injured in collision with heavy transport vehicle or bus in nontraffic accident**

X● **V14.1 Pedal cycle passenger injured in collision with heavy transport vehicle or bus in nontraffic accident**

X● **V14.2 Unspecified pedal cyclist injured in collision with heavy transport vehicle or bus in nontraffic accident**

X● **V14.3 Person boarding or alighting a pedal cycle injured in collision with heavy transport vehicle or bus**

X● **V14.4 Pedal cycle driver injured in collision with heavy transport vehicle or bus in traffic accident**

X● **V14.5 Pedal cycle passenger injured in collision with heavy transport vehicle or bus in traffic accident**

X● **V14.9 Unspecified pedal cyclist injured in collision with heavy transport vehicle or bus in traffic accident**

● **V15 Pedal cycle rider injured in collision with railway train or railway vehicle**

The appropriate 7th character is to be added to each code from category V15

A	initial encounter
D	subsequent encounter
S	sequela

X● **V15.0 Pedal cycle driver injured in collision with railway train or railway vehicle in nontraffic accident**

X● **V15.1 Pedal cycle passenger injured in collision with railway train or railway vehicle in nontraffic accident**

X● **V15.2 Unspecified pedal cyclist injured in collision with railway train or railway vehicle in nontraffic accident**

X● **V15.3 Person boarding or alighting a pedal cycle injured in collision with railway train or railway vehicle**

X● **V15.4 Pedal cycle driver injured in collision with railway train or railway vehicle in traffic accident**

X● **V15.5 Pedal cycle passenger injured in collision with railway train or railway vehicle in traffic accident**

X● **V15.9 Unspecified pedal cyclist injured in collision with railway train or railway vehicle in traffic accident**

● **V16 Pedal cycle rider injured in collision with other nonmotor vehicle**

Includes collision with animal-drawn vehicle, animal being ridden, streetcar

The appropriate 7th character is to be added to each code from category V16

A	initial encounter
D	subsequent encounter
S	sequela

X● **V16.0 Pedal cycle driver injured in collision with other nonmotor vehicle in nontraffic accident**

X● **V16.1 Pedal cycle passenger injured in collision with other nonmotor vehicle in nontraffic accident**

X● **V16.2 Unspecified pedal cyclist injured in collision with other nonmotor vehicle in nontraffic accident**

X● **V16.3 Person boarding or alighting a pedal cycle injured in collision with other nonmotor vehicle in nontraffic accident**

X● **V16.4 Pedal cycle driver injured in collision with other nonmotor vehicle in traffic accident**

X● **V16.5 Pedal cycle passenger injured in collision with other nonmotor vehicle in traffic accident**

X● **V16.9 Unspecified pedal cyclist injured in collision with other nonmotor vehicle in traffic accident**

● **V17 Pedal cycle rider injured in collision with fixed or stationary object**

The appropriate 7th character is to be added to each code from category V17

A	initial encounter
D	subsequent encounter
S	sequela

X● **V17.0 Pedal cycle driver injured in collision with fixed or stationary object in nontraffic accident**

X● **V17.1 Pedal cycle passenger injured in collision with fixed or stationary object in nontraffic accident**

X● **V17.2 Unspecified pedal cyclist injured in collision with fixed or stationary object in nontraffic accident**

X● **V17.3 Person boarding or alighting a pedal cycle injured in collision with fixed or stationary object**

X● **V17.4 Pedal cycle driver injured in collision with fixed or stationary object in traffic accident**

X● **V17.5 Pedal cycle passenger injured in collision with fixed or stationary object in traffic accident**

X● **V17.9 Unspecified pedal cyclist injured in collision with fixed or stationary object in traffic accident**

● **V18 Pedal cycle rider injured in noncollision transport accident**

Includes fall or thrown from pedal cycle (without antecedent collision)
overturning pedal cycle NOS
overturning pedal cycle without collision

The appropriate 7th character is to be added to each code from category V18

A	initial encounter
D	subsequent encounter
S	sequela

X● **V18.0** **Pedal cycle driver injured in noncollision transport accident in nontraffic accident**

X● **V18.1** **Pedal cycle passenger injured in noncollision transport accident in nontraffic accident**

X● **V18.2** **Unspecified pedal cyclist injured in noncollision transport accident in nontraffic accident**

X● **V18.3** **Person boarding or alighting a pedal cycle injured in noncollision transport accident**

X● **V18.4** **Pedal cycle driver injured in noncollision transport accident in traffic accident**

X● **V18.5** **Pedal cycle passenger injured in noncollision transport accident in traffic accident**

X● **V18.9** **Unspecified pedal cyclist injured in noncollision transport accident in traffic accident**

● **V19 Pedal cycle rider injured in other and unspecified transport accidents**

The appropriate 7th character is to be added to each code from category V19

A	initial encounter
D	subsequent encounter
S	sequela

● **V19.0** **Pedal cycle driver injured in collision with other and unspecified motor vehicles in nontraffic accident**

X● **V19.00** **Pedal cycle driver injured in collision with unspecified motor vehicles in nontraffic accident**

X● **V19.09** **Pedal cycle driver injured in collision with other motor vehicles in nontraffic accident**

● **V19.1** **Pedal cycle passenger injured in collision with other and unspecified motor vehicles in nontraffic accident**

X● **V19.10** **Pedal cycle passenger injured in collision with unspecified motor vehicles in nontraffic accident**

X● **V19.19** **Pedal cycle passenger injured in collision with other motor vehicles in nontraffic accident**

● **V19.2** **Unspecified pedal cyclist injured in collision with other and unspecified motor vehicles in nontraffic accident**

X● **V19.20** **Unspecified pedal cyclist injured in collision with unspecified motor vehicles in nontraffic accident**
Pedal cycle collision NOS, nontraffic

X● **V19.29** **Unspecified pedal cyclist injured in collision with other motor vehicles in nontraffic accident**

X● **V19.3** **Pedal cyclist (driver) (passenger) injured in unspecified nontraffic accident**
Pedal cycle accident NOS, nontraffic
Pedal cyclist injured in nontraffic accident NOS

● **V19.4** **Pedal cycle driver injured in collision with other and unspecified motor vehicles in traffic accident**

X● **V19.40** **Pedal cycle driver injured in collision with unspecified motor vehicles in traffic accident**

X● **V19.49** **Pedal cycle driver injured in collision with other motor vehicles in traffic accident**

● **V19.5** **Pedal cycle passenger injured in collision with other and unspecified motor vehicles in traffic accident**

X● **V19.50** **Pedal cycle passenger injured in collision with unspecified motor vehicles in traffic accident**

X● **V19.59** **Pedal cycle passenger injured in collision with other motor vehicles in traffic accident**

● **V19.6** **Unspecified pedal cyclist injured in collision with other and unspecified motor vehicles in traffic accident**

X● **V19.60** **Unspecified pedal cyclist injured in collision with unspecified motor vehicles in traffic accident**
Pedal cycle collision NOS (traffic)

X● **V19.69** **Unspecified pedal cyclist injured in collision with other motor vehicles in traffic accident**

● **V19.8** **Pedal cyclist (driver) (passenger) injured in other specified transport accidents**

X● **V19.81** **Pedal cyclist (driver) (passenger) injured in transport accident with military vehicle**

X● **V19.88** **Pedal cyclist (driver) (passenger) injured in other specified transport accidents**

X● **V19.9** **Pedal cyclist (driver) (passenger) injured in unspecified traffic accident**
Pedal cycle accident NOS

MOTORCYCLE RIDER INJURED IN TRANSPORT ACCIDENT (V20-V29)

Includes moped motorcycle with sidecar motorized bicycle motor scooter

Excludes1 three-wheeled motor vehicle (V30-V39)

● **V20 Motorcycle rider injured in collision with pedestrian or animal**

Excludes1 motorcycle rider collision with animal-drawn vehicle or animal being ridden (V26.-)

The appropriate 7th character is to be added to each code from category V20

A	initial encounter
D	subsequent encounter
S	sequela

X● **V20.0** **Motorcycle driver injured in collision with pedestrian or animal in nontraffic accident**

X● **V20.1** **Motorcycle passenger injured in collision with pedestrian or animal in nontraffic accident**

X● **V20.2** **Unspecified motorcycle rider injured in collision with pedestrian or animal in nontraffic accident**

X● **V20.3** **Person boarding or alighting a motorcycle injured in collision with pedestrian or animal**

X● **V20.4** **Motorcycle driver injured in collision with pedestrian or animal in traffic accident**

X● **V20.5** **Motorcycle passenger injured in collision with pedestrian or animal in traffic accident**

X● **V20.9** **Unspecified motorcycle rider injured in collision with pedestrian or animal in traffic accident**

● **V21 Motorcycle rider injured in collision with pedal cycle**

The appropriate 7th character is to be added to each code from category V21

A	initial encounter
D	subsequent encounter
S	sequela

X● **V21.0** **Motorcycle driver injured in collision with pedal cycle in nontraffic accident**

X● **V21.1** **Motorcycle passenger injured in collision with pedal cycle in nontraffic accident**

X● **V21.2** **Unspecified motorcycle rider injured in collision with pedal cycle in nontraffic accident**

X● **V21.3** **Person boarding or alighting a motorcycle injured in collision with pedal cycle**

X● **V21.4** **Motorcycle driver injured in collision with pedal cycle in traffic accident**

X● **V21.5** **Motorcycle passenger injured in collision with pedal cycle in traffic accident**

X● **V21.9** **Unspecified motorcycle rider injured in collision with pedal cycle in traffic accident**

● **V22 Motorcycle rider injured in collision with two- or three-wheeled motor vehicle**

The appropriate 7th character is to be added to each code from category V22

A initial encounter
D subsequent encounter
S sequela

X● V22.Ø Motorcycle **driver** injured in collision with two- or three-wheeled motor vehicle in **nontraffic accident**

X● V22.1 Motorcycle **passenger** injured in collision with two- or three-wheeled motor vehicle in **nontraffic accident**

X● V22.2 **Unspecified** motorcycle rider injured in collision with two- or three-wheeled motor vehicle in **nontraffic accident**

X● V22.3 Person **boarding or alighting** a motorcycle injured in collision with two- or three-wheeled motor vehicle

X● V22.4 Motorcycle **driver** injured in collision with two- or three-wheeled motor vehicle in **traffic accident**

X● V22.5 Motorcycle **passenger** injured in collision with two- or three-wheeled motor vehicle in **traffic accident**

X● V22.9 **Unspecified** motorcycle rider injured in collision with two- or three-wheeled motor vehicle in **traffic accident**

● **V23 Motorcycle rider injured in collision with car, pick-up truck or van**

The appropriate 7th character is to be added to each code from category V23

A initial encounter
D subsequent encounter
S sequela

X● V23.Ø Motorcycle **driver** injured in collision with car, pick-up truck or van in **nontraffic accident**

X● V23.1 Motorcycle **passenger** injured in collision with car, pick-up truck or van in **nontraffic accident**

X● V23.2 **Unspecified** motorcycle rider injured in collision with car, pick-up truck or van in **nontraffic accident**

X● V23.3 Person **boarding or alighting** a motorcycle injured in collision with car, pick-up truck or van

X● V23.4 Motorcycle **driver** injured in collision with car, pick-up truck or van in **traffic accident**

X● V23.5 Motorcycle **passenger** injured in collision with car, pick-up truck or van in **traffic accident**

X● V23.9 **Unspecified** motorcycle rider injured in collision with car, pick-up truck or van in **traffic accident**

● **V24 Motorcycle rider injured in collision with heavy transport vehicle or bus**

Excludes1 motorcycle rider injured in collision with military vehicle (V29.81)

The appropriate 7th character is to be added to each code from category V24

A initial encounter
D subsequent encounter
S sequela

X● V24.Ø Motorcycle **driver** injured in collision with heavy transport vehicle or bus in **nontraffic accident**

X● V24.1 Motorcycle **passenger** injured in collision with heavy transport vehicle or bus in **nontraffic accident**

X● V24.2 **Unspecified** motorcycle rider injured in collision with heavy transport vehicle or bus in **nontraffic accident**

X● V24.3 Person **boarding or alighting** a motorcycle injured in collision with heavy transport vehicle or bus

X● V24.4 Motorcycle **driver** injured in collision with heavy transport vehicle or bus in **traffic accident**

X● V24.5 Motorcycle **passenger** injured in collision with heavy transport vehicle or bus in **traffic accident**

X● V24.9 **Unspecified** motorcycle rider injured in collision with heavy transport vehicle or bus in **traffic accident**

● **V25 Motorcycle rider injured in collision with railway train or railway vehicle**

The appropriate 7th character is to be added to each code from category V25

A initial encounter
D subsequent encounter
S sequela

X● V25.Ø Motorcycle **driver** injured in collision with railway train or railway vehicle in **nontraffic accident**

X● V25.1 Motorcycle **passenger** injured in collision with railway train or railway vehicle in **nontraffic accident**

X● V25.2 **Unspecified** motorcycle rider injured in collision with railway train or railway vehicle in **nontraffic accident**

X● V25.3 Person **boarding or alighting** a motorcycle injured in collision with railway train or railway vehicle

X● V25.4 Motorcycle **driver** injured in collision with railway train or railway vehicle in **traffic accident**

X● V25.5 Motorcycle **passenger** injured in collision with railway train or railway vehicle in **traffic accident**

X● V25.9 **Unspecified** motorcycle rider injured in collision with railway train or railway vehicle in **traffic accident**

● **V26 Motorcycle rider injured in collision with other nonmotor vehicle**

Includes collision with animal-drawn vehicle, animal being ridden, streetcar

The appropriate 7th character is to be added to each code from category V26

A initial encounter
D subsequent encounter
S sequela

X● V26.Ø Motorcycle **driver** injured in collision with other nonmotor vehicle in **nontraffic accident**

X● V26.1 Motorcycle **passenger** injured in collision with other nonmotor vehicle in **nontraffic accident**

X● V26.2 **Unspecified** motorcycle rider injured in collision with other nonmotor vehicle in **nontraffic accident**

X● V26.3 Person **boarding or alighting** a motorcycle injured in collision with other nonmotor vehicle

X● V26.4 Motorcycle **driver** injured in collision with other nonmotor vehicle in **traffic accident**

X● V26.5 Motorcycle **passenger** injured in collision with other nonmotor vehicle in **traffic accident**

X● V26.9 **Unspecified** motorcycle rider injured in collision with other nonmotor vehicle in **traffic accident**

● **V27 Motorcycle rider injured in collision with fixed or stationary object**

The appropriate 7th character is to be added to each code from category V27

A initial encounter
D subsequent encounter
S sequela

X● V27.Ø Motorcycle **driver** injured in collision with fixed or stationary object in **nontraffic accident**

X● V27.1 Motorcycle **passenger** injured in collision with fixed or stationary object in **nontraffic accident**

X● V27.2 **Unspecified** motorcycle rider injured in collision with fixed or stationary object in **nontraffic accident**

X● V27.3 Person **boarding or alighting** a motorcycle injured in collision with fixed or stationary object

X● V27.4 Motorcycle **driver** injured in collision with fixed or stationary object in **traffic accident**

X● V27.5 Motorcycle **passenger** injured in collision with fixed or stationary object in **traffic accident**

X● V27.9 **Unspecified** motorcycle rider injured in collision with fixed or stationary object in **traffic accident**

● **V28 Motorcycle rider injured in noncollision transport accident**

Includes fall or thrown from motorcycle (without antecedent collision)
overturning motorcycle NOS
overturning motorcycle without collision

The appropriate 7th character is to be added to each code from category V28

A	initial encounter
D	subsequent encounter
S	sequela

X● **V28.0 Motorcycle driver injured in noncollision transport accident in nontraffic accident**

X● **V28.1 Motorcycle passenger injured in noncollision transport accident in nontraffic accident**

X● **V28.2 Unspecified motorcycle rider injured in noncollision transport accident in nontraffic accident**

X● **V28.3 Person boarding or alighting a motorcycle injured in noncollision transport accident**

X● **V28.4 Motorcycle driver injured in noncollision transport accident in traffic accident**

X● **V28.5 Motorcycle passenger injured in noncollision transport accident in traffic accident**

X● **V28.9 Unspecified motorcycle rider injured in noncollision transport accident in traffic accident**

● **V29 Motorcycle rider injured in other and unspecified transport accidents**

The appropriate 7th character is to be added to each code from category V29

A	initial encounter
D	subsequent encounter
S	sequela

Coding Clinic: 2015, Q3, P20

● **V29.0 Motorcycle driver injured in collision with other and unspecified motor vehicles in nontraffic accident**

X● **V29.00 Motorcycle driver injured in collision with unspecified motor vehicles in nontraffic accident**

X● **V29.09 Motorcycle driver injured in collision with other motor vehicles in nontraffic accident**

● **V29.1 Motorcycle passenger injured in collision with other and unspecified motor vehicles in nontraffic accident**

X● **V29.10 Motorcycle passenger injured in collision with unspecified motor vehicles in nontraffic accident**

X● **V29.19 Motorcycle passenger injured in collision with other motor vehicles in nontraffic accident**

● **V29.2 Unspecified motorcycle rider injured in collision with other and unspecified motor vehicles in nontraffic accident**

X● **V29.20 Unspecified motorcycle rider injured in collision with unspecified motor vehicles in nontraffic accident**
Motorcycle collision NOS, nontraffic

X● **V29.29 Unspecified motorcycle rider injured in collision with other motor vehicles in nontraffic accident**

X● **V29.3 Motorcycle rider (driver) (passenger) injured in unspecified nontraffic accident**
Motorcycle accident NOS, nontraffic
Motorcycle rider injured in nontraffic accident NOS

● **V29.4 Motorcycle driver injured in collision with other and unspecified motor vehicles in traffic accident**

X● **V29.40 Motorcycle driver injured in collision with unspecified motor vehicles in traffic accident**

X● **V29.49 Motorcycle driver injured in collision with other motor vehicles in traffic accident**

● **V29.5 Motorcycle passenger injured in collision with other and unspecified motor vehicles in traffic accident**

X● **V29.50 Motorcycle passenger injured in collision with unspecified motor vehicles in traffic accident**

X● **V29.59 Motorcycle passenger injured in collision with other motor vehicles in traffic accident**

● **V29.6 Unspecified motorcycle rider injured in collision with other and unspecified motor vehicles in traffic accident**

X● **V29.60 Unspecified motorcycle rider injured in collision with unspecified motor vehicles in traffic accident**
Motorcycle collision NOS (traffic)

X● **V29.69 Unspecified motorcycle rider injured in collision with other motor vehicles in traffic accident**

● **V29.8 Motorcycle rider (driver) (passenger) injured in other specified transport accidents**

X● **V29.81 Motorcycle rider (driver) (passenger) injured in transport accident with military vehicle**

X● **V29.88 Motorcycle rider (driver) (passenger) injured in other specified transport accidents**

X● **V29.9 Motorcycle rider (driver) (passenger) injured in unspecified traffic accident**
Motorcycle accident NOS

OCCUPANT OF THREE-WHEELED MOTOR VEHICLE INJURED IN TRANSPORT ACCIDENT (V30-V39)

Includes motorized tricycle
motorized rickshaw
three-wheeled motor car

Excludes1 all-terrain vehicles (V86.-)
motorcycle with sidecar (V20-V29)
vehicle designed primarily for off-road use (V86.-)

● **V30 Occupant of three-wheeled motor vehicle injured in collision with pedestrian or animal**

Excludes1 three-wheeled motor vehicle collision with animal-drawn vehicle or animal being ridden (V36.-)

The appropriate 7th character is to be added to each code from category V30

A	initial encounter
D	subsequent encounter
S	sequela

X● **V30.0 Driver of three-wheeled motor vehicle injured in collision with pedestrian or animal in nontraffic accident**

X● **V30.1 Passenger in three-wheeled motor vehicle injured in collision with pedestrian or animal in nontraffic accident**

X● **V30.2 Person on outside of three-wheeled motor vehicle injured in collision with pedestrian or animal in nontraffic accident**

X● **V30.3 Unspecified occupant of three-wheeled motor vehicle injured in collision with pedestrian or animal in nontraffic accident**

X● **V30.4 Person boarding or alighting a three-wheeled motor vehicle injured in collision with pedestrian or animal**

X● **V30.5 Driver of three-wheeled motor vehicle injured in collision with pedestrian or animal in traffic accident**

X● **V30.6 Passenger in three-wheeled motor vehicle injured in collision with pedestrian or animal in traffic accident**

X● **V30.7 Person on outside of three-wheeled motor vehicle injured in collision with pedestrian or animal in traffic accident**

X● **V30.9 Unspecified occupant of three-wheeled motor vehicle injured in collision with pedestrian or animal in traffic accident**

V31 Occupant of three-wheeled motor vehicle injured in collision with pedal cycle

The appropriate 7th character is to be added to each code from category V31

A	initial encounter
D	subsequent encounter
S	sequela

X V31.0 **Driver** of three-wheeled motor vehicle injured in collision with pedal cycle in **nontraffic accident**

X V31.1 **Passenger** in three-wheeled motor vehicle injured in collision with pedal cycle in **nontraffic accident**

X V31.2 **Person on outside** of three-wheeled motor vehicle injured in collision with pedal cycle in **nontraffic accident**

X V31.3 **Unspecified** occupant of three-wheeled motor vehicle injured in collision with pedal cycle in **nontraffic accident**

X V31.4 Person **boarding or alighting** a three-wheeled motor vehicle injured in collision with pedal cycle

X V31.5 **Driver** of three-wheeled motor vehicle injured in collision with pedal cycle in **traffic accident**

X V31.6 **Passenger** in three-wheeled motor vehicle injured in collision with pedal cycle in **traffic accident**

X V31.7 **Person on outside** of three-wheeled motor vehicle injured in collision with pedal cycle in **traffic accident**

X V31.9 **Unspecified** occupant of three-wheeled motor vehicle injured in collision with pedal cycle in **traffic accident**

V32 Occupant of three-wheeled motor vehicle injured in collision with two- or three-wheeled motor vehicle

The appropriate 7th character is to be added to each code from category V32

A	initial encounter
D	subsequent encounter
S	sequela

X V32.0 **Driver** of three-wheeled motor vehicle injured in collision with two- or three-wheeled motor vehicle in **nontraffic accident**

X V32.1 **Passenger** in three-wheeled motor vehicle injured in collision with two- or three-wheeled motor vehicle in **nontraffic accident**

X V32.2 **Person on outside** of three-wheeled motor vehicle injured in collision with two- or three-wheeled motor vehicle in **nontraffic accident**

X V32.3 **Unspecified** occupant of three-wheeled motor vehicle injured in collision with two- or three-wheeled motor vehicle in **nontraffic accident**

X V32.4 Person **boarding or alighting** a three-wheeled motor vehicle injured in collision with two- or three-wheeled motor vehicle

X V32.5 **Driver** of three-wheeled motor vehicle injured in collision with two- or three-wheeled motor vehicle in **traffic accident**

X V32.6 **Passenger** in three-wheeled motor vehicle injured in collision with two- or three-wheeled motor vehicle in **traffic accident**

X V32.7 **Person on outside** of three-wheeled motor vehicle injured in collision with two- or three-wheeled motor vehicle in **traffic accident**

X V32.9 **Unspecified** occupant of three-wheeled motor vehicle injured in collision with two- or three-wheeled motor vehicle in **traffic accident**

V33 Occupant of three-wheeled motor vehicle injured in collision with car, pick-up truck or van

The appropriate 7th character is to be added to each code from category V33

A	initial encounter
D	subsequent encounter
S	sequela

X V33.0 **Driver** of three-wheeled motor vehicle injured in collision with car, pick-up truck or van in **nontraffic accident**

X V33.1 **Passenger** in three-wheeled motor vehicle injured in collision with car, pick-up truck or van in **nontraffic accident**

X V33.2 **Person on outside** of three-wheeled motor vehicle injured in collision with car, pick-up truck or van in **nontraffic accident**

X V33.3 **Unspecified** occupant of three-wheeled motor vehicle injured in collision with car, pick-up truck or van in **nontraffic accident**

X V33.4 Person **boarding or alighting** a three-wheeled motor vehicle injured in collision with car, pick-up truck or van

X V33.5 **Driver** of three-wheeled motor vehicle injured in collision with car, pick-up truck or van in **traffic accident**

X V33.6 **Passenger** in three-wheeled motor vehicle injured in collision with car, pick-up truck or van in **traffic accident**

X V33.7 **Person on outside** of three-wheeled motor vehicle injured in collision with car, pick-up truck or van in **traffic accident**

X V33.9 **Unspecified** occupant of three-wheeled motor vehicle injured in collision with car, pick-up truck or van in **traffic accident**

V34 Occupant of three-wheeled motor vehicle injured in collision with heavy transport vehicle or bus

Excludes1 occupant of three-wheeled motor vehicle injured in collision with military vehicle (V39.81)

The appropriate 7th character is to be added to each code from category V34

A	initial encounter
D	subsequent encounter
S	sequela

X V34.0 **Driver** of three-wheeled motor vehicle injured in collision with heavy transport vehicle or bus in **nontraffic accident**

X V34.1 **Passenger** in three-wheeled motor vehicle injured in collision with heavy transport vehicle or bus in **nontraffic accident**

X V34.2 **Person on outside** of three-wheeled motor vehicle injured in collision with heavy transport vehicle or bus in **nontraffic accident**

X V34.3 **Unspecified** occupant of three-wheeled motor vehicle injured in collision with heavy transport vehicle or bus in **nontraffic accident**

X V34.4 Person **boarding or alighting** a three-wheeled motor vehicle injured in collision with heavy transport vehicle or bus

X V34.5 **Driver** of three-wheeled motor vehicle injured in collision with heavy transport vehicle or bus in **traffic accident**

X V34.6 **Passenger** in three-wheeled motor vehicle injured in collision with heavy transport vehicle or bus in **traffic accident**

X V34.7 **Person on outside** of three-wheeled motor vehicle injured in collision with heavy transport vehicle or bus in **traffic accident**

X V34.9 **Unspecified** occupant of three-wheeled motor vehicle injured in collision with heavy transport vehicle or bus in **traffic accident**

V35 Occupant of three-wheeled motor vehicle injured in collision with railway train or railway vehicle

The appropriate 7th character is to be added to each code from category V35

A	initial encounter
D	subsequent encounter
S	sequela

X **V35.0 Driver of three-wheeled motor vehicle injured in collision with railway train or railway vehicle in nontraffic accident**

X **V35.1 Passenger in three-wheeled motor vehicle injured in collision with railway train or railway vehicle in nontraffic accident**

X **V35.2 Person on outside of three-wheeled motor vehicle injured in collision with railway train or railway vehicle in nontraffic accident**

X **V35.3 Unspecified occupant of three-wheeled motor vehicle injured in collision with railway train or railway vehicle in nontraffic accident**

X **V35.4 Person boarding or alighting a three-wheeled motor vehicle injured in collision with railway train or railway vehicle**

X **V35.5 Driver of three-wheeled motor vehicle injured in collision with railway train or railway vehicle in traffic accident**

X **V35.6 Passenger in three-wheeled motor vehicle injured in collision with railway train or railway vehicle in traffic accident**

X **V35.7 Person on outside of three-wheeled motor vehicle injured in collision with railway train or railway vehicle in traffic accident**

X **V35.9 Unspecified occupant of three-wheeled motor vehicle injured in collision with railway train or railway vehicle in traffic accident**

V36 Occupant of three-wheeled motor vehicle injured in collision with other nonmotor vehicle

Includes collision with animal-drawn vehicle, animal being ridden, streetcar

The appropriate 7th character is to be added to each code from category V36

A	initial encounter
D	subsequent encounter
S	sequela

X **V36.0 Driver of three-wheeled motor vehicle injured in collision with other nonmotor vehicle in nontraffic accident**

X **V36.1 Passenger in three-wheeled motor vehicle injured in collision with other nonmotor vehicle in nontraffic accident**

X **V36.2 Person on outside of three-wheeled motor vehicle injured in collision with other nonmotor vehicle in nontraffic accident**

X **V36.3 Unspecified occupant of three-wheeled motor vehicle injured in collision with other nonmotor vehicle in nontraffic accident**

X **V36.4 Person boarding or alighting a three-wheeled motor vehicle injured in collision with other nonmotor vehicle**

X **V36.5 Driver of three-wheeled motor vehicle injured in collision with other nonmotor vehicle in traffic accident**

X **V36.6 Passenger in three-wheeled motor vehicle injured in collision with other nonmotor vehicle in traffic accident**

X **V36.7 Person on outside of three-wheeled motor vehicle injured in collision with other nonmotor vehicle in traffic accident**

X **V36.9 Unspecified occupant of three-wheeled motor vehicle injured in collision with other nonmotor vehicle in traffic accident**

V37 Occupant of three-wheeled motor vehicle injured in collision with fixed or stationary object

The appropriate 7th character is to be added to each code from category V37

A	initial encounter
D	subsequent encounter
S	sequela

X **V37.0 Driver of three-wheeled motor vehicle injured in collision with fixed or stationary object in nontraffic accident**

X **V37.1 Passenger in three-wheeled motor vehicle injured in collision with fixed or stationary object in nontraffic accident**

X **V37.2 Person on outside of three-wheeled motor vehicle injured in collision with fixed or stationary object in nontraffic accident**

X **V37.3 Unspecified occupant of three-wheeled motor vehicle injured in collision with fixed or stationary object in nontraffic accident**

X **V37.4 Person boarding or alighting a three-wheeled motor vehicle injured in collision with fixed or stationary object**

X **V37.5 Driver of three-wheeled motor vehicle injured in collision with fixed or stationary object in traffic accident**

X **V37.6 Passenger in three-wheeled motor vehicle injured in collision with fixed or stationary object in traffic accident**

X **V37.7 Person on outside of three-wheeled motor vehicle injured in collision with fixed or stationary object in traffic accident**

X **V37.9 Unspecified occupant of three-wheeled motor vehicle injured in collision with fixed or stationary object in traffic accident**

V38 Occupant of three-wheeled motor vehicle injured in noncollision transport accident

Includes fall or thrown from three-wheeled motor vehicle
overturning of three-wheeled motor vehicle NOS
overturning of three-wheeled motor vehicle without collision

The appropriate 7th character is to be added to each code from category V38

A	initial encounter
D	subsequent encounter
S	sequela

X **V38.0 Driver of three-wheeled motor vehicle injured in noncollision transport accident in nontraffic accident**

X **V38.1 Passenger in three-wheeled motor vehicle injured in noncollision transport accident in nontraffic accident**

X **V38.2 Person on outside of three-wheeled motor vehicle injured in noncollision transport accident in nontraffic accident**

X **V38.3 Unspecified occupant of three-wheeled motor vehicle injured in noncollision transport accident in nontraffic accident**

X **V38.4 Person boarding or alighting a three-wheeled motor vehicle injured in noncollision transport accident**

X **V38.5 Driver of three-wheeled motor vehicle injured in noncollision transport accident in traffic accident**

X **V38.6 Passenger in three-wheeled motor vehicle injured in noncollision transport accident in traffic accident**

X **V38.7 Person on outside of three-wheeled motor vehicle injured in noncollision transport accident in traffic accident**

X **V38.9 Unspecified occupant of three-wheeled motor vehicle injured in noncollision transport accident in traffic accident**

V39 Occupant of three-wheeled motor vehicle injured in other and unspecified transport accidents

The appropriate 7th character is to be added to each code from category V39

A	initial encounter
D	subsequent encounter
S	sequela

V39.Ø Driver of three-wheeled motor vehicle injured in collision with other and unspecified motor vehicles in nontraffic accident

X **V39.ØØ Driver of three-wheeled motor vehicle injured in collision with unspecified motor vehicles in nontraffic accident**

X **V39.Ø9 Driver of three-wheeled motor vehicle injured in collision with other motor vehicles in nontraffic accident**

V39.1 Passenger in three-wheeled motor vehicle injured in collision with other and unspecified motor vehicles in nontraffic accident

X **V39.1Ø Passenger in three-wheeled motor vehicle injured in collision with unspecified motor vehicles in nontraffic accident**

X **V39.19 Passenger in three-wheeled motor vehicle injured in collision with other motor vehicles in nontraffic accident**

V39.2 Unspecified occupant of three-wheeled motor vehicle injured in collision with other and unspecified motor vehicles in nontraffic accident

X **V39.2Ø Unspecified occupant of three-wheeled motor vehicle injured in collision with unspecified motor vehicles in nontraffic accident**

Collision NOS involving three-wheeled motor vehicle, nontraffic

X **V39.29 Unspecified occupant of three-wheeled motor vehicle injured in collision with other motor vehicles in nontraffic accident**

X **V39.3 Occupant (driver) (passenger) of three-wheeled motor vehicle injured in unspecified nontraffic accident**

Accident NOS involving three-wheeled motor vehicle, nontraffic

Occupant of three-wheeled motor vehicle injured in nontraffic accident NOS

V39.4 Driver of three-wheeled motor vehicle injured in collision with other and unspecified motor vehicles in traffic accident

X **V39.4Ø Driver of three-wheeled motor vehicle injured in collision with unspecified motor vehicles in traffic accident**

X **V39.49 Driver of three-wheeled motor vehicle injured in collision with other motor vehicles in traffic accident**

V39.5 Passenger in three-wheeled motor vehicle injured in collision with other and unspecified motor vehicles in traffic accident

X **V39.5Ø Passenger in three-wheeled motor vehicle injured in collision with unspecified motor vehicles in traffic accident**

X **V39.59 Passenger in three-wheeled motor vehicle injured in collision with other motor vehicles in traffic accident**

V39.6 Unspecified occupant of three-wheeled motor vehicle injured in collision with other and unspecified motor vehicles in traffic accident

X **V39.6Ø Unspecified occupant of three-wheeled motor vehicle injured in collision with unspecified motor vehicles in traffic accident**

Collision NOS involving three-wheeled motor vehicle (traffic)

X **V39.69 Unspecified occupant of three-wheeled motor vehicle injured in collision with other motor vehicles in traffic accident**

V39.8 Occupant (driver) (passenger) of three-wheeled motor vehicle injured in other specified transport accidents

X **V39.81 Occupant (driver) (passenger) of three-wheeled motor vehicle injured in transport accident with military vehicle**

X **V39.89 Occupant (driver) (passenger) of three-wheeled motor vehicle injured in other specified transport accidents**

X **V39.9 Occupant (driver) (passenger) of three-wheeled motor vehicle injured in unspecified traffic accident**

Accident NOS involving three-wheeled motor vehicle

CAR OCCUPANT INJURED IN TRANSPORT ACCIDENT (V4Ø-V49)

Includes a four-wheeled motor vehicle designed primarily for carrying passengers
automobile (pulling a trailer or camper)

Excludes1 bus (V5Ø-V59)
minibus (V5Ø-V59)
minivan (V5Ø-V59)
motorcoach (V7Ø-V79)
pick-up truck (V5Ø-V59)
sport utility vehicle (SUV) (V5Ø-V59)

V4Ø Car occupant injured in collision with pedestrian or animal

Excludes1 car collision with animal-drawn vehicle or animal being ridden (V46.-)

The appropriate 7th character is to be added to each code from category V4Ø

A	initial encounter
D	subsequent encounter
S	sequela

X **V4Ø.Ø Car driver injured in collision with pedestrian or animal in nontraffic accident**

X **V4Ø.1 Car passenger injured in collision with pedestrian or animal in nontraffic accident**

X **V4Ø.2 Person on outside of car injured in collision with pedestrian or animal in nontraffic accident**

X **V4Ø.3 Unspecified car occupant injured in collision with pedestrian or animal in nontraffic accident**

X **V4Ø.4 Person boarding or alighting a car injured in collision with pedestrian or animal**

X **V4Ø.5 Car driver injured in collision with pedestrian or animal in traffic accident**

X **V4Ø.6 Car passenger injured in collision with pedestrian or animal in traffic accident**

X **V4Ø.7 Person on outside of car injured in collision with pedestrian or animal in traffic accident**

X **V4Ø.9 Unspecified car occupant injured in collision with pedestrian or animal in traffic accident**

V41 Car occupant injured in collision with pedal cycle

The appropriate 7th character is to be added to each code from category V41

A	initial encounter
D	subsequent encounter
S	sequela

X **V41.Ø Car driver injured in collision with pedal cycle in nontraffic accident**

X **V41.1 Car passenger injured in collision with pedal cycle in nontraffic accident**

X **V41.2 Person on outside of car injured in collision with pedal cycle in nontraffic accident**

X **V41.3 Unspecified car occupant injured in collision with pedal cycle in nontraffic accident**

X **V41.4 Person boarding or alighting a car injured in collision with pedal cycle**

X **V41.5 Car driver injured in collision with pedal cycle in traffic accident**

X **V41.6 Car passenger injured in collision with pedal cycle in traffic accident**

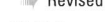

X● **V41.7** **Person on outside** of car injured in collision with pedal cycle in **traffic accident**

X● **V41.9** **Unspecified** car occupant injured in collision with pedal cycle in **traffic accident**

● **V42** Car occupant injured in collision with two- or three-wheeled motor vehicle

The appropriate 7th character is to be added to each code from category V42

A	initial encounter
D	subsequent encounter
S	sequela

X● **V42.0** Car **driver** injured in collision with two- or three-wheeled motor vehicle in **nontraffic accident**

X● **V42.1** Car **passenger** injured in collision with two- or three-wheeled motor vehicle in **nontraffic accident**

X● **V42.2** **Person on outside** of car injured in collision with two- or three-wheeled motor vehicle in **nontraffic accident**

X● **V42.3** **Unspecified** car occupant injured in collision with two- or three-wheeled motor vehicle in **nontraffic accident**

X● **V42.4** Person **boarding or alighting** a car injured in collision with two- or three-wheeled motor vehicle

X● **V42.5** Car **driver** injured in collision with two- or three-wheeled motor vehicle in **traffic accident**

X● **V42.6** Car **passenger** injured in collision with two- or three-wheeled motor vehicle in **traffic accident**

X● **V42.7** **Person on outside** of car injured in collision with two- or three-wheeled motor vehicle in **traffic accident**

X● **V42.9** **Unspecified** car occupant injured in collision with two- or three-wheeled motor vehicle in **traffic accident**

● **V43** Car occupant injured in collision with car, pick-up truck or van

The appropriate 7th character is to be added to each code from category V43

A	initial encounter
D	subsequent encounter
S	sequela

● **V43.0** Car **driver** injured in collision with car, pick-up truck or van in **nontraffic accident**

X● **V43.01** Car driver injured in collision with **sport utility vehicle** in nontraffic accident

X● **V43.02** Car driver injured in collision with **other type car** in nontraffic accident

X● **V43.03** Car driver injured in collision with **pick-up truck** in nontraffic accident

X● **V43.04** Car driver injured in collision with **van** in nontraffic accident

● **V43.1** Car **passenger** injured in collision with car, pick-up truck or van in **nontraffic accident**

X● **V43.11** Car passenger injured in collision with **sport utility vehicle** in nontraffic accident

X● **V43.12** Car passenger injured in collision with **other type car** in nontraffic accident

X● **V43.13** Car passenger injured in collision with **pick-up truck** in nontraffic accident

X● **V43.14** Car passenger injured in collision with **van** in nontraffic accident

● **V43.2** **Person on outside** of car injured in collision with car, pick-up truck or van in **nontraffic accident**

X● **V43.21** Person on outside of car injured in collision with **sport utility vehicle** in nontraffic accident

X● **V43.22** Person on outside of car injured in collision with **other type car** in nontraffic accident

X● **V43.23** Person on outside of car injured in collision with **pick-up truck** in nontraffic accident

X● **V43.24** Person on outside of car injured in collision with **van** in nontraffic accident

● **V43.3** **Unspecified** car occupant injured in collision with car, pick-up truck or van in **nontraffic accident**

X● **V43.31** Unspecified car occupant injured in collision with **sport utility vehicle** in nontraffic accident

X● **V43.32** Unspecified car occupant injured in collision with **other type car** in nontraffic accident

X● **V43.33** Unspecified car occupant injured in collision with **pick-up truck** in nontraffic accident

X● **V43.34** Unspecified car occupant injured in collision with **van** in nontraffic accident

● **V43.4** **Person boarding or alighting** a car injured in collision with car, pick-up truck or van

X● **V43.41** Person boarding or alighting a car injured in collision with **sport utility vehicle**

X● **V43.42** Person boarding or alighting a car injured in collision with **other type car**

X● **V43.43** Person boarding or alighting a car injured in collision with **pick-up truck**

X● **V43.44** Person boarding or alighting a car injured in collision with **van**

● **V43.5** Car **driver** injured in collision with car, pick-up truck or van in **traffic accident**

X● **V43.51** Car driver injured in collision with **sport utility vehicle** in traffic accident

X● **V43.52** Car driver injured in collision with **other type car** in traffic accident

X● **V43.53** Car driver injured in collision with **pick-up truck** in traffic accident

X● **V43.54** Car driver injured in collision with **van** in traffic accident

● **V43.6** Car **passenger** injured in collision with car, pick-up truck or van in **traffic accident**

X● **V43.61** Car passenger injured in collision with **sport utility vehicle** in traffic accident
Coding Clinic: 2015, Q1, P5-7

X● **V43.62** Car passenger injured in collision with **other type car** in traffic accident

X● **V43.63** Car passenger injured in collision with **pick-up truck** in traffic accident

X● **V43.64** Car passenger injured in collision with **van** in traffic accident

● **V43.7** **Person on outside** of car injured in collision with car, pick-up truck or van in **traffic accident**

X● **V43.71** Person on outside of car injured in collision with **sport utility vehicle** in traffic accident

X● **V43.72** Person on outside of car injured in collision with **other type car** in traffic accident

X● **V43.73** Person on outside of car injured in collision with **pick-up truck** in traffic accident

X● **V43.74** Person on outside of car injured in collision with **van** in traffic accident

● **V43.9** **Unspecified** car occupant injured in collision with car, pick-up truck or van in **traffic accident**

X● **V43.91** Unspecified car occupant injured in collision with **sport utility vehicle** in traffic accident

X● **V43.92** Unspecified car occupant injured in collision with **other type car** in traffic accident

X● **V43.93** Unspecified car occupant injured in collision with **pick-up truck** in traffic accident

X● **V43.94** Unspecified car occupant injured in collision with **van** in traffic accident

V44 Car occupant injured in collision with heavy transport vehicle or bus

Excludes1 car occupant injured in collision with military vehicle (V49.81)

The appropriate 7th character is to be added to each code from category V44

A	initial encounter
D	subsequent encounter
S	sequela

X **V44.0** Car **driver** injured in collision with heavy transport vehicle or bus in **nontraffic accident**

X **V44.1** Car **passenger** injured in collision with heavy transport vehicle or bus in **nontraffic accident**

X **V44.2** **Person on outside** of car injured in collision with heavy transport vehicle or bus in **nontraffic accident**

X **V44.3** **Unspecified** car occupant injured in collision with heavy transport vehicle or bus in **nontraffic accident**

X **V44.4** Person **boarding or alighting** a car injured in collision with heavy transport vehicle or bus

X **V44.5** Car **driver** injured in collision with heavy transport vehicle or bus in **traffic accident**

X **V44.6** Car **passenger** injured in collision with heavy transport vehicle or bus in **traffic accident**

X **V44.7** **Person on outside** of car injured in collision with heavy transport vehicle or bus in **traffic accident**

X **V44.9** **Unspecified** car occupant injured in collision with heavy transport vehicle or bus in **traffic accident**

V45 Car occupant injured in collision with railway train or railway vehicle

The appropriate 7th character is to be added to each code from category V45

A	initial encounter
D	subsequent encounter
S	sequela

X **V45.0** Car **driver** injured in collision with railway train or railway vehicle in **nontraffic accident**

X **V45.1** Car **passenger** injured in collision with railway train or railway vehicle in **nontraffic accident**

X **V45.2** **Person on outside** of car injured in collision with railway train or railway vehicle in **nontraffic accident**

X **V45.3** **Unspecified** car occupant injured in collision with railway train or railway vehicle in **nontraffic accident**

X **V45.4** Person **boarding or alighting** a car injured in collision with railway train or railway vehicle

X **V45.5** Car **driver** injured in collision with railway train or railway vehicle in **traffic accident**

X **V45.6** Car **passenger** injured in collision with railway train or railway vehicle in **traffic accident**

X **V45.7** **Person on outside** of car injured in collision with railway train or railway vehicle in **traffic accident**

X **V45.9** **Unspecified** car occupant injured in collision with railway train or railway vehicle in **traffic accident**

V46 Car occupant injured in collision with other nonmotor vehicle

Includes collision with animal-drawn vehicle, animal being ridden, streetcar

The appropriate 7th character is to be added to each code from category V46

A	initial encounter
D	subsequent encounter
S	sequela

X **V46.0** Car **driver** injured in collision with other nonmotor vehicle in **nontraffic accident**

X **V46.1** Car **passenger** injured in collision with other nonmotor vehicle in **nontraffic accident**

X **V46.2** **Person on outside** of car injured in collision with other nonmotor vehicle in **nontraffic accident**

X **V46.3** **Unspecified** car occupant injured in collision with other nonmotor vehicle in **nontraffic accident**

X **V46.4** Person **boarding or alighting** a car injured in collision with other nonmotor vehicle

X **V46.5** Car **driver** injured in collision with other nonmotor vehicle in **traffic accident**

X **V46.6** Car **passenger** injured in collision with other nonmotor vehicle in **traffic accident**

X **V46.7** **Person on outside** of car injured in collision with other nonmotor vehicle in **traffic accident**

X **V46.9** **Unspecified** car occupant injured in collision with other nonmotor vehicle in **traffic accident**

V47 Car occupant injured in collision with fixed or stationary object

The appropriate 7th character is to be added to each code from category V47

A	initial encounter
D	subsequent encounter
S	sequela

Coding Clinic: 2016, Q4, P73

X **V47.0** Car **driver** injured in collision with fixed or stationary object in **nontraffic accident**

X **V47.1** Car **passenger** injured in collision with fixed or stationary object in **nontraffic accident**

X **V47.2** **Person on outside** of car injured in collision with fixed or stationary object in **nontraffic accident**

X **V47.3** **Unspecified** car occupant injured in collision with fixed or stationary object in **nontraffic accident**

X **V47.4** Person **boarding or alighting** a car injured in collision with fixed or stationary object

X **V47.5** Car **driver** injured in collision with fixed or stationary object in **traffic accident**

X **V47.6** Car **passenger** injured in collision with fixed or stationary object in **traffic accident**

X **V47.7** **Person on outside** of car injured in collision with fixed or stationary object in **traffic accident**

X **V47.9** **Unspecified** car occupant injured in collision with fixed or stationary object in **traffic accident**

V48 Car occupant injured in noncollision transport accident

Includes overturning car NOS
overturning car without collision

The appropriate 7th character is to be added to each code from category V48

A	initial encounter
D	subsequent encounter
S	sequela

X **V48.0** Car **driver** injured in noncollision transport accident in **nontraffic accident**

X **V48.1** Car **passenger** injured in noncollision transport accident in **nontraffic accident**

X **V48.2** **Person on outside** of car injured in noncollision transport accident in **nontraffic accident**

X **V48.3** **Unspecified** car occupant injured in noncollision transport accident in **nontraffic accident**

X **V48.4** Person **boarding or alighting** a car injured in noncollision transport accident

X **V48.5** Car **driver** injured in noncollision transport accident in **traffic accident**

X **V48.6** Car **passenger** injured in noncollision transport accident in **traffic accident**

X **V48.7** **Person on outside** of car injured in noncollision transport accident in **traffic accident**

X **V48.9** **Unspecified** car occupant injured in noncollision transport accident in **traffic accident**

V49 Car occupant injured in other and unspecified transport accidents

The appropriate 7th character is to be added to each code from category V49

A	initial encounter
D	subsequent encounter
S	sequela

V49.Ø Driver injured in collision with other and unspecified motor vehicles in nontraffic accident

X **V49.ØØ Driver injured in collision with unspecified motor vehicles in nontraffic accident**

X **V49.Ø9 Driver injured in collision with other motor vehicles in nontraffic accident**

V49.1 Passenger injured in collision with other and unspecified motor vehicles in nontraffic accident

X **V49.1Ø Passenger injured in collision with unspecified motor vehicles in nontraffic accident**

X **V49.19 Passenger injured in collision with other motor vehicles in nontraffic accident**

V49.2 Unspecified car occupant injured in collision with other and unspecified motor vehicles in nontraffic accident

X **V49.2Ø Unspecified car occupant injured in collision with unspecified motor vehicles in nontraffic accident**

Car collision NOS, nontraffic

X **V49.29 Unspecified car occupant injured in collision with other motor vehicles in nontraffic accident**

X **V49.3 Car occupant (driver) (passenger) injured in unspecified nontraffic accident**

Car accident NOS, nontraffic
Car occupant injured in nontraffic accident NOS

V49.4 Driver injured in collision with other and unspecified motor vehicles in traffic accident

X **V49.4Ø Driver injured in collision with unspecified motor vehicles in traffic accident**

X **V49.49 Driver injured in collision with other motor vehicles in traffic accident**

V49.5 Passenger injured in collision with other and unspecified motor vehicles in traffic accident

X **V49.5Ø Passenger injured in collision with unspecified motor vehicles in traffic accident**

X **V49.59 Passenger injured in collision with other motor vehicles in traffic accident**

V49.6 Unspecified car occupant injured in collision with other and unspecified motor vehicles in traffic accident

X **V49.6Ø Unspecified car occupant injured in collision with unspecified motor vehicles in traffic accident**

Car collision NOS (traffic)

X **V49.69 Unspecified car occupant injured in collision with other motor vehicles in traffic accident**

V49.8 Car occupant (driver) (passenger) injured in other specified transport accidents

X **V49.81 Car occupant (driver) (passenger) injured in transport accident with military vehicle**

X **V49.88 Car occupant (driver) (passenger) injured in other specified transport accidents**

X **V49.9 Car occupant (driver) (passenger) injured in unspecified traffic accident**

Car accident NOS

Coding Clinic: 2015, Q1, P11

OCCUPANT OF PICK-UP TRUCK OR VAN INJURED IN TRANSPORT ACCIDENT (V5Ø-V59)

Includes a four- or six-wheel motor vehicle designed primarily for carrying passengers and property but weighing less than the local limit for classification as a heavy goods vehicle
minibus
minivan
sport utility vehicle (SUV)
truck
van

Excludes1 heavy transport vehicle (V6Ø-V69)

V5Ø Occupant of pick-up truck or van injured in collision with pedestrian or animal

Excludes1 pick-up truck or van collision with animal-drawn vehicle or animal being ridden (V56.-)

The appropriate 7th character is to be added to each code from category V5Ø

A	initial encounter
D	subsequent encounter
S	sequela

X **V5Ø.Ø Driver of pick-up truck or van injured in collision with pedestrian or animal in nontraffic accident**

X **V5Ø.1 Passenger in pick-up truck or van injured in collision with pedestrian or animal in nontraffic accident**

X **V5Ø.2 Person on outside of pick-up truck or van injured in collision with pedestrian or animal in nontraffic accident**

X **V5Ø.3 Unspecified occupant of pick-up truck or van injured in collision with pedestrian or animal in nontraffic accident**

X **V5Ø.4 Person boarding or alighting a pick-up truck or van injured in collision with pedestrian or animal**

X **V5Ø.5 Driver of pick-up truck or van injured in collision with pedestrian or animal in traffic accident**

X **V5Ø.6 Passenger in pick-up truck or van injured in collision with pedestrian or animal in traffic accident**

X **V5Ø.7 Person on outside of pick-up truck or van injured in collision with pedestrian or animal in traffic accident**

X **V5Ø.9 Unspecified occupant of pick-up truck or van injured in collision with pedestrian or animal in traffic accident**

V51 Occupant of pick-up truck or van injured in collision with pedal cycle

The appropriate 7th character is to be added to each code from category V51

A	initial encounter
D	subsequent encounter
S	sequela

X **V51.Ø Driver of pick-up truck or van injured in collision with pedal cycle in nontraffic accident**

X **V51.1 Passenger in pick-up truck or van injured in collision with pedal cycle in nontraffic accident**

X **V51.2 Person on outside of pick-up truck or van injured in collision with pedal cycle in nontraffic accident**

X **V51.3 Unspecified occupant of pick-up truck or van injured in collision with pedal cycle in nontraffic accident**

X **V51.4 Person boarding or alighting a pick-up truck or van injured in collision with pedal cycle**

X **V51.5 Driver of pick-up truck or van injured in collision with pedal cycle in traffic accident**

X **V51.6 Passenger in pick-up truck or van injured in collision with pedal cycle in traffic accident**

X **V51.7 Person on outside of pick-up truck or van injured in collision with pedal cycle in traffic accident**

X **V51.9 Unspecified occupant of pick-up truck or van injured in collision with pedal cycle in traffic accident**

V52 Occupant of pick-up truck or van injured in collision with two- or three-wheeled motor vehicle

The appropriate 7th character is to be added to each code from category V52

A	initial encounter
D	subsequent encounter
S	sequela

X V52.0 **Driver** of pick-up truck or van injured in collision with two- or three-wheeled motor vehicle in **nontraffic accident**

X V52.1 **Passenger** in pick-up truck or van injured in collision with two- or three-wheeled motor vehicle in **nontraffic accident**

X V52.2 **Person on outside** of pick-up truck or van injured in collision with two- or three-wheeled motor vehicle in **nontraffic accident**

X V52.3 **Unspecified** occupant of pick-up truck or van injured in collision with two- or three-wheeled motor vehicle in **nontraffic accident**

X V52.4 Person **boarding or alighting** a pick-up truck or van injured in collision with two- or three-wheeled motor vehicle

X V52.5 **Driver** of pick-up truck or van injured in collision with two- or three-wheeled motor vehicle in **traffic accident**

X V52.6 **Passenger** in pick-up truck or van injured in collision with two- or three-wheeled motor vehicle in **traffic accident**

X V52.7 **Person on outside** of pick-up truck or van injured in collision with two- or three-wheeled motor vehicle in **traffic accident**

X V52.9 **Unspecified** occupant of pick-up truck or van injured in collision with two- or three-wheeled motor vehicle in **traffic accident**

V53 Occupant of pick-up truck or van injured in collision with car, pick-up truck or van

The appropriate 7th character is to be added to each code from category V53

A	initial encounter
D	subsequent encounter
S	sequela

X V53.0 **Driver** of pick-up truck or van injured in collision with car, pick-up truck or van in **nontraffic accident**

X V53.1 **Passenger** in pick-up truck or van injured in collision with car, pick-up truck or van in **nontraffic accident**

X V53.2 **Person on outside** of pick-up truck or van injured in collision with car, pick-up truck or van in **nontraffic accident**

X V53.3 **Unspecified** occupant of pick-up truck or van injured in collision with car, pick-up truck or van in **nontraffic accident**

X V53.4 Person **boarding or alighting** a pick-up truck or van injured in collision with car, pick-up truck or van

X V53.5 **Driver** of pick-up truck or van injured in collision with car, pick-up truck or van in **traffic accident**

X V53.6 **Passenger** in pick-up truck or van injured in collision with car, pick-up truck or van in **traffic accident**

X V53.7 **Person on outside** of pick-up truck or van injured in collision with car, pick-up truck or van in **traffic accident**

X V53.9 **Unspecified** occupant of pick-up truck or van injured in collision with car, pick-up truck or van in **traffic accident**

V54 Occupant of pick-up truck or van injured in collision with heavy transport vehicle or bus

Excludes1 occupant of pick-up truck or van injured in collision with military vehicle (V59.81)

The appropriate 7th character is to be added to each code from category V54

A	initial encounter
D	subsequent encounter
S	sequela

X V54.0 **Driver** of pick-up truck or van injured in collision with heavy transport vehicle or bus in **nontraffic accident**

X V54.1 **Passenger** in pick-up truck or van injured in collision with heavy transport vehicle or bus in **nontraffic accident**

X V54.2 **Person on outside** of pick-up truck or van injured in collision with heavy transport vehicle or bus in **nontraffic accident**

X V54.3 **Unspecified** occupant of pick-up truck or van injured in collision with heavy transport vehicle or bus in **nontraffic accident**

X V54.4 Person **boarding or alighting** a pick-up truck or van injured in collision with heavy transport vehicle or bus

X V54.5 **Driver** of pick-up truck or van injured in collision with heavy transport vehicle or bus in **traffic accident**

X V54.6 **Passenger** in pick-up truck or van injured in collision with heavy transport vehicle or bus in **traffic accident**

X V54.7 **Person on outside** of pick-up truck or van injured in collision with heavy transport vehicle or bus in **traffic accident**

X V54.9 **Unspecified** occupant of pick-up truck or van injured in collision with heavy transport vehicle or bus in **traffic accident**

V55 Occupant of pick-up truck or van injured in collision with railway train or railway vehicle

The appropriate 7th character is to be added to each code from category V55

A	initial encounter
D	subsequent encounter
S	sequela

X V55.0 **Driver** of pick-up truck or van injured in collision with railway train or railway vehicle in **nontraffic accident**

X V55.1 **Passenger** in pick-up truck or van injured in collision with railway train or railway vehicle in **nontraffic accident**

X V55.2 **Person on outside** of pick-up truck or van injured in collision with railway train or railway vehicle in **nontraffic accident**

X V55.3 **Unspecified** occupant of pick-up truck or van injured in collision with railway train or railway vehicle in **nontraffic accident**

X V55.4 Person **boarding or alighting** a pick-up truck or van injured in collision with railway train or railway vehicle

X V55.5 **Driver** of pick-up truck or van injured in collision with railway train or railway vehicle in **traffic accident**

X V55.6 **Passenger** in pick-up truck or van injured in collision with railway train or railway vehicle in **traffic accident**

X V55.7 **Person on outside** of pick-up truck or van injured in collision with railway train or railway vehicle in **traffic accident**

X V55.9 **Unspecified** occupant of pick-up truck or van injured in collision with railway train or railway vehicle in **traffic accident**

V56 Occupant of pick-up truck or van injured in collision with other nonmotor vehicle

Includes collision with animal-drawn vehicle, animal being ridden, streetcar

The appropriate 7th character is to be added to each code from category V56

A	initial encounter
D	subsequent encounter
S	sequela

X **V56.0** **Driver** of pick-up truck or van injured in collision with other nonmotor vehicle in **nontraffic accident**

X **V56.1** **Passenger** in pick-up truck or van injured in collision with other nonmotor vehicle in **nontraffic accident**

X **V56.2** **Person on outside** of pick-up truck or van injured in collision with other nonmotor vehicle in **nontraffic accident**

X **V56.3** **Unspecified** occupant of pick-up truck or van injured in collision with other nonmotor vehicle in **nontraffic accident**

X **V56.4** Person **boarding or alighting** a pick-up truck or van injured in collision with other nonmotor vehicle

X **V56.5** **Driver** of pick-up truck or van injured in collision with other nonmotor vehicle in **traffic accident**

X **V56.6** **Passenger** in pick-up truck or van injured in collision with other nonmotor vehicle in **traffic accident**

X **V56.7** **Person on outside** of pick-up truck or van injured in collision with other nonmotor vehicle in **traffic accident**

X **V56.9** **Unspecified** occupant of pick-up truck or van injured in collision with other nonmotor vehicle in **traffic accident**

V57 Occupant of pick-up truck or van injured in collision with fixed or stationary object

The appropriate 7th character is to be added to each code from category V57

A	initial encounter
D	subsequent encounter
S	sequela

X **V57.0** **Driver** of pick-up truck or van injured in collision with fixed or stationary object in **nontraffic accident**

X **V57.1** **Passenger** in pick-up truck or van injured in collision with fixed or stationary object in **nontraffic accident**

X **V57.2** **Person on outside** of pick-up truck or van injured in collision with fixed or stationary object in **nontraffic accident**

X **V57.3** **Unspecified** occupant of pick-up truck or van injured in collision with fixed or stationary object in **nontraffic accident**

X **V57.4** Person **boarding or alighting** a pick-up truck or van injured in collision with fixed or stationary object

X **V57.5** **Driver** of pick-up truck or van injured in collision with fixed or stationary object in **traffic accident**

X **V57.6** **Passenger** in pick-up truck or van injured in collision with fixed or stationary object in **traffic accident**

X **V57.7** **Person on outside** of pick-up truck or van injured in collision with fixed or stationary object in **traffic accident**

X **V57.9** **Unspecified** occupant of pick-up truck or van injured in collision with fixed or stationary object in **traffic accident**

V58 Occupant of pick-up truck or van injured in noncollision transport accident

Includes overturning pick-up truck or van NOS
overturning pick-up truck or van without collision

The appropriate 7th character is to be added to each code from category V58

A	initial encounter
D	subsequent encounter
S	sequela

X **V58.0** **Driver** of pick-up truck or van injured in noncollision transport accident in **nontraffic accident**

X **V58.1** **Passenger** in pick-up truck or van injured in noncollision transport accident in **nontraffic accident**

X **V58.2** **Person on outside** of pick-up truck or van injured in noncollision transport accident in **nontraffic accident**

X **V58.3** **Unspecified** occupant of pick-up truck or van injured in noncollision transport accident in **nontraffic accident**

X **V58.4** Person **boarding or alighting** a pick-up truck or van injured in noncollision transport accident

X **V58.5** **Driver** of pick-up truck or van injured in noncollision transport accident in **traffic accident**

X **V58.6** **Passenger** in pick-up truck or van injured in noncollision transport accident in **traffic accident**

X **V58.7** **Person on outside** of pick-up truck or van injured in noncollision transport accident in **traffic accident**

X **V58.9** **Unspecified** occupant of pick-up truck or van injured in noncollision transport accident in **traffic accident**

V59 Occupant of pick-up truck or van injured in other and unspecified transport accidents

The appropriate 7th character is to be added to each code from category V59

A	initial encounter
D	subsequent encounter
S	sequela

V59.0 **Driver** of pick-up truck or van injured in collision with other and unspecified motor vehicles in **nontraffic accident**

X **V59.00** Driver of pick-up truck or van injured in collision with **unspecified** motor vehicles in nontraffic accident

X **V59.09** Driver of pick-up truck or van injured in collision with **other** motor vehicles in nontraffic accident

V59.1 **Passenger** in pick-up truck or van injured in collision with other and unspecified motor vehicles in **nontraffic accident**

X **V59.10** Passenger in pick-up truck or van injured in collision with **unspecified** motor vehicles in nontraffic accident

X **V59.19** Passenger in pick-up truck or van injured in collision with **other** motor vehicles in nontraffic accident

V59.2 **Unspecified** occupant of pick-up truck or van injured in collision with other and unspecified motor vehicles in **nontraffic accident**

X **V59.20** Unspecified occupant of pick-up truck or van injured in collision with **unspecified** motor vehicles in nontraffic accident

Collision NOS involving pick-up truck or van, nontraffic

X **V59.29** Unspecified occupant of pick-up truck or van injured in collision with **other** motor vehicles in nontraffic accident

X● V59.3 Occupant (driver) (passenger) of pick-up truck or van injured in **unspecified nontraffic accident**
Accident NOS involving pick-up truck or van, nontraffic
Occupant of pick-up truck or van injured in nontraffic accident NOS

● V59.4 **Driver** of pick-up truck or van injured in collision with other and unspecified motor vehicles in **traffic accident**

X● V59.40 Driver of pick-up truck or van injured in collision with **unspecified** motor vehicles in traffic accident

X● V59.49 Driver of pick-up truck or van injured in collision with **other** motor vehicles in traffic accident

● V59.5 **Passenger** in pick-up truck or van injured in collision with other and unspecified motor vehicles in **traffic accident**

X● V59.50 Passenger in pick-up truck or van injured in collision with **unspecified** motor vehicles in traffic accident

X● V59.59 Passenger in pick-up truck or van injured in collision with **other** motor vehicles in traffic accident

● V59.6 **Unspecified** occupant of pick-up truck or van injured in collision with other and unspecified motor vehicles in **traffic accident**

X● V59.60 Unspecified occupant of pick-up truck or van injured in collision with **unspecified** motor vehicles in traffic accident
Collision NOS involving pick-up truck or van (traffic)

X● V59.69 Unspecified occupant of pick-up truck or van injured in collision with **other** motor vehicles in traffic accident

● V59.8 Occupant (driver) (passenger) of pick-up truck or van injured in other specified transport accidents

X● V59.81 Occupant (driver) (passenger) of pick-up truck or van injured in transport accident with **military** vehicle

X● V59.88 Occupant (driver) (passenger) of pick-up truck or van injured in **other** specified transport accidents

X● V59.9 Occupant (driver) (passenger) of pick-up truck or van injured in **unspecified traffic accident**
Accident NOS involving pick-up truck or van

OCCUPANT OF HEAVY TRANSPORT VEHICLE INJURED IN TRANSPORT ACCIDENT (V60-V69)

Includes 18 wheeler
armored car
panel truck

Excludes1 bus
motorcoach

● V60 Occupant of heavy transport vehicle injured in collision with pedestrian or animal

Excludes1 heavy transport vehicle collision with animal-drawn vehicle or animal being ridden (V66.-)

The appropriate 7th character is to be added to each code from category V60

A	initial encounter
D	subsequent encounter
S	sequela

X● V60.0 **Driver** of heavy transport vehicle injured in collision with pedestrian or animal in **nontraffic accident**

X● V60.1 **Passenger** in heavy transport vehicle injured in collision with pedestrian or animal in **nontraffic accident**

X● V60.2 **Person on outside** of heavy transport vehicle injured in collision with pedestrian or animal in **nontraffic accident**

X● V60.3 **Unspecified** occupant of heavy transport vehicle injured in collision with pedestrian or animal in **nontraffic accident**

X● V60.4 Person **boarding or alighting** a heavy transport vehicle injured in collision with pedestrian or animal

X● V60.5 **Driver** of heavy transport vehicle injured in collision with pedestrian or animal in **traffic accident**

X● V60.6 **Passenger** in heavy transport vehicle injured in collision with pedestrian or animal in **traffic accident**

X● V60.7 **Person on outside** of heavy transport vehicle injured in collision with pedestrian or animal in **traffic accident**

X● V60.9 **Unspecified** occupant of heavy transport vehicle injured in collision with pedestrian or animal in **traffic accident**

● V61 Occupant of heavy transport vehicle injured in collision with pedal cycle

The appropriate 7th character is to be added to each code from category V61

A	initial encounter
D	subsequent encounter
S	sequela

X● V61.0 **Driver** of heavy transport vehicle injured in collision with pedal cycle in **nontraffic accident**

X● V61.1 **Passenger** in heavy transport vehicle injured in collision with pedal cycle in **nontraffic accident**

X● V61.2 **Person on outside** of heavy transport vehicle injured in collision with pedal cycle in **nontraffic accident**

X● V61.3 **Unspecified** occupant of heavy transport vehicle injured in collision with pedal cycle in **nontraffic accident**

X● V61.4 Person **boarding or alighting** a heavy transport vehicle injured in collision with pedal cycle while boarding or alighting

X● V61.5 **Driver** of heavy transport vehicle injured in collision with pedal cycle in **traffic accident**

X● V61.6 **Passenger** in heavy transport vehicle injured in collision with pedal cycle in **traffic accident**

X● V61.7 **Person on outside** of heavy transport vehicle injured in collision with pedal cycle in **traffic accident**

X● V61.9 **Unspecified** occupant of heavy transport vehicle injured in collision with pedal cycle in **traffic accident**

● V62 Occupant of heavy transport vehicle injured in collision with two- or three-wheeled motor vehicle

The appropriate 7th character is to be added to each code from category V62

A	initial encounter
D	subsequent encounter
S	sequela

X● V62.0 **Driver** of heavy transport vehicle injured in collision with two- or three-wheeled motor vehicle in **nontraffic accident**

X● V62.1 **Passenger** in heavy transport vehicle injured in collision with two- or three-wheeled motor vehicle in **nontraffic accident**

X● V62.2 **Person on outside** of heavy transport vehicle injured in collision with two- or three-wheeled motor vehicle in **nontraffic accident**

X● V62.3 **Unspecified** occupant of heavy transport vehicle injured in collision with two- or three-wheeled motor vehicle in **nontraffic accident**

X● V62.4 Person **boarding or alighting** a heavy transport vehicle injured in collision with two- or three-wheeled motor vehicle

X● V62.5 **Driver** of heavy transport vehicle injured in collision with two- or three-wheeled motor vehicle in **traffic accident**

X● V62.6 **Passenger** in heavy transport vehicle injured in collision with two- or three-wheeled motor vehicle in **traffic accident**

X● **V62.7** **Person on outside of heavy transport vehicle injured in collision with two- or three-wheeled motor vehicle in traffic accident**

X● **V62.9** **Unspecified occupant of heavy transport vehicle injured in collision with two- or three-wheeled motor vehicle in traffic accident**

● **V63** **Occupant of heavy transport vehicle injured in collision with car, pick-up truck or van**

The appropriate 7th character is to be added to each code from category V63

A	initial encounter
D	subsequent encounter
S	sequela

X● **V63.Ø** **Driver of heavy transport vehicle injured in collision with car, pick-up truck or van in nontraffic accident**

X● **V63.1** **Passenger in heavy transport vehicle injured in collision with car, pick-up truck or van in nontraffic accident**

X● **V63.2** **Person on outside of heavy transport vehicle injured in collision with car, pick-up truck or van in nontraffic accident**

X● **V63.3** **Unspecified occupant of heavy transport vehicle injured in collision with car, pick-up truck or van in nontraffic accident**

X● **V63.4** **Person boarding or alighting a heavy transport vehicle injured in collision with car, pick-up truck or van**

X● **V63.5** **Driver of heavy transport vehicle injured in collision with car, pick-up truck or van in traffic accident**

X● **V63.6** **Passenger in heavy transport vehicle injured in collision with car, pick-up truck or van in traffic accident**

X● **V63.7** **Person on outside of heavy transport vehicle injured in collision with car, pick-up truck or van in traffic accident**

X● **V63.9** **Unspecified occupant of heavy transport vehicle injured in collision with car, pick-up truck or van in traffic accident**

● **V64** **Occupant of heavy transport vehicle injured in collision with heavy transport vehicle or bus**

Excludes1 occupant of heavy transport vehicle injured in collision with military vehicle (V69.81)

The appropriate 7th character is to be added to each code from category V64

A	initial encounter
D	subsequent encounter
S	sequela

X● **V64.Ø** **Driver of heavy transport vehicle injured in collision with heavy transport vehicle or bus in nontraffic accident**

X● **V64.1** **Passenger in heavy transport vehicle injured in collision with heavy transport vehicle or bus in nontraffic accident**

X● **V64.2** **Person on outside of heavy transport vehicle injured in collision with heavy transport vehicle or bus in nontraffic accident**

X● **V64.3** **Unspecified occupant of heavy transport vehicle injured in collision with heavy transport vehicle or bus in nontraffic accident**

X● **V64.4** **Person boarding or alighting a heavy transport vehicle injured in collision with heavy transport vehicle or bus while boarding or alighting**

X● **V64.5** **Driver of heavy transport vehicle injured in collision with heavy transport vehicle or bus in traffic accident**

X● **V64.6** **Passenger in heavy transport vehicle injured in collision with heavy transport vehicle or bus in traffic accident**

X● **V64.7** **Person on outside of heavy transport vehicle injured in collision with heavy transport vehicle or bus in traffic accident**

X● **V64.9** **Unspecified occupant of heavy transport vehicle injured in collision with heavy transport vehicle or bus in traffic accident**

● **V65** **Occupant of heavy transport vehicle injured in collision with railway train or railway vehicle**

The appropriate 7th character is to be added to each code from category V65

A	initial encounter
D	subsequent encounter
S	sequela

X● **V65.Ø** **Driver of heavy transport vehicle injured in collision with railway train or railway vehicle in nontraffic accident**

X● **V65.1** **Passenger in heavy transport vehicle injured in collision with railway train or railway vehicle in nontraffic accident**

X● **V65.2** **Person on outside of heavy transport vehicle injured in collision with railway train or railway vehicle in nontraffic accident**

X● **V65.3** **Unspecified occupant of heavy transport vehicle injured in collision with railway train or railway vehicle in nontraffic accident**

X● **V65.4** **Person boarding or alighting a heavy transport vehicle injured in collision with railway train or railway vehicle**

X● **V65.5** **Driver of heavy transport vehicle injured in collision with railway train or railway vehicle in traffic accident**

X● **V65.6** **Passenger in heavy transport vehicle injured in collision with railway train or railway vehicle in traffic accident**

X● **V65.7** **Person on outside of heavy transport vehicle injured in collision with railway train or railway vehicle in traffic accident**

X● **V65.9** **Unspecified occupant of heavy transport vehicle injured in collision with railway train or railway vehicle in traffic accident**

● **V66** **Occupant of heavy transport vehicle injured in collision with other nonmotor vehicle**

Includes collision with animal-drawn vehicle, animal being ridden, streetcar

The appropriate 7th character is to be added to each code from category V66

A	initial encounter
D	subsequent encounter
S	sequela

X● **V66.Ø** **Driver of heavy transport vehicle injured in collision with other nonmotor vehicle in nontraffic accident**

X● **V66.1** **Passenger in heavy transport vehicle injured in collision with other nonmotor vehicle in nontraffic accident**

X● **V66.2** **Person on outside of heavy transport vehicle injured in collision with other nonmotor vehicle in nontraffic accident**

X● **V66.3** **Unspecified occupant of heavy transport vehicle injured in collision with other nonmotor vehicle in nontraffic accident**

X● **V66.4** **Person boarding or alighting a heavy transport vehicle injured in collision with other nonmotor vehicle**

X● **V66.5** **Driver of heavy transport vehicle injured in collision with other nonmotor vehicle in traffic accident**

X● **V66.6** **Passenger in heavy transport vehicle injured in collision with other nonmotor vehicle in traffic accident**

X● **V66.7** **Person on outside of heavy transport vehicle injured in collision with other nonmotor vehicle in traffic accident**

X● **V66.9** **Unspecified occupant of heavy transport vehicle injured in collision with other nonmotor vehicle in traffic accident**

● V67 **Occupant of heavy transport vehicle injured in collision with fixed or stationary object**

The appropriate 7th character is to be added to each code from category V67

A	initial encounter
D	subsequent encounter
S	sequela

X● V67.Ø **Driver of heavy transport vehicle injured in collision with fixed or stationary object in nontraffic accident**

X● V67.1 **Passenger in heavy transport vehicle injured in collision with fixed or stationary object in nontraffic accident**

X● V67.2 **Person on outside of heavy transport vehicle injured in collision with fixed or stationary object in nontraffic accident**

X● V67.3 **Unspecified occupant of heavy transport vehicle injured in collision with fixed or stationary object in nontraffic accident**

X● V67.4 **Person boarding or alighting a heavy transport vehicle injured in collision with fixed or stationary object**

X● V67.5 **Driver of heavy transport vehicle injured in collision with fixed or stationary object in traffic accident**

X● V67.6 **Passenger in heavy transport vehicle injured in collision with fixed or stationary object in traffic accident**

X● V67.7 **Person on outside of heavy transport vehicle injured in collision with fixed or stationary object in traffic accident**

X● V67.9 **Unspecified occupant of heavy transport vehicle injured in collision with fixed or stationary object in traffic accident**

● V68 **Occupant of heavy transport vehicle injured in noncollision transport accident**

Includes overturning heavy transport vehicle NOS
overturning heavy transport vehicle without collision

The appropriate 7th character is to be added to each code from category V68

A	initial encounter
D	subsequent encounter
S	sequela

X● V68.Ø **Driver of heavy transport vehicle injured in noncollision transport accident in nontraffic accident**

X● V68.1 **Passenger in heavy transport vehicle injured in noncollision transport accident in nontraffic accident**

X● V68.2 **Person on outside of heavy transport vehicle injured in noncollision transport accident in nontraffic accident**

X● V68.3 **Unspecified occupant of heavy transport vehicle injured in noncollision transport accident in nontraffic accident**

X● V68.4 **Person boarding or alighting a heavy transport vehicle injured in noncollision transport accident**

X● V68.5 **Driver of heavy transport vehicle injured in noncollision transport accident in traffic accident**

X● V68.6 **Passenger in heavy transport vehicle injured in noncollision transport accident in traffic accident**

X● V68.7 **Person on outside of heavy transport vehicle injured in noncollision transport accident in traffic accident**

X● V68.9 **Unspecified occupant of heavy transport vehicle injured in noncollision transport accident in traffic accident**

● V69 **Occupant of heavy transport vehicle injured in other and unspecified transport accidents**

The appropriate 7th character is to be added to each code from category V69

A	initial encounter
D	subsequent encounter
S	sequela

● V69.Ø **Driver of heavy transport vehicle injured in collision with other and unspecified motor vehicles in nontraffic accident**

X● V69.ØØ **Driver of heavy transport vehicle injured in collision with unspecified motor vehicles in nontraffic accident**

X● V69.Ø9 **Driver of heavy transport vehicle injured in collision with other motor vehicles in nontraffic accident**

● V69.1 **Passenger in heavy transport vehicle injured in collision with other and unspecified motor vehicles in nontraffic accident**

X● V69.1Ø **Passenger in heavy transport vehicle injured in collision with unspecified motor vehicles in nontraffic accident**

X● V69.19 **Passenger in heavy transport vehicle injured in collision with other motor vehicles in nontraffic accident**

● V69.2 **Unspecified occupant of heavy transport vehicle injured in collision with other and unspecified motor vehicles in nontraffic accident**

X● V69.2Ø **Unspecified occupant of heavy transport vehicle injured in collision with unspecified motor vehicles in nontraffic accident**
Collision NOS involving heavy transport vehicle, nontraffic

X● V69.29 **Unspecified occupant of heavy transport vehicle injured in collision with other motor vehicles in nontraffic accident**

X● V69.3 **Occupant (driver) (passenger) of heavy transport vehicle injured in unspecified nontraffic accident**
Accident NOS involving heavy transport vehicle, nontraffic
Occupant of heavy transport vehicle injured in nontraffic accident NOS

● V69.4 **Driver of heavy transport vehicle injured in collision with other and unspecified motor vehicles in traffic accident**

X● V69.4Ø **Driver of heavy transport vehicle injured in collision with unspecified motor vehicles in traffic accident**

X● V69.49 **Driver of heavy transport vehicle injured in collision with other motor vehicles in traffic accident**

● V69.5 **Passenger in heavy transport vehicle injured in collision with other and unspecified motor vehicles in traffic accident**

X● V69.5Ø **Passenger in heavy transport vehicle injured in collision with unspecified motor vehicles in traffic accident**

X● V69.59 **Passenger in heavy transport vehicle injured in collision with other motor vehicles in traffic accident**

● V69.6 **Unspecified occupant of heavy transport vehicle injured in collision with other and unspecified motor vehicles in traffic accident**

X● V69.60 **Unspecified occupant of heavy transport vehicle injured in collision with unspecified motor vehicles in traffic accident**
Collision NOS involving heavy transport vehicle (traffic)

X● V69.69 **Unspecified occupant of heavy transport vehicle injured in collision with other motor vehicles in traffic accident**

● V69.8 **Occupant (driver) (passenger) of heavy transport vehicle injured in other specified transport accidents**

X● V69.81 **Occupant (driver) (passenger) of heavy transport vehicle injured in transport accidents with military vehicle**

X● V69.88 **Occupant (driver) (passenger) of heavy transport vehicle injured in other specified transport accidents**

X● V69.9 **Occupant (driver) (passenger) of heavy transport vehicle injured in unspecified traffic accident**
Accident NOS involving heavy transport vehicle

BUS OCCUPANT INJURED IN TRANSPORT ACCIDENT (V7Ø-V79)

Includes motorcoach
Excludes1 minibus (V5Ø-V59)

● V7Ø **Bus occupant injured in collision with pedestrian or animal**
Excludes1 bus collision with animal-drawn vehicle or animal being ridden (V76.-)

The appropriate 7th character is to be added to each code from category V7Ø

A	initial encounter
D	subsequent encounter
S	sequela

X● V7Ø.Ø **Driver of bus injured in collision with pedestrian or animal in nontraffic accident**

X● V7Ø.1 **Passenger on bus injured in collision with pedestrian or animal in nontraffic accident**

X● V7Ø.2 **Person on outside of bus injured in collision with pedestrian or animal in nontraffic accident**

X● V7Ø.3 **Unspecified occupant of bus injured in collision with pedestrian or animal in nontraffic accident**

X● V7Ø.4 **Person boarding or alighting from bus injured in collision with pedestrian or animal**

X● V7Ø.5 **Driver of bus injured in collision with pedestrian or animal in traffic accident**

X● V7Ø.6 **Passenger on bus injured in collision with pedestrian or animal in traffic accident**

X● V7Ø.7 **Person on outside of bus injured in collision with pedestrian or animal in traffic accident**

X● V7Ø.9 **Unspecified occupant of bus injured in collision with pedestrian or animal in traffic accident**

● V71 **Bus occupant injured in collision with pedal cycle**

The appropriate 7th character is to be added to each code from category V71

A	initial encounter
D	subsequent encounter
S	sequela

X● V71.Ø **Driver of bus injured in collision with pedal cycle in nontraffic accident**

X● V71.1 **Passenger on bus injured in collision with pedal cycle in nontraffic accident**

X● V71.2 **Person on outside of bus injured in collision with pedal cycle in nontraffic accident**

X● V71.3 **Unspecified occupant of bus injured in collision with pedal cycle in nontraffic accident**

X● V71.4 **Person boarding or alighting from bus injured in collision with pedal cycle**

X● V71.5 **Driver of bus injured in collision with pedal cycle in traffic accident**

X● V71.6 **Passenger on bus injured in collision with pedal cycle in traffic accident**

X● V71.7 **Person on outside of bus injured in collision with pedal cycle in traffic accident**

X● V71.9 **Unspecified occupant of bus injured in collision with pedal cycle in traffic accident**

● V72 **Bus occupant injured in collision with two- or three-wheeled motor vehicle**

The appropriate 7th character is to be added to each code from category V72

A	initial encounter
D	subsequent encounter
S	sequela

X● V72.Ø **Driver of bus injured in collision with two- or three-wheeled motor vehicle in nontraffic accident**

X● V72.1 **Passenger on bus injured in collision with two- or three-wheeled motor vehicle in nontraffic accident**

X● V72.2 **Person on outside of bus injured in collision with two- or three-wheeled motor vehicle in nontraffic accident**

X● V72.3 **Unspecified occupant of bus injured in collision with two- or three-wheeled motor vehicle in nontraffic accident**

X● V72.4 **Person boarding or alighting from bus injured in collision with two- or three-wheeled motor vehicle**

X● V72.5 **Driver of bus injured in collision with two- or three-wheeled motor vehicle in traffic accident**

X● V72.6 **Passenger on bus injured in collision with two- or three-wheeled motor vehicle in traffic accident**

X● V72.7 **Person on outside of bus injured in collision with two- or three-wheeled motor vehicle in traffic accident**

X● V72.9 **Unspecified occupant of bus injured in collision with two- or three-wheeled motor vehicle in traffic accident**

● V73 **Bus occupant injured in collision with car, pick-up truck or van**

The appropriate 7th character is to be added to each code from category V73

A	initial encounter
D	subsequent encounter
S	sequela

X● V73.Ø **Driver of bus injured in collision with car, pick-up truck or van in nontraffic accident**

X● V73.1 **Passenger on bus injured in collision with car, pick-up truck or van in nontraffic accident**

X● V73.2 **Person on outside of bus injured in collision with car, pick-up truck or van in nontraffic accident**

X● V73.3 **Unspecified occupant of bus injured in collision with car, pick-up truck or van in nontraffic accident**

X● V73.4 **Person boarding or alighting from bus injured in collision with car, pick-up truck or van**

X● V73.5 **Driver of bus injured in collision with car, pick-up truck or van in traffic accident**

X● V73.6 **Passenger on bus injured in collision with car, pick-up truck or van in traffic accident**

X● V73.7 **Person on outside of bus injured in collision with car, pick-up truck or van in traffic accident**

X● V73.9 **Unspecified occupant of bus injured in collision with car, pick-up truck or van in traffic accident**

● V74 Bus occupant injured in collision with heavy transport vehicle or bus
Excludes1 bus occupant injured in collision with military vehicle (V79.81)
The appropriate 7th character is to be added to each code from category V74

A	initial encounter
D	subsequent encounter
S	sequela

X● V74.0 **Driver** of bus injured in collision with heavy transport vehicle or bus in **nontraffic accident**
X● V74.1 **Passenger** on bus injured in collision with heavy transport vehicle or bus in **nontraffic accident**
X● V74.2 **Person on outside** of bus injured in collision with heavy transport vehicle or bus in **nontraffic accident**
X● V74.3 **Unspecified** occupant of bus injured in collision with heavy transport vehicle or bus in **nontraffic accident**
X● V74.4 Person **boarding or alighting** from bus injured in collision with heavy transport vehicle or bus
X● V74.5 **Driver** of bus injured in collision with heavy transport vehicle or bus in **traffic accident**
X● V74.6 **Passenger** on bus injured in collision with heavy transport vehicle or bus in **traffic accident**
X● V74.7 **Person on outside** of bus injured in collision with heavy transport vehicle or bus in **traffic accident**
X● V74.9 **Unspecified** occupant of bus injured in collision with heavy transport vehicle or bus in **traffic accident**

● V75 Bus occupant injured in collision with railway train or railway vehicle
The appropriate 7th character is to be added to each code from category V75

A	initial encounter
D	subsequent encounter
S	sequela

X● V75.0 **Driver** of bus injured in collision with railway train or railway vehicle in **nontraffic accident**
X● V75.1 **Passenger** on bus injured in collision with railway train or railway vehicle in **nontraffic accident**
X● V75.2 **Person on outside** of bus injured in collision with railway train or railway vehicle in **nontraffic accident**
X● V75.3 **Unspecified** occupant of bus injured in collision with railway train or railway vehicle in **nontraffic accident**
X● V75.4 Person **boarding or alighting** from bus injured in collision with railway train or railway vehicle
X● V75.5 **Driver** of bus injured in collision with railway train or railway vehicle in **traffic accident**
X● V75.6 **Passenger** on bus injured in collision with railway train or railway vehicle in **traffic accident**
X● V75.7 **Person on outside** of bus injured in collision with railway train or railway vehicle in **traffic accident**
X● V75.9 **Unspecified** occupant of bus injured in collision with railway train or railway vehicle in **traffic accident**

● V76 Bus occupant injured in collision with other nonmotor vehicle
Includes collision with animal-drawn vehicle, animal being ridden, streetcar
The appropriate 7th character is to be added to each code from category V76

A	initial encounter
D	subsequent encounter
S	sequela

X● V76.0 **Driver** of bus injured in collision with other nonmotor vehicle in **nontraffic accident**
X● V76.1 **Passenger** on bus injured in collision with other nonmotor vehicle in **nontraffic accident**
X● V76.2 **Person on outside** of bus injured in collision with other nonmotor vehicle in **nontraffic accident**
X● V76.3 **Unspecified** occupant of bus injured in collision with other nonmotor vehicle in **nontraffic accident**
X● V76.4 Person **boarding or alighting** from bus injured in collision with other nonmotor vehicle
X● V76.5 **Driver** of bus injured in collision with other nonmotor vehicle in **traffic accident**
X● V76.6 **Passenger** on bus injured in collision with other nonmotor vehicle in **traffic accident**
X● V76.7 **Person on outside** of bus injured in collision with other nonmotor vehicle in **traffic accident**
X● V76.9 **Unspecified** occupant of bus injured in collision with other nonmotor vehicle in **traffic accident**

● V77 Bus occupant injured in collision with fixed or stationary object
The appropriate 7th character is to be added to each code from category V77

A	initial encounter
D	subsequent encounter
S	sequela

X● V77.0 **Driver** of bus injured in collision with fixed or stationary object in **nontraffic accident**
X● V77.1 **Passenger** on bus injured in collision with fixed or stationary object in **nontraffic accident**
X● V77.2 **Person on outside** of bus injured in collision with fixed or stationary object in **nontraffic accident**
X● V77.3 **Unspecified** occupant of bus injured in collision with fixed or stationary object in **nontraffic accident**
X● V77.4 Person **boarding or alighting** from bus injured in collision with fixed or stationary object
X● V77.5 **Driver** of bus injured in collision with fixed or stationary object in **traffic accident**
X● V77.6 **Passenger** on bus injured in collision with fixed or stationary object in **traffic accident**
X● V77.7 **Person on outside** of bus injured in collision with fixed or stationary object in **traffic accident**
X● V77.9 **Unspecified** occupant of bus injured in collision with fixed or stationary object in **traffic accident**

● V78 Bus occupant injured in noncollision transport accident
Includes overturning bus NOS
overturning bus without collision
The appropriate 7th character is to be added to each code from category V78

A	initial encounter
D	subsequent encounter
S	sequela

X● V78.0 **Driver** of bus injured in noncollision transport accident in **nontraffic accident**
X● V78.1 **Passenger** on bus injured in noncollision transport accident in **nontraffic accident**
X● V78.2 **Person on outside** of bus injured in noncollision transport accident in **nontraffic accident**
X● V78.3 **Unspecified** occupant of bus injured in noncollision transport accident in **nontraffic accident**
X● V78.4 Person **boarding or alighting** from bus injured in noncollision transport accident
X● V78.5 **Driver** of bus injured in noncollision transport accident in **traffic accident**
X● V78.6 **Passenger** on bus injured in noncollision transport accident in **traffic accident**
X● V78.7 **Person on outside** of bus injured in noncollision transport accident in **traffic accident**
X● V78.9 **Unspecified** occupant of bus injured in noncollision transport accident in **traffic accident**

● **V79 Bus occupant injured in other and unspecified transport accidents**

The appropriate 7th character is to be added to each code from category V79

A	initial encounter
D	subsequent encounter
S	sequela

● **V79.0 Driver of bus injured in collision with other and unspecified motor vehicles in nontraffic accident**

X● **V79.00 Driver of bus injured in collision with unspecified motor vehicles in nontraffic accident**

X● **V79.09 Driver of bus injured in collision with other motor vehicles in nontraffic accident**

● **V79.1 Passenger on bus injured in collision with other and unspecified motor vehicles in nontraffic accident**

X● **V79.10 Passenger on bus injured in collision with unspecified motor vehicles in nontraffic accident**

X● **V79.19 Passenger on bus injured in collision with other motor vehicles in nontraffic accident**

● **V79.2 Unspecified bus occupant injured in collision with other and unspecified motor vehicles in nontraffic accident**

X● **V79.20 Unspecified bus occupant injured in collision with unspecified motor vehicles in nontraffic accident**

Bus collision NOS, nontraffic

X● **V79.29 Unspecified bus occupant injured in collision with other motor vehicles in nontraffic accident**

X● **V79.3 Bus occupant (driver) (passenger) injured in unspecified nontraffic accident**

Bus accident NOS, nontraffic
Bus occupant injured in nontraffic accident NOS

● **V79.4 Driver of bus injured in collision with other and unspecified motor vehicles in traffic accident**

X● **V79.40 Driver of bus injured in collision with unspecified motor vehicles in traffic accident**

X● **V79.49 Driver of bus injured in collision with other motor vehicles in traffic accident**

● **V79.5 Passenger on bus injured in collision with other and unspecified motor vehicles in traffic accident**

X● **V79.50 Passenger on bus injured in collision with unspecified motor vehicles in traffic accident**

X● **V79.59 Passenger on bus injured in collision with other motor vehicles in traffic accident**

● **V79.6 Unspecified bus occupant injured in collision with other and unspecified motor vehicles in traffic accident**

X● **V79.60 Unspecified bus occupant injured in collision with unspecified motor vehicles in traffic accident**

Bus collision NOS (traffic)

X● **V79.69 Unspecified bus occupant injured in collision with other motor vehicles in traffic accident**

● **V79.8 Bus occupant (driver) (passenger) injured in other specified transport accidents**

X● **V79.81 Bus occupant (driver) (passenger) injured in transport accidents with military vehicle**

X● **V79.88 Bus occupant (driver) (passenger) injured in other specified transport accidents**

X● **V79.9 Bus occupant (driver) (passenger) injured in unspecified traffic accident**

Bus accident NOS

OTHER LAND TRANSPORT ACCIDENTS (V80-V89)

● **V80 Animal-rider or occupant of animal-drawn vehicle injured in transport accident**

The appropriate 7th character is to be added to each code from category V80

A	initial encounter
D	subsequent encounter
S	sequela

● **V80.0 Animal-rider or occupant of animal drawn vehicle injured by fall from or being thrown from animal or animal-drawn vehicle in noncollision accident**

● **V80.01 Animal-rider injured by fall from or being thrown from animal in noncollision accident**

● **V80.010 Animal-rider injured by fall from or being thrown from horse in noncollision accident**

● **V80.018 Animal-rider injured by fall from or being thrown from other animal in noncollision accident**

X● **V80.02 Occupant of animal-drawn vehicle injured by fall from or being thrown from animal-drawn vehicle in noncollision accident**

Overturning animal-drawn vehicle NOS
Overturning animal-drawn vehicle without collision

● **V80.1 Animal-rider or occupant of animal-drawn vehicle injured in collision with pedestrian or animal**

Excludes1 animal-rider or animal-drawn vehicle collision with animal-drawn vehicle or animal being ridden (V80.7)

X● **V80.11 Animal-rider injured in collision with pedestrian or animal**

X● **V80.12 Occupant of animal-drawn vehicle injured in collision with pedestrian or animal**

● **V80.2 Animal-rider or occupant of animal-drawn vehicle injured in collision with pedal cycle**

X● **V80.21 Animal-rider injured in collision with pedal cycle**

X● **V80.22 Occupant of animal-drawn vehicle injured in collision with pedal cycle**

● **V80.3 Animal-rider or occupant of animal-drawn vehicle injured in collision with two- or three-wheeled motor vehicle**

X● **V80.31 Animal-rider injured in collision with two- or three-wheeled motor vehicle**

X● **V80.32 Occupant of animal-drawn vehicle injured in collision with two- or three-wheeled motor vehicle**

● **V80.4 Animal-rider or occupant of animal-drawn vehicle injured in collision with car, pick-up truck, van, heavy transport vehicle or bus**

Excludes1 animal-rider injured in collision with military vehicle (V80.910)
occupant of animal-drawn vehicle injured in collision with military vehicle (V80.920)

X● **V80.41 Animal-rider injured in collision with car, pick-up truck, van, heavy transport vehicle or bus**

X● **V80.42 Occupant of animal-drawn vehicle injured in collision with car, pick-up truck, van, heavy transport vehicle or bus**

CHAPTER 20 (V00-Y99)

● V80.5 Animal-rider or occupant of animal-drawn vehicle injured in collision with other specified motor vehicle
X● V80.51 Animal-rider injured in collision with other specified motor vehicle
X● V80.52 Occupant of animal-drawn vehicle injured in collision with other specified motor vehicle
● V80.6 Animal-rider or occupant of animal-drawn vehicle injured in collision with railway train or railway vehicle
X● V80.61 Animal-rider injured in collision with railway train or railway vehicle
X● V80.62 Occupant of animal-drawn vehicle injured in collision with railway train or railway vehicle
● V80.7 Animal-rider or occupant of animal-drawn vehicle injured in collision with other nonmotor vehicles
● V80.71 Animal-rider or occupant of animal-drawn vehicle injured in collision with animal being ridden
● V80.710 Animal-rider injured in collision with other animal being ridden
● V80.711 Occupant of animal-drawn vehicle injured in collision with animal being ridden
● V80.72 Animal-rider or occupant of animal-drawn vehicle injured in collision with other animal-drawn vehicle
● V80.720 Animal-rider injured in collision with animal-drawn vehicle
● V80.721 Occupant of animal-drawn vehicle injured in collision with other animal-drawn vehicle
● V80.73 Animal-rider or occupant of animal-drawn vehicle injured in collision with streetcar
● V80.730 Animal-rider injured in collision with streetcar
● V80.731 Occupant of animal-drawn vehicle injured in collision with streetcar
● V80.79 Animal-rider or occupant of animal-drawn vehicle injured in collision with other nonmotor vehicles
● V80.790 Animal-rider injured in collision with other nonmotor vehicles
● V80.791 Occupant of animal-drawn vehicle injured in collision with other nonmotor vehicles
● V80.8 Animal-rider or occupant of animal-drawn vehicle injured in collision with fixed or stationary object
X● V80.81 Animal-rider injured in collision with fixed or stationary object
X● V80.82 Occupant of animal-drawn vehicle injured in collision with fixed or stationary object
● V80.9 Animal-rider or occupant of animal-drawn vehicle injured in other and unspecified transport accidents
● V80.91 Animal-rider injured in other and unspecified transport accidents
● V80.910 Animal-rider injured in transport accident with military vehicle
● V80.918 Animal-rider injured in other transport accident
● V80.919 Animal-rider injured in unspecified transport accident
Animal rider accident NOS
● V80.92 Occupant of animal-drawn vehicle injured in other and unspecified transport accidents
● V80.920 Occupant of animal-drawn vehicle injured in transport accident with military vehicle
● V80.928 Occupant of animal-drawn vehicle injured in other transport accident
● V80.929 Occupant of animal-drawn vehicle injured in unspecified transport accident
Animal-drawn vehicle accident NOS

● V81 Occupant of railway train or railway vehicle injured in transport accident
Includes derailment of railway train or railway vehicle
person on outside of train
Excludes1 streetcar (V82.-)

The appropriate 7th character is to be added to each code from category V81

A	initial encounter
D	subsequent encounter
S	sequela

X● V81.0 Occupant of railway train or railway vehicle injured in collision with motor vehicle in nontraffic accident
Excludes1 occupant of railway train or railway vehicle injured due to collision with military vehicle (V81.83)
X● V81.1 Occupant of railway train or railway vehicle injured in collision with motor vehicle in traffic accident
Excludes1 occupant of railway train or railway vehicle injured due to collision with military vehicle (V81.83)
X● V81.2 Occupant of railway train or railway vehicle injured in collision with or hit by rolling stock
X● V81.3 Occupant of railway train or railway vehicle injured in collision with other object
Railway collision NOS
X● V81.4 Person injured while boarding or alighting from railway train or railway vehicle
X● V81.5 Occupant of railway train or railway vehicle injured by fall in railway train or railway vehicle
X● V81.6 Occupant of railway train or railway vehicle injured by fall from railway train or railway vehicle
X● V81.7 Occupant of railway train or railway vehicle injured in derailment without antecedent collision
● V81.8 Occupant of railway train or railway vehicle injured in other specified railway accidents
X● V81.81 Occupant of railway train or railway vehicle injured due to explosion or fire on train
X● V81.82 Occupant of railway train or railway vehicle injured due to object falling onto train
Occupant of railway train or railway vehicle injured due to falling earth onto train
Occupant of railway train or railway vehicle injured due to falling rocks onto train
Occupant of railway train or railway vehicle injured due to falling snow onto train
Occupant of railway train or railway vehicle injured due to falling trees onto train
X● V81.83 Occupant of railway train or railway vehicle injured due to collision with military vehicle
X● V81.89 Occupant of railway train or railway vehicle injured due to other specified railway accident
X● V81.9 Occupant of railway train or railway vehicle injured in unspecified railway accident
Railway accident NOS

V82 Occupant of powered streetcar injured in transport accident

Includes interurban electric car
person on outside of streetcar
tram (car)
trolley (car)

Excludes1 bus (V7Ø-V79)
motorcoach (V7Ø-V79)
nonpowered streetcar (V76.-)
train (V81.-)

The appropriate 7th character is to be added to each code from category V82

A initial encounter
D subsequent encounter
S sequela

X **V82.Ø Occupant of streetcar injured in collision with motor vehicle in nontraffic accident**

X **V82.1 Occupant of streetcar injured in collision with motor vehicle in traffic accident**

X **V82.2 Occupant of streetcar injured in collision with or hit by rolling stock**

X **V82.3 Occupant of streetcar injured in collision with other object**

Excludes1 collision with animal-drawn vehicle or animal being ridden (V82.8)

X **V82.4 Person injured while boarding or alighting from streetcar**

X **V82.5 Occupant of streetcar injured by fall in streetcar**

Excludes1 fall in streetcar:
while boarding or alighting (V82.4)
with antecedent collision (V82.Ø-V82.3)

X **V82.6 Occupant of streetcar injured by fall from streetcar**

Excludes1 fall from streetcar:
while boarding or alighting (V82.4)
with antecedent collision (V82.Ø-V82.3)

X **V82.7 Occupant of streetcar injured in derailment without antecedent collision**

Excludes1 occupant of streetcar injured in derailment with antecedent collision (V82.Ø-V82.3)

X **V82.8 Occupant of streetcar injured in other specified transport accidents**

Streetcar collision with military vehicle
Streetcar collision with train or nonmotor vehicles

X **V82.9 Occupant of streetcar injured in unspecified traffic accident**

Streetcar accident NOS

V83 Occupant of special vehicle mainly used on industrial premises injured in transport accident

Includes battery-powered airport passenger vehicle
battery-powered truck (baggage) (mail)
coal-car in mine
forklift (truck)
logging car
self-propelled industrial truck
station baggage truck (powered)
tram, truck, or tub (powered) in mine or quarry

Excludes1 special construction vehicles (V85.-)
special industrial vehicle in stationary use or maintenance (W31.-)

The appropriate 7th character is to be added to each code from category V83

A initial encounter
D subsequent encounter
S sequela

X **V83.Ø Driver of special industrial vehicle injured in traffic accident**

X **V83.1 Passenger of special industrial vehicle injured in traffic accident**

X **V83.2 Person on outside of special industrial vehicle injured in traffic accident**

X **V83.3 Unspecified occupant of special industrial vehicle injured in traffic accident**

X **V83.4 Person injured while boarding or alighting from special industrial vehicle**

X **V83.5 Driver of special industrial vehicle injured in nontraffic accident**

X **V83.6 Passenger of special industrial vehicle injured in nontraffic accident**

X **V83.7 Person on outside of special industrial vehicle injured in nontraffic accident**

X **V83.9 Unspecified occupant of special industrial vehicle injured in nontraffic accident**

Special-industrial-vehicle accident NOS

V84 Occupant of special vehicle mainly used in agriculture injured in transport accident

Includes self-propelled farm machinery
tractor (and trailer)

Excludes1 animal-powered farm machinery accident (W3Ø.8-)
contact with combine harvester (W3Ø.Ø)
special agricultural vehicle in stationary use or maintenance (W3Ø.-)

The appropriate 7th character is to be added to each code from category V84

A initial encounter
D subsequent encounter
S sequela

X **V84.Ø Driver of special agricultural vehicle injured in traffic accident**

X **V84.1 Passenger of special agricultural vehicle injured in traffic accident**

X **V84.2 Person on outside of special agricultural vehicle injured in traffic accident**

X **V84.3 Unspecified occupant of special agricultural vehicle injured in traffic accident**

X **V84.4 Person injured while boarding or alighting from special agricultural vehicle**

X **V84.5 Driver of special agricultural vehicle injured in nontraffic accident**

X **V84.6 Passenger of special agricultural vehicle injured in nontraffic accident**

X **V84.7 Person on outside of special agricultural vehicle injured in nontraffic accident**

X **V84.9 Unspecified occupant of special agricultural vehicle injured in nontraffic accident**

Special-agricultural vehicle accident NOS

V85 Occupant of special construction vehicle injured in transport accident

Includes bulldozer
digger
dump truck
earth-leveller
mechanical shovel
road-roller

Excludes1 special industrial vehicle (V83.-)
special construction vehicle in stationary use or maintenance (W31.-)

The appropriate 7th character is to be added to each code from category V85

A initial encounter
D subsequent encounter
S sequela

X **V85.Ø Driver of special construction vehicle injured in traffic accident**

X **V85.1 Passenger of special construction vehicle injured in traffic accident**

X● V85.2 **Person on outside** of special construction vehicle injured **in traffic accident**

X● V85.3 **Unspecified** occupant of special construction vehicle injured in **traffic accident**

X● V85.4 Person injured while **boarding or alighting** from special construction vehicle

X● V85.5 **Driver** of special construction vehicle injured in **nontraffic accident**

X● V85.6 **Passenger** of special construction vehicle injured in **nontraffic accident**

X● V85.7 **Person on outside** of special construction vehicle injured in **nontraffic accident**

X● V85.9 **Unspecified** occupant of special construction vehicle injured in **nontraffic accident**
Special-construction-vehicle accident NOS

● V86 Occupant of special all-terrain or other off-road motor vehicle, injured in transport accident

Excludes1 special all-terrain vehicle in stationary use or maintenance (W31.-)
sport-utility vehicle (V5Ø-V59)
three-wheeled motor vehicle designed for on-road use (V3Ø-V39)

The appropriate 7th character is to be added to each code from category V86

A	initial encounter
D	subsequent encounter
S	sequela

● V86.Ø **Driver** of special all-terrain or other off-road motor vehicle injured in **traffic accident**

X● V86.Ø1 Driver of **ambulance or fire engine** injured in traffic accident

X● V86.Ø2 Driver of **snowmobile** injured in traffic accident

X● V86.Ø3 Driver of **dune buggy** injured in traffic accident

X● V86.Ø4 Driver of **military** vehicle injured in traffic accident

X● V86.Ø5 Driver of **3- or 4-wheeled all-terrain vehicle** (ATV) injured in traffic accident

X● V86.Ø6 Driver of **dirt bike or motor/cross bike** injured in traffic accident

X● V86.Ø9 Driver of **other off-road special all-terrain or other off-road vehicle** injured in traffic accident
~~Driver of dirt bike injured in traffic accident~~
Driver of go cart injured in traffic accident
Driver of golf cart injured in traffic accident

● V86.1 **Passenger** of special all-terrain or other off-road motor vehicle injured in **traffic accident**

X● V86.11 Passenger of **ambulance or fire engine** injured in traffic accident

X● V86.12 Passenger of **snowmobile** injured in traffic accident

X● V86.13 Passenger of **dune buggy** injured in traffic accident

X● V86.14 Passenger of **military** vehicle injured in traffic accident

X● V86.15 Passenger of **3- or 4-wheeled all-terrain vehicle** (ATV) injured in traffic accident

X● V86.16 Passenger of **dirt bike or motor/cross bike** injured in traffic accident

X● V86.19 Passenger of **other off-road special all-terrain or other off-road off-road motor vehicle** injured in traffic accident
~~Passenger of dirt bike injured in traffic accident~~
Passenger of go cart injured in traffic accident
Passenger of golf cart injured in traffic accident

● V86.2 **Person on outside** of special all-terrain or other off-road motor vehicle injured in **traffic accident**

X● V86.21 Person on outside of **ambulance or fire engine** injured in traffic accident

X● V86.22 Person on outside of **snowmobile** injured in traffic accident

X● V86.23 Person on outside of **dune buggy** injured in traffic accident

X● V86.24 Person on outside of **military** vehicle injured in traffic accident

X● V86.25 Person on outside of **3- or 4-wheeled all-terrain vehicle** (ATV) injured in traffic accident

X● V86.26 Person on outside of **dirt bike or motor/cross bike** injured in traffic accident

X● V86.29 Person on outside of **other special all-terrain or other off-road motor vehicle** injured in traffic accident
~~Person on outside of dirt bike injured in traffic accident~~
Person on outside of go cart in traffic accident
Person on outside of golf cart injured in traffic accident

● V86.3 **Unspecified** occupant of special all-terrain or other off-road motor vehicle injured in **traffic accident**

X● V86.31 Unspecified occupant of **ambulance or fire engine** injured in traffic accident

X● V86.32 Unspecified occupant of **snowmobile** injured in traffic accident

X● V86.33 Unspecified occupant of **dune buggy** injured in traffic accident

X● V86.34 Unspecified occupant of **military** vehicle injured in traffic accident

X● V86.35 Unspecified occupant of **3- or 4-wheeled all-terrain vehicle** (ATV) injured in traffic accident

X● V86.36 Unspecified occupant of **dirt bike or motor/cross bike** injured in traffic accident

X● V86.39 Unspecified occupant of **other special all-terrain or other off-road motor vehicle** injured in traffic accident
~~Unspecified occupant of dirt bike injured in traffic accident~~
Unspecified occupant of go cart injured in traffic accident
Unspecified occupant of golf cart injured in traffic accident

● V86.4 Person injured while **boarding or alighting** from special all-terrain or other off-road motor vehicle

X● V86.41 Person injured while boarding or alighting from **ambulance or fire engine**

X● V86.42 Person injured while boarding or alighting from **snowmobile**

X● V86.43 Person injured while boarding or alighting from **dune buggy**

X● V86.44 Person injured while boarding or alighting from **military** vehicle

X● V86.45 Person injured while boarding or alighting from a **3- or 4-wheeled all-terrain vehicle** (ATV)

X● V86.46 Person injured while boarding or alighting from a **dirt bike or motor/cross bike**

X● V86.49 Person injured while boarding or alighting from **other special all-terrain or other off-road motor vehicle**
~~Person injured while boarding or alighting from dirt bike~~
Person injured while boarding or alighting from go cart
Person injured while boarding or alighting from golf cart

● V86.5 **Driver of special all-terrain or other off-road motor vehicle injured in nontraffic accident**

X● V86.51 **Driver of ambulance or fire engine injured in nontraffic accident**

X● V86.52 **Driver of snowmobile injured in nontraffic accident**

X● V86.53 **Driver of dune buggy injured in nontraffic accident**

X● V86.54 **Driver of military vehicle injured in nontraffic accident**

X● V86.55 **Driver of 3- or 4-wheeled all-terrain vehicle (ATV) injured in nontraffic accident**

X● V86.56 **Driver of dirt bike or motor/cross bike injured in nontraffic accident**

X● V86.59 **Driver of other off-road special all-terrain or other off-road motor vehicle injured in nontraffic accident**

~~Driver of dirt bike injured in nontraffic accident~~
Driver of go cart injured in nontraffic accident
Driver of golf cart injured in nontraffic accident

● V86.6 **Passenger of special all-terrain or other off-road motor vehicle injured in nontraffic accident**

X● V86.61 **Passenger of ambulance or fire engine injured in nontraffic accident**

X● V86.62 **Passenger of snowmobile injured in nontraffic accident**

X● V86.63 **Passenger of dune buggy injured in nontraffic accident**

X● V86.64 **Passenger of military vehicle injured in nontraffic accident**

X● V86.65 **Passenger of 3- or 4-wheeled all-terrain vehicle (ATV) injured in nontraffic accident**

X● V86.66 **Passenger of dirt bike or motor/cross bike injured in nontraffic accident**

X● V86.69 **Passenger of other special all-terrain or other off-road vehicle injured in nontraffic accident**

~~Passenger of dirt bike injured in nontraffic accident~~
Passenger of go cart injured in nontraffic accident
Passenger of golf cart injured in nontraffic accident

● V86.7 **Person on outside of special all-terrain or other off-road motor vehicle injured in nontraffic accident**

X● V86.71 **Person on outside of ambulance or fire engine injured in nontraffic accident**

X● V86.72 **Person on outside of snowmobile injured in nontraffic accident**

X● V86.73 **Person on outside of dune buggy injured in nontraffic accident**

X● V86.74 **Person on outside of military vehicle injured in nontraffic accident**

X● V86.75 **Person on outside of 3- or 4-wheeled all-terrain vehicle (ATV) injured in nontraffic accident**

X● V86.76 **Person on outside of dirt bike or motor/cross bike injured in nontraffic accident**

X● V86.79 **Person on outside of other special all-terrain or other off-road motor vehicles injured in nontraffic accident**

~~Person on outside of dirt bike injured in nontraffic accident~~
Person on outside of go cart injured in nontraffic accident
Person on outside of golf cart injured in nontraffic accident

● V86.9 **Unspecified occupant of special all-terrain or other off-road motor vehicle injured in nontraffic accident**

X● V86.91 **Unspecified occupant of ambulance or fire engine injured in nontraffic accident**

X● V86.92 **Unspecified occupant of snowmobile injured in nontraffic accident**

X● V86.93 **Unspecified occupant of dune buggy injured in nontraffic accident**

X● V86.94 **Unspecified occupant of military vehicle injured in nontraffic accident**

X● V86.95 **Unspecified occupant of 3- or 4-wheeled all-terrain vehicle (ATV) injured in nontraffic accident**

X● V86.96 **Unspecified occupant of dirt bike or motor/cross bike injured in nontraffic accident**

X● V86.99 **Unspecified occupant of other special all-terrain or other off-road motor vehicle injured in nontraffic accident**

Off-road motor-vehicle accident NOS
Other motor-vehicle accident NOS
Unspecified occupant of go cart injured in nontraffic accident
Unspecified occupant of golf cart injured in nontraffic accident
Unspecified occupant of race car injured in nontraffic accident

● V87 **Traffic accident of specified type but victim's mode of transport unknown**

Excludes1 collision involving:
pedal cycle (V1Ø-V19)
pedestrian (VØ1-VØ9)

The appropriate 7th character is to be added to each code from category V87

A	initial encounter
D	subsequent encounter
S	sequela

X● V87.Ø **Person injured in collision between car and two- or three-wheeled powered vehicle (traffic)**

X● V87.1 **Person injured in collision between other motor vehicle and two- or three-wheeled motor vehicle (traffic)**

X● V87.2 **Person injured in collision between car and pick-up truck or van (traffic)**

X● V87.3 **Person injured in collision between car and bus (traffic)**

X● V87.4 **Person injured in collision between car and heavy transport vehicle (traffic)**

X● V87.5 **Person injured in collision between heavy transport vehicle and bus (traffic)**

X● V87.6 **Person injured in collision between railway train or railway vehicle and car (traffic)**

X● V87.7 **Person injured in collision between other specified motor vehicles (traffic)**

X● V87.8 **Person injured in other specified noncollision transport accidents involving motor vehicle (traffic)**

X● V87.9 **Person injured in other specified (collision) (noncollision) transport accidents involving nonmotor vehicle (traffic)**

● V88 **Nontraffic accident of specified type but victim's mode of transport unknown**

Excludes1 collision involving:
pedal cycle (V1Ø-V19)
pedestrian (VØ1-VØ9)

The appropriate 7th character is to be added to each code from category V88

A	initial encounter
D	subsequent encounter
S	sequela

X● V88.Ø **Person injured in collision between car and two- or three-wheeled motor vehicle, nontraffic**

X● V88.1 **Person injured in collision between other motor vehicle and two- or three-wheeled motor vehicle, nontraffic**

X● V88.2 **Person injured in collision between car and pick-up truck or van, nontraffic**

CHAPTER 2Ø (VØØ-Y99)

X V88.3 **Person injured in collision between car and bus, nontraffic**

X V88.4 **Person injured in collision between car and heavy transport vehicle, nontraffic**

X V88.5 **Person injured in collision between heavy transport vehicle and bus, nontraffic**

X V88.6 **Person injured in collision between railway train or railway vehicle and car, nontraffic**

X V88.7 **Person injured in collision between other specified motor vehicle, nontraffic**

X V88.8 **Person injured in other specified noncollision transport accidents involving motor vehicle, nontraffic**

X V88.9 **Person injured in other specified (collision) (noncollision) transport accidents involving nonmotor vehicle, nontraffic**

V89 **Motor- or nonmotor-vehicle accident, type of vehicle unspecified**

The appropriate 7th character is to be added to each code from category V89

A	initial encounter
D	subsequent encounter
S	sequela

X V89.0 **Person injured in unspecified motor-vehicle accident, nontraffic**
Motor-vehicle accident NOS, nontraffic

X V89.1 **Person injured in unspecified nonmotor-vehicle accident, nontraffic**
Nonmotor-vehicle accident NOS (nontraffic)

X V89.2 **Person injured in unspecified motor-vehicle accident, traffic**
Motor-vehicle accident [MVA] NOS
Road (traffic) accident [RTA] NOS

X V89.3 **Person injured in unspecified nonmotor-vehicle accident, traffic**
Nonmotor-vehicle traffic accident NOS

X V89.9 **Person injured in unspecified vehicle accident**
Collision NOS

WATER TRANSPORT ACCIDENTS (V00-V94)

V90 **Drowning and submersion due to accident to watercraft**

Excludes1 civilian water transport accident involving military watercraft (V94.81-)
fall into water not from watercraft (W16.-)
military watercraft accident in military or war operations (Y36.0-, Y37.0-)
water-transport–related drowning or submersion without accident to watercraft (V92.-)

The appropriate 7th character is to be added to each code from category V90

A	initial encounter
D	subsequent encounter
S	sequela

V90.0 **Drowning and submersion due to watercraft overturning**

X V90.00 **Drowning and submersion due to merchant ship overturning**

X V90.01 **Drowning and submersion due to passenger ship overturning**
Drowning and submersion due to ferry-boat overturning
Drowning and submersion due to liner overturning

X V90.02 **Drowning and submersion due to fishing boat overturning**

X V90.03 **Drowning and submersion due to other powered watercraft overturning**
Drowning and submersion due to hovercraft (on open water) overturning
Drowning and submersion due to jet ski overturning

X V90.04 **Drowning and submersion due to sailboat overturning**

X V90.05 **Drowning and submersion due to canoe or kayak overturning**

X V90.06 **Drowning and submersion due to (nonpowered) inflatable craft overturning**

X V90.08 **Drowning and submersion due to other unpowered watercraft overturning**
Drowning and submersion due to windsurfer overturning

X V90.09 **Drowning and submersion due to unspecified watercraft overturning**
Drowning and submersion due to boat NOS overturning
Drowning and submersion due to ship NOS overturning
Drowning and submersion due to watercraft NOS overturning

V90.1 **Drowning and submersion due to watercraft sinking**

X V90.10 **Drowning and submersion due to merchant ship sinking**

X V90.11 **Drowning and submersion due to passenger ship sinking**
Drowning and submersion due to ferry-boat sinking
Drowning and submersion due to liner sinking

X V90.12 **Drowning and submersion due to fishing boat sinking**

X V90.13 **Drowning and submersion due to other powered watercraft sinking**
Drowning and submersion due to hovercraft (on open water) sinking
Drowning and submersion due to jet ski sinking

X V90.14 **Drowning and submersion due to sailboat sinking**

X V90.15 **Drowning and submersion due to canoe or kayak sinking**

X V90.16 **Drowning and submersion due to (nonpowered) inflatable craft sinking**

X V90.18 **Drowning and submersion due to other unpowered watercraft sinking**

X V90.19 **Drowning and submersion due to unspecified watercraft sinking**
Drowning and submersion due to boat NOS sinking
Drowning and submersion due to ship NOS sinking
Drowning and submersion due to watercraft NOS sinking

V90.2 **Drowning and submersion due to falling or jumping from burning watercraft**

X V90.20 **Drowning and submersion due to falling or jumping from burning merchant ship**

X V90.21 **Drowning and submersion due to falling or jumping from burning passenger ship**
Drowning and submersion due to falling or jumping from burning ferry-boat
Drowning and submersion due to falling or jumping from burning liner

X V90.22 **Drowning and submersion due to falling or jumping from burning fishing boat**

X V90.23 **Drowning and submersion due to falling or jumping from other burning powered watercraft**
Drowning and submersion due to falling and jumping from burning hovercraft (on open water)
Drowning and submersion due to falling and jumping from burning jet ski

X V90.24 **Drowning and submersion due to falling or jumping from burning sailboat**

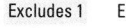

X● V90.25 **Drowning and submersion due to falling or jumping from burning canoe or kayak**

X● V90.26 **Drowning and submersion due to falling or jumping from burning (nonpowered) inflatable craft**

X● V90.27 **Drowning and submersion due to falling or jumping from burning water-skis**

X● V90.28 **Drowning and submersion due to falling or jumping from other burning unpowered watercraft**
Drowning and submersion due to falling and jumping from burning surf-board
Drowning and submersion due to falling and jumping from burning windsurfer

X● V90.29 **Drowning and submersion due to falling or jumping from unspecified burning watercraft**
Drowning and submersion due to falling or jumping from burning boat NOS
Drowning and submersion due to falling or jumping from burning ship NOS
Drowning and submersion due to falling or jumping from burning watercraft NOS

● V90.3 **Drowning and submersion due to falling or jumping from crushed watercraft**

X● V90.30 **Drowning and submersion due to falling or jumping from crushed merchant ship**

X● V90.31 **Drowning and submersion due to falling or jumping from crushed passenger ship**
Drowning and submersion due to falling and jumping from crushed ferry-boat
Drowning and submersion due to falling and jumping from crushed liner

X● V90.32 **Drowning and submersion due to falling or jumping from crushed fishing boat**

X● V90.33 **Drowning and submersion due to falling or jumping from other crushed powered watercraft**
Drowning and submersion due to falling and jumping from crushed hovercraft
Drowning and submersion due to falling and jumping from crushed jet ski

X● V90.34 **Drowning and submersion due to falling or jumping from crushed sailboat**

X● V90.35 **Drowning and submersion due to falling or jumping from crushed canoe or kayak**

X● V90.36 **Drowning and submersion due to falling or jumping from crushed (nonpowered) inflatable craft**

X● V90.37 **Drowning and submersion due to falling or jumping from crushed water-skis**

X● V90.38 **Drowning and submersion due to falling or jumping from other crushed unpowered watercraft**
Drowning and submersion due to falling and jumping from crushed surf-board
Drowning and submersion due to falling and jumping from crushed windsurfer

X● V90.39 **Drowning and submersion due to falling or jumping from crushed unspecified watercraft**
Drowning and submersion due to falling and jumping from crushed boat NOS
Drowning and submersion due to falling and jumping from crushed ship NOS
Drowning and submersion due to falling and jumping from crushed watercraft NOS

● V90.8 **Drowning and submersion due to other accident to watercraft**

X● V90.80 **Drowning and submersion due to other accident to merchant ship**

X● V90.81 **Drowning and submersion due to other accident to passenger ship**
Drowning and submersion due to other accident to ferry-boat
Drowning and submersion due to other accident to liner

X● V90.82 **Drowning and submersion due to other accident to fishing boat**

X● V90.83 **Drowning and submersion due to other accident to other powered watercraft**
Drowning and submersion due to other accident to hovercraft (on open water)
Drowning and submersion due to other accident to jet ski

X● V90.84 **Drowning and submersion due to other accident to sailboat**

X● V90.85 **Drowning and submersion due to other accident to canoe or kayak**

X● V90.86 **Drowning and submersion due to other accident to (nonpowered) inflatable craft**

X● V90.87 **Drowning and submersion due to other accident to water-skis**

X● V90.88 **Drowning and submersion due to other accident to other unpowered watercraft**
Drowning and submersion due to other accident to surf-board
Drowning and submersion due to other accident to windsurfer

X● V90.89 **Drowning and submersion due to other accident to unspecified watercraft**
Drowning and submersion due to other accident to boat NOS
Drowning and submersion due to other accident to ship NOS
Drowning and submersion due to other accident to watercraft NOS

● V91 **Other injury due to accident to watercraft**

Includes any injury except drowning and submersion as a result of an accident to watercraft

Excludes1 civilian water transport accident involving military watercraft (V94.81-)
military watercraft accident in military or war operations (Y36, Y37.-)

Excludes2 drowning and submersion due to accident to watercraft (V90.-)

The appropriate 7th character is to be added to each code from category V91

A	initial encounter
D	subsequent encounter
S	sequela

● V91.0 **Burn due to watercraft on fire**

Excludes1 burn from localized fire or explosion on board ship without accident to watercraft (V93.-)

X● V91.00 **Burn due to merchant ship on fire**

X● V91.01 **Burn due to passenger ship on fire**
Burn due to ferry-boat on fire
Burn due to liner on fire

X● V91.02 **Burn due to fishing boat on fire**

X● V91.03 **Burn due to other powered watercraft on fire**
Burn due to hovercraft (on open water) on fire
Burn due to jet ski on fire

X● V91.04 **Burn due to sailboat on fire**

X● V91.05 **Burn due to canoe or kayak on fire**

X● V91.06 **Burn due to (nonpowered) inflatable craft on fire**

X● V91.07 **Burn due to water-skis on fire**

X● V91.08 **Burn due to other unpowered watercraft on fire**

X● V91.09 **Burn due to unspecified watercraft on fire**
Burn due to boat NOS on fire
Burn due to ship NOS on fire
Burn due to watercraft NOS on fire

● **V91.1 Crushed between watercraft and other watercraft or other object due to collision**
Crushed by lifeboat after abandoning ship in a collision
Note: Select the specified type of watercraft that the victim was on at the time of the collision.

X● **V91.10 Crushed between merchant ship and other watercraft or other object due to collision**

X● **V91.11 Crushed between passenger ship and other watercraft or other object due to collision**
Crushed between ferry-boat and other watercraft or other object due to collision
Crushed between liner and other watercraft or other object due to collision

X● **V91.12 Crushed between fishing boat and other watercraft or other object due to collision**

X● **V91.13 Crushed between other powered watercraft and other watercraft or other object due to collision**
Crushed between hovercraft (on open water) and other watercraft or other object due to collision
Crushed between jet ski and other watercraft or other object due to collision

X● **V91.14 Crushed between sailboat and other watercraft or other object due to collision**

X● **V91.15 Crushed between canoe or kayak and other watercraft or other object due to collision**

X● **V91.16 Crushed between (nonpowered) inflatable craft and other watercraft or other object due to collision**

X● **V91.18 Crushed between other unpowered watercraft and other watercraft or other object due to collision**
Crushed between surfboard and other watercraft or other object due to collision
Crushed between windsurfer and other watercraft or other object due to collision

X● **V91.19 Crushed between unspecified watercraft and other watercraft or other object due to collision**
Crushed between boat NOS and other watercraft or other object due to collision
Crushed between ship NOS and other watercraft or other object due to collision
Crushed between watercraft NOS and other watercraft or other object due to collision

● **V91.2 Fall due to collision between watercraft and other watercraft or other object**
Fall while remaining on watercraft after collision
Note: Select the specified type of watercraft that the victim was on at the time of the collision.
Excludes1 crushed between watercraft and other watercraft and other object due to collision (V91.1-)
drowning and submersion due to falling from crushed watercraft (V90.3-)

X● **V91.20 Fall due to collision between merchant ship and other watercraft or other object**

X● **V91.21 Fall due to collision between passenger ship and other watercraft or other object**
Fall due to collision between ferry-boat and other watercraft or other object
Fall due to collision between liner and other watercraft or other object

X● **V91.22 Fall due to collision between fishing boat and other watercraft or other object**

X● **V91.23 Fall due to collision between other powered watercraft and other watercraft or other object**
Fall due to collision between hovercraft (on open water) and other watercraft or other object
Fall due to collision between jet ski and other watercraft or other object

X● **V91.24 Fall due to collision between sailboat and other watercraft or other object**

X● **V91.25 Fall due to collision between canoe or kayak and other watercraft or other object**

X● **V91.26 Fall due to collision between (nonpowered) inflatable craft and other watercraft or other object**

X● **V91.29 Fall due to collision between unspecified watercraft and other watercraft or other object**
Fall due to collision between boat NOS and other watercraft or other object
Fall due to collision between ship NOS and other watercraft or other object
Fall due to collision between watercraft NOS and other watercraft or other object

● **V91.3 Hit or struck by falling object due to accident to watercraft**
Hit or struck by falling object (part of damaged watercraft or other object) after falling or jumping from damaged watercraft
Excludes2 drowning or submersion due to fall or jumping from damaged watercraft (V90.2-, V90.3-)

X● **V91.30 Hit or struck by falling object due to accident to merchant ship**

X● **V91.31 Hit or struck by falling object due to accident to passenger ship**
Hit or struck by falling object due to accident to ferry-boat
Hit or struck by falling object due to accident to liner

X● **V91.32 Hit or struck by falling object due to accident to fishing boat**

X● **V91.33 Hit or struck by falling object due to accident to other powered watercraft**
Hit or struck by falling object due to accident to hovercraft (on open water)
Hit or struck by falling object due to accident to jet ski

X● **V91.34 Hit or struck by falling object due to accident to sailboat**

X● **V91.35 Hit or struck by falling object due to accident to canoe or kayak**

X● **V91.36 Hit or struck by falling object due to accident to (nonpowered) inflatable craft**

X● **V91.37 Hit or struck by falling object due to accident to water-skis**
Hit by water-skis after jumping off of waterskis

X● **V91.38 Hit or struck by falling object due to accident to other unpowered watercraft**
Hit or struck by surf-board after falling off damaged surf-board
Hit or struck by object after falling off damaged windsurfer

X● **V91.39 Hit or struck by falling object due to accident to unspecified watercraft**
Hit or struck by falling object due to accident to boat NOS
Hit or struck by falling object due to accident to ship NOS
Hit or struck by falling object due to accident to watercraft NOS

● V91.8 **Other injury due to other accident to watercraft**

X● V91.80 **Other injury due to other accident to merchant ship**

X● V91.81 **Other injury due to other accident to passenger ship**
Other injury due to other accident to ferry-boat
Other injury due to other accident to liner

X● V91.82 **Other injury due to other accident to fishing boat**

X● V91.83 **Other injury due to other accident to other powered watercraft**
Other injury due to other accident to hovercraft (on open water)
Other injury due to other accident to jet ski

X● V91.84 **Other injury due to other accident to sailboat**

X● V91.85 **Other injury due to other accident to canoe or kayak**

X● V91.86 **Other injury due to other accident to (nonpowered) inflatable craft**

X● V91.87 **Other injury due to other accident to water-skis**

X● V91.88 **Other injury due to other accident to other unpowered watercraft**
Other injury due to other accident to surf-board
Other injury due to other accident to windsurfer

X● V91.89 **Other injury due to other accident to unspecified watercraft**
Other injury due to other accident to boat NOS
Other injury due to other accident to ship NOS
Other injury due to other accident to watercraft NOS

● V92 **Drowning and submersion due to accident on board watercraft, without accident to watercraft**

Excludes1 civilian water transport accident involving military watercraft (V94.81-)
drowning or submersion due to accident to watercraft (V90-V91)
drowning or submersion of diver who voluntarily jumps from boat not involved in an accident (W16.711, W16.721)
fall into water without watercraft (W16.-)
military watercraft accident in military or war operations (Y36, Y37)

The appropriate 7th character is to be added to each code from category V92

A	initial encounter
D	subsequent encounter
S	sequela

● V92.0 **Drowning and submersion due to fall off watercraft**
Drowning and submersion due to fall from gangplank of watercraft
Drowning and submersion due to fall overboard watercraft

Excludes2 hitting head on object or bottom of body of water due to fall from watercraft (V94.0-)

X● V92.00 **Drowning and submersion due to fall off merchant ship**

X● V92.01 **Drowning and submersion due to fall off passenger ship**
Drowning and submersion due to fall off ferry-boat
Drowning and submersion due to fall off liner

X● V92.02 **Drowning and submersion due to fall off fishing boat**

X● V92.03 **Drowning and submersion due to fall off other powered watercraft**
Drowning and submersion due to fall off hovercraft (on open water)
Drowning and submersion due to fall off jet ski

X● V92.04 **Drowning and submersion due to fall off sailboat**

X● V92.05 **Drowning and submersion due to fall off canoe or kayak**

X● V92.06 **Drowning and submersion due to fall off (nonpowered) inflatable craft**

X● V92.07 **Drowning and submersion due to fall off water-skis**

Excludes1 drowning and submersion due to falling off burning water-skis (V90.27)
drowning and submersion due to falling off crushed water-skis (V90.37)
hit by boat while water-skiing NOS (V94.X)

X● V92.08 **Drowning and submersion due to fall off other unpowered watercraft**
Drowning and submersion due to fall off surf-board
Drowning and submersion due to fall off windsurfer

Excludes1 drowning and submersion due to fall off burning unpowered watercraft (V90.28)
drowning and submersion due to fall off crushed unpowered watercraft (V90.38)
drowning and submersion due to fall off damaged unpowered watercraft (V90.88)
drowning and submersion due to rider of nonpowered watercraft being hit by other watercraft (V94.-)
other injury due to rider of nonpowered watercraft being hit by other watercraft (V94.-)

X● V92.09 **Drowning and submersion due to fall off unspecified watercraft**
Drowning and submersion due to fall off boat NOS
Drowning and submersion due to fall off ship
Drowning and submersion due to fall off watercraft NOS

● V92.1 **Drowning and submersion due to being thrown overboard by motion of watercraft**

Excludes1 drowning and submersion due to fall off surf-board (V92.08)
drowning and submersion due to fall off water-skis (V92.07)
drowning and submersion due to fall off windsurfer (V92.08)

X● V92.10 **Drowning and submersion due to being thrown overboard by motion of merchant ship**

X● V92.11 **Drowning and submersion due to being thrown overboard by motion of passenger ship**
Drowning and submersion due to being thrown overboard by motion of ferry-boat
Drowning and submersion due to being thrown overboard by motion of liner

X● V92.12 **Drowning and submersion due to being thrown overboard by motion of fishing boat**

X● V92.13 **Drowning and submersion due to being thrown overboard by motion of other powered watercraft**
Drowning and submersion due to being thrown overboard by motion of hovercraft

X● V92.14 **Drowning and submersion due to being thrown overboard by motion of sailboat**

X● V92.15 **Drowning and submersion due to being thrown overboard by motion of canoe or kayak**

X● V92.16 **Drowning and submersion due to being thrown overboard by motion of (nonpowered) inflatable craft**

X● V92.19 **Drowning and submersion due to being thrown overboard by motion of unspecified watercraft**
Drowning and submersion due to being thrown overboard by motion of boat NOS
Drowning and submersion due to being thrown overboard by motion of ship NOS
Drowning and submersion due to being thrown overboard by motion of watercraft NOS

● V92.2 **Drowning and submersion due to being washed overboard from watercraft**
Code first any associated cataclysm (X37.Ø-)

X● V92.20 **Drowning and submersion due to being washed overboard from merchant ship**

X● V92.21 **Drowning and submersion due to being washed overboard from passenger ship**
Drowning and submersion due to being washed overboard from ferry-boat
Drowning and submersion due to being washed overboard from liner

X● V92.22 **Drowning and submersion due to being washed overboard from fishing boat**

X● V92.23 **Drowning and submersion due to being washed overboard from other powered watercraft**
Drowning and submersion due to being washed overboard from hovercraft (on open water)
Drowning and submersion due to being washed overboard from jet ski

X● V92.24 **Drowning and submersion due to being washed overboard from sailboat**

X● V92.25 **Drowning and submersion due to being washed overboard from canoe or kayak**

X● V92.26 **Drowning and submersion due to being washed overboard from (nonpowered) inflatable craft**

X● V92.27 **Drowning and submersion due to being washed overboard from water-skis**
Excludes1 drowning and submersion due to fall off water-skis (V92.Ø7)

X● V92.28 **Drowning and submersion due to being washed overboard from other unpowered watercraft**
Drowning and submersion due to being washed overboard from surf-board
Drowning and submersion due to being washed overboard from windsurfer

X● V92.29 **Drowning and submersion due to being washed overboard from unspecified watercraft**
Drowning and submersion due to being washed overboard from boat NOS
Drowning and submersion due to being washed overboard from ship NOS
Drowning and submersion due to being washed overboard from watercraft NOS

● V93 **Other injury due to accident on board watercraft, without accident to watercraft**
Excludes1 civilian water transport accident involving military watercraft (V94.81-)
other injury due to accident to watercraft (V91.-)
military watercraft accident in military or war operations (Y36, Y37.-)
Excludes2 drowning and submersion due to accident on board watercraft, without accident to watercraft (V92.-)

The appropriate 7th character is to be added to each code from category V93

A	initial encounter
D	subsequent encounter
S	sequela

● V93.Ø **Burn due to localized fire on board watercraft**
Excludes1 burn due to watercraft on fire (V91.Ø-)

X● V93.ØØ **Burn due to localized fire on board merchant vessel**

X● V93.Ø1 **Burn due to localized fire on board passenger vessel**
Burn due to localized fire on board ferry-boat
Burn due to localized fire on board liner

X● V93.Ø2 **Burn due to localized fire on board fishing boat**

X● V93.Ø3 **Burn due to localized fire on board other powered watercraft**
Burn due to localized fire on board hovercraft
Burn due to localized fire on board jet ski

X● V93.Ø4 **Burn due to localized fire on board sailboat**

X● V93.Ø9 **Burn due to localized fire on board unspecified watercraft**
Burn due to localized fire on board boat NOS
Burn due to localized fire on board ship NOS
Burn due to localized fire on board watercraft NOS

● V93.1 **Other burn on board watercraft**
Burn due to source other than fire on board watercraft
Excludes1 burn due to watercraft on fire (V91.Ø-)

X● V93.1Ø **Other burn on board merchant vessel**

X● V93.11 **Other burn on board passenger vessel**
Other burn on board ferry-boat
Other burn on board liner

X● V93.12 **Other burn on board fishing boat**

X● V93.13 **Other burn on board other powered watercraft**
Other burn on board hovercraft
Other burn on board jet ski

X● V93.14 **Other burn on board sailboat**

X● V93.19 **Other burn on board unspecified watercraft**
Other burn on board boat NOS
Other burn on board ship NOS
Other burn on board watercraft NOS

● V93.2 **Heat exposure on board watercraft**
Excludes1 exposure to man-made heat not aboard watercraft (W92)
exposure to natural heat while on board watercraft (X3Ø)
exposure to sunlight while on board watercraft (X32)
Excludes2 burn due to fire on board watercraft (V93.Ø-)

X● V93.2Ø **Heat exposure on board merchant ship**

X● V93.21 **Heat exposure on board passenger ship**
Heat exposure on board ferry-boat
Heat exposure on board liner

X● V93.22 **Heat exposure on board fishing boat**

X● V93.23 **Heat exposure on board other powered watercraft**
Heat exposure on board hovercraft

X● V93.24 **Heat exposure on board sailboat**

X● V93.29 **Heat exposure on board unspecified watercraft**
Heat exposure on board boat NOS
Heat exposure on board ship NOS
Heat exposure on board watercraft NOS

V93.3 Fall on board watercraft

Excludes1 fall due to collision of watercraft (V91.2-)

X V93.30 **Fall on board merchant ship**

X V93.31 **Fall on board passenger ship**
Fall on board ferry-boat
Fall on board liner

X V93.32 **Fall on board fishing boat**

X V93.33 **Fall on board other powered watercraft**
Fall on board hovercraft (on open water)
Fall on board jet ski

X V93.34 **Fall on board sailboat**

X V93.35 **Fall on board canoe or kayak**

X V93.36 **Fall on board (nonpowered) inflatable craft**

X V93.38 **Fall on board other unpowered watercraft**

X V93.39 **Fall on board unspecified watercraft**
Fall on board boat NOS
Fall on board ship NOS
Fall on board watercraft NOS

V93.4 Struck by falling object on board watercraft
Hit by falling object on board watercraft

Excludes1 struck by falling object due to accident to watercraft (V91.3)

X V93.40 **Struck by falling object on merchant ship**

X V93.41 **Struck by falling object on passenger ship**
Struck by falling object on ferry-boat
Struck by falling object on liner

X V93.42 **Struck by falling object on fishing boat**

X V93.43 **Struck by falling object on other powered watercraft**
Struck by falling object on hovercraft

X V93.44 **Struck by falling object on sailboat**

X V93.48 **Struck by falling object on other unpowered watercraft**

X V93.49 **Struck by falling object on unspecified watercraft**

V93.5 Explosion on board watercraft
Boiler explosion on steamship

Excludes2 fire on board watercraft (V93.Ø-)

X V93.50 **Explosion on board merchant ship**

X V93.51 **Explosion on board passenger ship**
Explosion on board ferry-boat
Explosion on board liner

X V93.52 **Explosion on board fishing boat**

X V93.53 **Explosion on board other powered watercraft**
Explosion on board hovercraft
Explosion on board jet ski

X V93.54 **Explosion on board sailboat**

X V93.59 **Explosion on board unspecified watercraft**
Explosion on board boat NOS
Explosion on board ship NOS
Explosion on board watercraft NOS

V93.6 Machinery accident on board watercraft

Excludes1 machinery explosion on board watercraft (V93.4-)
machinery fire on board watercraft (V93.Ø-)

X V93.60 **Machinery accident on board merchant ship**

X V93.61 **Machinery accident on board passenger ship**
Machinery accident on board ferry-boat
Machinery accident on board liner

X V93.62 **Machinery accident on board fishing boat**

X V93.63 **Machinery accident on board other powered watercraft**
Machinery accident on board hovercraft

X V93.64 **Machinery accident on board sailboat**

X V93.69 **Machinery accident on board unspecified watercraft**
Machinery accident on board boat NOS
Machinery accident on board ship NOS
Machinery accident on board watercraft NOS

V93.8 Other injury due to other accident on board watercraft
Accidental poisoning by gases or fumes on watercraft

X V93.80 **Other injury due to other accident on board merchant ship**

X V93.81 **Other injury due to other accident on board passenger ship**
Other injury due to other accident on board ferry-boat
Other injury due to other accident on board liner

X V93.82 **Other injury due to other accident on board fishing boat**

X V93.83 **Other injury due to other accident on board other powered watercraft**
Other injury due to other accident on board hovercraft
Other injury due to other accident on board jet ski

X V93.84 **Other injury due to other accident on board sailboat**

X V93.85 **Other injury due to other accident on board canoe or kayak**

X V93.86 **Other injury due to other accident on board (nonpowered) inflatable craft**

X V93.87 **Other injury due to other accident on board water-skis**
Hit or struck by object while waterskiing

X V93.88 **Other injury due to other accident on board other unpowered watercraft**
Hit or struck by object while surfing
Hit or struck by object while on board windsurfer

X V93.89 **Other injury due to other accident on board unspecified watercraft**
Other injury due to other accident on board boat NOS
Other injury due to other accident on board ship NOS
Other injury due to other accident on board watercraft NOS

V94 Other and unspecified water transport accidents

Excludes1 military watercraft accidents in military or war operations (Y36, Y37)

The appropriate 7th character is to be added to each code from category V94

A	initial encounter
D	subsequent encounter
S	sequela

X V94.Ø **Hitting object or bottom of body of water due to fall from watercraft**

Excludes2 drowning and submersion due to fall from watercraft (V92.Ø-)

V94.1 Bather struck by watercraft
Swimmer hit by watercraft

X V94.11 **Bather struck by powered watercraft**

X V94.12 **Bather struck by nonpowered watercraft**

V94.2 Rider of nonpowered watercraft struck by other watercraft

X V94.21 **Rider of nonpowered watercraft struck by other nonpowered watercraft**
Canoer hit by other nonpowered watercraft
Surfer hit by other nonpowered watercraft
Windsurfer hit by other nonpowered watercraft

X V94.22 **Rider of nonpowered watercraft struck by powered watercraft**
Canoer hit by motorboat
Surfer hit by motorboat
Windsurfer hit by motorboat

● V94.3 Injury to rider of (inflatable) watercraft being pulled behind other watercraft
X● V94.31 Injury to rider of (inflatable) recreational watercraft being pulled behind other watercraft
Injury to rider of inner-tube pulled behind motor boat
X● V94.32 Injury to rider of non-recreational watercraft being pulled behind other watercraft
Injury to occupant of dingy being pulled behind boat or ship
Injury to occupant of life-raft being pulled behind boat or ship
X● V94.4 Injury to barefoot water-skier
Injury to person being pulled behind boat or ship
● V94.8 Other water transport accident
● V94.81 Water transport accident involving military watercraft
● V94.810 Civilian watercraft involved in water transport accident with military watercraft
Passenger on civilian watercraft injured due to accident with military watercraft
● V94.811 Civilian in water injured by military watercraft
● V94.818 Other water transport accident involving military watercraft
X● V94.89 Other water transport accident
X● V94.9 Unspecified water transport accident
Water transport accident NOS

AIR AND SPACE TRANSPORT ACCIDENTS (V95-V97)

Excludes1 military aircraft accidents in military or war operations (Y36, Y37)

● V95 Accident to powered aircraft causing injury to occupant
The appropriate 7th character is to be added to each code from category V95

A	initial encounter
D	subsequent encounter
S	sequela

● V95.0 Helicopter accident injuring occupant
X● V95.00 Unspecified helicopter accident injuring occupant
X● V95.01 Helicopter crash injuring occupant
X● V95.02 Forced landing of helicopter injuring occupant
X● V95.03 Helicopter collision injuring occupant
Helicopter collision with any object, fixed, movable or moving
X● V95.04 Helicopter fire injuring occupant
X● V95.05 Helicopter explosion injuring occupant
X● V95.09 Other helicopter accident injuring occupant
● V95.1 Ultralight, microlight or powered-glider accident injuring occupant
X● V95.10 Unspecified ultralight, microlight or powered-glider accident injuring occupant
X● V95.11 Ultralight, microlight or powered-glider crash injuring occupant
X● V95.12 Forced landing of ultralight, microlight or powered-glider injuring occupant
X● V95.13 Ultralight, microlight or powered-glider collision injuring occupant
Ultralight, microlight or powered-glider collision with any object, fixed, movable or moving
X● V95.14 Ultralight, microlight or powered-glider fire injuring occupant
X● V95.15 Ultralight, microlight or powered-glider explosion injuring occupant
X● V95.19 Other ultralight, microlight or powered-glider accident injuring occupant
● V95.2 Other private fixed-wing aircraft accident injuring occupant
X● V95.20 Unspecified accident to other private fixed-wing aircraft, injuring occupant
X● V95.21 Other private fixed-wing aircraft crash injuring occupant
X● V95.22 Forced landing of other private fixed-wing aircraft injuring occupant
X● V95.23 Other private fixed-wing aircraft collision injuring occupant
Other private fixed-wing aircraft collision with any object, fixed, movable or moving
X● V95.24 Other private fixed-wing aircraft fire injuring occupant
X● V95.25 Other private fixed-wing aircraft explosion injuring occupant
X● V95.29 Other accident to other private fixed-wing aircraft injuring occupant
● V95.3 Commercial fixed-wing aircraft accident injuring occupant
X● V95.30 Unspecified accident to commercial fixed-wing aircraft injuring occupant
X● V95.31 Commercial fixed-wing aircraft crash injuring occupant
X● V95.32 Forced landing of commercial fixed-wing aircraft injuring occupant
X● V95.33 Commercial fixed-wing aircraft collision injuring occupant
Commercial fixed-wing aircraft collision with any object, fixed, movable or moving
X● V95.34 Commercial fixed-wing aircraft fire injuring occupant
X● V95.35 Commercial fixed-wing aircraft explosion injuring occupant
X● V95.39 Other accident to commercial fixed-wing aircraft injuring occupant
● V95.4 Spacecraft accident injuring occupant
X● V95.40 Unspecified spacecraft accident injuring occupant
X● V95.41 Spacecraft crash injuring occupant
X● V95.42 Forced landing of spacecraft injuring occupant
X● V95.43 Spacecraft collision injuring occupant
Spacecraft collision with any object, fixed, moveable or moving
X● V95.44 Spacecraft fire injuring occupant
X● V95.45 Spacecraft explosion injuring occupant
X● V95.49 Other spacecraft accident injuring occupant
X● V95.8 Other powered aircraft accidents injuring occupant
X● V95.9 Unspecified aircraft accident injuring occupant
Aircraft accident NOS
Air transport accident NOS

V96 Accident to nonpowered aircraft causing injury to occupant
The appropriate 7th character is to be added to each code from category V96

A	initial encounter
D	subsequent encounter
S	sequela

V96.0 Balloon accident injuring occupant
X **V96.00 Unspecified balloon accident injuring occupant**
X **V96.01 Balloon crash injuring occupant**
X **V96.02 Forced landing of balloon injuring occupant**
X **V96.03 Balloon collision injuring occupant**
Balloon collision with any object, fixed, moveable or moving
X **V96.04 Balloon fire injuring occupant**
X **V96.05 Balloon explosion injuring occupant**
X **V96.09 Other balloon accident injuring occupant**
V96.1 Hang-glider accident injuring occupant
X **V96.10 Unspecified hang-glider accident injuring occupant**
X **V96.11 Hang-glider crash injuring occupant**
X **V96.12 Forced landing of hang-glider injuring occupant**
X **V96.13 Hang-glider collision injuring occupant**
Hang-glider collision with any object, fixed, moveable or moving
X **V96.14 Hang-glider fire injuring occupant**
X **V96.15 Hang-glider explosion injuring occupant**
X **V96.19 Other hang-glider accident injuring occupant**
V96.2 Glider (nonpowered) accident injuring occupant
X **V96.20 Unspecified glider (nonpowered) accident injuring occupant**
X **V96.21 Glider (nonpowered) crash injuring occupant**
X **V96.22 Forced landing of glider (nonpowered) injuring occupant**
X **V96.23 Glider (nonpowered) collision injuring occupant**
Glider (nonpowered) collision with any object, fixed, moveable or moving
X **V96.24 Glider (nonpowered) fire injuring occupant**
X **V96.25 Glider (nonpowered) explosion injuring occupant**
X **V96.29 Other glider (nonpowered) accident injuring occupant**
X **V96.8 Other nonpowered-aircraft accidents injuring occupant**
Kite carrying a person accident injuring occupant
X **V96.9 Unspecified nonpowered-aircraft accident injuring occupant**
Nonpowered-aircraft accident NOS

V97 Other specified air transport accidents
The appropriate 7th character is to be added to each code from category V97

A	initial encounter
D	subsequent encounter
S	sequela

X **V97.0 Occupant of aircraft injured in other specified air transport accidents**
Fall in, on or from aircraft in air transport accident
Excludes1 accident while boarding or alighting aircraft (V97.1)
X **V97.1 Person injured while boarding or alighting from aircraft**
V97.2 Parachutist accident
X **V97.21 Parachutist entangled in object**
Parachutist landing in tree
X **V97.22 Parachutist injured on landing**
X **V97.29 Other parachutist accident**
V97.3 Person on ground injured in air transport accident
X **V97.31 Hit by object falling from aircraft**
Hit by crashing aircraft
Injured by aircraft hitting house
Injured by aircraft hitting car
X **V97.32 Injured by rotating propeller**
X **V97.33 Sucked into jet engine**
X **V97.39 Other injury to person on ground due to air transport accident**
V97.8 Other air transport accidents, not elsewhere classified
Excludes1 aircraft accident NOS (V95.9)
exposure to changes in air pressure during ascent or descent (W94.-)
V97.81 Air transport accident involving military aircraft
V97.810 Civilian aircraft involved in air transport accident with military aircraft
Passenger in civilian aircraft injured due to accident with military aircraft
V97.811 Civilian injured by military aircraft
V97.818 Other air transport accident involving military aircraft
X **V97.89 Other air transport accidents, not elsewhere classified**
Injury from machinery on aircraft

OTHER AND UNSPECIFIED TRANSPORT ACCIDENTS (V98-V99)

Excludes1 vehicle accident, type of vehicle unspecified (V89.-)

V98 Other specified transport accidents
The appropriate 7th character is to be added to each code from category V98

A	initial encounter
D	subsequent encounter
S	sequela

X **V98.0 Accident to, on or involving cable-car, not on rails**
Caught or dragged by cable-car, not on rails
Fall or jump from cable-car, not on rails
Object thrown from or in cable-car, not on rails
X **V98.1 Accident to, on or involving land-yacht**
X **V98.2 Accident to, on or involving ice yacht**
X **V98.3 Accident to, on or involving ski lift**
Accident to, on or involving ski chair-lift
Accident to, on or involving ski-lift with gondola
X **V98.8 Other specified transport accidents**

X **V99 Unspecified transport accident**
The appropriate 7th character is to be added to code V99

A	initial encounter
D	subsequent encounter
S	sequela

CHAPTER 20 (V00-Y99)

OTHER EXTERNAL CAUSES OF ACCIDENTAL INJURY (W00-X58)

SLIPPING, TRIPPING, STUMBLING AND FALLS (W00-W19)

Excludes1 assault involving a fall (Y01-Y02)
fall from animal (V80.-)
fall (in) (from) machinery (in operation) (W28-W31)
fall (in) (from) transport vehicle (V01-V99)
intentional self-harm involving a fall (X80-X81)

Excludes2 at risk for fall (history of fall) Z91.81
fall (in) (from) burning building (X00.-)
fall into fire (X00-X04, X08)

● **W00 Fall due to ice and snow**

Includes pedestrian on foot falling (slipping) on ice and snow

Excludes1 fall on (from) ice and snow involving pedestrian conveyance (V00.-)
fall from stairs and steps not due to ice and snow (W10.-)

The appropriate 7th character is to be added to each code from category W00

A	initial encounter
D	subsequent encounter
S	sequela

X● **W00.0 Fall on same level due to ice and snow**
Coding Clinic: 2016, Q2, P5

X● **W00.1 Fall from stairs and steps due to ice and snow**

X● **W00.2 Other fall from one level to another due to ice and snow**

X● **W00.9 Unspecified fall due to ice and snow**

● **W01 Fall on same level from slipping, tripping and stumbling**

Includes fall on moving sidewalk

Excludes1 fall due to bumping (striking) against object (W18.0-)
fall in shower or bathtub (W18.2-)
fall on same level NOS (W18.30)
fall on same level from slipping, tripping and stumbling due to ice or snow (W00.0)
fall off or from toilet (W18.1-)
slipping, tripping and stumbling NOS (W18.40)
slipping, tripping and stumbling without falling (W18.4-)

The appropriate 7th character is to be added to each code from category W01

A	initial encounter
D	subsequent encounter
S	sequela

X● **W01.0 Fall on same level from slipping, tripping and stumbling without subsequent striking against object**
Falling over animal

● **W01.1 Fall on same level from slipping, tripping and stumbling with subsequent striking against object**

X● **W01.10 Fall on same level from slipping, tripping and stumbling with subsequent striking against unspecified object**

● **W01.11 Fall on same level from slipping, tripping and stumbling with subsequent striking against sharp object**

● **W01.110 Fall on same level from slipping, tripping and stumbling with subsequent striking against sharp glass**

● **W01.111 Fall on same level from slipping, tripping and stumbling with subsequent striking against power tool or machine**

● **W01.118 Fall on same level from slipping, tripping and stumbling with subsequent striking against other sharp object**

● **W01.119 Fall on same level from slipping, tripping and stumbling with subsequent striking against unspecified sharp object**

● **W01.19 Fall on same level from slipping, tripping and stumbling with subsequent striking against other object**

● **W01.190 Fall on same level from slipping, tripping and stumbling with subsequent striking against furniture**

● **W01.198 Fall on same level from slipping, tripping and stumbling with subsequent striking against other object**

X● **W03 Other fall on same level due to collision with another person**
Fall due to non-transport collision with other person

Excludes1 collision with another person without fall (W51)
crushed or pushed by a crowd or human stampede (W52)
fall involving pedestrian conveyance (V00-V09)
fall due to ice or snow (W00)
fall on same level NOS (W18.30)

The appropriate 7th character is to be added to code W03

A	initial encounter
D	subsequent encounter
S	sequela

Coding Clinic: 2015, Q1, P9-10; 2012, Q4, P108

X● **W04 Fall while being carried or supported by other persons**
Accidentally dropped while being carried

The appropriate 7th character is to be added to code W04

A	initial encounter
D	subsequent encounter
S	sequel

● **W05 Fall from non-moving wheelchair, nonmotorized scooter and motorized mobility scooter**

Excludes1 fall from moving wheelchair (powered) (V00.811)
fall from moving motorized mobility scooter (V00.831)
fall from nonmotorized scooter (V00.141)

The appropriate 7th character is to be added to each code from category W05

A	initial encounter
D	subsequent encounter
S	sequela

X● **W05.0 Fall from non-moving wheelchair**
Coding Clinic: 2019, Q2, P27

X● **W05.1 Fall from non-moving nonmotorized scooter**

X● **W05.2 Fall from non-moving motorized mobility scooter**

X● **W06 Fall from bed**

The appropriate 7th character is to be added to code W06

A	initial encounter
D	subsequent encounter
S	sequela

X● **W07 Fall from chair**

The appropriate 7th character is to be added to code W07

A	initial encounter
D	subsequent encounter
S	sequela

X● W08 **Fall from other furniture**

The appropriate 7th character is to be added to code W08

A	initial encounter
D	subsequent encounter
S	sequela

● W09 **Fall on and from playground equipment**

Excludes1 fall involving recreational machinery (W31)

The appropriate 7th character is to be added to each code from category W09

A	initial encounter
D	subsequent encounter
S	sequela

X● W09.0 **Fall on or from playground slide**

X● W09.1 **Fall from playground swing**

X● W09.2 **Fall on or from jungle gym**

X● W09.8 **Fall on or from other playground equipment**

● W10 **Fall on and from stairs and steps**

Excludes1 fall from stairs and steps due to ice and snow (W00.1)

The appropriate 7th character is to be added to each code from category W10

A	initial encounter
D	subsequent encounter
S	sequela

X● W10.0 **Fall (on) (from) escalator**

X● W10.1 **Fall (on) (from) sidewalk curb**

X● W10.2 **Fall (on) (from) incline**

Fall (on) (from) ramp

X● W10.8 **Fall (on) (from) other stairs and steps**

X● W10.9 **Fall (on) (from) unspecified stairs and steps**

X● W11 **Fall on and from ladder**

The appropriate 7th character is to be added to code W11

A	initial encounter
D	subsequent encounter
S	sequela

X● W12 **Fall on and from scaffolding**

The appropriate 7th character is to be added to code W12

A	initial encounter
D	subsequent encounter
S	sequela

● W13 **Fall from, out of or through building or structure**

The appropriate 7th character is to be added to each code from category W13

A	initial encounter
D	subsequent encounter
S	sequela

X● W13.0 **Fall from, out of or through balcony**

Fall from, out of or through railing

X● W13.1 **Fall from, out of or through bridge**

X● W13.2 **Fall from, out of or through roof**

X● W13.3 **Fall through floor**

X● W13.4 **Fall from, out of or through window**

Excludes2 fall with subsequent striking against sharp glass (W01.110)

X● W13.8 **Fall from, out of or through other building or structure**

Fall from, out of or through viaduct
Fall from, out of or through wall
Fall from, out of or through flag-pole

X● W13.9 **Fall from, out of or through building, not otherwise specified**

Excludes1 collapse of a building or structure (W20.-)
fall or jump from burning building or structure (X00.-)

X● W14 **Fall from tree**

The appropriate 7th character is to be added to code W14

A	initial encounter
D	subsequent encounter
S	sequela

X● W15 **Fall from cliff**

The appropriate 7th character is to be added to code W15

A	initial encounter
D	subsequent encounter
S	sequela

● W16 **Fall, jump or diving into water**

Excludes1 accidental non-watercraft drowning and submersion not involving fall (W65-W74)
effects of air pressure from diving (W94.-)
fall into water from watercraft (V90-V94)
hitting an object or against bottom when falling from watercraft (V94.0)

Excludes2 striking or hitting diving board (W21.4)

The appropriate 7th character is to be added to each code from category W16

A	initial encounter
D	subsequent encounter
S	sequela

● W16.0 **Fall into swimming pool**

Fall into swimming pool NOS

Excludes1 fall into empty swimming pool (W17.3)

● W16.01 **Fall into swimming pool striking water surface**

● W16.011 **Fall into swimming pool striking water surface causing drowning and submersion**

Excludes1 drowning and submersion while in swimming pool without fall (W67)

● W16.012 **Fall into swimming pool striking water surface causing other injury**

CHAPTER 20 (V00-Y99)

W16.02 **Fall into swimming pool striking bottom**

W16.021 **Fall into swimming pool striking bottom causing drowning and submersion**

Excludes1 drowning and submersion while in swimming pool without fall (W67)

W16.022 **Fall into swimming pool striking bottom causing other injury**

W16.03 **Fall into swimming pool striking wall**

W16.031 **Fall into swimming pool striking wall causing drowning and submersion**

Excludes1 drowning and submersion while in swimming pool without fall (W67)

W16.032 **Fall into swimming pool striking wall causing other injury**

W16.1 **Fall into natural body of water**

Fall into lake
Fall into open sea
Fall into river
Fall into stream

W16.11 **Fall into natural body of water striking water surface**

W16.111 **Fall into natural body of water striking water surface causing drowning and submersion**

Excludes1 drowning and submersion while in natural body of water without fall (W69)

W16.112 **Fall into natural body of water striking water surface causing other injury**

W16.12 **Fall into natural body of water striking bottom**

W16.121 **Fall into natural body of water striking bottom causing drowning and submersion**

Excludes1 drowning and submersion while in natural body of water without fall (W69)

W16.122 **Fall into natural body of water striking bottom causing other injury**

W16.13 **Fall into natural body of water striking side**

W16.131 **Fall into natural body of water striking side causing drowning and submersion**

Excludes1 drowning and submersion while in natural body of water without fall (W69)

W16.132 **Fall into natural body of water striking side causing other injury**

W16.2 **Fall in (into) filled bathtub or bucket of water**

W16.21 **Fall in (into) filled bathtub**

Excludes1 fall into empty bathtub (W18.2)

W16.211 **Fall in (into) filled bathtub causing drowning and submersion**

Excludes1 drowning and submersion while in filled bathtub without fall (W65)

W16.212 **Fall in (into) filled bathtub causing other injury**

W16.22 **Fall in (into) bucket of water**

W16.221 **Fall in (into) bucket of water causing drowning and submersion**

W16.222 **Fall in (into) bucket of water causing other injury**

W16.3 **Fall into other water**

Fall into fountain
Fall into reservoir

W16.31 **Fall into other water striking water surface**

W16.311 **Fall into other water striking water surface causing drowning and submersion**

Excludes1 drowning and submersion while in other water without fall (W73)

W16.312 **Fall into other water striking water surface causing other injury**

W16.32 **Fall into other water striking bottom**

W16.321 **Fall into other water striking bottom causing drowning and submersion**

Excludes1 drowning and submersion while in other water without fall (W73)

W16.322 **Fall into other water striking bottom causing other injury**

W16.33 **Fall into other water striking wall**

W16.331 **Fall into other water striking wall causing drowning and submersion**

Excludes1 drowning and submersion while in other water without fall (W73)

W16.332 **Fall into other water striking wall causing other injury**

W16.4 **Fall into unspecified water**

X W16.41 **Fall into unspecified water causing drowning and submersion**

X W16.42 **Fall into unspecified water causing other injury**

W16.5 **Jumping or diving into swimming pool**

W16.51 **Jumping or diving into swimming pool striking water surface**

W16.511 **Jumping or diving into swimming pool striking water surface causing drowning and submersion**

Excludes1 drowning and submersion while in swimming pool without jumping or diving (W67)

W16.512 **Jumping or diving into swimming pool striking water surface causing other injury**

W16.52 **Jumping or diving into swimming pool striking bottom**

W16.521 **Jumping or diving into swimming pool striking bottom causing drowning and submersion**

Excludes1 drowning and submersion while in swimming pool without jumping or diving (W67)

W16.522 **Jumping or diving into swimming pool striking bottom causing other injury**

● **W16.53** **Jumping or diving into swimming pool striking wall**

● **W16.531** **Jumping or diving into swimming pool striking wall causing drowning and submersion**

Excludes1 drowning and submersion while in swimming pool without jumping or diving (W67)

● **W16.532** **Jumping or diving into swimming pool striking wall causing other injury**

● **W16.6** **Jumping or diving into natural body of water**

Jumping or diving into lake
Jumping or diving into open sea
Jumping or diving into river
Jumping or diving into stream

● **W16.61** **Jumping or diving into natural body of water striking water surface**

● **W16.611** **Jumping or diving into natural body of water striking water surface causing drowning and submersion**

Excludes1 drowning and submersion while in natural body of water without jumping or diving (W69)

● **W16.612** **Jumping or diving into natural body of water striking water surface causing other injury**

● **W16.62** **Jumping or diving into natural body of water striking bottom**

● **W16.621** **Jumping or diving into natural body of water striking bottom causing drowning and submersion**

Excludes1 drowning and submersion while in natural body of water without jumping or diving (W69)

● **W16.622** **Jumping or diving into natural body of water striking bottom causing other injury**

● **W16.7** **Jumping or diving from boat**

Excludes1 fall from boat into water - see watercraft accident (V9Ø-V94)

● **W16.71** **Jumping or diving from boat striking water surface**

● **W16.711** **Jumping or diving from boat striking water surface causing drowning and submersion**

● **W16.712** **Jumping or diving from boat striking water surface causing other injury**

● **W16.72** **Jumping or diving from boat striking bottom**

● **W16.721** **Jumping or diving from boat striking bottom causing drowning and submersion**

● **W16.722** **Jumping or diving from boat striking bottom causing other injury**

● **W16.8** **Jumping or diving into other water**

Jumping or diving into fountain
Jumping or diving into reservoir

● **W16.81** **Jumping or diving into other water striking water surface**

● **W16.811** **Jumping or diving into other water striking water surface causing drowning and submersion**

Excludes1 drowning and submersion while in other water without jumping or diving (W73)

● **W16.812** **Jumping or diving into other water striking water surface causing other injury**

● **W16.82** **Jumping or diving into other water striking bottom**

● **W16.821** **Jumping or diving into other water striking bottom causing drowning and submersion**

Excludes1 drowning and submersion while in other water without jumping or diving (W73)

● **W16.822** **Jumping or diving into other water striking bottom causing other injury**

● **W16.83** **Jumping or diving into other water striking wall**

● **W16.831** **Jumping or diving into other water striking wall causing drowning and submersion**

Excludes1 drowning and submersion while in other water without jumping or diving (W73)

● **W16.832** **Jumping or diving into other water striking wall causing other injury**

● **W16.9** **Jumping or diving into unspecified water**

X● **W16.91** **Jumping or diving into unspecified water causing drowning and submersion**

X● **W16.92** **Jumping or diving into unspecified water causing other injury**

● **W17** **Other fall from one level to another**

The appropriate 7th character is to be added to each code from category W17

A	initial encounter
D	subsequent encounter
S	sequela

X● **W17.Ø** **Fall into well**

X● **W17.1** **Fall into storm drain or manhole**

X● **W17.2** **Fall into hole**

Fall into pit

X● **W17.3** **Fall into empty swimming pool**

Excludes1 fall into filled swimming pool (W16.Ø-)

X● **W17.4** **Fall from dock**

● **W17.8** **Other fall from one level to another**

X● **W17.81** **Fall down embankment (hill)**

X● **W17.82** **Fall from (out of) grocery cart**

Fall due to grocery cart tipping over

X● **W17.89** **Other fall from one level to another**

Fall from cherry picker
Fall from lifting device
Fall from mobile elevated work platform [MEWP]
Fall from sky lift

Coding Clinic: 2Ø15, Q2, P6

CHAPTER 2Ø (VØØ-Y99)

● **W18 Other slipping, tripping and stumbling and falls**

The appropriate 7th character is to be added to each code from category W18

A	initial encounter
D	subsequent encounter
S	sequela

● **W18.0 Fall due to bumping against object**

Striking against object with subsequent fall

Excludes1 fall on same level due to slipping, tripping, or stumbling with subsequent striking against object (W01.1-)

X● **W18.00 Striking against unspecified object with subsequent fall**

X● **W18.01 Striking against sports equipment with subsequent fall**

X● **W18.02 Striking against glass with subsequent fall**

X● **W18.09 Striking against other object with subsequent fall**

● **W18.1 Fall from or off toilet**

X● **W18.11 Fall from or off toilet without subsequent striking against object**

Fall from (off) toilet NOS

X● **W18.12 Fall from or off toilet with subsequent striking against object**

X● **W18.2 Fall in (into) shower or empty bathtub**

Excludes1 fall in full bathtub causing drowning or submersion (W16.21-)

● **W18.3 Other and unspecified fall on same level**

X● **W18.30 Fall on same level, unspecified**

X● **W18.31 Fall on same level due to stepping on an object**

Fall on same level due to stepping on an animal

Excludes1 slipping, tripping and stumbling without fall due to stepping on animal (W18.41)

X● **W18.39 Other fall on same level**

● **W18.4 Slipping, tripping and stumbling without falling**

Excludes1 collision with another person without fall (W51)

X● **W18.40 Slipping, tripping and stumbling without falling, unspecified**

X● **W18.41 Slipping, tripping and stumbling without falling due to stepping on object**

Slipping, tripping and stumbling without falling due to stepping on animal

Excludes1 slipping, tripping and stumbling with fall due to stepping on animal (W18.31)

X● **W18.42 Slipping, tripping and stumbling without falling due to stepping into hole or opening**

X● **W18.43 Slipping, tripping and stumbling without falling due to stepping from one level to another**

X● **W18.49 Other slipping, tripping and stumbling without falling**

X● **W19 Unspecified fall**

Accidental fall NOS

The appropriate 7th character is to be added to code W19

A	initial encounter
D	subsequent encounter
S	sequela

Coding Clinic: 2012, Q4, P95

EXPOSURE TO INANIMATE MECHANICAL FORCES (W20-W49)

Excludes1 assault (X92-Y09)
contact or collision with animals or persons (W50-W64)
exposure to inanimate mechanical forces involving military or war operations (Y36.-, Y37.-)
intentional self-harm (X71-X83)

Coding Clinic: 2016, Q4, P129

● **W20 Struck by thrown, projected or falling object**

Code first any associated:
cataclysm (X34-X39)
lightning strike (T75.00)

Excludes1 falling object in machinery accident (W24, W28-W31)
falling object in transport accident (V01-V99)
object set in motion by explosion (W35-W40)
object set in motion by firearm (W32-W34)
struck by thrown sports equipment (W21.-)

The appropriate 7th character is to be added to each code from category W20

A	initial encounter
D	subsequent encounter
S	sequela

X● **W20.0 Struck by falling object in cave-in**

Excludes2 asphyxiation due to cave-in (T71.21)

X● **W20.1 Struck by object due to collapse of building**

Excludes1 struck by object due to collapse of burning building (X00.2, X02.2)

X● **W20.8 Other cause of strike by thrown, projected or falling object**

Excludes1 struck by thrown sports equipment (W21.-)

● **W21 Striking against or struck by sports equipment**

Excludes1 assault with sports equipment (Y08.0-)
striking against or struck by sports equipment with subsequent fall (W18.01)

The appropriate 7th character is to be added to each code from category W21

A	initial encounter
D	subsequent encounter
S	sequela

● **W21.0 Struck by hit or thrown ball**

X● **W21.00 Struck by hit or thrown ball, unspecified type**

X● **W21.01 Struck by football**

X● **W21.02 Struck by soccer ball**

X● **W21.03 Struck by baseball**

X● **W21.04 Struck by golf ball**

X● **W21.05 Struck by basketball**

X● **W21.06 Struck by volleyball**

X● **W21.07 Struck by softball**

X● **W21.09 Struck by other hit or thrown ball**

● **W21.1 Struck by bat, racquet or club**

X● **W21.11 Struck by baseball bat**

X● **W21.12 Struck by tennis racquet**

X● **W21.13 Struck by golf club**

X● **W21.19 Struck by other bat, racquet or club**

● **W21.2 Struck by hockey stick or puck**

● **W21.21 Struck by hockey stick**

● **W21.210 Struck by ice hockey stick**

● **W21.211 Struck by field hockey stick**

● **W21.22 Struck by hockey puck**

● **W21.220 Struck by ice hockey puck**

● **W21.221 Struck by field hockey puck**

W21.3 Struck by sports foot wear

X **W21.31 Struck by shoe cleats**

Stepped on by shoe cleats

X **W21.32 Struck by skate blades**

Skated over by skate blades

X **W21.39 Struck by other sports foot wear**

X **W21.4 Striking against diving board**

Use additional code for subsequent falling into water, if applicable (W16.-)

W21.8 Striking against or struck by other sports equipment

X **W21.81 Striking against or struck by football helmet**

X **W21.89 Striking against or struck by other sports equipment**

X **W21.9 Striking against or struck by unspecified sports equipment**

W22 Striking against or struck by other objects

Excludes1 striking against or struck by object with subsequent fall (W18.Ø9)

The appropriate 7th character is to be added to each code from category W22

A	initial encounter
D	subsequent encounter
S	sequela

W22.Ø Striking against stationary object

Excludes1 striking against stationary sports equipment (W21.8)

X **W22.Ø1 Walked into wall**

X **W22.Ø2 Walked into lamppost**

X **W22.Ø3 Walked into furniture**

W22.Ø4 Striking against wall of swimming pool

W22.Ø41 Striking against wall of swimming pool causing drowning and submersion

Excludes1 drowning and submersion while swimming without striking against wall (W67)

W22.Ø42 Striking against wall of swimming pool causing other injury

X **W22.Ø9 Striking against other stationary object**

W22.1 Striking against or struck by automobile airbag

X **W22.1Ø Striking against or struck by unspecified automobile airbag**

X **W22.11 Striking against or struck by driver side automobile airbag**

X **W22.12 Striking against or struck by front passenger side automobile airbag**

X **W22.19 Striking against or struck by other automobile airbag**

X **W22.8 Striking against or struck by other objects**

Striking against or struck by object NOS

Excludes1 struck by thrown, projected or falling object (W2Ø.-)

W23 Caught, crushed, jammed or pinched in or between objects

Excludes1 injury caused by cutting or piercing instruments (W25-W27)
injury caused by firearms malfunction (W32.1, W33.1-, W34.1-)
injury caused by lifting and transmission devices (W24.-)
injury caused by machinery (W28-W31)
injury caused by nonpowered hand tools (W27.-)
injury caused by transport vehicle being used as a means of transportation (VØ1-V99)
injury caused by struck by thrown, projected or falling object (W2Ø.-)

The appropriate 7th character is to be added to each code from category W23

A	initial encounter
D	subsequent encounter
S	sequela

X **W23.Ø Caught, crushed, jammed, or pinched between moving objects**

X **W23.1 Caught, crushed, jammed, or pinched between stationary objects**

W24 Contact with lifting and transmission devices, not elsewhere classified

Excludes1 transport accidents (VØ1-V99)

The appropriate 7th character is to be added to each code from category W24

A	initial encounter
D	subsequent encounter
S	sequela

X **W24.Ø Contact with lifting devices, not elsewhere classified**

Contact with chain hoist
Contact with drive belt
Contact with pulley (block)

X **W24.1 Contact with transmission devices, not elsewhere classified**

Contact with transmission belt or cable

X **W25 Contact with sharp glass**

Code first any associated:
injury due to flying glass from explosion or firearm discharge (W32-W4Ø)
transport accident (VØØ-V99)

Excludes1 fall on same level due to slipping, tripping and stumbling with subsequent striking against sharp glass (WØ1.11Ø)
striking against sharp glass with subsequent fall (W18.Ø2)

Excludes2 glass embedded in skin (W45)

The appropriate 7th character is to be added to code W25

A	initial encounter
D	subsequent encounter
S	sequela

● W26 Contact with other sharp objects

Excludes2 sharp object(s) embedded in skin (W45)

The appropriate 7th character is to be added to each code from category W26

A initial encounter
D subsequent encounter
S sequela

Coding Clinic: 2016, Q4, P73

X● W26.0 Contact with knife

Excludes1 contact with electric knife (W29.1)

X● W26.1 Contact with sword or dagger

X● W26.2 Contact with edge of stiff paper

Paper cut

Coding Clinic: 2016, Q4, P73

X● W26.8 Contact with other sharp object(s), not elsewhere classified

Contact with tin can lid

Coding Clinic: 2016, Q4, P73

X● W26.9 Contact with unspecified sharp object(s)

Coding Clinic: 2016, Q4, P73

● W27 Contact with nonpowered hand tool

The appropriate 7th character is to be added to each code from category W27

A initial encounter
D subsequent encounter
S sequela

X● W27.0 Contact with workbench tool

Contact with auger
Contact with axe
Contact with chisel
Contact with handsaw
Contact with screwdriver

X● W27.1 Contact with garden tool

Contact with hoe
Contact with nonpowered lawn mower
Contact with pitchfork
Contact with rake

X● W27.2 Contact with scissors

X● W27.3 Contact with needle (sewing)

Excludes1 contact with hypodermic needle (W46.-)

X● W27.4 Contact with kitchen utensil

Contact with fork
Contact with ice-pick
Contact with can-opener NOS

X● W27.5 Contact with paper-cutter

X● W27.8 Contact with other nonpowered hand tool

Contact with nonpowered sewing machine
Contact with shovel

X● W28 Contact with powered lawn mower

Powered lawn mower (commercial) (residential)

Excludes1 contact with nonpowered lawn mower (W27.1)

Excludes2 exposure to electric current (W86.-)

The appropriate 7th character is to be added to code W28

A initial encounter
D subsequent encounter
S sequela

● W29 Contact with other powered hand tools and household machinery

Excludes1 contact with commercial machinery (W31.82)
contact with hot household appliance (X15)
contact with nonpowered hand tool (W27.-)
exposure to electric current (W86)

The appropriate 7th character is to be added to each code from category W29

A initial encounter
D subsequent encounter
S sequela

X● W29.0 Contact with powered kitchen appliance

Contact with blender
Contact with can-opener
Contact with garbage disposal
Contact with mixer

X● W29.1 Contact with electric knife

X● W29.2 Contact with other powered household machinery

Contact with electric fan
Contact with powered dryer (clothes) (powered) (spin)
Contact with washing-machine
Contact with sewing machine

X● W29.3 Contact with powered garden and outdoor hand tools and machinery

Contact with chainsaw
Contact with edger
Contact with garden cultivator (tiller)
Contact with hedge trimmer
Contact with other powered garden tool

Excludes1 contact with powered lawn mower (W28)

X● W29.4 Contact with nail gun

X● W29.8 Contact with other powered hand tools and household machinery

Contact with do-it-yourself tool NOS

● W30 Contact with agricultural machinery

Includes animal-powered farm machine

Excludes1 agricultural transport vehicle accident (V01-V99)
explosion of grain store (W40.8)
exposure to electric current (W86.-)

The appropriate 7th character is to be added to each code from category W30

A initial encounter
D subsequent encounter
S sequela

X● W30.0 Contact with combine harvester

Contact with reaper
Contact with thresher

X● W30.1 Contact with power take-off devices (PTO)

X● W30.2 Contact with hay derrick

X● W30.3 Contact with grain storage elevator

Excludes1 explosion of grain store (W40.8)

● W30.8 Contact with other specified agricultural machinery

X● W30.81 Contact with agricultural transport vehicle in stationary use

Contact with agricultural transport vehicle under repair, not on public roadway

Excludes1 agricultural transport vehicle accident (V01-V99)

X● W30.89 Contact with other specified agricultural machinery

X● W30.9 Contact with unspecified agricultural machinery

Contact with farm machinery NOS

CHAPTER 20 (V00-Y99)

W31 Contact with other and unspecified machinery

Excludes1 contact with agricultural machinery (W3Ø.-)
contact with machinery in transport under own power or being towed by a vehicle (VØ1-V99)
exposure to electric current (W86)

The appropriate 7th character is to be added to each code from category W31

A	initial encounter
D	subsequent encounter
S	sequela

X **W31.Ø Contact with mining and earth-drilling machinery**
Contact with bore or drill (land) (seabed)
Contact with shaft hoist
Contact with shaft lift
Contact with undercutter

X **W31.1 Contact with metalworking machines**
Contact with abrasive wheel
Contact with forging machine
Contact with lathe
Contact with mechanical shears
Contact with metal drilling machine
Contact with milling machine
Contact with power press
Contact with rolling-mill
Contact with metal sawing machine

X **W31.2 Contact with powered woodworking and forming machines**
Contact with band saw
Contact with bench saw
Contact with circular saw
Contact with molding machine
Contact with overhead plane
Contact with powered saw
Contact with radial saw
Contact with sander

Excludes1 nonpowered woodworking tools (W27.Ø)

X **W31.3 Contact with prime movers**
Contact with gas turbine
Contact with internal combustion engine
Contact with steam engine
Contact with water driven turbine

W31.8 Contact with other specified machinery

X **W31.81 Contact with recreational machinery**
Contact with roller-coaster

X **W31.82 Contact with other commercial machinery**
Contact with commercial electric fan
Contact with commercial kitchen appliances
Contact with commercial powered dryer (clothes) (powered) (spin)
Contact with commercial washing-machine
Contact with commercial sewing machine

Excludes1 contact with household machinery (W29.-)
contact with powered lawn mower (W28)

X **W31.83 Contact with special construction vehicle in stationary use**
Contact with special construction vehicle under repair, not on public roadway

Excludes1 special construction vehicle accident (VØ1-V99)

X **W31.89 Contact with other specified machinery**

X **W31.9 Contact with unspecified machinery**
Contact with machinery NOS

W32 Accidental handgun discharge and malfunction

Includes accidental discharge and malfunction of gun for single hand use
accidental discharge and malfunction of pistol
accidental discharge and malfunction of revolver
handgun discharge and malfunction NOS

Excludes1 accidental airgun discharge and malfunction (W34.Ø1Ø, W34.11Ø)
accidental BB gun discharge and malfunction (W34.Ø1Ø, W34.11Ø)
accidental pellet gun discharge and malfunction (W34.Ø1Ø, W34.11Ø)
accidental shotgun discharge and malfunction (W33.Ø1, W33.11)
assault by handgun discharge (X93)
handgun discharge involving legal intervention (Y35.Ø-)
handgun discharge involving military or war operations (Y36.4-)
intentional self-harm by handgun discharge (X72)
Very pistol discharge and malfunction (W34.Ø9, W34.19)

The appropriate 7th character is to be added to each code from category W32

A	initial encounter
D	subsequent encounter
S	sequela

X **W32.Ø Accidental handgun discharge**

X **W32.1 Accidental handgun malfunction**
Injury due to explosion of handgun (parts)
Injury due to malfunction of mechanism or component of handgun
Injury due to recoil of handgun
Powder burn from handgun

W33 Accidental rifle, shotgun and larger firearm discharge and malfunction

Includes rifle, shotgun and larger firearm discharge and malfunction NOS

Excludes1 accidental airgun discharge and malfunction (W34.Ø1Ø, W34.11Ø)
accidental BB gun discharge and malfunction (W34.Ø1Ø, W34.11Ø)
accidental handgun discharge and malfunction (W32.-)
accidental pellet gun discharge and malfunction (W34.Ø1Ø, W34.11Ø)
assault by rifle, shotgun and larger firearm discharge (X94)
firearm discharge involving legal intervention (Y35.Ø-)
firearm discharge involving military or war operations (Y36.4-)
intentional self-harm by rifle, shotgun and larger firearm discharge (X73)

The appropriate 7th character is to be added to each code from category W33

A	initial encounter
D	subsequent encounter
S	sequela

W33.Ø Accidental rifle, shotgun and larger firearm discharge

X **W33.ØØ Accidental discharge of unspecified larger firearm**
Discharge of unspecified larger firearm NOS

X **W33.Ø1 Accidental discharge of shotgun**
Discharge of shotgun NOS

X **W33.Ø2 Accidental discharge of hunting rifle**
Discharge of hunting rifle NOS

X **W33.Ø3 Accidental discharge of machine gun**
Discharge of machine gun NOS

X **W33.Ø9 Accidental discharge of other larger firearm**
Discharge of other larger firearm NOS

● W33.1 **Accidental rifle, shotgun and larger firearm malfunction**
Injury due to explosion of rifle, shotgun and larger firearm (parts)
Injury due to malfunction of mechanism or component of rifle, shotgun and larger firearm
Injury due to piercing, cutting, crushing or pinching due to (by) slide trigger mechanism, scope or other gun part
Injury due to recoil of rifle, shotgun and larger firearm
Powder burn from rifle, shotgun and larger firearm

X● W33.10 **Accidental malfunction of unspecified larger firearm**
Malfunction of unspecified larger firearm NOS

X● W33.11 **Accidental malfunction of shotgun**
Malfunction of shotgun NOS

X● W33.12 **Accidental malfunction of hunting rifle**
Malfunction of hunting rifle NOS

X● W33.13 **Accidental malfunction of machine gun**
Malfunction of machine gun NOS

X● W33.19 **Accidental malfunction of other larger firearm**
Malfunction of other larger firearm NOS

● W34 **Accidental discharge and malfunction from other and unspecified firearms and guns**
The appropriate 7th character is to be added to each code from category W34

A	initial encounter
D	subsequent encounter
S	sequela

● W34.Ø **Accidental discharge from other and unspecified firearms and guns**

X● W34.ØØ **Accidental discharge from unspecified firearms or gun**
Discharge from firearm NOS
Gunshot wound NOS
Shot NOS
Coding Clinic: 2Ø15, Q1, P17

● W34.Ø1 **Accidental discharge of gas, air or spring-operated guns**

● W34.Ø1Ø **Accidental discharge of airgun**
Accidental discharge of BB gun
Accidental discharge of pellet gun

● W34.Ø11 **Accidental discharge of paintball gun**
Accidental injury due to paintball discharge

● W34.Ø18 **Accidental discharge of other gas, air or spring-operated gun**

X● W34.Ø9 **Accidental discharge from other specified firearms**
Accidental discharge from Very pistol [flare]

● W34.1 **Accidental malfunction from other and unspecified firearms and guns**

X● W34.10 **Accidental malfunction from unspecified firearms or gun**
Firearm malfunction NOS

● W34.11 **Accidental malfunction of gas, air or spring-operated guns**

● W34.11Ø **Accidental malfunction of airgun**
Accidental malfunction of BB gun
Accidental malfunction of pellet gun

● W34.111 **Accidental malfunction of paintball gun**
Accidental injury due to paintball gun malfunction

● W34.118 **Accidental malfunction of other gas, air or spring-operated gun**

X● W34.19 **Accidental malfunction from other specified firearms**
Accidental malfunction from Very pistol [flare]

X● W35 **Explosion and rupture of boiler**
Excludes1 explosion and rupture of boiler on watercraft (V93.4)
The appropriate 7th character is to be added to code W35

A	initial encounter
D	subsequent encounter
S	sequela

● W36 **Explosion and rupture of gas cylinder**
The appropriate 7th character is to be added to each code from category W36

A	initial encounter
D	subsequent encounter
S	sequela

X● W36.1 **Explosion and rupture of aerosol can**
X● W36.2 **Explosion and rupture of air tank**
X● W36.3 **Explosion and rupture of pressurized-gas tank**
X● W36.8 **Explosion and rupture of other gas cylinder**
X● W36.9 **Explosion and rupture of unspecified gas cylinder**

● W37 **Explosion and rupture of pressurized tire, pipe or hose**
The appropriate 7th character is to be added to each code from category W37

A	initial encounter
D	subsequent encounter
S	sequela

X● W37.Ø **Explosion of bicycle tire**
X● W37.8 **Explosion and rupture of other pressurized tire, pipe or hose**

X● W38 **Explosion and rupture of other specified pressurized devices**
The appropriate 7th character is to be added to code W38

A	initial encounter
D	subsequent encounter
S	sequela

X● W39 **Discharge of firework**
The appropriate 7th character is to be added to code W39

A	initial encounter
D	subsequent encounter
S	sequela

● W4Ø **Explosion of other materials**
Excludes1 assault by explosive material (X96)
explosion involving legal intervention (Y35.1-)
explosion involving military or war operations (Y36.Ø-, Y36.2-)
intentional self-harm by explosive material (X75)
The appropriate 7th character is to be added to each code from category W4Ø

A	initial encounter
D	subsequent encounter
S	sequela

X● W4Ø.Ø **Explosion of blasting material**
Explosion of blasting cap
Explosion of detonator
Explosion of dynamite
Explosion of explosive (any) used in blasting operations

X● W4Ø.1 **Explosion of explosive gases**
Explosion of acetylene
Explosion of butane
Explosion of coal gas
Explosion in mine NOS
Explosion of explosive gas
Explosion of fire damp
Explosion of gasoline fumes
Explosion of methane
Explosion of propane

X● **W40.8 Explosion of other specified explosive materials**
Explosion in dump NOS
Explosion in factory NOS
Explosion in grain store
Explosion in munitions
Excludes1 explosion involving legal intervention (Y35.1-)
explosion involving military or war operations (Y36.0-, Y36.2-)

X● **W40.9 Explosion of unspecified explosive materials**
Explosion NOS

● **W42 Exposure to noise**
The appropriate 7th character is to be added to each code from category W42

A	initial encounter
D	subsequent encounter
S	sequela

X● **W42.0 Exposure to supersonic waves**
X● **W42.9 Exposure to other noise**
Exposure to sound waves NOS

● **W45 Foreign body or object entering through skin**
Includes foreign body or object embedded in skin
nail embedded in skin
Excludes2 contact with hand tools (nonpowered) (powered) (W27-W29)
contact with other sharp object(s) (W26.-)
contact with sharp glass (W25.-)
struck by objects (W20-W22)
The appropriate 7th character is to be added to each code from category W45

A	initial encounter
D	subsequent encounter
S	sequela

X● **W45.0 Nail entering through skin**
X● **W45.8 Other foreign body or object entering through skin**
Splinter in skin NOS

● **W46 Contact with hypodermic needle**
The appropriate 7th character is to be added to each code from category W46

A	initial encounter
D	subsequent encounter
S	sequela

X● **W46.0 Contact with hypodermic needle**
Hypodermic needle stick NOS
X● **W46.1 Contact with contaminated hypodermic needle**

● **W49 Exposure to other inanimate mechanical forces**
Includes exposure to abnormal gravitational [G] forces
exposure to inanimate mechanical forces NEC
Excludes1 exposure to inanimate mechanical forces involving military or war operations (Y36.-, Y37.-)
The appropriate 7th character is to be added to each code from category W49

A	initial encounter
D	subsequent encounter
S	sequela

● **W49.0 Item causing external constriction**
X● **W49.01 Hair causing external constriction**
X● **W49.02 String or thread causing external constriction**
X● **W49.03 Rubber band causing external constriction**
X● **W49.04 Ring or other jewelry causing external constriction**
X● **W49.09 Other item causing external constriction**
X● **W49.9 Exposure to other inanimate mechanical forces**

EXPOSURE TO ANIMATE MECHANICAL FORCES (W50-W64)

Excludes1 toxic effect of contact with venomous animals and plants (T63.-)

● **W50 Accidental hit, strike, kick, twist, bite or scratch by another person**
Includes hit, strike, kick, twist, bite, or scratch by another person NOS
Excludes1 assault by bodily force (Y04)
struck by objects (W20-W22)
The appropriate 7th character is to be added to each code from category W50

A	initial encounter
D	subsequent encounter
S	sequela

X● **W50.0 Accidental hit or strike by another person**
Hit or strike by another person NOS
X● **W50.1 Accidental kick by another person**
Kick by another person NOS
X● **W50.2 Accidental twist by another person**
Twist by another person NOS
Coding Clinic: 2015, Q1, P8
X● **W50.3 Accidental bite by another person**
Human bite
Bite by another person NOS
X● **W50.4 Accidental scratch by another person**
Scratch by another person NOS

X● **W51 Accidental striking against or bumped into by another person**
Excludes1 assault by striking against or bumping into by another person (Y04.2)
fall due to collision with another person (W03)
The appropriate 7th character is to be added to code W51

A	initial encounter
D	subsequent encounter
S	sequela

X● **W52 Crushed, pushed or stepped on by crowd or human stampede**
Crushed, pushed or stepped on by crowd or human stampede with or without fall
The appropriate 7th character is to be added to code W52

A	initial encounter
D	subsequent encounter
S	sequela

● **W53 Contact with rodent**
Includes contact with saliva, feces or urine of rodent
The appropriate 7th character is to be added to each code from category W53

A	initial encounter
D	subsequent encounter
S	sequela

● **W53.0 Contact with mouse**
X● **W53.01 Bitten by mouse**
X● **W53.09 Other contact with mouse**
● **W53.1 Contact with rat**
X● **W53.11 Bitten by rat**
X● **W53.19 Other contact with rat**
● **W53.2 Contact with squirrel**
X● **W53.21 Bitten by squirrel**
X● **W53.29 Other contact with squirrel**
● **W53.8 Contact with other rodent**
X● **W53.81 Bitten by other rodent**
X● **W53.89 Other contact with other rodent**

● W54 Contact with dog

Includes contact with saliva, feces or urine of dog

The appropriate 7th character is to be added to each code from category W54

A	initial encounter
D	subsequent encounter
S	sequela

X● W54.0 **Bitten by dog**

X● W54.1 **Struck by dog**
Knocked over by dog

X● W54.8 **Other contact with dog**

● W55 Contact with other mammals

Includes contact with saliva, feces or urine of mammal

Excludes1 animal being ridden - see transport accidents
bitten or struck by dog (W54)
bitten or struck by rodent (W53.-)
contact with marine mammals (W56.X-)

The appropriate 7th character is to be added to each code from category W55

A	initial encounter
D	subsequent encounter
S	sequela

● W55.0 Contact with cat

X● W55.01 **Bitten by cat**

X● W55.03 **Scratched by cat**

X● W55.09 **Other contact with cat**

● W55.1 Contact with horse

X● W55.11 **Bitten by horse**

X● W55.12 **Struck by horse**

X● W55.19 **Other contact with horse**

● W55.2 Contact with cow
Contact with bull

X● W55.21 **Bitten by cow**

X● W55.22 **Struck by cow**
Gored by bull

X● W55.29 **Other contact with cow**

● W55.3 Contact with other hoof stock
Contact with goats
Contact with sheep

X● W55.31 **Bitten by other hoof stock**

X● W55.32 **Struck by other hoof stock**
Gored by goat
Gored by ram

X● W55.39 **Other contact with other hoof stock**

● W55.4 Contact with pig

X● W55.41 **Bitten by pig**

X● W55.42 **Struck by pig**

X● W55.49 **Other contact with pig**

● W55.5 Contact with raccoon

X● W55.51 **Bitten by raccoon**

X● W55.52 **Struck by raccoon**

X● W55.59 **Other contact with raccoon**

● W55.8 Contact with other mammals

X● W55.81 **Bitten by other mammals**

X● W55.82 **Struck by other mammals**

X● W55.89 **Other contact with other mammals**

● W56 Contact with nonvenomous marine animal

Excludes1 contact with venomous marine animal (T63.-)

The appropriate 7th character is to be added to each code from category W56

A	initial encounter
D	subsequent encounter
S	sequela

● W56.0 Contact with dolphin

X● W56.01 **Bitten by dolphin**

X● W56.02 **Struck by dolphin**

X● W56.09 **Other contact with dolphin**

● W56.1 Contact with sea lion

X● W56.11 **Bitten by sea lion**

X● W56.12 **Struck by sea lion**

X● W56.19 **Other contact with sea lion**

● W56.2 Contact with orca
Contact with killer whale

X● W56.21 **Bitten by orca**

X● W56.22 **Struck by orca**

X● W56.29 **Other contact with orca**

● W56.3 Contact with other marine mammals

X● W56.31 **Bitten by other marine mammals**

X● W56.32 **Struck by other marine mammals**

X● W56.39 **Other contact with other marine mammals**

● W56.4 Contact with shark

X● W56.41 **Bitten by shark**

X● W56.42 **Struck by shark**

X● W56.49 **Other contact with shark**

● W56.5 Contact with other fish

X● W56.51 **Bitten by other fish**

X● W56.52 **Struck by other fish**

X● W56.59 **Other contact with other fish**

● W56.8 Contact with other nonvenomous marine animals

X● W56.81 **Bitten by other nonvenomous marine animals**

X● W56.82 **Struck by other nonvenomous marine animals**

X● W56.89 **Other contact with other nonvenomous marine animals**

X● W57 Bitten or stung by nonvenomous insect and other nonvenomous arthropods

Excludes1 contact with venomous insects and arthropods (T63.2-, T63.3-, T63.4-)

The appropriate 7th character is to be added to code W57

A	initial encounter
D	subsequent encounter
S	sequela

● W58 Contact with crocodile or alligator

The appropriate 7th character is to be added to each code from category W58

A	initial encounter
D	subsequent encounter
S	sequela

● W58.0 Contact with alligator

X● W58.01 **Bitten by alligator**

X● W58.02 **Struck by alligator**

X● W58.03 **Crushed by alligator**

X● W58.09 **Other contact with alligator**

● W58.1 Contact with crocodile

X● W58.11 **Bitten by crocodile**

X● W58.12 **Struck by crocodile**

X● W58.13 **Crushed by crocodile**

X● W58.19 **Other contact with crocodile**

W59 Contact with other nonvenomous reptiles

Excludes1 contact with venomous reptile (T63.Ø-, T63.1-)

The appropriate 7th character is to be added to each code from category W59

A initial encounter
D subsequent encounter
S sequela

W59.Ø Contact with nonvenomous lizards

X **W59.Ø1 Bitten by nonvenomous lizards**

X **W59.Ø2 Struck by nonvenomous lizards**

X **W59.Ø9 Other contact with nonvenomous lizards**
Exposure to nonvenomous lizards

W59.1 Contact with nonvenomous snakes

X **W59.11 Bitten by nonvenomous snake**

X **W59.12 Struck by nonvenomous snake**

X **W59.13 Crushed by nonvenomous snake**

X **W59.19 Other contact with nonvenomous snake**

W59.2 Contact with turtles

Excludes1 contact with tortoises (W59.8-)

X **W59.21 Bitten by turtle**

X **W59.22 Struck by turtle**

X **W59.29 Other contact with turtle**
Exposure to turtles

W59.8 Contact with other nonvenomous reptiles

X **W59.81 Bitten by other nonvenomous reptiles**

X **W59.82 Struck by other nonvenomous reptiles**

X **W59.83 Crushed by other nonvenomous reptiles**

X **W59.89 Other contact with other nonvenomous reptiles**

X **W6Ø Contact with nonvenomous plant thorns and spines and sharp leaves**

Excludes1 contact with venomous plants (T63.X7-)

The appropriate 7th character is to be added to code W6Ø

A initial encounter
D subsequent encounter
S sequela

W61 Contact with birds (domestic) (wild)

Includes contact with excreta of birds

The appropriate 7th character is to be added to each code from category W61

A initial encounter
D subsequent encounter
S sequela

W61.Ø Contact with parrot

X **W61.Ø1 Bitten by parrot**

X **W61.Ø2 Struck by parrot**

X **W61.Ø9 Other contact with parrot**
Exposure to parrots

W61.1 Contact with macaw

X **W61.11 Bitten by macaw**

X **W61.12 Struck by macaw**

X **W61.19 Other contact with macaw**
Exposure to macaws

W61.2 Contact with other psittacines

X **W61.21 Bitten by other psittacines**

X **W61.22 Struck by other psittacines**

X **W61.29 Other contact with other psittacines**
Exposure to other psittacines

W61.3 Contact with chicken

X **W61.32 Struck by chicken**

X **W61.33 Pecked by chicken**

X **W61.39 Other contact with chicken**
Exposure to chickens

W61.4 Contact with turkey

X **W61.42 Struck by turkey**

X **W61.43 Pecked by turkey**

X **W61.49 Other contact with turkey**

W61.5 Contact with goose

X **W61.51 Bitten by goose**

X **W61.52 Struck by goose**

X **W61.59 Other contact with goose**

W61.6 Contact with duck

X **W61.61 Bitten by duck**

X **W61.62 Struck by duck**

X **W61.69 Other contact with duck**

W61.9 Contact with other birds

X **W61.91 Bitten by other birds**

X **W61.92 Struck by other birds**

X **W61.99 Other contact with other birds**
Contact with bird NOS

W62 Contact with nonvenomous amphibians

Excludes1 contact with venomous amphibians (T63.81-R63.83)

The appropriate 7th character is to be added to each code from category W62

A initial encounter
D subsequent encounter
S sequela

X **W62.Ø Contact with nonvenomous frogs**

X **W62.1 Contact with nonvenomous toads**

X **W62.9 Contact with other nonvenomous amphibians**

X **W64 Exposure to other animate mechanical forces**

Includes exposure to nonvenomous animal NOS

Excludes1 contact with venomous animal (T63.-)

The appropriate 7th character is to be added to code W64

A initial encounter
D subsequent encounter
S sequela

ACCIDENTAL NON-TRANSPORT DROWNING AND SUBMERSION (W65-W74)

Excludes1 accidental drowning and submersion due to fall into water (W16.-)
accidental drowning and submersion due to water transport accident (V9Ø.-, V92.-)

Excludes2 accidental drowning and submersion due to cataclysm (X34-X39)

X **W65 Accidental drowning and submersion while in bathtub**

Excludes1 accidental drowning and submersion due to fall in (into) bathtub (W16.211)

The appropriate 7th character is to be added to code W65

A initial encounter
D subsequent encounter
S sequela

X **W67 Accidental drowning and submersion while in swimming pool**

Excludes1 accidental drowning and submersion due to fall into swimming pool (W16.Ø11, W16.Ø21, W16.Ø31)
accidental drowning and submersion due to striking into wall of swimming pool (W22.Ø41)

The appropriate 7th character is to be added to code W67

A initial encounter
D subsequent encounter
S sequela

CHAPTER 2Ø (VØØ-Y99)

X● **W69 Accidental drowning and submersion while in natural water**
Accidental drowning and submersion while in lake
Accidental drowning and submersion while in open sea
Accidental drowning and submersion while in river
Accidental drowning and submersion while in stream
Excludes1 accidental drowning and submersion due to fall into natural body of water (W16.111, W16.121, W16.131)
The appropriate 7th character is to be added to code W69
A initial encounter
D subsequent encounter
S sequela

X● **W73 Other specified cause of accidental non-transport drowning and submersion**
Accidental drowning and submersion while in quenching tank
Accidental drowning and submersion while in reservoir
Excludes1 accidental drowning and submersion due to fall into other water (W16.311, W16.321, W16.331)
The appropriate 7th character is to be added to code W73
A initial encounter
D subsequent encounter
S sequela

X● **W74 Unspecified cause of accidental drowning and submersion**
Drowning NOS
The appropriate 7th character is to be added to code W74
A initial encounter
D subsequent encounter
S sequela

EXPOSURE TO ELECTRIC CURRENT, RADIATION AND EXTREME AMBIENT AIR TEMPERATURE AND PRESSURE (W85-W99)

Excludes1 exposure to:
failure in dosage of radiation or temperature during surgical and medical care (Y63.2-Y63.5)
lightning (T75.0-)
natural cold (X31)
natural heat (X30)
natural radiation NOS (X39)
radiological procedure and radiotherapy (Y84.2)
sunlight (X32)

X● **W85 Exposure to electric transmission lines**
Broken power line
The appropriate 7th character is to be added to code W85
A initial encounter
D subsequent encounter
S sequela

● **W86 Exposure to other specified electric current**
The appropriate 7th character is to be added to each code from category W86
A initial encounter
D subsequent encounter
S sequela

X● **W86.0 Exposure to domestic wiring and appliances**

X● **W86.1 Exposure to industrial wiring, appliances and electrical machinery**
Exposure to conductors
Exposure to control apparatus
Exposure to electrical equipment and machinery
Exposure to transformers

X● **W86.8 Exposure to other electric current**
Exposure to wiring and appliances in or on farm (not farmhouse)
Exposure to wiring and appliances outdoors
Exposure to wiring and appliances in or on public building
Exposure to wiring and appliances in or on residential institutions
Exposure to wiring and appliances in or on schools

● **W88 Exposure to ionizing radiation**
Excludes1 exposure to sunlight (X32)
The appropriate 7th character is to be added to each code from category W88
A initial encounter
D subsequent encounter
S sequela

X● **W88.0 Exposure to X-rays**
X● **W88.1 Exposure to radioactive isotopes**
X● **W88.8 Exposure to other ionizing radiation**

● **W89 Exposure to man-made visible and ultraviolet light**
Includes exposure to welding light (arc)
Excludes1 exposure to sunlight (X32)
The appropriate 7th character is to be added to each code from category W89
A initial encounter
D subsequent encounter
S sequela

X● **W89.0 Exposure to welding light (arc)**
X● **W89.1 Exposure to tanning bed**
X● **W89.8 Exposure to other man-made visible and ultraviolet light**
X● **W89.9 Exposure to unspecified man-made visible and ultraviolet light**

● **W90 Exposure to other nonionizing radiation**
Excludes1 exposure to sunlight (X32)
The appropriate 7th character is to be added to each code from category W90
A initial encounter
D subsequent encounter
S sequela

X● **W90.0 Exposure to radiofrequency**
X● **W90.1 Exposure to infrared radiation**
X● **W90.2 Exposure to laser radiation**
X● **W90.8 Exposure to other nonionizing radiation**

X● **W92 Exposure to excessive heat of man-made origin**
The appropriate 7th character is to be added to code W92
A initial encounter
D subsequent encounter
S sequela

● **W93 Exposure to excessive cold of man-made origin**
The appropriate 7th character is to be added to each code from category W93
A initial encounter
D subsequent encounter
S sequela

● **W93.0 Contact with or inhalation of dry ice**
X● **W93.01 Contact with dry ice**
X● **W93.02 Inhalation of dry ice**

● W93.1 **Contact with or inhalation of liquid air**

X● W93.11 **Contact with liquid air**
Contact with liquid hydrogen
Contact with liquid nitrogen

X● W93.12 **Inhalation of liquid air**
Inhalation of liquid hydrogen
Inhalation of liquid nitrogen

X● W93.2 **Prolonged exposure in deep freeze unit or refrigerator**

X● W93.8 **Exposure to other excessive cold of man-made origin**

● W94 **Exposure to high and low air pressure and changes in air pressure**

The appropriate 7th character is to be added to each code from category W94

A	initial encounter
D	subsequent encounter
S	sequela

X● W94.0 **Exposure to prolonged high air pressure**

● W94.1 **Exposure to prolonged low air pressure**

X● W94.11 **Exposure to residence or prolonged visit at high altitude**

X● W94.12 **Exposure to other prolonged low air pressure**

● W94.2 **Exposure to rapid changes in air pressure during ascent**

X● W94.21 **Exposure to reduction in atmospheric pressure while surfacing from deep-water diving**

X● W94.22 **Exposure to reduction in atmospheric pressure while surfacing from underground**

X● W94.23 **Exposure to sudden change in air pressure in aircraft during ascent**

X● W94.29 **Exposure to other rapid changes in air pressure during ascent**

● W94.3 **Exposure to rapid changes in air pressure during descent**

X● W94.31 **Exposure to sudden change in air pressure in aircraft during descent**

X● W94.32 **Exposure to high air pressure from rapid descent in water**

X● W94.39 **Exposure to other rapid changes in air pressure during descent**

X● W99 **Exposure to other man-made environmental factors**

The appropriate 7th character is to be added to code W99

A	initial encounter
D	subsequent encounter
S	sequela

EXPOSURE TO SMOKE, FIRE AND FLAMES (X00-X08)

Excludes1 arson (X97)

Excludes2 explosions (W35-W40)
lightning (T75.0-)
transport accident (V01-V99)

● X00 **Exposure to uncontrolled fire in building or structure**

Includes conflagration in building or structure

Code first any associated cataclysm

Excludes2 exposure to ignition or melting of nightwear (X05)
exposure to ignition or melting of other clothing and apparel (X06.-)
exposure to other specified smoke, fire and flames (X08.-)

The appropriate 7th character is to be added to each code from category X00

A	initial encounter
D	subsequent encounter
S	sequela

X● X00.0 **Exposure to flames in uncontrolled fire in building or structure**
Coding Clinic: 2016, Q2, P5-6; 2015, Q1, P19

X● X00.1 **Exposure to smoke in uncontrolled fire in building or structure**

X● X00.2 **Injury due to collapse of burning building or structure in uncontrolled fire**

Excludes1 injury due to collapse of building not on fire (W20.1)

X● X00.3 **Fall from burning building or structure in uncontrolled fire**

X● X00.4 **Hit by object from burning building or structure in uncontrolled fire**

X● X00.5 **Jump from burning building or structure in uncontrolled fire**

X● X00.8 **Other exposure to uncontrolled fire in building or structure**

● X01 **Exposure to uncontrolled fire, not in building or structure**

Includes exposure to forest fire

The appropriate 7th character is to be added to each code from category X01

A	initial encounter
D	subsequent encounter
S	sequela

X● X01.0 **Exposure to flames in uncontrolled fire, not in building or structure**

X● X01.1 **Exposure to smoke in uncontrolled fire, not in building or structure**

X● X01.3 **Fall due to uncontrolled fire, not in building or structure**

X● X01.4 **Hit by object due to uncontrolled fire, not in building or structure**

X● X01.8 **Other exposure to uncontrolled fire, not in building or structure**

● X02 **Exposure to controlled fire in building or structure**

Includes exposure to fire in fireplace exposure to fire in stove

The appropriate 7th character is to be added to each code from category X02

A	initial encounter
D	subsequent encounter
S	sequela

X● X02.0 **Exposure to flames in controlled fire in building or structure**

X● X02.1 **Exposure to smoke in controlled fire in building or structure**

X● X02.2 **Injury due to collapse of burning building or structure in controlled fire**

Excludes1 injury due to collapse of building not on fire (W20.1)

X● X02.3 **Fall from burning building or structure in controlled fire**

X● X02.4 **Hit by object from burning building or structure in controlled fire**

X● X02.5 **Jump from burning building or structure in controlled fire**

X● X02.8 **Other exposure to controlled fire in building or structure**

● X03 **Exposure to controlled fire, not in building or structure**

Includes exposure to bon fire exposure to camp fire
exposure to trash fire

The appropriate 7th character is to be added to each code from category X03

A	initial encounter
D	subsequent encounter
S	sequela

X● X03.0 **Exposure to flames in controlled fire, not in building or structure**
Coding Clinic: 2015, Q1, P19

X● X03.1 **Exposure to smoke in controlled fire, not in building or structure**

X● X03.3 **Fall due to controlled fire, not in building or structure**

X● X03.4 **Hit by object due to controlled fire, not in building or structure**

X● X03.8 **Other exposure to controlled fire, not in building or structure**

X ● **X04 Exposure to ignition of highly flammable material**
Exposure to ignition of gasoline
Exposure to ignition of kerosene
Exposure to ignition of petrol
Excludes2 exposure to ignition or melting of nightwear (X05)
exposure to ignition or melting of other clothing and apparel (X06)
The appropriate 7th character is to be added to code X04

A	initial encounter
D	subsequent encounter
S	sequela

Coding Clinic: 2016, Q2, P4

X ● **X05 Exposure to ignition or melting of nightwear**
Excludes2 exposure to uncontrolled fire in building or structure (X00.-)
exposure to uncontrolled fire, not in building or structure (X01.-)
exposure to controlled fire in building or structure (X02.-)
exposure to controlled fire, not in building or structure (X03.-)
exposure to ignition of highly flammable materials (X04.-)
The appropriate 7th character is to be added to code X05

A	initial encounter
D	subsequent encounter
S	sequela

● **X06 Exposure to ignition or melting of other clothing and apparel**
Excludes2 exposure to uncontrolled fire in building or structure (X00.-)
exposure to uncontrolled fire, not in building or structure (X01.-)
exposure to controlled fire in building or structure (X02.-)
exposure to controlled fire, not in building or structure (X03.-)
exposure to ignition of highly flammable materials (X04.-)
The appropriate 7th character is to be added to each code from category X06

A	initial encounter
D	subsequent encounter
S	sequela

X ● **X06.0 Exposure to ignition of plastic jewelry**
X ● **X06.1 Exposure to melting of plastic jewelry**
X ● **X06.2 Exposure to ignition of other clothing and apparel**
X ● **X06.3 Exposure to melting of other clothing and apparel**

● **X08 Exposure to other specified smoke, fire and flames**
The appropriate 7th character is to be added to each code from category X08

A	initial encounter
D	subsequent encounter
S	sequela

● **X08.0 Exposure to bed fire**
Exposure to mattress fire
X ● **X08.00 Exposure to bed fire due to unspecified burning material**
X ● **X08.01 Exposure to bed fire due to burning cigarette**
Coding Clinic: 2015, Q1, P19
X ● **X08.09 Exposure to bed fire due to other burning material**

● **X08.1 Exposure to sofa fire**
X ● **X08.10 Exposure to sofa fire due to unspecified burning material**
X ● **X08.11 Exposure to sofa fire due to burning cigarette**
X ● **X08.19 Exposure to sofa fire due to other burning material**
● **X08.2 Exposure to other furniture fire**
X ● **X08.20 Exposure to other furniture fire due to unspecified burning material**
X ● **X08.21 Exposure to other furniture fire due to burning cigarette**
X ● **X08.29 Exposure to other furniture fire due to other burning material**
X ● **X08.8 Exposure to other specified smoke, fire and flames**

CONTACT WITH HEAT AND HOT SUBSTANCES (X10-X19)

Excludes1 exposure to excessive natural heat (X30)
exposure to fire and flames (X00-X08)

● **X10 Contact with hot drinks, food, fats and cooking oils**
The appropriate 7th character is to be added to each code from category X10

A	initial encounter
D	subsequent encounter
S	sequela

X ● **X10.0 Contact with hot drinks**
X ● **X10.1 Contact with hot food**
X ● **X10.2 Contact with fats and cooking oils**

● **X11 Contact with hot tap-water**
Includes contact with boiling tap-water
contact with boiling water NOS
Excludes1 contact with water heated on stove (X12)
The appropriate 7th character is to be added to each code from category X11

A	initial encounter
D	subsequent encounter
S	sequela

X ● **X11.0 Contact with hot water in bath or tub**
Excludes1 contact with running hot water in bath or tub (X11.1)
X ● **X11.1 Contact with running hot water**
Contact with hot water running out of hose
Contact with hot water running out of tap
X ● **X11.8 Contact with other hot tap-water**
Contact with hot water in bucket
Contact with hot tap-water NOS

X ● **X12 Contact with other hot fluids**
Contact with water heated on stove
Excludes1 hot (liquid) metals (X18)
The appropriate 7th character is to be added to code X12

A	initial encounter
D	subsequent encounter
S	sequela

● **X13 Contact with steam and other hot vapors**
The appropriate 7th character is to be added to each code from category X13

A	initial encounter
D	subsequent encounter
S	sequela

X ● **X13.0 Inhalation of steam and other hot vapors**
X ● **X13.1 Other contact with steam and other hot vapors**

X14 Contact with hot air and other hot gases

The appropriate 7th character is to be added to each code from category X14

A	initial encounter
D	subsequent encounter
S	sequela

X **X14.0 Inhalation of hot air and gases**

X **X14.1 Other contact with hot air and other hot gases**

X15 Contact with hot household appliances

Excludes1 contact with heating appliances (X16)
contact with powered household appliances (W29.-)
exposure to controlled fire in building or structure due to household appliance (X02.8)
exposure to household appliances electrical current (W86.0)

The appropriate 7th character is to be added to each code from category X15

A	initial encounter
D	subsequent encounter
S	sequela

X **X15.0 Contact with hot stove (kitchen)**

X **X15.1 Contact with hot toaster**

X **X15.2 Contact with hotplate**

X **X15.3 Contact with hot saucepan or skillet**

X **X15.8 Contact with other hot household appliances**

Contact with cooker
Contact with kettle
Contact with light bulbs

X **X16 Contact with hot heating appliances, radiators and pipes**

Excludes1 contact with powered appliances (W29.-)
exposure to controlled fire in building or structure due to appliance (X02.8)
exposure to industrial appliances electrical current (W86.1)

The appropriate 7th character is to be added to code X16

A	initial encounter
D	subsequent encounter
S	sequela

X **X17 Contact with hot engines, machinery and tools**

Excludes1 contact with hot heating appliances, radiators and pipes (X16)
contact with hot household appliances (X15)

The appropriate 7th character is to be added to code X17

A	initial encounter
D	subsequent encounter
S	sequela

X **X18 Contact with other hot metals**

Contact with liquid metal

The appropriate 7th character is to be added to code X18

A	initial encounter
D	subsequent encounter
S	sequela

X **X19 Contact with other heat and hot substances**

Excludes1 objects that are not normally hot, e.g., an object made hot by a house fire (X00-X08)

The appropriate 7th character is to be added to code X19

A	initial encounter
D	subsequent encounter
S	sequela

EXPOSURE TO FORCES OF NATURE (X30-X39)

X **X30 Exposure to excessive natural heat**

Exposure to excessive heat as the cause of sunstroke
Exposure to heat NOS

Excludes1 excessive heat of man-made origin (W92)
exposure to man-made radiation (W89)
exposure to sunlight (X32)
exposure to tanning bed (W89)

The appropriate 7th character is to be added to code X30

A	initial encounter
D	subsequent encounter
S	sequela

X **X31 Exposure to excessive natural cold**

Excessive cold as the cause of chilblains NOS
Excessive cold as the cause of immersion foot or hand
Exposure to cold NOS
Exposure to weather conditions

Excludes1 cold of man-made origin (W93.-)
contact with or inhalation of dry ice (W93.-)
contact with or inhalation of liquefied gas (W93.-)

The appropriate 7th character is to be added to code X31

A	initial encounter
D	subsequent encounter
S	sequela

X **X32 Exposure to sunlight**

Excludes1 man-made radiation (tanning bed) (W89)

Excludes2 radiation-related disorders of the skin and subcutaneous tissue (L55-L59)

The appropriate 7th character is to be added to code X32

A	initial encounter
D	subsequent encounter
S	sequela

X **X34 Earthquake**

Excludes2 tidal wave (tsunami) due to earthquake (X37.41)

The appropriate 7th character is to be added to code X34

A	initial encounter
D	subsequent encounter
S	sequela

X **X35 Volcanic eruption**

Excludes2 tidal wave (tsunami) due to volcanic eruption (X37.41)

The appropriate 7th character is to be added to code X35

A	initial encounter
D	subsequent encounter
S	sequela

X36 Avalanche, landslide and other earth movements

Includes victim of mudslide of cataclysmic nature

Excludes1 earthquake (X34)

Excludes2 transport accident involving collision with avalanche or landslide not in motion (V01-V99)

The appropriate 7th character is to be added to each code from category X36

A	initial encounter
D	subsequent encounter
S	sequela

X **X36.0 Collapse of dam or man-made structure causing earth movement**

X **X36.1 Avalanche, landslide, or mudslide**

X37 Cataclysmic storm

The appropriate 7th character is to be added to each code from category X37

A initial encounter
D subsequent encounter
S sequela

X X37.0 **Hurricane**
Storm surge
Typhoon

X X37.1 **Tornado**
Cyclone
Twister

X X37.2 **Blizzard (snow) (ice)**

X X37.3 **Dust storm**

X37.4 **Tidalwave**

X X37.41 **Tidal wave due to earthquake or volcanic eruption**
Tidal wave NOS
Tsunami

X X37.42 **Tidal wave due to storm**

X X37.43 **Tidal wave due to landslide**

X X37.8 **Other cataclysmic storms**
Cloudburst
Torrential rain
Excludes2 flood (X38)

X X37.9 **Unspecified cataclysmic storm**
Storm NOS
Excludes1 collapse of dam or man-made structure causing earth movement (X36.0)

X X38 **Flood**
Flood arising from remote storm
Flood of cataclysmic nature arising from melting snow
Flood resulting directly from storm
Excludes1 collapse of dam or man-made structure causing earth movement (X36.0)
tidal wave NOS (X37.41)
tidal wave caused by storm (X37.42)

The appropriate 7th character is to be added to code X38

A initial encounter
D subsequent encounter
S sequela

X39 Exposure to other forces of nature

The appropriate 7th character is to be added to each code from category X39

A initial encounter
D subsequent encounter
S sequela

X39.0 **Exposure to natural radiation**
Excludes1 contact with and (suspected) exposure to radon and other naturally occurring radiation (Z77.123)
exposure to man-made radiation (W88-W90)
exposure to sunlight (X32)

X X39.01 **Exposure to radon**

X X39.08 **Exposure to other natural radiation**

X X39.8 **Other exposure to forces of nature**

OVEREXERTION AND STRENUOUS OR REPETITIVE MOVEMENTS (X50)

X50 Overexertion and strenuous or repetitive movements

The appropriate 7th character is to be added to each code from category X50

A initial encounter
D subsequent encounter
S sequela

Coding Clinic: 2016, Q4, P73-74

X X50.0 **Overexertion from strenuous movement or load**
Lifting heavy objects
Lifting weights
Coding Clinic: 2016, Q4, P74

X X50.1 **Overexertion from prolonged static or awkward postures**
Prolonged bending
Prolonged kneeling
Prolonged reaching
Prolonged sitting
Prolonged standing
Prolonged twisting
Static bending
Static kneeling
Static reaching
Static sitting
Static standing
Static twisting

X X50.3 **Overexertion from repetitive movements**
Use of hand as hammer
Excludes2 Overuse from prolonged static or awkward postures (X50.1)
Coding Clinic: 2016, Q4, P74

X X50.9 **Other and unspecified overexertion or strenuous movements or postures**
Contact pressure
Contact stress

ACCIDENTAL EXPOSURE TO OTHER SPECIFIED FACTORS (X52, X58)

X X52 **Prolonged stay in weightless environment**
Weightlessness in spacecraft (simulator)

The appropriate 7th character is to be added to code X52

A initial encounter
D subsequent encounter
S sequela

X X58 **Exposure to other specified factors**
Accident NOS
Exposure NOS

The appropriate 7th character is to be added to code X58

A initial encounter
D subsequent encounter
S sequela

INTENTIONAL SELF-HARM (X71-X83)

Purposely self-inflicted injury
Suicide (attempted)

X71 Intentional self-harm by drowning and submersion

The appropriate 7th character is to be added to each code from category X71

A initial encounter
D subsequent encounter
S sequela

X X71.0 **Intentional self-harm by drowning and submersion while in bathtub** A, D, S

X X71.1 **Intentional self-harm by drowning and submersion while in swimming pool** A, D, S

X X71.2 **Intentional self-harm by drowning and submersion after jump into swimming pool** A, D, S

CHAPTER 20 (V00-Y99)

X● **X71.3 Intentional self-harm by drowning and submersion in natural water** A, D, S

X● **X71.8 Other intentional self-harm by drowning and submersion** A, D, S

X● **X71.9 Intentional self-harm by drowning and submersion, unspecified** A, D, S

X● **X72 Intentional self-harm by handgun discharge** A, D, S

Intentional self-harm by gun for single hand use
Intentional self-harm by pistol
Intentional self-harm by revolver

Excludes1 Very pistol (X74.8)

The appropriate 7th character is to be added to code X72

A initial encounter
D subsequent encounter
S sequela

● **X73 Intentional self-harm by rifle, shotgun and larger firearm discharge**

Excludes1 airgun (X74.01)

The appropriate 7th character is to be added to each code from category X73

A initial encounter
D subsequent encounter
S sequela

X● **X73.0 Intentional self-harm by shotgun discharge** A, D, S

X● **X73.1 Intentional self-harm by hunting rifle discharge** A, D, S

X● **X73.2 Intentional self-harm by machine gun discharge** A, D, S

X● **X73.8 Intentional self-harm by other larger firearm discharge** A, D, S

X● **X73.9 Intentional self-harm by unspecified larger firearm discharge** A, D, S

● **X74 Intentional self-harm by other and unspecified firearm and gun discharge**

The appropriate 7th character is to be added to each code from category X74

A initial encounter
D subsequent encounter
S sequela

● **X74.0 Intentional self-harm by gas, air or spring-operated guns**

X● **X74.01 Intentional self-harm by airgun** A, D, S

Intentional self-harm by BB gun discharge
Intentional self-harm by pellet gun discharge

X● **X74.02 Intentional self-harm by paintball gun** A, D, S

X● **X74.09 Intentional self-harm by other gas, air or spring-operated gun** A, D, S

X● **X74.8 Intentional self-harm by other firearm discharge** A, D, S

Intentional self-harm by Very pistol [flare] discharge

X● **X74.9 Intentional self-harm by unspecified firearm discharge** A, D, S

X● **X75 Intentional self-harm by explosive material** A, D, S

The appropriate 7th character is to be added to code X75

A initial encounter
D subsequent encounter
S sequela

X● **X76 Intentional self-harm by smoke, fire and flames** A, D, S

The appropriate 7th character is to be added to code X76

A initial encounter
D subsequent encounter
S sequela

● **X77 Intentional self-harm by steam, hot vapors and hot objects**

The appropriate 7th character is to be added to each code from category X77

A initial encounter
D subsequent encounter
S sequela

X● **X77.0 Intentional self-harm by steam or hot vapors** A, D, S

X● **X77.1 Intentional self-harm by hot tap water** A, D, S

X● **X77.2 Intentional self-harm by other hot fluids** A, D, S

X● **X77.3 Intentional self-harm by hot household appliances** A, D, S

X● **X77.8 Intentional self-harm by other hot objects** A, D, S

X● **X77.9 Intentional self-harm by unspecified hot objects** A, D, S

● **X78 Intentional self-harm by sharp object**

The appropriate 7th character is to be added to each code from category X78

A initial encounter
D subsequent encounter
S sequela

X● **X78.0 Intentional self-harm by sharp glass** A, D, S

X● **X78.1 Intentional self-harm by knife** A, D, S

X● **X78.2 Intentional self-harm by sword or dagger** A, D, S

X● **X78.8 Intentional self-harm by other sharp object** A, D, S

X● **X78.9 Intentional self-harm by unspecified sharp object** A, D, S

X● **X79 Intentional self-harm by blunt object** A, D, S

The appropriate 7th character is to be added to code X79

A initial encounter
D subsequent encounter
S sequela

X● **X80 Intentional self-harm by jumping from a high place** A, D, S

Intentional fall from one level to another

The appropriate 7th character is to be added to code X80

A initial encounter
D subsequent encounter
S sequela

● **X81 Intentional self-harm by jumping or lying in front of moving object**

The appropriate 7th character is to be added to each code from category X81

A initial encounter
D subsequent encounter
S sequela

X● **X81.0 Intentional self-harm by jumping or lying in front of motor vehicle** A, D, S

X● **X81.1 Intentional self-harm by jumping or lying in front of (subway) train** A, D, S

X● **X81.8 Intentional self-harm by jumping or lying in front of other moving object** A, D, S

● **X82 Intentional self-harm by crashing of motor vehicle**

The appropriate 7th character is to be added to each code from category X82

A initial encounter
D subsequent encounter
S sequela

X● **X82.0 Intentional collision of motor vehicle with other motor vehicle** A, D, S

X● **X82.1 Intentional collision of motor vehicle with train** A, D, S

CHAPTER 20 (V00-Y99)

X● X82.2 **Intentional collision of motor vehicle with tree** A, D, S

X● X82.8 **Other intentional self-harm by crashing of motor vehicle** A, D, S

● X83 **Intentional self-harm by other specified means**

Excludes1 intentional self-harm by poisoning or contact with toxic substance - see Table of Drugs and Chemicals

The appropriate 7th character is to be added to each code from category X83

A	initial encounter
D	subsequent encounter
S	sequela

X● X83.0 **Intentional self-harm by crashing of aircraft** A, D, S

X● X83.1 **Intentional self-harm by electrocution** A, D, S

X● X83.2 **Intentional self-harm by exposure to extremes of cold** A, D, S

X● X83.8 **Intentional self-harm by other specified means** A, D, S

ASSAULT (X92-Y09)

Includes homicide injuries inflicted by another person with intent to injure or kill, by any means

Excludes1 injuries due to legal intervention (Y35.-)
injuries due to operations of war (Y36.-)
injuries due to terrorism (Y38.-)

● X92 **Assault by drowning and submersion**

The appropriate 7th character is to be added to each code from category X92

A	initial encounter
D	subsequent encounter
S	sequela

X● X92.0 **Assault by drowning and submersion while in bathtub**

X● X92.1 **Assault by drowning and submersion while in swimming pool**

X● X92.2 **Assault by drowning and submersion after push into swimming pool**

X● X92.3 **Assault by drowning and submersion in natural water**

X● X92.8 **Other assault by drowning and submersion**

X● X92.9 **Assault by drowning and submersion, unspecified**

X● X93 **Assault by handgun discharge**

Assault by discharge of gun for single hand use
Assault by discharge of pistol
Assault by discharge of revolver

Excludes1 Very pistol (X95.8)

The appropriate 7th character is to be added to code X93

A	initial encounter
D	subsequent encounter
S	sequela

● X94 **Assault by rifle, shotgun and larger firearm discharge**

Excludes1 airgun (X95.01)

The appropriate 7th character is to be added to each code from category X94

A	initial encounter
D	subsequent encounter
S	sequela

X● X94.0 **Assault by shotgun**

X● X94.1 **Assault by hunting rifle**

X● X94.2 **Assault by machine gun**

X● X94.8 **Assault by other larger firearm discharge**

X● X94.9 **Assault by unspecified larger firearm discharge**

● X95 **Assault by other and unspecified firearm and gun discharge**

The appropriate 7th character is to be added to each code from category X95

A	initial encounter
D	subsequent encounter
S	sequela

● X95.0 **Assault by gas, air or spring-operated guns**

X● X95.01 **Assault by airgun discharge**

Assault by BB gun discharge
Assault by pellet gun discharge

X● X95.02 **Assault by paintball gun discharge**

X● X95.09 **Assault by other gas, air or spring-operated gun**

X● X95.8 **Assault by other firearm discharge**

Assault by very pistol [flare] discharge

X● X95.9 **Assault by unspecified firearm discharge**

Coding Clinic: 2016, Q3, P24

● X96 **Assault by explosive material**

Excludes1 incendiary device (X97)
terrorism involving explosive material (Y38.2-)

The appropriate 7th character is to be added to each code from category X96

A	initial encounter
D	subsequent encounter
S	sequela

X● X96.0 **Assault by antipersonnel bomb**

Excludes1 antipersonnel bomb use in military or war (Y36.2-)

X● X96.1 **Assault by gasoline bomb**

X● X96.2 **Assault by letter bomb**

X● X96.3 **Assault by fertilizer bomb**

X● X96.4 **Assault by pipe bomb**

X● X96.8 **Assault by other specified explosive**

X● X96.9 **Assault by unspecified explosive**

X● X97 **Assault by smoke, fire and flames**

Assault by arson
Assault by cigarettes
Assault by incendiary device

The appropriate 7th character is to be added to code X97

A	initial encounter
D	subsequent encounter
S	sequela

● X98 **Assault by steam, hot vapors and hot objects**

The appropriate 7th character is to be added to each code from category X98

A	initial encounter
D	subsequent encounter
S	sequela

X● X98.0 **Assault by steam or hot vapors**

X● X98.1 **Assault by hot tap water**

X● X98.2 **Assault by hot fluids**

X● X98.3 **Assault by hot household appliances**

X● X98.8 **Assault by other hot objects**

X● X98.9 **Assault by unspecified hot objects**

X99 Assault by sharp object

Excludes1 assault by strike by sports equipment (Y08.0-)

The appropriate 7th character is to be added to each code from category X99

A	initial encounter
D	subsequent encounter
S	sequela

X **X99.0 Assault by sharp glass**

X **X99.1 Assault by knife**

X **X99.2 Assault by sword or dagger**

X **X99.8 Assault by other sharp object**

X **X99.9 Assault by unspecified sharp object**

Assault by stabbing NOS

X **Y00 Assault by blunt object**

Excludes1 assault by strike by sports equipment (Y08.0)

The appropriate 7th character is to be added to code Y00

A	initial encounter
D	subsequent encounter
S	sequela

X **Y01 Assault by pushing from high place**

The appropriate 7th character is to be added to code Y01

A	initial encounter
D	subsequent encounter
S	sequela

Y02 Assault by pushing or placing victim in front of moving object

The appropriate 7th character is to be added to each code from category Y02

A	initial encounter
D	subsequent encounter
S	sequela

X **Y02.0 Assault by pushing or placing victim in front of motor vehicle**

X **Y02.1 Assault by pushing or placing victim in front of (subway) train**

X **Y02.8 Assault by pushing or placing victim in front of other moving object**

Y03 Assault by crashing of motor vehicle

The appropriate 7th character is to be added to each code from category Y03

A	initial encounter
D	subsequent encounter
S	sequela

X **Y03.0 Assault by being hit or run over by motor vehicle**

X **Y03.8 Other assault by crashing of motor vehicle**

Y04 Assault by bodily force

Excludes1 assault by:
submersion (X92.-)
use of weapon (X93-X95, X99, Y00)

The appropriate 7th character is to be added to each code from category Y04

A	initial encounter
D	subsequent encounter
S	sequela

X **Y04.0 Assault by unarmed brawl or fight**

X **Y04.1 Assault by human bite**

X **Y04.2 Assault by strike against or bumped into by another person**

X **Y04.8 Assault by other bodily force**

Assault by bodily force NOS

OGCR Section I.C.19.f.

Adult and child abuse, neglect and other maltreatment

Sequence first the appropriate code from categories T74 or T76 for abuse, neglect and other maltreatment, followed by any accompanying mental health or injury code(s).

If the documentation in the medical record states abuse or neglect it is coded as confirmed (T74.-). It is coded as suspected if it is documented as suspected (T76.-).

For cases of confirmed abuse or neglect an external cause code from the assault section (X92-Y09) should be added to identify the cause of any physical injuries. A perpetrator code (Y07) should be added when the perpetrator of the abuse is known. For suspected cases of abuse or neglect, do not report external cause or perpetrator code.

If a suspected case of abuse, neglect or mistreatment is ruled out during an encounter code Z04.71, Encounter for examination and observation following alleged physical adult abuse, ruled out, or code Z04.72, Encounter for examination and observation following alleged adult rape, should be used, not a code from T76.

If a suspected case of alleged rape or sexual abuse is ruled out during an encounter code Z04.41, Encounter for examination and observation following alleged adult rape or code Z04.42, Encounter for examination and observation following alleged child rape should be used, not a code from T76.

Y07 Perpetrator of assault, maltreatment and neglect

Note: Codes from this category are for use only in cases of confirmed abuse (T74.-)

Selection of the correct perpetrator code is based on the relationship between the perpetrator and the victim

Includes perpetrator of abandonment
perpetrator of emotional neglect
perpetrator of mental cruelty
perpetrator of physical abuse
perpetrator of physical neglect
perpetrator of sexual abuse
perpetrator of torture

Coding Clinic: 2016, Q4, P129

Y07.0 Spouse or partner, perpetrator of maltreatment and neglect

Spouse or partner, perpetrator of maltreatment and neglect against spouse or partner

Y07.01 Husband, perpetrator of maltreatment and neglect

Y07.02 Wife, perpetrator of maltreatment and neglect

Y07.03 Male partner, perpetrator of maltreatment and neglect

Y07.04 Female partner, perpetrator of maltreatment and neglect

Y07.1 Parent (adoptive) (biological), perpetrator of maltreatment and neglect

Y07.11 Biological father, perpetrator of maltreatment and neglect

Y07.12 Biological mother, perpetrator of maltreatment and neglect

Y07.13 Adoptive father, perpetrator of maltreatment and neglect

Y07.14 Adoptive mother, perpetrator of maltreatment and neglect

Y07.4 Other family member, perpetrator of maltreatment and neglect

Y07.41 Sibling, perpetrator of maltreatment and neglect

Excludes1 stepsibling, perpetrator of maltreatment and neglect (Y07.435, Y07.436)

Y07.410 Brother, perpetrator of maltreatment and neglect

Y07.411 Sister, perpetrator of maltreatment and neglect

CHAPTER 20 (V00-Y99)

● Y07.42 **Foster parent**, perpetrator of maltreatment and neglect
Y07.420 **Foster father**, perpetrator of maltreatment and neglect
Y07.421 **Foster mother**, perpetrator of maltreatment and neglect
● Y07.43 **Stepparent or stepsibling**, perpetrator of maltreatment and neglect
Y07.430 **Stepfather**, perpetrator of maltreatment and neglect
Y07.432 **Male friend of parent** (co-residing in household), perpetrator of maltreatment and neglect
Y07.433 **Stepmother**, perpetrator of maltreatment and neglect
Y07.434 **Female friend of parent** (co-residing in household), perpetrator of maltreatment and neglect
Y07.435 **Stepbrother**, perpetrator or maltreatment and neglect
Y07.436 **Stepsister**, perpetrator of maltreatment and neglect
● Y07.49 **Other family member**, perpetrator of maltreatment and neglect
Y07.490 **Male cousin**, perpetrator of maltreatment and neglect
Y07.491 **Female cousin**, perpetrator of maltreatment and neglect
Y07.499 **Other family member**, perpetrator of maltreatment and neglect
● Y07.5 **Non-family member**, perpetrator of maltreatment and neglect
Y07.50 **Unspecified non-family member**, perpetrator of maltreatment and neglect
● Y07.51 **Daycare provider**, perpetrator of maltreatment and neglect
Y07.510 **At-home childcare provider**, perpetrator of maltreatment and neglect
Y07.511 **Daycare center childcare provider**, perpetrator of maltreatment and neglect
Y07.512 **At-home adultcare provider**, perpetrator of maltreatment and neglect
Y07.513 **Adultcare center provider**, perpetrator of maltreatment and neglect
Y07.519 **Unspecified daycare provider**, perpetrator of maltreatment and neglect
● Y07.52 **Healthcare provider**, perpetrator of maltreatment and neglect
Y07.521 **Mental health provider**, perpetrator of maltreatment and neglect
Y07.528 **Other therapist or healthcare provider**, perpetrator of maltreatment and neglect
Nurse perpetrator of maltreatment and neglect
Occupational therapist perpetrator of maltreatment and neglect
Physical therapist perpetrator of maltreatment and neglect
Speech therapist perpetrator of maltreatment and neglect
Y07.529 **Unspecified healthcare provider**, perpetrator of maltreatment and neglect
Y07.53 **Teacher or instructor**, perpetrator of maltreatment and neglect
Coach, perpetrator of maltreatment and neglect
Y07.59 **Other non-family member**, perpetrator of maltreatment and neglect
Y07.6 Multiple perpetrators of maltreatment and neglect
Y07.9 Unspecified perpetrator of maltreatment and neglect

● Y08 Assault by other specified means
The appropriate 7th character is to be added to each code from category Y08

A	initial encounter
D	subsequent encounter
S	sequela

● Y08.0 Assault by strike by sport equipment
X● Y08.01 **Assault by strike by hockey stick**
X● Y08.02 **Assault by strike by baseball bat**
X● Y08.09 **Assault by strike by other specified type of sport equipment**
● Y08.8 Assault by other specified means
X● Y08.81 **Assault by crashing of aircraft**
X● Y08.89 **Assault by other specified means**

● Y09 Assault by unspecified means
Assassination (attempted) NOS
Homicide (attempted) NOS
Manslaughter (attempted) NOS
Murder (attempted) NOS

EVENT OF UNDETERMINED INTENT (Y21-Y33)

Undetermined intent is only for use when there is specific documentation in the record that the intent of the injury cannot be determined. If no such documentation is present, code to accidental (unintentional)

● Y21 Drowning and submersion, undetermined intent
The appropriate 7th character is to be added to each code from category Y21

A	initial encounter
D	subsequent encounter
S	sequela

X● Y21.0 **Drowning and submersion while in bathtub, undetermined intent**
X● Y21.1 **Drowning and submersion after fall into bathtub, undetermined intent**
X● Y21.2 **Drowning and submersion while in swimming pool, undetermined intent**
X● Y21.3 **Drowning and submersion after fall into swimming pool, undetermined intent**
X● Y21.4 **Drowning and submersion in natural water, undetermined intent**
X● Y21.8 **Other drowning and submersion, undetermined intent**
X● Y21.9 **Unspecified drowning and submersion, undetermined intent**

X● Y22 **Handgun discharge, undetermined intent**
Discharge of gun for single hand use, undetermined intent
Discharge of pistol, undetermined intent
Discharge of revolver, undetermined intent
Excludes2 very pistol (Y24.8)
The appropriate 7th character is to be added to code Y22

A	initial encounter
D	subsequent encounter
S	sequela

● **Y23 Rifle, shotgun and larger firearm discharge, undetermined intent**

Excludes2 airgun (Y24.0)

The appropriate 7th character is to be added to each code from category Y23

A	initial encounter
D	subsequent encounter
S	sequela

X● **Y23.0 Shotgun discharge, undetermined intent**

X● **Y23.1 Hunting rifle discharge, undetermined intent**

X● **Y23.2 Military firearm discharge, undetermined intent**

X● **Y23.3 Machine gun discharge, undetermined intent**

X● **Y23.8 Other larger firearm discharge, undetermined intent**

X● **Y23.9 Unspecified larger firearm discharge, undetermined intent**

● **Y24 Other and unspecified firearm discharge, undetermined intent**

The appropriate 7th character is to be added to each code from category Y24

A	initial encounter
D	subsequent encounter
S	sequela

X● **Y24.0 Airgun discharge, undetermined intent**

BB gun discharge, undetermined intent
Pellet gun discharge, undetermined intent

X● **Y24.8 Other firearm discharge, undetermined intent**

Paintball gun discharge, undetermined intent
Very pistol [flare] discharge, undetermined intent

X● **Y24.9 Unspecified firearm discharge, undetermined intent**

X● **Y25 Contact with explosive material, undetermined intent**

The appropriate 7th character is to be added to code Y25

A	initial encounter
D	subsequent encounter
S	sequela

X● **Y26 Exposure to smoke, fire and flames, undetermined intent**

The appropriate 7th character is to be added to code Y26

A	initial encounter
D	subsequent encounter
S	sequela

● **Y27 Contact with steam, hot vapors and hot objects, undetermined intent**

The appropriate 7th character is to be added to each code from category Y27

A	initial encounter
D	subsequent encounter
S	sequela

X● **Y27.0 Contact with steam and hot vapors, undetermined intent**

X● **Y27.1 Contact with hot tap water, undetermined intent**

X● **Y27.2 Contact with hot fluids, undetermined intent**

X● **Y27.3 Contact with hot household appliance, undetermined intent**

X● **Y27.8 Contact with other hot objects, undetermined intent**

X● **Y27.9 Contact with unspecified hot objects, undetermined intent**

● **Y28 Contact with sharp object, undetermined intent**

The appropriate 7th character is to be added to each code from category Y28

A	initial encounter
D	subsequent encounter
S	sequela

X● **Y28.0 Contact with sharp glass, undetermined intent**

X● **Y28.1 Contact with knife, undetermined intent**

X● **Y28.2 Contact with sword or dagger, undetermined intent**

X● **Y28.8 Contact with other sharp object, undetermined intent**

X● **Y28.9 Contact with unspecified sharp object, undetermined intent**

X● **Y29 Contact with blunt object, undetermined intent**

The appropriate 7th character is to be added to code Y29

A	initial encounter
D	subsequent encounter
S	sequela

X● **Y30 Falling, jumping or pushed from a high place, undetermined intent**

Victim falling from one level to another, undetermined intent

The appropriate 7th character is to be added to code Y30

A	initial encounter
D	subsequent encounter
S	sequela

X● **Y31 Falling, lying or running before or into moving object, undetermined intent**

The appropriate 7th character is to be added to code Y31

A	initial encounter
D	subsequent encounter
S	sequela

X● **Y32 Crashing of motor vehicle, undetermined intent**

The appropriate 7th character is to be added to code Y32

A	initial encounter
D	subsequent encounter
S	sequela

X● **Y33 Other specified events, undetermined intent**

The appropriate 7th character is to be added to code Y33

A	initial encounter
D	subsequent encounter
S	sequela

LEGAL INTERVENTION, OPERATIONS OF WAR, MILITARY OPERATIONS, AND TERRORISM (Y35-Y38)

Y35 Legal intervention

Includes any injury sustained as a result of an encounter with any law enforcement official, serving in any capacity at the time of the encounter, whether on-duty or off-duty. Includes: injury to law enforcement official, suspect and bystander

The appropriate 7th character is to be added to each code from category Y35

A initial encounter
D subsequent encounter
S sequela

Y35.0 Legal intervention involving **firearm discharge**

Y35.00 Legal intervention involving **unspecified** firearm discharge
Legal intervention involving gunshot wound
Legal intervention involving shot NOS

Y35.001 Legal intervention involving unspecified firearm discharge, **law enforcement official injured**

Y35.002 Legal intervention involving unspecified firearm discharge, **bystander injured**

Y35.003 Legal intervention involving unspecified firearm discharge, **suspect injured**

▶ Y35.009 Legal intervention involving unspecified firearm discharge, unspecified person injured

Y35.01 Legal intervention involving injury by **machine gun**

Y35.011 Legal intervention involving injury by machine gun, **law enforcement official injured**

Y35.012 Legal intervention involving injury by machine gun, **bystander injured**

Y35.013 Legal intervention involving injury by machine gun, **suspect injured**

▶ Y35.019 Legal intervention involving injury by machine gun, unspecified person injured

Y35.02 Legal intervention involving injury by **handgun**

Y35.021 Legal intervention involving injury by handgun, **law enforcement official injured**

Y35.022 Legal intervention involving injury by handgun, **bystander injured**

Y35.023 Legal intervention involving injury by handgun, **suspect injured**

▶ Y35.029 Legal intervention involving injury by handgun, unspecified person injured

Y35.03 Legal intervention involving injury by **rifle pellet**

Y35.031 Legal intervention involving injury by rifle pellet, **law enforcement official injured**

Y35.032 Legal intervention involving injury by rifle pellet, **bystander injured**

Y35.033 Legal intervention involving injury by rifle pellet, **suspect injured**

▶ Y35.039 Legal intervention involving injury by rifle pellet, unspecified person injured

Y35.04 Legal intervention involving injury by **rubber bullet**

Y35.041 Legal intervention involving injury by rubber bullet, **law enforcement official injured**

Y35.042 Legal intervention involving injury by rubber bullet, **bystander injured**

Y35.043 Legal intervention involving injury by rubber bullet, **suspect injured**

▶ Y35.049 Legal intervention involving injury by rubber bullet, unspecified person injured

Y35.09 Legal intervention involving **other firearm** discharge

Y35.091 Legal intervention involving other firearm discharge, **law enforcement official injured**

Y35.092 Legal intervention involving other firearm discharge, **bystander injured**

Y35.093 Legal intervention involving other firearm discharge, **suspect injured**

▶ Y35.099 Legal intervention involving other firearm discharge, unspecified person injured

Y35.1 Legal intervention involving **explosives**

Y35.10 Legal intervention involving **unspecified** explosives

Y35.101 Legal intervention involving unspecified explosives, **law enforcement official injured**

Y35.102 Legal intervention involving unspecified explosives, **bystander injured**

Y35.103 Legal intervention involving unspecified explosives, **suspect injured**

▶ Y35.109 Legal intervention involving unspecified explosives, unspecified person injured

Y35.11 Legal intervention involving injury by **dynamite**

Y35.111 Legal intervention involving injury by dynamite, **law enforcement official injured**

Y35.112 Legal intervention involving injury by dynamite, **bystander injured**

Y35.113 Legal intervention involving injury by dynamite, **suspect injured**

▶ Y35.119 Legal intervention involving injury by dynamite, unspecified person injured

Y35.12 Legal intervention involving injury by **explosive shell**

Y35.121 Legal intervention involving injury by explosive shell, **law enforcement official injured**

Y35.122 Legal intervention involving injury by explosive shell, **bystander injured**

Y35.123 Legal intervention involving injury by explosive shell, **suspect injured**

▶ Y35.129 Legal intervention involving other explosives, unspecified person injured

Y35.19 Legal intervention involving **other explosives**
Legal intervention involving injury by grenade
Legal intervention involving injury by mortar bomb

Y35.191 Legal intervention involving other explosives, **law enforcement official injured**

Y35.192 Legal intervention involving other explosives, **bystander injured**

Y35.193 Legal intervention involving other explosives, **suspect injured**

Y35.199 Legal intervention involving other explosives, unspecified person injured

Y35.2 Legal intervention involving gas
Legal intervention involving asphyxiation by gas
Legal intervention involving poisoning by gas

Y35.20 Legal intervention involving **unspecified gas**

Y35.201 Legal intervention involving unspecified gas, **law enforcement official injured**

Y35.202 Legal intervention involving unspecified gas, **bystander injured**

Y35.203 Legal intervention involving unspecified gas, **suspect injured**

Y35.209 Legal intervention involving unspecified gas, unspecified person injured

Y35.21 Legal intervention involving injury by **tear gas**

Y35.211 Legal intervention involving injury by tear gas, **law enforcement official injured**

Y35.212 Legal intervention involving injury by tear gas, **bystander injured**

Y35.213 Legal intervention involving injury by tear gas, **suspect injured**

Y35.219 Legal intervention involving injury by tear gas, unspecified person injured

Y35.29 Legal intervention involving **other gas**

Y35.291 Legal intervention involving other gas, **law enforcement official injured**

Y35.292 Legal intervention involving other gas, **bystander injured**

Y35.293 Legal intervention involving other gas, **suspect injured**

Y35.299 Legal intervention involving other gas, unspecified person injured

Y35.3 Legal intervention involving blunt objects
Legal intervention involving being hit or struck by blunt object

Y35.30 Legal intervention involving **unspecified blunt objects**

Y35.301 Legal intervention involving unspecified blunt objects, **law enforcement official injured**

Y35.302 Legal intervention involving unspecified blunt objects, **bystander injured**

Y35.303 Legal intervention involving unspecified blunt objects, **suspect injured**

Y35.309 Legal intervention involving unspecified blunt objects, unspecified person injured

Y35.31 Legal intervention involving **baton**

Y35.311 Legal intervention involving baton, **law enforcement official injured**

Y35.312 Legal intervention involving baton, **bystander injured**

Y35.313 Legal intervention involving baton, **suspect injured**

Y35.319 Legal intervention involving baton, unspecified person injured

Y35.39 Legal intervention involving **other blunt objects**

Y35.391 Legal intervention involving other blunt objects, **law enforcement official injured**

Y35.392 Legal intervention involving other blunt objects, **bystander injured**

Y35.393 Legal intervention involving other blunt objects, **suspect injured**

Y35.399 Legal intervention involving other blunt objects, unspecified person injured

Y35.4 Legal intervention involving sharp objects
Legal intervention involving being cut by sharp objects
Legal intervention involving being stabbed by sharp objects

Y35.40 Legal intervention involving **unspecified sharp objects**

Y35.401 Legal intervention involving unspecified sharp objects, **law enforcement official injured**

Y35.402 Legal intervention involving unspecified sharp objects, **bystander injured**

Y35.403 Legal intervention involving unspecified sharp objects, **suspect injured**

Y35.409 Legal intervention involving unspecified sharp objects, unspecified person injured

Y35.41 Legal intervention involving **bayonet**

Y35.411 Legal intervention involving bayonet, **law enforcement official injured**

Y35.412 Legal intervention involving bayonet, **bystander injured**

Y35.413 Legal intervention involving bayonet, **suspect injured**

Y35.419 Legal intervention involving bayonet, unspecified person injured

Y35.49 Legal intervention involving **other sharp objects**

Y35.491 Legal intervention involving other sharp objects, **law enforcement official injured**

Y35.492 Legal intervention involving other sharp objects, **bystander injured**

Y35.493 Legal intervention involving other sharp objects, **suspect injured**

Y35.499 Legal intervention involving other sharp objects, unspecified person injured

Y35.8 Legal intervention involving other specified means

Y35.81 Legal intervention involving **manhandling**

Y35.811 Legal intervention involving manhandling, **law enforcement official injured**

Y35.812 Legal intervention involving manhandling, **bystander injured**

Y35.813 Legal intervention involving manhandling, **suspect injured**

Y35.819 Legal intervention involving manhandling, unspecified person injured

Y35.83 Legal intervention involving a conducted energy device
Electroshock device (taser)
Stun gun

Y35.831 Legal intervention involving a conducted energy device, law enforcement official injured

Y35.832 Legal intervention involving a conducted energy device, bystander injured

▶● Y35.833 Legal intervention involving a conducted energy device, suspect injured

▶● Y35.839 Legal intervention involving a conducted energy device, unspecified person injured

● Y35.89 Legal intervention involving other specified means

● Y35.891 Legal intervention involving other specified means, law enforcement official injured

● Y35.892 Legal intervention involving other specified means, bystander injured

● Y35.893 Legal intervention involving other specified means, suspect injured

Coding Clinic: 2018, Q1, P5

● Y35.9 Legal intervention, means unspecified

X● Y35.91 Legal intervention, means unspecified, law enforcement official injured

X● Y35.92 Legal intervention, means unspecified, bystander injured

X● Y35.93 Legal intervention, means unspecified, suspect injured

▶X● Y35.99 Legal intervention, means unspecified, unspecified person injured

● Y36 Operations of war

Includes injuries to military personnel and civilians caused by war, civil insurrection, and peacekeeping missions

Excludes1 injury to military personnel occurring during peacetime military operations (Y37.-)

military vehicles involved in transport accidents with non-military vehicle during peacetime (V09.01, V09.21, V19.81, V29.81, V39.81, V49.81, V59.81, V69.81, V79.81)

The appropriate 7th character is to be added to each code from category Y36

A	initial encounter
D	subsequent encounter
S	sequela

● Y36.0 War operations involving explosion of marine weapons

Weapons and military watercraft

● Y36.00 War operations involving explosion of unspecified marine weapon

War operations involving underwater blast NOS

● Y36.000 War operations involving explosion of unspecified marine weapon, military personnel

● Y36.001 War operations involving explosion of unspecified marine weapon, civilian

● Y36.01 War operations involving explosion of depth-charge

● Y36.010 War operations involving explosion of depth-charge, military personnel

● Y36.011 War operations involving explosion of depth-charge, civilian

● Y36.02 War operations involving explosion of marine mine

War operations involving explosion of marine mine, at sea or in harbor

● Y36.020 War operations involving explosion of marine mine, military personnel

● Y36.021 War operations involving explosion of marine mine, civilian

● Y36.03 War operations involving explosion of sea-based artillery shell

● Y36.030 War operations involving explosion of sea-based artillery shell, military personnel

● Y36.031 War operations involving explosion of sea-based artillery shell, civilian

● Y36.04 War operations involving explosion of torpedo

● Y36.040 War operations involving explosion of torpedo, military personnel

● Y36.041 War operations involving explosion of torpedo, civilian

● Y36.05 War operations involving accidental detonation of onboard marine weapons

● Y36.050 War operations involving accidental detonation of onboard marine weapons, military personnel

● Y36.051 War operations involving accidental detonation of onboard marine weapons, civilian

● Y36.09 War operations involving explosion of other marine weapons

● Y36.090 War operations involving explosion of other marine weapons, military personnel

● Y36.091 War operations involving explosion of other marine weapons, civilian

● Y36.1 War operations involving destruction of aircraft

● Y36.10 War operations involving unspecified destruction of aircraft

● Y36.100 War operations involving unspecified destruction of aircraft, military personnel

● Y36.101 War operations involving unspecified destruction of aircraft, civilian

● Y36.11 War operations involving destruction of aircraft due to enemy fire or explosives

War operations involving destruction of aircraft due to air to air missile

War operations involving destruction of aircraft due to explosive placed on aircraft

War operations involving destruction of aircraft due to rocket propelled grenade [RPG]

War operations involving destruction of aircraft due to small arms fire

War operations involving destruction of aircraft due to surface to air missile

● Y36.110 War operations involving destruction of aircraft due to enemy fire or explosives, military personnel

● Y36.111 War operations involving destruction of aircraft due to enemy fire or explosives, civilian

● Y36.12 War operations involving destruction of aircraft due to collision with other aircraft

● Y36.120 War operations involving destruction of aircraft due to collision with other aircraft, military personnel

● Y36.121 War operations involving destruction of aircraft due to collision with other aircraft, civilian

● Y36.13 War operations involving destruction of aircraft due to onboard fire

● Y36.130 War operations involving destruction of aircraft due to onboard fire, military personnel

● Y36.131 War operations involving destruction of aircraft due to onboard fire, civilian

Y36.14 War operations involving destruction of aircraft due to accidental detonation of onboard munitions and explosives

Y36.140 War operations involving destruction of aircraft due to accidental detonation of onboard munitions and explosives, military personnel

Y36.141 War operations involving destruction of aircraft due to accidental detonation of onboard munitions and explosives, civilian

Y36.19 War operations involving other destruction of aircraft

Y36.190 War operations involving other destruction of aircraft, military personnel

Y36.191 War operations involving other destruction of aircraft, civilian

Y36.2 War operations involving other explosions and fragments

Excludes1 war operations involving explosion of aircraft (Y36.1-)
war operations involving explosion of marine weapons (Y36.0-)
war operations involving explosion of nuclear weapons (Y36.5-)
war operations involving explosion occurring after cessation of hostilities (Y36.8-)

Y36.20 War operations involving unspecified explosion and fragments

War operations involving air blast NOS
War operations involving blast NOS
War operations involving blast fragments NOS
War operations involving blast wave NOS
War operations involving blast wind NOS
War operations involving explosion NOS
War operations involving explosion of bomb NOS

Y36.200 War operations involving unspecified explosion and fragments, military personnel

Y36.201 War operations involving unspecified explosion and fragments, civilian

Y36.21 War operations involving explosion of aerial bomb

Y36.210 War operations involving explosion of aerial bomb, military personnel

Y36.211 War operations involving explosion of aerial bomb, civilian

Y36.22 War operations involving explosion of guided missile

Y36.220 War operations involving explosion of guided missile, military personnel

Y36.221 War operations involving explosion of guided missile, civilian

Y36.23 War operations involving explosion of improvised explosive device [IED]

War operations involving explosion of person-borne improvised explosive device [IED]
War operations involving explosion of vehicle-borne improvised explosive device [IED]
War operations involving explosion of roadside improvised explosive device [IED]

Y36.230 War operations involving explosion of improvised explosive device [IED], military personnel

Y36.231 War operations involving explosion of improvised explosive device [IED], civilian

Y36.24 War operations involving explosion due to accidental detonation and discharge of own munitions or munitions launch device

Y36.240 War operations involving explosion due to accidental detonation and discharge of own munitions or munitions launch device, military personnel

Y36.241 War operations involving explosion due to accidental detonation and discharge of own munitions or munitions launch device, civilian

Y36.25 War operations involving fragments from munitions

Y36.250 War operations involving fragments from munitions, military personnel

Y36.251 War operations involving fragments from munitions, civilian

Y36.26 War operations involving fragments of improvised explosive device [IED]

War operations involving fragments of person-borne improvised explosive device [IED]
War operations involving fragments of vehicle-borne improvised explosive device [IED]
War operations involving fragments of roadside improvised explosive device [IED]

Y36.260 War operations involving fragments of improvised explosive device [IED], military personnel

Y36.261 War operations involving fragments of improvised explosive device [IED], civilian

Y36.27 War operations involving fragments from weapons

Y36.270 War operations involving fragments from weapons, military personnel

Y36.271 War operations involving fragments from weapons, civilian

Y36.29 War operations involving other explosions and fragments

War operations involving explosion of grenade
War operations involving explosions of land mine
War operations involving shrapnel NOS

Y36.290 War operations involving other explosions and fragments, military personnel

Y36.291 War operations involving other explosions and fragments, civilian

Y36.3 War operations involving fires, conflagrations and hot substances

War operations involving smoke, fumes, and heat from fires, conflagrations and hot substances

Excludes1 war operations involving fires and conflagrations aboard military aircraft (Y36.1-)
war operations involving fires and conflagrations aboard military watercraft (Y36.0-)
war operations involving fires and conflagrations caused indirectly by conventional weapons (Y36.2-)
war operations involving fires and thermal effects of nuclear weapons (Y36.53-)

Y36.30 War operations involving unspecified fire, conflagration and hot substance

Y36.300 War operations involving unspecified fire, conflagration and hot substance, military personnel

Y36.301 War operations involving unspecified fire, conflagration and hot substance, civilian

CHAPTER 20 (V00-Y99)

- Y36.31 War operations involving **gasoline bomb**
  War operations involving incendiary bomb
  War operations involving petrol bomb
  - Y36.310 War operations involving gasoline bomb, **military personnel**
  - Y36.311 War operations involving gasoline bomb, **civilian**
- Y36.32 War operations involving **incendiary bullet**
  - Y36.320 War operations involving incendiary bullet, **military personnel**
  - Y36.321 War operations involving incendiary bullet, **civilian**
- Y36.33 War operations involving **flamethrower**
  - Y36.330 War operations involving flamethrower, **military personnel**
  - Y36.331 War operations involving flamethrower, **civilian**
- Y36.39 War operations involving **other** fires, conflagrations and hot substances
  - Y36.390 War operations involving other fires, conflagrations and hot substances, **military personnel**
  - Y36.391 War operations involving other fires, conflagrations and hot substances, **civilian**

Y36.4 War operations involving firearm discharge and other forms of conventional warfare

- Y36.41 War operations involving **rubber bullets**
  - Y36.410 War operations involving rubber bullets, **military personnel**
  - Y36.411 War operations involving rubber bullets, **civilian**
- Y36.42 War operations involving **firearms pellets**
  - Y36.420 War operations involving firearms pellets, **military personnel**
  - Y36.421 War operations involving firearms pellets, **civilian**
- Y36.43 War operations involving **other firearms** discharge
  War operations involving bullets NOS
  Excludes1 war operations involving munitions fragments (Y36.25-)
  war operations involving incendiary bullets (Y36.32-)
  - Y36.430 War operations involving other firearms discharge, **military personnel**
  - Y36.431 War operations involving other firearms discharge, **civilian**
- Y36.44 War operations involving **unarmed hand to hand combat**
  Excludes1 war operations involving combat using blunt or piercing object (Y36.45-)
  war operations involving intentional restriction of air and airway (Y36.46-)
  war operations involving unintentional restriction of air and airway (Y36.47-)
  - Y36.440 War operations involving unarmed hand to hand combat, **military personnel**
  - Y36.441 War operations involving unarmed hand to hand combat, **civilian**
- Y36.45 War operations involving combat **using blunt or piercing object**
  - Y36.450 War operations involving combat using blunt or piercing object, **military personnel**
  - Y36.451 War operations involving combat using blunt or piercing object, **civilian**
- Y36.46 War operations involving **intentional restriction of air and airway**
  - Y36.460 War operations involving intentional restriction of air and airway, **military personnel**
  - Y36.461 War operations involving intentional restriction of air and airway, **civilian**
- Y36.47 War operations involving **unintentional restriction of air and airway**
  - Y36.470 War operations involving unintentional restriction of air and airway, **military personnel**
  - Y36.471 War operations involving unintentional restriction of air and airway, **civilian**
- Y36.49 War operations involving **other** forms of conventional warfare
  - Y36.490 War operations involving other forms of conventional warfare, **military personnel**
  - Y36.491 War operations involving other forms of conventional warfare, **civilian**

Y36.5 War operations involving **nuclear weapons**
War operations involving dirty bomb NOS

- Y36.50 War operations involving **unspecified effect** of nuclear weapon
  - Y36.500 War operations involving unspecified effect of nuclear weapon, **military personnel**
  - Y36.501 War operations involving unspecified effect of nuclear weapon, **civilian**
- Y36.51 War operations involving **direct blast effect** of nuclear weapon
  War operations involving blast pressure of nuclear weapon
  - Y36.510 War operations involving direct blast effect of nuclear weapon, **military personnel**
  - Y36.511 War operations involving direct blast effect of nuclear weapon, **civilian**
- Y36.52 War operations involving **indirect blast effect** of nuclear weapon
  War operations involving being thrown by blast of nuclear weapon
  War operations involving being struck or crushed by blast debris of nuclear weapon
  - Y36.520 War operations involving indirect blast effect of nuclear weapon, **military personnel**
  - Y36.521 War operations involving indirect blast effect of nuclear weapon, **civilian**
- Y36.53 War operations involving **thermal radiation** effect of nuclear weapon
  War operations involving direct heat from nuclear weapon
  War operation involving fireball effects from nuclear weapon
  - Y36.530 War operations involving thermal radiation effect of nuclear weapon, **military personnel**
  - Y36.531 War operations involving thermal radiation effect of nuclear weapon, **civilian**

Y36.54 **War operation involving nuclear radiation effects of nuclear weapon**
War operation involving acute radiation exposure from nuclear weapon
War operation involving exposure to immediate ionizing radiation from nuclear weapon
War operation involving fallout exposure from nuclear weapon
War operation involving secondary effects of nuclear weapons

Y36.54Ø **War operation involving nuclear radiation effects of nuclear weapon, military personnel**

Y36.541 **War operation involving nuclear radiation effects of nuclear weapon, civilian**

Y36.59 **War operation involving other effects of nuclear weapons**

Y36.59Ø **War operation involving other effects of nuclear weapons, military personnel**

Y36.591 **War operation involving other effects of nuclear weapons, civilian**

Y36.6 **War operations involving biological weapons**

Y36.6X **War operations involving biological weapons**

Y36.6XØ **War operations involving biological weapons, military personnel**

Y36.6X1 **War operations involving biological weapons, civilian**

Y36.7 **War operations involving chemical weapons and other forms of unconventional warfare**

Excludes1 war operations involving incendiary devices (Y36.3-, Y36.5-)

Y36.7X **War operations involving chemical weapons and other forms of unconventional warfare**

Y36.7XØ **War operations involving chemical weapons and other forms of unconventional warfare, military personnel**

Y36.7X1 **War operations involving chemical weapons and other forms of unconventional warfare, civilian**

Y36.8 **War operations occurring after cessation of hostilities**
War operations classifiable to categories Y36.Ø-Y36.8 but occurring after cessation of hostilities

Y36.81 **Explosion of mine placed during war operations but exploding after cessation of hostilities**

Y36.81Ø **Explosion of mine placed during war operations but exploding after cessation of hostilities, military personnel**

Y36.811 **Explosion of mine placed during war operations but exploding after cessation of hostilities, civilian**

Y36.82 **Explosion of bomb placed during war operations but exploding after cessation of hostilities**

Y36.82Ø **Explosion of bomb placed during war operations but exploding after cessation of hostilities, military personnel**

Y36.821 **Explosion of bomb placed during war operations but exploding after cessation of hostilities, civilian**

Y36.88 **Other war operations occurring after cessation of hostilities**

Y36.88Ø **Other war operations occurring after cessation of hostilities, military personnel**

Y36.881 **Other war operations occurring after cessation of hostilities, civilian**

Y36.89 **Unspecified war operations occurring after cessation of hostilities**

Y36.89Ø **Unspecified war operations occurring after cessation of hostilities, military personnel**

Y36.891 **Unspecified war operations occurring after cessation of hostilities, civilian**

Y36.9 Other and unspecified war operations

X Y36.9Ø **War operations, unspecified**

X Y36.91 **War operations involving unspecified weapon of mass destruction [WMD]**

X Y36.92 **War operations involving friendly fire**

Y37 Military operations

Includes Injuries to military personnel and civilians occurring during peacetime on military property and during routine military exercises and operations

Excludes1 military aircraft involved in aircraft accident with civilian aircraft (V97.81-)
military vehicles involved in transport accident with civilian vehicle (VØ9.Ø1, VØ9.21, V19.81, V29.81, V39.81, V49.81, V59.81, V69.81, V79.81)
military watercraft involved in water transport accident with civilian watercraft (V94.81-)
war operations (Y36.-)

The appropriate 7th character is to be added to each code from category Y37

A	initial encounter
D	subsequent encounter
S	sequela

Y37.Ø **Military operations involving explosion of marine weapons**

Y37.ØØ **Military operations involving explosion of unspecified marine weapon**
Military operations involving underwater blast NOS

Y37.ØØØ **Military operations involving explosion of unspecified marine weapon, military personnel**

Y37.ØØ1 **Military operations involving explosion of unspecified marine weapon, civilian**

Y37.Ø1 **Military operations involving explosion of depth-charge**

Y37.Ø1Ø **Military operations involving explosion of depth-charge, military personnel**

Y37.Ø11 **Military operations involving explosion of depth-charge, civilian**

Y37.Ø2 **Military operations involving explosion of marine mine**
Military operations involving explosion of marine mine, at sea or in harbor

Y37.Ø2Ø **Military operations involving explosion of marine mine, military personnel**

Y37.Ø21 **Military operations involving explosion of marine mine, civilian**

CHAPTER 2Ø (VØØ-Y99)

- Y37.03 Military operations involving explosion of sea-based artillery shell
  - Y37.030 Military operations involving explosion of sea-based artillery shell, military personnel
  - Y37.031 Military operations involving explosion of sea-based artillery shell, civilian
- Y37.04 Military operations involving explosion of torpedo
  - Y37.040 Military operations involving explosion of torpedo, military personnel
  - Y37.041 Military operations involving explosion of torpedo, civilian
- Y37.05 Military operations involving accidental detonation of onboard marine weapons
  - Y37.050 Military operations involving accidental detonation of onboard marine weapons, military personnel
  - Y37.051 Military operations involving accidental detonation of onboard marine weapons, civilian
- Y37.09 Military operations involving explosion of other marine weapons
  - Y37.090 Military operations involving explosion of other marine weapons, military personnel
  - Y37.091 Military operations involving explosion of other marine weapons, civilian

Y37.1 Military operations involving destruction of aircraft

- Y37.10 Military operations involving unspecified destruction of aircraft
  - Y37.100 Military operations involving unspecified destruction of aircraft, military personnel
  - Y37.101 Military operations involving unspecified destruction of aircraft, civilian
- Y37.11 Military operations involving destruction of aircraft due to enemy fire or explosives

  Military operations involving destruction of aircraft due to air to air missile
  Military operations involving destruction of aircraft due to explosive placed on aircraft
  Military operations involving destruction of aircraft due to rocket propelled grenade [RPG]
  Military operations involving destruction of aircraft due to small arms fire
  Military operations involving destruction of aircraft due to surface to air missile
  - Y37.110 Military operations involving destruction of aircraft due to enemy fire or explosives, military personnel
  - Y37.111 Military operations involving destruction of aircraft due to enemy fire or explosives, civilian
- Y37.12 Military operations involving destruction of aircraft due to collision with other aircraft
  - Y37.120 Military operations involving destruction of aircraft due to collision with other aircraft, military personnel
  - Y37.121 Military operations involving destruction of aircraft due to collision with other aircraft, civilian
- Y37.13 Military operations involving destruction of aircraft due to onboard fire
  - Y37.130 Military operations involving destruction of aircraft due to onboard fire, military personnel
  - Y37.131 Military operations involving destruction of aircraft due to onboard fire, civilian
- Y37.14 Military operations involving destruction of aircraft due to accidental detonation of onboard munitions and explosives
  - Y37.140 Military operations involving destruction of aircraft due to accidental detonation of onboard munitions and explosives, military personnel
  - Y37.141 Military operations involving destruction of aircraft due to accidental detonation of onboard munitions and explosives, civilian
- Y37.19 Military operations involving other destruction of aircraft
  - Y37.190 Military operations involving other destruction of aircraft, military personnel
  - Y37.191 Military operations involving other destruction of aircraft, civilian

Y37.2 Military operations involving other explosions and fragments

Excludes1 military operations involving explosion of aircraft (Y37.1-)
military operations involving explosion of marine weapons (Y37.0-)
military operations involving explosion of nuclear weapons (Y37.5-)

- Y37.20 Military operations involving unspecified explosion and fragments

  Military operations involving air blast NOS
  Military operations involving blast NOS
  Military operations involving blast fragments NOS
  Military operations involving blast wave NOS
  Military operations involving blast wind NOS
  Military operations involving explosion NOS
  Military operations involving explosion of bomb NOS
  - Y37.200 Military operations involving unspecified explosion and fragments, military personnel
  - Y37.201 Military operations involving unspecified explosion and fragments, civilian
- Y37.21 Military operations involving explosion of aerial bomb
  - Y37.210 Military operations involving explosion of aerial bomb, military personnel
  - Y37.211 Military operations involving explosion of aerial bomb, civilian
- Y37.22 Military operations involving explosion of guided missile
  - Y37.220 Military operations involving explosion of guided missile, military personnel
  - Y37.221 Military operations involving explosion of guided missile, civilian

● Y37.23 **Military operations involving explosion of improvised explosive device [IED]**
Military operations involving explosion of person-borne improvised explosive device [IED]
Military operations involving explosion of vehicle-borne improvised explosive device [IED]
Military operations involving explosion of roadside improvised explosive device [IED]

● Y37.230 **Military operations involving explosion of improvised explosive device [IED], military personnel**

● Y37.231 **Military operations involving explosion of improvised explosive device [IED], civilian**

● Y37.24 **Military operations involving explosion due to accidental detonation and discharge of own munitions or munitions launch device**

● Y37.240 **Military operations involving explosion due to accidental detonation and discharge of own munitions or munitions launch device, military personnel**

● Y37.241 **Military operations involving explosion due to accidental detonation and discharge of own munitions or munitions launch device, civilian**

● Y37.25 **Military operations involving fragments from munitions**

● Y37.250 **Military operations involving fragments from munitions, military personnel**

● Y37.251 **Military operations involving fragments from munitions, civilian**

● Y37.26 **Military operations involving fragments of improvised explosive device [IED]**
Military operations involving fragments of person-borne improvised explosive device [IED]
Military operations involving fragments of vehicle-borne improvised explosive device [IED]
Military operations involving fragments of roadside improvised explosive device [IED]

● Y37.260 **Military operations involving fragments of improvised explosive device [IED], military personnel**

● Y37.261 **Military operations involving fragments of improvised explosive device [IED], civilian**

● Y37.27 **Military operations involving fragments from weapons**

● Y37.270 **Military operations involving fragments from weapons, military personnel**

● Y37.271 **Military operations involving fragments from weapons, civilian**

● Y37.29 **Military operations involving other explosions and fragments**
Military operations involving explosion of grenade
Military operations involving explosions of land mine
Military operations involving shrapnel NOS

● Y37.290 **Military operations involving other explosions and fragments, military personnel**

● Y37.291 **Military operations involving other explosions and fragments, civilian**

● Y37.3 **Military operations involving fires, conflagrations and hot substances**
Military operations involving smoke, fumes, and heat from fires, conflagrations and hot substances
Excludes1 military operations involving fires and conflagrations aboard military aircraft (Y37.1-)
military operations involving fires and conflagrations aboard military watercraft (Y37.Ø-)
military operations involving fires and conflagrations caused indirectly by conventional weapons (Y37.2-)
military operations involving fires and thermal effects of nuclear weapons (Y36.53-)

● Y37.30 **Military operations involving unspecified fire, conflagration and hot substance**

● Y37.300 **Military operations involving unspecified fire, conflagration and hot substance, military personnel**

● Y37.301 **Military operations involving unspecified fire, conflagration and hot substance, civilian**

● Y37.31 **Military operations involving gasoline bomb**
Military operations involving incendiary bomb
Military operations involving petrol bomb

● Y37.310 **Military operations involving gasoline bomb, military personnel**

● Y37.311 **Military operations involving gasoline bomb, civilian**

● Y37.32 **Military operations involving incendiary bullet**

● Y37.320 **Military operations involving incendiary bullet, military personnel**

● Y37.321 **Military operations involving incendiary bullet, civilian**

● Y37.33 **Military operations involving flamethrower**

● Y37.330 **Military operations involving flamethrower, military personnel**

● Y37.331 **Military operations involving flamethrower, civilian**

● Y37.39 **Military operations involving other fires, conflagrations and hot substances**

● Y37.390 **Military operations involving other fires, conflagrations and hot substances, military personnel**

● Y37.391 **Military operations involving other fires, conflagrations and hot substances, civilian**

● Y37.4 **Military operations involving firearm discharge and other forms of conventional warfare**

● Y37.41 **Military operations involving rubber bullets**

● Y37.410 **Military operations involving rubber bullets, military personnel**

● Y37.411 **Military operations involving rubber bullets, civilian**

● Y37.42 **Military operations involving firearms pellets**

● Y37.420 **Military operations involving firearms pellets, military personnel**

● Y37.421 **Military operations involving firearms pellets, civilian**

● Y37.43 **Military operations involving other firearms discharge**
Military operations involving bullets NOS
Excludes1 military operations involving munitions fragments (Y37.25-)
military operations involving incendiary bullets (Y37.32-)

● Y37.430 **Military operations involving other firearms discharge, military personnel**

● Y37.431 **Military operations involving other firearms discharge, civilian**

● Y37.44 **Military operations involving unarmed hand to hand combat**
Excludes1 military operations involving combat using blunt or piercing object (Y37.45-)
military operations involving intentional restriction of air and airway (Y37.46-)
military operations involving unintentional restriction of air and airway (Y37.47-)
● Y37.44Ø **Military operations involving unarmed hand to hand combat, military personnel**
● Y37.441 **Military operations involving unarmed hand to hand combat, civilian**

● Y37.45 **Military operations involving combat using blunt or piercing object**
● Y37.45Ø **Military operations involving combat using blunt or piercing object, military personnel**
● Y37.451 **Military operations involving combat using blunt or piercing object, civilian**

● Y37.46 **Military operations involving intentional restriction of air and airway**
● Y37.46Ø **Military operations involving intentional restriction of air and airway, military personnel**
● Y37.461 **Military operations involving intentional restriction of air and airway, civilian**

● Y37.47 **Military operations involving unintentional restriction of air and airway**
● Y37.47Ø **Military operations involving unintentional restriction of air and airway, military personnel**
● Y37.471 **Military operations involving unintentional restriction of air and airway, civilian**

● Y37.49 **Military operations involving other forms of conventional warfare**
● Y37.49Ø **Military operations involving other forms of conventional warfare, military personnel**
● Y37.491 **Military operations involving other forms of conventional warfare, civilian**

● Y37.5 **Military operations involving nuclear weapons**
Military operation involving dirty bomb NOS

● Y37.5Ø **Military operations involving unspecified effect of nuclear weapon**
● Y37.5ØØ **Military operations involving unspecified effect of nuclear weapon, military personnel**
● Y37.5Ø1 **Military operations involving unspecified effect of nuclear weapon, civilian**

● Y37.51 **Military operations involving direct blast effect of nuclear weapon**
Military operations involving blast pressure of nuclear weapon
● Y37.51Ø **Military operations involving direct blast effect of nuclear weapon, military personnel**
● Y37.511 **Military operations involving direct blast effect of nuclear weapon, civilian**

● Y37.52 **Military operations involving indirect blast effect of nuclear weapon**
Military operations involving being thrown by blast of nuclear weapon
Military operations involving being struck or crushed by blast debris of nuclear weapon
● Y37.52Ø **Military operations involving indirect blast effect of nuclear weapon, military personnel**
● Y37.521 **Military operations involving indirect blast effect of nuclear weapon, civilian**

● Y37.53 **Military operations involving thermal radiation effect of nuclear weapon**
Military operations involving direct heat from nuclear weapon
Military operation involving fireball effects from nuclear weapon
● Y37.53Ø **Military operations involving thermal radiation effect of nuclear weapon, military personnel**
● Y37.531 **Military operations involving thermal radiation effect of nuclear weapon, civilian**

● Y37.54 **Military operation involving nuclear radiation effects of nuclear weapon**
Military operation involving acute radiation exposure from nuclear weapon
Military operation involving exposure to immediate ionizing radiation from nuclear weapon
Military operation involving fallout exposure from nuclear weapon
Military operation involving secondary effects of nuclear weapons
● Y37.54Ø **Military operation involving nuclear radiation effects of nuclear weapon, military personnel**
● Y37.541 **Military operation involving nuclear radiation effects of nuclear weapon, civilian**

● Y37.59 **Military operation involving other effects of nuclear weapons**
● Y37.59Ø **Military operation involving other effects of nuclear weapons, military personnel**
● Y37.591 **Military operation involving other effects of nuclear weapons, civilian**

● Y37.6 **Military operations involving biological weapons**
● Y37.6X **Military operations involving biological weapons**
● Y37.6XØ **Military operations involving biological weapons, military personnel**
● Y37.6X1 **Military operations involving biological weapons, civilian**

● Y37.7 **Military operations involving chemical weapons and other forms of unconventional warfare**
Excludes1 military operations involving incendiary devices (Y36.3-, Y36.5-)
● Y37.7X **Military operations involving chemical weapons and other forms of unconventional warfare**
● Y37.7XØ **Military operations involving chemical weapons and other forms of unconventional warfare, military personnel**
● Y37.7X1 **Military operations involving chemical weapons and other forms of unconventional warfare, civilian**

● Y37.9 Other and unspecified military operations

X● Y37.90 **Military operations, unspecified**

X● Y37.91 **Military operations involving unspecified weapon of mass destruction [WMD]**

X● Y37.92 **Military operations involving friendly fire**

● Y38 Terrorism

These codes are for use to identify injuries resulting from the unlawful use of force or violence against persons or property to intimidate or coerce a government, the civilian population, or any segment thereof, in furtherance of political or social objective

Use additional code for place of occurrence (Y92.-)

The appropriate 7th character is to be added to each code from category Y38

A	initial encounter
D	subsequent encounter
S	sequela

● Y38.0 Terrorism involving explosion of marine weapons
Terrorism involving depth-charge
Terrorism involving marine mine
Terrorism involving mine NOS, at sea or in harbor
Terrorism involving sea-based artillery shell
Terrorism involving torpedo
Terrorism involving underwater blast

● Y38.0X Terrorism involving explosion of marine weapons

● Y38.0X1 **Terrorism involving explosion of marine weapons, public safety official injured**

● Y38.0X2 **Terrorism involving explosion of marine weapons, civilian injured**

● Y38.0X3 **Terrorism involving explosion of marine weapons, terrorist injured**

● Y38.1 Terrorism involving destruction of aircraft
Terrorism involving aircraft burned
Terrorism involving aircraft exploded
Terrorism involving aircraft being shot down
Terrorism involving aircraft used as a weapon

● Y38.1X **Terrorism involving destruction of aircraft**

● Y38.1X1 **Terrorism involving destruction of aircraft, public safety official injured**

● Y38.1X2 **Terrorism involving destruction of aircraft, civilian injured**

● Y38.1X3 **Terrorism involving destruction of aircraft, terrorist injured**

● Y38.2 Terrorism involving other explosions and fragments
Terrorism involving antipersonnel (fragments) bomb
Terrorism involving blast NOS
Terrorism involving explosion NOS
Terrorism involving explosion of breech block
Terrorism involving explosion of cannon block
Terrorism involving explosion (fragments) of artillery shell
Terrorism involving explosion (fragments) of bomb
Terrorism involving explosion (fragments) of grenade
Terrorism involving explosion (fragments) of guided missile
Terrorism involving explosion (fragments) of land mine
Terrorism involving explosion of mortar bomb
Terrorism involving explosion of munitions
Terrorism involving explosion (fragments) of rocket
Terrorism involving explosion (fragments) of shell
Terrorism involving shrapnel
Terrorism involving mine NOS, on land

Excludes1 terrorism involving explosion of nuclear weapon (Y38.5)
terrorism involving suicide bomber (Y38.81)

● Y38.2X Terrorism involving **other explosions and fragments**

● Y38.2X1 **Terrorism involving other explosions and fragments, public safety official injured**

● Y38.2X2 **Terrorism involving other explosions and fragments, civilian injured**

● Y38.2X3 **Terrorism involving other explosions and fragments, terrorist injured**

● Y38.3 Terrorism involving fires, conflagration and hot substances
Terrorism involving conflagration NOS
Terrorism involving fire NOS
Terrorism involving petrol bomb

Excludes1 terrorism involving fire or heat of nuclear weapon (Y38.5)

● Y38.3X Terrorism involving **fires, conflagration and hot substances**

● Y38.3X1 **Terrorism involving fires, conflagration and hot substances, public safety official injured**

● Y38.3X2 **Terrorism involving fires, conflagration and hot substances, civilian injured**

● Y38.3X3 **Terrorism involving fires, conflagration and hot substances, terrorist injured**

● Y38.4 Terrorism involving firearms
Terrorism involving carbine bullet
Terrorism involving machine gun bullet
Terrorism involving pellets (shotgun)
Terrorism involving pistol bullet
Terrorism involving rifle bullet
Terrorism involving rubber (rifle) bullet

● Y38.4X Terrorism **involving firearms**

● Y38.4X1 **Terrorism involving firearms, public safety official injured**

● Y38.4X2 **Terrorism involving firearms, civilian injured**

● Y38.4X3 **Terrorism involving firearms, terrorist injured**

● Y38.5 Terrorism involving nuclear weapons
Terrorism involving blast effects of nuclear weapon
Terrorism involving exposure to ionizing radiation from nuclear weapon
Terrorism involving fireball effect of nuclear weapon
Terrorism involving heat from nuclear weapon

● Y38.5X Terrorism **involving nuclear weapons**

● Y38.5X1 **Terrorism involving nuclear weapons, public safety official injured**

● Y38.5X2 **Terrorism involving nuclear weapons, civilian injured**

● Y38.5X3 **Terrorism involving nuclear weapons, terrorist injured**

● Y38.6 Terrorism involving biological weapons
Terrorism involving anthrax
Terrorism involving cholera
A serious, often deadly, infectious disease of the small intestine
Terrorism involving smallpox

● Y38.6X Terrorism **involving biological weapons**

● Y38.6X1 **Terrorism involving biological weapons, public safety official injured**

● Y38.6X2 **Terrorism involving biological weapons, civilian injured**

● Y38.6X3 **Terrorism involving biological weapons, terrorist injured**

● Y38.7 Terrorism involving chemical weapons
Terrorism involving gases, fumes, chemicals
Terrorism involving hydrogen cyanide
Terrorism involving phosgene
Terrorism involving sarin

● Y38.7X Terrorism involving chemical weapons

● Y38.7X1 Terrorism involving chemical weapons, public safety official injured

● Y38.7X2 Terrorism involving chemical weapons, civilian injured

● Y38.7X3 Terrorism involving chemical weapons, terrorist injured

● Y38.8 Terrorism involving other and unspecified means

● Y38.8Ø Terrorism involving unspecified means
Terrorism NOS

● Y38.81 Terrorism involving suicide bomber

● Y38.811 Terrorism involving suicide bomber, public safety official injured

● Y38.812 Terrorism involving suicide bomber, civilian injured

● Y38.89 Terrorism involving other means
Terrorism involving drowning and submersion
Terrorism involving lasers
Terrorism involving piercing or stabbing instruments

● Y38.891 Terrorism involving other means, public safety official injured

● Y38.892 Terrorism involving other means, civilian injured

● Y38.893 Terrorism involving other means, terrorist injured

● Y38.9 Terrorism, secondary effects
Note: This code is for use to identify conditions occurring subsequent to a terrorist attack not those that are due to the initial terrorist attack.

● Y38.9X Terrorism, secondary effects

● Y38.9X1 Terrorism, secondary effects, public safety official injured

● Y38.9X2 Terrorism, secondary effects, civilian injured categories

COMPLICATIONS OF MEDICAL AND SURGICAL CARE (Y62-Y84)

Includes complications of medical devices surgical and medical procedures as the cause of abnormal reaction of the patient, or of later complication, without mention of misadventure at the time of the procedure

MISADVENTURES TO PATIENTS DURING SURGICAL AND MEDICAL CARE (Y62-Y69)

Excludes1 surgical and medical procedures as the cause of abnormal reaction of the patient, without mention of misadventure at the time of the procedure (Y83-Y84)

● Y62 Failure of sterile precautions during surgical and medical care

Y62.Ø Failure of sterile precautions during surgical operation

Y62.1 Failure of sterile precautions during infusion or transfusion

Y62.2 Failure of sterile precautions during kidney dialysis and other perfusion

Y62.3 Failure of sterile precautions during injection or immunization

Y62.4 Failure of sterile precautions during endoscopic examination

Y62.5 Failure of sterile precautions during heart catheterization

Y62.6 Failure of sterile precautions during aspiration, puncture and other catheterization

Y62.8 Failure of sterile precautions during other surgical and medical care

Y62.9 Failure of sterile precautions during unspecified surgical and medical care

● Y63 Failure in dosage during surgical and medical care
Excludes2 accidental overdose of drug or wrong drug given in error (T36-T5Ø)

Y63.Ø Excessive amount of blood or other fluid given during transfusion or infusion

Y63.1 Incorrect dilution of fluid used during infusion

Y63.2 Overdose of radiation given during therapy

Y63.3 Inadvertent exposure of patient to radiation during medical care

Y63.4 Failure in dosage in electroshock or insulin-shock therapy

Y63.5 Inappropriate temperature in local application and packing

Y63.6 Underdosing and nonadministration of necessary drug, medicament or biological substance

Y63.8 Failure in dosage during other surgical and medical care

Y63.9 Failure in dosage during unspecified surgical and medical care

● Y64 Contaminated medical or biological substances

Y64.Ø Contaminated medical or biological substance, transfused or infused

Y64.1 Contaminated medical or biological substance, injected or used for immunization

Y64.8 Contaminated medical or biological substance administered by other means

Y64.9 Contaminated medical or biological substance administered by unspecified means
Administered contaminated medical or biological substance NOS

● Y65 Other misadventures during surgical and medical care

Y65.Ø Mismatched blood in transfusion

Y65.1 Wrong fluid used in infusion

Y65.2 Failure in suture or ligature during surgical operation

Y65.3 Endotracheal tube wrongly placed during anesthetic procedure

Y65.4 Failure to introduce or to remove other tube or instrument

● Y65.5 Performance of wrong procedure (operation)

● Y65.51 Performance of wrong procedure (operation) on correct patient
Wrong device implanted into correct surgical site
Excludes1 performance of correct procedure (operation) on wrong side or body part (Y65.53)

● Y65.52 Performance of procedure (operation) on patient not scheduled for surgery
Performance of procedure (operation) intended for another patient
Performance of procedure (operation) on wrong patient

● Y65.53 Performance of correct procedure (operation) on wrong side or body part
Performance of correct procedure (operation) on wrong side
Performance of correct procedure (operation) on wrong site

Y65.8 Other specified misadventures during surgical and medical care
Coding Clinic: 2Ø19, Q2, P24

Y66 Nonadministration of surgical and medical care
Premature cessation of surgical and medical care
Excludes1 DNR status (Z66)
palliative care (Z51.5)

Y69 Unspecified misadventure during surgical and medical care

MEDICAL DEVICES ASSOCIATED WITH ADVERSE INCIDENTS IN DIAGNOSTIC AND THERAPEUTIC USE (Y7Ø-Y82)

Includes breakdown or malfunction of medical devices (during use) (after implantation) (ongoing use)
Excludes2 later complications following use of medical devices without breakdown or malfunctioning of device (Y83-Y84)
misadventure to patients during surgical and medical care, classifiable to (Y62-Y69)
surgical and other medical procedures as the cause of abnormal reaction of the patient, or of later complication, without mention of misadventure at the time of the procedure (Y83-Y84)

● **Y7Ø Anesthesiology devices associated with adverse incidents**
- Y7Ø.Ø **Diagnostic and monitoring anesthesiology devices associated with adverse incidents**
- Y7Ø.1 **Therapeutic (nonsurgical) and rehabilitative anesthesiology devices associated with adverse incidents**
- Y7Ø.2 **Prosthetic and other implants, materials and accessory anesthesiology devices associated with adverse incidents**
- Y7Ø.3 **Surgical instruments, materials and anesthesiology devices (including sutures) associated with adverse incidents**
- Y7Ø.8 **Miscellaneous anesthesiology devices associated with adverse incidents, not elsewhere classified**

● **Y71 Cardiovascular devices associated with adverse incidents**
- Y71.Ø **Diagnostic and monitoring cardiovascular devices associated with adverse incidents**
- Y71.1 **Therapeutic (nonsurgical) and rehabilitative cardiovascular devices associated with adverse incidents**
- Y71.2 **Prosthetic and other implants, materials and accessory cardiovascular devices associated with adverse incidents**
- Y71.3 **Surgical instruments, materials and cardiovascular devices (including sutures) associated with adverse incidents**
- Y71.8 **Miscellaneous cardiovascular devices associated with adverse incidents, not elsewhere classified**

● **Y72 Otorhinolaryngological devices associated with adverse incidents**
- Y72.Ø **Diagnostic and monitoring otorhinolaryngological devices associated with adverse incidents**
- Y72.1 **Therapeutic (nonsurgical) and rehabilitative otorhinolaryngological devices associated with adverse incidents**
- Y72.2 **Prosthetic and other implants, materials and accessory otorhinolaryngological devices associated with adverse incidents**
- Y72.3 **Surgical instruments, materials and otorhinolaryngological devices (including sutures) associated with adverse incidents**
- Y72.8 **Miscellaneous otorhinolaryngological devices associated with adverse incidents, not elsewhere classified**

● **Y73 Gastroenterology and urology devices associated with adverse incidents**
- Y73.Ø **Diagnostic and monitoring gastroenterology and urology devices associated with adverse incidents**
- Y73.1 **Therapeutic (nonsurgical) and rehabilitative gastroenterology and urology devices associated with adverse incidents**
- Y73.2 **Prosthetic and other implants, materials and accessory gastroenterology and urology devices associated with adverse incidents**
- Y73.3 **Surgical instruments, materials and gastroenterology and urology devices (including sutures) associated with adverse incidents**
- Y73.8 **Miscellaneous gastroenterology and urology devices associated with adverse incidents, not elsewhere classified**

● **Y74 General hospital and personal-use devices associated with adverse incidents**
- Y74.Ø **Diagnostic and monitoring general hospital and personal-use devices associated with adverse incidents**
- Y74.1 **Therapeutic (nonsurgical) and rehabilitative general hospital and personal-use devices associated with adverse incidents**
- Y74.2 **Prosthetic and other implants, materials and accessory general hospital and personal-use devices associated with adverse incidents**
- Y74.3 **Surgical instruments, materials and general hospital and personal-use devices (including sutures) associated with adverse incidents**
- Y74.8 **Miscellaneous general hospital and personal-use devices associated with adverse incidents, not elsewhere classified**

● **Y75 Neurological devices associated with adverse incidents**
- Y75.Ø **Diagnostic and monitoring neurological devices associated with adverse incidents**
- Y75.1 **Therapeutic (nonsurgical) and rehabilitative neurological devices associated with adverse incidents**
- Y75.2 **Prosthetic and other implants, materials and neurological devices associated with adverse incidents**
- Y75.3 **Surgical instruments, materials and neurological devices (including sutures) associated with adverse incidents**
- Y75.8 **Miscellaneous neurological devices associated with adverse incidents, not elsewhere classified**

● **Y76 Obstetric and gynecological devices associated with adverse incidents**
- Y76.Ø **Diagnostic and monitoring obstetric and gynecological devices associated with adverse incidents** ♀
- Y76.1 **Therapeutic (nonsurgical) and rehabilitative obstetric and gynecological devices associated with adverse incidents** ♀
- Y76.2 **Prosthetic and other implants, materials and accessory obstetric and gynecological devices associated with adverse incidents** ♀
- Y76.3 **Surgical instruments, materials and obstetric and gynecological devices (including sutures) associated with adverse incidents** ♀
- Y76.8 **Miscellaneous obstetric and gynecological devices associated with adverse incidents, not elsewhere classified** ♀

CHAPTER 2Ø (VØØ-Y99)

● Y77 Ophthalmic devices associated with adverse incidents
- Y77.0 Diagnostic and monitoring ophthalmic devices associated with adverse incidents
- Y77.1 Therapeutic (nonsurgical) and rehabilitative ophthalmic devices associated with adverse incidents
- Y77.2 Prosthetic and other implants, materials and accessory ophthalmic devices associated with adverse incidents
- Y77.3 Surgical instruments, materials and ophthalmic devices (including sutures) associated with adverse incidents
- Y77.8 Miscellaneous ophthalmic devices associated with adverse incidents, not elsewhere classified

● Y78 Radiological devices associated with adverse incidents
- Y78.0 Diagnostic and monitoring radiological devices associated with adverse incidents
- Y78.1 Therapeutic (nonsurgical) and rehabilitative radiological devices associated with adverse incidents
- Y78.2 Prosthetic and other implants, materials and accessory radiological devices associated with adverse incidents
- Y78.3 Surgical instruments, materials and radiological devices (including sutures) associated with adverse incidents
- Y78.8 Miscellaneous radiological devices associated with adverse incidents, not elsewhere classified

● Y79 Orthopedic devices associated with adverse incidents
- Y79.0 Diagnostic and monitoring orthopedic devices associated with adverse incidents
- Y79.1 Therapeutic (nonsurgical) and rehabilitative orthopedic devices associated with adverse incidents
- Y79.2 Prosthetic and other implants, materials and accessory orthopedic devices associated with adverse incidents
- Y79.3 Surgical instruments, materials and orthopedic devices (including sutures) associated with adverse incidents
- Y79.8 Miscellaneous orthopedic devices associated with adverse incidents, not elsewhere classified

● Y80 Physical medicine devices associated with adverse incidents
- Y80.0 Diagnostic and monitoring physical medicine devices associated with adverse incidents
- Y80.1 Therapeutic (nonsurgical) and rehabilitative physical medicine devices associated with adverse incidents
- Y80.2 Prosthetic and other implants, materials and accessory physical medicine devices associated with adverse incidents
- Y80.3 Surgical instruments, materials and physical medicine devices (including sutures) associated with adverse incidents
- Y80.8 Miscellaneous physical medicine devices associated with adverse incidents, not elsewhere classified

● Y81 General- and plastic-surgery devices associated with adverse incidents
- Y81.0 Diagnostic and monitoring general- and plastic-surgery devices associated with adverse incidents
- Y81.1 Therapeutic (nonsurgical) and rehabilitative general- and plastic-surgery devices associated with adverse incidents
- Y81.2 Prosthetic and other implants, materials and accessory general- and plastic-surgery devices associated with adverse incidents
- Y81.3 Surgical instruments, materials and general- and plastic-surgery devices (including sutures) associated with adverse incidents
- Y81.8 Miscellaneous general- and plastic-surgery devices associated with adverse incidents, not elsewhere classified

● Y82 Other and unspecified medical devices associated with adverse incidents
- Y82.8 Other medical devices associated with adverse incidents
- Y82.9 Unspecified medical devices associated with adverse incidents

SURGICAL AND OTHER MEDICAL PROCEDURES AS THE CAUSE OF ABNORMAL REACTION OF THE PATIENT, OR OF LATER COMPLICATION, WITHOUT MENTION OF MISADVENTURE AT THE TIME OF THE PROCEDURE (Y83-Y84)

Excludes1 misadventures to patients during surgical and medical care, classifiable to (Y62-Y69)

Excludes2 breakdown or malfunctioning of medical device (after implantation) (during procedure) (ongoing use) (Y70-Y82)

● Y83 Surgical operation and other surgical procedures as the cause of abnormal reaction of the patient, or of later complication, without mention of misadventure at the time of the procedure
- Y83.0 Surgical operation with transplant of whole organ as the cause of abnormal reaction of the patient, or of later complication, without mention of misadventure at the time of the procedure
- Y83.1 Surgical operation with implant of artificial internal device as the cause of abnormal reaction of the patient, or of later complication, without mention of misadventure at the time of the procedure
- Y83.2 Surgical operation with anastomosis, bypass or graft as the cause of abnormal reaction of the patient, or of later complication, without mention of misadventure at the time of the procedure
- Y83.3 Surgical operation with formation of external stoma as the cause of abnormal reaction of the patient, or of later complication, without mention of misadventure at the time of the procedure
- Y83.4 Other reconstructive surgery as the cause of abnormal reaction of the patient, or of later complication, without mention of misadventure at the time of the procedure
- Y83.5 Amputation of limb(s) as the cause of abnormal reaction of the patient, or of later complication, without mention of misadventure at the time of the procedure
- Y83.6 Removal of other organ (partial) (total) as the cause of abnormal reaction of the patient, or of later complication, without mention of misadventure at the time of the procedure
- Y83.8 Other surgical procedures as the cause of abnormal reaction of the patient, or of later complication, without mention of misadventure at the time of the procedure
- Y83.9 Surgical procedure, unspecified as the cause of abnormal reaction of the patient, or of later complication, without mention of misadventure at the time of the procedure

● Y84 Other medical procedures as the cause of abnormal reaction of the patient, or of later complication, without mention of misadventure at the time of the procedure
- Y84.0 Cardiac catheterization as the cause of abnormal reaction of the patient, or of later complication, without mention of misadventure at the time of the procedure
- Y84.1 Kidney dialysis as the cause of abnormal reaction of the patient, or of later complication, without mention of misadventure at the time of the procedure
- Y84.2 Radiological procedure and radiotherapy as the cause of abnormal reaction of the patient, or of later complication, without mention of misadventure at the time of the procedure
  Coding Clinic: 2019, Q1, P21; 2017, Q1, P34
- Y84.3 Shock therapy as the cause of abnormal reaction of the patient, or of later complication, without mention of misadventure at the time of the procedure
- Y84.4 Aspiration of fluid as the cause of abnormal reaction of the patient, or of later complication, without mention of misadventure at the time of the procedure
- Y84.5 Insertion of gastric or duodenal sound as the cause of abnormal reaction of the patient, or of later complication, without mention of misadventure at the time of the procedure
- Y84.6 Urinary catheterization as the cause of abnormal reaction of the patient, or of later complication, without mention of misadventure at the time of the procedure

Y84.7 **Blood-sampling** as the cause of abnormal reaction of the patient, or of later complication, without mention of misadventure at the time of the procedure

Y84.8 **Other medical procedures** as the cause of abnormal reaction of the patient, or of later complication, without mention of misadventure at the time of the procedure

Y84.9 Medical procedure, **unspecified** as the cause of abnormal reaction of the patient, or of later complication, without mention of misadventure at the time of the procedure

SUPPLEMENTARY FACTORS RELATED TO CAUSES OF MORBIDITY CLASSIFIED ELSEWHERE (Y90-Y99)

Note: These categories may be used to provide supplementary information concerning causes of morbidity. They are not to be used for single-condition coding.

● **Y90 Evidence of alcohol involvement determined by blood alcohol level**

Code first any associated alcohol related disorders (F10)

Y90.0 **Blood alcohol level of less than 20 mg/100 ml**

Y90.1 **Blood alcohol level of 20-39 mg/100 ml**

Y90.2 **Blood alcohol level of 40-59 mg/100 ml**

Y90.3 **Blood alcohol level of 60-79 mg/100 ml**

Y90.4 **Blood alcohol level of 80-99 mg/100 ml**

Y90.5 **Blood alcohol level of 100-119 mg/100 ml**

Y90.6 **Blood alcohol level of 120-199 mg/100 ml**

Y90.7 **Blood alcohol level of 200-239 mg/100 ml**

Y90.8 **Blood alcohol level of 240 mg/100 ml or more**

Y90.9 **Presence of alcohol in blood, level not specified**

OGCR Section I.C.20.b.

Place of Occurrence Guideline

Codes from category Y92, Place of occurrence of the external cause, are secondary codes for use after other external cause codes to identify the location of the patient at the time of injury or other condition.

Generally, a place of occurrence code is assigned only once, at the initial encounter for treatment. However, in the rare instance that a new injury occurs during hospitalization, an additional place of occurrence code may be assigned. No 7th characters are used for Y92. Only one code from Y92 should be recorded on a medical record.

Do not use place of occurrence code Y92.9 if the place is not stated or is not applicable.

● **Y92 Place of occurrence of the external cause**

The following category is for use, when relevant, to identify the place of occurrence of the external cause. Use in conjunction with an activity code.

Place of occurrence should be recorded only at the initial encounter for treatment

● Y92.0 **Non-institutional (private) residence as the place of occurrence of the external cause**

Excludes1 abandoned or derelict house (Y92.89)
home under construction but not yet occupied (Y92.6-)
institutional place of residence (Y92.1-)

● Y92.00 **Unspecified non-institutional (private) residence as the place of occurrence of the external cause**

Y92.000 **Kitchen of unspecified non-institutional (private) residence as the place of occurrence of the external cause**

Y92.001 **Dining room of unspecified non-institutional (private) residence as the place of occurrence of the external cause**

Y92.002 **Bathroom of unspecified non-institutional (private) residence single-family (private) house as the place of occurrence of the external cause**

Y92.003 **Bedroom of unspecified non-institutional (private) residence as the place of occurrence of the external cause**

Y92.007 **Garden or yard of unspecified non-institutional (private) residence as the place of occurrence of the external cause**

Y92.008 **Other place in unspecified non-institutional (private) residence as the place of occurrence of the external cause**

Y92.009 **Unspecified place in unspecified non-institutional (private) residence as the place of occurrence of the external cause**
Home (NOS) as the place of occurrence of the external cause

● Y92.01 **Single-family non-institutional (private) house as the place of occurrence of the external cause**
Farmhouse as the place of occurrence of the external cause

Excludes1 barn (Y92.71)
chicken coop or hen house (Y92.72)
farm field (Y92.73)
orchard (Y92.74)
single family mobile home or trailer (Y92.02-)
slaughter house (Y92.86)

Y92.010 **Kitchen of single-family (private) house as the place of occurrence of the external cause**

Y92.011 **Dining room of single-family (private) house as the place of occurrence of the external cause**

Y92.012 **Bathroom of single-family (private) house as the place of occurrence of the external cause**

Y92.013 **Bedroom of single-family (private) house as the place of occurrence of the external cause**

Y92.014 **Private driveway to single-family (private) house as the place of occurrence of the external cause**

Y92.015 **Private garage of single-family (private) house as the place of occurrence of the external cause**

Y92.016 **Swimming pool in single-family (private) house or garden as the place of occurrence of the external cause**

Y92.017 **Garden or yard in single-family (private) house as the place of occurrence of the external cause**

Y92.018 **Other place in single-family (private) house as the place of occurrence of the external cause**

Y92.019 **Unspecified place in single-family (private) house as the place of occurrence of the external cause**

● Y92.02 **Mobile home** as the place of occurrence of the external cause
- Y92.020 **Kitchen** in mobile home as the place of occurrence of the external cause
- Y92.021 **Dining room** in mobile home as the place of occurrence of the external cause
- Y92.022 **Bathroom** in mobile home as the place of occurrence of the external cause
- Y92.023 **Bedroom** in mobile home as the place of occurrence of the external cause
- Y92.024 **Driveway** of mobile home as the place of occurrence of the external cause
- Y92.025 **Garage** of mobile home as the place of occurrence of the external cause
- Y92.026 **Swimming pool** of mobile home as the place of occurrence of the external cause
- Y92.027 **Garden or yard** of mobile home as the place of occurrence of the external cause
- Y92.028 **Other place** in mobile home as the place of occurrence of the external cause
- Y92.029 **Unspecified** place in mobile home as the place of occurrence of the external cause

● Y92.03 **Apartment** as the place of occurrence of the external cause

Condominium as the place of occurrence of the external cause

Co-op apartment as the place of occurrence of the external cause

- Y92.030 **Kitchen** in apartment as the place of occurrence of the external cause
- Y92.031 **Bathroom** in apartment as the place of occurrence of the external cause
- Y92.032 **Bedroom** in apartment as the place of occurrence of the external cause
- Y92.038 **Other place** in apartment as the place of occurrence of the external cause
- Y92.039 **Unspecified** place in apartment as the place of occurrence of the external cause

● Y92.04 **Boarding-house** as the place of occurrence of the external cause
- Y92.040 **Kitchen** in boarding-house as the place of occurrence of the external cause
- Y92.041 **Bathroom** in boarding-house as the place of occurrence of the external cause
- Y92.042 **Bedroom** in boarding-house as the place of occurrence of the external cause
- Y92.043 **Driveway** of boarding-house as the place of occurrence of the external cause
- Y92.044 **Garage** of boarding-house as the place of occurrence of the external cause
- Y92.045 **Swimming pool** of boarding-house as the place of occurrence of the external cause
- Y92.046 **Garden or yard** of boarding-house as the place of occurrence of the external cause
- Y92.048 **Other place** in boarding-house as the place of occurrence of the external cause
- Y92.049 **Unspecified** place in boarding-house as the place of occurrence of the external cause

● Y92.09 **Other non-institutional residence** as the place of occurrence of the external cause
- Y92.090 **Kitchen** in other non-institutional residence as the place of occurrence of the external cause
- Y92.091 **Bathroom** in other non-institutional residence as the place of occurrence of the external cause
- Y92.092 **Bedroom** in other non-institutional residence as the place of occurrence of the external cause
- Y92.093 **Driveway** of other non-institutional residence as the place of occurrence of the external cause
- Y92.094 **Garage** of other non-institutional residence as the place of occurrence of the external cause
- Y92.095 **Swimming pool** of other non-institutional residence as the place of occurrence of the external cause
- Y92.096 **Garden or yard** of other non-institutional residence as the place of occurrence of the external cause
- Y92.098 **Other place** in other non-institutional residence as the place of occurrence of the external cause
- Y92.099 **Unspecified** place in other non-institutional residence as the place of occurrence of the external cause

  Coding Clinic: 2017, Q2, P10

● Y92.1 **Institutional** (nonprivate) **residence** as the place of occurrence of the external cause
- Y92.10 **Unspecified** residential institution as the place of occurrence of the external cause

● Y92.11 **Children's home and orphanage** as the place of occurrence of the external cause
- Y92.110 **Kitchen** in children's home and orphanage as the place of occurrence of the external cause
- Y92.111 **Bathroom** in children's home and orphanage as the place of occurrence of the external cause
- Y92.112 **Bedroom** in children's home and orphanage as the place of occurrence of the external cause
- Y92.113 **Driveway** of children's home and orphanage as the place of occurrence of the external cause
- Y92.114 **Garage** of children's home and orphanage as the place of occurrence of the external cause
- Y92.115 **Swimming pool** of children's home and orphanage as the place of occurrence of the external cause
- Y92.116 **Garden or yard** of children's home and orphanage as the place of occurrence of the external cause
- Y92.118 **Other place** in children's home and orphanage as the place of occurrence of the external cause
- Y92.119 **Unspecified** place in children's home and orphanage as the place of occurrence of the external cause

● **Y92.12** **Nursing home** as the place of occurrence of the external cause
Home for the sick as the place of occurrence of the external cause
Hospice as the place of occurrence of the external cause
- Y92.120 **Kitchen** in nursing home as the place of occurrence of the external cause
- Y92.121 **Bathroom** in nursing home as the place of occurrence of the external cause
- Y92.122 **Bedroom** in nursing home as the place of occurrence of the external cause
- Y92.123 **Driveway** of nursing home as the place of occurrence of the external cause
- Y92.124 **Garage** of nursing home as the place of occurrence of the external cause
- Y92.125 **Swimming pool** of nursing home as the place of occurrence of the external cause
- Y92.126 **Garden or yard** of nursing home as the place of occurrence of the external cause
- Y92.128 **Other place** in nursing home as the place of occurrence of the external cause
- Y92.129 **Unspecified** place in nursing home as the place of occurrence of the external cause
Coding Clinic: 2017, Q2, P10

● **Y92.13** **Military base** as the place of occurrence of the external cause
Excludes1 military training grounds (Y92.83)
- Y92.130 **Kitchen** on military base as the place of occurrence of the external cause
- Y92.131 **Mess hall** on military base as the place of occurrence of the external cause
- Y92.133 **Barracks** on military base as the place of occurrence of the external cause
- Y92.135 **Garage** on military base as the place of occurrence of the external cause
- Y92.136 **Swimming pool** on military base as the place of occurrence of the external cause
- Y92.137 **Garden or yard** on military base as the place of occurrence of the external cause
- Y92.138 **Other place** on military base as the place of occurrence of the external cause
- Y92.139 **Unspecified** place military base as the place of occurrence of the external cause

● **Y92.14** **Prison** as the place of occurrence of the external cause
- Y92.140 **Kitchen** in prison as the place of occurrence of the external cause
- Y92.141 **Dining room** in prison as the place of occurrence of the external cause
- Y92.142 **Bathroom** in prison as the place of occurrence of the external cause
- Y92.143 **Cell** of prison as the place of occurrence of the external cause
- Y92.146 **Swimming pool** of prison as the place of occurrence of the external cause
- Y92.147 **Courtyard** of prison as the place of occurrence of the external cause
- Y92.148 **Other place** in prison as the place of occurrence of the external cause
- Y92.149 **Unspecified** place in prison as the place of occurrence of the external cause

● **Y92.15** **Reform school** as the place of occurrence of the external cause
- Y92.150 **Kitchen** in reform school as the place of occurrence of the external cause
- Y92.151 **Dining room** in reform school as the place of occurrence of the external cause
- Y92.152 **Bathroom** in reform school as the place of occurrence of the external cause
- Y92.153 **Bedroom** in reform school as the place of occurrence of the external cause
- Y92.154 **Driveway** of reform school as the place of occurrence of the external cause
- Y92.155 **Garage** of reform school as the place of occurrence of the external cause
- Y92.156 **Swimming pool** of reform school as the place of occurrence of the external cause
- Y92.157 **Garden or yard** of reform school as the place of occurrence of the external cause
- Y92.158 **Other place** in reform school as the place of occurrence of the external cause
- Y92.159 **Unspecified** place in reform school as the place of occurrence of the external cause

● **Y92.16** **School dormitory** as the place of occurrence of the external cause
Excludes1 reform school as the place of occurrence of the external cause (Y92.15-)
school buildings and grounds as the place of occurrence of the external cause (Y92.2-)
school sports and athletic areas as the place of occurrence of the external cause (Y92.3-)
- Y92.160 **Kitchen** in school dormitory as the place of occurrence of the external cause
- Y92.161 **Dining room** in school dormitory as the place of occurrence of the external cause
- Y92.162 **Bathroom** in school dormitory as the place of occurrence of the external cause
- Y92.163 **Bedroom** in school dormitory as the place of occurrence of the external cause
- Y92.168 **Other place** in school dormitory as the place of occurrence of the external cause
- Y92.169 **Unspecified** place in school dormitory as the place of occurrence of the external cause

● Y92.19 **Other specified residential institution** as the place of occurrence of the external cause

Y92.19Ø **Kitchen** in other specified residential institution as the place of occurrence of the external cause

Y92.191 **Dining room** in other specified residential institution as the place of occurrence of the external cause

Y92.192 **Bathroom** in other specified residential institution as the place of occurrence of the external cause

Y92.193 **Bedroom** in other specified residential institution as the place of occurrence of the external cause

Y92.194 **Driveway** of other specified residential institution as the place of occurrence of the external cause

Y92.195 **Garage** of other specified residential institution as the place of occurrence of the external cause

Y92.196 **Pool** of other specified residential institution as the place of occurrence of the external cause

Y92.197 **Garden or yard** of other specified residential institution as the place of occurrence of the external cause

Y92.198 **Other place** in other specified residential institution as the place of occurrence of the external cause

Coding Clinic: 2Ø17, Q2, P11

Y92.199 **Unspecified** place in other specified residential institution as the place of occurrence of the external cause

Coding Clinic: 2Ø17, Q2, P1Ø

● Y92.2 School, other institution and public administrative area as the place of occurrence of the external cause

Building and adjacent grounds used by the general public or by a particular group of the public

Excludes1 building under construction as the place of occurrence of the external cause (Y92.6)
residential institution as the place of occurrence of the external cause (Y92.1)
school dormitory as the place of occurrence of the external cause (Y92.16-)
sports and athletics area of schools as the place of occurrence of the external cause (Y92.3-)

● Y92.21 **School** (private) (public) (state) as the place of occurrence of the external cause

Y92.21Ø **Daycare center** as the place of occurrence of the external cause

Y92.211 **Elementary school** as the place of occurrence of the external cause

Kindergarten as the place of occurrence of the external cause

Y92.212 **Middle school** as the place of occurrence of the external cause

Y92.213 **High school** as the place of occurrence of the external cause

Coding Clinic: 2Ø12, Q4, P1Ø8

Y92.214 **College** as the place of occurrence of the external cause

University as the place of occurrence of the external cause

Y92.215 **Trade school** as the place of occurrence of the external cause

Y92.218 **Other school** as the place of occurrence of the external cause

Y92.219 **Unspecified** school as the place of occurrence of the external cause

Y92.22 **Religious institution** as the place of occurrence of the external cause

Church as the place of occurrence of the external cause
Mosque as the place of occurrence of the external cause
Synagogue as the place of occurrence of the external cause

● Y92.23 **Hospital** as the place of occurrence of the external cause

Excludes1 ambulatory (outpatient) health services establishments (Y92.53-)
home for the sick as the place of occurrence of the external cause (Y92.12-)
hospice as the place of occurrence of the external cause (Y92.12-)
nursing home as the place of occurrence of the external cause (Y92.12-)

Y92.23Ø **Patient room** in hospital as the place of occurrence of the external cause

Y92.231 **Patient bathroom** in hospital as the place of occurrence of the external cause

Y92.232 **Corridor** of hospital as the place of occurrence of the external cause

Y92.233 **Cafeteria** of hospital as the place of occurrence of the external cause

Y92.234 **Operating room** of hospital as the place of occurrence of the external cause

Y92.238 **Other place** in hospital as the place of occurrence of the external cause

Y92.239 **Unspecified** place in hospital as the place of occurrence of the external cause

● Y92.24 **Public administrative building** as the place of occurrence of the external cause

Y92.24Ø **Courthouse** as the place of occurrence of the external cause

Y92.241 **Library** as the place of occurrence of the external cause

Y92.242 **Post office** as the place of occurrence of the external cause

Y92.243 **City hall** as the place of occurrence of the external cause

Y92.248 **Other public administrative building** as the place of occurrence of the external cause

● Y92.25 **Cultural building** as the place of occurrence of the external cause

Y92.25Ø **Art gallery** as the place of occurrence of the external cause

Y92.251 **Museum** as the place of occurrence of the external cause

Y92.252 **Music hall** as the place of occurrence of the external cause

Y92.253 **Opera house** as the place of occurrence of the external cause

Y92.254 **Theater (live)** as the place of occurrence of the external cause

Y92.258 **Other cultural public building** as the place of occurrence of the external cause

Y92.26 **Movie house or cinema** as the place of occurrence of the external cause

Y92.29 **Other specified public building** as the place of occurrence of the external cause

Assembly hall as the place of occurrence of the external cause
Clubhouse as the place of occurrence of the external cause

● **Y92.3 Sports and athletics area** as the place of occurrence of the external cause

● **Y92.31 Athletic court** as the place of occurrence of the external cause

Excludes1 tennis court in private home or garden (Y92.Ø9)

Y92.31Ø Basketball court as the place of occurrence of the external cause

Y92.311 Squash court as the place of occurrence of the external cause

Y92.312 Tennis court as the place of occurrence of the external cause

Y92.318 Other athletic court as the place of occurrence of the external cause

● **Y92.32 Athletic field** as the place of occurrence of the external cause

Y92.32Ø Baseball field as the place of occurrence of the external cause

Y92.321 Football field as the place of occurrence of the external cause

Y92.322 Soccer field as the place of occurrence of the external cause

Y92.328 Other athletic field as the place of occurrence of the external cause

Cricket field as the place of occurrence of the external cause

Hockey field as the place of occurrence of the external cause

● **Y92.33 Skating rink** as the place of occurrence of the external cause

Y92.33Ø Ice skating rink (indoor) (outdoor) as the place of occurrence of the external cause

Y92.331 Roller skating rink as the place of occurrence of the external cause

Y92.34 Swimming pool (public) as the place of occurrence of the external cause

Excludes1 swimming pool in private home or garden (Y92.Ø16)

Y92.39 Other specified sports and athletic area as the place of occurrence of the external cause

Golf-course as the place of occurrence of the external cause

Gymnasium as the place of occurrence of the external cause

Riding-school as the place of occurrence of the external cause

Stadium as the place of occurrence of the external cause

● **Y92.4 Street, highway and other paved roadways** as the place of occurrence of the external cause

Excludes1 private driveway of residence (Y92.Ø14, Y92.Ø24, Y92.Ø43, Y92.Ø93, Y92.113, Y92.123, Y92.154, Y92.194)

● **Y92.41 Street and highway** as the place of occurrence of the external cause

Y92.41Ø Unspecified street and highway as the place of occurrence of the external cause

Road NOS as the place of occurrence of the external cause

Y92.411 Interstate highway as the place of occurrence of the external cause

Freeway as the place of occurrence of the external cause

Motorway as the place of occurrence of the external cause

Y92.412 Parkway as the place of occurrence of the external cause

Y92.413 State road as the place of occurrence of the external cause

Y92.414 Local residential or business street as the place of occurrence of the external cause

Y92.415 Exit ramp or entrance ramp of street or highway as the place of occurrence of the external cause

● **Y92.48 Other paved roadways** as the place of occurrence of the external cause

Y92.48Ø Sidewalk as the place of occurrence of the external cause

Y92.481 Parking lot as the place of occurrence of the external cause

Y92.482 Bike path as the place of occurrence of the external cause

Y92.488 Other paved roadways as the place of occurrence of the external cause

● **Y92.5 Trade and service area** as the place of occurrence of the external cause

Excludes1 garage in private home (Y92.Ø15)
schools and other public administration buildings (Y92.2-)

● **Y92.51 Private commercial establishments** as the place of occurrence of the external cause

Y92.51Ø Bank as the place of occurrence of the external cause

Y92.511 Restaurant or café as the place of occurrence of the external cause

Y92.512 Supermarket, store or market as the place of occurrence of the external cause

Y92.513 Shop (commercial) as the place of occurrence of the external cause

● **Y92.52 Service areas** as the place of occurrence of the external cause

Y92.52Ø Airport as the place of occurrence of the external cause

Y92.521 Bus station as the place of occurrence of the external cause

Y92.522 Railway station as the place of occurrence of the external cause

Y92.523 Highway rest stop as the place of occurrence of the external cause

Y92.524 Gas station as the place of occurrence of the external cause

Petroleum station as the place of occurrence of the external cause

Service station as the place of occurrence of the external cause

● **Y92.53 Ambulatory health services establishments** as the place of occurrence of the external cause

Y92.53Ø Ambulatory surgery center as the place of occurrence of the external cause

Outpatient surgery center, including that connected with a hospital as the place of occurrence of the external cause

Same day surgery center, including that connected with a hospital as the place of occurrence of the external cause

Y92.531 Health care provider office as the place of occurrence of the external cause

Physician office as the place of occurrence of the external cause

Y92.532 Urgent care center as the place of occurrence of the external cause

Y92.538 Other ambulatory health services establishments as the place of occurrence of the external cause

Coding Clinic: 2019, Q1, P21

Y92.59 **Other trade areas as the place of occurrence of the external cause**
Office building as the place of occurrence of the external cause
Casino as the place of occurrence of the external cause
Garage (commercial) as the place of occurrence of the external cause
Hotel as the place of occurrence of the external cause
Radio or television station as the place of occurrence of the external cause
Shopping mall as the place of occurrence of the external cause
Warehouse as the place of occurrence of the external cause

● Y92.6 **Industrial and construction area as the place of occurrence of the external cause**

Y92.61 **Building [any] under construction as the place of occurrence of the external cause**

Y92.62 **Dock or shipyard as the place of occurrence of the external cause**
Dockyard as the place of occurrence of the external cause
Dry dock as the place of occurrence of the external cause
Shipyard as the place of occurrence of the external cause

Y92.63 **Factory as the place of occurrence of the external cause**
Factory building as the place of occurrence of the external cause
Factory premises as the place of occurrence of the external cause
Industrial yard as the place of occurrence of the external cause

Y92.64 **Mine or pit as the place of occurrence of the external cause**
Mine as the place of occurrence of the external cause

Y92.65 **Oil rig as the place of occurrence of the external cause**
Pit (coal) (gravel) (sand) as the place of occurrence of the external cause

Y92.69 **Other specified industrial and construction area as the place of occurrence of the external cause**
Gasworks as the place of occurrence of the external cause
Power-station (coal) (nuclear) (oil) as the place of occurrence of the external cause
Tunnel under construction as the place of occurrence of the external cause
Workshop as the place of occurrence of the external cause

● Y92.7 **Farm as the place of occurrence of the external cause**
Ranch as the place of occurrence of the external cause
Excludes1 farmhouse and home premises of farm (Y92.01-)

Y92.71 **Barn as the place of occurrence of the external cause**

Y92.72 **Chicken coop as the place of occurrence of the external cause**
Hen house as the place of occurrence of the external cause

Y92.73 **Farm field as the place of occurrence of the external cause**

Y92.74 **Orchard as the place of occurrence of the external cause**

Y92.79 **Other farm location as the place of occurrence of the external cause**

● Y92.8 **Other places** as the place of occurrence of the external cause

● Y92.81 **Transport vehicle as the place of occurrence of the external cause**
Excludes1 transport accidents (V00-V99)

Y92.810 **Car as the place of occurrence of the external cause**

Y92.811 **Bus as the place of occurrence of the external cause**

Y92.812 **Truck as the place of occurrence of the external cause**

Y92.813 **Airplane as the place of occurrence of the external cause**

Y92.814 **Boat as the place of occurrence of the external cause**

Y92.815 **Train as the place of occurrence of the external cause**

Y92.816 **Subway car as the place of occurrence of the external cause**

Y92.818 **Other transport vehicle as the place of occurrence of the external cause**

● Y92.82 **Wilderness area**

Y92.820 **Desert as the place of occurrence of the external cause**

Y92.821 **Forest as the place of occurrence of the external cause**

Y92.828 **Other wilderness area as the place of occurrence of the external cause**
Swamp as the place of occurrence of the external cause
Mountain as the place of occurrence of the external cause
Marsh as the place of occurrence of the external cause
Prairie as the place of occurrence of the external cause

● Y92.83 **Recreation area as the place of occurrence of the external cause**

Y92.830 **Public park as the place of occurrence of the external cause**

Y92.831 **Amusement park as the place of occurrence of the external cause**

Y92.832 **Beach as the place of occurrence of the external cause**
Seashore as the place of occurrence of the external cause

Y92.833 **Campsite as the place of occurrence of the external cause**

Y92.834 **Zoological garden (zoo) as the place of occurrence of the external cause**

Y92.838 **Other recreation area as the place of occurrence of the external cause**

Y92.84 **Military training ground as the place of occurrence of the external cause**

Y92.85 **Railroad track as the place of occurrence of the external cause**

Y92.86 **Slaughter house as the place of occurrence of the external cause**

Y92.89 **Other specified places as the place of occurrence of the external cause**
Derelict house as the place of occurrence of the external cause

OGCR Section I.C.20.b.

Do not use place of occurrence code Y92.9 if the place is not stated or is not applicable.

Y92.9 **Unspecified place or not applicable**

OGCR See Section I.C.20.c.

Activity Code

Assign a code from category Y93, Activity code, to describe the activity of the patient at the time the injury or other health condition occurred.

An activity code is used only once, at the initial encounter for treatment. Only one code from Y93 should be recorded on a medical record.

The activity codes are not applicable to poisonings, adverse effects, misadventures or sequela.

Do not assign Y93.9, Unspecified activity, if the activity is not stated.

A code from category Y93 is appropriate for use with external cause and intent codes if identifying the activity provides additional information about the event.

● **Y93 Activity codes**

Note: Category Y93 is provided for use to indicate the activity of the person seeking healthcare for an injury or health condition, such as a heart attack while shoveling snow, which resulted from, or was contributed to, by the activity. These codes are appropriate for use for both acute injuries, such as those from Chapter 19, and conditions that are due to the long-term, cumulative effects of an activity, such as those from Chapter 13. They are also appropriate for use with external cause codes for cause and intent if identifying the activity provides additional information on the event. These codes should be used in conjunction with codes for external cause status (Y99) and place of occurrence (Y92).

This section contains the following broad activity categories:

- Y93.0 Activities involving walking and running
- Y93.1 Activities involving water and water craft
- Y93.2 Activities involving ice and snow
- Y93.3 Activities involving climbing, rappelling, and jumping off
- Y93.4 Activities involving dancing and other rhythmic movement
- Y93.5 Activities involving other sports and athletics played individually
- Y93.6 Activities involving other sports and athletics played as a team or group
- Y93.7 Activities involving other specified sports and athletics
- Y93.A Activities involving other cardiorespiratory exercise
- Y93.B Activities involving other muscle strengthening exercises
- Y93.C Activities involving computer technology and electronic devices
- Y93.D Activities involving arts and handcrafts
- Y93.E Activities involving personal hygiene and interior property and clothing maintenance
- Y93.F Activities involving caregiving
- Y93.G Activities involving food preparation, cooking and grilling
- Y93.H Activities involving exterior property and land maintenance, building and construction
- Y93.I Activities involving roller coasters and other types of external motion
- Y93.J Activities involving playing musical instrument
- Y93.K Activities involving animal care
- Y93.8 Activities, other specified
- Y93.9 Activity, unspecified

● **Y93.0 Activities involving walking and running**

Excludes1 Activity, walking an animal (Y93.K1)
Activity, walking or running on a treadmill (Y93.A1)

Y93.01 Activity, walking, marching and hiking
Activity, walking, marching and hiking on level or elevated terrain
Excludes1 activity, mountain climbing (Y93.31)

Y93.02 Activity, running

● **Y93.1 Activities involving water and water craft**

Excludes1 activities involving ice (Y93.2-)

Y93.11 Activity, swimming

Y93.12 Activity, springboard and platform diving

Y93.13 Activity, water polo

Y93.14 Activity, water aerobics and water exercise

Y93.15 Activity, underwater diving and snorkeling
Activity, SCUBA diving

Y93.16 Activity, rowing, canoeing, kayaking, rafting and tubing
Activity, canoeing, kayaking, rafting and tubing in calm and turbulent water

Y93.17 Activity, water skiing and wake boarding

Y93.18 Activity, surfing, windsurfing and boogie boarding
Activity, water sliding

Y93.19 Activity, other involving water and watercraft
Activity involving water NOS
Activity, parasailing
Activity, water survival training and testing

● **Y93.2 Activities involving ice and snow**

Excludes1 activity, shoveling ice and snow (Y93.H1)

Y93.21 Activity, ice skating
Activity, figure skating (singles) (pairs)
Activity, ice dancing
Excludes1 activity, ice hockey (Y93.22)

Y93.22 Activity, ice hockey

Y93.23 Activity, snow (alpine) (downhill) skiing, snowboarding, sledding, tobogganing and snow tubing
Excludes1 activity, cross country skiing (Y93.24)

Y93.24 Activity, cross country skiing
Activity, nordic skiing

Y93.29 Activity, other activity involving ice and snow
Activity, activity involving ice and snow NOS

● **Y93.3 Activities involving climbing, rappelling and jumping off**

Excludes1 activity, hiking on level or elevated terrain (Y93.01)
activity, jumping rope (Y93.56)
activity, trampoline jumping (Y93.44)

Y93.31 Activity, mountain climbing, rock climbing and wall climbing

Y93.32 Activity, rappelling

Y93.33 Activity, BASE jumping
Activity, building, Antenna, Span, Earth jumping

Y93.34 Activity, bungee jumping

Y93.35 Activity, hang gliding

Y93.39 Activity, other activity involving climbing, rappelling and jumping off

● **Y93.4 Activities involving dancing and other rhythmic movement**

Excludes1 activity, martial arts (Y93.75)

Y93.41 Activity, dancing
Coding Clinic: 2012, Q4, P108

Y93.42 Activity, yoga

Y93.43 Activity, gymnastics
Activity, rhythmic gymnastics
Excludes1 activity, trampolining (Y93.44)

Y93.44 Activity, trampolining

Y93.45 Activity, cheerleading

Y93.49 Activity, other involving dancing and other rhythmic movements

CHAPTER 20 (V00-Y99)

● **Y93.5 Activities involving other sports and athletics played individually**
Excludes1 activity, dancing (Y93.41)
activity, gymnastic (Y93.43)
activity, trampolining (Y93.44)
activity, yoga (Y93.42)

Y93.51 Activity, roller skating (inline) and skateboarding
Y93.52 Activity, horseback riding
Y93.53 Activity, golf
Y93.54 Activity, bowling
Y93.55 Activity, bike riding
Y93.56 Activity, jumping rope
Y93.57 Activity, non-running track and field events
Excludes1 activity, running (any form) (Y93.Ø2)

Y93.59 Activity, other involving other sports and athletics played individually
Excludes1 activities involving climbing, rappelling, and jumping (Y93.3-)
activities involving ice and snow (Y93.2-)
activities involving walking and running (Y93.Ø-)
activities involving water and watercraft (Y93.1-)

● **Y93.6 Activities involving other sports and athletics played as a team or group**
Excludes1 activity, ice hockey (Y93.22)
activity, water polo (Y93.13)

Y93.61 Activity, American tackle football
Activity, football NOS
Y93.62 Activity, American flag or touch football
Y93.63 Activity, rugby
Y93.64 Activity, baseball
Activity, softball
Y93.65 Activity, lacrosse and field hockey
Coding Clinic: 2Ø15, Q1, P9
Y93.66 Activity, soccer
Y93.67 Activity, basketball
Y93.68 Activity, volleyball (beach) (court)
Y93.6A Activity, physical games generally associated with school recess, summer camp and children
Activity, capture the flag
Activity, dodge ball
Activity, four square
Activity, kickball
Y93.69 Activity, other involving other sports and athletics played as a team or group
Cricket

● **Y93.7 Activities involving other specified sports and athletics**
Y93.71 Activity, boxing
Y93.72 Activity, wrestling
Y93.73 Activity, racquet and hand sports
Activity, handball
Activity, racquetball
Activity, squash
Activity, tennis
Y93.74 Activity, frisbee
Activity, ultimate frisbee
Y93.75 Activity, martial arts
Activity, combatives
Y93.79 Activity, other specified sports and athletics
Excludes1 sports and athletics activities specified in categories Y93.Ø-Y93.6

● **Y93.A Activities involving other cardiorespiratory exercise**
Activities involving physical training
Y93.A1 Activity, exercise machines primarily for cardiorespiratory conditioning
Activity, elliptical and stepper machines
Activity, stationary bike
Activity, treadmill
Y93.A2 Activity, calisthenics
Activity, jumping jacks
Activity, warm up and cool down
Y93.A3 Activity, aerobic and step exercise
Y93.A4 Activity, circuit training
Y93.A5 Activity, obstacle course
Activity, challenge course
Activity, confidence course
Y93.A6 Activity, grass drills
Activity, guerilla drills
Y93.A9 Activity, other involving other cardiorespiratory exercise
Excludes1 activities involving cardiorespiratory exercise specified in categories Y93.Ø-Y93.7

● **Y93.B Activity involving other muscle strengthening exercises**
Y93.B1 Activity, exercise machines primarily for muscle strengthening
Y93.B2 Activity, push-ups, pull-ups, sit-ups
Y93.B3 Activity, free weights
Activity, barbells
Activity, dumbbells
Y93.B4 Activity, pilates
Y93.B9 Activity, other involving other muscle strengthening exercises
Excludes1 activities involving muscle strengthening specified in categories Y93.Ø-Y93.A

● **Y93.C Activities involving computer technology and electronic devices**
Excludes1 activity, electronic musical keyboard or instruments (Y93.J-)

Y93.C1 Activity, computer keyboarding
Activity, electronic game playing using keyboard or other stationary device
Y93.C2 Activity, hand held interactive electronic device
Activity, cellular telephone and communication device
Activity, electronic game playing using interactive device
Excludes1 activity, electronic game playing using keyboard or other stationary device (Y93.C1)

Y93.C9 Activity, other involving computer technology and electronic devices

● **Y93.D Activities involving arts and handcrafts**
Excludes1 activities involving playing musical instrument (Y93.J-)

Y93.D1 Knitting and crocheting
Y93.D2 Sewing
Y93.D3 Furniture building and finishing
Furniture repair
Y93.D9 Activity, other involving arts and handcrafts

● **Y93.E Activities involving personal hygiene and interior property and clothing maintenance**
Excludes1 activities involving cooking and grilling (Y93.G-)
activities involving exterior property and land maintenance, building and construction (Y93.H-)
activity involving caregiving (Y93.F-)
activity, dishwashing (Y93.G1)
activity, food preparation (Y93.G1)
activity, gardening (Y93.H2)

Y93.E1 Activity, **personal bathing and showering**
Y93.E2 Activity, **laundry**
Y93.E3 Activity, **vacuuming**
Y93.E4 Activity, **ironing**
Y93.E5 Activity, **floor mopping and cleaning**
Y93.E6 Activity, **residential relocation**
Activity, packing up and unpacking involved in moving to a new residence
Y93.E8 Activity, **other personal hygiene activity**
Y93.E9 Activity, **other household maintenance**

● **Y93.F Activities involving person providing caregiving**
Activity involving the provider of caregiving
Y93.F1 Activity, **caregiving involving bathing**
Y93.F2 Activity, **caregiving involving lifting**
Coding Clinic: 2016, Q4, P74
Y93.F9 Activity, **other caregiving**

● **Y93.G Activities involving food preparation, cooking and grilling**
Y93.G1 Activity, **food preparation and clean up**
Activity, dishwashing
Y93.G2 Activity, **grilling and smoking food**
Y93.G3 Activity, **cooking and baking**
Activity, use of stove, oven and microwave oven
Y93.G9 Activity, **other activity involving cooking and grilling**

● **Y93.H Activities involving property and land maintenance, building and construction**
Y93.H1 Activity, **digging, shoveling and raking**
Activity, dirt digging
Activity, raking leaves
Activity, snow shoveling
Y93.H2 Activity, **gardening and landscaping**
Activity, pruning, trimming shrubs, weeding
Y93.H3 Activity, **building and construction**
Y93.H9 Activity, **other activity involving property and land maintenance, building and construction**

● **Y93.I Activities involving roller coasters and other types of external motion**
Y93.I1 Activity, **rollercoaster riding**
Y93.I9 Activity, **other involving external motion**

● **Y93.J Activities involving playing musical instrument**
Activity involving playing electric musical instrument
Y93.J1 Activity, **piano playing**
Activity, musical keyboard (electronic) playing
Y93.J2 Activity, **drum and other percussion instrument playing**
Y93.J3 Activity, **string instrument playing**
Y93.J4 Activity, **winds and brass instrument playing**

● **Y93.K Activities involving animal care**
Excludes1 activity, horseback riding (Y93.52)
Y93.K1 Activity, **walking an animal**
Y93.K2 Activity, **milking an animal**
Y93.K3 Activity, **grooming and shearing an animal**
Y93.K9 Activity, **other activity involving animal care**

● **Y93.8 Other activity**
Coding Clinic: 2016, Q4, P74
Y93.81 Activity, **refereeing a sports activity**
Y93.82 Activity, **spectator at an event**
Y93.83 Activity, **rough housing and horseplay**
Coding Clinic: 2015, Q1, P8
Y93.84 Activity, **sleeping**
Y93.85 Activity, **choking game**
Activity, blackout game
Activity, fainting game
Activity, pass out game
Coding Clinic: 2016, Q4, P74-76
Y93.89 Activity, **other specified**

OGCR See Section I.C.20.c.

Do not assign Y93.9, Unspecified activity, if the activity is not stated.

● **Y93.9 Activity, unspecified**

Y95 Nosocomial condition

● **Y99 External cause status**
Note: A single code from category Y99 should be used in conjunction with the external cause code(s) assigned to a record to indicate the status of the person at the time the event occurred.
Coding Clinic: 2016, Q4, P74

Y99.0 Civilian activity done for income or pay
Civilian activity done for financial or other compensation
Excludes1 military activity (Y99.1)
volunteer activity (Y99.2)

Y99.1 Military activity
Excludes1 activity of off duty military personnel (Y99.8)

Y99.2 Volunteer activity
Excludes1 activity of child or other family member assisting in compensated work of other family member (Y99.8)

Y99.8 Other external cause status
Activity NEC
Activity of child or other family member assisting in compensated work of other family member
Hobby not done for income
Leisure activity
Off-duty activity of military personnel
Recreation or sport not for income or while a student
Student activity
Excludes1 civilian activity done for income or compensation (Y99.0)
military activity (Y99.1)
Coding Clinic: 2012, Q4, P108

Y99.9 Unspecified external cause status

CHAPTER 21

FACTORS INFLUENCING HEALTH STATUS AND CONTACT WITH HEALTH SERVICES (Z00-Z99)

OGCR Chapter-Specific Coding Guidelines

21. **Chapter 21: Factors influencing health status and contact with health services (Z00-Z99)**
Note: The chapter specific guidelines provide additional information about the use of Z codes for specified encounters.

a. **Use of Z codes in any healthcare setting**
Z codes are for use in any healthcare setting. Z codes may be used as either a first-listed (principal diagnosis code in the inpatient setting) or secondary code, depending on the circumstances of the encounter. Certain Z codes may only be used as first-listed or principal diagnosis.

b. **Z Codes indicate a reason for an encounter**
Z codes are not procedure codes. A corresponding procedure code must accompany a Z code to describe any procedure performed.

c. **Categories of Z Codes**

1) **Contact/Exposure**
Category Z20 indicates contact with, and suspected exposure to, communicable diseases. These codes are for patients who do not show any sign or symptom of a disease but are suspected to have been exposed to it by close personal contact with an infected individual or are in an area where a disease is epidemic.

Category Z77, Other contact with and (suspected) exposures hazardous to health, indicates contact with and suspected exposures hazardous to health.

Contact/exposure codes may be used as a first-listed code to explain an encounter for testing, or, more commonly, as a secondary code to identify a potential risk.

2) **Inoculations and vaccinations**
Code Z23 is for encounters for inoculations and vaccinations. It indicates that a patient is being seen to receive a prophylactic inoculation against a disease. Procedure codes are required to identify the actual administration of the injection and the type(s) of immunizations given. Code Z23 may be used as a secondary code if the inoculation is given as a routine part of preventive health care, such as a well-baby visit.

3) **Status**
Status codes indicate that a patient is either a carrier of a disease or has the sequelae or residual of a past disease or condition. This includes such things as the presence of prosthetic or mechanical devices resulting from past treatment. A status code is informative, because the status may affect the course of treatment and its outcome. A status code is distinct from a history code. The history code indicates that the patient no longer has the condition.

A status code should not be used with a diagnosis code from one of the body system chapters, if the diagnosis code includes the information provided by the status code. For example, code Z94.1, Heart transplant status, should not be used with a code from subcategory T86.2, Complications of heart transplant. The status code does not provide additional information. The complication code indicates that the patient is a heart transplant patient.

For encounters for weaning from a mechanical ventilator, assign a code from subcategory J96.1, Chronic respiratory failure, followed by code Z99.11, Dependence on respirator [ventilator] status.

The status Z codes/categories are:

Z14 Genetic carrier
Genetic carrier status indicates that a person carries a gene, associated with a particular disease, which may be passed to offspring who may develop that disease. The person does not have the disease and is not at risk of developing the disease.

Z15 Genetic susceptibility to disease Genetic susceptibility indicates that a person has a gene that increases the risk of that person developing the disease.

Codes from category Z15 should not be used as principal or first-listed codes. If the patient has the condition to which he/she is susceptible, and that condition is the reason for the encounter, the code for the current condition should be sequenced first. If the patient is being seen for follow-up after completed treatment for this condition, and the condition no longer exists, a follow-up code should be sequenced first, followed by the appropriate personal history and genetic susceptibility codes. If the purpose of the encounter is genetic counseling associated with procreative management, code Z31.5, Encounter for genetic counseling, should be assigned as the first-listed code, followed by a code from category Z15. Additional codes should be assigned for any applicable family or personal history.

Z16 Resistance to antimicrobial drugs
This code indicates that a patient has a condition that is resistant to antimicrobial drug treatment. Sequence the infection code first.

Z17 Estrogen receptor status

Z18 Retained foreign body fragments

Z19 Hormone sensitivity malignancy status

Z21 Asymptomatic HIV infection status This code indicates that a patient has tested positive for HIV but has manifested no signs or symptoms of the disease.

Z22 Carrier of infectious disease Carrier status indicates that a person harbors the specific organisms of a disease without manifest symptoms and is capable of transmitting the infection.

Z28.3 Underimmunization status

Z33.1 Pregnant state, incidental This code is a secondary code only for use when the pregnancy is in no way complicating the reason for visit. Otherwise, a code from the obstetric chapter is required.

Z66 Do not resuscitate

This code may be used when it is documented by the provider that a patient is on do not resuscitate status at any time during the stay.

Z67 Blood type

Z68 Body mass index (BMI)
BMI codes should only be assigned when the associated diagnosis (such as overweight or obesity) meets the definition of a reportable diagnosis (see Section III, Reporting Additional Diagnoses). Do not assign BMI codes during pregnancy. See Section I.B.14 for BMI documentation by clinicians other than the patient's provider.

Z74.01 Bed confinement status

Z76.82 Awaiting organ transplant status

Z78 Other specified health status

Code Z78.1, Physical restraint status, may be used when it is documented by the provider that a patient has been put in restraints during the current encounter. Please note that this code should not be reported when it is documented by the provider that a patient is temporarily restrained during a procedure.

Z79 Long-term (current) drug therapy

Codes from this category indicate a patient's continuous use of a prescribed drug (including such things as aspirin therapy) for the long-term treatment of a condition or for prophylactic use. It is not for use for patients who have addictions to drugs. This subcategory is not for use of medications for detoxification or maintenance programs to prevent withdrawal symptoms in patients with drug dependence (e.g., methadone maintenance for opiate dependence). Assign the appropriate code for the drug dependence instead.

Assign a code from Z79 if the patient is receiving a medication for an extended period as a prophylactic measure (such as for the prevention of deep vein thrombosis) or as treatment of a chronic condition (such as arthritis) or a disease requiring a lengthy course of treatment (such as cancer). Do not assign a code from category Z79 for medication being administered for a brief period of time to treat an acute illness or injury (such as a course of antibiotics to treat acute bronchitis).

Z88 Allergy status to drugs, medicaments and biological substances Except: Z88.9, Allergy status to unspecified drugs, medicaments and biological substances status

Z89 Acquired absence of limb

Z90 Acquired absence of organs, not elsewhere classified

Z91.0- Allergy status, other than to drugs and biological substances

Z92.82 Status post administration of tPA (rtPA) in a different facility within the last 24 hours prior to admission to a current facility Assign code Z92.82, Status post administration of tPA (rtPA) in a different facility within the last 24 hours prior to admission to current facility, as a secondary diagnosis when a patient is received by transfer into a facility and documentation indicates they were administered tissue plasminogen activator (tPA) within the last 24 hours prior to admission to the current facility. This guideline applies even if the patient is still receiving the tPA at the time they are received into the current facility. The appropriate code for the condition for which the tPA was administered (such as cerebrovascular disease or myocardial infarction) should be assigned first. Code Z92.82 is only applicable to the receiving facility record and not to the transferring facility record.

Z93	Artificial opening status
Z94	Transplanted organ and tissue status
Z95	Presence of cardiac and vascular implants and grafts
Z96	Presence of other functional implants
Z97	Presence of other devices
Z98	Other postprocedural states

Assign code Z98.85, Transplanted organ removal status, to indicate that a transplanted organ has been previously removed. This code should not be assigned for the encounter in which the transplanted organ is removed. The complication necessitating removal of the transplant organ should be assigned for that encounter.

See Section I.C.19. for information on the coding of organ transplant complications.

Z99	Dependence on enabling machines and devices, not elsewhere classified

Note: Categories Z89-Z90 and Z93-Z99 are for use only if there are no complications or malfunctions of the organ or tissue replaced, the amputation site or the equipment on which the patient is dependent.

4) History (of)

There are two types of history Z codes, personal and family. Personal history codes explain a patient's past medical condition that no longer exists and is not receiving any treatment, but that has the potential for recurrence, and therefore may require continued monitoring.

Family history codes are for use when a patient has a family member(s) who has had a particular disease that causes the patient to be at higher risk of also contracting the disease.

Personal history codes may be used in conjunction with follow-up codes and family history codes may be used in conjunction with screening codes to explain the need for a test or procedure. History codes are also acceptable on any medical record regardless of the reason for visit. A history of an illness, even if no longer present, is important information that may alter the type of treatment ordered.

The history Z code categories are:

Z80	Family history of primary malignant neoplasm
Z81	Family history of mental and behavioral disorders
Z82	Family history of certain disabilities and chronic diseases (leading to disablement)
Z83	Family history of other specific disorders
Z84	Family history of other conditions
Z85	Personal history of malignant neoplasm
Z86	Personal history of certain other diseases
Z87	Personal history of other diseases and conditions
Z91.4-	Personal history of psychological trauma, not elsewhere classified
Z91.5	Personal history of self-harm
Z91.81	History of falling
Z91.82	Personal history of military deployment
Z92	Personal history of medical treatment Except: Z92.0, Personal history of contraception Except: Z92.82, Status post administration of tPA (rtPA) in a different facility within the last 24 hours prior to admission to a current facility

5) Screening

Screening is the testing for disease or disease precursors in seemingly well individuals so that early detection and treatment can be provided for those who test positive for the disease (e.g., screening mammogram).

The testing of a person to rule out or confirm a suspected diagnosis because the patient has some sign or symptom is a diagnostic examination, not a screening. In these cases, the sign or symptom is used to explain the reason for the test.

A screening code may be a first-listed code if the reason for the visit is specifically the screening exam. It may also be used as an additional code if the screening is done during an office visit for other health problems. A screening code is not necessary if the screening is inherent to a routine examination, such as a pap smear done during a routine pelvic examination.

Should a condition be discovered during the screening then the code for the condition may be assigned as an additional diagnosis.

The Z code indicates that a screening exam is planned. A procedure code is required to confirm that the screening was performed.

The screening Z codes/categories:

Z11	Encounter for screening for infectious and parasitic diseases
Z12	Encounter for screening for malignant neoplasms
Z13	Encounter for screening for other diseases and disorders Except: Z13.9, Encounter for screening, unspecified
Z36	Encounter for antenatal screening for mother

6) Observation

There are three observation Z code categories. They are for use in very limited circumstances when a person is being observed for a suspected condition that is ruled out. The observation codes are not for use if an injury or illness or any signs or symptoms related to the suspected condition are present. In such cases the diagnosis/symptom code is used with the corresponding external cause code.

The observation codes are to be used as principal diagnosis only. The only exception to this is when the principal diagnosis is required to be a code from category Z38, Liveborn infants according to place of birth and type of delivery. Then a code from category Z05, Encounter for observation and evaluation of newborn for suspected diseases and conditions ruled out, is sequenced after the Z38 code. Additional codes may be used in addition to the observation code but only if they are unrelated to the suspected condition being observed.

Codes from subcategory Z03.7 Encounter for suspected maternal and fetal conditions ruled out, may either be used as a first-listed or as an additional code assignment depending on the case. They are for use in very limited circumstances on a maternal record when an encounter is for a suspected maternal or fetal condition that is ruled out during that encounter (for example, a maternal or fetal condition may be suspected due to an abnormal test result). These codes should not be used when the condition is confirmed. In those cases, the confirmed condition should be coded. In addition, these codes are not for use if an illness or any signs or symptoms related to the suspected condition or problem are present. In such cases the diagnosis/symptom code is used.

Additional codes may be used in addition to the code from subcategory Z03.7, but only if they are unrelated to the suspected condition being evaluated.

Codes from subcategory Z03.7 may not be used for encounters for antenatal screening of mother. *See Section I.C.21. Screening.*

For encounters for suspected fetal condition that are inconclusive following testing and evaluation, assign the appropriate code from category O35, O36, O40 or O41.

The observation Z code categories:

Z03	Encounter for medical observation for suspected diseases and conditions ruled out
Z04	Encounter for examination and observation for other reasons Except: Z04.9, Encounter for examination and observation for unspecified reason
Z05	Encounter for observation and evaluation of newborn for suspected diseases and conditions ruled out

7) Aftercare

Aftercare visit codes cover situations when the initial treatment of a disease has been performed and the patient requires continued care during the healing or recovery phase, or for the long-term consequences of the disease. The aftercare Z code should not be used if treatment is directed at a current, acute disease. The diagnosis code is to be used in these cases.

Exceptions to this rule are codes Z51.0, Encounter for antineoplastic radiation therapy, and codes from subcategory Z51.1, Encounter for antineoplastic chemotherapy and immunotherapy. These codes are to be first-listed, followed by the diagnosis code when a patient's encounter is solely to receive radiation therapy, chemotherapy, or immunotherapy for the treatment of a neoplasm. If the reason for the encounter is more than one type of antineoplastic therapy, code Z51.Ø and a code from subcategory Z51.1 may be assigned together, in which case one of these codes would be reported as a secondary diagnosis.

The aftercare Z codes should also not be used for aftercare for injuries. For aftercare of an injury, assign the acute injury code with the appropriate 7th character (for subsequent encounter).

The aftercare codes are generally first-listed to explain the specific reason for the encounter. An aftercare code may be used as an additional code when some type of aftercare is provided in addition to the reason for admission and no diagnosis code is applicable. An example of this would be the closure of a colostomy during an encounter for treatment of another condition.

Aftercare codes should be used in conjunction with other aftercare codes or diagnosis codes to provide better detail on the specifics of an aftercare encounter visit, unless otherwise directed by the classification. Should a patient receive multiple types of antineoplastic therapy during the same encounter, code Z51.Ø, Encounter for antineoplastic radiation therapy, and codes from subcategory Z51.1, Encounter for antineoplastic chemotherapy and immunotherapy, may be used together on a record. The sequencing of multiple aftercare codes depends on the circumstances of the encounter.

Certain aftercare Z code categories need a secondary diagnosis code to describe the resolving condition or sequelae. For others, the condition is included in the code title.

Additional Z code aftercare category terms include fitting and adjustment, and attention to artificial openings.

Status Z codes may be used with aftercare Z codes to indicate the nature of the aftercare. For example code Z95.1, Presence of aortocoronary bypass graft, may be used with code Z48.812, Encounter for surgical aftercare following surgery on the circulatory system, to indicate the surgery for which the aftercare is being performed. A status code should not be used when the aftercare code indicates the type of status, such as using Z43.Ø, Encounter for attention to tracheostomy, with Z93.Ø, Tracheostomy status.

The aftercare Z category/codes:

Z42	Encounter for plastic and reconstructive surgery following medical procedure or healed injury
Z43	Encounter for attention to artificial openings
Z44	Encounter for fitting and adjustment of external prosthetic device
Z45	Encounter for adjustment and management of implanted device
Z46	Encounter for fitting and adjustment of other devices
Z47	Orthopedic aftercare
Z48	Encounter for other postprocedural aftercare
Z49	Encounter for care involving renal dialysis
Z51	Encounter for other aftercare and medical care

8) Follow-up

The follow-up codes are used to explain continuing surveillance following completed treatment of a disease, condition, or injury. They imply that the condition has been fully treated and no longer exists. They should not be confused with aftercare codes, or injury codes with a 7th character for subsequent encounter, that explain ongoing care of a healing condition or its sequelae. Follow-up codes may be used in conjunction with history codes to provide the full picture of the healed condition and its treatment. The follow-up code is sequenced first, followed by the history code.

A follow-up code may be used to explain multiple visits. Should a condition be found to have recurred on the follow-up visit, then the diagnosis code for the condition should be assigned in place of the follow-up code.

The follow-up Z code categories:

ZØ8	Encounter for follow-up examination after completed treatment for malignant neoplasm
ZØ9	Encounter for follow-up examination after completed treatment for conditions other than malignant neoplasm
Z39	Encounter for maternal postpartum care and examination

9) Donor

Codes in category Z52, Donors of organs and tissues, are used for living individuals who are donating blood or other body tissue. These codes are only for individuals donating for others, not for self-donations. They are not used to identify cadaveric donations.

1Ø) Counseling

Counseling Z codes are used when a patient or family member receives assistance in the aftermath of an illness or injury, or when support is required in coping with family or social problems.

The counseling Z codes/categories:

Z3Ø.Ø-	Encounter for general counseling and advice on contraception
Z31.5	Encounter for procreative genetic counseling
Z31.6-	Encounter for general counseling and advice on procreation
Z32.2	Encounter for childbirth instruction
Z32.3	Encounter for childcare instruction
Z69	Encounter for mental health services for victim and perpetrator of abuse
Z7Ø	Counseling related to sexual attitude, behavior and orientation
Z71	Persons encountering health services for other counseling and medical advice, not elsewhere classified
Z76.81	Expectant mother prebirth pediatrician visit

11) Encounters for Obstetrical and Reproductive Services

See Section I.C.15. Pregnancy, Childbirth, and the Puerperium, for further instruction on the use of these codes.

Z codes for pregnancy are for use in those circumstances when none of the problems or complications included in the codes from the Obstetrics chapter exist (a routine prenatal visit or postpartum care). Codes in category Z34, Encounter for supervision of normal pregnancy, are always first listed and are not to be used with any other code from the OB chapter.

Codes in category Z3A, Weeks of gestation, may be assigned to provide additional information about the pregnancy. Category Z3A codes should not be assigned for pregnancies with abortive outcomes (categories OØØ-OØ8), elective termination of pregnancy (code Z33.2), nor for postpartum conditions, as category Z3A is not applicable to these conditions. The date of the admission should be used to determine weeks of gestation for inpatient admissions that encompass more than one gestational week.

The outcome of delivery, category Z37, should be included on all maternal delivery records. It is always a secondary code. Codes in category Z37 should not be used on the newborn record.

Z codes for family planning (contraceptive) or procreative management and counseling should be included on an obstetric record either during the pregnancy or the postpartum stage, if applicable.

Z codes/categories for obstetrical and reproductive services:

Z3Ø	Encounter for contraceptive management
Z31	Encounter for procreative management
Z32.2	Encounter for childbirth instruction
Z32.3	Encounter for childcare instruction
Z33	Pregnant state
Z34	Encounter for supervision of normal pregnancy
Z36	Encounter for antenatal screening of mother
Z3A	Weeks of gestation
Z37	Outcome of delivery
Z39	Encounter for maternal postpartum care and examination
Z76.81	Expectant mother prebirth pediatrician visit

12) Newborns and Infants

See Section I.C.16. Newborn (Perinatal) Guidelines, for further instruction on the use of these codes.

Newborn Z codes/categories:

Z76.1	Encounter for health supervision and care of foundling
ZØØ.1-	Encounter for routine child health examination
Z38	Liveborn infants according to place of birth and type of delivery

13) Routine and administrative examinations

The Z codes allow for the description of encounters for routine examinations, such as, a general check-up, or, examinations for administrative purposes, such as, a pre-employment physical. The codes are not to be used if the examination is for diagnosis of a suspected condition or for treatment purposes. In such cases the diagnosis code is used. During a routine exam, should a diagnosis or condition be discovered, it should be coded as an additional code. Pre-existing and chronic conditions and history codes may also be included as additional codes as long as the examination is for administrative purposes and not focused on any particular condition.

Some of the codes for routine health examinations distinguish between "with" and "without" abnormal findings. Code assignment depends on the information that is known at the time the encounter is being coded. For example, if no abnormal findings were found during the examination, but the encounter is being coded before test results are back, it is acceptable to assign the code for "without abnormal findings." When assigning a code for "with abnormal findings," additional code(s) should be assigned to identify the specific abnormal finding(s).

Pre-operative examination and pre-procedural laboratory examination Z codes are for use only in those situations when a patient is being cleared for a procedure or surgery and no treatment is given.

The Z codes/categories for routine and administrative examinations:

Z00	Encounter for general examination without complaint, suspected or reported diagnosis
Z01	Encounter for other special examination without complaint, suspected or reported diagnosis
Z02	Encounter for administrative examination Except: Z02.9, Encounter for administrative examinations, unspecified
Z32.0-	Encounter for pregnancy test

14) Miscellaneous Z codes

The miscellaneous Z codes capture a number of other health care encounters that do not fall into one of the other categories. Certain of these codes identify the reason for the encounter; others are for use as additional codes that provide useful information on circumstances that may affect a patient's care and treatment.

Prophylactic Organ Removal

For encounters specifically for prophylactic removal of an organ (such as prophylactic removal of breasts due to a genetic susceptibility to cancer or a family history of cancer), the principal or first-listed code should be a code from category Z40, Encounter for prophylactic surgery, followed by the appropriate codes to identify the associated risk factor (such as genetic susceptibility or family history).

If the patient has a malignancy of one site and is having prophylactic removal at another site to prevent either a new primary malignancy or metastatic disease, a code for the malignancy should also be assigned in addition to a code from subcategory Z40.0, Encounter for prophylactic surgery for risk factors related to malignant neoplasms. A Z40.0 code should not be assigned if the patient is having organ removal for treatment of a malignancy, such as the removal of the testes for the treatment of prostate cancer.

Miscellaneous Z codes/categories:

Z28	Immunization not carried out Except: Z28.3, Underimmunization status
Z29	Encounter for other prophylactic measures
Z40	Encounter for prophylactic surgery
Z41	Encounter for procedures for purposes other than remedying health state Except: Z41.9, Encounter for procedure for purposes other than remedying health state, unspecified
Z53	Persons encountering health services for specific procedures and treatment, not carried out
Z55	Problems related to education and literacy
Z56	Problems related to employment and unemployment
Z57	Occupational exposure to risk factors
Z58	Problems related to physical environment
Z59	Problems related to housing and economic circumstances
Z60	Problems related to social environment
Z62	Problems related to upbringing
Z63	Other problems related to primary support group, including family circumstances
Z64	Problems related to certain psychosocial circumstances
Z65	Problems related to other psychosocial circumstances
Z72	Problems related to lifestyle Note: These codes should be assigned only when the documentation specifies that the patient has an associated problem
Z73	Problems related to life management difficulty
Z74	Problems related to care provider dependency Except: Z74.01, Bed confinement status
Z75	Problems related to medical facilities and other health care
Z76.0	Encounter for issue of repeat prescription
Z76.3	Healthy person accompanying sick person
Z76.4	Other boarder to healthcare facility
Z76.5	Malingerer [conscious simulation]
Z91.1-	Patient's noncompliance with medical treatment and regimen
Z91.83	Wandering in diseases classified elsewhere
Z91.84-	Oral health risk factors
Z91.89	Other specified personal risk factors, not elsewhere classified

See Section I.B.14 for Z55-Z65 Persons with potential health hazards related to socioeconomic and psychosocial circumstances, documentation by clinicians other than the patient's provider.

15) Nonspecific Z codes

Certain Z codes are so non-specific, or potentially redundant with other codes in the classification, that there can be little justification for their use in the inpatient setting. Their use in the outpatient setting should be limited to those instances when there is no further documentation to permit more precise coding. Otherwise, any sign or symptom or any other reason for visit that is captured in another code should be used.

Nonspecific Z codes/categories:

Z02.9	Encounter for administrative examinations, unspecified
Z04.9	Encounter for examination and observation for unspecified reason
Z13.9	Encounter for screening, unspecified
Z41.9	Encounter for procedure for purposes other than remedying health state, unspecified
Z52.9	Donor of unspecified organ or tissue
Z86.59	Personal history of other mental and behavioral disorders
Z88.9	Allergy status to unspecified drugs, medicaments and biological substances status
Z92.0	Personal history of contraception

16) Z Codes That May Only Be Principal/First-Listed Diagnosis

The following Z codes/categories may only be reported as the principal/first-listed diagnosis, except when there are multiple encounters on the same day and the medical records for the encounters are combined:

Z00	Encounter for general examination without complaint, suspected or reported diagnosis Except: Z00.6
Z01	Encounter for other special examination without complaint, suspected or reported diagnosis
Z02	Encounter for administrative examination
Z03	Encounter for medical observation for suspected diseases and conditions ruled out
Z04	Encounter for examination and observation for other reasons
Z33.2	Encounter for elective termination of pregnancy
Z31.81	Encounter for male factor infertility in female patient
Z31.83	Encounter for assisted reproductive fertility procedure cycle
Z31.84	Encounter for fertility preservation procedure
Z34	Encounter for supervision of normal pregnancy
Z39	Encounter for maternal postpartum care and examination
Z38	Liveborn infants according to place of birth and type of delivery
Z40	Encounter for prophylactic surgery
Z42	Encounter for plastic and reconstructive surgery following medical procedure or healed injury
Z51.0	Encounter for antineoplastic radiation therapy
Z51.1-	Encounter for antineoplastic chemotherapy and immunotherapy
Z52	Donors of organs and tissues Except: Z52.9, Donor of unspecified organ or tissue
Z76.1	Encounter for health supervision and care of foundling
Z76.2	Encounter for health supervision and care of other healthy infant and child
Z99.12	Encounter for respirator [ventilator] dependence during power failure

CHAPTER 21

FACTORS INFLUENCING HEALTH STATUS AND CONTACT WITH HEALTH SERVICES (Z00-Z99)

Note: Z codes represent reasons for encounters. A corresponding procedure code must accompany a Z code if a procedure is performed. Categories Z00-Z99 are provided for occasions when circumstances other than a disease, injury or external cause classifiable to categories A00-Y89 are recorded as "diagnoses" or "problems." This can arise in two main ways:

(a) When a person who may or may not be sick encounters the health services for some specific purpose, such as to receive limited care or service for a current condition, to donate an organ or tissue, to receive prophylactic vaccination (immunization), or to discuss a problem which is in itself not a disease or injury.

(b) When some circumstance or problem is present which influences the person's health status but is not in itself a current illness or injury.

This chapter contains the following blocks:

Z00-Z13	Persons encountering health services for examination
Z14-Z15	Genetic carrier and genetic susceptibility to disease
Z16	Resistance to antimicrobial drugs
Z17	Estrogen receptor status
Z18	Retained foreign body fragments
Z19	Hormone sensitivity malignancy status
Z20-Z29	Persons with potential health hazards related to communicable diseases
Z30-Z39	Persons encountering health services in circumstances related to reproduction
Z40-Z53	Encounters for other specific health care
Z55-Z65	Persons with potential health hazards related to socioeconomic and psychosocial circumstances
Z66	Do not resuscitate status
Z67	Blood type
Z68	Body mass index (BMI)
Z69-Z76	Persons encountering health services in other circumstances
Z77-Z99	Persons with potential health hazards related to family and personal history and certain conditions influencing health status

PERSONS ENCOUNTERING HEALTH SERVICES FOR EXAMINATIONS (Z00-Z13)

Note: Nonspecific abnormal findings disclosed at the time of these examinations are classified to categories R70-R94.

Excludes1 examinations related to pregnancy and reproduction (Z30-Z36, Z39.-)

● **Z00 Encounter for general examination without complaint, suspected or reported diagnosis**

Excludes1 encounter for examination for administrative purposes (Z02.-)

Excludes2 encounter for pre-procedural examinations (Z01.81-)
special screening examinations (Z11-Z13)

● **Z00.0 Encounter for general adult medical examination**
Encounter for adult periodic examination (annual) (physical) and any associated laboratory and radiologic examinations

Excludes1 encounter for examination of sign or symptom - code to sign or symptom
general health check-up of infant or child (Z00.12.-)

Coding Clinic: 2016, Q4, P131

Z00.00 Encounter for general adult medical examination without abnormal findings A
Encounter for adult health check-up NOS
Coding Clinic: 2017, Q4, P95; 2016, Q1, P37

Z00.01 Encounter for general adult medical examination with abnormal findings A
Use additional code to identify abnormal findings
Coding Clinic: 2016, Q1, P36

● **Z00.1 Encounter for newborn, infant and child health examinations**

● **Z00.11 Newborn health examination**
Health check for child under 29 days old
Use additional code to identify any abnormal findings

Excludes1 health check for child over 28 days old (Z00.12-)

Z00.110 Health examination for newborn under 8 days old N
Health check for newborn under 8 days old

Z00.111 Health examination for newborn 8 to 28 days old N
Health check for newborn 8 to 28 days old
Newborn weight check

● **Z00.12 Encounter for routine child health examination**
Immunizations appropriate for age
Health check (routine) for child over 28 days old
Routine developmental screening of infant or child
Routine vision and hearing testing

Excludes1 health check for child under 29 days old (Z00.11-)
health supervision of foundling or other healthy infant or child (Z76.1-Z76.2)
newborn health examination (Z00.11-)

Z00.121 Encounter for routine child health examination with abnormal findings P
Use additional code to identify abnormal findings
Coding Clinic: 2017, Q4, P95; 2016, Q1, P34-35

Z00.129 Encounter for routine child health examination without abnormal findings P
Encounter for routine child health examination NOS
Coding Clinic: 2016, Q1, P34

Z00.2 Encounter for examination for period of rapid growth in childhood P

Z00.3 Encounter for examination for adolescent development state P
Encounter for puberty development state

Z00.5 Encounter for examination of potential donor of organ and tissue

Z00.6 Encounter for examination for normal comparison and control in clinical research program
Examination of participant or control in clinical research program

● **Z00.7 Encounter for examination for period of delayed growth in childhood**

Z00.70 Encounter for examination for period of delayed growth in childhood without abnormal findings P

Z00.71 Encounter for examination for period of delayed growth in childhood with abnormal findings P
Use additional code to identify abnormal findings

Z00.8 Encounter for other general examination
Encounter for health examination in population surveys

Z01 Encounter for other special examination without complaint, suspected or reported diagnosis

Includes routine examination of specific system

Note: Codes from category Z01 represent the reason for the encounter. A separate procedure code is required to identify any examinations or procedures performed.

Excludes1 encounter for examination for administrative purposes (Z02.-)
encounter for examination for suspected conditions, proven not to exist (Z03.-)
encounter for laboratory and radiologic examinations as a component of general medical examinations (Z00.0-)
encounter for laboratory, radiologic and imaging examinations for sign(s) and symptom(s) - code to the sign(s) or symptom(s)

Excludes2 screening examinations (Z11-Z13)

Z01.0 Encounter for examination of eyes and vision

Excludes1 examination for driving license (Z02.4)

Z01.00 Encounter for examination of eyes and vision without abnormal findings
Encounter for examination of eyes and vision NOS

Z01.01 Encounter for examination of eyes and vision with abnormal findings
Use additional code to identify abnormal findings
Coding Clinic: 2016, Q4, P21

Z01.02 Encounter for examination of eyes and vision following failed vision screening

Excludes1 examination for examination of eyes and vision with abnormal findings (Z01.01)
examination for examination of eyes and vision without abnormal findings (Z01.00)

Z01.020 Encounter for examination of eyes and vision following failed vision screening without abnormal findings

Z01.021 Encounter for examination of eyes and vision following failed vision screening with abnormal findings
Use additional code to identify abnormal findings

Z01.1 Encounter for examination of ears and hearing

Z01.10 Encounter for examination of ears and hearing without abnormal findings
Encounter for examination of ears and hearing NOS
Coding Clinic: 2016, Q4, P25

Z01.11 Encounter for examination of ears and hearing with abnormal findings
Coding Clinic: 2016, Q3, P18

Z01.110 Encounter for hearing examination following failed hearing screening
Coding Clinic: 2016, Q3, P18-19

Z01.118 Encounter for examination of ears and hearing with other abnormal findings
Use additional code to identify abnormal findings
Coding Clinic: 2016, Q3, P17

Z01.12 Encounter for hearing conservation and treatment

Z01.2 Encounter for dental examination and cleaning

Z01.20 Encounter for dental examination and cleaning without abnormal findings
Encounter for dental examination and cleaning NOS

Z01.21 Encounter for dental examination and cleaning with abnormal findings
Use additional code to identify abnormal findings

Z01.3 Encounter for examination of blood pressure

Z01.30 Encounter for examination of blood pressure without abnormal findings
Encounter for examination of blood pressure NOS

Z01.31 Encounter for examination of blood pressure with abnormal findings
Use additional code to identify abnormal findings

Z01.4 Encounter for gynecological examination

Excludes2 pregnancy examination or test (Z32.0-)
routine examination for contraceptive maintenance (Z30.4-)

Z01.41 Encounter for routine gynecological examination
Encounter for general gynecological examination with or without cervical smear
Encounter for gynecological examination (general) (routine) NOS
Encounter for pelvic examination (annual) (periodic)
Use additional code:
for screening for human papillomavirus, if applicable (Z11.51)
for screening vaginal pap smear, if applicable (Z12.72)
to identify acquired absence of uterus, if applicable (Z90.71-)

Excludes1 gynecologic examination status-post hysterectomy for malignant condition (Z08)
screening cervical pap smear not a part of a routine gynecological examination (Z12.4)

Z01.411 Encounter for gynecological examination (general) (routine) with abnormal findings ♀
Use additional code to identify any abnormal findings

Z01.419 Encounter for gynecological examination (general) (routine) without abnormal findings ♀

Z01.42 Encounter for cervical smear to confirm findings of recent normal smear following initial abnormal smear ♀

Z01.8 Encounter for other specified special examinations

Z01.81 Encounter for preprocedural examinations
Encounter for preoperative examinations
Encounter for radiological and imaging examinations as part of preprocedural examination

Z01.810 Encounter for preprocedural cardiovascular examination

Z01.811 Encounter for preprocedural respiratory examination

Z01.812 Encounter for preprocedural laboratory examination
Blood and urine tests prior to treatment or procedure

Z01.818 Encounter for other preprocedural examination
Encounter for preprocedural examination NOS
Encounter for examinations prior to antineoplastic chemotherapy

Z01.82 **Encounter for allergy testing**
Excludes1 encounter for antibody response examination (Z01.84)

Z01.83 **Encounter for blood typing**
Encounter for Rh typing

Z01.84 **Encounter for antibody response examination**
Encounter for immunity status testing
Excludes1 encounter for allergy testing (Z01.82)

Z01.89 **Encounter for other specified special examinations**

● Z02 **Encounter for administrative examination**

Z02.0 **Encounter for examination for admission to educational institution**
Encounter for examination for admission to preschool (education)
Encounter for examination for re-admission to school following illness or medical treatment

Z02.1 **Encounter for pre-employment examination**

Z02.2 **Encounter for examination for admission to residential institution**
Excludes1 examination for admission to prison (Z02.89)

Z02.3 **Encounter for examination for recruitment to armed forces**

Z02.4 **Encounter for examination for driving license**

Z02.5 **Encounter for examination for participation in sport**
Excludes1 blood-alcohol and blood-drug test (Z02.83)

Z02.6 **Encounter for examination for insurance purposes**

● Z02.7 **Encounter for issue of medical certificate**
Excludes1 encounter for general medical examination (Z00-Z01, Z02.0-Z02.6, Z02.8-Z02.9)

Z02.71 **Encounter for disability determination**
Encounter for issue of medical certificate of incapacity
Encounter for issue of medical certificate of invalidity

Z02.79 **Encounter for issue of other medical certificate**

● Z02.8 **Encounter for other administrative examinations**

Z02.81 **Encounter for paternity testing**

Z02.82 **Encounter for adoption services**

Z02.83 **Encounter for blood-alcohol and blood-drug test**
Use additional code for findings of alcohol or drugs in blood (R78.-)

Z02.89 **Encounter for other administrative examinations**
Encounter for examination for admission to prison
Encounter for examination for admission to summer camp
Encounter for immigration examination
Encounter for naturalization examination
Encounter for premarital examination
Excludes1 health supervision of foundling or other healthy infant or child (Z76.1-Z76.2)

Z02.9 **Encounter for administrative examinations, unspecified**

OGCR Section II.C.21.c.6.

Observation

There are three observation Z code categories. They are for use in very limited circumstances when a person is being observed for a suspected condition that is ruled out. The observation codes are not for use if an injury or illnesses or any signs or symptoms related to the suspected condition are present. In such cases the diagnosis/symptom code is used with the corresponding external cause code.

The observation codes are to be used as principal diagnosis only. The only exception to this is when the principal diagnosis is required to be a code from category Z38, Liveborn infants according to place of birth and type of delivery. Then a code from category Z05, Encounter for observation and evaluation of newborn for suspected diseases and conditions ruled out, is sequenced after the Z38 code. Additional codes may be used in addition to the observation code but only if they are unrelated to the suspected condition being observed.

Codes from subcategory Z03.7 Encounter for suspected maternal and fetal conditions ruled out, may either be used as a first listed or as an additional code assignment depending on the case. They are for use in very limited circumstances on a maternal record when an encounter is for a suspected maternal or fetal condition that is ruled out during that encounter (for example, a maternal or fetal condition may be suspected due to an abnormal test result). These codes should not be used when the condition is confirmed. In those cases, the confirmed condition should be coded. In addition, these codes are not for use if an illness or any signs or symptoms related to the suspected condition or problem are present. In such cases the diagnosis/symptom code is used.

Additional codes may be used in addition to the code from subcategory Z03.7, but only if they are unrelated to the suspected condition being evaluated.

Codes from subcategory Z03.7 may not be used for encounters for antenatal screening of mother. *See Section I.C.21. Screening.*

For encounters for suspected fetal condition that are inconclusive following testing and evaluation, assign the appropriate code from category O35, O36, O40 or O41.

The observation Z code categories:

Z03 Encounter for medical observation for suspected diseases and conditions ruled out

Z04 Encounter for examination and observation for other reasons
Except: Z04.9, Encounter for examination and observation for unspecified reason

Z05 Encounter for observation and evaluation of newborn for suspected diseases and conditions ruled out

● Z03 **Encounter for medical observation for suspected diseases and conditions ruled out**
This category is to be used when a person without a diagnosis is suspected of having an abnormal condition, without signs or symptoms, which requires study, but after examination and observation, is ruled out. This category is also for use for administrative and legal observation status.
Excludes1 contact with and (suspected) exposures hazardous to health (Z77.-)
encounter for observation and evaluation of newborn for suspected diseases and conditions ruled out (Z05.-)
person with feared complaint in whom no diagnosis is made (Z71.1)
signs or symptoms under study - code to signs or symptoms

Z03.6 **Encounter for observation for suspected toxic effect from ingested substance ruled out**
Encounter for observation for suspected adverse effect from drug
Encounter for observation for suspected poisoning

CHAPTER 21 (Z00-Z99)

● **Z03.7 Encounter for suspected maternal and fetal conditions ruled out**
Encounter for suspected maternal and fetal conditions not found
Excludes1 known or suspected fetal anomalies affecting management of mother, not ruled out (O26.-, O35.-, O36.-, O40.-, O41.-)

Z03.71 Encounter for suspected problem with amniotic cavity and membrane ruled out ♀ M
Encounter for suspected oligohydramnios ruled out
Encounter for suspected polyhydramnios ruled out

Z03.72 Encounter for suspected placental problem ruled out ♀ M

Z03.73 Encounter for suspected fetal anomaly ruled out ♀ M
Coding Clinic: 2016, Q4, P6

Z03.74 Encounter for suspected problem with fetal growth ruled out ♀ M

Z03.75 Encounter for suspected cervical shortening ruled out ♀ M

Z03.79 Encounter for other suspected maternal and fetal conditions ruled out ♀ M
Coding Clinic: 2016, Q4, P7

● **Z03.8 Encounter for observation for other suspected diseases and conditions ruled out**

● **Z03.81 Encounter for observation for suspected exposure to biological agents ruled out**

Z03.810 Encounter for observation for suspected exposure to anthrax ruled out

Z03.818 Encounter for observation for suspected exposure to other biological agents ruled out

Z03.89 Encounter for observation for other suspected diseases and conditions ruled out

● **Z04 Encounter for examination and observation for other reasons**
Includes encounter for examination for medicolegal reasons
This category is to be used when a person without a diagnosis is suspected of having an abnormal condition, without signs or symptoms, which requires study, but after examination and observation, is ruled-out. This category is also for use for administrative and legal observation status.

Z04.1 Encounter for examination and observation following transport accident
Excludes1 encounter for examination and observation following work accident (Z04.2)
Coding Clinic: 2019, Q2, P11

Z04.2 Encounter for examination and observation following work accident

Z04.3 Encounter for examination and observation following other accident

● **Z04.4 Encounter for examination and observation following alleged rape**
Encounter for examination and observation of victim following alleged rape
Encounter for examination and observation of victim following alleged sexual abuse
Coding Clinic: 2016, Q4, P129

Z04.41 Encounter for examination and observation following alleged adult rape A
Suspected adult rape, ruled out
Suspected adult sexual abuse, ruled out

Z04.42 Encounter for examination and observation following alleged child rape P
Suspected child rape, ruled out
Suspected child sexual abuse, ruled out

Z04.6 Encounter for general psychiatric examination, requested by authority

● **Z04.7 Encounter for examination and observation following alleged physical abuse**

Z04.71 Encounter for examination and observation following alleged adult physical abuse A
Suspected adult physical abuse, ruled out
Excludes1 confirmed case of adult physical abuse (T74.-)
encounter for examination and observation following alleged adult sexual abuse (Z04.41)
suspected case of adult physical abuse, not ruled out (T76.-)

Z04.72 Encounter for examination and observation following alleged child physical abuse P
Suspected child physical abuse, ruled out
Excludes1 confirmed case of child physical abuse (T74.-)
encounter for examination and observation following alleged child sexual abuse (Z04.42)
suspected case of child physical abuse, not ruled out (T76.-)

● **Z04.8 Encounter for examination and observation for other specified reasons**
Encounter for examination and observation for request for expert evidence

Z04.81 Encounter for examination and observation of victim following forced sexual exploitation

Z04.82 Encounter for examination and observation of victim following forced labor exploitation

Z04.89 Encounter for examination and observation for other specified reasons

Z04.9 Encounter for examination and observation for unspecified reason
Encounter for observation NOS

● **Z05 Encounter for observation and evaluation of newborn for suspected diseases and conditions ruled out**
This category is to be used for newborns, within the neonatal period (the first 28 days of life), who are suspected of having an abnormal condition, but without signs or symptoms, and which, after examination and observation, is ruled out.
Coding Clinic: 2019, Q2, P11; 2016, Q4, P54, 77, 126-127, 130

Z05.0 Observation and evaluation of newborn for suspected cardiac condition ruled out N

Z05.1 Observation and evaluation of newborn for suspected infectious condition ruled out N
Coding Clinic: 2019, Q2, P11

Z05.2 Observation and evaluation of newborn for suspected neurological condition ruled out N

Z05.3 Observation and evaluation of newborn for suspected respiratory condition ruled out N

● **Z05.4 Observation and evaluation of newborn for suspected genetic, metabolic or immunologic condition ruled out**

Z05.41 Observation and evaluation of newborn for suspected genetic condition ruled out N
Coding Clinic: 2016, Q4, P55

Z05.42 Observation and evaluation of newborn for suspected metabolic condition ruled out N

Z05.43 Observation and evaluation of newborn for suspected immunologic condition ruled out N

Z05.5 Observation and evaluation of newborn for suspected gastrointestinal condition ruled out N

Z05.6 Observation and evaluation of newborn for suspected genitourinary condition ruled out N

CHAPTER 21 (Z00-Z99)

● **Z05.7 Observation and evaluation of newborn for suspected skin, subcutaneous, musculoskeletal and connective tissue condition ruled out**

Z05.71 Observation and evaluation of newborn for suspected skin and subcutaneous tissue condition ruled out N

Z05.72 Observation and evaluation of newborn for suspected musculoskeletal condition ruled out N

Z05.73 Observation and evaluation of newborn for suspected connective tissue condition ruled out N

Z05.8 Observation and evaluation of newborn for other specified suspected condition ruled out N

Z05.9 Observation and evaluation of newborn for unspecified suspected condition ruled out N

OGCR See Section II.C.21.c.8.

The follow-up codes are used to explain continuing surveillance following completed treatment of a disease, condition, or injury. They imply that the condition has been fully treated and no longer exists. They should not be confused with aftercare codes, or injury codes with 7th character "D," that explain ongoing care of a healing condition or its sequelae. Follow-up codes may be used in conjunction with history codes to provide the full picture of the healed condition and its treatment. The follow-up code is sequenced first, followed by the history code.

A follow-up code may be used to explain multiple visits. Should a condition be found to have recurred on the follow-up visit, then the diagnosis code for the condition should be assigned in place of the follow-up code.

The follow-up Z code categories:

Z08 Encounter for follow-up examination after completed treatment for malignant neoplasm

Z09 Encounter for follow-up examination after completed treatment for conditions other than malignant neoplasm

Z39 Encounter for maternal postpartum care and examination

Z08 Encounter for follow-up examination after completed treatment for malignant neoplasm

Medical surveillance following completed treatment

Use additional code to identify any acquired absence of organs (Z90.-)

Use additional code to identify the personal history of malignant neoplasm (Z85.-)

Excludes1 aftercare following medical care (Z43-Z49, Z51)

Z09 Encounter for follow-up examination after completed treatment for conditions other than malignant neoplasm

Medical surveillance following completed treatment

Use additional code to identify any applicable history of disease code (Z86.-. Z87.-)

Excludes1 aftercare following medical care (Z43-Z49, Z51)
surveillance of contraception (Z30.4-)
surveillance of prosthetic and other medical devices (Z44-Z46)

Coding Clinic: 2017, Q1, P9; 2015, Q1, P8

OGCR Section II.C.21.c.5.

Screening

Screening is the testing for disease or disease precursors in seemingly well individuals so that early detection and treatment can be provided for those who test positive for the disease (e.g., screening mammogram).

The testing of a person to rule out or confirm a suspected diagnosis because the patient has some sign or symptom is a diagnostic examination, not a screening. In these cases, the sign or symptom is used to explain the reason for the test.

A screening code may be a first listed code if the reason for the visit is specifically the screening exam. It may also be used as an additional code if the screening is done during an office visit for other health problems. A screening code is not necessary if the screening is inherent to a routine examination, such as a pap smear done during a routine pelvic examination.

Should a condition be discovered during the screening then the code for the condition may be assigned as an additional diagnosis.

The Z code indicates that a screening exam is planned. A procedure code is required to confirm that the screening was performed.

The screening Z codes/categories:

Z11 Encounter for screening for infectious and parasitic diseases

Z12 Encounter for screening for malignant neoplasms

Z13 Encounter for screening for other diseases and disorders
Except: Z13.9, Encounter for screening, unspecified

Z36 Encounter for antenatal screening for mother

● **Z11 Encounter for screening for infectious and parasitic diseases**

Screening is the testing for disease or disease precursors in asymptomatic individuals so that early detection and treatment can be provided for those who test positive for the disease.

Excludes1 encounter for diagnostic examination - code to sign or symptom

Z11.0 Encounter for screening for intestinal infectious diseases
▶Encounter for screening for active tuberculosis disease

Z11.1 Encounter for screening for respiratory tuberculosis

Z11.2 Encounter for screening for other bacterial diseases

Z11.3 Encounter for screening for infections with a predominantly sexual mode of transmission

Excludes2 encounter for screening for human immunodeficiency virus [HIV] (Z11.4)
encounter for screening for human papillomavirus (Z11.51)

Z11.4 Encounter for screening for human immunodeficiency virus [HIV]

● **Z11.5 Encounter for screening for other viral diseases**

Excludes2 encounter for screening for viral intestinal disease (Z11.0)

Z11.51 Encounter for screening for human papillomavirus (HPV)

Z11.59 Encounter for screening for other viral diseases

Z11.6 Encounter for screening for other protozoal diseases and helminthiases

Diseases or infestations caused by parasitic worms

Excludes2 encounter for screening for protozoal intestinal disease (Z11.0)

▶**Z11.7 Encounter for testing for latent tuberculosis infection**

Z11.8 Encounter for screening for other infectious and parasitic diseases

Encounter for screening for chlamydia
Encounter for screening for rickettsial
Encounter for screening for spirochetal
Encounter for screening for mycoses

Z11.9 Encounter for screening for infectious and parasitic diseases, unspecified

CHAPTER 21 (Z00-Z99)

Z12 Encounter for screening for malignant neoplasms

Screening is the testing for disease or disease precursors in asymptomatic individuals so that early detection and treatment can be provided for those who test positive for the disease.

Use additional code to identify any family history of malignant neoplasm (Z80.-)

Excludes1 encounter for diagnostic examination - code to sign or symptom

Z12.0 Encounter for screening for malignant neoplasm of stomach

Z12.1 Encounter for screening for malignant neoplasm of intestinal tract

Z12.10 Encounter for screening for malignant neoplasm of intestinal tract, unspecified

Z12.11 Encounter for screening for malignant neoplasm of colon

Encounter for screening colonoscopy NOS

Coding Clinic: 2018, Q1, P7; 2017, Q1, P8-9

Z12.12 Encounter for screening for malignant neoplasm of rectum

Z12.13 Encounter for screening for malignant neoplasm of small intestine

Z12.2 Encounter for screening for malignant neoplasm of respiratory organs

Z12.3 Encounter for screening for malignant neoplasm of breast

Z12.31 Encounter for screening mammogram for malignant neoplasm of breast

Excludes1 inconclusive mammogram (R92.2)

Coding Clinic: 2015, Q1, P24

Z12.39 Encounter for other screening for malignant neoplasm of breast

Z12.4 Encounter for screening for malignant neoplasm of cervix ♀

Encounter for screening pap smear for malignant neoplasm of cervix

Excludes1 when screening is part of general gynecological examination (Z01.4-)

Excludes2 encounter for screening for human papillomavirus (Z11.51)

Z12.5 Encounter for screening for malignant neoplasm of prostate ♂

Z12.6 Encounter for screening for malignant neoplasm of bladder

Z12.7 Encounter for screening for malignant neoplasm of other genitourinary organs

Z12.71 Encounter for screening for malignant neoplasm of testis ♂

Z12.72 Encounter for screening for malignant neoplasm of vagina ♀

Vaginal pap smear status - post hysterectomy for non-malignant condition

Use additional code to identify acquired absence of uterus (Z90.71-)

Excludes1 vaginal pap smear status - post hysterectomy for malignant conditions (Z08)

Z12.73 Encounter for screening for malignant neoplasm of ovary ♀

Z12.79 Encounter for screening for malignant neoplasm of other genitourinary organs

Z12.8 Encounter for screening for malignant neoplasm of other sites

Z12.81 Encounter for screening for malignant neoplasm of oral cavity

Z12.82 Encounter for screening for malignant neoplasm of nervous system

Z12.83 Encounter for screening for malignant neoplasm of skin

Z12.89 Encounter for screening for malignant neoplasm of other sites

Z12.9 Encounter for screening for malignant neoplasm, site unspecified

Z13 Encounter for screening for other diseases and disorders

Screening is the testing for disease or disease precursors in asymptomatic individuals so that early detection and treatment can be provided for those who test positive for the disease.

Excludes1 encounter for diagnostic examination - code to sign or symptom

Z13.0 Encounter for screening for diseases of the blood and blood-forming organs and certain disorders involving the immune mechanism

Z13.1 Encounter for screening for diabetes mellitus

Z13.2 Encounter for screening for nutritional, metabolic and other endocrine disorders

Z13.21 Encounter for screening for nutritional disorder

Z13.22 Encounter for screening for metabolic disorder

Z13.220 Encounter for screening for lipoid disorders

Encounter for screening for cholesterol level

Encounter for screening for hypercholesterolemia

Encounter for screening for hyperlipidemia

Z13.228 Encounter for screening for other metabolic disorders

Z13.29 Encounter for screening for other suspected endocrine disorder

Excludes1 encounter for screening for diabetes mellitus (Z13.1)

Z13.3 Encounter for screening examination for mental health and behavioral disorders

Z13.30 Encounter for screening examination for mental health and behavioral disorders, unspecified

Z13.31 Encounter for screening for depression

Encounter for screening for depression, adult

Encounter for screening for depression for child or adolescent

Z13.32 Encounter for screening for maternal depression ♀

Encounter for screening for perinatal depression

Z13.39 Encounter for screening examination for other mental health and behavioral disorders

Encounter for screening for alcoholism

Encounter for screening for intellectual disabilities

Z13.4 Encounter for screening for certain developmental disorders in childhood P

Encounter for development testing of infant or child

Encounter for screening for developmental handicaps in early childhood

Excludes2 encounter for routine child health examination (Z00.12-)

Z13.40 Encounter for screening for unspecified developmental delays

Z13.41 Encounter for autism screening

Z13.42 Encounter for screening for global developmental delays (milestones)

Encounter for screening for developmental handicaps in early childhood

Z13.49 Encounter for screening for other developmental delays

CHAPTER 21 (Z00-Z99)

Z13.5 Encounter for screening for **eye and ear** disorders
Excludes2 encounter for general hearing examination (Z01.1-)
encounter for general vision examination (Z01.0-)
Coding Clinic: 2016, Q3, P17

Z13.6 Encounter for screening for **cardiovascular** disorders

● Z13.7 Encounter for screening for **genetic and chromosomal** anomalies
Excludes1 genetic testing for procreative management (Z31.4-)

Z13.71 Encounter for **nonprocreative** screening for genetic **disease carrier status**

Z13.79 Encounter for **other** screening for genetic and chromosomal anomalies

● Z13.8 Encounter for screening for **other specified** diseases and disorders
Excludes2 screening for malignant neoplasms (Z12.-)

● Z13.81 Encounter for screening for **digestive system** disorders

Z13.810 Encounter for screening for **upper** gastrointestinal disorder

Z13.811 Encounter for screening for **lower** gastrointestinal disorder
Excludes1 encounter for screening for intestinal infectious disease (Z11.0)

Z13.818 Encounter for screening for **other** digestive system disorders

● Z13.82 Encounter for screening for **musculoskeletal** disorder

Z13.820 Encounter for screening for **osteoporosis**

Z13.828 Encounter for screening for **other** musculoskeletal disorder

Z13.83 Encounter for screening for **respiratory** disorder NEC
Excludes1 encounter for screening for respiratory tuberculosis (Z11.1)

Z13.84 Encounter for screening for **dental** disorders

● Z13.85 Encounter for screening for **nervous system** disorders

Z13.850 Encounter for screening for **traumatic brain injury**

Z13.858 Encounter for screening for **other** nervous system disorders

Z13.88 Encounter for screening for **disorder due to exposure to contaminants**
Excludes1 those exposed to contaminants without suspected disorders (Z57-Z77.-)

Z13.89 Encounter for screening for **other** disorder
Encounter for screening for genitourinary disorders

Z13.9 Encounter for screening, **unspecified**

GENETIC CARRIER AND GENETIC SUSCEPTIBILITY TO DISEASE (Z14-Z15)

● Z14 Genetic carrier

● Z14.0 **Hemophilia A carrier**

Z14.01 **Asymptomatic** hemophilia A carrier

Z14.02 **Symptomatic** hemophilia A carrier

Z14.1 **Cystic fibrosis** carrier

Z14.8 Genetic carrier of **other** disease

● Z15 Genetic susceptibility to disease
Excludes1 chromosomal anomalies (Q90-Q99)
Includes confirmed abnormal gene
Use additional code, if applicable, for any associated family history of the disease (Z80-Z84)

● Z15.0 Genetic susceptibility to **malignant neoplasm**
Code first if applicable, any current malignant neoplasm (C00-C75, C81-C96)
Use additional code, if applicable, for any personal history of malignant neoplasm (Z85.-)

Z15.01 Genetic susceptibility to malignant neoplasm of **breast**

Z15.02 Genetic susceptibility to malignant neoplasm of **ovary** ♀

Z15.03 Genetic susceptibility to malignant neoplasm of **prostate** ♂

Z15.04 Genetic susceptibility to malignant neoplasm of **endometrium** ♀

Z15.09 Genetic susceptibility to **other** malignant neoplasm

● Z15.8 Genetic susceptibility to other disease

Z15.81 Genetic susceptibility to **multiple endocrine neoplasia** [MEN]
Excludes1 multiple endocrine neoplasia [MEN] syndromes (E31.2-)

Z15.89 Genetic susceptibility to **other** disease

RESISTANCE TO ANTIMICROBIAL DRUGS (Z16)

● Z16 Resistance to antimicrobial drugs
Note: The codes in this category are provided for use as additional codes to identify the resistance and non-responsiveness of a condition to antimicrobial drugs.
Code first the infection
Excludes1 Methicillin resistant Staphylococcus aureus infection (A49.02)
Methicillin resistant Staphylococcus aureus pneumonia (J15.212)
Sepsis due to Methicillin resistant Staphylococcus aureus (A41.02)

● Z16.1 Resistance to **beta lactam antibiotics**

Z16.10 Resistance to **unspecified** beta lactam antibiotics

Z16.11 Resistance to **penicillins**
Resistance to amoxicillin
Resistance to ampicillin

Z16.12 **Extended spectrum beta lactamase (ESBL)** resistance
Excludes2 Methicillin resistant Staphylococcus aureus infection in diseases classified elsewhere (B95.62)

Z16.19 Resistance to **other** specified beta lactam antibiotics
Resistance to cephalosporins

● Z16.2 Resistance to **other antibiotics**

Z16.20 Resistance to **unspecified** antibiotic
Resistance to antibiotics NOS

Z16.21 Resistance to **vancomycin**

Z16.22 Resistance to **vancomycin related** antibiotics

Z16.23 Resistance to **quinolones and fluoroquinolones**

Z16.24 Resistance to **multiple** antibiotics

Z16.29 Resistance to **other single** specified antibiotic
Resistance to aminoglycosides
Resistance to macrolides
Resistance to sulfonamides
Resistance to tetracyclines

● **Z16.3 Resistance to other antimicrobial drugs**
Excludes1 resistance to antibiotics (Z16.1-, Z16.2-)
Z16.30 **Resistance to unspecified antimicrobial drugs**
Drug resistance NOS
Z16.31 **Resistance to antiparasitic drug(s)**
Resistance to quinine and related compounds
Z16.32 **Resistance to antifungal drug(s)**
Z16.33 **Resistance to antiviral drug(s)**
● Z16.34 **Resistance to antimycobacterial drug(s)**
Resistance to tuberculostatics
Z16.341 **Resistance to single antimycobacterial drug**
Resistance to antimycobacterial drug NOS
Z16.342 **Resistance to multiple antimycobacterial drugs**
Z16.35 **Resistance to multiple antimicrobial drugs**
Excludes1 Resistance to multiple antibiotics only (Z16.24)
Z16.39 **Resistance to other specified antimicrobial drug**

ESTROGEN RECEPTOR STATUS (Z17)

● **Z17 Estrogen receptor status**
Code first malignant neoplasm of breast (C50.-)
Z17.0 **Estrogen receptor positive status [ER+]**
Z17.1 **Estrogen receptor negative status [ER-]**

RETAINED FOREIGN BODY FRAGMENTS (Z18)

● **Z18 Retained foreign body fragments**
Includes embedded fragment (status)
embedded splinter (status)
retained foreign body status
Excludes1 artificial joint prosthesis status (Z96.6-)
foreign body accidentally left during a procedure (T81.5-)
foreign body entering through orifice (T15-T19)
in situ cardiac device (Z95.-)
organ or tissue replaced by means other than transplant (Z96.-, Z97.-)
organ or tissue replaced by transplant (Z94.-)
personal history of retained foreign body fully removed Z87.821
superficial foreign body (non-embedded splinter) - code to superficial foreign body, by site
● Z18.0 **Retained radioactive fragments**
Z18.01 **Retained depleted uranium fragments**
Z18.09 **Other retained radioactive fragments**
Other retained depleted isotope fragments
Retained nontherapeutic radioactive fragments
● Z18.1 **Retained metal fragments**
Excludes1 retained radioactive metal fragments (Z18.01-Z18.09)
Z18.10 **Retained metal fragments, unspecified**
Retained metal fragment NOS
Z18.11 **Retained magnetic metal fragments**
Z18.12 **Retained nonmagnetic metal fragments**
Z18.2 **Retained plastic fragments**
Acrylics fragments
Diethylhexylphthalates fragments
Isocyanate fragments
● Z18.3 **Retained organic fragments**
Z18.31 **Retained animal quills or spines**
Z18.32 **Retained tooth**
Z18.33 **Retained wood fragments**
Z18.39 **Other retained organic fragments**
● Z18.8 **Other specified retained foreign body**
Z18.81 **Retained glass fragments**
Z18.83 **Retained stone or crystalline fragments**
Retained concrete or cement fragments
Z18.89 **Other specified retained foreign body fragments**
Coding Clinic: 2016, Q3, P24
Z18.9 **Retained foreign body fragments, unspecified material**

HORMONE SENSITIVITY MALIGNANCY STATUS (Z19)

● **Z19 Hormone sensitivity malignancy status**
Code first malignant neoplasm —*see* Table of Neoplasms, by site, malignant
Coding Clinic: 2016, Q4, P129
Z19.1 **Hormone sensitive malignancy status**
Coding Clinic: 2016, Q4, P76
Z19.2 **Hormone resistant malignancy status**
Castrate resistant prostate malignancy status
Coding Clinic: 2016, Q4, P76

PERSONS WITH POTENTIAL HEALTH HAZARDS RELATED TO COMMUNICABLE DISEASES (Z20-Z29)

● **Z20 Contact with and (suspected) exposure to communicable diseases**
Excludes1 carrier of infectious disease (Z22.-)
diagnosed current infectious or parasitic disease - see Alphabetic Index
Excludes2 personal history of infectious and parasitic diseases (Z86.1-)
● Z20.0 **Contact with and (suspected) exposure to intestinal infectious diseases**
Z20.01 **Contact with and (suspected) exposure to intestinal infectious diseases due to Escherichia coli (E. coli)**
Z20.09 **Contact with and (suspected) exposure to other intestinal infectious diseases**
Z20.1 **Contact with and (suspected) exposure to tuberculosis**
Z20.2 **Contact with and (suspected) exposure to infections with a predominantly sexual mode of transmission**
Z20.3 **Contact with and (suspected) exposure to rabies**
Z20.4 **Contact with and (suspected) exposure to rubella**
Z20.5 **Contact with and (suspected) exposure to viral hepatitis**
Z20.6 **Contact with and (suspected) exposure to human immunodeficiency virus [HIV]**
Excludes1 asymptomatic human immunodeficiency virus [HIV]
HIV infection status (Z21)
Z20.7 **Contact with and (suspected) exposure to pediculosis, acariasis and other infestations**
● Z20.8 **Contact with and (suspected) exposure to other communicable diseases**
● Z20.81 **Contact with and (suspected) exposure to other bacterial communicable diseases**
Z20.810 **Contact with and (suspected) exposure to anthrax**
Z20.811 **Contact with and (suspected) exposure to meningococcus**
Z20.818 **Contact with and (suspected) exposure to other bacterial communicable diseases**
● Z20.82 **Contact with and (suspected) exposure to other viral communicable diseases**
Z20.820 **Contact with and (suspected) exposure to varicella**
Z20.821 **Contact with and (suspected) exposure to Zika virus**
Z20.828 **Contact with and (suspected) exposure to other viral communicable diseases**
Coding Clinic: 2016, Q4, P6-7, 121
Z20.89 **Contact with and (suspected) exposure to other communicable diseases**
Z20.9 **Contact with and (suspected) exposure to unspecified communicable disease**

Z21 Asymptomatic human immunodeficiency virus [HIV] infection status (HCC)
HIV positive NOS
Code first Human immunodeficiency virus [HIV] disease complicating pregnancy, childbirth and the puerperium, if applicable (O98.7-)
Excludes1 acquired immunodeficiency syndrome (B2Ø)
contact with human immunodeficiency virus [HIV] (Z2Ø.6)
exposure to human immunodeficiency virus [HIV] (Z2Ø.6)
human immunodeficiency virus [HIV] disease (B2Ø)
inconclusive laboratory evidence of human immunodeficiency virus [HIV] (R75)
Coding Clinic: 2019, Q1, P1Ø-11

● **Z22 Carrier of infectious disease**
Includes colonization status
suspected carrier
Excludes2 carrier of viral hepatitis (B18.-)
- Z22.Ø **Carrier of typhoid**
- Z22.1 **Carrier of other intestinal infectious diseases**
- Z22.2 **Carrier of diphtheria**
- ● Z22.3 **Carrier of other specified bacterial diseases**
  - Z22.31 **Carrier of bacterial disease due to meningococci**
  - ● Z22.32 **Carrier of bacterial disease due to staphylococci**
    - Z22.321 **Carrier or suspected carrier of Methicillin susceptible Staphylococcus aureus**
      MSSA colonization
    - Z22.322 **Carrier or suspected carrier of Methicillin resistant Staphylococcus aureus**
      MRSA colonization
  - ● Z22.33 **Carrier of bacterial disease due to streptococci**
    - Z22.33Ø **Carrier of Group B streptococcus**
      Excludes1 Carrier of streptococcus group B (GBS) complicating pregnancy, childbirth and the puerperium (O99.82-)
    - Z22.338 **Carrier of other streptococcus**
  - Z22.39 **Carrier of other specified bacterial diseases**
- Z22.4 **Carrier of infections with a predominantly sexual mode of transmission**
- Z22.6 **Carrier of human T-lymphotropic virus type-1 [HTLV-1] infection**
- ▶ Z22.7 **Latent tuberculosis**
  ▶Latent tuberculosis infection (LTBI)
  ▶ **Excludes1** nonspecific reaction to cell mediated immunity measurement of gamma interferon antigen response without active tuberculosis (R76.12)
  ▶nonspecific reaction to tuberculin skin test without active tuberculosis (R76.11)
- Z22.8 **Carrier of other infectious diseases**
- Z22.9 **Carrier of infectious disease, unspecified**

Z23 Encounter for immunization
Code first any routine childhood examination
Note: Procedure codes are required to identify the types of immunizations given.

● **Z28 Immunization not carried out and underimmunization status**
Includes vaccination not carried out
- ● Z28.Ø **Immunization not carried out because of contraindication**
  - Z28.Ø1 **Immunization not carried out because of acute illness of patient**
  - Z28.Ø2 **Immunization not carried out because of chronic illness or condition of patient**
  - Z28.Ø3 **Immunization not carried out because of immune compromised state of patient**
  - Z28.Ø4 **Immunization not carried out because of patient allergy to vaccine or component**
  - Z28.Ø9 **Immunization not carried out because of other contraindication**
- Z28.1 **Immunization not carried out because of patient decision for reasons of belief or group pressure**
  Immunization not carried out because of religious belief
- ● Z28.2 **Immunization not carried out because of patient decision for other and unspecified reason**
  - Z28.2Ø **Immunization not carried out because of patient decision for unspecified reason**
  - Z28.21 **Immunization not carried out because of patient refusal**
  - Z28.29 **Immunization not carried out because of patient decision for other reason**
- Z28.3 **Underimmunization status**
  Delinquent immunization status
  Lapsed immunization schedule status
- ● Z28.8 **Immunization not carried out for other reason**
  - Z28.81 **Immunization not carried out due to patient having had the disease**
  - Z28.82 **Immunization not carried out because of caregiver refusal**
    Immunization not carried out because of guardian refusal
    Immunization not carried out because of parent refusal
    Excludes1 immunization not carried out because of caregiver refusal because of religious belief (Z28.1)
  - Z28.83 **Immunization not carried out due to unavailability of vaccine**
    Delay in delivery of vaccine
    Lack of availability of vaccine
    Manufacturer delay of vaccine
  - Z28.89 **Immunization not carried out for other reason**
- Z28.9 **Immunization not carried out for unspecified reason**

● **Z29 Encounter for other prophylactic measures**
Excludes1 desensitization to allergens (Z51.6)
prophylactic surgery (Z4Ø.-)
Coding Clinic: 2016, Q4, P13Ø
- ● Z29.1 **Encounter for prophylactic immunotherapy**
  Encounter for administration of immunoglobulin
  Coding Clinic: 2016, Q4, P78-79
  - Z29.11 **Encounter for prophylactic immunotherapy for respiratory syncytial virus (RSV)**
  - Z29.12 **Encounter for prophylactic antivenin**
  - Z29.13 **Encounter for prophylactic Rho(D) immune globulin**
  - Z29.14 **Encounter for prophylactic rabies immune globin**
- Z29.3 **Encounter for prophylactic fluoride administration**
  Coding Clinic: 2016, Q4, P79
- Z29.8 **Encounter for other specified prophylactic measures**
  Coding Clinic: 2016, Q4, P79
- Z29.9 **Encounter for prophylactic measures, unspecified**
  Coding Clinic: 2016, Q4, P79

CHAPTER 21 (ZØØ-Z99)

▶ New ▶ Revised ~~deleted~~ Deleted Excludes 1 Excludes 2 Includes Use additional Code first Code also Key words
OGCR Official Guidelines X Assign placeholder X ● Use Additional Character(s) Manifestation Code (HCC) Hierarchical Condition Category Coding Clinic

PERSONS ENCOUNTERING HEALTH SERVICES IN CIRCUMSTANCES RELATED TO REPRODUCTION (Z30-Z39)

● **Z30** Encounter for contraceptive management

● **Z30.0** Encounter for general counseling and advice on contraception

● **Z30.01** Encounter for initial prescription of contraceptives

Excludes1 encounter for surveillance of contraceptives (Z30.4-)

Z30.011 Encounter for initial prescription of contraceptive pills ♀

Z30.012 Encounter for prescription of emergency contraception ♀
Encounter for postcoital contraception

Z30.013 Encounter for initial prescription of injectable contraceptive ♀

Z30.014 Encounter for initial prescription of intrauterine contraceptive device ♀

Excludes1 encounter for insertion of intrauterine contraceptive device (Z30.430, Z30.432)

Z30.015 Encounter for initial prescription of vaginal ring hormonal contraceptive ♀
Coding Clinic: 2016, Q4, P78

Z30.016 Encounter for initial prescription of transdermal patch hormonal contraceptive device
Coding Clinic: 2016, Q4, P78

Z30.017 Encounter for initial prescription of implantable subdermal contraceptive
Coding Clinic: 2016, Q4, P78

Z30.018 Encounter for initial prescription of other contraceptives ♀
Encounter for initial prescription of barrier contraception
Encounter for initial prescription of diaphragm

Z30.019 Encounter for initial prescription of contraceptives, unspecified ♀

Z30.02 Counseling and instruction in natural family planning to avoid pregnancy

Z30.09 Encounter for other general counseling and advice on contraception
Encounter for family planning advice NOS

Z30.2 Encounter for sterilization

● **Z30.4** Encounter for surveillance of contraceptives

Z30.40 Encounter for surveillance of contraceptives, unspecified

Z30.41 Encounter for surveillance of contraceptive pills ♀
Encounter for repeat prescription for contraceptive pill

Z30.42 Encounter for surveillance of injectable contraceptive ♀

● **Z30.43** Encounter for surveillance of intrauterine contraceptive device

Z30.430 Encounter for insertion of intrauterine contraceptive device ♀

Z30.431 Encounter for routine checking of intrauterine contraceptive device ♀

Z30.432 Encounter for removal of intrauterine contraceptive device ♀

Z30.433 Encounter for removal and reinsertion of intrauterine contraceptive device ♀
Encounter for replacement of intrauterine contraceptive device

Z30.44 Encounter for surveillance of vaginal ring hormonal contraceptive device ♀
Coding Clinic: 2016, Q4, P78

Z30.45 Encounter for surveillance of transdermal patch hormonal contraceptive device ♀
Coding Clinic: 2016, Q4, P78

Z30.46 Encounter for surveillance of implantable subdermal contraceptive ♀
Encounter for checking, reinsertion or removal of implantable subdermal contraceptive
Coding Clinic: 2016, Q4, P78

Z30.49 Encounter for surveillance of other contraceptives ♀
Encounter for surveillance of barrier contraception
Encounter for surveillance of diaphragm

Z30.8 Encounter for other contraceptive management
Encounter for postvasectomy sperm count
Encounter for routine examination for contraceptive maintenance

Excludes1 sperm count following sterilization reversal (Z31.42)
sperm count for fertility testing (Z31.41)

Z30.9 Encounter for contraceptive management, unspecified

● **Z31** Encounter for procreative management

Excludes1 complications associated with artificial fertilization (N98.-)
female infertility (N97.-)
male infertility (N46.-)

Z31.0 Encounter for reversal of previous sterilization

● **Z31.4** Encounter for procreative investigation and testing

Excludes1 postvasectomy sperm count (Z30.8)

Z31.41 Encounter for fertility testing
Encounter for fallopian tube patency testing
Encounter for sperm count for fertility testing

Z31.42 Aftercare following sterilization reversal
Sperm count following sterilization reversal

● **Z31.43** Encounter for genetic testing of female for procreative management
Use additional code for recurrent pregnancy loss, if applicable (N96, O26.2-)

Excludes1 nonprocreative genetic testing (Z13.7-)

Z31.430 Encounter of female for testing for genetic disease carrier status for procreative management ♀

Z31.438 Encounter for other genetic testing of female for procreative management ♀

● **Z31.44** Encounter for genetic testing of male for procreative management

Excludes1 nonprocreative genetic testing (Z13.7-)

Z31.440 Encounter of male for testing for genetic disease carrier status for procreative management ♂

Z31.441 Encounter for testing of male partner of patient with recurrent pregnancy loss ♂ A

Z31.448 Encounter for other genetic testing of male for procreative management ♂ A

Z31.49 Encounter for other procreative investigation and testing

CHAPTER 21 (Z00-Z99)

Z31.5 Encounter for procreative genetic counseling

● Z31.6 Encounter for general counseling and advice on procreation

Z31.61 Procreative counseling and advice using natural family planning

Z31.62 Encounter for fertility preservation counseling
Encounter for fertility preservation counseling prior to cancer therapy
Encounter for fertility preservation counseling prior to surgical removal of gonads

Z31.69 Encounter for other general counseling and advice on procreation

Z31.7 Encounter for procreative management and counseling for gestational carrier ♀
Excludes1 pregnant state, gestational carrier (Z33.3)
Coding Clinic: 2016, Q4, P78

● Z31.8 Encounter for other procreative management

Z31.81 Encounter for male factor infertility in female patient ♀

Z31.82 Encounter for Rh incompatibility status ♀
Coding Clinic: 2015, Q3, P40

Z31.83 Encounter for assisted reproductive fertility procedure cycle ♀
Patient undergoing in vitro fertilization cycle
Use additional code to identify the type of infertility
Excludes1 pre-cycle diagnosis and testing - code to reason for encounter

Z31.84 Encounter for fertility preservation procedure
Encounter for fertility preservation procedure prior to cancer therapy
Encounter for fertility preservation procedure prior to surgical removal of gonads

Z31.89 Encounter for other procreative management

Z31.9 Encounter for procreative management, unspecified

● Z32 Encounter for pregnancy test and childbirth and childcare instruction

● Z32.0 Encounter for pregnancy test

Z32.00 Encounter for pregnancy test, result unknown ♀
Encounter for pregnancy test NOS

Z32.01 Encounter for pregnancy test, result positive ♀ M

Z32.02 Encounter for pregnancy test, result negative ♀

Z32.2 Encounter for childbirth instruction

Z32.3 Encounter for childcare instruction
Encounter for prenatal or postpartum childcare instruction

● Z33 Pregnant state

Z33.1 Pregnant state, incidental ♀ M
Pregnant state NOS
Excludes1 complications of pregnancy (O00-O9A)
pregnant state, gestational carrier (Z33.3)

Z33.2 Encounter for elective termination of pregnancy ♀ M
Excludes1 early fetal death with retention of dead fetus (O02.1)
late fetal death (O36.4)
spontaneous abortion (O03)
Coding Clinic: 2016, Q4, P130

Z33.3 Pregnant state, gestational carrier ♀
Excludes1 encounter for procreative management and counseling for gestational carrier (Z31.7)
Coding Clinic: 2016, Q4, P78

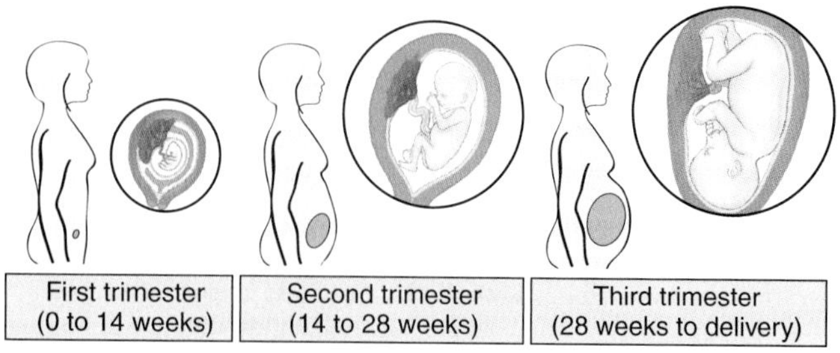

Figure 21-1 Trimesters. (From Shiland, Betsy J. Medical Terminology & Anatomy for ICD-10 Coding, ed 2, Mosby, 2015)

● Z34 Encounter for supervision of normal pregnancy
Excludes1 any complication of pregnancy (O00-O9A)
encounter for pregnancy test (Z32.0-)
encounter for supervision of high risk pregnancy (O09.-)
Coding Clinic: 2016, Q4, P6

● Z34.0 Encounter for supervision of normal first pregnancy

Z34.00 Encounter for supervision of normal first pregnancy, unspecified trimester ♀ M

Z34.01 Encounter for supervision of normal first pregnancy, first trimester ♀ M

Z34.02 Encounter for supervision of normal first pregnancy, second trimester ♀ M

Z34.03 Encounter for supervision of normal first pregnancy, third trimester ♀ M

● Z34.8 Encounter for supervision of other normal pregnancy

Z34.80 Encounter for supervision of other normal pregnancy, unspecified trimester ♀ M

Z34.81 Encounter for supervision of other normal pregnancy, first trimester ♀ M

Z34.82 Encounter for supervision of other normal pregnancy, second trimester ♀ M

Z34.83 Encounter for supervision of other normal pregnancy, third trimester ♀ M

● Z34.9 Encounter for supervision of normal pregnancy, unspecified

Z34.90 Encounter for supervision of normal pregnancy, unspecified, unspecified trimester ♀ M

Z34.91 Encounter for supervision of normal pregnancy, unspecified, first trimester ♀ M

Z34.92 Encounter for supervision of normal pregnancy, unspecified, second trimester ♀ M

Z34.93 Encounter for supervision of normal pregnancy, unspecified, third trimester ♀ M

● Z36 Encounter for antenatal screening of mother ♀
Includes Encounter for placental sample (taken vaginally)
Screening is the testing for disease or disease precursors in asymptomatic individuals so that early detection and treatment can be provided for those who test positive for the disease.
Excludes1 diagnostic examination - code to sign or symptom
encounter for suspected maternal and fetal conditions ruled out (Z03.7-)
suspected fetal condition affecting management of pregnancy - code to condition in Chapter 15
Excludes2 abnormal findings on antenatal screening of mother (O28.-)
genetic counseling and testing (Z31.43-, Z31.5)
routine prenatal care (Z34)

Z36.0 Encounter for antenatal screening for chromosomal anomalies ♀ M

Z36.1 Encounter for antenatal screening for **raised alphafetoprotein level** ♀ **M**
Encounter for antenatal screening for elevated maternal serum alphafetoprotein level

Z36.2 Encounter for other antenatal screening **follow-up** ♀ **M**
Non-visualized anatomy on a previous scan

Z36.3 Encounter for antenatal screening for **malformations** ♀ **M**
Screening for a suspected anomaly

Z36.4 Encounter for antenatal screening for **fetal growth retardation** ♀ **M**
Intrauterine growth restriction (IUGR)/small-for-dates

Z36.5 Encounter for antenatal screening for **isoimmunization** ♀ **M**

● Z36.8 Encounter for **other** antenatal screening

Z36.81 Encounter for antenatal screening for **hydrops fetalis** ♀ **M**

Z36.82 Encounter for antenatal screening for **nuchal translucency** ♀ **M**

Z36.83 Encounter for fetal screening for **congenital cardiac abnormalities** ♀ **M**

Z36.84 Encounter for antenatal screening for **fetal lung maturity** ♀ **M**

Z36.85 Encounter for antenatal screening for **Streptococcus B** ♀ **M**

Z36.86 Encounter for antenatal screening for **cervical length** ♀ **M**
Screening for risk of pre-term labor

Z36.87 Encounter for antenatal screening for **uncertain dates** ♀

Z36.88 Encounter for antenatal screening for **fetal macrosomia** ♀ **M**
Screening for large-for-dates

Z36.89 Encounter for **other specified** antenatal screening ♀ **M**

Z36.8A Encounter for antenatal screening for **other genetic defects** ♀ **M**

Z36.9 Encounter for antenatal screening, **unspecified** ♀ **M**

● Z3A Weeks of gestation

Note: Codes from category Z3A are for use, only on the maternal record, to indicate the weeks of gestation of the pregnancy, if known.

Code first complications of pregnancy, childbirth and the puerperium (O09-O9A)

Coding Clinic: 2016, Q4, P130; 2013, Q2, P33

● Z3A.0 Weeks of gestation of pregnancy, **unspecified or less than 10** weeks

Z3A.00 Weeks of gestation of pregnancy **not specified** ♀ **M**

Z3A.01 **Less than 8 weeks** gestation of pregnancy ♀ **M**

Z3A.08 **8 weeks** gestation of pregnancy ♀ **M**

Z3A.09 **9 weeks** gestation of pregnancy ♀ **M**

● Z3A.1 Weeks of gestation of pregnancy, weeks **10-19**

Z3A.10 **10 weeks** gestation of pregnancy ♀ **M**

Z3A.11 **11 weeks** gestation of pregnancy ♀ **M**

Z3A.12 **12 weeks** gestation of pregnancy ♀ **M**

Z3A.13 **13 weeks** gestation of pregnancy ♀ **M**

Z3A.14 **14 weeks** gestation of pregnancy ♀ **M**

Z3A.15 **15 weeks** gestation of pregnancy ♀ **M**

Z3A.16 **16 weeks** gestation of pregnancy ♀ **M**
Coding Clinic: 2016, Q4, P5

Z3A.17 **17 weeks** gestation of pregnancy ♀ **M**

Z3A.18 **18 weeks** gestation of pregnancy ♀ **M**
Coding Clinic: 2019, Q2, P11

Z3A.19 **19 weeks** gestation of pregnancy ♀ **M**

● Z3A.2 Weeks of gestation of pregnancy, weeks **20-29**

Z3A.20 **20 weeks** gestation of pregnancy ♀ **M**
Coding Clinic: 2016, Q4, P6

Z3A.21 **21 weeks** gestation of pregnancy ♀ **M**

Z3A.22 **22 weeks** gestation of pregnancy ♀ **M**
Coding Clinic: 2016, Q4, P6

Z3A.23 **23 weeks** gestation of pregnancy ♀ **M**

Z3A.24 **24 weeks** gestation of pregnancy ♀ **M**

Z3A.25 **25 weeks** gestation of pregnancy ♀ **M**

Z3A.26 **26 weeks** gestation of pregnancy ♀ **M**

Z3A.27 **27 weeks** gestation of pregnancy ♀ **M**

Z3A.28 **28 weeks** gestation of pregnancy ♀ **M**

Z3A.29 **29 weeks** gestation of pregnancy ♀ **M**

● Z3A.3 Weeks of gestation of pregnancy, weeks **30-39**

Z3A.30 **30 weeks** gestation of pregnancy ♀ **M**

Z3A.31 **31 weeks** gestation of pregnancy ♀ **M**

Z3A.32 **32 weeks** gestation of pregnancy ♀ **M**
Coding Clinic: 2016, Q4, P6

Z3A.33 **33 weeks** gestation of pregnancy ♀ **M**

Z3A.34 **34 weeks** gestation of pregnancy ♀ **M**

Z3A.35 **35 weeks** gestation of pregnancy ♀ **M**

Z3A.36 **36 weeks** gestation of pregnancy ♀ **M**

Z3A.37 **37 weeks** gestation of pregnancy ♀ **M**

Z3A.38 **38 weeks** gestation of pregnancy ♀ **M**
Coding Clinic: 2016, Q2, P34

Z3A.39 **39 weeks** gestation of pregnancy ♀ **M**

● Z3A.4 Weeks of gestation of pregnancy, weeks **40 or greater**

Z3A.40 **40 weeks** gestation of pregnancy ♀ **M**

Z3A.41 **41 weeks** gestation of pregnancy ♀ **M**

Z3A.42 **42 weeks** gestation of pregnancy ♀ **M**

Z3A.49 **Greater than 42 weeks** gestation of pregnancy ♀ **M**

● Z37 Outcome of delivery

This category is intended for use as an additional code to identify the outcome of delivery on the mother's record. It is not for use on the newborn record.

Excludes1 stillbirth (P95)

Z37.0 Single live birth ♀ **M**
Coding Clinic: 2016, Q2, P34

Z37.1 Single stillbirth ♀ **M**

Z37.2 Twins, both liveborn ♀ **M**

Z37.3 Twins, one liveborn and one stillborn ♀ **M**

Z37.4 Twins, both stillborn ♀ **M**

● Z37.5 Other multiple births, **all liveborn**

Z37.50 Multiple births, **unspecified**, all liveborn ♀ **M**

Z37.51 Triplets, all liveborn ♀ **M**

Z37.52 Quadruplets, all liveborn ♀ **M**

Z37.53 Quintuplets, all liveborn ♀ **M**

Z37.54 Sextuplets, all liveborn ♀ **M**

Z37.59 Other multiple births, all liveborn ♀ **M**

● Z37.6 **Other** multiple births, **some liveborn**

Z37.60 Multiple births, **unspecified**, some liveborn ♀ **M**

Z37.61 Triplets, some liveborn ♀ **M**

Z37.62 Quadruplets, some liveborn ♀ **M**

Z37.63 Quintuplets, some liveborn ♀ **M**

Z37.64 Sextuplets, some liveborn ♀ **M**

Z37.69 Other multiple births, some liveborn ♀ **M**

Z37.7 **Other** multiple births, **all stillborn** ♀ **M**

Z37.9 Outcome of delivery, **unspecified** ♀ **M**
Multiple birth NOS
Single birth NOS

● Z38 Liveborn infants according to place of birth and type of delivery

This category is for use as the principal code on the initial record of a newborn baby. It is to be used for the initial birth record only. It is not to be used on the mother's record.

Coding Clinic: 2017, Q2, P6-7; 2016, Q4, P126-127, 130; 2015, Q2, P15

● Z38.0 Single liveborn infant, **born in hospital**
Single liveborn infant, born in birthing center or other health care facility
Coding Clinic: 2017, Q2, P5-7

Z38.00 Single liveborn infant, **delivered vaginally** **N**
Coding Clinic: 2018, Q4, P26; 2016, Q4, P7, 55

Z38.01 Single liveborn infant, **delivered by cesarean** **N**
Coding Clinic: 2017, Q2, P7; 2016, Q3, P18

CHAPTER 21 (Z00-Z99)

Z38.1 Single liveborn infant, born outside hospital N
Z38.2 Single liveborn infant, unspecified as to place of birth N
Single liveborn infant NOS
● Z38.3 Twin liveborn infant, born in hospital
Z38.30 Twin liveborn infant, delivered vaginally N
Z38.31 Twin liveborn infant, delivered by cesarean N
Z38.4 Twin liveborn infant, born outside hospital N
Z38.5 Twin liveborn infant, unspecified as to place of birth N
● Z38.6 Other multiple liveborn infant, born in hospital
Z38.61 Triplet liveborn infant, delivered vaginally N
Z38.62 Triplet liveborn infant, delivered by cesarean N
Z38.63 Quadruplet liveborn infant, delivered vaginally N
Z38.64 Quadruplet liveborn infant, delivered by cesarean N
Z38.65 Quintuplet liveborn infant, delivered vaginally N
Z38.66 Quintuplet liveborn infant, delivered by cesarean N
Z38.68 Other multiple liveborn infant, delivered vaginally N
Z38.69 Other multiple liveborn infant, delivered by cesarean N
Z38.7 Other multiple liveborn infant, born outside hospital N
Z38.8 Other multiple liveborn infant, unspecified as to place of birth N

● Z39 Encounter for maternal postpartum care and examination
Z39.0 Encounter for care and examination of mother immediately after delivery ♀ M
Care and observation in uncomplicated cases when the delivery occurs outside a healthcare facility
Excludes1 care for postpartum complication - see Alphabetic index
Z39.1 Encounter for care and examination of lactating mother ♀ M
Encounter for supervision of lactation
Excludes1 disorders of lactation (O92.-)
Z39.2 Encounter for routine postpartum follow-up ♀ M

ENCOUNTERS FOR OTHER SPECIFIC HEALTH CARE (Z40-Z53)

Categories Z40-Z53 are intended for use to indicate a reason for care. They may be used for patients who have already been treated for a disease or injury, but who are receiving aftercare or prophylactic care, or care to consolidate the treatment, or to deal with a residual state

Excludes2 follow-up examination for medical surveillance after treatment (Z08-Z09)

● Z40 Encounter for prophylactic surgery
Excludes1 organ donations (Z52.-)
therapeutic organ removal - code to condition
Coding Clinic: 2016, Q4, P79
● Z40.0 Encounter for prophylactic surgery for risk factors related to malignant neoplasms
Admission for prophylactic organ removal
Use additional code to identify risk factor
Z40.00 Encounter for prophylactic removal of unspecified organ
Z40.01 Encounter for prophylactic removal of breast
Z40.02 Encounter for prophylactic removal of ovary(s) ♀
Encounter for prophylactic removal of ovary(s) and fallopian tube(s)
Z40.03 Encounter for prophylactic removal of fallopian tube(s) ♀
Z40.09 Encounter for prophylactic removal of other organ
Z40.8 Encounter for other prophylactic surgery
Z40.9 Encounter for prophylactic surgery, unspecified

● Z41 Encounter for procedures for purposes other than remedying health state
Z41.1 Encounter for cosmetic surgery
Encounter for cosmetic breast implant
Encounter for cosmetic procedure
Excludes1 encounter for plastic and reconstructive surgery following medical procedure or healed injury (Z42.-)
encounter for post-mastectomy breast implantation (Z42.1)
Z41.2 Encounter for routine and ritual male circumcision ♂
Z41.3 Encounter for ear piercing
Z41.8 Encounter for other procedures for purposes other than remedying health state
Z41.9 Encounter for procedure for purposes other than remedying health state, unspecified

● Z42 Encounter for plastic and reconstructive surgery following medical procedure or healed injury
Excludes1 encounter for cosmetic plastic surgery (Z41.1)
encounter for plastic surgery for treatment of current injury - code to relevent injury
Z42.1 Encounter for breast reconstruction following mastectomy A
Excludes1 deformity and disproportion of reconstructed breast (N65.1-)
Z42.8 Encounter for other plastic and reconstructive surgery following medical procedure or healed injury
Coding Clinic: 2017, Q1, P42

● Z43 Encounter for attention to artificial openings
Includes closure of artificial openings
passage of sounds or bougies through artificial openings
reforming artificial openings
removal of catheter from artificial openings
toilet or cleansing of artificial openings
Excludes1 complications of external stoma (J95.0-, K94.-, N99.5-)
Excludes2 fitting and adjustment of prosthetic and other devices (Z44-Z46)
Z43.0 Encounter for attention to tracheostomy HCC
Z43.1 Encounter for attention to gastrostomy HCC
Excludes2 artificial opening status only, without need for care (Z93.-)
Z43.2 Encounter for attention to ileostomy HCC
Coding Clinic: 2016, Q3, P5
Z43.3 Encounter for attention to colostomy HCC
Z43.4 Encounter for attention to other artificial openings of digestive tract HCC
Z43.5 Encounter for attention to cystostomy HCC
Z43.6 Encounter for attention to other artificial openings of urinary tract HCC
Encounter for attention to nephrostomy
Encounter for attention to ureterostomy
Encounter for attention to urethrostomy
Z43.7 Encounter for attention to artificial vagina
Z43.8 Encounter for attention to other artificial openings HCC
Z43.9 Encounter for attention to unspecified artificial opening HCC

Z44 Encounter for fitting and adjustment of external prosthetic device

Includes removal or replacement of external prosthetic device

Excludes1 malfunction or other complications of device - see Alphabetical Index presence of prosthetic device (Z97.-)

Z44.0 Encounter for fitting and adjustment of artificial arm

Z44.00 Encounter for fitting and adjustment of unspecified artificial arm

Z44.001 Encounter for fitting and adjustment of unspecified right artificial arm

Z44.002 Encounter for fitting and adjustment of unspecified left artificial arm

Z44.009 Encounter for fitting and adjustment of unspecified artificial arm, unspecified arm

Z44.01 Encounter for fitting and adjustment of complete artificial arm

Z44.011 Encounter for fitting and adjustment of complete right artificial arm

Z44.012 Encounter for fitting and adjustment of complete left artificial arm

Z44.019 Encounter for fitting and adjustment of complete artificial arm, unspecified arm

Z44.02 Encounter for fitting and adjustment of partial artificial arm

Z44.021 Encounter for fitting and adjustment of partial artificial right arm

Z44.022 Encounter for fitting and adjustment of partial artificial left arm

Z44.029 Encounter for fitting and adjustment of partial artificial arm, unspecified arm

Z44.1 Encounter for fitting and adjustment of artificial leg

Z44.10 Encounter for fitting and adjustment of unspecified artificial leg

Z44.101 Encounter for fitting and adjustment of unspecified right artificial leg

Z44.102 Encounter for fitting and adjustment of unspecified left artificial leg

Z44.109 Encounter for fitting and adjustment of unspecified artificial leg, unspecified leg

Z44.11 Encounter for fitting and adjustment of complete artificial leg

Z44.111 Encounter for fitting and adjustment of complete right artificial leg

Z44.112 Encounter for fitting and adjustment of complete left artificial leg

Z44.119 Encounter for fitting and adjustment of complete artificial leg, unspecified leg

Z44.12 Encounter for fitting and adjustment of partial artificial leg

Z44.121 Encounter for fitting and adjustment of partial artificial right leg

Z44.122 Encounter for fitting and adjustment of partial artificial left leg

Z44.129 Encounter for fitting and adjustment of partial artificial leg, unspecified leg

Z44.2 Encounter for fitting and adjustment of artificial eye

Excludes1 mechanical complication of ocular prosthesis (T85.3)

Z44.20 Encounter for fitting and adjustment of artificial eye, unspecified

Z44.21 Encounter for fitting and adjustment of artificial right eye

Z44.22 Encounter for fitting and adjustment of artificial left eye

Z44.3 Encounter for fitting and adjustment of external breast prosthesis

Excludes1 complications of breast implant (T85.4-)
encounter for adjustment or removal of breast implant (Z45.81-)
encounter for initial breast implant insertion for cosmetic breast augmentation (Z41.1)
encounter for breast reconstruction following mastectomy (Z42.1)

Z44.30 Encounter for fitting and adjustment of external breast prosthesis, unspecified breast

Z44.31 Encounter for fitting and adjustment of external right breast prosthesis

Z44.32 Encounter for fitting and adjustment of external left breast prosthesis

Z44.8 Encounter for fitting and adjustment of other external prosthetic devices

Z44.9 Encounter for fitting and adjustment of unspecified external prosthetic device

Z45 Encounter for adjustment and management of implanted device

Includes removal or replacement of implanted device

Excludes1 malfunction or other complications of device - see Alphabetical Index

Excludes2 encounter for fitting and adjustment of non-implanted device (Z46.-)

Z45.0 Encounter for adjustment and management of cardiac device

Z45.01 Encounter for adjustment and management of cardiac pacemaker

Encounter for adjustment and management of cardiac resynchronization therapy pacemaker (CRT-P)

Excludes1 encounter for adjustment and management of automatic implantable cardiac defibrillator with synchronous cardiac pacemaker (Z45.02)

Z45.010 Encounter for checking and testing of cardiac pacemaker pulse generator [battery]

Encounter for replacing cardiac pacemaker pulse generator [battery]

Z45.018 Encounter for adjustment and management of other part of cardiac pacemaker

Excludes1 presence of other part of cardiac pacemaker (Z95.0)

Excludes2 presence of prosthetic and other devices (Z95.1-Z95.5, Z95.811-Z97)

Z45.02 Encounter for adjustment and management of automatic implantable cardiac defibrillator

Encounter for adjustment and management of automatic implantable cardiac defibrillator with synchronous cardiac pacemaker

Encounter for adjustment and management of cardiac resynchronization therapy defibrillator (CRT-D)

Z45.09 Encounter for adjustment and management of other cardiac device

Z45.1 Encounter for adjustment and management of infusion pump

Z45.2 Encounter for adjustment and management of vascular access device

Encounter for adjustment and management of vascular catheters

Excludes1 encounter for adjustment and management of renal dialysis catheter (Z49.01)

● **Z45.3 Encounter for adjustment and management of implanted devices of the special senses**

Z45.31 **Encounter for adjustment and management of implanted visual substitution device**

● Z45.32 **Encounter for adjustment and management of implanted hearing device**

Excludes1 encounter for fitting and adjustment of hearing aide (Z46.1)

Z45.320 **Encounter for adjustment and management of bone conduction device**

Z45.321 **Encounter for adjustment and management of cochlear device**

Z45.328 **Encounter for adjustment and management of other implanted hearing device**

● **Z45.4 Encounter for adjustment and management of implanted nervous system device**

Z45.41 **Encounter for adjustment and management of cerebrospinal fluid drainage device**

Encounter for adjustment and management of cerebral ventricular (communicating) shunt

Z45.42 **Encounter for adjustment and management of neuropacemaker**

▶Encounter for adjustment and management of brain neurostimulator

▶Encounter for adjustment and management of gastric neurostimulator

▶Encounter for adjustment and management of peripheral nerve neurostimulator

▶Encounter for adjustment and management of sacral nerve neurostimulator

▶Encounter for adjustment and management of spinal cord neurostimulator

▶Encounter for adjustment and management of vagus nerve neurostimulator

Z45.49 **Encounter for adjustment and management of other implanted nervous system device**

● **Z45.8 Encounter for adjustment and management of other implanted devices**

● Z45.81 **Encounter for adjustment or removal of breast implant**

Encounter for elective implant exchange (different material) (different size)

Encounter removal of tissue expander with or without synchronous insertion of permanent implant

Excludes1 complications of breast implant (T85.4-)
encounter for initial breast implant insertion for cosmetic breast augmentation (Z41.1)
encounter for breast reconstruction following mastectomy (Z42.1)

Z45.811 **Encounter for adjustment or removal of right breast implant**

Z45.812 **Encounter for adjustment or removal of left breast implant**

Z45.819 **Encounter for adjustment or removal of unspecified breast implant**

Z45.82 **Encounter for adjustment or removal of myringotomy device (stent) (tube)**

Z45.89 **Encounter for adjustment and management of other implanted devices**

Z45.9 Encounter for adjustment and management of unspecified implanted device

● **Z46 Encounter for fitting and adjustment of other devices**

Includes removal or replacement of other device

Excludes1 malfunction or other complications of device - see Alphabetical Index

Excludes2 encounter for fitting and management of implanted devices (Z45.-)
issue of repeat prescription only (Z76.Ø)
presence of prosthetic and other devices (Z95-Z97)

Z46.Ø Encounter for fitting and adjustment of spectacles and contact lenses

Z46.1 Encounter for fitting and adjustment of hearing aid

Excludes1 encounter for adjustment and management of implanted hearing device (Z45.32-)

Z46.2 Encounter for fitting and adjustment of other devices related to nervous system and special senses

Excludes2 encounter for adjustment and management of implanted nervous system device (Z45.4-)
encounter for adjustment and management of implanted visual substitution device (Z45.31)

Z46.3 Encounter for fitting and adjustment of dental prosthetic device

Encounter for fitting and adjustment of dentures

Z46.4 Encounter for fitting and adjustment of orthodontic device

● **Z46.5 Encounter for fitting and adjustment of other gastrointestinal appliance and device**

Excludes1 encounter for attention to artificial openings of digestive tract (Z43.1-Z43.4)

Z46.51 **Encounter for fitting and adjustment of gastric lap band**

Z46.59 **Encounter for fitting and adjustment of other gastrointestinal appliance and device**

Z46.6 Encounter for fitting and adjustment of urinary device

Excludes2 attention to artificial openings of urinary tract (Z43.5, Z43.6)

● **Z46.8 Encounter for fitting and adjustment of other specified devices**

Z46.81 **Encounter for fitting and adjustment of insulin pump**

Encounter for insulin pump instruction and training

Encounter for insulin pump titration

Z46.82 **Encounter for fitting and adjustment of non-vascular catheter**

Z46.89 **Encounter for fitting and adjustment of other specified devices**

Encounter for fitting and adjustment of wheelchair

Z46.9 Encounter for fitting and adjustment of unspecified device

● **Z47 Orthopedic aftercare**

Excludes1 aftercare for healing fracture - code to fracture with 7th character D

Z47.1 Aftercare following joint replacement surgery

Use additional code to identify the joint (Z96.6-)

Z47.2 Encounter for removal of internal fixation device

Excludes1 encounter for adjustment of internal fixation device for fracture treatment - code to fracture with appropriate 7th character
encounter for removal of external fixation device - code to fracture with 7th character D
infection or inflammatory reaction to internal fixation device (T84.6-)
mechanical complication of internal fixation device (T84.1-)

CHAPTER 21 (ZØØ-Z99)

● Z47.3 **Aftercare following explantation of joint prosthesis**
Aftercare following explantation of joint prosthesis, staged procedure
Encounter for joint prosthesis insertion following prior explantation of joint prosthesis
Coding Clinic: 2015, Q1, P17

Z47.31 **Aftercare following explantation of shoulder joint prosthesis**
Excludes1 acquired absence of shoulder joint following prior explantation of shoulder joint prosthesis (Z89.23-)
shoulder joint prosthesis explantation status (Z89.23-)

Z47.32 **Aftercare following explantation of hip joint prosthesis**
Excludes1 acquired absence of hip joint following prior explantation of hip joint prosthesis (Z89.62-)
hip joint prosthesis explantation status (Z89.62-)
Coding Clinic: 2015, Q1, P17

Z47.33 **Aftercare following explantation of knee joint prosthesis**
Excludes1 acquired absence of knee joint following prior explantation of knee prosthesis (Z89.52-)
knee joint prosthesis explantation status (Z89.52-)

● Z47.8 **Encounter for other orthopedic aftercare**

Z47.81 **Encounter for orthopedic aftercare following surgical amputation**
Use additional code to identify the limb amputated (Z89.-)

Z47.82 **Encounter for orthopedic aftercare following scoliosis surgery**

Z47.89 **Encounter for other orthopedic aftercare**
Coding Clinic: 2015, Q1, P8

● Z48 **Encounter for other postprocedural aftercare**
Excludes1 encounter for aftercare following injury - code to Injury, by site, with appropriate 7th character for subsequent encounter
encounter for follow-up examination after completed treatment (Z08-Z09)
Excludes2 encounter for attention to artificial openings (Z43.-)
encounter for fitting and adjustment of prosthetic and other devices (Z44-Z46)

● Z48.0 **Encounter for attention to dressings, sutures and drains**
Excludes1 encounter for planned postprocedural wound closure (Z48.1)

Z48.00 **Encounter for change or removal of nonsurgical wound dressing**
Encounter for change or removal of wound dressing NOS

Z48.01 **Encounter for change or removal of surgical wound dressing**
Coding Clinic: 2019, Q2, P33; 2015, Q4, P38

Z48.02 **Encounter for removal of sutures**
Encounter for removal of staples
Coding Clinic: 2015, Q1, P6

Z48.03 **Encounter for change or removal of drains**

Z48.1 **Encounter for planned postprocedural wound closure**
Excludes1 encounter for attention to dressings and sutures (Z48.0-)

● Z48.2 **Encounter for aftercare following organ transplant**

Z48.21 **Encounter for aftercare following heart transplant**

Z48.22 **Encounter for aftercare following kidney transplant**

Z48.23 **Encounter for aftercare following liver transplant**

Z48.24 **Encounter for aftercare following lung transplant**

● Z48.28 **Encounter for aftercare following multiple organ transplant**

Z48.280 **Encounter for aftercare following heart-lung transplant**

Z48.288 **Encounter for aftercare following multiple organ transplant**

● Z48.29 **Encounter for aftercare following other organ transplant**

Z48.290 **Encounter for aftercare following bone marrow transplant**

Z48.298 **Encounter for aftercare following other organ transplant**

Z48.3 **Aftercare following surgery for neoplasm**
Use additional code to identify the neoplasm

● Z48.8 **Encounter for other specified postprocedural aftercare**

● Z48.81 **Encounter for surgical aftercare following surgery on specified body systems**
These codes identify the body system requiring aftercare. They are for use in conjunction with other aftercare codes to fully explain the aftercare encounter. The condition treated should also be coded if still present.
Excludes1 aftercare for injury - code the injury with 7th character D
aftercare following surgery for neoplasm (Z48.3)
Excludes2 aftercare following organ transplant (Z48.2-)
orthopedic aftercare (Z47.-)

Z48.810 **Encounter for surgical aftercare following surgery on the sense organs**

Z48.811 **Encounter for surgical aftercare following surgery on the nervous system**
Excludes2 encounter for surgical aftercare following surgery on the sense organs (Z48.810)

Z48.812 **Encounter for surgical aftercare following surgery on the circulatory system**
Coding Clinic: 2012, Q4, P96

Z48.813 **Encounter for surgical aftercare following surgery on the respiratory system**
Coding Clinic: 2019, Q2, P33

Z48.814 **Encounter for surgical aftercare following surgery on the teeth or oral cavity**

Z48.815 **Encounter for surgical aftercare following surgery on the digestive system**
Coding Clinic: 2015, Q4, P38

Z48.816 **Encounter for surgical aftercare following surgery on the genitourinary system**
Excludes1 encounter for aftercare following sterilization reversal (Z31.42)

CHAPTER 21 (Z00-Z99)

Z48.817 Encounter for surgical aftercare following surgery on the skin and subcutaneous tissue
Coding Clinic: 2015, Q1, P6

Z48.89 Encounter for other specified surgical aftercare

Z49 Encounter for care involving renal dialysis
Code also associated end stage renal disease (N18.6)

Z49.0 Preparatory care for renal dialysis
Encounter for dialysis instruction and training

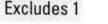

Z49.01 Encounter for fitting and adjustment of extracorporeal dialysis catheter
Removal or replacement of renal dialysis catheter
Toilet or cleansing of renal dialysis catheter

Z49.02 Encounter for fitting and adjustment of peritoneal dialysis catheter

Z49.3 Encounter for adequacy testing for dialysis

Z49.31 Encounter for adequacy testing for hemodialysis

Z49.32 Encounter for adequacy testing for peritoneal dialysis
Encounter for peritoneal equilibration test

Z51 Encounter for other aftercare and medical care
Code also condition requiring care
Excludes1 follow-up examination after treatment (Z08-Z09)
Coding Clinic: 2017, Q1, P49; 2016, Q4, P130

Z51.0 Encounter for antineoplastic radiation therapy
Coding Clinic: 2017, Q4, P103

Z51.1 Encounter for antineoplastic chemotherapy and immunotherapy
Excludes2 encounter for chemotherapy and immunotherapy for nonneoplastic condition-code to condition

Z51.11 Encounter for antineoplastic chemotherapy
Coding Clinic: 2015, Q3, P19

Z51.12 Encounter for antineoplastic immunotherapy

Z51.5 Encounter for palliative care
Coding Clinic: 2017, Q1, P48-49

Z51.6 Encounter for desensitization to allergens
Coding Clinic: 2016, Q4, P77-79

Z51.8 Encounter for other specified aftercare
Excludes1 holiday relief care (Z75.5)

Z51.81 Encounter for therapeutic drug level monitoring
Code also any long-term (current) drug therapy (Z79.-)
Excludes1 encounter for blood-drug test for administrative or medicolegal reasons (Z02.83)

Z51.89 Encounter for other specified aftercare
Coding Clinic: 2012, Q4, P96-97

Z52 Donors of organs and tissues
Includes autologous and other living donors
Excludes1 cadaveric donor - omit code
examination of potential donor (Z00.5)
Coding Clinic: 2012, Q4, P100

Z52.0 Blood donor

Z52.00 Unspecified blood donor
Z52.000 Unspecified donor, whole blood
Z52.001 Unspecified donor, stem cells
Z52.008 Unspecified donor, other blood

Z52.01 Autologous blood donor
Z52.010 Autologous donor, whole blood
Z52.011 Autologous donor, stem cells
Z52.018 Autologous donor, other blood

Z52.09 Other blood donor
Volunteer donor
Z52.090 Other blood donor, whole blood
Z52.091 Other blood donor, stem cells
Z52.098 Other blood donor, other blood

Z52.1 Skin donor
Z52.10 Skin donor, unspecified
Z52.11 Skin donor, autologous
Z52.19 Skin donor, other

Z52.2 Bone donor
Z52.20 Bone donor, unspecified
Z52.21 Bone donor, autologous
Z52.29 Bone donor, other

Z52.3 Bone marrow donor
Z52.4 Kidney donor
Z52.5 Cornea donor
Z52.6 Liver donor
Coding Clinic: 2012, Q4, P100

Z52.8 Donor of other specified organs or tissues

Z52.81 Egg (Oocyte) donor
Z52.810 Egg (Oocyte) donor under age 35, anonymous recipient ♀
Egg donor under age 35 NOS
Z52.811 Egg (Oocyte) donor under age 35, designated recipient ♀
Z52.812 Egg (Oocyte) donor age 35 and over, anonymous recipient ♀
Egg donor age 35 and over NOS
Z52.813 Egg (Oocyte) donor age 35 and over, designated recipient ♀
Z52.819 Egg (Oocyte) donor, unspecified ♀

Z52.89 Donor of other specified organs or tissues

Z52.9 Donor of unspecified organ or tissue
Donor NOS

Z53 Persons encountering health services for specific procedures and treatment, not carried out

Z53.0 Procedure and treatment not carried out because of contraindication
Z53.01 Procedure and treatment not carried out due to patient smoking
Z53.09 Procedure and treatment not carried out because of other contraindication

Z53.1 Procedure and treatment not carried out because of patient's decision for reasons of belief and group pressure

Z53.2 Procedure and treatment not carried out because of patient's decision for other and unspecified reasons
Z53.20 Procedure and treatment not carried out because of patient's decision for unspecified reasons
Z53.21 Procedure and treatment not carried out due to patient leaving prior to being seen by health care provider
Z53.29 Procedure and treatment not carried out because of patient's decision for other reasons

Z53.3 Procedure converted to open procedure
Coding Clinic: 2016, Q4, P79
Z53.31 Laparoscopic surgical procedure converted to open procedure
Coding Clinic: 2016, Q4, P100
Z53.32 Thoracoscopic surgical procedure converted to open procedure
Z53.33 Arthroscopic surgical procedure converted to open procedure
Z53.39 Other specified procedure converted to open procedure

Z53.8 Procedure and treatment not carried out for other reasons

Z53.9 Procedure and treatment not carried out, unspecified reason

CHAPTER 21 (Z00-Z99)

PERSONS WITH POTENTIAL HEALTH HAZARDS RELATED TO SOCIOECONOMIC AND PSYCHOSOCIAL CIRCUMSTANCES (Z55-Z65)

● **Z55 Problems related to education and literacy**
Excludes1 disorders of psychological development (F80-F89)
- **Z55.0 Illiteracy and low-level literacy**
- **Z55.1 Schooling unavailable and unattainable**
- **Z55.2 Failed school examinations**
- **Z55.3 Underachievement in school**
- **Z55.4 Educational maladjustment and discord with teachers and classmates**
- **Z55.8 Other problems related to education and literacy**
  Problems related to inadequate teaching
- **Z55.9 Problems related to education and literacy, unspecified**
  Academic problems NOS

● **Z56 Problems related to employment and unemployment**
Excludes2 occupational exposure to risk factors (Z57.-)
problems related to housing and economic circumstances (Z59.-)
- **Z56.0 Unemployment, unspecified**
- **Z56.1 Change of job** A
- **Z56.2 Threat of job loss**
- **Z56.3 Stressful work schedule**
- **Z56.4 Discord with boss and workmates**
- **Z56.5 Uncongenial work environment**
  Difficult conditions at work
- **Z56.6 Other physical and mental strain related to work**
- ● **Z56.8 Other problems related to employment**
  - **Z56.81 Sexual harassment on the job**
  - **Z56.82 Military deployment status**
    Individual (civilian or military) currently deployed in theater or in support of military war, peacekeeping and humanitarian operations
  - **Z56.89 Other problems related to employment**
- **Z56.9 Unspecified problems related to employment**
  Occupational problems NOS

● **Z57 Occupational exposure to risk factors**
- **Z57.0 Occupational exposure to noise**
- **Z57.1 Occupational exposure to radiation**
- **Z57.2 Occupational exposure to dust**
- ● **Z57.3 Occupational exposure to other air contaminants**
  - **Z57.31 Occupational exposure to environmental tobacco smoke**
    Excludes2 exposure to environmental tobacco smoke (Z77.22)
  - **Z57.39 Occupational exposure to other air contaminants**
- **Z57.4 Occupational exposure to toxic agents in agriculture**
  Occupational exposure to solids, liquids, gases or vapors in agriculture
- **Z57.5 Occupational exposure to toxic agents in other industries**
  Occupational exposure to solids, liquids, gases or vapors in other industries
- **Z57.6 Occupational exposure to extreme temperature**
- **Z57.7 Occupational exposure to vibration**
- **Z57.8 Occupational exposure to other risk factors**
- **Z57.9 Occupational exposure to unspecified risk factor**

● **Z59 Problems related to housing and economic circumstances**
Excludes2 problems related to upbringing (Z62.-)
- **Z59.0 Homelessness**
- **Z59.1 Inadequate housing**
  Lack of heating
  Restriction of space
  Technical defects in home preventing adequate care
  Unsatisfactory surroundings
  Excludes1 problems related to the natural and physical environment (Z77.1-)
- **Z59.2 Discord with neighbors, lodgers and landlord**
- **Z59.3 Problems related to living in residential institution**
  Boarding-school resident
  Excludes1 institutional upbringing (Z62.2)
- **Z59.4 Lack of adequate food and safe drinking water**
  Inadequate drinking water supply
  Excludes1 effects of hunger (T73.0)
  inappropriate diet or eating habits (Z72.4)
  malnutrition (E40-E46)
- **Z59.5 Extreme poverty**
- **Z59.6 Low income**
- **Z59.7 Insufficient social insurance and welfare support**
- **Z59.8 Other problems related to housing and economic circumstances**
  Foreclosure on loan
  Isolated dwelling
  Problems with creditors
- **Z59.9 Problem related to housing and economic circumstances, unspecified**

● **Z60 Problems related to social environment**
- **Z60.0 Problems of adjustment to life-cycle transitions**
  Empty nest syndrome
  Phase of life problem
  Problem with adjustment to retirement [pension]
- **Z60.2 Problems related to living alone**
- **Z60.3 Acculturation difficulty**
  Problem with migration
  Problem with social transplantation
- **Z60.4 Social exclusion and rejection**
  Exclusion and rejection on the basis of personal characteristics, such as unusual physical appearance, illness or behavior.
  Excludes1 target of adverse discrimination such as for racial or religious reasons (Z60.5)
- **Z60.5 Target of (perceived) adverse discrimination and persecution**
  Excludes1 social exclusion and rejection (Z60.4)
- **Z60.8 Other problems related to social environment**
- **Z60.9 Problem related to social environment, unspecified**

● **Z62 Problems related to upbringing**
Includes current and past negative life events in childhood
current and past problems of a child related to upbringing
Excludes2 maltreatment syndrome (T74.-)
problems related to housing and economic circumstances (Z59.-)
- **Z62.0 Inadequate parental supervision and control**
- **Z62.1 Parental overprotection**
- ● **Z62.2 Upbringing away from parents**
  Excludes1 problems with boarding school (Z59.3)
  - **Z62.21 Child in welfare custody** P
    Child in care of non-parental family member
    Child in foster care
    Excludes2 problem for parent due to child in welfare custody (Z63.5)
  - **Z62.22 Institutional upbringing**
    Child living in orphanage or group home
  - **Z62.29 Other upbringing away from parents**

Z62.3 **Hostility towards and scapegoating of child** P

Z62.6 **Inappropriate (excessive) parental pressure**

● Z62.8 **Other specified problems related to upbringing**

● Z62.81 **Personal history of abuse in childhood**

Z62.810 **Personal history of physical and sexual abuse in childhood**

Excludes1 current child physical abuse (T74.12, T76.12)
current child sexual abuse (T74.22, T76.22)

Z62.811 **Personal history of psychological abuse in childhood**

Excludes1 current child psychological abuse (T74.32, T76.32)

Z62.812 **Personal history of neglect in childhood**

Excludes1 current child neglect (T74.02, T76.02)

Z62.813 **Personal history of forced labor or sexual exploitation in childhood**

Z62.819 **Personal history of unspecified abuse in childhood**

Excludes1 current child abuse NOS (T74.92, T76.92)

● Z62.82 **Parent-child conflict**

Z62.820 **Parent-biological child conflict**
Parent-child problem NOS

Z62.821 **Parent-adopted child conflict**

Z62.822 **Parent-foster child conflict**

● Z62.89 **Other specified problems related to upbringing**

Z62.890 **Parent-child estrangement NEC**

Z62.891 **Sibling rivalry**

Z62.898 **Other specified problems related to upbringing**

Z62.9 **Problem related to upbringing, unspecified**

● Z63 **Other problems related to primary support group, including family circumstances**

Excludes2 maltreatment syndrome (T74.-, T76)
parent-child problems (Z62.-)
problems related to negative life events in childhood (Z62.-)
problems related to upbringing (Z62.-)

Z63.0 **Problems in relationship with spouse or partner**
Relationship distress with spouse or intimate partner

Excludes1 counseling for spousal or partner abuse problems (Z69.1)
counseling related to sexual attitude, behavior, and orientation (Z70.-)

Z63.1 **Problems in relationship with in-laws**

● Z63.3 **Absence of family member**

Excludes1 absence of family member due to disappearance and death (Z63.4)
absence of family member due to separation and divorce (Z63.5)

Z63.31 **Absence of family member due to military deployment**
Individual or family affected by other family member being on military deployment

Excludes1 family disruption due to return of family member from military deployment (Z63.71)

Z63.32 **Other absence of family member**

Z63.4 **Disappearance and death of family member**
Assumed death of family member
Bereavement

Z63.5 **Disruption of family by separation and divorce**
Marital estrangement

Z63.6 **Dependent relative needing care at home**

● Z63.7 **Other stressful life events affecting family and household**

Z63.71 **Stress on family due to return of family member from military deployment**
Individual or family affected by family member having returned from military deployment (current or past conflict)

Z63.72 **Alcoholism and drug addiction in family**

Z63.79 **Other stressful life events affecting family and household**
Anxiety (normal) about sick person in family
Health problems within family
Ill or disturbed family member
Isolated family

Z63.8 **Other specified problems related to primary support group**
Family discord NOS
Family estrangement NOS
High expressed emotional level within family
Inadequate family support NOS
Inadequate or distorted communication within family

Z63.9 **Problem related to primary support group, unspecified**
Relationship disorder NOS

● Z64 **Problems related to certain psychosocial circumstances**

Z64.0 **Problems related to unwanted pregnancy** ♀

Z64.1 **Problems related to multiparity** ♀

Z64.4 **Discord with counselors**
Discord with probation officer
Discord with social worker

● Z65 **Problems related to other psychosocial circumstances**

Z65.0 **Conviction in civil and criminal proceedings without imprisonment**

Z65.1 **Imprisonment and other incarceration**

Z65.2 **Problems related to release from prison**

Z65.3 **Problems related to other legal circumstances**
Arrest
Child custody or support proceedings
Litigation
Prosecution

Z65.4 **Victim of crime and terrorism**
Victim of torture

Z65.5 **Exposure to disaster, war and other hostilities**

Excludes1 target of perceived discrimination or persecution (Z60.5)

Z65.8 **Other specified problems related to psychosocial circumstances**
Religious or spiritual problem

Z65.9 **Problem related to unspecified psychosocial circumstances**

DO NOT RESUSCITATE STATUS (Z66)

Z66 **Do not resuscitate**
DNR status

BLOOD TYPE (Z67)

● Z67 **Blood type**
Coding Clinic: 2015, Q3, P40

● Z67.1 **Type A blood**

Z67.10 **Type A blood, Rh positive**

Z67.11 **Type A blood, Rh negative**

● Z67.2 **Type B blood**

Z67.20 **Type B blood, Rh positive**

Z67.21 **Type B blood, Rh negative**

Z67.3 Type AB blood
Z67.30 Type AB blood, Rh positive
Z67.31 Type AB blood, Rh negative
Z67.4 Type O blood
Z67.40 Type O blood, Rh positive
Z67.41 Type O blood, Rh negative
Z67.9 Unspecified blood type
Z67.90 Unspecified blood type, Rh positive
Z67.91 Unspecified blood type, Rh negative
Coding Clinic: 2015, Q3, P40

BODY MASS INDEX [BMI] (Z68)

OGCR Section I.B.14.

General Coding Guidelines

14. Documentation for BMI, Depth of Non-pressure ulcers, Pressure Ulcer Stages, Coma Scale, and NIH Stroke Scale

For the Body Mass Index (BMI), depth of non-pressure chronic ulcers, pressure ulcer stage, coma scale, and NIH stroke scale (NIHSS) codes, code assignment may be based on medical record documentation from clinicians who are not the patient's provider (i.e., physician or other qualified healthcare practitioner legally accountable for establishing the patient's diagnosis), since this information is typically documented by other clinicians involved in the care of the patient (e.g., a dietitian often documents the BMI, a nurse often documents the pressure ulcer stages, and an emergency medical technician often documents the coma scale). However, the associated diagnosis (such as overweight, obesity, acute stroke, or pressure ulcer) must be documented by the patient's provider. If there is conflicting medical record documentation, either from the same clinician or different clinicians, the patient's attending provider should be queried for clarification.

The BMI, coma scale, and NIHSS codes should only be reported as secondary diagnoses.

Z68 Body mass index [BMI]
Kilograms per meters squared
Note: BMI adult codes are for use for persons 20 years of age or older.
BMI pediatric codes are for use for persons 2-19 years of age.
These percentiles are based on the growth charts published by the Centers for Disease Control and Prevention (CDC)
Coding Clinic: 2018, Q4, P81; 2016, Q4, P129

Z68.1 Body mass index (BMI) 19.9 or less, adult A
Coding Clinic: 2017, Q1, P39
Z68.2 Body mass index (BMI) 20-29, adult
Z68.20 Body mass index (BMI) 20.0-20.9, adult A
Z68.21 Body mass index (BMI) 21.0-21.9, adult A
Z68.22 Body mass index (BMI) 22.0-22.9, adult A
Z68.23 Body mass index (BMI) 23.0-23.9, adult A
Z68.24 Body mass index (BMI) 24.0-24.9, adult A
Z68.25 Body mass index (BMI) 25.0-25.9, adult A
Z68.26 Body mass index (BMI) 26.0-26.9, adult A
Z68.27 Body mass index (BMI) 27.0-27.9, adult A
Z68.28 Body mass index (BMI) 28.0-28.9, adult A
Z68.29 Body mass index (BMI) 29.0-29.9, adult A
Z68.3 Body mass index (BMI) 30-39, adult
Z68.30 Body mass index (BMI) 30.0-30.9, adult A
Z68.31 Body mass index (BMI) 31.0-31.9, adult A
Z68.32 Body mass index (BMI) 32.0-32.9, adult A
Z68.33 Body mass index (BMI) 33.0-33.9, adult A
Z68.34 Body mass index (BMI) 34.0-34.9, adult A
Z68.35 Body mass index (BMI) 35.0-35.9, adult A
Z68.36 Body mass index (BMI) 36.0-36.9, adult A
Z68.37 Body mass index (BMI) 37.0-37.9, adult A
Z68.38 Body mass index (BMI) 38.0-38.9, adult A
Z68.39 Body mass index (BMI) 39.0-39.9, adult A
Z68.4 Body mass index (BMI) 40 or greater, adult
Z68.41 Body mass index (BMI) 40.0-44.9, adult A
Z68.42 Body mass index (BMI) 45.0-49.9, adult A
Z68.43 Body mass index (BMI) 50.0-59.9, adult A
Z68.44 Body mass index (BMI) 60.0-69.9, adult A
Z68.45 Body mass index (BMI) 70 or greater, adult A
Z68.5 Body mass index (BMI) pediatric
Coding Clinic: 2018, Q4, P81
Z68.51 Body mass index (BMI) pediatric, less than 5th percentile for age
Coding Clinic: 2018, Q4, P82
Z68.52 Body mass index (BMI) pediatric, 5th percentile to less than 85th percentile for age
Z68.53 Body mass index (BMI) pediatric, 85th percentile to less than 95th percentile for age
Z68.54 Body mass index (BMI) pediatric, greater than or equal to 95th percentile for age

PERSONS ENCOUNTERING HEALTH SERVICES IN OTHER CIRCUMSTANCES (Z69-Z76)

Z69 Encounter for mental health services for victim and perpetrator of abuse
Includes counseling for victims and perpetrators of abuse
Z69.0 Encounter for mental health services for child abuse problems
Z69.01 Encounter for mental health services for parental child abuse
Z69.010 Encounter for mental health services for victim of parental child abuse P
Encounter for mental health services for victim of child abuse by parent
Encounter for mental health services for victim of child neglect by parent
Encounter for mental health services for victim of child psychological abuse by parent
Encounter for mental health services for victim of child sexual abuse by parent
Z69.011 Encounter for mental health services for perpetrator of parental child abuse
Encounter for mental health services for perpetrator of parental child neglect
Encounter for mental health services for perpetrator of parental child psychological abuse
Encounter for mental health services for perpetrator of parental child sexual abuse
Excludes1 encounter for mental health services for non-parental child abuse (Z69.02-)
Z69.02 Encounter for mental health services for non-parental child abuse
Z69.020 Encounter for mental health services for victim of non-parental child abuse P
Encounter for mental health services for victim of non-parental child neglect
Encounter for mental health services for victim of non-parental child psychological abuse
Encounter for mental health services for victim of non-parental child sexual abuse

CHAPTER 21 (Z00-Z99)

Z69.021 Encounter for mental health services for perpetrator of non- parental child abuse
Encounter for mental health services for perpetrator of non-parental child neglect
Encounter for mental health services for perpetrator of non-parental child psychological abuse
Encounter for mental health services for perpetrator of non-parental child sexual abuse

● **Z69.1 Encounter for mental health services for spousal or partner abuse problems**

Z69.11 Encounter for mental health services for victim of spousal or partner abuse
Encounter for mental health services for victim of spouse or partner neglect
Encounter for mental health services for victim of spouse or partner psychological abuse
Encounter for mental health services for victim of spouse or partner violence, physical

Z69.12 Encounter for mental health services for perpetrator of spousal or partner abuse
Encounter for mental health services for perpetrator of spouse or partner neglect
Encounter for mental health services for perpetrator of spouse or partner psychological abuse
Encounter for mental health services for perpetrator of spouse or partner violence, physical
Encounter for mental health services for perpetrator of spouse or partner violence, sexual

● **Z69.8 Encounter for mental health services for victim or perpetrator of other abuse**

Z69.81 Encounter for mental health services for victim of other abuse
~~Encounter for mental health services for perpetrator of non-spousal adult abuse~~
Encounter for mental health services for victim of non-spousal adult abuse
Encounter for mental health services for victim of spouse or partner violence, sexual
Encounter for rape victim counseling

Z69.82 Encounter for mental health services for perpetrator of other abuse
▶Encounter for mental health services for perpetrator of non-spousal adult abuse

● **Z70 Counseling related to sexual attitude, behavior and orientation**
Includes encounter for mental health services for sexual attitude, behavior and orientation
Excludes2 contraceptive or procreative counseling (Z30-Z31)

Z70.0 Counseling related to sexual attitude

Z70.1 Counseling related to patient's sexual behavior and orientation
Patient concerned regarding impotence
Patient concerned regarding non-responsiveness
Patient concerned regarding promiscuity
Patient concerned regarding sexual orientation

Z70.2 Counseling related to sexual behavior and orientation of third party
Advice sought regarding sexual behavior and orientation of child
Advice sought regarding sexual behavior and orientation of partner
Advice sought regarding sexual behavior and orientation of spouse

Z70.3 Counseling related to combined concerns regarding sexual attitude, behavior and orientation

Z70.8 Other sex counseling
Encounter for sex education

Z70.9 Sex counseling, unspecified

● **Z71 Persons encountering health services for other counseling and medical advice, not elsewhere classified**
Excludes2 contraceptive or procreation counseling (Z30-Z31)
sex counseling (Z70.-)

Z71.0 Person encountering health services to consult on behalf of another person
Person encountering health services to seek advice or treatment for non-attending third party
Excludes2 anxiety (normal) about sick person in family (Z63.7)
expectant (adoptive) parent(s) pre-birth pediatrician visit (Z76.81)

Z71.1 Person with feared health complaint in whom no diagnosis is made
Person encountering health services with feared condition which was not demonstrated
Person encountering health services in which problem was normal state
"Worried well"
Excludes1 medical observation for suspected diseases and conditions proven not to exist (Z03.-)
Coding Clinic: 2016, Q4, P7

Z71.2 Person consulting for explanation of examination or test findings

Z71.3 Dietary counseling and surveillance
Use additional code for any associated underlying medical condition
Use additional code to identify body mass index (BMI), if known (Z68.-)

● **Z71.4 Alcohol abuse counseling and surveillance**
Use additional code for alcohol abuse or dependence (F10.-)

Z71.41 Alcohol abuse counseling and surveillance of alcoholic

Z71.42 Counseling for family member of alcoholic
Counseling for significant other, partner, or friend of alcoholic

● **Z71.5 Drug abuse counseling and surveillance**
Use additional code for drug abuse or dependence (F11-F16, F18-F19)

Z71.51 Drug abuse counseling and surveillance of drug abuser

Z71.52 Counseling for family member of drug abuser
Counseling for significant other, partner, or friend of drug abuser

Z71.6 Tobacco abuse counseling
Use additional code for nicotine dependence (F17.-)

Z71.7 Human immunodeficiency virus [HIV] counseling

● **Z71.8 Other specified counseling**
Excludes2 counseling for contraception (Z30.0-)

Z71.81 Spiritual or religious counseling

Z71.82 Exercise counseling

Z71.83 Encounter for nonprocreative genetic counseling
Excludes1 counseling for procreative genetics (Z31.5)
counseling for procreative management (Z31.6)

CHAPTER 21 (Z00-Z99)

Z71.84 **Encounter for health counseling related to travel**
Encounter for health risk and safety counseling for (international) travel
Code also, if applicable, encounter for immunization (Z23)
Excludes2 encounter for administrative examination (Z02.-)
encounter for other special examination without complaint, suspected or reported diagnosis (Z01.-)

Z71.89 **Other specified counseling**

Z71.9 **Counseling, unspecified**
Encounter for medical advice NOS

Z72 **Problems related to lifestyle**
Excludes2 problems related to life-management difficulty (Z73.-)
problems related to socioeconomic and psychosocial circumstances (Z55-Z65)
Coding Clinic: 2016, Q4, P130

Z72.0 **Tobacco use**
Tobacco use NOS
Excludes1 history of tobacco dependence (Z87.891)
nicotine dependence (F17.2-)
tobacco dependence (F17.2-)
tobacco use during pregnancy (O99.33-)

Z72.3 **Lack of physical exercise**

Z72.4 **Inappropriate diet and eating habits**
Excludes1 behavioral eating disorders of infancy or childhood (F98.2.-F98.3)
eating disorders (F50.-)
lack of adequate food (Z59.4)
malnutrition and other nutritional deficiencies (E40-E64)

Z72.5 **High risk sexual behavior**
Promiscuity
Excludes1 paraphilias (F65)

Z72.51 **High risk heterosexual behavior**

Z72.52 **High risk homosexual behavior**

Z72.53 **High risk bisexual behavior**

Z72.6 **Gambling and betting**
Excludes1 compulsive or pathological gambling (F63.0)

Z72.8 **Other problems related to lifestyle**

Z72.81 **Antisocial behavior**
Excludes1 conduct disorders (F91.-)

Z72.810 **Child and adolescent antisocial behavior** P
Antisocial behavior (child) (adolescent) without manifest psychiatric disorder
Delinquency NOS
Group delinquency
Offenses in the context of gang membership
Stealing in company with others
Truancy from school

Z72.811 **Adult antisocial behavior** A
Adult antisocial behavior without manifest psychiatric disorder

Z72.82 **Problems related to sleep**

Z72.820 **Sleep deprivation**
Lack of adequate sleep
Excludes1 insomnia (G47.0-)

Z72.821 **Inadequate sleep hygiene**
Bad sleep habits
Irregular sleep habits
Unhealthy sleep wake schedule
Excludes1 insomnia (F51.0-, G47.0-)

Z72.89 **Other problems related to lifestyle**
Self-damaging behavior

Z72.9 **Problem related to lifestyle, unspecified**

Z73 **Problems related to life management difficulty**
Excludes2 problems related to socioeconomic and psychosocial circumstances (Z55-Z65)

Z73.0 **Burn-out**

Z73.1 **Type A behavior pattern**

Z73.2 **Lack of relaxation and leisure**

Z73.3 **Stress, not elsewhere classified**
Physical and mental strain NOS
Excludes1 stress related to employment or unemployment (Z56.-)

Z73.4 **Inadequate social skills, not elsewhere classified**

Z73.5 **Social role conflict, not elsewhere classified**

Z73.6 **Limitation of activities due to disability**
Excludes1 care-provider dependency (Z74.-)

Z73.8 **Other problems related to life management difficulty**

Z73.81 **Behavioral insomnia of childhood**

Z73.810 **Behavioral insomnia of childhood, sleep-onset association type** P

Z73.811 **Behavioral insomnia of childhood, limit setting type** P

Z73.812 **Behavioral insomnia of childhood, combined type** P

Z73.819 **Behavioral insomnia of childhood, unspecified type** P

Z73.82 **Dual sensory impairment**

Z73.89 **Other problems related to life management difficulty**

Z73.9 **Problem related to life management difficulty, unspecified**

Z74 **Problems related to care provider dependency**
Excludes2 dependence on enabling machines or devices NEC (Z99.-)

Z74.0 **Reduced mobility**

Z74.01 **Bed confinement status**
Bedridden

Z74.09 **Other reduced mobility**
Chairridden
Reduced mobility NOS
Excludes2 wheelchair dependence (Z99.3)

Z74.1 **Need for assistance with personal care**

Z74.2 **Need for assistance at home and no other household member able to render care**

Z74.3 **Need for continuous supervision**

Z74.8 **Other problems related to care provider dependency**

Z74.9 **Problem related to care provider dependency, unspecified**

● Z75 **Problems related to medical facilities and other health care**

Z75.0 **Medical services not available in home**

Excludes1 no other household member able to render care (Z74.2)

Z75.1 **Person awaiting admission to adequate facility elsewhere**

Z75.2 **Other waiting period for investigation and treatment**

Z75.3 **Unavailability and inaccessibility of health care facilities**

Excludes1 bed unavailable (Z75.1)

Z75.4 **Unavailability and inaccessibility of other helping agencies**

Z75.5 **Holiday relief care**

Z75.8 **Other problems related to medical facilities and other health care**

Z75.9 **Unspecified problem related to medical facilities and other health care**

● Z76 **Persons encountering health services in other circumstances**

Z76.0 **Encounter for issue of repeat prescription**

Encounter for issue of repeat prescription for appliance
Encounter for issue of repeat prescription for medicaments
Encounter for issue of repeat prescription for spectacles

Excludes2 issue of medical certificate (Z02.7)
repeat prescription for contraceptive (Z30.4-)

Z76.1 **Encounter for health supervision and care of foundling**

Z76.2 **Encounter for health supervision and care of other healthy infant and child** P

Encounter for medical or nursing care or supervision of healthy infant under circumstances such as adverse socioeconomic conditions at home
Encounter for medical or nursing care or supervision of healthy infant under circumstances such as awaiting foster or adoptive placement
Encounter for medical or nursing care or supervision of healthy infant under circumstances such as maternal illness
Encounter for medical or nursing care or supervision of healthy infant under circumstances such as number of children at home preventing or interfering with normal care

Z76.3 **Healthy person accompanying sick person**

Z76.4 **Other boarder to healthcare facility**

Excludes1 homelessness (Z59.0)

Z76.5 **Malingerer [conscious simulation]**

Person feigning illness (with obvious motivation)

Excludes1 factitious disorder (F68.1-, F68.A)
peregrinating patient (F68.1-)

● Z76.8 **Persons encountering health services in other specified circumstances**

Z76.81 **Expectant parent(s) prebirth pediatrician visit**

Pre-adoption pediatrician visit for adoptive parent(s)

Z76.82 **Awaiting organ transplant status**

Patient waiting for organ availability

Z76.89 **Persons encountering health services in other specified circumstances**

Persons encountering health services NOS

PERSONS WITH POTENTIAL HEALTH HAZARDS RELATED TO FAMILY AND PERSONAL HISTORY AND CERTAIN CONDITIONS INFLUENCING HEALTH STATUS (Z77-Z99)

Code also any follow-up examination (Z08-Z09)

● Z77 **Other contact with and (suspected) exposures hazardous to health**

Includes contact with and (suspected) exposures to potential hazards to health

Excludes2 contact with and (suspected) exposure to communicable diseases (Z20.-)
exposure to (parental) (environmental) tobacco smoke in the perinatal period (P96.81)
newborn affected by noxious substances transmitted via placenta or breast milk (P04.-)
occupational exposure to risk factors (Z57.-)
retained foreign body (Z18.-)
retained foreign body fully removed (Z87.821)
toxic effects of substances chiefly nonmedicinal as to source (T51-T65)

● Z77.0 **Contact with and (suspected) exposure to hazardous, chiefly nonmedicinal, chemicals**

● Z77.01 **Contact with and (suspected) exposure to hazardous metals**

Z77.010 **Contact with and (suspected) exposure to arsenic**

Z77.011 **Contact with and (suspected) exposure to lead**

Z77.012 **Contact with and (suspected) exposure to uranium**

Excludes1 retained depleted uranium fragments (Z18.01)

Z77.018 **Contact with and (suspected) exposure to other hazardous metals**

Contact with and (suspected) exposure to chromium compounds
Contact with and (suspected) exposure to nickel dust

● Z77.02 **Contact with and (suspected) exposure to hazardous aromatic compounds**

Z77.020 **Contact with and (suspected) exposure to aromatic amines**

Z77.021 **Contact with and (suspected) exposure to benzene**

Z77.028 **Contact with and (suspected) exposure to other hazardous aromatic compounds**

Aromatic dyes NOS
Polycyclic aromatic hydrocarbons

● Z77.09 **Contact with and (suspected) exposure to other hazardous, chiefly nonmedicinal, chemicals**

Z77.090 **Contact with and (suspected) exposure to asbestos**

Z77.098 **Contact with and (suspected) exposure to other hazardous, chiefly nonmedicinal, chemicals**

Dyes NOS

● Z77.1 **Contact with and (suspected) exposure to environmental pollution and hazards in the physical environment**

● Z77.11 **Contact with and (suspected) exposure to environmental pollution**

Z77.110 **Contact with and (suspected) exposure to air pollution**

Z77.111 **Contact with and (suspected) exposure to water pollution**

Z77.112 **Contact with and (suspected) exposure to soil pollution**

Z77.118 **Contact with and (suspected) exposure to other environmental pollution**

● **Z77.12 Contact with and (suspected) exposure to hazards in the physical environment**

Z77.120 Contact with and (suspected) exposure to mold (toxic)

Z77.121 Contact with and (suspected) exposure to harmful algae and algae toxins
Contact with and (suspected) exposure to (harmful) algae bloom NOS
Contact with and (suspected) exposure to blue-green algae bloom
Contact with and (suspected) exposure to brown tide
Contact with and (suspected) exposure to cyanobacteria bloom
Contact with and (suspected) exposure to Florida red tide
Contact with and (suspected) exposure to pfiesteria piscicida
Contact with and (suspected) exposure to red tide

Z77.122 Contact with and (suspected) exposure to noise

Z77.123 Contact with and (suspected) exposure to radon and other naturally occurring radiation
Excludes2 radiation exposure as the cause of a confirmed condition (W88-W90, X39.0-)
radiation sickness NOS (T66)

Z77.128 Contact with and (suspected) exposure to other hazards in the physical environment

● **Z77.2 Contact with and (suspected) exposure to other hazardous substances**

Z77.21 Contact with and (suspected) exposure to potentially hazardous body fluids

Z77.22 Contact with and (suspected) exposure to environmental tobacco smoke (acute) (chronic)
Exposure to second hand tobacco smoke (acute) (chronic)
Passive smoking (acute) (chronic)
Excludes1 nicotine dependence (F17.-)
tobacco use (Z72.0)
Excludes2 occupational exposure to environmental tobacco smoke (Z57.31)

Z77.29 Contact with and (suspected) exposure to other hazardous substances
Coding Clinic: 2016, Q2, P34

Z77.9 Other contact with and (suspected) exposures hazardous to health

● **Z78 Other specified health status**
Excludes2 asymptomatic human immunodeficiency virus [HIV] infection status (Z21)
postprocedural status (Z93-Z99)
sex reassignment status (Z87.890)

Z78.0 Asymptomatic menopausal state ♀ A
Menopausal state NOS
Postmenopausal status NOS
Excludes2 symptomatic menopausal state (N95.1)

Z78.1 Physical restraint status
Excludes1 physical restraint due to a procedure - omit code

Z78.9 Other specified health status

● **Z79 Long term (current) drug therapy**
Includes long term (current) drug use for prophylactic purposes
Code also any therapeutic drug level monitoring (Z51.81)
Excludes2 drug abuse and dependence (F11-F19)
drug use complicating pregnancy, childbirth, and the puerperium (O99.32-)
long term (current) use of oral antidiabetic drugs (Z79.84)
long term (current) use of oral hypoglycemic drugs (Z79.84)

● **Z79.0 Long term (current) use of anticoagulants and antithrombotics/antiplatelets**
Excludes2 long term (current) use of aspirin (Z79.82)

Z79.01 Long term (current) use of anticoagulants

Z79.02 Long term (current) use of antithrombotics/antiplatelets

Z79.1 Long term (current) use of non-steroidal anti-inflammatories (NSAID)
Excludes2 long term (current) use of aspirin (Z79.82)

Z79.2 Long term (current) use of antibiotics

Z79.3 Long term (current) use of hormonal contraceptives
Long term (current) use of birth control pill or patch

Z79.4 Long term (current) use of insulin
Coding Clinic: 2016, Q4, P121-122, 126

● **Z79.5 Long term (current) use of steroids**

Z79.51 Long term (current) use of inhaled steroids

Z79.52 Long term (current) use of systemic steroids

● **Z79.8 Other long term (current) drug therapy**

● **Z79.81 Long term (current) use of agents affecting estrogen receptors and estrogen levels**
Code first, if applicable:
malignant neoplasm of breast (C50.-)
malignant neoplasm of prostate (C61)
Use additional code, if applicable, to identify:
estrogen receptor positive status (Z17.0)
family history of breast cancer (Z80.3)
genetic susceptibility to malignant neoplasm (cancer) (Z15.0-)
personal history of breast cancer (Z85.3)
personal history of prostate cancer (Z85.46)
postmenopausal status (Z78.0)
Excludes1 hormone replacement therapy (Z79.890)

Z79.810 Long term (current) use of selective estrogen receptor modulators (SERMs)
Long term (current) use of raloxifene (Evista)
Long term (current) use of tamoxifen (Nolvadex)
Long term (current) use of toremifene (Fareston)

Z79.811 Long term (current) use of aromatase inhibitors
Long term (current) use of anastrozole (Arimidex)
Long term (current) use of exemestane (Aromasin)
Long term (current) use of letrozole (Femara)

Z79.818 Long term (current) use of other agents affecting estrogen receptors and estrogen levels
Long term (current) use of estrogen receptor downregulators
Long term (current) use of fulvestrant (Faslodex)
Long term (current) use of gonadotropin-releasing hormone (GnRH) agonist
Long term (current) use of goserelin acetate (Zoladex)
Long term (current) use of leuprolide acetate (leuprorelin) (Lupron)
Long term (current) use of megestrol acetate (Megace)

CHAPTER 21 (Z00-Z99)

Z79.82 Long term (current) use of **aspirin**

Z79.83 Long term (current) use of **bisphosphonates**
Coding Clinic: 2016, Q4, P42

Z79.84 Long term (current) use of **oral hypoglycemic drugs**
Long term (current) use of oral antidiabetic drugs
Excludes2 long term (current) use of insulin (Z79.4)
Coding Clinic: 2016, Q4, P76, 121-122, 126

● Z79.89 Other long term (current) drug therapy

Z79.890 **Hormone replacement therapy**

Z79.891 Long term (current) use of **opiate analgesic**
Long term (current) use of methadone for pain management
Excludes1 methodone use NOS (F11.9-)
use of methodone for treatment of heroin addiction (F11.2-)

Z79.899 **Other** long term (current) drug therapy
Coding Clinic: 2015, Q4, P34, Q3, P21

● **Z80** Family history of primary malignant neoplasm

Z80.0 Family history of malignant neoplasm of **digestive organs**
Conditions classifiable to C15-C26
Coding Clinic: 2018, Q1, P7

Z80.1 Family history of malignant neoplasm of **trachea, bronchus and lung**
Conditions classifiable to C33-C34

Z80.2 Family history of malignant neoplasm of **other respiratory and intrathoracic organs**
Conditions classifiable to C30-C32, C37-C39

Z80.3 Family history of malignant neoplasm of **breast**
Conditions classifiable to C50.-

● Z80.4 Family history of malignant neoplasm of **genital organs**
Conditions classifiable to C51-C63

Z80.41 Family history of malignant neoplasm of **ovary**

Z80.42 Family history of malignant neoplasm of **prostate**

Z80.43 Family history of malignant neoplasm of **testis**

Z80.49 Family history of malignant neoplasm of **other** genital organs

● Z80.5 Family history of malignant neoplasm of **urinary tract**
Conditions classifiable to C64-C68

Z80.51 Family history of malignant neoplasm of **kidney**

Z80.52 Family history of malignant neoplasm of **bladder**

Z80.59 Family history of malignant neoplasm of **other** urinary tract organ

Z80.6 Family history of **leukemia**
Conditions classifiable to C91-C95

Z80.7 Family history of **other** malignant neoplasms of **lymphoid, hematopoietic and related tissues**
Conditions classifiable to C81-C90, C96.-

Z80.8 Family history of malignant neoplasm of **other organs or systems**
Conditions classifiable to C00-C14, C40-C49, C69-C79

Z80.9 Family history of malignant neoplasm, **unspecified**
Conditions classifiable to C80.1

● **Z81** Family history of mental and behavioral disorders

Z81.0 Family history of **intellectual disabilities**
Conditions classifiable to F70-F79

Z81.1 Family history of **alcohol abuse** and dependence
Conditions classifiable to F10.-

Z81.2 Family history of **tobacco abuse** and dependence
Conditions classifiable to F17.-

Z81.3 Family history of other **psychoactive substance abuse** and dependence
Conditions classifiable to F11-F16, F18-F19

Z81.4 Family history of **other substance abuse** and dependence
Conditions classifiable to F55

Z81.8 Family history of **other mental and behavioral disorders**
Conditions classifiable elsewhere in F01-F99

● **Z82** Family history of certain disabilities and chronic diseases (leading to disablement)

Z82.0 Family history of **epilepsy** and other **diseases of the nervous system**
Conditions classifiable to G00-G99

Z82.1 Family history of **blindness** and visual loss
Conditions classifiable to H54.-

Z82.2 Family history of **deafness** and hearing loss
Conditions classifiable to H90-H91

Z82.3 Family history of **stroke**
Conditions classifiable to I60-I64

● Z82.4 Family history of ischemic heart disease and other diseases of the circulatory system
Conditions classifiable to I00-I52, I65-I99

Z82.41 Family history of **sudden cardiac death**

Z82.49 Family history of **ischemic heart disease** and other diseases of the circulatory system

Z82.5 Family history of **asthma** and other chronic lower respiratory diseases
Conditions classifiable to J40-J47
Excludes2 family history of other diseases of the respiratory system (Z83.6)

● Z82.6 Family history of arthritis and other diseases of the musculoskeletal system and connective tissue
Conditions classifiable to M00-M99

Z82.61 Family history of **arthritis**

Z82.62 Family history of **osteoporosis**

Z82.69 Family history of **other** diseases of the musculoskeletal system and connective tissue

● Z82.7 Family history of congenital malformations, deformations and chromosomal abnormalities
Conditions classifiable to Q00-Q99

Z82.71 Family history of **polycystic kidney**

Z82.79 Family history of **other** congenital malformations, deformations and chromosomal abnormalities

Z82.8 Family history of **other disabilities and chronic diseases leading to disablement**, not elsewhere classified

● **Z83** Family history of other specific disorders
Excludes2 contact with and (suspected) exposure to communicable disease in the family (Z20.-)

Z83.0 Family history of **human immunodeficiency virus** [HIV] disease
Conditions classifiable to B20

Z83.1 Family history of **other infectious and parasitic diseases**
Conditions classifiable to A00-B19, B25-B94, B99

Z83.2 Family history of **diseases of the blood and blood-forming organs** and certain disorders involving the immune mechanism
Conditions classifiable to D50-D89

Z83.3 Family history of **diabetes mellitus**
Conditions classifiable to E08-E13

● **Z83.4 Family history of other endocrine, nutritional and metabolic diseases**
Conditions classifiable to E00-E07, E15-E88

Z83.41 Family history of multiple endocrine neoplasia [MEN] syndrome

Z83.42 Family history of familial hypercholesterolemia
Coding Clinic: 2016, Q4, P77

● **Z83.43 Family history of other disorder of lipoprotein metabolism and other lipidemias**

Z83.430 Family history of elevated lipoprotein(a)
Family history of elevated Lp(a)

Z83.438 Family history of other disorder of lipoprotein metabolism and other lipidemia
Family history of familial combined hyperlipidemia

Z83.49 Family history of other endocrine, nutritional and metabolic diseases

● **Z83.5 Family history of eye and ear disorders**

● **Z83.51 Family history of eye disorders**
Conditions classifiable to H00-H53, H55-H59
Excludes2 family history of blindness and visual loss (Z82.1)

Z83.511 Family history of glaucoma

Z83.518 Family history of other specified eye disorder

Z83.52 Family history of ear disorders
Conditions classifiable to H60-H83, H92-H95
Excludes2 family history of deafness and hearing loss (Z82.2)

Z83.6 Family history of other diseases of the respiratory system
Conditions classifiable to J00-J39, J60-J99
Excludes2 family history of asthma and other chronic lower respiratory diseases (Z82.5)

● **Z83.7 Family history of diseases of the digestive system**
Conditions classifiable to K00-K93

Z83.71 Family history of colonic polyps
Excludes2 family history of malignant neoplasm of digestive organs (Z80.0)

Z83.79 Family history of other diseases of the digestive system

● **Z84 Family history of other conditions**

Z84.0 Family history of diseases of the skin and subcutaneous tissue
Conditions classifiable to L00-L99

Z84.1 Family history of disorders of kidney and ureter
Conditions classifiable to N00-N29

Z84.2 Family history of other diseases of the genitourinary system
Conditions classifiable to N30-N99
Coding Clinic: 2016, Q4, P77

Z84.3 Family history of consanguinity

● **Z84.8 Family history of other specified conditions**

Z84.81 Family history of carrier of genetic disease

Z84.82 Family history of sudden infant death syndrome
Family history of SIDS

Z84.89 Family history of other specified conditions

● **Z85 Personal history of malignant neoplasm**
Code first any follow-up examination after treatment of malignant neoplasm (Z08)
Use additional code to identify:
alcohol use and dependence (F10.-)
exposure to environmental tobacco smoke (Z77.22)
history of tobacco dependence (Z87.891)
occupational exposure to environmental tobacco smoke (Z57.31)
tobacco dependence (F17.-)
tobacco use (Z72.0)
Excludes2 personal history of benign neoplasm (Z86.01-)
personal history of carcinoma-in-situ (Z86.00-)

● **Z85.0 Personal history of malignant neoplasm of digestive organs**

Z85.00 Personal history of malignant neoplasm of unspecified digestive organ

Z85.01 Personal history of malignant neoplasm of esophagus
Conditions classifiable to C15

● **Z85.02 Personal history of malignant neoplasm of stomach**

Z85.020 Personal history of malignant carcinoid tumor of stomach
Conditions classifiable to C7A.092

Z85.028 Personal history of other malignant neoplasm of stomach
Conditions classifiable to C16

● **Z85.03 Personal history of malignant neoplasm of large intestine**

Z85.030 Personal history of malignant carcinoid tumor of large intestine
Conditions classifiable to C7A.022-C7A.025, C7A.029

Z85.038 Personal history of other malignant neoplasm of large intestine
Conditions classifiable to C18

● **Z85.04 Personal history of malignant neoplasm of rectum, rectosigmoid junction, and anus**

Z85.040 Personal history of malignant carcinoid tumor of rectum
Conditions classifiable to C7A.026

Z85.048 Personal history of other malignant neoplasm of rectum, rectosigmoid junction, and anus
Conditions classifiable to C19-C21

Z85.05 Personal history of malignant neoplasm of liver
Conditions classifiable to C22

● **Z85.06 Personal history of malignant neoplasm of small intestine**

Z85.060 Personal history of malignant carcinoid tumor of small intestine
Conditions classifiable to C7A.01-

Z85.068 Personal history of other malignant neoplasm of small intestine
Conditions classifiable to C17

Z85.07 Personal history of malignant neoplasm of pancreas
Conditions classifiable to C25

Z85.09 Personal history of malignant neoplasm of other digestive organs

Z85.1 Personal history of malignant neoplasm of trachea, bronchus and lung
Z85.11 Personal history of malignant neoplasm of bronchus and lung
Z85.110 Personal history of malignant carcinoid tumor of bronchus and lung
Conditions classifiable to C7A.090
Z85.118 Personal history of other malignant neoplasm of bronchus and lung
Conditions classifiable to C34
Z85.12 Personal history of malignant neoplasm of trachea
Conditions classifiable to C33
Z85.2 Personal history of malignant neoplasm of other respiratory and intrathoracic organs
Z85.20 Personal history of malignant neoplasm of unspecified respiratory organ
Z85.21 Personal history of malignant neoplasm of larynx
Conditions classifiable to C32
Z85.22 Personal history of malignant neoplasm of nasal cavities, middle ear, and accessory sinuses
Conditions classifiable to C30-C31
Z85.23 Personal history of malignant neoplasm of thymus
Z85.230 Personal history of malignant carcinoid tumor of thymus
Conditions classifiable to C7A.091
Z85.238 Personal history of other malignant neoplasm of thymus
Conditions classifiable to C37
Z85.29 Personal history of malignant neoplasm of other respiratory and intrathoracic organs
Z85.3 Personal history of malignant neoplasm of breast
Conditions classifiable to C50.-
Z85.4 Personal history of malignant neoplasm of genital organs
Conditions classifiable to C51-C63
Z85.40 Personal history of malignant neoplasm of unspecified female genital organ ♀
Z85.41 Personal history of malignant neoplasm of cervix uteri ♀
Z85.42 Personal history of malignant neoplasm of other parts of uterus ♀
Z85.43 Personal history of malignant neoplasm of ovary ♀
Z85.44 Personal history of malignant neoplasm of other female genital organs ♀
Z85.45 Personal history of malignant neoplasm of unspecified male genital organ ♂
Z85.46 Personal history of malignant neoplasm of prostate ♂
Z85.47 Personal history of malignant neoplasm of testis ♂
Z85.48 Personal history of malignant neoplasm of epididymis ♂
Z85.49 Personal history of malignant neoplasm of other male genital organs ♂
Z85.5 Personal history of malignant neoplasm of urinary tract
Conditions classifiable to C64-C68
Z85.50 Personal history of malignant neoplasm of unspecified urinary tract organ
Z85.51 Personal history of malignant neoplasm of bladder
Z85.52 Personal history of malignant neoplasm of kidney
Excludes1 personal history of malignant neoplasm of renal pelvis (Z85.53)
Z85.520 Personal history of malignant carcinoid tumor of kidney
Conditions classifiable to C7A.093
Z85.528 Personal history of other malignant neoplasm of kidney
Conditions classifiable to C64
Z85.53 Personal history of malignant neoplasm of renal pelvis
Z85.54 Personal history of malignant neoplasm of ureter
Z85.59 Personal history of malignant neoplasm of other urinary tract organ
Z85.6 Personal history of leukemia
Conditions classifiable to C91-C95
Excludes1 leukemia in remission C91.0-C95.9 with 5th character 1
Z85.7 Personal history of other malignant neoplasms of lymphoid, hematopoietic and related tissues
Z85.71 Personal history of Hodgkin lymphoma
Conditions classifiable to C81
Z85.72 Personal history of non-Hodgkin lymphomas
Conditions classifiable to C82-C85
Z85.79 Personal history of other malignant neoplasms of lymphoid, hematopoietic and related tissues
Conditions classifiable to C88-C90, C96
Excludes1 multiple myeloma in remission (C90.01)
plasma cell leukemia in remission (C90.11)
plasmacytoma in remission (C90.21)
Z85.8 Personal history of malignant neoplasms of other organs and systems
Conditions classifiable to C00-C14, C40-C49, C69-C75, C7A.098, C76-C79
Z85.81 Personal history of malignant neoplasm of lip, oral cavity, and pharynx
Z85.810 Personal history of malignant neoplasm of tongue
Z85.818 Personal history of malignant neoplasm of other sites of lip, oral cavity, and pharynx
Z85.819 Personal history of malignant neoplasm of unspecified site of lip, oral cavity, and pharynx
Z85.82 Personal history of malignant neoplasm of skin
Z85.820 Personal history of malignant melanoma of skin
Conditions classifiable to C43
Z85.821 Personal history of Merkel cell carcinoma
Conditions classifiable to C4A
Z85.828 Personal history of other malignant neoplasm of skin
Conditions classifiable to C44
Z85.83 Personal history of malignant neoplasm of bone and soft tissue
Z85.830 Personal history of malignant neoplasm of bone
Z85.831 Personal history of malignant neoplasm of soft tissue
Excludes2 personal history of malignant neoplasm of skin (Z85.82-)

● Z85.84 **Personal history of malignant neoplasm of eye and nervous tissue**

Z85.840 **Personal history of malignant neoplasm of eye**

Z85.841 **Personal history of malignant neoplasm of brain**

Z85.848 **Personal history of malignant neoplasm of other parts of nervous tissue**

● Z85.85 **Personal history of malignant neoplasm of endocrine glands**

Z85.850 **Personal history of malignant neoplasm of thyroid**

Z85.858 **Personal history of malignant neoplasm of other endocrine glands**

Z85.89 **Personal history of malignant neoplasm of other organs and systems**

Z85.9 **Personal history of malignant neoplasm, unspecified**
Conditions classifiable to C7A.ØØ, C8Ø.1

● Z86 **Personal history of certain other diseases**
Code first any follow-up examination after treatment (ZØ9)

● Z86.Ø **Personal history of in-situ and benign neoplasms and neoplasms of uncertain behavior**

Excludes2 personal history of malignant neoplasms (Z85.-)

● Z86.ØØ **Personal history of in-situ neoplasm**
Conditions classifiable to DØØ-DØ9

Z86.ØØØ **Personal history of in-situ neoplasm of breast**
▶Conditions classifiable to DØ5

Z86.ØØ1 **Personal history of in-situ neoplasm of cervix uteri** ♀
▶Conditions classifiable to DØ6
Personal history of cervical intraepithelial neoplasia III [CIN III]

▶ Z86.ØØ2 **Personal history of in-situ neoplasm of other and unspecified genital organs**
▶Conditions classifiable to DØ7
▶Personal history of high-grade prostatic intraepithelial neoplasia III [HGPIN III]
▶Personal history of vaginal intraepithelial neoplasia III [VAIN III]
▶Personal history of vulvar intraepithelial neoplasia III [VIN III]

▶ Z86.ØØ3 **Personal history of in-situ neoplasm of oral cavity, esophagus and stomach**
▶Conditions classifiable to DØØ

▶ Z86.ØØ4 **Personal history of in-situ neoplasm of other and unspecified digestive organs**
▶Conditions classifiable to DØ1
▶Personal history of anal intraepithelial neoplasia (AIN III)

▶ Z86.ØØ5 **Personal history of in-situ neoplasm of middle ear and respiratory system**
▶Conditions classifiable to DØ2

▶ Z86.ØØ6 **Personal history of melanoma in-situ**
▶Conditions classifiable to DØ3
▶ **Excludes2** sites other than skin - code to personal history of in-situ neoplasm of the site

▶ Z86.ØØ7 **Personal history of in-situ neoplasm of skin**
▶Conditions classifiable to DØ4
▶Personal history of carcinoma in situ of skin

Z86.ØØ8 **Personal history of in-situ neoplasm of other site**
~~Personal history of vaginal intraepithelial neoplasia III [VAIN III]~~
~~Personal history of vulvar intraepithelial neoplasia III [VIN III]~~
▶Conditions classifiable to DØ9

● Z86.Ø1 **Personal history of benign neoplasm**
Coding Clinic: 2017, Q1, P14

Z86.Ø1Ø **Personal history of colonic polyps**
Coding Clinic: 2017, Q1, P9, P14

Z86.Ø11 **Personal history of benign neoplasm of the brain**

Z86.Ø12 **Personal history of benign carcinoid tumor**

Z86.Ø18 **Personal history of other benign neoplasm**
Coding Clinic: 2017, Q1, P14

Z86.Ø3 **Personal history of neoplasm of uncertain behavior**

● Z86.1 **Personal history of infectious and parasitic diseases**
Conditions classifiable to AØØ-B89, B99

Excludes1 personal history of infectious diseases specific to a body system sequelae of infectious and parasitic diseases (B9Ø-B94)

Coding Clinic: 2016, Q4, P5

Z86.11 **Personal history of tuberculosis**

Z86.12 **Personal history of poliomyelitis**

Z86.13 **Personal history of malaria**

Z86.14 **Personal history of Methicillin resistant Staphylococcus aureus infection**
Personal history of MRSA infection

▶ Z86.15 **Personal history of latent tuberculosis infection**

Z86.19 **Personal history of other infectious and parasitic diseases**

Z86.2 **Personal history of diseases of the blood and blood-forming organs and certain disorders involving the immune mechanism**
Conditions classifiable to D5Ø-D89

● Z86.3 **Personal history of endocrine, nutritional and metabolic diseases**
Conditions classifiable to EØØ-E88

Z86.31 **Personal history of diabetic foot ulcer**

Excludes2 current diabetic foot ulcer (EØ8.621, EØ9.621, E1Ø.621, E11.621, E13.621)

Z86.32 **Personal history of gestational diabetes** ♀
Personal history of conditions classifiable to O24.4-

Excludes1 gestational diabetes mellitus in current pregnancy (O24.4-)

Z86.39 **Personal history of other endocrine, nutritional and metabolic disease**

● Z86.5 **Personal history of mental and behavioral disorders**
Conditions classifiable to F4Ø-F59

Z86.51 **Personal history of combat and operational stress reaction** A

Z86.59 **Personal history of other mental and behavioral disorders**

CHAPTER 21 (ZØØ-Z99)

● Z86.6 **Personal history of diseases of the nervous system and sense organs**
Conditions classifiable to GØØ-G99, HØØ-H95

Z86.61 **Personal history of infections of the central nervous system**
Personal history of encephalitis
Personal history of meningitis

Z86.69 **Personal history of other diseases of the nervous system and sense organs**
Coding Clinic: 2016, Q4, P25

● Z86.7 **Personal history of diseases of the circulatory system**
Conditions classifiable to IØØ-I99
Excludes2 old myocardial infarction (I25.2)
personal history of anaphylactic shock (Z87.892)
postmyocardial infarction syndrome (I24.1)

● Z86.71 **Personal history of venous thrombosis and embolism**

Z86.711 **Personal history of pulmonary embolism**

Z86.718 **Personal history of other venous thrombosis and embolism**

Z86.72 **Personal history of thrombophlebitis**

Z86.73 **Personal history of transient ischemic attack (TIA), and cerebral infarction without residual deficits**
Personal history of prolonged reversible ischemic neurological deficit (PRIND)
Personal history of stroke NOS without residual deficits
Excludes1 personal history of traumatic brain injury (Z87.82Ø)
sequelae of cerebrovascular disease (I69.-)
Coding Clinic: 2012, Q4, P3

Z86.74 **Personal history of sudden cardiac arrest**
Personal history of sudden cardiac death successfully resuscitated

Z86.79 **Personal history of other diseases of the circulatory system**

● Z87 **Personal history of other diseases and conditions**
Code first any follow-up examination after treatment (ZØ9)

● Z87.Ø **Personal history of diseases of the respiratory system**
Conditions classifiable to JØØ-J99

Z87.Ø1 **Personal history of pneumonia (recurrent)**

Z87.Ø9 **Personal history of other diseases of the respiratory system**

● Z87.1 **Personal history of diseases of the digestive system**
Conditions classifiable to KØØ-K93

Z87.11 **Personal history of peptic ulcer disease**

Z87.19 **Personal history of other diseases of the digestive system**
Coding Clinic: 2017, Q1, P14

Z87.2 **Personal history of diseases of the skin and subcutaneous tissue**
Conditions classifiable to LØØ-L99
Excludes2 personal history of diabetic foot ulcer (Z86.31)

● Z87.3 **Personal history of diseases of the musculoskeletal system and connective tissue**
Conditions classifiable to MØØ-M99
Excludes2 personal history of (healed) traumatic fracture (Z87.81)

● Z87.31 **Personal history of (healed) nontraumatic fracture**

Z87.31Ø **Personal history of (healed) osteoporosis fracture**
Personal history of (healed) fragility fracture
Personal history of (healed) collapsed vertebra due to osteoporosis

Z87.311 **Personal history of (healed) other pathological fracture**
Personal history of (healed) collapsed vertebra NOS
Excludes2 personal history of osteoporosis fracture (Z87.31Ø)

Z87.312 **Personal history of (healed) stress fracture**
Personal history of (healed) fatigue fracture

Z87.39 **Personal history of other diseases of the musculoskeletal system and connective tissue**

● Z87.4 **Personal history of diseases of genitourinary system**
Conditions classifiable to NØØ-N99

● Z87.41 **Personal history of dysplasia of the female genital tract**
Excludes1 personal history of intraepithelial neoplasia III of female genital tract (Z86.ØØ1, Z86.ØØ8)
personal history of malignant neoplasm of female genital tract (Z85.4Ø-Z85.44)

Z87.41Ø **Personal history of cervical dysplasia** ♀

Z87.411 **Personal history of vaginal dysplasia** ♀

Z87.412 **Personal history of vulvar dysplasia** ♀

Z87.42 **Personal history of other diseases of the female genital tract** ♀

● Z87.43 **Personal history of diseases of male genital organs**

Z87.43Ø **Personal history of prostatic dysplasia** ♂
Excludes1 personal history of malignant neoplasm of prostate (Z85.46)

Z87.438 **Personal history of other diseases of male genital organs** ♂

● Z87.44 **Personal history of diseases of urinary system**
Excludes1 personal history of malignant neoplasm of cervix uteri (Z85.41)

Z87.44Ø **Personal history of urinary (tract) infections**

Z87.441 **Personal history of nephrotic syndrome**

Z87.442 **Personal history of urinary calculi**
Personal history of kidney stones

Z87.448 **Personal history of other diseases of urinary system**

● **Z87.5 Personal history of complications of pregnancy, childbirth and the puerperium**
Conditions classifiable to O00-O9A
Excludes2 recurrent pregnancy loss (N96)

Z87.51 Personal history of pre-term labor ♀
Excludes1 current pregnancy with history of pre-term labor (O09.21-)

Z87.59 Personal history of other complications of pregnancy, childbirth and the puerperium ♀
Personal history of trophoblastic disease

● **Z87.7 Personal history of (corrected) congenital malformations**
Conditions classifiable to Q00-Q89 that have been repaired or corrected
Excludes1 congenital malformations that have been partially corrected or repair but which still require medical treatment - code to condition
Excludes2 other postprocedural states (Z98.-)
personal history of medical treatment (Z92.-)
presence of cardiac and vascular implants and grafts (Z95.-)
presence of other devices (Z97.-)
presence of other functional implants (Z96.-)
transplanted organ and tissue status (Z94.-)

● **Z87.71 Personal history of (corrected) congenital malformations of genitourinary system**

Z87.710 Personal history of (corrected) hypospadias ♂

Z87.718 Personal history of other specified (corrected) congenital malformations of genitourinary system

● **Z87.72 Personal history of (corrected) congenital malformations of nervous system and sense organs**

Z87.720 Personal history of (corrected) congenital malformations of eye

Z87.721 Personal history of (corrected) congenital malformations of ear

Z87.728 Personal history of other specified (corrected) congenital malformations of nervous system and sense organs

● **Z87.73 Personal history of (corrected) congenital malformations of digestive system**

Z87.730 Personal history of (corrected) cleft lip and palate

Z87.738 Personal history of other specified (corrected) congenital malformations of digestive system

Z87.74 Personal history of (corrected) congenital malformations of heart and circulatory system

Z87.75 Personal history of (corrected) congenital malformations of respiratory system

Z87.76 Personal history of (corrected) congenital malformations of integument, limbs and musculoskeletal system

● **Z87.79 Personal history of other (corrected) congenital malformations**

Z87.790 Personal history of (corrected) congenital malformations of face and neck

Z87.798 Personal history of other (corrected) congenital malformations

● **Z87.8 Personal history of other specified conditions**
Excludes2 personal history of self harm (Z91.5)

Z87.81 Personal history of (healed) traumatic fracture
Excludes2 personal history of (healed) nontraumatic fracture (Z87.31-)

● **Z87.82 Personal history of other (healed) physical injury and trauma**
Conditions classifiable to S00-T88, except traumatic fractures

Z87.820 Personal history of traumatic brain injury
Excludes1 personal history of transient ischemic attack (TIA), and cerebral infarction without residual deficits (Z86.73)

Z87.821 Personal history of retained foreign body fully removed

Z87.828 Personal history of other (healed) physical injury and trauma

● **Z87.89 Personal history of other specified conditions**

Z87.890 Personal history of sex reassignment

Z87.891 Personal history of nicotine dependence
Excludes1 current nicotine dependence (F17.2-)
Coding Clinic: 2017, Q2, P27

Z87.892 Personal history of anaphylaxis
Code also allergy status such as:
allergy status to drugs, medicaments and biological substances (Z88.-)
allergy status, other than to drugs and biological substances (Z91.0-)

Z87.898 Personal history of other specified conditions
Coding Clinic: 2013, Q1, P21

● **Z88 Allergy status to drugs, medicaments and biological substances**
Excludes2 allergy status, other than to drugs and biological substances (Z91.0-)

Z88.0 Allergy status to penicillin

Z88.1 Allergy status to other antibiotic agents status

Z88.2 Allergy status to sulfonamides status
Coding Clinic: 2015, Q3, P23

Z88.3 Allergy status to other anti-infective agents status

Z88.4 Allergy status to anesthetic agent status

Z88.5 Allergy status to narcotic agent status

Z88.6 Allergy status to analgesic agent status

Z88.7 Allergy status to serum and vaccine status

Z88.8 Allergy status to other drugs, medicaments and biological substances status

Z88.9 Allergy status to unspecified drugs, medicaments and biological substances status

● Z89 Acquired absence of limb

Includes amputation status
postprocedural loss of limb
post-traumatic loss of limb

Excludes1 acquired deformities of limbs (M20-M21)
congenital absence of limbs (Q71-Q73)

● Z89.0 Acquired absence of **thumb and other finger(s)**

● Z89.01 Acquired absence of **thumb**

Z89.011 Acquired absence of **right** thumb
Z89.012 Acquired absence of **left** thumb
Z89.019 Acquired absence of **unspecified** thumb

● Z89.02 Acquired absence of other **finger(s)**

Excludes2 acquired absence of thumb (Z89.01-)

Z89.021 Acquired absence of **right** finger(s)
Z89.022 Acquired absence of **left** finger(s)
Z89.029 Acquired absence of **unspecified** finger(s)

● Z89.1 Acquired absence of **hand and wrist**

● Z89.11 Acquired absence of **hand**

Z89.111 Acquired absence of **right** hand
Z89.112 Acquired absence of **left** hand
Z89.119 Acquired absence of **unspecified** hand

● Z89.12 Acquired absence of **wrist**
Disarticulation at wrist

Z89.121 Acquired absence of **right** wrist
Z89.122 Acquired absence of **left** wrist
Z89.129 Acquired absence of **unspecified** wrist

● Z89.2 Acquired absence of **upper limb above wrist**

● Z89.20 Acquired absence of upper limb, **unspecified level**

Z89.201 Acquired absence of **right** upper limb, unspecified level
Z89.202 Acquired absence of **left** upper limb, unspecified level
Z89.209 Acquired absence of **unspecified** upper limb, unspecified level
Acquired absence of arm NOS

● Z89.21 Acquired absence of **upper limb below elbow**

Z89.211 Acquired absence of **right** upper limb below elbow
Z89.212 Acquired absence of **left** upper limb below elbow
Z89.219 Acquired absence of **unspecified** upper limb below elbow

● Z89.22 Acquired absence of **upper limb above elbow**
Disarticulation at elbow

Z89.221 Acquired absence of **right** upper limb above elbow
Z89.222 Acquired absence of **left** upper limb above elbow
Z89.229 Acquired absence of **unspecified** upper limb above elbow

● Z89.23 Acquired absence of **shoulder**
Acquired absence of shoulder joint following explantation of shoulder joint prosthesis, with or without presence of antibiotic-impregnated cement spacer

Z89.231 Acquired absence of **right** shoulder
Z89.232 Acquired absence of **left** shoulder
Z89.239 Acquired absence of **unspecified** shoulder

● Z89.4 Acquired absence of **toe(s), foot, and ankle**

● Z89.41 Acquired absence of **great toe**

Z89.411 Acquired absence of **right** great toe
Z89.412 Acquired absence of **left** great toe
Z89.419 Acquired absence of **unspecified** great toe

● Z89.42 Acquired absence of **other toe(s)**

Excludes2 acquired absence of great toe (Z89.41-)

Z89.421 Acquired absence of other **right** toe(s)
Z89.422 Acquired absence of other **left** toe(s)
Z89.429 Acquired absence of other toe(s), **unspecified** side

● Z89.43 Acquired absence of **foot**

Z89.431 Acquired absence of **right** foot
Z89.432 Acquired absence of **left** foot
Z89.439 Acquired absence of **unspecified** foot

● Z89.44 Acquired absence of **ankle**
Disarticulation of ankle

Z89.441 Acquired absence of **right** ankle
Z89.442 Acquired absence of **left** ankle
Z89.449 Acquired absence of **unspecified** ankle

● Z89.5 Acquired absence of leg below knee

● Z89.51 Acquired absence of **leg below knee**

Z89.511 Acquired absence of **right** leg below knee
Z89.512 Acquired absence of **left** leg below knee
Z89.519 Acquired absence of **unspecified** leg below knee

● Z89.52 Acquired absence of **knee**
Acquired absence of knee joint following explantation of knee joint prosthesis, with or without presence of antibiotic-impregnated cement spacer

Z89.521 Acquired absence of **right** knee
Z89.522 Acquired absence of **left** knee
Z89.529 Acquired absence of **unspecified** knee

● Z89.6 Acquired absence of leg above knee

● Z89.61 Acquired absence of **leg above knee**
Acquired absence of leg NOS
Disarticulation at knee

Z89.611 Acquired absence of **right** leg above knee
Z89.612 Acquired absence of **left** leg above knee
Z89.619 Acquired absence of **unspecified** leg above knee

● Z89.62 Acquired absence of **hip**
Acquired absence of hip joint following explantation of hip joint prosthesis, with or without presence of antibiotic-impregnated cement spacer
Disarticulation at hip

Z89.621 Acquired absence of **right** hip joint
Z89.622 Acquired absence of **left** hip joint
Z89.629 Acquired absence of **unspecified** hip joint

Z89.9 Acquired absence of limb, **unspecified**

Z90 Acquired absence of organs, not elsewhere classified
Includes postprocedural or post-traumatic loss of body part NEC
Excludes1 congenital absence - see Alphabetical Index
Excludes2 postprocedural absence of endocrine glands (E89.-)

Z90.0 Acquired absence of part of head and neck
Z90.01 Acquired absence of eye
Z90.02 Acquired absence of larynx
Z90.09 Acquired absence of other part of head and neck
Acquired absence of nose
Excludes2 teeth (K08.1)

Z90.1 Acquired absence of breast and nipple
Z90.10 Acquired absence of unspecified breast and nipple
Z90.11 Acquired absence of right breast and nipple
Z90.12 Acquired absence of left breast and nipple
Z90.13 Acquired absence of bilateral breasts and nipples

Z90.2 Acquired absence of lung [part of]
Z90.3 Acquired absence of stomach [part of]
Z90.4 Acquired absence of other specified parts of digestive tract
Z90.41 Acquired absence of pancreas
Code also exocrine pancreatic insufficiency (K86.81)
Use additional code to identify any associated:
diabetes mellitus, postpancreatectomy (E13.-)
insulin use (Z79.4)
Z90.410 Acquired total absence of pancreas
Acquired absence of pancreas NOS
Z90.411 Acquired partial absence of pancreas
Z90.49 Acquired absence of other specified parts of digestive tract

Z90.5 Acquired absence of kidney
Z90.6 Acquired absence of other parts of urinary tract
Acquired absence of bladder
Z90.7 Acquired absence of genital organ(s)
Excludes1 personal history of sex reassignment (Z87.890)
Excludes2 female genital mutilation status (N90.81-)
Z90.71 Acquired absence of cervix and uterus
Z90.710 Acquired absence of both cervix and uterus ♀
Acquired absence of uterus NOS
Status post total hysterectomy
Z90.711 Acquired absence of uterus with remaining cervical stump ♀
Status post partial hysterectomy with remaining cervical stump
Z90.712 Acquired absence of cervix with remaining uterus ♀
Z90.72 Acquired absence of ovaries
Z90.721 Acquired absence of ovaries, unilateral ♀
Z90.722 Acquired absence of ovaries, bilateral ♀
Z90.79 Acquired absence of other genital organ(s)
Z90.8 Acquired absence of other organs
Z90.81 Acquired absence of spleen
Z90.89 Acquired absence of other organs

Z91 Personal risk factors, not elsewhere classified
Excludes2 contact with and (suspected) exposures hazardous to health (Z77.-)
exposure to pollution and other problems related to physical environment (Z77.1-)
female genital mutilation status (N90.81-)
occupational exposure to risk factors (Z57.-)
personal history of physical injury and trauma (Z87.81, Z87.82-)

Z91.0 Allergy status, other than to drugs and biological substances
Excludes2 allergy status to drugs, medicaments, and biological substances (Z88.-)
Z91.01 Food allergy status
Excludes2 food additives allergy status (Z91.02)
Z91.010 Allergy to peanuts
Z91.011 Allergy to milk products
Excludes1 lactose intolerance (E73.-)
Z91.012 Allergy to eggs
Z91.013 Allergy to seafood
Allergy to shellfish
Allergy to octopus or squid ink
Z91.018 Allergy to other foods
Allergy to nuts other than peanuts
Z91.02 Food additives allergy status
Z91.03 Insect allergy status
Z91.030 Bee allergy status
Z91.038 Other insect allergy status
Z91.04 Nonmedicinal substance allergy status
Z91.040 Latex allergy status
Latex sensitivity status
Z91.041 Radiographic dye allergy status
Allergy status to contrast media used for diagnostic X-ray procedure
Z91.048 Other nonmedicinal substance allergy status
Z91.09 Other allergy status, other than to drugs and biological substances

Z91.1 Patient's noncompliance with medical treatment and regimen
Z91.11 Patient's noncompliance with dietary regimen
Z91.12 Patient's intentional underdosing of medication regimen
Code first underdosing of medication (T36-T50) with fifth or sixth character 6
Excludes1 adverse effect of prescribed drug taken as directed - code to adverse effect
poisoning (overdose) - code to poisoning
Z91.120 Patient's intentional underdosing of medication regimen due to financial hardship
Z91.128 Patient's intentional underdosing of medication regimen for other reason
Z91.13 Patient's unintentional underdosing of medication regimen
Code first underdosing of medication (T36-T50) with fifth or sixth character 6
Excludes1 adverse effect of prescribed drug taken as directed - code to adverse effect
poisoning (overdose) - code to poisoning
Z91.130 Patient's unintentional underdosing of medication regimen due to age-related debility
Z91.138 Patient's unintentional underdosing of medication regimen for other reason

Z91.14 **Patient's other noncompliance with medication regimen**
Patient's underdosing of medication NOS

Z91.15 **Patient's noncompliance with renal dialysis** HCC

Z91.19 **Patient's noncompliance with other medical treatment and regimen**
Nonadherence to medical treatment

● Z91.4 **Personal history of psychological trauma, not elsewhere classified**

● Z91.41 **Personal history of adult abuse**
Excludes2 personal history of abuse in childhood (Z62.81-)

Z91.410 **Personal history of adult physical and sexual abuse** A
Excludes1 current adult physical abuse (T74.11, T76.11)
current adult sexual abuse (T74.21, T76.11)

Z91.411 **Personal history of adult psychological abuse** A

Z91.412 **Personal history of adult neglect** A
Excludes1 current adult neglect (T74.Ø1, T76.Ø1)

Z91.419 **Personal history of unspecified adult abuse** A

Z91.42 **Personal history of forced labor or sexual exploitation**

Z91.49 **Other personal history of psychological trauma, not elsewhere classified**

Z91.5 **Personal history of self-harm**
Personal history of parasuicide
Personal history of self-poisoning
Personal history of suicide attempt

● Z91.8 **Other specified personal risk factors, not elsewhere classified**

Z91.81 **History of falling**
At risk for falling

Z91.82 **Personal history of military deployment** A
Individual (civilian or military) with past history of military war, peacekeeping and humanitarian deployment (current or past conflict)
Returned from military deployment

Z91.83 ***Wandering in diseases classified elsewhere***
Code first underlying disorder such as:
Alzheimer's disease (G3Ø.-)
autism or pervasive developmental disorder (F84.-)
intellectual disabilities (F7Ø-F79)
unspecified dementia with behavioral disturbance (FØ3.9-)

● Z91.84 **Oral health risk factors**

Z91.841 **Risk for dental caries, low**

Z91.842 **Risk for dental caries, moderate**

Z91.843 **Risk for dental caries, high**

Z91.849 **Unspecified risk for dental caries**

Z91.89 **Other specified personal risk factors, not elsewhere classified**
Coding Clinic: 2017, Q1, P46

● Z92 **Personal history of medical treatment**
Excludes2 postprocedural states (Z98.-)

Z92.Ø **Personal history of contraception**
Excludes1 counseling or management of current contraceptive practices (Z3Ø.-)
long term (current) use of contraception (Z79.3)
presence of (intrauterine) contraceptive device (Z97.5)

● Z92.2 **Personal history of drug therapy**
Excludes2 long term (current) drug therapy (Z79.-)

Z92.21 **Personal history of antineoplastic chemotherapy**

Z92.22 **Personal history of monoclonal drug therapy**

Z92.23 **Personal history of estrogen therapy**

● Z92.24 **Personal history of steroid therapy**

Z92.24Ø **Personal history of inhaled steroid therapy**

Z92.241 **Personal history of systemic steroid therapy**
Personal history of steroid therapy NOS

Z92.25 **Personal history of immunosupression therapy**
Excludes2 personal history of steroid therapy (Z92.24)

Z92.29 **Personal history of other drug therapy**

Z92.3 **Personal history of irradiation**
Personal history of exposure to therapeutic radiation
Excludes1 exposure to radiation in the physical environment (Z77.12)
occupational exposure to radiation (Z57.1)

● Z92.8 **Personal history of other medical treatment**
Coding Clinic: 2016, Q4, P72

Z92.81 **Personal history of extracorporeal membrane oxygenation (ECMO)**

Z92.82 **Status post administration of tPA (rtPA) in a different facility within the last 24 hours prior to admission to current facility**
Code first condition requiring tPA administration, such as:
acute cerebral infarction (I63.-)
acute myocardial infarction (I21.-, I22.-)

Z92.83 **Personal history of failed moderate sedation**
Personal history of failed conscious sedation
Excludes2 failed moderate sedation during procedure (T88.52)

Z92.84 **Personal history of unintended awareness under general anesthesia**
Excludes2 unintended awareness under general anesthesia during procedure (T88.53)
Coding Clinic: 2016, Q4, P72, 77

Z92.89 **Personal history of other medical treatment**

● Z93 **Artificial opening status**
Excludes1 artificial openings requiring attention or management (Z43.-)
complications of external stoma (J95.Ø-, K94.-, N99.5-)

Z93.Ø **Tracheostomy status** HCC

Z93.1 **Gastrostomy status** HCC

Z93.2 **Ileostomy status** HCC

Z93.3 **Colostomy status** HCC

Z93.4 **Other artificial openings of gastrointestinal tract status**

● Z93.5 **Cystostomy status**

Z93.50 **Unspecified cystostomy status**

Z93.51 **Cutaneous-vesicostomy status**

Z93.52 **Appendico-vesicostomy status**

Z93.59 **Other cystostomy status**

Z93.6 **Other artificial openings of urinary tract status**
Nephrostomy status
Ureterostomy status
Urethrostomy status

Z93.8 **Other artificial opening status**

Z93.9 **Artificial opening status, unspecified**

● Z94 **Transplanted organ and tissue status**

Includes organ or tissue replaced by heterogenous or homogenous transplant

Excludes1 complications of transplanted organ or tissue - see Alphabetical Index

Excludes2 presence of vascular grafts (Z95.-)

Z94.0 **Kidney transplant status**

Z94.1 **Heart transplant status**

Excludes1 artificial heart status (Z95.812)
heart-valve replacement status (Z95.2-Z95.4)

Z94.2 **Lung transplant status**

Z94.3 **Heart and lungs transplant status**

Z94.4 **Liver transplant status**

Z94.5 **Skin transplant status**
Autogenous skin transplant status

Z94.6 **Bone transplant status**

Z94.7 **Corneal transplant status**

● Z94.8 **Other transplanted organ and tissue status**

Z94.81 **Bone marrow transplant status**

Z94.82 **Intestine transplant status**

Z94.83 **Pancreas transplant status**

Z94.84 **Stem cells transplant status**

Z94.89 **Other transplanted organ and tissue status**

Z94.9 **Transplanted organ and tissue status, unspecified**

● Z95 **Presence of cardiac and vascular implants and grafts**

Excludes2 complications of cardiac and vascular devices, implants and grafts (T82.-)

Z95.0 **Presence of cardiac pacemaker**
Presence of cardiac resynchronization therapy (CRT-P) pacemaker

Excludes1 adjustment or management of cardiac device (Z45.0-)
adjustment or management of cardiac pacemaker (Z45.0)
presence of automatic (implantable) cardiac defibrillator with synchronous cardiac pacemaker (Z95.810)

Coding Clinic: 2019, Q1, P33

Z95.1 **Presence of aortocoronary bypass graft**
Presence of coronary artery bypass graft

Z95.2 **Presence of prosthetic heart valve**
Presence of heart valve NOS

Z95.3 **Presence of xenogenic heart valve**

Z95.4 **Presence of other heart-valve replacement**

Z95.5 **Presence of coronary angioplasty implant and graft**

Excludes1 coronary angioplasty status without implant and graft (Z98.61)

● Z95.8 **Presence of other cardiac and vascular implants and grafts**

● Z95.81 **Presence of other cardiac implants and grafts**

Z95.810 **Presence of automatic (implantable) cardiac defibrillator**
Presence of automatic (implantable) cardiac defribillator with synchronous cardiac pacemaker
Presence of cardiac resynchronization therapy defibrillator (CRT-D)
Presence of cardioverter-defribillator (ICD)

Z95.811 **Presence of heart assist device**

Z95.812 **Presence of fully implantable artificial heart**

Z95.818 **Presence of other cardiac implants and grafts**

● Z95.82 **Presence of other vascular implants and grafts**

Z95.820 **Peripheral vascular angioplasty status with implants and grafts**

Excludes1 peripheral vascular angioplasty without implant and graft (Z98.62)

Z95.828 **Presence of other vascular implants and grafts**
Presence of intravascular prosthesis NEC

Z95.9 **Presence of cardiac and vascular implant and graft, unspecified**

● Z96 **Presence of other functional implants**

Excludes2 complications of internal prosthetic devices, implants and grafts (T82-T85)
fitting and adjustment of prosthetic and other devices (Z44-Z46)

Z96.0 **Presence of urogenital implants**

Z96.1 **Presence of intraocular lens**
Presence of pseudophakia

● Z96.2 **Presence of otological and audiological implants**

Z96.20 **Presence of otological and audiological implant, unspecified**

Z96.21 **Cochlear implant status**

Z96.22 **Myringotomy tube(s) status**

Z96.29 **Presence of other otological and audiological implants**
Presence of bone-conduction hearing device
Presence of eustachian tube stent
Stapes replacement

Z96.3 **Presence of artificial larynx**

● Z96.4 **Presence of endocrine implants**

Z96.41 **Presence of insulin pump (external) (internal)**

Z96.49 **Presence of other endocrine implants**

Z96.5 **Presence of tooth-root and mandibular implants**

● Z96.6 **Presence of orthopedic joint implants**

Z96.60 **Presence of unspecified orthopedic joint implant**

● Z96.61 **Presence of artificial shoulder joint**

Z96.611 **Presence of right artificial shoulder joint**

Z96.612 **Presence of left artificial shoulder joint**

Z96.619 **Presence of unspecified artificial shoulder joint**

● Z96.62 **Presence of artificial elbow joint**

Z96.621 **Presence of right artificial elbow joint**

Z96.622 **Presence of left artificial elbow joint**

Z96.629 **Presence of unspecified artificial elbow joint**

CHAPTER 21 (Z00-Z99)

● Z96.63 Presence of artificial wrist joint
Z96.631 Presence of right artificial wrist joint
Z96.632 Presence of left artificial wrist joint
Z96.639 Presence of unspecified artificial wrist joint

● Z96.64 Presence of artificial hip joint
Hip-joint replacement (partial) (total)
Z96.641 Presence of right artificial hip joint
Coding Clinic: 2016, Q3, P17
Z96.642 Presence of left artificial hip joint
Coding Clinic: 2015, Q1, P16
Z96.643 Presence of artificial hip joint, bilateral
Z96.649 Presence of unspecified artificial hip joint

● Z96.65 Presence of artificial knee joint
Z96.651 Presence of right artificial knee joint
Z96.652 Presence of left artificial knee joint
Z96.653 Presence of artificial knee joint, bilateral
Z96.659 Presence of unspecified artificial knee joint

● Z96.66 Presence of artificial ankle joint
Z96.661 Presence of right artificial ankle joint
Z96.662 Presence of left artificial ankle joint
Z96.669 Presence of unspecified artificial ankle joint

● Z96.69 Presence of other orthopedic joint implants
Z96.691 Finger-joint replacement of right hand
Z96.692 Finger-joint replacement of left hand
Z96.693 Finger-joint replacement, bilateral
Z96.698 Presence of other orthopedic joint implants

Z96.7 Presence of other bone and tendon implants
Presence of skull plate

● Z96.8 Presence of other specified functional implants
Z96.81 Presence of artificial skin
▶ Z96.82 Presence of neurostimulator
▶Presence of brain neurostimulator
▶Presence of gastric neurostimulator
▶Presence of peripheral nerve neurostimulator
▶Presence of sacral nerve neurostimulator
▶Presence of spinal cord neurostimulator
▶Presence of vagus nerve neurostimulator
Z96.89 Presence of other specified functional implants

Z96.9 Presence of functional implant, unspecified

● Z97 Presence of other devices
~~Excludes1 complications of internal prosthetic devices, implants and grafts (T82-T85)~~
~~fitting and adjustment of prosthetic and other devices (Z44-Z46)~~
▶ **Excludes2** fitting and adjustment of prosthetic and other devices (Z44-Z46)
presence of cerebrospinal fluid drainage device (Z98.2)

Z97.0 Presence of artificial eye

● Z97.1 Presence of artificial limb (complete) (partial)
Z97.10 Presence of artificial limb (complete) (partial), unspecified
Z97.11 Presence of artificial right arm (complete) (partial)
Z97.12 Presence of artificial left arm (complete) (partial)
Z97.13 Presence of artificial right leg (complete) (partial)
Z97.14 Presence of artificial left leg (complete) (partial)
Z97.15 Presence of artificial arms, bilateral (complete) (partial)
Z97.16 Presence of artificial legs, bilateral (complete) (partial)

Z97.2 Presence of dental prosthetic device (complete) (partial)
Presence of dentures (complete) (partial)

Z97.3 Presence of spectacles and contact lenses

Z97.4 Presence of external hearing-aid

Z97.5 Presence of (intrauterine) contraceptive device ♀
Excludes1 checking, reinsertion or removal of implantable subdermal contraceptive (Z30.46)
checking, reinsertion or removal of intrauterine contraceptive device (Z30.43-)

Z97.8 Presence of other specified devices

● Z98 Other postprocedural states
Excludes2 aftercare (Z43-Z49, Z51)
follow-up medical care (Z08-Z09)
postprocedural complication - see Alphabetical Index

Z98.0 Intestinal bypass and anastomosis status
Excludes2 bariatric surgery status (Z98.84)
gastric bypass status (Z98.84)
obesity surgery status (Z98.84)

Z98.1 Arthrodesis status

Z98.2 Presence of cerebrospinal fluid drainage device
Presence of CSF shunt

Z98.3 Post therapeutic collapse of lung status
Code first underlying disease

● Z98.4 Cataract extraction status
Use additional code to identify intraocular lens implant status (Z96.1)
Excludes1 aphakia (H27.0)
Z98.41 Cataract extraction status, right eye
Z98.42 Cataract extraction status, left eye
Z98.49 Cataract extraction status, unspecified eye

● Z98.5 Sterilization status
Excludes1 female infertility (N97.-)
male infertility (N46.-)
Z98.51 Tubal ligation status ♀
Z98.52 Vasectomy status ♂ A

● Z98.6 Angioplasty status
Z98.61 Coronary angioplasty status
Excludes1 coronary angioplasty status with implant and graft (Z95.5)
Z98.62 Peripheral vascular angioplasty status
Excludes1 peripheral vascular angioplasty status with implant and graft (Z95.820)

● Z98.8 Other specified postprocedural states
Coding Clinic: 2016, Q4, P76
● Z98.81 Dental procedure status
Z98.810 Dental sealant status
Z98.811 Dental restoration status
Dental crown status
Dental fillings status
Z98.818 Other dental procedure status
Z98.82 Breast implant status
Excludes1 breast implant removal status (Z98.86)
Z98.83 Filtering (vitreous) bleb after glaucoma surgery status
Excludes1 inflammation (infection) of postprocedural bleb (H59.4-)

Z98.84 Bariatric surgery status
Gastric banding status
Gastric bypass status for obesity
Obesity surgery status
Excludes1 bariatric surgery status complicating pregnancy, childbirth, or the puerperium (O99.84)
Excludes2 intestinal bypass and anastomosis status (Z98.0)

Z98.85 Transplanted organ removal status
Transplanted organ previously removed due to complication, failure, rejection or infection
Excludes1 encounter for removal of transplanted organ - code to complication of transplanted organ (T86.-)

Z98.86 Personal history of breast implant removal

Z98.87 Personal history of in utero procedure

Z98.870 Personal history of in utero procedure during pregnancy ♀
Excludes2 complications from in utero procedure for current pregnancy (O35.7)
supervision of current pregnancy with history of in utero procedure during previous pregnancy (O09.82-)

Z98.871 Personal history of in utero procedure while a fetus

Z98.89 Other specified postprocedural states
Coding Clinic: 2016, Q4, P76

Z98.890 Other specified postprocedural states
Personal history of surgery, not elsewhere classified

Z98.891 History of uterine scar from previous surgery ♀
Excludes1 Maternal care due to uterine scar from previous surgery (O34.2-)
Coding Clinic: 2016, Q4, P52, P76

Z99 Dependence on enabling machines and devices, not elsewhere classified
Excludes1 cardiac pacemaker status (Z95.0)

Z99.0 Dependence on aspirator

Z99.1 Dependence on respirator
Dependence on ventilator

Z99.11 Dependence on respirator [ventilator] status
Coding Clinic: 2018, Q1, P14; 2015, Q1, P21

Z99.12 Encounter for respirator [ventilator] dependence during power failure
Excludes1 mechanical complication of respirator [ventilator] (J95.850)

Z99.2 Dependence on renal dialysis
Hemodialysis status
Peritoneal dialysis status
Presence of arteriovenous shunt for dialysis
Renal dialysis status NOS
Excludes1 encounter for fitting and adjustment of dialysis catheter (Z49.0-)
Excludes2 noncompliance with renal dialysis (Z91.15)
Coding Clinic: 2016, Q1, P13

Z99.3 Dependence on wheelchair
Wheelchair confinement status
Code first cause of dependence, such as:
muscular dystrophy (G71.0-)
obesity (E66.-)

Z99.8 Dependence on other enabling machines and devices

Z99.81 Dependence on supplemental oxygen
Dependence on long-term oxygen

Z99.89 Dependence on other enabling machines and devices
Dependence on machine or device NOS

CHAPTER 21 (Z00-Z99)